Clinical Anesthesia

Clinical Anesthesia

SIXTH EDITION

Paul G. Barash, MD

Professor, Department of Anesthesiology
Yale University School of Medicine
Attending Anesthesiologist
Yale-New Haven Hospital
New Haven, Connecticut

Bruce F. Cullen, MD

Emeritus Professor
Department of Anesthesiology
University of Washington
Seattle, Washington

Robert K. Stoelting, MD

Emeritus Professor and Past Chair
Department of Anesthesia
Indiana University School of Medicine
Indianapolis, Indiana

Michael K. Cahalan, MD

Professor and Chair, Department of Anesthesiology
The University of Utah School of Medicine
Salt Lake City, Utah

M. Christine Stock, MD

Professor and Chair, Department of Anesthesiology
Northwestern University
Feinberg School of Medicine
Chicago, Illinois

Wolters Kluwer | Lippincott Williams & Wilkins
Health

Philadelphia • Baltimore • New York • London
Buenos Aires • Hong Kong • Sydney • Tokyo

Acquisitions Editor: Brian Brown
Managing Editor: Nicole T. Dernoski
Marketing Manager: Angela Panetta
Production Editor: Bridgett Dougherty
Senior Manufacturing Manager: Benjamin Rivera
Design Coordinator: Stephen Druding
Compositor: Aptara, Inc.

© 2009 by LIPPINCOTT WILLIAMS & WILKINS, a WOLTERS KLUWER BUSINESS

530 Walnut Street
Philadelphia, PA 19106 USA
LWW.com

Printed in China

Library of Congress Cataloging-in-Publication Data

Clinical anesthesia / edited by Paul G. Barash . . . [et al.].—6th ed.
    p. ; cm.
  Includes bibliographical references and index.
  ISBN 978-0-7817-8763-5 (alk. paper)
  1. Anesthesiology. 2. Anesthesia. I. Barash, Paul G.
  [DNLM: 1. Anesthesiology. 2. Anesthesia. 3. Anesthetics. WO 200 C6398 2009]
  RD81.C58 2009
  617.9′6—dc22
                                                                  2008056102

Care has been taken to confirm the accuracy of the information presented and to
describe generally accepted practices. However, the authors, editors, and publisher are not
responsible for errors or omissions or for any consequences from application of the information in this book and make no warranty, expressed or implied, with respect to the currency,
completeness, or accuracy of the contents of the publication. Application of this information
in a particular situation remains the professional responsibility of the practitioner.

The authors, editors, and publisher have exerted every effort to ensure that drug selection and dosage set forth in this text are in accordance with current recommendations and
practice at the time of publication. However, in view of ongoing research, changes in government regulations, and the constant flow of information relating to drug therapy and drug
reactions, the reader is urged to check the package insert for each drug for any change in
indications and dosage and for added warnings and precautions. This is particularly important when the recommended agent is a new or infrequently employed drug.

Some drugs and medical devices presented in this publication have Food and Drug
Administration (FDA) clearance for limited use in restricted research settings. It is the
responsibility of the health care provider to ascertain the FDA status of each drug or device
planned for use in their clinical practice.

To purchase additional copies of this book, call our customer service department at
(800) 638-3030 or fax orders to (301) 223-2320. International customers should call
(301) 223-2300.

Visit Lippincott Williams & Wilkins on the Internet: at LWW.com. Lippincott Williams
& Wilkins customer service representatives are available from 8:30 am to 6 pm, EST.

10 9 8 7 6 5 4

ROBERT K. STOELTING, MD
EDITOR EMERITUS, *CLINICAL ANESTHESIA*

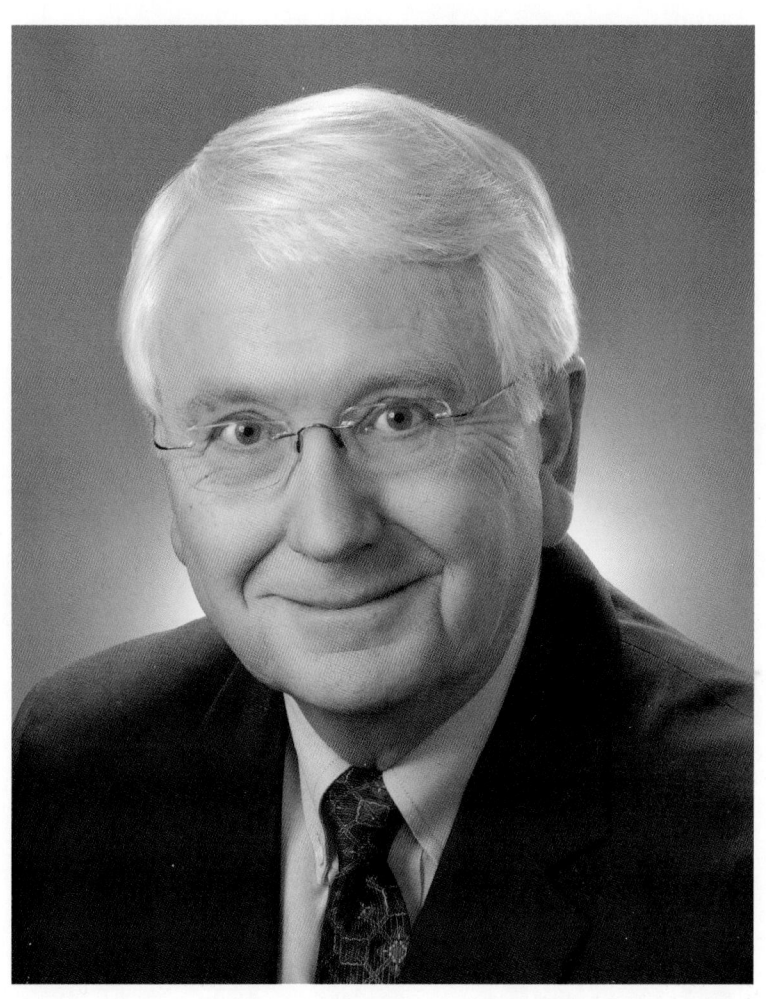

HIGHLY RESPECTED ANESTHESIOLOGIST,
DEDICATED EDUCATOR,
GIFTED AUTHOR AND EDITOR.

J. Jeffrey Andrews, MD
Professor and Chair
Department of Anesthesiology
University of Texas Health Science Center, San Antonio
San Antonio, Texas

Shamsuddin Akhtar, MBBS
Associate Professor
Department of Anesthesiology
Yale University School of Medicine
Attending Physician
Yale-New Haven Hospital
New Haven, Connecticut

Michael L. Ault, MD, FCCP, FCCM
Assistant Professor
Department of Anesthesiology
Northwestern University Feinberg School of Medicine
Associate Chief, Section of Critical Care Medicine
Northwestern Memorial Hospital
Chicago, Illinois

Douglas R. Bacon, MD
Professor
Department of Anesthesiology
Mayo Clinic
Rochester, Minnesota

Paul G. Barash, MD
Professor
Department of Anesthesiology
Yale University School of Medicine
Attending Anesthesiologist
Yale-New Haven Hospital
New Haven, Connecticut

Honorio T. Benzon, MD
Professor
Department of Anesthesiology
Northwestern University
Feinberg School of Medicine
Chief, Division of Pain Medicine
Northwestern Memorial Hospital
Chicago, Illinois

Christopher M. Bernards, MD
Anesthesiology Faculty
Department of Anesthesiology
Virginia Mason Medical
Seattle, Washington

Arnold J. Berry, MD, MPH
Professor
Department of Anesthesiology
Emory Univeristy School of Medicine
Emory University Hospital
Department of Anesthesiology
Atlanta, Georgia

David R. Bevan, MB
Professor
Department of Anesthesiology
University of Toronto
University Health Network
Toronto, Ontario, Canada

Barbara W. Brandom, MD
Professor
Department of Anesthesiology
University of Pittsburgh Medical Center
Attending Anesthesiologist
Children's Hospital of Pittsburgh
Pittsburgh, Pennsylvania

Ferne R. Braveman, MD, CM
Professor
Department of Anesthesiology
Yale University School of Medicine
Chief, Section of Obstetrical Anesthesiology
Attending Physician
Yale-New Haven Hospital
New Haven, Connecticut

Russell C. Brockwell, MD
Anesthesia Associates of Naples
Naples, Florida

Sorin J. Brull, MD
Professor
Department of Anesthesiology
Mayo Clinic College of Medicine
Mayo Clinic Hospital
Jacksonville, Florida

Michael K. Cahalan, MD
Professor and Chair
Department of Anesthesiology
The University of Utah School of Medicine
Salt Lake City, Utah

Levon M. Capan, MD
Professor of Anesthesiology
Vice Chair for Promotion
New York University School of Medicine
Associate Director of Anesthesia Service
Bellevue Hopital Center
New York, New York

C. Richard Chapman, PhD
Director
Pain Research Center
Department of Anesthesiology
Univeristy of Utah School
Salt Lake City, Utah

Amalia Cochran, MD
Assistant Professor
Adjunct Assistant Professor of Pediatrics
Department of Surgery
University of Utah
Salt Lake City, Utah

Barbara A. Coda, MD
Staff Anesthesiologist
Three Rivers Anesthesia
Oregon Urology Institute
Springfield, Oregon

Edmond Cohen, MD
Professor of Anesthesiology
The Mount Sinai School of Medicine
Director of Thoracic Anesthesia
The Mount Sinai Medical Center
New York, New York

Joseph P. Cravero, MD
Associate Professor of Anesthesiology
Dartmouth Hitchcock Medical Center
Lebanon, New Hampshire

C. Michael Crowder, MD, PhD
Assocaiate Professor of Anesthesiology and Molecular
    Biology/Pharmacology
Washington University School of Medicine
Barnes-Jewish Hospital
St. Louis, Missouri

Marie Csete, MD, PhD
Associate Professor
Department of Anesthesiology
Emory University
Atlanta, Georgia

Bruce F. Cullen, MD
Emeritus Professor
Department of Anesthesiology
University of Washington
Seattle, Washington

Steven Deem, MD
Associate Professor
Department of Anesthesiology and Medicine
University of Washington
Associate Director, Neurocritical Care Service
Harborview Medical Center
Seattle, Washington

Timothy R. Deer, MD
Clinical Professor
Department of Anesthesiology
West Virginia University School of Medicine
The Center for Pain Relief, Inc.
Charleston, West Virginia

Stephen F. Dierdorf, MD
Professor and Vice Chair
Department of Anesthesia
Indiana University School of Medicine
Indianapolis, Indiana

Karen B. Domino, MD, MPH
Professor
Department of Anesthesiology
University of Washington School of Medicine
Seattle, Washington

Francois Donati, MD, PhD, FRCPC
Professor
Department of Anesthesiology
University of Montreal
Hospital Maisonneuve-Rosemont
Montreal, Quebec, Canada

Michael B. Dorrough, MD
Resident Physician
Department of Anesthesiology
University of Utah School of Medicine
University Health Care
Salt Lake City, Utah

John C. Drummond, MD, FRCPC
Professor of Anesthesiology
The University of California, San Diego
Staff Anesthesiologist
VA Medical Center, San Diego
San Diego, California

Randal O. Dull, MD, PhD
Associate Professor
Department of Anesthesiology
University of Utah
Salt Lake City, Utah

Thomas J. Ebert, MD, PhD
Professor of Anesthesiology
Program Director
Medical College of Wisconsin
VA Medical Center, 112A
Milwaukee, Wisconsin

Jan Ehrenwerth, MD
Professor
Department of Anesthesiology
Yale University School of Medicine
Yale-New Haven Hospital
New Haven, Connecticut

John H. Eichhorn, MD
Professor
Department of Anesthesiology
University of Kentucky College of Medicine
Univeristy of Kentucky Medical Center
Lexington, Kentucky

James B. Eisenkraft, MD
Professor
Department of Anesthesiology
The Mount Sinai School of Medicine
Attending Anesthesiologist
The Mount Sinai Hospital
New York, New York

John E. Ellis, MD
Adjunct Professor
Department of Anesthesiology and Critical Care
University of Pennsylvania School of Medicine
Philadelphia, Pennsylvania

Matthew Eng, MD
Department of Anesthesiology
University of Texas Southwestern
Dallas, Texas Department of Anesthesiology
Cedars Sinai Medical Center
Los Angeles, California

Alex S. Evers, MD
Henry E. Mallinckrodt Professor and Chair
Department of Anesthesiology
Washington University School of Medicine
Anesthesiologist-in-Chief
Barnes-Jewish Hospital
St. Louis, Missouri

Lynne R. Ferrari, MD
Associate Professor of Anesthesiology
Department of Anesthesiology
Harvard Medical School
Chief, Perioperative Anesthesia
The Children's Hospital
Boston, Massachusetts

Scott M. Fishman, MD
Chief, Division of Pain Medicine
Professor of Clinical Anesthesiology
Department of Anesthesiology and Pain Medicine
University of California, Davis
Ellison Ambulatory Care Center
Sacramento, California

Michael A. Fowler, MD, MBA
Associate Professor
Department of Anesthesiology
Virginia Commonwealth University
Director, Post Anesthesia Care Unit
Virginia Commonwealth Medical Center
Richmond, Virginia

J. Sean Funston, MD
Assistant Professor
Department of Anesthesiology
University of Texas Medical Branch
Galveston, Texas

Steven I. Gayer, MD, MBA
Associate Professor
Departments of Anesthesiology and Ophthalmology
University of Miami Miller School of Medicine
Bascom Palmer Eye Institute
Miami, Florida

Ronald George, MD, FRCP
Department of Anesthesiology
Duke University Medical Center
Durham, North Carolina

Kathryn Glas, MD, FASE, MBA
Associate Professor
Department of Anesthesiology
Emory University School of Medicine
Co-Director, Cardiothoracic Anesthesiology
Crawford Long Hospital
Atlanta, Georgia

Alexander W. Gotta, MD
Emeritus Professor of Anesthesiology
State University of New York
Downstate Medical Center
Brooklyn, New York

Loreta Grecu, MD
Assistant Professor
Department of Anesthesiology
Yale University
Attending Physician
Yale-New Haven Hospital
New Haven, Connecticut

Steven B. Greenberg, MD
Assistant Professor
Department of Anesthesiology
NorthShore University HealthSystem
Evanston, Illinois

Dhanesh K. Gupta, MD
Associate Professor
Department of Anesthesiology and Neurological Surgery
Northwestern University Feinberg School of Medicine
Northwestern Memorial Hospital
Chicago, Illinois

Steven C. Hall, MD
Arthur C. King Professor of Pediatric Anesthesia
Department of Anesthesiology
Northwestern University Feinberg School of Medicine
Anesthesiologist-in-Chief
Department of Pediatric Anesthesia
Children's Memorial Hospital
Chicago, Illinois

Tara M. Hata, MD
Clinical Associate Professor
Department of Anesthesia
Carver College of Medicine
University of Iowa
University of Iowa Hospitals and Clinics
Iowa City, Iowa

Laurence M. Hausman, MD
Associate Professor
Department of Anesthesiology
Mount Sinai School of Medicine
Mount Sinai Medical Center
New York, New York

Thomas K. Henthorn, MD
Professor and Chair
Department of Anesthesiology
University of Colorado, Denver
University of Colorado Hospital
Aurora, Colorado

Simon C. Hillier, MB, ChB
Department of Anesthesia
Section of Pediatric Anesthesia and Critical Care
Indiana University School of Medicine
Indianapolis, Indiana

Harriet W. Hopf, MD
Professor
Department of Anesthesiology
University of Utah School of Medicine
University Health Care
Salt Lake City, Utah

Terese T. Horlocker, MD
Professor
Departments of Anesthesiology and Orthopedics
Mayo Clinic College of Medicine
Rochester, Minnesota

Robert W. Hurley, MD, PhD
Assistant Professor
Department of Anesthesiology and Critical Care
Johns Hopkins University
Medical Director, Pain Clinic
Johns Hopkins Medical Institutions
Baltimore, Maryland

Adam K. Jacob, MD, MS
Fellow
Department of Anesthesiology
Mayo Clinic
Rochester, Minnesota

Joel O. Johnson, MD, PhD
Russell D. Sheldon Professor and Chair
Department of Anesthesiology and Perioperative Medicine
University of Missouri
Missouri Univeristy Health
Columbia, Missouri

Zeev N. Kain, MD, MBA
Professor and Chair
Department of Anesthesiology
University of California, Irvine
Irvine, California

John P. Kampine, MD, PhD
Professor Emeritus
Department of Anesthesiology
Medical College of Wisconsin
Milwaukee, Wisconsin

Jonathan C. Katz, MD
Staff Anesthesiologist
Private Practice
Plantation, Florida

Jonathan D. Katz, MD
Clinical Professor
Department of Anesthesiology
Yale University School of Medicine
New Haven, Connecticut
Attending Anesthesiologist
Department of Anesthesiology
St. Vincent's Medical Center
Bridgeport, Connecticut

Brian S. Kaufman, MD
Associate Professor
Departments of Medicine, Anesthesiology
   and Neurosurgery
New York University School of Medicine
Director of Critical Care
NYU Langone Medical Center
New York, New York

M. Sean Kincaid, MD
Clinical Instructor
Department of Anesthesiology
University of Washington
Attending Physician
Department of Anesthesiology
Harborview Medical Center
Seattle, Washington

Sandra L. Kopp, MD
Assistant Professor
Department of Anesthesiology
Mayo Clinic
Rochester, Minnesota

Arthur M. Lam, MD, FRCPC
Anesthesiologist in Chief
Director of Cerebrovascular Laboratory Harborview Medical
   Center
Professor of Anesthesiology and Neurological Surgery
University of Washington
Seattle, Washington

Thomas A. Lane, MD
Professor of Pathology
University of California, San Diego
Medical Director
UCSD Transfusion Services and Stem Cell Processing Lab
San Diego, California

Noel W. Lawson, MD
Professor
Department of Anesthesiology
University of Missouri-Columbia
Staff Anesthesiologist
University of Missouri-Columbia Hospitals and Clinics
Columbia, Missouri

Wilton C. Levine, MD
Instructor in Anesthesia
Harvard Medical School
Assistant in Anesthesia
Departments of Anesthesiology and Critical Care
Massachusetts General Hospital
Boston, Massachusetts

Jerrold H. Levy, MD, FAHA
Professor and Deputy Chair for Research
Department of Anesthesiology
Emory University School of Medicine
Director of Cardiothoracic Anesthesiology and Critical Care
Emory Healthcare
Atlanta, Georgia

Adam D. Lichtman, MD
Assistant Professor of Anesthesiology
Department of Anesthesiology
Weill Cornell Medical Center
New York Presbyterian Hospital
New York, New York

J. Lance Lichtor, MD
Professor
Department of Anesthesiology
University of Massachusetts Medical School
Worcester, Massachusetts

Yi Lin, MD, PhD
Clinical Instructor of Anesthesiology
Department of Anesthesiology
Weill Medical College of Cornell University
Assistant Attending Anesthesiologist
Hospital for Special Surgery
New York, New York

Spencer S. Liu, MD
Clinical Professor
Department of Anesthesiology
Weill Medical College of Cornell University
Hospital for Special Surgery
New York, New York

David A. Lubarsky, MD, MBA
Emanuel M. Papper Professor and Chair
Department of Anesthesiology, Perioperative Medicine, and
    Pain Management
University of Miami Miller School of Medicine
Department of Anesthesiology
Jackson Memorial Hospital
Miami, Florida

Stephen M. Macres, PharmD, MD
Director, Postoperative Pain and Regional Anesthesia Service
Clinical Professor of Anesthesiology
Department of Anesthesiology and Pain Medicine
University of California, Davis
Sacramento, California

Srinivas Mantha, MD
Professor and Sub-Dean
Department of Anesthesiology and Intensive Care
Nizam's Institute of Medical Sciences
Hyderabad, India

Joseph P. Mathew, MD, MHSc
Professor
Department of Anesthesiology
Duke University
Chief, Division of Cardiothoracic Anesthesiology
Duke University Medical Center
Durham, North Carolina

Michael S. Mazurek, MD
Associate Professor
Department of Anesthesiology
Indiana University School of Medicine
Riley Hospital for Children
Indianapolis, Indiana

Kathryn E. McGoldrick, MD
Professor and Chair
Department of Anesthesiology
New York Medical College
Westchester Medical Center
Valhalla, New York

Sanford M. Miller, MD
Clinical Associate Professor
New York University School of Medicine
Assistant Director of Anesthesiology
Bellevue Hospital Center
New York, New York

Peter G. Moore, MB, BS, PhD, FANZCA
Professor and Chair
Department of Anesthesiology and Pain Medicine
University of California, Davis
University of California, Davis Medical Center
Sacramento, California

John R. Moyers, MD
Professor
Department of Anesthesia
Carver College of Medicine
University of Iowa
University of Iowa Hopsitals and Clinics
Iowa City, Iowa

Holly Muir, MD
Assistant Professor
Department of Anesthesiology
Duke University Medical Center
Durham, North Carolina

Glenn S. Murphy, MD
NorthShore University HealthSystem
Evanston, Illinois

Michael J. Murray, MD, PhD
Professor
Department of Anesthesiology
Mayo Clinic College of Medicine
Mayo Clinic Hospital
Jacksonville, Florida

Steven M. Neustein, MD
Associate Professor
Department of Anesthesiology
The Mount Sinai School of Medicine
Mount Sinai Hospital
New York, New York

E. Andrew Ochroch, MD, MSCE
Associate Professor of Anesthesiology and Critical Care
Director of Clinical Research
Director of Thoracic Anesthesiology
University of Pennsylvania Health System
Philadelphia, Pennsylvania

Babatunde O. Ogunnaike, MD
Associate Professor
Department of Anesthesiology and Pain Management
University of Texas Southwestern Medical Center
Chief of Anesthesia Services
Parkland Health and Hospital System
Dallas, Texas

Charles W. Otto, MD, FCCM
Professor
Department of Anesthesiology
University of Arizona College of Medicine
Arizona Health Sciences Center
Tucson, Arizona

Nathan Leon Pace, MD, Mstat
Professor
Department of Anesthesiology
University of Utah
Salt Lake City, Utah

Paul S. Pagel, MD, PhD
Professor
Department of Anesthesiology
Medical College of Wisconsin
Staff Anesthesiologist
Department of Anesthesia and Special Care
Zablocki VA Medcial Center
Milwaukee, Wisconsin

Albert C. Perrino, Jr., MD
Professor
Department of Anesthesiology
Yale University School of Medicine
Attending Physician
Yale-New Haven Hospital
New Haven, Connecticut

Charise Petrovitch, MD
Clinical Professor
Department of Anesthesia and Clinical Care Medicine
George Washington University Hospital
Chief, Anesthesia Section
VA Medical Center
Washington, DC

Mihai V. Podgoreanu, MD, FASE
Associate Professor
Department of Anesthesiology
Duke University
Director, Perioperatibe Genomics Program
Duke University Medical Center
Durham, North Carolina

Wanda M. Popescu, MD
Assistant Professor of Anesthesiology
Department of Anesthesiology
Yale University School of Medicine
Attending Physician
Yale-New Haven Hospital
New Haven, Connecticut

Karen L. Posner, PhD
Research Professor
Department of Anesthesiology
University of Washington
Seattle, Washington

Donald S. Prough, MD
Professor, and Chair
Department of Anesthesiology
University of Texas Medical Branch
Galveston, Texas

Kevin T. Riutort, MD
Chief Resident
Department of Anesthesiology
Mayo Clinic
Mayo Clinic Hospital
Jacksonville, Florida

J. David Roccoforte, MD
Assistant Professor
Department of Anesthesiology
New York University School of Medicine
New York, New York

Michael F. Roizen, MD
Professor
Division of Anesthesiology, Critical Care Medicine and
    Comprehensive Pain Management
Chair, Wellness Institute
Cleveland Clinical Foundation
Cleveland, Ohio

G. Alec Rooke, MD, PhD
Visiting Professor
Department of Anesthesiology
Beth Israel Deaconess Medical Center
Harvard Medical School
Boston, Massachusetts
Professor
Department of Anesthesiology and Critical Care
University of Washington
University of Washington Medical Center
Seattle, Washington

Stanley H. Rosenbaum, MD
Professor
Department of Anesthesiology
Yale University School of Medicine
Attending Physician
Yale-New Haven Hospital
New Haven, Connecticut

Henry Rosenberg, MD, CPE
Director
Department of Medical Education and Clinical Research
Saint Barnabas Medical Center
Livingston, New Jersey

Meg A. Rosenblatt, MD
Associate Professor
Department of Anesthesiology
Mount Sinai School of Medicine
New York, New York

William H. Rosenblatt, MD
Professor
Department of Anesthesiology
Yale University School of Medicine
Attending Physician
Yale New Haven Hospital
New Haven, Connecticut

Richard W. Rosenquist, MD
Professor
Department of Anesthesia
University of Iowa
Director, Pain Medicine Division
University of Iowa Hospital
Iowa City, Iowa

Carl E. Rosow, MD, PhD
Professor
Department of Anesthesia and Critical Care
Harvard Medical School
Massachusetts General Hospital
Boston, Massacusetts

Nyamkhishig Sambuughin, PhD
Assistant Professor
Department of Anesthesiology
Uniformed Services University
Bethesda, Maryland

Alan C. Santos, MD, MPH
Chairman of Anesthesiology
Ochsner Clinic Foundation
New Orleans, Louisiana

Barbara M. Scavone, MD
Associate Professor
Department of Anesthesiology
Northwestern University Feinberg School of Medicine
Northwestern Memorial Hospital
Chicago, Illinois

Philliip G. Schmid, MD
Department of Anesthesiology
St. Alphonsus Regional Medical Center
Boise, Idaho

Jeffrey J. Schwartz, MD
Associate Professor
Department of Anesthesiology
Yale University School of Medicine
Attending Physician
Yale-New Haven Hospital
New Haven, Connecticut

Harry A. Seifert, MD
Adjunct Assistant Professor of Clinical Anesthesiology
Department of Anesthesiology and Critical Care
The Children's Hospital of Philadelphia
Philadelphia, Pennsylvania

Aarti Sharma, MD
Assistant Professor
Department of Anesthesiology
Weill Cornell Medical Center
New York Presbyterian Hospital
New York, New York

Andrew Shaw, BSc, MBBS, FRCA, FCCM
Associate Professor
Department of Anesthesiology
Duke University
Attending Anesthesiologist
Duke University Medical Center
Durham, North Carolina

Nikolaos J. Skubas, MD, FASE
Associate Professor
Department of Anesthesiology
Weill Cornell Medical College
Associate Attending
New York Hospital-Weill Cornell Medical Center
New York, New York

Hugh M. Smith, MD, PhD
Instructor
Department of Anesthesiology
Mayo Clinic College of Medicine
Mayo Clinic
Rochester, Minnesota

Karen J. Souter, BBS, FRCA
Associate Professor
Department of Anesthesiology and Pain Medicine
University of Washington
Seattle, Washington

Bruce D. Spiess, MD, FAHA
Professor of Anesthesiology and Emergency Medicine
Director of Virginia Commonwealth University Reanimation
  Engineering Shock Center
Virginia Commonwealth University Medical Center
Richmond, Viginia

Mark Stafford-Smith, MD, CM, FRCP, FASE
Professor
Department of Anesthesiology,
Duke University Medical Center
Durham, North Carolina

M. Christine Stock, MD
Professor
Department of Anesthesiology
Northwestern University Feinberg School of Medicine
Northweston Memorial Hospital
Chicago, Illinois

Robert K. Stoelting, MD
Emeritus Professor and Past Chair
Department of Anesthesia
Indiana University School of Medicine
Indianapolis, Indiana

Karen J. Souter, BBS, FRCA
Associate Professor
Department of Anesthesiology and Pain Medicine
University of Washington
Seattle, Washington

David F. Stowe, MD, PhD
Professor
Despartment of Anesthesiology and Physiology
Medical College of Wisconsin
Froedtert Hospital & Zablocki VA Medical Center
Milwaukee Regional Medical Center
Milwaukee, Wisconsin

Wariya Sukhupragarn, MD, FRCAT
Assistant Professor
Department of Anesthesiology
Chiang Mai University
Maharaj Nakorn Chiang Mai Hospital
Chiang Mai, Thailand
Research Fellow in Airway Management
Department of Anesthesiology
Yale University School of Medicine
Yale-New Haven Hospital
New Haven, Connecticut

Santhanam Suresh, MD
Professor
Department of Anesthesiology
Northwestern University Feinberg School of Medicine
Children's Memorial Hospital
Chicago, Illinois

Christer H. Svensén, MD, PhD, DEAA, MBA
Associate Professor
Department of Anesthesiology
Weill Medical College of Cornell University
New York Presbyterian Hospital
New York, New York

Stephen J. Thomas, MD
Topkin-Van Poznak Professor and Vice-Chairman
Department of Anesthesiology
Weill Medical College of Cornell University
New York Presbyterian Hospital
New York, New York

Miriam M. Treggiari, MD, PhD, MPH
Associate Professor
Department of Anesthesiology and Pain Medicine
University of Washington
Harborview Medical Center
Seattle, Washington

Ban Tsui, BSc, MSc, MD, FRCPC
Professor
Department of Anesthesiology and Pain Medicine
University of Alberta
Director, Regional Anesthesia and Pain Service
University of Alberta Hospital
Stollery Children's Hospital
Edmonton, Alberta, Canada

Jeffrey S. Vender, MD, FCCM, FCCP
Department of Anesthesiology
NorthShore University HealthSystem
Evanston, Illinois

J. Scott Walton, MD
Associate Professor
Department of Anesthesia and Perioperative Medicine
Medical University of South Carolina
Charleston, South Carolina

Mark A. Warner, MD
Professor
Department of Anesthesiology
Mayo Clinic
Rochester, Minnesota

Denise J. Wedel, MD
Professor
Department of Anesthesiology
Mayo Clinic College of Medicine
Rochester, Minnesota

Paul F. White, PhD, MD
Professor and Holder of the Margaret Milam McDermott
    Distinguished Chair in Anesthesiology
Department of Anesthesiology & Pain Management
    University of Texas Southwestern Medical Center
Dallas, Texas

Charles W. Whitten, MD
Professor and Chair
Department of Anesthesiology and Pain Management
University of Texas Southwestern Medical Center
Dallas, Texas

Scott W. Wolf, MD
Assistant Professor
Department of Anesthesiology
Northwestern University Feinberg School of Medicine
Northwestern Memorial Hospital
Chicago, Illinois

Cynthia A. Wong, MD
Associate Professor
Department of Anesthesiology
Northwestern University Feinberg School of Medicine
Medical Director of Obstetric Anesthesia
Northwestern Memorial Hospital
Chicago, Illinois

James R. Zaidan, MD, MBA
Professor and Chair
Department of Anesthesiology
Emory University Hospital
Atlanta, Georgia

Welcome to the sixth edition of *Clinical Anesthesia*. The publication of this edition occurs at a time of great clinical, educational, and research advances. At no time in our specialty's history is the observation more true that the major achievements in surgery could not occur without the accompanying vision of skillful anesthesiologists. Everyday in operating rooms around the world anesthesiologists are challenged to meet exemplary levels of clinical care while ensuring the highest level of patient safety. To meet these needs new educational paradigms are being employed which require education in a variety of formats and settings.

The prime goal of *Clinical Anesthesia* from its inception has been:

"To develop a textbook that supports efficient and rapid acquisition of knowledge."

The editors have employed a variety of educational methods to achieve this objective making *Clinical Anesthesia*, in reality, a series of interconnected publications using the printed word, electronic medium, and the Internet. Our efforts have been recognized with numerous international awards. With the publication of each edition, we try to develop innovative and contemporary ways to disseminate knowledge to our reader. With this edition, we are the first anesthesia text to use podcasting as one of the newest methods to rapidly transmit clinically relevant information, while also assisting practiners who are preparing for Board examinations and recertification.

Starting with the cover, you will see major changes in the textbook. Drs. M. Christine Stock and Michael K. Cahalan have joined the Editors. Both Chris and Mike bring their unique talents to enhance our ability to deliver a forward-looking clinical text that enhances acquisition of clinically important information and aligns chapter content with contemporary educational goals. Dr. Robert Stoelting will assume Editor Emeritus status. Bob is instrumental in the success of the *Clinical Anesthesia* series. His writing and editing capabilities are legendary. The editors have benefited enormously from his insights into modern anesthesia, as well as his hands-on approach to the logistically complex task of editorial supervision.

Once the book is opened, the reader will be able to appreciate a unified graphic format. All illustrations and graphics are presented to augment the educational experience and rapidly transmit important information. In addition, to a re-ordered table of contents, two new chapters have been added: *Inflammation, Wound Healing and Infection,* and *Echocardiography.* Approximately a third of the contributors are new to this edition, incorporating a fresh point of view to important chapter content. We have encouraged contributors to develop clinically relevant themes and prioritize various clinical options considered by many to be the definitive strength of previous editions.

We realize that redundancies may exist in a book of this size. The editors have taken every opportunity to reduce repetition or even disagreement between chapters. However, clinical problems are managed differently by practiners, so this diversity of approach serves to enrich the educational experience.

We wish to express our appreciation to all our contributors whose knowledge, hard work, dedication and timely submissions have allowed us to maintain quality while working with a tight production schedule. Our readers have also been instrumental in providing comments that allow the editors to continually improve *Clinical Anesthesia* to meet the needs of our audience. Dr. Jorge Galvez deserves special recognition for his enormous input on the logistical management of our podcasting project. We also thank Christopher Cambic, MD who proofread for details, as well as our administrative assistants—Gail Norup, Ruby Wilson, Deanna Walker, and Victoria Ramos. We would like to thank our editors at Lippincott Williams & Wilkins-Wolters Kluwer, Brian Brown and Lisa McAllister, for their commitment to excellence. Finally, we owe a debt of gratitude to Nicole Dernoski—Managing Editor at LWW, Chris Miller—Production Manager at Aptara, Angela Panetta—Marketing at LWW, and Ed Schultes, Jr.—Media Assistant at LWW whose day-to-day management of this endeavor resulted in a publication that exceeded the Editor's expectations.

Paul G. Barash, MD
Bruce F. Cullen, MD
Robert K. Stoelting, MD
Michael K. Cahalan, MD
M. Christine Stock, MD

CONTENTS

SECTION VII ■ ANESTHESIA FOR SURGICAL SUBSPECIALTIES

SECTION VIII ■ PERIOPERATIVE AND CONSULTATIVE SERVICES

SECTION I ■ INTRODUCTION TO ANESTHESIOLOGY

CHAPTER 1 ■ THE HISTORY OF ANESTHESIA

ADAM K. JACOB, SANDRA L. KOPP, DOUGLAS R. BACON, AND HUGH M. SMITH

KEY POINTS

1 Anesthesiology is a young specialty historically, especially when compared with surgery or internal medicine.

2 Discoveries in anesthesiology have taken decades to build upon the observations and experiments of many people, and in some instances we are still searching. For example, the ideal volatile anesthetic has yet to be discovered.

3 Regional anesthesia is the direct outgrowth of a chance observation by an intern who would go on to become a successful ophthalmologist.

4 Pain medicine began as an outgrowth of regional anesthesia.

5 Much of our current anesthesia equipment is the direct result of anesthesiologists being unhappy with and needing better tools to properly anesthetize patients.

6 Many safety standards have been established through the work of anesthesiologists who were frustrated by the status quo.

7 Organizations of anesthesia professionals have been critical in establishing high standards in education and proficiency, which in turn has defined the specialty.

8 Respiratory critical care medicine started as the need by anesthesiologists to use positive pressure ventilation to help polio victims.

9 Surgical anesthesia and physician specialization in its administration have allowed for increasingly complex operations to be performed on increasingly ill patients.

Surgery without adequate pain control may seem cruel to the modern reader, and in contemporary practice we are prone to forget the realities of preanesthesia surgery. Fanny Burney, a well-known literary artist from the early 19th century, described a mastectomy she endured after receiving a "wine cordial" as her sole anesthetic. As seven male assistants held her down, the surgery commenced: "When the dreadful steel was plunged into the breast-cutting through veins-arteries-flesh-nerves-I needed no injunction not to restrain my cries. I began a scream that lasted unintermittently during the whole time of the incision—& I almost marvel that it rings not in my Ears still! So excruciating was the agony. Oh Heaven!—I then

felt the knife racking against the breast bone—scraping it! This performed while I yet remained in utterly speechless torture."[1] Burney's description illustrates the difficulty of overstating the impact of anesthesia on the human condition. An epitaph on a monument to William Thomas Green Morton, one of the founders of anesthesia, summarizes the contribution of anesthesia: "BEFORE WHOM in all time Surgery was **1** Agony."[2] Although most human civilizations evolved some method for diminishing patient discomfort, *anesthesia*, in its modern and effective meaning, is a comparatively recent discovery with traceable origins in the mid-19th century. How we have changed perspectives from one in which surgical pain was terrible and expected to one in which patients reasonably assume they will be safe, pain-free, and unaware during extensive operations is a fascinating story and the subject of this chapter.

Anesthesiologists are like no other physicians: we are experts at controlling the airway and at emergency resuscitation; we are real-time cardio pulmonologists achieving hemodynamic and respiratory stability for the anesthetized patient; we are pharmacologists and physiologists, calculating appropriate doses and desired responses; we are gurus of postoperative care and patient safety; we are internists performing perianesthetic medical evaluations; we are the pain experts across all medical disciplines and apply specialized techniques in pain clinics and labor wards; we manage the severely sick and injured in critical care units; we are neurologists, selectively blocking sympathetic, sensory, or motor functions with our regional techniques; we are trained researchers exploring scientific mystery and clinical phenomenon.

Anesthesiology is an amalgam of specialized techniques, equipment, drugs, and knowledge that, like the growth rings of a tree, have built up over time. Current anesthesia practice is the summation of individual effort and fortuitous discovery of centuries. Every component of modern anesthesia was at some point a new discovery and reflects the experience, knowledge, and inventiveness of our predecessors. Historical examination enables understanding of how these individual components of anesthesia evolved. Knowledge of the history of anesthesia enhances our appreciation of current practice and intimates where our specialty might be headed.

ANESTHESIA BEFORE ETHER

Physical and Psychological Anesthesia

The Edwin Smith Surgical Papyrus, the oldest known written surgical document, describes 48 cases performed by an Egyptian surgeon from 3000 to 2500 BC. While this remarkable surgical treatise contains no direct mention of measures to lessen patient pain or suffering, Egyptian pictographs from the same era show a surgeon compressing a nerve in a patient's antecubital fossa while operating on the patient's hand. Another image displays a patient compressing his own brachial plexus while a procedure is performed on his palm.[3] In the 16th century, military surgeon Ambroise Paré became adept at nerve compression as a means of creating anesthesia.

Medical science has benefited from the natural refrigerating properties of ice and snow as well. For centuries anatomical dissections were performed only in winter because colder temperatures delayed deterioration of the cadaver, and in the Middle Ages the anesthetic effects of cold water and ice were recognized. In the 17th century, Marco Aurelio Severino described the technique of "refrigeration anesthesia" in which snow was placed in parallel lines across the incisional plane such that the surgical site became insensate within minutes. The technique never became widely used, likely because of the challenge of maintaining stores of snow year-round.[4] Severino is also known to have saved numerous lives during an epidemic of diphtheria by performing tracheostomies and inserting trocars to maintain patency of the airway.[5]

Formal manipulation of the psyche to relieve surgical pain was undertaken by French physicians Charles Dupotet and Jules Cloquet in the late 1820s with hypnosis, then called *mesmerism*. Although the work of Anton Mesmer was discredited by the French Academy of Science after formal inquiry several decades earlier, proponents like Dupotet and Cloquet continued with mesmeric experiments and pleaded to the Academie de Medicine to reconsider its utility.[6] In a well-attended demonstration in 1828, Cloquet removed the breast of a 64-year-old patient while she reportedly remained in a calm, mesmeric sleep. This demonstration made a lasting impression on British physician John Elliotson, who became a leading figure of the mesmeric movement in England in the 1830s and 1840s. Innovative and quick to adopt new advances, Elliotson performed mesmeric demonstrations and in 1843 published *Numerous Cases of Surgical Operations without Pain in the Mesmeric State*. Support for mesmerism faded when in 1846 renowned surgeon Robert Liston performed the first operation using ether anesthesia in England and remarked, "This Yankee dodge beats mesmerism all hollow."[7]

Early Analgesics and Soporifics

Dioscorides, a Greek physician from the first century AD, commented on the analgesia of mandragora, a drug prepared from the bark and leaves of the mandrake plant. He observed that the plant substance could be boiled in wine, strained, and used "in the case of persons . . . about to be cut or cauterized, when they wish to produce anesthesia."[8] Mandragora was still being used to benefit patients as late as the 17th century. From the ninth to the thirteenth centuries, the *soporific sponge* was a dominant mode of providing pain relief during surgery. Mandrake leaves, along with black nightshade, poppies, and other herbs, were boiled together and cooked onto a sponge. The sponge was then reconstituted in hot water and placed under the patient's nose before surgery. Prior to the hypodermic syringe and routine venous access, ingestion and inhalation were the only known routes for administering medicines to gain systemic effects. Prepared as indicated by published reports of the time, the sponge generally contained morphine and scopolamine in varying amounts—drugs used in modern anesthesia.[9]

Alcohol was another element of the pre-ether armamentarium because it was thought to induce stupor and blunt the impact of pain. Although alcohol is a central nervous system depressant, in the amounts administered it produced little analgesia in the setting of true surgical pain. Fanny Burney's account underscores the ineffectiveness of alcohol as an anesthetic. Not only did the alcohol provide minimal pain control, it did nothing to dull her recollection of events. Laudanum was an alcohol-based solution of opium first compounded by Paracelsus in the 16th century. It was wildly popular in the Victorian and Romantic periods, and prescribed for a wide variety of ailments from the common cold to tuberculosis. Although appropriately used as an analgesic in some instances, it was frequently misused and abused. Laudanum was given by nursemaids to quiet wailing infants and abused by many upper-class women, poets, and artists who fell victim to its addictive potential.

Inhaled Anesthetics

Nitrous oxide was known for its ability to induce lightheadedness and was often inhaled by those seeking a thrill. It was not used as frequently as ether because it was more difficult to synthesize and store. It was made by heating ammonium nitrate in the presence of iron filings. The evolved gas was passed through water to eliminate toxic oxides of nitrogen before being stored. Nitrous oxide was first prepared in 1773 by Joseph Priestley, an English clergyman and scientist, who ranks among the great pioneers of chemistry. Without formal scientific training, Priestley prepared and examined several gases, including nitrous oxide, ammonia, sulfur dioxide, oxygen, carbon monoxide, and carbon dioxide.

At the end of the 18th century in England, there was a strong interest in the supposed wholesome effects of mineral waters and gases, particularly with regard to treatment of scurvy, tuberculosis, and other diseases. Thomas Beddoes opened his Pneumatic Institute close to the small spa of Hotwells, in the city of Bristol, to study the beneficial effects of inhaled gases. He hired Humphry Davy in 1798 to conduct research projects for the Institute. Davy performed brilliant investigations of several gases but focused much of his attention on nitrous oxide. His human experimental results, combined with research on the physical properties of the gas, were published in *Nitrous Oxide,* a 580-page book published in 1800. This impressive treatise is now best remembered for a few incidental observations. Davy commented that nitrous oxide transiently relieved a severe headache, obliterated a minor headache, and briefly quenched an aggravating toothache. The most frequently quoted passage was a casual entry: "As nitrous oxide in its extensive operation appears capable of destroying physical pain, it may probably be used with advantage during surgical operations in which no great effusion of blood takes place ."[10] This is perhaps the most famous of the "missed opportunities" to discover surgical anesthesia. Davy's lasting nitrous oxide legacy was coining the phrase "laughing gas" to describe its unique property.

Almost Discovery: Hickman, Clarke, Long, and Wells

② As the 19th century progressed, societal attitudes toward pain changed, perhaps best exemplified in the writings of the Romantic poets.[11] Thus, efforts to relieve pain were undertaken and several more near-breakthroughs occurred deserve mention. An English surgeon named Henry Hill Hickman searched intentionally for an inhaled anesthetic to relieve pain in his patients.[12] Hickman used high concentrations of carbon dioxide in his studies on mice and dogs. Carbon dioxide has some anesthetic properties, as shown by the absence of response to an incision in the animals of Hickman's study, but it was never determined if the animals were insensate because of hypoxia rather than anesthesia. Hickman's concept was magnificent; his choice of agent was regrettable.

The discovery of surgical anesthetics in the modern era remains linked to inhaled anesthetics. The compound now known as *diethyl ether* had been known for centuries; it may have been synthesized first by an eighth-century Arabian philosopher Jabir ibn Hayyam, or possibly by Raymond Lully, a 13th century European alchemist. But diethyl ether was certainly known in the 16th century, both to Valerius Cordus and Paracelsus who prepared it by distilling sulfuric acid (oil of vitriol) with fortified wine to produce an *oleum vitrioli dulce* (sweet oil of vitriol). One of the first "missed" observations on the effects of inhaled agents, Paracelsus observed that ether caused chickens to fall asleep and awaken unharmed. He must have been aware of its analgesic qualities because he reported that it could be recommended for use in painful illnesses.

For three centuries thereafter, this simple compound remained a therapeutic agent with only occasional use. Some of its properties were examined but without sustained interest by distinguished British scientists Robert Boyle, Isaac Newton, and Michael Faraday, none of whom made the conceptual link to surgical anesthesia. Its only routine application came as an inexpensive recreational drug among the poor of Britain and Ireland, who sometimes drank an ounce or two of ether when taxes made gin prohibitively expensive.[13] An American variation of this practice was conducted by groups of students who held ether-soaked towels to their faces at nocturnal "ether frolics."

William E. Clarke, a medical student from Rochester, New York, may have given the first ether anesthetic in January 1842. From techniques learned as a chemistry student in 1839, Clarke entertained his companions with nitrous oxide and ether. Emboldened by these experiences, he administered ether, from a towel, to a young woman named Hobbie. One of her teeth was then extracted without pain by a dentist named Elijah Pope.[14] However, it was suggested that the woman's unconsciousness was due to hysteria and Clarke was advised to conduct no further anesthetic experiments.[15]

Two months later, on March 30, 1842, Crawford Williamson Long administered ether with a towel for surgical anesthesia in Jefferson, Georgia. His patient, James M. Venable, was a young man who was already familiar with ether's exhilarating effects, for he reported in a certificate that he had previously inhaled it and was fond of its use. Venable had two small tumors on his neck but refused to have them excised because he feared the pain that accompanied surgery. Knowing that Venable was familiar with ether's action, Dr. Long proposed that ether might alleviate pain and gained his patient's consent to proceed. After inhaling ether from the towel and having the procedure successfully completed, Venable reported that he was unaware of the removal of the tumors.[16] In determining the first fee for anesthesia and surgery, Long settled on a charge of $2.00.[17]

A common mid-19th century problem facing dentists was that patients refused beneficial treatment of their teeth for fear of the pain of the procedure. From a dentist's perspective, pain was not so much life-threatening as it was livelihood-threatening. One of the first dentists to engender a solution was Horace Wells of Hartford, Connecticut, whose great moment of discovery came on December 10, 1844. He observed a lecture-exhibition on nitrous oxide by an itinerant "scientist," Gardner Quincy Colton, who encouraged members of the audience to inhale a sample of the gas. Wells observed a young man injure his leg without pain while under the influence of nitrous oxide. Sensing that it might provide pain relief during dental procedures, Wells contacted Colton and boldly proposed an experiment in which Wells was to be the subject. The following day, Colton gave Wells nitrous oxide before a fellow dentist, William Riggs, extracted a tooth.[18] Afterward Wells declared that he had not felt any pain and deemed the experiment a success. Colton taught Wells to prepare nitrous oxide, which the dentist administered with success to patients in his practice. His apparatus probably resembled that used by Colton: a wooden tube placed in the mouth through which nitrous oxide was breathed from a small bag filled with the gas.

Public Demonstration of Ether Anesthesia

Another New Englander, William Thomas Green Morton, briefly shared a dental practice with Wells in Hartford. Wells' daybook shows that he gave Morton a course of instruction in anesthesia, but Morton apparently moved to Boston without paying for the lessons.[19] In Boston, Morton continued his interest in anesthesia and sought instruction from chemist and physician Charles T. Jackson. After learning that ether dropped on the skin provided analgesia, he began experiments with inhaled ether, an agent that proved to be much more versatile than nitrous oxide. Bottles of liquid ether were easily transported, and the volatility of the drug permitted effective inhalation. The concentrations required for surgical anesthesia were so low that patients did not become hypoxic when breathing ether vaporized in air. It also possessed what would later be recognized as a unique property among all inhaled anesthetics: the quality of providing surgical anesthesia without causing respiratory depression. These properties, combined with a slow rate of induction, gave the patient a significant safety margin even in the hands of relatively unskilled anesthetists.[20]

After anesthetizing a pet dog, Morton became confident of his skills and anesthetized patients in his dental office.

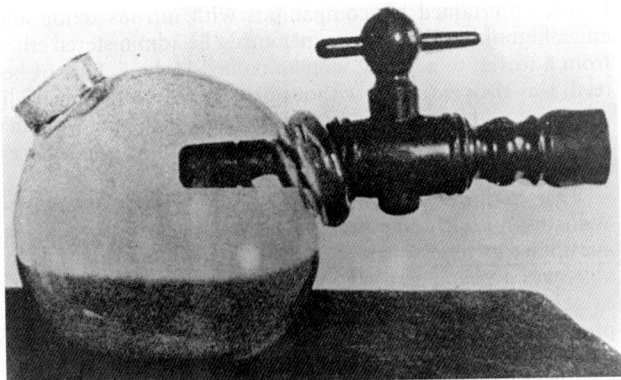

FIGURE 1-1.   Morton's ether inhaler (1846).

Encouraged by his success, Morton sought an invitation to give a public demonstration in the Bullfinch amphitheater of the Massachusetts General Hospital, the same site as Wells' failed demonstration. Many details of the October 16, 1846, demonstration are well known. Morton secured permission to provide an anesthetic to Edward Gilbert Abbott, a patient of surgeon John Collins Warren. Warren planned to excise a vascular lesion from the left side of Abbott's neck and was about to proceed when Morton arrived late. He had been delayed because he was obliged to wait for an instrument maker to complete a new inhaler (Fig. 1-1). It consisted of a large glass bulb containing a sponge soaked with colored ether and a spout that was placed in the patient's mouth. An opening on the opposite side of the bulb allowed air to enter and be drawn over the ether-soaked sponge with each breath.[21]

The conversations of that morning were not accurately recorded; however, popular accounts state that the surgeon responded testily to Morton's apology for his tardy arrival by remarking, "Sir, your patient is ready." Morton directed his attention to his patient and first conducted a very abbreviated preoperative evaluation. He inquired, "Are you afraid?" Abbott responded that he was not and took the inhaler in his mouth. After a few minutes, Morton turned to the surgeon and said, "Sir, your patient is ready." Gilbert Abbott later reported that he was aware of the surgery but experienced no pain. When the procedure ended, Warren immediately turned to his audience and uttered the statement, "Gentlemen, this is no humbug."[22]

What would be recognized as America's greatest contribution to 19th century medicine had occurred. However, Morton, wishing to capitalize on his "discovery," refused to divulge what agent was in his inhaler. Some weeks passed before Morton admitted that the active component of the colored fluid, which he had called "Letheon," was simple diethyl ether. Morton, Wells, Jackson, and their supporters soon became drawn into a contentious, protracted, and fruitless debate over priority for the discovery. This debate has subsequently been termed *the ether controversy*. In short, Morton had applied for a patent for Letheon, and when it was granted, tried to receive royalties for the use of ether as an anesthetic.

When the details of Morton's anesthetic technique became public knowledge, the information was transmitted by train, stagecoach, and coastal vessels to other North American cities, and by ship to the world. As ether was easy to prepare and administer, anesthetics were performed in Britain, France, Russia, South Africa, Australia, and other countries almost as soon as surgeons heard the welcome news of the extraordinary discovery. Even though surgery could now be performed with "pain put to sleep," the frequency of operations did not rise rapidly, and several years would pass before anesthesia was universally recommended.

Chloroform and Obstetrics

James Young Simpson was a successful obstetrician of Edinburgh, Scotland, and among the first to use ether for the relief of labor pain. Dissatisfied with ether, Simpson soon sought a more pleasant, rapid-acting anesthetic. He and his junior associates conducted a bold search by inhaling samples of several volatile chemicals collected for Simpson by British apothecaries. David Waldie suggested chloroform, which had first been prepared in 1831. Simpson and his friends inhaled it after dinner at a party in Simpson's home on the evening of November 4, 1847. They promptly fell unconscious and, when they awoke, were delighted with their success. Simpson quickly set about encouraging the use of chloroform. Within 2 weeks, he submitted his first account of its use to *The Lancet*.

In the 19th century, the relief of obstetric pain had significant social ramifications and made anesthesia during childbirth a controversial subject. Simpson argued against the prevailing view, which held that relieving labor pain opposed God's will. The pain of the parturient was viewed as both a component of punishment and a means of atonement for Original Sin. Less than a year after administering the first anesthesia during childbirth, Simpson addressed these concerns in a pamphlet entitled *Answers to the Religious Objections Advanced against the Employment of Anaesthetic Agents in Midwifery and Surgery and Obstetrics*. In it, Simpson recognized the Book of Genesis as being the root of this sentiment, and noted that God promised to relieve the descendants of Adam and Eve of the curse. Additionally, Simpson asserted that labor pain was a result of scientific and anatomic causes, and not the result of religious condemnation. He stated that the upright position of humans necessitated strong pelvic muscles to support the abdominal contents. As a result, he argued, the uterus necessarily developed strong musculature to overcome the resistance of the pelvic floor and that great contractile power caused great pain. Simpson's pamphlet probably did not have a significant impact on the prevailing attitudes, but he did articulate many concepts that his contemporaries were debating at the time.[23]

Chloroform gained considerable notoriety after John Snow used it to deliver the last two children of Queen Victoria. The Queen's consort, Prince Albert, interviewed John Snow before he was called to Buckingham Palace to administer chloroform at the request of the Queen's obstetrician. During the monarch's labor, Snow gave analgesic doses of chloroform on a folded handkerchief. This technique was soon termed *chloroform à la reine*. Victoria abhorred the pain of childbirth and enjoyed the relief that chloroform provided. She wrote in her journal, "Dr. Snow gave that blessed chloroform and the effect was soothing, quieting, and delightful beyond measure."[24] When the Queen, as head of the Church of England, endorsed obstetric anesthesia, religious debate over the management of labor pain terminated abruptly.

John Snow, already a respected physician, took an interest in anesthetic practice and was soon invited to work with many leading surgeons of the day. In 1848, Snow introduced a chloroform inhaler. He had recognized the versatility of the new agent and came to prefer it in his practice. At the same time, he initiated what was to become an extraordinary series of experiments that were remarkable in their scope and for anticipating sophisticated research performed a century later. Snow realized that successful anesthetics should abolish pain and unwanted movements. He anesthetized several species of animals with varying strengths of ether and chloroform to determine the concentration required to prevent reflex movement from sharp stimuli. This work approximated the modern concept of minimum alveolar concentration.[25] Snow assessed the anesthetic action of a large number of potential anesthetics but did not find any to rival chloroform or ether. His studies led him to recognize the relationship between solubility, vapor pressure, and anesthetic potency, which was not fully appreciated until after World War II. Snow published two remarkable books, *On the Inhalation of the Vapour of Ether* (1847) and *On Chloroform and Other Anaesthetics* (1858). The latter was almost completed when he died of a stroke at the age of 45.

ANESTHESIA PRINCIPLES, EQUIPMENT, AND STANDARDS

Control of the Airway

Definitive control of the airway, a skill anesthesiologists now consider paramount, developed only after many harrowing and apneic episodes spurred the development of safer airway management techniques. Preceding tracheal intubation, however, several important techniques were proposed toward the end of the 19th century that remain integral to anesthesiology education and practice. Joseph Clover was the first Englishman to urge the now universal practice of thrusting the patient's jaw forward to overcome obstruction of the upper airway by the tongue. Clover also published a landmark case report in 1877 in which he performed a surgical airway. Once his patient was asleep, Clover discovered that his patient had a tumor of the mouth that obstructed the airway completely, despite his trusted jaw-thrust maneuver. He averted disaster by inserting a small curved cannula of his design through the cricothyroid membrane. He continued anesthesia via the cannula until the tumor was excised. Clover, the model of the prepared anesthesiologist, remarked, "I have never used the cannula before although it has been my companion at some thousands of anaesthetic cases."[26]

Tracheal Intubation

The development of techniques and instruments for intubation ranks among the major advances in the history of anesthesiology. The first tracheal tubes were developed for the resuscitation of drowning victims, but were not used in anesthesia until 1878. The first use of elective oral intubation for an anesthetic was undertaken by Scottish surgeon William Macewan. He had practiced passing flexible metal tubes through the larynx of a cadaver before attempting the maneuver on an awake patient with an oral tumor at the Glasgow Royal Infirmary on July 5, 1878.[27] Because topical anesthesia was not yet known, the experience must have demanded fortitude on the part of Macewan's patient. Once the tube was correctly positioned, an assistant began a chloroform–air anesthetic via the tube. Once anesthetized, the patient soon stopped coughing. Unfortunately, Macewan abandoned the practice following a fatality in which a patient had been successfully intubated while awake but the tube became dislodged once the patient was asleep. After the tube was removed, an attempt to provide chloroform by mask anesthesia was unsuccessful and the patient died.

An American surgeon named Joseph O'Dwyer is remembered for his extraordinary dedication to the advancement of tracheal intubation. In 1885, O'Dwyer designed a series of metal laryngeal tubes, which he inserted blindly between the vocal cords of children suffering a diphtheritic crisis. Three years later, O'Dwyer designed a second rigid tube with a coni-

cal tip that occluded the larynx so effectively that it could be used for artificial ventilation when applied with the bellows and T-piece tube designed by George Fell. The Fell-O'Dwyer apparatus, as it came to be known, was used during thoracic surgery by Rudolph Matas of New Orleans. Matas was so pleased with it that he predicted, "The procedure that promises the most benefit in preventing pulmonary collapse in operations on the chest is . . . the rhythmical maintenance of artificial respiration by a tube in the glottis directly connected with a bellows."

After O'Dwyer's death, the outstanding pioneer of tracheal intubation was Franz Kuhn, a surgeon of Kassel, Germany. From 1900 until 1912, Kuhn published several articles and a classic monograph, *"Die perorale Intubation,"* which were not well known in his lifetime but have since become widely appreciated.[25] His work might have had a more profound impact if it had been translated into English. Kuhn described techniques of oral and nasal intubation that he performed with flexible metal tubes composed of coiled tubing similar to those now used for the spout of metal gasoline cans. After applying cocaine to the airway, Kuhn introduced his tube over a curved metal stylet that he directed toward the larynx with his left index finger. While he was aware of the subglottic cuffs that had been used briefly by Victor Eisenmenger, Kuhn preferred to seal the larynx by positioning a supralaryngeal flange near the tube's tip before packing the pharynx with gauze. Kuhn even monitored the patient's breath sounds continuously through a monaural earpiece connected to an extension of the tracheal tube by a narrow tube.

Intubation of the trachea by palpation was an uncertain and sometimes traumatic act; surgeons even believed that it would be anatomically impossible to visualize the vocal cords directly. This misapprehension was overcome in 1895 by Alfred Kirstein in Berlin who devised the first direct-vision laryngoscope.[28] Kirstein was motivated by a friend's report that a patient's trachea had been accidentally intubated during esophagoscopy. Kirstein promptly fabricated a handheld instrument that at first resembled a shortened cylindrical esophagoscope. He soon substituted a semicircular blade that opened inferiorly. Kirstein could now examine the larynx while standing behind his seated patient, whose head had been placed in an attitude approximating the "sniffing position." Although Alfred Kirstein's "autoscope" was not used by anesthesiologists, it was the forerunner of all modern laryngoscopes. Endoscopy was refined by Chevalier Jackson in Philadelphia, who designed a U-shaped laryngoscope by adding a handgrip that was parallel to the blade. The Jackson blade has remained a standard instrument for endoscopists but was not favored by anesthesiologists. Two laryngoscopes that closely resembled modern L-shaped instruments were designed in 1910 and 1913 by two American surgeons, Henry Janeway and George Dorrance, but neither instrument achieved lasting use despite their excellent designs.[29]

Before the introduction of muscle relaxants in the 1940s, intubation of the trachea could be challenging. This challenge was made somewhat easier, however, with the advent of laryngoscope blades specifically designed to increase visualization of the vocal cords. Robert Miller of San Antonio, Texas, and Robert Macintosh of Oxford University created their respectively named blades within an interval of 2 years. In 1941, Miller brought forward the slender, straight blade with a slight curve near the tip to ease the passage of the tube through the larynx. Although Miller's blade was a refinement, the technique of its use was identical to that of earlier models as the epiglottis was lifted to expose the larynx.[30]

The Macintosh blade, which is placed in the vallecula rather than under the epiglottis, was invented as an incidental result of a tonsillectomy. Sir Robert Macintosh later described the circumstances of its discovery in an appreciation of the career of his technician, Mr. Richard Salt, who constructed the blade. As Sir Robert recalled, "A Boyle-Davis gag, a size larger than intended, was inserted for tonsillectomy, and when the mouth was fully opened the cords came into view. This was a surprise since conventional laryngoscopy, at that depth of anaesthesia, would have been impossible in those pre-relaxant days. Within a matter of hours, Salt had modified the blade of the Davis gag and attached a laryngoscope handle to it; and streamlined (after testing several models), the end result came into widespread use."[31] Macintosh underestimated the popularity of the blade, as more than 800,000 have been produced and many special-purpose versions have been marketed.

The most distinguished innovator in tracheal intubation was the self-trained British anesthetist Ivan (later, Sir Ivan) Magill.[32] In 1919, while serving in the Royal Army as a general medical officer, Magill was assigned to a military hospital near London. Although he had only rudimentary training in anesthesia, Magill was obliged to accept an assignment to the anesthesia service, where he worked with another neophyte, Stanley Rowbotham.[33] Together, Magill and Rowbotham attended casualties disfigured by severe facial injuries who underwent repeated restorative operations. These procedures required that the surgeon, Harold Gillies, have unrestricted access to the face and airway. These patients presented formidable challenges, but both Magill and Rowbotham became adept at tracheal intubation and quickly understood its current limitations. Because they learned from fortuitous observations, they soon extended the scope of tracheal anesthesia.

They gained expertise with blind nasal intubation after they learned to soften semirigid insufflation tubes for passage through the nostril. Even though their original intent was to position the tips of the nasal tubes in the posterior pharynx, the slender tubes frequently ended up in the trachea. Stimulated by this chance experience, they developed techniques of deliberate nasotracheal intubation. In 1920, Magill devised an aid to manipulating the catheter tip, the "Magill angulated forceps," which continue to be manufactured according to his original design of nearly 90 years ago.

With the war over, Magill entered civilian practice and set out to develop a wide-bore tube that would resist kinking but be conformable to the contours of the upper airway. While in a hardware store, he found mineralized red rubber tubing that he cut, beveled, and smoothed to produce tubes that clinicians around the world would come to call "Magill tubes." His tubes remained the universal standard for more than 40 years until rubber products were supplanted by inert plastics. Magill also rediscovered the advantage of applying cocaine to the nasal mucosa, a technique that greatly facilitated awake blind nasal intubation.

In 1926, Arthur Guedel began a series of experiments that led to the introduction of the cuffed tube. Guedel transformed the basement of his Indianapolis home into a laboratory where he subjected each step of the preparation and application of his cuffs to a vigorous review.[34] He fashioned cuffs from the rubber of dental dams, condoms, and surgical gloves that were glued onto the outer wall of tubes. Using as his model animal tracheas donated by the family butcher, he considered whether the cuff should be positioned above, below, or at the level of the vocal cords. He recommended that the cuff be positioned just below the vocal cords to seal the airway. Waters later recommended that cuffs be constructed of two layers of soft rubber cemented together. These detachable cuffs were first manufactured by Waters' children, who sold them to the Foregger Company.

Guedel sought ways to show the safety and utility of the cuffed tube. He first filled the mouth of an anesthetized and intubated patient with water and showed that the cuff sealed the airway. Even though this exhibition was successful, he searched for a more dramatic technique to capture the atten-

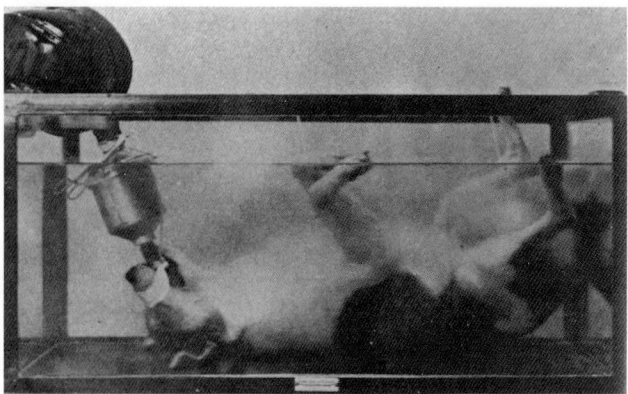

FIGURE 1-2.   The "dunked dog."

tion of those unfamiliar with the advantages of intubation. He reasoned that if the cuff prevented water from entering the trachea of an intubated patient, it should also prevent an animal from drowning, even if it were submerged under water. To encourage physicians attending a medical convention to use his tracheal techniques, Guedel prepared the first of several "dunked dog" demonstrations (Fig. 1-2). An anesthetized and intubated dog, Guedel's own pet, "Airway," was immersed in an aquarium. After the demonstration was completed, the anesthetic was discontinued before the animal was removed from the water. Airway awoke promptly, shook water over the onlookers, saluted a post, then trotted from the hall to the applause of the audience.

After a patient experienced an accidental endobronchial intubation, Ralph Waters reasoned that a very long cuffed tube could be used to ventilate the dependent lung while the upper lung was being resected.[35] On learning of his friend's success with intentional one-lung anesthesia, Arthur Guedel proposed an important modification for chest surgery, the double-cuffed single-lumen tube, which was introduced by Emery Rovenstine. These tubes were easily positioned, an advantage over bronchial blockers that had to be inserted by a skilled bronchoscopist. In 1953, single-lumen tubes were supplanted by double-lumen endobronchial tubes. The double-lumen tube currently most popular was designed by Frank Robertshaw of Manchester, England, and is prepared in both right- and left-sided versions. Robertshaw tubes were first manufactured from mineralized red rubber but are now made of extruded plastic, a technique refined by David Sheridan. Sheridan was also the first person to embed centimeter markings along the side of tracheal tubes, a safety feature that reduced the risk of the tube's being incorrectly positioned.

Advanced Airway Devices

Conventional laryngoscopes proved inadequate for patients with "difficult airways." A few clinicians credit harrowing intubating experiences as the incentive for invention. In 1928, a rigid bronchoscope was specifically designed for examination of the large airways. Rigid bronchoscopes were refined and used by pulmonologists. Although it was known in 1870 that a thread of glass could transmit light along its length, technological limitations were not overcome until 1964 when Shigeto Ikeda developed the first flexible fiberoptic bronchoscope. Fiberoptic-assisted tracheal intubation has become a common approach in the management of patients with difficult airways having surgery.

Roger Bullard desired a device to simultaneously examine the larynx and intubate the vocal cords. He had been frustrated by failed attempts to visualize the larynx of a patient with Pierre-Robin syndrome. In response, he developed the Bullard laryngoscope, whose fiberoptic bundles lie beside a curved blade. Similarly, the Wu-scope was designed by Tzu-Lang Wu in 1994 to combine and facilitate visualization and intubation of the trachea in patients with difficult airways.[36]

Dr. A. I. J. "Archie" Brain first recognized the principle of the laryngeal mask airway (LMA) in 1981 when, like many British clinicians, he provided dental anesthesia via a Goldman nasal mask. However, unlike any before him, he realized that just as the dental mask could be fitted closely about the nose, a comparable mask attached to a wide-bore tube might be positioned around the larynx. He not only conceived of this radical departure in airway management, which he first described in 1983,[37] but also spent years in single-handedly fabricating and testing scores of incremental modifications. Scores of Brain's prototypes are displayed in the Royal Berkshire Hospital, Reading, England, where they provide a detailed record of the evolution of the LMA. He fabricated his first models from Magill tubes and Goldman masks, then refined their shape by performing postmortem studies of the hypopharynx to determine the form of cuff that would be most functional. Before silicone rubber was selected, Brain had even mastered the technique of forming masks from liquid latex. Every detail of the LMA, the number and position of the aperture bars, the shape and the size of the masks, required repeated modification.

Early Anesthesia Delivery Systems

3 The transition from ether inhalers and chloroform-soaked handkerchiefs to more sophisticated anesthesia delivery equipment occurred gradually, with incremental advances supplanting older methods. One of the earliest anesthesia apparatus designs was that of John Snow, who had realized the inadequacies of ether inhalers through which patients rebreathed via a mouthpiece. After practicing anesthesia for only 2 weeks, Snow created the first of his series of ingenious ether inhalers.[38] His best-known apparatus featured unidirectional valves within a malleable, well-fitting mask of his own design, which closely resembles the form of a modern face mask. The face piece was connected to the vaporizer by a breathing tube, which Snow deliberately designed to be wider than the human trachea so that even rapid respirations would not be impeded. A metal coil within the vaporizer ensured that the patient's inspired breath was drawn over a large surface area to promote the uptake of ether. The device also incorporated a warm water bath to maintain the volatility of the agent (Fig. 1-3).

Snow did not attempt to capitalize on his creativity, in contrast to William Morton; he closed his account of its preparation with the generous observation, "There is no restriction respecting the making of it."[39]

Joseph Clover, another British physician, was the first anesthetist to administer chloroform in known concentrations through the "Clover bag." He obtained a 4.5% concentration of chloroform in air by pumping a measured volume of air with a bellows through a warmed evaporating vessel containing a known volume of liquid chloroform.[40] Although it was realized that nitrous oxide diluted in air often gave a hypoxic mixture, and that the oxygen-nitrous oxide mixture was safer, Chicago surgeon Edmund Andrews complained about the physical limitations of delivering anesthesia to patients in their homes. The large bag was conspicuous and awkward to carry along busy streets. He observed that, "In city practice, among the higher classes, however, this is no obstacle as the bag can always be taken in a carriage, without attracting attention."[41] In 1872, Andrews was delighted to report the availability of liquefied nitrous oxide compressed under 750 pounds of pressure, which allowed a supply sufficient for three patients to be carried in a single cylinder.

Critical to increasing patient safety was the development of a machine capable of delivering a calibrated amount of gas and volatile anesthetic. In the late 19th century, demands in dentistry instigated development of the first freestanding anesthesia machines. Three American dentist-entrepreneurs, Samuel S. White, Charles Teter, and Jay Heidbrink, developed the original series of U.S. instruments that used compressed cylinders of nitrous oxide and oxygen. Before 1900, the S. S. White Company modified Frederick Hewitt's apparatus and marketed its continuous-flow machine, which was refined by Teter in 1903. Heidbrink added reducing valves in 1912. In the same year, physicians initiated other important developments. Water-bubble flowmeters, introduced by Frederick Cotton and Walter Boothby of Harvard University, allowed the proportion of gases and their flow rate to be approximated. The Cotton and Boothby apparatus was transformed into a practical portable machine by James Tayloe Gwathmey of New York. The Gwathmey machine caught the attention of a London anesthetist Henry E. G. "Cockie" Boyle, who acknowledged his debt to the American when he incorporated Gwathmey's concepts in the first of the series of "Boyle" machines that were marketed by Coxeter and British Oxygen Corporation. During the same period in Lubeck, Germany, Heinrich Draeger and his son, Bernhaard, adapted compressed-gas technology, which they had originally developed for mine rescue equipment, to manufacture ether and chloroform-oxygen machines.

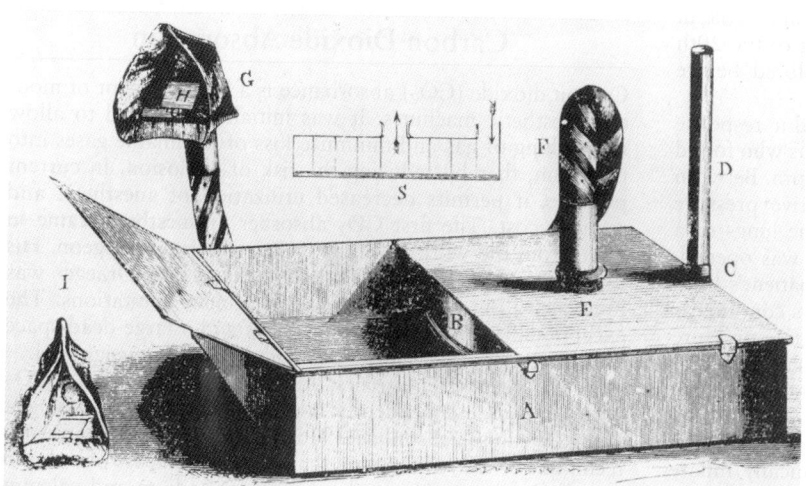

FIGURE 1-3. John Snow's inhaler (1847). The ether chamber (B) contained a spiral coil so that the air entering through the bross tube (D) was saturated by ether before ascending the flexible tube (F) to the face mask (G). The ether chamber rested in a bath of warm water (A).

In the years after World War I, several U.S. manufacturers continued to bring forward widely admired anesthesia machines. Richard von Foregger was an engineer who was exceptionally receptive to clinicians' suggestions for additional features for his machines. Elmer McKesson became one of the country's first specialists in anesthesiology in 1910 and developed a series of gas machines. In an era of flammable anesthetics, McKesson carried nitrous oxide anesthesia to its therapeutic limit by performing inductions with 100% nitrous oxide and thereafter adding small volumes of oxygen. If the resultant cyanosis became too profound, McKesson depressed a valve on his machine that flushed a small volume of oxygen into the circuit. Even though his techniques of primary and secondary saturation with nitrous oxide are no longer used, the oxygen flush valve is part of McKesson's legacy.

Alternative Circuits

A valveless device, the Ayre's T-piece, has found wide application in the management of intubated patients. Phillip Ayre practiced anesthesia in England when the limitations of equipment for pediatric patients produced what he described as "a protracted and sanguine battle between surgeon and anaesthetist, with the poor unfortunate baby as the battlefield."[42] In 1937, Ayre introduced his valveless T-piece to reduce the effort of breathing in neurosurgical patients. The T-piece soon became particularly popular for cleft palate repairs, as the surgeon had free access to the mouth. Positive pressure ventilation could be achieved when the anesthetist obstructed the expiratory limb. In time, this ingenious, lightweight, nonrebreathing device evolved through more than 100 modifications for a variety of special situations. A significant alteration was Gordon Jackson Rees' circuit, which permitted improved control of ventilation by substituting a breathing bag on the outflow limb.[43] An alternative method to reduce the amount of equipment near the patient is provided by the coaxial circuit of the Bain-Spoerel apparatus.[44] This lightweight tube-within-a-tube has served very well in many circumstances since its Canadian innovators described it in 1972.

Ventilators

Mechanical ventilators are now an integral part of the anesthesia machine. Patients are ventilated during general anesthesia by electrical or gas-powered devices that are simple to control yet sophisticated in their function. The history of mechanical positive pressure ventilation began with attempts to resuscitate victims of drowning by a bellows attached to a mask or tracheal tube. These experiments found little role in anesthetic care for many years. At the beginning of the 20th century, however, several modalities were explored before intermittent positive pressure machines evolved.

A series of artificial environments were created in response to the frustration experienced by thoracic surgeons who found that the lung collapsed when they incised the pleura. Between 1900 and 1910, continuous positive or negative pressure devices were created to maintain inflation of the lungs of a spontaneously breathing patient once the chest was opened. Brauer (1904) and Murphy (1905) placed the patient's head and neck in a box in which positive pressure was continually maintained. Sauerbruch (1904) created a negative-pressure operating chamber encompassing both the surgical team and the patient's body and from which only the patient's head projected.[45]

In 1907, the first intermittent positive pressure device, the Draeger "Pulmotor," was developed to rhythmically inflate the lungs. This instrument and later American models such as

the E & J Resuscitator were used almost exclusively by firefighters and mine rescue workers. In 1934 a Swedish team developed the "Spiropulsator," which C. Crafoord later modified for use during cyclopropane anesthesia.[46] Its action was controlled by a magnetic control valve called *the flasher*, a type first used to provide intermittent gas flow for the lights of navigational buoys. When Trier Morch, a Danish anesthesiologist, could not obtain a Spiropulsator during World War II, he fabricated the Morch "Respirator," which used a piston pump to rhythmically deliver a fixed volume of gas to the patient.[45]

A major stimulus to the development of ventilators came as a consequence of a devastating epidemic of poliomyelitis that struck Copenhagen, Denmark, in 1952. As scores of patients were admitted, the only effective ventilatory support that could be provided to patients with bulbar paralysis was continuous manual ventilation via a tracheostomy employing devices such as Waters' "to-and-fro" circuit. This succeeded only through the dedicated efforts of hundreds of volunteers. Medical students served in relays to ventilate paralyzed patients. The Copenhagen crisis stimulated a broad European interest in the development of portable ventilators in anticipation of another epidemic of poliomyelitis. At this time, the common practice in North American hospitals was to place polio patients with respiratory involvement in "iron lungs," metal cylinders that encased the body below the neck. Inspiration was caused by intermittent negative pressure created by an electric motor acting on a pistonlike device occupying the foot of the chamber.

Some early American ventilators were adaptations of respiratory-assist machines originally designed for the delivery of aerosolized drugs for respiratory therapy. Two types employed the Bennett or Bird "flow-sensitive" valves. The Bennett valve was designed during World War II when a team of physiologists at the University of Southern California encountered difficulties in separating inspiration from expiration in an experimental apparatus designed to provide positive pressure breathing for aviators at high altitude. An engineer, Ray Bennett, visited their laboratory, observed their problem, and resolved it with a mechanical flow-sensitive automatic valve. A second valving mechanism was later designed by an aeronautical engineer, Forrest Bird.

The use of the Bird and Bennett valves gained an anesthetic application when the gas flow from the valve was directed into a rigid plastic jar containing a breathing bag or bellows as part of an anesthesia circuit. These "bag-in-bottle" devices mimicked the action of the clinician's hand as the gas flow compressed the bag, thereby providing positive pressure inspiration. Passive exhalation was promoted by the descent of a weight on the bag or bellows.

Carbon Dioxide Absorption

Carbon dioxide (CO_2) absorbance is a basic element of modern anesthetic machines. It was initially developed to allow rebreathing of gas and minimize loss of flammable gases into the room, thereby reducing the risk of explosion. In current practice, it permits decreased utilization of anesthetic and reduced cost. The first CO_2 absorber in anesthesia came in 1906 from the work of Franz Kuhn, a German surgeon. His use of canisters developed for mine rescues by Draeger was innovative, but his circuit had unfortunate limitations. The exceptionally narrow breathing tubes and a large dead space explain its very limited use, and Kuhn's device was ignored.

A few years later, the first American machine with a CO_2 absorber was independently fabricated by a pharmacologist named Dennis Jackson. In 1915, Jackson developed an early technique of CO_2 absorption that permitted the use of a closed anesthesia circuit. He used solutions of sodium and calcium

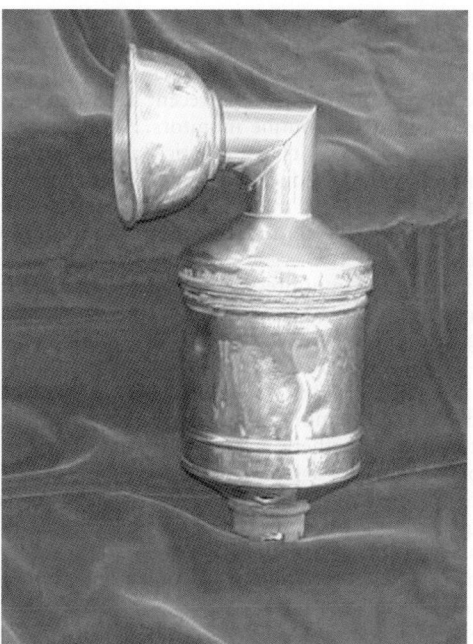

FIGURE 1-4.   Waters' carbon dioxide absorbance canister.

American equipment still featured nonrotating floats. The now universal practice of displaying gas flow in liters per minute was not a customary part of all American machines until more than a decade after World War II.

Vaporizers

The art of a smooth induction with a potent anesthetic was a great challenge, particularly if the inspired concentration could not be determined with accuracy. Even the clinical introduction of halothane after 1956 might have been similarly thwarted except for a fortunate coincidence: the prior development of calibrated vaporizers. Two types of calibrated vaporizers designed for other anesthetics had become available in the half decade before halothane was marketed. The prompt acceptance of halothane was in part because of an ability to provide it in carefully titrated concentrations.

The Copper Kettle was the first temperature-compensated, accurate vaporizer. It had been developed by Lucien Morris at the University of Wisconsin in response to Ralph Waters' plan to test chloroform by giving it in controlled concentrations.[50] Morris achieved this goal by passing a metered flow of oxygen through a vaporizer chamber that contained a sintered bronze disk to separate the oxygen into minute bubbles. The gas became fully saturated with anesthetic vapor as it percolated through the liquid. The concentration of the anesthetic inspired by the patient could be calculated by knowing the vapor pressure of the liquid anesthetic, the volume of oxygen flowing through the liquid, and the total volume of gases from all sources entering the anesthesia circuit. Although experimental models of Morris' vaporizer used a water bath to maintain stability, the excellent thermal conductivity of copper was substituted in later models. When first marketed, the Copper Kettle did not feature a mechanism to indicate changes in the temperature (and vapor pressure) of the liquid. Shuh-Hsun Ngai proposed the incorporation of a thermometer, a suggestion that was later added to all vaporizers of that class.[51] The Copper Kettle (Foregger Company) and the Vernitrol (Ohio Medical Products) were universal vaporizers that could be charged with any anesthetic liquid, and, provided that its vapor pressure and temperature were known, the inspired concentration could be calculated quickly.

When halothane was first marketed in Britain, an effective temperature-compensated, agent-specific vaporizer had recently been placed in clinical use. The TECOTA (TEmperature COmpensated Trichloroethylene Air) vaporizer featured a bimetallic strip composed of brass and a nickel–steel alloy, two metals with different coefficients of expansion. As the anesthetic vapor cooled, the strip bent to move away from the orifice, thereby permitting more fresh gas to enter the vaporizing chamber. This maintained a constant inspired concentration despite changes in temperature and vapor pressure. After their TECOTA vaporizer was accepted into anesthetic practice, the technology was used to create the "Fluotec," the first of a series of agent-specific "tec" vaporizers for use in the operating room.

hydroxide to absorb CO_2. As his laboratory was located in an area of St. Louis, Missouri, heavily laden with coal smoke, Jackson reported that the apparatus allowed him the first breaths of absolutely fresh air he had ever enjoyed in that city. The complexity of Jackson's apparatus limited its use in hospital practice, but his pioneering work in this field encouraged Ralph Waters to introduce a simpler device using soda lime granules 9 years later. Waters positioned a soda lime canister (Fig. 1-4) between a face mask and an adjacent breathing bag to which was attached the fresh gas flow. As long as the mask was held against the face, only small volumes of fresh gas flow were required and no valves were needed.[47]

Waters' device featured awkward positioning of the canister close to the patient's face. Brian Sword overcame this limitation in 1930 with a freestanding machine with unidirectional valves to create a circle system and an in-line CO_2 absorber.[48] James Elam and his coworkers at the Roswell Park Cancer Institute in Buffalo, New York, further refined the CO_2 absorber, increasing the efficiency of CO_2 removal with a minimum of resistance for breathing.[49] Consequently, the circle system introduced by Sword in the 1930s, with a few refinements, became the standard anesthesia circuit in North America.

Flow Meters

As closed and semiclosed circuits became practical, gas flow could be measured with greater accuracy. Bubble flowmeters were replaced with dry bobbins or ball-bearing flowmeters, which, although they did not leak fluids, could cause inaccurate measurements if they adhered to the glass column. In 1910, M. Neu had been the first to apply rotameters in anesthesia for the administration of nitrous oxide and oxygen, but his machine was not a commercial success, perhaps because of the great cost of nitrous oxide in Germany at that time. Rotameters designed for use in German industry were first employed in Britain in 1937 by Richard Salt; but as World War II approached, the English were denied access to these sophisticated flowmeters. After World War II rotameters became regularly employed in British anesthesia machines, although most

Patient Monitors

In many ways, the history of late-nineteenth and early-20th century anesthesiology is the quest for the safest anesthetic. The discovery and widespread use of electrocardiography, pulse oximetry, blood gas analysis, capnography, and neuromuscular blockade monitoring have reduced patient morbidity and mortality and revolutionized anesthesia practice. While safer machines assured clinicians that appropriate gas mixtures were delivered to the patient, monitors provided an early warning of acute physiologic deterioration before patients suffered irrevocable damage.

Joseph Clover was one of the first clinicians to routinely perform basic hemodynamic monitoring. Clover developed the habit of monitoring his patients' pulse but surprisingly, this was a contentious issue at the time. Prominent Scottish surgeons scorned Clover's emphasis on the action of chloroform on the heart. Baron Lister and others preferred that senior medical students give anesthetics and urged them to "strictly carry out certain simple instructions, among which is that of never touching the pulse, in order that their attention may not be distracted from the respiration."[52] Lister also counseled, "it appears that preliminary examination of the chest, often considered indispensable, is quite unnecessary, and more likely to induce the dreaded syncope, by alarming the patients, than to avert it."[53] Little progress in anesthesia could come from such reactionary statements. In contrast, Clover had observed the effect of chloroform on animals and urged other anesthetists to monitor the pulse at all times and to discontinue the anesthetic temporarily if any irregularity or weakness was observed in the strength of the pulse.

Two American surgeons, George W. Crile and Harvey Cushing, developed a strong interest in measuring blood pressure during anesthesia. Both men wrote thorough and detailed examinations of blood pressure monitoring; however, Cushing's contribution is better remembered because he was the first American to apply the Riva Rocci cuff, which he saw while visiting Italy. Cushing introduced the concept in 1902 and had blood pressure measurements recorded on anesthesia records.[54] In 1894, Cushing and a fellow student at Harvard Medical School, Charles Codman, initiated a system of recording patients' pulses to assess the course of the anesthetics they administered. In 1902, Cushing continued the practice of monitoring and recording patient blood pressures and pulses. The transition from manual to automated blood pressure devices, which first appeared in 1936 and operate on an oscillometric principle, has been gradual.

The first precordial stethoscope was believed to have been used by S. Griffith Davis at Johns Hopkins University.[38] He adapted a technique developed by Harvey Cushing in a laboratory in which dogs with surgically induced valvular lesions had stethoscopes attached to their chest wall so that medical students might listen to bruits characteristic of a specific malformation. Davis' technique was forgotten but was rehabilitated by Dr. Robert Smith, an energetic pioneer of pediatric anesthesiology in Boston in the 1940s. A Canadian contemporary, Albert Codesmith, of the Hospital for Sick Children, Toronto, became frustrated by the repeated dislodging of the chest piece under the surgical drapes and fabricated his first esophageal stethoscope from urethral catheters and Penrose drains. His brief report heralded its clinical role as a monitor of both normal and adventitious respiratory and cardiac sounds.[55]

Electrocardiography, Pulse Oximetry, and Capnography

Clinical electrocardiography began with Willem Einthoven's application of the string galvanometer in 1903. Within two decades, Thomas Lewis had described its role in the diagnosis of disturbances of cardiac rhythm, while James Herrick and Harold Pardee first drew attention to the changes produced by myocardial ischemia. After 1928, cathode ray oscilloscopes were available, but the risk of explosion owing to the presence of flammable anesthetics forestalled the introduction of the electrocardiogram into routine anesthetic practice until after World War II. At that time, the small screen of the heavily shielded "bullet" oscilloscope displayed only 3 seconds of data, but that information was highly prized.

Pulse oximetry, the optical measurement of oxygen saturation in tissues, is one of the more recent additions to the anesthesiologist's array of routine monitors. Although research in this area began in 1932, its first practical application came during World War II. An American physiologist, Glen Millikan, responded to a request from British colleagues in aviation research. Millikan set about preparing a series of devices to improve the supply of oxygen that was provided to pilots flying at high altitude in unpressurized aircraft. To monitor oxygen delivery and to prevent the pilot from succumbing to an unrecognized failure of his oxygen supply, Millikan created an oxygen-sensing monitor worn on the pilot's earlobe, and coined the name *oximeter* to describe its action. Before his tragic death in a climbing accident in 1947, Millikan had begun to assess anesthetic applications of oximetry. Refinements of oximetry by a Japanese engineer, Takuo Aoyagi, led to the development of pulse oximetry. As John Severinghaus recounted the episode, Aoyagi had attempted to eliminate the changes in a signal caused by pulsatile variations when he realized that this fluctuation could be used to measure both the pulse and oxygen saturation.[53]

Anesthesiologists have recognized a need for breath-by-breath measurement of respiratory and anesthetic gases. After 1954, infrared absorption techniques gave immediate displays of the exhaled concentration of CO_2. The ability to confirm endotracheal intubation and monitor ventilation, as reflected by concentrations of CO_2 in respired gas, began in 1943. At that time, K. Luft described the principle of infrared absorption by CO_2 and he developed an apparatus for measurement.[56] Routine application of capnography in anesthesia practice was pioneered by Dr. Bob Smalhout and Dr. Zden Kalenda in the Netherlands. Breath-to-breath continuous monitoring and a waveform display of CO_2 levels help anesthesiologists recognize abnormalities in metabolism, ventilation, and circulation. More recently, infrared analysis has been perfected to enable breath-by-breath measurement of anesthetic gases as well. This technology has largely replaced mass spectrometry, which initially had only industrial applications before Albert Faulconer of the Mayo Clinic first used it to monitor the concentration of an exhaled anesthetic in 1954.

Safety Standards

The introduction of safety features was coordinated by the American National Standards Institute (ANSI) Committee Z79, which was sponsored from 1956 until 1983 by the American Society of Anesthesiologists. Since 1983, representatives from industry, government, and health care professions have met on Committee Z79 of the American Society for Testing and Materials. They establish voluntary goals that may become accepted national standards for the safety of anesthesia equipment.

Ralph Tovell voiced the first call for standards during World War II while he was the U.S. Army Consultant in Anesthesiology for Europe. Tovell found that, as there were four different dimensions for connectors, tubes, masks, and breathing bags, supplies dispatched to field hospitals might not match their anesthesia machines. As Tovell observed, "When a sudden need for accessory equipment arose, nurses and corpsmen were likely to respond to it by bringing parts that would not fit."[57] Although Tovell's reports did not gain an immediate response, after the war Vincent Collins and Hamilton Davis took up his concern and formed the ANSI Committee Z79. One of the committee's most active members, Leslie Rendell-Baker, wrote an account of the committee's domestic and international achievements.[58] He reported that Tovell encouraged all manufacturers to select the now uniform orifice of 22 mm for all adult and pediatric face masks and to make every tracheal tube connector 15 mm in diameter. For the first time, a Z79-designed mask-tube elbow adapter would fit every mask and tracheal tube connector.

The Z79 Committee introduced other advances. Tracheal tubes of nontoxic plastic bear a Z79 or IT (Implantation Tested) mark. The committee also mandated touch identification of oxygen flow control at the suggestion of Roderick Calverley,[59] which reduced the risk that the wrong gas would be selected before internal mechanical controls prevented the selection of an hypoxic mixture. Pin indexing reduced the hazard of attaching a wrong cylinder in the place of oxygen. Diameter indexing of connectors prevented similar errors in high-pressure tubing. For many years, however, errors committed in reassembling hospital oxygen supply lines led to a series of tragedies before polarographic oxygen analyzers were added to the inspiratory limb of the anesthesia circuit.

THE HISTORY OF ANESTHETIC AGENTS AND ADJUVANTS

Inhaled Anesthetics

Throughout the second half of the 19th century, other compounds were examined for their anesthetic potential. The pattern of fortuitous discovery that brought nitrous oxide, diethyl ether, and chloroform forward between 1844 and 1847 continued. The next inhaled anesthetics to be used routinely, ethyl chloride and ethylene, were also discovered as a result of unexpected observations. Ethyl chloride and ethylene were first formulated in the 18th century. Ethyl chloride was used as a topical anesthetic and counterirritant; it was so volatile that the skin transiently "froze" after ethyl chloride was sprayed on it. Its rediscovery as an anesthetic came in 1894, when a Swedish dentist named Carlson sprayed ethyl chloride into a patient's mouth to "freeze" a dental abscess. Carlson was surprised to discover that his patient suddenly lost consciousness.

As the mechanisms to deliver drugs were refined, entirely new classes of medications were also developed, with the intention of providing safer, more pleasant pain control. Ethylene gas was the first alternative to ether and chloroform, but it had some major disadvantages. The rediscovery of ethylene in 1923 also came from a serendipitous observation. After it was learned that ethylene gas had been used to inhibit the opening of carnation buds in Chicago greenhouses, it was speculated that a gas that put flowers to sleep might also have an anesthetic action on humans. Arno Luckhardt was the first to publish a clinical study in February 1923. Within a month, Isabella Herb in Chicago and W. Easson Brown in Toronto presented two other independent studies. Ethylene was not a successful anesthetic because high concentrations were required and it was explosive. An additional significant shortcoming was a particularly unpleasant smell, which could only be partially disguised by the use of oil of orange or a cheap perfume. When cyclopropane was introduced, ethylene was abandoned.

The anesthetic action of cyclopropane was inadvertently discovered in 1929.[60] Brown and Henderson had previously shown that propylene had desirable properties as an anesthetic when freshly prepared, but after storage in a steel cylinder, it deteriorated to create a toxic material that produced nausea and cardiac irregularities in humans. Velyien Henderson, a professor of pharmacology at the University of Toronto, suggested that the toxic product be identified. After a chemist, George Lucas, identified cyclopropane among the chemicals in the tank, he prepared a sample in low concentration with

oxygen and administered it to two kittens. The animals fell asleep quietly but quickly recovered unharmed. Rather than being a toxic contaminant, Lucas saw that cyclopropane was a potent anesthetic. After its effects in other animals were studied and cyclopropane proved to be stable after storage, human experimentation began.

Henderson was the first volunteer; Lucas followed. They then arranged a public demonstration in which Frederick Banting, a Nobel laureate for the discovery of insulin, was anesthetized before a group of physicians. Despite this promising beginning, further research was abruptly halted. Several anesthetic deaths in Toronto had been attributed to ethyl chloride, and concern about Canadian clinical trials of cyclopropane prevented human studies from proceeding. Rather than abandon the study, Henderson encouraged an American friend, Ralph Waters, to use cyclopropane at the University of Wisconsin. The Wisconsin group investigated the drug thoroughly and reported their clinical success in 1934.[61]

In 1930, Chauncey Leake and MeiYu Chen performed successful laboratory trials of vinethene (divinyl ether) but were thwarted in its further development by a professor of surgery in San Francisco. Ironically, Canadians, who had lost cyclopropane to Wisconsin, learned of vinethene from Leake and Chen in California and conducted the first human study in 1932 at the University of Alberta, Edmonton. International research collaboration enabled early anesthetic use of both cyclopropane and divinyl ether, advances that may not have occurred independently in either the United States or Canada.

All potent anesthetics of this period were explosive save for chloroform, whose hepatic and cardiac toxicity limited use in America. Anesthetic explosions remained a rare but devastating risk to both anesthesiologist and patient. To reduce the danger of explosion during the incendiary days of World War II, British anesthetists turned to trichloroethylene. This nonflammable anesthetic found limited application in America, as it decomposed to release phosgene when warmed in the presence of soda lime. By the end of World War II, however, another class of noninflammable anesthetics was prepared for laboratory trials. Ten years later, fluorinated hydrocarbons revolutionized inhalation anesthesia.

Fluorine, the lightest and most reactive halogen, forms exceptionally stable bonds. These bonds, although sometimes created with explosive force, resist separation by chemical or thermal means. For that reason, many early attempts to fluorinate hydrocarbons in a controlled manner were frustrated by the marked chemical activity of fluorine. In 1930, the first commercial application of fluorine chemistry came in the form of the refrigerant, Freon. This was followed by the first attempt to prepare a fluorinated anesthetic by Harold Booth and E. May Bixby in 1932. Although their drug, monochlorodifluoromethane, was devoid of anesthetic action, as were other drugs studied that decade, their report predicted future developments. "A survey of the properties of 166 known gases suggested that the best possibility of finding a new noncombustible anesthetic gas lay in the field of organic fluoride compounds. Fluorine substitution for other halogens lowers the boiling point, increases stability, and generally decreases toxicity."[62]

After the war, a team at the University of Maryland under Professor of Pharmacology John C. Krantz, Jr., investigated the anesthetic properties of dozens of hydrocarbons over a period of several years, but only one, ethyl vinyl ether, entered clinical use in 1947. Because it was flammable, Krantz requested that it be fluorinated. In response, Julius Shukys prepared several fluorinated analogs. One of these, trifluoroethyl vinyl ether, or fluroxene, became the first fluorinated anesthetic. Fluroxene was marketed from 1954 until 1974.

In 1951, Charles Suckling, a British chemist of Imperial Chemical Industries, was asked to create a new anesthetic.

Suckling, who already had an expert understanding of fluorination, began by asking clinicians to describe the properties of an ideal anesthetic. He learned from this inquiry that his search must consider several limiting factors, including the volatility, inflammability, stability, and potency of the compounds. After 2 years of research and testing, Charles Suckling created halothane. He first determined that halothane possessed anesthetic action by anesthetizing mealworms and houseflies before he forwarded it to pharmacologist James Raventos. Suckling also made accurate predictions as to the concentrations required for anesthesia in higher animals. After Raventos completed a favorable review, halothane was offered to Michael Johnstone, a respected anesthetist of Manchester, England, who recognized its great advantages over other anesthetics available in 1956. After Johnstone's endorsement, halothane use spread quickly and widely within the practice of anesthesia.[63]

Halothane was followed in 1960 by methoxyflurane, an anesthetic that remained popular for a decade. By 1970, however, it was learned that dose-related nephrotoxicity following protracted methoxyflurane anesthesia was caused by inorganic fluoride. Similarly, because of persisting concern that rare cases of hepatitis following anesthesia might be a result of a metabolite of halothane, the search for newer inhaled anesthetics focused on the resistance to metabolic degradation.

Two fluorinated liquid anesthetics, enflurane and its isomer isoflurane, were results of the search for increased stability. They were synthesized by Ross Terrell in 1963 and 1965, respectively. Because enflurane was easier to create, it preceded isoflurane. Its application was restricted after it was shown to be a marked cardiovascular depressant and to have some convulsant properties. Isoflurane was nearly abandoned because of difficulties in its purification, but after Louise Speers overcame this problem, several successful trials were published in 1971. The release of isoflurane for clinical use was delayed again for more than half a decade by calls for repeated testing in lower animals, owing to an unfounded concern that the drug might be carcinogenic. As a consequence, isoflurane received more thorough testing than any other drug heretofore used in anesthesia. The era when an anesthetic could be introduced following a single fortuitous observation had given way to a cautious program of assessment and reassessment. Remarkably, no anesthetics were introduced into clinical use for another 20 years. Finally, desflurane was released in 1992 and sevoflurane was released in 1994. Xenon, a gas having many properties of the ideal anesthetic, was administered to a few patients in the early 1950s but it never gained popularity because of the extreme costs associated with its removal from air. However, interest in xenon has been renewed now that gas concentrations can be accurately measured when administered at low flows, and devices are available to scavenge and reuse the gas.

Intravenous Anesthetics

Prior to William Harvey's description of a complete and continuous intravascular circuit in *De Motu Cordis* (1628), it was widely held that blood emanated from the heart and was propelled to the periphery where it was consumed. The idea that substances could be injected intravascularly and travel systemically probably originated with Christopher Wren. In 1657, Wren injected aqueous opium into a dog through a goose quill attached to a pig's bladder, rendering the animal "stupefied."[64] Wren similarly injected intravenous *crocus metallorum*, an impure preparation of antimony, and observed the animals to vomit and then die. Knowledge of a circulatory system and intravascular access spurred investigations in other areas, and Wren's contemporary, Richard Lower, performed the first

blood transfusions of lamb's blood into dogs and other animals.

In the mid-19th century, equipment necessary for effective intravascular injections was conceived. Vaccination lancets were used in the 1830s to puncture the skin and force morphine paste subcutaneously for analgesia.[65] The hollow needle and hypodermic syringe were developed in the following decades but were not initially designed for intravenous use. In 1845, Dublin surgeon Francis Rynd created the hollow needle for injection of morphine into nerves in the treatment of "neuralgias." Similarly, Charles Gabriel Pravaz designed the first functional syringe in 1853 for perineural injections. Alexander Wood, however, is generally credited with perfecting the hypodermic glass syringe. In 1855, Wood published an article on the injection of opiates into painful spots by use of hollow needle and his glass syringe.[66]

In 1872, Pierre Oré of Lyons performed what is perhaps the first successful intravenous surgical anesthetic by injecting chloral hydrate immediately prior to incision. His 1875 publication describes its use in 36 patients but several postoperative deaths lent little to recommend this method to other practitioners.[67] In 1909, Ludwig Burkhardt produced surgical anesthesia by intravenous injections of chloroform and ether in Germany. Seven years later, Elisabeth Bredenfeld of Switzerland reported the use of intravenous morphine and scopolamine. The trials failed to show an improvement over inhaled techniques. Intravenous anesthesia found little application or popularity, primarily because of a lack of suitable drugs. In the following decades, this would change.

The first barbiturate, barbital, was synthesized in 1903 by Fischer and von Mering. Phenobarbital and all other successors of barbital had very protracted action and found little use in anesthesia. After 1929, oral pentobarbital was used as a sedative before surgery, but when it was given in anesthetic concentrations, long periods of unconsciousness followed. The first short-acting oxybarbiturate was hexobarbital (Evipal), available clinically in 1932. Hexobarbital was enthusiastically received by the anesthesia communities in Europe and North America because its abbreviated induction time was unrivaled by any other technique. A London anesthetist, Ronald Jarman, found that it had a dramatic advantage over inhalation inductions for minor procedures. Jarman instructed his patients to raise one arm while he injected hexobarbital into a vein of the opposite forearm. When the upraised arm fell, indicating the onset of hypnosis, the surgeon could begin. Patients were also amazed in that many awoke unable to believe they had been anesthetized.[68]

Even though the prompt action of hexobarbital had a dramatic effect on the conduct of anesthesia, it was soon replaced by two thiobarbiturates. In 1932, Donalee Tabern and Ernest H. Volwiler of the Abbott Company synthesized thiopental (Pentothal) and thiamylal (Surital). The sulfated barbiturates proved to be more satisfactory, potent, and rapid acting than were their oxybarbiturate analogs. Thiopental was first administered to a patient at the University of Wisconsin in March 1934, but the successful introduction of thiopental into clinical practice followed a thorough investigation conducted by John Lundy and his colleagues at the Mayo Clinic in June 1934.

When first introduced, thiopental was often given in repeated increments as the primary anesthetic for protracted procedures. Its hazards were soon appreciated. At first, depression of respiration was monitored by the simple expedient of observing the motion of a wisp of cotton placed over the nose. Only a few skilled practitioners were prepared to pass a tracheal tube if the patient stopped breathing. Such practitioners realized that thiopental without supplementation did not suppress airway reflexes, and they therefore encouraged the prophylactic provision of topical anesthesia of the airway beforehand. The vasodilatory effects of thiobarbiturates were widely appreciated only when thiopental caused cardiovascular collapse in hypovolemic burned civilian and military patients in World War II. In response, fluid replacement was used more aggressively and thiopental administered with greater caution.

In 1962, ketamine was synthesized by Dr. Calvin Stevens at the Parke Davis Laboratories in Ann Arbor, Michigan. One of the cyclohexylamine compounds that includes phencyclidine, ketamine was the only drug of this group that gained clinical utility. The other compounds produced undesirable postanesthetic delirium and psychomimetic reactions. In 1966, the neologism "dissociative anesthesia" was created by Guenter Corrsen and Edward Domino to describe the trancelike state of profound analgesia produced by ketamine.[69] It was released for use in 1970, and although it remains primarily an agent for anesthetic induction, its analgesic properties are increasingly studied and used by pain specialists.

Etomidate was first described by Paul Janssen and his colleagues in 1964, and originally given the name Hypnomidate. Its key advantages, minimal hemodynamic depression and lack of histamine release, account for its ongoing utility in clinical practice. It was released for use in 1974 and despite its drawbacks (pain on injection, myoclonus, postoperative nausea and vomiting, and inhibition of adrenal steroidogenesis), etomidate is often the drug of choice for anesthetizing hemodynamically unstable patients.

Propofol, or 2,-6 di-isopropyl phenol, was first synthesized by Imperial Chemical Industries and tested clinically in 1977. Investigators found that it produced hypnosis quickly with minimal excitation and that patients awoke promptly once the drug was discontinued. In addition to its excellent induction characteristics, the antiemetic action of propofol made it an agent of choice in patient populations prone to nausea and emesis. Regrettably, Cremophor EL, the solvent with which it was formulated, produced several severe anaphylactic reactions and it was withdrawn from use. Once propofol was reformulated with egg lecithin, glycerol, and soybean oil, the drug re-entered clinical practice and gained great success. Its popularity in Britain coincided with the introduction of the LMA, and it was soon noted that propofol suppressed pharyngeal reflexes to a degree that permitted the insertion of an LMA without a need for either muscle relaxants or potent inhaled anesthetics.

Local Anesthetics

Centuries after the conquest of Peru, Europeans became aware of the stimulating properties of a local, indigenous plant that the Peruvians called *khoka*. *Khoka*, which meant *the plant*, quickly became known as *coca* in Europe. In 1860, shortly after the Austrian Carl von Scherzer imported enough coca leaves to allow for analysis, German chemists Albert Niemann and Wilhelm Lossen isolated the main alkaloid and named it *cocaine*. Twenty-five years later, at the recommendation of his friend Sigmund Freud, Carl Koller became interested in the effects of cocaine. After several animal experiments, Koller successfully demonstrated the analgesic properties of cocaine applied to the eye in a patient with glaucoma.[70] Unfortunately, nearly simultaneous with the first reports of cocaine use, there were reports of central nervous system and cardiovascular toxicity.[71,72] As the popularity of cocaine grew, so did the frequency of toxic reactions and cocaine addictions.[73] Skepticism about the use of cocaine quickly grew within the medical community, forcing the pharmacological industry to develop alternative local anesthetics.

In 1898, Alfred Eihorn synthesized nivaquine, the first amino amide local anesthetic.[74] Nirvaquine proved to be an irri-tant to tissues and its use was immediately stopped. Returning his attention toward the development of amino ester local anesthetics, Eihorn synthesized benzocaine in 1900 and procaine (novocaine) shortly after in 1905. Amino esters were commonly used for local infiltration and spinal anesthesia despite their low potency and high likelihood to cause allergic reactions. Tetracaine, the last (and probably safest) amino ester local anesthetic developed, proved to be quite useful for many years.

In 1944, Nils Löfgren and Bengt Lundquist developed lidocaine, an amino amide local anesthetic.[73] Lidocaine gained immediate popularity because of its potency, rapid onset, decreased incidence of allergic reactions, and overall effectiveness for all types of regional anesthetic blocks. Since the introduction of lidocaine, all local anesthetics developed and marketed have been of the amino amide variety.

Because of the increase in lengthy and sophisticated surgical procedures, the development of a long-acting local anesthetic took precedence. From that demand, bupivacaine was introduced in 1965. Synthesized by B. Ekenstam in 1957,[76] bupivacaine was initially discarded after it was found to be highly toxic. By 1980, several years after being introduced to the United States, there were several reports of almost simultaneous seizures *and* cardiovascular collapse following unintended intravascular injection.[77] Shortly after this, as a result of the cardiovascular toxicity associated with bupivacaine and the profound motor block associated with etidocaine, the pharmaceutical industry began searching for a new long-acting alternative. Introduced in 1996, ropivacaine is structurally similar to mepivacaine and bupivacaine, although it is prepared as a single levorotatory isomer rather than a racemic mixture. The levorotatory isomer has less potential for toxicity than the dextrorotatory isomer.[78] The potential safety of ropivacaine is controversial because ropivacaine is approximately 25% less potent than bupivacaine. Therefore, at equalpotent doses the margin of safety between ropivacaine and bupivacaine becomes less apparent, although systemic toxicity with ropivacaine may respond more quickly to conventional resuscitation.[79]

Each local anesthetic developed has had its own positive and negative attributes, which is why some are still used today and others have fallen out of favor. Currently, the pharmaceutical industry is in the process of developing extended-release local anesthetics using liposomes and microspheres.[80,81]

Opioids

Opioids (historically referred to as *narcotics*, although semantically incorrect—see Chapter 19) remain the analgesic workhorse in anesthesia practice. They are used routinely in the perioperative period, in the management of acute pain, and in a variety of terminal and chronic pain states. The availability of short-, medium-, and long-acting opioids, as well as the many routes of administration, gives physicians considerable flexibility in the use of these agents. The analgesic and sedating properties of opium have been known for more than two millennia. Certainly the Greeks and Chinese civilizations harnessed these properties in medical and cultural practices. Opium is derived from the seeds of the poppy (*Papaver somniferum*), and is an amalgam of more than 25 pharmacologic alkaloids. The first alkaloid isolated, morphine, was extracted by Prussian chemist Freidrich A. W. Sertürner in 1803. He named this alkaloid after the Greek god of dreams, Morpheus. Morphine became commonly used as a supplement to inhaled anesthesia and for postoperative pain control during the latter half of the 19th century. Codeine, another alkaloid of opium, was isolated in 1832 by Robiquet but its relatively weaker analgesic potency and nausea at higher doses limits its role in managing moderate-to-severe perioperative surgical pain.

Meperidine was the first synthetic opioid and was developed in 1939 by two German researchers at IG Farben, Otto Eisleb and O. Schaumann. Although many pharmacologists are remembered for the introduction of a single drug, one prolific researcher, Paul Janssen, has since 1953 brought forward more than 70 agents from among 70,000 chemicals created in his laboratory. His products have had profound effects on disciplines as disparate as parasitology and psychiatry. The pace of productive innovation in Janssen's research laboratory is astonishing. Chemical R4263 (fentanyl), synthesized in 1960, was followed only a year later by R4749 (droperidol), and then etomidate in 1964. Innovar, the fixed combination of fentanyl and droperidol, is less popular now but Janssen's phenylpiperidine derivatives, fentanyl, sufentanil and alfentanil, are staples in the anesthesia pharmacopoeia. Remifentanil, an ultra short-acting opioid introduced by Glaxo-Wellcome in 1996, is a departure from other opioids in that it has very rapid onset and equally rapid offset due to metabolism by nonspecific tissue esterases. Ketorolac, a nonsteroidal antiinflammatory drug (NSAID) approved for use in 1990, was the first parenteral NSAID indicated for postoperative pain. With a 6- to 8-mg morphine equivalent analgesic potency, Ketorolac provides significant postoperative pain control and has particular use when an opioid-sparing approach is essential. Ketorolac use is limited by side effects and may be inappropriate in patients with underlying renal dysfunction, bleeding problems, or compromised bone healing.

Muscle Relaxants

Muscle relaxants entered anesthesia practice nearly a century after inhalational anesthetics (Table 1-1). Curare, the first known neuromuscular blocking agent, was originally used in hunting and tribal warfare by native peoples of South America. The curares are alkaloids prepared from plants native to equatorial rain forests. The refinement of the harmless sap of several species of vines into toxins that were lethal only when injected was an extraordinary triumph introduced by paleopharmacologists in loincloths. Their discovery was the more remarkable because it was independently repeated on three separate continents—South America, Africa, and Asia. These jungle tribes also developed nearly identical methods of delivering the toxin by darts, which, after being dipped in curare, maintained their potency indefinitely until they were propelled through blowpipes to strike the flesh of monkeys and other animals of the treetops. Moreover, the American Indians knew of the juice of an herb that would counteract the effects of the poison if administered in time.[82]

The earliest clinical use of curare in humans was to ameliorate the tortuous muscle spasms of infectious tetanus. In 1858, New York physician Louis Albert Sayres reported two cases in which he attempted to treat severe tetanus with curare at the Bellevue Hospital. Both of his patients died. Similar efforts were undertaken to use muscle relaxants to treat epilepsy, rabies, and choreiform disorders. Treatment of Parkinson-like rigidity and the prevention of trauma from seizure therapy also preceded the use of curare in anesthesia.[83]

Interestingly, curare antagonists were developed well before muscle relaxants were ever used in surgery. In 1900, Jacob Pal, a Viennese physician, recognized that curare could be antagonized by physostigmine. This substance had been isolated from the calabar bean some 36 years earlier by Scottish pharmacologist Sir T. R. Fraser. Neostigmine methylsulphate was synthesized in 1931 and was significantly more potent in antagonizing the effects of curare.[84]

In 1938, Richard and Ruth Gill returned to New York from South America, bringing with them 11.9 kg of crude curare collected near their Ecuadorian ranch. Their motivation was a mixture of personal and altruistic goals. Some months before, while on an earlier visit to the United States, Richard Gill learned that he had multiple sclerosis. His physician, Dr. Walter Freeman, mentioned the possibility that curare might have a therapeutic role in the management of spastic disorders. When the Gills returned to the United States with their supply of crude curare, they encouraged scientists at E. R. Squibb & Co. to take an interest in its unique properties. Squibb soon offered semirefined curare to two groups of American anesthesiologists, who assessed its action but quickly abandoned their studies when it caused total respiratory paralysis in two patients and the death of laboratory animals.

The earliest effective clinical application of curare in medicine occurred in physiatry. After A. R. McIntyre refined a portion of the raw curare in 1939, Abram E. Bennett of Omaha, Nebraska, injected it into children with spastic disorders. While no persistent benefit could be observed in these patients, he next administered it to patients about to receive Metrazol, a precursor to electroconvulsive therapy. Because it eliminated seizure-induced fractures, they termed it a "shock absorber." By 1941, other psychiatrists followed this practice and, when they found that the action of curare was protracted, occasionally used neostigmine as an antidote.

Curare was used initially in surgery by Arthur Lawen in 1912, but the published report was written in German and was ignored for decades. Lawen, a physiologist and physician from Leipzig, used curare in his laboratory before boldly producing abdominal relaxation at a light level of anesthesia in a surgical patient. Lawen's efforts were not appreciated for decades, and while his pioneering work anticipated later clinical application, safe use would have to await the introduction of regular intubation of the trachea and controlled ventilation of the lungs.[85]

Thirty years after Lawen, Harold Griffith, the chief anesthetist of the Montreal Homeopathic Hospital, learned of A. E. Bennett's successful use of curare and resolved to apply it in anesthesia. As Griffith was already a master of tracheal intubation, he was much better prepared than were most of his contemporaries to attend to potential complications. On January 23, 1942, Griffith and his resident, Enid Johnson, anesthetized and intubated the trachea of a young man before injecting curare early in the course of his appendectomy. Satisfactory abdominal relaxation was obtained and the surgery proceeded without incident. Griffith and Johnson's report of the successful use of curare in the 25 patients of their series launched a revolution in anesthetic care.[86]

Anesthesiologists who practiced before muscle relaxants recall the anxiety they felt when a premature attempt to intubate the trachea under cyclopropane caused persisting laryngospasm. Before 1942, abdominal relaxation was possible only if the patient tolerated high concentrations of an inhaled anesthetic, which might bring profound respiratory depression and protracted recovery. Curare and the drugs that followed transformed anesthesia profoundly. Because intubation of the trachea could now be taught in a deliberate manner, a neophyte could fail on a first attempt without compromising the safety of the patient. For the first time, abdominal relaxation could be attained when curare was supplemented by light planes of inhaled anesthetics or by a combination of intravenous agents providing "balanced anesthesia." New frontiers opened. Sedated and paralyzed patients could now successfully undergo the major physiologic trespasses of cardiopulmonary bypass, deliberate hypothermia, or long-term respiratory support after surgery.

Credit for successful and safe introduction of curare and d-tubocurarine into anesthesia must in part be given to a Squibb researcher named H. A. Holaday. Crude, unstandardized preparations of curare produced uncertain clinical effects and undesirable side effects related to various impurities. Isolation

TABLE 1-1

EVENTS IN THE DEVELOPMENT OF MUSCLE RELAXANTS

YEAR	EVENT
1516	Peter Martyr d'Anghera, *De orbe novo*, published account of South American Indian arrow poisons
1596	Sir Walter Raleigh provides detailed account of arrow poison effects and antidote
1745	Charles-Marie de la Condamine returns from Ecuador and conducts curare experiments with chickens and attempted to use sugar as an antidote
1780	Abbe Felix Fontana inserts curare directly into exposed sciatic nerve of rabbit without effect, concludes that mechanism is the destruction of the irritability of voluntary muscles. Publishes *On the American Poison Ticunas* (name of South American tribe)
1811	Benjamin Collins Brodie demonstrates that animals mechanically ventilated may survive significant doses of curare
1812	William Sewell suggests use of curare in "hydrophobia" (rabies) and tetanus
1844	Claude Bernard determines that death occurs by respiratory failure, motor nerves are unable to transmit stimuli from higher centers, differential effect on muscles with peripheral and thoracic muscles being affected before respiratory muscles. Bernard concludes that the site of action is the junction between muscles and nerves, neuromuscular junction
1858	Louis Albert Sayres, New York physician, uses curare to treat tetanus in two patients
1864	Physostigmine isolated from Calabar beans by Sir T. R. Fraser, a Scottish pharmacologist
1886–1897	R. Boehm, a German chemist, demonstrated three separate classes of alkaloids in each of three types of indigenous containers: tube-curares, pot-curares, and calabash-curares
1900	Jacob Pal recognizes that physostigmine can antagonize the effects of curare
1906	Succinylcholine prepared by Reid Hunt and R. Taveau, experimented on rabbits pretreated with curare to learn of cardiac effects and so paralysis went unrecognized
1912	Arthur Lawen uses curare in surgery but report published in German so it goes largely unrecognized
1938	Richard and Ruth Gill bring large quantity of curare to New York for further study by pharmaceutical company
1939	Abram E. Bennett uses curare in children with spastic disorders and to prevent trauma from Metrazol therapy (precursor to ECT)
1942	Harold Griffith and Enid Johnson use curare for abdominal relaxation in surgery
1942	H. A. Halody develops rabbit head-drop assay for standardization and large-scale production of curare and d-tubocurarine
1948	Decamethonium, a depolarizing relaxant, is synthesized
1949	Succinylcholine prepared by Daniel Bovet, and the following year by J. C. Castillo and Edwin de Beer
1956	Distinction between depolarizing and nondepolarizing neuromuscular blockade is made by William D. M. Paton
1964	Pancuronium released for use in humans, synthesized by Savage and Hewett
1979	Vecuronium introduced, specifically designed to be more hepatically metabolized than pancuronium
1993	Mivacurium released for clinical use
1994	Rocuronium introduced to clinical practice

of d-tubocurarine in 1935 renewed clinical interest but a method for standardizing "Intocostrin" and its purer derivative, d-tubocurarine, had yet to be devised. In the early 1940s, in part as a result of Griffith and Johnson's successful trials, Squibb embarked on wide-scale production. Holaday developed a reliable, easily reproducible method for standardizing curare doses that became known as the rabbit head-drop assay (Fig. 1-5). The assay consisted of aqueous curare solution injected intravenously in 0.1-mL doses every 15 seconds until the end point, when the rabbit became unable to raise its head, was reached.[87]

Successful clinical use of curare led to the introduction of other muscle relaxants. By 1948, gallamine and decamethonium had been synthesized. Metubine, a curare "rediscovered" in the 1970s, was used clinically in the same year. Succinylcholine was prepared by the Nobel laureate Daniel Bovet in 1949 and was in wide international use before historians noted that the drug had been synthesized and tested long beforehand. In 1906, Reid Hunt and R. Taveaux prepared succinylcholine among a series of choline esters, which they had injected into rabbits to observe their cardiac effects. If their rabbits had not been previously paralyzed with curare, the

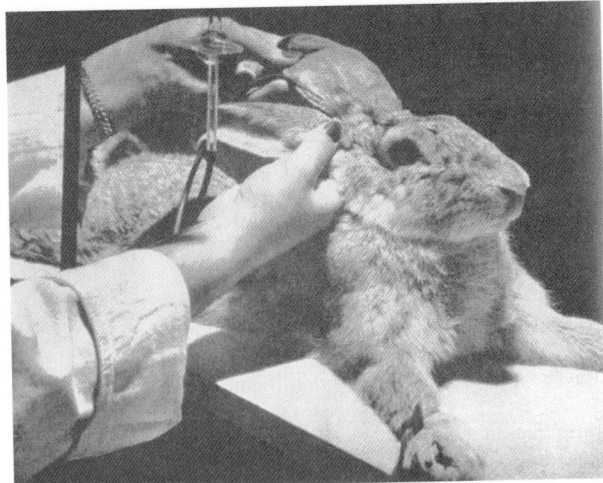
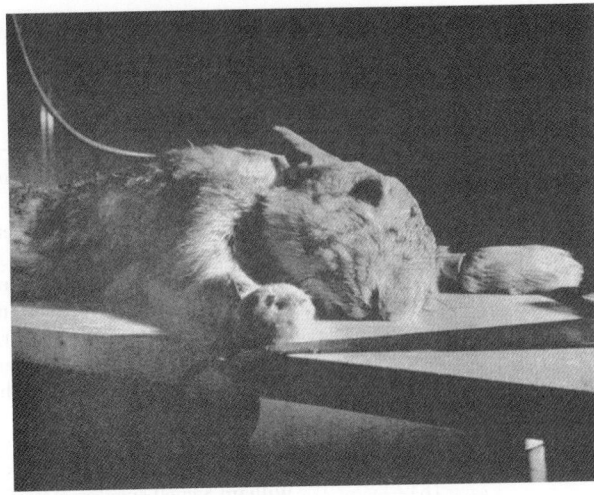

A   **B**

FIGURE 1-5. The Rabbit head-drop assay. H. A. Halloday of Squibb pharmaceutical company developed a method of standardizing doses of curare and d-tubocurarine a normal rabbit (**A**) had 0.1 ml of aqueous cecurane solution injected every 15 seconds until it could no longer raise its head (**B**).

depolarizing action of succinylcholine might have been recognized decades earlier.

The ability to monitor intraoperative neuromuscular blockade with nerve stimulators began in 1958. Working at St. Thomas' Hospital in London, T. H. Christie and H. Churchill-Davidson developed a method for monitoring peripheral neuromuscular blockade during anesthesia. It was not until 1970, however, that H. H. Ali and colleagues devised the technique of delivering four supramaximal impulses delivered at 2 Hz (0.5 seconds apart), or a "Train of Four," as a method of quantifying the degree of residual neuromuscular blockade.[88]

Research in relaxants was rekindled in 1960 when researchers became aware of the action of maloetine, a relaxant from the Congo basin. It was remarkable in that it had a steroidal nucleus. Investigations of maloetine led to pancuronium in 1968. In the 1970s and 1980s, research shifted toward identification of specific receptor biochemistry and development of receptor-specific drugs. From these isoquinolines, four related products emerged: vecuronium, pipecuronium, rocuronium, and rapacuronium. Rapacuronium, released in the early 1990s, was withdrawn from clinical use after several cases of intractable bronchospasm led to brain damage or death. Four clinical products based on the steroid parent drug d-tubocurarine (atracurium, mivacurium, doxacurium, and cis-atracurium) also made it to clinical use. Recognition that atracurium and cis-atracurium undergo spontaneous degradation by Hoffmann elimination has defined a role for these muscle relaxants in patients with liver and renal insufficiency.

Antiemetics

Effective treatment for postoperative nausea and vomiting (PONV) evolved relatively recently and has been driven by incentives to limit hospitalization expenses and improve patient satisfaction. But PONV is an old problem for which late 19th century practitioners recognized many causes including anxiety, severe pain, sudden changes in blood pressure, ileus, ingestion of blood, and the residual effects of opioids and inhalational anesthetics. Risk of pulmonary aspiration of gastric contents and subsequent death from asphyxia or aspiration pneumonia was a feared consequence of anesthetics, especially those preceding use of cuffed endotracheal tubes. Vomiting and aspiration during anesthesia led to the practice of maintaining an empty stomach preoperatively, a policy that

continues today despite evidence that clear fluids up to 3 hours before surgery do not increase gastric volumes, change gastric pH, or increase the risk of aspiration.

A variety of treatments for nausea and vomiting were proposed by early anesthetists. James Gwathemy's 1914 publication, *Anesthesia*, commented that British surgeons customarily gave tincture of iodine in a teaspoonful of water every half hour for three or four doses. Inhalation of vinegar fumes, and rectal injection of 30 to 40 drops of tincture of opium with 60 grains of sodium bromide, were also thought to quiet the vomiting center.[89] Other practitioners attempted olfactory control by placing a piece of gauze moistened with essence of orange or an aromatic oil on the upper lip of the patient.[90] A 1937 anesthesia textbook encouraged treatment of PONV with lateral positioning, "iced soda water, strong black coffee, and chloretone."[91] Counterirritation, such as mustard leaf on the epigastrium, was also believed useful in limiting emesis.[92] As late as 1951, anesthesia texts recommended oxygen administration, whiffs of ammonia spirits, and control of blood pressure and positioning.[93] The complex central mechanisms of nausea and vomiting were largely unaffected by most of these treatments. Newer drugs capable of intervening at specific pathways were needed to have an impact on PONV. As more short-acting anesthetics were developed, the problem received sharper focus in awake postoperative patients in the recovery room. The nausea attending use of newer chemotherapy agents provided additional impetus to the development of antiemetic medications.

In 1955, a nonrandomized study using the antihistamine cyclizine showed a reduction in PONV from 27% to 21% in a group of 3,000 patients. The following year, a more rigorous study by Knapp and Beecher reported a significant benefit from prophylaxis with the neuroleptic chlorpromazine. In 1957, promethazine (Phenergan) and chlorpromazine were both found to reduce PONV when used prophylactically. Thirteen years later, a double-blind study evaluating metoclopramide was published and that drug became a first-line drug in the management of PONV. Droperidol, released in the early 1960s, became widely used until 2001 when concerns regarding prolongation of QT intervals prompted a warning from the Food and Drug Administration about its continued use.

The antiemetic effects of corticosteroids were first recognized by oncologists treating intracranial edema from tumors.[94] Subsequent studies have borne out the antiemetic properties of this class of drugs in treating PONV. Recognition of the serotonin 5-HT3 pathway in PONV has led to a unique class of drugs devoted only to addressing this particular problem. Ondansetron, the first representative of this drug class, was approved by the Food and Drug Administration in 1991. Additional serotonin 5-HT3 antagonists have been approved and are available today.

ANESTHESIA SUBSPECIALTIES

Regional Anesthesia

5 Cocaine, an extract of the coca leaf, was the first effective local anesthetic. After Albert Niemann refined the active alkaloid and named it *cocaine*, it was used in experiments by a few investigators. It was noted that cocaine provided topical anesthesia and even produced local insensibility when injected, but Carl Koller, a Viennese surgical intern, first recognized the utility of cocaine in clinical practice.

In 1884, Carl Koller was completing his medical training at a time when many operations on the eye were performed without general anesthesia. Almost four decades after the discovery of ether, general anesthesia by mask still had limitations for ophthalmic surgery: lack of patient cooperation, interference of the anesthesia apparatus with surgical access, and the high incidence of PONV. At that time, since fine sutures were not available and surgical incisions of the eye were not closed, postoperative vomiting threatened the extrusion of the globe's contents, putting the patient at risk for irrevocable blindness.[95]

While a medical student, Koller had worked in a Viennese laboratory in a search of a topical ophthalmic anesthetic to overcome the limitations of general anesthesia. Unfortunately, the suspensions of morphine, chloral hydrate, and other drugs that he had used had been ineffectual. In 1884, Koller's friend, Sigmund Freud, became interested in the cerebral-stimulating effects of cocaine and gave him a small sample in an envelope, which he placed in his pocket. When the envelope leaked, a few grains of cocaine stuck to Koller's finger and he absent-mindedly licked his tongue. When his tongue became numb, Koller instantly realized that he had found the object of his search. In his laboratory, he made a suspension of cocaine crystals that he and a laboratory associate tested in the eyes of a frog, a rabbit, and a dog. Satisfied with the anesthetic effects seen in the animal models, Koller dropped the solution onto his own cornea. To his amazement, his eyes were insensitive to the touch of a pin.[96] As an intern, Carl Koller could not afford to attend a Congress of German Ophthalmologists in Heidelberg on September 15, 1884. However, a friend presented his article at the meeting and a revolution in ophthalmic surgery and other surgical disciplines began. Within the next year, more than 100 articles supporting the use of cocaine appeared in European and American medical journals. In 1888, Koller immigrated to New York, where he practiced ophthalmology for the remainder of his career.

American surgeons quickly developed new applications for cocaine. Its efficacy in anesthetizing the nose, mouth, larynx, trachea, rectum, and urethra was described in October 1884. The next month, the first reports of its subcutaneous injection were published. In December 1884, two young surgeons, William Halsted and Richard Hall, described blocks of the sensory nerves of the face and arm. Halsted even performed a brachial plexus block but did so under direct vision while the patient received an inhaled anesthetic.[97] Unfortunately, self-experimentation with cocaine was hazardous, as both surgeons became addicted.[98] Addiction was an ill-understood but frequent problem in the late 19th century, especially when cocaine and morphine were present in many patent medicines and folk remedies.

Other regional anesthetic techniques were attempted before the end of the 19th century. The term *spinal anesthesia* was coined in 1885 by Leonard Corning, a neurologist who had observed Hall and Halsted. Corning wanted to assess the action of cocaine as a specific therapy for neurologic problems. After first assessing its action in a dog, producing a blockade of rapid onset that was confined to the animal's rear legs, he performed a neuraxial block using cocaine on a man "addicted to masturbation." Corning administered one dose without effect, then after a second dose, the patient's legs "felt sleepy." The man had impaired sensibility in his lower extremity after about 20 minutes and left Corning's office "none the worse for the experience."[99] Although Corning did not describe escape of cerebrospinal fluid (CSF) in either case, it is likely that the dog had a spinal anesthetic and that the man had an epidural anesthetic. No therapeutic benefit was described, but Corning closed his account and his attention to the subject by suggesting that cocainization might in time be "a substitute for etherization in genito-urinary or other branches of surgery."[100]

Two other authors, August Bier and Theodor Tuffier, described authentic spinal anesthesia, with mention of CSF, injection of cocaine, and an appropriately short onset of action. In a comparative review of the original articles by Bier, Tuffier, and Corning, it was concluded that Corning's injection was extradural, and Bier merited the credit for introducing spinal anesthesia.[101]

Fourteen years passed before spinal anesthesia was performed for surgery. In the interval, Heinrich Quincke of Kiel, Germany, had described his technique of lumbar puncture. He offered the valuable observation that it was most safely performed at the level of the third or fourth lumbar interspace because entry at that level was below the termination of the spinal cord. Quincke's technique was used in Kiel for the first deliberate cocainization of the spinal cord in 1899 by his surgical colleague, August Bier. Six patients received small doses of cocaine intrathecally, but because some cried out during surgery while others vomited and experienced headaches, Bier considered it necessary to conduct further experiments before continuing this technique for surgery.

Professor Bier permitted his assistant, Dr. Hildebrandt, to perform a lumbar puncture, but after the needle penetrated the dura, Hildebrandt could not fit the syringe to the needle and a large volume of the professor's spinal fluid escaped. They were at the point of abandoning the study when Hildebrandt volunteered to be the subject of a second attempt. Their persistence was rewarded with an astonishing success. Twenty-three minutes after the spinal injection, Bier noted: "A strong blow with an iron hammer against the tibia was not felt as pain. After 25 minutes: Strong pressure and pulling on a testicle were not painful."[94] They celebrated their success with wine and cigars. That night, both developed violent headaches, which they attributed at first to their celebration. Bier's headache was relieved after 9 days of bed rest. Hildebrandt, as a house officer, did not have the luxury of continued rest. Bier postulated that their headaches were a result of the loss of large volumes of CSF and urged that this be avoided if possible. The high incidence of complications following lumbar puncture with wide-bore needles and the toxic reactions attributed to cocaine explain his later loss of interest in spinal anesthesia.[102]

Surgeons in several other countries soon practiced spinal anesthesia and progress occurred by many small contributions to the technique. Theodor Tuffier published the first series of 125 spinal anesthetics from France and he later counseled that the solution should not be injected before CSF was seen. The first American report was by Rudolph Matas of New Orleans, whose first patient developed postanesthetic meningismus, a frequent complication that was overcome in part by the use of hermetically sealed sterile solutions recommended by E. W. Lee of Philadelphia and sterile gloves as advocated by Halsted. During 1899, Dudley Tait and Guidlo Caglieri of San Francisco performed experimental studies in animals and therapeutic spinals for orthopaedic patients. They encouraged the use of fine needles to lessen the escape of CSF and urged that the skin and deeper tissues be infiltrated beforehand with local anesthesia.[103] This had been suggested earlier by William Halsted and the foremost advocate of infiltration anesthesia, Carl Ludwig Schleich of Berlin. An early American specialist in anesthesia, Ormond Goldan, published an anesthesia record appropriate for recording the course of "intraspinal cocainization" in 1900. In the same year, Heinrich Braun learned of a newly described extract of the adrenal gland, epinephrine, which he used to prolong the action of local anesthetics with great success. Braun developed several new nerve blocks, coined the term *conduction anesthesia*, and is remembered by European writers as the "father of conduction anesthesia." Braun was the first person to use procaine, which, along with stovaine, was one of the first synthetic local anesthetics produced to reduce the toxicity of cocaine.

Before 1907, anesthesiologists were sometimes disappointed to observe that their spinal anesthetics were incomplete. Most believed that the drug spread solely by local diffusion before the property of baricity was investigated by Arthur Barker, a London surgeon.[104] Barker constructed a glass tube shaped to follow the curves of the human spine and used it to demonstrate the limited spread of colored solutions that he had injected through a T-piece in the lumbar region. Barker applied this observation to use solutions of stovaine made hyperbaric by the addition of 5% glucose, which worked in a more predictable fashion. After the injection was complete, Barker placed his patient's head on pillows to contain the anesthetic below the nipple line. Lincoln Sise acknowledged Barker's work in 1935 when he introduced the use of hyperbaric solutions of tetracaine (Pontocaine). John Adriani advanced the concept further in 1946 when he used a hyperbaric solution to produce "saddle block," or perineal anesthesia. Adriani's patients remained seated after injection as the drug descended to the sacral nerves.

Tait, Jonnesco, and other early masters of spinal anesthesia used a cervical approach for thyroidectomy and thoracic procedures, but this radical approach was supplanted in 1928 by the lumbar injection of hypobaric solutions of "light" nupercaine by G. P. Pitkin. Although the use of hypobaric solutions is now limited primarily to patients positioned in the jackknife position, their former use for thoracic procedures demanded skill and precise timing. The enthusiasts of hypobaric anesthesia devised formulas to attempt to predict the time in seconds needed for a warmed solution of hypobaric nupercaine to spread in patients of varying size from its site of injection in the lumbar area to the level of the fourth thoracic dermatome.

The recurring problem of inadequate duration of single-injection spinal anesthesia led a Philadelphia surgeon, William Lemmon, to devise an apparatus for continuous spinal anesthesia in 1940.[105] Lemmon began with the patient in the lateral position. The spinal tap was performed with a malleable silver needle, which was left in position. As the patient was turned supine, the needle was positioned through a hole in the mattress and table. Additional injections of local anesthetic could be performed as required. Malleable silver needles also found a less cumbersome and more common application in 1942 when Waldo Edwards and Robert Hingson encouraged the use of Lemmon's needles for continuous caudal anesthesia in obstetrics. In 1944 Edward Tuohy of the Mayo Clinic introduced two important modifications of the continuous spinal techniques. He developed the now familiar Tuohy needle[106] as a means of improving the ease of passage of lacquered silk ureteral catheters through which he injected incremental doses of local anesthetic.[107]

In 1949, Martinez Curbelo of Havana, Cuba, used Tuohy's needle and a ureteral catheter to perform the first continuous epidural anesthetic. Silk and gum elastic catheters were difficult to sterilize and sometimes caused dural infections before being superseded by disposable plastics. Yet, deliberate single-injection peridural anesthesia had been practiced occasionally for decades before continuous techniques brought it greater popularity. At the beginning of the 20th century, two French clinicians experimented independently with caudal anesthesia. The neurologist Jean Athanase Sicard applied the technique for a nonsurgical purpose, the relief of back pain. Fernand Cathelin used caudal anesthesia as a less dangerous alternative to spinal anesthesia for hernia repairs. He also demonstrated that the epidural space terminated in the neck by injecting a solution of India ink into the caudal canal of a dog. The lumbar approach was first used solely for multiple paravertebral nerve blocks before the Pagés-Dogliotti single-injection technique became accepted. As they worked separately, the technique carries the names of both men. Captain Fidel Pagés prepared an elegant demonstration of segmental single-injection peridural anesthesia in 1921, but died soon after his article appeared in a Spanish military journal.[108] Ten years later, Achille M. Dogliotti of Turin, Italy, wrote a classic study that made the epidural technique well known.[73] Whereas Pagés used a tactile approach to identify the epidural space, Dogliotti identified it by the loss-of-resistance technique.

Surgery on the extremities lent itself to other regional anesthesia techniques. In 1902, Harvey Cushing coined the phrase *regional anesthesia* for his technique of blocking either the brachial or sciatic plexus under direct vision during general anesthesia to reduce anesthesia requirements and provide postoperative pain relief.[75] Fifteen years before his publication, George Crile advanced a similar approach to reduce the stress and shock of surgery. Crile, a dedicated advocate of regional and infiltration techniques during general anesthesia, coined the term *anoci-association*.[109]

An intravenous regional technique with procaine was reported in 1908 by August Bier, the surgeon who had pioneered spinal anesthesia. Bier injected procaine into a vein of the upper limb between two tourniquets. Even though the technique is termed the *Bier block*, it was not used for many decades until it was reintroduced 55 years later by Mackinnon Holmes, who modified the technique by exsanguination before applying a single proximal cuff. Holmes used lidocaine, the very successful amide local anesthetic synthesized in 1943 by Lofgren and Lundquist of Sweden.

Several investigators achieved upper extremity anesthesia by percutaneous injections of the brachial plexus. In 1911, based on his intimate knowledge of the anatomy of the axillary area, Hirschel promoted a "blind" axillary injection. In the same year, Kulenkampff described a supraclavicular approach in which the operator sought out paresthesias of the plexus while keeping the needle at a point superficial to the first rib and the pleura. The risk of pneumothorax with Kulenkampff's approach led Mulley to attempt blocks more proximally by a lateral paravertebral approach, the precursor of what is now popularly known as the *Winnie block*.

Heinrich Braun wrote the earliest textbook of local anesthesia, which appeared in its first English translation in 1914. After 1922, Gaston Labat's *Regional Anesthesia* dominated the American market. Labat migrated from France to the Mayo Clinic in Minnesota, where he served briefly before taking a permanent position at the Bellevue Hospital in New York. He formed the first American Society for Regional Anesthesia.[110] After Labat's death, Emery A. Rovenstine was recruited to Bellevue to continue Labat's work, among other responsibilities. Rovenstein created the first American clinic for the treatment of chronic pain, where he and his associates refined techniques of lytic and therapeutic injections and used the American Society of Regional Anesthesia to further the knowledge of pain management across the United States.[111]

❻ The development of the multidisciplinary pain clinic was one of many contributions to anesthesiology made by John J. Bonica, a renowned teacher of regional techniques. During his periods of military, civilian, and university service at the University of Washington, Bonica formulated a series of improvements in the management of patients with chronic pain. His classic text *The Management of Pain,* now in its third edition, is regarded as a standard of the literature of anesthesia.

Cardiovascular Anesthesia

The earliest attempts to operate on the heart were limited to repairing cardiac wounds. These attempts generally failed until German surgeon Ludwig Rehn repaired a right ventricular stab wound in September 1896.[112] Despite this success, the field was not ready to advance. The taboo of cardiac surgery was summarized by Theodore Billroth when he supposedly said "any surgeon who would attempt an operation on the heart should lose the respect of his colleagues."[113] The resistance to such operations was partly because of fledgling anesthetic medications, lack of adequate monitors, and even a clear understanding of cardiovascular physiology that pervades modern anesthesia practice.

Fortunately, the turn of the 20th century saw many advances in anesthesia practice, blood typing and transfusion, anticoagulation, antibiosis, as well as surgical instrumentation and technique. Some continued to attempt procedures like closed mitral valvotomy in the midst of these technological advancements, but outcomes were still very poor with mortality rates exceeding 80%. Many believe that the successful ligation of a 7-year-old girl's patent ductus arteriosus by Robert Gross in 1938 served as the landmark case for modern cardiac surgery. Soon after Gross' achievement, a host of new procedures were developed for repairing congenital cardiac lesions, including the first Blalock-Taussig shunt performed on a 15 month-old "blue baby" in 1944.[114] Although the shunt had been successfully demonstrated in animal models, Austin Lamont, Chief of Anesthesia at Johns Hopkins, was not supportive of the procedure. He emphatically stated "I will not put that child to death" and left the open drop ether-oxygen anesthetic to resident anesthesiologist Merel Harmel.[115] Lamont attended on the second Blalock-Taussig shunt 2 months later. Together, Harmel and Lamont would publish the first article on anesthesia for cardiac surgery in 1946 based on 100 cases with Alfred Blalock and repair of congenital pulmonic stenosis.[116]

Closed cardiac surgery ensued and anesthesia pioneers like William McQuiston and Kenneth Keown worked side-by-side with surgeons during procedures like the first aortic-pulmonary anastomosis and the first transmyocardial mitral commissurotomy. Never before had anesthesia providers worked as intimately with surgeons for the patient's welfare. Anesthesiologist and World War II physician Max Samuel Sadove remarked "the small-arms fire of the anesthesiologist joins the spy system of the lab to back up the surgeon's big artillery in a coordinated attack to conquer disease."[117]

Through the 1930s and 1940s, John Gibbon had been experimenting with several extracorporeal circuit designs and by 1947 was able to successfully place dogs on heart-lung bypass. The first successful use of Gibbon's cardiopulmonary bypass machine in humans in May 1953 was a monumental advance in the surgical treatment of complex cardiac pathology that stimulated international interest in open heart surgery and the specialty of cardiac anesthesia.

Over the next decade, rapid growth and expanded applications of cardiac surgery, including artificial valves and coronary artery bypass grafting, required many more anesthesiologists acquainted with these specialized techniques. In 1967, J. Earl Waynards published one of the first articles on anesthetic management of patients undergoing surgery for coronary artery disease.

As cardiac surgery evolved, so did the perioperative monitoring and care of patients undergoing cardiac surgery. Postoperative mechanical ventilation and surgical intensive care units appeared by the late 1960s. Devices like the left atrial pressure monitor and the intra-aortic balloon pump offered new methods of understanding cardiopulmonary physiology and treating postoperative ventricular failure. Cardiac anesthesiologists were quick to bring the pulmonary artery catheter (PAC) into the operating room, permitting more precise hemodynamic monitoring and intervention. Joel Kaplan, already known for using the V_5 lead to monitor for myocardial ischemia and nitroglycerin infusions to treat ischemia, popularized the use of the PAC to detect myocardial ischemia. At Texas Heart Institute, Slogoff and Keats demonstrated the negative impact of myocardial ischemia on clinical outcome. By the end of the 1980s, the same duo would reveal that the choice of anesthetic agent had little impact on outcome, challenging the earlier paradigm of isoflurane steal proposed by Reiz.

Developments like cold potassium cardioplegia, monitoring and reversal of heparin, and reduction of blood loss with aprotinin would change the practice of cardiac anesthesia. Transesophageal echocardiography, introduced into cardiac surgery by Roizen, Cahalan, and Kremer in the 1980s, helped to further define the subspecialty of cardiac anesthesia.

Neuroanesthesia

Brain surgery is considered by some to be the oldest of the practiced medical arts. Evidence of trepanation, a form of neurosurgery in which a hole is drilled or scraped into the skull to access the dura, was discovered in skulls dating back to 6500 BC at a French burial site. Prehistoric brain surgery was also practiced by civilizations in South America, Africa, and Asia.[118]

With the introduction of inhalational anesthesia in the mid-1800s, Scottish surgeon and neurosurgery pioneer Sir William Macewen used this novel practice while performing the first successful craniotomy for tumor removal in 1879. Macewen, well known for introducing the technique of orotracheal intubation, promoted the idea of teaching medical students at Glasgow Royal Infirmary the art of chloroform anesthesia.

Like Macewen, Sir Victor Horsely was a neurosurgeon with an interest in anesthesia. His experiments of how ether, chloroform, and morphine affected intracranial contents led him to conclude that "the agent of choice was chloroform and that morphine had some value because of its cerebral constriction effects."[119] He first published his anesthetic technique for brain surgery in the *British Medical Journal* in 1886.[120] Later, he omitted morphine from his regimen after discovering its tendency to produce respiratory depression.

Meanwhile, Harvard medical student and aspiring neurosurgeon Harvey Cushing developed the first charts to record heart rate, temperature, and respiration during anesthesia. Soon after, he would add blood pressure readings to the record. Cushing was one of the first surgeons to recognize the importance of dedicated, specially trained anesthesia personnel versed in neurosurgery. Charles Frazier, a neurosurgical contemporary of Cushing, also recognized this need, stating that "no [cranial] operation be undertaken unless the services of a skilled anesthetizer are available."[121]

Since ether and chloroform anesthesia had significant drawbacks, beginning in 1918 Cushing and his contemporaries explored the advantages of regional or local anesthesia for intracranial surgery. Part of the motivation driving this change was the increased duration in surgical time. Cushing and colleagues used a "slow" surgical technique for most surgical procedures, where the average duration for cranial operations was 5 hours.[122] In contrast, early neurosurgeons like Horseley and Sir Percy Sargeant could perform similar procedures in less than 90 minutes. Therefore, prolonged patient exposure to chloroform or ether anesthesia were likely to result in increased bleeding, postoperative headache, confusion, and/or vomiting. Cushing and contemporaries thought the use of local or regional anesthesia lessened the risk of these complications.

After a decade, it was realized that the remote positioning of the anesthetist was troublesome when managing the airway of an awake or lightly sedated patient undergoing cranial surgery with regional anesthesia. Also, endotracheal tubes, although introduced at the beginning of the century, had become popular instruments for securing a patient's airway and providing inhalation anesthesia. Combined, these circumstances led to the rapid resurgence of popularity in general anesthesia for cranial surgery, a trend that would continue to present day.

While the introduction of agents like thiopental, curare, and halothane advanced the practice of anesthesiology in general, the development of methods to measure brain electrical activity, cerebral blood flow and metabolic rate by Kety and Schmidt, and intracranial pressure by Lundburg "put neuroanesthesia practice on a scientific foundation and opened doors to neuroanesthesia research."[123] Clinician-scientists like John D. (Jack) Michenfelder, later known as the father of neuroanesthesia, conducted basic science and clinical research on cerebral blood flow and brain function and protection in response to various anesthetic agents and techniques. Many lessons learned during this period of groundbreaking research are still commonly used in modern neuroanesthesia practice.

Obstetric Anesthesia

Social attitudes about pain associated with childbirth began to change in the 1860s and women started demanding anesthesia for childbirth. Societal pressures were so great that physicians, although unconvinced of the benefits of analgesia, felt obligated to offer this service to their obstetric patients.[124] In 1907 an Austrian physician, Richard von Steinbüchel used a combination of morphine and scopolamine to produce *Dämmerschlaff* or "Twilight Sleep."[125] Although these two drugs were well known, physicians remained skeptical that Twilight Sleep was essential to labor and delivery, which unfortunately contrasted with the opinion of most women. This method gained popularity after German obstetricians Carl Gauss and Bernhardt Krőnig widely publicized the technique. Numerous advertisements touted the benefits of Twilight Sleep (analgesia, partial pain relief, and amnesia) as compared to ether and chloroform, which resulted in total unconsciousness.[126] Gauss recognized the narrow therapeutic margin of these medications and gave precise instructions on its use: the first injection (morphine 10 mg and scopolamine) was to be given shortly after active labor began—this was intended to blunt the pain of labor—and subsequent injections consisted of only scopolamine, which was dosed to obliterate the memory of labor. Because of the effects of scopolamine, many patients became disoriented and would scream and thrash about during labor and delivery. Gauss believed that he could minimize this reaction by decreasing the sensory input; therefore, he would put patients in a dark room, cover their eyes with gauze, and insert oil-soaked cotton into their ears. The patients were often confined to a padded bed and restrained with leather straps during the delivery.[127] Over time, the doses of morphine administered seemed to increase, although there were few, if any, reports of adverse neonatal effects. Virginia Apgar's system for

evaluating newborns, developed in 1953, demonstrated that there actually was a difference in the neonates of mothers who had been anesthetized.[128]

The bulk of the interest in this technique appears to have been popular rather than medical and, for a brief period, was intensely followed in the United States.[129] Public enthusiasm for Twilight Sleep quickly subsided after a prominent advocate of the method died during childbirth. Her physicians claimed her death was not related to complications from the method of Twilight Sleep that was used.[130]

The first articles describing the obstetric application of spinal, epidural, caudal, paravertebral, parasacral, and pudendal nerve blocks appeared between 1900 and 1930. However, their benefits were underappreciated for many years because the obstetricians seldom used these techniques.[130] Continuous caudal anesthesia was introduced in 1944 by Hingson and Edwards[131] and spinal anesthesia became popular shortly thereafter. Initially, spinal anesthesia could be administered by inexperienced personnel without monitoring. The combination of inexperienced providers and lack of patient monitoring led to higher rates of morbidity and mortality than those observed for general anesthesia.[132] Therefore, the use of spinal anesthesia was highly discouraged in the 1950s, leading to the "dark ages of obstetric anesthesia" when pain relief in obstetrics was essentially abandoned and women were forced to endure "natural childbirth" to avoid serous anesthesia-related complications.[133]

With an increased understanding of neuraxial anesthesia, involvement by well-trained anesthesiologists, and an appreciation for the physiologic changes during pregnancy, maternal and fetal safety greatly improved. In the past decade, anesthesia-related deaths during cesarean sections under general anesthesia have become more likely than neuraxial anesthesia-related deaths, making regional anesthesia the method of choice.[134,135] With the availability of safe and effective options for pain relief during labor and delivery, today's focus is improving the quality of the birth experience for expectant parents.

Transfusion Medicine

Paleolithic cave drawings found in France depict a bear losing blood from multiple spear wounds, indicating that primitive man understood the simple relationship between blood and life.[136] More than 10,000 years later, modern anesthesiologists attempt to preserve this intimate relationship by replacing fluids and blood products when faced with intravascular volume depletion or diminished oxygen-carrying capacity from blood loss.

Blood transfusion was first attempted in 1667 by physician to Louis XIV, Jean Baptiste Denis. Denis had learned of Richard Lower's transfusion of lamb's blood into a dog the previous year. Lamb's blood was most frequently used because the donating animal's essential qualities were thought to be transferred to the recipient. Despite this dangerous transspecies transfusion, Denis' first patient got better, however, and his next two patients were not as fortunate, and Denis avoided further attempts. Given the poor outcomes of these early blood transfusions, and heated religious controversy regarding the implications of transferring animal-specific qualities across species, blood transfusion in humans was banned for more than a hundred years in both France and England beginning in 1670.[114]

In 1900, Karl Landsteiner and Samuel Shattock independently helped lay the scientific basis of all subsequent transfusions by recognizing that blood compatibility was based on different blood groups. Landsteiner, an Austrian physician, originally organized human blood into three groups based on substances present on the red blood cells. The fourth type, AB group, was identified in 1902 by two students, A. Decastrello and A. Sturli. Based on these findings, Reuben Ottenberg performed the first type-specific blood transfusion in 1907. Transfusion of physiologic solutions occurred in 1831, independently performed by O'Shaughnessy and Lewins in Great Britain. In his letter to *The Lancet*, Lewins described transfusing large volumes of saline solutions into patients with cholera. He reported that he would inject into adults from 5 to 10 pounds of saline solution and repeat as needed.[137] Despite its publication in a prominent journal, Lewins' technique was apparently overlooked for decades, and balanced physiologic solution availability would have to await the coming of analytical chemistry.

PROFESSIONALISM AND ANESTHESIA PRACTICE

Organized Anesthesiology

7 Physician anesthetists sought to obtain respect among their surgical colleagues by organizing professional societies and improving the quality of training. The first American organization was founded by nine members on October 6, 1905, and called the Long Island Society of Anesthetists with annual dues of $1.00. In 1911, the annual assessment rose to $3.00 when the Long Island Society became the New York Society of Anesthetists. Although the new organization still carried a local title, it drew members from several states and had a membership of 70 physicians in 1915.[138]

One of the most noteworthy figures in the struggle to professionalize anesthesiology was Francis Hoffer McMechan. McMechan had been a practicing anesthesiologist in Cincinnati until 1911, when he suffered a severe first attack of rheumatoid arthritis, which eventually left him confined to a wheelchair and forced his retirement from the operating room in 1915. McMechan had been in practice only 15 years, but he had written 18 clinical articles in this short time. A prolific researcher and writer, McMechan did not permit his crippling disease to sideline his career. Instead of pursuing goals in clinical medicine, he applied his talents to establishing anesthesiology societies.[139]

McMechan supported himself and his devoted wife through editing the *Quarterly Anesthesia Supplement* from 1914 until August 1926. He became editor of the first journal devoted to anesthesia, *Current Researches in Anesthesia and Analgesia*, the precursor of *Anesthesia and Analgesia*, the oldest journal of the specialty. As well as fostering the organization of the International Anesthesia Research Society (IARS) in 1925, McMechan and his wife, Laurette, became overseas ambassadors of American anesthesia. Since Laurette was French, it was understandable that McMechan combined his own ideas about anesthesiology with concepts from abroad.[123]

In 1926, McMechan held the Congress of Anesthetists in a joint conference with the Section on Anaesthetics of the British Medical Association. Subsequently, he traveled throughout Europe, giving lectures and networking physicians in the field. On his final return to America, he was gravely ill and was confined to bed for 2 years. His hard work and constant travel paid dividends, however: in 1929, the IARS, which McMechan founded in 1922, had members not only from North America but also from several European countries, Japan, India, Argentina, and Brazil.[122]

In the 1930s, McMechan expanded his mission from organizing anesthesiologists to promoting the academic aspects of the specialty. In 1931, work began on what would become the International College of Anesthetists. This body began to award fellowships in 1935. For the first time, physicians were recognized as specialists in anesthesiology. The certification qualifications were universal, and fellows were recognized as specialists in several countries. Although the criteria for certification were not strict, the College was a success in raising the standards of anesthesia practice in many nations.[140] In 1939, McMechan finally succumbed to illness, and the anesthesia world lost its tireless leader.

Other Americans promoted the growth of organized anesthesiology. Ralph Waters and John Lundy, among others, participated in evolving organized anesthesia. Waters' greatest contribution to the specialty was raising its academic standards. After completing his internship in 1913, he entered medical practice in Sioux City, Iowa, where he gradually limited his practice to anesthesia. His personal experience and extensive reading were supplemented by the only postgraduate training available, a 1-month course conducted in Ohio by E. I. McKesson. At that time, the custom of becoming a self-proclaimed specialist in medicine and surgery was not uncommon. Waters, who was frustrated by low standards and who would eventually have a great influence on establishing both anesthesia residency training and the formal examination process, recalled that, before 1920, "The requirements for specialization in many Midwestern hospitals consisted of the possession of sufficient audacity to attempt a procedure and persuasive power adequate to gain the consent of the patient or his family."[141]

Academic Anesthesia

In an effort to improve anesthetic care, Waters regularly corresponded with Dennis Jackson and other scientists. In 1925, he relocated to Kansas City with a goal of gaining an academic post at the University of Kansas, but the professor of surgery failed to support his proposal. The larger city did allow him to initiate his freestanding outpatient surgical facility, "The Downtown Surgical Clinic," which featured one of the first postanesthetic recovery rooms.[130] In 1927, Erwin Schmidt, professor of surgery at the University of Wisconsin's medical school, encouraged Dean Charles Bardeen to recruit Waters.

In accepting the first American academic position in anesthesia, Waters described four objectives that have been since adopted by many other academic departments. His goals were as follows: "(1) to provide the best possible service to patients of the institution; (2) to teach what is known of the principles of Anesthesiology to all candidates for their medical degree; (3) to help long-term graduate students not only to gain a fundamental knowledge of the subject and to master the art of administration, but also to learn as much as possible of the effective methods of teaching; (4) to accompany these efforts with the encouragement of as much cooperative investigation as is consistent with achieving the first objectives."[129]

Waters' personal and professional qualities impressed talented young men and women who sought residency posts in his department. He encouraged residents to initiate research interests in which they collaborated with two pharmacologists whom Waters had known before arriving in Wisconsin, Arthur Loevenhart and Chauncey Leake, as well as others with whom he became associated in Madison. Clinical concerns were also investigated. As an example, anesthesia records were coded onto punch cards to form a database that was used to analyze departmental activities. Morbidity and mortality meetings, now a requirement of all training programs, also originated in Madison. Members of the department and distinguished visitors from other centers attended these meetings. As a consequence of their critical reviews of the conduct of anesthesia, responsibility for an operative tragedy gradually passed from the patient to the physician. In more casual times, a practitioner could complain, "The patient died because he did not take a good anesthetic." Alternatively, the death might be attributed to a mysterious force such as "status lymphaticus," of which Arthur Guedel, a master of sardonic humor, observed, "Certainly status lymphaticus is at times a great help to the anesthetist. When he has a fatality under anesthesia with no other cleansing explanation he is glad to recognize the condition as an entity."[129]

In 1929, John Lundy at the Mayo Clinic organized the Anaesthetists' Travel Club, whose members were leading American or Canadian teachers of anesthesia. Each year one member was the host for a group of 20 to 40 anesthesiologists who gathered for a program of informal discussions. There were demonstrations of promising innovations for the operating room and laboratory, which were all subjected to what is remembered as a "high-spirited, energetic, critical review."[127] The Travel Club would be critical in the upcoming battle to form the American Board of Anesthesiology.

Even during the lean years of the Depression, international guests also visited Waters' department. For Geoffrey Kaye of Australia, Torsten Gordh of Sweden, Robert Macintosh and Michael Nosworthy of England, and scores of others, Waters' department was their "mecca of anesthesia." Ralph Waters trained 60 residents during the 22 years he was the "Chief." From 1937 onward, the alumni, who declared themselves the "Aqualumni" in his honor, returned annually for a professional and social reunion. Thirty-four Aqualumni took academic positions and, of these, 14 became chairpersons of departments of anesthesia. They maintained Waters' professional principles and encouraged teaching careers for many of their own graduates.[142] His enduring legacy was once recognized by the dean who had recruited him in 1927, Charles Bardeen, who observed, "Ralph Waters was the first person the University hired to put people to sleep, but, instead, he awakened a world-wide interest in anesthesia."[143]

Establishing a Society

Waters and Lundy, along with Paul Wood of New York City, had an important role in establishing organized anesthesia and the definition of the specialty. In the heart of the Great Depression, these three physicians realized that anesthesiology needed to have a process to determine who was an anesthetic specialist with American Medical Association (AMA) backing. Using the New York Society of Anesthetists, of which Paul Wood was secretary-treasurer, a new class of members, "Fellows," was created. The Fellows criteria followed established AMA guidelines for specialty certification. However, the AMA wanted a national organization to sponsor a specialty board. The New York Society of Anesthetists changed its name to the American Society of Anesthetists (ASA) in 1936. Combined with the American Society of Regional Anesthesia, whose president was Emery Rovenstein, the American Board of Anesthesiology (ABA) was organized as a subordinate board to the American Board of Surgery in 1938. With McMechan's death in 1939, the AMA favored independence for the ABA, and in 1940, independence was granted.[126,131]

A few years later, the officers of the American Society of Anesthetists were challenged by Dr. M. J. Seifert, who wrote, "An Anesthetist is a technician and an Anesthesiologist is the specific authority on anesthesia and anesthetics. I cannot understand why you do not term yourselves the American Society of Anesthesiologists."[133] Ralph Waters was declared the first president of the newly named ASA in 1945. In that year, when World War II ended, 739 (37%) of 1,977 ASA members were in the armed forces. In the same year, the ASA's first Distinguished Service Award was presented to Paul M.

Wood for his tireless service to the specialty, one element of which can be examined today in the extensive archives preserved in the Society's Wood Library Museum at ASA headquarters, Park Ridge, Illinois.[143]

CONCLUSIONS

This overview of the development of anesthesiology is but a brief outline of our current roles in which anesthesiologists serve in hospitals, clinics, and laboratories. The operating room and obstetric delivery suite remain the central interest of most specialists. Aside from being the location where the techniques described in this chapter find regular application, service in these areas brings us into regular contact with new advances in pharmacology and bioengineering.

After surgery, patients are transported to the postanesthesia care unit or recovery room, an area that is now considered the anesthesiologist's "ward." Fifty years ago, patients were carried directly from the operating room to a surgical ward to be attended only by a junior nurse. That person lacked both the skills and equipment to intervene when complications occurred. After the experiences of World War II taught the value of centralized care, physicians and nurses created recovery rooms, which were soon mandated for all major hospitals. By 1960 the evolution of critical care progressed through the use of mechanical ventilators. Patients who required many days of intensive medical and nursing management were cared for in a curtained corner of the recovery room. In time, curtains drawn about one or two beds gave way to fixed partitions and the relocation of those areas to form intensive care units. The principles of resuscitative and supportive care established by anesthesiologists transformed critical care medicine.

The future of anesthesiology is a bright one. The safer drugs that once revolutionized the care of patients undergoing surgery are constantly being improved. The role of the anesthesiologist continues to broaden as physicians with backgrounds in the specialty have developed clinics for chronic pain control and outpatient surgery. Anesthesia practice will continue to increase in scope, both inside and outside the operating suite, such that anesthesiologists will become an integral part of the entire perioperative experience.

References

1. Joyce H: The Journals and Letters of Fanny Burney. Oxford, Clarendon 1975. As quoted in: Papper EM: Romance, Poetry, and Surgical Sleep. Westport, CT, Greenwood Press, 1995, p. 12
2. Epitaph to W.T.G. Morton on a memorial from the Mt. Auburn Cemetery, Cambridge, Massachusetts
3. These Egyptian Pictographs are dated approximately 2500 B.C. See Ellis ES: Ancient Anodynes: Primitive Anaesthesia and Allied Conditions. London, WM Heinemann Medical Books, 1946, p 80
4. Bacon DR: Regional anesthesia and chronic pain therapy: A history. In: Brown DL (ed): Regional Anesthesia and Analgesia. Philadelphia, WB Saunders, 1996, p 11
5. Rutkow I: Surgery, An Illustrated History. St. Louis, Mosby, 1993, p 215
6. Winter A: Mesmerized: Powers of Mind in Victorian Britain. Chicago, University of Chicago Press, 1998, p 42
7. Marmer MJ: Hypnosis in Anesthesiology. Springfield, IL, Charles C. Thomas, 1959, p 10
8. Dioscorides: On mandragora. In: Dioscorides Opera Libra. Quoted in: Bergman N: The Genesis of Surgical Anesthesia. Park Ridge, IL, Wood Library-Museum of Anesthesiology, 1998, p 11
9. Infusino M, Viole O'Neill Y, Calmes S: Hog beans, poppies, and mandrake leaves—A test of the efficacy of the soporific sponge In: Atkinson RS, Boulton TB, eds. The History of Anaesthesia. London, Parthenon Publishing Group, 1989, p 31
10. Davy H: Researches Chemical and Philosophical Chiefly Concerning Nitrous Oxide or Dephlogisticated Nitrous Air, and Its Respiration. London, J Johnson, 1800, p 533.
11. Papper EM: Romance, Poetry, and Surgical Sleep. Westport, CT, Greenwood Press, 1995

12. Hickman HH: A letter on suspended animation, containing experiments showing that it may be safely employed during operations on animals, with the view of ascertaining its probable utility in surgical operations on the human subject, addressed to T.A. Knight, Esq. Imprint Ironbridge, W. Smith, 1824

13. Strickland RA: Ether drinking in Ireland. Mayo Clin Proc 1996;71:1015, 1996

14. Lyman HM: Artificial Anaesthesia and Anaesthetics. New York, William Hood, 1881, p 6

15. Stetson JB, William E: Clarke and the discovery of anesthesia. In: Fink BR, Morris L, Stephen ER (eds): The History of Anesthesia: Third International Symposium Proceedings. Park Ridge, IL, Wood Library-Museum of Anesthesiology, 1992, p 400

16. Long CW: An account of the first use of sulphuric ether by inhalation as an anaesthetic in surgical operations. South Med Surg J 1849;5:705

17. Robinson V: Victory Over Pain. New York, Henry Schuman 1946, p 91

18. Smith GB, Hirsch NP: Gardner Quincy Colton: Pioneer of nitrous oxide anesthesia. Anesth Analg 1991;72:382

19. Menczer LF: Horace Wells's "day book A": A transcription and analysis. In: Wolfe RJ, Menczer LF (eds): I Awaken to Glory. Boston, Boston Medical Library, 1994, p 112

20. Greene NM: A consideration of factors in the discovery of anesthesia and their effects on its development. Anesthesiology 1971; 35:515

21. Fenster J: Ether Day. New York, Harper Collins, 2001, p 77

22. Duncum BM: The Development of Inhalation Anaesthesia. London, Oxford University Press, 1947, p 86

23. Caton D: What a Blessing She had Chloroform. New Haven, Yale University Press, 1999, p 103

24. Journal of Queen Victoria, In: Strauss MB (ed): Familiar Medical Quotations. Boston, Little Brown, 1968, p 17

25. Kuhn F: Nasotracheal intubation (trans). In: Faulconer A, Keys TE (eds): Foundations of Anesthesiology. Springfield, IL, Charles C Thomas, 1965, p 677

26. Clover JT: Laryngotomy in chloroform anesthesia. Br Med J 1877;1:132

27. Macewan W: Clinical observations on the introduction of tracheal tubes by the mouth instead of performing tracheotomy or laryngotomy. Br Med J 1880;2:122, 163

28. Hirsch NP, Smith GB, Hirsch PO: Alfred Kirstein, pioneer of direct laryngoscopy. Anaesthesia 1986; 41:42

29. Burkle CM, Zepeda FA, Bacon DR, et al: A historical perspective on use of the laryngoscope as a tool in anesthesiology. Anesthesiology. 2004; 100:1003

30. Miller RA: A new laryngoscope. Anesthesiology 1941; 2:317

31. Macintosh RR: Richard Salt of Oxford, anaesthetic technician extraordinary. Anaesthesia 1976;31:855

32. Thomas KB: Sir Ivan Whiteside Magill, KCVO, DSc, MB, BCh, BAO, FRCS, FFARCS (Hon), FFARCSI (Hon), DA: A review of his publications and other references to his life and work. Anaesthesia 1978; 33:628

33. Condon HA, Gilchrist E: Stanley Rowbotham: Twentieth century pioneer anaesthetist. Anaesthesia 1986; 41:46

34. Calverley RK: Classical file. Surv Anesth 1984; 28:70

35. Gale JW, Waters RM: Closed endobronchial anesthesia in thoracic surgery: Preliminary report. Curr Res Anesth Analg 1932;11:283

36. Wu TL, Chou HC: A new laryngoscope: the combination intubating device (letter). Anesthesiology 1994; 81:1085

37. Brain AIJ: The laryngeal mask: A new concept in airway management. Br J Anaesthesia 1983;55:801

38. Calverley RK: An early ether vaporizer designed by John Snow, a Treasure of the Wood Library-Museum of Anesthesiology. In: Fink BR, Morris LE, Stephen CR (eds): The History of Anesthesia. . Park Ridge, IL, Wood Library-Museum of Anesthesiology, 1992, p 91

39. Snow J: On the Inhalation of the Vapour of Ether (reprinted by the Wood Library-Museum of Anesthesiology). London, J Churchill, 1847, p 23

40. Calverley RK, J. T. Clover: A giant of Victorian anaesthesia. In: Rupreht J, van Lieburg MJ, Lee JA, Erdmann W (eds): Anaesthesia: Essays on Its History. Berlin, Springer-Verlag, 1985, p 21

41. Andrews E: The oxygen mixture, a new anaesthetic combination. Chicago Medical Examiner 1868;9:656

42. Obituary of T. Philip Ayre. Br Med J 1980;280:125

43. Rees GJ: Anaesthesia in the newborn. Br Med J 1950; 2:1419

44. Bain JA, Spoerel WE: A stream-lined anaesthetic system. Can Anaesth Soc J 1972;19:426

45. Mushin WW, Rendell-Baker L: Thoracic Anaesthesia Past and Present (reprinted by the Wood Library Museum of Anesthesiology 1991). Springfield, IL, Charles C Thomas, 1953, p 44

46. Shephard DAE: Harvey Cushing and anaesthesia. Can Anaesth Soc J 1965; 12:431

47. Waters RM: Clinical scope and utility of carbon dioxide filtration in inhalation anesthesia. Curr Res Anesth Analg 1923; 3:20

48. Sword BC: The closed circle method of administration of gas anesthesia. Curr Res Anesth Analg 1930; 9:198

49. Sands RP, Bacon DR: An inventive mind: The career of James O. Elam, M.D. (1918–1995). Anesthesiology 1998; 88:1107

50. Morris LE: A new vaporizer for liquid anesthetic agents. Anesthesiology 1952;13:587

51. Sands R, Bacon DR: The copper kettle: A historical perspective. J Clin Anesthesiology 1996;8:528

52. Duncum BM: The Development of Inhalation Anaesthesia. London, Oxford University Press, 1947, p 538

53. Severinghaus JC, Honda Y: Pulse oximetry. Int Anesthesiol Clin 1987; 25:205

54. Cushing H: On the avoidance of shock in major amputations by cocainization of large nerve trunks preliminary to their division: With observations on blood-pressure changes in surgical cases. Ann Surg 1902; 36:321

55. Codesmith A: An endo-esophageal stethoscope. Anesthesiology 1954; 15:566

56. Luft K: Methode der registrieren gas analyse mit hilfe der absorption ultraroten Strahlen ohne spectrale Zerlegung. Z Tech Phys 1943; 24:97

57. Tovell RM: Problems in supply of anesthetic gases in the European theater of operations. Anesthesiology 1947; 8:303

58. Rendell-Baker L: History of standards for anesthesia equipment. In: Rupreht J, van Lieburg MJ, Lee JA, Erdmann W (eds): Anaesthesia: Essays on Its History. Berlin, Springer-Verlag, 1985, p 161

59. Calverley RK: A safety feature for anaesthesia machines: Touch identification of oxygen flow control. Can Anaesth Soc J 1971; 18:225

60. Lucas GH: The discovery of cyclopropane. Curr Res Anesth Analg 1961; 40:15

61. Seevers MH, Meek WJ, Rovenstine EA, et al: Cyclopropane study with espical reference to gas concentration, respiratory and electrocardiographic changes. J Pharmacol Exp Ther 1934; 51:1

62. Calverley RK: Fluorinated anesthetics: I. The early years. Surv Anesth 1986; 29:170

63. Suckling CW: Some chemical and physical factors in the development of Fluothane. Br J Anaesth 1957; 29:466

64. Wren PC: Philosophical Transactions, Vol I. London, Anno, 1665 and 1666

65. Keys TE: The History of Surgical Anesthesia. New York, Dover Publications, 1945, p 38

66. Dundee J, Wyant G: Intravenous Anesthesia. Hong Kong, Churchill Livingstone, 1974, p 1

67. Oré PC: Etudes, cliniques sur l'anesthésie chirurgicale par la methode des injection de choral dans les veines. Paris, JB Balliere et Fils, 1875. As quoted in: Hemelrijck JV, Kissin I: History of intravenous anesthesia. White PF (ed): Textbook of Intravenous Anesthesia. Baltimore, Williams & Wilkins, 1997, p 3

68. Macintosh RR: Modern anaesthesia, with special reference to the chair of anaesthetics in Oxford. In: Rupreht J, van Lieburg MJ, Lee JA, Erdmann W (eds): Anaesthesia: Essays on Its History. Berlin, Springer-Verlag, 1985, p 352

69. Hemelrijck JV, Kissin I: History of intravenous anesthesia. In: White PF (ed): Textbook of Intravenous Anesthesia. Baltimore, Williams & Wilkins, 1997, p 3

70. Fink BR: Leaves and needles: the introduction of surgical local anesthesia. Anesthesiology, 1985; 63:77-83

71. Koller C: Über die Verwendung des Cocain zur Anästhesirung am Auge. Wein Med Wochenschr. 1884; 34:1276

72. Calatayud J, Gonzalez A: History of the development and evolution of local anesthesia since the coca leaf. Anesthesiology 2003; 98:1503

73. Fink BR: History of local anesthesia. In: Cousins MJ, Bridenbaugh PO (eds): Neural Blockade. Philadelphia, JB Lippincott, 1980, p 12

74. Ruetsch YA, Boni T, Borgeat A: From cocaine to ropivacaine: the history of local anesthetic drugs. Curr Top Med Chem, 2001; 1:175

75. Cushing H: On the avoidance of shock in major amputations by cocainization of large nerve trunks preliminary to their division: With observations on blood-pressure changes in surgical cases. Ann Surg 1902;36:321

76. Ekenstam B, Egnev B, Pettersson G: Local anesthetics: I. N-alkyl pyrrolidine and N-alkyl piperidine carboxylic acid amides. Acta Chem Scand, 1957;11:1183

77. Albright GA: Cardiac arrest following regional anesthesia with etidocaine or bupivacaine. Anesthesiology, 1979; 51:285,

78. Aberg G: Toxicological and local anaesthetic effects of optically active isomers of two local anaesthetic compounds. Acta Pharmacol Toxicol (Copenh), 1972;31:273,

79. Polley LS, Santos AC: Cardiac arrest following regional anesthesia with ropivacaine: here we go again! Anesthesiology, 2003; 99:1253,

80. Castillo J, Curley J, Hotz J, et al: Glucocorticoids prolong rat sciatic nerve blockade in vivo from bupivacaine microspheres. Anesthesiology, 1996; 85:1157

81. Mowat JJ, Mok MJ, MacLeod BA, et al: Liposomal bupivacaine. Extended duration nerve blockade using large unilamellar vesicles that exhibit a proton gradient. Anesthesiology, 1996; 85:635

82. McIntyre AR: Curare, Its History, Nature, and Clinical Use. Chicago, University of Chicago Press, 1947, p 6, 131

83. Thomas BK: Curare: Its History and Usage. Philadelphia, JB Lippincott Company, 1963, p 90

84. Rushman GB, Davies NJH, Atkinson RS: A Short History of Anaesthesia. Oxford, Butterworth-Heinemann, 1996, p 78

85. Knoefel PK: Felice Fontana: Life and Works. Trento, Societa de Studi Trentini, 1985, p 284

86. Griffith HR, Johnson GE: The use of curare in general anesthesia. Anesthesiology 1942;3:418

87. McIntyre AR: Historical background, early use and development of muscle relaxants. Anesthesiology 1959; 20:412

88. Ali HH, Utting JE, Gray C: Quantitative assessment of residual antidepolarizing block (part II). Br J Anaesthesia 1971;43:478
89. Gwathmey JT: Anesthesia. New York, Appleton and Company, 1914, p 379
90. Flagg PJ: The Art of Anaesthesia. Philadelphia, JB Lippincott Company, 1918, p 80
91. Chloretone (chlorobutanol) is prepared by mixing chloroform and acetone, and has a camphor-like odor that some find pleasant. Chloretone is now commonly used for euthanizing reptiles and amphibians
92. Hewer CL: Recent Advances in Anaesthesia and Analgesia. Philadelphia: P Blakiston's Son & Co. Inc., 1937, p 237
93. Collins VJ: Principles and Practice of Anesthesiology. Philadelphia, Lea & Febiger, 1952, p 327
94. Raeder J: History of Postoperative Nausea and Vomiting. Int Anesthesiol Clin 2003;41:1
95. Koller C: Personal reminiscences of the first use of cocaine as local anesthetic in eye surgery. Curr Res Anesth Analg 1928; 7:9
96. Becker HK: Carl Koller and cocaine. Psychoanal Q 1963;32:309
97. Halstead WS: Practical comments on the use and abuse of cocaine; suggested by its in variably successful employment in more than a thousand minor surgical operations. NY Med J 1885; 42:294
98. Olch PD, William S: Halstead and local anesthesia: Contributions and complications. Anesthesiology 1975; 42:479
99. Marx G: The first spinal anesthesia: Who deserves the laurels? Reg Anesth 1994; 19:429
100. Corning JL: Spinal anaesthesia and local medication of the cord. NY Med J 1885; 42:483
101. Bier AKG: Experiments in cocainization of the spinal cord, 1899. In: Faulconer A, Keys TE (trans): Foundations of Anesthesiology. Springfield, IL, Charles C Thomas, 1965, p 854
102. Goerig M, Agarwal K, Schulte am Esch J: The versatile August Bier (1861-1949), father of spinal anesthesia. J Clin Anesth 2000; 12:561
103. Larson MD: Tait and Caglieri. The first spinal anesthetic in America. Anesthesiology. 1996; 85:913
104. Lee JA: Arthur Edward James Barker, 1850-1916: British pioneer of regional anaesthesia. Anaesthesia 1979;34:885
105. Lemmon WT: A method for continuous spinal anesthesia: A preliminary report. Ann Surg 1940; 111:141
106. Martini JA, Bacon DR, Vasdev GM: Edward Tuohy: The man, his needle, and its place in obstetric anesthesia. Reg Anesth Pain Med 2002; 27:520
107. Tuohy EB: Continuous spinal anesthesia: Its usefulness and technique involved. Anesthesiology 1944; 5:142
108. Pagés F: Metameric anesthesia, 1921. In: Faulconer A, Keys TE (trans): Foundations of Anesthesiology. Springfield, IL, Charles C Thomas, 1965, p 927
109. Crile GW, Lower WE: Anoci-Association. Philadelphia, WB Saunders Company, 1915
110. Brown DL, Winnie AP: Biography of Louis Gaston Labat, M.D. Regional Anesthesia 1992; 17:248
111. Bacon DR, Darwish H: Emery Rovenstine and regional anesthesia. Reg Anesth 1997; 22:273
112. Rehn L: On Penetrating Cardiac Injuries and Cardiac Suturing. Arch Klin Chir 1897; 55:315
113. Naef AP: The Mid-Century Revolution in Thoracic and Cardiovascular Surgery: Part 1. Interact Cardiovasc Thor Surg 2003; 2:219
114. Keys TE: The History of Surgical Anesthesia. New York, Dover Publications, 1945, p 38
115. Baum VC: Pediatric Cardiac Surgery: An Historical Appreciation. Pediatr Anesth 2006; 16:1213
116. Harmel M, Lamont A: Anesthesia in the Treatment of Congenital Pulmonary Stenosis. Anesthesiology 1948; 7:477
117. [Anon.] With Gas & Needle." Time. Monday, October 19, 1953
118. Tracy PT, Hanigan WC: The history of neuroanesthesia. In: Greenblatt SH (ed): The History of Neurosurgery. Thieme, 1997, p 213
119. Samuels SI: The history of neuroanesthesia: A contemporary review. Int Anesthesiol Clin 1996; 34:1
120. Horsley V: Brain surgery. Br Med J 1886;2:670
121. Frazier C:. Problems and procedures in cranial surgery. JAMA 1909; 52:1805
122. Bacon DR: The world federation of societies of anesthesiologists: McMechan's final legacy? Anesth Analg 1997; 84:1131
123. Seldon TH: Francis Hoeffer McMechan. In: Volpitto PP, Vandam LD (eds): Genesis of American Anesthesiology. Springfield, IL, Charles C Thomas, 1982, p 5
124. Canton D: The history of obstetric anesthesia. In: Chestnut DH (ed): Obstetric Anesthesia: Principles and Practice. Philadelphia, Elsevier Mosby, 2004
125. Barnett R: A horse named 'Twilight Sleep': The language of obstetric anaesthesia in 20th century Britain. Int J Obstet Anesth, 2005; 14:310
126. Canton D: What a blessing she had cloroform. New Haven, Yale University Press, 1999
127. MacKenzie RA, Bacon DR, Martin DP: Anaesthetists' Travel Club: A transformation of the society of clinical surgery? Bull Anesth Hist. 2004; 22:7
128. Apgar V: A proposal for a new method of evaluation of the newborn infant. Curr Res Anesth Analg, 1953; 32:260
129. Guedel AE: Inhalation Anesthesia: A Fundamental Guide. New York, MacMillan, 1937, p 129
130. Waters RM: The down-town anesthesia clinic. Am J Surg 1919;33:71
131. Hingson RA: Continuous caudal analgesia in obstetrics, surgery, and therapeutics. Br Med J, 1949;2:777
132. Gogarten W, Van Aken H: A century of regional analgesia in obstetrics. Anesth Analg, 2000;91:773
133. Little DM Jr, Betcher AM: The Diamond Jubilee 1905-1980. Park Ridge, IL, American Society of Anesthesiologists, 1980, p 8
134. Hawkins JL, Koonin LM, Palmer SK, et al: Anesthesia-related deaths during obstetric delivery in the United States, 1979-1990. Anesthesiology, 1997; 86:277
135. Hawkins JL: Anesthesia-related maternal mortality. Clin Obstet Gynecol, 2003; 46:679
136. Gottlieb AM: A Pictorial History of Blood Practices and Transfusion. Scottsdale, AZ, Arcane Publications, 1992, p 2
137. Jenkins MT: Epochs in intravenous fluid therapy: from the goose quill and pig bladder to balanced salt solutions. Park Ridge, IL, The Lewis H. Wright Memorial Lecture, Wood Library-Museum Collection, 1993, p 4
138. Betcher AM, Ciliberti BJ, Wood PM, et al: The jubilee year of organized anesthesia. Anesthesiology. 1956;17:226
139. Bacon DR: The promise of one great anesthesia society. Anesthesiology. 1994; 80:929
140. Bacon DR, Lema MJ: To define a specialty: A brief history of the American Board of Anesthesiology's first written examination. J Clin Anesth 1992; 4:489
141. Waters RM: Pioneering in anesthesiology. Postgrad Med 1948; 4:265
142. Bacon DR, Ament R: Ralph Waters and the beginnings of academic anesthesiology in the United States: The Wisconsin template. J Clin Anesth 1995; 7:534
143. Bamforth BJ, Siebecker KL: Ralph M. Waters. In: Volpitto PP, Vandam LD (eds): Genesis of American Anesthesiology. Springfield, IL, Charles C Thomas, 1982

CHAPTER 2 ■ SCOPE OF PRACTICE

JOHN H. EICHHORN

KEY POINTS

1 Anesthesia trainees, and many postgraduates also, tend to lack sufficient knowledge (with sometimes unfortunate results) about modes of practice or employment, financial matters of all types, and contracting in particular. They must educate themselves and also seek expert advice and counsel to survive (and hopefully flourish) in today's exceedingly complex medical practice milieu.

2 There are several very helpful detailed information resources concerning practice and OR management available from the American Society of Anesthesiologists and other sources. Factors influencing anesthesiology practice conditions are changing rapidly, and today's anesthesia professionals must be armed with detailed information about concepts (such as "pay for performance") that did not exist just a few years ago.

3 Securing hospital privileges is far more than a bureaucratic annoyance and must be taken seriously by anesthesiologists.

4 Anesthesiology is the leading medical specialty in establishing and promulgating standards of practice that have significantly influenced practice in a positive manner.

5 The immediate response to a major adverse anesthesia event is critical to the eventual result. An extremely valuable protocol is available at www.apsf.org, "Resource Center: Clinical Safety Tools."

6 Anesthesiologists need to be involved, concerned, active participants and leaders in their institution and medical community in order to enhance their practice function and image.

7 Managed care's influence has waxed and waned but it must always be considered by modern anesthesia professionals. While cost, value, outcome, and quality issues are certainly central to all anesthesiology practices, difficulties in constructing and applying definitive measurements and rigorous statistical analysis of these parameters have prevented, so far at least, some of the potential negative influences of the core features of fully managed health care on anesthesiology practice.

8 Anesthesiologists must participate in operating room (OR) management in their facilities and should play a central leadership role. OR scheduling, staffing, utilization, and patient flow issues are complex, and anesthesiologists should work hard both to thoroughly understand and positively influence them.

9 Anesthesiology personnel issues involve an elaborate balancing act and groups/departments should give these issues, as well as their constituent personnel, more attention and energy than has been done traditionally in the past or the anesthesia provider shortage will likely continue to worsen.

10 Attention to the many often-underemphasized details of infrastructure, organization, and administration can transform a merely endurable anesthesia practice into one that is efficient, effective, productive, collegial, and even fun.

Medical practice, including its infrastructure and functional details, is evolving rapidly in the United States. Anesthesia practice is no exception. In the past, anesthesia professionals traditionally were little involved in the management of many components of their practice beyond the strictly medical ele-

ments of applied physiology and pharmacology, pathophysiology, and therapeutics. This was perhaps somewhat understandable because anesthesia professionals traditionally spent most of their usually very long work hours in a hospital operating room (OR). Business matters were often left to the one or two group members who were interested or willing to deal with an outside-contractor billing agency. In that era, very little formal teaching in practice management of any kind occurred in anesthesia training programs. Today the Anesthesiology Residency Review Committee of the Accreditation Council on Graduate Medical Education requires that the didactic curricula of anesthesiology residencies include material on practice management. Most training programs offer at least a cursory introduction to issues of practice management, but these can be insufficient to prepare satisfactorily the professional being graduated for the real infrastructure, administrative, business, and management challenges of the modern practice of anesthesiology.

This chapter presents a wide variety of topics that, until recently, were not included in anesthesiology textbooks. Several basic components are outlined of the background, administrative, organizational (including both practice arrangements and daily functioning of the OR), and financial aspects of anesthesiology practice in the complex modern environment. Although many issues are undergoing almost constant change, it is important to understand the basic vocabulary and principles in this dynamic universe. Lack of understanding of these issues may put anesthesia professionals at a disadvantage when attempting to maximize the efficiency and impact of their daily activities, to create and execute practice arrangements, and to secure fair compensation in an increasingly complex health care system with greater and greater competition for scarcer and scarcer resources.

ADMINISTRATIVE COMPONENTS OF ANESTHESIOLOGY PRACTICE

Operational and Information Resources

Overview summaries such as this chapter are intended as an introduction to practice management. Further, fortunately, the American Society of Anesthesiologists (ASA), the professional association for physician anesthesiologists in the United States, for many years has made available to its members extensive resource material regarding practice in general and specific arrangements for its execution. Citation and availability of this material can be found on the ASA Web site, www.asahq.org. Elements are updated periodically by the ASA through its physician officers, committees, task forces, administrative and support staff, and its various offices. Although many of the documents generated and even the advice given in response to members' questions contain broad-brush generalities that must be interpreted in each individual practice situation, these nonetheless stand as a solid foundation on which many anesthesiology practices can be formulated. Prospective familiarity with the principles outlined in the ASA material likely could help avoid some of the problems leading to calls for help. Selected key documents have been compiled and bound into one volume.[1] Also, each spring, the ASA offers a Practice Management Conference, following which the lecture materials are published in an annual volume (see www.asahq.org, "Publications and Services," "Publications on Practice Management").

Background

The ASA *Guidelines for the Ethical Practice of Anesthesiology*[1] includes sections on the principles of medical ethics; the definition of medical direction of nonphysician personnel (including the specific statement that an anesthesiologist engaged in medical direction should not personally be administering another anesthetic); the anesthesiologist's relationship to patients and other physicians; the anesthesiologist's duties, responsibilities, and relationship to the hospital; and the anesthesiologist's relationship to nurse anesthetists and other nonphysician personnel. Further, the ASA publishes *The Organization of an Anesthesia Department*[1] and states through it that the ASA "has adopted a Statement of Policy, which contains principles that the Society urges its members to consider in structuring their own individual medical practices." This document has sections on physician responsibilities for medical care and on medical-administrative organization and responsibilities. Beyond summaries such as this chapter, reference to the considerable body of material created and presented by the ASA (which includes a thick volume specifically on the details of business arrangements[2]) is an excellent starting point to help young anesthesia professionals during training prepare for the increasing rigors of starting and managing a career in practice. Likewise, there is a great deal of information on the ASA Web site concerning the most recent governmental regulations, rulings, and billing codes. The ASA *Newsletter* contains the monthly columns "Washington Report" and "Practice Management," which disseminate related current developments.

In addition to the ASA and the American Association of Nurse Anesthetists, most anesthesiology subspecialty societies and interest groups have Web locations, as do most journals. Particularly, the Web site of the Anesthesia Patient Safety Foundation, www.apsf.org, has been cited as especially useful in promoting safe clinical practice. Electronic bulletin boards allow anesthesiology practitioners from around the world to immediately exchange ideas on diverse topics, both medical and administrative. Traditionally, the ASA has not maintained one. However, one of the original sites that remains very popular is www.gasnet.org, and a Web search ("anesthesiology + bulletin board") using a search engine such as www.google.com reveals a great number of sites that contain a variety of discussions about all manner of anesthesiology-related topics, including practice organization, administration, and management. Additionally, references to the entirety of the medical literature are readily accessible to any practitioner (such as by starting with www.nlm.nih.gov to access Medline). A modern anesthesiology practice cannot reasonably exist without readily available high-speed Internet connections.

The Credentialing Process and Clinical Privileges

The system of credentialing a health care professional and granting clinical privileges in a health care facility is motivated by a fundamental assumption that appropriate education, training, and experience, along with the absence of excessive numbers of bad patient outcomes, increase the chances that the individual will deliver acceptable-quality care. The process of credentialing health care professionals has been the focus of considerable public attention (particularly in the mass media), in part the result of very rare incidents of untrained persons (impostors) infiltrating the health care system and sometimes harming patients. The more common situation, however, involves health professionals who exaggerate past experience and credentials or fail to disclose adverse past experiences. There has been some justified publicity concerning physicians who lost their licenses sequentially in several states and simply moved on each time to start practice elsewhere (which should be much, much more difficult now).

Intense public and political pressure has been brought to bear on various law-making bodies, regulatory and licensing agencies, and health care institution administrations to discover and purge both (1) fraudulent, criminal, and deviant health care providers, and (2) incompetent or simply poor-quality practitioners whose histories show sufficient poor patient outcomes to attract attention, usually through malpractice suits. Identifying and avoiding or correcting an incompetent practitioner is the goal. Verification of appropriate education, training, and experience on the part of a candidate for a position rendering anesthesia care assumes special importance in light of the legal doctrine of *vicarious liability*, which can be described as: if an individual, group, or institution hires an anesthesia provider or even simply approves of that person (e.g., by granting clinical privileges through a hospital medical staff), those involved in the decision may later be held liable in the courts, along with the individual, for the individual's actions. This would be especially true if it were later discovered that the offending practitioner's past adverse outcomes had not been adequately investigated during the credentialing process.

Out of these various long-standing concerns has arisen the sometimes cumbersome process of obtaining state licenses to practice and of obtaining hospital privileges. The stringent credentialing process for health care practice is intended both to protect patients and to safeguard the integrity of the profession. Recently, central credentialing systems have been developed, including those affiliated with the American Medical Association, American Osteopathic Association, and, particularly, the Federation Credentials Verification Service of the Federation of State Medical Boards. These systems verify a physician's basic credentials (e.g., identity, citizenship or immigration status, medical education, postgraduate training, licensure examination history, prior licenses, and board actions) once, and then thereafter can certify the validity of these credentials to a state licensing board or medical facility. A few states do not yet accept this verification and most states seek specific supplemental information.

There are checklists of the requirements for the granting of medical staff privileges by hospitals (see the American Hospital Association Resource Center, www.aharc.library.net). In addition, the National Practitioner Data Bank and reporting system administered by the U.S. government now contains many years' worth of information. This data bank is a central repository of licensing and credentials information about physicians. Many adverse situations involving a physician—particularly instances of substance abuse, malpractice litigation, or the revocation, suspension, or limitation of that physician's license to practice medicine or ability to hold hospital privileges—must be reported (via the state board of medical registration/licensure) to the National Practitioner Data Bank. It is a statutory requirement that all applications for hospital staff privileges be cross-checked against this national data bank. The potential medicolegal liability on the part of a facility's medical staff, and the anesthesiology group in particular, for failing to do so is significant. The Data Bank, however, is not a complete substitute for direct documentation and background checking. Often, practitioners reach private negotiated solutions following quality-driven medical staff problems, thereby avoiding the mandatory public reporting. In such cases, a suspect physician may be given the option to resign medical staff privileges and avoid Data Bank reporting rather than undergo full involuntary privilege revocation (although most applications contain a question specifically about this).

Documentation

The documentation for the credentialing process for each anesthesia practitioner must be complete. Privileges to administer anesthesia must be officially granted and delineated in writing.[1] This can be straightforward or it can be more complex to accommodate institutional needs to identify practitioners specially qualified to practice in designated anesthesia subspecialty areas such as cardiac, infant/pediatric, obstetric,

intensive care, or pain management. Specific documentation of the process of granting or renewing clinical privileges is required and, unlike some other records, the documentation likely is protected as confidential peer review information. Any questions about complex sensitive issues such as this should be referred to an experienced attorney familiar with applicable federal and state law. Verification of an applicant's credentials and experience is mandatory. Because of another type of legal case, some examples of which have been highly publicized, medical practitioners may be hesitant to give an honest evaluation (or any evaluation at all) of individuals known to them who are seeking a professional position elsewhere. Obviously, someone writing a reference for a current or former coworker should be honest. Sticking to clearly documentable facts is advisable. Stating a fact that is in the public record (such as a malpractice case lost at trial) should not justify an objection from the subject of the reference. Whether such potentially "negative" facts can be omitted by a reference writer is complex. Including positive opinions and enthusiastic recommendations, of course, is no problem. Some fear that including facts that may be perceived as negative (e.g., the lost malpractice case or personal problems such as a history of treatment for substance abuse) and/or negative opinions will provoke a retaliatory lawsuit (such as for libel, defamation of character, or loss of livelihood) from the subject of the reference. Further, however, there have been cases of the facility doing the hiring suing reference writers for failing to mention (perceived as concealing) negative information about an applicant who later was charged with substandard practice. Because of the complexities and even apparent contradictions, many reference writers in these questionable situations confine their written material to brief, simple facts such as dates employed and position held. As always, questions about complex sensitive issues such as this should be referred to an experienced attorney familiar with applicable federal and state law.

Because there should be no hesitation for a reference writer to include positive facts and opinions, receipt of a reference that includes nothing more than dates worked and position held can be a suggestion that there may be more to the story (although some entities have adopted such a policy in all cases simply to eliminate any value judgments as to what is positive or negative information). Receipt of such a "dates/position only" reference about a person applying for a position should usually provoke a telephone call to the writer. A telephone call is likely advisable in all cases, independent of whatever the written reference contains. Frequently, pertinent questions over the telephone can elicit more candid information. In rare instances, there may be dishonesty through omission by the reference giver even at this level. This may involve an applicant who an individual, a department or group, or an institution would like to see leave.

In all cases, new personnel in an anesthesia practice environment must be given a thorough orientation and checkout. Policy, procedures, and equipment may be unfamiliar to even the most thoroughly trained, experienced, and safe practitioner. This may occasionally seem tedious, but it is sound and critically important safety policy. Being in the midst of a crisis situation caused by unfamiliarity with a new setting is not the optimal orientation session.

After the initial granting of clinical privileges to practice anesthesia, anesthesia professionals must periodically renew their privileges within the institution or facility (e.g., annually or every other year). There are moral, ethical, and societal obligations on the part of the privilege-granting entity to take this process seriously. State licensing bodies often become aware of problems with health professionals very late in the evolution of any difficulties. An anesthesia professional's peers in the hospital or facility are much more likely to notice untoward developments as they first appear. However, privilege renewals are often essentially automatic and receive little of the necessary attention. Judicious checking of renewal applications and awareness of relevant peer review information is absolutely necessary. The anesthesia professionals or administrators responsible for evaluating staff members and reviewing their practices and privileges may be justifiably concerned about retaliatory legal action by a staff member who is censured or denied privilege renewal. Accordingly, such evaluating groups must be thoroughly objective (totally eliminating any hint of political or financial motives) and must have documentation that the staff person in question is in fact practicing below the standard of care. Court decisions have found liability by a hospital, its medical staff group, or both, when the incompetence of a staff member was known or should have been known and was not acted upon.[3] Again, questions about complex sensitive issues such as this should be referred to an experienced attorney familiar with applicable federal and state law.

A major issue in the granting of clinical privileges, especially in procedure-oriented specialties such as anesthesiology, is whether it is reasonable to continue the common practice of "blanket" privileges. This process in effect authorizes the practitioner to attempt any treatment or procedure normally considered within the purview of the applicant's medical specialty. These considerations may have profound political and economic implications within medicine, such as which type of surgeon should be doing carotid endarterectomies or lumbar discectomies. More important, however, is whether the practitioner being evaluated is qualified to do everything traditionally associated with the specialty. Specifically, should the granting of privileges to practice anesthesia automatically approve the practitioner to handle pediatric cardiac cases, critically ill newborns (such as a day-old premature infant with a large diaphragmatic hernia), ablative pain therapy (such as an alcohol celiac plexus block under fluoroscopy), high-risk obstetric cases, and so forth? This question raises the issue of procedure-specific or limited privileges. The quality assurance (QA) and risk management considerations in this question are weighty if inexperienced or insufficiently qualified practitioners are allowed or even expected, because of peer or scheduling pressures, to undertake major challenges for which they are not prepared. The likelihood of complications and adverse outcome will be higher, and the difficulty of defending the practitioner against a malpractice claim in the event of catastrophe will be significantly increased.

There is no clear answer to the question of procedure-specific credentialing and granting of privileges. Ignoring issues regarding qualifications to undertake complex and challenging procedures has clear negative potential. On the other hand, stringent procedure-specific credentialing is impractical in smaller groups, and in larger groups encourages many small "fiefdoms," with a consequent further atrophy of the clinical skills outside the practitioner's specific area(s). Each anesthesia department or group needs to address these issues. At the very least, the common practice of every applicant for privileges (new or renewal) checking off every line on the printed list of anesthesia procedures should be reviewed. Additionally, board certification for physicians is now essentially a standard of quality assurance of the minimum skills required for the consultant practice of anesthesiology. Subspecialty boards, such as those in pain management, critical care, and transesophageal echocardiography, further objectify the credentialing process. This is now significant because initial board certification after the year 2000 by the American Board of Anesthesiology (ABA) is time-limited and subject to periodic testing and recertification. Clearly, this will encourage an ongoing process of continuing medical education. Many states, some institutions, even some regulatory bodies have requirements for a minimum number of hours of continuing medical education. Doc-

umentation of meeting such a standard again acts as one type of quality assurance mechanism for the individual practitioner, while providing another objective credentialing measurement for those granting licenses or privileges.

Professional Staff Participation and Relationships

All medical care facilities and practice settings depend on their professional staffs, of course, for daily activities of the delivery of health care but, very importantly, they also depend on those staffs to provide administrative structure and support. Medical staff activities are increasingly important in achieving favorable accreditation status (e.g., from the Joint Commission for the Accreditation of Healthcare Organizations [JCAHO]), now often known as the "Joint Commission," and in meeting a wide variety of governmental regulations and reviews. Principal medical staff activities involve sometimes time-consuming efforts, such as duties as a staff officer or committee member. Anesthesiologists should be participants in—in fact, should play a significant role in—credentialing, peer review, tissue review, transfusion review, OR management, and medical direction of same-day surgery units, postanesthesia care units (PACUs), intensive care units (ICUs), and pain management units. Also, it is very important that anesthesiology personnel be involved in fund-raising activities, benefits, community outreach projects sponsored by the facility, and social events of the facility staff.

Anesthesia professionals as a group have a reputation for lack of involvement in medical staff and facility issues because of lack of time (because of long hours in the OR) or simply lack of interest. In fact, anesthesiology personnel are all too often perceived in a facility as the ones who slip in and out of the building essentially anonymously (often dressed very casually or even in the pajamalike comfort of scrub suits) and virtually unnoticed. This is an unfortunate state of affairs, and it has frequently come back in various painful ways to haunt those who have not been involved, or even noticed. Anesthesia professionals sometimes respond that the demands for anesthesiology service are so great that they simply never have the time or the opportunity to become involved in their facility and with their peers. If this is really true, it is clear that more anesthesia professionals must be added at that facility, even if doing so slightly reduces the income of those already there.

If anesthesia professionals are not involved and not perceived as interested, dedicated "team players," they will be shut out of critical negotiations and decisions. Although one obvious instance in which others will make decisions for anesthesia professionals is the distribution of capitated or bundled practice fee income collected by a central "umbrella" organization, there are many such situations, and the anesthesia professionals will be forced to comply with the resulting mandates.

Similarly, involvement with a facility, a professional staff, or a multispecialty group goes beyond formal organized governance and committee activity. Collegial relationships with professional of other specialties and with administrators are central to maintenance of a recognized position and avoidance of the situation of exclusion previously described. Being readily available for formal and informal consults, particularly regarding preoperative patient workup and the maximally efficient way to get surgeons' patients to the OR in a timely, expedient manner, is extremely important. No one individual can be everywhere all the time, but an anesthesiology group or department should strive to be always responsive to any request for help from physicians or administrators. It often appears that anesthesia professionals fail to appreciate just how great a positive impact a relatively simple involvement (starting an intravenous line for a pediatrician, helping an internist manage an ICU ventilator, or helping a facility administrator unclog a jammed recovery room) may have.

Establishing Standards of Practice and Understanding the Standard of Care

The increasing frequency and intensity of "production pressure,"[4] with the tacit (or even explicit) directive to anesthesia professionals to "go fast" no matter what and to "do more with less," creates situations in which anesthesia professionals may conclude that they must cut corners and compromise maximally safe patient care just to stay in business. This type of pressure has become even greater with the implementation of more and more protocols or parameters for practice, some from professional societies such as the ASA and some mandated by or developed in conjunction with purchasers of health care (government, insurance companies, or managed care organizations). Many of these protocols are devised to fast-track patients through the medical care system, especially when an elective procedure is involved, in as absolutely little time as possible, thus minimizing costs. Do these fast-track protocols constitute standards of care that health care providers are mandated to implement? What are the implications of doing so? Of not doing so?

To better understand answers to such questions, it is important to have a basic background in the concept of the standard of care.

The *standard of care* is the conduct and skill of a prudent practitioner that can be expected by a reasonable patient. This is a very important medicolegal concept because a bad medical result due to failure to meet the standard of care is malpractice. Courts have traditionally relied on medical experts knowledgeable about the point in question to give opinions as to what is the standard of care and if it has been met in an individual case. This type of standard is somewhat different from the standards promulgated by various standard-setting bodies regarding, for example, the color of gas hoses connected to an anesthesia machine or the inability to open two vaporizers on that machine simultaneously. However, ignoring the equipment standards and tolerating an unsafe situation is a violation of the standard of care. Promulgated standards, such as the various safety codes and anesthesia machine specifications, rapidly become the standard of care because patients (through their attorneys, in the case of an untoward event) expect the published standards to be observed by the prudent practitioner.

Ultimately, the standard of care is what a jury says it is. However, it is possible to anticipate, at least in part, what knowledge and actions will be expected. There are two main sources of information as to exactly what is the expected standard of care. Traditionally, the beliefs offered by expert witnesses in medical liability lawsuits regarding what is actually being done in real life (de facto standards of care) were the main input juries had in deciding what was reasonable to expect from the defendant. The resulting problem is well known: except in the most egregious cases, it is usually possible for the lawyers to find experts who will support each of the two opposing sides, making the process more subjective than objective. (Because of this, there are even ASA *Guidelines for Expert Witness Qualifications and Testimony* and an equivalent document from the American Association of Nurse Anesthetists). Of course, there can be legitimate differences of opinion among thoughtful, insightful experts, but even in these cases the jury still must decide who is more believable, looks better, or sounds better. The second, much more objective, source for defining certain component parts of the standard of care is the published standards of care, guidelines, practice parameters, and protocols now becoming more common. These serve as hard evidence of what can be reasonably expected of practitioners and can make it easier for a jury evaluating whether a malpractice defendant failed to meet the applicable standard of care. Several types of documents exist and have differing implications.

Leading the Way

4 Anesthesiology may be the medical specialty most involved with published standards of care. It has been suggested that the nature of anesthesia practice (having certain central critical functions relatively clearly defined and common to all situations and also having an emphasis on technology) makes it the most amenable of all the fields of medicine to the use of published standards. The original intraoperative monitoring standards[5] are a classic example. The ASA first adopted its own set of basic intraoperative monitoring standards in 1986 and has modified them several times. The text of all ASA standards, guidelines, and statements is readily available (see www.asahq.org, "Clinical Information," and "Standards, Guidelines, and Statements").

This monitoring standards document (www.asahq.org/publicationsAndServices/standards/02.pdf) includes clear specifications for the presence of personnel during an anesthetic episode and for continual evaluation of oxygenation, ventilation, circulation, and temperature. These ASA monitoring standards very quickly became part of the accepted standard of care in anesthesia practice. This means they are important to practice management because they have profound medicolegal implications: a catastrophic accident occurring while the standards are being actively ignored is very difficult to defend in the consequent malpractice suit, whereas an accident that occurs during well-documented full compliance with the standards will automatically have a strong defense because the standard of care was being met. Several states in the United States have made compliance with these ASA standards mandatory under state regulations or even statutes. Various malpractice insurance companies offer discounts on malpractice insurance policy premiums for compliance with these standards, something quite natural to insurers because they are familiar with the idea of managing known risks to help minimize financial loss to the company. The ASA monitoring standards have been widely emulated in other medical specialties and even in fields outside medicine.

With many of the same elements of thinking, the ASA adopted "Basic Standards for Preanesthesia Care" (www.asahq.org/publicationsAndServices/standards/03.pdf). This was supplemented significantly by another type of document, the ASA *Practice Advisory for Preanesthesia Evaluation* (see www.asahq.org, "Publications and Services," and "Practice Parameters"), a 40-page meta-analysis of clinical aspects of preoperative evaluation. Also, the ASA adopted "Standards for Postanesthesia Care," in which there was consideration of and collaboration with the very detailed standards of practice for PACU care published by the American Society of Post Anesthesia Nurses (another good example of the sources of standards of care). This also was later supplemented by an extensive *Practice Guideline*.[6]

A slightly different situation exists with regard to the standards for conduct of anesthesia in obstetrics. These standards were originally passed by the ASA in 1988, in the same manner as the other ASA standards, but the ASA membership eventually questioned whether they reflected a realistic and desirable standard of care. Accordingly, the obstetric anesthesia standards were downgraded in 1990 to guidelines, specifically to remove the mandatory nature of the document. Because there was no agreement as to what should be prescribed as the standard of care, the medicolegal imperative of published standards in this instance has been temporarily set aside. From a management perspective, this makes the guidelines (www.asahq.org/publicationsAndServices/standards/45.pdf) no less valuable because the intent of optimizing care through the avoidance of complications is no less operative. However, in the event of the need to defend against a malpractice claim in this area, it is clear from this sequence of events that the exact standard of care is debatable and not yet finally established (an extremely important medicolegal consideration). A different ASA document has been generated, *Practice Guidelines for Obstetrical Anesthesia*, with more detail and specificity as well as an emphasis on the meta-analytic approach.[7]

Practice Guidelines

An important type of related ASA document is the *Practice Guideline* (formerly "Practice Parameter"). This has some of the same elements as a standard of practice but is more intended to guide judgment, largely through algorithms with some element of guidelines, in addition to directing the details of specific procedures as would a formal standard. Beyond the details of the minimum standards for carrying out the procedure, these practice parameters set forth algorithms and guidelines for helping to determine under what circumstances and with what timing to perform it. Understandably, purchasers of health care (government, insurance companies, and managed care organizations [MCOs]) with a strong desire to limit the costs of medical care have great interest in practice parameters as potential vehicles for helping to eliminate "unnecessary" procedures and limit even the necessary ones.

The ASA has been very active in creating and publishing practice guidelines. The first published parameter (since revised) concerned the use of pulmonary artery (PA) catheters.[8] It considered the clinical effectiveness of PA catheters, public policy issues (costs and concerns of patients and providers), and recommendations (indications and practice settings). Also, the ASA *Difficult Airway Algorithm* was published (also since revised).[9] This thoughtful document synthesized a strategy summarized in a decision tree diagram for dealing acutely with airway problems. It has great clinical value and it is reasonable to anticipate that it will be used to help many patients. However, all these documents are readily noticed by plaintiffs' lawyers, the difficult airway parameter from the ASA being an excellent example.

An important and so-far undecided question is whether guidelines and practice parameters from recognized entities such as the ASA *define* the standard of care. There is no simple answer. This will be decided over time by practitioners' actions, debates in the literature, mandates from malpractice insurers, and, of course, court decisions. Some guidelines, such as the U.S. Food and Drug Administration (FDA) preanesthetic apparatus checkout, are accepted as the standard of care. There will be debate among experts, but the practitioner must make the decision as to how to apply practice parameters and guidelines such as those from the ASA. Practitioners have incorrectly assumed that they *must* do everything specified. This is clearly not true, yet there is a valid concern that these will someday be held up as defining the standard of care. Accordingly, prudent attention within the bounds of reason to the principles outlined in guidelines and parameters will put the practitioner in at least a reasonably defensible position, whereas radical deviation from them should be based on obvious exigencies of the situation at that moment or clear, defensible alternative beliefs (with documentation).

The most recent type of document has been the "practice advisory," which can seem functionally similar, but appears to have the implication of more consensus compromise than previous documents. Examples of practice advisories include: "Intraoperative Awareness and Brain Function Monitoring,"

"Perioperative Management of Patients with Cardiac Rhythm Management Devices: Pacemakers and Implantable Cardioverter-Defibrillators," and "Perioperative Visual Loss Associated with Spine Surgery." The potential quality assurance and medicolegal implications of these documents are so important to anesthesia professionals and their practices, the ASA has what is essentially a guideline for the guidelines in its 2007 update of the "Policy Statement on Practice Parameters" (see www.asahq.org, "Publications and Services," and "Standards, Guidelines, and Statements") in which the distinction is made between evidence-based documents and consensus-based documents with explanations of the background and formulation processes for each.

On the other hand, practice protocols, such as those for the fast-track management of coronary artery bypass graft patients, that are handed down by MCOs or health insurance companies are a different matter. Even though the desired implication is that practitioners must observe (or at least strongly consider) them, they do not have the same implications in defining the standard of care as the other documents. Practitioners must avoid getting trapped. It may well not be a valid legal defense to justify action or the lack of action because of a company protocol. As difficult as it may be to reconcile with the payer, the practitioner still is subject to the classic definitions of standard of care.

The other type of standards associated with medical care are those of the Joint Commission, which is the best-known medical care quality regulatory agency. As noted, these standards were for many years concerned largely with structure (e.g., gas tanks chained down) and process (e.g., documentation complete), but in recent years they have been expanded to include reviews of the *outcome* of care. Joint Commission standards also focus on credentialing and privileges, verification that anesthesia services are of uniform quality throughout an institution, the qualifications of the director of the service, continuing education, and basic guidelines for anesthesia care (need for preoperative and postoperative evaluations, documentation, and so forth). Full Joint Commission accreditation of a health care facility is usually for 3 years. Even the best hospitals and facilities receive some citations of problems or deficiencies that are expected to be corrected, and an interim report of efforts to do so is required. If there are enough problems, accreditation can be conditional for 1 year, with a complete reinspection at that time. Preparing for Joint Commission inspections starts with verification that essential group/department structure is in place; excellent examples exist.[1] The process ultimately involves a great deal of work, but because the standards usually do promote high-quality care, the majority of this work is highly constructive and of benefit to the institution and its medical staff.

Review Implications

Another type of regulatory agency is the peer review organization. Professional standards review organizations (PSROs) were established in 1972 as utilization review/QA overseers of the care of federally subsidized patients (Medicare and Medicaid). Despite their efforts to deal with quality of care, these groups were seen by all involved as primarily interested in cost containment. Various negative factors led to the PSROs being replaced in 1984 with the peer review organization (PRO).[10] There is a PRO in each state, many being associated with a state medical association. The objectives of a PRO include 14 goals related to hospital admissions (e.g., to shift care to an outpatient basis as much as possible) and 5 related to quality of care (e.g., to reduce avoidable deaths and avoidable complications). The PROs comprise full-time support staff and physician reviewers paid as consultants or directors. Ideally, PRO monitoring will discover suboptimal care, which will lead to specific recommendations for improvement in quality. There is a perception that quality of care efforts are hampered by the lack of realistic objectives and also that these PRO groups, like others before them, will largely or entirely function to limit the cost of health care services.

The practice management implications have become clear. Aside from the as-yet unrealized potential for quality improvement efforts and the occasional denial of payment for a procedure, the most likely interaction between the local PRO and anesthesia professionals will involve a request for perioperative admission of a patient whose care is mandated to be outpatient surgery (this could also occur in dealing with an MCO). If the anesthesiologist feels, for example, that either (1) preoperative admission for treatment to optimize cardiac, pulmonary, diabetic, or other medical status or (2) postoperative admission for monitoring of labile situations such as uncontrolled hypertension will reduce clear anesthetic risks for the patient, an application to the PRO for approval of admission must be made and vigorously supported. All too often, however, such issues surface a day or so before the scheduled procedure in a preanesthesia screening clinic or even in a preoperative holding area outside the OR on the day of surgery. This will continue to occur until anesthesia providers educate their constituent surgeon community as to what types of associated medical conditions may disqualify a proposed patient from the outpatient (ambulatory) surgical schedule. If adequate notice is given by the surgeon, the patient can be seen far enough in advance by an anesthesiologist to allow appropriate planning.

In the circumstance in which the first knowledge of a questionable patient comes 1 or 2 days before surgery, the anesthesiologist can try to have the procedure postponed, if possible, or can undertake the time-consuming task of multiple telephone calls to get the surgeon's agreement, get PRO approval, and make the necessary arrangements. Because neither alternative is particularly attractive, especially from administrative and reimbursement perspectives, there may be a strong temptation to "let it slide" and try to deal with the patient as an outpatient even though this may be questionable. In almost all cases, it is likely that there would be no adverse result (the "get away with it" phenomenon). However, the patient might well be exposed to an avoidable risk. Both because of the workings of probability and because of the inevitable tendency to let sicker and sicker patients slip by as lax practitioners repeatedly get away with it and are lulled into a false sense of security, sooner or later there will be an unfortunate outcome or some preventable major morbidity or even mortality.

The situation is worsened when the first contact with a questionable ambulatory patient is preoperatively (possibly even already in the OR) on the day of surgery. There may be intense pressure from the patient, the surgeon, or the OR administrator and staff to proceed with a case for which the anesthesia practitioner believes the patient is poorly prepared. The arguments made regarding patient inconvenience and anxiety are valid. However, they should not outweigh the best medical interests of the patient. Although this is a point in favor of screening all outpatients before the day of surgery, the anesthesia professional facing this situation on the day of operation should state clearly to all concerned the reasons for postponing the surgery, stressing the issue of avoidable risk and standards of care, and then help with alternative arrangements (including, if necessary, dealing with the PRO or managed care organization).

Potential liability in this regard is the other side of the standard of care issue. Particularly concerning is the question of postoperative admission of ambulatory patients who have been unstable. It is an extremely poor defense against a malpractice claim to state that the patient was discharged home, only later to suffer a complication, because the PRO/managed care organization deemed that operative procedure outpatient and not inpatient surgery. As bureaucratically annoying as it may be, it is a prudent management strategy to admit the patient if there is any legitimate question, thus minimizing the chance for complications, and later haggle with the PRO or directly with the involved third-party payer.

Policy and Procedure

One important organizational point that is often overlooked is the need for a complete policy and procedure manual. Such a compilation of documents is necessary for all practices, from the largest departments covering multiple hospitals to a single-room outpatient facility with one anesthesia provider. Such a manual can be extraordinarily valuable, as, for example, when it provides crucial information during an emergency. Some suggestions for the content of this compendium exist[11] but, at minimum, organizational and procedural elements must be included.

The organizational elements that should be present include a chart of organization and responsibilities that is not just a call schedule but a clear explanation of who is responsible for what functions of the department and when, with attendant details such as expectations for the practitioner's presence within the institution at designated hours, telephone availability, pager availability, the maximum permissible distance from the institution when on call, and so forth. Experience suggests it is especially important for there to be an absolutely clear specification of the availability of qualified anesthesiology personnel for emergency cesarean section, particularly in practice arrangements in which there are several people on call covering multiple locations. Sadly, these issues often are only considered after a disaster has occurred that involved miscommunication and the mistaken belief by one or more people that someone else would take care of an acute problem.

The organizational component of the policy and procedure manual should also include a clear explanation of the orientation and checkout procedure for new personnel, continuing medical education requirements and opportunities, the mechanisms for evaluating personnel and for communicating this evaluation to them, disaster plans (or reference to a separate disaster manual or protocol), QA activities of the department, and the format for statistical record keeping (number of procedures, types of anesthetics given, types of patients anesthetized, number and types of invasive monitoring procedures, number and type of responses to emergency calls, complications, or whatever the group/department decides).

The procedural component of the policy and procedure manual should give both handy practice tips and specific outlines of proposed courses of action for particular circumstances; it also should store little-used but valuable information. Reference should be made to the statements, guidelines, practice parameters, and standards appearing on the ASA Web site. Also included should be references to or specific protocols for the areas mentioned in the JCAHO standards: preanesthetic evaluation, immediate preinduction re-evaluation, safety of the patient during the anesthetic period, release of the patient from any PACU, recording of all pertinent events during anesthesia, recording of postanesthesia visits, guidelines defining the role of anesthesia services in hospital infection control, and guidelines for safe use of general anesthetic agents. Other appropriate topics include the following:

1. Recommendations for preanesthesia apparatus checkout, such as from the FDA[12] (see Chapter 26)
2. Guidelines for admission to, minimal monitoring and duration of stay of an infant, child, or adult in, and then discharge from the PACU
3. Procedures for transporting patients to/from the OR, PACU, or ICU

4. Policy on ambulatory surgical patients—for example, screening, use of regional anesthesia, discharge home criteria
5. Policy on evaluation and processing of same-day admissions
6. Policy on ICU admission and discharge
7. Policy on physicians responsible for writing orders in recovery room and ICU
8. Policy on informed consent for anesthesia and its documentation
9. Policy on the use of patients in clinical research (if applicable)
10. Guidelines for the support of cadaveric organ donors and its termination (plus organ donation after cardiac death)
11. Guidelines on environmental safety, including pollution with trace gases and electrical equipment inspection, maintenance, and hazard prevention
12. Procedure for change of personnel during an anesthetic and documentation (particularly if a printed hand-off protocol is used)
13. Procedure for the introduction of new equipment, drugs, or clinical practices
14. Procedure for epidural and spinal narcotic administration and subsequent patient monitoring (e.g., type, minimum time, nursing units)
15. Procedure for initial treatment of cardiac or respiratory arrest (updated Advanced Cardiac Life Support guidelines)
16. Policy for handling patient's refusal of blood or blood products, including the mechanism to obtain a court order to transfuse
17. Procedure for the management of malignant hyperthermia
18. Procedure for the induction and maintenance of barbiturate coma
19. Procedure for the evaluation of suspected pseudocholinesterase deficiency
20. Protocol for responding to an adverse anesthetic event (such as a copy of the update of the "Adverse Event Protocol"[13])
21. Policy on resuscitation of do-not-resuscitate patients in the OR

Individual departments will add to these suggestions as dictated by their specific needs. A thorough, carefully conceived policy and procedure manual is a valuable tool. The manual should be reviewed and updated as needed but at least annually, with a particularly thorough review preceding each Joint Commission inspection. Each member of a group or department should review the manual at least annually and sign off in a log indicating familiarity with current policies and procedures.

Meetings and Case Discussion

There must be regularly scheduled departmental or group meetings. Although didactic lectures and continuing education meetings are valuable and necessary, there also must be regular opportunities for open clinical discussion about interesting cases and problem cases. Also, the Joint Commission requires that there be at least monthly meetings at which risk management and QA activities are documented and reported. Whether these meetings are called case conferences, morbidity and mortality conferences, or deaths and complications conferences, the entire department or group should gather for an interchange of ideas. More recently these gatherings have been called *QA meetings*. An open review of departmental statistics should be done, including all complications, even those that may appear trivial. Unusual patterns of small events may point toward a larger or systematic problem, especially if they are more frequently associated with one individual practitioner.

A problem case presented at the departmental meeting might be an overt accident, a near accident (critical incident), or an untoward outcome of unknown origin. Honest but constructive discussion, even of an anesthesia professional's technical deficiencies or lack of knowledge, should take place in the spirit of constructive peer review. The classic question, "What would you do differently next time?" is a good way to start the discussion. There may be situations in which inviting the surgeon or the internist involved in a specific case would be advantageous. The opportunity for each type of provider to hear the perspective of another discipline is not only inherently educational, but also can promote communication and cooperation in future potential problem cases.

Records of these meetings must be kept for accreditation purposes, but the enshrining of overly detailed minutes (potentially subject to discovery by a plaintiff's attorney at a later date) may inhibit true educational and corrective interchanges about untoward events. In the circumstance of discussion of a case that seems likely to provoke litigation, it is appropriate to be certain that the meeting is classified as official "peer review" and possibly even invite the hospital attorney or legal counsel from the relevant malpractice insurance carrier (to guarantee the privacy of the discussion and minutes).

Support Staff

There is a fundamental need for support staff in every anesthesia practice. Even independent practitioners rely in some measure on facilities, equipment, and services provided by the organization maintaining the anesthetizing location. In large, well-organized departments, reliance on support staff is often very great. What is often overlooked, however, is a process analogous to that of credentialing and privileges for anesthesia professionals, although at a slightly different level. The people expected to provide clinical anesthesia practice support must be qualified and must at all times understand what they are expected to do and how to do it. It is singularly unfortunate to realize only after an anesthesia catastrophe has occurred that basic details of simple work assignments, such as the changing of carbon dioxide absorbent, were routinely ignored. This indicates the need for supervision and monitoring of the support staff by the involved practitioners. Further, such support personnel are favorite targets of cost-cutting administrators who do not understand the function of anesthesia technicians or their equivalent. In the modern era, many administrators seem driven almost exclusively by the "bottom line" and cannot appreciate the connection between valuable workers such as these and the "revenue stream." Even though it is obvious to all who work in an OR that the anesthesia support personnel make it possible for there to be patients flowing through the OR, it is their responsibility to convince the facility's fiscal administrator that elimination of such positions is genuinely false economy because of the attendant loss in efficiency, particularly in turning over the room between surgeries. Further, it is also false economy to reduce the number of personnel below that genuinely needed to retrieve, clean, sort, disassemble, sterilize, reassemble, store, and distribute the tools of daily anesthesia practice. Vigorous defense (or initiation of new positions if the staff is inadequate) by the anesthesia professionals should be undertaken, always with the realization that it may be necessary in some circumstances for them to supplement the budget from the facility with some of their practice income to guarantee an adequate complement of competent workers.

Business and organizational issues in the management of an anesthesia practice are also critically dependent on the existence of a sufficient number of appropriately trained support staff. One frequently overlooked issue that contributes to the negative impression generated by some anesthesiology practices centers on being certain there is someone available to answer the telephone *at all times* during the hours surgeons, other physicians, and OR scheduling desks are likely to call. This seemingly trivial component of practice management is very important to the success of an anesthesiology practice as a business whose principal customers are the surgeons. Certainly there is a commercial server–client relationship both with the patient and the purchaser of health care; however, the uniquely symbiotic nature of the relationship between surgeons and anesthesiologists is such that availability even for simple "just wanted to let you know" telephone calls is genuinely important. The person who answers the telephone is the representative of the practice to the world and must take that responsibility seriously. From a management standpoint, significant impact on the success of the practice as a business often hinges on such details. Further, anesthesiologists should always have permanent personal electronic pagers and reliable mobile telephones (or the radio equivalent) to facilitate communications from other members of the department or group and from support personnel. This may sound intrusive, but the unusual position of anesthesia professionals in the spectrum of health care workers mandates this feature of managing an anesthesiology practice. Anesthesiology professionals should have no hesitation about spending their own practice income to do so. The symbolism alone is obvious.

Anesthesia Equipment and Equipment Maintenance

Problems with anesthesia equipment have been discussed for some time.[14–16] However, compared with human error, overt equipment failure rarely causes intraoperative critical incidents[17] or deaths resulting from anesthesia care. Aside from the obvious human errors involving misuse of or unfamiliarity with the equipment, when the rare equipment failure does occur, it often appears that correct maintenance and servicing of the apparatus has not been done. These issues become the focus of anesthesia practice management efforts, which could have significant liability implications because there can often be confusion or even disputes about precisely who is responsible for arranging maintenance of the anesthesia equipment—the facility or the practitioners who use it and collect practice income from that activity. In many cases, the facility assumes the responsibility. In situations in which that is not true, however, it is necessary for the practitioners to recognize that responsibility and seek help securing a service arrangement, because this is likely an unfamiliar obligation for clinicians.

Programs for anesthesia equipment maintenance and service have been outlined.[1,18] A distinction is made between failure resulting from progressive deterioration of equipment, which should be preventable because it is observable and should provoke appropriate remedial action, and catastrophic failure, which, realistically, often cannot be predicted. Preventive maintenance for mechanical parts is critical and involves periodic performance checks every 4 to 6 months. Also, an annual safety inspection of each anesthetizing location and the equipment itself is necessary. For equipment service, an excellent mechanism is a relatively elaborate cross-reference system (possibly kept handwritten in a notebook but ideal for maintenance on an electronic spreadsheet program) to identify both the device needing service and also the mechanism to secure the needed maintenance or repair.

Equipment-handling principles are straightforward. Before purchase, it must be verified that a proposed piece of equipment meets all applicable standards, which will usually be true when dealing with recognized major manufacturers. The renewed efforts of some facility administrators to save money by attempting to find "refurbished" anesthesia machines and monitoring systems should provoke thorough review by the involved practitioners. On arrival, electrical equipment must be checked for absence of hazard (especially leakage of current) and compliance with applicable electrical standards. Complex equipment such as anesthesia machines and ventilators should be assembled and checked out by a representative from the manufacturer or manufacturer's agent. There are potential adverse medicolegal implications when relatively untrained personnel certify a particular piece of new equipment as functioning within specification, even if they do it perfectly. On arrival, a sheet or section in the departmental master equipment log must be created with the make, model, serial number, and in-house identification for each piece of capital equipment. This not only allows immediate identification of any equipment involved in a future recall or product alert, but also serves as the permanent repository of the record of every problem, problem resolution, maintenance, and servicing occurring until that particular equipment is scrapped. This log must be kept up-to-date at all times. There have been rare but frightening examples of potentially lethal problems with anesthesia machines leading to product alert notices requiring immediate identification of certain equipment and its service status. It is also very important to involve the manufacturer's representative in pre- and in-service training for those who will use the new equipment. Anesthesia systems with their ventilation and monitoring components have become significantly more integrated and more complex, particularly as they are increasingly electronic and less mechanical. Accordingly, it is critical that anesthesia professionals are properly trained to use their equipment safely. The perception that inadequate training is common and that this represents a threat to patient safety has led the Anesthesia Patient Safety Foundation to initiate a campaign urging anesthesia departments and groups to ensure organized verified complete training of all professionals who will use this new technology.[19]

Service

Beyond the administrative liability implications, precisely what type of support personnel should maintain and service major anesthesia equipment has been widely debated. Some groups or departments rely on factory service representatives from the equipment manufacturers for all attention to equipment, others engage independent service contractors, and still other (often larger) departments have access to personnel (either engineers and/or technicians) permanently within their facility. The single underlying principle is clear: the person(s) doing preventive maintenance and service on anesthesia equipment must be qualified. Anesthesia practitioners may wonder how they can assess these qualifications. The best way is to unhesitatingly ask pertinent questions about the education, training, and experience of those involved, including asking for references and speaking to supervisors and managers responsible for those doing the work. Whether an engineering technician who spent a week at a course at a factory can perform the most complex repairs depends on a variety of factors, which can be investigated by the practitioners ultimately using the equipment in the care of patients. Failure to be involved in this oversight function exposes the practice to increased liability in the event of an untoward outcome associated with improperly maintained or serviced equipment.

Replacement of obsolete anesthesia machines and monitoring equipment is a key element of a risk-modification program. Ten years is often cited as an estimated useful life for an anesthesia machine, but although an ASA statement repeats that idea, it also notes that the ASA promulgated "Guidelines for Determining Anesthesia Machine Obsolescence" in 2004 that does not subscribe to any specific time interval. Anesthesia machines considerably more than 20 years old likely do not meet certain of the safety standards now in force for new machines (such as vaporizer lockout, fresh gas ratio protection, and automatic enabling of the oxygen analyzer) and, unless extensively retrofitted, do not incorporate the new technology that advanced very rapidly during the 1980s, much of it directly related to the effort to prevent untoward incidents. Further, it appears that this technology will continue to advance, particularly because of the adoption of anesthesia workstation standards by the European Economic Union that are affecting anesthesia machine design worldwide. Note that some anesthesia equipment manufacturers, anxious to minimize their own potential liability, have refused to support (with parts and service) some of the oldest of their pieces (particularly gas machines) still in use. This disowning of equipment by its own manufacturer is a very strong message to practitioners that such equipment must be replaced as soon as possible.

Should a piece of equipment fail, it must be removed from service and a replacement substituted. Groups, departments, and facilities are obligated to have sufficient backup equipment to cover any reasonable incidence of failure. The equipment removed from service must be clearly marked with a prominent label (so it is not returned into service by a well-meaning technician or practitioner) containing the date, time, person discovering, and the details of the problem. The responsible personnel must be notified so they can remove the equipment, make an entry in the log, and initiate the repair. As indicated in the protocol for response to an adverse event,[13] a piece of equipment involved or suspected in an anesthesia accident must be immediately sequestered and not touched by anybody—particularly not by any equipment service personnel. If a severe accident occurred, it may be necessary for the equipment in question to be inspected at a later time by a group consisting of qualified representatives of the manufacturer, the service personnel, the plaintiff's attorney, the insurance companies involved, and the practitioner's defense attorney. The equipment should thus be impounded following an adverse event and treated similarly to any object in a forensic "chain of evidence," with careful documentation of parties in contact with and responsible for securing the equipment in question following such an event. Also, major equipment problems may, in some circumstances, reflect a pattern of failure due to a design or manufacturing fault. These problems should be reported to the FDA's Medical Device Problem Reporting system[20] via MedWatch on Form 3500 (found at www.fda.gov/medwatch/index.html, or telephone 800-FDA-1088). This system accepts voluntary reports from users and requires reports from manufacturers when there is knowledge of a medical device being involved in a serious incident. Whether or not filing such a report will have a positive impact in subsequent litigation is impossible to know, but it is a worthwhile practice management point that needs to be considered in the unlikely but important instance of a relevant event involving equipment failure.

Malpractice Insurance

All practitioners need liability insurance coverage specific for the specialty and role in which they are practicing. It is absolutely critical that applicants for medical liability insurance be completely honest in informing the insurer what duties and procedures they perform. Failure to do so, either from carelessness or from a foolishly misguided desire to reduce the resulting premium, may well result in retrospective denial of insurance coverage in the event of an untoward outcome from an activity the insurer did not know the insured engaged in.

Proof of adequate insurance coverage is usually required to secure or renew privileges to practice at a health care facility. The facility may specify certain minimum policy limits in an attempt to limit its own liability exposure. It is difficult to suggest specific dollar amounts for policy limits because the details of practice vary so much among situations and locations. The malpractice crisis of the 1980s eased significantly in the early 1990s for anesthesia professionals, largely because of the decrease in number and severity of malpractice claims resulting from anesthesia catastrophes as anesthesia care in the United States became safer.[21–23] The exact analysis of this phenomenon can be debated,[24,25] but it is a simple fact that malpractice insurance risk ratings have been decreased and premiums for anesthesia professionals have not been increased at the same rate as for other specialties over the past 15 years and, in many cases, have actually decreased. In 2008, coverage limits of $1 million/$3 million are still common and would seem the minimum advisable. This policy specification usually means that the insurer will cover up to $1 million liability per claim and up to $3 million total per year, but this terminology is not necessarily universal. Therefore, anesthesia professionals must be absolutely certain what they are buying when they apply for malpractice insurance. Even though anesthesiologists have not recently suffered a great number of very large malpractice payments or jury verdicts,[26] in specific parts of the United States known for a pattern of exorbitant settlements and jury verdicts, liability coverage limits of $2 million/$5 million or even greater may be prudent. An additional feature in this regard is the potential to employ "umbrella" liability coverage above the limits of the base policy, as will be noted.

Background

The fundamental mechanism of medical malpractice insurance changed significantly in the last 3 decades because of the need for insurance companies to have better ways to predict their losses (amounts paid in settlements and judgments). Traditionally, medical liability insurance was sold on an "occurrence" basis, meaning that if the insurance policy was in force at the time of the occurrence of an incident resulting in a claim, whenever within the statute of limitations that claim might be filed, the practitioner would be covered. Occurrence insurance was somewhat more expensive than the alternative "claims made" policies, but was seen as worth it by some (many) practitioners. These policies created some open-ended exposure for the insurer that sometimes led to unexpected large losses, even some large enough to threaten the existence of the insurance company. As a result, medical malpractice insurers have converted almost exclusively to claims-made insurance, which covers claims that are filed while the insurance is in force. Premium rates for the first year a physician is in practice are relatively low because there is less likelihood of a claim coming in (a majority of malpractice suits are filed 1 to 3 years after the event in question). The premiums usually increase yearly for the first 5 years and then the policy is considered "mature." The issue comes when the physician later, for whatever reason, must change insurance companies (e.g., because of relocation to another state). If the physician simply discontinues the policy and a claim is filed the next year, there will be no insurance coverage. Therefore, the physician must secure "tail coverage," sometimes for a minimum number of years (e.g., 5) or, more often, indefinitely to guarantee liability insurance protection for claims filed after the physician is no longer primarily covered by that insurance policy. It may be possible in some circumstances to purchase tail coverage from a different insurer than was involved with the primary policy, but by far the most common thing done is to simply extend the existing insurance coverage for the period of the tail. This very often yields a bill for the entire tail coverage premium, which can be quite sizable, potentially staggering a physician who simply wants to move to another state where his or her existing insurance company is not licensed to or refuses to do business. Individual situations will vary widely, but it is reasonable for anesthesiologists organized into a fiscal entity to consider this issue at the time of the inception of the group and record their policy decisions in writing, rather than facing the potentially difficult question of how to treat one individual later. Other strategies have occasionally been employed when insuring the tail period, including converting the previous policy to part-time status for a period of years, and purchasing "nose" coverage from the new insurer—that is, paying an initial higher yearly premium with the new insurer, who then will cover claims that may occur during the tail period. Whatever strategy is adopted, it is critical that the individual practitioner is absolutely certain though personal verification that he or she is thoroughly covered at the time of any transition. The potential stakes are much too great to leave such important issues solely to an office clerk. Further, a practitioner arriving in a new location is often filling a need or void and is urged to begin clinical work as soon as possible by others who have been shouldering an increased load. It is essential that the new arrival verify with confirmation in writing (often called a "binder") that malpractice liability insurance coverage is in force before there is any patient contact.

Another component to the liability insurance situation is consideration of the advisability of purchasing yet another type of insurance called *umbrella coverage*, which is activated at the time of the need to pay a claim that exceeds the limits of coverage on the standard malpractice liability insurance policy. Because such an enormous claim is extremely unlikely, many practitioners are tempted to forgo the comparatively modest cost of such insurance coverage in the name of economy. As before, it is easy to see that this is potentially a very false economy—if there is a huge claim. Practitioners should consult with their financial managers and advisors, but it is likely that it would be considered wise management to purchase "umbrella" liability insurance coverage.

Medical malpractice insurers are becoming increasingly active in trying to prevent incidents that will lead to insurance claims. They often sponsor risk-management seminars to teach practices and techniques to lessen the chances of liability claims and, in some cases, suggest (or even mandate) specific practices, such as strict documented compliance with the ASA "Standards for Basic Anesthetic Monitoring." In return for attendance at such events and/or the signing of contracts stating that the practitioner will follow certain guidelines or standards, the insurer often gives a discount on the liability insurance premium. Clearly, it is sound practice management strategy for practitioners to participate maximally in such programs. Likewise, some insurers make coverage conditional on the consistent implementation of certain strategies such as minimal monitoring, even stipulating that the practitioner will not be covered if it is found that the guidelines were being consciously ignored at the time of an untoward event. Again, it is obviously wise from a practice management standpoint to cooperate fully with such stipulations.

Response to an Adverse Event

⑤ In spite of the decreased incidence of anesthesia catastrophes, even with the very best of practice, it is statistically likely that each anesthesiologist at least once in his or her professional life will be involved in a major anesthesia accident (see Chapter 4). Precisely because such an event is rare, very few are prepared for it. It is probable that the involved personnel will have no relevant past experience regarding what to do. Although an obvious resource is another anesthetist who has had some exposure or

experience, one of these may not be available either. Various authors have discussed what to do in that event.[27–29] Cooper, et al.[30] have thoughtfully presented the appropriate immediate response to an accident in a straightforward, logical, compact format (that has been updated[13]) that should periodically be reviewed by all anesthesiology practitioners and should be included in all anesthesia policy and procedure manuals. This "adverse events protocol" is also always immediately available at www.apsf.org ("Resource Center," and "Clinical Safety Tools"). Unfortunately, however, the principal personnel involved in a significant untoward event may react with such surprise or shock as to temporarily lose sight of logic. At the moment of recognition that a major anesthetic complication has occurred or is occurring, help must be called. A sufficient number of people to deal with the situation must be assembled on site as quickly as possible. For example, in the unlikely but still possible event that an esophageal intubation goes unrecognized long enough to cause a cardiac arrest, the immediate need is for enough skilled personnel to conduct the resuscitative efforts, including making the correct diagnosis and replacing the tube into the trachea. Whether the anesthesiologist apparently responsible for the complication should direct the immediate remedial efforts will depend on the person and the situation. In such a circumstance, it would seem wise for a senior or supervising anesthesiologist quickly to evaluate the scenario and make a decision. This person becomes the "incident supervisor" and has responsibility for helping prevent continuation or recurrence of the incident, for investigating the incident, and for ensuring documentation while the original and helping anesthesiologists focus on caring for the patient. As noted, involved equipment must be sequestered and not touched until such time as it is certain that it was not involved in the incident.

If the accident is not fatal, continuing care of the patient is critical. Measures may be instituted to help limit damage from brain hypoxia. Consultants may be helpful and should be called without hesitation. If not already involved, the chief of anesthesiology must be notified as well as the facility administrator, risk manager, and the anesthesiologist's insurance company. These latter are critical to allow consideration of immediate efforts to limit later financial loss. (Likewise, there are often provisions in medical malpractice insurance policies that might limit or even deny insurance coverage if the company is not notified of any reportable event immediately.) If there is an involved surgeon of record, he or she probably will first notify the family, but the anesthesiologist and others (risk manager, insurance loss control officer, or even legal counsel) might appropriately be included at the outset. Full disclosure of facts as they are best known—with no confessions, opinions, speculation, or placing of blame—is currently still believed to be the best presentation. Any attempt to conceal or shade the truth will only later confound an already difficult situation. Obviously, comfort and support should be offered, including, if appropriate, the services of facility personnel such as clergy, social workers, and counselors. There is a new movement in medical risk management and insurance advocating immediate full disclosure to the victim or survivors, including "confessions" of medical judgment and performance errors with attendant sincere apologies. If indicated, early offers of reasonable compensation may be included. There have been instances when this overall strategy has prevented the filing of a malpractice lawsuit and has been applauded by all involved as an example of a shift from the "culture of blame" with punishment to a "just culture" with restitution. A widespread movement to implement immediate disclosure and apology has received support.[31,32]

Certain states have enacted or proposed so-called "I'm sorry!" legislation intended to prevent any explanation or apology from being used as plaintiff's evidence in a subsequent malpractice suit. The importance of the patient's perspective on a serious adverse anesthesia event was highlighted in a riveting account of the stories of both survivors of anesthesia catastrophes and the families of patients who died.[33] In each case, one main message was the enormous negative impact of the perceived failure of the involved anesthesia professionals and their institutions to share detailed information about what exactly happened. A recent review summarizes what patients want and expect following an adverse event.[34] Laudable as this policy of immediate full disclosure and apology may sound, it would be mandatory for an individual practitioner to check with the involved liability insurance carrier, the practice group, and the facility administration before attempting it.

The primary anesthesia provider and any others involved must document relevant information. Never, ever change any existing entries in the medical record. Write an amendment note if needed, with careful explanation of why amendment is necessary, particularly stressing explanations of professional judgments involved. State only facts as they are known. Make no judgments about causes or responsibility and do not "point fingers." The same guidelines hold true for the filing of the incident report in the facility, which should be done as soon as is practical. Further, all discussions with the patient or family should be carefully documented in the medical record. Recognizing that detailed memories of the events may fade in the 1 to 3 years before the practitioner may face deposition questions about exactly what happened, it is possible that it will be recommended, immediately after the incident, that the involved clinical personnel sit down as soon as practical and write out their own personal notes, which will include opinions and impressions as well as maximally detailed accounts of the events as they unfolded. These personal notes are not part of the medical record or the facility files. These notes should be written in the physical presence of an involved attorney representing the practitioner, even if this is not yet the specific defense attorney secured by the malpractice insurance company, and then that attorney should take possession of and keep those notes as case material. This strategy is intended to make the personal notes "attorney–client work product," and thus not subject to forced "discovery" (revelation) by other parties to the case.

Follow-up after the immediate handling of the incident will involve the primary anesthesiologist but should again be directed by a senior supervisor, who may or may not be the same person as the incident supervisor. The "follow-up supervisor" verifies the adequacy and coordination of ongoing care of the patient and facilitates communication among all involved, especially with the risk manager. Lastly, it is necessary to verify that adequate postevent documentation is taking place.

Of course, it is expected that such an adverse event will be discussed in the applicable morbidity and mortality meeting. It is necessary, however, to coordinate this activity with the involved risk manager and attorney so as to be completely certain that the contents and conclusions of the discussion are clearly considered peer review activity, and thus are shielded from discovery by the plaintiffs' attorney.

Unpleasant as this is to contemplate, it is better to have a clear plan and execute it in the event of an accident causing injury to a patient. Vigorous immediate intervention may improve the outcome for all concerned.

PRACTICE ESSENTIALS

The "Job Market" for Anesthesia Professionals

While it is true that in the mid-1990s, for the first time, uncertainty faced residents finishing anesthesiology training because of a perception that there were not enough jobs for physician anesthesiologists available, that concept faded quickly. A tension between supply and demand developed, with a significant ongoing component of the idea that there is an overall shortage of anesthesia professionals. It appears that late in the first decade of the 2000s this fundamental paradigm will persist. With the fading of the concept that managed care would significantly reduce the demand for medical services and also the aging of the Baby Boom population, it is clear that there is a significant shortage of all medical professionals in the United States, and this especially includes anesthesia professionals.

Types of Practice

At least through the first decade of the 21st century, residents finishing anesthesiology training will still need to choose among three fundamental possibilities: academic practice in a teaching hospital environment; a practice exclusively of patient care in the private practice marketplace; and a practice exclusively of patient care as an employee of a health care system, organization, or facility.

Teaching hospitals with anesthesiology residency programs constitute only a very small fraction of the total number of facilities requiring anesthesia services. These academic departments tend to be among the largest groups of anesthesiologists, but the aggregate fraction of the entire anesthesiologist population is small. It is interesting, however, that by the nature of the system, most residents finishing their training have almost exclusively been exposed only to academic anesthesiology. Accordingly, finishing residents in the past often were comparatively unprepared to evaluate and enter the anesthesiology job market.

Specialty certification by the ABA should be the goal of all anesthesia residency graduates. Some finishing residents who know they are eventually headed for private practice have started their attending careers as full-time junior faculty in an academic department. This allows them to obtain some clinical practice and supervisory experience and offers them the opportunity to prepare for the ABA examinations in the nurturing, protected academic environment with which they are familiar. Most residents, however, do not become junior faculty; they accept practice positions immediately. But such newly trained residents should take into account the need to become ABA-certified and build into their new practice arrangements the stipulation that there will be time and consideration given toward this goal.

Academic Practice

For those who choose to stay in academic practice, a number of specific characteristics of academic anesthesia departments can be used as screening questions.

How big is the department? Junior faculty sometimes can get lost in very big departments and be treated as little better than glorified senior residents. On the other hand, the availability of subspecialty service opportunities and significant research and educational resources can make large departments extremely attractive. In smaller academic departments, there may be fewer resources, but the likelihood of being quickly accepted as a valued and contributing member of the teaching faculty (and research team, if appropriate) may be higher. In very small departments, the number of expectations, projects, and involvements could potentially be overwhelming. Additionally, a small department may lack a dedicated research infrastructure, so it may be necessary for the faculty in this situation to collaborate with other, larger departments to accomplish meaningful academic work.

What exactly is expected of junior faculty? If teaching one resident class every other week is standard, the candidate must enthusiastically accept that assignment and the attendant preparation work and time up front. Likewise, if it is expected that junior faculty will, by definition, be actively involved in publishable research, specific plans for projects to which the candidate is amenable must be made. In such situations, clear stipulations about startup research funding and nonclinical time to carry out the projects should be obtained as much as possible (although clinical workload demands and revenue generation expectations may make this very difficult in some settings). Particularly important is determining what the expectation is concerning outside funding. For example, it can be a rude shock to realize that projects will suddenly halt after 2 years if extramural funding has not been secured.

What are the prospects for advancement? Many new junior faculty directly out of residency start with medical school appointments as instructors unless there is something else in their background that immediately qualifies them as assistant professors. It is wise to understand from the beginning what it takes in that department and medical school to facilitate academic advancement. There may be more than one academic "track"; the tenure track, for example, usually depends on published research whereas the clinical or teacher track relies more heavily on one's value in patient care and as a clinical educator. The criteria for promotion may be clearly spelled out by the institution—number of papers needed, involvement and recognition at various levels, grants submitted and funded, and so on—or the system may be less rigid and depend more heavily on the department chairman's and other faculty evaluations and recommendations. In either case, careful inquiry before accepting the position can avert later surprise and disappointment.

How much does it pay? Traditionally, academic anesthesiologists have not earned quite as much as those in private practice—in return for the advantage of more predictable schedules, continued intellectual stimulation, and the intangible rewards of academic success. There is now great activity and attention concerning reimbursement of anesthesiologists, and it is difficult to predict future income for any anesthesiology practice situation. However, all of the forces influencing payment for anesthesia care may significantly diminish the traditional income differential between academic and private practice. In some cases, a faculty member is exclusively an employee of the institution, which bills and collects or negotiates group contracts for the patient care rendered by the faculty member, and then pays a negotiated amount (either an absolute dollar figure or a floating amount based on volume and/or collections—or a combination of the two) that constitutes the faculty person's entire income. Under other much less common arrangements, faculty members themselves may be able to bill and collect or negotiate contracts for their clinical work. Some institutions have a (comparatively small) academic salary from the medical school for being on the faculty, but many do not; some channel variable amounts of money (from so-called Part A clinical revenue) into the academic practice in recognition of teaching and administration or simply as a subsidy for needed service. A salary from the medical school, if extant, is then supplemented significantly by the practice income. Usually, the faculty will be members of some type of group or practice plan (either for the anesthesia department alone or the entire faculty as a whole) that bills and collects or negotiates contracts and then distributes the practice income to the faculty under an arrangement that must be examined by the candidate. In most academic institutions, practice expenses such as all overhead and malpractice insurance as well as reasonable benefits, including discretionary funds for meetings, subscriptions, books, dues, and so forth, are automatically part of the compensation package, which often may not be true in private practice and must be counted

in making any comparison. An important corollary issue is that of the source of the salaries of the department's primary anesthesia providers—residents and, in some cases, nurse anesthetists. Although the hospital usually pays for at least some of these, arrangements vary, and it is important to ascertain whether the faculty practice income is also expected to cover the cost of the primary providers. Overall, it is reasonable to sound out faculty, both anesthesiology and others, regarding the past and likely future commitment of the institution to the establishment and maintenance of reasonable compensation for the expected involvement.

Private Practice in the Marketplace

Obviously, rotations to a private practice hospital in the final year of anesthesia residency could help greatly in this regard, but not all residency programs offer such opportunities. In that case, the finishing resident who is certain about going into private practice must seek information on career development and mentors from the private sector.

Armed with as much information as possible, one fundamental initial choice is between independent individual practice and a position with a group (either a sole proprietorship, partnership, or corporation) that functions as a single financial entity. Independent practice may become increasingly less viable in many locations because of the need to be able to bid for contracts with managed care entities. However, where independent practice is possible, it usually first involves attempting to secure clinical privileges at a number of hospitals or facilities in the area in which one chooses to live. This may not always be easy, and this issue has been the subject of many (frequently unsuccessful) antitrust suits over recent years (see "Antitrust Considerations"). Then the anesthesiologist makes it known to the respective surgeon communities that he or she is available to render anesthesia services and waits until there is a request for his or her services. The anesthesiologist obtains the requisite financial information from the patient and then either individually bills and collects for services rendered or employs a service to do billing and collection for a percentage fee (which will vary depending on the circumstances, especially the volume of business; for billing [without scheduling services] it would be unlikely to be >7% or, at the most, 8% of actual collections).

How much of the needed equipment and supplies will be provided by the hospital or facility and how much by the independent anesthesiologist varies widely. If an anesthesiologist spends considerable time in one operating suite, he or she may purchase an anesthesia machine exclusively for his or her own use and move it from room to room as needed. It is likely to be impractical to move a fully equipped anesthesia machine from hospital to hospital on a day-to-day basis. Among the features of this style of practice are the collegiality and relationships of a genuine private practice based on referrals and also the ability to decide independently how much time one wants to be available to work. The downside is the potential unpredictability of the demand for service and the time needed to establish referral patterns and obtain bookings sufficient to generate a livable income.

When seeking a position with a private group, the applicant should search for potential practice opportunities through word of mouth, recruiting letters sent to the training program supervisor, journal advertisements, and placement services (either commercial or professional, such as that provided at the ASA annual meeting). Some of the screening questions are the same as for an academic position, but there must be even more emphasis on the exact details of clinical expectations and financial arrangements. Some residents finish residency (or fellowship training to an even greater extent) very highly skilled in complex, difficult anesthesia procedures. They can be surprised to find that in some private practice group situations, the junior-most anesthesiologist must wait some time, perhaps even years, before being eligible to do, for example, open heart anesthesia, and in the meantime will mostly be assigned more routine or less challenging anesthetics.

Financial arrangements in private group practices vary widely. Some groups are loose organizational alliances of independent practitioners who bill and collect separately and rotate clinical assignments and call for mutual convenience. Many groups act also as a fiscal entity, and there are many possible variations on this theme. In many circumstances in the past, new junior members started out as functional employees of the group for a probationary interval before being considered for full membership or partnership. This is not a classic employment situation because it is intended to be temporary as a prelude to full financial participation in the group. However, there have been enough instances of established groups abusing this arrangement that the ASA includes in its fundamental "Statement of Policy" the proviso: "Exploitation of anesthesiologists by other anesthesiologists is improper."[1] This goes on to say that after a reasonable trial period, income should reflect services rendered. Unfortunately, these statements may have little meaning or impact on groups in the marketplace. Some groups have a history of demanding excessively long trial periods during which the junior anesthesiologist's income is artificially low and then denying partnership and terminating the relationship to go on to employ a new probationer and start the cycle over again. Accordingly, new junior staff attempting to join groups should try to have such an arrangement spelled out carefully in the agreement drafted by an expert representing the anesthesiologist. Another variation of this, in an attempt to disguise the fundamentally unethical nature of the practice, is to employ anesthesiologists on a fixed salary with the false incentive of no night or weekend call. This is disingenuous, as most income is usually generated during routine scheduled day work, for which the anesthesiologist-employee is poorly compensated. Yet another usurious scheme is for a group to employ an anesthesiologist for a period of years at a low salary and then require a further cash outlay to purchase partnership in the corporation. As the cash outlay can be quite substantial, it is frequently borrowed from the corporation, leading to a sophisticated form of indentured servitude. Sadly, when the job market conditions are poor as they were some years ago, the tendency is for there to be less likelihood of securing a prospective commitment of partnership at a specified future time.

Private Practice as an Employee

There has been some trend toward anesthesiologists becoming permanent employees of any one of various fiscal entities. The key difference is that there is no intention or hope of achieving an equity position (share of ownership, usually of a partnership, thus becoming a full partner). Hospitals, outpatient surgery centers, multidisciplinary clinics, other facilities tied to a specific location where surgery is performed, physician groups that have umbrella fiscal entities specifically created to serve as the employer of physicians, and even surgeons may seek to hire anesthesiologists as permanent employees. The common thread in this system is that these fiscal entities see the anesthesiologists as additional ways of generating profits. Again, in many cases it would appear that employees are not paid a salary that is commensurate with their production of receivables. That is, the fiscal entity will pay a salary substantially below collections generated plus appropriate overhead. These arrangements are particularly favored by some large MCOs in certain cities that view anesthesiologists simply as expensive necessities that prevent hospitals from realizing maximum profit (although sometimes there is a promise of a lighter or more manageable schedule in these positions compared with marketplace private practice).

Negotiating for a position as a permanent full-time employee is somewhat simpler and more straightforward than it is in marketplace private practice. It parallels the usual understandings that apply to most regular employer–employee situations: job description, role expectations, working conditions, hours, pay, and benefits. The idea of anesthesiologists functionally becoming shift workers disturbs many in the profession because it contradicts the traditional professional model. Again, the complex nature and multiple levels of such considerations make it a personal issue that must be carefully evaluated by each individual with full awareness and consideration of the issues outlined here and commensurate research of ASA resources and available data about common regional circumstances and details of any specific medical community.

Practice for a Management Company. One prominent newer development is the growth and impact of large state, regional, or even national management companies that advertise the provision of comprehensive anesthesia services on a contract basis with hospitals, surgery centers, and clinics. These companies, some started and/or managed by anesthesia professionals, promise the facility availability of anesthesia care during the specified hours in return for a lucrative contract to do so. This relieves the facility from any concern about recruiting, hiring/contracting, and retaining anesthesia professionals, virtually eliminating concern about disruption of OR schedules due to limited availability of anesthesia care. The only requirement of the facility is approval of the already prepared credentialing information for each anesthesia professional. Unlike many locum tenens companies in which anesthesia professionals are considered independent contractors and paid fixed contract amounts per hour, per day, or per job for a limited interval with no benefits, some of the management companies may employ anesthesia professionals full-time on a salary with benefits (paid vacation, health insurance, retirement contribution, and so forth). The employment agreement would stipulate whether travel for assignments in locations away from the employee's permanent home would be required as a condition of the full-time job or the position will always be in the practitioner's home community.

Practice as a Hospital Employee. While certified registered nurse anesthetists in some locations have traditionally practiced as hospital employees, until recently, it was less common outside full vertically integrated MCOs for physician anesthesiologists to be hospital (or facility) employees. In recent years, one of the responses of hospitals to requests for subsidies from exclusive-contract practice groups of anesthesiologists has been to offer the anesthesiologists full-time employment status rather than subsidize an independent practice group that has its own significant administrative and overhead costs.[35] The hospital likely suggests that integrating the billing, collecting, and management functions as well as major overhead costs such as malpractice insurance into the existing larger hospital operation would be very cost-efficient, allowing more financial resources to go to physician salaries, and also with possibly a somewhat greater predictability in uncertain times. The hospital can also guarantee the availability of anesthesia care (a requirement to sustain the OR, one of the main hospital revenue sources) in an era when some anesthesiologist groups may simply walk away from a hospital in search of greater income elsewhere, leaving the hospital to seek a contract probably with one of the large and very expensive anesthesia management companies (previously described). Of course, in return for employee status, the anesthesiologists surrender some degree of independence and also, for the group's partners, their equity stake in sharing in any subsequent increased practice revenue. A hospital might counter that concern with the contention that traditional fee-for-service practice that has been so common for so long for private-practice anesthesiologists will *never again* yield enough revenue to maintain the income levels anesthesiologists have come to expect, so they will not be losing anything.

Billing and Collecting

In practices in which anesthesiologists are directly involved with the financial management, they need to understand as much as possible about the complex world of health care reimbursement. This significant task has been made easier by the ASA, which some time ago added a significant component to its Washington, D.C., office (see www.asahq.org/government.htm) by adding a practice management coordinator to the staff. One of the associated assignments is helping ASA members understand and work with the sometimes confusing and convoluted issues of effective billing for anesthesiologists' services. There are often updates with the latest information and codes in the monthly ASA *Newsletter*.

There continue to be proposals for significant changes in billing for anesthesiology care. However, the basics have changed only slightly in recent years. It is important to understand that many of the most contentious issues, such as the requirement for physician supervision of nurse anesthetists and the implications of that for reimbursement, apply in many circumstances mostly to Medicare and, in some states, Medicaid. Thus, the fraction of the patient population covered by these government payers is important in any consideration. Different practice situations have different arrangements regarding the financial relationships between anesthesiologists and nurse anesthetists, and this can affect the complex situation of who bills for what. The nurses may be employees of a hospital, of the anesthesiologists who medically direct them, or of no one in that they are independent contractors billing separately (even in cases in which physician supervision—not medical direction—is required but where those physicians do not bill for that component). In 1998, Medicare mandated that an anesthesia care team of a nurse anesthetist medically directed by an anesthesiologist could bill as a team no more than 100% of the fee that would apply if the anesthesiologist did the case alone. The implications of this change are complex and variable among anesthesiology practices, particularly because there is another trend for health care facilities that traditionally had employed nurse anesthetists to seek to shift total financial responsibility for them to the anesthesiologist practice group. Also, complex related issues played out in the early 2000 years. The federal government issued a new regulation allowing individual states to "opt out" of the requirement that nurse anesthetists be supervised by physicians and several states did so. This was opposed by the ASA. Because perioperative patient care, one component of which is administering anesthesia, is traditionally considered the practice of medicine, the implications of this change as far as the role of surgeons supervising nurse anesthetists and the malpractice liability status of nurse anesthetists practicing independently were unclear. Further, the implications of all this for billing insurers other than Medicare and Medicaid are exceedingly complex.

Classic Methodology

Because there is still widespread application of the traditional method of billing for anesthesiology services, understanding it is very important for anesthesiologists starting practice. In this system, each anesthetic generates a value of so many "units," which represent effort and time. A conversion factor (dollars per unit) that can vary widely multiplied by the number of units generates an amount to be billed. Each anesthetic has a base value number of units (e.g., 8 for a cholecystectomy) and then the time taken for the anesthetic is divided into units, usually 15 minutes per unit. Thus, a cholecystectomy with anesthesia time of 1 hour and 50 minutes would have 8 base units and 7.33 time units for a total of 15.33 units. In some practice settings, it may be allowed to add modifiers, such as extra units for complex patients with multiple problems as reflected by an ASA physical status classification of 3–5 and/or E ("emergency") or for insertion of an arterial or PA catheter. The sum is the total billing unit value. Determining the base value for an anesthetic in units depends on full and correct understanding of what operation was done. Although this sounds easy, it is the most difficult component of traditional anesthesia billing. The process of determining the procedure done is known as *coding* because the procedure name listed on the anesthesia record is assigned an identifying code number from the universally used current procedural terminology (CPT)-4 coding book. This code is then translated through the ASA "Relative Value Guide," which assigns a base unit value to the type of procedure identified by the CPT-4 code. In the past, some anesthesiologists failed to understand the importance of correct coding to the success of the billing process. Placing this task in the hands of someone unfamiliar with the system and with surgical terminology can easily lead to incorrect coding. This can fail to capture charges and the resulting income to which the anesthesiologist is entitled or, worse, can systematically overcharge the payers, which will bring sanctions, penalties and, in certain cases, criminal prosecution.

In recent years a prevailing official attitude has been that there are no simple, innocent coding errors. All upcoding (charging for more expensive services than were actually delivered) is considered to be prima facie evidence of fraud and is subject to severe disciplinary and legal action. All practices should have detailed compliance programs in place to ensure correct coding for services rendered.[36] Outside expert help (such as from a health care law firm that specializes in compliance programs) is highly desirable for the process of formulating and implementing a compliance plan regarding correct coding.

Assembly and transfer of the information necessary to generate bills must be efficient and complete. Traditionally, this involved depositing in a secure central location a paper extra copy of the anesthesia record and often a "billing sheet" with it, on which was inscribed the names of all the involved personnel and any additional information about other potentially billable services, such as invasive monitors. Any practice involved with a comprehensive electronic perioperative information management system in the facility should be using that to assemble this "front end" billing information. Short of that, some practices collect electronic information specifically generated by the anesthesia providers for that purpose. They have equipped each staff member with a hand-held organizer into which data are entered and then the device is synched with a departmental computer at the end of the day. If the OR suite has "Wi-Fi" (wireless electronic connection), the same function could be accomplished in real time with the providers entering the requisite information into a miniprogram on a laptop computer affixed to each anesthesia machine (or one carried by each staff member). Once the information has been secured, a mechanism must be employed to generate the actual bill and communicate it to the payer (on paper, on disk, or, usually, directly computer-to-computer: "electronic claims submission"). The possible exact arrangements for doing this vary widely.

Whether an anesthesia practice that will be billing and collecting for anesthesia services should employ its own in-house clerical and bookkeeping personnel to perform this function or should contract with an outside company whose sole function is medical billing and collecting (possibly, ideally, for anesthesiology only) can be debated endlessly. Whichever is chosen, knowledgeable oversight by the anesthesia professionals who ultimately will derive income from the revenue collected is required. Ultimately, the entity actually submitting the bill will verify that it has been paid (posting of receipts) and may or may not actually handle the incoming money. Very often, anesthesia practices or individuals who use a billing service (and even some who have in-house billing staffs) will arrange that the actual payments go directly to a bank lockbox, which is a post office box (better individual than shared, even if more expensive) to which the payments come and then go directly into a bank account. This system avoids the situation of having the people who generate the bill actually handle the incoming receipts, a practice that has led to theft and fraud in a few cases. Eventual decisions about how hard to try to collect from payers who deny coverage and then from patients directly will depend on the circumstances, including local customs.

Detailed summary statistics of the work done by an anesthesiology practice group are critical for logistic management of personnel, scheduling, and financial analysis. Spreadsheet and database computer programs customized for an individual practice's characteristics will be invaluable. A summary of the types of data an anesthesia practice should track is shown in

TABLE 2-1

TYPES OF DATA AN ANESTHESIOLOGY GROUP SHOULD TRACK AND MAINTAIN CONCERNING ITS OWN PRACTICE

Types of Data the Anesthesiology Group's Computer System Should Track
- Transaction-based system (track each case and charge as separate record)
  - Track individual charges by CPT-4 code
  - Track individual payments by payer
- Track all data elements on an interrelated basis
  - By place of service
  - By charge, broken down
    - by number of units (time and base)
    - by ASA modifiers
    - by number of lines
  - By CPT-4 code
  - By payer
  - By payment code (full payment, discount, write-off, or refund)
  - By diagnosis (ICD-9 code)
  - By surgeon
  - By anesthesiologist
  - By anesthesia care team provider
  - By start and stop times
  - By age
  - By gender
  - By employer
  - By ZIP code

Type of Information to Generate From These Data
- Aggregate number of cases per year for the group
- Total number of cases per year for each provider within the group
  - Number of cases performed by anesthesiologists
  - Number of cases performed by the anesthesia care team
- Average number of units per case (as one measure of intensity per case)
- Average number of units per CPT-4 code
- Average time units per case and per CPT-4 code
  - Group should be able to calculate time units per individual surgeon
- Average line charge per case
- Charges per case by CPT-4 code
- Payments per case by payer
- Patient mix
  - Percent traditional indemnity
  - Percent managed care (broken down by each MCO for which services are provided)
  - Percent self-pay
  - Percent Medicare
  - Percent Medicaid
- Collection rate for each population served
- Overall collection rate
- Costs per unit (total costs, excluding compensation ÷ total units) (costs include liability insurance, rent, collection costs, and legal and accounting fees)
- Compensation costs per unit (total compensation ÷ total units) for MCO populations, utilization patterns by age, gender, and diagnosis

CPT, current procedural terminology; ASA, American Society of Anesthesiologists; ICD-9, International Classification of Diseases, ninth revision; MCO, managed care organization.
Reprinted from Managed Care Reimbursement Mechanisms: A Guide for Anesthesiologists. Park Ridge, IL, American Society of Anesthesiologists, 1994, with permission.

Table 2-1. Once all the data are assembled and reviewed, at least monthly analysis by a business manager or equivalent as well as officers/leaders of the practice group can spot trends very early in their development and allow appropriate correction or planning. Often the responsible members of an anesthesiology group question how effective their financial services operation is, particularly regarding net collections. This is a complex issue[37] that, again, often requires outside help. Routine internal audits can be useful but could be self-serving. No billing office or company that is honest and completely above board should ever object to a client, in this case the anesthesiology practice group, engaging an independent outside auditor to come in and thoroughly examine both the efficiency of the operation and also "the books" concerning correctness and completeness of collections.

Anesthesia billing and collecting are among the most complex challenges in the medical reimbursement field. Traditional anesthesia reimbursement is unique in all of medicine. The experience of many people over the years has suggested that it often is well advised to deal with an entity that is not only very experienced in anesthesia billing, but also does anesthesia billing exclusively or as a large fraction of its efforts. It is very difficult for an anesthesiologist or a family member to do billing and collecting as a side activity to a normal life. This has led to inefficient and inadequate efforts in many cases, illustrating the value of paying a reasonable fee to a professional who will devote great time and energy to this challenging endeavor.

Antitrust Considerations

There can be antitrust implications of business arrangements involving anesthesiologists—particularly with all the realignments, consolidations, mergers, and contracts associated with the attempted implementation of managed care. The applicable statutes and regulations are often poorly understood. Contrary to popular belief, the antitrust laws do not involve the rights of individuals to engage in business. Rather, the laws are concerned solely with the preservation of competition within a defined marketplace and the rights of the consumer, independent of whether any one vendor or provider of service is involved. When an anesthesiologist has been excluded from a particular hospital's staff or anesthesia group and then sues based on an alleged antitrust violation, the anesthesiologist loses virtually automatically. This is because there is still significant competition in the relevant medical care marketplace (community or region) and competition in that market is not threatened by the exclusion of one physician from one staff.

In essence, if there are *several* hospitals offering relatively similar services to an immediate community (the market), denial of privileges to one physician by one hospital is not anticompetitive. If, on the other hand, there is only *one* hospital in a smaller market, then the same act, the same set of circumstances, could be seen very differently. In that case, there would be a limitation of competition because the hospital dominates and, in fact, may control the market for hospital services. Exclusion of one physician, then, could limit access by the consumers to alternative competing services and hence would likely be judged an antitrust violation.

The Sherman Antitrust Act is a federal law more than 100 years old. Section 1 deals with contracts, combinations, conspiracy, and restraint of trade. By definition, two or more separate economic entities must be involved in an agreement that is challenged as illegal for this section to apply. Section 2 prohibits monopolies or conspiracy to create a monopoly, and it is possible that this could apply to a single economic entity that has illegally gained domination of a market. Consideration of possible monopolistic domination of a market involves a situation in which a single entity controls at least 50% of the business in that market. The stakes are high in that the antitrust legislation provides for triple damages if a lawsuit is successful. The U.S. Department of Justice and the Federal Trade Commission are keenly interested in the current rapid evolution in the health care industry, and thus are actively involved in evaluating situations of possible antitrust violations.

There are two ways to judge violations. Under the *per se rule*, which is applied relatively rarely, conduct that is obviously limiting competition in a market is automatically illegal. The other type of violation is based on the *rule of reason*, which involves a careful analysis of the market and the state of competition. The majority of complaints against physicians are judged by this rule. The more competitors there are in a market, the less likely that any one act is anticompetitive. In a community with two hospitals, one smaller than the other, with an anesthesiology group practice exclusively at each, if the larger anesthesiology practice group buys out and absorbs the smaller, leaving only one group for the only two hospitals in the community, that may be anticompetitive, particularly if a new anesthesiologist seeks to practice solo at those hospitals.

Legal Implications

In the current era of rapidly evolving practice arrangements, the antitrust laws are important. If physicians (individuals or groups) who normally would be competitors because they are separate economic entities meet and agree on the prices they will charge or the terms they will seek in a managed care or institutional contract, that can be anticompetitive, monopolistic, and hence possibly illegal. Note that sharing a common office and common billing service alone is not enough to constitute a true group. If, on the other hand, the same physicians join in a true economic partnership to form a new group (total integration) that is a single economic entity (and meets certain other criteria) that will set prices and negotiate contracts, that is perfectly legal. The other criteria are critical. There must be capital investment and also risk sharing (if there is a profit or loss, it is distributed among the group members)—that is, total integration into a genuine partnership (that is usually incorporated, some times as a limited liability corporation). This issue is very important in considering the drive for new organizations to put together networks of physicians that then seek contracts with major employers to provide medical care. Sometimes, hospitals or clinics attempt to form a network comprising all the members of the medical staff so that the resulting entity can bid globally for total care contracts. Any network is a joint venture of independent practitioners. If the participating physicians of one specialty in a network are separate economic entities and the network advertises one price for their services, this would seem to suggest an antitrust violation (horizontal price fixing). In the past, if a network involved fewer than 20% of one type of medical specialist in a market, that was called a *safe harbor*, meaning that it was permissible for nonpartners to get together and negotiate prices. The federal government has tried to encourage formation of such networks to help reduce health care costs, and as a result made some relevant exceptions to the application of these rules. As long as the network is nonexclusive (other nonnetwork physicians of a given specialty are free to practice in the same facilities and compete for the same patients), the network can comprise up to 30% of the physicians of one specialty in a market. Note specifically that this does not allow a local specialty society in a big city to serve as a bargaining agent on fees for its members because it is very likely that >30% of the specialists in an area will be members of the society. The only real exception to this provision is in thinly populated rural areas where there may be just one physician network. In such cases (which are, so far, rare because the major managed care and network activity has occurred mainly in heavily populated urban areas), there is no limit on how many of one specialty can become network members and have the network negotiate fees, as long as the network is nonexclusive.

Relevant legislation, regulations, and court actions all happen rapidly and often. Mergers among anesthesiology groups in a market area for the purposes of both efficiency and strength in negotiating fees have been very popular as a response to the rapidly changing marketplace. A list of questions must be answered to determine if such a merger would have anticompetitive implications. Although compendia of relevant information are available to anesthesiologists,[38–40] they cannot substitute for expert advice and help. Obviously, anesthesiologists contemplating a merger or facing any one of a great number of other situations in the modern health care arena must secure assistance from professional advisors, usually attorneys, whose job it is to be aware of the most recent developments, how they apply, and how best to forge agreements in formal contracts. Anesthesiologists hoping to find reputable advisors can start their search with word-of-mouth referrals from colleagues who have used such services. Local or state medical societies frequently know of attorneys who specialize in this area. Finally, the ASA Washington, D.C., office has compiled a state-by-state list of advisors who have worked successfully with anesthesiologists in the past.

Exclusive Service Contracts

Often, one of the larger issues faced by anesthesiologists seeking to define practice arrangements concerns the desirability of considering an exclusive contract with a health care facility to provide anesthesia services. An exclusive contract states that anesthesiologists seeking to practice at a given facility must be members of the group holding the exclusive contract and, usually, that members of the group will practice nowhere else. A hospital may want to give an exclusive contract in return for a guarantee of coverage as part of the contract. Also, the hospital may believe that such a contract can help ensure the quality of practitioner because the contract can contain credentialing and performance criteria. It is important to understand that the hospital likely will exercise a degree of control over the anesthesiologists with such a contract in force, such as requiring them to participate as providers in any contracts the hospital makes with third-party payers and also tying hospital privileges to the existence of the contract (the so-called clean-sweep provision that bypasses any due process of the medical staff should the hospital terminate the contract). Certain of these types of provisions constitute *economic credentialing*, which is defined as the use of economic criteria unrelated to the quality of care or professional competency of physicians in granting or renewing hospital privileges (such as the acceptance of below-market fees associated with a hospital-negotiated care contract or even requiring financial contributions in some form to the hospital).

The ASA in 1993 issued a statement condemning economic credentialing.[1] The anesthesiologists involved may accept such an exclusive services contract to guarantee that they alone will get the business from the surgeons on staff at that hospital, and hence the resulting income. There may be other considerations on both sides, and these have been outlined in extensive relevant ASA publications that also include a sample contract for information purposes only.[36,39] Although many exclusive contracts with anesthesiology groups are in force, the sentiment, particularly from the ASA, is against them. As stated, it is critical that anesthesiologists faced with important practice management decisions such as whether to enter into an exclusive contract must seek outside advice and counsel. There are a great many nuances to these issues,[39–43] and anesthesiologists are at risk attempting to negotiate such complex matters alone, just as patients would be at risk if a contract attorney attempted to induce general anesthesia.

Denial of hospital privileges as a result of the existence of an exclusive contract with the anesthesiologists in place at the facility has been the source of many lawsuits, including the well-known Louisiana case of *Hyde v Jefferson Parish*. In that case, the court found for the defendant anesthesiologists and the hospital, saying that there was no antitrust violation because there was no real adverse effect on competition as far as patients were concerned because there were several other hospitals within the market to which they could go, and therefore they could exercise their rights to take advantage of competition in the relevant market. Thus, existence of an exclusive contract only in the rare setting where anticompetitive effects on patients can be proved might lead to a legitimate antitrust claim by a physician denied privileges. This was proven true in the *Kessel v Monongalia County General Hospital* case in West Virginia in which an exclusive anesthesiology contract was held illegal. Therefore, again, these arrangements are by definition complex and fraught with hazard. Accordingly, outside advice and counsel are always necessary.

Hospital Subsidies

Modern economic realities have forced a great number of anesthesiology practice groups (in both private and academic settings) to recognize that their patient care revenue, after overhead is paid, does not provide sufficient compensation to attract and retain the number and quality of staff necessary to provide the expected clinical service (and fulfill any other group/department missions). Attempting to do the same (or more) work with fewer staff may temporarily provide increased financial compensation. Cutting benefits (discretionary personal professional expenses, retirement contributions, or even insurance coverage) may also be a component of a response to inadequate practice revenue. However, the resulting decrements in personal security, in convenience, and in quality of life as far as acute and chronic fatigue, decreased family and recreation time, and tension among colleagues fearful someone else is getting a "better deal" will quickly overcome any brief advantage of a somewhat higher income. Therefore, many practice groups in such situations are requesting their hospital (or other health care facility where they practice) to pay them a direct cash subsidy that is used to augment practice revenue in order to maintain benefits and amenities while maintaining or even increasing the direct compensation to staff members, hopefully to a market-competitive level that will promote recruitment and retention of group members.

Obviously, requests by a practice group for a direct subsidy must be thoroughly justified to the facility administration receiving the petition. The group's business operation should already have been examined carefully for any possible defects or means to enhance revenue generation. Explanation of the general trend of declining reimbursements for anesthesia services should be carefully documented. Facts and figures on that and also the shortage of anesthesia providers can be obtained from journal articles and ASA publications, particularly the *Newsletter*. Demand for anesthesia coverage for the surgical schedule is a key component of this proposal. Scheduling and utilization, particularly if early-morning staffing is required for many ORs that are routinely unused later during the traditional work day, is a major issue to be understood and presented. Any other OR inefficiencies created by hospital support staff and previous efforts to deal with them should also be highlighted. Unfavorable payer mix, impact of contracts, and programs initiated by the hospital also often are major factors

6 in situations of inadequate practice revenue. Always, the group's good will with the surgeons and the community in general should be emphasized, as well as of the indirect or "behind the scenes" services and benefits the anesthesiology group provides to the hospital. Note that the necessity for such a subsidy request is precisely the time when the anesthesia professionals will benefit from being perceived as "good citizens" of the health care facility. An overly aggressive effort beyond the bounds of logic could provoke the facility to consider alternative arrangements, even up to the point of putting out a request for proposal from other anesthesiology practice groups. Therefore, thoughtful calculations are required and a careful balance must be sought, seeking enough financial support to supplement practice revenues so that members' compensation is competitive but not so much as to be excessive. Supporting statements and documents about offers and potential earnings elsewhere must be completely honest and not exaggerated or credibility and good faith will be lost. Further, part of any agreement will be the full sharing of the group's detailed financial information with the facility administration, both at the time of the request and on an ongoing basis if the payment is more than a one-time "bail out." Plans for review and renewal should be made once a subsidy is paid.

Any subsidy will likely require a formal contract. There may be concern about malpractice liability implications for the hospital even though the practice group stays an independent entity as before. There may be "inurement" or "private benefit" concerns that could be perceived as a threat to the tax-exempt status of a nonprofit hospital. Lack of understanding of the applicable laws may lead to fears that a subsidy could be an illegal "kickback" or a violation of the Stark II self-referral prohibition. As is almost always the case, expert outside professional consultant advice, usually from an attorney who specializes exclusively in health care finance contracting, is mandatory in such circumstances. The ASA Washington, D.C., office maintains lists of consultants who have helped other anesthesiologists or groups in the past with various subjects, and the ASA has some basic information on subsidies to anesthesiology practice groups.[44–46]

New Practice Arrangements

Even though the impact of managed care plans has waned somewhat over the first decade of the 21st century, various iterations still exist and have ongoing impact on anesthesiology practice. Further, renewed concern at the end of the decade about disproportionate increases in health care spending as a percentage of U.S. gross domestic product and the fear of the postulated bankruptcy of Medicare and Medicaid again raise the specter of new efforts to impose managed care.

7 In the initial stages of the evolution of a managed care marketplace, the MCO usually seeks contracts with providers based on discounted fee-for-service arrangements. This preserves the basic traditional idea of production-based physician reimbursement (do more, bill more) but the price of each act of services is lower (the providers are induced to give deep discounts with the promise of significant volumes of patients); also, the MCO gatekeeper primary care physicians and the MCO reviewers are strongly encouraged to limit complex and costly services as much as possible. There are other features intermittently along the way, such as global fees and negotiated fee schedules (agreed-upon single prices for individual procedures, independent of length or complexity). In an application of the concept of risk-sharing (spend too much for patient care and lose income), this usually is initially manifest in the form of "withholds," the practice of the MCO holding back a fraction of the agreed-upon payment to the providers (e.g., 10 or 15%) and keeping this money until the end of the

fiscal year. At that time, if there is any money left in the risk pool or withhold account after all the (partial) provider fees and MCO expenses are paid, it is distributed to the providers in proportion to their degree of participation during the year. This is a clever and powerful incentive to providers to reduce health care expenses. It is not as powerful as the stage of full risk-sharing, however. As the managed care marketplace matures and MCOs grow and succeed, the existing organizations and, especially any new ones, shift to prospective capitated payments for providers.

Prospective Payments

Prospective capitated payments constitutes an entirely new world to health care providers, involving prospective capitated payments for large populations of patients, in which each group of providers in the MCO receives a fixed amount per enrolled covered life (member) per month (PMPM) and agrees, except in the most unusual circumstances, to provide whatever care is needed by that population for that prospective payment. The most unusual circumstances involve "carve-out" arrangements in which specific very costly and unusual conditions or procedures (such as the birth of a child with disastrous multiple congenital anomalies) are covered separately on a discounted fee-for-service basis. With full capitation, the entire financial underpinning of American medical care does a complete about-face from the traditional rewards for giving more care and doing more procedures to new rewards for giving and doing less. Some managed care contracts contain other features intended to protect the providers against unexpected overutilization by patients that would stretch the providers beyond the bounds of the original contract with the MCO. The provisions setting the boundaries are called *risk corridors*, and the "stop-loss clauses" add some discounted fee-for-service payment for the excess care beyond the risk corridor (capitated contract limit). Providers who were used to getting paid more for doing more can suddenly find themselves getting paid a fixed amount no matter how much or how little they do with regard to a specified population—hence, the perceived incentive to do, and consequently spend, less. If the providers render too much care within the defined boundary of the contract, they essentially will be working for free, the ultimate in risk-sharing.

There are clearly potential internal conflicts in such a system,[47] and how patients reacted initially to this radical change in attitude on the part of physicians demonstrated that this overall mechanism is unlikely to be readily embraced by the general public. Health care providers (physicians, other health care professionals, and facilities), in turn, allied themselves in a wide variety of organizations to create strength and desirable resources to present to the MCOs in contract negotiations. Management service organizations are joint-venture network arrangements that do not involve true economic integration among the practitioners, but merely offer common services to physicians who may, as a loosely organized informal group, elect to seek MCO contracts. Preferred provider organizations are network arrangements of otherwise economically independent physicians who form a new corporate entity to seek managed care contracts in which there are significant financial incentives to patients to use the network providers and financial penalties for going to out-of-network providers. This has proved a relatively popular model and appears to be gaining wide acceptance. Physician–hospital organizations are similar entities but involve understandings between groups of physicians and a hospital so that a large package or bundle of services can be constructed as essentially one-stop points of care. Independent practice associations are like preferred provider organizations but are specifically oriented toward capitated contracts for covered lives with significant risk-sharing by the providers. Groups (or clinics) "without walls" are collections of practitioners who fully integrate economically into a single fiscal entity (true partnership) and then compete for MCO contracts on the basis of risk-sharing incentives among the partners. Fully integrated groups or health maintenance organizations (such as Kaiser Permanente in California or Harvard Pilgrim Health in New England) house the group of partner provider physicians and associated support staff at a single location for the convenience of patients, a big selling point when they seek MCO or employer contracts.

Changing Paradigm

The era of solo independent practitioners may be ending in some locations where MCOs dominate because the organizations simply will not contract with one person. Independent hospital-based groups (likely still the most common private practice model) may face growing similar difficulties.[48] These smaller groups of anesthesiologists may find themselves at a competitive disadvantage unless they become part of a vertically integrated (multispecialty) or horizontally integrated (with other anesthesiologists) organization. An extensive compendium of relevant information has been prepared by the ASA.[38] Because it appears likely that many anesthesiologists in the United States will be affected by evolving changes in practice arrangements, the information in this and related publications[49] is very important. Negotiations with MCOs require expert advice, probably even more so than the traditional exclusive contracts with hospitals as previously noted. Before any negotiation can even be considered, the MCO must provide significant amounts of information about the covered patient population. The projected health care utilization pattern of a large group of white-collar workers (and their families) from major upscale employers in an urban area will be quite different from that of a relatively rural Medicaid population. Specific demographics and past utilization histories are absolutely mandatory for each proposed population to be covered, and this information should go directly to the advising experts for evaluation, whether the proposed negotiation is for discounted fee-for-service, a fee schedule, global bundled fees, or full capitation.

Significant questions were pointedly raised about the reimbursement implications for anesthesiologists of the putative managed care/practice reorganization revolution. Again, the ASA has assembled relevant information, the understanding of which is essential to successful negotiations.[38] Table 2-1 has a list of information an anesthesia practice should have about its activities. Initial consideration of a capitated contract should involve an attempt to take all the data about the existing practice and the proposed MCO-covered population from a "capitation checklist"[38] and translate back from the proposed capitated rate to income figures that would correlate with the existing practice structure, to allow a comparison and an understanding of the relationship of the projected work in the contract the to projected income from it. It is, of course, impossible to suggest dollar values for capitated rates for anesthesiology care because details and conditions vary so widely. One ASA publication[38] used examples, purely for illustrative purposes, involving $2.50 or $4.00 PMPM, but there were unconfirmed reports at the peak of the managed care bubble of capitated rates as low as $0.75 PMPM for anesthesiology.

Discounted fee-for-service arrangements are easier for anesthesiologists to understand because these are directly referable to existing fee structures. Reports of groups instituting 10 to 50% discounts off the starting point of 80% of usual and customary reimbursement in various practice circumstances were circulated at national meetings of anesthesiologists. Were rigidly controlled fully mature managed care to dominate the practice community, it would be likely that the average income

for anesthesiologists would decrease from past levels. However, it likely also would be true that anesthesia professionals would continue to have incomes still above average among all health care professionals in that market.

Another recent feature of this discussion is the tendency of private (nongovernmental) contracting organizations to attempt to tie their payments for professional services to the government's Medicare rate for specific CPT-4 codes. It is common for both commercial indemnity insurance entities (e.g., Blue Shield, Aetna, Humana, United Health) as well as MCOs to offer primary care physicians, for example, 125% of the Medicare payment rate for specific services. Although groups of primary care physicians may view this as somewhat reasonable and, thus, they sign such contracts, anesthesiologists face unique challenges in this regard. Even with the most recent promise from the responsible offices within Medicare of a reimbursement upgrade for anesthesia services, most anesthesia professionals still believe that the Medicare reimbursement rate is unfairly low for the work involved in providing anesthesia care. The new rate would still be less than half the per unit "conversion factor" that the large indemnity carriers have been paying for anesthesia care in recent years. Therefore, 125% of what many anesthesia professionals consider woefully inadequate would still be inadequate. Thus, in spite of sometimes intense pressure, anesthesia professionals in many markets have been reluctant to accept indemnity insurance contract rates tied to Medicare rates. As always, anesthesia professionals faced with complex reimbursement situations and decisions should seek expert advice from the national offices of their professional practice organizations and from knowledgeable paid consultants and attorneys.

"Pay for Performance"

Commercial indemnity insurance entities (e.g., Blue Shield, Aetna, Humana, United Health), MCOs, and particularly, the federal Center for Medicare and Medicaid Services (CMS) are all currently fixated on the concept of "performance-based payments" as a significant new way to limit the growth of (and even reduce) health care costs,[50] especially by reducing expensive complications of medical care. This "pay for performance" movement began with the federal Tax Relief and Healthcare Act of 2006 and continues with the Physician Quality Reporting Initiative in 2008. The potential implications for anesthesia practice have been summarized.[51]

In general, CMS made strenuous efforts to attempt to define and promulgate objective quality measures that could be documented as indicators of the "quality" of health care delivered. The main issue is the promotion of specific care elements that help avoid expensive outcomes or complications that currently generate a disproportionate (preventable) fraction of health care costs. The administration of aspirin and beta-blockers within a fixed brief interval after the arrival of an acute myocardial infarction patient is a good example, as are various parameters in the care of patients with community-acquired pneumonia or congestive heart failure. Defining and validating objective and easily quantifiable so-called quality measures that will prevent expensive complications of anesthesia care proved to be more difficult. The initial targeted parameter was somewhat indirect: the timing of the administration of prophylactic antibiotics prior to surgical incision. The anesthesia professional is judged to be in compliance when the antibiotic is administered within the 1 hour (2 hours for vancomycin and fluoroquinolones) prior to incision. This must be verifiably documented on the anesthesia record. Benchmark criteria such as an initial 80% compliance (but likely increasing to at least 95%) for a specific financial entity billing Medicare and Medicaid must be met or the reimbursement for anesthesia services by that financial entity will be reduced by a specific fraction (or a promised "bonus" will be withheld) as a compliance incentive, but also somewhat as an offset to the increased cost of the consequent complications associated with failure to comply. If performance is in compliance, CMS will pay the maximum allowable reimbursement (pay for performance).

The second target is catheter-related bloodstream infection, and the performance behavior expected of anesthesia professionals is observance of strict aseptic protocol during central vascular catheter placement (and avoiding the femoral route if at all possible). As of this writing, the third objective parameter of anesthesia care quality is scheduled to target temperature management of the surgical patient with the compliance behavior being met by achieving one of three possible goals: use of active warming intraoperative or documented temperature $\geq 36°C$ either in the last 30 minutes of anesthesia or the first 30 minutes in the PACU. Future potential objective performance criteria intended to encourage avoidance of costly complications of anesthesia care may include glucose control in major surgery, use of pencil-point spinal needles in obstetric anesthesia, use of electronic medical records, preoperative screening for sleep apnea, preoperative fasting instructions, meperidine administration for postoperative shivering, and several others. In all cases when a parameter is adopted, benchmark criteria for degree of compliance will be established and reimbursement will be reduced one way or another for failure to comply, as documented on the relevant records and self-reported by the billing financial entity (subject to audit, of course).

Hospitals will have even more at stake in the sense that the pay for performance movement is creating paradigms in which hospitals will not receive reimbursements for care associated with preventable complications such as catheter-related sepsis, ventilator-acquired pneumonia, and decubitus ulcers. This concept has several implications. One is that smaller hospitals often populated by less acute patients will be more likely and quicker to transfer sicker patients to larger referral facilities in order to avoid losing reimbursement associated with the development of patient complications. Concomitantly, documentation of the timing of the development of complications will become critical. If a hospital or department has documented the pre-existing presence of a complication at the time of a patient's admission, it should not be penalized for the development of that condition. In this context, anesthesia professionals can have an important role documenting the existence of pneumonia or sacral decubitus ulcers in their records when they first see a newly admitted patient, usually for preoperative evaluation. This will be perceived as excellent institutional citizenship by the anesthesia professional because it may prevent significant reimbursement reduction to the hospital.

HIPAA

The 2003 implementation of the Privacy Rule of the Health Insurance Portability and Accountability Act (HIPAA) of 1996 required significant changes in how medical records and patient information are handled in the day-to-day delivery of health care. The impact on and requirements for anesthesiologists are summarized in a comprehensive publication from the ASA[52] that followed two educational summaries.[53,54]

Attention is focused on "protected health information" (identifiable as from a specific patient by name). Patients must be notified of their privacy rights. Usually this will be covered by the health care facility in which anesthesiologists work, but if separate private records are maintained, separate notification may be necessary. Privacy policies must be created, adopted, and promulgated to all practitioners, all of whom then must be trained in application of those policies. Often,

anesthesiology groups can combine with the facilities in which they practice as an "organized health care arrangement" so that the anesthesia practitioners can be covered in part by the HIPAA compliance activities of the facility. A "privacy officer" must be appointed for the practice group. Finally, and most importantly, medical records containing protected health information must be secured so they are not readily available to those who do not need them to render care.

One of the most obvious applications for many anesthesiologists is concern about the assembled preoperative information and charts for tomorrow's cases that frequently were placed prominently in the OR holding area at the end of one work day in readiness for the next day's cases. HIPAA provisions require that all that patient information be locked away overnight. Another classic example is what many ORs refer to as "the board." Often, a large white dry-marker board occupies a prominent wall near the front desk of an OR suite, and the rooms, cases, and personnel assignments are inscribed thereon at the beginning of the day and modified or crossed off as the day progresses. Under HIPAA, patients' names may not be used on such a board if there is any chance that anyone not directly involved in their care could see them. Alternatively, some facilities tape a copy of the day's OR schedule (including patients' names, ages, and operations) on the wall, which would also be a violation. The same is true for similar boards or posted schedules in OR holding areas and PACUs. Another issue often overlooked that is very problematic and probably the one that concerns patients the most is the obtaining of history information in a location, such as a "bed slot" behind just a curtain in the OR holding area, where sensitive medical and personal information is spoken out loud within earshot of other patients, other patients' families, and noninvolved caregivers. This concern is difficult to address and there is no one universally applicable suggestion. However, anesthesia professionals who interact with patients in such environments should be as sensitive as physically possible to being overheard and also should bring such concerns to the attention of the facility administrators.

Further, many anesthesiology practices also must apply HIPAA provisions to their billing operations; the details will vary depending on the mechanisms used and a great deal will depend on which type of electronic claims submission software is being used by the billing entity actually submitting the claims.[55] Telephone calls and faxes into offices must be handled specially if containing identifiable patient information. Presentation of patient information for QA or teaching purposes must be free of all identifiers unless specific individual permission has been obtained on prescribed printed forms. Requests for patient information from a wide variety of outside entities, including insurance companies and collection agencies, must be processed in HIPAA-compliant ways. HIPAA policy and actions, as well as enforcement activities, are being developed over time and as situations develop. This system depends in part on patient complaints for both enforcement and policy evolution. In many practices and practice locations, there have been few or even no formal complaints of violations of patient privacy, indicating the initial implementation of HIPAA compliance may have largely had the desired effect.

Electronic Medical Records

Databases, spreadsheets, and electronic transfer of information are nonspecific features that have been applied to health care. The classic medical record, on the other hand, has required the creation of entirely new software in an attempt to duplicate the function of the handwritten or dictated traditional "chart." This has afforded opportunities to multiple competing commercial entities to attempt to fill this need. Usually, competing proprietary systems are incompatible and do not "talk to each other." This fact severely limits one of the highly touted benefits of medical practices "going electronic." Cost is another great barrier, as is the formidable task of entering the required information from the old paper records into the electronic system. There has been governmental and public pressure for health care institutions, facilities, and practices to adopt electronic records because of the potential for increased legibility causing reduction in errors and confusion, greater speed of filing and retrieval, easy transmission of large amounts of information (such as from a surgeon's office to an anesthesia practice's booking office and also to a hospital's preoperative clinic or OR holding area), and QA monitoring of vast databases. Increased ease of transmission and filing of reimbursement claims and cost savings from clerical staff down-sizing are claims intended to encourage physician practice groups to adopt electronic medical records (EMRs). However, experience to date has suggested that the commercially available software systems (both for institutions and practice groups) are not as robust or reliable as advertised by their often aggressive manufacturers. Accordingly, the expected benefits have not materialized quite as predicted, particularly in that costs have been great, often far in excess of estimates, and cost savings have been minimal at best. Practice groups of anesthesia professionals should consider all of these noted points prior to investing in an EMR system. At minimum, careful study and evaluation of the same system already in place in another anesthesiology practice should be undertaken.

If basic EMR implementation has been problematic for practices, true electronic anesthesia information management systems have been even more difficult. These include preoperative, intraoperative, postoperative, billing, and QA components. For the actual OR anesthesia record, several commercial versions are available. Different anesthesia professionals have various opinions about ease of implementation and subsequent use. Unless one massive bolus of fully integrated new technology from a single manufacturer is installed all at one time, integration of a new EMR with the existing anesthesia machines and monitors to ensure full accurate capture of all data parameters can often be difficult and frustrating. The function and value of electronic anesthesia records can be debated endlessly. All of them today will require computers on or in the anesthesia machine. These computers should be Internet-enabled so that demographic and billing information can be automatically uploaded to the facility's and the practice's database. Any such system must also integrate with the billing systems of the facility and the practice or the touted benefits will be largely negated. Again, the best, and in some senses, the only way to evaluate seriously and thoroughly a proposed major investment of money, effort, and time is to visit a fully up-and-working installation of that electronic anesthesia information management system and talk directly in detail with the users. The costs, in all senses of the word, are so great that it remains a significant gamble to be the first to purchase and implement such a system.

Expansion Into Perioperative Medicine, Hospital Care, and Hyperbaric Medicine

Some anesthesiologists now function at least some of the time in preoperative screening clinics because of the great fraction of OR patients who do not spend the night before surgery in the hospital or who do not come to a hospital at all. In such settings, these anesthesiologists frequently assume a role analogous to that of a primary care physician, planning and executing a workup of one or more significant medical or surgical

problems before the patient can reasonably be expected to undergo surgery. Likewise, this concept would be excellent for the postoperative period. An anesthesiologist, completely free of OR or other duties, could not only make at least twice-daily rounds of patients after surgery and provide exceedingly comprehensive pain-management service, but also could follow the surgical progress and make reports (likely via an EMR or e-mail) to the surgeon's office or alphanumeric pocket communicator. A fundamental aspect of the practice of anesthesiology is the management of acute problems in the hospital setting. It is logical that anesthesiologists would be among the physicians best suited to provide primary care for patients in the hospital setting.

An additional evolving opportunity is the creation and implementation of "rapid response teams" within acute care hospitals. In essence, studies have revealed that patients on general care nursing floors sometimes begin to deteriorate and, for one reason or another but often because of the responsible physician being unavailable or at a considerable distance at that moment, the patients are not evaluated or treated in a timely manner and often not until they have further deteriorated, sometimes to a critical status. Therefore, a national trend has developed in which hospitals create a team of knowledgeable professionals (who have other regular responsibilities) who usually have no prior knowledge of the deteriorating patient but who will respond within a very few minutes to the call from (usually) a floor nurse who detects a deteriorating patient (e.g., increasing fever, relative hypotension and tachycardia, absent urine output). Frequently, the rapid response team institutes immediate symptomatic treatment, arranges for a higher acuity level of care, and contacts the primary responsible physician. Importantly, in larger hospitals, it has been suggested that the in-house anesthesiologists are uniquely qualified to be key members of the rapid response team because the interventions almost always involve acute "bread-and-butter" resuscitative care. Although many anesthesiologists may believe they already have plenty of work in the OR, such participation when possible would be an outstanding and highly visible contribution to the hospital's mission of enhanced patient care. Also, such interventions could be separately billable encounters as consultations or, alternatively, excellent support for the maintenance or even increase of the hospital's financial subsidy to its anesthesia professional group.

Finally, anesthesiologists in some locations have become involved in the practice of hyperbaric medicine and wound care. This is likely related to the familiarity of anesthesiologists with concepts of gas laws and physics, along with their constant presence in the hospital. The treatment of various medical conditions by the application of oxygen under increased pressure, usually 2 to 3 atmospheres absolute, at one time was one of the more rapidly growing hospital services. Anesthesiologists are among the leaders of this field, with unlimited opportunities for clinical care, teaching, and research. Even a brief discussion of this field is outside the scope of this chapter, and interested readers are referred to the Undersea and Hyperbaric Medical Society (www.umhs.org).

OPERATING ROOM MANAGEMENT

The role of anesthesiologists in OR management has changed dramatically in the past few years. With the current climate of a considerable shortage of anesthesia professionals, hospitals subsidizing many anesthesiology group practices, and an increasing workload, participation in OR management is essentially mandatory. The current emphasis on cost containment and efficiency will force anesthesiologists to take an active role in eliminating many dysfunctional aspects of OR practice that were previously ignored. First-case morning start times have changed from a suggestion to a mandate. Delays of any sort are now often tracked electronically in real time and carefully scrutinized to eliminate waste and inefficiency. Together, anesthesiologists, surgeons, OR nurses and technicians, and increasingly, professional administrators/managers need to determine who is best qualified to be a leader in the day-to-day management of the OR.[56] Clearly, different groups have different perspectives. However, anesthesiologists are in the best position to see the "big picture," both overall and on any given day. Surgeons are commonly elsewhere before and after their individual cases (and sometimes for the beginning and the end of their cases); nurses and administrators may lack the medical knowledge to make appropriate, timely decisions, often "on the fly." It is the anesthesiologist with the insight, overview, and unique perspective who is best qualified to provide leadership in an OR community. The subsequent recognition and appreciation from the other groups (especially hospital administration) will clearly establish the anesthesiologists as concerned physicians genuinely interested in the welfare of the OR and the institution.

Organization

The symbiotic relationship between anesthesia professionals and surgeons remains unchanged. Both groups recognize this fact and also the common goal of having the OR function in a safe, expeditious manner. The age-old question, "Who is in charge of the operating room?" still confronts many hospitals/institutions. Because some anesthesiology groups are subsidized by the hospital, the OR organization in such cases has changed accordingly. Many hospital administrators want to have input regarding who is in charge of the OR with an eye to increasing efficiency and throughput while reducing cost. Their wishes have an even added significance when more of their dollars are involved through the anesthesiology group subsidy. Sometimes there can be no real answer to, "Who's in charge?" because of the complexity of the interpersonal relationships in the OR. Some institutions have a professional manager (often a former OR registered nurse) whose sole job is to organize and run the OR. This individual may be vested with enough authority to be recognized by all as the person in charge. Other institutions ostensibly have a "medical director of the OR." However, the implications to the surgeons that an anesthesiologist is in charge, or vice versa, have caused many institutions to abandon the title or retain the position but assign no authority to it. In such instances, institutions usually resolve disputes through some authority with a physician's perspective. If there is no medical director with authority to make decisions stick, central authority usually resides with the OR committee, most often populated by physicians, senior nurses, and administrators. Every OR has this forum for major policy and fiscal decisions. As part of committee function, the standard practices of negotiation, diplomacy, and lobbying for votes are regularly carried out. The impact of such an OR committee varies widely among institutions.

Despite the constantly changing dynamics of the OR management and the frequent major frustrations, anesthesiologists should pursue a greater role in day-to-day management in every possible applicable practice setting. An anesthesiologist who is capable of facilitating the start of cases with minimal delays and solving problems "on the fly" as they arise will be in an excellent position to serve his or her department. Succeeding in this role will have a dramatic positive impact on all the OR constituents. The surgeons will be less concerned about who is in charge because their cases are getting done. The hospital administration will welcome the effort because they want something extra in return for any money they are now giving to the anesthesiology groups as a subsidy. Furthermore, the OR committee (or whatever system for dispute resolution is in place) is still functional and has not been circumvented (and will be thankful for the absence of disputes needing resolution).

Some institutions use the term *Clinical Director of the OR*. The person awarded this designation should be a senior-level individual with first-hand knowledge of the OR environment and function. Anesthesiologists have a better understanding of the perioperative process. They possess the medical knowledge to make appropriate decisions. Their intimate association with surgeons and their patients allows them to best allocate resources. The American Association of Clinical Directors in 2002 reported that 71% of survey respondents stated that an anesthesiologist was designated as the Clinical Director of the OR.

Contact and Communication

An important issue for the anesthesia professionals in any OR setting is who among the group will be the contact person to interact with the OR and its related administrative functions. In situations in which everyone is an independent contractor, there may be a titular chief who by design is the contact person. The anesthesiologist in this role commonly changes yearly to spread the duties among all the members. Large groups or departments that function as the sole providing entity for that hospital/facility often identify an individual as the contact person to act as the voice for the department. Furthermore, these same groups delineate someone on a daily basis to be the clinical director, or the person "running the board." Frequently, this position is best filled by one of a small dedicated fraction of the group (e.g., three people) rather than rotating the responsibility among every member of the group. Experienced "board runners" have an instinctually derived better perspective on the nuances of managing the operating schedule in real time. Certain procedures may require specific training (e.g., transesophageal echocardiography skills) that not all members of the group possess. Clearly, changes sometimes have to be made to match the ability of the anesthesia provider and the requirements of the procedure when urgent or emergent cases are posted.

Another benefit of a very small number of daily clinical directors is a relative consistency in the application of OR policies, particularly in relationship to the scheduling of cases, especially add-ons. One of the most frustrating aspects to both surgeons and OR personnel is unpredictability and inconsistency in the decisions made by the anesthesia group/department members. A patient deemed unacceptable for surgery by anesthesiologist X on Monday may be perfectly acceptable, in the same medical condition, for anesthesiologist Y on Tuesday. Disagreements are inevitable in any large group. However, day-to-day OR function may be hampered by a large number of these types of circumstances. Having one member of a very small group in charge will lead to more consistency in this process, especially if the board runner/clinical director has the authority to switch personnel to accommodate the situation. Without stifling individual practices, philosophies, and comfort levels, a certain amount of consistency applied to similar clinical scenarios will improve OR function immeasurably. These few dedicated directors should be able to accomplish both goals better than a large rotating group.

A newer potential component of intra-OR communications is the concept of checklists and team briefings. Analogous to the now-required "time out" in each OR prior to surgical incision when the correct identity of the patient, the intended procedure, and any laterality involved is verified, some ORs are attempting to have a similar interprofessional communication involving all relevant OR personnel (the team) prior to the patient entering the actual OR, during which the involved surgeon, anesthesia professional, circulating nurse, scrub person, and support persons as indicated each acknowledge a summary of what is projected to take place in this case, any anticipated need for extra or unusual resources or equipment, any anticipated difficulties or increased risks, and specific plans to deal with any feature of any of these points that would require intervention. In many models, a printed single-page checklist with routine prompts and fill-in boxes is used to facilitate the process. One study reported a two-thirds' reduction in "communication failures" that have otherwise likely caused problems, risks, or inefficiencies.[57]

Materials Management

Usually, the institutional component of the anesthesia service staffs and maintains a location containing the specific supplies unique to the practice of anesthesia ("the workroom"). Objectives necessary for efficient materials management include the standardization of equipment, drugs, and supplies. Avoidance of duplication, volume purchasing, and inventory reduction are also worthwhile. There needs to be coordination with the OR staff as to who is responsible for acquisition of routine hospital supplies such as syringes, needles, tubing, and intravenous fluids. Decisions as to which brands of which supplies to purchase ideally should be made as a group. Often, when several companies compete against each other in an open market, lower prices are negotiable. These negotiations may occur between the anesthesia professionals and the hospital administration, or by the physician components of the OR committee. In many cases, however, hospitals belong to large buying groups that determine what brands and models of equipment and supplies will be available, with no exceptions possible except at greatly increased cost. Sometimes, this is false economy if the provided items are inferior (cheap) or annoying and, for example, if it routinely takes opening three or four intravenous cannulae in the process of starting a preoperative intravenous line as opposed to the higher quality and reliable single one that may cost more per cannula but is less expensive overall because far fewer will be used. Dispassionate presentation of such logic by a respected team-player senior anesthesiologist to the OR committee or director of materials management may help resolve such conundrums.

Scheduling Cases

Anesthesiologists need to participate in the OR scheduling process at their facility or institution. In some facilities the scheduling office and the associated clerical personnel work under the anesthesia group. Commonly, scheduling falls under the OR staff's responsibility. Direct control of the schedule usually resides with the OR supervisor or charge person, frequently a nurse. Whatever the arrangements, the anesthesia group must have a direct line of communication with the scheduling system. The necessary number of anesthesia professionals that must be supplied often changes on a daily basis per the caseload and sometimes because of institutional policy decisions. After-hours call must be arranged, policy changes factored in, and additions/subtractions to the surgical load (day-to-day, week-to-week, and long-term as surgical practices come and go in that OR) dealt with as well. These issues are important even when all the anesthesia professionals are independently contracted and are not affiliated with each other. In such situations, the titular chief of anesthesia should be the one to act as the link to the scheduling system. When the anesthesia group/department functions as a single entity, the chairman/chief, clinical director, or appointed spokesperson will be the individual who represents his or her group at meetings in which scheduling decisions are made in conjunction with the OR supervisors, surgeons, and hospital administrators.

There are as many different ways to create scheduling policies as there are OR suites. Most hospitals/facilities follow patterns established over the years. Despite all the efforts directed toward its creation, the OR schedule (both weekly time allotments and day-to-day scheduling of specific cases) remains one of the most contentious subjects for the OR. Recognizing the fact that it is impossible to satisfy everyone, the anesthesia group should endeavor to facilitate the process as much as possible. Initially, anesthesiologists need to be sympathetic toward all the surgeons' desires/demands (stated or implied) and attempt to coordinate these requests with the institution's ability to provide rooms, equipment, and staff. Secondly, the anesthesia group should make every possible effort to provide enough anesthesia services and personnel to realistically meet the goals of the institution. In light of the current shortage of anesthesia professionals in this country, these efforts need to be made with a great deal of open communication among all contingencies of the OR committee as well as every member of the anesthesia group.

Regarding scheduling, surgeons essentially fall into one of three groups. One group wants to operate any time they can get their cases scheduled. This group wants the OR open 24/7. Another larger group wants "first case of the day" as often as possible so they can get to their offices. A smaller third group wants either the first time slot or an opening following that time slot, a several-hour hiatus, then to return to the OR after office hours to complete additional cases; usually starting after 5 PM. Clearly a compromise among these disparate constituencies must be reached. Anesthesiologists who approach the OR committee regarding this dilemma with a nonconfrontational attitude will greatly facilitate agreement on a compromise.

Types of Schedules

The majority of ORs use either block scheduling (preassigned guaranteed OR time for a surgeon or surgical service to schedule cases prior to an agreed-upon cut-off time; e.g., 24 or 48 hours before) or open scheduling (first come, first serve). Most large institutions have a combination of both. Block scheduling inherently contains several advantageous aspects for creating a schedule. Block scheduling allows for more predictability in the daily OR function as well as an easy review of utilization of allotted time. Historic utilization data should be reviewed with surgeons, OR staff, and the OR committee to determine its validity. Many operating suites have found it useful to assemble rather comprehensive statistics about what occurs in each OR. Some computerized scheduling systems (see following discussion) are part of a larger computerized perioperative information management system that automatically generates statistics. Graphic examples are 13-month "statistical control charts" or "run charts" that show the number of cases, number of OR minutes used for those cases (and when, such as in block, exceeding block, evenings, nights, weekends, and so forth), number of cancellations (and multiple other related parameters if desired) by service, by individual surgeon, and total for the current month and the 12 prior months, always with "control limits" (usually 2 SD from the 13-month moving average) clearly indicated. All these data are valuable in that they generate a clear picture of what is actually going on in the OR. It is also extremely valuable in that block time allocation should be reviewed periodically and adjusted based on changes, degree of utilization, and projected needs. Inflexible block time scheduling can create a major point of contention if the assigned blocks are not regularly reevaluated. The surgeon or surgical service with the early starting block that habitually runs beyond his or her block time will create problems for the following cases. If this surgeon were made to schedule into the later block on a rotating basis, delays in his or her start caused by others may provoke improved accuracy of his or her subsequent early case postings. Adjustments in availability of block time can also be made in the setting of the "release time," the time prior to the operative date that a given block is declared not full and becomes available for open scheduling. Surgeons prefer as late a release time as possible in order to maintain their access to their OR block time. However, unused reserved block time wastes resources and prevents another service from scheduling. A single release time rarely fits all circumstances, but negotiating service-specific release times may lead to improved satisfaction for all. In the ideal system, enough OR time and equipment should exist to provide for each surgical service's genuine needs while retaining the ability to add to the schedule (via open scheduling) as needed. Such an environment does not exist. Invariably, in busy environments, surgical demand exceeds available block and open time, leading services to request additional block time. When this time is not granted, services perversely then schedule procedures in open time before filling their block time. Surgeons who prefer open time would then be shut out of OR time. Open scheduling may reward those surgeons who run an efficient service, but it also may be a source of problems to those surgeons who have a significant portion of their service arrive unscheduled, such as orthopaedic surgeons. Some degree of flexibility will be necessary whichever system is used. The anesthesia group should adopt a neutral position in these discussions while being realistic about what can be accomplished given the number of ORs and the length of the normal operating day.

The handling of the urgent/emergent case posting precipitates a great deal of discussion in most OR environments. No studies allow determination of exactly what rate of OR utilization is the most cost-effective. However, many institutions subscribe to following parameters: adjusted utilization rates averaging below 70% are not associated with full use of available block time, wasting resources, while rates above 90% are frequently associated with the need for overtime hours.[58] Different OR constituencies have different comfort zones for degrees of utilization (Table 2-2). Most institutions cannot afford to have one or two ORs staffed and waiting unless there is a reliable steady supply of late open-schedule additions, that is, urgent cases/emergencies, during the regular work day. A previously agreed-upon, clear algorithm for the acceptance and ordering of these cases will need to be adopted. In general, critical life-threatening emergencies and elective add-ons are fairly straightforward and at the two ends of the spectrum. The critical emergency goes in the next available room, whereas the elective case gets added to the end of the schedule.

The so-called urgent patient requires the most judgment. Individual services should provide guidelines and limitations for their expected urgent cases. These "add-on case policy" guidelines[59] should be common knowledge to everyone involved in running the OR. Consequently, these cases, such as ectopic pregnancies, open fractures, the patient with obstructed bowel, and eye injuries, can then be triaged and inserted into the elective schedule as needed with minimal discussion from the delayed surgeon. The surgeons whose urgent case is presented as one that must immediately bump another service's patient, yet could wait several hours if it is their own patient that will be delayed, will have to face their own previously agreed-upon standards in a future OR committee meeting. A simple way to express one logical policy for urgent cases (e.g., acute appendicitis, unruptured ectopic pregnancy, intestinal obstruction) is: 1) bump the same surgeon's elective scheduled case; 2) if none, bump a scheduled case on the same service (gynecology, general A, and so forth); 3) if none, bump a scheduled case from an open-schedule surgical service; and 4), if none, bump a scheduled case from a block schedule service.[59] Some institutions require the attending surgeon of the posted urgent/emergent patient to speak personally with the surgeon of any bumped case.

Another area of burgeoning growth that must be accounted for in the daily work schedule is the non-OR "off site" diagnostic test, or therapeutic intervention that requires anesthesia care. In many instances these procedures replace operations that, in the recent past, would have been posted on the OR schedule as urgent/emergency cases. For example, cerebral aneurysm coiling and computed tomography-guided abscess drainage, among other procedures, are done in imaging suites; some patients, adult as well as pediatric, require deep sedation or even general anesthesia for magnetic resonance imaging or computed tomography in radiology or for invasive procedures in catheterization laboratories. Additionally, depending on distances involved and logistics, it may even be necessary to assign two people, a primary provider and an attending, exclusively to that one remote location when, had the case come to the OR, the attending may have been able to cover another or other cases also. Hospital administration or the OR committee may try to view these cases as unrelated to OR function and, thus, purely a problem for the anesthesia group to solve. These cases must be treated with the same methodology regarding access and prioritization as all other OR procedures.

In order to apportion hospital-based anesthesia resources reasonably, these off-site procedures should be subject to the same guidelines and processes as any other OR posting. Most institutions have added at least one extra anesthetizing location to their formal operating schedule to designate these off-site

---

TABLE 2-2

OPERATING ROOM (OR) UTILIZATION: "COMFORT ZONES" OF THE OPERATING ROOM PERSONNEL CONSTITUENCIES

■ BLOCK TIME UTILIZATION (%)	■ FACILITY ADMINISTRATION	■ ANESTHESIOLOGY GROUP	■ OR STAFF	■ SURGEONS
>100	++	− −	− − −	− − − −
85–100	++++	++	−	− − −
70–84	+++	++++	+	+ /−
53–69	+	+++	+++	++
<55	− −	−	++	++++

"+", favorable; "−", unfavorable.
Reprinted from Mazzei WJ: OR management: State of the art. Proceedings of the 2003 Conference on Practice Management. Park Ridge, IL, American Society of Anesthesiologists, 2003, p. 65 with permission.

procedures (occasionally with an imaginative name such as "road show," "outfield," or "safari"). For many of these off-site cases, there is little or no reimbursement for anesthesia care. Most government plans and insurance carriers will probably not pay for the claustrophobic adult to receive monitored anesthesia care or even a general anesthetic for an obviously needed diagnostic magnetic resonance image, even though the patient, the surgeon, and the hospital benefit from the test results. The anesthesia group, the OR committee, and the hospital administration need to reach compromises regarding off-site procedures, regarding scheduling, allocation of anesthesia resources that would otherwise go to the OR, and even subsidization of the personnel costs in order to continue this obviously beneficial service.

Computerization

Computerized scheduling will likely benefit every OR regardless of size. Whether this scheduling function should be one component of a comprehensive EMR system is a complex question, as previously noted. In the OR, however, computerization allows for a faster, more efficient method of case posting than any hand-written system. Changes to the schedule can be made quickly without any loss of information. Rearranging the daily schedule is much simpler on a computer than erasing and rewriting on a ledger. Furthermore, most hospitals have adopted a computer-determined average time for a given surgical procedure for that particular surgeon. Commonly, this time is the average of the last 10 (or 10 of the last 12, with the longest and shortest discarded) of the specific procedure (e.g., total knee replacement) with the potential to add a modifier (e.g., it is a repeat surgery) that shows a material difference in the projected time length (almost always longer) for one particular patient type. Suppose surgeon X has block time of 8 hours on a given day and wants to schedule four procedures in that allotted time. The computerized scheduling program looks at surgeons X's past performances and determines a projected length for each of the procedures that are identified to the computer usually by CPT-4 codes or possibly some other code developed locally for frequent procedures done by surgeon X. (Note that the recorded time length includes the turnover time, thus making the case time definition from the time the patient enters the OR until the time any following patient enters that OR [unless an "exception" is entered specifically for an unusual circumstance].) The use of agreed-upon codes instead of just text descriptions helps ensure accuracy because it eliminates any need for the scheduling clerk to guess what the surgeon intends to do. Bookings in most circumstances should not be taken without the accompanying codes (surgeons' offices objections not withstanding). The computer then decides whether surgeon X will finish the four procedures in the allotted block time. If the computer concludes that the fourth case would finish significantly (the definition of which can be determined and entered into the program) beyond the available block time, it will not accept the fourth case into that room's schedule on that particular day. The surgeon will accept the computer's assigned times and adjust accordingly, planning only three cases, or appeal for an "exception" based on some factor not in the booking that is claimed will materially decrease the time needed for at least one of the four cases, which the surgeon must explain to the "exception czar" (anesthesiology clinical director or OR charge nurse) of the day. An alternative method has the computer simply add (to each case except the last) a projected turnover time that is agreed upon by all involved at an (often contentious) OR committee meeting. Computerizing the scheduling process significantly reduces any personal biases and smoothes out the entire operating day. The long-standing ritual of late-afternoon disputes between the surgeons and the

anesthesia group and/or OR staff whether or not to start the last case may be eliminated or at least reduced by this more realistic prospective OR scheduling method.

There are many variables to consider in any OR scheduling system. The patient population served and the nature of the institution dictate the overall structure of the OR schedule. Inner-city level 1 trauma centers must accommodate emergencies on a regular basis, 24 hours a day. These centers are unlikely to create a workable schedule more than a day in advance. An ambulatory surgery center serving plastic surgery patients may see only the rare emergency bring-back bleeding patient. Their schedule may be accurate many days in advance, with a high degree of expectation that the patient will arrive on time properly prepared for surgery. The anesthesia group at this ambulatory center may rarely have to make changes to the schedule, allowing them to proceed with a fairly predictable daily workload. At the inner-city trauma hospital, a great deal of flexibility and constant communication with the surgeons will be required in an attempt to get the cases done in a reasonable time frame with the inherent constraints placed on the OR staff's resources and the time available. These two extreme examples from opposite ends of the scheduling-process spectrum can provide guidelines for the majority of the institutions that fall somewhere in between. Beyond open communication, how best to work toward this mutual understanding depends on the particulars of the people involved and the environment, but some ORs report benefits from team-building exercises, leadership retreats, and even OR-wide social events. ORs with a particularly malignant history of finger-pointing and bad feelings among the personnel groups may constitute one of the few instances an outside consultant really may be valuable in that there are workplace psychologists who specialize in analyzing dysfunctional work environments and implementing changes to improve the situation for all involved.

Preoperative Clinic

An anesthesia preoperative evaluation clinic (APEC) that provides a comprehensive perioperative medical evaluation usually results in a more efficient running of the OR schedule.[60,61] Unanticipated cancellations or delays are avoided when the anesthesia group evaluates complex patients prior to surgery. Even if the patient arrives to the OR on time the day of surgery, inadequate preoperative clearance mandating the ordering of additional tests will consume precious OR time during the delay waiting for results. Cancellations or delays adversely affect the efficiency of any OR. Subsequent cases in the delayed room, whether for the same or a different surgeon, may get significantly delayed or forced to be squeezed into an already busy schedule on another day. The financial impact of delays or cancellations on the institution is considerable. Revenue is lost with no offsetting absence of expenses. Worse, expenses may actually increase when overtime has to be paid, or the sterile equipment has to be repackaged after having been opened for the canceled procedure. Even worse, the inconvenienced patient and/or surgeon may go to another facility.

Optimal timing for preoperative evaluation should be related to the institution's scheduling preferences, patient convenience, and the overall health of the patient. Earlier completion of the preoperative evaluation may not reduce the overall cancellation rate when compared with a more proximate evaluation. However, an early evaluation and clearance may well provide a larger pool of patients available to place on the OR schedule (block or open) resulting in a more efficient use of OR time. Additionally, a protocol-driven evaluation process can anticipate possible need for time-consuming investigations (such as a cardiology evaluation for the patient with probable angina). Early recognition of a failed preoperative test allows time for another patient to be moved into the now-vacant time slot. Also, early identification of certain problems requiring special care on the day of surgery (e.g., preoperative epidural or PA catheter placement) should lead to fewer unanticipated delays. Unfortunately, many issues precipitating delays are discovered on the day of surgery. Some of these preventable delays are unrelated to the patients' health status. Seemingly simple issues such as verification of a ride home or incomplete financial information also contribute to unexpected delays. A properly functioning APEC may be able to eliminate a majority of these annoying causes of preventable delays.

Regardless of the institutional specifics surrounding the service provided by the APEC, further cost savings can be obtained through its proper usage by the anesthesia group. The APEC frequently reduces dramatically the number of preoperative tests performed by focusing on which diagnostic tests and medical consults are really required for any specific patient. In some circumstances, the APEC may also function as an additional source of revenue for the anesthesia group when a formal preoperative consult on a complicated patient is ordered well in advance by the surgeon, in the same manner as would have otherwise been directed to a primary care physician for "clearance for surgery." The ability to centralize pertinent information including admission precertification/clearance, financial data, diagnostic and laboratory results, consult reports, and preoperative recommendations improves OR function by decreasing the time spent searching for all these items after changes have been made to the schedule. Patient and family education performed by the APEC frequently leads to an increase in patients' overall satisfaction of the perioperative experience. In addition, patient anxiety may be reduced secondary to the more in-depth contact possible inherent in the APEC process when compared with anesthesia practitioners meeting an ambulatory outpatient for the first time in an OR holding area immediately prior to surgery. The APEC model enables the anesthesia group to be more active and proactive in the perioperative process, improving their relations with the other OR constituents.

Anesthesiology Personnel Issues

In light of the current and future shortage of anesthesia care providers, creating, managing, and maintaining a stable supply of anesthesia practitioners promises to dominate the OR landscape for years to come.[62] Active recruiting for anesthesiologists appears to be widespread and intense, sometimes involving creative marketing and incentives.[63] The lean resident recruiting years of the mid to late 1990s continue to impact the profession. Even though applications to anesthesiology residencies from highly qualified applicants rebounded significantly,[62] it will take many more years of relatively large numbers of anesthesia residency graduates to even begin to address actual needs.[64] Further, just as the overall projected dramatic shortage of physicians in general has led to the opening and planning of several new medical schools in the United States, perhaps the shortage of anesthesiologists (still estimated at several thousand) will provoke the establishment of new residency training programs. Furthermore, the supply of nonphysician anesthesia professionals is also dwindling. With the aging population of nurse anesthetists and the limited number of applications to schools in that profession, as well as the very limited number of training facilities for anesthesiology assistants, the overall supply of anesthesia professionals remains inadequate to meet current and, at least, short-term future demands. The need for anesthesia groups to create a flexible, attractive work environment in order to retain providers who might leave or retire will continue to increase.

A related issue is consideration of what is a reasonable work load for an anesthesiologist and how best to measure, if possible, the clinical productivity of an anesthesia group/department. These questions have been the subject of considerable discussion.[65–68] Beyond the simple number of full-time equivalents, cases, and OR minutes, consideration of factors such as the nature of the facility, types of surgical practice, patient acuity, and speed of the surgeons must be incorporated to allow fair comparisons. Thoughtful filtering of resulting data should take place before dissemination of the aggregate information to all members of a group because of the understandable extreme sensitivity among stressed and fatigued anesthesiologists to a suggestion that they are not working as hard as their group/department peers.

Except in highly unusual circumstances, flexible scheduling of anesthesia professionals and also fulfilling the demands placed on the group by the institution continues to be a constant balancing act. This demand assumes added significance because institutions now subsidize many anesthesia groups. Even when a majority of providers in a facility are independent contractors where it is required that a specific surgeon request their services, there are time conflicts ranging from no one at all being available to unwanted down time. When the anesthesia group/department accepts the responsibility of providing anesthesia services for an institution, they must schedule enough providers for that OR suite on each given day. Ideally, a sufficient number of professionals would be hired so that there would always be enough personnel to staff the minimum number of rooms scheduled on any given day, as well as after-hours call duty. This situation rarely exists because it would be financially disadvantageous to have an excess number of providers with no clinical activity. Having exactly the right number of anesthesia professionals in a group for the clinical load works well until one (or more) of them is out with an unplanned absence such as an extended illness or a family emergency. Many academic departments have a natural buffer with some clinicians assigned intervals of nonclinical time for research, teaching, or administrative duties. However, repeated loss of these nonclinical days because of inadequate clinical staffing in the OR leads to undermining the academic/research mission of the department. Continued loss of this time will eventually lead to faculty resignations (and possible migration to private practice), thus eliminating the original buffer. Consequently, anesthesia groups/departments need to anticipate available clinical personnel and match them to the OR demands. Ideally, this information should be accurate for several months into the future. Meeting this specification has become more difficult in the recent past. Hospital administrators must offer reasonable assurances to the anesthesia group providing service that a given OR utilization rate is likely, as well as accurate data regarding reimbursement (payer mix and any package contracts negotiated by the hospital). These data must be provided accurately and updated frequently if a health care institution is to acquire and retain an anesthesia group staffed with the personnel to meet the expected demands.

Timing

Each operating environment has its own personnel scheduling system and expectations for the anesthesia group. Daily coordination between the anesthesia group's clinical director and the OR supervisor permits the construction of a reasonable schedule showing the number of ORs that day and when the schedule expects each of them to finish. Invariably, some cases take longer than anticipated or add-ons are posted, requiring the OR to run into the late afternoon or early evening. Many anesthesia professionals accept this occurrence as a matter of course. Few anesthesia professionals will tolerate this sequence of events as an essentially daily routine whether they are paid overtime or not. These practitioners become exhausted and resent the burdens continuously placed on them. If the OR schedule is such that add-ons frequently occur and elective cases run well into the evening, many anesthesia professionals will opt to protect their personal and family time and cut back their working hours or resign. Neither would be welcome in such a tight market. Under these circumstances, hiring additional personnel who are scheduled to arrive at a later time, for example, 11: 00 AM, and then providing lunch relief and staying late (e.g., 7: 30 PM or later if needed) to finish the schedule may well be a very worthwhile investment.

Another possible solution to the demands of an extended OR schedule on an anesthesia group's personnel may revolve around employing part-time anesthesia professionals. Part-time opportunities could enhance a group's ability to attract additional staff. In the past, a disproportionately high percentage of women chose anesthesiology as a career. In 1970, women represented 7.6% of the physician population but were 14% of anesthesiologists; much more recently, they make up 45% of the physician population and only 20% of anesthesiologists, proportionately a significant reduction.[69] Beyond the basic demographic shift among all physicians, one likely partial explanation for the decreased number of women anesthesiologists may be the lack of part-time positions, which will hamper an anesthesia group's ability to attract and keep at least some of the female anesthesia professionals.

Scheduling after-hours coverage also adds to the personnel difficulties facing the anesthesia group. The variations of call schemes are endless. The nature of the institution and the workload determine the degree of late-night coverage. Major referral centers and level 1 trauma centers require in-house primary providers. If these providers include residents and/or nurse anesthetists, then the supervising attending staff will also be in-house 24 hours a day. A common solution employed at many institutions is to staff the evening/night call shifts for an average workload, recognizing that on some occasions there will be idle ORs, and on other nights, the surgical demand will exceed the call team's numbers.

There are also medicolegal issues surrounding the call team's availability. At a small community hospital with a limited number of independent attending practitioners, the practitioners may agree to cover call on a rotating basis. The individuals not on call are usually not obligated to the OR and may well be truly unreachable. What happens then when the on-call anesthesiologist is administering an anesthetic and another true emergency case arrives in the OR suite and the remaining staff anesthesiologists are legitimately unavailable? Does that anesthesiologist leave his or her current patient under the care of an OR nurse and go next door to tend to a more acutely (possibly critically) ill patient? Should the patient be transferred from the emergency department to another (hopefully nearby) hospital? These questions have no easy answers. Clearly, those practitioners on the scene have to assess in real time the relative risks and benefits and make the difficult decisions. If the call duty requires the practitioner(s) frequently to work much or all of the night, leaving the individual(s) stressed and fatigued, they should not be required to work the next day during normal working hours.

A more complicated answer involves what to do when the call assignment rarely requires a long night's work and the on-call anesthesia professionals routinely have rooms assigned to them the next day, but at least one person has just finished a difficult 24-hour shift being awake and working all night. Anesthesia groups need to decide how to handle the possible call shift scenarios, with permutations and combinations, and clearly communicate prospectively their decisions to the OR committee before any difficult decision has to be made one morning. As always, the medicolegal aspects of any decision such as this need to be taken into consideration. Whether or not fatigue was a factor, the practitioner who worked throughout the night before and appeared to contribute to an anesthetic catastrophe the next morning would have a very difficult defense in court. Further, the anesthesiology group may also be held liable in that their practice/policy was in place, allegedly authorizing the supposedly dangerous conduct.

COST AND QUALITY ISSUES

One of the more pervasive aspects of American medical care in today's environment is the drive to maintain and improve high-quality health care while reducing the cost of that care. Health care costs account for a remarkable 16% of the gross domestic product, nearly triple the fraction a generation ago. Even more alarming, if costs continue to increase at the current rate, by 2016, it will be 20% of the gross domestic product. Consequently, all physicians, including anesthesiologists, are urged constantly to include cost-consciousness in decisions balancing the natural desire to provide the highest possible quality of care with the overall priorities of both the health care system and the individual patient, all while facing increasingly limited resources.[70] Anesthesiologists remain a target for limiting health care expenditures. Anesthesia professionals (directly and indirectly) have represented 3 to 5% of the total health care costs in the country.[71] Complicated decisions are required regarding which patients are suitable for ambulatory surgery, what preoperative studies to order, what anesthetic drugs or technique is best for the patient, what monitors or equipment are reasonably required to run an OR, and the list goes on and on. With this as background, anesthesiologists legitimately can include economic considerations in their decision processes. When presented with multiple options to provide for therapeutic intervention or patient assessment, one should not automatically choose the more expensive approach (just to "cover all the bases") unless there is compelling evidence proving its value. Decisions that clearly materially increase cost should only be pursued when the benefit outweighs the risk. In anesthesia care as well as medicine in general, such decisions can be difficult regarding interventions that provide marginal benefit but contain significant cost increases.[72] Because cost containment initially requires accurate cost awareness, anesthesiologists need to find out the actual costs and benefits of their anesthesia care techniques. Details will be unique to each practice setting. Because they will be excited that the anesthesiologists actually care, usually it is possible to get the cooperation of the facility administration's financial department members in researching and calculating the actual cost of anesthesia care so that thoughtful evaluations of potential reductions can be initiated.

Anesthesia drug expenses represent a small portion of the total perioperative costs. However, the great number of doses actually administered contributes substantially to aggregate total cost to the institution in actual dollars. Prudent drug selection combined with appropriate anesthetic technique can result in substantial savings. Reducing fresh gas flow from 5 L/min to 2 L/min wherever possible would save approximately $100 million annually in the United States.[73] A majority of anesthesia professionals usually attempt a practical approach to cost savings, but they are more frequently faced with difficult choices regarding methods of anesthesia that likely produce similar outcomes but at substantially different cost. When comparing the total costs of more expensive anesthetic drugs and techniques to lesser expensive ones, many variables need to be added to the formula. The cost of anesthetic drugs needs to include the costs of additional equipment such as special vaporizers or extra infusion pumps and the associated maintenance. There are other indirect costs that may be difficult to quantitate and are commonly overlooked. Some of these indirect costs include increased set-up time, possibly increasing room turnover time, extended PACU recovery time, and additional expensive drugs required to treat side effects. Sometimes, more expensive techniques reduce indirect costs. A propofol infusion, although more expensive than vapor, commonly results in a decreased PACU stay for a short noninvasive procedure. If fewer PACU staff are needed or patient throughput is increased, the more expensive drug can reduce overall cost. Conversely, using comparatively expensive propofol for a long procedure definitely requiring postoperative admission to an ICU is hardly justified. The impact of shorter-acting drugs and those with fewer side effects is context-specific. During long surgical procedures, such drugs may offer limited benefits over older, less expensive, longer-acting alternatives.[74] Under these conditions, advocating cost containment using educational efforts may decrease drug expenditures for several categories of drugs.[75] Drugs in the same therapeutic class have widely varying costs. The acquisition expenses may vary as much as 50-fold in some pharmacologic categories. It is estimated that the 10 highest expenditure drugs account for >80% of the anesthetic drug costs at some institutions.[76] Although newer, more expensive drugs may be easier to use, no data exist to support or refute the hypothesis that these drugs provide a "better" anesthetic experience when compared with carefully titrated older, less expensive, longer-acting drugs in the same class.

Evaluation of outcomes and their subsequent application to cost analysis can be derived from two principle sources: data published in the literature and data collected from experience. As noted, computerized information management systems are useful tools to track outcomes and analyze the impact on the cost/benefit ledger. Using the collated data in the same manner as for OR utilization and case load, practitioners can readily apply a statistical process to evaluate outcomes in their practice, possibly including correlation with cost. This information may take on added importance in that published incidence studies may not exist for the specific outcome an anesthesia group is searching for. Cause-and-effect diagrams can track the parameters involved in the process and relate them to the various outcomes desired. Multiple pertinent examples could be constructed from the now-extensive body of literature on the factors contributing to postoperative nausea and vomiting and the various possible preventions and treatments, many of which involve very expensive medications. Of course, this can be done locally within an institution. Information would be collected and stored in the database. Ideally, the database would identify and track as many variables as needed/possible to delineate sources for possible improvement and its ultimate cost analysis. Once these sources for improvement and the ensuing cost impact are known, the anesthesia group can determine whether or not to pursue changing their practice. Outcomes related to adverse effects can also be monitored. If analysis reveals a significant difference in an adverse outcome among practitioners, after all the other variables such as surgeon, patient mix, and so forth are eliminated, the outcome database can investigate the anesthetic technique used by that practitioner. If significant variations are identified, that practitioner would be able to learn of these variations in a nonthreatening manner because computer-derived data is used as opposed to a specific case analysis, which might lead that practitioner to feel singled out for public criticism. The database becomes a tool both for QA and professional education.

CONCLUSION

🔟 Practice and OR management in anesthesiology today is more complex and more important than ever before. Attention to details that previously either did not exist or were perceived as unimportant can likely make the difference between success and failure in anesthesiology practice.

Outlined here are basic descriptions and understandings of many different administrative, organizational, financial, and personnel components and factors in the practice of anesthesiology. Ongoing significant changes in the health care system will provide a continuing array of challenges. Application of the principles presented here will allow anesthesiologists to extrapolate creatively from these basics to their own individual circumstances and then forge ahead in anesthesiology practice that is efficient, effective, productive, collegial, and even fun.

References

1. American Society of Anesthesiologists: 2003–04 Manual for Anesthesia Department Organization and Management. Park Ridge, IL, American Society of Anesthesiologists, 2003
2. American Society of Anesthesiologists: Anatomy of the Bargain: Sword, Shield, or Shackle? Park Ridge, IL, American Society of Anesthesiologists, 1999
3. Peters JD, Fineberg KS, Kroll DA, et al: Anesthesiology and the Law. Ann Arbor, MI, Health Administration Press, 1983
4. Gaba DM, Howard SK, Jump B: Production pressure in the work environment. Anesthesiology 1994; 81: 488
5. Eichhorn JH, Cooper JB, Cullen DJ, et al: Anesthesia practice standards at Harvard: A review. J Clin Anesth 1988; 1: 56
6. American Society of Anesthesiologists Task Force on Postanesthetic Care: Practice Guidelines for Postanesthetic Care. Anesthesiology 2002; 96: 742
7. Hawkins JL (Chair), et al: Practice guidelines for obstetrical anesthesia. Anesthesiology 2007; 106: 843
8. American Society of Anesthesiologists Task Force on Pulmonary Artery Catheterization: Practice guidelines for pulmonary artery catheterization: An updated report by the American Society of Anesthesiologists Task Force on Pulmonary Artery Catheterization. Anesthesiology 2003; 99: 988
9. American Society of Anesthesiologists Task Force on Management of the Difficult Airway: Practice guidelines for management of the difficult airway: An updated report by the American Society of Anesthesiologists Task Force on Management of the Difficult Airway. Anesthesiology 2003; 98: 1269
10. Dans PE, Weiner JP, Otter SE: Peer review organizations: Promises and potential pitfalls. N Engl J Med 1985; 313: 1131
11. Peer review in anesthesiology, Park Ridge, IL, American Society of Anesthesiologists, 1993, pp 105
12. Eichhorn JH: Anesthesia equipment: Checkout and quality assurance. Anesthesia Equipment: Principles and Applications, Edited by Ehrenwerth J, Eisenkraft JB. St. Louis, Mosby–Yearbook, 1992, p 473
13. Eichhorn JH: Organized response to major anesthesia accident will help limit damage: Update of "Adverse Event Protocol" provides valuable plan. Anesthesia Patient Safety Foundation Newsletter 2006; 21: 11
14. Spooner RB, Kirby RR: Equipment-related anesthetic incidents. Analysis of Anesthetic Mishaps. Edited by Pierce EC, Cooper JB. Boston: International Anesthesiology Clinics 1984; 22: 133
15. Cooper JB, Newbower RS, Kitz RJ: An analysis of major errors and equipment failures in anesthesia management: Considerations for prevention and detection. Anesthesiology 1984; 60: 34
16. Caplan RA, Vistica M, Posner KL, et al: Adverse anesthetic outcomes arising from gas delivery equipment: A closed claims analysis. Anesthesiology 1997; 87: 741
17. Cooper JB, Newbower RS, Long CD, et al: Preventable anesthesia mishaps: A study of human factors. Anesthesiology 1978; 49: 399
18. Duberman S, Wald A: An integrated quality control program for anesthesia equipment, Risk Management and Quality Assurance: Issues and Interactions. Edited by Chapman-Cliburn G. Chicago, Joint Commission on the Accreditation of Hospitals, 1986, p 105
19. Olympio MA, Reinke B, Abramovich A: Challenges ahead in technology training: A report on the training initiative of the Committee on Technology. APSF Newsletter 2006; 21: 43
20. HHS Publication No. (FDA) 85-4196. Food and Drug Administration, Center for Devices and Radiologic Health, Rockville, MD 20857, p 10
21. Eichhorn JH: Influence of practice standards on anesthesia outcome, Outcome After Anesthesia and Surgery. Edited by Desmonts JM. Bailliere's Clinical Anaesthesiology—International Practice and Research. 1992; 6: 663
22. Eichhorn JH: Prevention of intraoperative anesthesia accidents and related severe injury through safety monitoring. Anesthesiology 1989; 70: 572
23. Keats AS: Anesthesia mortality in perspective. Anesth Analg 1990; 71: 113
24. Lagasse RS: Anesthesia safety: Model or myth? Anesthesiology 2002; 97: 1609

25. Cooper JB, Gaba DM: No myth: Anesthesia is a model for addressing patient safety. Anesthesiology 2002; 97: 1335
26. Peterson GN: Malpractice insurance: What are the limits? ASA Newsletter 2007; 71: 14
27. Bacon AK: Death on the table: Some thoughts on how to handle an anaesthetic-related death. Anaesthesia 1989; 44: 245
28. Runciman WB, Webb RK, Klepper ID, et al: Crisis management: Validation of an algorithm by analysis of 2000 incident reports. Anaesth Intensive Care 1993; 21: 579
29. Davies JM, Webb RK: Adverse events in anaesthesia: The wrong drug. Can J Anaesth 1994; 41: 83
30. Cooper JB, Cullen DJ, Eichhorn JH, et al: Administrative guidelines for response to an adverse anesthesia event. J Clin Anesth 1993; 5: 79
31. Kraman SS, Hamm G: Risk management: Extreme honesty may be the best policy. Ann Intern Med 1999; 131: 963
32. Lazare A: Apology in medical practice: An emerging clinical skill. JAMA 2006; 296: 1401
33. Eichhorn JH: Patient perspective personalizes patient safety. APSF Newsletter 2005; 20: 61
34. Cox W: The five A's: What do patients want after an adverse event? J Healthcare Risk Management 2007; 27: 25
35. Semo JJ: Our hospital wants to employ us: Now what? Proceedings of the American Society of Anesthesiologists 2008 Conference on Practice Management. Park Ridge, IL, American Society of Anesthesiologists, 2008, p 48
36. Practice management: Compliance with Medicare and other payor billing requirements. Park Ridge, IL, American Society of Anesthesiologists, 1997
37. Locke J: The net collections fallacy and other performance metric myths. Proceedings of the American Society of Anesthesiologists 2003 Conference on Practice Management. Park Ridge, IL, American Society of Anesthesiologists, 2003, p 141
38. Managed Care Reimbursement Mechanisms: A Guide for Anesthesiologists. Park Ridge, IL, American Society of Anesthesiologists, 1994
39. Contracting Issues: A Primer for Anesthesiologists. Park Ridge, IL, American Society of Anesthesiologists, 1999
40. Willett DE: Exclusive contracts: Update on legal issues. Proceedings of the American Society of Anesthesiologists 2001 Conference on Practice Management. Park Ridge, IL, American Society of Anesthesiologists, 2001, p 8
41. Scott SJ, Blough GG: Exclusive contracts: Survey of hospital contracts. Proceedings of the American Society of Anesthesiologists 2001 Conference on Practice Management. Park Ridge, IL, American Society of Anesthesiologists, 2001, p 9
42. Practice Management: Managed Care Contracting. Park Ridge, IL, American Society of Anesthesiologists, 1996
43. Bierstein K: Pros and cons of exclusive contracts. ASA Newsletter 2006; 70(8): 36
44. Everett PC: Securing a hospital stipend: The business-like approach. Proceedings of the American Society of Anesthesiologists 2003 Conference on Practice Management. Park Ridge, IL, American Society of Anesthesiologists, 2003, p 189
45. Semo JJ: Hospital stipend negotiations: Practical and legal issues. Proceedings of the American Society of Anesthesiologists 2004 Conference on Practice Management. Park Ridge, IL, American Society of Anesthesiologists, 2004, p 51
46. Laden J, Monea M: Preparing the financial case for hospital support. Proceedings of the American Society of Anesthesiologists 2008 Conference on Practice Management. Park Ridge, IL, American Society of Anesthesiologists, 2008, p 258
47. Rodin MA: Conflicts in managed care. N Engl J Med 1995; 332: 604
48. Adessa A: The vulnerability and potential extinction of independent, hospital-based practices. Proceedings of the American Society of Anesthesiologists 2008 Conference on Practice Management. Park Ridge, IL, American Society of Anesthesiologists, 2008, p 65
49. Hetrick WD: Health care reform: Implications for the anesthesiologist. Adv Anesth 1995; 12: 1
50. Epstein AM, Lee TH, Hamel MB: Paying physicians for high-quality care. N Engl J Med 2004; 350: 406
51. Hannenberg AA: Progress report: Quality incentives in anesthesiology. Proceedings of the American Society of Anesthesiologists 2008 Conference on Practice Management. Park Ridge, IL, American Society of Anesthesiologists, 2008, p 57
52. The HIPAA Privacy Rule in Anesthesia and Pain Medicine Practices. Park Ridge, IL, American Society of Anesthesiologists, 2003
53. Semo JJ: HIPAA privacy: What you need to know, what you need to do. Proceedings of the American Society of Anesthesiologists 2003 Conference on Practice Management. Park Ridge, IL, American Society of Anesthesiologists, 2003, p 96
54. Semo, JJ: HIPAA privacy update. Proceedings of the American Society of Anesthesiologists 2004 Conference on Practice Management. Park Ridge, IL, American Society of Anesthesiologists, 2004, p 123
55. Johnson JF: Questions to ask your billing software vendor. Proceedings of the American Society of Anesthesiologists 2003 Conference on Practice Management. Park Ridge, IL, American Society of Anesthesiologists, 2003, p 130
56. Sexton J, Makary M, Tersigni, et al: Teamwork in the operating room. Anesthesiology 2006; 105: 877
57. Lingard L, Regehr G, Orser B, et al: Evaluation of a preoperative checklist and team briefing among surgeons, nurses, and anesthesiologists to reduce failures in communication. Arch Surg 2008; 143: 12
58. Mazzei WJ: OR management. Proceedings of the American Society of Anesthesiologists 2001 Conference on Practice Management. Park Ridge, IL, American Society of Anesthesiologists ASA, 2001, 12-1
59. Malhotra V: Practical issues in OR management: The obvious and the not so obvious. Proceedings of the American Society of Anesthesiologists 2004 Conference on Practice Management. Park Ridge, IL, American Society of Anesthesiologists, 2004, p 43
60. Pollard JB, Zboray AL, Mazze RI: Economic benefits attributed to opening a preoperative evaluation clinic for outpatients. Anesth Analg 1996; 83: 407
61. Fischer SP: Development and effectiveness of an anesthesia preoperative evaluation clinic in a teaching hospital. Anesthesiology 1996; 85: 196
62. Schubert A: Implications of a changing anesthesia workforce. Proceedings of the American Society of Anesthesiologists 2008 Conference on Practice Management. Park Ridge, IL, American Society of Anesthesiologists, 2008, p 297
63. Blough GG, Scott SJ: Creative scheduling for anesthesiologists: Physician retention in a tight market. Proceedings of the American Society of Anesthesiologists 2003 Conference on Practice Management. Park Ridge, IL, American Society of Anesthesiologists, 2003, p 71
64. Schubert A: Anesthesiology resident class sizes and graduation rates. ASA Newsletter 2007; 71(12): 24
65. Abouleish AE, Prough DS, Zornow MH, et al: Designing meaningful industry metrics for clinical productivity for anesthesiology departments. Anesth Analg 2001; 93: 309
66. Abouleish AE, Prough DS, Whitten CW, et al: Comparing clinical productivity of anesthesiology departments. Anesthesiology 2002; 97: 608
67. Abouleish AE, Prough DS, Barker SJ et al.: Organizational factors affect comparisons of clinical productivity of academic anesthesiology departments. Anesth Analg 96: 802, 2003
68. Abouleish AE: Working hard: Hardly working; comparing clinical productivity of anesthesiology groups. Proceedings of the American Society of Anesthesiologists 2004 Conference on Practice Management. Park Ridge, IL, American Society of Anesthesiologists, 2004, p 195
69. Calmes SH: Anesthesiology Demographics: Women's Changing Specialty Choices and Implications for Anesthesiology Workforce Shortage. ASA Newsletter 2001; 65(8): 22
70. Tuman KJ, Ivankovich AD: High cost, high tech medicine—are we getting our money's worth? J Clin Anesth 1993; 5: 168
71. Johnstone RE, Martinec CL: Costs of anesthesia. Anesth Analg 1993; 76: 840
72. Eddy DM: Applying cost-effectiveness analysis: The inside story. JAMA 1992; 268: 2575
73. Baum JA: Low flow anaesthesia: The sensible and judicious use of inhalation anaesthetics. Acta Anaesthiol Scand 1997; 111: 264
74. Szocik JF, Learned DW: Impact of a cost containment program on the use of volatile anesthetics and neuromuscular blocking drugs. J Clin Anesth 1994; 6: 378
75. Barclay LP, Hatton RC, Doering PL, et al: Physicians' perceptions and knowledge of drug costs: Results of a survey. Formulary 1995; 30: 268
76. Johnstone R, Jozefczyk KG: Costs of anesthetic drugs: Experiences with a cost education trial. Anesth Analg 1994; 78: 766

CHAPTER 3 ■ OCCUPATIONAL HEALTH

ARNOLD J. BERRY AND JONATHAN D. KATZ

PHYSICAL HAZARDS
Anesthetic Gases
Chemicals
Allergic Reactions
Radiation
Noise Pollution
Human Factors
Work Hours and Night Call
INFECTION HAZARDS
Respiratory Viruses
Herpes Viruses
Rubella
Measles (Rubeola)
Severe Acute Respiratory Syndrome
Viral Hepatitis

Pathogenic Human Retroviruses
Occupational Safety and Health Administration Standards, Standard Precautions, and Transmission-Based Precautions
Creutzfeldt-Jakob Disease
Tuberculosis
Viruses in Smoke Plumes
EMOTIONAL CONSIDERATIONS
Stress
Substance Use, Abuse, and Addiction
Impairment and Disability
The Aging Anesthesiologist
Mortality Among Anesthesiologists
Suicide

KEY POINTS

1 With the use of scavenging equipment, routine machine maintenance, and appropriate work practices, exposure to waste anesthetic gases can be reduced to levels below those recommended by National Institute for Occupational Safety and Health (NIOSH).

2 Twenty-four percent of anesthesia personnel manifest evidence of contact dermatitis in response to latex exposure and approximately 15% are sensitized and vulnerable to allergic reactions.

3 Vigilance is one of the most critical tasks performed by anesthesiologists. The vigilance task is adversely affected by several factors including poor equipment engineering and design, excessive noise in the operating room, impediments to interpersonal communication, production pressure, and fatigue.

4 Sleep deprivation and fatigue are common among anesthesiologists. Sleep deprivation can have deleterious effects on cognition, performance, mood, and health.

5 The risk of exposure to infectious pathogens can be reduced by the routine use of standard precautions, transmission-based precautions for infected patients, and safety devices designed to prevent needlestick injuries.

6 Hepatitis B vaccine is recommended for all anesthesia personnel because of the increased risk for occupational transmission of this blood-borne pathogen.

7 Many consider chemical dependency to be the primary occupational hazard among anesthesiologists. An incidence of 1 to 2% of controlled substance abuse has been repeatedly reported within anesthesia training programs.

8 It remains controversial whether anesthesiologists are, on average, vulnerable to premature death. However, by correcting for the fact that living anesthesiologists are, on average, younger than most other specialists, it is apparent that anesthesiologists do not die younger.

Anesthesia personnel spend long hours, in fact, most of their waking days, in an environment filled with many potential hazards—the operating room. This setting is unique among workplaces as a result of the potential exposure to chemical vapors, ionizing radiation, and infectious agents. Additionally, anesthesia personnel are subject to heightened levels of psychological stress engendered by the high-stakes nature of the practice and the long periods of sustained time on duty. Although such physical hazards as fires and explosions from flammable anesthetic agents are currently of limited concern, occupational

illnesses, such as alcohol and drug abuse, are well recognized as significant within the anesthesia community. Some hazards, such as exposure to trace levels of waste anesthetic gases, have been extensively studied. Others, like suicide, have been recognized but not adequately pursued. Only within the past few decades have epidemiologic surveys been conducted to assess the health of anesthesia personnel. In general, the potential health risks to those working in the operating room may be significant, but with awareness of the problems and the use of proper precautions, they are not formidable.

PHYSICAL HAZARDS

Anesthetic Gases

Although the inhalation anesthetics diethyl ether, nitrous oxide, and chloroform were first used in the 1840s, the biologic effects of occupational exposure to anesthetic agents were not investigated until the 1960s. Reports on the effects of chronic environmental exposure to anesthetics have included epidemiologic surveys, in vitro studies, cellular research, and studies in laboratory animals and humans. Areas addressed include the potential influence of trace anesthetic concentrations on the incidence in affected populations of the following: death, infertility, spontaneous abortion, congenital malformations, cancer, hematopoietic diseases, liver disease, neurologic disease, psychomotor, and behavioral changes.

Anesthetic Levels in the Operating Room

The first report of occupational exposure to modern anesthetics was by Linde and Bruce in 1969.[1] They sampled air at various distances from the "pop-off" valve of anesthesia machines and noted an average concentration of halothane of 10 parts per million (ppm) and of nitrous oxide of 130 ppm. (Parts per million is a volume-per-volume unit of measurement; 10,000 ppm equals 1%.) End-expired air samples taken from 24 anesthesiologists after work revealed 0 to 12 ppm of halothane. It was later demonstrated that with appropriate scavenging equipment integrated with the anesthesia breathing circuit and with adequate air exchange in the operating room, levels of waste anesthetic gases could be significantly reduced.

Waste anesthetic concentrations in modern operating rooms where routine scavenging is performed are considerably less than those found in the early studies.[2,3] This raises the questions of whether chronic exposure to these low levels of waste anesthetic gases actually constitutes a significant occupational hazard and whether results from studies performed in "unscavenged" operating rooms are applicable to current practice.

Epidemiologic Studies

Epidemiologic surveys were among the first studies to suggest the possibility of a hazard resulting from exposure to trace levels of anesthetics. Although epidemiologic studies may be useful in assessing problems of this type, they have the potential for errors associated with the collection of data and their interpretation. Valid epidemiologic studies require appropriate design strategies including the presence of an appropriate control group for the cohort being studied. When questionnaires are used to obtain personal medical information, the data may be misleading because individuals may knowingly or unknowingly give incorrect information based solely on remembered data (recall bias). Cause-and-effect relationships or causality cannot be documented by epidemiologic observational studies unless all other possible etiologies (confounders) can be ruled out or other lines of evidence are used for substantiation. Few epidemiologic studies on the effects of occupational exposure to waste anesthetic gases fulfill these design criteria.

Reproductive Outcome.   One of the largest epidemiologic studies to assess the effects of trace anesthetics on reproductive outcome was conducted by the American Society of Anesthesiologists (ASA).[4] Questionnaires were sent to 49,585 operating room personnel who had potential exposure to waste anesthetic gases (members of the ASA, the American Association of Nurse Anesthetists, the Association of Operating Room Nurses, and the Association of Operating Room Technicians). A nonexposed group of 23,911 from the American Academy of Pediatrics and the American Nurses' Association served as controls. Analyses of these data indicated that there was an increased risk of spontaneous abortion and congenital abnormalities in children of women who worked in the operating room and an increased risk of congenital abnormalities in offspring of unexposed wives of male operating room personnel. Several reviews have identified inconsistencies in the data used to compare exposed and unexposed groups and to make within-group comparisons. Expected levels of anesthetic exposure did not correlate with reproductive outcome.

The ASA subsequently commissioned a group of epidemiologists and biostatisticians to evaluate and assess conflicting data from published epidemiologic surveys.[5] After analysis of methods, they found only five studies on spontaneous abortion and congenital abnormalities in offspring of anesthesia personnel that were free of errors in study design or statistical analysis. From these studies, the relative risks (the ratio of the rate of disease among those exposed to that found in those not exposed) of spontaneous abortion for female physicians and female nurses working in the operating room were 1.4 and 1.3, respectively (a relative risk of 1.3 represents a 30% increase in risk when compared with the risk of the control population). The increased relative risk for congenital abnormalities was of borderline statistical significance for exposed physicians only. Although they found a statistically significant relative risk of spontaneous abortion and congenital abnormalities in women working in the operating room, the relative risk was small compared with other, better-documented environmental hazards. They also pointed out that duration and level of anesthetic exposure were not measured in any of the studies and that other confounding factors, such as stress, infections, and radiation exposure, were not considered as confounders.

Because personnel working in some dental operatories have exposure to nitrous oxide, the dental literature has also addressed these issues. One pertinent study used data collected via telephone interviews with 418 female dental assistants to assess the effect of nitrous oxide exposure on fertility.[6] Fecundability (the ability to conceive) was significantly reduced in women with 5 or more hours of exposure to unscavenged nitrous oxide per week. In another study of 7,000 female dental assistants, questionnaires were used to determine rates of spontaneous abortion.[7] There was an increased rate of spontaneous abortion among women who worked for 3 or more hours per week in offices not using scavenging devices for nitrous oxide (relative risk [RR] = 2.6, adjusted for age, smoking, and number of amalgams prepared per week). These findings must be viewed with caution because the estimates of nitrous oxide exposure were based solely on respondents' reports, and measurements of nitrous oxide concentrations in the work space were not performed. Therefore, dose-effect relationships cannot be confirmed. It is important to note that in both studies of female dental assistants, use of nitrous oxide in offices with scavenging devices was not associated with an increased risk for adverse reproductive outcomes.[6,7]

A meta-analysis of 19 epidemiologic studies, which included hospital workers, dental assistants, and veterinarians and veterinary assistants, demonstrated an increased risk of spontaneous abortion in women with occupational exposure to anesthetic gases (RR = 1.48; 95% confidence interval, 1.40 to 1.58).[8] Additional analysis demonstrated that the relative risk of 1.48 corresponded to an increased absolute risk of abortion of 6.2%. Stratification by job category indicated that the relative risk was greatest for veterinarians (RR = 2.45), followed by dental assistants (RR = 1.89) and hospital workers (RR = 1.30). When the meta-analysis was confined to five studies that controlled for several nonoccupational confounding variables, had appropriate control groups, and had sufficient response rate, the relative risk for spontaneous abortion was 1.90 (95% confidence interval, 1.72 to 2.09). The author noted that the routine use of scavenging devices has been implemented since the time that most of the studies in this analysis were performed and that there was no risk of spontaneous abortion in studies of personnel who worked in scavenged environments.

Retrospective surveys of large numbers of women who worked during pregnancy indicate that adverse reproductive outcomes may be related to job-associated conditions other than exposure to trace anesthetic gases. A survey of 3,985 Swedish midwives demonstrated that night work was significantly associated with spontaneous abortions after the 12th week of pregnancy (odds ratio = 3.33), while exposure to nitrous oxide appeared to have no effect.[9] Using a case-control study design, Luke et al[10] found that increased work hours, hours worked while standing, and occupational fatigue were associated with preterm birth in obstetric and neonatal nurses. These and other studies have provided data that link spontaneous abortion in women working in health care to job-related factors other than exposure to trace anesthetic gases. This casts doubt on the validity of earlier studies that did not control for occupational stresses such as fatigue, long work hours, and night shifts.

Although many of the existing epidemiologic studies have potential flaws in design, the evidence taken as a whole suggests that there is a slight increase in the relative risk of spontaneous abortion and congenital abnormalities in offspring for female physicians working in the operating room.[11] Whether these findings are attributable to anesthetic exposure or other work-related conditions cannot be definitely determined from this type of investigation. Well-designed surveys of large numbers of personnel and appropriate control groups, controlled for other factors such as work hours and night shifts, are necessary to link trace anesthetic exposures to adverse reproductive outcomes. The routine use of scavenging techniques has generally lowered environmental anesthetic levels in the operating room and may make it more difficult to prove any adverse reproductive effects using epidemiologic data. Although it is easy to measure and quantify the levels of anesthetic in the operating room air, it is harder to measure and assess the effect of other possible factors, such as stress, alterations in working schedule, and fatigue.

Neoplasms and Other Nonreproductive Diseases. Early surveys enumerating causes of death among anesthesiologists indicated that male anesthesiologists had a greater risk of malignancies of the lymphoid and reticuloendothelial tissues and from suicide, but a lower death rate from lung cancer and coronary artery disease.[12] Data from a subsequent prospective study provided no evidence to support the previous conclusion that lymphoid malignancies were an occupational hazard for anesthesiologists.[13]

An ASA-sponsored study, published in 1974, found no differences in cancer rates between men exposed and those not exposed to trace concentrations of anesthetic gases.[4] For women respondents, there was a 1.3-fold to 2-fold increase in the occurrence of cancer in the exposed group, resulting predominantly from an increase in leukemia and lymphoma. The analysis of Buring et al[5] of these data confirmed an increase in relative risk of cancer in exposed women (RR = 1.4) but attributed the increase solely to cervical cancer (RR = 2.8). They also noted that the ASA study did not assess the effect of confounding variables, such as sexual history or smoking, that may have contributed to the findings. It is doubtful that the

carcinogenic effect of anesthetics would be sex-related, and the conflicting results for men and women, especially in light of the low statistical significance of the data, cast doubt that anesthetics were the causative agents.

Another ASA-sponsored mortality study of anesthesiologists, covering the period from 1976 to 1995, used data on cause of death from the National Death Index.[14] The mortality risks of a cohort of 40,242 anesthesiologists were compared with a matched cohort of internists. There was no difference between the two groups in overall mortality risk or mortality from cancer or heart disease, but the mean age at death was significantly lower for anesthesiologists compared with internists (66.5 years vs. 69.0 years). In a subsequent study, Katz[15] used data from the American Medical Association (AMA) to conclude that there was no statistical difference in age-specific mortality among anesthesiologists, internists, and other physicians when ages of the living members of the physician groups were considered in the analyses.

Epidemiologic observational studies are useful tools for attempting to identify adverse effects of the operating room environment, including exposure to many substances, of which waste anesthetic gases comprise but one factor. The data from observational surveys can, at best, identify associations but can never prove cause-and-effect relationships between an exposure to a condition or substance and a disease process. Many surveys that attempt to assess the effects of waste anesthetic gases have method design flaws such as failure to control for possible confounding factors, and these have resulted in conflicting conclusions. Overall, there appears to be some evidence that the operating room environment produces a slight increase in the rate of spontaneous abortion and cancer in female anesthesiologists and nurses.[5] Mortality risks from cancer and heart disease for anesthesiologists do not differ from those for other medical specialists.

Laboratory Studies

Along with epidemiologic studies, investigators have been active in the laboratory, assessing the effects of anesthetic agents on cell, tissue, and animal models. It is thought that this work might provide the scientific evidence linking anesthetic exposure to the adverse effects that have been suggested by some observational studies.

Cellular Effects. Nitrous oxide administered in clinically useful concentrations affects hematopoietic and neural cells by irreversibly oxidizing the cobalt atom of vitamin B_{12} from an active to inactive state. This inhibits methionine synthetase and prevents the conversion of methyltetrahydrofolate to tetrahydrofolate, which is required for DNA synthesis, assembly of the myelin sheath, and methyl substitutions in neurotransmitters. Inhibition of methionine synthetase in individuals exposed to high concentrations of nitrous oxide may result in anemia and polyneuropathy, but chronic exposure to trace levels found in scavenged operating rooms does not appear to produce these effects.

Many studies have been performed in animals to assess the carcinogenicity of anesthetics. Because of the extreme variability of study protocols, use of animals of differing species, and failure to consider possible confounders in study design, a definitive link between anesthetics and cancer has not been proven.

Several investigators have used the Ames bacterial assay system for studying the mutagenicity of anesthetics. This assay is rapid, inexpensive, and has a high true-positive rate when compared with in vivo tests. Halothane, enflurane, methoxyflurane, isoflurane, sevoflurane and urine from patients anesthetized with these agents was not mutagenic using this assay. Urine from people working in scavenged or unscavenged operating rooms was also negative for mutagens.

Other studies have used analyses of sister chromatid exchanges or formation of micronucleated lymphocytes to assess for genotoxicity in association with anesthetic exposure. These tests may be of interest because there may be an association between these genetic changes and cancer. The majority of studies using sister chromatid exchange testing have been negative for enflurane, isoflurane, and sevoflurane exposure.[16]

Anesthetists at an institution where waste gas scavenging was not used had an increased fraction of micronucleated lymphocytes compared with those practicing in a hospital where waste anesthetic gases were scavenged.[17] Low-level exposure as occurs in scavenged operating rooms was not associated with increased formation of micronucleated lymphocytes. The predictive value for the association of this test to the incidence of cancer is unclear.

The data from several lines of evidence indicate that occupational exposure to the low levels of anesthetics found with effective waste gas scavenging is not associated with significant cellular effects.

Reproductive Outcome. Because of the suggestion from epidemiologic data that occupational exposure to waste anesthetic gases may have resulted in an increased rate of spontaneous abortion and congenital abnormalities, numerous studies have been performed in laboratory animals to assess reproductive outcome. Most animal experiments fail to demonstrate alterations in female or male fertility or reproductive outcome with exposure to the subanesthetic concentrations of the currently used anesthetic agents achievable with scavenging and appropriate work practices. It is important to realize that data from laboratory investigations in animals may not be directly applicable to humans.

Effects of Trace Anesthetic Levels on Psychomotor Skills

Several studies have been conducted to attempt to clarify whether low concentrations of anesthetics alter the psychomotor skills required for providing high-quality care. In one investigation, psychomotor tests were used to assess the effect of nitrous oxide (500, 50, or 25 ppm) alone or with halothane (10, 1.0, or 0.5 ppm).[18] After exposure to the highest concentrations of nitrous oxide and halothane, subjects' performance declined on four of the seven tests. Interestingly, there was a decrease in ability in six of seven tests after exposure to the same level of nitrous oxide alone. Exposure to the lowest concentrations studied, 25 ppm nitrous oxide and 0.5 ppm halothane, produced no effects as measured by this battery of tests.

Other investigators using similar protocols have found no effect on psychomotor test performance after exposure to trace concentrations of halothane or nitrous oxide. The reason for differences in outcome between studies is unclear, but Bruce and Stanley,[19] among the original investigators, have attributed the psychological effects of low levels of anesthetics to unusual sensitivity in the group of paid volunteers used in the study.

Recommendations of the National Institute for Occupational Safety and Health

The National Institute for Occupational Safety and Health (NIOSH) is the federal agency responsible for ensuring that workers have a safe and healthful working environment. It meets these goals through the conduct and funding of research, through education of employers and employees about occupational illnesses, and through establishing occupational health standards. A second federal agency, the Occupational Safety and Health Administration (OSHA), is responsible for enacting job health standards, investigating work sites to detect violation of standards, and enforcing the standards by citing violators. In 1977, NIOSH published a criteria document that included recommended exposure limits (REL) for waste anesthetic gases of 2 ppm (1-hour ceiling) for halogenated anesthetic agents (halothane, enflurane) when used alone or 0.5 ppm of a halogenated agent and 25 ppm of nitrous oxide (time-weighted average during the period of anesthetic administration).[20] In addition, it stated that operating room employees should be advised of the potential harmful effects of anesthetics. The guidelines proposed that annual medical and occupational histories be obtained from all personnel and that any abnormal outcomes of pregnancies should be documented. The publication also included information on scavenging procedures and equipment and methods for monitoring concentrations of waste anesthetic gases in the air.

The 1977 NIOSH criteria document has not been adopted by OSHA, which has not set a standard permissible exposure limit for waste anesthetic gases. Some states, however, have instituted regulations calling for routine measurement of ambient nitrous oxide in operating rooms and have mandated that levels not exceed an arbitrary maximum. In 1994, NIOSH published an alert to warn health care personnel that exposure to nitrous oxide may produce "harmful effects."[21] In this document, NIOSH recommends the following to reduce nitrous oxide exposure: (1) monitoring the air in operating rooms; (2) implementation of appropriate engineering controls, work practices, and equipment maintenance procedures; and (3) institution of a worker education program.

NIOSH has not developed RELs for the agents most commonly used in current practice (isoflurane, sevoflurane, and desflurane). These volatile agents have potencies, chemical characteristics, and rates and products of metabolism that differ significantly from older anesthetics. In 2006, NIOSH issued a request for information to permit the agency to evaluate possible health risks of occupational exposure to isoflurane, sevoflurane, and desflurane and to establish RELs.

It is important to note that other organizations both in and outside the United States have set occupational exposure limits for waste anesthetic gases and, in most cases, these are greater than those recommended by NIOSH. For example, the American Conference of Governmental Industrial Hygienists has recommended a threshold limit value–time-weighted average (calculated for an 8-hour shift) for nitrous oxide of 50 ppm, for enflurane of 75 ppm, and for halothane of 50 ppm.

In view of the conflicting scientific data and published recommendations, it is reasonable to ask what is an acceptable exposure level for waste anesthetic gases. Although it may be difficult to be certain of a threshold concentration below which chronic exposure is "safe," it is prudent to institute measures that reduce waste anesthetic levels in the operating room environment to as low as possible without compromising patient safety.

Methods for reducing and monitoring waste gases in the operating room have been suggested.[3,21] Through the use of scavenging equipment, equipment maintenance procedures, appropriate anesthetic work practices, and efficient operating room ventilation systems, the environmental anesthetic concentration can be reduced to minimal levels. To ensure reduced occupational exposure, departmental programs should incorporate the ability to monitor for detection of leaks in the high- and low-pressure systems of anesthetic machines, contamination as a result of faulty anesthetic techniques such as poor mask fit or leaks around the cuffs of endotracheal tubes and

TABLE 3-1

SOURCES OF OPERATING ROOM CONTAMINATION

■ **ANESTHETIC TECHNIQUES**

- Failure to turn off gas flow control valves at the end of an anesthetic
- Turning gas flow on before placing mask on patient
- Poorly fitting masks, especially with mask induction of anesthesia
- Flushing of the circuit
- Filling of anesthesia vaporizers
- Uncuffed or leaking tracheal tubes (e.g., pediatric) or poorly fitting laryngeal mask airways
- Pediatric circuits (e.g., Jackson-Rees version of the Mapleson D system)
- Sidestream sampling carbon dioxide and anesthetic gas analyzers

■ **ANESTHESIA MACHINE DELIVERY SYSTEM AND SCAVENGING SYSTEM**

- Open/closed system
- Occlusion/malfunction of hospital disposal system
- Maladjustment of hospital disposal system vacuum
- Leaks
   High-pressure hoses or connectors
   Nitrous oxide tank mounting
   O rings
   CO_2 absorbent canisters
   Low-pressure circuit

■ **OTHER SOURCES**

- Cryosurgery units
- Cardiopulmonary bypass circuits

Modified from Task Force on Trace Anesthetic Gases of the Committee on Occupational Health of Operating Room Personnel: Waste Anesthetic Gases: Information for Management in Anesthetizing Areas and the Postanesthesia Care Unit (PACU). Park Ridge, IL, American Society of Anesthesiologists, 1999, with permission from the American Society of Anesthesiologists. A copy of the full text can be obtained from the ASA, 520 N. Northwest Highway, Park Ridge, IL 60068-2573.

laryngeal mask airways, and scavenging system malfunctions (Table 3-1). When there have been leaks of anesthetic gases, dispersion and removal of the pollutants depend on the adequacy of room ventilation. Standards for operating room construction from the American Institute of Architects require 15 to 21 air exchanges per hour with 3 bringing in outside air.[22] Environmental levels of anesthetics can be measured using instantaneously collected samples, continuous air monitoring, or time-weighted averages.[3] With appropriate care, environmental levels of anesthetics in the operating room can be reduced to comply with the RELs established by NIOSH.

Anesthetic Levels in the Postanesthesia Care Unit

Patients who have received volatile anesthetics release these gases into the environment as they awaken from general anesthesia in the postanesthesia care unit (PACU). In a 1998 study, the time-weighted average concentrations for isoflurane, desflurane, and nitrous oxide were 1.1 ppm, 2.1 ppm, and 29 ppm, respectively, in the breathing zone of PACU nurses.[23] Half of the patients were intubated on arrival in the PACU, suggesting that they were still partially anesthetized and were exhaling a greater concentration of anesthetic gases than if they had already awakened. In contrast, other investigators reported time-weighted nitrous oxide levels <2.0 ppm from two PACUs.[24] The practice in these institutions was to routinely discontinue nitrous oxide at the end of surgery,

approximately 5 minutes before the patient left the operating room. Also, there was adequate air exchange documented in the PACUs. NIOSH threshold limits for anesthetic gases can be obtained in the PACU by ensuring adequate room ventilation and fresh gas exchange and by discontinuing the anesthetic gases in sufficient time prior to leaving the operating room.

Chemicals

Methyl Methacrylate

Methyl methacrylate is commonly used to cement prostheses to bone or to repair bone defects. Known cardiovascular complications of methyl methacrylate in surgical patients include hypotension, bradycardia, and cardiac arrest. The effects of occupational exposure are less well documented. Reported risks from repeated occupational exposure to methyl methacrylate include skin irritation and burns, allergic reactions and asthma, eye irritation including possible corneal ulceration, headache, and neurologic signs. Airborne concentrations greater than 170 ppm have been associated with chronic lung, liver, and kidney damage. In one report, a health care worker (HCW) suffered significant lower limb neuropathy after repeated occupational exposure to methyl methacrylate.[25] OSHA has established an 8-hour, time-weighted average allowable exposure of 100 ppm. Concentrations as high as 280 ppm have been measured when methyl methacrylate is prepared for use in the operating room, but peak environmental concentration can be decreased by 75% when scavenging devices are properly used.

Allergic Reactions

In addition to concerns about toxic effects associated with exposure to volatile anesthetics or chemicals, anesthesiologists may develop sensitivities or allergic reactions to substances found in the health care environment.

Halothane

Allergic reactions to volatile anesthetic agents have been associated with contact dermatitis, hepatitis, and anaphylaxis in individual anesthesiologists.[26,27] Analyses of sera from pediatric and general anesthesiologists demonstrated that exposure to halothane was associated with an increased prevalence of autoantibodies to cytochrome P450 2E1 and hepatic endoplasmic reticulum protein (ERp58).[28] Despite the presence of these autoantibodies, only 1 of 105 pediatric anesthesiologists had symptoms of hepatic injury. These data suggest that although autoantibodies may occur in anesthesiologists exposed to volatile anesthetics, they do not appear to be the cause of anesthetic-induced hepatitis.

Latex

Latex in surgical and examination gloves has become a common source of allergic reactions among operating room personnel. In many cases, HCWs who are allergic to latex experience their first adverse reactions while they are patients undergoing surgery. The prevalence of latex sensitivity among anesthesiologists is approximately 15%.[29,30]

The latex found in medical products is actually a composite of many substances including proteins, polyisoprenes,

lipids and phospholipids combined with preservatives, accelerators, antioxidants, vulcanizing compounds, and lubricating agents (such as cornstarch or talc). The protein content is responsible for most of the generalized allergic reactions to latex-containing surgical gloves. These reactions are exacerbated by the presence of powder that enhances the potential of latex particles to aerosolize and to spread to the respiratory system of personnel and to environmental surfaces during the donning or removal of gloves.

Irritant or contact dermatitis accounts for the majority of reactions resulting from wearing latex-containing gloves. (Table 3-2). True allergic reactions present as T-cell–mediated contact dermatitis (type IV) or as an immunoglobulin E-mediated anaphylactic reaction.

Anesthesiologists who believe that they are allergic to latex should take immediate steps to assess this possibility.[31] If a diagnosis of allergy has been established, the affected anesthesiologist must avoid all direct contact with latex-containing products. It is also important that coworkers wear nonlatex or powderless, low latex-allergen gloves to limit the levels of ambient allergens. Because sensitization is an irreversible process, limited exposure and primary prevention of allergy is the best overall strategy. Anaphylactic reactions to latex can be life-threatening.

Radiation

Many modern surgical procedures rely heavily on fluoroscopic guidance techniques. As a result, anesthesiologists are at risk for being exposed to excessive radiation. The magnitude of radiation absorbed by individuals is a function of three variables: (1) total radiation exposure intensity and time, (2) distance from the source of radiation, and (3) the use of radiation shielding. The latter two are amenable to modification by the

TABLE 3-2

TYPES OF REACTIONS TO LATEX GLOVES

REACTION	SIGNS/SYMPTOMS	CAUSE	MANAGEMENT
Irritant contact dermatitis	Scaling, drying cracking of skin	Direct skin irritation by gloves, powder, soaps	Identify reaction, avoid irritant, possible use of glove liner, use of alternative product
Type IV—delayed hypersensitivity	Itching, blistering, crusting (delayed 6–72 hours)	Chemical additives used in manufacturing (such as accelerators)	Identify offending chemical, possible use of alternative product without chemical additive, possible use of glove liner
Type I—immediate hypersensitivity	—	Proteins found in latex	Identify reaction; avoid latex-containing products; use of nonlatex or powder-free, low-protein gloves by co-workers
A. Localized contact urticaria	Itching, hives in area of contact with latex (immediate)		Antihistamines, topical/systemic steroids
B. Generalized reaction	Runny nose, swollen eyes, generalized rash or hives, bronchospasm, anaphylaxis		Anaphylaxis protocol

Reproduced from American Society of Anesthesiologists Task Force on Latex Sensitivity of the Committee on Occupational Health of Operating Room Personnel: Natural Rubber Latex Allergy: Considerations for Anesthesiologists. Park Ridge, IL, American Society of Anesthesiologists, 2005 (http://www.asahq.org/publicationsAndServices/latexallergy.pdf) with permission from the American Society of Anesthesiologists. A copy of the full text can be obtained from the ASA, 520 N. Northwest Highway, Park Ridge, IL 60068-2573.

anesthesiologist. Unfortunately, the lead aprons and thyroid collars commonly worn leave exposed many vulnerable sites, such as the long bones of the extremities, the cranium, the skin of the face, and the eyes. Because radiation exposure is inversely proportional to the square of the distance from the source, increasing this distance is more universally protective. Radiation exposure becomes minimal at a distance greater than 36 inches from the source, a distance that is easily attainable in most anesthetizing locations.

The U.S. Regulatory Commission has established an occupational exposure limit of 5,000 mrem/year. Occupational exposures among anesthesia personnel have been reported to be considerably below this limit.[32] However, these studies were conducted before the introduction of many of the modern surgical procedures that rely heavily on fluoroscopic guidance techniques. A more recent study reported a doubling of the aggregate radiation exposure to the members of a department of anesthesiology in the year following the introduction of an electrophysiology laboratory.[33] Pregnant workers present special concerns, and the dose to the fetus should be <500 mrem during the gestation period.

Oncogenesis, teratogenesis, and long-term genetic defects can occur with sufficiently high exposure to radiation. The risks associated with radiation vary considerably, depending on age, gender, and specific organ site exposure.[34] However, even low levels of radiation exposure are not inconsequential. The stochastic biologic effects of radiation are cumulative and permanent.[a] There are no published data that define the lower threshold for radiation-induced disease. Therefore, the general admonition regarding occupational radiation exposure, and the basis of protection programs, is as low as reasonably achievable.

Noise Pollution

Noise pollution is a potential health hazard that is virtually uncontrolled in the modern hospital and specifically in the operating room. Noise is quantified by determining both the intensity of the sound in decibels (dB) and the duration of the exposure. NIOSH has determined that the maximum level for safe noise exposure is 90 dB for 8 hours.[35] Each increase in noise of 5 dB halves the permissible exposure time, so that 100 dB is acceptable for just 2 hours per day. The maximum allowable exposure in an industrial setting is 115 dB.

The noise level in many operating rooms is surprisingly close to what constitutes a health hazard.[36] Ventilators, suction equipment, music, and conversation produce background noise at a level of 75 to 90 dB. Superimposed on this are sporadic and unexpected noises caused by dropped equipment, surgical saws and drills, and monitor alarms. Resultant noise levels frequently exceed 120 dB and are comparable to the clamor of a busy freeway.[37]

Excessive levels of noise can have an adverse influence on the anesthesiologist's capacity to perform clinical tasks. Noise can interfere with the ability to discern conversational speech and to hear auditory alarms. Mental efficiency and short-term memory are diminished by exposure to excess noise.[36] Complex psychomotor tasks associated with anesthesiology, such as monitoring and vigilance, are particularly sensitive to the adverse influences of noise pollution.

There are also chronic ramifications of long-term exposure to excessive noise in the workplace. At the very least, noise pollution is an important factor in decreased worker produc-

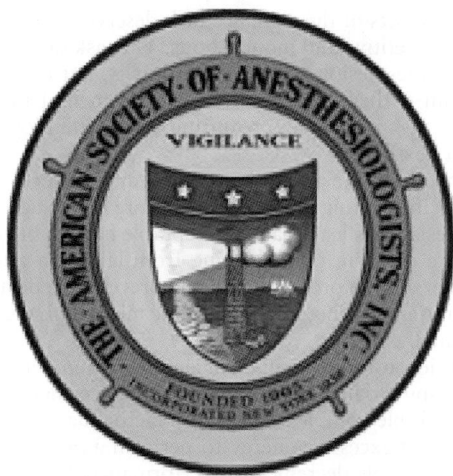

FIGURE 3-1.   Official seal of the American Society of Anesthesiologists. "VIGILANCE" has always been recognized as the most critical of the anesthesiologist's tasks.

tivity. At higher noise levels, workers are likely to show signs of irritability and demonstrate evidence of stress, such as elevated blood pressure. Ultimately, hearing loss may ensue.[38]

On the other hand, one form of background noise, music, can provide a number of beneficial effects. Music has proved advantageous as a supplement to sedation and analgesia for surgical patients.[39,40] Self-selected background music can contribute to reducing autonomic responses in surgeons and improving their performance.[41] The beneficial effects are less pronounced when the music is chosen by a third party. The selection of music, and the volume at which it is played, should be by mutual agreement of all parties present in the operating room.

Human Factors

The work performed by an anesthesiologist can be intricate and includes a number of complex tasks. Extensive research and marketing efforts have been directed toward finding high-technology solutions to assist the anesthesiologist in managing this demanding workload. Less attention has been given to applying human factor technology to improve the workplace and ensure patient safety. Human error has been identified as a significant cause of patient morbidity and mortality.[42]

A number of human factor difficulties potentially exist in the operating room. For example, anesthesia equipment is often poorly designed or positioned. Anesthesia monitors and record-keeping equipment are frequently placed so that attention must be directed away from the patient and surgical field. This was well demonstrated by observations that the insertion and monitoring of a transesophageal echocardiograph added significantly to the anesthesiologist's workload and diverted attention away from other patient-specific tasks.[43]

The ability to respond to critical incidents and to sustain complex monitoring tasks, such as maintaining vigilance[b] are among those tasks that are most vulnerable to the distractions created by poor equipment design or placement. The critical importance of the vigilance task to the practice of anesthesiology is evidenced by the fact that the seal of the ASA bears as its only motto, "Vigilance" (Fig. 3-1).

---

[a]A *stochastic* effect is one for which the probability of the occurrence increases with an increasing dose but the severity of the resulting disease does not depend on the magnitude of the dose.

[b]Vigilance is the ability to detect changes in a stimulus during prolonged monitoring tasks when the subject has no prior knowledge of whether or when any changes might occur.

Several aspects of the vigilance task deserve attention. This function is repetitive and monotonous. The task does not fully occupy the anesthesiologist's mental activity, but neither does it leave him or her free to perform other mental functions. Finally, the task is complex, requiring visual attention as well as manual dexterity.

Vigilance tasks are generally performed at the level of 90% accuracy.[44] In a setting where the stakes are high, such as during anesthesia, this leaves an unacceptable margin of error. In fact, human error, in part resulting from lapses in attention, accounts for a large proportion of the preventable deaths and serious injuries resulting from anesthetic mishaps in the United States annually.

In addition to poor equipment design, a number of other factors conspire to hamper the ability of the anesthesiologist to perform multiple complex tasks. Any factor that requires the expenditure of excessive energy to perform a given task produces a predictable decrement in performance. Even the most trivial aspect of an operator's performance plays a significant role over the course of time. For example, if the anesthesiologist must make frequent rapid changes in observation from a dim, distant screen to a bright, nearby one, the continuous muscular activity required for pupil dilation and constriction and lens accommodation promotes fatigue and hinders performance.

The detrimental effects of unnecessary energy expenditure can be mental as well as physical. As more functions are monitored and more data processed during the course of a surgical procedure, increasingly larger amounts of mental work are expended. The mental work varies directly with the difficulty encountered in extracting information from the monitors and displays competing for the anesthesiologist's attention. Poor engineering of the monitor displays, so that mode of presentation, signal frequency, or strength is suboptimal, can adversely influence the operator's performance.

Even the alarms that have been developed with the specific goal of supplementing the task of vigilance can have considerable drawbacks. In general, alarms are nonspecific (the same alarm signaling as many as 12 different deviations from "normal") and can be a source of frustration and confusion. They are frequently susceptible to artifacts and frequent false-positive alarms that can distract the observer from more clinically significant information. It is not unusual for frequently distractive alarms to be inactivated. In 2005, the ASA revised its Standards for Basic Monitoring to mandate that pulse oximeter and capnography alarms should not be turned off.[c]

Noise can have a detrimental influence on the anesthesiologist working at multiple tasks. The average noise level of 77 decibels found in operating rooms can reduce mental efficiency and short-term memory. In general, obtrusive noises, such as loud talking, excessive clanging of instruments, and "broadband" noise, are associated with decrements in performance.

Organizational issues, such as failed communication among team members, can have a detrimental effect on an anesthesiologist's performance. The potential for disaster as a result of poor communication has been well illustrated in a number of airline catastrophes.[45] The possibility for miscommunication and resultant accident is heightened in the operating room where, in contrast to the structure inherent in an airline crew, there is an absence of a well-defined hierarchical organization and there are overlaps in areas of expertise and responsibility. Poor communication can lead to conflict, compromised patient safety,[46] and has been identified as a root cause of 35% of anesthesia-related sentinel events.[47]

Effective conflict resolution is an important element of the team work necessary for successful surgical outcomes. Conflict and unpleasant interpersonal interactions among team members are among the most stressful aspects of the job of an anesthesiologist and can hinder safe anesthetic care.[48] Conflict occurs during the management of as many as 78% of patients in high-intensity areas such as operating rooms or critical care units.[49]

Successful resolution of conflict is a skill that can be learned.[50] The airline industry has successfully implemented crew resource management programs to improve the performance of cockpit teams.[51] Fundamentally, mutual respect is required among team members along with a willingness to carefully listen and recognize the differences of opinion. Intervention by a neutral third party is frequently helpful in finding an innovative solution.[52]

"Production pressure" is an organizational concern that has the potential to create an environment in which issues of productivity supersede those of safety.[53] Production pressure has been associated with the commission of errors resulting from haste and/or deliberate deviations from known safe practices.

The application of simulation technology is gaining acceptance as a tool to study and teach human performance issues in anesthesiology.[54] It appears to be particularly suited to training nontechnical skills such as resource management, teamwork, and communication.[55]

Work Hours and Night Call

Prolonged work hours that result in sleep deprivation and fatigue are a ubiquitous component of many anesthesiologists' professional lives. Ten- to 12-hour workdays are common. Additional emergency and on-call coverage frequently result in 24- to 32-hour shifts. Gravenstein et al[56] reported the average anesthesiologist's work week was 56 hours. Seventy-four percent of the study respondents reported that they had worked without a break for longer periods than they personally thought was safe and 64% attributed an error in anesthetic management to fatigue. Howard et al[57] demonstrated that residents in their routine, non–postcall state suffered from chronic sleep deprivation and had the same degree of sleepiness as measured in residents finishing 24 hours of in-house call.

Long hours of work and night call are especially challenging for the aging anesthesiologist. Older individuals are particularly sensitive to disturbances of the sleep–wake cycle and are in general better suited to phase advances (morning work) than phase delays (nocturnal work).[58] Demands associated with night call have been identified as the most stressful aspect of practice and most frequently cited impetus toward retirement.[58]

Sleep deprivation and circadian disruption have deleterious effects on cognition, performance, mood, and health.[59] Both acute sleep loss (24 hours of on-call duty) and chronic partial sleep deprivation (<6 hours of sleep per night) result in a similar degree of neurobehavioral impairment. The nature and degree of impairment on psychomotor testing with acute sleep deprivation bears a striking similarity to that seen with alcohol intoxication.[60]

The deleterious effect of sleep loss and fatigue on work efficiency and accuracy is well documented in many industries.[54,61] Sleep deprivation has been implicated as a contributing factor in many well-publicized industrial accidents such as those that occurred at Chernobyl and Three Mile Island. Data collected from residents in many clinical settings demonstrate that work shifts of greater than 24 hours are associated with an increased risk of attentional failures, significant medical errors, and adverse patient events.[62] Other studies indicate that residents working extended duration shifts

---

had an increased risk of percutaneous injuries and were more likely to report motor vehicle crashes or near-miss incidents during their commute from work.

Complex cognitive tasks that are specific to anesthesiology, such as monitoring and accurate clinical decision-making, may be adversely affected by sleep deprivation. Surveys of anesthesia personnel have linked fatigue and anesthetic errors, but these contain self-reported data that may not be verifiable.[56] In a study of performance on an anesthesia simulator, residents in the sleep-deprived condition demonstrated progressive impairment of alertness, mood, and performance and had longer response latency to vigilance probes.[54] In spite of this, there were no significant differences in the clinical management of the simulated patients between the rested and sleep-deprived groups. Subsequent to a period of sleep deprivation, performance does not return to normal levels until 24 hours of rest and recovery has occurred. An interesting phenomenon is the "end-spurt," in which previously deteriorated performance shows improvement when the subject realizes that the task is 90% completed. The converse undoubtedly also occurs, a "let-down" with additional deterioration in performance when the procedure is unexpectedly prolonged.

The sleep-loss pattern experienced by anesthesiologists who take night call is complex and includes elements of each of the three general classes of sleep deprivation: total, partial, and selective sleep deprivation. Selective sleep deprivation resulting from frequent interruptions is most disruptive to important components of sleep including slow-wave sleep (associated with "body repair") and rapid eye movement sleep ("mind repair"). Indicators of psychosocial distress, including irritability, displaced anger, depression, and anxiety, have all been identified in house officers suffering from sleep deprivation.[63] An additional area of concern is the potential effect of sleep deprivation and chronic fatigue on health and psychosocial adjustment. Work schedules that disrupt circadian rhythms are associated with impaired health, emotional problems, and a decline in performance.

National attention was focused on the problems associated with sleep-deprived medical housestaff by the well-publicized Libby Zion case. A large portion of this claim hinged on the allegation that fatal, avoidable mistakes were made by exhausted, unsupervised residents. A number of medical organizations and state legislatures subsequently took action to limit excessive work hours and resultant sleep deprivation among physicians, especially trainees. For example, the Accreditation Council for Graduate Medical Education (ACGME) has set universal standards that limit resident duty hours to an average of 80 hours per week and no more than 30 hours at any one time, limit the frequency of in-house call, and mandate that "off-duty" time be provided. Unfortunately, no regulations pertain to the practicing anesthesiologist or nurse anesthetist. In this area, medicine remains significantly behind other industries, most notably the transport and airline industries, in identifying and regulating work practices that permit excessively long shifts.[59]

After ACGME set duty hour limits for residents in 2003, investigators have attempted to assess the effects. Although studies suggest that residents' quality of life has generally improved, the effect on education is uncertain because many of the studies contain significant method flaws.[64] There have been conflicting reports on whether duty hour limits have resulted in improved patient outcome.[65,66] Although it was expected that reducing resident fatigue would be associated with fewer medical errors, duty hour limits may have created unintended consequences, such as the loss of continuity of care, an increased likelihood for failure to transmit critical information when responsibility for care is transferred at the end of shifts, and the allocation of many medical tasks typically performed by residents to nonphysician extenders.

Several strategies can be used to prevent fatigue and the effects of sleep deprivation during long work periods.[59] Personnel should be educated on the problems associated with poor sleep habits outside the hospital. Naps prior to the start of call as well as the use of caffeine can improve alertness during long shifts. Modafinil may be useful to treat sleepiness in individuals with shift-work sleep disorder.[67]

INFECTION HAZARDS

Anesthesia personnel are at risk for acquiring infections both from patients and from other personnel. Viral infections, reflecting their prevalence in the community, are the most significant threat to HCWs. Most commonly, these are spread through the respiratory route—a mechanism that is, unfortunately, the most difficult to control effectively. Other infections are propagated by hand-to-hand transmission, and hand washing is considered the single most important intervention for protection against this form of contagion.[68] Immunity against some viral pathogens can be provided through vaccination.[69] Blood-borne pathogens such as hepatitis and human immunodeficiency virus (HIV) cause serious infections, but transmission can be prevented with mechanical barriers blocking portals of entry or, in the case of hepatitis B, by producing immunity by vaccination.[70] Current recommendations from the Centers for Disease Control and Prevention (CDC) for pre-employment screening, infection control practices, vaccination, postexposure treatment, and work restrictions for infected personnel should be consulted for specific information related to each pathogen.[70–72]

Respiratory Viruses

Respiratory viruses, which are responsible for many community-acquired infections, are usually transmitted by two routes. Small-particle aerosols produced by coughing, sneezing, or talking can propel viruses over large distances. The influenza and measles viruses are spread in this way. The second mechanism involves large droplets produced by coughing or sneezing, contaminating the donor's hands or an inanimate surface, whereupon the virus is transferred to the oral, nasal, or conjunctival mucous membranes of a susceptible person by self-inoculation. Rhinovirus and respiratory syncytial virus (RSV) are spread by this process.

Influenza Viruses

Because influenza viruses are easily transmitted, community epidemics of influenza are common, with large outbreaks occurring annually. Acutely ill patients shed virus through small-particle aerosols by coughing or sneezing for as long as 5 days after the onset of symptoms. Respiratory isolation precautions can be used for the duration of the clinical illness in an attempt to prevent spread to susceptible individuals. Because of their contact with nasopharyngeal secretions, anesthesiologists can play a role in the spread of influenza virus in hospitals.

Influenza rarely produces significant morbidity in healthy personnel but can result in high rates of absenteeism. Hospital staff, especially those who care for patients in high-risk groups, should be immunized annually (October or November) with the inactivated (killed virus) influenza virus vaccine.[72] Antigenic variation of influenza viruses occurs over time, so that new viral strains (usually two type A and one type B) are selected for inclusion in each year's vaccine.

In the United States, there are four antiviral agents for chemoprophylaxis and treatment of influenza: amantadine, rimantadine, zanamivir, and oseltamivir.[72] Because of a high likelihood of influenza A viral resistance, amantadine and rimantadine are not currently recommended. The neuraminidase inhibitors zanamivir and oseltamivir have been shown to be effective in preventing and treating both influenza A and B. During hospital outbreaks of influenza, the antiviral agents zanamivir and oseltamivir are about 80% effective in preventing influenza infection in unvaccinated hospital personnel and, if administered within 48 hours of the onset of illness, can reduce the duration and severity of illness. Because of possible morbidity to hospitalized patients and to hospital personnel, it is recommended that during community influenza epidemics, hospitals should consider limiting elective admissions and surgery.

Influenza Pandemic. In the past century, there have been three influenza pandemics (1918, 1957, and 1968) with the "Great Influenza" in 1918 killing between 40 and 50 million people worldwide. Although the timing and severity cannot be predicted, another influenza pandemic is likely and represents one of the greatest public health threats.[d] In the event of a pandemic, the large number of infected patients would strain global resources such as health care facilities and equipment (respirators for personnel and ventilators for patients). Containment to prevent the spread of infection requires early identification and isolation of infected individuals to limit disease transmission. For patients requiring hospitalization, specific wards should be established with dedicated staff. NIOSH-certified respirators (N95 or higher) should be used by personnel during activities or procedures likely to generate infectious respiratory aerosols.

Avian Influenza A. Avian influenza virus occurs naturally in birds, but there have been outbreaks in humans.[73] The first human cases were reported from Asia, but the virus has been identified in Europe, the Near East, and Africa. Avian influenza A type H5N1 has a human mortality of over 50%. Clinical illness begins as a severe pneumonia that may rapidly progress to acute respiratory distress syndrome. Outbreaks of avian flu have usually occurred in people who have had close contact with infected poultry. Human-to-human transmission is uncommon, but because influenza viruses have the ability to mutate, there is concern that future H5N1 viruses may be capable of spread from one person to another. There is variable susceptibility of the virus to currently available antiviral agents. A vaccine for prophylaxis against avian influenza H5N1 was approved for use in the United States in 2007.

Respiratory Syncytial Virus

RSV is the most common cause of serious bronchiolitis and lower respiratory tract disease in infants and young children worldwide. During periods when RSV is prevalent in the community (usually late November through May in the United States), many hospitalized infants and children may carry the virus. Large numbers of virus are present in respiratory secretions of infected children, and although viable virus can be recovered for up to 6 hours on contaminated environmental surfaces, it is readily inactivated with soap and water and dis-

infectants. Infection of susceptible people occurs by self-inoculation when RSV in secretions is transferred to the hands, which then contact the mucous membranes of the eyes or nose.[74] Although most children have been exposed to RSV early in life, immunity is not permanent and reinfection is common.

RSV may also be a significant cause of illness in healthy elderly patients and those with chronic cardiac or pulmonary disease.[75] RSV is shed for approximately 7 days after infection. Hospitalized patients with the virus should be isolated, but during seasonal outbreaks large numbers of patients may make isolation impractical.[76] Careful hand washing and the use of gowns, gloves, masks, and goggles (standard precautions) have all been shown to reduce RSV infection in hospital personnel.

Herpes Viruses

Varicella-zoster virus (VZV), herpes simplex virus types 1 and 2, and cytomegalovirus (CMV) are members of the Herpetoviridine family. Close personal contact is required for transmission of all the herpes viruses except for VZV, which is spread by direct contact or small-particle aerosols. After primary infection with herpes viruses, the organism becomes latent and may reactivate at a later time. Most people in the United States have been infected with all of the herpes viruses by middle age. Therefore, nosocomial transmission is uncommon except in the pediatric population and in immunosuppressed patients.

Varicella-Zoster Virus

VZV produces both chicken pox and herpes zoster (shingles). Although the primary infection (chicken pox) is usually uncomplicated in healthy children, VZV infection in adults may be associated with major morbidity or death. Infection during pregnancy may result in fetal death or, rarely, in congenital defects. Health care workers with active VZV infection can transmit the virus to others.

After the primary infection, VZV remains latent in dorsal root or extramedullary cranial ganglia. Herpes zoster results from reactivation of the VZV infection and produces a painful vesicular rash in the innervated dermatome. Anesthesiologists working in pain clinics may be exposed to VZV when caring for patients who have discomfort from herpes zoster.

VZV is highly contagious, especially from patients with chicken pox or disseminated zoster. The CDC estimates that the period of communicability begins 1 to 2 days before the onset of the rash and ends when all the lesions are crusted, usually 4 to 6 days after the rash appears.[77] Because VZV may be spread through airborne transmission, respiratory isolation should be used for patients with chicken pox or disseminated herpes zoster.[76] Use of gloves to avoid contact with vesicular fluid is adequate to prevent VZV spread from patients with localized herpes zoster.

Most adults in the United States have protective antibodies to VZV. Because there have been many reports of nosocomial transmission of VZV, it is recommended that all HCWs have immunity to the virus. Anesthesia personnel should be questioned about prior VZV infection, and those with a negative or unknown history of infection should be serologically tested.[77] All employees with negative titers should be restricted from caring for patients with active VZV infection and should be offered immunization with two doses of the live, attenuated varicella vaccine.

Susceptible personnel with a significant exposure to an individual with VZV infection are potentially infective from 10 to 21 days after exposure and should not contact patients

---

[d]U.S. Department of Health and Human Services, www.hhs.gov/pandemicflu/plan.

during this period. They should be offered vaccination within 3 to 5 days of the exposure since it might modify the disease. Varicella-zoster immune globulin can also be considered but it is most effective when administered within 96 hours after exposure.[77] Personnel without VZV immunity should be reassigned to alternative locations so that they do not care for patients who have active VZV infections.

Herpes Simplex

Herpes simplex virus (HSV) infection is quite common in adults. After viral entry through the mucous membranes of the mouth, the primary infection with HSV type 1 is usually clinically inapparent but may involve severe oral lesions, fever, and adenopathy. In healthy people, the primary infection subsides and the virus persists in a latent state within the sensory nerve ganglion innervating the site of infection. Any of several mechanisms can reactivate the virus to produce recurrent infection, which manifests in the vicinity of the primary lesion.

A second HSV, type 2, is usually associated with genital infections and is spread by sexual contact. Newborns may become infected with HSV type 2 during vaginal delivery.

Health care personnel may be inoculated by direct contact with body fluids carrying either HSV type 1 or 2.

Herpetic infection of the finger, herpetic paronychia or herpetic whitlow, is an occupational hazard for anesthesia personnel. The infection usually begins at the portal of viral entry, a site on the distal finger where the integrity of the skin has been broken, and results in vesicle formation. Within 3 weeks, the throbbing pain lessens and the lesions begin to heal. Use of acyclovir, an antiviral drug that inhibits replication of HSV, may shorten the course of the primary cutaneous viral infection. Personnel with HSV infections of the fingers or hands should not contact patients until their lesions are healed.

Cytomegalovirus

CMV infects between 50 and 85% of individuals in the United States before age 40, with most infections producing minimal symptoms. After the primary infection, the virus remains dormant, and recurrent disease only occurs with compromise of the individual's immune system. Transmission of CMV can take place through close contact with an individual excreting the virus or through contact with contaminated saliva or urine. It is unlikely that aerosols or small droplets play a role in CMV transmission.

Primary or recurrent CMV infection during pregnancy results in fetal infection in up to 2.5% of occurrences. Congenital CMV syndrome may be found in up to 10% of infected infants. Thus, although CMV infection usually does not result in morbidity in healthy adults, it may have significant sequelae in pregnant women. CMV infection can also be deadly in immunocompromised patients, such as those undergoing bone marrow transplantation.

The two major populations with CMV infection in the hospital include infected infants and immunocompromised patients, such as those who have undergone organ transplants or those on oncology units. Routine infection control procedures (standard precautions) are sufficient to prevent CMV infection in HCWs (Tables 3-3 and 3-4).[71] Pregnant personnel should be made aware of the risks associated with CMV infection during pregnancy and of appropriate infection control precautions to be used when caring for high-risk patients. There is no evidence to indicate that it is necessary to reassign pregnant women from patient care areas in which they may have contact with CMV-positive patients.

Rubella

Outbreaks of rubella, or German measles, in hospital personnel have resulted in significant loss in employee working time, employee morbidity, and cost to the hospital. Although most adults in the United States are immune to rubella, up to 20% of women of childbearing age are still susceptible. Rubella infection during the first trimester of pregnancy is associated with congenital malformations or fetal death.

Rubella is transmitted by contact with nasopharyngeal droplets spread by infected individuals coughing or sneezing. Patients are most contagious while the rash is erupting but can transmit the virus from 1 week before to 5 to 7 days after the onset of the rash. Droplet precautions should be used to prevent transmission (Table 3-4).[76]

TABLE 3-3

PREVENTION OF OCCUPATIONALLY ACQUIRED INFECTIONS

■ INFECTIOUS AGENT	■ PREVENTIVE MEASURES[a]
Cytomegalovirus	Standard precautions
Hepatitis A	Vaccine in some cases; contact precautions
Hepatitis B	Vaccine; hepatitis B immune globulin, standard precautions
Hepatitis C	Standard precautions
Herpes simplex	Standard precautions; contact precautions if disseminated disease
Human immunodeficiency virus	Standard precautions; postexposure prophylactic antiretrovirals
Influenza, human	Vaccine; prophylactic antiretrovirals; droplet precautions
Measles	Vaccine; airborne precautions
Rubella	Vaccine; droplet precautions
Severe acute respiratory syndrome	Standard precautions; airborne precautions
Tuberculosis	Airborne precautions; isoniazid ± ethambutol for purified protein derivative conversion
Varicella-zoster	Vaccine; varicella-zoster immune globulin; airborne and contact precautions; standard precautions if localized disease

Data derived from reference 76.
[a]Isolation precautions outlined in Table 3-4.

TABLE 3-4

HEALTH CARE ISOLATION PRECAUTIONS*a*

■ STANDARD PRECAUTIONS

These are to be used for the care of all patients regardless of their diagnosis or presumed infection status.
Standard precautions should be used in conjunction with other forms of transmission-based precautions (described later in table) for the care of specific patients.

1. *Hand washing (hand hygiene)*
   After touching blood, body fluids, or contaminated items and environmental surfaces even if gloves are worn.
2. *Gloves*
   Wear gloves when it is reasonably anticipated that there will be contact with blood or infectious material, mucous membranes, nonintact skin, or contaminated intact skin.
   Change gloves between tasks on the same patient when the hands will move from a contaminated body-site to a clean one.
   Remove gloves after use, before touching noncontaminated items and environmental surfaces.
3. *Mask, eye protection, face shield*
   Use during procedures likely to generate splashes of blood or body fluids that may contaminate face or mucous membranes.
4. *Gown*
   Use during procedures likely to generate splashes of blood or body fluids that may contaminate clothing or arms.
5. *Respiratory hygiene/cough etiquette*
   Educate health care personnel and implement methods to contain respiratory secretions in patients and visitors especially during seasonal outbreaks of viral respiratory tract infections.
6. *Patient-care equipment and instruments/devices*
   Use PPE when handling soiled devices to prevent contamination of skin, mucous membranes, or clothing.
7. *Environmental control*
   Contaminated environmental surfaces should routinely be cleaned and/or disinfected.
8. *Linen*
   Soiled linen should be handled in a manner that prevents contamination of personnel, other patients, and environmental surfaces.
9. *Occupational health and blood-borne pathogens*
   Use care to prevent injuries when using or disposing of needles and sharp devices.
   Contaminated needles should not be recapped or manipulated by using both hands. If recapping is necessary for the procedure being performed, a one-handed scoop technique or mechanical device for holding the needle sheath should be used.
   Contaminated needles should not be removed from disposable syringes by hand.
   Do not break or bend contaminated needles before disposal.
   After use, disposable syringes and needles and other sharp devices should be placed in appropriate puncture-resistant containers located as close as practical to the area in which the items were used.
   Mouthpieces, resuscitation bags, or other ventilation devices should be available for use as an alternative to mouth-to-mouth ventilation.
10. *Patient placement*
    Single-patient rooms should be used for patients who pose a risk for transmission of infectious agents to others.

■ TRANSMISSION-BASED PRECAUTIONS

These should be used along with standard precautions for patients known or suspected to be infected or colonized with highly transmissible pathogens requiring additional precautions.

■ AIRBORNE PRECAUTIONS

These should be used for patients known or suspected to be infected with micro-organisms transmitted by airborne droplet nuclei (particles 5 μm or smaller in size) that can be dispersed over large distances by air currents.

1. *Patient placement*
   The patient should be placed in a single-patient room with (1) documented negative air pressure relative to surrounding areas, (2) 6 to 12 air changes per hour, (3) discharge of air outdoors or monitored high-efficiency filtration of room air before the air is circulated to other areas in the hospital.
   The door to the room should be kept closed and the patient should remain in the room.
2. *Respiratory protection*
   A fit-tested NIOSH-approved N95 or higher level respirator should be worn when entering the room of a patient with known or suspected infectious pulmonary or laryngeal tuberculosis or smallpox.
   Susceptible personnel should not enter the room of patients known or suspected to have measles, varicella, disseminated zoster, or smallpox if other immune caregivers are available. If susceptible persons must enter the room of a patient known or suspected to have measles or varicella, they should wear respiratory protection. Persons known to be immune to measles or varicella need not wear respiratory protection.
3. *Patient transport*
   Patients should be transported from the isolation room only for medically necessary purposes. When transport is necessary, a surgical mask should be placed on the patient to prevent dispersal of droplets and the patient should be instructed to follow respiratory hygiene/cough etiquette.
4. *Patients with tuberculosis*
   Current CDC guidelines should be consulted for additional precautions.[76]

(continued)

TABLE 3-4

Continued

■ DROPLET PRECAUTIONS

These should be used for patients known or suspected to be infected with microorganisms transmitted by large-particle droplets (particles larger than 5 μm) that can be generated during coughing, sneezing, talking, or by performing certain procedures.

1. *Patient placement*
   The patient should be placed in a single-patient room.
2. *Respiratory protection*
   Personnel should wear a mask when entering the patient's room.
3. *Patient transport*
   Patients should be transported from the isolation room only for medically necessary purposes. When transport is necessary, a surgical mask should be placed on the patient and they should be instructed to follow respiratory hygiene/cough etiquette. No mask is required for the person transporting the patient.

■ CONTACT PRECAUTIONS

These should be used for patients known or suspected to be infected or colonized with epidemiologically important micro-organisms transmitted by direct contact with the patient or indirect contact with environmental surfaces or patient-care items.

1. *Patient placement*
   The patient should be placed in a single-patient room.
2. *Gloves and hand washing*
   In addition to wearing gloves as outlined under standard precautions, gloves should be worn when entering the patient's room. Gloves should be changed after contacting infective material or environmental surfaces that may contain high concentrations of micro-organisms.
   Gloves should be removed before leaving the patient's environment and hands should be washed immediately with an antimicrobial agent or a waterless antiseptic agent.
   After removal of gloves and hand washing, care should be taken so that contaminated environmental surfaces should not be touched to avoid transfer of microorganisms to other patients.
3. *Gown*
   In addition to wearing a gown as outlined under standard precautions, a gown (nonsterile) should be worn when entering the room when it is anticipated that clothing will have contact with the patient, environmental surfaces, or contaminated items or if the patient is incontinent or has diarrhea, an ileostomy, a colostomy, or wound drainage not contained by a dressing.
   The gown should be removed before leaving the patient's environment.
   Clothing should not contact potentially contaminated surfaces after removal of the gown.
4. *Patient transport*
   The patient should be transported from the room for only medically necessary purposes.
   If it is necessary to transport the patient, infected or colonized areas of the patient's body should be covered to prevent transmission of micro-organisms to other patients and contamination of environmental surfaces or equipment.
   Remove contaminated PPE prior to transporting patients and don clean PPE to handle the patient at the transport destination.
5. *Patient-care equipment*
   Use disposable noncritical patient-care equipment (e.g., blood pressure cuffs) or dedicate nondisposable equipment to a single patient to avoid transmission of micro-organisms to another patient. If use of common equipment is unavoidable, then items should be adequately cleaned or disinfected before use on another patient.

PPE, personal protective equipment such as gloves, gown, eye-shield, or face mask; NIOSH, National Institute for Occupational Safety and Health; CDC, Centers for Disease Control.
^{a}This table summarizes isolation precautions, but the complete guideline should be consulted for more detailed information.[76]

Ensuring immunity at the time of employment (evidence of prior vaccination with live rubella vaccine or serologic confirmation) should prevent nosocomial transmission of rubella to personnel. It has been shown that history is a poor indicator of immunity. A live, attenuated rubella virus vaccine, contained in measles, mumps, rubella vaccine, is available to produce immunity in susceptible personnel.[69,78] Many state or local health departments mandate rubella immunity for all HCWs, and local regulations should be consulted.

Measles (Rubeola)

Measles virus is highly transmissible both by large droplets and by the airborne route. The virus is found in the mucus of the nose and pharynx of the infected individual and is spread by coughing and sneezing. The disease can be transmitted from 4 days prior to the onset of the rash to 4 days after its onset. Airborne precautions should be used for infected patients (Table 3-4).[71,76] Introduction of the measles vaccine in the United States has successfully eliminated indigenous cases of measles but importation of measles from other countries continues to occur.

HCWs are at increased risk for acquiring measles and transmitting the virus to susceptible coworkers and patients. The CDC recommends that medical personnel have adequate immunity to measles, as documented by one of the following: evidence of two doses of live measles vaccine, a record of physician-diagnosed measles, or serologic evidence of measles immunity (Table 3-3).[69] Susceptible personnel born in or after 1957 should receive two doses of the live measles vaccine at the time of employment.[78]

Severe Acute Respiratory Syndrome

Severe acute respiratory syndrome (SARS) is a respiratory tract infection produced by a coronavirus, SARS-associated coronavirus (SARS-CoV). After the first cases were reported from Asia in late 2002, the disease quickly spread globally in 2003 before being controlled. Since then, global surveillance for SARS-CoV has detected no confirmed cases. Because of the rapid spread and the significant morbidity and mortality associated with the infection, there is a need to understand the disease. Health care facilities should be prepared to rapidly implement control measures if new outbreaks occur.

SARS typically presents with a high fever, greater than 38.0° C, and is followed with symptoms of headache, generalized aches, and cough. Severe pneumonia may lead to acute respiratory distress syndrome and death. SARS is spread by close person-to-person contact through virus carried in large respiratory droplets and possibly by airborne transmission. The virus can also be spread when an individual touches a contaminated object and then inoculates the mouth, nose, or eyes. Aerosolization of respiratory secretions during coughing or endotracheal suctioning has been associated with transmission of the disease to HCWs, including anesthesiologists and critical care nurses.

One of the most important interventions to prevent the spread of SARS in the health care setting is early detection and isolation of patients who may be infected with SARS-CoV.[79] Gloves, gown, respiratory protection (as a minimum, use a NIOSH-certified N95 filtering respirator), and eye protection should be donned before entering a SARS patient's room or during procedures likely to generate respiratory aerosols.[79]

Viral Hepatitis

Although many viruses may produce hepatitis, the most common are type A or infectious hepatitis, type B (HBV) or serum hepatitis, and type C (HCV), which is responsible for most cases of parenterally transmitted non-A, non-B hepatitis (NANBH) in the United States. Delta hepatitis, caused by an incomplete virus, occurs only in people infected with HBV. Outbreaks of an enterically transmitted NANBH (hepatitis E) have been reported from outside the United States and are usually caused by contaminated water. The greatest risks of occupational transmission to anesthesia personnel are associated with HBV and HCV.

Hepatitis A

About 20 to 40% of viral hepatitis in adults in the United States is caused by the type A virus. Hepatitis A is usually a self-limited illness, and no chronic carrier state exists. Spread is predominantly by the fecal–oral route, either by person-to-person contact or by ingestion of contaminated food or water. Outbreaks are usually found in institutions or other closed groups where there has been a breakdown in normal sanitary conditions. Hospital personnel do not appear to be at increased risk for hepatitis A and nosocomial transmission is rare. Personnel exposed to patients with hepatitis A should receive immune globulin intramuscularly as soon as possible but not more than 2 weeks after the exposure to reduce the likelihood of infection.[80] Immune globulin provides protection against hepatitis A through passive transfer of antibodies and is used for postexposure prophylaxis. Hepatitis A vaccine is not routinely recommended for HCWs except for those that may be working in countries where hepatitis A is endemic.[69,80]

Hepatitis B

Hepatitis B is a significant occupational hazard for nonimmune anesthesiologists and other medical personnel who have frequent contact with blood and blood products. The prevalence (the proportion of people who have or have had the condition at the time of the survey) of hepatitis B in the general population of the United States is 3 to 5%, and the carrier rate is 0.2 to 0.9% based on serologic screening. Serosurveys conducted in the United States and several other countries in the 1980s included more than 2,400 unvaccinated anesthesia personnel and demonstrated a mean prevalence of HBV serologic markers of 17.8% (range, 3.2 to 48.6%).[81.] Before the widespread usage of hepatitis B vaccine the prevalence of hepatitis B serologic markers in anesthesia personnel ranged from 19 to 49% and reflected the prevalence of HBV carriers in the referral population for the area.

Acute HBV infection may be asymptomatic and usually resolves without significant hepatic damage. Less than 1% of acutely infected patients develop fulminant hepatitis. Approximately 10% become chronic carriers of HBV (i.e., serologic evidence demonstrated for >6 months). Within 2 years, half of the chronic carriers resolve their infection without significant hepatic impairment. Chronic active hepatitis, which may progress to cirrhosis and is linked to hepatocellular carcinoma, is found most commonly in individuals with chronic viral infection for >2 years.

The diagnosis and classification of the stage of HBV infection can be made on the basis of serologic testing. Antibody to the surface antigen (anti-HBs) appears with resolution of the acute infection and confers lasting immunity against subsequent HBV infections. Chronic HBV carriers are likely to have hepatitis B surface antigen (HBsAg) and antibody to the core antigen (anti-HBc) present in serum samples. The presence of hepatitis B e antigen (HBeAg) in serum is indicative of active viral replication in hepatocytes.

Anesthesia personnel are at risk for occupationally acquired HBV infection as a result of accidental percutaneous or mucosal contact with blood or body fluids from infected patients. Patient groups with a high prevalence of HBV include immigrants from endemic areas, users of illicit parenteral drugs, homosexual men, and patients on hemodialysis.[70] Carriers are frequently not identified during hospitalization because the clinical history and routine preoperative laboratory tests may be insufficient for diagnosis. The risk for infection after an HBV-contaminated percutaneous exposure, such as an accidental needle stick, is 37 to 62% if the source patient is HBeAg-positive and 23 to 37% if HBeAg-negative. HBV can be found in saliva, but the rate of transmission is significantly less after mucosal contact with infected oral secretions than after percutaneous exposures to blood. HBV is a hardy virus that may be infectious for at least 1 week in dried blood on environmental surfaces.

Hepatitis B is now a preventable and a treatable disease. The implementation of routine vaccination has dramatically reduced the incidence of new cases in the U.S. population. In addition to vaccination, use of standard precautions, use of safety devices, and postexposure prophylaxis have significantly reduced the risk of occupationally acquired HBV infection and its sequelae in HCW.

Hepatitis B Vaccine. Use of hepatitis B vaccine is the primary strategy to prevent occupational transmission of HBV to anesthesia personnel and other HCWs at increased risk.[70] Administration of three doses of vaccine into the deltoid muscle results in the production of protective antibodies (anti-HBs) in >90% of healthy HCWs. Hospitals or anesthesia departments should have policies for educating, screening, and counseling personnel about their risk of acquiring HBV infection and should make vaccination available for susceptible personnel.[70,82]

To ensure adequate postvaccination immunity, serologic testing for anti-HBs should take place within 1 to 2 months after the third dose of vaccine.[70] Protective antibodies develop in 30 to 50% of nonresponders (i.e., anti-HBs <10 mIU/mL) with a second three-dose vaccine series. Nonresponders to vaccination, who are HBsAg-negative, remain at risk for HBV infection and should be counseled on strategies to prevent infections and the need for postexposure prophylaxis.

Vaccine-induced antibodies decline over time, with maximum titers after vaccination correlating directly with duration of antibody persistence. The CDC states that for vaccinated adults with normal immune status, routine booster doses are not necessary and periodic monitoring of antibody concentration is not recommended.[70]

When susceptible or nonvaccinated anesthesia personnel have a documented exposure to a contaminated needle or to blood from an HBsAg-positive patient, postexposure prophylaxis with HBV hyperimmune globulin is recommended.[70] Hepatitis B vaccine should be offered to any unvaccinated, susceptible person who sustains a blood or body fluid exposure.

Hepatitis C

HCV causes most cases of parenterally transmitted NANBH and is a leading cause of chronic liver disease in the United States. Although antibody to HCV (anti-HCV) can be detected in most patients with hepatitis C, its presence does not correlate with resolution of the acute infection or progression of hepatitis, and it does not confer immunity against HCV infection.[83] Seropositivity for HCV RNA is a marker of chronic infection and continued viral presence. Six major genotypes of HCV have been identified with the specific genotype being predictive for the response to and the needed duration of antiviral therapy.

Most cases of acute HCV infection are asymptomatic, and up to 40% will clear the infection within 6 months. Chronically infected individuals have a high rate of progression to chronic hepatitis with about 20% developing cirrhosis. Hepatocellular carcinoma occurs in 1 to 4% of cirrhotic patients per year. Combination therapy with interferon alpha (standard or pegylated) and ribavirin has been effective in the treatment of some cases of acute and chronic hepatitis C.[84]

Like HBV, HCV is transmitted through blood, but the rate of occupational HCV infection is less than for HBV. Although HCV transmission has been documented in health care settings, the prevalence of anti-HCV in HCWs in the United States is not greater than that found in the general population (1.6%). The greatest risk of occupational HCV transmission is associated with exposure to blood from an HCV-positive source, and the average rate of seroconversion after accidental percutaneous exposure is 1.8%.[70] HCV has been transmitted through blood splashes to the eye and with exposure via nonintact skin. HCV in dried blood on environmental surfaces may remain infectious for up to 16 hours, but environmental contamination does not appear to be a common route of transmission. Although HCV can be found in the saliva of infected individuals, it is not believed to represent a great risk for occupational transmission.[70]

There is no vaccine or effective postexposure prophylaxis available to prevent HCV infection, and use of immune globulin is no longer recommended after a known exposure.[70] Antiviral agents like interferon or ribavirin are not recommended as effective prophylaxis after occupational exposure. Prevention of exposures remains as the primary strategy for protecting HCWs against HCV infection. Personnel who have had a percutaneous or mucosal exposure to HCV-positive blood should have serologic testing for anti-HCV and alanine aminotransferase and counseling at the time of the exposure and at 6 months.[70]

Pathogenic Human Retroviruses

HIV Infection and Acquired Immunodeficiency Syndrome

The agent that produces acquired immunodeficiency syndrome (AIDS) is the human immunodeficiency virus (HIV), one of several pathogenic human retroviruses. Current estimates suggest that 650,000 to 900,000 people in the United States are infected with HIV, and one of four is unaware that they are HIV-positive. According to CDC data, from 1981 through December 2005 there have been about 956,000 cases of AIDS in the United States.[85] In 2005, it is estimated that globally there are 38.6 million persons living with HIV.

The initial infection with HIV presents clinically as a mononucleosis-like syndrome with lymphadenopathy and rash. Although the patient then enters an asymptomatic period, monocyte-macrophage cells serve as a reservoir for the virus throughout the body, and CD4+ T cells harbor the virus in the blood. Within a few weeks after infection, an antibody may be detected by the enzyme immunoassay or a rapid HIV antibody test, but a positive result must be confirmed using the more specific Western blot or immunofluorescent assay. After a variable length period of asymptomatic HIV infection, there is an increase in viral titer and impaired host immunity, resulting in opportunistic infections and malignancies characteristic of AIDS. As the use of highly active antiretroviral therapy became widespread in the United States in 1996, the average time of survival after HIV infection increased.

HIV is spread by sexual contact (especially homosexual males), perinatally from infected mother to neonate, and through infected blood (transfusion or shared needles) and blood products. Although the virus can be found in saliva, tears, and urine, these body fluids have a low risk for viral transmission. Many HIV-infected patients in health care settings may not be identified as such by their initial or presenting diagnosis.

Risk of Occupational HIV Infection. Although there are several modes of transmission for HIV infection in the community, the most important source for occupational transmission of HIV to the HCW is blood contact.[70] The rate of seroconversion in HCWs sustaining a percutaneous exposure (needlestick injury) to HIV-infected blood is estimated to be 0.3%,[86] while the rate after a mucous membrane exposure is 0.09%.[87] Transmission has occurred after blood exposure to nonintact skin, but although the rate is unknown, it is likely less than for mucous membrane exposure.

A case-control study has demonstrated that specific factors are associated with an increased rate of HIV transmission after a percutaneous injury.[88] Increased risk was associated with a deep injury, visible blood on the device producing the injury, a procedure in which the needle was placed in an artery or vein, and terminal illness (death from AIDS within 2 months) in the source patient. Therefore, the risk of occupational HIV transmission is greatest after a deep injury with a blood-filled, large-gauge, hollow-bore needle used on a patient in the terminal phase of AIDS.

The occupational risk of HIV infection is a function of the annual number of blood exposures, the rate of HIV transmission with each exposure to infected blood, and the prevalence of HIV infection in the specific patient population. Greene et al[89] prospectively collected data on 138 contaminated percutaneous injuries to anesthesia personnel. The rate of contaminated percutaneous injuries per year per full-time equivalent anesthesia worker was 0.42, and the average annual risk of HIV and HCV infection was estimated to be 0.0016 and 0.015%, respectively.

Anesthesia personnel are frequently exposed to blood and body fluids during invasive procedures such as insertion of vascular catheters, arterial punctures, and endotracheal intubation.[89,90] Although many exposures are mucocutaneous and can be prevented by the use of gloves and protective clothing, these barriers do not prevent percutaneous exposures such as needlestick injuries, which carry a greater risk for pathogen transmission. Because of the tasks they perform, anesthesia personnel are likely to use and be injured by large-bore, hollow needles such as intravenous catheter stylets and needles on syringes.[89,91] Needleless or protected needle safety devices can be used to replace standard devices to reduce the risk of needlestick injuries. Although safety devices usually are more expensive than a comparable nonsafety item, they may be more cost-effective when the cost of needlestick injury investigation and medical care for infected personnel is considered.

Percutaneous injuries have now been accepted as a significant occupational risk for HCWs. The Needlestick Safety and Prevention Act of 2000 mandated that OSHA update its Bloodborne Pathogen Standard to require that exposure control plans include a process for evaluating and implementing the use of commercially available safety medical devices.[82] Employers were also required to maintain a "sharps" injury log to collect data to evaluate exposure risks and the effectiveness of safety devices. Because federal regulations require the use of safety devices, as new technologies become available, clinicians must assess these within their practice to determine which are most effective for specific tasks.

Postexposure Treatment and Prophylactic Antiretroviral Therapy.

When personnel have been exposed to patients' blood or body fluids, the incident should immediately be reported to the employee health service or the designated individual within the institution. Based on the nature of the injury, the exposed worker and the source individual should be tested for serologic evidence of HIV, HBV, and HCV infection.[70] Current local laws must be consulted to determine policies for testing the source patient, and confidentiality must be maintained. When the source patient is found to be HIV-positive, the employee should be retested for HIV antibodies at 6 and 12 weeks and at 6 months after exposure, although most infected people are expected to undergo seroconversion within the first 6 to 12 weeks. During this period, the exposed employee should follow CDC recommendations for preventing transmission of HIV to family members and patients.[70] If the source patient is found to be HIV-negative, no additional treatment is required.

The U.S. Public Health Service recommends that antiretroviral postexposure prophylaxis (PEP) be offered to HCWs who have incurred a significant percutaneous exposure to HIV-infected blood.[92] The specific antiretroviral regimen is based on the severity of exposure and the source patient. Because protocols for chemoprophylaxis are likely to change with additional research and the introduction of new antiretroviral drugs, the most current recommendations should be consulted prior to instituting postexposure prophylactic therapy. To be most effective, PEP should be initiated as soon as possible after exposure (<24 hours) and continued for 4 weeks. HCWs should be counseled on the potential toxic effects of antiretrovirals so that they can make an informed decision on the risks associated with PEP. Failure of PEP has been attributed to large viral inoculum, use of a single antiviral agent, drug resistance in the virus from the source patient, and delayed initiation or short duration of PEP therapy.

Occupational Safety and Health Administration Standards, Standard Precautions, and Transmission-Based Precautions

In the late 1980s the CDC formulated recommendations, or universal precautions, for preventing transmission of blood-borne infections (including HIV, HBV, and HCV) to HCWs. The guidelines were based on the epidemiology of HBV as a worst-case model for transmission of blood-borne infections and available knowledge of the epidemiology of HIV and HCV. Because some carriers of blood-borne viruses could not be identified, universal precautions were recommended for use during all patient contact. Although exposure to blood carries the greatest risk of occupationally related transmission of HIV, HBV, and HCV, it was recognized that universal precautions should also be applied to semen, vaginal secretions, human tissues, and the following body fluids: cerebrospinal, synovial, pleural, peritoneal, pericardial, and amniotic. Subsequently, the CDC synthesized the major features of universal precautions into standard precautions, a single set of precautions that should be applied to all patients since every person is potentially infected or colonized with an organism that might be transmitted during care (Table 3-4).[76] Standard precautions were included in a more complete set of isolation precautions, which contain guidelines (contact precautions, droplet precautions, and airborne precautions) to reduce the risk of transmission of blood-borne and other pathogens in health care settings.[76]

Standard precautions include the appropriate application and use of hand washing, personal protective equipment (PPE), and respiratory hygiene/cough etiquette. The selection of specific barriers or PPE should be commensurate with the task being performed. Gloves should be worn during any contact with mucous membranes and oral fluids, such as during endotracheal intubation and pharyngeal suctioning. Gloves may be all that is necessary during insertion of a peripheral intravenous catheter, whereas gloves, gown, mask, and face shield may be required during endotracheal intubation in a patient with hematemesis or during bronchoscopy or endotracheal suctioning. Gloves should be removed after they become contaminated to prevent dissemination of blood or body fluids to equipment or other items that may be contacted by ungloved personnel. Waterless antiseptics should be available to permit anesthesia personnel to wash their hands without leaving the operating room after glove removal. Respiratory hygiene/cough etiquette, to contain respiratory secretions in patients, has been added to standard precautions to prevent droplet transmission of respiratory pathogens, especially during seasonal outbreaks.

OSHA has promulgated standards to protect employees from occupational exposure to blood-borne pathogens.[82] Employers subject to OSHA must comply with these federal regulations. The standard requires that there must be an exposure control plan specifically detailing the methods that the employer is providing to reduce employees' risk of exposure to blood-borne pathogens. The employer must evaluate engineering controls such as needleless devices to eliminate hazards. Work practice controls are encouraged to reduce blood exposures by altering the manner in which personnel perform tasks (e.g., an instrument rather than fingers should be used to handle needles). The employer must furnish appropriate PPE (e.g., gloves, gowns) in various sizes to permit employees to comply with standard precautions. The HBV vaccine must be offered at no charge to personnel. A mechanism for postexposure treatment and follow-up must be provided. An annual educational program should inform employees of their risk for blood-borne infection and the resources available to prevent blood exposures. Implementation of standard precautions and OSHA regulations have been effective in decreasing the number of exposure incidents that result in HCW contact with patient blood and body fluids.

Creutzfeldt-Jakob Disease

Creutzfeldt-Jakob disease (CJD), caused by an infectious protein or prion, may be unsuspected in patients presenting with dementia.[93] The prion protein enters brain cells and induces abnormal folding of cellular proteins leading to irreversible damage with loss of neurons. More recently, it has been recognized that the prion strain associated with bovine spongiform encephalopathy may infect humans to produce a variant CJD (vCJD). There have been no reported cases of direct human-to-human transmission of CJD or vCJD by casual or environmental contact, droplet, or airborne routes. Iatrogenic transmission of CJD or vCJD to patients has taken place through contaminated biologic products and neurosurgical instruments and via blood transfusion. The risk of transmission to hospital personnel is unknown because surveillance is complicated by the long period from the time of infection until the onset of symptoms. Standard precautions should be used. Tissues with greatest risk of infectivity are brain, spinal cord, and eyes.

The prion is difficult to eradicate from equipment, and special sterilization methods are required for instruments that come into contact with high-infectivity tissues. The World Health Organization has developed infection control and sterilization guidelines for CJD.[e]

Tuberculosis

The incidence of tuberculosis (TB) in U.S.-born residents has declined since 1992 while the rate among foreign-born individuals living in the United States has increased over the same period. Although most individuals infected with TB are treated on an outpatient basis, undiagnosed patients may be hospitalized for the workup of pulmonary pathology or unrelated causes. Hospital personnel are especially at risk for infection from unrecognized cases.[94,95] Groups with a higher prevalence of TB include (1) personal contacts of people with active TB, (2) people from countries with a high prevalence of TB, and (3) certain populations such as the medically underserved or those living in congregate settings like homeless shelters or correctional facilities.[94] Global surveillance has documented the emergence of multidrug-resistant TB (resistance to at least two of the primary treatments, isoniazid and rifampin) as well as extensively drug-resistant organisms (resistance to at least two of the primary treatments, isoniazid and rifampin, and to any fluoroquinolone and at least one of three injectable drugs). Several hospital outbreaks of multidrug-resistant *Mycobacterium tuberculosis* infection have been reported.[95,96] Mortality associated with these outbreaks is high.

Mycobacterium tuberculosis can be transmitted over great distances through viable bacilli carried on airborne particles, 1 to 5 μm in size, by coughing, speaking, or sneezing. Airborne precautions should be used for individuals suspected of having TB until they are confirmed as nontransmitters by repeat sputum examination that demonstrates no bacilli.[94] Outbreaks of TB in health care facilities have been attributed to delayed diagnosis of TB in the source patient, delayed initiation of or inadequate airborne precautions, lapses in precautions during aerosol-generating procedures, and lack of adequate respiratory protection in HCWs. Administration of appropriate chemotherapy for sufficient duration is required to cure the individual patient, but treatment also benefits the community by preventing spread of the infection.[97]

A decrease in the health care-associated transmission of TB has been attributed to the rigorous implementation of infection-control measures. Effective prevention of spread to HCWs requires early identification of infected patients and immediate initiation of airborne infection isolation (negative-pressure rooms with air vented outside; see Table 3-4).[94] Patients must remain in isolation until adequate treatment is documented. If patients with TB must leave their rooms, they should wear face masks to prevent spread of organisms into the air. HCWs should wear fit-tested respiratory protective devices when they enter an isolation room or when performing procedures that may induce coughing, such as endotracheal intubation or tracheal suctioning.[94] The CDC recommends that respiratory protective devices worn to protect against *M. tuberculosis* should be able to filter 95% of particles 1 mm in size at flow rates of 50 L/min and should fit the face with a leakage rate around the seal of <10% documented by fit testing.[94] High-efficiency particulate air respirators (classified as N95) are NIOSH-approved devices that meet the CDC criteria for respiratory protective devices against *M. tuberculosis*.[98] Elective surgery should be postponed until infected patients have had an adequate course of chemotherapy. If surgery is required, bacterial filters (high-efficiency particulate filters) should be used on the anesthetic breathing circuit for patients with TB.[94] Patients must be recovered in a room that meets all the requirements for airborne precautions.

Routine periodic screening of employees for TB should be included as part of a hospital's employee health policy with the frequency of screening dependent on the prevalence of infected patients in the hospitalized population. When a new conversion is detected by skin testing, a history of exposure should be sought to determine the source patient. Treatment or preventive therapy is based on the drug-susceptibility pattern of the *M. tuberculosis* in the source patient, if known.

Viruses in Smoke Plumes

The laser is commonly used for vaporizing carcinomatous tumors and lesions that may contain active viruses. Use of lasers and electrosurgical devices is associated with several hazards, both to patients and to operating room personnel. Risks include thermal burns, eye injuries, electrical hazards, and fires and explosions. There is evidence that the smoke plumes resulting from tissue vaporization contain toxic chemicals such as benzene and formaldehyde, and in 1996, NIOSH released a health hazard alert on the dangers of smoke plumes.[99]

Clinical and laboratory studies have demonstrated that when the carbon dioxide laser is used to treat verrucae (papilloma and warts), intact viral DNA could be recovered from the plume. Viable viruses can be found in plumes produced by both carbon dioxide and argon laser vaporization of a virus-loaded culture plate, but viable viruses are carried on larger particles that travel <100 mm from the site being vaporized.[100]

A case report describes laryngeal papillomatosis in a surgeon who had used a laser to remove anogenital condylomas from several patients.[101] Although DNA analysis of the surgeon's papillomas revealed a viral type similar to that of the condylomas, proof of transmission is lacking.

To protect operating room personnel from exposure to the viral and chemical content of the laser plume, it is recommended that a smoke evacuation system with a high-efficiency filter be used with the suction nozzle being held as close as possible to the tissue being vaporized.[102] In addition, operating room personnel working in the vicinity of the laser plume should wear gloves, goggles, and high-efficiency filter masks (N95 respirators).[90,102]

EMOTIONAL CONSIDERATIONS

Stress

Stress is a well-recognized element of the operating room workplace. However, there is very little objective information specifically directed toward understanding the nature of job-related stress among anesthesiologists.[103,104] Stress is a nonspecific response to any change, demand, pressure, challenge, threat, or trauma.[48] There are three distinct components of the stress response: the initiating stressors, the psychological filters that process and evaluate the stressors, and the coping mechanisms that are employed in an attempt to control the stressful situation.

Stress on the job is unavoidable and to a certain degree is desirable. A moderate, manageable level of stress is the fuel necessary for individual achievement. Hans Seyle,[105] a pioneer in the modern study of stress, described a beneficial effect resulting from mild, brief, and controllable episodes of stress. As succinctly stated by Seyle,[105] "The absence of stress is death." On the other hand, extreme degrees of stress, especially in the workplace, can result in mental or physical disease.[106] Exactly how an individual responds to a particular stressor is the product of a number of factors, including age, gender, experience, pre-existing personality style, available defense and coping mechanisms, support systems, and concomitant events (such as sleep deprivation).

The workplace of an anesthesiologist frequently mirrors the circumstances that classically define a stressful workplace. There is a background of chronic, low-level stress punctuated by intermittent episodes of extreme stress. The demands are externally paced, usually out of the anesthesiologist's control. Habituation to the demands is difficult. Perturbations are intermittently but continuously inserted into the system. Finally, failure to meet the demands imposed by the workplace can result in serious consequences.

Certain stressors are specific to the practice of anesthesiology. Concerns about liability, long working hours and night call, production pressures, economic uncertainty, and interpersonal relations are frequently cited as sources of chronic stress for anesthesiologists. The process of inducing anesthesia (particularly with a difficult airway) can be among the most profound sources of acute stress to anesthesiologists. Physiologic changes, including heart rate and rhythm, elevations in blood pressure, and myocardial ischemia, are not uncommon. One study reported increases in the blood pressure and heart rate of anesthesiologists during all stages of the anesthetic procedure, especially during the induction.[107] There was an inverse relationship between the years of experience of the anesthesiologist and the degree of stress as manifested by heart rate change.

Interpersonal relationships impose a set of demands that can be a major source of stress to an anesthesiologist. The operating room is unique as one of the few hospital sites where two co-equal physicians simultaneously share responsibility for the care of a patient. As a result, there exist overlapping realms of clinical responsibility that can upset the customary hierarchy of command. To many anesthesiologists, as well as surgeons, this shared responsibility is the source of greatest conflict and professional stress.[50] Other workplace settings, most notably the airline industry, have made better progress in identifying and correcting sources of interpersonal friction that facilitate stress and lead to professional errors.[108]

Several personality traits, in many cases identifiable before entrance to medical school, can be predictive of the potential toward maladaptive responses to stress. Prominent among these is the obsessive-compulsive, dependent character structure. These individuals typically manifest pessimism, passivity, self-doubt, and feelings of insecurity. They commonly respond to stress by internalizing anger and becoming hypochondriacal and depressed. Undergraduate students who demonstrate these characteristics were more likely to have their medical careers disrupted by alcoholism or drug abuse, psychiatric illness, and marital disturbances.[109,110] A number of adaptive coping functions are useful for successful stress management.[48] Only when appropriate coping mechanisms become overwhelmed by the magnitude of the stress do the defenses tend to become inappropriate. This situation can give rise to maladaptive behavior and the personal and professional deterioration that can lead to disorders such as drug addiction, professional burnout, and suicide.

Substance Use, Abuse, and Addiction

Illicit drug use remains one of our society's major afflictions. It is estimated that 20 million Americans are drug abusers, with some 5 million addicted. *Substance abuse* is characterized by significant adverse consequences resulting from the repeated use of a substance.[111] With *addiction*, the individual continues to use a substance in spite of having significant substance-related problems including symptoms of withdrawal, the need for larger amounts of the substance, unsuccessful attempts to control its use, and the need to spend increasing amounts of time seeking the substance. With time, addiction leads to health, social, and economic problems. The term, *chemical dependence*, is sometimes used rather than addiction, but it is a more generic term covering physical or psychological dependency to a psychoactive substance.

Epidemiology

The abuse of drugs and consequent addiction by physicians has attracted considerable media attention and notoriety. Recognition of the problem of substance abuse among physicians is not new. In the first edition of *The Principles and Practice of Medicine*, edited by Sir William Osler and published in 1892, it is stated: "The habit (morphia) is particularly prevalent among women and physicians who use the hypodermic syringe for the alleviation of pain, as in neuralgia or sciatica."

It is debatable whether substance abuse is more prevalent among physicians than the general population. Hughes et al[112] found that physicians abused alcohol, minor opiates, and benzodiazepine tranquilizers more frequently than the general population. In many cases, the prescription drugs were self-prescribed and were considered by the physician to be "self-treatment." On the other hand, physicians were less likely to use tobacco or illicit substances. A report from the National Institute on Drug Abuse concludes that HCWs suffer from chemical dependency (including alcohol abuse) at a rate roughly equivalent to that of the general population (8 to 12%).[113]

In the event that a drug-related problem does exist, physicians are less likely than the population in general to seek professional assistance. Denial plays a major role in this reluctance to undergo counseling or therapy. Medical students learn early in their education to use denial to enable them to endure long, sleepless nights and the personal shortcomings that inevitably accompany the practice of medicine. These well-developed denial mechanisms enable the physician-addict to conclude that his or her problem is minor and that self-treatment is possible. Physicians typically enter programs for treatment only after they have reached the end stages of their illness.

It is commonly reported that chemical dependency is a specific problem for the specialty of anesthesiology and represents its primary occupational hazard.[114] One example of the increased incidence of substance abuse among anesthesiologists comes from early reports from the Medical Association of Georgia Disabled Doctors' Program.[115] Anesthesiologists constituted 12% of physician patients treated at the center although they represented only 3.9% of American physicians. On the other hand, other studies have failed to identify an overall excess prevalence of substance abuse among anesthesiologists with the notable exception of major opiates.[116,117]

One very troubling aspect of this problem is the increased incidence of substance abuse reported among anesthesiology residents. In the report from the Medical Association of Georgia Disabled Doctors' Program,[115] anesthesiology residents constituted 33.7% of the resident population of the treatment group, despite representing only 4.6% of the resident population. The incidence of controlled substance abuse within anesthesiology training programs is estimated to be 1 to 2%.[118] This statistic is particularly significant because it has persisted despite an increased emphasis placed on education and accountability of controlled substances. ACGME requirements mandate that anesthesiology residency programs have a written policy and an educational program regarding substance abuse, but these efforts have not successfully addressed the problem of substance abuse in training programs.

The Disease of Addiction

What accounts for this unacceptably high prevalence of substance abuse and addiction among anesthesiologists? To answer this, it is important to understand addiction as a chronic psychosocial, biogenetic disease.[119] Addiction shares many characteristics with other common chronic illnesses: it is a primary condition (not a symptom), it has established causes, it is associated with specific anatomic and physiologic changes, it has a set of recognizable signs and symptoms, and if left untreated, it has a predictable, progressive course.

The causative factors in this disease process involve a genetic predisposition as well as the environment. The disease results from a dynamic interplay between a susceptible host and a "favorable" environment. Vulnerability in the host is an important factor and may account for 40 to 60% of the risk for addiction. What constitutes an instigating exposure to a drug in one person may have absolutely no effect on another. Unfortunately, there is not a predictive tool to identify the susceptible individual until he or she gets the disease.

Causative factors thought to be specific to certain anesthesiologists include job stress, an orientation toward self-medication, lack of external recognition and self-respect, the availability of addicting drugs, and a susceptible premorbid personality. Self-prescription and recreational use of drugs are commonly seen as a prelude to more extensive substance abuse and dependence. Of concern is the increasing recreational use of drugs among younger physicians and medical students and the choice of more potent drugs with enhanced potential for addiction, such as cocaine, the synthetic opioids, and some of the newer inhalation anesthetics. Most notable has been the significant increase in propofol abuse among residents.[120] This may be attributable to the lack of pharmacy accounting or control of this drug in many centers.

Anesthesiologists work in a climate in which large quantities of powerful psychoactive drugs are readily available and are unique among physicians because they usually prescribe as well as personally administer these drugs. In contrast, physicians in most other specialties prescribe medications while other personnel administer them. Because availability of drugs plays a role in the onset of this disease, attention has been directed toward programs to enforce increased accountability and regulation of controlled substances.[121] However, despite widespread application of protocols to enforce greater accountability, such as satellite pharmacies for operating suites, the frequency of substance abuse has changed little, if at all, in recent years.[118]

There is an apparent association between behavior before entering medical school and subsequent development of substance abuse.[122] Personality profiles of anesthesiologists have suggested a disturbingly high proportion that may be associated with a predisposition toward maladaptive behavior. Talbott et al[115] have observed that many of the anesthesia residents in their treatment program specifically chose the specialty of anesthesiology because of the known availability of powerful drugs.

The consequences of untreated addiction are ultimately devastating. There is a gradual and inexorable deterioration in professional, family, and social relationships. The substance abuser becomes increasingly withdrawn and isolated, first in his or her personal life, and ultimately in his or her professional existence (Table 3-5). Every attempt is made to maintain a facade of normality at work because discovery means isolation from the source of the abused drug. When professional conduct is finally impaired such that it is apparent to the physician's colleagues, the disease is approaching its end stage.

If not detected and treated, addiction is often a fatal illness. Using mortality data collected between 1979 and 1995, Alexander et al[14] calculated a relative risk of 2.79 for drug-related deaths among anesthesiologists compared to a matched cohort of internists. Menk et al[123] found 14 drug-related deaths among the 79 drug abusers who had been re-enrolled in anesthesiology residencies after treatment. Using data from a more recent survey, Collins et al[124] reported that there were nine deaths in 100 residents who returned to and remained in anesthesiology training programs after treatment for chemical dependence. In addition to health hazards, there are significant legal and medicolegal considerations that may affect chemically dependent physicians.[114] Laws and regulations vary by state but they detail the necessary steps for handling the drug-abusing physician. In many states disciplinary action and criminal penalties can be imposed on physicians who knowingly fail to report an impaired colleague. Disciplinary action taken against an impaired physician must also be reported to the National Practitioner Data Bank to be in compliance with federal law. Most state medical societies have sanctioned physicians health programs. When chemically dependent physicians seek treatment through this venue, the legal impact may be mitigated, and the disease can be effectively treated.

Debate continues regarding the issue of compulsory random drug testing of physicians.[125] Pre-employment and/or random drug screening is already well established in various industries, especially those with high public health profiles (nuclear, aviation, military). Many chairs of academic anesthesiology programs have indicated a willingness to initiate a program of random drug screening of their staff.[118] Although random drug testing is an established element of most re-entry contracts for recovering anesthesiologists, serious questions remain about the legality of this approach and its effectiveness in preventing substance abuse. Because fentanyl and sufentanil are the drugs abused by many chemically dependent anesthesiologists and because routine drug screens do not detect these agents, tests that effectively identify their use are expensive and have limited availability.

When there are sufficient data to identify an anesthesiologist as having the disease of addiction, an intervention should be conducted by an experienced individual. The purpose of the intervention is to demonstrate to the anesthesiologist that he or she has the disease and to immediately have the person

TABLE 3-5

SIGNS OF SUBSTANCE ABUSE AND DEPENDENCE

▪ WHAT TO LOOK FOR OUTSIDE THE HOSPITAL

1. Addiction is a disease of loneliness and isolation. Addicts quickly withdraw from family, friends, and leisure activities.
2. Addicts have unusual changes in behavior, including wide mood swings and periods of depression, anger, and irritability alternating with periods of euphoria.
3. Unexplained overspending, legal problems, gambling, extramarital affairs, and increased problems at work are commonly seen in addicts.
4. An obvious physical sign of alcoholism is the frequent smell of alcohol on the breath.
5. Domestic strife, fights, and arguments may increase in number and intensity.
6. Sexual drive may significantly decrease.
7. Children may develop behavioral problems.
8. Some addicts frequently change jobs over a period of several years in an attempt to find a "geographic cure" for their disease or to hide it from coworkers.
9. Addicts need to be near their drug source. For a health care professional, this means long hours at the hospital, even when off duty. For alcoholics, it means calling in sick to work. Alcoholics may disappear without any explanation to bars or hiding places to drink secretly.
10. Addicts may suddenly develop the habit of locking themselves in the bathroom or other rooms while they are using drugs.
11. Addicts frequently hide pills, syringes, or alcohol bottles around the house.
12. Persons who inject drugs may leave bloody swabs and syringes containing blood-tinged liquid in conspicuous places.
13. Addicts may display evidence of withdrawal, especially diaphoresis (sweating) and tremors.
14. Narcotic addicts often have pinpoint pupils.
15. Weight loss and pale skin are also common signs of addiction.
16. Addicts may be seen injecting drugs.
17. Tragically, some addicts are found comatose or dead before any of these signs have been recognized by others.

▪ WHAT TO LOOK FOR INSIDE THE HOSPITAL

1. Addicts sign out ever-increasing quantities of narcotics.
2. Addicts frequently have unusual changes in behavior, such as wide mood swings and periods of depression, anger, and irritability alternating with periods of euphoria.
3. Charting becomes increasingly sloppy and unreadable.
4. Addicts often sign out narcotics in inappropriately high doses for the operation being performed.
5. They refuse lunch and coffee relief.
6. Addicts like to work alone in order to use anesthetic techniques without narcotics, falsify records, and divert drugs for personal use.
7. They volunteer for extra cases, often where large amounts of narcotics are available (e.g., cardiac cases).
8. They frequently relieve others.
9. They are often at the hospital when off duty, staying close to their drug supply to prevent withdrawal.
10. They volunteer frequently for extra call.
11. They are often difficult to find between cases, taking short naps after using.
12. Addicted anesthesia personnel may insist on personally administering narcotics in the recovery room.
13. Addicts make frequent requests for bathroom relief. This is usually where they use drugs.
14. Addicts may wear long-sleeved gowns to hide needle tracks and also to combat the subjective feeling of cold they experience when using narcotics.
15. Narcotic addicts often have pinpoint pupils.
16. An addict's patients may come into the recovery room complaining of pain out of proportion to the amount of narcotic charted on the anesthesia records.
17. Weight loss and pale skin are also common signs of addiction.
18. Addicts may be seen injecting drugs.
19. Untreated addicts are found comatose.
20. Undetected addicts are found dead.

Adapted from Farley WJ, Arnold WP: Videotape: Unmasking addiction: Chemical Dependency in Anesthesiology. Produced by Davids Productions, Parsippany, NJ, funded by Janssen Pharmaceutica, Piscataway, NJ, 1991.
Reprinted with permission from American Society of Anesthesiologists: Task Force on Chemical Dependence of the Committee on Occupational Health of Operating Room Personnel: Chemical Dependence in Anesthesiologists: What You Need to Know When You Need to Know It. Park Ridge, IL, American Society of Anesthesiologists, 1998.

enter a facility for evaluation and treatment. The physician, or his or her colleagues, should consider referral to a state-affiliated physicians health program.[f] Treatment usually begins with inpatient therapy progressing to outpatient sessions. The

family is actively involved with treatment, and the individual begins association with Alcoholics Anonymous (AA) or Narcotics Anonymous (NA).

Controversy remains about the ultimate career path of the anesthesiologist in recovery. Within the general population, the recidivism rate approaches 60% for patients who have been treated for addiction. However, physicians are highly

---

[f]Federation of State Physician Health Programs: http://www.fsphp.org/.

motivated and better rehabilitation rates might be expected. Early reports provided optimism that in many cases anesthesiologists could be successfully rehabilitated and safely returned to their practices. In a study that examined relapse in addicted physicians, the rate of relapse among anesthesiologists was 40% and that of control physicians was 44%.[126] Sustained recovery for longer than 2 years occurred in 81 and 86%, respectively. Although these data suggested that the outcome for recovering anesthesiologists was similar to other physicians, a study by Menk and colleagues[123] drew a different conclusion. Among 79 opioid-dependent anesthesiology residents, there was a 66% (52 of 79) failure rate for successful rehabilitation and return to practice. Even more discouraging, there were 14 suicide or overdose deaths among the 79 returning trainees. Their conclusion was that redirection into another specialty is the safer course after rehabilitation of narcotic-dependent residents. Using survey data from U.S. training programs, Collins et al[124] found that only 46% of anesthesia residents treated for substance abuse successfully completed their anesthesiology training, 34% chose to enter a training program in another medical specialty, and 16% left medicine. There were 9 deaths among the 100 anesthesia residents that continued in anesthesia training programs after treatment.

Data from a retrospective study of health care professionals has identified three factors associated with relapse after completion of treatment for chemical dependency.[127] Although the overall rate for relapse was 25%, the risk was increased when there was a family history of substance abuse (hazard ratio [HR] = 2.3) and when a major opioid was the abused drug in an individual with a coexisting psychiatric disorder (dual diagnosis, [HR = 5.8]). The risk of relapse was greatest (HR = 13.3) when all three factors were present, that is, family history, major opioid use, and dual diagnosis. Treated anesthesiologists who returned to the practice of anesthesiology had a greater risk of relapse (HR = 8.5) compared with those who did not return. Because of the small sample size, a more detailed analysis of risk factors for anesthesiologists could not be performed.

No universal recommendations can be made about re-entry into the practice of anesthesia after treatment. To re-enter practice, the recovering physician must qualify for a valid license to practice medicine and must be recredentialed at their medical facility. This must be done in compliance with their state laws and regulations that detail the circumstances under which a recovering physician can return to practice. Federal laws, such as the Americans with Disabilities Act, impose additional considerations. Additionally, a carefully worded contract is an important first step in the re-entry process to define the obligations of the physician and the department.[114,128] Contracts usually include an agreement to refrain from self-prescription of medication, submit to random urine drug screens, and directly observed administration of naltrexone or disulfiram for at least 6 months. There should also be regular meetings with the departmental supervisor to monitor the return process. It is also generally recommended that the returning anesthesiologist not take night or weekend call or handle opioids without direct supervision for at least the first 3 months. Monitoring and treatment for an extended period is more likely to reduce the risk for relapse. Despite all of these precautions, the potential for relapse must be anticipated.

Guidelines from physician treatment centers may be helpful to assist in the decisions surrounding re-entry.[111] Individuals who, in most situations, can successfully return to the practice of anesthesiology immediately after treatment (Category I) accept and understand their disease and have no evidence of accompanying psychiatric disorders. They have strong support from their family, demonstrate a balanced lifestyle, are committed to their recovery contract, and bond with AA or NA. Their anesthesiology department and hospital must be sup-

portive of their return, and the individual must have a sponsor that supports the return to anesthesiology.

Category II includes those individuals who could possibly return to anesthesiology within a few years. They must have no or minimal denial regarding their disease and have no other psychiatric diagnoses. Their recovery skills are continually improving and they are involved, but not necessarily bonded, with AA/NA. Although their family situation may be characterized as dysfunctional, there should be tangible evidence of improvement.

Individuals who should not return to anesthesiology and would best be redirected into another medical specialty are included in Category III. These individuals may have had a history of prolonged intravenous substance use and have experienced relapses and prior treatment failures. Their disease remains active, and they have coexisting severe psychiatric diagnoses.

Impairment and Disability

Impairment[g] and disability[h] can arise from physical, mental, emotional, sensory or developmental causes. The onset can be sudden, as occurs with injury or acute illness, or more gradual, as is the case with many chronic diseases.

Data regarding the prevalence of disabling disorders among physicians are difficult to obtain. Substance related disorders (see "Substance Use, Abuse, and Addiction") occurs as frequently among physicians as in the general population[113] (8% to 12%) and accounts for many cases of physician impairment.[i] It has been questioned whether, with the notable exception of opioid abuse, substance-related disease is more common among anesthesiologists than other physicians.[124] However, unpublished data collected from one large insurance underwriter indicate that the rate of substance related disability among anesthesiologists is 3 times that seen among other physicians (personal communication, UnumProvident). Other factors that may lead to impairment include physical or mental illness and deterioration associated with aging. Unwillingness or inability to keep up with current literature and techniques can be considered a form of impairment.

Among physicians who are impaired as a result of emotional illness, depression is a prominent finding. In one study, approximately 30% of medical interns were clinically depressed.[129] Indeed, when exaggerated, many of the personality traits that ensure success in the physician's world, such as self-sacrifice, competitiveness, achievement orientation, denial of feelings, and intellectualization of emotions, may also serve as risk factors for depression. Several studies on alcoholic physicians have provided some insight into this link between achievement orientation and emotional disturbance. In one study, more than half of the alcoholic physicians graduated in the upper one third of their medical school class, 23% were in the upper one tenth of their class, and only 5% were in the lower one third of their class.[130] Similarly, a report on alcohol use in medical school demonstrated better first-year grades and higher scores on Part I National Board of Medical Examiners tests among those students identified as alcohol abusers.[131]

It can be difficult to appropriately respond to the problems imposed by the impaired or unsafe anesthesiologist.[132]

---

[g]Impairment is any loss of use of any body part, organ system or organ function.
[h]Disability is an impairment that substantially limits one or more major life activities.
[i]An impaired physician is one whose performance as a professional person and as a practitioner of the healing arts is impaired because of alcoholism, drug abuse, mental illness, senility, or disabling disease.

Fortunately, many state legislatures and medical societies have formal protocols that address the impaired physician in a therapeutic and nonpunitive fashion. The license suspension power of the state board of medical examiners is usually exercised only in cases in which there is a substantial risk to the public welfare and the involved physician is unwilling to voluntarily suspend practice. Management protocols for dealing with the impaired physician are covered in a series of articles by Canavan and Baxter.[133]

The Aging Anesthesiologist

Little attention has been given to the challenges faced by older anesthesiologists.[58] This is in contrast to the situation in most other industries in which much consideration is directed toward the competence and well-being of older workers. For example, commercial pilots are required to take regular medical examinations and conform to policies regarding hours of work.

Advancing chronologic age is predictably accompanied by changes in most organ systems. Most notable for the safe practice of anesthesiology are the changes commonly observed in the central nervous system. Neuronal density and brain weight decrease from 1,375 g at age 20 years to 1,200 g at age 80 years.[134] There is an age related decline in training-dependent plasticity in the motor cortex accompanied by a diminished ability to reorganize in response to training.[135]

These and other anatomic changes are associated with common decrements in physiologic function. There are measurable decreases in hearing, vision, short-term memory, creative thinking and problem-solving abilities. Learning is slower and requires more effort. Intellectual quickness and on-the-spot reasoning and reaction time slow. These have the potential of adversely affecting the older anesthesiologist's ability to assimilate and apply new knowledge and to instantaneously process information, rapidly make complex decisions, and initiate the appropriate response.[136] These deficiencies are especially exposed in a stressful environment such as the operating room.[137]

The cardiovascular and musculoskeletal systems also undergo age-related changes that can affect the ability to practice anesthesiology. One area of particular difficulty for anesthesiologists is maintaining the stamina required for long work shifts and night call. Superimposed on a propensity to sleep disturbance, the demands of night call and associated sleep deprivation are particularly difficult for older anesthesiologists. Night call is considered one of the most stressful aspects of practice and is often cited as a reason for retirement among older anesthesiologists.[58,138]

The physiologic changes that accompany the normal aging process are often compensated by advantages conferred by older age. These include wisdom, judgment, and the experience acquired by a lifelong practice of the specialty. There is a strong correlation between experience and performance.[139,140] However, this correlation does not necessarily exist between experience and complex cognitive skills. As pointed out by Weinger,[141] experience is not synonymous with expertise.

Aging among anesthesiologists raises interesting legal issues. There are no age-specific conditions placed on state medical licensure or on the practice of anesthesiology. In most cases, the decision to limit practice or retire remains at the discretion of the individual anesthesiologist based on his or her self-evaluation. A number of federal laws impact the aging anesthesiologist's rights and responsibilities regarding continuation of work. These include the Age Discrimination Act, Title VII of the Civil Rights Act ("Equal Pay Act"), the Medical and Family Leave Act, the Fair Labor Standards Act, and the Employee Retirement Income Security Act (ERISA).

Anesthesiology, similar to other high-stress professions, is commonly considered a young person's specialty. Anesthesiologists tend to retire at a younger age than do many other specialists.[142] The decision to retire for an anesthesiologist is frequently precipitated by the growing burdens of night call or concerns about deteriorating clinical skills. In many cases, the retiring anesthesiologist just "felt it was time."[138] A growing number of practices are establishing phased retirement plans that permit senior anesthesiologists to avoid some of the more onerous aspects while remaining vital members of a practice.[143]

As a result of a number of demographic factors, including the smaller residency class sizes observed during the mid-1990s, the mean age of the anesthesiology workforce is increasing. The greatest number (30%) of anesthesiologists are between age 45 and 54 years of age, and 56% are age 45 and older (up from 49% 10 years ago).[15]

Mortality Among Anesthesiologists

8 A number of studies have examined mortality among anesthesiologists. Employing different databases and methods, these studies have reported conflicting conclusions including a shortened,[14,144] an average,[15,145] or a prolonged[146,147] life expectancy. A 2006 study reported a significant increase in life expectancy among anesthesiologists during the last decade, such that the average age at death in 2001 (the last year of the study) was 78 years, the same as the national average for all Americans.[148]

The cause of death among anesthesiologists has also been extensively studied. Earlier work found an increased incidence of certain types of cancer, including leukemia and lymphoma.[4,12] A more recent report by Alexander et al[14] found no increased risk of cancer-related deaths among anesthesiologists as compared with the control group (internists). Significantly increased risks for anesthesiologists resulted from drug-related death, suicide, drug-related suicide, other external causes, HIV-related, and cerebrovascular disease. The risk to anesthesiologists of drug-related deaths was highest in the first 5 years after graduation from medical school and remained increased for entire professional careers.

Suicide

It has been well documented that the rate of suicide ranks disproportionately high as a cause of death among both male[149] and female[150] physicians. Several reports have singled out anesthesiologists as being particularly vulnerable.[14,147,151] However, this conclusion has been questioned as the result of the methodological difficulties in collecting accurate data on suicide and the frequent failure to adequately correct for confounding variables in the study populations.[152]

Why might there be a high rate of suicide among anesthesiologists? A partial explanation lies with the high degree of stress that is an integral part of the job.[48] There is a close association in many individuals between stressful life events and major depressive disorders.[153] In susceptible individuals, feelings of inability to cope resulting from the stress-induced depression can give way to despair and suicide ideation.

Extensive personality profiles collected from suicide-susceptible individuals indicate characteristics such as high anxiety, insecurity, low self-esteem, impulsiveness, and poor self-control. It is disturbing to note that in the study of personality traits of anesthesiologists by Reeve,[154] some 20% manifested psychological profiles that reflected a predisposition to behavioral disintegration and attempted suicide when placed under extremes of stress. This study raises the discomforting notion that "premorbid" personality characteristics exist before entering specialty training and are not being identified in the admissions process.

One specific type of stress, that resulting from a malpractice lawsuit, may have a direct causative association with suicide among physicians in general and anesthesiologists in particular. Newspaper reports have described the emotional deterioration and ultimate suicide of experienced physicians who have become involved in a malpractice suit. One study reported that 4 of 185 anesthesiologists being sued for medical malpractice attempted or committed suicide.[151] Substance abuse among anesthesia personnel is another potential contributor to the increased suicide rate. Individuals with chemical dependence, who are not identified and are in the end stages of the disease, may die of drug overdose, a cause of death that can be difficult to distinguish from suicide. In one recent study, drug abuse was among the highest causes of death and the most frequent method of suicide among anesthesiologists.[14] Drug overdose and death was the initial relapse symptom in 16% (13 of 79) of the parenteral opioid abusers who had re-entered their residency in anesthesiology.[123] Physicians who are impaired from chemical dependence and whose privileges to practice medicine have been revoked are also at heightened risk for attempting suicide. Crawshaw et al[155] reported 8 successful and 2 near-miss suicide attempts among 43 physicians placed on probation for drug-related disability.

References

1. Linde HW, Bruce DL: Occupational exposure of anesthetists to halothane, nitrous oxide and radiation. Anesthesiology 1969; 30:363–368
2. Panni MK, Corn SB: Scavenging in the operating room. Curr Opin Anaesthesiol 2003; 16: 611
3. Task Force on Trace Anesthetic Gases of the Committee on Occupational Health of Operating Room Personnel: Waste Anesthetic Gases: Information for Management in Anesthetizing Areas and the Postanesthesia Care Unit (PACU). Park Ridge, IL, American Society of Anesthesiologists, 1999
4. American Society of Anesthesiologists Ad Hoc Committee on the Effect of Trace Anesthetics on the Health of Operating Room Personnel: Occupational disease among operating room personnel: A national study. Anesthesiology 1977; 41: 321
5. Buring JE, Hennekens CH, Mayrent SL , Rosner B, Greenberg ER, Colton T: Health experiences of operating room personnel. Anesthesiology 1985; 62: 325–330
6. Rowland AS, Baird DD, Weinberg CR, et al: Reduced fertility among women employed as dental assistants exposed to high levels of nitrous oxide. N Engl J Med 1992; 327: 993
7. Rowland AS, Baird DD, Shore DL, et al: Nitrous oxide and spontaneous abortion in female dental assistants. Am J Epidemiol 1995; 141: 531
8. Boivin JF: Risk of spontaneous abortion in women occupationally exposed to anaesthetic gases: a meta-analysis. Occup Environ Med 1997; 54: 541
9. Axelsson G, Ahlborg G, Jr., Bodin L: Shift work, nitrous oxide exposure, and spontaneous abortion among Swedish midwives. Occup Environ Med 1996; 53: 374
10. Luke B, Mamelle N, Keith L, et al: The association between occupational factors and preterm birth: a United States nurses' study. Research Committee of the Association of Women's Health, Obstetric, and Neonatal Nurses. Am J Obstet Gynecol 1995; 173: 849
11. Ebi KL, Rice SA: Reproductive and developmental toxicity of anesthetics in humans, Anesthetic Toxicity. Edited by Rice SA, Fish KJ. New York, Raven Press, 1994
12. Bruce DL, Eide KA, Linde HW, et al: Causes of death among anesthesiologists: a 20-year survey. Anesthesiology 1968; 29: 565
13. Bruce DL, Eide KA, Smith NJ, et al: A prospective survey of anesthesiologist mortality, 1967–1971. Anesthesiology 1974; 41: 71–74
14. Alexander BH, Checkoway H, Nagahama SI, et al: Cause-specific mortality risks of anesthesiologists. Anesthesiology 2000; 93: 922
15. Katz JD: Do anesthesiologists die at a younger age than other physicians? Age-adjusted death rates. Anesth Analg 2004; 98: 1111
16. Byhahn C, Wilke HJ, Westpphal K: Occupational exposure to volatile anaesthetics: epidemiology and approaches to reducing the problem. CNS Drugs 2001; 15: 197
17. Wiesner G, Hoerauf K, Schroegendorfer K, et al: High-level, but not low-level, occupational exposure to inhaled anesthetics is associated with genotoxicity in the micronucleus assay. Anesth Analg 2001; 92: 118

18. Bruce DL, Bach MJ: Effects of trace anaesthetic gases on behavioural performance of volunteers. Br J Anaesth 1976; 48: 871
19. Bruce DL, Stanley TH: Research replication may be subject specific. Anesth Analg 1983; 62: 617
20. National Institute for Occupational Safety and Health (NIOSH): Criteria for a Recommended Standard . . . Occupational Exposure to Waste Anesthetic Gases and Vapors. Cincinnati, Ohio, Department of Health, Education, and Welfare (NIOSH), Publication No. 77-140
21. NIOSH Alert: Request for assistance in controlling exposures to nitrous oxide during anesthetic administration. Cincinnati, Ohio, DHHS (NIOSH) Publication No. 94-100, 1994
22. American Institute of Architects Academy of Architecture for Health, U.S. Department of Health and Human Services: 1996–1997 Guidelines for design and construction of hospital and health care facilities. Washington, DC, The American Institute of Architects Press, 1996
23. Sessler DI, Badgwell JM: Exposure of postoperative nurses to exhaled anesthetic gases. Anesth Analg 1998; 87: 1083
24. McGregor DG, Senjem DH, Mazze RI: Trace nitrous oxide levels in the postanesthesia care unit. Anesth Analg 1999; 89: 472
25. Sadoh DR, Sharief MK, Howard RS: Occupational exposure to methyl methacrylate monomer induces generalised neuropathy in a dental technician. Br Dent J 1999; 186: 380
26. Vellore AD, Drought VJ, Sherwood-Jones D, et al: Occupational asthma and allergy to sevoflurane and isoflurane in anaesthetic staff. Allergy 2006; 61: 1485
27. Klatskin G, Kimberg DV: Recurrent hepatitis attributable to halothane sensitization in an anesthetist. N Engl J Med 1969; 280: 515
28. Njoku DB, Greenberg RS, Bourdi M, et al: Autoantibodies associated with volatile anesthetic hepatitis found in the sera of a large cohort of pediatric anesthesiologists. Anesth Analg 2002; 94: 243
29. Brown RH, Schauble JF, Hamilton RG: Prevalence of latex allergy among anesthesiologists: identification of sensitized but asymptomatic individuals. Anesthesiology 1998; 89: 292
30. Konrad C, Fieber T, Gerber H, et al: The prevalence of latex sensitivity among anesthesiology staff. Anesth Analg 1997; 84: 629
31. Task Force on Latex Sensitivity of the Committee on Occupational Health of Operating Room Personnel: Natural Rubber Latex Allergy: Considerations for Anesthesiologists. Park Ridge, Illinois, American Society of Anesthesiologists, 2005 http://www.asahq.org/publicationsAndServices/latexallergy.pdf
32. McGowan C, Heaton B, Stephenson RN: Occupational x-ray exposure of anaesthetists. Br J Anaesth 1996; 76: 868
33. Katz JD: Radiation exposure to anesthesia personnel: the impact of an electrophysiology laboratory. Anesth Analg 2005; 101: 1725
34. Einstein AJ, Henzlova MJ, Rajagopalan S: Estimating risk of cancer associated with radiation exposure from 64-slice computed tomography coronary angiography. JAMA 2007; 298: 317
35. NIOSH recommendations for occupational safety and health standards 1988. MMWR Morb Mortal Wkly Rep 1988; 37 Suppl 7: 1
36. Murthy VS, Malhotra SK, Bala I, et al: Detrimental effects of noise on anaesthetists. Can J Anaesth 1995; 42: 608
37. Kracht JM, Busch-Vishniac IJ, West JE: Noise in the operating rooms of Johns Hopkins Hospital. J Acoust Soc Am 2007; 121: 2673
38. Consensus conference. Noise and hearing loss. JAMA 1990; 263: 3185
39. Nilsson U, Unosson M, Rawal N: Stress reduction and analgesia in patients exposed to calming music postoperatively: a randomized controlled trial. Eur J Anaesthesiol 2005; 22: 96
40. Koch ME, Kain ZN, Ayoub C, et al: The sedative and analgesic sparing effect of music. Anesthesiology 1998; 89: 300
41. Allen K, Blascovich J: Effects of music on cardiovascular reactivity among surgeons. JAMA 1994; 272: 882
42. Gaba DM: Human error in anesthetic mishaps. Int Anesthesiol Clin 1989; 27: 137
43. Weinger MB, Herndon OW, Gaba DM: The effect of electronic record keeping and transesophageal echocardiography on task distribution, workload, and vigilance during cardiac anesthesia. Anesthesiology 1997; 87: 144
44. Paget NS, Lambert TF, Sridhar K: Factors affecting an anaesthetist's work: some findings on vigilance and performance. Anaesth Intensive Care 1981; 9: 359
45. Davies JM: Team communication in the operating room. Acta Anaesthesiol Scand 2005; 49: 898–901
46. Awad SS, Fagan SP, Bellows C, et al: Bridging the communication gap in the operating room with medical team training. Am J Surg 2005; 190: 770
47. Joint Commission on Accreditation of Healthcare Organizations: Sentinel Event Alert. Oak Brooks, Ill. Joint Commission on Accreditation of Healthcare Organizations 2004
48. Jackson SH: The role of stress in anaesthetists' health and well- being. Acta Anaesthesiologica Scandinavica 1999; 43: 583
49. Breen CM, Abernethy AP, Abbott KH, et al: Conflict associated with decisions to limit life-sustaining treatment in intensive care units. J Gen Intern Med 2001; 16: 283
50. Katz JD: Conflict and its resolution in the operating room. J Clin Anesth 2007; 19: 152
51. Helmreich RL, Merritt AC, Wilhelm JA: The evolution of Crew Resource Management training in commercial aviation. Int J Aviat Psychol 1999; 9: 19

52. Schneiderman LJ, Gilmer T, Teetzel HD: Impact of ethics consultations in the intensive care setting: a randomized, controlled trial. Crit Care Med 2000; 28: 3920

53. Gaba DM, Howard SK, Jump B: Production pressure in the work environment: California Anesthesiologists' attitudes and experiences. Anesthesiology 1994; 81: 488

54. Howard SK, Gaba DM, Smith BE, et al: Simulation study of rested versus sleep-deprived anesthesiologists. Anesthesiology 2003; 98: 1345

55. Gaba DM, Howard SK, Fish KJ, et al: Simulation-based training in anesthesia crisis resource management (ARCM): A decade of experience. Simul Gaming 2001; 32: 175

56. Gravenstein JS, Cooper JB, Orkin FK: Work and rest cycles in anesthesia practice. Anesthesiology 1990; 72: 737

57. Howard SK, Gaba DM, Rosekind MR, et al: The risks and implications of excessive daytime sleepiness in resident physicians. Acad Med 2002; 77: 1019

58. Katz J: Issues of concern for the aging anesthesiologist. Anesth Analg 2001; 92: 1487

59. Howard SK, Rosekind MR, Katz JD, et al: Fatigue in anesthesia: implications and strategies for patient and provider safety. Anesthesiology 2002; 97: 1281

60. Dawson D, Reid K: Fatigue, alcohol and performance impairment. Nature 1997; 388: 235

61. Weinger MB, Ancoli-Israel S: Sleep deprivation and clinical performance. JAMA 2002; 287: 955

62. Barger LK, Ayas NT, Cade BE, et al: Impact of extended-duration shifts on medical errors, adverse events, and attentional failures. PLoS Med 2006; 3: e487

63. Veasey S, Rosen R, Barzansky B, et al: Sleep loss and fatigue in residency training: a reappraisal. JAMA 2002; 288: 1116

64. Fletcher KE, Underwood W, Davis SQ, et al: Effects of work hour reduction on residents' lives: a systematic review. JAMA 2005; 294: 1088

65. Volpp KG, Rosen AK, Rosenbaum PR, et al: Mortality among patients in VA hospitals in the first 2 years following ACGME resident duty hour reform. JAMA 2007; 298: 984

66. Salim A, Teixeira PG, Chan L, et al: Impact of the 80-hour workweek on patient care at a level I trauma center. Arch Surg 2007; 142: 708

67. Czeisler CA, Walsh JK, Roth T, et al: Modafinil for excessive sleepiness associated with shift-work sleep disorder. N Engl J Med 2005; 353: 476

68. Katz JD: Hand washing and hand disinfection: more than your mother taught you. Anesthesiol Clin North America 2004; 22: 457

69. Recommended adult immunization schedule: United States, October 2007–September 2008. Ann Intern Med 2007; 147: 725

70. Updated U.S. Public Health Service Guidelines for the Management of Occupational Exposures to HBV, HCV, and HIV and Recommendations for Postexposure Prophylaxis. MMWR Recomm Rep 2001; 50: 1

71. Bolyard EA, Tablan OC, Williams WW, et al: Guideline for infection control in healthcare personnel, 1998. Hospital Infection Control Practices Advisory Committee. Infect Control Hosp Epidemiol 1998; 19: 407

72. Fiore AE, Shay DK, Haber P, et al: Prevention and control of influenza. Recommendations of the Advisory Committee on Immunization Practices (ACIP), 2007. MMWR Recomm Rep 2007; 56: 1

73. Abdel-Ghafar AN, Chotpitayasunondh T, Gao Z, et al: Update on avian influenza A (H5N1) virus infection in humans. N Engl J Med 2008; 358: 261

74. Tablan OC, Anderson LJ, Besser R, et al: Guidelines for preventing healthcare—associated pneumonia, 2003: recommendations of CDC and the Healthcare Infection Control Practices Advisory Committee. MMWR Recomm Rep 2004; 53: 1

75. Falsey AR, Hennessey PA, Formica MA, et al: Respiratory syncytial virus infection in elderly and high-risk adults. N Engl J Med 2005; 352: 1749

76. Siegel JD, Rhinehart E, Jackson M, et al: 2007 Guideline for isolation precautions: Preventing transmission of infectious agents in health care settings. Am J Infect Control 2007; 35: S65

77. Marin M, Guris D, Chaves SS, et al: Prevention of varicella: recommendations of the Advisory Committee on Immunization Practices (ACIP). MMWR Recomm Rep 2007; 56: 1

78. Watson JC, Hadler SC, Dykewicz CA, et al: Measles, mumps, and rubella—vaccine use and strategies for elimination of measles, rubella, and congenital rubella syndrome and control of mumps: recommendations of the Advisory Committee on Immunization Practices (ACIP). MMWR Recomm Rep 1998; 47: 1

79. Centers for Disease Control and Prevention: In the absence of SARS-CoV transmission worldwide: Guidance for surveillance, clinical and laboratory evaluation, and reporting version. http://www.cdc.gov/ncidod/sars/guidance/index.htm

80. Centers for Disease Control and Prevention: Protection of hepatitis A through active or passive immunization: Recommendations of the Immunization Practices Advisory Committee (ACIP). MMWR 55(no. RR-7):1, 2006

81. Berry AJ, Greene ES: The risk of needlestick injuries and needlestick-transmitted diseases in the practice of anesthesiology. Anesthesiology 1992; 77: 1007

82. Department of Labor, Occupational Safety and Health Administration: Occupational exposure to bloodborne pathogens: Needle-sticks and other sharp injuries: Final rule (29 CFR Part 1910.1030). Federal Register 66:5318, 2001

83. Scott JD, Gretch DR: Molecular diagnostics of hepatitis C virus infection: a systematic review. JAMA 2007; 297: 724

84. Hoofnagle JH, Seeff LB: Peginterferon and ribavirin for chronic hepatitis C. N Engl J Med 2006; 355: 2444

85. Centers for Disease Control and Prevention: HIV/AIDS surveillance report, 2005. Vol. 17. Rev ed. Atlanta: U.S. Department of Health and Human Services, Centers for Disease Control and Prevention, 2007

86. Bell DM: Occupational risk of human immunodeficiency virus infection in healthcare workers: an overview. Am J Med 1997; 102: 9

87. Ippolito G, Puro V, De Carli G: The risk of occupational human immunodeficiency virus infection in health care workers. Italian Multicenter Study. The Italian Study Group on Occupational Risk of HIV infection. Arch Intern Med 1993; 153: 1451

88. Cardo DM, Culver DH, Ciesielski CA, et al: A case-control study of HIV seroconversion in health care workers after percutaneous exposure. Centers for Disease Control and Prevention Needlestick Surveillance Group. N Engl J Med 1997; 337: 1485

89. Greene ES, Berry AJ, Jagger J, et al: Multicenter study of contaminated percutaneous injuries in anesthesia personnel. Anesthesiology 1998; 89: 1362

90. Task Force on Infection Control of the Committee on Occupational Health of Operating Room Personnel: Recommendations for Infection Control for the Practice of Anesthesiology, 2nd ed. Park Ridge, Illinois, American Society of Anesthesiologists, 1998

91. Greene ES, Berry AJ, Arnold WP, 3rd, et al: Percutaneous injuries in anesthesia personnel. Anesth Analg 1996; 83: 273

92. Panlilio AL, Cardo DM, Grohskopf LA, et al: Updated U.S. Public Health Service guidelines for the management of occupational exposures to HIV and recommendations for postexposure prophylaxis. MMWR Recomm Rep 2005; 54: 1

93. Johnson RT, Gibbs CJ, Jr.: Creutzfeldt-Jakob disease and related transmissible spongiform encephalopathies. N Engl J Med 1998; 339: 1994

94. Jensen PA, Lambert LA, Iademarco MF, et al: Guidelines for preventing the transmission of Mycobacterium tuberculosis in health-care settings, 2005. MMWR Recomm Rep 2005; 54: 1

95. Menzies D, Fanning A, Yuan L, et al: Tuberculosis among health care workers. N Engl J Med 1995; 332: 92

96. Jereb JA, Klevens RM, Privett TD, et al: Tuberculosis in health care workers at a hospital with an outbreak of multidrug-resistant Mycobacterium tuberculosis. Arch Intern Med 1995; 155: 854

97. Blumberg HM, Burman WJ, Chaisson RE, et al: American Thoracic Society/Centers for Disease Control and Prevention/Infectious Diseases Society of America: treatment of tuberculosis. Am J Respir Crit Care Med 2003; 167: 603

98. United States Department of Health and Human Services: 42 CRF Part 84: Respiratory protective devices; final rule and notice. Federal Register 60:30336, 1995

99. Control of Smoke from Laser/Electric Surgical Procedures, DHHS (NIOSH) Publication No. 96-128, National Institute for Occupational Safety and Health, Cincinnati, Ohio September 1996

100. Matchette LS, Faaland RW, Royston DD, et al: In vitro production of viable bacteriophage in carbon dioxide and argon laser plumes. Lasers Surg Med 1991; 11: 380

101. Hallmo P, Naess O: Laryngeal papillomatosis with human papillomavirus DNA contracted by a laser surgeon. Eur Arch Otorhinolaryngol 1991; 248: 425

102. Sehulster L, Chinn RY: Guidelines for environmental infection control in health-care facilities. Recommendations of CDC and the Healthcare Infection Control Practices Advisory Committee (HICPAC). MMWR Recomm Rep 2003; 52: 1

103. Nyssen AS, Hansez I, Baele P, et al: Occupational stress and burnout in anaesthesia. Br J Anaesth 2003; 90: 333

104. Lindfors PM, Nurmi KE, Meretoja OA, et al: On-call stress among Finnish anaesthetists. Anaesthesia 2006; 61: 856

105. Seyle H: The stress of life. New York, NY, McGraw-Hill Book Co., 1984

106. Aboa-Eboule C, Brisson C, Maunsell E, et al: Job strain and risk of acute recurrent coronary heart disease events. JAMA 2007; 298: 1652

107. Kain ZN, Chan KM, Katz JD, et al: Anesthesiologists and acute perioperative stress: a cohort study. Anesth Analg 2002; 95: 177

108. Sexton JB, Thomas EJ, Helmreich RL: Error, stress, and teamwork in medicine and aviation: cross sectional surveys. BMJ 2000; 320: 745

109. Vaillant GE, Brighton JR, McArthur C: Physicians' use of mood-altering drugs. A 20-year follow-up report. N Engl J Med 1970; 282: 365

110. McDonald JS, Lingam RP, Gupta B, et al: Psychologic testing as an aid to selection of residents in anesthesiology. Anesth Analg 1994; 78: 542

111. Angres DH, Talbott GD, Bettinardi-Angres K: Anesthesiologist's Return to Practice, in Healing the Healer: The Addicted Physician. Madison, CT, Psychosocial Press, 1998

112. Hughes PH, Brandenburg N, Baldwin DC, Jr., et al: Prevalence of substance use among US physicians. JAMA 1992; 267: 2333

113. Prescription Drugs: Abuse and Addiction. Bethesda, M.D., National Institute on Drug Abuse, 2001

114. Silverstein JH, Silva DA, Iberti TJ: Opioid addiction in anesthesiology. Anesthesiology 1993; 79: 354

115. Talbott GD, Gallegos KV, Wilson PO, et al: The Medical Association of Georgia's Impaired Physicians Program. Review of the first 1000 physicians: analysis of specialty. JAMA 1987; 257: 2927

116. Lutsky I, Hopwood M, Abram SE, et al: Use of psychoactive substances in three medical specialties: anaesthesia, medicine and surgery. Can J Anaesth 1994; 41: 561
117. Hughes PH, Storr CL, Brandenburg NA, et al: Physician substance use by medical specialty. J Addict Dis 1999; 18: 23
118. Booth JV, Grossman D, Moore J, et al: Substance abuse among physicians: a survey of academic anesthesiology programs. Anesth Analg 2002; 95: 1024
119. Cami J, Farre M: Drug addiction. N Engl J Med 2003; 349: 975
120. Wischmeyer PE, Johnson BR, Wilson JE, et al: A survey of propofol abuse in academic anesthesia programs. Anesth Analg 2007; 105: 1066
121. Epstein RH, Gratch DM, Grunwald Z: Development of a scheduled drug diversion surveillance system based on an analysis of atypical drug transactions. Anesth Analg 2007; 105: 1053
122. Moore RD, Mead L, Pearson TA: Youthful precursors of alcohol abuse in physicians. Am J Med 1990; 88: 332
123. Menk EJ, Baumgarten RK, Kingsley CP, et al: Success of reentry into anesthesiology training programs by residents with a history of substance abuse. JAMA 1990; 263: 3060
124. Collins GB, McAllister MS, Jensen M, et al: Chemical dependency treatment outcomes of residents in anesthesiology: results of a survey. Anesth Analg 2005; 101: 1457
125. Scott M, Fisher KS: The evolving legal context for drug testing programs. Anesthesiology 1990; 73: 1022
126. Paris RT, Canavan DI: Physician substance abuse impairment: anesthesiologists vs. other specialties. J Addict Dis 1999; 18: 1
127. Domino KB, Hornbein TF, Polissar NL, et al: Risk factors for relapse in health care professionals with substance use disorders. JAMA 2005; 293: 1453
128. Task Force on Chemical Dependence of the Committee on Occupational Health of Operating Room Personnel: Chemical Dependence in Anesthesiologists: What You Need to Know When You Need to Know It. Park Ridge, Ill., American Society of Anesthesiologists, 1998
129. Clark DC, Salazar-Grueso E, Grabler P, et al: Predictors of depression during the first 6 months of internship. Am J Psychiatry 1984; 141: 1095
130. Bissell L, Jones RW: The alcoholic physician: a survey. Am J Psychiatry 1976; 133: 1142
131. Clark DC, Eckenfels EJ, Daugherty SR, et al: Alcohol-use patterns through medical school. A longitudinal study of one class. JAMA 1987; 257: 2921
132. Atkinson RS: The problem of the unsafe anaesthetist. British Journal of Anaesthesia 1994; 73: 29
133. Canavan DI, Baxter LE, Sr.: The twentieth anniversary of the Physicians' Health Program of the Medical Society of New Jersey. N J Med 2003; 100: 27
134. Brody H: The aging brain. Acta Neurol. Scand. Supplement 1992; 137: 40
135. Sawaki L, Yaseen Z, Kopylev L, et al: Age-dependent changes in the ability to encode a novel elementary motor memory. Ann Neurol 2003; 53: 521
136. Eva KW: The aging physician: changes in cognitive processing and their impact on medical practice. Acad Med 2002; 77: S1
137. Eyraud MY, Borowsky MS: Age and pilot performance. Aviation, Space, and Environmental Medicine 1985; 56: 553
138. Travis KW, Mihevc NT, Orkin FK, et al: Age and anesthetic practice: a regional perspective. Journal of Clinical Anesthesia 1999; 11: 175
139. Dimick JB, Birkmeyer JD, Upchurch GR, Jr.: Measuring surgical quality: what's the role of provider volume? World J Surg 2005; 29: 1217
140. See WA, Cooper CS, Fisher RJ: Predictors of laparoscopic complications after formal training in laparoscopic surgery. JAMA 1993; 270: 2689
141. Weinger MB: Experience [not equal to] expertise: can simulation be used to tell the difference? Anesthesiology 2007;107:691–694
142. McNamee R, Keen RI, Corkill CM: Morbidity and early retirement among anaesthetists and other specialists. Anaesthesia 1987; 42: 133
143. Lowes R: The graceful goodbye: how groups phase out their older doctors. Medical Economics 1998: 72
144. Svardsudd K, Wedel H, Gordh T: Mortality rates among Swedish physicians: a population-based nationwide study with special reference to anesthesiologists. Acta Anaesthesiol Scand 2002; 46: 1187
145. Mostafa MS, Freeman RA: The specialty of physicians in relation to longevity and mortality, 1978–1979. Ala Med 1985; 54: 13
146. Carpenter LM, Swerdlow AJ, Fear NT: Mortality of doctors in different specialties: findings from a cohort of 20,000 NHS hospital consultants. Occup Environ Med 1997; 54: 388
147. Lew EA: Mortality experiences among anesthesiologists, 1954–1976. Anesthesiology 1979; 51: 195
148. Katz JD, Slade MD: Anesthesiologists are living longer: mortality experience 1992 to 2001. J Clin Anesth 2006; 18: 405
149. Center C, Davis M, Detre T, et al: Confronting depression and suicide in physicians: a consensus statement. JAMA 2003; 289: 3161
150. North CS, Ryall JE: Psychiatric illness in female physicians. Are high rates of depression an occupational hazard? Postgrad Med 1997; 101: 233
151. Birmingham PK, Ward RJ: A high-risk suicide group: the anesthesiologist involved in litigation. Am J Psychiatry 1985; 142: 1225
152. Boxer PA, Burnett C, Swanson N: Suicide and occupation: a review of the literature. J Occup Environ Med 1995; 37: 442
153. Hammen C: Stress and depression. Annu Rev Clin Psychol 2005; 1: 293
154. Reeve PE: Personality characteristics of a sample of anaesthetists. Anaesthesia 1980; 35: 559
155. Crawshaw R, Bruce JA, Eraker PL, et al: An epidemic of suicide among physicians on probation. JAMA 1980; 243: 1915

CHAPTER 4 ■ ANESTHETIC RISK, QUALITY IMPROVEMENT AND LIABILITY

KAREN L. POSNER AND KAREN B. DOMINO

KEY POINTS

1 Anesthetic mortality has decreased, but accidental deaths and disabling complications still occur.

2 Risk management programs are broadly oriented toward reducing the liability exposure of the organization. Risk management programs complement quality improvement programs in minimizing liability exposure while maximizing quality of patient care.

3 Quality improvement programs are generally guided by the requirements of the Joint Commission that accredits healthcare organizations. Quality improvement programs focus on improving the structure, process, and outcome of care.

4 Continuous quality improvement (CQI) is a systems approach to identifying and improving quality of care.

5 Medical malpractice refers to the legal concept of professional negligence. The patient-plaintiff must prove that the anesthesiologist owed the patient a duty, failed to fulfill this duty, that the anesthesiologist's actions caused an injury, and that the injury resulted from a breach in the standard of anesthesia care.

6 The most common lawsuits against anesthesiologists (excluding dental injuries) are for death, brain damage, nerve damage, and airway injury.

In anesthesia, as in other areas of life, everything does not always go as planned. Undesirable outcomes occur regardless of the quality of care provided. An anesthesia risk management program can work in conjunction with a program for quality improvement to minimize the liability risk of practice, while assuring the highest quality of care for patients. Payers such as Medicare are increasingly depending on accreditation through bodies such as the Joint Commission to ensure that mechanisms are in place to deliver quality and safe care to all patients. In addition, there has been a move toward performance measurement linked to reimbursement. The legal aspects of American medical practice have also become increasingly important as the public has turned to the courts for economic redress when their expectations of medical treatment are not met.

This chapter discusses anesthetic mortality and morbidity, risk management, continuous quality improvement, performance measurement, and medical liability. The chapter provides background for the practitioner concerning the role of risk management activity in minimizing and managing liability exposure. Also described is the medical legal system, the most frequent causes of lawsuits for anesthesiologists, and appropriate actions for physicians to take in the event of a malpractice suit.

ANESTHESIA RISK

Mortality and Major Morbidity Related to Anesthesia

Estimates of anesthesia-related morbidity and mortality are difficult to quantify. Not only are there difficulties obtaining data on complications, but different methods yield different estimates of anesthesia risk. Studies differ in their definitions of complications, length of follow-up, and especially in approaches to evaluation of the contribution of anesthesia care to patient outcomes. A comprehensive review of anesthesia complications is beyond the scope of this chapter. A sampling of studies of anesthesia mortality and morbidity will be presented to provide historical perspective plus a limited overview of relatively recent findings.

Early studies estimated the anesthesia-related mortality rate as 1 per 1,560 anesthetics.[1] More recent studies using data from the 1990s estimate the anesthesia-related death rate in the United States to be <1 per 10,000 anesthetics.[2–5] Some examples of modern estimates of anesthesia-related death from throughout the world are provided in Table 4-1.[2–13] Differences in estimates may be influenced by different reporting

TABLE 4-1

ESTIMATES OF ANESTHESIA-RELATED DEATH

REFERENCE	COUNTRY	TIME	DATA SOURCES/METHODS	RATE OF DEATH
Flick et al[4]	USA	1988–2005	Perioperative cardiac arrest in pediatric patients at a tertiary referral hospital (n = 92,881 anesthetics)	Anesthesia-attributed deaths = 0.22/10,000 anesthetics
Biboulet et al[8]	France	1989–1995	ASA 1–4 patients undergoing anesthesia (n = 101,769 anesthetics); cardiac arrest within 12 hr postanesthesia (n = 24)	Anesthesia-related death = 0.6/10,000 anesthetics
Newland et al[2]	USA	1989–1999	Cardiac arrests within 24 hr of surgery (n = 72,959 anesthetics) in a teaching hospital	Death related to anesthesia-attributable perioperative cardiac arrest = 0.55/10,000 anesthetics
Eagle and Davis[6]	Western Australia	1990–1995	Deaths within 48 hr or deaths in which anesthesia was considered a contributing factor (n = 500 deaths)	Anesthesia-related death = 1/40,000 anesthetics
Lagasse[3]	USA	(a) 1992–1994	(a) Suburban teaching hospital (n = 115 deaths; n = 37,924 anesthetics)	Anesthesia-related death = (a) 0.79/10,000 anesthetics
		(b) 1995–1999	(b) Urban teaching hospital (n = 232 deaths; n = 146,548 anesthetics)	(b) 0.75/10,000 anesthetics
Davis[7]	Australia	1994–1996	Deaths reported to the committee (n = 8,500,000 anesthetics)	Anesthesia-related death = 0.16/10,000 anesthetics
Morray et al[5]	USA	1994–1997	Pediatric patients from 63 hospitals (n = 1,089,200 anesthetics)	Anesthesia-related death = 0.36/10,000 anesthetics
Kawashima et al[10]	Japan	1994–1998	Questionnaires to training hospitals (n = 2,363,038 anesthetics)	Death totally attributable to anesthesia = 0.21/10,000 anesthetics
Arbous et al[9]	Holland	1995–1997	All deaths within 24 hr or patients who remained unintentionally comatose 24 hr postanesthesia (n = 811 in 869,483 anesthetics)—64 hospitals	Anesthesia-related death = 1.4/10,000 anesthetics
Lienhart et al[13]	France	1999	Nationwide survey of anesthesia-related deaths	Death totally related to anesthesia = 0.069/10,000 Death partially related to anesthesia = 0.47/10,000
Kawashima et al[11]	Japan	1999	Questionnaires to training hospitals (n = 793,840 anesthetics)	Death totally attributable to anesthesia = 0.13/10,000 anesthetics
Irita et al[12]	Japan	1999–2002	Deaths as a result of life-threatening events in the operating room (n = 3,855,384 anesthetics) in training hospitals	Death totally attributable to anesthetic management = 0.1/10,000 anesthetics

methods, definitions, anesthesia practices, patient population, as well as actual differences in underlying complication rates. Nevertheless, it is generally accepted that anesthesia safety has improved over the past 50 years.

Other complications related to anesthesia that have received relatively recent attention include postoperative nerve injury, awareness during general anesthesia, eye injuries and visual deficits, dental injury, and postoperative cognitive dysfunction in elderly patients. Ulnar neuropathy is one of the most common nerve injuries leading to anesthesia malpractice claims in the United States.[14] The incidence of ulnar neuropathy has been estimated between 3.7 and 50 per 10,000 patients (Table 4-2).[15–17] Lower extremity neuropathy following

surgery in the lithotomy position was observed in 2.7 per 10,000 patients (Table 4-2).[18] Permanent neurologic injury following neuraxial anesthesia was estimated at 0 to 4.2 per 10,000 spinal anesthetics and 0 to 7.6 per 10,000 epidural anesthetics.[19] Awareness during general anesthesia has been estimated to occur in 1 to 2 per 1,000 patients in tertiary care settings,[20,21] but may occur with lower frequency in ambulatory patients.[22]

Eye injuries are a risk of anesthesia, including corneal abrasions as well as more rare complications such as blindness from ischemic optic neuropathy or central retinal artery occlusion (Table 4-2).[23–24] Eye injury after nonocular surgery was observed in 5.6 per 10,000 patients.[23] New-onset blurred

TABLE 4-2

RATES OF SELECTED ANESTHESIA COMPLICATIONS

■ COMPLICATION	■ REFERENCE	■ COUNTRY	■ TIME	■ SPECIFIC COMPLICATION	■ RESULTS
Nerve injury	Warner et al[18]	USA	1957–1991	Lower extremity motor neuropathy following surgery in lithotomy position	1/3,608 procedures
	Warner et al[16]	USA	1957–1991	Persistent ulnar neuropathy following diagnostic or noncardiac procedures with anesthesia	1/2,729 patients
	Alvine and Schurrer[15]	USA	1980–1981	Ulnar neuropathy after general anesthesia	0.26%
	Brull et al[19]	Various	1987–1999	Radiculopathy or peripheral neuropathy after spinal anesthesia	3.78/10,000 anesthetics
				Radiculopathy or peripheral neuropathy after epidural anesthesia	2.19/10,000 anesthetics
				Permanent neurologic injury after spinal anesthesia	0–4.2/10,000 anesthetics
				Permanent neurologic injury after epidural anesthetic	0–7.6/10,000 anesthetics
			Varies	Transient neurologic deficit after interscalene block	2.84/10,000 anesthetics
	Warner et al[17]	USA	1995	Ulnar neuropathy in adults following noncardiac surgery	0.5%
Awareness and recall	Sandin et al[20]	Sweden	1997–1998	Awareness and recall associated with general anesthesia	18/11,785 procedures
	Sebel et al[21]	USA	2001–2002	Awareness with recall in patients ≥ 18 yr old in seven academic medical centers	0.13%
	Pollard et al[22]	USA	2002–2004	Awareness and recall in a regional medical center	1/14,560 patients
Eye injuries and visual changes	Warner et al[23]	USA	1986–1998	New-onset visual loss or visual changes lasting >30 days after noncardiac surgery	1/125,234 patients
	Warner et al[24]	USA	1999	New-onset blurred vision lasting ≥ 3 days	4.2%
Dental injury	Warner et al[25]	USA	1987–1997	Dental injuries within 7 days of anesthesia that required intervention	1/4,537 patients

vision has been observed in 4.2% of patients (Table 4-2).[24] New-onset visual loss or changes lasting more than 30 days after noncardiac surgery were observed in 1 per 125,234 patients.[24]

Damage to teeth or dentures is perhaps the most common injury leading to anesthesia malpractice claims. Dental injury complaints are usually resolved by a hospital risk management department. Dental injuries requiring intervention were observed in 1 per 4,537 patients.[25]

Cognitive dysfunction is observed in many adult patients after major surgery, but only the elderly are at significant risk for long-term cognitive problems.[26] The cause for postoperative cognitive dysfunction is unknown.

Risk Management

Conceptual Introduction

Risk management and quality improvement programs work hand in hand in minimizing liability exposure while maximizing quality of patient care. Although the functions of these programs vary from one institution to another, they overlap in their focus on patient safety. They can generally be distinguished by their basic difference in orientation. A hospital risk management program is broadly oriented toward reducing the liability exposure of the organization. This includes not only professional liability (and therefore patient safety) but also contracts, employee safety, public safety, and any other liability exposure of the institution. Quality improvement programs have as their main goal the continuous maintenance and improvement of the quality of patient care. These programs may be broader in their patient safety focus than strictly risk management. Quality improvement (sometimes called *patient safety*) departments are responsible for providing the resources to provide safe, patient-centered, timely, efficient, effective, and equitable patient care.[27]

Risk Management in Anesthesia

Those aspects of risk management that are most directly relevant to the liability exposure of the anesthesiologist include prevention of patient injury, adherence to standards of care, documentation, and patient relations.

The key factors in the prevention of patient injury are vigilance, up-to-date knowledge, and adequate monitoring.[28] Physiologic monitoring of cardiopulmonary function, combined with monitoring of equipment function, might be expected to reduce anesthetic injury to a minimum. This was the rationale for the adoption by the American Society of Anesthesiologists (ASA) of *Standards for Basic Anesthetic Monitoring.*[a]

The ASA Web site should be reviewed yearly for any changes in these standards. It would also be reasonable to review the *Guidelines and Statements* published on the ASA Web site. It should be noted that, although membership in the ASA is not required for the practice of anesthesiology, expert witnesses will, with virtual certainty, hold any practitioner to the ASA standards. It is also possible that, as a risk management strategy, a professional liability insurer or hospital may hold an individual anesthesiologist to standards higher than those promulgated by the ASA.

Another risk management tool is the use of checklists prior to each case, or at least daily, in an attempt to reduce equipment-related mishaps.[29–31] A regular schedule of equipment maintenance should be established as well as procedures to follow whenever equipment malfunction is suspected of contributing to patient injury. The ASA Web site has recommendations for preanesthesia checkout procedures[b] as well as guidelines for determining anesthesia machine obsolescence.[c] If equipment malfunction is suspected to have contributed to a complication, the device should be impounded and examined concurrently by the representatives of the hospital, the anesthesiologist, and the manufacturer.

Although it may seem obvious, qualified anesthesia personnel should be in continuous attendance during the conduct of all anesthetics. The only exceptions should be those that lay people (i.e., judge and jury) can understand, such as radiation hazards or an unexpected life-threatening emergency elsewhere. Even then, provisions should be made for monitoring the patient adequately. Adequate supervision of nurse anesthetists and residents is also important, as is good communication with surgeons when adverse anesthetic outcomes occur.

Informed Consent

Informed consent regarding anesthesia should be documented with a general surgical consent, which should include a statement to the effect that, "I understand that all anesthetics involve risks of complications, serious injury, or, rarely, death from both known and unknown causes." In addition, there should be a note in the patient's record that the risks of anesthesia and alternatives were discussed, and that the patient accepted the proposed anesthetic plan. A brief documentation in the record that the common complications of the proposed technique were discussed is helpful. In some institutions, a separate written anesthesia consent form may be used, which may include more detail about risks. If it is necessary to change the agreed-on anesthesia plan significantly after the patient is premedicated or anesthetized, the reasons for the change should be documented in the record.

Record Keeping

Good records can form a strong defense if they are adequate; however, records can be disastrous if inadequate. The anesthesia record itself should be as accurate, complete, and as neat as possible. The use of automated anesthesia records may be helpful in the defense of malpractice cases,[32] but they may also serve as damaging evidence for the lack of vigilance prior to an adverse event. In addition to documenting vital signs at least every 5 minutes, special attention should be paid to ensure that the patient's ASA classification, the monitors used, fluids administered, and doses and times of all administered drugs are accurately charted. Because the principal causes of hypoxic brain damage and death during anesthesia are related to ventilation and/or oxygenation, all respiratory variables that are monitored should be documented accurately. It is important to note when there is a change of anesthesia personnel during the conduct of a case. Sloppy, inaccurate anesthesia records, with gaps during critical events, can be extremely damaging to the defense when enlarged and placed before a jury.

What To Do After an Adverse Outcome

If a critical incident occurs during the conduct of an anesthetic, the anesthesiologist should document, in narrative form, what happened, which drugs were used, the time sequence, and who was present. This should be documented in the patient's progress notes, as a catastrophic intra-anesthetic event cannot be summarized adequately in a small amount of space on the usual anesthesia record. The critical incident note should be written as soon as possible. The report should be as consistent as possible with concurrent records, such as the anesthesia, operating room, recovery room, and cardiac arrest records. If significant inconsistencies exist, they should be explained. Records should never be altered after the fact. If an error is made in record keeping, a line should be drawn through the error, leaving it legible, and the correction should be initialed and timed. Litigation is a lengthy process, and a court appearance to explain the incident to a jury may be years away, when memories have faded.

If anesthetic complications occur, the anesthesiologist should be honest with both the patient and family about the cause. The providers should provide the facts about the event, express regret to the patient and family about the outcome, and give a formal apology if the unanticipated outcome is the result of an error or system failure.[33] Some states have laws mandating disclosure of serious adverse events to patients, and disclosure has been incorporated into quality reporting. Some states prohibit use of disclosure discussions as evidence in malpractice litigation. Whenever an anesthetic complication becomes apparent, appropriate consultation should be obtained quickly, and the departmental or institutional risk management group should be notified. If the complication is apt to lead to prolonged hospitalization or permanent injury, the liability insurance carrier should be notified. The patient should be followed closely while in the hospital, with telephone follow-up, if indicated, after discharge. The anesthesiologist(s), surgeon(s), consulting physicians and the institution should coordinate and be consistent in their explanations to the patient or the patient's family as to the cause of any complication.

Special Circumstances: "Do Not Attempt Resuscitation" and Jehovah's Witnesses

It is important to recognize that patients have well-established rights, and that among these is the right to refuse specific treatments. Two situations most relevant to anesthesia care are "Do Not Attempt Resuscitation" (DNAR) orders and the special circumstance of blood transfusion for Jehovah's Witnesses.

Patients with severe medical conditions may elect to forgo resuscitation attempts in the event of cardiac arrest. Such DNAR orders may be specified at hospital admission or may

---

[a]http://www.asahq.org/publicationsAndServices/sgstoc.htm
[b]http://www.asahq.org/clinical/FINALCHECKOUTDESIGNGUIDE-LINES11-27-2007.pdf
[c]http://www.asahq.org/publicationsAndServices/machineobsolescence.pdf

be in place in the form of an advance directive prior to admission. DNAR orders or advance directives may be general or specific, such as refusal of tracheal intubation or mechanical ventilation. When a patient with DNAR status presents for anesthesia care, it is important to discuss this with the patient or patient's surrogate to clarify the patient's intentions. In many hospitals, the institutional policy is to suspend the DNAR order during the immediate perioperative period since the cause for a cardiac arrest may be easily identified and treated. In other institutions, the patient may choose to suspend the DNAR order during the entire perioperative period. It should be clarified when the DNAR order should be reinstated (e.g., discharge from recovery or possibly later, when the patient has recovered from the procedure) and documented in the patient's chart. The perioperative status of DNAR orders should also be clarified with the surgeon and other providers who will be involved in the patient's perioperative care. The ASA has published *Ethical Guidelines of the Anesthesia Care of Patients with Do-Not-Resuscitate Orders.*[d]

In the case of Jehovah's Witnesses, the treatment that may be refused is the administration of blood or blood products. A central religious belief of many Jehovah's Witnesses is that the faithful will be forbidden the pleasures of the afterlife if they receive blood or blood products. Thus, for them to receive a transfusion is a mortal sin, and many Jehovah's Witnesses would actually rather die in grace than live with no possibility of salvation. Anesthesiologists must recognize and respect these beliefs, but may also be cognizant that these convictions may conflict with their own personal, religious, or ethical codes.

As a general rule, physicians are not obligated to treat all patients who apply for treatment in elective situations. It is well within the rights of a physician to decline to care for any patient who wishes to place burdensome constraints on the physician or to unacceptably limit the physician's ability to provide optimal care. When presented with the opportunity to provide elective care for a Jehovah's Witness, the physician may decline to provide any care or may limit, by mutual consent with the patient, his or her obligation to adhere to the patient's religious beliefs. If such an agreement is reached, it must be documented clearly in the medical record, and it is desirable to have the patient co-sign the note. Not all Jehovah's Witnesses have identical beliefs regarding blood transfusions or which methods of blood preservation or sequestration will be allowed. Some patients will not allow any blood that has left the body to be reinfused, yet others will accept autotransfusion if their blood remains in constant contact with the body (via tubing). Therefore, it is important to reach a clear understanding of which techniques for blood preservation are to be used and to document this plan in the record. Parents of a minor child may not legally prevent that child from receiving blood. It may be necessary to obtain a court order in this circumstance.

National Practitioner Data Bank

It is usually the obligation of the hospital risk management department to make reports and inquiries to the National Practitioner Data Bank (NPDB), a nationwide information system that theoretically allows licensing boards and hospitals a means of detecting adverse information about physicians.[34] Simply moving into another state would no longer provide safe haven for incompetent physicians.

The NPDB requires input from five sources: (1) medical malpractice payments, (2) license actions by medical boards,

(3) professional review or clinical privilege actions taken by hospitals and other health care entities (including professional societies), (4) actions taken by the Drug Enforcement Agency, and (5) Medicare/Medicaid exclusions. There has been a great deal of effort to establish a minimum malpractice payment below which no report is necessary, but to date, any payment made on behalf of a physician in response to a written complaint or claim must be reported. Settlements made by cancellation of bills or settlements made on verbal complaints are not considered a reportable payment.

Once a report has been submitted, the physician is notified and may dispute the accuracy of the report. At this time, the reporting entity may correct the form or void it. Failing that, the physician has the option of putting a brief statement in the file or appealing to the U.S. Secretary of Health and Human Services, who may also either correct or void the form. A practitioner may make a query about his or her file at any time. A physician may also add a statement to a report at any time. Such statements will be included in any reports that are sent in response to inquiries. The existence of the NPDB reporting requirements has made physicians reluctant to allow settlement of nuisance suits because it will cause their names to be added to the data bank.

QUALITY IMPROVEMENT AND PATIENT SAFETY IN ANESTHESIA

Quality is a concept that has continued to elude precise definition in medical practice. However, it is generally accepted that attention to quality will improve patient safety and satisfaction with anesthesia care. The field of quality improvement is continually evolving, as is the terminology used to describe such efforts. A more recent trend is emphasis on patient safety, the prevention of harm from medical care. At the time of this writing, patient safety initiatives are evolving and a movement toward "pay for performance" (direct linkage between care processes and outcomes and reimbursement) is on the horizon. These will be discussed in a separate section.

❸ Anesthesia quality improvement programs at the service level are generally guided by requirements of the Joint Commission that accredits hospitals and health care organizations. Quality improvement programs are basically oriented toward improvement of the structure, process, and outcome of health care delivery. An understanding of the fundamental principles of quality improvement may clarify the relationship between the continually evolving Joint Commission requirements and mandated quality improvement and other reporting initiatives.

Structure, Process, and Outcome: The Building Blocks of Quality

Although quality of care is difficult to define, it is generally accepted that it is composed of three components: structure, process, and outcome.[35] *Structure* refers to the setting in which care was provided; for example, personnel and facilities used to provide health care services and the manner in which they are organized. This includes the qualifications and licensing of personnel, ratio of practitioners to patients, standards for the facilities and equipment used to provide care, and the organizational structure within which care is delivered. The *process* of care includes the sequence and coordination of patient care activities; that is, what was actually done. Was a preanesthetic evaluation performed and documented? Was the patient continuously attended and monitored throughout the anesthetic? *Outcome* of care refers to changes in health status of the patient following the delivery of medical care. A quality

---

[d]http://www.asahq.org/publicationsAndServices/standards/09.html

improvement program focuses on measuring and improving these basic components of care.

Continuous quality improvement (CQI) takes a systems approach to identifying and improving quality of care.[36,37] The operator is just one part of a complex system. An important underlying premise is that poor results may be a result of either random or systematic error. Random errors are inherently difficult to prevent and programs focused in this direction are misguided. System errors, however, should be controllable and strategies to minimize them should be within reach. CQI is basically the process of continually evaluating anesthesia practice to identify systematic problems (opportunities for improvement) and implementing strategies to prevent their occurrence.

A CQI program may focus on undesirable outcomes as a way to identify opportunities for improvement in the structure and process of care. The focus is not on blame but rather on identification of the causes of undesirable outcomes. Instead of asking which practitioners have the highest patient mortality rates, a CQI program may focus on the relationship between the process of care and patient mortality. What proportion of deaths was related to the patient's disease process or debilitated condition? Are these patients being appropriately evaluated for anesthesia and surgery? Were there any controllable causes, such as a lack of extra help during resuscitation? The latter may lead to a modification of personnel resources (structure) or assignments (process) to be sure that adequate personnel are available at all times.

Formally, the process of CQI involves the identification of opportunities for improvement through the continual assessment of important aspects of care. It is a process that is instituted from the bottom up, by those who are actually involved in the process to be improved, rather than from the top down by administrators. Identification of opportunities for improvement may be carried out by various means, from brainstorming sessions focusing on a systematic evaluation of care activities to the careful measurement of indicators of quality (such as morbidity and mortality). In any event, once areas are identified for improvement, their current status is measured and documented. This may involve measurement of outcomes, such as delayed recovery from anesthesia or peripheral nerve injury. The process of care leading to these problems is then analyzed. If a change is identified that should lead to improvement, it is implemented. After an appropriate time, the status is then measured again to determine whether improvement actually resulted. Attention may then be directed to continuing to improve this process or turning to a different process to target for improvement.

Difficulty of Outcome Measurement in Anesthesia

Improvement in quality of care is often measured by a reduction in the rate of adverse outcomes. However, adverse outcomes are relatively rare in anesthesia, making measurement of improvement difficult. For example, if an institution lowers its mortality rate of surgery patients from 1 in 1,000 to 0.5 in 1,000, this difference may not be statistically significant. In other words, it may be impossible to know if the change in outcome resulted from changes in care, or are simply random fluctuations. Many adverse outcomes in anesthesia are sufficiently rare to render them problematic as quality improvement measures.

To complement outcome measurement, anesthesia CQI programs can focus on critical incidents, sentinel events, and human errors. Critical incidents are events that cause, or have the potential to cause, patient injury if not noticed and corrected in a timely manner. For example, a partial disconnect of the breathing circuit may be corrected before patient injury occurs, yet has the potential for causing hypoxic brain injury or death. Critical incidents are more common than adverse outcomes. Measurement of the occurrence rate of important critical incidents may serve as a proxy measure for rare outcomes in anesthesia in a CQI program designed to improve patient safety and prevent injury.

Sentinel events are single, isolated events that may indicate a systemic problem. The Joint Commission has a specific definition of sentinel events that will be discussed later. In general, a sentinel event may be a significant or alarming critical incident that did not result in patient injury, such as a syringe swap and administration of a potentially lethal dose of medication that was noted and treated promptly, avoiding catastrophe. Or a sentinel event may be an unexpected significant patient injury such as intraoperative death. In either case, a CQI program may investigate sentinel events in an attempt to uncover systemic problems in the delivery of care that can be corrected. For example, a syringe swap may be analyzed for confusing or unclear labeling of medications or unnecessary medications routinely stocked on the anesthesia cart, setting the scene for unintended mix-up. In the case of death, all aspects of the patient's hospital course from selection for surgery to anesthetic management may be analyzed to determine if similar deaths can be prevented by a change in the care delivery system.

Human error has garnered much attention since a government report that 98,000 Americans may die annually from medical errors in hospitals.[38] Human errors are inevitable yet potentially preventable by appropriate system safeguards. Errors of planning involve use of a wrong plan to achieve an aim.[39] Errors of execution are the failure of a planned action to be completed as intended.[39] Modern anesthesia equipment is designed with safeguards such as alarm systems to detect errors that could lead to patient injury. Other anesthesia care processes are also amenable to human factors design principles, such as color coding of drug labels. A quality improvement program may identify human errors and institute safety systems to aid in error prevention.

Joint Commission Requirements for Quality Improvement

Joint Commission requirements for quality improvement activities are updated on an annual basis. In general, a hospital must adopt a method for systematically assessing and improving important functions and processes of care and their outcomes in a cyclical fashion. The general outline for this CQI cycle is the design of a process or function, measurement of performance, assessment of performance measures through statistical analysis or comparison with other data sources, and improvement of the process or function. Then the cycle repeats. The Joint Commission provides specific standards that must be met, with examples of appropriate measures of performance. The goal of this cycle of design, measurement, assessment, and improvement of performance of important functions and processes is to improve patient safety and quality of care.

Anesthesia care is one important function of the care of patients monitored by the Joint Commission. It is important that policies and procedures for administration of anesthesia be consistent in all locations within the organization.

The Joint Commission has adopted and annually updates patient safety goals for accredited organizations. Recent patient safety goals include improved accuracy of patient identification, improved effectiveness of communication among caregivers including handoffs, improved safety of medication usage including anticoagulation therapy, reduction of health care-associated infections, and improved recognition and response to changes in a patient's condition. Joint Commission accreditation visits are unannounced, and involve the inspector watching patient care to see that safe and acceptable practices are routinely implemented. In the intraoperative environment, this may involve such processes as timely administration of antibiotics and proper labeling of all syringes on the anesthesia cart. The Joint Commission also requires all sentinel events (any unexpected occurrences involving death or serious physical or psychological injury or risk thereof) to undergo *root cause analysis*.[e] A root cause analysis is typically facilitated by the hospital and includes everyone involved in the care of the affected patient in reconstructing the events to identify system process flaws that facilitated medical error. Any surgery on the wrong patient or wrong body part is included in this policy. The Joint Commission publishes a sentinel event alert so health care organizations can learn from the experiences of others and prevent future medical errors.

Pay for Performance

A relatively recent development related to quality improvement is P4P or "pay for performance." P4P programs provide monetary incentives for implementation of safe practices, measuring performance, and/or achieving performance goals. This is a recent and evolving trend, so only a conceptual introduction will be provided here. Anesthesia providers and service groups will need to be cognizant of any P4P initiatives that are operative in their location and with their payers.

At the time of this writing, P4P is being driven by the Leapfrog Group, the Institute of Healthcare Improvement, the Center for Medicare and Medicaid Services (CMS), and the National Quality Forum. The basic concept involves payment for quality rather than simply payment for services. In some cases, quality incentive payments are provided for simply measuring processes. However, as measurement systems are implemented, it is expected that benchmarks for quality performance will be established and providers will need to show that they are meeting such performance benchmarks to receive incentive payments. Eventually, providers falling short of benchmark performance may see their reimbursements reduced. P4P is being implemented at both the hospital and specific provider level. CMS and other payers may eventually link reimbursement to individual provider profiles.

A multitude of performance measures are being developed to meet the benchmarking challenge. At present, individual institutions are not being held to particular benchmarks but are expected to adopt some of the major quality indicators for measurement and improvement. These include "never events," which are serious adverse events that should never occur. Never events include surgery on the wrong patient or location, unintentional retention of a foreign body after surgery, patient death resulting from a medication error, and perioperative death of an ASA 1 patient. At the end of 2007, there were 28 never events established by the National Quality Forum. Many, but not all of these events are relevant to anesthesia care. The list of never events is periodically updated.[f]

PROFESSIONAL LIABILITY

This section addresses the basic concepts of medical liability. A more detailed discussion of the steps of the lawsuit process and appropriate actions for physicians to take when sued is available from the ASA.[g]

The Tort System

Although physicians may become involved in the criminal law system in a professional capacity, they more commonly become involved in the legal system of civil laws. Civil law is broadly divided into *contract law* and *tort law*. A tort may be loosely defined as a civil wrongdoing; negligence is one type of tort. *Malpractice* actually refers to any professional misconduct but its use in legal terms typically refers to professional negligence.

To be successful in a malpractice suit, the patient–plaintiff must prove four things:

1. Duty: that the anesthesiologist owed the patient a duty;
2. Breach of duty: that the anesthesiologist failed to fulfill his or her duty;
3. Causation: that a reasonably close causal relation exists between the anesthesiologist's acts and the resultant injury; and
4. Damages: that actual damage resulted because of a breach of the standard of care.

Failure to prove any one of these four elements will result in a decision for the defendant–anesthesiologist.

Duty

As a physician, the anesthesiologist establishes a duty to the patient when a doctor–patient relationship exists. When the patient is seen preoperatively, and the anesthesiologist agrees to provide anesthesia care for the patient, a duty to the patient has been established. In the most general terms, the duty the anesthesiologist owes to the patient is to adhere to the *standard of care* for the treatment of the patient. Because it is virtually impossible to delineate specific standards for all aspects of medical practice and all eventualities, the courts have created the concept of the *reasonable and prudent* physician. For all specialties, there is a national standard that has displaced the local standard.

There are certain general duties that all physicians have to their patients, and breaching these duties may also serve as the basis for a lawsuit. One of these general duties is that of obtaining informed consent for a procedure. Consent may be written, verbal, or implied. Oral consent is just as valid, albeit harder to prove years after the fact, as written consent. Implied consent for anesthesia care may be present in circumstances in which the patient is unconscious or unable, for any reason, to give his or her consent, but where it is presumed that any reasonable and prudent patient would give consent.

Although there are exceptions to the requirement that consent be obtained, anesthesiologists should be sure to obtain consent whenever possible. Failure to do so could, in theory, expose the anesthesiologist to possible prosecution for battery.

The requirement that the consent be *informed* is somewhat more opaque. The guideline is determining whether the patient received a fair and reasonable account of the proposed procedures and the risks inherent in these procedures. Most states

[e]The Joint Commission. Sentinel Event Policy and Procedures, Updated: July 2007. http://www.jointcommission.org/SentinelEvents/PolicyandProcedures/se_pp.htm.
[f]National Quality Forum. http://www.qualityforum.org/

[g]Kroll DA: Professional Liability and the Anesthesiologist. Park Ridge, IL, American Society of Anesthesiologists, 1992. Available at: http://www.asahq.org/publicationsAndServices/professional.pdf

have adopted a "reasonable patient" standard, which requires that the physician disclose risks that a reasonable patient under similar circumstances would want to know to make an informed decision. Besides disclosure of common risks, risks that would be important in deciding whether or not to undertake the proposed therapy should also be discussed. For regional anesthesia, these should include both the common risks (e.g., local pain/discomfort, infection, headache, transient neuropathy), as well as those that are rare, but of major consequence (e.g., seizure, cardiac arrest, permanent neuropathy, paralysis, and death).

Breach of Duty

In a malpractice action, expert witnesses will review the medical records of the case and determine whether the anesthesiologist acted in a reasonable and prudent manner in the specific situation and fulfilled his or her duty to the patient. If they find that the anesthesiologist either did something that should not have been done, or failed to do something that should have been done, then the duty to adhere to the standard of care has been breached. Therefore, the second requirement for a successful suit will have been met.

Causation

Judges and juries are interested in determining whether the breach of duty was the *proximate cause* of the injury. If the odds are better than even that the breach of duty led, however circuitously, to the injury, this requirement is met.

There are two common tests employed to establish causation. The first is the *but for* test, and the second is the *substantial factor* test. If the injury would not have occurred but for the action of the defendant-anesthesiologist, or if the act of the anesthesiologist was a substantial factor in the injury despite other causes, then proximate cause is established.

Although the burden of proof of causation ordinarily falls on the patient-plaintiff, it may, under special circumstances, be shifted to the physician-defendant under the doctrine of *res ipsa loquitur* (literally, "the thing speaks for itself"). Applying this doctrine requires proving that:

1. the injury is of a kind that typically would not occur in the absence of negligence,
2. the injury must be caused by something under the exclusive control of the anesthesiologist,
3. the injury must not be attributable to any contribution on the part of the patient, and
4. the evidence for the explanation of events must be more accessible to the anesthesiologist than to the patient.

Because anesthesiologists render patients insensible to their surroundings and unable to protect themselves from injury, the doctrine of *res ipsa loquitur* may be invoked in anesthesia malpractice cases. While this argument was commonly used in the past in lawsuits for nerve injuries, it is less commonly used successfully today.

Damages

The law allows for three different types of damages. *General damages* are those such as pain and suffering that directly result from the injury. *Special damages* are those actual damages that are a consequence of the injury, such as medical expenses, lost income, and funeral expenses. *Punitive damages* are intended to punish the physician for negligence that was reckless, wanton, fraudulent, or willful. Punitive damages are exceedingly rare in medical malpractice cases. More likely in the case of gross negligence is a loss of the license to practice anesthesia. In extreme cases, criminal charges may

be brought against the physician, although this is rare. Determination of the dollar amount is usually based on some assessment of the plaintiff's condition versus the condition he or she would have been in had there been no negligence. Plaintiffs' attorneys generally charge a percentage of the damages and will, therefore, seek to maximize the award given.

Standard of Care

Because medical malpractice usually involves issues beyond the comprehension of lay jurors and judges, the court establishes the standard of care in a particular case by the testimony of *expert witnesses*. These witnesses differ from factual witnesses mainly in that they may give opinions. The trial court judge has sole discretion in determining whether a witness may be qualified as an expert. Although any licensed physician may be an expert, information will be sought regarding the witness's education and training, the nature and scope of the person's practice, memberships and affiliations, and publications. The purpose in gathering this information is not only to establish the qualifications of the witness to provide expert testimony, but also to determine the weight to be given to that testimony by the jury. In many cases the success of a lawsuit depends primarily on the stature and believability of the expert witnesses.

Unfortunately, there is a tendency for experts to link severe injury with inappropriate care (i.e., a bias that "bad outcomes mean bad care"). To investigate the influence of the severity of the injury on the assessment of standard of care, a group of 112 practicing anesthesiologists judged appropriateness of care in 21 cases involving adverse anesthetic outcomes.[40] The original outcome in each case was either temporary or permanent. For each original case, a matching alternate case was created that was identical to the original in every respect, except that a plausible outcome of the opposite severity was substituted. Reviewers judged the standard of care in each case. Knowledge of the severity of injury produced a significant inverse effect on the judgment of appropriateness of care (Fig. 4-1).[40] The proportion of ratings for appropriate care decreased when the outcome was changed from temporary to permanent, and increased when the outcome was changed from permanent to temporary. These results suggest that outcome bias in the assessment of standard of care may contribute to the frequency and size of payments.

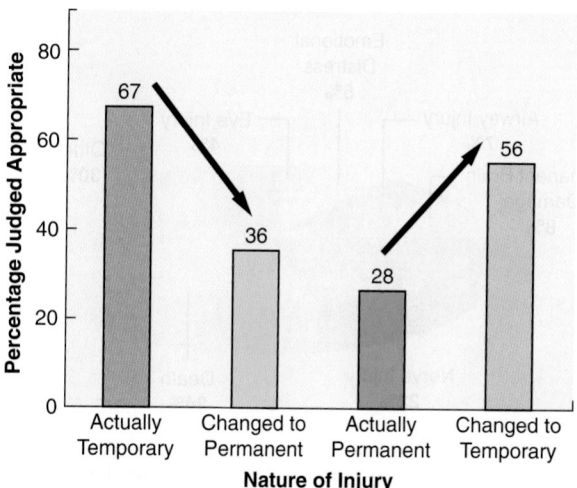

FIGURE 4-1. Effect of outcome on physician judgments of appropriateness of care. (Adapted from Caplan et al. Effect of outcome on physician judgements of appropriateness of care. JAMA 1991;265: 1957–1960.)

In certain circumstances, the standard of care may also be determined from published societal guidelines, written policies of a hospital or department, or textbooks and monographs. Some medical specialty societies have carefully avoided applying the term *standards* to their guidelines in the hope that no binding behavior or mandatory practices have been created. The essential difference between standards and guidelines is that guidelines *should* be adhered to and standards *must* be adhered to. The ASA publishes standards and guidelines for a variety of anesthesia-related activities.

Causes of Anesthesia-Related Lawsuits

Relatively few adverse outcomes end up in a malpractice suit. It has been estimated that less than 1 of 25 patient injuries result in malpractice litigation.[41] The ASA Committee on Professional Liability has conducted a nationwide analysis of malpractice claims against anesthesiologists, excluding dental damage, since 1985 (i.e., the *Closed Claims Project*).[42,43] The leading injuries in malpractice claims in the 1990s were death (24%), nerve damage (22%), permanent brain damage (8%), and airway injury (7%; Fig. 4-2). The causes of death and permanent brain damage were predominantly problems in airway management (e.g., inadequate ventilation, difficult intubation, premature extubation) and other complications such as pulmonary embolism, inadequate fluid therapy, stroke, hemorrhage, and myocardial infarction.[44] Nerve damage, especially to the ulnar nerve, often occurs despite apparently adequate positioning.[14,16] Spinal cord injury was the most common cause of nerve damage claims against anesthesiologists in the 1990s.[14] Chronic pain management is an increasing source of malpractice claims against anesthesiologists.[45]

The anesthesiologist is likely to be the target of a lawsuit if an untoward outcome occurs because the physician–patient relationship is usually tenuous at best. The patient rarely chooses the anesthesiologist, the preoperative visit is brief, and the anesthesiologist who sees the patient preoperatively may not actually anesthetize the patient. Communication between anesthesiologists and surgeons about complications is often lacking and the tendency is for the surgeon to "blame anesthesia." In addition, anesthesiologists are often sued along with

the surgeon in the case of an adverse outcome. This may occur even if the outcome was in no way related to the anesthetic care.

What to Do When Sued

A lawsuit begins when the patient-plaintiff's attorney files a *complaint* and demand for jury trial with the court. The anesthesiologist is then served with the complaint and a summons requiring an answer to the complaint. Until this happens, no lawsuit has been filed. Insurance carriers must be notified immediately after the receipt of the complaint. The anesthesiologist will need assistance in answering the complaint, and there is a time limit placed on the response.

Specific actions at this point include the following:

1. Do not discuss the case with anyone, including colleagues who may have been involved, operating room personnel, or friends.
2. Never alter any records.
3. Gather together all pertinent records, including a copy of the anesthetic record, billing statements, and correspondence concerning the case.
4. Make notes recording all events recalled about the case.
5. Cooperate fully with the attorney provided by the insurer.

The first task the anesthesiologist must perform with an attorney is to prepare an answer to the complaint. The complaint contains certain facts and allegations with which the defense may either agree or disagree. Defense attorneys rely on the frank and totally candid observations of the physician in preparing an answer to the complaint. Physicians should be willing to educate their attorneys about the medical facts of the case, although most medical malpractice attorneys will be knowledgeable and medically sophisticated.

The next phase of the malpractice suit is called *discovery*. The purpose of discovery is the gathering of facts and clarification of issues in advance of the trial. In all likelihood the anesthesiologist will initially receive a written interrogatory, which will request factual information. In consultation with the defense attorney, the interrogatory should be answered in writing because carelessly or inadvertently misstated facts can become troublesome later.

Depositions are a second mechanism of discovery. The defendant–anesthesiologist will be deposed as a fact witness, and depositions will be obtained from other anesthesiologists who will act as expert witnesses. A nationally recognized expert in the area in question, recommended by the defendant but who is not a personal friend, and who agrees with the defense position, may be very valuable.

The plaintiff's attorney, not the defense attorney, will depose the anesthesiologist. Despite the apparent informality of the deposition, the anesthesiologist must be constantly aware that what is said during the deposition carries as much weight as what would be said in court. It is important to be factually prepared for the deposition by review of personal notes, the anesthetic record, and the medical record. The physician should dress conservatively and professionally because appearance and image are very important. The opposition is assessing the physician to see how he or she will appear to a jury. Answer only the question asked, and do not volunteer information. Rely on one's attorney for assistance when preparing for a deposition.

There will be depositions from expert witnesses, both for the plaintiff and for the defense. The anesthesiologist should work with his or her attorney to suggest questions and rebuttals. The better educated the attorney is about the medical facts, the reasons the anesthesiologist did what was done, and

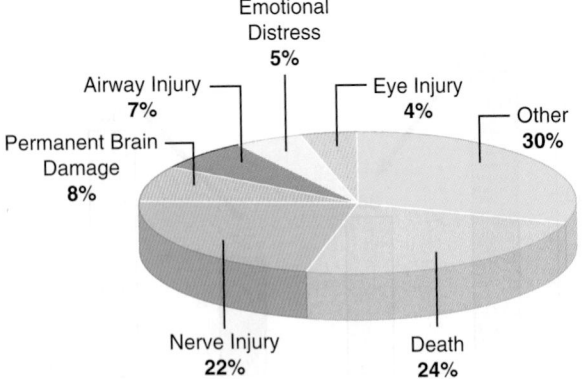

FIGURE 4-2.   Most common injuries leading to anesthesia malpractice claims. Other category includes 3% each for newborn injury, pneumothorax, myocardial infarction, stroke, burns, headache, and back pain; and 1.5% for awareness/recall. Damage to teeth and dentures excluded. American Society of Anesthesiologists' Closed Claims Project (N = 7,328).

INTRODUCTION TO ANESTHESIOLOGY

the alternative approaches, the better able the attorney will be to conduct these expert depositions.

If there is some merit in the case but the damages are minimal, or if proof of innocence will be difficult, there will probably be a settlement offer. There is a high cost incurred by both plaintiffs and defendants in pursuing a malpractice claim up through a jury trial. Unless there is a strong probability of a large dollar award, reputable plaintiffs' attorneys are not likely to pursue the claim. Thus, even if physicians believe that they are totally innocent of any wrongdoing, they should not be offended or angered about settling of the case: this is solely a matter of money, not medicine.

If a settlement is not reached during the discovery phase, a trial will occur. Only about 1 in 20 malpractice cases ever reach the point of a jury trial. Only those cases in which both sides think they can win, and which are likely to have significant financial impact, will proceed to trial.

The discussion of deposition testimony also applies to testimony in court, but there are a few additional points to consider during the trial. The members of the jury will not be as sophisticated medically as the attorneys who deposed the anesthesiologist during discovery. However, do not underestimate the intelligence of the jury. Talking down to them will create an unfavorable impression. If the answer to a question is not known, avoid guessing. If specific facts cannot be remembered, say so. Nobody expects total recall of events that may have occurred years before.

The defendant-physician should be present during the entire trial, even when not testifying, and should dress professionally. Displays of anger, remorse, relief, or hostility will hurt the physician in court. The physician should be able to give his or her testimony without using notes or documents. When it is necessary to refer to the medical record, it will be admitted into evidence. The anesthesiologist's goal is to convince the jury that he or she behaved in this case as any other competent and prudent anesthesiologist would have behaved.

It is important to keep in mind that *proof* in a malpractice case means only "more likely than not." The patient-plaintiff must "prove" the four elements of negligence, not to absolute certainty, but only to a probability greater than 50%. On the positive side, this means that the defendant-anesthesiologist must only show that his or her actions were, more likely than not, within an acceptable standard of care.

ACKNOWLEDGMENTS

The authors wish to thank F. W. Cheney, MD, and D. A. Kroll, MD, whose material from previous editions of this chapter has been retained in the current edition. The authors also thank Gene Peterson, MD, PhD for his helpful suggestions on this revision.

References

1. Beecher HK, Todd DP: A study of the deaths associated with anesthesia and surgery: based on a study of 599,548 anesthesias in 10 institutions 1948–1952, inclusive. Ann Surg 1954; 140:2
2. Newland MC, Ellis SJ, Lydiatt CA, et al: Anesthetic-related cardiac arrest and its mortality: A report covering 72,959 anesthetics over 10 years from a US teaching hospital. Anesthesiology 2002; 97: 108
3. Lagasse RS: Anesthesia safety: model or myth? A review of the published literature and analysis of current original data. Anesthesiology 2002; 97: 1609
4. Flick RP, Sprung J, Harrison TE, et al: Perioperative cardiac arrests in children between 1988 and 2005 at a tertiary referral center: a study of 92,881 patients. Anesthesiology 2007; 106: 226
5. Morray JP, Geiduschek JM, Ramamoorthy C, et al: Anesthesia-related cardiac arrest in children: initial findings of the Pediatric Perioperative Cardiac Arrest (POCA) Registry. Anesthesiology 2000; 93: 6
6. Eagle CC, Davis NJ: Report of the Anaesthetic Mortality Committee of Western Australia 1990–1995. Anaesth Intensive Care 1997; 25: 51
7. Davis NJ (ed): Anaesthesia related mortality in Australia 1994. Report of the Committee convened under the auspices of the Australian and New Zealand College of Anaesthetists. Capitol Press, 1999
8. Biboulet P, Aubas P, Dubourdieu J, et al: Fatal and non fatal cardiac arrests related to anesthesia. Can J Anaesth 2001; 48: 326–332
9. Arbous MS, Grobbee DE, van Kleef JW, et al: Mortality associated with anaesthesia: a qualitative analysis to identify risk factors. Anaesthesia 2001; 56: 1141
10. Kawashima Y, Takahashi S, Suzuki M, et al: Anesthesia-related mortality and morbidity over a 5-year period in 2,363,038 patients in Japan. Acta Anaesthesiol Scand 2003; 47: 809
11. Kawashima Y, Seo N, Morita K, et al: Annual study of perioperative mortality and morbidity for the year of 1999 in Japan: the outlines report of the Japan Society of Anesthesiologists Committee on Operating Room Safety (in Japanese). Masui 2001; 50: 1260
12. Irita K, Kawashima Y, Iwao Y, et al: Annual mortality and morbidity in operating rooms during 2002 and summary of morbidity and mortality between 1999 and 2002 in Japan: a brief review (in Japanese). Masui 2004; 53: 320
13. Lienhart A. Auroy Y, Pequignot F, et al: Survey of anesthesia-related mortality in France. Anesthesiology 2006; 105: 1087
14. Cheney FW, Domino KB, Caplan RA, et al: Nerve injury associated with anesthesia: a closed claims analysis. Anesthesiology 1999; 90: 1062
15. Alvine FG, Schurrer ME: Postoperative ulnar-nerve palsy. Are there predisposing factors? J Bone Joint Surg Am 1987; 69: 255
16. Warner MA, Warner ME, Martin JT: Ulnar neuropathy. Incidence, outcome, and risk factors in sedated or anesthetized patients. Anesthesiology 1994; 81: 1332–1340
17. Warner MA, Warner DO, Matsumoto JY, et al: Ulnar neuropathy in surgical patients. Anesthesiology 1999; 90: 54
18. Warner MA, Martin JT, Schroeder DR, et al: Lower-extremity motor neuropathy associated with surgery performed on patients in a lithotomy position. Anesthesiology 1994; 81: 6
19. Brull R, McCartney CJ, Chan VW, et al: Neurological complications after regional anesthesia: contemporary estimates of risk. Anesth Analg 2007; 104: 965
20. Sandin RH, Enlund G, Samuelsson P, et al: Awareness during anaesthesia: a prospective case study. Lancet 2000; 355: 707
21. Sebel PS, Bowdle TA, Ghoneim MM, et al: The incidence of awareness during anesthesia: a multicenter United States study. Anesth Analg 2004; 99: 833
22. Pollard RJ, Coyle JP, Gilber RL, et al: Intraoperative awareness in a regional medical system: a review of 3 years' data. Anesthesiology 2007; 106: 269
23. Warner ME, Warner MA, Garrity JA, et al: The frequency of perioperative vision loss. Anesth Analg 2001; 93: 1417
24. Warner ME, Fronapfel PJ, Hebl JR, et al: Perioperative visual changes. Anesthesiology 2002; 96: 855
25. Warner ME, Benenfeld SM, Warner MA, et al: Perianesthetic dental injuries: frequency, outcomes, and risk factors. Anesthesiology 1999; 90: 1302
26. Monk TG, Weldon BC, Garvan CW, et al: Predictors of cognitive dysfunction after major noncardiac surgery. Anesthesiology 2008; 108: 18
27. Committee on Quality of Health Care in America, Institute of Medicine: Crossing the Quality Chasm, A New Health System for the 21st Century. Washington, DC, National Academy Press, 2001
28. Gaba DM, Maxwell M, DeAnda A: Anesthetic mishaps: breaking the chain of accident evolution. Anesthesiology 1987; 66: 670
29. Petty C: The Anesthesia Machine. New York, Churchill-Livingstone, 1987, p 213
30. Spooner RB, Kirby RR: Equipment-related anesthetic incidents. Int Anesthesiol Clin 1984; 22: 133
31. Food and Drug Administration: Anesthesia Apparatus Checkout Recommendations, 1993. Rockville, MD, Food and Drug Administration, 1994
32. Feldman JM: Do anesthesia information systems increase malpractice exposure? Results of a survey. Anes Analg 2004; 99: 840
33. Gallagher TH, Studdert D, Levinson W: Disclosing harmful medical errors to patients. N Engl J Med 2007; 356: 2713
34. Baldwin LM, Hart LG, Oshel RE, et al: Hospital peer review and the National Practitioner Data Bank: clinical privileges action reports. JAMA 1999; 282: 349
35. Donabedian A: The quality of care. How can it be assessed? JAMA 1988; 260: 1743
36. Deming WE: Out of the Crisis. Cambridge, MA, Massachusetts Institute of Technology, 1986
37. Juran JM: Juran on Planning for Quality. New York, Free Press, 1988
38. Kohn LT, Corrigan JM, Donaldson MS (eds): Committee on Quality of Health Care in America, Institute of Medicine. To Err is Human: Building a Safer Health System. Washington, DC, National Academy Press, 1999

39. Reason JT: Human Error. Cambridge, Cambridge University Press, 1990

40. Caplan RA, Posner KL, Cheney FW: Effect of outcome on physician judgments of appropriateness of care. JAMA 1991; 265: 1957–1960

41. Localio AR, Lawthers AG, Brennan TA, et al: Relation between malpractice claims and adverse events due to negligence. Results of the Harvard Medical Practice Study III. N Engl J Med 1991; 325: 245

42. Cheney FW, Posner K, Caplan RA, et al: Standard of care and anesthesia liability. JAMA 1989; 261: 1599

43. Cheney FW: The American Society of Anesthesiologists Closed Claims Project: What have we learned, how has it affected practice, and how will it affect practice in the future? Anesthesiology 1999; 91: 552

44. Cheney FW, Posner KL, Lee LA, et al: Trends in anesthesia-related death and brain damage: a closed claims analysis. Anesthesiology 2006; 105:1081

45. Fitzgibbon DR, Posner KL, Domino KB, et al: Chronic pain management: American Society of Anesthesiologists Closed Claims Project. Anesthesiology 2004; 100: 98

SECTION II ■ SCIENTIFIC FOUNDATIONS OF ANESTHESIA

SECTION I. SCIENTIFIC FOUNDATIONS
OF ANESTHESIA

CHAPTER 5 ■ MECHANISMS OF ANESTHESIA AND CONSCIOUSNESS

ALEX S. EVERS AND C. MICHAEL CROWDER

KEY POINTS

1 The components of the anesthetic state include unconsciousness, amnesia, analgesia, immobility, and attenuation of autonomic responses to noxious stimulation.

2 Minimum alveolar concentration (MAC) remains the most robust measurement and the standard for determining the potency of volatile anesthetics.

3 Anesthetic actions on the spinal cord cannot produce either amnesia or unconsciousness. However, several lines of evidence indicate that the spinal cord is probably the site at which anesthetics act to inhibit purposeful responses to noxious stimulation.

4 A developing body of evidence indicates that inhalational anesthetics can depress the excitability of thalamic neurons, thus blocking thalamocortical communication and potentially resulting in loss of consciousness.

5 Whereas certain anesthetic effects may be attributable to specific anatomic locations (e.g., purposeful response to noxious stimulation maps to the spinal cord), existing evidence provides no basis for a single anatomic site responsible for anesthesia.

6 While current data still support the prevailing view that neuronal excitability is only slightly affected by general anesthetics, this small effect may nevertheless contribute significantly to the clinical actions of volatile anesthetics.

7 The synapse is generally thought to be the most likely relevant site of anesthetic action. Existing evidence indicates that even at this one site, anesthetics produce various effects, including presynaptic inhibition of neurotransmitter release,

inhibition of excitatory neurotransmitter effect, and enhancement of inhibitory neurotransmitter effect. Furthermore, the effects of anesthetics on synaptic function differ among various anesthetic agents, neurotransmitters, and neuronal preparations.

8 Existing evidence suggests that most voltage-dependent calcium channels (VDCCs) are modestly sensitive or insensitive to anesthetics. However, some sodium channels subtypes are inhibited by volatile anesthetics and this effect may be responsible in part for a reduction in neurotransmitter release at some synapses.

9 A large body of evidence shows that clinical concentrations of many anesthetics potentiate GABA-activated currents in the central nervous system. Other members of the ligand-activated ion channel family, including glycine receptors, neuronal nicotinic receptors, and 5-HT$_3$ receptors, are also affected by clinical concentrations of anesthetics and remain plausible anesthetic targets.

10 Activation of background K$^+$ channels in mammalian vertebrates could be an important and general mechanism through which inhalational and gaseous anesthetics regulate neuronal resting membrane potential and thereby excitability.

11 Direct interactions of anesthetic molecules with proteins would not only satisfy the Meyer-Overton rule, but would also provide the simplest explanation for compounds that deviate from this rule.

12 Current evidence strongly indicates protein rather than lipid as the molecular target for anesthetic action.

13 All anesthetic actions cannot be localized to a specific anatomic site in the central nervous system; indeed, some evidence suggests that different components of the anesthetic state may be mediated by actions at disparate anatomic sites.

14 At a molecular level, volatile anesthetics show some selectivity, but still affect the function of multiple ion channels and synaptic proteins. The intravenous anesthetics, etomidate, propofol, and barbiturates, are more specific with the $GABA_A$ receptor as their major target.

The introduction of general anesthetics into clinical practice over 150 years ago stands as one of the seminal innovations of medicine. This single discovery facilitated the development of modern surgery and spawned the specialty of anesthesiology. Despite the importance of general anesthetics and despite more than 100 years of active research, the molecular mechanisms responsible for anesthetic action remain one of the unsolved mysteries of pharmacology.

Why have mechanisms of anesthesia been so difficult to elucidate? Anesthetics, as a class of drugs, are challenging to study for three major reasons:

1. Anesthesia, by definition, is a change in the responses of an *intact animal* to external stimuli. Making a definitive link between anesthetic effects observed in vitro and the anesthetic state observed and defined *in vivo* has proven difficult.
2. No structure–activity relationships are apparent among anesthetics; a wide variety of structurally unrelated compounds, ranging from steroids to elemental xenon, are capable of producing clinical anesthesia. This suggests that there are multiple molecular mechanisms that can produce clinical anesthesia.
3. Anesthetics work at very high concentrations in comparison to drugs, neurotransmitters, and hormones that act at specific receptors. This implies that if anesthetics do act by binding to specific receptor sites, they must bind with very low affinity and probably stay bound to the receptor for very short periods of time. Low-affinity binding is much more difficult to observe and characterize than high-affinity binding.

Despite these difficulties, molecular and genetic tools are now available that should allow for major insights into anesthetic mechanisms in the next decade. The aim of this chapter is to provide a conceptual framework for the reader to catalog current knowledge and integrate future developments about mechanisms of anesthesia. Five specific questions will be addressed in this chapter:

1. What is anesthesia and how do we measure it?
2. What is the anatomic site of anesthetic action in the central nervous system?
3. What are the cellular neurophysiologic mechanisms of anesthesia (e.g., effects on synaptic function vs. effects on action potential generation) and what anesthetic effects on ion channels and other neuronal proteins underlie these mechanisms?
4. What are the molecular targets of anesthetics?
5. How are the molecular and cellular effects of anesthetics linked to the behavioral effects of anesthetics observed in vivo?

WHAT IS ANESTHESIA?

General anesthesia can broadly be defined as a drug-induced reversible depression of the central nervous system (CNS) resulting in the loss of response to and perception of all external stimuli. Unfortunately, such a broad definition is inadequate for two reasons. First, the definition is not actually broad enough. Anesthesia is not simply a deafferented state; amnesia and unconsciousness are important aspects of the anesthetic state. Second, the definition is too broad, as all general anesthetics do not produce equal depression of all sensory modalities. For example, barbiturates are considered to be anesthetics, but they are not particularly effective analgesics. These conflicting problems with definition can be bypassed by a more practical description of the anesthetic state as a collection of "component" changes in behavior or perception. The components of the anesthetic state include unconsciousness, amnesia, analgesia, immobility, and attenuation of autonomic responses to noxious stimulation.

Regardless of which definition of anesthesia is used, essential to anesthesia are rapid and reversible drug-induced changes in behavior or perception. As such, anesthesia can only be defined and measured in the intact organism. Changes in behavior such as unconsciousness or amnesia can be intuitively understood in higher organisms such as mammals, but become increasingly difficult to define as one descends the phylogenetic tree. Thus, while anesthetics have effects on organisms ranging from worms to man, it is difficult to map with certainty the effects of anesthetics observed in lower organisms to any of our behavioral definitions of anesthesia. This contributes to the difficulty of using simple organisms as models in which to study the molecular mechanisms of anesthesia. Similarly, any cellular or molecular effects of anesthetics observed in higher organisms can be extremely difficult to link with the constellation of behaviors that constitute the anesthetic state. The absence of a simple and concise definition of anesthesia is clearly one of the stumbling blocks to elucidating the mechanisms of anesthesia at a molecular and cellular level.

An additional difficulty in defining anesthesia is that our understanding of the mechanisms of consciousness is rather amorphous at present. One cannot easily define anesthesia when the neurobiological phenomena ablated by anesthesia are not well understood. Nevertheless, recent advances in the study of sleep and attention have identified what may form the anatomic and neurophysiological basis for sleep and perhaps other forms of unconsciousness.[1] Central to the mechanism of sleep is a set of hypothalamic nuclei that appear to form an awake/sleep switch mechanism (Fig. 5-1). The ventrolateral preoptic nucleus (VLPO) in the anterior hypothalamus promotes sleep while the tuberomammillary nucleus (TMN) in the posterior hypothalamus promotes wakefulness. Importantly, the VLPO and the TMN are mutually inhibitory. Thus, for example, if by influence of other modulatory sleep-promoting nuclei the activity of the VLPO gains ground relative to the TMN, the VLPO will ultimately shut down the output of the TMN and sleep will be favored. On the other hand during wakefulness, the TMN is dominant and silences the VLPO. Modulatory influences on the TMN and VLPO include orexinergic neurons in the lateral hypothalamus, the circadian clock, which is directly modulated by light and contained within the hypothalamic suprachiasmatic nucleus, and multiple brainstem nuclei, in particular the locus coeruleus and dorsal raphe. These brainstem nuclei as a whole promote arousal and are a part of the reticular activating formation. In addition to synaptic modulators, adenosine has been proposed as a neurohumoral factor that promotes sleep by disinhibiting the VLPO. The TMN and the VLPO are thought to promote the awake or sleep state by acting on thalamic and cortical circuits, either directly or through the reticular activating formation. The thalamus and cortex maintain wakefulness and consciousness through complex interactions that may involve

SCIENTIFIC FOUNDATIONS
OF ANESTHESIA

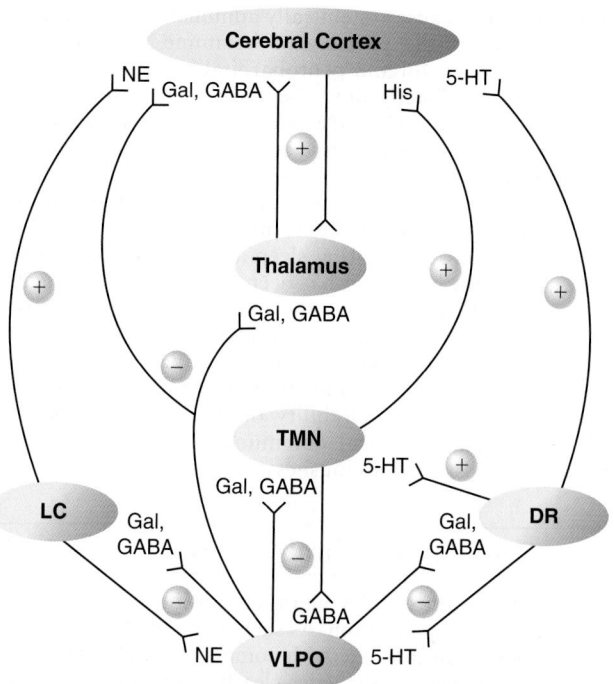

FIGURE 5-1.   Simplified sleep/wake control circuit. The wake/sleep switch is composed of the mutually-inhibitory ventrolateral preoptic nucleus (VLPO) and the tuberomammillary nucleus (TMN) hypothalamic neurons. The direction of this switch is influenced by humoral factors such as adenosine, the circadian clock, other hypothalamic neurons releasing orexin (not shown), and brainstem arousal nuclei such as the dorsal raphe (DR) and the locus coeruleus (LC). Both the wake/sleep switch and the brainstem arousal system act on higher order circuits in the thalamus and cerebral cortex. General anesthetics appear to act on multiple components of the sleep/wake control system. 5-HT, 5-hydroxytryptamine/serotonin; Gal, galanin; NE, norepinephrine; His, histamine; GABA, γ-aminobutyric acid.

intrinsic oscillators and widespread synaptic communication. Awareness and consciousness is thought to emerge from communication between the prefrontal cortex and multiple cortical and subcortical areas that have distributed representations of a perception. Again, the precise mechanisms of the emergent properties of consciousness are unclear. As discussed later, some recent evidence implicates components of the sleep switch as anatomic targets of certain general anesthetics.

HOW IS ANESTHESIA MEASURED?

In order to study the pharmacology of anesthetic action, quantitative measurements of anesthetic potency are absolutely essential. To this end, Quasha and colleagues[2] have defined the concept of MAC, or minimum alveolar concentration. MAC is defined as the alveolar partial pressure of a gas at which 50% of humans do not respond to a surgical incision. In animals, MAC is defined as the alveolar partial pressure of a gas at which 50% of animals do not respond to a noxious stimulus, such as tail clamp,[3] or at which they lose their righting reflex. The use of MAC as a measure of anesthetic potency has two major advantages. First, it is an extremely reproducible measurement that is remarkably constant over a wide range of species.[2] Second, the use of end-tidal gas concentration provides an index of the "free" concentration of drug required to produce anesthesia since the end-tidal gas concentration is in equilibrium with the free concentration in plasma. The MAC

concept has several important limitations, particularly when trying to relate MAC values to anesthetic potency observed in vitro. First, the end point in a MAC determination is quantal: a subject is either anesthetized or unanesthetized; it cannot be partially anesthetized. Furthermore, MAC represents the average response of a whole population of subjects rather than the response of a single subject. The quantal nature of the MAC measurement makes it very difficult to compare MAC measurements to concentration–response curves obtained in vitro, where the graded response of a single preparation is measured as a function of anesthetic concentration. The second limitation of MAC measurements is that they can only be directly applied to anesthetic gases. Parenteral anesthetics (barbiturates, neurosteroids, propofol) cannot be assigned a MAC value, making it difficult to compare the potency of parenteral and volatile anesthetics. A MAC equivalent for parental anesthetics is the free concentration of the drug in plasma required to prevent response to a noxious stimulus in 50% of subjects; this value has been estimated for several parenteral anesthetics.[4] A third limitation of MAC is that it is highly dependent on the anesthetic end point used to define it. For example, if loss of response to a verbal command is used as an anesthetic end point, the MAC values obtained (MAC$_{awake}$) will be much lower than classic MAC values based on response to a noxious stimulus. Indeed, each behavioral component of the anesthetic state will likely have a different MAC value. Despite its limitations, MAC remains the most robust measurement and the standard for determining the potency of volatile anesthetics.

Because of the limitations of MAC, monitors that measure some correlate of anesthetic depth have been introduced into clinical practice.[5] The most popular of these monitors converts spontaneous electroencephalogram waveforms into a single value that correlates with anesthetic depth for some general anesthetics. Anesthetic depth monitors have great potential. They may reduce the incidence of awareness during anesthesia, which is estimated to be approximately 0.1 to 0.2%.[6] They may also reduce the amount of anesthetic used and may hasten emergence and recovery room discharge. However, at this time whether any of the available anesthetic depth monitors is superior to MAC, to standardized dosing of intravenous anesthetics, or to clinical indicators of anesthetic depth is controversial and is still an active area of investigation.

WHERE IN THE CENTRAL NERVOUS SYSTEM DO ANESTHETICS WORK?

In principle, general anesthesia could result from interruption of nervous system activity at myriad levels. Plausible targets include peripheral sensory receptors, spinal cord, brainstem, and cerebral cortex. Of these potential sites, only peripheral sensory receptors can be eliminated as an important site of anesthetic action. Animal studies have shown that fluorinated volatile anesthetics have no effect on cutaneous mechanosensors in cats[7] and can even sensitize nociceptors in monkeys.[8] Furthermore, selective perfusion studies in dogs have shown that MAC for isoflurane is unaffected by the presence or absence of isoflurane at the site of noxious stimulation, provided that the CNS is perfused with blood containing isoflurane.[9]

Spinal Cord

Clearly, anesthetic actions on the spinal cord cannot produce either amnesia or unconsciousness. However, several lines of evidence indicate that the spinal cord is probably the site at which anesthetics act to inhibit purposeful responses to noxious stimulation. This is, of course, the end point used in most measurements of anesthetic potency. Rampil and colleagues[10,11] have shown that MAC values for fluorinated volatile anesthetics are unaffected in the rat by either decerebration[10] or cervical spinal cord transection.[11] Antognini and Schwartz[12] have used the strategy of isolating the cerebral circulation of goats to explore the contribution of brain and spinal cord to the determination of MAC. They found that when isoflurane is administered only to the brain, MAC is 2.9%, whereas when it is administered to the entire body, MAC is 1.2%. Surprisingly, when isoflurane was preferentially administered to the body and not to the brain, isoflurane MAC was reduced to 0.8%.[13] The actions of volatile anesthetics in the spinal cord are mediated, at least in part, by direct effects on the excitability of spinal motor neurons. This conclusion has been substantiated by experiments in rats,[14] goats,[15] and humans[16] showing that volatile anesthetics depress the amplitude of the F wave in evoked potential measurements (F-wave amplitude correlates with motor neuron excitability). These provocative results suggest not only that anesthetic action at the spinal cord underlies MAC, but also that anesthetic action on the brain may actually sensitize the cord to noxious stimuli. The plausibility of the spinal cord as a locus for anesthetic immobilization is also supported by several electrophysiological studies showing inhibition of excitatory synaptic transmission in the spinal cord.[17–20]

Brainstem, Hypothalamic, and Thalamic Arousal Systems

The reticular activating system, a diffuse collection of brainstem neurons involved in arousal behavior, has long been speculated to be a site of general anesthetic action on consciousness. Evidence to support this notion came from early whole-animal experiments showing that electrical stimulation of the reticular activating system could induce arousal behavior in anesthetized animals.[21] A role for the brainstem in anesthetic action is also supported by studies examining somatosensory evoked potentials. Generally, these studies show that anesthetics produce increased latency and decreased amplitude of cortical potentials, indicating that anesthetics inhibit information transfer through the brainstem.[22] In contrast, studies using brainstem auditory evoked potentials have shown variable effects ranging from depression to enhancement of information transfer through the reticular formation.[23–25] While there is evidence that the reticular formation of the brainstem is a locus for anesthetic effects, it cannot be the only anatomic site of anesthetic action for two reasons. First, as discussed, the brainstem is not even required for anesthetics to inhibit responsiveness to noxious stimuli. Second, the reticular formation can be largely ablated without eliminating awareness.[26]

Within the reticular formation is a set of pontine noradrenergic neurons called the *locus coeruleus*. The locus coeruleus widely innervates targets in the cortex, thalamus, and hypothalamus including the sleep-promoting VLPO. As discussed previously, the mutually inhibitory VLPO and TMN may form a sleep/awake switch circuit. This switch was directly implicated in anesthetic action by a set of elegant experiments from Nelson et al.[27] They showed that the application of a GABAergic antagonist directly onto the TMN diminished the efficacy of the anesthetics propofol and pentobarbital. Indeed, discrete application of the GABAergic antagonist gabazine onto the TMN markedly reduced the duration of sedation produced by systemically administered propofol or pentobarbital. This effect is unlikely to be a consequence of a nonspecific increase in arousal state because systemically administered gabazine did not antagonize the potency of ketamine whereas it did antagonize propofol and pentobarbital in a manner similar to application directly onto the TMN. This result strongly implicates the VLPO/TMN sleep switch as a site for the sedative action of GABAergic anesthetics like propofol and barbiturates. However, general anesthesia is clearly not equivalent to sleep. By definition, one cannot be aroused from general anesthesia. Thus, additional neuroanatomical loci besides those mediating sleep are likely to be targeted. One area of the brain that has been postulated as a potential site of anesthetic action is the thalamus. The thalamus is important in relaying sensory modalities and motor information to the cortex via thalamocortical pathways. A developing body of evidence indicates that inhalational anesthetics can depress the excitability of thalamic neurons, thus blocking thalamocortical communication and potentially resulting in loss of consciousness.

Cerebral Cortex

The cerebral cortex is the major site for integration, storage, and retrieval of information. As such, it is a likely site at which anesthetics might interfere with complex functions like memory and awareness. Anesthetics clearly alter cortical electrical activity, as evidenced by the changes in surface electroencephalogram patterns recorded during anesthesia. Anesthetic effects on patterns of cortical electrical activity vary widely among anesthetics,[28] providing an initial suggestion that all anesthetics are not likely to act through identical mechanisms. More detailed in vitro electrophysiological studies examining anesthetic effects on different cortical regions support the notion that anesthetics can differentially alter neuronal function in various cortical preparations. For example, volatile anesthetics have been shown to inhibit excitatory transmission at some synapses in the olfactory cortex[29] but not at others.[30] Similarly, whereas volatile anesthetics inhibit excitatory transmission in the dentate gyrus of the hippocampus,[31] these same drugs can actually enhance excitatory transmission at other synapses in the hippocampus.[32] Anesthetics also produce a variety of effects on inhibitory transmission in the cortex. A variety of parenteral and inhalation anesthetics have been shown to enhance inhibitory transmission in olfactory cortex[30] and in the hippocampus.[33] Conversely, volatile anesthetics have also been reported to depress inhibitory transmission in hippocampus.[34]

Summary

Anesthetics produce effects on a variety of anatomic structures in the CNS, including spinal cord, brainstem, hypothalamus, and cerebral cortex. Whereas certain anesthetic effects may be attributable to specific anatomic locations (*e.g.*, purposeful response to noxious stimulation maps to the spinal cord), existing evidence provides no basis for a single anatomic site responsible for anesthesia. This difficulty in identifying a site for anesthesia might plausibly result from the various components of the anesthetic state being produced by anesthetic effects on different regions of the CNS. Nevertheless, despite the difficulty in identifying a common anatomic site for anesthesia, investigators have continued to look for other unifying principles in anesthetic action. Specifically, attention has been focused on identifying common cellular or molecular anesthetic targets that may have a wide anatomic distribution, explaining the ability of anesthetic to affect nervous system function in an anatomically diffuse manner.

HOW DO ANESTHETICS INTERFERE WITH THE ELECTROPHYSIOLOGIC FUNCTION OF THE NERVOUS SYSTEM?

In the simplest terms anesthetics inhibit or "turn off" vital CNS functions. They must do this by acting at specific physiologic "switches." A great deal of investigative effort has been devoted to identifying these switches. In principle, the CNS could be switched off by several means:

1. By depressing those neurons or pattern generators that subserve a pacemaker function in the CNS.
2. By reducing overall neuronal excitability, either by changing resting membrane potential or by interfering with the processes involved in generating an action potential.
3. By reducing communication between neurons; specifically, by either inhibiting excitatory synaptic transmission or enhancing inhibitory synaptic transmission.

Pattern Generators

Information concerning the effects of anesthetics on pattern-generating neuronal circuits in the CNS is limited, but clinical concentrations of anesthetics are likely to have significant effects on these circuits. The simplest evidence for this is the observation that most anesthetics exert profound effects on respiratory rate and rhythm, strongly suggesting an effect on respiratory pattern generators in the brainstem. Invertebrate studies suggest that volatile anesthetics can selectively inhibit the spontaneous (pacemaker) firing of specific neurons. As shown in Figure 5-2, halothane (1 MAC) completely inhibits spontaneous action potential generation by one neuron in the right parietal ganglion of the great pond snail while producing no observable effect on the firing frequency of adjacent neurons.[35]

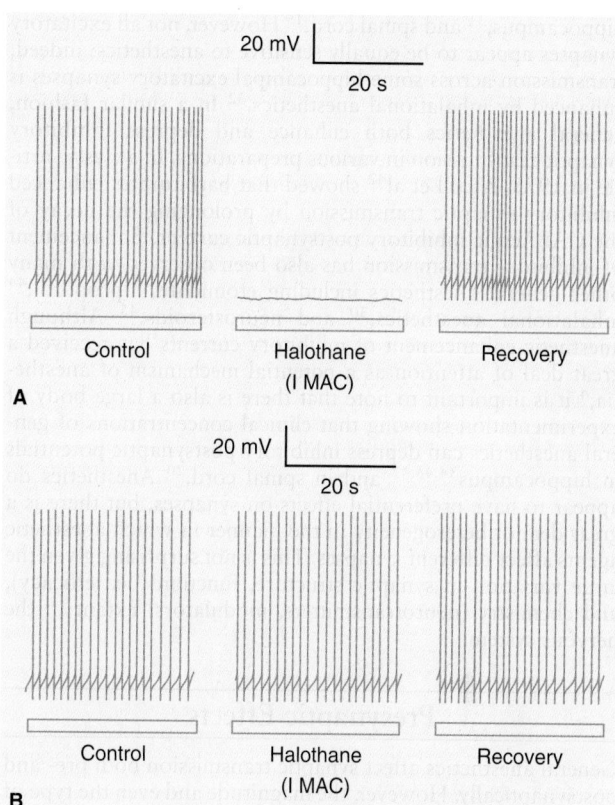

FIGURE 5-2. Selectivity of volatile anesthetic inhibition of neuronal automaticity. **A:** Halothane (1 MAC) reversibly inhibits the spontaneous firing activity of a neuron from the parietal ganglion of *Lymnaea stagnalis*). **B:** The same concentration of halothane has no effect on the firing activity of an adjacent, and apparently identical, neuron). Note that in A, halothane markedly reduces resting membrane potential in addition to inhibiting firing. (Reprinted with permission from Franks NP, Lieb WR: Mechanisms of general anesthesia. Environ Health Perspect 87:204, 1990.)

Neuronal Excitability

The ability of a neuron to generate an action potential is determined by three parameters: resting membrane potential, the threshold potential for action potential generation, and the function of voltage-gated sodium channels. Anesthetics can hyperpolarize (create a more negative resting membrane potential) both spinal motor neurons and cortical neurons,[36,37] and this ability to hyperpolarize neurons correlates with anesthetic potency. In general, the increase in resting membrane potential produced by anesthetics is small in magnitude and is unlikely to have an effect on axonal *propagation* of an action potential. Small changes in resting potential may, however, inhibit the *initiation* of an action potential either at a postsynaptic site or in a spontaneously firing neuron. Indeed, hyperpolarization is responsible for the inhibition of spontaneous action potential generation shown in Figure 5-2. Recent evidence also indicates that isoflurane hyperpolarizes thalamic neurons, leading to an inhibition of tonic firing of action potentials.[38] There is no evidence indicating that anesthetics alter the threshold potential of a neuron for action potential generation. However, the data are conflicting on whether the size of the action potential, once initiated, is diminished by general anesthetics. A classic article by Larabee and Posternak[39] demonstrated that concentrations of ether and chloroform that completely block synaptic transmission in mammalian sympathetic ganglia have no effect on presynaptic action potential amplitude. Similar results have been obtained with fluorinated volatile anesthetics in mammalian brain preparations.[29,31] This dogma that the action potential is relatively resistant to general anesthetics has been challenged by more recent reports that volatile anesthetics at clinical concentrations produce a small but significant reduction in the size of the action potential in mammalian neurons.[40,41] In one case, the reduction in the action potential was shown to be amplified at the presynaptic terminal resulting in a large reduction in neurotransmitter release.[41] Thus, while current data still support the prevailing view that neuronal excitability is only slightly affected by general anesthetics, this small effect may nevertheless contribute significantly to the clinical actions of volatile anesthetics.

Synaptic Function

Synaptic function is widely considered to be the most likely subcellular site of general anesthetic action. Neurotransmission across both excitatory and inhibitory synapses is markedly altered by general anesthetics. General anesthetics inhibit excitatory synaptic transmission in a variety of preparations, including sympathetic ganglia,[39] olfactory cortex,[29] hippocampus,[31] and spinal cord.[19] However, not all excitatory synapses appear to be equally sensitive to anesthetics; indeed, transmission across some hippocampal excitatory synapses is enhanced by inhalational anesthetics.[32] In a similar fashion, general anesthetics both enhance and depress inhibitory synaptic transmission in various preparations. In a classic article in 1975, Nicoll et al[42] showed that barbiturates enhanced inhibitory synaptic transmission by prolonging the decay of the GABAergic inhibitory postsynaptic current. Enhancement of inhibitory transmission has also been observed with many other general anesthetics including etomidate,[43] propofol,[44] inhalational anesthetics,[30] and neurosteroids.[45] Although anesthetic enhancement of inhibitory currents has received a great deal of attention as a potential mechanism of anesthesia,[4] it is important to note that there is also a large body of experimentation showing that clinical concentrations of general anesthetics can depress inhibitory postsynaptic potentials in hippocampus[34,46,47] and in spinal cord.[20] Anesthetics do appear to have preferential effects on synapses, but there is a great deal of heterogeneity in the manner in which anesthetic agents affect different synapses. This is not surprising given the large variation in synaptic structure, function (i.e., efficacy), and chemistry (neurotransmitters, modulators) extant in the nervous system.

Presynaptic Effects

General anesthetics affect synaptic transmission both pre- and postsynaptically. However, the magnitude and even the type of effect vary according to the type of synapse and the particular anesthetic. Presynaptically, neurotransmitter release from glutamatergic synapses has consistently been found to be inhibited by clinical concentrations of volatile anesthetics. For example, a study by Perouansky and colleagues[48] conducted in mouse hippocampal slices showed that halothane inhibited excitatory postsynaptic potentials elicited by presynaptic electrical stimulation, but not those elicited by direct application of glutamate. This indicates that halothane must be acting to prevent the release of glutamate, the major excitatory neurotransmitter in the brain. MacIver and colleagues extended these observations by finding that the inhibition of glutamate release from hippocampal neurons is not due to effects at GABAergic synapses that could indirectly decrease transmitter release from glutamatergic neurons.[32] Effects of intravenous anesthetics on glutamate release have also been demonstrated, but the evidence is more limited and the effects potentially indirect.[49,50] The data for anesthetic effects on inhibitory neurotransmitter release is mixed. Inhibition,[51] stimulation,[52,53] and no effect[54] have been reported for volatile anesthetic and intravenous anesthetic action on GABA (γ-aminobutyric acid) release. In a brain synaptosomal preparation where effects on both GABA and glutamate release could be studied simultaneously, Westphalen and Hemmings[55] found that glutamate and, to a lesser degree, GABA release were inhibited by clinical concentrations of isoflurane. The mechanism underlying anesthetic effects on transmitter release has not been established. The effects of anesthetics on neurotransmitter release do not appear to be mediated by reduced neurotransmitter synthesis or storage, but rather by a direct effect on the process of neurosecretion. A variety of evidence argues that at some synapses a substantial portion of the anesthetic effect is upstream of the transmitter release machinery, perhaps on presynaptic sodium channels or potassium leak channels (see later discussion). However, genetic data in *Caenorhabditis elegans* shows that the transmitter release machinery strongly influences volatile anesthetic sensitivity[56]; at present, it is unclear whether these findings represent species differences or different aspects of the same mechanism.

Postsynaptic Effects

Anesthetics alter the postsynaptic response to released neurotransmitter. The effects of general anesthetics on excitatory neurotransmitter receptor function vary depending on neurotransmitter type, anesthetic agent, and preparation. Richards and Smaje[57] examined the effects of several anesthetic agents on the response of olfactory cortical neurons to application of glutamate, the major excitatory neurotransmitter in the CNS. They found that while pentobarbital, diethyl ether, methoxyflurane, and alphaxalone depressed the electrical response to glutamate, halothane was without effect. In contrast, when acetylcholine was applied to the same olfactory cortical preparation, halothane and methoxyflurane stimulated the electrical response whereas pentobarbital had no effect; only alphaxalone depressed the electrical response to acetylcholine.[58] The effects of anesthetics on neuronal responses to inhibitory neurotransmitters are more consistent. A wide variety of anesthetics, including barbiturates, etomidate, neurosteroids, propofol, and the fluorinated volatile anesthetics, have been shown to enhance the electrical response to exogenously applied GABA (for a review, see ref. 59). For example, Figure 5-3 illustrates the ability of enflurane to increase both the amplitude and the duration of the current elicited by application of GABA to hippocampal neurons.[60]

Summary

Attempts to identify a physiologic switch at which anesthetics act have suffered from their own success. Anesthetics produce a variety of effects on many physiologic processes that might logically contribute to the anesthetic state, including neuronal automaticity, neuronal excitability, and synaptic function. The synapse is generally thought to be the most likely relevant site of anesthetic action. Existing evidence indicates that even at this one site, anesthetics produce various effects, including presynaptic inhibition of neurotransmitter release, inhibition of excitatory neurotransmitter effect, and enhancement of inhibitory neurotransmitter effect. Furthermore, the effects of anesthetics on synaptic function differ among various anesthetic agents, neurotransmitters, and neuronal preparations.

ANESTHETIC ACTIONS ON ION CHANNELS

Ion channels are one likely target of anesthetic action. The advent of patch clamp techniques in the early 1980s made it possible to directly measure the currents from single ion channel proteins. It was attractive to think that anesthetic effects on a small number of ion channels might help to explain the complex physiologic effects of anesthetics that we have already described. Accordingly, during the 1980s and 1990s a major effort was directed at describing the effects of anesthetics on the various kinds of ion channels. The following section summarizes and distills this effort. For the purposes of this discussion, ion channels are cataloged according to the stimuli to which they respond by opening or closing (i.e., their mechanism of gating).

Anesthetic Effects on Voltage-Dependent Ion Channels

A variety of ion channels can sense a change in membrane potential and respond by either opening or closing their pore. These channels include voltage-dependent sodium, potassium,

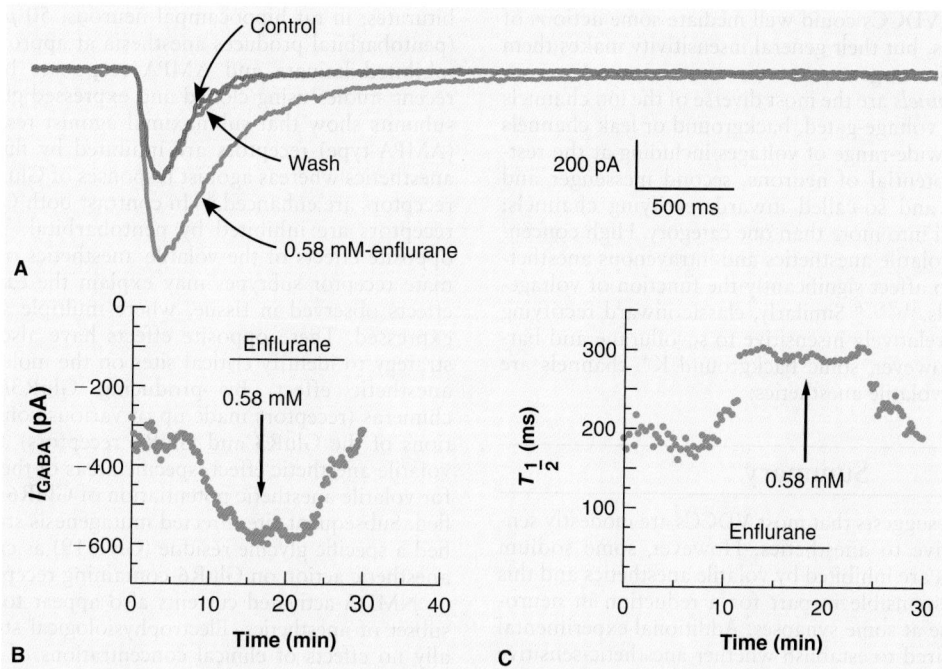

FIGURE 5-3. Enflurane potentiates the ability of GABA (γ-aminobutyric acid) to activate a chloride current in cultured rat hippocampal cells. This potentiation is rapidly reversed by removal of enflurane (wash; **A**). Enflurane increases both the amplitude of the current (**B**) and the time ($\tau_{1/2}$) it takes for the current to decay (**C**). (Reproduced with permission from Jones MV, Brooks PA, Harrison L: Enhancement of γ-aminobutyric acid-activated Cl⁻ currents in cultured rat hippocampal neurones by three volatile anaesthetics. J Physiol 449:289, 1992.)

and calcium channels, all of which share significant structural homologies. Voltage-dependent sodium and potassium channels are largely involved in generating and shaping action potentials. The effects of anesthetics on these channels have been extensively studied by Haydon and Urban[61] in the squid giant axon. These studies show that these invertebrate sodium channels and potassium channels are remarkably insensitive to volatile anesthetics. For example, 50% inhibition of the peak sodium channel current required halothane concentrations 8 times those required to produce anesthesia. The delayed rectifier potassium channel was even less sensitive, requiring halothane concentrations more than 20 times those required to produce anesthesia. Similar results have been obtained in a mammalian cell line (GH₃ pituitary cells) where both sodium and potassium currents were inhibited by halothane only at concentrations greater than 5 times those required to produce anesthesia.[62] However, a number of recent studies with volatile anesthetics have challenged the notion that voltage-dependent sodium channels are insensitive to anesthetics. Rehberg and colleagues[63] expressed rat brain IIA sodium channels in a mammalian cell line, and showed that clinically relevant concentrations of a variety of inhalational anesthetics suppressed voltage-elicited sodium currents. Ratnakumari and Hemmings[64] showed that sodium flux mediated by rat brain sodium channels was significantly inhibited by clinical concentrations of halothane. Shiraishi and Harris[65] documented the effects of isoflurane on a variety of sodium channel subtypes and found that several but not all subtypes are sensitive to clinical concentrations. Finally, as previously described, in a rat brainstem neuron, Wu and colleagues[41] found that a small inhibition of sodium currents by isoflurane resulted in a large inhibition of synaptic activity. Thus, sodium channel activity not only appears to be inhibited by volatile anesthetics, but this inhibition results in a significant reduction in synaptic

function, at least at some mammalian synapses. Intravenous anesthetics have also been shown to inhibit sodium channels, but the concentrations for this effect are supra-clinical.[66,67]

Voltage-dependent calcium channels (VDCCs) serve to couple electrical activity to specific cellular functions. In the nervous system, VDCCs located at presynaptic terminals respond to action potentials by opening. This allows calcium to enter the cell, activating calcium-dependent secretion of neurotransmitter into the synaptic cleft. At least six types of calcium channels (designated L, N, P, Q, R, and T) have been identified on the basis of electrophysiological properties and a larger number based on amino acid sequence similarities. N-, P-, Q-, and R-type channels, as well as some of the untitled channels, are preferentially expressed in the nervous system and are thought to play a major role in synaptic transmission. L-type calcium channels, although expressed in brain, have been best studied in their role in excitation–contraction coupling in cardiac, skeletal, and smooth muscle and are thought to be less important in synaptic transmission. The effects of anesthetics on L- and T-type currents have been well characterized,[62,68,69] and there are some reports concerning the effects of anesthetics on N- and P-type currents.[70–72] As a general rule, these studies have shown that volatile anesthetics inhibit VDCCs (50% reduction in current) at concentrations 2 to 5 times those required to produce anesthesia in humans, with less than a 20% inhibition of calcium current at clinical concentrations of anesthetics. However, some studies have found VDCCs that are extremely sensitive to anesthetics. Takenoshita and Steinbach[73] reported a T-type calcium current in dorsal root ganglion neurons that was inhibited by subanesthetic concentrations of halothane. Additionally, ffrench-Mullen and colleagues[74] have reported a VDCC of unspecified type in guinea pig hippocampus that is inhibited by pentobarbital at concentrations identical to those required to produce anesthesia. Thus, VDCCs could well mediate some actions of general anesthetics, but their general insensitivity makes them unlikely to be major targets.

Potassium channels are the most diverse of the ion channels types and include voltage-gated, background or leak channels that open over a wide-range of voltages including at the resting membrane potential of neurons, second messenger and ligand-activated, and so-called inward rectifying channels; some channels fall into more than one category. High concentrations of both volatile anesthetics and intravenous anesthetics are required to affect significantly the function of voltage-gated K$^+$ channels.[61,75,76] Similarly, classic inward rectifying K$^+$ channels are relatively insensitive to sevoflurane and barbiturates.[77–79] However, some background K$^+$ channels are quite sensitive to volatile anesthetics.

Summary

8 Existing evidence suggests that most VDCCs are modestly sensitive or insensitive to anesthetics. However, some sodium channels subtypes are inhibited by volatile anesthetics and this effect may be responsible in part for a reduction in neurotransmitter release at some synapses. Additional experimental data will be required to establish whether anesthetic-sensitive VDCCs are localized to specific synapses at which anesthetics have been shown to inhibit neurotransmitter release.

Anesthetic Effects on Ligand-Gated Ion Channels

Fast excitatory and inhibitory neurotransmission is mediated by the actions of ligand-gated ion channels. Synaptically released glutamate or GABA diffuse across the synaptic cleft and bind to channel proteins that open as a consequence of neurotransmitter release. The channel proteins that bind GABA (GABA$_A$ receptors) are members of a superfamily of structurally related ligand-gated ion channel proteins that include nicotinic acetylcholine receptors, glycine receptors, and 5-HT$_3$ receptors. Based on the structure of the nicotinic acetylcholine receptor, each ligand-gated channel is thought to be composed of five nonidentical subunits. The glutamate receptors also comprise a family, each receptor thought to be a tetrameric protein composed of structurally related subunits. The ligand-gated ion channels provide a logical target for anesthetic action because selective effects on these channels could inhibit fast excitatory synaptic transmission and/or facilitate fast inhibitory synaptic transmission. The effects of anesthetic agents on ligand-gated ion channels are thoroughly cataloged in a review by Krasowski and Harrison.[59] The following section provides a brief summary of this large body of work.

Glutamate-Activated Ion Channels

Glutamate-activated ion channels have been classified, based on selective agonists, into three categories: AMPA receptors, kainate receptors, and NMDA receptors. AMPA and kainate receptors are relatively nonselective monovalent cation channels involved in fast excitatory synaptic transmission, whereas NMDA channels conduct not only Na$^+$ and K$^+$ but also Ca^{++} and are involved in long-term modulation of synaptic responses (long-term potentiation). Studies from the early 1980s in mouse and rat brain preparations showed that AMPA- and kainate-activated currents are insensitive to clinical concentrations of halothane,[80] enflurane,[81] and the neurosteroid allopregnanolone.[82] In contrast, kainate- and AMPA-activated currents were shown to be sensitive to barbiturates; in rat hippocampal neurons, 50 μM pentobarbital (pentobarbital produces anesthesia at approximately 50 μM) inhibited kainate and AMPA responses by 50%.[82] More recent studies using cloned and expressed glutamate receptor subunits show that submaximal agonist responses of GluR3 (AMPA-type) receptors are inhibited by fluorinated volatile anesthetics whereas agonist responses of GluR6 (kainate-type) receptors are enhanced.[83] In contrast both GluR3 and GluR6 receptors are inhibited by pentobarbital. The directionally opposite effects of the volatile anesthetics on different glutamate receptor subtypes may explain the earlier inconclusive effects observed in tissue, where multiple subunit types are expressed. These opposite effects have also been used as a strategy to identify critical sites on the molecules involved in anesthetic effect. By producing GluR3/GluR6 receptor chimeras (receptors made up of various combinations of sections of the GluR3 and GluR6 receptors) and screening for volatile anesthetic effect, specific areas of the protein required for volatile anesthetic potentiation of GluR6 have been identified. Subsequent site-directed mutagenesis studies have identified a specific glycine residue (Gly-819) as critical for volatile anesthetic action on GluR6-containing receptors.[84]

NMDA-activated currents also appear to be sensitive to a subset of anesthetics. Electrophysiological studies show virtually no effects of clinical concentrations of volatile anesthetics,[80,81] neurosteroids, or barbiturates[82] on NMDA-activated currents. It should be noted that there is some evidence from flux studies that volatile anesthetics may inhibit NMDA-activated channels. A study in rat brain microvesicles showed that anesthetic concentrations (0.2 to 0.3 mM) of halothane and enflurane inhibited NMDA-activated calcium flux by 50%.[85] In contrast, ketamine is a potent and selective inhibitor of NMDA-activated currents. Ketamine stereoselectively inhibits NMDA currents by binding to the phencyclidine site on the NMDA receptor protein.[86–88] The anesthetic effects of ketamine in intact animals show the same stereoselectivity as that observed in vitro,[89] suggesting that the NMDA receptor may be the principal molecular target for the anesthetic actions of ketamine. Two other recent findings suggest that NMDA receptors may be an important target for nitrous oxide and xenon. These studies show that N$_2$O[90,91] and xenon[92] are potent and selective inhibitors of NMDA-activated currents. This is illustrated in Figure 5-4, showing that N$_2$O inhibits NMDA-elicited, but not GABA-elicited, currents in hippocampal neurons.

GABA-Activated Ion Channels

GABA is the most important inhibitory neurotransmitter in the mammalian CNS. GABA-activated ion channels (GABA$_A$ receptors) mediate the postsynaptic response to synaptically released GABA by selectively allowing chloride ions to enter and thereby hyperpolarizing neurons. GABA$_A$ receptors are multi-subunit proteins consisting of various combinations of α, β, δ and ε subunits, and there are many subtypes of each of these subunits. The function of GABA$_A$ receptors is modulated by a wide variety of pharmacologic agents including convulsants, anticonvulsants, sedatives, anxiolytics, and anesthetics.[93] The effects of these various drugs on GABA$_A$ receptor function varies across brain regions and cell types. The following section briefly reviews the effects of anesthetics on GABA$_A$ receptor function.

Barbiturates, anesthetic steroids, benzodiazepines, propofol, etomidate, and the volatile anesthetics all modulate GABA$_A$ receptor function.[60,93–96] These drugs produce three kinds of effects on the electrophysiological behavior of the GABA$_A$ receptor channels: potentiation, direct gating, and inhibition. *Potentiation* refers to the ability of anesthetics to increase markedly the current elicited by low concentrations of GABA, but to produce

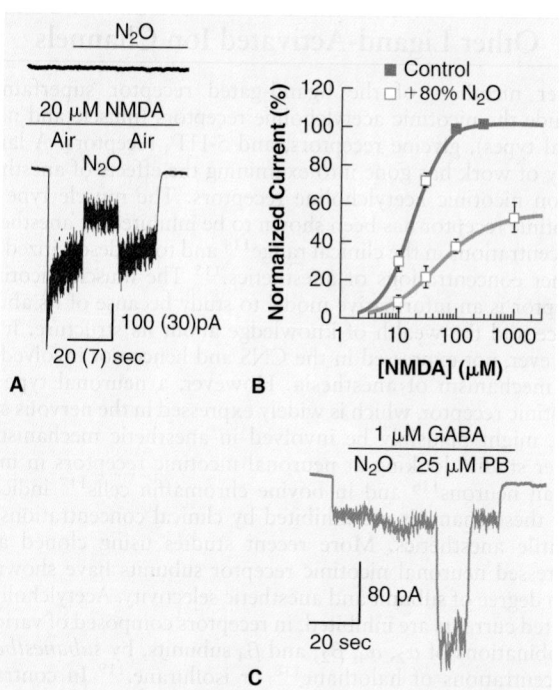

FIGURE 5-4. Nitrous oxide inhibits NMDA-elicited, but not GABA-elicited, currents in rat hippocampal neurons. **A:** Eighty percent N_2O has no effect on holding current (upper trace), but inhibits the current elicited by NMDA. **B:** N_2O causes a rightward and downward shift of the NMDA concentration–response curve, indicating a mixed competitive/noncompetitive antagonism. **C:** Eighty percent N_2O has little effect on GABA-elicited currents. In contrast, an equipotent anesthetic concentration of pentobarbital markedly enhances the GABA-elicited current. (Reproduced with permission from Jevtovic-Todorovic V, Todorovic SM, Mennerick S *et al*: Nitrous oxide (laughing gas) is an NMDA antagonist, neuroprotectant, and neurotoxin. Nat Med 4:460, 1998.)

no increase in the current elicited by a maximally effective concentration of GABA. Potentiation is illustrated in Figure 5-5, showing the effects of halothane on currents elicited by a range of GABA concentrations in dissociated cortical neurons. Anesthetic potentiation of $GABA_A$ currents generally occurs at concentrations of anesthetics within the clinical range. *Direct gating* refers to the ability of anesthetics to activate $GABA_A$ channels in the absence of GABA. Generally, direct gating of $GABA_A$ currents occurs at anesthetic concentrations higher than those used clinically, but the concentration–response curves for potentiation and for direct gating can overlap. It is not known whether direct gating of $GABA_A$ channels is either required for or contributes to the effects of anesthetics on GABA-mediated inhibitory synaptic transmission in vivo. In the case of anesthetic steroids, strong evidence indicates that potentiation, rather than direct gating of $GABA_A$ currents, is required for producing anesthesia.[97] Anesthetics can also inhibit GABA-activated currents. *Inhibition* refers to the ability of anesthetics to prevent GABA from initiating current flow through $GABA_A$ channels, and has generally been observed at high concentrations of both GABA and anesthetic.[98,99] Inhibition of $GABA_A$ channels may help to explain why volatile anesthetics have, in some cases, been observed to inhibit rather than facilitate inhibitory synaptic transmission.[34]

Effects of anesthetics have also been observed on the function of single $GABA_A$ channels. These studies show that barbiturates,[94] propofol,[96] and volatile anesthetics[100] do not alter the conductance (rate at which ions traverse the open channel) of the channel, but that they increase the frequency with which the channel opens and/or the average length of time that the channel remains open. Collectively, the whole cell and single channel data are most consistent with the idea that clinical concentrations of anesthetics produce a change in the conformation of $GABA_A$ receptors that increases the affinity of the receptor for GABA. This is consistent with the ability of anesthetics to increase the duration of inhibitory postsynaptic potentials, since higher affinity binding of GABA would slow the dissociation of GABA from postsynaptic $GABA_A$ channels. It would not be expected that anesthetics would increase the peak amplitude of a GABAergic inhibitory postsynaptic potential since synaptically

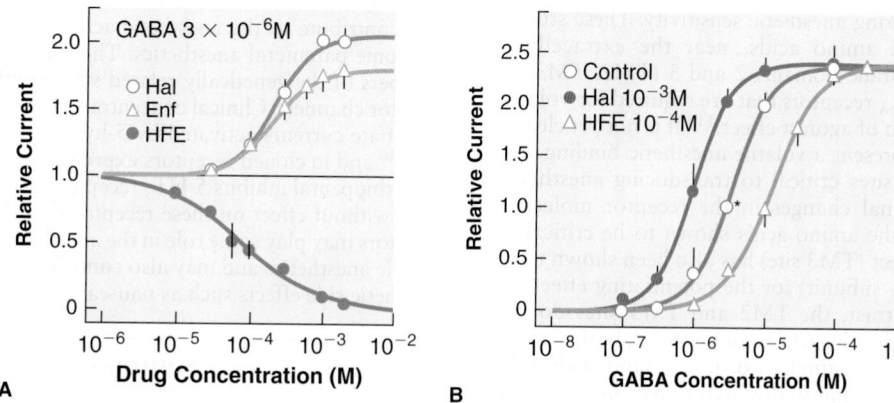

FIGURE 5-5. The effects of halothane (Hal), enflurane (Enf), and fluorothyl (HFE) on GABA-activated chloride currents in dissociated rat CNS neurons. **A:** Clinical concentrations of halothane and enflurane potentiate the ability of GABA to elicit a chloride current. The convulsant fluorothyl antagonizes the effects of GABA (γ-aminobutyric acid). **B:** GABA causes a concentration-dependent activation of a chloride current. Halothane shifts the GABA concentration–response curve to the left (increases the apparent affinity of the channel for GABA), whereas fluorothyl shifts the curve to the right (decreases the apparent affinity of the channel for GABA). (Reproduced with permission from Wakamori M, Ikemoto Y, Akaike N: Effects of two volatile anesthetics and a volatile convulsant on the excitatory and inhibitory amino acid responses in dissociated CNS neurons of the rat. J Neurophysiol 66:2014, 1991.)

released GABA probably reaches very high concentrations in the synapse. Higher concentrations of anesthetics can produce additional effects, either directly activating or inhibiting GABA$_A$ channels. Consistent with these ideas, a study by Banks and Pearce[101] showed that isoflurane and enflurane simultaneously increased the duration and decreased the amplitude of GABAergic inhibitory postsynaptic currents in hippocampal slices.

Despite the similar effects of many anesthetics on GABA$_A$ receptor function, there is significant evidence that the various anesthetics do not act by binding to a single common binding site on the channel protein. First, even anesthetics that directly activate the channel probably do not bind to the GABA binding site. This is most clearly demonstrated by molecular biologic studies in which the GABA binding site is eliminated from the channel protein but pentobarbital can still activate the channel.[102] Direct radioligand binding studies have demonstrated that benzodiazepines bind to the GABA$_A$ receptor at nanomolar concentrations and that other anesthetics can modulate binding but do not bind directly to the benzodiazepine site.[93,103] A series of more complex studies examining the interactions between barbiturates, anesthetic steroids, and benzodiazepines indicates that these three classes of drugs cannot be acting at the same sites.[93] The actions of anesthetics on GABA$_A$ receptors are further complicated by the observation that steroid anesthetics can produce different effects on GABA$_A$ receptors in different brain regions.[104] This suggests the possibility that the specific subunit composition of a GABA$_A$ receptor may encode pharmacologic selectivity. This is well illustrated by benzodiazepine sensitivity, which requires the presence of the $\gamma2$ subunit subtype.[105] Similarly, sensitivity to etomidate has been shown to require the presence of a $\beta2$ or $\beta3$ subunit.[106] More recently, it has been shown that the presence of a δ or ε subunit in a GABA$_A$ receptor confers insensitivity to the potentiating effects of some anesthetics.[107,108]

Interestingly, GABA$_A$ receptors composed of ρ-type subunits (referred to as *GABA$_C$ receptors*) have been shown to be inhibited rather than potentiated by volatile anesthetics.[109] This property has been exploited, using molecular biologic techniques, by constructing chimeric receptors composed of part of the ρ-receptor coupled to part of an α, β, or glycine receptor subunit. By screening these chimeras for anesthetic sensitivity, regions of the α, β, and glycine subunits responsible for anesthetic sensitivity have been identified. Based on the results of these chimeric studies, site-directed mutagenesis studies were performed to identify the specific amino acids responsible for conferring anesthetic sensitivity. These studies revealed two critical amino acids, near the extracellular regions of transmembrane domains 2 and 3 (TM2, TM3) of the glycine and GABA$_A$ receptors that are required for volatile anesthetic potentiation of agonist effect.[110] It is not yet clear if these amino acids represent a volatile anesthetic binding site, or whether they are sites critical to transducing anesthetic-induced conformational changes in the receptor molecule. Interestingly, one of the amino acids shown to be critical to volatile anesthetic effect (TM3 site) has also been shown to be required (in the β_2/β_3 subunit) for the potentiating effects of etomidate.[111] In contrast, the TM2 and TM3 sites do not appear to be required for the actions of propofol, barbiturates, or neurosteroids.[112] Interestingly, a distinct amino acid in the TM3 region of the β_1 subunit of the GABA$_A$ receptor has been shown to selectively modulate the ability of propofol to potentiate GABA agonist effects.[112] Recent evidence also indicates that neurosteroids actions on GABA$_A$ receptors occur via interactions with specific sites within the transmembrane spanning regions of the α_1 and β_2 subunits that are distinct from those with which benzodiazepines and pentobarbital act.[113] Collectively, these molecular biologic data provide strong evidence that there are multiple unique binding sites for anesthetics on the GABA$_A$ receptor protein.

Other Ligand-Activated Ion Channels

Other members of the ligand-gated receptor superfamily include the nicotinic acetylcholine receptors (muscle and neuronal types), glycine receptors, and 5-HT$_3$ receptors. A large body of work has gone into examining the effects of anesthetics on nicotinic acetylcholine receptors. The muscle type of nicotinic receptor has been shown to be inhibited by anesthetic concentrations in the clinical range[114] and to be desensitized by higher concentrations of anesthetics.[115] The muscle nicotinic receptor is an informative model to study because of its abundance and the wealth of knowledge about its structure. It is, however, not expressed in the CNS and hence not involved in the mechanism of anesthesia. However, a neuronal type of nicotinic receptor, which is widely expressed in the nervous system, might plausibly be involved in anesthetic mechanisms. Older studies looking at neuronal nicotinic receptors in molluscan neurons[116] and in bovine chromaffin cells[117] indicate that these channels are inhibited by clinical concentrations of volatile anesthetics. More recent studies using cloned and expressed neuronal nicotinic receptor subunits have shown a high degree of subunit and anesthetic selectivity. Acetylcholine-elicited currents are inhibited, in receptors composed of various combinations of α_2, α_4, β_2, and β_4 subunits, by *subanesthetic* concentrations of halothane[118] or isoflurane.[119] In contrast, these receptors are relatively insensitive to propofol. Most interestingly, receptors composed of α_7 subunits are completely insensitive to both isoflurane and propofol.[119,120] Subsequent pharmacologic experiments using selective inhibitors of neuronal nicotinic receptors led to the conclusion that these receptors are unlikely to have a major role in immobilization by volatile anesthetics.[121,122] However, they might play a role in the amnestic or hypnotic effects of volatile anesthetics.[123]

Glycine is an important inhibitory neurotransmitter, particularly in the spinal cord and brainstem. The glycine receptor is a member of the ligand-activated channel superfamily that, like the GABA$_A$ receptor, is a chloride-selective ion channel. A large number of studies have shown that clinical concentrations of volatile anesthetics potentiate glycine-activated currents in intact neurons[80] and in cloned glycine receptors expressed in oocytes.[124,125] The volatile anesthetics appear to produce their potentiating effect by increasing the affinity of the receptor for glycine.[125] Propofol,[96] alphaxalone, and pentobarbital also potentiate glycine-activated currents, whereas etomidate and ketamine do not.[124] Potentiation of glycine receptor function may contribute to the anesthetic action of volatile anesthetics and some parenteral anesthetics. The 5-HT$_3$ receptors are also members of the genetically related superfamily of ligand-gated receptor channels. Clinical concentrations of volatile anesthetics potentiate currents activated by 5-hydroxytryptamine in intact cells[126] and in cloned receptors expressed in oocytes.[127] In contrast, thiopental inhibits 5-HT$_3$ receptor currents[126] and propofol is without effect on these receptor channels.[127] The 5-HT$_3$ receptors may play some role in the anesthetic state produced by volatile anesthetics and may also contribute to some unpleasant anesthetic side effects such as nausea and vomiting.

Summary

Several ligand-gated ion channels are modulated by clinical concentrations of anesthetics. Ketamine, N$_2$O, and xenon inhibit NMDA-type glutamate receptors, and this effect may play a major role in their mechanism of action. A large body of evidence shows that clinical concentrations of many anesthetics potentiate GABA-activated currents in the CNS. This suggests that GABA$_A$ receptors are a probable molecular target of anesthetics. Other members of the ligand-activated ion channel family, including glycine receptors, neuronal nicotinic receptors, and 5-HT$_3$ receptors, are also affected by clinical concentrations of anesthetics and remain plausible anesthetic targets.

Anesthetic Effects on Background Potassium Ion Channels

Certain potassium channels called *background* or *leak channels* are activated by both volatile and gaseous anesthetics.[128] Background or leak channels are so named because they tend to be open at all voltages including the resting membrane potential of neurons, producing a "leak current." Leak currents can significantly regulate the excitability of neurons in which they are expressed. Anesthetic activation of a leak channel was first observed in a ganglion of the pond snail, *Lymnea stagnalis*. [129] Clinical concentrations of halothane activated this channel called I$_{K(AN)}$, resulting in silencing of the spontaneous bursting of these neurons (Fig. 5-6A). A similar anesthetic-activated background potassium channel was subsequently found by Winegar and Yost[130] in the marine mollusk *Aplysia*. The importance of volatile anesthetic activation of these invertebrate potassium channels has now become apparent with the discovery of a large family of background potassium channels in mammals. These mammalian potassium channels have a unique structure with two pore-forming domains in tandem plus four transmembrane segments (2P/4TM; Fig. 5-6C).[131] Patel et al[132] have studied the effects of volatile anesthetics on several members of the mammalian 2P/4TM family. They have shown that TREK-1 channels are activated by clinical concentrations of chloroform, diethyl ether, halothane, and isoflurane (Fig. 5-6B). In contrast, closely related TRAAK channels are insensitive to all the volatile anesthetics, and TASK channels are activated by halothane and isoflurane, inhibited by diethyl ether, and unaffected by chloroform. These authors went on to show that the C-terminal regions of TASK and TREK-1 contain amino acids essential for anesthetic action.[132] More recently, TREK-1 but not TASK was found to be activated by clinical concentrations of the gaseous anesthetics: xenon, nitrous oxide, and cyclopropane.[133] Thus, activation of background K$^+$ channels in mammalian vertebrates could be an important and general mechanism through which inhalational and gaseous anesthetics regulate neuronal resting membrane potential and thereby excitability. Indeed, genetic evidence argues for a role of these channels in producing anesthesia (see later discussion).

Summary

Recent evidence suggests that members of the 2P/4TM family of background potassium channels may be important in producing some components of the anesthetic state.

WHAT IS THE CHEMICAL NATURE OF ANESTHETIC TARGET SITES?

The Meyer-Overton Rule

More than 100 years ago, Meyer[134] and Overton[135] independently observed that the potency of gases as anesthetics was strongly correlated with their solubility in olive oil (Fig. 5-7).

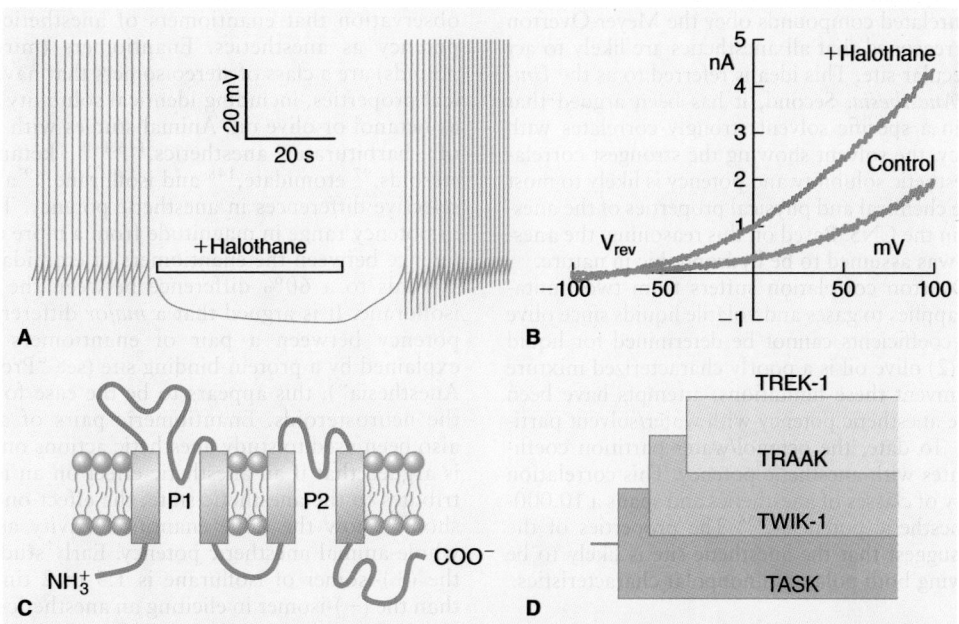

FIGURE 5-6. Volatile anesthetics activate background K$^+$ channels. **A:** Halothane reversibly hyperpolarizes a pacemaker neuron from *Lymnaea stagnalis* (the pond snail) by activating I$_{Kan}$. **B:** Halothane (300 μM) activates human recombinant TREK-1 channels expressed in COS cells. The figure shows current–voltage relationships with reversal potential (V_{rev}) of –88 mV, indicative of a K$^+$ channel. **C:** Predicted structure of a typical subunit of the mammalian background K$^+$ channels. Note the four transmembrane spanning segments (in black) and the two pore-forming domains (P1 and P2). Some but not all of these 2P/4TM K$^+$ channels are activated by volatile anesthetics. **D:** Phylogenetic tree for the 2P/4TM family. (Reproduced with permission from Franks NP, Lieb WR: Background K$^+$ channels: An important target for anesthetics? Nat Neurosci 2:395, 1999.)

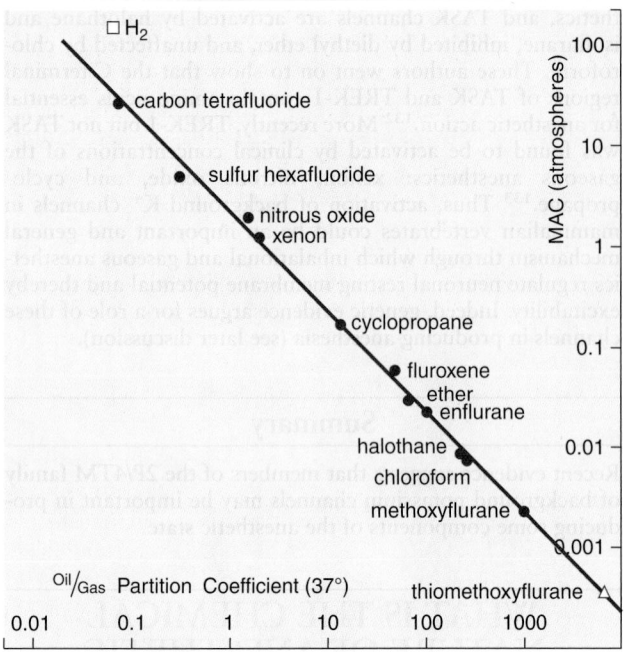

FIGURE 5-7. The Meyer-Overton rule. There is a linear relationship (on a log–log scale) between the oil/gas partition coefficient and the anesthetic potency (minimum alveolar concentration, MAC) of a number of gases. The correlation between lipid solubility and MAC extends over a 70,000-fold difference in anesthetic potency. (Reproduced with permission from Tanfuji Y, Eger EI, Terrell RC: Some characteristics of an exceptionally potent inhaled anesthetic: thiomethoxyflurane. Anesth Analg 56:387, 1977.)

This observation has significantly influenced thinking about anesthetic mechanisms in two ways. First, since a wide variety of structurally unrelated compounds obey the Meyer-Overton rule, it has been reasoned that all anesthetics are likely to act at the same molecular site. This idea is referred to as the *Unitary Theory of Anesthesia*. Second, it has been argued that since solubility in a specific solvent strongly correlates with anesthetic potency, the solvent showing the strongest correlation between anesthetic solubility and potency is likely to most closely mimic the chemical and physical properties of the anesthetic target site in the CNS. Based on this reasoning, the anesthetic target site was assumed to be hydrophobic in nature.

The Meyer-Overton correlation suffers from two limitations: (1) it only applies to gases and volatile liquids since olive oil/gas partition coefficients cannot be determined for liquid anesthetics, and (2) olive oil is a poorly characterized mixture of oils. To circumvent these limitations, attempts have been made to correlate anesthetic potency with water/solvent partition coefficients. To date, the octanol/water partition coefficient best correlates with anesthetic potency. This correlation holds for a variety of classes of anesthetics and spans a 10,000-fold range of anesthetic potencies.[136] The properties of the solvent octanol suggest that the anesthetic site is likely to be amphipathic, having both polar and nonpolar characteristics.

Exceptions to the Meyer-Overton Rule

Halogenated compounds exist that are structurally similar to the inhaled anesthetics yet are convulsants rather than anesthetics.[137] There are also convulsant barbiturates[138] and neurosteroids.[139] One convulsant compound, fluorothyl (hexafluorodiethyl ether) has been shown to cause seizures in 50% of mice at 0.12 vol%, but to produce anesthesia at higher concentrations (EC$_{50}$ = 1.22 vol%).[140] The concentration of fluorothyl required to produce anesthesia is approximately predicted by the Meyer-Overton rule. In contrast, several polyhalogenated alkanes have been identified that are convulsants, but that do not produce anesthesia. Based on the olive oil/gas partition coefficients of these compounds, anesthesia should have been achieved within the range of concentrations studied.[141] The end point used to determine the anesthetic effect of these compounds was movement in response to a noxious stimulus (MAC). Interestingly, some of these polyhalogenated compounds do produce amnesia in animals.[142] These compounds are thus referred to as *nonimmobilizers* rather than as nonanesthetics. Several polyhalogenated alkanes have also been identified that anesthetize mice, but only at concentrations 10 times those predicted by their oil/gas partition coefficients[141]; these compounds are referred to as *transitional* compounds. The nonimmobilizers and transitional compounds have been proposed as a "litmus test" for the relevance of anesthetic effects observed in vitro to those observed in the whole animal.

In several homologous series of anesthetics, anesthetic potency increases with increasing chain length until a certain critical chain length is reached. Beyond this critical chain length, compounds are unable to produce anesthesia, even at the highest attainable concentrations. In the series of *n*-alkanols, for example, anesthetic potency increases from methanol through dodecanol; all longer alkanols are unable to produce anesthesia.[143] This phenomenon is referred to as the *cutoff effect*. Cutoff effects have been described for several homologous series of anesthetics including *n*-alkanes, *n*-alkanols, cycloalkanemethanols,[144] and perfluoroalkanes.[145] While the anesthetic potency in each of these homologous series of anesthetics shows a cutoff, a corresponding cutoff in octanol/water or oil/gas partition coefficients has not been demonstrated. Therefore, compounds above the cutoff represent a deviation from the Meyer-Overton rule.

A final deviation from the Meyer-Overton rule is the observation that enantiomers of anesthetics differ in their potency as anesthetics. Enantiomers (mirror-image compounds) are a class of stereoisomers that have identical physical properties, including identical solubility in solvents such as octanol or olive oil. Animal studies with the enantiomers of barbiturate anesthetics,[146,147] ketamine,[89] neurosteroids,[97] etomidate,[148] and isoflurane[149] all show enantioselective differences in anesthetic potency. These differences in potency range in magnitude from a more than tenfold difference between the enantiomers of etomidate or the neurosteroids to a 60% difference between the enantiomers of isoflurane. It is argued that a *major* difference in anesthetic potency between a pair of enantiomers could only be explained by a protein-binding site (see "Protein Theories of Anesthesia"); this appears to be the case for etomidate and the neurosteroids. Enantiomeric pairs of anesthetics have also been used to study anesthetic actions on ion channels. It is argued that if an anesthetic effect on an ion channel contributes to the anesthetic state, the effect on the ion channel should show the same enantioselectivity as is observed in whole-animal anesthetic potency. Early studies showed that the (+)-isomer of isoflurane is 1.5 to 2 times more potent than the (−)-isomer in eliciting an anesthetic-activated potassium current, in potentiating GABA$_A$ currents, and in inhibiting the current mediated by a neuronal nicotinic acetylcholine receptor.[99,116] In contrast, the stereoisomers of isoflurane are equipotent in their effects on a voltage-activated potassium current and in their effects on lipid phase-transition temperature.[116] Studies with the neurosteroids[97] and etomidate[148] show that these anesthetics exert enantioselective effects on GABA$_A$ currents that parallel the enantioselective effects observed for anesthetic potency.

The exceptions to the Meyer-Overton rule do not obviate the importance of the rule. They do, however, indicate that the properties of a solvent such as octanol describe some, but not all, of the properties of an anesthetic binding site. Compounds that deviate from the Meyer-Overton rule suggest that anesthetic target site(s) are also defined by other properties including size and shape.

In defining the molecular target(s) of anesthetic molecules one must be able to account both for the Meyer-Overton rule and for the well-defined exceptions to this rule. It has sometimes been suggested that a correct molecular mechanism of anesthesia should also be able to account for pressure reversal. *Pressure reversal* is a phenomenon whereby the concentration of a given anesthetic needed to produce anesthesia is greatly increased if the anesthetic is administered to an animal under hyperbaric conditions. The idea that pressure reversal is a useful tool for elucidating mechanisms of anesthesia is based on the assumption that pressure reverses the specific physicochemical actions of the anesthetic that are responsible for producing anesthesia; that is to say, pressure and anesthetics act on the same molecular targets. However, recent evidence suggests that pressure reverses anesthesia by producing excitation that physiologically counteracts anesthetic depression, rather than by acting as an anesthetic antagonist at the anesthetic site of action.[150] Therefore, in the following discussion of molecular targets of anesthesia, pressure reversal will not be further mentioned.

Lipid versus Protein Targets

Anesthetics might interact with several possible molecular targets to produce their effects on the *function* of ion channels and other proteins. Anesthetics might dissolve in the *lipid* bilayer, causing physicochemical changes in membrane structure that alter the ability of embedded membrane proteins to undergo conformational changes important for their function. Alternatively, anesthetics could bind directly to *proteins* (either ion channel proteins or modulatory proteins), thus either (1) interfering with binding of a ligand (e.g., a neurotransmitter, a substrate, a second messenger molecule) or (2) altering the ability of the protein to undergo conformational changes important for its function. The following section summarizes the arguments for and against lipid theories and protein theories of anesthesia.

Lipid Theories of Anesthesia

The elucidation of the Meyer-Overton rule suggested that anesthetics interact with a hydrophobic target. To investigators in the early part of the 20th century, the most logical hydrophobic target was a lipid. In its simplest incarnation, the lipid theory of anesthesia postulates that anesthetics dissolve in the lipid bilayers of biological membranes and produce anesthesia when they reach a critical concentration in the membrane. Consistent with this hypothesis, the membrane/gas partition coefficients of anesthetic gases in pure lipid bilayers correlate strongly with anesthetic potency.[151] Also, consistent with the lipid theories, various membrane perturbations are produced by general anesthetics; however, the magnitude of these changes produced by clinical concentrations of anesthetics are quite small and are thought to be very unlikely to disrupt nervous system function.[152] While some of the more sophisticated lipid theories can account for the cutoff effect and impotence of nonimmobilizers, no lipid theory can plausibly explain all anesthetic pharmacology. Thus, most investigators do not consider membranes/lipids as the most likely target of general anesthetics.

Protein Theories of Anesthesia

The Meyer-Overton rule could also be explained by the direct interaction of anesthetics with hydrophobic sites on proteins. Three types of hydrophobic sites on proteins might interact with anesthetics:

1. Hydrophobic amino acids comprise the core of water-soluble proteins. Anesthetics could bind in hydrophobic pockets that are fortuitously present in the protein core.
2. Hydrophobic amino acids also form the lining of binding sites for hydrophobic ligands. For example, there are hydrophobic pockets in which fatty acids tightly bind on proteins such as albumin and the low-molecular-weight fatty acid–binding proteins. Anesthetics could compete with endogenous ligands for binding to such sites on either water-soluble or membrane proteins.
3. Hydrophobic amino acids are major constituents of the α-helices, which form the membrane-spanning regions of membrane proteins; hydrophobic amino acid side chains form the protein surface that faces the membrane lipid. Anesthetic molecules could interact with the hydrophobic surface of these membrane proteins, disrupting normal lipid–protein interactions and possibly directly affecting protein conformation. This last possibility would involve the interaction of many anesthetic molecules with each membrane protein molecule and would probably be a nonselective interaction between anesthetic molecules and *all* membrane proteins.

Direct interactions of anesthetic molecules with proteins would not only satisfy the Meyer-Overton rule, but would also provide the simplest explanation for compounds that deviate from this rule. Any protein-binding site is likely to be defined by properties such as size and shape in addition to its solvent properties. Limitations in size and shape could reduce the binding affinity of compounds beyond the cutoff, thus explaining their lack of anesthetic effect. Enantioselectivity is also most easily explained by a direct binding of anesthetic molecules to defined sites on proteins; a protein-binding site of defined dimensions could readily distinguish between enantiomers on the basis of their different shape. Protein-binding sites for anesthetics could also explain the convulsant effects of some polyhalogenated alkanes. Different compounds binding (in slightly different ways) to the same binding pocket can produce different effects on protein conformation and hence on protein function. For example, there are three kinds of compounds that can bind at the benzodiazepine binding site on the $GABA_A$ channel: *agonists*, which potentiate GABA effects and produce sedation and anxiolysis; *inverse agonists*, which promote channel closure and produce convulsant effects; and *antagonists*, which produce no effect on their own but can competitively block the effects of agonists and inverse agonists. By analogy, polyhalogenated alkanes could be inverse agonists, binding at the same protein sites at which halogenated alkane anesthetics are agonists. The evidence for direct interactions between anesthetics and proteins is briefly reviewed in the following section.

Evidence for Anesthetic Binding to Proteins

A breakthrough in protein theories of anesthesia was the demonstration that a purified water-soluble protein, firefly luciferase, could be inhibited by general anesthetics. This provided the important proof-of-principle that anesthetics could bind to proteins in the absence of membranes. Numerous studies have extensively characterized anesthetic inhibition of firefly luciferase activity and have revealed the following[153,154]:

1. Anesthetics inhibit firefly luciferase activity at concentrations very similar to those required to produce clinical anesthesia.
2. The potency of anesthetics as inhibitors of firefly luciferase activity correlates strongly with their potency as anesthetics, in keeping with the Meyer-Overton rule.
3. Halothane inhibition of luciferase activity is competitive with respect to the substrate D-luciferin.
4. Inhibition of firefly luciferase activity shows a cutoff in anesthetic potency for both *n*-alkanes and *n*-alkanols.

Based on these studies it can be inferred that a wide variety of anesthetics can bind in the luciferin-binding pocket of firefly luciferase. The fact that anesthetic inhibition of luciferase activity is consistent with the Meyer-Overton rule, occurs at clinical anesthetic concentrations, and explains the cutoff effect suggests that the luciferin-binding pocket may have physical and chemical characteristics similar to those of a putative anesthetic binding site in the CNS.

More direct approaches to study anesthetic binding to proteins have included NMR spectroscopy and photoaffinity labeling. Based on early studies by Wishnia and Pinder,[155,156] it was suspected that anesthetics could bind to several fatty acid–binding proteins, including β-lactoglobulin and bovine serum albumin (BSA). ^{19}F-NMR spectroscopic studies confirmed[157] this, and demonstrated that isoflurane binds to approximately three saturable binding sites on BSA. Isoflurane binding is eliminated by coincubation with oleic acid, suggesting that isoflurane binds to the fatty acid–binding sites on albumin. Other anesthetics, including halothane, methoxyflurane, sevoflurane, and octanol, compete with isoflurane for binding to BSA.[158] The studies with BSA provide direct evidence that a variety of anesthetics can compete for binding to the same site on a protein. Using this BSA model, it was subsequently shown that anesthetic binding sites could be identified and characterized using a photoaffinity labeling technique. The anesthetic halothane contains a carbon–bromine bond. This bond can be broken by ultraviolet light generating a free radical. That free radical allows the anesthetic to permanently (covalently) label the anesthetic binding site. Eckenhoff and Shuman[159] used ^{14}C-labeled halothane to photoaffinity-label anesthetic binding sites on BSA, and obtained results virtually identical to those obtained using NMR spectroscopy. Eckenhoff[160] subsequently has identified the specific amino acids that are photoaffinity-labeled by [^{14}C]halothane. NMR and photoaffinity-labeling techniques have also been applied to several other proteins. For example, saturable binding of halothane to the luciferin-binding site on firefly luciferase has been directly confirmed using NMR and photoaffinity-labeling techniques.[161] Most recently, Husain and colleagues[162] have developed a general anesthetic that is an analog of octanol and functions as a photoaffinity label. This compound, 3-diazyrinyloctanol, binds to specific sites on the nicotinic acetylcholine receptor.

Although NMR and photoaffinity techniques can provide extensive information about anesthetic binding sites on proteins, they cannot reveal the details of the three-dimensional structure of these sites. X-Ray diffraction crystallography can provide this kind of three-dimensional detail and has been used to study anesthetic interactions with a small number of proteins. To date, it has been difficult to crystallize membrane proteins; thus, these studies have been limited to water-soluble proteins. Firefly luciferase has been crystallized in the presence and absence of the anesthetic bromoform. X-Ray diffraction studies of these crystals showed that the anesthetic does bind in the luciferin-binding pocket, as had been inferred from functional studies. Interestingly, two molecules of bromoform bind in the luciferin pocket—one that is likely to compete directly with luciferin for binding and one that is not.[163] The binding data with firefly luciferase is of particular interest because it demonstrates that anesthetics can bind to endogenous ligand binding sites and that this binding strongly correlates with anesthetic inhibition of protein function. The same group has also crystallized human serum albumin in the presence of either propofol or halothane. The x-ray crystallographic data demonstrate binding of both anesthetics to preformed pockets that had been shown previously to bind fatty acids.[164] Given that both of these anesthetics bind to serum albumin at clinical concentrations, these data give the best insight yet into the structure of an anesthetic binding pocket.

A recent approach to study anesthetic interactions with proteins has been to employ site-directed mutagenesis of candidate anesthetic targets, coupled with molecular modeling to make predictions about the location and structure of anesthetic binding sites. For example, Wick and colleagues[165] have used this approach to predict the location and structure of the alcohol binding site on GABA$_A$ and glycine receptors. Similarly, the likely neurosteroid binding sites for activation and potentiation of the GABA$_A$ receptor were found by extensive site-directed mutagenesis experiments.[113] A related approach has been to develop model proteins to define the structural requirements for an anesthetic binding site. Using this approach, Johansson et al[166] have shown that a four–α-helix bundle with a hydrophobic core can bind volatile anesthetics at concentrations (K_D) similar to those required to produce anesthesia.[166]

Summary

Unequivocal evidence from studies using water-soluble proteins demonstrates that anesthetics can bind to hydrophobic pockets on proteins. Functional and binding studies with firefly luciferase demonstrate that anesthetics can bind to a protein site at clinically relevant concentrations in a manner that can account for the Meyer-Overton rule and deviations from it. Evidence that direct anesthetic–protein binding interactions may be responsible for anesthetic effects on ion channels in the CNS remains indirect; stereoselectivity currently offers the strongest indirect argument.

Overall, current evidence strongly indicates protein rather than lipid as the molecular target for anesthetic action. While the long-standing controversy between lipid and protein theories of anesthesia may be behind us, numerous unanswered questions remain about the details of anesthetic–protein interactions, including:

1. What is the stoichiometry of anesthetic binding to a protein (i.e., Do many anesthetic molecules interact with a single protein molecule or only a few)?
2. Do anesthetics compete with endogenous ligands for binding to hydrophobic pockets on protein targets or do they bind to fortuitous cavities in the protein?
3. Do all anesthetics bind to the same pocket on a protein or are there multiple hydrophobic pockets for different anesthetics?
4. How many proteins have hydrophobic pockets in which anesthetics can bind at clinically used concentrations?

HOW ARE THE MOLECULAR EFFECTS OF ANESTHETICS LINKED TO ANESTHESIA IN THE INTACT ORGANISM?

The previous sections have described how anesthetics affect the function of a number of ion channels and signaling proteins, probably via direct anesthetic–protein interactions. It is unclear which, if any, of these effects of anesthetics on protein function are necessary and/or sufficient to produce anesthesia in an intact organism. A number of approaches have been employed to try to link anesthetic effects observed at a molecular level to anesthesia in intact animals. These approaches and their pitfalls are briefly explored in the following section.

Pharmacologic Approaches

An experimental paradigm frequently used to study anesthetic mechanisms is to administer a drug thought to act specifically at a putative anesthetic target (e.g., a receptor agonist or antagonist, an ion channel activator or antagonist), then determine whether the drug has either increased or decreased the animal's sensitivity to a given anesthetic. The underlying assumption is that if a change in anesthetic sensitivity is observed, then the anesthetic is likely to act via an action on the specific target of the administered drug. This is a largely flawed strategy that has nonetheless produced a huge literature. The drugs used to modulate anesthetic sensitivity usually have their own direct effects on CNS excitability and thus *indirectly* affect anesthetic requirements. For example, while α_2-adrenergic agonists decrease halothane MAC,[167] they are profound CNS depressants in their own right and produce anesthesia by mechanisms distinct from those used by volatile anesthetics. Thus, the "MAC-sparing" effects of α_2-agonists provide little insight into how halothane works. A more useful pharmacologic strategy would be to identify drugs that have no effect on CNS excitability but prevent the effects of given anesthetics. Currently, however, there are no such anesthetic antagonists. Development of specific antagonists for anesthetic agents would provide a major tool for linking anesthetic effects at the molecular level to anesthesia in the intact organism, and might also be of significant clinical utility.

An alternative pharmacologic approach is to develop "litmus tests" for the relevance of anesthetic effects observed in vitro. One such test takes advantage of compounds that are nonanesthetic despite the predictions of the Meyer-Overton rule. It is argued that "a site affected by these nonanesthetic compounds is unlikely to be relevant to the production of anesthesia."[141] A similar argument uses stereoselectivity as the discriminator and argues that a site that does not show the same stereoselectivity as that observed for whole animal anesthesia is unlikely to be relevant to the production of anesthesia.[168] Although these tests may be useful, they are very dependent on the assumption that anesthesia is produced via drug action at a *single* site. For example, a nonanesthetic might depress CNS excitability via its actions on an important anesthetic target site while simultaneously producing counterbalancing excitatory effects at a second site. In this case the "litmus test" would incorrectly eliminate the anesthetic site as irrelevant to whole-animal anesthesia. This example is quite plausible given the convulsant effects of many of the nonanesthetic polyhalogenated hydrocarbons. Another sort of litmus test is to selectively antagonize the putative anesthetic target so that this target is no longer functional. If anesthetic effects are mediated through this target, inactivation of the target by the antagonist should result in anesthetic resistance. Using this logic, the modest MAC-sparing effects of GABA$_A$ and glycine receptor antagonists were used to argue that both GABA$_A$ and glycine receptors mediate some but not all of the immobilizing effects of volatile anesthetics in rodents.[169,170] This same group used the lack of effect of neuronal nicotinic antagonists on isoflurane MAC to conclude that these receptors had no role in volatile anesthetic immobilization.[122] As with many pharmacologic results, the issues of specificity and efficacy of the antagonists prevent these experiments from being definitive. Nevertheless, these results are consistent with the findings

that volatile anesthetics affect the function of a large number of important neuronal proteins and no one target is likely to mediate all of the effects of these drugs.

Genetic Approaches

An alternative approach to study the relationship between anesthetic effects observed in vitro and whole-animal anesthesia is to alter the structure or abundance of putative anesthetic targets and determine how this affects whole-animal anesthetic sensitivity. Genetic techniques provide the most reliable and versatile methods for changing the structure or abundance of putative anesthetic targets. The first true genetic screen for mutants with altered general anesthetic sensitivity was performed in the nematode C. elegans by Phil Morgan and Margaret Sedensky.[171] They screened for altered sensitivity to supraclinical concentrations of halothane. High halothane concentrations were used because they are required to immobilize C. elegans. The first mutant isolated had a threefold reduction in its EC$_{50}$ for halothane. The mutation was genetically mapped and found to be a loss-of-function allele of the unc-79 gene, which encodes a large neuronal protein very similar in sequence to a human protein.[172] The cellular function of either the C. elegans or human protein is unknown. In the absence of anesthetics, unc-79 mutants have an interesting locomotion defect called *fainting*. Normal C. elegans worms crawl almost continuously whereas unc-79 mutants appear to faint where they spontaneously stop moving for extended periods of time. In testing other such mutants, Humphrey et al[172] and Morgan and Sedensky[173] found that, in general, "fainters" were hypersensitive to halothane. Subsequent extensive genetic screens and mapping of fainting mutants have led to a focus on a novel presumptive cation channel, NCA-1/NCA-2, that controls halothane sensitivity in both C. elegans and in the fruit fly Drosophila.[172] This remarkable conservation of the anesthetic hypersensitivity phenotype across such divergent species argues for a fundamental role of NCA-1/NCA-2 in the action of halothane.

Clinical concentrations of volatile anesthetics do not immobilize C. elegans, but they do produce behavioral effects including loss of coordinated movement.[174] Crowder and colleagues[174] have screened for mutants that are resistant to anesthetic-induced uncoordination and found that mutations in a set of genes encoding proteins regulating neurotransmitter release control anesthetic sensitivity. The gene with the largest effect encoded syntaxin 1A, a neuronal protein highly conserved from C. elegans to humans and essential for fusion of neurotransmitter vesicles with the presynaptic membrane.[175] Importantly, some syntaxin mutations produced hypersensitivity to volatile anesthetics while others conferred resistance. These allelic differences in anesthetic sensitivity could not be accounted for by effects on the process of transmitter release itself[56,175]; rather, the genetic data argued that syntaxin interacts with a protein critical for volatile anesthetic action, perhaps an anesthetic target. Recently, a highly evolutionarily conserved presynaptic protein called UNC-13 in C. elegans was implicated in this presynaptic volatile anesthetic mechanism.[176] UNC-13 is required for normal isoflurane sensitivity, unc-13 mutants are fully resistant to the effects of clinical concentration of isoflurane, and isoflurane prevents the normal synaptic localization of UNC-13. Whether UNC-13 is a direct target of volatile anesthetics is unknown. This same laboratory has also shown by mutant analysis that an NMDA glutamate receptor subunit is essential for nitrous oxide sensitivity in C. elegans[177] and that another glutamate receptor subunit is required for the effects of Xenon.[178]

In Drosophila, clinical concentrations of volatile anesthetics disrupt negative geotaxis behavior and response to a noxious light or heat stimulus.[179-181] Using one or more of these anesthetics effects, Krishnan and Nash[179] performed a forward genetic screen for halothane resistance. The results of this screen have led to a focus on the *Drosophila* homolog of *nca-1/2*. As previously discussed, mutants in the *Drosophila* homolog of *nca-1/2* are hypersensitive to halothane like the *C. elegans* mutants.[172] The synergy of both *Drosophila* and *C. elegans* genetics should lead to an understanding of how this channel controls volatile anesthetic sensitivity.

In mammals, the most powerful genetic model organism is mouse, where techniques have been developed to alter or delete any gene of interest. The GABA$_A$ receptor has been extensively studied using mouse genetic techniques.[182,183] The genes encoding for various subunits of the GABA$_A$ receptor have been mutated so that they are either nonfunctional (gene knockouts) or so that they have altered amino acids that might produce altered function (gene knockins). Knockouts of three α subunits of the GABA$_A$ receptor have been tested for their anesthetic sensitivity. Deletion of the $\alpha1$ subunit does not alter sensitivity of mice to the hypnotic effects of pentobarbital.[184] Similarly, $\alpha6$ subunit knockout mice are normally sensitive to halothane and enflurane.[185] However, $\alpha5$ knockout mice are resistant to learning impairment by etomidate.[186] Knockin mouse strains have been generated for several of the α-subunits, primarily for examining benzodiazepine action. The loss of various aspects of benzodiazepine action in these strains demonstrated that the $\alpha1$ subunit mediates the sedative and amnestic actions, and is partially required for its anticonvulsant properties. Similarly, the $\alpha2$ subunit has been shown to be essential for anxiolysis by diazepam, and $\alpha3$ and $\alpha5$ knockin strains are partially resistant to its myorelaxant effects. Finally, a mouse expressing a double mutated $\alpha1$ subunit, $\alpha1$(S270H, L277A), has recently been tested for its anesthetic sensitivity.[187,188] The $\alpha1$S270H mutation has been shown to block GABA potentiation by volatile anesthetics, but the mutation also increases native sensitivity to GABA, confounding interpretation of the data. Moreover, $\alpha1$S270H single-mutant mice are quite abnormal behaviorally and are prone to anesthetic-induced seizure activity.[189] Thus, a second mutation, L277A, was introduced into the $\alpha1$ subunit that compensated for the change in native gating properties. The $\alpha1$(S270H, L277A) mice are viable and behaviorally normal. These mice are mildly resistant to the ataxic effects of isoflurane and enflurane; however, the potency of the drugs in MAC and fear-conditioning assays (a measure of learning) are not altered by the double-mutant $\alpha1$ subunit.

In vitro electrophysiological experiments show that a specific $\beta3$ subunit point mutation, $\beta3$(N265M), blocks the action of etomidate and propofol on the GABA$_A$ receptor without greatly altering receptor function in the absence of drug.[111,190] A $\beta3$(N265M) knockin strain was generated and found to be insensitive to the immobilizing effects of etomidate, propofol, and pentobarbital.[191,192] However, the $\beta3$(N265M) mice are not completely resistant to the loss-of-righting reflex by these anesthetics, indicating that other targets mediate this behavioral effect. Interestingly, the respiratory depressant effects of etomidate and propofol are also blocked by the $\beta3$(N265M) mutation, but the cardiovascular and hypothermic actions of the drugs are not.[193] The $\beta3$(N265M) mice show a slightly reduced sensitivity to the immobilizing actions of volatile anesthetics, suggesting that the $\beta3$ subunit may play a minor role in immobilization, but the mutant has unaltered sensitivity to the amnestic effects of isoflurane.[194] A similar approach for the $\beta2$ subunit has shown that it is critical for the sedating but not anesthetic action of etomidate.[195,196] Finally, strains carrying a knockout mutation of the δ subunit of the GABA$_A$ receptor have a shorter duration of neurosteroid-induced loss-of-righting reflex whereas their sensitivity to other intravenous and volatile anesthetics is unchanged.[197] Thus, the δ subunit may play a relatively specific role in neurosteroid action.

The roles in anesthetic sensitivity of two of the background potassium channels have been tested in limited mouse genetic studies. A TREK-1 knockout mouse was found to be significantly resistant to multiple volatile anesthetics for MAC and loss-of-righting reflex endpoints.[198] The volatile anesthetic resistance of the TREK-1 knockout is substantial, particularly for halothane where MAC was increased by 48%. Importantly, the TREK-1 knockout mice have a normal sensitivity to pentobarbital, indicating specificity for volatile anesthetics consistent with previous electrophysiological data. Recently, Westphalen et al[199] of the Hemmings laboratory has used the TREK-1 knockout strain to test the hypothesis that TREK-1 mediates some of the presynaptic inhibitory effects of volatile anesthetics. Indeed, glutamate release from synaptosomes prepared from the TREK-1 knockout strain is significantly resistant to inhibition by halothane compared to release from wild type control synaptosomes. The role of TASK-2, another two-pore background potassium channel, has been similarly tested by measuring the MAC of a TASK-2 knockout mouse. However, unlike for TREK-1, the TASK-2 knockout has MAC values similar to wild type controls for desflurane, halothane, and isoflurane.[77] This result is somewhat surprising given that TASK-2 is strongly activated by halothane and isoflurane and may be explained by an overall reduced expression in the nervous system compared to TREK-1.[128]

Summary

Results from both invertebrate and vertebrate genetics indicate that multiple proteins control volatile anesthetic sensitivity. Some of these may be anesthetic targets and some not. Certain GABA$_A$ receptor subunits and the TREK-1 background potassium channel are very likely to be targets relevant to general anesthesia, but are probably not the only ones. The mammalian electrophysiological data and the genetic evidence in *C. elegans* both implicate the NMDA glutamate receptor as the primary target of nitrous oxide. Similarly, elegant electrophysiological and genetic experiments have shown that the GABA$_A$ receptor is the primary mediator for immobilization by etomidate, propofol, and pentobarbital.

CONCLUSIONS

In this chapter evidence has been reviewed concerning the anatomic, physiologic, and molecular loci of anesthetic action. It is clear that all anesthetic actions cannot be localized to a specific anatomic site in the CNS; indeed, some evidence suggests that different components of the anesthetic state may be mediated by actions at disparate anatomic sites. The actions of anesthetics also cannot be localized to a specific physiologic process. While there is consensus that anesthetics ultimately affect synaptic function as opposed to intrinsic neuronal excitability, the effects of anesthetics depend on the agent and synapse studied and can affect presynaptic and/or postsynaptic function. At a molecular level, volatile anesthetics show some selectivity, but still affect the function of multiple ion channels and synaptic proteins. The intravenous anesthetics, etomidate, propofol, and barbiturates, are more specific with the GABA$_A$ receptor as their major target. Although it is likely that these effects are mediated via direct protein–anesthetic interactions, it appears that there are numerous proteins that can directly interact with anesthetics. Genetic data plainly demonstrate that the unitary theory of anesthesia is not correct. No single mechanism is responsible for the effects of all general anesthetics, nor does a single mechanism account for all of the effects of a single anesthetic, at least where it has been examined. Figure 5-8 provides a simple model of the molecular

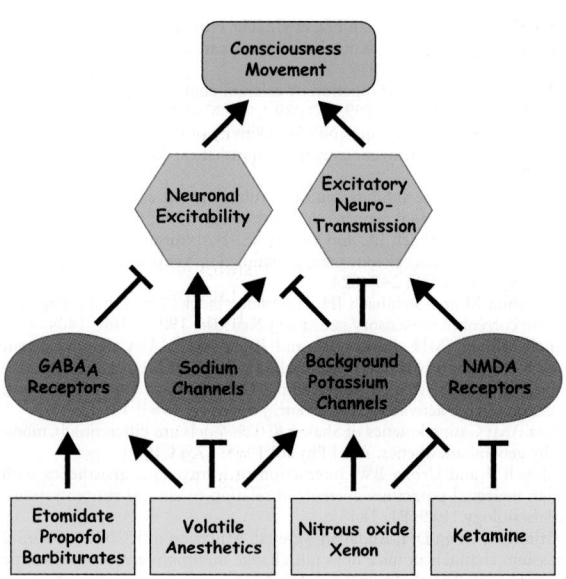

FIGURE 5-8. A multisite model for anesthesia. Anesthetics are grouped according to similarity of mechanism. Arrows indicate activation or potentiation and "T's" indicate inhibition or antagonism. The neurophysiological effects of general anesthetics are lumped into neuronal excitability (the probability of a neuron firing and propagating an axon potential) and excitatory neurotransmission (synaptic activity at excitatory synapses such as glutamatergic). Neuronal excitability in this context is the sum of both intrinsic and extrinsic factors (e.g., GABAergic inhibition).

SCIENTIFIC FOUNDATIONS OF ANESTHESIA

and cellular effects of general anesthetics. This cartoon is not meant to include all potential targets of general anesthetics. Rather, only those molecules with strong evidence for importance in anesthetic action from multiple different approaches are shown.

Although the precise molecular interactions responsible for producing anesthesia have not been fully elucidated, it has become clear that anesthetics do act via selective effects on specific molecular targets. The technologic revolutions in molecular biology, genetics, and cell physiology make it likely that the next decade will provide some answers to the century-old pharmacologic puzzle of the molecular mechanism of anesthesia.

ACKNOWLEDGMENT

The authors acknowledge generous ongoing funding support from National Institute of General Medical Sciences, Bethesda, Maryland, for ASE-P01 GM047969 and CMC-R01 GM59781.

References

1. Pace-Schott EF, Hobson JA: The neurobiology of sleep: genetics, cellular physiology and subcortical networks. Nat Rev Neurosci 591
2. Quasha AL, Eger EI, Tinker JH: Determination and applications of MAC. Anesthesiology 1980; 53: 315
3. White PF, Johnston RR, Eger II EI: Determination of anesthetic requirement in rats. Anesthesiology 1974; 40: 52
4. Franks NP, Lieb WR: Molecular and cellular mechanisms of general anesthesia. Nature 1994; 367: 607
5. Bowdle TA: Depth of anesthesia monitoring. Anesthesiol Clin 2006; 24: 793
6. Sackel DJ: Anesthesia awareness: an analysis of its incidence, the risk factors involved, and prevention. J Clin Anesth 2006; 18: 483
7. De Jong RH and Nace RA: Nerve impulse conduction and cutaneous receptor responses during general anesthesia. Anesthesiology 1967; 28: 851
8. Campbell JN, Raja SN, and Meyer RA: Halothane sensitizes cutaneous nociceptors in monkeys. J Neurophysiol 1984; 52: 762
9. Antognini JF and Kien ND: Potency (minimum alveolar anesthetic concentration) of isoflurane is independent of peripheral anesthetic effects. Anesth Analg 1995; 81: 69
10. Rampil IJ, Mason P, and Singh H: Anesthetic potency (MAC) is independent of forebrain structures in the rat. Anesthesiology 1993; 78: 707
11. Rampil IJ: Anesthetic potency is not altered after hypothermic spinal cord transection in rats. Anesthesiology 1994; 80: 606
12. Antognini JF and Schwartz K: Exaggerated anesthetic requirements in the preferentially anesthetized brain. Anesthesiology 1993; 79: 1244
13. Borges M and Antognini JF: Does the brain influence somatic responses to noxious stimuli during isoflurane anesthesia? Anesthesiology 1994; 81: 1511
14. Rampil IJ and King BS: Volatile anesthetics depress spinal motor neurons. Anesthesiology 1996; 85(1): 129
15. Antognini JF, Carstens E, and Buzin V: Isoflurane depresses motoneuron excitability by a direct spinal action: an F-wave study. Anesth Analg 1999; 88(3): 681
16. Zhou HH, Mehra M, and Leis AA: Spinal cord motoneuron excitability during isoflurane and nitrous oxide anesthesia. Anesthesiology 1997; 86: 302
17. Zorychta E, Esplin DW, and Capek R: Action of halothane on transmitter release in the spinal monosynaptic pathway. Fed Proc Am Soc Exp Biol 1975; 34: 2999
18. Fujiwara N, Higashi H, and Fujita S: Mechanism of halothane action on synaptic transmission in motoneurons of the newborn rat spinal cord *in vitro*. J Physiol 1988; 412: 155
19. Kullmann DM, Martin RL, and Redman SJ: Reduction by general anaesthetics of group Ia excitatory postsynaptic potentials and currents in the cat spinal cord. J Physiol (Lond) 1989; 412: 277
20. Takenoshita M and Takahashi T: Mechanisms of halothane action on synaptic transmission in motoneurons of the newborn rat spinal cord *in vitro*. Brain Res 1987; 402: 303
21. French JD, Verzeano M, and Magoun HW: A neural basis of the anesthetic state. Arch Neurol Psychiatry 1953; 69: 519
22. Angel A: Central neuronal pathways and the process of anaesthesia. Br J Anaesth 1993; 71: 148
23. Mori K and Winters WD: Neural background of sleep and anesthesia. Int Anesthesiol Clin 1975; 13: 67
24. Darbinjan TM, Golovchinsky VB, and Plehotinka SI: The effects of anesthetics on reticular and cortical activity. Anesthesiology 1971; 34: 219
25. Thornton C, Heneghan CP, James MF, et al.: Effects of halothane or enflurane with controlled ventilation on auditory evoked potentials. Br J Anaesth 1984; 56: 315
26. Feldman SM and Waller HJ: Dissociation of electrocortical activation and behavioral arousal. Nature 1962; 196: 1320
27. Nelson LE, Guo TZ, Lu J, et al.: The sedative component of anesthesia is mediated by GABA_A receptors in an endogenous sleep pathway. Nat Neurosci 2002; 5(10): 979
28. Frost EAM: Electroencephalography and evoked potential monitoring. In: Saidman LJ, Smith NT (eds): Monitoring in Anesthesia, p 203. Boston, Butterworth-Heinemann, 1993
29. Richards CD, Russel WJ, and Smaje JC: The action of ether and methoxyflurane on synaptic transmission in isolated preparations of the mammalian cortex. J Physiol (Lond) 1975; 248: 121
30. Nicoll RA: The effects of anaesthetics on synaptic excitation and inhibition in the olfactory bulb. J Physiol (Lond) 1972; 223: 803
31. Richards CD and White AN: The actions of volatile anaesthetics on synaptic transmission in the dentate gyrus. J Physiol (Lond) 1975; 252: 241
32. MacIver MB and Roth SH: Inhalational anaesthetics exhibit pathway-specific and differential actions on hippocampal synaptic responses in vitro. Br J Anaesth 1988; 60: 680
33. Gage PW and Robertson B: Prolongation of inhibitory postsynaptic currents by pentobarbitone, halothane and ketamine in CA1 pyramidal cells in rat hippocampus. Br J Pharmacol 1985; 85: 675
34. Fujiwara M, Higashi H, Nishi S, et al.: Changes in spontaneous firing patterns of rat hippocampal neurones induced by volatile anaesthetics. J Physiol (Lond) 1988; 402: 155

35. Franks NP and Lieb WR: Mechanisms of general anesthesia. Environ Health Perspect 1990; 87: 199

36. Madison DV and Nicoll RA: General anesthetics hyperpolarize neurons in the vertebrate central nervous system. Science 1982; 217: 1055

37. MacIver MB and Kendig JJ: Anesthetic effects on resting membrane potential are voltage-dependent and agent-specific. Anesthesiology 1991; 74: 83

38. Ries CR and Puil E: Mechanism of anesthesia revealed by shunting actions of isoflurane on thalamocortical neurons. J Neurophysiol 1999; 81: 1795

39. Larrabee MG and Posternak JM: Selective action of anesthetics on synapses and axons in mammalian sympathetic ganglia. J Neurophysiol 1952; 15: 91

40. Langmoen IA, Larsen M, and Berg-Johnsen J: Volatile anaesthetics: Cellular mechanisms of action. Eur J Anaesthesiol 1995; 12: 51

41. Wu XS, Sun JY, Evers AS, et al.: Isoflurane inhibits transmitter release and the presynaptic action potential. Anesthesiology 2004; 100: 663

42. Nicoll RA, Eccles JC, Oshima T, et al.: Prolongation of inhibitory postsynaptic potentials by barbiturates. Nature 1975; 258: 625

43. Proctor WR, Mynlieff M, and Dunwiddie TV: Facilitatory action of etomidate and pentobarbital on recurrent inhibition in rat hippocampal pyramidal neurons. J Neurosci 1986; 6: 3161

44. Collins GG: Effects of the anaesthetic 2,6-diisopropylphenol on synaptic transmission in the rat olfactory cortex slice. Br J Pharmacol 1988; 95: 939

45. Harrison NL, Vicini S, and Barker JL: A steroid anesthetic prolongs inhibitory postsynaptic currents in cultured rat hippocampal neurons. J Neurosci 1987; 7: 604

46. Yoshimura M, Higashi H, Fujita S, et al.: Selective depression of hippocampal inhibitory postsynaptic potentials and spontaneous firing by volatile anesthetics. Brain Res 1985; 340: 363

47. Mui P and Puil E: Isoflurane-induced impairment of synaptic transmission in hippocampal neurons. Exp Brain Res 1989; 75: 354

48. Perouansky M, Baranov D, Salman M, et al.: Effects of halothane on glutamate receptor-mediated excitatory post-synaptic currents: A patch-clamp study in adult mouse hippocampal slices. Anesthesiology 1995; 83: 109

49. Buggy DJ, Nicol B, Rowbotham DJ, et al.: Effects of intravenous anesthetic agents on glutamate release: a role for GABAA receptor-mediated inhibition. Br J Pharmacol 1988; 95: 939

50. Kendall TJ and Minchin MC: The effects of anaesthetics on the uptake and release of amino acid neurotransmitters in thalamic slices. Br J Pharmacol 1982; 75: 219

51. Larsen M, Haugstad TS, Berg-Johnsen J, et al.: Effect of isoflurane on release and uptake of gamma-aminobutyric acid from rat cortical synaptosomes. Br J Anaesth 1998; 80: 634

52. Collins GGS: Release of endogenous amino acid neurotransmitter candidates from rat olfactory cortex slices: possible regulatory mechanisms and the effects of pentobarbitone. Brain Res 1980; 190: 517

53. Murugaiah KD and Hemmings Jr. HC: Effects of intravenous general anesthetics on [3H]GABA release from rat cortical synaptosomes. Anesthesiology 1998; 89: 919

54. Mantz J, Lecharny JB, Laudenbach V, et al.: Anesthetics affect the uptake but not the depolarization-evoked release of GABA in rat striatal synaptosomes. Anesthesiology 1995; 82: 502

55. Westphalen RI and Hemmings Jr. HC: Selective depression by general anesthetics of glutamate versus GABA release from isolated cortical nerve terminals. J Pharmacol Exp Ther 2003; 304: 1188

56. Hawasli AH, Saifee O, Liu C, et al.: Resistance to volatile anesthetics by mutations enhancing excitatory neurotransmitter release in Caenorhabditis elegans. Genetics 2004; 168: 831

57. Richards CD and Smaje JC: Anaesthetics depress the sensitivity of cortical neurones to L-glutamate. Br J Pharmacol 1976; 58: 347

58. Smaje JC: General anaesthetics and the acetylcholine-sensitivity of cortical neurones. Br J Pharmacol 1976; 58: 359

59. Krasowski MD and Harrison NL: General anaesthetic actions on ligand-gated ion channels. Cell Mol Life Sci 1999; 55: 1278

60. Jones MV, Brooks PA, and Harrison NL: Enhancements of gamma-aminobutyric acid-activated Cl⁻ currents in cultured rat hippocampal neurones by three volatile anesthetics. J Physiol 1992; 449: 279

61. Haydon DA and Urban BW: The actions of some general anaesthetics on the potassium current of the squid giant axon. J Physiol 1986; 373: 311

62. Herrington J, Stern RC, Evers AS, et al.: Halothane inhibits two components of calcium current in clonal (GH₃) pituitary cells. J Neurosci 1991; 11(7): 2226

63. Rehberg B, Xiao YH, and Duch DS: Central nervous system sodium channels are significantly suppressed at clinical concentrations of volatile anesthetics. Anesthesiology 1996; 84: 1223

64. Ratnakumari L and Hemmings Jr. HC: Inhibition of presynaptic sodium channels by halothane. Anesthesiology 1998; 88: 1043

65. Shiraishi M and Harris RA: Effects of alcohols and anesthetics on recombinant voltage-gated Na+ channels. J Pharmacol Exp Ther 2004; 309: 987

66. Frenkel C, Weckbecker K, Wartenberg HC, et al.: Blocking effects of the anaesthetic etomidate on human brain sodium channels. Neurosci Lett 1998; 249: 131

67. Rehberg B and Duch DS: Suppression of central nervous system sodium channels by propofol. Anesthesiology 1999; 91(2): 512

68. Eskinder H, Rusch NJ, Supan FD, et al.: The effects of volatile anesthetics on L- and T-type calcium channel currents in canine cardiac Purkinje cells. Anesthesiology 1991; 74: 919

69. Terrar DA: Structure and function of calcium channels and the actions of anaesthetics. Br J Anaesth 1993; 71: 39

70. Hall AC, Lieb WR, and Franks NP: Insensitivity of P-type calcium channels to inhalational and intravenous general anesthetics. Anesthesiology 1994; 81: 117

71. Study RE: Isoflurane inhibits multiple voltage-gated calcium currents in hippocampal pyramidal neurons. Anesthesiology 1994; 81: 104

72. Gundersen CB, Umbach JA, and Swartz BE: Barbiturates depress currents through human brain calcium channels studied in Xenopus oocytes. J Pharmacol Exp Ther 1988; 247: 824

73. Takenoshita M and Steinbach JH: Halothane blocks low-voltage-activated calcium current in rat sensory neurons. J Neurosci 1991; 11(5): 1404

74. ffrench-Mullen JMH, Barker JL, and Rogawski MA: Calcium current block by (−)-pentobarbital, phenobarbital, and CHEB but not (+)-pentobarbital in acutely isolated hippocampal CA1 neurons: Comparison with effects on GABA-activated Cl⁻ current. J Neurosci 1993; 13: 3211

75. Correa AM: Gating kinetics of Shaker K+ channels are differentially modified by general anesthetics. Am J Physiol 1998; 275: C1009

76. Friederich P and Urban BW: Interaction of intravenous anesthetics with human neuronal potassium currents in relation to clinical concentrations. Anesthesiology 1999; 91: 1853

77. Gerstin KM, Gong DH, Abdallah M, et al. Mutation of KCNK5 or Kir3.2 potassium channels in mice does not change minimum alveolar anesthetic concentration. Anesth Analg 2003; 96: 1345

78. Gibbons SJ, Nunez-Hernandez R, Maze G, et al.: Inhibition of a fast inwardly rectifying potassium conductance by barbiturates. Anesth Analg 1996; 82: 1242

79. Stadnicka A, Bosnjak ZJ, Kampine JP, et al.: Effects of sevoflurane on inward rectifier K+ current in guinea pig ventricular cardiomyocytes. Am J Physiol 1997; 273: H324

80. Wakamori M, Ikemoto Y, and Akaike N: Effects of two volatile anesthetics and a volatile convulsant on the excitatory and inhibitory amino acid responses in dissociated CNS neurons of the rat. J Neurophysiol 1991; 66: 2014

81. Lin L, Chen LL, and Harris RA: Enflurane inhibits NMDA,AMPA and kainate-induced currents in Xenopus oocytes expressing mouse and human brain mRNA. FASEB J 1992; 7: 479

82. Weight FF, Lovinger DM, White G, et al.: Alcohol and anesthetic actions on excitatory amino acid-activated ion channels. Ann N Y Acad Sci 1991; 625: 97

83. Dildy-Mayfield JE, Eger EI, 2nd, and Harris RA: Anesthetics produce subunit-selective actions on glutamate receptors. J Pharmacol Exp Ther 1996; 276: 1058

84. Minami K, Wick MJ, Stern-Bach Y, et al.: Sites of volatile anesthetic action on kainate (glutamate receptor 6) receptors. J Biol Chem 1998; 273: 8248

85. Aronstam RS, Martin DC, and Dennison RL: Volatile anesthetics inhibit NMDA-stimulated ⁴⁵Ca uptake by rat brain microvesicles. Neurochem Res 1994; 19: 1515

86. Lodge D, Anis NA, and Burton NR: Effects of optical isomers of ketamine on excitation of cat and rat spinal neurons by amino acids and acetylcholine. Neurosci Lett 1982; 29: 281

87. Anis NA, Berry SC, Burton NR, et al.: The dissociative anaesthetics, ketamine and phencyclidine, selectively reduce excitation of central mammalian neurones by N-methyl-aspartate. Br J Pharmacol 1983; 79: 565

88. Zeilhofer HU, Swandulla D, Geisslinger G, et al.: Differential effects of ketamine enantiomers on NMDA receptor currents in cultured neurons. Eur J Pharmacol 1992; 213: 155

89. Ryder S, Way WL, and Trevor AJ: Comparative pharmacology of the optical isomers of ketamine in mice. Eur J Pharmacol 1978; 49: 15

90. Mennerick S, Jevtovic-Todorovic V, Todorovic SM, et al.: Effect of nitrous oxide on excitatory and inhibitory synaptic transmission in hippocampal cultures. J Neurosci 1998; 18: 9716

91. Jevtovic-Todorovic V, Todorovic SM, Mennerick S, et al.: Nitrous oxide (laughing gas) is an NMDA antagonist, neuroprotectant and neurotoxin. Nat Med 1998; 4: 460

92. Franks NP, Dickinson R, de Sousa SL, et al.: How does xenon produce anaesthesia? [letter]. Nature 1998; 396: 324

93. Macdonald RL and Olsen RW: GABA_A receptor channels. Annu Rev Neurosci 1994; 17: 569

94. Macdonald RL, Rogers CJ, and Twyman RE: Barbiturate regulation of kinetic properties of the GABAA receptor channels of mouse spinal neurones in culture. J Physiol 1989; 417: 483

95. Barker JL, Harrison NL, Lange GD, et al: Potentiation of gamma-aminobutyric-acid-activated chloride conductance by a steroid anesthetic in cultured rat spinal neurons. J Physiol 1987; 386: 485

96. Hales TH and Lambert JJ: Modulation of the GABA_A receptor by propofol. Br J Pharmacol 1988; 93: 84P

97. Wittmer LL, Hu Y, Kalkbrenner M, Evers AS, Zorumski CF, and Covey DF: Enantioselectivity of steroid-induced gamma-aminobutyric acid A receptor modulation and anesthesia. Mol Pharmacol 1996; 50: 1581

98. Nakahiro M, Yeh JZ, Brunner E, et al.: General anesthetics modulate GABA receptor channel complex in rat dorsal root ganglion neurons. FASEB J 1989; 3: 1850

99. Hall AC, Lieb WR, and Franks NP: Stereoselective and non-stereoselective actions of isoflurane on the GABA$_A$ receptor. Br J Pharmacol 1994; 112: 906

100. Yeh JZ, Quandt FN, Tanguy J, et al.: General anesthetic action on gamma-aminobutyric acid-activated channels. Ann N Y Acad Sci 1991; 625: 155

101. Banks MI and Pearce RA: Dual actions of volatile anesthetics on GABA(A) IPSCs: Dissociation of blocking and prolonging effects. Anesthesiology 1999; 90: 120

102. Amin J and Weiss DS: GABA$_A$ receptors need two homologous domains of the beta-subunit for activation by GABA but not by pentobarbital. Nature 1993; 366: 565

103. Tanelian DL, Kosek P, Mody I, et al.: The role of the GABA$_A$ receptor/chloride channel complex in anesthesia. Anesthesiology 1993; 78: 757

104. Sapp DW, Witte U, Turner DM, et al.: Regional variation in steroid anesthetic modulation of [^{35}S]TBPS binding to gamma-aminobutyric acid receptors in rat brain. J Pharmacol Exp Ther 1992; 262: 801

105. Pritchett DB, Sontheimer H, and Shivers BD: Importance of a novel GABA$_A$ receptor subunit for benzodiazepine pharmacology. Nature 1989; 338: 582

106. Hill-Venning C, Belelli D, Paters JA, et al.: Subunit-dependent interaction of the general anaesthetic etomidate with the gamma-aminobutyric acid type A receptor. Br J Pharmacol 1997; 120: 749

107. Zhu WJ, Wang JF, Krueger KE, et al.: Delta subunit inhibits neurosteroid modulation of GABA$_A$ receptors. J Neurosci 1996; 16: 6648

108. Davies PA, Hanna MC, Hales TG, et al.: Insensitivity to anaesthetic agents conferred by a class of GABA$_A$ receptor subunit. Nature 1997; 385: 820

109. Mihic SJ and Harris RA: Inhibition of rho1 receptor GABAergic currents by alcohols and volatile anesthetics. J Pharmacol Exp Ther 1996; 277: 411

110. Mihic SJ, Ye Q, Wick MJ, et al.: Sites of alcohol and volatile anaesthetic action on GABA(A) and glycine receptors. Nature 1997; 389: 385

111. Belelli D, Lambert JJ, Peters JA, et al.: The interaction of the general anesthetic etomidate with the gamma-aminobutyric acid type A receptor is influenced by a single amino acid. Proc Natl Acad Sci USA 1997; 92: 11031

112. Krasowski MD, Koltchine VV, Rick CE, Ye Q, Finn SE, and Harrison NL: Propofol and other intravenous anesthetics have sites of action on the gamma-aminobutyric acid type A receptor distinct from that for isoflurane. Mol Pharmacol 1998; 53: 530

113. Hosie AM, Wilkins ME, da Silva HM, et al: Endogenous neurosteroids regulate GABA$_A$ receptors through two discrete transmembrane sites. Nature 2006; 444: 486

114. Dilger JP, Vidal AM, Mody HI, et al.: Evidence for direct actions of general anesthetics on an ion channel protein. An new look at a unified mode of action. Anesthesiology 1994; 81: 431

115. Firestone LL, Sauter JF, Braswell LM, et al.: Actions of general anesthetics on acetylcholine receptor-rich membranes from Torpedo californica. Anesthesiology 1986; 64: 694

116. Franks NP and Lieb WR: Stereospecific effects of inhalational general anesthetic optical isomers on nerve ion channels. Science 1991; 254: 427

117. Charlesworth P and Richards CD: Anaesthetic modulation of nicotinic ion channel kinetics in bovine chromaffin cells. Br J Pharmacol 1995; 114: 909

118. Violet JM, Downie DL, Nakisa RC, et al.: Differential sensitivities of mammalian neuronal and muscle nicotinic acetylcholine receptors to general anesthetics. Anesthesiology 1997; 86(4): 866

119. Flood P, Ramirez-Latorre J, and Role L: Alpha 4 beta 2 neuronal nicotinic acetylcholine receptors in the central nervous system are inhibited by isoflurane and propofol, but alpha 7-type nicotinic acetylcholine receptors are unaffected. Anesthesiology 1997; 86: 859

120. Evers AS and Steinbach JH: Supersensitive sites in the central nervous system: Anesthetics block brain nicotinic receptors. Anesthesiology 1997; 86: 760

121. Wong SM, Sonner JM, and Kendig JJ: Acetylcholine receptors do not mediate isoflurane's actions on spinal cord in vitro. Anesth Analg 2002; 94: 1495

122. Eger II EI, Zhang Y, Laster M, et al.: Acetylcholine receptors do not mediate the immobilization produced by inhaled anesthetics. Anesth Analg 2002; 94: 1500

123. Raines DE, Claycomb RJ, and Forman SA: Nonhalogenated anesthetic alkanes and perhalogenated nonimmobilizing alkanes inhibit alpha(4)beta(2) neuronal nicotinic acetylcholine receptors. Anesth Analg 2002; 95: 573

124. Mascia MP, Machu TK, and Harris RA: Enhancement of homomeric glycine receptor function by long-chain alcohols and anaesthetics. Br J Pharmacol 1996; 119(7): 1331

125. Downie DL, Hall AC, Lieb WR, et al.: Effects of inhalational general anaesthetics on native glycine receptors in rat medullary neurons and recombinant glycine receptors in Xenopus oocytes. Br J Pharmacol 1996; 118: 493

126. Jenkins A, Franks NP, and Lieb WR: Actions of general anaesthetics on 5-HT3 receptors in N1E-115 neuroblastoma cells. Br J Pharmacol 1996; 117: 1507

127. Machu TK and Harris RA: Alcohols and anesthetics enhance the function of 5-hydroxytryptamine3 receptors expressed in Xenopus laevis oocytes. J Pharmacol Exp Ther 1994; 271: 898

128. Patel AJ and Honore E: Anesthetic-sensitive 2P domain K+ channels. Anesthesiology 2001; 95: 1013

129. Franks NP and Lieb WR: Volatile general anaesthetics activate a novel neuronal K+ current. Nature 1988; 333: 662

130. Winegar BD and Yost CS: Volatile anesthetics directly activate baseline S K$^+$ channels in aplysia neurons. Brain Res 1998; 807: 255

131. Honore E: The neuronal background K2P channels: focus on TREK1. Nat Rev Neurosci 2007; 8: 251

132. Patel AJ, Honore E, Lesage F, et al.: Inhalational anesthetics activate two-pore-domain background K$^+$ channels. Nat Neurosci 1999; 2: 422

133. Gruss M, Bushell TJ, Bright DP, et al.: Two-pore-domain K+ channels are a novel target for the anesthetic gases xenon, nitrous oxide, and cyclopropane. Mol Pharmacol 2004; 65: 443

134. Overton CE, Studies of narcosis. 1st ed., London, Chapman and Hall, 1991

135. Meyer H: Theorie der alkoholnarkose. Arch Exp Pathol Pharmakol 1899; 42: 109

136. Franks NP and Lieb WR: Where do general anaesthetics act? Nature 1978; 274: 339

137. Larsen ER: Fluorine compounds in anesthesiology. 1960: 1

138. Andrews PR, Jones JG, and Pulton DB: Convulsant, anticonvulsant and anaesthetic barbiturates. In vivo activities of oxo- and thiobarbiturates related to pentobarbitone. Eur J Pharmacol 1982; 79: 61

139. Paul SM and Purdy RH: Neuroactive steroids. FASEB J 1992; 6: 2311

140. Koblin DD, Eger II EI, Johnson BH, et al.: Are convulsant gases also anesthetics? Anesth Analg 1981; 60: 464

141. Koblin DD, Chortkoff BS, Laster MJ, et al.: Polyhalogenated and perfluorinated compounds that disobey the Meyer-Overton hypothesis. Anesth Analg 1994; 79: 1043

142. Kandel L, Chortkoff BS, Sonner J, et al: Nonanesthetics can suppress learning. Anesth Analg 1996; 82: 321

143. Alifimoff JK, Firestone LL, and Miller KW: Anaesthetic potencies of primary alkanols: Implications for the molecular dimensions of the anaesthetic site. Br J Pharmacol 1989; 96: 9

144. Raines DE, Korten SE, Hill WAG, et al.: Anesthetic cutoff in cycloalkanemethanols. A test of current theories. Anesthesiology 1993; 78: 918

145. Liu J, Laster MJ, Koblin DD, et al.: A cutoff in potency exists in the perfluoroalkanes. Anesth Analg 1994; 79: 238

146. Andrews PR and Mark LC: Structural specificity of barbiturates and related drugs. Anesthesiology 1982; 57: 314

147. Richter JA and Holtman JR: Barbiturates: their in vivo effects and potential biochemical mechanisms. Prog Neurobiol 1982; 18: 275

148. Tomlin SL, Jenkins A, Lieb WR, et al.: Stereoselective effects of etomidate optical isomers on gamma-aminobutyric acid type A receptors and animals. Anesthesiology 1998; 88: 708

149. Lysko GS, Robinson JL, Casto R, et al.: The stereospecific effects of isoflurane isomers in vivo. Eur J Pharmacol 1994; 263: 25

150. Kendig JJ, Grossman Y, and MacIver MB: Pressure reversal of anaesthesia: a synaptic mechanism. Br J Anaesth 1988; 60: 806

151. Smith RA, Porter EG, and Miller KW: The solubility of anesthetic gases in lipid bilayers. Biochim Biophys Acta 1981; 645: 327

152. Franks NP: Molecular targets underlying general anaesthesia. Br J Pharmacol 2006; 147 Suppl 1: S72

153. Franks NP and Liebs WR: Do general anaesthetics act by competitive binding to specific receptors? Nature 1984; 310: 599

154. Franks NP and Lieb WR: Mapping of general anaesthetic target sites provides a molecular basis for cutoff effects. Nature 1985; 316: 149

155. Wishnia A and Pinder TW: Hydrophobic interactions in proteins. The alkane binding site of β-lactoglobulins A and B. Biochemistry 1966; 5: 1534

156. Wishnia A and Pinder T: Hydrophobic interactions in proteins: Conformation changes in bovine serum albumin below pH 5. Biochemistry 1964; 3: 1377

157. Dubois BW and Evers AS: An ^{19}F-NMR spin-spin relaxation (T_2) method for characterizing volatile anesthetic binding to proteins. Analysis of isoflurane binding to serum albumin. Biochemistry 1992; 31: 7069

158. Dubois BW, Cherian SF, and Evers AS: Volatile anesthetics compete for common binding sites on bovine serum albumin: A ^{19}F-NMR study. Proc Natl Acad Sci USA 1993; 90: 6478

159. Eckenhoff RG and Shuman H: Halothane binding to soluble proteins determined by photoaffinity labeling. Anesthesiology 1993; 79: 96

160. Eckenhoff RG: Amino acid resolution of halothane binding sites in serum albumin. J Biol Chem 1996; 271: 15521

161. Burris KE, Dubois BW, and Evers AS: Direct observation of saturable halothane binding to firefly luciferase: A photoaffinity labeling and ^{19}F-NMR study. Anesthesiology 1993; 79: A700

162. Husain SS, Forman SA, Kloczewiak MA, et al.: Synthesis and properties of 3-(2-hydroxyethyl)-3-n-pentyldiazirine, a photoactivable general anesthetic. J Med Chem 1999; 41: 3300

163. Franks NP, Jenkins A, Conti E, et al.: Structural basis for the inhibition of firefly luciferase by a general anesthetic. Biophys J 1998; 75: 2205

164. Bhattacharya AA, Curry S, and Franks NP: Binding of the general anesthetics propofol and halothane to human serum albumin. High resolution crystal structures. J Biol Chem 2000; 275: 38731

165. Wick MJ, Mihic SJ, Ueno S, et al.: Mutations of gamma-aminobutyric acid and glycine receptors change alcohol cutoff: evidence for an alcohol receptor? Proc Natl Acad Sci USA 1998; 95: 6504

166. Johansson JS, Gibney BR, Rabanal F, et al.: A designed cavity in the hydrophobic core of a four-alpha-helix bundle improves volatile anesthetic binding affinity. Biochemistry 1998; 37: 1421

167. Segal IS, Vickery RG, Walton JK, et al.: Dexmedetomidine diminishes halothane anesthetic requirements in rats through a postsynaptic alpha 2 adrenergic receptor. Anesthesiology 1988; 69: 818

168. Moody EJ, Harris BD, and Skolnick P: The potential for safer anaesthesia using stereoselective anaesthetics. Trends Pharmacol Sci 1994; 15: 387

169. Zhang Y, Laster MJ, Hara K, et al.: Glycine receptors mediate part of the immobility produced by inhaled anesthetics. Anesth Analg 2003; 96: 97

170. Zhang Y, Wu S, Eger II EI, et al.: Neither GABA(A) nor strychnine-sensitive glycine receptors are the sole mediators of MAC for isoflurane. Anesth Analg 2001; 92: 123

171. Morgan PG and Cascorbi HF: Effect of anesthetics and a convulsant on normal and mutant *Caenorhabditis elegans*. Anesthesiology 1985; 62: 738

172. Humphrey JA, Hamming KS, Thacker CM, et al.: A Putative Cation Channel and Its Novel Regulator: Cross-Species Conservation of Effects on General Anesthesia. Current Biology 2007; 17: 624

173. Sedensky MM and Meneely PM: Genetic analysis of halothane sensitivity in *Caenorhabditis elegans*. Science 1987; 236: 952

174. Crowder CM, Shebester LD, and Schedl T: Behavioral effects of volatile anesthetics in Caenorhabditis elegans. Anesthesiology 1996; 85: 901

175. van Swinderen B, Saifee O, Shebester L, et al.: A neomorphic syntaxin mutation blocks volatile-anesthetic action in Caenorhabditis elegans. Proc Natl Acad Sci USA 1999; 96: 2479

176. Metz LB, Dasgupta N, Liu C, et al.: An evolutionarily conserved presynaptic protein is required for isoflurane sensitivity in Caenorhabditis elegans. Anesthesiology 2007; 107: 971

177. Nagele P, Metz LB, and Crowder CM: Nitrous oxide (N2O) requires the N-methyl-D-aspartate receptor for its action in Caenorhabditis elegans. Proc Natl Acad Sci USA 2004; 101: 8791

178. Nagele P, Metz LB, and Crowder CM: Xenon acts by inhibition of non-N-methyl-D-aspartate receptor-mediated glutamatergic neurotransmission in Caenorhabditis elegans. Anesthesiology 2005; 103: 508

179. Krishnan KS and Nash HA: A genetic study of the anesthetic response: mutants of *Drosophila melanogaster* altered in sensitivity to halothane. Proc Natl Acad Sci USA 1990; 87: 8632

180. Campbell DB and Nash HA: Use of *Drosophila* mutants to distinguish among volatile general anesthetics. Proc Natl Acad Sci USA 1994; 91: 2135

181. Campbell JL and Nash HA: The visually-induced jump response of *Drosophila melanogaster* is sensitive to volatile anesthetics. Proc Natl Acad Sci USA 1998; 12: 241

182. Rudolph U and Mohler H: Analysis of GABAA receptor function and dissection of the pharmacology of benzodiazepines and general anesthetics through mouse genetics. Annu Rev Pharmacol Toxicol 2004; 44: 475

183. Solt K and Forman SA: Correlating the clinical actions and molecular mechanisms of general anesthetics. Curr Opin Anaesthesiol 2007; 20: 300

184. Blednov YA, Jung S, Alva H, et al.: Deletion of the alpha1 or beta2 subunit of GABAA receptors reduces actions of alcohol and other drugs. J Pharmacol Exp Ther 2003; 304: 30

185. Homanics GE, Ferguson C, Quinlan JJ, et al.: Gene knockout of the alpha6 subunit of the gamma-aminobutyric acid type A receptor: lack of effect on responses to ethanol, pentobarbital, and general anesthetics. Mol Pharmacol 1997; 51: 588

186. Cheng VY, Martin LJ, Elliott EM, et al.: {alpha}5GABAA Receptors Mediate the Amnestic But Not Sedative-Hypnotic Effects of the General Anesthetic Etomidate. J Neurosci 2006; 26: 3713

187. Borghese CM, Werner DF, Topf N, et al.: An Isoflurane- and Alcohol-Insensitive Mutant GABAA Receptor {alpha}1 Subunit with Near-Normal Apparent Affinity for GABA: Characterization in Heterologous Systems and Production of Knockin Mice. J Pharmacol Exp Ther 2006; 319: 208

188. Sonner JM, Werner DF, Elsen FP, et al.: Effect of isoflurane and other potent inhaled anesthetics on minimum alveolar concentration, learning, and the righting reflex in mice engineered to express alpha1 gamma-aminobutyric acid type A receptors unresponsive to isoflurane. Anesthesiology 2007; 106: 107

189. Homanics GE, Elsen FP, Ying SW, et al.: A gain-of-function mutation in the GABA receptor produces synaptic and behavioral abnormalities in the mouse. Genes Brain Behav 2005; 4: 10

190. Siegwart R, Jurd R, and Rudolph U: Molecular determinants for the action of general anesthetics at recombinant alpha(2)beta(3)gamma(2)gamma-aminobutyric acid(A) receptors. J Neurochem 2002; 80: 140

191. Jurd R, Arras M, Lambert S, et al.: General anesthetic actions *in vivo* strongly attenuated by a point mutation in the GABA(A) receptor beta3 subunit. FASEB J 2003; 17: 250

192. Zeller A, Arras M, Jurd R, et al.: Identification of a molecular target mediating the general anesthetic actions of pentobarbital. Mol Pharmacol 2007; 71: 852

193. Zeller A, Arras M, Lazaris A, et al.: Distinct molecular targets for the central respiratory and cardiac actions of the general anesthetics etomidate and propofol. Faseb J 2005; 19: 1677

194. Liao M, Sonner JM, Jurd R, et al.: Beta3-containing gamma-aminobutyric acidA receptors are not major targets for the amnesic and immobilizing actions of isoflurane. Anesth Analg 2005; 101: 412

195. O'Meara GF, Newman RJ, Fradley RL, et al.: The GABA-A beta3 subunit mediates anaesthesia induced by etomidate. Neuroreport 2004; 15: 1653

196. Reynolds DS, Rosahl TW, Cirone J, et al.: Sedation and anesthesia mediated by distinct GABA(A) receptor isoforms. J Neurosci 2003; 23: 8608

197. Mihalek RM, Banerjee PK, Korpi ER, et al.: Attenuated sensitivity to neuroactive steroids in gamma-aminobutyrate type A receptor delta subunit knockout mice. Proc Natl Acad Sci USA 1999; 96: 12905

198. Heurteaux C, Guy N, Laigle C, et al.: TREK-1, a K(+) channel involved in neuroprotection and general anesthesia. Embo J 2004; 23: 2684

199. Westphalen RI, Krivitski M, Amarosa A, et al.: Reduced inhibition of cortical glutamate and GABA release by halothane in mice lacking the K+ channel, TREK-1. Br J Pharmacol 2007; 152: 939

CHAPTER 6 ■ GENOMIC BASIS OF PERIOPERATIVE MEDICINE

MIHAI V. PODGOREANU AND JOSEPH P. MATHEW

KEY POINTS

1. Genetic variation can significantly modulate risk of adverse perioperative events.
2. Several methodological approaches are used to study the genetic architecture of perioperative outcomes.
3. Current perioperative risk profiling has limited ability to explain individual variability in adverse outcomes.
4. Genetic variants in inflammatory and coagulation pathways are associated with susceptibility to perioperative myocardial infarction.
5. Biomarkers associated with perioperative atrial fibrillation were identified through genetic association studies and gene expression analysis.
6. Variants in inflammation and platelet activation pathways modify susceptibility to perioperative cerebral injury.
7. A genetic basis for perioperative acute kidney injury has been identified.

8. Pharmacogenomics describes the relationship between inherited variations in genes modulating drug actions and individual variability in drug response.
9. Individual variability in response to anesthetic agents is as high as 24% and has a genetic component.
10. Individual variability in analgesic responsiveness is attributed to genetic control of peripheral nociceptive pathways and descending central pain modulatory pathways.
11. Host responses to injury and the clinical trajectory of critically ill injured patients are genetically determined.
12. Genomic technology applications are beginning to fulfill the "Five Ps" of perioperative medicine and pain management (personalized, preventive, predictive, participatory, and prospective).

GENETIC BASIS OF DISEASE

Human biological diversity involves interindividual variability in morphology, behavior, physiology, development, susceptibility to disease, and response to stressful stimuli and drug therapy (i.e., *phenotypes*). This phenotypic variation is determined, at least in part, by differences in the specific genetic makeup (i.e., *genotype*) of an individual. In 2003, the 50th anniversary of Watson and Crick's description of the DNA double-helix structure also marked the completion of the Human Genome Project.[1] This major accomplishment provides the discipline of genomics with basic resources to study the functions and interactions of all genes in a systematic fash-ion, including their interaction with environmental factors, and translate the findings into clinical and societal benefits. *Functional genomics* employs large-scale experimental methods and statistical analyses to investigate the regulation of gene expression in response to physiological, pharmacologic, and pathologic changes. It also uses genetic information from clinical studies to examine the impact of genetic variability on disease characterization and outcome.[2]

Many common diseases like atherosclerosis, coronary artery disease, hypertension, diabetes, cancer, asthma, and our responses to injury, drugs, and nonpharmacologic therapies are genetically complex, characteristically involving an interplay of many genetic variations in molecular and biochemical pathways (i.e., *polygenic*) and genetic-environmental interactions (i.e., *multifactorial*). In other words, complex phenotypes can be viewed as the integrated effect of many susceptibility genes and many environmental exposures. The proportion of phenotypic variance explained by genetic factors is referred to as *heritability*, and can be estimated by examining the increased similarity of a phenotype in related as compared with unrelated individuals. One of the major challenges and ongoing research efforts facing the postgenomic period are to connect the nearly 25,000 protein-coding genes of mammalian organisms to the genetic basis of complex polygenic diseases and the integrated function of complex biological systems. According to the "common-disease/common-variants hypothesis,"[3] individual susceptibility to common complex diseases and the manifestation, severity, and prognosis of the disease process is modulated by multiple common functional polymorphisms, each with only modest effect on disease risk. However, it is likely that rare modest-risk alleles are important as well in polygenic disease, but their detection is more difficult because of sample size and sequencing constraints.

The perioperative period represents a unique and extreme example of such gene-environment interaction. As we appreciate in our daily practice in the operating rooms and intensive care units, one hallmark of perioperative physiology is the striking variability in patient responses to the acute, robust, and generalized perioperative (environmental) perturbations induced by surgical injury, hemodynamic challenges, vascular cannulation, extracorporeal circulation, intra-aortic balloon counterpulsation, mechanical ventilation, partial/total organ resection, transient limb/organ ischemia, transfusions, anesthetic agents, and the pharmacopoeia used in the perioperative period. This translates into substantial interindividual variability in immediate perioperative adverse events (mortality or incidence/severity of organ dysfunction), as well as long-term outcomes (Table 6-1). For decades we have attributed this variability to many complexities such as age, nutritional state,

comorbidities—what we colloquially call *protoplasm*. Now we are beginning to appreciate that genetic variation is also partly responsible for this observed variability in outcomes. Overall, an individual's genetic susceptibility to adverse perioperative events stems not only from genetic contributions to the development of comorbid risk factors (like coronary artery disease [CAD] and reduced preoperative cardiopulmonary reserve) during the patient's lifetime, but also from genetic variability in specified biological pathways participating in pathophysiological events during and after surgery (Fig. 6-1). With increasing evidence suggesting that genetic variation can significantly modulate risk of adverse perioperative events,[4–7] the emerging field of *perioperative genomics* aims to apply functional genomic approaches to discover underlying biological mechanisms. These approaches will explain why similar patients have such dramatically different outcomes after surgery, and is justified by a unique combination of environmental insults and postoperative phenotypes that characterize surgical and critically ill patient populations.

To integrate this new generation of genetic results into clinical practice, perioperative physicians need to understand the patterns of human genome variation, the methods of population-based genetic investigation, and the principles of gene and protein expression analysis. This chapter reviews general genetic/genomic concepts and highlights current and future applications of genomic technologies for perioperative risk stratification, outcome prediction, mechanistic understanding of surgical stress responses, as well as identification and validation of novel targets for perioperative organ protection.

Overview of Human Genetic Variation

Although the human DNA sequence is 99.9% identical between individuals, the variations may greatly affect a

---

TABLE 6-1

CATEGORIES OF PERIOPERATIVE PHENOTYPES

Immediate perioperative outcomes	• In-hospital mortality • Perioperative myocardial infarction • Perioperative low cardiac output syndrome/acute decompensated heart failure • Perioperative vasoplegic syndrome • Perioperative arrhythmias (atrial fibrillation) • Postoperative bleeding • Perioperative venous thrombosis • Acute postoperative stroke • Postoperative delirium • Perioperative acute kidney injury • Acute perioperative lung injury/prolonged postoperative mechanical ventilation • Acute allograft dysfunction/rejection • Postoperative sepsis • Multiple organ dysfunction syndrome • Variability in response to anesthetics, analgesics and other perioperative drugs • Intermediate phenotypes (plasma biomarker levels)
Long-term postoperative outcomes	• Event-free survival/major adverse cardiac events • Progression of vein graft disease • Chronic allograft dysfunction/rejection • Postoperative cognitive dysfunction • Postoperative depression • Quality of life

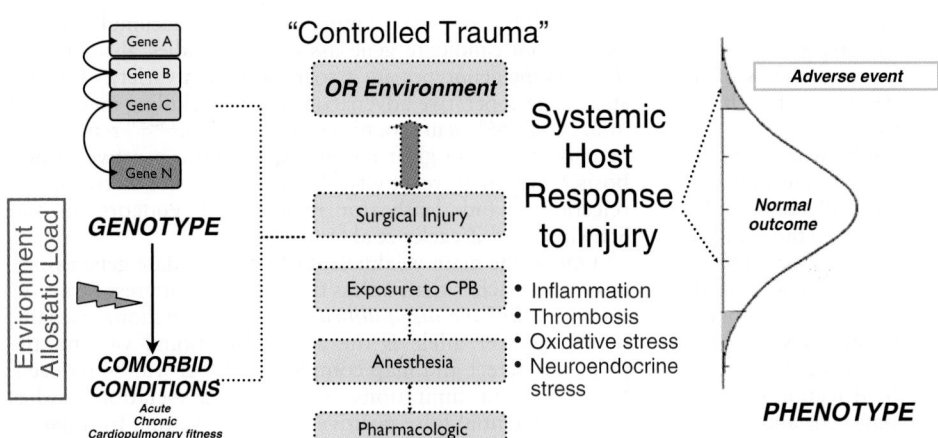

FIGURE 6-1. Perioperative adverse events are complex traits, characteristically involving an interaction between robust operative environmental perturbations (surgical trauma, hemodynamic challenges, exposure to extracorporeal circulation, drug administration) and multiple susceptibility genes. The observed variability in perioperative outcomes can be partly attributed to genetic variability modulating the host response to surgical injury. OR, operating room; CPB, cardiopulmonary bypass.

person's disease susceptibility. In elucidating the genetic basis of disease, much of what has been investigated in the pre-Human Genome Project era focused on identifying rare genetic variants (*mutations*) responsible for >1,500 monogenic disorders such as hypertrophic cardiomyopathy, long-QT syndrome, sickle cell anemia, cystic fibrosis, or familial hypercholesterolemia, which are highly penetrant (carriers of the mutant gene will likely have the disease) and inherited in mendelian fashion (hence, termed *mendelian diseases*). However, most of the genetic diversity in the population is attributable to more widespread DNA sequence variations (*polymorphisms*), typically single nucleotide base substitutions (*single nucleotide polymorphisms* [SNPs]) or to a broader category of previously overlooked *structural genetic variants*. These structural variants include short sequence repeats (*microsatellites*), insertion/deletion of one or more nucleotides (*indels*), inversions, and the recently discovered copy number variants (*CNVs*, large segments of DNA that vary in number of copies),[8] all of which may or may not be associated with a specific phenotype (Fig. 6-2). To be classified as a polymorphism, the DNA sequence alternatives (i.e., *alleles*) must exist with a frequency of at least 1% in the population. About 15 million SNPs are estimated to exist in the human genome, approximately once every 300 base pairs, located in genes, as well as in the surrounding regions of the genome. Polymorphisms may directly alter the amino acid sequence and therefore potentially alter protein function, or alter regulatory DNA sequences that modulate protein expression. Sets of nearby SNPs on a chromosome are inherited in blocks, referred to as *haplotypes*. As will be shown later, haplotype analysis is a useful way of applying genotype information in disease gene discovery. On the other hand, CNVs involve approximately 12% of the human genome, often encompass genes (especially regulating inflammation and brain development), and may influence disease susceptibility through dosage imbalances. The year 2007 was marked by the realization that DNA differs from person to person much more than previously suspected; equipped with faster and cheaper DNA sequencing technologies, researchers have catalogued >3 million SNPs as part of the HapMap Project,[9] published the first diploid genome sequence of an individual human,[10] launched the 1000 Genomes Project (sequencing the genomes of 1,000 people from around the world), and begun charting CNVs and other structural variants, thus making understanding of human genetic variation the 2007 *Science* magazine "Breakthrough of the Year." In the following section we review the common strategies used to incorporate genetic analysis into clinical studies.

Methodologic Approaches to Study the Genetic Architecture of Common Complex Diseases

Most ongoing research on complex disorders focuses on identifying genetic polymorphisms that enhance susceptibility to

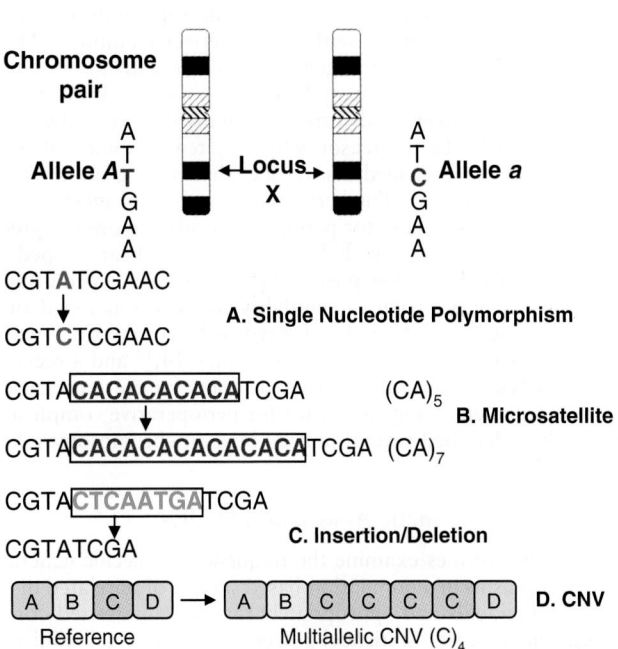

FIGURE 6-2. Categories of common human genetic variation. **A.** *Single nucleotide polymorphisms (SNP)* can be silent or have functional consequences: changes in amino acid sequence or premature termination of protein synthesis (if they occur in the coding regions of the gene) or alterations in the expression of the gene, resulting in more or less protein (if they occur in regulatory regions of the gene such as the promoter region or the intron/exon boundaries). Structural genetic variants include *Microsatellites* with varying number of dinucleotide (CA)n repeats (**B**); *Insertions/deletions* (**C**); and Copy number variation (CNV; **D**). A–D are long DNA segments, segment C shows variation in copy number. Glossary: *locus*, the location of a gene/genetic marker in the genome; *alleles*, alternative forms of a gene/genetic marker; *genotype*, the observed alleles for an individual at a genetic locus; *heterozygous*, two different alleles are present at a locus; *homozygous*, two identical alleles are present at a locus. A SNP at position 1691 of a gene with alleles G and A would be written as 1691G>A.

given conditions. Often the design of such studies is complicated by the presence of multiple risk factors, gene-environment interactions, and a lack of even rough estimates of the number of genes underlying such complex traits. Two broad strategies are being employed to identify complex trait loci. The *candidate gene* approach is motivated by what is known about the trait biologically and can be characterized as a hypothesis-testing approach, but is intrinsically biased. The second strategy is the *genomewide scan*, in which thousands of markers uniformly distributed throughout the genome are used to locate regions that may harbor genes influencing the phenotypic variability. This is a hypothesis-free and unbiased approach, in the sense that no prior assumptions are being made about the biological processes involved and no weight is given to known genes, thus allowing the detection of previously unknown trait loci. Both the candidate gene and genome scan approaches can be implemented using one of two fundamental methods of identifying polymorphisms affecting common diseases: linkage analysis or association studies in human populations.

Linkage Analysis

Linkage analysis is used to identify the chromosomal location of gene variants related to a given disease by studying the distribution of disease alleles in affected individuals throughout a pedigree and has successfully mapped hundreds of genes for rare, monogenic disorders. However, common complex diseases are characterized by a multitude of genes with rare and/or common alleles, which create an apparently chaotic pattern of heterogeneity within and between families. The overall effect of this heterogeneity, together with the potentially weak influence of many loci, places a heavy burden on the statistical power needed to detect individual contributing genes, and may be the reason why very few genome linkage scans so far have yielded disease loci that meet genomewide significance criteria.[11] Furthermore, the nature of most complex diseases (especially for perioperative adverse events) precludes the study of extended multigenerational family pedigrees. Nevertheless, a few positive findings have emerged using this approach: a stroke susceptibility locus was mapped on chromosome 5q12,[12] risk of myocardial infarction was mapped to a single region on chromosome 14,[13] and a recent meta-analysis of several genomewide scans for pulse pressure variation, an emerging risk factor for perioperative complications, has identified several linkage bins on chromosomes 22 and 10.[14]

Genetic Association Studies

Association studies examine the frequency of specific genetic polymorphisms in a population-based sample of unrelated diseased individuals and appropriately matched unaffected controls. The increased statistical power to uncover small clinical effects of multiple genes[15] and the fact that they do not require family-based sample collections are the main advantages of this approach over linkage analysis. Until very recently, most significant results in dissecting common complex diseases were gathered from candidate gene association studies, with genes selected because of a priori hypotheses about their potential etiologic role in disease based on current understanding of the disease pathophysiology.[16] For example, genetic variants within the renin-angiotensin system,[17] nitric oxide synthase,[18] and β_2-adrenergic receptors,[19] known to modulate vascular tone, were tested and found to be associated with hypertension. Similarly, the possible effects of polymorphisms on genetic predisposition for CAD[20] or restenosis after angioplasty[21] have been extensively investigated; more recently, two large-scale association studies have identified gene variants that might affect susceptibility to myocardial infarction.[22]

As will be presented in more detail later, accumulating evidence from candidate gene association studies also suggests that specific genotypes are associated with a variety of organ-specific perioperative adverse outcomes, including myocardial infarction,[23,24] neurocognitive dysfunction,[25–27] renal compromise,[28–30] vein graft restenosis,[31,32] postoperative thrombosis,[33] vascular reactivity,[34] severe sepsis,[35,36] transplant rejection,[37] and death (for reviews, see Podgoreanu and Schwinn[4] and Ziegeler et al.[7]).

One of the main weaknesses of the candidate gene association approach is that, unless the marker of interest "travels" (i.e., is in *linkage disequilibrium*) with a functional variant, or the marker allele *is* the actual functional variant, the power to detect and map complex trait loci will be reduced. Other known limitations of genetic association studies include potential false-positive findings resulting from population stratification (i.e., admixture of different ethnic or genetic backgrounds in the case and control groups), and multiple comparison issues when large numbers of candidate genes are being assessed.[38] Replication of findings across different populations or related phenotypes remains the most reliable method of validating a true relationship between genetic polymorphisms and disease,[16] but poor reproducibility in subsequent studies has been one of the main criticisms of the candidate gene association approach.[39] However, a recent meta-analysis suggested that lack of statistical power may be the main contributor to this inconsistent replication, and proposed more stringent statistical criteria to exclude false-positive results and the design of large collaborative association studies.[40]

At last, after several decades of frustrating limitations in the ability to find genetic variations responsible for common disease risk, with the completion of the second phase of the International HapMap Project (a high-resolution maps of human genetic variation and haplotypes)[9] and advances in high-throughput genotyping technologies, the year 2007 marked an explosion of adequately powered and successfully replicated *genomewide association studies* (GWAS) that identified very significant genetic contributors to risk for common polygenic diseases like CAD,[41–43] myocardial infarction,[44] diabetes (type I and II),[45,46] atrial fibrillation,[47] obesity,[48] asthma, common cancers, rheumatoid arthritis, Crohn disease, and others. GWAS make use of the known linkage disequilibrium pattern between SNPs from the human HapMap and the new high-density SNP chip technology to comprehensively interrogate between 65 and 80% of common variation across the genome, with even higher coverage being possible using statistical imputation techniques. The largest, most comprehensive GWAS to date was conducted by the Wellcome Trust Case-Control Consortium, investigating the association between 500,000 SNPs and seven common diseases in 2,000 cases and 3,000 shared controls. This study identified 25 independent association signals at stringent levels of significance ($p < 5 \times 10^{-7}$).[41] Interestingly, variants in or near *CDKN2A/B* (cyclin-dependent kinase inhibitor 2 A/B) conferred increased risk for both type II diabetes (odds ratio [OR], 1.2; $p = 7.8 \times 10^{-15}$) and myocardial infarction (OR, 1.64; $p = 1.2 \times 10^{-20}$), which may lead to a mechanistic explanation for the link between the two disorders. This finding also highlights the power of GWAS to identify variants outside described genes: while one of the signals occurs in the *CDKN2A/B* region, the other much stronger association signal occurs >200 kB from these genes, in a gene desert, and thus would not have been picked up by a candidate gene approach. Identifying the mechanism by which this variant may affect *CDKN2A/B* expression will provide new insights into the regulation of these important genes.

Large-Scale Gene and Protein Expression Profiling: Static versus Dynamic Genomic Markers of Perioperative Outcomes

Genomic approaches are anchored in the "central dogma" of molecular biology, the concept of transcription of messenger RNA (mRNA) from a DNA template, followed by translation of RNA into protein (Fig. 6-3). Since transcription is a key regulatory step that may eventually signal many other cascades of events, the study of RNA levels in a cell or organ (i.e., quantifying gene expression) can improve the understanding of a wide variety of biological systems. Furthermore, while the human genome contains only about 25,000 genes, functional variability at the protein level is far more diverse, resulting from extensive posttranscriptional, translational, and posttranslational modifications. It is believed that there are approximately 200,000 distinct proteins in humans, which are further modified posttranslationally by phosphorylation, glycosylation, oxidation, and disulfide structures. There is increasing evidence that variability in gene expression levels underlies complex disease and is determined by regulatory DNA polymorphisms affecting transcription, splicing, and translation efficiency in a tissue- and stimulus-specific manner.[49] Thus, in addition to the assessment of genetic variability at the DNA sequence level using various genotyping techniques as described in previous sections (*static genomics*), analysis of large-scale variability in the pattern of RNA and protein expression both at baseline and in response to the multidimensional perioperative stimuli (*dynamic genomics*) using microarray and proteomic approaches provides a much needed complementary understanding of the overall regulatory networks involved in the pathophysiology of adverse postoperative outcomes. Such dynamic genomic markers can be incorporated in genomic classifiers and used clinically to improve perioperative risk stratification or monitor postoperative recovery.[50] This emergent concept of *molecular classification* involves the description of informational features in a training data set using changes in relative RNA and protein abundance in the context of genetic predisposition and apply-

ing to a test data set to recognize a defined "fingerprint" characteristic of a particular perioperative phenotype (Table 6-2). For example, Feezor et al.[51] used a combined genomic and proteomic approach to identify expression patterns of 138 genes from peripheral blood leukocytes and the concentrations of 7 circulating plasma proteins that discriminated patients who developed multiple organ dysfunction syndrome after thoracoabdominal aortic aneurysm repair from those who did not. More importantly, these patterns of genomewide gene expression and plasma protein concentration were observed before surgical trauma and visceral ischemia-reperfusion injury, suggesting that patients who developed multiple organ dysfunction syndrome differed in either their genetic predisposition or their pre-existing inflammatory state.[51]

Alternatively, dynamic genomic markers can be used to improve mechanistic understanding of perioperative stress and to evaluate and catalogue organ-specific responses to surgical stress and severe systemic stimuli such as cardiopulmonary bypass (CPB) and endotoxemia, which can be subsequently used to identify and validate novel targets for organ protective strategies.[52] Using a similar integrated approach of transcriptomic and proteomic analyses, Tomic et al.[53] characterized the molecular response signatures in peripheral blood to cardiac surgery with and without CPB, a robust trigger of systemic inflammation. The authors demonstrated that, rather than being the primary source of serum cytokines, peripheral blood leukocytes only assume a "primed" phenotype on contact with the extracorporeal circuit, which facilitates their trapping and subsequent tissue-associated inflammatory response. Interestingly, many inflammatory mediators achieved similar systemic levels following off-pump surgery but with delayed kinetics, offering novel insights into the concepts of contact activation and compartmentalization of inflammatory responses to major surgery. Several studies have profiled myocardial gene expression in the ischemic heart, demonstrating alterations in the expression of immediate-early genes (c-*fos*, *jun*B), as well as genes coding for calcium-handling proteins (calsequestrin, phospholamban), extracellular matrix and cytoskeletal proteins.[54]

Up-regulation of transcripts mechanistically involved in cytoprotection (heat shock proteins), resistance to apoptosis, and cell growth has been found in stunned myocardium.[55] Moreover, cardiac gene expression profiling after CPB and cardioplegic arrest has identified the up-regulation of inflammatory and transcription activators, apoptotic genes, and stress genes,[56] which appear to be age-related.[57] Microarray technology has also been used in the quest for novel cardioprotective genes, with the ultimate goal of designing strategies to activate these genes and prevent myocardial injury. Preconditioning is one of such well-studied models of cardioprotection, which can be induced by various triggers including intermittent ischemia, osmotic or redox stress, heat shock, toxins, and inhaled anesthetics. The main functional categories of genes identified as potentially involved in cardioprotective pathways include a host of transcription factors, heat shock proteins, antioxidant genes (heme-oxygenase, glutathione peroxidase), and growth factors, but different gene programs appear to be activated in ischemic versus anesthetic preconditioning, resulting in two distinct cardioprotective phenotypes.[58] More recently, a transcriptional response pattern consistent with late preconditioning has been reported in peripheral blood leukocytes following sevoflurane administration in healthy volunteers, characterized by reduced expression of L selectin as well as down-regulation of genes involved in fatty acid oxidation and the PCG1α (peroxisome-activated receptor gamma coactivator 1α) pathway,[59] which mirrors changes observed in the myocardium from patients undergoing off-pump coronary artery bypass surgery (CABG; Table 6-2).[60] Deregulation of these novel survival pathways

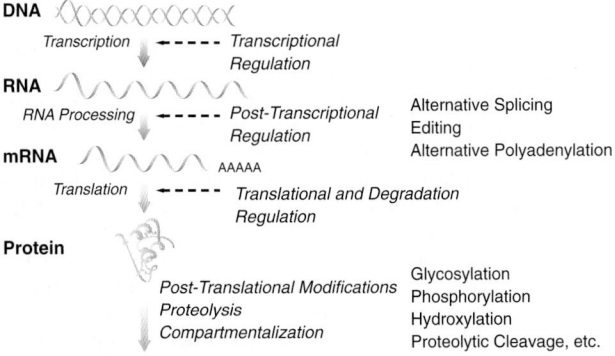

DNA

Transcription → Transcriptional Regulation

RNA

RNA Processing → Post-Transcriptional Regulation — Alternative Splicing / Editing / Alternative Polyadenylation

mRNA AAAAA

Translation → Translational and Degradation Regulation

Protein

Post-Translational Modifications — Glycosylation / Phosphorylation / Hydroxylation / Proteolytic Cleavage, etc.
Proteolysis
Compartmentalization

BIOLOGICAL EFFECTS

FIGURE 6-3.   Central dogma of molecular biology. Protein expression involves two main processes, RNA synthesis (*transcription*) and protein synthesis (*translation*), with many intermediate regulatory steps. A single gene can give rise to multiple protein products (isoforms) via alternative splicing and RNA editing. Thus, functional variability at the protein level, ultimately responsible for biological effects, is the cumulative result of genetic variability as well as extensive posttranscriptional, translational, and posttranslational modifications.

TABLE 6-2

SUMMARY OF GENE EXPRESSION STUDIES WITH IMPLICATIONS FOR PERIOPERATIVE CARDIOVASCULAR OUTCOMES

TISSUE (SPECIES)	STIMULUS/METHOD	GENOMIC SIGNATURE: NUMBER/TYPES OF GENES	REFERENCE
Myocardium (rat)	Ischemia/μA	14 (wound-healing, Ca-handling)	54
Myocardium (human)	CPB/circulatory arrest/ μA	58 (inflammation, transcription activators, apoptosis, stress response)—adults	56
		50 (cardioprotective, antiproliferative, antihypertrophic)—neonates	57
Myocardium (rat)	IPC vs APC/μA	566 differentially regulated/56 jointly regulated (cell defense)	58
Myocardium (rat)	APC vs ApostC/μA	Opposing genomic profiles, 8 gene clusters, <2% jointly regulated genes	184
Myocardium (human)	APC, OPCAB, postoperative LV function/μA	319 up-regulated and 281 down-regulated gene sets in response to OPCAB; deregulation of fatty acid oxidation, DNA-damage signaling and G-CSF survival (perioperative) and PGC-1α (constitutive) pathways predict improved LV function in sevoflurane-treated patients	60
PBMC (human)	APC, sevoflurane/μA	Deregulation of late preconditioning, PGC-1α, fatty acid oxidation, and L selectin pathways	59
Atrial myocardium (pig)	Pacing-induced AF/μA + P	81 (MCL-2 ventricular/atrial isoform shift)	185
Atrial myocardium (human)	AF/μA	1,434 (ventricularlike genomic signature)	101
PBMC (human)	Cardiac surgery, PoAF/ μA	1,302 genes uniquely deregulated in PoAF/401 up-regulated (oxidative stress), 902 down-regulated	102
PBMC (human)	Cardiac surgery, POCD/μA	1,201 genes uniquely deregulated in POCD/531 Up-regulated, 670 down-regulated (inflammation, antigen presentation, cell adhesion, and apoptosis)	122
PBMC (human)	Heart transplant/μA	30 (profile correlated with biopsy-proven rejection; persistent immune activation in response to treatment)	186
PBMC (human)	Heart transplant /RT-PCR	20 (AlloMap, AlloMap score)	187
Myocardium (human)	Heart transplant/P	2 (increased B-crystallin and tropomyosin serum levels)	188
PBMC, plasma (human)	TAAA/μA + P	138 genes and 7 plasma proteins predicted MODS	51

μA, microarray; CPB, cardiopulmonary bypass; IPC, ischemic preconditioning; APC, anesthetic preconditioning; APostC, anesthetic postconditioning; OPCAB, off-pump coronary artery bypass; LV, left ventricle; G-CSF granulocyte colony-stimulating factor; PGC-1α, peroxisome proliferators-activated receptor γ cofactor-1α; AF, atrial fibrillation; MCL-2, myosin light chain 2; P, proteomics; PBMC, peripheral blood mononuclear cells; PoAF, postoperative atrial fibrillation; POCD, postoperative cognitive decline; RT-PCR, real time polymerase chain reaction; TAAA, thoracoabdominal aortic aneurysm repair; MODS, multiple organ dysfunction syndrome.

thus appears to generalize across tissues, making them important targets for cardioprotection, but further studies are needed to correlate perioperative gene expression response patterns in end organs such as the myocardium to those in readily available potential surrogate tissues such as peripheral blood leukocytes.

The *transcriptome* (the complete collection of transcribed elements of the genome) is not fully representative of the *proteome* (the complete complement of proteins encoded by the genome) because many transcripts are not targeted for translation, as evidenced recently with the concept of gene silencing by RNA interference. Alternative splicing, a wide variety of posttranslational modifications, and protein-protein interactions responsible for biological function, therefore would remain undetected by gene expression profiling (Fig. 6-3). This has led to the emergence of a new field, *proteomics*, studying the sequence, modification, and function of many proteins in a biological system at a given time. Rather than focusing on "static" DNA, proteomic studies examine dynamic protein products with the goal of identifying proteins that undergo changes in abundance, modification, or localization in response to a particular disease state, trauma, stress, or therapeutic intervention (for a review, see Atkins

and Johansson[61]). Thus, proteomics offers a more global and integrated view of biology, complementing other functional genomic approaches. Currently available methods for proteomic analysis include protein extraction, separation by two-dimensional gel electrophoresis or chromatography, followed by identification using mass spectrometry. Although rapidly improving, these methods are currently limited by sensitivity, specificity, and throughput. Several preclinical proteomic studies relevant to perioperative medicine have characterized the temporal changes in brain protein expression in response to various inhaled anesthetics,[62,63] or following cardiac surgery with hypothermic circulatory arrest.[64] This may focus further studies aimed to identify new anesthetic binding sites, and the development of neuroprotective strategies. Furthermore, detailed knowledge of the plasma proteome has profound implications in perioperative transfusion medicine,[65] particularly those related to peptide and protein changes that occur during storage of blood products. The development of protein arrays and real-time proteomic analysis technologies has the potential to allow the use of these versatile and rigorous high-throughput methods for clinical applications, and is the object of intense investigation.

GENOMICS AND PERIOPERATIVE RISK PROFILING

More than 40 million patients undergo surgery annually in the United States at a cost of $450 billion. Each year approximately 1 million patients sustain medical complications after surgery, resulting in costs of $25 billion annually. The proportion of the U.S. population older than 65 is estimated to double in the next two decades, leading to a 25% increase in the number of surgeries, a 50% increase in surgery-related costs, and a 100% increase in complications from surgery. Recognizing the significant increase in surgical burden due to accelerated aging of the population and increased reliance on surgery for treatment of disease, the National Heart, Blood and Lung Institute has recently convened a Working Group on perioperative medicine. The group concluded that perioperative complications are significant, costly, variably reported, and often imprecisely detected, and identified a critical need for accurate comprehensive perioperative outcome databases. Furthermore, presurgical risk profiling is inconsistent and deserves further attention, especially for noncardiac, nonvascular surgery and older patients[66] (see Chapter 35).

3 Although many preoperative predictors have been identified and are constantly being refined, risk stratification based on clinical, procedural, and biological markers explains only a small part of the variability in the incidence of perioperative complications. As previously mentioned, it is becoming increasingly recognized that perioperative morbidity arises as a direct result of the environmental stress of surgery occurring on a landscape of susceptibility that is determined by an individual's clinical and genetic characteristics, and may even occur in otherwise healthy individuals. Such adverse outcomes will develop only in patients whose combined burden of genetic and environmental risk factors exceeds a certain threshold, which may vary with age. Identification of such genetic contributions to not only disease causation and susceptibility, but also influencing the *response* to disease and drug therapy and incorporation of genetic risk information in clinical decision-making, may lead to improved health outcomes and reduced costs. For instance, understanding the gene-environment interactions involved in atherosclerotic cardiovascular disease and neurologic injury may facilitate preoperative patient optimization and resource utilization. Furthermore, understanding the role of allotypic variation in proinflammatory and prothrombotic pathways, the main pathophysiological mechanisms responsible for perioperative complications, may contribute to the development of target-specific therapies, thereby limiting the incidence of adverse events in high-risk patients. To increase clinical relevance for the practicing perioperative physician, we summarize existing evidence by specific outcome while highlighting candidate genes in relevant mechanistic pathways (Tables 6-3 to 6-5).

Genetic Susceptibility to Adverse Perioperative Cardiovascular Outcomes

Perioperative Myocardial Infarction

4 As part of the preoperative evaluation, anesthesiologists are involved in assessing the risks of perioperative complications. It is commonly accepted that patients who have underlying cardiovascular disease are at risk for adverse cardiac events after surgery, and several multifactorial risk indices have been developed and validated for patients undergoing both noncardiac surgical procedures (such as the Goldman or the Lee Cardiac Risk Index), as well as cardiac surgery (such as the Han-

nan or Sergeant scores). However, identifying patients at the highest risk of perioperative infarction remains difficult. Risk scores, while potentially valuable for population studies, are not an ideal tool for directing care in an individual patient.[67] Genomic approaches have been used in the search for a better assessment of the individual coronary risk profile. Numerous reports from animal models, linkage analysis, family, twin, and population association studies have definitely proven the role of genetic influences in the incidence and progression of CAD, with a heritability of death from CAD as high as 0.58. Furthermore, hazardous patterns of angiographic CAD (left main and proximal disease), known major risk factors for perioperative cardiac complications, are also highly heritable. Similarly, genetic susceptibility to myocardial infarction has been established through multiple lines of evidence,[13,22] including a recent well-powered and replicated GWAS.[44] Although these studies do not directly address the heritability of adverse perioperative myocardial events, they do suggest a strong genetic contribution to the risk of adverse cardiovascular outcomes in general.

Despite advances in surgical, cardioprotective, and anesthetic techniques, the incidence of perioperative myocardial infarction (PMI) following cardiac and vascular surgery in several large randomized clinical trials has been reported at 7 to 19%[68,69] and is consistently associated with reduced short- and long-term survival. In the setting of cardiac surgery, PMI involves three major converging pathophysiological processes, including systemic and local inflammation, "vulnerable" blood, and neuroendocrine stress[4] (see Chapter 12). In noncardiac surgery, pathophysiology of PMI is not so clearly understood, but a combination of two mechanisms appears predominant: (1) plaque rupture and coronary thrombosis triggered by perioperative endothelial injury from catecholamine surges, proinflammatory and prothrombotic states; and (2) prolonged stress-induced ischemia and tachycardia in the setting of compromised perfusion. Extensive genetic variability exists in each of these mechanistic pathways, which may combine to modulate the magnitude of myocardial injury. However, only a paucity of studies exists relating genetic risk factors to adverse perioperative myocardial outcomes, mainly following CABG surgery (Table 6-3).[31,70,71]

Inflammation Variability and Perioperative Myocardial Outcomes. Consistent with the "inflammatory hypothesis" in the pathogenesis of perioperative organ injury, our group has recently identified three inflammatory gene polymorphisms that are independently predictive of PMI following cardiac surgery with CPB (see Chapter 41). These include the proinflammatory cytokine *IL6*-572G>C (OR 2.47) and two adhesion molecules: intercellular adhesion molecule 1 (*ICAM1* Lys469Glu, OR 1.88) and E selectin (*SELE* 98G>T, OR 0.16).[23] Importantly, inclusion of genotypic information from these SNPs improves prediction models for postcardiac surgery myocardial infarction based on traditional risk factors alone. Using a similar definition of PMI, Collard et al.[24] have reported that a combined haplotype in the mannose-binding lectin gene (*MBL2* LYQA secretor haplotype), an important recognition molecule in the lectin complement pathway, is independently associated with PMI in a cohort of white patients undergoing primary CABG with CPB. Furthermore, genetic variants in *IL6* and *TNFA* are associated with increased incidence of postoperative cardiovascular complications (a composite outcome that included PMI) following lung resection for cancer.[72] Other genetic variants modulating the magnitude of postoperative inflammatory response have been identified. Polymorphisms in the promoter of the interleukin 6 (*IL6*) gene (−572G>C and −174G>C) significantly increase the inflammatory response after heart surgery with CPB,[73] and have been associated with length of hospitalization after CABG.[74] Furthermore, apolipoprotein E genotype (the ε4

TABLE 6-3

REPRESENTATIVE GENETIC POLYMORPHISMS ASSOCIATED WITH ALTERED SUSCEPTIBILITY TO ADVERSE PERIOPERATIVE CARDIOVASCULAR EVENTS

■ GENE	■ POLYMORPHISM	■ TYPE OF SURGERY	■ OR	■ REFERENCE
Perioperative Myocardial Infarction/Dysfunction, Early Vein Graft Failure				
IL6	−572G>C, −174G>C	Cardiac/CPB, thoracic	2.47, 1.8	23, 72
ICAM-1	E469L	Cardiac/CPB	1.88	23
SELE	98G>T		0.16	23
MBL2	LYQA secretor haplotype	CABG/CPB	3.97	24
ITGB3	L33P (Pl$_{A1}$/Pl$_{A2}$)	CABG/CPB, major vascular	2.5[a], 2.4	83, 85
GP1BA	T145M	Major vascular	3.4	85
TNFA	−308G>A	Thoracic	2.5	72
TNFB (LTA)	TNFB2	Cardiac/CPB	3.84	78
IL10	−1082G>A	Cardiac/CPB	n.r.	79
F5	R506Q(FVL)	CABG/CPB	3.29	87
CMA1	−1905A>G	CABG/CPB	n.r.	31
PAI-1	4G/5G	CABG	n.r.	81
Perioperative Vasoplegia, Vascular Reactivity, Coronary Tone				
DDAH II	−449G>C	Cardiac/CPB	0.4	93
NOS3	E298D		n.r.	90, 189
ACE	In/del		n.r.	34, 91
ADRB2	Q27E	Tracheal intubation	11.7[b]	92
GNB3	825C>T	Response to α-AR agonists	n.r.	189
PON1	Q192R	Resting coronary tone	n.r.	189
Postoperative Arrhythmias: Atrial Fibrillation, QTc Prolongation				
IL6	−174G>C	CABG/CPB beta-blocker failure,	3.25 n.r. 1.8	96, 98
		Thoracic		190, 72
RANTES	−403G>A	Beta-blocker failure	n.r.	190
TNFA	−308G>A	Thoracic	2.5	72
IL1B	−511T>C 5810G>A	Cardiac/CPB	1.44, 0.66	191
Postoperative MACE, Late Vein Graft Failure				
ADRB1	R389G	Noncardiac with spinal block	1.87[c]	89
ACE	In/del	CABG/CPB	3.1[d]	71
ITGB3	L33P		4.7	84
MTHFR	A222V	PTCA and CABG/CBP	2.8	192
ADRB2	R16G, Q27E	Cardiac surgery/CPB	1.96, 2.82	105
HP	Hp1/Hp2	CABG	n.r.	70
CR1,KDR, MICA				
HLA-DPB1, VTN		CABG/CPB	n.r.	32
LPL	HindIII		n.r.	193
Cardiac Allograft Rejection				
TNFA	−308G>A	Cardiac transplant	n.r.	194
IL10	−1082G>A		n.r.	194
ICAM1	K469E		n.r.	195
IL1RN	86-bp VNTR	Thoracic transplant	2.02	196
IL1B	3953C>T		20.5[e]	196

OR, odds ratio; IL6, interleukin 6; CPB, cardiopulmonary bypass; ICAM-1, intercellular adhesion molecule 1; SELE, E selectin; MBL2, mannose binding lectin 2; CABG, coronary artery bypass graft; ITGB3, glycoprotein IIIa; GP1BA, glycoprotein Ibα; TNFA, tumor necrosis factor-α; TNFB, tumor necrosis factor-β; LTA, lymphotoxin-α; IL10, interleukin 10; n.r., not reported; F5, factor V; FVL, factor V Leiden; CMA1, heart chymase; PAI-1, plasminogen activator inhibitor 1; DDAH II, dimethylarginine dimethyl aminohydrolase II; NOS3, endothelial nitric oxide synthase; ACE, angiotensin-converting enzyme; In/del, insertion/deletion; ADRB2, β$_2$-adrenergic receptor; GNB3, G-protein β3 subunit; α-AR, α-adrenergic receptor; PON1, paraoxonase 1; RANTES, regulated on activation normally T-expressed and secreted; IL1B, interleukin 1β; ADRB1, β$_1$-adrenergic receptor; MTHFR, methylenetetrahydrofolate reductase; PTCA, percutaneous transluminal coronary angioplasty; HP, haptoglobin; CR1, complement component 3b/4b; KDR, kinase inert domain receptor; MICA, MHC I polypeptide; HLA-DPB1, β chain of class II major histocompatibility complex; VTN, vitronectin; LPL, lipoprotein lipase; IL1RN, interleukin 1 receptor antagonist; VNTR, variable number tandem repeat.
[a]Relative risk.
[b]F-value.
[c]Hazard ratio.
[d]β-coefficient.
[e]In haplotype with IL1RN VNTR.

allele),[75] several variants in the tumor necrosis factor genes (*TNFA*-308G>A, *LTA*+250G>A),[76] and a functional SNP in the macrophage migration inhibitory factor[77] have been associated with proinflammatory effects in patients undergoing CPB, and in some instances with postoperative ventricular dysfunction.[78] In addition, a genetic variant modulating the release of the anti-inflammatory cytokine interleukin 10 (*IL10*) in response to CPB has been reported (*IL10*-1082G>A),[79] with high levels of IL10 being associated with postoperative ventricular dysfunction.[79]

Coagulation Variability and Perioperative Myocardial Outcomes. In addition to robust inflammatory activation, the host response to surgery is also characterized by an increase in fibrinogen concentration, platelet adhesiveness, and plasminogen activator inhibitor-1 (PAI-1) production (see Chapter 16). During cardiac surgery, alterations in the hemostatic system are even more complex and multifactorial, including the effects of hypothermia, hemodilution, and CPB-induced activation of coagulation, fibrinolytic, and inflammatory pathways. Perioperative thrombotic outcomes following cardiac surgery (e.g., coronary graft thrombosis, myocardial infarction, stroke, pulmonary embolism) represent one extreme on a continuum of coagulation dysfunction, with coagulopathy at the other end of the spectrum (see Chapter 16). Pathophysiologically, the balance between bleeding, normal hemostasis, and thrombosis is markedly influenced by the rate of thrombin formation and platelet activation. Recent evidence suggests that genetic variability modulates the activation of each of these mechanistic pathways,[80] suggesting significant heritability of the prothrombotic state (see Table 6-5 for an overview of genetic variants associated with postoperative bleeding).

Several genotypes have been associated with increased risk of coronary graft thrombosis and myocardial injury following CABG. PAI-1 is an important negative regulator of fibrinolytic activity; a variant in the promoter of the *PAI-1* gene, consisting of an insertion (5G)/deletion (4G) polymorphism at position −675, has been consistently associated with changes in the plasma levels of PAI-1. The 4G allele is associated with increased risk of early graft thrombosis after CABG[81] and, in a recent meta-analysis, with increased incidence of myocardial infarction.[82] Similarly, a polymorphism in the platelet glycoprotein IIIa gene (*ITGB3*), resulting in increased platelet aggregation (Pl[A2] polymorphism), is associated with higher postoperative levels of troponin I following CABG[83] and increased risk for 1-year thrombotic coronary graft occlusion, myocardial infarction, and death following CABG.[84] On the other hand, in patients undergoing major vascular surgery, two SNPs in platelet glycoprotein receptors (*ITGB3* and *GP1BA*) are independent risk predictors of PMI and result in improved discrimination of an ischemia risk assessment tool when added to historic and procedural risk factors.[85] One of the most common inherited prothrombotic risk factors is a point mutation in coagulation factor V (1691G>A) resulting in resistance to activated protein C, and referred to as factor V Leiden (FVL). FVL has been associated with various postoperative thrombotic complications following noncardiac surgery (for a review, see Donahue[33]), but interestingly, also associated with a significant reduction in postoperative blood loss and overall risk of transfusion in cardiac surgery patients.[86] In a prospective study of CABG patients with routine 3-month postoperative angiographic follow-up, a higher proportion of FVL carriers had graft occlusion compared to noncarriers.[87]

Genetic Variability and Perioperative Vascular Reactivity. Perioperative stress responses are also characterized by robust sympathetic nervous system activation, known to play a role in the pathophysiology of PMI, thus patients with CAD and specific adrenergic receptor (AR) genetic polymorphisms may be particularly susceptible to catecholamine toxicity and cardiac complications. Several functionally important SNPs modulating AR pathways have been characterized (for review, see Zaugg et al.[88]). One such variant, the Arg389Gly polymorphism in β1-AR gene (*ADRB1*), was recently associated with increased risk of a composite cardiovascular morbidity outcome at 1 year following noncardiac surgery under spinal anesthesia, while perioperative beta-blockade had no significant effect.[89] The authors suggest that proper analysis of future perioperative beta-blocker trials should be stratified by AR genotype, which may help identify patients likely to benefit from this therapy. Significantly increased vascular responsiveness to α-adrenergic stimulation (phenylephrine) was found in carriers of the endothelial nitric oxide synthase 894G>T polymorphism,[90] and angiotensin-converting enzyme (ACE) insertion/deletion (I/D) polymorphism[34,91] undergoing cardiac surgery with CPB. Two studies have reported on the role of β2-AR (*ADRB2*) genetic variants in perioperative vascular reactivity. Increased blood pressure responses to endotracheal intubation have been associated with a common functional *ADRB2* SNP (Glu27).[92] The second study, conducted in the obstetric population, showed that incidence and severity of maternal hypotension following spinal anesthesia for cesarean delivery, as well as the response to treatment, was affected by *ADRB2* genotype (Gly16 and/or Glu27 led to lower vasopressor use for the treatment of hypotension). In cardiac surgery patients, the development of vasoplegic syndrome is one manifestation of the perioperative systemic inflammatory response, but remains poorly predicted by clinical and procedural risk factors. Vasopressor requirement after surgery is associated with a common polymorphism in the dimethylarginine dimethyl aminohydrolase II (*DDAH II*) gene, an important regulator of nitric oxide synthase activity.[93]

Perioperative Atrial Fibrillation

New-onset perioperative atrial fibrillation (PoAF) remains a common complication of cardiac and major noncardiac thoracic surgical procedures (incidence 27 to 40%), and is associated with increased morbidity, hospital length of stay, rehospitalization, health care costs, and reduced survival. Several large prospective multicenter trials have developed and validated comprehensive risk indices for occurrence of PoAF based on demographic, clinical, electrocardiographic, and procedural risk factors, but their predictive accuracy remains at best moderate,[94] suggesting an inherent genetic preoperative risk. Heritable forms of AF occur in the ambulatory nonsurgical population, and it appears that both monogenic forms like "lone" AF as well as polygenic predisposition to more common acquired forms like PoAF do exist.[95] Recently, a team led by researchers at deCODE genetics (Reykjavik, Iceland) reported the results of a genomewide association study for AF; two polymorphisms on chromosome 4q25 demonstrated a highly significant association ($p = 3.3 \times 10^{-41}$) with AF,[47] with findings replicated in other populations from Sweden, the United States, and Hong Kong, although the mechanism of action for these variants remains unknown. On the other hand, candidate susceptibility genes for PoAF include those determining action, potential duration (voltage-gated ion channels, ion transporters), responses to extracellular factors (adrenergic and other hormone receptors, heat shock proteins), remodeling processes, and magnitude of inflammatory and oxidative stress. In particular, a role for inflammation for PoAF is suggested by the fact that baseline C-reactive protein (CRP) levels in male patients and exaggerated postoperative leukocytosis both predict PoAF, whereas postoperative administration of non-steroidal anti-inflammatory drugs shows a protective effect. However, specific evidence for a genetic role in PoAF is sparse. A functional SNP in the *IL6* promoter (−174G>C) is associated with plasma perioperative IL-6 levels and several clinical outcomes after CABG surgery, including PoAF[96,97], and independently validated.[98] Additionally, polymorphisms in two inflammatory genes (*IL6* and *TNFA*) are associated with composite postoperative morbidity (including new-onset arrhythmias) following lung resection procedures.[72] There is however a contradictory lack of association between CRP levels (strongly regulated by IL-6) and PoAF in women undergoing cardiac surgery.[99] On the other hand, a recent study reported that of 21 serum biomarkers investigated in relationship with PoAF, both pre- and postoperative PAI-1 levels are independently associated with development of PoAF following cardiac surgery.[100]

Several groups have investigated transcriptional responses to AF in human atrial appendage myocardium obtained at the time of cardiac surgery or in preclinical animal models (Table 6-2), and identified a ventricularlike genomic signature in fibrillating atria, with increased ratios of ventricular to atrial isoforms, suggesting dedifferentiation.[101] Although it remains unclear whether this "ventricularization" of atrial gene expression reflects cause or effect of AF, it nevertheless seems to represent an adaptive energy-saving process to the high metabolic demand of fibrillating atrial myocardium, akin to chronic hibernation. A recent study investigating gene expression changes in peripheral blood leukocytes in relationship to PoAF following cardiac surgery has suggested that patients who exhibit PoAF display a differential genomic response to CPB, characterized by up-regulation of oxidative stress genes, which correlated with a significantly larger increase in oxidant stress both systemically (as measured by total peroxide levels) as well as at the myocardial level (as measured in the right atrium).[102]

Cardiac Allograft Rejection

Identification of peripheral blood gene- and protein-based biomarkers to noninvasively monitor, diagnose, and predict perioperative cardiac allograft rejection is an area of rapid scientific growth (see Chapter 54). While several polymorphisms in genes involved in alloimmune interactions, the renin-angiotensin-aldosterone system and the transforming growth factor-β superfamily have been associated with cardiac transplant outcomes, their relevance as useful clinical monitoring tools remains uncertain. However, peripheral blood mononuclear cell-based molecular assays have shown much promise for monitoring the dynamic responses of the immune system to the transplanted heart, discriminating immunologic allograft quiescence and predicting future rejection.[103] A noninvasive molecular test to identify patients at risk for acute cellular rejection is commercially available (AlloMap, XDx Brisbane, CA), in which the expression levels of 20 genes is measured by quantitative real-time polymerase chain reaction (qRT-PCR) and translated using a mathematical algorithm into a clinically actionable AlloMap score that enhances the ability to deliver personalized monitoring and treatment to heart transplant patients. Furthermore, several clinically available protein-based biomarkers of alloimmune activation, microvascular injury (troponins), systemic inflammation (CRP), and wall stress and remodeling (brain natriuretic peptide) correlate well with allograft failure and vasculopathy and have good negative predictive values, but require additional studies to guide their clinical use. Similarly, molecular signatures of functional recovery in end-stage heart failure following left ventricular assist device support using gene expression profiling have been reported,[104] and could be used to monitor patients who received a left ventricular assist device as destination therapy or assess the timing of potential device explantation.

Genetic Variability and Postoperative Event-Free Survival

Several large randomized clinical trials examining the benefits of CABG surgery and percutaneous coronary interventions relative to medical therapy and/or to one another have refined our knowledge of early and long-term survival after CABG. While these studies have helped define the subgroups of patients who benefit from surgical revascularization, they also demonstrated a substantial variability in long-term survival after CABG, altered by important demographic and environmental risk factors. Increasing evidence suggests that the *ACE* gene indel polymorphism may influence post-CABG complications, with carriers of the *D* allele having higher mortality and restenosis rates after CABG surgery compared with the *I* allele.[71] As previously discussed, a prothrombotic amino acid alteration in the β3-integrin chain of the glycoprotein IIb/IIIa platelet receptor (the Pl^{A2} polymorphism) is associated with an increased risk (OR 4.7) for major adverse cardiac events (a composite of myocardial infarction, coronary bypass graft occlusion, or death) following CABG surgery (Table 6-3).[84] We found preliminary evidence for association of two functional polymorphisms modulating β$_2$-adrenergic receptor activity (Arg16Gly and Gln27Glu) with incidence of death or major adverse cardiac events following cardiac surgery,[105] and recently identified two functional polymorphisms in apolipoprotein E (*APOE*-219G>T, OR 0.46) and thrombomodulin (*THBD* Ala455Val, OR 2.64) genes associated with altered 5-year mortality after CABG independent of EuroSCORE.[106]

Genetic Susceptibility to Adverse Perioperative Neurologic Outcomes

6 Despite advances in surgical and anesthetic techniques, significant neurologic morbidity continues to occur following cardiac surgery, ranging in severity from coma and focal stroke (incidence 1 to 3%) to more subtle cognitive deficits (incidence up to 69%), with a substantial impact on the risk of perioperative death, quality of life, and resource utilization. Variability in the reported incidence of both early and late neurologic deficits remains poorly explained by procedural risk factors, suggesting that environmental (operative) and genetic factors may interact to determine disease onset, progression, and recovery (see Chapter 41). The pathophysiology of perioperative neurologic injury is thought to involve complex interactions between primary pathways associated with atherosclerosis and thrombosis, and secondary response pathways like inflammation, vascular reactivity, and direct cellular injury. Many functional genetic variants have been reported in each of these mechanistic pathways involved in modulating the magnitude and the response to neurologic injury, which may have implications in chronic as well as acute perioperative neurocognitive outcomes. For example, Grocott at al.[107] examined 26 SNPs in relationship to the incidence of acute postoperative ischemic stroke in 1,635 patients undergoing cardiac surgery and found that the interaction of minor alleles of the CRP (1846C>T) and IL-6 promoter SNP-174G>C significantly increases the risk of acute stroke. Similarly, a recent study suggests that P selectin and *CRP* genes both contribute to modulating the susceptibility to postoperative cognitive decline (POCD) following cardiac surgery.[27] Specifically, the loss-of-function minor alleles of *CRP* 1059G>C and *SELP* 1087G>A are independently associated with a *reduction* in the observed incidence of POCD after adjustment for known clinical and demographic covariates (Table 6-4).

TABLE 6-4

REPRESENTATIVE GENETIC POLYMORPHISMS ASSOCIATED WITH ALTERED SUSCEPTIBILITY TO ADVERSE PERIOPERATIVE NEUROLOGIC EVENTS

■ GENE	■ POLYMORPHISM	■ TYPE OF SURGERY	■ OR	■ REFERENCE
Perioperative Stroke				
IL6	−174G>C	Cardiac/CPB	3.3	107
CRP	1846C>T			
Perioperative Cognitive Dysfunction, Neurodevelopmental Dysfunction				
SELP	E298D	Cardiac/CPB	0.51	27
CRP	1059G>C	Cardiac/CPB	0.37	27
ITGB3	L33P (Pl$_{A1}$/Pl$_{A2}$)	Cardiac/CPB	n.r.	26
APOE	ε4	CABG/CPB (adults)	n.r. 7,	25,
	ε2	Cardiac/CPB (children)	11	115, 116
Postoperative Delirium				
APOE	ε4	Major noncardiac, critically ill	3.64, 7.32	113, 114

OR, odds ratio; IL6, interleukin 6; CPB, cardiopulmonary bypass; CRP, C-reactive protein; SELP, P selectin; ITGB3, platelet glycoprotein IIIa; n.r., not reported; APOE, apolipoprotein E; CABG, coronary artery bypass graft.

SCIENTIFIC FOUNDATIONS OF ANESTHESIA

Our group has demonstrated a significant association between the apolipoprotein E (*APOE*) E4 genotype and adverse cerebral outcomes in cardiac surgery patients.[25,108] This is consistent with the role of the *APOE* genotype in recovery from acute brain injury, such as intracranial hemorrhage,[109] closed head injury,[110] and stroke,[111] as well as experimental models of cerebral ischemia-reperfusion injury[112]; two subsequent studies in CABG patients, however, have not replicated these initial findings. Furthermore, the incidence of postoperative delirium following major noncardiac surgery in the elderly[113] and in critically ill patients[114] is increased in carriers of the *APOE* ε4 allele. Unlike adult cardiac surgery patients, infants possessing the *APOE* ε2 allele are at increased risk for developing adverse neurodevelopmental sequelae following cardiac surgery.[115,116] The mechanisms by which the *APOE* genotypes might influence neurologic outcomes have yet to be determined, but do not seem to be related to alterations in global cerebral blood flow of oxygen metabolism during CPB[117]; however, genotypic effects in modulating the inflammatory response,[75] extent of aortic atheroma burden,[118] and risk for premature coronary atherosclerosis[119] may play a role.

Recent studies have suggested a role for platelet activation in the pathophysiology of adverse neurologic sequelae. Genetic variants in surface platelet membrane glycoproteins, important mediators of platelet adhesion and platelet-platelet interactions, have been shown to increase the susceptibility to prothrombotic events. Among these, the Pl^{A2} polymorphism in glycoprotein IIb/IIIa has been related to various adverse thrombotic outcomes, including acute coronary thrombosis[120] and atherothrombotic stroke.[121] We found the Pl^{A2} allele to be associated with more severe neurocognitive decline after CPB,[26] which could represent exacerbation of platelet-dependent thrombotic processes associated with plaque embolism.

Cardiac surgical patients who develop POCD demonstrate inherently different genetic responses to CPB from those without POCD, as evidenced by acute deregulation in peripheral blood leukocytes of gene expression pathways involving inflammation, antigen presentation, and cellular adhesion.[122] These findings corroborate with proteomic changes, in which patients with POCD similarly have significantly higher serologic inflammatory indices compared with those patients without POCD,[123,124] and add to the increasing level of evidence that CPB does not cause an indiscriminate variation in gene expression, but rather distinct patterns in specific pathways that are highly associated with the development of postoperative complications such as POCD. The implications for perioperative medicine include identifying populations at risk who might benefit not only from an improved informed consent, stratification, and resource allocation, but also from targeted anti-inflammatory strategies.

Genetic Susceptibility to Adverse Perioperative Renal Outcomes

Acute renal dysfunction is a common, serious complication of cardiac surgery; about 8 to 15% of patients develop moderate renal injury (>1.0 mg/dL peak creatinine rise), and up to 5% of them develop renal failure requiring dialysis.[125] Acute renal failure is independently associated with in-hospital mortality rates, exceeding 60% in patients requiring dialysis.[125] Several studies have demonstrated that inheritance of genetic polymorphisms in the *APOE* gene (ε4 allele)[30] and in the promoter region of the *IL6* gene (−174C allele)[97] are associated with acute kidney injury following CABG surgery (Table 6-5). Stafford-Smith et al.[28] have reported that major differences in peak postoperative serum creatinine rise after CABG are predicted by possession of combinations of polymorphisms that interestingly differ by race: the angiotensinogen (*AGT*) 842T>C and *IL6* −572G>C variants in whites, and the endothelial nitric oxide synthase (*NOS3*) 894G>T and angiotensin-converting enzyme (*ACE*) insertion/deletion in African Americans are associated with more than 50% reduction in postoperative glomerular filtration rate. Further identification of genotypes predictive of adverse perioperative renal outcomes may facilitate individually tailored therapy, risk stratify the patients for interventional trials targeting the gene product itself, and aid in medical decision-making (e.g., selecting medical over surgical management; see Chapter 52).

Genetic Variants and Risk for Prolonged Postoperative Mechanical Ventilation

Prolonged mechanical ventilation (inability to extubate patient by 24 hours postoperatively) is a significant complication following cardiac surgery, occurring in 5.6% and 10.5% of

TABLE 6-5

REPRESENTATIVE GENETIC POLYMORPHISMS ASSOCIATED WITH OTHER ADVERSE PERIOPERATIVE OUTCOMES

▪ GENE	▪ POLYMORPHISM	▪ TYPE OF SURGERY	▪ OR	▪ REFERENCE
Perioperative Thrombotic Events				
F5	FVL	Noncardiac, Cardiac	n.r.	33
Perioperative Bleeding				
F5	R506Q(FVL)	Cardiac/CPB	-1.25^a	86
PAI-1	4G/5G		10^b	197
ITGA2	−52C>T, 807C>T		-0.15^a	198
GP1BA	T145M		-0.22^a	198
TF	−603A>G		-0.03^a	198
TFPI	−399C>T	CABG/CPB	-0.05^a	198
F2	20210G>A		0.38^a	198
ACE	In/del		0.15^a	198
ITGB3	L33P (Pl$_{A1}$/Pl$_{A2}$)		n.r.	199
PAI-1	4G/5G	Cardiac/CPB	10^b	197
TNFA	−238G>A	Brain AVM treatment	3.5^c	200
APOE	ε2		10.9^c	200
Perioperative Acute Kidney Injury				
IL6	−572G>C		20.04^d	28
AGT	M235T	CABG/CPB	32.19^d	28
NOS3	E298D		4.29^d	28
APOE	ε4		-0.13^a	28, 30
Perioperative Severe Sepsis				
APOE	ε3		0.28^e	36

OR, odds ratio; F5, factor V; FVL, factor V Leiden; n.r., not reported; CPB, cardiopulmonary bypass; PAI-1, plasminogen activator inhibitor 1; ITGA2, glycoprotein IaIIa; GP1BA, glycoprotein Ibα; TF, tissue factor; TFPI, tissue factor pathway inhibitor; CABG, coronary artery bypass graft; F2, prothrombin; ACE, angiotensin-converting enzyme; In/del, insertion/deletion; ITGB3, glycoprotein IIIa; TNFA, tumor necrosis factor-α; AVM, arteriovenous malformation; APOE, apolipoprotein E; IL6, interleukin 6; AGT, angiotensinogen; NOS3, endothelial nitric oxide synthase.
^{a}β coefficient.
^{b}Odds ratio.
^{c}Hazard ratio.
^{d}F-value.
^{e}Relative risk.

patients undergoing first and repeat CABG surgery, respectively.[126] Several pulmonary and nonpulmonary causes have been identified, and scoring systems based on preoperative and procedural risk factors have been proposed and validated. Recently, genetic variants in the renin-angiotensin pathway and in proinflammatory cytokine genes have been associated with respiratory complications post-CPB. The D allele of a common functional insertion/deletion polymorphism in the angiotensin-converting enzyme (ACE) gene, accounting for 47% of variance in circulating ACE levels,[127] is associated with prolonged mechanical ventilation following CABG[128] and with susceptibility to and prognosis of acute respiratory distress syndrome.[129] Furthermore, a hyposecretory haplotype in the neighboring genes tumor necrosis factor-α (TNFA) and lymphotoxin-α (LTA) on chromosome 6 (TNFA-308G/LTA+250G haplotype)[130] and a functional polymorphism modulating postoperative IL-6 levels (IL6-174G>C)[97] are independently associated with higher risk of prolonged mechanical ventilation post-CABG. The association is more dramatic in patients undergoing conventional CABG than in those undergoing off-pump CABG, suggesting that in high-risk patients identified by preoperative genetic screening, off-pump CABG may be the optimal surgical procedure.

A next crucial step in understanding the complexity of adverse perioperative outcomes is to assess the contribution of variations in many genes simultaneously and their interaction with traditional risk factors to the longitudinal prediction of outcomes in individual patients. The use of such outcome predictive models incorporating genetic information may help stratify mortality and morbidity in surgical patients, improve prognostication, direct medical decision-making both intraoperatively and during postoperative follow-up, and even suggest novel targets for therapeutic intervention in the perioperative period.

PHARMACOGENOMICS AND ANESTHESIA

Interindividual variability in response to drug therapy, both in terms of efficacy and safety, is a rule by which anesthesiologists live. In fact, much of the art of anesthesiology is the astute clinician being prepared to deal with outliers. The term *pharmacogenomics* is used to describe how inherited variations in genes modulating drug actions are related to interindividual variability in drug response (see Chapter 7). Such variability in drug action may be *pharmacokinetic* or *pharmacodynamic* (Fig. 6-4). Pharmacokinetic variability refers to variability in a drug's absorption, distribution, metabolism, and excretion that mediates its efficacy and/or toxicity. The molecules involved in these processes include drug-metabolizing enzymes (such as members of the cytochrome P450, or CYP superfamily), and drug-transport molecules that mediate drug uptake into, and efflux from, intracellular sites. Pharmacodynamic variability refers to variable drug effects despite equivalent drug delivery to molecular sites of action. This may reflect variability in the function of the molecular target of the drug, or in the pathophysiological context in which the drug

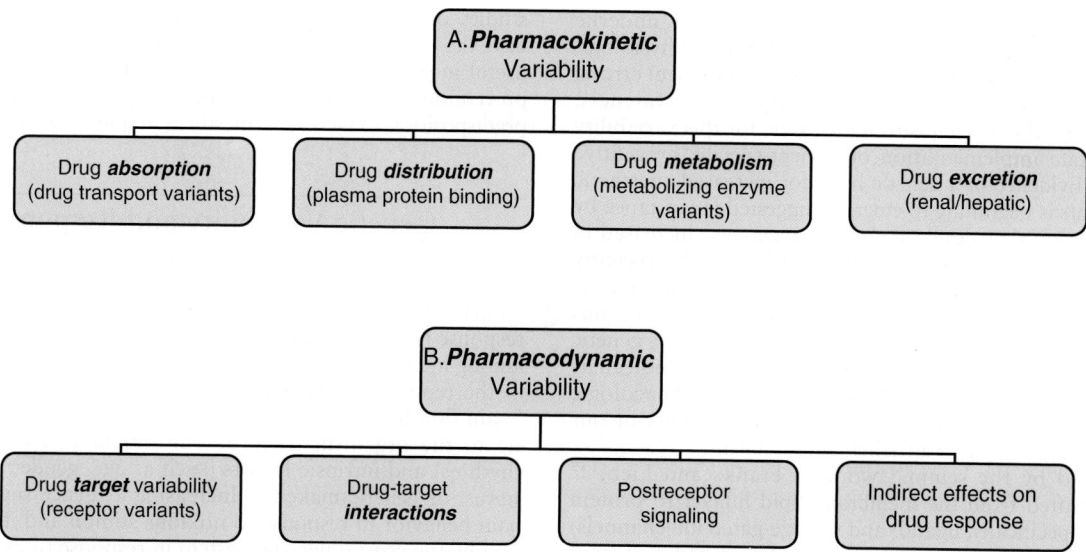

FIGURE 6-4.   Pharmacogenomic determinants of individual drug response operate by pharmacokinetic and pharmacodynamic mechanisms. **A.** Genetic variants in *drug transporters* (e.g., ATP-binding cassette subfamily B member 1 or *ABCB1* gene) and *drug-metabolizing enzymes* (e.g., cytochrome P450 2D6 or *CYP2D6* gene, *CYP2C9* gene, *N*-acetyltransferase or *NAT2* gene, plasma cholinesterase or *BCHE* gene) are responsible for *pharmacokinetic* variability in drug response. **B.** Polymorphisms in *drug targets* (e.g., β_1- and β_2–adrenergic receptor *ADRB1*, *ADRB2* genes; angiotensin-I converting enzyme *ACE* gene), *postreceptor signaling molecules* (e.g., guanine nucleotide binding protein $\beta3$ or *GNB3* gene), or *molecules indirectly affecting drug response* (e.g., various ion channel genes involved in drug-induced arrhythmias) are sources of *pharmacodynamic* variability.

interacts with its receptor-target (e.g., affinity, coupling, expression).[131] Thus, pharmacogenomics investigates complex, polygenically determined phenotypes of drug efficacy or toxicity, with the goal of identifying novel therapeutic targets and customizing drug therapy.

Pseudocholinesterase Deficiency

Historically, characterization of the genetic basis for plasma pseudocholinesterase deficiency in 1956 was of fundamental importance to anesthesia and the further development and understanding of genetically determined differences in drug response.[132] Individuals with an atypical form of pseudocholinesterase resulting in a markedly reduced rate of drug metabolism are at risk for excessive neuromuscular blockade and prolonged apnea. More than 20 variants have since been identified in the butyrylcholinesterase gene (*BCHE*), the most common of which are the A-variant (209A>G) and the K-variant (1615G>A), with various and somewhat poorly defined phenotypic consequences on prolonged neuromuscular blockade. Therefore, pharmacogenetic testing is currently not recommended in the population at large, but only as an explanation for an adverse event.[133]

Genetics of Malignant Hyperthermia

Malignant hyperthermia (MH) is a rare autosomal dominant genetic disease of skeletal muscle calcium metabolism, triggered by administration of general anesthesia with volatile anesthetic agents or succinylcholine in susceptible individuals. The clinical MH syndrome is characterized by skeletal muscle hypermetabolism and manifested as skeletal muscle rigidity, tachycardia, tachypnea, hemodynamic instability, increased oxygen consumption and CO_2 production, lactic acidosis and

fever, progressing to malignant ventricular arrhythmias, disseminated intravascular coagulation, and myoglobinuric renal failure. MH susceptibility has been initially linked to the ryanodine receptor (*RYR1*) gene locus on chromosome 19q.[134] However, subsequent studies have shown that MH may represent a common severe phenotype that originates not only from point mutations in the *RYR1* gene (Arg614Cys), but also within its functionally and/or structurally associated proteins regulating excitation-contraction coupling (such as $\alpha 1DHPR$ and *FKBP12*). It is becoming increasingly apparent that MH susceptibility results from a complex interaction between multiple genes and environment (such as environmental toxins), suggested by the heterogeneity observed in the clinical MH syndrome and the variable penetrance of the MH phenotype.[135] Current diagnostic methods (the caffeine-halothane contracture test) are invasive and potentially nonspecific. Unfortunately, because of the polygenic determinism and variable penetrance, direct DNA testing in the general population for susceptibility to MH is currently not recommended; in contrast, testing in individuals from families with affected individuals has the potential to greatly reduce mortality and morbidity.[133] Furthermore, genomic approaches may help elucidate the molecular mechanisms involved in altered RYR1-mediated calcium signaling and identify novel, more specific therapeutic targets.

Genetic Variability and Response to Anesthetic Agents

Anesthetic potency, defined by the minimum alveolar concentration (MAC) of an inhaled anesthetic that abolishes purposeful movement in response to a noxious stimulus, varies among individuals, with a coefficient of variation (the ratio of standard deviation to the mean) of approximately 10%[36] (see Chapter 7). This observed variability may be explained by interindividual differences in multiple genes that underlie responsiveness to anesthetics, by environmental or physiological factors (brain temperature, age), or by measurement errors. With growing public concern over intraoperative awareness, understanding the mechanisms responsible for this variability may facilitate implementation of patient-specific preventive strategies. Evidence of a genetic basis for increased anesthetic requirements is beginning to emerge, suggested for instance by the observation that desflurane requirements are increased in subjects with red hair versus dark hair,[137] and by recently reported variability in the immobilizing dose of sevoflurane (as much as 24%) in populations with different ethnic (and thus genetic) backgrounds.[138] Several studies evaluating the genetic control of anesthetic responses, coupled with molecular modeling, proteomic, neurophysiology, and pharmacologic approaches, have provided important developments in our understanding of general anesthetic mechanisms.

Triggered by the seminal work of Franks and Lieb,[139] research shifted from the membrane lipid bilayer to protein receptors (specifically, ligand- and voltage-gated ion channels) as potential anesthetic targets, ending a few decades of stagnation that were primarily due to an almost universal acceptance of the dogma of nonspecific anesthetic action (the so-called lipid theory). Some of the genes responsible for phenotypic differences in anesthetic effects have been mapped in various animal models and, following genomic manipulation of plausible candidate receptors to investigate their function in vitro, were evaluated in genetically engineered animals for their relationship to various anesthetic end points, such as immobility (i.e., MAC), hypnosis, amnesia, and analgesia (for review, see Sonner et al.[140]). Several thousand different strains of knockout mice have been created and are used to investigate specific functions of particular genes and mechanisms of drug action, including the sensitivity to general anesthetic in animals lacking the $\beta3$ subunit[141] or the $\alpha6$ subunit[142] of the GABA$_A$ receptor. On the other hand, *knockin* animals express a site-directed mutation in the targeted gene that remains under the control of endogenous regulatory elements, allowing the mutated gene to be expressed in the same amount, at the same time, and in the same tissues as the normal gene. This method has provided remarkable insight into the mechanisms of action of benzodiazepines[143] and intravenous anesthetics. In a seminal study by Jurd et al.,[145] a point mutation in the gene encoding the $\beta3$ subunit of the GABA$_A$ receptor previously known to render the receptor insensitive to etomidate and propofol in vitro,[144] was validated in vivo by creating a knockin mouse strain that proved also essentially insensitive to the immobilizing actions of etomidate and propofol. A point mutation in the $\beta2$ subunit of the GABA$_A$ receptor results in a knockin mouse with reduced sensitivity to the sedative[146] and hypothermic effects[147] of etomidate. Knockin mice harboring point mutations in the α_2A-adrenergic receptor have enabled the elucidation of the role of this receptor in anesthetic-sparing, analgesic, and sedative responses to dexmedetomidine.[148]

The situation is far more complex for inhaled anesthetics, which appear to mediate their effects by acting on several receptor targets. Based on combined pharmacologic and genetic *in vivo* studies to date, several receptors are unlikely to be direct mediators of MAC, including the GABA$_A$ (despite their compelling role in intravenous anesthetic-induced immobility), 5-HT3, AMPA, kainate, acetylcholine and α2-adrenergic receptors, and potassium channels.[149] Glycine, NMDA receptors and sodium channels remain likely candidates.[140] These conclusions, however, do not apply to other anesthetic endpoints, such as hypnosis, amnesia and analgesia. Several preclinical proteomic analyses have identified in a more unbiased way a group of potential anesthetic targets for halothane,[61] desflurane,[62] and sevoflurane,[63] which should provide the basis for more focused

studies of anesthetic binding sites. Such "omic" approaches have the potential to evolve into preoperative screening profiles useful in guiding individualized therapeutic decisions, such as prevention of anesthetic awareness in patients with a genetic predisposition to increased anesthetic requirements.

Genetic Variability and Response to Pain

Similar to the observed variability in anesthetic potency, the response to painful stimuli and analgesic manipulations varies among individuals (see Chapter 57). The sources of variability in the report and experience of pain and analgesia (i.e., the "pain threshold") are multifactorial, including factors extrinsic to the organism (such as cultural factors or circadian rhythms) and intrinsic factors (such as age, gender, hormonal status, or genetic makeup). Increasing evidence suggests that pain behavior in response to noxious stimuli and its modulation by the central nervous system in response to drug administration or environmental stress, as well as the development of persistent pain conditions through pain amplification, are strongly influenced by genetic factors.[150–152]

Results from studies in twins[153] and inbred mouse strains[154] indicate a moderate heritability for chronic pain syndromes and nociceptive sensitivity, which appears to be mediated by multiple genes (see Chapter 58). Various strains of knockout mice lacking target genes like neurotrophins and their receptors (e.g., nerve growth factor), peripheral mediators of nociception and hyperalgesia (e.g., substance P), opioid and nonopioid transmitters and their receptors, and intracellular signaling molecules have significantly contributed to the understanding of pain-processing mechanisms.[155] A locus responsible for 28% of phenotypic variance in magnitude of systemic morphine analgesia in mice has been mapped to chromosome 10, in or near the *OPRM* (μ-opioid receptor) gene. The μ-opioid receptor is also subject to pharmacodynamic variability; polymorphisms in the promoter region of the *OPRM* gene modulating interleukin-4–mediated gene expression have been correlated with morphine antinociception. The much quoted *OPRM* 188A>G polymorphism is associated with decreased responses to morphine-6-glucuronide, resulting in altered analgesic requirements, but also reduced incidence of postoperative nausea and vomiting, and reduced risks of toxicity in patients with renal failure. Conversely, variants of the melanocortin 1 receptor (*MC1R*) gene, which produce a red hair-fair skin phenotype, are associated with increased analgesic responses to κ-opioid agonists in women but not men, providing evidence for a gene-by-gender interaction in regulating analgesic response (for a review, see Somogyi et al.[156]). Very recent reports suggest that peripherally located β_2-adrenergic receptors (*ADRB2*) also contribute to basal pain sensitivity, the development of chronic pain states, as well as opioid-induced hyperalgesia.[152] Functionally important haplotypes in the *ADRB2*(151) and catechol-O-methyltransferase (*COMT*)[157] genes are associated with enhanced pain sensitivity in humans.

In addition to the genetic control of peripheral nociceptive pathways, considerable evidence exists for genetic variability in the descending central pain modulatory pathways, further explaining the interindividual variability in analgesic responsiveness. One good example relevant to analgesic efficacy is cytochrome P450D6 (*CYP2D6*), a member of the superfamily of microsomal enzymes that catalyze phase I drug metabolism, and responsible for the metabolism of a large number of therapeutic compounds. The relationship between the *CYP2D6* genotype and the enzyme metabolic rate has been extensively characterized, with at least 12 known mutations leading to a tetramodal distribution CYP2D6 activity: ultrarapid metabolizers (5 to 7% of the population), extensive metabolizers (60%), intermediate metabolizers (25%), and poor metabolizers (10%). Currently, pharmacogenomic screening tests predict CYP2D6 phenotype with >95% reliability. The consequences of inheriting an allele that compromises CYP2D6 function include the inability to metabolize codeine (a prodrug) to morphine by O-demethylation, leading to lack of analgesia but increased side effects from the parent drug (e.g., fatigue) in poor metabolizers.[133,150]

Genetic Variability in Response to Other Drugs Used Perioperatively

A wide variety of drugs used in the perioperative period display significant pharmacokinetic or pharmacodynamic variability that is genetically modulated (Table 6-6.). Although such genetic variation in drug-metabolizing enzymes or drug targets usually result in unusually variable drug response, genetic markers associated with rare but life-threatening side effects have also been described. Of note, the most commonly cited categories of drugs involved in adverse drug reactions include cardiovascular, antibiotic, psychiatric, and analgesic medications; interestingly, each category has a known genetic basis for increased risk of adverse reactions.

There are more than 30 families of drug-metabolizing enzymes in humans, most with genetic polymorphisms shown to influence enzymatic activity. Of special importance to the anesthesiologist is the CYP2D6, one of the most intensively studied and best understood examples of pharmacogenetic variation, involved in the metabolism of several drugs including analgesics (codeine, dextromethorphan), beta-blockers, antiarrhythmics (flecainide, propafenone,

quinidine), and diltiazem. Another important pharmacogenetic variation has been described in cytochrome P450C9 (CYP2C9), involved in metabolizing anticoagulants (warfarin), anticonvulsants (phenytoin), antidiabetic agents (glipizide, tolbutamide), and nonsteroidal anti-inflammatory drugs (celecoxib, ibuprofen), among others. Three known CYP2C9 variant alleles result in different enzyme activities (extensive, intermediate, and slow metabolizer phenotypes), and have clinical implications in the increased risk of life-threatening bleeding complications in slow metabolizers during standard warfarin therapy. This illustrates the concept of "high-risk pharmacokinetics," which applies to drugs with low therapeutic ratios eliminated by a single pathway (in this case, CYP2C9-mediated oxidation); genetic variation in that pathway may lead to large changes in drug clearance, concentrations, and effects.[131] Dose adjustments based on the pharmacogenetic phenotype have been proposed for drugs metabolized via both CYP2D6 and CYP2C9 pathways,[133] and a commercially available, Food and Drug Administration (FDA)-approved test (CYP450 AmpliChip, Roche Molecular Diagnostics) allows clinicians for the first time to test patients for a wide spectrum of genetic variation in drug-metabolizing enzymes. Using this technology, Candiotti et al.[158] showed that patients carrying either three copies of the CYP2D6 gene, a genotype consistent with ultrarapid metabolism, or both, have an increased risk of ondansetron failure for the prevention of postoperative vomiting but not nausea.[158] The strongest evidence to date for use of pharmacogenomic testing is to aid in the determination of warfarin dosage by using genotypes in the CYP2C9 and vitamin K epoxide reductase complex 1 (VKORC1) genes, and at least four FDA-approved tests are now commercially available.

Genetic variation in drug targets (receptors) can have profound effect on drug efficacy, and more than 25 examples have

TABLE 6-6

EXAMPLES OF GENETIC POLYMORPHISMS INVOLVED IN VARIABLE RESPONSES TO DRUGS USED IN THE PERIOPERATIVE PERIOD

■ DRUG CLASS	■ GENE NAME (GENE SYMBOL)	■ EFFECT OF POLYMORPHISM
Pharmacokinetic variability		
Beta-blockers	Cytochrome P450 2D6 (CYP2D6)	Enhanced drug effect
Codeine, dextromethorphan	CYP2D6	Decreased drug effect
Ca-channel blockers	Cytochrome P450 3A4 (CYP3A4)	Uncertain
Alfentanil	CYP3A4	Enhanced drug response
Angiotensin-II receptor type 1 blockers	Cytochrome P450 2C9 (CYP2C9)	Enhanced blood pressure response
Warfarin	CYP2C9	Enhanced anticoagulant effect, risk of bleeding
Phenytoin	CYP2C9	Enhanced drug effect
ACE-inhibitors	Angiotensin-I converting enzyme (ACE)	Blood pressure response
Procainamide	N-acetyltransferase 2 (NAT2)	Enhanced drug effect
Succinylcholine	Butyrylcholinesterase (BCHE)	Enhanced drug effect
Digoxin	P-glycoprotein (ABCB1, MDR1)	Increased bioavailability
Pharmacodynamic variability		
Beta-blockers	β_1- and β_2-adrenergic receptors (ADRB1, ADRB2)	Blood pressure and heart rate response, airway responsiveness to β_2-agonists
QT-prolonging drugs (e.g., antiarrhythmics, cisapride, erythromycin)	Sodium and potassium ion channels (SCN5A, KCNH2, KCNE2, KCNQ1)	Long QT-syndrome, risk of torsade de pointes
Aspirin, glycoprotein IIb/IIIa inhibitors	Glycoprotein IIIa subunit of platelet glycoprotein IIb/IIIa (ITGB3)	Variability in antiplatelet effects
Phenylephrine	Endothelial nitric oxide synthase (NOS3)	Blood pressure response

already been identified. For example, functional polymorphisms in the β2-AR (Arg16Gly, Gln27Glu) influence the bronchodilator and vascular responses to β-agonists, and β1-AR variants (Arg389Gly) modulate responses to beta-blockers and may impact postoperative cardiovascular adverse events.[88,89]

Finally, clinically important genetic polymorphisms with indirect effects on drug response have been described. These include variants in candidate genes like sodium (SCN5A) and potassium ion channels (KCNH2, KCNE2, KCNQ1), which alter susceptibility to drug-induced long-QT syndrome and ventricular arrhythmias (torsade de pointes) associated with the use of drugs like erythromycin, terfenadine, disopyramide, sotalol, cisapride, or quinidine. Carriers of such susceptibility alleles have no manifest QT-interval prolongation or family history of sudden death until QT-prolonging drug challenge is superimposed.[131] Predisposition to QT-interval prolongation (considered a surrogate for risk of life-threatening ventricular arrhythmias) has been responsible for more drug withdrawals from the market than any other category of adverse event in recent times, so understanding genetic predisposing factors constitutes one of the highest priorities of current pharmacogenomic efforts.

Pharmacogenomics is emerging as an additional modifying component to anesthesia along with age, gender, comorbidities, and medication usage. Specific testing and treatment guidelines allowing clinicians to appropriately modify drug utilization (e.g., adjust dose or change drug) already exist for a few compounds,[133] and will likely be expanded to all relevant therapeutic compounds, together with identification of novel therapeutic targets.

GENOMICS AND CRITICAL CARE

Genetic Variability in Response to Injury

⑪ Systemic injury (including trauma and surgical stress), shock, or infection trigger physiological responses of fever, tachycardia, tachypnea, and leukocytosis that collectively define the systemic inflammatory response syndrome (see Chapter 12). This can progress to severe sepsis, septic shock, and multiple organ dysfunction syndrome, the pathophysiology of which remains poorly understood. With the genomic revolution, a new paradigm has emerged in critical care medicine: outcomes of critical illness are determined by the interplay between the *injury* and *repair* processes triggered by the initial insults.[159] Negative outcomes are thus the combined result of direct tissue injury, the side effects of resulting repair processes, and secondary injury mechanisms leading to suboptimal repair. This concept forms the basis of the new PIRO (Predisposition, Infection/Insult, Response, Organ dysfunction) staging system in critical illness.[160] Genomic factors play a role along this continuum, from inflammatory gene variants and modulators of pathogen-host interaction, to microbial genomics and rapid detection assays to identify pathogens, to biomarkers differentiating infection from inflammation, to dynamic measures of cellular responses to insult, apoptosis, cytopathic hypoxia, and cell stress. Regulation of these mechanisms is currently being extensively investigated at the genomic, proteomic, and pharmacogenomic levels, aiming to model adaptive and maladaptive responses to injury, aid in development of diagnostic indices predictive of injury, monitor progress of repair, and eventually design novel therapeutic modalities that take into account the individual genetic makeup.

The large interindividual variability in the magnitude of response to injury, including activation of inflammatory and coagulation cascades, apoptosis and fibrosis, suggests the involvement of genetic regulatory factors. Several functional genetic polymorphisms in molecules involved in various components of the inflammatory response have been associated

with differences in susceptibility to and mortality from sepsis of different etiologies, including postoperative sepsis. These include polymorphisms in bacterial recognition molecules like lipopolysaccharide binding protein (LBP), bactericidal/permeability increasing protein (BPI), CD14, toll-like receptors (TLR2, TLR4), mannose-binding lectin (MBL), and proinflammatory cytokines like tumor necrosis-α (TNFA), lymphotoxin alpha (LTA), interleukin-1 (IL1) and IL-1 receptor antagonist (IL1RN), and interleukin-6 (IL6) (for reviews, see Lin and Albertson[161] and De Maio et al.[162]). Similarly, functional genetic variants in the PAI-1 (PAI-1) and angiotensin I converting enzyme (ACE) genes have been associated with poor outcomes in sepsis, reflecting the complex interaction between inflammation, coagulation, endothelial function, and vascular tone in the pathogenesis of sepsis-induced organ dysfunction.

This continuing effort to identify initial SNP-disease associations is followed by a process of selecting reliable predictive SNPs by validation in independent populations and determining which and how many markers will maximize the power to predict risk for sepsis or mortality following injury.

Functional Genomics of Injury

At a cellular level, injurious stimuli trigger adaptive stress responses determined by quantitative and qualitative changes in interdigitating cascades of biological pathways interacting in complex, often redundant ways. As a result, numerous clinical trials attempting to block single inflammatory mediators, such as TNFα in sepsis, have been largely unsuccessful.[163] Given these complex interconnections, the standard "single gene" paradigm is insufficient to adequately describe the tissue response to severe systemic stimuli. Instead, organ injury might better be defined by patterns of altered gene and protein expression.[164] As previously discussed, DNA microarray technology has become a powerful high-throughput method of analyzing changes induced by various injuries on a genomewide scale, by quantifying mRNA abundance and generating an expression profile for the cell or tissue of interest. Several studies have reported the gene expression profiles in both critically ill patients and in animal models of sepsis,[165,166] acute lung injury,[167] and burn injury.[168] Using gene expression profiling in peripheral blood neutrophils, Tang et al.[169] have identified a set of 50 signature genes that correctly identified sepsis with a prediction accuracy of 91%. Importantly, this genomic classifier was a stronger predictor of sepsis than physiologic indices and cytokines, such as procalcitonin. Once gene lists are identified, extracting biological information has proven to be one of the most perplexing challenges. In human subjects administered endotoxin, the number of genes whose expression changed in blood leukocytes was >4,000,[170] and in severely traumatized patients, the expression of >6,000 genes changed in peripheral blood leukocytes.[171] It thus became evident that tools had to be developed that could categorize these genes and responses into "functional modules," "interactome maps," and signaling pathways.[170] Two large-scale national programs are using gene and protein expression profiles in circulating leukocytes to investigate the biological reasons behind the extreme variability in patient outcomes after similar traumatic insults (the National Institutes of Health-funded Trauma Glue Grant[a]), and to elucidate regulatory mechanisms in response to septic challenge in high-risk patients (the German National Genome Research Network[b]).[164] Analytical and organizational approaches to a systematic evaluation of the variance associated with genomewide expression analysis in human blood leukocytes in

---

[a]See www.gluegrant.org.
[b]See www.ngfn.de/ngfn_en/index.html.

the "real world" have been reported by these groups, and are very informative in the study of critical illness.[172]

Since only less than half of the changes at mRNA level are usually translated into changes in protein expression, transcriptional profiling has to be complemented by characterizing the injury proteome, for a more complete understanding of the host response to injury. Integrated analysis of neutrophils transcriptome and proteome in response to lipopolysaccharide stimulation has identified up-regulation of a variety of genes, including transcriptional regulators (NF-κB), cytokines (TNFα, IL-6, IL-1β), and chemokines (MCP-1, MIP-3α), and confirmed the poor concordance between transcriptional and translational responses.[173] A recent study has established an extensive reference protein database for trauma patients, providing a foundation for future high-throughput quantitative plasma proteomic investigations of the mechanisms underlying systemic inflammatory responses.[174] Changes in serum proteome associated with sepsis and septic shock have been reported,[175] and may allow rapid subclassification of sepsis syndrome into variants that may better predict responsiveness to fluid resuscitation, intravenous steroids, activated protein C, anti-TNF drugs, or specific antibiotics.[61]

Modeling disease entities like sepsis and multiple organ dysfunction syndrome, which are complex, nonlinear systems, requires not only the ability to measure many diverse molecular events simultaneously, but also to integrate the data using novel analytical tools based on complex systems theory and nonlinear dynamics.[176] Such analysis might help identify the key signaling nodes against which therapeutics can be directed.

FUTURE DIRECTIONS

Systems Biology Approach to Perioperative Medicine: The "Perioptome"

Systems biology is a conceptual framework within which scientists attempt to correlate massive amounts of apparently unrelated data into a single unifying explanation of how biological processes occur.[177] This evolving discipline that merges experimental and computational approaches to observe, record, and integrate information from the molecular, cellular, tissue, and whole organism levels into testable models of a dynamic biological process can be applied to understand the way patients respond to a multidimensional stimulus such as a surgical procedure and the mechanistic basis of perioperative morbidity (Fig. 6-5). Such an approach involves multiple levels

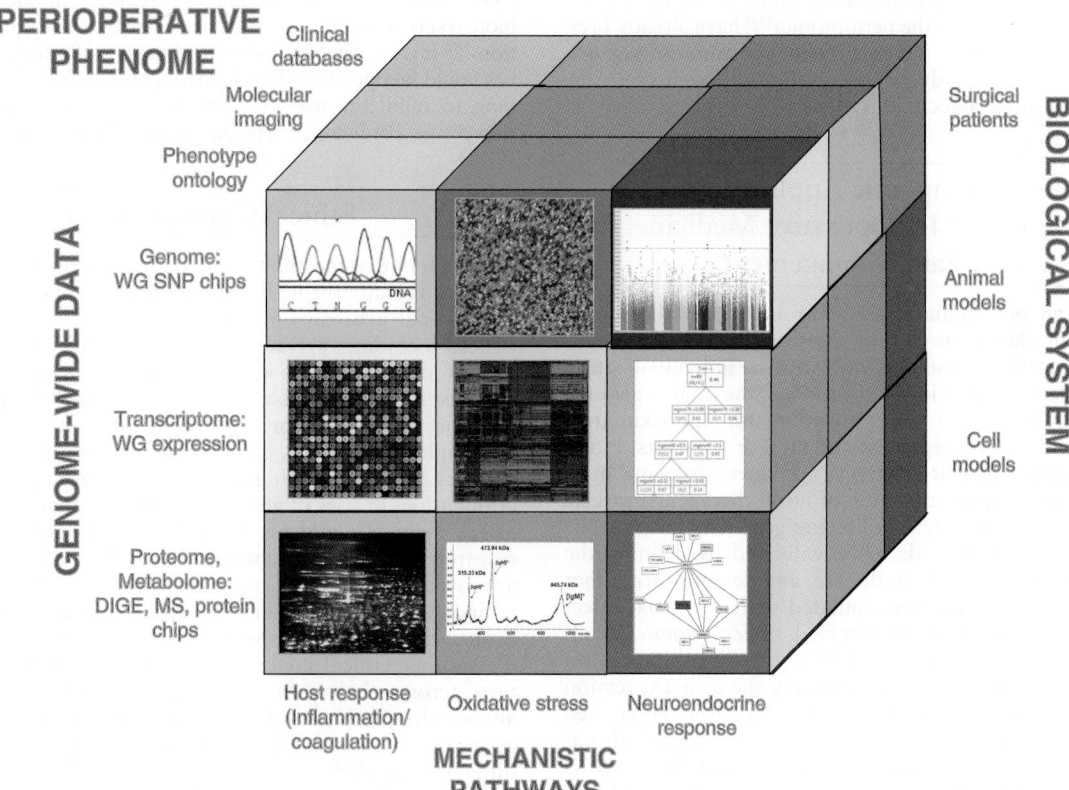

FIGURE 6-5. Levels of integration in perioperative systems biology: the "perioptome." Cellular function is organized as a multilayered set of interdependent processes controlled at the level of the *genome* (DNA), *transcriptome* (messenger RNA), *proteome* (the collection of all proteins encoded within the DNA of a genome), and *metabolome* (the complete set of small-molecule metabolites to be found in a biological system), which can all be interrogated using high-throughput technologies. Accurate representation of the perioperative *phenome* (the set of all perioperative phenotypes expressed by an individual patient) requires integration of standardized phenotype definitions (phenotype ontology), state-of-the-art imaging technologies, and comprehensive clinical data warehousing. Relating genome variability to specific perioperative phenotypes through systems biology approaches involves the orthogonal integration of multiple levels of biological organization provided by genomewide data sets with clinical data and literature data, modeling the regulatory networks involved in adverse perioperative outcomes, and identifying critical regulatory nodes for therapeutic manipulation. WG, whole-genome; SNP, single nucleotide polymorphisms; DIGE, differential in-gel electrophoresis; MS, mass spectrometry.

of data integration. First, delineating the composition of the *perioperative phenome* (the representation of all perioperative phenotypes expressed by a given patient) requires standardized definitions, controlled vocabularies, and data dictionaries (a perioperative phenotype ontology), new (molecular) imaging technologies, and the availability of comprehensive data warehousing capabilities that will allow cataloguing individual perioperative phenotypes as well as correlations between combinations of phenotypes (organ cross-talk, multiple organ failure). Second, orthogonal integration of whole-genome genotypic, transcriptomic, proteomic, and metabolomic data, augmented by more recent functional genomic and proteomic approaches including protein-protein, protein-DNA, or other "component-component" interaction mapping (*interactome*), transcript or protein three-dimensional localization mapping (*localizome*),[178] and literature data within individual biological systems involved in perioperative morbidity. This highest level of data integration is the mapping of the integrated high-throughput static and dynamic genomic data into regulatory networks in order to model interactions of the different components of the system, identify modules of highly interconnected genes, and hub points that can be prioritized as therapeutic targets. Ultimately, mathematical models require experimental validation in animal models of disease or tissue culture, in an iterative process that is one of the core characteristics of systems biology.[179] Such integrative approaches to study cardiovascular function (the Cardiome Project), but also perioperative morbidity (the perioptome)[180] have already been outlined and promise to increase the identification of key drivers of perioperative adverse events beyond what could be achieved by genetic associations alone.

Targeted Therapeutic Applications: The "Five Ps" of Perioperative Medicine and Pain Management

Genomic and proteomic approaches are rapidly becoming platforms for all aspects of drug discovery and development, from target identification and validation to individualization of drug therapy. As previously mentioned, the human genome contains about 25,000 genes encoding for approximately 200,000 proteins that represent potential drug targets. However, only about 120 drug targets are currently being marketed, thus making identification of novel therapeutic targets an area of intense research. Following gene identification, its therapeutic potential needs to be validated by defining the sequence function, its role in disease, and demonstrating that the gene product can be manipulated with beneficial effect and no toxic effects. A developing field, *toxicogenomics*, studies the influence of toxic or potentially toxic substances on different model organisms by evaluating the gene expression changes induced by novel drugs in a given tissue. Sponsored by the National Institutes of Health, a nationwide collaborative effort called the Pharmacogenetics Research Network[c] is aiming to establish a strong pharmacogenomics knowledge base[d], as well as create a shared computational and experimental infrastructure, required to connect human sequence variation with drug responses and translate information into novel therapeutics.

The epidemiologic framework for assessing the applicability of previously identified biomarkers of perioperative morbidity and the successful implementation of molecular diagnostics in perioperative medicine is contingent on demon-

strating their *clinical validity*, *analytical validity*, and *clinical utility*.[181] Perioperative genomic investigators are currently conducting replication studies in different surgical patient populations to formally assess the clinical validity of the markers reported so far. For genomic classifiers, the emphasis during external validation is placed on prospectively testing the accuracy of the entire molecular fingerprint in a new patient population rather than corroborating results in individual genes. In perioperative and critical care settings it is vital to have fast turnaround time (several hours) and easy-to-use testing capabilities, so that meaningful therapeutic interventions can take place. In this regard, new molecular diagnostic systems based on the random access technology such as the GeneXpert (Cepheid, Sunnyvale, CA), eSensor (Osmetech, Pasadena, CA), and Liat Analyzer (Iquum, Marlborough, MA) are already becoming available. Clinical utility (targeted interventions to reduce perioperative morbidity among patients with a certain genomic profile) remains to be evaluated in future genomically stratified perioperative trials. Indeed, a landmark study on the effects of a 5-lipoxygenase-activating protein (FLAP) inhibitor on biomarkers associated with the risk of myocardial infarction demonstrates that by defining at-risk patients for two genes in the leukotriene pathway, one can predict who will respond to targeted drug therapy. Specifically, in patients carrying the at-risk variants in the FLAP and in the leukotriene A4 hydrolase genes, use of a FLAP inhibitor in a randomized controlled trial resulted in significant and dose-dependent suppression of biomarkers associated with increased risk of myocardial infarction.[182] It is expected that similar principles of targeted therapeutics could be operational in the perioperative period, thus beginning to fulfill the five Ps of modern medicine (Personalized, Preventive, Predictive, Participatory, and Prospective).

Ethical Considerations

Although one of the aims of the Human Genome Project is to improve therapy through genome-based prediction, the birth of personal genomics opens up a Pandora's box of ethical issues, including privacy and the risk for discrimination against individuals who are genetically predisposed for a medical disorder. Such discrimination may include barriers to obtaining health, life, or long-term care insurance, or obtaining employment. Thus, extensive efforts are made to protect patients participating in genetic research from prejudice, discrimination, or uses of genetic information that will adversely affect them. To address the concerns of both biomedical research and health communities, the U.S. Senate has approved in 2003 the Genetic Information and Nondiscrimination Act, which provides the strong safeguards required to protect the public participating in human genome research.

Another ethical concern is the transferability of genetic tests across ethnic groups, particularly in the prediction of adverse drug responses. It is known that most polymorphisms associated with variability in drug response show significant differences in allele frequencies among populations and racial groups. Furthermore, the patterns of linkage disequilibrium are markedly different between ethnic groups, which may lead to spurious findings when markers, instead of causal variants, are used in diagnostic tests extrapolated across populations. In exploring racial disparities in health and disease outcomes, considerable debate has focused on whether race and ethnic identity are primarily social or biological constructs, and the contribution of genetic variability in explaining observed differences in the rates of disease between racial groups. With the goal of personalized medicine being the prediction of risk and treatment of disease on the basis of an individual's genetic profile, some have argued that biological consideration of race will become obsolete. However, in this discovery phase of the

---

[c]See http://www.nigms.nih.gov/pharmacogenetics/.
[d]See http://www.pharmgkb.org/.

postgenome era, continuing to incorporate racial information in genetic studies should improve our understanding of the architecture of the human genome and its implications for novel strategies aiming at identifying variants protecting against, or conferring susceptibility to, common diseases and modulating drug effects.[183]

CONCLUSIONS

The Human Genome Project has revolutionized all aspects of medicine, allowing us to assess the impact of genetic variability on disease taxonomy, characterization, and outcome, and individual responses to various drugs and injuries. Mechanistically, information gleaned through genomic approaches is already unraveling long-standing mysteries behind general anesthetic action and adverse responses to drugs used perioperatively. However, a strong need remains for prospective, well-powered genetic studies in highly phenotyped surgical populations, which require the development of multidimensional perioperative databases. For the anesthesiologist, this may soon translate into prospective risk assessment incorporating genetic profiling of markers important in thrombotic, inflammatory, vascular, and neurologic responses to perioperative stress, with implications ranging from individualized additional preoperative testing and physiological optimization, to choice of perioperative monitoring strategies and critical care resource utilization. Furthermore, genetic profiling of drug-metabolizing enzymes, carrier proteins, and receptors, using currently available high-throughput molecular technologies, will enable personalized choice of drugs and dosage regimens tailored to suit a patient's pharmacogenetic profile. At that point, perioperative physicians will have far more robust information to use in designing the most appropriate and safest anesthetic plan for given patient.

Future trends and challenges in perioperative genomics are still being defined, but mainly concern interdisciplinary studies designed to combine an analytical system approach, mathematical modeling, and engineering principles with the multiple molecular and genetic factors and stimuli, and the macroscale interactions that determine the pathophysiological response to surgery.

Acknowledgments

Supported in part by National Institutes of Health grants HL075273 and HL092071 to MVP.

References

1. Collins FS, Green ED, Guttmacher AE, et al: A vision for the future of genomics research. Nature 2003; 422: 835
2. Schwinn DA, and Booth JV: Genetics infuses new life into human physiology: implications of the human genome project for anesthesiology and perioperative medicine. Anesthesiology 2002; 96: 261
3. Lander ES: The new genomics: Global views of biology. Science 1996; 274: 536
4. Podgoreanu MV, Schwinn DA: New paradigms in cardiovascular medicine: Emerging technologies and practices: perioperative genomics. J Am Coll Cardiol 2005; 46: 1965
5. Fox AA, Shernan SK, Body SC: Predictive genomics of adverse events after cardiac surgery. Semin Cardiothorac Vasc Anesth 2004; 8: 297
6. Stuber F, Hoeft A. The influence of genomics on outcome after cardiovascular surgery. Curr Opin Anaesthesiol 2002; 15: 3
7. Ziegeler S, Tsusaki BE, Collard CD. Influence of genotype on perioperative risk and outcome. Anesthesiology 2003; 99: 212
8. Redon R, Ishikawa S, Fitch KR, et al: Global variation in copy number in the human genome. Nature 2006; 444: 444
9. Frazer KA, Ballinger DG, Cox DR, et al: A second generation human haplotype map of over 3.1 million SNPs. Nature 2007; 449: 851
10. Levy S, Sutton G, Ng PC, et al: The diploid genome sequence of an individual human. PLoS Biol 2007; 5: e254.
11. Podgoreanu MV, Schwinn DA: Genomics and the circulation. Br J Anaesth 2004; 93: 140
12. Gretarsdottir S, Sveinbjornsdottir S, Jonsson HH, et al: Localization of a susceptibility gene for common forms of stroke to 5q12. Am J Hum Genet 2002; 70: 593
13. Broeckel U, Hengstenberg C, Mayer B, et al: A comprehensive linkage analysis for myocardial infarction and its related risk factors. Nat Genet 2002; 30: 210
14. Zintzaras E, Kitsios G, Kent D, et al: Genome-wide scans meta-analysis for pulse pressure. Hypertension 2007; 50: 557
15. Risch N, Merikangas K: The future of genetic studies of complex human diseases. Science 1996; 273: 1516
16. Tabor HK, Risch NJ, Myers RM. Opinion: Candidate-gene approaches for studying complex genetic traits: practical considerations. Nat Rev Genet 2002; 3: 391
17. Zhu X, Chang YP, Yan D, et al: Associations between hypertension and genes in the renin-angiotensin system. Hypertension 2003; 41: 1027
18. Jachymova M, Horky K, Bultas J, et al: Association of the Glu298Asp polymorphism in the endothelial nitric oxide synthase gene with essential hypertension resistant to conventional therapy. Biochem Biophys Res Commun 2001; 284: 426
19. Tomaszewski M, Brain NJ, Charchar FJ, et al: Essential hypertension and beta2-adrenergic receptor gene: linkage and association analysis. Hypertension 2002; 40: 286
20. Winkelmann BR, Hager J: Genetic variation in coronary heart disease and myocardial infarction: methodological overview and clinical evidence. Pharmacogenomics 2000; 1: 73
21. Agema WR, Jukema JW, Pimstone SN, et al: Genetic aspects of restenosis after percutaneous coronary interventions: towards more tailored therapy. Eur Heart J 2001; 22: 2058
22. Ozaki K, Ohnishi Y, Iida A, et al: Functional SNPs in the lymphotoxin-alpha gene that are associated with susceptibility to myocardial infarction. Nat Genet 2002; 32: 650
23. Podgoreanu MV, White WD, Morris RW, et al: Inflammatory gene polymorphisms and risk of postoperative myocardial infarction after cardiac surgery. Circulation 2006; 114: I275
24. Collard CD, Shernan SK, Fox AA, et al: The MBL2 'LYQA secretor' haplotype is an independent predictor of postoperative myocardial infarction in whites undergoing coronary artery bypass graft surgery. Circulation 2007; 116: I106
25. Tardiff BE, Newman MF, Saunders AM, et al: Preliminary report of a genetic basis for cognitive decline after cardiac operations. The Neurologic Outcome Research Group of the Duke Heart Center. Ann Thorac Surg 1997; 64: 715
26. Mathew JP, Rinder CS, Howe JG, et al: Platelet PlA2 polymorphism enhances risk of neurocognitive decline after cardiopulmonary bypass. Multicenter Study of Perioperative Ischemia (McSPI) Research Group. Ann Thorac Surg 2001; 71: 663
27. Mathew JP, Podgoreanu MV, Grocott HP, et al: Genetic variants in P-selectin and C-reactive protein influence susceptibility to cognitive decline after cardiac surgery. J Am Coll Cardiol 2007; 49: 1934
28. Stafford-Smith M, Podgoreanu M, Swaminathan M, et al: Association of genetic polymorphisms with risk of renal injury after coronary bypass graft surgery. Am J Kidney Dis 2005; 45: 519
29. Chew ST, Newman MF, White WD, et al: Preliminary report on the association of apolipoprotein E polymorphisms, with postoperative peak serum creatinine concentrations in cardiac surgical patients. Anesthesiology 2000; 93: 325
30. MacKensen GB, Swaminathan M, Ti LK, et al: Preliminary report on the interaction of apolipoprotein E polymorphism with aortic atherosclerosis and acute nephropathy after CABG. Ann Thorac Surg 2004; 78: 520
31. Ortlepp JR, Janssens U, Bleckmann F, et al: A chymase gene variant is associated with atherosclerosis in venous coronary artery bypass grafts. Coron Artery Dis 2001; 12: 493
32. Ellis SG, Chen MS, Jia G, et al: Relation of polymorphisms in five genes to long-term aortocoronary saphenous vein graft patency. Am J Cardiol 2007; 99: 1087
33. Donahue BS: Factor V Leiden and perioperative risk. Anesth Analg 2004; 98: 1623
34. Lasocki S, Iglarz M, Seince PF, et al: Involvement of renin-angiotensin system in pressure-flow relationship: role of angiotensin-converting enzyme gene polymorphism. Anesthesiology 2002; 96: 271
35. Stuber F, Petersen M, Bokelmann F, et al: A genomic polymorphism within the tumor necrosis factor locus influences plasma tumor necrosis factor-alpha concentrations and outcome of patients with severe sepsis. Crit Care Med 1996; 24: 381
36. Moretti EW, Morris RW, Podgoreanu M, et al: APOE polymorphism is associated with risk of severe sepsis in surgical patients. Crit Care Med 2005; 33: 2521
37. Slavcheva E, Albanis E, Jiao Q, et al: Cytotoxic T-lymphocyte antigen 4 gene polymorphisms and susceptibility to acute allograft rejection. Transplantation 2001; 72: 935
38. Cardon LR, Bell JI. Association study designs for complex diseases. Nat Rev Genet 2001; 2: 91

39. Hirschhorn JN, Lohmueller K, Byrne E, Hirschhorn K: A comprehensive review of genetic association studies. Genet Med 2002; 4: 45

40. Lohmueller KE, Pearce CL, Pike M, et al: Meta-analysis of genetic association studies supports a contribution of common variants to susceptibility to common disease. Nat Genet 2003; 33: 177

41. Wellcome Trust Case Control Consortium. Genome-wide association study of 14,000 cases of seven common diseases and 3,000 shared controls. Nature 2007; 447: 661

42. Samani NJ, Erdmann J, Hall AS, et al: Genomewide association analysis of coronary artery disease. N Engl J Med 2007; 357: 443

43. McPherson R, Pertsemlidis A, Kavaslar N, et al: A common allele on chromosome 9 associated with coronary heart disease. Science 2007; 316: 1488

44. Helgadottir A, Thorleifsson G, Manolescu A, et al: A common variant on chromosome 9p21 affects the risk of myocardial infarction. Science 2007; 316: 1491

45. Todd JA, Walker NM, Cooper JD, et al: Robust associations of four new chromosome regions from genome-wide analyses of type 1 diabetes. Nat Genet 2007; 39: 857

46. Saxena R, Voight BF, Lyssenko V, et al: Genome-wide association analysis identifies loci for type 2 diabetes and triglyceride levels. Science 2007; 316: 1331

47. Gudbjartsson DF, Arnar DO, Helgadottir A, et al: Variants conferring risk of atrial fibrillation on chromosome 4q25. Nature 2007; 448: 353

48. Scuteri A, Sanna S, Chen WM, et al: Genome-Wide Association Scan Shows Genetic Variants in the FTO Gene Are Associated with Obesity-Related Traits. PLoS Genet 2007; 3: e115.

49. Stranger BE, Nica AC, Forrest MS, et al: Population genomics of human gene expression. Nat Genet 2007; 39: 1217

50. Hopf HW: Molecular diagnostics of injury and repair responses in critical illness: what is the future of "monitoring" in the intensive care unit? Crit Care Med 2003; 31: S518

51. Feezor RJ, Baker HV, Xiao W, et al: Genomic and proteomic determinants of outcome in patients undergoing thoracoabdominal aortic aneurysm repair. J Immunol 2004; 172: 7103

52. Hughes TR, Marton MJ, Jones AR, et al: Functional discovery via a compendium of expression profiles. Cell 2000; 102: 109

53. Tomic V, Russwurm S, Moller E, et al: Transcriptomic and proteomic patterns of systemic inflammation in on-pump and off-pump coronary artery bypass grafting. Circulation 2005; 112: 2912

54. Sehl PD, Tai JT, Hillan KJ, et al: Application of cDNA microarrays in determining molecular phenotype in cardiac growth, development, and response to injury. Circulation 2000; 101: 1990

55. Depre C, Tomlinson JE, Kudej RK, et al: Gene program for cardiac cell survival induced by transient ischemia in conscious pigs. Proc Natl Acad Sci USA 2001; 98: 9336

56. Ruel M, Bianchi C, Khan TA, et al: Gene expression profile after cardiopulmonary bypass and cardioplegic arrest. J Thorac Cardiovasc Surg 2003; 126: 1521

57. Konstantinov IE, Coles JG, Boscarino C, et al: Gene expression profiles in children undergoing cardiac surgery for right heart obstructive lesions. J Thorac Cardiovasc Surg 2004; 127: 746

58. Sergeev P, da Silva R, Lucchinetti E, et al: Trigger-dependent gene expression profiles in cardiac preconditioning: evidence for distinct genetic programs in ischemic and anesthetic preconditioning. Anesthesiology 2004; 100: 474

59. Lucchinetti E, Aguirre J, Feng J, et al: Molecular evidence of late preconditioning after sevoflurane inhalation in healthy volunteers. Anesth Analg 2007; 105: 629

60. Lucchinetti E, Hofer C, Bestmann L, et al: Gene regulatory control of myocardial energy metabolism predicts postoperative cardiac function in patients undergoing off-pump coronary artery bypass graft surgery: inhalational versus intravenous anesthetics. Anesthesiology 2007; 106: 444

61. Atkins JH, Johansson JS: Technologies to shape the future: proteomics applications in anesthesiology and critical care medicine. Anesth Analg 2006; 102: 1207

62. Futterer CD, Maurer MH, Schmitt A, et al: Alterations in rat brain proteins after desflurane anesthesia. Anesthesiology 2004; 100: 302

63. Kalenka A, Hinkelbein J, Feldmann RE, Jr., et al: The effects of sevoflurane anesthesia on rat brain proteins: a proteomic time-course analysis. Anesth Analg 2007; 104: 1129

64. Sheikh AM, Barrett C, Villamizar N, et al: Proteomics of cerebral injury in a neonatal model of cardiopulmonary bypass with deep hypothermic circulatory arrest. J Thorac Cardiovasc Surg 2006; 132: 820

65. Queloz PA, Thadikkaran L, Crettaz D, et al: Proteomics and transfusion medicine: future perspectives. Proteomics 2006; 6: 5605

66. Mangano DT: Perioperative medicine: NHLBI working group deliberations and recommendations. J Cardiothorac Vasc Anesth 2004; 18: 1

67. Howell SJ, Sear JW: Perioperative myocardial injury: individual and population implications. Br J Anaesth 2004; 93: 3

68. Mangano DT: Effects of acadesine on myocardial infarction, stroke, and death following surgery. A meta-analysis of the 5 international randomized trials. The Multicenter Study of Perioperative Ischemia (McSPI) Research Group. Jama 1997; 277: 325

69. Mahaffey KW, Roe MT, Kilaru R, et al: Creatine kinase-MB elevation after coronary artery bypass grafting surgery in patients with non-ST-segment elevation acute coronary syndromes predict worse outcomes: results from four large clinical trials. Eur Heart J 2007; 28: 425

70. Delanghe J, Cambier B, Langlois M, et al: Haptoglobin polymorphism, a genetic risk factor in coronary artery bypass surgery. Atherosclerosis 1997; 132: 215

71. Volzke H, Engel J, Kleine V, et al: Angiotensin I-converting enzyme insertion/deletion polymorphism and cardiac mortality and morbidity after coronary artery bypass graft surgery. Chest 2002; 122: 31

72. Shaw AD, Vaporciyan AA, Wu X, et al: Inflammatory gene polymorphisms influence risk of postoperative morbidity after lung resection. Ann Thorac Surg 2005; 79: 1704

73. Brull DJ, Montgomery HE, Sanders J, et al: Interleukin-6 gene −174g>c and −572g>c promoter polymorphisms are strong predictors of plasma interleukin-6 levels after coronary artery bypass surgery. Arterioscler Thromb Vasc Biol 2001; 21: 1458

74. Burzotta F, Iacoviello L, Di Castelnuovo A, et al: Relation of the −174 G/C polymorphism of interleukin-6 to interleukin-6 plasma levels and to length of hospitalization after surgical coronary revascularization. Am J Cardiol 2001; 88: 1125

75. Grocott HP, Newman MF, El-Moalem H, et al: Apolipoprotein E genotype differentially influences the proinflammatory and anti-inflammatory response to cardiopulmonary bypass. J Thorac Cardiovasc Surg 2001; 122: 622

76. Roth-Isigkeit A, Hasselbach L, Ocklitz E, et al: Inter-individual differences in cytokine release in patients undergoing cardiac surgery with cardiopulmonary bypass. Clin Exp Immunol 2001; 125: 80

77. Lehmann LE, Schroeder S, Hartmann W, et al: A single nucleotide polymorphism of macrophage migration inhibitory factor is related to inflammatory response in coronary bypass surgery using cardiopulmonary bypass. Eur J Cardiothorac Surg 2006; 30: 59

78. Tomasdottir H, Hjartarson H, Ricksten A, et al: Tumor necrosis factor gene polymorphism is associated with enhanced systemic inflammatory response and increased cardiopulmonary morbidity after cardiac surgery. Anesth Analg 2003; 97: 944

79. Galley HF, Lowe PR, Carmichael RL, et al: Genotype and interleukin-10 responses after cardiopulmonary bypass. Br J Anaesth 2003; 91: 424

80. Voetsch B, Loscalzo J: Genetic determinants of arterial thrombosis. Arterioscler Thromb Vasc Biol 2004; 24: 216

81. Rifon J, Paramo JA, Panizo C, et al: The increase of plasminogen activator inhibitor activity is associated with graft occlusion in patients undergoing aorto-coronary bypass surgery. Br J Haematol 1997; 99: 262

82. Iacoviello L, Burzotta F, Di Castelnuovo A, et al: The 4G/5G polymorphism of PAI-1 promoter gene and the risk of myocardial infarction: a meta-analysis. Thromb Haemost 1998; 80: 1029

83. Rinder CS, Mathew JP, Rinder HM, et al: Platelet PlA2 polymorphism and platelet activation are associated with increased troponin I release after cardiopulmonary bypass. Anesthesiology 2002; 97: 1118

84. Zotz RB, Klein M, Dauben HP, et al: Prospective analysis after coronary-artery bypass grafting: platelet GP IIIa polymorphism (HPA-1b/PIA2) is a risk factor for bypass occlusion, myocardial infarction, and death. Thromb Haemost 2000; 83: 404

85. Faraday N, Martinez EA, Scharpf RB, et al: Platelet gene polymorphisms and cardiac risk assessment in vascular surgical patients. Anesthesiology 2004; 101: 1291

86. Donahue BS, Gailani D, Higgins MS, et al: Factor V Leiden protects against blood loss and transfusion after cardiac surgery. Circulation 2003; 107: 1003

87. Moor E, Silveira A, van't Hooft F, et al: Coagulation factor V (Arg506—>Gln) mutation and early saphenous vein graft occlusion after coronary artery bypass grafting. Thromb Haemost 1998; 80: 220

88. Zaugg M, Schaub MC: Genetic modulation of adrenergic activity in the heart and vasculature: implications for perioperative medicine. Anesthesiology 2005; 102: 429

89. Zaugg M, Bestmann L, Wacker J, et al: Adrenergic receptor genotype but not perioperative bisoprolol therapy may determine cardiovascular outcome in at-risk patients undergoing surgery with spinal block: the Swiss Beta Blocker in Spinal Anesthesia (BBSA) study: a double-blinded, placebo-controlled, multicenter trial with 1-year follow-up. Anesthesiology 2007; 107: 33

90. Philip I, Plantefeve G, Vuillaumier-Barrot S, et al: G894T polymorphism in the endothelial nitric oxide synthase gene is associated with an enhanced vascular responsiveness to phenylephrine. Circulation 1999; 99: 3096

91. Henrion D, Benessiano J, Philip I, et al: The deletion genotype of the angiotensin I-converting enzyme is associated with an increased vascular reactivity in vivo and in vitro. J Am Coll Cardiol 1999; 34: 830

92. Kim NS, Lee IO, Lee MK, et al: The effects of beta2 adrenoceptor gene polymorphisms on pressor response during laryngoscopy and tracheal intubation. Anaesthesia 2002; 57: 227

93. Ryan R, Thornton J, Duggan E, et al: Gene polymorphism and requirement for vasopressor infusion after cardiac surgery. Ann Thorac Surg 2006; 82: 895

94. Mathew JP, Fontes ML, Tudor IC, et al: A multicenter risk index for atrial fibrillation after cardiac surgery. Jama 2004; 291: 1720

95. Brugada R: Is atrial fibrillation a genetic disease? J Cardiovasc Electrophysiol 2005; 16: 553

96. Gaudino M, Andreotti F, Zamparelli R, et al: The −174G/C interleukin-6 polymorphism influences postoperative interleukin-6 levels and postopera-

tive atrial fibrillation. Is atrial fibrillation an inflammatory complication? Circulation 2003; 108 Suppl 1: II195

97. Gaudino M, Di Castelnuovo A, Zamparelli R, et al: Genetic control of postoperative systemic inflammatory reaction and pulmonary and renal complications after coronary artery surgery. J Thorac Cardiovasc Surg 2003; 126: 1107

98. Motsinger AA, Donahue BS, Brown NJ, et al: Risk factor interactions and genetic effects associated with post-operative atrial fibrillation. Pac Symp Biocomput 2006: 584

99. Hogue CW, Jr., Palin CA, Kailasam R, et al: C-reactive protein levels and atrial fibrillation after cardiac surgery in women. Ann Thorac Surg 2006; 82: 97

100. Pretorius M, Donahue BS, Yu C, et al: Plasminogen activator inhibitor-1 as a predictor of postoperative atrial fibrillation after cardiopulmonary bypass. Circulation 2007; 116: I1

101. Barth AS, Merk S, Arnoldi E, et al: Reprogramming of the human atrial transcriptome in permanent atrial fibrillation: expression of a ventricular-like genomic signature. Circ Res 2005; 96: 1022

102. Ramlawi B, Otu H, Mieno S, et al: Oxidative stress and atrial fibrillation after cardiac surgery: a case-control study. Ann Thorac Surg 2007; 84: 1166–1172; discussion 1172

103. Mehra MR, Feller E, Rosenberg S: The promise of protein-based and gene-based clinical markers in heart transplantation: from bench to bedside. Nat Clin Pract Cardiovasc Med 2006; 3: 136

104. Hall JL, Birks EJ, Grindle S, et al: Molecular signature of recovery following combination left ventricular assist device (LVAD) support and pharmacologic therapy. Eur Heart J 2007; 28: 613

105. Podgoreanu MV, Booth JV, White WD, et al: Beta adrenergic receptor polymorphisms and risk of adverse events following cardiac surgery. Circulation 2003; 108: IV-434.

106. Lobato RL, Mathew JP, Schwinn DA, et al: Genomic predictors of long-term mortality following coronary artery bypass graft surgery. Anesthesiology 2007; 107: A1440 (abstract).

107. Grocott HP, White WD, Morris RW, et al: Genetic polymorphisms and the risk of stroke after cardiac surgery. Stroke 2005; 36: 1854

108. Newman MF, Booth JV, Laskowitz DT, et al: Genetic predictors of perioperative neurological and cognitive injury and recovery. Best Practice and Research Clinical Anesthesiology 2001; 15: 247

109. Alberts MJ, Graffagnino C, McClenny C, et al: ApoE genotype and survival from intracerebral haemorrhage. Lancet 1995; 346: 575.

110. Teasdale GM, Nicoll JA, Murray G, et al: Association of apolipoprotein E polymorphism with outcome after head injury. Lancet 1997; 350: 1069

111. Slooter AJ, Tang MX, van Duijn CM, et al: Apolipoprotein E epsilon4 and the risk of dementia with stroke. A population-based investigation. Jama 1997; 277: 818

112. Sheng H, Laskowitz DT, Bennett E, et al: Apolipoprotein E isoform-specific differences in outcome from focal ischemia in transgenic mice. J Cereb Blood Flow Metab 1998; 18: 361

113. Leung JM, Sands LP, Wang Y, et al: Apolipoprotein E e4 allele increases the risk of early postoperative delirium in older patients undergoing noncardiac surgery. Anesthesiology 2007; 107: 406

114. Ely EW, Girard TD, Shintani AK, et al: Apolipoprotein E4 polymorphism as a genetic predisposition to delirium in critically ill patients. Crit Care Med 2007; 35: 112

115. Gaynor JW, Gerdes M, Zackai EH, et al: Apolipoprotein E genotype and neurodevelopmental sequelae of infant cardiac surgery. J Thorac Cardiovasc Surg 2003; 126: 1736

116. Zeltser I, Jarvik GP, Bernbaum J, et al: Genetic factors are important determinants of neurodevelopmental outcome after repair of tetralogy of Fallot. J Thorac Cardiovasc Surg 2008; 135: 91

117. Ti LK, Mathew JP, Mackensen GB, et al: Effect of apolipoprotein E genotype on cerebral autoregulation during cardiopulmonary bypass. Stroke 2001; 32: 1514

118. Ti LK, Mackensen GB, Grocott HP, et al: Apolipoprotein E4 increases aortic atheroma burden in cardiac surgical patients. J Thorac Cardiovasc Surg 2003; 125: 211

119. Newman MF, Laskowitz DT, White WD, et al: Apolipoprotein E polymorphisms and age at first coronary artery bypass graft. Anesth Analg 2001; 92: 824

120. Weiss EJ, Bray PF, Tayback M, et al: A polymorphism of a platelet glycoprotein receptor as an inherited risk factor for coronary thrombosis. N Engl J Med 1996; 334: 1090

121. Carter AM, Catto AJ, Bamford JM, et al: Platelet GP IIIa PlA and GP Ib variable number tandem repeat polymorphisms and markers of platelet activation in acute stroke. Arterioscler Thromb Vasc Biol 1998; 18: 1124

122. Ramlawi B, Otu H, Rudolph JL, et al: Genomic expression pathways associated with brain injury after cardiopulmonary bypass. J Thorac Cardiovasc Surg 2007; 134: 996

123. Ramlawi B, Rudolph JL, Mieno S, et al: C-Reactive protein and inflammatory response associated to neurocognitive decline following cardiac surgery. Surgery 2006; 140: 221

124. Ramlawi B, Rudolph JL, Mieno S, et al: Serologic markers of brain injury and cognitive function after cardiopulmonary bypass. Ann Surg 2006; 244: 593

125. Mangano CM, Diamondstone LS, Ramsay JG, et al: Renal dysfunction after myocardial revascularization: risk factors, adverse outcomes, and

126. Yende S, Wunderink R: Causes of prolonged mechanical ventilation after coronary artery bypass surgery. Chest 2002; 122: 245

127. Rigat B, Hubert C, Alhenc-Gelas F, et al: An insertion/deletion polymorphism in the angiotensin I-converting enzyme gene accounting for half the variance of serum enzyme levels. J Clin Invest 1990; 86: 1343

128. Yende S, Quasney MW, Tolley EA, et al: Clinical relevance of angiotensin-converting enzyme gene polymorphisms to predict risk of mechanical ventilation after coronary artery bypass graft surgery. Crit Care Med 2004; 32: 922

129. Marshall RP, Webb S, Bellingan GJ, et al: Angiotensin converting enzyme insertion/deletion polymorphism is associated with susceptibility and outcome in acute respiratory distress syndrome. Am J Respir Crit Care Med 2002; 166: 646

130. Yende S, Quasney MW, Tolley E, et al: Association of tumor necrosis factor gene polymorphisms and prolonged mechanical ventilation after coronary artery bypass surgery. Crit Care Med 2003; 31: 133

131. Roden DM: Cardiovascular pharmacogenomics. Circulation 2003; 108: 3071

132. Lehmann H, Ryan E: The familial incidence of low pseudocholinesterase level. Lancet 1956; 271: 124.

133. Bukaveckas BL, Valdes R, Jr., Linder MW: Pharmacogenetics as related to the practice of cardiothoracic and vascular anesthesia. J Cardiothorac Vasc Anesth 2004; 18: 353

134. McCarthy TV, Healy JM, Heffron JJ, et al: Localization of the malignant hyperthermia susceptibility locus to human chromosome 19q12-13.2. Nature 1990; 343: 562

135. Pessah IN, Allen PD: Malignant hyperthermia. Best Practice and Research Clinical Anesthesiology 2001; 15: 277

136. Eger EI, 2nd: Anesthetic uptake and action. Baltimore,: Williams and Wilkins, 1974.

137. Liem EB, Lin CM, Suleman MI, et al: Anesthetic requirement is increased in redheads. Anesthesiology 2004; 101: 279

138. Ezri T, Sessler D, Weisenberg M, et al: Association of ethnicity with the minimum alveolar concentration of sevoflurane. Anesthesiology 2007; 107: 9

139. Franks NP, Lieb WR: Molecular and cellular mechanisms of general anaesthesia. Nature 1994; 367: 607

140. Sonner JM, Antognini JF, Dutton RC, et al: Inhaled anesthetics and immobility: mechanisms, mysteries, and minimum alveolar anesthetic concentration. Anesth Analg 2003; 97: 718

141. Wong SM, Cheng G, Homanics GE, Kendig JJ: Enflurane actions on spinal cords from mice that lack the beta3 subunit of the GABA(A) receptor. Anesthesiology 2001; 95: 154

142. Homanics GE, Ferguson C, Quinlan JJ, et al: Gene knockout of the alpha6 subunit of the gammaaminobutyric acid type A receptor: lack of effect on responses to ethanol, pentobarbital, and general anesthetics. Mol Pharmacol 1997; 51: 588

143. Rudolph U, Crestani F, Benke D, et al: Benzodiazepine actions mediated by specific gamma-aminobutyric acid(A) receptor subtypes. Nature 1999; 401: 796

144. Belelli D, Lambert JJ, Peters JA, et al: The interaction of the general anesthetic etomidate with the gamma-aminobutyric acid type A receptor is influenced by a single amino acid. Proc Natl Acad Sci USA 1997; 94: 11031

145. Jurd R, Arras M, Lambert S, et al: General anesthetic actions in vivo strongly attenuated by a point mutation in the GABA(A) receptor beta3 subunit. Faseb J 2003; 17: 250

146. Reynolds DS, Rosahl TW, Cirone J, et al: Sedation and anesthesia mediated by distinct GABA(A) receptor isoforms. J Neurosci 2003; 23: 8608

147. Cirone J, Rosahl TW, Reynolds DS, et al: Gamma-aminobutyric acid type A receptor beta 2 subunit mediates the hypothermic effect of etomidate in mice. Anesthesiology 2004; 100: 1438

148. Lakhlani PP, MacMillan LB, Guo TZ, et al: Substitution of a mutant alpha2a-adrenergic receptor via "hit and run" gene targeting reveals the role of this subtype in sedative, analgesic, and anesthetic-sparing responses in vivo. Proc Natl Acad Sci USA 1997; 94: 9950

149. Gerstin KM, Gong DH, Abdallah M, et al: Mutation of KCNK5 or Kir3.2 potassium channels in mice does not change minimum alveolar anesthetic concentration. Anesth Analg 2003; 96: 1345

150. Sternberg WF, Mogil JF: Genetic and hormonal basis of pain states. Best Practice and Research Clinical Anesthesiology 2001; 15: 229

151. Diatchenko L, Anderson AD, Slade GD, et al: Three major haplotypes of the beta2 adrenergic receptor define psychological profile, blood pressure, and the risk for development of a common musculoskeletal pain disorder. Am J Med Genet B Neuropsychiatr Genet 2006; 141: 449

152. Diatchenko L, Nackley AG, Tchivileva IE, et al: Genetic architecture of human pain perception. Trends Genet 2007; 23: 605

153. Bengtsson B, Thorson J: Back pain: a study of twins. Acta Genet Med Gemellol (Roma) 1991; 40: 83

154. Mogil JS, Wilson SG, Bon K, et al: Heritability of nociception I: responses of 11 inbred mouse strains on 12 measures of nociception. Pain 1999; 80: 67

155. Lacroix-Fralish ML, Ledoux JB, Mogil JS: The Pain Genes Database: An interactive web browser of pain-related transgenic knockout studies. Pain 2007; 131: 3 e1

156. Somogyi AA, Barratt DT, Coller JK: Pharmacogenetics of opioids. Clin Pharmacol Ther 2007; 81: 429

157. Diatchenko L, Nackley AG, Slade GD, et al: Catechol-O-methyltransferase gene polymorphisms are associated with multiple pain-evoking stimuli. Pain 2006; 125: 216

158. Candiotti KA, Birnbach DJ, Lubarsky DA, et al: The impact of pharmacogenomics on postoperative nausea and vomiting: do CYP2D6 allele copy number and polymorphisms affect the success or failure of ondansetron prophylaxis? Anesthesiology 2005; 102: 543

159. Lin LH, Hopf HW: Paradigm of the injury-repair continuum during critical illness. Crit Care Med 2003; 31: S493

160. Angus DC, Burgner D, Wunderink R, et al: The PIRO concept: P is for predisposition. Crit Care 2003; 7: 248

161. Lin MT, Albertson TE: Genomic polymorphisms in sepsis. Crit Care Med 2004; 32: 569

162. De Maio A, Torres MB, Reeves RH: Genetic determinants influencing the response to injury, inflammation, and sepsis. Shock 2005; 23: 11

163. Zeni F, Freeman B, Natanson C: Anti-inflammatory therapies to treat sepsis and septic shock: a reassessment. Crit Care Med 1997; 25: 1095

164. Cobb JP, O'Keefe GE: Injury research in the genomic era. Lancet 2004; 363: 2076

165. Prucha M, Ruryk A, Boriss H, et al: Expression profiling: toward an application in sepsis diagnostics. Shock 2004; 22: 29

166. Cobb JP, Laramie JM, Stormo GD, et al: Sepsis gene expression profiling: murine splenic compared with hepatic responses determined by using complementary DNA microarrays. Crit Care Med 2002; 30: 2711

167. Leikauf GD, McDowell SA, Wesselkamper SC, et al: Acute lung injury: functional genomics and genetic susceptibility. Chest 2002; 121: 70S

168. Dasu MR, Cobb JP, Laramie JM, et al: Gene expression profiles of livers from thermally injured rats. Gene 2004; 327: 51

169. Tang BM, McLean AS, Dawes IW, et al: The use of gene-expression profiling to identify candidate genes in human sepsis. Am J Respir Crit Care Med 2007; 176: 676

170. Calvano SE, Xiao W, Richards DR, et al: A network-based analysis of systemic inflammation in humans. Nature 2005; 437: 1032

171. Laudanski K, Miller-Graziano C, Xiao W, et al: Cell-specific expression and pathway analyses reveal alterations in trauma-related human T cell and monocyte pathways. Proc Natl Acad Sci U S A 2006; 103: 15564

172. Cobb JP, Mindrinos MN, Miller-Graziano C, et al: Application of genome-wide expression analysis to human health and disease. Proc Natl Acad Sci USA 2005; 102: 4801

173. Fessler MB, Malcolm KC, Duncan MW, et al: A genomic and proteomic analysis of activation of the human neutrophil by lipopolysaccharide and its mediation by p38 mitogen-activated protein kinase. J Biol Chem 2002; 277: 31291

174. Liu T, Qian WJ, Gritsenko MA, et al: High dynamic range characterization of the trauma patient plasma proteome. Mol Cell Proteomics 2006; 5: 1899

175. Kalenka A, Feldmann RE, Jr., Otero K, et al: Changes in the serum proteome of patients with sepsis and septic shock. Anesth Analg 2006; 103: 1522

176. Buchman TG, Cobb JP, Lapedes AS, et al: Complex systems analysis: a tool for shock research. Shock 2001; 16: 248

177. Strange K: The end of "naive reductionism": rise of systems biology or renaissance of physiology? Am J Physiol Cell Physiol 2005; 288: C968

178. Ge H, Walhout AJ, Vidal M: Integrating 'omic' information: a bridge between genomics and systems biology. Trends Genet 2003; 19: 551

179. Lusis AJ: A thematic review series: systems biology approaches to metabolic and cardiovascular disorders. J Lipid Res 2006; 47: 1887

180. Shaw A: Exploring the perioptome: the role of genomics in thoracic surgery and anaesthesia. Curr Opin Anaesthesiol 2007; 20: 32

181. Khoury MJ, Yang Q, Gwinn M, et al: An epidemiologic assessment of genomic profiling for measuring susceptibility to common diseases and targeting interventions. Genet Med 2004; 6: 38

182. Hakonarson H, Thorvaldsson S, Helgadottir A, et al: Effects of a 5-lipoxygenase-activating protein inhibitor on biomarkers associated with risk of myocardial infarction: a randomized trial. JAMA 2005; 293: 2245

183. Phimister EG: Medicine and the racial divide. N Engl J Med 2003; 348: 1081

184. Lucchinetti E, da Silva R, Pasch T, et al: Anaesthetic preconditioning but not postconditioning prevents early activation of the deleterious cardiac remodeling programme: evidence of opposing genomic responses in cardioprotection by pre- and postconditioning. Br J Anaesth 2005; 95: 140

185. Lai LP, Lin JL, Lin CS, et al: Functional genomic study on atrial fibrillation using cDNA microarray and two-dimensional protein electrophoresis techniques and identification of the myosin regulatory light chain isoform reprogramming in atrial fibrillation. J Cardiovasc Electrophysiol 2004; 15: 214

186. Horwitz PA, Tsai EJ, Putt ME, et al: Detection of cardiac allograft rejection and response to immunosuppressive therapy with peripheral blood gene expression. Circulation 2004; 110: 3815

187. Mehra MR, Kobashigawa JA, Hunt SA, et al: Molecular testing and prediction of clinical outcome in heart transplantation: a prospective multicenter trial. J Heart Lung Transplant 2004; 23: S106 (abstr).

188. Borozdenkova S, Westbrook JA, Patel V, et al: Use of proteomics to discover novel markers of cardiac allograft rejection. J Proteome Res 2004; 3: 282

189. Heusch G, Erbel R, Siffert W: Genetic determinants of coronary vasomotor tone in humans. Am J Physiol Heart Circ Physiol 2001; 281: H1465

190. Donahue BS, Roden D: Inflammatory cytokine polymorphisms are associated with beta-blocker failure in preventing postoperative atrial fibrillation. Anesth Analg 2005; 100: SCA30 (abstract).

191. Podgoreanu MV, Morris R, Zhang Q, et al: Gene variants in Interleukin 1-beta are associated with early QTc prolongation after cardiac surgery. Anesthesiology 2007; 107: A1287 (abstract).

192. Botto N, Andreassi MG, Rizza A, et al: C677T polymorphism of the methylenetetrahydrofolate reductase gene is a risk factor of adverse events after coronary revascularization. Int J Cardiol 2004; 96: 341

193. Taylor KD, Scheuner MT, Yang H, et al: Lipoprotein lipase locus and progression of atherosclerosis in coronary-artery bypass grafts. Genet Med 2004; 6: 481

194. Holweg CT, Weimar W, Uitterlinden AG, et al: Clinical impact of cytokine gene polymorphisms in heart and lung transplantation. J Heart Lung Transplant 2004; 23: 1017

195. Borozdenkova S, Smith J, Marshall S, et al: Identification of ICAM-1 polymorphism that is associated with protection from transplant associated vasculopathy after cardiac transplantation. Hum Immunol 2001; 62: 247

196. Vamvakopoulos JE, Taylor CJ, Green C, et al: Interleukin 1 and chronic rejection: possible genetic links in human heart allografts. Am J Transplant 2002; 2: 76

197. Duggan E, O'Dwyer MJ, Caraher E, et al: Coagulopathy after cardiac surgery may be influenced by a functional plasminogen activator inhibitor polymorphism. Anesth Analg 2007; 104: 1343

198. Welsby IJ, Podgoreanu MV, Phillips-Bute B, et al: Genetic factors contribute to bleeding after cardiac surgery. J Thromb Haemost 2005; 3: 1206

199. Morawski W, Sanak M, Cisowski M, et al: Prediction of the excessive perioperative bleeding in patients undergoing coronary artery bypass grafting: role of aspirin and platelet glycoprotein IIIa polymorphism. J Thorac Cardiovasc Surg 2005; 130: 791

200. Achrol AS, Kim H, Pawlikowska L, et al: Association of tumor necrosis factor-alpha-238G>A and apolipoprotein E2 polymorphisms with intracranial hemorrhage after brain arteriovenous malformation treatment. Neurosurgery 2007; 61: 731

CHAPTER 7 ■ PHARMACOLOGIC PRINCIPLES

DHANESH K. GUPTA AND THOMAS K. HENTHORN

SCIENTIFIC FOUNDATIONS OF ANESTHESIA

KEY POINTS

1. Most drugs must pass through cell membranes to reach their sites of action. Consequently, drugs tend to be relatively lipophilic, rather than hydrophilic.

2. The highly lipophilic anesthetic drugs have a rapid onset of action because they rapidly diffuse into the highly perfused brain tissue. They have a very short duration of action because of redistribution of drug from the central nervous system to the blood.

3. The cytochrome P450 (CYP) superfamily is the most important group of enzymes involved in drug metabolism. It and other drug-metabolizing enzymes exhibit genetic polymorphism.

4. The kidneys eliminate hydrophilic drugs and relatively hydrophilic metabolites of lipophilic drugs. Renal elimination of lipophilic compounds is negligible.

5. The liver is the most important organ for metabolism of drugs. Hepatic drug clearance depends on three factors: the intrinsic ability of the liver to metabolize a drug, hepatic blood flow, and the extent of binding of the drug to blood components.

6. The volume of distribution quantifies the extent of drug distribution. The greater the affinity of tissues for a drug relative to blood, the greater its volume of distribution (i.e., lipophilic drugs have greater volumes of distribution).

7. Elimination clearance is the parameter that characterizes the ability of drug-eliminating organs to irreversibly remove drugs from the body. The efficiency of the body to remove a drug from the body is proportional to the elimination clearance.

8. All else being equal, an increase in the volume of distribution of a drug will increase its elimination half-life; an increase in elimination clearance will decrease elimination half-life.

9. Most drugs bring about a pharmacologic effect by binding to a specific receptor that brings about a change in cellular function to produce the pharmacologic effect.

10. Although most pharmacologic effects can be characterized by both dose-response curves and concentration-response curves, the dose-response curves are unable to determine whether variations in pharmacologic response are caused by differences in pharmacokinetics, pharmacodynamics, or both.

11. Integrated pharmacokinetic-pharmacodynamic models allow temporal characterization of the relationship between dose, plasma concentration, and pharmacologic effect.

12. Simulations of multicompartmental pharmacokinetic models that describe intravenous anesthetics demonstrate that for most anesthetic dosing regimens, the distribution of drug from the plasma to the pharmacologically inert peripheral tissues has a greater influence on the plasma concentration profile of the drug than the elimination of drug from the body.

13. Target-controlled infusions are achieved with computer-controlled infusion pumps worldwide (not yet approved by the Food and Drug Administration [FDA] in the United States) and permit clinicians to make use of the drug concentration–effect relationship, optimally accounting for pharmacokinetics and predicting the offset of drug effect.

14. By understanding the interactions between the opioids and the sedative-hypnotics (e.g., response surface models), it is possible to select target concentration pairs of the two drugs that produce the desired clinical effect while minimizing unwanted side effects associated with high concentrations of a single drug.

15. The time until a patient regains responsiveness from a single drug anesthetic is determined by the pharmacokinetics of the individual drug, the concentration-effect relationship, and the duration of administration of the drug (context-sensitive decrement time). For two-drug anesthetics, the time to awakening not only depends on the individual drug pharmacokinetics and the duration of administration of the anesthetics, but it also depends on the pharmacodynamic interactions of the two drugs.

In 1943, Halford[1] labeled thiopental as "an ideal method of euthanasia" for war surgical patients and pronounced that "open drop ether still retains primacy!" Based on this recount of the experience with thiopental at Pearl Harbor, it is impressive that cooler heads prevailed—Adams and Gray[2] detailed a case of a civilian gunshot wound in which they carefully titrated incremental doses of thiopental without any adverse respiratory or cardiovascular events. To highlight the importance of the quiet case report versus the animated condemnation of intravenous anesthesia for patients with hemorrhagic shock, an anonymous editorial appeared in the same issue of *Anesthesiology* that attempted to give some scientific justification for the discrepancy in opinions.[3] As the editorial detailed, thiopental had a small therapeutic index and the tolerance to normal doses was decreased in extreme physical conditions (e.g., blood loss, sepsis). Therefore, as with open-drop ether, small doses of thiopental should be titrated to achieve the desired affects and avoid side effects associated with overdose. Fortuitously, the anesthesia community did not simply abandon the use of thiopental, and in 1960, Price[4] used mathematical models in order to describe the effects of hypovolemia on thiopental distribution.

Anesthetic drugs are administered with the goal of rapidly establishing and maintaining a therapeutic effect while minimizing undesired side effects. Although open-drop ether and chloroform were administered using knowledge of a dose-effect relationship, the more potent volatile agents, along with the intravenous hypnotics, neuromuscular junction blocking agents, and intravenous opioids, require a sound knowledge of pharmacokinetics and pharmacodynamics in order to accurately achieve the desired the pharmacologic effect for the desired period of time without any drug toxicity.

This chapter attempts to guide the reader through the fundamental knowledge of what the body does to a drug (i.e., pharmacokinetics) and what a drug does to the body (i.e., pharmacodynamics). The initial section of this chapter discusses the biologic and pharmacologic factors that influence the absorption, distribution, and elimination of a drug from the body. Where necessary, quantitative analyses of these processes are discussed to give readers insight into the intricacies of pharmacokinetics that cannot be easily described by text alone. The second section concentrates on the factors that determine the relationship between drug concentration and pharmacologic effect. Once again, mathematical models are presented as needed in order to clarify pharmacodynamic concepts. The final section builds on the reader's knowledge gained from the first two sections to apply the principles of pharmacokinetics and pharmacodynamics to determine the target concentration of intravenous anesthetics required and the dosing strategies necessary to produce an adequate anesthetic state. Understanding these concepts should allow the reader to integrate the anesthetic drugs of the future into a rational anesthetic regimen. Although specific drugs are used to illustrate pharmacokinetic and pharmacodynamic principles throughout this chapter, detailed pharmacologic information of anesthetic pharmacopeia are presented in subsequent chapters of this book.

PHARMACOKINETIC PRINCIPLES

Drug Absorption and Routes of Administration

Transfer of Drugs Across Membranes

For even the simplest drug that is directly administered into the blood to exert its action, it must move across at least one cell membrane to its site of action. Because biologic membranes are lipid bilayers composed of a lipophilic core sandwiched between two hydrophilic layers, only small lipophilic drugs can passively diffuse across the membrane down its concentration gradient. In order for water-soluble drugs to passively diffuse across the membrane down its concentration gradient, transmembrane proteins that form a hydrophilic channel are required. Because of the abundance of these nonspecific hydrophilic channels in the capillary endothelium of all organs except for the central nervous system (CNS), where the blood–brain barrier capillary endothelial cells have very limited numbers of transmembrane hydrophilic channels, *passive transport* of drugs from the intravascular space into the interstitium of various organs is limited by blood flow, not by the lipid solubility of the drug.[5]

Hydrophilic drugs can only enter the CNS after binding to drug-specific transmembrane proteins that actively transport the hydrophilic drug across the capillary endothelium into the CNS interstitium. When these transmembrane carrier proteins require energy to transport the drug across the membrane, they are able to shuttle proteins against their concentration gradients, a process called *active transport*. In contrast, when these carrier proteins do not require energy to shuttle drugs, they cannot overcome concentration gradients, a process called *facilitated diffusion*. Therefore, active transport is not limited to the CNS but is also found in the organs related to drug elimination (e.g., hepatocytes, renal tubular cells, pulmonary capillary endothelium), where the ability to transport drugs against the concentration gradient has specific biologic advantages. Both active transport and facilitated diffusion of drugs are saturable processes that are limited only by the number of carrier proteins available to shuttle a specific drug.[5]

For lipophilic compounds, transporters are not needed for the drug to diffuse across the capillary wall into tissues, but the presence of transporters does affect the concentration gradients that exist. For instance, some lipophilic drugs are transported out of tissues by adenosine triphosphate-dependent transporters such as p-glycoprotein. The lipophilic potent μ-opioid agonist, loperamide, used for the treatment of diarrhea, has limited bioavailability because of p-glycoprotein transporters at the intestine-portal capillary interface, and then what does reach the circulation has its CNS penetrance limited by p-glycoprotein at the blood–brain barrier.[6] Conversely, lipophilic compounds can be transported into tissues, increasing the tissue concentration of the drug beyond what would be accomplished by passive diffusion. The class of transporters called *organic anion polypeptide transporters*, like p-glycoprotein, is located in the microvascular endothelium of the brain and transport endogenous opioids into the brain.[7,8] These organic anion polypeptide transporters also transport drugs. The degree to which transporter proteins may account for intra- and interindividual responses to anesthetic drugs has not been well studied to date.[9]

Intravenous Administration

In order for a drug to be delivered to the site of drug action, the drug must be absorbed into the systemic circulation. Therefore, intravenous administration results in rapid increases in drug concentration. Although this can lead to a very rapid onset of drug effect, for drugs that have a low *therapeutic index* (the ratio of the intravenous dose that produces a toxic effect in 50% of the population to the intravenous dose that produces a therapeutic effect in 50% of the population), rapid overshoot of the desired plasma concentration can potentially result in immediate and severe side effects. Except for intravenous administration, the absorption of a drug into the systemic circulation is an important determinant of the time course of drug action and the maximum drug effect produced. As the absorption of drug is slowed, the maximum plasma concentration achieved—and therefore the maximum drug effect achieved—is limited. However, as long as the plasma concentration is maintained at a level above the minimum effective plasma concentration, the drug will produce a drug effect.[10] Therefore, nonintravenous methods of drug administration can produce a sustained and significant drug effect that may be more advantageous than administering drugs by the intravenous route.[11]

Bioavailability is the *relative amount* of a drug dose that reaches the systemic circulation unchanged and the *rate* at which this occurs. For most intravenously administered drugs, the absolute bioavailability of drug available is close to unity and the rate is nearly instantaneous. However, the pulmonary endothelium can slow the rate at which intravenously administered drugs reach the systemic circulation if distribution into the alveolar endothelium is extensive, such as occurs with the pulmonary uptake of fentanyl. The pulmonary endothelium also contains enzymes that may metabolize intravenously administered drugs (e.g., propofol) on first pass and reduce their absolute bioavailability.[12]

Oral Administration

For almost all therapeutic agents in all fields of medicine, oral administration is the safest and most convenient method of administration. However, this route is not used significantly in anesthetic practice because of the limited and variable rate of bioavailability. The absorption rate in the gastrointestinal tract is highly variable because the main determinant of the timing of absorption is gastric emptying into the small intestines where the surface area for absorption is several orders of magnitude greater than that of the stomach or large intestines. Additionally, the active metabolism of drug by the small intestine mucosal epithelium, and the obligatory path through the portal circulation before entering the systemic circulation, contribute to decreased bioavailability of orally administered drugs.[13] In fact, the metabolic capacity of the liver for drugs is so high that only a small fraction of most lipophilic drugs actually reach the systemic circulation. Because of this extensive *first-pass metabolism*, the oral dose of most drugs must be significantly higher to generate a therapeutic plasma concentration. Coupled with the prolonged and variable time until peak concentrations are usually achieved from oral administration (between tens of minutes to hours), it is nearly impractical to use this mode to administer perioperative anesthetic agents.

Highly lipophilic drugs that can maintain a high contact time with nasal or oral (sublingual) mucosa can be absorbed without needing to traverse the gastrointestinal tract. Sublingual administration of drug has the additional advantage over gastrointestinal absorption in that absorbed drug directly enters the systemic venous circulation and therefore is able to bypass the metabolically active intestinal mucosa and the hepatic first-pass metabolism. Therefore, small amounts of drug can rapidly produce a significant plasma concentration and therapeutic effect.[14] However, because of formulation limitations and the small amount of surface area available for absorption, sublingual administration is limited to drugs that fortuitously meet these requirements and require a rapid onset of drug action (e.g., nitroglycerin, fentanyl).

Transcutaneous Administration

A few lipophilic drugs have been manufactured in formulations that are sufficient to allow penetration of intact skin. Although scopolamine, nitroglycerin, opioids, and clonidine all produce therapeutic systemic plasma concentrations when administered as "drug patches," the extended amount of time that it takes to achieve an effective therapeutic concentration

limits practical application except for maintenance therapy. Attempts to speed the passive diffusion of these drugs using an electric current has been described for fentanyl,[15] but is still limited in its practicality.

Intramuscular and Subcutaneous Administration

Absorption of drugs from the depots in the subcutaneous tissue or in muscle tissue is directly dependent on the drug formulation and the blood flow to the depot. Because of the high blood flow to muscles in most physiologic states, intramuscular absorption of drugs in solution is relatively rapid and complete. Therefore, some aqueous drugs can be administered as intramuscular injection with rapid and predictable effects (e.g., neuromuscular junction blocking agents). The subcutaneous route of drug absorption is more variable in its onset because of the variability of subcutaneous blood flow during varying physiologic states—this is the primary reason that subcutaneous regular insulin administered in the operating room has a variable time of onset and maximum effect.

Intrathecal, Epidural, and Perineural Injection

Because the spinal cord is the primary site of action of many anesthetic agents, direct injection of local anesthetics and opioids directly into the intrathecal space bypasses the limitations of drug absorption and drug distribution of any other route of administration. This is not the case for epidural and perineural administration of local anesthetics because not delivering the drug directly into the cerebrospinal fluid necessitates that the drug be absorbed through the dura or nerve sheath in order to reach the site of drug action. The major downside to all of these techniques is the relative expertise required to perform regional anesthetics relative to oral, intravenous, and inhalational administration of drug.

Inhalational Administration

The large surface area of the pulmonary alveoli available for exchange with the large volumetric flow of blood found in the pulmonary capillaries makes inhalational administration an extremely attractive method by which to administer drugs.[16] New technologies have been developed that can rapidly and predictably aerosolize a wide range of drugs and thus approximate intravenous administration.[17] These devices are currently in phase 2 FDA trials.

Drug Distribution

Once the drug has entered the systemic circulation, it is transported through bulk flow of blood to all of the organs throughout the body. The relative distribution of cardiac output among organ vascular beds determines the speed at which organs are exposed to the drug. The highly perfused core circulatory components—the brain, lungs, heart, and kidneys—receive the highest relative distribution of cardiac output and therefore are the initial organs to reach equilibrium with plasma drug concentrations.[4] Drug concentrations then equilibrate with the less well-perfused muscles and liver and then, finally, with the relatively poorly perfused splanchnic vasculature, adipose tissue, and bone.

Whether by passive diffusion or transporter-mediation, drug transport at the capillaries is not usually saturable, so the amount of drug uptake by tissues and organs is limited by the blood flow they receive (i.e., flow-limited drug uptake).

Although the rate of initial drug delivery may depend on the relative blood flow of the organ, the rate of drug equilibration by the tissue depends on the ratio of blood flow to tissue content. Therefore, drug uptake rapidly approaches equilibrium in the highly perfused but low-volume brain, kidneys, and lungs in a matter of minutes, whereas drug transfer to the less well perfused, intermediate volume muscle tissue may take hours to approach equilibrium, and drug transfer to the poorly perfused, large cellular volumes of adipose tissue does not equilibrate for days.[11]

Redistribution

2 Highly lipophilic drugs such as thiopental and propofol rapidly begin to diffuse into the highly perfused brain tissue usually less than a minute after intravenous injection (see Chapter 18). Because of the low tissue volume but high perfusion of the brain, the drug concentration in the cerebral arterial blood rapidly equilibrates, usually within 3 minutes, with the concentration in the brain tissue. As drug continues to be taken up by other tissues with lower blood flows and higher tissue mass, the plasma concentration of the drug continues to decrease rapidly. Once the concentration of drug in the brain tissue is higher than the plasma concentration of drug, there is a reversal of the drug concentration gradient so that the lipophilic drug readily diffuses back into the blood and is *redistributed* to the other tissues that are still taking up drug.[4,18,19] This process continues for each of the organ beds until, ultimately, the adipose tissue will contain the majority of the lipophilic drug that has not been removed from the body by metabolism or excretion. However, after a single bolus of a highly lipophilic drug, the brain's tissue concentration rapidly decreases below therapeutic levels because of redistribution of drug to muscle tissue, which has a larger perfusion than adipose tissue.[4,19] Although single, moderate doses of highly lipophilic drugs have a very short CNS duration of action because of redistribution of drug from the CNS to the blood and other, less well-perfused tissues, repeated injections of a drug allows the rapid establishment of significant peripheral tissue concentrations. When the tissue concentrations of a drug are high enough, the decrease in plasma drug concentration below therapeutic threshold becomes solely dependent on drug elimination from the body.[20]

Drug Elimination

Besides being excreted unchanged from the body, a drug can be biotransformed (metabolized) into one or more new compounds that are then eliminated from the body. Either mechanism of elimination will decrease the drug concentration in the body such that the concentration will eventually be negligible and therefore unable to produce drug effect. *Elimination* is the pharmacokinetic term that describes all the processes that remove a drug from the body. Although the liver and the kidneys are considered the major organs of drug elimination, drug metabolism can occur at many other locations that contain active drug-metabolizing enzymes (e.g., pulmonary vasculature, red blood cells) and drug can be excreted unchanged from other organs (e.g., lungs).

Elimination clearance (drug clearance) is the theoretical volume of blood from which drug is completely and irreversibly removed in a unit of time.[21] Elimination clearance has the units of flow—[volume per time]. *Total* drug clearance can be calculated with pharmacokinetic models of blood concentration versus time data.

Biotransformation Reactions

Most drugs that are excreted unchanged from the body are hydrophilic and therefore readily passed into urine or stool. Drugs that are not sufficiently hydrophilic to be able to be excreted unchanged require modification into more hydrophilic, excretable compounds. Enzymatic reactions that metabolize drugs can be classified into phase I and phase II biotransformation reactions. Phase I reactions tend to transform a drug into one or more polar, and hence potentially excretable compounds. Phase II reactions transform the original drug by conjugating a variety of endogenous compounds to a polar functional group of the drug, making the metabolite even more hydrophilic. Often drugs will undergo a phase I reaction to produce a new compound with a polar functional group that will then undergo a phase II reaction. However, it is possible for a drug to undergo either a phase I reaction alone or a phase II reaction alone.

Phase I Reactions

Phase I reactions may hydrolyze, oxidize, or reduce the parent compound. *Hydrolysis* is the insertion of a molecule of water into another molecule, which forms an unstable intermediate compound that subsequently splits apart. Thus, hydrolysis cleaves the original substance into two separate molecules. Hydrolytic reactions are the primary way amides, such as lidocaine and other amide local anesthetics, and esters, such as succinylcholine, are metabolized.

Many drugs are biotransformed by oxidative reactions. *Oxidations* are defined as reactions that remove electrons from a molecule. The common element of most, if not all, oxidations is an enzymatically mediated reaction that inserts a hydroxyl group (OH) into the drug molecule. In some instances, this produces a chemically stable, more polar hydroxylated metabolite. However, hydroxylation usually creates unstable compounds that spontaneously split into separate molecules. Many different biotransformations are affected by this basic mechanism. Dealkylation (removal of a carbon-containing group), deamination (removal of nitrogen-containing groups), oxidation of nitrogen-containing groups, desulfuration, dehalogenation, and dehydrogenation all follow an initial hydroxylation. Hydrolysis and hydroxylation are comparable processes. Both have an initial, enzymatically mediated step that produces an unstable compound that rapidly dissociates into separate molecules.

Some drugs are metabolized by *reductive reactions*, that is, reactions that add electrons to a molecule. In contrast to oxidations, where electrons are transferred from nicotinamide adenine dinucleotide phosphate (NADPH) to an oxygen atom, the electrons are transferred to the drug molecule. Oxidation of xenobiotics requires oxygen, but reductive biotransformation is inhibited by oxygen, so it is facilitated when the intracellular oxygen tension is low.

Cytochrome P450 Enzymes

3 The cytochromes P450 (CYP) is the superfamily of constitutive and inducible enzymes that catalyze most phase I biotransformations. CYP3A4 is the single most important enzyme, accounting for 40 to 45% of all CYP-mediated drug metabolism. CYPs are incorporated into the smooth endoplasmic reticulum of hepatocytes and the membranes of the upper intestinal enterocytes in high concentrations. CYPs are also found in the lungs, kidneys, and skin, but in much smaller amounts. CYP isoenzymes oxidize their substrates primarily by the insertion of an atom of oxygen in the form of a hydroxyl group, while another oxygen atom is reduced to water.

Several constitutive CYPs are involved in the production of various endogenous compounds, such as cholesterol, steroid hormones, prostaglandins, and eicosanoids. In addition to the constitutive forms, production of various CYPs can be induced by a wide variety of xenobiotics. CYP drug-metabolizing activity increases after exposure to various exogenous chemicals,

TABLE 7-1

SUBSTRATES FOR CYTOCHROME P450 (CYP) ISOENZYMES ENCOUNTERED IN ANESTHESIA

CYP3A4	CYP2D6	CYP2C9	CYP2C19
Acetaminophen	Captopril	Diclofenac	Diazepam
Alfentanil	Codeine	Ibuprofen	Omeprazole
Alprazolam	Hydrocodone	Indomethacin	Propranolol
Bupivacaine	Metoprolol		Warfarin
Cisapride	Ondansetron		
Codeine	Propranolol		
Diazepam	Timolol		
Digitoxin	Captopril		
Diltiazem	Codeine		
Fentanyl	Hydrocodone		
Lidocaine			
Methadone			
Midazolam			
Nicardipine			
Nifedipine			
Omeprazole			
Ropivacaine			
Statins			
Sufentanil			
Verapamil			
Warfarin			

including many drugs. The number and type of CYPs present at any time depends on exposure to different xenobiotics. The CYP system is able to protect the organism from the deleterious effects of accumulation of exogenous compounds because of its two fundamental characteristics—broad substrate specificity and the capability to adapt to exposure to different substances by induction of different CYP isoenzymes. Table 7-1 groups drugs encountered in anesthetic practice according to the CYP isoenzymes responsible for their biotransformation.

Biotransformations can be inhibited if different substrates compete for the drug-binding site on the same CYP member. The effect of two competing substrates on each other's metabolism depends on their relative affinities for the enzyme. Biotransformation of the compound with the lower affinity is inhibited to a greater degree. This is the mechanism by which the H_2 receptor antagonist cimetidine inhibits the metabolism of many drugs, including meperidine, propranolol, and diazepam. The newer H_2 antagonist ranitidine has a different structure and causes fewer clinically significant drug interactions. Other drugs, notably calcium channel blockers and antidepressants, also inhibit oxidative drug metabolism in humans. This information allows clinicians to predict which combinations of drugs are more likely to lead to clinically significant interactions because of altered drug metabolism by the cytochrome P450 system.

Phase II Reactions

Phase II reactions are also known as *conjugation* or *synthetic reactions*. Many drugs do not have a polar chemical group suitable for conjugation, so conjugation occurs only after a phase I reaction. Other drugs, such as morphine, already have a polar group that serves as a "handle" for conjugation, and they undergo these reactions directly. Various endogenous compounds can be attached to parent drugs or their phase I metabolites to form different conjugation products. These endogenous substrates include glucuronic acid, acetate, and

amino acids. Mercapturic acid conjugates result from the binding of exogenous compounds to glutathione. Other conjugation reactions produce sulfated or methylated derivatives of drugs or their metabolites. Like the cytochrome P450 system, the enzymes that catalyze phase II reactions are inducible. Phase II reactions produce conjugates that are polar, water-soluble compounds. This facilitates the ultimate excretion of the drug via the kidneys or hepatobiliary secretion. Like CYP, there are different families and superfamilies of the enzymes that catalyze phase II biotransformations.

Genetic Variations in Drug Metabolism

For most enzymes involved in phase I and phase II reactions, there are several biologically available isoforms. Drug metabolism varies substantially among individuals because of variability in the genes controlling the numerous enzymes responsible for biotransformation (see Chapter 6). For most drugs, individual subjects' rates of metabolism have a unimodal distribution. However, distinct subpopulations with different rates of elimination of some drugs have been identified. The resulting multimodal distribution of individual rates of metabolism is known as *polymorphism*. For example, different genotypes result in either normal, low, or (rarely) absent plasma pseudocholinesterase activity, accounting for the well-known differences in individuals' responses to succinylcholine, which is hydrolyzed by this enzyme. Many drug-metabolizing enzymes exhibit genetic polymorphism, including CYP and various transferases that catalyze phase II reactions. However, none of these have a sex-related difference.

Chronologic Variations in Drug Metabolism

The activity and capacity of the CYP enzymes increase from subnormal levels in the fetal and neonatal period to reach normal levels at about 1 year of age. Although age is a covariate in mathematical models of drug elimination, it is not clear if these changes are related to chronologic changes in organ function (age-related organ dysfunction) or a decrease in CYP levels with increasing age. In contrast, it is clear that the neonate has a limited ability to perform phase II conjugation reactions, but after normalizing phase II activity over the initial year of life, advanced age does not affect the capacity to perform phase II reactions.

Renal Drug Clearance

④ The primary role of the kidneys in drug elimination is to excrete into urine the unchanged, hydrophilic drugs, and the hepatic-derived metabolites from phase I and phase II reactions of lipophilic drugs. The passive elimination of drugs by passive glomerular filtration is a very inefficient process—any significant degree of binding of the drug to plasma proteins or erythrocytes will decrease the renal clearance below the glomerular filtration rate of 20% of renal blood flow. In order to make renal elimination more efficient, discrete active transporters of organic acids and bases exist in the proximal renal tubular cells. Although these transporters are saturable, they allow for the renal clearance of drugs to approach the entire renal blood flow.

In reality, renal drug clearance of actively secreted drugs can be inhibited by both passive tubular reabsorption of lipophilic drugs and active, carrier-mediated tubular reabsorption of hydrophilic drugs. Therefore, the small amount of filtered and secreted lipophilic drug is easily reabsorbed in the distal tubules, making the net renal clearance negligible. In contrast, the large amount of filtered and secreted hydrophilic drug can be passively reabsorbed if renal tubular flow decreases substantially (e.g., oliguria) and/or the urine pH favors the un-ionized form of the hydrophilic drug. Because overall renal function is readily estimated by clearance of endogenous creatinine, renal drug clearance, even for drugs eliminated primarily by tubular secretion, depends on renal function. Therefore, in patients with acute and chronic causes of decreased renal function, including age, low cardiac output states, and hepatorenal syndrome, drug dosing must be altered in order to avoid accumulation of parent compounds and potentially toxic metabolites (e.g., lidocaine, meperidine; Table 7-2; see Chapter 52).

Hepatic Drug Clearance

⑤ Drug elimination by the liver depends on the intrinsic ability of the liver to metabolize the drug (intrinsic clearance, Cl_l), and the amount of drug available to diffuse into the liver. Many types of mathematical models have been developed to attempt to accurately model the relationship between hepatic artery blood flow, portal artery blood flow, intrinsic clearance, and drug binding to plasma proteins.[22,23] According to these models, the unbound concentration of drug in the hepatic venous blood (C_v) is in equilibrium with the drug within the liver that

---

TABLE 7-2

DRUGS WITH SIGNIFICANT RENAL EXCRETION ENCOUNTERED IN ANESTHESIOLOGY

Aminoglycosides	Nor-meperidine
Atenolol	Pancuronium
Cephalosporins	Penicillins
Digoxin	Procainamide
Edrophonium	Pyridostigmine
Nadolol	Quinolones
Neostigmine	Rocuronium

---

is available for elimination. These models also make the assumption that all of the drugs delivered to the liver are available for elimination and that the elimination is a first-order process—a constant *fraction* of the available drug is eliminated per unit time. The fraction of the drug removed from the blood passing through the liver is the hepatic extraction ratio, *E*:

$$E = \frac{C_a - C_v}{C_a} \tag{7-1}$$

where C_a is the mixed hepatic arterial–portal venous drug concentration and C_v is the mixed hepatic venous drug concentration. The total hepatic drug clearance, Cl_H, is:

$$Cl_H = Q \cdot E \tag{7-2}$$

where Q is hepatic blood flow. Therefore, hepatic clearance is a function of hepatic blood flow and the ability of the liver to extract drug from the blood.

The ability to extract drug depends on the activity of drug-metabolizing enzymes and the capacity for hepatobiliary excretion—the intrinsic clearance of the liver (Cl_l).

Intrinsic clearance represents the ability of the liver to remove drug from the blood in the absence of any limitations imposed by blood flow or drug binding. The relationship of total hepatic drug clearance to the extraction ratio and intrinsic clearance, Cl_l, is:

$$Cl_H = Q \cdot E = Q\left(\frac{Cl_l}{Q + Cl_l}\right) \tag{7-3}$$

The right-hand side of Equation 7-3 indicates that if intrinsic clearance is very high (many times larger than hepatic blood flow, $Cl_l >> Q$), total hepatic clearance approaches hepatic blood flow. On the other hand, if intrinsic clearance is very small ($Q + Cl_l \approx Q$), hepatic clearance will be similar to intrinsic clearance. These relationships are shown in Figure 7-1.

Thus, hepatic drug clearance and extraction are determined by two independent variables, intrinsic clearance and hepatic blood flow. Changes in either will change hepatic clearance. However, the extent of the change depends on the initial relationship between intrinsic clearance and hepatic blood flow, according to the nonlinear relationship:

$$E = \frac{Cl_l}{Q + Cl_l} \tag{7-4}$$

If the initial intrinsic clearance is small relative to hepatic blood flow, then the extraction ratio is also small, and Equation 7-4 reduces to the following relationship:

$$E = \frac{Cl_l}{Q} \ll 1 \tag{7-4a}$$

Equation 7-4a indicates that doubling intrinsic clearance will produce an almost proportional increment in the extraction ratio, and, consequently, hepatic elimination clearance (Fig. 7-1, inset). However, if intrinsic clearance is much greater than hepatic blood flow, Equation 7-4 reduces to the following relationship:

$$E = \frac{Cl_l}{Cl_l} \approx 1 \tag{7-4b}$$

Equation 7-4b demonstrates that the extraction ratio is independent of intrinsic clearance and therefore a change in

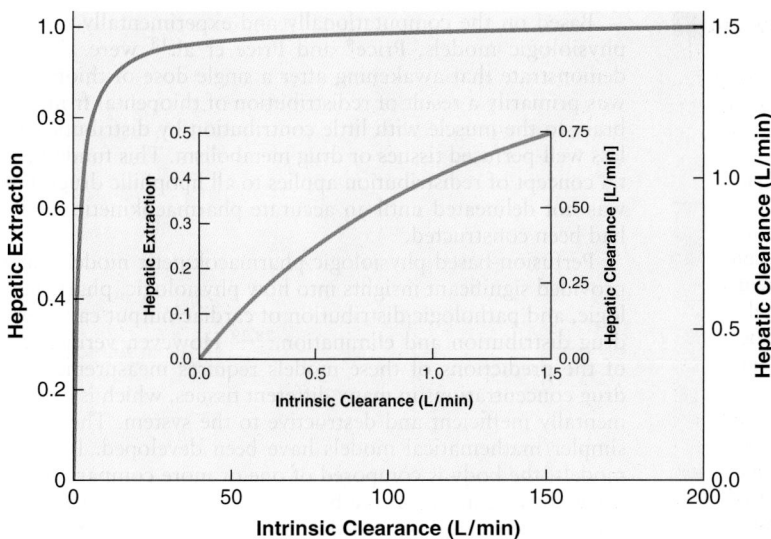

FIGURE 7-1. The relationship between hepatic extraction ratio (E, right y-axis), intrinsic clearance (Cl_I, x-axis), and hepatic clearance (Cl_H, left y-axis) at the normal hepatic blood flow (Q) of 1.5 L/min. For drugs with a high intrinsic clearance ($Cl_I \gg Q$), increasing intrinsic clearance has little effect on hepatic extraction and total hepatic clearance and total hepatic clearance approaches hepatic blood flow. In contrast, if the intrinsic clearance is small ($Cl_I \le Q$), the extraction ratio is similar to the intrinsic clearance (inset). (Adapted from Wilkinson GR, Shand DG: A physiologic approach to hepatic drug clearance. *Clin Pharmacol Ther* 1975; 18: 377.)

SCIENTIFIC FOUNDATIONS OF ANESTHESIA

intrinsic clearance has a negligible effect on the extraction ratio and hepatic drug clearance (Fig. 7-1). In nonmathematical terms, high intrinsic clearance indicates efficient hepatic elimination. It is hard to enhance an already efficient process, whereas it is relatively easy to improve on inefficient drug clearance because of low intrinsic clearance.

For drugs with a high extraction ratio and a high intrinsic clearance, hepatic elimination clearance is directly proportional to hepatic blood flow. Therefore, any manipulation of hepatic blood flow will be directly reflected by a proportional change in hepatic elimination clearance (Fig. 7-2). In contrast, when the intrinsic clearance is low, changes in hepatic blood flow produce inversely proportional changes in extraction

ratio (Fig. 7-3), and therefore the hepatic elimination clearance is essentially independent of hepatic blood flow and exquisitely related to intrinsic clearance (Fig. 7-3). Therefore, classifying drugs as having either low, intermediate, or high extraction ratios (Table 7-3), allows predictions to be made on how intrinsic hepatic clearance and hepatic blood flow effect hepatic elimination clearance. This allows gross adjustments to be made in hepatically metabolized drug dosing to avoid excess accumulation of drugs (decreased hepatic elimination without dose adjustment) or subtherapeutic dosing strategies (increased hepatic elimination without dose adjustment).

Pharmacologic and pathologic manipulations of cardiac output with its consequences on hepatic/splanchnic blood flow

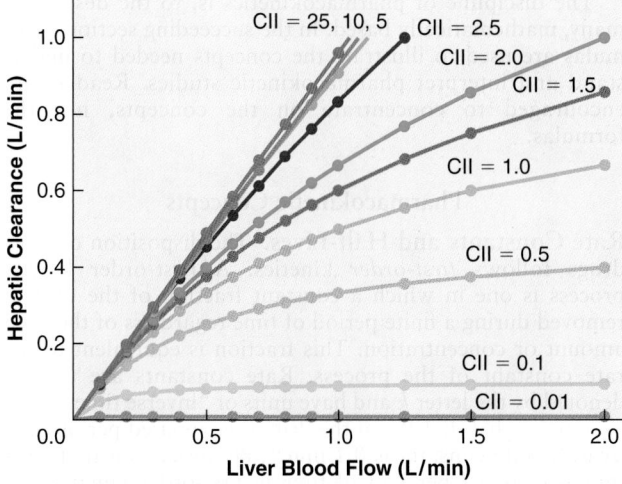

FIGURE 7-2. The relationship between liver blood flow (Q, x-axis) and hepatic clearance (Cl_H, y-axis) for different values of intrinsic clearance (Cl_I). When the intrinsic clearance is low, hepatic elimination clearance is independent of liver blood flow—the drug elimination limited by the capacity of the liver to metabolize the drug (i.e., the intrinsic clearance). In contrast, as intrinsic clearance increases, the hepatic elimination becomes more dependent on hepatic blood flow—the liver is able to metabolize all of the drug that it is exposed to and therefore only limited by the amount of drug that is delivered to the liver (i.e., flow limited metabolism).

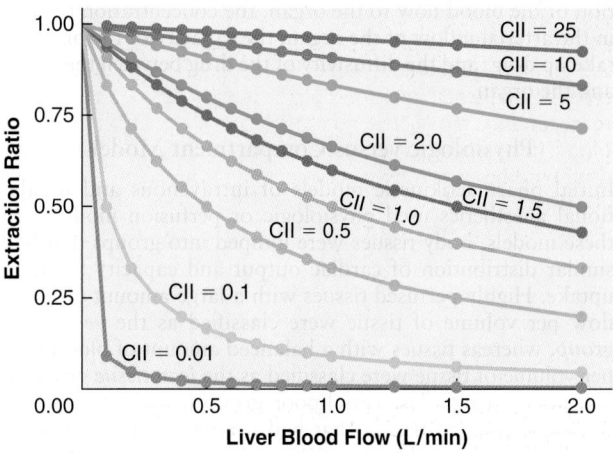

FIGURE 7-3. The relationship between liver blood flow (Q, x-axis) and hepatic extraction ratio (E, y-axis) for different values of intrinsic clearance (Cl_I). When the intrinsic clearance is low, increases in hepatic blood flows cause a decrease in the extraction ratio because the liver has limited metabolic capabilities. In contrast, when the intrinsic clearance is high, the extraction ratio is essentially independent of hepatic blood flow because the liver's ability to eliminate drug is well above the amount of drug provided by normal hepatic blood flow.

TABLE 7-3

CLASSIFICATION OF DRUGS ENCOUNTERED IN ANESTHESIOLOGY ACCORDING TO HEPATIC EXTRACTION RATIOS

■ LOW	■ INTERMEDIATE	■ HIGH
Diazepam	Alfentanil	Alprenolol
Lorazepam	Methohexital	Bupivacaine
Methadone	Midazolam	Diltiazem
Phenytoin	Vecuronium	Fentanyl
Rocuronium		Ketamine
Theophylline		Lidocaine
Thiopental		Meperidine
		Metoprolol
		Morphine
		Naloxone
		Nifedipine
		Propofol
		Propranolol
		Sufentanil

and renal blood flow are important covariates when designing drug-dosing strategies.[24] As previously detailed, in states where cardiac output is decreased (e.g., heart failure, shock, spinal anesthesia), high extraction-rate drugs will have a decrease in hepatic elimination, whereas low extraction-rate drugs will have minimal change in clearance.[25,26] In contrast, autoregulation of renal blood flow maintains a relatively constant renal elimination clearance until low urine output states eventually allow increased reabsorption of drugs from the distal tubules.[27]

Pharmacokinetic Models

The concentration of drug at its site or sites of action is the fundamental determinant of a drug's pharmacologic effects. Although the blood is rarely the site of action of drug effect, the tissue drug concentration of an individual organ is a function of the blood flow to the organ, the concentration of drug in the arterial inflow of the organ, the capacity of the organ to take up drug, and the diffusivity of the drug between the blood and the organ.

Physiologic versus Compartment Models

Initial pharmacokinetic models of intravenous and inhalational anesthetics used physiologic or perfusion models.[4] In these models, body tissues were lumped into groups that had similar distribution of cardiac output and capacity for drug uptake. Highly perfused tissues with a large amount of blood flow per volume of tissue were classified as the *vessel-rich group*, whereas tissues with a balanced amount of blood flow per volume of tissue were classified as the *lean tissue group* or *fast tissue group*. The vessel-poor group (slow tissue group) was composed of tissues that had a large capacity for drug uptake but a limited tissue perfusion. Although identification of the exact organs that made up each tissue group was not possible from the mathematical model, it was apparent that the highly perfused tissues were composed of the brain, lungs, kidneys, and a subset of muscle, the fast equilibrating tissue would be consistent with the majority of muscle and some of the splanchnic bed (e.g., liver), and the slowly equilibrating tissues contained the majority of the adipose tissue and the remainder of the splanchnic organs.

Based on the computationally and experimentally intense physiologic models, Price[4] and Price et al.[18] were able to demonstrate that awakening after a single dose of thiopental was primarily a result of redistribution of thiopental from the brain to the muscle with little contribution by distribution to less well-perfused tissues or drug metabolism. This fundamental concept of redistribution applies to all lipophilic drugs and was not delineated until an accurate pharmacokinetic model had been constructed.

Perfusion-based physiologic pharmacokinetic models have provided significant insights into how physiologic, pharmacologic, and pathologic distribution of cardiac output can effect drug distribution and elimination.[28,29] However, verification of the predictions of these models requires measurement of drug concentrations in many different tissues, which is experimentally inefficient and destructive to the system. Therefore, simpler mathematical models have been developed. In these models, the body is composed of one or more compartments. Drug concentrations in the blood are used to define the relationship between dose and the time course of changes in the drug concentration. The compartments of the compartmental pharmacokinetic models cannot be equated with the tissue groups that make up physiologic pharmacokinetic models because the compartments are theoretical entities that are used to mathematically characterize the blood concentration profile of a drug. These models allow the derivation of pharmacokinetic parameters that can be used to quantify drug distribution and elimination—volume of distribution, clearance, and half-lives.

Although the simplicity of compartmental models, compared with physiologic pharmacokinetic models, has its advantages, it also has some disadvantages. For example, cardiac output is not a parameter of compartmental models, and compartmental models therefore cannot be used to predict directly the effect of cardiac failure on drug disposition.[30] However, compartmental pharmacokinetic models can still quantify the effects of reduced cardiac output on the disposition of a drug if a group of patients with cardiac failure is compared with a group of otherwise healthy subjects.

The discipline of pharmacokinetics is, to the despair of many, mathematically based. In the succeeding sections, formulas are used to illustrate the concepts needed to understand and interpret pharmacokinetic studies. Readers are encouraged to concentrate on the concepts, not the formulas.

Pharmacokinetic Concepts

Rate Constants and Half-Lives. The disposition of most drugs follows *first-order* kinetics. A first-order kinetic process is one in which a constant fraction of the drug is removed during a finite period of time regardless of the drug amount or concentration. This fraction is equivalent to the rate constant of the process. Rate constants are usually denoted by the letter k and have units of "inverse time," such as $\min^{-1}$ or h^{-1}. If 10% of the drug is eliminated per minute, then the rate constant is 0.1 $\min^{-1}$. Because a constant fraction is removed per unit of time in first-order kinetics, the absolute amount of drug removed is proportional to the concentration of the drug. It follows that, in first-order kinetics, the rate of change of the amount of drug at any given time is proportional to the concentration present at that time. When the concentration is high, more drugs will be removed than when it is low. First-order kinetics apply not only to elimination, but also to absorption and distribution. Rather than using rate constants, the rapidity of pharmacokinetic processes is often described with half-lives—the time required for the concentration to change by a factor of 2. Half-lives are calculated directly from the corresponding rate constants with this simple equation:

$$t_{1/2} = \frac{\ln 2}{k} = \frac{0.693}{k} \qquad (7\text{-}6)$$

Thus, for a rate constant (k) of 0.1 min^{-1}

$$t_{1/2} = \frac{\ln 2}{k} = \frac{\ln 2}{0.1 \text{ min}^{-1}} = 6.93 \text{ min} \qquad (7\text{-}6a)$$

the half-life is 6.93 minutes. The half-life of any first-order kinetic process, including drug absorption, distribution, and elimination, can be calculated. First-order processes asymptotically approach completion because a constant fraction of the drug, not an absolute amount, is removed per unit of time. However, after five half-lives, the process will be almost 97% complete (Table 7-4). For practical purposes, this is essentially 100% and therefore there is a negligible amount of drug remaining in the body.

6 **Volume of Distribution.** The volume of distribution quantifies the extent of drug distribution. The physiologic factor that governs the extent of drug distribution is the overall capacity of tissues versus the capacity of blood for that drug. Overall tissue capacity for uptake of a drug is in turn a function of the total mass of the tissues into which a drug distributes and their average affinity for the drug. In compartmental pharmacokinetic models, drugs are envisaged as distributing into one or more "boxes," or compartments. These compartments cannot be equated directly with specific tissues. Rather, they are hypothetical entities that permit analysis of drug distribution and elimination and description of the drug concentration versus time profile.

The volume of distribution is an "apparent" volume because it represents the size of these hypothetical boxes, or compartments, that are necessary to explain the concentration of drug in a reference compartment, usually called the *central* or *plasma compartment*. The volume of distribution, V_d, relates the total amount of drug present to the concentration observed in the central compartment:

$$V_d = \frac{\text{amount of drug administered}}{\text{initial drug plasma concentration}} \qquad (7\text{-}7)$$

If a drug is extensively distributed, then the concentration will be lower relative to the amount of drug present, which equates to a larger volume of distribution. For example, if a total of 10 mg of drug is present and the concentration is 2 mg/L, then the apparent volume of distribution is 5 L. On the other hand, if the concentration was 4 mg/L, then the volume of distribution would be 2.5 L.

Simply stated, the apparent volume of distribution is a numeric index of the extent of drug distribution that does not have any relationship to the actual volume of any tissue or group of tissues. It may be as small as plasma volume, or, if overall tissue uptake is extensive, the apparent volume of distribution may greatly exceed the actual total volume of the body. In general, lipophilic drugs have larger volumes of distribution than hydrophilic drugs. Because the volume of distribution is a mathematical construct to model the distribution of a drug in the body, the volume of distribution cannot provide any information regarding the actual tissue concentration in any specific real organ in the body. However, this simple mathematical construct provides a useful summary description of the behavior of the drug in the body. In fact, the loading dose of drug required to achieve a target plasma concentration can be easily calculated by rearranging Equation 7-7 as follows:

$$\text{Loading Dose} = V_d \times \text{Target Concentration} \qquad (7\text{-}7a)$$

Based on this equation, it is clear that an increase in the volume of distribution means that a larger loading dose will be required to "fill up the box" and achieve the same concentration. Therefore any change in state because of changes in physiologic and pathologic conditions can alter the volume of distribution, necessitating therapeutic adjustments.

7 **Total Drug (Elimination) Clearance.** *Elimination clearance* (drug clearance) is the theoretical volume of blood from which drug is completely and irreversibly removed in a unit of time. Elimination clearance has the units of flow—[volume per time]. *Total* drug clearance can be calculated with pharmacokinetic models of blood concentration versus time data. Drug clearance is often corrected for weight or body surface area, in which case the units are mL/min/kg or mL/min/m^2, respectively.

Elimination clearance, Cl, can be calculated from the declining blood levels observed after an intravenous injection, as follows:

$$Cl = \frac{\text{amount of drug administered}}{\text{area under the concentration versus time curve}} \qquad (7\text{-}8)$$

If a drug is rapidly removed from the plasma, its concentration will fall more quickly than the concentration of a drug that is less readily eliminated. This results in a smaller area under the concentration versus time curve, which equates to greater clearance (Fig. 7-4).

TABLE 7-4

HALF-LIVES AND PERCENT OF DRUG REMOVED

NUMBER OF HALF-LIVES	PERCENT OF DRUG REMAINING	PERCENT OF DRUG REMOVED
0	100	0
1	50	50
2	25	75
3	12.5	87.5
4	6.25	93.75
5	3.125	96.875

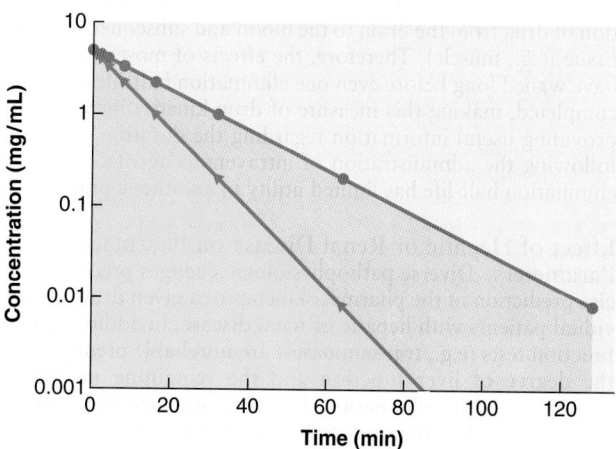

FIGURE 7-4. The plasma concentration (y-axis) versus time (x-axis) curve for two drugs that differ only in their elimination clearance. Notice that the areas under the curves are different, signifying that the drug that has the smaller area under the curve is more rapidly eliminated from the body than the drug that has the slower elimination clearance.

Without additional organ-specific data (e.g., urine drug concentration measurements, drug arterial inflow concentration), calculating elimination clearance from compartmental pharmacokinetic models usually does not specify the relative contribution of different organs to drug elimination. Nonetheless, estimation of drug clearance with these models has made important contributions to clinical pharmacology. In particular, these models have provided a great deal of clinically useful information regarding altered drug elimination in various pathologic conditions.

Elimination Half-Life. Although the elimination clearance is the pharmacokinetic parameter that best describes the physiologic process of drug elimination (i.e., drug delivery to organs of elimination coupled with the capacity of the organ to eliminate the drug), the pharmacokinetic variable most often reported in textbooks and literature is the *elimination half-life* of a drug ($t_{1/2_\beta}$). The elimination half-life is the time during which the amount of drug in the body decreases by 50%. Although this parameter appears to be a simple summary of the physiology of drug elimination, it is actually a complex parameter, influenced by the distribution and the elimination of the drug, as follows:

$$t_{1/2_\beta} = \frac{\ln 2}{k_\beta} = 0.693 \times \frac{V_d}{Cl_E} \qquad (7\text{-}9)$$

Therefore, when a physiologic or pathologic perturbation changes the elimination half-life of a drug, it is not a simple reflection of the change in the body's ability to metabolize or eliminate the drug. For example, the elimination half-life of thiopental is prolonged in the elderly; however, the elimination clearance is unchanged and the volume of distribution is increased.[31] Therefore, elderly patients need dosing strategies that accommodate for the change in the distribution of the drug rather than a decreased metabolism of the drug. In contrast, in patients with renal insufficiency, the increase in the elimination half-life of pancuronium is due to a simple decrease in renal elimination of the drug and the volume of distribution is unchanged.[32]

Besides its inability to give insight into the mechanism by which a drug is retained in the body, the elimination half-life is unable to give insight into the time that it takes for a single or a series of repeated drug doses to terminate its effect. Although elimination of drug from the body begins the moment the drug is delivered to the organs of elimination, the rapid termination of effect of a bolus of an intravenous agent is due to redistribution of drug from the brain to the blood and subsequently other tissue (e.g., muscle). Therefore, the effects of most anesthetics have waned long before even one elimination half-life has been completed, making this measure of drug kinetics incapable of providing useful information regarding the duration of action following the administration of intravenous agents. Thus the elimination half-life has limited utility in anesthetic practice.[10]

Effect of Hepatic or Renal Disease on Pharmacokinetic Parameters. Diverse pathophysiologic changes preclude precise prediction of the pharmacokinetics of a given drug in individual patients with hepatic or renal disease. In addition, liver function tests (e.g., transaminases) are unreliable predictors of the degree of liver function and the remaining metabolic capacity for drug elimination. However, some generalizations can be made. In patients with hepatic disease, the elimination half-life of drugs metabolized or excreted by the liver is often increased because of decreased clearance, and, possibly, increased volume of distribution caused by ascites and altered protein binding.[10,33] Drug concentration at steady-state is inversely proportional to elimination clearance. Therefore, when hepatic drug clearance is reduced, repeated bolus dosing or continuous infusion of such drugs as benzodiazepines, opi-

oids, and barbiturates may result in excessive accumulation of drug as well as excessive and prolonged pharmacologic effects. Since recovery from small doses of drugs such as thiopental and fentanyl is largely the result of redistribution, recovery from conservative doses will be minimally affected by reductions in elimination clearance. In patients with renal failure, similar concerns apply to the administration of drugs excreted by the kidneys. It is almost always better to underestimate a patient's dose requirement, observe the response, and give additional drug if necessary.

Nonlinear Pharmacokinetics. The physiologic and compartmental models thus far discussed are based on the assumption that drug distribution and elimination are first-order processes. Therefore, their parameters, such as clearance and elimination half-life, are independent of the dose or concentration of the drug. However, the rate of elimination of a few drugs is dose-dependent, or *nonlinear.*

Elimination of drugs involves interactions with either enzymes catalyzing biotransformation reactions or carrier proteins for transmembrane transport. If sufficient drug is present, the capacity of the drug-eliminating systems can be exceeded. When this occurs, it is no longer possible to excrete a constant fraction of the drug present to the eliminating system, and a constant amount of drug is excreted per unit time. Phenytoin is a well-known example of a drug that exhibits nonlinear elimination at therapeutic concentrations,[34] whereas in anesthetic practice, the extremely high doses of thiopental used for cerebral protection can demonstrate zero-order elimination.[35] In theory, all drugs are cleared in a nonlinear fashion. In practice, the capacity to eliminate most drugs is so great that this is usually not evident, even with toxic concentrations.

Compartmental Pharmacokinetic Models

One-Compartment Model. Although for most drugs the one-compartment model is an oversimplification, it does serve to illustrate the basic relationships among clearance, volume of distribution, and the elimination half-life. In this model, the body is envisaged as a single homogeneous compartment. Drug distribution after injection is assumed to be instantaneous, so there are no concentration gradients within the compartment. The concentration can decrease only by elimination of drug from the system. The plasma concentration versus time curve for a hypothetical drug with one-compartment kinetics is shown in Figure 7-5. The decrease in plasma concentration (C) with time from the initial concentration (C_0) can be characterized by the simple monoexponential function:

$$C(t) = C_0 \times e^{-k_e \times t} \qquad (7\text{-}10)$$

With the concentration plotted on a logarithmic scale, the concentration versus time curve becomes a straight line. The slope of the logarithm of concentration versus time is equal to the first-order elimination rate constant (k_e).

In the one-compartment model, drug clearance, Cl, is equal to the product of the elimination rate constant, k_e, and the volume of distribution:

$$Cl = k_e \cdot V_d \qquad (7\text{-}11)$$

Combining Equations 6 and 10 yields Equation 7-9 (where $k_e = k_\beta$):

$$t_{1/2_\beta} = \frac{\ln 2}{k_e} = 0.693 \times \frac{V_d}{Cl_E} \qquad (7\text{-}9)$$

Therefore, when it is appropriate to make the simplifying assumption of instantaneous mixing of drug into a single compartment, the elimination half-life is inversely proportional to the slope of the concentration time curve. For drugs that require

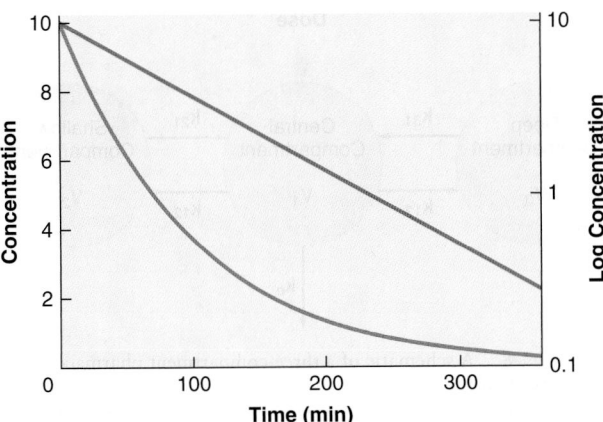

FIGURE 7-5. The plasma concentration versus time profile plotted on both linear (*dashed line*, left y-axis) and logarithmic (*dotted line*, right y-axis) scales for a hypothetical drug exhibiting one-compartment, first-order pharmacokinetics. Note that the slope of the logarithmic concentration profile is equal to the elimination rate constant (k_e) and related to the elimination half-life ($t_{1/2\beta}$) as described in Equation 7-9.

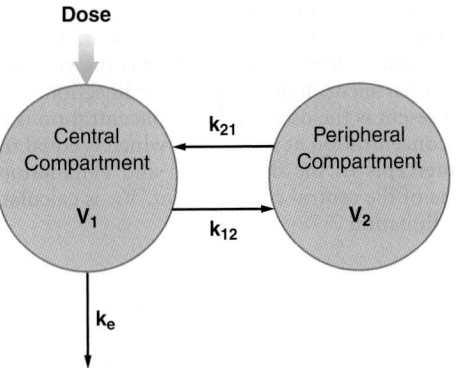

FIGURE 7-7. A schematic of a two-compartment pharmacokinetic model. See text for explanation.

⑧ consideration of their multicompartmental pharmacokinetics, the relationship among clearance, volume of distribution, and the elimination half-life is not a simple linear one such as Equation 7-9. However, the same principles apply. All else being equal, the greater the clearance, the shorter the elimination half-life; the larger the volume of distribution, the longer the elimination half-life. Thus, the elimination half-life depends on two other variables, clearance and volume of distribution, that characterize, respectively, the extent of drug distribution and efficiency of drug elimination.

Two-Compartment Model. For many drugs, a graph of the logarithm of the plasma concentration versus time after an intravenous injection is similar to the schematic graph shown in Figure 7-6. There are two discrete phases in the decline of the

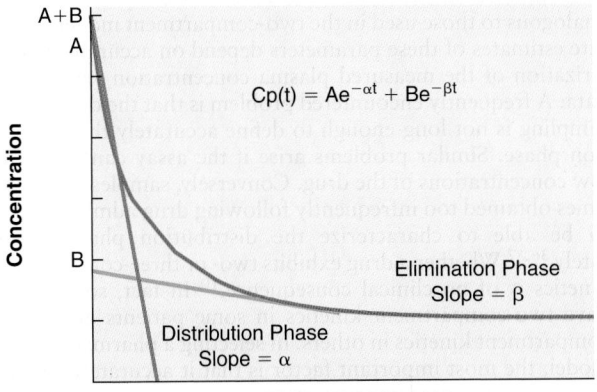

Time After IV Injection

FIGURE 7-6. The logarithmic plasma concentration versus time profile for a hypothetical drug exhibiting two-compartment, first-order pharmacokinetics. Note that the distribution phase has a slope that is significantly larger than that of the elimination phase, indicating that the process of distribution is not only more rapid than elimination of the drug from the body, but also responsible for the majority of the decline in plasma concentration in the several minutes after drug administration. IV, intravenous.

plasma concentration. The first phase after injection is characterized by a very rapid decrease in concentration. The rapid decrease in concentration during this "distribution phase" is largely caused by passage of drug from the plasma into tissues. The distribution phase is followed by a slower decline of the concentration owing to drug elimination. Elimination also begins immediately after injection, but its contribution to the drop in plasma concentration is initially much smaller than the fall in concentration because of drug distribution.

To account for this biphasic behavior, one must consider the body to be made up of two compartments, a central compartment, which includes the plasma, and a peripheral compartment (Fig. 7-7). This two-compartment model assumes that it is the central compartment into which the drug is injected and from which the blood samples for measurement of concentration are obtained, and that drug is eliminated only from the central compartment. Drug distribution within the central compartment is considered to be instantaneous. In reality, this last assumption cannot be true. However, drug uptake into some of the highly perfused tissues is so rapid that it cannot be detected as a discrete phase on the plasma concentration versus time curve.

The distribution and elimination phases can be characterized by graphic analysis of the plasma concentration versus time curve, as shown in Figure 7-6. The elimination phase line is extrapolated back to time zero (the time of injection). In Figure 7-6, the zero time intercepts of the distribution and elimination lines are points A and B, respectively. The *hybrid rate constants*, α and β, are equal to the slopes of the two lines, and are used to calculate the distribution and elimination half-lives; α and β are called *hybrid rate constants* because they depend on both distribution and elimination processes.

At any time after an intravenous injection, the plasma concentration of drugs with two-compartment kinetics is equal to the sum of two exponential terms:

$$C_p(t) = Ae^{-\alpha t} + Be^{-\beta t} \qquad (7\text{-}12)$$

where t = time, $C_p(t)$ = plasma concentration at time t, A = y-axis intercept of the distribution phase line, α = hybrid rate constant of the distribution phase, B = y-axis intercept of the elimination phase line, and β = hybrid rate constant of the elimination phase. The first term characterizes the distribution phase and the second term characterizes the elimination phase. Immediately after injection, the first term represents a much larger fraction of the total plasma concentration than the second term. After several distribution half-lives, the value of the first term approaches zero, and the plasma concentration is essentially equal to the value of the second term (see Fig. 7-6).

In multicompartmental models, the drug is initially distributed only within the central compartment. Therefore, the initial apparent volume of distribution is the volume of the central compartment. Immediately after injection, the amount of drug present is the dose, and the concentration is the extrapolated concentration at time $t = 0$, which is equal to the sum of the intercepts of the distribution and elimination lines. The volume of the central compartment, V_1, is calculated by modifying Equation 7-7:

$$V_1 = \frac{dose}{initial\ plasma\ concentration} = \frac{dose}{A + B} \quad (7\text{-}13)$$

The volume of the central compartment is important in clinical anesthesiology because it is the pharmacokinetic parameter that determines the peak plasma concentration after an intravenous bolus injection. Hypovolemia, for example, reduces the volume of the central compartment. If doses are not correspondingly reduced, the higher plasma concentrations will increase the incidence of adverse pharmacologic effects.

Immediately after intravenous injection, all of the drug is in the central compartment. Simultaneously, three processes begin. Drug moves from the central to the peripheral compartment, which also has a volume, V_2. This intercompartmental transfer is a first-order process, and its magnitude is quantified by the rate constant k_{12}. As soon as drug appears in the peripheral compartment, some passes back to the central compartment, a process characterized by the rate constant k_{21}. The transfer of drug between the central and peripheral compartments is quantified by the *distributional* or *intercompartmental clearance*:

$$Intercompartmental\ Clearance = Cl_{12} = Cl_{21} = V_1 \times k_{12}$$
$$= V_2 \times k_{21} \quad (7\text{-}14)$$

The third process that begins immediately after administration of the drug is irreversible removal of drug from the system via the central compartment. As in the one-compartment model, the elimination rate constant is k_e, and *elimination clearance* is:

$$Elimination\ Clearance = Cl_E = V_1 \times k_e \quad (7\text{-}15)$$

The rapidity of the decrease in the central compartment concentration after intravenous injection depends on the magnitude of the compartmental volumes, the intercompartmental clearance, and the elimination clearance.

At equilibrium, the drug is distributed between the central and the peripheral compartments, and by definition, the drug concentrations in the compartments are equal. Therefore, the ultimate volume of distribution, termed the *volume of distribution at steady-state* (V_{ss}), is the sum of V_1 and V_2. Extensive tissue uptake of a drug is reflected by a large volume of the peripheral compartment, which, in turn, results in a large V_{ss}. Consequently, V_{ss} can greatly exceed the actual volume of the body.

As in the single-compartment model, in multicompartment models the elimination clearance is equal to the dose divided by the area under the concentration versus time curve. This area, as well as the compartmental volumes and intercompartmental clearances, can be calculated from the intercepts and hybrid rate constants, without having to reach steady-state conditions.

Three-Compartment Model. After intravenous injection of some drugs, the initial, rapid distribution phase is followed by a second, slower distribution phase before the elimination phase becomes evident. Therefore, the plasma concentration is the sum of three exponential terms:

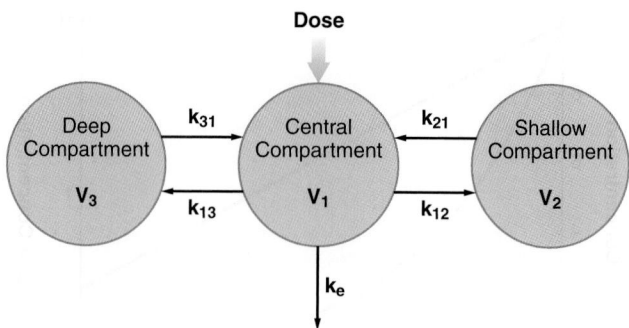

FIGURE 7-8. A schematic of a three-compartment pharmacokinetic model. See text for details.

$$C_p(t) = Ae^{-\alpha t} + Be^{-\beta t} + Ge^{-\gamma t} \quad (7\text{-}16)$$

where t = time, $C_p(t)$ = plasma concentration at time t, A = intercept of the rapid distribution phase line, α = hybrid rate constant of the rapid distribution phase, B = intercept of the slower distribution phase line, β = hybrid rate constant of the slower distribution phase, G = intercept of the elimination phase line, and γ = hybrid rate constant of the elimination phase. This triphasic behavior is explained by a three-compartment pharmacokinetic model (Fig. 7-8). As in the two-compartment model, the drug is injected into and eliminated from the central compartment. Drug is reversibly transferred between the central compartment and two peripheral compartments, which accounts for two distribution phases. Drug transfer between the central compartment and the more rapidly equilibrating, or "shallow," peripheral compartment is characterized by the first-order rate constants k_{12} and k_{21}. Transfer in and out of the more slowly equilibrating, "deep" compartment is characterized by the rate constants k_{13} and k_{31}. In this model, there are three compartmental volumes: V_1, V_2, and V_3, whose sum equals V_{ss}; and three clearances: the rapid intercompartmental clearance, the slow intercompartmental clearance, and elimination clearance.

The pharmacokinetic parameters of interest to clinicians, such as clearance, volumes of distribution, and distribution and elimination half-lives, are determined by calculations analogous to those used in the two-compartment model. Accurate estimates of these parameters depend on accurate characterization of the measured plasma concentration versus time data. A frequently encountered problem is that the duration of sampling is not long enough to define accurately the elimination phase. Similar problems arise if the assay cannot detect low concentrations of the drug. Conversely, samples are sometimes obtained too infrequently following drug administration to be able to characterize the distribution phases accurately.[36,37] Whether a drug exhibits two- or three-compartment kinetics is of no clinical consequence.[10] In fact, some drugs have two-compartment kinetics in some patients and three-compartment kinetics in others. In selecting a pharmacokinetic model, the most important factor is that it accurately characterizes the measured concentrations.

In general, the model with the smallest number of compartments or exponents that accurately reflects the data is used. However, it is good to consider that the data collected in a particular study may not be reflective of the clinical pharmacologic issues of concern in another situation, making published pharmacokinetic model parameters potentially irrelevant. For instance, new data indicate that hypotension following intravenous administration of drug X is related to peak arterial plasma drug X concentrations

1 minute after injection, but previous pharmacokinetic models are based on venous plasma drug X concentrations beginning 5 minutes after the dose. In this case, the pharmacokinetic models will not be of use in designing dosing regimens for drug X that avoid toxic drug concentrations at 1 minute.[10,38,39]

Almost all earlier pharmacokinetic studies used *two-stage modeling*. With this technique, pharmacokinetic parameters were estimated independently for each subject and then averaged to provide estimates of the typical parameters for the population. One problem with this approach is that if outliers are present, averaging parameters could result in a model that does not accurately predict typical drug concentrations. Currently, most pharmacokinetic models are developed using *population pharmacokinetic modeling*, which has been made feasible because of advances in modeling software and increased computing power. With these techniques, the pharmacokinetic parameters are estimated using all the concentration versus time data from the entire group of subjects in a single stage, using sophisticated nonlinear regression methods. This modeling technique provides single estimates of the typical parameter values for the population.

Noncompartmental (Stochastic) Pharmacokinetic Models

Often investigators performing pharmacokinetic analyses of drugs want to avoid the experimental requirements of a physiologic model—data or empirical estimations of individual organ inflow and outflow concentration profiles and organ tissue drug concentrations are required in order to identify the components of the model.[40] Although compartmental models do not assume any physiologic or anatomic basis for the model structure, investigators often attribute anatomic and physiologic function to these empiric models.[41] Even if the disciplined clinical pharmacologist avoids overinterpretation of the meaning of compartment models, the simple fact that several competing models can provide equally good descriptions of the mathematical data or that some subjects in a data set may be better fit with a three-compartment model rather than the two-compartment model that provides the best fit for the other data set subjects leads many to question whether there is a true best model architecture for any given drug. Therefore, some investigators choose to employ mathematical techniques to characterize a pharmacokinetic data set that attempt to avoid any preconceived notion of structure and yet yield the pharmacokinetic parameters that summarize drug distribution and elimination. These techniques are classified as *noncompartmental* techniques or *stochastic* techniques and are similar to the methods based on moment analysis used in process analysis of chemical engineering systems. Although these techniques are often called *model-independent*, like any mathematical construct, assumptions must be made to simplify the mathematics. The basic assumptions of noncompartmental analysis are that all of the elimination clearance occurs directly from the plasma, the distribution and elimination of drug is a linear and first-order process, and the pharmacokinetics of the system does not vary over the time of the data collection (time-invariant). All of these assumptions are also made in the basic compartmental and most physiologic models. Therefore, the main advantage of the noncompartmental pharmacokinetic methods is that a general description of drug absorption, distribution, and elimination can be made without resorting to more complex mathematical modeling techniques.[40]

Another appealing facet of noncompartmental analysis is that the parameters that describe drug distribution (volume of distribution at steady-state, Vd_{ss}) and drug elimination (elimination clearance, Cl_E) are analogous to parameters found in other pharmacokinetic techniques. In fact, when properly defined, the estimates of these parameters from the noncompartmental approach and a well-defined compartmental model yield similar values. The main unique parameter of noncompartmental analysis is the mean residence time (MRT), which is the average time a drug molecule spends in the body before being eliminated.[42] The MRT unfortunately suffers from the main failings of the elimination half-life derived from compartmental models—not only does it fail to capture the contribution of extensive distribution versus limited elimination to allow a drug to linger in the body, but both parameters also fail to describe the situation in which the drug effect can dissipate by redistribution of drug from the site of action back into blood and then into other, less well-perfused tissues.[43]

PHARMACODYNAMIC PRINCIPLES

Much of the clinical pharmacology efforts of the late 1980s through 1990s were devoted to applying new computational power of desktop personal computers to deciphering the pharmacokinetics of intravenous anesthetics. However, the premise behind developing models to better characterize and understand the effects of various physiologic and pathologic states on drug distribution and elimination was that the efforts of the previous 30 years had clearly characterized the relationship between a dose of drug and its effect(s). As computational power and drug assay technology grew, it became possible to characterize the relationship between a drug concentration and the associated pharmacologic effect. As a result, pharmacodynamic studies since the 1990s have focused on the quantitative analysis of the relationship between the drug concentration in the blood and the resultant effects of the drug on physiologic processes.

Drug-Receptor Interactions

Most pharmacologic agents produce their physiologic effects by binding to a drug-specific receptor, which brings about a change in cellular function. The majority of pharmacologic receptors are cell membrane-bound proteins, although some receptors are located in the cytoplasm or the nucleoplasm of the cell.

Binding of drugs to receptors, like the binding of drugs to plasma proteins, is usually reversible, and follows the law of Mass Action:

$$[drug] + [receptor] \leftrightarrow [drug - receptor\ complex] \quad (7\text{-}17)$$

This relationship demonstrates that the higher the concentration of free drug or unoccupied receptor, the greater the tendency to form the drug-receptor complex. Plotting the percentage of receptors occupied by a drug against the logarithm of the concentration of the drug yields a sigmoid curve, as shown in Figure 7-9.[44]

The percentage of receptors occupied by a drug is not equivalent to the percentage of maximal effect produced by the drug. In fact, most receptor systems have more receptors than required to obtain the maximum drug effect.[45] The presence of "extra" unoccupied receptors will promote the formation of the drug-receptor complex (law of Mass Action, Equation 7-17), therefore, near-maximal drug effects can occur at very low drug concentrations. This not only allows

FIGURE 7-9.   A schematic curve of the effect of a drug plotted against dose. In the left panel, the response data are plotted against the dose data on a linear scale. In the right panel, the same response data are plotted against the dose data on a logarithmic scale yielding a sigmoid dose-response curve that is linear between 20 and 80% of the maximal effect.

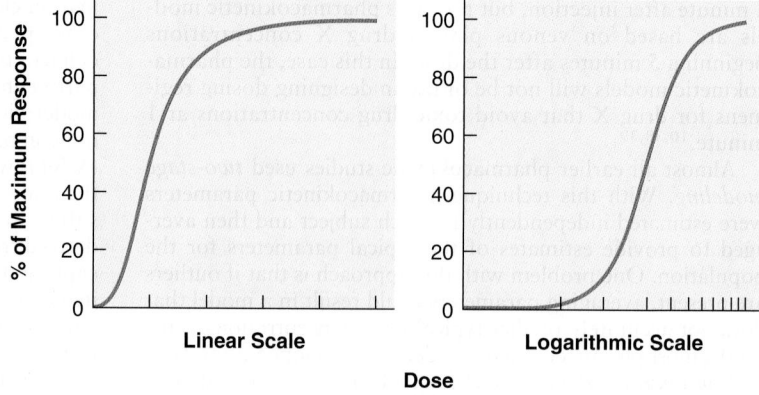

extremely efficient responses to drugs, but it provides a large margin of safety—an extremely large number of a drugs receptors must be bound to an antagonist before the drug is unable to produce its pharmacologic effect. For example, at the neuromuscular junction, only 20 to 25% of the postjunctional nicotinic cholinergic receptors need to bind acetylcholine to produce contraction of all the fibers in the muscle whereas 75% of the receptors must be blocked by a nondepolarizing neuromuscular antagonist to produce a significant drop in muscle strength. This accounts for the "margin of safety" of neuromuscular transmission[45] (see Chapter 20).

The binding of drugs to receptors and the resulting changes in cellular function are the last two steps in the complex series of events between administration of the drug and production of its pharmacologic effects. There are two primary schemes by which the binding of an agonist to a receptor changes cellular function: receptor-linked membrane ion channels called *ionophores,* and guanine nucleotide binding proteins, referred to as *G-proteins.* The nicotinic cholinergic receptor in the neuromuscular postsynaptic membrane is one example of a receptor-ionophore complex. Binding of acetylcholine opens the cation ionophore, leading to an influx of Na^+ ions, propagation of an action potential, and, ultimately, muscle contraction. The β-amino butyric acid (GABA) receptor–chloride ionophore complex is another example of this type of effector mechanism. Binding of either endogenous neurotransmitters (GABA) or exogenous agonists (benzodiazepines and intravenous anesthetics) increases Cl^- conductance, which hyperpolarizes the neuron and decreases its excitability. Adrenergic receptors are the prototypical G protein coupled receptors. G proteins change the intracellular concentrations of various so-called *second messengers,* such as Ca^{2+} and cyclic AMP in order to transducer their signal and produce modify cellular behavior (see Chapter 15).

Desensitization and Down-Regulation of Receptors

Receptors are not static entities. Rather, they are dynamic cellular components that adapt to their environment. Prolonged exposure of a receptor to its agonist leads to desensitization; subsequent doses of the agonist will produce lower maximal effects. With sustained elevation of the cytosolic second messengers downstream of the G-proteins, pathways to prevent further G protein signaling are activated. Phosphorylation by G-protein receptor kinases and arrestin-mediated blockage of the coupling site needed to form the active heterotrimeric G-protein complex prevents G protein-coupled receptors from becoming active. Arrestins and other cell membrane proteins

can tag receptors that have sustained activity so that these non–G protein receptors are internalized and sequestered so they are no longer accessible to agonists. Similar mechanisms will prevent the trafficking of stored receptors to the cell membrane. The combined increased rate of internalization and decreased rate of replenishing of receptor results in *down-regulation*—a decrease in the total number of receptors. Signals that produce down-regulation with sustained receptor activation are essentially reversed in the face of constant receptor inactivity. Therefore, chronically denervated neuromuscular junctions just like cardiac tissue constantly bathed with adrenergic antagonists will both up-regulate the specific receptors in an attempt to produce a signal in the face of lower concentrations of agonists.

Agonists, Partial Agonists, and Antagonists

Drugs that bind to receptors and produce an effect are called *agonists.* Drugs may be capable of producing the same maximal effect (E_{MAX}), although they may differ in concentration that produces the effect (i.e., potency). Agonists that differ in potency but bind to the same receptors will have parallel concentration-response curves (curves *A* and *B* in Fig. 7-10). Differences in potency of agonists reflect differences in affinity for the receptor. *Partial agonists* are drugs that are not capable of producing the maximal effect, even at very high concentrations (curve *C* in Fig. 7-10).

Compounds that bind to receptors without producing any changes in cellular function are referred to as *antagonists*—antagonists blocking the active binding site(s) inhibit agonist binding to the receptors. *Competitive antagonists* bind reversibly to receptors, and their blocking effect can be overcome by high concentrations of an agonist (i.e., competition). Therefore, competitive antagonists produce a parallel shift in the dose-response curve, but the maximum effect is not altered (see curves *A* and *B* in Fig. 7-10). *Noncompetitive antagonists* bind irreversibly to receptors. This has the same effect as reducing the number of receptors and shifts the dose-response curve downward and to the right, decreasing both the slope and the maximum effect (curves *A* and *C* in Fig. 7-10). The effect of noncompetitive antagonists is reversed only by synthesis of new receptor molecules.

Agonists produce a structural change in the receptor molecule that initiates changes in cellular function. Partial agonists may produce a qualitatively different change in the receptor, whereas antagonists bind without producing a change in the receptor that results in altered cellular function. The underlying mechanisms by which different compounds that bind to the same receptor act as agonists, partial agonists, or antagonists are not fully understood.

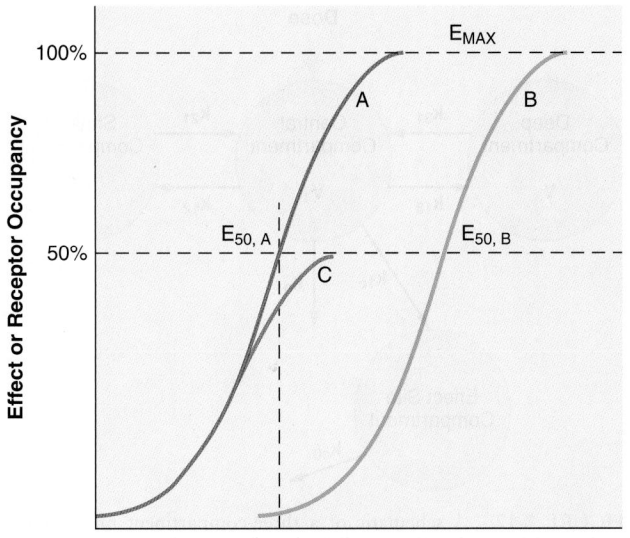

FIGURE 7-10. Schematic pharmacodynamic curves, with dose or concentration on the x-axis and effect or receptor occupancy on the y-axis, that illustrate agonism, partial agonism, and antagonism. Drug A produces a maximum effect, E_{MAX}, and a 50% of maximal effect at dose or concentration $E_{50,A}$. Drug B, a full agonist, can produce the maximum effect, E_{MAX}; however, it is less potent ($E_{50,B} > E_{50,A}$). Drug C, a partial agonist, can only produce a maximum effect of approximately 50% E_{MAX}. If a competitive antagonist is given to a patient, the dose response for the agonist would shift from curve A to curve B. Although the receptors would have the same affinity for the agonist, the presence of the competitor would necessitate an increase in agonist in order to produce an effect. In fact, the agonist would still be able to produce a maximal effect if a sufficient overdose was given to displace the competitive antagonist. However, the competitive antagonist would not change the binding characteristics of the receptor for the agonist and so curve B is simply shifted to the right but remains parallel to curve A. In contrast, if a noncompetitive antagonist binds to the receptor, the agonist would no longer be able to produce a maximal effect, no matter how much of an overdose is administered (curve C).

Dose-Response Relationships

Dose-response studies determine the relationship between increasing doses of a drug and the ensuing changes in pharmacologic effects. Schematic dose-response curves are shown in Figure 7-9, with the dose plotted on both linear and logarithmic scales. There is a curvilinear relationship between dose and the intensity of response. Low doses produce little pharmacologic effect. Once effects become evident, a small increase in dose produces a relatively large change in effect. At near-maximal response, large increases in dose produce little change in effect. Usually the dose is plotted on a logarithmic scale (see Fig. 7-9, right panel), which demonstrates the linear relationship between the logarithm of the dose and the intensity of the response between 20 and 80% of the maximum effect.

Acquiring the pharmacologic effect data from a population of subjects exposed to a variety of doses of a drug provides four key characteristics of the drug dose-response relationship: potency, drug-receptor affinity, efficacy, and population pharmacodynamic variability. The *potency* of the drug—the dose required to produce a given effect—is usually expressed as the dose required to produce a given effect in 50% of subjects, the ED_{50}. The *slope* of the curve between 20 and 80% of the maximal effect indicates the rate of increase in effect as the dose is

increased and is a reflection of the affinity of the receptor for the drug. The maximum effect is referred to as the *efficacy* of the drug. Finally, if curves from multiple subjects are generated, the *variability* in potency, efficacy, and the slope of the dose-response curve can be estimated.

The dose needed to produce a given pharmacologic effect varies considerably, even in "normal" patients. The patient most resistant to the drug usually requires a dose two- to threefold greater than the patient with the lowest dose requirements. This variability is caused by differences among individuals in the relationship between drug concentration and pharmacologic effect, superimposed on differences in pharmacokinetics. Dose-response studies have the disadvantage of not being able to determine whether variations in pharmacologic response are caused by differences in pharmacokinetics, pharmacodynamics, or both.

Concentration-Response Relationships

The onset and duration of pharmacologic effects depend not only on pharmacokinetic factors but also on the pharmacodynamic factors governing the degree of temporal disequilibrium between changes in concentration and changes in effect. The magnitude of the pharmacologic effect is a function of the amount of drug present at the site of action, so increasing the dose increases the peak effect. Larger doses have a more rapid onset of action because pharmacologically active concentrations at the site of action occur sooner. Increasing the dose also increases the duration of action because pharmacologically effective concentrations are maintained for a longer time.

Ideally, the concentration of drug at its site of action should be used to define the concentration-response relationship. Unfortunately, these data are rarely available, so the relationship between the concentration of drug in the blood and pharmacologic effect is studied instead. This relationship is easiest to understand if the changes in pharmacologic effect that occur during and after an intravenous infusion of a hypothetical drug are considered. If a drug is infused at a constant rate, the plasma concentration initially increases rapidly and asymptotically approaches a steady-state level after approximately five elimination half-lives have elapsed (Fig. 7-11). The effect of the drug initially increases very slowly, then more rapidly, and eventually also reaches a steady state. When the infusion is discontinued, indicated by point C in Figure 7-11, the plasma concentration immediately decreases because of drug distribution and elimination. However, the effect stays the same for a short period, and then also begins to decrease;

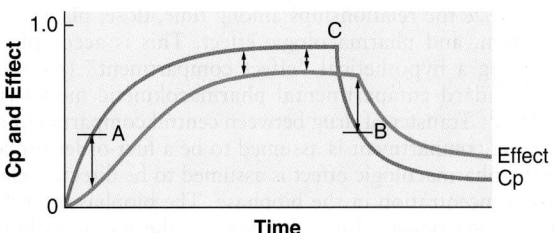

FIGURE 7-11. The changes in plasma drug concentration (C_p) and pharmacologic effect during and after an intravenous infusion. See text for explanation. (Reprinted with permission from Stanski DR, Sheiner LB. Pharmacokinetics and pharmacodynamics of muscle relaxants. Anesthesiology 1979; 51: 103.)

there is always a time lag between changes in plasma concentration and changes in pharmacologic response. Figure 7-11 also demonstrates that the same plasma concentration is associated with different responses if the concentration is changing. At points *A* and *B* in Figure 7-11, the plasma concentrations are the same, but the effects at each time differ. When the concentration is increasing, there is a concentration gradient from blood to the site of action. When the infusion is discontinued, the concentration gradient is reversed. Therefore, at the same plasma concentration, the concentration at the site of action is higher after, compared with during, the infusion. This is associated with a correspondingly greater effect.

In theory, there must be some degree of temporal disequilibrium between plasma concentration and drug effect for all drugs with extravascular sites of action. However, for some drugs, the time lag may be so short that it cannot be demonstrated. The magnitude of this temporal disequilibrium depends on several factors:

1. The perfusion of the organ on which the drug acts
2. The tissue:blood partition coefficient of the drug
3. The rate of diffusion or transport of the drug from the blood to the cellular site of action
4. The rate and affinity of drug–receptor binding
5. The time required for processes initiated by the drug-receptor interaction to produce changes in cellular function

The consequence of this time lag between changes in concentration and changes in effects is that the plasma concentration will have an unvarying relationship with pharmacologic effect only under steady-state conditions. At steady state, the plasma concentration is in equilibrium with the concentrations throughout the body, and is thus directly proportional to the steady-state concentration at the site of action. Plotting the logarithm of the steady-state plasma concentration versus response generates a curve identical in appearance to the dose-response curve shown in the right panel of Figure 7-9. The $Cp_{ss}50$, the steady-state plasma concentration producing 50% of the maximal response, is determined from the concentration-response curve. Like the ED_{50}, the $Cp_{ss}50$ is a measure of sensitivity to a drug, but the $Cp_{ss}50$ has the advantage of being unaffected by pharmacokinetic variability. Because it takes five elimination half-lives to approach steady-state conditions, it is not practical to determine the $Cp_{ss}50$ directly. For drugs with long elimination half-lives, the pseudoequilibrium during the elimination phase can be used to approximate steady-state conditions because the concentrations in plasma and at the site of action are changing very slowly.

Combined Pharmacokinetic-Pharmacodynamic Models

⑪ Integrated pharmacokinetic-pharmacodynamic models fully characterize the relationships among time, dose, plasma concentration, and pharmacologic effect. This is accomplished by adding a hypothetical "effect compartment" (biophase) to a standard compartmental pharmacokinetic model (Fig. 7-12).[46,47] Transfer of drug between central compartment and the effect compartment is assumed to be a first-order process, and the pharmacologic effect is assumed to be directly related to the concentration in the biophase. The biophase is a "virtual" compartment, although linked to the pharmacokinetic model, does not actually receive or return drug to the model and, therefore, ensures that the effect-site processes do not influence the pharmacokinetics of the rest of the system. By simultaneously characterizing the pharmacokinetics of the drug and the time course of drug effect, the combined pharmacokinetic-pharmacodynamic model is able to quantify the temporal dissociation between the plasma (central compart-

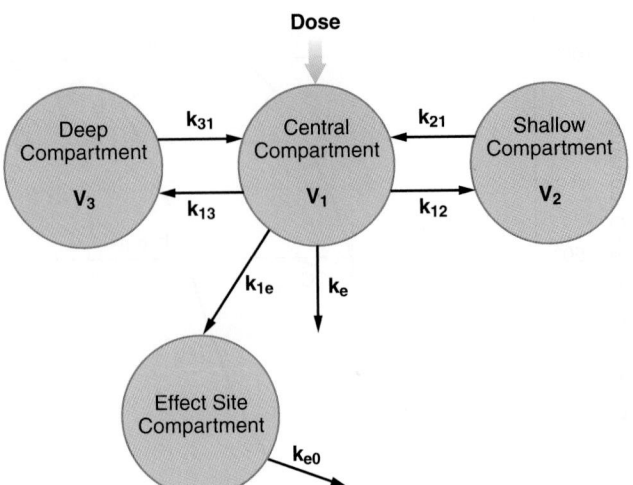

FIGURE 7-12. A schematic of a three-compartment pharmacokinetic model with the effect site linked to the central compartment. The rate constant for transfer between the plasma (central compartment) and the effect site, k_{1e}, and the volume of the effect site are both presumed to be negligible to ensure that the effect site does not influence the pharmacokinetic model. The rate constant for drug removal from the effect site, which relates the concentration in the central compartment to the pharmacologic effect, is k_{e0}.

ment) concentration and effect with the rate constant for equilibration between the plasma and the biophase, k_{e0}. By quantifying the time lag between changes in plasma concentration and changes in pharmacologic effect, these models can also define the $Cp_{ss}50$, even without steady-state conditions. These models have contributed greatly to our understanding of factors influencing the response to intravenous anesthetics,[48–50] opioids,[20,51–53] and nondepolarizing muscle relaxants[47,54,55] in humans.

The rate of equilibration between the plasma and the biophase, k_{e0}, can also be characterized by the half life of effect site equilibration ($T_{1/2ke0}$) using the formula:

$$T_{1/2ke0} = \frac{\ln2}{k_{e0}} = \frac{0.693}{k_{e0}} \qquad (7\text{-}18)$$

$T_{1/2ke0}$ is the time for the effect site concentration to reach 50% of the plasma concentration when the plasma concentration is held constant. For anesthetics with a short $T_{1/2ke0}$ (high k_{e0}), equilibration between the plasma and the biophase is rapid and therefore there is little delay before an effect is reached when a bolus of drug is administered or an infusion of drug is initiated. However, because the decline in the effect site concentration will also depend on the concentration gradient between the effect site and the plasma, drugs that rapidly equilibrate with the biophase may take longer to redistribute away.[56] Therefore, the offset of drug effect is more dependent on the pharmacokinetics of the body than on the rapidity of biophase-plasma equilibration.[20,56]

Drug Interactions

Taking into account premedication, perioperative antibiotics, intravenous agents used for induction or maintenance, inhalational anesthetics, opioids, muscle relaxants, the drugs used to restore neuromuscular transmission, and postoperative analgesics, 10 or more drugs may be given for a relatively "routine" anesthetic. Consequently, thorough understanding of the mechanisms of drug interactions and knowledge of specific interactions with drugs used in anesthesia are essential to the safe practice of anesthesiology (see Chapter 22). Indeed, anesthesiologists often deliberately take advantage of drug interactions. For example, moderate to high doses of opioid are often used to decrease the amount of volatile anesthetic required to provide immobility and hemodynamic stability to surgical incision (e.g., MAC^a and $MAC_{BAR}{}^b$), thereby avoiding the side effects of higher concentrations of inhaled anesthetics (e.g., vasodilation, prolonged awakening; see Chapter 17).

Drug interactions because of physicochemical properties can occur in vitro. Mixing acidic drugs, such as thiopental, and basic drugs, such as opioids or muscle relaxants, results in the formation of insoluble salts that precipitate. Another type of in vitro reaction is absorption of drugs by plastics. Examples include the uptake of nitroglycerin by polyvinyl chloride infusion sets and the absorption of fentanyl by the apparatus used for cardiopulmonary bypass.

Drugs can alter each other's absorption, distribution, and elimination. Drugs like ranitidine, which alters gastric pH, and metoclopramide, which speeds gastric emptying, alter absorption from the gastrointestinal tract. Vasoconstrictors are added to local anesthetic solutions to prolong their duration of action at the site of injection and to decrease the risk of systemic toxicity from rapid absorption.

Drugs that inhibit or induce the enzymes that catalyze biotransformation reactions can affect clearance of other concomitantly administered drugs. For example, the anticonvulsant phenytoin shortens the duration of action of the nondepolarizing neuromuscular junction blocking agents by inducing CYP and therefore increasing elimination clearance of the drug.[55] Clearance can also be affected by drug-induced changes in hepatic blood flow. Drugs that are cleared by the kidneys and have similar physicochemical characteristics compete for the transport mechanisms involved in renal tubular secretion.

Pharmacodynamic interactions fall into two broad classifications. Drugs can interact, either directly or indirectly, at the same receptors. Opioid antagonists directly displace opioids from opiate receptors. Cholinesterase inhibitors indirectly antagonize the effects of neuromuscular blockers by increasing the amount of acetylcholine, which displaces the blocking drug from nicotinic receptors. Pharmacodynamic interactions can also occur if two drugs affect a physiologic system at different sites.[57,58] Hypnotics and opioids, each acting on their own specific receptors, appear to interact synergistically.[59] The pharmacodynamic interaction between two drugs can be characterized using response surface models.[60–65] The three-dimensional models are useful in delineating the concentration pairs of a hypnotic (e.g., volatile anesthetic, propofol, midazolam) and an opioid (e.g., remifentanil, alfentanil, fentanyl) that produce adequate anesthesia while minimizing undesired side effects.[66] (See "Response Surface Models of Drug-Drug Interactions.")

---

^{a}MAC: Minimum Alveolar Concentration—the steady state end-tidal alveolar concentration at which 50% of patients do not move in response to surgical incision (see Chapter 17).
^{b}MACBAR = Minimum Alveolar Concentration that Blocks Autonomic Responses—the steady state end-tidal alveolar concentration at which 50% of patients do not have an increase in heart rate or blood pressure in response to surgical incision (see Chapter 15).

CLINICAL APPLICATIONS OF PHARMACOKINETIC AND PHARMACODYNAMICS TO THE ADMINISTRATION OF INTRAVENOUS ANESTHETICS

Although no new inhaled anesthetics have been synthesized since the 1970s,[67] intravenous drugs that act on the CNS continue to be developed. Anesthesiologists have become accustomed to the exquisite control of anesthetic blood (and effect site) concentrations afforded by modern volatile anesthetic agents and their vaporizers, coupled to end-tidal anesthetic gas monitoring. Although pharmacokinetic and pharmacodynamic principles and data have contributed greatly to our understanding of the behavior of intravenous anesthetics, their primary utility and ultimate purpose are to determine optimal dosing with as much mathematical precision and clinical accuracy as possible. In most pharmacotherapeutic scenarios outside anesthesia care, the time scales for onset of drug effect, its maintenance, and its offset are measured in days, weeks, or even years. In such cases, global pharmacokinetic variables (and one-compartment models) such as total volume of distribution (V_{SS}), elimination clearance (Cl_e), and half-life ($t_{1/2}$) are sufficient and utilitarian parameters for calculating dose regimens. However, in the operating room and intensive care unit, the temporal tolerances for onset and offset of desired drug effects are measured in minutes.[38,39] Consequently, these global variables are insufficient to describe the details of kinetic behavior of drugs in the minutes following intravenous administration. This is particularly true of lipid-soluble hypnotics and opioids that rapidly and extensively distribute throughout the various tissues of the body because distribution processes dominate pharmacokinetic behavior during the time frame of most anesthetics. Additionally, the therapeutic indices of many intravenous anesthetic drugs are small and two-tailed (i.e., an underdose, resulting in awareness, which is a "toxic" effect). Optimal dosing in these situations requires use of all the variables of a multicompartmental pharmacokinetic model to account for drug distribution in blood and other tissues.

It is not easy to intuit the pharmacokinetic behavior of a multicompartmental system by simple examination of the kinetic variables.[10] Computer simulation is required to meaningfully interpret dosing or to accurately devise new dosing regimens. In addition, there are several pharmacokinetic concepts that are uniquely applicable to intravenous administration of drugs with multicompartmental kinetics and must be taken into account when administering intravenous infusions.

To achieve similar degrees of control of intravenously administered anesthetic drug concentrations in blood and in the CNS, new technologies aimed at improving intravenous infusion devices, as well as new software to manage the daunting pharmacokinetic principles involved, are needed. This section examines the current state of infusion devices and the pharmacokinetic and pharmacodynamic principles specifically required for precise delivery of anesthetic agents.

Rise to Steady-State Concentration

The drug concentration versus time profile for the rise to steady state is the mirror image of its elimination profile. In a one-compartment model with a decline in concentration versus time that is monoexponential following a single dose, the rise of drug concentration to the steady-state concentration (C_{SS}) is likewise monoexponential during a continuous infusion. That is, in one elimination half-life an infusion is halfway to its eventual steady-state concentration, in another half-life it reaches half of what remains between halfway and steady state (i.e., 75% of the eventual steady state is reached in two elimination half-lives), and so on for each half-life increment. The equation describing this behavior is:

$$C_p(t) = C_{SS}[1 - e^{-kt}] \qquad (7\text{-}19)$$

where $C_p(t)$ = the concentration at time t, k is the rate constant related to the elimination half-life, and t is the time from the start of the infusion. This relationship can also be described by:

$$C_p(n) = C_{SS}[1 - (1/2)^n] \qquad (7\text{-}20)$$

in which $C_p(n)$ is the concentration at n half-lives. Equation 7-20 indicates that during a constant infusion, the concentration reaches 90% of C_{SS} after 3.3 half-lives, which is usually deemed close enough for clinical purposes.

However, for a drug such as propofol, which partitions extensively to pharmacologically inert body tissues (e.g., muscle, gut), a monoexponential equation, or single-compartment model, is insufficient to describe the time course of propofol concentrations in the first minutes and hours after beginning drug administration. Instead, a multicompartmental or multiexponential model must be used. With such a model, the picture changes drastically for the plasma drug concentration rise toward steady state. The rate of rise toward steady state is determined by the distribution rate constants to the degree that their respective exponential terms contribute to the total area under the concentration versus time curve. Thus, for the three-compartment model describing the pharmacokinetics of propofol, Equation 7-19 becomes:

$$
\begin{aligned}
C_p(t) = C_{SS}[& \frac{A}{A + B + G}(1 - e^{-\alpha t}) \\
& + \frac{B}{A + B + G}(1 - e^{-\beta t}) \\
& + \frac{G}{A + B + G}(1 - e^{-\gamma t})]
\end{aligned}
\qquad (7\text{-}21)
$$

in which t = time; $C_p(t)$ = plasma concentration at time; A = coefficient of the rapid distribution phase and α = hybrid rate constant of the rapid distribution phase; B = coefficient of the slower distribution phase, and β = hybrid rate constant of the slower distribution; and G = coefficient of elimination phase and γ = hybrid rate constant of the elimination phase. $A + B + G$ is the sum of the coefficients of all the exponential terms. For most lipophilic anesthetics and opioids, A is typically one order of magnitude greater than B, and B is in turn an order of magnitude greater than G. Therefore, distribution-phase kinetics for intravenous anesthetics have a much greater influence on the time to reach C_{SS} than do elimination-phase kinetics.[56]

For example, with propofol having an elimination half-life of approximately 6 hours, the simple one-compartment rule in Equation 7-20 tells us that it would take 6 hours from the start of a constant rate infusion to reach even 50% of the eventual steady-state propofol plasma concentration and 12 hours to reach 75%. In contrast, with a full three-compartment propofol kinetic model, Equation 7-21 accurately predicts that 50% of steady state is reached in <30 minutes and 75% will be reached in <4 hours. This example emphasizes the necessity of using multicompartment models to describe the clinical pharmacokinetics of intravenous anesthetics.

Manual Bolus and Infusion Dosing Schemes

Based on a one-compartment pharmacokinetic model, a stable steady-state plasma concentration ($C_{p,SS}$) can be maintained by administering an infusion at a rate (I) that is proportional to the elimination of drug from the body (Cl_E):

$$I = C_{p,SS} \times Cl_E \qquad (7\text{-}22)$$

However, if the drug was administered only by initiating and maintaining this infusion, it would take one elimination half-time to reach 50% of the target plasma concentration and three times that long to reach 90% of the target plasma concentration. In order to decrease the time until the target plasma concentration is achieved, an initial bolus (loading dose) of drug can be administered that would produce the target plasma concentration:

$$Bolus = C_{p,SS} \times V_{d,SS} \qquad (7\text{-}23)$$

Although this method is very efficient in achieving and maintaining the target plasma concentration of a drug that instantaneously mixes and equilibrates throughout the tissues of the body (e.g., drugs modeled with a one-compartment pharmacokinetic model), using the steady-state elimination clearance and volume of distribution to calculate the loading dose and maintenance infusion rate will result in plasma drug concentrations that are higher throughout the initial distribution phase (see Fig. 7-13).

Using Equations 7-22 and 7-23 and $V_{d,SS}$ = 262 L and Cl_E = 1.7 L/min (for a 50-year-old man who is 178 cm tall and weighs 70 kg from Schnider et al.[49]), the loading dose and infusion rate of propofol that is needed to achieve a steady-state plasma concentration of 5 μg/mL is 1,300 mg (18 mg/kg) and 120 μg/kg/min. Obviously, the loading dose of propofol is too high, compared with clinically used doses (1 to 2 mg/kg) while the infusion rate appears to be a clinically acceptable dose. The erroneous estimate of the loading dose is because the initial bolus of drug is not instantaneously mixed and equilibrated with the entire volume of tissue that will eventually take up drug. Therefore,

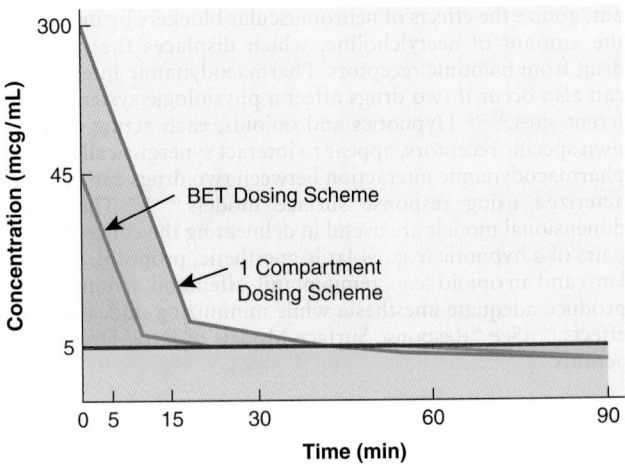

FIGURE 7-13. A computer simulation of the plasma propofol concentration profile during and after the administration of a single bolus and infusion scheme calculated using the steady-state, one-compartment pharmacokinetic parameters (*solid line*) and the BET scheme from Table 7-5 (*dashed line*) to achieve a plasma concentration of 5 mcg/mL. $V_{d,SS}$ = 262 L and Cl_E = 1.7 L/min for a 50-year-old man who is 178 cm tall and weighs 70 kg. See text for description of BET scheme.

TABLE 7-5

BET^a SCHEME TO ACHIEVE C_p 5 μg/mL FOR 120 MINUTES

■ DOSE	■ AMOUNT	■ TIME (min)
Bolus	2.8 mg/kg	
Infusion	238 μg/kg/min	0–10
	187 μg/kg/min	10–20
	136 μg/kg/min	20–60
	112 μg/kg/min	60–120

^{a}B is the loading bolus dose, E is the infusion to replace drug removed by elimination clearance, and T is a continuously decreasing infusion that compensates for transfer of drug to the peripheral tissues.

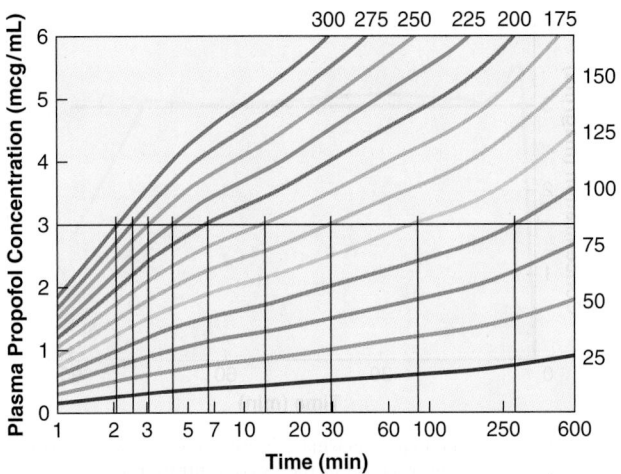

FIGURE 7-14. Isoconcentration nomogram for determining propofol infusion rates designed to maintain a desired plasma propofol concentration. This nomogram is based on the pharmacokinetics of Schnider et al. and plotted on a log–log scale to better delineate the early time points. *Curved lines* represent the plasma propofol concentration versus time plots, resulting from the various continuous infusion rates indicated along the right and upper borders (units in μg/kg/min). A horizontal line is placed at the desired target plasma propofol concentration (3 μg/mL in this case) and vertical lines are placed at each intersection of a curved concentration time plot. The vertical lines indicate the times that the infusion rate should be set to the one represented by the next intersected curve as one moves from left to right along the horizontal line drawn at 3 μg/mL. In this example the infusion rate would be reduced from 300 to 275 μg/kg/min at 2.5 minutes, to 250 μg/kg/min at 3 minutes, to 225 μg/kg/min at 4.5 minutes, and so on until it is turned to 100 μg/kg/min at 260 minutes.

manual dosing strategies for intravenous anesthetics need to be modified to account for the fact that when a bolus of drug is administered, it rapidly mixes and equilibrates with the blood and only a small volume of tissue (e.g., the central compartment), and then will distribute over time into other tissues.

To design a manual bolus that more precisely achieves the desired target plasma concentration, it is necessary to choose a bolus that is based on the small, initial volume of distribution (V_c). To maintain the target plasma concentration, a series of infusions of decreasing rate can be used to match the elimination clearance and compensates for drug loss from the central to the peripheral compartments during the initial period of extensive drug distribution and the second period of moderate drug distribution. This manual dosing scheme has been termed the *BET scheme*, where B is the loading bolus dose, E is the infusion to replace drug removed by elimination clearance, and T is a continuously decreasing infusion that compensates for transfer of drug to the peripheral tissues (i.e., distribution).[68] An example of a BET scheme for propofol to achieve a target plasma concentration of 5 μg/mL is shown in Table 7-5.

Isoconcentration Nomogram

To make the calculations of the various infusion rates required to maintain a target plasma concentration for a drug that follows multicompartment pharmacokinetics, a clinician would need access to a basic computer and the software to perform the appropriate simulations. With the appropriate formulas, this is quite feasible to do on any basic computer with any basic spreadsheet. However, even with more sophisticated pharmacokinetic software (e.g., SAAM II, WinNonLin, RugLoop, Stanpump), this is a time-consuming process that diverts the clinician's attention from the patient. In 1994, Shafer[69] introduced an isoconcentration nomogram for propofol that used the rise toward steady state described by a multicompartmental system (Fig. 7-14). This graphical tool allows users to employ concentration-effect, rather than dose-effect, relationships when determining optimal dosing of intravenous anesthetic agents. The nomogram is constructed by calculating the plasma drug concentration versus time curve for a constant-rate infusion from a set of pharmacokinetic variables for a particular drug. From this single simulation, one can readily visualize (and estimate) the rise toward steady-state plasma drug concentration described by the drug's pharmacokinetic model. By simulating a range of potential infusion rates, a series of curves of identical shape are then plotted on a single graph with drug concentrations at any time that are directly proportional to the infusion rate.

By placing a horizontal line at the desired plasma drug concentration (y-axis) the times (x-axis) at which the horizontal intersects the line for a particular infusion rate will represent

the times at which the infusion rate should be set to the rate on the intercepting line. In the example shown (see Fig. 7-14) with 25 mcg/kg/min increments, the predicted plasma propofol concentrations remain within 10% of the target from 2 minutes onward with a bias of underestimation. If never allowing the estimated concentration to fall below the target is desired, then the time to decrease to the next lower infusion should be at the midpoint of the subsequent interval. Extending the infusions to the subsequent midpoint times will introduce a maximum overestimation bias of approximately 17% with the illustrated infusion increments (Fig. 7-14). Biases would be increased or decreased by constructing nomograms with larger or smaller infusion increments, respectively.

The nomogram can also be used to increase or reduce the targeted plasma propofol concentration. To target a new plasma drug concentration, a new horizontal line can be drawn at the desired concentration. The infusion rate that is closest to the current time intersect is the one that should be used initially, followed by the decremented rates dictated by the subsequent intercept times. For best results when increasing the target concentration, a bolus equal to the product of V_c (the central compartment volume) and the incremental change in concentration should be administered. Likewise, when decreasing the concentration the best strategy is to turn off the infusion for the duration predicted by the applicable context-sensitive decrement time and resume the infusion rate predicted for the current time plus the context-sensitive decrement time. For instance, if after 30 minutes one wishes to decrease the target plasma propofol concentration from 3 μg/mL to 2 μg/mL (a 33% decrement at a time context of 30 minutes), one would shut off the infusion for 1 minute and 10 seconds to let the concentration fall by 33% and then restart at 75 μg/kg/min. The estimated plasma

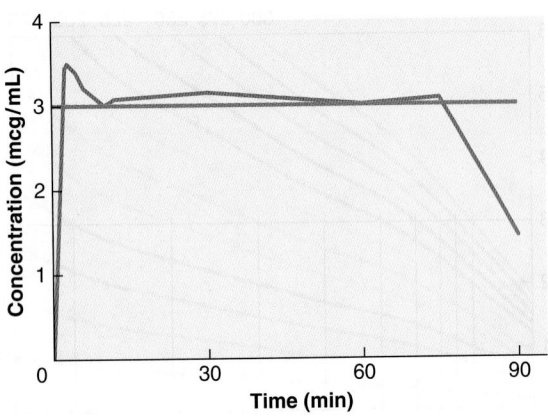

FIGURE 7-15. Simulated plasma propofol concentration history resulting from the information in the isoconcentration nomogram in Figure 7-14 and extending the times to switch the infusion to the next lower increment to the midpoint of the subsequent time segment (i.e., the switch from 250 to 225 μg/kg/min was at 5 minutes, rather than at 4.5 minutes). Note that for the first 30 minutes, this sequence predicts plasma propofol concentrations that are always slightly above 3 μg/mL (see text). The infusion is stopped at 90 minutes in this case.

propofol concentrations from this nomogram-guided dosing scheme are shown in Figure 7-15.

Context-Sensitive Decrement Times

During an infusion, drug is taken up by the inert, peripheral tissues.[18] Once drug delivery is terminated, recovery occurs when the effect site concentration decreases below a threshold concentration for producing a pharmacologic effect (e.g., MAC$_{AWAKE}$—the concentration where 50% of patients follow commands).[56,65] Although the rate of elimination of the drug from the body can give some indication for the time required to reach a subtherapeutic effect site drug concentration, distribution to and from the peripheral tissues also contributes to the time course of decreasing drug concentrations of the central and the effect site. For drugs with multicompartmental kinetics, the elimination half-life will always overestimate the time to recovery from anesthetic drugs. This is best understood by considering the limiting condition of steady state. With a steady-state infusion the amount of drug being infused into the central compartment exactly matches the amount of drug being removed by the eliminating organs, and there is no net transfer between tissue compartments and plasma (central) as their drug concentrations are in equilibrium. When the infusion stops, the elimination clearance rapidly decreases only the central compartment drug concentrations on which it is operating. The compartments thus become "disequilibrated" and drug returns from the tissues to the plasma compartment in amounts determined by the distribution clearances, the concentration gradients, and the size of the peripheral compartment depots. This return of drug from the tissue will gradually slow the rate of decrease in plasma drug concentration until pseudoequilibrium is reached and the process can then proceed at the rate of the elimination half-life. For drugs with large elimination clearances relative to the peripheral drug depot size, the time to reach a concentration half the steady-state concentration (or half-time) will be much shorter than the elimination half-life. Propofol fits this category with an initial half-time of 30 minutes as compared with its half-life of 6 hours even after an infinitely long infusion. For infusions of shorter duration than infinity the tissue depots will contribute drug back to the

plasma to a lesser degree, depending on how long the infusion had run, that is, how close to equilibration with the central compartment they were, and the half-times will get progressively shorter until the condition of an infinitely short infusion (bolus dose) is reached.[20] Therefore, the contribution of redistribution to the rate of decay of the plasma concentration depends on the duration of infusion of a drug. Note that here redistribution describes the drug returning from all tissue compartments, not just from the brain, into plasma as opposed to the previous usage that described redistribution of drug from brain to blood and into inert tissues.

To characterize the contribution of redistribution to the time required to reach a subtherapeutic drug concentration, the duration of infusion must be taken into account. Multicompartment pharmacokinetic models of anesthetic drugs can be used to simulate the time required for a decrease in the plasma or effect site concentration by different percentages after terminating infusions of various durations.[20] The time required for the drug concentration of the plasma to decrease by 50% increases as the duration of infusion increases. Once the tissue drug concentrations are completely equilibrated with the plasma, redistribution plays a negligible role in decreasing the plasma concentration, and the time required for a 50% drop in plasma concentration is equal to the elimination half-life. The *context-sensitive half-time* is defined as the time required for the drug concentration of the plasma to decrease by 50%, where the context is the duration of the infusion.[51] The context-sensitive half-time for the common synthetic opioids fentanyl, alfentanil, sufentanil, and remifentanil is illustrated in Figure 7-16.

Although a 50% decrease in plasma concentration is an appealing and comprehensible parameter, larger or smaller decreases in plasma concentrations may be required for recovery from the drug. Simulations show that the time for different percent decreases in plasma concentration is not linear.[10,20] Therefore, if a 25% or 75% decrease in plasma concentration is required, simulations must be performed to calculate the context-sensitive 25% decrement time or context sensitive 75% decrement time (Fig. 7-17). In addition, if the concentration of interest is the effect-site concentration rather than the plasma concentration, simulations can be performed to calculate the context-sensitive effect-site decrement time. Finally, if a constant plasma or effect-site concentration is not maintained throughout the delivery of the drug (which is typically the case with manual bolus and infusion schemes and also with varying drug requirements depending on surgical stimulation and so forth), the context-sensitive decrement times are guidelines of recovery rather than an absolute prediction of the

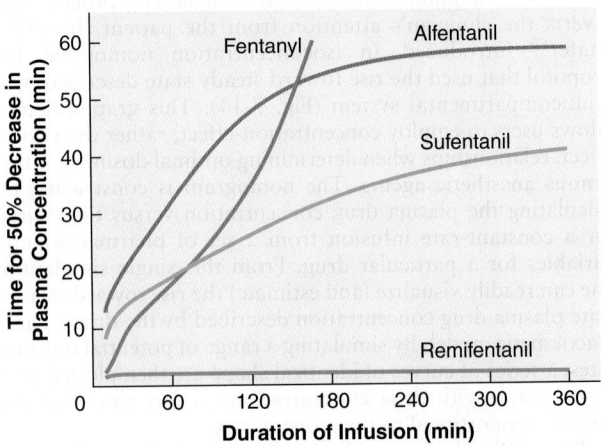

FIGURE 7-16. The context-sensitive plasma half-time for fentanyl, alfentanil, sufentanil, and remifentanil.

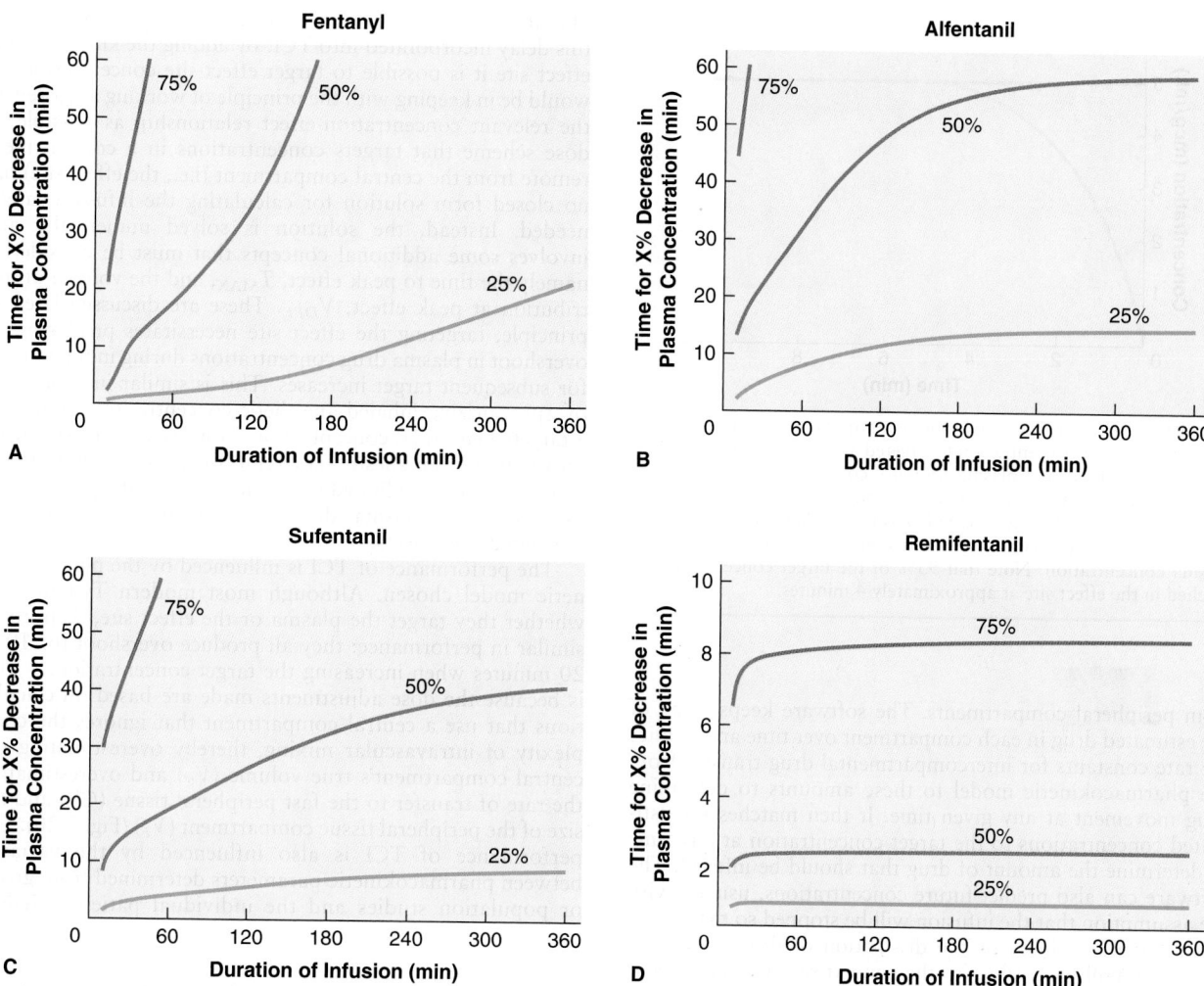

FIGURE 7-17. The context-sensitive 25%, 50%, and 75% plasma decrement times for fentanyl (A), alfentanil (B), sufentanil (C), and remifentanil (D).

decay in drug concentration. If precise drug administration data are known, it is possible to compute the context-sensitive decrement time for the individual situation or context. Even though the context-sensitive decrement times are limited, this concept has changed the way that intravenous anesthetics are described and has helped foster an increase in accurately and safely administering intravenous anesthetics.

Target-Controlled Infusions

Prior to performing an administering, it is possible to perform the calculations presented here and derive a BET scheme targeted to a predetermined plasma or effect-site concentration. However, in the operating room, once the anesthetic has commenced, without the help of a computer, software, and possibly an assistant, it is laborious and difficult to make any calculations to determine how to adjust the infusion or how to bolus (or stop the infusion) to increase or decrease the target plasma concentration.[70] By linking a computer with the appropriate pharmacokinetic model to an infusion pump, it is possible for the physician to enter the desired target plasma concentration of a drug and for the computer to nearly instantaneously calculate the appropriate infusion scheme to achieve this target in a matter of seconds.[71] Because drug accumulates at various rates among the

various tissues and organs in the body, the computer continually calculates the current drug concentration and adjusts the infusion pump in order to account for the current status of drug uptake, distribution, and elimination. Therefore, the computer-driven BET scheme can in fact control the infusion pump in order to achieve a steady target concentration (Fig. 7-18).

The success of this approach is influenced by the extent to which the drug pharmacokinetic and pharmacodynamic parameters programmed into the computer match those of the particular patient at hand. While this same limitation applies to the more rudimentary (non–target-controlled infusions [TCIs]) dosing done routinely in every clinical setting, we must examine the special ramifications of pharmacokinetic–pharmacodynamic model misspecification with TCI in any discussion of its future importance in the clinical setting.

The mathematical principles governing TCI are actually quite simple. For a computer-control pump to produce and maintain a plasma drug concentration it must first administer a dose equal to the product of the central compartment, V_1, and the target concentration (Fig. 7-19). Then for each moment after that, the amount of drug to be administered into the central compartment to maintain the target concentration is equal to drug eliminated from the central compartment *plus* drug distributed from the central compartment to peripheral compartments *minus* drug returning to the central compartment

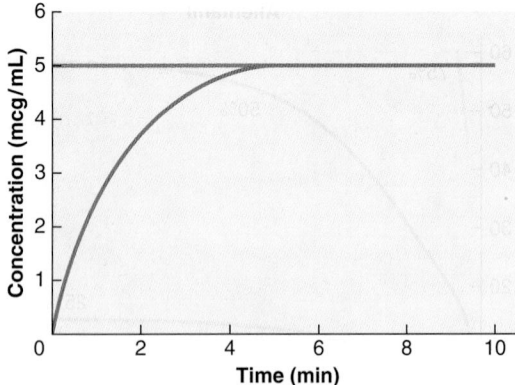

FIGURE 7-18.   This is a simulation of a target-controlled infusion in which the plasma concentration is targeted at 5 $\mu g/mL$. The *solid line* represents the predicted plasma propofol concentration of 5 $\mu g/mL$, which in theory is attained at time $t = 0$ and is then maintained by a variable rate infusion. The *dashed line* is the predicted effect site concentration under the conditions of a constant pseudo–steady-state plasma concentration. Note that 95% of the target concentration is reached in the effect site at approximately 4 minutes.

from peripheral compartments. The software keeps track of the estimated drug in each compartment over time and applies the rate constants for intercompartmental drug transfer from the pharmacokinetic model to these amounts to determine drug movement at any given time. It then matches the estimated concentrations to the target concentration at any time to determine the amount of drug that should be infused. The software can also predict future concentrations, usually with the assumption that the infusion will be stopped so that emergence from anesthesia or the dissipation of drug effect will occur optimally according to the context-sensitive decrement time.

Because there is a delay or hysteresis between the attainment of a drug concentration in the plasma and the production

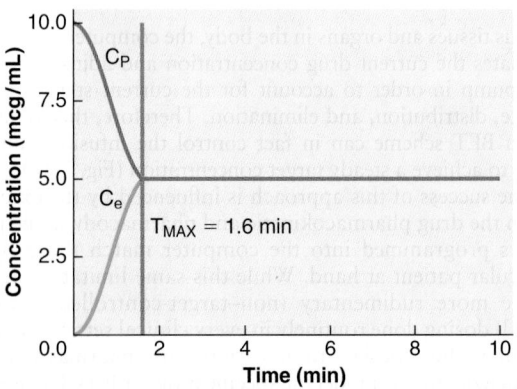

FIGURE 7-19.   This is a simulation of a target controlled infusion in which the effect-site concentration (C_e) is targeted at 5 $\mu g/mL$. The *solid line* represents the predicted plasma propofol concentration (C_p) that results from a bolus dose, given at time $t = 0$, that is predicted to purposely overshoot the plasma propofol concentration target until time $t = T_{MAX}$ (1.6 minutes). At T_{MAX} pseudoequilibration between the effect site and the plasma occurs and both concentrations are then predicted to be the same until the target is changed. Note that the effect site attains the target in less than half the time with effect-site targeting compared to the plasma concentration targeting seen in Figure 7-18.

of a drug effect, it is advantageous to have the mathematics of this delay incorporated into TCI. By adding the kinetics of the effect site it is possible to target effect-site concentrations as would be in keeping with the principle of working as closely to the relevant concentration-effect relationship as possible. A dose scheme that targets concentrations in a compartment remote from the central compartment (i.e., the effect site) has no closed form solution for calculating the infusion rate(s) needed. Instead, the solution is solved numerically and involves some additional concepts that must be considered, namely the time to peak effect, T_{MAX}, and the volume of distribution at peak effect, V_{DPE}. These are discussed later. In principle, targeting the effect site necessitates producing an overshoot in plasma drug concentrations during induction and for subsequent target increases. This is similar in concept to overpressurizing inhaled anesthetic concentrations to achieve a targeted end-tidal concentration. However, unlike the inspiratory limb of an anesthesia circuit, the plasma compartment seems to be closely linked to cardiovascular effects, and large overshoots in plasma drug concentration may produce unwanted side effects.

The performance of TCI is influenced by the pharmacokinetic model chosen. Although most modern TCI models, whether they target the plasma or the effect site, seem to be similar in performance: they all produce overshoot for 10 to 20 minutes when increasing the target concentration.[36] This is because the dose adjustments made are based on calculations that use a central compartment that ignores the complexity of intravascular mixing, thereby overestimating the central compartment's true volume (V_C) and overestimating the rate of transfer to the fast peripheral tissue (Cl_F) and the size of the peripheral tissue compartment (V_F) (Fig. 7-20). The performance of TCI is also influenced by the variance between pharmacokinetic parameters determined from group or population studies and the individual patient. Median

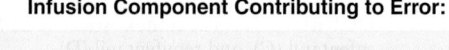

Infusion Component Contributing to Error:

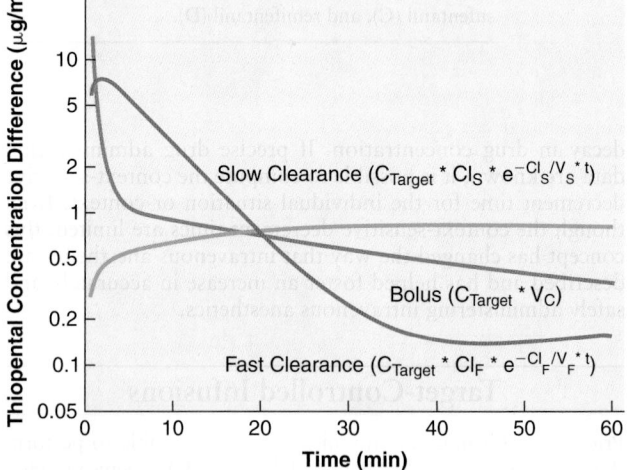

FIGURE 7-20.   The influence of the misspecification of each of the components of the traditional three-compartment pharmacokinetic models on the prolonged discrepancy (overshoot) between predicted and targeted concentrations with target-controlled infusions (TCIs). The error resulting from elimination clearance was negligible and therefore not illustrated. Notice that the loading dose (based on V_C) produces a large amount of error in the initial minutes; however, from 1 to 20 minutes, the deviation from the target concentration is largely due to the overestimation of Cl_F. The equations listed are for the respective BET infusions of the TCI system. See text for description of BET. (From Avram MJ, Krejcie TC: Using front-end kinetics to optimize target-controlled drug infusions. Anesthesiology 2003; 99: 1078.)

absolute performance errors for fentanyl,[72] alfentanil,[73] sufentanil,[74] midazolam,[75,76] and propofol[76,77] are in the range of $\pm30\%$ when literature values for pharmacokinetic parameters are used to drive the TCI device and fall to approximately $\pm7\%$ when the average kinetics of the test subjects themselves are used.[73] Divergence (the percentage change of the absolute performance error) is generally quite low (approximately 1%) when target concentrations remain relatively stable, but increase to nearly 20% when the frequency of concentration steps is as frequent as every 12 minutes.[36,77] These data suggest that while a considerable error may exist ($\pm30\%$) between the targeted drug concentration and the one actually achieved in a patient, the concentration attained will not vary much over time. Thus, incremental adjustments in the target should result in incremental and stable new concentrations in the patient as long as the incremental adjustments are not too frequent.

The introduction of the concept of TCIs was first described by Schwilden et al. in early 1980s. Other software systems were developed in North America by groups at Stanford University and Duke University. By the late 1990s a commercially available TCI system for propofol (Diprifusor) was introduced. This greatly increased both anesthesiologists' interest in this mode of delivery and their understanding of the concentration-effect relationships for hypnotics and opioids. In most of the world, devices for delivering propofol by TCI are commercially available from at least three companies (Graseby, Alaris, and Fresenius) with similar performance parameters.[78] In the United States, there are still no FDA-approved devices. For investigational purposes, STANPUMP[c] (developed by Steve Shafer at Stanford University) can be interfaced via an RS232 port to an infusion pump. STANPUMP currently provides pharmacokinetic parameters for 19 different drugs, but has the ability to accept any kinetic model for any drug provided by the user. RUGLOOP[d] is TCI software (developed by Michel Struys of Ghent University), which is similar to STANPUMP but operates in Windows rather than DOS and is capable of controlling multiple drug infusions simultaneously.

Although the pharmacologic principle of relating a concentration rather than a dose is scientifically sound, few studies have actually attempted to determine whether TCI improves clinical performance or outcome. Only a few limited studies have actually compared manual infusion control versus TCI. Some have shown better control and a more predictable emergence with TCI,[78,79] whereas others have simply shown no advantage.[80,81]

TCI principles continue to be developed beyond the scope of intravenous anesthesia techniques. TCI has been used to provide postoperative analgesia with alfentanil.[82,83] In this system, a desired target plasma alfentanil concentration was set in the range of 40 to 100 ng/mL. A demand by the patient automatically increased the target level by 5 ng/mL. Lack of a demand caused the system to gradually reduce the targeted level. The quality of analgesia was judged to be superior to standard morphine patient-controlled analgesia.

Similarly, TCI has been used to provide patient-controlled sedation with propofol.[84,85] The TCI was set to 1 μg/mL and a demand by the patient increased the level by 0.2 μg/mL. As with the TCI analgesia system, the lack of a demand caused the system to gradually reduce the targeted plasma propofol concentration. The timing and increment of the decrease were adjusted by the clinician. Over 90% of patients were satisfied with this method of sedation.

Time to Maximum Effect Compartment Concentration

Earlier in this chapter, the delay between attaining a plasma concentration and an effect-site concentration was described (Fig. 7-11). This delay, or hysteresis, is presumed to be a result of transfer of drug between the plasma compartment, V_C, and an effect compartment, V_e, as well as the time required for a cellular response. By simultaneously modeling the plasma drug concentration versus time data (pharmacokinetics) and the measured drug effect (pharmacodynamics), an estimate of the drug transfer rate constant, k_{e0}, between plasma and the putative effect site can be estimated.[47] However, estimates of k_{e0}, like all rate constants, are model-specific.[86,87] That is, k_{e0} cannot be transported from one set of kinetic parameters determined in one specific pharmacokinetic–pharmacodynamic study to any another set of pharmacokinetic parameters. Likewise, it is not valid to compare estimates of k_{e0} among studies of the same drug or across different drugs; therefore, one should not be surprised that reported values for k_{e0} for the same drug vary markedly among studies. The model-independent parameter that characterizes the delay between the plasma and effect site is the time to maximal effect, or T_{MAX}.[87] Accordingly, if the T_{MAX} and the pharmacokinetics for a drug are known from independent studies, a k_{e0} can be estimated by numeric techniques for the independent kinetic set that would produce the known effect-site T_{MAX}.

The concept of a transportable, model-independent parameter that characterizes the kinetics of the effect site is important for robust effect-site–targeted, computer-controlled infusions. This is because there are many more pharmacokinetic studies characterizing a wider variety of patient types and groups in the literature than there are complete pharmacokinetic-pharmacodynamic studies. By making the generally valid assumption that intraindividual differences are small in a drug's rate of effect site equilibration, it is possible with a known T_{MAX} to estimate effect-site kinetics for a drug across a wide variety of patient groups in which only the pharmacokinetics are known. This cannot be done in a valid manner using k_{e0} or $t_{1/2ke0}$ alone.[86,87]

Volume of Distribution at Peak Effect

Although the plasma concentration can be brought rapidly to the targeted drug concentration by administering a bolus dose to the central compartment ($C \times V_C$) and then held there by a computer-controlled infusion (Fig. 7-18), the time for the effect site to reach the target concentration will be much longer than T_{MAX} (4 minutes for propofol effect-site concentration to reach 95% of that targeted). It is possible to calculate a bolus dose that will attain the estimated effect site concentration at T_{MAX} without overshoot in the effect site. However, plasma drug concentration will overshoot (Fig. 7-19). This is done by combining the concept of describing drug distribution as an expanding volume of distribution that starts at V_C and approaches V_β (the apparent volume of distribution during the elimination phase) over time with the concept of T_{MAX}.[88,89]

Volume of distribution over time is calculated by dividing the total amount of drug remaining in the body by the plasma drug concentration at each time, t. The time-dependent volume at the time of peak effect (or T_{MAX}) is V_{DPE}. The product

---

[c]Information regarding STANPUMP is available at http://anesthesia.stanford.edu/ pkpd/

[d]Information regarding RUGLOOP is available at http://www.demed.be/index.html

of the targeted effect-site concentration and V_{DPE} plus the amount lost to elimination in the time to T_{MAX} becomes the proper bolus dose that will attain the target concentration at the effect site as rapidly as possible without overshoot. In practical terms this bolus is given at time $t = 0$, after which the infusion stops until time $t = T_{MAX}$. It then resumes infusing drug in its normal "stop loss" manner.

Some software programs for controlling target-controlled infusions include this concept in their algorithms. In the case of the propofol kinetics used to construct the isoconcentration nomogram in Figure 7-14, the pharmacokinetic-pharmacodynamic parameter set of Schnider et al.,[49] predicts a T_{MAX} of 1.6 minutes, a V_{DPE} of 16.62 L, and an elimination loss of 23.8% of the dose over 1.6 minutes in a 70-kg man. Thus, the proper propofol bolus for a targeted effect-site propofol concentration of 5 μg/mL is 109 mg. The computer-controlled infusion pump will deliver this dose as rapidly as possible and then begin a targeted infusion for 5 μg/mL at $t = 1.6$ minutes (see Fig. 7-19).

Front-End Pharmacokinetics

The term *front-end pharmacokinetics* refers to the intravascular mixing, pulmonary uptake, and recirculation events that occur in the first few minutes during and after intravenous drug administration.[39] These kinetic events and the drug concentration versus time profile that results are important because the peak effect of rapidly acting drugs occurs during this temporal window.[17,90–93] Although it has been suggested that front-end pharmacokinetics be used to guide drug dosing,[36] current TCI does not incorporate front-end kinetics into the models from which drug infusion rates are calculated. As previously described, not doing so introduces further error.

TCI relies on pharmacokinetic models that are based on the simplifying assumption of instantaneous and complete mixing within V_C. However, the determination of V_C is routinely overestimated in most pharmacokinetic studies. Overestimation of V_C, when used to calculate TCI infusion rates, results in plasma drug concentrations that overshoot the desired target concentration, especially in the first few minutes after beginning TCI. Furthermore, correct description of drug distribution to tissues depends on an accurate V_C estimate, so inaccuracies caused by not taking front-end pharmacokinetics into account may be persistent and result in undershoot as well as overshoot. Simulation indicates that pharmacokinetic parameters derived from studies in which the drug is administered by a short (approximately 2 minutes) infusion better estimate V_C and tissue-distribution kinetics than those from a rapid intravenous bolus infusion.[36,37] When the latter drug administration method is used, full characterization of the front-end recirculatory pharmacokinetics is required to obtain valid estimates of V for use in TCI.[36,37]

Closed-Loop Infusions

When a valid, and nearly continuous, measure of drug effect is available, drug delivery can be automatically titrated by feedback control. Such systems have been used experimentally for control of blood pressure,[94] oxygen delivery,[95] blood glucose,[96] neuromuscular blockade,[97] and depth of anesthesia.[98–104] A target value for the desired effect measure (the output of the system) is selected and the rate of drug delivery (the input into the system) depends on whether the effect measure is above, below, or at the target value. Thus, the output feeds back and controls the input. Standard controllers (referred to as *proportional-integral-derivative* [or PID] *controllers*) adjust drug delivery based on both the integral, or magnitude, of the deviation from target and the rate of deviation, or the derivative.

Under a range of responses, standard PID controllers work quite well. However, they have been shown to develop unstable characteristics in situations in which the output may vary rapidly and widely. Schwilden et al.[105] have proposed a controller in which the output (measured response) controls not only the input (drug infusion rate), but also the pharmacokinetic model driving the infusion rate. This is a so-called *model-driven* or *adaptive* closed-loop system. Such a system has performed well in clinical trials,[99] and in a simulation of extreme conditions it was demonstrated to outperform a standard PID controller.[102]

Closed-loop systems for anesthesia are the most difficult to design and implement because the precise definition of "anesthesia" remains elusive, as does a robust monitor for "anesthetic depth."[65] Because modification of consciousness must accompany anesthesia, processed electroencephalographic parameters that correlate with level of consciousness, such as the bispectral index, electroencephalographic entropy, and auditory-evoked potentials, make it possible to undertake closed-loop control of anesthesia. There is keen interest in further developing these tools to make them more reliable because advances in pharmacokinetic modeling, including the effect compartment, the implementation of such models into drug-delivery systems, and the creation of adaptive controllers based on these models, have made routine closed-loop delivery of anesthesia imaginable.[98] So far it has been difficult to bring a true closed-loop system to market in medical applications because of the regulatory agency hurdles. From a regulatory point of view, an open-loop TCI system is much easier to attain and offers many of the benefits of actual closed-loop systems. Unless there is a regulatory or a design "breakthrough," closed-loop systems for anesthesia will likely remain in the theoretical and experimental realms.

Response Surface Models of Drug-Drug Interactions

During the course of an operation, the level of anesthetic drug administered is adjusted to ensure amnesia to ongoing events, provide immobility to noxious stimulation, and blunt the sympathetic response to noxious stimulation. Although it is possible to achieve an adequate anesthetic state with a high dose of a sedative-hypnotic alone (i.e., a volatile anesthetic or propofol), the effect-site drug concentration necessary is often associated with excessive hemodynamic depression[58] and excessively deep plane of hypnosis that may be associated with long-standing morbidity or mortality.[106,107] Therefore, to limit side effects, an opioid and a sedative-hypnotic are administered together. Although the administration of two volatile anesthetics or a volatile anesthetic and propofol produce a net-additive effect, the combination of an opioid and a sedative-hypnotic are synergistic for most pharmacologic effects. By understanding the interactions between the opioids and the sedative-hypnotics, it is possible to select target concentration pairs of the two drugs that produce the desired clinical effect while minimizing unwanted side effects associated with high concentrations of a single drug (e.g., hemodynamic instability, prolonged respiratory depression).

Studies designed to evaluate the pharmacodynamic interactions between an opioid and a sedative-hypnotic have traditionally focused on the effects of adding one or two fixed doses or concentrations of the opioid to several defined concentrations or doses of the sedative-hypnotic.[57,58,108–115] Graphical demonstration of these interaction data are most commonly performed

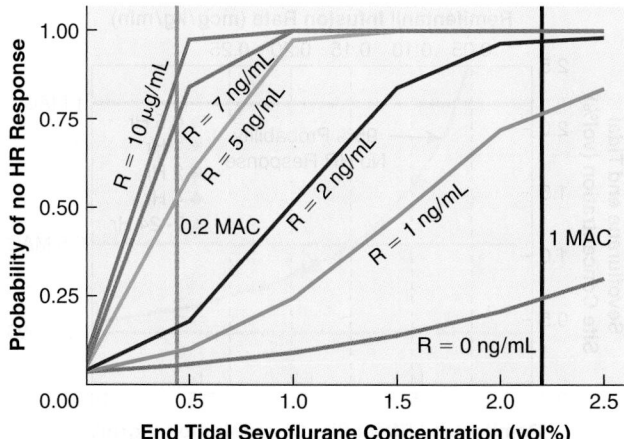

FIGURE 7-21. The effect of adding remifentanil on the concentration-effect curve for sevoflurane-induced analgesia (no hemodynamic response to a 5-second, 50 mA tetanic stimulation in volunteers). Each curve represents the concentration-effect relation for sevoflurane with a fixed effect-site concentration of remifentanil. The leftward shift in the curves indicates that remifentanil decreases the amount of sevoflurane needed to produce adequate analgesia. The changes in the slopes of the concentration-response curves indicate that there is significant pharmacodynamic synergy between sevoflurane-remifentanil. Also note that there is a ceiling effect to this pharmacodynamic interaction—the magnitude of the leftward shift decreases as the remifentanil concentration increases. HR, heart rate; MAC, minimum alveolar concentration. (Adapted from Manyam SC, Gupta DK, Johnson KB, White JL, Pace NL, Westenskow DR, Egan TD: Opioid-volatile anesthetic synergy: A response surface model with remifentanil and sevoflurane as prototypes. Anesthesiology 2006; 105: 267.)

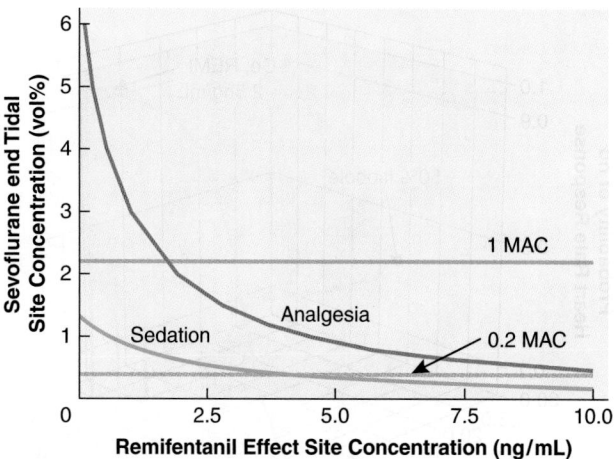

FIGURE 7-22. Remifentanil-sevoflurane interaction for sedation (*dashed line*) and analgesia to electrical tetanic stimulation (*solid line*) for volunteers. The respective 95% isoboles demonstrate the myriad of target concentration pairs of remifentanil and sevoflurane that have a 95% probability of producing the desired pharmacodynamic end point. (Adapted from Manyam SC, Gupta DK, Johnson KB, White JL, Pace NL, Westenskow DR, Egan TD: Opioid-volatile anesthetic synergy: A response surface model with remifentanil and sevoflurane as prototypes. Anesthesiology 2006; 105: 267.)

by demonstrating a shift of parallel dose-response curves (Fig. 7-21). An alternative mathematical model is the isobologram—isoeffect curves that show dose combinations that result in equal effect (Fig. 7-22). Isobolographic analysis has the additional benefit of characterizing the interaction between the two drugs as additive, antagonistic, or synergistic (Fig. 7-23), whereas shifts of dose-response curves requires more complex concentrations to determine if the interaction demonstrated by a leftward shift in the curve is more than additive.

An alternative mathematical model that can fully characterize the complete spectrum of interaction between two drugs for all possible levels of concentration and effects is the response surface model.[61,64] The surface morphology of a response surface not only demonstrates whether the interaction is additive, synergistic, or antagonistic, but the model itself can quantitatively describe the degree of interaction between the two drugs. Furthermore, isobolograms can be derived from the projection of the response surface onto the appropriate horizontal effect plane (Fig. 7-24) and concentration-response curves can be derived from taking a vertical slice through a response surface in the plane perpendicular to the fixed-opioid concentration of interest (Fig. 7-24).[61,64,65] Therefore, response surface models can be viewed as generalizations of the traditional pharmacodynamic methods of analysis. The major limitation of response surface models is that they require a large number of pharmacodynamic measurements across all possible concentration pair combinations to accurately characterize the entire surface.[116] This is most efficiently done in the laboratory setting using volunteers who can be exposed to subtherapeutic (e.g., below the level that guarantees amnesia) and supratherapeutic drug

concentration pairs. However, because response surface models characterize the drug concentration pairs that provide adequate anesthesia and also adequate recovery from anesthesia, these models provide information that are not normally available from studies that generate an isobologram from surgical patients.

Isobolograms and response surface models clearly demonstrate that there are multiple target concentration pairs of an opioid and a sedative-hypnotic that can provide adequate anesthesia—a 95% probability of no hemodynamic response to a noxious stimulus and 95% probability of clinically

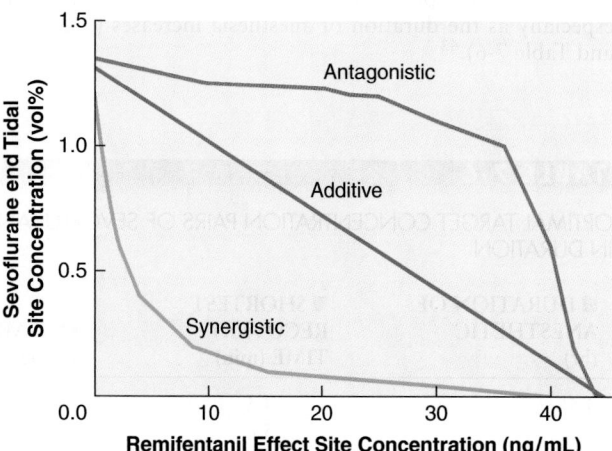

FIGURE 7-23. Isoboles to demonstrate additive (*solid line*), synergistic (*dashed line*), and antagonistic (*dotted line*) interactions between Drug A and Drug B.

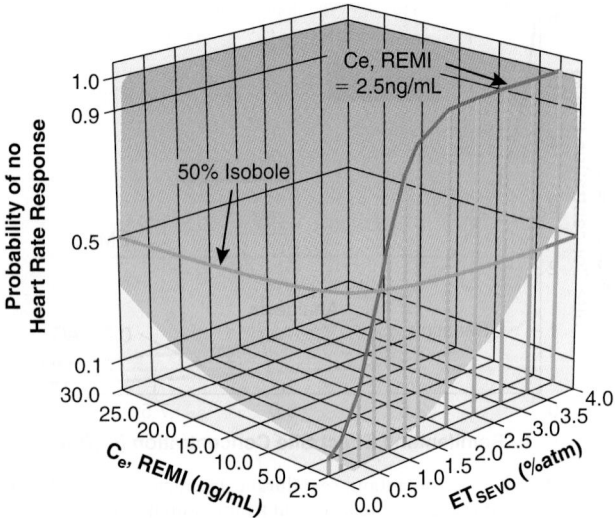

FIGURE 7-24. A response surface model characterizing the remifentanil-sevoflurane interaction for analgesia to electrical tetanic stimulation. The projection of the response surface onto the 50% probability horizontal plane results in the 50% effect isobole while the projection of the response surface onto the 2.5 ng/mL remifentanil effect-site concentration vertical plane results in the sevoflurane concentration-response curve under 2.5 ng/mL of remifentanil. (Adapted from Manyam SC, Gupta DK, Johnson KB, White JL, Pace NL, Westenskow DR, Egan TD: Opioid-volatile anesthetic synergy: A response surface model with remifentanil and sevoflurane as prototypes. Anesthesiology 2006; 105: 267.)

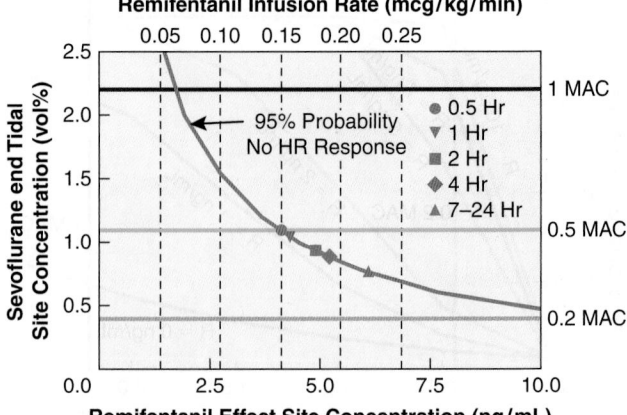

FIGURE 7-25. The optimal target concentration pairs of remifentanil and sevoflurane to maintain adequate analgesia (95% isobole for analgesia to electrical tetanic stimulation) and result in the most rapid emergence for anesthetics of various durations. For example, for a 2-hour anesthetic, target concentrations of 0.93 vol% sevoflurane and 4.9 ng/mL remifentanil would result in a 5.8-minute time to awakening. As the duration of anesthesia increases, a minimum sevoflurane target concentration of 0.75 vol% is reached. (Adapted from Manyam SC, Gupta DK, Johnson KB, White JL, Pace NL, Westenskow DR, Egan TD: Opioid-volatile anesthetic synergy: A response surface model with remifentanil and sevoflurane as prototypes. Anesthesiology 2006; 105: 267.)

⑮ adequate sedation.[62,63,66] Combining the response surface pharmacodynamic models with pharmacokinetic models allows computer simulations to be performed to identify the target concentration pair of the opioid and the sedative-hypnotic that produces an adequate anesthetic and yet optimizes one or more pharmacodynamic end points, such as the speed of awakening from anesthesia, drug-induced respiratory depression, or drug acquisition costs.[59,63] For sevoflurane-remifentanil anesthetics, these types of pharmacokinetic-pharmacodynamic simulations demonstrate the benefit of minimizing the administered dose of even the low solubility volatile anesthetic sevoflurane to near 0.5 MAC to take advantage of the pharmacokinetic efficiency of remifentanil, especially as the duration of anesthesia increases (Fig. 7-25 and Table 7-6).[63]

CONCLUSION

Since World War II, we have moved from characterizing all anesthetics by a dose-response relationship to developing sophisticated models to characterize the synergistic interaction between sedative-hypnotics and opioids and having the physical devices and the computer support to accurately administer drugs to achieve the desired concentrations at the effect site of drug action. The rational selection of drug target concentrations required to achieve adequate anesthesia and minimize side effects (e.g., prolonged awakening, hemodynamic depression) and the methods by which to efficiently achieve those concentration targets with minimal overshoot requires a solid understanding of the clinical pharmacology of anesthetics. As new drugs enter the anesthetic armamentarium, careful characterization of their pharmacokinetic and pharmacodynamic properties will allow them to be safely and appropriately used as part of a balanced anesthetic.[65]

TABLE 7-6

OPTIMAL TARGET CONCENTRATION PAIRS OF SEVOFLURANE AND REMIFENTANIL FOR ANESTHETICS 30 TO 900 MINUTES IN DURATION

■ DURATION OF ANESTHETIC (hr)	■ SHORTEST RECOVERY TIME (min)	■ REMIFENTANIL C_e (ng/mL)	■ REMIFENTANIL INFUSION RATE (μg/kg/min)	■ SEVOFLURANE ET (vol%)
0.5	4.5	4.1	0.15	1.1
1	5.0	4.3	0.16	1.05
2	5.8	4.9	0.18	0.93
4	6.7	5.2	0.19	0.88
7–24	7.2–7.7	6.1	0.22	0.75

References

1. Halford FJ: A critique of intravenous anesthesia in war surgery. Anesthesiology 1943; 4: 67
2. Adams RC, Gray HK: Intravenous anesthesia with pentothal sodium in the case of gunshot wound associated with accompanying severe traumatic shock and loss of blood: Report of a case. Anesthesiology 1943; 4: 70
3. The question of intravenous anesthesia in war surgery. Anesthesiology 1943; 4: 74
4. Price HL: A dynamic concept of the distribution of thiopental in the human body. Anesthesiology 1960; 21: 40
5. Pratt WB, Taylor P: Principles of Drug Action: The Basis of Pharmacology, 3rd edition. New York, Churchill Livingstone, 1990
6. Johnstone RW, Ruefli AA, Smyth MJ: Multiple physiological functions for multidrug transporter P-glycoprotein? Trends Biochem Sci 2000; 25: 1
7. Gao B, Hagenbuch B, Kullak-Ublick GA, et al: Organic anion-transporting polypeptides mediate transport of opioid peptides across blood-brain barrier. J Pharmacol Exp Ther 2000; 294: 73
8. Hagenbuch B, Gao B, Meier PJ: Transport of xenobiotics across the blood-brain barrier. News Physiol Sci 2002; 17: 231
9. Upton RN: Cerebral uptake of drugs in humans. Clin Exp Pharmacol Physiol 2007; 34: 695
10. Shafer SL, Stanski DR: Improving the clinical utility of anesthetic drug pharmacokinetics. Anesthesiology 1992; 76: 327
11. Stanski DR, Greenblatt DJ, Lowenstein E: Kinetics of intravenous and intramuscular morphine. Clin Pharmacol Ther 1978; 24: 52
12. Kuipers JA, Boer F, Olieman W, Burm AG, Bovill JG: First-pass lung uptake and pulmonary clearance of propofol: assessment with a recirculatory indocyanine green pharmacokinetic model. Anesthesiology 1999; 91: 1780
13. Ding X, Kaminsky LS: Human extrahepatic cytochromes P450: function in xenobiotic metabolism and tissue-selective chemical toxicity in the respiratory and gastrointestinal tracts. Annu Rev Pharmacol Toxicol 2003; 43: 149
14. Stanley TH, Hague B, Mock DL, Streisand JB, Bubbers S, Dzelzkalns RR, et al: Oral transmucosal fentanyl citrate (lollipop) premedication in human volunteers. Anesth Analg 1989; 69: 21
15. Ashburn MA, Streisand J, Zhang J, Love G, Rowin M, Niu S, et al. The iontophoresis of fentanyl citrate in humans. Anesthesiology 1995; 82: 1146
16. Eger EI, 2nd, Severinghaus JW: Effect of Uneven Pulmonary Distribution of Blood and Gas on Induction with Inhalation Anesthetics. Anesthesiology 1964; 25: 620
17. Avram MJ, Henthorn TK, Spyker DA, Krejcie TC, Lloyd PM, Cassella JV, Rabinowitz JD: Recirculatory pharmacokinetic model of the uptake, distribution, and bioavailability of prochlorperazine administered as a thermally generated aerosol in a single breath to dogs. Drug Metab Dispos 2007; 35: 262
18. Price HL, Kovnat PJ, Safer JN, et al: The uptake of thiopental by body tissues and its relationship to the duration of narcosis. Clin Pharmacol Ther 1960; 1: 16
19. Saidman LJ, Eger EI, 2nd: The effect of thiopental metabolism on duration of anesthesia. Anesthesiology 1966; 27: 118
20. Shafer SL, Varvel JR: Pharmacokinetics, pharmacodynamics, and rational opioid selection. Anesthesiology 1991; 74: 53
21. Wilkinson GR: Clearance approaches in pharmacology. Pharmacol Rev 1987; 39: 1
22. Ahmad AB, Bennett PN, Rowland M: Models of hepatic drug clearance: discrimination between the 'well stirred' and 'parallel-tube' models. J Pharm Pharmacol 1983; 35: 219
23. Wilkinson GR, Shand DG: Commentary: a physiological approach to hepatic drug clearance. Clin Pharmacol Ther 1975; 18: 377
24. Weiss M, Krejcie TC, Avram MJ: Transit time dispersion in pulmonary and systemic circulation: effects of cardiac output and solute diffusivity. Am J Physiol Heart Circ Physiol 2006; 291: H861
25. Nies AS, Shand DG, Wilkinson GR: Altered hepatic blood flow and drug disposition. Clin Pharmacokinet 1976; 1: 135
26. Wilkinson GR: Pharmacokinetics of drug disposition: hemodynamic considerations. Annu Rev Pharmacol 1975; 15: 11
27. Rane A, Villeneuve JP, Stone WJ, Nies AS, Wilkinson GR, Branch RA: Plasma binding and disposition of furosemide in the nephrotic syndrome and in uremia. Clin Pharmacol Ther 1978; 24: 199
28. Ebling WF, Wada DR, Stanski DR: From piecewise to full physiologic pharmacokinetic modeling: applied to thiopental disposition in the rat. J Pharmacokinet Biopharm 1994; 22: 259
29. Wada DR, Bjorkman S, Ebling WF, Harashima H, Harapat SR, Stanski DR: Computer simulation of the effects of alterations in blood flows and body composition on thiopental pharmacokinetics in humans. Anesthesiology 1997; 87: 884
30. Henthorn TK, Avram MJ, Krejcie TC: Intravascular mixing and drug distribution: the concurrent disposition of thiopental and indocyanine green. Clin Pharmacol Ther 1989; 45: 56
31. Homer TD, Stanski DR: The effect of increasing age on thiopental disposition and anesthetic requirement. Anesthesiology 1985; 62: 714
32. Miller RD, Stevens WC, Way WL: The effect of renal failure and hyperkalemia on the duration of pancuronium neuromuscular blockade in man. Anesth Analg 1973; 52: 661
33. Patwardhan RV, Johnson RF, Hoyumpa A, Jr., Sheehan JJ, Desmond PV, Wilkinson GR, et al: Normal metabolism of morphine in cirrhosis. Gastroenterology 1981; 81: 1006
34. Lund L, Alvan G, Berlin A, Alexanderson B: Pharmacokinetics of single and multiple doses of phenytoin in man. Eur J Clin Pharmacol 1974; 7: 81
35. Stanski DR, Mihm FG, Rosenthal MH, Kalman SM: Pharmacokinetics of high-dose thiopental used in cerebral resuscitation. Anesthesiology 1980; 53: 169
36. Avram MJ, Krejcie TC: Using front-end kinetics to optimize target-controlled drug infusions. Anesthesiology 2003; 99: 1078
37. Chiou WL, Peng GW, Nation RL: Rapid estimation of volume of distribution after a short intravenous infusion and its application to dosing adjustments. J Clin Pharmacol 1978; 18: 266
38. Fisher DM: (Almost) everything you learned about pharmacokinetics was (somewhat) wrong! Anesth Analg 1996; 83: 901
39. Krejcie TC, Avram MJ: What determines anesthetic induction dose? It's the front-end kinetics, doctor! Anesth Analg 1999; 89: 541
40. Weiss M, Krejcie TC, Avram MJ: A minimal physiological model of thiopental distribution kinetics based on a multiple indicator approach. Drug Metab Dispos 2007; 35: 1525
41. Hull CJ: How far can we go with compartmental models? Anesthesiology 1990; 72: 399
42. Kong AN, Jusko WJ: Definitions and applications of mean transit and residence times in reference to the two-compartment mammillary plasma clearance model. J Pharm Sci 1988; 77: 157
43. Jacobs JR, Shafer SL, Larsen JL, Hawkins ED: Two equally valid interpretations of the linear multicompartment mammillary pharmacokinetic model. J Pharm Sci 1990; 79: 331
44. Norman J: Drug-receptor reactions. Br J Anaesth 1979; 51: 595
45. Waud BE, Waud DR: The margin of safety of neuromuscular transmission in the muscle of the diaphragm. Anesthesiology 1972; 37: 417
46. Segre G: Kinetics of interaction between drugs and biological systems. Farmaco [Sci] 1968; 23: 907
47. Sheiner LB, Stanski DR, Vozeh S, Miller RD, Ham J: Simultaneous modeling of pharmacokinetics and pharmacodynamics: application to d-tubocurarine. Clin Pharmacol Ther 1979; 25: 358
48. Avram MJ, Krejcie TC, Henthorn TK: The relationship of age to the pharmacokinetics of early drug distribution: the concurrent disposition of thiopental and indocyanine green. Anesthesiology 1990; 72: 403
49. Schnider TW, Minto CF, Gambus PL, Andresen C, Goodale DB, Shafer SL, Youngs EJ: The influence of method of administration and covariates on the pharmacokinetics of propofol in adult volunteers. Anesthesiology 1998; 88: 1170
50. Stanski DR, Maitre PO: Population pharmacokinetics and pharmacodynamics of thiopental: the effect of age revisited. Anesthesiology 1990; 72: 412
51. Hughes MA, Glass PS, Jacobs JR: Context-sensitive half-time in multicompartment pharmacokinetic models for intravenous anesthetic drugs. Anesthesiology 1992; 76: 334
52. Minto CF, Schnider TW, Egan TD, Youngs E, Lemmens HJ, Gambus PL, et al: Influence of age and gender on the pharmacokinetics and pharmacodynamics of remifentanil. I. Model development. Anesthesiology 1997; 86: 10
53. Minto CF, Schnider TW, Shafer SL: Pharmacokinetics and pharmacodynamics of remifentanil. II. Model application. Anesthesiology 1997; 86: 24
54. Wright PM, Brown R, Lau M, Fisher DM: A pharmacodynamic explanation for the rapid onset/offset of rapacuronium bromide. Anesthesiology 1999; 90: 16
55. Wright PM, McCarthy G, Szenohradszky J, Sharma ML, Caldwell JE: Influence of chronic phenytoin administration on the pharmacokinetics and pharmacodynamics of vecuronium. Anesthesiology 2004; 100: 626–633
56. Jacobs JR, Reves JG: Effect site equilibration time is a determinant of induction dose requirement. Anesth Analg 1993; 76: 1
57. Zbinden AM, Maggiorini M, Petersen-Felix S, Lauber R, Thomson DA, Minder CE: Anesthetic depth defined using multiple noxious stimuli during isoflurane/oxygen anesthesia. I. Motor reactions. Anesthesiology 1994; 80: 253
58. Zbinden AM, Petersen-Felix S, Thomson DA: Anesthetic depth defined using multiple noxious stimuli during isoflurane/oxygen anesthesia. II. Hemodynamic responses. Anesthesiology 1994; 80: 261
59. Vuyk J, Mertens MJ, Olofsen E, Burm AG, Bovill JG: Propofol anesthesia and rational opioid selection: determination of optimal EC50-EC95 propofol-opioid concentrations that assure adequate anesthesia and a rapid return of consciousness. Anesthesiology 1997; 87: 1549
60. Bouillon TW, Bruhn J, Radulescu L, Andresen C, Shafer TJ, Cohane C, Shafer SL: Pharmacodynamic interaction between propofol and remifentanil regarding hypnosis, tolerance of laryngoscopy, bispectral index, and electroencephalographic approximate entropy. Anesthesiology 2004; 100: 1353

61. Greco WR, Bravo G, Parsons JC: The search for synergy: a critical review from a response surface perspective. Pharmacol Rev 1995; 47: 331

62. Kern SE, Xie G, White JL, Egan TD: A response surface analysis of propofol-remifentanil pharmacodynamic interaction in volunteers. Anesthesiology 2004; 100: 1373

63. Manyam SC, Gupta DK, Johnson KB, White JL, Pace NL, Westenskow DR, Egan TD: Opioid-volatile anesthetic synergy: a response surface model with remifentanil and sevoflurane as prototypes. Anesthesiology 2006; 105: 267

64. Minto CF, Schnider TW, Short TG, Gregg KM, Gentilini A, Shafer SL: Response surface model for anesthetic drug interactions. Anesthesiology 2000; 92: 1603

65. Shafer SL, Stanski DR: Defining depth of anesthesia. Handb Exp Pharmacol 2008; 409

66. Manyam SC, Gupta DK, Johnson KB, White JL, Pace NL, Westenskow DR, Egan TD: When is a bispectral index of 60 too low?: Rational processed electroencephalographic targets are dependent on the sedative-opioid ratio. Anesthesiology 2007; 106: 472

67. Terrell RC: The invention and development of enflurane, isoflurane, sevoflurane, and desflurane. Anesthesiology 2008; 108: 531

68. Schuttler J, Schwilden H, Stoekel H: Pharmacokinetics as applied to total intravenous anaesthesia. Practical implications. Anaesthesia 1983; 38 Suppl: 53

69. Shafer SL: towards optimal intravenous dosing strategies. Semin Anesth 1994; 12: 222

70. Maitre PO, Shafer SL: A simple pocket calculator approach to predict anesthetic drug concentrations from pharmacokinetic data. Anesthesiology 1990; 73: 332

71. Egan TD: Target-controlled drug delivery: progress toward an intravenous "vaporizer" and automated anesthetic administration. Anesthesiology 2003; 99: 1214

72. Shafer SL, Varvel JR, Aziz N, Scott JC: Pharmacokinetics of fentanyl administered by computer-controlled infusion pump. Anesthesiology 1990; 73: 1091

73. Barvais L, Cantraine F, D'Hollander A, Coussaert E: Predictive accuracy of continuous alfentanil infusion in volunteers: variability of different pharmacokinetic sets. Anesth Analg 1993; 77: 801

74. Barvais L, Heitz D, Schmartz D, Maes V, Coussaert E, Cantraine F, d'Hollander A: Pharmacokinetic model-driven infusion of sufentanil and midazolam during cardiac surgery: assessment of the prospective predictive accuracy and the quality of anesthesia. J Cardiothorac Vasc Anesth 2000; 14: 402

75. Barvais L, D'Hollander AA, Cantraine F, Coussaert E, Diamon G: Predictive accuracy of midazolam in adult patients scheduled for coronary surgery. J Clin Anesth 1994; 6: 297

76. Veselis RA, Glass P, Dnistrian A, Reinsel R: Performance of computer-assisted continuous infusion at low concentrations of intravenous sedatives. Anesth Analg 1997; 84: 1049

77. Vuyk J, Engbers FH, Burm AG, Vletter AA, Bovill JG: Performance of computer-controlled infusion of propofol: an evaluation of five pharmacokinetic parameter sets. Anesth Analg 1995; 81: 1275

78. Schraag S, Flaschar J: Delivery performance of commercial target-controlled infusion devices with Diprifusor module. Eur J Anaesthesiol 2002; 19: 357

79. Passot S, Servin F, Allary R, Pascal J, Prades JM, Auboyer C, Molliex S: Target-controlled versus manually-controlled infusion of propofol for direct laryngoscopy and bronchoscopy. Anesth Analg 2002; 94: 1212–1216, table of contents

80. Gale T, Leslie K, Kluger M: Propofol anaesthesia via target controlled infusion or manually controlled infusion: effects on the bispectral index as a measure of anaesthetic depth. Anaesth Intensive Care 2001; 29: 579

81. Suttner S, Boldt J, Schmidt C, Piper S, Kumle B: Cost analysis of target-controlled infusion-based anesthesia compared with standard anesthesia regimens. Anesth Analg 1999; 88: 77

82. Checketts MR, Gilhooly CJ, Kenny GN: Patient-maintained analgesia with target-controlled alfentanil infusion after cardiac surgery: a comparison with morphine PCA. Br J Anaesth 1998; 80: 748

83. van den Nieuwenhuyzen MC, Engbers FH, Burm AG, Vletter AA, van Kleef JW, Bovill JG: Target-controlled infusion of alfentanil for postoperative analgesia: contribution of plasma protein binding to intra-patient and inter-patient variability. Br J Anaesth 1999; 82: 580

84. Campbell L, Imrie G, Doherty P, Porteous C, Millar K, Kenny GN, Fletcher G: Patient maintained sedation for colonoscopy using a target controlled infusion of propofol. Anaesthesia 2004; 59: 127

85. Irwin MG, Thompson N, Kenny GN: Patient-maintained propofol sedation. Assessment of a target-controlled infusion system. Anaesthesia 1997; 52: 525

86. Gentry WB, Krejcie TC, Henthorn TK, Shanks CA, Howard KA, Gupta DK, Avram MJ: Effect of infusion rate on thiopental dose-response relationships. Assessment of a pharmacokinetic-pharmacodynamic model. Anesthesiology 1994; 81: 316–324; discussion 25A

87. Minto CF, Schnider TW, Gregg KM, Henthorn TK, Shafer SL: Using the time of maximum effect site concentration to combine pharmacokinetics and pharmacodynamics. Anesthesiology 2003; 99: 324

88. Henthorn TK, Krejcie TC, Shanks CA, Avram MJ: Time-dependent distribution volume and kinetics of the pharmacodynamic effector site. J Pharm Sci 1992; 81: 1136

89. Shafer SL, Gregg KM: Algorithms to rapidly achieve and maintain stable drug concentrations at the site of drug effect with a computer-controlled infusion pump. J Pharmacokinet Biopharm 1992; 20: 147

90. Avram MJ, Krejcie TC, Henthorn TK: The concordance of early antipyrine and thiopental distribution kinetics. J Pharmacol Exp Ther 2002; 302: 594

91. Kuipers JA, Boer F, Olofsen E, Bovill JG, Burm AG: Recirculatory pharmacokinetics and pharmacodynamics of rocuronium in patients: the influence of cardiac output. Anesthesiology 2001; 94: 47

92. Kuipers JA, Boer F, Olofsen E, Olieman W, Vletter AA, Burm AG, Bovill JG: Recirculatory and compartmental pharmacokinetic modeling of alfentanil in pigs: the influence of cardiac output. Anesthesiology 1999; 90: 1146

93. Niemann CU, Henthorn TK, Krejcie TC, Shanks CA, Enders-Klein C, Avram MJ: Indocyanine green kinetics characterize blood volume and flow distribution and their alteration by propranolol. Clin Pharmacol Ther 2000; 67: 342

94. Woodruff EA, Martin JF, Omens M: A model for the design and evaluation of algorithms for closed-loop cardiovascular therapy. IEEE Trans Biomed Eng 1997; 44: 694

95. Tehrani F, Rogers M, Lo T, Malinowski T, Afuwape S, Lum M, et al: Closed-loop control if the inspired fraction of oxygen in mechanical ventilation. J Clin Monit Comput 2002; 17: 367

96. Renard E: Implantable closed-loop glucose-sensing and insulin delivery: the future for insulin pump therapy. Curr Opin Pharmacol 2002; 2: 708

97. O'Hara DA, Hexem JG, Derbyshire GJ, Overdyk FJ, Chen B, Henthorn TK, Li KJ: The use of a PID controller to model vecuronium pharmacokinetics and pharmacodynamics during liver transplantation. Proportional-integral-derivative. IEEE Trans Biomed Eng 1997; 44: 610

98. De Smet T, Struys MM, Greenwald S, Mortier EP, Shafer SL: Estimation of optimal modeling weights for a Bayesian-based closed-loop system for propofol administration using the bispectral index as a controlled variable: a simulation study. Anesth Analg 2007; 105: 1629–1638, table of contents

99. Mortier E, Struys M, De Smet T, Versichelen L, Rolly G: Closed-loop controlled administration of propofol using bispectral analysis. Anaesthesia 1998; 53: 749

100. Schwilden H, Schuttler J, Stoeckel H: Closed-loop feedback control of methohexital anesthesia by quantitative EEG analysis in humans. Anesthesiology 1987; 67: 341

101. Schwilden H, Stoeckel H: Effective therapeutic infusions produced by closed-loop feedback control of methohexital administration during total intravenous anesthesia with fentanyl. Anesthesiology 1990; 73: 225

102. Struys MM, De Smet T, Greenwald S, Absalom AR, Binge S, Mortier EP: Performance evaluation of two published closed-loop control systems using bispectral index monitoring: a simulation study. Anesthesiology 2004; 100: 640

103. Struys MM, De Smet T, Mortier EP: Closed-loop control of anaesthesia. Curr Opin Anaesthesiol 2002; 15: 421

104. Struys MM, De Smet T, Versichelen LF, Van De Velde S, Van den Broecke R, Mortier EP: Comparison of closed-loop controlled administration of propofol using Bispectral Index as the controlled variable versus "standard practice" controlled administration. Anesthesiology 2001; 95: 6

105. Tzabazis A, Ihmsen H, Schywalsky M, Schwilden H: EEG-controlled closed-loop dosing of propofol in rats. Br J Anaesth 2004; 92: 564

106. Monk TG, Saini V, Weldon BC, Sigl JC: Anesthetic management and one-year mortality after noncardiac surgery. Anesth Analg 2005; 100: 4

107. Monk TG, Weldon BC, Garvan CW, Dede DE, van der Aa MT, Heilman KM, Gravenstein JS: Predictors of cognitive dysfunction after major non-cardiac surgery. Anesthesiology 2008; 108: 18

108. Katoh T, Ikeda K: The effects of fentanyl on sevoflurane requirements for loss of consciousness and skin incision. Anesthesiology 1998; 88: 18

109. Katoh T, Kobayashi S, Suzuki A, Iwamoto T, Bito H, Ikeda K: The effect of fentanyl on sevoflurane requirements for somatic and sympathetic responses to surgical incision. Anesthesiology 1999; 90: 398

110. Katoh T, Nakajima Y, Moriwaki G, Kobayashi S, Suzuki A, Iwamoto T, et al: Sevoflurane requirements for tracheal intubation with and without fentanyl. Br J Anaesth 1999; 82: 561

111. Katoh T, Uchiyama T, Ikeda K: Effect of fentanyl on awakening concentration of sevoflurane. Br J Anaesth 1994; 73: 322

112. McEwan AI, Smith C, Dyar O, Goodman D, Smith LR, Glass PS: Isoflurane minimum alveolar concentration reduction by fentanyl. Anesthesiology 1993; 78: 864

113. Sebel PS, Glass PS, Fletcher JE, Murphy MR, Gallagher C, Quill T: Reduction of the MAC of desflurane with fentanyl. Anesthesiology 1992; 76: 52

114. Vuyk J, Lim T, Engbers FH, Burm AG, Vletter AA, Bovill JG: Pharmacodynamics of alfentanil as a supplement to propofol or nitrous oxide for lower abdominal surgery in female patients. Anesthesiology 1993; 78: 1036–1045; discussion 23A

115. Vuyk J, Lim T, Engbers FH, Burm AG, Vletter AA, Bovill JG: The pharmacodynamic interaction of propofol and alfentanil during lower abdominal surgery in women. Anesthesiology 1995; 83: 8

116. Short TG, Ho TY, Minto CF, Schnider TW, Shafer SL: Efficient trial design for eliciting a pharmacokinetic-pharmacodynamic model-based response surface describing the interaction between two intravenous anesthetic drugs. Anesthesiology 2002; 96: 400

CHAPTER 8 ■ ELECTRICAL AND FIRE SAFETY

JAN EHRENWERTH AND HARRY A. SEIFERT

SCIENTIFIC FOUNDATIONS OF ANESTHESIA

KEY POINTS

1. A basic principle of electricity is known as *Ohm's law* (Voltage = Current × Resistance).
2. To have the completed circuit necessary for current flow, a closed loop must exist and a voltage source must drive the current through the impedance.
3. To receive a shock, one must contact the electrical circuit at two points, and there must be a voltage source that causes the current to flow through an individual.
4. In electrical terminology, *grounding* is applied to two separate concepts: the grounding of electrical power and the grounding of electrical equipment.
5. To provide an extra measure of safety from gross electrical shock (macroshock), the power supplied to most operating rooms (ORs) is ungrounded.
6. The line isolation monitor is a device that continuously monitors the integrity of an isolated power system.
7. The ground fault circuit interrupter is a popular device used to prevent individuals from receiving an electrical shock in a grounded power system.

8. An electrically susceptible patient (i.e., one who has a direct, external connection to the heart) they may be at risk from very small currents; this is called *microshock*.
9. Problems can arise if the electrosurgical return plate is improperly applied to the patient or if the cord connecting the return plate to the electrosurgical unit (ESU) is damaged or broken.
10. Fires in the OR are just as much a danger today as they were 100 years ago when patients were anesthetized with flammable anesthetic agents.
11. The necessary components for a fire consist of the triad of heat or an ignition source, a fuel, and an oxidizer.
12. The two major ignition sources for OR fires are the ESU and the laser.
13. It is known that desiccated carbon dioxide absorbent can, in rare circumstances, react with sevoflurane to produce a fire.
14. All OR personnel should be familiar with the location and operation of the fire extinguishers.

The myriad of electrical and electronic devices in the modern operating room (OR) greatly improve patient care and safety. However, these devices also subject both the patient and OR personnel to increased risks. To reduce the risk of electrical shock, most ORs have electrical systems that incorporate special safety features. It is incumbent upon the anesthesiologist to have a thorough understanding of the basic principles of electricity and an appreciation of the concepts of electrical safety applicable to the OR environment.

PRINCIPLES OF ELECTRICITY

1. A basic principle of electricity is known as *Ohm's law,* which is represented by the equation:

$$E = I \times R$$

where E is electromotive force (in volts), I is current (in amperes), and R is resistance (in ohms). Ohm's law forms the basis for the physiologic equation $BP = CO \times SVR$; that is, blood pressure (BP) is equal to the cardiac output (CO) times the systemic vascular resistance (SVR). In this case, the blood pressure of the vascular system is analogous to voltage, the cardiac output to current, and the systemic vascular resistance to the forces opposing the flow of electrons. Electrical power is measured in watts. Wattage (W) is the product of the voltage (E) and the current (I), as defined by the formula:

$$W = E \times I$$

The amount of electrical work done is measured in watts multiplied by a unit of time. The watt-second (a joule, J) is a common designation for electrical energy expended in doing work. The energy produced by a defibrillator is measured in watt-seconds (or joules). The kilowatt-hour is used by electrical utility companies to measure larger quantities of electrical energy.

Wattage can be thought of as a measure not only of work done but also of heat produced in any electrical circuit. Substituting Ohm's law in the formula:

$$W = E \times I$$
$$W = (I \times R) \times I$$
$$W = I^2 \times R$$

Thus, wattage is equal to the square of the current I^2 (amperage) times the resistance R. Using these formulas, it is possible to calculate the number of amperes and the resistance of a given device if the wattage and the voltage are known. For example, a 60-watt light bulb operating on a household 120-volt circuit would require 0.5 ampere of current for operation. Rearranging the formula so that:

$$I = W/E$$

we have:

$$I = (60 \text{ watts})/(120 \text{ volts})$$
$$I = 0.5 \text{ ampere}$$

Using this in Ohm's law:

$$R = E/I$$

the resistance can be calculated to be 240 ohms:

$$R = (120 \text{ volts})/(0.5 \text{ ampere})$$
$$R = 240 \text{ ohms}$$

It is obvious from the previous discussion that 1 volt of electromotive force (EMF) flowing through a 1-ohm resistance will generate 1 ampere of current. Similarly, 1 ampere of current induced by 1 volt of electromotive force will generate 1 watt of power.

Direct and Alternating Currents

Any substance that permits the flow of electrons is called a *conductor*. Current is characterized by electrons flowing through a conductor. If the electron flow is always in the same direction, it is referred to as *direct current* (DC). However, if the electron flow reverses direction at a regular interval, it is termed *alternating current* (AC). Either of these types of current can be pulsed or continuous in nature.

The previous discussion of Ohm's law is accurate when applied to DC circuits. However, when dealing with AC circuits, the situation is more complex because the flow of the current is opposed by a more complicated form of resistance, known as *impedance*.

Impedance

Impedance, designated by the letter Z, is defined as the sum of the forces that oppose electron movement in an AC circuit. Impedance consists of resistance (ohms) but also takes capacitance and inductance into account. In actuality, when referring to AC circuits, Ohm's law is defined as:

$$E = I \times Z$$

An *insulator* is a substance that opposes the flow of electrons. Therefore, an insulator has a high impedance to electron flow, whereas a conductor has a low impedance to electron flow.

In AC circuits the capacitance and inductance can be important factors in determining the total impedance. Both capacitance and inductance are influenced by the frequency (cycles per second or hertz, Hz) at which the AC current

reverses direction. The impedance is directly proportional to the frequency (f) times the inductance (IND):

$$Z \alpha\, (f \times \text{IND})$$

and the impedance is inversely proportional to the product of the frequency (f) and the capacitance (CAP):

$$Z \alpha 1/(f \times \text{CAP})$$

As the AC current increases in frequency, the net effect of both capacitance and inductance increases. However, because impedance and capacitance are inversely related, total impedance decreases as the product of the frequency and the capacitance increases. Thus, as frequency increases, impedance falls and more current is allowed to pass.

Capacitance

A *capacitor* consists of any two parallel conductors that are separated by an insulator (Fig. 8-1). A capacitor has the ability to store charge. *Capacitance* is the measure of that substance's ability to store charge. In a DC circuit the capacitor plates are charged by a voltage source (i.e., a battery) and there is only a momentary current flow. The circuit is not completed and no further current can flow unless a resistance is connected between the two plates and the capacitor is discharged.

In contrast to DC circuits, a capacitor in an AC circuit permits current flow even when the circuit is not completed by a resistance. This is because of the nature of AC circuits, in which the current flow is constantly being reversed. Because current flow results from the movement of electrons, the capacitor plates are alternately charged—first positive and then negative with every reversal of the AC current direction—resulting in an effective current flow as far as the remainder of the circuit is concerned, even though the circuit is not completed.

Because the effect of capacitance on impedance varies directly with the AC frequency in hertz, the greater the AC frequency, the lower the impedance. Therefore, high-frequency currents (0.5 to 2 million Hz), such as those used by electrosurgical units (ESUs), will cause a marked decrease in impedance.

Electrical devices use capacitors for various beneficial purposes. There is, however, a phenomenon known as *stray capacitance*—capacitance that was not designed into the system but is incidental to the construction of the equipment. All AC-operated equipment produces stray capacitance. An ordinary power cord, for example, consisting of two insulated wires running next to each other will generate significant capacitance simply by being plugged into a 120-volt circuit, even though the piece of equipment is not turned on. Another example of stray capacitance is found in electric motors. The circuit wiring in electric motors generates stray capacitance to the metal housing of the motor. The clinical importance of capacitance will be emphasized later in the chapter.

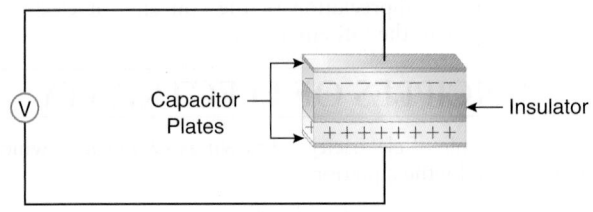

FIGURE 8-1.   A capacitor consists of two parallel conductors separated by an insulator. The capacitor is capable of storing charge supplied by a voltage source.

Inductance

Whenever electrons flow in a wire, a magnetic field is induced around the wire. If the wire is coiled repeatedly around an iron core, as in a transformer, the magnetic field can be very strong. *Inductance* is a property of AC circuits in which an opposing EMF can be electromagnetically generated in the circuit. The net effect of inductance is to increase impedance. Because the effect of inductance on impedance also depends on AC frequency, increases in frequency will increase the total impedance. Therefore, the total impedance of a coil will be much greater than its simple resistance.

ELECTRICAL SHOCK HAZARDS

Alternating and Direct Currents

Whenever an individual contacts an external source of electricity, an electrical shock is possible. An electrical current can stimulate skeletal muscle cells to contract, and thus can be used therapeutically in devices such as pacemakers or defibrillators. However, casual contact with an electrical current, whether AC or DC, can lead to injury or death. Although it takes approximately 3 times as much DC as AC to cause ventricular fibrillation, this by no means renders DC harmless. Devices such as an automobile battery or a DC defibrillator can be sources of direct current shocks.

In the United States, utility companies supply electrical energy in the form of alternating currents of 120 volts at a frequency of 60 Hz. The 120 volts of EMF and 1 ampere of current are the effective voltage and amperage in an AC circuit. This is also referred to as *RMS* (root-mean-square). It takes 1.414 amperes of peak amperage in the sinusoidal curve to give an effective amperage of 1 ampere. Similarly, it takes 170 volts (120 × 1.414) at the peak of the AC curve to get an effective voltage of 120 volts. The 60 Hz refers to the number of times in 1 second that the current reverses its direction of flow. Both the voltage and current waveforms form a sinusoidal pattern (Fig. 8-2).

To have the completed circuit necessary for current flow, a closed loop must exist and a voltage source must drive the current through the impedance. If current is to flow in the electrical circuit, there has to be a *voltage differential*, or a drop in the driving pressure across the impedance. According to Ohm's law, if the resistance is held constant, then the greater the current flow, the larger the voltage drop must be.

The power company attempts to maintain the line voltage constant at 120 volts. Therefore, by Ohm's law the current flow is inversely proportional to the impedance. A typical power cord consists of two conductors. One, designated as *hot* carries the current to the impedance; the other is *neutral*, and it returns the current to the source. The potential difference between the two is effectively 120 volts (Fig. 8-3). The amount

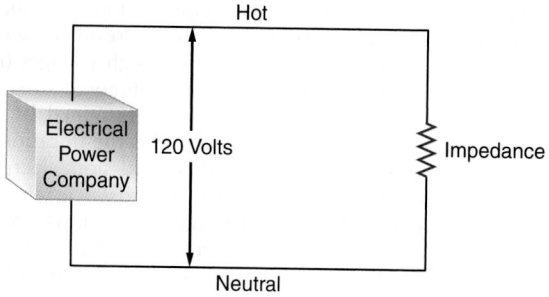

FIGURE 8-3. A typical alternating current (AC) circuit where there is a potential difference of 120 volts between the hot and neutral sides of the circuit. The current flows through a resistance, which in AC circuits is more accurately referred to as *impedance*, and then returns to the electrical power company.

of current flowing through a given device is frequently referred to as the *load*. The load of the circuit depends on the impedance. A very high impedance circuit allows only a small current to flow and thus has a small load. A very low impedance circuit will draw a large current and is said to be a large load. A *short circuit* occurs when there is a zero impedance load with a very high current flow.[1]

Source of Shocks

Electrical accidents or shocks occur when a person becomes part of, or completes, an electrical circuit. To receive a shock, one must contact the electrical circuit at two points, and there must be a voltage source that causes the current to flow through an individual (Fig. 8-4).

When an individual contacts a source of electricity, damage occurs in one of two ways. First, the electrical current can disrupt the normal electrical function of cells. Depending on its magnitude, the current can contract muscles, alter brain function, paralyze respiration, or disrupt normal heart function, leading to ventricular fibrillation. The second mechanism involves the dissipation of electrical energy throughout the body's tissues. An electrical current passing through any resistance raises the temperature of that substance. If enough thermal energy is released, the

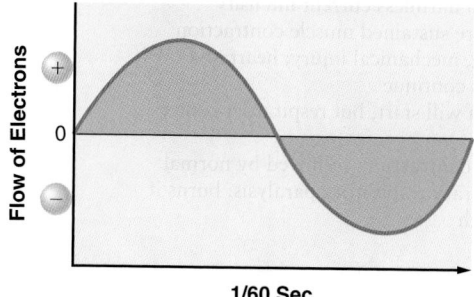

FIGURE 8-2. Sine wave flow of electrons in a 60-Hz alternating current.

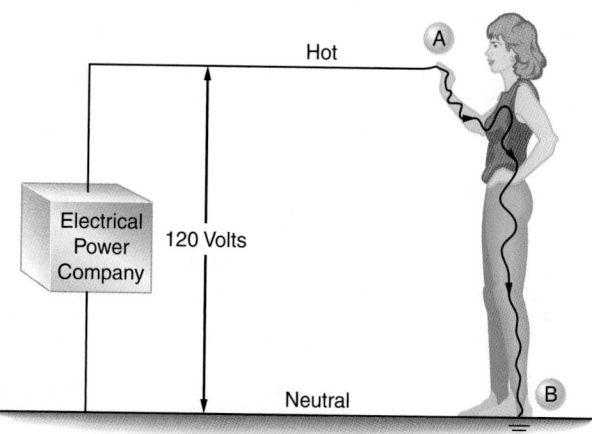

FIGURE 8-4. An individual can complete an electric circuit and receive a shock by coming in contact with the hot side of the circuit (point *A*). This is because he or she is standing on the ground (point *B*) and the contact point *A* and the ground point *B* provide the two contact points necessary for a completed circuit. The severity of the shock that the individual receives depends on his or her skin resistance.

temperature will rise sufficiently to produce a burn. Accidents involving household currents usually do not result in severe burns. However, in accidents involving very high voltages (i.e., power transmission lines), severe burns are common.

The severity of an electrical shock is determined by the amount of current (number of amperes) and the duration of the current flow. For the purposes of this discussion, electrical shocks are divided into two categories. *Macroshock* refers to large amounts of current flowing through a person, which can cause harm or death. *Microshock* refers to very small amounts of current and applies only to the electrically susceptible patient. This is an individual who has an external conduit that is in direct contact with the heart. This can be a pacing wire or a saline-filled catheter such as a central venous or pulmonary artery catheter. In the case of the electrically susceptible patient, even minute amounts of current (microshock) may cause ventricular fibrillation.

Table 8-1 shows the effects typically produced by various currents following a 1-second contact with a 60-Hz current. When an individual contacts a 120-volt household current, the severity of the shock will depend on his or her skin resistance, the duration of the contact, and the current density. Skin resistance can vary from a few thousand to 1 million ohms. If a person with a skin resistance of 1,000 ohms contacts a 120-volt circuit, he or she would receive 120 milliamperes (mA) of current, which would probably be lethal. However, if that same person's skin resistance is 100,000 ohms, the current flow would be 1.2 mA, which would barely be perceptible.

$$I = E/R = (120 \text{ volts})/(1,000 \text{ ohms}) = 120 \text{ mA}$$

$$I = E/R = (120 \text{ volts})/(100,000 \text{ ohms}) = 1.2 \text{ mA}$$

The longer an individual is in contact with the electrical source, the more dire the consequences because more energy will be released and more tissue damaged. Also, there will be a greater chance of ventricular fibrillation from excitation of the heart during the vulnerable period of the electrocardiogram (ECG) cycle.

Current density is a way of expressing the amount of current that is applied per unit area of tissue. The diffusion of current in the body tends to be in all directions. The greater the current or the smaller the area to which it is applied, the higher the current density. In relation to the heart, a current of 100 mA (100,000 μA) is generally required to produce ventricular fibrillation when applied to the surface of the body. However, only 100 μA (0.1 mA) is required to produce ventricular fibrillation when that minute current is applied directly to the myocardium through an instrument having a very small contact area, such as a pacing wire electrode. In this case, the current density is 1,000-fold greater when applied directly to the heart; therefore, only 1/1,000 of the energy is required to cause ventricular fibrillation. In this case, the electrically susceptible patient can be electrocuted with currents well below 1 mA, which is the threshold of perception for humans. The frequency at which the current reverses is also an important factor in determining the amount of current an individual can safely contact. Utility companies in the United States produce electricity at a frequency of 60 Hz. They use 60 Hz because higher frequencies cause greater power loss through transmission lines and lower frequencies cause a detectable flicker from light sources.[2] The "let-go" current is defined as that current above which sustained muscular contraction occurs and at which an individual would be unable to let go of an energized wire. The let-go current for a 60-Hz AC power is 10 to 20 mA,[1,3,4] whereas at a frequency of 1 million Hz, up to 3 amperes (3,000 mA) is generally considered safe. It should be noted that very high frequency currents do not excite contractile tissue; consequently, they do not cause cardiac dysrhythmias.

It can be seen that Ohm's law governs the flow of electricity. For a completed circuit to exist, there must be a closed loop with a driving pressure to force a current through a resistance, just as in the cardiovascular system there must be a blood pressure to drive the cardiac output through the peripheral resistance. Figure 8-5 illustrates that a hot wire carrying a 120-volt pressure through the resistance of a 60-watt light bulb produces a current flow of 0.5 ampere. The voltage in the neutral wire is approximately 0 volts, while the current in the neutral wire remains at 0.5 ampere. This correlates with our cardiovascular analogy, where a mean blood pressure decrease of 80 mm Hg between the aortic root and the right atrium forces a cardiac output of 6 L/min through a systemic vascular resistance of 13.3 resistance units. However, the flow (in this case, the cardiac output, or in the case of the electrical model, the current) is still the same everywhere in the circuit. That is, the cardiac output on the arterial side is the same as the cardiac output on the venous side.

TABLE 8-1

EFFECTS OF 60-Hz CURRENT ON AN AVERAGE HUMAN FOR A 1-SECOND CONTACT

■ CURRENT	■ EFFECT
Macroshock	
1 mA (0.001 A)	Threshold of perception
5 mA (0.005 A)	Accepted as maximum harmless current intensity
10–20 mA (0.01–0.02 A)	"Let-go" current before sustained muscle contraction
50 mA (0.05 A)	Pain, possible fainting, mechanical injury; heart and respiratory functions continue
100–300 mA (0.1–0.3 A)	Ventricular fibrillation will start, but respiratory center remains intact
6,000 mA (6 A)	Sustained myocardial contraction, followed by normal heart rhythm; temporary respiratory paralysis; burns if current density is high
Microshock	
100 μA (0.1 mA)	Ventricular fibrillation
10 μA (0.01 mA)	Recommended maximum 60-Hz leakage current

A, amperes; mA, milliamperes; μA, microamperes.

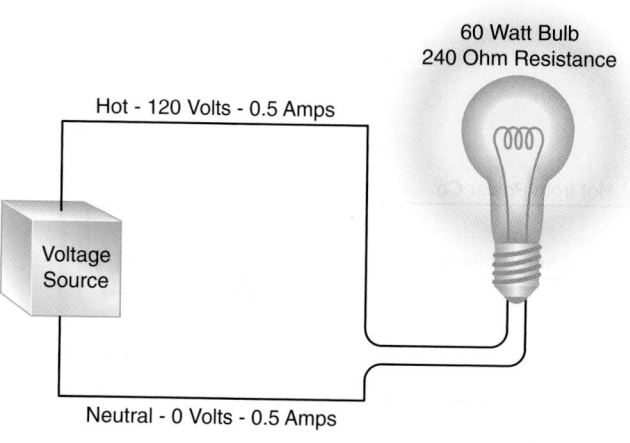

FIGURE 8-5.   A 60-watt light bulb has an internal resistance of 240 ohms and draws 0.5 ampere of current. The voltage drop in the circuit is from 120 in the hot wire to 0 in the neutral wire, but the current is 0.5 ampere in both the hot and neutral wires.

Grounding

To fully understand electrical shock hazards and their prevention, one must have a thorough knowledge of the concepts of grounding. These concepts of grounding probably constitute the most confusing aspects of electrical safety because the same term is used to describe several different principles. In electrical terminology, grounding is applied to two separate concepts. The first is the grounding of electrical *power,* and the second is the grounding of electrical *equipment.* Thus, the concepts that (1) power can be grounded or ungrounded and that (2) power can supply electrical devices that are themselves grounded or ungrounded are not mutually exclusive. It is vital to understand this point as the basis of electrical safety (*Table 8-2*). Whereas electrical *power* is grounded in the home, it is usually ungrounded in the OR. In the home, electrical *equipment* may be grounded or ungrounded, but it should always be grounded in the OR.

ELECTRICAL POWER: GROUNDED

Electrical utilities universally provide power that is grounded (by convention, the earth-ground potential is zero, and all voltages represent a difference between potentials). That is, one of the wires supplying the power to a home is intentionally connected to the earth. The utility companies do this as a safety measure to prevent electrical charges from building up in their wiring during electrical storms. This also prevents the very high voltages used in transmitting power by the utility from entering the home in the event of an equipment failure in their high-voltage system.

The power enters the typical home via two wires. These two wires are attached to the main fuse or the circuit breaker box at the service entrance. The "hot" wire supplies power to the "hot" distribution strip. The neutral wire is connected to the neutral distribution strip and to a service entrance ground (i.e., a pipe buried in the earth; Fig. 8-6). From the fuse box, three wires leave to sup-

ply the electrical outlets in the house. In the United States, the hot wire is color-coded black and carries a voltage 120 volts above ground potential. The second wire is the neutral wire color-coded white; the third wire is the ground wire, which is either color-coded green or is uninsulated (bare wire). The ground and the neutral wires are attached at the same point in the circuit breaker box and then further connected to a cold-water pipe (Figs. 8-7 and 8-8). Thus, this grounded power system is also referred to as a *neutral grounded power system.* The black wire is not connected to the ground, as this would create a short circuit. The black wire is attached to the hot (i.e., 120 volts above ground) distribution strip on which the circuit breakers or fuses are located. From here, numerous branch circuits supply electrical power to the outlets in the house. Each branch circuit is protected by a circuit breaker or fuse that limits current to a specific maximum amperage. Most electrical circuits in the house are 15- or 20-ampere circuits. These typically supply power to the electrical outlets and lights in the house. Several higher amperage circuits are also provided for devices such as an electric stove or an electric clothes dryer. These devices are powered by 240-volt circuits, which can draw from 30 to 50 amperes of current. The circuit breaker or fuse will interrupt the flow of current on the hot side of the line in the event of a short circuit or if the demand placed on that circuit is too high. For example, a 15-ampere branch circuit will be capable of supporting 1,800 watts of power.

$$W = E/I$$

$$W = 120 \text{ volts} \times 15 \text{ amperes}$$

$$W = 1,800 \text{ watts}$$

Therefore, if two 1,500-watt hair dryers were simultaneously plugged into one outlet, the load would be too great for a 15-ampere circuit, and the circuit breaker would open (trip) or the fuse would melt. This is done to prevent the supply wires in the circuit from melting and starting a fire. The amperage of the circuit breaker on the branch circuit is determined by the thickness of the wire that it supplies. If a 20-ampere breaker is used with wire rated for only 15 amperes, the wire could melt and start a fire before the circuit breaker would trip. It is important to note that a 15-ampere circuit breaker does not protect an individual from lethal shocks. The 15 amperes of current that would trip the circuit breaker far exceeds the 100 to 200 mA that will produce ventricular fibrillation.

The wires that leave the circuit breaker supply the electrical outlets and lighting for the rest of the house. In older homes the electrical cable consists of two wires, a hot and a neutral, which supply power to the electrical outlets (Fig. 8-9). In newer homes, a third wire has been added to the electrical cable (Fig. 8-10). This third wire is either green or uninsulated (bare) and serves as a ground wire for the power receptacle

TABLE 8-2

DIFFERENCES BETWEEN POWER AND EQUIPMENT GROUNDING IN THE HOME AND THE OPERATING ROOM

	■ POWER	■ EQUIPMENT
Home	+	±
Operating room	−	+

+, grounded; −, ungrounded; ±, may or may not be grounded.

FIGURE 8-6. In a neutral grounded power system, the electric company supplies two lines to the typical home. The neutral wire is connected to ground by the power company and again connected to a service entrance ground when it enters the fuse box. Both the neutral and ground wires are connected together in the fuse box at the neutral bus bar, which is also attached to the service entrance ground.

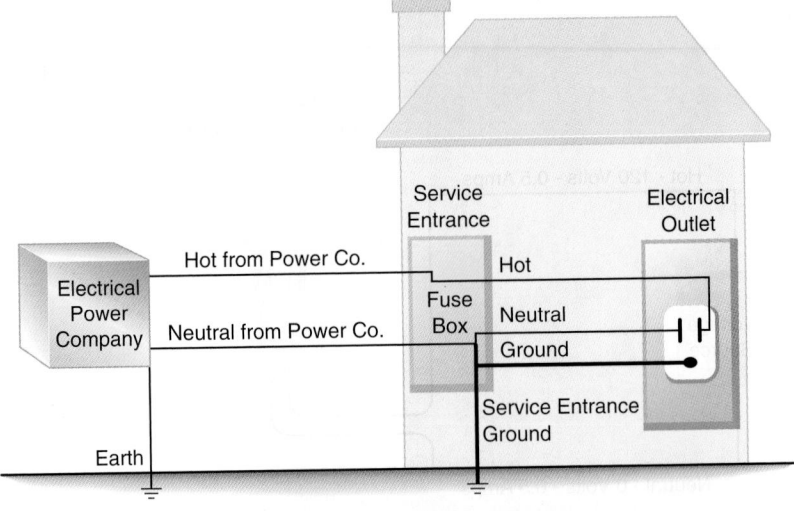

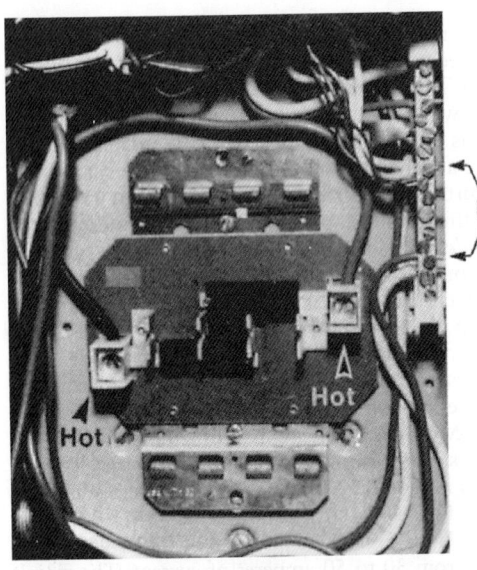

FIGURE 8-7. Inside a fuse box with the circuit breakers removed. The *arrowheads* indicate the hot wires energizing the strips where the circuit breakers are located. The *arrows* point to the neutral bus bar where the neutral and ground wires are connected.

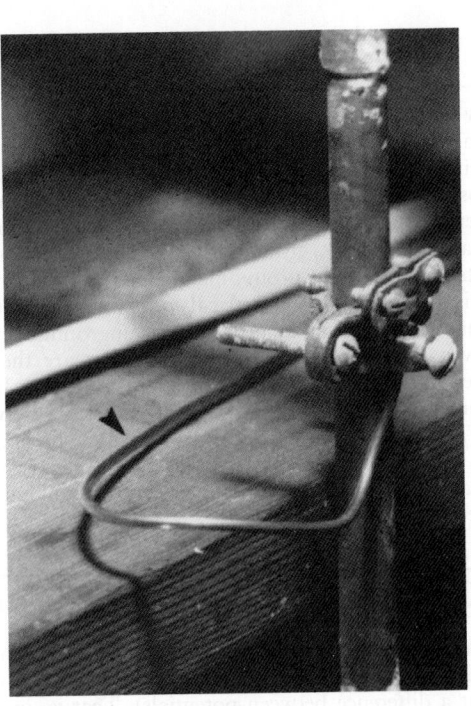

FIGURE 8-8. The *arrowhead* indicates the ground wire from the fuse box attached to a cold-water pipe.

FIGURE 8-9. An older style electrical outlet consisting of just two wires (a hot and a neutral). There is no ground wire.

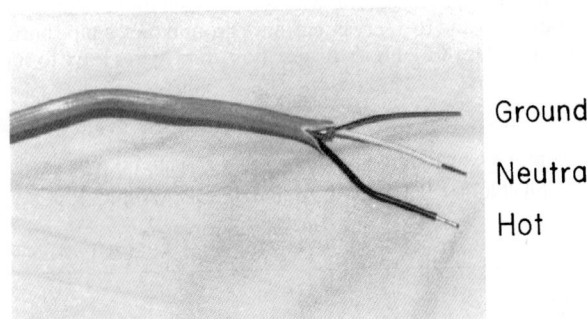

FIGURE 8-10. Modern electrical cable in which a third, or ground, wire has been added.

FIGURE 8-11.   Modern electrical outlet in which the ground wire is present. The *arrowhead* points to the part of the receptacle where the ground wire connects.

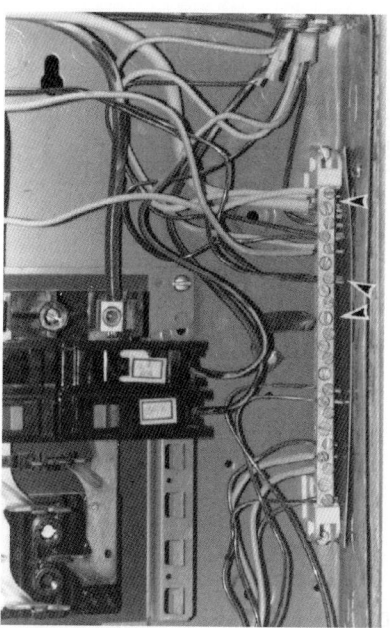

FIGURE 8-13.   The ground wires from the power outlet are run to the neutral bus bar, where they are connected with the neutral wires (*arrowheads*).

(Fig. 8-11). On one end, the ground wire is attached to the electrical outlet (Fig. 8-12); on the other, it is connected to the neutral distribution strip in the circuit breaker box along with the neutral (white) wires (Fig. 8-13).

It should be realized that in both the old and new situations, the power is grounded. That is, a 120-volt potential exists between the hot (black) and the neutral (white) wire and between the hot wire and ground. In this case, the ground is the earth (Fig. 8-14). In modern home construction, there is still a 120-volt potential difference between the hot (black) and the neutral (white) wire as well as a 120-volt difference

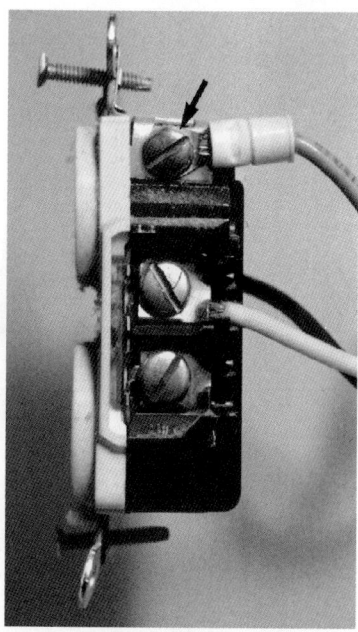

FIGURE 8-12.   Detail of modern electrical power receptacle. The *arrow* points to the ground wire, which is attached to the grounding screw on the power receptacle.

between the equipment ground wire (which is the third wire), and between the hot wire and earth (Fig. 8-15).

A 60-watt light bulb can be used as an example to further illustrate this point. Normally, the hot and neutral wires are connected to the two wires of the light bulb socket, and throwing the switch will illuminate the bulb (Fig. 8-16). Similarly, if the hot wire is connected to one side of the bulb socket and the other wire from the light bulb is connected to the equipment ground wire, the bulb will illuminate. If there is no equipment ground wire, the bulb will still light if the second wire is connected to any grounded metallic object such as a water pipe or a faucet. This illustrates the fact that the 120-volt potential difference exists not only between the hot and the neutral wires but also between the hot wire and any grounded object. Thus, in a grounded power system, the current will flow between the hot wire and any conductor with an earth ground.

As previously stated, current flow requires a closed loop with a source of voltage. For an individual to receive an electric shock, he or she must contact the loop at two points. Because we may be standing on ground or be in contact with an object that is referenced to ground, only one additional contact point is necessary to complete the circuit and thus receive an electrical shock. This is an unfortunate and inherently dangerous consequence of grounded power systems. Modern wiring systems have added the third wire, the equipment ground wire, as a safety measure to reduce the severity of a potential electrical shock. This is accomplished by providing an alternate, low-resistance pathway through which the current can flow to ground.

Over time the insulation covering wires may deteriorate. It is then possible for a bare, hot wire to contact the metal case or frame of an electrical device. The case would then become energized and constitute a shock hazard to someone coming in contact with it. Figure 8-17 illustrates a typical short circuit, where the individual has come in contact with the hot case of an instrument. This illustrates the type of wiring found in older homes. There is no ground wire in the electrical outlet, nor is the electrical apparatus equipped with a ground wire. Here, the individual completes the circuit and receives a severe

FIGURE 8-14. Diagram of a house with older style wiring that does not contain a ground wire. A 120-volt potential difference exists between the hot and the neutral wires, as well as between the hot wire and the earth.

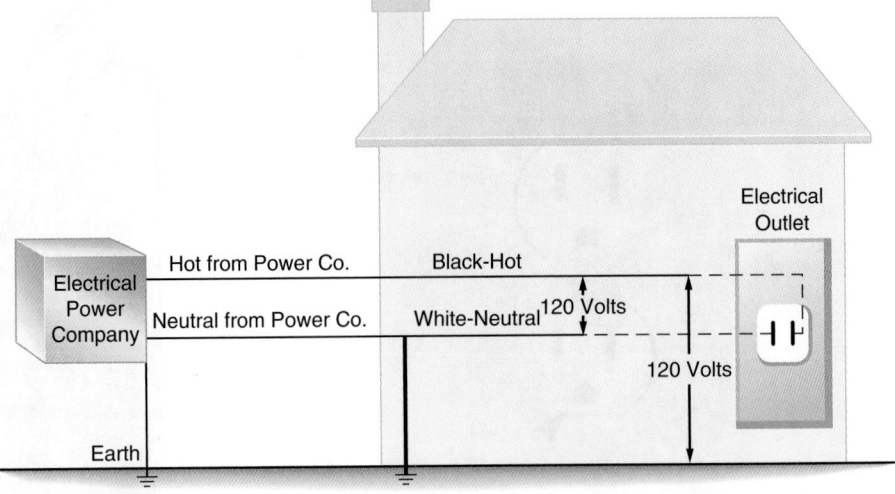

FIGURE 8-15. Diagram of a house with modern wiring in which the third, or ground, wire has been added. The 120-volt potential difference exists between the hot and neutral wires, the hot and the ground wires, and the hot wire and the earth.

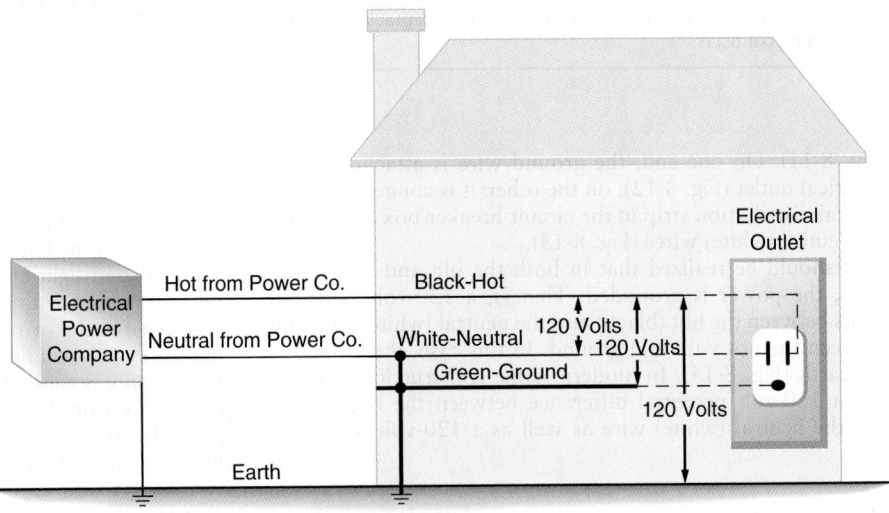

FIGURE 8-16. A simple light bulb circuit in which the hot and neutral wires are connected with the corresponding wires from the light bulb fixture.

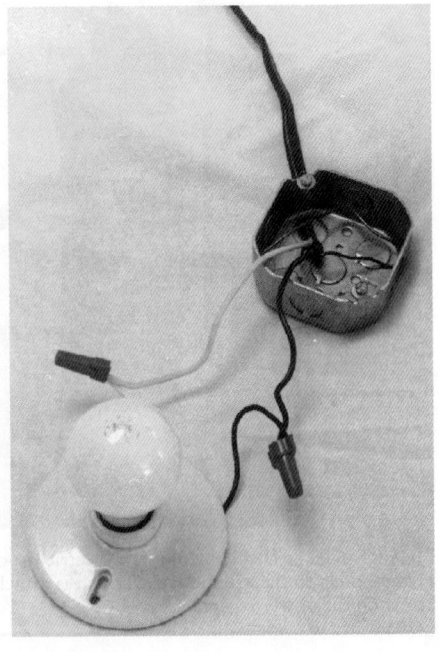

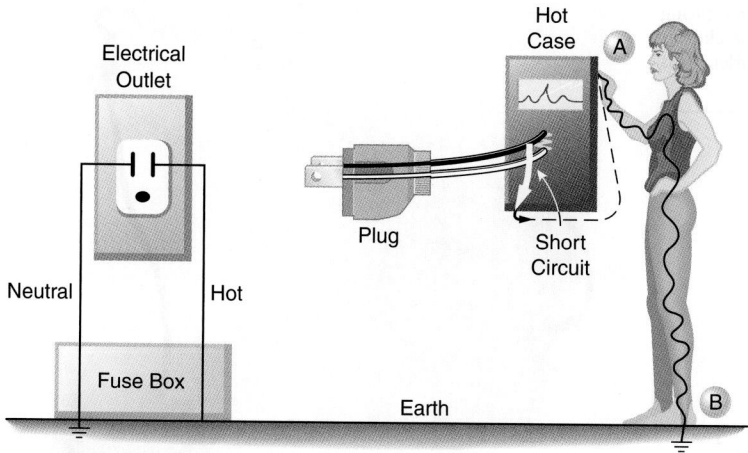

FIGURE 8-17. When a faulty piece of equipment without an equipment ground wire is plugged into an electrical outlet not containing a ground wire, the case of the instrument will become hot. An individual touching the hot case (point *A*) will receive a shock because he or she is standing on the earth (point *B*) and completes the circuit. The current (*dashed line*) will flow from the instrument through the individual touching the hot case.

shock. Figure 8-18 illustrates a similar example, except that now the equipment ground wire is part of the electrical distribution system. In this example, the equipment ground wire provides a pathway of low impedance through which the current can travel; therefore, most of the current would travel through the ground wire. In this case, the person may get a shock, but it is unlikely to be fatal.

The electrical power supplied to homes is always grounded. A 120-volt potential always exists between the hot conductor and ground or earth. The third or equipment ground wire used in modern electrical wiring systems does not normally have current flowing through it. In the event of a short circuit, an electrical device with a three-prong plug (i.e., a ground wire connected to its case) will conduct the majority of the short-circuited or "fault" current through the ground wire and away from the individual. This provides a significant safety benefit to someone accidentally contacting the defective device. If a large enough fault current exists, the ground wire also will provide a means to complete the short circuit back to the circuit breaker or fuse, and this will either melt the fuse or trip the circuit breaker. Thus, in a grounded power system, it is possible to have either grounded or ungrounded equipment, depending on when the wiring was installed and whether the electrical device is equipped with a three-prong plug containing a ground wire. Obviously, attempts to bypass the safety system of the equipment ground should be avoided. Devices such as a "cheater plug" (Fig. 8-19) should never be used because they defeat the safety feature of the equipment ground wire.

ELECTRICAL POWER: UNGROUNDED

Numerous electronic devices, together with power cords and puddles of saline solutions on the floor, make the OR an electrically hazardous environment for both patients and personnel. Bruner et al.[5] found that 40% of electrical accidents in hospitals occurred in the OR. The complexity of electrical equipment in the modern OR demands that electrical safety be a factor of paramount importance. To provide an extra measure of safety from macroshock, the power supplied to most ORs is ungrounded. In this ungrounded power system, the current is isolated from ground potential. The 120-volt potential difference exists only between the two wires of the isolated power system, but no circuit exists between the ground and either of the isolated power lines.

Supplying ungrounded power to the OR requires the use of an *isolation transformer* (Fig. 8-20). This device uses electromagnetic induction to induce a current in the ungrounded or secondary winding of the transformer from energy supplied to the primary winding. There is no direct electrical connection between the power supplied by the utility company on the primary side and the power induced by the transformer on the ungrounded or secondary side. Thus, the power supplied to the OR is isolated from ground (Fig. 8-21). Because the 120-volt potential exists only between the two wires of the isolated circuit, neither wire is hot or neutral with reference to ground. In this case, they are simply referred to as line 1 and

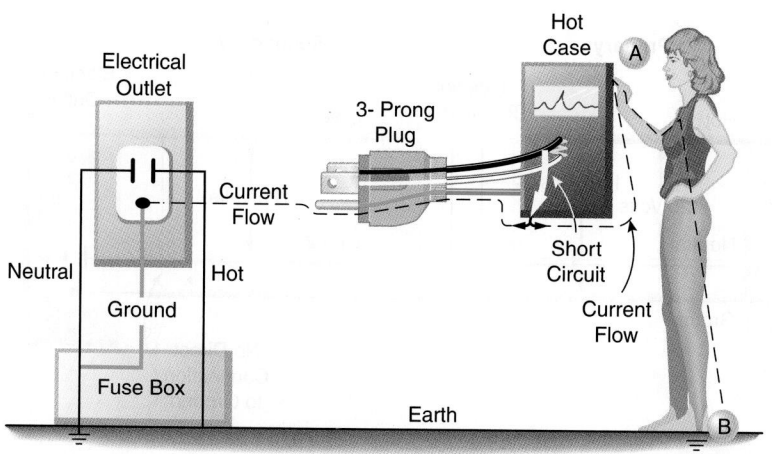

FIGURE 8-18. When a faulty piece of equipment containing an equipment ground wire is properly connected to an electrical outlet with a grounding connection, the current (*dashed line*) will preferentially flow down the low-resistance ground wire. An individual touching the case (point *A*) while standing on the ground (point *B*) will still complete the circuit; however, only a small part of the current will go through the individual.

FIGURE 8-19. **Right.** A "cheater plug" that converts a three-prong power cord to a two-prong cord. **Left.** The wire attached to the cheater plug is rarely connected to the screw in the middle of the outlet. This totally defeats the purpose of the equipment ground wire.

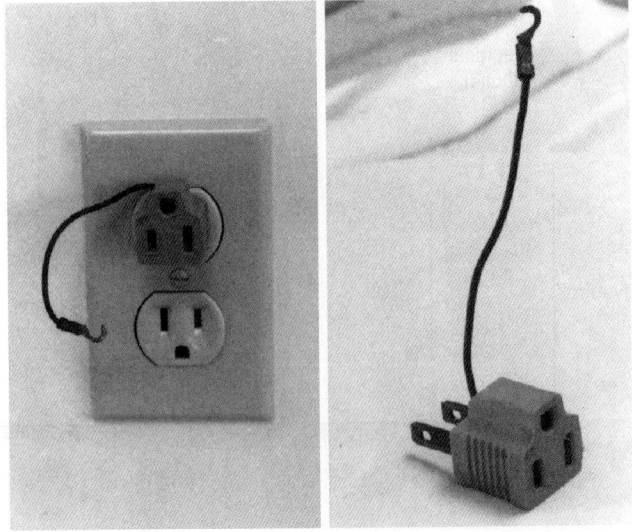

FIGURE 8-20. **A.** Isolated power panel showing circuit breakers, line isolation monitor, and isolation transformer (*arrow*). **B.** Detail of an isolation transformer with the attached warning lights. The arrow points to ground wire connection on the primary side of the transformer. Note that no similar connection exists on the secondary side of the transformer.

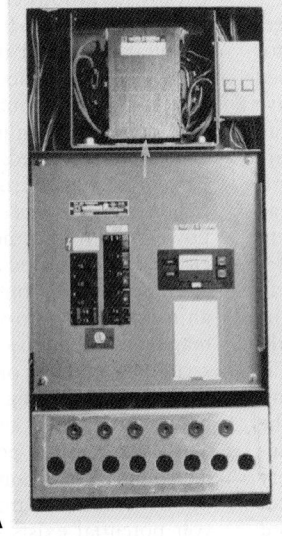

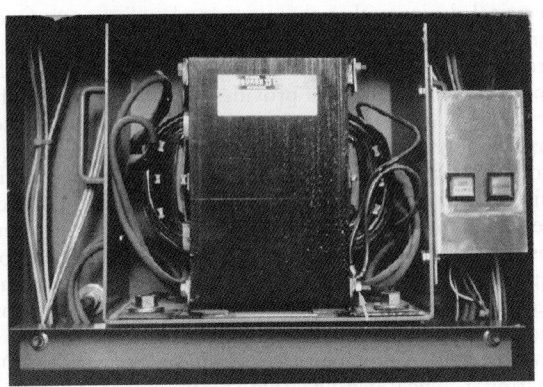

A   B

FIGURE 8-21. In the operating room, the isolation transformer converts the grounded power on the primary side to an ungrounded power system on the secondary side of the transformer. A 120-volt potential difference exists between line 1 and line 2. There is no direct connection from the power on the secondary side to ground. The equipment ground wire, however, is still present.

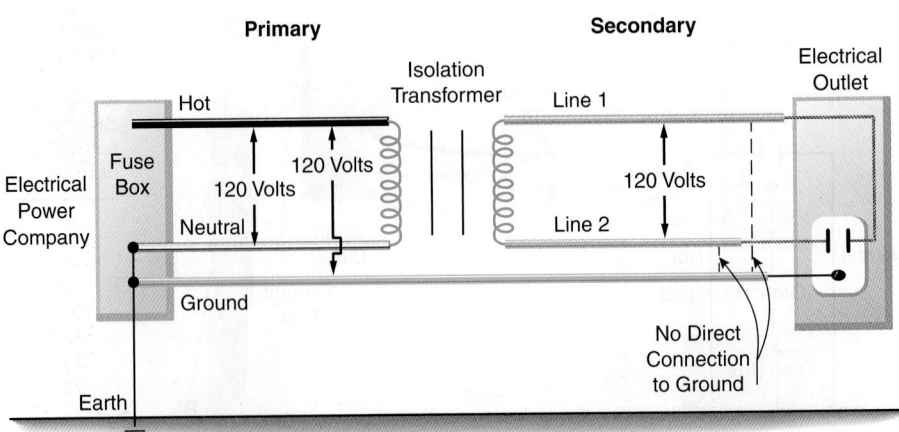

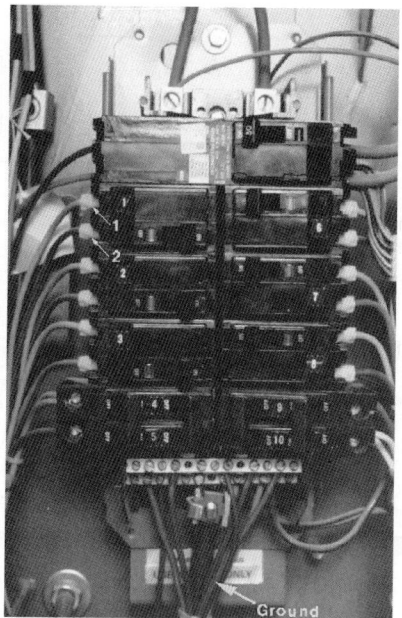

FIGURE 8-22.   Detail of the inside of a circuit breaker box in an isolated power system. The *bottom arrow* points to ground wires meeting at the common ground terminal. *Arrows 1* and *2* indicate lines 1 and 2 from the isolated power circuit breaker. Neither line 1 nor line 2 is connected to the same terminals as the ground wires. This is in marked contrast to Figure 8-13, where the neutral and ground wires are attached at the same point.

line 2 (Fig. 8-22). Using the example of the light bulb, if one connects the two wires of the bulb socket to the two wires of the isolated power system, the light will illuminate. However, if one connects one of the wires to one side of the isolated power and the other wire to ground, the light will not illuminate. If the wires of the isolated power system are connected, the short circuit will trip the circuit breaker. In comparing the two systems, the standard grounded power has a direct connection to ground, whereas the isolated system imposes a very high impedance to any current flow to ground. The added safety of this system can be seen in Figure 8-23. In this case, a person has come in contact with one side of the isolated power system (point A). Because standing on ground (point B) does not constitute a part of the isolated circuit, the individual does not complete the loop and will not receive a shock. This is because the ground is part of the primary circuit (*solid lines*), and the person is contacting only one side of the isolated secondary circuit (*cross-hatched lines*). The person does not complete either circuit (i.e., have two contact points); therefore, this situation does not pose an electric shock hazard. Of course, if the person contacts both lines of the isolated power system (an unlikely event), he or she would receive a shock.

If a faulty electrical appliance with an intact equipment ground wire is plugged into a standard household outlet, and the home wiring has a properly connected ground wire, then the amount of electrical current that will flow through the individual is considerably less than what will flow through the low-resistance ground wire. Here, an individual would be fairly well protected from a serious shock. However, if that ground wire were broken, the individual might receive a lethal shock. No shock would occur if the same faulty piece of equipment were plugged into the isolated power system, even if the equipment ground wire were broken. Thus, the isolated power system provides a significant amount of protection from macroshock. Another feature of the isolated power system is that the faulty piece of equipment, even though it may be partially short-circuited, will not usually trip the circuit breaker. This is an important feature because the faulty piece of equipment may be part of a life-support system for a patient. It is important to note that even though the power is isolated from ground, the case or frame of all electrical equipment is still connected to an equipment ground. The third wire (equipment ground wire) is necessary for a total electrical safety program.

Figure 8-24 illustrates a scenario involving a faulty piece of equipment connected to the isolated power system. This does not represent a hazard; it merely converts the isolated power back to a grounded power system as exists outside the OR. In fact, a *second* fault is necessary to create a hazard.

The previous discussion assumes that the isolated power system is perfectly isolated from ground. Actually, perfect isolation is impossible to achieve. All AC-operated power systems and electrical devices manifest some degree of capacitance. As previously discussed, electrical power cords, wires, and electrical motors exhibit capacitive coupling to the ground wire and metal conduits and "leak" small amounts of current to ground (Fig. 8-25). This so-called *leakage current* partially ungrounds the isolated power system. This does not usually amount to more than a few milliamperes in an OR. So an individual coming in contact with one side of the isolated power system would receive only a very small shock (1 to 2 mA). Although this amount of current would be perceptible, it would not be dangerous.

THE LINE ISOLATION MONITOR

The *line isolation monitor* (LIM) is a device that continuously monitors the integrity of an isolated power system. If a faulty

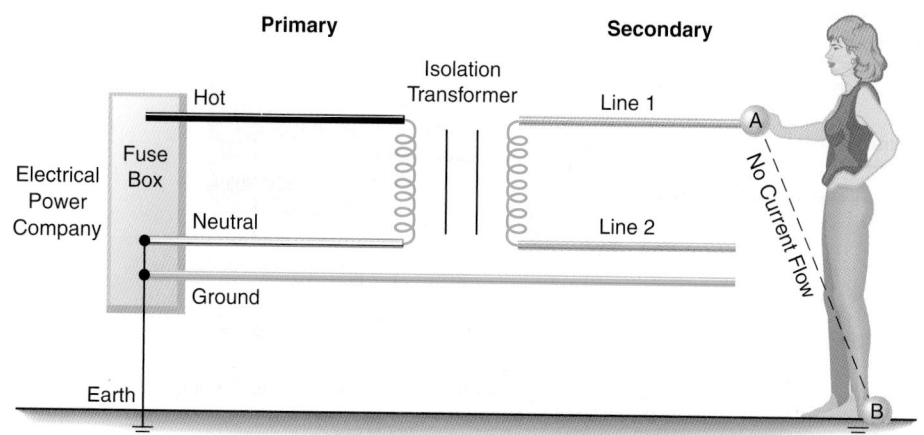

FIGURE 8-23.   A safety feature of the isolated power system is illustrated. An individual contacting one side of the isolated power system (point A) and standing on the ground (point B) will not receive a shock. In this instance, the individual is not contacting the circuit at two points and thus is not completing the circuit. Point A (*cross-hatched lines*) is part of the isolated power system, and point B is part of the primary or grounded side of the circuit (*solid lines*).

FIGURE 8-24. A faulty piece of equipment plugged into the isolated power system does not present a shock hazard. It merely converts the isolated power system into a grounded power system. The figure inset illustrates that the isolated power system is now identical to the grounded power system. The *dashed line* indicates current flow in the ground wire.

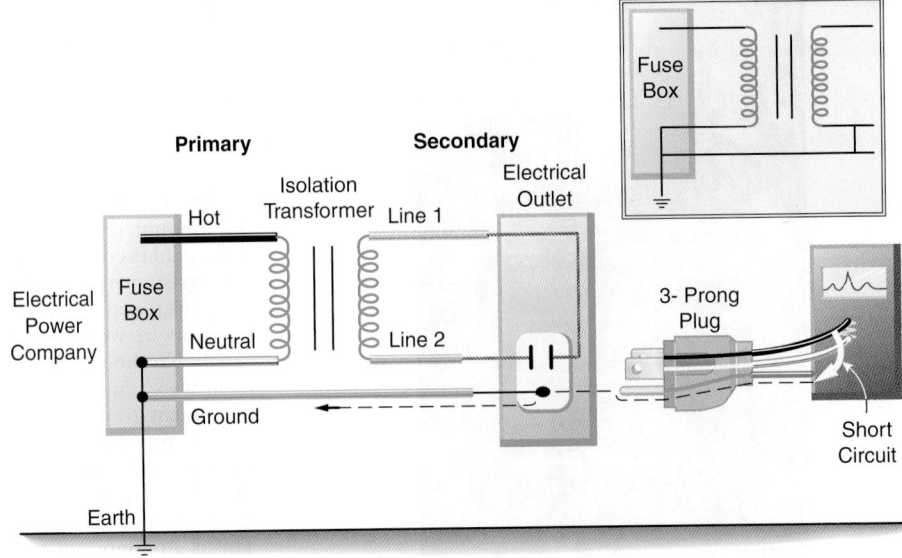

piece of equipment is connected to the isolated power system, this will, in effect, change the system back to a conventional grounded system. Also, the faulty piece of equipment will continue to function normally. Therefore, it is essential that a warning system be in place to alert the personnel that the power is no longer ungrounded. The LIM continuously monitors the isolated power to ensure that it is indeed isolated from ground, and the device has a meter that displays a continuous indication of the integrity of the system (Fig. 8-26). The LIM is actually measuring the impedance to ground of each side of the isolated power system. As previously discussed, with perfect isolation, impedance would be infinitely high and there would be no current flow in the event of a first fault situation ($Z = E/I$; if $I = 0$, then $Z = \infty$). Because all AC wiring and all AC-operated electrical devices have some capacitance, small leakage currents are present that partially degrade the isolation of the system. The meter of the LIM will indicate (in milliamperes) the total amount of leakage in the system resulting from capacitance, electrical wiring, and any devices plugged into the isolated power system.

The reading on the LIM meter does not mean that current is actually flowing; rather, it indicates how much current would flow in the event of a first fault. The LIM is set to alarm at 2 or 5 mA, depending on the age and brand of the system. Once this preset limit is exceeded, visual and audible alarms are triggered to indicate that the isolation from ground has been degraded beyond a predetermined limit (Fig. 8-27). This does not necessarily mean that there is a hazardous situation, but rather that the system is no longer totally isolated from ground. It would require a second fault to create a dangerous situation.

For example, if the LIM were set to alarm at 2 mA, using Ohm's law, the impedance for either side of the isolated power system would be 60,000 ohms:

$$Z = E/I$$

$$Z = (120 \text{ volts})/(0.002 \text{ ampere})$$

$$Z = 60,000 \text{ ohms}$$

Therefore, if either side of the isolated power system had less than 60,000 ohms impedance to ground, the LIM would trigger an alarm. This might occur in two situations. In the first situation, a faulty piece of equipment is plugged into the isolated power system. In this case, a true fault to ground exists

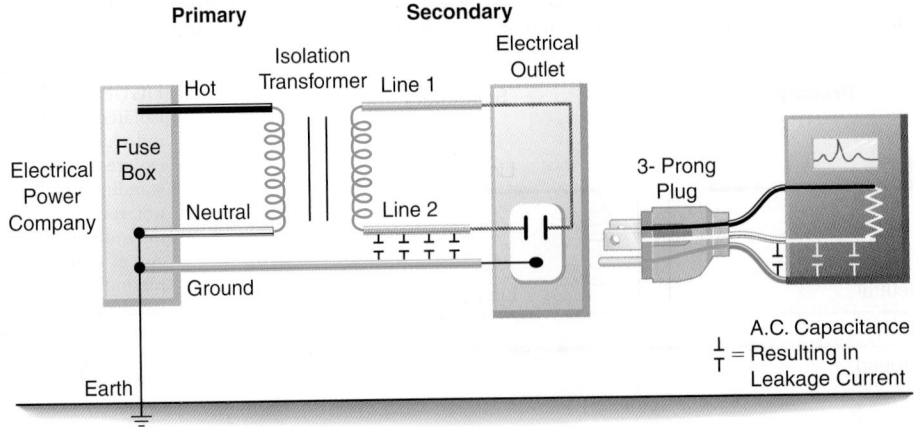

FIGURE 8-25. The capacitance that exists in alternating current (AC) power lines and AC-operated equipment results in small "leakage currents" that partially degrade the isolated power system.

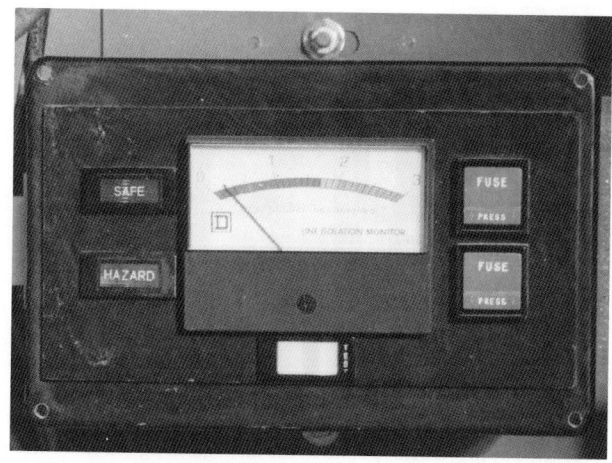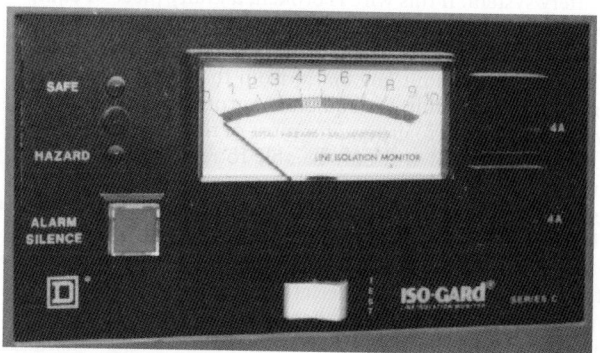

A   **B**

FIGURE 8-26.   The meter of the line isolation monitor (LIM) is calibrated in milliamperes. If the isolation of the power system is degraded such that >2 mA (5 mA in newer systems) of current could flow, the hazard light will illuminate and a warning buzzer will sound. Note the button for testing the hazard warning system. **A.** Older LIM that will trigger an alarm at 2 mA. **B.** Newer LIM that will trigger an alarm at 5 mA.

from one line to ground. Now the system would be converted to the equivalent of a grounded power system. This faulty piece of equipment should be removed and serviced as soon as possible. However, this piece of equipment could still be used safely if it were essential for the care of the patient. It should be remembered, however, that continuing to use this faulty piece of equipment would create the potential for a serious electrical shock. This would occur if a second faulty piece of equipment were simultaneously connected to the isolated power system.

The second situation involves connecting many perfectly normal pieces of equipment to the isolated power system. Although each piece of equipment has only a small amount of leakage current, if the total leakage exceeds 2 mA, the LIM will trigger an alarm. Assume that in the same OR there are 30 electrical devices, each having 100 μA of leakage current. The total leakage current (30 × 100 μA) would be 3 mA. The impedance to ground would still be 40,000 ohms (120/0.003). The LIM alarm would sound because the 2-mA set point was violated. However, the system is still safe and represents a state signifi-

cantly different from that in the first situation. For this reason, the newer LIMs are set to alarm at 5 mA instead of 2 mA.

The newest LIMs are referred to as *third-generation monitors*. The first-generation monitor, or static LIM, was unable to detect balanced faults (i.e., a situation in which there are equal faults to ground from both line 1 and line 2). The second-generation, or dynamic, LIM did not have this problem but could interfere with physiologic monitoring. Both of these monitors would trigger an alarm at 2 mA, which led to annoying "false" alarms. The third-generation LIM corrects the problems of its predecessors and has the alarm threshold set at 5 mA.[6] Proper functioning of the LIM depends on having both intact equipment ground wires as well as its own connection to ground. First- and second-generation LIMs could not detect the loss of the LIM ground connection. The third-generation LIM can detect this loss of ground to the monitor. In this case the LIM alarm would sound and the red hazard light would illuminate, but the LIM meter would read zero. This condition will alert the staff that the LIM needs to be repaired. However, the LIM still cannot detect broken equipment ground wires.

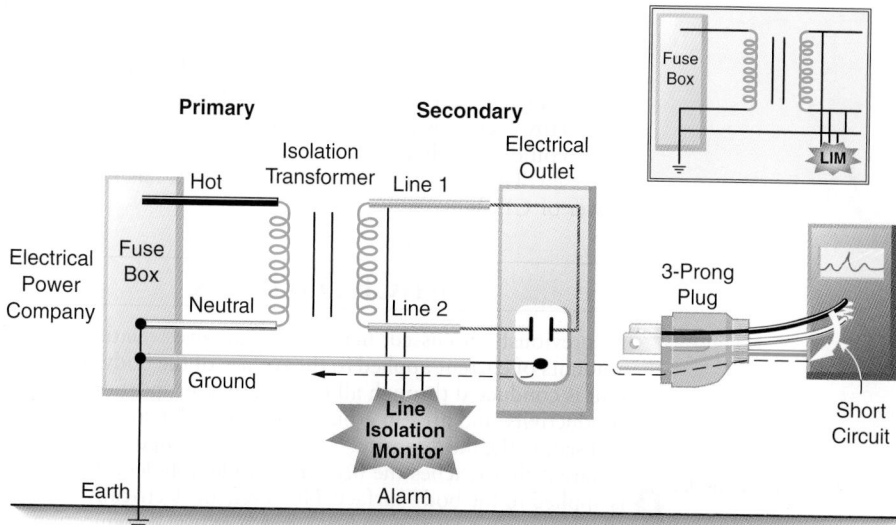

FIGURE 8-27.   When a faulty piece of equipment is plugged into the isolated power system, it will markedly decrease the impedance from line 1 or line 2 to ground. This will be detected by the line isolation monitor, which will sound an alarm.

An example of the third-generation LIM is the *Iso-Gard* made by the Square D Company (Monroe, NC).

The equipment ground wire is again an important part of the safety system. If this wire is broken, a faulty piece of equipment that is plugged into an outlet would operate normally, but the LIM would not alarm. A second fault could therefore cause a shock, without any alarm from the LIM. Also, in the event of a second fault, the equipment ground wire provides a low-resistance path to ground for most of the fault current (see Fig. 8-24). The LIM will only be able to register leakage currents from pieces of equipment that are connected to the isolated power system and have intact ground wires.

If the LIM alarm is triggered, the first thing to do is to check the gauge to determine if it is a true fault. The other possibility is that too many pieces of electrical equipment have been plugged in and the 2-mA limit has been exceeded. If the gauge is between 2 and 5 mA, it is probable that too much electrical equipment has been plugged in. If the gauge reads >5 mA, most likely there is a faulty piece of equipment present in the OR. The next step is to identify the faulty equipment, which is done by unplugging each piece of equipment until the alarm ceases. If the faulty piece of equipment is not of a life-support nature, it should be removed from the OR. If it is a vital piece of life-support equipment, it can be safely used. However, it must be remembered that the protection of the isolated power system and the LIM is no longer operative. Therefore, if possible, no other electrical equipment should be connected during the remainder of the case, or until the faulty piece of equipment can be safely removed.

GROUND FAULT CIRCUIT INTERRUPTER

7 The ground fault circuit interrupter (GFCI, or occasionally abbreviated as GFI) is another popular device used to prevent individuals from receiving an electrical shock in a grounded power system. Electrical codes for most new construction require that a GFCI circuit be present in potentially hazardous (e.g., wet) areas such as bathrooms, kitchens, or outdoor electrical outlets. The GFCI may be installed as an individual power outlet (Fig. 8-28) or may be a special circuit breaker to which all the individual protected outlets are connected at a

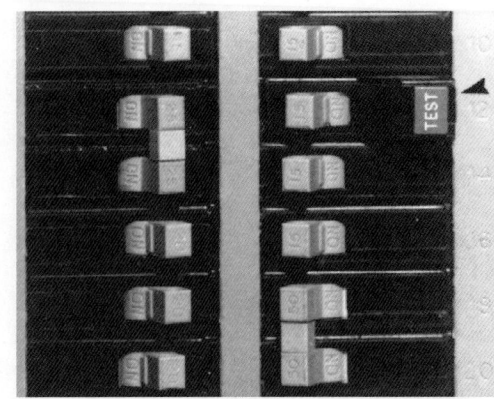

FIGURE 8-29. Special ground fault circuit interrupter circuit breaker. The *arrowhead* points to the distinguishing red test button.

single point. The special GFCI circuit breaker is located in the main fuse/circuit breaker box and can be distinguished by its red test button (Fig. 8-29). As Figure 8-5 demonstrates, the current flowing in both the hot and neutral wires is usually equal. The GFCI monitors both sides of the circuit for the equality of current flow; if a difference is detected, the power is immediately interrupted. If an individual should contact a faulty piece of equipment such that current flowed through the individual, an imbalance between the two sides of the circuit would be created, which would be detected by the GFCI. Because the GFCI can detect very small current differences (in the range of 5 mA), the GFCI will open the circuit in a few milliseconds, thereby interrupting the current flow before a significant shock occurs. Thus, the GFCI provides a high level of protection at a very modest cost.

The disadvantage of using a GFCI in the OR is that it interrupts the power without warning. A defective piece of equipment could no longer be used, which might be a problem if it were of a life-support nature, whereas if the same faulty piece of equipment were plugged into an isolated power system, the LIM would alarm but the equipment could still be used.

DOUBLE INSULATION

There is one instance in which it is acceptable for a piece of equipment to have only a two-prong and not a three-prong plug. This is permitted when the instrument has what is termed *double insulation*. These instruments have two layers of insulation and usually have a plastic exterior. Double insulation is found in many home power tools and is seen in hospital equipment such as infusion pumps. Double-insulated equipment is permissible in the OR with isolated power systems. However, if water or saline should get inside the unit, there could be a hazard because the double insulation is bypassed. This is even more serious if the OR has no isolated power or GFCIs.[7]

MICROSHOCK

As previously discussed, macroshock involves relatively large amounts of current applied to the surface of the body. The current is conducted through all the tissues in proportion to their conductivity and area in a plane perpendicular to the current. Consequently, the "density" of the current (amperes per meter squared) that reaches the heart is considerably less than what is applied to the body surface. However, an electrically susceptible patient (i.e., one who has a direct, external connection to

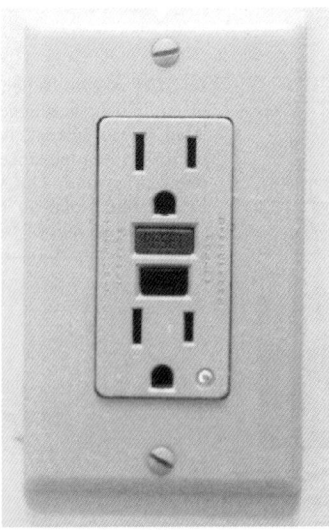

FIGURE 8-28. A ground fault circuit interrupter electrical outlet with integrated test and reset buttons.

8

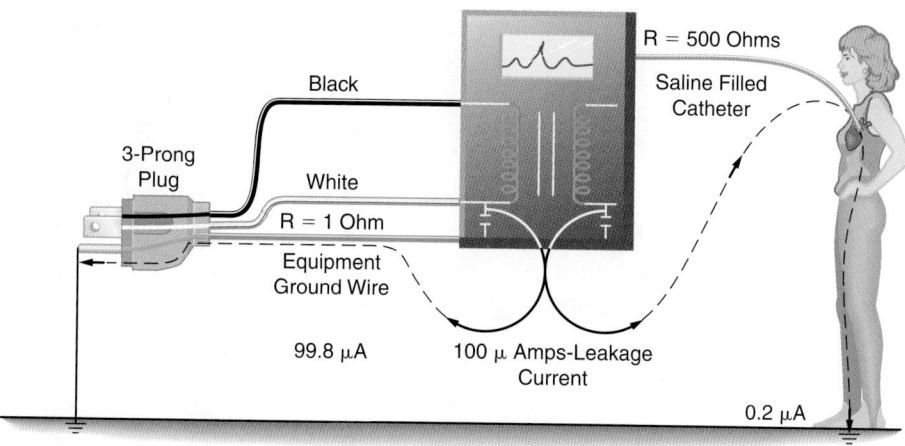

FIGURE 8-30. The electrically susceptible patient is protected from microshock by the presence of an intact equipment ground wire. The equipment ground wire provides a low-impedance path in which the majority of the leakage current (*dashed lines*) can flow. R, resistance.

the heart, such as through a central venous pressure catheter or transvenous cardiac pacing wires) may be at risk from very small currents; this is called *microshock*.[8] The catheter orifice or electrical wire with a very small surface area in contact with the heart produces a relatively large current density at the heart.[9] Stated another way, even very small amounts of current applied directly to the myocardium will cause ventricular fibrillation. Microshock is a particularly difficult problem because of the insidious nature of the hazard.

In the electrically susceptible patient, ventricular fibrillation can be produced by a current that is below the threshold of human perception. The exact amount of current necessary to cause ventricular fibrillation in this type of patient is unknown. Whalen et al.[10] were able to produce fibrillation with 20 μA of current applied directly to the myocardium of dogs. Raftery et al.[11] produced fibrillation with 80 μA of current in some patients. Hull[12] used data obtained by Watson et al.[13] to show that 50% of patients would fibrillate at currents of 200 μA. Because 1,000 μA (1 mA) is generally regarded as the threshold of human perception with 60-Hz AC, the electrically susceptible patient can be electrocuted with one-tenth the normally perceptible currents. This is not only of academic interest but also of practical concern because many cases of ventricular fibrillation from microshock have been reported.[14–18]

The stray capacitance that is part of any AC-powered electrical instrument may result in significant amounts of charge buildup on the case of the instrument. If an individual simul-

taneously touches the case of an instrument where this has occurred and the electrically susceptible patient, he or she may unknowingly cause a discharge to the patient that results in ventricular fibrillation. Once again, the equipment ground wire constitutes the major source of protection against microshock for the electrically susceptible patient. In this case, the equipment ground wire provides a low-resistance path by which most of the leakage current is dissipated instead of stored as a charge.

Figure 8-30 illustrates a situation involving a patient with a saline-filled catheter in the heart with a resistance of ~500 ohms. The ground wire with a resistance of 1 ohm is connected to the instrument case. A leakage current of 100 μA will divide according to the relative resistances of the two paths. In this case, 99.8 μA will flow through the equipment ground wire and only 0.2 μA will flow through the fluid-filled catheter. This extremely small current does not endanger the patient. However, if the equipment ground wire were broken, the electrically susceptible patient would be at great risk because all 100 μA of leakage current could flow through the catheter and cause ventricular fibrillation (Fig. 8-31). Currently, electronic equipment is permitted 100 μA of leakage current.

Modern patient monitors incorporate another mechanism to reduce the risk of microshock for electrically susceptible patients.[19] This mechanism involves electrically isolating all direct patient connections from the power supply of the monitor by placing a very high impedance between the patient and

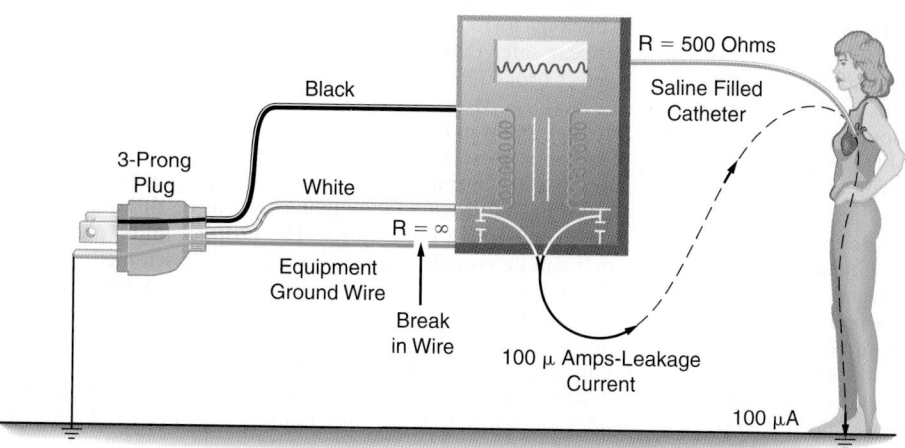

FIGURE 8-31. A broken equipment ground wire results in a significant hazard to the electrically susceptible patient. In this case, the entire leakage current can be conducted to the heart and may result in ventricular fibrillation. R, resistance.

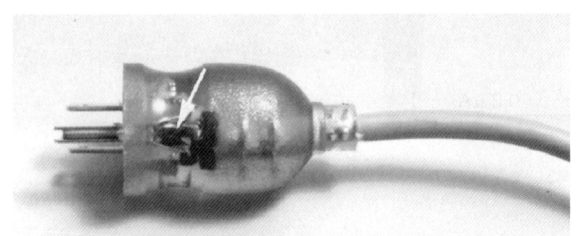
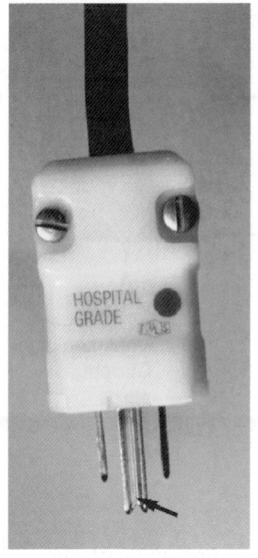
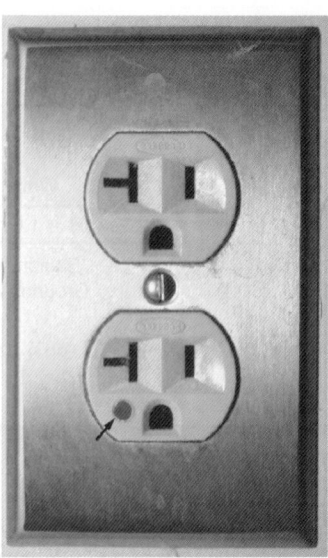

FIGURE 8-32.   **A.** A hospital-grade plug that can be visually inspected. The *arrow* points to the equipment ground wire whose integrity can be readily verified. **B.** A hospital-grade plug that can be easily disassembled for inspection. Note that the prong for the ground wire (*arrow*) is longer than the hot or neutral prong, so that it is the first to enter the receptacle. **C.** The *arrow* points to the green dot denoting a hospital-grade power outlet.

any device. This limits the amount of internal leakage through the patient connection to a very small value. The standard currently is <10 μA. For instance, the output of an ECG monitor's power supply is electrically isolated from the patient by placing a very high impedance between the monitor and the patient's ECG leads.[20] Isolation techniques are designed to inhibit hazardous electrical pathways between the patient and the monitor while allowing the passage of the physiologic signal.

An intact equipment ground wire is probably the most important factor in preventing microshock. There are, however, other things that the anesthesiologist can do to reduce the incidence of microshock. One should never simultaneously touch an electrical device and a saline-filled central catheter or external pacing wires. Whenever one is handling a central catheter or pacing wires, it is best to insulate oneself by wearing rubber gloves. Also, one should never let any external current source, such as a nerve stimulator, come into contact with the catheter or wires. Finally, one should be alert to potential sources of energy that can be transmitted to the patient. Even stray radiofrequency current from the ESU (cautery) can, with the right conditions, be a source of microshock.[21] It must be remembered that the LIM is not designed to provide protection from microshock. The microampere currents involved in microshock are far below the LIM threshold of protection. In addition, the LIM does not register the leakage of individual monitors, but rather indicates the status of the total system. The LIM reading indicates the total amount of leakage current resulting from the entire capacitance of the system. This is the amount of current that would flow to ground in the event of a first-fault situation.

The essence of electrical safety is a thorough understanding of all the principles of grounding. The objective of electrical safety is to make it difficult for electrical current to pass through people. For this reason, both the patient and the anesthesiologist should be isolated from ground as much as possible. That is, their resistance to current flow should be as high as is technologically feasible. In the inherently unsafe electrical environment of an OR, several measures can be taken to help protect against contacting hazardous current flows. First, the

grounded power provided by the utility company can be converted to ungrounded power by means of an isolation transformer. The LIM will continuously monitor the status of this isolation from ground and warn that the isolation of the power (from ground) has been lost in the event that a defective piece of equipment is plugged into one of the isolated circuit outlets. In addition, the shock that an individual could receive from a faulty piece of equipment is determined by the capacitance of the system and is limited to a few milliamperes. Second, all equipment plugged into the isolated power system has an equipment ground wire that is attached to the case of the instrument. This equipment ground wire provides an alternative low-resistance pathway enabling potentially dangerous currents to flow to ground. Thus, the patient and the anesthesiologist should be as insulated from ground as possible and all electrical equipment should be grounded.

The equipment ground wire serves three functions. First, it provides a low-resistance path for fault currents to reduce the risk of macroshock. Second, it dissipates leakage currents that are potentially harmful to the electrically susceptible patient. Third, it provides information to the LIM on the status of the ungrounded power system. If the equipment ground wire is broken, a significant factor in the prevention of electrical shock is lost. Additionally, the isolated power system will appear safer than it actually is because the LIM is unable to detect broken equipment ground wires.

Because power cord plugs and receptacles are subjected to greater abuse in the hospital than in the home, the Underwriters Laboratories (Melville, NY) has issued a strict specification for special "hospital-grade" plugs and receptacles (Fig. 8-32). The plugs and receptacles that conform to this specification are marked by a green dot.[22] The hospital-grade plug is one that can be visually inspected or easily disassembled to ensure the integrity of the ground wire connection. Molded opaque plugs are not acceptable. Edwards[23] reported that of 3,000 nonhospital-grade receptacles installed in a new hospital building, 1,800 (60%) were defective after 3 years. When 2,000 of the nonhospital-grade receptacles were replaced with ones of hospital grade, no failures had occurred after 18 months of use.

ELECTROSURGERY

On that fateful October day in 1926 when Dr. Harvey W. Cushing first used an electrosurgical machine invented by Professor William T. Bovie to resect a brain tumor, the course of modern surgery and anesthesia was forever altered.[24] The ubiquitous use of electrosurgery attests to the success of Professor Bovie's invention. However, this technology was not adopted without a cost. The widespread use of electrocautery has, at the very least, hastened the elimination of explosive anesthetic agents from the OR. In addition, as every anesthesiologist is aware, few things in the OR are immune to interference from the "Bovie." The high-frequency electrical energy generated by the ESU interferes with everything from the ECG signal to cardiac output computers, pulse oximeters, and even implanted cardiac pacemakers.[25]

The ESU operates by generating very-high-frequency currents (radiofrequency range) of anywhere from 500,000 to 1 million Hz. Heat is generated whenever a current passes through a resistance. The amount of heat (H) produced is proportional to the square of the current and inversely proportional to the area through which the current passes ($H = I^2/A$).[26] By concentrating the energy at the tip of the "Bovie pencil," the surgeon can produce either a cut or a coagulation at any given spot. This very-high-frequency current behaves differently from the standard 60-Hz AC current and can pass directly across the precordium without causing ventricular fibrillation.[26] This is because high-frequency currents have a low tissue penetration and do not excite contractile cells.

The large amount of energy generated by the ESU can pose other problems to the operator and the patient. Dr. Cushing became aware of one such problem. He wrote, "Once the operator received a shock which passed through a metal retractor to his arm and out by a wire from his headlight, which was unpleasant to say the least."[27] The ESU cannot be safely operated unless the energy is properly routed from the ESU through the patient and back to the unit. Ideally, the current generated by the active electrode is concentrated at the ESU tip, constituting a very small surface area. This energy has a high current density and is able to generate enough heat to produce a therapeutic cut or coagulation. The energy then passes through the patient to a dispersive electrode of large surface area that returns the energy safely to the ESU (Fig. 8-33).

One unfortunate quirk in terminology concerns the return (dispersive) plate of the ESU. This plate, often incorrectly referred to as a *ground plate*, is actually a dispersive electrode of large surface area that safely returns the generated energy to the ESU via a low current density pathway. When inquiring whether the dispersive electrode has been attached to the patient, OR personnel frequently ask, "Is the patient grounded?" Because the aim of electrical safety is to isolate the patient from ground, this expression is worse than erroneous; it can lead to confusion. Because the area of the return plate is large, the current density is low; therefore, no harmful heat is generated and no tissue destruction occurs. In a properly functioning system, the only tissue effect is at the site of the active electrode that is held by the surgeon.

Problems can arise if the electrosurgical return plate is improperly applied to the patient or if the cord connecting the return plate to the ESU is damaged or broken. In these instances, the high-frequency current generated by the ESU will seek an alternate return pathway. Anything attached to the patient, such as ECG leads or a temperature probe, can provide this alternate return pathway. The current density at the ECG pad will be considerably higher than normal because its surface area is much less than that of the ESU return plate. This may result in a serious burn at this alternate return site. Similarly, a burn may occur at the site of the ESU return plate if it is not properly applied to the patient or if it becomes partially dislodged during the operation (Fig. 8-34). This is not merely a theoretical possibility but is evidenced by the numerous case reports involving patients who have received ESU burns.[28–33]

The original ESUs were manufactured with the power supply connected directly to ground by the equipment ground wire. These devices made it extremely easy for ESU current to return by alternate pathways. The ESU would continue to operate normally even without the return plate connected to the patient. In most modern ESUs, the power supply is isolated from ground to protect the patient from burns. It was hoped that by isolating the return pathway from ground, the only route for current flow would be via the return electrode. Theoretically, this would eliminate alternate return pathways and greatly reduce the incidence of burns. However, Mitchell[34] found two situations in which the current could return via alternate pathways, even with the isolated ESU circuit. If the return plate were left either on top of an uninsulated ESU cabinet or in contact with the bottom of the OR table, then the ESU could operate fairly normally and the current would return via alternate pathways. It will be recalled that the impedance is inversely proportional to the capacitance times the current frequency. The ESU operates at 500,000 to >1,000,000 Hz, which greatly enhances the effect of capacitive coupling and causes a marked reduction in impedance. Therefore, even with isolated ESUs, the decrease in impedance allows the current to return to the ESU by alternate pathways. In addition, the isolated ESU does not protect the patient from burns if the return electrode does not make proper contact with the patient. Although the isolated ESU does provide additional

SCIENTIFIC FOUNDATIONS OF ANESTHESIA

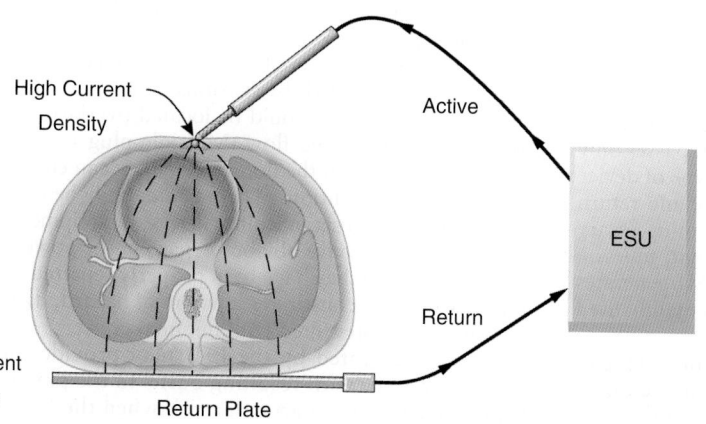

FIGURE 8-33. A properly applied electrosurgical unit (ESU) return plate. The current density at the return plate is low, resulting in no danger to the patient.

FIGURE 8-34.   An improperly applied electro-surgical unit (ESU) return plate. Poor contact with the return plate results in a high current density and a possible burn to the patient.

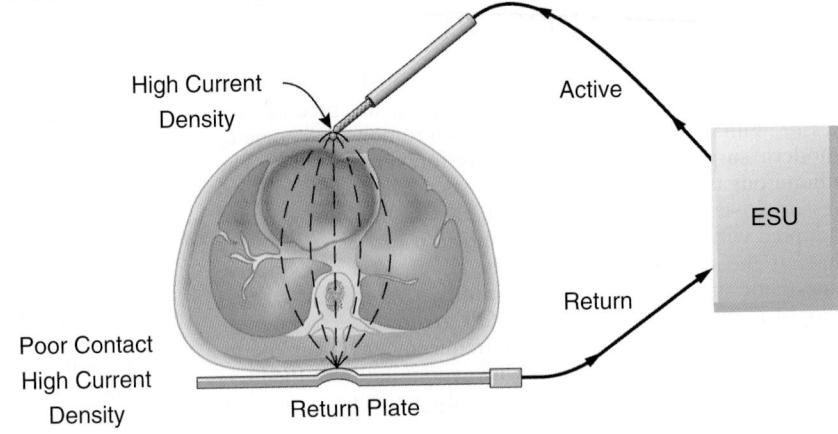

High Current Density

Active

ESU

Poor Contact High Current Density

Return

Return Plate

patient safety, it is by no means foolproof protection against the patient receiving a burn.

Preventing patient burns from the ESU is the responsibility of all professional staff in the OR. Not only the circulating nurse, but also the surgeon and the anesthesiologist must be aware of proper techniques and be vigilant to potential problems. The most important factor is the proper application of the return plate. It is essential that the return plate has the appropriate amount of electrolyte gel and an intact return wire. Reusable return plates must be properly cleaned after each use, and disposable plates must be checked to ensure that the electrolyte has not dried out during storage. In addition, it is prudent to place the return plate as close as possible to the site of the operation. ECG pads should be placed as far from the site of the operation as is feasible. OR personnel must be alert to the possibility that pools of flammable "prep" solutions such as alcohol and acetone can ignite when the ESU is used. If the ESU must be used on a patient with a demand pacemaker, the return electrode should be located below the thorax, and preparations for treating potential dysrhythmias should be available, including a magnet to convert the pacemaker to a fixed rate, a defibrillator, and an external pacemaker. It is best to keep the pacemaker out of the path between the surgical site and the dispersal plate.

The ESU has also caused other problems in patients with pacemakers, including reprogramming and microshock.[35,36] If the surgeon requests higher than normal power settings on the ESU, this should alert both the circulating nurse and the anesthesiologist to a potential problem. The return plate and cable must be immediately inspected to ensure that it is functioning and properly positioned. If this does not correct the problem, the return plate should be replaced.[37,38] If the problem remains, the entire ESU should be taken out of service. Finally, an ESU that is dropped or damaged must be removed immediately from the OR and thoroughly tested by a qualified biomedical engineer. Following these simple safety steps will prevent most patient burns from the ESU.

The previous discussion concerned only *unipolar* ESUs. There is a second type of ESU, in which the current passes only between the two blades of a pair of forceps. This type of device is referred to as a *bipolar* ESU. Because the active and return electrodes are the two blades of the forceps, it is not necessary to attach another dispersive electrode to the patient, unless a unipolar ESU is also being used. The bipolar ESU generates considerably less power than the unipolar and is mainly used for ophthalmic and neurologic surgery.

In 1980 Mirowski et al.[39] reported the first human implantation of a device to treat intractable ventricular tachydysrhythmias. This device, known as the *automatic implantable*

cardioverter-defibrillator (AICD), is capable of sensing ventricular tachycardia and ventricular fibrillation and then automatically defibrillating the patient. Since 1980 thousands of patients have received AICD implants.[40,41] Because some of these patients may present for noncardiac surgery, it is important that the anesthesiologist be aware of potential problems.[42] The use of a unipolar ESU may cause electrical interference that could be interpreted by the AICD as a ventricular tachydysrhythmia. This would trigger a defibrillation pulse to be delivered to the patient and would likely cause an actual episode of ventricular tachycardia or ventricular fibrillation. The patient with an AICD is also at risk for ventricular fibrillation during electroconvulsive therapy.[42] In both cases, the AICD should be disabled by placing a magnet over the device or by use of a specific protocol to shut it off. Therefore, it is best to consult with someone experienced with the device before starting surgery. The device can be reactivated by reversing the process. Also, an external defibrillator and a noninvasive pacemaker should be in the OR whenever a patient with an AICD is anesthetized.

Electrical safety in the OR is a matter of combining common sense with some basic principles of electricity. Once OR personnel understand the importance of safe electrical practice, they are able to develop a heightened awareness to potential problems. All electrical equipment must undergo routine maintenance, service, and inspection to ensure that it conforms to designated electrical safety standards. Records of these test results must be kept for future inspection because human error can easily compound electrical hazards. Starmer et al.[43] cited one case concerning a newly constructed laboratory where the ground wire was not attached to a receptacle. In another study Albisser et al.[44] found a 14% (198/1,424) incidence of improperly or incorrectly wired outlets. Furthermore, potentially hazardous situations should be recognized and corrected before they become a problem. For instance, electrical power cords are frequently placed on the floor where they can be crushed by various carts or the anesthesia machine. These cords could be located overhead or placed in an area of low traffic flow. Multiple-plug extension boxes should not be left on the floor where they can come in contact with electrolyte solutions. These could easily be mounted on a cart or the anesthesia machine. Pieces of equipment that have been damaged or have obvious defects in the power cord must not be used until they have been properly repaired. If everyone is aware of what constitutes a potential hazard, dangerous situations can be prevented with minimal effort.

Sparks generated by the ESU may provide the ignition source for a fire with resulting burns to the patient and OR personnel. This is a particular risk when the ESU is used in an oxygen-enriched environment as may be present in the patient's airway or in close proximity to the patient's face. The administration of high-flow nasal oxygen to a sedated patient during procedures on the face and eye is particularly hazardous. Most plastics such as tracheal tubes and components of the anesthetic breathing system that would not burn in room air will ignite in the presence of oxygen and/or nitrous oxide. Tenting of the drapes to allow dispersion of any accumulated oxygen and/or its dilution by room air or use of a circle anesthesia breathing system with minimal to no leak of gases around the anesthesia mask will decrease the risk of ignition from a spark generated by a nearby ESU.

Conductive Flooring

In past years, conductive flooring was mandated for ORs where flammable anesthetic agents were being administered. This would minimize the buildup of static charges that could cause a flammable anesthetic agent to ignite. The standards have now been changed to eliminate the necessity for conductive flooring in anesthetizing areas where flammable agents are no longer used.

ENVIRONMENTAL HAZARDS

There are a number of potential electrically related hazards in the OR that are of concern to the anesthesiologist. There is the potential for electrical shock not only to the patient but also to OR personnel. In addition, cables and power cords to electrical equipment and monitoring devices can become hazardous. Finally, all OR personnel should have a plan of what to do in the event of a power failure.

In today's OR there are literally dozens of pieces of electrical equipment. It is not uncommon to have numerous power cords lying on the floor, where they are vulnerable to damage. If the insulation on the power cable becomes damaged, it is fairly easy for the hot wire to come in contact with a piece of metal equipment. If the OR did not have isolated power, that piece of equipment would become energized and a potential electrical shock hazard.[45] Having isolated power minimizes the risk to the patient and OR personnel. Clearly, getting electrical power cords off the floor is desirable. This can be accomplished by having electrical outlets in the ceiling or by having ceiling-mounted articulated arms that contain electrical outlets. Also, the use of multi-outlet extension boxes that sit on the floor can be hazardous. These can be contaminated with fluids, which could easily trip the circuit breaker. In one case, it apparently tripped the main circuit breaker for the entire OR, resulting in a loss of all electrical power except for the overhead lights.[46]

Modern monitoring devices have many safety features incorporated into them. Virtually all of them have isolated the patient input from the power supply of the device. This was an important feature that was lacking from the original ECG monitors. In the early days, patients could actually become part of the electrical circuit of the monitor. There have been relatively few problems with patients and monitoring devices since the advent of isolated inputs. However, between 1985 and 1994, the Food and Drug Administration (FDA) received approximately 24 reports in which infants and children had received an electrical shock, including five children who died by electrocution.[47,48] These electrical accidents occurred because the electrode lead wires from either an ECG monitor or an apnea monitor were plugged directly into a 120-volt electrical outlet instead of the appropriate patient cable. In

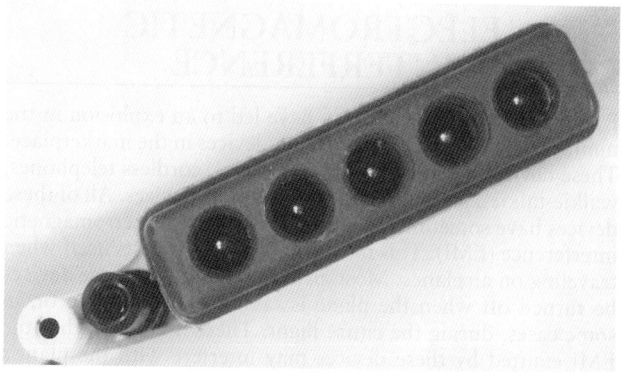

FIGURE 8-35. The current standard for patient lead wires (**left**) requires a female connector. The patient cable (**right**) has shielded connector pins that the lead wires plug into.

1997, the FDA issued a new performance standard for electrode lead wires and patient cables that requires that the exposed male connector pins from the electrode lead wires be eliminated. Therefore, the lead wires must have female connections and the connector pins must be housed in a protected patient cable (Fig. 8-35). This effectively eliminates the possibility of the patient being connected directly to an alternating current source since there are no exposed connector pins on the lead wires.

All health care facilities are required to have a source of emergency power. This generally consists of one or more electrical generators. These generators are configured to start up automatically and provide power to the facility within 10 seconds after detecting the loss of power from the utility company. The facility is required to test these generators on a regular basis. However, in the past, not all health care facilities tested them under actual load. There are numerous anecdotal reports of generators not functioning properly during an actual power failure. If the generators are not tested under actual load, it is possible that many years will pass before a real power outage puts a severe demand on the generator. If the facility has several generators and one of them fails, the increased demand on the others may be enough to cause them to fail in rapid succession. Hospitals (under the current National Fire Protection Association [NFPA] 99 standards) must test their emergency power supply systems (generators) under connected load once a month for at least 30 minutes. If the generator is oversized for the application and cannot be loaded to at least 30% of its rating, it must be load-banked and run for a total of 2 hours every year. A fairly recent requirement is for emergency power supply systems to be tested once every 3 years for 4 continuous hours, with a recommendation this be performed during peak usage of the system.[49,50]

It is vitally important that each OR have a contingency plan for a power failure. In most cases, the emergency generator will take over, but that is not always going to happen. There should be a supply of battery-operated light sources available in each OR. A laryngoscope can serve as a readily available source of light that allows one to find flashlights and other pieces of equipment. The overhead lights in the OR should also be connected to some sort of battery-operated lighting system. A supply of battery-operated monitoring devices and pneumatically powered ventilators and anesthesia machines would enable life-support functions to continue. The cost of these contingencies is relatively small but the benefits can be incomparable in an emergency.

ELECTROMAGNETIC INTERFERENCE

Rapid advances in technology have led to an explosion in the number of wireless communication devices in the marketplace. These devices include cellular telephones, cordless telephones, walkie-talkies, and wireless Internet access devices. All of these devices have something in common: they emit electromagnetic interference (EMI). This most commonly manifests itself when traveling on airplanes. Most airlines require that these devices be turned off when the plane is taking off or landing or, in some cases, during the entire flight. There is concern that the EMI emitted by these devices may interfere with the plane's navigation and communication equipment.

In recent years, the number of people who own these devices has increased exponentially. Indeed, in some hospitals, they form a vital link in the regular or emergency communication system. It is not uncommon for physicians, nurses, paramedics, and other personnel to have their own cellular telephones. In addition, patients and visitors may also have cellular telephones and other types of communication devices. Hospital maintenance and security personnel frequently have walkie-talkie–type radios and some hospitals have even instituted an in-house cellular telephone network that augments or replaces the paging system. There has been concern that the EMI emitted by these devices may interfere with implanted pacemakers or various types of monitoring devices and ventilators in critical care areas.[51] One case of a patient death has been reported when a ventilator malfunctioned secondary to EMI.[52]

Several studies have been done to find out if cellular telephones cause problems with cardiac pacemakers. One report by Hayes et al.[53] studied 980 patients with five different types of cellular telephones. They conducted more than 5,000 tests and found that in more than 20% of the cases they could detect some interference from the cellular telephone. Patients were symptomatic in 7.2% of the cases, and clinically significant interference occurred in 6.6% of the cases. When the telephone was held in the normal position over the ear, clinically significant interference was not detected. In fact, the interference that caused clinical symptoms occurred only if the telephone was directly over the pacemaker. Other studies have demonstrated changes such as erroneous sensing and pacer inhibition.[54,55] Again, these occurred only when the telephone was close to the pacemaker. The changes were temporary, and the pacemaker reverted to normal when the cellular telephone was moved to a safe distance. Currently, the FDA guidelines are that the cellular telephones be kept at least 6 inches from the pacemaker. Therefore, a patient with a pacemaker should not carry a cellular telephone in the shirt pocket, which is adjacent to the pacemaker. There appears to be little risk if hospital personnel carry a cellular telephone and if they ensure that it is kept at a reasonable distance from patients with a pacemaker.

AICDs comprise another group of devices of concern to biomedical engineers. Fetter et al.[56] conducted a study of 41 patients who had AICDs. They concluded that the cellular telephones did not interfere with the AICDs. They did, however, recommend keeping the cellular telephone at least 6 inches from the device.

EMI extends well beyond that of cellular telephones. Walkie-talkies, which are frequently used by hospital maintenance and security personnel, paging systems, police radios, and even televisions all emit EMI, which could potentially interfere with medical devices of any nature. Although there are many anecdotal reports, the amount of available scientific information on this problem is scant. Reports of interference include ventilator and infusion pumps that have been shut down or reprogrammed, interference with ECG monitors, and even an electronic wheelchair that was accidentally started because of EMI. It is a difficult problem to study because there are many different types of devices that emit EMI and a vast array of medical equipment that has the potential to interact with these devices. Even though a device may seem "safe" in the medical environment, if two or three cellular telephones or walkie-talkies are brought together in the same area at the same time, there may be unanticipated problems or interference.

Any time a cellular telephone is turned on, it is actually communicating with the cellular network, even though a call is not in progress. Therefore, the potential to interfere with devices exists. The Emergency Care Research Institute (ECRI) reported in October 1999 that walkie-talkies were far more likely to cause problems with medical devices than cellular telephones.[57] This is because they operate on a lower frequency than cellular telephones and have a higher power output. The ECRI recommends that cellular telephones be maintained at a distance of 1 meter from medical devices, while walkie-talkies be kept at a distance of 6 to 8 meters.

Some hospitals have made restrictive policies on the use of cellular telephones, particularly in critical care areas.[58] These policies are supported by little scientific documentation and are nearly impossible to enforce. The ubiquitous presence of cellular telephones carried by hospital personnel and visitors makes enforcing a ban virtually impossible. Even when people try to comply with the ban, failure is nearly inevitable because the general public is usually unaware that a cellular telephone in the standby mode is still communicating with the tower and generating EMI.

The real solution is to "harden" devices against EMI. This is difficult to do because of the many different frequencies on which these devices operate. Education of medical personnel is essential. When working in an OR or critical care area, all personnel must be alert to the fact that electronic devices and pacemakers can be interfered with by EMI. Creating a restrictive policy would certainly irritate personnel and visitors, and, in some cases, may actually compromise emergency communications.[59]

CONSTRUCTION OF NEW OPERATING ROOMS

Frequently, an anesthesiologist is asked to consult with hospital administrators and architects in designing new, or remodeling older, ORs. In the past a strict electrical code was enforced because of the use of flammable anesthetic agents. This code included a requirement for isolated power systems and LIMs. The NFPA revised its standard for health care facilities in 1984 (NFPA 99-1984). These standards do not require isolated power systems or LIMs in areas designated for use of nonflammable anesthetic agents only.[60,61] Although not mandatory, NFPA standards are usually adopted by local authorities when revising their electrical codes.

This change in the standard creates a dilemma. The NFPA 99—Standard for Health Care Facilities, 2005 edition, mandates that "wet location patient care areas be provided with special protection against electrical shock." Section 3-4.1.2.6 further states that "this special protection shall be provided by a power distribution system that inherently limits the possible ground fault current due to a first fault to a low value, without interrupting the power supply; or by a power distribution system in which the power supply is interrupted if the ground fault current does, in fact, exceed a value of 6 milliamperes."

The decision of whether to install isolated power hinges on two factors. The first is whether or not the OR is considered a wet location, and, if so, whether an interruptible power supply is tolerable. Where power interruption is tolerable, a GFCI is permitted as the protective means. However, the standard also states that "the use of an isolated power system (IPS) shall be permitted as a protective means capable of limiting ground fault current without power interruption."

Most people who have worked in an OR would attest to its being a wet location. The presence of blood, body fluids, and saline solutions spilled on the floor all contribute to making this a wet environment. The cystoscopy suite serves as a good example.

Once the premise that the OR is a wet location is accepted, it ⑩ must be determined whether a GFCI can provide the means of protection. The argument against using GFCIs in the OR is illustrated by the following example. Assume that during an open heart procedure the cardiopulmonary bypass pump and the patient monitors are plugged into outlets on the same branch circuit. Also assume that during bypass, the circulating nurse now plugs in a faulty headlight. If there is a GFCI protecting the circuit, the fault will be detected and the GFCI will interrupt all power to the pump and the monitors. This undoubtedly would cause a great deal of confusion and consternation among the OR personnel and may place the patient at risk for injury. The pump would have to be manually operated while the problem was being resolved. In addition, the GFCI could not be reset (and power restored) until the headlight was identified as the cause of the fault and unplugged from the outlet. However, if the OR were protected with an isolated power system and LIM, the same scenario would cause the LIM to alarm, but the pump and patient monitors would continue to operate normally. There would be no interruption of power and the problem could be resolved without risk to the patient.

It should be realized that a GFCI is an active system. That is, a potentially hazardous current is already flowing and must be actively interrupted, whereas the isolated power system (with LIM) is designed to be safe during a first-fault situation. Thus, it is a passive system because no mechanical action is required to activate the protection.[62]

It is likely that hospital administrators may want to eliminate isolated power systems in new OR construction as a cost-saving measure. Others, however, have advocated the retention of isolated power systems.[62–64] Not to do this would be a short-sighted, foolhardy measure. This is especially true because the cost of adding isolated power is estimated to be 1% of the cost of constructing an OR.[62] Although not perfect,[65] the isolated power system and LIM do provide both the patient and OR personnel with a significant amount of protection in an electrically hazardous environment. Isolated power systems provide clean stable voltages, which is important for sensitive diagnostic equipment.[66] Also, modern LIMs, which are microprocessor-based, require only yearly instead of monthly testing.

The value of the isolated power system is illustrated in a report by Day[67] in 1994. He reported four instances of electrical shock to OR personnel in a 1-year period. The operating suite had been renovated and the isolated power system removed, and it was not until the OR personnel received a shock that a problem was discovered.

Anesthesiologists need to be aware of this cost-saving attitude and strongly encourage that new ORs be constructed with isolated power systems. The relatively small cost savings that the alternative would represent do not justify the elimination of such a useful safety system. The use of GFCIs in the OR environment can be acceptable if carefully planned and engineered. In order to avoid the loss of power to multiple instruments and monitors at one time, each outlet must be an individual GFCI. If that is done, then a fault will result in only one piece of equipment losing power. Using GFCIs also precludes the use of multiple plug strips in the OR.

Electrical safety should be the concern of everyone in the OR. Accidents can be prevented only if proper installation and maintenance of the appropriate safety equipment in the OR have occurred and the OR personnel understand the concepts of electrical safety and are vigilant in their efforts to detect new hazards.[68]

FIRE SAFETY

Fires in the OR are just as much a danger today as they were ⑩ 100 years ago when patients were anesthetized with flammable anesthetic agents.[69,70] Because the potential consequences of a fire or explosion with ether or cyclopropane were well known and potentially devastating, OR fire safety practices were routinely followed.[71,72]

Today, the risk of an OR fire is probably as great or greater than the days when ether and cyclopropane were used, in part because of the routine use of potential sources of ignition (including electrosurgical cauteries) in an environment rich in fuel sources (i.e., flammable materials) and oxidizers (e.g., oxygen and nitrous oxide). Although the number of OR fires that occur annually in the United States is unknown, some estimates suggest that there are 50 to 200 fires each year, with as many as 20% associated with serious injury or death. In contrast to the era of flammable anesthetics, there currently appears to be a lack of awareness of the potential for an OR fire. In response to the risks presented by this situation, in 2008 the American Society of Anesthesiologists released a Practice Advisory on the Prevention and Management of Operating Room Fires[73] (Table 8-3).

For a fire to start, three components are necessary. The ⑪ limbs of the "fire triad" are a heat or ignition source, fuel, and an oxidizer.[74] A fire occurs when there is a chemical reaction of a fuel rapidly combining with an oxidizer to release energy in the form of heat and light. In the OR, there are many heat or ignition sources, such as the ESU, lasers, and the ends of fiberoptic light cords. The main oxidizers in the OR are air, oxygen, and nitrous oxide. Oxygen and nitrous oxide function equally well as oxidizers, so a combination of 50% oxygen and 50% nitrous oxide would support combustion, as would 100% oxygen. Fuel for a fire can be found everywhere in the OR. Paper drapes, which have largely replaced cloth drapes, are much easier to ignite and can burn with greater intensity.[75,76] Other sources of fuel include gauze dressings, endotracheal tubes, gel mattress pads, and even facial or body hair[77] (Table 8-4).

Fire prevention is accomplished by not allowing all three of the elements of the fire triad to come together at the same time.[78] The challenge in the OR is that frequently each of the limbs of the fire triad is controlled by a different individual. For instance, the surgeon is frequently in charge of the ignition source, the anesthesiologist is usually administering the oxidizer, and the OR nurse frequently controls the fuel sources. It is not always evident to any one individual that all of these elements may be coming together at the same time. This is especially true in any case in which there is the possibility of oxygen or an oxygen-nitrous oxide mixture being delivered around the surgical site. In these circumstances, the risk of an OR fire is markedly increased and the need for communication among the surgeon, the anesthesiologist, and the OR nurses throughout the procedure is essential.

There are several dangers that may result from an OR fire. The most obvious is that the patient and OR personnel can suffer severe burns. However, a less obvious but potentially more deadly risk can be posed by the products of combustion (called *toxicants*). When materials, such as plastics burn, a variety of injurious compounds can be produced. These include carbon monoxide, ammonia, hydrogen chloride, and

TABLE 8-3

RECOMMENDATIONS FOR THE PREVENTION AND MANAGEMENT OF OPERATING ROOM FIRES

Preparation
- Train personnel in OR fire management
- Practice responses to fires (fire drills)
- Assure that fire-management equipment is readily available
- Determine if a high-risk situation exists
- Team decides how to prevent/manage a fire
- Each person assigned a task (e.g., remove endotracheal tube or disconnect circuit)

Prevention
- Allow flammable skin preparations to dry before draping
- Configure surgical drapes to avoid buildup of oxidizer
- Anesthesiologist collaborates with team throughout the procedure to minimize oxidizer-enriched environment near ignition source
  - Keep O_2 concentration as low as clinically possible
  - Avoid N_2O
- Notify surgeon if oxidizer ↔ ignition source are in proximity to each other
- Moisten gauze and sponges that are near an ignition source

Management
- Look for early warning sign of a fire (e.g., pop, flash, or smoke)
- Stop procedure and each team member immediately carries out assigned task

Airway fire
- *Simultaneously* remove the endotracheal tube and stop gases/disconnect circuit
- Pour saline into airway
- Remove burning materials
- Mask ventilate patient, assess injury, consider bronchoscopy, reintubate

Fire *on* the patient
- Turn off gases
- Remove drapes and burning materials
- Extinguish flames with water, saline, or fire extinguisher
- Assess patient's status, devise care plan, assess for smoke inhalation

Failure to extinguish
- Use CO_2 fire extinguisher
- Activate fire alarm
- Consider evacuation of room: close door and do not reopen
- Turn off medical gas supply to room

Risk management
- Preserve scene
- Notify hospital risk manager
- Follow local regulatory reporting requirements
- Treat fire as an adverse event
- FIRE DRILLS

Adapted from Practice Advisory for the Prevention and Management of Operating Room Fires, Park Ridge, IL, American Society of Anesthesiologists. Approved by the ASA House of Delegates in October 2007; published in *Anesthesiology*, May 2008.

TABLE 8-4

FUEL SOURCES COMMONLY FOUND IN THE OPERATING ROOM

"Prep" agents
  Alcohol
  Degreasers (acetone, ether)
  Adhesives (tincture of benzoin, Aeroplast)™
  Chlorhexidine digluconate (Hibitane)™
  Iodophor (Dura-Prep)™
Drapes and covers
  Patient drapes (paper, plastic, cloth)
  Equipment drapes (paper, plastic, cloth)
  Blankets and sheets
  Pillows, mattresses, and padding
  Gowns
  Masks
  Shoe covers
  Gloves (latex, nonlatex)
  Clothing
  Compression (anti-embolism) stockings
Patient
  Hair
  Alimentary tract gases (methane, hydrogen)
  Desiccated tissue
Dressings
  Gauze and sponges
  Petrolatum-impregnated dressings
  Xeroform™
  Adhesive tape (cloth, plastic, paper)
  Elastic bandages
  Stockinettes
  Sutures
  Steri-Strips
  Collodion
Ointments
  Petrolatum
  Antibiotics (bacitracin, neomycin, polymyxin B)
  Nitropaste (Nitro-Bid)™
  EMLA™
  Lip balms
Anesthesia equipment
  Breathing circuit hoses
  Masks
  Endotracheal tubes
  Oral and nasal airways
  Laryngeal mask airways
  Nasogastric tubes
  Suction catheters and tubing
  Scavenger hoses
  Volatile anesthetics
  CO_2 absorbers
  Intravenous tubing
  Pressure monitor tubing and plastic transducers
Other equipment
  Charts and records
  Cardboard, wooden, and particleboard boxes and cabinets
  Packing materials (cardboard, expanded polystyrene [Styrofoam])
  Fiberoptic cable covers
  Wire covers and insulation
  Fiberoptic endoscope coverings
  Sphymomanometer cuffs and tubing
  Pneumatic tourniquet cuffs and tubing
  Stethoscope tubing™
  Vascular shunts (Gore-tex, Dacron)™
  Dialysis and extracorporeal circulation circuits
  Wound drains and collection systems
  Mops and brooms
  Textbooks and instruction manuals

even cyanide. Toxicants can produce injury by damaging airways and lung tissue, and can cause asphyxia. OR fires can often produce significant amounts of smoke and toxicants, but may not cause enough heat to activate overhead sprinkler systems. If enough smoke is produced, the OR personnel may have to evacuate the area. Thus, it is essential to have a prethought-out evacuation plan for both the OR personnel and the patient.

OR fires can be divided into two different types. The more common type of fire occurs *in* or *on* the patient, especially during high-risk procedures in which an ignition source is used in an oxidizer-rich environment. These would include airway fires (including endotracheal tube fires, fires in the oropharynx, which may occur during a tonsillectomy, and fires in the breathing circuit), and fires during laparoscopy. Fires occurring on the patient mainly involve head and neck surgery done under regional anesthesia or monitored anesthesia care when the patient is receiving high flows of supplemental oxygen. Because these fires occur in an oxygen-enriched environment, items such as surgical towels, drapes, or even the body hair can be readily ignited and produce a severe burn. The other type of OR fire is one that is remote from the patient. This would include an electrical fire in a piece of equipment, or a carbon dioxide (CO_2) absorber fire.

12 The two major ignition sources for OR fires are the ESU and the laser. However, the ends of some fiberoptic light cords can also become hot enough to start a fire if they are placed on paper drapes. Although the ESU is responsible for igniting the majority of the fires,[79] it is the laser that has generated the most attention and research. Laser is the acronym for *l*ight *a*mplification by *s*timulated *e*mission of *r*adiation. A laser consists of an energy source and material that the energy excites to emit light.[80–82] The material that the energy excites is called the *lasing medium* and provides the name of the particular type of laser. The important property of laser light is that it is coherent, meaning that is monochromatic (or even of a single wavelength). This coherent light can be focused into very small spots that have very-high-power density.

There are many different types of medical lasers, and each has a specific application. The argon laser is used in eye and dermatologic procedures because it is absorbed by hemoglobin and has a modest tissue penetration of between 0.05 and 2.0 mm. The potassium-titanyl-phosphate (KTP) or frequency-doubled yttrium aluminum garnet (YAG) lasers are also absorbed by hemoglobin and have tissue penetrations similar to that of the argon laser. The Dilaser has a wavelength that is easily changed and can be used in different applications, particularly in dermatologic procedures. The neodymium-doped yttrium aluminum garnet (Nd:YAG) laser is the most powerful of the medical lasers. Since the tissue penetration is between 2 and 6 mm, it can be used for tumor debulking, particularly in the trachea and main stem bronchi, or in the upper airway. The energy can be transmitted through a fiberoptic cable that is placed down the suction port of a fiberoptic bronchoscope. The laser can then be used in a contact mode to treat a tumor mass. The CO_2 laser has very little tissue penetration and can be used where great precision is needed. It is also absorbed by water, so that minimal heat is dispersed to surrounding tissues. The CO_2 laser is used primarily for procedures in the oropharynx and in and around the vocal cords. The helium-neon laser (He-Ne) produces an intense red light and thus can be used for aiming the CO_2 and the Nd:YAG lasers. It has very low power and thus will present no significant danger to OR personnel.

One of the most devastating types of OR fires occurs when an endotracheal tube is ignited *in* the patient.[83–88] If the patient is being ventilated with oxygen and/or nitrous oxide, the endotracheal tube will essentially emit a blowtorch type of flame that can result in severe injury to the trachea, lungs, and surrounding tissues. Red rubber, polyvinyl chloride, and sili-

cone endotracheal tubes all have oxygen-flammability indices (defined as the minimum O_2 fraction in N_2 that will just support a candlelike flame for a given fuel source using a standard ignition source)[89] of <26%.[90] Historically, anesthesiologists attempted to improve the safety of these tubes by wrapping red rubber or polyvinyl chloride tubes with some sort of reflective tape. However, taped-wrapped tubes often became kinked, gaps in the tape exposed areas of the tube to the laser, and non–laser-resistant tape was sometimes unintentionally used. To prevent these problems during high-risk procedures, "laser-resistant" endotracheal tubes have been developed.[91–93] Anesthesiologists can now use an endotracheal tube that is designed to be resistant to ignition by the specific type of laser that will be used during surgery. For instance, when using the CO_2 laser, the LaserFlex (Mallinckrodt, Pleasanton, CA) is an excellent choice. This is a flexible metal tube that has two cuffs that can be inflated with saline colored with methylene blue. The methylene blue enables the surgeon to easily recognize if he or she has accidentally penetrated one of the cuffs. The LaserFlex™ tube is highly resistant to being struck by the laser. If the Nd:YAG laser is being used, then the Lasertubus™ (Rüsch Inc., Duluth, GA) can be used. The Lasertubus™ has a soft rubber shaft that is covered by a corrugated silver foil that is in turn covered in a Merocel sponge jacket. In order to provide maximum protection, the Merocel must be kept moist with saline.

Another potential source of ignition for an OR fire is the ESU.[94,95] A typical example of how an ESU could cause ignition would be during a tonsillectomy in a child in whom the anesthesiologist was using an uncuffed, flammable endotracheal tube. In this case, the oxygen or oxygen-nitrous oxide mixture could leak around the endotracheal tube and pool at the operative site, providing an oxider-enriched environment. When the surgeon uses the ESU (or laser) to cauterize the tonsil bed, the combination of a high concentration of oxidizer (oxygen or oxygen-nitrous oxide mixture), fuel (endotracheal tube), and ignition source (the ESU or laser) could easily start a fire.[96,97]

The best way to prevent this type of fire is to take steps to prevent the three legs of the fire triad from coming together. For example, mixing the oxygen with air will keep the inspired oxygen concentration as low as possible, thus reducing the available oxidizer. Another possibility would be to place wet pledgets around the endotracheal tube, which would prevent the escape of oxygen or oxygen-nitrous oxide mixture from the trachea into the operative field. This reduces the available oxidizer and would keep the endotracheal tube and tissues from becoming desiccated, thus reducing their suitability as fuel sources. However, the pledgets must be kept moist, lest they dry out and become an additional source of fuel for a fire.

A related situation that requires a different solution can arise when a critically ill patient requires a tracheostomy.[98,99] These patients may require very high concentrations of inspired oxygen to maintain tissue oxygenation so that any decrease in inspired oxygen concentration or interruption of ventilation would not be tolerated. In this circumstance, the best option for preventing a fire would be to avoid the use of electrocautery (ignition source) when the surgeon enters the trachea.

The Nd:YAG laser can be used to treat tumors of the lower trachea and main stem bronchi. Most commonly, the surgeon will use a fiberoptic bronchoscope (FOB) and pass the laser fiber through the suction port of the bronchoscope. The fiberoptic bronchoscope can be used in conjunction with a rigid metal bronchoscope or passed through an 8.5- or 9.0-mm polyvinyl chloride endotracheal tube. A special laser-resistant tube would not be used in this circumstance because the FOB and laser fiber pass through the endotracheal tube and focus on tissue distal to the tube. Fire safety precautions available in this setting include titrating the concentration of inspired oxygen to as low a concentration as the patient can tolerate while maintaining a saturation of between 90 and 95% (ideally keeping the inspired oxygen below 30%), keeping the tip of the endotracheal tube and FOB away from the site of surgery and out of the "line of fire" of the laser, and removing charred and desiccated tissue from the surgical field.

The use of a rigid metal bronchoscope instead of an endotracheal tube will eliminate the possibility of setting the tube on fire but does not eliminate the possibility of setting the FOB on fire. This would also necessitate the use of a jet venturi system to ventilate the patient, which would, in turn, deliver an inspired oxygen concentration of between 40 and 60%.

There are a number of basic safety precautions that should be taken whenever a laser is used in surgery. Since laser light can be reflected off any metal surface, it is important that all OR personnel wear protective goggles that are specific to the type of laser being used. The anesthesiologist needs to be aware that the laser goggles may make it difficult to read certain monitor displays. In addition, it is important that the patient's eyes be covered with wet gauze or eye packs. OR personnel should also wear high filtration masks because the laser "plume" may contain vaporized virus particles or chemical toxins. Finally, all doors to the OR should have warning signs that a laser is in use, and all windows should be covered with black window shades.

Laparoscopic surgery in the abdomen is another potential risk for a surgically related fire. Ordinarily, the abdomen is inflated with CO_2, which does not support combustion. It is important to verify that, indeed, only CO_2 is being used, as erroneous inclusion of oxygen can be disastrous.[100] Also, nitrous oxide administered to the patient as part of the anesthetic can, over 30 minutes, diffuse into the abdominal cavity and attain a concentration that could support combustion.[101] In fact, when sampling the abdominal gas contents after 30 minutes, the mean nitrous oxide concentration was 36%; however, in certain patients it reached a concentration of 47%. Both methane and hydrogen are flammable gases that are frequently present in bowel gas in significant concentrations. Methane concentration in bowel gas can be up to 56% and hydrogen has been reported as high as 69%. With the maximum abdominal concentration of 47% nitrous oxide mixed with CO_2, it would require the maximum of 56% of methane to be flammable. Therefore, this represents a relatively small hazard. In contrast, a concentration of 69% hydrogen is flammable if the nitrous oxide concentration is >29%. Therefore, a fire is possible if the surgeon, while using the ESU, enters the bowel with a high concentration of hydrogen and the intra-abdominal nitrous oxide content is >29%.

In recent years, fires *on* the patient seem to have become the most frequent type of OR fire. These cases occur most often during surgery in and around the head and neck, where the patient is receiving monitored anesthesia care and supplemental oxygen is being administered by either a face mask or nasal cannulae.[102–106] In these cases, the oxygen can collect under the drapes if not properly vented, and when the surgeon uses the ESU or the laser, a fire can easily start. There are many things that can act as fuel, such as the surgical towels, paper drapes, disinfecting preparation solutions, sponges, plastic tubing from the oxygen face mask, and even the body hair. These fires start very quickly and can turn into an intense blaze in only a few seconds. Even if the fire is quickly extinguished, the patient will usually sustain a significant burn.

The most important principle that the anesthesiologist has to keep in mind to minimize the risk of fire is to titrate the inspired oxygen to the lowest amount necessary to keep patient's oxygenation within safe levels. If the anesthesia machine has the ability to deliver air, then the nasal cannula or face mask can be attached to the anesthesia circuit by using a small no. 3 or no. 4, 15-mm endotracheal tube adapter. This is attached to the right-angle elbow of the circuit. If the anesthesia machine is equipped with an auxiliary oxygen flowmeter that has a removable nipple adapter, then a humidifier can be installed in place of the nipple adapter. The humidifier has a Venturi mechanism through which room air is entrained and thus the oxygen concentration that is delivered to the face mask can be varied from 28 to 100%. Finally, if this machine has a common gas outlet that is easily accessible, a nasal cannula or face mask can be attached at this point using the same small 3- or 4-mm endotracheal tube adaptor. If it is not possible to dilute the oxygen with air, then it is important that the drapes be arranged in such a manner that there is no oxygen buildup beneath them. Tenting the drapes and having the surgeon use an adhesive sticky drape that seals the operative site from the oxygen flow are steps that will help reduce the risk of a fire.

It is potentially possible to discontinue the use of oxygen before the surgeon plans to use the electrocautery or laser. This would have to be done several minutes beforehand in order to allow any oxygen that has built up to dissipate. If the surgeon is planning to use the electrocautery or laser during the entire case, this may not be practical.

Some newer surgical preparation solutions can contribute to surgically related fires. These solutions typically come prepackaged in a "paint stick" applicator with a sponge on the end (e.g., DuraPrep™, St. Paul, MN). It consists of Iodophor mixed with 74% isopropyl alcohol. This is highly flammable and can easily be the fuel for an OR fire. In 2001, Barker and Polson[102] reported just such a case. In a laboratory re-creation, they found that if the DuraPrep™ had been allowed to dry completely (4 to 5 minutes), the fire did not occur (Fig. 8-36). The other problem with these types of preparation solutions is that small pools of the solution can accumulate if the person doing the preparation is not careful. The alcohol in these small puddles will continue to evaporate for a period of time, and the alcohol vapors are also extremely flammable. Flammable skin preparation solutions should be allowed to dry and puddles removed before the site is draped (Fig. 8-37).

It is important to bear in mind that halogenation of hydrocarbon anesthetics confers relative, but not absolute, resistance to combustion. Even the newer, "nonflammable" volatile anesthetics can, under certain circumstances, present fire hazards. For example, sevoflurane is nonflammable in air, but can serve as a fuel at concentrations as low as 11% in oxygen and 10% in nitrous oxide.[107] In addition, sevoflurane and desiccated CO_2 absorbent (either soda lime or Baralyme) can undergo exothermic chemical reactions that have been implicated in several fires that involved the anesthesia breathing circuit.[108–111] In 2003, the manufacturer of sevoflurane published a "Dear Health Care Provider" letter and advisory alert.[112] To prevent futures fires, the manufacturer of sevoflurane has recommended that anesthesiologists employ several measures, including avoiding the use of desiccated CO_2 absorbent and monitoring the temperature of the absorbers and the inspired concentration of sevoflurane; if elevated temperature or an inspired sevoflurane concentration that differed unexpectedly from the vaporizer setting is detected, it is recommended that the patient be disconnected from the anesthesia circuit and monitored for signs of thermal or chemical injury, and that the CO_2 absorbent is removed from the circuit and/or replaced.

Another way to prevent this type of fire is to use a CO_2 absorbent that does not contain a strong alkali, as do soda lime and Baralyme™ (Chemetron Medical Division, Allied Healthcare Products, St. Louis, Missouri). Amsorb™ (Amstrong Medical Limited, Coleraine, Northern Ireland) is a CO_2 absorbent that contains calcium hydroxide and calcium chloride, but no strong alkali.[113] In experimental studies, it was found that Amsorb is unreactive with currently used volatile anesthetics

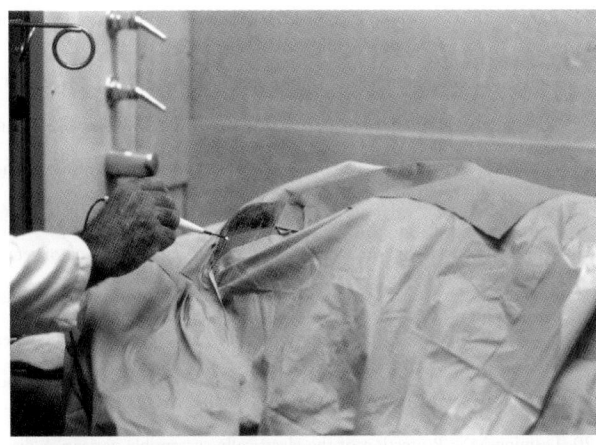 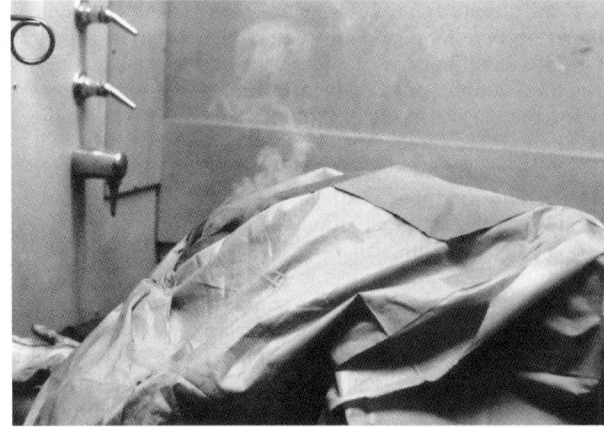

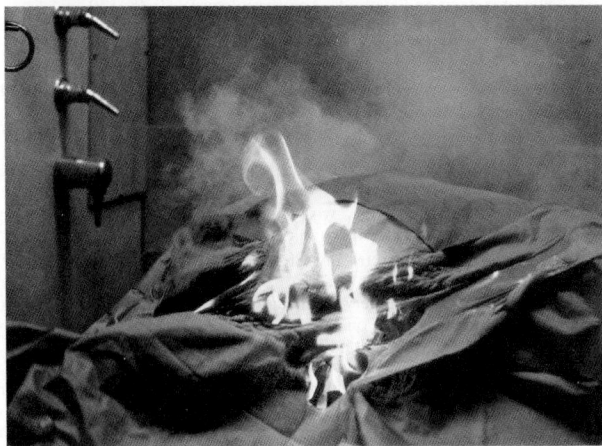 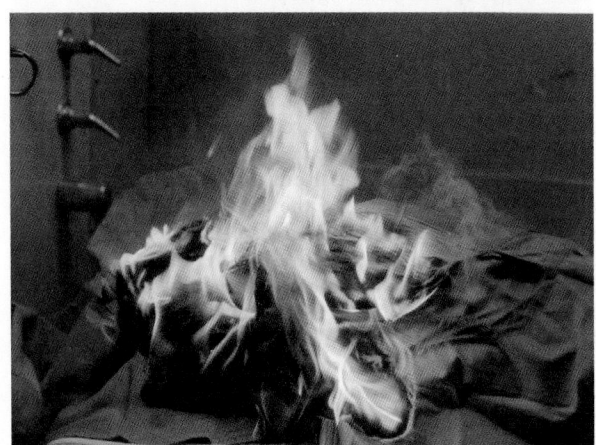

FIGURE 8-36. Simulation of fire caused by ESU electrode during surgery. **A.** Mannequin prepared and draped for surgery. Electrosurgical unit monopolar pencil electrode applied to operative site at start of surgery. **B.** Six seconds after electrosurgical unit application. Smoke appears from under the drapes. **C.** Fourteen seconds after electrosurgical unit application. Flames burst through the drapes. **D.** Twenty-four seconds after electrosurgical unit application. Entire patient head and drapes in flames. (From Barker SJ, Polson JS: Fire in the operating room: A case report and laboratory study. Anesth Analg 2001; 93: 960, with permission.)

and does not produce carbon monoxide or Compound A with desiccated absorbent. Therefore, it would not interact with sevoflurane and undergo an exothermic chemical reaction.

If a fire does occur, it is important to extinguish it as soon as possible. The first step is to interrupt the fire triad by remov-

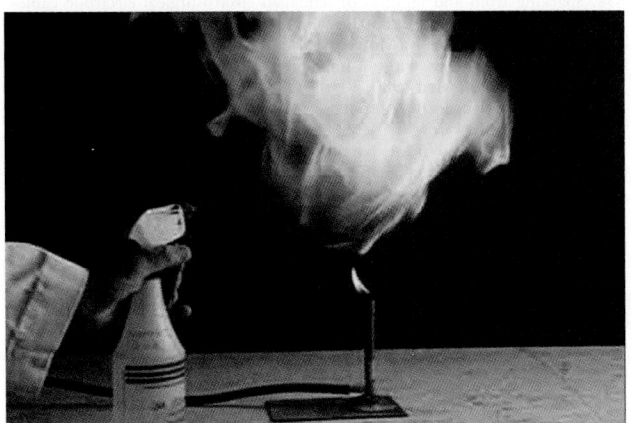

FIGURE 8-37. A demonstration of the intense heat and flame that is present in an alcohol fire. (Photograph courtesy of Marc Bruley of Emergency Care Research Institute. Reprinted with permission, Copyright 2009, ECRI Institute. www.ecri.org.)

ing one component. This is usually best accomplished by removing the oxidizer from the fire. Therefore, if an endotracheal tube is on fire, disconnecting the circuit from the tube or disconnecting the inspiratory limb of the circuit will usually result in the fire immediately going out. Simultaneously the surgeon should remove the burning endotracheal tube. Once the fire is extinguished, the airway inspected via bronchoscopy, and the patient reintubated.

If the fire is on the patient, then extinguishing it with a basin of saline may be the most rapid and effective method to deal with this type of fire. There is also a method to use a sheet or towel to extinguish the fire. If the drapes are burning, particularly if they are paper drapes, then they must be removed and placed on the floor. Paper drapes are impervious to water; thus, throwing water or saline on them will do little to extinguish the fire. Once the burning drapes are removed from the patient, the fire can then be extinguished with a fire extinguisher. In most OR fires, the sprinkler system is not activated. This is because the sprinklers are not located directly over the OR table and because OR fires seldom get hot enough to activate the sprinklers.

All OR personnel should receive OR fire safety education, which should include training in institutional fire safety protocols and learning the location and operation of the fire extinguishers. Fire safety education, including fire drills, allows each member of the OR team to learn and practice what his or her responsibilities and actions should be if a fire were to

SCIENTIFIC FOUNDATIONS OF ANESTHESIA

occur. Fire drills are an important part of the plan and can help personnel become familiar with the exits, evacuation routes, location of fire extinguishers, and how to shut off medical gas and electrical supplies. Although institutional fire safety protocols vary, the general principles of responding to an OR fire can be summarized by the mnemonic ERASE: *extinguish, rescue, activate, shut,* and *evaluate.* In sequence: First, the team should generally attempt to *extinguish* a fire on, in, or near the patient. Depending on the situation, this may include the use of saline or a CO_2 fire extinguisher (see later discussion). If the initial attempts at extinguishing the fire are unsuccessful, the patient and all other persons at risk should be *rescued* and the OR evacuated, if possible, and the fire *alarm* should be activated. Once the OR is emptied of personnel, the doors should be *shut* and the medical gas supply to the room should be *shut* off. The patient should then be *evaluated* and any injuries should be appropriately managed.

Fire extinguishers are divided into three classes, termed *A*, *B*, and *C*, based on the types of fires for which they are best suited. Class A extinguishers are used on paper, cloth, and plastic materials; Class B extinguishers are used for fires when liquids or grease are involved; Class C extinguishers are used for energized electrical equipment. A single fire extinguisher may be useful for any one, two, or all three types of fires. Probably the best fire extinguisher for the OR is the CO_2 extinguisher. This can be used on Class B and C fires and some Class A fires. Other extinguishers are water mist and new environmentally friendly fluorocarbons that replaced the Halon fire extinguisher. Finally, many ORs are equipped with a fire hose that supplies pressurized water at a rate of 50 gallons per minute. Such equipment is best left to the fire department to use, unless there is a need to rescue someone from a fire. In order to effectively use a fire extinguisher, the acronym "PASS" can be used. This stands for *pull* the pin to activate the fire extinguisher, *aim* at the base of the fire, *squeeze* the trigger, and *sweep* the extinguisher back and forth across the base of the fire. When responding to a fire, the acronym RACE is useful. This stands for *rescue; alarm; confine; extinguish.* Clearly, having a plan that everyone is familiar with will greatly facilitate extinguishing the fire and minimize the harm to the patient and equipment.

However, neither fire drills nor the presence and use of fire extinguishers should be relied on to provide a fire-safe operating environment. Only through heightened awareness, continuing education, and ongoing communication can the legs of the fire triad be kept apart and the risk of an OR fire minimized.

References

1. Harpell TR: Electrical shock hazards in the hospital environment: Their causes and cures. Can Hosp 1970; 47: 48
2. Buczko GB, McKay WPS: Electrical safety in the operating room. Can J Anaesth 1987; 34: 315
3. Wald A: Electrical safety in medicine, Handbook of Bioengineering. Edited by Skalak R, Chien S. New York, McGraw-Hill, 1987, pp 34.1
4. Dalziel CF, Massoglia FP: Let-go currents and voltages. AIEE Trans 1956; 75: 49
5. Bruner JMR, Aronow S, Cavicchi RV: Electrical incidents in a large hospital: A 42 month register. JAAMI 1972; 6: 222
6. Bernstein MS: Isolated power and line isolation monitors. Biomed Instrum Technol 1990; 24: 221
7. Gibby GL: Shock and electrocution, Complications in Anesthesiology. Edited by Lobato EB, Gravenstein N, Kirby RR. Philadelphia, Wolters Kluwer/Lippincott Williams & Wilkins, 2008, pp 780
8. Weinberg DI, Artley JL, Whalen RE, et al.: Electric shock hazards in cardiac catheterization. Circ Res 1962; 11: 1004
9. Starmer CF, Whalen RE: Current density and electrically induced ventricular fibrillation. Med Instrum 1973; 7: 158
10. Whalen RE, Starmer CF, McIntosh HD: Electrical hazards associated with cardiac pacemaking. Ann NY Acad Sci 1964; 111: 922
11. Raftery EB, Green HL, Yacoub MH: Disturbances of heart rhythm produced by 50-Hz leakage currents in human subjects. Cardiovasc Res 1975; 9: 263
12. Hull CJ: Electrocution hazards in the operating theatre. Br J Anaesth 1978; 50: 647
13. Watson AB, Wright JS, Loughman J: Electrical thresholds for ventricular fibrillation in man. Med J Aust 1973; 1: 1179
14. Furman S, Schwedel JB, Robinson G, et al.: Use of an intracardiac pacemaker in the control of heart block. Surgery 1961; 49: 98
15. Noordijk JA, Oey FJI, Tebra W: Myocardial electrodes and the danger of ventricular fibrillation. Lancet 1961; 1: 975
16. Pengelly LD, Klassen GA: Myocardial electrodes and the danger of ventricular fibrillation. Lancet 1961; 1: 1234
17. Rowe GG, Zarnstorff WC: Ventricular fibrillation during selective angiocardiography. JAMA 1965; 192: 947
18. Hopps JA, Roy OS: Electrical hazards in cardiac diagnosis and treatment. Med Electr Biol Eng 1963; 1: 133
19. Baas LS, Beery TA, Hickey CS: Care and safety of pacemaker electrodes in intensive care and telemetry nursing units. Am J Crit Care 1997; 6: 301
20. Leeming MN: Protection of the electrically susceptible patient: A discussion of systems and methods. Anesthesiology 1973; 38: 370
21. McNulty SE, Cooper M, Staudt S: Transmitted radiofrequency current through a flow directed pulmonary artery catheter. Anesth Analg 1994; 78: 587
22. Cromwell L, Weibell FJ, Pfeiffer EA: Biomedical Instrumentation and Measurements, 2nd ed. Englewood Cliffs, NJ: Prentice-Hall, 1980, pp. 430
23. Edwards NK: Specialized electrical grounding needs. Clin Perinatol 1976; 3: 367
24. Goldwyn RM: Bovie: The man and the machine. Ann Plast Surg 1979; 2: 135
25. Lichter I, Borrie J, Miller WM: Radio-frequency hazards with cardiac pacemakers. Br Med J 1965; 1: 1513
26. Dornette WHL: An electrically safe surgical environment. Arch Surg 1973; 107: 567
27. Cushing H: Electro-surgery as an aid to the removal of intracranial tumors: With a preliminary note on a new surgical-current generator by W.T. Bovie. Surg Gynecol Obstet 1928; 47: 751
28. Meathe EA: Electrical safety for patients and anesthetists. In Saidman LJ, Smith NT (eds): Monitoring in Anesthesia, 2nd ed. Boston, Butterworth, 1984, pp 497
29. Rolly G: Two cases of burns caused by misuse of coagulation unit and monitoring. Acta Anaesthesiol Belg 1978; 29: 313
30. Parker EO: Electrosurgical burn at the site of an esophageal temperature probe. Anesthesiology 1984; 61: 93
31. Schneider AJL, Apple HP, Braun RT: Electrosurgical burns at skin temperature probes. Anesthesiology 1977; 47: 72
32. Bloch EC, Burton LW: Electrosurgical burn while using a battery-operated Doppler monitor. Anesth Analg 1979; 58: 339
33. Becker CM, Malhotra IV, Hedley-Whyte J: The distribution of radiofrequency current and burns. Anesthesiology 1973; 38: 106
34. Mitchell JP: The isolated circuit diathermy. Ann R Coll Surg Engl 1979; 61: 287
35. Titel JH, El Etr AA: Fibrillation resulting from pacemaker electrodes and electrocautery during surgery. Anesthesiology 1968; 29: 845
36. Domino KB, Smith TC: Electrocautery-induced reprogramming of a pacemaker using a precordial magnet. Anesth Analg 1983; 62: 609
37. Damaged reusable ESU return electrode cables. Health Devices. 1985; 14: 214
38. Sparking from and ignition of damaged electrosurgical electrode cables. Health devices. 1998; 27: 301
39. Mirowski M, Reid PR, Mower MM et al: Termination of malignant ventricular arrhythmias with an implanted automatic defibrillator in human beings. N Engl J Med 1980; 303: 322
40. Crozier IG, Ward DE: Automatic implantable defribrillators. Br J Hosp Med 1988; 40: 136
41. Elefteriades JA, Biblo LA, Batsford WP et al: Evolving patterns in the surgical treatment of malignant ventricular tachyarrhythmias. Ann Thorac Surg 1990; 49: 94
42. Carr CME, Whiteley SM: The automatic implantable cardioverter-defibrillator. Anaesthesia 1991; 46: 737
43. Starmer CF, McIntosh HD, Whalen RE: Electrical hazards and cardiovascular function. N Engl J Med 1971; 284: 181
44. Albisser AM, Parson ID, Pask BA: A survey of the grounding systems in several large hospitals. Med Instrum 1973; 7: 297
45. McLaughlin AJ, Campkin NT: Electrical safety: A reminder (letter). Anaesthesia 1998; 53: 608
46. Nixon MC, Ghurye M: Electrical failure in theatre—A consequence of complacency? Anaesthesia 1997; 52: 88
47. Medical Devices; Establishment of a Performance Standard for Electrode Lead Wires and Patient Cables, Federal Register 1997; 62: 25477
48. Emergency Care Research Institute: FDA establishes performance standards for electrode lead wires. Health Devices 1998; 27: 34
49. National Fire Protection Association: NFPA 99, Standard for Health Care Facilities, 2005 Edition, Article 4.4.4.1.1.2 Inspection and Testing of Alternate Power Source and Transfer Switches

50. National Fire Protection Association: NFPA 110, Standard for Emergency and Standby Power Systems, Chapter 8

51. Jones RP, Conway DH: The effect of electromagnetic interference from mobile communication on the performance of intensive care ventilators. Eur J Anaesthesiol 2005; 22: 578

52. Lawrentschuk N, Bolton DM: Mobile phone interference with medical equipment and its clinical relevance: A systematic review. Med J Aust 2004; 181: 145

53. Hayes DL, Wang PJ, Reynolds DW et al: Interference with cardiac pacemakers by cellular telephones. N Engl J Med 1997; 336: 1473

54. Schlegel RE, Grant FH, Raman S, Reynolds D: Electromagnetic compatibility study of the in vitro interaction of wireless phones with cardiac pacemakers. Biomed Instrum Technol 1998; 32: 645

55. Chen WH, Lau CP, Leung SK et al: Interference of cellular phones with implanted permanent pacemakers. Clin Cardiol 1996; 19: 881

56. Fetter JG, Ivans V, Benditt DG, Collins J: Digital cellular telephone interaction with implantable cardioverter-defibrillators. J Am Coll Cardiol 1998; 21: 623

57. Emergency Care Research Institute: Cell phones and walkie-talkies: Is it time to relax your restrictive policies? Health Devices 1999; 28: 409

58. Adler D, Margulies L, Mahler Y, Israeli A: Measurements of electromagnetic fields radiated from communication equipment and of environmental electromagnetic noise: Impact on the use of communication equipment within the hospital. Biomed Instrum Technol 1998; 32: 581

59. Schwartz JJ, Ehrenwerth J: Electrical safety, Clinical Monitoring: Practical Applications for Anesthesia and Critical Care. Edited by Lake CL, Hines RH, Blitt C. Philadelphia, WB Saunders, 2000

60. Kermit E, Staewen WS: Isolated power systems: Historical perspective and update on regulations. Biomed Tech Today 1986; 1: 86

61. National Fire Protection Association: National electric code (ANSI/NFPA 70-1984). Quincy, MA, National Fire Protection Association, 1984

62. Bruner JMR, Leonard PF: Electricity, Safety and the Patient. Chicago, Year Book Medical Publishers, 1989, pp 300

63. Matjasko MJ, Ashman MN: All you need to know about electrical safety in the operating room, ASA Refresher Courses in Anesthesiology, vol 18. Edited by Barash PG, Deutsch S, Tinker J. Philadelphia, JB Lippincott, 1990, pp 251

64. Lennon RL, Leonard PF: A hitherto unreported virtue of the isolated power system (letter). Anesth Analg 1987; 66: 1056

65. Gilbert TB, Shaffer M, Matthews M: Electrical shock by dislodged spark gap in bipolar electrosurgical device. Anesth Analg 1991; 73: 355

66. Van Kerchhove K: Re-Evaluating the isolated power equation: Electrical Products and Solutions: March 2008, pp 24–28

67. Day FJ: Electrical safety revisited: A new wrinkle. Anesthesiology 1994; 80: 220

68. Litt L, Ehrenwerth J: Electrical safety in the operating room: Important old wine, disguised in new bottles. Anesth Analg 1994; 78: 417

69. Seifert HA: Fire safety in the operating room, Progress in Anesthesiology. Edited by Eisenkraft JB. Philadelphia, WB Saunders, 1994

70. Neufeld GR: Fires and explosions, Complications in Anesthesiology. Edited by Orkin K, Cooperman LH. Philadelphia, Lippincott, 1983, pp 671

71. Moxon MA: Fire in the operating room. Anaesthesia 1986; 41: 543

72. Vickers MD: Fire and explosion hazards in operating theatres. Br J Anaesth 1978; 50: 659

73. Practice Advisory for the Prevention and Management of Operating Room Fires. A Report by the American Society of Anesthesiologists Task Force on Operating Room Fires. Anesthesiology 2008; 108: 786

74. de Richemond AL: The patient is on fire! Health Devices 1992; 21: 19

75. Cameron BG, Ingram GS: Flammability of drape materials in nitrous oxide and oxygen. Anesthesiology 1971; 26: 218

76. Johnson RM, Smith CV, Leggett K: Flammability of disposable surgical drapes. Arch Ophthalmol 1976; 94: 1327

77. Simpson JI, Wolf GL: Flammability of esophageal stethoscopes, nasogastric tubes, feeding tubes, and nasopharyngeal airways in oxygen- and nitrous oxide-enriched atmospheres. Anesth Analg 1988; 67: 1093

78. Ponath RE: Preventing surgical fires. JAMA 1984; 252: 1762

79. Food and Drug Administration: Surgical Fires Reported January 1995—June 1998. FDA Databases MDR/MAUDE, 1999

80. Rampil IJ: Anesthetic considerations for laser surgery. Anesth Analg 1992; 74: 424

81. Pashayan AG, Ehrenwerth J: Lasers and electrical safety in the operating room, Anesthesia Equipment: Principles and Applications. Edited by Ehrenwerth J, Eisenkraft JB. St. Louis, Mosby, 1993

82. Emergency Care Research Institute: Lasers in medicine—An introduction. Health Devices 1984; 13: 151

83. Casey KR, Fairfax WR, Smith SJ et al: Intratracheal fire ignited by the Nd:YAG laser during treatment of tracheal stenosis. Chest 1983; 84: 295

84. Burgess GE, LeJeune FE: Endotracheal tube ignition during laser surgery of the larynx. Arch Otolaryngol 1979; 105: 561

85. Cozine K, Rosenbaum LM, Askanazi J et al: Laser induced endotracheal tube fire. Anesthesiology 1981; 55: 583

86. Geffin B, Shapshay SM, Bellack GS et al: Flammability of endotracheal tubes during Nd:YAG laser application in the airway. Anesthesiology 1986; 65: 511

87. Hirshman CA, Smith J: Indirect ignition of the endotracheal tube during carbon dioxide laser surgery. Arch Otolaryngol 1980; 106: 639

88. Krawtz S, Mehta AC, Weidemann HP et al: Nd:YAG laser-induced endobronchial burn. Chest 1989; 95: 916

89. Goldblum KB; Oxygen index: Key to precise flammability ratings. Society of Plastics Engineers Journal 1969; 25: 50–52

90. Wolf GL, Simpson JI: Flammability of endotracheal tubes in oxygen and nitrous oxide enriched atmosphere. Anesthesiology 1987; 67: 236

91. de Richemond AL: Laser resistant endotracheal tubes—Protection against oxygen-enriched airway fires during surgery? Flammability and Sensitivity of Material in Oxygen-Enriched Atmospheres, vol 5 (ASTM STP 1111). Edited by Stoltzfus JM, McIlroy K. Philadelphia, American Society for Testing and Materials, 1991, pp 157

92. Emergency Care Research Institute: Airway fires: Reducing the risk during laser surgery. Health Devices 1990; 19: 109

93. Emergency Care Research Institute: Laser-resistant tracheal tubes (evaluation). Health Devices 1992; 21: 4

94. Aly A, McIlwain M, Ward M: Electrosurgery-induced endotracheal tube ignition during tracheotomy. Ann Otol Rhinol Laryngol 1991; 100: 31

95. Simpson JI, Wolf GL: Endotracheal tube fire ignited by pharyngeal electrocautery. Anesthesiology 1986; 65: 76

96. Gupte SR: Gauze fire in the oral cavity: A case report. Anesth Analg 1972; 51: 645

97. Snow JC, Norton ML, Saluja TS et al: Fire hazard during CO_2 laser microsurgery on the larynx and trachea. Anesth Analg 1975; 55: 146

98. Lew EO, Mittleman RE, Murray D: Tube ignition by electrocautery during tracheostomy: Case report with autopsy findings. J Forensic Sci 1991; 36: 1586

99. Marsh B, Riley DH: Double-lumen tube fire during tracheostomy. Anesthesiology 1992; 76: 480

100. Neuman GG, Sidebotham G, Negoianu E et al: Laparoscopy explosion hazards with nitrous oxide. Anesthesiology 1993; 78: 875

101. Greilich PE, Froelich EG et al: Intraabdominal fire during laparoscopic cholecystectomy. Anesthesiology 1995; 83: 871

102. Barker SJ, Polson JS: Fire in the operating room: A case report and laboratory study. Anesth Analg 2001; 93: 960

103. Bruley ME, Lavanchy C: Oxygen-enriched fires during surgery of the head and neck, Symposium on Flammability and Sensitivity of Material in Oxygen-Enriched Atmospheres (ASTM STP 1040). Philadelphia, American Society for Testing and Materials, 1989, pp 392

104. de Richemond AL, Bruley ME: Head and neck surgical fires, Complications in Head and Neck Surgery. Edited by Eisele DW. St. Louis, Mosby, 1993

105. Emergency Care Research Institute: Fires during surgery of the head and neck area (hazard). Health Devices 1979; 9: 50

106. Ramanathan S, Capan L, Chalon J et al: Mini-environmental control under the drapes during operations on eyes of conscious patients. Anesthesiology 1978; 48: 286

107. Wallin RF, Regan BM, Napoli MD, Stern IJ: Sevoflurane: A new inhalational anesthetic agent. Anesth Analg 1975; 54: 758

108. Fatheree RS, Leighton BL: Acute respiratory syndrome after an exothermic baralymeR-sevoflurane reaction. Anesthesiology 2004; 101: 531

109. Castro BA, Freedman LA, Craig WL, Lynch C: Explosion within an anesthesia machine: BaralymeR, high fresh gas flows and sevoflurane concentration. Anesthesiology 2004; 101: 537

110. Wu J, Previte JP, Adler E et al: Spontaneous ignition, explosion and fire with sevoflurane and barium hydroxide lime. Anesthesiology 2004; 101: 534

111. Abbott A: Dear healthcare provider (letter). November 17, 2003. [www.fda.gov/medwatch/SAFETY/2003/ultane_deardoc.pdf]

112. Murray JM, Renfrew CW, Bedi A, et al: Amsorb: A new carbon dioxide absorbent for use in anesthetic breathing systems. Anesthesiology 1999; 91: 1342

113. Laster M, Roth P, Eger EI: Fires from the interaction of anesthetics with desiccated absorbent. Anesth Analg 2004; 99: 769

SCIENTIFIC FOUNDATIONS OF ANESTHESIA

CHAPTER 9 ■ EXPERIMENTAL DESIGN AND STATISTICS

NATHAN LEON PACE

DESIGN OF RESEARCH STUDIES
    Sampling
    Experimental Constraints
    Control Groups
    Random Allocation of Treatment Groups
    Blinding
    Types of Research Design
DATA AND DESCRIPTIVE STATISTICS
    Data Structure
    Descriptive Statistics
    Central Location
    Spread or Variability
HYPOTHESES AND PARAMETERS
    Hypothesis Formulation
    Logic of Proof
    Sample Size Calculations

    Inferential Statistics
    Confidence Intervals
    Confidence Intervals on Proportions
STATISTICAL TESTS AND MODELS
    Dichotomous Data Testing
    Interval Data Testing
    t Test
    Analysis of Variance
    Robustness and Nonparametric Tests
    Linear Regression
    Systematic Reviews and Meta-Analyses
    Interpretation of Results
CONCLUSIONS
    Guidelines for Reading Journal Articles
    Statistical Resources
    Statistics and Anesthesia

KEY POINTS

1 Statistics and mathematics are the language of scientific medicine.

2 Good research planning includes a clear biologic hypothesis, the specification of outcome variables, the choice of anticipated statistical methods, and sample size planning.

3 To avoid bias in the performance of clinical research, the crucial elements of good research design include concurrent control groups, random allocation of subjects to treatment groups, and blinding of random allocation to patients, caregivers, and outcome assessors.

4 Descriptive (e.g., mean, standard deviation) and inferential statistics (e.g., *t* test, confidence interval) are both essential methods for the presentation of research results.

5 The central limit theorem allows the use of parametric statistics for most statistical testing.

6 Systematic review and meta-analysis can synthesize and summarize the results of smaller, nonsignificant individual studies and permit more powerful inferences.

---

1 Medical journals are replete with numbers. These include weights, lengths, pressures, volumes, flows, concentrations, counts, temperatures, rates, currents, energies, and forces. The analysis and interpretation of these numbers require the use of statistical techniques. The design of the experiment to acquire these numbers is also part of statistical competence. The need for these statistical techniques is mandated by the nature of our universe, which is both orderly and random at the same time. The methods of probability and statistics have been formulated to solve concrete problems, such as betting on cards, understanding biologic inheritance, and improving food processing. Studies in anesthesia have even inspired new statistics. The development of statistical techniques is manifest in the increasing use of more sophisticated research designs and statistical tests in anesthesia research.

If a physician is to be a practitioner of scientific medicine, he or she must read the language of science to be able to independently assess and interpret the scientific report. Without exception, the language of the medical report is increasingly statistical. Readers of the anesthesia literature, whether in a

community hospital or a university environment, cannot and should not totally depend on the editors of journals to banish all errors of statistical analysis and interpretation. In addition, there are regularly questions about simple statistics in examinations required for anesthesiologists. Finally, certain statistical methods have everyday applications in clinical medicine. This chapter briefly scans some elements of experimental design and statistical analysis.

DESIGN OF RESEARCH STUDIES

2 The scientific investigator should view himself or herself as an experimenter and not merely as a naturalist. The naturalist goes out into the field ready to capture and report the numbers that flit into view; this is a worthy activity, typified by the *case report*. Case reports engender interest, suspicion, doubt, wonder, and perhaps the desire to experiment; however, the case report is not sufficient evidence to advance scientific medicine. The experimenter attempts to constrain and control, as much as possible, the environment in which he or she collects numbers to test a hypothesis. The elements of experimental design are intended to prevent and minimize the possibility of bias, that is, a deviation of results or inferences from the truth.

Sampling

Two words of great importance to statisticians are *population* and *sample*. In statistical language, each has a specialized meaning. Instead of referring only to the count of individuals in a geographic or political region, population refers to any target group of things (animate or inanimate) in which there is interest. For anesthesia researchers, a typical target population might be mothers in the first stage of labor or head-trauma victims undergoing craniotomy. A target population could also be cell cultures, isolated organ preparations, or hospital bills. A sample is a subset of the target population. Samples are taken because of the impossibility of observing the entire population; it is generally not affordable, convenient, or practical to examine more than a relatively small fraction of the population. Nevertheless, the researcher wishes to generalize from the results of the small sample group to the entire population.

Although the subjects of a population are alike in at least one way, these population members are generally quite diverse in other ways. Because the researcher can work only with a subset of the population, he or she hopes that the sample of subjects in the experiment is representative of the population's diversity. Head-injury patients can have open or closed wounds, a variety of coexisting diseases, and normal or increased intracranial pressure. These subgroups within a population are called *strata*. Often the researcher wishes to increase the sameness or homogeneity of the target population by further restricting it to just a few strata; perhaps only closed and not open head injuries will be included. Restricting the target population to eliminate too much diversity must be balanced against the desire to have the results be applicable to the broadest possible population of patients.

The best hope for a representative sample of the population would be realized if every subject in the population had the same chance of being in the experiment; this is called *random sampling*. If there were several strata of importance, random sampling from each stratum would be appropriate. Unfortunately, in most clinical anesthesia studies researchers are limited to using those patients who happen to show up at their hospitals; this is called *convenience sampling*. Convenience sampling is also subject to the nuances of the surgical schedule, the goodwill of the referring physician and attending surgeon, and the willingness of the patient to cooperate. At best, the convenience sample is representative of patients at that institution, with no assurance that these patients are similar to those elsewhere. Convenience sampling is also the rule in studying new anesthetic drugs; such studies are typically performed on healthy, young volunteers.

Experimental Constraints

The researcher must define the conditions to which the sample members will be exposed. Particularly in clinical research, one must decide whether these conditions should be rigidly standardized or whether the experimental circumstances should be adjusted or individualized to the patient. In anesthetic drug research, should a fixed dose be given to all members of the sample or should the dose be adjusted to produce an effect or to achieve a specific end point? Standardizing the treatment groups by fixed doses simplifies the research work. There are risks to this standardization, however: (1) a fixed dose may produce excessive numbers of side effects in some patients,

(2) a fixed dose may be therapeutically insufficient in others, and (3) a treatment standardized for an experimental protocol may be so artificial that it has no broad clinical relevance, even if demonstrated to be superior. The researcher should carefully choose and report the adjustment/individualization of experimental treatments.

Control Groups

Even if a researcher is studying just one experimental group, the results of the experiment are usually not interpreted solely in terms of that one group but are also contrasted and compared with other experimental groups. Examining the effects of a new drug on blood pressure during anesthetic induction is important, but what is more important is comparing those results with the effects of one or more standard drugs commonly used in the same situation. Where can the researcher obtain these comparative data? There are several possibilities: (1) each patient could receive the standard drug under identical experimental circumstances at another time, (2) another group of patients receiving the standard drug could be studied simultaneously, (3) a group of patients could have been studied previously with the standard drug under similar circumstances, and (4) literature reports of the effects of the drug under related but not necessarily identical circumstances could be used. Under the first two possibilities, the control group is contemporaneous—either a *self-control* (crossover) or *parallel control* group. The second two possibilities are examples of the use of *historical controls*.

Because historical controls already exist, they are convenient and seemingly cheap to use. Unfortunately, the history of medicine is littered with the "debris" of therapies enthusiastically accepted on the basis of comparison with past experience. A classic example is operative ligation of the internal mammary artery for the treatment of angina pectoris—a procedure now known to be of no value. Proposed as a method to improve coronary artery blood flow, the lack of benefit was demonstrated in a trial where some patients had the procedure and some had a sham procedure; both groups showed benefit.[1] There is now firm empirical evidence that studies using historical controls usually show a favorable outcome for a new therapy, whereas studies with concurrent controls, that is, parallel control group or self-control, less often reveal a benefit.[2] Nothing seems to increase the enthusiasm for a new treatment as much as the omission of a concurrent control group. If the outcome with an old treatment is not studied simultaneously with the outcome of a new treatment, one cannot know if any differences in results are a consequence of the two treatments, or of unsuspected and unknowable differences between the patients, or of other changes over time in the general medical environment. One possible exception would be in studying a disease that is uniformly fatal (100% mortality) over a very short time.

Random Allocation of Treatment Groups

Having accepted the necessity of an experiment with a control group, the question arises as to the method by which each subject should be assigned to the predetermined experimental groups. Should it depend on the whim of the investigator, the day of the week, the preference of a referring physician, the wish of the patient, the assignment of the previous subject, the availability of a study drug, a hospital chart number, or some other arbitrary criterion? All such methods have been used and are still used, but all can ruin the purity and usefulness of the experiment. It is important to remember the purpose of sampling: by exposing a small number of subjects from the target population to the various experimental conditions, one hopes to make conclusions about the entire population. Thus, the experimental groups should be as similar as possible to each other in reflecting the target population; if the groups are different, bias is introduced into the experiment. Although randomly allocating subjects of a sample to one or another of the experimental groups requires additional work, this principle prevents selection bias by the researcher, minimizes (but cannot always prevent) the possibility that important differences exist among the experimental groups, and disarms the critics' complaints about research methods. Random allocation is most commonly accomplished by the use of computer-generated random numbers.

Blinding

Blinding refers to the masking from the view of patient and experimenters the experimental group to which the subject has been or will be assigned. In clinical trials, the necessity for blinding starts even before a patient is enrolled in the research study; this is called the *concealment of random allocation*. There is good evidence that, if the process of random allocation is accessible to view, the referring physicians, the research team members, or both are tempted to manipulate the entrance of specific patients into the study to influence their assignment to a specific treatment group[3]; they do so having formed a personal opinion about the relative merits of the treatment groups and desiring to get the "best" for someone they favor. This creates bias in the experimental groups.

Each subject should remain, if possible, ignorant of the assigned treatment group after entrance into the research protocol. The patient's expectation of improvement, a placebo effect, is a real and useful part of clinical care. But when studying a new treatment, one must ensure that the fame or infamy of the treatments does not induce a bias in outcome by changing patient expectations. A researcher's knowledge of the treatment assignment can bias his or her ability to administer the research protocol and to observe and record data faithfully; this is true for clinical, animal, and in vitro research. If the treatment group is known, those who observe data cannot trust themselves to record the data impartially and dispassionately. The appellations *single-blind* and *double-blind* to describe blinding are commonly used in research reports, but often applied inconsistently; the researcher should carefully plan and report exactly who is blinded.

Types of Research Design

Ultimately, research design consists of choosing what subjects to study, what experimental conditions and constraints to enforce, and which observations to collect at what intervals. A few key features in this research design largely determine the strength of scientific inference on the collected data. These key features allow the classification of research reports (Table 9-1). This classification reveals the variety of experimental approaches and indicates strengths and weaknesses of the same design applied to many research problems.

The first distinction is between *longitudinal* and *cross-sectional* studies. The former is the study of changes over time, whereas the latter describes a phenomenon at a certain point in time. For example, reporting the frequency with which certain drugs are used during anesthesia is a cross-sectional study, whereas investigating the hemodynamic effects of different drugs during anesthesia is a longitudinal one.

Longitudinal studies are next classified by the method with which the research subjects are selected. These methods for choosing research subjects can be either *prospective* or *retro-*

TABLE 9-1

CLASSIFICATION OF CLINICAL RESEARCH REPORTS

I.   Longitudinal studies
   A. Prospective (cohort) studies
      1. Studies of deliberate intervention
         a. Concurrent controls
         b. Historical controls
      2. Observational studies
   B. Retrospective (case-control) studies
II. Cross-sectional studies

spective; these two approaches are also known as *cohort* (prospective) or *case-control* (retrospective). A prospective study assembles groups of subjects by some input characteristic that is thought to change an output characteristic; a typical input characteristic would be the opioid drug administered during anesthesia; for example, remifentanil or fentanyl. A retrospective study gathers subjects by an output characteristic; an output characteristic is the status of the subject after an event; for example, the occurrence of a myocardial infarction. A prospective (cohort) study would be one in which a group of patients undergoing neurologic surgery was divided in two groups, given two different opioids (remifentanil or fentanyl), and followed for the development of a perioperative myocardial infarction. In a retrospective (case-control) study, patients who suffered a perioperative myocardial infarction would be identified from hospital records; a group of subjects of similar age, gender, and disease who did not suffer a perioperative myocardial infarction also would be chosen, and the two groups would then be compared for the relative use of the two opioids (remifentanil or fentanyl). Retrospective studies are a primary tool of epidemiology. A case-control study can often identify an association between an input and output characteristic, but the causal link or relationship between the two is more difficult to specify.

Prospective studies are further divided into those in which the investigator performs a deliberate intervention and those in which the investigator merely observes. In a study of *deliberate intervention,* the investigator would choose several anesthetic maintenance techniques and compare the incidence of postoperative nausea and vomiting. If it was performed as an *observational study,* the investigator would observe a group of patients receiving anesthetics chosen at the discretion of each patient's anesthesiologist and compare the incidence of postoperative nausea and vomiting among the anesthetics used. Obviously, in this example of an observational study, there has been an intervention; an anesthetic has been given. The crucial distinction is whether the investigator controlled the intervention. An observational study may reveal differences among treatment groups, but whether such differences are the consequence of the treatments or of other differences among the patients receiving the treatments will remain obscure.

Studies of deliberate intervention are further subdivided into those with concurrent controls and those with historical controls. Concurrent controls are either a simultaneous parallel control group or a self-control study; historical controls include previous studies and literature reports. A *randomized controlled trial* is thus a longitudinal, prospective study of deliberate intervention with concurrent controls.

Although most of this discussion about experimental design has focused on human experimentation, the same principles apply and should be followed in animal experimentation. The randomized, controlled clinical trial is the most potent scientific tool for evaluating medical treatment; randomization into treatment groups is relied on to equally weight the subjects of the treatment groups for baseline attributes that might predispose or protect the subjects from the outcome of interest.

DATA AND DESCRIPTIVE STATISTICS

Statistics is a method for working with *sets* of numbers, a set being a group of objects. Statistics involves the description of number sets, the comparison of number sets with theoretical models, comparison between number sets, and comparison of recently acquired number sets with those from the past. A typical scientific hypothesis asks which of two methods (treatments), *X* and *Y*, is better. A statistical hypothesis is formulated concerning the sets of numbers collected under the conditions of treatments *X* and *Y*. Statistics provides methods for deciding if the set of values associated with *X* are different from the values associated with *Y*. Statistical methods are necessary because there are sources of variation in any data set, including random biologic variation and measurement error. These errors in the data cause difficulties in avoiding bias and in being precise. Bias keeps the true value from being known and fosters incorrect decisions; precision deals with the problem of the data scatter and with quantifying the uncertainty about the value in the population from which a sample is drawn. These statistical methods are relatively independent of the particular field of study. Regardless of whether the numbers in sets *X* and *Y* are systolic pressures, body weights, or serum chlorides, the approach for comparing sets *X* and *Y* is usually the same.

Data Structure

Data collected in an experiment include the defining characteristics of the experiment and the values of events or attributes that vary over time or conditions. The former are called *explanatory variables* and the latter are called *response variables*. The researcher records his or her observations on data sheets or case record forms, which may be one to many pages in length, and assembles them together for statistical analysis. Variables such as gender, age, and doses of accompanying drugs reflect the variability of the experimental subjects. Explanatory variables, it is hoped, explain the systematic variations in the response variables. In a sense, the response variables depend on the explanatory variables.

Response variables are also called *dependent variables*. Response variables reflect the primary properties of experimental interest in the subjects. Research in anesthesiology is particularly likely to have repeated measurement variables; that is, a particular measurement recorded more than once for each individual. Some variables can be both explanatory and response; these are called *intermediate response variables*. Suppose an experiment is conducted comparing electrocardiography and myocardial responses between five doses of an opioid. One might analyze how ST segments depended on the dose of opioids; here, maximum ST segment depression is a response variable. Maximum ST segment depression might also be used as an explanatory variable to address the subtler question of the extent to which the effect of an opioid dose on postoperative myocardial infarction can be accounted for by ST segment changes.

The mathematical characteristics of the possible values of a variable fit into five classifications (Table 9-2). Properly assigning a variable to the correct data type is essential for choosing the correct statistical technique. For *interval variables*, there is equal distance between successive intervals; the difference between 15 and 10 is the same as the difference between 25 and 20. *Discrete interval data* can have only integer values; for example, number of living children. *Continuous interval data* are measured on a continuum and can be a decimal fraction; for example, blood pressure can be described as accurately as desired (e.g., 136, 136.1, or 136.14 mm Hg). The same statistical techniques are used for discrete and continuous data.

Putting observations into two or more discrete categories derives *categorical variables*; for statistical analysis, numeric values are assigned as labels to the categories. *Dichotomous data* allow only two possible values; for example, male versus female. *Ordinal data* have three or more categories that can logically be ranked or ordered; however, the ranking or ordering of the variable indicates only relative and not absolute differences between values; there is not necessarily the same difference between American Society of Anesthesiologists Physical Status score I and II as there is between III and IV. Although ordinal data are often treated as interval data in choosing a statistical technique, such analysis may be suspect; alternative techniques for ordinal data are available. *Nominal variables* are placed into categories that have no logical ordering. The eye colors blue, hazel, and brown might be assigned the numbers 1, 2, and 3, but it is nonsense to say that blue < hazel < brown.

TABLE 9-2

DATA TYPES

■ DATA TYPE	■ DEFINITION	■ EXAMPLES
Interval		
Discrete	Data measured with an integer only scale	Parity, number of teeth
Continuous	Data measured with a constant scale interval	Blood pressure, temperature
Categorical		
Dichotomous	Binary data	Mortality, gender
Nominal	Qualitative data that cannot be ordered or ranked	Eye color, drug category
Ordinal	Data ordered, ranked, or measured without a constant scale interval	ASA physical status score, pain score

ASA, American Society of Anesthesiologists.

Descriptive Statistics

❹ A typical hypothetical data set could be a sample of ages (the response or dependent variable) of 12 residents in an anesthesia training program (the population). Although the results of a particular experiment might be presented by repeatedly showing the entire set of numbers, there are concise ways of summarizing the information content of the data set into a few numbers. These numbers are called *sample* or *summary statistics;* summary statistics are calculated using the numbers of the sample. By convention, the symbols of summary statistics are roman letters. The two summary statistics most frequently used for interval variables are the *central location* and the *variability,* but there are other summary statistics. Other data types have analogous summary statistics. Although the first purpose of descriptive statistics is to describe the sample of numbers obtained, there is also the desire to use the summary statistics from the sample to characterize the population from which the sample was obtained. For example, what can be said about the age of all anesthesia residents from the information in a sample? The population also has measures of central location and variability called the *parameters* of the population; Greek letters denote population parameters. Usually, the population parameters cannot be directly calculated because data from all population members cannot be obtained. The beauty of properly chosen summary statistics is that they are the best possible estimators of the population parameters.

These sampling statistics can be used in conjunction with a probability density function to provide additional descriptions of the sample and its population. Also commonly described as a probability distribution, a probability density function is an algebraic equation, $f(x)$, which gives a theoretical percentage distribution of x. Each value of x has a probability of occurrence given by $f(x)$. The most important probability distribution is the *normal* or *Gaussian function*

$$f(x) = \frac{1}{\sqrt{2\pi\sigma^2}} \exp\left[-\frac{1}{2}\left(\frac{x - \mu}{\sigma}\right)^2\right].$$ There are two parameters (population mean and population variance) in the equation of the normal function that are denoted μ and σ^2. Often called the *normal equation*, it can be plotted and produces the familiar bell-shaped curve. Why are the mathematical properties of this curve so important to biostatistics? First, it has been empirically noted that when a biologic variable is sampled repeatedly, the pattern of the numbers plotted as a histogram resembles the normal curve; thus, most biologic data are said to follow or to obey a normal distribution. Second, if it is reasonable to assume that a sample is from a normal population, the mathematical properties of the normal equation can be used with the sampling statistic estimators of the population parameters to describe the sample and the population. Third, a mathematical theorem (the central limit theorem) allows the use of the assumption of normality for certain purposes, even if the population is not normally distributed.

Central Location

The three most common summary statistics of central location for interval variables are the arithmetic *mean,* the *median,* and the *mode.* The mean is merely the average of the numbers in the data set. Being a summary statistic of the sample, the arithmetic mean is denoted by the Roman letter x under a bar or

$$\bar{x} = \frac{1}{n} \sum_{i=1}^{n} x_i$$ where i is the index of summation and n is the count of objects in the sample. If all values in the population

could be obtained, then the population mean μ could be calculated similarly. Because all values of the population cannot be obtained, the sample mean is used. (Statisticians describe the sample mean as the unbiased, consistent, minimum variance, sufficient estimator of the population mean. Estimators are denoted by a hat over a roman letter; for example, $\hat{x}$. Thus, the sample mean $\bar{x}$ is the estimator $\hat{x}$ of the population mean μ.)

The median is the middlemost number or the number that divides the sample into two equal parts—first, ranking the sample values from lowest to highest and then counting up halfway to obtain the median. The concept of ranking is used in nonparametric statistics. A virtue of the median is that it is hardly affected by a few extremely high or low values. The mode is the most popular number of a sample; that is, the number that occurs most frequently. A sample may have ties for the most common value and be bi- or polymodal; these modes may be widely separated or adjacent. The raw data should be inspected for this unusual appearance. The mode is always mentioned in discussions of descriptive statistics, but it is rarely used in statistical practice.

Spread or Variability

Any set of interval data has variability unless all the numbers are identical. The range of ages from lowest to highest expresses the largest difference. This spread, diversity, and variability can also be expressed in a concise manner. Variability is specified by calculating the *deviation* or *deviate* of each individual x_i from the center (mean) of all the x_i's. The *sum of the squared deviates* is always positive unless all set values are identical. This sum is then divided by the number of individual measurements. The result is the *averaged squared deviation*; the average squared deviation is ubiquitous in statistics.

The concept of describing the spread of a set of numbers by calculating the average distance from each number to the center of the numbers applies to both a sample and a population; this average squared distance is called the *variance.* The population variance is a parameter and is represented by σ^2. As with the population mean, the population variance is not usually known and cannot be calculated. Just as the sample mean is used in place of the population mean, the sample variance is used in place of the population variance. The sample variance is

$$VAR = SD^2 = \frac{\sum_{i=1}^{n}(x_i - \bar{x})^2}{(n - 1)}.$$

Statistical theory demonstrates that if the divisor in the formula for SD^2 is $(n - 1)$ rather than n, the sample variance is an unbiased estimator of the population variance. While the variance is used extensively in statistical calculations, the units of variance are squared units of the original observations. The square root of the variance has the same units as the original observations; the square roots of the sample and population variances are called the *sample (SD)* and *population (σ)* standard deviations.

It was previously mentioned that most biologic observations appear to come from populations with normal distributions. By accepting this assumption of a normal distribution, further meaning can be given to the sample summary statistics (mean and SD) that have been calculated. This involves the use of the expression $\bar{x} \pm k \times SD$, where $k = 1, 2, 3$, and so forth. If the population from which the sample is taken is unimodal and roughly symmetric, then the bounds for 1, 2, and 3 encompasses roughly 68%, 95%, and 99% of the sample and population members.

HYPOTHESES AND PARAMETERS

Hypothesis Formulation

The researcher starts work with some intuitive feel for the phenomenon to be studied. Whether stated explicitly or not, this is the *biologic hypothesis*; it is a statement of experimental expectations to be accomplished by the use of experimental tools, instruments, or methods accessible to the research team. An example would be the hope that isoflurane would produce less myocardial ischemia than fentanyl; the experimental method might be the electrocardiography determination of ST segment changes. The biologic hypothesis of the researcher becomes a *statistical hypothesis* during research planning. The researcher measures quantities that can vary—variables such as heart rate or temperature or ST segment change—in samples from populations of interest. In a statistical hypothesis, statements are made about the relationship among parameters of one or more populations. (To restate, a *parameter* is a number describing a variable of a population; Greek letters are used to denote parameters.) The typical statistical hypothesis can be established in a somewhat rote fashion for every research project, regardless of the methods, materials, or goals. The most frequently used method of setting up the algebraic formulation of the statistical hypothesis is to create two mutually exclusive statements about some parameters of the study population (Table 9-3); estimates for the values for these parameters are acquired by sampling data. In the hypothetical example comparing isoflurane and fentanyl, ϕ_1 and ϕ_2 would represent the ST segment changes with isoflurane and with fentanyl. The *null hypothesis* is the hypothesis of no difference of ST segment changes between isoflurane and fentanyl. The *alternative hypothesis* is usually nondirectional, that is, either $\phi_1 < \phi_2$ or $\phi_1 > \phi_2$; this is known as a *two-tail alternative hypothesis*. This is a more conservative alternative hypothesis than assuming that the inequality can only be either less than or greater than.

Logic of Proof

One particular decision strategy is used most commonly to choose between the null and alternative hypothesis. The decision strategy is similar to a method of indirect proof used in

TABLE 9-3

ALGEBRAIC STATEMENT OF STATISTICAL HYPOTHESES

H_0: $\phi_1 = \phi_2$ (null hypothesis)
H_a: $\phi_1 \neq \phi_2$ (alternative hypothesis)
ϕ_1 = Parameter estimated from sample of first population
ϕ_2 = Parameter estimated from sample of second population

mathematics called *reductio ad absurdum* (proof by contradiction). If a theorem cannot be proved directly, assume that it is not true; show that the falsity of this theorem will lead to contradictions and absurdities; thus, reject the original assumption of the falseness of the theorem. For statistics, the approach is to assume that the null hypothesis is true even though the goal of the experiment is to show that there is a difference. One examines the consequences of this assumption by examining the actual sample values obtained for the variable(s) of interest. This is done by calculating what is called a *sample test statistic*; sample test statistics are calculated from the sample numbers. Associated with a sample test statistic is a *probability*. One also chooses the *level of significance*; the level of significance is the probability level considered too low to warrant support of the null hypothesis being tested. If sample values are sufficiently unlikely to have occurred by chance (i.e., the probability of the sample test statistic is less than the chosen level of significance), the null hypothesis is rejected; otherwise, the null hypothesis is not rejected.

Because the statistics deal with probabilities, not certainties, there is a chance that the decision concerning the null hypothesis is erroneous. These errors are best displayed in table form (Table 9-4); condition 1 and condition 2 could be different drugs, two doses of the same drug, or different patient groups. Of the four possible outcomes, two decisions are clearly undesirable. The error of wrongly rejecting the null hypothesis (false-positive) is called the *type I* or *alpha error*. The experimenter should choose a probability value for alpha before collecting data; the experimenter decides how cautious to be against falsely claiming a difference. The most common choice for the value of alpha is 0.05. What are the consequences of choosing an alpha of 0.05? Assuming that there is, in fact, no difference between the two conditions and that the experiment is to be repeated 20 times, then during one of these

TABLE 9-4

ERRORS IN HYPOTHESIS TESTING: THE TWO-WAY TRUTH TABLE

		REALITY (POPULATION PARAMETERS)	
		CONDITIONS 1 AND 2 EQUIVALENT	CONDITIONS 1 AND 2 NOT EQUIVALENT
CONCLUSION FROM SAMPLE (SAMPLE STATISTICS)	CONDITIONS 1 AND 2 EQUIVALENT[a]	Correct conclusion	False-negative type II error (beta error)
	CONDITIONS 1 AND 2 NOT EQUIVALENT[b]	False-positive type I error (alpha error)	Correct conclusion

[a]Do not reject the null hypothesis: condition 1 = condition 2.
[b]Reject the null hypothesis: condition 1 ≠ condition 2.

experimental replications (5% of 20) a mistaken conclusion that there is a difference would be made. The probability of a type I error depends on the chosen level of significance and the existence or nonexistence of a difference between the two experimental conditions. The smaller the chosen alpha, the smaller will be the risk of a type I error.

The error of failing to reject a false null hypothesis (false-negative) is called a *type II* or *beta error*. (The power of a test is 1 minus beta). The probability of a type II error depends on four factors. Unfortunately, the smaller the alpha, the greater the chance of a false-negative conclusion; this fact keeps the experimenter from automatically choosing a very small alpha. Second, the more variability there is in the populations being compared, the greater the chance of a type II error. This is analogous to listening to a noisy radio broadcast; the more static there is, the harder it will be to discriminate between words. Next, increasing the number of subjects will lower the probability of a type II error. The fourth and most important factor is the magnitude of the difference between the two experimental conditions. The probability of a type II error goes from very high, when there is only a small difference, to extremely low, when the two conditions produce large differences in population parameters.

Sample Size Calculations

Formerly, researchers typically ignored the latter error in experimental design. The practical importance of worrying about type II errors reached the consciousness of the medical research community several decades ago. Some controlled clinical trials that claimed to find no advantage of new therapies compared with standard therapies lacked sufficient statistical power to discriminate between the experimental groups and would have missed an important therapeutic improvement. There are four options for decreasing type II error (increasing statistical power): (1) raise alpha, (2) reduce population variability, (3) make the sample bigger, and (4) make the difference between the conditions greater. Under most circumstances, only the sample size can be varied. Sample size planning has become an important part of research design for controlled clinical trials. Some published research still fails the test of adequate sample size planning.

Inferential Statistics

The testing of hypotheses or *significance testing* has been the main focus of inferential statistics. Hypothesis testing allows the experimenter to use data from the sample to make inferences about the population. Statisticians have created formulas that use the values of the samples to calculate test statistics.

Statisticians have also explored the properties of various theoretical probability distributions. Depending on the assumptions about how data are collected, the appropriate probability distribution is chosen as the source of critical values to accept or reject the null hypothesis. If the value of the test statistic calculated from the sample(s) is greater than the critical value, the null hypothesis is rejected. The critical value is chosen from the appropriate probability distribution after the magnitude of the type I error is specified.

There are parameters within the equation that generate any particular probability distribution; for the normal probability distribution, the parameters are μ and σ^2. For the normal distribution, each set of values for μ and σ^2 will generate a different shape for the bell-like normal curve. All probability distributions contain one or more parameters and can be plotted as curves; these parameters may be discrete (integer only) or continuous. Each value or combination of values for these parameters will create a different curve for the probability distribution being used. Thus, each probability distribution is actually a family of probability curves. Some additional parameters of theoretical probability distributions have been given the special name *degrees of freedom* and are represented by Latin letters such as *m, n*, and *s*.

Associated with the formula for computing a test statistic is a rule for assigning integer values to the one or more parameters called degrees of freedom. The number of degrees of freedom and the value for each degree of freedom depend on (1) the number of subjects, (2) the number of experimental groups, (3) the specifics of the statistical hypothesis, and (4) the type of statistical test. The correct curve of the probability distribution from which to obtain a critical value for comparison with the value of the test statistic is obtained with the values of one or more degrees of freedom.

To accept or reject the null hypothesis, the following steps are performed: (1) confirm that experimental data conform to the assumptions of the intended statistical test; (2) choose a significance level (alpha); (3) calculate the test statistic; (4) determine the degree(s) of freedom; (5) find the critical value for the chosen alpha and the degree(s) of freedom from the appropriate probability distribution; (6) if the test statistic exceeds the critical value, reject the null hypothesis; (7) if the test statistic does not exceed the critical value, do not reject the null hypothesis. There are general guidelines that relate the variable type and the experimental design to the choice of statistical test (Table 9-5).

Confidence Intervals

The other major areas of statistical inference are the estimation of parameters with associated *confidence intervals* (CIs). In statistics, a CI is an interval estimate of a population parameter. A CI describes how likely it is that the population

---

TABLE 9-5

WHEN TO USE WHAT

■ VARIABLE TYPE	■ ONE-SAMPLE TESTS	■ TWO-SAMPLE TESTS	■ MULTIPLE-SAMPLE TESTS
Dichotomous or nominal	Binomial distribution	Chi-square test, Fisher's exact test	Chi-square test
Ordinal	Chi-square test	Chi-square test, nonparametric tests	Chi-square test, nonparametric tests
Continuous or discrete	*z* distribution or *t* distribution	Unpaired *t* test, paired *t* test, nonparametric tests	Analysis of variance, nonparametric analysis of variance

parameter is estimated by any particular sample statistic such as the mean. (The technical definition of the CI of the mean is more rigorous. A 95% CI implies that if the experiment were done over and over again, 95 of each 100 CIs would be expected to contain the true value of the mean.) CIs are a range of the following form: summary statistic ± (confidence factor) × (precision factor).

The *precision factor* is derived from the sample itself, whereas the *confidence factor* is taken from a probability distribution and also depends on the specified confidence level chosen. For a sample of interval data taken from a normally distributed population for which CIs are to be chosen for $\bar{x}$, the precision factor is called the *standard error of the mean* and is obtained by dividing SD by the square root of the sample size

or $SE = \dfrac{SD}{\sqrt{n}} = \sqrt{\sum_{i=1}^{n}(x_i - \bar{x})^2/n(n-1)}$.

The confidence factors are the same as those used for the dispersion or spread of the sample and are obtained from the normal distribution. The CIs for confidence factors 1, 2, and 3 have roughly a 68%, 95%, and 99% chance of containing the population mean. Strictly speaking, when the SD must be estimated from sample values, the confidence factors should be taken from the *t distribution*, another probability distribution. These coefficients will be larger than those used previously. This is usually ignored if the sample size is reasonable; for example, $n > 25$. Even when the sample size is only five or greater, the use of the coefficients 1, 2, and 3 is simple and sufficiently accurate for quick mental calculations of CIs on parameter estimates.

5 Almost all research reports include the use of SE, regardless of the probability distribution of the populations sampled. This use is a consequence of the *central limit theorem*, one of the most remarkable theorems in all of mathematics. The central limit theorem states that the SE can always be used, if the sample size is sufficiently large, to specify CIs around the sample mean. These CIs are calculated as previously described. This is true even if the population distribution is so different from normal that SD cannot be used to characterize the dispersion of the population members. Only rough guidelines can be given for the necessary sample size; for interval data, 25 and above is large enough and 4 and below is too small.

Although the SE is often discussed along with other descriptive statistics, it is really an inferential statistic. SE and SD are usually mentioned together because of their similarities of computation, but there is often confusion about their use in research reports in the form "mean ± number." Some confusion results from the failure of the author to specify whether the number after the ± sign is the one or the other. More important, the choice between using SD and using SE has become controversial. Because SE is always less than SD, it has been argued that authors seek to deceive by using SE to make the data look better than they really are. The choice is actually simple. When describing the spread, scatter, or dispersion of the sample, use SD; when describing the precision with which the population mean is known, use SE.

Confidence Intervals on Proportions

Categorical binary data, also called *enumeration data*, provide counts of subject responses. Given a sample of subjects of whom some have a certain characteristic (e.g., death, female sex), a ratio of responders to the number of subjects can be easily calculated as $p = x/n$; this ratio or rate can be expressed as a decimal fraction or as a percentage. It should be clear that this is a measure of central location of a binary data in the same way that μ was a measure of central location for continuous data. In the population from which the sample is taken,

the ratio of responders to total subjects is a population parameter, denoted π; π is the measure of central location for the population. (This is not related to the geometry constant $\pi = 3.14159...$). As with other data types, π is usually not known, but must be estimated from the sample. The sample ratio p is the best estimate of π. The probability of binary data is provided by the *binomial distribution function*.

Because the population is not generally known, the experimenter usually wishes to estimate π by the sample ratio p and to specify with what confidence π is known. If the sample is sufficiently large ($n \times p \geq 5$; $n \times (1 - p) \geq 5$), advantage is taken of the central limit theorem to derive an SE analogous to that derived for interval data or $SE = \sqrt{\dfrac{p \times (1 - p)}{n}}$. This sample SE is exactly analogous to the sample SE of the mean for interval data, except that it is an SE of the proportion. Just as a 95% CI of the mean was calculated, so may a CI on the proportion be obtained. Larger samples will make the CI more precise.

STATISTICAL TESTS AND MODELS

Dichotomous Data Testing

In the experiment negating the value of mammary artery ligation, five of eight patients (62.5%) having ligation showed benefit while five of nine patients (55.6%) having sham surgery also had benefit.[1] Is this difference real? This experiment sampled patients from two populations—those having the real procedure and those having the sham procedure. A variety of statistical techniques allow a comparison of the success rate. These include *Fisher's exact test* and (Pearson's) *chi-square test*. The chi-square test offers the advantage of being computationally simpler; it can also analyze contingency tables with more than two rows and two columns; however, certain assumptions of sample size and response rate are not achieved by this experiment. Fisher's exact test fails to reject the null hypothesis for this data.

The results of such experiments are often presented as rate ratios. The rate of improvement for the experimental group (5/8 = 62.5%) is divided by the rate of improvement for the control group (5/9 = 55.6%). A rate ratio of 1.00 (100%) fails to show a difference of benefit or harm between the two groups. In this example the rate ratio is 1.125. Thus, the experimental group had a 12.5% greater chance of improvement compared with the control group. A CI can be calculated for the rate ratio; in this example it is (0.40, 3.13), thus widely spread to either side of the rate ratio of no difference. (If such experiment were performed now, the sample size would be much larger to have adequate statistical power.)

Interval Data Testing

Parametric statistics are the usual choice in the analysis of interval data, both discrete and continuous. The purpose of such analysis is to test the hypothesis of a difference between population means. The population means are unknown and are estimated by the sample means. A typical example would be the comparison of the mean heart rates of patients receiving and not receiving atropine. Parametric test statistics have been developed by using the properties of the normal probability distribution and two related probability distributions, the t and the F distributions. In using such parametric methods, the assumption is made that the sample or samples is/are drawn from population(s) with a normal distribution. The parametric test statistics that have been created for interval data all have the form of a ratio. In general terms, the numerator of this ratio is the variability of the means of the samples; the denominator of this ratio is the variability among all the members of the samples. These variabilities are similar to the variances developed for descriptive statistics. The test statistic is thus a ratio of variabilities or variances. All parametric test statistics are used in the same fashion; if the test statistic ratio becomes large, the null hypothesis of no difference is rejected. The critical values against which to compare the test statistic are taken from tables of the three relevant probability distributions (normal, t, or F). In hypothesis testing at least one of the population means is unknown, but the population variance(s) may or may not be known. Parametric statistics can be divided into two groups according to whether or not the population variances are known. If the population variance is known, the test statistic used is called the z score; critical values are obtained from the normal distribution. In most biomedical applications, the population variance is rarely known and the z score is little used.

t Test

An important advance in statistical inference came early in the 20th century with the creation of *Student's t test statistic* and the *t distribution*, which allowed the testing of hypotheses when the population variance is not known. The most common use of Student's t test is to compare the mean values of two populations. There are two types of t test. If each subject has two measurements taken, for example, one before (x_i) and one after (y_i) a drug, then a one sample or *paired t test* procedure is used; each control measurement taken before drug administration is paired with a measurement in the same patient after drug administration. Of course, this is a self-control experiment. This pairing of measurements in the same patient reduces variability and increases statistical power. The difference $d_i = x_i - y_i$ of each pair of values is calculated and the average $\bar{d}$ is calculated. In the formula for Student's t statistic, the numerator is $\bar{d}$, whereas the denominator is the SE of $\bar{d}$ denoted $(SE_{\bar{d}})$ so the test statistic is $t = \dfrac{\bar{d}}{SE_{\bar{d}}}$.

All t statistics are created in this way; the numerator is the difference of two means, whereas the denominator is the SE of the two means. If the difference between the two means is large compared with their variability, then the null hypothesis of no difference is rejected. The critical values for the t statistic are taken from the t probability distribution. The t distribution is symmetric and bell-shaped but more spread out than the normal distribution. The t distribution has a single integer parameter; for a paired t test, the value of this single degree of freedom is the sample size minus one. There can be some confusion about the use of the letter t. It refers both to the value of the test statistic calculated by the formula and to the critical value from the theoretical probability distribution. The critical t value is determined by looking in a t table after a significance level is chosen and the degree of freedom is computed.

More commonly, measurements are taken on two separate groups of subjects. For example, one group receives blood pressure treatment with sample values x_i, whereas no treatment is given to a control group with sample values y_i. The number of subjects in each group might or might not be identical; regardless of this, in no sense is an individual measurement in the first group matched or paired with a specific measurement in the second group. An *unpaired* or *two-sample t test* is used to compare the means of the two groups. The numerator of the t statistic is $\bar{x} - \bar{y}$. The denominator is a weighted average of the SDs of each sample so that the test statistic t is $t = \dfrac{\bar{x} - \bar{y}}{\sqrt{\left(\sqrt{\dfrac{1}{n_x} + \dfrac{1}{n_y}}\right)\left(\dfrac{(n_x - 1)s_x^2 + (n_y - 1)s_y^2}{n_x + n_y - 2}\right)}}$.

The degree of freedom for an unpaired t test is calculated as the sum of the subjects of the two groups minus two. As with the paired t test, if the t ratio becomes large, the null hypothesis is rejected.

Analysis of Variance

Experiments in anesthesia, whether they are with humans or with animals, may not be limited to one or two groups of data for each variable. It is very common to follow a variable longitudinally; heart rate, for example, might be measured five times before and during anesthetic induction. These are also called *repeated measurement experiments*; the experimenter will wish to compare changes between the initial heart rate measurement and those obtained during induction. The experimental design might also include several groups receiving different induction drugs; for example, comparing heart rate across groups immediately after laryngoscopy. Researchers have mistakenly handled these analysis problems with just the t test. If heart rate is collected five times, these collection times could be labeled A, B, C, D, and E. Then A could be compared with B, C, D, and E; B could be compared with C, D, and E; and so forth. The total of possible pairings is ten; thus, ten paired t tests could be calculated for all the possible pairings of A, B, C, D, and E. A similar approach can be used for comparing more than two groups for unpaired data.

The use of t tests in this fashion is inappropriate. In testing a statistical hypothesis, the experimenter sets the level of type I error; this is usually chosen to be 0.05. When using many t tests, as in the example given earlier, the chosen error rate for performing all these t tests is much higher than 0.05, even though the type I error is set at 0.05 for each individual comparison. In fact, the type I error rate for all t tests simultaneously; that is, the chance of finding at least one of the multiple t test statistics significant merely by chance is given by the formula $\alpha = 1 - 0.95^\kappa$. If 13 t tests are performed ($\kappa = 13$), the real error rate is 49%. Applying t tests over and over again to all the possible pairings of a variable will misleadingly identify statistical significance when in fact there is none.

The most versatile approach for handling comparisons of means between more than two groups or between several measurements in the same group is called *analysis of variance* and is frequently cited by the acronym ANOVA. Analysis of variance consists of rules for creating test statistics on means when there are more than two groups. These test statistics are called *F ratios*, after Ronald Fisher; the critical values for the F test statistic are taken from the F probability distribution that Fisher derived.

Suppose that data for three groups are obtained. What can be said about the mean values of the three target populations? The F test is actually asking several questions simultaneously: is group 1 different from group 2; is group 2 different from group 3; and is group 1 different from group 3? As with the t test, the F test statistic is a ratio; in general terms, the numerator expresses the variability of the mean values of the three groups, whereas the denominator expresses the average variability or difference of each sample value from the mean of all sample values. The formulas to create the test statistic are computationally elegant but are rather hard to appreciate intuitively. The F statistic has two degrees of freedom, denoted m and n; the value of m is a function of the number of experimental groups; the value for n is a function of the number of subjects in all experimental groups. The analysis of multigroup data is not necessarily finished after the ANOVAs are calculated. If the null hypothesis is rejected and it is accepted that there are differences among the groups tested, how can it be decided where the differences are? A variety of techniques are available to make what are called *multiple comparisons* after the ANOVA test is performed.

Robustness and Nonparametric Tests

Most statistical tests depend on certain assumptions about the nature of the distribution of values in the underlying populations from which experimental samples are taken. For the parametric statistics, that is, t tests and analysis of variance, it is assumed that the populations follow the normal distribution. However, for some data, experience or historical reasons suggests that these assumptions of a normal distribution do not hold; some examples include proportions, percentages, and response times. What should the experimenter do if he or she fears that the data are not normally distributed?

The experimenter might choose to ignore the problem of nonnormal data and inhomogeneity of variance, hoping that everything will work out. Such insouciance is actually a very practical and reasonable approach to the problem. Parametric statistics are called *robust* statistics; they stand up to much adversity. To a statistician, robustness implies that the magnitude of type I errors is not seriously affected by ill-conditioned data. Parametric statistics are sufficiently robust that the accuracy of decisions reached by means of t tests and analysis of variance remains very credible, even for moderately severe departures from the assumptions.

Another possibility would be to use statistics that do not require any assumptions about probability distributions of the populations. Such statistics are known as *nonparametric tests*; they can be used whenever there is very serious concern about the shape of the data. Nonparametric statistics are also the tests of choice for ordinal data. The basic concept behind nonparametric statistics is the ability to rank or order the observations; nonparametric tests are also called *order statistics*.

Most nonparametric statistics still require the use of theoretical probability distributions; the critical values that must be exceeded by the test statistic are taken from the binomial, normal, and chi-square distributions, depending on the nonparametric test being used. The *nonparametric sign test, Mann-Whitney rank sum test,* and *Kruskal-Wallis one-way analysis of variance* are analogous to the paired t test, unpaired t test, and one-way analysis of variance, respectively. The currently available nonparametric tests are not used more commonly because they do not adapt well to complex statistical models and because they are less able than parametric tests to distinguish between the null and alternative hypotheses if the data are, in fact, normally distributed.

Linear Regression

Often the goal of an experiment is to predict the value of one characteristic from knowledge of another characteristic; the most commonly used technique for this purpose is regression analysis. Experiments for this purpose capture data pairs (x, y); these data should be displayed in a scatter plot. In the simplest type, a straight line (linear relationship) is assumed between two variables; one (y), the response or dependent variable, is considered a function of the other (x), the explanatory or independent variable. This is expressed as the linear regression equation $y = a + bx$; the parameters of the regression equation are a and b. The parameter b is the slope of the straight line relating x and y; for each 1 unit change in x, there is a b unit change in y. The parameter a is the intercept (value of y when x equals 0). Estimates of the parameters are obtained from a least squares method that sets the slope b value to minimize the distances from the data pairs to the regression line: $b = \dfrac{\sum_{i=1}^{n}(x_i - \bar{x})(y_i - \bar{y})}{\sum_{i=1}^{n}(x_i - \bar{x})^2}$; $a = \bar{y} - b\bar{x}$. The parameter of greatest interest in regression is usually the slope, especially whether the slope is nonzero; a zero valued slope implies that x and y are not related. A t test statistic is used to check the statistical significance of the slope.

While there is an additional assumption, the same (x, y) data pairs are usually subjected to correlation analysis. The correlation coefficient r is a measure of the covariation of x and y; r ranges from -1 to 1. There is no correlation for a zero valued r.

It is estimated by: $r = \dfrac{\sum_{i=1}^{n}(x_i - \bar{x})(y_i - \bar{y})}{\sqrt{\sum_{i=1}^{n}(x_i - \bar{x})^2}\sqrt{\sum_{i=1}^{n}(y_i - \bar{y})^2}}$.

The test of the statistical significance of r is equivalent to the test for the significance of the regression slope b. The squared value of r or coefficient of determination (r^2) has a very useful interpretation: the fraction of the variation of y explained by the variation of x.

Regression methods can be extended to data sets in which one response variable is thought to be linearly related to many explanatory variables; this is called *multiple variable linear regression*. This regression includes methods for choosing which of the explanatory variables have a statistically significant regression slope. Other extensions of regression include the typically sigmoidally shaped regression of a binary outcome (e.g., movement) versus anesthetic dose. There are multiple methods for regression of binary outcomes, the most common being logistic regression.

A researcher or reader should not be satisfied to see only the statistical results of regression and correlation. The statistician Anscombe[4] created four hypothetical data sets to illustrate the importance of visual inspection of data. Each data set has 11 paired (x, y) observations (Fig. 9-1). For the data (x_2, y_2), the relationship between x and y is curvilinear; for (x_4, y_4), there is no relationship between x and y; for (x_3, y_3), there is a near perfect correlation between x and y except for one (x, y) pair. All regression and correlation values of the four data sets including means, SDs, slopes, intercepts, standard errors of regression parameters, statistical significance of regression parameters, and correlation coefficients are equal. Yet, these are clearly four different patterns that can only be detected by visual inspection. Even this simplest form of linear regression is based on the strong assumption of an underlaying linear relationship between x and y; failure of that assumption leads to erroneous statistical inference.

Systematic Reviews and Meta-Analyses

Reports using a new type of research method—the systematic review (SR) with an accompanying meta-analysis (MA)—have become commonplace over the last 25 years in anesthesia journals.[5] (As of November 2007, a literature search for "('systematic review' OR meta-analysis) AND anesthesia" in PubMed at the National Library of Medicine returned 334 citations of a total of all 36,026 citations for SRs or MAs[a].) In systematic reviews, a focused question drives the research, for example, (1) *Transient neurologic symptoms (TNS) following spinal*

[a]See www.ncbi.nlm.nih.gov/sites/entrez.

FIGURE 9-1. Four scatter plots from the Anscombe data sets.[4] For each data set, $n = 11$, $\bar{x} = 9.00$, $SD_x = 3.31$, $\bar{y} = 7.50$, $SD_y = 2.03$, $y = 3.00 + 0.50x$, $SE_a = 1.12$, $SE_b = 0.12$, $r^2 = 0.67$, and so forth. All statistics are equal up to the fourth decimal place.

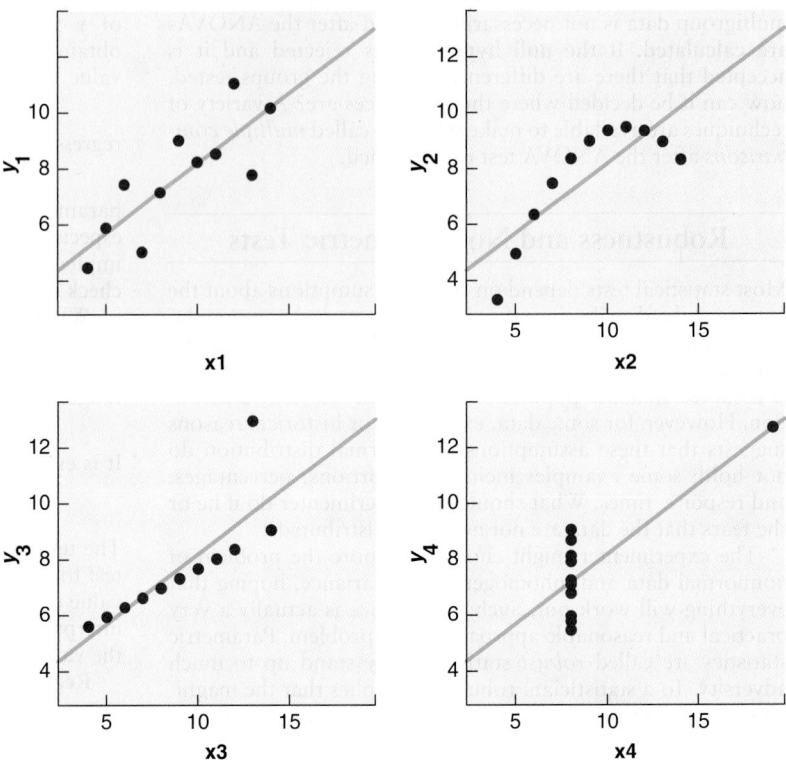

Anscombe's 4 Regression Data Sets

anaesthesia with lidocaine versus other local anaesthetics[6] or (2) Ventilation with lower tidal volumes versus traditional tidal volumes in adults for acute lung injury and acute respiratory distress syndrome.[7] These titles reveal some of the research design of a systematic review. There is a population of interest: (1) patients having spinal anesthesia and (2) adults (with) acute lung injury and acute respiratory distress syndrome. There is a comparison of two interventions: (1) lidocaine versus other local anaesthetics and (2) ventilation with lower tidal volumes versus traditional tidal volumes. There is an outcome for choosing success or failure of the interventions: (1) occurrence of TNS and (2) 28-day mortality (listed in text).

To answer the experimental question, data are obtained from controlled trials (usually randomized) already in the medical literature rather than from newly conducted clinical trials; the basic unit of analysis of this observational research is the published study. The researchers, also called the review authors, proceed through a structured protocol, which includes in part: (1) choice of study inclusion/exclusion criteria, (2) explicitly defined literature searching, (3) abstraction of data from included studies, (4) appraisal of data quality, (5) systematic pooling of data, and (6) discussion of inferences. This structured protocol is intended to minimize bias. Even randomized controlled trials may have sources of bias such as (1) selection bias: systematic differences between the patients receiving each intervention; (2) performance bias: systematic differences in care being given to study patients other than the preplanned interventions being evaluated; (3) attrition bias: systematic differences in the withdrawal of patients from each of the two intervention groups; and (4) detection bias: systematic differences in the ascertainment and recording of outcomes. The main focus of bias detection in the trials incorporated into a SR is (1) the randomization process, (2) the concealment of random allocation, (3) the use of blinding, and (4) the reporting/analysis of dropouts.[8]

Binary outcomes (yes/no, alive/dead, presence/absence) within a study are usually compared by the relative risk (rate ratio) statistic. If there is sufficient clinical similarity among the included studies, a summary relative risk of the overall effect of the comparison treatments is estimated by meta-analysis; meta-analysis is a set of statistical techniques for combining results from different studies.[8] The calculations for the statistical analyses of a meta-analysis are unfamiliar to most, but are not difficult. The results of a meta-analysis are usually present in a figure called a forest plot (Fig. 9-2). The far left column identifies the included studies and the observed data. The horizontal lines and diamond shapes are graphical representations of individual study relative risk and summary relative risk, respectively; the far right column of the figure lists the relative risks with 95% CIs for the individual studies and the summary statistics. There are also descriptive and inferential statistics concerning the statistical heterogeneity of the meta-analysis and the significance of the summary statistics.

An examination of Figure 9-2 shows that many of the individual studies (11 of 14) had wide, nonsignificant confidence intervals that touch or cross the relative risk of identity (RR = 1). However, the overall relative risk calculated from all studies was 7.16 with a 95% CI [4.2, 12.75]. The power of summary statistics to combine evidence is clear. The review authors concluded: "Lidocaine can cause transient neurologic symptoms (TNS) in every seventh patient who receives spinal anesthesia. The relative risk of developing TNS is about seven times higher for lidocaine than for bupivacaine, prilocaine, and procaine. These painful symptoms disappear completely by the tenth postoperative day."[6]

The production of SRs comes from several sources. Many come from the individual initiative of researchers who publish their results as stand-alone reports in the journals of medicine and anesthesia. The American Society of Anesthesiologists has

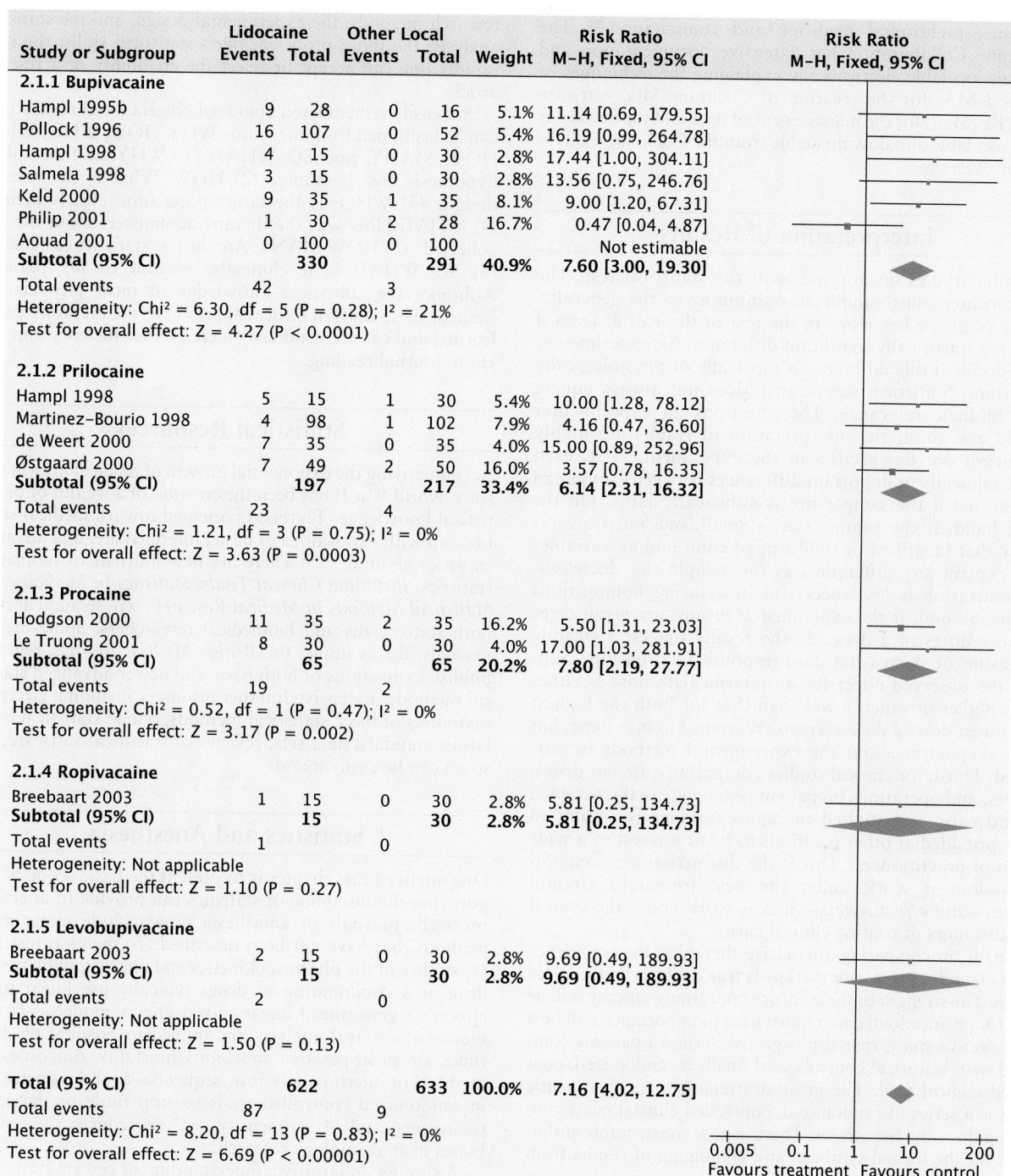

FIGURE 9-2. Forest plot. (Modified from Graph 02/01 in Zaric D, Christiansen C, Pace NL, Punjasawadwong Y: Transient neurologic symptoms (TNS) following spinal anaesthesia with lidocaine versus other local anaesthetics (Cochrane Review). In: *The Cochrane Library*, Issue 3. Chichester, UK, John Wiley & Sons, Ltd., 2004. Copyright Cochrane Library, reproduced with permission.)

developed a process for the creation of practice parameters that includes among other things a variant form of SRs. The most prominent proponent of SRs is the Cochrane Collaboration, Oxford, United Kingdom. "The Cochrane Collaboration is an international not-for-profit and independent organization, dedicated to making up-to-date, accurate information about the effects of healthcare readily available worldwide. It produces and disseminates systematic reviews of healthcare interventions and promotes the search for evidence in the form of clinical trials and other studies of interventions. The

Cochrane Collaboration was founded in 1993 and named after the British epidemiologist, Archie Cochrane."[b]

There are more than 50 collaborative review groups that provide the editorial control and supervision of SRs; one of these, located in Copenhagen,[9] ". . . produce(s) and disseminate systematic reviews of healthcare interventions in anesthesia, perioperative medicine, intensive care medicine, emergency

[b]See cochrane.org/docs/descrip.htm.

medicine, prehospital medicine and resuscitation."[c] The Cochrane Collaboration has extensive documentation and tutorials available electronically explaining the techniques of SRs and MA; for the creation of Cochrane SRs, software (titled RevMan) for the management of data and for the MA is freely available and downloadable from the Cochrane Collaboration Web site.

Interpretation of Results

Scientific studies do not end with the statistical test. The experimenter must submit an opinion as to the generalizability of his or her work to the rest of the world. Even if there is a statistically significant difference, the experimenter must decide if this difference is medically or physiologically important. Statistical significance does not always equate with biologic relevance. The questions an experimenter should ask about the interpretation of results are highly dependent on the specifics of the experiment. First, even small, clinically unimportant differences between groups can be detected if the sample size is sufficiently large. On the other hand, if the sample size is small, one must always worry that identified or unidentified confounding variables may explain any difference; as the sample size decreases, randomization is less successful in assuring homogenous groups. Second, if the experimental groups are given three or more doses of a drug, do the results suggest a steadily increasing or decreasing dose-response relationship? Suppose the observed effect for an intermediate dose is either much higher or much lower than that for both the highest and lowest dose; a dose-response relationship may exist, but some skepticism about the experimental methods is warranted. Third, for clinical studies comparing different drugs, devices, and operations on patient outcome, are the patients, clinical care, and studied therapies sufficiently similar to those provided at other locations to be of interest to a wide group of practitioners? This is the distinction between *efficacy*—does it work under the best (research) circumstances—and *effectiveness*—does it work under the typical circumstances of routine clinical care?

Finally, in comparing alternative therapies, the confidence that a claim for a superior therapy is true depends on the study design. The strength of the evidence concerning efficacy will be least for an anecdotal case report; next in importance will be a retrospective study, then a prospective series of patients compared with historical controls, and finally a randomized, controlled clinical trial. The greatest strength for a therapeutic claim is a series of randomized, controlled clinical trials confirming the same hypothesis. There is now considerable enthusiasm for the formal synthesis and combining of results from two or more trials in a systematic review.

CONCLUSIONS

Guidelines for Reading Journal Articles

Thousands of words are written each year in journal articles relevant to anesthesia. No one can read them all. How should the clinician determine which articles are useful? All that is possible is to learn to rapidly skip over most articles and concentrate on the few selected for their importance to the reader. Those few should be chosen according to their relevance and credibility. Relevance is determined by the specifics of one's anesthetic practice. Credibility is a function of the merits of the

research methods, the experimental design, and the statistical analysis; the more proficient one's statistical skills, the more rapidly one can accept or reject the credibility of a research article.

Six easily remembered appraisal criteria for clinical studies can be fashioned from the words WHY, HOW, WHO, WHAT, HOW MANY, and SO WHAT: (1) WHY: Is the biologic hypothesis clearly stated? (2) HOW: What is the research design? (3) WHO: Is the target population clearly defined? (4) WHAT: How was the therapy administered and the data collected? (5) HOW MANY: Are the test statistics convincing? (6) SO WHAT: Is it clinically relevant to my patients? Although the statistical knowledge of most physicians is limited, these skills of critical appraisal of the literature can be learned and can tremendously increase the efficiency and benefit of journal reading.

Statistical Resources

Accompanying the exponential growth of medical information since World War II has been the creation of a wealth of biostatistical knowledge. Textbooks oriented toward medical statistics and with expositions of basic, intermediate, and advanced statistics abound.[10–15] There are new journals of biomedical statistics, including *Clinical Trials, Statistics in Medicine,* and *Statistical Methods in Medical Research,* whose audiences are both statisticians and biomedical researchers. Some medical journals, for example, the *British Medical Journal,* regularly publish expositions of both basic and newer advanced statistical methods. Extensive Internet resources including electronic textbooks of basic statistical methods, online statistical calculators, standard data sets, reviews of statistical software, and so on can be easily found.

Statistics and Anesthesia

One intent of this chapter is to present the basic scope of support that the discipline of statistics can provide to anesthesia research. Journals of anesthesia now include many newer methods that have not been described. To mention just four: (1) studies of the pharmacokinetics and pharmacokinetics of a drug or a combination of drugs typically use linear mixed effects or generalized linear mixed effects models, (2) techniques of survival analysis are applied to hospital discharge times or postoperative morbidity/mortality outcomes, (3) methods of interim analysis or sequential trial design are used in randomized controlled trials to stop futile or dangerous treatments, and (4) propensity analysis reduces the possible biases in epidemiology research.

Although an intuitive understanding of certain basic principles is emphasized, these basic principles are not necessarily simple and have been developed by statisticians with great mathematical rigor. Academic anesthesia needs more workers to immerse themselves in these statistical fundamentals. Having done so, these statistically knowledgeable academic anesthesiologists will be prepared to improve their own research projects, to assist their colleagues in research, to efficiently seek consultation from the professional statistician, to strengthen the editorial review of journal articles, and to expound to the clinical reader the whys and wherefores of statistics. The clinical reader also needs to expend his or her own effort to acquire some basic statistical skills. Journals are increasingly difficult to understand without some basic statistical understanding. Some clinical problems can be best understood with a perspective based on probability. Finally, understanding principles of experimental design can prevent premature acceptances of new therapies from faulty studies.

---

[c]See www.carg.cochrane.org/en/index.html.

References

1. Cobb LA, Thomas GI, Dillard DH, et al: An evaluation of internal-mammary-artery ligation by a double-blind technic. N Engl J Med 1959; 260: 1115
2. Sacks H, Chalmers TC, Smith HJ: Randomized versus historical controls for clinical trials. Am J Med 1982; 72: 233
3. Schulz KF, Chalmers I, Hayes RJ, et al: Empirical evidence of bias. Dimensions of methodological quality associated with estimates of treatment effects in controlled trials. JAMA 1995; 273: 408
4. Anscombe FJ. Graphs in statistical analysis. Am Stat 1973; 27: 17
5. Carlisle JB. Systematic reviews: How they work and how to use them. Anaesthesia 2007; 62: 702
6. Zaric D, Christiansen C, Pace NL, et al: Transient neurologic symptoms (TNS) following spinal anaesthesia with lidocaine versus other local anaesthetics. Cochrane Database Syst Rev 2005, Oct 19; CD003006
7. Petrucci N, Iacovelli W: Lung protective ventilation strategy for the acute respiratory distress syndrome. Cochrane Database Syst Rev 2007, Jul 18; CD003844
8. Pace N: The meta-analysis of a systematic review, Evidence-Based Anaesthesia and Intensive Care. Edited by Møller A, Pedersen T, Cracknell J. New York, Cambridge University Press, 2006, pp 46
9. Pedersen T, Møller A: The Cochrane Collaboration and the Cochrane Anaesthesia Review Group, Evidence-Based Anaesthesia and Intensive Care. Edited by Møller A, Pedersen T, Cracknell J. New York, Cambridge University Press, 2006, pp 77
10. Altman DG, Trevor B, Gardner MJ, et al: Statistics with Confidence: Confidence Intervals and Statistical Guidelines. New York, John Wiley & Sons, 2000
11. Campbell MJ, Machin D: Medical Statistics: A Commonsense Approach. New York, John Wiley & Sons, 1999
12. Dawson B, Trapp RG, Trapp R: Basic & Clinical Biostatistics. New York, McGraw-Hill Medical, 2004
13. Riffenburgh RH: Statistics in Medicine. San Diego, Academic Press, 2005
14. Glantz SA: Primer of Biostatistics. New York, McGraw-Hill Medical, 2005
15. Rennie D, Guyatt G: Users' Guides to the Medical Literature: A Manual for Evidence-Based Clinical Practice. Edited by Gordon Guyatt and Drummond Rennie. Chicago, IL: American Medical Association, 2002

SECTION III ■ ANATOMY AND PHYSIOLOGY

CHAPTER 10 ■ CARDIOVASCULAR ANATOMY AND PHYSIOLOGY

JOHN P. KAMPINE, DAVID F. STOWE, AND PAUL S. PAGEL

KEY POINTS

1 The left ventricle (LV) is capable of tolerating large increases in arterial pressure without a substantial reduction in stroke volume, but the right ventricle may acutely decompensate with even modest increases in pulmonary vascular resistance.

2 Atrial contraction establishes final ventricular stroke volume at end-diastole and normally contributes between 15 and 20% of this volume.

3 Diastolic dysfunction may independently cause heart failure, even in the presence of relatively normal contractile function. This "heart failure with normal systolic function" has been increasingly recognized as a major underlying cause for as many as 50% of patients admitted to the hospital with congestive heart failure.

4 According to Starling's law, the force of LV contraction and volume of blood ejected from the chamber during systole (stroke volume) is directly related to the end-diastolic myofilament length, and hence, the end-diastolic volume.

5 The distensibility of the aorta, the resistance of the peripheral arterial vasculature, and the actions of reflected waves on the central aortic circulation are the principle determinants of afterload. Systemic vascular resistance (the ratio of pressure to cardiac output, P/Q) is the most commonly used nonparametric expression of peripheral resistance and is primarily affected by autonomic nervous system activity.

6 The primary determinant of myocardial oxygen consumption is heart rate because the heart completes an entire cycle with each beat, and hence, the more frequently the

heart performs pressure-volume work, the more oxygen must be consumed.

7 The fundamental contractile unit of cardiac muscle is the sarcomere. The myofilaments within each sarcomere are arranged in parallel cross-striated bundles of thin (containing actin, tropomyosin, and the troponin complex) and thick (primarily composed of myosin and its supporting proteins) fibers. Sarcomeres are connected in series, thereby producing characteristic shortening and thickening of the long and short axes of each myocyte, respectively, during contraction.

8 Attachment of myosin to its binding site on the actin molecule releases the phosphate anion from the myosin head, thereby producing a molecular conformation within this cross-bridge structure that generates tension in both myofilaments. Release of adenosine diphosphate (ADP) and the stored potential energy from this activated conformation produce rotation of the cross-bridge ("power stroke") at the hinge point separating the helix tail region from the globular myosin head and its associated light chain proteins.

9 The QRS complex records potentials at the body surface when the wave of depolarization is distributed throughout ventricular myocardium. The QRS complex is much larger in magnitude than the P wave because ventricular mass is greater than the atrial mass. Rapid conduction through the His-Purkinje system spreads the wave of depolarization quickly to the ventricles.

10 Short-duration regulation of mean arterial pressure occurs through the arterial, and to a lesser extent, intracardiac baroreceptors. Arterial baroreceptors are located at the bifurcation of the common carotid arteries and in the aortic arch.

11 Blood supply to the LV is directly dependent on the difference between the aortic pressure and LV end-diastolic pressure (coronary perfusion pressure) and inversely related to the vascular resistance to flow, which varies to the fourth power of the radius of the vessel (Poiseuille's law).

12 Metabolic factors are the major physiological determinants of coronary vascular tone and, hence, myocardial perfusion.

13 Myocardial infarction may occur without evidence of major coronary thromboses, emboli, or stenosis. This form of infarction is caused by excessive metabolic demands resulting from severe LV hypertrophy (e.g., critical aortic stenosis) or vasoactive drug ingestion (e.g., amphetamines, cocaine) or it may also result from coronary artery vasospasm.

14 The lung is richly innervated by the parasympathetic and sympathetic nervous system, but the dominant effect of the autonomic nervous system occurs primarily at the level of alveolar and bronchial smooth muscle.

15 Cerebral blood flow remains relatively constant when mean arterial pressure varies between 50 and 150 mm Hg in healthy subjects. This autoregulation of cerebral blood flow is shifted to the right in patients with chronic, poorly controlled essential hypertension.

16 Arterial CO_2 tension is a major regulator of cerebral blood flow within the physiologic range of arterial CO_2 tension. Cerebral blood flow linearly increases 1 to 2 mL/100 g/min for each 1 mm Hg increase in Pa_{CO_2}. Below an arterial CO_2 tension of 25 mm Hg, the cerebral blood flow response to Pa_{CO_2} is attenuated.

FUNCTIONAL ANATOMY OF THE HEART

The left and right atria consist of two, thin overlying sheaths of muscle oriented at right angles to each other. The two thicker-walled ventricles consist of three interdigitating muscle layers: the deep sinospiral, the superficial sinospiral, and the superficial bulbospiral muscles (Fig. 10-1). The two outer muscle layers are oriented obliquely from the base of the heart to the apex. Constriction of these fibers shortens the longitudinal axis of the left ventricle (LV) by moving the base toward the apex. The circumferential deep sinospiral muscles reduce the LV diameter (Fig. 10-2). Thus, synchronous contraction of the LV muscles shortens the long axis of the heart, decreases the circumference of the LV chamber, and lifts the apex toward the anterior chest wall. This latter action produces the familiar palpable point of maximum impulse, which is normally located in the fifth or sixth intercostal space in the midclavicular line.[1,2] The LV pumps blood from the low-pressure venous into the high-pressure arterial system. The right ventricle (RV) receives venous blood from the right atrium via the superior and inferior vena cavae at low pressure (2 to 10 mm Hg) and oxygen saturation (60 to 75%). The RV is crescent-shaped and contains embryologically distant inflow and outflow tracts that contract in a peristaltic sequence to propel blood into the pulmonary arterial tree. Blood flow through the pulmonary circulation functions primarily as a gas exchanger, providing for the elimination of carbon dioxide (CO_2; a major product of cellular metabolism) and the uptake of oxygen (O_2). The pulmonary vasculature is characterized by lower pressure than the systemic circulation and has shorter, larger-bore blood vessels with relatively thinner walls than systemic resistance vessels. Thus, the pulmonary circulation is a low-pressure, low-resistance system into which the RV transfers blood. The LV is

1 capable of tolerating large increases in arterial pressure without a substantial reduction in stroke volume; the RV may acutely decompensate with even modest increases in pulmonary vascular resistance. The RV free wall occupies a more right-sided, anterior position within the mediastinum compared with the position of the thicker-walled LV that is located in a left-sided, posterior orientation (Fig. 10-3, A and B). During contraction, the RV moves toward the interventricular septum with a "bellows-like" action. The atrioventricular (AV) groove

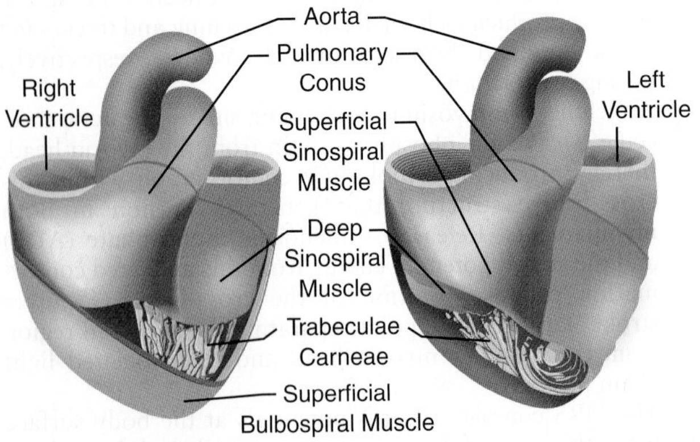

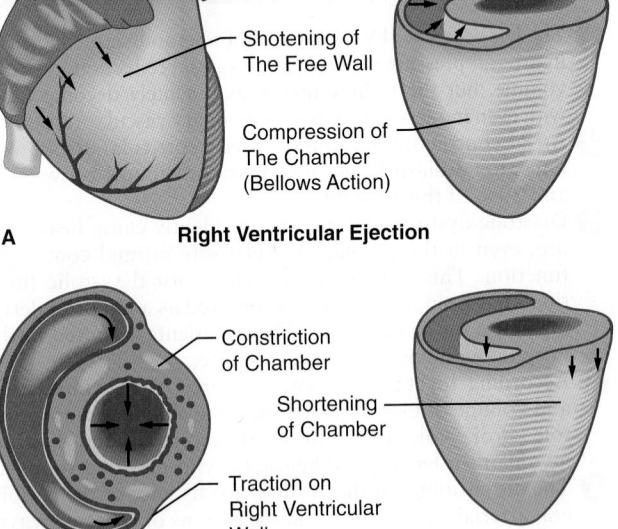

A   **Right Ventricular Ejection**

- Shotening of The Free Wall
- Compression of The Chamber (Bellows Action)

B   **Left Ventricular Ejection**

- Constriction of Chamber
- Shortening of Chamber
- Traction on Right Ventricular Wall

FIGURE 10-2.   Ventricular volume ejection. Contraction characteristics and modes of emptying. The volumes ejected by each ventricle is equal but the left ventricle requires a more circumferential muscular wall to eject its volume at a pressure that is approximately 4 to 5 times greater than that in the right ventricle. (Reproduced with permission from Rushmer RF: Cardiovascular Dynamics. Philadelphia, WB Saunders, 1976, Fig. 3-12, p 92.)

FIGURE 10-1.   Components of the myocardium. The outer muscle layers pull the apex of the heart toward the base. The inner circumferential layers constrict the lumen, particularly of the left ventricle. (Reproduced with permission from Rushmer RF: Cardiovascular Dynamics. Philadelphia, WB Saunders, 1976, Fig. 3-2, p 78.)

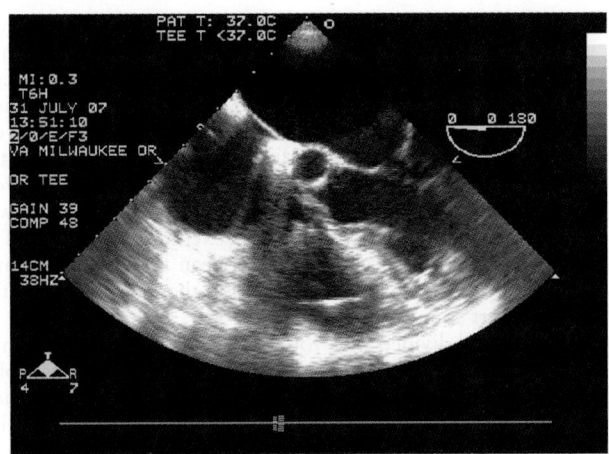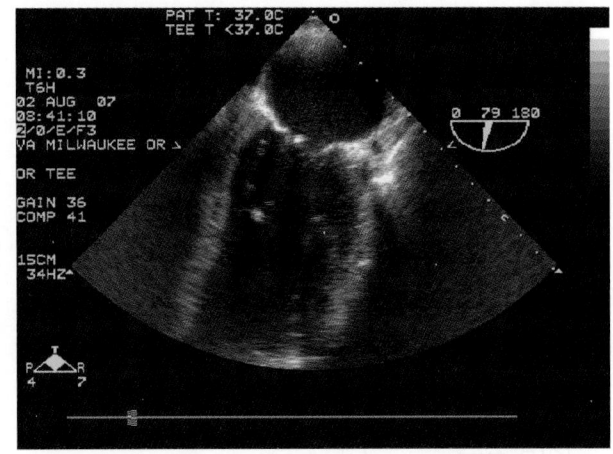

A   B

FIGURE 10-3.   Transesophageal echocardiography demonstrates the thickness and motion of atrial and ventricular walls mid esophageal five-chamber and two chamber views (**A** and **B** respectively).

separating the right atrium and RV shortens toward the apex during contraction. This anatomic configuration permits the more flexible RV wall to eject a large volume of blood with a minimal amount of shortening. The echocardiographic depiction of ventricular contraction is shown in Figure 10-3.

The LV has a cylindrical endocardial border, and this anatomic configuration provides a mechanical advantage over the RV in generating stroke work and power because a reduction in the cross-sectional area of the cylinder a (function of the square of the radius) is partially responsible for LV stroke volume. The LV also provides a splint against which the outer wall of the RV is pulled during contraction. The O_2 content and saturation of blood within the LV (O_2 20 mL/dL and 98%, respectively) is very high compared with blood in the RV. Left ventricular O_2 saturation is incomplete because a small quantity of coronary venous return through thebesian veins empties directly into the left side of the heart. During contraction, LV pressure increases from end-diastolic values of 10 to 12 mm Hg to a peak pressure of 120 to 140 mm Hg during systole. The peak pressures generated by the LV reflect the requirement to circulate blood through the high-resistance systemic circulation that is composed of thicker blood vessels containing larger quantities of vascular smooth muscle than their counterparts in the pulmonary arterial tree. Resistance to blood flow is especially high in small arterioles and precapillary vessels, and blood flow in these vessels requires that the LV generate higher perfusion pressure than the RV. The volume of blood pumped by RV and LV is identical (stroke volume), but the pressure-volume work (stroke work) performed by the LV is 5 to 7 times greater than that of the RV. Left ventricular ejection is associated with a wall tension gradient from the apex to the base of the heart (aortic outflow tract), thereby producing the intraventricular gradient required to transfer stroke volume from the LV into the aorta.

Efficient pumping action of the heart requires two pairs of unidirectional valves. One pair is located at the outlets of the RV and LV (pulmonic and aortic valves, respectively). These three-leaflet valves operate passively with changes in pressure gradients. The aortic valve leaflets do not flatten against the aortic wall during LV ejection because a modest dilation of the aortic root located immediately distal to each leaflet establishes an eddy current of blood flow. These dilated regions are termed the *sinuses of Valsalva* and permit blood flow through the right and left main coronary arteries whose openings are located in the aortic wall directly behind the valve cusps. The AV valves separating the atria from the ventricles are the tri-

cuspid and mitral valve on the right and left sides of the heart, respectively. The mitral valve is the only cardiac valve with two leaflets. Both tricuspid and mitral valves are thin, fibrous structures that are supported by chordae tendinae attachments to papillary muscles that are part of the ventricular musculature and contract during systole. The tricuspid and mitral valves open and close with alternations in the pressure gradients between the corresponding atrial and ventricular chambers.

The RV and LV are the major cardiac pumping chambers, but the atria play critically important supporting roles. The atria function as reservoirs, conduits, and contractile chambers and facilitate the transition between continuous, low-pressure venous to phasic, high-pressure arterial blood flow. The normal atrial pressure curve has three positive reflections. Shortly after the onset of atrial depolarization (indicated by the P wave of the electrocardiogram), the atria contract, producing a positive pressure wave (the A wave) late in diastole. At the onset of systole, ventricular contraction produces another pressure wave that is transmitted through the AV valves to the atria, resulting in the C wave. During the remainder of systole, the AV valves remain closed, atrial filling continues from peripheral and pulmonary veins, and atrial pressures rise, thereby producing a positive pressure deflection known as the *V wave* (Fig. 10-4). Atrial contraction establishes final ventricular stroke volume at end-diastole and normally contributes between 15 and 20% of this volume. When atrial contraction is absent or ineffective (e.g., atrial failure, atrial fibrillation or flutter), the heart may be capable of compensating for the loss of the atrial contractile function and continue to function effectively under resting conditions. However, during increased physical activity or stress, the absence of the atrial pump may substantially limit cardiac output, thereby causing a marked reduction in arterial blood pressure accompanied by syncope, exertional dyspnea, easy fatigability, or acute heart failure.

The Cardiac Cycle

The cardiac cycle is traditionally defined based on events occurring before, during, and after LV contraction. Left ventricular systole is commonly divided into three parts: isovolumic contraction, rapid ejection, and slower ejection.[2-3] Closure of both the tricuspid and mitral valves occurs when RV and LV pressures exceed corresponding atrial pressure and is the source of the first heart sound (S_1; Fig. 10-4). Isovolumic

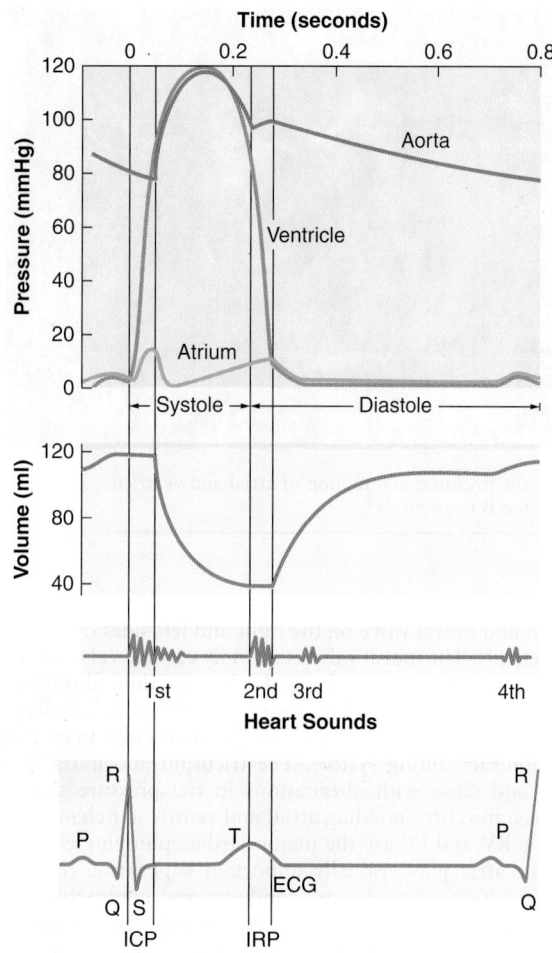

FIGURE 10-4. Mechanical and electrical events of the cardiac cycle showing also the ventricular volume curve and the heart sounds. Note the isovolumic contraction (ICP) and the relaxation period (IRP) during which there is no change in ventricular volume because all valves are closed. The ventricle decreases in volume as it ejects its contents into the aorta. During the first third of systolic ejection—the rapid ejection period—the curve of emptying is steep. ECG, electrocardiogram. (Reproduced with permission from Smith JJ, Kampine JP: Circulatory Physiology—The Essentials, 3rd edition. Baltimore, Williams & Wilkins, 1990, Fig. 3-5, p 40.)

contraction is the interval between closure of the mitral valve and the opening of the aortic valve. Left ventricular volume remains constant during this period of the cardiac cycle. The rate of increase of LV pressure (dP/dt, an index of myocardial contractility) reaches its maximum during isovolumic contraction. True isovolumic contraction does not occur in the RV because the sequential nature of inflow followed by outflow tract RV contraction. Pressure in the aortic root declines to its minimum value immediately before the aortic valve opens. Rapid ejection occurs when LV pressure exceeds aortic pressure and the aortic valve opens. Approximately two thirds of the LV end-diastolic volume is ejected into the aorta during this rapid ejection phase of systole. Aortic dilation occurs in response to this rapid increase in volume as the kinetic energy of LV contraction is transferred to the systemic arterial circulation as potential energy. The compliance of the aorta and proximal great vessels determines the amount of potential energy that can be stored and subsequently released to the arterial vasculature during diastole. The normal LV end-diastolic volume is about 120 mL. The average ejected stroke volume is 80 mL, and the normal ejection fraction is approxi-

mately 67%. A decrease in ejection fraction below 40% is typically observed when the myocardium is affected by ischemia, infarction, or cardiomyopathic disease processes (e.g., myocarditis, amyloid infiltration). Contractile dysfunction may also occur as a result of chronic pressure or volume overload, diabetes, or hypothyroidism. As aortic pressure peaks and resists further LV ejection, transfer of further stroke volume slows and eventually stops. During this period of slower ejection, aortic pressure may briefly exceed LV pressure. The reversal of the pressure gradient between the aortic root and the LV causes the aortic valve to close, thereby producing the second heart sound (S_2).

Diastole is divided into four phases in the LV: isovolumic relaxation, early filling, diastasis, and atrial systole. Isovolumic relaxation defines the period between aortic valve closure and mitral valve opening during which LV volume remains constant. LV pressure falls precipitously as the myofilaments relax. When LV pressure falls below left atrial pressure, the mitral valve opens, and blood volume stored in the left atrium rapidly enters the LV driven by the pressure gradient between these chambers. This early-filling phase of diastole accounts for approximately 70 to 75% of total LV stroke volume available for the subsequent contraction. Delays in LV relaxation occur as a consequence of aging or disease process (e.g., myocardial ischemia) and may attenuate early ventricular filling. After left atrial and LV pressures have equalized, the mitral valve remains open and pulmonary venous return continues to flow through the left atrium into the LV. This phase of diastole is known as *diastasis*, during which the left atrium functions as a conduit. Tachycardia progressively shortens and may completely eliminate this phase of diastole. Diastasis accounts for no more than 5% of total LV end-diastolic volume under normal circumstances. The final phase of diastole is atrial systole. Contraction of the left atrium contributes the remaining blood volume (approximately 15 to 20%) used in the subsequent LV systole. Disease processes known to reduce LV compliance (e.g., myocardial ischemia, pressure-overload hypertrophy) attenuate early filling and increase the importance of atrial systole to overall LV filling. Thus, loss of normal sinus rhythm may precipitate catastrophic decreases in cardiac output in patients with symptomatic coronary artery disease, critical aortic stenosis, or poorly controlled chronic essential hypertension.[6]

The importance of diastole to overall cardiac performance cannot be understated. The rate and extent of relaxation, the viscoelastic properties of LV myocardium, the pericardium, and the structure and function of the left atrium, pulmonary venous circulation, and mitral valve determine the timing, rate, and degree of LV filling. The ability of the LV to adequately collect blood from the low-pressure pulmonary venous circulation is critical in determining the stroke volume that can be transferred to the arterial circulation during systole. Thus, diastolic dysfunction may independently cause heart failure, even in the presence of relatively normal contractile function. This "heart failure with normal systolic function" has been increasingly recognized as a major underlying cause for as many as 50% of patients admitted to the hospital with congestive heart failure.[8,9]

Determinants of Cardiac Output

Cardiac output is the amount of blood pumped by the heart per minute. It is the product of heart rate and stroke volume and may be normalized to the body surface area (cardiac index). Cardiac output (Q) is directly related to pressure (P) and inversely related to peripheral vascular resistance (R) using an equation analogous to Ohm's law: $Q = P/R$. Cardiac output is a function of preload, afterload, myocardial contractility (inotropic state), and heart rate. Preload is defined by LV end-diastolic volume in the intact heart and reflects the stretch of ventricular myofilaments produced by this end-diastolic volume immediately before the onset of contraction. According to Starling's law, the force of LV contraction and volume of blood ejected from the chamber during systole (stroke volume) is directly related to the end-diastolic myofilament length, and hence, the end-diastolic volume.[10,11] Thus, the ventricular myocardium behaves similar to skeletal muscle in that an increase in initial stretch determines the subsequent force of contraction. Afterload may be simplistically represented as the aortic pressure against which the LV must propel blood. The distensibility of the aorta, the resistance of the peripheral arterial vasculature, and the actions of reflected waves on the central aortic circulation are the principle determinants of afterload. Systemic vascular resistance (the ratio of pressure to cardiac output, P/Q) is the most commonly used nonparametric expression of peripheral resistance and is primarily affected by autonomic nervous system activity. For example, an increase in sympathetic nervous system tone produces vasoconstriction of peripheral resistance arterioles through activation of α_1-adrenoceptors in vascular smooth muscle, thereby augmenting afterload. A brief, large increase in afterload may cause a transient decrease in stroke volume, but a compensatory increase in preload during successive cardiac cycles restores cardiac output by increasing LV force of contraction.

Inotropic state is the intrinsic force of myocardial contraction independent of changes in preload, afterload, or heart rate. The number of cross bridges between the contractile elements and the relative sensitivity of the contractile elements to activator Ca^{2+} play important roles in determining inotropic state. In the intact heart, a positive inotropic effect is reflected by an increase in pressure-volume work at each end-diastolic volume. Such an increase in inotropic state may occur in response to an increase in cardiac sympathetic nerve activity through stimulation of β_1-adrenoceptors. Pharmacologic increases in contractility may be produced by drugs that activate β_1-adrenoceptors (e.g., dobutamine) or by those that prevent metabolism of the intracellular second messenger cyclic adenosine monophosphate (cAMP; e.g., milrinone). Cardiac output is also influenced by heart rate. The primary determinant of myocardial oxygen consumption is heart rate because the heart completes an entire cycle with each beat, and hence, the more frequently the heart performs pressure-volume work, the more oxygen must be consumed. The upper and lower limits of heart rate may influence cardiac output. At low heart rates (except in trained athletes), there simply may not be adequate cardiac output to meet the body's oxygen requirements, deliver substrates for metabolism, or remove products of cellular metabolism. In contrast, at high heart rates, particularly in patients with heart disease, there may not be adequate diastolic filling time to maintain cardiac output and coronary artery perfusion, the latter of which is particularly dependent on duration of diastole. Thus, shortened diastolic time during profound tachycardia may reduce stroke volume and cardiac output, contribute to hypotension, and decrease the duration of coronary perfusion. Such events may cause acute myocardial ischemia or infarction.

Measures of Cardiac Function

Clinical indicators of contractile performance include cardiac output, ejection fraction, fractional shortening or area change of the LV short axis, and LV systolic wall thickening. These indices of contractility are heart rate-, preload-, and afterload-dependent, but nevertheless may be measured with reasonable reliability using echocardiographic techniques and remain use-

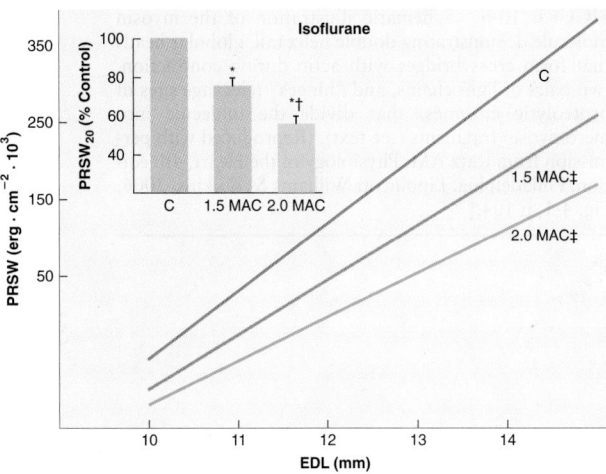

FIGURE 10-5. Preload recruitable stroke work (PRSW) relationship for control (C) and 1.5 and 2 minimal alveolar concentrations (MAC) of isoflurane. PRSW is plotted against end diastolic length (EDL). The inset depicts PRSW done at a constant end-diastolic length of 20 mm (PRSW$_{20}$) and is represented as a percent of control. *Significantly ($p < 0.05$) different than control; †significantly ($p < 0.05$) different than 1.5 MAC isoflurane; ‡significantly ($p < 0.05$) different slope than control. (Reproduced with permission from Pagel PS, Kampine JP, Schmeling WT, Warltier DC: Comparison of end-systolic pressure-length relations and preload recruitable stroke work as indices of myocardial contractility in the conscious and anesthetized, chronically instrumented dog. Anesthesiology 1990; 73: 278.)

ful indices of contractile performance, especially in the presence of chronic heart disease, during recovery after an acute ischemic event, and in patients undergoing cardiac surgery. More sophisticated methods of assessing myocardial contractility in vivo, including the LV end-systolic pressure-volume relations and preload recruitable stroke work, require invasive measurement of continuous LV pressure and volume.[10,12–16] Preload recruitable stroke work and the effects of isoflurane are shown in Figure 10-5. These techniques are usually assessed only in a laboratory setting, but may also be obtained using echocardiography (automated border detection) combined with invasive determination of continuous LV pressure during cardiac catheterization. Discussion of indices of contractile state derived from pressure-volume relations are beyond the scope of the current chapter.

CELLULAR AND MOLECULAR BIOLOGY OF CARDIAC MUSCLE CONTRACTION

Ultrastructure of the Cardiac Myocyte

The heart contracts and relaxes nearly 3 billion times during an average lifetime, based on a heart rate of 70 beats per minute and a life expectancy of 75 years. A review of cardiac myocyte ultrastructure provides important insights into how the heart accomplishes this astonishing performance. The sarcolemma is the external membrane of the cardiac muscle cell. The sarcolemma contains ion channels (e.g., Na^+, K^+, Ca^{2+}), ion pumps and exchangers (e.g., Na^+-K^+ ATPase, Ca^{2+}-ATPase, Na^+-Ca^{2+} or -H^+ exchangers), G protein-coupled and other receptors (e.g., β_1-adrenergic, adenosine, opioid), and transporter enzymes that regulate intracellular ion concentrations, facilitate signal transduction, and provide metabolic substrates

FIGURE 10-6. Schematic illustration of the myosin molecule demonstrating double helix tail, globular heads that form cross bridges with actin during contraction, two pairs of light chains, and "hinges" (cleavage sites of proteolytic enzymes) that divide the molecule into meromyosin fragments (see text). (Reproduced with permission from Katz AM: Physiology of the Heart, 4th edition. Philadelphia, Lippincott Williams & Wilkins, 2006, Fig. 4-1, p 104.)

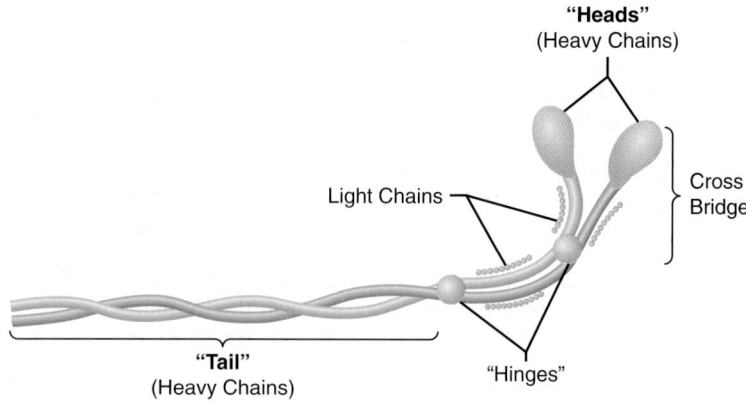

required for energy production. Deep invaginations of the sarcolemma, known as *transverse ("T") tubules*, penetrate the internal structure of the myocyte at regular intervals, thereby assuring rapid, uniform transmission of the depolarizing impulses that initiate contraction to be simultaneously distributed throughout the cell. Unlike the skeletal muscle cell, the cardiac myocyte is densely packed with mitochondria, which are responsible for generation of the large quantities of high-energy phosphates (e.g., adenosine triphosphate [ATP]) required for the heart's phasic cycle of contraction and relaxation. The fundamental contractile unit of cardiac muscle is the sarcomere. The myofilaments within each sarcomere are arranged in parallel cross-striated bundles of thin (containing actin, tropomyosin, and the troponin complex) and thick (primarily composed of myosin and its supporting proteins) fibers. Sarcomeres are connected in series, thereby producing characteristic shortening and thickening of the long and short axes of each myocyte, respectively, during contraction.

The structure of each sarcomere is described based on observations from light and electron microscopy. The area of overlap of thick and thin fibers characterizes the "A" band. This band lengthens as the sarcomere shortens during contraction. The "I" band represents the region of the sarcomere that contains thin filaments alone, and this band is reduced in width as the cell contracts. Each "I" band is bisected by a "Z" (from the German *zuckung* [twitch]) line, which delineates the border between two adjacent sarcomeres. Thus, the length of each sarcomere contains a complete "A" band and two one-half "I" band units located between "Z" lines. A central "M" band is also present within the "A" band and is composed of thick filaments spatially constrained in a cross-sectional hexagonal matrix by myosin binding protein C. An extensively intertwined network of sarcoplasmic reticulum (SR) invests each bundle of contractile proteins and functions as a Ca^{2+} reservoir, thereby assuring homogenous distribution and reuptake of activator Ca^{2+} throughout the myofilaments during contraction and relaxation, respectively. The subsarcolemmal cisternae of the SR are specialized structures located immediately adjacent to, but not continuous with, the sarcolemmal and transverse tubular membranes and contain large numbers of ryanodine receptors that function as the primary Ca^{2+} release channel for the SR. The contractile machinery and the mitochondria that power it occupy >80%, whereas the cytosol and nucleus fill <15%, of the total volume of the cardiac myocyte. It is abundantly clear based on this simple observation that contraction and relaxation, and not new protein synthesis, are the predominant functions of the cardiac myocyte. Intercalated discs mechanically connect adjacent myocytes through the fascia adherens and desmosomes, which link actin and other proteins between cells, respectively. The

intercalated discs also provide a seamless electrical connection between myocytes via large, nonspecific ion channels known as *gap junctions* that facilitate intercellular cytosolic diffusion of ions and small molecules.

Proteins of the Contractile Apparatus

Myosin, actin, tropomyosin, and the three-protein troponin complex compose the six major components of the contractile apparatus. Myosin (molecular weight of approximately 500 kDa; length, 0.17 μm) contains two interwoven chain helices with two globular heads that bind to actin and two additional pairs of light chains. Enzymatic digestion of myosin divides the structure into light (containing the tail section of the complex) and heavy (composed of the globular heads and the light chains) meromyosin. The elongated tail section of the myosin complex functions as the architectural support of the molecule (Fig. 10-6). The globular heads of the myosin dimer contain two "hinges" located at the junction of the distal light chains and the tail helix that play a critical role in myofilament shortening during contraction. These globular structures bind to actin, thereby activating an ATPase that plays a central role in hinge rotation and release of actin during contraction and relaxation, respectively. The maximum velocity of sarcomere shortening has been shown to be dependent on the activity of this actin-activated myosin ATPase. Notably, adult and neonatal atrial and ventricular myocardium contain several different myosin ATPase isoforms that are distinguished by their relative ATPase activity. The myosin molecules are primarily arranged in series along the length of the thick filament, but are abutted "tail-to-tail" in the center of the thick filament. This orientation facilitates shortening of the distance between Z lines during contraction as the thin filaments are drawn progressively toward the center of the sarcomere.

The light chains contained within the myosin complex serve either "regulatory" or "essential" roles. Regulatory myosin light chains may favorably modulate myosin-actin interaction through Ca^{2+}-dependent protein kinase phosphorylation, whereas essential light chains serve an as yet undefined obligate function in myosin activity, as their removal denatures the myosin molecule. Discussion of myosin light chain isoforms is beyond the scope of the current chapter, but isoform switches from ventricular to atrial forms have been observed in left ventricular hypertrophy that may contribute to contractile dysfunction.[17] In addition to myosin and its binding protein, thick filaments contain titin, a long elastic protein that attaches myosin to the Z lines. Titin has been postulated to be a "length sensor" similar to a bidirectional spring that establishes progressively greater passive restoring forces as sarcomere length approaches

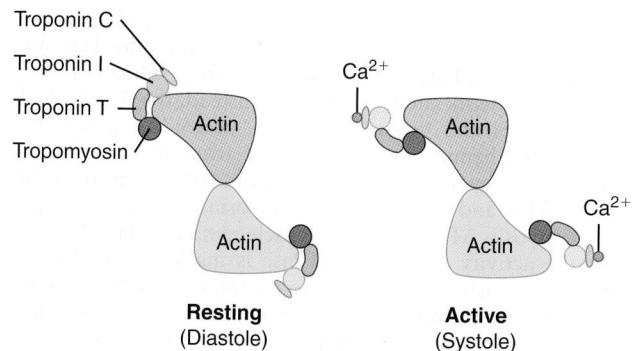

Resting
(Diastole)

Active
(Systole)

FIGURE 10-7. Cross-sectional schematic illustration demonstrating the structural relationship between the troponin-tropomyosin complex and actin under resting conditions (**left**) and after Ca^{2+} binding to troponin C (**right**; see text). (Reproduced with permission from Katz AM: Physiology of the Heart, 4th edition. Philadelphia, Lippincott Williams & Wilkins, 2006, Fig. 4-15, p 117.)

its maximum or minimum.[18] Compression and stretching of titin occur during decreases and increases in muscle load, thereby resisting further sarcomere shortening and lengthening, respectively. Thus, titin is a third important elastic element (in addition to actin and myosin) that contributes to the stress-strain biomechanical properties of cardiac muscle.[19]

Actin is the major component of the thin filament. Actin is a 42-kDa, ovoid-shaped, globular protein ("G" form; 5.5 nm in diameter) that exists in a polymerized filamentous ("F") form in cardiac muscle. F-actin binds adenosine diphosphate (ADP) and a divalent cation (Ca^{2+} or Mg^{2+}), but unlike myosin, the molecule does not directly hydrolyze high-energy nucleotides such as ATP. F-actin is wound in double-stranded helical chains of G-actin monomers that resemble two intertwined strands of pearls (each G-actin monomer; Fig. 10-6). A single complete helical revolution of filamentous actin is approximately 77 nm in length and contains 14 G-actin monomers. Actin derives its name from its function as the "activator" of myosin ATPase through its reversible binding with myosin. The hydrolysis of ATP by this actin-myosin complex provides the chemical energy required to produce the conformational changes in the myosin heads that drive the cycle of contraction and relaxation within the sarcomere. Tropomyosin is one of two major inhibitors of actin-myosin interaction. Tropomyosin (length of 40 nm; weight between 68 and 72 kDa) is a rigid double-stranded α-helix protein linked by a single disulfide bond. Human tropomyosin contains both α and β isoforms (34 and 36 kDa, respectively) and may be present as either a homo- or heterodimer.[20] Tropomyosin stiffens the thin filament through its position within the longitudinal cleft between intertwined F-actin polymers (Fig. 10-7), but its Ca^{2+}-dependent interaction with troponin complex proteins is the mechanism that links sarcolemmal membrane depolarization to actin-myosin interaction in the cardiac myocyte (excitation-contraction coupling). The

thin filaments are anchored to Z lines by cytoskeletal proteins including α- and β-actinin and nebulette.[21,22]

The troponin proteins serve complementary but distinct roles as critical regulators of the contractile apparatus.[23] The troponin complexes are arranged at 40-nm intervals along the length of the thin filament. Troponin C (so named because this molecule binds Ca^{2+}) exists in a highly conserved, single isoform in cardiac muscle. Troponin C is composed of a central nine-turn α-helix separating two globular regions that contain four discrete amino acid sequences capable of binding divalent cations including Ca^{2+} and Mg^{2+}. Of this quartet of amino acid-cation binding sequences, two (termed *sites I and II*) are Ca^{2+}-specific, thereby allowing the troponin C molecule to respond to the acute changes in intracellular Ca^{2+} concentration that accompany contraction and relaxation. Troponin I ("inhibitor") is a 23-kDa protein that exists in a single isoform in cardiac muscle. Troponin I alone weakly prevents the interaction between actin and myosin, but when combined with tropomyosin, the troponin I-tropomyosin complex becomes the major inhibitor of actin-myosin binding. The troponin I molecule contains a serine residue that may be phosphorylated by protein kinase A (PKA) via the intracellular second messenger cAMP, thereby reducing troponin C-Ca^{2+} binding and enhancing relaxation during administration of β-adrenoceptor agonists (e.g., dobutamine) or phosphodiesterase fraction III inhibitors (e.g., milrinone). Troponin T (so denoted because it binds other *t*roponin molecules and *t*ropomyosin) is the largest of the troponin proteins and exists in four major isoforms in human cardiac muscle. Troponin T anchors the other troponin molecules and may also influence the relative Ca^{2+} sensitivity of the complex.[24]

Calcium-Myofilament Interaction

Binding of Ca^{2+} to troponin C precipitates a series of conformational changes in the troponin-tropomyosin complex that lead to the exposure of the myosin binding site on the actin molecule. During conditions in which intracellular Ca^{2+} concentration is low (10^{-7} M; diastole), very little Ca^{2+} is bound to troponin C, and each tropomyosin molecule is constrained to the outer region of the groove between F-actin filaments by a troponin complex (Fig. 10-8). This structural configuration prevents myosin-actin interaction by effectively blocking cross-bridge formation. Thus, an inhibitory state produced by the troponin-tropomyosin complex exists in cardiac muscle under resting conditions. A 100-fold increase in intracellular Ca^{2+} concentration (10^{-5} M; systole) occurs as a consequence of sarcolemmal depolarization, which opens L- and T-type sarcolemmal Ca^{2+} channels, thereby allowing Ca^{2+} influx into the myocyte from the extracellular compartment and stimulating Ca^{2+}-dependent Ca^{2+} release from the SR via its ryanodine receptors. When Ca^{2+} is bound to troponin C under these conditions, the shape of the troponin C protein becomes elongated and its interactions with troponin I and T are enhanced. These Ca^{2+}-induced allosteric rearrangements in troponin complex structure weaken the interaction between troponin I and actin, allow repositioning of the tropomyosin

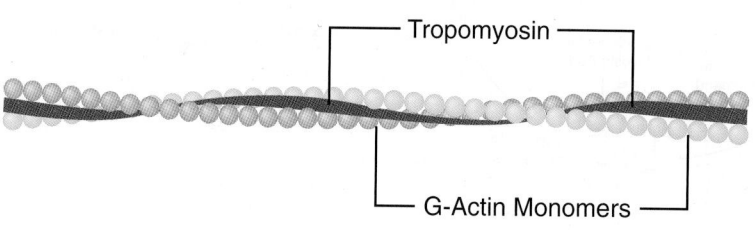

FIGURE 10-8. Schematic illustration demonstrating the location of tropomyosin interlaced within the groove formed by two F-actin chains. (Reproduced with permission from Katz AM: Physiology of the Heart, 4th edition. Philadelphia, Lippincott Williams & Wilkins, 2006, Fig. 4-16, p 108.)

ANATOMY AND PHYSIOLOGY

molecule along the F-actin filaments, and reverse the baseline inhibition of actin-myosin binding by tropomyosin.[25] In this way, Ca^{2+} binding to troponin C may be directly linked to a series of changes in regulatory protein chemical structure that block inhibition of the binding site for myosin on the actin molecule and allow cross-bridge formation and contraction to occur. This antagonism of inhibition is fully reversible, as relaxation is facilitated by dissociation of Ca^{2+} from troponin C concomitant with rapid restoration of the original conformation of the troponin-tropomyosin complex on F-actin.

Most Ca^{2+} ions are removed from the myofilaments and the cytosol after membrane repolarization by a Ca^{2+}-ATPase located in the SR membrane (sarcoendoplasmic reticulum Ca^{2+}-ATPase, SERCA). This Ca^{2+} is stored (concentration of approximately 10^{-3} M) in the SR bound to calsequestrin and calreticulin until the subsequent sarcolemmal depolarization is initiated. The Na^+/Ca^{2+} exchanger and a Ca^{2+}-ATPase located within the sarcolemmal membrane also remove a small quantity of Ca^{2+}, similar to that which originally entered the myocyte from the extracellular space during depolarization. Phospholamban is a small protein (6 kDa) located in the SR membrane that partially inhibits the activity of the dominant form (type 2a) of cardiac SERCA under baseline conditions. However, phosphorylation of this protein by PKA blocks this inhibition and enhances the rate of SERCA uptake of Ca^{2+} into the SR,[26] thereby increasing the rate and extent of relaxation (positive lusitropic effect) and augmenting the amount of Ca^{2+} stored for the next cycle of contraction (positive inotropic effect). Thus, SERCA activity is regulated by a cAMP-dependent PKA that is responsive to β-adrenoceptor stimulation or phosphodiesterase fraction III inhibition. In addition to PKA-mediated phosphorylation of troponin I that facilitates Ca^{2+} release from troponin C, these observations explain why positive inotropic drugs such as dobutamine and milrinone also augment relaxation.

Myosin-Actin Contraction Biochemistry

The biochemistry of cardiac muscle contraction is most often described using a simplified four-component model (Fig. 10-9).[27] Binding of ATP with high affinity to the catalytic domain of myosin initiates the series of chemical and mechanical events that cause contraction of the sarcomere to occur. The myosin ATPase enzyme hydrolyzes the ATP molecule into ADP and inorganic phosphate, but these reaction products do not immediately dissociate from myosin. Instead, the ATP hydrolysis products and myosin form an "active" complex that retains the chemical energy released from the reaction as potential energy. In the absence of actin, subsequent dissociation of ADP and phosphate from myosin is the rate-limiting step of myosin ATPase and the muscle remains relaxed. However, the activity of myosin ATPase is markedly accelerated when the myosin-ADP-phosphate complex is bound to actin, and under these circumstances, the chemical energy obtained from ATP hydrolysis becomes directly transferred into mechanical work. Attachment of myosin to its binding site on the actin molecule releases the phosphate anion from the myosin head, thereby producing a molecular conformation within this cross-bridge structure that generates tension in both myofilaments.[28] Release of ADP and the stored potential energy from this activated conformation produce rotation of the cross-bridge ("power stroke") at the hinge point separating the helix tail region from the globular myosin head and its associated light chain proteins. Each cross-bridge rotation generates 3 to 4×10^{-12} newtons of force[29] and moves myosin approximately 11 nm along the actin molecule. Completion of myosin head rotation and ADP release does not dissociate the myosin-active complex, but leaves it in a low-energy bound ("rigor") state. Separation of myosin and actin occurs when a new ATP molecule binds to myosin, and the process is subsequently repeated, provided that energy supply is adequate and the myosin-binding site on actin remains unimpeded by troponin-tropomyosin inhibition.

Several factors may affect the efficiency of cross-bridge biochemistry and myocardial contractility independent of autonomic nervous system tone or administration of exogenous vasoactive drugs. There is a direct relationship between myosin ATPase activity and the maximal velocity of unloaded muscle shortening (V_{max}), and the normal increase in intracellular Ca^{2+} concentration (from 10^{-7} to 10^{-5} M) that occurs after sarcolemmal depolarization enhances baseline myosin ATPase activity fivefold before it interacts with actin, thereby increasing V_{max}. Contractile force depends on sarcomere length immediately before sarcolemmal depolarization. This

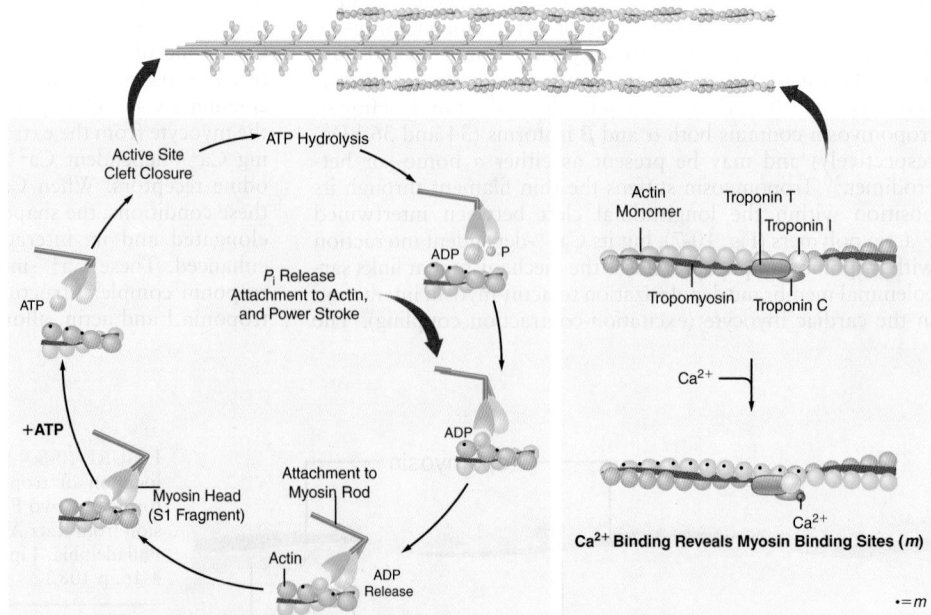

FIGURE 10-9. Schematic illustration of the actin filaments and its individual monomers and active myosin bindings sites (*m*; **left panel**). The myosin head is dissociated from actin by binding with adenosine triphosphate (ATP). Subsequent ATP hydrolysis and release of inorganic phosphate (*P_i*) "cocks" the head group into a tension-generating configuration. Attachment of the myosin head to actin allows the head to apply tension to the myosin rod and the actin filament. The **right panel** illustrates calcium binding to troponin C, which causes troponin I to decrease its affinity for actin. As a result in a conformational shift in tropomyosin position (see text), seven sites on actin monomers are revealed.

length-dependent activation (Frank-Starling effect) may be related to an increase in myofilament sensitivity to Ca^{2+}, favorable alterations in spacing between myofilaments, or titin-induced elastic recoil. Abrupt increases in load during contraction (Anrep effect) or those that occur after a prolonged pause between beats (Woodworth phenomenon) causes transient increases in contractile force through a length-dependent activation mechanism. An increase in cardiac muscle stimulation frequency also augments contractile force (treppe phenomenon) via enhanced myofilament Ca^{2+} sensitivity and greater SR Ca^{2+} release.

ELECTRICAL PROPERTIES OF THE HEART

The Clinical Electrocardiogram

The clinical electrocardiogram (ECG) consists of a regular series of deflections from the isoelectric line. The first deflection of the ECG is the P wave (Einthoven began his depiction of the ECG in the middle of the alphabet). The P wave is a positive deflection that occurs as a consequence of atrial depolarization. The initial electrical event is depolarization of the sinoatrial (SA) node pacemaker cells and is followed almost immediately by progressive depolarization of both atria. The SA node pacemaker activity is not observed on the ECG because the node is too small to generate electrical potential differences large enough to be recorded from the body surface. The duration of the P wave is the time required for depolarization to spread over the atria and may be prolonged by atrial enlargement or a conduction delay. The SA node is located in the wall of the right atrium at the junction of this chamber and the superior vena cava. Propagation of the depolarizing impulse throughout the atria is not uniform, as a slightly higher conduction velocity occurs through the anterior, middle, and posterior internodal pathways between the SA and the AV nodes. Activation and depolarization of the AV node begins during the P wave before depolarization of the atria is completed (Fig. 10-10).[7,30,31]

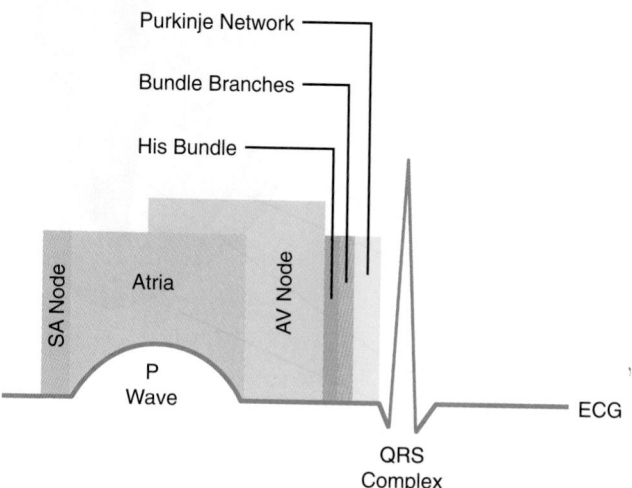

FIGURE 10-10. The electrocardiogram (ECG). Major waves (P, QRS, and T) of the ECG are indicated as well as the timing of the activation of some of the key conductive structures. SA, sinoatrial. (Reproduced with permission from Katz AM: Physiology of the Heart, 4th edition. Philadelphia, Lippincott Williams & Wilkins, 2006, Fig. 15-10, p 436.)

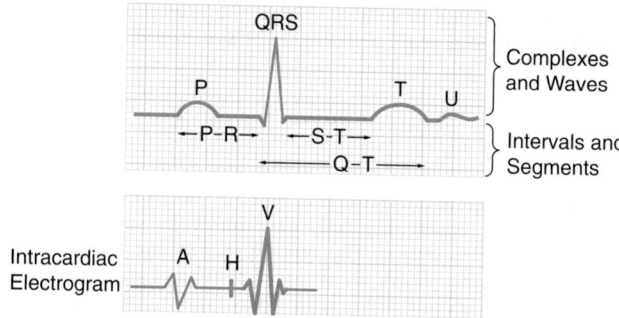

FIGURE 10-11. Top: Electrocardiogram recorded from the body surface. Bottom: Intracardiac electrogram. (Reproduced with permission from Katz AM: Physiology of the Heart, 4th edition. Philadelphia, Lippincott Williams & Wilkins, 2006, Fig. 15-9, p 435.)

The P wave is followed by a brief interval returning to the isoelectric line. The PR interval is the duration between the onset of the P wave and the beginning of ventricular depolarization signified by the onset of the QRS complex (Fig. 10-11). Prolongation of the PR interval usually indicates a conduction delay between atrial and ventricular conduction. After the P wave is complete, the ECG becomes isoelectric because changing potential differences within the heart are no longer recorded at the body surface as a result of the relatively small mass of tissue that continues the depolarization-conduction process. During this apparent "silent" interval between atrial and ventricular depolarization, the wave of depolarization is being conducted through the AV node, AV bundle, right and left bundle branches, and His-Purkinje fiber network. The conduction velocity through the AV node is relatively slow. In contrast, conduction velocity is very rapid in the His-Purkinje system (H in Fig. 10-11), approaching the velocity observed in small nerves. The QRS complex records potentials at the body surface when the wave of depolarization is distributed throughout ventricular myocardium. The QRS complex is much larger in magnitude than the P wave because ventricular mass is greater than the atrial mass. Rapid conduction through the His-Purkinje system spreads the wave of depolarization quickly to the ventricles. Delays in this conduction distal to the AV node most often result from intrinsic myocardial disease (most notably, ischemia) and may have profound consequences on cardiac rhythm and LV contractile synchrony.

The ST segment is the interval between the end of the QRS complex and the T wave. The ST segment is normally isoelectric because all of the ventricular myocardium is depolarized. The ST segment also reflects the long plateau phase of the cardiac action potential. The injury current of an elevated or depressed ST segment observed during myocardial ischemia or infarction may occur as a result of an abbreviated action potential within the ischemic region or because depolarizing currents propagate more slowly through the ischemic zone. Repolarization of the ventricles generates the T wave, which corresponds to the end of phase 2 and all of phase 3 of the cardiac action potential (see later discussion). The duration of the T wave is considerably longer than the QRS complex because, unlike the rapidly transmitted, nearly homogenous ventricular depolarization, repolarization occurs more slowly and is less synchronous. The QT interval is the duration between the onset of ventricular depolarization (indicated by the QRS complex) and completion of repolarization (as signified by the end of the T wave). The QT interval varies inversely with heart rate, and may precipitate malignant ventricular arrhythmias when shortened or prolonged by administration of vasoactive drugs (e.g., volatile anesthetics) or in the presence of intrinsic cardiac pathology (e.g., prolonged QT syndrome).[30,31]

Role of Ion Channels

The action potentials of individual groups of excitable cardiac myocytes are quite different (Fig. 10-12). The SA and AV nodes and accessory pacemaker cells have unstable, spontaneously depolarizing properties. The resting membrane potential of these cells is not –90 mV, as observed in typical atrial and ventricular myocytes or His-Purkinje fibers. Spontaneous, phase 4 slow depolarization of SA and AV node cells is initiated at membrane potentials between –55 and –66 mV. The SA node, AV node, and the remaining specialized conduction tissue of the heart are all characterized as potential pacemakers, but the SA node is the normal cardiac pacemaker because of its intrinsically faster discharge rate. Cells within the SA node are not homogenous, and some of these pacemaker cells have faster discharge frequencies than others. The resting membrane potential of cardiac pacemaker cells is unstable and displays a slow depolarization of the membrane during diastole (Fig. 10-12). The rate of rise of the action potential from threshold (phase 1) is relatively slow in SA nodal cells compared with atrial and ventricular muscle cells. The magnitude and slope of spontaneous depolarization (also known as *automaticity*) of SA node cells are important in the regulation of heart rate and depend on the activity of the sympathetic and vagal (parasympathetic) neural innervation. Slowing the rate of depolarization increases the time to reach the threshold potential (TP) and decreases heart rate (SA node rate of discharge; Fig. 10-13). The heart rate may also slow as a result of a shift in threshold potential to a higher level (TP1 to TP2) or a more negative resting potential.[2] These effects are usually observed during vagal stimulation via parasympathetic nerve or administration of acetylcholine agonists. In contrast, a sharp rise in the diastolic depolarization of the pacemaker cell (resulting in tachycardia) occurs during stimulation of the cardiac sympathetic nerves or administration of exogenous catecholamines. The SA node pacemaker may be displaced by a latent pacemaker elsewhere in the heart during myocardial ischemia because of primary suppression of the SA node or because of spontaneous discharge of a latent pacemaker at a higher intrinsic rate. When the frequency of excitation is higher in a group of latent pacemakers, the rate of firing of the other pacemakers is suppressed. This process is known as *overdrive suppression*.

The ion channels that are active in the SA node cell membrane during depolarization and repolarization are depicted in Figure 10-14.[7] Two decreasing outward currents and two increasing inward currents are observed during depolarization.

FIGURE 10-12. Cardiac action potentials throughout the conductance system from the sinoatrial node (SA) through the ventricular muscle during one cardiac cycle. Note the automatic pacemaker activity (slow spontaneous depolarization) of the SA and atrioventricular nodal cells and the lack of spontaneous activity of atrial, Purkinje, and ventricular muscle cells. (Reproduced with permission from Lynch C III, Lake CL: Cardiovascular anatomy and physiology, Cardiac Vascular, and Thoracic Anesthesia. Edited by Youngberg JA, Lake CL, Roizen MF, Wilson RS. New York, Churchill Livingstone, 1999, p 87.)

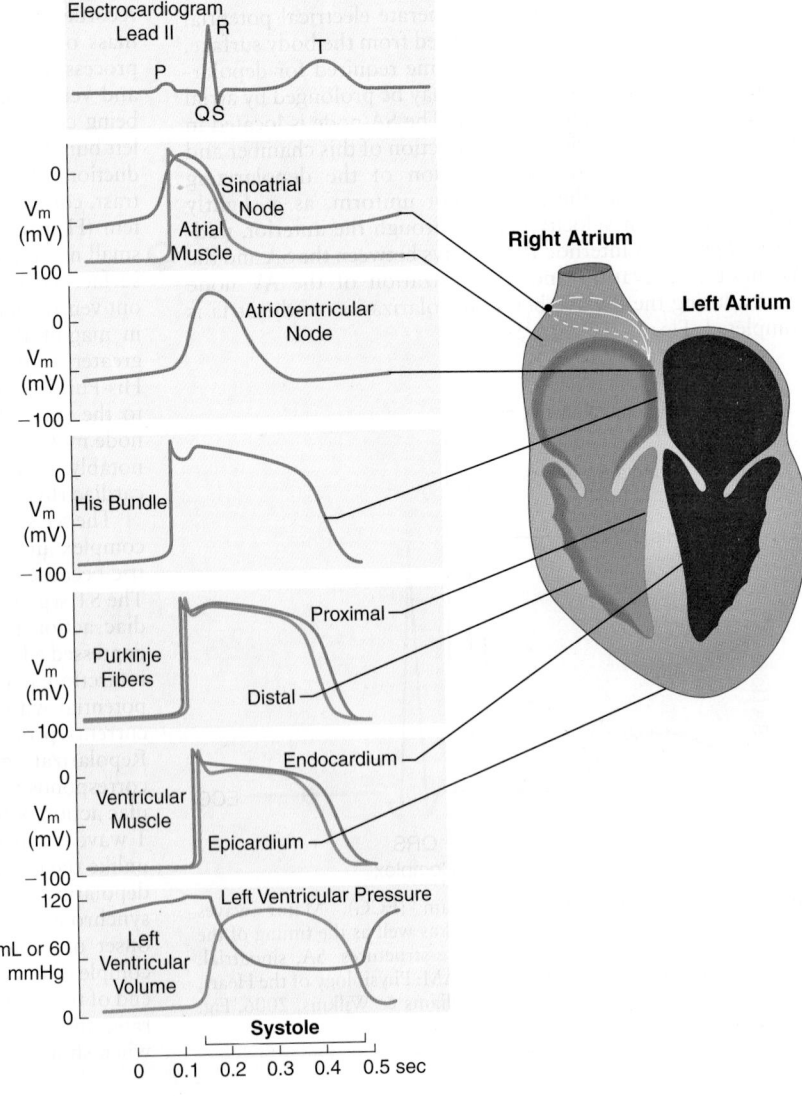

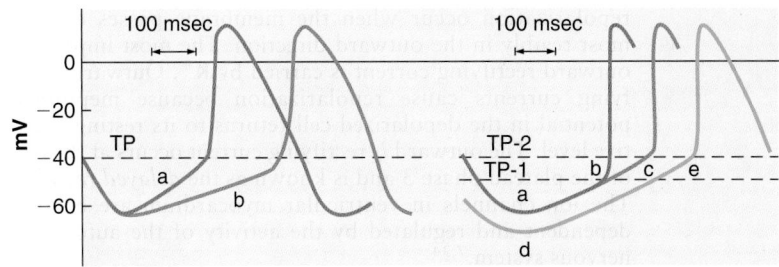

FIGURE 10-13. Pacemaker potentials in sinoatrial node illustrating the effect of diastolic depolarization slopes and potentials on heart rate. The action potential begins when the depolarization potential reaches the threshold potential (TP). A slowing of the rate of depolarization from *a* to *b* increases the time required to reach the TP, whereas an increase of the TP level (*b, c*) or a greater resting potential (*d*) slows the heart rate. (Reproduced with permission from Hoffman BF, Cranefield PF: Electrophysiology of the Heart. New York, McGraw-Hill. 1960, Fig. 4.5, p 57.)

Pacemaker activity is partly due to decay of the delayed rectifier current (i_K, an outward current), which is permissive by allowing other currents to depolarize the pacemaker. An anomalous rectifier current (i_{k1}, a second outward current) also permissively contributes to pacemaker activity. The first inward current is i_{Ca}. This slow inward Ca^{2+} current is primarily responsible for the action potential upstroke in pacemaker cells, and its continuation after initial depolarization contributes to early diastolic depolarization. The inward Na^+ current (i_f) most likely plays an important role in the control of heart rate by the autonomic nervous system. This inward i_f current occurs through a channel that conducts both Na^+ and Ca^{2+} ions. This "f" or "funny" channel mediates autonomic-dependent modulation of heart rate.[33] The inward current i_f is activated by cAMP. Thus, β_1-adrenergic stimulation accelerates, whereas vagal stimulation slows, heart rate by increasing and decreasing, respectively, the intracellular cAMP concentration and the degree of activation of the f channel. The f channel is thought to be responsible for generating spontaneous activity.

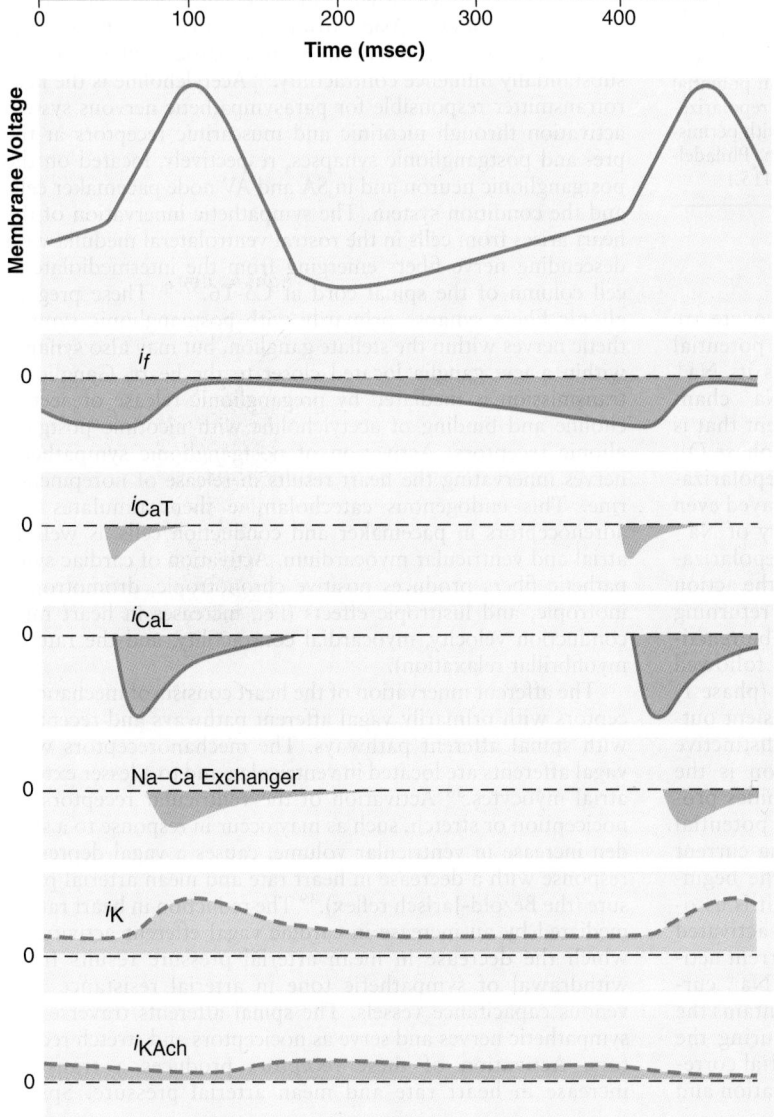

Time (msec)

FIGURE 10-14. Changes in four ionic currents responsible for action potential depolarization and repolarization in a sinoatrial nodal pacemaker cell. Two are increasing inward currents (i_i and i_{Ca}) and two are decreasing outward currents (i_K, delayed rectifier and i_{K1}, inward rectifier). (Reproduced with permission from Katz AM: Physiology of the Heart, 4th edition. Philadelphia, Lippincott Williams & Wilkins, 2006, Fig. 14-14, p 417.)

ANATOMY AND PHYSIOLOGY

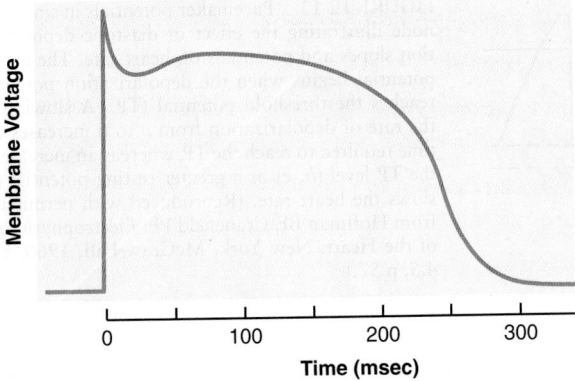

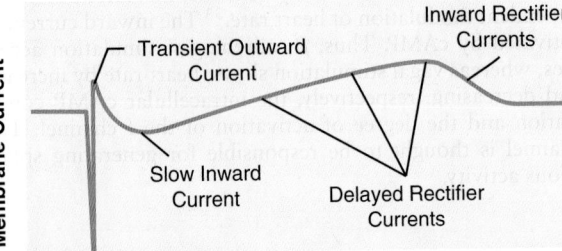

FIGURE 10-15. Membrane potential and current in a voltage-clamped ventricular cell. Note that the rapid and transient influx of Na$^+$ ions induces the rapid depolarization (phase 0); this is followed by a longer inward Ca^{2+} current that prolongs the plateau potential (phase 1) and then a slow outward K$^+$ current the leads to repolarization (phase 3). Resting potential is phase 4. (Reproduced with permission from Katz AM: Physiology of the Heart, 4th edition. Philadelphia, Lippincott Williams & Wilkins, 2006, Fig. 14-12, p 415.)

Alterations in ion currents in the ventricular myocyte are illustrated in Figure 10-15. The resting membrane potential of the myocyte is –90 mV; this potential controls its Na$^+$ channel. Above this threshold, activation of the Na$^+$ channel produces a sharp increase in inward Na$^+$ current that is primarily responsible for myocyte depolarization (phase O). These Na$^+$ channels are rapidly inactivated by depolarization, but their ability to reopen (reactivation) is delayed even after the myocyte is fully repolarized. The inability of Na$^+$ channels to respond to a second stimulus after depolarization occurs as a result of the prolonged plateau of the action potential that prevents membrane potential from returning to the resting levels at which Na$^+$ channels may be reactivated. The rapid depolarization of the myocyte is followed by a brief, rapid repolarization of small magnitude (phase 1) caused by a reduction in Na$^+$ permeability, a transient outward K$^+$ current, and an outward Cl$^-$ current. A distinctive feature of ventricular myocardium depolarization is the plateau (phase 2) of the action potential that signifies prolonged stabilization of the myocyte near zero potential (duration ≥100 ms). An inward Ca^{2+} depolarizing current through Ca^{2+} conductance channels appears at the beginning of the plateau. This slow inward Ca^{2+} current is associated with opening of slow Ca^{2+} channels that are activated at a membrane potential of −50 mV. The Ca^{2+} current activates and inactivates much more slowly than the Na$^+$ current, thereby providing an inward current that maintains the sarcolemmal membrane in a depolarized state during the plateau phase. Phase 3 of the cardiac action potential corresponds to the T wave of the ECG. Outward rectification and

repolarization occur when the membrane passes current most readily in the outward direction. The most important outward rectifying current is carried by K$^+$. Outward rectifying currents cause repolarization because membrane potential in the depolarized cell returns to its resting negative level. The outward i_k rectifying current occurs at the end of the plateau phase 3 and is known as the *delayed rectifier*. The ion channels in ventricular myocardium are energy-dependent and regulated by the activity of the autonomic nervous system.[7,34]

NEURAL INNERVATION OF THE HEART AND BLOOD VESSELS

Baroreflex Regulation of Blood Pressure

The heart is innervated by the parasympathetic and the sympathetic nervous systems. Parasympathetic innervation arises in the motor nucleus of the vagus and the nucleus ambiguous in the medulla.[35] As observed with other parasympathetic nerves, long preganglionic fibers synapse with short postganglionic fibers within the heart. The postganglionic fibers innervate pacemaker cells and conducting pathways. When activated, these fibers produce slowing of pacemaker cells and reduce conduction velocity. Aside from their effects on heart rate, excitability, and conduction, parasympathetic fibers do not substantially influence contractility.[36] Acetylcholine is the neurotransmitter responsible for parasympathetic nervous system activation through nicotinic and muscarinic receptors at the pre- and postganglionic synapses, respectively, located on the postganglionic neuron and in SA and AV node pacemaker cells and the condition system. The sympathetic innervation of the heart arises from cells in the rostral ventrolateral medulla with descending nerve fibers emerging from the intermediolateral cell column of the spinal cord at C5-T6.[37,38] These preganglionic fibers synapse primarily with postganglionic sympathetic nerves within the stellate ganglion, but may also synapse within a few ganglia located closer to the heart. Ganglionic transmission is mediated by preganglionic release of acetylcholine and binding of acetylcholine with nicotinic postganglionic receptors. Activation of postganglionic sympathetic nerves innervating the heart results in release of norepinephrine. This endogenous catecholamine then stimulates β$_1$-adrenoceptors in pacemaker and conduction cells as well as atrial and ventricular myocardium. Activation of cardiac sympathetic fibers produces positive chronotropic, dromotropic, inotropic, and lusitropic effects (i.e., increases in heart rate, conduction velocity, myocardial contractility, and the rate of myofibrillar relaxation).

The afferent innervation of the heart consists of mechanoreceptors with primarily vagal afferent pathways and receptors with spinal afferent pathways. The mechanoreceptors with vagal afferents are located in ventricular, and to a lesser extent, atrial myocytes.[36] Activation of the ventricular receptors by nociception or stretch, such as may occur in response to a sudden increase in ventricular volume, causes a vagal depressor response with a decrease in heart rate and mean arterial pressure (the Bezold-Jarisch reflex).[39] The reduction in heart rate is mediated by an increase in cardiac vagal efferent activity, in which the decrease in mean arterial pressure results from withdrawal of sympathetic tone in arterial resistance and venous capacitance vessels. The spinal afferents traverse the sympathetic nerves and serve as nociceptors and stretch receptors. Activation of these receptors produces a transient increase in heart rate and mean arterial pressure. Spinal afferent-mediated nociceptors may be stimulated by events such as acute myocardial ischemia. Both the cardiac vagal and spinal afferent fibers project centrally to the nucleus tractus solitarius, similar to aortic and carotid baroreceptors and chemoreceptors.

The majority of the peripheral vascular system derives its sympathetic innervation from the thoracolumbar section of the spinal cord. In contrast, the sympathetic innervation of the coronary vasculature, lung, and cerebral circulation is derived from the superior cervical and stellate ganglia. α-Adrenoceptors mediate most sympathetic nerve vascular responses, but β-adrenoceptors uniquely modulate sympathetic innervation of the adrenal gland, thereby causing the release of epinephrine and norepinephrine. Sympathetic innervation of small arterioles and metarterioles produces vasoconstriction, thereby increasing systemic vascular resistance and mean arterial pressure. Sympathetic innervation of small veins and venules causes constriction of these vessels. This action reduces the volume of blood stored in capacitance vessels, transiently increases preload, and subsequently decreases blood flow in the splanchnic circulation and, to a lesser extent, the lower extremities. Thus, activation of peripheral sympathetic nerves increases mean arterial pressure by arterial vasoconstriction combined with an increase in preload due to a reduction in venous capacitance while simultaneously increasing heart rate and myocardial contractility. These effects are critical compensatory responses to hypovolemia resulting from acute blood loss. α- and β-adrenoceptor antagonists may attenuate sympathetically mediated cardiovascular effects.

10 Short-duration regulation of mean arterial pressure occurs through the arterial, and to a lesser extent, intracardiac baroreceptors. Arterial baroreceptors are located at the bifurcation of the common carotid arteries and in the aortic arch. These receptors, particularly those in the carotid arteries, display tonic activity under normal conditions. An acute rise in arterial pressure activates baroreceptors through stretch-sensitive Na^+ channels. Receptor activation increases afferent nerve traffic in the carotid sinus nerve, which is centrally transmitted by a unique branch of the glossopharyngeal nerve that first synapses in the nucleus tractus solitarius. The postsynaptic neurons activate the vagal motor nucleus and nucleus ambiguous, thereby causing a reduction in heart rate.[38,40,41] The postsynaptic baroreceptor neurons also synapse with γ-aminobutyric acid–mediated inhibitory neurons in the caudal ventrolateral medulla that innervate medullary sympathetic neurons and produce a decrease in sympathetic nervous system activity via the rostral ventrolateral medulla.[38,41,42] The resultant effect is a decrease in cardiac output and systemic vascular resistance concomitant with an increase in vascular capacitance.

The aortic baroreceptors and cardiac vagal receptors produce similar hemodynamic effects. Cardiac receptors have been theorized to be responsible for radiocontrast-induced bradycardia and hypotension during coronary angiography. Low-pressure baroreceptors located in the vena cavae, right atrium, RV, and pulmonary vein-left atrial junction respond to decreases in right atrial filling pressure by activating sympathetic tone in the arterial vasculature. Interestingly, baroreceptor activation does not influence all peripheral vascular beds. For example, the cutaneous circulation does not appear to respond to baroreceptor stimulation or inhibition. Instead, the cutaneous circulation is primarily affected by peripheral and central thermoregulatory mechanisms that produce vasoconstriction or vasodilation in a cold or warm environment to prevent or facilitate heat loss, respectively. Thermoreceptor-mediated central nervous system responses originate in the supraoptic region of the hypothalamus.

Other Cardiovascular Reflexes

Other reflexogenic areas within the cardiovascular system regulate hemodynamics through arterial chemoreceptors and the central nervous system response to ischemia. High-pressure sensitive receptors in the LV and low-pressure responsive elements in the atria and RV consist of stretch-induced mechanoreceptors that respond to pressure or volume changes. Three sets of receptors have been identified. First, discrete receptors in the endocardium are located at the junctions of the vena cavae with the right atrium and the pulmonary veins with the left atrium. These receptors activate myelinated vagal afferent fibers that project to the nucleus tractus solitarius and increase sympathetic nerve activity to the SA node but not to the ventricles, thereby increasing heart rate but not contractility. Distention of these mechanoreceptors also increases renal excretion of free water by inhibition of antidiuretic hormone secretion from the posterior lobe of the pituitary gland.[43] It appears highly likely that the Bainbridge reflex may be mediated by distention of these mechanoreceptors.[4] Second, a diffuse receptor network is distributed throughout the cardiac chambers that projects via unmyelinated vagal afferent neurons to the nucleus tractus solitarius. These receptors behave like the carotid and aortic mechanoreceptors and produce a vasodepressor response consisting of vagus activation concomitant with inhibition of sympathetic innervation of the heart and peripheral circulation. These actions cause reductions in heart rate, inotropic state, and systemic vascular resistance concomitant with a simultaneous increase in venous capacitance. This intracardiac receptor network plays a relatively minor role in the normal physiological control of the cardiovascular system compared with the arterial baroreceptors. Lastly, sympathetic afferent fibers are activated by receptors that respond rhythmically during the cardiac cycle. Some of these neurons convey visceral pain sensations and may be activated during myocardial ischemia. Stimulation of these fibers produces a transient increase in heart rate and mean arterial pressure by activating central nervous system sympathetic efferent fibers innervating the heart and peripheral circulation.[4,44,45]

The arterial baroreceptors located in the carotid sinus and aortic arch play the major role in cardiovascular homeostasis. Arterial baroreceptor reflex-induced regulation of heart rate is inhibited by volatile and many intravenous anesthetics.[32,46] This inhibition of high-pressure baroreceptor reflexes by anesthetics involves several discrete sites including sympathetic ganglionic transmission, end-organ responses, and central nervous system pathways, and appears to be especially important in short-term regulation of arterial pressure.[5,47] These reflexes demonstrate accommodation or adaptation to the level of arterial blood pressure and may be reset in patients with hypertension. Cardiopulmonary reflexes also appear to be inhibited by potent inhaled anesthetics and have a crucial role in short-term regulation of arterial pressure, primarily by modulating arterial baroreceptor reflex activity.[32] The peripheral chemoreceptors located in the carotid and aortic bodies are sensitive to increases in arterial CO_2 tension and decreases in pH. The carotid body receptors project centrally through Herring's nerve, which travels with the glossopharyngeal nerve to the nucleus tractus solitarius. In contrast, the aortic body receptors have vagal afferent fibers that also project to the nucleus tractus solitarius. The carotid body reflex appears to be more important than its aortic counterpart in the regulation of respiration in humans. Activation of the carotid and aortic chemoreceptors produces an increase in respiratory drive manifested by an increase in respiratory rate, tidal volume, and minute ventilation. These chemoreceptors may also cause activation of sympathetic nervous system fibers in the heart and peripheral circulation, thereby increasing heart rate and mean arterial pressure. The peripheral chemoreceptor reflex is an important protective mechanism in response to pathophysiological conditions including high-altitude hypoxia, chronic lung disease, and profound hypovolemia.

In addition to the baroreceptor responses, severe hypotension also causes arterial vaso- and venoconstriction in response to brainstem hypoxia. This central nervous system ischemic response may be activated when mean arterial pressure is reduced below 50 mm Hg. An analogous mechanism may also mediate the Cushing reflex. This sympathetically mediated hypertension occurs in response to an acute elevation of intracranial pressure and a consequent reduction in cerebral perfusion pressure. Under these circumstances, arterial pressure rises progressively in an effort to exceed elevated intracranial pressure and maintain cerebral perfusion and oxygen delivery. The Cushing reflex may also be activated by brainstem compression, acute traumatic brain injury, or intracranial hemorrhage resulting from aneurysm rupture.

In animals, the diving reflex redistributes blood flow and oxygen delivery to the heart and brain as a survival defense of the submerged vertebrate against asphyxia. This reflex enables whales to remain submerged for as long as 2 hours. The residual counterpart of the diving reflex in humans may be activated by immersion of the face in cold water, which produces a comparable, albeit less intense, diving response characterized by rapid reduction in heart rate and cutaneous and skeletal muscle blood flow concomitant with an increase in arterial pressure. Stimulation of receptors in the face or upper airway initiates the diving reflex and causes apnea by inhibiting the medullary respiratory center. The hyperventilation stimuli of hypoxemia and hypercapnia are also suppressed. The cardiovascular limbs of the chemoreceptor reflex are partially retained, resulting in generalized systemic vasoconstriction, except in the coronary and cerebral circulations. The diving reflex response is distinctly different from the cold-pressor reflex. This latter reflex is activated by complete immersion of one hand in ice water. The cold-pressor reflex increases heart rate and mean arterial pressure by stimulating both pain and cold receptors. A cold environment directly causes vasoconstriction to prevent heat loss and also stimulates reflex central nervous system thermoregulatory receptors in the hypothalamic preoptic region. This latter effect produces sympathetically mediated vasoconstriction. A warm, ambient environment or an increase in metabolically induced heat production produces an opposite response to dissipate accumulated heat.

Somatic pain increases heart rate and mean arterial pressure by activation of sympathetic efferent nerves. In contrast, visceral pain or distention of a hollow viscus (e.g., small intestine, bladder) may produce reflex vagal bradycardia and hypotension. The oculocardiac reflex is activated by pressure on the ocular globe and causes pronounced bradycardia and hypotension by activation of vagal nerve fibers innervating the SA node. The Valsalva maneuver consists of forced expiration against a closed glottis. This maneuver reduces venous return to the right heart, decreases cardiac output and mean arterial pressure, and increases heart rate. The reflex tachycardia occurs because of reduced activity of arterial baroreceptors and LV mechanoreceptors. Release of the forced expiration by glottic opening acutely increases venous return, cardiac output, and mean arterial pressure while simultaneously causing reflex bradycardia mediated by vagal innervation of the SA node triggered by the arterial baroreceptors.

CORONARY CIRCULATION

Anatomy of the Coronary Arterial and Venous Systems

The heart is the only organ that furnishes its own blood supply. The left main and right coronary arteries arise from the aorta behind the left and right aortic valve leaflets (Fig. 10-16). The coronary ostia remain patent throughout systole because eddy currents prevent the valve leaflets from contacting the aortic walls. The left main coronary artery divides almost immediately into the left anterior descending (LAD) artery and left circumflex coronary artery (LCCA). The LAD further divides into several branches along the anterior interventricular groove toward the apex of the heart where they supply the anterior wall of the LV and the anterior two thirds of the

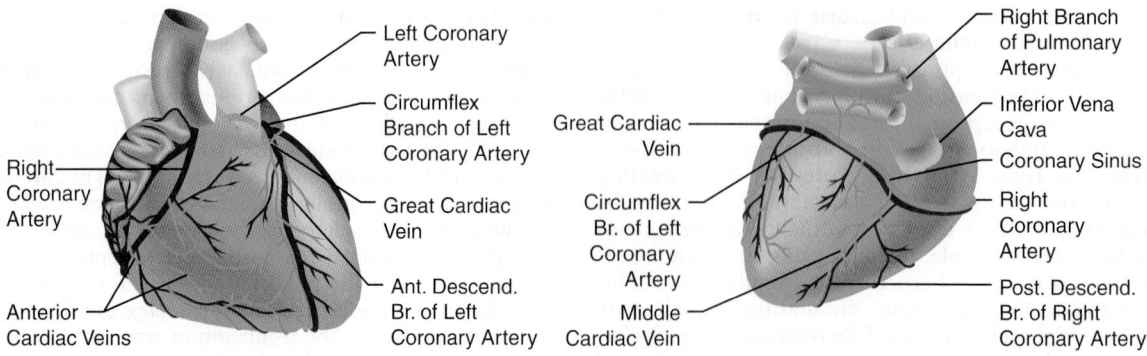

FIGURE 10-16. Anterior view (**left**) shows right coronary and left anterior descending arteries. Posterior view (**right**) shows left circumflex and posterior descending arteries. Note that the right coronary or left circumflex artery may form the latter artery. The anterior cardiac veins from the right ventricle and the coronary sinus, which drain primarily the left ventricle, empty into the right atrium. (Reproduced with permission from Smith JJ, Kampine JP: Circulatory Physiology—The Essentials, 3rd edition. Baltimore, Williams & Wilkins, 1990, Fig. 3-1, p 32.)

interventricular septum (Fig. 10-16). The LCCA marks a pathway along the base of the LV within the coronary sulcus and terminates in the left posterior descending branch. The LCCA supplies the LV lateral wall and part of the LV posterior wall. The right coronary artery (RCA) courses along the AV groove toward the right chambers of the heart and frequently extends along the posterior interventricular sulcus to give rise to the right posterior descending branch (Fig. 10-16). The RCA supplies the anterior and posterior walls of the RV except for the apex (supplied by the LAD), the right atrium including the SA node, the upper half of the atrial septum, the posterior third of the interventricular septum, the inferior wall of the LV, the AV node, and the posterior base of the LV. A branch of the LCCA occasionally supplies the SA node. Because either the RCA or the LCCA may supply the posterior descending coronary artery, the coronary circulation is described as right or left dominant, respectively, based on the source of this vessel's blood supply.

The proximal branches of the RCA, LCCA, and LAD are located on the epicardial surface of the heart and give rise to multiple intramural vessels that penetrate perpendicularly or obliquely deep into the ventricular walls. Except for the thin tissue layer on the endocardial surface, the nutritive blood supply is almost entirely derived from these major coronary arteries. The penetrating branches divide into dense capillary networks located roughly along the courses of the myocardial bundles. Arterial branches with diameters between 50 and 500 μm form interconnecting anastomoses throughout the endocardium of the ventricular walls (Fig. 10-17, A and B). Another network of subendocardial vessels between 100 and 200 μm in diameter forms a plexus of deep anastomoses. A coronary collateral circulation may also arise from different branches of the same coronary artery or from branches of two different coronary arteries. Flow through such coronary collaterals is usually negligible because the driving pressure at the two ends of the anastomoses is nearly equal. However, if the artery supplying one branch of this collateral circulation becomes severely stenotic or occluded, the large pressure reduction will divert blood flow through the patent artery and into the distribution of the occluded artery through these collateral vessels. Thus, the coronary collateral circulation may be especially important to patients with coronary artery disease.[48–50]

Most of the coronary venous system remains unnamed with the exception of the great cardiac vein (that runs along the AV groove and the LAD), the anterior cardiac vein (located with the RCA), and the middle cardiac vein (associated with the posterior descending branch of the RCA; Fig. 10-16). Thus, the main coronary venous drainage tends to retrace the course of the major coronary arteries along the AV and interventricular grooves. In general, there are two coronary veins located along either side of each coronary arterial branch. The coronary veins converge and terminate in the coronary sinus, which empties into the posterior aspect of the right atrium. Approximately 85% of the total coronary blood flow to the LV drains into the coronary sinus. The remaining blood flow empties directly into the atrial and ventricular cavities by the thebesian veins. The RV veins drain into the anterior cardiac veins; these empty individually into the right atrium just above the tricuspid valve.

Coronary Microcirculation

The coronary capillary network has an organizational structure that is similar to that observed in other tissue beds. Myocardium has a very high density of capillary blood vessels to myofibrils, approximately 1:1 (Fig. 10-18); this is because of the exceptionally high metabolic demand of the heart. On

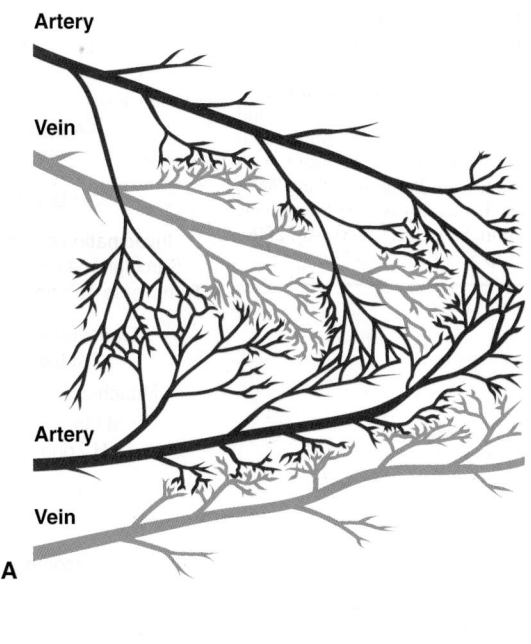

Artery

Vein

Artery

Vein

A

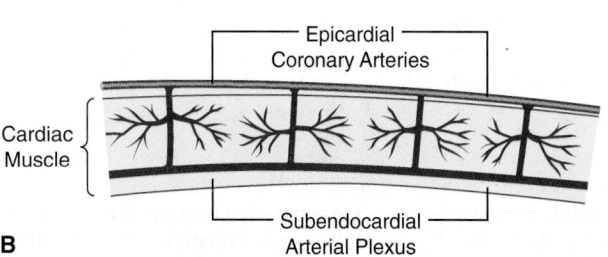

Epicardial
Coronary Arteries

Cardiac
Muscle

Subendocardial
Arterial Plexus

B

FIGURE 10-17.   **A.** Diagram of the minute arterial-to-arterial and venous-to-venous anastomoses of the coronary arterial system, which allows diversion of flow if one distribution becomes blocked. (Reproduced with permission from Guyton AC, Hall JE: Human Physiology and Mechanisms of Disease, 6th edition. Philadelphia, WB Saunders, 1997, Fig. 18-4, pp 185.) **B.** Diagram of the epicardial coronary vessels lying on the cardiac muscle surface, the penetrating deep vessels, and the subendocardial arterial plexus connecting the deep vessels. (Reproduced with permission from Guyton AC: Textbook of Medical Physiology, 6th edition. Philadelphia, WB Saunders, 1997, Fig. 25-3, p 299.)

average, adjacent capillaries are separated by the diameter of approximately one myocyte. The distribution of capillaries is quite uniform and ranges between 3,000 and 4,000/mm² of tissue. Interestingly, capillary density is reduced in the interventricular septum and AV nodal tissue, and this observation may explain why the specialized conducting system is more vulnerable to ischemia than the myocardium itself. As in other capillary beds, coronary capillaries are the sites for exchange of O_2, CO_2, and for the movement of larger molecules across the endothelial cell lining, where it is devoid of vascular smooth muscle.

Mechanics of Coronary Blood Flow

⑪ Blood supply to the LV is directly dependent on the difference between the aortic pressure and LV end-diastolic pressure (coronary perfusion pressure) and inversely related to the vascular resistance to flow, which varies to the fourth power of the radius of the vessel (Poiseuille's law). Two other determinants of coronary flow are vessel length and viscosity of the

FIGURE 10-18.   Diagram of an electron micrograph of cardiac muscle showing large numbers of mitochondria and the intercalated disks with nexi (gap junction), transverse tubules, and longitudinal tubules surrounding capillary endothelium. (Reproduced with permission from Berne RM, Levy MN: Chapter 3: Cardiovascular Physiology, 8th edition. St. Louis, CV Mosby, 2000, Fig. 3-1, p 56.)

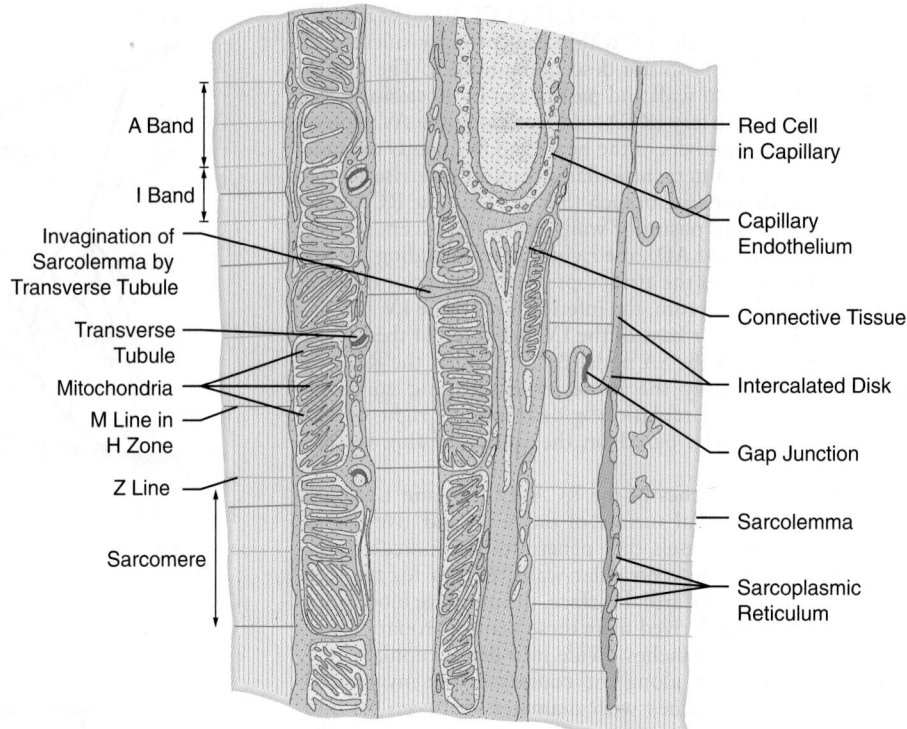

blood, but these factors are generally constant. Resting coronary blood flow in the adult is approximately 250 mL/min (1 mL/g), representing approximately 5% of cardiac output. The changes in aortic pressure and the impedance to flow due to physical compression of the intramural coronary arteries during the contraction-relaxation cycle (Fig. 10-4) govern the pulsatile pattern of coronary flow in the LV. Aortic pressure is slightly less than LV pressure during systole. As a result, blood flow in the LV subendocardium occurs only during diastole (Fig. 10-19). Overall coronary flow does not cease completely during the early part of systole because of this extravascular compression, but most of the flow occurs during diastole when impedance to flow is minimal and aortic pressure remains sufficient to maintain adequate coronary perfusion pressure.

During systole, LV subendocardium is exposed to a higher pressure than the subepicardial layer. Indeed, the systolic intraventricular pressure may be higher than the peak LV systolic pressure. Because of these differences in tissue pressure, the subendocardial layer is more susceptible to ischemia in the presence of coronary artery disease, pressure-overload hypertrophy, or pronounced tachycardia concomitant with compromised regional myocardial perfusion flow, a greater intraventricular-aortic pressure gradient, or reduced total diastolic flow, respectively. Coronary blood flow is also compromised when aortic diastolic pressure is reduced (e.g., severe aortic insufficiency), and this observation may also adversely affect perfusion, particularly in the presence of a critical coronary stenosis.[51] Elevated LV end-diastolic pressure, as observed during acute heart failure, also reduces coronary blood flow because of decreased coronary perfusion pressure. In contrast to left coronary blood flow, RCA flow is continuous throughout the cardiac cycle because the lower pressure in the RV compared with the LV causes substantially less extravascular compression (Fig. 10-19). Coronary sinus (venous) blood flow is maximal during late systole because of the extravascular compression and the low right atrial pressure.

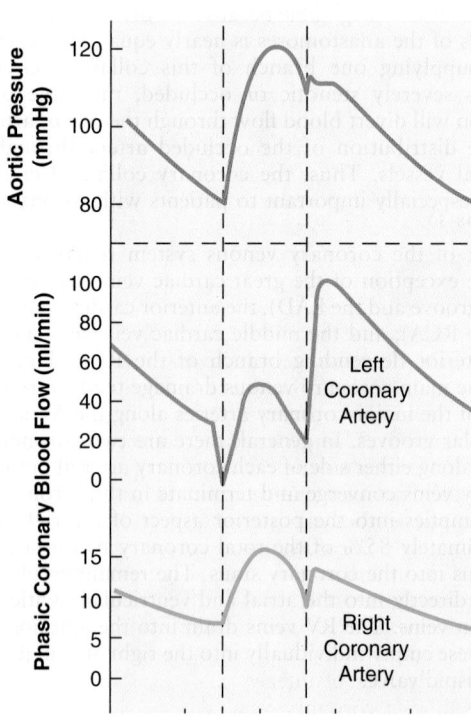

FIGURE 10-19.   Schematic representation of blood flow in the left and right coronary arteries during phases of the cardiac cycle. Note that most left coronary flow occurs during diastole while right coronary flow (and coronary sinus flow) occurs mostly during late systole and early diastole. (Reproduced with permission from Berne RM, Levy MN: Chapter 10: Cardiovascular Physiology, 8th edition. St. Louis, CV Mosby, 2000, Fig. 10-3, p 231.)

Regulation of Coronary Blood Flow

The two major determinants of coronary blood flow (perfusion pressure and vascular resistance) vary substantially during the cardiac cycle (Fig. 10-4). Coronary perfusion pressure certainly varies with changes in aortic, intramyocardial, and coronary venous pressures during systole and diastole, but the major factor that regulates coronary blood flow is the variable resistance produced by coronary vascular smooth muscle. Sympathetic nervous system innervation modulates the contractile state of coronary vascular smooth muscle. In addition, smooth muscle tone is affected by stretch of the muscle (termed the *myogenic factor*). However, metabolic factors are the major physiological determinants of coronary vascular tone and, hence, myocardial perfusion. The ratio of epicardial to endocardial blood flow ratio remains near 1.0 throughout the cardiac cycle despite systolic compressive forces exerted on the subendocardium. The more pronounced resistance to flow in the subendocardium is offset by β-adrenoceptor–mediated vasodilation and by local metabolic autocrine factors (e.g., adenosine during hypoxia) produced by the myocardium itself. The relative maintenance of subendocardial blood flow may also be related to the extensive number of redundant arteriolar and capillary anastomoses in the subendocardium.[1]

Oxygen Delivery and Demand

The heart normally extracts between 75 and 80% of arterial O_2 content, by far the greatest O_2 extraction of all organs. The majority of O_2 demand is derived from the development of LV pressure during isovolumic contraction. Oxygen consumption is also affected by the rate of LV pressure development (dP/dt) and the diameter of the LV (Laplace's law). An increase in myocardial contractility enhances O_2 consumption, but heart rate is the primarily determinant of O_2 consumption. Cardiac O_2 extraction is near maximal under resting conditions and cannot be substantially increased during exercise. Thus, the primary mechanism by which myocardium meets its O_2 demand is through enhanced O_2 delivery, which is proportional to coronary blood flow at constant hemoglobin concentration. Coronary blood flow and O_2 consumption increase four- to fivefold during strenuous physical exercise. The difference between maximal and resting coronary blood flow is known as *coronary reserve*. Myocardial O_2 consumption is a major determinant of coronary blood flow. For example, coronary vascular resistance is greater in the rested, perfused heart than in the contracting heart, indicating that coronary blood flow increases in response to a higher rate of O_2 consumption. The mechanism(s) responsible for the correlation between myocardial work, O_2 consumption, and coronary vessel dilatation has yet to be precisely determined. In addition to metabolically induced vasodilation, the factors responsible for coronary autoregulation (maintenance of coronary blood flow with a change in perfusion pressure) and reactive hyperemia (the several-fold increase in blood flow above baseline after a brief period of ischemia) are also not well understood.

Despite decades of intense research into the mediators of local metabolic coronary vasodilation, surprisingly little is known about the details of this phenomenon. To date, it has been established that metabolic coronary vasodilation is at least partly the result of activation of the sympathetic nerves to the heart and coronary vasculature during an increase in heart rate and myocardial contractility. Sympathetic nerve activation produces a feed-forward β-adrenoceptor–induced vasodilation, primarily of small coronary arterioles. This feed-forward mechanism operates without an error signal, indicating that there is a direct and apparently unregulated relationship between heart rate and inotropic state and the activation of β-adrenoceptor-mediated vasodilation.[49,50,52] There also appears to be a feed-forward, sympathetically mediated, α-adrenoceptor–induced vasoconstriction in larger coronary arteries during exercise. This vasoconstriction occurs upstream from coronary small coronary arterioles and serves two important functions: reduction of vascular compliance and attenuation of systolic minus diastolic flow oscillations during the cardiac cycle. These actions assist in the preservation of blood flow to the more vulnerable LV endocardium when heart rate, contractility, and O_2 consumption are elevated. Interestingly, cardiac parasympathetic nerves have a prominent role in regulating heart rate, but these nerves appear to have a negligible direct effect on the regulation of coronary blood flow.

The conclusions about sympathetic nervous system control of the coronary circulation are based on alterations in the slope of the O_2 consumption-coronary venous O_2 tension relation during graded exercise in the presence of exogenous α- or β-adrenoceptor blockade (Fig. 10-20). The current evidence implicating the β-adrenoceptor in coronary vasodilation accounts for only about one fourth of the total coronary vasodilation observed during exercise-induced hyperemia.[53] These data suggest that the other three fourths of coronary vasodilation during exercise may be produced by as yet undefined local metabolic factors that act on coronary vascular smooth muscle with or without the influence of endothelium. Many metabolic factors have been proposed to individually or collectively modulate coronary flow at the arterial or capillary level, including adenosine, nitric oxide, arterial oxygen or CO_2 tension, pH, osmolarity, K^+, Ca^{2+}, and prostaglandins. Many of these factors exert predictable direct effects. For example, hypoxia or ischemia decreases arterial oxygen tension and pH and increases CO_2 tension, adenosine, K^+, and Ca^{2+} concentrations, and serum osmolarity. Many of these changes may indeed increase coronary blood flow, but none appear to be crucial determinants of vasodilation during exercise. For example, adenosine receptor blockade does not alter coronary blood flow under resting conditions or during exercise. Similarly, inhibition of nitric oxide production or ATP-sensitive K^+ (K_{ATP}) channels also does not alter the O_2 consumption-coronary venous O_2 slope during graded exercise. Nevertheless, nitric oxide and K_{ATP} channels have been shown to regulate the balance between O_2 supply and demand under resting conditions.

There is very strong evidence however, that adenosine released during hypoxia or ischemia causes coronary vasodilation and that this effect is mediated by activation of K_{ATP} channels. Adenosine and K_{ATP} channels have also been implicated during reactive hyperemia after ischemia, but these mediators do not appear to be required for coronary autoregulation. Moreover, the K_{ATP} channel probably maintains a lower vascular smooth muscle tone and thus, a higher basal coronary flow during resting conditions. While not acting as a local metabolic vasodilator, nitric oxide may react to increased downstream arterial dilation by dilating larger, upstream epicardial coronary arteries to prevent excessive sheer stress on coronary endothelial cells.

Myocardial Ischemia and Infarction

Ischemic heart disease remains the leading cause of death in the United States. Global ischemia results from insufficient total coronary blood flow for the overall metabolic needs of the heart.[54,55] Regional ischemia results from insufficient coronary blood flow to a region of the heart supplied by its vascular limb. A large, acute coronary artery occlusion produces acute myocardial ischemia and often contributes to the

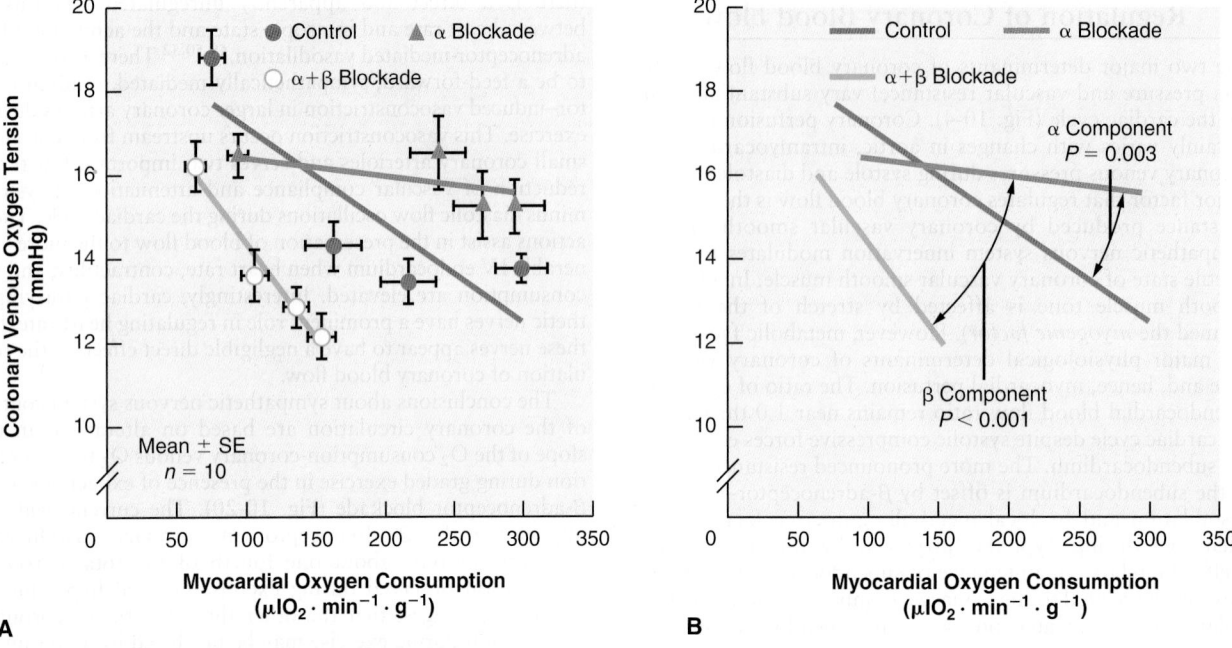

FIGURE 10-20. Coronary venous oxygen (O_2) tension at rest and during three levels of exercise plotted as a function of myocardial O_2 consumption with individual regression lines for α blockade alone and with β blockade. The steep slope of combined α + β blockade indicates a modest match by local metabolic factors in the absence of adrenergic mechanisms. The differences in slopes between α + β blockade and α blockade demonstrates β-adrenergic–mediated coronary vasodilation, whereas the difference in slopes between β blockade and control demonstrates α–mediated coronary vasoconstriction. Note that β-adrenergic vasodilation accounts for only about 25% of the increase in coronary flow during exercise. (Reproduced with permission from Gorman MW, Tune JD, Richmond MW, Feigl EO: Feedforward sympathetic coronary vasodilation in exercising dogs. J Appl Physiol 2000; 89: 1892.)

development of a malignant ventricular arrhythmia because blood flow through coronary collaterals fails to provide sufficient perfusion to the ischemic zone.[49,51] Thus, many patients with acute coronary syndrome succumb to sudden cardiac death before or during the evolution of a myocardial infarction. If the coronary artery occlusion develops more slowly, collateral formation in the watershed region may reduce the degree of myocardial damage associated with acute coronary occlusion. New collateral development (known as *vasculogenesis*) into the occluded vascular bed will result in the independence of this region from its original blood supply.

An atherosclerotic plaque is the most frequent cause of obstructed blood flow in large, epicardial coronary artery vessels.[56] The most common site for development of an atherosclerotic plaque is the first several centimeters of the major and coronary arteries and their primary branches. The position of atherosclerotic plaques facilitates their palliation by coronary artery bypass graft surgery.[57] Atherosclerotic plaques typically develop very slowly, eventually protruding into the vessel and partially or completely blocking flow. The atherosclerotic plaque may also precipitate thrombus formation, which more rapidly occludes the coronary artery. A thrombus usually develops when the plaque has broken through the vascular intima, thereby exposing vascular smooth muscle or adventitia to clotting factors and platelets contained in blood. When fibrin and platelets begin to be deposited, blood cells become entrapped and form a thrombus that grows rapidly until it produces a critical stenosis or complete occlusion of the coronary artery. The thrombus may also embolize by detaching from its original site of formation and flow to a more peripheral branch of the coronary arterial bed. Atherosclerotic plaques are composed of cholesterol and other lipids that

become deposited beneath the intima and fibrous tissue, which also frequently becomes calcified. These calcium deposits are located predominantly at the junction of the intimal and medial layers of the blood vessel.

An acute occlusion of a major epicardial coronary artery causes almost immediate, maximal dilation of existing small collateral vessels supplying blood flow to the ischemic zone. Unfortunately, blood flow through these minute collaterals is generally insufficient to nourish all of the myocardium that they supply. Collateral perfusion through these anastomoses temporally increases and may double within 24 hours after acute coronary occlusion. Eventually, the affected myocardium will be supplied by a normal quantity of blood flow, albeit from a different source. During the gradual development of an atherosclerotic plaque, collateral vessels may develop at a rate similar to, and thereby compensate for, the slow occlusion of the vessel lumen. This redistribution of myocardial blood flow from a partially occluded to a collateral vascular supply may prevent an acute episode of ischemia when the original coronary artery becomes occluded. Only when the atherosclerotic process develops more rapidly than the formation of an adequate collateral blood supply will the O_2 demand exceed delivery and produce myocardial dysfunction. This type of ischemic cardiomyopathy is the most common cause of heart failure. Myocardial necrosis and apoptosis (programmed cell death) occur as a consequence of ischemia and infarction. However, cellular demise usually will not occur in a region unless coronary blood flow falls below 65% of resting values. Myocytes in this region may be viable, but their contractile ability may be severely impaired because of the lack of O_2 and nutrients. Critically stenotic atherosclerotic plaques may produce a pressure gradient across the stenosis and substantially reduce the perfusion pressure in distal branches of the affected vessel. Such gradients are especially important when stenoses occur in coronary arteries of smaller caliber. There may be compensatory vasodilation of the coronary distal bed, but progressive diminution of distal blood flow may occur despite this response.

Myocardial infarction may also occur without evidence of major coronary thromboses, emboli, or stenosis. This form of infarction is caused by excessive metabolic demands resulting from severe LV hypertrophy (e.g., critical aortic stenosis) or vasoactive drug ingestion (e.g., amphetamines, cocaine) or may also result from coronary artery vasospasm. Either of these mechanisms may lead to ischemia by adversely affecting myocardial O_2 supply-demand relations. Clearly, the presence of coronary stenoses that would otherwise be asymptomatic (<70%) may exacerbate O_2 demand-mediated myocardial ischemia. Such causes for myocardial infarction are relatively uncommon, and coronary artery disease remains the primary cause of transmural necrosis. Subendocardial infarction may have a different etiology than the transmural infarction caused by an acute coronary occlusion. Subendocardial infarction may occur when coronary perfusion pressure is adversely reduced by decline in diastolic aortic pressure or increases in LV end-diastolic pressure. Thus, patients with severe aortic insufficiency or end-stage heart failure may be especially prone to subendocardial injury.

Along with the severity of coronary artery stenosis, the metabolic activity of the heart during ischemia is a critical factor in determining the extent of cell death. If an area of the heart has reduced blood supply due to ischemia, the region distal to this coronary stenosis is maximally vasodilated, and an increase in O_2 demand causes vasodilation of adjacent coronary vessels that supply surrounding normal myocardium. This metabolically induced vasodilation may inadvertently redistribute blood flow away from the ischemic zone through coronary collateral vessels. This phenomenon is known as *coronary steal*.[58,59] Despite original arguments to the contrary, most experimental and clinical evidence collected to date indicates that volatile anesthetics do not cause coronary steal unless profound hypotension (<50 mm Hg) is present. Volatile anesthetics are not potent vasodilators, unlike drugs such as adenosine and sodium nitroprusside that are known to produce coronary steal.

A potentially lethal complication of acute coronary occlusion is the development of malignant ventricular arrhythmias (e.g., ventricular tachycardia, fibrillation). Ventricular arrhythmias are most likely to occur during the first 10 minutes after an acute coronary occlusion, especially if the coronary blood flow to the conduction system becomes ischemic. Myocytes distal to occluded coronary artery may become electrically dysfunctional and fail to temporally repolarize with surrounding normal myocardium. This repolarization dyssynchrony is a frequent cause of arrhythmogenesis during acute myocardial ischemia. Compensatory activation of the sympathetic nervous system in response to marked reductions in cardiac output may also contribute to the development of ventricular arrhythmias. Left ventricular dilatation or formation of an LV aneurysm late after myocardial infarction may also provide a substrate for arrhythmogenesis by increasing the duration of impulse conduction and creating abnormal conduction pathways around the infarcted zone. These consequences of infarction may predispose to circuitous electrical activity and result in an impulse re-entering a section of the myocardium that is still recovering from its refractory period, thereby initiating an abnormal subsequent cycle of excitation and reentry.

A central zone of myocardial necrosis develops within 1 hour after acute coronary artery occlusion, which is eventually replaced by scar as the infarcted myocardium heals. A border zone characterized by profoundly reduced contractility due to inadequate coronary collateral perfusion surrounds this central necrotic zone. Some of this border zone also develops scar tissue; other regions surrounding the central necrotic region hypertrophy as a compensatory response to increased workload. This postinfarction ventricular hypertrophy serves to maintain cardiac output, but may also contribute to the late development of heart failure as a result of progressive diastolic dysfunction.[1,50,52,60]

PULMONARY CIRCULATION

Comparison with the Systemic Circulation

The pulmonary circulation receives the blood pumped by the RV. Total pulmonary blood flow is equivalent to cardiac output. There are major differences in hemodynamics between the systemic and pulmonary circulations (Fig. 10-21).[61] There is a greater decrease in mean pressure across systemic arteries to arterioles compared with vessels of similar caliber in the pulmonary circulation. The precapillary and capillary vessels of the pulmonary vasculature are located in close proximity to the alveolar membranes, thereby facilitating gas exchange. The lung is richly innervated by the parasympathetic and sympathetic nervous system, but the dominant effect of the autonomic nervous system occurs primarily at the level of alveolar and bronchial smooth muscle. Vagal innervation of muscarinic receptors in airway smooth muscle produces bronchoconstriction and is an important contributing factor to bronchospasm in atopic pulmonary disease, pneumonia, and inhalation of noxious substances. The sympathetic innervation of the lung is derived from upper thoracic sympathetic fibers that innervate both airway and pulmonary vascular smooth muscle. Sympathetic stimulation of airway smooth muscle produces bronchodilation by activation of β_2-adrenoceptors. The sympathetic innervation of the pulmonary vascular system provides a physiological response to gravitational effects on the intrapulmonary distribution of blood flow and partially counteracts alterations in regional ventilation/perfusion (V/Q) ratio differences produced by such gravitational forces.[62]

Regional Differences in Perfusion and V/Q Matching

The V/Q distribution within the lung in an upright position varies because of the effect of gravity (Fig. 10-22). In the upper lung (zone 1), V/Q ratio is >1.0, indicating that alveolar ventilation occurs in excess of pulmonary blood flow. Because

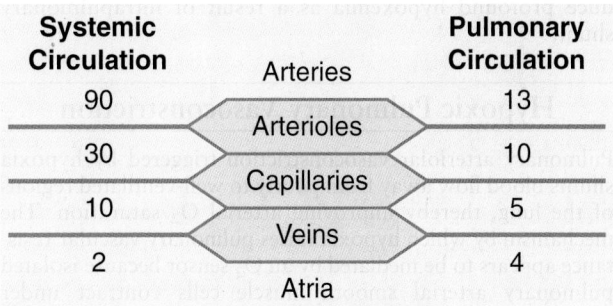

Systemic Circulation		Pulmonary Circulation
90	Arteries	13
30	Arterioles	10
10	Capillaries	5
2	Veins	4
	Atria	

FIGURE 10-21. Comparison of pressure gradients (in mm Hg) along the high-pressure systemic and low-pressure pulmonary circulation. (Reproduced with permission from Nunn JF: Applied Respiratory Physiology. London, Butterworth, 1971, p 213.)

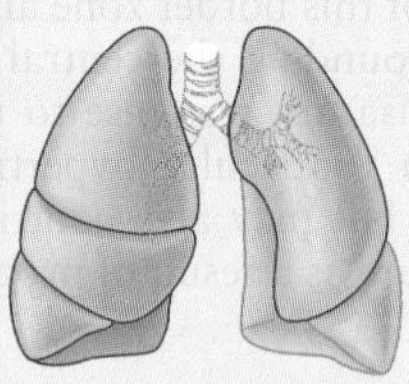

Percentage of Lung Volume Studied		Alveolar Ventilation (l./min.)	Pulmonary Blood Flow (l./min.)	Ventilation Perfusion Ratio
25		1.0	0.6	1.7
36		1.8	2.0	0.9
39		2.3	3.4	0.7
100	Total	5.1	6.0	0.85

FIGURE 10-22. Relative ventilation and perfusion (V/Q) distribution in different areas of the lungs (upright position). The left side shows the percentage distribution of the total lung volume and the right side shows the alveolar ventilation, pulmonary blood flow, and V/Q ratio of each horizontal slice of lung volume. Note the upper zone is relatively overventilated and the lower zone is relatively overperfused. (Reproduced with permission from Nunn JF: Applied Respiratory Physiology. London, Butterworth, 1971, p 234.)

part of this zone is ventilated but not perfused, zone 1 contributes to dead space ventilation. In the middle region of the lung (zone 2), the V/Q ratio is close to 1.0, indicating a balance between ventilation and perfusion. In the lower regions of the lung (zone 3), the V/Q ratio is substantially lower than 1.0. Under these conditions, ventilation inadequately matches perfusion and intrapulmonary shunt occurs. The overall V/Q ratio of the lung is between .85 and .90. Thus, there are large gradients in ventilation and perfusion from the top to bottom of the lung in standing position, and as a result of gravitational effects, the blood volume and blood flow are substantially greater at the lung base compared with the apex. However, ventilation may be more effective in the lung base because the diaphragm exerts a greater influence in this region.

The distribution of ventilation and perfusion throughout the lung also affects the relationships between pulmonary arterial, venous, and alveolar pressures within different lung zones. In the upper zone (zone 1), pulmonary arterial pressure of compressible vessels remains less than the pulmonary alveolar pressure and is insufficient to open the vessels, which remain collapsed during some of inspiration. In the middle zone (zone 2), the pressure at the arterial end of the compressible vessels exceeds pulmonary venous and pulmonary alveolar pressure; therefore, the blood flow becomes dependent on the pressure gradient between the pulmonary artery and alveolus, both of which exceed pulmonary venous pressure. In zone 3, the pulmonary venous pressure exceeds pulmonary alveolar pressure. Thus, blood flow depends on the pressure gradient between arterial to venous ends of the capillaries, similar to the situation observed in the systemic circulation. As intravascular pressures increase, progressively lower resistance to pulmonary blood flow is observed in this zone. In the supine position, similar V/Q distributions are observed over smaller pressure gradients (compared with the upright position) between anterior and posterior thorax. From this discussion, it is clear how pathologic conditions may reduce arterial O_2 tension. For example, alveolar collapse in areas of atelectasis in which perfusion persists despite compensatory hypoxic pulmonary vasoconstriction may produce profound hypoxemia as a result of intrapulmonary shunt.[63,64]

Hypoxic Pulmonary Vasoconstriction

Pulmonary arteriolar vasoconstriction triggered by hypoxia shunts blood flow away from poorly to well-ventilated regions of the lung, thereby improving arterial O_2 saturation. The mechanism by which hypoxia raises pulmonary vascular resistance appears to be mediated by an O_2 sensor because isolated pulmonary arterial smooth muscle cells contract under hypoxic conditions.[65,66] The O_2 sensor has yet to be identified, but may be mediated by smooth muscle mitochondria and pulmonary vascular endothelium. Pulmonary arterial strips with intact endothelium are more sensitive to hypoxia than skinned fiber preparations in vitro. Hypoxia also inhibits an outward

K^+ current; the resulting depolarization augments a Ca^{2+} influx into pulmonary vascular smooth muscle, thereby initiating contraction. The contractile mechanism of hypoxic pulmonary vasoconstriction appears to be mediated by the Ca^{2+}-calmodulin system and causes phosphorylation of vascular smooth muscle myosin light chains. Chronic hypoxia causes proliferation of vascular smooth muscle and thickens the pulmonary arterial tree. This response increases pulmonary vascular resistance and may also produce irreversible pulmonary hypertension.

Physiologic Modulation of the Pulmonary Circulation

The blood volume stored in the pulmonary circulation is substantial ($\geq$900 mL), and when combined with the blood volume contained within the heart and proximal great vessels, this pulmonary blood volume provides a crucial, rapidly available source of reserve intravascular volume during acute, massive hemorrhage. The mechanisms by which blood volume is shifted to central compartments in response to hypovolemia is poorly understood, but activation of regional sympathetic innervation of the volume-containing reservoirs, vasoconstriction of arterial resistance vessels, and the systemic action of epinephrine released from the adrenal gland clearly play important roles. Angiotensin, prostaglandins and other arachidonic acid metabolites, and nitric oxide are also critical regulators of pulmonary vascular resistance and the distribution of blood flow within the lung parenchyma.[67-69] Nitric oxide has proven benefits in the treatment of acquired and congenital pulmonary hypertension, often with life-saving results. For example, inhaled nitric oxide is a selective pulmonary vasodilator at doses <40 to 80 parts per million, and reductions in pulmonary arterial pressure produced by this drug are often essential to preserve RV function in patients undergoing heart or lung transplantation.

CEREBRAL CIRCULATION

Anatomy and Cerebral Autoregulation

Blood flow to the brain is provided through the internal carotid and vertebral arteries. The vertebral arteries join to form the basilar artery, which, along with branches of the internal carotid arteries, forms the circle of Willis. The brain is approximately 2% of total body weight, yet this organ receives approximately 15% of cardiac output. This remarkably large cerebral blood flow (45 to 55 mL/100 g/min) reflects the high metabolic rate of the brain. Cerebral oxygen consumption averages 3.5 mL/100 g/min and accounts for 20% of total body oxygen consumption at rest. Regional cerebral blood flow and metabolic rate vary substantially throughout the brain. Cerebral blood flow and metabolic rate are closely linked and are approximately 4 times greater in gray compared with white matter. Thus, the cerebral cortex has a substantially greater blood flow and metabolic rate than subcortical regions. Motor activity or sensory stimulation is associated with increased neuronal activity in the contralateral activated areas of brain and is closely coupled to regional increases in blood flow and metabolic rate in corresponding regions.[70,71] The mechanism of coupling of the activity-metabolism-blood flow relationship is most likely related to local metabolic vasodilators (e.g., lactic acid), alterations in electrolyte (e.g., K^+, Ca^{2+}) concentrations, and other substances (e.g., adenosine, released neurotransmitters). To date, no single causative molecule has yet been identified as the primary factor linking regional metabolic rate and blood flow to neuronal activity.[72,73]

Regulation of Cerebral Blood Flow: Hypercarbia, Hypoxia, and Arterial Pressure

(15) Cerebral blood flow remains relatively constant when mean arterial pressure varies between 50 and 150 mm Hg in healthy subjects (Fig. 10-23). This autoregulation of cerebral blood flow shifts to the right in patients with chronic, poorly controlled essential hypertension. For example, the autoregulation curve may range between 80 and 200 mm Hg in a patient with hypertension, and reducing the mean arterial pressure below 80 mm Hg may precipitate cerebral ischemia. This observation emphasizes that effective treatment of hypertension readjusts the autoregulation curve to its normal pressure range. Cerebral autoregulation is inhibited by hypercarbia and higher end-tidal concentrations of volatile anesthetics. In contrast, a reduction in arterial CO_2 tension counteracts the direct cerebral vasodilator actions of many drugs, including those of volatile anesthesia agents.[74]

(16) Arterial CO_2 tension is a major regulator of cerebral blood flow within the physiologic range of arterial CO_2 tensions. Cerebral blood flow linearly increases 1 to 2 ml/100 g/min for each 1 mmHg increase in PaCO$_2$. Below an arterial CO_2 tension of 25 mmHg (Fig. 23), the cerebral blood flow response to PaCO$_2$ is attenuated. The mechanism responsible for the cerebral blood flow-arterial CO_2 tension relationship is related to extracellular H^+ concentration. Carbon dioxide rapidly diffuses across the vascular endothelium, and changes in local pH are governed by the Henderson-Hasselbach equation. Notably, alterations in cerebral produced by changes in arterial CO_2 tension are not sustained blood flow because bicarbonate is eventually transported out of the brain extracellular fluid, thereby returning pH to a normal value. In contrast to the effects of respiratory acidosis on cerebral blood flow, the actions of metabolic acidosis are more gradual because the blood–brain barrier is relatively impermeable to H^+. Hypoxia-induced increases in cerebral blood flow occur at arterial O_2 tensions below 60 mm Hg (Fig. 10-23). The increase in cerebral blood flow at PaO$_2$ levels below 60 mm Hg is very rapid. The mechanism of this hypoxia-induced increase in cerebral blood flow may be related to the vasodilator effect of neuronal acidosis. Several other mediators and chemoreceptor activation have also been proposed as potential signaling mechanisms responsible for cerebral vasodilation during hypoxia. In contrast to the marked increases in cerebral blood flow observed during hypoxia, little change in cerebral blood flow occurs under normoxic or hyperbaric conditions (PaO$_2$ of 60 to 300 mm Hg).

Neural control of the cerebral circulation plays a relatively minor role in regulation of cerebral blood flow despite the extensive sympathetic nervous system innervation of cerebral blood vessels. Sympathetic postganglionic neurons originate in the cervical sympathetic ganglia, and vasoconstriction produced by sympathetic stimulation is largely exerted on the medium to larger-sized cerebral arteries. This response is primarily manifested during intense sympathetic nervous system activation that accompanies profound hypovolemia. The net effect of this sympathetic activation is a downward shift in the cerebral autoregulation curve, indicating a lower cerebral blood flow than predicted at a given level of mean arterial pressure. The cerebral blood vessels are also innervated by cholinergic and serotonergic fibers. Administration of exogenous vasodilators (e.g., sodium nitroprusside, adenosine, Ca^{2+} channel blockers, volatile anesthetics) increases cerebral blood flow. In contrast, catecholamines such as epinephrine do not substantially affect cerebral blood flow when these drugs are used to alter a systemic hemodynamics unless cerebral perfusion pressure is affected at the extremes of the autoregulation curve. It is important to recognize that autoregulation of cerebral blood flow is not effective and cerebral perfusion becomes pressure-dependent in areas of regional cerebral ischemia.

Effects of Increased Intracranial Pressure

Along with the brain, the cerebral circulation is entirely constrained within the rigid cranial cavity. This unique anatomic arrangement infers that increases in cerebral arterial blood flow must be matched by comparable increases in venous flow from the skull because the volume of blood and extracellular fluid within the brain is relatively constant. Thus, an intracranial mass (e.g., tumor, hematoma) is inevitably accompanied by an increase in intracranial pressure. Under these circumstances, the resistance to cerebral blood flow increases and cerebral perfusion is no longer determined by the difference between mean arterial pressure and cerebral venous pressure, but rather the difference between arterial pressure and intracranial pressure. If intracranial pressure continues to increase, a compensatory increase in arterial pressure occurs (Cushing reflex) that acts as a protective mechanism to maintain cerebral perfusion.

RENAL CIRCULATION

Anatomy of the Renal Circulation: Determinants of Glomerular Blood Flow

The primary branches of the renal artery divide into several interlobar arteries that traverse the parenchyma in a radial fashion from the hilum to the cortical-medullary junction that

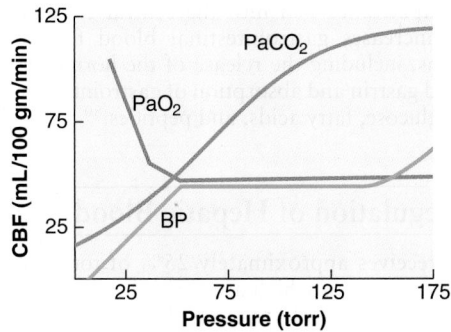

FIGURE 10-23. Cerebral blood flow (CBF) is autoregulated (relatively unchanged) as mean systemic blood pressure rises between 50 to 150 mm Hg. However, flow is nearly linearly increased with a rise in PaCO$_2$ and increased if PaO$_2$ falls below 50 mm Hg. (Modified and reproduced with permission from Michenfelder JD: Anesthesia and the brain, Clinical, Functional and Vascular Coordinates. New York, Churchill Livingstone, 1988, pp 94–113.)

separates the kidney into an outer cortex and an inner medulla where urine is primarily concentrated in the renal tubules. As an interlobar artery approaches the cortical-medullary junction, it branches into a series of arcuate arteries that are located over the bases of the adjacent medullary pyramids in the zone between the cortex and the medulla, but do not interconnect with adjacent interlobar arteries. This lack of collateral blood supply indicates that acute occlusion of an interlobar artery will produce a pyramid-shaped renal infarction. Interlobular branches from the arcuate arteries travel toward the capsular surface and form the afferent arterial supply to the glomeruli. The kidney has approximately 1 million glomeruli that filter plasma from circulating blood into Bowman's capsule that surround each glomerulus capillary tuft. The afferent arteriole to each glomerulus divides into several vessels that form discrete capillary loops. The proximal and distal limbs of each loop are interconnected by many smaller capillaries, thereby forming the capillary tuft. Plasma filtration occurs within these capillary networks. After exiting the capillary network, the distal ends of each capillary loop within the glomerulus rejoin to form the efferent arterioles. The diameter of efferent arterioles is usually substantially less than the afferent arteriole. The entire glomerular capillary tuft is enveloped by Bowman's capsule, which collects the glomerular filtrate and transports it to the renal tubules where urine is concentrated. The efferent arterioles subsequently divide into another capillary network, the peritubular capillaries, some of which surround relatively short renal tubules located almost entirely in the renal cortex. Most of the peritubular capillaries form the long hairpin loops of Henle extending deep into the renal medulla. These vasa recta capillaries are important components of the renal countercurrent exchange mechanism that is responsible for urine concentration.[75]

Renal Hemodynamics

The mean arterial pressure in the glomerular capillaries is normally between 50 and 60 mm Hg, thereby favoring the outward filtration of plasma water along the entire length of the capillary loop. Approximately 20% of the plasma water that enters the glomerular capillaries is filtered into Bowman's capsule. The efferent arterioles provide greatest vascular resistance in the renal circulation and reduce the pressure in the peritubular capillaries to values between 10 and 20 mm Hg. These relatively low pressures favor the net reabsorption of the large quantities of fluid that pass from the renal tubules into the interstitium. The permeability of the peritubular capillaries is also considerably higher than other capillaries in the body, a feature that substantially facilitates the primary diffusion function of the kidney. Renal blood flow is approximately 20% of cardiac output and is heavily balanced toward perfusion of the renal cortex. The inner medulla and papillae usually receive only approximately one tenth of cortical blood flow.[76]

The kidney has a very high metabolic rate, but the organ extracts less than 10% of O_2 present in renal arterial blood because renal perfusion far exceeds metabolic requirements. Renal blood flow is very important for the delivery of the large volumes of blood to the glomeruli required for ultrafiltration. Renal blood flow remains relatively constant between mean arterial pressures of 75 and 170 mm Hg, but becomes pressure-dependent beyond this range of autoregulation. Alterations in afferent arteriole resistance autoregulate glomerular filtration rate (GFR) by constricting the diameter of afferent arterioles in response to increases in driving pressure. The two primary mechanisms of renal autoregulation are myogenic (vascular smooth muscle intrinsically responds to stretch by constriction) and tubular-glomerular feedback. This later mechanism is mediated by a feedback loop in which

an alteration in renal tubular filtrate flow is detected by the macula densa of the juxtaglomerular apparatus, which signals the afferent arterioles to restore basal levels of renal blood flow and GFR. The signal that regulates the caliber of the afferent arterioles in tubular-glomerular feedback has yet to be precisely defined, but many vasoactive substances have been implicated, including products of arachidonic acid metabolism, catecholamines, adenosine, nitric oxide, and components of the renin-angiotensin system.[77–79] The role of atrial natriuretic factor, a 28 amino-acid peptide with potent diuretic and natriuretic properties in the renal circulation, has also been elucidated. This peptide is synthesized and released primarily from the cardiac atria, and distention of the atria causes renal vasodilation, increased filtration, inhibition of sodium reabsorption, natriuresis, and a resultant reduction of extracellular fluid volume. The sympathetic nervous system innervates the kidney and may control tubular transport of Na^+ during modest reductions in intravascular volume. Under conditions of profound hypovolemia, sympathetic activation causes renal vasoconstriction, lowers GFR, and reduces renal capillary hydrostatic pressure, thereby producing compensatory water retention that increases plasma volume. As a result of the distribution of blood flow within the kidney, perfusion to cortical compared with medullary nephrons is primary affected by sympathetic nervous system-induced renal vasoconstriction.

SPLANCHNIC AND HEPATIC CIRCULATION

Regulation of Gastrointestinal Blood Flow

The splanchnic circulation is unique. Arterial branches of the abdominal aorta supply blood to the gastrointestinal tract, spleen, and pancreas, whereas the liver has a dual blood supply consisting of the portal venous circulation and the hepatic artery. The intestinal circulation is weakly autoregulated compared with the cerebral, coronary, and renal vascular beds. Intestinal autoregulation appears to be primarily metabolic in origin. Adenosine is a likely mediator of this autoregulation, but other evidence suggests that K^+ concentration and serum osmolality may also play contributing roles. The sympathetic nervous system innervates the gastrointestinal tract and the consequences of sympathetic activation are mediated by α-adrenoceptors. Pronounced sympathetic stimulation during acute hypovolemia produces gastrointestinal arterial constriction and venoconstriction, thereby shifting blood from a large vascular capacitance bed into the central circulation. Food ingestion increases gastrointestinal blood flow by several mechanisms, including the release of the hormones cholecystokinin and gastrin and absorption of gastrointestinal contents including glucose, fatty acids, and peptides.[80]

Regulation of Hepatic Blood Flow

The liver receives approximately 25% of total cardiac output, three quarters of which are derived from the portal vein that contains venous blood from the gastrointestinal tract, spleen, and pancreas. The remaining 25% of hepatic blood flow is provided by the hepatic artery, which supplies the majority of oxygen to the liver. Mean portal venous and hepatic arterial pressures are 10 and 90 mm Hg, respectively.[38,81] The downstream resistance in the hepatic sinusoids is relatively low under normal circumstances, but may be elevated in RV failure or hepatic cirrhosis. A rise in sinusoidal and portal vein pressures accompanying these pathologic conditions may produce transudation of fluid into the peritoneal space (ascites) or dilate alternative routes of venous drainage, such as those located in the lower esophageal veins (esophageal varices). Blood flow in the portal venous and hepatic arterial systems tends to vary reciprocally, but these respective hepatic blood supplies do not fully interact. Thus, a reduction of blood flow in the portal vein may be not fully compensated by an increase in hepatic arterial flow. The hepatic arterial but not the portal venous system is autoregulated. The most important response of hepatic arterial circulation to sympathetic stimulation is constriction of the presinusoidal resistance vessels.[82] The liver contains about 15% of the total body blood volume and is an important volume reservoir that may be rapidly mobilized in response to sympathetic nervous system activation during acute hypovolemia. The reflex responses and response to hypoxia in small mesenteric capacitance vessels are inhibited by potent volatile anesthetics.[83,84]

References

1. Katz AM: Physiology of the Heart, 4th edition. Philadelphia, Lippincott Williams & Wilkins, 2006
2. Smith JJ, Kampine JP: The Heart: Structure and Function, Circulatory Physiology—The Essentials, 3rd edition. Baltimore, Williams & Wilkins, 1990
3. Berne RM, Levy MN: Cardiovascular Physiology, 8th edition. St. Louis, CV Mosby, 2001
4. Ledsome JHR, Lunden RJ: A reflex increase in heart rate from distention of the pulmonary vein atrial junction. J Physiol 1964; 170: 456
5. Seagard JL, Elegbe EO, Hopp FA, Bosnjak ZJ, von Colditz JH, Kalbfleisch JH, Kampine JP: Effects of isoflurane on the baroreceptor reflex. Anesthesiology 1983; 59: 511–520
6. Braunwald E. Sonenblick EH, Ross J: Contraction of the normal heart, Textbook of Cardiovascular Medicine, 2nd edition. Edited by Braunwald E. Philadelphia, WB Saunders, 1983, pp 409
7. Katz AM. The cardiac action potential, Physiology of the Heart, 2nd edition. New York, Raven Press, 1992, pp 438
8. Pagel PS, Grossman W, Haering JM, Warltier DC: Left ventricular diastolic function in the normal and diseased heart. Anestheiology 1993; 79: 1104
9. Pagel PS, Kampine JP, Schmeling WT, Warltier DC: Alteration of left ventricular diastolic function by desflurane, isoflurane, halothane in the chronically instrumented dog. Anesthesiology 1991; 74: 1103
10. Pagel PS, Kampine JP, Schmeling WT, Warltier DC: Comparison of end systolic pressure length relations and preload recruitable stroke work as indices of myocardial contractility in the conscious and anesthetized chronically instrumented dog. Anesthesiology 1990; 73: 278
11. Starling EF: The Linacre Lecture on the Law of the Heart. London, Logmans Green, 1918
12. Crohogini A, Barra J, Rodriquez CM, et al: Area beneath the end systolic pressure-volume relationship as an index of inotropic state in intact dogs. J Mol Cell Cardiol 1986; 18 (Suppl III) 20
13. Kass DA, Maaughan WL, Guo ZM, Kono A, Sunagawa K, Sagawa K: Comparative influence of load versus inotropic states on indexes of ventricular contractility. Experimental and theoretical analysis based on pressure-volume relationships. Circulation 1987; 76: 1422
14. Sagawa K: The ventricular pressure volume diagram revisited. Arc Res 1978; 43: 677
15. Sarnoff SJ: Myocardial contractility as described by ventricular function curves. Physiol Rev 1995; 35: 107
16. Suga H, Sagawa K, Shoukas AA: Load independence of the instantaneous pressure–volume ratio of the canine left ventricle and effects of epinephrine and heart rate on the ratio. Circ Res 1973; 32: 314
17. Schaub MC, Hefti MA, Zuellig RA, Morano I: Modulation of contractility in human cardiac hypertrophy by myosin essential light chain isoforms. Cardiovasc Res 1998; 37: 381
18. Cazorla O, Vassort G, Garnier D, Le Guennc JY: Length modulation of active force in rat cardiac myocytes: in titin the sensor? J Mol Cell Cardiol 1999; 31: 1215
19. Helmes M, Trombitas K, Ganzier H: Titin develops restoring force in rat cardiac myocytes. Circ Res 1996; 79: 619
20. Schiaffino S, Reggiani C: Molecular diversity of myofibrillar proteins: gene regulation and molecular significance. Physiol Rev 1996; 76: 371
21. Goldstein MA, Schroeter JP, Michael LH: Role of the Z band in the mechanical properties of the heart. FASEB J 1977; 5: 2167–2174
22. Moncman CL, Wang K: Nebulette: A 107 kD nebulin-like protein in cardiac muscle. Cell Motil Cytoskel 1995; 32: 205

23. Solaro RJ, Rarick HM: Troponin and tropomyosin. Proteins that switch on and tune in the activity of cardiac myofilaments. Circ Res 1998; 83: 417
24. Tobacman LS: Thin filament-mediated regulation of cardiac contraction. Ann Rev Physiol 1996; 58: 447
25. Solaro RJ, Van Eyk J: Altered interactions among thin filaments proteins modulate cardiac function. J Mol Cell Cardiol 1999; 28: 217
26. Luo W, Grupp IL, Harrer J, Ponniah S, Grupp G, Duffy JJ, Doetschman T, Kranias EG: Targeted ablation of the phospholamban gene is associated with markedly enhanced myocardial contractility and loss of β-agonist stimulation. Circ Res 1994; 75: 401
27. Rayment I, Holden HM, Whittaker M: Structure of the actin-myosin complex and its implications for muscle contraction. Science 1993; 261: 58
28. Dominguez R, Freyzon Y, Trybus KM, Cohen C: Crystal structure of a vertebrate smooth muscle myosin motor domain and its complex with the essential light chain: visualization of the pre-power stroke state. Cell 1998; 94: 559
29. Finer JT, Simmons RM, Spudich JA: Single myosin molecule mechanics: pico-newton forces and nanometer steps. Nature 1994; 368: 113
30. Katz AM. The electrocardiogram, Physiology of the Heart, 2nd edition. New York. Raven Press, 1992, p 472
31. Smith JJ, Kampine JP: Electrical properties of the heart, Circulatory Physiology—The Essentials, 3rd edition. Baltimore, Williams & Wilkins, 1990
32. Ebert TJ, Kotrly, KJ, Vucins EJ, Pattison CZ, Kampine JP: Effects of halothane anesthesia on cardiopulmonary baroreflex function in man. Anesthesiology 1985; 61: 668
33. Baruscotti M, Bucchi A, Di Francesco D: Physiology and pharmacology of the cardiac pacemaker ("funny") current. Pharmacol Ther 2005; 107: 59
34. Nerbonne JM, Kass RS: Molecular physiology of cardiac repolarization. Physiol Rev 2005; 85: 1205
35. McAllen RM, Spyer KM: The location of cardiac vagal preganglionic motoneurons in the medulla. J Physiol 1976; 258: 187
36. Kampine JP: General cardiovascular regulation, International Practice of Anaesthesia. Edited by Prys-Roberts C, Brown BR Jr. Oxford, Butterworth-Heinemann, 1996
37. Lipski J, Kanjhan R, Kruszewska B, Rong W: Properties of presympathetic neurons in the rostral ventrolateral medullar in the rat: An intracellular study "in vivo". J Physiol 1996; 490: 729
38. Guyenent PJ: Role of the ventral medulla oblongate in blood pressure regulation, Central Regulation of Autonomic Functions. Edited by Loewy AD, Spyer KM. New York, Oxford University Press, 1990
39. Jarisch A, Richter H: Die afferention bahnen des veratrius effektes in dem herz nerven. Arch Exp Path Pharmacol 1939; 193: 355
40. Dampney RA: Functional organization of central pathways regulating the cardiovascular system. Physiol Rev 1994; 74: 323
41. Spyer KM: The central nervous organization of reflex circulatory control, Central Regulation of Autonomic Function. Edited by Loewy AD, Spyer KM. New York, Oxford University Press, 1990
42. Ross CA, Ruggerio DA, Park DH, Joh TH, Sved AF, Fernandez-Pardal J, Saavedra JM, Reis DJ: Tonic vasomotor control of the rostral ventrolateral medulla: effect of electrical or chemical stimulation of the area containing C1 neurons on arterial blood pressure, heart rate, and plasma catecholamines and vasopressin. J Neurosci 1984; 4: 474
43. Gauer OH, Henry JP: Neurohumoral control of plasma volume, Cardiovascular Physiology II International Review of Physiology, Vol 9. Edited by Guyton AC, Cowley AW. Baltimore, University Park Press 1976, pp 145
44. Linden RJ: Atrial receptors and heart rate, Cardiac Receptors. Edited by Hainsworth R, Kidd C, Linden RJ. London, Cambridge University Press, 1979
45. Longhurst JC: Cardiac receptors: Their function in health and disease. Prog Cardiovasc Dis 1984; 27: 201
46. Kotrly KJ, Ebert TJ, Vucins EJ, Roerig DL, Kampine JP: Baroreceptor reflex control of heart rate during morphine sulfate, diazepam N_2O/O_2 anesthesia in man. Anesthesiology 1984; 61: 558
47. Seagard JL, Hopp FA, Donegan JH, Kampine JP: Halothane and the carotid sinus reflex: Evidence for multiple sites of action. Anesthesiology 1982; 57: 191
48. Crawford MH: Current Diagnosis and Treatment in Cardiology. Norwalk, CT, Appleton & Lange, 1995, pp 1
49. Libby PP, Bronow RO, Mann DL, et al: Braunwald's Heart Disease: A Textbook of Cardiovascular Medicine, 8th edition. Philadelphia, Elsevier Saunders, 2001
50. Marcus M: The Coronary Circulation in Health and Disease. New York, McGraw Hill, 1983, pp 465
51. Lance KL: Coronary Artery Stenosis. New York, Elsevier, 1991
52. Lilly LS: Pathophysiology of Heart Disease: A Collaborative Project of Medical Students and Faculty, 4th edition. Philadelphia, Lippincott Williams & Wilkins, 2007
53. Tune JD, Richmond KN, Gorman MW, Feigl EO: Control of coronary blood flow during exercise. Exp Biol Med 2002; 227: 238
54. Cardiac Vascular, and Thoracic Anesthesia. Edited by Youngberg JA, Lake CL, Roisen MF, Wilson RS. Elsevier, 2000, pp 1
55. Topol EJ, Califf RM, Prystowsky EN, et al: Textbook of Cardiovascular Medicine, 3rd edition. Philadelphia, Lippincott, Williams & Wilkins, 2007, pp 1628

56. King SB, Yeung AC: Interventional Cardiology. New York, McGraw-Hill Medical, 2007

57. Frazier OH, Westaby S: Ischemia Heart Disease: Surgical Management. London, Mosby, 1999, pp 1

58. Opie LH: Heart Physiology: From Cell to Circulation, 4th edition. Philadelphia, Lippincott, Williams & Wilkins, 2004, pp 648

59. Phibbs B: The Human Heart: A Basic Guide to Heart Disease, 2nd edition. Philadelphia, Lippincott, Williams & Wilkins, 2007, pp 229

60. Gerstenblith G: Cardiovascular Disease in the Elderly. Totowa, NJ, Humana Press, 2005

61. Nunn JF: Applied Respiratory Physiology. London, Butterworth, 1971, pp 213

62. Szidon JP, Fishmann AP: Autonomic control of the pulmonary circulation, The Pulmonary Circulation and Interstitial Space. Edited by Fishman AP, Hecht HH, Chicago, The University of Chicago Press, 1969, pp 239

63. West JB, Collery CT: Distribution of blood flow and the pressure-flow relations of the whole lung. J App Physiol 1965; 20: 175

64. West JB, Naimark AA: Distribution of blood flow in isolated lung; relation to vascular and alveolar pressures. J Appl Physiol 1964; 19: 713

65. Mauban JR, Reillard CV, Yuan JZ: Hypoxic pulmonary vasoconstriction: Role of ion channels. J Appl Physiol 2005; 98: 415

66. Waypa GB, Shumacker PT: Hypoxic pulmonary vasoconstriction: Redox events in oxygen sensing. J Appl Physiol 2005; 98: 404

67. Buzzard CJ, Pfister SL, Campbell WB: Endothelium-dependent contractions in rabbit pulmonary artery are mediated by thromboxaine A_2. Circ Res 1993; 72: 1023

68. Pfister SL, Campbell WB: Role of endothelium derived metabolites of arachidonic acid in enhanced pulmonary artery contractions in female rabbit. Hypertension 1996; 27: 43

69. Zhu D, Medhora M, Campbell WB, Spitzbarth N, Baker JE, Jacobs ER: Chronic hypoxia activates lung 15-lipoxygenase which catalyzes production of 15-HETE and enhances constriction in neonatal pulmonary arteries. Circ Res 2003; 92: 992

70. Greenberg J, Hand P, Sylverstro A, et al: Localized metabolic flow couple during functional activity. Acta Neurol Scand 1979; 60(Suppl 72): 12

71. Olsen J: Contralateral local increase in cerebral blood flow in man during arm work. Brain 1972; 94: 635

72. Gebrenedin D, Lange A, Lowry T, Taheri MR, Birks EK, Hudetz AG, Narayanan J, Falck JR, Okamoto H, Roman RJ, Nithipatikom K, Campbell WB, Harder DR: Production of 20-HETE and its role in autoregulation of cerebral blood flow. Circ Res 2000; 87: 60

73. Lou HC, Edvinsson L, MacKenzie ET: The concept of coupling blood flow to brain function: revision required? Ann Neurol 1987; 22: 289

74. Faraci FM, Heistad DD: Regulation of the cerebral circulation: Role of endothelium and potassium channels. Physiol Rev 1998; 78: 53

75. Levy MN, Pappano AJ: Cardiovascular Physiology. Philadelphia, Mosby Elsevier, 2007

76. Hall JE. Regulation of renal hemodynamics, Cardiovascular Physiology II. International Review of Physiology, Vol. 2. Edited by Guyton EC, Hall JE. Baltimore, University Park Press, 1982, pp 243

77. Benner BM: Glomerular ultrafiltration, The Kidney, Vol 1, 3rd edition. Edited by Brenner BM, Bector FC. Philadelphia, WB Saunders, 1986

78. Naraayanan J, Imig M. Roman R, Harder D. Pressurization of isolated renal arterial increases inositol tripghosphate and diacylglycerol. Am J Physiol Heart Circ Physiol 1994; 35: H1840

79. Roman RR: P-450 metabolites of arachadonic acid in the control of cardiovascular function. Physiol Rev 2002; 82: 131

80. Jacobson Ed, Tepperman BL, editors: Splanchnic circulation (symposium). Fed Proc 1982; 41, 2079

81. Greenway CV, Laut WW. Hepatic circulation, Handbook of Physiology, Section 6: The Gastrointestinal System—Motility and Circulation, Vol. 1. Edited by Schultz SG. Bethesda, MD, American Physiological Society, 1989

82. Ozono K, Bosnjak ZJ, Kampine JP. Reflex control of mesenteric venous capacitance in the rabbit: Direct measurement of vein diameter and intravenous pressure in the situ preparation. Am J Physiol 1989; 256: H1066

83. Stadnicka A, Stekiel TA, Bosnjak ZJ, Kampine JP: Hypoxic contractions of isolated rabbit small mesenteric capacitance veins: Contributions of endothelium and attenuation by volatile anesthetics. Anesthesiology 1995; 82: 550

84. Stekiel TA, Ozono K, McCallum JB, Bosnjak ZJ, Stekiel WJ, Kampine JP: The inhibitory action of halothane on reflex constriction in mesenteric capacitance veins. Anesthesiology 1990; 73: 1169

CHAPTER 11 ■ RESPIRATORY FUNCTION

MICHAEL L. AULT AND M. CHRISTINE STOCK

KEY POINTS

1 In a person with normal lungs, both breathing and coughing can be performed exclusively by the diaphragm.

2 In the adult, the tip of an orotracheal tube moves an average of 3.8 cm with flexion and extension of the neck, but can travel as much as 6.4 cm. In infants and children, displacement of even 1 cm can move the tube above the vocal cords or below the carina.

3 The following anatomy should be considered when contemplating the use of a double-lumen tube. The adult right main stem bronchus is ~2.5 cm long before it branches into lobar bronchi. In 10% of adults, the right upper lobe bronchus departs from the right main stem bronchus <2.5 cm below the carina. In 2 to 3% of adults, the right upper lobe bronchus opens into the trachea, above the carina.

4 When lung compliance is reduced, larger changes in pleural pressure are needed to create the same tidal volume (V_T). Patients with low lung compliance breathe with smaller V_T and more rapidly, making spontaneous respiratory rate the most sensitive clinical index of lung compliance.

5 Carotid and aortic bodies are stimulated by PaO_2 values less than 60 to 65 mm Hg. Thus, patients who depend on hypoxic ventilatory drive do not have PaO_2 values >65 mm Hg. The peripheral receptors' response will not reliably increase ventilatory rate or minute ventilation to herald the onset of hypoxemia during general anesthesia or recovery.

6 There are three causes of hyperventilation: arterial hypoxemia, metabolic acidemia, and central etiologies (e.g., intracranial hypertension, hepatic cirrhosis, anxiety, pharmacologic agents).

7 Increases in dead space ventilation primarily affect CO_2 elimination (with minimal influence on arterial oxygenation), and physiologic shunt increase primarily affects arterial oxygenation (with minimal influence on CO_2 elimination).

8 During spontaneous ventilation, the ratio of alveolar ventilation to dead space ventilation is 2:1. The alveolar-to-dead space ventilation ratio during positive-pressure ventilation is 1:1. Thus, minute ventilation during mechanical ventilatory support must be greater than that during spontaneous ventilation to achieve the same $PaCO_2$.

9 $PaCO_2 \geq PETCO_2$ unless the patient inspires or receives exogenous CO_2. The difference between $PaCO_2$ and $PETCO_2$ is because of dead space ventilation. The most common reason for an acute increase in dead space ventilation is decreased cardiac output.

10 The best evaluation of the efficiency with which the lungs oxygenate the arterial blood is the calculation of shunt fraction. It is the only index of oxygenation that takes into account the contribution of mixed venous blood to arterial oxygenation.

11 When functional residual capacity is reduced, lung compliance falls and results in tachypnea, and venous admixture increases, creating arterial hypoxemia.

12 There is no compelling evidence that defines rules or parameters for ordering preoperative pulmonary function tests. Rather, they should be obtained to ascertain the presence of the reversible pulmonary dysfunction (bronchospasm) or to define the severity of advanced pulmonary disease.

13 Smoking patients should be advised to *stop* smoking at least 2 months prior to an elective operation to decrease the risk of postoperative pulmonary complications (PPCs).

14 The operative site is one of the most important determinants of the risk of PPC. The highest risk for PPC is associated with nonlaparoscopic upper abdominal operations, followed by lower abdominal and intrathoracic operations.

15 The single most important aspect of postoperative pulmonary care and prevention of PPC is getting the patient out of bed, preferably walking.

Anesthesiologists directly manipulate pulmonary function. Thus, a sound and thorough working knowledge of applied pulmonary physiology is essential to the safe conduct of anesthesia. This chapter discusses pulmonary anatomy, the control of ventilation, oxygen and carbon dioxide transport, ventilation–perfusion relationships, lung volumes and pulmonary function testing, abnormal physiology and anesthesia, the effect of smoking on pulmonary function, and assessing risk for postoperative pulmonary complications (PPCs).

FUNCTIONAL ANATOMY OF THE LUNGS

This section emphasizes functional lung anatomy, with structure described as it applies to the mechanical and physiologic function of the lungs.

Thorax

The thoracic cage is shaped like a truncated cone, with a small superior aperture and a larger inferior opening to which the diaphragm is attached. The sternal angle is located in the horizontal plane that passes through the vertebral column at the T4 or T5 level. This plane separates the superior from the inferior mediastinum. During ventilation, the predominant changes in thoracic diameter occur in the anteroposterior direction in the upper thoracic region and in the lateral or transverse direction in the lower thorax.

Muscles of Ventilation

Work of breathing is the energy expenditure of ventilatory muscles. Like other skeletal muscles, the ventilatory muscles are endurance muscles that are subject to fatigue from inadequate oxygen delivery, poor nutrition, increased work secondary to chronic obstructive pulmonary disease (COPD) with gas trapping, or increased airway resistance. The ventilatory muscles include the diaphragm, intercostal muscles, abdominal muscles, cervical strap muscles, sternocleidomastoid muscles, and the large back and intervertebral muscles of the shoulder girdle. During breathing the diaphragm performs most of the muscle work. Work contribution from the intercostal muscles is minor. Normally, at rest, inspiration requires work and exhalation is passive. As work of breathing increases, abdominal muscles assist with rib depression and increase intra-abdominal pressure to facilitate forced exhalation causing the "stitch" athletes experience when they actively exhale. With further increases in work, the cervical strap muscles help elevate the sternum and upper portions of the chest. Finally, during periods of maximal work, the large back and paravertebral muscles of the shoulder girdle contribute to ventilatory effort. The muscles of the abdominal wall, the most powerful muscles of expiration, are important for expulsive efforts such as coughing.[1]

1 With normal lungs, both breathing and coughing can be performed solely by the diaphragm.

Breathing is an endurance phenomenon involving fatigue-resistant muscle fibers, characterized by a slow-twitch response to electrical stimulation that must create sufficient force to lift the ribs and generate subatmospheric pressure in the intrapleural space. These fatigue-resistant fibers comprise approximately 50% of the total diaphragmatic muscle fibers. The high oxidative capacity of theses fibers creates endurance units.[2] Fast-twitch muscle fibers, more susceptible to fatigue, have rapid responses to electrical stimulation imparting strength and allowing greater force over less time. The combination of fast-twitch fibers useful during brief maximal ventilatory effort periods (coughing, sneezing) and slow-twitch fibers providing endurance (breathing without rest) belie its unique duplicitous function as a muscle.[3]

A working muscle like the diaphragm must be firmly anchored at both its origin and insertion. However, its unique insertion is mobile—a central tendon originates from fibers attached to the vertebral bodies as well as the lower ribs and sternum. Diaphragmatic contraction results in descent of the diaphragmatic dome and expansion of the thoracic base creating decreases in intrathoracic and intrapleural pressure and an increase in intra-abdominal pressure.

The cervical strap muscles, active even during breathing at rest, are the most important inspiratory accessory muscles. When diaphragm function is impaired, as in patients with cervical spinal cord transection, they can become the primary inspiratory muscles.

Lung Structures

In an intact respiratory system, the expandable lung tissue fills the pleural cavity. The visceral and parietal pleurae oppose each other, creating a potential intrapleural space where pressure decreases when the diaphragm descends and the rib cage expands. At the end of inspiration, the resultant subatmospheric intrapleural pressure is a reflection of the opposing and equal forces between the tendency of the lung to collapse and the chest wall musculature to remain expanded to create subatmospheric pleural pressure. These equal and opposing forces at end inspiration result in the functional residual capacity (FRC), the volume of gas in the lungs at passive end expiration. At FRC the intrapleural space normally has a slightly subambient pressure (-2 to -3 mm Hg). Major divisions of the right and left lung are listed in Table 11-1. Knowledge of the bronchopulmonary segments is important for localizing lung pathology, interpreting lung radiographs, identifying lung regions during bronchoscopy, and operating on the lung. Each bronchopulmonary segment is separated from its adjacent segments by well-defined connective tissue planes that often anatomically confine initial primary lung pathologies.

The lung parenchyma can be subdivided into three airway categories based on functional lung anatomy (Table 11-2). The conductive airways allow or conduct basic gas transport without gas exchange. The next group of airways, which have smaller diameters, are transitional airways. Transitional airways are not only conduits for gas movement, but also allow limited gas diffusion and exchange. Finally, the primary function of the smallest respiratory airways is gas exchange.

Conventionally, large airways with diameters of >2 mm create 90% of total airway resistance. The number of alveoli increases progressively from approximately 24 million at birth to the final adult count of 300 million at the age of 8 or 9 years. These alveoli are associated with about 250 million

TABLE 11-1

MAJOR DIVISIONS OF THE LUNG

■ LUNG SIDE/LOBE	■ BRONCHOPULMONARY SEGMENT
RIGHT	
Upper	Apical
	Anterior
	Posterior
Middle	Medial
	Lateral
Lower	Superior
	Medial basal
	Lateral basal
	Anterior basal
	Posterior basal
LEFT	
Upper	Apical posterior
	Anterior
Lingula	Superior
	Inferior
Lower	Superior
	Posterior basal
	Anteromedial basal
	Lateral basal

precapillaries and 280 billion capillary segments, resulting in a surface area of ~70 m² for gas exchange.

Conductive Airways

In the adult, the trachea is a fibromuscular tube ~10 to 12 cm long with an outside diameter of ~20 mm. Structural support is provided by 20 U-shaped hyaline cartilages, with the open part of the U facing posteriorly. The cricoid membrane tethers the trachea to the cricoid cartilage at the level of the sixth cervical vertebral body. The trachea enters the superior mediastinum and bifurcates at the sternal angle (the lower border of the fourth thoracic vertebral body). Normally, half of the trachea is intrathoracic and half is extrathoracic. Because both ends of the trachea are attached to mobile structures, the adult carina can move superiorly as much as 5 cm from its normal resting position. Awareness of airway "motion" is essential to proper care of the intubated patient. In the adult, the tip of an orotracheal tube moves an average of 3.8 cm with flexion and extension of the neck but can travel as far as 6.4 cm.[4] In infants and children, tracheal tube movement with respect to the trachea is even more critical: displacement of even 1 cm can result in unintentional extubation or bronchial intubation.

The next airway generation is composed of the right and left main stem bronchi. The diameter of the right bronchus is generally greater than that of the left. In the adult, the right bronchus leaves the trachea at ~25 degrees from the vertical tracheal axis, whereas the angle of the left bronchus is ~45 degrees. Thus,

inadvertent endobronchial intubation or aspiration of foreign material is more likely to occur on the right than the left. Furthermore, the right upper lobe bronchus dives almost directly posterior at ~90 degrees from the right main bronchus facilitating aspiration of foreign bodies and fluid into the right upper lobe in the supine patient. In children younger than 3 years of age, the angles created by the right and left main stem bronchi are approximately equal, with takeoff angles of about 55 degrees.

The adult right main bronchus is ~2.5 cm long before it initially branches into lobar bronchi. However, in 10% of adults, the right upper lobe bronchus departs from the right main stem bronchus <2.5 cm from the carina. Furthermore, in ~2 to 3% of adults, the right upper lobe bronchus opens into the trachea, superior to the carina. Patients with these anomalies require special consideration when placing double-lumen tracheal tubes, especially if one contemplates inserting a right-sided endobronchial tube. After the right upper and middle lobe bronchi divide from the right main bronchus, the main channel becomes the right lower lobe bronchus.

The left main bronchus is ~5 cm long before its initial branching point to the left upper lobe and the lingula; it then continues as the left lower lobe bronchus.

The bronchioles, typically 1 mm in diameter, are devoid of cartilaginous support and have the highest proportion of smooth muscle in their walls. Of the three to four bronchiolar generations, the final generation is the terminal bronchiole, which is the last airway component incapable of gas exchange.

Transitional Airways

The respiratory bronchiole, which follows the terminal bronchiole, is the first site in the tracheobronchial tree where gas exchange occurs. In adults, two or three generations of respiratory bronchioles lead to alveolar ducts, of which there are four to five generations, each with multiple openings into alveolar sacs. The final divisions of alveolar ducts terminate in alveolar sacs that open into alveolar clusters.

Respiratory Airways and the Alveolar–Capillary Membrane

The alveolar-capillary membrane has two primary functions: transport of respiratory gases (oxygen and carbon dioxide) and the production of a wide variety of local and humoral substances. Gas transport is facilitated by the pulmonary capillary beds that logically are the densest capillary networks in the body. This extensive vascular branching system starts with pulmonary arterioles in the region of the respiratory bronchioles. Each alveolus is closely associated with ~1,000 short capillary segments.

The alveolar-capillary interface is complicated but well designed to facilitate gas exchange. Viewed with electron microscopy, the alveolar wall consists of a thin capillary epithelial cell, a basement membrane, a pulmonary capillary endothelial cell, and a surfactant lining layer. The flattened, squamous type I alveolar cells cover ~80% of the alveolar surface. Type I cells contain flattened nuclei and extremely thin

TABLE 11-2

FUNCTIONAL AIRWAY DIVISIONS

■ TYPE	■ FUNCTION	■ STRUCTURE
Conductive	Bulk gas movement	Trachea to terminal bronchioles
Transitional	Bulk gas movement	Respiratory bronchioles
	Limited gas exchange	Alveolar ducts
Respiratory	Gas exchange	Alveoli
		Alveolar sacs

cytoplasmic extensions that provide the surface for gas exchange. Type I cells are highly differentiated and metabolically limited, which makes them highly susceptible to injury. When type I cells are damaged severely (during acute lung injury or adult respiratory distress syndrome), type II cells replicate and modify to form new type I cells.[5]

Type II alveolar cells are interspersed among type I cells, primarily at alveolar–septal junctions. These polygonal cells have vast metabolic and enzymatic activity and manufacture surfactant. The enzymatic activity required to produce surfactant is only 50% of the total enzymatic activity present in type II alveolar cells.[6] The remaining enzymatic activity modulates local electrolyte balance, as well as endothelial and lymphatic cell functions. Both type I and type II alveolar cells have tight intracellular junctions, providing a relatively impermeable barrier to fluids.

Type III alveolar cells, alveolar macrophages, are an important element of immunologic lung defense. Their migratory and phagocytic activities permit ingestion of foreign materials within alveolar spaces.[7] Although functional pulmonary macrophages reduce the incidence of lung infection,[8] they are also an integral part of the organwide pulmonary inflammatory response. Thus, it is highly controversial whether the presence of these cells is beneficial (reducing the sequelae of infection) or harmful (contributing to the inflammatory response).[9]

Pulmonary Vascular Systems

Two major circulatory systems supply blood to the lungs: the pulmonary and bronchial vascular networks. The pulmonary vascular system delivers mixed-venous blood from the right ventricle to the pulmonary capillary bed via two pulmonary arteries. After gas exchange occurs in the pulmonary capillary bed, blood is returned to the left atrium via four pulmonary veins. The pulmonary veins run independently along the intralobar connective tissue planes. The pulmonary capillary system adequately provides for the metabolic and oxygen needs of the alveolar parenchyma. The bronchial arterial system provides oxygen to the conductive airways and pulmonary vessels. Anatomic connections between the bronchial and pulmonary venous circulations create an absolute shunt of ~2 to 5% of the total cardiac output, and represents "normal" shunt.

LUNG MECHANICS

Lung movement occurs secondary to forces external to the lungs. During spontaneous ventilation, the external forces are produced by ventilatory muscles. The lungs' response is governed by two main categories: ease of elastic recoil of the chest wall and by resistance to gas flow within airways.

Elastic Work

The natural tendency of the lungs is to collapse because of elastic recoil; thus, expiration at rest is normally passive as gas flows out of the lungs. The thoracic cage exerts an outward-directed force and the lungs exert an inward-directed force, and because the outward force of the thoracic cage exceeds the inward force of the lung, the overall tendency of the lung within the thoracic cage is to remain inflated. FRC represents the gas volume in the lungs when the outward and inward forces on the lung are equal. Gravitational forces create a more subatmospheric pressure in nondependent areas of the lung than in dependent areas. In the upright adult, the difference in intrapleural pressure from the top to the bottom of the lung is ~7 cm H_2O.

Surface tension at an air–fluid interface produces forces that tend to further reduce the area of interface. For a bubble to remain inflated the gas pressure within a bubble that is contained by surface tension must be higher than the surrounding gas pressure. Alveoli resemble bubbles in this respect, but unlike a bubble, alveolar gas communicates with the atmosphere via the airways. The Laplace equation describes this phenomenon: $P = 2T/R$, where P is the pressure within the bubble (dyne $\cdot$ cm^{-2}), T is the surface tension of the liquid (dyne $\cdot$ cm^{-1}), and R is the radius of the bubble (in centimeters).

During inspiration, the surface tension of the liquid in the lung increases to 40 mN/m, a value close to that of plasma. During expiration, this surface tension falls to 19 mN/m, a value lower than that of most other fluids. This change in surface tension creates hysteresis of the alveoli, different pressure-volume relationships of the alveoli during inspiration and expiration. Unlike a bubble, the pressure within an alveolus decreases as the radius of curvature decreases, creating gas flow from larger to smaller alveoli, which maintains structural stability and prevents lung collapse.

The alveolar transmural pressure gradient, or transpulmonary pressure, is the difference between intrapleural and alveolar pressure and is directly proportional to lung volume. Intrapleural pressure can be safely measured with a percutaneously inserted catheter[10]; however, clinicians rarely perform this technique. When measured with an esophageal balloon in the midesophagus, esophageal pressure can be used as a reflection of intrapleural pressure.[11] Commercially available esophageal pressure monitors increase the ease and accuracy of measuring esophageal pressure as a reflection of intrapleural pressure.[12] These monitors are useful for estimating the elastic work performed by the patient during spontaneous ventilation, mechanical ventilation, or a combination of spontaneous and mechanical ventilation. By estimating intrapleural pressure on a real-time basis, it is possible to quantitate the patient's work of breathing and changes secondary to intervention. Low levels of inspiratory pressure support can compensate for the work of breathing imposed by the endotracheal tube.[13]

Physiologic work of breathing includes elastic work (inspiratory work required to overcome the elastic recoil of the pulmonary system) and resistive work (work to overcome resistance to gas flow in the airway). For a patient in whom breathing apparatus is employed, the concept of total work of breathing encompasses physiologic work plus equipment-imposed ventilatory work to overcome the resistance imposed by the breathing apparatus; such as an endotracheal tube or a ventilator demand valve.

If the lungs are slowly inflated and deflated, the pressure–volume curve during inflation differs from that obtained during deflation. The two curves form a hysteresis loop that becomes progressively broader as the tidal volume is increased (Fig. 11-1). To inflate the lungs, pressure greater than the recoil pressure of deflation is needed, which means that the lung accepts deformation poorly and, once deformed, reforms to its original shape slowly. Elastic hysteresis is important for the maintenance of normal lung compliance but is not clinically significant.

The sum of the pressure-volume relationships of the thorax and lung results in a sigmoidal curve (Fig. 11-2). The vertical line drawn at end expiration coincides with FRC. Normally, humans breathe on the steepest part of the sigmoidal curve, where compliance ($\Delta V/\Delta P$) or slope is highest. In restrictive pulmonary diseases, the compliance curve shifts to the right, has decreased slope, or both. This decreased lung compliance results in smaller FRCs. When lung compliance is reduced, larger changes in intrapleural pressure are needed to create the same tidal volume; that is, the thorax has to work harder to get the same volume of gas into the lungs. The body, being an energy-conserving organism, prefers to move less gas with each breath rather than working harder to achieve the same tidal volume. Thus, patients with restrictive lung disease typically breathe with smaller tidal volumes at more rapid rates, making the spontaneous ventilatory rate one of the most sensitive indices of

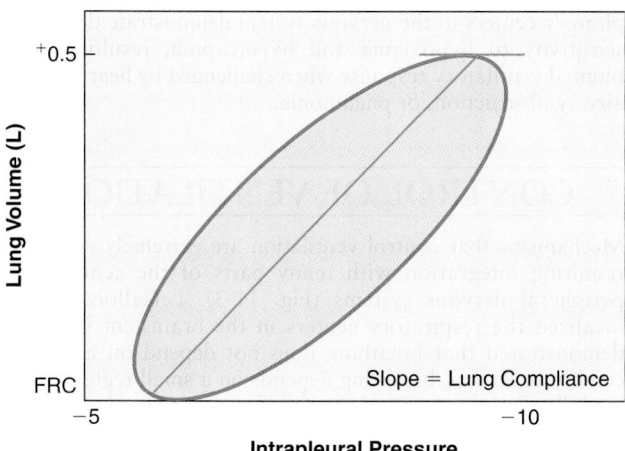

FIGURE 11-1. Dynamic pressure–volume loop of resting tidal volume. Quiet, normal breathing is characterized by hysteresis of the pressure–volume loop. The lung is more resistant to deformation than expected and returns to its original configuration less easily than expected. The slope of the line connecting the zenith and nadir lung volumes is lung compliance, ~500 mL/3 cm H_2O = 167 mL/cm H_2O.

lung compliance. When lung compliance is decreased, continuous positive airway pressure (CPAP) will shift the vertical line to the right, allowing the patient to breathe on a steeper, more efficient portion of the volume–pressure curve, resulting in a slower ventilatory rate with a larger tidal volume.

At the other end of the spectrum, patients with diseases that increase lung compliance expend less elastic work to inspire but have decreased elastic recoil creating larger than normal FRC (gas trapping), and their pressure–volume curves shift to the left and steepen. Chronic obstructive lung disease and acute asthma are the most common examples of diseases with high lung compliance. If lung compliance and FRC are sufficiently high that elastic recoil is minimal, the patient must use ventilatory muscles to actively exhale. The difficulty these

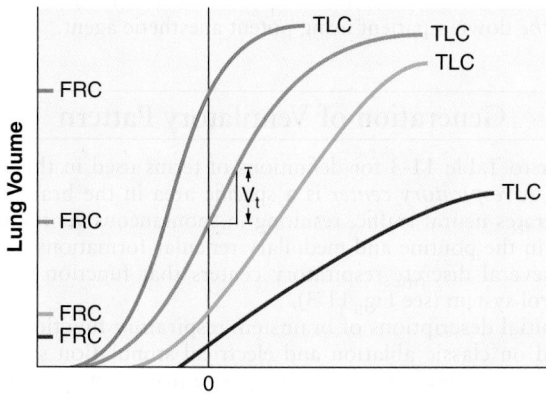

FIGURE 11-2. Pulmonary pressure–volume relationships at different values of total lung capacity (TLC), ignoring hysteresis. The *blue line* depicts the normal pulmonary pressure–volume relationships. Humans normally breathe on the linear, steep part of this sigmoidal curve, where the slope, which is equal to compliance, is greatest. The *vertical line* at zero defines functional residual capacity (FRC), regardless of the position of the curve on the graph. Mild restrictive lung disease, indicated by the *green line*, shifts the curve to the right with little change in slope. However, with restrictive disease, the patient breathes on a lower FRC, at a point on the curve where the slope is less. Severe restrictive pulmonary disease profoundly depresses the FRC and diminishes the slope of the entire curve (*red line*). Obstructive disease (*orange line*) elevates both FRC and compliance.

patients experience in emptying the lungs is compounded by the increased airway resistance.

Both compliance and inspiratory elastic work can be measured for a single breath by measuring airway (Paw), intrapleural (Ppl) pressures, and tidal volume. If esophageal pressure is measured correctly, the esophageal pressure values can be substituted for Ppl values. Lung compliance, C_L, the slope of the volume–pressure curve, is given by the equation:

$$C_L = \frac{\Delta V}{\Delta P_L} + \frac{V_T}{P_{L_i} - P_{L_e}} = \frac{V_T}{(Paw_i - Ppl_i) - (Paw_e - Ppl_e)}$$

(11-1)

where P_L is transpulmonary pressure, P_{L_i} and P_{L_e} are transpulmonary pressure at end-inspiratory and end-expiratory, V_T is tidal volume, Paw_e and Paw_i are expiratory and inspiratory airway pressures, and Ppl_e and Ppl_i are expiratory and inspiratory intrapleural pressures.

Elastic work (W_{el}) is performed during inspiration only because expiration is passive during normal breathing. The area within the triangle in Figure 11-2 describes the work required to inspire. The equation that yields elastic work (and the area of the triangle) is:

$$W_{el} = \frac{1}{2}(V_T)(P_{L_i} - P_{L_e})$$
$$= \frac{1}{2}(V_T)(Paw_i - Ppl_i) - (Paw_e - Ppl_{le})$$

(11-2)

Resistance to Gas Flow

Both laminar and turbulent flows exist within the respiratory tract, usually in mixed patterns. The physics of each, however, is significantly different and worth consideration.

Laminar Flow

Below critical flow rates that create turbulent flow, gas proceeds through a straight tube as a series of concentric cylinders that slide over one another. Fully developed flow has a parabolic profile with a velocity of zero at the cylinder wall and a maximum velocity at the center of the advancing "cone." This type of streamlined flow is usually inaudible. The advancing conical front means that some fresh gas reaches the end of the tube before the tube has been completely filled with fresh gas. Thus, laminar flow in the airways results in alveolar ventilation which can occur even when the tidal volume (V_T) is less than anatomic dead space. This phenomenon certainly has significant clinical implications, and as noted by Rohrer[14] in 1915 it allows high-frequency ventilation to achieve adequate alveolar ventilation.

Resistance to laminar gas flows in a straight, unbranched tube can be calculated by the following equation:

$$R = \frac{8 \times length \times viscosity}{\pi \times (radius)^4} = \frac{P_B - P_A}{flow}$$

(11-3)

where P_B and P_A are barometric and alveolar pressures. It is essential to note that as radius decreases in narrowed airways, resistance will increase by a power of four. Viscosity is the only physical gas property that is relevant under conditions of laminar flow. Helium has a low density, but its viscosity is close to that of air. Therefore, helium will not improve gas flow if the flow is laminar. Flow is usually turbulent when there is critical airway narrowing or abnormally high airway resistance, making low-density helium useful therapy (see next section).

Turbulent Flow

High flow rates, particularly through branched or irregularly shaped tubes, disrupt the orderly flow of laminar gas. When resistance to gas flow is significant, turbulent flow occurs and is usually audible. Turbulent flow usually presents with a square front so fresh gas will not reach the end of the tube until the amount of gas entering the tube is almost equal to the volume of the tube. Thus, turbulent flow effectively purges the contents of a tube. Four conditions that will change laminar flow to turbulent flow are high gas flows, sharp angles within the tube, branching in the tube, and a decrease in the tube's diameter. During laminar flow, resistance is inversely proportional to gas flow rate. Conversely, during turbulent flow, resistance increases significantly in proportion to the flow rate. A detailed description of these phenomena is beyond the scope of this chapter, but the reader is referred to descriptions by Nunn.[15]

Increased Airway Resistance

Bronchiolar smooth muscle hyperreactivity (true bronchospasm), mucosal edema, mucous plugging, epithelial desquamation, tumors, and foreign bodies all increase airway resistance. The conscious subject can detect small increases in inspiratory resistance.[16] The normal response to increased inspiratory resistance is increased inspiratory muscle effort, with little change in FRC.[17] Emphysematous patients retain remarkable ability to preserve an adequate alveolar ventilation, even with gross airway obstruction. In patients with preoperative values of forced expiratory volume in the first second of expiration (FEV_1) that are <1 L, $PaCO_2$ is normal in most patients. Furthermore, asthmatic patients compensate well for increased airway resistance and also keep the mean $PaCO_2$ in the lower end of normal range.[18] Thus, an increased $PaCO_2$ in the setting of increased airway resistance warrants serious attention as it may signal that the patient's compensatory mechanisms are nearly exhausted. Mild expiratory resistance does not result in muscle use for active exhalation in conscious or anesthetized subjects. Instead, the initial work to overcome expiratory resistance is performed by augmenting inspiratory force until a sufficiently high lung volume is achieved that allows elastic recoil to overcome expiratory resistance.[19] When expiratory resistance becomes excessive, accessory muscles are used to force gas from the lungs. During acute increases in expiratory resistance, this response can be well tolerated by most patients. However, chronic use of accessory muscles to exhale significantly increases the risk of ventilatory failure if work of breathing is further increased. When work of breathing exceeds physiologic reserves, work of breathing becomes detrimental to physiologic homeostasis and impending ventilatory failure secondary to ventilatory muscle fatigue becomes acute ventilatory failure evidenced by an acute increase in arterial carbon dioxide. Commonly, this is precipitated by pneumonia or heart failure.

Physiologic Changes in Respiratory Function Associated With Aging

Physiologic aging of the lung is associated with dilation of the alveoli, enlargement of the airspaces, decrease in exchange surface area, and loss of supporting tissue.[20] Changes in the aging lung and chest wall result in decreased lung recoil (elastance), creating an increased residual volume and FRC. Additionally, compliance of the chest wall diminishes, thereby increasing the work of breathing compared with younger subjects. Respiratory muscle strength decreases with aging and is strongly correlated with nutritional status and cardiac index. Expiratory flow rates decrease with a flow–volume curve suggestive of small airway resistance. Despite these changes, the respiratory system is normally able to maintain adequate gas exchange at rest and during exertion throughout life, with only modest decrements in PaO_2 and no change in $PaCO_2$. With aging, respiratory centers in the nervous system demonstrate decreased sensitivity to hypoxemia and hypercapnia, resulting in a blunted ventilatory response when challenged by heart failure, airway obstruction, or pneumonia.

CONTROL OF VENTILATION

Mechanisms that control ventilation are extremely complex, requiring integration with many parts of the central and peripheral nervous systems (Fig. 11-3). LeGallois,[21] who localized the respiratory centers in the brainstem in 1812, demonstrated that breathing does not depend on an intact cerebrum. Rather, breathing depends on a small region of the medulla near the origin of the vagus nerves. Countless studies in the past two centuries have greatly increased our knowledge and understanding of the anatomic components of ventilatory control. However, experimental work performed in animals is difficult to apply to humans because of interspecies variation.

Terminology

Breathing, ventilation, and respiration are often used interchangeably. However, it is important to realize that these terms have distinct meanings. The term *breathing* refers to the act of inspiring and exhaling, which requires energy utilization for muscle work and thus is limited by energy reserves. *Ventilation*, on the other hand, is the movement of gas in and out of the lungs. When spontaneous, ventilation requires energy for muscle work and is, thus, breathing. *Respiration* occurs when energy is released from organic molecules. Such energy release depends on the movement of gas molecules such as carbon dioxide and oxygen across membranes, whether alveolar or mitochondrial. Thus, humans breathe to ventilate and ventilate to respire. Despite what appears to be clear distinctions in terminology, vernacular use of these terms are often confused in daily dialog. For example: *respirators* are used to treat those who have succumbed to *respiratory* arrest and do not have a *respiratory* rate, and residents are sometimes advised to *breathe* down a patient using potent anesthetic agent.

Generation of Ventilatory Pattern

Refer to Table 11-3 for definitions of terms used in this section. A *respiratory center* is a specific area in the brain that integrates neural traffic, resulting in spontaneous ventilation. Within the pontine and medullary reticular formations, there are several discrete respiratory centers that function as the control system (see Fig. 11-3).

Initial descriptions of brainstem respiratory functions are based on classic ablation and electrical stimulation studies. Another method for localizing respiratory centers entails recording action potentials from different areas of the brainstem with microelectrodes. This method is based on the assumption that local brain activity that occurs in phase with respiratory activity is evidence that the area under study has "respiratory neurons."[22] These techniques are imperfect for precisely localizing discrete respiratory centers.

Medullary Centers

The medulla oblongata contains the most basic ventilatory control centers in the brain. Specific medullary areas are primarily active during inspiration or during expiration, with many neural inspiratory or expiratory interconnections. The inspiratory centers that reside in the dorsal respiratory group

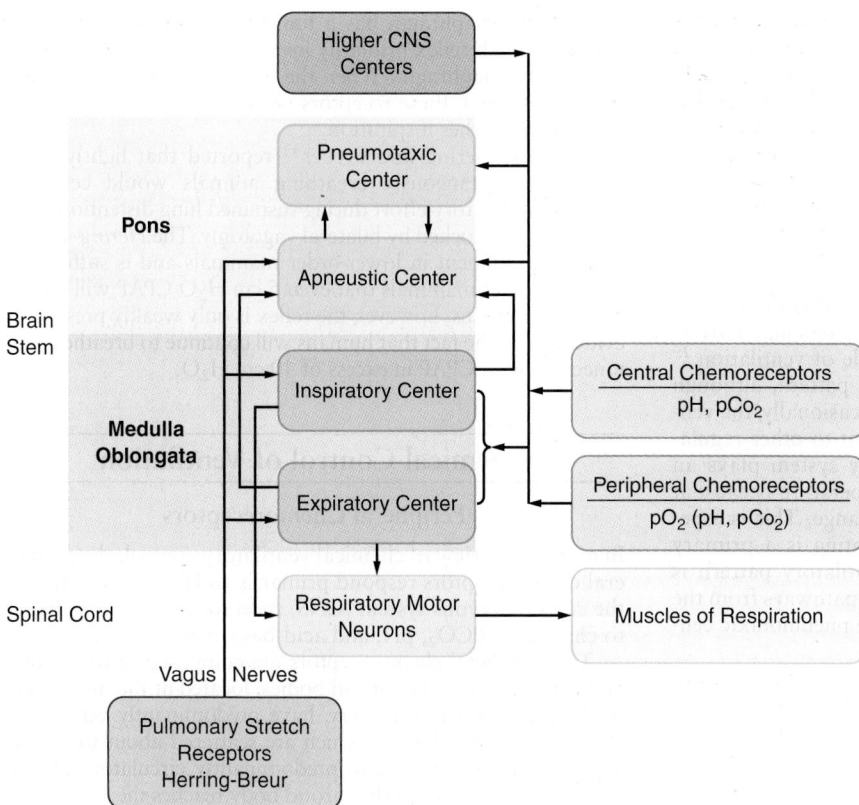

FIGURE 11-3. Classic central nervous system (CNS) respiratory centers. Diagram illustrates major respiratory centers, neurofeedback circuits, primary neurohumoral sensory inputs, and mechanical outputs.

(DRG) are located in the dorsal medullary reticular formation. The DRG is the source of elementary ventilatory rhythmicity[23,24] and serves as the "pacemaker" for the respiratory system.[25] Whereas resting lung volume occurs at end expiration, the electrical activity of the ventilatory centers is at rest at end inspiration. The rhythmic activity of the DRG persists even when all incoming peripheral and interconnecting nerves are sectioned or blocked completely. Isolating the DRG in this manner results in ataxic, gasping ventilation with frequent maximum inspiratory efforts: apneustic breathing.

The ventral respiratory group (VRG), which is located in the ventral medullary reticular formation, serves as the expiratory coordinating center. The inspiratory and expiratory neurons function by a system of reciprocal innervation, or negative feedback.[22] When the DRG creates an impulse to inspire, inspiration occurs and the DRG impulse is quenched by a reciprocating VRG impulse. This VRG transmission prohibits further use of the inspiratory muscles, thus allowing passive expiration to occur.

Pontine Centers

The pontine centers process information that originates in the medulla. The apneustic center is located in the middle or lower pons. With activation, this center sends impulses to inspiratory DRG neurons and is designed to sustain inspiration. Electrical stimulation of this area results in inspiratory spasm.[26] The middle and lower pons contain specific areas for phase-spanning neurons.[27] These neurons assist with the transition between inspiration and expiration, and do not exert direct control over ventilatory muscles.

The pneumotaxic respiratory center is in the rostral pons. A simple transection through the brainstem that isolates this portion of the pons from the upper brainstem reduces ventilatory

---

TABLE 11-3

DEFINITION OF RESPIRATORY PATTERN TERMINOLOGY

■ WORD	■ DEFINITION
Eupnea	"Good breathing": continuous inspiratory and expiratory movement without interruption
Apnea	"No breathing": cessation of ventilatory effort at passive end-expiration (lung volume = FRC)
Apneusis	Cessation of ventilatory effort with lungs filled at TLC
Apneustic ventilation	Apneusis with periodic expiratory spasms
Biot	Ventilatory gasps interposed between periods of ventilation apnea; *also* "agonal ventilation"

FRC, functional residual capacity; TLC, total lung capacity.

rate and increases tidal volume. If both vagus nerves are additionally transected, apneusis results.[28] Thus, the primary function of the pneumotaxic center is to limit the depth of inspiration. When maximally activated, the pneumotaxic center secondarily increases ventilatory frequency. However, the pneumotaxic center performs no pacemaking function and has no intrinsic rhythmicity.

Higher Respiratory Centers

Many higher brain structures clearly affect ventilatory control processes. In the midbrain, stimulation of the reticular activating system increases the rate and amplitude of ventilation.[29] The cerebral cortex also affects breathing pattern, although precise neural pathways are not known. Occasionally, the ventilatory control process becomes subservient to other regulatory centers. For example, the respiratory system plays an important role in the control of body temperature because it supplies a large surface area for heat exchange. This is especially important in animals in which panting is a primary means of dissipating heat. Thus, the, ventilatory pattern is influenced by neural input from descending pathways from the anterior and posterior hypothalamus to the pneumotaxic center of the upper pons.

Vasomotor control and certain respiratory responses are closely linked. Stimulation of the carotid sinus not only decreases vasomotor tone, but also inhibits ventilation. Alternatively, stimulation of the carotid body chemoreceptors (see "Chemical Control of Ventilation") results in an increase in both ventilatory activity and vasomotor tone.

Reflex Control of Ventilation

Reflexes that directly influence ventilatory pattern usually do so to prevent airway obstruction. *Deglutition*, or swallowing, involves the glossopharyngeal and vagus nerves. Stimulation of the anterior and posterior pharyngeal pillars of the posterior pharynx induces swallowing. During swallowing, inspiration ceases momentarily, is usually followed by a single large breath, and briefly increases ventilation.

Vomiting significantly modifies normal ventilatory activity.[30] Swallowing, salivation, gastrointestinal reflexes, rhythmic spasmodic ventilatory movements, and significant diaphragmatic and abdominal muscular activity must be coordinated over a very brief interval. Because of the obvious risk of aspirating gastric contents, it is advantageous to inhibit inspiration during vomiting. Input into the respiratory centers occurs from both cranial and spinal cord nerves.

Coughing results from stimulation of the tracheal subepithelium, especially along the posterior tracheal wall and carina.[31] Coughing also requires coordination of both airway and ventilatory muscle activity. An effective cough requires deep inspiration and then forced exhalation against a momentarily closed glottis to increase intrathoracic pressure, thus allowing an expulsive expiratory maneuver.

Proprioception in the pulmonary system, the qualitative knowledge of the gas volume within the lungs, probably arises from smooth muscle spindle receptors. These proprioceptors, which are located within the smooth muscle of all airways, are sensitive to pressure changes. Airway stretch reflexes can be demonstrated during distention of isolated airways so airway pressure, rather than volume distention, appears to be the primary stimulation.[32] Clinical conditions in which pulmonary airway stretch receptors are stimulated include pulmonary edema and atelectasis.

Golgi tendon organs (tendon spindles), which occur in series arrangements within ventilatory muscles, facilitate proprioception. The intercostal muscles are rich in tendon spindles,

whereas the diaphragm has a limited number. Thus, the pulmonary stretch reflex primarily involves the intercostal muscles but not the diaphragm. When the lungs are full and the chest wall is stretched, these receptors send signals to the brainstem that inhibit further inspiration.

In 1868, Hering and Breuer[33] reported that lightly anesthetized, spontaneously breathing animals would cease or decrease ventilatory effort during sustained lung distention. This response was blocked by bilateral vagotomy. The *Hering–Breuer reflex* is prominent in lower-order mammals and is sufficiently active in lower mammals that even 5 cm H_2O CPAP will induce apnea. In humans, however, the reflex is only weakly present, as evidenced by the fact that humans will continue to breathe spontaneously with CPAP in excess of 40 cm H_2O.

Chemical Control of Ventilation

Peripheral Chemoreceptors

In a simplistic view of chemical ventilatory control, the peripheral chemoreceptors respond primarily to lack of oxygen, and the central nervous system (CNS) receptors respond primarily to changes in PCO_2, pH, and acid-base disturbances.

The peripheral chemoreceptors are composed of the carotid and aortic bodies. The carotid bodies, located at the bifurcation of the common carotid artery, have predominantly ventilatory effects. The aortic bodies, which are scattered about the aortic arch and its branches, have predominantly circulatory effects. The neural output from the carotid body reaches the central respiratory centers via the afferent glossopharyngeal nerves. Output from the aortic bodies travels to the medullary centers via the vagus nerve. Both carotid and aortic bodies are stimulated by decreased PaO_2, but not by decreased SaO_2 or CaO_2. When PaO_2 falls to <100 mm Hg, neural activity from these receptors begins to increase. However, it is not until the PaO_2 reaches 60 to 65 mm Hg that neural activity increases sufficiently to substantially augment minute ventilation. Thus, patients who depend on hypoxic ventilatory drive have PaO_2 values in the middle 60s. Once these patients' PaO_2 values exceed 60 to 65 mm Hg, ventilatory drive diminishes and PaO_2 falls until ventilation is again stimulated by arterial hypoxemia. Thus, during withdrawal of mechanical ventilatory support in the patient who depends on hypoxic ventilatory drive, the PaO_2 must fall to <65 mm Hg for spontaneous ventilation to resume (see Chapter 56.)

The carotid bodies are also sensitive to decreased pH_a, but this response is minor. Similarly, changes in $PaCO_2$ do not stimulate these receptors sufficiently to alter minute ventilation. Increases in blood temperature, hypoperfusion of the carotid bodies themselves, and some chemicals will stimulate these receptors. Sympathetic ganglion stimulation by nicotine or acetylcholine will stimulate the carotid and aortic bodies; this effect is blocked by hexamethonium. Blockade of the cytochrome electron transport system by cyanide will prevent oxidative metabolism and will also stimulate these receptors.

Ventilatory effects resulting from stimulation of these receptors are increased ventilatory rate and tidal volume. Hemodynamic changes resulting from stimulation of these receptors include bradycardia, hypertension, increases in bronchiolar tone, and increases in adrenal secretion. The carotid body chemical receptors have been termed *ultimum moriens* ("last to die"). Although the response of peripheral receptors to hypoxemia was formerly believed to be resistant to the influences of anesthesia, potent inhaled anesthetics appear to depress hypoxic ventilatory response by depressing carotid body response to hypoxemia.[34] The response of the peripheral receptors is not sufficiently robust to reliably increase ventilatory rate or minute ventilation to herald the onset of arterial hypoxemia during general anesthesia or recovery from anesthesia. Furthermore, flumazenil, in a 1-mg intravenous dose, only partially reversed the diazepam-induced depression of hypoxic ventilatory drive.[35] The data of Mora et al.[35] further suggest that humans may develop tolerance to respiratory depressant effects of diazepam.

Central Chemoreceptors

Approximately 80% of the ventilatory response to inhaled carbon dioxide originates in the central medullary centers. Acid-base regulation involving carbon dioxide, H^+, and bicarbonate is related primarily to chemosensitive receptors located in the medulla close to or in contact with the cerebrospinal fluid (CSF). The chemosensitive areas of the brainstem are in the inferolateral aspects of the medulla near the origin of cranial nerves IX and X. The area just beneath the surface of the ventral medulla is exquisitely sensitive to the extracellular fluid H^+ concentration.[36] Although the central response is the major factor in the regulation of breathing by carbon dioxide, carbon dioxide has little direct stimulating effect on these chemosensitive areas. These receptors are primarily sensitive to changes in H^+ concentration. Carbon dioxide has a potent but indirect effect by reacting with water to form carbonic acid, which dissociates into hydrogen and bicarbonate ions.[37]

An acute increase in $PaCO_2$ is a more potent ventilatory stimulus than an acute increase in arterial protons concentration from a metabolic source. Carbon dioxide, but not H^+, passes readily through the blood–brain and blood–CSF barriers. Local buffering systems immediately neutralize H^+ in arterial blood and body fluids. In contrast, the CSF has minimal buffering capacity. Thus, once carbon dioxide crosses into the CSF, H^+ are created and trapped in the CSF, resulting in a CSF H^+ concentration considerably greater than that found in the blood. Because carbon dioxide crosses the blood–brain barrier readily, the $PaCO_2$ values in the CSF, cerebral tissue, and jugular venous blood rise quickly and to the same degree as the $PaCO_2$, although the central values are ~10 mm Hg higher than those measured in arterial blood.

The ventilatory response to changes in $PaCO_2$ (increased V_T, increased respiratory rate) is rapid and peaks within 1 to 2 minutes after an acute change in $PaCO_2$. With the same, persistent level of carbon dioxide stimulation, the resultant increase in ventilation declines over a period of several hours, probably as a result of bicarbonate ions that are actively transported from the blood into the CSF through the arachnoid villi.[38] This phenomenon explains the differing effects of acute hypercapnia versus chronic hypercapnia on the CNS-mediated ventilatory response. Finally, central medullary chemoreceptors also respond to temperature change. Cold CSF (with normal pH) or local anesthetic applied to the medullary surface will depress ventilation.

Ventilatory Response to Altitude

Ventilatory response and adaptation to high altitude are good examples of the integration of peripheral and central chemoreceptor control of ventilation. The following mechanism of acclimatization was proposed by Severinghaus et al.[39] in 1963 and has since been confirmed.

Following ascent from sea level to 4,000 m, acute exposure to high altitude and low PIO_2 results in arterial hypoxemia. This decrease in PaO_2 activates the peripheral hypoxemic ventilatory drive by stimulating the carotid and aortic bodies, and causes increased minute ventilation. As minute ventilation increases, $PaCO_2$ and CSF PCO_2 decrease, causing concomitant increases in pH_a and CSF pH. The alkaline shift of the CSF decreases ventilatory drive via medullary chemoreceptors, partially offsetting hypoxemic drive. A temporary equilibrium is attained within minutes, with $PaCO_2$ only 2 to 5 mm Hg less than normal and PaO_2 approximately 45 mm Hg. This initially profound hypox-

emia probably causes the acute respiratory distress and other associated symptoms (headache, diarrhea) associated with rapid ascent. However, the CNS is able to restore CSF pH to normal (7.326) by pumping bicarbonate ions out of the CSF over 2 to 3 days. In 2 to 3 days, CSF bicarbonate concentration decreases approximately 5 mEq/L and restores CSF pH to within 0.01 pH unit of values at sea level. Then, centrally mediated ventilatory drive returns to normal, and hypoxic drive and stimulation of peripheral receptors can proceed unopposed. Thus, after 3 days' exposure to 4,000 m altitude, ventilatory adaptation would result in a new equilibrium, with $PaCO_2$ approximately 30 mm Hg and PaO_2 approximately 55 mm Hg. Following descent to sea level, the low CSF bicarbonate concentration persists for several days, and the climber "overbreathes" until CSF bicarbonate and pH values return to normal.

Breath-Holding

Most adults with normal lungs and gas exchange can hold their breath for ~1 minute when breathing room air without previously hyperventilating. After 1 minute of breath-holding under these circumstances, PaO_2 decreases to ~65 to 70 mm Hg and $PaCO_2$ increases by ~12 mm Hg. In the absence of supplemental oxygen and hyperventilation, the "breakpoint" at which normal people are compelled to breathe is remarkably constant at a $PaCO_2$ of 50 mm Hg.[40,41] However, if the individual breathes 100% oxygen prior to breath-holding, he or she should be able to hold his or her breath for 2 to 3 minutes, or until $PaCO_2$ rises to 60 mm Hg. Hyperventilation sufficient to reduce $PaCO_2$ to 20 mm Hg can lengthen the period of breath-holding to 3 to 4 minutes.[42] Hyperventilation with 100% oxygen prior to breath-holding should extend the apneic period to 6 to 10 minutes. The $PaCO_2$ rate of rise in awake, preoxygenated adults with normal lungs who hold their breath without previous hyperventilation is 7 mm Hg/min in the first 10 seconds, 2 mm Hg/min in the next 10 seconds, and 6 mm Hg/min thereafter.[41]

The duration of voluntary breath-holding is directly proportional to lung volume at onset and is probably related both to oxygen stores in the alveoli and to the rate at which $PaCO_2$ rises. With smaller lung volumes, the same amount of carbon dioxide is emptied into a smaller volume during the apneic period, thus increasing the carbon dioxide concentration more rapidly than occurs with larger lung volumes. Of note, apneic patients during general anesthesia actually "breath-hold" at FRC rather than at vital capacity, which would tend to accelerate the rate of rise of carbon dioxide. Despite this difference in lung volume, the rate of rise of $PaCO_2$ in apneic anesthetized patients is 12 mm Hg during the first minute and 3.5 mm Hg/min thereafter, significantly lower than in the awake state.[42,43] During anesthesia, metabolic rate and carbon dioxide production are significantly less than during ambulatory wakefulness, which probably accounts for the different rates of rise in carbon dioxide levels.

Hyperventilation with room air prior to prolonged breath-holding during exercise is inadvisable. During underwater swimming after poolside hyperventilation, the urge to breathe is first stimulated by a rising $PaCO_2$. Because an increased arterial carbon dioxide tension provides the stimulus to inspire, swimmers who hyperventilate with room air prior to swimming long distances frequently lose consciousness from arterial hypoxemia before the $PaCO_2$ is sufficiently increased to stimulate the "need" to breathe.

Hyperventilation is rarely followed by an apneic period in awake humans, despite a markedly depressed $PaCO_2$. However, minute ventilation may decrease significantly. Aggressive intermittent positive-pressure breathing treatments for patients with COPD who continue to have a carbon dioxide-based ventilatory drive can depress minute ventilation sufficiently to create arterial hypoxemia if they breathe room air after cessation of therapy.[44] In contrast, even mild hyperventilation during general anesthesia will produce prolonged apneic periods.[45]

Quantitative Aspects of Chemical Control of Breathing

The ventilatory responses to oxygen and carbon dioxide can be assessed quantitatively. Unfortunately, the quantitative indices of hypoxemic sensitivity are not clinically useful because the normal range is wide and confounded by many environmental factors. The reader is referred to a classic discussion of the quantitative indices of hypoxemic sensitivity.[46]

Ventilatory responses to $PaCO_2$ changes are measured in several ways, provided that carbon dioxide production remains constant. When subjects voluntarily increase minute ventilation to a prescribed level, the $PaCO_2$ decreases hyperbolically. The plot of minute ventilation (independent variable) and $PaCO_2$ (dependent variable) is the metabolic hyperbola (Fig. 11-4). The metabolic hyperbola is cumbersome to evaluate and difficult to use clinically.

The curve more commonly used is the $PaCO_2$ ventilatory response curve (see Fig. 11-4). It describes the effect of changing $PaCO_2$ on the resultant minute ventilation. Usually, subjects inspire carbon dioxide to raise $PaCO_2$, and the effect on minute ventilation is measured. Creating these curves and observing how they change in various circumstances allow quantitative study of factors that affect the chemical carbon dioxide control of ventilation. The carbon dioxide response curve approaches linearity in the range most often encountered in life: at $PaCO_2$ values between 20 and 80 mm Hg. Once the $PaCO_2$ exceeds 80 mm Hg, the curve becomes parabolic, with its peak ventilatory response at a $PaCO_2$ between 100 and 120 mm Hg. Increasing the $PaCO_2$ to higher than 100 mm Hg allows carbon dioxide to act as a ventilatory and CNS depressant, the origin of the term carbon dioxide narcosis, with 1 minimum alveolar concentration being approximately 200 mm Hg.

The slope of the carbon dioxide response curve is considered to represent carbon dioxide sensitivity. When $PaCO_2$ reaches 100 mm Hg, carbon dioxide sensitivity is at its peak. The *set point*, the point of intersection of the carbon dioxide response curve and the metabolic hyperbola, defines normal resting $PaCO_2$. Extrapolation of the carbon dioxide response curve to the x-intercept (where minute ventilation is 0) defines the apneic threshold. In awake, normal adults, the apneic threshold normally occurs at a $PaCO_2$ of ~32 mm Hg, although awake adults usually continue to breathe when they achieve the apneic threshold because the sensation of apnea is disturbing. The slope of the curve is a measure of the response of the entire ventilatory mechanism to carbon dioxide stimulation.

Once PaO_2 exceeds 100 mm Hg, it no longer influences the carbon dioxide response curve. When the PaO_2 is between 65 and 100 mm Hg, its effect on the carbon dioxide response curve is small. However, when PaO_2 falls to <65 mm Hg, the carbon dioxide response curve shifts to the left and its slope increases, probably as a result of increased ventilatory drive stimulated by the peripheral chemoreceptors. Thus, during measurements of carbon dioxide ventilatory response, the subject should breathe supplemental oxygen to prevent hypoxic ventilatory drive interference.

The carbon dioxide response curve can be generated rapidly by increasing the fraction of inspired carbon dioxide ($FICO_2$) by requiring the subject to rebreathe exhaled gas. The results obtained with this technique are less pure because the $FICO_2$ is not controlled.

Three clinical states result in a left shift and/or a steepened slope of the carbon dioxide response curve. These same three situations are the only causes of true hyperventilation; that is, an increase in minute ventilation such that the decreased $PaCO_2$ creates respiratory alkalemia (either primary or compensatory). The three causes of hyperventilation (enhanced carbon dioxide response) are arterial hypoxemia, metabolic acidemia, and CNS etiologies. Examples of central causes that cause hyperventilation include drug administration, intracranial hypertension, hepatic cirrhosis, and nonspecific arousal states such as anxiety and fear. Aminophylline, doxapram, salicylates, and norepinephrine stimulate ventilation independent of peripheral chemoreceptors. Opioid antagonists, given in the absence of opioids, do not stimulate ventilation. However, when given after opioid administration, they do reverse the effects of opioids on the carbon dioxide response curve.

Ventilatory depressants displace the carbon dioxide response curve to the right or decrease its slope or both. Changes in physiology that depress ventilation include metabolic alkalemia, denervation of peripheral chemoreceptors, normal sleep, and drugs. During normal sleep, the carbon dioxide response curve is displaced to the right, with the degree of displacement depending on the depth of sleep. Usually, $PaCO_2$ increases up to 10 mm Hg during deep sleep. Hypoxemic responses are not impaired by sleep, which is convenient for continued survival at high altitude while sleeping.

Opioids displace the carbon dioxide response curve to the right with little change in slope at sedative doses (see Chapter 19.) With higher, "anesthetic" doses, the curve shifts farther to the right and its slope is depressed, simulating the effect of potent inhalation agents on the carbon dioxide response curve (see Fig. 11-4). In the absence of other ventilatory-depressant drugs, opioids induce pathognomonic changes in ventilatory patterns: a decreased ventilatory rate with an increased tidal volume. Not until opioids nearly induce apnea is tidal volume decreased. Large narcotic doses usually result in apnea responsive to verbal encouragement before consciousness is lost.

Barbiturates in sedative or light hypnotic doses have little effect on the carbon dioxide response curve. However, in doses adequate to allow skin incision, barbiturates shift the carbon dioxide response curve to the right. The ventilatory pattern

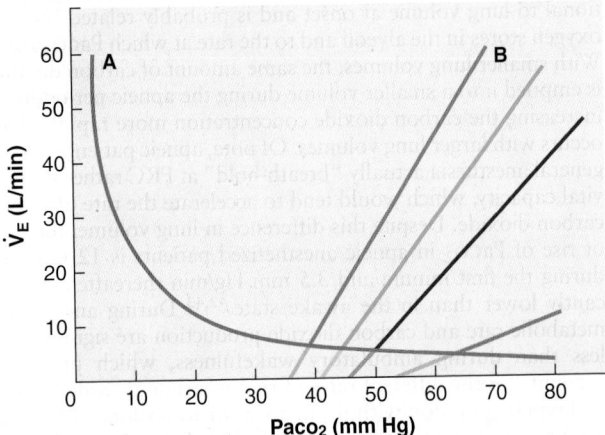

FIGURE 11-4. Carbon dioxide–ventilatory response curve. The metabolic hyperbola, curve A, is generated by varying $\dot{V}A/\dot{Q}E$ and measuring changes in carbon dioxide concentration. The hyperbolic configuration makes it cumbersome for clinical use. The carbon dioxide–ventilatory response curve, B, is linear between approximately 20 and 80 mm Hg. It is generated by varying $PaCO_2$ (usually by controlling inspired carbon dioxide concentration) and measuring the resultant $\dot{V}A/\dot{Q}E$. This is the most commonly used test of ventilatory response. The slope defines "sensitivity"; the set point, or resting $PaCO_2$, occurs at the intersection of the metabolic hyperbola and the carbon dioxide–ventilatory response curve; the apneic threshold can be obtained by extrapolating the carbon dioxide–ventilatory response curve to the x-intercept. In the absence of surgical stimulation, increasing doses of potent inhaled anesthesia or opioids will shift the curve to the right and eventually depress the slope (*dashed lines*). Painful stimulation will reverse these changes to varying and unpredictable degrees.

resulting from barbiturate administration is characterized by decreased tidal volume and increased ventilatory rate. Potent inhaled anesthetics displace the carbon dioxide response curve to the right and decrease the slope, the degree of which depends on the anesthetic dose and the level of surgical stimulation. Like barbiturates, the ventilatory pattern following administration of potent inhaled anesthetics is initially represented by a decreased tidal volume and increased ventilatory rate. As more potent anesthetic agent is administered, however, ventilatory rate decreases toward an apneic end point. This clinical response occurs when the carbon dioxide response curve eventually becomes horizontal (slope = 0), resulting in essentially no ventilatory response to $PaCO_2$ changes.

Potent inhaled anesthetics and opioids displace the setpoint to the right, implying that the resting, steady-state $PaCO_2$ is higher and minute ventilation lower. Furthermore, when the carbon dioxide response curve shifts to the right, the apneic threshold also increases (see Fig. 11-4). Surgical stimulation reverses the ventilatory response changes induced by inhaled anesthetics and opioids, but the degree of reversal is not predictable.

OXYGEN AND CARBON DIOXIDE TRANSPORT

This chapter discusses only external respiration, in which oxygen moves from the ambient environment into the pulmonary capillaries and carbon dioxide leaves the pulmonary capillaries to enter the atmosphere. The movement of gas across the alveolar-capillary membrane depends on the integrity of the pulmonary and cardiac systems. Unless it is otherwise stated, the reader should assume the ventilation and perfusion of alveolar-capillary units are normal. Abnormal distribution of ventilation or perfusion of the lungs is discussed later (see "Ventilation-Perfusion Relationships").

Bulk Flow of Gas (Convection)

Convection, in which all gas molecules move in the same direction, is the primary mechanism responsible for gas flow in large and most small airways, down to the bronchi and bronchiolar airways of the 14th or 15th generation. Because the cross-sectional area of the airways progressively increases as gas moves toward the lung periphery, the average velocity of gas particles decreases as they travel toward the alveoli. Because resistance depends on flow, the greatest part of airway resistance occurs in the larger airways, where gas molecules travel more quickly. During normal quiet ventilation, gas flow within convective airways is mainly laminar.

Gas Diffusion

Diffusion within a gas-filled space is random molecular motion that results in complete mixing of all gases. In the distal airways of the lung beginning with the terminal bronchioles (16th airway generation), diffusion becomes the predominant mode of gas transport. Once gas reaches the small alveolar ducts, alveolar sacs, and alveoli, both diffusion and regional ($\dot{V}_A/\dot{Q}$) relationships influence gas transport. Historically, clinicians assumed defects in gas diffusion were responsible for arterial hypoxemia. However, the most frequent cause of arterial hypoxemia is physiologic shunt (see "Ventilation-Perfusion Relationships").[47]

The other usage of "diffusion" refers to the passive movement of molecules across a membrane that is governed primarily by concentration gradient. In this sense, carbon dioxide is 20 times more diffusible across human membranes than is oxygen; therefore, carbon dioxide crosses alveoli easily. As a result, hypercapnia is *never* the result of defective diffusion; rather, it is the result of inadequate alveolar ventilation with respect to carbon dioxide production.

True diffusion defects that create arterial hypoxemia are rare. The most common reason for a measured decrease in diffusing capacity (see "Pulmonary Function Tests") is mismatched ventilation and perfusion, which functionally results in a decreased surface area available for diffusion.

Distribution of Ventilation and Perfusion

The efficiency with which oxygen and carbon dioxide exchange at the alveolar–capillary level highly depends on the matching of capillary perfusion and alveolar ventilation. At this level, the marriage between the lung and the circulatory system must be well matched and intimate.

Distribution of Blood Flow

Blood flow within the lung is mainly gravity-dependent. Because the alveolar–capillary beds are not composed of rigid vessels, the pressure of the surrounding tissues can influence the resistance to flow through the individual capillaries. Thus, blood flow depends on the relationship between pulmonary artery pressure (Ppa), alveolar pressure (PA), and pulmonary venous pressure (Ppv; Fig. 11-5). West et al.[47] and West and Dollery[48] created a lung model that divides the lung into three zones. Zone 1 conditions occur in the most gravity-independent part of the lung. Because alveolar pressure is approximately equal to atmospheric pressure; and pulmonary artery pressure,

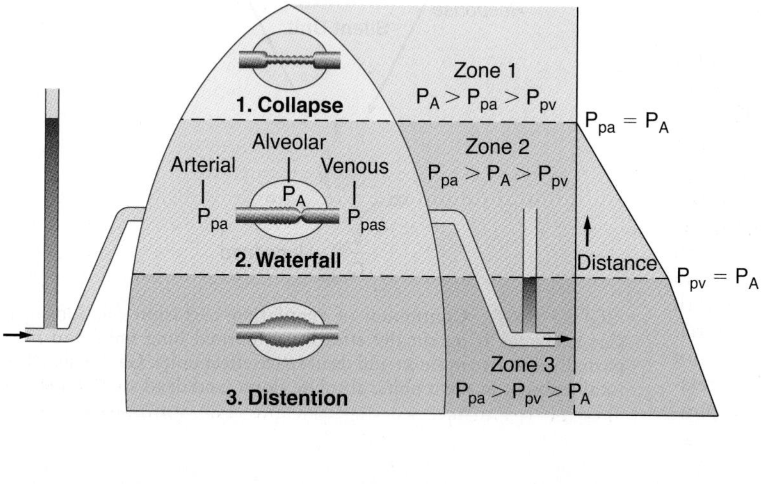

FIGURE 11-5. Distribution of blood flow in the isolated lung. In zone 1, alveolar pressure (P_A) exceeds pulmonary artery pressure (P_{pa}), and no flow occurs because the vessels are collapsed. In zone 2, arterial pressure exceeds alveolar pressure, but alveolar pressure exceeds pulmonary venous pressure (P_{pv}). Flow in zone 2 is determined by the arterial–alveolar pressure difference ($P_{pa} - P_A$), which steadily increases down the zone. In zone 3, pulmonary venous pressure exceeds alveolar pressure and flow is determined by the arterial–venous pressure difference ($P_{pa} - P_{pv}$), which is constant down this pulmonary zone. However, the pressure across the vessel walls increases down the zone so their caliber increases, as does flow. (From West JB, Dollery CT, Naimark A: Distribution of blood flow in isolated lung: Relation to vascular and alveolar pressures. J Appl Physiol 1964;19: 713, with permission.)

which is always in excess of pulmonary venous pressure, is subatmospheric in zone 1, then zone 1 is described by the following relationship: $P_A > P_{pa} > P_{pv}$. In zone 1 alveolar pressure that is transmitted to the pulmonary capillaries promotes their collapse, with a consequent theoretical blood flow of zero to this lung region. Thus, zone 1 receives ventilation in the absence of perfusion. This relationship is alveolar dead space ventilation. Normally, zone 1 areas exist only to a limited extent. However, in conditions of decreased pulmonary artery pressure such as hypovolemic shock, zone 1 enlarges.

Zone 2 occurs from the lower limit of zone 1 to the upper limit of zone 3, where $P_{pa} > P_A > P_{pv}$. The pressure difference between pulmonary artery and alveolar pressure determines blood flow in zone 2. Pulmonary venous pressure has little influence. Well-matched ventilation and perfusion occur in zone 2, which contains the majority of alveoli.

Finally, zone 3 occurs in the most gravity-dependent areas of the lung, where $P_{pa} > P_{pv} > P_A$ and blood flow is primarily governed by the pulmonary arterial to venous pressure difference. Because gravity also increases pulmonary venous pressure, the pulmonary capillaries become distended. Thus, perfusion in zone 3 is lush, resulting in capillary perfusion in excess of ventilation, or physiologic shunt.

Distribution of Ventilation

Alveolar pressure is the same throughout the lung; therefore, the more negative intrapleural pressure at the apex (or the least gravity-dependent area) results in larger, more distended apical alveoli than in other areas of the lung. The transpulmonary pressure (Paw – Ppl), or distending pressure of the lung, is greater at the top and lower at the bottom, where intrapleural pressure is less negative. Despite the smaller alveolar size, more ventilation is delivered to dependent pulmonary areas. The decrease in intrapleural pressure at the base of the lungs during inspiration is greater than at the apex because of diaphragmatic proximity. Thus, because the dependent area of the lung generates the greatest change in transpulmonary pressure, more gas is sucked into dependent areas of the lung.

Ventilation–Perfusion Relationships

As discussed previously, the majority of blood flow is distributed to the gravity-dependent part of the lung. Also, during a spontaneous breath, the largest portion of the tidal volume also reaches the gravity-dependent part of the lung. Thus, the nondependent area of the lung receives a lower proportion of both ventilation and perfusion, and dependent lung receives greater proportions of ventilation and perfusion. Nevertheless, ventilation and perfusion are not matched perfectly, and various $\dot{V}_A/\dot{Q}$ ratios result throughout the lung. The ideal $\dot{V}_A/\dot{Q}$ ratio of 1 is believed to occur at approximately the level of the third rib. Above this level, ventilation occurs slightly in excess of perfusion, whereas below the third rib the $\dot{V}_A/\dot{Q}$ ratio becomes less than 1 (Fig. 11-6).

In a simplified model, gas exchange units can be divided into normal ($\dot{V}_A/\dot{Q} = 1:1$), dead space ($\dot{V}_A/\dot{Q} = 1:0$), shunt ($\dot{V}_A/\dot{Q} = 0:1$), or a silent unit ($\dot{V}_A/\dot{Q} = 0:0$; Fig. 11-7). Although this model is helpful in understanding $\dot{V}_A/\dot{Q}$ relationships and their influences on gas exchange, $\dot{V}_A/\dot{Q}$ really occurs as a continuum. In the lungs of a healthy, upright, spontaneously breathing individual, the majority of alveolar-capillary units are normal gas exchange units. The $\dot{V}_A/\dot{Q}$ ratio varies between absolute shunt (in which $\dot{V}_A/\dot{Q} = 0$) to absolute dead space (in which $\dot{V}_A/\dot{Q} = \infty$). Rather than absolute shunt, most units with low $\dot{V}_A/\dot{Q}$ mismatch receive a small amount of ventilation relative to blood flow. Similarly, most dead space units are not absolute, but rather are characterized by low blood flow relative to ventilation. During acute lung injury and adult respira-

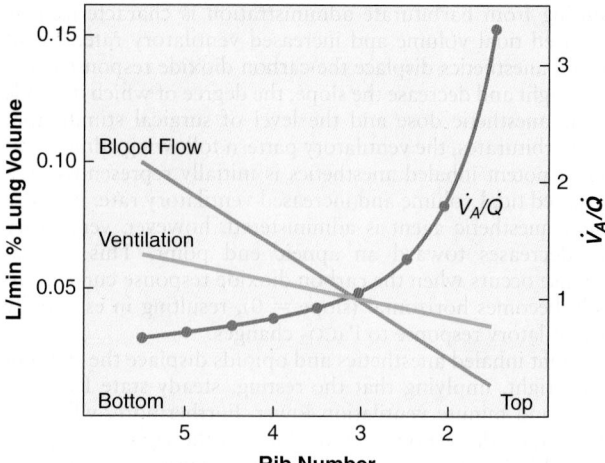

FIGURE 11-6. Distribution of ventilation, blood flow, and ventilation–perfusion ratio in the normal, upright lung. Straight lines have been drawn through the ventilation and blood flow data. Because blood flow falls more rapidly than ventilation with distance up the lung, ventilation–perfusion ratio rises, slowly at first, then rapidly. (From West JB: Ventilation/Blood Flow and Gas Exchange, 4th ed. Oxford, England, Blackwell Scientific, 1985, with permission.)

tory distress syndrome, areas of low $\dot{V}_A/\dot{Q}$ matching commonly lie adjacent to areas of high $\dot{V}_A/\dot{Q}$ matching.[49] Thus, the lung zone model proposed by West and coworkers[47,48] should be used to aid the understanding of pulmonary physiology and not be regarded as an incontrovertible anatomic truism.

Hypoxic pulmonary vasoconstriction and bronchoconstriction allow the lungs to maintain optimal $\dot{V}_A/\dot{Q}$ matching (see Chapter 40.) Hypoxic pulmonary vasoconstriction,

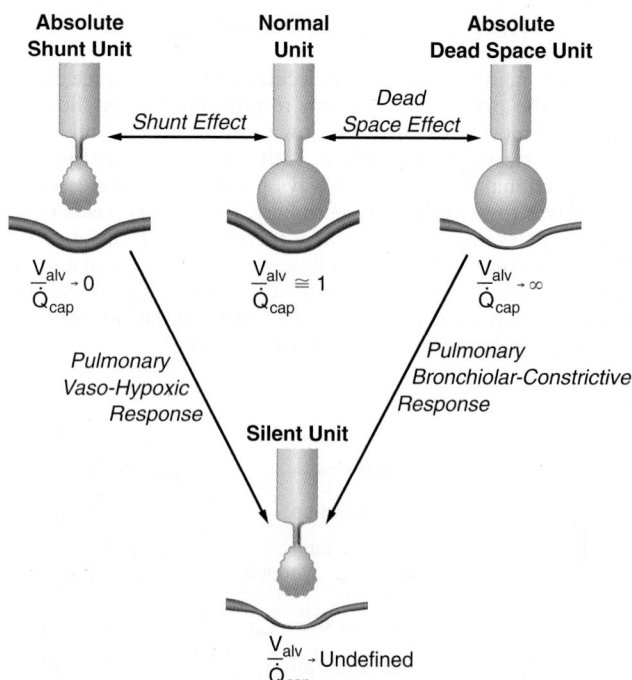

FIGURE 11-7. Continuum of ventilation–perfusion relationships. Gas exchange is maximally effective in normal lung units and only partially effective in shunt and dead space effect units. Gas exchange is totally absent in silent units, absolute shunt, and dead space units.

stimulated by alveolar hypoxia, severely decreases blood flow. Thus, poorly ventilated alveoli also receive minuscule blood flow. Furthermore, decreased regional pulmonary blood flow results in bronchiolar constriction and diminishes the degree of dead space ventilation.[50,51] When either phenomena occurs, the shunt or dead space units effectively become silent units in which little ventilation or perfusion occurs.

Many pulmonary diseases result in both physiologic shunt and dead space abnormalities. However, most disease processes can be characterized as producing either primarily shunt or dead space in their early stages. Increases in dead space ventilation primarily affect carbon dioxide elimination and have little influence on arterial oxygenation until dead space ventilation exceeds 80 to 90% of minute ventilation ($\dot{V}_E$). Similarly, physiologic shunt primarily affects arterial oxygenation with little effect on carbon dioxide elimination until the physiologic shunt fraction exceeds 75 to 80% of the cardiac output. Defective to absent gas exchange can be the net effect of either abnormality in the extreme.

Physiologic Dead Space

Each inspired breath is composed of gas that contributes to alveolar ventilation (V_A) and gas that becomes dead space ventilation (V_D). Thus, tidal volume (V_T) = V_A + V_D. In the normal, spontaneously breathing person, the ratio of alveolar-to-dead space ventilation for each breath is 2:1. Conveniently, the rule of "1, 2, 3" applies to normal, spontaneously breathing persons. For each breath, 1 mL/lb (lean body weight) becomes V_D, 2 mL · lb^{-1} becomes V_a, and 3 mL · lb^{-1} constitutes the V_T.

Physiologic dead space consists of anatomic and alveolar dead space. Anatomic dead space ventilation, approximately 2 mL/kg ideal body weight, accounts for the majority of physiologic dead space. It arises from ventilation of structures that do not exchange respiratory gases: the oronasopharynx to the terminal and respiratory bronchioles. Clinical conditions that modify anatomic dead space include tracheal intubation, tracheostomy, and large lengths of ventilator tubing between the tracheal tube and the ventilator Y-piece. It is important to note that ventilation occurs because gas flows into and out of the alveoli. In contrast, the inspiratory or expiratory limb of anesthesia circle system has unidirectional flow, and therefore is not a component of anatomic dead space ventilation.

Alveolar dead space ventilation arises from ventilation of alveoli where there is little or no perfusion. Because disease produces little change in anatomic dead space, physiologic dead space is primarily influenced by changes in alveolar dead space. Rapid changes in physiologic dead space ventilation most often arise from changes in pulmonary blood flow, resulting in decreased perfusion to ventilated alveoli. The most common cause of acutely increased physiologic dead space is an abrupt decrease in cardiac output. Another pathologic condition that interferes with pulmonary blood flow, and thereby creates dead space, is pulmonary embolism, whether due to thrombus or to fat, air, or amniotic fluid. Although there may be obstruction to blood flow with some types of pulmonary emboli, the greatest decrease in pulmonary blood flow is due to vasoconstriction induced by locally released vasoactive substances such as leukotrienes.

Chronic pulmonary diseases create dead space ventilation by irreversibly changing the relationship between alveolar ventilation and blood flow; this alteration is especially prominent in patients with COPD. Furthermore, acute diseases such as adult respiratory distress syndrome can cause an increase in dead space ventilation owing to intense pulmonary vasoconstriction. Finally, therapeutic or supportive manipulations such as positive-pressure ventilation or positive airway pressure therapy can

increase alveolar dead space because depressed venous return to the right heart will decrease cardiac output, which can usually be overcome by intravenous fluid administration. Occasionally, therapeutics that create intrapulmonary positive pressure may increase physiologic shunt when blood flow to a previously silent area of $\dot{V}_A/\dot{Q}$ matching now receives blood redistributed by positive pressure from more compliant areas of the lung.

Assessment of Physiologic Dead Space

Because the lung receives nearly 100% of the cardiac output, assessment of physiologic dead space ventilation in the acute setting yields valuable information about pulmonary blood flow and, ultimately, about cardiac output. If pulmonary blood flow decreases, the most likely cause is a decreased cardiac output. Thus, it is clinically useful to be able to readily assess the degree of physiologic dead space ventilation.

There are two easy and several difficult ways to assess dead space ventilation. A comparison of minute ventilation and $PaCO_2$ allows a gross qualitative assessment of physiologic dead space ventilation. The $PaCO_2$ is determined only by alveolar ventilation and $\dot{V}CO_2$. If $\dot{V}CO_2$ remains constant, $PaCO_2$ also will remain constant as long as minute ventilation supplies the same degree of alveolar ventilation. If the spontaneously breathing individual must increase minute ventilation to maintain the same $PaCO_2$, he or she has experienced an increase in dead space ventilation because less of the minute ventilation is contributing to alveolar ventilation. Alternatively, a mechanically ventilated patient with a fixed minute ventilation and no increase in $\dot{V}CO_2$ also experiences an increased dead space ventilation if the $PaCO_2$ rises. Hence, when $PaCO_2$ in a mechanically ventilated patient increases, it is necessary to determine if the cause is increased dead space ventilation or an increased $\dot{V}CO_2$.

Because positive pressure ventilation increases alveolar pressure, the mechanically ventilated patient with normal lungs has a dead space to alveolar ventilation ratio (V_D/V_a) of 1:1 (more West zone 1) rather than 1:2, as during spontaneous ventilation. If mechanical V_T is 1,000 mL, 500 mL contributes to V_A, and 500 mL contributes to V_D. At rest, the required $\dot{V}_A$ with normal $\dot{V}CO_2$ is approximately 60 mL/kg/min. A 70-kg man would then require a $\dot{V}_A$ of 4,200 mL/min. During spontaneous breathing, the required $\dot{V}_E$ would be 6,300 mL/min, but during mechanical ventilation $\dot{V}_E$ would have to be 8,400 mL/min. Using this calculation, if a 70-kg resting patient requires $\dot{V}_E$ much in excess of 8,400 mL/min, either $\dot{V}_D$ or $\dot{V}CO_2$ is increased. A rule of thumb for mechanically ventilated patients is that doubling baseline minute ventilation decreases $PaCO_2$ from 40 to 30 mm Hg, and quadrupling minute ventilation decreases $PaCO_2$ from 40 to 20 mm Hg.

The $PaCO_2$ will be greater than or equal to end-tidal $PaCO_2$ ($PETCO_2$) unless the patient inspires or receives exogenous carbon dioxide (e.g., from peritoneal insufflation). The difference between $PETCO_2$ and $PaCO_2$ is because of dead space ventilation. The most common reason for an acute increase in dead space ventilation is decreased cardiac output. Measurement of this difference—which is simple, readily obtainable, and fairly inexpensive—yields reliable information relative to the degree of dead space ventilation. Clinical situations that change pulmonary blood flow sufficiently to increase dead space ventilation can be detected by comparing $PETCO_2$ with temperature-corrected $PaCO_2$. Yamanaka and Sue[52] found that the $PETCO_2$ in ventilated patients varied linearly with the dead space to tidal volume ratio (V_D/V_T) and that $PETCO_2$ correlated poorly with $PaCO_2$. Thus, in the critically ill, mechanically ventilated patient, and in anesthetized patients, monitoring $PETCO_2$ gives far more information about ventilatory efficiency or dead space ventilation than it does about the absolute value of $PaCO_2$.

Anesthesiologists commonly measure $P_{ET}CO_2$ to detect venous air embolism during anesthesia. A lowered cardiac output alone, in the absence of venous air embolism, may sufficiently decrease pulmonary perfusion so dead space ventilation increases and $P_{ET}CO_2$ falls. Thus, a depressed $P_{ET}CO_2$ is sensitive for decreased cardiac output but nonspecific pulmonary embolism. Air in the pulmonary arteries mechanically interferes with blood flow and also causes pulmonary arterial constriction, further decreasing pulmonary blood flow. A decreased $P_{ET}CO_2$ suggests that a physiologically significant air embolism has occurred. The same physiologic considerations apply to detecting pulmonary thromboembolism.

Some clinicians use the divergence of $P_{ET}CO_2$ from $PaCO_2$ as a reflection of pulmonary blood flow for other applications. During intentional pharmacologic or surgical manipulation of pulmonary blood flow, the difference between $PaCO_2$ and $P_{ET}CO_2$ serves as a useful physiologic monitor of the effectiveness of these interventions. Furthermore, $P_{ET}CO_2$ as a reflection of pulmonary perfusion is a useful tool for studying and monitoring the effectiveness of resuscitation efforts and may provide a marker for survival after resuscitation.[53]

The most quantitative technique used to measure physiologic dead space uses a modification of the Bohr equation:

$$\frac{V_D}{V_T} = \frac{PaCO_2 - P\bar{E}CO_2}{PaCO_2} \qquad (11\text{-}4)$$

where $P\bar{E}CO_2$ is the PCO_2 from the mixture of all expired gases over the period of time during which measurements are made. This calculation estimates the fraction of each breath that does not contribute to gas exchange. In spontaneously breathing patients, normal V_D/V_T is between 0.2 and 0.4, or ~0.33. In patients receiving positive-pressure ventilation, V_D/V_T becomes ~0.5. The major limitation of performing this calculation is the difficulty in collecting exhaled gas for $P\bar{E}CO_2$ measurement. Exhaled gases, collected in cumbersome 50 L bags, can easily be contaminated with inspired air or supplemental oxygen. The measurement will also be inaccurate if the patient does not maintain a steady ventilatory pattern. Therefore, extreme care must be taken to ensure all measurements are performed accurately. In practice, this measurement is rarely performed.

Physiologic Shunt

Whereas physiologic dead space ventilation applies to areas of the lung that are ventilated but poorly perfused, physiologic shunt occurs in lung that is perfused but poorly ventilated. The physiologic shunt ($\dot{Q}_{SP}$) is that portion of the total cardiac output ($\dot{Q}_T$) that returns to the left heart and systemic circulation without receiving oxygen in the lung. When pulmonary blood is not exposed to alveoli or when those alveoli are devoid of ventilation, the result is *absolute or true shunt*, in which $\dot{V}_A/\dot{Q} = 0$. *Shunt effect*, or *venous admixture*, is the more common clinical phenomenon and occurs in areas where alveolar ventilation is deficient compared with the degree of perfusion: $0 < \dot{V}_A/\dot{Q} < 1$.

Because blood passing through areas of absolute shunt receives no oxygen, arterial hypoxemia resulting from absolute shunt is minimally reversed with supplemental oxygen. Alternatively, supplemental oxygen supplied to patients with arterial hypoxemia due to venous admixture will increase the PaO_2. Although ventilation to these alveoli is deficient, they do carry a small amount of oxygen to the capillary bed. Thus, assessment of arterial oxygen responsiveness to supplemental oxygen administration is a helpful diagnostic tool.

A small percentage of venous blood normally bypasses the right ventricle and empties directly into the left atrium. This anatomic, absolute, or true shunt arises from the venous return from the pleural, bronchiolar, and thebesian veins. This venous drainage accounts for 2 to 5% of total cardiac output and explains the small shunt that normally occurs. Anatomic shunts of greatest magnitude are usually associated with congenital heart disease that causes right-to-left shunt. Intrapulmonary anatomic shunts can also cause anatomic shunt. For example, the arterial hypoxemia associated with advanced hepatic failure (hepatopulmonary syndrome) is partly due to arteriovenous malformations.[54,55] Diseases that may cause absolute or true shunt include acute lobar atelectasis, extensive acute lung injury, advanced pulmonary edema, and consolidated pneumonia. Disease entities that tend to produce venous admixture include mild pulmonary edema, postoperative atelectasis, and COPD.

Assessment of Arterial Oxygenation and Physiologic Shunt

The simplest assessment of oxygenation is qualitative comparison of the patient's FIO_2 and PaO_2. The highest possible PaO_2 for any given FIO_2 (and $PaCO_2$) can be calculated from the alveolar gas equation:

$$P_{AO_2} = F_{IO_2}(P_B - P_{H_2O}) - \frac{P_{ACO_2}}{R} \qquad (11\text{-}5)$$

where P_{AO_2} and P_{ACO_2} are alveolar PO_2 and PCO_2, P_{H_2O} is water vapor pressure at 100% saturation and 37°C, P_b is barometric pressure, and R is respiratory quotient. Assuming one makes the calculation for a well-perfused alveolus, the alveolar and arterial PCO_2 are equal. Therefore, $PaCO_2$ can be substituted for P_{ACO_2}. Respiratory quotient (R) is the ratio of O_2 consumed ($\dot{V}O_2$) to CO_2 produced ($\dot{V}CO_2$):

$$\frac{\dot{V}_{CO_2}}{\dot{V}_{O_2}} = \frac{200 \text{ mL/min}}{250 \text{ mL/min}} = 0.8 \qquad (11\text{-}6)$$

Oxygen tension–based indices do not reflect mixed venous contribution to arterial oxygenation and can be misleading.[56] Even if venous admixture is small, mixed venous blood with very low oxygen content will magnify the effect of a small shunt. Oxygen tension–based indices, for example, PaO_2/FIO_2, alveolar to arterial PO_2 difference ($P_{(A-a)}O_2$), and ratio PaO_2/P_{AO_2}, do not take into account the influence of $C\bar{v}O_2$ on arterial oxygenation. Therefore, in critically ill patients who are hypoxemic, the insertion of a pulmonary artery catheter to assess shunt and to measure cardiac output may be essential to understanding the influence of cardiac function on arterial oxygenation.

$P_{(A-a)}O_2$ is a useful quantitative assessment of arterial oxygenation mainly when arterial hemoglobin is well saturated when normal DA-aO_2 is <5 mm Hg. When PaO_2 is <150 mm Hg (and certainly when it is <100 mm Hg), the relationship between oxygen content and oxygen tension is nonlinear, thus making DA-aO_2 more difficult to interpret.

The assessment of arterial oxygenation requires, at least, knowledge of FIO_2 and either PaO_2 or SaO_2. Oxygen tension–based indices of oxygenation are useful, but they do not take into account the contribution of mixed venous blood to arterial oxygenation. Mixed venous blood can become extremely desaturated in the critically ill patient owing to inadequate cardiac output, anemia, arterial hypoxemia, or increased $\dot{V}O_2$. The best knowledge of the efficiency with which the lungs oxygenate the arterial blood can be obtained only by calculating shunt fraction or ventilation–perfusion index (VQI).

Physiologic Shunt Calculation

The clinical reference standard for the calculation of physiologic shunt fraction is derived from a two-compartment pulmonary blood flow model where one compartment performs ideal gas exchange and contains perfectly married alveolar–capillary units. The other compartment is the shunt compartment and contains pulmonary capillaries that have no exposure to ventilated alveoli. Using the Fick relationship, the following equation can be derived:

$$\frac{\dot{Q}_{SP}}{\dot{Q}_T} = \frac{Cc'O_2 - Cao_2}{Cc'O_2 - C\bar{v}o_2} \qquad (11\text{-}7)$$

where $\dot{Q}_{SP}/\dot{Q}_T$ is the shunt fraction, $\dot{Q}_{SP}$ is blood flow through the physiologic shunt compartment, $\dot{Q}_T$ is total cardiac output, and $Cc'O_2$ and $C\bar{v}O_2$ are end-capillary and mixed-venous oxygen contents, respectively. Normal intrapulmonary shunt is approximately 5%. Because this equation is based on an artificial two-compartment model, the absolute value is physically meaningless. A calculated $\dot{Q}_{SP}/\dot{Q}_T$ of 25% means that if the lung existed in two compartments, 25% of the cardiac output would travel through the shunt compartment. Because the lung does not exist in two compartments, this equation only grossly estimates pulmonary oxygen exchange defects. Nevertheless, it remains our best tool for clinically evaluating the efficiency with which the lungs oxygenate arterial blood. Observing shunt fraction change with therapeutic intervention or with the progress of disease is more valuable than knowing the absolute value per se.

Because hemoglobin concentration is uniform throughout the vascular system, the oxygen contents in the shunt equation are determined primarily by oxyhemoglobin saturation. Thus, the shunt equation can be approximated by substituting saturation values for each term; the new value, called *ventilation–perfusion ratio* (VQI),[55] is determined as follows:

$$VQI = \frac{Sc'O_2 - SaO_2}{Sc'O_2 - S\bar{v}O_2} \cong \frac{1 - Sao_2}{1 - S\bar{v}O_2} \qquad (11\text{-}8)$$

If the patient is neither breathing a hypoxic gas mixture nor has a methemoglobin or carboxyhemoglobin value in excess of 5 to 6%, $Sc'O_2$ must equal 1 because the model requires a perfect alveolar–capillary interface. This substitution results in the final expression in the previous equation. The absolute values of VQI are meaningless, although "normal" should be 0 to 4%. Like $\dot{Q}_{SP}/\dot{Q}_T$, the importance of these values lies in their trend as disease and treatment progress.

Sao_2 and $S\bar{v}O_2$ can be estimated continuously with pulse oximetry and by using a pulmonary artery catheter with oximetry capability. By interfacing the outputs of these two devices with a computer, VQI can be calculated continuously. The greatest advantage of calculating $\dot{Q}_{SP}/\dot{Q}_T$ or VQI to assess arterial oxygenation efficiency is that these values include the contribution of mixed venous blood.

PULMONARY FUNCTION TESTING

Anesthesiologists frequently care for patients with significant pulmonary dysfunction (see Chapter 23). It is important for the anesthesiologist to be able to interpret tests of pulmonary function intelligently and to know which tests will help define dysfunction if the patient's history and physical are suggestive of disease. This section discusses lung volumes, tests of pulmonary mechanics, and diffusing capacity.

Lung Volumes and Capacities

Known, reproducible pulmonary gas volumes and capacities provide a reliable basis for comparison between normal and abnormal measurements.[57] Because normal measurements vary with size, height is most frequently used to define "normal." Lung capacities are composed of two or more lung volumes. Lung volumes and capacities are schematically illustrated in Figure 11-8.

Tidal volume is the volume of gas that moves in and out of the lungs during quiet breathing and is ~6 to 8 mL/kg. Tidal volume falls with decreased lung compliance or when the patient has reduced ventilatory muscle strength.

Vital capacity is usually ~60 mL/kg but may vary as much as 20% from normal in healthy individuals. Vital capacity correlates well with the capability for deep breathing and effective coughing. It is decreased by restrictive pulmonary disease such as pulmonary edema or atelectasis. Vital capacity may also be reduced by the mechanically induced extrapulmonary restriction seen in pleural effusion, pneumothorax, pregnancy, large ascites, or ventilatory muscle weakness.

The *inspiratory capacity* is the largest volume of gas that can be inspired from the resting expiratory level and is frequently decreased in the presence of significant extrathoracic airway obstruction. This measurement is one of the few simple tests that can detect extrathoracic airway obstruction. Most routine pulmonary function tests measure only exhaled flows and volumes, which may be relatively unaffected by extrathoracic obstruction until it is severe. Changes in the absolute volume of inspiratory capacity usually parallel changes in vital capacity. *Expiratory reserve volume* is not of great diagnostic value.

Functional residual capacity (FRC) is the volume of gas remaining in the lungs at passive end expiration. *Residual volume* is that gas remaining within the lungs at the end of forced maximal expiration. The FRC serves two primary physiologic functions. It determines the point on the

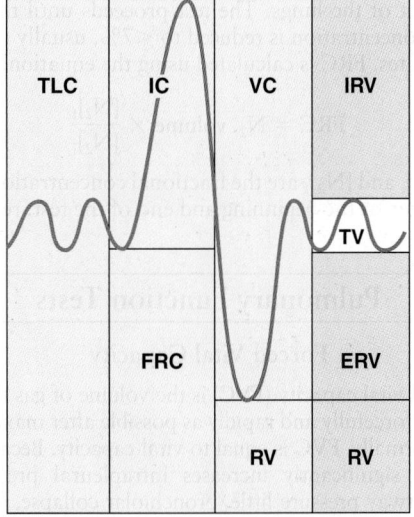

FIGURE 11-8. Lung volumes and capacities. The darkest bar on the far right depicts the four basic lung volumes that sum to create total lung capacity (TLC). Other lung capacities are composed of two or more lung volumes. The overlying spirographic tracing orients the reader to the relationship between the lung volumes and capacities and the spirogram. ERV, expiratory reserve volume; FRC, functional residual capacity; IC, inspiratory capacity; IRV, inspiratory reserve volume; RV, residual volume; VC, vital capacity; TV, tidal volume.

10

ANATOMY AND PHYSIOLOGY

pulmonary volume–pressure curve for resting ventilation (see Fig. 11-2). The tangent defined by the midportion pulmonary volume–pressure curve at FRC defines lung compliance. Thus, FRC determines the elastic pressure–volume relationships within the lung. Furthermore, FRC is the resting expiratory volume of the lung and is the primary determinant of oxygen reserve in humans when apnea occurs. As such, it greatly influences ventilation–perfusion relationships within the lung. When FRC is reduced, venous admixture (low $\dot{V}_A/\dot{Q}$) increases and results in arterial hypoxemia (see "Oxygen and Carbon Dioxide Transport" and "Lung Mechanics").

Further, the FRC may be used to quantify the degree of pulmonary restriction. Disease processes that reduce FRC and lung compliance include acute lung injury, pulmonary edema, pulmonary fibrotic processes, and atelectasis. Mechanical factors also reduce FRC; examples include pregnancy, obesity, pleural effusion, and posture. The FRC decreases 10% when a healthy subject lies down. Ventilatory muscle weakness or paralysis will also decrease FRC. In contrast, patients with COPD have excessively compliant lungs that recoil less forcibly. Their lungs retain an abnormally large volume at the end of passive expiration, a phenomenon called *gas trapping*.

Functional Residual Capacity Measurement

The FRC and residual volume must be measured indirectly because residual volume cannot be removed from the lung. The multiple-breath nitrogen washout test is performed by having the subject breathe 100% oxygen for several minutes so alveolar nitrogen is gradually "washed out." With each breath, the volume of gas and the concentration of nitrogen in the exhaled gas are measured. A rapid nitrogen analyzer coupled to a spirometer or pneumotachometer provides a breath-by-breath analysis of nitrogen washout. Electronic signals proportional to nitrogen concentrations and exhaled volumes (or flow, if a pneumotachometer is used) are integrated to derive the exhaled volume of nitrogen for each breath. Then the values for all breaths are summed to provide a total volume of nitrogen washed out of the lungs. The test proceeds until the alveolar nitrogen concentration is reduced to <7%, usually requiring 7 to 10 minutes. FRC is calculated using the equation:

$$FRC = N_2 \text{ volume} \times \frac{[N_2]_f}{[N_2]_i} \qquad (11\text{-}9)$$

where $[N_2]_i$ and $[N_2]_f$ are the fractional concentrations of alveolar nitrogen at the beginning and end of the test, respectively.

Pulmonary Function Tests

Forced Vital Capacity

The forced vital capacity (FVC) is the volume of gas that can be expired as forcefully and rapidly as possible after maximal inspiration. Normally, FVC is equal to vital capacity. Because forced expiration significantly increases intrapleural pressures but changes airway pressure little, bronchiolar collapse, obstructive lesions, and gas trapping are exaggerated. Thus, FVC may be reduced in chronic obstructive diseases even when the vital capacity appears near normal. FVC is nearly always decreased by restrictive diseases. FVC values <15 mL/kg are associated with an increased incidence of PPCs, probably because patients in this condition cough ineffectively.[58] FVC reduced to this level represents a profound defect, most commonly seen in quadriplegic patients or patients with severe neuromuscular disease. Finally, FVC is largely dependent on patient effort and cooperation.

Forced Expiratory Volume

FEV_T is the forced expiratory volume of gas over a given time interval during the FVC maneuver. The interval, described by the subscript T, is the time elapsed in seconds from the onset of expiration. Because FEV_T records a volume of gas expired over time, it is actually a measure of flow. By measuring expiratory flow at specific intervals, the severity of airway obstruction can be ascertained. Decreased FEV_T values are common in both obstructive and restrictive disease patterns. The most important application of FEV_T is its comparison with the patient's FVC. Normal subjects can expire at least three fourths of FVC within the first second of the forced expiratory maneuver. The FEV_1, the most frequently employed value, is normally ≥75% of the FVC, or $FEV_1/FVC \geq 0.75$.

Normally, an individual can expire 50 to 60% of FVC in 0.5 second, 75 to 85% in 1 second, 94% in 2 seconds, and 97% in 3 seconds. Cooperative patients with obstructive disease will exhibit a reduced FEV_1/FVC in most cases. However, patients with restrictive disease usually have normal FEV_1/FVC ratios. The validity of the evaluation of the FEV_1/FVC is highly dependent on patient cooperation and effort. It is possible to deliberately produce an artificially low FEV_1/FVC.

Forced Expiratory Flow

$FEF_{25-75\%}$ is the average forced expiratory flow during the middle half of the FEV maneuver. This test is also called *maximum midexpiratory flow rate*. The length of time required for a subject to expire the middle half of the FVC is divided into 50% of the FVC. The spirogram in Figure 11-9 marks the place from 25 to 75% of FVC, constituting the middle 50% of FVC. The straight line connecting the 25% and 75% volumes has a slope approximately equal to average flow. A normal value for a healthy 70-kg man is approximately 4.7 L/sec (or 280 mL/min). Normally, both the absolute value and the percentage of predicted value for the individual being studied are recorded. A normal value is 100 ± 25% of predicted value. Decreased flow rates from this middle 50% of FVC anatomically represent flow in medium-sized airways, and when decreased, there is obstructive disease of medium-sized airways. This value is typically normal in restrictive diseases. This test is fairly sensitive in the early stages of obstructive airway disease. Decreased $FEV_{25-75\%}$ frequently will be observed

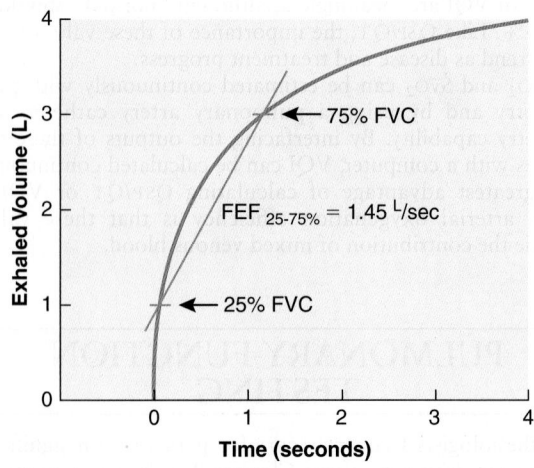

FIGURE 11-9. Forced expiratory flow, 25 to 75% ($FEF_{25-75\%}$). The spirogram depicts a 4-L forced vital capacity (FVC) on which the points representing 25% and 75% FVC are marked. The slope of the line connecting these points is the $FEF_{25-75\%}$.

before other obstructive manifestations occur. Although somewhat effort-dependent, the test is much more reliable and reproducible than FEV$_1$/FVC.

Maximum Voluntary Ventilation

Maximum voluntary ventilation (MVV) is the largest volume of gas that can be breathed in 1 minute by voluntary effort. The MVV is measured by having the subject breathe as deeply and as rapidly as possible for 10, 12, or 15 seconds. The results are extrapolated to 1 minute. The subject is instructed to set his or her own ventilatory rate and move more than tidal volume but less than vital capacity in each breath.

MVV measures the endurance of the ventilatory muscles and indirectly reflects lung–thorax compliance and airway resistance. MVV is the best ventilatory endurance test that can be performed in the laboratory. Values that vary by as much as 30% from predicted values may be normal, so only large reductions in MVV are significant. Healthy, young adults average ~170 L/min. Values are lower in women and decrease with age in both sexes. Because this maneuver exaggerates air trapping and exerts the ventilatory muscles, MVV is decreased greatly in patients with moderate-to-severe obstructive disease. MVV is usually normal in patients with restrictive disease.

Flow–Volume Loops

The flow–volume loop graphically demonstrates the flow generated during a forced expiratory maneuver followed by a forced inspiratory maneuver, plotted against the volume of gas expired (Fig. 11-10; see Chapter 40). The subject forcefully exhales completely, then immediately and forcefully inhales to vital capacity. The expired and inspired volumes are plotted on the abscissa and flow is plotted on the ordinate. Although various numbers can be generated from the flow–volume loop, the configuration of the loop itself is probably the most informative part of the test.

Flow–volume loops were formerly useful in the diagnosis of large airway and extrathoracic airway obstruction prior to the availability of precise imaging techniques. Imaging techniques such as magnetic resonance imaging give more precise and useful information in the diagnosis of upper airway and extrathoracic obstruction and superseded the use of flow–volume loops

for diagnosis of these conditions. Therefore, it is rare that flow–volume loops are useful for preoperative pulmonary evaluation in the modern era of imaging.

Carbon Monoxide Diffusing Capacity

Because PO$_2$ in the pulmonary capillary blood varies with time as it moves through the pulmonary capillary bed, oxygen cannot be used to assess diffusing capacity. A gas mixture containing carbon monoxide is the traditional diagnostic gas used to measure diffusing capacity. Its partial pressure in the blood is nearly zero, and its affinity for hemoglobin is 200 times that of oxygen.[59] Carbon monoxide diffusing capacity (D$_{LCO}$) collectively measures all the factors that affect the diffusion of gas across the alveolar–capillary membrane. The D$_{LCO}$ is recorded in mL CO/min/mm Hg at STPD (standard temperature and pressure, dry). In persons with normal hemoglobin concentrations and normal $\dot{V}_A/\dot{Q}$ matching, the main factor limiting diffusion is the alveolar–capillary membrane. Small amounts of carbon dioxide and inspired gas can produce measurable changes in the concentration of inspired gas compared with expired gas. There are several methods for determining D$_{LCO}$, but all methods measure diffusing capacity according to the equation:

$$D_{LCO} = \frac{mL\ CO\ transferred/min}{Mean\ P_{ACO} - mean\ capillary\ P_{CO}}$$

(11-10)

The average value for resting subjects when the single-breath method is used is 25 mL CO/min/mm Hg. D$_{LCO}$ values can increase to 2 or 3 times normal during exercise.

The D$_{LO_2}$ may be estimated from the D$_{LCO}$ by multiplying D$_{LCO}$ by 1.23, although the D$_{LCO}$ is usually the reported value. D$_{LCO}$ can be divided by the lung volume at which the measurement was made to obtain an expression of diffusing capacity per unit lung volume.

Some of the other factors that can influence D$_{LCO}$ are as follows:

1. Hemoglobin concentration: decreased hemoglobin concentration decreases the D$_{LCO}$.
2. Alveolar P$_{CO}$: an increased P$_{ACO}$ raises D$_{LCO}$.
3. Body position: the supine position increases D$_{LCO}$.
4. Pulmonary capillary blood volume.

Diffusing capacity is decreased in alveolar fibrosis associated with sarcoidosis, asbestosis, berylliosis, oxygen toxicity, and pulmonary edema. These states are frequently categorized as *diffusion defects*, but low D$_{LCO}$ is probably more closely related to loss of lung volume or capillary bed perfusion. D$_{LCO}$ is decreased in obstructive disease because of the decreased alveolar surface area, loss of capillary bed, the increased distance from the terminal bronchiole to the alveolar–capillary membrane, and $\dot{V}_A/\dot{Q}$ mismatching. In short, few disease states truly inhibit oxygen diffusion across the alveolar–capillary membrane.

Practical Application of Pulmonary Function Tests

Although we have a host of pulmonary function tests from which to choose, spirometry is the most useful, cost-effective, and commonly used test.[60] Screening spirometry yields vital capacity (VC), FVC, and FEV$_1$. From these values, two basic types of pulmonary dysfunction can be identified and quantitated: obstructive defects and restrictive defects. The primary criterion for airflow obstruction is decreased FEV$_1$/FCV ratio. Other measurements such as FEF$_{25-75\%}$ can be used to support

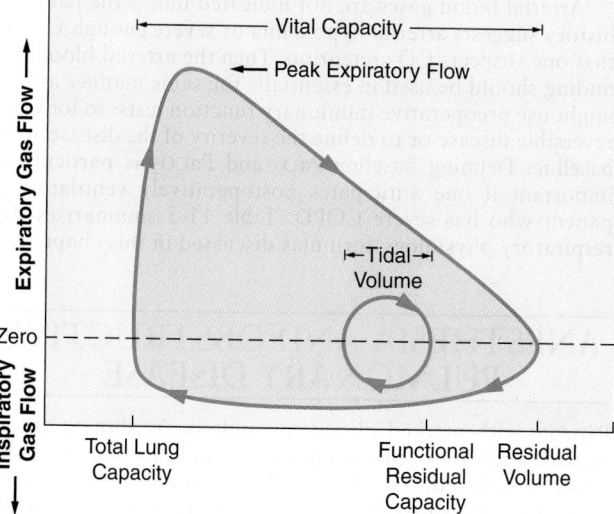

FIGURE 11-10. Flow–volume loop. The figure depicts a normally configured adult flow–volume loop. The slope of the loop after the subject reaches peak expiratory flow is nearly linear.

ANATOMY AND PHYSIOLOGY

TABLE 11-4

PULMONARY FUNCTION TESTS IN RESTRICTIVE AND OBSTRUCTIVE LUNG DISEASE

■ VALUE	■ RESTRICTIVE DISEASE	■ OBSTRUCTIVE DISEASE
Definition	Proportional decreases in all lung volumes	Small airway obstruction to expiratory flow
FVC	↓↓↓	Normal or slightly ↑
FEV_1	↓↓↓	Normal or slightly ↓
FEV_1/FVC	Normal	↓↓↓
$FEF_{25-75\%}$	Normal	↓↓↓
FRC	↓↓↓	Normal or ↑ if gas trapping
TLC	↓↓↓	Normal or ↑ if gas trapping

FVC, forced vital capacity; ↓↓↓, ↑↑↑ = large decrease or increase, respectively; ↓, ↑ = small/moderate decrease or increase, respectively; FEV, forced expiratory volume; FRC, functional residual capacity; TLC, total lung capacity.

the diagnosis of an obstructive defect or to assist in making decisions (e.g., whether to institute bronchodilation). A restrictive defect is a proportional decrease in all lung volumes; thus, VC, FVC, and FEV_1 all are reduced, but FEV_1/FVC remains normal. When there is a question about whether a decreased VC is due to restriction, total lung capacity should be measured. Reduced total lung capacity defines a restrictive defect but is not necessary unless VC on screening spirometry is reduced. The American Thoracic Society published an experts' consensus concerning interpretation of lung function tests.[61] Table 11-4 summarizes the distinction between pulmonary function results obtained from those with restrictive and obstructive defects. Refer to "Pulmonary Function Postoperatively" for a discussion of the use of pulmonary testing.

Preoperative Pulmonary Assessment

Markedly impaired pulmonary function is likely in patients who have the following:

1. Any chronic disease that involves the lung
2. Smoking history, persistent cough, and/or wheezing
3. Chest wall and spinal deformities
4. Morbid obesity
5. Requirement for single-lung anesthesia or lung resection
6. Severe neuromuscular disease

Preoperative pulmonary evaluation must include history and physical examination and may include chest radiograph, arterial blood gas analysis, and screening spirometry, depending on the patient's history. A history of sputum production, wheezing or dyspnea, exercise intolerance, or limited daily activities may yield more practical information than does formal testing. Arterial blood analysis, which should be sampled while the patient breathes room air, adds information regarding gas exchange and acid-base balance. Arterial blood gas sampling is primarily useful if the patient's history suggests that he or she may be chronically hypoxemic or may "retain" CO_2 (i.e., a patient with a chronic, compensated arterial acidemia) and be used to guide ventilatory management goals.

The goals one might hope to achieve through preoperative pulmonary function would be to predict the likelihood of pulmonary complications, obtain quantitative baseline information concerning pulmonary function that guides decision making, and identify patients who may benefit from therapy to improve pulmonary function preoperatively. For patients who will have lung resections, pulmonary function testing does provide some predictive benefit.[62] For all other patients, however, overwhelming evidence suggests that preoperative pul-

monary function testing does not predict or assign risk for PPCs.[63,64]

In 2002, the American Society of Anesthesiologists' Task Force on Preanesthetic Evaluation published a practice advisory[65] wherein they recommended that "there is insufficient evidence to identify explicit decision parameters or rules for ordering preoperative tests on the basis of specific clinical characteristics." Review of the literature[66] also reveals that specific measurements of lung function do not predict PPCs. Rather, they should be obtained to ascertain the presence of reversible pulmonary disease (bronchospasm) or to define the severity of advanced pulmonary disease. Instead, the clinician obtains more information from the patient's history. In a series of 272 adults undergoing nonthoracic surgery, McAlister et al.[67] found that the following historical factors independently increased the risk of PPC: age >65 years, smoking >40 packyears, COPD, asthma, productive cough, and exercise tolerance of less than one flight of stairs.

The need to obtain baseline pulmonary function data should be reserved for those patients with severely impaired preoperative pulmonary function, such as tetraplegics or myasthenics, so assessment for liberation from mechanical ventilation and/or tracheal extubation might be based on the patient's baseline pulmonary function.

Arterial blood gases are not indicated unless the patient's history suggests arterial hypoxemia or severe enough COPD that one suspects CO_2 retention. Then the arterial blood gas finding should be used in essentially the same manner as one might use preoperative pulmonary function tests: to look for reversible disease or to define the severity of the disease at its baseline. Defining baseline PaO_2 and $PaCO_2$ is particularly important if one anticipates postoperatively ventilating a patient who has severe COPD. Table 11-5 summarizes the respiratory physiology formulas discussed in this chapter.

ANESTHESIA AND OBSTRUCTIVE PULMONARY DISEASE

Patients with marked obstructive pulmonary disease are at increased risk for both intraoperative and PPCs. For example, patients with reduced FEV_1/FVC or reduced midexpiratory flow not only suffer airway obstruction, but also usually exhibit increased airway reactivity. Because of the hazard of provoking reflex bronchoconstriction during laryngoscopy and tracheal intubation, patients with COPD or asthma should receive aggressive bronchodilator therapy preoperatively.

TABLE 11-5

RESPIRATORY FORMULAS

■ FORMULA	■ NORMAL VALUES (70 KG)
Alveolar oxygen tension $PAO_2 = (PB - 47) FIO_2 -; (PACO_2/R)$	110 mm Hg ($FIO_2 = 0.21$)
Alveolar-arterial oxygen gradient $(A-aO_2) = PAO_2 - PaO_2$	<10 mm Hg ($FIO_2 = 0.21$)
Arterial-to-alveolar oxygen ratio, PaO_2/PAO_2 ratio	>0.75
Arterial oxygen content $CaO_2 = (SaO_2)(Hb \times 1.34) + PaO_2 (0.0031)$	20 mL/100 mL blood
Mixed venous oxygen content $C\bar{v}O_2 = (S\bar{v}O_2)(Hb \times 1.34) + P\bar{v}O_2 (0.0031)$	15 mL/100 mL blood
Arterial-venous oxygen content difference $C(a-\bar{v})O_2 = CaO_2 - C\bar{v}O_2$	4–6 mL/100 mL blood
Intrapulmonary shunt $\dot{Q}sp/\dot{Q}T = (Cc'O_2 - CaO_2)/(Cc'O_2 - C\bar{v}O_2)$ where $Cc'O_2 = (Hb \times 1.34) + (PAO_2 \times 0.0031)$	<5%
Physiologic dead space $VD/V_T = (PaCO_2 - P\bar{E}CO_2)/PaCO_2$	0.33
Oxygen consumption $VO_2 = CO(CaO_2 - C\bar{v}O_2)$	250 mL/min
Oxygen transport $DO_2 = CO(CaO_2)$	1,000 mL/min
Respiratory quotient $VCO_2/\dot{V}O_2 = R$	0.8

PAO_2, alveolar oxygen tension; PB, barometric pressure; FIO_2, fraction inspired oxygen; $PACO_2$, alveolar carbon dioxide tension; R, respiratory quotient; PaO_2, arterial oxygen tension; CaO_2, arterial oxygen content; SaO_2, arterial oxygen saturation; Hb, hemoglobin concentration; $C\bar{v}O_2$, mixed venous oxygen content; $S\bar{v}O_2$, mixed venous oxygen saturation; $P\bar{v}O_2$, mixed venous oxygen tension; Qsp/QT, intrapulmonary shunt; $Cc'O_2$, end-pulmonary capillary oxygen content; VD, dead space gas volume; V_T, tidal volume; $PaCO_2$, arterial carbon dioxide tension; $P\bar{E}CO_2$, mixed expired carbon dioxide tension; VO_2, oxygen consumption (mL/min); CO, cardiac output; $\dot{V}CO_2$, carbon dioxide production (mL/min); DO_2, oxygen transport.

High alveolar concentrations of most potent inhalational anesthetics will blunt airway reflexes and reflex bronchoconstriction, but require a fairly robust cardiovascular system. Adjunctive intravenous administration of opioids and lidocaine prior to airway instrumentation will decrease airway reactivity by deepening anesthesia. Furthermore, a single dose of corticosteroids may help prevent postoperative increases in airway resistance.

Spontaneous ventilation during general anesthesia in patients with severe obstructive disease is more likely to result in hypercapnia than in patients with normal pulmonary function.[68] Preoperative FEV_1 reduction correlates with the $PaCO_2$ increase during anesthesia. Slower rates of mechanical ventilation (8 to 10 breaths · min^{-1}) should be used to allow time for exhalation. Low ventilatory rates necessitate larger tidal volume if one desires a normal $PaCO_2$, but larger V_T and resultant higher peak airway pressure may predispose the patient to pulmonary barotrauma. Tidal volume and inspiratory flows should be adjusted to keep peak airway pressure less than 40 cm H_2O,[69,70] if possible. Higher inspiratory flows produce a shorter inspiratory time and, usually, a high peak airway pressure. Thus, a balance that avoids high peak airway pressure and excessively large V_T that allows the longest possible expiratory time should be sought.

Ideally, depending on the procedure and the duration of anesthesia, one would extubate the patient's trachea at the end of the operation. The irritating tracheal tube increases both airway resistance and reflex bronchoconstriction, limits the ability of the patient to clear secretions effectively, and increases the risk of iatrogenic infection. For some patients with obstructive disease (e.g., the young asthmatic patient),

many advocate tracheal extubation during deep anesthesia at the conclusion of the operation.

ANESTHESIA AND RESTRICTIVE PULMONARY DISEASE

Restrictive disease is characterized by proportional decreases in all lung volumes. The decreased FRC produces low lung compliance and also results in arterial hypoxemia because of low $\dot{V}A/\dot{Q}$ mismatching. Patients with this disease typically breathe rapidly and shallowly.

Positive-pressure ventilation of patients with restrictive disease is fraught with high peak airway pressures because more pressure is required to expand stiff lungs. Lower mechanical tidal volumes at more rapid rates reduce the risk of barotrauma but augment ventilation-induced cardiovascular depression and increase the chances of developing atelectasis. Larger tidal volumes should be avoided because of the increased risk of both barotrauma[71] and volutrauma.[72] Various lung-protective strategies have been developed to ventilate patients with profound restrictive lung disease (see Chapter 56).

Because the FRC is reduced, a lower oxygen store is available during apneic periods. Even preoxygenation with an FIO_2 of 1.0 can result in arterial hypoxemia seconds after the cessation of breathing or disconnection from a ventilator circuit. Patients with severe restrictive diseases tolerate apnea poorly. Because arterial hypoxemia develops so rapidly, transportation of these patients within the hospital should be performed with a pulse oximeter.

Even healthy individuals develop mild restrictive defects during anesthesia. FRC decreases 10 to 15% when healthy, spontaneously breathing individuals lie supine. Tracheal intubation further reduces FRC only slightly. General anesthesia consistently decreases FRC by a further 5 to 10%,[73] which usually results in decreased lung compliance.[74] The FRC reaches its nadir within the first 10 minutes of anesthesia[73,75,76] and is independent of whether ventilation is spontaneous or controlled. The diminished FRC persists in the postoperative period but may be restored postoperatively by the use of positive end-expiratory pressure or CPAP.[73,77,78] However, once positive airway pressure is removed, FRC plummets to previously diminished levels, which reach a postoperative nadir 12 hours after operation.[79]

EFFECTS OF CIGARETTE SMOKING ON PULMONARY FUNCTION

Smoking affects pulmonary function in many ways (see Chapter 23). The irritant smoke decreases ciliary motility and increases sputum production. Thus, these patients have a high volume of sputum and decreased ability to clear it effectively. As smoking habits persist, airway reactivity and the development of obstructive disease become problematic. Studies of the pathogenesis of COPD suggest that smoking results in an excess of pulmonary proteolytic enzymes, which directly cause damage to the lung parenchyma.[80] Exposure to smoke increases synthesis and release of elastolytic enzymes from alveolar macrophages—cells instrumental in the genesis of COPD from smoking. Further damage to the lung tissue is probably caused by reactive metabolites of oxygen, such as hydroxyl radicals and hydrogen peroxide, which are usually used by the macrophages to kill micro-organisms. The immunoregulatory function of the macrophages is also changed by cigarette smoking, with changes occurring in the presentation of antigens and interaction with T lymphocytes.[81] Other direct effects on lung tissue caused by smoking include increased epithelial permeability[82] and changed pulmonary surfactant.[83] The airway irritation or small airway reactivity evoked by inhaling cigarette smoke is the result of activation of sensory endings located in the central airways, which is primarily caused by nicotine.[84]

Early in the disease, mild $\dot{V}_A/\dot{Q}$ mismatch, bronchitic disease, and airway hyperreactivity are primary problems. Later, these problems are accompanied by the hallmarks of COPD: gas trapping, flattened diaphragmatic configuration (which decreases the efficiency with which the diaphragm functions), and barrel-chest deformity. Lung compliance increases significantly so limited elastic recoil prevents complete passive emptying. As a result, many patients exhale forcibly to reduce gas trapping.

With gas trapping, ventilation and perfusion become increasingly mismatched. Large areas of dead space ventilation and venous admixture occur. Carbon dioxide elimination is inefficient because of dead space ventilation. The typical minute ventilation for patients with advanced obstructive lung disease can be 1.5 to 2 times normal. In addition, venous admixture produces arterial hypoxemia that is exquisitely sensitive to low concentrations of supplemental oxygen. Gas exchange is further impaired by the increased carboxyhemoglobin concentration that results from inspiring smoke. Normal carboxyhemoglobin concentration in nonsmokers is approximately 1%; in smokers, however, it can be as high as 8 to 10%. Cessation of smoking, even for 12 to 24 hours preoperatively, can decrease CO concentration to near normal.

Smoking is one of the main and most prevalent risk factors associated with postoperative morbidity.[85] COPD patients who smoke have a two- to sixfold[86] risk of developing postoperative pneumonia compared with nonsmokers.

Further, smokers' relative risk of PPC is doubled, even if they do not have evidence of clinical pulmonary disease or abnormal pulmonary function.[87] The incidence of PPC in smokers can be reduced by abstinence from smoking, although there is no consensus on the minimal or optimal duration of preoperative smoking abstinence.[88–90] Warner et al.[85] studied 200 patients undergoing coronary artery bypass grafting and found that patients who continued to smoke or stopped <8 weeks before the operation had a complication rate nearly 4 times that of patients who had quit smoking more than 8 weeks preoperatively. These data further demonstrated that those who quit smoking <8 weeks preoperatively had a higher rate of complication than those who continued to smoke. Normalization of mucociliary function requires 2 to 3 weeks of abstinence from smoking, during which time sputum increases. Several months of smoking abstinence is required to return sputum clearance to normal.[91] In a study of bupropion-assisted smoking cessation, Hurt et al.[92] demonstrated decreased risk of postoperative complications even after 4 weeks of abstinence from smoking.

Nonetheless, Public Health Service guidelines published in 2000 emphasize the responsibility of health care facilities to coordinate interventions aimed at tobacco-dependence treatment. In addition to the guidelines noting that tobacco dependence often necessitates repeated interventions, "every patient who uses tobacco should be offered at least brief treatment" as brief tobacco-dependence therapy has been shown to be effective. These guidelines recognize five first-line pharmacologic adjuncts that increase smoking cessation success: bupropion SR, nicotine gum, nicotine inhaler, nicotine nasal spray and nicotine patch. Additionally, clonidine and nortriptyline were identified as second-line pharmacologic adjuncts.[93]

Following publication of these 2000 guidelines, a randomized controlled trial using the partial nicotinic acetylcholine agonist, varenicline, showed improved smoking abstinence rates at all times evaluated during the study when compared with bupropion SR treatment.[94] Based on this information, the utilization of varenicline in a smoking-cessation program should be considered.

Smokers who decrease, but do not stop, cigarette consumption without the aid of nicotine-replacement therapy continue to acquire equal amounts of nicotine from fewer cigarettes by changing their technique of smoking to maximize nicotine intake.[95] Levels of serum nicotine and cotinine and urinary mutagenesis levels remain unchanged. Thus, *reduction* in the number of cigarettes smoked will likely have little effect on the risk of developing PPCs.[86] Smoking patients should be advised to *stop* smoking 2 months prior to elective operations to maximize the effect of smoking cessation,[85] or for at least 4 weeks to benefit from improved mucociliary function and some reduction in PPC rate. If patients cannot stop smoking for 4 to 8 weeks preoperatively, it is controversial whether they should be advised to stop smoking 24 hours preoperatively. A 24-hour smoking abstinence would allow carboxyhemoglobin levels to fall to normal but may increase the risk of PPC.

PULMONARY FUNCTION POSTOPERATIVELY

Risk of Postoperative Pulmonary Complications

Postoperative Pulmonary Function

The changes in pulmonary function that occur postoperatively are primarily restrictive, with proportional decreases in all lung volumes and no change in airway resistance. The decrease in FRC, however, is the yardstick by which the severity of the restrictive defect is gauged. This defect is generated by abdominal contents that impinge on and prevent normal movement of the diaphragm and by an abnormal respiratory pattern devoid of sighs and characterized by shallow, rapid respirations. The normal resting respiratory rate for adults is 12 breaths per minute, whereas the postoperative patient usually breathes approximately 20 breaths per minute. Furthermore, most (but not all) factors that tend to make the restrictive defect worse are also those associated with a higher risk of PPCs.

The operative site is one of the single most important determinants of the degree of pulmonary restriction and the risk of PPCs. Nonlaparoscopic upper abdominal operations cause the most profound restrictive defect, precipitating a 40 to 50% decrease in FRC compared with preoperative levels, when conventional postoperative analgesia is employed. Lower abdominal and thoracic operations cause the next most severe change in pulmonary function, with decreases in FRC to 30% of preoperative levels. Most other operative sites—intracranial, peripheral vascular, otolaryngologic—have approximately the same effect on FRC, with reductions to 15 to 20% of preoperative levels.

Postoperative Pulmonary Complications

Two problems confound interpretation of the literature examining PPCs (see Chapter 65). First, there is no clear definition of what constitutes a PPC. For example, some clinical studies include only pneumonia, whereas others add atelectasis and/or ventilatory failure. Thus, to interpret data concerning rates of PPCs, it is important to discern what complications are specifically being addressed. Second, the criteria by which the diagnosis of postoperative pneumonia or atelectasis is made vary from study to study. For this discussion, PPCs include atelectasis and pneumonia only. Reasonable, well-accepted diagnostic criteria for these diagnoses include change in the color and quantity of sputum, oral temperature exceeding 38.5°C, and a new infiltrate on chest radiograph.

The operative site is an important risk factor for the development of PPCs. Nonlaparoscopic upper abdominal operations increase risk for PPC at least twofold,[89] with rates of occurrence varying from 20 to 70%.[95] Lower abdominal and intrathoracic operations are associated with slightly less risk, but still higher risk than extremity, intracranial, and head/neck operations.

Patients with COPD are at risk for PPC. Their risks can be minimized by ensuring they do not have an active pulmonary infection and any increased resistance associated with reactive airways disease is minimized by the use of bronchodilator therapy. Interestingly, those with asthma are not at increased risk for atelectasis or pneumonia. However, exacerbation of asthma in the postoperative period can be problematic. Careful attention must be given to ensuring the continuation of bronchodilating regimens and steroid administration (either inhaled or systemic) through the perioperative period.

There are several strategies by which it is possible to reduce risk of PPC: the use of lung-expanding therapies postoperatively, choice of analgesia,[96] and cessation of smoking. After upper abdominal operations, which are associated with the highest incidence of PPCs, FRC recovers over 3 to 7 days. With the use of intermittent CPAP by mask, FRC will recover within 72 hours.[97] Patients correctly use incentive spirometers only 10% of the time unless therapy is supervised.[98] Stir-up regimens are as effective as incentive spirometry at preventing PPCs[99] and they are less expensive than supervised incentive spirometry; thus, they are preferred over incentive spirometry therapy.

After median sternotomy for cardiac operations, FRC does not return to normal for several weeks, regardless of postoperative pulmonary therapy.[100] The persistently low FRC in this population is probably due to mechanical factors such as a widened mediastinum, intrapleural fluid, and altered chest wall compliance. The single most important aspect of postoperative pulmonary care is getting the patient out of bed, preferably walking.

The choice of anesthetic technique for intraoperative anesthesia does not change the risk for PPC independent of the operative site or duration of the operation. Operations exceeding 3 hours are associated with a higher rate of PPC. Choice of postoperative analgesia strongly influences the risk of PPC.[89] The use of postoperative epidural analgesia, particularly for abdominal and thoracic operations, markedly decreases the risk of PPC and appears to decrease length of stay in the hospital.

Although obesity is associated with marked restrictive defects, some studies demonstrate that obesity does not independently increase the risk of PPC, whereas others do demonstrate increased independent risk for PPCs in the obese population.[101] However, there are data to support[101] advanced age as an independent risk factor for PPCs.

Several authors have attempted to assess the influence of overall health on PPC risk. The use of indices that weight and score various aspects of physiology and health shows that patients who are in a poor state of health preoperatively tend to be at higher risk of PPC.[90]

Patients with obstructive airway disease and decreased expiratory flows may benefit from preoperative bronchodilator therapy and formal pulmonary toilet.[102] High-risk patients with COPD who receive bronchodilation, chest physical therapy, deep breathing, forced oral fluids (>3 L/day), and preoperative instruction in postoperative respiratory techniques, as well as those who stop smoking for more than 2 months preoperatively, experience a PPC rate approximately equal to that observed in normal patients.[103] Interestingly, although a regimen of this nature significantly reduces the incidence of PPCs,[104] airway obstruction and arterial hypoxemia are not measurably reversed during the 48 to 72 hours of preoperative therapy.[105] It is possible that the reduced complication rate results from the additional attention that these patients receive rather than from the specific regimen employed.

References

1. Lieberman DA, Falkner JA, Craig AB Jr et al: Performance and histochemical composition of guinea pig and human diaphragm. J Appl Physiol 1973; 34: 233
2. Roussos C, Macklin PT: Diaphragmatic fatigue in man. J Appl Physiol 1977; 43: 189
3. Campbell EJM, Green JH: The behaviour of the abdominal muscles and intra-abdominal pressure during quiet breathing and increased pulmonary ventilation: A study in man. J Physiol (Lond) 1955; 127: 423
4. Conrardy PA, Goodman CR, Lainge F et al: Alteration of endotracheal tube position: Flexion and extension of the neck. Crit Care Med 1976; 4: 8
5. Bachoven M, Weibel ER: Basic pattern of tissue repair in human lungs following unspecific injury. Chest 1974; 65: 145
6. Fishman AP: Non-respiratory function of lung. Chest 1977; 72: 84
7. Hocking WG, Golden DW: The pulmonary-alveolar macrophage. N Engl J Med 1979; 301: 580
8. Whitehead TC, Zhang H, Mullen B, Slutsky AS: Effect of mechanical ventilation on cytokine response to intratracheal lipopolysaccharide. Anesthesiology 2004; 101: 1
9. Dreyfuss D, Rouby J-J: Mechanical ventilation-induced lung release of cytokines: A key for the future or Pandora's box? Anesthesiology 2004; 101: 1
10. Downs JB: A technique for direct measurement of intrapleural pressure. Crit Care Med 1976; 4: 207
11. Baydur A, Behrakis P, Zin WA: A simple method for assessing the validity of the esophageal balloon technique. Am Rev Respir Dis 1982; 126: 788
12. Blanch MJ, Kirby RR, Gabrielli A et al: Partially and totally unloading respiratory muscles based on real time measurements of work of breathing. A clinical approach. Chest 1994; 106: 1835
13. Brochard L, Rua F, Lorino H: Inspiratory pressure support compensates for the additional work of breathing caused by the endotracheal tube. Anesthesiology 1991; 75: 739
14. Rohrer F: Der Strömungswiderstand in den menschlichen Atemwegen. Pflugers Arch 1915; 162: 225

15. Nunn JF: Resistance to gas flow and airway closure. In: Applied Respiratory Physiology. Boston, Butterworths, 1987, pp 50

16. Campbell EJM, Freedman S, Smith PS, Taylor ME: The ability of man to detect added elastic loads to breathing. Clin Sci 1961; 20: 223

17. Fink BR, Ngai SH, Holiday DA: Effect of air flow resistance on ventilation and respiratory muscle activity. JAMA 1958; 168: 2245

18. Palmer KNV, Diament ML: Effect of aerosol isoprenaline on blood-gas tensions in severe bronchial asthma. Lancet 1967; 2: 1232

19. Campbell EJM: The effects of increased resistance to expiration on the respiratory behaviour of the abdominal muscles and intra-abdominal pressure. J Physiol 1957; 136: 556

20. Janssens JP, Pache JC, Nicod LP: Physiologic changes in respiratory function associated with aging. Eur Respir J 1999; 13: 107

21. LeGallois CJJ: Expériences sur le Principe de la Vie. Paris, D'Hautel, 1812, p 325

22. Salmoiraghi GC, Burns BD: Localization and patterns of discharge of respiratory neurones in brain-stem of cat. J Neurophysiol 1960; 23: 2

23. Cohen MI: Neurogenesis of respiratory rhythm in the mammal. Physiol Rev 1979; 59: 1105

24. Guz A: Regulation of respiration in man. Ann Respir Physiol 1975; 37: 303

25. Pitts RF, Magoun HW, Ranson SW: The origin of respiratory rhythmicity. Am J Physiol 1939; 127: 654

26. Lumsden TL: Observations on the respiratory centers in the cat. J Physiol (Lond) 1923; 57: 153

27. Cohen MI, Wang SC: Respiratory neuronal activity in the pons of the cat. J Neurophysiol 1959; 22: 33

28. Stella G: On the mechanism of production and the physiologic significance of "apneusis." J Physiol (Lond) 1938; 93: 10

29. Kabat H: Electrical stimulation of points in the forebrain and mid-brain: The resultant alterations in respiration. J Comp Neurol 1936; 63: 211

30. Wang SC, Borison HL: The vomiting center: A critical experimental analysis. Arch Neurol Psychiatry 1950; 63: 928

31. Gaylor JB: The intrinsic nervous mechanisms of the human lung. Brain 1934; 57: 143

32. Davis HL, Fowler WS, Lambert EH: Effect of volume and rate of inflation and deflation on transpulmonary pressure and response of pulmonary stretch receptors. Am J Physiol 1956; 187: 558

33. Hering E, Breuer J: Die Sebsteuerung der Atmung durch den Nervus vagus. Stizber Akad Wiss Wien 1868; 57: 672

34. Ide T, Sakurai Y, Aono M, Nishino T: Contribution of peripheral chemoreception to the depression of the hypoxic ventilatory response during halothane anesthesia in cats. Anesthesiology 1998; 90: 1084

35. Mora CT, Torjman M, White PF: Effects of diazepam and flumazenil on sedation and hypoxic ventilatory response. Anesth Analg 1989; 68: 473

36. Leusen I: Regulation of cerebrospinal fluid composition with reference to breathing. Physiol Rev 1972; 52: 1

37. Cohen MI: Discharge patterns of brain-stem respiratory neurons in relation to carbon dioxide tension. J Neurophysiol 1968; 31: 142

38. Heinemann HO, Golaring RM: Bicarbonate and the regulation of ventilation. Am J Med 1974; 57: 361

39. Severinghaus JW, Mitchell RA, Richardson BW et al: Respiratory control at high altitude suggesting active transport regulation of CSF pH. J Appl Physiol 1963; 18: 1155

40. Ferris EB, Engel GL, Stevens CD, Webb J: Voluntary breath holding. J Clin Invest 1946; 25: 734

41. Stock MC, Downs JB, McDonald JS et al: The carbon dioxide rate of rise in awake apneic humans. J Clin Anesth 1988; 1: 96

42. Eger EI, Severinghaus JW: The rate of rise of $PaCO_2$ in the apneic anesthetized patient. Anesthesiology 1961; 22: 419

43. Stock MC, Schisler JQ, McSweeney TD: The $PaCO_2$ rate of rise in anesthetized patients with airway obstruction. J Clin Anesth 1989; 1: 328

44. Wright FG, Foley MF, Downs JB et al: Hypoxemia and hypocarbia following intermittent positive-pressure breathing. Anesth Analg 1976; 55: 555

45. Fink BR: The stimulant effect of wakefulness on respiration: Clinical aspects. Br J Anaesth 1961; 33: 97

46. Berger AJ, Mitchell RA, Severinghaus JW: Regulation of respiration: III. N Engl J Med 1977; 297: 194

47. West JB, Dollery CT, Naimark A: Distribution of blood flow in isolated lung: Relation to vascular and alveolar pressures. J Appl Physiol 1964; 19: 713

48. West JB, Dollery CT: Distribution of blood flow and the pressure-flow relations of the whole lung. J Appl Physiol 1965; 20: 175

49. Gattinoni L, Pesent A, Avalli L et al: Pressure-volume curve of total respiratory system in acute respiratory failure. Computed tomographic scan study. Am Rev Respir Dis 1987; 136: 730

50. Benumof JL, Pirla AF, Johanson I et al: Interaction of PVO_2 with PAO_2 on hypoxic pulmonary vasoconstriction. J Appl Physiol 1981; 51: 871

51. Swenson EW, Finley TN, Guzman SV: Unilateral hypoventilation in man during temporary occlusion of one pulmonary artery. J Clin Invest 1961; 40: 828

52. Yamanaka MK, Sue DY: Comparison of arterial-end-tidal PCO_2 difference and deadspace/tidal volume ratio in respiratory failure. Chest 1987; 92: 832

53. Tyburski JG, Collinge JD, Wilson RF, Carlin AM, Albaran RG, Steffes CP: End-tidal CO_2-derived values during emergency trauma surgery correlated with outcome: A prospective study. J Trauma 2002; 53: 738

54. Huffmyer JL, Nemergut EC: Respiratory dysfunction and pulmonary disease in cirrhosis and other hepatic disorders. Respir Care 2007; 52: 1030

55. Gaines DI, Fallon MB: Hepatopulmonary syndrome. Liver Int 2004; 24: 397

56. Räsänen J, Downs JB, Malec DJ, Oates K: Oxygen tensions and oxyhemoglobin saturations in the assessment of pulmonary gas exchange. Crit Care Med 1987; 15: 1058

57. Christi RV: Lung volume and its subdivisions. I. Methods of measurement. J Clin Invest 1932; 11: 1099

58. Tisi GM: Preoperative evaluation of pulmonary function. Validity, indications and benefits. [Review] Am Rev Respir Dis 1979; 119: 293

59. Apthorp GH, Marshall R: Pulmonary diffusing capacity: A comparison of breath-holding and steady-state methods using carbon monoxide. J Clin Invest 1961; 40: 1775

60. Crapo RO: Pulmonary function testing. N Engl J Med 1994; 331: 25

61. American Thoracic Society: Lung function testing: Selection of reference values and interpretive strategies. Am Rev Respir Dis 1991; 144: 1202

62. Kearney DJ, Lee TH, Reilly JJ et al: Assessment of operative risk in patients undergoing lung resection: Importance of predicted pulmonary function. Chest 1994; 105: 753

63. Ferguson MK: Preoperative assessment of pulmonary risk. Chest 1999; 115: 58S

64. Bapoje SR, Whitaker JF, Schulz T et al: Preoperative evaluation of the patient with pulmonary disease. Chest 2007; 132: 1637

65. Task Force on Preanesthetic Evaluation. Practice advisory for preanesthetia evaluation: A report by the American Society of Anesthesiologists. Anesthesiology 2002; 96: 485

66. Zollinger A, Hofer C, Pasch T: Preoperative pulmonary evaluation: Fact and myth. Curr Opin Anaesth 2001; 14: 59

67. McAlister FA, Khan NA, Strauss SE, Papaioakim M, Fisher BW, Majumdar SR, et al: Accuracy of the preoperative assessment in predicting pulmonary risk after nonthoracic surgery. Am J Respir Crit Care Med 2003; 167: 741

68. Pietak W, Weenig CS, Hickey RF et al: Anesthetic effects on ventilation in patients with chronic obstructive pulmonary disease. Anesthesiology 1975; 42: 160

69. Connors AF, McAferee D, Gray BA: Effect of inspiratory flow rate on gas exchange during mechanical ventilation. Am Rev Respir Dis 1981; 124: 537

70. Tuxen DV, Lane S: The effects of ventilatory pattern on hyperinflation, airway pressures, and circulation in mechanical ventilation of patients with severe airflow obstruction. Am Rev Respir Dis 1987; 136: 872

71. Petersen GW, Baier H: Incidence of pulmonary barotrauma in a medical ICU. Crit Care Med 1983; 11: 67

72. Gattinoni L, Pesenti A: The concept of "baby lung." Intensive Care Med 2005; 31: 776

73. Brisner B, Hedenstierna G, Lundquist H et al: Pulmonary densities during anesthesia with muscular relaxation: A proposal of atelectasis. Anesthesiology 1985; 62: 422

74. Don HF, Robson JG: The mechanics of the respiratory system during anesthesia. The effects of atropine and carbon dioxide. Anesthesiology 1965; 26: 168

75. Don HF, Wahba M, Cuadrado L et al: The effects of anesthesia and 100 per cent oxygen on the functional residual capacity of the lungs. Anesthesiology 1970; 32: 251

76. Westbrook PR, Stubbs SE, Sessler AD et al: Effects of anesthesia and muscle paralysis on respiratory mechanics in normal man. J Appl Physiol 1973; 34: 81

77. Wyche MQ, Teichner RL, Kallost T et al: Effects of continuous positive-pressure breathing on functional residual capacity and arterial oxygenation during intra-abdominal operation: studies in man during nitrous oxide and d-tubocurarine anesthesia. Anesthesiology 1973; 38: 68

78. Rose DM, Downs JB, Heenen TJ: Temporal responses of functional residual capacity and oxygen tension to changes in positive end-expiratory pressure. Crit Care Med 1981; 9: 79

79. Craig DB: Postoperative recovery of pulmonary function. Anesth Analg 1981; 60: 46

80. Diamond L, Lai YL: Augmentation of elastase-induced emphysema by cigarette smoke: effects of reducing tar and nicotine content. J Toxicol Environ Health 1987; 20: 287

81. deShazo RD, Banks DE, Diem JE, et al. Broncho-alveolar lavage cell–lymphocyte interactions in normal nonsmokers and smokers. Am Rev Respir Dis 1983; 127: 545

82. Hogg JC: The effect of smoking on airway permeability. Chest 1983; 83: 1

83. Clements JA: Smoking and pulmonary surfactant. N Engl J Med 1972; 286: 261

84. Lee L-Y, Gerhardstein DC, Wang AL, Burki NK: Nicotine is responsible for airway irritation evoked by cigarette smoke inhalation in men. J Appl Physiol 1993; 75: 1955

85. Warner MA, Divertie MB, Tinker JH: Preoperative cessation of smoking and pulmonary complications in coronary artery bypass patients. Anesthesiology 1984; 60: 380

86. Bluman LG, Mosca L, Newman N, Simon DG: Preoperative smoking habits and postoperative pulmonary complications. Chest 1998; 113: 883

87. Chalon J, Tayyab MA, Ramanathan S: Cytology of respiratory complications after operation. Chest 1975; 67: 32

88. Theadom A, Copley M: Effects of preoperative smoking cessation on the incidence and risk of intraoperative and postoperative complications in adult smokers: a systematic review. Tob Control 2006; 15: 352

89. Quraishi SA, Orkin FK, Roizen MF: The anesthesia preoperative assessment: an opportunity for smoking cessation intervention. J Clin Anesth 2006; 18: 635

90. Warner MA, Offord KP, Warner ME *et al:* Role of postoperative cessation of smoking and other factors in postoperative pulmonary complications: A blinded prospective study of coronary artery bypass patients. Mayo Clin Proc 1989; 64: 609

91. Beckers S, Camu F. The anesthetic risk of tobacco smoking. Acta Anaesthesiol Belg 1991; 42: 45

92. Hurt RD, Sachs DPL, Gover ED *et al:* A comparison of sustained-release bupropion and placebo of smoking cessation. N Engl J Med 1997; 337: 1195

93. Fiore MC; Bailey WC, Cohen SJ *et al:* US public health service clinical practice guideline: treating tobacco use and dependence. Respir Care 2000; 45: 1200

94. Gonzales D, Rennard SI, Nides M *et al:* Varenicline, an alpha4beta2 nicotinic acetylcholine receptor partial agonist, vs sustained-release bupropion and placebo for smoking cessation: a randomized controlled trial. JAMA 2006; 296: 47

95. Benowitz NL, Jacob P, Kozlowski LT *et al:* Influence of smoking fewer cigarettes on exposure to tar, nicotine and carbon monoxide. N Engl J Med 1986; 3115: 1310

96. Liu SS, Wu CL: Effect of postoperative analgesia on major postoperative complications: a systematic update of the evidence. Anesth Analg 2007; 104: 689

97. Gust R, Pecher S, Gust A *et al:* Effect of patient-controlled analgesia on pulmonary complications after coronary artery bypass grafting. Crit Care Med 1999; 27: 2218

98. Stock MC, Downs JB, Gauer PK *et al:* Prevention of postoperative pulmonary complications with CPAP, incentive spirometry and conservative therapy. Chest 1985; 87: 151

99. Lyager S, Wernberg M, Rajani N *et al:* Can postoperative pulmonary complications be improved by treatment with BartlettEdwards incentive spirometer after upper abdominal surgery? Acta Anaesthesiol Scand 1979; 23: 312

100. Stock MC, Downs JB, Cooper RB *et al:* Comparison of continuous positive airway pressure, incentive spirometry, and conservative therapy after cardiac operations. Crit Care Med 1984; 12: 969

101. Smetana GW, Lawrence VA, Cornell JE: Preoperative pulmonary risk stratification for noncardiothoracic surgery: systematic review for the American College of Physicians. Ann Intern Med 2006; 144: 581

102. Chumillas S, Pace JL, Delgado F *et al:* Prevention of postoperative pulmonary complications through respiratory rehabilitation: A controlled clinical trial. Arch Phys Med Rehab 1998; 79: 5

103. Brooks-Brunn JA: Validation of a predictive model for postoperative pulmonary complications. Heart Lung 1998; 27: 151

104. Gracey DR, Divertie MB, Didier EP: Preoperative pulmonary preparation of patients with chronic obstructive pulmonary disease: A prospective study. Chest 1979; 76: 123

105. Petty TL, Brink GA, Miller NW, Corsello PR: Objective functional improvement in chronic airway obstruction. Chest 1970; 57: 216

ANATOMY AND PHYSIOLOGY

CHAPTER 12 ■ IMMUNE FUNCTION AND ALLERGIC RESPONSE

JERROLD H. LEVY

KEY POINTS

1. Anesthesiologists routinely manage patients during their perioperative medical care during which they are exposed to foreign substances, including drugs (antibiotics, anesthetic agents, neuromuscular-blocking agents [NMBAs], sedative/hypnotics), polypeptides (e.g., protamine, aprotinin), blood products, and environmental antigens (e.g., latex).

2. Antibodies are specific proteins called *immunoglobulins* that can recognize and bind to a specific antigen.

3. Cytokines are inflammatory cell activators that are synthesized to act as secondary messengers and activate endothelial cells and white cells.

4. Immune competence during surgery can be affected by direct and hormonal effects of anesthetic drugs, by immunologic effects of other drugs used, by the surgery, by coincident infection, and by transfused blood products.

5. More than 90% of the allergic reactions evoked by intravenous drugs occur within 5 minutes of administration. In the anesthetized patient, the most common life-threatening manifestation of an allergic reaction is circulatory collapse, reflecting vasodilation with resulting decreased venous return.

6. Many diverse molecules administered during the perioperative period release histamine in a dose-dependent, nonimmunologic fashion.

7. A plan for treating anaphylactic reactions must be established before the event. Airway maintenance, 100% oxygen administration, intravascular volume expansion, and epinephrine are essential to treat the hypotension and hypoxia that result from vasodilation, increased capillary permeability, and bronchospasm. Vasopressin should be considered for refractory shock.

8. After an anaphylactic reaction, it is important to identify the causative agent to prevent readmission.

9. Health care workers and children with spina bifida, urogenital abnormalities, or certain food allergies have been recognized as people at increased risk for anaphylaxis to latex.

10. NMBAs have several unique molecular features that make them potential antigens.

Allergic reactions represent an important cause of perioperative complications. Anesthesiologists routinely manage patients during their perioperative medical care during which they are exposed to foreign substances, including drugs (i.e., antibiotics, anesthetic agents, neuromuscular-blocking agents [NMBAs], sedative hypnotics), polypeptides (protamine, aprotinin), blood products, and environmental antigens (i.e., latex). Anesthesiologists must be able to rapidly recognize and treat anaphylaxis, the most life-threatening form of an allergic reaction.[1]

The allergic response represents just one limb of the pathologic response that the immune system can mount against foreign substances. As part of normal host surveillance mechanisms, a series of cellular and humoral elements oversees foreign structures called *antigens* to provide host defense. These foreign substances (antigens) consist of molecular arrangements found on cells, bacteria, viruses, proteins, or complex macromolecules.[1-4] Immunologic mechanisms (1) involve antigen interaction with antibodies or specific effector cells; (2) are reproducible; and (3) are specific and adaptive, distinguishing foreign substances and amplifying reactivity through a series of inflammatory cells and proteins. The immune system serves to protect the body against external micro-organisms and toxins, as well as internal threats from neoplastic cells; however, it can respond inappropriately to cause hypersensitive (allergic) reactions. Life-threatening allergic reactions to drugs and other foreign substances observed perioperatively may represent different expressions of the immune response.[1,2]

BASIC IMMUNOLOGIC PRINCIPLES

Host defense can be divided into cellular and humoral elements.[1–4] The humoral system includes antibodies, complement, cytokines, and other circulating proteins, whereas cellular immunity is mediated by specific lymphocytes of the T-cell series. Lymphocytes have receptors that distinguish between antigens of host and foreign origin. When lymphocytes react with foreign antigens, they respond to orchestrate immunosurveillance, regulate immunospecific antibody synthesis, and destroy foreign invaders. Individual aspects of the immune response and their importance are considered separately.

Antigens

Molecules stimulating an immune response (antibody production or lymphocyte stimulation) are called *antigens*.[4] Only a few drugs used by anesthesiologists, such as polypeptides (protamine) and other large macromolecules (dextrans), are complete antigens (Table 12-1). Most commonly used drugs are simple organic compounds of low molecular weight (around 1,000 daltons). For such a small molecule to become immunogenic, it must form a stable bond with circulating proteins or tissue micromolecules to result in an antigen (hapten-macromolecular complex). Small-molecular-weight substances such as drugs or drug metabolites that bind to host proteins or cell membranes to sensitize patients are called *haptens*. Haptens are not antigenic by themselves. Often, a reactive drug metabolite (e.g., penicilloyl derivative of penicillin) is believed to bind with macromolecules to become antigens, but for most drugs this phenomenon has not been proved.

Thymus-Derived (T-Cell) and Bursa-Derived (B-Cell) Lymphocytes

The thymus of the fetus differentiates immature lymphocytes into thymus-derived cells (T cells). T cells have receptors that are activated by binding with foreign antigens and secrete mediators that regulate the immune response. The subpopulations of T cells that exist in humans include helper, suppressor, cytotoxic, and killer cells.[5] The two types of regulatory T cells are helper cells (OKT4) and suppressor cells (OKT8). Helper cells are important for key effector cell responses, whereas suppressor cells inhibit immune function. Infection of helper T cells with a retrovirus, the human immunodeficiency virus, produces a specific increase in the number of suppressor cells. Cytotoxic T cells destroy mycobacteria, fungi, and viruses. Other lymphocytes, called *natural killer cells*, do not need specific antigen stimulation to set up their role. Both the cytotoxic

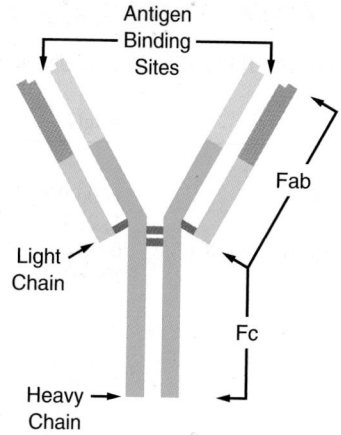

FIGURE 12-1. Basic structural configuration of the antibody molecule representing human immunoglobulin G. Immunoglobulins are composed of two heavy chains and two light chains bound by disulfide linkages (represented by *crossbars*). Papain cleaves the molecule into two Fab fragments and one Fc fragment. Antigen binding occurs on the Fab fragments, whereas the Fc segment is responsible for membrane binding or complement activation. (Reprinted with permission from Levy JH: Anaphylactic Reactions in Anesthesia and Intensive Care, 2nd edition. Boston, Butterworth-Heinemann, 1992.)

T cells and natural killer cells take part in defense against tumor cells and in transplant rejection. T cells produce mediators that influence the response of other cell types involved in the recognition and destruction of foreign substances.

B cells represent a specific lymphocyte cell line that can differentiate into specific plasma cells that synthesize antibodies, a step controlled by both helper and suppressor T-cell lymphocytes.[5] B cells are also called *bursa-derived cells* because in birds, the bursa of Fabricius is important in producing cells responsible for antibody synthesis.

Antibodies

Antibodies are specific proteins called *immunoglobulins* (Ig) that can recognize and bind to a specific antigen.[6] The basic structure of the antibody molecule is illustrated in Figure 12-1. Each antibody has at least two heavy chains and two light chains that are bound together by disulfide bonds. The Fab fragment has the ability to bind antigen, and the Fc, or crystallizable, fragment is responsible for the unique biological properties of the different classes of immunoglobulins (cell binding and complement activation). Antibodies function as specific receptor molecules for immune cells and proteins. When antigen binds covalently to the Fab fragments, the antibody undergoes

TABLE 12-1

AGENTS ADMINISTERED DURING ANESTHESIA THAT ACT AS ANTIGENS

■ HAPTENS	■ MACROMOLECULES
Penicillin and its derivatives	Aprotinin
	Blood products
Anesthetic drugs (?)	Chymopapain
	Colloid volume expanders
	Neuromuscular blocking agents
	Protamine
	Latex

TABLE 12-2

BIOLOGICAL CHARACTERISTICS OF IMMUNOGLOBULINS (Igs)

	■ IgG	■ IgM	■ IgA	■ IgE	■ IgD
Heavy chain	γ	μ	A	ϵ	δ
Molecular weight	160,000	900,000	170,000	188,000	184,000
Subclasses	1, 2, 3, 4	1, 2	1, 2		
Serum concentration (mg/dL)	6–14	0.5–1.5	1–3	$< -0.5 \times 10^3$	<0.1
Complement activation	All but IgG$_4$	+	−	−	−
Placental transfer	+	−	−	−	−
Serum half-life (days)	23	5	6	1–5	2–8
Cell binding	Mast cells (IgG$_4$) Neutrophils Lymphocytes Mononuclear cells Platelets	Lymphocytes		Mast cells Basophils	Neutrophils Lymphocytes

Modified from Levy JH: Anaphylactic Reactions in Anesthesia and Intensive Care, 2nd edition. Boston, Butterworth-Heinemann, 1992.

conformational changes to activate the Fc receptor. The results of antigen-antibody binding depend on the cell type, which causes a specific type of activation (e.g., lymphocyte proliferation and differentiation into antibody-secreting cells, mast cell degranulation, and complement activation).

Five major classes of antibodies occur in humans: IgG, IgA, IgM, IgD, and IgE. The heavy chain determines the structure and the function of each molecule. The basic properties of each antibody are listed in Table 12-2.

Effector Cells and Proteins of the Immune Response Cells

Monocytes, neutrophils (polymorphonuclear leukocytes [PMNs]), and eosinophils represent important effector cells that migrate into areas of inflammation in response to specific chemotactic factors, including lymphokines, cytokines, and complement-derived mediators. The deposition of antibody or complement fragments on the surface of foreign cells is called *opsonization*, a process that promotes killing foreign cells by effector cells. In addition, lymphokines and cytokines produce chemotaxis of other inflammatory cells in a manner described in the following sections.

Monocytes and Macrophages. Macrophages regulate immune responses by processing and presenting antigens to effect inflammatory, tumoricidal, and microbicidal functions. Macrophages arise from circulating monocytes or may be confined to specific organs such as the lung. They are recruited and activated in response to micro-organisms or tissue injury. Macrophages ingest antigens before they interact with receptors on the lymphocyte surface to regulate their action. Macrophages synthesize mediators to facilitate both B-lymphocyte and T-lymphocyte responses.

Polymorphonuclear Leukocytes (Neutrophils). The first cells to appear in acute inflammatory reaction are neutrophils that contain acid hydrolases, neutral proteases, and lysosomes. Once activated, they produce hydroxyl radicals, superoxide, and hydrogen peroxide, which aid in microbial killing.

Eosinophils. The exact function of the eosinophil in host defense is unclear; however, inflammatory cells recruit eosinophils to collect at sites of parasitic infections, tumors, and allergic reactions.[1]

Basophils. Basophils comprise 0.5 to 1% of circulating granulocytes in the blood.[1] The surface of basophils contain IgE receptors, which function similarly to those on mast cells.

Mast Cells. Mast cells are important cells for immediate hypersensitivity responses. They are tissue fixed and located in the perivascular spaces of the skin, lung, and intestine.[1] The surface of mast cells contain IgE receptors, which bind to specific antigens. Once activated, these cells release physiologically active mediators important to immediate hypersensitivity responses (see "IgE-Mediated Pathophysiology"). Mast cells can be activated by a series of both immune and nonimmune stimuli.

Proteins

Cytokines/Interleukins. Cytokines are inflammatory cell activators that are synthesized by macrophages to act as secondary messengers and activate endothelial cells and white cells.[7] Interleukin-1 and tumor necrosis factor are examples of cytokines considered to be important mediators of the biological responses to infection and other inflammatory reactions. Liberation of interleukin-1 and tumor necrosis factor produces fever, neuropeptide release, endothelial cell activation, increased adhesion molecule expression, neutrophil priming, hypotension, myocardial suppression, and a catabolic state.[7] The term *interleukin* was coined for a group of cytokines that promotes communication between and among ("inter") leukocytes ("leukin"). Interleukins are a group of different regulatory proteins that act to control many aspects of the immune and inflammatory responses. The interleukins are polypeptides synthesized in response to cellular activation; they produce their inflammatory effects by activating specific receptors on inflammatory cells and vasculature. T-cell lymphocytes influence the activity of other immunologic and nonimmunologic cells by producing an array of interleukins that they secrete. Different interleukins of this class have been isolated and characterized; they function as short-range or intracellular soluble mediators of the immune and inflammatory responses. The interleukin family of cytokines has been rapidly growing in number because of advances in gene cloning.

Complement. The primary humoral response to antigen and antibody binding is activation of the complement system.[8] The complement system consists of around 20 different proteins that bind to activated antibodies, other complement proteins, and cell membranes. The complement system is an important effector system of inflammation. Complement activation can be initiated

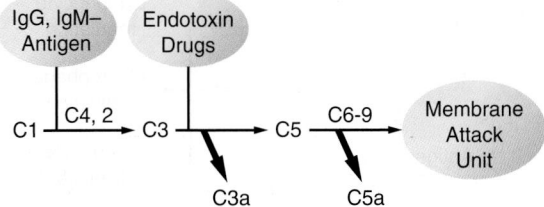

FIGURE 12-2. Diagram of complement activation. Complement system can be activated by either the classic pathway (immunoglobulin [Ig] G, IgM–antigen interaction) or the alternate pathway (endotoxin, drug interaction). Small peptide fragments of C3 and C5 called *anaphylatoxins* (C3a, C5a) that are released during activation are potent vasoactive mediators. Formation of the complete complement cascade produces a membrane attack unit that lyses cell walls and membranes. An inhibitor of the complement cascade, the C1 esterase inhibitor, ensures the complement system is turned off most of the time.

by IgG or IgM binding to antigen, by plasmin through the classic pathway, by endotoxin, or by drugs through the alternate (properdin) pathway[8] (Fig. 12-2). Specific fragments released during complement activation include C3a, C4a, and C5a, which have important humoral and chemotactic properties (see "Non–IgE-Mediated Reactions"). The major function of the complement system is to recognize bacteria both directly and indirectly by attracting phagocytes (chemotaxis), as well as the increased adhesion of phagocytes to antigens (opsonization), and cell lysis by activation of the complete cascade.

A series of inhibitors regulates activation to ensure regulation of the complement system. Hereditary (autosomal dominant) or acquired (associated with lymphoma, lymphosarcoma, chronic lymphocytic leukemia, and macroglobulinemia) angioneurotic edema is an example of a deficiency in an inhibitor of the C1 complement system (C1 esterase deficiency). This syndrome is characterized by recurrent increased vascular permeability of specific subcutaneous and serosal tissues (angioedema), which produces laryngeal obstruction and respiratory and cardiovascular abnormalities after tissue trauma and surgery, or even without any obvious precipitating factor.[9] One of the important pathologic manifestations of complement activation is acute pulmonary vasoconstriction associated with protamine administration.[1]

Effects of Anesthesia on Immune Function

Anesthesia and surgery depress nonspecific host resistance mechanisms, including lymphocyte activation and phagocytosis.[6] Immune competence during surgery can be affected by direct and hormonal effects of anesthetic drugs, by immunologic effects of other drugs used, by the surgery, by coincident infections, and by transfused blood products. Blood represents a complex of humoral and cellular elements that may alter immunomodulation to various antigens. Although multiple studies demonstrate in vitro changes of immune function, no studies have ever proved their importance.[6]

Besides, such changes are likely of minor importance compared with the hormonal aspects of stress responses.

HYPERSENSITIVITY RESPONSES (ALLERGY)

Gell et al.[3] first described a scheme for classifying immune responses to understand specific diseases mediated by immunologic processes. The immune pathway functions as a protective mechanism, but can also react inappropriately to produce a

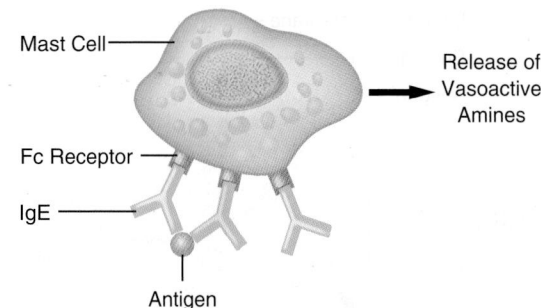

FIGURE 12-3. Type I immediate hypersensitivity reactions (anaphylaxis) involve immunoglobulin E (IgE) antibodies binding to mast cells or basophils by way of their Fc receptors. On encountering immunospecific antigens, the IgE becomes cross-linked, inducing degranulation, intracellular activation, and release of mediators. This reaction is independent of complement.

hypersensitivity or allergic response. They defined four basic types of hypersensitivity, types I to IV. It is useful first to review all four mechanisms to understand the different immune reactions that occur in humans.

Type I Reactions

Type I reactions are anaphylactic or immediate-type hypersensitivity reactions (Fig. 12-3). Physiologically active mediators are released from mast cells and basophils after antigen binding to IgE antibodies on the membranes of these cells. Type I hypersensitivity reactions include anaphylaxis, extrinsic asthma, and allergic rhinitis.

Type II Reactions

Type II reactions are also known as *antibody-dependent cell-mediated cytotoxic hypersensitivity* or *cytotoxic reactions* (antibody-dependent cell-mediated cytotoxic; Fig. 12-4). These reactions are mediated by either IgG or IgM antibodies directed

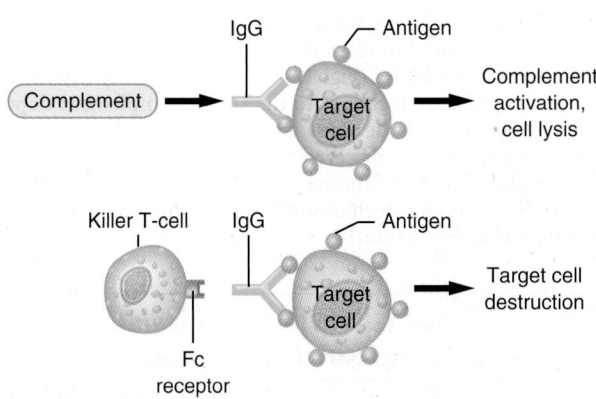

FIGURE 12-4. Type II or cytotoxic reactions. Antibody of an immunoglobulin (Ig) G or IgM class is directed against antigens on an individual's own cells (target cell). The antigens may be integral membrane components or foreign molecules that have been absorbed. This physiologic choice may lead to complement activation, including cell lysis (*upper figure*) or to cytotoxic action by killer T-cell lymphocytes (*lower figure*).

ANATOMY AND PHYSIOLOGY

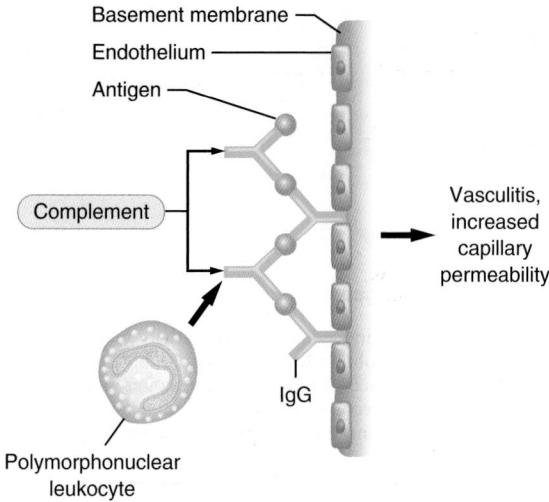

FIGURE 12-5. Type III immune complex reactions. Antibodies of an immunoglobulin (Ig) G or IgM type bind to the antigen in the soluble base and are subsequently deposited in the microvasculature. Complement is activated, resulting in chemotaxis and activation of polymorphonuclear leukocytes at the site of antigen-antibody complexes and subsequent tissue injury.

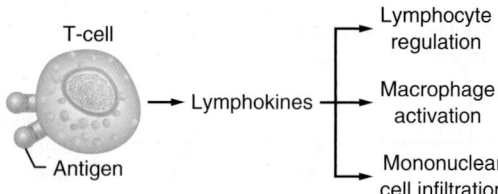

FIGURE 12-6. Type IV immune complex reactions (delayed hypersensitivity or cell-mediated immunity). Antigen binds to sensitized T-cell lymphocytes to release lymphokines after a second contact with the same antigen. This reaction is independent of circulating antibody or complement activation. Lymphokines induce inflammatory reactions and activate, as well as attract, macrophages and other mononuclear cells to produce delayed tissue injury.

against antigens on the surface of foreign cells. These antigens may be either integral cell membrane components (A or B blood group antigens in ABO incompatibility reactions) or haptens that absorb to the surface of a cell, stimulating the production of antihapten antibodies (autoimmune hemolytic anemia). The cell damage in type II reactions is produced by (1) direct cell lysis after complete complement cascade activation, (2) increased phagocytosis by macrophages, or (3) killer T-cell lymphocytes producing antibody-dependent cell-mediated cytotoxic effects. Examples of type II reactions in humans are ABO-incompatible transfusion reactions, drug-induced immune hemolytic anemia, and heparin-induced thrombocytopenia.

Type III Reactions (Immune Complex Reactions)

Type III reactions result from circulating soluble antigens and antibodies that bind to form insoluble complexes that deposit in the microvasculature (Fig. 12-5). Complement is activated, and neutrophils are localized to the site of complement deposition to produce tissue damage. Type III reactions include classic serum sickness observed after snake antisera or antithymocyte globulin, and immune complex vascular injury, and may occur through mechanisms of protamine-mediated pulmonary vasoconstriction.[1]

Type IV Reactions (Delayed Hypersensitivity Reactions)

Type IV reactions result from the interactions of sensitized lymphocytes with specific antigens (Fig. 12-6). Delayed hypersensitivity reactions are mainly mononuclear, manifest in 18 to 24 hours, peak at 40 to 80 hours, and disappear in 72 to 96 hours. Antigen-lymphocyte binding produces lymphokine synthesis, lymphocyte proliferation, generation of cytotoxic T cells, and attracts macrophages and other inflammatory cells. Cytotoxic T cells are produced specifically to kill target cells that bear antigens identical with those that triggered the reac-

tion. This form of immunity is important in tissue rejection, graft-versus-host reactions, contact dermatitis (e.g., poison ivy), and tuberculin immunity.

Intraoperative Allergic Reactions

Intraoperative allergic reactions occur once in every 5,000 to 25,000 anesthetics, with a 3.4% mortality rate.[10,11] More than 90% of the allergic reactions evoked by intravenous drugs occur within 5 minutes of administration. In the anesthetized patient, the most common life-threatening manifestation of an allergic reaction is circulatory collapse, reflecting vasodilation with resulting decreased venous return (Table 12-3). The only manifestation of an allergic reaction may be refractory hypotension.[12] Portier and Richet[13] first used the word *anaphylaxis* (from *ana*, "against," and *prophylaxis*, "protection") to describe the profound shock and resulting death that sometimes occurred in dogs immediately after a second challenge with a foreign antigen. When life-threatening allergic reactions mediated by antibodies occur, they are defined as anaphylactic. Although the term *anaphylactoid* has been used in the past to describe nonimmunologic reactions, this term is now rarely used.[14]

ANAPHYLACTIC REACTIONS

IgE-Mediated Pathophysiology

Antigen binding to IgE antibodies initiates anaphylaxis (Fig. 12-7). Prior exposure to the antigen or to a substance of similar structure is needed to produce sensitization, although an allergic history may be unknown to the patient. On re-exposure, binding of the antigen to bridge two immunospecific IgE antibodies found on the surfaces of mast cells and basophils releases stored mediators, including histamine, tryptase, and chemotactic factors.[15–17] Arachidonic acid metabolites (leukotrienes and prostaglandins), kinins, and cytokines are subsequently synthesized and released in response to cellular activation.[18] The released mediators produce a symptom complex of bronchospasm and upper airway edema in the respiratory system, vasodilation and increased capillary permeability in the cardiovascular system, and urticaria in the cutaneous system. Different mediators are released from mast cells and basophils after activation.

Chemical Mediators of Anaphylaxis

Histamine stimulates H_1, H_2, and H_3 receptors. H_1 receptor activation releases endothelium-derived relaxing factor (nitric oxide) from vascular endothelium, increases capillary permeability, and contracts airway and vascular smooth

TABLE 12-3

RECOGNITION OF ANAPHYLAXIS DURING REGIONAL AND GENERAL ANESTHESIA

■ SYSTEMS	■ SYMPTOMS	■ SIGNS
Respiratory	Dyspnea	Coughing
	Chest discomfort	Wheezing
		Sneezing
		Laryngeal edema
		Decreased pulmonary compliance
		Fulminant pulmonary edema
		Acute respiratory failure
Cardiovascular	Dizziness	Disorientation
	Malaise	Diaphoresis
	Retrosternal oppression	Loss of consciousness
		Hypotension
		Tachycardia
		Dysrhythmias
		Decreased systemic vascular resistance
		Cardiac arrest
		Pulmonary hypertension
Cutaneous	Itching	Urticaria (hives)
	Burning	Flushing
	Tingling	Periorbital edema
		Perioral edema

Reprinted with permission from Levy JH: Anaphylactic Reactions in Anesthesia and Intensive Care, 2nd edition. Boston, Butterworth-Heinemann, 1992.

muscle.[1,19,20] H_2 receptor activation causes gastric secretion, inhibits mast cell activation, and contributes to vasodilation.[19] When injected into skin, histamine produces the classic wheal (increased capillary permeability producing tissue edema) and flare (cutaneous vasodilation) response in humans.[21] Histamine undergoes rapid metabolism in humans by the enzymes histamine N-methyltransferase and diamine oxidase found in endothelial cells.[1]

Peptide Mediators of Anaphylaxis

Factors are released from mast cells and basophils that cause granulocyte migration (chemotaxis) and collection at the site of the inflammatory stimulus.[18] Eosinophilic chemotactic factor of anaphylaxis (ECF-A) is a small-molecular-weight peptide chemotactic for eosinophils.[22] Although the exact role of ECF-A or the eosinophil in acute allergic response is unclear,

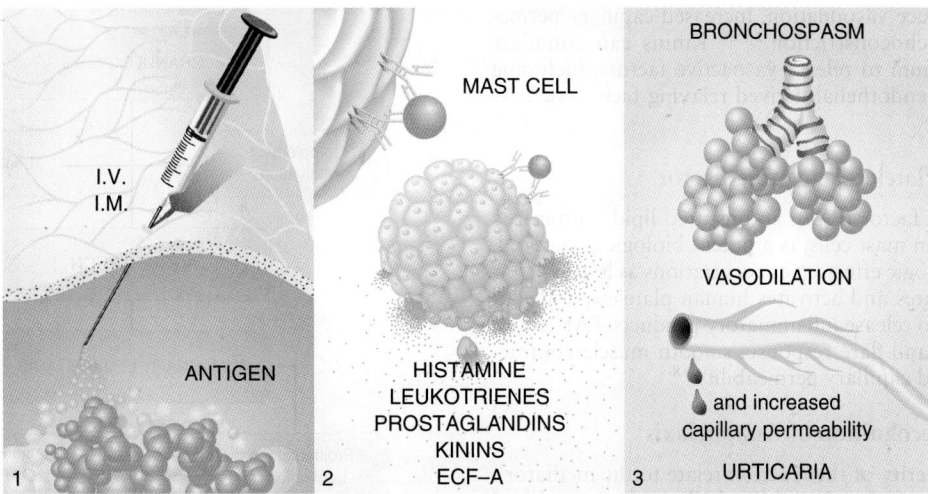

FIGURE 12-7.   During anaphylaxis (type I immediate hypersensitivity reaction), (1) antigen enters a patient during anesthesia through a parenteral route. (2) It bridges two immunoglobulin E antibodies on the surface of mast cells or basophils. In a calcium-dependent and energy-dependent process, cells release various substances—histamine, eosinophilic chemotactic factor of anaphylaxis (ECF-A), leukotrienes, prostaglandins, and kinins. (3) These released mediators produce the characteristic effects in the pulmonary, cardiovascular, and cutaneous systems. The most severe and life-threatening effects of the vasoactive mediators occur in the respiratory and cardiovascular systems. I.V., intravenous; I.M., intramuscular. (Reprinted with permission from Levy JH: Identification and Treatment of Anaphylaxis: Mechanisms of Action and Strategies for Treatment Under General Anesthesia. Chicago, Smith Laboratories, 1983.)

TABLE 12-4

BIOLOGICAL EFFECTS OF ANAPHYLATOXINS

■ BIOLOGICAL EFFECTS	■ C32	■ C52
Histamine release	+	+
Smooth muscle contraction	+	+
Increased vascular permeability	+	+
Chemotaxis		+
Leukocyte and platelet aggregation		+
Interleukin release	+	+

eosinophils release enzymes that can inactivate histamine and leukotrienes.[18] In addition, a neutrophilic chemotactic factor is released that causes chemotaxis and activation.[18,23] Neutrophil activation may be responsible for recurrent manifestations of anaphylaxis.

Arachidonic Acid Metabolites

Leukotrienes and prostaglandins are both synthesized after mast cell activation from arachidonic acid metabolism of phospholipid cell membranes through either lipoxygenase or cyclo-oxygenase pathways.[24,25] The classic slow-reacting substance of anaphylaxis is a combination of leukotrienes C_4, D_4, and E_4.[25] Leukotrienes produce bronchoconstriction (more intense than that produced by histamine), increased capillary permeability, vasodilation, coronary vasoconstriction, and myocardial depression.[25] Prostaglandins are potent mast cell mediators that produce vasodilation, bronchospasm, pulmonary hypertension, and increased capillary permeability.[18,25] Prostaglandin D_2, the major metabolite of mast cells, produces bronchospasm and vasodilation.[25] Elevated plasma levels of thromboxane B_2 (the metabolite of thromboxane A_2), also a prostaglandin synthesized by mast cells as well as by PMNs, have been demonstrated after protamine reactions associated with pulmonary hypertension.[26,27]

Kinins

Small peptides called *kinins* are synthesized in mast cells and basophils to produce vasodilation, increased capillary permeability, and bronchoconstriction.[18,28] Kinins can stimulate vascular endothelium to release vasoactive factors, including prostacyclin, and endothelial-derived relaxing factors such as nitric oxide.[1]

Platelet-Activating Factor

Platelet-activating factor (PAF), an unstored lipid synthesized in activated human mast cells, is a potent biological material, producing physiologic effects at concentrations as low as 10^{-10} M.[18] PAF aggregates and activates human platelets, and perhaps leukocytes, to release inflammatory products. PAF causes an intense wheal-and-flare response, smooth muscle contraction, and increased capillary permeability.[18]

Recognition of Anaphylaxis

The onset and severity of the reaction relate to the mediator's specific end-organ effects. Antigenic challenge in a sensitized individual usually produces immediate clinical manifestations of anaphylaxis, but the onset may be delayed 2 to 20 minutes.[29,30] The reaction may include some or all the symptoms and signs listed in Table 12-3. Individuals vary in their manifestations and course of anaphylaxis.[31,32] A spectrum of reactions exists, ranging from minor clinical changes to the full-blown syndrome leading to death.[31,33] The enigma of anaphylaxis lies in the unpredictability of when it happens, the severity of the attack, and the lack of a prior allergic history.

Non–IgE-Mediated Reactions

Other immunologic and nonimmunologic mechanisms release many of the mediators previously discussed, independent of IgE, creating a clinical syndrome identical with anaphylaxis. Specific pathways important in producing the same clinical manifestations are considered later.

Complement Activation

Complement activation follows both immunologic (antibody-mediated; i.e., classic pathway) or nonimmunologic (alternative) pathways to include a series of multimolecular, self-assembling proteins that release biologically active complement fragments of C3 and C5.[10,34] C3a and C5a are called *anaphylatoxins* because they release histamine from mast cells and basophils, contract smooth muscle, increase capillary permeability, and cause interleukin synthesis (Table 12-4). C5a interacts with specific high-affinity receptors on PMNs and platelets, causing leukocyte chemotaxis, aggregation, and activation.[35] Aggregated leukocytes embolize to various organs, producing microvascular occlusion and liberation of inflammatory products such as arachidonic acid metabolites, oxygen free radicals, and lysosomal enzymes (Fig. 12-8). Antibodies of the IgG class directed against antigenic determinants or granulocyte surfaces can also produce leukocyte aggregation.[36] These

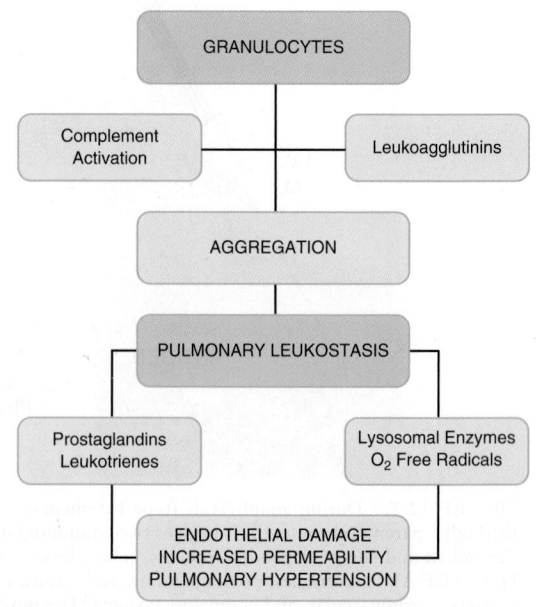

FIGURE 12-8.   Sequence of events producing granulocyte aggregation, pulmonary leukostasis, and cardiopulmonary dysfunction. (Reprinted from Levy JH: Anaphylactic Reactions in Anesthesia and Intensive Care, 2nd edition. Boston, Butterworth-Heinemann, 1992.)

TABLE 12-5

DRUGS CAPABLE OF NONIMMUNOLOGIC HISTAMINE RELEASE

Antibiotics (vancomycin, pentamidine)
Basic compounds
Hyperosmotic agents
Muscle relaxants (*d*-tubocurarine, metocurine, atracurium, mivacurium, doxacurium)
Opioids (morphine, meperidine, codeine)
Thiobarbiturates

antibodies are called *leukoagglutinins*. Investigators have associated complement activation and PMN aggregation in producing the clinical expression of transfusion reactions,[36,37] pulmonary vasoconstriction after protamine reactions,[27] adult respiratory distress syndrome,[36] and septic shock.[38]

Nonimmunologic Release of Histamine

Many diverse molecules administered during the perioperative period release histamine in a dose-dependent, nonimmunologic fashion[39–43] (Table 12-5 and Fig. 12-9). The mechanisms involved in nonimmunologic histamine release are not well understood, but represent selective mast cell and not basophil activation.[43,44] (Fig. 12-10). Human cutaneous mast cells are the only cell population that releases histamine in response to both drugs and endogenous stimuli (neuropeptides).[1] Nonimmunologic histamine release may involve mast cell activation through specific cell-signaling activation.[40] (Fig. 12-11). Different molecular structures release histamine in humans, which suggests that different mechanisms are involved. Histamine release does not depend on the μ receptor because fentanyl and sufentanil, the most potent μ receptor agonists clinically available, do not release histamine in human skin.[39] Although the newer muscle relaxants may be more potent at the neuromuscular junction, drugs that are mast cell degranulators are equally capable of releasing histamine.[39,40] On an equimolar basis, atracurium is as potent as *d*-tubocurarine or metocurine in its ability to degranulate mast cells.[40] At clinically recommended doses, newer aminosteroidal agents (such as rocuronium and rapacuronium) have minimal effects on histamine release.[44,45]

Antihistamine pretreatment before administration of drugs that are known to release histamine in humans does not inhibit histamine release; rather, the antihistamines compete with histamine at the receptor and may attenuate decreases in systemic vascular resistance.[1] However, the effect of any drug on systemic vascular resistance may depend on other factors in addition to histamine release.[46,47]

Treatment Plan

A plan for treating anaphylactic reactions must be established before the event. Airway maintenance, 100% oxygen administration, intravascular volume expansion, and epinephrine are essential to treat the hypotension and hypoxia that result from vasodilation, increased capillary permeability, and bronchospasm.[1] Table 12-6 lists a protocol for managing anaphylaxis during general anesthesia, with representative doses for a 70-kg adult. The treatment plan is the same for life-threatening anaphylactic or anaphylactoid reactions. Therapy must be titrated to needed effects with careful monitoring.[1] Severe reactions need aggressive therapy and may be protracted, with persistent hypotension, pulmonary hypertension, lower respiratory obstruction, or laryngeal obstruction that may persist 5 to 32 hours despite vigorous therapy.[48] All patients who have experienced an anaphylactic reaction should be admitted to an intensive care unit for 24 hours of monitoring because manifestations may recur after successful treatment.

ANATOMY AND PHYSIOLOGY

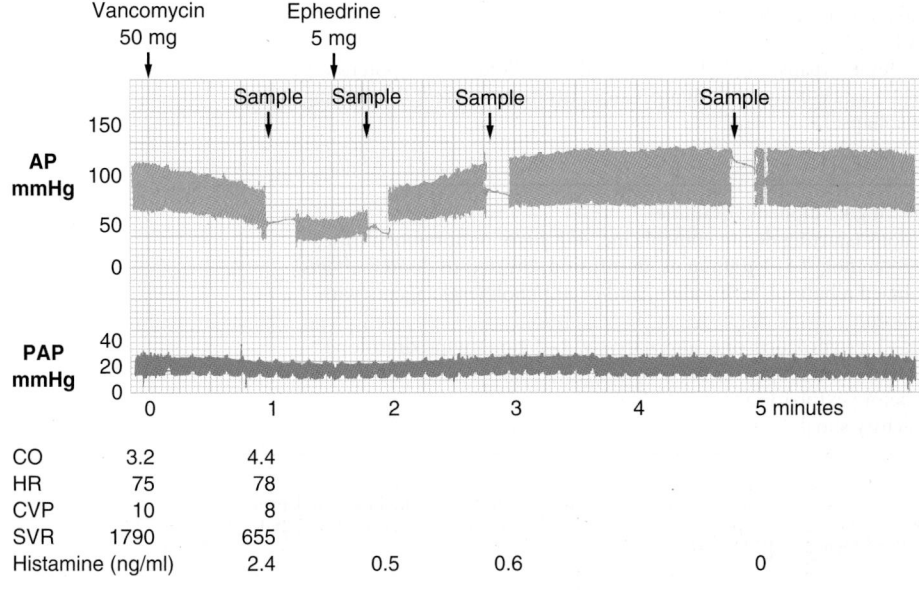

FIGURE 12-9. Example of an anaphylactic reaction after rapid vancomycin administration in a patient. Hypotension is associated with an increased cardiac output and decreased calculated systemic vascular resistance. Plasma histamine levels 1 minute after the vancomycin administration were 2.4 ng/mL and subsequently decreased to zero. The patient was given ephedrine, 5 mg, and blood pressure returned to baseline values. AP, arterial pressure; PAP, pulmonary arterial pressure; CO, cardiac output; HR, heart rate; CVP, central venous pressure; SVR, systemic vascular resistance. (Reprinted from Levy JH, Kettlekamp N, Goertz P, Hermens J, Hirshman CA: Histamine release by vancomycin: A mechanism for hypotension in man. Anesthesiology 1987; 67: 122–125.)

CO	3.2	4.4		
HR	75	78		
CVP	10	8		
SVR	1790	655		
Histamine (ng/ml)		2.4	0.5	0.6	0

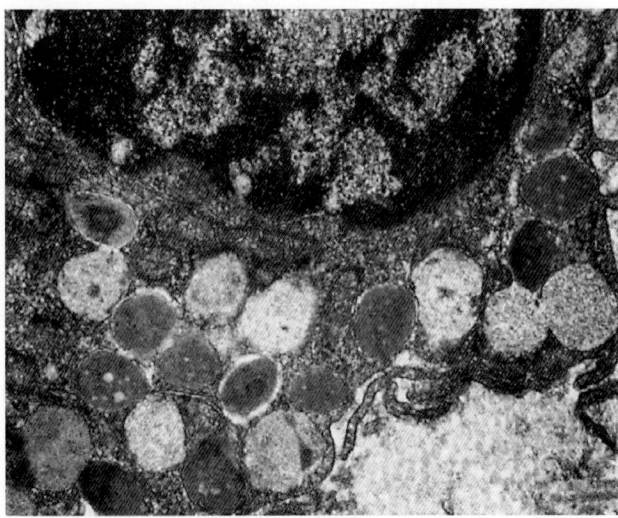

FIGURE 12-10. Electron micrograph of human cutaneous mast cell after injection of dynorphin, a κ opioid agonist. The cell outline is rounded and most of the cytoplasmic granules are swollen, exhibiting varying degrees of decreased electron density and flocculence consistent with ongoing degranulation. The perigranular membranes of the adjacent granules at the periphery of the cell are fused to each other and to plasma membrane. Original magnification ×72,000. (Reprinted with permission from Casale TB, Bowman S, Kaliner M: Induction of human cutaneous mast cell degranulation by opiates and endogenous opioid peptides: Evidence for opiate and nonopiate receptor participation. J Allergy Clin Immunol 1984; 73: 778–781.)

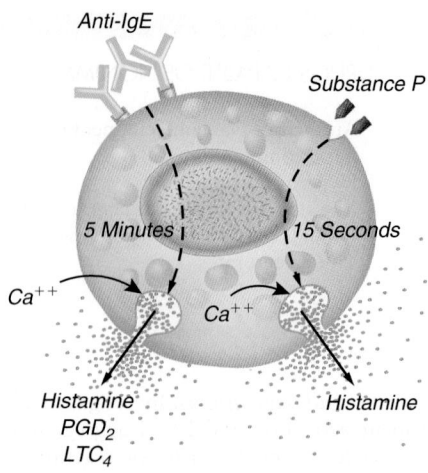

FIGURE 12-11. Different mechanisms of mediator release from human cutaneous mast cells stimulated immunologically by anti-immunoglobulin (Ig) E and by nonimmunologic stimuli with substance P. Anti-IgE stimulation, like antigen stimulation, initiates the release of histamine, prostaglandin D_2 (PGD_2), or leukotriene C_4 (LTC_4) by a mechanism that takes 5 minutes to reach completion and requires the influx of intracellular calcium. Nonimmunologic activation with drugs or substance P releases histamine but not PGD_2 or LTC_4 by a mechanism that is complete within 15 seconds and uses calcium mobilized from intracellular sources. (Reprinted with permission from Caulfield JP, El-Lati S, Thomas G, Church MK: Dissociated human foreskin mast cells degranulate in response to anti-IgE and substance P. Lab Invest 1990; 63: 502–510.)

Initial Therapy

Although it may not be possible to stop the administration of antigen, limiting antigen administration may prevent further mast cell and basophil activation.

Maintain Airway and Administer 100% Oxygen. Profound ventilation–perfusion abnormalities producing hypoxemia can occur with anaphylactic reactions.[49] Always administer 100% oxygen, with ventilatory support as needed. Arterial blood gas values may be useful to follow during resuscitation (see Chapter 59).

Discontinue All Anesthetic Drugs. Inhalational anesthetic drugs are not the bronchodilators of choice to treat bronchospasm during anaphylaxis, especially if the patient is hypotensive.

TABLE 12-6

MANAGEMENT OF ANAPHYLAXIS DURING GENERAL ANESTHESIA

■ INITIAL THERAPY

1. Stop administration of antigen.
2. Maintain airway and administer 100% O_2.
3. Discontinue all anesthetic agents.
4. Start intravascular volume expansion (2–4 L of crystalloid/colloid with hypotension).
5. Give epinephrine (5–10 μg IV bolus with hypotension, titrate as needed; 0.1–1.0 mg IV with cardiovascular collapse).

■ SECONDARY TREATMENT

1. Antihistamines (0.5–1 mg/kg diphenhydramine)
2. Catecholamine infusions (starting doses: epinephrine, 4–8 μg/min; norepinephrine, 4–8 μg/min; or isoproterenol, 0.5–1 μg/min as an infusion; titrated to desired effects)
3. Bronchodilators: inhaled albuterol, terbutaline, and/or anticholinergic agents with persistent bronchospasm)
4. Corticosteroids (0.25–1 g hydrocortisone; alternatively, 1–2 g methylprednisolone)[a]
5. Sodium bicarbonate (0.5–1 mEq/kg with persistent hypotension or acidosis)
6. Airway evaluation (before extubation)
7. Vasopressin for refractory shock

IV, intravenous(ly).
[a]Methylprednisolone may be the drug of choice if the reaction is suspected to be mediated by complement.
Reprinted with permission from Levy JH: Anaphylactic Reactions in Anesthesia and Intensive Care, 2nd edition, Boston, Butterworth-Heinemann, 1992; p 162.

These drugs interfere with the body's compensatory response to cardiovascular collapse, and halothane sensitizes the myocardium to epinephrine.

Provide Volume Expansion. Hypovolemia rapidly develops during anaphylactic shock.[50] Fisher[50] reported up to 40% loss of intravascular fluid into the interstitial space during reactions. Therefore, volume expansion and epinephrine are important in correcting the acute hypotension. Initially, 2 to 4 L of lactated Ringer solution, colloid, or normal saline should be administered, keeping in mind that an additional 25 to 50 mL/kg may be necessary if hypotension persists. Refractory hypotension after intravascular volume and epinephrine administration requires additional hemodynamic monitoring. The use of transesophageal echocardiography for rapid assessment of intraventricular volume and ventricular function, and to determine other occult causes of acute cardiovascular dysfunction, can be important for accurate assessment of intravascular volume and guidance of rational therapeutic interventions.[51] Fulminant noncardiogenic pulmonary edema with loss of intravascular volume can occur after anaphylaxis. This condition requires intravascular volume repletion with careful hemodynamic monitoring until the capillary defect improves. Colloid volume expansion has not proved to be more effective than crystalloid volume expansion for treating anaphylactic shock.

Administer Epinephrine. Epinephrine is the drug of choice when resuscitating patients during anaphylactic shock. Epinephrine's α-adrenergic effects vasoconstrict to reverse hypotension; β_2 receptor stimulation bronchodilates and inhibits mediator release by increasing cyclic adenosine monophosphate in mast cells and basophils.[52-54] The route of epinephrine administration and the dose depend on the patient's condition. Rapid and timely intervention is important when treating anaphylaxis. Furthermore, patients under general anesthesia may have altered sympathoadrenergic responses to acute anaphylactic shock, whereas patients under spinal or epidural anesthesia may not be able to mount the appropriate vasoconstrictive sympathetic response and may need even larger doses of catecholamines.

In hypotensive patients, 5- to 10-μg intravenous doses of epinephrine should be administered incrementally to restore blood pressure. Additional volume and incrementally increased doses of epinephrine should be administered until hypotension is corrected. Infusion is an ideal method of administering epinephrine; it is best to infuse epinephrine through central intravenous access lines during acute volume resuscitation. If cardiovascular collapse ensues, intravenous cardiopulmonary resuscitative doses of epinephrine, 0.1 to 1.0 mg, should be administered and repeated until hemodynamic stability resumes. Patients with laryngeal edema without hypotension should receive subcutaneous epinephrine. Intravenous epinephrine should not be administered to patients with normal blood pressures.

Secondary Treatment

Antihistamines. Because H_1 receptors mediate many of the adverse effects of histamine, the intravenous administration of 0.5 to 1 mg/kg of an H_1 antagonist such as diphenhydramine may be useful in treating acute anaphylaxis. Antihistamines do not inhibit anaphylactic reactions or histamine release, but compete with histamine at receptor sites after it is released. H_1 antagonists are indicated in all forms of anaphylaxis. The H_1 antagonists available for parenteral administration may have antidopaminergic effects and should be given slowly to prevent precipitous hypotension in potentially hypovolemic patients.[1] The indications for

administering an H_2 antagonist once anaphylaxis has occurred remain unclear.

Catecholamines. Epinephrine infusions may be useful in patients with persistent hypotension or bronchospasm after initial resuscitation.[1] Epinephrine infusions should be started at 0.05 to 0.1 μg/kg/min (5 to 10 μg/min) and titrated to correct hypotension. Norepinephrine infusions may be needed in patients with refractory hypotension due to decreased systemic vascular resistance. It may be started at 0.05 to 0.1 μg/kg/min and adjusted to correct hypotension.[51]

Bronchodilators. Inhaled β-adrenergic agents, including inhaled albuterol or terbutaline, if bronchospasm is a major feature.[54] Inhaled ipratropium may be especially useful for treatment of bronchospasm in patients receiving β-adrenergic blockers.[54] Special adapters allow administration of bronchodilators through the endotracheal tube (see Chapter 2).

Corticosteroids. Corticosteroids have a series of anti-inflammatory effects mediated by multiple mechanisms, including altering the activation and migration of other inflammatory cells (e.g., PMNs) after an acute reaction.[53,54] One should consider infusing high-dose corticosteroids early in the course of therapy, although beneficial effects are delayed at least 4 to 6 hours.[54] Despite their unproven usefulness in treating acute reactions, corticosteroids are often administered as adjuncts to therapy when refractory bronchospasm or refractory shock occurs after resuscitative therapy.[55] Although the exact corticosteroid dose and preparation are unclear, investigators have recommended 0.25 to 1 g intravenously of hydrocortisone in IgE-mediated reactions. Alternately, 1 to 2 g of methylprednisolone (30 to 35 mg/kg) intravenously may be useful in reactions believed to be complement-mediated, such as catastrophic pulmonary vasoconstriction after protamine transfusion reactions.[56] Administering corticosteroids after an anaphylactic reaction may also be important in attenuating the late-phase reactions reported to occur 12 to 24 hours after anaphylaxis.[48]

Bicarbonate. Acidosis develops rapidly in patients with persistent hypotension. This acidemia reduces the effect of epinephrine on the heart and systemic vasculature. Therefore, with refractory hypotension or acidemia, sodium bicarbonate, 0.5 to 1 mEq/kg, may be given and repeated every 5 minutes or as dictated by arterial blood gas values.

Airway Evaluation. Because profound laryngeal edema can occur, the airway should be evaluated before extubation of the trachea.[29] Persistent facial edema suggests airway edema. The trachea of these patients should remain intubated until the edema subsides. Developing a significant air leak after endotracheal tube cuff deflation and before extubation of the trachea is useful in assessing airway patency. If there is any question of airway edema, direct laryngoscopy should be performed before the trachea is extubated.

Refractory Hypotension—Vasopressin. Vasopressin is an important drug for refractory shock, including vasodilatory shock associated with anaphylaxis. Vasodilatory shock is characterized by hypotension association with a high cardiac output, and is thought to be due to the multiple activation of vasodilator mechanisms and the inability of α-adrenergic mechanisms to compensate.[51] Starting doses to consider are 0.01 units/min as an infusion, although bolus administration is part of Advanced Cardiopulmonary Life Support guidelines. Vasopressin may attenuate pathologic-induced vasodilation. Further, additional monitoring, including echocardiography and preferably transesophageal, should be considered in patients with refractory hypotension to better evaluate cardiac function or hypovolemia.

PERIOPERATIVE MANAGEMENT OF THE PATIENT WITH ALLERGIES

Allergic drug reactions account for 6 to 10% of all adverse reactions.[57] DeSwarte[58] suggested that the risk of an allergic drug reaction occurring is approximately 1 to 3% for most drugs, and that around 5% of adults in the United States may be allergic to one or more drugs. Unfortunately, patients often refer to adverse drug effects as being allergic in nature. For example, opioid administration can produce nausea, vomiting, or even local release of histamine along the vein of administration. Patients will say they are "allergic" to a specific drug when, in fact, their adverse reaction is independent of allergy. Nearly 15% of adults in the United States believe they are allergic to specific medication(s) and therefore may be denied treatment with an indicated drug. To understand allergic reactions, the spectrum of adverse reactions to drugs needs to be considered.

Predictable adverse drug reactions account for about 80% of adverse drug effects. They are often dose-dependent, related to known pharmacologic actions of the drug, and typically occur in normal patients. Most serious, predictable adverse drug reactions are toxic and are directly related to the drug in the body (overdosage) or to an unintentional route of administration (e.g., unintended intravenous bupivacaine-induced seizures and cardiovascular collapse). Side effects are the most common adverse drug reactions and are undesirable pharmacologic actions of the drugs occurring at usual prescribed dosages. Most anesthetic drugs present multiple side effects that can produce precipitous hypotension. For example, morphine dilates the venous capacitance bed, thereby decreasing preload; releases histamine from cutaneous mast cells, thereby producing arterial and venous dilation; slows the heart rate; and decreases sympathetic tone. However, the net effects of morphine on blood pressure and myocardial function depend on the patient's blood volume, sympathetic tone, and ventricular function. Hypotension rapidly develops in a volume-depleted trauma patient in pain who is given morphine. Drug interactions also represent important predictable adverse drug reactions. Intravenous fentanyl administration to a patient who has just received intravenous benzodiazepines or other sedative-hypnotic drugs may produce precipitous hypotension that results from decreased sympathetic tone or direct vasodilation from propofol administration.[59] This phenomenon represents a dose-dependent, predictable adverse drug reaction that is independent of allergy.

Unpredictable adverse drug reactions are usually dose-independent and usually not related to the drug's pharmacologic actions, but are often related to the immunologic response (allergy) of the individual. On occasion, adverse reactions can be related to genetic differences (i.e., idiosyncratic) in a susceptible individual who has an isolated genetic enzyme deficiency. In most allergic drug reactions, an immunologic mechanism is present or, more often, presumed. Providing that the causal event involves a reaction between the drug or drug metabolites with drug-specific antibodies or sensitized T lymphocytes is often impractical. Without direct immunologic evidence, attributes that may be helpful in distinguishing an allergic reaction from other adverse reactions include (1) allergic reactions occur in only a small percentage of patients receiving the drug, and (2) the clinical manifestations do not resemble known pharmacologic actions. In the absence of prior drug exposure, allergic symptoms rarely appear after <1 week of continuous treatment. After sensitization, the reaction develops rapidly on re-exposure to the drug. In general, drugs that have been administered without complications for several months or longer are rarely responsible for producing drug allergy. The time span between exposure to the drug and noticed manifestations is often the most vital information in deciding which drugs administered were the cause of a suspected allergic reaction.

Although the reaction may produce a life-threatening response in the cardiopulmonary system (anaphylaxis), various cutaneous manifestations, fever, and pulmonary reactions have been attributed to drug hypersensitivity. Usually, the reaction may be reproduced by small doses of the suspected drug or other agents having similar or cross-reacting chemical structures. On occasion, drug-specific antibodies or lymphocytes have been identified that react with the suspected drug, although the relationship is seldom diagnostically useful in practice. Even when an immune response to a drug is demonstrated, it may not be associated with a clinical allergic reaction. As with adverse drug reactions in general, the reaction usually subsides within several days of discontinuation of the drug.

Immunologic Mechanisms of Drug Allergy

Different immunologic responses to any antigen can occur. Drugs have been associated with all the immunologic mechanisms proposed by Gell et al.[3] Although more than one mechanism may contribute to a particular reaction, any one can occur. Penicillin may produce different reactions in different patients or a spectrum of reactions in the same patient. In one patient, penicillin can produce anaphylaxis (type I reaction), hemolytic anemia (type II reaction), serum sickness (type III reaction), and contact dermatitis (type IV reaction).[58] Therefore, any one antigen has the ability to produce a diffuse spectrum of allergic responses in humans. Why some patients have localized rashes or angioneurotic edema in response to penicillin whereas others suffer complete cardiopulmonary collapse is unknown. Most anesthetic drugs and agents administered perioperatively have been reported to produce anaphylactic reactions.[31,39-45,60-81] Muscle relaxants are the most common drugs responsible for evoking intraoperative allergic reactions.[67] In this regard, there is cross-sensitivity between succinylcholine and the nondepolarizing muscle relaxants. Unexplained intraoperative cardiovascular collapse has been attributed to anaphylaxis triggered by latex (natural rubber), and certain patients, including those with a history of spina bifida, are at a greater risk for reactions.[1,68] Even vascular graft material has been reported as a cause of intraoperative allergic reactions.[69]

Life-threatening allergic reactions are more likely to occur in patients with a history of allergy, atopy, or asthma. Nevertheless, because the incidence is low, the history is not a reliable predictor that an allergic reaction will occur and does not mandate that such patients should be investigated or pretreated, or that specific drugs be selected or avoided.[60] Although different mechanisms have been proposed, no one theory has been proved.[1] The drugs and foreign substances listed in Table 12-7 may have both immunologic and nonimmunologic mechanisms for adverse drug reactions in humans.

Evaluation of Patients With Allergic Reactions

Identifying the drug responsible for a suspected allergic reaction still depends on circumstantial evidence, suggesting the temporal sequence of drug administration. Conventional *in vivo* and *in vitro* methods of diagnosing allergic reactions to most anesthetic drugs are unavailable or not applicable. The

TABLE 12-7

AGENTS IMPLICATED IN ALLERGIC REACTIONS DURING ANESTHESIA

■ **ANESTHETIC AGENTS**

Induction agents (cremophor-solubilized drugs, barbiturates, etomidate, propofol)
Local anesthetics (para-aminobenzoic ester agents)
Muscle relaxants (succinylcholine, gallamine, pancuronium, *d*-tubocurarine, metocurine,
  atracurium, vecuronium, mivacurium, doxacurium)
Opioids (meperidine, morphine, fentanyl)

■ **OTHER AGENTS**

Antibiotics (cephalosporins, penicillin, sulfonamides, vancomycin)
Aprotinin
Blood products (whole blood, packed cells, fresh-frozen plasma, platelets, cryoprecipitate,
  fibrin glue, γ-globulin)
Bone cement
Chymopapain
Corticosteroids
Cyclosporin
Drug additives (preservatives)
Furosemide
Insulin
Mannitol
Methylmethacrylate
Nonsteroidal anti-inflammatory drugs
Protamine
Radiocontrast dye
Latex (natural rubber)
Streptokinase
Vascular graft material
Vitamin K
Colloid volume expanders (dextrans, protein fractions, albumin, hydroxyethyl starch)

Reprinted with permission from Levy JH: Anaphylactic Reactions in Anesthesia and Intensive Care, 2nd
edition. Boston, Butterworth-Heinemann, 1992.

ANATOMY AND PHYSIOLOGY

most important factor in diagnosis is the awareness of the physician that an untoward event may be related to a drug the patient received. The physician must always be aware of the capacity of any drug to produce an allergic reaction. The history is important when evaluating whether an adverse drug reaction is allergic and whether the drug can be readministered. Although a prior allergic reaction to the drug in question is important, it will rarely be conclusive. Direct challenge of a patient with a test dose of drug is the only way to prove a reaction, but this is potentially dangerous and not recommended. Although the anesthesiologist commonly gives small test doses of anesthetic drugs, these are pharmacologic test doses and have nothing to do with immunologic dosages. The demonstration of drug-specific IgE antibodies is accepted as evidence the patient may be at risk for anaphylaxis if the drug is administered.[58] Different clinical tests are available to confirm or diagnose drug allergy; several are considered in the following section.

Testing for Allergy

8 After an anaphylactoid reaction, it is important to identify the causative agent to prevent readministration. When one particular drug has been administered and there is a clear correlation between the time of administration and the occurrence of a reaction, testing may be unnecessary, and general avoidance of the drug should be instituted. However, when patients have simultaneously received multiple drugs (e.g., an opioid, muscle relaxant, hypnotic, and antibiotic), it is often difficult to prove which particular drug caused the reaction. Further, the reaction might have

been caused by the vehicle or by one of the preservatives. For patients who want to know which drug was responsible and for patients scheduled for subsequent procedures, some degree of allergy evaluation should be undertaken to evaluate the drug at risk. Unfortunately, few *laboratory* tests exist for anesthetic drugs; therefore, the available allergy tests are discussed.

Leukocyte Histamine Release. Leukocyte histamine release is performed by incubating the patient's leukocytes with the offending drug and measuring histamine release as a marker for basophil activation, although false-positive results can occur.[31] This test is not easy to perform, although variations allow the use of whole blood instead of isolated PMNs, and is generally not available.[76,82]

Radioallergosorbent Test. The radioallergosorbent test (RAST) allows *laboratory* detection of specific IgE directed toward particular antigens.[83] In this test, antigens are linked to insoluble material to make an immunoabsorbent.[83,84] When incubated with the serum in question, antibodies of different classes directed toward the antigen bind to it. After washing, the antigen-antibody complex on the immunoabsorbent is incubated with radiolabeled antibodies directed against human IgE and counted in a scintillation counter. The concentration of specific IgE in the patient's serum directed toward the allergen is measured. The RAST is more quantitative than skin tests and avoids the potential of reexposure.[84] RAST testing has been used to detect the presence of antibodies to meperidine,[49] succinylcholine,[85] and thiopental.[86] Two major limitations to this test include the commercial availability of the drug prepared as an antigen and false-positive test results in patients with high IgE levels.[87]

Enzyme-Linked Immunosorbent Assay. The enzyme-linked immunosorbent assay (ELISA) measures antigen-specific antibodies. The basis of the ELISA is similar to that of the RAST; however, immunospecific IgE directed against the antigen in question is determined by adding an anti-IgE coupled to an enzyme such as peroxidase that acts as a chromogen.[5] A colorless substrate is acted on by peroxidase to produce a colored byproduct. The ELISA has been used to prove IgE antibodies to chymopapain and protamine, and has been developed to screen for other antibodies to diverse agents.

Intradermal Testing (Skin Testing). Skin testing is the method most often used in patients after anaphylactic reaction to anesthetic drugs after the history has suggested the relevant antigens for testing.[88,89] Within minutes after antigen introduction, histamine released from cutaneous mast cells causes vasodilation (flare) and localized edema from increased vascular permeability (wheal). Fisher and Munro[67] and Fisher[88] suggested that this is a simple, safe, and useful method of establishing a diagnosis in most cases of anaphylactic reactions occurring in the perioperative period. If the strict protocols established by Fisher[88] are used, intradermal reactions are helpful. Intradermal testing is of no value in reactions to contrast media or colloid volume expanders. Cross-sensitivity between drugs of similar structures can often be evaluated based on skin testing. Skin testing to local anesthetics is considered a direct challenge or provocative dose testing.[90] Local anesthetic drugs are injected in increasing quantities under controlled circumstances. This testing decides if the person can safely receive amide derivatives (e.g., lidocaine) and can also be used to decide if the person is sensitive to the paraaminobenzoic ester agents (e.g., procaine, tetracaine).

Agents Implicated in Allergic Reactions

Multiple agents—including antibiotics, induction agents, muscle relaxants, nonsteroidal anti-inflammatory drugs, protamine, colloid volume expanders, and blood products—are the etiologic agents often responsible for anaphylaxis in surgical patients.[1] However, any agent the patient receives as an injection, infusion, or environmental antigen has the potential to produce an allergic reaction.[1] Almost everything has been reported to produce an allergic reaction at some time, but usually from a case report or small series. The agents most often implicated include antibiotics, blood products, colloid volume expanders, latex, polypeptides, and NMBAs. If patients are allergic to a muscle relaxant, there is a potential for cross-reactivity because of the similarity of the active site, a quaternary ammonium molecule, among the different types of relaxants, and alternatives cannot be chosen without some degree of immunologic testing. Because of the ubiquity of latex as a perioperative environmental antigen, latex allergy is considered separately.

Latex Allergy

For the anesthesiologist, latex represents an environmental agent often implicated as an important cause of perioperative anaphylaxis.[91-99] Latex is the milky sap derived from the tree *Hevea brasiliensis* to which multiple agents, including preservatives, accelerators, and antioxidants are added to make the final rubber product. Latex is present in a variety of different products. In March 1991, the U.S. Food and Drug Administration alerted health care professionals about the potential of severe allergic reactions to medical devices made of latex. The first case of an

allergic reaction because of latex was reported in 1979 and was manifested by contact urticaria. In 1989, the first reports of intraoperative anaphylaxis because of latex were reported.

Health care workers and children with spina bifida, urogenital abnormalities, or certain food allergies have also been recognized as people at increased risk for anaphylaxis to latex.[91-99] Brown et al.[95] reported a 24% incidence of irritant or contact dermatitis and a 12.5% incidence of latex-specific IgE positivity in anesthesiologists. Of this group, 10% were clinically asymptomatic, although IgE-positive. A history of atopy was also a significant risk factor for latex sensitization. Brown et al.[95] suggested that these people are in their early stages of sensitization and their progression to symptomatic disease may be prevented by avoiding latex exposure. Patients allergic to bananas, avocados, and kiwis have also been reported to have antibodies that cross-react with latex.[96,97] Multiple attempts are being made to reduce latex exposure to both health care workers and patients. If latex allergy occurs, then strict avoidance of latex from gloves and other sources needs to be considered, following recommendations as reported by Holzman.[91] Because latex is such a common environmental antigen, this represents a daunting task.

More important, anesthesiologists must be prepared to treat the life-threatening cardiopulmonary collapse that occurs after anaphylaxis, as previously discussed. The most important preventive therapy is to avoid antigen exposure; although clinicians have used pretreatment with antihistamine (diphenhydramine and cimetidine) and corticosteroids, there are no data in the literature to suggest that pretreatment prevents anaphylaxis or decreases its severity.[1] Two patients in a series reported by Gold et al.[93] were pretreated, yet still had life-threatening reactions to latex. Patients in whom latex allergy is suspected should be referred to an allergist for proper evaluation and potential in vitro testing (RAST) for definitive diagnosis. When this is not possible, patients should be treated as if they were latex-allergic, and the antigen avoided. Patients with a documented history of latex allergy should wear Medic Alert bracelets.

Muscle Relaxants

NMBAs have several unique molecular features that make them potential allergens. All NMBAs are functionally divalent and are thus capable of cross-linking cell-surface IgE and causing mediator release from mast cells and basophils without binding or haptenating to larger carrier molecules. NMBAs have also been implicated in epidemiologic studies of anesthetic drug-induced anaphylaxis. Epidemiologic data from France suggest that NMBAs are responsible for 62 to 81% of reactions, depending on the period evaluated.[100-105]

In more recent years, NMBAs, especially steroid-derived agents, have been reported as potential causative agents of anaphylactic reactions during anesthesia. The data associating NMBAs in the most recent reports from France are mainly based on skin testing; however, studies have previously reported the steroidal-derived NMBAs and other molecules produce false-positive skin tests (i.e., wheal and flare). One of the major problems is that anaphylaxis to NMBAs is rare in the United States, but has been reported more often in Europe.[105-107] Although suggestions have been made that this is because of underreporting, the severity of anaphylaxis and its sequelae to produce adverse outcomes clearly make this unlikely based on the current medicolegal climate that exists in the United States. One of the only ways to explain this widely divergent perspective is to understand how the diagnosis is made because the recommended threshold test concentrations have not been defined, resulting in unreliable results.

We previously reported in several studies that steroid-derived agents could induce positive wheal and flare responses independent of mast cell degranulation, even at low concentrations, following intradermal injection. This effect is likely because of a direct effect on the cutaneous vasculature that occurs for most NMBAs at concentrations as low as 10^{-5} M using intradermal skin tests in 30 volunteers.[106] A positive cutaneous reaction without evidence of mast cell degranulation was noted at low concentrations (100 μg/mL) of rocuronium in almost all the volunteers. Levy et al.[106] have used intradermal injections to compare cutaneous effects of anesthetic and other agents.

Other investigators have also reported similar results. Because prick tests are often used for authenticating NMBAs as causative drugs, Dhonneur et al.[105] evaluated 30 volunteers, using prick testing. Each subject received 10 prick tests (50 μL) on both forearms. The investigators studied the wheal and flare responses to prick tests with rocuronium and vecuronium, using four dilutions (1/1,000, 1/100, 1/10, and 1) and two controls, and measured wheal and flare immediately after and at 15 minutes. They noted 50 and 40% of the subjects had a positive skin reaction to undiluted rocuronium and vecuronium, respectively.[105] To avoid false-positive results, they suggested that prick testing with rocuronium and vecuronium should be performed in subjects who have experienced a hypersensitivity reaction during anesthesia, with concentrations below that commonly inducing positive reactions in anesthesia-naive, healthy subjects (i.e., for men in a dilution of 1/10 and for women in a dilution of 1/100). Guidelines for prick testing that are internationally agreed on need to be established. Many of these differences may explain the various incidences of allergy to NMBAs among countries. Concentration–skin response curves to rocuronium and vecuronium have showed that prick tests should be performed with dilution of the commercially available preparation. Female volunteers significantly ($p < 01$) reacted to lower vecuronium and rocuronium concentrations than male volunteers. In female subjects, positive skin reactions were reported with dilutions of 1/100 of both relaxants. In male subjects, positive skin reactions were noted with the undiluted concentration, except for one volunteer who reacted to rocuronium (1/10 dilution).

SUMMARY

Although the immune system functions to provide host defense, it can respond inappropriately to produce hypersensitivity or allergic reactions. A spectrum of life-threatening allergic reactions to any drug or agent can occur in the perioperative period.[100] The enigma of these reactions lies in their unpredictable nature. Certain patients undergoing high risk procedures with multiple blood product exposures are also at higher risk.[52] However, a high index of suspicion, prompt recognition, and appropriate and aggressive therapy can help avoid a disastrous outcome.

References

1. Levy JH: Anaphylactic Reactions in Anesthesia and Intensive Care, 2nd edition. Boston, Butterworth-Heinemann, 1992
2. deShazo RD, Kemp SF: Allergic reactions to drugs and biologic agents. JAMA 1997; 278: 1895
3. Gell PGH, Coombs RRA, Lachmann PJ: Clinical Aspects of Immunology, 3rd edition. Oxford, Blackwell Scientific Publications, 1975
4. Delves PJ, Roitt IM: The immune system (two parts). N Engl J Med 2000; 343: 37, 108
5. Kay AB: Allergy and allergic diseases (two parts). N Engl J Med 2001; 344: 30, 109
6. Stevenson GW, Hall SC, Rudnick S, et al: The effects of anesthetic agents on the human immune response. Anesthesiology 1990; 72: 144
7. Pober JS, Cotran RS: Cytokines and endothelial cell biology. Physiol Rev 1990; 70: 427

8. Walport MJ. Complement (first and second parts). N Engl J Med 2001; 344: 1058, 1140
9. Wall RT, Frank M, Hahn M: A review of 25 patients with hereditary angioedema requiring surgery. Anesthesiology 1989; 71: 309
10. Fisher MMD, More DG: The epidemiology and clinical features of anaphylactic reactions in anaesthesia. Anaesth Intensive Care 1981; 9: 226
11. Weiss ME, Adkinson NF, Hirshman CA: Evaluation of allergic reactions in the perioperative period. Anesthesiology 1989; 71: 438
12. Mertes PM, Laxenaire MC, Alla F; Groupe d'Etudes des Reactions Anaphylactoides Peranesthesiques: Anaphylactic and anaphylactoid reactions occurring during anesthesia in France in 1999–2000. Anesthesiology 2003; 99: 536
13. Portier MM, Richet C: De l'action anaphylactique de certains venins. C R Seances Soc Biol Fil 1902; 54: 170
14. Watkins J: Anaphylactoid reactions to IV substances. Br J Anaesth 1979; 51: 51
15. Costa JJ, Weller PF, Galli SJ: The cells of the allergic response: Mast cells, basophils, and eosinophils. JAMA 1997; 278: 1815
16. Galli SJ, Wedemeyer J, Tsai M: Analyzing the roles of mast cells and basophils in host defense and other biological responses. Int J Hematol 2002; 75: 363
17. Winslow CM, Austen KF: Enzymatic regulation of mast cell activation and secretion by adenylate cyclase and cyclic AMP-dependent protein kinases. Fed Proc 1982; 41: 22
18. Galli SJ: Mast cells and basophils. Curr Opin Hematol 2000; 7: 32
19. MacGlashan D Jr. Histamine: A mediator of inflammation. J Allergy Clin Immunol 2003; 112(4 Suppl): S53
20. Marone G, Bova M, Detoraki A, et al: The human heart as a shock organ in anaphylaxis. Novartis Found Symp 2004; 257: 133
21. Majno G, Palade GE: Studies on inflammation: I. The effect of histamine and serotonin on vascular permeability. An electron microscopic study. J Biophys Biochem Cytol 1961; 11: 571
22. Gould HJ, Sutton BJ, Beavil AJ, et al: The biology of IGE and the basis of allergic disease. Ann Rev Immunol 2003; 21: 579
23. Mathe AA, Hedqvist P, Strandberg K, et al: Aspects of prostaglandin function in the lung. N Engl J Med 1977; 296: 850, 910
24. Holgate ST, Peters-Golden M, Panettieri RA, Henderson WR: Roles of cysteinyl leukotrienes in airway inflammation, smooth muscle function, and remodeling. J Allergy Clin Immunol 2003; 111(1 Suppl): S18
25. Lazarus SC: Inflammation, inflammatory mediators, and mediator antagonists in asthma. J Clin Pharmacol 1998; 38: 577
26. Schulman ES, Newball HH, Demers LM, et al: Anaphylactic release of thromboxane A2, prostaglandin D2, and prostacyclin from human lung parenchyma. Am Rev Respir Dis 1981; 124: 402
27. Morel DR, Zapol WM, Thomas SJ, et al: C5a and thromboxane generation associated with pulmonary vaso- and bronchoconstriction during protamine reversal of heparin. Anesthesiology 1987; 66: 597
28. Tanaka KA, Katori N, Szlam F, Vega JD, Levy JH: Evaluation of a novel kallikrein inhibitor on hemostatic activation in vitro. Thromb Res 2004; 113: 333
29. Delage C, Irey NS: Anaphylactic deaths: A clinicopathologic study of 43 cases. J Forensic Sci 1972; 17: 525
30. Smith Laboratories: Chymodiactin Post Marketing Surveillance Report. Chicago, Smith Laboratories, 1984
31. Laxenaire MC, Moneret-Vautrin DA, Vervloet D, et al: Accidents anaphylactoides graves peranesthesiques. Ann Fr Anesth Reanim 1985; 4: 30
32. Pumphrey R. Anaphylaxis: Can we tell who is at risk of a fatal reaction? Curr Opin Allergy Clin Immunol 2004; 4: 285
33. Pavek K, Wegmann A, Nordström L, et al: Cardiovascular and respiratory mechanisms in anaphylactic and anaphylactoid shock reactions. Klin Wochenschr 1982; 60: 941
34. Atkinson JP, Frank MM: Role of complement in the pathophysiology of hematologic disease. Prog Hematol 1977; 10: 211
35. Jacobs HS, Craddock PR, Hammerschmidt DE, et al: Complement-induced granulocyte aggregation: An unsuspected mechanism of disease. N Engl J Med 1980; 302: 789
36. Sheppard CA, Logdberg LE, Zimring JC, et al.: Transfusion-related acute lung injury. Hematol Oncol Clin North Am 2007; 21: 163
37. Teissner B, Brandslund I, Grunnet N, et al: Acute complement activation during an anaphylactoid reaction to blood transfusion and the disappearance rate of C3c and C3d from the circulation. J Clin Lab Immunol 1983; 12: 63
38. Hammerschmidt DE, Weaver LJ, Hudson LD, et al: Association of complement activation and elevated plasma-C5a with adult respiratory distress syndrome. Lancet 1980; 1: 947
39. Levy JH, Brister NW, Shearin A, et al: Wheal and flare responses to opioids in humans. Anesthesiology 1989; 70: 756
40. Levy JH, Adelson DM, Walker BF: Wheal and flare responses to muscle relaxants in humans. Agents Actions 1991; 34: 302
41. Veien M, Holdin J, Szlam F, et al: Mechanisms of non-immunological histamine and tryptase release from human cutaneous mast cells. Anesthesiology 2000; 92: 1074
42. Levy JH, Kettlekamp N, Goertz P, et al: Histamine release by vancomycin: A mechanism for hypotension in man. Anesthesiology 1987; 67: 122
43. Caulfield JP, El-Lati S, Thomas G, et al.: Dissociated human foreskin mast cells degranulate in response to anti-IgE and substance P. Lab Invest 1990; 63: 502

44. Casale TB, Bowman S, Kaliner M: Induction of human cutaneous mast cell degranulation by opiates and endogenous opioid peptides: Evidence for opiate and nonopiate receptor participation. J Allergy Clin Immunol 1984; 73: 775

45. Levy JH, Davis GK, Duggan J, Szlam F: Determination of the hemodynamics and histamine release of rocuronium (Org 9426) when administered in increased doses under N$_2$O/O$_2$-sufentanil anesthesia. Anesth Analg 1994; 78: 318

46. Levy JH, Pitts M, Thanopoulos A, et al: The effects of rapacuronium on histamine release and hemodynamics in adult patients undergoing general anesthesia. Anesth Analg 1999; 89: 290

47. Hirshman CA, Downes H, Butler J: Relevance of plasma histamine levels to hypotension. Anesthesiology 1982; 57: 424

48. Stark BJ, Sullivan TJ: Biphasic and protracted anaphylaxis. J Allergy Clin Immunol 1986; 78: 76

49. Levy JH, Rockoff MR: Anaphylaxis to meperidine. Anesth Analg 1982; 61: 301

50. Fisher MM: Blood volume replacement in acute anaphylactic cardiovascular collapse related to anaesthesia. Br J Anaesth 1977; 49: 1023

51. Levy JH, Adkinson NF: Anaphylaxis during cardiac surgery: implications for clinicans. Anesth Analg 2008, In Press

52. Levy JH: Anaphylactic-anaphylactoid reactions during cardiac surgery. J Clin Anesthesiol 1989; 1: 426

53. Schwartz LB. Effector cells of anaphylaxis: Mast cells and basophils. Novartis Found Symp 2004; 257: 65

54. 2005 American Heart Association Guidelines for Cardiopulmonary Resuscitation and Emergency Cardiovascular Care Part 10.6: Anaphylaxis. Circulation 2005; 112: IV-143

55. Sin DD, Man J, Sharpe H, Gan WQ, Man SF: Pharmacological management to reduce exacerbations in adults with asthma: A systematic review and meta-analysis. JAMA 2004; 292: 367

56. Sheagren JN: Septic shock and corticosteroids (editorial). N Engl J Med 1981; 305: 456

57. Gruchalla RS: Drug allergy. J Allergy Clin Immunol 2003; 111: S548

58. DeSwarte RD: Drug allergy: Problems and strategies. J Allergy Clin Immunol 1984; 74: 209

59. Reich DL, Hossain S, Krol M, et al: Predictors of hypotension after induction of general anesthesia. Anesth Analg 2005; 101: 622

60. Fisher MM, Outhred A, Bowey CJ: Can clinical anaphylaxis to anaesthetic drugs be predicted from allergic history? Br J Anaesth 1987; 59: 690

61. Christman D: Immune reaction to propanidid. Anaesthesia 1984; 39: 470

62. Watkins J, Clarke SJ: Report of a symposium: Adverse responses to intravenous agents. Br J Anaesth 1978; 50: 1159

63. Driggs RL, O'Day RA: Acute allergic reaction associated with methohexital anaesthesia: Report of six cases. J Oral Surg 1972; 30: 906

64. Watkins J, Salo M, eds. Incidence of immediate adverse response to intravenous anaesthetic drugs, Trauma, Stress and Immunity in Anaesthesia and Surgery. London, Butterworth, 1982, pp 272

65. Schwartz HJ, Sher TH: Bisulfite sensitivity manifesting as allergy to local dental anaesthesia. J Allergy Clin Immunol 1985; 75: 525

66. Brown DT, Beamins D, Wildsmith JAW: Allergic reaction to an amide local anesthetic. Br J Anaesth 1981; 53: 435

67. Fisher MM, Munro I: Life-threatening anaphylactoid reactions to muscle relaxants. Anesth Analg 1983; 62: 559

68. Swartz J, Braude BM, Gilmour RF, et al: Intraoperative anaphylaxis to latex. Can J Anaesth 1990; 37: 589

69. Roizen MF, Rodgers GM, Valone FH, et al: Anaphylactoid reactions to vascular graft material presenting with vasodilation and subsequent disseminated intravascular coagulation. Anesthesiology 1989; 71: 331

70. Laxenaire MC, Moneret-Vautrin DA, Watkins J: Diagnosis of the causes of anaphylactoid anaesthetic reactions. Anaesthesia 1983; 38: 147

71. Vervloet D, Nizankowska E, Arnaud A, et al: Adverse reactions to suxamethonium and other muscle relaxants under general anesthesia. J Allergy Clin Immunol 1983; 71: 552

72. Harle DG, Baldo BA, Fisher MM: Detection of IgE antibodies to suxamethonium after anaphylactoid reactions during anaesthesia. Lancet 1984; 1: 930

73. Zucker-Pinchoff B, Ramanathan S: Anaphylactic reaction to epidural fentanyl. Anesthesiology 1989; 71: 599

74. Gilstad CW. Anaphylactic transfusion reactions. Curr Opin Hematol 2003; 10: 419

75. Sheffer AL, Pennoyer DS: Management of adverse drug reactions. J Allergy Clin Immunol 1984; 74: 580

76. Levy JH, Zaidan JR, Faraj B: Prospective evaluation of risk of protamine reactions in NPH insulin-dependent diabetics. Anesth Analg 1986; 65: 739

77. Levy JH, Schwieger IM, Zaidan JR, et al: Evaluation of patients at risk for protamine reactions. J Thorac Cardiovasc Surg 1989; 98: 200

78. Lasser EC: The radiocontrast molecule in anaphylaxis: A surprising antigen. Novartis Found Symp 2004; 257: 211

79. Isbister JP, Fisher MM: Adverse effects of plasma volume expanders. Anaesth Intensive Care 1980; 8: 145

80. Colman WR: Paradoxical hypotension after volume expansion with plasma protein fraction. N Engl J Med 1978; 299: 97

81. Ring K, Messmer K: Incidence and severity of anaphylactoid reactions to colloid volume substitutes. Lancet 1977; 1: 466

82. Levy JH: Hemostatic agents and their safety. J Cardiothorac Vasc Anesth 1999; 13(4 Suppl 1): 6

83. Thong BY, Yeow-Chan C: Anaphylaxis during surgical and interventional procedures. Ann Allergy Asthma Immunol 2004; 92: 619

84. Fisher MM, Baldo BA: Immunoassays in the diagnosis of anaphylaxis to neuromuscular blocking drugs: The value of morphine for the detection of IgE antibodies in allergic subjects. Anaesth Intensive Care 2000; 28: 167

85. Baldo BA, Fisher MM: Detection of serum IgE antibodies that react with alcuronium and tubocurarine after life-threatening reactions to muscle relaxants. Anaesth Intensive Care 1983; 11: 194

86. Harle DG, Baldo BA, Smal MA, et al: Detection of thiopentone-reactive IgE antibodies following anaphylactoid reactions during anesthesia. Clin Allergy 1986; 16: 493

87. Dueck R, O'Connor RD: Thiopental: False positive RAST in patient with elevated serum IgE. Anesthesiology 1984; 61: 337

88. Fisher MM: Intradermal testing after anaphylactoid reaction to anaesthetic drugs: Practical aspects of performance and interpretation. Anaesth Intensive Care 1984; 12: 115

89. Fisher MM, Bowey CJ: Intradermal compared with prick testing in the diagnosis of anaesthetic allergy. Br J Anaesth 1997; 79: 59

90. Shatz M: Skin testing and incremental challenge in the evaluation of adverse reactions to local anesthetics. J Allergy Clin Immunol 1984; 74: 606

91. Holzman RB: Clinical management of latex-allergic children. Anesth Analg 1997; 85: 529

92. Kibby T, Akl M: Prevalence of latex sensitization in a hospital employee population. Ann Allergy Asthma Immunol 1997; 78: 41

93. Gold M, Swartz JS, Braude BM, et al: Intraoperative anaphylaxis: An association with latex sensitivity. J Allergy Clin Immunol 1991; 87: 662

94. Holzman RS: Latex allergy: An emerging operating room problem. Anesth Analg 1993; 76: 635

95. Brown RH, Schauble JF, Hamilton RG: Prevalence of latex allergy among anesthesiologists: Identification of sensitized but asymptomatic individuals. Anesthesiology 1998; 89: 292

96. Lavaud F, Prevost A, Cossart C, et al: Allergy to latex, avocado, pear, and banana: Evidence for a 30 kd antigen in immunoblotting. J Allergy Clin Immunol 1995; 95: 557

97. Blanco C, Carrillo T, Castillo R, et al: Latex allergy: Clinical features and cross-reactivity with fruits. Ann Allergy 1994; 73: 309

98. Lebenbom-Mansour MH, Oesterle JR, Ownsby DR, et al: The incidence of latex sensitivity in ambulatory surgical patients: A correlation of historical factors with positive serum immunoglobin E levels. Anesth Analg 1997; 85: 44

99. Suli C, Parziale M, Lorini M, et al: Prevalence and risk factors for latex allergy: A cross sectional study on health-care workers of an Italian hospital. J Investig Allergol Clin Immunol 2004; 14: 64

100. Sampson HA, Munoz-Furlong A, Block SA, et al: Symposium on the definition and management of anaphylaxis: Summary report. J Allergy Clin Immunol 2005; 115: 584

101. Laxenaire MC: Drugs and other agents involved in anaphylactic shock occurring during anaesthesia. A French multicenter epidemiologic inquiry. Ann Fr Anesth Réanim 1993; 12: 91

102. Mertes PM, Laxenaire MC, Alla F: Groupe d'Etudes des Reactions Anaphylactoides Peranesthesiques. Anaphylactic and anaphylactoid reactions occurring during anesthesia in France in 1999–2000. Anesthesiology 2003; 99: 536

103. Moneret-Vautrin DA, Mouton C: Anaphylaxie aux myorelaxants: Valeur prédictive des intrader-journal moréactions et recherche de l'anaphylaxie croisée. Ann Fr Anesth Réanim 1985; 4: 186

104. Monnet-Vautrin DA: Cutaneous tests in anaphylactic reactions to muscular blocking agents. In reducing the risk of anaphylaxis during anaesthesia: Guidelines for clinical practice. Ann Fr Anesth Réanim 2002; 21: 97

105. Dhonneur G, Zoffer R, McCall C, et al: Skin sensitivity to rocuronium and vecuronium: A randomized controlled prick-testing study in healthy volunteers. Anesth Analg 2004; 88: 986

106. Levy JH, Gottge M, Szlam F, et al: Wheal and flare responses to intradermal rocuronium and cisatracurium in humans. Br J Anaesth 2000; 85: 844

107. Levy JH: Anaphylactic reactions to neuromuscular blocking drugs: Are we making the correct diagnosis? Anesth Analg 2004; 98: 881

CHAPTER 13 ■ INFLAMMATION, WOUND HEALING AND INFECTION

HARRIET W. HOPF, C. RICHARD CHAPMAN, AMALIA COCHRAN, MICHAEL B. DORROUGH, AND RANDAL O. DULL

ANATOMY AND PHYSIOLOGY

KEY POINTS

1. The most crucial component of infection prevention is frequent and effective hand hygiene.
2. The ideal hand hygiene agent kills a broad spectrum of microbes, has antimicrobial activity that persists for at least 6 hours after application, is simple to use, and has few side effects.
3. Wearing gloves does not reduce the need for hand hygiene.
4. Antibiotic prophylaxis has become standard for surgeries in which there is more than a minimum risk of infection. The most commonly used antibiotic for surgical prophylaxis is cefazolin, a first-generation cephalosporin, as the potential pathogens for most surgeries are Gram-positive cocci from the skin.
5. The exact timing for the administration of the antibiotic, ideally within 30 minutes to 1 hour of incision, depends on the pharmacology and half-life of the drug. Prophylactic antibiotics should be discontinued by 24 hours following surgery if postoperative dosing is selected at all. Prolonging the course of prophylactic antibiotics does not reduce the risk of infection but does increase the risk of adverse consequences of antibiotic administration, including resistance, *Clostridium difficile* infection, and sensitization.
6. Anesthesiologists should work in consultation with the surgeon to use guidelines determined by the local infection control committee to take initiative for administering prophylactic antibiotics because they have access to the patient during the 60 minutes prior to incision and can optimize timing of administration.
7. The standard teaching that oxygen delivery depends more on hemoglobin-bound oxygen (oxygen content) than on arterial PO_2 may be true of working muscle, but it is not true of wound healing.
8. Although oxygen consumption is relatively low in wounds, it is consumed by processes that require oxygen at a high concentration.
9. High oxygen tensions (>100 mm Hg) can be reached in wounds but only if perfusion is rapid and arterial PO_2 is high.
10. Peripheral vasoconstriction, which results from central sympathetic control of subcutaneous vascular tone, is probably the most frequent and clinically the most important impediment to wound oxygenation.
11. Prevention or correction of hypothermia and blood volume deficits has been shown to decrease wound infections and increase collagen deposition in patients undergoing major abdominal surgery.
12. Modifiable risks include smoking, malnutrition, hyperglycemia, hypercholesterolemia, and hypertension. These should be assessed and corrected when possible prior to surgery.
13. Maintenance of a high room temperature or forced air warming before, during, and after the operation is significantly more effective than other methods of warming, such as circulating water blankets placed under the patient and humidification of the breathing circuit.
14. Optimizing the volume of perioperative fluid administration to minimize morbidity and mortality remains a significant and controversial challenge.
15. Current best recommendations for volume management include replacing fluid losses based on standard recommendations for the type of surgery, replacement of blood loss, and replacement of other ongoing fluid losses (e.g., high urine output due to diuretic or dye administration, hyperglycemia, or thermoregulatory vasoconstriction).
16. Wounds are most vulnerable in the first few hours after surgery.
17. All vasoconstrictive stimuli must be corrected simultaneously to allow optimal healing.
18. Local perfusion is not assured until patients have a normal blood volume, are warm and pain-free, and are receiving no vasoconstrictive drugs; that is, until the sympathetic nervous system is inactivated.
19. Urine output is a poor, often misleading guide to peripheral perfusion.
20. Physical examination of the patient is a better guide to hypovolemia and vasoconstriction.

㉑ Administration of supplemental oxygen via face mask or nasal cannulae increases safety in patients receiving systemic opioids. As a side benefit, it may also improve wound healing, although this has not been formally studied. Pain control also appears important since it favorably influences both pulmonary function and vascular tone.

㉒ In patients with moderate to high risk of surgical site infection, anesthesiologists have the opportunity to enhance wound healing and reduce the incidence of wound infections by simple, inexpensive, and readily available means.

Despite major advances in the management of patients undergoing surgery—including aseptic technique, prophylactic antibiotics, and advances in surgical approaches such as laparoscopic surgery—surgical wound infection and wound failure remain common complications of surgery (Fig. 13-1). Wound complications are associated with prolonged hospitalization, increased resource consumption, and even increased mortality. More than 300,000 surgical site infections (SSIs; Table 13-1) occur each year in the United States at an estimated cost of more than $1 billion.[1] A growing body of literature supports the concept that patient factors are a major determinant of wound outcome following surgery. Comorbidities such as diabetes and cardiac disease clearly contribute, but environmental stressors as well the individual response to stress may be equally important. In particular, wounds are exquisitely sensitive to hypoxia, which is both common and preventable. Perioperative management can be adapted to promote postoperative wound healing and resistance to infection. Along with aseptic technique and prophylactic antibiotics, maintaining perfusion and oxygenation of the wound is paramount. This chapter discusses how knowledge of the principles of infection control and the biology and physiology of wound repair and resistance to infection can improve outcomes.

INFECTION CONTROL

Hand Hygiene

① Perhaps the most crucial component of infection prevention is frequent and effective hand hygiene. In 1847 Ignaz Semmelweis made the observation that women who delivered their babies in the First Clinic at the General Hospital of Vienna, staffed by medical students and physicians, had a mortality rate of 5 to

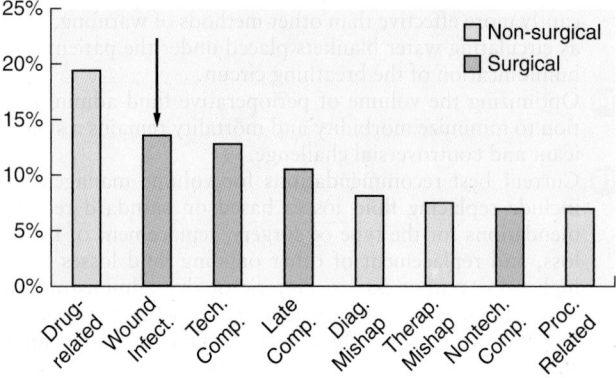

FIGURE 13-1. Brennan et al.[148] reviewed the records or 30,121 patients at 51 acute care hospitals in New York State in 1984 and found that surgical site infection was the most common adverse surgical event (and the second most common adverse event overall). Infect., infection; Tech. comp., technique complication; Diag., diagnosis; Therap, therapeutic; Proc., procedure. From Brennan TA, Leape LL, Laird NM, et al. Incidence of adverse events and negligence in hospitalized patients. Results of the Harvard Medical Practice Study. NEJM 1991;324:370, with permission.

15%, largely the result of puerperal infections; this was substantially higher than the 2% rate of women who delivered at Clinic 2, which was staffed by midwife students and midwives.[2] Students and physicians at Clinic 1 usually started the day performing autopsies (including on patients who died of puerperal fever) and then moved on to the Clinic, where they performed examinations on women in labor. Semmelweis made the connection, and although germ theory was some years off, he insisted that physicians and medical students wash their hands in a chlorinated solution when leaving the pathology laboratory. This reduced the rate of puerperal fever to the same rate as at Clinic 2. Soon, Semmelweis identified cases of transmission from an infected to an uninfected patient, and instituted the use of chlorinated solution hand washing between cases as well. He also demonstrated that the chlorinated solution was more effective than soap and water. Unfortunately, his innovation was not widely adopted, resulting from a combination of his delay in publishing his results, the reluctance of his colleagues to accept that they might be responsible for transmitting disease, and his lack of tact in trying to convince health care workers to adopt his measures. Despite our current knowledge of germ theory, hand hygiene remains an inexplicably neglected component of infection control: studies consistently demonstrate about a 40% rate of adherence (range, 5 to 81%) to hand-hygiene guidelines.[3]

Bacteria are resident in the skin and can never be completely eliminated.[3] Resident flora are embedded in the deeper folds of the skin and are more resistant to removal, but are also infrequently pathogenic. Coagulase-negative staphylococci and diphtheroids are the most common. Transient flora colonize the superficial layers of the skin and thus are easier to remove with hand hygiene. Transient flora are also the source of most health care-associated infections, as health care worker skin can become contaminated from patient contact or contact with contaminated surfaces. Contamination from surfaces is most commonly with organisms such as staphylococci and enterococci, which are resistant to drying. Even "clean" activities such as taking a patient's pulse or applying monitors can lead to hand contamination: 100 to 1,000 colony-forming units of *Klebsiella* species were measured on nurses' hands following such activities in one study.[4] No studies have related hand contamination to actual transmission of infection to patients; however, numerous studies, starting with those of Semmelweis, have demonstrated a reduction in health care-associated infections following institution of hand hygiene or improved adherence to hand hygiene.[3]

② A number of products are available for hand hygiene. The ideal agent kills a broad spectrum of microbes, has antimicrobial activity that persists for at least 6 hours after application, is simple to use, and has few side effects. The most commonly used and efficacious agents are reviewed here.

Plain (not antiseptic) soap and water are generally the least effective at reducing hand contamination.[5] Although obvious dirt is removed by the detergent effect of soap and the mechanical action of washing, bacterial load is not greatly reduced. Further, soap and water hand hygiene is associated with high rates of skin irritation and drying, both of which are risk factors for an increased bacterial load. Soap and water are, however, the most effective at removing spores, and therefore should be used when contamination with *Clostridium difficile* or *Bacillus anthracis* is a concern.[3]

TABLE 13-1

CRITERIA FOR DEFINING A SURGICAL SITE INFECTION (SSI)

Superficial Incisional SSI
- Infection occurs within 30 days after the operation
  and
- Infection involves only skin or subcutaneous tissue of the incision
  and
- At least *one* of the following:
  1. Purulent drainage, with or without laboratory confirmation, from the superficial incision
  2. Organisms isolated from an aseptically obtained culture of fluid or tissue from the superficial incision
  3. At least one of the following signs or symptoms of infection: pain or tenderness, localized swelling, redness, or heat *and* superficial incision is deliberately opened by the surgeon, *unless* incision is culture-negative
  4. Diagnosis of superficial incisional SSI by the surgeon or attending physician
- Do *not* report the following conditions as superficial incisional SSI:
  1. Stitch abscess (minimal inflammation and discharge confined to the points of suture penetration)
  2. Infection of an episiotomy or newborn circumcision site
  3. Infected burn wound
  4. Incisional SSI that extends into the facial and muscle layers (see "Deep Incisional SSI")
  Note: Specific criteria are used for identifying infected episiotomy and circumcision sites and burn wounds

Deep Incisional SSI
- Infection occurs within 30 days after the operation if no implant is left in place or within 1 year if implant is in place and the infection appears to be related to the operation
  and
- Infection involves deep soft tissues (e.g., fascial and muscle layers) of the incision
  and
- At least *one* of the following:
  1. Purulent drainage from the deep incision but not from the organ/space component of the surgical site
  2. A deep incision spontaneously dehisces or is deliberately opened by a surgeon when the patient has at least one of the following signs or symptoms: fever (>38°C), localized pain, or tenderness, unless site is culture-negative
  3. An abscess or other evidence of infection involving the deep incision is found on direct examination, during reoperation, or by histopathologic or radiologic examination
  4. Diagnosis of a deep incisional SSI by a surgeon or attending physician
  Notes:
  1. Report infection that involves both superficial and deep incision sites as deep incisional SSI
  2. Report an organ/space SSI that drains through the incision as a deep incisional SSI

Organ/Space SSI
- Infection occurs within 30 days after the operation if no implant is left in place or within 1 year if implant is in place and the infection appears to be related to the operation
  and
- Infection involves any part of the anatomy (e.g., organs or spaces), other than the incision, which was opened or manipulated during an operation
  and
- At least *one* of the following:
  1. Purulent drainage from a drain that is placed through a stab wound into the organ/space
  2. Organisms isolated from an aseptically obtained culture of fluid or tissue in the organ/space
  3. An abscess or other evidence of infection involving the organ/space that is found on direct examination, during reoperation, or by histopathologic or radiologic examination
  4. Diagnosis of an organ/space SSI by a surgeon or attending physician

From Mangram AJ, Horan TC, Pearson ML, et al: Guideline for prevention of surgical site infection, 1999. Centers for Disease Control and Prevention (CDC) Hospital Infection Control Practices Advisory Committee. Am J Infect Control 1999;27:97, with permission.

Alcohol-based rinses and gels denature proteins, and this confers their antimicrobial activity.[3] Ethanol is most commonly used because it has more antiviral activity than isopropanol. Antiseptics containing 60 to 95% ethanol with a water base are germicidal and effective against Gram-positive and Gram-negative bacteria, lipophilic viruses such as herpes simplex, human immunodeficiency, influenza, respiratory syncytial, and vaccinia viruses, and hepatitis B and C viruses. They have little persistent activity, although regrowth of bacteria does occur slowly after use of alcohol-based products. Combination with low doses of other agents such as chlorhexidine, quaternary ammonium compounds, or triclosan can confer persistent activity. Efficacy depends on volume applied (3 mL is superior to 1 mL) and duration of contact (ideally, 30 seconds).

Chlorhexidine is a cationic bisbiguanide that disrupts cytoplasmic membranes, resulting in precipitation of cellular contents.[3] It is germicidal against Gram-positive bacteria and lipophilic viruses, with somewhat less activity against Gram-negative bacteria and fungi, and minimal against tubercle bacilli. It has substantial persistence on the skin, and the Centers for Disease Control and Prevention (CDC) has identified it as the topical agent of choice for skin preparation in central venous catheter insertion. It may cause severe corneal damage after direct contact with the eye, ototoxicity after direct contact with the inner or middle ear, and neurotoxicity after direct contact with the brain or meninges. There are reports of bacteria that have acquired reduced susceptibility to chlorhexidine, but these are of questionable clinical pertinence since the concentrations at which resistance was found were substantially lower than that of commercially available products.

Iodine and iodophors (iodine with a polymer carrier) penetrate the cell wall and impair protein synthesis and cell membrane function.[3] They are bactericidal against Gram-positive, Gram-negative, and some spore-forming bacteria including clostridia and *Bacillus* species, although inactive against spores. They also have activity against mycobacteria, viruses, and fungi. Their persistence is generally fairly poor. They cause more contact dermatitis than other commonly used agents, and allergies to this class of topical agent are common. Iodophors generally cause fewer side effects than iodine agents.

The choice of an antiseptic depends on the expected pathogens, acceptability by health care workers, and cost. In general, antiseptics cost about $1 per patient day, far less than the cost of health care-associated infections. In nine studies that examined the effect of improved hand hygiene adherence on health care-associated infections, the majority demonstrated that as hand hygiene practices improved, infection rates decreased.[3]

Barriers to hand hygiene include skin irritation and fear of skin irritation, inaccessibility, time, and health care worker acceptance (largely related to the other factors mentioned). Although alcohol-based agents have long been believed to cause more skin irritation, several recent trials have demonstrated less skin irritation and better acceptance with emollient-containing, alcohol-based hand rubs compared with either antimicrobial or nonantimicrobial soap. The use of appropriate (glove-compatible) lotions twice a day also reduces skin irritation—as well as leading to a 50% increase in hand hygiene frequency in one study.[3] Alcohol-based gels are

also generally more accessible than antiseptic soap and water, as the dispenser may be pocket-sized or placed conveniently near sites of patient care. It has been estimated that alcohol-based gels require only about 25% of the time of going to a sink to wash one's hands. However, soap and water should be used to remove particulate matter including blood and other body fluids or after five to ten applications of alcohol-based agent.

Adherence to hand hygiene guidelines (Tables 13-2 through 13-4) generally decreases as the frequency of indicated hand washing increases, as the workload increases, and as staffing decreases. In an intensive care unit (ICU), hand hygiene for nurses is generally indicated about 20 times per hour, as compared with a normal ward where this number decreases to 8 per hour.[3] In the operating room (OR), frequent patient contact by the anesthesiologist requires frequent hand hygiene, probably at about the level of nurses in the ICU, while accessibility is often quite limited. Sinks are available only outside the OR. Therefore, alcohol-based agents should be available within hand's reach of the anesthesia machine. Loftus et al.[6] studied bacterial contamination of the anesthesia work area (adjustable pressure limiting valve complex and agent flowmeter) and cross-contamination of the sterile anesthesia stopcock during 61 first cases in their operating room. They found an average increase in bacterial contamination of the work area of 115 colonies per surface area sampled during cases (95% confidence interval: 62–169; $p < 0.001$). Transmission of bacteria from the work area to the sterile stopcock in the patients' intravenous tubing occurred in 32% of cases, including transmission of methicillin-resistant *Staphylococcus aureus* (MRSA) in two cases and vancomycin-resistant *Enterococcus* in one case. A high level of contamination of the work area (>100 colonies per surface area sampled) increased the risk of stopcock contamination 4.7 fold (95% confidence interval: 1.42–15.42; $p = 0.011$). Thus, transmission of bacterial contamination by the anesthesia provider appears to be common,

---

TABLE 13-2

INDICATIONS FOR HAND HYGIENE

- When hands are visibly dirty or contaminated with proteinaceous material or are visibly soiled with blood or other body fluids, wash hands with either a nonantimicrobial soap and water or an antimicrobial soap and water.
- If hands are not visibly soiled, use an alcohol-based hand rub for routinely decontaminating hands. Alternatively, wash hands with an antimicrobial soap and water.
- Decontaminate hands before having direct contact with patients.
- Decontaminate hands before donning sterile gloves when inserting a central intravascular catheter.
- Decontaminate hands before inserting indwelling urinary catheters, peripheral vascular catheters, or other invasive devices that do not require a surgical procedure.
- Decontaminate hands after contact with a patient's intact skin (e.g., applying monitors, moving patient).
- Decontaminate hands after contact with body fluids or excretions, mucous membranes, nonintact skin, and wound dressings if hands are not visibly soiled.
- Decontaminate hands if moving from a contaminated-body site (e.g., mouth during tracheal intubation) to a clean-body site (e.g., adjusting gas flow, turning on ventilator, starting IV) during patient care.
- Decontaminate hands after contact with inanimate objects (including medical equipment) in the immediate vicinity of the patient. Take care to reduce contamination of the anesthesia machine (e.g., after tracheal intubation) as well!
- Decontaminate hands after removing gloves.
- Before eating and after using a restroom, wash hands with a nonantimicrobial soap and water or with an antimicrobial soap and water.
- Antimicrobial-impregnated wipes (i.e., towelettes) may be considered as an alternative to washing hands with nonantimicrobial soap and water. Because they are not as effective as alcohol-based hand rubs or washing hands with an antimicrobial soap and water for reducing bacterial counts on the hands of HCWs, they are not a substitute for using an alcohol-based hand rub or antimicrobial soap.

IV, intravenous (tube); HCW, health care worker.
Modified from Boyce JM, Pittet D: Guideline for hand hygiene in health-care settings. Recommendations of the Healthcare Infection Control Practices Advisory Committee and the HIPAC/SHEA/APIC/IDSA Hand Hygiene Task Force. Am J Infect Control 2002; 30(8): S1.

TABLE 13-3

HAND HYGIENE TECHNIQUE

- When decontaminating hands with an alcohol-based hand rub, apply the recommended volume of product to palm of one hand and rub hands together, covering all surfaces of hands and fingers, until hands are dry.
- When washing hands with soap and water, wet hands first with water, apply an amount of product recommended by the manufacturer to hands, and rub hands together vigorously for at least 15 seconds, covering all surfaces of the hands and fingers. Rinse hands with water and dry thoroughly with a disposable towel. Use towel to turn off the faucet. Avoid using hot water because repeated exposure to hot water may increase the risk of dermatitis.
- Liquid, bar, leaflet, or powdered forms of plain soap are acceptable when washing hands with a nonantimicrobial soap and water. When bar soap is used, soap racks that facilitate drainage and small bars of soap should be used.

Modified from Boyce JM, Pittet D: Guideline for hand hygiene in health-care settings. Recommendations of the Healthcare Infection Control Practices Advisory Committee and the HIPAC/SHEA/APIC/IDSA Hand Hygiene Task Force. Am J Infect Control 2002; 30(8): S1.

a potential source of nosocomial infections, and largely preventable.[6]

3 Wearing gloves does not reduce the need for hand hygiene. Although gloves provide protection, bacterial flora from patients may be cultured from up to 30% of health care workers who wear gloves during patient contact.[3] Therefore, hand hygiene should be practiced both before putting on gloves and immediately after removal. Moreover, gloves should be removed or changed immediately after each procedure, including vascular access, intubation, and neuraxial anesthesia, because gloves become contaminated by patient contact just as hands do.

Artificial and long fingernails, as well as chipped fingernail polish, are associated with higher concentrations of bacteria on the hands of health care workers. Artificial nails have been identified as a source in several hospital-associated outbreaks of infection with Gram-negative bacilli and yeast, and CDC guidelines discourage wearing of artificial nails by health care workers in high-risk settings; many hospitals have banned wearing of artificial nails by any employee who has direct

TABLE 13-4

SKIN CARE

- Provide health care workers with hand lotions or creams to minimize the occurrence of irritant contact dermatitis associated with hand antisepsis or handwashing.
- Solicit information from manufacturers regarding any effects that hand lotions, creams, or alcohol-based hand antiseptics may have on the persistent effects of antimicrobial soaps being used in the institution, as well as on glove integrity. Select a combination of products that minimizes these effects.

Modified from Boyce JM, Pittet D: Guideline for hand hygiene in health-care settings. Recommendations of the Healthcare Infection Control Practices Advisory Committee and the HIPAC/SHEA/APIC/IDSA Hand Hygiene Task Force. Am J Infect Control 2002; 30(8): S1.

patient contact.[3] It may also be appropriate to counsel patients scheduled for surgery that artificial nails may increase their risk of infection, although this has not been investigated. Large quantities of bacteria are typically trapped under the fingernails, and 2002 CDC guidelines recommend that health care workers keep their nail tips trimmed to less than ¼ inch.[3]

Bacteria may be cultured at higher concentrations from the skin beneath a ring. On the other hand, wearing a ring does not increase overall bacterial levels measured on the hands of health care workers. Therefore, it remains unclear whether transmission of infection could be reduced by prohibiting health care workers from wearing rings.[3]

Antisepsis

Masks have long been advocated as preventing surgical site infection, and are used almost universally in U.S. operating rooms. Tunevall[7] studied the rate of wound infections in 3,088 patients over 115 weeks. In alternating weeks, OR personnel either wore masks or did not (personnel with active respiratory infections continued to wear masks). There was no difference in the rate of surgical wound infections (4.7 vs. 3.5%, respectively) in the two groups, nor in bacterial species cultured from the wounds. Friberg et al.[8] demonstrated comparable air and surface contamination during sham surgery in a horizontal laminar air flow unit whether OR personnel wore a nonsterile hood and mask or a sterilized helmet aspirator system. When the head covering but not the mask was omitted, however, contamination increased three- to fivefold. These data suggest that wearing a head cover is useful for preventing SSI, while wearing a mask is not. Nonetheless, the study by Tunevall is a small one, and most hospital personnel continue to require a mask in the OR while surgical instruments are open. Moreover, the mask does serve the purpose of protecting the health care provider, particularly when combined with eye protection, and thus should most likely be used during tracheal intubation and at other times when protection from body fluids is appropriate.

Although the preponderance of postoperative surgical infections is caused by flora that are endogenous to the patient, environmental and airborne contaminants may also play a causative role. An important, but frequently overlooked, consideration is the role that traffic patterns into an OR can play in patient exposure to airborne organisms. A recent Israeli study of risk factors for surgical infection after total knee replacement demonstrated a trend toward increased infection rates with in increased number of orthopaedic surgeons or anesthetists present in the OR.[9] This study reconfirmed a prior study showing a trend toward increased incidence of surgical site infection as the number of people in the operating suite increases.[10] However, it has been noted in one audit that physicians and nurses did little to limit the number of people through ORs during procedures.[11] Current recommended practices are that traffic patterns should limit the flow of people through an OR that is in use, and that no more people than necessary should be in an OR during a procedure.[12] The anesthesiologist is clearly in a position to play a leadership role in controlling human traffic through the OR.

Mermel et al.[13] in 1991 demonstrated that central venous lines placed by the anesthesiologist in the OR became infected more often (relative risk [RR], 2.1; $p = 0.03$) than those placed by surgeons or other providers, whether in or out of the OR. Contributing factors appeared to be site of placement and the stringency of aseptic technique. Internal jugular vein insertion has a greater risk of infection (RR, 4.3; $p < 0.01$) compared with subclavian vein, although its other benefits may outweigh this risk. Raad et al.[14] demonstrated that use of a maximal sterile barrier technique versus sterile gloves and small sterile drapes led to a significant reduction in central venous catheter-related infection from 7.2 to 2.2% ($p = 0.03$). Therefore, gowning and gloving, careful aseptic technique, and use of a wide sterile field should be routine.[15] In anesthetized patients, the central line is ideally placed before the surgical site is draped in order to avoid contamination of the wire on the underside of the surgical drape.

Epidural abscess formation is an extremely rare but potentially catastrophic complication of neuraxial anesthesia and epidural catheter placement. Therefore, careful attention to aseptic technique and infection control is required. The most important consideration is to prevent contamination of the needle and catheter. Thus, hand washing, skin preparation, draping, and maintenance of a sterile field should be carefully observed. Gowning and wearing a mask, however, are unlikely to reduce the risk of infection. Finally, epidurals should probably be avoided in patients known or suspected to have bacteremia or deferred until after appropriate antibiotics are administered.

Antibiotic Prophylaxis

After antibiotics came into widespread use in the 1940s and 1950s, there was much debate over the possibility that antibiotic prophylaxis might prevent SSI. In 1957 Miles et al.[16] used a guinea pig model for the proof of principle that administration of an antibiotic prior to contamination (incision) could reduce the risk of surgical site infection. When appropriate antibiotics were given within 2 hours before or after intradermal injection of bacteria they were effective in preventing invasive infection and necrosis. When given outside this window, they were not effective. This gave rise to the concept of a "decisive period" in which antibiotics will be effective, which remains a guiding principle of antibiotic prophylaxis. Miles et al. also demonstrated that injection of epinephrine intradermally prior to administration of antibiotics led to antibiotic failure, as demonstrated in an increased wound infection rate. This demonstrated the crucial role of local perfusion in delivering antibiotics to the site. Knighton et al.,[17] using the same model, demonstrated that increased inspired oxygen was equally as effective as antibiotics in preventing infection, and that the two effects were additive (Fig. 13-2). Knighton et al.[18] also delayed the administration of oxygen for up to 6 hours after inoculation and demonstrated no reduction in effect. Thus, the decisive period for oxygen is considerably longer than that of antibiotics.

Two surgeons at Washington University in St. Louis, Harvey Bernard and William Cole,[19] reported on the first controlled clinical trial of the efficacy of antibiotic prophylaxis in 1964 and demonstrated a benefit in abdominal operations. Thereafter, numerous clinical trials were performed with somewhat variable results. Eventually these served to define the timing and population in which prophylactic antibiotics work. By the 1970s antibiotic prophylaxis for high-risk surgery—meaning clean-contaminated and contaminated cases—was becoming well accepted and widely used, although some skeptics remained. In 1992, Classen et al.[20] published their prospective series including 2,847 patients undergoing clean or clean-contaminated surgical procedures at LDS Hospital in Salt Lake City, UT (Fig. 13-3). They demonstrated that the decisive period for SSI in humans undergoing surgery was essentially the same as for experimental infections in guinea pigs. That is, they found the lowest infection rate when antibiotics were given within 2 hours before or after incision and a rapid increase in SSI rate when they were given outside that range. The best results, though only by a small margin and not statistically significant, were within 0 to 60 minutes of surgery, and this subsequently became the clinical standard.

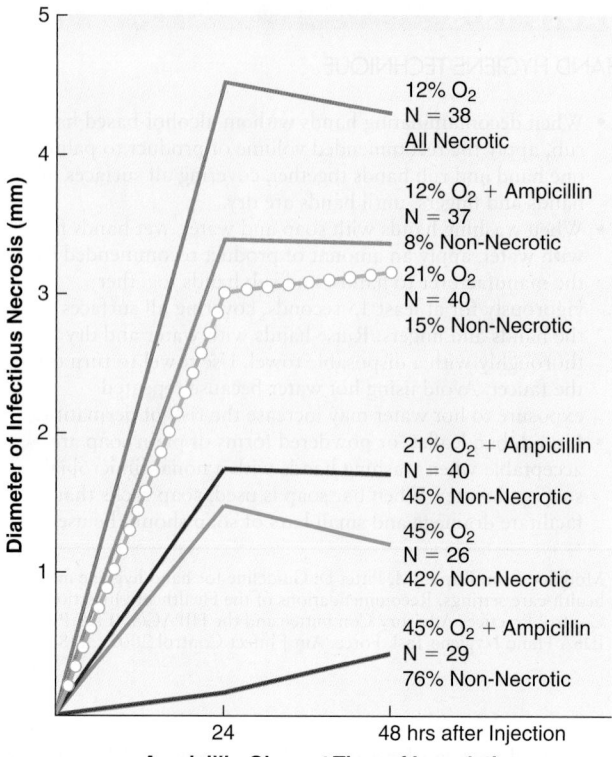

FIGURE 13-2. The effect of oxygen and/or antibiotics on lesion diameter after intradermal injection of bacteria into guinea pigs. Note that at every level, oxygen adds to the effect of antibiotics and that increasing oxygen in the breathing mixture from 12 to 20% or from 20 to 45% exerts an effect comparable to that of appropriately timed antibiotics. (From Rabkin J, Hunt TK: Infection and oxygen, Problem wounds: The Role of Oxygen. Edited by Davis J, Hunt TK. New York, Elsevier, 1988, pp 1, with permission.)

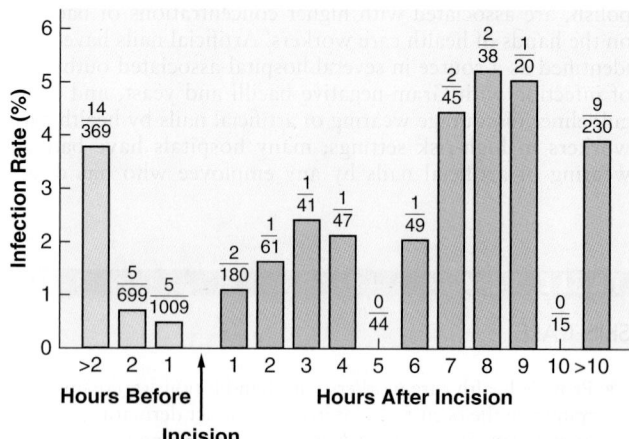

FIGURE 13-3. The figure demonstrates rates of surgical wound infection corresponding to the temporal relation between antibiotic administration and the start of surgery. The number of infections and the number of patients for each hourly interval appear as the numerator and denominator, respectively, of the fraction for that interval. The trend toward higher rates of infection for each hour that antibiotic administration was delayed after the surgical incision was significant (z score = 2.00; $p < 0.05$ by the Wilcoxon test). (From Classen D, Evans R, Pestotni KS, et al: The timing of prophylactic administration of antibiotics and the risk of surgical wound infection. NEJM 1992:326;281, with permission.)

(4) Antibiotic prophylaxis has now become standard for surgeries in which there is more than a minimum risk of infection. Although not every surgery and situation has been studied, a strong rationale for the approach to prophylactic antibiotics has emerged. Several groups separately developed guidelines for use, culminating in recommendations published in 2004 by the National Surgical Infection Prevention Project.[21] These guidelines emphasize timing and choice of appropriate agents. Guidelines generally do not specify antibiotic agents, although they give rationales for various choices.[21] The agent for antibiotic prophylaxis must cover the most likely spectrum of bacteria presented in the surgical field (see Table 13-5). The most commonly used antibiotic for surgical prophylaxis is cefazolin, a first-generation cephalosporin, as the potential pathogens for most surgeries are Gram-positive cocci from the skin.[21,22]

(5) By definition, prophylactic antibiotics are given pre- or intraoperatively. The exact timing for the administration of the antibiotic depends on the pharmacology and half-life of the drug. Ideally, administration of the prophylaxis should be within 30 minutes to 1 hour of incision.[16,20,22,23] This is uncomplicated for antibiotics that can be given as a bolus dose (e.g., cephalosporins) or as an infusion over a few minutes (e.g., clindamycin) and thus provide tissue levels within minutes. For drugs like vancomycin that require infusion over an hour, coordination of administration is more complex. In general, it is considered acceptable if the infusion is started prior to incision. When a tourniquet is used, the infusion must be complete prior to inflation of the tourniquet. An appropriate dose based on body weight and volume of distribution should be given. Depending on the half-life, antibiotics should be repeated during long operations or operations with large blood loss.[24] For example, cefazolin is normally dosed every 8 hours but the dose should be repeated every 4 hours intraoperatively.[24] Finally, prophylactic antibiotics should be discontinued by 24 hours following surgery if postoperative dosing is selected at all. Prolonging the course of prophylactic antibiotics does not reduce the risk of infection but does increase the risk of adverse consequences of antibiotic administration,[21] including resistance, *Clostridium difficile* infection, and sensitization.

Unfortunately, MRSA is becoming a more common pathogen. Although it varies by country, region, and hospital, about 60% of *S. aureus* are MRSA. Independent risk factors identified for MRSA infection include prolonged use of prophylaxis, use of drains for more than 24 hours, and increasing number of procedures performed on the patient. Hand hygiene is among the most effective means of preventing development of MRSA since alcohol-based gel used properly kills over 99.9% of all transient pathogens including MRSA. There does not appear to be a justification for using antibiotics effective against MRSA for prophylaxis in most clinical settings.

(6) Because they have access to the patient during the 60 minutes prior to incision and can optimize timing of administration, anesthesiologists should work in consultation with the surgeon to use guidelines determined by the local infection control committee to take initiative for administering prophylactic antibiotics. In this way, anesthesiologists can make a major contribution to preventing surgical site infection. The Centers for Medicare and Medicaid Services has identified timely and appropriate antibiotic prophylaxis administration as a cornerstone of surgical site infection prevention. Physician and hospital reimbursements are increasingly tied to such performance measures, meaning anesthesiologists also have an economic interest in ensuring adherence to guidelines.

MECHANISMS OF WOUND REPAIR

Wound healing is a complex process, requiring a coordinated repair response including inflammation, matrix production, angiogenesis, epithelization, and remodeling (Fig. 13-4). Many factors may impair wound healing. Systemic factors such as medical comorbidities, nutrition,[25,26] sympathetic nervous system activation,[27] and age[28–30] have a substantial effect on the repair process. Local environmental factors in and around the wound including bacterial load,[31] degree of inflammation, moisture content,[32] oxygen tension,[33] and vascular perfusion[34] also have a profound effect on healing. Although all of these factors are important, perhaps the most critical element is oxygen supply to the wound. Wound hypoxia impairs each of the components of healing.[35]

Although the role of oxygen is usually thought of in terms of aerobic respiration and energy production via oxidative phosphorylation, in wound healing oxygen is required as a cofactor for enzymatic processes and for cell-signaling mechanisms. Oxygen is a rate-limiting component in leukocyte-mediated bacterial killing and collagen formation because specific enzymes require oxygen at a partial pressure of at least 40 mm Hg.[36,37] The mechanisms by which the other processes are oxygen-dependent are less clear, but these processes also require oxygen at a concentration much above that required for cellular respiration.[38–41]

The Initial Response to Injury

A surgical incision disrupts the skin barrier, creating an acute wound, and an effective initial response to injury depends on the ability to clean foreign material and to resist infection. This response initiates a sequence of events that starts with any source of injury that disrupts homeostasis in the local environment and eventually leads to healing.

Wound healing has traditionally been described in four separate phases: hemostasis, inflammation, proliferation, and remodeling.[42] Considerable overlap exists between each of these phases, and differentiating precisely when one phase ends and the next begins is virtually impossible. Each phase is composed of complex interactions between host cells, contaminants, cytokines and other chemical mediators that, when functioning properly, lead to repair of injury. These processes are highly conserved across species,[43] indicating the critical importance of the inflammatory response that directs the process of cellular/tissue repair. When any component of healing is disturbed and interrupts the orderly progression of repair, wound failure may result.[44]

Injury damages the local circulation and causes platelets to aggregate and release a variety of substances, including chemoattractants and growth factors.[42] The initial result is coagulation, which prevents exsanguination but also widens the area that is no longer perfused. Platelet degranulation releases platelet-derived growth factor, transforming growth factorbeta (TGF-β), epidermal growth factor, and insulinlike growth factor-1 (IGF-1), which conjointly initiate the inflammatory process.[42] Bradykinin, complement, and histamine released by mast cells cause vasodilation and increased vascular permeability. Polymorphonuclear leukocytes arrive at the wound almost immediately and are followed by macrophages at 24 to 48 hours. These inflammatory cells activate in response to endothelial integrins, selectins, cell adhesion molecules, cadherins, fibrin, lactate, hypoxia, foreign bodies, infectious agents, and growth factors.[42] In turn, macrophages and lymphocytes produce more lactate[45] and growth factors, including IGF-1, leukocyte growth factor, interleukins (ILs) 1 and 2, TGF-β, and vascular endothelial growth factor

TABLE 13-5

UCSF GUIDELINES FOR PROPHYLACTIC ANTIBIOTICS IN ADULT PATIENTS TO REDUCE SURGICAL SITE INFECTION

■ DRUG	■ DOSE	■ TIMING	■ ADDITIONAL DOSE
Hip and Knee Arthroplasty, Extradural Ortho and Neuro Spine, Cardiothoracic, Vascular Surgery and Kidney Transplantation			
Cefazolin*	<80 kg: 1 gm ≥80 kg: 2 gm	<60 min before incision as a bolus over 3–5 min; with bolus dose, tissue levels are adequate in a few minutes	Q 4 hours Exclude Kidney Tx
Neurosurgery (Cranial and Intradural Spine)			
Ceftriaxone*	<80 kg: 1 gm ≥80 kg: 2 gm	<60 min before incision as a bolus over 3–5 min	Q 12 hours
Liver Transplantation			
Ceftriaxone*	<80 kg: 1 gm ≥80 kg: 2 gm	<60 min before incision as a bolus over 3–5 min	Q 12 hours
For Significant Beta Lactam Allergy (anaphylaxis to penicillins)			
Vancomycin or	1 gm	Start infusion on arrival in OR (once monitors are attached); infuse over 30–60 min	Q 12 hours
Clindamycin	<100 kg: 600 mg ≥100 kg: 900 mg	<60 min before incision as infusion over 10–15 min	Q 6 hours
Colon Surgery			
Cefotetan*	<80 kg: 1 gm ≥80 kg: 2 gm	<60 min before incision as a bolus over 3–5 min	Q 6 hours
For significant Beta Lactam Allergy (anaphylaxis to penicillins)			
Ciprofloxacin and	400 mg	<60 min before incision as infusion over 30 min	Q 6 hours
Metronidazole	500 mg		
Vaginal and Abdominal Hysterectomy			
Cefazolin or	<80 kg: 1 gm	<60 min before incision as a bolus over 3–5 min	Q 4 hours
Cefotetan (if bowel involved)	≥80 kg: 2 gm		Q 6 hours
For Significant Beta Lactam Allergy (anaphylaxis to penicillins)			
Ciprofloxacin and	400 mg	<60 min before incision as infusion over 30 min	Q 6 hours
Metronidazole or	500 mg		
Clindamycin and	600 mg	<60 min before incision as infusion over 10–15 min	Q 6 hours
Gentamicin	1.5 mg/kg		

Pediatric Patients—Suggested Dosing

■ DRUG	■ DOSE
Cefazolin	20–30 mg/kg
Ceftriaxone	25 mg/kg
Cefotetan	20–30 mg/kg
Cefuroxime	50 mg/kg
Vancomycin	15 mg/kg (as an infusion over 30–60 min)
Gentamicin	2 mg/kg
Clindamycin	15 mg/kg
Metronidazole	10 mg/kg
Ciprofloxacin	Not recommended

NOTES:
- Always confirm with surgeons at the Time-Out or earlier; in some cases they may wish to delay antibiotics until after culture.
- Make sure dose is in before tourniquet goes up.
- Additional intra-operative dose should also be given in circumstances of significant blood loss.

Used with permission from the University of California, San Francisco Department of Anesthesia and Perioperative Care.

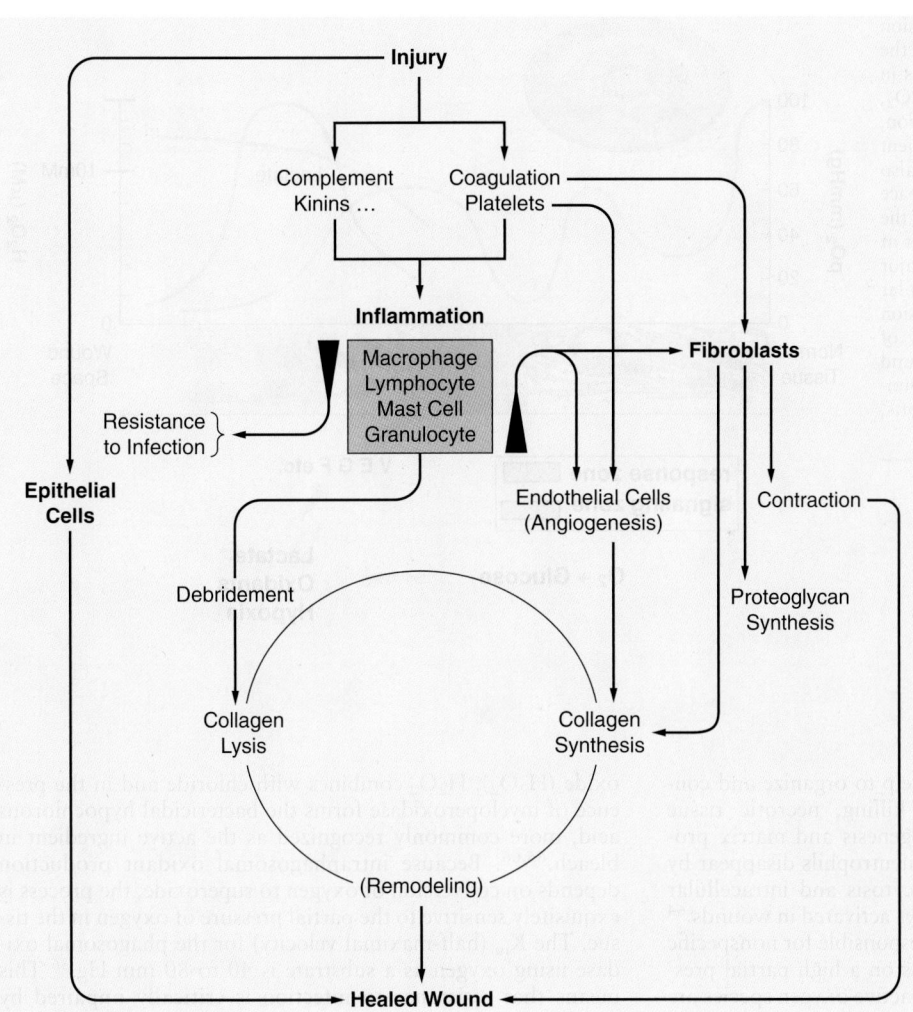

FIGURE 13-4. Schematic of the processes of wound healing. (From Hunt T: Fundamentals of wound management in surgery, Wound Healing: Disorders of Repair. South Plainfield, NJ, Chirugecom, Inc, 1976, with permission.)

ANATOMY AND PHYSIOLOGY

(VEGF).[46] This early inflammatory phase is characterized by erythema and edema of the wound edges.

Activated neutrophils and macrophages also release proteases, including neutrophil elastase, neutrophil collagenase, matrix metalloproteinase, and macrophage metalloelastase.[42] These proteases degrade damaged extracellular matrix components to allow their replacement. Proteases also degrade the basement membrane of capillaries to enable inflammatory cells to migrate into the wound.

In wounds, local blood supply is compromised at the same time that metabolic demand is increased. As a result, the wound environment becomes hypoxic and acidotic with high lactate levels.[47,48] This represents the sum of three effects: (1) decreased oxygen supply due to vascular damage and coagulation, (2) increased metabolic demand due to the heightened cellular response (anaerobic glycolysis), and (3) aerobic glycolysis by inflammatory cells.[49,50] Leukocytes contain few mitochondria and therefore acquire energy from glucose, primarily by production of lactate and even in the presence of adequate oxygen supply.[50] In activated neutrophils, the respiratory burst, in which oxygen and glucose are converted to superoxide, hydrogen ion, and lactate, accounts for up to 98% of oxygen consumption; in the setting of injury, this activity increases by up to 50-fold over baseline.[51,52]

Local hypoxia is a normal and inevitable result of tissue injury.[53,54] Hypoxia acts as a stimulus to repair,[55] but also leads to poor healing[33] and increased susceptibility to infec-

tion.[56,57] Numerous experimental models[16,56–59] as well as human clinical experience[60–62] have led to the conclusion that wound healing is delayed in hypoxic wounds. The partial pressure of oxygen in dermal wounds is heterogeneous, ranging from 0 to 10 mm Hg in the central ("dead space") portion of the wound, to 80 to 100 mm Hg (near arterial) adjacent to perfused arterioles and capillaries[53] (Fig. 13-5). The PO_2 of a given area depends on diffusion of oxygen from perfused capillaries, and thus wound PO_2 depends on capillary density, arterial PO_2, and the metabolic activity of the cells, with some contribution from shifts in the oxyhemoglobin dissociation curve associated with wound pH and temperature.

Resistance to Infection

After a disruption of the normal skin barrier, successful wound healing requires the ability to clear foreign material and resist infection. Neutrophils provide nonspecific immunity and prevent infection. Leukocytes migrate in tissue toward the site of injury via chemotaxis, defined as locomotion oriented along a chemical gradient.[42] Chemical gradients can be produced both exogenously and endogenously. Exogenous gradients result from bacterial products present in contaminated tissues. Endogenous mediators include components of the complement system (C5a), products of lipoxygenase pathway (leukotriene B4), and cytokines (IL-1, 8), along with lactate.[63]

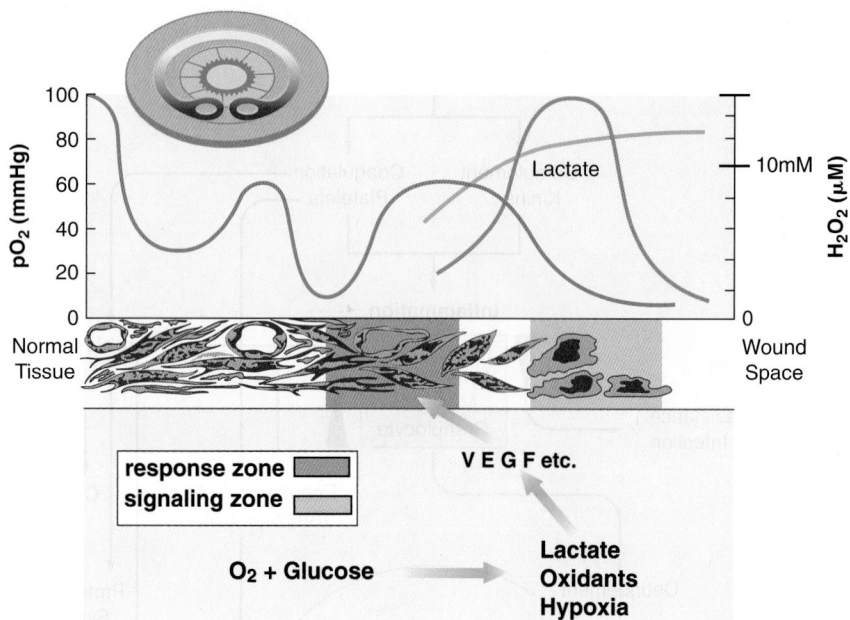

FIGURE 13-5. The varying oxygen tension in the wound module. Cross-section of the wound module in a rabbit ear chamber is in left upper corner of figure. Note that PO₂, depicted graphically above the cross-section, is highest next to the vessels, with a gradient down to zero at the wound edge. Note also the lactate gradient, high in the dead space and lower (but still above plasma) toward the vasculature. Hydrogen peroxide is present at fairly high concentrations and is also a major stimulus to wound repair.[73] VEGF, vascular endothelial growth factor. (Modified version reprinted from IA Silver: The physiology of wound healing, Fundamentals of Wound Management. Edited by TK Hunt, JE Dunphy. New York, Appleton-Century-Crofts, 1980, p 30, with permission.)

Together, these chemical mediators help to organize and control leukocyte invasion, bacterial killing, necrotic tissue removal, and the initiation of angiogenesis and matrix production. In the absence of infection, neutrophils disappear by about 48 hours. Nonspecific phagocytosis and intracellular killing are the major immune pathways activated in wounds.[64]

Neutrophils are the primary cell responsible for nonspecific immunity, and their function depends on a high partial pressure of oxygen.[36,65] This is because reactive oxygen species are the major component of the bactericidal defense against wound pathogens.[64] Phagocytosis of the pathogen activates the phagosomal oxidase (also known as the primary oxidase or nicotinamide adenine dinucleotide phosphate-oxidase [NADPH]-linked oxygenase), present in the phagocytic membrane, which uses oxygen as the substrate to catalyze the formation of superoxide. Superoxide itself is bactericidal, but more importantly it initiates a series of cascades that produce other oxidants within the phagosome that increase bacterial-killing capacity (Fig. 13-6). For example, in the presence of superoxide dismutase, superoxide is reduced to hydrogen per-

oxide (H_2O_2). H_2O_2 combines with chloride and in the presence of myeloperoxidase forms the bactericidal hypochlorous acid, more commonly recognized as the active ingredient in bleach.[65,66] Because intraphagosomal oxidant production depends on conversion of oxygen to superoxide, the process is exquisitely sensitive to the partial pressure of oxygen in the tissue. The K_m (half-maximal velocity) for the phagosomal oxidase using oxygen as a substrate is 40 to 80 mm Hg.[36] This means that resistance to infection is critically impaired by wound hypoxia and becomes more efficient as PO₂ increases even to very high levels (500 to 1,000 mm Hg).[36] Such levels do not occur naturally in tissue, but can be achieved by the administration of hyperbaric oxygen.[67–70] This is one mechanism for the proposed benefit of hyperbaric oxygen therapy as an adjunctive treatment for necrotizing infections and chronic refractory osteomyelitis.[71,72]

Oxidants produced by inflammatory cells have a dual role in wound repair. Not only are they central to resistance to infection, but they also play a major role in initiating and directing the healing process. Oxidants, and in particular

FIGURE 13-6. Schematic of superoxide and other oxidant production within the phagosome. NADPH, nicotinamide adenine dinucleotide phosphate-oxidase; NADP, nicotinamide adenine dinucleotide phosphate; SOD, superoxide dismutase; MP, myeloperoxidase. (From Hunt TK, Hopf HW: Wound healing and wound infection. What surgeons and anesthesiologists can do. Surg Clin North Am 1997; 77(3): 587, with permission.)

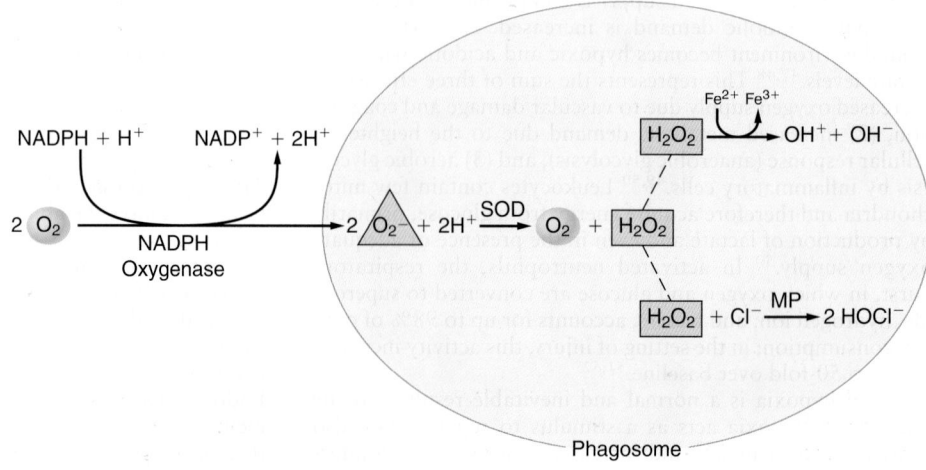

hydrogen peroxide produced via the respiratory burst, increase neovascularization and collagen deposition in vitro and in vivo.[73]

Proliferation

The proliferative phase normally begins approximately 4 days after injury, concurrent with a waning of the inflammatory phase. It consists of granulation tissue formation and epithelization. Granulation involves neovascularization and synthesis of collagen and connective tissue proteins.

Neovascularization

New blood vessels must replace the injured microcirculation. Neovascularization in wounds proceeds both by angiogenesis and vasculogenesis. Angiogenesis is the phenomenon of new vessel growth via budding from existing vessels. In the setting of wounds, new vessels grow from mature vessels, usually intact, postcapillary venules in the undamaged tissue immediately adjacent to the site of injury. Normally, the oxygen tension in adjacent tissue is sufficient to support this process. The new vessel growth extends and enters into the damaged areas that are typically high in lactate and have a low partial pressure of oxygen. Mature extracellular matrix is required for ingrowth of mature vessels.[74]

In vasculogenesis, bone marrow-derived endothelial precursor cells (EPCs) populate the tissue and differentiate and grow into new vessel tubules. In wounds, these tubules appear in the damaged area before any direct anastomosis with preexisting vessels is made. These tubules must connect with existing vasculature to establish an intact blood supply in the wound. Angiogenesis has long been held to be the primary mechanism for new blood vessel growth in granulation tissue. Recent research, however, has demonstrated that as many as 15 to 20% of new blood vessels in wounds are derived from hematopoietic stem cells.[74–76]

Angiogenesis and vasculogenesis both occur in response to similar stimuli, consisting of some combination of redox stress, hypoxia, and lactate. However, the specific mechanisms by which they proceed appear to differ somewhat. Angiogenesis involves the movement of endothelial cells in response to three waves of growth factors. The first wave of growth factors comes with the release by platelets of platelet-derived growth factor, TGF-β, IGF-1, and others during the inflammatory phase. The second wave comes from fibroblast growth factor released from normal binding sites on connective tissue molecules. The third and dominant wave comes from VEGF, delivered largely by macrophages stimulated by fibrinopeptides, hypoxia, and lactate.[77] Although it is usually present, hypoxia is not required for granulation because of constitutive (aerobic) lactate production by inflammatory cells and fibroblasts. Too little lactate leads to inadequate granulation, while levels in excess of about 15 mM—usually associated with inflammation or infection—delay granulation.[78] The capillary endothelial response to angiogenic agents requires oxygen so that angiogenesis progresses in proportion to blood perfusion and arterial PO_2.[79]

Vasculogenesis occurs in response to similar stressors as angiogenesis. EPCs are mobilized from the bone marrow into the circulation via a nitric oxide-mediated mechanism. Tissue hypoxia induces release of VEGF-A, which activates bone marrow stromal nitric oxide synthase. Increased bone marrow nitric oxide leads to release of EPCs into the circulation. These circulating EPCs home to the wound via tissue-hypoxia–induced up-regulation of stromal cell-derived factor 1-α. Within the wound, EPCs undergo differentiation and participate in the formation of new blood vessels.[75]

Collagen and Extracellular Matrix Deposition

New blood vessels grow into the matrix that is produced by fibroblasts. Although fibroblasts replicate and migrate mainly in response to growth factors and chemoattractants, production of mature collagen requires oxygen.[37,80,81] Lactate, hypoxia, and some growth factors induce collagen mRNA synthesis and procollagen production. Posttranslational modification by prolyl and lysyl hydroxylases is required to allow collagen peptides to aggregate into triple helices. Collagen can only be exported from the cell when it is in this triple helical structure. The helical configuration is also primarily responsible for tissue strength. The activity of the hydroxylases is critically dependent on vitamin C and tissue oxygen tension, with a K_m for oxygen of about 25 mm Hg.[37,80–82] Wound strength, which results from collagen deposition, is therefore highly vulnerable to wound hypoxia.[33]

Neovascularization and extracellular matrix (primarily collagen) production are closely linked. Fibroblasts cannot produce mature collagen in the absence of mature blood vessels that deliver oxygen to the site. New blood vessels cannot mature without a strong collagen matrix. Mice kept in a hypoxic environment of 13% inspired oxygen develop some new blood vessels in a test wound with the addition of exogenous VEGF or lactate, but these vessels are immature with little surrounding matrix and demonstrate frequent areas of hemorrhage.[41]

Epithelization

Epithelization is characterized by replication and migration of epithelial cells across the skin edges in response to growth factors. Cell migration may begin from any site that contains living keratinocytes, including remnants of hair follicles, sebaceous glands, islands of living epidermis, or the normal wound edge. In acute wounds that are primarily closed, epithelization is normally completed in 1 to 3 days. In open wounds healing by secondary intention, epithelization is the final phase of healing and cannot progress until the wound bed is fully granulated. Like immunity and granulation, epithelization depends on growth factors and oxygen. Silver[83] and Medawar[40] demonstrated in vivo that the rate of epithelization depends on local oxygen. Topical oxygen applied in a manner that does not dry out epithelial cells has been advocated as a method to increase the rate of epithelization.[84] Ngo et al.[85] demonstrated oxygen-dependent differentiation and cell growth in human keratinocyte culture. In contrast, O'Toole et al.[86] demonstrated that hypoxia increases epithelial migration in vitro. This may be explained, at least in part, by the dependence of epithelization on the presence of a bed of healthy granulation tissue, which is known to be oxygen-dependent.

Maturation and Remodeling

The final phase of wound repair is maturation, which involves ongoing remodeling of the granulation tissue and increasing wound tensile strength. As the matrix becomes denser with thicker, stronger collagen fibrils, it becomes stiffer and less compliant. Fibroblasts are capable of adapting to changing mechanical stress and loading. Fibroblasts migrate throughout the matrix to help mold the wound to new stresses. Matrix metalloproteinases and other proteases help with fibroblast migration and continued matrix remodeling in response to mechanical stress. Some fibroblasts differentiate into myofibroblasts under the influence of TGF-β, resulting in contractile cells. As the myofibroblasts contract, the collagenous matrix cross-links in the shortened position. This helps to strengthen the matrix and minimize scar size. Contraction is inhibited by the use of high doses of corticosteroids.[87] Even steroids given several days after injury have this effect. In those wounds where contraction is detrimental, this effect can be used for benefit.

Net collagen synthesis continues for at least 6 weeks and up to 6 months after wounding. Over time, the initial collagen threads are reabsorbed and deposited along stress lines, conferring greater tensile strength. Collagen found in granulation tissue is biochemically different from collagen of uninjured skin, and a scar never achieves the tensile strength of uninjured skin. Hydroxylation and glycosylation of lysine residues in granulation tissue collagen lead to thinner collagen fibers. At 1 week, a wound closed by primary intention has only reached 3% of the tensile strength of normal skin. By 3 weeks it is at 30%, and it only reaches 80% after 3 to 6 months.

Some wounds heal to excess. Hypertrophic scar and keloid are common forms of abnormal scar due to abnormal responses to healing. Hypertrophic scarring may be thought of as "exuberant" scarring in which the inflammatory process that allows wound healing remains excessively active, resulting in stiff, rubbery, nonmobile scar tissue. Hypertrophic scars are most commonly seen following burns and are thought to correlate with the length of time required to close the wound, although other factors are also believed to play a role and are being actively explored. Keloids are scars that outgrow the boundaries of the initial scar, and are most typically seen following surgical incisions. Keloid formation is most likely due to a genetic predisposition, although exogenous inflammatory factors may also play a role.

WOUND PERFUSION AND OXYGENATION

Complications of wounds include failure to heal, infection, and excessive scarring or contracture. Rapid repair has the least potential for infection and excess scarring. The perioperative physician's goals, therefore, are to avoid contamination, ensure rapid tissue synthesis, and optimize the immune response. All surgical procedures lead to some degree of contamination that must be controlled by local host defenses. The initial hours after contamination represent a decisive period during which inadequate local defenses may allow an infection to become established.

Normally, wounds on the extremities and trunk heal more slowly than those on the face. The major difference in these wounds is the degree of tissue perfusion and thus the wound tissue oxygen tension. As a rule, repair proceeds most rapidly and immunity is strongest when wound oxygen levels are high, and this is only achieved by maintaining perfusion of injured tissue.[88] Ischemic or hypoxic tissue, on the other hand, is highly susceptible to infection and heals poorly, if at all. Wound tissue oxygenation is complex and depends on the interaction of blood perfusion, arterial oxygen tension, hemoglobin dissociation conditions, carrying capacity, mass transfer resistances, and local oxygen consumption. Wound oxygen delivery depends on vascular anatomy, the degree of vasoconstriction, and arterial PO_2.

7 The standard teaching that oxygen delivery depends more on hemoglobin-bound oxygen (oxygen content) than on arterial PO_2 may be true of working muscle, but it is not true of wound healing. In muscle, intercapillary distances are small and oxygen consumption is high. In contrast, intercapillary distances are large and oxygen consumption is relatively low in subcutaneous tissue.[38] In wounds, where the microvasculature is damaged, diffusion distances are substantially increased. Peripheral vasoconstriction further increases diffusion distance.[53] The driving force of diffusion is partial pressure. Hence, a high PO_2 is needed to force oxygen into injured and healing tissues, particularly in subcutaneous tis-

sue, fascia, tendon, and bone, the tissues most at risk for poor healing.

8 Although oxygen consumption is relatively low in wounds, it is consumed by processes that require oxygen at a high concentration. Inflammatory cells use little oxygen for respiration, producing energy largely via the hexose-monophosphate shunt.[36] Most of the oxygen consumed in wounds is used for oxidant production (bacterial killing), with a significant contribution as well for collagen synthesis, angiogenesis, and epithelization. The rate constants (K_m) for oxygen for these components of repair all fall within the physiologic range of 25 to 100 mm Hg.[36,37,40,65,80,89]

Because of the high rate constants for oxygen substrate for the components of repair, the rate at which repair proceeds varies according to tissue PO_2 from zero to at least 250 mm Hg. In vitro fibroblast replication is optimal at a PO_2 of about 40 to 60 mm Hg. Neutrophils lose their ability to kill bacteria in vitro below a PO_2 of about 40 mm Hg.[90,91] These in vitro observations are clinically relevant. "Normal" subcutaneous PO_2, measured in test wounds in uninjured, euthermic, euvolemic volunteers breathing room air, is 65 ± 7 mm Hg.[92] Thus, any reduction in wound PO_2 may impair immunity and repair. In surgical patients, the rate of wound infections is inversely proportional[56] and collagen deposition is directly proportional[33] to postoperative subcutaneous wound tissue oxygen tension.

9 High oxygen tensions (>100 mm Hg) can be reached in wounds but only if perfusion is rapid and arterial PO_2 is high.[33,88] This is because subcutaneous tissue serves a reservoir function, so there is normally flow in excess of nutritional needs and wound cells consume relatively little oxygen, about 0.7 mL/100 mL of blood flow at a normal perfusion rate.[38,39] When arterial oxygen tension (PaO_2) is high, this small volume can be carried by plasma alone. Contrary to popular belief, therefore, oxygen-carrying capacity, that is, hemoglobin concentration, is not particularly important to wound healing, provided that perfusion is normal.[93,94] Wound PO_2 and collagen synthesis remain normal in individuals who have hematocrit levels as low as 15 to 18% provided they can appropriately increase cardiac output and vasoconstriction is **10** prevented.[94,95]

Peripheral vasoconstriction, which results from central sympathetic control of subcutaneous vascular tone, is probably the most frequent and clinically the most important impediment to wound oxygenation. Subcutaneous tissue is both a reservoir to maintain central volume and a major site of thermoregulation. There is little local regulation of blood flow, except by local heating.[96,97] Therefore, subcutaneous tissue is particularly vulnerable to vasoconstriction. Sympathetically induced peripheral vasoconstriction is stimulated by cold, pain, fear, and blood volume deficit,[98,99] and by various pharmacologic agents including nicotine,[92] β-adrenergic antagonists, and α_1-agonists, all commonly present in the perioperative environment. Perioperative hypothermia is common and results from anesthetic drugs, exposure to cold, and redistribution of body heat from the core to the periphery.[100] Blood loss and increases in insensible losses increase fluid requirements in the perioperative period, thereby leaving the patient vulnerable to inadequate fluid replacement. Thus, vasomotor tone is, to a large degree, under the perioperative physician's control.[98,99]

11 Prevention or correction of hypothermia[101] and blood volume deficits[102] have been shown to decrease wound infections and increase collagen deposition in patients undergoing major abdominal surgery. Preoperative systemic (forced air warmer) or local (warming bandage) warming have also been shown to decrease wound infections, even in clean, low-risk surgeries such as breast surgery and inguinal hernia repair.[103] Subcutaneous tissue oxygen tension is significantly higher in patients with good pain control than those with poor pain control after arthroscopic knee surgery.[104] Stress also causes wound hypoxia and significantly impairs wound healing and resistance to infection.[105,106] These effects are clearly mediated, in large part, by changes in the partial pressure of oxygen in the injured tissue.

Greif et al.[107] demonstrated in a randomized, controlled, double-blind trial including 500 patients that in warm, volume-replete patients with good pain control undergoing major colon surgery, administration of 80% versus 30% oxygen intraoperatively and for the first 2 postoperative hours significantly reduced the wound infection rate by 50%. Belda et al.[108] replicated these results (significant 40% reduction in surgical site infection) in a randomized, controlled, double-blind trial in 300 colon surgery patients randomized to 80% versus 30% oxygen intraoperatively and during the first 6 postoperative hours. Surgical and anesthetic management were standardized and intended to support optimal perfusion. Myles et al.[109] demonstrated a significant reduction in major postoperative complications, as well as specifically wound infections in 2,050 major surgery patients randomized to 80% oxygen versus 30% oxygen in 70% nitrous oxide intraoperatively. A smaller (n = 165) randomized, controlled study by Pryor et al.,[110] demonstrated a doubling of surgical site infection in patients randomized to 80% versus 35% oxygen intraoperatively. There were a number of methodologic flaws in the study, but, more importantly, the two groups of patients were not equivalent, which likely explained the increase in infections seen in the 80% oxygen group. Thus, the preponderance of evidence indicates that use of high inspired oxygen intraoperatively and providing supplemental oxygen postoperatively in *well-perfused* patients undergoing major abdominal surgery will reduce the risk of wound infection.

Delivery of antibiotics also depends on perfusion. Parenteral antibiotics given so that high levels are present in the blood at the time of wounding clearly diminish but do not eliminate wound infections.[20] In about one third of all wound infections, the bacteria cultured from the wound are sensitive to the prophylactic antibiotic given to the patient, even when the antibiotics were given according to standard procedure.[20] The vulnerable third of patients appear to be the hypoxic and vasoconstricted group. When antibiotics are present in the wound at the time of injury, they are trapped in the fibrin clot at the wound site where they may have efficacy against contaminating organisms. Antibiotics diffuse poorly into the fibrin clot, however, so that later administration, whether more than 2 hours after injury or in response to wound infection, will have little effect. On the other hand, oxygen diffuses easily through the fibrin clots and is effective even 6 hours after contamination.[18]

Role of Dysregulation in Impaired Wound Healing

Human beings challenged by adverse physical or psychosocial events mount a coordinated, adaptive reaction characterized by physiological arousal. This response is often associated psychologically with the experience of threat or other negative affect. The term for such an arousal reaction is *stress response*, and any event that triggers such a response is a stressor. The major mechanisms of the stress response are the hypothalamo-pituitary-adrenocortical (HPA) axis and the sympatho-adrenomedullary (SAM) axis.[111] Psychosocial stressors evoke cognitive responses such as appraisal, memory, expectation, and the attribution of meaning. These endogenous processes heavily involve the prefrontal and frontal cortices of the brain, and these cortices exert control over aspects of the hypothalamus, including the periventricular nucleus (PVN). The PVN initiates the HPA stress response and controls it through nega-

tive feedback mechanisms. The PVN triggers further stress response in the SAM axis by recruiting catecholaminergic cells in the rostral ventrolateral medulla. This structure is a cardiovascular regulatory area involved, together with the solitary nucleus, in the control of blood pressure. The rostral ventrolateral medulla activates the solitary nucleus and, together with it, provides tonic excitatory drive to sympathetic vasoconstrictor nerves that maintain resting blood pressure levels. A normal stress response involves a complex pattern of autonomic arousal that includes increased blood pressure followed by a period of recovery when blood pressure and other aspects of arousal return to normal.

Human life is complex and often involves repetitive stressors or a series of stressors. When the HPA axis must mount a new stress response before the previous stress response has fully recovered, it incurs risk of system dysregulation. That is, processes normally self-regulating through negative feedback become unregulated and dysfunctional, with maladaptive consequences. SAM dysregulation, which may involve altered medullary GABAergic neurotransmission,[112] can result in abnormal blood flow of indefinite duration. This, in turn, can compromise oxygenation of the healing wound.

PATIENT MANAGEMENT

Preoperative Preparation

Given knowledge of the physiology of wound healing, what are the best strategies to ensure optimal healing? Wound infection, healing failure, and dehiscence are dreaded complications of surgery. To the degree they are predictable, interventions can be targeted at those patients most at risk (Table 13-6).

The CDC, in the "Study of the Effect of Nosocomial Infection Control" (SENIC),[113] developed a remarkably useful and simple predictive tool based on a score of 0 or 1 for each of the following four patient factors: an abdominal operation, an operation that lasts 2 hours or more, a surgical site that is contaminated or infected, and a patient who will have three or more diagnoses at discharge, exclusive of wound infection. The risk of infection with a score of 0 is 1%, with a score of 1 is 3.6%, with a score of 2 is 9%, with a score of 3 is 17%, and with a score of 4 is 27%. These percentages may seem high, but this index was constructed on 3% of the American surgical patients in 1975–1976 and 1983, and the overall results are

TABLE 13-6

PREOPERATIVE CHECKLIST

- Assess and optimize cardiopulmonary function. Correct hypertension.
- Treat vasoconstriction: Attend to blood volume, thermoregulatory vasoconstriction, pain, and anxiety.
- Assess recent nutrition and treat as appropriate.
- Treat existing infection. Among other actions, clean and treat skin infections.
- Assess wound risk by SENIC[a] score in order to decide on the extent to which prophylactic measures should be taken.
- Start vitamin A or anabolic steroids in patients taking prednisone.
- Improve or maintain blood sugar control.

[a]See text and reference 113.
From Hunt TK, Hopf HW: Wound healing and wound infection. What surgeons and anesthesiologists can do. Surgical Clinics of North America 1997;77:587, with permission.

consistent with numerous other studies. More recent risk analyses by the same group, based on simpler predictors (e.g., American Society of Anesthesiologists Physical Status Classification) have yielded less sensitivity, but about the same overall infection rate.[114]

12 Modifiable risks include smoking, malnutrition, hyperglycemia, hypercholesterolemia, and hypertension. These should be assessed and corrected when possible prior to surgery. The decision to delay surgery must take into account both the urgency of the surgery and the severity of the risk.

Stress dysregulation also predisposes to poor wound healing. Human and murine studies are consistent in showing that exposing a subject to a stressor delays wound repair. Animal stress models typically involve restraint or social disruption, while human models usually employ a public speaking challenge.[115] Laboratory stress is short term and associated with increased cortisol and corticosterone levels that down-regulate the early inflammatory response. This directly implicates the HPA axis, but the background processes are more extensive. Human studies can also take advantage of naturally occurring stressors such as academic examination or marital discord. Such studies compare stressed and non-stressed populations in rate of healing following a punch biopsy or induced blister. This approach allows investigators to study chronic conditions associated with dysregulation such as depression.

The mechanisms behind wound healing are more extensive than altered HPA axis function alone, and so negative clinical outcomes can take multiple forms. The nervous, endocrine, and immune systems operate interdependently through a common chemical language composed of neurotransmitters, hormones, cytokines, peptides, and endocannabinoids.[111] Simple stress can slow wound healing, but stress-induced dysregulation can lead to enduring dysfunction in autonomic nervous system, endocrine function, and/or immune function. Immune complications include impaired bacterial clearance at the wound,[105] the sickness responses associated with proinflammatory cytokines,[116] and systemic imbalance in the T-helper 1/T-helper 2 (Th1/Th2) cytokine profile. This profile represents balance in the contributions of helper T-cell subsets: Th1 is proinflammatory and Th2 anti-inflammatory. Th1-dominant imbalance indicates excessive inflammation with resultant fatigue, aching joints, and loss of appetite. Surgery sometimes creates a Th2 imbalance, which puts the patient at risk for sepsis, edema, and other complications such as poor sleep. Th1/Th2 balance normally recovers after surgery, but some patients come to surgery already chronically dysregulated in cytokine profile, which may predispose them to poor wound healing and other negative outcomes.

Adverse psychosocial circumstances at the time of surgery may put patients at risk for poor wound healing. Kiecolt-Glaser et al.[117] studied the impact of hostile marital interactions on the healing of experimental blister wounds. High-hostile couples produced more proinflammatory cytokines and healed more slowly than low-hostile couples. Using a tape-stripping model, Muizzuddin et al.[118] investigated the effect of marital dissolution on skin barrier recovery and found that high stress was associated with slower recovery. Bosch and colleagues[119] studied the healing of a circular wound on the oral hard palate in subjects who varied in depression and/or dysphoria. High-dysphoric individuals had higher wound sizes from day 2 onward and depressive symptoms predicted slower wound healing. Collectively, these studies point to links between psychosocial distress, dysregulation at the system level, and impaired capacity for wound healing. It seems likely that stress-reduction techniques will reduce wound complications, and well-designed clinical trials are needed in this area.

Intraoperative Management

Careful surgical technique is fundamental to optimal wound healing (Table 13-7). Delicate handling of the tissue, adequate hemostasis, and surgeon experience lead to healthier wounds. Incisions should be planned with regard to blood supply, particularly when operating near or in old incisions. Mechanical retractors should be released from time to time to allow perfusion to the wound edges. Judicious antibiotic irrigation of contaminated areas may be effective. Because dried wounds lose perfusion, wounds should be kept moist, especially during long operations. Not all wounds can be anatomically closed. Edema, obesity, the possibility of unacceptable respiratory compromise, or need to debride grossly contaminated or necrotic soft tissues can all interfere with closure of the wound.

As the operation proceeds, new wounds are made and contamination continues. All anesthetic agents tend to cause hypothermia—first, by causing vasodilation, which redistributes heat from core to periphery in previously vasoconstricted patients, and secondly by increasing heat loss and decreasing heat production.[100] Vasoconstriction is uncommon intraoperatively, as the threshold for thermoregulatory vasoconstriction is decreased, but is often severe in the immediate postoperative period when anesthesia is discontinued and the thermoregulatory threshold returns to normal in the face of core hypothermia. The onset of pain with emergence from anesthesia adds to this vasoconstriction because of the associated catecholamine release.[104] Rapid rewarming using a forced air warmer for hypothermic patients in the postanesthesia care unit (PACU) does appear to be effective,[120] although prevention of
13 hypothermia is clearly the goal.[101] Maintenance of a high room temperature or forced air warming before, during, and after the operation is significantly more effective than other methods of warming such as circulating water blankets placed under the patient and humidification of the breathing circuit.[121]

Volume Management

Surgical stress results in increased intravenous fluid requirements. The increased fluid requirement may be partly due to substances like IL-6, TNF, substance-P, and bradykinin, which are released in response to, and in proportion to, surgical stress.[122] These inflammatory mediators cause both vasodilation and an

---

TABLE 13-7

INTRAOPERATIVE MANAGEMENT

- Appropriate prophylactic antibiotics should be given at the start of any procedure in which infection is highly probable and/or has potentially disastrous consequences. Maintain antibiotic levels during long operations.
- Keep patients warm.
- Observe gentle surgical technique with minimal use of ties and cautery.
- Keep wounds moist.
- Antibiotic irrigation in contaminated cases.
- Elevate PaO_2.
- Delayed closure for heavily contaminated wounds.
- Use appropriate sutures (and skin tapes).
- Use appropriate dressings.

From Hunt TK, Hopf HW: Wound healing and wound infection. What surgeons and anesthesiologists can do. Surgical Clinics of North America 1997;77:587, with permission.

increase in vascular permeability.[123] This loss of functional intravascular volume is in addition to other known causes of perioperative hypovolemia or fluid loss. These include preoperative mechanical bowel preparation, lack of oral intake, fever, pre-existing medical conditions, and medications such as diuretics, as well surgical fluid losses, which include evaporation and blood loss.

There are known serious complications of both hypervolemia and hypovolemia, particularly in the perioperative period. The major complications associated with hypervolemia include pulmonary edema, congestive heart failure, edema of gut with prolonged ileus, and possibly an increase in cardiac arrhythmias.[124] The major complications of hypovolemia, aside from hemodynamic instability, include decreased oxygenation of surgical wounds (which predisposes to wound infection),[33,56,88,125–127] decreased collagen formation,[33,102] impaired wound healing, and increased wound breakdown.

14 Optimizing the volume of perioperative fluid administration to minimize morbidity and mortality remains a significant and controversial challenge. Estimates of blood loss, third-space fluid losses, and maintenance requirements are notoriously inaccurate and may lead to either over- or underreplacement if used as guides. Currently, most practitioners rely on clinical acumen, vital signs such as heart rate and blood pressure, and urine output to manage perioperative fluids. Surgical patients can be markedly hypovolemic without a change in any one of these variables because of the compensatory action of peripheral vasoconstriction,[33,88,127] Unfortunately, this shunts blood away from skin, increases wound hypoxemia, and increases the risk of surgical wound infection.[56] Kabon et al.[128] performed a randomized, controlled trial to compare standard (8 mL/kg/hr) versus high (16 to 18 mL/kg/hr) volume administration in 253 patients undergoing elective colon resection. They found a trend toward reduced wound infections in the group that received high volume (8.5 vs. 11.3%), which would be a clinically significant reduction. Unfortunately, the study was terminated early, so it had inadequate power. Patients at high risk for heart failure or with end-stage renal disease were excluded, so the study also has limited generalizability.

A number of methods, both invasive and minimally invasive, have been investigated as more sensitive measures of volume status. Hartmann et al.[102] used subcutaneous PO_2 to guide perioperative volume management in a randomized controlled trial in abdominal surgery patients. Patients randomized to the intervention group (vs. usual management) received more fluid, had significantly higher wound oxygen tension, and deposited more collagen in a test wound.

Pulmonary arterial catheters have also been used in an attempt to optimize volume management, generally with little success. Most of these studies were performed in an ICU setting, rather than during surgery. In one study in 4,059 patients undergoing abdominal surgery,[123] those who received a pulmonary artery (PA) catheter had worse outcomes than those who did not. In fact, the rate of major postoperative cardiac events was 15.4% in the PA catheter group versus 3.6% in the control group. This could be partly due to the observation that many clinicians misinterpret PA data.[129] With recent studies demonstrating a lack of patient benefit with PA catheters and the increase in use and availability of less invasive monitors like echocardiography, the future of these catheters is uncertain.[130]

Esophageal doppler has been advocated as a useful monitor of intraoperative volume status. Mythen and Webb[131] used esophageal doppler to optimize intraoperative volume management in 60 cardiac patients and demonstrated that the patients with esophageal doppler-guided fluid management received more IV fluid and had decreased gut hypoperfusion (7 vs. 56%) compared with traditional management. There were also fewer "major complications" (0 vs. 6), although the study was too small to achieve statistical significance. Sinclair et al.[132] randomized 40 patients undergoing surgical repair of proximal femoral fractures to esophageal doppler-guided volume management or traditional management. The patients with the doppler-guided fluid management had faster recoveries and more rapid hospital discharge. Esophageal doppler can be difficult to use reliably. However, the same principles that are used in esophageal doppler are available in much more advanced technologies like transesophageal echocardiography. Thus, TEE shows promise for guiding volume management in both cardiac and non-cardiac surgeries. Identification of the appropriate markers and interventions, however, remains inadequately studied.

A final topic of debate is whether colloids or crystalloids are preferable for intraoperative fluid administration. Synthetic colloids have been associated with coagulopathy when large volumes are delivered, which appears to be in large part mediated by dilution of coagulation factors.[133] Crystalloids, on the other hand, may cause a hypercoagulable state.[134] The intravascular half-life of colloids, either albumin or synthetic colloids, is much longer than that of crystalloids, allowing the total volume of fluid administered to be reduced by including colloids in surgical fluid resuscitation.[135] Edema formation may also be decreased. A number of studies[124,135,136] purport to evaluate intraoperative or postoperative fluid administration in terms of restrictive versus traditional fluid management. Virtually all have compared colloid ("restrictive" group) with crystalloid ("traditional" group) administration. Thus, the "restricted" volume group likely received a larger amount of effective intravascular volume than the traditional or "liberal" group. In general, these studies have demonstrated improved outcomes (reduction in SSI, earlier return of bowel function) for the colloid group. The mechanism for the benefit is unclear, however, as on the basis of effective intravascular volume delivered, the crystalloid groups might actually have been less well volume replaced than the colloid groups.

15 Current best recommendations include replacing fluid losses based on standard recommendations (Table 13-8) for the type of surgery, replacement of blood loss, and replacement of other ongoing fluid losses (e.g., high urine output due to diuretic or dye administration, hyperglycemia, or thermoregulatory vasoconstriction). Maintenance of normothermia is

TABLE 13-8

STANDARD VOLUME MANAGEMENT GUIDELINES FOR SURGICAL PATIENTS

Fluid Requirement = Deficit + Maintenance (baseline plus replacement) + estimated blood loss and other sensible fluid losses

Deficit = Maintenance (1.5 mL/kg/hr) × hours NPO
Adjust for fever, high NG output, bowel preparation, and other sources of ongoing preoperative increased fluid loss
Replace EBL 3: 1 with crystalloid, 1: 1 with colloid

Maintenance requirements for different surgeries:
Superficial surgical trauma: 1–2 mL/kg/hr
    Peripheral surgery
Minimal Surgical Trauma: 3–4 mL/kg/hr
    Head and neck, hernia, knee surgery
Moderate Surgical Trauma: 5–6 mL/kg/hr
    Major surgery without exposed abdominal contents
Severe surgical trauma: 8–10 mL/kg/hr (or more)
    Major abdominal, especially with exposed abdominal contents

NPO, nothing by mouth; NG, nasogastric; EBL, estimated blood loss.

also critical to optimal volume management. Warm patients are unlikely to develop pulmonary edema with a high rate of fluid administration because they have excess capacitance due to vasodilation. Cold patients, on the other hand, are highly susceptible to pulmonary edema even after relatively small fluid boluses. Thermoregulatory vasoconstriction increases afterload, causing increased cardiac work. Moreover, administered fluid cannot open up constricted vessels until the hypothermic stimulus is removed; thus, there is virtually no excess capacitance in the system.

Pain control should be addressed intraoperatively so that patients do not have severe pain on emergence. Achieving the goal is more important than the technique used to do so. Although regional anesthesia and analgesia may provide superior pain relief, the effects of specific analgesic regimens on wound outcome have not yet been adequately studied.

Postoperative Management

16 Wounds are most vulnerable in the first few hours after surgery (Table 13-9). Although antibiotics lose their effectiveness after the first hours, oxygen-mediated natural wound immunity lasts longer.[17] Even a short period of vasoconstriction during the first day is sufficient to reduce oxygen supply and increase infection risk.[56] Correction and prevention of vasoconstriction in the first 24 to 48 hours after surgery will have significant beneficial effects.[56] Strict glycemic control is also important,[137] although the best method to achieve this in the non-ICU setting has not yet been established.

17 All vasoconstrictive stimuli must be corrected simultaneously to allow optimal healing. Volume is the last to be corrected because vasoconstriction for other reasons induces diuresis and renders the patient relatively hypovolemic (peripherally, not centrally). These measures are particularly important in any patients at high risk for wound complications for other reasons (e.g., malnutrition, steroid use, diabetes), or when vasoconstrictive drugs such as beta-blockers and α-agonists are required for other reasons.

18 Local perfusion is not assured until patients have a normal blood volume, are warm and pain-free, and are receiving no vasoconstrictive drugs; that is, until the sympathetic nervous system is inactivated. Warming should continue until patients are thoroughly awake and active and can maintain their own

TABLE 13-9

POSTOPERATIVE MANAGEMENT

- Keep patients warm.
- Provide analgesia to keep patients comfortable, if not pain-free. Patient report and the ability to move freely are the best signs of adequate pain relief.
- Only one more dose of antibiotic unless an infection is present or contamination continues.
- Keep up with third-space losses. Remember that fever increases fluid losses.
- Assess perfusion and react to abnormalities.
- Avoid diuresis until pain is gone and patient is warm.
- Assess losses (including thermal losses) if wound is open.
- Assess need for parenteral or enteral nutrition and respond.
- Continue to control hypertension and hyperglycemia.

From Hunt TK, Hopf HW: Wound healing and wound infection. What surgeons and anesthesiologists can do. Surgical Clinics of North America 1997;77:587, with permission.

thermal balance. After major operations, warming may be useful for many hours or even days. The goal is to achieve warmth at the skin; wound vasoconstriction due to cold surroundings often coexists with core hyperthermia. Moderate hyperthermia is not, itself, a problem. When extensive wounds are left open, warmth should be continued, and heat losses due to evaporation should be prevented to avoid vasoconstriction and to minimize caloric losses.

19 Assessing perfusion, especially in the PACU, is critical. Unfortunately, urine output is a poor, often misleading guide to peripheral perfusion.[126] Markedly low output may indicate decreased renal perfusion, but normal or even high urine output has little correlation to wound or tissue PO_2. Many factors commonly present in the perioperative period, including hyperglycemia, dye administration, thermoregulatory vasoconstriction, adrenal insufficiency, and various drugs, may cause inappropriate diuresis in the face of mild hypovolemia.

20 Physical examination of the patient is a better guide to hypovolemia and vasoconstriction. Assess vasoconstriction by a capillary return time of >2 to 3 seconds at the forehead and >5 seconds over the patella. Eye turgor is another good measure of volume status. Finally, patients can usually distinguish thirst from a dry mouth. Skin should be warm and dry.

After major abdominal surgery, third-space losses continue for about 12 to 24 hours, so that increased fluid requirements continue. In general, for large abdominal cases, 2 to 3 mL/kg/hr of IV fluids is sufficient for the first 12 to 24 postoperative hours. After that period, the IV rate should be decreased below calculated maintenance levels because edema fluid begins to be mobilized, thus increasing circulating intravascular volume.

When excessive tissue fluids have accumulated, diuresis should be undertaken gently so that transcapillary refill can maintain blood volume. This applies to patients who need renal dialysis as well. The average dialysis patient vasoconstricts sufficiently to lower tissue PO_2 by 30% or more during dialysis and needs about 24 hours to return vasomotor tone and wound and tissue PO_2 to normal.[138] Fluid losses from the vascular system are not necessarily replaced from the tissues as rapidly as they are sustained. Tissue edema may be the price paid for adequate intravascular volume. Edema increases intracapillary distance, so that there may be a delicate balance between excessive edema and peripheral vasoconstriction (which worsens the hypoxia caused by edema).

Vasoconstrictive drugs should be avoided. The most common and most avoidable is nicotine in the form of cigarettes. Beta-blockers should be used only when clearly medically indicated.[139] Both are known to reduce wound and tissue PO_2. Clonidine is an alternative drug for heart rate control[140-142] that also induces vasodilation and may increase wound PO_2.[143] High-dose α-adrenergic agonists or other vasopressors may cause harm by decreasing tissue PO_2, but in a limited experience we have found that lower doses have little or no effect on wound/tissue PO_2. It is important to remember that decreasing cardiac output may also reduce wound perfusion. Thus, a balance must be maintained between minimizing use of vasopressors and maintaining adequate cardiac output.

21 Maintenance of tissue PO_2 requires attention to pulmonary function postoperatively. Administration of supplemental oxygen via face mask or nasal cannulae increases safety in patients receiving systemic opioids.[144] As a side benefit it may also improve wound healing, although this has not been formally studied. Pain control also appears important since it favorably influences both pulmonary function and vascular tone. This is particularly true in patients at high risk for pulmonary complications postoperatively, such as morbidly obese patients and those with pulmonary disease.[145] Epidural analgesia may be the route of choice in these patients. It has several advantages over parenterally administered opioids in that it generally achieves lower pain scores with less sedation. Nonetheless, opioid-induced pruritus is more common with epidural administration, and in some patients may be severe enough to counteract the benefits of pain control.

Patient-controlled analgesia is also quite effective at achieving low pain scores. It also has the benefit of giving control to the patient, leading to patient satisfaction as high as with epidural analgesia in many cases.[146] Nurse-administered, as-needed doses of IV or intramuscular opioids should be avoided as inadequate pain control often exceeds 50% using this approach.[147] The key to pain control is recognition of the need for analgesia and attention to the patient's complaints of pain. Opioid requirements vary enormously and are not always predictable, but even tolerant patients (IV drug abusers or those with cancer pain) can be given adequate pain relief with sufficient attention.

SUMMARY

22 In patients with moderate to high risk of surgical site infection, anesthesiologists have the opportunity to enhance wound healing and reduce the incidence of wound infections by simple, inexpensive, and readily available means. Intraoperatively, appropriate antibiotic use, prevention of vasoconstriction through volume and warming, and maintenance of a high PaO_2 (300 to 500 mm Hg) are key. Postoperatively, the focus should remain on prevention of vasoconstriction through pain relief, warming, and adequate volume administration in the PACU. The addition of measures to reduce and prevent the stress response is likely to be effective as well, although further study is required.

Areas for Future Research

- When and why should a mask be worn in the OR?
- Should IVs be placed using sterile technique? A-lines?
- Is delay of antibiotics for culture justified?
- Can you modulate more than the sympathetic nervous system?
- Psychological preparation and intervention can modulate both HPA axis and SAM axis aspects of the stress response. Will this reduce wound complications?
- Do nonsteroidal anti-inflammatory agents increase risk of wound complications?
- Does dexamethasone for postoperative nausea and vomiting prophylaxis increase the risk of wound complications?
- Do epidurals reduce the risk of SSI? Are they cost-effective (vs. time and risk)?
- Who should get a high FIO_2? Is there potential toxicity?
- Does postoperative oxygen reduce wound complications? How long should patients receive supplemental oxygen postoperatively?

References

1. Kaye KS, Sands K, Donahue JG, et al: Preoperative drug dispensing as predictor of surgical site infection. Emerg Infect Dis 2001; 7(1): 57
2. Noakes TD, Borresen J, Hew-Butler T, Lambert MI, Jordaan E: Semmelweis and the aetiology of puerperal sepsis 160 years on: An historical review. Epidemiol Infect 2008; 136: 1
3. Boyce JM, Pittet D: Guideline for hand hygiene in health-care settings. Recommendations of the Healthcare Infection Control Practices Advisory Committee and the HIPAC/SHEA/APIC/IDSA Hand Hygiene Task Force. Am J Infect Control 2002; 30(8): S1
4. Casewell M, Phillips I. Hands as route of transmission for Klebsiella species. Br Med J 1977; 2(6098): 1315
5. Ehrenkranz NJ, Alfonso BC. Failure of bland soap handwash to prevent hand transfer of patient bacteria to urethral catheters. Infect Control Hosp Epidemiol, 1991; 12(11): 654
6. Loftus RW, Koff MD, Burchman CC, et al: Transmission of pathogenic bacterial organisms in the anesthesia work area. Anesthesiology 2008; 109: 399
7. Tunevall TG. Postoperative wound infections and surgical face masks: a controlled study. World J Surg, 1991; 15(3): 383–387; discussion 387
8. Friberg S, Ostensson R, Burman LG, et al: Surgical area contamination—comparable bacterial counts using disposable head and mask and helmet aspirator system, but dramatic increase upon omission of head-gear: an experimental study in horizontal laminar air-flow. J Hosp Infect, 2001; 47(2): 110
9. Babkin Y, Raveh D, Lifschitz M, et al: Incidence and risk factors for surgical infection after total knee replacement. Scand J Infect Dis 2007; 39(10): 890
10. Pryor F, Messmer PR. The effect of traffic patterns in the OR on surgical site infections. AORN Journal, 1998; 68(4): 649
11. Moro ML. Health Care-Associated Infections. Surg Infect 2006; 7(supplement 2): s-21
12. Allo MD, Tedesco M. Operating Room Management: Operative Suite Considerations, Infection Control. Surg Clin North Am 2005; 85(6): 1291
13. Mermel LA, McCormick RD, Springman SR, et al: The pathogenesis and epidemiology of catheter-related infection with pulmonary artery Swan-Ganz catheters: a prospective study utilizing molecular subtyping. Am J Med 1991; 91(3B): 197S
14. Raad II, Horn DC, Gilbreath BJ, et al: Prevention of central venous catheter-related infections by using maximal sterile barrier precautions during insertion. Infect Control Hosp Epidemiol 1994; 15(4 Pt 1): 231
15. O'Grady NP, Alexander M, Dellinger EP, et al: Guidelines for the prevention of intravascular catheter-related infections. Infect Control Hosp Epidemiol, 2002; 23(12): 759
16. Miles A, Miles E, Burke J. The value and duration of defence reactions of the skin to the primary lodgment of bacteria. Br J Exp Pathol 1957; 38: 79
17. Knighton DR, Halliday B, Hunt TK. Oxygen as an antibiotic: The effect of inspired oxygen on infection. Arch Surg 1984; 119: 199
18. Knighton DR, Halliday B, Hunt TK. Oxygen as an antibiotic. A comparison of the effects of inspired oxygen concentration and antibiotic administration on in vivo bacterial clearance. Arch Surg, 1986; 121(2): 191
19. Bernard HR, Cole WR. The Prophylaxis of Surgical Infection: the Effect of Prophylactic Antimicrobial Drugs on the Incidence of Infection Following Potentially Contaminated Operations. Surgery 1964; 56: 151
20. Classen D, Evans R, Pestotni KS, et al: The timing of prophylactic administration of antibiotics and the risk of surgical wound infection. NEJM 1992; 326(5): 281
21. Bratzler DW, Houck PM. Antimicrobial prophylaxis for surgery: an advisory statement from the National Surgical Infection Prevention Project. Clin Infect Dis 2004; 38(12): 1706
22. Nichols RL, Condon RE, Barie PS. Antibiotic prophylaxis in surgery—2005 and beyond. Surg Infect (Larchmt), 2005; 6(3): 349
23. Burke JP. Maximizing appropriate antibiotic prophylaxis for surgical patients: an update from LDS Hospital, Salt Lake City. Clin Infect Dis, 2001; 33(Suppl 2): S78
24. Scher K. Studies on the duration of antibiotic administration for surgical prophylaxis. Am Surg, 1997; 63: 59
25. Arnold M, Barbul A. Nutrition and wound healing. Plast Reconstr Surg, 2006; 117(7 Suppl): 42S
26. Hunt T, Hopf H. Nutrition in Wound Healing, in Nutrition and Metabolism in the Surgical Patient. Fischer J, Editor. Boston, Little, Brown and Company, 1996, pp 423
27. Jensen JA, Jonsson K, Goodson WH, et al: Epinephrine lowers subcutaneous wound oxygen tension. Curr Surg, 1985; 42(6): 472
28. Mogford JE, Sisco M, Bonomo SR, et al: Impact of aging on gene expression in a rat model of ischemic cutaneous wound healing. J Surg Res, 2004; 118(2): 190
29. Mogford JE, Tawil N, Chen A, et al: Effect of age and hypoxia on TGF-beta1 receptor expression and signal transduction in human dermal fibroblasts: impact on cell migration. J Cell Physiol, 2002; 190(2): 259
30. Lenhardt R, Hopf HW, Marker E, et al: Perioperative collagen deposition in elderly and young men and women. Arch Surg 2000; 135(1): 71
31. Robson MC, Mannari RJ, Smith PD, et al: Maintenance of wound bacterial balance. Am J Surg, 1999; 178(5): 399
32. Winter GD. Formation of the scab and the rate of epithelisation of superficial wounds in the skin of the young domestic pig. 1962. J Wound Care, 1995; 4(8): 366–367; discussion 368
33. Jonsson K, Jensen J, Goodson W, et al: Tissue oxygenation, anemia, and perfusion in relation to wound healing in surgical patients. Ann Surg 1991; 214: 605
34. Hopf HW, Ueno C, Aslam R, et al: Guidelines for the treatment of arterial insufficiency ulcers. Wound Repair Regen 2006; 14(6): 693
35. Ueno C, Hunt TK, Hopf HW. Using physiology to improve surgical wound outcomes. Plast Reconstr Surg, 2006; 117(7 Suppl): 59S
36. Allen DB, Maguire JJ, Mahdavian J, et al: Wound hypoxia and acidosis limit neutrophil bacterial killing mechanisms. Arch Surg 1997; 132(9): 991
37. DeJong L, Kemp A. Stoicheiometry and kinetics of the prolyl 4-hydroxylase partial reaction. Biochim Biophys Acta 1984; 787(1): 105
38. Evans NTS, Naylor PFD. Steady states of oxygen tension in human dermis. Resp Physiol 1966; 2: 46

ANATOMY AND PHYSIOLOGY

39. Hopf H, Hunt T, Jensen J. Calculation of Subcutaneous Tissue Blood Flow. Surgical Forum, 1988; 39: 33

40. Medawar PS. The behavior of mammalian skin epithelium under strictly anaerobic conditions. Q J Microsc Sci 1947; 88: 27

41. Hopf HW, Gibson JJ, Angeles AP, et al: Hyperoxia and angiogenesis. Wound Repair Regen, 2005; 13(6): 558

42. Schulz G. Molecular regulation of wound healing, in Acute and Chronic Wounds: Current Management Concepts. Edited by Bryant R, Nix D. St. Louis, Mosby Elsevier, 2006, pp 82

43. Adams JC. Functions of the conserved thrombospondin carboxy-terminal cassette in cell-extracellular matrix interactions and signaling. Int J Biochem Cell Biol, 2004; 36(6): 1102

44. Mast B, Shulz G. Interactions of cytokines, growth factors, and proteases in acute and chronic wounds. Wound Rep Regen, 1996; 4: 411

45. Constant J, Suh D, Hussain M, et al: Wound healing Angiogenesis: The metabolic basis of repair., in Molecular, Cellular, and Clinical Aspects of Angiogenesis. New York, Plenum Press, 1996, pp 151

46. Dvonch VM, Murphey RJ, Matsuoka J, et al: Changes in growth factor levels in human wound fluid. Surgery, 1992; 112(1): 18

47. Heppenstall RB, Littooy FN, Fuchs R, et al: Gas tensions in healing tissues of traumatized patients. Surgery 1974; 75(6): 874

48. Zabel DD, Feng JJ, Scheuenstuhl H, et al: Lactate stimulation of macrophage-derived angiogenic activity is associated with inhibition of poly(ADP-ribos) synthesis. Lab Invest, 1996; 74: 644

49. Caldwell MD, Shearer J, Morris A, et al: Evidence for aerobic glycolysis in lambda-carrageenan-wounded skeletal muscle. J Surg Res 1984; 37(1): 63

50. Trabold O, Wagner S, Wicke C, et al: Lactate and oxygen constitute a fundamental regulatory mechanism in wound healing. Wound Repair Regen, 2003; 11(6): 504

51. Remensnyder JP, Majno G. Oxygen gradients in healing wounds. Am J Pathol 1968; 52(2): 301

52. Klebanoff S. Oxygen metabolism and the toxic properties of phagocytes. Ann Intern Med 1980; 93: 480

53. Silver IA. Cellular microenvironment in healing and non-healing wounds, in Soft and Hard Tissue Repair. Hunt TK, Heppenstall RB, Pines E, Editors. New York, Praeger, 1984, pp 50

54. Niinikoski J, Hunt TK, Dunphy JE: Oxygen supply in healing tissue. Am J Surg 1972; 123(3): 247

55. Falcone PA and Caldwell MD: Wound metabolism. Clin Plast Surg 1990; 17(3): 443

56. Hopf HW, Hunt TK, West JM, et al: Wound tissue oxygen tension predicts the risk of wound infection in surgical patients. Arch Surg 1997; 132(9): 997 discussion 1005

57. Chang N, Mathes SJ: Comparison of the effect of bacterial inoculation in musculocutaneous and random-pattern flaps. Plast Reconstr Surg 1982; 95: 527

58. Schwentker A, Evans SM, Partington M, et al: A model of wound healing in chronically radiation-damaged rat skin. Cancer Lett 1998; 128(1): 71

59. Bauer SM, Goldstein LJ, Bauer RJ, et al: The bone marrow-derived endothelial progenitor cell response is impaired in delayed wound healing from ischemia. J Vasc Surg 2006; 43(1): 134

60. Wütschert R and Bounameaux H: Determination of amputation level in ischemic limbs. Reappraisal of the measurement of TcPo2. Diabetes Care 1997; 20(8): 1315

61. Dowd GS: Predicting stump healing following amputation for peripheral vascular disease using the transcutaneous oxygen monitor. Ann R Coll Surg Engl 1987; 69(1): 31

62. Ito K, Ohgi S, Mori T, et al: Determination of amputation level in ischemic legs by means of transcutaneous oxygen pressure measurement. Int Surg 1984; 69(1): 59

63. Beckert S, Farrahi F, Aslam RS, et al: Lactate stimulates endothelial cell migration. Wound Repair Regen 2006; 14(3): 321

64. Babior BM: Oxygen-dependent microbial killing by phagocytes. N Engl J Med 1978; 198: 659

65. Edwards S, Hallett M, and Campbell A: Oxygen-radical production during inflammation may be limited by oxygen concentration. Biochem J 1984; 217: 851

66. Gabig TG, Bearman SI, and Babior BM: Effects of oxygen tension and pH on the respiratory burst of human neutrophils. Blood 1979; 53(6): 1133

67. Sheffield PJ: Measuring tissue oxygen tension: a review. Undersea Hyperb Med 1998; 25(3): 179

68. Fife CE, Buyukcakir C, Otto GH, et al: The predictive value of transcutaneous oxygen tension measurement in diabetic lower extremity ulcers treated with hyperbaric oxygen therapy: a retrospective analysis of 1,144 patients. Wound Repair Regen 2002; 10(4): 198

69. Smith B, Desvigne L, Slade J et al: Transcutaneous oxygen measurements predict healing of leg wounds with hyperbaric therapy. Wound Rep Reg 1996; 4: 224

70. Rollins MD, Gibson JJ, Hunt TK: Wound oxygen levels during hyperbaric oxygen treatment in healing wounds. Undersea Hyperb Med 2006; 33(1): 17

71. Mader JT: Phagocytic killing and hyperbaric oxygen: Antibacterial mechanisms. HBO Reviews 1981; 2: 37

72. Mader JT, Brown GL, Guckian JC, et al: A mechanism for the amelioration by hyperbaric oxygen of experimental staphylococcal osteomyelitis in rabbits. J Infect Dis 1980; 142(6): 915

73. Sen CK, Khanna S, Babior BM, et al: Oxidant-induced vascular endothelial growth factor expression in human keratinocytes and cutaneous wound healing. J Biol Chem 2002; 277(36): 33284

74. Hunt TK, Aslam RS, Beckert S, et al: Aerobically Derived Lactate Stimulates Revascularization and Tissue Repair via Redox Mechanisms. Antioxid Redox Signal 2007; 9(8): 1115

75. Velazquez OC: Angiogenesis and vasculogenesis: inducing the growth of new blood vessels and wound healing by stimulation of bone marrow-derived progenitor cell mobilization and homing. J Vasc Surg 2007; 45 Suppl A: A39

76. Capla JM, Ceradini DJ, Tepper OM, et al: Skin graft vascularization involves precisely regulated regression and replacement of endothelial cells through both angiogenesis and vasculogenesis. Plast Reconstr Surg 2006; 117(3): 836

77. Schultz G, Grant M: Neovascular growth factors. Eye 1991; 5: 170

78. Beckert S, Hierlemann H, Muschenborn N, et al: Experimental ischemic wounds: correlation of cell proliferation and insulin-like growth factor I expression and its modification by different local IGF-I release systems. Wound Repair Regen 2005; 13(3): 278

79. Knighton DR, Silver IA, Hunt TK: Regulation of wound-healing angiogenesis-effect of oxygen gradients and inspired oxygen concentration. Surgery 1981; 90(2): 262

80. Myllyla R, Tuderman L, and Kivirikko KI: Mechanism of the prolyl hydroxylase reaction. 2. Kinetic analysis of the reaction sequence. Eur J Biochem 1977; 80(2): 349

81. Prockop DJ, Kivirikko KI, Tunderman L, et al: The biosynthesis of collagen and its disorders (first of two parts). N Engl J Med 1979; 301(1): 13

82. Uitto J and Prockop DJ: Synthesis and secretion of under-hydroxylated procollagen at various temperatures by cells subject to temporary anoxia. Biochem Biophys Res Commun, 1974; 60: 414

83. Silver IA: Oxygen tension and epithelialization, Epidermal Wound Healing. Edited by Maibach HI and Rovee DT. Chicago, Year Book Medical Publishers, 1972. pp 291

84. Feldmeier JJ, Hopf HW, Warriner RA, et al: UHMS position statement: topical oxygen for chronic wounds. Undersea Hyperb Med 2005; 32(3): 157

85. Ngo MA, Sinitsyna NN, Qin Q, et al: Oxygen-dependent differentiation of human keratinocytes. J Invest Dermatol 2007; 127(2): 354

86. O'Toole EA, Marinkovich MP, Peavey CL, et al: Hypoxia increases human keratinocyte motility on connective tissue. J Clin Invest, 1997; 100(11): 2881

87. Doughty DB: Preventing and managing surgical wound dehiscence. Adv Skin Wound Care, 2005; 18(6): 319

88. Gottrup F, Firmin R, Rabkin J, et al: Directly measured tissue oxygen tension and arterial oxygen tension assess tissue perfusion. Crit Care Med, 1987; 15(11): 1030

89. Hutton JJ, Tappel AL, Udenfriend S: Cofactor and substrate requirements of collagen proline hydroxylase. Arch Biochem Biophys 1967; 118: 231

90. Hohn DC, Mackey RD, Haliday B, et al: Effect of O2 tension on microbicidal function of leukocytes in wounds and in vitro. Surg Forum, 1976; 27(62): 18

91. Jonsson K, Hunt TK, Mathes SJ: Oxygen as an isolated variable influences resistance to infection. Ann Surg, 1988; 208: 783

92. Jensen JA, Goodson WH, Hopf HW et al: Cigarette smoking decreases tissue oxygen. Arch Surg 1991; 126: 1131

93. Hopf H and Hunt T: Does—and if so, to what extent—normovolemic dilutional anemia influence post-operative wound healing? Chirugische Gastroenterologie, 1992; 8: 148

94. Hopf HW, Viele M, Watson JJ, et al: Subcutaneous perfusion and oxygen during acute severe isovolemic hemodilution in healthy volunteers. Arch Surg, 2000; 135(12): 1443

95. Jensen JA, Goodson WH, Vasconez LD, et al: Wound healing in anemia. West J Med 1986; 144(4): 465

96. Sheffield C, Sessler D, Hopf H, et al: Centrally and locally mediated thermoregulatory responses alter subcutaneous oxygen tension. Wound Repair Regen 1996; 4(3): 339

97. Rabkin JM and Hunt TK: Local heat increases blood flow and oxygen tension in wounds. Arch Surg, 1987; 122(2): 221

98. Derbyshire D and Smith G, Sympathoadrenal responses to anaesthesia and surgery. Br J Anaesth, 1984; 56: 725

99. Halter J, Pflug A, Porte D: Mechanism of plasma catecholamine increases during surgical stress in man. J Clin Endocrin Metab, 1977; 45(5): 936

100. Matsukawa T, Sessler DI, Sessler AM, et al: Heat flow and distribution during induction of general anesthesia. Anesthesiology, 1995; 82: 662

101. Kurz A, Sessler DI, Lenhardt R: Perioperative normothermia to reduce the incidence of surgical-wound infection and shorten hospitalization. Study of Wound Infection and Temperature Group. N Engl J Med 1996; 334(19): 1209

102. Hartman M, Jonsson K, Zederfeldt B: Effect of tissue perfusion and oxygenation on accumulation of collagen in healing wounds. Randomized study in patients after major abdominal operations. Eur J Surg, 1992; 158(10): 521

103. Melling AC, Ali B, Scott EM, et al: Effects of preoperative warming on the incidence of wound infection after clean surgery: a randomised controlled trial. Lancet 2001; 358(9285): 876

104. Akça O, Melischek M, Scheck T, et al: Postoperative pain and subcutaneous oxygen tension [letter]. Lancet, 1999; 354(9172): 41

105. Rojas IG, Padgett DA, Sheridan JF, et al: Stress-induced susceptibility to bacterial infection during cutaneous wound healing. Brain Behav Immun, 2002; 16(1): 74

106. Horan MP, Quan N, Subramanian SV, et al: Impaired wound contraction and delayed myofibroblast differentiation in restraint-stressed mice. Brain Behav Immun 2005; 19(3): 207

107. Greif R, Akca O, Horn EP, et al: Supplemental perioperative oxygen to reduce the incidence of surgical-wound infection. Outcomes Research Group. N Engl J Med 2000; 342(3): 161

108. Belda FJ, Aguilera L, Garcia de la Asuncion J, et al: Supplemental perioperative oxygen and the risk of surgical wound infection: a randomized controlled trial. AMA 2005; 294(16): 2035

109. Myles PS, Leslie K, Chan MT, et al: Avoidance of Nitrous Oxide for Patients Undergoing Major Surgery: A Randomized Controlled Trial. Anesthesiology 2007; 107(2): 221

110. Pryor KO, Fahey TJ, 3rd, Lein CA, et al: Surgical site infection and the routine use of perioperative hyperoxia in a general surgical population: a randomized controlled trial. JAMA 2004; 291(1): 79

111. Chapman CR, Tuckett RP, Song CW: Pain and stress in a systems perspective: reciprocal neural, endocrine, and immune interactions. J Pain 2008; 9: 122

112. Buck BJ, Kerman IA, Burghardt PR, et al: Upregulation of GAD65 mRNA in the medulla of the rat model of metabolic syndrome. Neurosci Lett 2007; 419(2): 178

113. Haley RW, Culver DH, Morgan WM, et al: Identifying patients at high risk of surgical wound infection: A simple multivariate index of patient susceptibility and wound contamination. Am J Epidem, 1985; 121(2): 206

114. Culver D, Horan TC, Gaynes RP, et al: Surgical wound infection rates by wound class, operative procedure, and patient risk index. Am J Med, 1991; 91: 152S

115. Sheridan JF, Padgett DA, Avitsur R, et al: Experimental models of stress and wound healing. World J Surg, 2004; 28(3): 327

116. Dantzer R, and Kelley KW: Twenty years of research on cytokine-induced sickness behavior. Brain Behav Immun, 2007; 21(2): 153

117. Kiecolt-Glaser JK, Loving TJ, Stowell JR, et al: Hostile marital interactions, proinflammatory cytokine production, and wound healing. Arch Gen Psychiatry 2005; 62(12): 1377

118. Muizzuddin N, Matsui MS, Marenus KD, et al: Impact of stress of marital dissolution on skin barrier recovery: tape stripping and measurement of trans-epidermal water loss (TEWL). Skin Res Technol, 2003; 9(1): 34

119. Bosch JA, Engeland CG, Cacioppo JT, et al: Depressive symptoms predict mucosal wound healing. Psychosom Med, 2007; 69(7): 597

120. West J, Hopf H, Sessler D, et al: The effect of rapid postoperative rewarming on tissue oxygen. Wound Repair Regen 1993; 1(2): 93

121. Kurz A, Kurtz M, Poeschi G, et al: Forced-air warming maintains intraoperative normothermia better than circulating water mattresses. Anesth Analg, 1993; 77: 89

122. Kehlet H: Surgical stress response: does endoscopic surgery confer an advantage? World J Surg 1999; 23(8): 801

123. Holte K, Sharrock NE, Kehlet H: Pathophysiology and clinical implications of perioperative fluid excess. Br J Anaesth 2002; 89(4): 622

124. Nisanevich V, Feisenstein I, Almogy G, et al: Effect of intraoperative fluid management on outcome after intraabdominal surgery. Anesthesiology 2005; 103(1): 25

125. Arkilic CF, Taguchi A, Sharma N, et al: Supplemental perioperative fluid administration increases tissue oxygen pressure. Surgery 2003; 133(1): 49

126. Jonsson K, Jensen JA, Goodson WH, et al: Assessment of perfusion in postoperative patients using tissue oxygen measurements. Br J Surg, 1987; 74(4): 263

127. Gosain A, Rabkin J, Reynond J-P, et al: Tissue oxygen tension and other indicators of blood loss or organ perfusion during graded hemorrhage. Surgery 1991; 109(4): 523

128. Kabon B, Akça O, Taguchi A, et al: Supplemental intravenous crystalloid administration does not reduce the risk of surgical wound infection. Anesth Analg 2005; 101(5): 1546

129. Iberti TJ, Fischer EP, Leibowitz AB, et al: A multicenter study of physicians' knowledge of the pulmonary artery catheter. Pulmonary Artery Catheter Study Group. AMA 1990; 264(22): 2928

130. Rubenfeld GD, McNamara-Aslin E, Rubinson L: The pulmonary artery catheter, 1967–2007: rest in peace? AMA 2007; 298(4): 458

131. Mythen MG and Webb AR: Perioperative plasma volume expansion reduces the incidence of gut mucosal hypoperfusion during cardiac surgery. Arch Surg, 1995; 130(4): 423

132. Sinclair S, James S, Singer M: Intraoperative intravascular volume optimisation and length of hospital stay after repair of proximal femoral fracture: randomised controlled trial. BMJ 1997; 315: 909

133. Grocott MP, Mythen MG, Gan TJ: Perioperative fluid management and clinical outcomes in adults. Anesth Analg, 2005; 100(4): 1093

134. Ruttmann TG, James MF, Aronson I: In vivo investigation into the effects of haemodilution with hydroxyethyl starch (200/0.5) and normal saline on coagulation. Br J Anaesth, 1998; 80(5): 612

135. Lang K, Boldt J, Suttner S, et al: Colloids versus crystalloids and tissue oxygen tension in patients undergoing major abdominal surgery. Anesth Analg, 2001; 93(2): 405

136. Lobo DN, Bostock KA, Neal KR, et al: Effect of salt and water balance on recovery of gastrointestinal function after elective colonic resection: a randomised controlled trial. Lancet 2002; 359(9320): 1812

137. Mangram AJ, Horan TC, Pearson ML, et al: Guideline for Prevention of Surgical Site Infection, 1999. Centers for Disease Control and Prevention (CDC) Hospital Infection Control Practices Advisory Committee. Am J Infect Control 1999; 27(2): 97; quiz 133 discussion 96.

138. Jensen JA, Goodson WH, 3rd, Omachi RS, et al: Subcutaneous tissue oxygen tension falls during hemodialysis. Surgery, 1987; 101(4): 416

139. Mangano D, Layug E, Wallace A, et al: Effect of Atenolol on Mortality and Cardiovascular Morbidity After Noncardiac Surgery. NEJM, 1996; 335(23): 1713

140. Stuhmeier K, Mainzer B, Cierpka J, et al: Small, oral dose of clonidine reduces the incidence of intraoperative myocardial ischemia in patients having vascular surgery. Anesthesiology 1996; 85: 706

141. McSPI Europe Research Group: Perioperative sympatholysis: beneficial effects of the alpha-2-adrenoreceptor agonist mivazerol on hemodynamic stability and myocardial ischemia. Anesthesiology, 1997; 86: 346

142. Wallace AW, Galindez D, Salahieh A, et al: Effect of clonidine on cardiovascular morbidity and mortality after noncardiac surgery. Anesthesiology, 2004; 101(2): 284

143. Hopf H, West J, Hunt T: Clonidine increases tissue oxygen in patients with local tissue hypoxia in non-healing wounds. Wound Repair Regen 1996; 4(1): A129

144. Stone JG, Cozine KA, Wald A: Nocturnal oxygenation during patient-controlled analgesia. Anesth Analg, 1999; 89(1): 104

145. Wisner D: A stepwise logistic regression analysis of factors affecting morbidity and mortality after thoracic trauma: Effect of epidural analgesia. J Trauma 1990; 30(7): 799

146. Owen H, McMillan V, Rogowski D: Postoperative pain therapy: a survey of patients' expectations and their experiences. Pain 1990; 41: 303

147. Donovan M, Dillon P, McGuire L: Incidence and characteristics of pain in a sample of medical-surgical inpatients. Pain 1987; 30: 69

148. Brennan TA, Leape LL, Laird NM, et al: Incidence of adverse events and negligence in hospitalized patients. Results of the Harvard Medical Practice Study I. N Engl J Med 1991; 324(6): 370

ANATOMY AND PHYSIOLOGY

CHAPTER 14 ■ FLUIDS, ELECTROLYTES, AND ACID-BASE PHYSIOLOGY

DONALD S. PROUGH, J. SEAN FUNSTON, CHRISTER H. SVENSÉN, AND SCOTT W. WOLF

ACID-BASE INTERPRETATION AND TREATMENT
    Overview of Acid-Base Equilibrium
    Metabolic Alkalosis
    Metabolic Acidosis
    Respiratory Alkalosis
    Respiratory Acidosis
PRACTICAL APPROACH TO ACID-BASE
    INTERPRETATION
    Examples
FLUID MANAGEMENT
    Physiology

    Fluid Replacement Therapy
    Surgical Fluid Requirements
    Colloids, Crystalloids, and Hypertonic Solutions
    Fluid Status: Assessment and Monitoring
ELECTROLYTES
    Sodium
    Hypernatremia
    Potassium
    Calcium
    Phosphate
    Magnesium

KEY POINTS

1. The Henderson-Hasselbalch equation describes the relationship between pH, $PaCO_2$, and serum bicarbonate. The Henderson equation defines the previous relationship but substitutes hydrogen concentration for pH.

2. The pathophysiology of metabolic alkalosis is divided into generating and maintenance factors. A particularly important maintenance factor is renal hypoperfusion, often due to hypovolemia.

3. The addition of iatrogenic respiratory alkalosis to metabolic alkalosis can produce severe alkalemia.

4. Metabolic acidosis occurs as a consequence of the use of bicarbonate to buffer endogenous organic acids or as a consequence of external bicarbonate loss. The former causes an increase in the anion gap ($Na^+ - [Cl^- + [HCO_3^-]]$).

5. When substituting mechanical ventilation for spontaneous ventilation in a patient with severe metabolic acidosis, it is important to maintain an appropriate level of ventilatory compensation, pending effective treatment of the primary cause for the metabolic acidosis.

6. Sodium bicarbonate, never proved to alter outcome in patients with lactic acidosis, should be reserved for those patients with severe acidemia.

7. Tight control of blood glucose in critically ill surgical patients has been associated with substantial improvements in mortality.

8. In patients undergoing moderate surgical procedures, generous administration of fluids is associated with fewer minor complications, such as nausea, vomiting, and drowsiness.

9. In patients undergoing colon surgery, careful perioperative fluid restriction has been associated with lower mortality and better wound healing.

10. Homeostatic mechanisms are usually adequate for the maintenance of electrolyte balance. However, critical illnesses and their treatment strategies can cause significant perturbations in electrolyte status, possibly leading to worsened patient outcome.

11. Disorders of the concentration of sodium, the principal extracellular cation, depend on the total body water concentration and can lead to neurologic dysfunction. Disorders of potassium, the principal intracellular cation, are influenced primarily by insults that result in increased total body losses of potassium or changes in distribution.

12. Calcium, phosphorus, and magnesium are all essential for maintenance and function of the cardiovascular system. In addition, they also provide the milieu that ensures neuromuscular transmission. Disorders affecting any one of these electrolytes may lead to significant dysfunction and possibly result in cardiopulmonary arrest.

As a consequence of underlying diseases and of therapeutic manipulations, surgical patients develop potentially harmful disorders of acid-base equilibrium, intravascular and extravascular volume, and serum electrolytes. Precise perioperative management of acid-base status, fluids, and electrolytes may limit perioperative morbidity and mortality. Recent data provide provocative insights regarding appropriate perioperative fluid management in patients undergoing both ambulatory and major inpatient surgery or the possibility of chronic hypercapnia.

ACID-BASE INTERPRETATION AND TREATMENT

Management of perioperative acid-base disturbances requires an understanding of the four simple acid-base disorders—metabolic alkalosis, metabolic acidosis, respiratory alkalosis, and respiratory acidosis—as well as more complex combinations of disturbances. This section will review the pathogenesis, major complications, physiologic compensatory mechanisms, and treatment of common perioperative acid-base abnormalities.

Overview of Acid-Base Equilibrium

❶ Conventionally, acid-base equilibrium is described using the Henderson-Hasselbalch equation:

$$pH = 6.1 + \log \frac{[HCO_3^-]}{0.03 \times Pa_{CO_2}} \quad (14\text{-}1)$$

where 6.1 = the pK_a of carbonic acid and 0.03 is the solubility coefficient in blood of carbon dioxide (CO_2). Within this context, pH is the dependent variable while the bicarbonate concentration [HCO_3^-] and Pa_{CO_2} are independent variables; therefore, metabolic alkalosis and acidosis are defined as disturbances in which [HCO_3^-] is primarily increased or decreased and respiratory alkalosis and acidosis are defined as disturbances in which Pa_{CO_2} is primarily decreased or increased. pH, the negative logarithm of the hydrogen ion concentration ([H^+]), defines the acidity or alkalinity of solutions or blood. The simpler Henderson equation, after conversion of pH to [H^+], also describes the relationship between the three major variables measured or calculated in blood gas samples:

$$[H^+] = \frac{24 \times Pa_{CO_2}}{[HCO_3^-]} \quad (14\text{-}2)$$

To approximate the logarithmic relationship of pH to [H^+], assume that [H^+] is 40 mmol/L at a pH of 7.4; that an increase in pH of 0.10 pH units reduces [H^+] to 0.8 × the starting [H^+] concentration; that a decrease in pH of 0.10 pH units increases the [H^+] by a factor of 1.25; and that small changes (i.e., <0.05 pH units) produce reciprocal increases or decreases of approximately 1.0 mmol/L in [H^+] for each 0.01 decrease or increase pH units.

The alternative "Stewart" approach to acid-base interpretation distinguishes between the independent variables and dependent variables that determine pH.[1,2] The independent variables are Pa_{CO_2}, the strong (i.e., highly dissociated) ion difference, and the concentration of proteins, which usually are not strong ions. The strong ions include sodium (Na^+),

potassium (K^+), chloride (Cl^-), and lactate. The strong ion difference, calculated as ($Na^+ + K^+ - Cl^-$), under normal circumstances is approximately 42 mEq/L. In general, the Stewart approach provides more insight into the mechanisms underlying acid-base disturbances, in contrast to the more descriptive Henderson-Hasselbalch approach. However, the clinical interpretation or treatment of common acid-base disturbances is rarely handicapped by the simpler constructs of the conventional Henderson-Hasselbalch or Henderson equations.

Metabolic Alkalosis

Metabolic alkalosis, characterized by hyperbicarbonatemia (>27.0 mEq/L) and usually by an alkalemic pH (>7.45), occurs frequently in postoperative patients and critically ill patients. **❷** Factors that generate metabolic alkalosis include vomiting and diuretic administration (Table 14-1).[3] Maintenance of metabolic alkalosis depends on a continued stimulus, such as renal hypoperfusion, hypokalemia, hypochloremia or hypovolemia, for distal tubular reabsorption of [HCO_3^-] (Table 14-2).[3]

Metabolic alkalosis is associated with hypokalemia, ionized hypocalcemia, secondary ventricular arrhythmias, increased digoxin toxicity, and compensatory hypoventilation (hypercarbia), although compensation rarely results in Pa_{CO_2} >55 mm Hg (Table 14-3). Alkalemia may reduce tissue oxygen availability by shifting the oxyhemoglobin dissocia- **❸** tion curve to the left and by decreasing cardiac output. During anesthetic management, inadvertent addition of iatrogenic respiratory alkalosis to pre-existing metabolic alkalosis may produce severe alkalemia and precipitate cardiovascular depression, dysrhythmias, hypokalemia, and the complications.

In patients in whom arterial blood gases have not yet been obtained, serum electrolytes and a history of major risk factors, such as vomiting, nasogastric suction, or chronic diuretic use, can suggest metabolic alkalosis. Total CO_2 (usually abbreviated on electrolyte reports as CO_2) should be about 1.0 mEq/L greater than [HCO_3^-] on simultaneously obtained arterial blood gases. If either calculated [HCO_3^-] on the arterial blood gases or "CO_2" on the serum electrolytes exceeds normal (24 and 25 mEq/L, respectively) by >4.0 mEq/L, either the patient has a primary metabolic alkalosis or has conserved bicarbonate in response to chronic hypercarbia. Recognition

---

TABLE 14-1

GENERATION OF METABOLIC ALKALOSIS

■ GENERATION	■ EXAMPLES
I. Loss of acid from extracellular space	
A. Loss of gastric fluid (HCl)	Vomiting
B. Acid loss in the urine: increased distal Na delivery in presence of hyperaldosteronism	Primary aldosteronism plus diuretic
C. Acid shifts into cells	Potassium deficiency
D. Loss of acid into stool	Congenital chloride-losing diarrhea
II. Excessive HCO_3^- loads	
A. Absolute	
1) Oral or parenteral HCO_3^-	Milk Alkali syndrome
2) Metabolic conversion of the salts of organic acids to HCO	Lactate, acetate, or citrate administration
B. Relative	NaHCO$_3$ dialysis
III. Posthypercapnic states	Correction (e.g., by mechanical ventilatory support) of chronic hypercapnia

Modified from Khanna A, Kurtzman NA: Metabolic alkalosis. J Nephrol 2006; 19(Suppl 9): S86, with permission.

ANATOMY AND PHYSIOLOGY

TABLE 14-2

FACTORS THAT MAINTAIN METABOLIC ALKALOSIS

■ FACTOR	■ PROPOSED MECHANISM
Decreased GFR	Increases fractional HCO_3^- reabsorption and prevents the elevated plasma $[HCO_3^-]$ from exceeding Tm
Volume contraction	Stimulates proximal tubular HCO_3 reabsorption
Hypokalemia	Decreases GFR and increases proximal tubular HCO_3^- reabsorption; stimulates Na-independent/K-dependent (low) secretion in CCT.
Hypochloremia[a]	Increases renin, decreases GFR, and decreases distal chloride delivery ($\uparrow$ proton secretion in MCT)
Passive backflux of HCO_3^-	Creates a favorable concentration gradient for passive HCO_3^- movement from proximal tubular lumen to blood
Aldosterone	Increases Na-dependent proton secretion in CCT and Na-independent proton secretion in CCT and MCT

All factors decrease urinary HCO_3 excretion in vivo.
GFR, glomerular filtration rate; CCT, cortical collecting tubule; MCT, medullary collecting tubule.
[a]Animal models are associated with hypokalemia; thus, the precise role of chloride in humans is not clearly understood.
Modified from Khanna A, Kurtzman NA: Metabolic alkalosis. J Nephrol 2006; 19(Suppl 9): S86–S96, with permission.

of hyperbicarbonatemia on the preoperative serum electrolytes justifies arterial blood gas analysis and should alert the anesthesiologist to the likelihood of factors that generate or maintain metabolic alkalosis (see Tables 14-1 and 14-2).

Treatment of metabolic alkalosis consists of etiologic and nonetiologic therapy. Etiologic therapy consists of measures such as expansion of intravascular volume or the administration of potassium. Infusion of 0.9% saline will dose-dependently increase serum $[Cl^-]$ and decrease serum $[HCO_3^-]$.[4] Nonetiologic therapy includes administration of acetazolamide (a carbonic anhydrase inhibitor that causes renal bicarbonate wasting), infusion of $[H^+]$ in the form of ammonium chloride, arginine hydrochloride, or 0.1 N hydrochloric acid (100 mmol/L), or dialysis against a high-chloride/low bicarbonate dialysate.[3] Of the previously mentioned factors, 0.1 N hydrochloric acid most rapidly corrects life-threatening metabolic alkalosis but must be infused into a central vein; peripheral infusion will cause severe tissue damage.

Metabolic Acidosis

Metabolic acidosis, characterized by hypobicarbonatemia (<21 mEq/L) and usually by an acidemic pH (<7.35), can be innocuous or reflect a life-threatening emergency. Metabolic acidosis occurs as a consequence of buffering by bicarbonate of endogenous or exogenous acid loads or as a consequence of abnormal external loss of bicarbonate.[5–7] Approximately 70 mmol of acid metabolites are produced, buffered, and excreted daily; these include about 25 mmol of sulfuric acid from amino acid metabolism, 40 mmol of organic acids, and phosphoric and other acids. Extracellular volume in a 70-kg adult contains 336 mmol of bicarbonate buffer (24 mEq/L × 14 L of extracellular volume). Glomerular filtration of plasma volume necessitates reabsorption of 4,500 mmol of bicarbonate daily, of which 85% is reabsorbed in the proximal tubule, 10% in the thick ascending limb, and the remainder is titrated by proton secretion in the collecting duct.

Calculation of the anion gap $[(Na^+ - ([Cl^-] + [HCO_3^-]))]$ distinguishes between two types of metabolic acidosis (Table 14-4).[8] The anion gap is normal (<13 mEq/L) in situations such as diarrhea, biliary drainage, and renal tubular acidosis

TABLE 14-3

RESPIRATORY COMPENSATION IN RESPONSE TO METABOLIC ALKALOSIS AND METABOLIC ACIDOSIS

Metabolic alkalosis
1. $PaCO_2$ increases ~0.5–0.6 mm Hg per 1.0 mEq/L increase in $[HCO_3^-]$
2. The last two digits of the pH should approximate the $[HCO_3^-] + 15$

Metabolic acidosis
1. $PaCO_2 \sim [HCO_3^-] \times 1.5 + 8$
2. $PaCO_2$ decreases 1.2 mm Hg per 1.0 mEq/L in $[HCO_3^-]$ to a minimum of 10–15 mm Hg
3. The last two digits of the pH ~ $[HCO_3^-] + 15$

TABLE 14-4

DIFFERENTIAL DIAGNOSIS OF METABOLIC ACIDOSIS

■ ELEVATED ANION GAP[a]	■ NORMAL ANION GAP[b]
Three Diseases	
1. Uremia	1. Renal tubular acidosis
2. Ketoacidosis	2. Diarrhea
3. Lactic acidosis	3. Carbonic anhydrase inhibition
	4. Ureteral diversions
Toxins	5. Early renal failure
1. Methanol	6. Hydronephrosis
2. Ethylene glycol	7. HCl administration
3. Salicylates	8. Saline administration
4. Paraldehyde	

[a]Correction of the anion gap for hypoalbuminemia is essential for effective perioperative use.
[b]To correct the anion gap for hypoalbuminemia, add to the calculated anion gap twice the difference between normal serum albumin (4.0 g/L) and actual serum albumin.

in which bicarbonate is lost externally. The anion gap also is normal or reduced in hyperchloremic acidosis associated with perioperative infusion of substantial quantities of 0.9% saline.[4,9] Metabolic acidosis associated with a high anion gap (>13 mEq/L) occurs because of excess production or decreased excretion of organic acids or ingestion of one of several toxic compounds (Table 14-4). In metabolic acidosis associated with a high anion gap, bicarbonate ions are consumed in buffering hydrogen ions, while the associated anion replaces bicarbonate in serum. Because three quarters of the normal anion gap consists of albumin, the calculated anion gap should be corrected for hypoalbuminemia by adding to the calculated anion gap the difference between measured serum albumin and a normal albumin concentration of 4.0 g/dL multiplied by 2.0 to 2.5.[10] In general, an increase in the albumin-corrected anion gap (ΔAG) should be approximately matched by a decrease in the serum [HCO_3^-] (ΔHCO_3^-).[11] A ratio of ΔAG:ΔHCO_3^- that is <0.8 or >1.2 should prompt consideration of a mixed acid-base disturbance.

Sufficient reductions in pH may reduce myocardial contractility, increase pulmonary vascular resistance, and decrease systemic vascular resistance. It is particularly important to note that failure of a patient to appropriately hyperventilate in response to metabolic acidosis is physiologically equivalent to respiratory acidosis and suggests clinical deterioration. If a patient with metabolic acidosis requires mechanical ventilation, for example, during general anesthesia, every attempt should be made to maintain an appropriate level of ventilatory compensation (see Table 14-3) until the primary process can be corrected. Table 14-5 illustrates failure to maintain compensatory hyperventilation.

The anesthetic implications of metabolic acidosis are proportional to the severity of the underlying process. Although a patient with hyperchloremic metabolic acidosis may be relatively healthy, those with lactic acidosis, ketoacidosis, uremia, or toxic ingestions will be chronically or acutely ill. Preoperative assessment should emphasize volume status and renal function. If shock has caused metabolic acidosis, direct arterial pressure monitoring and preload may require assessment via echocardiography or pulmonary arterial catheterization. Intraoperatively, one should be concerned about the possibility of exaggerated hypotensive responses to drugs and positive pressure ventilation. In planning intravenous fluid therapy, consider that balanced salt solutions tend to increase [HCO_3^-] (e.g., by metabolism of lactate to bicarbonate) and pH and 0.9% saline tends to decrease [HCO_3^-] and pH.

The treatment of metabolic acidosis consists of the treatment of the primary pathophysiologic process, that is, hypoperfusion, hypoxia, and if pH is severely decreased, administration of $NaHCO_3^-$. Hyperventilation, although an important compensatory response to metabolic acidosis, is not definitive therapy for metabolic acidosis. The initial dose of $NaHCO_3$ can be calculated as:

$$NaHCO_3(mEq/L) = \frac{Wt(kg) \times 0.3(24 \text{ mEq/L} - Actual HCO_3^-)}{2} \qquad (14\text{-}3)$$

where 0.3 = the assumed distribution space for bicarbonate and 24 mEq/L is the normal value for [HCO_3^-] on arterial blood gas determination. The calculation markedly underestimates dosage in severe metabolic acidosis. In infants and children, a customary initial dose is 1.0 to 2.0 mEq/kg of body weight.

Both evidence and opinion suggest that $NaHCO_3$ should rarely be used to treat acidemia induced by metabolic acidosis.[5,6,12] In critically ill patients with lactic acidosis, there were no important differences between the physiologic effects (other than changes in pH) of 0.9 M $NaHCO_3$ and 0.9 M sodium chloride.[13] Importantly, $NaHCO_3$ did not improve the cardiovascular response to catecholamines and actually reduced plasma ionized calcium.[13] Although many clinicians continue to administer $NaHCO_3$ to patients with persistent lactic acidosis and ongoing deterioration, neither $NaHCO_3$ nor dichloroacetate[14] has improved outcome. The buffer THAM (*tris*-hydroxymethyl aminomethane) effectively reduces [H^+], does not increase plasma [Na^+], does not generate CO_2 as a byproduct of buffering, and does not decrease plasma [K+][15]; however, there is no generally accepted indication for THAM.

Respiratory Alkalosis

Respiratory alkalosis, always characterized by hypocarbia ($PaCO_2 \leq 35$ mm Hg) and usually characterized by an alkalemic pH (>7.45), results from an increase in minute ventilation that is greater than that required to excrete metabolic CO_2 production. Because respiratory alkalosis may be a sign of pain, anxiety, hypoxemia, central nervous system disease, or systemic sepsis, the development of spontaneous respiratory alkalosis in a previously normocarbic patient requires prompt evaluation. The hyperventilation syndrome, a diagnosis of exclusion, is most often encountered in the emergency department.[16]

Respiratory alkalosis, like metabolic alkalosis, may produce hypokalemia, hypocalcemia, cardiac dysrhythmias, bronchoconstriction, and hypotension, and may potentiate the toxicity of digoxin. In addition, both brain pH and cerebral blood flow are tightly regulated and respond rapidly to changes in systemic pH.[17] Doubling minute ventilation reduces $PaCO_2$ to 20 mm Hg and halves cerebral blood flow; conversely, halving minute ventilation doubles $PaCO_2$ and doubles cerebral blood

---

TABLE 14-5

FAILURE TO MAINTAIN APPROPRIATE VENTILATORY COMPENSATION FOR METABOLIC ACIDOSIS[a]

		SPONTANEOUS VENTILATION		MECHANICAL HYPOVENTILATION
Arterial blood gases	pH	7.29		7.13
	$PaCO_2$ (mm Hg)	29	$\rightarrow \rightarrow \rightarrow \rightarrow \rightarrow \rightarrow \rightarrow$	49
	[HCO_3^-] (mEq/L)	14		16

[a]In the presence of metabolic acidosis, an otherwise modest increase in $PaCO_2$ may create a life-threatening decrease in pH.

flow. Therefore, acute hyperventilation may be useful in neurosurgical procedures to reduce brain bulk and to control intracranial pressure (ICP) during emergent surgery for noncranial injuries associated with acute closed head trauma. In those situations, intraoperative monitoring of arterial blood gases, correlated with capnography, will document adequate reduction of $PaCO_2$. Acute profound hypocapnia (<20 mm Hg) may produce electroencephalographic evidence of cerebral ischemia. If $PaCO_2$ is maintained at abnormally high or low levels for 8 to 24 hours, cerebral blood flow will return toward previous levels, associated with a return of cerebrospinal fluid $[HCO_3^-]$ toward normal.

Treatment of respiratory alkalosis per se is often not required. The most important steps are recognition and treatment of the underlying cause.[16] For instance, correction of hypoxemia or hypoperfusion-induced lactic acidosis should result in resolution of the associated increases in respiratory drive. Preoperative recognition of chronic hyperventilation necessitates intraoperative maintenance of a similar $PaCO_2$.

Respiratory Acidosis

Respiratory acidosis, always characterized by hypercarbia ($PaCO_2 \leq 45$ mm Hg) and usually characterized by a low pH (<7.35), occurs because of a decrease in minute alveolar ventilation (V_A), an increase in production of carbon dioxide (V_{CO_2}) or both, from the equation:

$$Pa_{CO_2} = K \frac{V_{CO_2}}{V_A} \qquad (14\text{-}4)$$

where K = constant (rebreathing of exhaled, carbon dioxide-containing gas may also increase $PaCO_2$). Respiratory acidosis may be either acute, without compensation by renal $[HCO_3^-]$ retention, or chronic, with $[HCO_3^-]$ retention offsetting the decrease in pH (Table 14-6). A reduction in V_A may be due to an overall decrease in minute ventilation (V_E) or to an increase in the amount of wasted ventilation (V_D), according to the equation:

$$V_A = V_E - V_D \qquad (14\text{-}5)$$

TABLE 14-6

CHANGES OF $[HCO_3^-]$ AND pH IN RESPONSE TO ACUTE AND CHRONIC CHANGES IN $PaCO_2$

Decreased $PaCO_2$
1. pH increases 0.10 per 10 mm Hg decrease in $PaCO_2$
2. $[HCO_3^-]$ decreases 2 mEq/L per 10 mm Hg decrease in $PaCO_2$
3. pH will nearly normalize if hypocarbia is sustained
4. $[HCO_3^-]$ will decrease 5 to 6 mEq/L per 10 mm Hg chronic ↓ in $PaCO_2^a$

Increased $PaCO_2$
1. pH will decrease 0.05 per acute 10 mm Hg increase in $PaCO_2$
2. $[HCO_3^-]$ will increase 1.0 mEq/L per 10 mm Hg increase in $PaCO_2$
3. pH will return toward normal if hypercarbia is sustained
4. $[HCO_3^-]$ will increase 4–5 mEq/L per chronic 10 mm Hg increase in $PaCO_2$

^{a}Hospitalized patients rarely develop chronic compensation for hypocarbia because of stimuli that enhance distal tubular reabsorption of sodium.

Decreases in V_E may occur because of central ventilatory depression by drugs or central nervous system injury because of increased work of breathing, or because of airway obstruction or neuromuscular dysfunction. Increases in V_D occur with chronic obstructive pulmonary disease, pulmonary embolism, and most acute forms of respiratory failure. V_{CO_2} may be increased by sepsis, high-glucose parenteral feeding, or fever.

Patients with chronic hypercarbia due to intrinsic pulmonary disease require careful preoperative evaluation. The ventilatory restriction imposed by upper abdominal or thoracic surgery may aggravate ventilatory insufficiency after surgery. Administration of narcotics and sedatives, even in small doses, may cause hazardous ventilatory depression. Preoperative evaluation should consider direct arterial pressure monitoring and frequent intraoperative blood gas determinations, as well as strategies to manage postoperative pain with minimal doses of systemic opioids. Intraoperatively, a patient with chronically compensated hypercapnia should be ventilated to maintain a normal pH. Inadvertent restoration of normal V_A may result in profound alkalemia. Postoperatively, prophylactic ventilatory support may be required for selected patients with chronic hypercarbia. Epidural narcotic administration represents one potential alternative that may provide adequate postoperative analgesia while limiting depression of ventilatory drive.

The treatment of respiratory acidosis depends on whether the process is acute or chronic. Acute respiratory acidosis may require mechanical ventilation unless a simple etiologic factor (i.e., narcotic overdosage or residual muscular blockade) can be treated quickly. Bicarbonate administration rarely is indicated unless severe metabolic acidosis is also present or unless mechanical ventilation is ineffective in reducing acute hypercarbia. In contrast, chronic respiratory acidosis is rarely managed with ventilation but rather with efforts to improve pulmonary function. In patients requiring mechanical ventilation for acute respiratory failure, ventilation with a lung-protective strategy may result in hypercapnia, which occasionally may require administration of buffers to avoid excessive acidemia.[18]

PRACTICAL APPROACH TO ACID-BASE INTERPRETATION

Rapid interpretation of a patient's acid-base status involves the integration of three sets of data: arterial blood gases, electrolytes, and history. A systematic, sequential approach facilitates interpretation (Table 14-7). Acid-base assessment usually can be completed before initiating therapy; however, inspection of arterial blood gas data may disclose disturbances (e.g., respiratory acidosis or metabolic acidosis with pH <7.1) that require immediate attention.

The second step is to determine whether a patient is acidemic (pH <7.35) or alkalemic (pH >7.45). The pH status will usually indicate the predominant primary process, that is, acidosis produces acidemia; and alkalosis produces alkalemia. Note that the suffix "-osis" indicates a primary process that, if unopposed, will produce the corresponding pH change. The suffix "-emia" refers to the pH. A compensatory process is not considered an "-osis." Of course, a patient may have mixed "-oses," that is, more than one primary process.

The third step is to determine whether the entire arterial blood gas picture is consistent with a simple acute respiratory alkalosis or acidosis (see Table 14-6). For example, a patient with acute hypocapnia ($PaCO_2$ 30 mm Hg) would have a pH increase of 0.10 units to a pH of 7.50 and a decrease of calculated $[HCO_3^-]$ to 22 mEq/L.

As the fourth step, if changes in $PaCO_2$, pH, and $[HCO_3^-]$ are not consistent with a simple acute respiratory disturbance, chronic respiratory acidosis ($\geq$24 hours) or metabolic acidosis

TABLE 14-7

SEQUENTIAL APPROACH TO ACID-BASE INTERPRETATION

1. Is the pH life-threatening, requiring immediate intervention?
2. Is the pH acidemic or alkalemic?
3. Could the entire arterial blood gas picture represent only an acute increase or decrease in $Paco_2$?
4. If the answer to question 3 is "No," is there evidence of a chronic respiratory disturbance or of an acute metabolic disturbance?
5. If an acute metabolic disturbance is present, is it accompanied by appropriate respiratory compensatory changes?
6. Is an anion gap present?
7. Are the clinical data consistent with the proposed interpretation?

TABLE 14-8

HYPERCHLOREMIC METABOLIC ACIDOSIS DURING PROLONGED SURGERY

Arterial blood gases	pH	7.40
	$Paco_2$	32 mm Hg
	$[HCO_3^-]$	19 mEq/L
Electrolytes	$[Na^+]$	140 mEq/L
	$[Cl^-]$	114 mEq/L
	CO_2	20 mEq/L
	Anion gap	8 mEq/L
Serum albumin		3.0 g/dL

or alkalosis should be considered. In chronic respiratory acidosis, pH returns to nearly normal as bicarbonate is retained by the kidneys (Table 14-6), usually at a ratio of 4 to 5 mEq/L per 10 mm Hg chronic increase in $Paco_2$.[19] For example, chronic hypoventilation at a $Paco_2$ of 60 mm Hg would be associated with an increase in $[HCO_3^-]$ of 8 to 10 mEq/L so that $[HCO_3^-]$ would be expected to range from 32 to 34 mEq/L and pH would be expected to be within the low normal range (7.35 to 7.38). If neither an acute nor chronic respiratory change appears to explain the arterial blood gas data, then a metabolic disturbance must also be present.

The fifth question addresses respiratory compensation for metabolic disturbances. Respiratory compensation for metabolic disturbances occurs more rapidly than renal compensation for respiratory disturbances (Table 14-3). Several general rules describe compensation. First, overcompensation is rare. Second, inadequate or excessive compensation suggests an additional primary disturbance. Third, hypobicarbonatemia associated with an increased anion gap is never compensatory.

The sixth question, whether an anion gap is present, should be assessed even if the arterial blood gases appear straightforward. The simultaneous occurrence of metabolic alkalosis and metabolic acidosis may result in an unremarkable pH and $[HCO_3^-]$; therefore, the combined abnormality may only be appreciated by examining the anion gap (if the cause of the metabolic acidosis is associated with a high anion gap). As noted previously, correct assessment of the anion gap requires correction for hypoalbuminemia.[10] Metabolic acidoses associated with increased anion gaps require specific treatments, thus necessitating a correct diagnosis and differentiation from hyperchloremic metabolic acidosis. For instance, if metabolic acidosis results from administration of large volumes of 0.9% saline, no specific treatment of metabolic acidosis would usually be necessary.

The seventh and final question is whether the clinical data are consistent with the proposed acid-base interpretation. Failure to integrate clinical findings with arterial blood gas and plasma electrolyte data may lead to serious errors in interpretation and management.

Examples

The following two hypothetical cases illustrate the use of the algorithm and rules of thumb previously discussed.

Example Number 1

A 65-year-old woman has undergone 12 hours of an expected 16-hour radical neck dissection and flap construction. Estimated blood loss is 1,000 mL. She has received three units of packed red blood cells and six L of 0.9 % saline. Her blood pressure and heart rate have remained stable while anesthetized with 0.5% to 1.0% isoflurane in 70:30 nitrous oxide and oxygen. Urinary output is adequate. Arterial blood gas levels are shown in Table 14-8.

The step-by-step interpretation is as follows:

1. The pH requires no immediate treatment.
2. The pH is normal.
3. The arterial blood gases cannot be adequately explained by acute hypocarbia. The predicted pH would be 7.48 and the predicted $[HCO_3^-]$ would be 22 mEq/L (see Table 14-6).
4. A metabolic acidosis appears to be present.
5. Patients under general anesthesia with controlled mechanical ventilation cannot compensate for metabolic acidosis. However, spontaneous hypocapnia of this magnitude would represent slight overcompensation for metabolic acidosis (see Table 14-3) and would suggest the presence of a primary respiratory alkalosis.
6. Metabolic acidosis occurring during prolonged anesthesia and surgery could suggest lactic acidosis and prompt additional fluid therapy or other attempts to improve perfusion. However, serum electrolytes reveal an anion gap that is slightly less than normal (Table 14-8), indicating that the metabolic acidosis is probably the result of dilution of the extracellular volume with a high-chloride fluid. Correction of the anion gap for the serum albumin of 3.0 g/dL only increases the anion gap to 10 to 11 mEq/L, again consistent with hyperchloremic metabolic acidosis. After differentiation from high anion-gap metabolic acidoses, hyperchloremic acidosis secondary to infusion of high-chloride fluid usually requires no treatment. The arterial blood gases and serum electrolytes are compatible with the clinical picture.

Example Number 2

A 35-year-old man, 3 days after appendectomy, develops nausea with recurrent emesis persisting for 48 hours. An arterial blood gas reveals the results shown in the middle column of Table 14-9.

1. The pH of 7.50 requires no immediate intervention.
2. The pH is alkalemic, suggesting a primary alkalosis.
3. An acute $Paco_2$ of 46 mm Hg would yield a pH of approximately 7.37; therefore, this is not simply an acute ventilatory disturbance.
4. The patient has a primary metabolic alkalosis as suggested by the $[HCO_3^-]$ of 35 mEq/L.
5. The limits of respiratory compensation for metabolic alkalosis are wide and difficult to predict for individual patients. The rules of thumb, summarized in Table 14-3, suggest that $[HCO_3^-]$ + 15 should equal the last two digits of the pH and that the $Paco_2$ should increase 5 to 6 mm Hg

TABLE 14-9

METABOLIC ALKALOSIS SECONDARY TO NAUSEA AND VOMITING WITH SUBSEQUENT LACTIC ACIDOSIS SECONDARY TO HYPOVOLEMIA

		NORMAL	METABOLIC ALKALOSIS	METABOLIC ACIDOSIS
Blood gases	PH	7.40	7.50	7.40
	$PaCO_2$ (mm Hg)	40	46	40
	$[HCO_3^-]$ (mEq/L)	24	35	24
Serum electrolytes	$[Na^+]$ (mEq/L)	140	140	140
	$[Cl^-]$ (mEq/L)	105	94	94
	CO_2 (mEq/L)	25	36	25
	Anion gap (mEq/L)	10	10	21

for every 10 mEq/L change in serum $[HCO_3^-]$, that is, a pH of 7.50 and a $PaCO_2$ of 46 mm Hg are within the expected range.

6. The anion gap is 10 mEq/L.
7. The diagnosis of a primary metabolic alkalosis with compensatory hypoventilation is consistent with the history of recurrent vomiting. Consider how the arterial blood gases could change if vomiting were sufficiently severe to produce hypovolemic shock and lactic acidosis (third column, Table 14-9).

This sequence illustrates the important concept that the final pH, $PaCO_2$ and $[HCO_3^-]$ represent the result of all of the vectors operating on acid-base status. Complex or "triple disturbances" can only be interpreted using a thorough, stepwise approach.

FLUID MANAGEMENT

Physiology

Body Fluid Compartments

Accurate replacement of fluid deficits necessitates an understanding of the expected distribution spaces of water, sodium, and colloid. The sum of intracellular volume (ICV), which constitutes 40% of total body weight, and extracellular volume (ECV), which constitutes 20% of body weight, comprises total body water (TBW), which therefore approximates 60% of total body weight. Plasma volume (PV), equals about one fifth of ECV, the remainder of which is interstitial fluid volume (IFV). Red cell volume, approximately 2 L, is part of ICV.

The distribution volume of sodium-free water is TBW. The distribution volume of infused sodium is ECV, which contains equal sodium concentrations ($[Na^+]$) in the PV and IF. Plasma $[Na^+]$ is approximately 140 mEq/L. The predominant intracellular cation, potassium, has an intracellular concentration ($[K^+]$) approximating 150 mEq/L. Albumin, the most important oncotically active constituent of ECV, is unequally distributed in PV (~4 g/dL) and IFV (~1 g/dL). The IFV concentration of albumin varies greatly among tissues; however, ECV is the distribution volume for colloid solutions.

Distribution of Infused Fluids

Conventionally, clinical prediction of plasma volume expansion after fluid infusion assumes that body fluid spaces are static. Kinetic analysis of plasma volume expansion replaces the static assumption with a dynamic description. As an example

of the static approach, assume that a 70-kg patient has suffered an acute blood loss of 2,000 mL, approximately 40% of the predicted 5-L blood volume. The formula describing the effects of replacement with 5% dextrose in water (D5W), lactated Ringer solution, or 5% or 25% human serum albumin is as follows:

$$\text{Expected PV increment} = \text{volume infused} \times \text{normal PV/ distribution volume} \quad (14\text{-}6)$$

Rearranging the equation yields the following:

$$\text{Volume infused} = \text{expected PV increment} \times \text{distribution volume/normal PV} \quad (14\text{-}7)$$

To restore blood volume using D5W, assuming a distribution volume for sodium-free water of TBW, requires 28 L:

$$28 \text{ L} = 2 \text{ L} \times 42 \text{ L}/3 \text{ L} \quad (14\text{-}8)$$

where 2 L is the desired PV increment, 42 L = TBW in a 70-kg person, and 3 L is the normal estimated PV.

To restore blood volume using lactated Ringer solution requires 9.1 L:

$$9.1 \text{ L} = 2 \text{ L} \times 14 \text{ L}/3 \text{ L} \quad (14\text{-}9)$$

where 14 L = ECV in a 70-kg person.

If 5% albumin, which exerts colloid osmotic pressure similar to plasma, were infused, the infused volume initially would remain in the PV, perhaps attracting additional interstitial fluid intravascularly. Twenty-five percent human serum albumin, a concentrated colloid, expands PV by approximately 400 mL for each 100 mL infused.

However, these static analyses are simplistic. Infused fluid does not simply equilibrate throughout an assumed distribution volume but is added to a highly regulated system that attempts to maintain intravascular, interstitial, and intracellular volume. A more comprehensive kinetic model was proposed by Svensen and Hahn.[20] Kinetic models of intravenous fluid therapy allow clinicians to predict more accurately the time course of volume changes produced by infusions of fluids of various compositions. Kinetic analysis permits estimation of peak volume expansion and rates of clearance of infused fluid and complements analysis of "pharmacodynamic" effects, such as changes in cardiac output or cardiac filling pressures.

Using a kinetic approach to fluid therapy permits analysis of the effects of common physiologic and pharmacologic influences on fluid distribution in experimental animals or humans. For example, in chronically instrumented sheep, isoflurane anesthesia and the conscious state were associated with similar kinetics of PV expansion after fluid infusion, but reduced urinary output in anesthetized sheep demonstrated

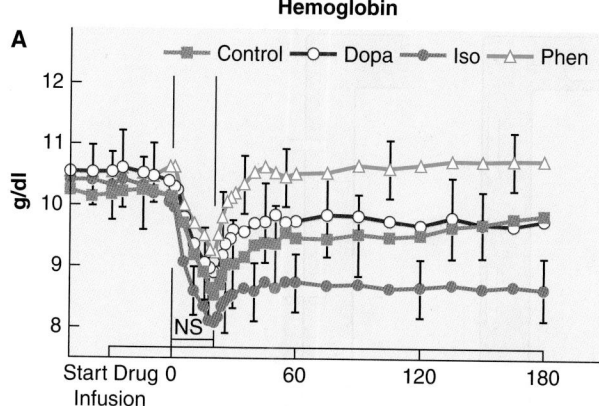

Hemoglobin

A

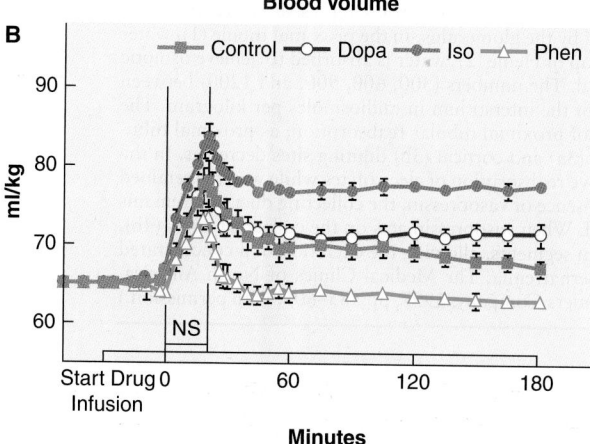

Blood Volume

B

Minutes

FIGURE 14-1. **A.** Blood hemoglobin (mean ± SEM) sampled at three baseline periods during a 30-minute catecholamine infusion and for 3 hours after starting a 20-minute 0.9% NaCl bolus of 24 mL/kg. Catecholamine protocols are dopamine (Dopa, *open diamonds*), isoproterenol (Iso, *closed circles*), phenylephrine (Phen, *open triangles*), and no-drug control (Control, *closed squares*). The 0.9% NaCl bolus decreased hemoglobin in all protocols at the end of the 20-minute 0.9% NaCL infusion and in all protocols except the Phen protocol thereafter. Postinfusion protocol differences were Phen > Dopa = Control > Iso. **B.** Calculated blood volume (mean ± SEM) at three baseline periods during a catecholamine infusion and for 3 hours after starting a 20-minute 0.9% NaCl bolus of 24 mL/kg. The 0.9% NaCl bolus increased blood volume in all protocols at T20 and in all protocols except the Phen protocol thereafter. Postinfusion protocol differences were Iso > Dopa = Control > Phen. NS, normal saline bolus. (From Vane LA, Prough DS, Kinsky MA, Williams CA, Grady JJ, Kramer GC: Effects of different catecholamines on the dynamics of volume expansion of crystalloid infusion. Anesthesiology 2004; 101: 1136–1144, with permission).

---

that expansion of extravascular volume was relatively greater during anesthesia[21]; subsequent experiments demonstrated that this effect was attributable to isoflurane and not to mechanical ventilation during anesthesia.[22] Also in chronically instrumented sheep, administration of catecholamine infusions before and during fluid infusions profoundly altered intravascular fluid retention, with phenylephrine diminishing and isoproterenol enhancing intravascular fluid retention (Fig. 14-1).[23]

Regulation of Extracellular Fluid Volume

Total body water content is regulated by the intake and output of water. Water intake includes ingested liquids plus an average of 750 mL ingested in solid food and 350 mL that is gen-

erated metabolically. Insensible losses are normally 1 L/day and gastrointestinal losses are 100 to 150 mL/day. Thirst, the primary mechanism of controlling water intake, is triggered by an increase in body fluid tonicity or by a decrease in extracellular volume.

Reabsorption of filtered water and sodium is enhanced by changes mediated by the hormonal factors antidiuretic hormone (ADH), atrial natriuretic peptide (ANP), and aldosterone. Renal water handling has three important components: (1) delivery of tubular fluid to the diluting segments of the nephron, (2) separation of solute and water in the diluting segment, and (3) variable reabsorption of water in the collecting ducts. In the descending loop of Henle, water is reabsorbed while solute is retained to achieve a final osmolality of tubular fluid of approximately 1,200 mOsm/kg (Fig. 14-2). This concentrated fluid is then diluted by the active reabsorption of electrolytes in the ascending limb of the loop of Henle and in the distal tubule, both of which are relatively impermeable to water. As fluid exits the distal tubule and enters the collecting duct, osmolality is approximately 50 mOsm/kg. Within the collecting duct, water reabsorption is modulated by ADH (also called *vasopressin*). Vasopressin binds to V_2 receptors along the basolateral membrane of the collecting duct cells, then stimulates the synthesis and insertion of the aquaporin-2 water channel into the luminal membrane of collecting duct cells.[24]

Plasma hypotonicity suppresses ADH release, resulting in excretion of dilute urine. Hypertonicity stimulates ADH secretion, which increases the permeability of the collecting duct to water and enhances water reabsorption. In response to changing plasma [Na^+], changing secretion of ADH can vary urinary osmolality from 50 to 1,200 mOsm/kg and urinary volume from 0.4 to 20 L/day (Fig. 14-3).[25] Other factors that stimulate ADH secretion, although none as powerfully as plasma tonicity, include hypotension, hypovolemia, and nonosmotic stimuli such as nausea, pain, and medications, including opiates.

Two powerful hormonal systems regulate total body sodium. The natriuretic peptides, ANP, brain natriuretic peptide, and C-type natriuretic peptide, defend against sodium overload[26–28] and the renin-angiotensin-aldosterone axis defends against sodium depletion and hypovolemia. ANP, released from the cardiac atria in response to increased atrial stretch, exerts vasodilatory effects and increases the renal excretion of sodium and water. ANP secretion is decreased during hypovolemia. Even in patients with chronic (nonoliguric) renal insufficiency, infusion of ANP in low, nonhypotensive doses increased sodium excretion and augmented urinary losses of retained solutes.[29]

Aldosterone is the final common pathway in a complex response to decreased effective arterial volume, whether decreased effective arterial volume is true or relative, as in edematous states or hypoalbuminemia. In this pathway, decreased stretch in the baroreceptors of the aortic arch and carotid body and stretch receptors in the great veins, pulmonary vasculature, and atria result in increased sympathetic tone. Increased sympathetic tone, in combination with decreased renal perfusion, leads to renin release and formation of angiotensin I from angiotensinogen. Angiotensin-converting enzyme (ACE) converts angiotensin I to angiotensin II, which stimulates the adrenal cortex to synthesize and release aldosterone.[30] Acting primarily in the distal tubules, high concentrations of aldosterone cause sodium reabsorption and may reduce urinary excretion of sodium nearly to zero. Intrarenal physical factors are also important in regulating sodium balance. Sodium loading decreases colloid osmotic pressure, thereby increasing the glomerular filtration rate (GFR), decreasing net sodium reabsorption and increasing distal sodium delivery, which, in turn, suppresses renin secretion.

ANATOMY AND PHYSIOLOGY

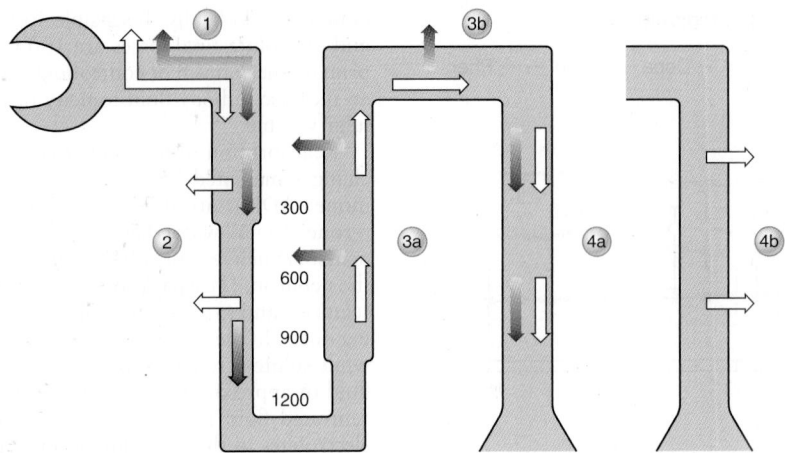

FIGURE 14-2.   Renal filtration, reabsorption, and excretion of water. *Open arrows* represent water and *solid arrows* represent electrolytes. Water and electrolytes are filtered by the glomerulus. In the proximal tubule (1), water and electrolytes are absorbed isotonically. In the descending loop of Henle (2), water is absorbed to achieve osmotic equilibrium with the interstitium while electrolytes are retained. The numbers (300, 600, 900, and 1200) between the descending and ascending limbs represent the osmolality of the interstitium in milliosmoles per kilogram. The delivery of solute and fluid to the distal nephron is a function of proximal tubular reabsorption; as proximal tubular reabsorption increases, delivery of solute to the medullary (3a) and cortical (3b) diluting sites decreases. In the diluting sites, electrolyte-free water is generated through selective reabsorption of electrolytes while water is retained in the tubular lumen, generating a dilute tubular fluid. In the absence of vasopressin, the collecting duct (4a) remains relatively impermeable to water and a diluted urine is excreted. When vasopressin acts on the collecting ducts (4b), water is reabsorbed from these vasopressin-responsive nephron segments, allowing the excretion of a concentrated urine. (From Fried LF, Palevsky PM: Hyponatremia and hypernatremia, The Medical Clinics of North America. Renal Disease. Edited by Saklayen MG. Philadelphia, WB Saunders Company, 1997, pp 585–609, with permission.)

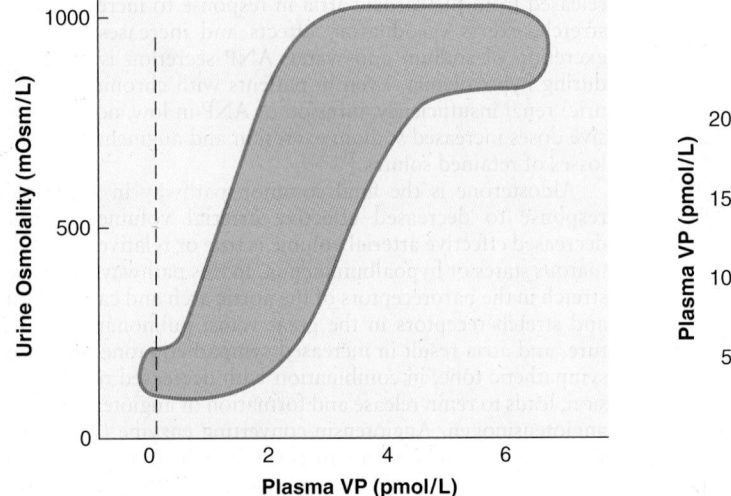
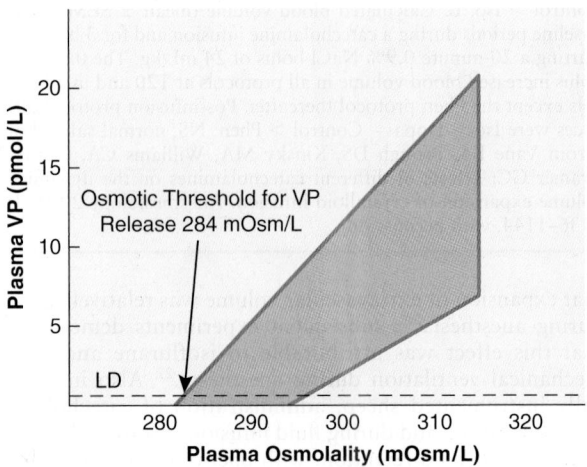

FIGURE 14-3.   **Left.** The sigmoid relationship between plasma vasopressin (VP) and urinary osmolality. Data were obtained during water loading and fluid restriction in a group of healthy adults. Maximum urinary concentration is achieved by plasma VP values of 3 to 4 pmol/L. **Right.** The linear relationship between plasma osmolality and plasma VP. Increases in VP in response to hypertonicity induced by infusion of 855 mmol/L saline in a group of healthy adults. The shaded area represents the reference range response. LD represents the limit of detection of the VP assay, 0.3 pmol/L. (From Ball SG: Vasopressin and disorders of water balance: the physiology and pathophysiology of vasopressin. Ann Clin Biochem 2007; 44: 417–431, with permission.)

Fluid Replacement Therapy

Maintenance Requirements for Water, Sodium, and Potassium

Calculation of maintenance fluid requirements is of limited value in determining intraoperative fluid requirements. However, calculation of maintenance fluid requirements (Table 14-10) is useful for estimating water and electrolyte deficits that result from preoperative restriction of oral food and fluids and for estimating the ongoing requirements for patients with prolonged postoperative bowel dysfunction. In healthy adults, sufficient water is required to balance gastrointestinal losses of 100 to 200 mL/day, insensible losses of 500 to 1,000 mL/day (half of which is respiratory and half is cutaneous), and urinary losses of 1,000 mL/day. Urinary losses exceeding 1,000 mL/day may represent an appropriate physiologic response to ECV expansion or pathophysiologic inability to conserve salt or water.

Daily adult requirements for sodium and potassium are approximately 75 and 40 mEq/kg, respectively, although wider ranges of sodium intake than potassium intake are physiologically tolerated because renal sodium conservation and excretion are more efficient than potassium conservation and excretion. Therefore, healthy, 70-kg adults require 2,500 mL/day of water containing a $[Na^+]$ of 30 mEq/L and a $[K^+]$ of 15 to 20 mEq/L. Intraoperatively, fluids containing sodium-free water (i.e., $[Na^+] < 130$ mEq/L) are rarely used in adults because of the necessity for replacing isotonic losses and the risk of postoperative hyponatremia.

Dextrose

Traditionally, glucose-containing intravenous fluids have been given in an effort to prevent hypoglycemia and limit protein catabolism. However, because of the hyperglycemic response associated with surgical stress, only infants and patients receiving insulin or drugs that interfere with glucose synthesis are at risk for hypoglycemia. Iatrogenic hyperglycemia can limit the effectiveness of fluid resuscitation by inducing an osmotic diuresis and, in animals, may aggravate ischemic neurologic injury.[31] Although associated with worsened outcome after subarachnoid hemorrhage[32] and traumatic brain injury[33] in humans, hyperglycemia may also constitute a hormonally mediated response to more severe injury. In critically ill patients, some evidence suggests that tight control of plasma glucose (maintenance of plasma glucose between 80 and 110 mg/dL) is associated with reduced mortality and morbidity, but other evidence does not.[34–37] Evidence also suggests that tight glucose control improves outcome in surgical patients.[38]

Surgical Fluid Requirements

Water and Electrolyte Composition of Fluid Losses

Surgical patients require replacement of PV and ECV losses secondary to wound or burn edema, ascites, and gastrointesti-

nal secretions. Wound and burn edema and ascitic fluid are protein-rich and contain electrolytes in concentrations similar to plasma. Although gastrointestinal secretions vary greatly in composition, the composition of replacement fluid need not be closely matched if ECV is adequate and renal and cardiovascular functions are normal. Substantial loss of gastrointestinal fluids requires more accurate replacement of electrolytes (i.e., potassium, magnesium, phosphate). Chronic gastric losses may produce hypochloremic metabolic alkalosis that can be corrected with 0.9% saline; chronic diarrhea may produce hyperchloremic metabolic acidosis that may be prevented or corrected by infusion of fluid containing bicarbonate or bicarbonate substrate (e.g., lactate). If cardiovascular or renal function is impaired, more precise replacement may require frequent assessment of serum electrolytes.

Influence of Perioperative Fluid Infusion Rates on Clinical Outcomes

Conventionally, intraoperative fluid management has included replacement of fluid that is assumed to accumulate extravascularly in surgically manipulated tissue. Until recently, perioperative clinical practice included, in addition to maintenance fluids and replacement of estimated blood loss, 4 to 6 mL/kg/hr for procedures involving minimal tissue trauma, 6 to 8 mL/kg/hr for those involving moderate trauma, and 8 to 12 mL/kg/hr for those involving extreme trauma.

However, recent clinical trials strongly link perioperative fluid management to potentially important alterations of both minor and major morbidity. Moreover, the influence of fluid volume may be specific to the type of surgery and to the types of fluid used. Maharaj et al.[39] randomized 80 ASA I-II patients scheduled for gynecologic laparoscopy either to large volume, defined as 2.0 mL/kg/hr of fasting over 20 minutes preoperatively (e.g., 1,440 mL/60 kg in a patient who had been fasting for 12 hours) or small volume, defined as total fluid of 3.0 mL/kg over 20 minutes preoperatively. In patients receiving the higher dose, postoperative nausea and vomiting and pain were significantly reduced (Fig. 14-4).[39] Holte et al.[40] randomized 48 ASA I-II patients undergoing laparoscopic cholecystectomy to receive either 15 or 40 mL/kg of lactated Ringer solution intraoperatively; the higher dose of fluid was associated with improved postoperative pulmonary function and exercise capacity, reduced neurohumoral stress response, and improvements in nausea, general sense of well-being, thirst, dizziness, drowsiness, fatigue, and balance function. Holte et al.[41] randomized 48 ASA I-III patients undergoing fast-track elective knee arthroplasty under intraoperative epidural/spinal anesthesia and postoperative epidural analgesia to either liberal or restricted fluids. Median intravenous fluid administered intraoperatively and in the postanesthesia care unit in the restrictive group was 1,740 mL (range, 1,100 to 2,165 mL) of lactated Ringer solution and in the liberal group was 3,275 mL (range, 2,400 to 4,000 mL). Restrictive fluid administration was associated with a higher incidence of vomiting but less hypercoagulability and no difference in short-term postoperative mobility or ileus. Therefore, fluid restriction appears to be less well tolerated than more liberal fluid therapy in patients undergoing surgery of limited scope, but perhaps at the expense of hypercoagulability.

In patients undergoing major intra-abdominal surgery, recent randomized controlled trials also suggest that restrictive fluid administration is associated with a combination of positive and negative effects. Brandstrup et al.[42] randomized 172 elective colon surgery patients to either restrictive perioperative fluid management or standard perioperative fluid management, with the primary goal of maintaining preoperative body weight in the fluid-restricted group. By design, the fluid-restricted group received less perioperative fluid and

TABLE 14-10

HOURLY AND DAILY MAINTENANCE WATER REQUIREMENTS

WEIGHT (kg)	WATER (mL/kg/hr)	WATER (mL/kg/day)
1–10	4	100
11–20	2	50
21–n+	1	20

FIGURE 14-4. **Top.** Mean postoperative verbal analog scale (VAS) nausea scores in each group over the first 72 postoperative hours. Mean VAS nausea scores were significantly lower in the group that received the large-volume intravenous fluid infusion compared with the control group at 1, 4, 24, and 72 hours postoperatively. **Bottom.** Mean postoperative VAS pain scores in each group over the first 72 postoperative hours. Mean VAS pain scores were significantly lower in the group that received the large-volume intravenous fluid infusion compared with the control group at 0, 1, 24, and 72 hours postoperatively. *Significantly higher ($p < 0.05$, t-test postanalysis of variance) VAS score compared with the large volume group. PACU, postanesthesia care unit. (From Maharaj CH, Kallam SR, Malik A, Hassett P, Grady D, Laffey JG: Preoperative intravenous fluid therapy decreases postoperative nausea and pain in high risk patients. Anesth Analg 2005; 100: 675–682, with permission.)

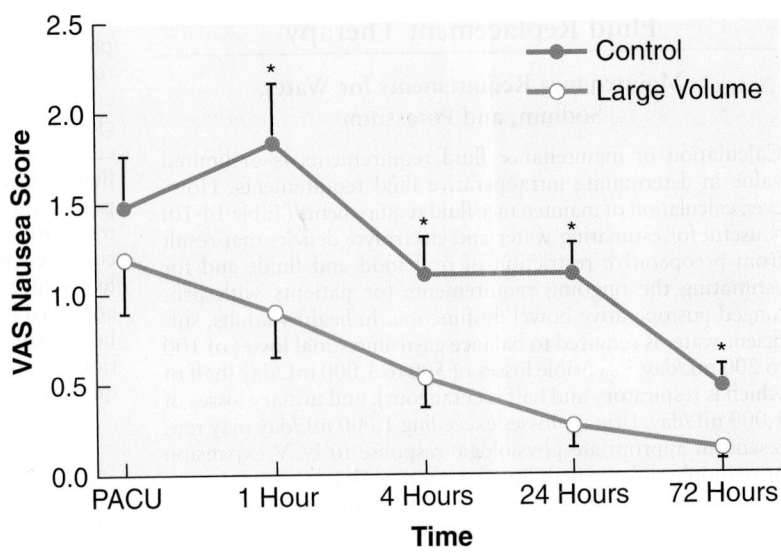

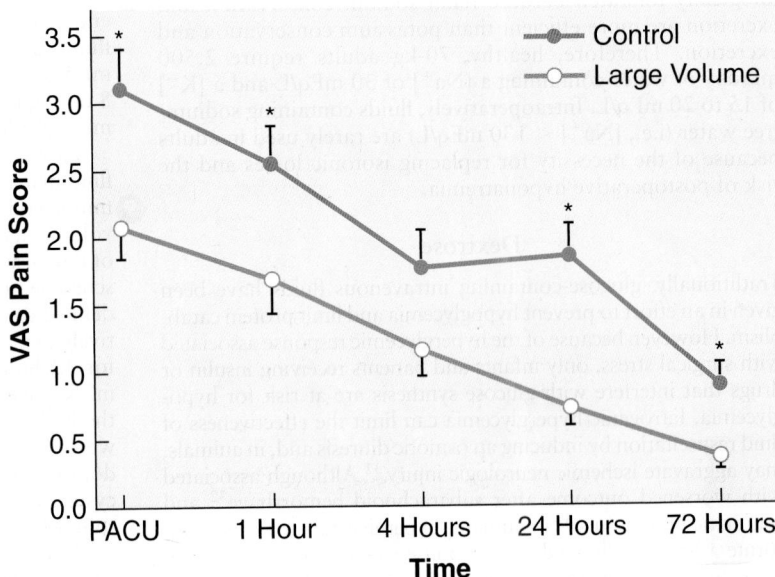

acutely gained <1 kg in contrast to >3 kg in the standard therapy group. More importantly, cardiopulmonary complications, tissue-healing complications, and total postoperative complications were significantly fewer in the fluid-restricted group. In 152 patients undergoing intra-abdominal surgery, including colon surgery, Nisanevich et al.[43] reported less prompt return of gastrointestinal function and longer hospital stays in patients receiving conventional fluid therapy (10 mL/kg/hr of lactated Ringer solution) than in patients receiving restricted fluid therapy (4.0 mL/kg/hr). In a small clinical trial comparing gastric emptying in patients randomized to receive postoperative fluids at a restricted (≤2.0 L/day of water; ≤77 mEq/day) or liberal regimen (≥3.0 L/day of water; ≥154 mEq/day), gastric emptying time for both liquids and solids was significantly reduced in patients receiving restricted fluids (Fig. 14-5).[44] Khoo et al.[45] randomized 70 ASA I-III patients undergoing elective colorectal surgery to conventional perioperative management, including intraoperative fluid management at the discretion of the anesthesiologist, or to multimodal perioperative management, including intraoperative fluid restriction, unrestricted postoperative oral intake, prokinetic agents, early ambulation, and postoperative epidural analgesia. Multimodal perioperative multimodal management was associated with a reduced median stay (5 vs. 7 days) and fewer cardiorespiratory and anastomotic complications, but more hospital readmissions. Holte et al.[46] randomized 32 ASA I-III patients undergoing "fast-track" colon resection under combined epidural/general anesthesia to intraoperative fluid administration using either a restrictive (median, 1,640 mL; range, 935 to 2,250 mL) or liberal (median, 5,050 mL; range, 3,563 to 8,050 mL) regimen. Fluid-restricted patients had significantly improved postoperative forced vital capacity and fewer, less severe episodes of oxygen saturation but at the expense of increased stress responses (aldosterone, antidiuretic hormone and angiotensin II measurements) and a statistically insignificantly increased number of complications.

Critically ill patients with acute lung injury represent an important group that may benefit from careful regulation of fluid intake. The ARDS Clinical Trials Network[47] random-

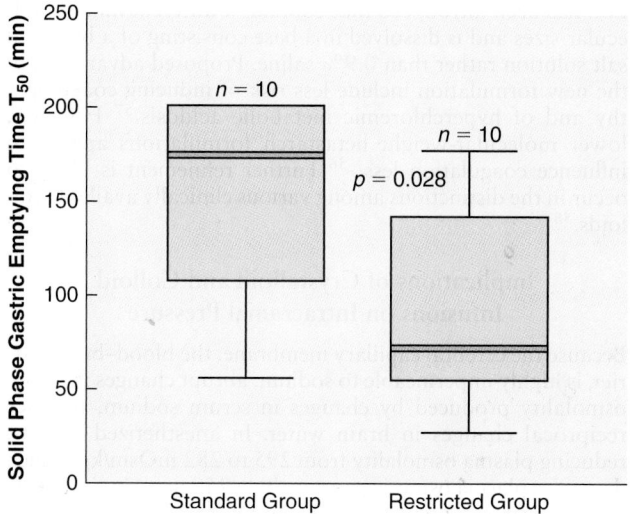

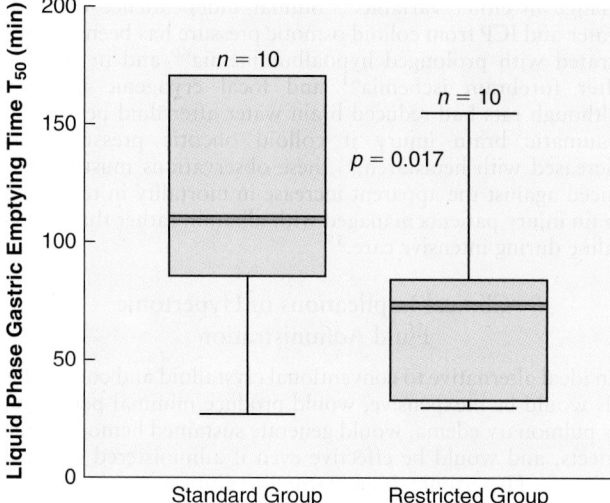

FIGURE 14-5. Solid and liquid phase gastric emptying times (T_{50}) after 4 days of standard or restricted intravenous postoperative fluid therapy. Solid lines are medians, shaded areas interquartile ranges, and whiskers represent extreme values. Differences between medians for solid and liquid phase T_{50} were 56 minutes (95% confidence interval: 12 to 132 minutes) and 52 minutes (9 to 95 mn), respectively. (Reprinted with permission from Lobo DN, Bostock KA, Neal KR, Perkins AC, Rowlands BJ, Allison SP: Effect of salt and water balance on recovery of gastrointestinal function after elective colonic resection: a randomised controlled trial. Lancet 2002; 359: 1812).

ized 1,000 patients with acute lung injury to a 7-day trial comparing a conservative fluid strategy with a liberal fluid strategy. Over the course of the trial the conservative strategy group had a cumulative net fluid balance that was slightly negative in comparison to a mean net cumulative fluid balance in the liberal group of nearly 7.0 L. Although overall mortality was no different in the two groups, the conservative fluid group had improved oxygenation and required fewer days of mechanical ventilation and intensive care. Despite achieving a negative fluid balance, the conservative strategy group had no greater incidence of acute renal failure.

Colloids, Crystalloids, and Hypertonic Solutions

Physiology and Pharmacology

Osmotically active particles attract water across semipermeable membranes until equilibrium is attained. The *osmolarity* of a solution refers to the number of osmotically active particles per *liter* of solvent; *osmolality*, a measurement of the number of osmotically active particles per *kilogram*, can be estimated as follows:

$$\text{Osmolality} = ([Na^+] \times 2) + (\text{Glucose}/18) + (\text{BUN}/2.3) \qquad (14\text{-}10)$$

where osmolality is expressed in mmol/kg, $[Na^+]$ is expressed in mEq/L, serum glucose is expressed in mg/dL, and BUN is blood urea nitrogen expressed in mg/dL. Sugars, alcohols, and radiographic dyes increase measured osmolality, generating an increased "osmolal gap" between the measured and calculated values.

A hyperosmolar state occurs whenever the concentration of osmotically active particles is high. Both uremia (increased BUN) and hypernatremia (increased serum sodium) increase serum osmolality. However, because urea distributes throughout TBW, an increase in BUN does not cause *hypertonicity*. Sodium, largely restricted to the ECV, causes hypertonicity, that is, osmotically mediated redistribution of water from ICV to ECV. The term *tonicity* is also used colloquially to compare the osmotic pressure of a parenteral solution to that of plasma.

Although only a small proportion of the osmotically active particles in blood consist of plasma proteins, those particles are essential in determining the equilibrium of fluid between the interstitial and plasma compartments of ECV. The reflection coefficient (σ) describes the permeability of capillary membranes to individual solutes, with 0 representing free permeability and 1.0 representing complete impermeability. The reflection coefficient for albumin ranges from 0.6 to 0.9 in various capillary beds. Because capillary protein concentrations exceed interstitial concentrations, the osmotic pressure exerted by plasma proteins (termed *colloid osmotic pressure* or *oncotic pressure*) is higher than interstitial oncotic pressure and tends to preserve PV. The filtration rate of fluid from the capillaries into the interstitial space is the net result of a combination of forces, including the gradient from intravascular to interstitial colloid osmotic pressures and the hydrostatic gradient between intravascular and interstitial pressures. The net fluid filtration at any point within a systemic or pulmonary capillary is represented by Starling's law of capillary filtration, as expressed in the equation:

$$Q = \underline{k}\underline{A}\,[(P_c - P_i) + \sigma(\pi_i - \pi_c)] \qquad (14\text{-}11)$$

where Q = fluid filtration, $\underline{k}$ = capillary filtration coefficient (conductivity of water), $\underline{A}$ = the area of the capillary membrane, P_c = capillary hydrostatic pressure, P_i = interstitial hydrostatic pressure, σ = reflection coefficient for albumin, π_i = interstitial colloid osmotic pressure, and π_c = capillary colloid osmotic pressure.

The IFV is determined by the relative rates of capillary filtration and lymphatic drainage. P_c, the most powerful factor promoting fluid filtration, is determined by capillary flow, arterial resistance, venous resistance, and venous pressure. If capillary filtration increases, the rates of water and sodium filtration usually exceed protein filtration, resulting in preservation of π_c, dilution of π_i, and preservation of the oncotic pressure gradient, the most powerful factor opposing fluid filtration. When coupled with increased lymphatic drainage, preservation of the oncotic pressure gradient limits the accumulation of IF. If P_c increases at a time when lymphatic drainage is maximal, then IFV accumulates, forming edema.

Clinical Implications of Choices Between Alternative Fluids

If membrane permeability is intact, colloids such as albumin or hydroxyethyl starch preferentially expand PV rather than IFV. Concentrated colloid-containing solutions (e.g., 25% albumin) exert sufficient oncotic pressure to translocate substantial volumes of IFV into the PV, thereby increasing PV by a volume that exceeds the original infused volume. PV expansion unaccompanied by IFV expansion offers apparent advantages: lower fluid requirements, less peripheral and pulmonary edema accumulation, and reduced concern about the cardiopulmonary consequences of later fluid mobilization (Table 14-11).

However, exhaustive research has failed to establish the superiority of either colloid-containing or crystalloid-containing fluids for either intraoperative or postoperative use. Moretti et al.[48] reported that patients who were randomized to receive 6% hetastarch had less postoperative nausea and vomiting than those who received lactated Ringer solution without colloid. In addition, colloid administration appears to have been an essential component of perioperative management strategies that demonstrated improved morbidity after colon surgery[42] and after major surgery in conjunction with goal-directed fluid challenges.[49,50]

In critically ill patients and patients undergoing more extensive surgery, systematic reviews of available comparisons of colloid versus crystalloid[51] and albumin versus crystalloid[52] suggested that the choice of fluid did not influence mortality. A recent randomized controlled trial comparing 4% albumin with 0.9% saline for fluid maintenance in 6,997 critically ill patients supports the conclusion that choice of colloid or crystalloid does not influence mortality.[53] Baseline serum albumin concentration did not alter the lack of effect of albumin management on outcome.[54] However, subgroup analyses suggested that crystalloid treatment could be superior in patients after trauma and that colloid could be superior in patients with severe sepsis.[53] Subsequent 2-year follow-up of a subset of 460 patients with traumatic brain injury (Glasgow Coma Scale score ≤13) demonstrated a nearly twofold increased risk of death in patients receiving colloid fluid management.[55]

Although hydroxyethyl starch, the most commonly used synthetic colloid, is less expensive than albumin, large doses (exceeding 20 mL/kg/day) produce laboratory evidence of coagulopathy.[56] Recently, a new hydroxyethyl starch formulation has been introduced that contains a different mix of molecular sizes and is dissolved in a base consisting of a balanced salt solution rather than 0.9% saline. Proposed advantages of the new formulation include less risk of inducing coagulopathy and of hyperchloremic metabolic acidosis.[57] However, lower molecular-weight hetastarch formulations appear to influence coagulation less.[56] Further refinement is likely to occur in the distinctions among various clinically available colloids.[58]

Implications of Crystalloid and Colloid Infusions on Intracranial Pressure

Because the cerebral capillary membrane, the blood–brain barrier, is highly impermeable to sodium, abrupt changes in serum osmolality produced by changes in serum sodium, produce reciprocal changes in brain water. In anesthetized rabbits, reducing plasma osmolality from 295 to 282 mOsm/kg (which decreases plasma osmotic pressure by ~250 mm Hg) increased cortical water content and ICP; in contrast reducing colloid osmotic pressure from 20 to 7 mm Hg produced no significant change in either variable.[59] Similar independence of brain water and ICP from colloid osmotic pressure has been demonstrated with prolonged hypoalbuminemia[60] and in animals after forebrain ischemia[61] and focal cryogenic injury.[62] Although rats had reduced brain water after fluid percussion traumatic brain injury if colloid oncotic pressure was increased with hetastarch,[63] these observations must be balanced against the apparent increase in mortality in traumatic brain injury patients managed with albumin rather than 0.9% saline during intensive care.[55]

Clinical Implications of Hypertonic Fluid Administration

An ideal alternative to conventional crystalloid and colloid fluids would be inexpensive, would produce minimal peripheral or pulmonary edema, would generate sustained hemodynamic effects, and would be effective even if administered in small volumes. Hypertonic, hypernatremic solutions, with or without added colloid, appear to fulfill some of these criteria (Table 14-12).

Current enthusiasm for hypertonic resuscitation was stimulated by the work of Velasco et al.,[64] who successfully used small volumes (6.0 mL/kg) of 7.5% hypertonic saline as the sole resuscitative measure in dogs after severe hemorrhage. Hypertonic solutions exert favorable effects on cerebral hemodynamics, in part because of the reciprocal relationship

TABLE 14-11

CLAIMED ADVANTAGES AND DISADVANTAGES OF COLLOID VERSUS CRYSTALLOID INTRAVENOUS FLUIDS

■ SOLUTION	■ ADVANTAGES	■ DISADVANTAGES
Colloid	Smaller infused volume Prolonged increase in plasma volume Less peripheral edema	Greater cost Coagulopathy (dextran > HES) Pulmonary edema (capillary leak states) Decreased GFR Osmotic diuresis (low-molecular-weight dextran) Greater duration of excessive volume expansion
Crystalloid	Lower cost Greater urinary flow Interstitial fluid replacement	Transient increase in intravascular volume Transient hemodynamic improvement Peripheral edema (protein dilution) Pulmonary edema (protein dilution plus high PAOP)

HES, hydroxyethyl starch; GFR, glomerular filtration rate; PAOP, pulmonary arterial occlusion pressure.

TABLE 14-12

HYPERTONIC RESUSCITATION FLUIDS: ADVANTAGES AND DISADVANTAGES

■ SOLUTION	■ ADVANTAGES	■ DISADVANTAGES
Hypertonic crystalloid	Inexpensive Promotes urinary flow Small initial volume Arteriolar dilation Reduced peripheral edema Lower intracranial pressure	Hypertonicity Subdural hemorrhage Transient effect Potential rebound intracranial hypertension
Hypertonic crystalloid plus colloid (in comparison to hypertonic crystalloid alone)	Sustained hemodynamic response Reduced subsequent volume requirements	Added expense Osmotic diuresis Hypertonicity

From Prough DS, Johnston WE: Fluid resuscitation in septic shock: No solution yet. Anesth Analg 1989; 69: 699–704, with permission.

between plasma osmolality and brain water.[59] ICP increased during resuscitation from hemorrhagic shock with lactated Ringer solution but remained unchanged if 7.5% saline was infused in a sufficient volume to comparably improve systemic hemodynamics.[65] However, improvements in ICP gradually are lost. Delayed increases in ICP were reported after hypertonic resuscitation from hypovolemic shock accompanied by an intracranial mass lesion.[66] In addition, systemic hemodynamic improvement produced by hypertonic resuscitation is short-lived.[65] Strategies to prolong the therapeutic effects beyond 30 to 60 minutes include continued infusion of hypertonic saline, subsequent infusion of blood or conventional fluids, or addition of colloid to hypertonic resuscitation.

Despite concerns about central nervous system dysfunction due to hypertonicity and hypernatremia associated with hypertonic saline, acute increases in serum sodium to 155 to 160 mEq/L produced no apparent harm in humans resuscitated with hypertonic saline.[67] Central pontine myelinolysis, which follows rapid correction of severe, chronic hyponatremia, has not been observed in clinical trials of hypertonic resuscitation. Despite theoretical considerations favoring the use of hypertonic saline in resuscitation of patients with traumatic brain injury, a recent randomized trial failed to demonstrate an improvement in outcome.[68]

Will clinicians routinely use hypertonic or combination hypertonic/hyperoncotic fluids for resuscitation in the future? Pending further preclinical work, the theoretical advantages of such fluids appear most attractive in the acute resuscitation of hypovolemic patients who have decreased intracranial compliance.[69]

Fluid Status: Assessment and Monitoring

For most surgical patients, conventional clinical assessment of the adequacy of intravascular volume is appropriate. For high-risk patients, goal-directed hemodynamic management may be superior.

Conventional Clinical Assessment.

Clinical quantification of blood volume and ECV begins with recognition of deficit-generating settings such as bowel obstruction, preoperative bowel preparation, chronic diuretic use, sepsis, burns, and trauma. Physical signs that suggest hypovolemia include oliguria, supine hypotension, and a positive tilt test. Oliguria implies hypovolemia, although hypovolemic patients may be nonoliguric and normovolemic

patients may be oliguric because of renal failure or stress-induced endocrine responses.[70] Supine hypotension implies a blood volume deficit exceeding 30%, although arterial blood pressure within the normal range could represent relative hypotension in an elderly or chronically hypertensive patient.

In the tilt test, a positive response is defined as an increase in heart rate ≥20 beats per minute and a decrease in systolic blood pressure ≥20 mm Hg when the subject assumes the upright position. However, young, healthy subjects can withstand acute loss of 20% of blood volume while exhibiting only postural tachycardia and variable postural hypotension. In contrast, orthostasis may occur in 20 to 30% of elderly patients despite normal blood volume. In volunteers, withdrawal of 500 mL of blood[71] was associated with a greater increase in heart rate on standing than before blood withdrawal, but with no significant difference in the response of blood pressure or cardiac index.

Laboratory evidence that suggests hypovolemia or ECV depletion includes azotemia, low urinary sodium, metabolic alkalosis (if hypovolemia is mild), and metabolic acidosis (if hypovolemia is severe). Hematocrit is virtually unchanged by acute hemorrhage until fluids are administered or until fluid shifts from the interstitial to the intravascular space. BUN, normally 8.0 to 20 mg/dL, is increased by hypovolemia, high-protein intake, gastrointestinal bleeding, or accelerated catabolism and decreased by severe hepatic dysfunction. Serum creatinine (SCr), a product of muscle catabolism, may be misleadingly low in elderly adults, females, and debilitated or malnourished patients. In contrast, in muscular or acutely catabolic patients, SCr may exceed the normal range (0.5 to 1.5 mg/dL) because of greater muscle protein metabolism. A ratio of BUN to SCr exceeding the normal range (10 to 20) suggests dehydration. In prerenal oliguria, enhanced sodium reabsorption should reduce urinary $[Na^+]$ to ≤20 mEq/L and enhanced water reabsorption should increase urinary concentration (i.e., urinary osmolality >400, urine/plasma creatinine ratio >40:1). However, the sensitivity and specificity of measurements of urinary variables may be misleading. Although hypovolemia does not generate metabolic alkalosis, ECV depletion is a potent stimulus for the maintenance of metabolic alkalosis. Severe hypovolemia may result in systemic hypoperfusion and lactic acidosis.

Intraoperative Clinical Assessment.

Visual estimation, the simplest technique for quantifying intraoperative blood loss, assesses the amount of blood absorbed by gauze squares and laparotomy pads and adds an estimate of blood accumulation on the floor and surgical drapes and in suction containers. Both surgeons and anesthesia providers tend to underestimate losses.

Assessment of the adequacy of intraoperative fluid resuscitation integrates multiple clinical variables, including heart rate, blood pressure, urinary output, arterial oxygenation, and pH. Tachycardia is an insensitive, nonspecific indicator of hypovolemia. In patients receiving potent inhalational agents, maintenance of a satisfactory blood pressure implies adequate intravascular volume. Preservation of blood pressure, accompanied by a CVP of 6 to 12 mm Hg, more strongly suggests adequate replacement. During profound hypovolemia, indirect measurements of blood pressure may significantly underestimate true blood pressure. In patients undergoing extensive procedures, direct arterial pressure measurements are more accurate than indirect techniques and provide convenient access for obtaining arterial blood samples. An additional advantage of direct arterial pressure monitoring may be recognition of increased systolic blood pressure variation accompanying positive pressure ventilation in the presence of hypovolemia.[72,73]

Urinary output usually declines precipitously during moderate to severe hypovolemia. Therefore, in the absence of glycosuria or diuretic administration, a urinary output of 0.5 to 1.0 mL/kg hr during anesthesia suggests adequate renal perfusion. Arterial pH may decrease only when tissue hypoperfusion becomes severe. Cardiac output can be normal despite severely reduced regional blood flow. Mixed venous hemoglobin desaturation, a specific indicator of poor systemic perfusion, reflects average perfusion in multiple organs and cannot supplant regional monitors such as urinary output.

A promising technique for assessing the adequacy of cardiac preload during high-risk surgical procedures is the use of esophageal Doppler that measures blood flow in the descending thoracic aorta and that also measures the duration of aortic systole, which, if corrected for heart rate, correlates with left ventricular preload.[74,81] In general, a corrected flow time <0.35 second suggests that volume expansion should improve cardiac output, while a corrected flow time >0.40 second suggests that further volume expansion will be ineffective.

Oxygen Delivery as a Goal of Management

No intraoperative monitor is sufficiently sensitive or specific to detect hypoperfusion in all patients. One key variable that has been associated with improved outcome in high-risk surgical patients and critically ill patients is a systemic oxygen delivery (Do_2) $\geq$ 600mL O_2/m^2 min (equivalent to a cardiac index [CI] of 3.0 L/m^2 min, a [Hgb] of 14 g/dL, and 98% oxyhemoglobin saturation). At present, available data are consistent with two inferences. First, there is no apparent benefit for patients other than surgical patients[75] and patients undergoing initial resuscitation from septic shock in the emergency department.[76] In surgical patients, early initiation of goal-directed resuscitation is associated with better outcome than delayed initiation.[77] Second, outcome may be strongly influenced by the choice of methods to increase oxygen delivery, that is, the choice of fluid administration or various inotropic agents. Lobo et al.[78] randomized 50 high-risk patients, defined as elderly patients with coexistent pathologies who were undergoing major elective surgery, to goal-directed hemodynamic therapy either with fluids alone or with fluids plus dobutamine. Hemodynamic goals intraoperatively and for the first 24 hours postoperatively consisted of DO$_2$I >600 mL O$_2$/m^2 min. Postoperative cardiovascular complications occurred significantly more frequently in the group receiving fluids alone (13/25, 52%, vs. 4/25, 16%; relative risk, 3.25; 95% CI, 1.22–8.60; $p < 0.05$) and mortality was greater, but not statistically significantly greater in this small series.

Increased fluid given as part of goal-oriented resuscitation has been associated with an increased incidence of abdominal compartment syndrome in trauma patients.[79] Wilson et al.[80] randomized 138 patients undergoing major elective surgery into three groups. One group received routine perioperative care; one received fluid and dopexamine preoperatively, intraoperatively, and postoperatively to maintain oxygen delivery $\geq$600 mL O_2/m^2 min; and the third received fluid plus epinephrine preoperatively, intraoperatively, and postoperatively to achieve the same end points. In the two groups in which oxygen delivery was supported, only 3 of 92 died, compared with 8 of 46 control patients. However, the complication rate was significantly lower in the dopexamine group than in the epinephrine group.

Recently, several studies have reported improved outcome based on adjustment of perioperative fluids through the use of an esophageal Doppler monitor.[81] Using the esophageal Doppler to guide administration of colloid boluses, Venn et al.[49] and Gan et al.[50] have reported shortened length of hospital stay after hip surgery and major surgery, respectively. Of note, Horowitz and Kumar[82] speculated that the infusion of colloid rather than the monitor-driven algorithm was responsible for the improved results.

ELECTROLYTES

Sodium

Physiologic Role

10 Sodium, the principal extracellular cation and solute, is essential for generation of action potentials in neurologic and cardiac tissue. Disorders (pathologic increases or decreases) of *total body sodium* are associated with corresponding increases or decreases of ECV and PV. Disorders of sodium *concentration*, that is, hyponatremia and hypernatremia, usually result from relative excesses or deficits, respectively, of water. Regulation of total body sodium and [Na$^+$] is accomplished primarily by the endocrine and renal systems (Table 14-13). Secretion of aldosterone and ANP control *total body sodium*. ADH, which is secreted in response to increased osmolality or decreased blood pressure, primarily regulates [Na$^+$]. Therefore, primary hyperaldosteronism is associated with hypervolemia and with hypertension, but not with abnormal [Na$^+$].[83,84]

Hyponatremia

Hyponatremia, defined as [Na$^+$] < 130 mEq/L, is the most common electrolyte disturbance in hospitalized patients. In the majority of hyponatremic patients, total body sodium is normal or increased. The most common clinical scenarios associated with hyponatremia include the postoperative state, acute intracranial disease, malignant disease, medications, and acute pulmonary disease. Hyponatremia is associated with increased mortality, both as a direct effect of hyponatremia and because of the association between hyponatremia and severe systemic disease.

The signs and symptoms of hyponatremia depend on both the rate and severity of the decrease in plasma [Na$^+$]. Symptoms that can accompany severe hyponatremia ([Na$^+$] < 120 mEq/L) include loss of appetite, nausea, vomiting, cramps, weakness, altered level of consciousness, coma, and seizures.

Acute central nervous system manifestations of hyponatremia result from brain overhydration. Because the blood–brain barrier is poorly permeable to sodium but freely permeable to water, a rapid decrease in plasma [Na$^+$] promptly increases both extracellular and intracellular brain

TABLE 14-13

REGULATION OF TOTAL BODY ELECTROLYTE MASS AND PLASMA CONCENTRATIONS

▧ ELECTROLYTE	▧ REGULATED BY
Sodium	Total body sodium regulated by aldosterone, ANP, $[Na^+]$ altered by ADH
Potassium	Total body potassium regulated by aldosterone, intrinsic renal mechanisms; $[K^+]$ regulated by epinephrine, insulin
Calcium	Both total body calcium and $[Ca^{++}]$ regulated by PTH, vitamin D
Phosphate	Both total body phosphate and $[HPO_4^{--}]$ regulated primarily by renal mechanisms with a minor contribution from PTH
Magnesium	Both total body magnesium and $[Mg^{++}]$ regulated primarily by renal mechanisms with a minor contribution from PTH and vitamin D

ANP, atrial natriuretic peptide; $[Na^+]$, sodium concentration; ADH, antidiuretic hormone; PTH, parathyroid hormone.

water. Because the brain rapidly compensates for changes in osmolality, acute hyponatremia produces more severe symptoms than chronic hyponatremia. The symptoms of chronic hyponatremia probably relate to depletion of brain electrolytes. Once brain volume has compensated for hyponatremia, rapid increases in $[Na^+]$ may lead to abrupt brain dehydration.

In hyponatremic patients, serum osmolality may be normal, high or low (Fig. 14-6). Hyponatremia with a normal or high serum osmolality results from the presence of a nonsodium solute, such as glucose or mannitol, which holds water within the extracellular space and results in dilutional hyponatremia. The presence of a nonsodium solute may be inferred if measured osmolality exceeds calculated osmolality by >10 mOsm/kg. For example, plasma $[Na^+]$ decreases approximately 2.4 mEq/L for each 100 mg/dL rise in glucose concentration with perhaps even greater decreases as glucose concentration >400 mg/dL.[85] In anesthesia practice, a common cause of hyponatremia associated with a normal osmolality is the absorption of large volumes of sodium-free irrigating solutions (containing mannitol, glycerine, or sorbitol as the solute) during transurethral resection of the prostate.[86] Neurologic symptoms are minimal if mannitol is used because the agent does not cross the blood–brain barrier and is excreted with water in the urine. In contrast, as glycine or sorbitol is metabolized, hyposmolality will gradually develop and cerebral edema may appear as a late complication, that is, hypoosmolality is more important in generating symptoms than hyponatremia per se.[86] Hyponatremia with a normal or elevated serum osmolality also may accompany renal insufficiency. BUN, included in the calculation of total osmolality, distributes throughout both ECV and ICV. Calculation of *effective* osmolality ($2[Na^+]$ + glucose/18) excludes the contribution of urea to tonicity and demonstrates true hypotonicity.

Hyponatremia with low serum osmolality may be associated with a high, low, or normal total body sodium and PV. Therefore, hyponatremia with hyposmolality (Fig. 14-6) is evaluated by assessing total body sodium content, BUN, SCr, urinary osmolality, and urinary $[Na^+]$. Hyponatremia with increased total body sodium is characteristic of edematous states, that is, congestive heart failure, cirrhosis, nephrosis, and renal failure. Aquaporin 2, the vasopressin-regulated water channel, is up-regulated in experimental congestive heart failure,[87] and cirrhosis[88] and decreased by chronic vasopressin stimulation.[89] In patients with renal insufficiency, reduced urinary diluting capacity can lead to hyponatremia if excess free water is given. In general, diseases that prompt hos-

pitalization generate numerous stimuli for secretion of arginine vasopressin (AVP), which has prompted some experts to suggest that hyponatremic fluids rarely be given to hospitalized patients.[90]

The underlying mechanism of hypovolemic hyponatremia is secretion of AVP synonymous with ADH in response to volume contraction in association with ongoing oral or intravenous intake of hypotonic fluid.[91] Angiotensin II also decreases renal free water clearance. Thiazide diuretics, unlike loop diuretics, promote hypovolemic hyponatremia by interfering with urinary dilution in the distal tubule.[91] Hypovolemic hyponatremia associated with a urinary $[Na^+]$ >20 mmol/L suggests mineralocorticoid deficiency, especially if serum $[K^+]$, BUN, and SCr are increased.[91]

The cerebral salt-wasting syndrome is an often severe, symptomatic salt-losing diathesis that appears to be mediated by brain natriuretic peptide and in which, in contrast to the syndrome of inappropriate antidiuretic hormone secretion (SIADH), secretion of arginine vasopressin is *appropriate*[91]; patients at risk for the cerebral salt wasting syndrome include those with cerebral lesions due to trauma, subarachnoid hemorrhage, tumors, and infection. In patients after subarachnoid hemorrhage, administration of hydrocortisone 1,200 mg/day prevented the cerebral salt-wasting syndrome.[92]

Euvolemic hyponatremia most commonly is associated with nonosmotic vasopressin secretion, for example, glucocorticoid deficiency, hypothyroidism, thiazide-induced hyponatremia, SIADH, and the reset osmostat syndrome. Total body sodium and ECV are relatively normal and edema is rarely evident. SIADH may be idiopathic but also is associated with diseases of the central nervous system and with pulmonary disease (Table 14-14). Euvolemic hyponatremia is usually associated with exogenous AVP administration, pharmacologic potentiation of AVP action, drugs that mimic the action of AVP in the renal tubules, or excessive ectopic AVP secretion. Tissues from some small cell lung cancers, duodenal cancers, and pancreatic cancers increase AVP production in response to osmotic stimulation.[91]

At least 4.0% of postoperative patients develop plasma $[Na^+]$ <130 mEq/L. Although neurologic manifestations usually do not accompany postoperative hyponatremia, signs of hypervolemia are occasionally present. Much less frequently, postoperative hyponatremia is accompanied by mental status changes, seizures and transtentorial herniaton,[93] attributable in part to intravenous administration of hypotonic fluids, secretion of AVP, and other factors, including drugs and altered renal function, that influence perioperative water balance.

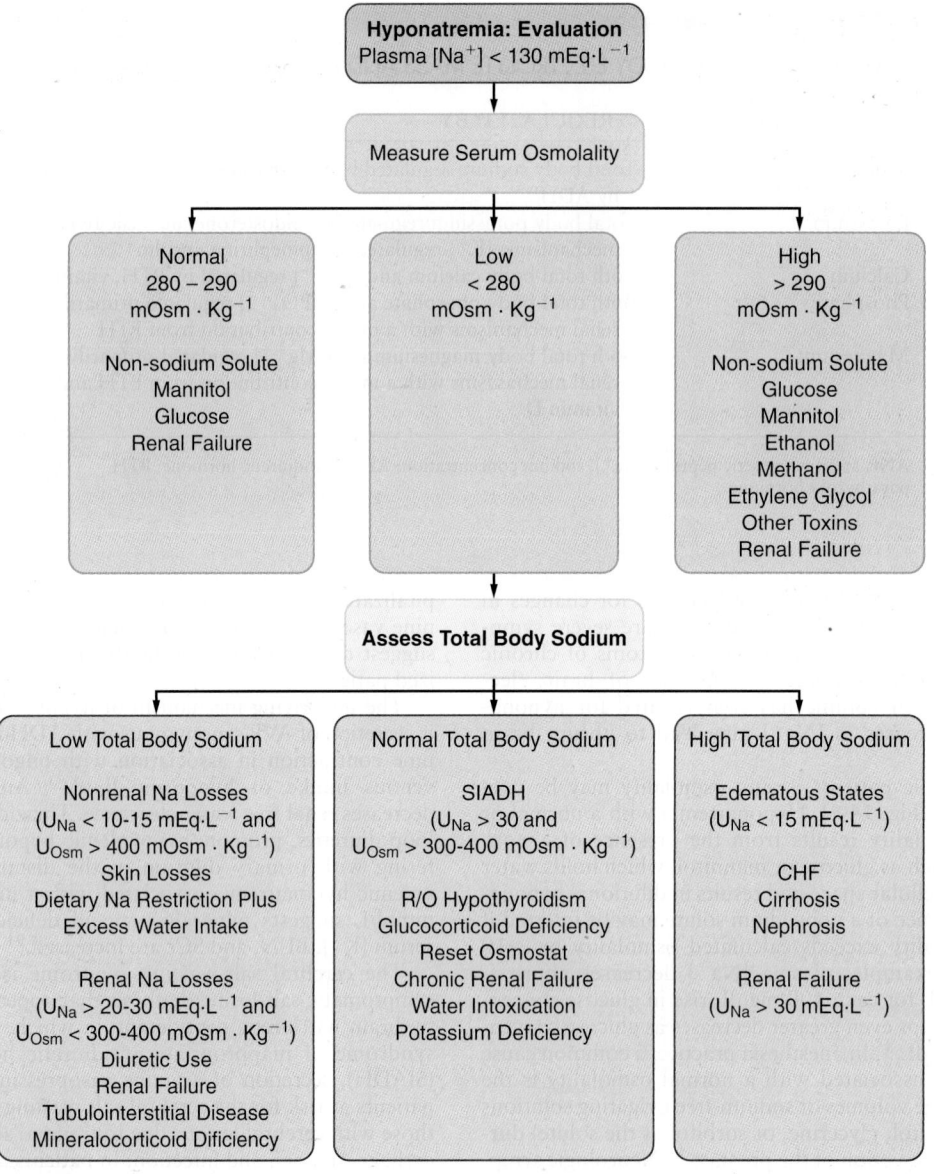

FIGURE 14-6.   Algorithm by which hyponatremia can be evaluated. SIADH, syndrome of inappropriate antidiuretic hormone secretion; R/O, rule out; CHF, congestive heart failure.

Women appear to be more vulnerable than men and premenopausal women appear to be more vulnerable than postmenopausal women to brain damage secondary to postoperative hyponatremia.[94] Postoperative hyponatremia can develop even with infusion of isotonic fluids if AVP is persistently increased. Twenty-four hours after surgery, mean plasma $[Na^+]$ in 22 women (mean age, 42 years) undergoing uncomplicated gynecologic surgery had decreased from 140 ± 1 to 136 ± 0.5 mEq/L.[95] Although the patients retained sodium perioperatively, they retained proportionately more water (an average of 1.1 L of electrolyte-free water). Careful postoperative attention to fluid and electrolyte balance may minimize the occurrence of symptomatic hyponatremia.

If both $[Na^+]$ and measured osmolality are below the normal range, hyponatremia is further evaluated by first assessing volume status using physical findings and laboratory data. In hypovolemic patients or edematous patients, the ratio of BUN to SCr should be >20:1. Urinary $[Na^+]$ is generally <15 mEq/L in edematous states and volume depletion and >20 mEq/L in hyponatremia secondary to renal salt wasting or renal failure with water retention.

The criteria for the diagnosis of SIADH are listed in Table 14-15. Urinary $[Na^+]$ should be >20 mEq/L unless fluids have been restricted. Arieff[96] has argued that the diagnosis of SIADH may be inaccurately applied to functionally hypovolemic postoperative patients, in whom, by definition, AVP secretion would be "appropriate."

Treatment of hyponatremia associated with a normal or high serum osmolality requires reduction of the elevated concentrations of the responsible solute, for example, urea or mannitol. Uremic patients are treated by free water restriction or dialysis. Treatment of edematous (hypervolemic) patients necessitates restriction of both sodium and water, usually accompanied by efforts to improve cardiac output and renal perfusion and to use diuretics to inhibit sodium reabsorption (Fig. 14-7). In hypovolemic, hyponatremic patients, blood volume must be restored, usually by infusion of 0.9% saline, and excessive sodium losses must be curtailed. Correction of hypovolemia usually results in removal of the stimulus for AVP release, accompanied by a rapid water diuresis.

The cornerstone of SIADH management is free water restriction and elimination of precipitating causes. Water

TABLE 14-14

COMMON ASSOCIATIONS WITH THE SYNDROME OF INAPPROPRIATE ANTIDIURETIC HORMONE SECRETION

Neoplastic disease
Carcinoma (e.g., lung)
Thymoma
Mesothelioma
Lymphoma, leukemia
Ewing sarcoma
Carcinoid
Bronchial adenoma

Neurologic disorders
Head injury, neurosurgery
Brain abscess or tumor
Meningitis, encephalitis
Cerebral hemorrhage
Guillain-Barré syndrome
Hydrocephalus

Alcohol withdrawal
Peripheral neuropathy
Seizures
Subdural hematoma

Chest disorders
Pneumonia
Tuberculosis
Empyema
Cystic fibrosis
Pneumothorax
Aspergillosis

Drugs
Sulphonylureas
Opiates
Thiazides and loop diuretics
Dopamine antagonists
Anticonvulsants
Tricyclic antidepressants
SSRIs

Miscellaneous
Idiopathic
Psychosis
Porphyria

SSRI, selective serotonin reuptake inhibitor.
Modified from Ball SG: Vasopressin and disorders of water balance: The physiology and pathophysiology of vasopressin. Ann Clin Biochem 2007; 44: 417–431, with permission.

restriction, sufficient to decrease TBW by 0.5 to 1.0 L per day, decreases ECV even if excessive AVP secretion continues. The resultant reduction in GFR enhances proximal tubular reabsorption of salt and water, thereby decreasing free water generation, and stimulates aldosterone secretion. As long as free water losses (i.e., renal, skin, gastrointestinal) exceed free water intake, plasma [Na^+] will increase. During treatment of hyponatremia, increases in plasma [Na^+] are determined both by the composition of the infused fluid and by the rate of renal free water excretion.[97] Free water excretion can be increased by administering furosemide.

Recently, vasopressin receptor blocking agents have been developed that inhibit the action of AVP on the renal collecting ducts.[98–101] In phase 3 clinical trials, these agents have proven to be safe and efficacious in hyponatremic patients, appearing to have particular value in patients with hypervolemic hypona-

TABLE 14-15

DIAGNOSTIC CRITERIA FOR SYNDROME OF INAPPROPRIATE ANTIDIURETIC HORMONE SECRETION

Hyponatremia with appropriately low plasma osmolality
Urinary osmolality greater than plasma osmolality
Renal sodium excretion >20 mmol/L
Absence of hypotension, hypovolemia, and edematous states
Normal renal and adrenal function
Absence of drugs that directly influence renal water and sodium handling

Modified from Ball SG: Vasopressin and disorders of water balance: The physiology and pathophysiology of vasopressin. Ann Clin Biochem 2007; 44: 417–431, with permission.

tremia secondary to congestive heart failure.[98] Conivaptan, which inhibits both $V_{1\alpha}$ and V_2 receptors, has been approved for treatment of normovolemic and hypervolemic hyponatremic patients.[100] However, potential decreases in blood pressure associated with $V_{1\alpha}$ receptor blockade necessitate caution in patients with borderline low blood pressure.[101] Tolvaptan, a selective V_2 receptor antagonist, also has proven effective in clinical trials.[102] Within a few years, vaptans will likely become a mainstay of therapy for normovolemic and hypervolemic hypernatremia.[101]

Neurologic symptoms or profound hyponatremia ([Na^+] <115 to 120 mEq/L) requires more aggressive therapy. Hypertonic (3%) saline is most clearly indicated in patients who have seizures or patients who acutely develop symptoms of water intoxication secondary to intravenous fluid administration. In such cases, 3% saline may be administered at a rate of 1 to 2 mL/kg/hr, to increase plasma [Na^+] by 1 to 2 mEq/L/hr; however, this treatment should not continue for more than a few hours. Three percent saline may only transiently increase plasma [Na^+] because ECV expansion results in increased urinary sodium excretion. Intravenous furosemide, combined with quantitative replacement of urinary sodium losses with 0.9% or 3.0% saline, can rapidly increase plasma [Na^+], in part by increasing free water clearance.

The rate of treatment of hyponatremia continues to generate controversy, extending from "too fast, too soon" to "too slow, too late." Although delayed correction may result in neurologic injury, inappropriately rapid correction may result in abrupt brain dehydration (Fig. 14-8) or permanent neurologic sequelae (i.e., osmotic demyelination syndrome),[103] cerebral hemorrhage, or congestive heart failure. The symptoms of the osmotic demyelination syndrome vary from mild (transient behavioral disturbances or seizures) to severe (including pseudobulbar palsy and quadriparesis).

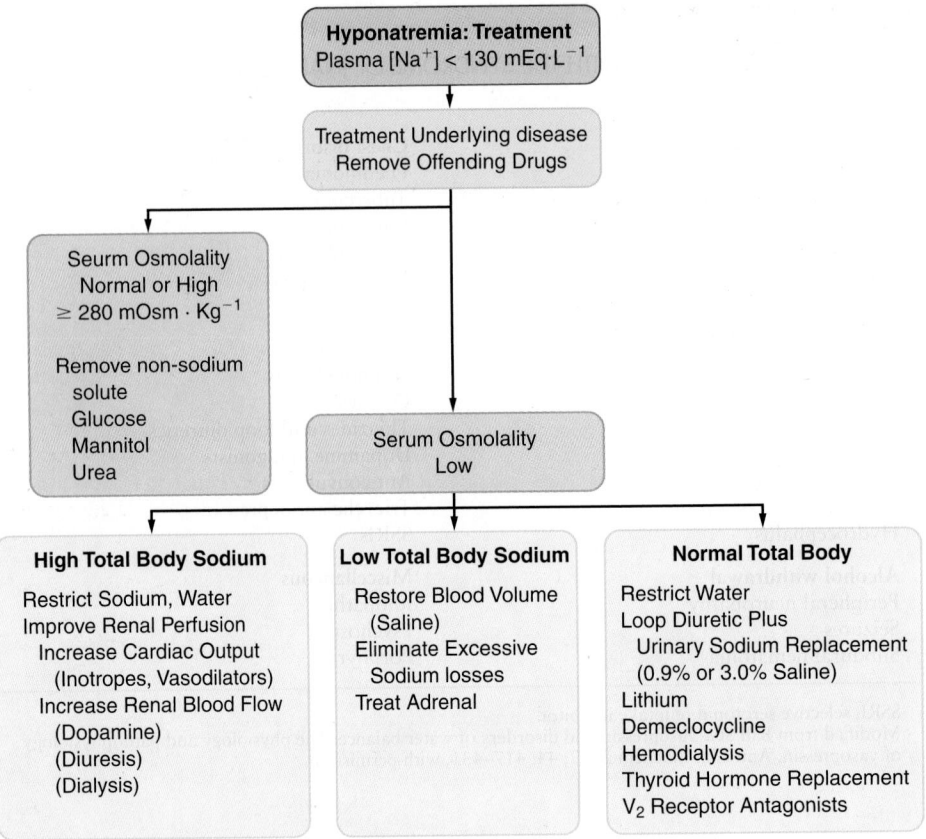

FIGURE 14-7.   Hyponatremia is treated according to the etiology of the disturbance, the level of serum osmolality, and a clinical estimation of total body sodium.

FIGURE 14-8.   Brain water and solute in concentrations in hyponatremia. If normal plasma sodium (Na; **A**) suddenly decreased, the increase in brain water theoretically would be proportional to the decrease in plasma Na (**B**). However, because of adaptive loss of cerebral intracellular solute, cerebral edema is minimized in chronic hyponatremia (**C**). Once adaptation has occurred, a rapid return of plasma Na concentration toward a normal level results in brain dehydration (**D**). (From Sterns RH: Vignettes in clinical pathophysiology. Neurological deterioration following treatment for hyponatremia. Am J Kidney Dis 1989; XIII: 434–437, with permission.)

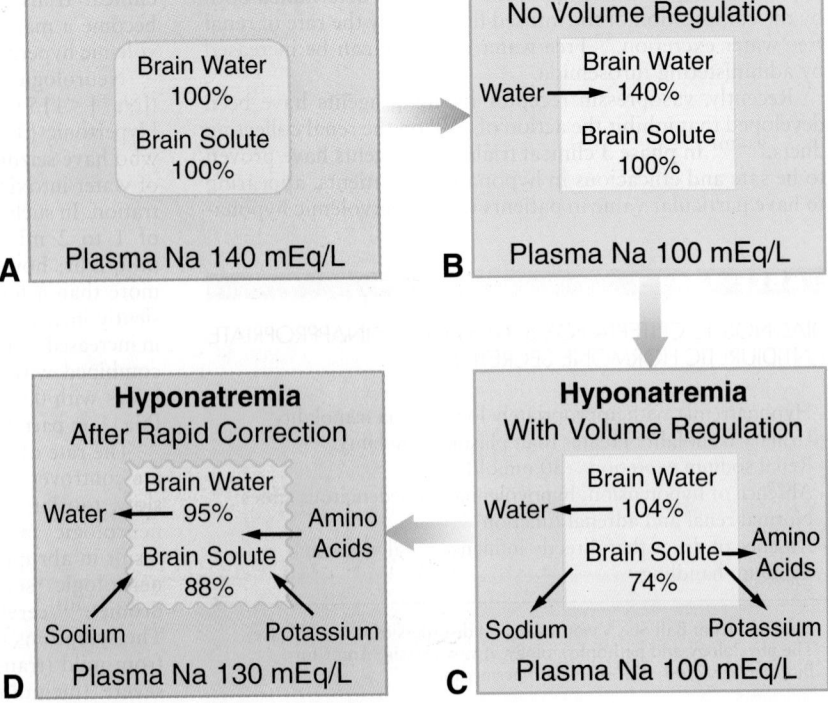

The principal determinants of neurologic injury appear to be the magnitude and chronicity of hyponatremia and the rate of correction. The osmotic demyelination syndrome is more likely when hyponatremia has persisted >48 hours. Most patients in whom the osmotic demyelination syndrome is fatal have undergone correction of plasma $[Na^+]$ of more than 20 mEq/L/day. Other risk factors for the development of the osmotic demyelination syndrome include alcoholism, poor nutritional status, liver disease, burns, and hypokalemia.

The clinician faces formidable difficulties in predicting the rate at which plasma $[Na^+]$ will increase because increases in plasma $[Na^+]$ are determined both by the composition of the infused fluid and by the rate of renal free water excretion. The expected change in plasma $[Na^+]$ resulting from 1 L of selected infusate can be estimated using the following equation[104]:

$$\Delta [Na^+]_s = \frac{[Na^+]_{inf} - [Na^+]_s}{TBW + 1} \quad (14\text{-}12)$$

where $\Delta[Na^+]_s$ = the change in the patient's serum $[Na^+]$, $[Na^+]_{inf}$ = $[Na^+]$ of the infusate, $[Na^+]_s$ = the patient's serum $[Na^+]$, TBW = the patient's estimated total body water in liters, and 1 = a factor added to take into account the volume of infusate.

Treatment should be interrupted or slowed when symptoms improve. Frequent determinations of $[Na^+]$ are important to prevent correction at a rate >1 to 2 mEq/L in any 1 hour and >8 mEq/L in 24 hours.[105] Initially, plasma $[Na^+]$ may be increased by 1 to 2 mEq/L/hr; however, the rate of correction should then be slowed to avoid excessively rapid correction. Hypernatremia should be avoided. Once plasma $[Na^+]$ exceeds 120 to 125 mEq/L, water restriction alone is usually sufficient to normalize $[Na^+]$. As acute hyponatremia is corrected, central nervous system signs and symptoms usually improve within 24 hours, although 96 hours may be necessary for maximal recovery.

For patients who require long-term pharmacologic therapy of hyponatremia, demeclocycline is currently the drug of choice.[106] Although better tolerated than lithium, demeclocycline may induce nephrotoxicity, a particular concern in patients with hepatic dysfunction. Hemodialysis is occasionally necessary in severely hyponatremic patients who cannot be adequately managed with drugs or hypertonic saline. Once hyponatremia has improved, careful fluid restriction is necessary to avoid recurrence of hyponatremia. In the future, oral receptor antagonists may be used to treat chronic hyponatremia.

Hypernatremia

Hypernatremia ($[Na^+] >150$ mEq/L) indicates an absolute or relative water deficit. Normally, slight increases in tonicity or $[Na^+]$ stimulate thirst and AVP secretion. Therefore, severe, persistent hypernatremia occurs only in patients who cannot respond to thirst by voluntary ingestion of fluid, that is, obtunded patients, anesthetized patients, and infants.

Hypernatremia produces neurologic symptoms (including stupor, coma, and seizures), hypovolemia, renal insufficiency (occasionally progressing to renal failure), and decreased urinary concentrating ability. Because hypernatremia frequently results from diabetes insipidus (DI) or osmotically induced losses of sodium and water, many patients are hypovolemic or bear the stigmata of renal disease. Postoperative neurosurgical patients who have undergone pituitary surgery are at particular risk of developing transient or prolonged DI. Polyuria may be present for only a few days within the first week of surgery, may be permanent, or may demonstrate a triphasic sequence: early DI, return of urinary concentrating ability, then recurrent DI.[107]

The clinical consequences of hypernatremia are most serious at the extremes of age and when hypernatremia develops abruptly. Geriatric patients are at increased risk of hypernatremia because of decreased renal concentrating ability and decreased thirst. Brain shrinkage secondary to rapidly developing hypernatremia may damage delicate cerebral vessels, leading to subdural hematoma, subcortical parenchymal hemorrhage, subarachnoid hemorrhage, and venous thrombosis. Polyuria may cause bladder distention, hydronephrosis, and permanent renal damage. Although the mortality of hypernatremia is 40 to 55%, it is unclear whether hypernatremia contributes to mortality or is simply a marker of severe associated disease.

Surprisingly, if plasma $[Na^+]$ is initially normal, moderate acute increases in plasma $[Na^+]$ do not appear to precipitate central pontine myelinolysis. However, larger accidental increases in plasma $[Na^+]$ have produced severe consequences in children. In experimental animals, acute severe hypernatremia (acute increase from 146 to 170 mEq/L) caused neuronal damage at 24 hours, suggestive of early central pontine myelinolysis.[108]

By definition, hypernatremia indicates an absolute or relative water deficit and is always associated with hypertonicity. Hypernatremia can be generated by hypotonic fluid loss, as in burns, gastrointestinal losses, diuretic therapy, osmotic diuresis, renal disease, mineralocorticoid excess or deficiency, and iatrogenic causes or can be generated by isolated water loss, as in central or nephrogenic DI. The acquired form of

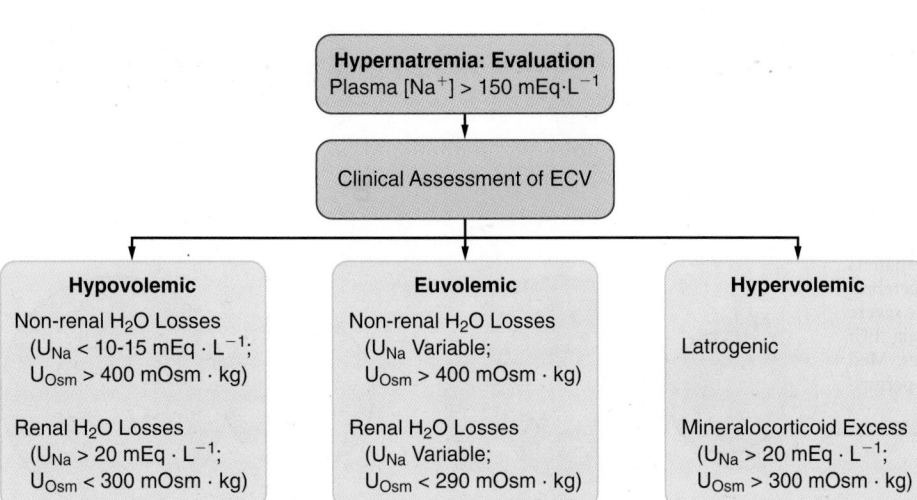

FIGURE 14-9. Severe hypernatremia is evaluated by first separating patients into hypovolemic, euvolemic, and hypervolemic groups based on assessment of extracellular volume (ECV). Next, potential etiologic factors are diagnostically assessed. $[Na^+]$, serum sodium concentration; U_{Na}, urinary sodium concentration; U_{OSm}, urinary osmolality.

nephrogenic DI is more common and usually less severe than the congenital form. As chronic renal failure advances, most patients have defective concentrating ability, resulting in resistance to AVP associated with hypotonic urine. Because hypovolemia accompanies most pathologic water loss, signs of hypoperfusion also may be present. In many patients, before the development of hypernatremia, an increased volume of hypotonic urine suggests an abnormality in water balance. Although uncommon as a cause of hypernatremia, isolated sodium gain occasionally occurs in patients who receive large quantities of sodium, such as treatment of metabolic acidosis with 8.4% sodium bicarbonate, in which [Na$^+$] is approximately 1,000 mEq/L, or perioperative or prehospital treatment with hypertonic saline resuscitation solutions.

Hypernatremic patients can be separated into three groups, based on clinical assessment of ECV (Fig. 14-9). Note that plasma [Na$^+$] does not reflect total body sodium, which must be estimated separately based on signs of the adequacy of ECV. Polyuric, hypernatremic patients may be undergoing solute diuresis or may have DI. Measurement of urinary sodium and osmolality can help to differentiate the various causes. A urinary osmolality <150 mOsm/kg in the setting of hypertonicity and polyuria is diagnostic of DI.

Treatment of hypernatremia produced by water loss requires repletion of water as well of associated deficits in total body sodium and other electrolytes (Table 14-16). Common errors in treating hypernatremia include excessively rapid correction as well as failing to appreciate the magnitude of the water deficit and failing to account for ongoing maintenance requirements and continued fluid losses in planning therapy.

The first step in treating hypernatremia is to estimate the TBW deficit, which can be accomplished by inserting the measured plasma [Na$^+$] into the equation:

$$\text{TBW deficit} = 0.6 \times \text{body weight (kg)} \times [([\text{Na}^+] - 140)/140] \quad (14\text{-}13)$$

where 140 is the middle of the normal range for [Na$^+$]. Adrogue and Madias[109] proposed an equation (see Eq. 14-12) that can be used in hypernatremic patients as it can be in

TABLE 14-16

HYPERNATREMIA: ACUTE TREATMENT

Sodium depletion (hypovolemia)
Hypovolemia correction (0.9% saline)
Hypernatremia correction (hypotonic fluids)

Sodium overload (hypervolemia)
Enhance sodium removal (loop diuretics, dialysis)
Replace water deficit (hypotonic fluids)

Normal total body sodium (euvolemia)
Replace water deficit (hypotonic fluids)
Control diabetes insipidus
  Central diabetes insipidus:
    DDAVP, 10-20 μg intranasally; 2–4 μg SC
Aqueous vasopressin, 5 U q 2–4 hr IM or SC
  Nephrogenic diabetes insipidus:
    Restrict sodium, water intake
    Thiazide diuretics

DDAVP, desmopressin.

hyponatremic patients to predict the expected decrease in serum [Na$^+$] produced by infusion of 1 L of infusate.[104] The accuracy of this equation has recently been validated in a large clinical series of hypernatremic and hyponatremic patients.[110]

Hypernatremia must be corrected slowly because of the risk of neurologic sequelae such as seizures or cerebral edema (Fig. 14-10). At the cellular level, restoration of cell volume occurs remarkably quickly after tonicity is altered; as a consequence, acute treatment of hypertonicity may result in overshooting the original, normotonic cell volume. The water deficit should be replaced over 24 to 48 hours, and the plasma [Na$^+$] should not be reduced by more than 1 to 2 mEq/L/hr. Reversible underlying causes should be treated. Hypovolemia should be corrected promptly with 0.9% saline. Although the

FIGURE 14-10. **A.** The concentration of sodium is reflected in the intensity of the stippling: the upper figure, representing extracellular volume (smaller circle) and intracellular volume (larger circle), is more heavily stippled, that is, serum sodium is higher. **B.** In response to an acute increase in serum sodium resulting from water loss, both intracellular and extracellular volume substantially decrease. The brain (schematically illustrated) shrinks in proportion to the reduction in intracellular volume in other tissues. **C.** However, owing to the production of idiogenic osmoles, the brain rapidly restores its intracellular volume, despite the persistent reduction in intracellular volume in other tissues and in extracellular volume. **D.** With excessively rapid correction of hypernatremia (the reduction in serum sodium is reflected in the decrease in the intensity of stippling), the brain expands to greater than its original size. The resulting increase in cerebral edema and intracranial pressure can cause severe neurologic damage. (Modified from Feig PU: Hypernatremia and hypertonic syndromes. Med Clin North Am 1981; 65: 271–290, with permission.)

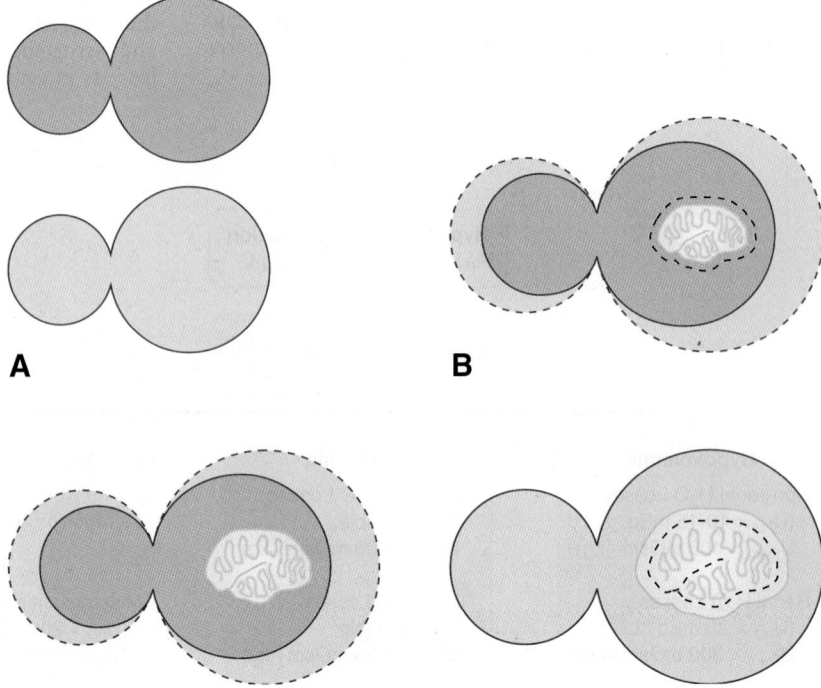

A   B

[Na$^+$] of 0.9% saline is 154 mEq/L, the solution is effective in treating volume deficits and will reduce [Na$^+$] that exceeds 154 mEq/L in hypovolemic hypernatremic patients. Once hypovolemia is corrected, water can be replaced orally or with intravenous hypotonic fluids, depending on the ability of the patient to tolerate oral hydration. In the occasional sodium-overloaded patient, sodium excretion can be accelerated using loop diuretics or dialysis.

The management of hypernatremia secondary to DI varies according to whether the cause is central or nephrogenic (see Table 14-16). The two most suitable agents for correcting central DI (an AVP deficiency syndrome) are desmopressin (DDAVP) and aqueous vasopressin. DDAVP, given subcutaneously in a dose of 1 to 4 μg or intranasally in a dose of 5 to 20 μg every 12 to 24 hours, is effective in most patients. DDAVP is preferred because it has a longer duration of action than AVP and lacks vasoconstrictor effects.[111] Incomplete AVP deficits (partial DI) often are effectively managed with pharmacologic agents that stimulate AVP release or enhance the renal response to AVP. Chlorpropamide, which potentiates the renal effects of vasopressin, and carbamazepine, which enhances vasopressin secretion, have been used to treat partial central DI, but are associated with clinically important side effects. In nephrogenic DI, salt and water restriction or thiazide diuretics induce contraction of ECV, thereby enhancing fluid reabsorption in the proximal tubules. If less filtrate passes through into the collecting ducts, less water will be excreted.

Potassium

Physiologic Role

11 Potassium plays an important role in cell membrane physiology, especially in maintaining resting membrane potentials and in generating action potentials in the central nervous system and heart. Potassium is actively transported into cells by a Na/K adenosine triphosphatase (ATPase) pump, which maintains an intracellular [K$^+$] that is at least 30-fold greater than extracellular [K$^+$]. Intracellular potassium concentration ([K$^+$]) is normally 150 mEq/L while the extracellular concentration is only 3.5 to 5.0 mEq/L. Serum [K$^+$] measures about 0.5 mEq/L higher than plasma [K$^+$] because of cell lysis during clotting. Total body potassium in a 70-kg adult is approximately 4,256 mEq, of which 4,200 mEq is intracellular; of the

56 mEq in the ECV, only 12 mEq is located in the PV. The ratio of intracellular to extracellular potassium contributes to the resting potential difference across cell membranes and therefore to the integrity of cardiac and neuromuscular transmission. The primary mechanism that maintains potassium inside cells is the negative voltage created by the transport of three sodium ions out of the cell for every two potassium ions transported in. Both insulin and β agonists promote potassium entry into cells.[112,113] Metabolic and respiratory acidosis tends to shift potassium out of cells, while metabolic and respiratory alkalosis favors movement into cells.

Usual potassium intake varies between 50 and 150 mEq/day. Freely filtered at the glomerulus, most potassium excretion is urinary, with some fecal elimination. Most filtered potassium is reabsorbed; usually, excretion is approximately equal to daily intake. As long as GFR is >8 mL/min, dietary potassium intake, unless greater than normal, can be excreted. Assuming a plasma [K$^+$] of 4.0 mEq/L and a normal GFR of 180 L/day, 720 mEq of potassium is filtered daily, of which 85 to 90% is reabsorbed in the proximal convoluted tubule and loop of Henle. The remaining 10 to 15% reaches the distal convoluted tubule, which is the major site at which potassium excretion is regulated. Excretion of potassium ions is a function of open potassium channels and the electrical driving force in the cortical collecting duct.

The two most important regulators of potassium excretion are plasma [K$^+$] and aldosterone. Potassium secretion into the distal convoluted tubules and cortical collecting ducts is increased by hyperkalemia, aldosterone, alkalemia, increased delivery of Na$^+$ to the distal tubule and collecting duct, high urinary flow rates, and the presence in luminal fluid of nonreabsorbable anions such as carbenicillin, phosphates, and sulfates. As sodium reabsorption increases, the electrical driving force opposing reabsorption of potassium is increased. Aldosterone increases sodium reabsorption by inducing a more open configuration of the epithelial sodium channel; potassium-sparing diuretics (amiloride and triamterene) and trimethoprim block the epithelial sodium channel, thereby increasing potassium reabsorption. Magnesium depletion contributes to renal potassium wasting.

Hypokalemia

Uncommon among healthy persons, hypokalemia ([K$^+$] <3.5 mEq/L) is a frequent complication of treatment with diuretic drugs and occasionally complicates other diseases and treatment regimens (Table 14-17). Plasma [K$^+$] poorly reflects

---

TABLE 14-17

CAUSES OF RENAL POTASSIUM LOSS

Drugs	**Bicarbonaturia**
Diuretics	Distal renal tubular acidosis
Thiazide diuretics	Treatment of proximal renal tubular acidosis
Loop diuretics	Correction phase of metabolic alkalosis
Osmotic diuretics	**Magnesium deficiency**
Antibiotics	**Other less common causes**
Penicillin and penicillin analogues	Cisplatin
Amphotericin B	Carbonic anhydrase inhibitors
Aminoglycosides	Leukemia
Hormones	Diuretic phase of acute tubular necrosis
Aldosterone	**Intrinsic renal transport defects**
Glucocorticoids	Barter syndrome
	Gitelman syndrome

Modified from Weiner ID, Wingo CS: Hypokalemia consequences, causes, and correction. J Am Soc Nephrol 1997; 8: 1179–1188, with permission.

total body potassium; hypokalemia may occur with normal, low, or high total body potassium. However, as a general rule, a chronic decrement of 1.0 mEq/L in the plasma $[K^+]$ corresponds to a total body deficit of approximately 200 to 300 mEq. In uncomplicated hypokalemia, the total body potassium deficit exceeds 300 mEq if plasma $[K^+]$ is <3.0 mEq/L and 700 mEq if plasma $[K^+]$ is <2.0 mEq/L.

The symptoms and signs of hypokalemia primarily relate to neuromuscular and cardiovascular function. Hypokalemia causes muscle weakness and, when severe, may even cause paralysis. With chronic potassium loss, the ratio of intracellular to extracellular $[K^+]$ remains relatively stable; in contrast, acute redistribution of potassium from the extracellular to the intracellular space substantially changes resting membrane potentials. Cardiac rhythm disturbances are among the most dangerous complications of potassium deficiency. Acute hypokalemia causes hyperpolarization of the cardiac cell and may lead to ventricular escape activity, re-entrant phenomena, ectopic tachycardias, and delayed conduction. In patients treated with digoxin, hypokalemia increases toxicity by increasing myocardial digoxin binding and pharmacologic effectiveness. Hypokalemia contributes to systemic hypertension, especially when combined with a high-sodium diet. In diabetic patients, hypokalemia impairs insulin secretion and end-organ sensitivity to insulin. Although no clear threshold has been defined for a level of hypokalemia below which safe conduct of anesthesia is compromised, $[K^+]$ <3.5 mEq/L in cardiac surgical patients has been associated with an increased incidence of perioperative dysrhythmias, especially atrial fibrillation/flutter.[114]

Potassium depletion also induces defects in renal concentrating ability, resulting in polyuria and a reduction in GFR. Potassium replacement improves GFR, although the concentrating deficit may not improve for several months after treatment. If hypokalemia is sufficiently prolonged, chronic renal interstitial damage may occur. In experimental animals, hypokalemia was associated with intrarenal vasoconstriction and a pattern of renal injury similar to that produced by ischemia.[115]

Hypokalemia may result from chronic depletion of total body potassium or from acute redistribution of potassium from the ECV to the ICV. Redistribution of potassium into cells occurs when the activity of the sodium-potassium ATPase pump is acutely increased by extracellular hyperkalemia or increased intracellular concentrations of sodium, as well as by insulin, carbohydrate loading (which stimulates release of endogenous insulin), β_2 agonists, and aldosterone. Both metabolic and respiratory alkalosis lead to decreases in plasma $[K^+]$.

Causes of chronic hypokalemia include those etiologies associated with renal potassium conservation (extrarenal potassium losses; low urinary $[K^+]$) and those with renal potassium wasting (Fig. 14-11).[116] A low urinary $[K^+]$ suggests inadequate dietary intake or extrarenal depletion (in the absence of recent diuretic use). Diuretic-induced urinary potassium losses are frequently associated with hypokalemia, secondary to increased aldosterone secretion, alkalemia, and increased renal tubular flow. Aldosterone does not cause renal potassium wasting unless sodium ions are present; that is, aldosterone primarily controls sodium reabsorption, not potassium excretion. Renal tubular damage due to nephrotoxins such as aminoglycosides or amphotericin B may also cause renal potassium wasting.

Initial evaluation of hypokalemia includes a medical history (e.g., diarrhea, vomiting, diuretic or laxative use), physical

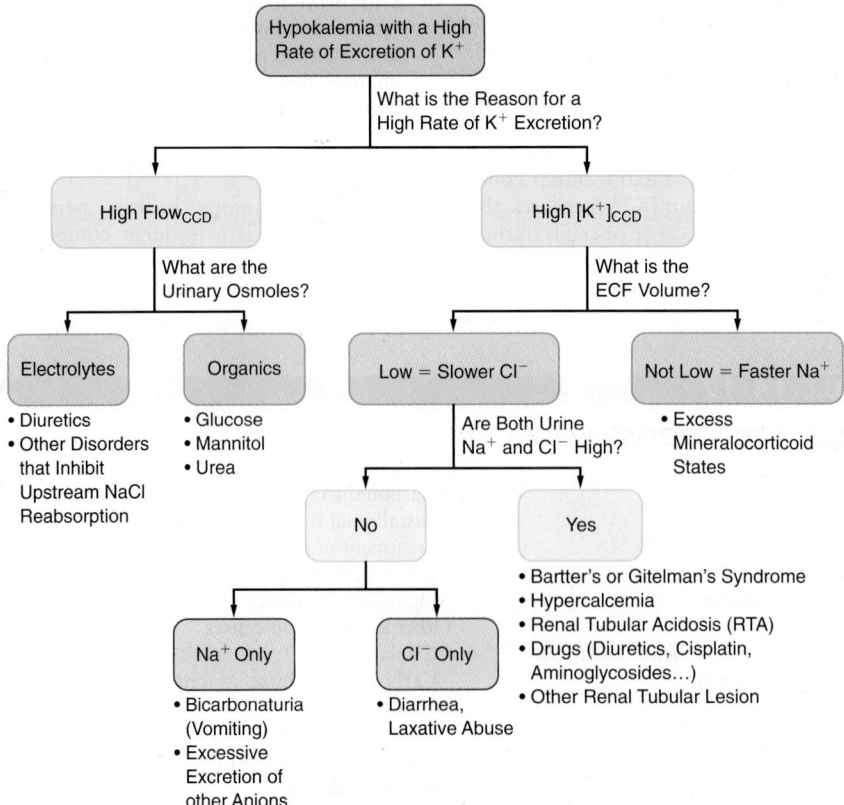

FIGURE 14-11. A diagnostic flow chart for hypokalemia with a high rate of K^+ excretion. ECF, extracellular fluid. (From Lin SH, Halperin ML: Hypokalemia: a practical approach to diagnosis and its genetic basis. Curr Med Chem 2007; 14: 1551–1565, with permission.)

TABLE 14-18

HYPOKALEMIA: TREATMENT

Correct precipitating factors
Increased pH
Decreased $[Mg^{2+}]$
Drugs

Mild hypokalemia ($[K^+]$ >2.0 mEq/L)
Intravenous KCl infusion ≤10 mEq/hr

Severe hypokalemia ($[K^+]$ ≤2.0 mEq/L, paralysis or ECG changes)
Intravenous KCl infusion ≤40 mEq/hr
Continuous ECG monitoring
If life-threatening, 5–6 mEq bolus

ECG, electrocardiographic.

examination (e.g., hypertension, cushingoid features, edema), measurement of serum electrolytes (e.g., magnesium), arterial pH assessment, and evaluation of the electrocardiogram (ECG). Measurement of 24-hour urinary excretion of sodium and potassium may distinguish extrarenal from renal causes. Magnesium deficiency, associated with aminoglycoside and cisplatin therapy, can generate hypokalemia that is resistant to replacement therapy. Plasma renin and aldosterone levels may be helpful in the differential diagnosis of hypokalemia of unclear origin, especially if primary hyperaldosteronism is suspected.[117] Characteristic electrocardiographic changes associated with hypokalemia include flat or inverted T waves, prominent U waves, and ST segment depression.

The treatment of hypokalemia consists of potassium repletion, correction of alkalemia, and removal of offending drugs (Table 14-18). Hypokalemia secondary only to acute redistribution (e.g., secondary to acute alkalemia) may not require treatment. There is no urgent need for potassium replacement therapy in mild-to-moderate hypokalemia (3 to 3.5 m Eq/L) in patients who have no symptoms. If total body potassium is decreased, oral potassium supplementation is preferable to intravenous replacement. Potassium is usually replaced as the chloride salt because coexisting chloride deficiency may limit the ability of the kidney to conserve potassium.

Intravenous potassium repletion, when necessary, must be performed cautiously (i.e., usually at a rate ≤10 to 20 mEq/hr) because the magnitude of potassium deficits is unpredictable. The plasma $[K^+]$ and the ECG must be monitored during rapid repletion (10 to 20 mEq/hr) to avoid hyperkalemic complications. The plasma $[K^+]$ and ECG should be monitored to detect inadvertent hyperkalemia. Particular care should be taken in patients who have concurrent acidemia, type IV renal tubular acidosis, diabetes mellitus, or in those patients receiving nonsteroidal anti-inflammatory agents, ACE inhibitors, or β_2 blockers, all of which delay movement of extracellular potassium into cells. Beta$_1$-blockers do not delay movement of extracellular potassium into cells or predispose patients to hyperkalemia.[118]

However, in patients with life-threatening dysrhythmias secondary to hypokalemia, serum $[K^+]$ must be rapidly increased. Assuming that PV in a 70-kg adult is 3.0 L, administration of 6.0 mEq/L of potassium in 1.0 minute will acutely increase serum $[K^+]$ by no more than 2.0 mEq/L because redistribution into interstitial fluid and intracellular volume will decrease the quantity remaining in the plasma volume.

Hypokalemia associated with hyperaldosteronemia (e.g., primary aldosteronism, Cushing syndrome) usually responds favorably to reduced sodium intake and increased potassium intake. Hypomagnesemia, if present, aggravates the effects of hypokalemia, impairs potassium conservation, and should be treated. Potassium supplements or potassium-sparing diuretics should be given cautiously to patients who have diabetes mellitus or renal insufficiency, which limit compensation for acute hyperkalemia. In patients such as those who have diabetic ketoacidosis, who are both hypokalemic and acidemic, potassium administration should precede correction of acidosis to avoid a precipitous decrease in plasma $[K^+]$ as pH increases.

In patients with normal serum potassium accompanied by symptoms of potassium depletion (e.g., muscle fatigue), history of potassium loss or insufficient intake, or in patients in whom potassium depletion may be of special threat (e.g., patients on diuretics, digitalis, or β_2 agonists), muscle biopsy with measurement of muscle potassium concentration may be a useful procedure to detect and quantify potassium depletion.

Hyperkalemia

The most lethal manifestations of hyperkalemia ($[K^+]$ >5.0 mEq/L) involve the cardiac conducting system and include dysrhythmias, conduction abnormalities, and cardiac arrest. In anesthesia practice, the classic example of hyperkalemic cardiac toxicity is associated with the administration of succinylcholine to paraplegic, quadriplegic or severely burned[119] patients. If plasma $[K^+]$ is <6.0 mEq/L, cardiac effects are negligible. As the concentration increases further, the electrocardiogram shows tall, peaked T waves, especially in the precordial leads. With further increases, the PR interval becomes prolonged, followed by a decrease in the amplitude of the P wave. Finally, the QRS complex widens into a pattern resembling a sine wave, as a prelude to cardiac standstill (Fig. 14-12).[112] Hyperkalemic cardiotoxicity is enhanced by hyponatremia, hypocalcemia, or acidosis. Because progression to fatal cardiotoxicity is unpredictable and often swift, the presence of hyperkalemic ECG changes mandates immediate therapy. The life-threatening cardiac effects usually require more urgent treatment than other manifestations of hyperkalemia. However, ascending muscle weakness appears when plasma $[K^+]$ approaches 7.0 mEq/L, and may progress to flaccid paralysis, inability to phonate, and respiratory arrest.

The most important diagnostic issues are medical history, emphasizing recent drug therapy, and assessment of renal function. Although the ECG may provide the first suggestion of hyperkalemia in some patients, and despite the well-described effects of hyperkalemia on cardiac conduction and rhythm, the ECG is an insensitive and nonspecific method of detecting hyperkalemia. If hyponatremia is also present, adrenal function should be evaluated.

Hyperkalemia may occur with normal, high, or low total body potassium stores. A deficiency of aldosterone, a major regulator of potassium excretion, leads to hyperkalemia in adrenal insufficiency and hyporeninemic hypoaldosteronism, a state associated with diabetes mellitus, renal insufficiency, and advanced age. Because the kidneys excrete potassium, severe renal insufficiency commonly causes hyperkalemia. Patients with chronic renal insufficiency can maintain normal plasma $[K^+]$ despite markedly decreased GFR because urinary potassium excretion depends on tubular secretion rather than glomerular filtration if GFR exceeds 8 mL/min.

Drugs are now the most common cause of hyperkalemia, especially in elderly patients. Drugs that may limit potassium excretion include nonsteroidal anti-inflammatory drugs, ACE inhibitors, cyclosporin, and potassium-sparing diuretics such as triamterene. Drug-induced hyperkalemia most commonly occurs in patients with other predisposing factors, such as diabetes mellitus, renal insufficiency, advanced age, or hyporeninemic hypoaldosteronism. ACE inhibitors are

ANATOMY AND PHYSIOLOGY

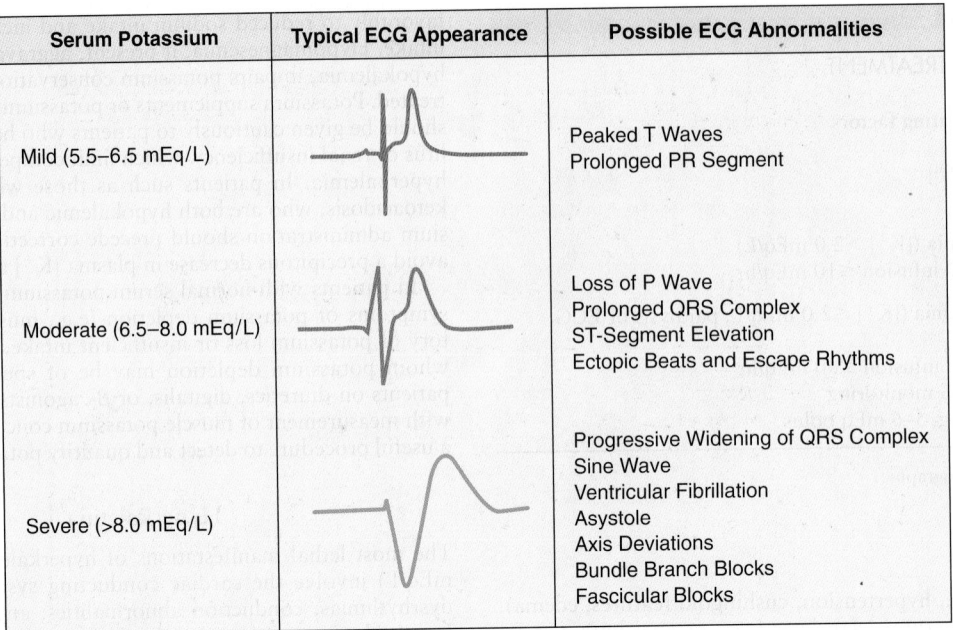

Serum Potassium	Typical ECG Appearance	Possible ECG Abnormalities
Mild (5.5–6.5 mEq/L)		Peaked T Waves Prolonged PR Segment
Moderate (6.5–8.0 mEq/L)		Loss of P Wave Prolonged QRS Complex ST-Segment Elevation Ectopic Beats and Escape Rhythms
Severe (>8.0 mEq/L)		Progressive Widening of QRS Complex Sine Wave Ventricular Fibrillation Asystole Axis Deviations Bundle Branch Blocks Fascicular Blocks

FIGURE 14-12. Electrocardiographic (ECG) manifestations of hyperkalemia. (From Sood MM, Sood AR, Richardson R: Emergency management and commonly encountered outpatient scenarios in patients with hyperkalemia. Mayo Clin Proc 2007; 82: 1553–1561, with permission.)

particularly likely to produce hyperkalemia in patients who have congestive heart failure.[120]

In patients who have normal total body potassium, hyperkalemia may accompany a sudden shift of potassium from the ICV to the ECV because of acidemia, increased catabolism, or rhabdomyolysis. Metabolic acidosis and respiratory acidosis tend to cause an increase in plasma [K+]. However, organic acidoses (i.e., lactic acidosis, ketoacidosis) have little effect on [K+], whereas mineral acids cause significant cellular shifts. In response to increased hydrogen ion activity because of addition of acids, potassium will increase if the anion remains in the extracellular volume. Neither lactate nor ketoacids remain in the extracellular fluid. Therefore, hyperkalemia in these circumstances reflects tissue injury or lack of insulin. Pseudohyperkalemia, which occurs when potassium is released from cells in blood collection tubes, can be diagnosed by comparing serum and plasma K+ levels from the same blood sample. Hyperkalemia usually accompanies malignant hyperthermia.

The treatment of hyperkalemia is aimed at eliminating the cause, reversing membrane hyperexcitability, and removing potassium from the body (Fig. 14-13).[112,113,120,121] Mineralocorticoid deficiency can be treated with 9-α-fludrocortisone (0.025 to 0.10 mg/day). Hyperkalemia secondary to digitalis intoxication may be resistant to therapy because attempts to shift potassium from the ECV to the ICV are often ineffective. In this situation, use of digoxin-specific antibodies has been successful.

Emergent management of severe hyperkalemia is described in detail in Table 14-19. Membrane hyperexcitability can be antagonized by translocating potassium from the ECV to the ICV, removing excess potassium, or (transiently) by infusing calcium chloride to depress the membrane threshold potential. Pending definitive treatment, rapid infusion of calcium chloride (1 g of CaCl2 over 3 minutes, or two to three ampules of 10% calcium gluconate over 5 minutes) may stabilize cardiac rhythm (Table 14-19). Calcium should be given cautiously if digitalis intoxication is likely. Insulin, in a dose-dependent fashion, causes cellular uptake of potassium by increasing the

activity of the sodium/potassium ATPase pump. Insulin increases cellular uptake of potassium best when high insulin levels are achieved by intravenous injection of 5 to 10 units of regular insulin, accompanied by 50 mL of 50% glucose.[112,120] β2-Adrenergic drugs such as salbutamol and albuterol also increase potassium uptake by skeletal muscle and reduce plasma [K+], an action that may explain hypokalemia with severe, acute illness. Salbutamol, a selective β2 agonist, decreases serum potassium acutely by 1 mEq/L or more when given by inhalation or intravenously, although cardiac dysrhythmias may occasionally complicate treatment with selective β2 agonists.[112] Although administration of sodium bicarbonate has long been considered a part of the treatment of hyperkalemia, bicarbonate, when used alone, is relatively ineffective and is no longer favored.[120]

Potassium may be removed from the body by the renal or gastrointestinal routes. Furosemide promotes kaliuresis in a dose-dependent fashion. Sodium polystyrene sulfonate resin (Kayexalate), which exchanges sodium for potassium, can be given orally (30 g) or as a retention enema (50 g in 200 mL of 20% sorbitol). However, sodium overload and hypervolemia are potential risks. Rarely, when temporizing measures are insufficient, emergency hemodialysis may remove 25 to 50 mEq/hr. Peritoneal dialysis is less efficient.

Calcium

Physiologic Role

Calcium is a divalent cation found primarily in the extracellular fluid. The free calcium concentration [Ca2+] in ECV is approximately 1 mM, whereas the free [Ca2+] in the ICV approximates 100 mM, a gradient of 10,000 to 1. Circulating calcium consists of a protein-bound fraction (40 to 50%), a fraction bound to inorganic anions (10 to 15%), and an ionized fraction (45 to 50%), which is the physiologically active and homeostatically regulated component. Acute acidemia increases and acute alkalemia decreases ionized calcium.[122]

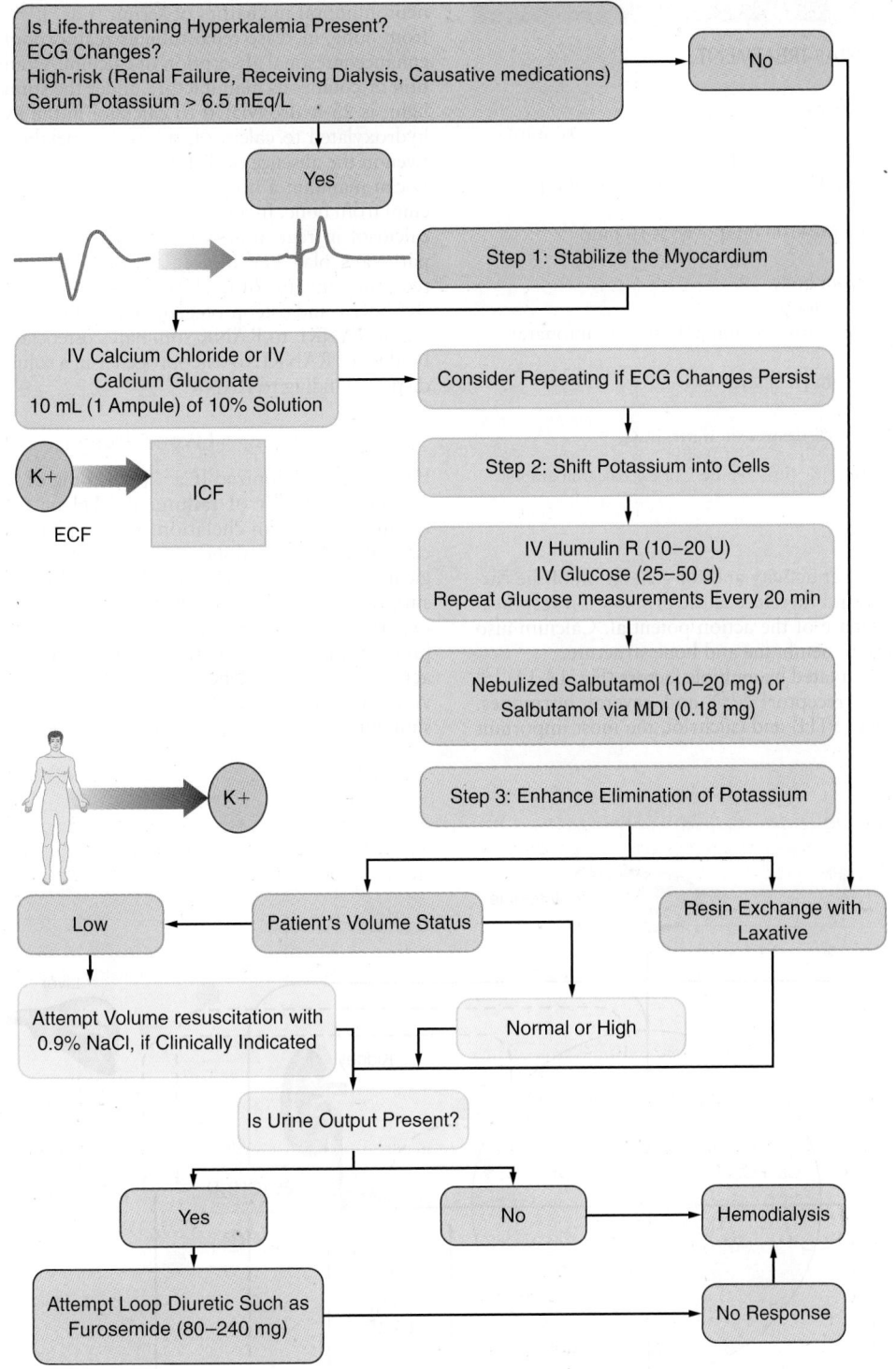

FIGURE 14-13.   Algorithmic management of hyperkalemia. ECG, electrocardiographic; IV, intravenous; K, potassium; ECF, extracellular fluid; ICF, intracellular fluid; MDI, metered-dose inhaler; NaCl, sodium chloride. (From Sood MM, Sood AR, Richardson R: Emergency management and commonly encountered outpatient scenarios in patients with hyperkalemia. Mayo Clin Proc 2007; 82: 1553–1561, with permission.)

Because mathematical formulae that "correct" total calcium measurements for albumin concentration are inaccurate in critically ill patients,[123] ionized calcium should be directly measured.

In general, calcium is essential for all movement that occurs in mammalian systems. Essential for normal excitation-contraction coupling, calcium is also necessary for proper function of

muscle tissue, ciliary movement, mitosis, neurotransmitter release, enzyme secretion, and hormonal secretion. Cyclic adenosine monophosphate (cAMP) and phosphoinositides, which are major second messengers regulating cellular metabolism, function primarily through the regulation of calcium movement. Activation of numerous intracellular enzyme systems requires calcium. Calcium is important both for generation

TABLE 14-19

SEVERE HYPERKALEMIA*a* TREATMENT

Reverse membrane effects
   Calcium (10 mL of 10% calcium chloride IV over 10 min)
Transfer extracellular [K⁺] into cells
   Glucose and insulin (D10W + 5–10 U regular insulin per
     25–50 g glucose)
   Sodium bicarbonate (50–100 mEq over 5–10 min)
   β_2 Agonists
Remove potassium from body
   Diuretics, proximal or loop
   Potassium-exchange resins (sodium polystyrene sulfonate)
   Hemodialysis
Monitor ECG and serum [K⁺] level

IV, intravenous; D10W, 10% dextrose in water; ECG,
electrocardiogram.
*a*Potassium concentration ([K⁺]) >7.0 mEq/L or electrocardiographic
changes.

of the cardiac pacemaker activity and for generation of the cardiac action potential and therefore is the primary ion responsible for the plateau phase of the action potential. Calcium also plays vital functions in membrane and bone structure.

Serum [Ca²⁺] is regulated by multiple factors (Fig. 14-14),[124] including a calcium receptor[124,125] and several hormones. Parathyroid hormone (PTH) and calcitriol, the most important neurohumoral mediators of serum [Ca²⁺],[126] mobilize calcium from bone, increase renal tubular reabsorption of calcium, and enhance intestinal absorption of calcium. Vitamin D, after ingestion or cutaneous manufacture under the stimulus of ultraviolet light, is 25-hydroxylated to calcidiol in the liver and then is 1-hydroxylated to calcitriol, the active metabolite, in the kidney. Even in the absence of dietary calcium intake, PTH and vitamin D can maintain a normal circulating [Ca²⁺] by mobilizing calcium from bone. In addition to the key roles played by PTH and calcitriol in regulating serum [Ca²⁺], other recently described pathways play key molecular roles in bone resorption. The receptor activator of nuclear factor κB (RANK), RANK ligand (RANKL), and osteoprotegenerin play key molecular roles; binding of RANKL to RANK stimulates osteoclast activity, whereas binding of RANKL to osteoprogenerin, a soluble decoy receptor, disrupts binding to RANK.[127]

Hypocalcemia

Hypocalcemia (ionized [Ca²⁺] <4.0 mg/dL or <1.0 mmol/L) occurs as a result of failure of PTH or calcitriol action or because of calcium chelation or precipitation, not because of calcium deficiency alone. PTH deficiency can result from surgical damage or removal of the parathyroid glands or from suppression of the parathyroid glands by severe hypo- or hypermagnesemia. Burns, sepsis, and pancreatitis may suppress parathyroid function and interfere with vitamin D action. Vitamin D deficiency may result from lack of dietary vitamin D or vitamin D malabsorption in patients who lack sunlight exposure. Hyperphosphatemia-induced hypocalcemia

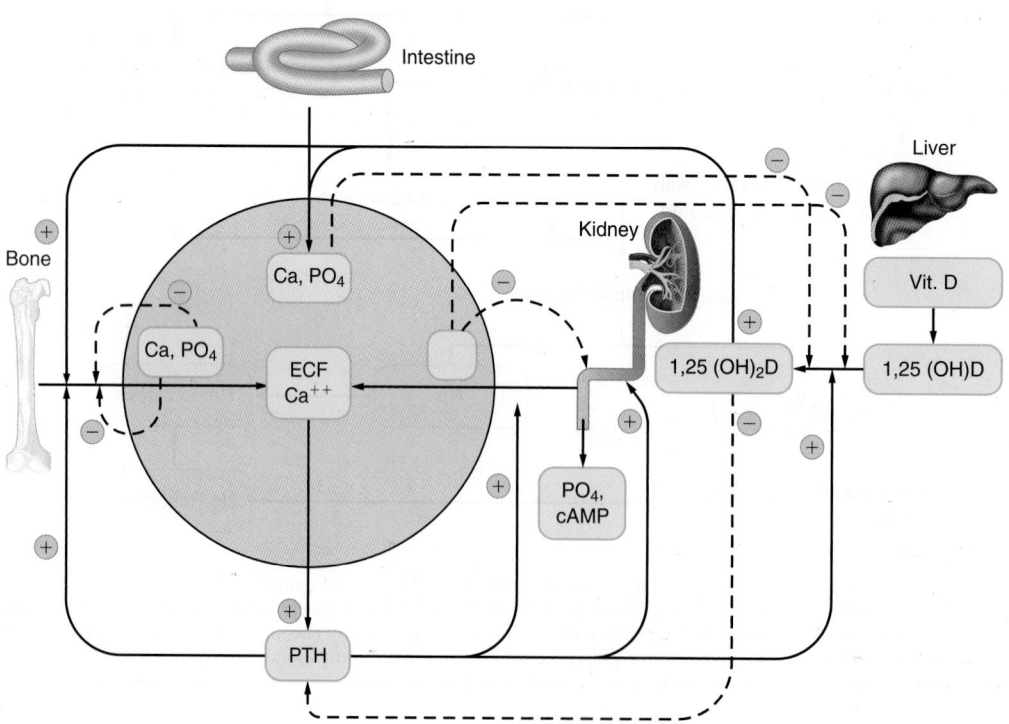

FIGURE 14-14. Schematic representation of the regulatory system maintaining Ca²⁺ homeostasis. The *solid arrows* and *lines* delineate effects of parathyroid hormone (PTH) and 1,25 (OH)₂D₃ (dihydroxyvitamin D) on their target tissues; *dashed arrows* and *lines* show examples of how extracellular Ca²⁺ or phosphate ions act directly on tissues regulating mineral ion metabolism. Ca, calcium; PO₄, phosphate; ECF, extracellular fluid; cAMP, cyclic adenosine monophosphate; 25(OH)D = 25-hydroxyvitamin D; negative signs indicate inhibitory actions and plus signs indicate stimulatory effects. (Reprinted with permission from Brown EM, Pollak M, Hebert SC: The extracellular calcium-sensing receptor: its role in health and disease. Ann Rev Med 1998; 49: 15–29).

TABLE 14-20

HYPOCALCEMIA: CLINICAL MANIFESTATIONS

Cardiovascular	**Respiratory**
Dysrhythmias	Apnea
Digitalis insensitivity	Laryngeal spasm
ECG changes	Bronchospasm
Heart failure	
Hypotension	**Psychiatric**
	Anxiety
Neuromuscular	Dementia
Tetany	Depression
Muscle spasm	Psychosis
Papilledema	
Seizures	
Weakness	
Fatigue	

ECG, electrocardiographic.

TABLE 14-21

HYPOCALCEMIA: ACUTE TREATMENT

Administer calcium
  IV: 10 mL 10% calcium gluconate[a] over 10 min, followed
    by elemental calcium 0.3–2.0 mg/kg/hr
  Oral: 500–100 mg elemental calcium q 6 hr
Administer vitamin D
  Ergocalciferol, 1,200 μg/day ($T_{1/2}$ = 30 days)
  Dihydrotachysterol, 200–400 μg/day ($T_{1/2}$ = 7 days)
  1,25-dihydroxycholecalciferol, 0.25–1.0 μg/day ($T_{1/2}$ = 1 day)
Monitor electrocardiogram

IV, intravenous; $T_{1/2}$, half-life.
[a]Calcium gluconate contains 93 mg elemental calcium per 10-ml vial.

may occur as a consequence of overzealous phosphate therapy, from cell lysis secondary to chemotherapy, or as a result of cellular destruction from rhabdomyolysis. Precipitation of $CaHPO_4$ complexes occurs with hyperphosphatemia. However, ionized $[Ca^{2+}]$ only decreases approximately 0.019 mM for each 1.0 mM increase in phosphate concentration. In massive transfusion, citrate may produce hypocalcemia by chelating calcium; however, decreases are usually transient and produce negligible cardiovascular effects, unless citrate clearance is decreased (e.g., by hepatic or renal disease or hypothermia) or blood transfusion exceeds 5 units of packed red blood cells.[128] Alkalemia resulting from hyperventilation or sodium bicarbonate injection can acutely decrease $[Ca^{2+}]$.

The hallmark of hypocalcemia is increased neuronal membrane irritability and tetany (Table 14-20). Early symptoms include sensations of numbness and tingling involving fingers, toes, and the circumoral region. In frank tetany, tonic contraction of respiratory muscles may lead to laryngospasm, bronchospasm, or respiratory arrest. Smooth muscle spasm can result in abdominal cramping and urinary frequency. Mental status alterations include irritability, depression, psychosis, and dementia. Hypocalcemia may impair cardiovascular function and has been associated with heart failure, hypotension, dysrhythmias, insensitivity to digitalis, and impaired β-adrenergic action.

Reduced *ionized* serum calcium occurs in as many as 88% of critically ill patients, 66% of less severely ill intensive care unit patients and 26% of hospitalized non–intensive care unit patients.[129] Patients at particular risk include patients after multiple trauma and cardiopulmonary bypass. In most such patients, ionized hypocalcemia is clinically mild ($[Ca^{2+}]$ 0.8 to 1.0 mmol/L).

Initial diagnostic evaluation should concentrate on history and physical examination, laboratory evaluation of renal function, and measurement of serum phosphate concentration. Latent hypocalcemia can be diagnosed by tapping on the facial nerve to elicit Chvostek sign or by inflating a sphygmomanometer to 20 mm Hg above systolic pressure, which produces radial and ulnar nerve ischemia and causes carpal spasm known as *Trousseau sign*. The differential diagnosis of hypocalcemia can be approached by addressing four issues: age of the patient, serum phosphate concentration, general clinical status, and duration of hypocalcemia.[130] Low or normal phosphate concentrations imply vitamin D or magnesium deficiency. An otherwise healthy patient with chronic hypocalcemia probably is hypoparathyroid. High phosphate concentrations suggest renal failure or hypoparathyroidism. In renal insufficiency, reduced phosphorus excretion results in hyperphosphatemia, which down-regulates the 1α-hydroxylase responsible for the renal conversion of calcidiol to calcitriol. This, in combination with decreased production of calcitriol secondary to reduced renal mass, causes reduced intestinal absorption of calcium and hypocalcemia.[126] Chronically ill adults with hypocalcemia often have disorders such as malabsorption, osteomalacia, or osteoblastic metastases.

The definitive treatment of hypocalcemia necessitates identification and treatment of the underlying cause (Table 14-21). Symptomatic hypocalcemia usually occurs when serum ionized $[Ca^{2+}]$ is <0.7 mM.

Unnecessary offending drugs should be discontinued. Hypocalcemia resulting from hypomagnesemia or hyperphosphatemia is treated by repletion of magnesium or removal of phosphate. Treatment of a patient who has tetany and hyperphosphatemia requires coordination of therapy to avoid the consequences of metastatic soft-tissue calcification.[131] Potassium and other electrolytes should be measured and abnormalities should be corrected. Hyperkalemia and hypomagnesemia potentiate hypocalcemia-induced cardiac and neuromuscular irritability. In contrast, hypokalemia protects against hypocalcemic tetany; therefore, correction of hypokalemia without correction of hypocalcemia may provoke tetany.

Mild, ionized hypocalcemia should not be overtreated. For instance, in most patients after cardiac surgery, administration of calcium only increases blood pressure and actually attenuates the β-adrenergic effects of epinephrine. In normocalcemic dogs, calcium chloride primarily acts as a peripheral vasoconstrictor, with transient reduction of myocardial contractility; in hypocalcemic dogs, calcium infusion significantly improves contractile performance and blood pressure.[132] Therefore, calcium infusions should be of limited value in surgical patients unless there is demonstrable evidence of ionized hypocalcemia. Calcium salts appear to confer no benefit to patients already receiving inotropic or vasoactive agents.

The cornerstone of therapy for confirmed, symptomatic, ionized hypocalcemia ($[Ca^{2+}]$ <0.7 mM) is calcium administration. In patients who have severe hypocalcemia or hypocalcemic symptoms, calcium should be administered intravenously. In emergency situations, in an averaged-sized adult, the "rule of 10s" advises infusion of 10 mL of 10% calcium gluconate (93 mg elemental calcium) over 10 minutes, followed by a continuous infusion of elemental calcium, 0.3 to 2 mg/kg/hr (i.e., 3 to 16 mL/hr of 10% calcium gluconate for a 70-kg adult). Calcium salts should be diluted in 50 to 100 mL D5W (to limit venous irritation and thrombosis), should not be mixed with bicarbonate (to prevent precipitation), and must be given cautiously to digitalized patients because calcium increases the toxicity of digoxin. Continuous ECG monitoring during initial therapy will detect cardiotoxicity (e.g., heart block, ventricular fibrillation). During calcium replacement, the clinician should monitor serum calcium, magnesium, phosphate, potassium, and creatinine. Once the ionized $[Ca^{2+}]$ is stable in the range of 4 to 5 mg/dL (1.0 to 1.25 mM), oral calcium supplements can substitute for parenteral therapy. Urinary calcium should be monitored in an attempt to avoid hypercalciuria (>5 mg/kg per 24 hours) and urinary tract stone formation.

When supplementation fails to maintain serum calcium within the normal range, or if hypercalciuria develops, vitamin D or vitamin D analogs may be added. Although the principal effect of vitamin D is to increase enteric calcium absorption, osseous calcium resorption is also enhanced. When rapid changes in dosage are anticipated or an immediate effect is required (e.g., postoperative hypoparathyroidism), shorter-acting calciferols such as dihydrotachysterol may be preferable. Because the effect of vitamin D is not regulated, the dosages of calcium and vitamin D should be adjusted to raise the serum calcium into the low normal range.

Adverse reactions to calcium and vitamin D include hypercalcemia and hypercalciuria. If hypercalcemia develops, calcium and vitamin D should be discontinued and appropriate therapy given. The toxic effects of vitamin D metabolites persist in proportion to their biologic half-lives (ergocalciferol, 20 to 60 days; dihydrotachysterol, 5 to 15 days; calcitriol, 2 to 10 days). Glucocorticoids antagonize the toxic effects of vitamin D metabolites.

Hypercalcemia

Although ionized $[Ca^{2+}]$ most accurately defines hypercalcemia (ionized $[Ca^{2+}]$ >1.5 mmol/L or total serum calcium >10.5 mg/dL), hypercalcemia customarily is discussed in terms of total serum calcium. In hypoalbuminemic patients, total serum calcium can be estimated (albeit inaccurately) by assuming an increase of 0.8 mg/dL for every 1 g/dL of albumin concentration below 4.0 g/dL. Patients in whom total serum calcium is <11.5 mg/dL are usually asymptomatic. Patients with moderate hypercalcemia (total serum calcium 11.5 to 13 mg/dL) may show symptoms of lethargy, anorexia, nausea, and polyuria. Severe hypercalcemia (total serum calcium >13 mg/dL) is associated with more severe neuromyopathic symptoms, including muscle weakness, depression, impaired memory, emotional lability, lethargy, stupor, and coma. The cardiovascular effects of hypercalcemia include hypertension, arrhythmias, heart block, cardiac arrest, and digitalis sensitivity. Skeletal disease may occur secondary to direct osteolysis or humoral bone resorption.

Hypercalcemia impairs urinary concentrating ability and renal excretory capacity for calcium by irreversibly precipitating calcium salts within the renal parenchyma and by reducing renal blood flow and GFR. In response to hypovolemia, renal tubular reabsorption of sodium enhances renal calcium reabsorption. Effective treatment of severe hypercalcemia is necessary to prevent progressive dehydration and renal failure leading to further increases in total serum calcium, because volume depletion exacerbates hypercalcemia.[133] Hypercalcemia occurs when calcium enters the ECV more rapidly than the kidneys can excrete the excess. Clinically, hypercalcemia most commonly results from an excess of bone resorption over bone formation, usually secondary to malignant disease, hyperparathyroidism, hypocalciuric hypercalcemia, thyrotoxicosis, immobilization, and granulomatous diseases. Granulomatous diseases produce hypercalciuria and hypercalcemia because of conversion by granulomatous tissue of calcidiol to calcitriol.[126]

Malignancy may produce hypercalcemia either through bone destruction or secretion by malignant tissue of hormones that promote hypercalcemia. Examples of malignancy-associated

hormonal effects include secretion by solid tumors of parathormonelike peptides and derangement of the RANKL/osteoprogenerin system in multiple myeloma.[134] Primary hyperparathyroidism is associated with weakness, weight loss, and anemia, symptoms that suggest malignancy but may result simply from hyperparathyroidism. Hypercalcemia associated with granulomatous diseases (e.g., sarcoidosis) results from the production of calcitriol by granulomatous tissue. To compensate for increased gut absorption or bone resorption of calcium, renal excretion can readily increase from 100 to more than 400 mg/day. Factors that promote hypercalcemia may be offset by coexisting disorders, such as pancreatitis, sepsis, or hyperphosphatemia, that cause hypocalcemia.

Although definitive treatment of hypercalcemia requires correction of underlying causes, temporizing therapy may be necessary to avoid complications and to relieve symptoms. Total serum calcium exceeding 14 mg/dL represents a medical emergency. General supportive treatment includes hydration, correction of associated electrolyte abnormalities, removal of offending drugs, dietary calcium restriction, and increased physical activity. Because anorexia and antagonism by calcium of ADH action invariably lead to sodium and water depletion, infusion of 0.9% saline will dilute serum calcium, promote renal excretion, and can reduce total serum calcium by 1.5 to 3 mg/dL. Urinary output should be maintained at 200 to 300 mL/hr. As GFR increases, sodium ions increase calcium excretion by competing with calcium ions for reabsorption in the proximal renal tubules and loop of Henle.

Furosemide further enhances calcium excretion by increasing tubular sodium. Patients who have renal impairment may require higher doses of furosemide. During saline infusion and forced diuresis, careful monitoring of cardiopulmonary status and electrolytes, especially magnesium and potassium, is required. Intensive diuresis and saline administration can achieve net calcium excretion rates of 2,000 to 4,000 mg per 24 hours, a rate 8 times greater than saline alone, but still somewhat less than the 6,000 mg every 8 hours that can be removed by hemodialysis. Patients treated with phosphates for hypercalcemia should be well hydrated.

Bone resorption, the primary cause of hypercalcemia, can be minimized by increasing physical activity and initiating drug therapy with biphosphonates, calcitonin, glucocorticoids, or calcimetrics.[135] Bisphosphonates, currently the first-line therapy for acute hypercalcemia, inhibit osteoclast function and viability. Bisphosphonates are the principal drugs for the management of hypercalcemia mediated by osteoclastic bone resorption.[134] Pamidronate, unlike earlier biphosphonates, does not appear to worsen renal insufficiency. More recently released biphosphonates include alendronate, risedronate. and zoledronate. Risedronate has been associated with less gastrointestinal morbidity than alendronate.[136,137] Zoledronate has the most rapid onset of action among the biphosphonates and prolongs the duration before relapse of hypercalcemia; however, zoledronate has been associated with compromised renal function.[135] Biphosphonates also are used to control osteoporosis in both men and women.[138,139]

Calcitonin, usually reserved as a secondary treatment for life-threatening hypercalcemia, lowers serum calcium within 24 to 48 hours and is more effective when combined with glucocorticoids.[134,135] Usually calcitonin reduces total serum calcium by only 1 to 2 mg/dL. Although calcitonin is relatively nontoxic, more than 25% of patients may not respond. Thus, calcitonin is unsuitable as a first-line drug during life-threatening hypercalcemia. Hydrocortisone is effective in treating hypercalcemic patients with lymphatic malignancies, vitamin D or A intoxication, and diseases associated with production by tumor or granulomas of $1,25(OH)_2D$ or osteoclast-activating factor. Glucocorticoids rarely improve hypercalcemia secondary to malignancy or hyperparathyroidism.

In the near future, calcimetics may become the treatment of choice for suppressing primary, secondary, and tertiary hyperparathyroidism. With the first agent, cinacalcet, recently released for clinical use in the United States and others undergoing clinical trials, calcimetic agents also reduce inorganic phosphate concentration (Pi) and the calcium × phosphate product.[140–142] Although hyperparathyroidectomy remains the treatment of choice for primary hyperparathyroidism, calcimetics represent an alternative for patients who are not acceptable candidates for surgery.[142] In hyperparathyroidism secondary to chronic renal failure, conventional treatment with calcium supplements, phosphate binders, and vitamin D analogs reduces the associated secondary hyperparathyroidism but also generate undesirable side effects, including hypercalcemia.[140] In effect, such patients develop a variation of the milk-alkali syndrome.[143] In chronic renal failure patients, calcimetics reduce serum calcium, Pi and the calcium × phosphate product by sensitizing the parathyroid calcium receptor to calcium.[141] In addition, calcimetics appear to be effective in tertiary hyperparathyroidism, which develops after renal transplantation in 25 to 50% of renal allograft recipients.[142]

Phosphates lower serum calcium by causing deposition of calcium in bone and soft tissue. Because the risk of extraskeletal calcification of organs such as the kidneys and myocardium is less if phosphates are given orally, the intravenous route should be reserved for patients with life-threatening hypercalcemia and those in whom other measures have failed.

Phosphate

Physiologic Role

Phosphorus, in the form of inorganic phosphate (Pi), is distributed in similar concentrations throughout intracellular and extracellular fluid. Of total body phosphorus, 90% exists in bone, 10% is intracellular, and the remainder, <1%, is found in the extracellular fluid. Phosphate circulates as the free ion (55%), complexed ion (33%), and in a protein-bound form (12%). Blood levels vary widely: the normal total Pi ranges from 2.7 to 4.5 mg/dL in adults.

Control of Pi is achieved by altered renal excretion and redistribution within the body compartments. Absorption occurs in the duodenum and jejunum and is largely unregulated. Phosphate reabsorption in the kidney is primarily regulated by PTH, dietary intake, and insulinlike growth factor. Phosphate is freely filtered at the glomerulus and its concentration in the glomerular ultrafiltrate is similar to that of plasma. The filtered phosphate is then reabsorbed in the proximal tubule where it is cotransported with sodium. Proximal tubular reabsorption of phosphorus occurs by passive cotransport with sodium. Cotransport is regulated by phosphorus intake and PTH. Phosphate excretion is increased by volume expansion and decreased by respiratory alkalosis.

Phosphates provide the primary energy bond in ATP and creatine phosphate. Therefore, severe phosphate depletion results in cellular energy depletion. Phosphorus is an essential element of second-messenger systems, including cAMP and phosphoinositides, and a major component of nucleic acids, phospholipids, and cell membranes. As part of 2,3-diphosphoglycerate, phosphate promotes release of oxygen from the hemoglobin molecule. Phosphorus also functions in protein phosphorylation and acts as a urinary buffer.

Hypophosphatemia

Hypophosphatemia is characterized by low levels of phosphate-containing cellular components, including ATP, 2,3-diphospho-glycerate, and membrane phospholipids. Serious life-threatening organ dysfunction may occur when the serum Pi falls below 1 mg/dL. Neurologic manifestations of hypophosphatemia include paresthesias, myopathy, encephalopathy, delirium, seizures, and coma.[144] Hematologic abnormalities include dysfunction of erythrocytes, platelets, and leukocytes. Because hypophosphatemia limits the chemotactic, phagocytic, and bactericidal activity of granulocytes, associated immune dysfunction may contribute to the susceptibility of hypophosphatemic patients to sepsis.[145] Muscle weakness and malaise are common. Respiratory muscle failure and myocardial dysfunction are potential problems of particular concern to anesthesiologists. Rhabdomyolysis is a complication of severe hypophosphatemia.

Common in postoperative and traumatized patients, hypophosphatemia (Pi <2.5 mg/dL) is caused by three primary abnormalities in Pi homeostasis: an intracellular shift of Pi, an increase in renal Pi loss, and a decrease in gastrointestinal Pi absorption. Carbohydrate-induced hypophosphatemia (the "refeeding syndrome"),[146] mediated by insulin-induced cellular Pi uptake, is the type most commonly encountered in hospitalized patients. Hypophosphatemia may also occur as catabolic patients become anabolic and during medical management of diabetic ketoacidosis. Acute alkalemia, which may reduce serum Pi to 1 to 2 mg/dL, increases intracellular consumption of Pi by increasing the rate of glycolysis. Hyperventilation significantly reduces Pi and, importantly, the effect is progressive after cessation of hyperventilation.[147] Acute correction of respiratory acidemia may also result in severe hypophosphatemia. Respiratory alkalosis probably explains the hypophosphatemia associated with Gram-negative bacteremia and salicylate poisoning. Excessive renal loss of Pi explains the hypophosphatemia associated with hyperparathyroidism, hypomagnesemia, hypothermia, diuretic therapy, and renal tubular defects in Pi absorption. Excess gastrointestinal loss of Pi is most commonly secondary to the use of Pi-binding antacids or to malabsorption syndromes.

Measurement of urinary Pi aids in differentiation of hypophosphatemia due to renal losses from that are due to excessive gastrointestinal losses or redistribution of Pi into cells. Extrarenal causes of hypophosphatemia cause avid renal tubular Pi reabsorption, reducing urinary excretion to <100 mg/day.

Patients who have severe (<1 mg/dL) or symptomatic hypophosphatemia require intravenous phosphate administration (Table 14-22).[144,147] In chronically hypophosphatemic patients, 0.2 to 0.68 mmol/kg (5 to 16 mg/kg elemental phosphorus) should be infused over 12 hours. For moderately hypophosphatemic adult patients suffering from critical illness, the use of 15 mmol boluses (465 mg) mixed with 100 mL of 0.9% sodium chloride and given over a 2-hour period safely repletes phosphate.[148] The dosage is then adjusted as indicated by the serum Pi level because the cumulative deficit cannot be predicted accurately. Oral therapy can be substituted for parenteral Pi once the serum Pi level exceeds 2.0 mg/dL. Continued therapy with Pi supplements is required for 5 to 10 days in order to replenish body stores.

TABLE 14-22

HYPOPHOSPHATEMIA: ACUTE TREATMENT

Parenteral phosphate, 0.2 mM to 0.68 mM/kg (5–16 mg/kg) over 12 hr
Potassium phosphate (93 mg/mL of phosphate)
Sodium phosphate (93 mg/mL of phosphate)

Phosphate should be administered cautiously to hypocalcemic patients because of the risk of precipitating more severe hypocalcemia. In hypercalcemic patients, Pi may cause soft-tissue calcification. Phosphorus must be given cautiously to patients with renal insufficiency because of impaired excretory ability. During treatment, close monitoring of serum Pi, calcium, magnesium, and potassium is essential to avoid complications.

Hyperphosphatemia

The clinical features of hyperphosphatemia (Pi >5.0 mg/dL) relate primarily to the development of hypocalcemia and ectopic calcification. Hyperphosphatemia is caused by three basic mechanisms: inadequate renal excretion, increased movement of Pi out of cells, and increased Pi or vitamin D intake. Rapid cell lysis from chemotherapy, rhabdomyolysis, and sepsis can cause hyperphosphatemia, especially when renal function is impaired. Renal failure is the most common cause of hyperphosphatemia.

Renal excretion of Pi remains adequate until the GFR falls below 20 to 25 mL/min. Accumulation of Pi in patients with chronic renal failure merits the inclusion of Pi as a uremic toxin.[149]

Measurements of BUN, creatinine, GFR, and urinary Pi are helpful in the differential diagnosis of hyperphosphatemia. Normal renal function accompanied by high Pi excretion (>1,500 mg/day) indicates an oversupply of Pi. An elevated BUN, elevated creatinine, and low GFR suggest impaired renal excretion of Pi. Normal renal function and Pi excretion <1,500 mg/day suggest increased Pi reabsorption (i.e., hypoparathyroidism).

Hyperphosphatemia is corrected by eliminating the cause of the Pi elevation and correcting the associated hypocalcemia. Calcium supplementation of hypocalcemic patients should be delayed until serum phosphate has fallen below 2.0 mmol/L (6.0 mg/dL).[126] The serum concentration of Pi is reduced by restricting intake, increasing urinary excretion with saline and acetazolamide (500 mg every 6 hours), and increasing gastrointestinal losses by enteric administration of aluminum hydroxide (30 to 45 mL every 6 hours).

Although calcimetics may replace Pi-binders for managing hyperphosphatemia in patients with chronic renal failure, several remain in common use. Calcium-based binders may contribute to hypercalcemia, sevelamer hydrochloride binds bile acids, and lanthanum carbonate offers the advantage of requiring patients to ingest fewer pills.[150] Hemodialysis and peritoneal dialysis are effective in removing Pi in patients who have renal failure.

Magnesium

Physiologic Role

Magnesium is an important, multifunctional, divalent cation located primarily in the intracellular space. Approximately 50% of the typical adult's 24 g of magnesium is located in bone, 12 g is located intracellularly (approximately one-half or 6 g in muscle), and <1% (<240 mg) of total body magnesium circulates in the serum.[151] Of the normal circulating total magnesium concentration (1.5 to 1.9 mEq/L or 0.75 to 0.95 mmol/L or 1.5 to 1.9 mg/dL), there are three components: protein-bound (30%), anion-bound (15%), and ionized (55%), of which only ionized magnesium is active.

Magnesium is necessary for enzymatic reactions involving DNA and protein synthesis, energy metabolism, glucose utilization, and fatty acid synthesis and breakdown.[152] As a primary regulator or cofactor in many enzyme systems, magnesium is important for the regulation of the sodium-potassium

pump, Ca-ATPase enzymes, adenyl cyclase, proton pumps, and slow calcium channels. Magnesium has been called an *endogenous calcium antagonist* because regulation of slow calcium channels contributes to maintenance of normal vascular tone, prevention of vasospasm, and perhaps the prevention of calcium overload in many tissues. Because magnesium partially regulates PTH secretion and is important for the maintenance of end-organ sensitivity to both PTH and vitamin D, abnormalities in ionized magnesium concentration ($[Mg^{2+}]$) may result in abnormal calcium metabolism. Magnesium functions in potassium metabolism primarily through regulating sodium-potassium ATPase, an enzyme that controls potassium entry into cells, especially in potassium-depleted states, and controls reabsorption of potassium by the renal tubules. In addition, magnesium functions as a regulator of membrane excitability and serves as a structural component in both cell membranes and the skeleton.

Because magnesium stabilizes axonal membranes, hypomagnesemia decreases the threshold of axonal stimulation and increases nerve conduction velocity. Magnesium also influences the release of neurotransmitters at the neuromuscular junction by competitively inhibiting the entry of calcium into the presynaptic nerve terminals. The concentration of calcium required to trigger calcium release and the rate at which calcium is released from the sarcoplasmic reticulum are inversely related to the ambient magnesium concentration. Thus, the net effect of hypomagnesemia is muscle that contracts more in response to stimuli and is tetany-prone.

Magnesium is widely available in foods and is absorbed through the gastrointestinal tract, although dietary consumption appears to have decreased over several decades.[152] Seventy percent of plasma magnesium is filtered through the glomerular membrane; of the filtered magnesium, 30% is absorbed in the proximal tubule, 60% in the thick ascending loop of Henle, and 10 to 15 % in the distal tubule.[151] While both magnesium and Pi are primarily regulated by intrinsic renal mechanisms, PTH exerts a greater effect on renal loss of Pi.

Magnesium has been used to help manage an impressive array of clinical problems in patients who are not hypomagnesemic. Therapeutic hypermagnesemia is used to treat patients with premature labor, pre-eclampsia, and eclampsia. Because magnesium blocks the release of catecholamines from adrenergic nerve terminals and the adrenal glands, magnesium has been used reduce the effects of catecholamine excess in patients with tetanus and pheochromocytoma.[153] In patients awaiting liver transplantation, one study showed that administration of magnesium significantly reversed hypocoagulability.[154] Although clinical data are inconsistent, magnesium also may exert an analgesic effect on postoperative pain,[153,155] perhaps in part due to magnesium's antagonism of the N-methyl-D-aspartate glutamate receptor.[153] Magnesium has been proposed as part of an antivasospasm regimen after subarachnoid hemorrhage, but its efficacy may be limited by induction of increasing magnesium levels of hypocalcemia, which in turn could aggravate cerebral vasospasm.[156] Surprisingly, redistribution of magnesium after subarachnoid hemorrhage has been correlated with ECG changes.[157]

Magnesium administration may influence dysrhythmias by direct effects on myocardial membranes, by altering cellular potassium and sodium concentrations, by inhibiting cellular calcium entry, by improving myocardial oxygen supply and demand, by prolonging the effective refractory period, by depressing conduction, by antagonizing catecholamine action on the conducting system, and by preventing vasospasm. Administration of magnesium reduces the incidence of dysrhythmias after myocardial infarction and in patients with congestive heart failure.[158] In humans with ischemic myocardium, magnesium prevented ischemic increases in action potential duration and membrane repolarization.[159]

After acute myocardial infarction, intravenous magnesium administration decreased short-term mortality.[160] In addition, magnesium may be useful as treatment for torsades de pointes, even in normomagnesemic patients.[161] Treatment of hypomagnesemia during cardiopulmonary bypass decreased the incidence of postoperative ventricular tachycardia from 30 to 7% and increased the frequency of continuous sinus rhythm from 5 to 34%.[162]

Hypomagnesemia

The clinical features of hypomagnesemia ($[Mg^{2+}]$ <1.8 mg/dL), like those of hypocalcemia, are characterized by increased neuronal irritability and tetany (Table 14-23).[151] Symptoms are rare when the serum $[Mg^{2+}]$ is 1.5 to 1.7 mg/dL; in most symptomatic patients serum $[Mg^{2+}]$ is <1.2 mg/dL. Patients frequently complain of weakness, lethargy, muscle spasms, paresthesias, and depression. When severe, hypomagnesemia may induce seizures, confusion, and coma. Cardiovascular abnormalities include coronary artery spasm, cardiac failure, dysrhythmias, and hypotension. Severe hypomagnesemia may reduce the response of adenylate cyclase to stimulation of the PTH receptor.[163] Hypomagnesemia can aggravate digoxin toxicity and congestive heart failure.

Rarely resulting from inadequate dietary intake, hypomagnesemia most commonly is caused by inadequate gastrointestinal absorption, excessive magnesium losses, or failure of renal magnesium conservation. Hypomagnesemia is particularly frequent in alcoholic patients.[151] Of alcoholic patients admitted to the hospital, 30% are hypomagnesemic.[164] Excessive loss of magnesium is associated with prolonged nasogastric suctioning, gastrointestinal or biliary fistulas, and intestinal drains.

Inability of the renal tubules to conserve magnesium complicates a variety of systemic and renal diseases, although advanced renal disease with a decreased GFR may lead to magnesium retention. Polyuria, whether secondary to ECV expansion or to pharmacologic or pathologic diuresis, may result in excessive urinary magnesium excretion. Various drugs, including aminoglycosides, cis-platinum, cardiac glycosides, and diuretics, enhance urinary magnesium excretion. Intracellular shifts of magnesium as a result of thyroid hormone or insulin administration may also decrease serum $[Mg^{2+}]$.

Because the sodium-potassium pump is magnesium-dependent, hypomagnesemia increases myocardial sensitivity to digitalis preparations and may cause hypokalemia as a result of renal potassium wasting. Attempts to correct potassium deficits with potassium-replacement therapy alone may not be successful without simultaneous magnesium therapy. Magnesium is important in the regulation of potassium channels. The interrelationships of magnesium and potassium in cardiac tissue have probably the greatest clinical relevance in terms of dysrhythmias, digoxin toxicity, and myocardial infarction. Both severe hypomagnesemia and hypermagnesemia suppress PTH secretion and can cause hypocalcemia. Severe hypomagnesemia may also impair end-organ response to PTH.

Hypomagnesemia is associated with hypokalemia, hyponatremia, hypophosphatemia, and hypocalcemia. The reported prevalence of hypomagnesemia in hospitalized and critically ill patients varies from 11 to 61%, with the variability attributable to differences in measurement technique.[165] Recent development of a specific electrode to measure ionized $[Mg^{2+}]$ has demonstrated an association between hypomagnesemia, use of

TABLE 14-23

MANIFESTATIONS OF ALTERED SERUM MAGNESIUM CONCENTRATIONS

MAGNESIUM LEVEL			
mg/dL	mEq/L	mmol/L	MANIFESTATION
<1.2	<1	<0.5	Tetany Seizures Arrhythmias
1.2–1.8	1.0–1.5	0.5–0.75	Neuromuscular irritability Hypocalcemia Hypokalemia
1.8–2.5	1.5–2.1	0.75–1.05	Normal magnesium level
2.5–5.0	2.1–4.2	1.05–2.1	Typically asymptomatic
5.0–7.0	4.2–5.8	2.1–2.9	Lethargy Drowsiness Flushing Nausea and vomiting Diminished deep tendon reflex
7.0–12	5.8–10	2.9–5	Somnolence Loss of deep tendon reflexes Hypotension ECG changes
>12	>10	>5	Complete heart block Cardiac arrest Apnea Paralysis Coma

ECG, electrocardiographic.
Reprinted from Topf JM, Murray PT: Hypomagnesemia and hypermagnesemia. Rev Endocr Metab Disord 2003; 4: 195–206, with permission.

TABLE 14-24

HYPOMAGNESEMIA: ACUTE TREATMENT

Intravenous Mg[a]: 8–16 mEq (1–2 g MgSO$_4$) bolus over 1 hr, followed by 2–4 mEq/hr (250–500 mg/hr MgSO$_4$) as continuous infusion

Intramuscular Mg[a]: 10 mEq q 4–6 hr

[a]MgSO$_4$: 1 g = 8 mEq/mg; MgCl$_2$: 1 g = 10 mEq/mg.

diuretics, and development of sepsis.[165] Patients who develop hypomagnesemia while in intensive care have an increased mortality.[165] Serum [Mg^{2+}] may not reflect intracellular magnesium content. Peripheral lymphocyte magnesium concentration correlates well with skeletal and cardiac magnesium content.

Measurement of 24-hour urinary magnesium excretion is useful in separating renal from nonrenal causes of hypomagnesemia. Normal kidneys can reduce magnesium excretion to <1 to 2 mEq/day in response to magnesium depletion. Hypomagnesemia accompanied by high urinary excretion of magnesium (>3 to 4 mEq/day) suggests a renal etiology. In the magnesium-loading test, urinary [Mg^{2+}] excretion is measured for 24 hours after an intravenous magnesium load.[166]

Magnesium deficiency is treated by the administration of magnesium supplements (Table 14-24). One gram of magnesium sulfate provides approximately 4 mmol (8 mEq, or 98 mg) of elemental magnesium. Mild deficiencies can be treated with diet alone. Replacement must be added to daily magnesium requirements (0.3 to 0.4 mEq/kg/day). Symptomatic or severe hypomagnesemia ([Mg^{2+}] <1.0 mg/dL) should be treated with parenteral magnesium: 1 to 2 g (8 to 16 mEq) of magnesium sulfate as an intravenous bolus over the first hour, followed by a continuous infusion of 2 to 4 mEq/hr. Therapy should be guided subsequently by the serum magnesium level. The rate of infusion should not exceed 1 mEq/min, even in emergency situations, and the patient should receive continuous cardiac monitoring to detect cardiotoxicity. Because magnesium antagonizes calcium, blood pressure and cardiac function should be monitored, although blood pressure and cardiac output usually change little during magnesium infusion.

During repletion, patellar reflexes should be monitored frequently and magnesium withheld if they become suppressed. Patients who have renal insufficiency have a diminished ability to excrete magnesium and require careful monitoring during therapy. Repletion of systemic magnesium stores usually requires 5 to 7 days of therapy, after which daily maintenance doses of magnesium should be provided. Magnesium can be given orally, usually in a dose of 60 to 90 mEq/day of magnesium oxide. Hypocalcemic, hypomagnesemic patients should receive magnesium as the chloride salt because the sulfate ion can chelate calcium and further reduce the serum [Ca^{2+}].

Hypermagnesemia

Most cases of hypermagnesemia ([Mg^{2+}] >2.5 mg/dL) are iatrogenic, resulting from the administration of magnesium in antacids, enemas, or parenteral nutrition, especially to patients with impaired renal function. Other rarer causes of mild hypermagnesemia are hypothyroidism, Addison disease, lithium intoxication, and familial hypocalciuric hypercalcemia. Hypermagnesemia is rarely detected in routine electrolyte determinations.[151] Hypermagnesemia antagonizes the release and effect of acetylcholine at the neuromuscular junction. The result is depressed skeletal muscle function and neu-

romuscular blockade. Magnesium potentiates the action of nondepolarizing muscle relaxants and decreases potassium release in response to succinylcholine. The clinical features of progressive hypermagnesemia are listed in Table 14-23.[151]

The neuromuscular and cardiac toxicity of hypermagnesemia can be acutely, but transiently, antagonized by giving intravenous calcium (5 to 10 mEq) to buy time while more definitive therapy is instituted.[151] All magnesium-containing preparations must be stopped. Urinary excretion of magnesium can be increased by expanding ECV and inducing diuresis with a combination of saline and furosemide. In emergency situations and in patients with renal failure, magnesium may be removed by dialysis.

References

1. Corey HE: Stewart and beyond: new models of acid-base balance. Kidney Int 2004; 64: 777
2. Moviat M, van Haren F, van der Hoeven H: Conventional or physicochemical approach in intensive care unit patients with metabolic acidosis. Crit Care 2003; 7: 219
3. Khanna A, Kurtzman NA: Metabolic alkalosis. J Nephrol 2006; 19(Suppl 9): S86
4. Prough DS, Bidani A: Hyperchloremic metabolic acidosis is a predictable consequence of intraoperative infusion of 0.9% saline. Anesthesiology 1999; 90: 1247
5. Adrogue HJ: Metabolic acidosis: pathophysiology, diagnosis and management. J Nephrol 2006; 19(Suppl 9): S62
6. Morris CG, Low J: Metabolic acidosis in the critically ill: part 2. Causes and treatment. Anaesthesia 2008; 63: 396
7. Morris CG, Low J: Metabolic acidosis in the critically ill: part 1. Classification and pathophysiology. Anaesthesia 2008; 63: 294
8. Kraut JA, Madias NE: Serum anion gap: its uses and limitations in clinical medicine. Clin J Am Soc Nephrol 2007; 2: 162
9. Scheingraber S, Rehm M, Sehmisch C, et al: Rapid saline infusion produces hyperchloremic acidosis in patients undergoing gynecologic surgery. Anesthesiology 1999; 90: 1265
10. Carvounis CP, Feinfeld DA: A simple estimate of the effect of the serum albumin level on the anion Gap. Am J Nephrol 2000; 20: 369
11. Rastegar A: Use of the DeltaAG/DeltaHCO3$^-$ ratio in the diagnosis of mixed acid-base disorders. J Am Soc Nephrol 2007; 18: 2429
12. Gehlbach BK, Schmidt GA: Bench-to-bedside review: treating acid-base abnormalities in the intensive care unit—the role of buffers. Crit Care 2004; 8: 259
13. Cooper DJ, Walley KR, Wiggs BR, et al: Bicarbonate does not improve hemodynamics in critically ill patients who have lactic acidosis. A prospective, controlled clinical study. Ann Intern Med 1990; 112: 492
14. Stacpoole PW, Wright EC, Baumgartner TG, et al: Dichloroacetate-Lactic Acidosis Study Group: A controlled clinical trial of dichloroacetate for treatment of lactic acidosis in adults. N Engl J Med 1992; 327: 1564
15. Hoste EA, Colpaert K, Vanholder RC, et al: Sodium bicarbonate versus THAM in ICU patients with mild metabolic acidosis. J Nephrol 2005; 18: 303
16. Foster GT, Vaziri ND, Sassoon CSH: Respiratory alkalosis. Respir Care 2001; 46: 384
17. Chesler M: Regulation and modulation of pH in the brain. Physiol Rev 2003; 83: 1183
18. Kallet RH, Liu K, Tang J: Management of acidosis during lung-protective ventilation in acute respiratory distress syndrome. Respir Care Clin North Am 2003; 9: 437
19. Martinu T, Menzies D, Dial S: Re-evaluation of acid-base prediction rules in patients with chronic respiratory acidosis. Can Respir J 2003; 10: 311
20. Svensén C, Hahn RG: Volume kinetics of Ringer solution, dextran 70, and hypertonic saline in male volunteers. Anesthesiology 1997; 87: 204
21. Brauer KI, Svensen C, Hahn RG, et al: Volume kinetic analysis of the distribution of 0.9% saline in conscious versus isoflurane-anesthetized sheep. Anesthesiology 2002; 96: 442
22. Connolly CM, Kramer GC, Hahn RG, et al: Isoflurane but not mechanical ventilation promotes extravascular fluid accumulation during crystalloid volume loading. Anesthesiology 2003; 98: 670
23. Vane LA, Prough DS, Kinsky MA, et al: Effects of Different Catecholamines on the Dynamics of Volume Expansion of Crystalloid Infusion. Anesthesiology 2004; 101: 1136
24. Schrier RW: The sea within us: disorders of body water homeostasis. Curr Opin Investig Drugs 2007; 8: 304
25. Ball SG: Vasopressin and disorders of water balance: the physiology and pathophysiology of vasopressin. Ann Clin Biochem 2007; 44: 417
26. Martinez-Rumayor A, Richards AM, Burnett JC, et al: Biology of the natriuretic peptides. Am J Cardiol 2008; 101: 3

27. Akashi YJ, Springer J, Lainscak M, et al: Atrial natriuretic peptide and related peptides. Clin Chem Lab Med 2007; 45: 1259

28. Silver MA: The natriuretic peptide system: kidney and cardiovascular effects. Curr Opin Nephrol Hypertens 2006; 15: 14

29. Conte G, Bellizzi V, Cianciaruso B, et al: Physiologic role and diuretic efficacy of atrial natriuretic peptide in health and chronic renal disease. Kidney Int 1997; 51: S28

30. Atlas SA: The renin-angiotensin aldosterone system: pathophysiological role and pharmacologic inhibition. J Manag Care Pharm 2007; 13: 9

31. Baughman VL: Brain protection during neurosurgery. Anesthesiol Clin North America 2002; 20: 315

32. Lanzino G, Kassell NF, Germanson T, et al: Plasma glucose levels and outcome after aneurysmal subarachnoid hemorrhage. J Neurosurg 1993; 79: 885

33. Rovlias A, Kotsou S: The influence of hyperglycemia on neurological outcome in patients with severe head injury. Neurosurgery 2000; 46: 335

34. Weiner RS, Weiner DC, Larson RJ: Benefits and risks of tight glucose control in critically ill adults: a meta-analysis. JAMA 2008; 300: 933

35. Finer S. Delancy A: Tight glycemic control in critically ill adults. JAMA 2008; 300:963

36. Van den Berghe G, Wouters P, Weekers F, et al: Intensive insulin therapy in critically ill patients. N Engl J Med 2001; 345: 1359

37. Pittas AG, Siegel RD, Lau J: Insulin therapy for critically ill hospitalized patients: a meta-analysis of randomized controlled trials. Arch Intern Med 2004; 164: 2005

38. Clement S, Braithwaite SS, Magee MF, et al: Management of diabetes and hyperglycemia in hospitals. Diabetes Care 2004; 27: 553

39. Maharaj CH, Kallam SR, Malik A, et al: Preoperative intravenous fluid therapy decreases postoperative nausea and pain in high risk patients. Anesth Analg 2005; 100: 675

40. Holte K, Klarskov B, Christensen DS, et al: Liberal versus restrictive fluid administration to improve recovery after laparoscopic cholecystectomy: a randomized, double-blind study. Ann Surg 2004; 240: 892

41. Holte K, Kristensen BB, Valentiner L, et al: Liberal versus restrictive fluid management in knee arthroplasty: a randomized, double-blind study. Anesth Analg 2007; 105: 465

42. Brandstrup B, Tonnesen H, Beier-Holgersen R, et al: Effects of intravenous fluid restriction on postoperative complications: Comparison of two perioperative fluid regimens—A randomized assessor-blinded multicenter trial. Ann Surg 2003; 238: 641

43. Nisanevich V, Felsenstein I, Almogy G, et al: Effect of intraoperative fluid management on outcome after intraabdominal surgery. Anesthesiology 2005; 103: 25

44. Lobo DN, Bostock KA, Neal KR, et al: Effect of salt and water balance on recovery of gastrointestinal function after elective colonic resection: a randomised controlled trial. Lancet 2002; 359: 1812

45. Khoo CK, Vickery CJ, Forsyth N, et al: A prospective randomized controlled trial of multimodal perioperative management protocol in patients undergoing elective colorectal resection for cancer. Ann Surg 2007; 245: 867

46. Holte K, Foss NB, Andersen J, et al: Liberal or restrictive fluid administration in fast-track colonic surgery: a randomized, double-blind study. Br J Anaesth 2007; 99: 500

47. Wiedemann HP, Wheeler AP, Bernard GR, et al: Comparison of two fluid-management strategies in acute lung injury. N Engl J Med 2006; 354: 2564

48. Moretti EW, Robertson KM, El Moalem H, et al: Intraoperative colloid administration reduces postoperative nausea and vomiting and improves postoperative outcomes compared with crystalloid administration. Anesth Analg 2003; 96: 611

49. Venn R, Steele A, Richardson P, et al: Randomized controlled trial to investigate influence of the fluid challenge on duration of hospital stay and perioperative morbidity in patients with hip fractures. Br J Anaesth 2002; 88: 65

50. Gan TJ, Soppitt A, Maroof M, et al: Goal-directed intraoperative fluid administration reduces length of hospital stay after major surgery. Anesthesiology 2002; 97: 820

51. Roberts I, Alderson P, Bunn F, et al: Colloids versus crystalloids for fluid resuscitation in critically ill patients. Cochrane Database Syst Rev 2004; 18: CD000567.

52. The Albumin Reviewers, Alderson P, Bunn F, Lefebvre C, et al: Human albumin solution for resuscitation and volume expansion in critically ill patients. Cochrane Database Syst Rev 2004; 18: CD001208.

53. Finfer S, Bellomo R, Boyce N, et al: A comparison of albumin and saline for fluid resuscitation in the intensive care unit. N Engl J Med 2004; 350: 2247

54. Finfer S, Bellomo R, McEvoy S, et al: Effect of baseline serum albumin concentration on outcome of resuscitation with albumin or saline in patients in intensive care units: analysis of data from the saline versus albumin fluid evaluation (SAFE) study. BMJ 2006; 333: 1044

55. Myburgh J, Cooper DJ, Finfer S, et al: Saline or albumin for fluid resuscitation in patients with traumatic brain injury. N Engl J Med 2007; 357: 874

56. Boldt J, Haisch G, Suttner S, et al: Effects of a new modified, balanced hydroxyethyl starch preparation (Hextend) on measures of coagulation. Br J Anaesth 2002; 89: 722

57. Gan TJ, Bennett-Guerrero E, Phillips-Bute B, et al: Hextend, a physiologically balanced plasma expander for large volume use in major surgery: a randomized phase III clinical trial. Anesth Analg 1999; 88: 992

58. Boldt J: Fluid choice for resuscitation of the trauma patient: a review of the physiological, pharmacological, and clinical evidence. Can J Anaesth 2004; 51: 500

59. Zornow MH, Todd MM, Moore SS: The acute cerebral effects of changes in plasma osmolality and oncotic pressure. Anesthesiology 1987; 67: 936

60. Kaieda R, Todd MM, Warner DS: Prolonged reduction in colloid oncotic pressure does not increase brain edema following cryogenic injury in rabbits. Anesthesiology 1989; 71: 554

61. Warner DS, Boehland LA: Effects of iso-osmolal intravenous fluid therapy on post-ischemic brain water content in the rat. Anesthesiology 1988; 68: 86

62. Zornow MH, Scheller MS, Todd MM, et al: Acute cerebral effects of isotonic crystalloid and colloid solutions following cryogenic brain injury in the rabbit. Anesthesiology 1988; 69: 180

63. Drummond JC, Patel PM, Cole DJ, et al: The effect of the reduction of colloid oncotic pressure, with and without reduction of osmolality, on post-traumatic cerebral edema. Anesthesiology 1998; 88: 993

64. Velasco IT, Pontieri V, Rocha E Silva M, Jr., et al: Hyperosmotic NaCl and severe hemorrhagic shock. Am J Physiol 1980; 239: H664

65. Prough DS, Whitley JM, Taylor CL, et al: Regional cerebral blood flow following resuscitation from hemorrhagic shock with hypertonic saline: Influence of a subdural mass. Anesthesiology 1991; 75: 319

66. Prough DS, Whitley JM, Taylor CL, et al: Rebound intracranial hypertension in dogs after resuscitation with hypertonic solutions from hemorrhagic shock accompanied by an intracranial mass lesion. J Neurosurg Anesth 1999; 11: 102

67. Vassar MJ, Fischer RP, O'Brien PE, et al: A multicenter trial for resuscitation of injured patients with 7.5% sodium chloride: The effect of added dextran 70. Arch Surg 1993; 128: 1003

68. Cooper DJ, Myles PS, McDermott FT, et al: Prehospital hypertonic saline resuscitation of patients with hypotension and severe traumatic brain injury: a randomized controlled trial. JAMA 2004; 291: 1350

69. Chesnut RM: Avoidance of hypotension: conditio sine qua non of successful severe head-injury management. J Trauma 1997; 42: S4

70. Zaloga GP, Hughes SS: Oliguria in patients with normal renal function. Anesthesiology 1990; 72: 598

71. Wong DH, O'Connor D, Tremper KK, et al: Changes in cardiac output after acute blood loss and position change in man. Crit Care Med 1989; 17: 979

72. Perel A: Assessing fluid responsiveness by the systolic pressure variation in mechanically ventilated patients. Anesthesiology 1998; 89: 1309

73. Stoneham MD: Less is more . . . using systolic pressure variation to assess hypovolaemia. Br J Anaesth 1999; 83: 550

74. Madan AK, UyBarreta VV, Aliabadi-Wahle S, et al: Esophageal Doppler ultrasound monitor versus pulmonary artery catheter in the hemodynamic management of critically ill surgical patients. J Trauma 1999; 46: 607

75. Heyland DK, Cook DJ, King D, et al: Maximizing oxygen delivery in critically ill patients: a methodologic appraisal of the evidence. Crit Care Med 1996; 24: 517

76. Rivers E, Nguyen B, Havstad S, et al: Early goal-directed therapy in the treatment of severe sepsis and septic shock. N Engl J Med 2001; 345: 1368

77. Kern JW, Shoemaker WC: Meta-analysis of hemodynamic optimization in high-risk patients. Crit Care Med 2002; 30: 1686

78. Lobo SM, Lobo FR, Polachini CA, et al: Prospective, randomized trial comparing fluids and dobutamine optimization of oxygen delivery in high-risk surgical patients. Crit Care 2006; 10: R72.

79. Balogh Z, McKinley BA, Cocanour CS, et al: Supranormal trauma resuscitation causes more cases of abdominal compartment syndrome. Arch Surg 2003; 138: 637

80. Wilson J, Woods I, Fawcett J, et al: Reducing the risk of major elective surgery: randomised controlled trial of preoperative optimisation of oxygen delivery. BMJ 1999; 318: 1099

81. DiCorte CJ, Latham P, Greilich PE, et al: Esophageal Doppler monitor determinations of cardiac output and preload during cardiac operations. Ann Thorac Surg 2000; 69: 1782

82. Horowitz P, Kumar A: It's the Colloid, Not the Esophageal Doppler Monitor. Anesthesiology 2003; 99: 238

83. Young WF: Primary aldosteronism: renaissance of a syndrome. Clin Endocrinol (Oxf) 2007; 66: 607

84. Karagiannis A, Tziomalos K, Papageorgiou A, et al: Spironolactone versus eplerenone for the treatment of idiopathic hyperaldosteronism. Expert Opin Pharmacother 2008; 9: 509

85. Kashyap AS: Hyperglycemia-induced hyponatremia: is it time to correct the correction factor? Arch Intern Med 1999; 159: 2745

86. Gravenstein D: Transurethral resection of the prostate (TURP) syndrome: a review of the pathophysiology and management. Anesth Analg 1997; 84: 438

87. Xu DL, Martin PY, Ohara M, et al: Upregulation of aquaporin-2 water channel expression in chronic heart failure rat. J Clin Invest 1997; 99: 1500

ANATOMY AND PHYSIOLOGY

88. Fujita N, Ishikawa SE, Sasaki S, et al: Role of water channel AQP-CD in water retention in SIADH and cirrhotic rats. Am J Physiol 1995; 269: F926

89. Ecelbarger CA, Nielsen S, Olson BR, et al: Role of renal aquaporins in escape from vasopressin-induced antidiuresis in rat. J Clin Invest 1997; 99: 1852

90. Moritz ML, Ayus JC: Hospital-acquired hyponatremia—why are hypotonic parenteral fluids still being used? Nat Clin Pract Nephrol 2007; 3: 374

91. Verbalis JG, Goldsmith SR, Greenberg A, et al: Hyponatremia treatment guidelines 2007: expert panel recommendations. Am J Med 2007; 120: S1

92. Katayama Y, Haraoka J, Hirabayashi H, et al: A randomized controlled trial of hydrocortisone against hyponatremia in patients with aneurysmal subarachnoid hemorrhage. Stroke 2007; 38: 2373

93. Fraser CL, Arieff AI: Fatal central diabetes mellitus and insipidus resulting from untreated hyponatremia: A new syndrome. Ann Intern Med 1990; 112: 113

94. Lien YH, Shapiro JI: Hyponatremia: clinical diagnosis and management. Am J Med 2007; 120: 653

95. Steele A, Gowrishankar M, Abrahamson S, et al: Postoperative hyponatremia despite near-isotonic saline infusion: a phenomenon of desalination. Ann Intern Med 1997; 126: 20

96. Arieff AI: Postoperative hyponatraemic encephalopathy following elective surgery in children. Paediatr Anesth 1998; 8: 1

97. Karmel KS, Bear RA: Treatment of hyponatremia: A quantitative analysis. Am J Kidney Dis 1994; 21: 439

98. Kumar S, Rubin S, Mather PJ, et al: Hyponatremia and vasopressin antagonism in congestive heart failure. Clin Cardiol 2007; 30: 546

99. Decaux G: V2-antagonists for the treatment of hyponatraemia. Nephrol Dial Transplant 2007; 22: 1853

100. Cawley MJ: Hyponatremia: current treatment strategies and the role of vasopressin antagonists. Ann Pharmacother 2007; 41: 840

101. Madias NE: Effects of tolvaptan, an oral vasopressin V2 receptor antagonist, in hyponatremia. Am J Kidney Dis 2007; 50: 184

102. Schrier RW, Gross P, Gheorghiade M, et al: Tolvaptan, a selective oral vasopressin V2-receptor antagonist, for hyponatremia. N Engl J Med 2006; 355: 2099

103. Sterns RH, Riggs JE, Schochet SS, Jr.: Osmotic demyelination syndrome following correction of hyponatremia. N Engl J Med 1986; 314: 1535

104. Adrogué HJ, Madias NE: Aiding fluid prescription for the dysnatremias. Intensive Care Med 1997; 23: 309

105. Biswas M, Davies JS: Hyponatraemia in clinical practice. Postgrad Med J 2007; 83: 373

106. Kumar S, Beri T: Sodium. Lancet 1998; 352: 220

107. Loh JA, Verbalis JG: Disorders of water and salt metabolism associated with pituitary disease. Endocrinol Metab Clin North Am 2008; 37: 213

108. Ayus JC, Armstrong DL, Arieff AI: Effects of hypernatraemia in the central nervous system and its therapy in rats and rabbits. J Physiol 1996; 492: 243

109. Adrogué HJ, Madias NE: Hypernatremia. N Engl J Med 2000; 342: 1493

110. Liamis G, Kalogirou M, Saugos V, et al: Therapeutic approach in patients with dysnatraemias. Nephrol Dial Transplant 2006; 21: 1564

111. Adler SM, Verbalis JG: Disorders of body water homeostasis in critical illness. Endocrinol Metab Clin North Am 2006; 35: 873

112. Sood MM, Sood AR, Richardson R: Emergency management and commonly encountered outpatient scenarios in patients with hyperkalemia. Mayo Clin Proc 2007; 82: 1553

113. Gilligan P, Pountney A, Wilson B, et al: SOCRATES Episode II (synopsis of Cochrane reviews applicable to emergency services Episode II): the return of Series III. Emerg Med J 2007; 24: 489

114. Wahr JA, Parks R, Boisvert D, et al: Preoperative serum potassium levels and perioperative outcomes in cardiac surgery patients. JAMA 1999; 281: 2203

115. Suga SI, Phillips MI, Ray PE, et al: Hypokalemia induces renal injury and alterations in vasoactive mediators that favor salt sensitivity. Am J Physiol Renal Physiol 2001; 281: F620

116. Lin SH, Halperin ML: Hypokalemia: a practical approach to diagnosis and its genetic basis. Curr Med Chem 2007; 14: 1551

117. Khosla S, Hogan D: Mineralocorticoid hypertension and hypokalemia. Semin Nephrol 2006; 26: 434

118. Furgeson SB, Chonchol M: Beta-blockade in chronic dialysis patients. Semin Dial 2008; 21: 43

119. Gronert GA: Succinylcholine hyperkalemia after burns. Anesthesiology 1999; 91: 320

120. Kim HJ, Han SW: Therapeutic approach to hyperkalemia. Nephron 2002; 92 Suppl 1: 33

121. Putcha N, Allon M: Management of hyperkalemia in dialysis patients. Semin Dial 2007; 20: 431

122. Shepard MM, Smith JW, III: Hypercalcemia. Am J Med Sci 2007; 334: 381

123. Slomp J, van der Voort PHJ, Gerritsen RT, et al: Albumin-adjusted calcium is not suitable for diagnosis of hyper-and hypocalcemia in the critically ill. Crit Care Med 2003; 31: 1389

124. Brown EM, Pollak M, Hebert SC: The extracellular calcium-sensing receptor: its role in health and disease. Ann Rev Med 1998; 49: 15

125. Brown EM, Pollak M, Seidman CE, et al: Calcium-ion-sensing cell-surface receptors. N Engl J Med 1995; 333: 234

126. Bushinsky DA, Monk RD: Calcium. Lancet 1998; 352: 306

127. Blair JM, Zheng Y, Dunstan CR: RANK ligand. Int J Biochem Cell Biol 2007; 39: 1077

128. Dickerson RN: Treatment of hypocalcemia in critical illness—part 1. Nutrition 2007; 23: 358

129. Zivin JR, Gooley T, Zager RA, et al: Hypocalcemia: a pervasive metabolic abnormality in the critically ill. Am J Kidney Dis 2001; 37: 689

130. Guise TA, Mundy GR: Evaluation of hypocalcemia in children and adults. J Clin Endocrinol Metab 1995; 80: 1473

131. Sutters M, Gaboury CL, Bennett WM: Severe hyperphosphatemia and hypocalcemia: a dilemma in patient management. J Am Soc Nephrol 1996; 7: 2055

132. Mathru M, Rooney MW, Goldberg SA, et al: Separation of myocardial versus peripheral effects of calcium administration in normocalcemic and hypocalcemic states using pressure-volume (conductance) relationships. Anesth Analg 1993; 77: 250

133. Bilezikian JP: Management of acute hypercalcemia. N Engl J Med 1992; 326: 1196

134. Zojer N, Ludwig H: Hematological emergencies. Ann Oncol 2007; 18(Suppl 1): i45

135. Ariyan CE, Sosa JA: Assessment and management of patients with abnormal calcium. Crit Care Med 2004; 32: S146

136. Kane S, Borisov NN, Brixner D: Pharmacoeconomic evaluation of gastrointestinal tract events during treatment with risedronate or alendronate: a retrospective cohort study. Am J Managed Care 2004; 10: S216

137. Miller RG, Bolognese M, Worley K, et al: Incidence of gastrointestinal events among bisphosphonate patients in an observational setting. Am J Managed Care 2004; 10: S207

138. Valverde P: Pharmacotherapies to manage bone loss-associated diseases: a quest for the perfect benefit-to-risk ratio. Curr Med Chem 2008; 15: 284

139. Olszynski WP, Davison KS: Alendronate for the treatment of osteoporosis in men. Expert Opin Pharmacother 2008; 9: 491

140. Ogata H, Koiwa F, Ito H, et al: Therapeutic strategies for secondary hyperparathyroidism in dialysis patients. Ther Apher Dial 2006; 10: 355

141. Shahapuni I, Monge M, Oprisiu R, et al: Drug Insight: renal indications of calcimimetics. Nat Clin Pract Nephrol 2006; 2: 316

142. Wuthrich RP, Martin D, Bilezikian JP: The role of calcimimetics in the treatment of hyperparathyroidism. Eur J Clin Invest 2007; 37: 915

143. Felsenfeld AJ, Levine BS: Milk alkali syndrome and the dynamics of calcium homeostasis. Clin J Am Soc Nephrol 2006; 1: 641

144. Peppers MP, Geheb M, Desai T: Hypophosphatemia and hyperphosphatemia. Crit Care Clin 1991; 7: 201.

145. Giovannini I, Chiarla C, Nuzzo G: Pathophysiologic and clinical correlates of hypophosphatemia and the relationship with sepsis and outcome in postoperative patients after hepatectomy. Shock 2002; 18: 111

146. Brooks MJ, Melnik G: The refeeding syndrome: an approach to understanding its complications and preventing its occurrence. Pharmacology 1995; 15: 713

147. Paleologos M, Stone E, Braude S: Persistent, progressive hypophosphataemia after voluntary hyperventilation. Clin Sci (Lond) 2000; 98: 619

148. Rosen GH, Boullata JI, O'Rangers EA, et al: Intravenous phosphate repletion regimen for critically ill patients with moderate hypophosphatemia. Crit Care Med 1995; 23: 1204

149. Burke SK: Phosphate is a uremic toxin. J Ren Nutr 2008; 18: 27

150. Sprague SM: A comparative review of the efficacy and safety of established phosphate binders: calcium, sevelamer, and lanthanum carbonate. Curr Med Res Opin 2007; 23: 3167

151. Topf JM, Murray PT: Hypomagnesemia and hypermagnesemia. Rev Endocr Metab Disord 2003; 4: 195

152. Gums JG: Magnesium in cardiovascular and other disorders. Am J Health Syst Pharm 2004; 61: 1569

153. Dube L, Granry JC: The therapeutic use of magnesium in anesthesiology, intensive care and emergency medicine: a review. Can J Anaesth 2003; 50: 732

154. Choi JH, Lee J, Park CM: Magnesium therapy improves thromboelastographic findings before liver transplantation: a preliminary study. Can J Anaesth 2005; 52: 156

155. Lysakowski C, Dumont L, Czarnetzki C, Tramer MR: Magnesium as an adjuvant to postoperative analgesia: a systematic review of randomized trials. Anesth Analg 2007; 104: 1532

156. Van De Water JM, van den Bergh WM, Hoff RG, et al: Hypocalcaemia may reduce the beneficial effect of magnesium treatment in aneurysmal subarachnoid haemorrhage. Magnes Res 2007; 20: 130

157. van den Bergh WM, Algra A, Rinkel GJ: Electrocardiographic abnormalities and serum magnesium in patients with subarachnoid hemorrhage. Stroke 2004; 35: 644

158. Sueta CA, Clarke SW, Dunlap SH, et al: Effect of acute magnesium administration on the frequency of ventricular arrhythmias in patients with heart failure. Circulation 1994; 89: 660

159. Redwood SR, Taggart PI, Sutton PM, et al: Effect of magnesium on the monophasic action potential during early ischemia in the in vivo human heart. J Am Coll Cardiol 1996; 28: 1765

160. Teo KK, Yusuf S, Collins R, et al: Effects of intravenous magnesium in suspected acute myocardial infarction: overview of randomised trials. BMJ 1991; 303: 1499

161. Tzivoni D, Banai S, Schuger C, et al: Treatment of torsade de pointes with magnesium sulfate. Circulation 1988; 77: 392.

162. Wilkes NJ, Mallett SV, Peachey T, et al: Correction of ionized plasma magnesium during cardiopulmonary bypass reduces the risk of postoperative cardiac arrhythmia. Anesth Analg 2002; 95: 828

163. Abbott LG, Rude RK: Clinical manifestations of magnesium deficiency. Miner Electrolyte Metab 1993; 19: 314

164. Elisaf M, Merkouropoulos M, Tsianos EV, et al: Pathogenetic mechanisms of hypomagnesemia in alcoholic patients. J Trace Elem Med Biol 1995; 9: 210

165. Soliman HM, Mercan D, Lobo SS, et al: Development of ionized hypomagnesemia is associated with higher mortality rates. Crit Care Med 2003; 31: 1082

166. Hebert P, Mehta N, Wang J, et al: Functional magnesium deficiency in critically ill patients identified using a magnesium-loading test. Crit Care Med 1997; 25: 749

ANATOMY AND PHYSIOLOGY

CHAPTER 15 ■ AUTONOMIC NERVOUS SYSTEM

JOEL O. JOHNSON, LORETA GRECU, AND NOEL W. LAWSON

KEY POINTS

1. The autonomic nervous system (ANS) includes that part of the central and peripheral nervous system concerned with involuntary regulation of cardiac muscle, smooth muscle, glandular, and visceral functions.

2. The sympathetic and parasympathetic nervous systems (SNS, PNS) affect cardiac pump function in three ways: (1) by changing the rate (chronotropism), (2) by changing the strength of contraction (inotropism), and (3) by modulating coronary blood flow.

3. SNS nerves are by far the most important regulators of the peripheral circulation.

4. The ANS can be pharmacologically subdivided by the neurotransmitter secreted at the effector cell: acetylcholine (ACh) released by the PNS and the catecholamines epinephrine (EPI) and norepinephrine (NE) are considered the mediators of peripheral SNS activity.

5. An agonist is a substance that interacts with a receptor to evoke a biologic response. An antagonist is a substance that interferes with the evocation of a response at a receptor site by an agonist.

6. The adrenergic receptors are termed *adrenergic* or *noradrenergic*, depending on their responsiveness to epinephrine or norepinephrine.

7. The numbers and sensitivity of adrenergic receptors can be influenced by normal, genetic, and developmental factors.

8. The autonomic nervous system reflex has (1) sensors, (2) afferent pathways, (3) central nervous system integration, and (4) efferent pathways to the receptors and efferent organs.

9. The clinical application of ANS pharmacology is based on knowledge of ANS anatomy, physiology, and molecular pharmacology.

10. Clinically, anticholinesterase drugs may be divided into two types: the reversible and nonreversible cholinesterase inhibitors.

11. The net physiologic effect of a sympathomimetic is usually defined by the relative actions on the α, β, and dopamine receptors.

12. Dexmedetomidine is a more selective α_2 agonist than clonidine.

13. Drugs that bind selectively to α-adrenergic receptors block the action of endogenous catecholamines or moderate the effects of exogenous adrenergics.

14. Calcium channel blockers are not true pharmacologic antagonists of calcium. They interact with the cell membrane to control the intracellular concentration of calcium.

ANESTHESIA AND THE AUTONOMIC NERVOUS SYSTEM

Anesthesiology is the practice of autonomic medicine. Drugs that produce anesthesia also produce potent autonomic side effects.

The greater part of our training and practice is spent acquiring skills in averting or using the autonomic nervous system (ANS) side effects of anesthetic drugs under a variety of pathophysiologic conditions. The success of any anesthetic depends on how well homeostasis is maintained. The numbers that we faithfully record during the course of anesthesia reflect ANS function.

1 The ANS includes that part of the central and peripheral nervous system concerned with involuntary regulation of cardiac muscle, smooth muscle, glandular, and visceral functions. ANS activity refers to visceral reflexes that function below the conscious level. The ANS is also responsive to changes in somatic motor and sensory activities of the body. The physiologic evidence of visceral reflexes as a result of somatic events is abundantly clear. The ANS is therefore not as distinct an entity as the term suggests. Neither somatic nor ANS activity occurs in isolation.[1] The ANS organizes visceral support for somatic behavior and adjusts body states in anticipation of emotional behavior or responses to the stress of disease (i.e., fight or flight).

Afferent fibers from visceral structures are the first link in the reflex arcs of the ANS whether relaying visceral pain or changes in vessel stretch. Most ANS efferent fibers are accompanied by sensory fibers that are now commonly recognized as components of the ANS. However, the afferent components of the ANS cannot be as distinctively divided, as can the efferent nerves. ANS visceral sensory nerves are anatomically indistinguishable from somatic sensory nerves. The clinical importance of visceral afferent fibers is more closely associated with chronic pain management.

FUNCTIONAL ANATOMY

The ANS falls into two divisions by anatomy, physiology, and pharmacology. Langley divided this nervous system into two parts in 1921. He retained the term *sympathetic* nervous system (SNS) introduced by Willis in 1665 for the first part and introduced the term *parasympathetic* (parasympathetic nervous system, PNS) for the second. The term *autonomic nervous system* was adopted as a comprehensive name for both. Table 15-1 lists the complementary effects of SNS (adrenergic, sympathetic) and PNS (cholinergic, parasympathetic) activity of organ systems.

Central Autonomic Organization

Pure central ANS or somatic centers are not known. Integration of ANS activity occurs at all levels of the cerebrospinal axis. Efferent ANS activity can be initiated locally and by centers located in the spinal cord, brainstem, and hypothalamus. The cerebral cortex is the highest level of ANS integration. Fainting at the sight of blood is an example of this higher level of somatic and ANS integration. ANS function has also been

ANATOMY AND PHYSIOLOGY

TABLE 15-1

HOMEOSTATIC BALANCE BETWEEN ADRENERGIC AND CHOLINERGIC EFFECTS

	■ RESPONSE	
■ ORGAN SYSTEM	■ ADRENERGIC	■ CHOLINERGIC
HEART		
Sinoatrial node	Tachycardia	Bradycardia
Atrioventricular node	Increased conduction	Decreased conduction
His-Purkinje	Increased automaticity and conduction velocity	Minimal
Myocardium	Increased contractility, conduction velocity, automaticity	Minimal decrease in contractility
Coronary vessels	Constriction (α_1) and dilation (β_1)	Dilation and constriction?[a]
BLOOD VESSELS		
Skin and mucosa	Constriction	Dilation
Skeletal muscle	Constriction (α_1) > dilation (β_2)	Dilation
Pulmonary	Constriction	?Dilation
BRONCHIAL SMOOTH MUSCLE	Relaxation	Contraction
GASTROINTESTINAL TRACT		
Gallbladder and ducts	Relaxation	Contraction
Gut motility	Decreased	Increased
Secretions	Decreased	Increased
Sphincters	Constriction	Relaxation
BLADDER		
Detrusor	Relaxes	Contracts
Trigone	Contracts	Relaxes
GLANDS		
Nasal	Vasoconstriction and reduced secretion	Stimulation of secretions
Lacrimal		
Parotid		
Submandibular		
Gastric		
Pancreatic		
SWEAT GLANDS	Diaphoresis (cholinergic)	None
APOCRINE GLANDS	Thick, odiferous secretion	None
EYE		
Pupil	Mydriasis	Miosis
Ciliary muscle	Relaxation for far vision	Contraction for near vision

[a]See "Interaction of Autonomic Nervous System Receptors."

FIGURE 15.1.   Schematic distribution of the craniosacral (parasympathetic) and thoracolumbar (sympathetic) nervous systems. Parasympathetic preganglionic fibers pass directly to the organ that is innervated. Their postganglionic cell bodies are situated near or within the innervated viscera. This limited distribution of parasympathetic postganglionic fibers is consistent with the discrete and limited effect of parasympathetic function. The postganglionic sympathetic neurons originate in either the paired sympathetic ganglia or one of the unpaired collateral plexuses. One preganglionic fiber influences many postganglionic neurons. Activation of the sympathetic nervous system produces a more diffuse physiologic response rather than discrete effects.

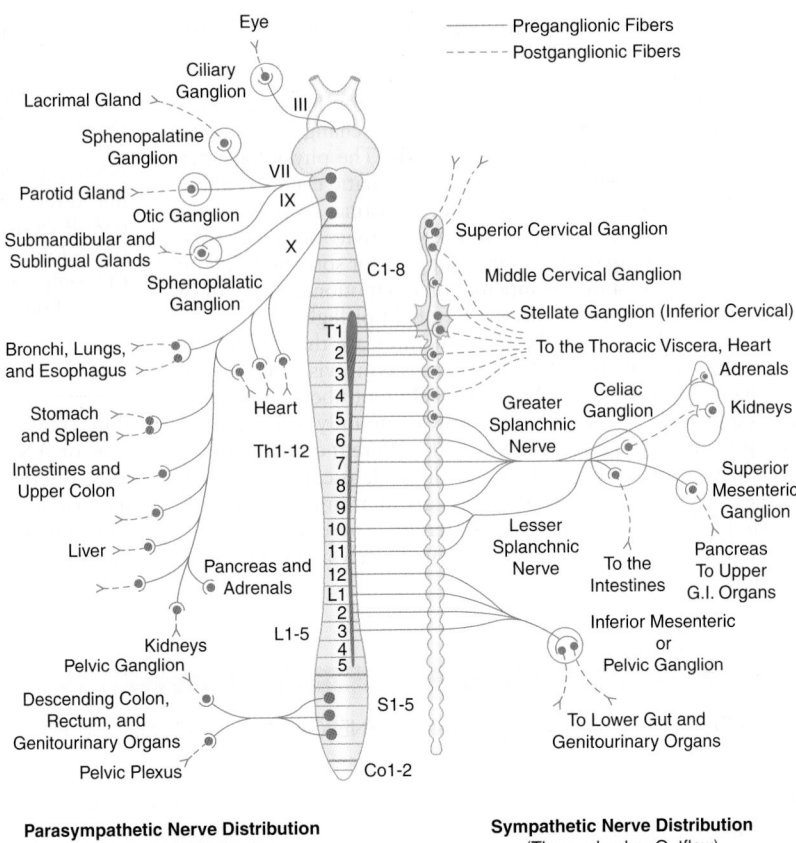

Parasympathetic Nerve Distribution
(Craniosacral Outflow)

Sympathetic Nerve Distribution
(Thoracolumbar Outflow)

successfully modulated through conscious, intentional efforts demonstrating that somatic responses are always accompanied by visceral responses and vice versa.

The principal site of ANS organization is the *hypothalamus*. SNS functions are controlled by nuclei in the posterolateral hypothalamus. Stimulation of these nuclei results in a massive discharge of the sympathoadrenal system. PNS functions are governed by nuclei in the midline and some anterior nuclei of the hypothalamus. The anterior hypothalamus is involved with regulation of temperature. The supraoptic hypothalamic nuclei regulate water metabolism and are anatomically and functionally associated with the posterior lobe of the pituitary (see "Interaction of Autonomic Nervous System Receptors"). This hypothalamic-neurohypophyseal connection represents a central ANS mechanism that affects the kidney by means of antidiuretic hormone. Long-term blood pressure control, reactions to physical and emotional stress, sleep, and sexual reflexes are regulated through the hypothalamus.

The *medulla oblongata* and *pons* are the vital centers of acute ANS organization. Together they integrate momentary hemodynamic adjustments and maintain the sequence and automaticity of ventilation. Integration of afferent and efferent ANS impulses at this central nervous system (CNS) level is responsible for the tonic activity exhibited by the ANS. Tonicity holds visceral organs in a state of intermediate activity that can either be diminished or augmented by altering the rate of nerve firing. The nucleus tractus solitarius, located within the medulla, is the primary area for relay of afferent chemoreceptor and baroreceptor information from the glossopharyngeal and vagus nerves. Increased afferent impulses from these two nerves inhibits peripheral SNS vascular tone, producing vasodilation and increasing vagal tone, producing bradycardia. Studies of patients with high spinal cord lesions show that a number of reflex changes are mediated at the spinal or seg-

mental level. ANS hyperreflexia is an example of spinal cord mediation of ANS reflexes without integration of function from higher inhibitory centers.[1]

Peripheral Autonomic Nervous System Organization

The peripheral ANS is the efferent (motor) component of the ANS and consists of the same two complementary parts, the SNS and the PNS. Most organs receive fibers from both divisions (Fig. 15-1). In general, activities of the two systems produce opposite but complementary effects (Table 15-1). A few tissues, such as sweat glands and spleen, are innervated only by SNS fibers. Although the anatomy of the somatic and ANS sensory pathways is identical, the motor pathways are characteristically different. The efferent somatic motor system, like somatic afferents, is composed of a single (unipolar) neuron with its cell body in the ventral gray matter of the spinal cord. Its myelinated axon extends directly to the voluntary striated muscle unit. In contrast, the efferent (motor) ANS is a two-neuron (bipolar) chain from the CNS to the effector organ. The first neuron of both the SNS and PNS originates within the CNS but does not make direct contact with the effector organ. Instead, it relays the impulse to a second station known as an *ANS ganglion*, which contains the cell body of the second ANS (postganglionic) neuron. Its axon contacts the effector organ. Thus, the motor pathways of both divisions of the ANS are schematically a serial, two-neuron chain consisting of a preganglionic neuron and a postganglionic effector neuron (Fig. 15-2).

Preganglionic fibers of both subdivisions are myelinated with diameters of <3 mm.[1] Impulses are conducted at a speed of 3 to 15 m/s. The postganglionic fibers are unmyelinated and conduct impulses at slower speeds of <2 m/s. They are similar

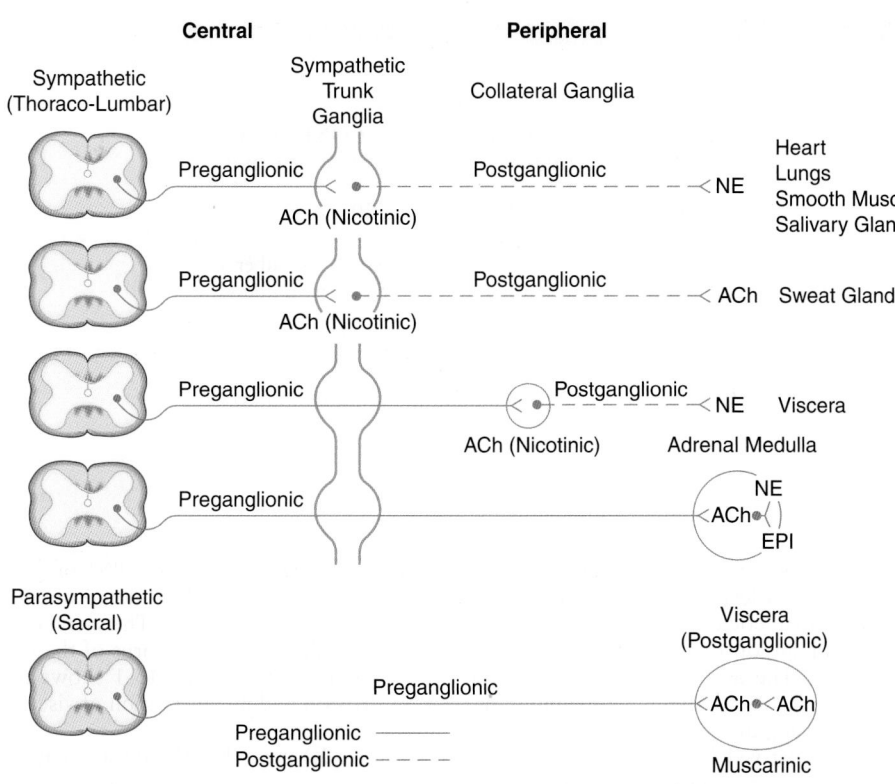

FIGURE 15.2. Schematic diagram of the efferent autonomic nervous system. Afferent impulses are integrated centrally and sent reflexly to the adrenergic and cholinergic receptors. Sympathetic fibers ending in the adrenal medulla are preganglionic, and acetylcholine (ACh) is the neurotransmitter. Stimulation of the chromaffin cells, acting as postganglionic neurons, releases epinephrine (EPI) and norepinephrine (NE).

to unmyelinated visceral and somatic afferent C fibers (Table 15-2). Compared with the myelinated somatic nerves, the ANS conducts impulses at speeds that preclude its participation in the immediate phase of a somatic response.

Sympathetic Nervous System

The efferent SNS is referred to as the *thoracolumbar nervous system.* Figure 15–1 demonstrates the distribution of the SNS and its innervation of visceral organs. The preganglionic fibers

of the SNS (thoracolumbar division) originate in the intermediolateral gray column of the 12 thoracic (T1 through T12) and the first three lumbar segments (L1 through L3) of the spinal cord. The myelinated axons of these nerve cells leave the spinal cord with the motor fibers to form the white (myelinated) communicating rami (Fig. 15-3). The rami enter one of the paired 22 sympathetic ganglia at their respective segmental levels. On entering the paravertebral ganglia of the lateral sympathetic chain, the preganglionic fiber may follow one of three courses: (1) synapse with postganglionic fibers in ganglia

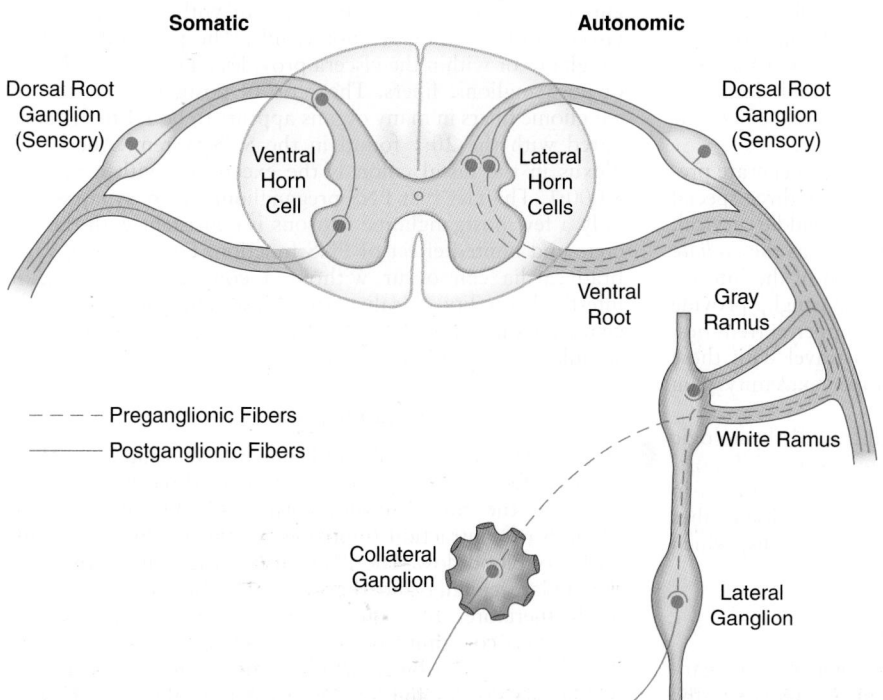

FIGURE 15.3. The spinal reflex arc of the somatic nerves is shown on the left. The different arrangements of neurons in the sympathetic system are shown on the right. Preganglionic fibers coming out through white rami may make synaptic connections following one of three courses: (1) synapse in ganglia at the level of exit, (2) course up or down the sympathetic chain to synapse at another level, or (3) exit the chain without synapsing to an outlying collateral ganglion.

ANATOMY AND PHYSIOLOGY

TABLE 15-2

CLASSIFICATION OF NERVE FIBERS

■ DESCRIPTION OF NERVE FIBERS	■ GROUP	■ DIAMETER (μm)	■ CONDUCTION VELOCITY (m/s)
Myelinated somatic	A { Alpha α Beta β Gamma γ Delta δ Epsilon ε	20 3–4 2	120 5–40 (pain fibers) 5–40 (pain fibers) 5
Myelinated visceral (preganglionic autonomic)	B	<3	3–15
Unmyelinated somatic	C	<2	0.5–2 (pain fibers)

at the level of exit, (2) course upward or downward in the trunk of the SNS chain to synapse in ganglia at other levels, or (3) track for variable distances through the sympathetic chain and exit without synapsing to terminate in an outlying, unpaired, SNS collateral ganglion (Fig. 15-3). The adrenal gland is an exception to the rule. Preganglionic fibers pass directly into the adrenal medulla without synapsing in a ganglion (Fig. 15-2). The cells of the medulla are derived from neuronal tissue and are analogous to postganglionic neurons.

The sympathetic postganglionic neuronal cell bodies are located in ganglia of the paired lateral SNS chain or unpaired collateral ganglia in more peripheral plexuses. Collateral ganglia, such as the celiac and inferior mesenteric ganglia (plexus), are formed by the convergence of preganglionic fibers with many postganglionic neuronal bodies. SNS ganglia are almost always located closer to the spinal cord than to the organs they innervate. The sympathetic postganglionic neuron can therefore originate in either the paired lateral paravertebral SNS ganglia or one of the unpaired collateral plexus. The unmyelinated postganglionic fibers then proceed from the ganglia to terminate within the organs they innervate. Many of the postganglionic fibers pass from the lateral SNS chain back into the spinal nerves, forming the gray (unmyelinated) communicating rami at all levels of the spinal cord (Fig. 15-2). They are distributed distally to sweat glands, pilomotor muscle, and blood vessels of the skin and muscle. These nerves are unmyelinated C type fibers (Table 15-2) and are carried within the somatic nerves. Approximately 8% of the fibers in the average somatic nerve are sympathetic.

The first four or five thoracic spinal segments generate preganglionic fibers that ascend in the neck to form three special paired ganglia. These are the superior cervical, middle cervical, and cervicothoracic ganglia. The last is known as the *stellate ganglion* and is actually formed by the fusion of the inferior cervical and first thoracic SNS ganglia. These ganglia provide sympathetic innervation of the head, neck, upper extremities, heart, and lungs. Afferent pain fibers also travel with these nerves, accounting for chest, neck, or upper extremity pain with myocardial ischemia.

Activation of the SNS produces a diffused physiologic response (mass reflex) rather than discrete effects. SNS postganglionic neurons outnumber the preganglionic neurons in an average ratio of 20:1 to 30:1.[2] One preganglionic fiber influences a larger number of postganglionic neurons, which are dispersed to many organs.

Parasympathetic Nervous System

The PNS, like the SNS, has both preganglionic and postganglionic neurons. The preganglionic cell bodies originate in the brainstem and sacral segments of the spinal cord. PNS preganglionic fibers are found in cranial nerves III (oculomotor), VII (facial), IX (glossopharyngeal), and X (vagus). The sacral outflow originates in the intermediolateral gray horns of the second, third, and fourth sacral nerves. Figure 15-1 shows the distribution of the PNS division and its innervation of visceral organs.

The vagus (cranial nerve X) nerve has the most extensive distribution of all the PNS, accounting for more than 75% of PNS activity. The paired vagus nerves supply PNS innervation to the heart, lungs, esophagus, stomach, small intestine, proximal half of the colon, liver, gallbladder, pancreas, and upper portions of the ureters. The sacral fibers form the pelvic visceral nerves, or nervi erigentes. These nerves supply the remainder of the viscera that are not innervated by the vagus. They supply the descending colon, rectum, uterus, bladder, and lower portions of the ureters, and are primarily concerned with emptying. Various sexual reactions are also governed by the sacral PNS. The PNS is responsible for penile erection, but SNS stimulation governs ejaculation.

In contrast to the SNS division, PNS preganglionic fibers pass directly to the organ that is innervated. The postganglionic cell bodies are situated near or within the innervated viscera and generally are not visible. The proximity of PNS ganglia to or within the viscera provides a limited distribution of postganglionic fibers. The ratio of postganglionic to preganglionic fibers in many organs appears to be 1:1 to 3:1 compared with the 20:1 found in the SNS system. Auerbach's plexus in the distal colon is the exception, with a ratio of 8,000:1. The fact that PNS preganglionic fibers synapse with only a few postganglionic neurons is consistent with the discrete and limited effect of PNS function. For example, vagal bradycardia can occur without a concomitant change in intestinal motility or salivation. Mass reflex action is not a characteristic of the PNS. The effects of organ response to PNS stimulation are outlined in Table 15-1.

Autonomic Innervation

Heart. The heart is well supplied by the SNS and PNS. These nerves affect cardiac pump function in three ways: (1) by changing the rate (chronotropism), (2) by changing the strength of contraction (inotropism), and (3) by modulating coronary blood flow. The PNS cardiac vagal fibers approach the stellate ganglia and then join the efferent cardiac SNS fibers; therefore, the vagus nerve to the heart and lungs is a mixed nerve containing both PNS and SNS efferent fibers. The PNS fibers are distributed mainly to the sinoatrial and atrioventricular (AV) nodes and to a lesser extent to the atria. There is little or no distribution to the ventricles. Therefore, the main effect of vagal cardiac stimulation to the heart is chronotropic. Vagal stimulation decreases the rate of sinoatrial node discharge and decreases excitability of the AV junctional fibers, slowing impulse conduction to the ventricles. A strong vagal discharge can completely arrest sinoatrial node firing and block impulse conduction to the ventricles.[3]

The physiologic importance of the PNS on myocardial contractility is not as well understood as that of the SNS. Cholinergic blockade can double the heart rate (HR) without altering contractility of the left ventricle. Vagal stimulation of the heart can reduce left ventricular maximum rate of tension development (dP/dT) and decrease contractile force by as much as 10 to 20%. However, PNS stimulation is relatively unimportant in this regard compared with its predominant effect on HR. The SNS has the same supraventricular distribution as the PNS, but with stronger representation to the ventricles. SNS efferents to the myocardium funnel through the paired stellate ganglia. The right stellate ganglion distributes primarily to the anterior epicardial surface and the interventricular septum. Right stellate stimulation decreases systolic duration and increases HR. The left stellate ganglion supplies the posterior and lateral surfaces of both ventricles. Left stellate stimulation increases mean arterial pressure and left ventricular contractility without causing a substantial change in HR. Normal SNS tone maintains contractility approximately 20% above that in the absence of any SNS stimulation.[4] Therefore, the dominant effect of the ANS on myocardial contractility is mediated primarily through the SNS. Intrinsic mechanisms of the myocardium, however, can maintain circulation quite well without the ANS, as evidenced by the success of cardiac transplants (see Chapter 54). Early investigations, performed in anesthetized, open-chest animals, demonstrated that cardiac ANS nerves exert only slight effects on the coronary vascular bed; however, more recent studies on chronically instrumented, intact, conscious animals show considerable evidence for a strong SNS regulation of the small coronary resistance and larger conductance vessels.[5,6]

Different segments of the coronary arterial tree react differently to various stimuli and drugs. Normally, the large conductance vessels contribute little to overall coronary vascular resistance (see Chapter 10). Fluctuations in resistance reflect changes in lumen size of the small, precapillary vessels. Blood flow through the resistance vessels is regulated primarily by the local metabolic requirements of the myocardium. The larger conductance vessels, however, can constrict markedly because of neurogenic stimulation. Neurogenic influence also assumes a greater role in the resistance vessels when they become hypoxic and lose autoregulation.

❸ Peripheral Circulation. The SNS nerves are by far the most important regulators of the peripheral circulation. The PNS nerves play only a minor role in this regard. The PNS dilates vessels, but only in limited areas such as the genitals. SNS stimulation produces both vasodilation and vasoconstriction, with vasoconstrictor effects predominating. The SNS effect on the vascular bed is determined by the type of receptors on which the SNS fiber terminates (see "Adrenergic Receptors"). SNS constrictor receptors are distributed to all segments of the circulation. Blood vessels in the skin, kidneys, spleen, and mesentery have an extensive SNS distribution, whereas those in the heart, brain, and muscle have less SNS innervation.

Basal vasomotor tone is maintained by impulses from the lateral portion of the vasomotor center in the medulla oblongata that continually transmits impulses through the SNS, maintaining partial arteriolar and venular constriction. Circulating epinephrine (EPI) from the adrenal medulla has additive effects. This basal ANS tone maintains arteriolar constriction

at an intermediate diameter. The arteriole, therefore, has the potential for either further constriction or dilation. If the basal tone were not present, the SNS could only effect vasoconstriction and not vasodilation.[7] The SNS tone in the venules produces little resistance to flow compared with the arterioles and the arteries. The importance of SNS stimulation of veins is to reduce or increase their capacity. By functioning as a reservoir for approximately 80% of the total blood volume, small changes in venous capacitance produce large changes in venous return and, thus, cardiac preload.

Lungs. The lungs are innervated by both the SNS and PNS. Postganglionic SNS fibers from the upper thoracic ganglia (stellate) pass to the lungs to innervate the smooth muscles of the bronchi and pulmonary blood vessels. PNS innervation of these structures is via the vagus nerve. SNS stimulation produces bronchodilation and pulmonary vasoconstriction.[8] Little else has been proven conclusively about the vasomotor control of the pulmonary vessels other than that they adjust to accommodate the output of the right ventricle. The effect of stimulation of the pulmonary SNS nerves on pulmonary vascular resistance is not ideal but may be important in maintaining hemodynamic stability during stress and exercise by balancing right and left ventricular output. Stimulation of the vagus nerve produces almost no vasodilation of the pulmonary circulation. Hypoxic pulmonary vasoconstriction is a local phenomenon capable of providing a faster adjustment to the organism needs.

Both the SNS and the vagus nerve provide active bronchomotor control. SNS stimulation causes bronchodilation, whereas vagal stimulation produces constriction. PNS stimulation may also increase secretions of the bronchial glands. Vagal receptor endings in the alveolar ducts also play an important role in the reflex regulation of the ventilation cycle. The lung has important nonventilatory activity as well. It serves as a metabolic organ that removes local mediators such as norepinephrine (NE) from the circulation and converts others, such as angiotensin 1, to active compounds.[9]

Autonomic Nervous System Transmission

Transmission of excitation across the terminal junctional sites (synaptic clefts) of the peripheral ANS occurs through the mediation of liberated chemicals (Fig. 15-4). Transmitters interact with a receptor on the end organ to evoke a biologic response. The ANS can be pharmacologically subdivided by the neurotransmitter secreted at the effector cell.

❹ Pharmacologic parlance designates the SNS and PNS as adrenergic and cholinergic, respectively. The terminals of the PNS postganglionic fibers release acetylcholine (ACh). With the exception of sweat glands, NE is considered the principal neurotransmitter released at the terminals of the sympathetic postganglionic fibers (see Fig. 15-2). Cotransmission of adenosine triphosphate (ATP), neuropeptide Y, and NE has been demonstrated at vascular sympathetic nerve terminals in a number of different tissues including muscle, intestine, kidney, and skin (see "Sympathetic Nervous System Neurotransmission"). The preganglionic neurons of both systems secrete ACh.

The terminations of the postganglionic fibers of both ANS subdivisions are anatomically and physiologically similar. The terminations are characterized by multiple branchings called *terminal effector plexuses*, or reticulae. These filaments surround the elements of the effector unit "like a mesh stocking."[7] Thus, one SNS postganglionic neuron, for example, can innervate ~25,000 effector cells (e.g., vascular smooth

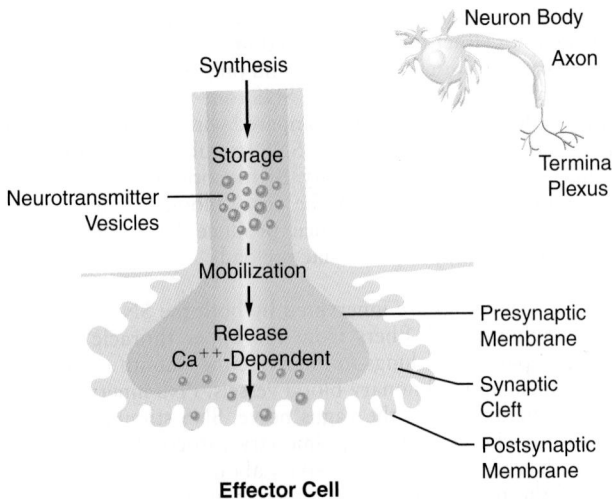

FIGURE 15.4. The anatomy and physiology of the terminal postganglionic fibers of sympathetic and parasympathetic fibers are similar.

muscle). The terminal filaments end in presynaptic enlargements called *varicosities*. Each varicosity contains vesicles, ~500 μm in diameter, in which the neurotransmitters are stored (Fig. 15-4). The rate of synthesis depends on the level of ANS activity and is regulated by local feedback. The distance between the varicosity and the effector cell (synaptic or junctional cleft) varies from 100 μm in ganglia and arterioles to as much as 20,000 μm in large arteries. The time for diffusion is directly proportional to the width of the synaptic gap. Depolarization on the nerve releases the vesicular contents into the synaptic cleft by exocytosis.

Parasympathetic Nervous System Transmission

Synthesis. ACh is considered the primary neurotransmitter of the PNS. ACh is formed in the presynaptic terminal by acetylation of choline with acetyl coenzyme A. This step is catalyzed by choline acetyl transferase (Fig. 15-5). ACh is then stored in a concentrated form in presynaptic vesicles. A continual release of small amounts of ACh, called *quanta*, occurs during the resting state. Each quantum results in small changes in the electrical potential of the synaptic end plate without producing depolarization. These are known as miniature endplate potentials. Arrival of an action potential causes a synchronous release of hundreds of quanta, resulting in depolarization of the end plate. Release of ACh from the vesicles

depends on influx of calcium (Ca^{2+}) from the interstitial space. ACh is not reused like NE; therefore, it must be synthesized constantly.

Metabolism. The ability of a receptor to modulate function of an effector organ depends on rapid recovery to its baseline state after stimulation. For this to occur, the neurotransmitter must be quickly removed from the vicinity of the receptor. ACh removal occurs by rapid hydrolysis by acetylcholinesterase (Fig. 15-5). This enzyme is found in neurons, at the neuromuscular junction, and in various other tissues of the body. A similar enzyme, pseudocholinesterase or plasma cholinesterase, is also found throughout the body but only to a limited extent in nervous tissue. It does not appear to be physiologically important in termination of the action of ACh. Both acetylcholinesterase and pseudocholinesterase hydrolyze ACh as well as other esters (such as the ester-type local anesthetics), and they may be distinguished by specific biochemical tests.[3]

Sympathetic Nervous System Transmission. Traditionally, the catecholamines EPI and NE are considered the mediators of peripheral SNS activity. NE is released from localized presynaptic vesicles of nearly all postganglionic sympathetic nerves. Vascular SNS nerve terminals, though, also release ATP. Thus, ATP and NE are coneurotransmitters. They are released directly into the site where they act. Their postjunctional effects appear to be synergistic in tissues.

The SNS fibers ending in the adrenal medulla are preganglionic, and ACh is the neurotransmitter (see Fig. 15-2). It interacts with the chromaffin cells in the adrenal medulla, causing release of EPI and NE. The chromaffin cells take the place of the postganglionic neurons. Stimulation of the sympathetic nerves innervating the adrenal medulla, however, causes the release of large quantities of a mixture of EPI and NE into the circulation. The greater portion of this hormonal surge is normally EPI. Nevertheless, EPI and NE, when released into the circulation, are classified as hormones in that they are synthesized, stored, and released from the adrenal medulla to act at distant sites.

Hormonal EPI and NE have almost the same effects on effector cells as those caused by local direct sympathetic stimulation; however, the hormonal effects, although brief, last about 10 times as long as those caused by direct stimulation. EPI has a greater metabolic effect than NE. It can increase the metabolic rate of the body as much as 100%. It also increases glycogenolysis in the liver and muscle with glucose release into the blood. These functions are all necessary to prepare the body for fight or flight.

FIGURE 15.5. Synthesis and metabolism of acetylcholine.

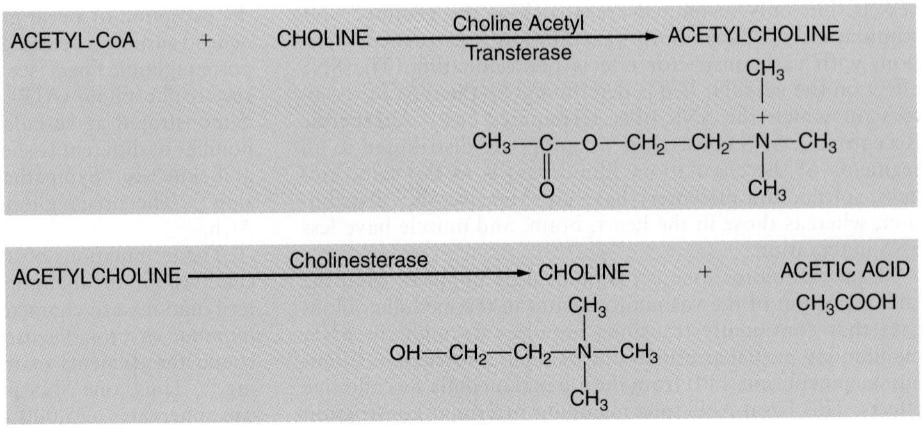

$$ACETYL\text{-}CoA \quad + \quad CHOLINE \xrightarrow{\text{Choline Acetyl Transferase}} ACETYLCHOLINE$$

$$CH_3\text{—}\underset{\underset{O}{\|}}{C}\text{—}O\text{—}CH_2\text{—}CH_2\text{—}\underset{\underset{CH_3}{|}}{\overset{\overset{CH_3}{|}}{\overset{+}{N}}}\text{—}CH_3$$

$$ACETYLCHOLINE \xrightarrow{\text{Cholinesterase}} CHOLINE \quad + \quad ACETIC\ ACID$$
$$CH_3COOH$$

$$OH\text{—}CH_2\text{—}CH_2\text{—}\underset{\underset{CH_3}{|}}{\overset{\overset{CH_3}{|}}{N}}\text{—}CH_3$$

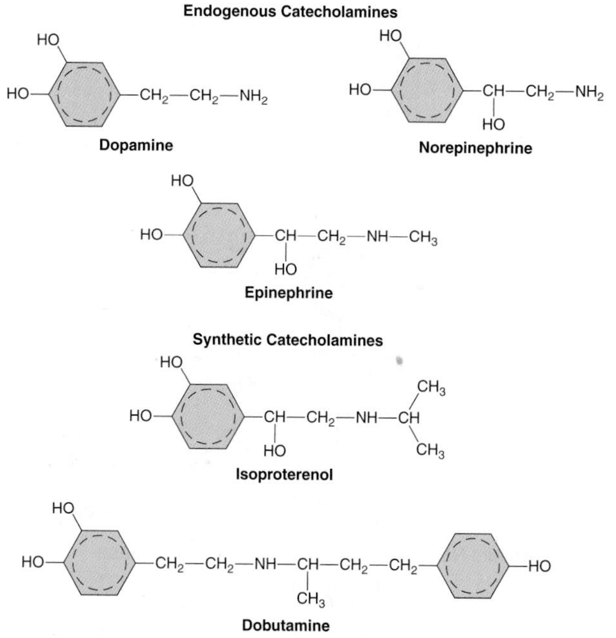

FIGURE 15.6. The chemical configurations of three endogenous catecholamines are compared with those of two synthetic catecholamines. Sympathomimetic drugs differ in their hemodynamic effects largely because of differences in substitution of the amine group on the catechol nucleus.

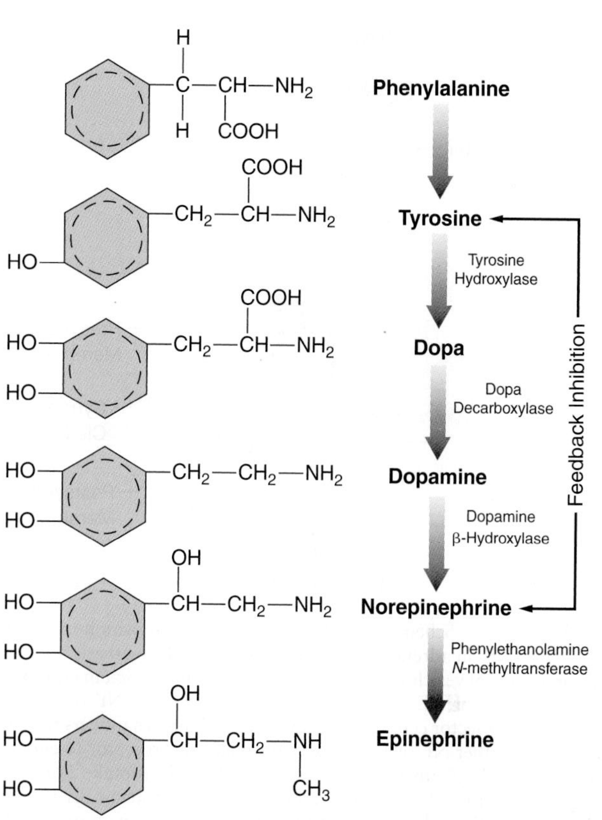

FIGURE 15.7. Schematic of the synthesis of catecholamines. The conversion of tyrosine to DOPA by tyrosine hydroxylase is inhibited by increased norepinephrine synthesis. Epinephrine is shown in these steps but is primarily synthesized in the adrenal medulla.

ANATOMY AND PHYSIOLOGY

Catecholamines: The First Messenger. A catecholamine is any compound of a catechol nucleus (a benzene ring with two adjacent hydroxyl groups) and an amine-containing side chain. The chemical configuration of five of the more common catecholamines in clinical use is demonstrated in Figure 15-6. The endogenous catecholamines in humans are dopamine (DA), NE, and EPI. DA is a neurotransmitter present in the CNS. It is primarily involved in coordinating motor activity in the brain. It is the precursor of NE. NE is synthesized and stored in nerve endings of postganglionic SNS neurons. It is also synthesized in the adrenal medulla and is the chemical precursor of EPI. Stored EPI is located chiefly in chromaffin cells of the adrenal medulla. Eighty to eighty-five percent of the catecholamine content of the adrenal medulla is EPI and 15–20% is NE. The brain contains both noradrenergic and dopaminergic receptors, but circulating catecholamines do not cross the blood–brain barrier. The catecholamines present in the brain are synthesized there.

Catecholamines are often referred to as adrenergic drugs because their effector actions are mediated through receptors specific for the SNS. Sympathomimetics can activate these same receptors because of their structural similarity. For example, clonidine is a α_2-receptor agonist that does not possess a catechol nucleus and even has two ring systems that are aplanar to each other. However, clonidine enjoys a remarkable spatial similarity to NE that allows it to activate the receptor. Drugs that produce sympathetic-like effects but lack the basic catecholamine structure are defined as sympathomimetics. All clinically useful catecholamines are sympathomimetics, but not all sympathomimetics are catecholamines. The effects of endogenous or synthetic catecholamines on adrenergic receptors can be direct or indirect Indirect-acting catecholamines

(i.e. ephedrine) have little intrinsic effect on adrenergic receptors but produce their effects by stimulating release of the stored neurotransmitter from SNS nerve terminals. Some synthetic and endogenous catecholamines stimulate adrenergic receptor sites directly, whereas others have a mixed mode of action. The actions of direct-acting catecholamines are independent of endogenous NE stores; however, the indirect-acting catecholamines are totally dependent on adequate neuronal stores of endogenous NE.

Synthesis. The main site of NE synthesis is in or near the postganglionic nerve endings. Some synthesis does occur in vesicles near the cell body that pass to the nerve endings. Phenylalanine or tyrosine is taken up into the axoplasm of the nerve terminal and synthesized into either NE or EPI. Figure 15-7 demonstrates this synthesis cascade. Tyrosine hydroxylase catalyzes the conversion of tyrosine to dihydroxyphenylalanine. This is the rate-limiting step at which NE synthesis is controlled through feedback inhibition. Dopamine (DA) synthesis occurs in the cytoplasm of the neuron. The vesicles of peripheral postganglionic neurons contain the enzyme dopamine-b-hydroxylase, which converts DA to NE. The adrenal medulla additionally contains phenylethanolamine-*N*-methyltransferase, which converts NE to EPI. This reaction takes place outside the medullary vesicles, and the newly formed EPI then enters the vesicle for storage (Fig. 15-8). All the endogenous catecholamines are stored in presynaptic vesicles and released on arrival of an action potential. Excitation-secretion coupling in sympathetic neurons is Ca^{2+}-dependent.

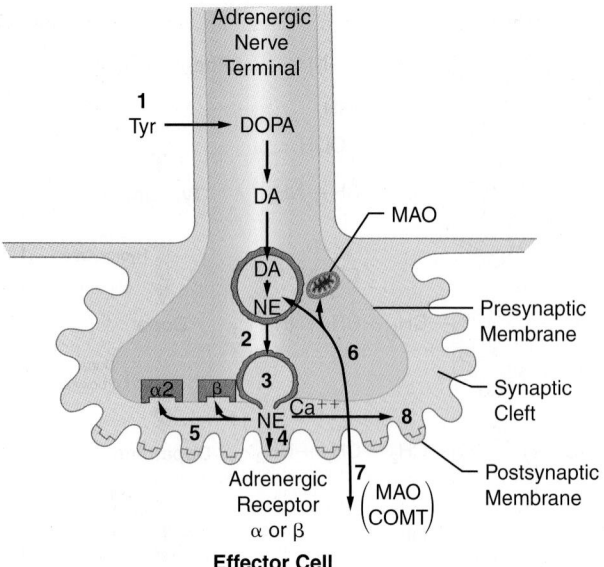

FIGURE 15.8. Schematic of the synthesis and disposition of norepinephrine (NE) in adrenergic neurotransmission. (1) Synthesis and storage in neuronal vesicles; (2) action potential permits calcium entry with (3) exocytosis of NE into synaptic gap. (4) Released NE reacts with receptor on effector cell. NE (5) may react with presynaptic α_2 receptor to inhibit further NE release or with presynaptic β receptor to enhance reuptake of NE (6; uptake 1). Extraneuronal uptake (uptake 2) absorbs NE into effector cell (7) with overflow occurring systemically (8). Tyr, tyrosine; DOPA, dihydroxyphenylalanine; DA, dopamine; MAO, monoamine oxidase; COMT, catechol-*O*-methyltransferase.

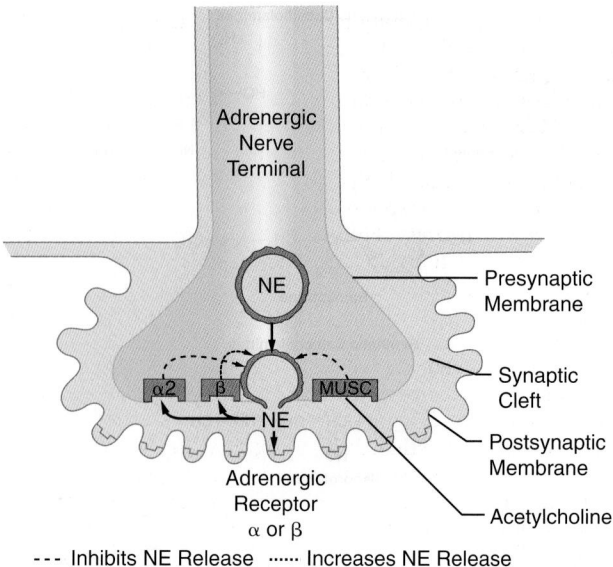

FIGURE 15.9. This schematic demonstrates just a few of the presynaptic adrenergic receptors thought to exist. Agonist and antagonist drugs are clinically available for these receptors (see Table 15-5). The α_2 receptors serve as a negative feedback mechanism whereby norepinephrine (NE) stimulation inhibits its own release. Presynaptic β stimulation increases NE uptake, augmenting its availability. Presynaptic muscarinic (MUSC) receptors respond to acetylcholine (ACh) diffusing from nearby cholinergic terminals. They inhibit NE release and can be blocked by atropine.

Regulation. Increased SNS nervous activity, as in congestive heart failure or chronic stress, stimulates the synthesis of catecholamines. Glucocorticoids from the adrenal cortex stimulate an increase in phenylethanolamine-*N*-methyltransferase that methylates NE to EPI.

The release of NE depends on depolarization of the nerve and an increase in calcium ion permeability. This release is inhibited by colchicine and prostaglandin E$_2$, suggesting a contractile mechanism. NE inhibits its own release by stimulating presynaptic (prejunctional) α_2 receptors. Phenoxybenzamine and phentolamine, α-receptor antagonists, increase the release of NE by blocking inhibitory presynaptic α_2 receptors (Fig. 15-9). Other receptors are also important in NE regulation.

Inactivation. The catecholamines are removed from the synaptic cleft by three mechanisms (Fig. 15-8). These are reuptake into the presynaptic terminals, extraneuronal uptake, and diffusion. Termination of NE at the effector site is almost entirely by reuptake of NE into the terminals of the presynaptic neuron. This is an active, energy-requiring, and temperature-dependent process. The reuptake of NE in the presynaptic terminals is also a stereospecific process. Structurally similar compounds (guanethidine, metaraminol) may enter the vesicles and displace the neurotransmitter. Tricyclic antidepressants and cocaine inhibit the reuptake of NE, resulting in high synaptic NE concentrations and accentuated receptor response. In addition, evidence suggests that NE reuptake is mediated by a presynaptic β-adrenergic mechanism because beta-blockade causes marked elevations of EPI and NE[10] (see Figs. 15-8 and 15-9). Extraneuronal uptake is a minor pathway for inactivating NE. Effector cells and other extraneuronal tissues take up NE. The NE that is taken up by the extraneuronal tissue is metabolized by monoamine oxidase (MAO) and by catechol-*O*-methyltransferase to form vanillylmandelic acid. The minute amount of catecholamine that escapes these two mechanisms diffuses into the circulation, where it is metabolized by the liver and kidney. The same enzymes inactivate EPI. Reuptake is the predominant pathway for inactivation of the endogenous catecholamines, while metabolism by the liver and kidney is the predominant pathway for catecholamines given exogenously. This accounts for the longer duration of action of the exogenous catecholamines than that noted at the local synapse.

The final metabolic product of the catecholamines is vanillylmandelic acid. Vanillylmandelic acid constitutes the major metabolite (80 to 90%) of NE found in the urine. Less than 5% of released NE appears unchanged in the urine. The metabolic products excreted in the urine provide a gross estimate of SNS activity and can facilitate the clinical diagnosis of pheochromocytoma (see "Endocrine Function").

RECEPTORS

5 An agonist is a substance that interacts with a receptor to evoke a biologic response. ACh, NE, EPI, DA, and ATP are the major agonists of the ANS. An antagonist is a substance that interferes with the evocation of a response at a receptor site by an agonist. Receptors are therefore regarded as target sites that, when activated by an agonist, will lead to a response by the effector cell. Receptors are protein macromolecules and are located in the plasma membrane. Several thousand receptors have been demonstrated in a single cell. The enormity of this network is realized when it is considered that ~25,000 single cells can be innervated by a single neuron.

Cholinergic Receptors

ACh is the neurotransmitter for three distinct classes of receptors. These receptors can be differentiated by their anatomic location and their affinity to bind various agonists and antagonists. ACh mediates the "first messenger" function of transmitting impulses within the PNS, the ganglia of the SNS, and the neuroeffector junction of striated, voluntary muscle (Fig. 15-2). Cholinergic receptors are further subdivided into muscarinic and nicotinic receptors because muscarine and nicotine stimulate them selectively.[3] However, both muscarinic and nicotinic receptors respond to ACh (see "Cholinergic Drugs"). Muscarine activates cholinergic receptors at the postganglionic PNS junctions of cardiac and smooth muscle throughout the body. Muscarinic stimulation is characterized by bradycardia, decreased inotropism, bronchoconstriction, miosis, salivation, gastrointestinal hypermotility, and increased gastric acid secretion (Table 15-1). Muscarinic receptors can be blocked by atropine without effect on nicotinic receptors (see "Cholinergic Drugs"). Muscarinic receptors are known to exist in sites other than PNS postganglionic junctions. They are found on the presynaptic membrane of sympathetic nerve terminals in the myocardium, coronary vessels, and peripheral vasculature (Fig. 15-9). These are referred to as *adrenergic muscarinic receptors* because of their location; however, ACh stimulates them also. Stimulation of these receptors inhibits release of NE in a manner similar to α_2-receptor stimulation. Muscarinic blockade removes inhibition of NE release, augmenting SNS activity. Atropine, the prototypical muscarinic blocker, may produce sympathomimetic activity in this manner as well as vagal blockade. Neuromuscular blocking drugs that cause tachycardia are thought to have a similar mechanism of action. ACh acting on presynaptic adrenergic muscarinic receptors is a potent inhibitor of NE release.[10] The prejunctional muscarinic receptor may play an important physiologic role because several autonomically innervated tissues (e.g., the heart) possess ANS plexuses in which the SNS and PNS nerve terminals are closely associated. In these plexuses, ACh, released from the nearby PNS nerve terminals (vagus nerve), can inhibit NE release by activation of presynaptic adrenergic muscarinic receptors (Fig. 15-9).

Nicotinic receptors are found at the synaptic junctions of both SNS and PNS ganglia. Because both junctions are cholinergic, ACh or ACh-like substances such as nicotine will excite postganglionic fibers of both systems (see Fig. 15-2). Low doses of nicotine produce stimulation of ANS ganglia, whereas high doses produce blockade. This dualism is referred to as the *nicotinic effect* (see "Ganglionic Drugs"). Nicotinic stimulation of the SNS ganglia produces hypertension and tachycardia by causing the release of EPI and NE from the adrenal medulla. Adrenal hormone release is mediated by ACh in the chromaffin cells, which are analogous to postganglionic neurons (Fig. 15-2). A further increase in nicotine concentration produces hypotension and neuromuscular weakness, as it becomes a ganglionic blocker. The cholinergic neuroeffector junction of skeletal muscle also contains nicotinic receptors, although they are not identical to the nicotinic receptors in ANS ganglia.

Adrenergic Receptors

6 The adrenergic receptors are termed *adrenergic* or *noradrenergic*, depending on their responsiveness to EPI or NE. The dissimilarities of these two drugs led Ahlquist in 1948 to propose two types of opposing adrenergic receptors, termed *alpha* (α) and *beta* (β). The development of new agonists and antagonists with relatively selective activity allowed subdivision the β receptors into β_1 and β_2. α-Receptors were subsequently divided into α_1 and α_2, and later further subdivided using molecular cloning. The sympathomimetic adrenergic drugs in current use differ from one another in their effects largely because of differences in substitution on the amine group, which influences the relative α or β effect (Fig. 15-6).

Another major peripheral adrenergic receptor specific for DA is termed the *dopaminergic* receptor. Further studies have revealed not only subsets of the α and β receptors but also the DA receptor. These DA receptors have been identified in the CNS and in renal, mesenteric, and coronary vessels. The physiologic importance of these receptors is a matter of controversy because there are no identifiable peripheral DA neurons. DA measured in the circulation is assumed to result from spillover from the brain.

The function of DA in the CNS has long been known, but the peripheral DA receptor has been elucidated only within the past 25 years. The presence of the peripheral DA receptor was obscured because DA does not affect the DA receptor exclusively. It also stimulates α and β receptors in a dose-related manner. However, DA receptors function independently of α or β blockade and are modified by DA antagonists such as haloperidol, droperidol, and phenothiazines. Thus, there is a necessity for the addition of the DA receptor and its subsets (DA_1 and DA_2).

The distribution of adrenergic receptors in organs and tissues is not uniform and their function differs not only by their location but also in their numbers and/or distribution. Adrenergic receptors are found in two loci in the sympathetic neuroeffector junction. They are found in both the presynaptic (prejunctional) and postsynaptic (postjunctional) sites as well as extrasynaptic sites (Fig. 15-10). Table 15-3 is a review of the function and synaptic location of some of the clinically important receptors and their subtypes.

Alpha-Adrenergic Receptors

The α-adrenergic receptors have been further subdivided into two clinically important classes α_1 and α_2. This classification is based on their response to the α-antagonists yohimbine and prazosin. Prazosin is a more potent antagonist of α_1 receptors, whereas α_2 receptors are more sensitive to yohimbine. Recently, the pharmacologic experiments have demonstrated the existence of two subtypes within the α_1 group, namely α_{1A} and α_{1B}, and at least two subtypes within the α_2, respectively α_{2A}, and α_{2B}. The importance of these subsets is still emerging with evidence that the spleen, and liver contain mainly α_{1B} receptors, and the heart, neocortex, kidney, vas deferns, and hippocampus containing equal amounts of α_{1A} and α_{1B} receptors. The α_1-adrenergic receptors are found in the smooth muscle cells of the peripheral vasculature of the coronary arteries, skin, uterus, intestinal mucosa, and splanchnic beds[11] (Table 15-4). The α_1 receptors serve as postsynaptic activators of vascular and intestinal smooth muscle as well as of endocrine glands. Their activation results in either decreased or increased tone, depending on the effector organ. The response in resistance and capacitance vessels is constriction, whereas in the intestinal tract it is relaxation. There is now a large body of evidence documenting the presence of postjunctional α_1 adrenoceptors in the mammalian heart. α_1–Adrenergic receptors have been shown to have a positive inotropic effect on cardiac tissues from most mammals studied, including humans. Experimental work strongly supports the concept that enhanced myocardial α_1 responsiveness plays a primary role in the genesis of malignant arrhythmias induced by catecholamines during myocardial ischemia and reperfusion. Drugs possessing potent α_1 antagonist activity such as prazosin and phentolamine provide significant antiarrhythmic activity. The clinical mechanism and significance of these findings are not yet clear. However, there is no doubt that α_1-adrenergic antagonists prevent catecholamine-induced ventricular arrhythmias.[12] In contrast, studies of the effects of β antagonists in experimental and clinical myocardial infarction have provided conflicting results.

The discovery of presynaptic α adrenoreceptors and their role in the modulation of NE transmission provided the stimulus for the subclassification of α receptors into α_1 and α_2 subtypes.

FIGURE 15.10. Loci of several known adrenergic receptors. The presynaptic α_2 and dopamine (DA) receptors serve as a negative feedback mechanism, whereby stimulation of norepinephrine (NE) inhibits its own release. Presynaptic β_2 stimulation increases NE uptake, augmenting its availability. Postsynaptic α_2 and β_2 receptors are extrasynaptic and are considered noninnervated hormonal receptors.

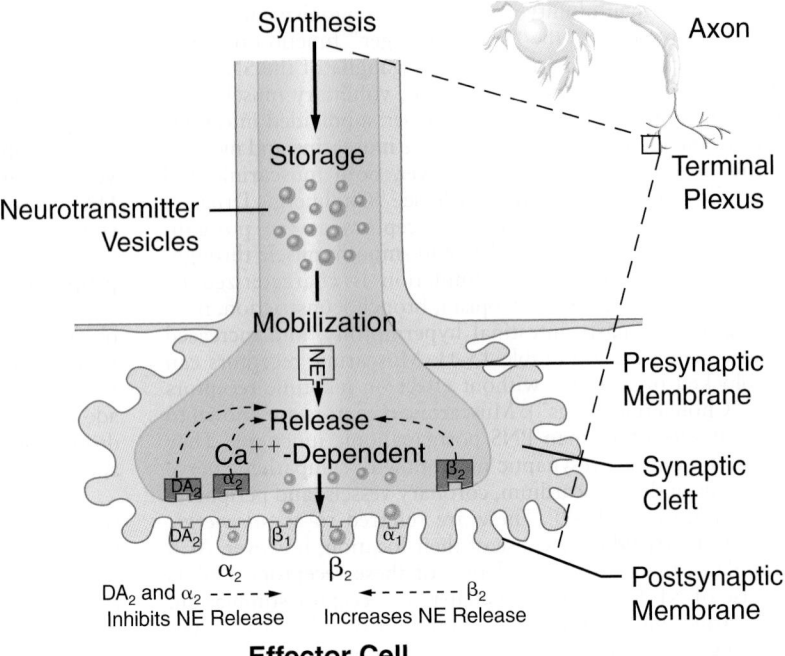

Presynaptic α_1 receptors have not been identified and they appear confined only to the postsynaptic membrane. On the other hand, α_2 receptors are found on both presynaptic and postsynaptic membranes of the adrenergic neuroeffector junction. Table 15-4 reviews these sites. Postsynaptic membranes contain a near equal mix of α_1 and α_2 receptors.

The α_2 adrenoreceptors may be subdivided even further into as many as four possible subtypes. The postsynaptic α_2 receptors have many actions, which include arterial and venous vasoconstriction, platelet aggregation, inhibition of insulin release, inhibition of bowel motility, stimulation of growth hormone release, and inhibition of antidiuretic hormone release.

α_2 Receptors can be found in cholinergic pathways as well as in adrenergic pathways. They can significantly modulate parasympathetic activity as well. Current research implies that α_2 stimulation of the parasympathetic pathways plays a role in the modulation of the baroreceptor reflex (increased sensitivity), vagal mediation of HR (bradycardia), bronchoconstriction, and salivation (dry mouth). However, cholinergic receptors can also be found in adrenergic pathways; thus, muscarinic and nicotinic receptors have been found in presynaptic and postsynaptic locations, where in turn they modulate sympathetic activity (Fig. 15-9). There is speculation that the features that are so desirable to the anesthesiologist, such as sedation, anxiolysis, analgesia, and hypnosis, are mediated through this site.

Stimulation of presynaptic α_2 receptors mediates inhibition of NE release into the synaptic cleft, serving as a negative feedback mechanism. The central effects are primarily related to a reduction in sympathetic outflow with a concomitantly enhanced parasympathetic outflow (e.g., enhanced baroreceptor activity). These results in a decreased systemic vascular resistance, decreased cardiac output (CO), decreased inotropic state in the myocardium, and decreased HR. The peripheral presynaptic α_2 effects are similar, and NE release is inhibited in postganglionic neurons. However, stimulation of postsynaptic α_2 receptors, like the α_1 postsynaptic receptor, affects vasoconstriction. NE acts on

both α_1 and α_2 receptors. Thus, NE not only activates smooth muscle vasoconstriction (postsynaptic α_1 and α_2 receptors) but also stimulates presynaptic α_2 receptors and inhibits its own release. Selective stimulation of the presynaptic α_2 receptor could produce a beneficial reduction of peripheral vascular resistance. Unfortunately, most known presynaptic α_2 agonists also stimulate the postsynaptic α_2 receptors, causing vasoconstriction. Blockade of α_2 presynaptic receptors, however, ablates normal inhibition of NE, causing vasoconstriction. Vasodilation occurs with the blockade of postsynaptic α_1 and α_2 receptors.

Alpha-Adrenergic Receptors in the Cardiovascular System. Postsynaptic α_1 and α_2 receptors in the mammalian myocardium and coronary arteries mediate a number of responses.

Coronary Arteries. The presence of postsynaptic α_1 and α_2 receptors in mammalian models has been demonstrated. Sympathetic nerves cause coronary vasoconstriction, which is mediated more by postsynaptic α_2 than α_1 receptors. The larger epicardial arteries possess mainly α_1 receptors, whereas α_2 receptors and some α_1 receptors are present in the small coronary artery resistance vessels.[13] Epicardial vessels contribute only 5% to the total resistance of the coronary circulation; therefore, α_1 agonists such as phenylephrine have little influence on coronary resistance.[14,15] Myocardial ischemia has been shown to increase α_2 receptor density in the coronary arteries. Ischemia has also been shown to cause a reflex increase in sympathetic activity mediated by α mechanisms. This cascade may further increase coronary constriction. Postsynaptic α_1 receptors do not rely upon extracellular Ca^{2+} to constrict the vessel, whereas the α_2-constrictor response is highly dependent on extracellular influx and exquisitely sensitive to calcium channel inhibitors.[16]

Myocardium. The role of β receptors in mediating catecholamine induced inotropism and arrhythmogenesis is well known (see "Beta-Adrenergic Receptors"). Studies have shown the presence of postsynaptic myocardial α_1 receptors,

TABLE 15-3

ADRENERGIC RECEPTORS: ORDER OF POTENCY OF AGONISTS AND ANTAGONISTS

■ RECEPTOR		■ AGONISTS[a]	■ ANTAGONISTS	■ LOCATION	■ ACTION
α_1	++++	Norepinephrine	Phenoxybenzamine[b]	Smooth muscle (vascular, iris, radial, ureter, pilomotor, uterus, trigone, gastrointestinal, and bladder sphincters)	Contraction
	+++	Epinephrine	Phentolamine[b]		Vasoconstriction
	++	Dopamine	Ergot alkaloids[b]		
	+	Isoproterenol	Prazosin		
			Tolazoline[b]	Brain	Neurotransmission
			Labetalol[b]	Smooth muscle (gastrointestinal)	Relaxation
				Heart	Glycogenolysis
				Salivary glands	Increased force,[c] glycolysis
				Adipose tissue	Secretion (K^+, H_2O)
				Sweat glands (localized)	Glycogenesis
				Kidney (proximal tubule)	Secretion
					Gluconeogenesis
					Na^+ reabsorption
α_2	++++	Clonidine	Yohimbine	Adrenergic nerve endings	Inhibition
	+++	Norepinephrine	Piperoxan	Presynaptic—CNS	norepinephrine release
	++	Epinephrine	Phentolamine[b]		
	++	Norepinephrine	Phenoxybenzamine[b]	Platelets	Aggregation, granule release
	+	Phenylephrine	Tolazoline[b]		
			Labetalol[b]	Adipose tissue	Inhibition lypolysis
				Endocrine pancrease	Inhibition insulin release
				Vascular smooth muscle—?	Contraction
				Kidney	Inhibition renin disease
				Brain	Neurotransmission
β_1	++++	Isoproterenol[b]	Acebutolol	Heart	Increased rate, contractility, conduction velocity
	+++	Epinephrine	Practolol		
	++	Norepinephrine	Propranolol[b]		Coronary vasodilation
	+	Dopamine	Alprenolol[b]	Adipose tissue	Lipolysis
			Metoprolol		
			Esmolol		
β_2	++++	Isoproterenol[a]	Propranolol[b]	Liver	Glycogenolysis, gluconeogenesis
	+++	Epinephrine	Butoxamine		
	+++	Norepinephrine	Alprenolol		
	+	Dopamine	Esmolol	Skeletal muscle	Glycogenolysis, lactate release
			Nadolol		
			Timolol	Smooth muscle (bronchi, uterus, vascular, gastrointestinal, detrusor, spleen capsule)	Relaxation
			Labetalol		
				Endocrine pancreas	Insulin secretion
				Salivary glands	Amylase secretion
DA$_1$	++++	Fenoldopam		Vascular smooth muscle	Vasodilation
	++	Dopamine	Haloperidol	Renal and mesentery	
	+	Epinephrine	Droperidol		
	+	Metaclopramide	Phenothiazines		
DA$_2$	++	Dopamine	Domperidone	Presynaptic—adrenergic nerve endings	Inhibits norepinephrine release
	+	Bromocriptine			

DA, dopamine.
[a]Listed in decreasing order of potency.
[b]Nonselective.
[c]β_1-adrenergic responses are greater.
Pluses indicate strength of potency.

ANATOMY AND PHYSIOLOGY

TABLE 15-4

ADRENERGIC RECEPTORS

■ RECEPTOR	■ SYNAPTIC SITE	■ ANATOMIC SITE	■ ACTION	■ LV FUNCTION AND STROKE VOLUME
α_1	Postsynaptic	Peripheral vascular smooth muscle	Constriction	Decreased
		Renal vascular smooth muscle	Constriction	
		Coronary arteries, epicardial	Constriction	
		Myocardium 30–40% of resting tone	Positive inotropism	Improved
		Renal tubules	Antidiuresis	
α_2	Presynaptic	Peripheral vascular smooth muscle release	Inhibit NE	
			Secondary vasodilation	Improved
		Coronaries	?	
		CNS	Inhibition of CNS activity Sedation Decrease MAC	
	Postsynaptic	Coronaries, endocardial	Constriction	Decreased
		CNS	Inhibition of insulin release Decreased bowel motility Inhibition of antidiuretic hormone Analgesia	
		Renal tubule	Promotes Na^{2+} and H_2O excretion	
β_1	Postsynaptic NE sensitive	Myocardium	Positive inotropism and chronotropism	Improved
		Sinoatrial (SA) node Ventricular conduction		
		Kidney	Renin release	
		Coronaries	Relaxation	
β_2	Presynaptic NE sensitive	Myocardium	Accelerates NE release	Improved
		SA node ventricular conduction vessels	Opposite action to presynaptic α_2 agonism Constriction	
	Postsynaptic (extrasynaptic) (EPI sensitive)	Myocardium	Positive inotropism and chronotropism	
		Vascular smooth muscle	Relaxation	Improved
		Bronchial smooth muscle	Relaxation	Improved
		Renal vessels	Relaxation	Improved
DA_1	Postsynaptic	Blood vessels (renal, mesentery, coronary)	Vasodilation	Improved
		Renal tubules	Natriuresis Diuresis	
		Juxtaglomerular cells	Renin release (modulates diuresis)	
		Sympathetic ganglia	Minor inhibition	
DA_2	Presynaptic	Postganglionic sympathetic nerves	Inhibit NE release	Improved
			Secondary vasodilation	
	Postsynaptic	Renal and mesenteric vasculature	? Vasoconstriction	

LV, left ventricular; NE, norepinephrine; MAC, EPI, epinephrine; DA, dopamine.

which also exert a major, facilitory, positive inotropic effect on the myocardium of several species of mammals including humans. Their contribution to malignant reperfusion arrhythmogenesis has also been recognized.

Phenylephrine, an α_1 agonist, can increase myocardial contractility two- to threefold compared with a six- to sevenfold increase produced by isoproterenol, a pure β agonist. Myocardial postsynaptic α_1 receptors mediate perhaps as much as 30 to 50% of the basal inotropic tone of the normal heart.

Postsynaptic myocardial α_1 receptors play a more prominent inotropic role in the failing heart by serving as a reserve to the normally predominant β_1 receptors. Although the response to both α_1 and β_1 agonists is reduced in the failing myocardium, the interaction between the two receptors is more apparent. Chronic heart failure is known to produce a reduced density (down-regulation) of myocardial β_1 receptors as a result of high levels of circulating catecholamines. However, there is no evidence of down-regulation of either α_1 or β_2 receptors due to cardiac failure. The increase in density of myocardial α_1 adrenoreceptors shows a relative increase with failure and myocardial ischemia.[17] Thus, enhanced myocardial α_1-receptor numbers, and sensitivity, may contribute to positive inotropism seen during ischemia as well as to the malignant arrhythmias that occur with reperfusion. Intracellular mobilization of cytosolic Ca^{2+} by the activated α_1-myocardial receptors during ischemia appears to contribute to these arrhythmias. The α_1 receptor also increases the sensitivity of the contractile elements to Ca^{2+}. Drugs possessing potent α_1 antagonism such as prazosin and phentolamine have been shown to possess significant antiarrhythmic activity, although of limited usefulness because of hypotension. Enhanced α_1 activity with myocardial ischemia may explain why the antiarrhythmic benefits of β antagonists in patients with acute myocardial infarction are far from certain. The contribution of β receptors to positive inotropism and arrhythmogenesis during ischemia and reperfusion may be overshadowed by the α receptors during acute failure and ischemia.

Peripheral Vessels. Activation of the presynaptic α_2-vascular receptors produces vasodilation, whereas the postsynaptic α_1- and α_2-vascular receptors subserve vasoconstriction. Presynaptic vascular α_2 receptors inhibit NE release. This represents a negative feedback mechanism by which NE inhibits its own release via the prejunctional receptor. Presynaptic α_2 agonists, such as clonidine, inhibit NE release at the neurosympathetic junction producing vasodilatation. The effect of selective presynaptic α_2-receptor agonists to ameliorate coronary vasoconstriction in humans is unclear. Excitation of the inhibitory presynaptic α_2 receptors by endogenous or synthetic catecholamines also inhibits NE release. However, most sympathomimetics are nonselective α agonists that will excite equally presynaptic α_2 vasodilators and vasoconstrictive postsynaptic α_1 and α_2 receptors. Postsynaptic α_1 and α_2 receptors coexist in both the arterial and venous sides of the circulation with the relative distribution of α_2 receptors being greater on the venous side.[11] This may explain why pure α_1 agonists, such as methoxamine, produce little venoconstriction, whereas many nonselective agonists such as phenylephrine produce significant venoconstriction. NE is the most potent venoconstrictor of all the catecholamines. Clinically, venoconstriction would have the effect of preloading by shifting venous capacitance centrally, whereas stimulation of arterial postsynaptic α_1 and α_2 receptors would effect afterloading by increasing arterial resistance.

Alpha-Adrenergic Receptors in the Central Nervous System. All subtypes of the α, β, and DA receptors have been found in various regions of the brain and spinal cord. The functional role of the cerebral α and β receptors suggests a close association with blood pressure and HR control. Cerebral and spinal cord presynaptic α_2 receptors are also involved in inhibition of presynaptic NE release. Although the brain contains adrenergic and dopaminergic receptors, circulating catecholamines do not cross the blood–brain barrier. The catecholamines in the brain are synthesized there. Many actions have been attributed to the cerebral postsynaptic α_2 receptor. This includes inhibition of insulin release, inhibition of bowel motility, stimulation of growth hormone release, and inhibition of antidiuretic hormone release. Central neuraxis injection of α_2 agonists, such as clonidine, induces analgesia, sedation, and cardiovascular depression. The increased duration of epidural or intrathecal anesthesia by the addition of nonselective α agonists to the local anesthetic may produce additional analgesia through this mechanism.

Alpha Receptors in the Kidney. The kidney has an extensive and exclusive adrenergic innervation of the afferent and efferent glomerular arterioles, proximal and distal renal tubules, ascending loop of Henle, and juxtaglomerular apparatus. The greatest density of innervation is in the thick ascending loop of Henle, followed by the distal convoluted tubules and proximal tube. Both α_1 and α_2 subtypes are found in the kidney with the α_2 receptor dominating. The α_1 receptor is predominant in the renal vasculature and elicits vasoconstriction, which modulates renal blood flow. Tubular α_1 receptors enhance sodium and water reabsorption, leading to antinatriuresis, whereas tubular α_2 receptors promote sodium and water excretion.

Beta-Adrenergic Receptors

The β-adrenergic receptors, like the α receptor, have been divided into subtypes. They are designated as the β_1 and β_2 subtypes. Recently, molecular cloning has demonstrated the existence of a third subtype, namely β_3 receptor. Activation of all these receptors subtypes induces the activation of adenylyl cyclase and increased conversion of ATP to cyclic adenosine-3', 5'-monophosphate (cAMP). β_1 receptors predominate in the myocardium, the sinoatrial node, and the ventricular conduction system. The β_1 receptors also mediate the effects of the catecholamines on the myocardium. These receptors are equally sensitive to EPI and NE, which distinguishes them from the β_2 receptors. Effects of β_1 stimulation are outlined in Table 15-4, which includes their effects specifically on the cardiovascular system.

The β_2 receptors are located in the smooth muscles of the blood vessels in the skin, muscle, mesentery, and in bronchial smooth muscle. Stimulation produces vasodilation and bronchial relaxation. The β_2 receptors are more sensitive to EPI than NE. β Receptors are found in both presynaptic and postsynaptic membranes of the adrenergic neuro effector junction (Table 15-4). β_1 Receptors are distributed to postsynaptic sites and have not been identified on the presynaptic membrane. Presynaptic β receptors are of the β_2 subtype. The effects of activation of the presynaptic β_2 receptor are diametrically opposed to those of the presynaptic α_2 receptor. The presynaptic β_2 receptor accelerates endogenous NE release, whereas blockade of this receptor will inhibit NE release. Antagonism of the presynaptic β_2 receptors produces a physiological result similar to activation of the presynaptic α_2 receptor. The postsynaptic β_1 receptors are located on the synaptic membrane and respond primarily to neuronal NE. The postsynaptic β_2 receptors, like the postsynaptic α_2 receptor, respond primarily to circulating EPI.

Beta Receptors in the Cardiovascular System
Myocardium. Myocardial β receptors were originally classified as β_1 receptors. Those in the vascular and bronchial smooth muscle were called the β_2 subtype. However, studies have confirmed the coexistence of β_1 and β_2 receptors in the myocardium.[18] Both β_1 and β_2 receptors are functionally coupled to adenylate cyclase, suggesting a similar involvement in the regulation of inotropism and chronotropism. Postsynaptic β_1 receptors are distributed predominantly to the myocardium, the sinoatrial node, and the ventricular conduction system. The β_2 receptors have the same distribution but are presynaptic. Activation of the presynaptic β_2 receptor accelerates the release of NE into the synaptic cleft. The β_2 receptor approximates 20 to 30% of the β receptors in the ventricular myocardium and up to 40% of the β receptors in the atrium.

The effect of NE on inotropism in the normal heart is mediated entirely through the postsynaptic β_1 receptor, whereas the inotropic effects of EPI are mediated through both the β_1- and

β_2-myocardial receptors. The β_2 receptors may also mediate the chronotropic responses to EPI, which explains why selective β_1 antagonists are less effective in suppressing induced tachycardia than the nonselective β_1 antagonist propranolol.

Peripheral Vessels. The postsynaptic vascular β receptors are virtually all of the β_2 subtype. The β_2 receptors are located in the smooth muscle of the blood vessels of the skin, muscle, mesentery, and bronchi. Stimulation of the postsynaptic β_2 receptor produces vasodilation and bronchial relaxation. Modest vasoconstriction occurs when subjected to blockade because the actions of the vascular postsynaptic β_2 receptors no longer oppose the actions of the α_1-and α-postsynaptic receptors.

Beta Receptors in the Kidney. The kidney contains both β_1 and β_2 receptors, with the β_1 being predominant. Renin release from the juxtaglomerular apparatus is enhanced by β stimulation. The β_1 receptor evokes renin release in humans. Renal β_2 receptors also appear to regulate renal blood flow at the vascular level. They have been identified pharmacologically and mediate a vasodilatory response.

Dopaminergic Receptors

DA, synthesized in 1910, was recognized in 1959 not only as a vasopressor and the precursor of NE and EPI, but also as an important central and peripheral neurotransmitter. DA receptors have been localized in the CNS, on blood vessels, and postganglionic sympathetic nerves (Table 15-4). Two clinically important types of DA receptors have been recognized DA$_1$ and DA$_2$, while other subtypes like DA$_4$, and DA$_5$, are still being investigated. The DA$_1$ receptors are postsynaptic, whereas the DA$_2$ receptors are both presynaptic and postsynaptic. The presynaptic DA$_2$ receptors, like the presynaptic α_2 receptor, inhibit NE release and can produce vasodilatation. The postsynaptic DA$_2$ receptor may subserve vasoconstriction similar to that of the postsynaptic α_2 receptor. This effect is opposite to that of the postsynaptic DA$_1$ renal vascular receptor. The zona glomerulosa of the adrenal cortex also contains DA$_2$ receptors, which inhibit the release of aldosterone.

Myocardium

Defining specific dopaminergic receptors has been difficult because DA also exerts effects on the α and β receptors. DA receptors have not been described in the myocardium. Effects of DA are those related to activation of β_1 receptors, which promote positive inotropism and chronotropism. β_2 Activation would produce some systemic vasodilatation.

Peripheral Vessels

The greatest numbers of DA$_1$-postsynaptic receptors are found on vascular smooth muscle cells of the kidney and mesentery, but are also found in the other systemic arteries including coronary, cerebral, and cutaneous arteries. The vascular receptors are, like the β_2 receptors, linked to adenylate cyclase and mediate smooth muscle relaxation. Activation of these receptors produces vasodilatation, increasing blood flow to these organs. Concurrent activation of vascular presynaptic DA$_2$ receptors also inhibits NE release at presynaptic α_2 receptors, which may also contribute to peripheral vasodilatation. Higher doses of DA can mediate vasoconstriction via the postsynaptic α_1 and α_2 receptors. The constrictive effect is relatively weak in the cardiovascular system where the action of DA on adrenergic receptors is 1/35 and 1/50 as potent as that of EPI and NE, respectively.[19,20]

Central Nervous System

DA receptors have been identified in the hypothalamus where they are involved in prolactin release. They are also found in the basal ganglia where they coordinate motor function. Degeneration of dopaminergic neurons in the substantia nigra is the source of Parkinson disease. Another central action of DA is to stimulate the chemoreceptor trigger zone of the medulla, producing nausea and vomiting. DA antagonists such as haloperidol and droperidol are clinically effective in countering this action.

Kidney and Mesentery

Apart from their effect on the vessels of the kidney and mesentery, DA receptors on the smooth muscle of the esophagus, stomach, and small intestine enhance secretion production and reduce intestinal motility.[19,20] Metoclopramide, a DA antagonist, is useful for aspiration prophylaxis by promoting gastric emptying. The distribution of DA receptors in the renal vasculature is well known, but DA receptors have other functions within the kidney. DA$_1$ receptors are located on renal tubules, which inhibit sodium reabsorption with subsequent natriuresis and diuresis. The natriuresis may be the result of a combined renal vasodilatation, improved CO, and tubular action of the DA$_1$ receptors. Juxtaglomerular cells also contain DA$_1$ receptors, which increase renin release when activated. This action modulates the diuresis produced by DA$_1$ activation of the tubules.

DA has unique autonomic effects by activating specific peripheral dopaminergic receptors, which promote natriuresis and reduce afterload via dilatation of the renal and mesenteric arterial beds. Peripheral dopaminergic activity serves as a natural antihypertensive mechanism. Its actions are overshadowed by the opposite effect of its main biologic partner, NE. Plasma NE levels are known to increase with aging, likely the result of reduced clearance, while peripheral dopaminergic activity is known to diminish. Subtle changes in the DA-NE balance with aging may account for the diminished ability of the aged kidney to excrete a salt load.

Other Receptors

Adenosine Receptors

Adenosine produces inhibition of NE release. The effect of adenosine is blocked by caffeine and other methylxanthines. The physiologic function of these receptors may be the reduction of sympathetic tone under hypoxic conditions when adenosine production is enhanced. As a consequence of reduced NE release, cardiac work would be decreased and oxygen demand reduced. Adenosine has been effectively used to produce controlled hypotension.[21]

Serotonin

Serotonin (5-hydroxytryptamine) depresses the response of isolated blood vessels to SNS stimulation and decreases release of labeled NE in these preparations. Raising the external calcium ion concentration antagonizes this inhibitory action of serotonin. Thus, serotonin may inhibit neuronal NE release by a mechanism that limits the availability of calcium ions at the nerve terminal.

Prostaglandin E2, Histamine, and Opioids

Prostaglandin E$_2$, histamine, and several opioids have been reported to act on prejunctional receptor sites to inhibit NE release in certain sympathetically innervated tissue. However, these inhibitory receptors are unlikely to play a physiologic role in limiting NE release since their direct antagonists, compounds like inhibitors of cyclo-oxygenase, histamine antagonists, and naloxone do not increase a NE release.

Histamine acts in a manner similar to the neurotransmitters of the SNS. Cell membrane has specific receptors for histamine, with the individual response being determined by the type of cell being stimulated (see Chapter 13). Two receptors for histamine have been determined. These have been designated H_1 and H_2, for which it has been possible to develop specific agonists and antagonists. Stimulation of the H_1 receptors produces bronchoconstriction and intestinal contraction. The major role of the H_2 receptors is related to acid production by the parietal cells of the stomach; however, histamine is present in relatively high concentrations in the myocardium and cardiac conducting tissue, where it exerts positive inotropic and chronotropic effects while depressing dromotropism. The positive inotropic and chronotropic effects of histamine are H_2 receptor effects that are not blocked by β antagonism. These effects are blocked by H_2 antagonists, such as cimetidine, which accounts for the occasional report of cardiovascular collapse following the use of cimetidine. The negative dromotropic effect and that of coronary spasm caused by histamine are H_1 receptor effects.

Adrenergic Receptor Numbers and Sensitivity

Receptors, once thought to be static entities, are now thought to be dynamically regulated by a variety of conditions and to be in a constant state of flux. Receptors are synthesized in the sarcoplasmic reticulum of the parent cell, where they may remain extrasynaptic or externalize to the synaptic membranes where they may cluster. Membrane receptors may be removed or internalized to intracellular sites for either dehydration or recycling.

7 The numbers and sensitivity of adrenergic receptors can be influenced by normal, genetic, and developmental factors. Changes in the number of receptors alter the response to catecholamines. Alteration in the number, or density, of receptors is referred to as either *up-regulation* or *down-regulation*. As a rule, the number of receptors is inversely proportional to the ambient concentration of the catecholamines. Extended exposure of receptors to their agonists markedly reduces, but does not ablate, the biologic response to catecholamines. For example, increased adrenergic activity occurs in response to reduced perfusion as a result of acute or chronic myocardial dysfunction. Plasma catecholamines are increased. Subsequently, the myocardial postsynaptic β_1 receptors "down regulate" (see Chapter 6). This is thought to explain the diminished inotropic and chronotropic response to β_1 agonists and exercise in patients with chronic heart failure. However, calcium-induced inotropism is not impaired because β_2-receptor (extrasynaptic) numbers remain relatively intact. The β_2 receptors may account for up to 40% of the inotropism of the failing heart compared with 20% in the normal heart.[17,22] Tachyphylaxis to infused catecholamines is also thought to be the result of acute "down-regulation" of receptor numbers. There appears to be a reduction in numbers or sensitivity of β receptors in hypertensive patients who also have elevated plasma catecholamines. Down-regulation is the presumptive explanation for the lack of correlation between plasma catecholamine levels and the blood pressure elevation in patients with pheochromocytoma. Chronic use of β agonists such as terbutaline, isoproterenol, or EPI for the treatment of asthma can result in tachyphylaxis because of down-regulation. Even short-term use (1 to 6 hours) of β agonists may cause down-regulation of receptor numbers. Down-regulation is reversible on termination of the agonist. Chronic treatment of animals with nonselective beta-blockade causes a 100% increase in the number of β receptors. This accounts for the propranolol withdrawal syndrome in which the acute discontinuation of the β antagonist leaves the α receptors unopposed plus an increased number of β receptors. Clonidine withdrawal can be explained by the same mechanism. Up- or down-regulation of receptor numbers may not alter sensitivity of the receptor. Likewise, sensitivity may be increased or decreased in the presence of normal numbers of receptors. The pharmacologic factors affecting up- or down-regulation of the α and β receptors are similar.

AUTONOMIC NERVOUS SYSTEM REFLEXES AND INTERACTIONS

8 The ANS reflex has been compared to the computer circuit. This control system, as in all reflex systems, has (1) sensors, (2) afferent pathways, (3) CNS integration, and (4) efferent pathways to the receptors and efferent organs. Fine adjustments are made at the local level according to positive and negative feedback mechanisms. The baroreceptor is an example. The variable to be controlled (blood pressure) is sensed (carotid sinus), integrated (medullary vasomotor center), and adjusted through specific effector-receptor sites. Drugs or disease can interrupt this circuit at any point. Beta-blockers may attenuate the effector response, whereas an α agonist such as clonidine may alter both the effector and the integrator functions of blood pressure control.

Baroreceptors

There are several reflexes in the cardiovascular system, which help control arterial blood pressure, CO, and HR. The aim of the circulation is to provide blood flow to all the body organs (see Chapter 10). Yet, the most important controlled variable to which the sensors are attuned is blood pressure, a product of the blood flow and vascular resistance. Etienne Marey noted in 1859 that the pulse rate is inversely proportional to the blood pressure, and this is known as *Marey's law*. Subsequently, Hering, Koch, and others demonstrated that the alterations in HR evoked by changes in blood pressure depend on baroreceptors located in the aortic arch and the carotid sinuses. These pressure sensors react to alterations in stretch caused by blood pressure. Impulses from the carotid sinus and aortic arch reach the medullary vasomotor center by the glossopharyngeal and vagus nerves, respectively. Increased sensory traffic from the baroreceptors, caused by increased blood pressure, inhibits SNS effector traffic. The relative increase in vagal tone produces vasodilation, slowing of the HR, and a lowering of blood pressure. Real increases in vagal tone occur when blood pressure exceeds normal limits. The Valsalva maneuver can best demonstrate the arterial baroreceptor reflex (Fig. 15-11). The Valsalva maneuver

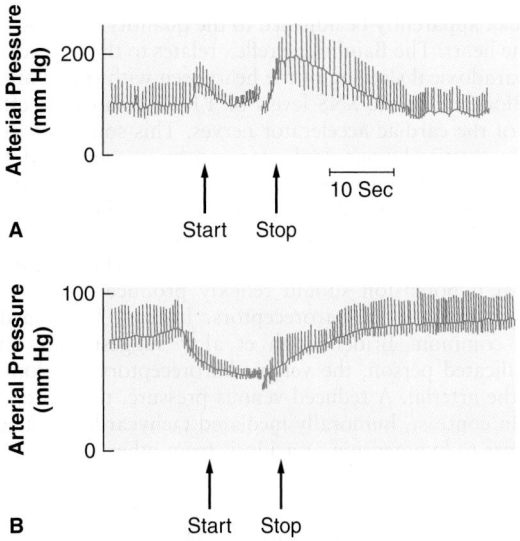

FIGURE 15.11. **A.** The normal blood pressure response to the Valsalva maneuver is demonstrated. Pulse rate moves in a reciprocal direction according to Marey's law of the heart. **B.** An abnormal Valsalva response is shown in a patient with C5 quadriplegia.

raises the intrathoracic pressure by forced expiration against a closed glottis. The arterial blood pressure rises momentarily as the intrathoracic blood is forced into the heart (preload). Sustained intrathoracic pressure diminishes venous return, reduces the CO, and drops the blood pressure. Reflex vasoconstriction and tachycardia ensue. Blood pressure returns to normal with release of the forced expiration, but then briefly "overshoots" because of the vasoconstriction and increased venous return. A slowing of the HR accompanies the overshoot in pressure. The cardiovascular responses to the Valsalva maneuver require an intact ANS circuit from peripheral sensor to peripheral adrenergic receptors. The Valsalva maneuver has been used to identify patients at risk for anesthesia because of ANS instability (Fig. 15-11). This was once a major concern in patients receiving drugs that depleted catecholamines, such as reserpine. Dysfunction of the SNS is implicated if exaggerated and prolonged hypotension develops during the forced expiration phase (50% from resting mean arterial pressure). In addition, the overshoot at the end of the Valsalva maneuver is absent. Dysfunction of the PNS can be assumed if the HR does not respond appropriately to the blood pressure changes.

Venous baroreceptors may be more dominant in the moment-to-moment regulation of CO. Baroreceptors in the right atrium and great veins produce an increase in HR when stretched by increased right atrial pressure. Reduced venous pressure decreases HR. Unlike the arterial baroreceptors, venous sensors are not thought to alter vascular tone; however, venoconstriction is postulated to occur when atrial pressures decline. Stretch of the venous receptors produces changes in HR opposite those produced when the arterial pressure sensors are stimulated. The arterial and venous pressure receptors are separately monitoring two of the four major determinants of CO, afterload and preload, respectively. Venous baroreceptors sample preload by stretch of the atrium. Arterial baroreceptors survey resistance, or afterload, as reflected in the mean arterial pressure. Afterload and preload produce opposite effects on CO; thus, one should not be surprised that the venous and arterial baroreceptors produce effects opposite those of a similar stretch stimulus, pressure.

Bainbridge described the venous baroreceptor reflex and demonstrated that it can be abolished by vagal resection. Numerous investigators have confirmed the acceleration of the HR in response to volume. However, the magnitude and direction of the HR response depend on the prevailing HR at the time of stimulation. The denervated, transplanted mammalian heart also accelerates in response to volume loading. HR, like CO, can apparently be adjusted to the quantity of blood entering the heart. The Bainbridge reflex relates to the characteristic but paradoxical slowing of the heart seen with spinal anesthesia. Blockade of the SNS levels of T1-T4 ablates the efferent limb of the cardiac accelerator nerves. This source of cardiac deceleration is obvious, as the vagus nerve is unopposed. However, bradycardia during spinal anesthesia is more related to the development of arterial hypotension than to the height of the block. The primary defect in the development of spinal hypotension is a decrease in venous return. Theoretically, the arterial hypotension should reflexly produce a tachycardia through the arterial baroreceptors. Instead, bradycardia is more common. Bridenbaugh et al.[23] suggest that, in the unmedicated person, the venous baroreceptors are dominant over the arterial. A reduced venous pressure, therefore, slows HR. In contrast, humorally mediated tachycardia is the usual response to hypotension or acidosis from other causes.

Denervated Heart

Reflex modulation of the adrenergic agonists is best seen in the denervated transplant heart, which retains the recipient's innervated sinoatrial node and the donor's denervated sinoatrial node[24] (see Chapter 54). NE infusion in the transplanted heart produces a slowing of the recipient's atrial rate through vagal feedback as the blood pressure rises. In the unmodulated donor heart, atrial rate increases. The baroreceptors are therefore not operant in the transplanted heart. Isoproterenol, a pure β agonist, increases the discharge rate of both the recipient and donor node by direct action, with the donor rate near doubling that of the recipient node. Atropine accelerates the recipient's atrial rate, whereas no effect is seen on the donor rate, which now controls HR.

Beta blockade produces comparable slowing of the sinoatrial node of both recipient and donor. The exercise capability of the denervated heart is conspicuously reduced by beta-blockade, presumably because of its reliance on circulating catecholamines. Propranolol has also been demonstrated to reduce the β response to chronotropic effects of NE and isoproterenol in the transplanted heart. The CO of the transplanted heart varies appropriately with changes in preload and afterload.

Interaction of Autonomic Nervous System Receptors

Strong interactions have been noted between SNS and PNS nerves in organs that receive dual, antagonistic innervation. Release of NE at the presynaptic terminal is modified by the PNS. For example, vagal inhibition of left ventricular contractility is accentuated as the level of SNS activity is raised. This interaction is termed *accentuated antagonism* and is mediated by a combination of presynaptic and postsynaptic mechanisms. The coronary arteries present an example of this phenomenon and deserve special attention.

The myocardium and coronary vessels are abundantly supplied with adrenergic and cholinergic fibers. Strong activity of both α and β receptors has been demonstrated in the coronary vascular bed. Selective stimulation of both the α_1 and postsynaptic α_2 receptors increases coronary vascular resistance, whereas selective α blockade eliminates this effect. Therefore, both β_1 and α_1 adrenoreceptors are present on coronary arteries and accessible to NE released by sympathetic nerves.[5,14]

The presynaptic adrenergic terminals of the myocardium and coronary vessels, like all blood vessels examined, contain muscarinic receptors.[10] Recent observations confirm that muscarinic agents and vagal stimulation, acting on the presynaptic, SNS muscarinic receptor, inhibit the release of NE in a manner similar to that of the presynaptic α_2 and DA_2 receptors (Fig. 15-9). Conversely, blockade of the muscarinic receptors with atropine markedly augments the positive inotropic responses to catecholamines.[5] Suppression of NE release explains, in part, vagal-induced attenuation of the inotropic response to strong SNS stimulation (accentuated antagonism) and only a weak negative inotropic effect of vagal stimulation when there is low background SNS activity. This may also explain why vagal activity reduces the vulnerability of the myocardium to fibrillation during infusions of NE.

ACh may cause coronary spasm during periods of high SNS tone.[5] Inhibition of NE release by presynaptic adrenergic muscarinic receptors of the smooth muscle of coronary vessels would lessen the coronary relaxation normally produced by NE on the β_1 receptor (Fig. 15-9). In anesthetized dogs, the rate of NE outflow into the coronary sinus blood, evoked by cardiac SNS stimulation, is markedly diminished by simultaneous vagal efferent stimulation.[25] This action is known to be prevented by atropine, which also causes coronary vasodilation.

Interaction with Other Regulatory Systems

The ANS is integrally related to several endocrine systems that ultimately summate to control blood pressure and regulate homeostasis. These include the renin-angiotensin system,

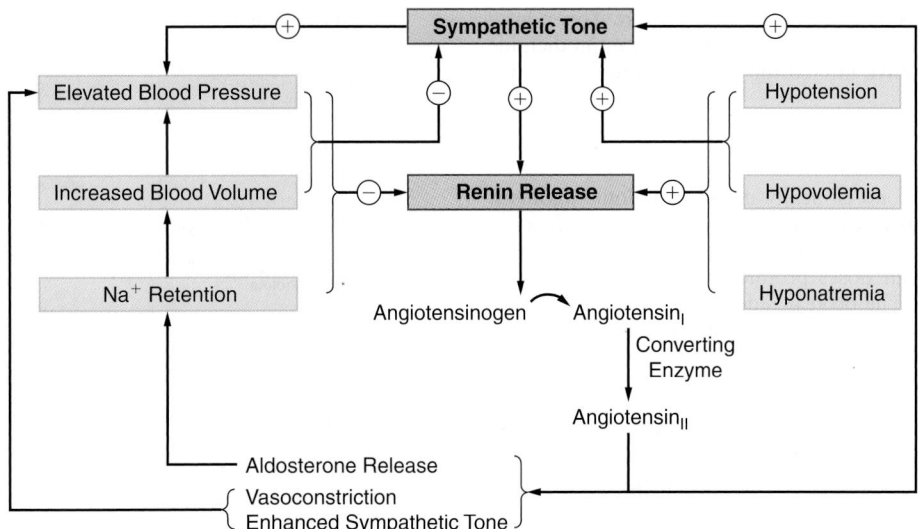

FIGURE 15.12.   The interactions of the renin–angiotensin and sympathetic nervous system in regulating homeostasis are shown schematically along with the physiologic variables that modulate their function. Arrows with a plus sign (+) represent stimulation, and those with a minus sign (−) represent inhibition.

antidiuretic hormone, glucocorticoids, and insulin (see Chapter 49). Both α and β receptors have been found in the endocrine pancreas and modulate insulin release (Table 15-4). β Stimulation increases insulin release, whereas α stimulation decreases it. The overall importance of this interaction is not entirely clear, but decreased tolerance to glucose and potassium has been noted in subjects taking beta-blocking drugs. The renin-angiotensin system is a complex endocrine system that modulates both blood pressure and water-electrolyte homeostasis (Fig. 15-12). Renin is a proteolytic enzyme contained within the cells of the juxtaglomerular apparatus of the renal cortex. When released, it acts on plasma angiotensinogen to form angiotensin I. Angiotensin I is then converted to angiotensin II by converting enzyme in the lung. Angiotensin II is a powerful direct arterial vasoconstrictor. It also acts on the adrenal cortex to release aldosterone and on the adrenal medulla to release EPI. In addition to its direct effects on vascular smooth muscle, angiotensin II augments NE release via presynaptic receptors, thus enhancing peripheral SNS tone. Captopril, enalapril, and lisinopril inhibit the action of converting enzyme, thus preventing the conversion of angiotensin I to angiotensin II. Renin is released in response to hyponatremia, decreased renal perfusion pressure, and ANS stimulation via β receptors on juxtaglomerular cells. Changes in sympathetic tone may thus alter renin release and affect homeostasis in a variety of ways. The ANS is also intimately related to adrenocortical function. As previously outlined, glucocorticoid release modulates phenylethanolamine-N-methyltransferase formation and thus synthesis of EPI. Glucocorticoids are also important in regulating the response of peripheral tissues to changes in SNS tone. Thus, the ANS is intimately related to other homeostatic mechanisms.

CLINICAL AUTONOMIC NERVOUS SYSTEM PHARMACOLOGY

9 The clinical application of ANS pharmacology is based on knowledge of ANS anatomy, physiology, and molecular pharmacology. Drugs that modify ANS activity can be classified by their site of action, mechanism of action, or pathology for which they are most commonly used. Antihypertensive drugs

are an example of the third category. This classification is a matter of degree because considerable functional overlap occurs. An example of classification by site relates to the ganglionic agonists or blocking agents. ANS drugs can be further categorized as those that act at the prejunctional membrane and those acting postjunctionally. They can then be more specifically classified by the predominant receptor or receptors on which they act.

Mode of Action

ANS drugs may be broadly classified by mode of action according to their mimetic or lytic actions. This may also be termed *agonist* or *antagonist*. A sympathomimetic, such as ephedrine, mimics SNS sympathetic activity by stimulation of adrenergic receptor sites both directly and indirectly. Sympatholytic drugs cause dissolution of SNS activity at these same receptor sites. β Receptor blockers are examples of sympatholytic drugs. Several modes of ANS drug action become evident when one follows the cascade of neurotransmission. Drugs that act on prejunctional membranes may therefore (1) interfere with transmitter synthesis (α-methyl paratyrosine), (2) interfere with transmitter storage (reserpine), (3) interfere with transmitter release (clonidine), (4) stimulate transmitter release (ephedrine), or (5) interfere with reuptake of transmitter (cocaine). Drugs may also (6) modify metabolism of the neurotransmitter in the synaptic cleft (anticholinesterase). Drugs acting at postjunctional sites may (7) directly stimulate postjunctional receptors and (8) interfere with transmitter agonist at the postjunctional receptor.

The ultimate response of an effector organ to an agonist or antagonist depends on (1) the drug, (2) its plasma concentration, (3) the number of receptors in the effector organ, (4) binding by the receptor, (5) the concurrent activities of other drugs and hormones, (6) the cellular metabolic status, and (7) reflex adjustments by the organism.

Ganglionic Drugs

SNS and PNS ganglia are pharmacologically similar in that transmission through these ANS ganglia is effected by ACh (Fig. 15-2). Most ganglionic agonists and antagonists are not selective and affect SNS and PNS ganglia equally. This nonselective property creates many undesirable and unpredictable side effects, which have limited the clinical usefulness of this category of drug.

Agonists

There are essentially no clinically useful ganglionic agonists. Nicotine is the prototypical ganglionic agonist. In low doses, it stimulates ANS ganglia and the neuromuscular junction of striated muscle. High doses produce ganglionic and neuromuscular blockade. The protean side effects of nicotinic stimulation render it useful only as an investigative tool.

Antagonists

Drugs that interfere with neurotransmission at ANS ganglia are known as *ganglionic blocking agents*. Nicotine in high doses is the prototypical ganglionic blocking agent also; however, early stimulatory nicotinic activity can be blocked both at the ganglia and muscle end plates with other ganglionic blockers and muscle relaxants, respectively, without blocking muscarinic effects. Ganglionic blockers produce their nicotinic effects by competing, mimicking, or interfering with ACh metabolism. Hexamethonium, trimethaphan, and pentolinium produce a selective nondepolarizing blockade of neurotransmission at ANS ganglia without producing nicotinic neuromuscular blockade. They compete with ACh in the ganglia without stimulating the receptors. The introduction of drugs that produce vasodilation directly or by action on the SNS vasomotor center has made the ganglionic blockers obsolete. d-Tubocurare produces a competitive nondepolarizing block of both motor end plates and ANS ganglia. The action of motor paralysis predominates, but the concomitant ganglionic blockade at higher doses explains part of the hypotensive effect often seen with the use of d-tubocurare for muscle relaxation. Anticholinesterase drugs may produce nicotinic type ganglionic blockade by competition with ACh as well as by persistent depolarization via accumulated ACh.

Trimethaphan produces blockade by competition with ACh for receptors, thus stabilizing the postsynaptic membrane. However, side effects and rapid onset tachyphylaxis have markedly reduced its use in anesthesia.[26] The patient's pupils become fixed and dilated during administration, which obscures eye signs, an important consideration for neurosurgery. In this regard, it is distinctly inferior to nitroprusside. The major advantage of trimethaphan is its short duration of action, which is the result of pseudocholinesterase hydrolysis.

Cholinergic Drugs

Muscarinic Agonists

The cholinomimetic muscarinic drugs act at sites in the body where ACh is the neurotransmitter of the nerve impulse. These drugs may be divided into three groups, the first two of which are direct muscarinic agonists. The third group acts indirectly. These groups are choline esters (ACh, methacholine, carbamylcholine, bethanechol), alkaloids (pilocarpine, muscarine), and anticholinesterases (physostigmine, neostigmine, pyridostigmine, edrophonium, echothiophate).

Direct Cholinomimetics. ACh has virtually no therapeutic applications because of its diffuse action and rapid hydrolysis by cholinesterase (see Fig. 15-5). One may encounter the use of topical ACh (1%) drops during cataract extraction when a rapid miosis is desired. Systemic effects are not usually seen because of the rapidity of ACh hydrolysis. Derivatives of ACh, other choline esters have been synthesized, which possess more

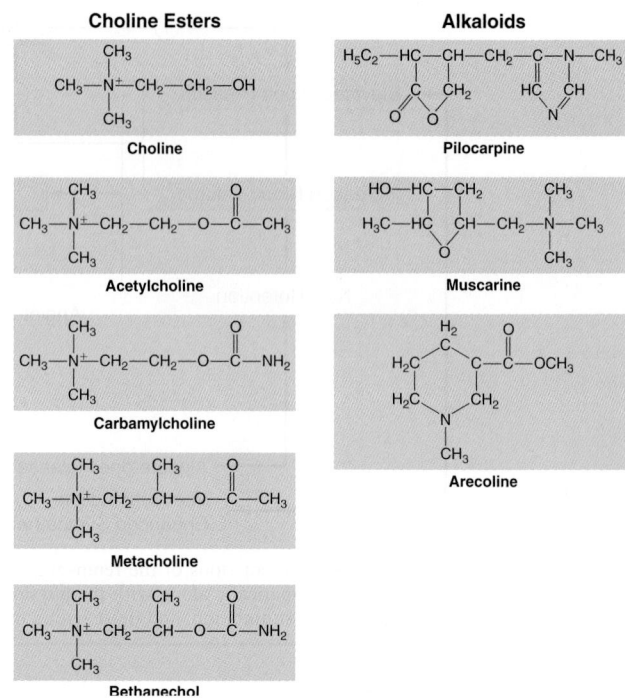

FIGURE 15.13. Chemical structures of direct-acting cholinomimetic esters and alkaloids.

selective muscarinic activity than ACh. They differ from ACh in being more resistant to inactivation by cholinesterase and thus having a more prolonged and useful action. They also differ from ACh in their relative muscarinic and nicotinic activities. The best studied of these drugs are methacholine, bethanechol, and carbamylcholine. The chemical structures of ACh and these choline esters are shown in Figure 15-13. Their pharmacologic actions are compared with those of ACh in Table 15-5. These are not important drugs in anesthesiology practice but anesthesiologists may encounter patients who are receiving them.

ACh is a quaternary ammonium compound that interacts with postsynaptic receptors, causing conformational membrane changes. This results in increased permeability to small ions and, thus, depolarization. All the receptors translate the reversible binding of ACh into openings of discrete channels in excitable membranes, allowing Na^+ and K^+ ions to flow along their electrochemical gradients. Structure-activity relationships point to the presence of two important binding sites on the receptor, an esteratic site that binds the ester end of the molecule and an ionic site that binds the quaternary amine portion (Fig. 15-5). Subtle changes in the structure of the compound can markedly alter the responses among different tissue groups. The degree of muscarinic activity falls if the acetyl group is replaced, but this confers a resistance to enzymatic hydrolysis. Bethanechol is resistant to hydrolysis but possesses mainly muscarinic activity. β-Methyl substitution produces methacholine, which is less resistant to hydrolysis and is primarily a muscarinic agonist. Methacholine slows the heart and dilates peripheral blood vessels. It is used to terminate supraventricular tachydysrhythmias, especially paroxysmal tachycardia, when other measures have failed. It also increases intestinal tone. Methacholine should not be given to patients with asthma. Hypertensive patients may also develop marked hypotension. Side effects are those of PNS stimulation such as nausea, vomiting, and flushed sweating. Overdose is treated with atropine. Bethanechol is relatively selective for the

TABLE 15-5

COMPARATIVE MUSCARINIC ACTIONS OF DIRECT CHOLINOMIMETIC AGENTS

	SYSTEMIC				
	ACETYL-CHOLINE	METHA-CHOLINE	CARBAMYL-CHOLINE	BETHANECHOL	PILOCARPINE
Esterase Hydrolysis	+++	+	0	0	0
Eye (Topical)					
Iris	++	++	+++	+++	+++
Ciliary	++	++	+++	+++	++
Heart					
Rate	—	—	—	—	?
Contractility	—	—	—	—	
Conduction	—	—	—	—	
Smooth Muscle					
Vascular	—	—	—	—	— —
Bronchial	++	++	+	+	++
Gastrointestinal motility	++	++	+++	+++	++
Gastrointestinal sphincters	—	—	—	—	++
Biliary	++	++	+++	+++	++
Bladder					
Detrusor	++	++	+++	+++	++
Sphincter	—	—	—	—	—
Exocrine Glands					
Respiratory	+++	++	+++	++	++++
Salivary	++	++	++	++	+++++
Pharyngeal	++	++	++	++	++++
Lacrimal	++	++	++	++	++++
Sweat	++	++	++	++	+++++
Gastrointestinal acid and secretions	++	++	++	++	++++
Nicotinic Actions	+++	+	+++	—	+++

+, stimulation; –, inhibition.

gastrointestinal and urinary tracts. In usual doses it does not slow the heart or lower the blood pressure. Bethanecol is of value in treating postoperative abdominal distention (nonobstructive paralytic ileus), gastric atony following bilateral vagotomy, congenital megacolon, nonobstructive urinary retention, and some cases of neurogenic bladder.

Direct-acting cholinomimetic alkaloids include muscarine and pilocarpine. They act at the same sites as ACh, and their effects are similar to those of ACh as described in Table 15-5. There are no uses for these drugs in anesthesiology. Pilocarpine is the only drug of this group used therapeutically in the United States. Its sole use is for the treatment of glaucoma, for which it is the standard. It is used as a topical miotic drug in ophthalmologic practice to reduce intraocular pressure in glaucoma.

Muscarinic agonists are particularly dangerous in patients with myasthenia gravis (who are receiving anticholinesterases), bulbar palsy, cardiac disease, asthma, peptic ulcer, progressive muscular atrophy, or mechanical intestinal obstruction or urinary retention because they intensify these conditions.

Indirect Cholinomimetics. The indirect-acting cholinomimetic drugs are of greater importance to the anesthesiologist than are the direct-acting drugs. These drugs produce cholinomimetic effects indirectly as a result of inhibition or inactivation of the enzyme acetylcholinesterase, which normally destroys ACh by hydrolysis. They are referred to as *cholinesterase inhibitors* or *anticholinesterases*. Most of these drugs inhibit both acetyl-

cholinesterase and pseudocholinesterase. Inhibition of acetylcholinesterase permits the accumulation of ACh transmitter in the synapse, resulting in intense PNS activity similar to that of the direct cholinomimetic agents. The accumulation of ACh by the anticholinesterases potentially can produce all of the following: (1) stimulation of muscarinic receptors at ANS effect organs, (2) stimulation followed by depression of all ANS ganglia and skeletal muscle (nicotinic), and (3) stimulation with later depression of cholinergic receptor sites in the CNS. All of these effects may be seen with lethal doses of anticholinesterase drugs, but therapeutic doses only produce the first two.

Actions of therapeutic significance of the anticholinesterase drugs to the anesthesiologist concern the eye, the intestine, and the neuromuscular junction. The effects of anticholinesterases are useful in the treatment of myasthenia gravis, glaucoma, and atony of the gastrointestinal and urinary tracts. Anticholinesterase drugs are used routinely in anesthesia to reverse nondepolarizing neuromuscular block. The most prominent pharmacologic effects of the anticholinesterase drugs are muscarinic. Their most useful actions are their nicotinic effects. Muscarinic activity is evoked by lower concentrations of ACh than are necessary to produce the desired nicotinic effect. For example, the anticholinesterase neostigmine reverses neuromuscular blockade by increasing ACh concentration at the muscle end plate, a nicotinic receptor. Nicotinic reversal of neuromuscular blockade can usually be produced safely only when the patient has been protected by atropine or other muscarinic

ANATOMY AND PHYSIOLOGY

blockers. This prevents the untoward muscarinic effects of bradycardia, hypotension, bronchospasm, or intestinal spasm. Reversal of neuromuscular blockade in patients who have had bowel anastomosis was at one time a major controversy (see "Neuromuscular Blockers"). Some thought that the muscarinic effects of anticholinesterase drugs (hypermotility) increased the risk of anastomotic leakage whereas others found no association between their use and subsequent breakdown. National experience has favored the latter opinion.

⑩ Clinically, anticholinesterase drugs may be divided into two types: the reversible and nonreversible cholinesterase inhibitors.[26] Reversible cholinesterase inhibitors delay the hydrolysis of ACh from 1 to 8 hours. Nonreversible drugs are so named because their inhibitory effects may last from days to weeks. The differences in duration of various anticholinesterases apparently depend on whether they inhibit the anionic or esteratic site of acetylcholinesterase. Therefore, the anticholinesterase drugs have also been pharmacologically subdivided. Drugs that inhibit the anionic site are called *competitive inhibitors*. Their action is due to competition between the anticholinesterase and ACh for the anionic site. These drugs tend to be short-acting. Edrophonium is an example of this type. Drugs that inhibit the esteratic site are called *acid-transferring inhibitors*. These drugs include the longer-acting neostigmine, pyridostigmine, and physostigmine.

Most of the reversible cholinesterase inhibitors are quaternary ammonium compounds and do not cross the blood–brain barrier. Physostigmine is a tertiary amine that readily passes into the CNS (Fig. 15-14). It produces central muscarinic stim-

Physostigmine

Neostigmine

Edrophonium

Pyridostigmine

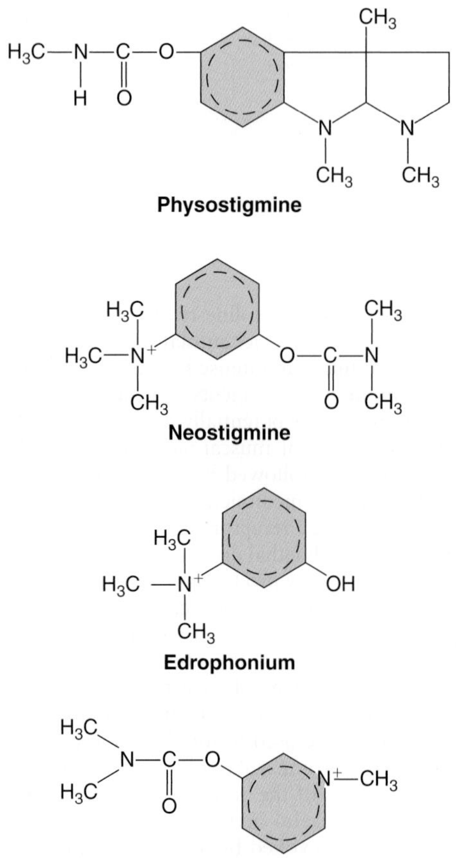

FIGURE 15.14.   Structural formulas of clinically useful reversible anticholinesterase drugs. Physostigmine is a tertiary amine and crosses the blood–brain barrier. It is useful in treating the central anticholinergic syndrome.

ulation and, thus, is not used to reverse neuromuscular blockade but can be used to treat atropine poisoning. Conversely, atropine is used to treat physostigmine poisoning. Physostigmine has also been found to be a specific antidote in the treatment of postoperative delirium (see "Central Anticholinergic Syndrome").[3]

The irreversible cholinesterase inhibitors are mostly organophosphate compounds. The organophosphate compounds are highly lipid-soluble, readily pass into the CNS, and are rapidly absorbed through the skin. They are used as the active ingredient in potent insecticides and chemical warfare agents known as *nerve gases* (see Chapter 60). The only therapeutic drug of this group is echothiophate, which is available in the form of topical drops for the treatment of glaucoma. Its primary advantage is its prolonged duration of action. Topical absorption is variable but considerable. Echothiophate can remain effective for 2 or 3 weeks following cessation of therapy. A history of use of echothiophate is important in avoiding prolonged action of succinylcholine, which requires pseudocholinesterase for its hydrolysis. Organophosphate poisoning manifests all the signs and symptoms of excess ACh. The antidote cartridges dispensed to troops to counter the effects of anticholinesterase nerve gases contain only atropine, which would effectively counter the muscarinic effects of the gas; however, atropine does little to counter the high-dose nicotinic muscle paralysis or the central ventilation depression that contributes to death from nerve gases. Treatment requires high doses of atropine, 35 to 70 mg/kg intravenously (IV) every 3 to 10 minutes until muscarinic symptoms abate. Lower doses at less frequent intervals may be required for several days. Central ventilatory depression and weakness require respiratory support and specific therapy of the cholinesterase lesion. Pralidoxime has been reported to reactivate cholinesterase activity by hydrolysis of the phosphate enzyme complex. It is particularly effective with parathion poisoning and is the only cholinesterase reactivator available in the United States.[26]

Muscarinic Antagonists

Muscarinic antagonist refers to a specific drug action for which the term *anticholinergic* is widely used. Any drug that interferes with the action of ACh as a transmitter can be considered an anticholinergic agent. The term anticholinergic refers to a broader classification that also includes the nicotinic antagonists.

Atropine-Like Drugs.   Atropine, scopolamine, and glycopyrrolate are the most commonly used muscarinic antagonists used in anesthesia (Fig. 15-15). The actions of these drugs include inhibition of salivary, bronchial, pancreatic, and gastrointestinal secretions and antagonism the muscarinic side effects of anticholinesterases during reversal of muscle relaxants. Historically, atropine was introduced to anesthesia practice to prevent excessive secretions during ether anesthesia and to prevent vagal bradycardia during the administration of chloroform.[26] Antimuscarinic agents do not inhibit transmission equally, and there are marked variations in sensitivity at different muscarinic sites owing to differences in penetration and affinities of the various receptors. Differences in relative potency between the different antimuscarinics are outlined in Table 15-6. Atropine and scopolamine are tertiary amines (Fig. 15-15) and easily penetrate the blood–brain barrier and placenta. Glycopyrrolate is a quaternary amine that, like the reversible anticholinesterase drugs, does not easily penetrate these barriers. Glycopyrrolate, a synthetic antimuscarinic, has gained popularity because it avoids the central effects of the other two drugs. Atropine and scopolamine have notable CNS effects that are dissimilar. Scopolamine differs from atropine mainly in its central depressant effects, which produce

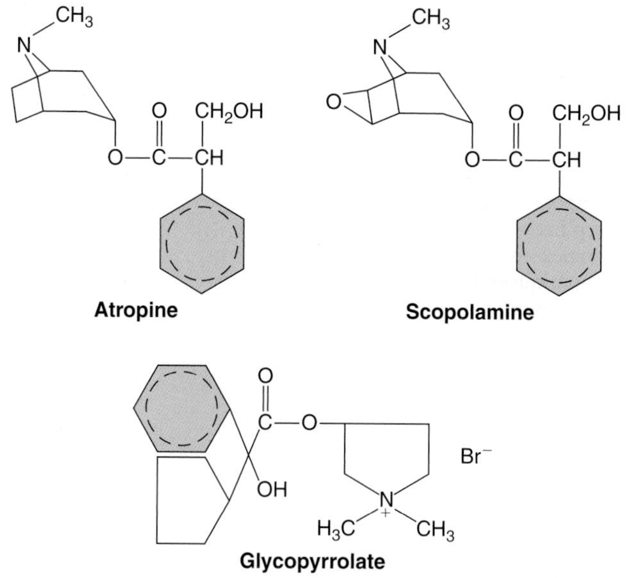

FIGURE 15.15.   Structural formulas of the clinically useful antimuscarinic drugs.

inhibition (see "Cholinergic Receptors: Muscarinic"). Atropinelike drugs that cross the blood–brain barrier also produce dilation of the pupil (mydriasis) and paralysis of accommodation (cycloplegia). Atropine-like drugs are widely used in ophthalmology as mydriatics and cycloplegics. Atropine is contraindicated in patients with narrow-angle glaucoma (see Chapter 51). Pupillary dilation thickens the peripheral part of the iris, which narrows the iridocorneal angle. This leads to impaired drainage of aqueous humor and increase of the intraocular pressure. Doses of atropine used for premedication have little effect in this regard, whereas equal doses of scopolamine cause mydriasis. Prudence would dictate avoidance of either agent in patients with narrow-angle glaucoma. The need for antimuscarinic premedication is questionable in this situation.

Atropine and scopolamine also possess antiemetic action. Atropine, however, reduces the opening pressure of the lower esophageal sphincter, which theoretically increases the risk of passive regurgitation. The belladonna alkaloids (atropine and scopolamine) also block ACh transmission to sweat glands, which, although they are cholinergic, are innervated by the SNS. Antimuscarinic agents produce antinicotinic actions at higher doses and result in important actions on CNS transmission that are pharmacologically similar to the postganglionic cholinergic function. Atropine is best avoided where tachycardia would be harmful, as may occur in thyrotoxicosis, pheochromocytoma, or obstructive coronary artery disease. Atropine should be avoided in hyperpyrexial patients because it inhibits sweating.

Central Anticholinergic Syndrome. The belladonna alkaloids have long been known to produce undesirable side effects ranging from stupor (scopolamine) to delirium (atropine). This syndrome has been called *postoperative delirium*, *atropine toxicity*, and the *central anticholinergic syndrome*. Biochemical studies have demonstrated abundant muscarinic ACh receptors in the brain that can be affected by any drug possessing antimuscarinic activity and capable of crossing the blood–brain barrier. Hundreds of drugs exist that meet these criteria with which this syndrome has been associated. Table 15-7 lists some of those drugs.[3] High doses of atropinic alkaloids rapidly produce dryness of the mouth, blurred vision with photophobia (mydriasis), hot and dry skin (flushed), and fever. Mental symptoms range from sedation, stupor, and coma to anxiety, restlessness, disorientation, hallucinations, and delirium. Convulsions may occur if lethal poisoning has occurred. Although an alarming reaction may occur, fatalities are rare. Intoxication is usually short-lived and followed by amnesia. These reactions can be controlled by the intravenous injection of physostigmine. Physostigmine is an anticholinesterase that, by virtue of being a tertiary amine, readily passes into the CNS to counter antimuscarinic activity. It should be given slowly in 1-mg doses,

sedation, amnesia, and euphoria. Such properties are widely used for premedication for cardiac patients in combination with morphine and a major tranquilizer. It also has been used to induce amnesia in patients who have a high risk for intraoperative awareness, such as trauma victims who are hemodynamically unstable and cannot receive adequate anesthesia. Atropine, as a premedicant, has slight effects on the CNS, including mild stimulation. Higher doses such as those given for reversal of muscle relaxants (1 to 2 mg) may produce restlessness, disorientation, hallucinations, and delirium (see "Central Anticholinergic Syndrome").

Atropine is useful in increasing CO when sinus bradycardia due to vagal stimulation is present. Atropine and scopolamine are noted to produce a paradoxical bradycardia when given in low doses. Scopolamine (0.1 to 0.2 mg) usually causes more slowing than atropine but also produces less cardiac acceleration at higher doses. The usual intramuscular premedicant doses of scopolamine cause either a decrease or no change in HR. Atropine may also produce sympathomimetic effects by blocking presynaptic muscarinic receptors found on adrenergic nerve terminals.[27] ACh stimulation of these receptors inhibits NE release, and blockade by atropine releases this

TABLE 15-6

COMPARISON OF ANTIMUSCARINIC DRUGS

	DURATION		CNS	GI TONE	GASTRIC ACID	AIRWAY SECRETIONS[a]	HEART RATE
	IV	IM					
Atropine	15–30 min	2–4 hr	++	--	-	--	+++[c]
Scopolamine	30–60 min	4–6 hr	+++[b]	-	-	----	−0[c]
Glycopyrrolate	2–4 hr	6–8 hr	0	---	---	---	+0

IV, intravenous; IM, intramuscular; GI, gastrointestinal.
[a]Secretions may be reduced by inspissation.
[b]CNS effect often manifest as sedation before stimulation.
[c]May decelerate initially.

TABLE 15-7

ANTIMUSCARINIC COMPOUNDS ASSOCIATED WITH CENTRAL
ANTICHOLINERGIC SYNDROME

Belladonna Alkaloids
Atropine sulfate
Scopolamine hydrobromide
**Synthetic and Natural Tertiary Amine
  Compounds**
Dicyclomine antispasmodic with local
  anesthetic activity
Thiphenamil antispasmodic with local
  anesthetic activity
Procaine
Cocaine
Cyclopentolate mydriatic
**Quaternary Derivatives of Belladonna
  Alkaloids**
Methscopolamine bromide—antispasmodic
Homatropine methylbromide—sedative,
  antispasmodic
Homatropine hydrobromide—ophthalmic
  solution—mydriatic
Synthetic Quaternary Compounds
Methantheline bromide
Propantheline bromide
Antihistamines
Chlorpheniramine
Diphenhydramine
Plants
Deadly nightshade (atropine)
Bittersweet
Potato leaves and sprouts
Jimson or loco weed
Coca plant (cocaine)

Over-the-Counter
Asthma-Dor—atropine-like
Compoz—scopolamine sedation
Sleep Eze—scopolamine sedation
Sominex—scopolamine sedation
Antiparkinson Drugs
Benztropine
Trihexphenidyl
Biperiden
Ethopropazine
Procyclidine
Antipsychotic Drugs
Chlorpromazine
Thioriazine
Haloperidol
Droperidol
Promethazine
Tricyclic Antidepressants
Amitriptyline
Imipramine
Desipramine
Synthetic Opioids
Meperidine
Methadone

not exceeding 3 mg, to avoid producing peripheral cholinergic activity. Neostigmine, pyridostigmine, and edrophonium are not effective because they cannot pass into the CNS. The duration of physostigmine action may be shorter than that of the offending antimuscarinic agent and require repeated injection if symptoms recur. Physostigmine appears safe when used within dose recommendations and when indications are established. Central disorientation alone does not establish a diagnosis. Peripheral signs of antimuscarinic activity should be present in addition to a central anticholinergic syndrome.

Physostigmine has been reported to reverse the CNS effects of many of the drugs listed in Table 15-7, including antihistamines, tricyclic antidepressants, and tranquilizers. Reversal of the sedative effects of opioids and benzodiazepines has also been reported.[28] However, anticholinesterase agents potentiate cholinergic synaptic transmission and increase neuronal activity, even if no receptor antagonist is present. Thus, arousal may not be a function independent of its cholinesterase activity, and claims that physostigmine is a nonspecific CNS stimulant may not be warranted and could, in fact, be dangerous. These considerations, in association with possible significant bradycardia, made the use of physostigmine fairly rare in the modern recovery rooms.

Sympathomimetic Drugs

The selection of vasoactive drugs requires knowledge of both the hemodynamic disturbance and pharmacology of the available drugs. The catecholamines and sympathomimetic drugs continue to be the pharmacologic mainstay of cardiovascular support for the low-flow state. Sustained interest in the catecholamines is related to their predictable pharmacodynamics and favorable pharmacokinetic profiles. The half-life of most is short, ranging from 2 to 3 minutes. Undesirable side effects dissipate within minutes of lowering or stopping the infusion. Sympathomimetics, as a group, produce a wide range of hemodynamic effects and can be used in combination to achieve a yet wider spectrum of effects. As a result, one needs to become familiar with only a few agents to manage most clinical situations (Table 15-8).

The goal for managing the low-output or high-output shock syndrome is to establish and maintain adequate tissue perfusion. Sympathomimetics are not a substitute for volume, and are to be used in hypotensive emergencies, in order to preserve cerebral and coronary blood flow, that may be due to severe hemorrhage, spinal cord injury, antihypertensive overdose, or central nervous system depressant medication, just to name a few circumstances. Therefore, while intravascular volume is optimized, a vasoactive drug may be required to sustain CO. Aggressive fluid therapy will suffice in most instances. If, on the other hand, adequate fluid resuscitation has been achieved and hemodynamic status still requires sympathomimetics to maintain a normal arterial blood pressure, one must consider alternative causes for hypotension such as septic shock, and seek the most adequate therapy. The term *inodilator* has entered our lexicon during the early 1990s to supplant the more archaic term *vasopressor*. This neologism reflects a change in philosophy in managing low-flow states, particularly those characterized by heart failure. The new synthetic sympathomimetics have been chemically engineered to obtain inotropism and

TABLE 15-8

DOSE SCHEDULE AND HEMODYNAMIC EFFECTS OF THE ADRENERGIC AGONISTS

HEMODYNAMICS (↑ INCREASE; ↓ DECREASE; — = NO CHANGE)

DRUG LISTED FROM α TO β	DOSAGES IV PUSH ADULTS	DOSAGES IV INFUSION[a]	SITE OF ACTIVITY α1A	α1V	β1	β2	DA	CO	INOTROP	HR	VR	TPR	RBF
Phenylephrine	50–100 μg	a. 10 mg/250 mL b. 40 μg/mL c. 0.15–0.75 μg/kg/min d. 0.15 μg/kg/min	+++	+++	0	0	0	→↓	—	Reflex	↑↑↑	↑↑	— →
Norepinephrine	N/R	a. 4 mg/250 mL b. 16 μg/mL c. 0.01–0.1 μg/kg/min d. 0.1 μg/kg/min	++++	++++	++++	0	0	→↓	↑	Reflex ↓	↑↑↑	↑↑↑	↓↓↓
Epinephrine	0.3–0.5 mL 1:1000 (0.3–0.5 mg) SC—Asthma IV—Anaphylaxis 5 mL 1:10,000 (0.5 mg) cardiac arrest every 5 min	a. 1 mg/250 mL b. 4 μg/mL 0.01–0.03 μg/kg/min c. 0.03–0.15 μg/kg/min 0.15–0.30 μg/kg/min d. 0.015 μg/kg/min	++ +++ ++++	++ +++ ++++	++++ ++++ +++	+++ ++ +	0	↑→	↑	Reflex ↓	↑↑↑	↑↑↑	↓↓↓
Ephedrine	5–10 mg	N/R ++	+++	+++	+++	++	0	↑↑	↑↑	↑↑	↑↑	→↑	↑
Dopamine[c]	N/R	a. 200 mg/250 mL b. 800 μg/mL 0.05–5 μg/kg/min c. 2–10 μg/kg/min 10 μg/kg/min[b] d. 2 μg/kg/min	+→++++	+→++++	+++	+	↑↑	↑↑ —↑ ↑↑	↑↑↑ ↑↑↑ ↑	↑↑ ↑↑ ↑	↑↑ ↑↑ ↑	↓↓ ↑↑ ↑↑↑	↑ ↑→ ↑
Dobutamine[c]	N/R	a. 250 mg/250 mL b. 1,000 μg/mL c. 2–30 μg/kg/min d. 5 μg/kg/min	+	+	++++	++	0	↑↑	↑	↑	→↓	→↓	↑→
Isoproterenol	0.004 mg (0.2 mL of 0.2 mg/mL solution) Third-degree heart block	a. 1 mg/250 mL b. 4 μg/mL c. 0.15 μg/kg/min to desired effect d. 0.015 μg/kg/min	0–+	?	++++	+++	0	↑↑ →↑ ↑↑	↑ ↑↑ —	—↑ ↑↑ —	— — ↓↓	→↑ —↑ ↑	↑ ↑ →

IV, intravenous; DA, dopamine; CO, cardiac output; Inotrop, contractility; HR, heart rate; VR, venous return (preload); TPR, peripheral resistance (afterload); RBF, renal blood flow; N/R, not recommended.

[a]a. Mixture
b. Concentration μg/mL.
c. Dose range μg/kg/min.
d. Standard rate infusion.
[b]"Rule of six."
[c]Dopamine and dobutamine employ the same doses. Dosage of either may quickly be calculated by multiplying patient's weight (kg) × 6 = mg added to 100 mL D5%W. The number of drops delivered through a calibrated infusor (60 drops = 1 mL) is the number of μg/kg/min infused into the patient. Example: 70 kg × 6 = 420; 420 mg/100 mL = 4,200 μg/kg or 70 μg gtt; 5 μg/kg/min = 5 gtt/min.
From Lawson NW, Wallfisch HK: Cardiovascular pharmacology: A new look at the "pressors," Advances in Anesthesia. Edited by Stoelting RK, Barash PG, Gallagher TJ. Chicago, Year Book Medical Publishers, 1986, p 195, with permission.

TABLE 15-9

ACTIONS OF ADRENERGIC AGONISTS

■ SYMPATHO-MIMETICS	■ RECEPTORS						■ DOSE DEPENDENCE (α, β, or DA)
	■ α_1	■ α_2	■ β_1	■ β_2	■ DA$_1$	■ DA$_2$	
Phenylephrine	+++++	?	±	0	0		++
Norepinephrine	+++++	+++++	+++	0	0		+++
Epinephrine	+++++	+++	++++	++	0		++++
Ephedrine	++	?	+++	++	0		++
Dopamine	+ to +++++	?	++++	++	+++	?	+++++
Dobutamine	0 to +	?	++++	++	0		++
Isoproterenol	0	0	+++++	+++++	0		0

DA, dopamine.

vasodilation rather than for pressor effects. The potential for benefit or harm can best be understood in terms of receptor characteristics. For example, activation of the inotropic β_1 and β_2 receptors results in positive inotropism and chronotropism. Selective stimulation of the vascular β_2 receptors causes vasodilatation. Left ventricular outflow may improve as a function of afterload reduction and inotropism. However, chronotropism may not be a desirable feature in a patient with mitral (valvular) stenosis or coronary artery disease.

Catecholamine Receptor-Effector Coupling

11 The net physiologic effect of a sympathomimetic is usually defined as the algebraic sum of its relative actions on the α, β, and DA receptors. Most adrenergic drugs activate or block these receptors to varying degrees. Each catecholamine has a distinctive effect, qualitatively and quantitatively, on the myocardium and peripheral vasculature. Table 15-9 demonstrates the relative potency of the adrenergic amines on the various myocardial and vascular receptors. This relative potency is also dose-related, adding yet another variable. For many years, the emphasis on catecholamines was focused almost entirely on their actions on the myocardium and on arteriolar resistance vessels. Changes in venous resistance contribute little to total vascular resistance and blood pressure. However, small changes in venous capacitance result in large changes in venous return because 60 to 70% of the circulating blood volume is the venous circulation.[4] The effect of the sympathomimetic amines on the venous circulation appears to be distributive in that acute venular constriction increases the central blood volume (preload), whereas dilatation decreases venous return by the promotion of peripheral pooling.[4] The distributive effect of a catecholamine may be as important as its inotropic action and more important than its arteriolar effect.[10] Further definition should elucidate some of the complex and confusing data in the literature generated when clinical observations are limited solely to adrenergic effects on the myocardium and arteriolar vasculature.

Intravenous and intra-arterial infusions of EPI in humans have been shown to cause marked constriction of the veins. Arteriolar vasoconstriction may or may not precede venoconstriction; however, stroke volume does not increase until the onset of venoconstriction. The initial increase in CO seen with the infusion of EPI is more an effect of increased preload than an arteriolar or direct cardiac effect. NE produces a similar effect, but the onset of venoconstriction is slower. The peripheral receptors of both resistance and capacitance vessels subserve vasoconstriction, but with divergent effects on afterload and preload; therefore, the α_1 receptors have been subdivided into α_1 arterial (α_{1a})

and α_1 venous (α_{1v}). DA has potent venoconstrictor (α_{1v}) effect at doses at which few α_{1a} or β_1 effects are noted.

Adverse Effects

The major adverse effects of the sympathomimetic amines are related to excessive α or β activity. The potential for harm can be understood in terms of receptor characteristics. Excessive β_1 activity may increase contractility but increase HR and myocardial oxygen consumption beyond supply. Severe dysrhythmias are a frequent companion of excess β_1 activity as a result of increased conduction velocity, automaticity, and ischemia. The β_2 activity has the potential to increase CO by reducing resistance (afterload) while reducing blood pressure. An excessive decrease in diastolic pressure, however, reduces coronary perfusion pressure and may further aggravate myocardial ischemia. Unfortunately, it is difficult to separate the inotropic, dromotropic, and chronotropic effects in the clinical setting. The characteristics of the ideal positive inotropic agent are listed in Table 15-9 for comparison with each drug as it is discussed.

Drugs with prominent α_1 agonist effects may produce an increase in blood pressure but at the same time can reduce total flow due to increases in arteriolar resistance (afterload). A more prominent α_1 venous constriction may improve CO by increasing preload or precipitate failure if preload exceeds the contractile limits of the myocardium. In general, the α effects of the sympathomimetics are of benefit only when used for specific indications such as significant vasodilation due to different mechanisms. Other measures like fluid resuscitation are usually more effective in improving flow and are indicated before a pressor should be used. Cardiopulmonary resuscitation is the primary example where a pressor effect is necessary to create diastolic coronary perfusion during closed or open heart massage. Any drug with strong α agonist properties seems equally effective in this regard. EPI, with its added β properties, has been the first-line agent for this situation. Vasopressin has recently been added as an important agent in cardiopulmonary resuscitation.[29]

Adrenergic Agonists

Phenylephrine. Tables 15-8 and 15-9 list adrenergic agonists to be discussed in this section. Phenylephrine, is considered a pure α drug, increases both venous constriction and arterial constriction in a dose-related manner. Venous constriction may be its most redeeming feature when compared with the purely arteriolar effect of methoxamine. One cannot discount the possibility of an inotropic effect now that α_1 receptors are known to exist in the myocardium. Acutely, venoconstriction favors venous return (preload), and even though arterial resistance (afterload) also increases, one may observe a rise in the arterial blood pressure. Because phenylephrine does increase the venous return and stroke volume, but at the same time induces reflex bradycardia secondary to a vagal reflex, one must be aware that CO is not increased. Phenylephrine does not change CO in normal individuals but can cause a decreased output in patients with ischemic heart disease.[30] Phenylephrine is useful in reversing right-to-left shunt in tetralogy of Fallot when patients are having "spells" during anesthesia. Phenylephrine has continued to be favored in operating rooms to increase blood pressure during cardiopulmonary bypass as well as during intracranial, vascular procedures and to reverse significant vasodilatory states related to regional blocks like spinal and epidural analgesia. Its efficacy, the fact that it can be used either as a bolus, or as a peripheral infusion, made this drug one of the most commonly used medications in the operating room to reverse anesthetic hypotension from a multitude of causes. In addition, it can be used in primary vasodilatory conditions, such as incipient phases of septic shock.[31]

Norepinephrine. NE is the naturally occurring mediator of the SNS and the immediate precursor of EPI. It produces direct-acting hemodynamic effects on the α and β receptors in a dose-related manner when given by infusion. NE produces increased CO and blood pressure when given in low doses (Table 15-8). Higher doses reduce flow because α arteriolar constriction supersedes the β effects. Reflex baroreceptor-mediated bradycardia may occur despite active β stimulation. Increased plasma levels of the endogenous catecholamines NE and EPI are the sympathetic milieu in which exogenous sympathomimetics are ordinarily given. NE is the catecholamine standard against which other catecholamines are compared. Intravenous NE has received an unseemly reputation over the years that is not merited. Studies indicate that NE was being used in doses that are orders of magnitude greater than that necessary to obtain its best response. Complications such as tissue necrosis may be expected when NE is used. A resurgence of interest in this agent is noted and it has remained clinically useful because its effects are predictable, prompt, and potent. Objections to the use of NE for the treatment of cardiogenic shock are based on two considerations: (1) vasoconstriction increases the pressure work of the left ventricle, with an adverse effect on the oxygen economy of the ischemic pump, and (2) these drugs cause further vasoconstriction and organ ischemia in a syndrome in which intense constriction may already have occurred. For management of cardiogenic shock, other drugs are more appropriate (dobutamine and milrinone). However, the predictability of NE pharmacologic effects makes it one of the most useful drugs when intense α activity is intended. Reduced vascular tone states with or without cardiogenic shock, including separation from cardiopulmonary bypass, or situations when other vasopressors such as phenylephrine fail to maintain a steady hemodynamic state, render NE one of the most commonly used drugs.[10,32] Additional undesirable effects associated with NE include renal arteriolar constriction and oliguria. These effects are secondary to persistent and untreated hypovolemia. Recently, clinicians who manage oliguria in intensive care units, after adequate fluid resuscitation to control prerenal causes, do use NE to maintain renal perfusion pressure, especially in cases of vasodilated hypotension.[33]

NE should only be administered in a centrally placed IV to avoid tissue necrosis from extravasation. It can be used for its inotropic effect at low doses and titrated to effect while monitoring CO. Monitoring of blood pressure alone, or titrating to a predetermined effect, is often detrimental to CO. Blood pressure increases are usually due to increases in systemic vascular resistance, and excessive increases of the afterload can diminish forward flow and contribute to cardiac failure. Even moderate doses of NE may have a detrimental effect on end-organ perfusion, which has given the drug an ill-gotten reputation when used to titrate to pressure rather than flow. However, in those clinical conditions characterized by high-ouput, low-tone states with a low perfusion pressure, NE has been shown to improve renal and splanchnic blood flow by increasing pressure, provided the patient has been volume resuscitated.

Epinephrine. EPI is the prototypical endogenous catecholamine. It is synthesized, stored, and released from the adrenal medulla and is the key hormonal element in the fight-or-flight response. It is the most widely used catecholamine in medicine and, to date, it remains the drug of choice in cases of cardiac arrest. It is used to treat asthma, anaphylaxis, cardiac arrest, bleeding, and to prolong regional anesthesia. The cardiovascular effects of EPI, when given systemically, result from its direct stimulation of both α and β receptors. This is dose-dependent and is outlined in Table 15-8.

The effect of EPI on the peripheral vasculature is mixed. It has predominantly α-stimulating effects in some beds (skin, mucosa, and kidney) and β-stimulating actions in others (skeletal muscle). These effects are also dose-dependent. At therapeutic doses, β-adrenergic effects predominate in the peripheral vessels, and total resistance may be reduced. However, constriction is maintained in the renal and cutaneous areas because of its dominant α effect in these areas. An increase in CO with EPI may be due to a redistribution of blood to low-resistance vessels in the muscle, but with further reduction in flow to vital organs. Cardiac dysrhythmias are a prominent hazard, and the strong chronotropic effects of EPI have limited its use in the treatment of cardiogenic shock.

EPI is commonly used in the perioperative period in anesthesia. It is often used to produce a bloodless field in dentistry, otolaryngology, and skin grafting either topically or in local and field blocks. Anesthesiologists often use it to prolong regional anesthesia (see Chapter 21). The addition of EPI to arthroscopic infusions to attain a bloodless field is another area of increased EPI usage with the development of these techniques. These infusions are usually safe in maintaining a dry operative field because the solutions are very dilute at around 1:3,000,000. However, the large volumes infused, the unpredictable absorption of the EPI, especially in denuded cancellous bone, offers the opportunity of exposure of the patient to an excessive amount of EPI over a short period despite the dilution. The dose of submuscoally injected EPI necessary to produce ventricular cardiac dysrhythmia in 50% of patients anesthetized with a 1.25 minimal alveolar concentration (MAC) of a volatile anesthetic was 10.9, 10.9, and 6.7 μg/kg during administration of halothane, enflurane, and isoflurane, respectively.[34] The incidence of cardiac dysrhythmia is eliminated when this dose is halved in patients anesthetized with halothane or isoflurane. In contrast with adults, children seem to tolerate higher doses of subcutaneous EPI without developing cardiac dysrhythmia.[35] EPI infusion maintains positive chronotropism in circumstances of symptomatic bradycardia when single doses of atropine do not suffice.[36] At low doses, the use of EPI infusion may also induce a benefic bronchodilation effects due to its effect on β_2 receptors. Nevertheless, EPI can be used at higher doses, which induces a significant increase in the arterial blood pressure and CO. Unfortunately, these relative high doses of EPI can be followed by increases in arrhythmogenic properties, including supraventricular and tachycardia, which impose an increase in the myocardial oxygen consumption; therefore, many clinicians find other alternatives.[36]

ANATOMY AND PHYSIOLOGY

TABLE 15-10

COMPARISON OF RELATIVE α_1 CATECHOLAMINE RESPONSES ON PERIPHERAL RESISTANCE AND CAPACITANCE VESSELS[a]

	■ VASOCONSTRICTION	
	■ α_1 ARTERIAL (α_{1a})	■ α_1 VENOUS (α_{1v})
Norepinephrine	+++++	++++
Phenylephrine	++++	+++++
Epinephrine	0/++++[b]	0/++++[b]
Dopamine	0/++++[c]	+++
Ephedrine	++	+++
Dobutamine	+/0	?
Isoproterenol	0	0

[a]Drugs are listed in descending order of potency within each vascular region.
[b]Dose-dependent; β effects of epinephrine predominate at low doses.
[c]Dose-dependent; dopamine and β effects predominate at low doses.
Reprinted with permission from Lawson NW, Wallfisch HK: Cardiovascular pharmacology: A new look at the "pressors," Advances in Anesthesia. Edited by Stoelting RK, Barash PG, Gallagher TJ. Chicago, Year Book Medical Publishers, 1986, p 195.

Ephedrine. Ephedrine is one of the most commonly used noncatecholamine sympathomimetic agents. It is used extensively for treating hypotension following spinal or epidural anesthesia. Ephedrine stimulates both α and β receptors by direct and indirect actions. It is predominantly an indirect-acting pressor, producing its effects by causing NE release. Tachyphylaxis develops rapidly and is probably related to the depletion of NE stores with repeated injection. The cardiovascular effects of ephedrine (Table 15-8) are nearly identical to those of EPI, but are less potent. Its effects are sustained about 10 times longer than those of EPI. Ephedrine remains the pressor of choice in obstetrics because uterine blood flow improves linearly with blood pressure (see Chapter 43).[23] This effect is probably not related to its arteriolar vasoconstriction but rather to its venoconstrictive action. Ephedrine is a weak, indirect-acting sympathomimetic agent that produces venoconstriction to a greater degree than arteriolar constriction (Table 15-10). This may be its most important and unappreciated effect. It causes a redistribution of blood centrally, improves venous return (preload), increases CO, and restores uterine perfusion. The mild β action restores HR simultaneously with improved venous return. An increased blood pressure is noted as a result rather than a cause of these events. Mild α_1-arteriolar constriction does occur, but the net effect of improving venous return and HR is increased CO. Uterine blood flow is spared. This response, however, depends on the patient's state of hydration.

Isoproterenol. Isoproterenol is a potent balanced β_1 and β_2 receptor agonist with no vasoconstrictor effects. It increases HR and contractility while decreasing systemic vascular resistance. Although it can increase CO, it is not useful in shock because it redistributes blood to nonessential areas by its preferential effect on the cutaneous and muscular vessels. As a result, it produces variable and unpredictable results on CO and blood pressure. Isoproterenol is a potent dysrhythmogenic drug and extends myocardial ischemic areas. Deleterious effects on an evolving cardiac ischemic process include cardiac dysrhythmias, tachycardia, and reduced diastolic coronary perfusion pressure and time. Increased myocardial oxygen demand makes it an unattractive drug for patients in cardio-

genic shock. However, isoproterenol is helpful in managing cardiac failure associated with bradycardia, asthma, and cor pulmonale. It is also a useful chemical pacemaker in third-degree heart block until an artificial pacemaker can be inserted or the cause can be removed, and may be one of the most important drugs used for denervated heart in cases of significant bradycardia (see Chapter 54). Isoproterenol might be useful in treating both idiopathic and secondary pulmonary hypertension. It has also been reported as useful in improving the forward flow in patients with regurgitant aortic valvular disease, but it should not be used if there is an accompanying stenosis.

Dobutamine. Dobutamine (DBT) is a synthetic catecholamine modified from the classic inodilator isoproterenol. Isoproterenol was, in turn, synthesized from DA. Variations and similarities in structure can be seen in Figure 15-6. DBT has clear advantages over isoproterenol and DA in many clinical situations. It acts directly on β_1 receptors but exerts much weaker β_2 stimulation than isoproterenol. It does not cause NE release or stimulate DA receptors. DBT possesses weak α_1 agonism, which can be unmasked by beta-blockade as a prompt and dramatic increase in blood pressure. DBT increases HR more than EPI for a given increase in CO.[32,37]

DBT may decrease diastolic coronary filling pressure because of its vasodilation. However, it appears to produce coronary vasodilation in contrast to the constriction produced by DA. Dobutamine has been used effectively to improve coronary flow to differentiate, by echocardiography, responsive or unresponsive areas of dyskinesia in patients following myocardial infarction. DBT does not have any clinically important venoconstrictor activity, in contrast to DA, in which an increase in ventricular filling pressure can be noted at low doses. Clinical studies suggest that DBT is less likely to increase HR than DA for a given dose, a major concern in the patient with coronary artery disease. DBT is a coronary artery dilator, whereas DA is not. A DA-induced tachycardia, however, may be of less concern in the septic patient who commonly has a maldistribution of volume, low vascular resistance, a pre-existing refractory tachycardia, but a

TABLE 15-11

AUTONOMIC EFFECTS OF CALCIUM ENTRY BLOCKERS IN INTACT HUMANS

	■ VERAPAMIL	■ DILTIAZEM	■ NIFEDIPINE
Negative inotropic	+	0/+	0
Negative chronotropic	+	0/+	0
Negative dromotropic	++++	+++	0
Coronary vasodilation	++	+++	++++
Systemic vasodilation	++	++	++++
Bronchodilation	0/+		0/+

previously healthy heart. The empiric preference of DA in surgical units and DBT in coronary units has been observed and is perhaps well founded. DA and DBT also have contrasting effects on the pulmonary vasculature. DA has been noted to increase pulmonary artery pressure and does not inhibit the pulmonary hypoxic response. It is not recommended for patients in right heart failure. DBT does vasodilate the pulmonary vasculature and is helpful in treating right heart failure and cor pulmonale.[38,39] DBT is highly controllable, with a half-life of 2 minutes. Tachyphylaxis is rare but may be noted if given over 72 hours. The net hemodynamic effects of DBT include an increase in CO, a decrease in left ventricular filling pressure, and a decrease in systemic vascular resistance without a significant increase in chronotropism at lower doses.[40]

Dopamine.   DA offers advantages over many sympathomimetics in treating the low-output syndrome. It is a dose-related agonist to all three types of adrenoceptors, and the desired action can be selected by changing the infusion rate. The DA receptors are most sensitive followed by the β, and then α receptors. DA dosage regimens have been traditionally, and arbitrarily, divided into low, medium, and high doses according to its dose-receptor sensitivity (Table 15-11). Renal and mesenteric vascular dilatation and tubular cell natriuresis are mediated through the DA receptors at low-dose infusion rates of 0.5 to 2.0 μg/kg. This is often referred to as *renal dose* DA because of the purported enhanced renal blood flow and diuresis. However, the concept of renal dose DA may be more imagined than real, and is now considered outdated.[41,42] The hemodynamic effects of low-dose DA are primarily related to vasodilatation by activation of the DA_1 and DA_2 receptors. Activation of presynaptic DA_2 adrenoceptors adds to the vasodilating effect of the DA_1 receptors by inhibiting presynaptic NE release in the renal and mesenteric vessels. The reduction of total systemic vascular resistance would be significant when one considers that 25% of the CO goes to the kidneys alone. A reduced diastolic blood pressure is often noted with a slight reflex increase in HR. Increasing the infusion rate of DA to 2 to 5 μg/kg/min begins to activate β receptors increasing the CO by increasing chronotropism and contractility with early venoconstriction (preload) and systemic vasodilatation (afterload reduction). Blood pressure may not increase despite significant increases in CO. This dose range would appear optimal for managing congestive heart and lung failure because it combines inotropism and afterload reduction with possible diuresis, but for this specific reason, inotropes without α activity are better used. Further increases in dose activate α receptors, which will increase vascular resistance and blood pressure, but further improvements in CO may be attenuated. Infusion rates of greater than 10 μg/kg/min produce intense α activity, which may override any beneficial DA or β vasodilation effect on total flow. High-dose DA behaves much like NE and, in fact, causes NE release at this dose range.

Despite the apparent dose-response divisions of DA, a wide variability of individual responses has been noted. The α-adrenergic effects can be seen in some individuals in doses as low as 5 μg/kg/min, whereas doses as high as 20 μg/kg/min may be required to obtain this effect in shocked patients. This wide variation in dose response has led to a re-examination of DA as a primary adrenergic for patients in cardiogenic shock or failure. Increased venous return may not be desirable in this situation, but DA's hemodynamic versatility continues to be useful in cardiogenic shock when combined with other complementary catecholamines such as DBT. The venoconstriction, or distributive effects, of DA are useful in surgical patients in whom third-space edema and sepsis are the most common abnormalities. DA increases mean pulmonary arterial pressure and is not recommended for sole support in patients with right heart failure, adult respiratory distress syndrome, or pulmonary hypertension.

Combination Therapy.   The studied use of adrenergic combinations in patients with cardiac failure has been proposed because pathophysiology cannot be approached with the attitude that β agonism is all good and β agonism is all bad. The objective is to increase coronary perfusion and CO while decreasing afterload. No single vasoactive agent can achieve this, but these conditions can be approached with combination therapy. Because of receptor summation during combination therapy, standard rates of infusion (as outlined in Table 15-8) no longer apply. Invasive hemodynamic monitoring is mandatory for success; otherwise, iatrogenic disasters can be expected. Other conditions necessary for success with vasoactive drugs also require that the failing myocardium or vasculature must have functional reserve, the reserve can be stimulated, and perfusion can be maintained. The adrenergic effects of combined sympathomimetics, like the solo drugs, also appear to be additive and competitive for receptor sites. Summation is more consistent with current receptor pharmacology and can be used to advantage in avoiding unwanted side effects of one drug while supplementing its desired attributes with another. The summation principle obviates the necessity of knowing a large number of drugs. One need only become familiar with a few agents to manage most clinical situations. Because of summation, many combinations of vasoactive drugs have been found useful in making fine hemodynamic adjustments in the critically ill. The available sympathomimetic agents provide a wide range of hemodynamic effects particularly when combined with vasodilators. For example, if a larger positive inotropic action and less vasoconstriction are desired, DBT could be added to DA. Also, nitroprusside could be added to DA or combined with any other appropriate inodilator.[43]

DA and DBT are two of the most popular inodilators in use today. A comparison of these two drugs will underscore the importance of the extracardiac side effects in selecting a drug either for use alone or in combination.[39,44-46] This comparison is particularly appropriate because DA and DBT are considered equipotent inotropic agents, and are effective in the same dose range of 2 to 15 μg/kg/min. Their differences can be compared at low (0.5 to 4 μg/kg/min), medium (5 to 9 μg/kg/min), and high (10 to 15 μg/kg/min) doses. This comparison will illustrate the divergent effects of two drugs on preload and afterload while sharing the property of inotropism. Although they share several clinical indications, these drugs are pharmacologically distinct and not interchangeable. Their divergent properties, however, make them particularly valuable when administered in combination. Although frequently combined previously, this combination therapy is falling out of favor since they act on the same receptors and they have so many similarities of action. Therefore, most clinicians now combine an inotrope, such as DBT or milrinone, with the more potent α agonists phenylephrine, NE, or even EPI infusions, in order to compensate for the vasodilation induced by the inotropes, and to maintain an adequate perfusion pressure. DBT is a direct-acting catecholamine that produces a positive inotropic β_1 effect but with minimal changes in β_2 HR or vascular resistance (β_2, α_1 counteraction). Thus, DBT may not alter blood pressure even though CO is markedly improved (see Chapter 10).

DBT and/or milrinone are the mainstay for the treatment of decompensated cardiac failure. Although these agents do improve the CO, their use is associated with increase in the cardiac oxygen consumption, cardiac arrhythmias, and even mortality. Therefore, for patients with normal blood pressure and no evidence of hypoperfusion, there is little role for the inotropic therapy. Nevertheless, in patients with evidence of impaired organ perfusion (hypotension, decreased renal function) and low-output state, with or without congestion or pulmonary edema refractory to diuretics and vasodilators at optimal doses, there is a role for these agents, at least for short-term stabilization. Recently, a new class of drugs was developed, namely calcium sensitizing agents (levosimendan). These drugs are a unique class of positive inotropic agents that increase the sensitivity of the cardiomyocyte contractile apparatus to intracellular calcium. These may prove to be beneficial either alone or in combination with the classic inotropes in management of decompensated heart failure, but more studies are necessary to evaluate their overall benefit and long-term outcome.[45,46]

Fenoldopam. Fenoldopam, a benzazepine derivative, is a selective DA$_1$ agonist with no α or β receptor activity compared to DA[41] (see Chapter 56). Intravenous fenoldopam has direct natriuretic and diuretic properties and promotes an increase in creatinine clearance. It offers advantages in the acute resolution of severe hypertension compared to sodium nitroprusside, particularly if the patient has pre-existing renal impairment.[47] Preservation or augmentation of renal blood flow during blood pressure reduction presents a potential for use during several situations in the perioperative period. Fenoldopam has an elimination half-life of 5 minutes. This property might well lend itself in the producing hypotensive anesthesia while preserving renal function. Human studies have demonstrated that fenoldopam is a potent direct renal vasodilator. Intravenous fenoldopam may prove to be ideal for treating conditions in which renal vasoconstriction is an expected complication. Since it has renal vasodilatory effects and it promotes increased urine output, fenoldopam has been employed in vascular anesthesia as a renal protector, especially in cases when renal arteries have been temporarily clamped. Its role in preventing development of renal dysfunction is still debatable because there are conflicting results in different studies. Therefore, Stone et al.[48] and Zacharias et al.[49] show in a 315-patient population that fenoldopam is not useful in preventing further deterioration of the renal function after contrast administration. A large meta-analysis concluded that there is no pharmacologic intervention that is effective in treat-

ment of patients with acute renal injury. On the other hand, Landoni et al.,[50] in a more recent and complete meta-analysis, suggest that fenoldopam reduces the risk of acute tubular necrosis, the need for renal replacement therapy, and overall mortality in patients with acute kidney injury. It is obvious that in such circumstances of conflicting results, large randomized studies are necessary to reach a valid conclusion.

The onset of action with IV fenoldopam is about 5 minutes, reaching a steady state in about 20 minutes. The drug is rapidly metabolized in the liver and excreted in the urine. The elimination half-life is about 5 minutes. There has been no evidence of tolerance in reducing blood pressure for up to 24 hours. No rebound on withdrawal has been noted. The most common adverse effects of fenoldopam are related to vasodilation, which include hypotension, flushing, dizziness, headache, and increases in HR, nausea, and hypokalemia have occurred. It should be used cautiously in patients with glaucoma as it can increase intraocular pressure. No significant drug interactions have been reported. Concomitant use with beta-blockers will reduce the effective dose of fenoldopam.

Fenoldopam is diluted in normal saline or 5% dextrose is given by continuous infusion without a bolus dose. The effective dosage range is 0.1 to 1.6 μg/kg/min. A reflex tachycardia may be produced. The dosage is titrated upward every 15 minutes according to patient response. Any change in infusion rate should be detectable within 15 minutes.

Clonidine. Clonidine is a centrally acting selective partial α_2 adrenergic agonist (220:1 α_2 to α_1). It is an antihypertensive drug because of its ability to decrease central sympathetic outflow. Stimulation of α_2 receptors in the vasomotor centers of the medulla oblongata is thought to produce this effect.[51] It is not clear whether these are pre-or postsynaptic receptors; however, the end result is decreased SNS tone and enhanced vagal tone. Peripherally, there is decreased plasma renin activity as well as decreased EPI and NE levels. This drug has been proven to be effective in the treatment of severe hypertension and renin-dependent hypertensive disease.

Clonidine is not available for IV use. The usual daily adult oral dose is 0.2 to 0.3 mg. A transdermal clonidine patch is available for use on a weekly basis for surgical patients unable to take oral medication. Clonidine is clinically useful in anesthesiology in other ways. It has been found to produce dose-dependent analgesia when introduced into the epidural or subarachnoid space in doses of 150 to 450 μg (see Chapter 57). Clonidine can be added to local anesthetics for epidural, spinal, or regional blocks, and therefore intensifies the anesthesia. It can also be used postoperatively as it reduces the dose of other regional anesthetic components, and subsequently the possible side effects. One must be aware that clonidine can produce hypotension, bradycardia, and sedation.[52] Oral clonidine (5 μg/kg) when used as a premedicant enhances the postoperative analgesia provided by intrathecal morphine without adding to the side effects of the morphine. Other additional benefits noted from a clonidine premedication include (1) blunted reflex tachycardia for intubation, (2) reduction of vasomotor liability, (3) decreased plasma catecholamines, and (4) dramatic decreases in MAC for inhaled gases or injected drugs.

Clonidine is rapidly absorbed by mouth and reaches peak plasma levels within 60 to 90 minutes. The elimination half-life is between 9 and 12 hours. It is equally excreted in the liver and kidneys. The duration of the hypotensive effect after a single dose is about 8 hours. The transdermal administration of clonidine requires about 48 hours to achieve therapeutic levels. The decrease in systolic blood pressure is more prominent than the decrease in diastolic blood pressure. There seems to be no effect on glomerular filtration rate. The perioperative administration of clonidine either as an oral doses or as a patch for total of 4 days, has significantly reduced the incidence of myocardial ischemia and mortality up to 2 years postoperatively.

The most common side effects are sedation and a dry mouth. However, skin rashes are frequent with chronic use. Impotence may be seen occasionally, and orthostatic hypotension is rare. One of the more worrisome complications of chronic clonidine use is a withdrawal syndrome on acute discontinuation of the drug. This usually occurs about 18 hours after discontinuation. The symptoms are hypertension, tachycardia, insomnia, flushing, headache, apprehension, sweating, and tremulousness. This condition lasts for 24 to 72 hours and is most likely to occur in patients taking more than 1.2 mg/day of clonidine. The withdrawal syndrome has been noted postoperatively in patients who were withdrawn from clonidine before surgery. It can be confused with anesthesia emergence symptoms, particularly in a patient with uncontrolled hypertension.[53] Absent the availability of the oral route in the surgical patient, withdrawal can be treated with clonidine transdermally or more rapidly with rectal clonidine.

⑫ Dexmedetomidine. Dexmedetomidine is a more selective α_2 agonist than clonidine (see Chapter 56).[54] Its potent α_2 agonism is 1,620:1 α_2 to α_1. Compared with clonidine, dexmedetomidine is 7 times more selective for α_2 receptors and has a shorter half-life of 1.5 hours. The loading dose (1 μg/kg) is given over 10 minutes or longer. Then an infusion is begun at 0.2 to 0.7 μg/kg/hr. Because of hemodynamic side effects, some centers omit the loading dose and start the continuous infusion. It has a more rapid onset of action (<5 minutes). The time to peak effect is 15 minutes. It can be given intravenously and has many uses in anesthesiology. It provides excellent sedation, reduces blood pressure, HR, and profoundly decreases plasma catecholamines. Little respiratory depression accompanies weaning from mechanical ventilation. It can be administered as a premedicant in cases of difficult intubations where awake fiberoptic intubation is employed. In the intensive care unit the use of clonidine is employed because of its sedating and analgesic effects without the respiratory depressive actions of other agents. There is concern for possible rebound hypertension, rebound hyperexcitability, and arrhythmias in infusions longer than 24 hours; ultimately, clinical trials are required to clarify these questions.[55] A recent meta-analysis demonstrated a trend toward improved cardiac outcomes in noncardiac surgical patients who have been treated perioperatively with dexmedetomidine.[56] Dexmedetomidine has been shown to be an effective anxiolytic and sedative when used as premedication. Pretreatment with dexmedetomidine, like clonidine, attenuates hemodynamic responses to intubation. Likewise, it decreases the MAC for volatile anesthetics from 35 to 50% but increases the likelihood of hypotension. Dexmedetomidine, like clonidine, increases the range of temperatures not triggering thermoregulatory defenses. It is likely to promote perioperative hypothermia, but also is effective against shivering.

Nonadrenergic Sympathomimetic Agents

Nonadrenergic sympathomimetic drugs also act indirectly by influencing the cAMP-calcium cascade, exclusive of the receptors (Fig. 15-10). The function of the second messenger (Ca^{2+}) nearly always goes together. This concept reinforces the recent appreciation of the homogeneity of action of a wide variety of drugs previously thought to be unrelated. Sympathomimetics have more pharmacologic similarities than differences.

Vasopressin. Vasopressin, and its congener (desmopressin) are exogenous preparations of the endogenous antidiuretic hormone (ADH). ADH and oxytocin are the two principle hormones secreted by the posterior pituitary. Target sites for ADH are the renal collecting ducts, vascular smooth muscle, and cardiac myocytes. Water absorption is passively reabsorbed from renal collecting ducts into extracellular fluid. Nonrenal actions include inotropism and intense vasoconstriction accounting for its alternative designation as vasopressin.[57] Arginine vasopressin is the most active form of ADH. Historically, vasopressin has been used for (1) treatment of diabetes insipidus, (2) diagnosis of diabetes insipidus, (3) abdominal distention, and (4) as an adjunct in the treatment of gastrointestinal hemorrhage and esophageal varices. Recently, three new indications for the use of vasopressin have emerged: (1) pressure support for septic shock, (2) cardiac arrest secondary to ventricular fibrillation/ventricular tachycardia, or (3) pulseless electrical activity/asystole.[58–61] Animal studies have shown, both in open- and closed-chest models, vasopressin caused larger increases in systemic vascular resistance, cerebral perfusion pressure, and coronary perfusion pressure than EPI. Vasopressin is a more effective vasoconstrictor than EPI in the presence of hypoxia and acidosis. In contrast to EPI, vasopressin does not seem to increase myocardial oxygen consumption or lactate production.[61,62] The 2005 guidelines for Advanced Cardiac Life Support (ACLS) of the American Heart Association recommend that vasopressin may be used to replace the first or second dose of EPI during the pulseless arrest algorithm[63] (see Chapter 59). EPI is class IIb recommendation, and vasopressin, which did not show any improvement in survival when compared with EPI, may be used instead of the first or the second dose of EPI and is considered class-indeterminate[36] (see Chapter 59). Vasopressin administered for cardiac arrest is known as *vasopressin injection USP*. The dose in cardiac arrest is 40 IU in 40 mL IV as a single dose in a peripheral IV line. Extravasation may cause local tissue necrosis. Its use in vasodilated sepsis is by infusion pump starting at 0.04 IU/min. There are suggestions that vasopressin may be useful in addition to potent α agonists for treatment of shock, especially from relative sparing of the mesenteric vessels; these data are supported by rat studies.[64] Despite a theoretical advantage of using vasopressin to decrease the catecholamines dosage in septic patients, the use of vasopressin failed to decrease mortality when compared with NE.[58] In such circumstances it seems that timing of initiation of therapy is the most important parameter for survival.[65,66]

Adenosine. Adenosine, available for more than 50 years, has been recognized recently as a clinically useful drug. It is an endogenous nucleotide and is found in every cell in the body. It is composed of adenine and a pentose sugar. Production can be increased by stimuli such as hypoxia and ischemia. This ubiquitous nucleotide has potent electrophysiological effects in addition to having a major role in regulation of vasomotor tone. Adenosine is believed to have a cardioprotective effect by regulating oxygen supply and demand (see Chapter 59). The receptors in the myocardial conduction system are the most sensitive and mediate sinoatrial node slowing and AV nodal conduction delay. Adenosine hyperpolarizes atrial myocytes and decreases their action potential duration via an increase in outward K^+ current. These are the ACh-regulated K^+ channels.

Adenosine mimics the effects of ACh in many ways, including an extremely short plasma half-life of mere seconds. Adenosine also antagonizes the inward Ca^{2+} current produced by catecholamines. This antidysrhythmic mechanism of Ca^{2+} channel blockade is thought to be an indirect effect and important only when β stimulation is present. The primary antidysrhythmic effect of adenosine is to interrupt re-entrant AV nodal tachycardia, which most likely relates to its K^+ current, rather than Ca^{2+} current effects. The chief indication for adenosine is paroxysmal supraventricular tachycardia, which it may terminate in a matter of seconds, adenosine being the recommended as first line of treatment.[36,67] Adenosine is to be used only cautiously in patients with Wolff-Parkinson-White syndrome with narrow complex tachycardia, and should be avoided in Wolff-Parkinson-White syndrome with atrial fibrillation as its use may increase the conduction via the atrioventricular node and induce ventricular fibrillation. One may use adenosine for re-entrant tachycardias involving the AV node, as well as right ventricular tachycardia.[68] The same characteristics that make adenosine an effective therapeutic agent may also make it an ideal agent for diagnosing other types of dysrhythmia. The incidence of incorrect diagnosis of supraventricular dysrhythmia has been reported to be as high as 15% using conventional means. Approximately 10% of supraventricular tachycardias do not involve AV nodal re-entry. Adenosine will nevertheless slow AV nodal conduction in these cases, decrease the ventricular rate, and allow inspection of P waves. Thus, adenosine may be useful in unmasking atrial fibrillation or flutter when fast ventricular responses are noted.

A number of side effects have been reported with the use of adenosine, including flushing, headache, dyspnea, bronchospasm, and chest pain. The majority of these are brief (seconds) and not clinically significant. Transient new dysrhythmias (65%) will be noted at the time of cardioversion, but these disappear during the half-life of the drug. Major hemodynamic changes are rare but consist of hypotension and bradycardia. Adenosine should be given by means of a rapid IV bolus with flush because of its extremely short half-life of <10 seconds. The initial adult dose is 6 mg (100 to 150 μg/kg for pediatrics), which can be followed by 12 mg within 1 to 2 minutes if the initial dose is without effect.[51] The 12-mg dose may be repeated once. The antidysrhythmic effect of adenosine occurs as soon as the drug reaches the AV node. Although both adenosine and verapamil are as effective in treating the paroxysmal supraventricular tachycardia, one must be aware of side effects before choosing one versus the other. Nevertheless, adenosine seems to be a better choice because of fewer side effects, a view that is recommended by the recent ACLS Guidelines[36,69] (see Chapter 59).

Phosphodiesterase Inhibitors. Phosphodiesterase inhibitors have pharmacologic properties approaching the characteristics of the ideal inotropic agent.[70–72] They do not rely on stimulation of β and/or α receptors. These drugs combine positive inotropism with vasodilator activity by selectively inhibiting phosphodiesterase (PDE) III. PDE I and II hydrolyze all cyclic nucleotides, whereas PDE III acts specifically on cAMP. The PDE III inhibitors interact with PDE III at the cell membrane and impede the breakdown of cAMP. cAMP levels increase and protein kinase is activated to promote phosphorylation. In cardiac muscle, phosphorylation increases the slow inward movement of calcium current, promoting increased intracellular calcium stores. Thus, inotropism increases. In vascular smooth muscle, increased cAMP activity accounts for the vasodilation, decreased peripheral vascular resistance, and lusitropism. Amrinone (currently termed *inamrinone*) is the prototypical PDE III inhibitor, and like nitroprusside and nitroglycerin, promotes diastolic relaxation, which promotes ventricular filling.[73] Milrinone is currently the most popular PDE inhibitor released for clinical use in the United States. The degree of hemodynamic effect of these drugs depends on the dose, degree of inotropic reserve, and state of cAMP depletion.

Milrinone. Milrinone is a derivative of amrinone. (In most centers milrinone has replaced amrinone; in general, their hemodynamic actions are similar.) It has nearly 20 times the inotropic potency of the parent compound. Milrinone is active both intravenously and orally and has beneficial short-term hemodynamic effects in patients with severe refractory conges-

tive heart failure. Improvement of CO appears to result from a combination of enhanced myocardial contractility and peripheral vasodilation. Treatment with oral milrinone for up to 11 months has been effective and well tolerated without evidence of fever, thrombocytopenia, or gastrointestinal effects. Milrinone has been approved for short-term IV therapy of congestive heart failure.[70–72] It is administered with a loading dose of 50 μg/kg over 10 minutes. The maintenance IV infusion rate ranges from a minimum of 0.375 μg/kg/min to a maximum of 0.75 μg/kg/min (not to exceed 1.13 μg/kg/day). Dosage must be adjusted in renal failure patients as milrinone is excreted in the urine, primarily in unconjugated form. Peak response with an IV dose occurs after 5 minutes and reveals no evidence of tolerance over short-term trials (24 hours); it is compatible with other adrenergic agonists. It is an effective inotropic agent in patients receiving beta-blockers. Its efficacy in the patient who has been digitalized has been demonstrated. Milrinone and DBT have become the mainstay of treatment for decompensated heart failure patients who require IV vasodilators and positive inotropic agents. Nevertheless, the use of such agents significantly increases mortality[74] and one must be aware that these drugs may increase the risk of arrhythmias in these patients who may in fact require implantable cardioverter defibrillators.[75]

Glucagon. Glucagon is a single-chain polypeptide of 29 amino acids that is secreted by pancreatic cells in response to hypoglycemia (see Chapter 49). The liver and kidney are responsible for its degradation. Known effects of this hormone in humans include the following: (1) inhibition of gastric motility, (2) enhanced urinary excretion of inorganic electrolytes, (3) increased insulin secretion, (4) hepatic glycogenolysis and gluconeogenesis, (5) anorexia, (6) inotropic and chronotropic cardiac effects, and (7) relaxation of smooth muscle (biliary, i.e., sphincters).[76] Little attention was given to glucagon until 1968, when it was demonstrated to produce positive inotropic and chronotropic effects in the canine heart. Glucagon enhances the activation of adenyl cyclase in a manner similar to that of NE, EPI, and isoproterenol. These cardiac actions of glucagon are not blocked by β blockade or catecholamine depletion. Glucagon, in contrast to the xanthines, rarely causes dysrhythmia, even in the face of ischemic heart disease, hypokalemia, and digitalis toxicity. Glucagon may possess antidysrhythmic activity in digitalis toxicity because it has been shown to enhance AV nodal conduction in patients with varying degrees of AV block. An IV dose of 1 to 5 mg of glucagon increases cardiac index, mean arterial pressure, and ventricular contractility, even in the presence of digitalis therapy. After a bolus dose, its action dissipates in approximately 30 minutes. Nausea and vomiting are common side effects in the awake patient, especially following a bolus dose. Hypokalemia, hypoglycemia, and hyperglycemia are also seen. Glucagon is also useful in treating insulin-induced hypoglycemia.

Despite the obvious benefits of glucagon in cardiac patients, its use has not become popular. This pancreatic hormone may be of hemodynamic benefit when more conventional approaches have proved refractory in the following settings: (1) low CO syndrome following cardiopulmonary bypass, (2) low CO syndrome with myocardial infarction, (3) chronic congestive heart failure, and (4) excessive β-adrenergic blockade. In cases of anaphylactic shock with significant and refractory hypotension, glucagon is extremely useful alternative agent in reversing the decreased blood pressure.[77]

Digitalis Glycosides. The most important actions of the digitalis glycosides are those affecting myocardial contractility, conduction, and rhythm. The glycoside most likely to be used by the anesthesiologist is digoxin. The principal uses of digoxin are for the treatment of congestive heart failure and to control supraventricular cardiac dysrhythmia such as atrial fibrillation. Digoxin is one of the few positive inotropes that does not increase HR. Digoxin enhances myocardial inotropism and automaticity but slows impulse propagation through the conduction tissues.[51] Despite nearly two centuries of use, its mechanism of action is only modestly certain. Digitalis reciprocally facilitates calcium entry into the myocardial cell by blocking the Na^+,K^+ adenosine triphosphatase pump. This calcium influx may account for its positive inotropic action because this inotropic response is not catecholamine- or β receptor-dependent, and is therefore effective in patients taking β-blocking drugs. The inhibition of this enzyme transport mechanism also results in a net K^+ loss from the myocardial cell. This contributes to digitalis toxicity with hypokalemia. Calcium potentiates the toxic effects of digitalis. Extreme caution should be observed when calcium is given to a patient taking digitalis or when digitalis administration is contemplated in the patient with hypercalcemia. Digitalis has been of little use in cardiogenic shock and has proved potentially injurious in patients with uncomplicated myocardial infarction because of its vasoconstrictive properties and effects on myocardial oxygen consumption in the absence of cardiomegaly. Care must be taken to rule out conditions in which the use of digitalis is of no benefit and is potentially harmful. These include mitral stenosis with normal sinus rhythm and constrictive pericarditis with tamponade. Signs and symptoms of idiopathic hypertrophic subaortic stenosis are often exacerbated by digitalis. With increased strength of contraction, the muscular obstruction can be markedly increased. The same is true for the use of digitalis in patients with infundibular pulmonic stenosis, as occurs with tetralogy of Fallot. Any augmentation of contractility may further reduce an already diminished pulmonary blood flow. Beware of digitalis toxic reactions in the older age group and in patients suffering from arterial hypoxemia, acidosis, renal compromise, hypothyroidism, hypokalemia, or hypomagnesemia, as well as in patients receiving quinidine or calcium channel blockers.

When entertaining the possibility of perioperative digitalis administration, the following points must be considered.

1. Myocardial oxygen consumption is increased in the non-failing, nondilated heart.
2. The therapeutic-to-toxic ratio of digitalis is narrow.
3. Inotropic drugs that are less toxic and reversible are readily available.
4. Verapamil or beta-blockers are more efficacious for supraventricular tachydysrhythmias not initiated by heart failure.
5. Digitalis may cause serious dysrhythmia in the unstable patient.
6. Serum potassium concentrations may fluctuate in the surgical patient.
7. Any cardiac dysrhythmia that occurs in the presence of digitalis must be considered a toxic phenomenon.
8. Digitalis-induced cardiac dysrhythmias are difficult to treat.
9. Renal compromise will result in toxic effects with standard maintenance doses.
10. Cardioversion may be dangerous after digitalis administration.
11. After initiation of digitalis therapy, the administration of alternative drugs becomes more complicated.

Digoxin, beta-blockers, and calcium channel blockers such as diltiazem and verapamil may be used in patients with heart failure and normal ejection fraction to control the HR, especially if patients do have supraventricular tachyarrhythmias such as atrial fibrillation. Nevertheless, digoxin is not recommended for patients with heart failure, but with normal ejection fraction, as it may increase the left ventricular filling pressure, and subsequently aggravate their heart failure.[78]

Calcium Salts. Calcium is of great importance in the genesis of the cardiac action potential and is the key to controlling intracellular energy storage and utilization. Movement of extracellular calcium across membranes also governs the function of uterine smooth muscle as well as the smooth muscle of the blood vessels. The sympathomimetic drugs promote the transmembrane influx of calcium, whereas the beta-blockers and calcium channel blockers inhibit such movement. The American Heart Association has recommended against the use of calcium during cardiac arrest except when hyperkalemia, hypocalcemia, or calcium-channel blocker toxicity is present.[79] Subsequently, the indications for calcium use are now limited to only few clinical applications (see Chapter 59). Calcium chloride is often given at the termination of cardiopulmonary bypass to offset the myocardial depression associated with hypothermic potassium cardioplegia.[80] There is newer evidence that the use of calcium in the early postbypass period may induce spasm of the coronaries, including the newly grafted internal mammary artery, also causes hypercontracture of the heart cells, and therefore increases the risk for myocardial ischemia, reperfusion injury, and even myocardial infarction.[81-83] The use of calcium salts is clearly indicated during rapid or massive transfusions of citrated blood.[80]

Citrate binds calcium, and rapid infusion rates of citrated blood result in myocardial depression that is reversible by calcium. Two forms of calcium salts are commonly available: calcium chloride and calcium gluconate. Traditionally, calcium gluconate has been preferred in pediatric patients and calcium chloride in adult patients. Previous data held that calcium chloride produced consistently higher and more predictable levels of ionized calcium.[84] Studies have shown, however, that ionization of any of the preparations is immediate and equally effective (see Chapter 14). Calcium chloride produces only transient increases in CO and blood pressure. Bolus doses of 2 to 10 mg/kg (1.5 mg/kg/min) of calcium chloride can produce moderate improvement in contractility. The rapid administration of calcium salts, if the heart is beating, can produce bradycardia and must be used cautiously in the patient who is digitalized because of the hazard of producing toxic effects. Calcium salts will precipitate as calcium carbonate if mixed with sodium bicarbonate.

Antidepressant Drugs

Monoamine Oxidase Inhibitors

Monoamine oxidase inhibitors (MAOIs) and the tricyclic antidepressants are used to treat psychotic depression. These drugs are not used in the practice of anesthesia but are a source of potentially serious anesthetic interactions in patients who are taking them chronically (see Chapter 23). Their use is rapidly declining as the nontricyclic antidepressants such as Prozac are more efficacious and produce fewer side effects. Few of the MAOIs or tricyclic antidepressants will be encountered in an anesthesia practice today, with the exceptions of phenelzine (Nardil) and amitriptyline (Amitril, Elavil). Their pharmacologic actions and side effects are a direct result of their effect on the cascade of catecholamine metabolism. MAOIs block the oxidative deamination of endogenous catecholamines into inactive vanillylmandelic acid. They do not inhibit synthesis. Thus, blockade of MAO would produce an accumulation of NE, EPI, DA, and 5-hydroxytryptamine in adrenergically active tissues, including the brain. The action of sympathomimetic amines is potentiated in patients taking MAOIs. Indirect-acting sympathomimetics (ephedrine, tyramine) produce an exaggerated response as they trigger the release of accumulated catecholamines. Foods containing a high tyramine content such as cheese, red Italian wine, and pickled herring can also precipitate hypertensive crises.[26] Meperidine has been reported to produce hypertensive crisis, convulsions, and coma with MAOIs. Hepatotoxicity has been reported that does not seem to be related to dosage or duration of treatment. Its incidence is low but remains a factor in selecting anesthesia.

The anesthetic management of patients taking MAOIs remains controversial. Currently, recommendations for management include discontinuation of the drugs for at least 2 weeks before surgery; however, this recommendation is not based on controlled studies but rather is the result of limited case reports that suggest potent drug interactions.

Tricyclic Antidepressants

This group of antidepressant drugs is referred to as *tricyclic antidepressants* because of their structure. These drugs have almost replaced the MAOIs because of fewer side effects. All of these agents block uptake of NE into adrenergic nerve endings. Just as with the MAOIs, high doses of the tricyclic antidepressants can induce seizure activity that is responsive to diazepam. Neuroleptic drugs may potentiate the effects of tricyclic antidepressants by competition with metabolism in the liver. Chronic barbiturate use increases metabolism of the tricyclic antidepressants by microsomal enzyme induction. Other sedatives, however, potentiate the tricyclic antidepressants in a manner similar to that occurring with the MAOIs. Atropine also has an exaggerated effect because of the anticholinergic effect of tricyclic antidepressants. Prolonged sedation from thiopental has been reported. Ketamine may also be dangerous in patients taking tricyclic antidepressants by producing acute hypertension and cardiac dysrhythmia. Despite these serious interactions, discontinuation of these drugs before surgery is probably not necessary. The latency of onset of these drugs is from 2 to 5 weeks; however, the excretion of tricyclic antidepressants is rapid, with approximately 70% of a dose appearing in the urine during the first 72 hours. The long latency period for resumption of treatment militates against interrupted treatment. A thorough knowledge of the possible drug interactions and autonomic countermeasures now available obviates postponement.

Selective Serotonin Reuptake Inhibitors

The mechanism of action of selective serotonin reuptake inhibitors appears to be the selective inhibition of neuronal uptake of serotonin. This potentiates the behavioral changes induced by the serotonin precursor, 5-hydroxytryptophan.[85] The availability of sympathetic antagonists for possible side effects during anesthesia weighs in favor of continuation of therapy versus the risk of exacerbation of a severe depression. Prozac (fluoxetine) is a popular oral nontricyclic antidepressant. Unlike desyrel, the elimination half-life of Prozac is 1 to 3 days and can lead to significant accumulation of the drug. Prozac's metabolism, like that of other compounds including tricyclic antidepressants, phenobarbital, ethanol, and pentothal, involves the P450 II D6 system. Therefore concomitant therapy with drugs also metabolized by this enzyme system may lead to drug interactions and prolongation of effect of the benzodiazepines. Buproprion is used as an antidepressant, whereas a sustained release drug is marketed as a nonnicotine aid to smoking cessation. The neurochemical mechanism of the antidepressant effect of buproprion is not known. It does not inhibit monoamine oxidase and is a weak blocker of the neuronal uptake of serotonin and NE. It also inhibits the neuronal uptake of DA to some extent. No systematic data have been collected on the interactions of bupropion and other drugs.

Sympatholytics Drugs

Alpha Antagonists

13 Drugs that bind selectively to α-adrenergic receptors block the action of endogenous catecholamines or moderate the effects of exogenous adrenergics. The resultant effects may be ascribed together the blockade effect to α-adrenergic agonists or to unopposed α-adrenergic receptor activity. The effect is smooth muscle relaxation. The response to the vasculature may vary over a wide range in a single vascular bed, depending on its intrinsic state of constriction. Vessels with higher initial tone have a greater response to α blockade. Prominent clinical effects of α blockers include hypotension, orthostatic hypotension, tachycardia and miosis, nasal stuffiness, diarrhea, and inhibition of ejaculation. The α blockers may be classified according to binding characteristics. Phenoxybenzamine is an oral α blocker that produces and irreversible blockade. It is a relatively nonselective α blocker. Phentolamine, tolazoline, and prazosin are characterized by reversible binding and antagonism. When patients are taking these drugs chronically, one should keep in mind that the normal autonomic response to stress, inhalation anesthetics, or extensive regional anesthesia may be blunted. Elevations of catecholamines will not reflexly increase peripheral vascular resistance and may actually decrease if vascular β receptors are unopposed. α Blockers are often used in combination with diuretics and other antihypertensives. Volume depletion may not be evident on preoperative examination but become unmasked with the induction of anesthesia, resulting in the onset of a marked hypotension. This hypotension is usually responsive to volume repletion and the temporary use of a direct acting α agonist such as neosynephrine. There is no cause for discontinuation of these drugs before surgery but preloading with IV fluids is suggested to ensure adequate central volume.

Phentolamine.   Phentolamine is used almost exclusively in the presurgical treatment of pheochromocytoma (see Chapter 49). It is a competitive antagonist at α_1 and α_2 receptors. Phentolamine may also have some antihistaminic and cholinomimetic activity. The cholinomimetic activity may result in abdominal cramping and diarrhea, both of which are blocked by atropine. Tachycardia and hypotension are also common side effects.

Intravenously, phentolamine produces peripheral vasodilatation and a decrease in systemic blood pressure within 2 minutes and lasting from 10 to 15 minutes. Blood pressure reduction elicits baroreceptor reflexes and NE release. Cardiac arrhythmias and angina pectoris may accompany phentolamine administration. It can be given in doses of 30 to 70 μg/kg IV to produce a transient decrease in blood pressure. It can also be used as a continuous infusion to maintain blood pressure during resection of a pheochromocytoma.

Phenoxybenzamine.   Phenoxybenzamine acts as a nonselective α-adrenergic antagonist (see Chapter 49). α Blockade is 100 times more potent on postsynaptic α_1 receptors than at α_2 receptors. Preoperatively in preparation for removal of a pheochromocytoma, the dug is administered orally starting at 10 mg twice daily.[86] The onset of α blockade is slow. This is related to the time required for structural modification of the phenoxybenzamine molecule to become active. The elimination half-life is about 24 hours. Orthostatic hypotension is prominent, especially in the presence of pre-existing hypertension or hypovolemia. CO is often increased and renal blood flow is not greatly altered except in pre-existing renal vasoconstriction or stenosis. Coronary and cerebral vascular resistance is not changed.

Prazosin.   Prazosin is relatively selective for α_1 receptors, leaving the inhibiting effect of α_2 receptor activity on NE release intact. As a result, it is less likely than nonselective α antagonists to evoke reflex tachycardia. The initial oral dose is 1 mg twice daily, then titrated to effect. Prazosin dilates both arterioles and veins. Cardiovascular effects include total body reductions in systemic vascular resistance and venous return. When combined with a diuretic it is an effective antihypertensive drug. It should not be used with clonidine or α-methyldopa, as it appears to decrease their effectiveness. Prazosin may also cause bronchodilation.

Oral α_1 blockers have been found useful for benign prostatic hypertrophy and hypertension. The anesthesiologist may encounter patients taking these medications on a chronic basis and must be aware of their possible interactions with anesthetics (see Chapter 23). Doxazosin is a long-acting selective α_1 blocker used for treating benign prostate hyperplasia and hypertension. The most common side effect, as with all α blockers, is orthostatic hypotension and dizziness. Tamsulosin is another α blocker that is used for benign prostate hyperplasia. It is not indicated for hypertension but it is capable of producing orthostatic hypotension.

Beta Antagonists

β-Adrenergic blockers were introduced in the 1960s. These sympatholytic agents have dominated cardiovascular pharmacology. They are among the most common drugs used in the treatment of cardiac disease and hypertension. A variety of drugs are available with β-blocking activity that may be distinguished by differing pharmacokinetic and pharmacodynamic properties. Examples of some of the drugs available and their diversity of actions are listed in Table 15-12. Beta-blockers can be classified according to whether they are selective or nonselective on the β_1 or β_2 receptor and whether they possess intrinsic sympathomimetic activity. For example, a beta-blocker with selective properties for the β_1 receptor would bind to the cardiac receptors, whereas a nonselective beta-blocker would bind to both β_1 (cardiac) and β_2 (vascular, bronchial smooth muscle and metabolic) receptors. Nonselective β-antagonists are referred to as *first-generation beta-blockers*. These include propranolol, nadolol, sotalol, and timolol. Second-generation drugs are those considered selective for β_1-adrenergic blockade. These include atenolol, esmolol, and metoprolol. Over the past decade, and because of their selectivity, the use of beta-blockers has expanded to include the treatment of congestive heart failure. Recently, a new beta-blocker subcategory has been developed, respectively, beta-blocker with vasodilatory properties, such as in a new beta-blocker, nebivolol.[87]

Beta-blockers are an important class of agents that are indicated for treatment of coronary artery disease, hypertension, heart failure, and tachyarrhythmias. They have a primary role in treatment of patients after a myocardial infarction.[88] Beta-blockers have a direct effect on reducing the mortality in patients with heart failure due to left ventricular systolic dysfunction (bisoprolol, carvedilol, and metoprolol). Recently, a fourth agent has been used with similar favorable results, and this is nebivolol.[89,90] Nebivolol is a beta-blocker with an excellent β selectivity, and endothelium-dependent vasodilation secondary to L-arginine/nitric oxide pathway. Therefore, this novel drug has hemodynamic advantages and a better profile for side effects. Recent trials demonstrated a reduced morbidity and mortality in elderly patients with chronic heart failure, which makes this drug a very interesting option for the future treatment of cardiac disease because it is currently only available in Europe.[87,91] Beta-blockers reduce the incidence of

perioperative myocardial infarction; there is an increased interest in using these agents perioperatively in high-risk patients undergoing vascular and other high-risk surgical procedures[92] (see Chapter 42).

Selective β-blockade is of great benefit in treatment of patients with obstructive airway disease, diabetes, or peripheral vascular disease. However, it must be emphasized that *specificity* is a relative term and not absolute. Nonselective blocking effects may be seen in all tissues if higher blood levels are reached with "selective" drugs. For example, the use of β_1-selective blockers in patients with obstructive or reactive airway disease remains controversial. Patients with reactive airway disease may develop serious reductions in ventilatory function even with β_1-selective antagonists, but these circumstances are rare, so these drugs can be employed for large categories of patients. Other drugs are available for treatment of supraventricular arrhythmias and hypertension in asthmatic patients. Sympathetic activation generally results in increased circulating glucose levels secondary to enhanced glycogenolysis, lipolysis, and gluconeogenesis. Administration of β_2 blockers to insulin-dependent diabetics reduces their ability to recover from hypoglycemic episodes (see Chapter 49).

In patients receiving chronic beta-blocker therapy, the drug should be continued throughout the perioperative and postoperative period[92] (see Chapter 42). Acute withdrawal of β-antagonists may produce a hemodynamic withdrawal syndrome and induce tachycardia.[26] HR is a major determinant of myocardial oxygen demands. Tachycardia is known to increase the risk of poor outcome in patients with ischemic heart disease; therefore, hemodynamic control of HR and blood pressure (work) is important in reducing perioperative risk. Several studies have shown the benefits of prophylactic β-blockade with atenolol in patients at risk for ischemic cardiac disease.[93] The reduction in perioperative morbidity and mortality in these groups of patients was significant.[94–99] Recent data suggest that the use of beta-blocker alone is not effective, unless tight HR control is present (<80 beats per minute perioperatively). For this purpose a combination of drugs may be required; further studies are underway that may indeed establish the best clinical practice.[95,97,100–104]

Several of the β blockers listed in Table 15-12 also have a local anestheticlike effect on myocardial membranes at high doses. This effect is similar to that of quinidine in that phase 0 of the cardiac action potential is depressed slowing conduction. This membrane-stabilizing activity is caused by the D-isomer, whereas the L-isomer is responsible for β blocking activity. The clinical significance of membrane-stabilizing activity is unclear.

Propranolol.   Propranolol is the prototypical β-blocking drug against which all others are compared. It is nonselective and has no intrinsic sympathomimetic activity but does have membrane-stabilizing activity at higher doses. It is available in both IV and oral forms. The IV dose is usually 0.5 to 1 mg repeated every 5 minutes up to a total of 5 mg with careful titration to effect.[51] It is highly lipophilic and is metabolized by the liver to more water-soluble metabolites, one of which, 17-OH propranolol, has weak β-blocking activity. There is a significant first-pass effect by the liver after oral administration of the drug. It is highly protein-bound, and the free drug level may be altered by other highly bound drugs. The elimination half-life is approximately 4 hours, but the pharmacologic half-life is around 10 hours. Hemodynamic effects include decreased HR and contractility. The major factors contributing to the decrease in blood pressure by propranolol are decreased CO and renin release. Systemic vascular resistance may increase on acute administration owing to blockade of β_2 receptors in the peripheral vasculature. With chronic administration, however, peripheral vascular resistance decreases. This is thought to be secondary to decreased renin release and, possibly, decreased

TABLE 15-12

β-ADRENERGIC BLOCKING DRUGS

DRUG	RELATIVE β_1 SELECTIVITY	MEMBRANE-STABILIZING ACTIVITY	INTRINSIC SYMPATHO-MIMETIC ACTIVITY	PLASMA HALF-LIFE (hr)	ORAL AVAILABILITY (%)	LIPID SOLUBILITY	ELIMINATION	PREPARATIONS
Propranolol	0	+	0	3-4	36	+++	Hepatic	Oral, IV
Metoprolol	++	0	0	3-4	38	+	Hepatic	
Atenolol	++	0	0	6-9	57	0	Renal	Oral, eye drops
Esmolol	++	0	0	0-16	—	?	RBC esterase	Oral
Timolol	0	0	0	4-5	50	+	Hepatic and renal	IV

RBC, red blood cells.
[a]Primarily hepatic, but active metabolites are formed that must be renally excreted.

central SNS outflow. Complications with the use of propranolol include bradycardia, heart block, worsening of congestive heart failure, bronchospasm, and sedation.[105] During anesthesia with halothane, it may cause severe bradydysrhythmias. Because it is not cardioselective, most clinicians are moving away from using propranolol, and instead are using the selective alternatives such as metoprolol, or atenolol.

Metoprolol. Metoprolol is a relatively selective β-blocking drug with β-blocking effects at moderate and high doses. It has neither intrinsic sympathomimetic activity nor membrane-stabilizing activity. It has a possible advantage in patients with reactive airway disease at oral doses up to 100 mg/day. The initial IV dose is 1.25-5 mg every 6 to 12 hours. For myocardial infarction the dose is 2 to 5 mg every 2 minutes for three doses, followed by 50 mg orally every 6 hours, with careful monitoring of the heart rate while the loading dose is being administered.[51] It is mostly metabolized in the liver, with only about 5% excreted unchanged in the urine. The elimination half-life is 3.5 hours. It is available in IV as well as oral form; therefore, it is commonly recommended prior to surgery and anesthesia.[89]

Atenolol. Atenolol is similar to metoprolol in that it is relatively cardioselective and has no intrinsic sympathomimetic activity or membrane-stabilizing activity. It is less lipophilic, however, and is eliminated primarily by renal excretion. The starting dose is 5 mg over 5 minutes IV, and 25 to 50 mg/day oral administration.[51] The elimination half-life is 6 to 7 hours. The lack of first-pass metabolism results in more predictable blood levels after oral dosing. The main advantage of this drug is its once a day dosing.[93,106]

Esmolol. Esmolol has several uses in the perioperative period.[107] The most unique feature of the drug is the ester function incorporated into the phenoxypropanolamine structure. This allows for rapid degradation by esterases in the red blood cells and a resultant pharmacologic half-life of 10 to 20 minutes. Esmolol is cardioselective and appears to have little effect on bronchial or vascular tone at doses that decrease HR in humans. It has been used successfully in low doses in patients with asthma but caution is again advised when using beta-blockers in these patients. The IV bolus dose is 0.25 to 0.5 mg/kg, and a continuous infusion loading dose is 500 μg/kg/min over 1 to 2 minutes, with a maintenance dose of 50 to 200 μg/kg/min.[51]

Esmolol is metabolized rapidly in the blood by an esterase located in the red blood cell cytoplasm. It is different from the plasma cholinesterase and is not inhibited to a significant degree by physostigmine or echothiophate but is markedly inhibited by sodium fluoride. There are no apparent important clinical interactions between esmolol and other ester-containing drugs. At the highest infusion rates (500 μg/kg/min), esmolol does not prolong neuromuscular blockade by succinylcholine. Esmolol has proven to be useful in the perioperative period because of its capability to be administered intravenously and its short half-life. This feature permits a trial of β blockade in doubtful situations. Esmolol has been shown to blunt the response to intubation of the trachea and is moderately effective in treating postoperative hypertension.[108–110] Most reported studies in humans have used doses of 50 to 500 μg/kg/min. The most beneficial approach seems to be a loading dose of 500 μg/kg over 30 seconds, followed by continuous infusion of 50 to 300 μg/kg/min. Peak blockade appears to occur within 5 minutes. On discontinuation of the infusion, serum levels decline with an elimination half-life of 9 minutes.

Timolol. Timolol is also noncardioselective with little intrinsic sympathomimetic activity and no membrane-stabilizing activity. It is the only beta-blocker used as the L-isomer rather than the racemic mixture. It is 5 to 10 times as potent as propranolol. Hepatic metabolism accounts for approximately 66% of its elimination, and another 20% is found unchanged in the urine. The elimination half-life is 5.6 hours, and the pharmacologic half-life is approximately 15 hours. It was first used topically for treatment of glaucoma but is now used in hypertension and has been shown to decrease the risk of reinfarction and death following myocardial infarction. Its hemodynamic effects and side effects are similar to those of other beta-blockers. The anesthesiologist should also be aware that timolol eye drops may be absorbed systemically and cause bradycardia and hypotension that are refractory to treatment with atropine.[111]

Other Beta-Blockers

Other beta-blockers include drugs such as nadolol (noncardioselective beta-blocker), acebutolol (cardioselective beta-blocker with intrinsic sympathomimetic activity and membrane-stabilizing activity), pindolol (nonselective beta-blocker with membrane-stabilizing activity and intrinsic sympathomimetic activity), betaxolol (cardiac selective), penbutolol (nonselective with some intrinsic sympathetic activity), carteolol (nonselective) are used for treatment of hypertension or HR control.

Mixed Antagonists

Labetalol

Labetalol is an antihypertensive drug with blocking activity at both α and β receptors. The relative α/β-blocking effects depend on the route of administration. After oral administration, the ratio of α/β effectiveness is 1:3; however, when given intravenously, it is 1:7. The α effects are primarily on α_1 receptors, whereas the β effects on nonselective. Hemodynamic effects consist primarily of decreased peripheral resistance and decreased or unchanged HR with little change in CO. Serum renin activity is decreased. Maintenance of lower HRs in the presence of decreased systemic blood pressure is beneficial in controlling the myocardial oxygen supply/demand ratio and is a major benefit of labetalol in patients with coronary artery disease.

Labetalol is eliminated by hepatic glucuronide conjugation. The elimination half-life after IV administration is 5.5 hours and 6 to 8 hours after oral use. Elimination is not markedly prolonged in-patients with hepatic or renal failure. Another advantage of the drug is the ability to convert from IV to oral forms of the same drug after the patient is stable. For treatment of hypertension when used as a bolus, the initial dose is 2.5 to 10 mg IV over 2 minutes, then repeat every 10 minutes to a total of 30 mg. When used as a continuous infusion, it is usually started at 0.5 to 2.0 mg/min and titrated to effect. Because there is an enhanced effect by inhalation anesthetics, these doses should be decreased when used intraoperatively.

Complications and contraindications are similar to those for the beta-blockers. Labetalol should be used with caution in patients with compromised myocardial function because it may worsen heart failure. Also, owing to β-blocking activity, the drug may induce bronchospasm in asthmatics. As with other beta-blockers, abrupt withdrawal is not recommended. Labetalol is one of the favorites of many anesthesiologists for use in the perioperative period because it rapidly decreases both blood pressure, and to some extent, also the HR, it can be used as a bolus, and ultimately achieves normotension within a few minutes of initial administration.[112,113]

Calcium Channel Blockers

Calcium is regarded as the universal messenger in cells and plays a critical role in a number of biologic processes. It is

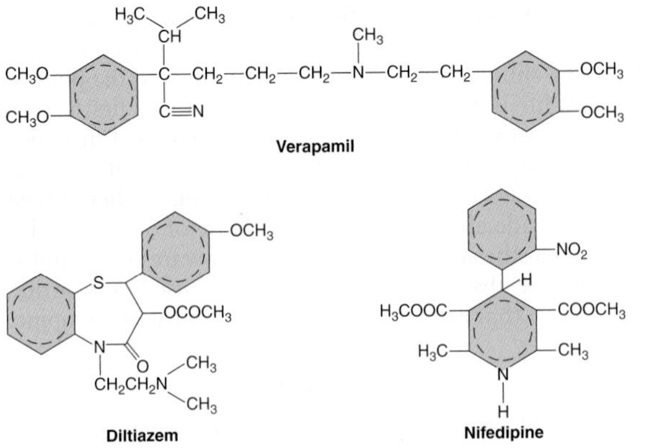

FIGURE 15.16. Structural formulas of the calcium entry blockers demonstrate dissimilar structures consistent with their dissimilar electrophysiologic and pharmacologic properties. They also share some similarities but cannot be considered therapeutically interchangeable. Nifedipine and nitrendipine are structurally similar and are both potent vasodilators.

involved in blood coagulation, a broad array of enzymatic reactions, the metabolism of bone, neuromuscular transmission, the electrical activation of various excitable membranes, as well as endocrine secretion and muscle contraction. Calcium initiates several physiologic events in the specialized automatic and conducting cells in the heart. It is involved in the genesis of the cardiac action potential and it links excitation to contraction and controls energy stores and utilization. Movement of extracellular calcium across membranes also governs the function of smooth muscle in bronchi and in coronary, pulmonary,

and systemic arterioles. Its roles in adrenergic effector response have been outlined in detail (see Adrenergic Receptors). Membrane calcium channels are known to provide a pathway for calcium influx across cell membranes that differ from calcium efflux movements associated with active pumps or exchange. The inward calcium channel exhibits two distinguishing properties: (1) selectivity in that they have the ability to distinguish between ion species, and (2) excitability in that they have the property of responding to changes in membrane potential. Separate, ion-specific channels for sodium and calcium influx exist. The status of these channels can vary to produce three kinetic states: resting, activated, and inactivated.

Classification of calcium channel blockers has been difficult since their discovery. They were initially thought to be β-adrenergic blocking drugs because of their sympatholytic action. Later they were called *calcium antagonists*. It is clear, however, that these drugs are not true pharmacologic antagonists of calcium. Instead, they interact with the cell membrane to control the intracellular concentration of calcium. The correct terminology for this group of drugs appears to be *calcium channel blockers*. The molecular structures of three clinically useful calcium entry blockers are seen in Figure 15-16. These drugs produce vasodilatation, depress cardiac conduction velocity (dromotropism), depress contractility (inotropism), and decrease HR (chronotropism). All calcium channel blockers do this, but with varying degrees of potency in the intact human and in vitro (Table 15-11). Thus, despite their similarities, these drugs cannot be considered therapeutically interchangeable. The useful pharmacologic effects of the calcium channel blockers have been confined almost solely to the cardiovascular system.[99] The drugs are all absorbed via the gastrointestinal tract, but the extensive first-pass hepatic extraction of verapamil limits its bioavailability orally (Table 15-13). Onset of action is equivalent for all three

TABLE 15-13

COMPARATIVE PHARMACOLOGY OF CALCIUM ENTRY BLOCKERS

	■ VERAPAMIL	■ DILTIAZEM	■ NIFEDIPINE
Dose			
Oral	80–160 mg tid	60–90 mg tid	10–20 mg tid
IV	75–150 µg/kg	75–150 µg/kg	5–15 µg/kg
Absorption			
Oral (%)	>90%	>90%	>90%
Bioavailability			
Oral (%)	<20%	?<20%	60–70%[a]
Onset			
Oral	15–20 min	20–30 min	15–20 min
IV	1 min	?	1 min
Sublingual	—	—	3 min
Peak Effect			
Oral	5 hr	30 min	1–2 hr
IV	5–30 min	?	1–3 hr
Elimination half-life	2–7 hr	4 hr	4–5 hr
Plasma protein binding	90%	80%	90%
Metabolism	70%	Deacetylated	80% to lactone
	First-pass hepatic		
Elimination			
Renal	75%	35%	70%
Gastrointestinal (liver)	15%	75%	<15%
Side effects	Constipation, headache, vertigo, hypotension, atrioventricular conduction disturbances	Headache, dizziness, flushing, atrioventricular conduction disturbances, constipation	Headache, hypotension, flushing, digital dysesthesias, leg edema

IV, intravenous.
[a]Light-sensitive.

drugs and is consistent with rapid membrane transport. All three drugs are extensively protein-bound and subject to the effect of changes in plasma protein concentration and competition from other protein-bound drugs and metabolites, but final elimination of verapamil and nifedipine is primarily renal.

Verapamil

Verapamil is a calcium channel blocker that is administered intravenously for terminating supraventricular tachydysrhythmias. Nearly all forms of supraventricular tachydysrhythmias are caused by re-entry using either the sinoatrial or the AV node as part of the circuit. Verapamil terminates these cardiac dysrhythmias by decreasing nodal conductivity and converting the unidirectional block of re-entry to a bidirectional block. Verapamil does not alter the action potential upstroke in fibers whose resting membrane potential is more negative than –60 mV, that is, fast-action potentials. (It does slow or prevent depolarization in cardiac tissue with a resting membrane potential that is less negative than –50 mV, that is, calcium-dependent upstroke.) Verapamil, therefore, has profound effects on pacemaker cells, which depend on the calcium current for depolarization. It depresses the rate of sinus discharge, reduces conduction velocity, and increases refractoriness of the AV node. A dose-dependent increase in the PR interval and AV interval is produced on the electrocardiogram. This has been described as a quinidinelike effect similar to that produced by class IA antidysrhythmic drugs (e.g., procainamide), which are also effective for supraventricular dysrhythmia. In contrast to procainamide, verapamil does not increase the QRS or QT interval because it lacks activity on the sodium-dependent action potentials.

Verapamil is a first-line drug for treatment of supraventricular tachydysrhythmias (Table 15-11) (see Chapter 59). The incidence of successful termination of paroxysmal atrial tachycardia with verapamil in adults has approached 90%. It is also effective in treating atrial fibrillation and atrial flutter by either converting to a sinus rhythm or slowing the ventricular response. The ventricular rate will slow as a result of decreased conduction velocity through the AV node even when conversion is not produced. Caution must be exercised in treating patients when the underlying cause of the atrial tachycardia, atrial fibrillation, or atrial flutter is the Wolff-Parkinson-White syndrome.[36] Verapamil may terminate the tachydysrhythmia by its specific depressant effects on the AV node, which is one limb of the re-entrant pathway. It may also increase conduction velocity in the accessory tract, in which case the HR may actually increase. Verapamil has no adverse effects on bronchial asthma or obstructive lung disease and may be selected over propranolol in patients with these conditions. It should be avoided in patients with sick sinus syndrome, AV block, and the presence of heart failure, unless the heart failure is the result of a supraventricular tachycardia. Verapamil has been effective in terminating ventricular tachycardias and premature depolarizations in about two thirds of the treatment trials when other drugs have failed, and can be used also as an antihypertensive.[78,114]

The important side effects of verapamil are directly related to its predominant pharmacologic action (Table 15-11). It may produce unwanted AV conduction delays and bradycardia, resulting in cardiovascular collapse. Verapamil must be used carefully, if at all, in the presence of propranolol. The combined effect has produced complete heart block in animals and humans. It must be used carefully in digitalized patients for the same reason. No such interactions exist with nifedipine. The combination of β blockade and nifedipine may be beneficial in patients with ischemic heart disease because the reflex tachycardia seen with nifedipine can be countered with β blockade.

Nifedipine

Nifedipine is the most potent calcium entry blocker when tested in isolated tissue preparations. It is an equipotent cardiac depressant and vasodilator. Depression of inotropism and cardiac conduction, however, is not evident in the intact human. It does not affect baroreflex mechanisms and, as a result, the marked vasodilation is accompanied by increased SNS tone and afterload reduction (Table 15-11).[26] A compensatory tachycardia may result, and CO may actually increase as a result of the afterload reduction. The most specific therapeutic application for nifedipine is coronary vasospasm (variant of Prinzmetal's angina; see Chapter 41). It has been more successful than nitroglycerin for this purpose because it produces a more profound and predictable coronary vasodilation. It has also been extremely useful in other types of ischemic heart disease ranging from unstable angina to myocardial infarction. The decrease in myocardial oxygen demand that results from the reduced afterload and reduced left ventricular volume appears to be the mechanism for the relief of angina. Coronary vasodilation is another factor, but it is not known if this is the antianginal effect in patients with coronary artery disease. The dilating effect may last only 5 minutes, but the antianginal effect may last more than 1 hour. As an antihypertensive the usual dosage is oral administration of 10 to 20 mg/day.[51]

Diltiazem

The hemodynamic effects of diltiazem lie somewhere between those of verapamil and nifedipine. It is less potent than either of these two agents. Diltiazem is a good coronary artery dilator but a poor peripheral vasodilator. It often produces bradycardia and delayed conduction, and reflex tachycardia is not a problem. It appears to be an effective oral drug for the treatment of coronary disease in which cardiac dysrhythmias are troublesome. Cardiac dysrhythmias are noticeably a part of the clinical picture in patients suffering from coronary spasm. Intravenous administration of diltiazem is effective therapy for supraventricular tachycardias including paroxysmal supraventricular tachycardia, atrial fibrillation, atrial flutter, and re-entrant tachycardias. Like verapamil, diltiazem acts by prolonging AV nodal conduction. The peripheral vascular effects of diltiazem, though, are less severe, making it a more desirable therapeutic choice in most cases. A bolus dose of 0.25 mg/kg is administered over 2 minutes and may be repeated at 0.35 mg/kg if necessary after 15 minutes. An infusion of 5 to 15 mg/hr may be necessary to maintain the reduction of HR The new 2005 ACLS Guidelines recommends use of calcium channel blockers for a variety of supraventricular arrhythmias, and because of diminished peripheral vasodilation, which implies limited effect on the arterial blood pressure, diltiazem appears to be one of the best options for management of tachyarrhythmias[36] (see Chapter 59).

Nicardipine

Nicardipine hydrochloride is a calcium channel blocker that can be administered orally and intravenously. It is the only calcium channel blocker that can be titrated intravenously to be used as an antihypertensive agent, the usual dose being 1 to 2 $\mu g/kg/min$ or 5 mg/hr.[51] Nicardipine is a smooth muscle relaxant producing vasodilation of peripheral and coronary arteries. It has a rapid onset of action, and the major effects last 10 to 15 minutes. Toxic metabolic products are not produced. It has minimal cardiodepressant effects and does not decrease the rate of the sinus node pacemaker or slow conduction through the AV node, but one should use it cautiously in patients having acute myocardial ischemia. Renal failure does not affect the dosage, but the dosage should be reduced in the elderly and those with hepatic dysfunction. It is compatible with most

ANATOMY AND PHYSIOLOGY

crystalloid solutions. Side effects of nicardipine include headache, lightheadedness, flushing, and hypotension. Reflex tachycardia is not a frequent finding with nicardipine, as is the case with nitroprusside, hydralazine, or nifedipine.[112,113,115]

Nimodipine

Nimodipine is highly lipophilic. It has a greater vasodilating effect on cerebral arteries than on vessels elsewhere because of its lipophilism, which promotes crossing the blood–brain barrier. Clinical studies demonstrate a favorable effect on the severity of neurologic deficits caused by cerebral vasospasm following subarachnoid hemorrhage. However, no radiographic evidence has been presented that nimodipine either prevents or relieves spasm of these arteries. The mechanism for clinical improvement is not known. It is an oral drug that is rapidly absorbed, with a T-terminal half-life of approximately 8 to 9 hours. The usual dose is 60 mg every 4 hours for 21 days.[51] Earlier elimination rates are much more rapid, which results in a need to redose every 4 hours. The bioavailability of an oral dose is only 13%. Dosage should be reduced in patients with hepatic dysfunction. The primary indication for nimodipine is for the improvement of neurologic deficits caused by vasospasm following subarachnoid hemorrhage from a ruptured cerebral aneurysm.[112,113,116]

Calcium Channel Blockers and Anesthesia

Evidence indicates that halothane depresses slow-channel kinetics. All of the potent inhalation anesthetics behave in a similar fashion in that they depress myocardial contractility and vascular tone in a dose-related manner. Most studies indicate that the calcium entry blockers and inhalation anesthetics exert additive effects on the inward calcium current.[117] Opioid anesthetics do not appear to add anything to the effects of the calcium entry blockers. Calcium channel blockers appear to augment the effects of both depolarizing and nondepolarizing muscle relaxants.[118] These observations serve as a word of caution because their clinical significance has not been defined. Prolonged apnea and relaxation have been reported when verapamil was used to treat a supraventricular tachycardia in a patient with Duchenne's muscular dystrophy.[119] One must be aware that calcium channel blockers may have side effects such as hypotension, in cases of overdosage, headaches, facial flushing, dizziness, ankle edema, constipation, and may even induce angina; therefore, their administration in perioperative period, when dehydration is a common occurrence, should be closely monitored.[120] Calcium entry blockers should be continued until the time of surgery to maintain control of angina pectoris, hypertension, or cardiac dysrhythmia.[101] In addition, the use of calcium channel blockers in the perioperative period appears to induce a beneficial effect of decreasing cardiac complications unrelated to cardiac surgical procedures[121] (see Chapter 23). Verapamil may increase the toxicity of digoxin, the benzodiazepines, carbamazepine, oral hypoglycemics, and possibly quinidine and theophylline.[122] Cardiac failure, AV conduction disturbances, and sinus bradycardia may be more frequent with concurrent use of beta-blockers, and severe hypotension and bradycardia may occur with bupivacaine. Decreased lithium effect and lithium neurotoxicity have both been reported with the concurrent use of verapamil.[123] The effects of verapamil may also be increased by cimetidine.

Vasodilators

Most antihypertensive drugs blunt the ANS or its effector organs or cause reflex increases in ANS outflow. Anesthetic agents may also inhibit ANS tone to some degree and might therefore have additive effects with antihypertensive drugs. In addition, patients with hypertension may exhibit greater lability in blood pressure intraoperatively and rebound hypertension in the postoperative period. A rational approach to their perioperative use includes decisions as to holding or continuing them preoperatively, possible interactions with anesthetic drugs, and resumption of treatment postoperatively.

Angiotensin-Converting Enzyme Inhibitors

The renin-angiotensin system is integrally related to the ANS in controlling blood pressure (Fig. 15-12; see Chapter 49). The central role of the renin-angiotensin-aldosterone system in the regulation of fluid balance and hemodynamics was not fully appreciated until the discovery and clinical application of inhibitors of the angiotensin-converting enzyme (ACE). Captopril, enalapril, and lisinopril inhibit converting enzyme and thereby prevent the conversion of angiotensin I to the active angiotensin II. These drugs have been highly effective in the treatment of all levels of essential hypertension as well as renovascular and malignant hypertension. The cardiovascular effects normally involve only decreased peripheral vascular resistance. CO may remain normal or increase while the filling pressure remains unchanged. Thus, these drugs have been effective in the management of congestive heart failure as well.[40] There is usually no increase in SNS tone in response to the lowered blood pressure. ACE inhibition generally results in reductions in angiotensin-aldosterone, NE, and plasma antidiuretic hormone. This suppression is accompanied by a decrease in aldosterone and an improvement in cumulative plasma potassium levels, which are beneficial in both congestive heart failure and hypertension. It can be concluded that the major humoral responses to chronic congestive heart failure, even overlooking the effects of the diuretics, are affected by the release of angiotensin, aldosterone, and increased SNS tone. Captopril, the first orally active compound, has proven highly effective in the treatment of all levels of hypertension and congestive heart. Enalapril is a second-generation (nonsulfhydryl) ACE inhibitor. The omission of the sulfhydryl group possibly diminishes side effects. Both captopril and enalapril combine a high degree of clinical efficacy with a low rate of side effects. Both are eliminated via renal excretion and should be given in reduced doses in patients with renal dysfunction. Captopril has a shorter half-life and requires more frequent dosing than enalapril. Enalapril has to be converted by esterase in the liver and other tissues into the active compound enalaprilat. Lisinopril is one of these ACE inhibitors that is absorbed as the active form and is very long acting.

The ACE inhibitors are associated with few side effects and are popular in treating hypertension. Captopril may produce reversible neutropenia, dermatitis, and angioedema. Enalapril produces syncope, headache, and dizziness in about 1% of elderly patients. All ACE inhibitors may cause hypotension in patients who are hypovolemic and taking diuretic therapy. The hypotensive effects are also enhanced by the concomitant use of calcium channel blockers. The ACE inhibitors blunt the hypokalemic effects of thiazide diuretics and may magnify the potassium-sparing effects of spironolactone, triamterene, and amiloride. In addition, nonsteroidal anti-inflammatory drugs, including aspirin, may magnify the potassium-retaining effects of ACE inhibitors. ACE-I is now a mainstay in treatment of patients with heart failure and decreased ejection fraction, since it increases their survival.[74] For patients with heart failure and normal left ventricular ejection fraction, the first line of treatment is loop diuretics in combination with beta-blockers and (ACE) inhibitors.[99] In the perioperative period, the ACE inhibitors have been associated with significant hypotension, which at times such as when separating from cardiopulmonary bypass requires additional vasopressors to sustain systemic blood pressure.[124]

A new class of drugs, namely angiotensin–receptor blockers, was developed by inhibiting directly the effects of the hormone angiotensin II. These medications have been developed with the hope that, being similar to an ACE inhibitor, one could expect the same effectiveness, with fewer side effects such as cough, angioneurotic edema, and rash.[125] Alternatively, there are data that this class of drugs may have some beneficial effects on decreasing the renal deterioration in diabetic patients.[126]

Hydralazine

Hydralazine is the most commonly used vasodilator and can be given by the intramuscular, intravenous, and oral routes to achieve an optimum blood pressure control. It relaxes smooth muscle tone directly, without interacting with adrenergic or cholinergic receptors. The mechanism of action is unknown. It is most potent in coronary, splanchnic, renal, and cerebral vessels, causing increased blood flow in each of these organs. The decrease in cardiac afterload is beneficial, but, unfortunately, there is usually a concomitant reflex tachycardia that may be severe. It is commonly combined with a beta-blocker such as propranolol. Hydralazine is metabolized by hepatic acetylation, and oral bioavailability may be low owing to first-pass metabolism. The elimination half-life is about 4 hours, but the pharmacologic half-life is much longer as a result of avid binding of the drug to smooth muscle. The effective half-life is approximately 100 hours. Side effects include a lupuslike syndrome, drug fever, skin rash, pancytopenia, and peripheral neuropathy. The IV dose for perioperative use is 5 to 10 mg in an IV bolus every 15 to 20 minutes until blood pressure control is achieved. It may also be given 10 to 40 mg intramuscularly, but the response is slower.[78,112,127]

Sodium Nitroprusside

Sodium nitroprusside is an extremely potent vasodilator that is available only for IV administration (see Chapter 41). It acts directly on smooth muscle, causing both arterial and venous dilation. The action of sodium nitroprusside on both venous and arterial sides of the circulation causes decreases in cardiac preload as well as afterload.[99,128] This results in decreased cardiac work; however, it has been suggested that sodium nitroprusside may further compromise ischemic myocardium in the presence of occlusive coronary artery disease by shunting blood away from the ischemic zone.[129] Other potential and deleterious side effects include pulmonary vasodilation with an increased ventilation-perfusion mismatch and with resultant hypoxia, and temporary decrease in platelet function.[51,130] Sodium nitroprusside is useful during the perioperative period. It lowers blood pressure within 1 to 2 minutes, with the effect dissipating within 2 minutes after infusion is stopped. It is extremely potent and should be administered through a central venous line by infusion pump while continuously monitoring arterial pressure. The starting dose is 0.25 to 0.5 μg/kg/min. It can be increased slowly as needed to control blood pressure, but chances for toxicity are greater if the dose of 2 μg/kg/min is exceeded. The dose required for steady-state-induced hypotension is variable. The hypotensive effects of sodium nitroprusside may be potentiated by inhalation anesthetics and blood loss; therefore, close perioperative monitoring is essential. It is commonly used to induce hypotension for decreasing blood loss in patients predisposed to major hemorrhage.[112]

Chemically, sodium nitroprusside consists of a ferrous iron atom bound with five cyanide molecules and one nitric group. The ferrous iron reacts with sulfhydryl groups in red blood cells and releases cyanide. Cyanide is reduced to thiocyanate in the liver and excreted in the urine. The half-life of thiocyanate is 4 days, and it accumulates in the presence of renal failure.

Administration of high doses of sodium nitroprusside can result in cyanide toxicity. The cyanide molecule binds to cytochrome oxidase, interfering with electron transport and causing cellular hypoxia. Toxicity can be recognized by the triad of tachyphylaxis (increasing tolerance to the drug dose), elevated mixed venous PaO_2, and metabolic acidosis. The possible treatments of cyanide toxicity consist of (1) administration of amyl nitrate (by inhalation or directly into the anesthesia circuit), (2) infusion of sodium nitrite, and (3) administration of sodium thiosulfate.

Nitroglycerin

Nitroglycerin, or glyceryl trinitrate, is a venodilator used to treat myocardial ischemia (see Chapter 41). Its predominant action is on venules, causing increased venous capacitance and decreased cardiac preload. Effects on the arterial side are minimal except at very high doses. The usual IV dose is 1 to 3 μg/kg/min. On IV administration, effects can be seen within 2 minutes, and they usually resolve within 5 minutes of discontinuing the drug. Side effects are minimal, and there is no potential for cyanide toxicity as with nitroprusside. Use of nitroglycerin for control of perioperative hypertension has been reported but because of its relatively weak arteriolar action it is not as useful as other drugs as an antihypertensive agent.[99,128] In obstetric patients with pre-eclampsia, however, it may be chosen over nitroprusside to circumvent potential cyanide toxicity to the fetus.[131]

Nesiritide

Nesiritide is a recombinant form of a human B-type natriuretic peptide. It is identical with the endogenous hormone liberated by the ventricles in situations characterized by volume overload and increased wall tension. Nesiritide acts on guanylate cyclase similar to nitric oxide, and therefore induces beneficial effects on hemodynamics by venous and arterial vasodilation, including coronary vasodilation. It is more effective than nitroglycerin in decreasing the right atrial pressure, pulmonary capillary wedge pressure, systemic vascular resistance, and ultimately improves the CO. The possible side effects include hypotension, headache, and renal dysfunction. The dose is 2 μg/kg bolus, continued with continuous infusion of 0.01 μg/kg/min that may be increased to a maximum of 0.03 μg/kg/min, with the most significant side effect being hypotension. The biologic effects last longer than expected from the drug's half-life. Nesiritide is beneficial for rapid improvement of dyspnea, and can be used in patients with decompensated heart failure, in addition to diuretic therapy for rapid improvement of symptoms; but again the possibility of worsening renal function, together with possible worsening 30-day mortality in a recent study, made its safety questionable.[31,40,128]

References

1. Guyton AC, Hall JE: The autonomic nervous system and the adrenal medulla, Textbook of Medical Physiology, 11th edition. Edited by Guyton AC, Hall JE. Philadelphia, Elsevier & Saunders, 2006, pp 748
2. Eisenhofer G: Sympathetic nerve function—assessment by radioisotope dilution analysis. Clin Autonom Res 2005; 15: 264
3. Flacke WE, Flacke JW: Cholinergic and anticholinergic agents, Drug interactions in anesthesia, 2nd edition. Edited by Smith NT, Corbascio AN. Philadelphia, Lea & Febiger, 1986, pp 160
4. Guyton AC, Hall JE: Cardiac output, venous return, and their regulation, Textbook of Medical Physiology. Edited by Guyton AC, Hall JE. Philadelphia, Elsevier & Saunders, 2006, pp 232

5. Ajani AE, Yan BP: The mystery of coronary artery spasm. Heart Lung Circ 2007; 16: 10

6. Kawano H, Ogawa H: Endothelial dysfunction and coronary artery spasm. Curr Drug Targets Cardiovasc Haematol Dis 2004; 4: 23

7. Bevan JA: Some bases of differences in vascular response to sympathetic activity. Circ Res 1979; 45: 161

8. O'Rourke ST, Vanhoutte PM: Adrenergic and cholinergic regulation of bronchial vascular tone. Am Rev Respir Dis 1992; 146: S11

9. Pearl RG, Maze M, Rosenthal MH: Pulmonary and systemic hemodynamic effects of central venous and left atrial sympathomimetic drug administration in the dog. J Cardiothorac Anesth 1987; 1: 29

10. Sinski M, Lewandowski J, Abramczyk P, et al: Why study sympathetic nervous system? J Physiol Pharmacol 2006; 57(Suppl 11): 79

11. Civantos Calzada B, Aleixandre de Artinano A: Alpha-adrenoceptor subtypes. Pharmacol Res 2001; 44: 195

12. Aubry ML, Davey MJ, Petch B: Cardioprotective and antidysrhythmic effects of alpha 1-adrenoceptor blockade during myocardial ischaemia and reperfusion in the dog. J Cardiovasc Pharmacol 1985; 7(Suppl 6): S93

13. Cohen RA, Shepherd JT, Vanhoutte PM: Effects of the adrenergic transmitter on epicardial coronary arteries. Fed Proc 1984; 43: 2862–2866.

14. Baumgart D, Haude M, Gorge G, et al: Augmented alpha-adrenergic constriction of atherosclerotic human coronary arteries. Circulation 1999; 99: 2090

15. DM Griggs Jr WC, RB Boatwright: Evidence against significant resting alpha-adrenergic coronary vasoconstrictor tone. Fed Proc 1984; 43: 2873

16. Heusch G, Baumgart D, Camici P, et al: Alpha-adrenergic coronary vasoconstriction and myocardial ischemia in humans. Circulation 2000; 101: 689

17. Lymperopoulos A, Rengo G, Koch WJ, et al: Adrenal adrenoceptors in heart failure: fine-tuning cardiac stimulation. Trends Molec Med 2007; 13: 503

18. Vanhoutte PM: Endothelial adrenoceptors. J Cardiovasc Pharmacol 2001; 38: 796

19. Tobata D, Takao K, Mochizuki M, et al: Effects of dopamine, dobutamine, amrinone and milrinone on regional blood flow in isoflurane anesthetized dogs. J Vet Med Sci 2004; 66: 1097

20. M Hilberman JM, EB Stinson: The diuretic properties of dopamine in patients after open-heart surgery. Anesthesiology 1984; 61: 489

21. Owall A, Gordon E, Lagerkranser M, et al: Clinical experience with adenosine for controlled hypotension during cerebral aneurysm surgery. Anesth Analg 1987; 66: 229

22. Brodde OE: Beta-adrenoceptors in cardiac disease. Pharmacol Ther 1993; 60: 405

23. Bridenbaugh PO, Greene NM, Brull SJ: Spinal (subarahnoid) neural blockade, Neural Blockade in Clinical Anesthesia, and management of pain, 3rd Edition. Edited by Cousins MJ, Bridenbaugh PO. Philadelphia-New York, Lippincott Williams & Wilkins, 1997.

24. Valantine H: Cardiac allograft vasculopathy after heart transplantation: risk factors and management. J Heart Lung Transplant 2004; 23: S187

25. Levy MN, Blattberg B: Effect of vagal stimulation on the overflow of norepinephrine into the coronary sinus during cardiac sympathetic nerve stimulation in the dog. Circ Res 1976; 38: 81

26. Stoelting RK, Hillier S: Pharmacology & physiology in anesthetic practice, 4th Edition. Philadelphia, Lippincott Williams & Wilkins, 2006.

27. Dampney RA, Coleman MJ, Fontes MA, et al: Central mechanisms underlying short- and long-term regulation of the cardiovascular system. Clin Exp Pharmacol Physiol 2002; 29: 261

28. Spaulding BC, Choi SD, Gross JB, et al: The effect of physostigmine on diazepam-induced ventilatory depression: a double-blind study. Anesthesiology 1984; 61: 551

29. Miano TA, Crouch MA: Evolving role of vasopressin in the treatment of cardiac arrest. Pharmacotherapy 2006; 26: 828

30. Rooke GA, Freund PR, Jacobson AF: Hemodynamic response and change in organ blood volume during spinal anesthesia in elderly men with cardiac disease. Anesth Analg 1997; 85: 99

31. Poole-Wilson PA, Opie LH: Digitalis, acute inotropes, and inotropic dilators. Acute and chronic heart failure, Drugs for the heart, 6th Edition. Edited by Opie LH, Gersh BJ. Philadelphia, Elsevier Saunders, 2005, pp 149

32. Dellinger RP, Levy MM, Carlet JM, et al: International Surviving Sepsis Campaign Guidelines C, American Association of Critical-Care N, American College of Chest P, American College of Emergency P, Canadian Critical Care S, European Society of Clinical Microbiology and Infectious D, European Society of Intensive Care M, European Respiratory S, International Sepsis F, Japanese Association for Acute M, Japanese Society of Intensive Care M, Society of Critical Care M, Society of Hospital M, Surgical Infection S, World Federation of Societies of Intensive and Critical Care M,: Surviving Sepsis Campaign: International Guidelines for Management of Severe Sepsis and Septic Shock: 2008. Crit Care Med 2008; 36: 296

33. Sladen RN: Oliguria in the ICU. Systematic approach to diagnosis and treatment. Anesthesiol Clin North Am 2000; 18: 739

34. Johnston RR, Eger EI, II, Wilson C: A comparative interaction of epinephrine with enflurane, isoflurane, and halothane in man. Anesth Analg 1976; 55: 709

35. Karl HW, Swedlow DB, Lee KW, et al: Epinephrine-halothane interactions in children. Anesthesiology 1983; 58: 142

36. 2005 American Heart Association Guidelines for Cardiopulmonary Resuscitation and Emergency Cardiovascular Care. Circulation 2005; 112: IV1

37. Butterworth JFt, Prielipp RC, Royster RL, et al: Dobutamine increases heart rate more than epinephrine in patients recovering from aortocoronary bypass surgery. J Cardiothorac Vasc Anesth 1992; 6: 535

38. Zamanian RT, Haddad F, Doyle RL, et al: Management strategies for patients with pulmonary hypertension in the intensive care unit. Crit Care Med 2007; 35: 2037

39. Asfar P, Hauser B, Radermacher P, et al: Catecholamines and vasopressin during critical illness. Crit Care Clin 2006; 22: 131

40. Shin DD, Brandimarte F, De Luca L, et al: Review of current and investigational pharmacologic agents for acute heart failure syndromes. Am J Cardiol 2007; 99: 4A

41. Venkataraman R: Can we prevent acute kidney injury? Crit Care Med 2008; 36: S166

42. Friedrich JO, Adhikari N, Herridge MS, et al: Meta-analysis: low-dose dopamine increases urine output but does not prevent renal dysfunction or death. Ann Intern Med 2005; 142: 510

43. Banic A, Krejci V, Erni D, et al: Effects of sodium nitroprusside and phenylephrine on blood flow in free musculocutaneous flaps during general anesthesia. Anesthesiology 1999; 90: 147

44. Bayram M, De Luca L, Massie MB, et al: Reassessment of dobutamine, dopamine, and milrinone in the management of acute heart failure syndromes. Am J Cardiol 2005; 96: 47G

45. Parissis J, Farmakis D, Nieminen M: Classical inotropes and new cardiac enhancers. Heart Failure Reviews 2007; 12: 149

46. Petersen JW, Felker GM: Inotropes in the management of acute heart failure. Crit Care Med 2008; 36: S106

47. Feneck R: Drugs for the perioperative control of hypertension: current issues and future directions. Drugs 2007; 67: 2023

48. Stone GW, McCullough PA, Tumlin JA, et al: Fenoldopam mesylate for the prevention of contrast-induced nephropathy: a randomized controlled trial. Jama 2003; 290: 2284

49. Zacharias M, Gilmore IC, Herbison GP, et al: Interventions for protecting renal function in the perioperative period. Cochrane Database Syst Rev 2005: CD003590.

50. Landoni G, Biondi-Zoccai GG, Tumlin JA, et al: Beneficial impact of fenoldopam in critically ill patients with or at risk for acute renal failure: a meta-analysis of randomized clinical trials. Am J Kidney Dis 2007; 49: 56

51. Brunton LL, Lazo J, Parker KL: The Goodman and Gilman's The Pharmacological Basis of Therapeutics. 11th edition, New York, McGraw-Hill, 2006.

52. Buvanendran A, Kroin JS, Buvanendran A, et al: Useful adjuvants for postoperative pain management. Best Pract Res Clin Anaesthesiol 2007; 21: 31

53. Wallace AW GD, Salahieh A: Effect of Clonidine on Cardiovascular Morbidity and Mortality after Noncardiac Surgery. . Anesthesiology 2004; 101: 284

54. Aantaa R, Kanto J, Scheinin M, et al: Dexmedetomidine, an alpha 2-adrenoceptor agonist, reduces anesthetic requirements for patients undergoing minor gynecologic surgery. Anesthesiology 1990; 73: 230

55. Szumita PM, Baroletti SA, Anger KE, et al: Sedation and analgesia in the intensive care unit: evaluating the role of dexmedetomidine. Am J Health Syst Pharm 2007; 64: 37

56. Biccard BM, Goga S, de Beurs J: Dexmedetomidine and cardiac protection for non-cardiac surgery: a meta-analysis of randomised controlled trials. Anaesthesia 2008; 63: 4

57. Lee CR, Watkins ML, Patterson JH, et al: Vasopressin: a new target for the treatment of heart failure. Am Heart J 2003; 146: 9

58. Russell JA: Vasopressin in septic shock. Crit Care Med 2007; 35: S609

59. Diamond LM: Cardiopulmonary resuscitation and acute cardiovascular life support–a protocol review of the updated guidelines. Crit Care Clin 2007; 23: 873

60. Russell JA, Walley KR, Singer J, et al: Vasopressin versus norepinephrine infusion in patients with septic shock. N Engl J Med 2008; 358: 877

61. Barrett LK, Singer M, Clapp LH: Vasopressin: mechanisms of action on the vasculature in health and in septic shock. Crit Care Med 2007; 35: 33

62. Craig RL, Michael LW, Patterson JH, et al: Vasopressin: a new target for the treatment of heart failure. Am Heart J 2003; 146: 9

63. Wyer PC, Perera P, Jin Z, et al: Vasopressin or epinephrine for out-of-hospital cardiac arrest. Ann Emerg Med 2006; 48: 86

64. Studer W, Wu X, Siegemund M, et al: Resuscitation from cardiac arrest with adrenaline/epinephrine or vasopressin: effects on intestinal mucosal tonometer pCO(2) during the postresuscitation period in rats. Resuscitation 2002; 53: 201

65. Parrillo JE: Septic shock—vasopressin, norepinephrine, and urgency. N Engl J Med 2008; 358: 954

66. Rivers E, Nguyen B, Havstad S, et al: Early goal-directed therapy in the treatment of severe sepsis and septic shock. N Engl J Med 2001; 345: 1368

67. Delacretaz E: Clinical practice. Supraventricular tachycardia. N Engl J Med 2006; 354: 1039

68. Chiu C, Sequeira IB: Diagnosis and treatment of idiopathic ventricular tachycardia. AACN Clin Issues 2004; 15: 449

69. Holdgate A, Foo A: Adenosine versus intravenous calcium channel antagonists for the treatment of supraventricular tachycardia in adults. Cochrane Database Syst Rev 2006: CD005154.

70. Gillies M, Bellomo R, Doolan L, et al: Bench-to-bedside review: Inotropic drug therapy after adult cardiac surgery — a systematic literature review. [see comment]. Crit Care (London, England) 2005; 9: 266

71. McBride BF, White CM: Acute decompensated heart failure: a contemporary approach to pharmacotherapeutic management. Pharmacotherapy 2003; 23: 997

72. Shakar SF, Linseman JV, Lowes BD: Inotropes and beta-blockers: is there a need for new guidelines? J Cardiac Failure 2001; 7: 8

73. Endoh M, Hori M: Acute heart failure: inotropic agents and their clinical uses. Exp Opin Pharmacother 2006; 7: 2179

74. Aronow WS: Treatment of heart failure with abnormal left ventricular systolic function in the elderly. Heart Fail Clin 2007; 3: 423

75. Rosen D, Decaro MV, Graham MG: Evidence-based treatment of chronic heart failure. Compr Ther 2007; 33: 2

76. Zaloga G, Chernow B: Insulin, glucagon and growth hormone, The Pharmacologic Approach to the Critically Ill Patient. Edited by Chernow B, Lake C. Baltimore, Williams & Wilkins, 1983, pp 562

77. Sampson HA, Munoz-Furlong A, Campbell RL, et al: Second symposium on the definition and management of anaphylaxis: summary report—Second National Institute of Allergy and Infectious Disease/Food Allergy and Anaphylaxis Network Symposium. J Allergy Clin Immunol 2006; 117: 391

78. Aronow WS: Treatment of heart failure with normal left ventricular ejection fraction. Compr Ther 2007; 33: 223

79. Ariyan CE, Sosa JA: Assessment and management of patients with abnormal calcium. Crit Care Med 2004; 32: S146

80. Aguilera IM, Vaughan RS: Calcium and the anaesthetist. [see comment]. Anaesthesia 2000; 55: 779

81. Shapira N, Schaff HV, White RD, et al: Hemodynamic effects of calcium chloride injection following cardiopulmonary bypass: response to bolus injection and continuous infusion. Ann Thorac Surg 1984; 37: 133

82. Janelle GM, Urdaneta F, Martin TD, et al: Effects of calcium chloride on grafted internal mammary artery flow after cardiopulmonary bypass. J Cardiothorac Vasc Anesth 2000; 14: 4

83. Yellon DM, Hausenloy DJ: Myocardial reperfusion injury. N Engl J Med 2007; 357: 1121

84. White RD, Goldsmith RS, Rodriguez R, et al: Plasma ionic calcium levels following injection of chloride, gluconate, and gluceptate salts of calcium. J Thorac Cardiovasc Surg 1976; 71: 609

85. Bhatara VS, Magnus RD, Paul KL, et al: Serotonin syndrome induced by venlafaxine and fluoxetine: a case study in polypharmacy and potential pharmacodynamic and pharmacokinetic mechanisms. Ann Pharmacother 1998; 32: 432

86. Pacak K: Preoperative management of the pheochromocytoma patient. J Clin Endocrinol Metab 2007; 92: 4069

87. Weber MA: The role of the new beta-blockers in treating cardiovascular disease. Am J Hypertens 2005; 18: 169S

88. Pratt CM: Three decades of clinical trials with beta-blockers: the contribution of the CAPRICORN trial and the effect of carvedilol on serious arrhythmias. J Am Coll Cardiol 2005; 45: 531

89. Effect of metoprolol CR/XL in chronic heart failure: Metoprolol CR/XL Randomised Intervention Trial in Congestive Heart Failure (MERIT-HF). Lancet 1999; 353: 2001

90. Cleland JG, Loh H, Windram J: Are there clinically important differences between beta-blockers in heart failure? Heart Fail Clin 2005; 1: 57

91. Flather MD, Shibata MC, Coats AJ, et al: Randomized trial to determine the effect of nebivolol on mortality and cardiovascular hospital admission in elderly patients with heart failure (SENIORS). Eur Heart J 2005; 26: 215

92. Baxter AD, Kanji S: Protocol implementation in anesthesia: beta-blockade in non-cardiac surgery patients. Can J Anaesth 2007; 54: 114

93. Wallace A, Layug B, Tateo I, et al: Prophylactic atenolol reduces postoperative myocardial ischemia. McSPI Research Group. Anesthesiology 1998; 88: 7

94. Beattie WS, Wijeysundera DN, Karkouti K, et al: Does tight heart rate control improve beta-blocker efficacy? An updated analysis of the noncardiac surgical randomized trials. Anesth Analg 2008; 106: 1039

95. Feringa HH, Bax JJ, Boersma E, et al: High-dose beta-blockers and tight heart rate control reduce myocardial ischemia and troponin T release in vascular surgery patients. Circulation 2006; 114: I344

96. London MJ: Beta blockers and alpha2 agonists for cardioprotection. Best Pract Res Clin Anaesthesiol 2008; 22: 95

97. POISE Study Group. Effects of extended-release metoprolol succinate in patients undergoing non-cardiac surgery (POISE trial): a randomised controlled trial. Lancet 2008; 371: 1839

98. Poldermans D, Boersma E: Beta-blocker therapy in noncardiac surgery. N Engl J Med 2005; 353: 412

99. Trujillo TC, Dobesh PP: Traditional management of chronic stable angina. Pharmacotherapy 2007; 27: 1677

100. Fleisher LA: Perioperative beta-blockade: how best to translate evidence into practice. Anesth Analg 2007; 104: 1

101. Fleisher LA, Beckman JA, Brown KA, Calkins H, Chaikof E, Fleischmann KE, et al: ACC/AHA 2007 guidelines on perioperative cardiovascular evaluation and care for noncardiac surgery: executive summary: a report of the American College of Cardiology/American Heart Association Task Force on Practice Guidelines (Writing Committee to Revise the 2002 Guidelines on Perioperative Cardiovascular Evaluation for Noncardiac Surgery). Anesth Analg 2008; 106: 685

102. Fleisher LA, Beckman JA, Brown KA, Calkins H, Chaikof E, Fleischmann KE, et al: a report of the American College of Cardiology/American Heart Association Task Force on Practice Guidelines (Writing Committee to Update the 2002 Guidelines on Perioperative Cardiovascular Evaluation for Noncardiac Surgery): developed in collaboration with the American Society of Echocardiography, American Society of Nuclear Cardiology, Heart Rhythm Society, Society of Cardiovascular Anesthesiologists, Society for Cardiovascular Angiography and Interventions, and Society for Vascular Medicine and Biology. Circulation 2006; 113: 2662

103. Wetterslev J, Juul AB: Benefits and harms of perioperative beta-blockade. Best Pract Res Clin Anaesthesiol 2006; 20: 285

104. Fleisher LA, Poldermans D. Perioperative β blockade: where do we go from here? Lancet 2008; 371: 1813

105. Norbury WB, Jeschke MG, Herndon DN: Metabolism modulators in sepsis: propranolol. Crit Care Med 2007; 35: S616

106. Mangano DT, Layug EL, Wallace A, et al: Effect of atenolol on mortality and cardiovascular morbidity after noncardiac surgery. Multicenter Study of Perioperative Ischemia Research Group. [see comment][erratum appears in N Engl J Med 1997 Apr 3;336(14):1039]. New England Journal of Medicine 1996; 335: 1713

107. Degoute C-S: Controlled hypotension: a guide to drug choice. Drugs 2007; 67: 1053

108. Frakes MA: Rapid sequence induction medications: an update. J Emerg Nurs 2003; 29: 533

109. Frakes MA: Esmolol: a unique drug with ED applications. J Emerg Nurs 2001; 27: 47

110. Tafreshi MJ, Weinacker AB: Beta-adrenergic-blocking agents in bronchospastic diseases: a therapeutic dilemma. Pharmacotherapy 1999; 19: 974

111. Nieminen T, Lehtimaki T, Maenpaa J, et al: Ophthalmic timolol: plasma concentration and systemic cardiopulmonary effects. Scand J Clin Lab Invest 2007; 67: 237

112. Ezzeddine MA, Suri MF, Hussein HM, et al: Blood pressure management in patients with acute stroke: pathophysiology and treatment strategies. Neurosurg Clin N Am 2006; 17 Suppl 1: 41

113. Mocco J, Zacharia BE, Komotar RJ, et al: A review of current and future medical therapies for cerebral vasospasm following aneurysmal subarachnoid hemorrhage. Neurosurg Focus 2006; 21: E9.

114. Weck M: Treatment of hypertension in patients with diabetes mellitus: relevance of sympathovagal balance and renal function. Clin Res Cardiol 2007; 96: 707

115. Curran MP, Robinson DM, Keating GM: Intravenous nicardipine: its use in the short-term treatment of hypertension and various other indications. Drugs 2006; 66: 1755

*116. Pantoni L, del Ser T, Soglian AG, et al: Efficacy and safety of nimodipine in subcortical vascular dementia: a randomized placebo-controlled trial. Stroke 2005; 36: 619

117. Reves JG, Kissin I, Lell WA, et al: Calcium entry blockers: uses and implications for anesthesiologists. Anesthesiology 1982; 57: 504

118. Carpenter RL, Mulroy MF: Edrophonium antagonizes combined lidocaine-pancuronium and verapamil-pancuronium neuromuscular blockade in cats. Anesthesiology 1986; 65: 506

119. Zalman F, Perloff JK, Durant NN, et al: Acute respiratory failure following intravenous verapamil in Duchenne's muscular dystrophy. Am Heart J 1983; 105: 510

120. Opie LH: Calcium Channel Blockers (calcium antagonists), Drugs for the heart. 6th edition. Edited by Opie LH, Gersh BJ. Philadelphia, Elsevier Saunders, 2005, pp 50

121. Wijeysundera DN, Beattie WS: Calcium channel blockers for reducing cardiac morbidity after noncardiac surgery: a meta-analysis. Anesth Analg 2003; 97: 634

122. Zhou SF, Xue CC, Yu XQ, et al: Clinically important drug interactions potentially involving mechanism-based inhibition of cytochrome P450 3A4 and the role of therapeutic drug monitoring. Ther Drug Monit 2007; 29: 687

123. Price WA, Giannini AJ: Neurotoxicity caused by lithium-verapamil synergism. J Clin Pharmacol 1986; 26: 717

124. Tuman KJ, McCarthy RJ, O'Connor CJ, Holm WE, Ivankovich AD: Angiotensin-converting enzyme inhibitors increase vasoconstrictor requirements after cardiopulmonary bypass. Anesth Analg 1995; 80: 473

125. Cohn JN, Tognoni G: A randomized trial of the angiotensin-receptor blocker valsartan in chronic heart failure. N Engl J Med 2001; 345: 1667

126. Lewis EJ, Hunsicker LG, Clarke WR, Berl T, Pohl MA, Lewis JB, et al: Renoprotective effect of the angiotensin-receptor antagonist irbesartan in patients with nephropathy due to type 2 diabetes. N Engl J Med 2001; 345: 851

ANATOMY AND PHYSIOLOGY

127. Vigil-De Gracia P, Ruiz E, Lopez JC, et al: Management of severe hypertension in the postpartum period with intravenous hydralazine or labetalol: a randomized clinical trial. Hypertens Preg 2007; 26: 163

128. Elkayam U, Janmohamed M, Habib M, et al: Vasodilators in the management of acute heart failure. Crit Care Med 2008; 36: S95

129. Chiariello M, Gold HK, Leinbach RC, et al: Comparison between the effects of nitroprusside and nitroglycerin on ischemic injury during acute myocardial infarction. Circulation 1976; 54: 766

130. Harris SN, Rinder CS, Rinder HM, et al: Nitroprusside inhibition of platelet function is transient and reversible by catecholamine priming. Anesthesiology 1995; 83: 1145

131. Dufour P, Vinatier D, Puech F: The use of intravenous nitroglycerin for cervico-uterine relaxation: a review of the literature. Arch Gynecol Obstet 1997; 261: 1

CHAPTER 16 ■ HEMOSTASIS AND TRANSFUSION MEDICINE

JOHN C. DRUMMOND, CHARISE T. PETROVITCH, AND THOMAS A. LANE

ANATOMY AND PHYSIOLOGY

KEY POINTS

1 In terms of transfusion-transmitted infectious diseases, the American blood supply has never been safer than it is today.

2 Clerical and patient identification errors are the most common causes of ABO incompatibility and a large fraction of these errors typically occur in the operating theater.

3 The three leading causes of transfusion-related death in the United States are ABO incompatibility, transfusion-related acute lung injury, and sepsis caused by bacterial infections.

4 In the setting of massive transfusion, assuming maintenance of isovolemia and the absence of a consumptive coagulopathy, critical dilution of clotting factors and platelets is likely to occur after an average replacement of 140% and 230% of blood volume, respectively.

5 With the possible exception of trauma resuscitation, coagulation factor and platelet replacement should be determined by laboratory assessment and/or observation of clinical coagulopathy and *not* estimated blood loss-driven formulas.

6 The red blood cell (RBC) transfusion "trigger" for most patients will lie between hemoglobin values of 7 and 10 g/dL.

7 Platelet administration thresholds relevant to anesthesiologists usually will lie between 50,000 and 100,000/uL.

8 Normal coagulation can be achieved with clotting factor levels of 20 to 30% of normal. Those levels can usually be achieved by administration of 10 to 15 mL/kg of fresh-frozen plasma.

9 Recipient or donor unit identification errors will result in an acute hemolytic transfusion reaction for one of every three packed RBC (PRBC) units mistransfused.

10 A patient who has received 10 to 12 units of group O RBCs should not be switched back to his or her own ABO group until testing has been performed to confirm that significant titers of anti-A or anti-B antibodies are not present.

11 The classic, dual-cascade (intrinsic and extrinsic pathway) model of coagulation is an inadequate representation of coagulation, as it occurs in vivo.

12 In vivo, coagulation is initiated principally by contact of factor VII with extravascular tissue factor leading first to platelet activation followed by the generation of large amounts of thrombin by activated clotting factors acting on the phospholipid surface provided by activated platelets.

13 Under normal conditions, plasmin is generated only at the site of clot formation and is destroyed rapidly once released into the circulation. This localization process fails at times of accelerated fibrinolysis (disseminated intravascular coagulation, primary fibrinolysis).

14 von Willebrand disease is the most common hereditary bleeding disorder. Some form of the disease, which may be subclinical prior to surgery, is present in approximately 1% of the population.

15 Factors II, VII, IX, and X and proteins C and S depend on vitamin K for their synthesis. Vitamin K deficiency occurs frequently in hospitalized patients because of dietary insufficiency, gut sterilization, and malabsorption. A high index of suspicion for vitamin K deficiency should be maintained.

16 As many as 5% of patients who receive heparin therapy for 5 days will develop heparin-induced thrombocytopenia/thrombosis. The clinical manifestations are more often the result of thrombosis and thromboembolism than thrombocytopenia.

In the year 2004, 14.2 million units of packed red blood cells (PRBCs), 9.9 million units of platelets (84% of which were apheresis units), and 4.1 million units of fresh-frozen plasma (FFP) were administered in the United States.[1] At the University of California, San Diego (UCSD) Medical Center, approximately 40% of all transfused units are administered to surgical patients by anesthesia personnel. An extrapolation of these numbers suggests that anesthesia providers may be involved in as many as 8.3 million donor unit exposures per year in the United States. Accordingly, no specialty group, save those who collect, process, and deliver blood products, has a greater incentive to have a broad grasp of the principles of transfusion medicine.

This chapter begins with a review of the risks associated with the administration of blood products, followed by a discussion of the factors that determine the necessity for the administration of the three most commonly used components, RBCs, FFP, and platelets, and then a discussion of conservation techniques for minimizing the necessity for transfusion. The remainder of the chapter presents a description of the preparation of blood products, a discussion of the physiology of hemostasis, a description of tests of the hemostatic mechanism, and finally a review of common bleeding disorders, including a discussion of the effects of pharmacologic agents on hemostasis.

THE RISKS OF BLOOD PRODUCT ADMINISTRATION

The recognition that the human immunodeficiency virus (HIV) is transmissible by blood generated public fear of transfusion and led to dramatic changes in transfusion practices (see Chapter 13). While the transfusion-related transmission of HIV is now vanishingly rare, there remain numerous other hazards associated with blood products. The risks can be subdivided into those of infectious and noninfectious etiologies. Transfusion-transmissible infections, in particular viral infections, have generated the greatest concern and will therefore be addressed first. However, in reality, the morbidity and mortality associated with nonviral hazards are far greater concerns.

Infectious Risks Associated with Blood Product Administration

The potentially transmittable diseases/agents in blood are numerous. They include several viruses (hepatitis A, B, C, D, E), the human T-cell lymphotropic viruses (HTLV-1, HTLV-2), the human immunodeficiency viruses 1 and 2, cytomegalovirus (CMV), West Nile virus (WNV), the Epstein-Barr virus, human herpes virus-8 (the agent of Kaposi sarcoma), parvovirus B19, the GBV-C virus (also called hepatitis G), transfusion-transmitted virus, and the SEN virus. Other diseases/agents include prions (Creutzfeldt-Jakob disease [CJD] and variant Creutzfeldt-Jakob disease [vCJD]), Lyme disease, contaminating bacteria, parasites (malaria, Chagas' disease, ehrlichiosis, babesiosis), and syphilis.[2,3] Several of these will not be considered further. Although GBV-C, transfusion-transmitted virus, and SEN virus are transmitted by transfusion, they do not appear to cause clinical disease; the rate of transmission of parvovirus B19 is very low and clinical disease is extremely infrequent[2]; there have been no reported instances of transfusion-transmitted Lyme disease and only one instance of ehrlichiosis.[4]

Estimates of the frequency of infectious agents in the North American blood supply are presented in Table 16-1. The rate of viral infectivity has decreased dramatically in the last 2 decades. The advent of universal (in the United States) nucleic

TABLE 16-1

ESTIMATES OF THE RATE (PER DONOR EXPOSURE) OF TRANSFUSION-TRANSMITTED INFECTIOUS DISEASE IN NORTH AMERICA

■ DISEASE	■ RATE
• Hepatitis B (HBV)	1/269,000
• Hepatitis C (HCV)	1/1,600,000
• Human immunodeficiency virus (HIV)	1/1,780,000
• Human T-cell lymphotrophic virus (HTLV)	1/2,900,000
• West Nile Virus (WNV)	Indeterminate/very low
• Cytomegalovirus (CMV)—Nonleukoreduced random donor	7%
• Leukoreduced random donor	2–4%
• CMV seronegative donor	1–2%
• Epstein-Barr virus (EBV)	0–5%
• Chagas'; malaria; other parasites	< 1/1,000,000
Bacterial sepsis	
• Platelets (apheresis, culture tested)	1/50,000
• Platelets (whole-blood derived, surrogate tested)	1/33,000
• Platelets (untested)	1/2,500–13,400

Data derived from several sources (Refs. 5, 7, 14, 17–19, 52, and 276).

acid testing (NAT) for HIV and hepatitis C (HCV) has reduced the frequency of transmission of those agents to very low levels, approximately 1 in 1.7 million units transfused. Hepatitis B (HBV) remains the greatest risk, currently with about 1/269,000 donor exposures.[5] All of these estimates are derived from the observed rates of seropositivity among donors and the statistical likelihood of administration of blood from donors whose infection is in the window period between contracting the virus and detectability by the available assays. The window periods from infection to detection by 16-unit minipool NAT testing for HIV and HCV are estimated to be 9 and 7.4 days, respectively.[6] Minipool testing entails analysis of pooled aliquots from 6 to 24 units. It is estimated that the more expensive individual donor testing could reduce the window period for HIV and HCV to 5.6 and 4.9 days, respectively.[6] For HBV, using hepatitis B surface antigen testing, the window period is 38 days.[7] A NAT test for HBV is available. However, when performed on minipools rather than on individual donations, it will probably add little to the detection sensitivity achieved with the combination of hepatitis B surface antigen and the anti-hepatitis B core antigen.[7–9]

1   In terms of transfusion-transmitted infectious diseases, the North American blood supply has never been safer than it is today.

Hepatitis C

The significance of HCV is that, despite its commonly mild initial presentation, it progresses to a chronic state in 85% with significant associated morbidity and mortality of patients. Twenty percent of chronic carriers develop cirrhosis and 1 to 5% develop hepatocellular carcinoma.[10,11]

Hepatitis B

It is estimated that only 35% of HBV-exposed patients will develop acute disease,[12] although approximately 1% will develop fulminant acute hepatitis. In approximately 85% of patients, the disease resolves spontaneously, 9% develop chronic persistent hepatitis, 3% develop chronic active hepatitis, 1% develop cirrhosis with or without chronic active hepatitis, and 1% develop hepatocellular carcinoma.

Hepatitis A

Transmission of hepatitis A virus (HAV) by transfusion has been very rare. Blood banks screen for HAV by history only and there is no carrier state for this virus. The infectious period is limited to 1 to 2 weeks. The diagnosis depends on hepatitis antibody seroconversion.

Human Immunodeficiency Virus

HIV is a retrovirus, so called because its propagation requires translation of RNA to DNA. Current screening tests are directed at both HIV-1 and HIV-2, though the latter has been an extremely infrequent cause of human disease. The incidence of transfusion-related HIV infection has decreased dramatically. As a testimonial to the effectiveness of our blood delivery system's response to the emergence of HIV, the risk of transfusion-related transmission, which was approximately 1:100 in the early 1980s and 1:400,000 in 1997,[13] is currently approximately 1 per 1.7 million donor exposures.

Human T-Cell Lymphotropic Virus

HTLV-1 and HTLV-2 belong to the same retrovirus family as HIV. The incidence of clinical disease resulting from transmitted virus appears to be very low. They are associated with T-cell leukemia and lymphoma rather than the generalized immunodeficiency of the acquired immune deficiency syndrome (AIDS). In the United States, all donor units are screened for the presence of antibody to HTLV-I and HTLV-2.

Cytomegalovirus

Transfusion-associated CMV infections are usually benign and self-limited. However, CMV may cause serious, even fatal, infections in immunocompromised patients. Patients at risk include premature neonates, CMV-seronegative bone marrow transplant recipients, pregnant females, and those patients with severely depressed immune function. Leukoreduction and/or the use of blood from CMV-seronegative donors reduce, but do not prevent, CMV transmission.[14] Restriction of immunocompromised patients to leukoreduced blood from CMV-seronegative donors is standard in many centers.

West Nile Virus

WNV is a mosquito-borne flavivirus (as is dengue fever) that became epidemic in midwestern states in 2002 and has since occurred nationwide. Although the majority of infected individuals are either asymptomatic or develop only a mild illness, encephalitis/meningitis can occur and the death rate among confirmed cases is 5 to 10%.[15,16] Transmission by transfusion and organ transplantation has been confirmed. Fortunately, the window period between infection and clinical symptoms is short, approximately 3 days, and the period of infectivity also appears to be relatively brief. Universal minipool NAT testing for WNV began in 2003, with discretionary selective individual donor NAT testing in areas of high incidence.[17] Transfusion transmission has subsequently been very infrequent.[17]

Parasitic Diseases

Transfusion-transmitted malaria is relatively common in regions where the disease is endemic but has been rare in the United States.[3] Because the parasite resides within the red cell, the hazard is associated almost exclusively with RBC transfusion. Chagas' disease is caused by a protozoan (*Trypanosoma cruzi*) that is endemic to South and Central America (including Mexico). Significant clinical disease has been rare in North America and has occurred almost exclusively in immunocompromised transfusion recipients. Donor screening for Chagas' disease by immunoassay is now standard in all Red Cross collection centers and is increasing among other U.S. agencies, especially in the southwest and Florida.[3]

Bacterial Contamination of Blood Components

Bacterial contamination occurs at a much higher frequency (Table 16-1) than any of the other infections discussed in this section and is associated with substantial mortality.[18,19] The incidence of sepsis is substantially greater with platelet than RBC administration because the former are stored at room temperature. The risk is less with apheresis platelets (obtained from a single donor with one venipuncture) than with whole blood-derived platelet administration, which entails pools derived from six to ten separate donor units. The source of the bacteria can be donor skin flora, donor bacteremia, or contaminants introduced during collection, processing, and storage. Numerous Gram-positive and -negative organisms can occur in platelets including *Staphylococcus aureus*, *Klebsiella pneumoniae*, *Serratia marcescens*, and *Staphylococcus epidermidis*.[12] Only a limited number of bacteria, including *Yersinia enterocolitica* and certain *Serratia* and *Pseudomonas* species can grow at RBC storage temperatures.[2] Fatal sepsis is usually the result of Gram-negative organisms, and *Y. enterocolitica* is the most frequently implicated.

There is considerable current attention being given to the prevention of platelet-transmitted bacterial infection. Careful skin preparation is the norm and some collection centers divert and discard the first few milliliters of the draw. In 2004, bacterial testing of all platelets became a requirement for achieving AABB (formerly, the American Association of Blood Banks) certification, and the majority of agencies now culture apheresis units. However, culture is not practical for whole blood-derived pools, and less sensitive surrogate methods (based on measurements of pH, glucose, PO$_2$, or assay for bacterial RNA[20]) are employed. These measures have reduced but not eliminated transfusion of contaminated units (Table 16-1).[18,19,21]

The patient who receives contaminated blood transfusion will rapidly experience some combination of fever, chills, tachycardia, dyspnea, emesis, shock, and may develop disseminated intravascular coagulation (DIC) and acute renal failure. The reactions are variable in severity, and an index of suspicion should be maintained in order to distinguish these reactions from other major and minor transfusion reactions. The transfusion should be stopped immediately, blood cultures obtained, and the patient treated with broad-spectrum antibiotics. The blood bank should be notified immediately in order that it may interdict administration of other components made from the same donation and perform diagnostic testing (Gram stain and unit culture).

Prion-Related Diseases

Prions are the causative agents of CJD and vCJD. The latter is the human disease caused by the agent responsible for bovine spongiform encephalitis. All three are fatal, degenerative neurologic diseases caused by an abnormally folded variant of a protein that is constitutively present. Since the emergence of bovine spongiform encephalitis in England in 1984, approximately 200 cases of vCJD had been reported, with the large majority occurring in the United Kingdom.[22] The risk of transfusion-related vCJD is undefined. CJD has never been known to have been transmitted by transfusion but there have been three reported cases of apparently transfusion-related vCJD.[22] The incubation period of vCJD may be as long as 6 years. Accordingly, the true transmission rate may as yet be underrecognized. NAT testing is not feasible (prions have no nucleic acids) and there are no known antigenic or immune response markers. Therefore, it must be hoped that changes in animal husbandry practices combined with exclusion of donors who have spent time in high-risk areas will minimize whatever risk exists.

Other Infectious Risks

Many additional microbial agents can be transmitted by blood components. They include *Borrelia*, *Babesia*, dengue, the viral agent of severe acute respiratory syndrome, and other herpes viruses. Transmission of these agents is apparently extremely rare. However, the recent experience with WNV reveals, once again, the potential for new agents to become a sudden threat to the blood supply and serves as a reminder of the continuing need to administer blood components only when absolutely indicated.

Noninfectious Risks Associated with Blood Product Administration

The noninfectious risks associated with blood product administration, the majority of which are immunologically mediated, and their approximate incidences are presented in Table 16-2.

TABLE 16-2

THE NONINFECTIOUS ADVERSE REACTIONS ASSOCIATED WITH BLOOD PRODUCT ADMINISTRATION, IN THE APPROXIMATE ORDER OF THEIR AVERAGE FREQUENCIES IN THE PUBLISHED LITERATURE[a]

ADVERSE REACTION	INCIDENCE	COMMENT
• TRIM	100%	
• Inflammatory response	(?) 100%	Increases with duration of storage
• Alloimmunization		
• RBCs	0.5%	
• Plts	10%	Reduced by leukoreduction[25]
• Minor allergic reactions (urticaria, flushing)	0.5–4%	Plts and FFP > RBCs
• Febrile reactions	0.1–2%	Probably reduced by leukoreduction
• DHTR	1/2,000	Most often Kell, Kidd, and Rhesus (E) antibodies
• TRALI	1/5,000	All plasma containing products; FFP and Plts > PRBCs
• Anaphylactic/toid reactions	1/25,000	Plts > PRBCs IgA deficiency increases risk
• AHTR	1/25,000	Usually patient ID error; 2% mortality; Plasma-incompatible Plts are a rare cause
• GVHD	Rare	Immunocompromised patients, especially marrow transplant recipients

TRIM, transfusion-related immunomodulation; RBCs, red blood cells; Plts, platelets; FFP, fresh-frozen plasma; DHTR, delayed hemolytic transfusion reaction; TRALI, transfusion-related acute lung injury; PRBCs, packed RBCs; IgA, immunoglobulin A; AHTR, acute hemolytic transfusion reaction; ID, identification; GVHD, graft-versus-host disease.
[a]The frequencies are presented as percentages when >0.1% and otherwise as ratios.
This table draws extensively from information presented by Eder et al.[26] and Klein et al.[277] as well as other sources.[24,278]

Immunologically Mediated Transfusion Reactions

Reactions to transfused blood products can occur as a result of the presence of antibodies that are constitutive (e.g., anti-A, anti-B) or that have been formed as a result of exposure to donor RBCs, white blood cells, platelets and/or proteins, or as a consequence of the effects of transfused white cells.

Reactions to RBC Antigens

Acute Hemolytic Transfusion Reactions. The most hazardous of the immune reactions is the immediate acute hemolytic transfusion reaction (AHTR) against foreign RBCs. Hemolysis of donor RBCs can lead to acute renal failure and DIC. The mortality rate is 2%.[23] There are more than 300 antigens on human red cells, but most are weak immunogens that usually do not elicit a clinically detectable antibody response. The antibodies that fix complement and commonly produce immediate intravascular hemolysis include those against A, B, Kell, Kidd, Duffy, and Ss antigens. Rh antibodies (i.e., anti-D, anti-Cc, and anti-Ee), although typically not complement binding, are also capable of causing serious acute hemolytic reactions. Transfusion of incompatible FFP to A, B, or AB patients, resulting in hemolysis of recipient red cells, has also been a rare cause of AHTRs.[23]

ABO incompatibility, in company with transfusion-related acute lung injury (TRALI) and bacterial contamination, is among the three leading causes of transfusion-related deaths in the United States. Clerical and patient identification errors are the most common causes of ABO incompatibility and a large fraction of these errors typically occur in the operating theater. It is an uncomfortable irony that one of principal hazards of transfusion resides not in the blood supply per se, but rather in the process whereby it is delivered to the patient.

When incompatible blood is administered, antibodies and complement in recipient plasma attack the corresponding antigens on donor RBCs. Hemolysis ensues. The hemolytic reaction will take place in the intravascular space and it may also occur extravascularly within the reticuloendothelial system (spleen, liver, bone marrow). The antigen-antibody complexes activate Hageman factor (factor XII), which in turn acts on the kinin system to produce bradykinin (see Chapter 13). The release of bradykinin increases capillary permeability and dilates arterioles, both of which contribute to hypotension. Activation of the complement system results in the release of histamine and serotonin from mast cells, resulting in bronchospasm. Thirty to 50% of patients develop DIC.

Hemolysis releases hemoglobin (Hb) into the blood. Initially it is bound to haptoglobin and albumin. When those binding sites are saturated, it circulates unbound until it is excreted by the kidneys. Renal damage occurs for several reasons. Blood flow to the kidneys is reduced in the presence of systemic hypotension and renal vasoconstriction. Free Hb in the form of acid hematin or red cell stroma may damage renal tubules. Antigen-antibody complexes may be deposited in the glomeruli. If the patient develops DIC, fibrin thrombi will also be deposited in the renal vasculature, further compromising perfusion and/or causing acute cortical necrosis, which is frequently irreversible.

The signs and symptoms of a hemolytic transfusion reaction include fever, chills, nausea and vomiting, diarrhea, and rigors. The patient is hypotensive and tachycardic (bradykinin effects) and may appear flushed and dyspneic (histamine). Chest and back pains occur and have been attributed to cytokine release. The patient is often restless, has a headache, and a sense of impending doom. Hemoglobinuria will occur if plasma Hb rises above the renal threshold (about 25 mg/dL). Diffuse bleeding occurs with the development of DIC. With renal failure, oliguria develops. During general anesthesia, many of the signs are masked. Hypotension and microvascular

bleeding may be the only initial clues that a hemolytic transfusion reaction has occurred, and the diagnosis may not be suspected until hemoglobinuria is observed. A reasonable index of suspicion should be maintained during administration of RBCs to anesthetized patients in order to avoid critical delay in diagnosis.

If a reaction is suspected, the transfusion should be stopped and the identity of the patient and the labeling of the blood rechecked. Examination of the patient's plasma after brief centrifugation for the pinkish discoloration caused by free Hb is a simple, rapid screening test when a hemolytic transfusion reaction is suspected. Hemolysis can be due to other causes, but should be assumed to indicate a hemolytic transfusion reaction until proven otherwise. Management has three main objectives: maintenance of systemic blood pressure, preservation of renal function, and the prevention of DIC. Systemic blood pressure should be supported by administration of volume, pressors, and inotropes as required. Urine output should be promoted by administration of fluids and the use of diuretics, either mannitol or furosemide, or both. Sodium bicarbonate can be administered to alkalinize the urine. There is currently no specific therapy to prevent the development of DIC. However, preventing hypotension and supporting cardiac output to prevent stasis and hypoperfusion, both of which contribute to the evolution of DIC, are important.

The response should include immediate notification of the blood bank, to which the suspected unit of blood should be returned, aseptically sealed, along with a posttransfusion EDTA blood specimen. The blood bank will determine whether the unit of blood had been correctly released to the patient. Immediate tests on the posttransfusion specimen will include (1) a visual check for hemoglobinemia and (2) a direct antiglobulin (Coombs) test. The direct antiglobulin test examines recipient RBCs for the presence of surface immunoglobulins and complement. If positive, an acute hemolytic reaction may have occurred and additional testing is indicated to ascertain the cause, including repeat ABO/Rh type, antibody screen, cross-matching, and other tests as indicated. Serum haptoglobin level, plasma, and urine Hb and bilirubin assays are usually performed. However, these are evidence of hemolysis only, not specifically of an immune reaction. The unit should be cultured if bacterial sepsis, usually associated with temperature elevation, is in the differential diagnosis. Laboratory tests to establish baseline coagulation status including platelet count, prothrombin time (PT), activated partial thromboplastin time (aPTT), thrombin time (TT), fibrinogen level, and fibrin degradation products should be performed, as should baseline studies of renal function.

Delayed Hemolytic Transfusion Reactions. Numerous instances have been reported in which transfused red cells are rapidly eliminated from the circulation at a short interval (days) after an apparently "compatible" crossmatch. These delayed hemolytic transfusion reactions can be the result of a donor RBC antigen to which the recipient has been previously exposed by either transfusion or pregnancy. Over time, the recipient antibodies fall to levels too low to be detected by compatibility testing. With re-exposure, an anamnestic response results in antibody that eventually lyses the foreign RBCs. In other instances, de novo alloimmunization may be responsible. Typically, the antibody-coated RBC is sequestered extravascularly and lysis occurs in the spleen and reticuloendothelial system. Because the RBC destruction occurs extravascularly, symptoms are less severe and the reaction is unlikely to be fatal. Unlike AHTRs, which usually involve antibodies in the ABO system, delayed hemolytic transfusion reactions commonly involve antibodies against Kell, Kidd, and Rhesus antigens.[24] While alloimmunization and the appearance of new antibodies occurs with approximately 1 per 200 units transfused, clinically detectable delayed hemolytic reactions occur at a rate of only 1 per 2,000 to 2,500 transfusions[24] (Table 16-2).

Evidence of hemolysis is usually detected by the first or second week following transfusion. The reaction should be suspected in the event of a low-grade fever, increased indirect bilirubin with or without mild jaundice, and/or an unexplained reduction in Hb concentration. Serum haptoglobin may also be decreased. The diagnosis is confirmed by a positive direct antiglobulin test (Coombs test) and the identification of a new antibody in the patient's plasma. The reaction is typically mild and self-limiting and the clinical manifestations resolve as the transfused cells are removed from the circulation. Supportive care includes monitoring of Hb, maintenance of hydration, and provision of compatible blood if necessary.

Reactions to Donor Proteins

Minor Allergic Reactions. Allergic reactions to proteins in donor plasma cause urticarial reactions in 0.5 to 4% of all transfusions.[2,23] The reaction is most frequently associated with the transfusion of FFP or platelets. The patient may have itching, swelling, and a rash (histamine release). These mild symptoms can be treated with diphenhydramine (Chapter 12). Most mild urticarial reactions are isolated events that do not recur. Patients who experience repeated reactions or a single severe urticarial reaction may benefit from the use of saline-washed red cells. The washing of platelets is generally ineffective, and susceptible patients who require platelets or FFP can be managed by administration of antihistamine and steroids (e.g., prednisone, 1 mg/kg or equivalent) 1 hour prior to transfusion.

Anaphylactic Reactions. Infrequently, more severe, anaphylactic reactions including dyspnea, bronchospasm, angioedema, and hypotension may occur (Chapter 12). Classically, these occur when patients with hereditary immunoglobulin (Ig) A deficiency who have been sensitized by previous transfusions or pregnancy are exposed to blood with foreign IgA protein. However, other plasma protein polymorphisms (e.g., haptoglobin) may cause similar reactions. Treatment consists of discontinuation of the transfusion and administration of epinephrine and methylprednisolone. Washed red cells, frozen deglycerolized red cells, or in appropriate cases, red cells from IgA-deficient donors should subsequently be used for these patients. Platelet and FFP transfusion may be managed with pretransfusion administration of prednisone (see previous discussion), careful monitoring, and epinephrine at the bedside.

White Cell-Related Transfusion Reactions

Febrile Reactions. Patients who receive multiple transfusions of RBCs or platelets commonly develop antibodies (alloimmunization) to the human leukocyte antigens (HLAs) on the passenger leukocytes in these products. During subsequent RBC transfusions, febrile reactions may occur as a result of antibody attack on donor leukocytes. These febrile responses occur in up to 2% of platelet, FFP, and RBC transfusions (Table 16-2). Typically, the patient experiences a temperature increase of more than 1°C within 4 hours of a blood transfusion and defervesces within 48 hours. The fever is sometimes accompanied by chills, respiratory distress, anxiety, headache, myalgias, nausea, and a nonproductive cough. Febrile reactions can be treated with acetaminophen. A leukocyte-mediated febrile transfusion reaction should be distinguished from a hemolytic transfusion reaction (direct Coombs test). Leukoreduction (see later) reduces or prevents these reactions.[25]

Transfusion-Related Acute Lung Injury. TRALI is a noncardiogenic form of pulmonary edema occurring after blood product administration (see Chapter 12). It has been associated with all plasma-containing blood components, with platelet concentrates and FFP being implicated much more commonly than PRBCs or other products.[26,27] The incidence (Table 16-2) is frequently estimated to be 1:5,000 units transfused, although it has been recently reported to be as high as 1 per 1,271 transfused units in a carefully observed, at-risk intensive care unit (ICU) patient population.[28] It is likely that TRALI, which carries a mortality of at least 5%,[29] has historically been both underrecognized and underreported. Awareness is increasing, and according to a report by Holness and Epstein, TRALI was responsible for 46.5% of deaths reported to the Food and Drug Administration (FDA) in the first half of 2006.[30]

Detailed reviews of TRALI are available.[29,31] In most instances (>90%), TRALI occurs when mediators present in the plasma phase of donor blood activate leukocytes in the host. Those mediators are usually anti-HLA (Class I or Class II) or antigranulocyte antibodies in donor plasma formed as a result of previous transfusion or pregnancy. In a small percentage of instances, the inverse reaction, aggregation of donor leukocytes by recipient antibodies, may be the cause when the recipient has been alloimmunized against leukocyte antigens. In either circumstance, the activated leukocytes are sequestrated in the lung and the mediators they release cause capillary endothelial damage and increased permeability.

Because antileukocyte antibodies cannot be demonstrated in all instances of TRALI, it seems certain that other mechanisms are sometimes operative. A double insult, or "two-hit," theory proposes that the humoral response to various physiologic stresses (e.g., trauma, surgery, sepsis, systemic inflammatory response) may first "prime" native granulocytes, causing the appearance of surface adhesion sites, which in turn results in lung sequestration. Transfusion is proposed to be the wielder of the second hit. The mediators are thought to be biologically active lipids, sometimes referred to as *biological response modifiers* (BRMs) that accumulate as a result of the breakdown of membranes of the cellular elements in stored blood products. It is the BRMs, notably various lysophosphatidylcholines, that activate the sequestered leukocytes. Consistent with this theory is that TRALI has been reported to be more likely to occur with longer product storage times.[32] A merging of these two theories may occur, if for instance it is demonstrated that the combination of antibodies and BRMs in donor blood collaborate in some way to effect the two hits.

The clinical appearance is very similar to that of acute lung injury of other etiologies, although the mortality rate should be substantially less. Beginning within 6 hours of transfusion, and often more rapidly, the patient develops dyspnea, chills, fever, and noncardiogenic pulmonary edema. Both hypotension and hypertension may occur. Chest x-ray reveals bilateral infiltrates. Severe pulmonary insufficiency can develop. Specific diagnostic criteria for the diagnosis of TRALI have been established (Table 16-3).[33]

Treatment is largely supportive. The transfusion should be stopped if the reaction is recognized in time. Transfusion-associated circulatory overload ("TACO" in the vernacular of blood bankers) should be considered and ruled out. Supplemental oxygen and ventilatory support should be provided as necessary, ideally using the same low tidal volume lung protective strategies that are employed in the acute respiratory distress syndrome.[34] The pulmonary edema is noncardiogenic. Accordingly, diuretics are nonwarranted. Glucocorticoids have been administered but there are no data to support the practice.

There are preventive standards at the time of this writing (April 2008). It is anticipated that universal leukoreduction

TABLE 16-3

DIAGNOSTIC CRITERIA FOR TRANSFUSION-RELATED ACUTE LUNG INJURY

1. Acute onset of hypoxemia (within 6 hours of conclusion of transfusion)
2. Bilateral CXR infiltrates consistent with ALI
3. Absence of evidence of left atrial hypertension
4. Absence of other temporally related causes of ALI

CXR, chest x-ray; ALI, acute lung injury.
From Kleinman S, Caulfield T, Chan P, et al: Toward an understanding of transfusion-related acute lung injury: statement of a consensus panel. Transfusion 2004; 44: 1774 with permission.

will decrease the presence of antileukocyte antibodies in both donors and recipients.[35] Multiparous female donors have been identified as the most common source of the antileukocyte antibodies in TRALI fatalities.[23] Beginning in 2003, the United Kingdom substantially restricted the use of plasma-containing products from this donor subgroup. A program to similarly limit the preparation of high plasma-volume components (FFP, TP, FP24, or plasma frozen within 24 hours after phlebotomy [see later discussion], apheresis platelets, whole blood) from donors known to be leukocyte-alloimmunized or at increased risk of leukocyte alloimmunization (pregnancy or prior transfusion), or to perform HLA antibody testing, is in the process of implementation in the United States.[1]

Graft-versus-Host Disease. PRBCs and platelets both contain a significant number of viable donor lymphocytes. When transfused into immunocompromised patients, the donor lymphocytes may become engrafted, proliferate, and establish an immune response against the recipient (see Chapter 54). In essence, the engrafted lymphocytes reject the host.[36]

Patients at risk for graft-versus-host disease (GVHD) include organ transplant recipients, neonates who have undergone a blood-exchange transfusion, and patients immunocompromised by many other disease processes (but not AIDS; Table 16-4). GVHD typically progresses rapidly to pancytope-

TABLE 16-4

IRRADIATION OF CELLULAR BLOOD PRODUCTS FOR PATIENTS AT RISK OF GRAFT-VERSUS-HOST DISEASE

Widely recommended:
  Bone marrow transplant recipients
  Transfusion from consanguineous donor
  Hodgkin's disease
  Intrauterine transfusions
  HLA-matched platelet or granulocytes transfusion
  Ongoing treatment with purine analog antimetabolites
  Severe combined immunodeficiency syndrome
Lesser risk/practices vary with intensity of
  immunosuppression:
  Acute leukemias
  Non-Hodgkin's lymphoma
  Solid tumors
  Solid organ transplant recipients

Modified from Schroeder ML: Transfusion-associated graft-versus-host disease. Br J Haematol 2002; 117: 275.

nia. The fatality rate is very high. Transfusion-associated GVHD has also been reported in apparently immunocompetent patients when a genetic relationship exists between the donor and the recipient. In these circumstances, the recipient may share HLA antigen haplotypes with the donor lymphocytes. The patients, although immunologically competent, fail to reject the transfused cells because they do not recognize them as foreign. The transfused donor lymphocytes, however, recognize the host as foreign and a GVHD reaction takes place.

GVHD has been reported only after the transfusion of cellular blood components. It has not occurred following transfusion of FFP or cryoprecipitate. The AABB recommends that HLA-matched platelets and directed donations from first-degree relatives be irradiated to inactivate donor lymphocytes.[a] Leukoreduction may reduce the incidence of GVHD, but it does not prevent it[2] or reduce the mortality if it occurs. Irradiation remains the only effective means for preventing GVHD.[37] Anesthesiologists will encounter patients in operating rooms and ICUs who are at risk for GVHD; they should be prepared to ask, "Should the blood we administer to this patient be gamma irradiated?"

③ *The three leading causes of transfusion-related death in the United States are TRALI, ABO incompatibility, and sepsis caused by bacterial contamination.*

Transfusion-Related Immunomodulation (TRIM). Allogeneic transfusion has long been known to cause alteration of immune responsiveness. The initial observations were of decreased rates of transplant rejection[38] and decreased rates of spontaneous abortion among patients who had received allogeneic transfusions. That some modification of immune surveillance occurs seems inescapable, and the occurrence of numerous transfusion-associated changes in immune-related processes, including T-lymphocyte helper/suppressor ratio, the function of killer T cells, lymphocyte responsiveness, and delayed hypersensitivity has been demonstrated.[39] While transfused mononuclear white cells are thought to be principally responsible, other mechanisms may be involved.[39] Numerous adverse effects, presumed to reflect this attenuation of immunocompetence, have been reported, including increased mortality, accelerated recurrence of malignancy, increased rates of infection, and more rapid progression of HIV/AIDS. Although many of the typical observational studies have left it less than absolutely clear whether transfusion was the *cause* of the adverse outcome or merely a reflection of the concomitant processes that necessitated blood product administration, the weight of the accumulated investigations, including some that have controlled carefully for confounding variables,[40–43] argue that the adverse effect of transfusion on infection rates and mortality is a real one in at least some contexts.[44] One investigation is particularly revealing. Hebert et al.[45] prospectively compared transfusion strategies based on a liberal (10 g/dL) versus a restrictive (7 g/dL) transfusion threshold in an ICU population in whom the potential confounders were balanced at the time of patient enrollment. They observed lesser severity of multiple-organ dysfunction, reduced length of ICU and hospital stay, and reduced mortality at all follow-up intervals in the restrictive group. Although this investigation is strongly suggestive of an adverse effect of allogeneic blood and further supports the importance of avoiding unnecessary transfusion, it should be acknowledged that there is no certainty that the adverse effect was entirely a function of immune *suppression* (see next section).

[a]See AABB Association Bulletins no. 06-07 and no. 07-03 at www.AABB.org.

ANATOMY AND PHYSIOLOGY

Transfusion-Induced Inflammatory Response. It seems probable that, in addition to any TRIM effect, transfusion induces an inflammatory response in the recipient. (Note that "TRIM" is now sometimes used to encompass *both* the immune suppressant and proinflammatory effects of transfusion.)

Numerous bioactive substances, including cytokines, membrane lipid breakdown products, and complement, accumulate during blood product storage and are suspected of contributing to an inflammatory response in the recipient and to the progression of multiorgan dysfunction.[39,46,47] It is possible that some of the adverse effects of transfusion on mortality are a function of a proinflammatory rather than an immune suppressant effect. Because the concentrations of these mediators increase during storage, several investigations have sought to determine whether the duration of storage has any relation to outcome. A correlation between the age of transfused PRBCs and the severity of multiorgan failure in trauma patients,[48] life-threatening outcomes and mortality in an ICU population,[49] and mortality, renal dysfunction, and length of stay in cardiac surgical patients[50,51] have been reported. If these results are borne out by larger prospective trials, it will bring pressure on our blood delivery system to achieve shorter "shelf times" (which currently average about 20 days[52]), at least for patients in the more critical circumstances.

Leukoreduction. The suspicion that transfused leukocytes are the mediators of the immunity-attenuating effects of transfusion mentioned previously led to the development and progressive application of techniques for leukocyte depletion of donor blood products. If leukocytes are responsible for TRIM, leukoreduction should attenuate the adverse effects. However, meta-analysis of studies comparing white blood cell (WBC)-reduced and non–WBC-reduced blood has revealed a reduction of mortality that is evident only in the context of cardiac surgery.[53] A recent retrospective comparison of patients who received allogeneic blood after the onset of acute lung injury subsequently reported increased mortality among patients who received nonleukoreduced blood.[43] That study was limited by some noncurrency of the leukoreduced and nonleukoreduced groups. Further meta-analysis, limited to the most carefully performed investigations, also revealed an effect on the rate of postoperative infections.[53] However, when the impact of leukoreduction on the progression of HIV/AIDS was studied in a blinded prospective manner, no effect was identified.[54]

Albeit that the extent to which white cells are responsible for the adverse immunologic effects of transfusion is not absolutely clear, for that and other reasons, many countries—including Canada, France, Portugal, and the United Kingdom—and certain states and regions within the United States have already adopted the practice of leukoreduction of 100% of their blood supplies. The entire United States is moving towards that objective. At present (2008), about 70% of platelets and 40 to 50% of FFP and PRBCs are leukoreduced. There are several other well-confirmed benefits of leukoreduction[25] including reduction in the development of alloimmunization and platelet refractoriness, reduction in the incidence of febrile nonhemolytic transfusion reactions, and reduction in (but not prevention of[14]) the transmission of CMV. However, it has been argued that (less expensive) selective leukoreduction could readily be applied for the patients to whom these benefits are relevant. The advocacy of universal leukoreduction is based on the premise that it might serve to accomplish the various unconfirmed benefits listed in Table 16-5, and/or that selective leukocyte reduction might result in many patients receiving nonleukoreduced blood before the indication for leukocyte reduction became apparent e.g., a severely anemic, undiagnosed, acute leukemic patient. In individual institutions with dual inventories, it will be the responsibility

---

TABLE 16-5

THE BENEFITS OF LEUKOREDUCTION

- Confirmed benefits
  - Decreased alloimmunization/platelet refractoriness in multiply transfused leukemics
  - Prevention of febrile reactions to RBC transfusions
  - Reduction of CMV transmission
  - Reduced inflammatory mediator accumulation during storage
- Reported but unconfirmed benefits:
  - Shortened hospitalization
  - Decreased postoperative mortality in cardiac surgery
  - Decreased postoperative infections
  - Prevention of transfusion-related increase in tumor recurrence
- Suggested but unconfirmed:
  - Reduced incidence of GVHD

RBC, red blood cell; CMV, cytomegalovirus; GVHD, graft-versus-host disease.

---

of the clinician at the bedside to request leukoreduced blood when he or she perceives it to be in the patient's best interest.

While many of the putative benefits are unconfirmed, additional reports of benefits attributed to leukoreduction are being added to the literature.[55,56] Although skepticism persists, the common view is that, in spite of the associated costs, because the hazards of leukoreduction are minimal, the possible benefits justify proceeding with universal leukoreduction. Universal leukoreduction, when fully implemented, will employ prestorage depletion rather than bedside leukoreduction filters at the time of administration. Prestorage depletion avoids the accumulation of cytokines released by WBCs during storage. Clinicians should also be attentive to the possibility of severe, apparently bradykinin-mediated hypotension in patients who receive bedside-filtered blood. The reaction appears to occur more frequently, although not exclusively, in patients receiving angiotensin-converting enzyme inhibitors (which reduce breakdown of bradykinin).[57]

Other Noninfectious Risks Associated with Transfusion

Massive Transfusion

The rapid transfusion of large volumes of stored blood can have several consequences (Table 16-6). Some of these are functions of properties of the blood itself, some of the agents used to preserve and anticoagulate it, and some of the biochemical reactions that occur during storage (see Chapter 36). Other complications are not unique to blood transfusions, but may occur with the rapid transfusion of large volumes of any fluid.

Hypothermia. Hypothermia slows hemostasis (as it does all enzymatically mediated processes) and causes sequestration of platelets. The administration of one unit of PRBCs at 4°C will reduce the core temperature of a 70-kg patient approximately 0.25°C. At 29°C (the temperature at which the risk of cardiac dysrhythmias is critical), PT and aPTT will increase approximately 50% over normothermic values, and platelet count will decrease by approximately 40%.[58] Dysrhythmias may be seen at higher core temperatures if unwarmed blood is administered

TABLE 16-6

HAZARDS ASSOCIATED WITH MASSIVE TRANSFUSION

- Hypothermia
- Volume overload
- Dilutional coagulopathy
- Reduced oxygen-carrying capacity (decreased 2,3-DPG)
- Metabolic acidosis
- Hyperkalemia
- Citrate intoxication

2,3-DPG, 2,3-diphosphoglycerate.

rapidly; in particular, through central catheters. With decreasing body temperature, cardiac output declines, tissue perfusion is impaired (as a consequence of both vasoconstriction and a left shift of the oxygen-hemoglobin [O_2-Hb] dissociation curve), and metabolic acidosis may develop. Shivering on emergence can increase oxygen consumption by 400%.

A meta-analysis concluded that even mild hypothermia increases blood loss.[59] Hypothermia, after attempting to correct for covariates, is an independent predictor of mortality in trauma patients.[60,61] Hypothermia has been associated with increased postoperative morbidity and mortality including increased rates of postoperative infection.[62] However, in studies of this nature, it is difficult to separate the effects of the common clinical concomitants of hypothermia (e.g., acidosis, shock, massive transfusion, massive tissue injury) from those of hypothermia per se. Furthermore, the significance of hypothermia may lie in the interaction with other variables as suggested by the observation that temperatures of 33°C have been used extensively in elective neurosurgery without clinically apparent coagulopathy. Nonetheless, hypothermia should be carefully avoided and aggressively corrected in the patient receiving massive transfusion. Accordingly, transfusions administered rapidly or in substantial volume should be warmed.

Volume Overload. Circulatory volume overload occurs when blood or fluid is transfused too rapidly for compensatory fluid redistribution to take place.

In the setting of massive transfusion, assuming maintenance of isovolemia and the absence of a consumptive coagulopathy, critical dilution of clotting factors and platelets is likely to occur after an average replacement of 140% and 230% of blood volume, respectively.

Dilutional Coagulopathy. Administration of large volumes of fluid deficient in platelets and clotting factors will result in a coagulopathy as a consequence of dilution. In contemporary practice, in which patients receive principally PRBCs with only very limited amounts of residual plasma, factor deficiencies develop before thrombocytopenia. With large-volume isovolemic dilution, clinically significant dilution of fibrinogen, factors II, V, and VIII, and platelets would be expected to occur after volume exchanges of approximately 140%, 200 to 230% and 230% (i.e., 1.4, 2, and 2.3 blood volumes), respectively.[63] However, fibrinogen is an acute phase reactant, and levels will often be greater than would be predicted by dilution calculations. Resuscitation from hypovolemia will result in reaching these thresholds at smaller percentage volume exchanges. Note that calculations of this nature should not be used as a guide to blood product administration but merely as a means of anticipating clinically relevant occurrences. The decision to administer FFP or platelets will depend on clinical and laboratory evidence of coagulopathy, or frequently on the uncertain-

ties associated with rapid and ongoing blood loss. In the setting of trauma, PT/international normalized ratio (INR) has been shown to reveal factor deficiencies with greater sensitivity than aPTT.[64] This is probably because the aPTT assay is very FVIII-sensitive, and FVIII, like fibrinogen, is an acute phase reactant that is often increased in the setting of trauma. The most common initial factor deficiencies in the setting of trauma are FV and FX.[64]

With the possible exception of trauma resuscitation, coagulation factor and platelet replacement should be determined by laboratory assessment and/or observation of clinical coagulopathy and *not* estimated blood loss-driven formulas.

Decreases in 2,3-Diphosphoglycerate. Storage of RBCs is associated with a progressive decrease in intracellular ATP and 2,3-diphosphoglycerate (2,3-DPG) with a resultant left shift of the O_2-Hb dissociation curve. Accordingly, transfusion of the 2,3-DPG–depleted blood, while increasing the patient's Hb value, will result in less efficient oxygen delivery than would occur with native Hb at the same hematocrit. After transfusion, 2,3-DPG levels return toward normal over 12 to 24 hours.[65]

Acid-Base Changes. When citrate-phosphate- dextrose (CPD) solution is added to a unit of freshly drawn blood, pH decreases to approximately 7.0 to 7.1 (see Chapter 14). Further reduction of pH will occur during storage as a consequence of ongoing metabolism of glucose to lactate. At the end of 21 days, the pH may be as low as 6.9, but much of this is the result of the production of CO_2 that is rapidly eliminated following the transfusion. Whether rapid infusion of this acidic bank blood leads to metabolic acidosis is debated. When the liver is adequately perfused, citrate from the CPD solution is metabolized to bicarbonate and any acid-base disturbance should therefore be self-correcting. Clinically, in the injured patient who is hypotensive, poorly perfused, and has inadequate tissue oxygenation, it will be difficult to differentiate what portion of the metabolic acidosis is due to rapid transfusion, and what portion is due to the production of lactic acid. The appropriate course is to base bicarbonate therapy on blood gas analysis.

Hyperkalemia. During storage, potassium moves out of the RBCs, in part to maintain electrochemical neutrality as hydrogen ions generated during storage redistribute. The potassium concentration in plasma may reach levels variously reported to be between 19 and 35 mEq/L in blood stored for 21 days. Hazard exists if large volumes of stored blood are administered rapidly. While there are only 20 to 60 mL of plasma in a unit of PRBCs, contemporary infusion devices allow blood to be transfused at rates of 500 to 1,000 mL/min. At these infusion rates, critical hyperkalemia can occur and intraoperative arrests have been documented.[66] Premature neonates are especially susceptible to hyperkalemia, and typically therefore receive either fresh (<8 day old), plasma-reduced, or washed PRBCs if rapid transfusion (>10 to 15 mL/kg per 2 hours) is required.

Citrate Intoxication. When large volumes of stored blood (more than one blood volume) are administered rapidly, the citrate can cause a temporary reduction in ionized calcium levels. Citrate is normally metabolized efficiently by the liver and decreased ionized calcium levels should not occur unless the rate of transfusion exceeds 1 mL/ kg per minute or about 1 unit of blood per 5 minutes in an average-sized adult. The now-common additive solution blood preservatives have a much smaller citrate content than citrate-phosphate-dextrose-adenine (CPDA). This should further reduce the hazard of citrate intoxication with PRBC administration. However, most of the citrate administered during massive transfusion is in the FFP rather than the PRBCs. Impaired liver function or perfusion will lower the rate threshold for developing citrate intoxication. Note also that critical cardiac consequences that occur before hypocalcemia have significant implications for coagulation. Signs of citrate intoxication (hypocalcemia) include hypotension, narrow pulse pressure, and elevated intraventricular end-diastolic pressure and central venous pressure, prolonged QT interval, widened QRS complexes, and flattened T waves.

Microaggregate Delivery. Stored blood contains microaggregates. Platelet aggregates form during the second to fifth day of storage and after approximately 10 days, larger aggregates composed of fibrin, degenerated white cells, and platelets appear. Macroaggregates of RBCs also develop. Standard fluid administration sets contain 170 micron filters, which will remove these larger aggregates, and are appropriate for RBCs, FFP, cryoprecipitate, and platelet administration. Microaggregates have been suspected in the pathogenesis of pulmonary insufficiency after large-volume transfusion. However, concomitant physiologic disturbances (hypotension, sepsis, tissue injury) may be the actual causes, and some of what has been attributed to microaggregates may in fact be TRALI. Micropore filters, typically with a 40-micron pore size, were once advocated for RBC administration but were of no demonstrated benefit (with the exception of the arterial cannula of the cardiopulmonary bypass [CPB] circuit).

RBCs are frequently diluted with crystalloid solutions to increase the rate at which the blood can be transfused. In the ideal situation, normal saline, Normosol, or other diluents accepted by the FDA and AABB should be used in preference to lactated Ringer solution (LR). In fact, the amount of citrate present in stored blood is more than sufficient to bind the small amounts of calcium in the 100 to 300 mL of LR typically used for dilution.[67] There is no evidence that any clinically significant sequelae have resulted from the use of LR as an RBC diluent.[68]

BLOOD PRODUCTS AND TRANSFUSION THRESHOLDS

Red Blood Cells

The question of what hemoglobin/hematocrit (Hb/Hct) level justifies the risks associated with the administration of blood has been widely discussed. The once all but inviolable "10–30" rule has been abandoned. Experience with several patient subpopulations (renal failure, military casualties, Jehovah's Witnesses) and systematic study has revealed that considerable greater degrees of anemia can be well tolerated and that, in many situations, morbidity and mortality rates did not increase until Hb levels fell below 7 g/dL.[45,69] As significant as the identification of a 7-g/dL threshold for increased morbidity was the observation that stable general medical-surgical managed to a target Hb of 10 g/dL fared less well than a parallel group managed with a transfusion trigger of 7g/dL.[45] That observation implies an adverse effect of transfusion (see "Transfusion-Related Immunomodulation"). Accordingly, the contemporary transfusion trigger for stable general medical-surgical patients is 21%/7.0 g/dL (Hb/Hct). However, there is evidence that the threshold for patients with cardiac disease should be higher.[45] That evidence includes an investigation supporting a threshold of 30%/10 g/dL (Hb/Hct) in patients who have suffered a recent acute myocardial infarction (MI),[70] and an observational study suggests better outcomes in patients with several cardiac diagnoses (cardiac and vascular surgery, ischemic heart disease, dysrhythmias) above a threshold of 9.5 g/dL[71] (see Chapter 42). *The Practice Guidelines for Blood Component Therapy* developed by the American Society of Anesthesiologists (ASA) state that "red blood cell transfusion is rarely indicated when the hemoglobin concentration is greater than 10 g/dL and is almost always indicated when it is less than 6 g/dL. The indications for autologous transfusion may be more liberal than for allogeneic (homologous) transfusion."[72]

The clinician's responsibility is to anticipate, on a patient-by-patient basis, the minimum Hb level (probably in the range of 7 to 10 g/dL) that will avoid organ damage due to oxygen deprivation. Determining this individual "transfusion trigger" requires reference to the many elements of patient condition that determine demand for the delivery of oxygen and the physiologic reserve (Table 16-7),[73] including ongoing blood loss and the potential for sudden blood loss. Ultimately, the decision to transfuse RBCs should be made on the basis of the clinical judgment that the oxygen-carrying capacity of the blood must be increased to prevent oxygen consumption from outstripping oxygen delivery. That judgment is based on an understanding of the physiologic mechanisms that compensate for anemia and the limits of those mechanisms.

6 The RBC transfusion "trigger" for most patients will lie between hemoglobin values of 7 and 10 g/dL.

TABLE 16-7

CONDITIONS THAT MAY DECREASE TOLERANCE FOR ANEMIA AND INFLUENCE THE RED BLOOD CELL TRANSFUSION THRESHOLD

- Increased oxygen demand
  - Hyperthermia
  - Hyperthyroidism
  - Sepsis
  - Pregnancy
- Limited ability to increase cardiac output
  - Coronary artery disease
  - Myocardial dysfunction (infarction, cardiomyopathy)
  - β-Adrenergic blockade
  - Inability to redistribute cardiac output
  - Low SVR states
    - Sepsis
    - Post–cardiopulmonary bypass
- Occlusive vascular disease (cerebral, coronary)
- Left shift of the O_2-Hb curve
  - Alkalosis
  - Hypothermia
- Abnormal hemoglobins
  - Presence of recently transfused Hb (decreased 2,3-DPG)
  - Hb S (sickle cell disease)[a]
  - Acute anemia (limited 2,3-DPG compensation)
- Impaired oxygenation
  - Pulmonary disease
  - High altitude
- Ongoing or imminent blood loss
  - Traumatic/surgical bleeding
  - Placenta previa or accreta, abruption, uterine atony
  - Clinical coagulopathy

SVR, systemic vascular resistance; O_2-Hb, oxygen-hemoglobin; 2,3-DPG, 2,3-diphosphoglycerate.
[a]Total Hb should not be increased to >10 g/dL unless Hb S <30%.[73]

Compensatory Mechanisms During Anemia

When anemia develops, but blood volume is maintained (isovolemic hemodilution), four compensatory mechanisms serve to maintain oxygen delivery: (1) an increase in cardiac output, (2) a redistribution of blood flow to organs with greater oxygen requirements, (3) increases in the extraction ratios of some vascular beds, and (4) alteration of oxygen-Hb binding to allow the Hb to deliver oxygen at lower oxygen tensions.

1. Increased cardiac output.

   With isovolemic hemodilution, cardiac output increases primarily because of an increase in stroke volume brought about by reductions in systemic vascular resistance (SVR). The two principal determinants of SVR are vascular tone and blood viscosity.[74] As Hct decreases, reduction of blood viscosity decreases SVR. This decrease in SVR increases stroke volume and consequently cardiac output and blood flow to the tissues. Over a wide range of Hcts, isovolemic hemodilution is self-correcting. Linear decreases in the oxygen-carrying capacity of the blood are matched by improvements in oxygen transport. Because oxygen transport is optimal at Hcts of 30%, oxygen delivery may remain constant between the Hcts of 45 and 30%.[74] Further reductions in Hct are accompanied by increases in cardiac output, which reach 180% of control as the Hct approaches 20%. The exact Hb value at which cardiac output rises varies among individuals and is influenced by age and whether the anemia is acute or develops slowly.

2. Redistribution of cardiac output.

   With isovolemic hemodilution, blood flow to the tissues increases, but this increased flow is not distributed equally to all tissue beds. Organs with higher extraction ratios (brain and heart) receive disproportionately more of the increase in blood flow than organs with low extraction ratios (muscle, skin, viscera). Because basal extraction ratio (ER) is already high in the coronary circulation (see next paragraph), increased flow must be the principal means by which the healthy heart compensates for anemia.[74] Coronary blood flow can increase by as much as 500%.[75] When the heart can achieve no further increase in cardiac output and coronary blood flow, the limits of isovolemic hemodilution have been reached. Thereafter, further decreases in oxygen delivery will result in myocardial injury. Acute isovolemic Hb reductions to 5 g/dL can occur without impairment of total-body oxygen delivery in healthy, otherwise unstressed adults.[76] However, in the same experimental paradigm (acute isovolemic reduction), reversible impairment of cognitive function occurred when Hb concentrations fell below 7.0 g/dL.[77] The latter observation serves as a reminder that measures of global oxygen delivery may conceal critical occurrences in individual circulatory beds.

3. Increased oxygen extraction.

   Increasing oxygen ER is a critical compensatory mechanism when Hct drops below 25%. As isovolemic Hct decreases to 15%, the whole-body oxygen ER increases from 38 to 60%, and the mixed venous oxygen saturation decreases from 70 to 50% or less.[68] Some organs (brain and heart) already have high ERs under basal conditions, and have a limited capacity to further increase oxygen delivery by this mechanism. The heart, under basal conditions, extracts between 55 and 70% of the oxygen delivered.[78,79] The brain's ER is 30 to 35%. This contrasts with ERs of 7 to 30%, in most other tissues. In clinical practice, the measurement of the ERs of individual organs is usually not feasible. Because the heart has the highest ER, it is commonly said to be the organ at greatest risk under conditions of isovolemic anemia (although the work of Weiskopf et al.[76,77] cited in the previous paragraph argues that it may in fact be the brain).

4. Changes in oxygen-hemoglobin affinity.

   The sigmoid O_2-Hb dissociation curve describes the relationship between the partial pressure of oxygen (PO_2) in the blood and the percentage saturation of the Hb molecule (see Chapter 11). The P50, the PO_2 at which the Hb molecule is 50% saturated with oxygen at 37°C and a pH of 7.4, is 27 mm Hg. When the curve is shifted to the left (hypothermia, alkalosis), the P50 is reduced. The Hb molecule is more "stingy" and requires lower PO_2 to release oxygen to the tissues; that is, the Hb molecule does not release 50% of its oxygen until an ambient PO_2 <27 mm Hg is reached. This may impair tissue oxygenation. Right-shifting of the curve (increased temperature, acidosis) results in an increase of P50, decreased Hb affinity for the oxygen molecules and release of oxygen to tissues at higher partial pressures of oxygen.

   When anemia develops slowly, the affinity of Hb for oxygen may be decreased, that is, the curve is right-shifted as a result of the accumulation of 2,3-DPG in RBCs. Synthesis of supranormal levels of 2,3-DPG begins at a Hb of 9 g/dL. Stored RBCs become depleted of 2,3-DPG. Temperature reduction and storage-related pH decreases also reduce the P_{50} of stored blood. These changes, however, are reversed in vivo, but the resynthesis of 2,3-DPG by RBCs will require from 12 to 24 hours.

Isovolemic Anemia Versus Acute Blood Loss

Although the same compensatory mechanisms are operative in acute and chronic anemias, they have different degrees of importance and occur at different Hb concentrations. In chronically anemic patients, the accumulation of 2,3-DPG in the RBCs, thereby increasing the P_{50} of Hb, is the important first mechanism for compensation. Cardiac output increases as Hb decreases to approximately 7 to 8 g/dL. With acute blood loss, vasoconstriction occurs and cardiac output does not increase. Redistribution and increased extraction are the compensatory mechanisms.

Platelets

While published guidelines for platelet administration are available, there is once again a substantial requirement for clinician judgment. The indications for platelet administration presented in Table 16-8 are an amalgam of recommendations presented by the ASA in 1996 and 2006, the British Committee for Standards in Haematology in 2003 and 2006, and the French Safety Agency for Health Products in 2003.[27,72,80–82]

Table 16-8 makes it apparent that the platelet administration thresholds that will most often be relevant to anesthesiologists will lie between 50,000 and 100,000/uL.[83,84] The threshold within that range at which platelets are administered should be based on the likelihood of the intended procedure to cause bleeding, the hazard of bleeding should it occur (e.g., intracranial neurosurgery > peripheral orthopaedics), and the presence or possibility of additional causes of coagulation disturbance (e.g., recent administration of antiplatelet agents, CPB, DIC, dilution due to large-volume administration). Bleeding manifestations can vary substantially from patient to patient in the face of similar platelet counts. This occurs because some platelets are more effective than others. When thrombocytopenia results from peripheral destruction of platelets, the bone marrow continues to produce normal, young, large platelets that are hemostatically very effective. A patient with these platelets may have more effective primary hemostasis than a patient with the same platelet count but whose platelets were produced by a less active, less healthy bone marrow.

TABLE 16-8

INDICATIONS, EXPRESSED AS PLATELET COUNT THRESHOLDS OR TARGET LEVELS, COMMONLY WARRANTING THE ADMINISTRATION OF PLATELETS

• Nonbleeding patients without other abnormalities of hemostasis[25]	10,000/μL
• Lumbar puncture, epidural anesthesia,[a] central line placement, endoscopy with biopsy, liver biopsy or laparotomy in patients without other abnormalities of hemostasis, vaginal delivery	50,000/μL
• To maintain platelet count during ongoing bleeding and transfusion not less than	50,000/μL
• To maintain platelet count during DIC with ongoing bleeding not less than	50,000/μL
• To maintain platelets during management of massive blood loss	75,000/μL
• Intended procedures in which closed cavity bleeding might be especially hazardous (e.g., neurosurgery)	100,000/μL
• Microvascular bleeding attributed to platelet dysfunction such as uremia,[b] post–cardiopulmonary bypass, or in association with massive transfusion.	Clinician judgment

DIC, disseminated intravascular coagulation.
[a]The French Safety Agency for Health Products recommends 50,000/μL for spinal and 80,000/μL for epidural anesthesia.[82]
[b]After a trial of DDAVP, if permitted by the clinical situation.[83,84]

7   Platelet administration thresholds relevant to anesthesiologists will lie usually between 50,000 and 100,000/μL.

A platelet concentrate derived from a single unit of donor blood will increase the platelet count of a 70-kg recipient by 5,000 to 10,000/μL. However, the majority of platelets (>70%) are now obtained by apheresis (see "Collection and Preparation of Blood Products"). One apheresis unit will increase platelet count by 30,000 to 60,000/μL. A common practice is to administer either one unit of apheresis platelets to an adult or one unit of platelet concentrate/10 kg of body weight. The increase in platelet count must be verified by platelet count, especially in patients who may have been alloimmunized by frequent platelet administration.

Fresh-Frozen Plasma

In spite of the fact that over 2,000,000 units of FFP are administered annually in the United States, there is remarkably little systematically-derived evidence of efficacy.[85] Nonetheless, the use of FFP to restore coagulation factor levels is inevitably valid in many clinical circumstances. The indications for FFP administration presented in Table 16-9 are an amalgam of recommendations presented by the ASA in 1996 and 2006, and the British Committee for Standards in Haematology in 2004.[72,80,86] Effective coagulation can usually occur with clotting factor levels of 20 to 30% of normal. Levels that are 30% of normal can usually be achieved by administration of 10 to 15 mL/kg of FFP.[80]

Fresh-Frozen Plasma/Thawed Plasma in Trauma Resuscitation

It is the traditional dogma that administration of blood products, in particular FFP and platelets, should not be formula-driven, but should occur in response to a clinical coagulopathy, ideally with laboratory demonstration of abnormality. However, there is an evolving sentiment in the area of trauma resuscitation that this approach results in "falling behind" in the struggle against the tightening spiral of bleeding, hypotension, stasis, acidosis, hypothermia, and DIC[87–89] (see Chapter 36). Because of the very high incidence of coagulopathy in multiple trauma victims,[87,88,90] empiric approaches that involve the once-taboo formulas (e.g., two units of FFP or

TABLE 16-9

INDICATIONS FOR THE ADMINISTRATION OF FRESH-FROZEN PLASMA

- Correction of multiple coagulation factor deficiencies (e.g., DIC) with evidence of microvascular bleeding and PT and/or aPTT >1.5 times normal
- Correction of microvascular bleeding during massive transfusion (more than one blood volume) when PT/aPTT cannot be obtained in a timely manner
- Urgent reversal of warfarin therapy[a]
- Heparin resistance (antithrombin III [AT] deficiency) in a patient requiring heparin when AT concentrate is not available
- Thrombotic thrombocytopenic purpura or hemolytic uremic syndrome
- Correction of single coagulation factor deficiencies for which specific concentrates are not available (principally factor V)
- ? Formula management of trauma/massive blood loss (see text)

DIC, disseminated intravascular coagulation; PT, prothrombin time; aPTT, activated partial thromboplastin time.
[a]Prothrombin complex concentrate (II, VII, IX, X) is an alternative that has been reported to be more effective than fresh-frozen plasma.

TABLE 16-10

INDICATIONS FOR THE ADMINISTRATION OF CRYOPRECIPITATE

- Microvascular bleeding when there is a disproportionate decrease in fibrinogen, such as DIC and very massive transfusion,[a] with fibrinogen <80–100 mg/dL (or assay result not available)
- Fibrin sealant (if virus-inactivated concentrate is unavailable)
- Bleeding due to uremia that is unresponsive to DDAVP
- Prophylaxis before surgery or treatment of bleeding in hemophilia A and vWD (if virus-inactivated concentrates are unavailable or ineffective)
- Prophylaxis before surgery or treatment of bleeding in patients with congenital dysfibrinogenemias
- FXIII deficiency

DIC, disseminated intravascular coagulation; vWD, von Willebrand disease.
[a]Fresh-frozen plasma is the first-line component for the factor depletion associated with massive transfusion.

TABLE 16-11

BLOOD CONSERVATION TECHNIQUES

- Preoperative autologous donation
- Acute normovolemic hemodilution
- Intraoperative blood salvage
- Postoperative blood salvage
- Pharmacologic agents
  - Erythropoietin
  - Blood substitutes (hemoglobin- and nonhemoglobin-based)
  - DDAVP
  - Anti-fibrinolytics

thawed plasma [TP; see later for description of TP] with every five units of PRBC) when massive transfusion is anticipated or ongoing are already in routine use.[87,88,91] An RBC-to-plasma ratio of 1:1 has been advocated and reported effective in military trauma.[89] Formula-driven administration of platelets is also occurring. However, platelet administration may be less urgent because, as Ho and colleagues[88] have observed, thrombocytopenia is not a central element of the insidious spiral just mentioned, and it may be easier to "catch up" from the consequences of a low platelet count than from coagulopathy-driven bleeding and the associated hypovolemia.

8   Normal coagulation can be achieved with clotting factor levels of 20 to 30% of normal. Those levels can usually be achieved by administration of 10 to 15 mL/kg of FFP.

Cryoprecipitate

Cryoprecipitate contains factor VIII, the von Willebrand factor (vWF), fibrinogen, fibronectin, and factor XIII. Virally inactivated factor VIII concentrates, some of which contain clinically effective concentrations of vWF (e.g., Haemate P, Alphanate) are now available. As a result, hemophilia A and von Willebrand disease (vWD) are usually treated (in consultation with a hematologist) with those concentrates[92] rather than cryoprecipitate, which is now generally used for fibrinogen-deficient states. The remaining indications for cryoprecipitate are presented in Table 16-10.

BLOOD CONSERVATION STRATEGIES

Because of the many hazards of blood product administration, numerous techniques and alternatives have been explored (Table 16-11).

Autologous Donation

Preoperative donation and perioperative salvage of autologous blood have been used extensively as part of programs to reduce allogeneic blood administration. Autologous blood may be collected days to weeks prior to surgery (predonation); it may be collected immediately prior to surgery (isovolemic hemodilution); or it may be salvaged from the surgical field or wound drains and reinfused (blood salvage). In spite of the demonstration of modest efficacy,[93] enthusiasm for many of these approaches has declined pari passu with the progressive reduction of the risk of transfusion-transmitted infections.

Preoperative Autologous Donation

Preoperative donation of autologous blood (PAD) has been applied principally in patients undergoing major orthopaedic procedures (total hip and knee replacement, scoliosis procedures) and prostatic and cardiac surgery. However, with limited exception,[94] the systematic experience has generally failed to demonstrate a reduction in allogeneic blood exposure.[95] Effectiveness has probably been limited because the patients' erythropoietic response is often not vigorous, in which case the process may simply result in an anemia at the time of surgery. Furthermore, the PAD procedure is more expensive than the collection of allogeneic blood, and if autologous blood is not transfused it is usually discarded. The wastage rate was 59% in 2004.[1] Note also that the transfusion of autologous blood does not eliminate the chance of human error during blood collection, processing, and reinfusion or the risk of bacterial contamination or the adverse effects of the storage lesion (bioactive lipids, cytokines). The use of PAD has decreased substantially since the initial enthusiasm for the technique.[95–97] PAD nonetheless may be a useful alternative in alloimmunized patients for whom compatible allogeneic blood is difficult to obtain.

The medical condition of the patient must be considered prior to recommending PAD. Severe aortic stenosis, significant coronary disease or myocardial dysfunction, low initial Hct and blood volume (body weight <50 kg) are relative contraindications to PAD. If the patient's Hb level, cardiac status, and general condition permit, blood can be donated at weekly intervals prior to surgery. Four units is typically the maximum donation because of the shelf life of the first unit collected. Patients making PAD should receive supplemental iron (e.g., 2 mg/kg/day for 3 weeks). In addition, PAD can be supplemented with administration of recombinant erythropoietin (Epo).

Erythropoietin

The effectiveness of Epo in hastening recovery of Hct in conjunction with PAD and in improving Hct in patients not submitted to PAD has been demonstrated.[98–104] However, the practice has not become widespread in part because of the expense of the agent and in part because of the necessity for frequent (e.g., weekly injections for 3 weeks and two additional injections in the final week) parenteral (subcutaneous or intravenous) administration. Administration of Epo to presurgical patients has resulted in reduction in allogeneic blood administration,[105] and selective administration to anemic patients has been more obviously effective[106,107] than has administration to "all comers."[108,109] Epo, a recombinant product, is often accepted by Jehovah's Witnesses, and its efficacy in that population has been demonstrated.[110,111] The demonstration of the reduction by Epo of transfusion requirements in critically ill patients[112] may increase awareness and encourage its systematic use in anemic elective surgical patients. Erythropoietic agents with longer half-lives (e.g., darbepoetin alpha) are under development and may serve to overcome one of the logistic limitations (frequent parenteral administration) to the preoperative use of Epo.[113]

Acute Normovolemic Hemodilution

Acute normovolemic hemodilution (ANH) entails withdrawal of the patient's blood early in the intraoperative period with simultaneous administration of crystalloids or colloids to maintain normovolemia. The rationale is that during the ensuing surgery, the patient will lose blood of low Hct, and the withdrawn blood will be available for reinfusion at the end of the operation. The end point for the initial withdrawal is a Hct of 27 to 33%, depending on the patient's cardiovascular and respiratory reserve. Selection for this technique should rely on careful evaluation of the patient for coronary or cerebral vascular disease. ANH evolved in the anticipation that it would reduce total red cell loss and allogeneic blood administration. However, both mathematical modeling and empiric experience have revealed only a modest benefit.[114] By way of example, Goodnough[115] calculated that, in a 100-kg patient from whom three units of blood is withdrawn and replaced by asanguinous fluid, if the subsequent blood loss is 2,800 mL, 215 mL of RBCs (about one unit) will be saved. For patients of limited body size, low starting Hct, or blood loss <70% of one blood volume,[116] avoidance of allogeneic blood might be difficult to achieve. A recent meta-analysis reported that ANH does not achieve complete avoidance of allogeneic blood, but that when transfusion is necessary the amount transfused is reduced by one to two units per patient. The authors concluded that "widespread adoption of ANH cannot be encouraged."[114] Nonetheless, there are reports of favorable experiences in liver resection, prostatectomy, total hip arthroplasty, and abdominal aortic surgery.[101,117–120] It is possible that in the future the efficacy of ANH will be enhanced by administration of preoperative erythropoietics and/or by the use of either Hb-based oxygen-carrying compounds or perfluorocarbon emulsions to permit withdrawal of larger volumes of blood.

ANH has also been employed for the purpose of making fresh autologous blood available at the end of procedures in which either a dilutional or CPB-related coagulopathy may occur. The efficacy in this context has not been confirmed by systematic study. Blood collected and reinfused for this purpose should not be passed through a 40-micron filter in order to avoid platelet elimination.

Perioperative Blood Salvage

Perioperative blood salvage refers to the recovery of shed blood from the surgical field or wound drains and readministration to the patient. In most instances, the process involves "washing" of the salvaged material with return of only the RBC component of blood. In some instances, usually those involving wound drainage, blood is returned filtered but otherwise unprocessed.

Intraoperative Blood Salvage

Intraoperative blood salvage (IBS) is employed with many surgical procedures that have the potential to require allogeneic transfusion. Contemporary cell-salvage devices anticoagulate the salvaged blood as it leaves the surgical field, separate the RBCs from other liquid and cellular elements by centrifugation, and then wash the salvaged RBCs extensively with saline. The RBCs are typically returned to the patient suspended in saline in aliquots of 125 or 225 mL with a Hct of 45 to 65%.[121] Higher Hcts can be achieved at the expense of the additional time required for slower filling of the centrifuge chamber.

IBS has been used commonly during cardiovascular surgical procedures, aortic reconstruction, spinal instrumentation, joint arthroplasty, liver transplantation, resection of arteriovenous malformations,[122] and occasionally in the management of trauma patients.[123] There have been numerous demonstrations that IBS can reduce total blood loss and/or the use of allogeneic RBCs.[124–126] The presence of infection, malignant cells, urine, bowel contents, and amniotic fluid in the operative field have been viewed as contraindications. However, although malignant cells are known to be retained with RBCs after the washing process, IBS has been applied in the management of hepatic and urologic malignancies without evidence of metastasis.[127,128] At least one IBS washing device has also been shown to remove the critical procoagulant factors present in amniotic fluid[129] and IBS has been employed successfully in cesarean section.[130] However, the safety of IBS use in that context is unconfirmed and should not be routine.[131]

The potential complications of IBS are largely a function of the reinfusion of materials that might remain after the washing process. These include fat, microaggregates such as platelets and leukocytes, air, red cell stroma, free Hb, heparin, bacteria, and debris from the surgical field. Most of these are removed quite efficiently by contemporary cell-salvage equipment. Bacteria are the exception, and contamination of cell salvage return with skin organisms is relatively common.[124] Leukocyte-reduction filters have been shown to remove most bacteria[132] and may be relevant to the use of IBS in trauma and cesarean section. Massive air embolism has occurred as a result of user error. Direct return from the cell-salvage apparatus has now been largely abandoned in favor of return via an intermediary bag under the control of the anesthesiologist. Care should still be taken in the event that pressure infuser devices are applied to these bags.

A dilutional coagulopathy in association with large-volume IBS is to be expected because essentially all clotting factors and most platelets are removed by the washing process. A DIC-like coagulopathy was once associated with IBS; however, it seems likely that this syndrome was the result of inadequate preparation of blood by older cell-salvage devices. Unwashed, salvaged blood has been shown to contain numerous constituents that influence the coagulation process: thromboplastic material, interleukins, complement, fibrin-degradation products, and factors released from activated leukocytes and platelets[122] and to activate the coagulation process in recipients.[133] The majority of these are quite efficiently removed by contemporary IBS processing devices. However, their presence is used as an argument against the return of unprocessed blood from wound drains (see "Postoperative Blood Salvage").[134] Similar elements, including lipids and cytokines, in blood shed into the mediastinum during CPB are suspected of contributing to postprocedure morbidity, including cognitive dysfunction.[135] Accordingly, it is an increasingly common practice to return mediastinal blood to the patient via IBS devices rather than the CPB reservoir.

An additional coagulopathy risk arises with the use of thrombin and microfibrillar collagen or cellulose products in the surgical field.[136] These agents are not reliably removed by the washing process, and suctioning of blood into the IBS device should be discontinued during the use of these agents and resumed after the field has been irrigated.

The clinician should appreciate that the efficiency of the recovery of shed RBCs by the IBS process is on the order of 50%. Allogeneic blood will therefore frequently be necessary in spite of the IBS, and blood and fluid replacement calculations should take this into account.[137,138] The efficiency of RBC recovery is improved by prompt recovery of blood from the surgical field (i.e., before clotting occurs) by limiting the negative pressure used, and by minimizing the mechanical air-blood interface during suctioning.[139]

Postoperative Blood Salvage

Postoperative recovery of blood from mediastinal chest tubes and wound drains after hip and knee replacement with immediate reinfusion of the "unwashed" blood has been employed quite commonly. The many substances present in the unprocessed blood (see previous section) suggest that coagulation dysfunction might result, and many are skeptical regarding the wisdom of this practice[121,134] (with one editorialist going so far as to characterize the technique as "repugnant"[140]). However, there have been several reports of efficacy in reducing allogeneic blood exposure without apparent adverse effects,[141–143] and only occasional reports of apparent adverse consequences.[144] This may reflect the fact that the reinfused volumes are usually small.

Hemoglobin-Based Oxygen-Carrying Solutions

Hemoglobin-based oxygen-carrying solutions would offer numerous advantages: long shelf live, minimal infection hazard, absence of alloimmunization, immediate availability (no typing), little likelihood of TRIM, and no storage lesion/inflammatory response. However, while numerous polymerized Hb products have been studied, only one, Hemopure (Biopure Inc Evanston IL), is approved for human use (in South Africa) and only one, PolyHeme (Northfield Laboratories Cambridge, MA) is currently in phase III trial in the United States.[145] One additional product is at the phase II trial stage (Hemospan, Sangart, San Diego, CA). The many products studied have used bovine, outdated human, or recombinant Hb that has been entirely separated from red cell membranes (stroma) and polymerized to increase half-life. The initial difficulties with renal failure caused by residual stroma and excessive free Hb have been overcome. However, there are several remaining difficulties with which clinicians will probably have to contend including methemoglobinemia, interference with some calorimetrically based laboratory assays (including creatinine, total bilirubin, and lactate dehydrogenase), some degree of vasoconstriction caused by nitric oxide binding by free Hb, and a relatively short half-life. The nitric oxide effect is probably the basis for the failure of the several products that have been withdrawn from clinical trials. Polymerization increases half-life to 18 to 36 hours but that period is sufficiently short such that oxygen-carrying capacity will usually become inadequate before native reticulocytosis can compensate.[146] Perfluorocarbon emulsions[146] appear to be further from potential clinical application than hemoglobin-based oxygen-carrying solutions and will not be discussed here.

Jehovah's Witnesses

In general, on the basis of New Testament admonitions (Acts 15: 20, 29), Jehovah's Witnesses will accept neither administration of most allogeneic blood products nor the readministration of autologous products that have left the circulation. According to a recent Jehovah's Witness publication, "they reject all transfusions involving whole blood or the four primary components—red cells, plasma, white cells, and platelets. As for the various fractions, derived from those components—and products that contain such fractions—the Bible does not comment on these. Therefore each Witness makes his own personal decision on such matters."[147] Accordingly, the wishes of each patient must be clarified carefully. Few will permit the administration of PRBCs, FFP, platelets, or granulocytes, but other components and fractions may be acceptable. The majority will decline PAD. However, many will accept procedures that maintain extracorporeal blood in continuity with the circulation. The acceptability of CPB, acute normovolemic hemodilution, and perioperative cell salvage must be clarified with each patient individually. Most will permit administration of Epo.

COLLECTION AND PREPARATION OF BLOOD PRODUCTS FOR TRANSFUSION

Red Blood Cells

Whole blood is first collected in bags containing CPDA or CPD solution. The citrate chelates the calcium present in blood and prevents coagulation. Sequential centrifugation at various spin speeds and durations is used to separate whole blood into components including PRBCs, platelet concentrates, cryoprecipitate, and cell-free plasma. The two common PRBC preparations ultimately delivered to the clinician have either CPDA or so-called additive solution as the preservative. CPDA blood has an Hct of about 70 to 75%, contains 50 to 70 mL of residual plasma in a total volume of 250 to 275 mL, and has a shelf life of 35 days. With the additive solution preparation, the original preservative and most of the plasma (10 to 15 mL remains) is removed and replaced with 100 mL of additive solution. This results in a lower Hct (60%) in a total volume of 250 to 350 mL, less citrate per unit, 75 to 80% fewer microaggregates, and a longer shelf life (42 days). Additive solution RBCs are thought to regenerate 2,3-DPG more rapidly. The pH and K+ content of the two preparations are similar. The smaller plasma volume in additive solution blood results in smaller amounts of coagulation factors in PRBCs but also a potentially lesser risk of minor allergic reactions and TRALI (Table 16-2).

There are alternative RBC preparations that eliminate the various "passengers." Saline-washed RBCs may be used for patients who experience reactions to foreign proteins. RBCs can be frozen and stored indefinitely. Preservatives to prevent freeze-thaw–associated damage must be added and subsequently removed before administration, which must occur within 24 hours of thawing. The process is expensive and therefore not widely used. Lymphocytes can be rendered incapable of division (and therefore unable to induce GVHD) by irradiation.

The administration of one unit of PRBCs will increase the Hb and Hct of a 70-kg adult by approximately 1 g/dL and 3%, respectively. However, both the freeze-thaw process and washing to reduce allergic reactions result in an RBC wastage of at least 20%.

Compatibility Testing

Compatibility testing involves three separate procedures: ABO Rhesus blood type identification, antibody screening of donor and recipient plasma, and the donor/recipient crossmatch.

ABO, Rhesus Typing

The first step is to determine the ABO blood group type and the Rh status of both donor and recipient blood. This is a critical step because most of the fatal hemolytic transfusion reactions result from the transfusion of ABO-incompatible blood. Blood types are defined according to the antigens present on the surface of the RBCs. Patients with type A blood have type A antigens on the surface of their red cells. Type B blood has B antigens. When both antigens are present the patient is said to have type AB blood, and when both are lacking the patient is has type O blood. By 6 to 12 months of age, the serum constitutively contains antibodies to the A and B antigens that are lacking on the RBC. Patients with type A blood have antibodies against the B antigen and vice versa. Patients with no antigens on their cells, type O blood, will have both anti-A and anti-B antibodies in the plasma.

Patients with the D antigen of the Rhesus group of antigens are said to be Rh-positive. Approximately 85% of the population is Rh-positive. In contrast to the A and B blood groups, anti-D antibodies are not constitutively present in the serum of an Rh-negative patient. However, 60 to 70% of Rh-negative patients exposed to donor Rh-positive RBCs will develop anti-D antibodies. There is a latency before these antibodies are synthesized. As a consequence, the reaction between the Rh-positive donor cells and the anti-D evolves slowly and may not be clinically apparent on first exposure. This process whereby a foreign antigen stimulates the synthesis of the corresponding antibody is termed *alloimmunization*. Subsequent exposure of these Rh-negative individuals to Rh-positive cells may result in an AHTR.

AHTRs are most often caused by antibodies in recipient plasma directed against A, B, or D antigens on donor RBCs. The antibody-antigen interaction activates complement and leads to intravascular hemolysis. "O-positive" recipients (type O, Rh[D]-positive) will have both anti-A and anti-B antibodies, but not the anti-D antibody in their plasma. These patients must not receive type A, type B, or type AB blood. They must receive type O blood, but it may be Rh-positive or Rh-negative. In contrast, patients with blood type AB-negative (type AB, Rh-negative) will lack both the A and B antibodies in their plasma and may or may not have the anti-D antibody in their plasma. They can receive A−, B−, AB−, or O− blood. Individuals with the greatest number of antigens on their RBCs (i.e., type AB-positive) have the fewest constitutive antibodies in their plasma and can receive all blood types (types A+, A−, B+, B−, AB+, AB−, O+, and O−) and are referred to as *universal recipients*. Individuals with the fewest antigens on their cells (type O) have the greatest number of antibodies in their plasma. Type O-negative RBCs can be administered to all ABO, Rh types and these individuals are referred to as *universal donors*. The distribution of A, B, O, and D phenotypes in the U.S. population is presented in Table 16-12. A derivative of those distributions is that, assuming the same representation among donors and recipients (and the absence of superimposed alloimmunization that would compound the risk), random administration of blood (or recipient identification errors) will result in an AHTR with one of every three PRBC units administered.

The Antibody Screen

The antibody screen, an indirect Coombs test, is performed to identify recipient antibodies against RBC antigens. Commercially supplied RBCs, selected for strong expression of 25 to 30 potentially hemolytic antigens, are mixed with recipient serum. Only about 4 in 1,000 potential recipients demonstrate unexpected antibodies. The likelihood that the antibody screen will miss a potentially dangerous antibody has been estimated to be much less than 1 in 10,000. If the recipient plasma screen is positive, the antibody must be identified and appropriate antigen-negative donor units selected. The antibody screening of recipient plasma should be repeated at 3-day intervals if the patient is receiving ongoing transfusion.

The Crossmatch

The predictive power of a negative antibody screen is such that most hospitals perform no further crossmatch procedures in patients who have no history of antibody formation. In institutions with validated blood bank computer systems, eligible patients may receive blood solely on the basis of an "electronic [computer database] crossmatch" of the recipient and the available units. Alternatively, some institutions perform an "immediate spin" (30 seconds at room temperature) crossmatch of recipient plasma and donor RBCs and examine for gross agglutination, which is predictive of ABO incompatibility. The requisite time for ABO/Rh typing and antibody screen, from sample arrival in the blood bank to blood release, is 30 to 45 minutes when the antibody screen is negative.

A formal crossmatch is performed if an antibody is identified, if the patient has a history of antibody formation, or if the patient is deemed to be at high risk for alloimmunization. Current procedures, which use a variety of enhancement techniques (e.g., low ionic strength solutions, polyethylene glycol, gels, or solid phase technology) allow antibody screens and/or crossmatches to be accomplished in approximately 20 minutes. The various incubation phases that were once used, necessitating 2 hours for a complete crossmatch, are no longer performed in the majority of institutions. Crossmatch procedures vary, but at a minimum will entail incubation of recipient plasma with donor RBCs at 37°C for 10 to 15 minutes followed by an indirect antiglobulin test and examination for agglutination.

In patients who have been transfused previously or who may have been exposed to foreign RBC antigens during pregnancy, the rate of development of an anti-RBC antibody to other than the A, B antigens is about 1 per 200 exposures (and is cumulative with multiple exposures).[24] Determining the ABO and Rh status alone is sufficient to assure that the transfusion will be compatible in 99.8% of patients who have not previously been transfused or pregnant (i.e., the likelihood of incompatible transfusion is about 1 in 1,000). That latter rate will rise in proportion to the number of prior donor exposures or pregnancies. The addition of the 30-to 45-minute antibody screen further increases the likelihood of a compatible transfusion (to >99.9% in UCSD Medical Center's experience with >50,000 transfused units). These data reveal that the administration, in emergency situations, of type-specific, uncrossmatched blood to patients with no history of pregnancy or transfusion should entail relatively little risk.

Type and Screen Orders

When blood is ordered preoperatively for surgical cases in which it is unlikely that the blood will actually be transfused, the orders should be for "type and screen" only. The ABO,

TABLE 16-12

MAJOR RED BLOOD CELL SURFACE ANTIGEN INCIDENCE (%) IN THE U.S. POPULATION

GROUP	WHITES	BLACKS
O	45	49
A	40	27
B	11	20
AB	4	4
Rh (D)	85	92

Rh status of the patient is determined and the antibody screen (see previous discussion) is performed to determine the presence of antibodies other than ABO in the potential recipient's plasma. If the antibody screen is negative, type-specific otherwise uncrossmatched blood will result in a hemolytic reaction in <1/50,000 units. If the screen is positive, the blood bank will proceed to identify a pool of potentially compatible units.

Emergency Transfusions

The exsanguinating patient may require RBCs before complete compatibility testing can be performed. If testing is to be abbreviated, there is a preferred order for selecting partially tested blood (see Chapter 36). The first choice is to transfuse type-specific partially crossmatched blood or type-specific uncrossmatched blood (although verification of blood type by analysis of two separately drawn specimens must be performed before releasing any uncrossmatched blood). In urgent situations in which the patient's ABO and Rh type is unknown, group O RBCs should be administered until there is time to complete ABO and Rh testing. Rh-negative blood is preferable, particularly if the patient is a woman of child-bearing age. If Rh-negative blood is not available for a critically ill, bleeding Rh-negative patient, Rh-positive blood is frequently used. If a non–group O patient receives a large volume of group O red cells, the combined amount of anti-A and/or anti-B present in small amounts in the residual plasma of each PRBC unit may react with the patient's own A, B, or AB red cells and cause some hemolysis. For this reason, a non–group O patient who has received group O red cells approximating one patient blood volume (10 to 12 units) during the period of acute blood loss should not be switched back to his or her own ABO group until testing has been performed to confirm that significant titres of anti-A or anti-B antibodies are not present. That testing is typically performed automatically by contemporary blood banks. When FFP or TP (see later discussion) are administered prior to ABO typing, type AB plasma is preferable,[90] although sometimes not feasible because of limited supply (Table 16-12).

Platelets

Platelets are separated from plasma by centrifugation.[25] More than 70% of the platelets used in the United States are now derived by apheresis. A single apheresis unit (referred to as *apheresis platelets*), which is obtained from a single donor at a single session, supplies 3×10^{11} platelets in a volume of 200 to 400 mL. An apheresis unit supplies the equivalent of the platelets derived by concentrating platelets from six to eight individual donor units of whole blood. The latter, when combined, are referred to as platelet *packs* or *concentrates*. The use of apheresis platelets substantially reduces donor exposures with the attendant risks of alloimmunization and infection (viral and bacterial). Platelet viability is optimal at 22°C. Although platelets are potentially viable for as long as 10 days (the normal in vivo lifespan), by FDA mandate, storage is limited to 5 days because of the time-related risk of bacterial growth.[25] Platelets should be delivered through the standard 170-micron blood set filter. A micropore filter should *not* be used.

Platelets bear ABO, HLA, and other platelet-specific antigens. ABO compatibility is ideal, although not absolutely required. ABO incompatibility reduces platelet survival. In addition, it appears to increase immune responsiveness to HLA and other platelet surface antigens, thereby increasing the incidence of alloimmunization.[25] ABO/HLA-matched platelets, crossmatched platelets, and HLA antigen-negative platelets can be used for patients who become refractory to random donor platelets. Platelets do not carry the Rh antigen. However, administration of platelets from an Rh-positive donor to an Rh-negative female of child-bearing age should be avoided if delay does not impose hazard in order to prevent sensitization as a result of passenger RBCs in the platelet preparation. The sensitization risk is small because of the very limited number of RBCs in contemporary platelet preparations and is effectively prevented by Rh immune globulin, which should be administered. ABO compatibility of platelets is also desirable because the antibodies present in the plasma phase can cause hemolysis of recipient RBCs.[148] Hemolytic events have invariably involved administration of O type platelets to a non-O recipient, and blood bank procedures typically avoid large-volume administration of those pairings.[148]

Fresh-Frozen Plasma/Thawed Plasma

Plasma is separated from the RBC component of whole blood by centrifugation. One unit has a volume of 200 to 250 mL. It will contain the preservative added at the time of collection, usually CPDA. To preserve the two labile clotting factors (V and VIII), FFP is frozen promptly and thawed only immediately prior to administration. FFP must be ABO compatible. Avoiding Rh-positive plasma in Rh-negative patients seems unnecessary because there has been no reported instance of alloimmunization in over 40 years.

TP is being ever more widely used in lieu of FFP, especially in the management of trauma. (Many of the readers of this chapter may discover that they have already been administering TP.) It is obtained from thawed FFP that is maintained at 6°C for a maximum of 5 days. Its advantage is immediate availability (and reduction of wastage of thawed FFP not administered within 24 hours). Levels of FV and FVIII decline during storage. However, it is believed that there is sufficient residual FV even after 5 days to achieve FV levels of 25 to 30% readily. Factor VIII is an acute phase reactant that is usually present in sufficient amounts in trauma victims. TP can be used interchangeably with FFP in most situations, with the exception of patients with specific deficiencies of FV or FVIII, in DIC, and in neonates. Some clinicians will encounter FP24 (plasma frozen within 24 hours after phlebotomy), which is typically used interchangeably with FFP.

Solvent Detergent Plasma

One of the principal hazards of FFP administration has been virus transmission. Three procedures—pasteurization, photochemical treatment, and solvent detergent (SD) treatment—have been used to inactivate viruses. The SD technique is highly effective in inactivating all of the lipid encapsulated viruses (i.e., HIV, HCV, HBV, and HTLV). The disadvantage of the SD technique is that the process involves pooling of large numbers of single FFP units (>1,000) and is not effective against non–lipid-enveloped viruses (HAV, parvovirus) or the agent of CJD. The concern with SD plasma is that the pooling process might result in wide dissemination of an infectious agent. The incidence of parvovirus viremia among donors is estimated to be nearly 1.0%.[149] Parvovirus B19 infection has been reported as a consequence of transfusion. While the disease is usually self-limited, significant morbidity, such as red cell aplasia and/or meningitis, especially in immunocompromised patents can occur.[150] SD plasma is now tested for B19 and HAV and is widely used in Europe but is no longer available in the United States.

Cryoprecipitate

Cryoprecipitate is the precipitate that remains when FFP is thawed slowly at 4°C. It is a concentrated source of FVIII, FXIII, vWF, and fibrinogen. One unit of cryoprecipitate (the yield from one unit of FFP) contains sufficient fibrinogen to increase fibrinogen levels by 5 to 7 mg/dL.[151] Accordingly, it is usually provided in bags that contain 10 or 20 units. ABO compatibility is not essential because of the limited antibody content of the associated plasma vehicle (10 to 20 mL). Viruses can be transmitted with cryoprecipitate. It is stored at −20°C and thawed immediately prior to use.

Factor VIII and IX

Recombinant and virally inactivated plasma-derived FVIII and FIX concentrates are available.[152]

Antithrombin III

Virus-treated antithrombin III (AT) concentrates are available. They can be used in the treatment of congenital and acquired AT deficiencies, including heparin resistance, DIC, and fulminant hepatic failure.[153–155]

THE HEMOSTATIC MECHANISM

Normal hemostasis involves a series of physiologic checks and balances that assure that blood remains invariably in a liquid state as it circulates throughout the body but, once the vascular network is violated, transforms rapidly to a solid state. That transformation to a solid state (i.e., coagulation) must inevitably be complemented by processes for eliminating clot that is no longer needed for hemostasis. The latter is accomplished by fibrinolysis.

The Nomenclature of Coagulation

The nomenclature of coagulation is unfortunately complex. The first 4 of the 12 originally identified factors are usually referred to by their common names—fibrinogen, prothrombin, tissue factor (TF), and calcium—and not by their Roman numerals. FVI no longer exists; it proved to be activated FV. The more recently discovered clotting factors (e.g., prekallikrein and high-molecular-weight kininogen) have not been assigned Roman numerals. Some factors have more than one name (Table 16-13).

The Coagulation Mechanism

⑪ The classic dual cascade (intrinsic and extrinsic pathway) model of coagulation (Fig. 16-1) is now recognized to be an inadequate representation of in vivo coagulation. It fails to explain several clinical phenomena. First, persons lacking FXII, prekallikrein, or high-molecular-weight kininogen do not bleed abnormally, suggesting that contact activation is not critical for in vivo hemostasis. Second, patients with only trace quantities of FXI withstand major trauma without unusual bleeding, and those completely lacking factor XI (hemophilia C) have only a mild hemorrhagic disorder. FXI therefore appears to have a more minor role in coagulation than ascribed to it by classic theory. Next, deficiencies of FVIII and FIX (both intrinsic pathway factors) lead to hemophilia A and B, respectively. However, the classic description of two pathways of coagulation leaves it unclear clear why either type of hemophiliac could not simply clot via the unaffected pathway. Most importantly, it is now appreciated that while the classic theories may provide a reasonable model of in vitro coagulation tests (i.e., the aPTT and PT), they fail to incorporate the central role of cell-based surfaces in the in vivo coagulation process. The three stages of that process that have been thoroughly defined and described by Hoffman and

TABLE 16-13

FACTOR NOMENCLATURE AND HALF-LIVES

■ FACTOR	■ SYNONYMS	■ IN VIVO HALF-LIFE (hours)
I	Fibrinogen	100–150
II	Prothrombin	50–80
III	Tissue factor, thromboplastin	
IV	Calcium ion	
V	Proaccelerin, labile factor	24
VII	Serum prothrombin conversion accelerator, stable factor	6
VIII	Antihemophilic factor (AHF), AHF-A, factor VIII:C	12
vWF	von Willebrand factor	24
IX	Christmas factor, AHF-B	24
X	Stuart-Prower factor, Stuart factor, Autoprothrombin	25–60
XI	Plasma thromboplastin antecedent, AHF-C	40–80
XII	Hageman factor, contact factor	50–70
XIII	Fibrin stabilizing factor	150
Prekallikrein	Fletcher factor	35
HMW kininogen	Fitzgerald, Flaujeac, or Williams factor; contact activation cofactor	150

HMW, high molecular weight.

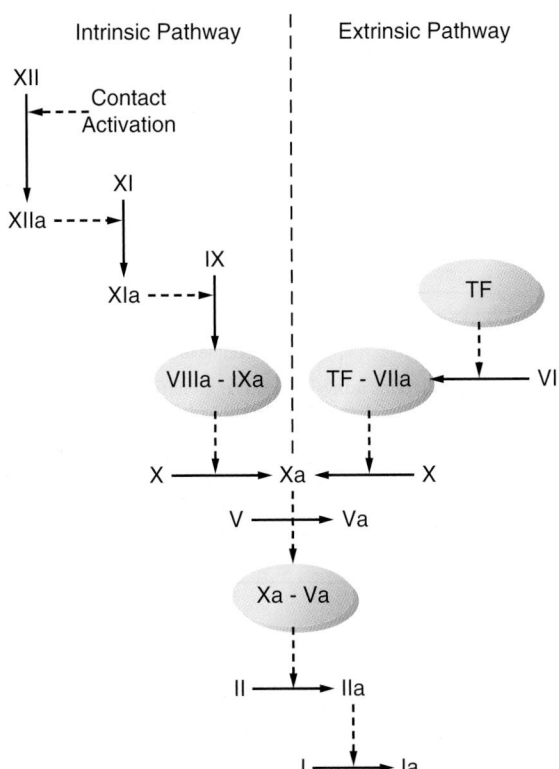

FIGURE 16-1.   The classic intrinsic and extrinsic pathways of coagulation. Intrinsic pathway (**left**). A cascade initiated by contact with a foreign surface (contact activation) leads to the formation of fibrin (Ia). Extrinsic pathway (**right**). This pathway, also leading to fibrin formation, is depicted as it was originally thought to occur, that is, largely extravascularly and independent of the classic intrinsic pathway (cf: Fig. 16-2). The *dotted arrows* indicate the occurrence of an enzymatically mediated conversion of an inactive factor to its active form. The *shaded spheroids* represent the procoagulant surfaces provided in the extrinsic pathway both in vivo and in vitro by tissue factor (TF) and, in the intrinsic pathway, by phospholipids in vitro and platelets in vivo.

Monroe[156] are summarized in the following sections and in Figure 16-2.

Activation

Activation of the coagulation process begins when a breach in the vascular endothelium exposes blood to TF. TF is a membrane-bound protein, with adjacent membrane phospholipids, that is constitutively expressed in extravascular tissue, principally on fibroblasts (Fig. 16-2A). TF also appears on the surface of vascular endothelium and circulating monocytes in response to mechanical injury or inflammation.[157] TF activates FVII (Fig. 16-2B) to yield a complex of TF and activated FVII (FVIIa) on the phospholipid surface. The TF-VIIa in turn activates FX, yielding a complex of TF-VIIa-Xa (Fig. 16-2C). The FXa, still on the phospholipid surface, then binds with FVa to form the "prothrombinase complex." The FVa that participates in this reaction is liberated from the alpha granules of platelets that were activated at the site of injury as a result of binding to subendothelial vWF (Figs. 16-2E and 16-3). The prothrombinase complex catalyzes the conversion of prothrombin (FII) to thrombin (FIIa; Fig. 16-2E). However, generation of IIa by this pathway is limited by tissue factor pathway inhibitor (TFPI). TFPI, a protein that is constitutively present in endothelium and platelets,[158] binds to and inhibits the Xa component of the TF-VIIa-Xa complex and, once bound, inhibits adjacent TF-VIIa complexes from further activation of FX[158] (Fig. 16-2D). As a consequence, only very limited amounts of thrombin can be generated by this mechanism (which explains why hemophiliacs bleed in spite of an intact intrinsic pathway). But this initial formation of small amounts of thrombin is sufficient to advance the coagulation process to the more efficient "amplification" phase that follows.

Amplification

While it was the surface provided by membrane-bound TF and adjacent phospholipid that initiated the coagulation process, it is now the phospholipid surface provided by platelets that serves to perpetuate it. The breach in the vascular tree that

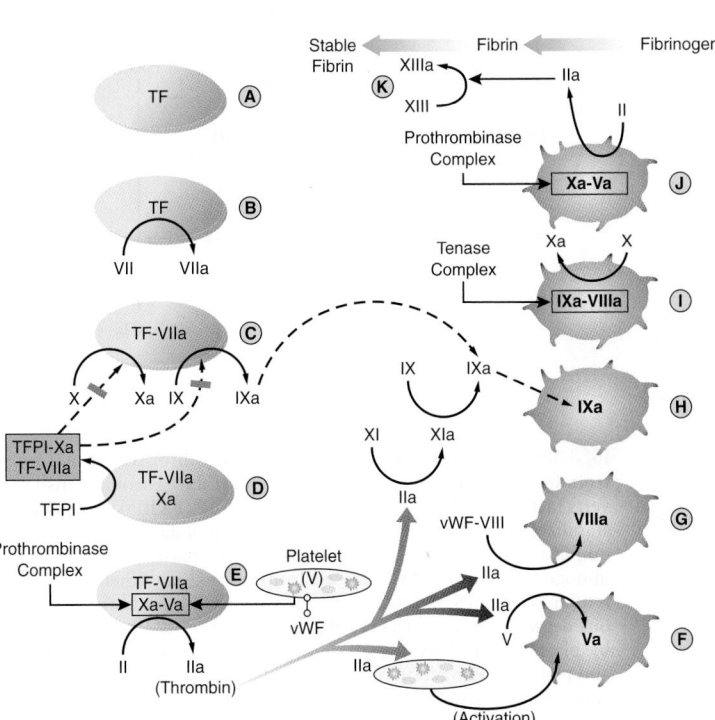

FIGURE 16-2.   The coagulation mechanism. See text for details. TF, membrane-bound tissue factor on a extravascular cell surface; TFPI, tissue factor pathway inhibitor; vWF-VIII:C, circulating factor VIII bound to its carrier protein, the von Willebrand factor.

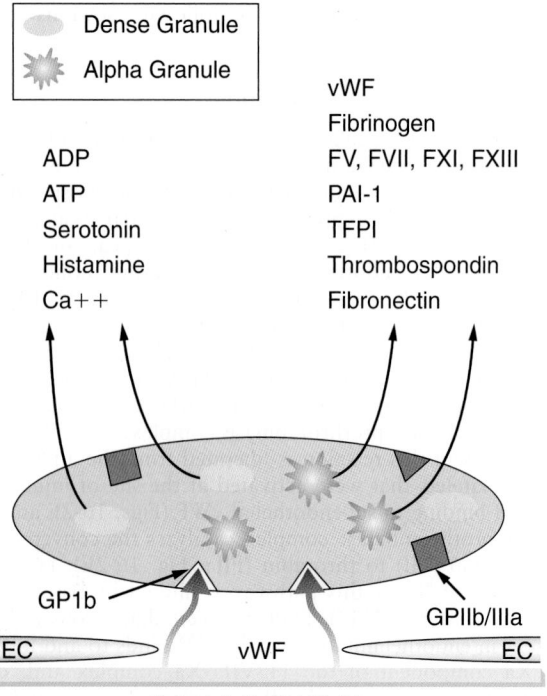

FIGURE 16-3. Platelet release reaction. Platelets undergo a release reaction in response to adherence to the subendothelium or to physiologic agonists including epinephrine, adenosine diphosphate (ADP), and thrombin. The numerous substances released from the alpha and dense granules of platelets contribute to additional platelet activation (ADP, Ca++, serotonin), platelet aggregation (von Willebrand factor [vWF], fibronectin, thrombospondin, fibrinogen), and clot formation (calcium, fibrinogen, factors V, XI and XIII, plasminogen activator inhibitor [PAI-1]). ATP, adenosine triphosphate; TFPI, tissue factor pathway inhibitor; GP, glycoprotein; EC, endothelial cell.

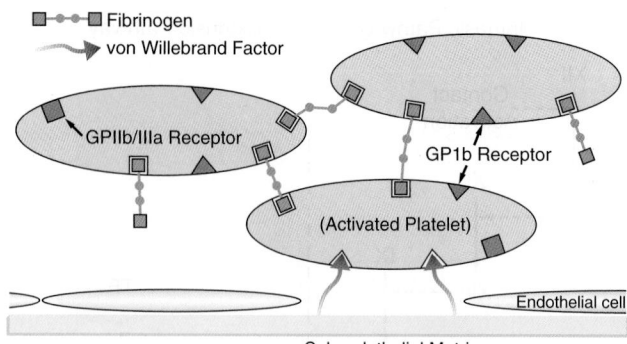

FIGURE 16-4. Platelet adhesion and aggregation. When the endothelium is denuded, platelets adhere to the collagen in the subendothelium via their glycoprotein glycoprotein (GP) 1b receptors and von Willebrand factor, present in both plasma and the subendothelial matrix. Platelets aggregate to one another by cross-linking via fibrinogen (or von Willebrand factor, not shown) between GPIIb/IIIa receptors expressed on the platelet surface during the process of platelet activation.

Propagation

The platelet then provides the phospholipid surface on which two coagulation factor complexes form and act to produce the explosive generation of thrombin. First, FVIIIa and FIXa form the "tenase complex," which activates FX (Fig. 16-2H). The resultant FXa forms additional prothrombinase complex (Xa-Va), and large amounts of thrombin are elaborated (Fig. 16-2J). (For mnemonic purposes it is "eight-nine and nickel-dime" that together are responsible for the thrombin burst.) Thrombin (FIIa) catalyzes the formation of fibrin from fibrinogen, and fibrin acts to crosslink the platelets, largely via the IIb/IIIa receptors (Fig. 16-4), to reinforce the friable platelet plug. Thrombin also activates FXIII (Figs. 16-2K and 16-5) and thrombin-activatable fibrinolysis inhibitor (TAFI; Fig. 16-5). Fibrin

began the activation process also exposed platelets to collagen to which they become bound via vWF and the GPIb receptor on the platelet surface (Fig. 16-4). That binding results in platelet surface changes, most notably the appearance of the GPIIb/IIIa receptor, and in the release of the contents of alpha and dense platelet granules (Fig. 16-3).[159] The latter contain numerous substances that contribute to additional platelet activation (adenosine diphosphate [ADP], Ca++, serotonin), platelet aggregation (vWF, fibronectin, thrombospondin, fibrinogen), clot formation and stabilization (calcium, fibrinogen, factors V, XI and XIII, plasminogen activator inhibitor [PAI-1]), and to adhesion and activation of additional platelets. The thrombin just generated by the TF-bound prothrombinase complex supports the amplification of the coagulation process in four ways. First, thrombin, a serine protease, further activates the adjacent platelets (Fig. 16-2F) via protease-activated surface receptors.[160] Thrombin's second effect is to promote the activation FV in plasma to FVa (Fig. 16-2F). Third, thrombin releases circulating FVIII from its carrier molecule (vWF) and activates it (Fig. 16-2G). Fourth, thrombin activates FXI. FXIa in turn activates FIX (Fig. 16-2H). Note that some FIXa was also generated by the TF-VIIa during the activation phase (Fig. 16-2C). This may explain why FXI deficiency results in such a minor coagulation disturbance. The net result of this amplification stage is the availability of additional activated platelets and activated Factors V, VIII, and IX.

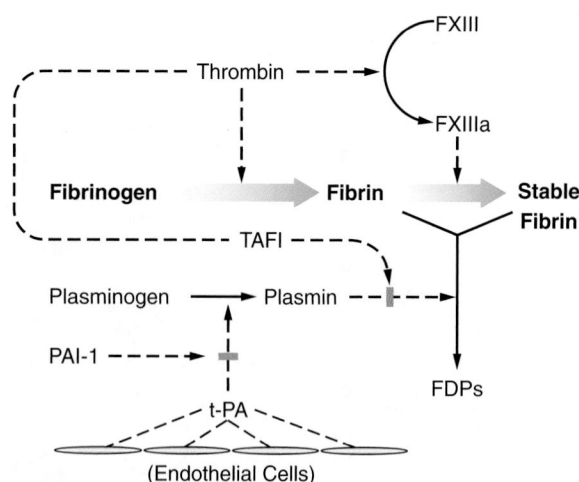

FIGURE 16-5. The formation and lysis of fibrin. Fibrin is formed from fibrinogen by the action of thrombin (FIIa). Thrombin also converts factor XIII (FXIII) to activated factor XIII (FXIIIa), which in turn stabilizes the evolving fibrin clot by cross-linkage. Circulating plasminogen binds to fibrin and is converted to plasmin by tissue plasminogen activator (tPA) released from normal endothelium in areas remote from sites of vascular injury. Plasmin digests fibrin to its various degradation products (FDPs). The action of tPA can be inhibited by plasminogen activator inhibitor (PAI-1) released by endothelium and platelets. The action of plasmin is also inhibited by thrombin-activated fibrinolysis inhibitor (TAFI).

monomers initially aggregate relatively loosely to form clot composed of fibrin S (soluble), which is held together only by hydrogen bonds. FXIII (fibrin-stabilizing factor) mediates the formation of covalent peptide bonds between the fibrin monomers. FXIII may be an underappreciated cause of clinical coagulation disturbance.[161] TAFI functions to prevent lysis of the newly formed clot (Fig. 16-5). In the presence of subnormal amounts of thrombin, although fibrin clot can form, it may not achieve normal strength and stability[162] and may not be protected by adequate concentrations of TAFI.[163]

In vivo, coagulation is initiated principally by contact of factor VII with extravascular TF leading first to the generation of small amounts of thrombin. Thereafter, activated clotting factors, acting intravascularly on the phospholipid surface provided by activated platelets, lead to the generation of large amounts of thrombin.

Additional Principles of Coagulation

A few additional facts will aid in achieving a broader understanding of coagulation.

1. Most clotting factors circulate in an inactive proenzyme, or zymogen, form. During the process of coagulation, a portion of the molecule is cleaved off, resulting in active enzymes (designated by the addition of a lower case "a" after the Roman numeral, e.g., Xa), most of which are serine proteases.

2. Most clotting factors are synthesized by the liver. The probable exception is factor VIII, which probably also has some extrahepatic synthesis.

3. Factor VIII is actually a large, two-molecule complex (vWF and coagulant factor VIII). Factor VIII circulates as a very large complex of two distinct protein components. The high-molecular-weight portion (VIIIR:Ag) encompasses both the FVIII antigen and vWF. The vWF portion serves as a carrier protein for the second and smaller component of this macromolecular complex, VIIIC, which contains the factor VIII coagulant activity. The vWF has a second function. During the process of primary hemostasis, when the endothelial lining has been denuded, vWF in the subendothelial matrix mediates adhesion of platelets to collagen. Absence of the smaller portion of the factor VIII complex (VIII:C), results in hemophilia A. vWF deficiency causes two hemostatic abnormalities: (1) a defect in primary hemostasis because of a failure of platelet adhesion to the sites of vascular injury, and (2) the clinical equivalent of hemophilia A because of deficiency of circulating factor VIII:C. Restoration of vWF levels restores normal hemostasis. Synthesis of the vWF occurs in endothelial cells and megakaryocytes. The site of synthesis of the coagulant portion of factor VIII is unknown but may be located in the hepatic sinusoidal endothelial cells.

4. Four clotting factors are vitamin K-dependent. Factors II, VII, IX, and X require vitamin K for completion of their synthesis in the liver. Each undergoes a final enzymatic addition of a carboxyl group that requires the presence of vitamin K. The carboxyl group enables these factors to bind (using calcium as a cofactor) to phospholipid surfaces. Without vitamin K, factors II, VII, IX, and X are produced in normal amounts but are nonfunctional.

   The anticoagulant action of vitamin K antagonists is the result of their ability to inhibit this final carboxylation step. The warfarin-like drugs compete with vitamin K for binding sites on the hepatocyte. With sufficient warfarin administration, vitamin K is displaced and the vitamin K-dependent factors are not carboxylated. Of the four vitamin K-dependent factors, factor VII has the shortest half-life. It is the first clotting factor to disappear from the circulation when a patient is given warfarin or begins to develop vitamin K deficiency.

5. Factors V and VIII have short storage half-lives. Factors V and VIII are also referred to as the *labile factors* because their coagulant activity is not durable in stored blood. While PRBCs contain some residual plasma with clotting factors, massive transfusion with stored blood will nonetheless lead to a dilutional coagulopathy because of diminished activity of factors V and VIII.

Fibrinolysis

Fibrinolysis serves to dissolve or remodel fibrin clots and thereby "recanalize" vessels that have been occluded by thrombosis.

The Formation of Plasmin

Plasminogen is the inactive form of the fibrinolytic enzyme plasmin. Conversion of plasminogen to plasmin is accomplished principally by tissue plasminogen activator (tPA; Fig. 16-5). Plasmin is rapidly degraded by circulating antiplasmins and therefore cannot circulate freely. Plasminogen, however, can circulate. It binds to fibrin on contact and is incorporated in the evolving fibrin clot where it is converted to plasmin by tPA. While bound plasmin is protected from attack by circulating antiplasmins, any plasmin that is released from the clot is immediately neutralized by circulating α_2-antiplasmin. Thus, like the coagulation cascade, the fibrinolytic system relies on surface-mediated reactions that limit both plasmin formation and fibrinolysis to the site of vascular injury.

Plasminogen Activation

The principal activator of plasmin is tPA. tPA is synthesized by vascular endothelial cells. In the event of clot formation (which requires the presence of thrombin), thrombin forms a complex with thrombomodulin (present on the vascular endothelial surface) that activates protein C. Activated protein C (APC) stimulates the release of tPA. tPA is also released from the endothelium in response to venous occlusion, physical activity, stress, or vasoactive drugs (such as epinephrine, vasopressin, and DDAVP).[164] tPA binds to the adjacent fibrin and converts plasminogen to plasmin (Fig. 16-5). This mechanism serves to localize fibrinolysis to the site of vascular injury, thereby preventing vascular injury at a single location from initiating widespread fibrinolysis. As a further "check" on the fibrinolytic process, the vascular endothelium and platelets also synthesize an inhibitor of tPA, PAI-1, which reduces the amount of plasmin formed and serves to slow the fibrinolytic process (Fig. 16-5). Some patients with thrombotic disorders have been found to have increased levels of this inhibitor.[164] A similar inhibitor is found in placental tissue, and it may be that the progressive hypercoagulable state associated with pregnancy is related to increased levels of this tPA inhibitor.[164]

There are other plasminogen activators. Urokinase is present in prostatic tissue and urine but not in circulating blood. Physiologic activators of the fibrinolytic system include vigorous exercise, anoxia, and stress. Exogenous plasminogen activators include streptokinase, urokinase, and recombinant tPA. These fibrinolytic agents all differ with respect to their action, clot specificity, systemic fibrinolytic effect, antigenic effect, and efficacy. Proteins derived from streptococci and staphylococci have also been found to be activators of the fibrinolytic system. The therapeutic fibrinolytic agents, streptokinase and urokinase, differ from tPA in that they will activate circulating plasminogen. These lead to more widespread fibrinolysis. Fibrinolytic therapy has been used in the treatment of unstable angina, acute thrombotic stroke, acute peripheral arterial occlusions, deep vein thrombosis, pulmonary embolism (PE), and occluded indwelling catheters and arteriovenous shunts.

Plasmin Inactivation/Inhibition

Under normal circumstances, free plasmin is rapidly inactivated by antiplasmins. In the event of deficiency of α_2-antiplasmin or when antiplasmin capacity is exceeded in primary fibrinolysis or DIC, plasmin circulates. Circulating plasmin will contribute to the bleeding diathesis because plasmin, in addition to degrading fibrin, is a serine protease that can also degrade other coagulation process components including fibrinogen, FV, FVIII, FXIII, vWF, and the GPIb platelet receptor.[164]

Fibrin Degradation Products

The structure of the products of fibrin breakdown, called *fibrin degradation products* (FDPs) or *fibrin split products* (FSPs), varies according to whether plasmin cleaves fibrinogen, fibrin that is cross-linked, or fibrin that is not cross-linked. FDPs are removed from the blood by the liver, kidney, and reticuloendothelial system. If they are produced at a rate that exceeds their normal clearance, they will accumulate. In high concentrations, FDPs impair platelet function, inhibit thrombin, and prevent the cross-linking of fibrin strands. The defective polymerization of the fibrin monomers results in a clot that is more readily degraded by plasmin.[164]

Under normal conditions, plasmin is generated only at the site of clot formation and is destroyed rapidly once released into the circulation. This localization process fails at times of accelerated fibrinolysis (DIC, primary fibrinolysis).

Control of Coagulation—The Checks and Balances

Coagulation must be precisely regulated to prevent rampant, uncontrolled clotting, such as that which occurs with DIC. Several mechanisms regulate and control coagulation.

Endothelial Inhibition

The first line of defense is the vascular endothelium. The intact endothelium has antithrombotic properties that serve to limit both platelet aggregation and coagulation and to induce fibrinolysis should a clot begin to form on normal endothelium. These properties are summarized in Table 16-14.

TABLE 16-14

ENDOTHELIAL CONTROL OF PLATELET AGGREGATION, COAGULATION, AND FIBRINOLYSIS

- Endothelial control of platelet aggregation
  - Synthesis of prostacyclin
  - Synthesis of ADPases and nitric oxide
- Endothelial inhibition of coagulation
  - Synthesis of thrombomodulin
  - Synthesis of heparan sulfate
- Endothelial control of fibrinolysis
  - Synthesis of tPA

ADPase, adenosine diphosphatase; tPA, tissue plasminogen activator.

1. The thromboxane-prostacyclin balance. Primary hemostasis is, in part, controlled by the balance between the effects of two prostaglandins, thromboxane A_2 (TxA$_2$) and prostacyclin. TxA$_2$ is synthesized at the site of vascular damage by activated platelets. TxA$_2$ has two hemostatic effects: (1) it is a potent vasoconstrictor that limits flow to the site of injury, and (2) it stimulates additional ADP release from platelets, thereby recruiting additional platelets. Remote from the site of vascular damage, normal endothelial cells synthesize prostacyclin (Fig. 16-6). Prostacyclin has actions opposite those of TxA$_2$. Prostacyclin inhibits platelet activation, secretion, and aggregation and is a potent vasodilator and thereby serves to prevent platelet aggregation and clot formation on the endothelial surface beyond the site of injury.

2. Nitric oxide and adenosine diphosphatase (ADPase). The effects of prostacyclin are potentiated by nitric oxide, which is constitutively synthesized by normal endothelium and which also has vasodilatory and platelet antiaggregant effects (Fig. 16-6). As an additional means of preventing clot formation on the surface of normal endothelium, ADPases are expressed on the outer membrane of endothelial cells and serve to degrade "surplus" ADP that might otherwise initiate platelet aggregation on normal surfaces.

3. Heparan sulfate. One of the constituents of the mucopolysaccharide glycocalyx that covers normal endothelium is a naturally occurring heparinlike substance, heparan sulfate (Fig. 16-6). Like heparin, heparan has the ability to accelerate the binding of AT to thrombin and the other activated clotting factors of the classic intrinsic pathway. This heparan sulfate is well positioned because it is at this blood-endothelial interface that activated factors of the coagulation cascade are being generated.

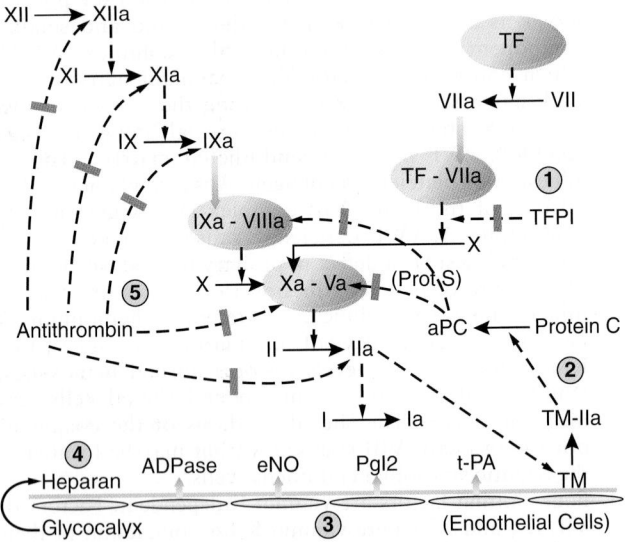

FIGURE 16-6. Five antithrombotic mechanisms. Five mechanisms that serve to prevent unrestrained coagulation are depicted. 1. Tissue factor pathway inhibitor (TFPI) inhibits the initial activation of factor X by the extrinsic pathway. 2. A complex of thrombomodulin (TM) and thrombin (IIa) activates protein C, which, with protein S (Prot S) as a cofactor, inhibits activated factors V and VIII. 3. Intact vascular endothelium releases several substances that have a platelet-inhibiting or clot-lysing effect, including nitric oxide (eNO), prostacyclin (PgI2), adenosine diphosphatase (ADPase), and tissue plasminogen activator (tPA). 4. In addition to TM, other coagulation-inhibiting substances including heparan sulphate and dermatan sulphate (latter not shown) are present in the intact glycocalyx. 5. Antithrombin III binds, and thereby inhibits, several activated clotting factors (XIIa, XIa, IXa, Xa, and IIa).

4. Thrombin, thrombomodulin, and proteins C and S. Thrombin, in a negative feedback process, can decrease its own synthesis by inhibition of factors V and VIII. That inhibition is accomplished via protein C. Protein C circulates in plasma as an inactive precursor. Thrombomodulin is a glycoprotein located on the vascular endothelial cell surface (Fig. 16-6). The binding of thrombin to thrombomodulin alters the thrombin molecule such that it can no longer directly activate clotting factors V and VIII or catalyze the conversion of fibrinogen to fibrin. In addition, the thrombin-thrombomodulin complex rapidly converts protein C to activated protein C (APC). APC, with protein S as a cofactor, cleaves and inactivates factors Va and VIIIa (Fig. 16-6). Like protein C, protein S is vitamin K-dependent. Where the endothelium is intact, the thrombomodulin-thrombin-protein C interaction will inhibit coagulation and maintain the "nonthrombogenic" property of the endothelial lining. Where the endothelium has been stripped away or damaged, this anticoagulant mechanism will be absent and clotting can continue unopposed.

5. Endothelial synthesis of tPA. Endothelial synthesis of tPA is one of several mechanisms by which the normal endothelial surface is maintained in a nonthrombogenic state (Fig. 16-6). Should clot begin to form on the normal endothelial surface, the associated thrombin induces the release of tPA, which, in the absence of other promoters of coagulation, leads rapidly to dissolution of the incipient clot.

Other Modulators of Coagulation

Several additional factors serve to limit and localize clot formation. First, the clotting factors themselves circulate in an inactive form. Once activated at an injury site, normal blood flow dilutes their concentration and clears them away from sites of injury, limiting clot formation. Activated clotting factors are preferentially removed from the circulation by the liver and the reticuloendothelial system. Finally, most of the interactions of the coagulation pathway require the presence of a phospholipid surface, which localizes clot formation to those surfaces (TF, activated platelets). Several specific coagulation-inhibiting systems are operative. Five of them are depicted in Figure 16-6. TFPI and AT are described later. The others have been previously described in "Endothelial Inhibition."

1. Tissue Factor Pathway Inhibitor (TFPI). Superficially, the description of the cell-based coagulation mechanism still leaves in place one of the inadequacies of the classic cascade theories of coagulation, that is, if activated factor X, and subsequently thrombin, can be formed via the direct action of the VIIa/TF complex, why is it that hemophiliacs bleed? Why do they appear to be dependent on factors VIII and IX to produce activated factor X? The answer lies in a feedback inhibitor of the extrinsic pathway known as TFPI (Figs. 16-2 and 16-6). TFPI, the precursor molecule of activated TFPI (TFPIa), is constitutively present on the endothelial surface and bound to circulating lipoproteins.[158] It is activated by contact with the Xa-VIIa-TF complex, that is, it is not activated until coagulation has been initiated. It inactivates factor Xa and causes internalization of membrane bound VIIa/TF complexes.[158] In the presence of TFPI, extensive activation of factor X appears to require the reaction sequences of the classic intrinsic pathway. The TF pathway can initiate the first flurry of thrombin generation—enough to activate platelets and stimulate cofactors V and VIII. Thereafter, continued thrombin production appears to require the action of factors VIIIa and IXa.[165]

2. Antithrombin (AT). AT is a circulating serine protease inhibitor that binds to thrombin and thereby inactivates it.

AT can bind and inactivate each of the activated clotting factors of the classic "intrinsic" coagulation cascade—factors XIIa, XIa, IXa, and Xa (see Fig. 16-6). The AT molecule has two critical binding sites, one of which reacts with thrombin and the other activated clotting factors and a second to which heparin can bind (see Chapter 41). In the absence of heparin, AT has a relatively low affinity for thrombin. Heparin binding to AT increases the efficiency of binding of AT to thrombin and the other factors dramatically. Congenital AT deficiency (levels 40 to 50% of normal) can lead to a prothrombotic diathesis. Acquired AT deficiency can occur with liver disease, prolonged heparin administration, nephrotic syndrome, DIC, sepsis, preeclampsia, fatty liver of pregnancy, oral contraceptive use, and during CPB.[166, 167] AT concentrates have been used in AT deficiency states, including heparin resistance.[167–169]

3. Thrombin Activatable Fibrinolysis Inhibitor (TAFI). An additional feedback mechanism to prevent excessive fibrinolysis and premature clot breakdown exists in the form of TAFI (Fig. 16-5). TAFI is activated by low concentrations of thrombin when thrombomodulin is present or directly by greater concentrations. TAFI's role in abnormalities of hemostasis is not well-defined.[163]

The Complexities of the Hemostatic Mechanism

Many mechanisms interact to maintain the liquid state of the blood under normal circumstances and to transform blood into a solid clot when injury occurs. These mechanisms include numerous feedback processes. The complexity is revealed by the existence of "double agents," which act at some times as procoagulants and at other times as anticoagulants. Chief among them is thrombin. Thrombin is primarily a procoagulant. It promotes primary hemostasis by activating platelets, and promotes coagulation by direct activation of factors V, VIII, and XIII. Thrombin, in the final step of the coagulation cascade, cleaves fibrinogen to fibrin. However, it also has anticoagulant effects. It inhibits coagulation through its interaction with thrombomodulin and protein C. APC stimulates the release of tPA from endothelial cells, and by this mechanism thrombin has a fibrinolytic effect while simultaneously activating the fibrinolysis inhibitor TAFI. Accordingly, thrombin through its effects at many stages of the feedback-controlled hemostasis process, functions as platelet proaggregant, a procoagulant, an anticoagulant, a profibrinolytic, and an anti-fibrinolytic.

The Hemostatic Mechanism: Summary

Under normal circumstances, the hemostatic mechanism is quiescent with many of the potential participants circulating in an inactive form. Only when the endothelial lining is breached is the hemostatic mechanism set in motion. With collagen and TF exposed, the intertwined processes of platelet-mediated primary hemostasis and factor-mediated coagulation begin. Vascular injury is sealed rapidly by a platelet mass into which are incorporated fibrinogen, thrombin, plasminogen, and tPA. The completion of the coagulation process converts fibrinogen into fibrin and the platelet plug is transformed into a fibrin clot. Simultaneously, several properties of adjacent intact endothelium (elaboration of ADPases, prostacyclin, thrombomodulin, heparans, and tPA) serve to prevent extension of the clot beyond the site of injury. Within the clot, plasmin, generated by the action of tPA on the trapped plasminogen, begins the process of fibrinolysis. Over time, the entire fibrin clot dissolves, new endothelial cells line the vessel, and flow is restored.

ANATOMY AND PHYSIOLOGY

LABORATORY EVALUATION OF THE HEMOSTATIC MECHANISM

Laboratory Evaluation of Primary Hemostasis

Platelet Count

A platelet count should be the first test ordered in the evaluation of primary hemostasis. The platelet count is quick, accurate, and reproducible. However, it reveals only platelet numbers and gives no information regarding their function. Normal platelet counts range between 150,000 and 440,000/mm^3. Counts below 150,000/mm^3 are defined as *thrombocytopenia*. Spontaneous bleeding is unlikely in patients with platelet counts >10,000 to 20,000/mm^3. With counts from 40,000 to 70,000/ mm^3, bleeding induced by surgery, may be severe. A detailed review of the many methods for testing platelet function is available.[170] Only the more widely used methods are mentioned here.

Bleeding Time

The Ivy bleeding time (BT) is the most widely accepted clinical test of platelet function. A blood pressure cuff is placed around the upper arm and inflated to 40 mm Hg. A cut is made on the volar surface of the forearm and the wound blotted at 30-second intervals until bleeding stops. The Simplate Bleeding Time (Organon Telenika Corp., Durham, NC) device, which uses a spring-loaded lancet, standardizes the size and depth of the cut. The normal range is 2 to 9 minutes. Variations in venous pressure, blotting technique, and patient cooperation result in a lack of precision and reproducibility that make this test somewhat less reliable than other coagulation tests. The BT is purported to evaluate the time necessary for a platelet plug to form following vascular injury. This requires a normal number of circulating platelets, platelets with normal function (which can adhere and aggregate), and an appropriate platelet interaction with the blood vessel wall. A prolongation of the BT may be because of (1) thrombocytopenia, (2) platelet dysfunction (adhesion, aggregation), and (3) vascular abnormalities such as scurvy or the Ehlers-Danlos syndrome. BTs are prolonged in patients with many conditions that cause platelet dysfunction (e.g., use of aspirin, uremia). However, prolonged BTs have been observed with numerous disorders that are not associated with platelet dysfunction, such as vitamin K deficiency of the newborn, amyloidosis, congenital heart disease, the presence of factor VIII inhibitors, or anemia.[171] Whether or not the BT test represents a specific measure of in vivo platelet function is much debated. The test is unpleasant for the patient and leaves a small scar. In spite of the correlation of BT with conditions known to influence platelet function, and in spite of BT quite reliably becoming progressively prolonged as platelet count falls below 80,000/μL, there are no convincing data to confirm that BT is a reliable predictor of the bleeding that will occur in association with surgical procedures.

Platelet Aggregometry

Platelet aggregometry quantifies platelet aggregation either spectrophotometrically or by impedance changes in response to stimulation with ADP, epinephrine, collagen, arachidonic acid, or ristocetin. The tests are sufficiently well standardized to allow distinctions among normal function, drug-related impairment of function, and intrinsic platelet defects. However, the tests are time-consuming and require absolutely fresh blood, and are therefore not widely used in acute patient management.[170]

The Platelet Function Analyser

The PFA-100 (Dade-Behring, Marburg, Germany) is a point of care, flow cytometry device. The test is based on the time to occlusion as the specimen passes through a small aperture impregnated with platelet activators (e.g., collagen, ADP). In one investigation, it proved less sensitive to the effect of aspirin than aggregometry.[172] The PFA-100 has also been reported to be very insensitive to the platelet-inhibiting effect of clopidogrel.[172,173] Its predictive value has not been well confirmed, and a report by the Platelet Physiology Subcommittee of the Scientific and Standardization Committee of the International Society on Thrombosis and Hemostasis offered the opinion that, "Although the PFA-100 closure time is abnormal in some forms of platelet disorders, the test does not have sufficient sensitivity or specificity to be used as a screening tool for platelet disorders."[174]

Clot Retraction

Clot retraction is another function of platelets that can be assessed grossly and by thromboelastography. When maintained at 37°C, a clot should begin to retract within 2 to 4 hours. This test is difficult to quantify and only qualitative results (retraction vs. no retraction) are usually reported.

Laboratory Evaluation of Coagulation

When blood is placed in a glass test tube, clot formation occurs in response to contact with the foreign surface. No exogenous reagents are required because all of the factors necessary for contact initiated coagulation are "intrinsic" to blood. The time to formation of a clot via this pathway can be prolonged by deficiencies of any factors in the classic intrinsic pathway. However, the observation that, even in hemophiliacs, the addition of thromboplastin (now more commonly called TF) to the test tube could shorten the time to clot formation suggested the presence of an alternative pathway of fibrin formation. That pathway required the addition of something "extrinsic to blood" and did not require the presence of factors VIII or IX. In 1936, when Quick introduced the prothrombin time (PT) to clinical medicine, sufficient "thromboplastin" was used to yield a clot formation time of approximately 12 seconds. Under these circumstances, even patients lacking factors VIII or IX showed normal clot formation times.[175] However, when "dilute" (partial) thromboplastin, which lacked the TF-equivalent activity necessary to activate FVII, was used in lieu of the "12-second reagent," hemophiliacs showed much longer clotting times than did healthy controls. The two different pathways could be tested individually. With "complete thromboplastin," coagulation proceeds via reactions that are independent of factors VIIIa and IXa. With "partial thromboplastin," coagulation must proceed via a sequence of reactions that requires factors VIII and IX. For both tests, calcium is added because of the chelating agent in the blood specimen container. The time to fibrin strand formation is then measured.

Prothrombin Time

The PT measures the time to fibrin strand formation via a short sequence of reactions involving only TF, factors VII, X, V, II (prothrombin) and I (fibrinogen), that is, the classic extrinsic coagulation pathway (Fig. 16-1). The normal PT is 10 to 12 seconds and will be prolonged by deficiencies, abnormalities, or inhibitors of factors VII, X, V, II, or I. The PT has limitations. First, it is not very sensitive to deficiencies of any of these factors. The coagulant activity of these factors must drop to 30% of normal before the PT is prolonged. The PT is most sensitive to a decrease in FVII and least sensitive to changes in prothrombin (FII). When prothrombin levels are only 10% of normal, the increase in the PT may be only 2 seconds. PT will not be prolonged until the fibrinogen level is below 100 mg/dL. If the aPTT (see later discussion) is normal, then a prolonged PT is most likely to represent a deficiency or abnormality of factor VII. Because FVII has the shortest half-life among the clotting factors synthesized in the liver, it is the factor that first becomes deficient with liver disease, vitamin K deficiency, or warfarin therapy. Prolongation of the PT may also be due to deficiencies of multiple factors. However, when multiple factor deficiencies occur, the aPTT is usually also prolonged.

International Normalized Ratio. The variation in thromboplastin reagents used resulted in wide variation in normal values and made comparison of PT results between laboratories difficult. The INR was introduced to circumvent this difficulty.[176] Each thromboplastin is compared with an internationally accepted standard thromboplastin and assigned an International Sensitivity Index. PT test times obtained with individual reagents can thereby be normalized and reported as an INR.[177]

Activated Partial Thromboplastin Time

The aPTT assesses the function of the classic intrinsic and final common pathways (Fig. 16-1). Patient blood is combined with three reagents. In addition to calcium, there is a contact activator (e.g., diatomaceous earth, kaolin, celite, and ellagic acid) on the basis of which the test is called an *activated* PTT; and a *partial thromboplastin* (often a phospholipid extracted from rabbit brain or human placenta), which substitutes for the phospholipid surface provided by platelets in vivo. The aPTT will reveal deficiencies, abnormalities, or inhibitors of one or more coagulation factors: high-molecular-weight kininogen (HMWK), prekallikrein, XII, XI, IX, VIII, X, V, II, and I. Surface activation in the laboratory parallels the (clinically relatively unimportant) contact activation phase involving factors XII and XI, prekallikrein, and HMWK that initiates the intrinsic pathway in vivo. Normal aPTT values are between 25 and 35 seconds. The aPTT is prolonged when there is a deficiency, abnormality, or inhibitor of factors XII, XI, IX, VIII, X, V, II, and I (i.e., all factors except VII and XIII). The aPTT is most sensitive to deficiencies of factors VIII and IX, but, as is the case with the PT, levels of these factors must be reduced to approximately 30% of normal values, before the test is prolonged. The assay is also very sensitive to inhibition of thrombin (e.g., by unfractionated heparin and direct thrombin inhibitors). Heparin initially prolongs the aPTT, but with high levels will also prolong PT. As with the PT, the level of fibrinogen must be reduced to 100 mg/dL before the aPTT is prolonged. FXII deficiency, which is a relatively common cause of aPTT prolongation, does not cause a clinical coagulopathy. FXIII deficiency, which *is* associated with a significant bleeding diathesis, does not alter aPTT (or any other common coagulation test). aPTT results (like those of the PT) vary from laboratory to laboratory because of nonstandardization of the phospholipids and activators.

Activated Clotting Time

The activated clotting time (ACT) is similar to the aPTT in that it depends on factors that are all "intrinsic" to blood (the classic intrinsic pathway of coagulation; see Chapter 41). Fresh whole blood is added to a test tube that contains a particulate surface activator of factors XII and XI. The time to clot formation is measured. Neither partial thromboplastin nor phospholipid substitute is added. Coagulation therefore depends on adequate amounts of platelet phospholipid being present in the blood sample. The automated ACT is widely used to monitor heparin therapy in the operating room. Normal values are in the range of 90 to 120 seconds. The ACT is less sensitive than the aPTT to factor deficiencies in the classic intrinsic coagulation pathway.

Thrombin Time

TT, also called *thrombin clotting time*, is a measure of the ability of thrombin to convert fibrinogen to fibrin. This test, which is performed by adding exogenous thrombin to citrated plasma, bypasses all the preceding reactions. TT may be prolonged by conditions that affect either the substrate, fibrinogen, or the action of the enzyme, thrombin. TT is prolonged when there is an inadequate amount of fibrinogen (<100 mg/dL) or fibrinogen is abnormal (dysfibrinogenemia), as in advanced liver disease. Thrombin's enzymatic function can be inhibited by heparin (complexed to antithrombin III), direct thrombin inhibitors (see later discussion), FDPs (see previous discussion), or by inhibitors that may occur in patients with plasma cell myeloma and other immunoproliferative conditions.[178] The normal TT is 10 to 15 seconds.

Reptilase Time

When TT is prolonged, the reptilase time can be used to differentiate between the effects of heparin and FDPs. Reptilase, which is derived from snake venom, converts fibrinogen to fibrin. The action of reptilase is unaffected by heparin but is inhibited by FDPs. A prolonged TT and a normal reptilase time suggest the presence of heparin. Prolongation of both TT and reptilase time will occur in the presence of FDPs, or when fibrinogen level is low. The normal reptilase time is 14 to 21 seconds.

Ecarin Clotting Time

Direct thrombin inhibitors (DTIs) such as hirudin, lepirudin, argatroban, and bivalirudin are frequently used in patients with heparin-induced thrombocytopenia/thrombosis (HIT/T). At low DTI concentrations, TT, aPTT, and ACT provide reasonable correlations with DTI concentration, and on the limited occasions when monitoring is deemed necessary (most often patients in renal failure), the aPTT is commonly used. But with the levels required for CPB, the correlation becomes poor and the risk of overdose with these agents, for which there are no antagonists, becomes significant. The ecarin clotting time provides a better correlation and can be used for monitoring in that context.[179] The test employs the venom of the saw-scaled (also known as sawtooth) viper (*Echis carinatus*). A metalloprotease in the venom converts normal prothrombin to a form (meizothrombin) that is still capable of converting fibrinogen to fibrin but that is inhibited by DTIs in a reliably dose-dependent manner.[180] A thromboelastographic method in which ecarin is used to initiate coagulation has also been reported to provide a much better correlation with bivalirudin levels than the ACT.[181]

Anti-Xa Activity Assay

The anti-Xa activity assay is used to monitor the effects of low-molecular-weight heparins, indirect Xa inhibitors and occasionally unfractionated heparin. Patient plasma is mixed with a reagent containing a known amount of Xa and excess antithrombin. A chromogenic substrate of Xa is added, and a color change reaction occurs in proportion to the Xa not bound by anti-Xa activity in the patient's serum.

Fibrinogen Level

Normal fibrinogen values are between 160 and 350 mg/dL. Below 100 mg/dL, fibrinogen may be inadequate. Fibrinogen is rapidly depleted during DIC. A marked increase in fibrinogen may occur in response to stress, including surgery and trauma. Levels in excess of 700 mg/dL may occur. Because of this increase, in spite of rapid fibrinogen consumption during a hypercoagulable state such as DIC, the fibrinogen level may still appear to be "normal."

Evaluation of Fibrinolysis-Fibrin Degradation Products and D-Dimer

The FDP test identifies the breakdown products of fibrin (cross-linked or uncross-linked) and fibrinogen. The D-dimer assay is specific for breakdown products of cross-linked fibrin. FDPs will be increased in any state of accelerated fibrinolysis, including advanced liver disease, fibrinolysis associated with CPB, exogenous thrombolytics (e.g., streptokinase), and DIC. D-dimer is specific to conditions in which extensive lysis of the cross-linked fibrin of a mature thrombus is occurring, as occurs in DIC, but also with deep vein thrombosis (DVT) and PE.

The Thromboelastogram

Thromboelastography provides a measure of the mechanical properties of evolving clot as a function of time. A principal advantage is that the processes it measures require the integrated action of all the elements of the hemostatic process: platelet aggregation, coagulation, and fibrinolysis. The thromboelastogram is obtained by placing a specimen of blood in a rotating cuvette containing a contact activator and calcium. (Heparinase can also be added to eliminate heparin effect.) A "piston" is lowered into the cuvette. As clot formation begins, the piston rotates as a function of the adherence of the evolving fibrin clot to the piston. The rotation of the piston results in a to-and-fro excursion of a stylus, the amplitude of which is proportional to the speed of piston rotation.

Figure 16-7 depicts a normal thromboelastogram. Several parameters are derived from the thromboelastogram. The most commonly used ones and their interpretation are as follows.[182] R, the reaction time, is the interval until initial clot formation. It requires thrombin formation, and prolongation is usually indicative of an intrinsic pathway factor deficiency. K, the clot formation time, is the interval required after R for the thromboelastogram to achieve a width of 20 mm. Prolongation occurs with deficiencies of thrombin formation or generation of fibrin from fibrinogen. The alpha angle, like K, is a measure of the speed of clot formation. A decrease of the alpha angle has similar significance to a prolongation of K. MA, the maximum amplitude, is a measure of the strength of the fully formed clot. It reflects primarily platelet number and function, although it also requires proper fibrin formation to achieve normal values. MA typically occurs between 30 and 60 min-

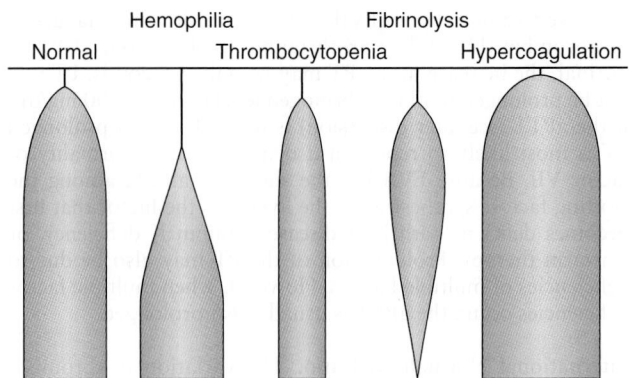

FIGURE 16-8.   Thromboelastogram patterns seen in normal subjects and in subjects with four abnormalities of hemostasis. (From Kang Y: Monitoring and treatment of coagulation, Hepatic Transplantation: Anesthetic and Periperative Management. Edited by Winter K, Kang Y. New York, Praeger, 1986, pp 151, with permission.)

utes. The (MA + x)/MA, is the ratio of the amplitude at a specific time interval (x) after MA divided by MA, is used as a measure of the rate of fibrinolysis. The (MA + 60)/MA ratio has been used most widely.[183] A ratio of <0.85 is evidence of abnormal fibrinolysis.[184] In clinical practice, particularly in liver transplantation, a nonquantitative appreciation of the typical teardrop shape (Fig. 16-8) is used more often to support a diagnosis of increased fibrinolysis than are specific numerical values. F, the interval from MA to return to a zero amplitude, is a measure of the rate of fibrinolysis. F is sufficiently long in normal subjects so that the test is usually terminated before this time elapses.

The thromboelastogram has been employed in cardiac surgery, major trauma, and hepatic transplantation. It is in the latter that it is used most frequently. Commonly, in that context, an increased R prompts the administration of FFP, a decreased MA leads to platelet administration, and the teardrop configuration of fibrinolysis leads to the administration of antifibrinolytics. The use of the thromboelastogram to guide transfusion in liver transplantation has been shown to decrease the amounts of RBCs and FFP administered.[185]

Interpretation of Tests of the Hemostatic Mechanism

An effective approach to the interpretation of coagulation tests is to appreciate in advance the constellation of test results (the coagulation "profile") that is likely to occur with each of the common bleeding disorders (Table 16-15). The most commonly ordered coagulation tests are the platelet count, PT, aPTT, and occasionally BT. When a greater disruption of the hemostatic mechanism is suspected, further tests including fibrinogen, TT, and assays for FDPs and D-dimer may be ordered. Note that some significant clinical bleeding diatheses, including deficiencies of FXIII and α_2-antiplasmin and mild degrees of vWD, will not be revealed by routine coagulation testing.

Because the coagulation defects that appear most often are revealed by abnormal values of PT and/or aPTT, Figure 16-9 provides an algorithm for the evaluation of those abnormalities.

Common Coagulation Profiles

1. Platelet count decreased (normal aPTT and PT). Differential diagnosis: decreased platelet production (see later discussion), excess consumption, platelet destruction, or sequestration in the spleen (see bleeding disorders, thrombocytopenia).

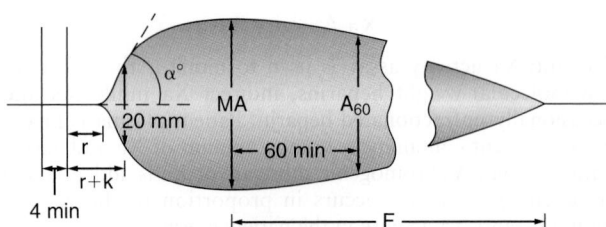

FIGURE 16-7.   The normal thromboelastogram and the variables commonly derived from it. See text for details. (From Kang Y, Lewis JH, Navalgund A, et al: Epsilon-aminocaproic acid for treatment of fibrinolysis during liver transplantation. Anesthesiology 1987; 66: 766, with permission.)

TABLE 16-15

INTERPRETATION OF COAGULATION TESTS

PLATELET COUNT	BLEEDING TIME	aPTT	PT	TT	FIBRINOGEN	FDPs	POSSIBLE CAUSE	EXAMPLE
↓	N or ↓	N	N	N	N	N	↓ Production sequestration ↑ Consumption Immune destruction	Radiation, chemotherapy Splenomegaly Extensive tissue damage H.I.T.
N	↑	N	N	N	N	N	Platelet dysfunction	Drugs: ASA, NSAIDs, Clopidogrel, IIb/IIIa inhibitors; uremia; mild vWD
N	↑	↑	N	N	N	N	Severe vWF deficiency	vWD
N	N	↑	N	N	N	N	Factor deficiency Factor inhibition Antiphospholipid antibody	Hemophilia A or B Low-dose heparin, LMWH[a] Poor collection technique Lupus anticoagulant
N	N	N	↑	N	N	N	Factor VII deficiency	Early liver disease Early vitamin K deficiency Early Coumadin therapy
N	N	↑	↑	↑	N	N	Multiple factor deficiencies	Late vitamin K deficiency Late Coumadin therapy Heparin therapy[b]
↓	↑	↑	↑	↑	↓	N	Dilution of factors and platelets	Massive transfusion
↓	↑	↑	↑	↑	↓	↑	Hypercoagulable state ± ↓ production of factors	DIC[c] Advanced liver disease

↑, increased; ↓, decreased; N, normal; ASA, aspirin; aPTT, "activated" partial thromboplastin time; PT, prothrombin time; TT, thrombin time; FDPs, fibrin degradation products; HIT, heparin-induced thrombocytopenia; vWF, von Willebrand factors; vWD, von Willebrand's disease; LMWH, low–molecular-weight heparin; NSAIDs, nonsteroidal anti-inflammatory drugs; DIC, disseminated intravascular coagulation; H.I.T., heparin induced thrombocytopenia.
[a]aPTT prolongation is more likely to occur with LMWHs with lower Xa/IIa effect ratios, for example, tinzaparin, than with greater ratios, for example, enoxaparin.
[b]Bleeding time may also be prolonged in association with a marked aPTT increase.
[c]DIC may be distinguished by the presence of D-dimers.

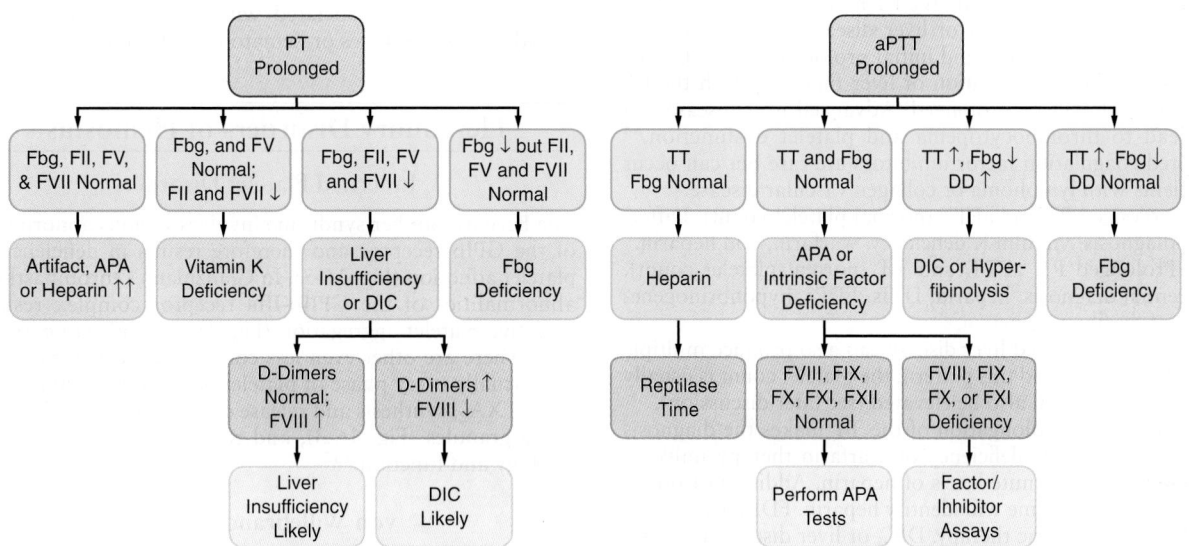

FIGURE 16-9. An approach to the evaluation of prolonged prothrombin time (PT) and/or activated partial thromboplastin time (aPTT). TT, thrombin time; Fbg, fibrinogen; DD, D-dimers; APA, antiphospholipid antibody (e.g., lupus anticoagulant, anticardiolipin, and anti-B2-GPI antibodies); DIC, disseminated intravascular coagulation. (Modified from Bombeli T, Spahn DR: Updates in perioperative coagulation: physiology and management of thromboembolism and haemorrhage. Br J Anaesth 2004; 93: 275, with permission.)

2. Prolonged BT (normal platelet count, aPTT, PT). Differential diagnosis: antiplatelet drug ingestion (e.g., nonsteroidal anti-inflammatory drugs, acetylsalicylic acid, clopidogrel), uremia, vWD (although factor VIII:C levels may be decreased with vWD [type 1], only 25 to 30% of VIII:C coagulant activity is necessary to produce a normal aPTT).

3. Prolonged aPTT (normal platelet count and PT). Differential diagnosis: heparin, the lupus anticoagulant or other antiphospholipid antibodies such as anticardiolipin and anti-B2-GPI antibodies,[186] deficiency of FXII, HMWK, or prekallikrein, hemophilia A or B, vWD, acquired factor inhibitors, and poor collection technique.

Disorders that produce this combination affect factors of the intrinsic pathway (prekallikrein, HMWK, factors XII, XI, IX, and VIII) and/or the common pathway (X, V, II, and I). With heparin therapy, initially only the aPTT is prolonged. At higher doses both the aPTT and PT are prolonged. Note that some common causes of a prolonged aPTT are not associated with a bleeding diathesis. The aPTT prolongation caused by the lupus "anticoagulant" and other antiphospholipid antibodies is the result of the binding of the phospholipid used to support coagulation in vitro. These patients actually have a prothrombotic tendency. Deficiencies of FXII, HMWK, or prekallikrein, in particular FXII, are also common causes of aPTT prolongation. They are not usually associated with a significant clinical hemostatic defect. Collection technique can prolong the aPTT either by heparin contamination or because factors V and VIII, the labile factors, may be consumed if the blood becomes partially clotted prior to delivery to the laboratory. The aPTT is very sensitive to factor VIII deficiency. When the aPTT is prolonged in isolation, is it less likely to be due to a bleeding disorder that involves multiple factor deficiencies (such as liver disease, vitamin K deficiency, the administration of warfarin, or the coagulopathy associated with massive transfusion or DIC). Heparin therapy or congenital disorders of hemostasis are more probable.

4. Prolonged PT (normal platelet count and aPTT). Differential diagnosis: vitamin K deficiency, warfarin administration, early liver dysfunction, FVII deficiency, and acquired coagulation factor inhibitors.

Because factor VII has the shortest half-life among the vitamin K-dependent factors, depletion of the vitamin K-dependent factors will first prolong the PT and only later the aPTT. Similarly, the development of liver disease will lead to deficiencies of factor VII first and initial prolongation of only the PT. With further deterioration of liver function, both the PT and the aPTT will be prolonged. Advanced liver disease can also lead to thrombocytopenia and platelet dysfunction.[84] Acquired coagulation factor inhibitors are rare but can occur in patients with lymphoma or collagen vascular disease.

5. Prolonged PT and aPTT (normal platelet count). Differential diagnosis: vitamin K deficiency, warfarin, and heparin.

6. Prolonged PT, aPTT, and TT (normal platelet count). Differential diagnosis: heparin, DTIs, FDPs, hypofibrinogenemia, and dysfibrinogenemia.

Although advanced liver disease can also produce multiple factor deficiencies and this pattern, the platelet count is usually decreased. FDPs will also be elevated (see later discussion).

Simultaneous prolongation of the TT makes the diagnosis of simple vitamin K deficiency or warfarin therapy unlikely. TT is sensitive to minute levels of heparin. Addition of protamine or a reptilase time will identify heparin. FDPs may be elevated with fibrinolytic therapy, DIC, or liver disease. DIC and liver disease usually result in thrombocytopenia as well. A normal platelet count makes heparin or extensive fibrinolysis more likely.

7. Prolonged PT, aPTT, TT, decreased platelet count. Differential diagnosis: DIC, dilution by massive transfusion, liver disease, and heparin therapy.

FDPs and D-dimer are elevated in DIC and allow differentiation from dilutional effects and excess heparin. Heparin causes thrombocytopenia only when prolonged exposure results in HIT/T. FDPs, but not D-dimer, are elevated in severe liver disease.

The interpretation of coagulation tests may be made more difficult by the fact that patients who develop a bleeding diathesis in the perioperative period may have more than one bleeding disorder (e.g., DIC and coagulopathy related to massive transfusion) and may also have a surgical cause for bleeding.

DISORDERS OF HEMOSTASIS: DIAGNOSIS AND TREATMENT

The hemostatic mechanism involves an intricate balance that serves to limit blood loss in the event of vascular injury while maintaining the liquid character of blood at other times. Under normal circumstances, an equilibrium between clotting and bleeding is maintained with the help of multiple activators, inhibitors, cofactors, and feedback loops, both positive and negative. Under pathologic circumstances, that equilibrium may be lost, leading to either hemorrhagic or thrombotic complications. Accordingly, disorders of hemostasis can be broadly classified into those that lead to abnormal bleeding and those that lead to abnormal clotting. The disorders may be further categorized according to whether they involve platelets, clotting factors, and/or the presence or absence of inhibitors (such as FDPs). Finally, disorders may be hereditary or acquired. Treatment may require administration of hemostatic blood products (platelets and/or clotting factors) or pharmacologic agents. The latter may be chosen for effects on platelets (desmopressin, antiplatelet drugs), on clotting factors (vitamin K, warfarin, heparin), or on naturally occurring inhibitors (antifibrinolytic agents, protamine, fibrinolytics).

The preoperative history is invaluable. Abnormalities of primary hemostasis, usually caused by reduced platelet number or function, will be revealed by evidence of "superficial" (skin and mucosal) bleeding including easy bruising, petechiae, prolonged bleeding from minor skin lacerations, recurrent epistaxis, and menorrhagia (see Chapter 23). Coagulation abnormalities are associated with "deep" bleeding events including hemarthroses or hematomas after blunt trauma.

Hereditary Disorders of Hemostasis

Inherited Platelet Disorders

The Bernard-Soulier syndrome involves various abnormalities of the GPIb receptor and therefore results in deficiencies of platelet adhesion (Fig. 16-3). In Glanzmann's thrombasthenia, abnormalities of the GPIIb-IIIa receptor complex result in defective platelet aggregation (Fig. 16-4). Both are extremely rare. There are other even less common abnormalities affecting virtually every phase of platelet function including synthesis of TXA_2, synthesis and release of the contents of alpha and dense granules (Fig. 16-3), and receptor (ADP, TXA_2) morphology and function.[187]

von Willebrand Disease

vWD is the most common hereditary bleeding disorder. Some form of the disease is present in approximately 1% of the general population, although it is overtly symptomatic in only about 10% of those afflicted.[188] vWD is the result of the synthesis of an abnormal vWF or normal vWF in reduced amount. The vWF is a protein synthesized by endothelial cells, megakaryocytes, and platelets. It is important for both primary hemostasis, that is, the binding of platelets to sites of vascular injury, and for coagulation, the latter through its role as a carrier protein/stabilizer for FVIII. vWF has several distinct binding domains responsible for its several hemostatic functions. Those domains include sites that are specific for collagen (for adherence to the subendothelium), for the platelet GPIb receptor (for platelet adhesion to collagen), for the platelet GP IIb/IIIa receptor (for platelet aggregation), and for factor VIII:C (for vWF's carrier protein function). There are at least 50 genetic variations of vWD, which accounts for its phenotypic heterogeneity. There are three principal subtypes. Type 1, which comprises 70 to 80% of vWD, is a quantitative defect. vWF is present but is secreted in reduced amount. Patients with type 1 vWD present with a pattern of bleeding that is characteristic of abnormalities of primary hemostasis. Type 2 vWD, which comprises 20 to 30% of patients with vWD, includes a host of qualitative defects of vWF. Some mutations affect the platelet interactions of vWF and others the factor VIII interaction. Type 2 is subdivided into four subtypes. Type 2B is characterized by a variant of the vWF that causes abnormal aggregation of platelets and thrombocytopenia. The abnormal vWF has a high affinity for the platelet GPIb receptor. The bleeding diathesis is probably the result of formation and clearance of vWF-platelet complexes and the resultant thrombocytopenia. In the 2N (Normandy) subtype, the vWF has a markedly reduced affinity for factor VIII. These patients demonstrate normal platelet function, but bleed because of decreased factor VIII coagulant activity. These patients are readily misdiagnosed as having mild hemophilia A. Type 3 vWD, which is very rare, entails a complete absence of vWF, resulting in a severe abnormality of both primary hemostasis and coagulation.

The Role of vWF in Hemostasis. vWF is essential for platelet plug formation. It mediates platelet adhesion to the subendothelial surface of blood vessels. After binding to the subendothelium, vWF undergoes a conformational change that only then allows platelets to adhere via their glycoprotein GPIb receptors. The antibiotic, ristocetin, can induce the platelet GPIb-vWF interaction and, accordingly, is the basis for one laboratory test of platelet function. vWF also participates in platelet to platelet aggregation. Platelet aggregation occurs by binding of vWF molecules to the GPIIb/IIIa receptors on the surface of several platelets. The vWF also acts as a carrier protein for the coagulant activity of factor VIII, referred to as *VIII:C*, with which it circulates in a complexed form that prolongs the circulation time of VIII:C.

Diagnosis and Treatment of vWD. History will commonly reveal abnormal bleeding from mucosal surfaces. Sixty percent of the patients will report epistaxis, 50 will report menorrhagia, and 35 will acknowledge gingival bleeding, easy bruising, and hematomas.[189] vWD should be considered in patients who give a history of unexplained postoperative bleeding, particularly following tonsillectomy or dental extraction. Although vWD is a hereditary disease, a clear family history is not always evident because disease severity varies substantially.

Specialized laboratory tests, ideally directed by a hematologist, may be required to confirm the diagnosis and type of vWD. One or more vWF markers, including vWF factor antigen (vWF:Ag), vWF ristocetin cofactor activity (vWF:RCo), and/or vWF collagen binding activity (vWF:CB) will be diminished or absent. Because vWD is a carrier protein/stabilizer of FVIII, FVIII half-life is diminished, and FVIII levels are characteristically also decreased. What is important for the anesthesiologist to appreciate is that the results of the most commonly ordered coagulation tests, the platelet count, the aPTT,

and the PT, may be normal in the patient with vWD. Although the half-life of VIII:C is diminished in vWD, there is usually sufficient VIII:C to yield a normal aPTT in basal conditions.

The two established treatments for vWD are DDAVP (1-deamino-8-D-arginine vasopressin) and factor concentrates.[190,191] DDAVP, which promotes release of vWF, is effective first-line therapy for the large majority (approximately 80%) of patients with vWD, including those with type 1 and type 2A disease.[192] However, the recognition of subtype 2B (see previous discussion) is important because DDAVP will cause thrombocytopenia in these patients.[193] DDAVP, given intravenously in a dose of 0.3 μg/kg, increases factor VIII:C and vWF two to fivefold in most patients. Its effect is maximal after 30 minutes, and elevated levels persist for 6 to 8 hours[189,192] (see "Pharmacologic Therapy: Desmopressin"). For the 20% of patients who do not respond adequately to DDAVP, virally inactivated factor concentrates (e.g., Haemate-P) will be appropriate. Their efficacy is well confirmed.[194,195] Antifibrinolytic agents, ε-aminocaproic acid (EACA) and tranexamic acid (TXA), are sometimes used in combination with DDAVP to manage these patients during the perioperative period.[193] These drugs may be given intravenously or orally. They have also been administered topically, as mouthwashes, in patients with vWD undergoing dental extractions. Oral contraceptives (estrogens) have been used to treat patients with vWD who have menorrhagia, or who are undergoing elective surgery.[193] The mechanism of action of the estrogens is not well understood, although a connection with vWF synthesis is suspected. Antiplatelet drugs should be avoided in patients with vWD.

The Hemophilias

Hemophilia A results from mutations that lead to either deficient or functionally defective factor VIII:C. Hemophilia B (Christmas disease) and hemophilia C are caused by deficiency or abnormality of factors IX and XI, respectively.[196] The relative frequencies of the three hemophilias are factor VIII:C, 85%; factor IX, 14%; and factor XI, 1%. Rare inherited deficiencies of factors II, VII, V, and X also occur.[196] Both hemophilia A and B are sex-linked recessive disorders, which therefore occur almost exclusively in males. Hemophilia C is an autosomal recessive disorder that occurs almost exclusively in Ashkenazi Jews.[196] About 50% of operations in hemophiliacs are orthopaedic procedures required for treatment of the arthritic consequences of hemarthroses.

Hemophilia A. Factor VIII:C circulates bound to and protected by vWF. In hemophilia A, patients have normal levels of vWF but have reduced or defective factor VIII:C. Hemophilia A occurs in approximately 1 in 10,000 males. Hemophiliacs experience deep tissue bleeding, hemarthroses, and hematuria most commonly. Patients with mild disease have factor levels of 5 to 30% of normal and usually bleed abnormally only following trauma. Patients with moderate disease have factor levels of 1 to 5% and occasionally bleed spontaneously. The great majority of hemophiliacs have the severe form of the disease. Factor VIII:C levels are <1% of normal and they frequently experience spontaneous bleeding episodes. The severity of clinical symptoms usually correlates with the level of clotting factor activity. Like the patient with vWD, hemophiliacs should avoid aspirin and other platelet-inhibiting agents.

Diagnosis and Treatment. Patients with hemophilia A will commonly report a history that reveals the X-linked recessive pattern of disease inheritance. Diagnosis is made on the basis of a prolonged aPTT and specific factor assays demonstrating a deficiency of factor VIII coagulant activity with normal levels of vWF, factor IX, and factor XI. PT and BT will be

ANATOMY AND PHYSIOLOGY

normal. Hemophilia A is treated with plasma-derived, virally attenuated concentrates or with recombinant factor VIII.[196]

In the event of an episode of spontaneous bleeding (most often a hemarthrosis), a procoagulant level of 25% is a common target. For elective surgical procedures, the level of factor VIII:C activity is usually raised to 50 to 100% of normal by administration of virally inactivated factor concentrate. Many hemophiliacs develop inhibitors to factor VIII:C, which increases the amount of concentrate that will be required. Recombinant activated FVIIa (see later discussion) may be necessary for the patient with inhibitors.

DDAVP will also increase plasma factor VIII:C and vWF concentrations and is often effective in mild hemophilia A. The effect may be partly the result of "protection" of available FVIII by increased concentrations of the carrier molecule, vWF. However, DDAVP is also thought to cause the release of factor VIII:C from liver endothelial cells.[197] There is a large variation in patient response to DDAVP, and it is most effective in patients with factor VIII:C levels >5%.[83,192,198] It is given intravenously in a dose of 0.3 μg/kg in 50 mL of saline over 15 to 30 minutes. It causes a prompt increase in factor VIII:C. However, tachyphylaxis does develop, which limits its usefulness. The antifibrinolytics EACA and TXA have been used to treat hemophiliac patients prior to dental procedures. The agents are contraindicated in bleeding episodes involving joints or the urinary tract because the clots that do form may not be lysed for a long period of time.

Hemophilia B. Factor IX deficiency is also an X-linked recessive disorder, occurring in approximately 1/25,000 males.[196] It produces a bleeding diathesis that is clinically indistinguishable from hemophilia A. Typically, minor hemorrhage is managed by achieving FIX levels of 20 to 30% of normal. Levels of 50 to 100% are sought for more severe hemorrhage and in anticipation of surgery. Recombinant and virally attenuated FIX factor concentrates are available and are the preferred treatment.

Protein C and Protein S Deficiency

Hereditary deficiencies of protein C and protein S are associated with thromboembolic events originating on the venous side of the circulation (e.g., DVT, PE, and paradoxical embolization causing stroke). The complete absence of protein C is associated with death in infancy. Patients who experience thromboembolic events and have decreased levels of protein C or protein S should remain on anticoagulant therapy indefinitely.

Acquired Disorders of Hemostasis

For mnemonic purposes, it is helpful to classify bleeding disorders according to which of the three hemostatic processes is involved: primary hemostasis (platelet disorders), coagulation (clotting factor disorders), fibrinolysis (production of inhibitors such as FDPs), or some combination of the three. Similarly, it is useful to use the results of coagulation tests to determine whether the clinical problem involves primary hemostasis (e.g., decreased platelet count, increased BT), coagulation (e.g., prolonged PT and aPTT, decreased factor levels), fibrinolysis (increased FDPs, increased D-dimer), or some combination of the three. Ultimately, therapeutic decisions (e.g., administration of platelets, FFP, or an antifibrinolytic agent) will similarly be oriented to treatment of one or more of these processes.

Acquired Disorders of Platelets

The clinical conditions that cause an isolated disorder of primary hemostasis typically involve abnormalities of either platelet number or function.

Thrombocytopenia. Platelets are derived from megakaryocytes in the bone marrow in response to thrombopoietin, which is synthesized by the liver. The causes of thrombocytopenia may be categorized as (1) inadequate production by the bone marrow, (2) increased peripheral consumption or destruction (non–immune-mediated), (3) increased peripheral destruction (immune-mediated), (4) dilution of circulating platelets, and (5) sequestration.

1. Bone marrow production of platelets can be impaired in many ways. Physical and chemical agents (radiation and chemotherapy), various drugs (thiazide diuretics, sulfonamides, diphenylhydantoin, alcohol), infectious agents (hepatitis B, TB, overwhelming sepsis), and chronic disease states (uremia, liver disease) can all cause bone marrow suppression. Infiltration of the bone marrow by cancer cells or replacement by fibrosis will also result in inadequate platelet production.
2. Accelerated nonimmunologically mediated consumption can occur in many conditions that cause extensive activation of coagulation with or without the occurrence of DIC. After extensive tissue damage (e.g., burns, crush injuries), which denude vascular endothelium, the normal process of hemostasis activates platelets and leads to their consumption and to thrombocytopenia. In a similar fashion, the interaction of platelets with nonendothelialized structures such as large vascular grafts can also lead to a transient thrombocytopenia. Platelets are consumed in patients with an extensive vasculitis such as occurs with toxemia of pregnancy. The many conditions that cause DIC (see later discussion) will also cause platelets to be consumed or destroyed more rapidly than they can be produced.
3. Immunologically mediated consumption can be caused by various drugs (heparin, quinidine, cephalosporins, vancomycin) and autoimmune disorders (systemic lupus erythematosus, rheumatoid arthritis, thrombotic thrombocytopenic purpura). Alloimmunization resulting from previous transfusions or pregnancy can cause refractoriness to platelet transfusions.
4. Dilution of platelets will occur in the context of massive transfusion (see later discussion and "Massive Transfusion").
5. Under normal conditions, approximately one third of platelets are sequestered in the spleen. When the spleen enlarges, an increasing number of platelets are sequestered and thrombocytopenia may result. This may occur with the splenomegaly associated with myelodysplastic syndromes and cirrhosis of the liver, although in the latter condition, decreased production also contributes to thrombocytopenia.

Disorders of Platelet Function

Uremia. Platelet dysfunction is common in uremia. Thorough reviews are available.[84,199] The accumulation of several metabolites is thought to interfere with vWF formation and release and to cause abnormal function of the GPIIb-IIIa receptor. Synthesis of prostacyclin and nitric oxide synthesis, both of which have platelet inhibitory effects, is increased in uremia. Dialysis frequently improves the hemostatic defect. There are several other potential treatment modalites.[84,200] Cryoprecipitate (a source of vWF) was once used for uremic bleeding but has now been supplanted by DDAVP, which induces immediate release of vWF from endothelial cells and rapidly improves platelet adhesiveness. Severe anemia, per se, contributes to bleeding because in the lower viscosity state, platelets have a reduced tendency to travel in the periphery of the blood column, along the endothelial surface. Improvement of the hemostatic defect associated with uremia has been observed with administration of erythropoietin (probably by correction of anemia[201]) and conjugated estrogens[84] (perhaps by reduction of nitric oxide formation). When life-threatening bleeding occurs in the uremic patient, platelet concentrates should be administered.

Antiplatelet Agents. Numerous medications are administered expressly for the purpose of platelet inhibition to reduce the risk of MI, stroke, and other thromboembolic complications. They induce platelet dysfunction by several mechanisms, which include inhibition of cyclo-oxygenase (Cox), inhibition of phosphodiesterase, ADP receptor antagonism, and blockade of the GP IIb/IIIa receptor.

Cyclo-oxygenase Inhibitors. Aspirin is the prototype. Aspirin produces irreversible inhibition of platelet Cox, which prevents synthesis of TxA_2, a potent platelet proaggregant and vasoconstrictor. In moderate doses, there is selective sparing of the synthesis of prostacyclin (antiaggregant, vasodilator), which results in "tilting" the balance substantially in favor of platelet inhibition. The platelet-inhibiting effectiveness of aspirin varies substantially. Increased rates of new platelet synthesis, simultaneous administration of other drugs that temporarily bind and thereby protect Cox-1 (e.g., ibuprofen), and polymorphisms of the Cox-1 enzyme may be responsible.[202]

Indomethacin, phenylbutazone, and all the nonsteroidal anti-inflammatory agents (e.g., Naprosyn, ibuprofen) also inhibit Cox. However, unlike aspirin, their inhibition is promptly reversible with clearance of the drug. The more recent Cox-2 inhibitors selectively inhibit Cox-2, the isoform responsible for generating the mediators of pain and inflammation, while sparing Cox-1, the inhibition of which causes both gastric damage and decreased renal blood flow and inhibition of platelet TxA_2. Accordingly, platelet function should not be impaired. However, it has become apparent that Cox-2 inhibitors reduce prostacyclin generation by vascular endothelial cells and may thereby tilt the natural balance toward platelet aggregation. That procoagulant effect is not uniform among Cox-2 inhibitors. Celecoxib simultaneously decreases endothelial expression of TF and may thereby produce a compensatory "counter-tilt."[203] An increased rate of myocardial ischemic events resulted in the withdrawal of some Cox-2 inhibitors from the market in 2004.

Phosphodiesterase Inhibitors. Cyclic adenosine monophosphate is an inhibitor of platelet aggregation, and levels are increased by inhibition of phosphodiesterase. Dipyridamole, which is used for stroke prophylaxis (usually in combination with aspirin), and cilostazol appear to act primarily by this mechanism. Caffeine, aminophylline, and theophylline will also similarly produce mild, reversible platelet inhibition.

ADP Receptor Antagonists. Activation of the platelet ADP receptor leads to surface expression of the IIb/IIIa receptor. Clopidogrel, which is administered for prevention of stent occlusion as well as stroke and MI prophylaxis, blocks the ADP receptor in a noncompetitive and irreversible manner.

Glycoprotein IIb/IIIa Receptor Antagonists. The GPIIb/IIIa platelet surface receptor, by which fibrinogen cross-links platelets, is the final common pathway for platelet aggregation. The IIb/IIIa antagonists have been used principally for the management of acute coronary syndromes. They include abciximab (ReoPro), a monoclonal antibody, tirofiban (Aggrastat), and eptifibatide (Integrilin). These agents all require intravenous administration. Their effect is reversible. The half-lives are approximately 2.5 hours for tirofiban and eptifibatide (both increased with renal dysfunction) and 12 hours for abciximab.[204] However, abciximab has a relatively high affinity for the IIb/IIIa receptor, and platelet dysfunction lasts longer (approximately 48 hours) than implied by half-life. All of these agents have also been associated with thrombocytopenia, the incidence of which has been greater for abciximab (2.5%) than tirofiban and eptifibatide (0.5%).[205] The thrombocytopenia caused by abciximab can be either delayed (antibody mediated) or immediate.[174] Note that these agents cause prolongation of the ACT.[204]

Herbal Medications and Vitamins. Several herbal medications may cause inhibition of platelet function[84] (see Chapter 22). Among the more common agents identified by the ASA Practice Advisory are feverfew, flaxseed oil, garlic, ginger, gingko biloba, grape seed extract, and saw palmetto.[80] Because the actual risks are not well defined, they should be discontinued before surgery, and in particular, before cardiac, neurologic, and cosmetic surgical procedures. Vitamin E and ginseng are also platelet/coagulation inhibitors and should similarly be discontinued.[206,207]

Other Conditions. Myeloproliferative and myelodysplastic syndromes can produce intrinsic defects in platelets. In these disorders, the platelets may be abnormal in both morphology and function. Platelet dysfunction occurs in conjunction with conditions that also cause other hemostatic abnormalities (liver disease, fibrinolytic states including DIC, storage defects), which are discussed in the following section.

Acquired Disorders of Clotting Factors (Including Anticoagulant Therapy)

Vitamin K Deficiency

Hepatic synthesis of clotting factors II, VII, IX, and X as well as protein C and protein S requires the presence of vitamin K. Vitamin K is necessary for the enzymatic carboxylation of these factors. The carboxyl group enables binding to phospholipid surfaces during the coagulation process. With vitamin K deficiency, these factors are depleted in an order determined by their half-lives. Factor VII has the shortest half-life and is the first to be depleted, followed by FIX, FX, and finally FII (prothrombin). Vitamin K deficiency occurs frequently in hospitalized patients because of dietary insufficiency, gut sterilization, and malabsorption. A high index of suspicion should be maintained.

Vitamin K occurs naturally in two forms.[206] Vitamin K_1 (phylloquinone) is found in leafy green vegetables. The greatest concentrations occur in brussels sprouts. Vitamin K_2 (menaquinone) is synthesized by the normal intestinal flora. It is uncommon for patients to develop vitamin K deficiency solely because of dietary deficiency, but it may occur in patients who are receiving parenteral nutrition without vitamin K supplementation, and who are being treated concurrently with broad-spectrum antibiotics that destroy the gut flora. Because the body has no appreciable stores of vitamin K, deficiencies can develop in as little as 7 days. Newborns, who have a sterile gut at birth, have been noted to develop vitamin K deficiency. Vitamin K is fat-soluble and therefore requires bile salts for absorption from the jejunum. Biliary obstruction, malabsorption syndromes, gastrointestinal obstruction, or rapid gastrointestinal transit can result in vitamin K deficiency because of inadequate absorption.

Diagnosis and Treatment of Vitamin K Deficiency. Vitamin K deficiency will cause prolongation of the PT. PT is an FVII-sensitive assay and with vitamin K deficiency, FVII is the first factor to be depleted. With more prolonged deficiency, aPTT (a very FIX-sensitive assay) will also increase. Platelet count will be normal. Vitamin K may be administered orally, intramuscularly, or intravenously. Urgent treatment of vitamin K deficiency is best accomplished by the intramuscular or intravenous administration of vitamin K (Aquamephyton), usually in doses of 1 to 5 mg. Vitamin K should be administered slowly to avoid the occurrence of hypotension. Improvement of the coagulation disturbance will begin to be apparent in 6 to 8 hours.

Warfarin Therapy

Warfarin is administered for the prevention of DVT and PE and to patients with atrial fibrillation, some prosthetic heart valves, and ventricular mural thrombi in the setting of acute MI. Patients with protein S or protein C deficiency may also be treated with long-term anticoagulation with warfarin. Warfarin produces its anticoagulant effect by competition with vitamin K for the carboxylation binding sites and leads to the depletion of factors II, VII, IX, X, protein C, and protein S. As with vitamin K deficiency (previous paragraph), FVII is the first factor to be depleted and initially only the PT will be prolonged. With higher doses, FIX levels will decrease and the aPTT will increase. Warfarin therapy is adjusted according to the INR (see "Tests of the Hemostatic Mechanism"). The primary untoward effect of warfarin therapy is bleeding. Rapid reversal (12 to 24 hours) of warfarin effect[208] can be accomplished by intravenous administration of vitamin K. Doses of 5 to 10 mg intravenously are recommended for urgent situations.[209] Smaller doses, 0.5 to 3 mg, and the oral route should be used in less urgent situations when the objective is to reduce rather than normalize INR. INR should be rechecked at 6-hour intervals. Vitamin K administration may have to be repeated at 12-hour intervals. In situations of greater urgency, FFP, TP (which is immediately available in facilities that provide it), or prothrombin complex concentrate (PCC) will all provide the relevant factors and can be employed. In patients who might not tolerate the requisite volume of FFP or TP (>15 mL/kg), PCC, which contains FII, FVII, FIX, and FX, is an alternative. PCC dosing recommendations vary. However, 15 IU/kg when INR is <5 and 30 IU/kg for INR >5 appear reasonable.[210] Recombinant FVIIa (rFVIIa; see later discussion) has also been used to achieve rapid normalization of INR.[211] Note, however, that the action of rFVIIa requires the participation of FX and FII (prothrombin), both of which are depleted at greater degrees of warfarin effect (as witnessed by aPTT prolongation). In this circumstance, rFVIIa may not provide effective reversal of anticoagulation. PCC contains FII, VII, FIX, and FX and is more likely to be effective.[212] Thrombotic events have occurred with the administration of both PCC and rFVIIa.[212,213] If FFP, TP, PCC, or rFVIIa are administered for rapid reversal and sustained reversal is desired, vitamin K should be administered simultaneously[209] because of the short half-life of FVII (6 hours for native FVII, 2 hours for rFVIIa).

Heparin Therapy

Unfractionated heparin (UFH) is used widely for anticoagulation in vascular surgery and in procedures requiring CPB. It inhibits coagulation principally through its interaction with AT (see Chapter 41). UFH binds to AT, and in so doing causes a conformational change that greatly increases AT's inhibitory activity. In spite of its name, anti-"thrombin," AT also inhibits several activated factors including, in addition to IIa (thrombin), Xa, IXa, XIa, and XIIa (Fig. 16-6). It is most active against thrombin and Xa. UFH also increases the activity of a second native antithrombin, heparin cofactor II. Heparin cofactor II inhibits thrombin and not the other activated factors. Its contribution to the clinical effects of UFH is not clear. Resistance to UFH can occur in patients who are deficient in AT on either a hereditary or an acquired basis. The latter may occur in patients on sustained UFH therapy, in the presence of depletion by a consumptive coagulopathy or during CPB.

UFH responsiveness can be restored by administration of AT concentrates[168,169] or FFP.

Low-Molecular-Weight Heparin. Low-molecular-weight fractions of heparin (LMWH) have been employed principally for DVT prophylaxis and treatment, and are supplanting subcutaneous UFH and warfarin for these indications.[214] There are several available agents including certoparin, dalteparin, enoxaparin, reviparin, and tinzaparin. These agents do not appear to differ in their efficacy,[215] and enoxaparin is used most widely in the United States. LMWHs, which also act via AT, have greater activity against FXa than thrombin (FIIa). However, the ratio of that activity varies among the agents (e.g., enoxaparin, 3.8:1; tinzaparin, 1.9:1).[216] Accordingly, the effect of these agents on standard coagulation tests will vary (minimal for enoxaparin[217]) as will the effect of protamine neutralization, which is very incomplete for enoxaparin. Monitoring is usually not required or performed. If it is deemed necessary (e.g., renal failure, extreme obesity), the anti-Xa activity level (see previous discussion) is the appropriate test. The LMWHs cause less platelet inhibition and are associated with a lesser incidence of HIT/T than UFH.[218] While twice-daily dosing with enoxaparin has been common in North America, once-daily regimens are usually sufficient. Because of the relatively long half-life of enoxaparin, twice-daily dosing poses a problem with respect to removal of epidural catheters because there is no anticoagulant nadir (see Chapter 53.)

Heparin Induced Thrombocytopenia/Thrombosis (HIT/T). One to five percent of patients who receive UFH therapy for 5 days will develop thrombocytopenia as a result of antibodies (usually IgG) directed against platelet factor 4 (PF4)-heparin complexes on the platelet surface.[219,220] Onset requires several days in the heparin-naive patient but can occur much more quickly (10 to 12 hours) in those who have been exposed within the preceding 100 days. Occurrence appears to be dose-related and is more common with bovine than porcine heparin. HIT/T is relatively uncommon with LMWH and requires longer periods of exposure.[218,221] When LMWH does induce antibodies, they are more commonly of the IgM or IgA type and often do not cause thrombocytopenia. However, patients who have developed IgG antibodies and HIT/T in response to UFH will frequently develop HIT/T on exposure to LMWH.[218] Although HIT/T is most often identified because of thrombocytopenia, not all patients become markedly thrombocytopenic. Thrombotic and thromboembolic events including DVT, PE, limb or acral ischemia, MI, or stroke frequently reveal the occurrence of HIT/T. Diagnosis is complicated by the fact that not all patients who develop antiplatelet antibodies have clinical HIT/T. A hematologist should be consulted.

Treatment entails withdrawal of heparin and administration of a nonheparin anticoagulant. The DTIs (lepirudin, argatroban, and bivalirudin) and the indirect Xa inhibitor danaparoid are approved for this use in various countries (although danaparoid is not available in the United States). Several other anticoagulants are under development, including orally administered DTIs and direct inhibitors of FXa and FXIa.[222] A LMWH is not appropriate. Fondaparinux (an indirect Xa inhibitor; see later discussion) has a negligible (perhaps zero) incidence of antiheparin/PF4 cross-reactivity but is not formally approved. Warfarin is contraindicated because the combination of protein C and S inhibition by warfarin in the face of ongoing platelet clumping may aggravate thrombosis. Platelets similarly should not be administered unless thrombocytopenia is extreme.

Cardiac Surgery and HIT/T. Several alternatives have been employed for the patient with HIT/T who requires CPB[180] (see

Chapter 41). The most common, when antiheparin/PF4 antibodies are still present, is the use of nonheparin anticoagulants, usually a DTI (see later discussion). An alternative is to provide profound inhibition of platelet activation with either iloprost (synthetic prostacyclin) or a IIb/IIIa inhibitor (tirofiban at UCSD) during CPB and proceed with UFH administration, protamine reversal, and a nonheparin anticoagulant in the postoperative period.[223] When antiheparin/PF4 antibodies have decreased to undetectable levels in a patient with a history of HIT/T, heparin may be employed during CPB, although it must be rigidly avoided during the remainder of the hospitalization. Antibody generation requires 5 days by which time heparin will be absent.[219]

As many as 5% of patients who receive UFH therapy for 5 days will develop heparin-induced thrombocytopenia/thrombosis. The clinical manifestations are more often the result of thrombosis and thromboembolism than thrombocytopenia.

Heparin in Cardiopulmonary Bypass. A comprehensive discussion of this topic is beyond the scope of this chapter. Extensive reviews are available[224] (see Chapter 41). In brief, the common practice is to maintain ACT >480 to 500 seconds for the duration of bypass. There is substantial variation in the UFH-ACT dose-response relationship, probably because of variability in UFH binding to many native surfaces including platelets, WBCs, endothelium, and plasma proteins including the vWF and AT.[224] There is hazard, in terms of activation of both platelets and coagulation, in allowing ACT to be on the "low side." Platelet and coagulation activation can be demonstrated at ACT levels of 400 seconds.[225] Evidence of activation is less apparent when longer ACTs are maintained.[226] Protamine is administered for reversal of UFH effect. Many clinicians employ a "milliliter for milliliter" technique. However, a more careful titration of protamine against ACT is ideal to avoid excessive administration of protamine, which has inherent anticoagulant effects including platelet inhibition, stimulation of tPA release from endothelium, and inhibition of fibrinogen cleavage by thrombin.[227]

Direct Thrombin Inhibitors

DTIs produce their anticoagulant effect by directly binding to thrombin.[180] Hirudin is a naturally occurring compound; lepirudin is its recombinant equivalent. Argatroban and bivalirudin are synthetic. By contrast with UFH, LMWH, and fondaparinux, all of which act via AT to inhibit only unbound thrombin, DTIs inhibit both unbound and fibrin-bound thrombin. DTIs therefore inhibit *all* of thrombin's numerous effects on hemostasis (Figs. 16-2 and 16-5). Clot-bound thrombin can continue to promote coagulation by activation of platelets, by activation of FV, FVIII, FXI, and FXIII, and by conversion of fibrinogen to fibrin.[228] There is no antidote to the anticoagulant effect of DTIs. Termination of the effect of hirudin and lepirudin (half-life, 80 minutes) depends on renal elimination. Argatroban (half-life, 40 to 50 minutes) is metabolized by the liver. Bivalirudin (half-life, 25 minutes) is largely cleared by proteolysis by plasma proteases with some contribution by renal clearance.

DTIs do not bind to PF4 and are widely used to anticoagulate patients with HIT/T, in particular those who require CPB. For the latter, bivalirudin is the most widely used agent because of its relative independence of hepatic and renal clearance and a relatively short half-life. Monitoring of anticoagulation is problematic. As noted in the section "Laboratory Evaluation of Coagulation," with the greater degrees of anticoagulation required for CPB, the correlation between ACT and DTI serum level is poor, and unnecessary overdose can occur easily. The ecarin clotting time (see previous discussion) is the preferred test. However, it is not widely available. Fixed dosage regimens have therefore been employed (e.g., loading dose, 1.0 to 1.5 mg/kg; infusion, 2.5 mg/kg/hr).[229,230] ACT should be >400. Note that the relatively short half-life and enzymatic degradation mean that blood that is static (CPB or cell salvage reservoirs) may clot. The technique has to be adjusted accordingly. In the patient with renal failure or in urgent situations, elimination can be accomplished by dialysis or hemofiltration.[231]

Ximelagatran is a direct thrombin inhibitor. It has been withdrawn from the market on the basis of hepatotoxicity.

Indirect Inhibitors of Xa

Fondaparinux and idraparinux are synthetic agents that act via AT to produce a highly specific inhibition of FXa.[232] Fondaparinux is an increasingly popular alternative for DVT prophylaxis, in part because of its very predictable uptake (after once daily subcutaneous administration) and kinetics that make monitoring and dosage adjustment unnecessary. Fondaparinux can form a complex with PF4. However, heparin/PF4 antibodies do not react with that complex in a manner that produces platelet activation and HIT/T.[233] Nonetheless, fondaparinux is not yet approved for use in HIT/T. These agents have long half-lives (fondaparinux, 17 hours; idraparinux, 80 hours), and there is no antidote. Excretion is via the kidneys. With therapeutic doses PT, aPTT, and ACT remain within the normal range.

Danaparoid, which is not available in the United States, is a mixture of three glycosaminoglycans (heparan sulphate, dermatan sulfate, and chondroitin sulfate) derived from porcine intestine. Anti-Xa to anti-IIa activity occurs in a ratio of 22:1. Half-life is 25 hours. Elimination is renal. PT and aPTT are unaffected by therapeutic doses. Cross-reactivity with heparin/PF4 antibodies occurs infrequently, and danaparoid is approved for use in HIT/T.[180]

Acquired Combined Disorders of Platelets and Clotting Factors with Increased Fibrinolysis

Liver Disease. Chronic liver disease is associated with abnormalities of all three phases of hemostasis: primary hemostasis, coagulation, and fibrinolysis. Table 16-16 provides an overview of these abnormalities.

TABLE 16-16

THE ETIOLOGY OF HEMOSTATIC ABNORMALITIES IN LIVER DISEASE

- Thrombocytopenia
  - Decreased production
  - Hypersplenism
  - Increased consumption (DIC)
- Impaired platelet function
  - Decreased FDP clearance
- Decreased factor synthesis
  - Decreased hepatocyte function
  - Vitamin K deficiency (diet, malabsorption)
- Increased factor consumption
  - Decreased clearance of activated factors
  - Decreased synthesis of inhibitors (protein C, protein S)
- Increased fibrinolysis
  - Decreased synthesis of α_2-antiplasmin
  - Decreased clearance of tPA
  - Decreased synthesis of PAI-1

DIC, disseminated intravascular coagulation; FDP, fibrin degradation product; tPA, tissue plasminogen activator; PAI-1, plasminogen activator inhibitor-1.

Impaired Primary Hemostasis. Impaired primary hemostasis occurs as a result of both thrombocytopenia and impaired platelet function. The former is largely the result of decreased production, which in turn is probably the result of decreased thrombopoietin secretion by the liver. Hypersplenism may also contribute, but its role has been overemphasized. Platelet dysfunction can occur when liver disease is sufficiently advanced that clearance of FDPs is impaired, or when DIC complicates the coagulation disturbance. The FDPs coat the surface of platelets and impair aggregation.[84] Ethanol can also directly contribute to platelet dysfunction by inhibition of the synthesis of ADP, ATP, and TxA_2.[84] Accordingly, when faced with a patient with liver disease who is bleeding, a normal platelet count cannot be assurance of intact primary hemostasis. DDAVP may be helpful, but transfusion of platelet concentrates may be necessary.

Disturbances of Coagulation. With liver disease, factor production decreases and consumption increases. The liver synthesizes all of the clotting factors (with the probable exception of factor VIII). As with vitamin K deficiency, hepatic disease first leads to a deficiency of factor VII as it has the shortest half-life. Thereafter, deficiencies will develop in factors IX, X, and II. Dietary deficiency of vitamin K, as may occur in alcoholics, combined with diminished secretion of bile salts leading to malabsorption, will exaggerate these deficiencies. If impaired coagulation is the result of vitamin K deficiency and not hepatic damage, then parenteral vitamin K may be helpful in restoring factor levels of II, VII, IX, and X. Further deterioration of hepatic function will affect the remaining factors, I, V, XI, XII, and XIII.

Impaired liver function can also cause a thrombotic tendency, which leads to increased consumption of clotting factors. This occurs for two reasons. First, synthesis of the natural anticoagulants, AT, protein C, and protein S, may be diminished, thereby altering the balance of pro- and anticoagulant forces. Second, clearance of activated clotting factors from the circulation may be impaired, thereby allowing persistent activation of the coagulation cascade.

Increased Fibrinolysis. Increased fibrinolysis occurs as a result of decreased clearance of tPA from the circulation by the impaired liver and decreased hepatic synthesis of α_2-antiplasmin. Production of the natural inhibitor of the plasmin system, PAI-1, is also diminished.[234] The combination of accelerated coagulation and increased fibrinolysis in patients with advanced liver disease can lead to a persistent, low-grade DIC. The release into the circulation of the breakdown products of necrotic hepatocytes may contribute to the development of DIC.[235]

Diagnosis and Treatment of Coagulation Abnormalities Associated with Liver Disease. The initial laboratory evaluation should include platelet count, PT, aPTT, fibrinogen level, and D-dimer. In the event of thrombocytopenia and clinical bleeding or pending surgery, platelet transfusion may be appropriate. If the PT is prolonged (>1.5 times control), vitamin K should be administered speculatively. In the absence of a response to vitamin K (which requires a minimum of 8 hours), factor deficiencies should be treated with FFP, with attention to the possibility of volume overload. Cryoprecipitate is appropriate in the event of hypofibrinogenemia (fibrinogen <100 to 125 g/dL). While antifibrinolytics have been applied in the context of liver transplantation, they should not otherwise be used for bleeding associated with liver disease because of the catastrophic consequences of administering these agents in the face of an unrecognized DIC. However, making the diagnosis of DIC (see later discussion) is often difficult because the laboratory tests used to identify DIC are already abnormal in patients with liver dysfunction. Thrombocytopenia, prolonged PT and aPTT, decreased fibrinogen level, and circulating FDPs will commonly occur in the absence of DIC. Elevated D-dimer is somewhat more specific for the occurrence of DIC.

DIC. Detailed reviews of DIC are available.[236–238] DIC is characterized by excessive deposition of fibrin throughout the vascular tree, with simultaneous depression of the normal coagulation inhibitory mechanisms and impaired fibrin degradation (see Chapter 56). It is triggered by the appearance of procoagulant material (TF or equivalent) in the circulation in amounts sufficient to overwhelm the mechanisms that normally restrain and localize clot formation. That appearance may be the result of either extensive endothelial injury, which exposes TF, or the release of TF into the circulation as occurs with amniotic fluid embolus, extensive soft-tissue damage, severe head injury, or any cause of a systemic inflammatory response. The native pathways that inhibit coagulation are either inhibited or overwhelmed: AT levels are depleted by excess thrombin formation, as reflected by elevated levels of thrombin-AT complexes; thrombomodulin expression in vascular endothelium is reduced in response to inflammation thereby reducing protein C formation; and the capacity of TFPI to restrain the TF-driven extrinsic pathway may be exceeded because of excessive TF.[238] The accelerated process of clot formation causes both tissue ischemia and, ultimately, critical depletion of platelets and factors. Simultaneously, the fibrinolytic system is activated, and plasmin is generated to lyse the extensive fibrin clots. FDPs appear in the circulation. FDPs stimulate release of PAI-1 from the endothelium, and thrombolysis becomes impaired. The FDPs also inhibit platelet aggregation and prevent the normal cross-linking of fibrin monomers. Depleted of platelets and clotting factors and inhibited by FDPs, the coagulation system fails and the patient bleeds. Simultaneously, the microvascular occlusion by fibrin causes both cutaneous (purpura fulminans) and deep tissue ischemia, with the latter contributing to multiorgan failure.

Table 16-17 lists the numerous clinical conditions that have been associated with DIC. It reveals that several clinical entities that are encountered frequently in anesthetic and critical

TABLE 16-17

CLINICAL CONDITIONS ASSOCIATED WITH DISSEMINATED INTRAVASCULAR COAGULOPATHY

- Sepsis (Gram-positive or -negative)
- Viremias
- Obstetric conditions
  - Amniotic fluid embolus
  - Fetal death in utero
  - Abruptio placentae
  - Pre-eclampsia
- Extensive tissue damage
  - Burns
  - Trauma
- Liver failure
- Extensive cerebral injury
  - Head injury
  - Stroke
- Extensive vascular endothelial damage
  - Vasculitis
  - Pre-eclampsia
- Hemolytic transfusion reactions
- Metastatic malignancies
- Leukemia
- Snake venoms

care practice are associated with the development of DIC. Sepsis is the most common. Endotoxins or lipopolysaccharide breakdown products from Gram-negative and positive bacteria, respectively, incite an inflammatory response that includes the generation of cytokines (tumor necrosis factor-α, various interleukins). These cytokines in turn stimulate the release or expression of TF by endothelial cells and monocytes, and the DIC sequence is initiated.

Several obstetric conditions can cause DIC. Amniotic fluid embolism, placental abruption, and fetal death in utero result in the direct release of TF-equivalent material into the circulation. Pre-eclampsia is characterized by a systemic vasculitis. The associated endothelial damage causes an initially low-grade DIC that accelerates as vasculitis-related damage leads to release of TF from ischemic tissues, in particular, placenta.

Large burns, extensive traumatic soft-tissue injuries, severe brain injury, and hemolytic transfusion reactions can also liberate TF-equivalent material into the circulation and incite DIC. Certain malignancies, most notably promyelocytic leukemia and adenocarcinomas, are associated with DIC. However, with malignancy-associated DIC, thrombotic manifestations are more likely to appear first, whereas with the others mentioned here, the hemorrhagic diathesis is often the first clinical manifestation.

A few general conditions such as acidosis, shock, and hypoxia are associated with DIC. Shock promotes coagulation because one of the control mechanisms (rapid blood flow) is compromised. Clearance of activated clotting factors is reduced when blood flow is decreased. Acidosis and hypoxia may contribute to both tissue and endothelial damage.

The clinical manifestations of DIC are a consequence of both thrombosis and bleeding. Bleeding is a more common clinical presentation in patients with acute, fulminant DIC. Petechiae, ecchymoses, epistaxis, gingival/mucosal bleeding, hematuria, and bleeding from wounds and puncture sites may be evident. With the chronic forms of DIC, thrombotic manifestations are more likely. Organs with the greatest blood flow (e.g., kidney and brain) typically sustain the greatest damage. Pulmonary function may deteriorate as a consequence of microthrombus accumulation.

Diagnosis of DIC. There is no absolutely consistent constellation of laboratory findings among routine tests. Increased PT, aPTT, thrombocytopenia, decreased fibrinogen level, and the presence of FDPs and D-dimer may all be noted. The peripheral smear may reveal schistocytes (fragmented RBCs reflecting the microangiopathy that occurs as a consequence of widespread fibrin deposition). Thrombocytopenia ($<100,000 /\mu L$) is not always evident early in the process, but true DIC without sequential reduction in platelet count is very unlikely. PT and aPTT may remain normal in spite of decreasing factor levels because of the presence of high levels of activated factors including thrombin and Xa. Fibrinogen levels may not be decreased, that is, <100 mg/dL, initially. Fibrinogen is an "acute phase reactant" that increases in response to stress, and the early consumption of fibrinogen may simply reduce its levels to "normal". FDPs are a sensitive measure of fibrinolytic activity although they are not specific for DIC. D-dimer (a breakdown product of the cross-linked fibrin in a mature clot) is somewhat more specific for DIC, but not entirely so, and should be measured when that diagnosis is suspected. The 3-P (plasma-protamine-paracoagulation) test is a relatively specific, although not very sensitive, assay sometimes used to confirm a diagnosis of DIC. It tests for the presence of soluble complexes composed of fibrin monomers (generated by excess thrombin) and FDPs. The addition of protamine desolublizes these complexes resulting in a precipitate.

Various other laboratory assays have been employed to support a diagnosis of DIC[236] but should probably not be considered part of the anesthesiologist's routine. They include levels of prothrombin fragments F1 + F2 (a marker of prothrombin conversion to thrombin—increased), thrombin-AT complexes (increased), AT (decreased), α$_2$-antiplasmin (decreased by binding to excess plasmin), protein C (decreased), plasminogen (decreased), and factor VIII (decreased in DIC but normal with hepatic failure without DIC).

Treatment of DIC. Treatment should focus on management of the underlying condition. Septicemia will require antibiotic therapy. The obstetric conditions are frequently self-limited, although evacuation of the uterus or hysterectomy may be warranted. Hypovolemia, acidosis, and hypoxemia should be corrected to prevent their contribution to the DIC process. When bleeding is or may become life-threatening, the consumptive coagulopathy must be treated. Platelets will be required for thrombocytopenia (e.g., $<50,000/mm^3$). FFP will replace the clotting factor deficiencies. Fibrinogen level should be raised to >100 mg/dL. When hypofibrinogenemia is severe (<50 mg/dL), cryoprecipitate may be required. Six units of cryoprecipitate will increase fibrinogen level by approximately 50 mg/dL in a 70-kg patient.[239]

Heparin has been advocated. However, the contemporary practice is to restrict its use to only those situations where thrombosis is clinically problematic, principally DIC associated with malignancies. There is no proven benefit in situations in which bleeding is the predominant manifestation. Administration of antifibrinolytics in the face of widespread thrombosis is potentially disastrous, and they should not be used. AT concentrates have been administered. The hope is that its administration will serve to slow the runaway coagulation process. However, a beneficial effect on outcome from DIC has not been confirmed (see data review by Levi[237]), and its use should be viewed as experimental. An insufficiency in the protein C endogenous coagulation inhibition system is thought to contribute to the prothrombotic state in DIC (see previous discussion). APC has been shown to decrease mortality and organ failure in patients with severe sepsis, and that improvement is also evident among patients with sepsis with overt DIC.[240] Its use should be considered in any sustained episode of DIC.[240]

Cardiopulmonary Bypass and Coagulation. Limited mention of this topic has been made in the earlier sections "Heparin in Cardiopulmonary Bypass, Cardiac Surgery, and HIT/T" and "Direct Thrombin Inhibitors." The management of anticoagulation and post-CPB bleeding is addressed in detail in Chapter 41.

Pharmacologic Therapy

Recombinant Factor VIIa

Recombinant FVIIa (rFVIIa) (NovoSeven) was developed for the treatment of patients with hemophilia A or B and inhibitors to exogenous FVIII or FIX preparations. The only current "on-label" indications for rFVIIa in the United States are those two conditions plus congenital FVII deficiency. Glanzmann's thrombasthenia is an approved indication in some other countries. However, rFVIIa has become a hemostatic agent of last (and sometimes earlier) resort in many clinical situations. Its use has been reported in trauma, hepatic failure, gastrointestinal bleeding, obstetric hemorrhage, acute intracerebral hemorrhage, and in cardiac, prostatic, hepatic, spinal, neurologic, and hepatic transplantation surgery. It has been used to reverse the anticoagulant effect of warfarin,

LMWHs, and selective Xa inhibitors. It has been administered to patients with vWD, FXI deficiency, thrombocytopenia, and with both congenital (Bernard-Soulier syndrome, Glanzmann's thrombasthenia) and acquired (uremia, aspirin, ADP and IIb/IIIa antagonists) platelet abnormalities.[211,241,242] However, most of these uses are supported by only anecdotal reports, among which there may be significant publication bias; that is, apparent success is reported more often than obvious failure. Of the off-label applications, only the use in prostate surgery, trauma, cardiac surgery (a very small series), and intracerebral hemorrhage are supported by randomized, blinded prospective trials.[243–246]

The mechanism of action is more than an augmentation of the native functions of FVII. Were that the case, rFVIIa would not be effective in hemophilia (Fig. 16-2). It seems probable that rFVIIa directly activates FX on platelet surfaces and thereby effects, without the participation of factors VIII, IX, and XI, the generation of the large amounts of thrombin necessary to produce a firm fibrin clot.[247] While the preferred ligand of FVIIa is TF, it also undergoes low-affinity binding to activated platelets. The serum concentrations achieved by typical rFVIIa dosing are several hundred times those that occur physiologically and are probably sufficient to activate FX on the platelet surface.

In a survey of experience with trauma patients, it was reported that acidosis (pH <7.20) appeared to decrease the efficacy of rFVIIa but that moderate hypothermia did not.[248] Note that while several reports speak to the efficacy of rFVIIa in reversing the effects of warfarin, LMWH, and fondaparinux, production of the fibrin burst in response to rFVIIa requires the availability of some FX. Warfarin, LMWH, and fondaparinux, all either inhibit the synthesis or the activity of FX. It seems reasonable to expect that in severe overdoses, rFVIIa may not be effective.

The appropriate dosing of this expensive agent (approximately US $1 per microgram at UCSD) is not well defined. The dose used most often in hemophilia has been 90 μg/kg and that dose has widely, and arbitrarily, we think, been adopted in other clinical situations. Doses as low as 20 μg/kg have been effective in some reports including the prostate surgery investigation just mentioned[243] and the reversal of warfarin effect.[249] In the prospective trauma investigation by Boffard et al.,[244] the initial dose was 200 μg/kg, although others have reported apparent efficacy in trauma patients with doses of 75 μg/kg.[250] It seems reasonable that the appropriate dosage may vary with the clinician's perception of the severity of the physiologic disturbance and the urgency of the situation. A one unit per hour gastrointestinal bleed and an exsanguinating trauma patient with escalating acidosis and hypothermia may warrant different doses. The current, somewhat arbitrary, algorithm in place at UCSD provides for the administration of 60 μg/kg for profuse bleeding that is unresponsive to conventional therapy. That dose is rounded to the nearest 1,200 μg in recognition that the agent is supplied in vials of 1.2 mg. A U.S. consensus panel recommended 20 to 40 μg/kg for "non-emergent reversal" and 41 to 90 μg/kg "for all other scenarios."[251] The half-life is approximately 2 hours and repeat dosing at that interval may be required.

Because rVIIa is an active procoagulant only when it is in contact with TF or activated platelets, thrombosis in locations remote from sites of vessel disruption has been infrequent. However, thrombotic complications, some fatal, have been reported,[213] and the use of rFVIIa should be undertaken with an awareness of that hazard. When the exigencies of the clinical situation permit, modest initial doses of 20 to 40 μg/kg with supplementary doses at 15-minute intervals as warranted by clinical response seem prudent. rFVIIa should probably be viewed as relatively contraindicated in clinical states in which

TF may be widely exposed or circulating freely, that is, in most of the conditions associated with DIC.

The effectiveness of available laboratory tests in monitoring the clinical effect of rFVIIa is uncertain.[241] It has not been confirmed that the effect of high serum concentrations of rFVIIa on in vitro tests (PT, PTT) will reflect effects on coagulation in vivo. Furthermore, the use of "normal values" as a comparator for post-rFVIIa aPTT values may have little meaning if, in vitro, rFVIIa directly activates FX on the phospholipid reagent, and thereby bypasses contact activation and all the earlier steps of the intrinsic pathway (Fig. 16-1).

Desmopressin

Desmopressin, 1-deamino-8-D-arginine vasopressin (DDAVP), is a synthetic analogue of the natural hormone vasopressin.[192,197] The actions of vasopressin are mediated by two general classes of receptors: V1, which mediate smooth muscle contraction in the peripheral vasculature, and V2, which regulate water reabsorption in the collecting ducts of the nephron. DDAVP is active only at V2 receptors. Accordingly, it is a potent antidiuretic with no vasoconstrictor effect. DDAVP was used primarily for clinical conditions such as diabetes insipidus until its hemostatic effects were recognized. DDAVP causes rapid release of vWF and tPA from vascular endothelium via stimulation of endothelial V2 receptors. DDAVP also causes increases in serum levels of FVIII, perhaps by release from hepatic sinusoidal endothelial cells,[197] and increased expression of platelet surface GP1b receptors.[252] In vWD, the DDAVP-induced increases in FVIII level are mediated in part by increased serum life of FVIII because of the availability of its protective carrier protein vWF. In mild hemophilia A, DDAVP can increase the circulating factor VIII:C concentration two- to sixfold. DDAVP increases platelet adhesiveness and shortens the BT.

Indications. DDAVP is effective treatment for type I and some type II variants of vWD and for mild hemophilia A (see "von Willebrand Disease" and "Hemophilia A"). DDAVP has been shown to reduce BT in several conditions associated with platelet dysfunction, including uremia (see "Uremia") and advanced liver disease.[84] DDAVP also decreases the prolonged BTs caused by many drugs including aspirin, nonsteroidal anti-inflammatory drugs, dextran, ticlopidine, and heparin. It is effective for some congenital platelet abnormalities, including the Bernard-Soulier syndrome (but not Glanzmann's thrombasthenia).[192]

Because platelet dysfunction and thrombocytopenia are common in cardiac surgery, studies of prophylactic administration of DDAVP have been performed. Those that have revealed decreased blood loss or blood product administration have involved principally patients who were predisposed to blood loss (e.g., those having repeat procedures[253–256]) and patients receiving aspirin.[257] It has not proven effective at reducing blood loss in unselected surgical populations.[258]

Dosage. DDAVP, when given for its procoagulant effect, is usually administered intravenously in a dose of 0.3 μg/kg. (Note that this dose is _not_ appropriate for the management of acute central diabetes insipidus, for which the total initial intravenous dose should be 0.2 to 0.4 μg.) Administration over 30 minutes is recommended because DDAVP induces endothelial release of nitric oxide, and mild degrees of hypotension may occur. Peak levels of factor VIII:C and vWF are achieved within 30 to 60 minutes, and the effect lasts for several hours. DDAVP administration may be repeated after 8 to 12 hours. When used in cardiac surgery, the drug should be administered after termination of CPB. Water balance should be monitored. However, while congestive cardiac failure and hyponatremia and seizures in children have been reported, clinically significant water retention is relatively uncommon.

Antifibrinolytics

Antifibrinolytic agents have been used frequently in situations in which exaggerated fibrinolysis is suspected of contributing to intraoperative bleeding. The situations in which favorable effects on blood loss and replacement have been reported include CPB procedures, hepatic transplantation, scoliosis surgery, total joint replacement, and prostate surgery[259–262] (see Chapter 41). The use of antifibrinolytic mouthwashes in the context of dental procedures in patients with hemophilia has been mentioned elsewhere in this chapter. Three antifibrinolytics have been widely employed: the lysine analogues, EACA, and TXA, and the serine protease inhibitor aprotinin (AP). AP was withdrawn from the market in November 2007 because of reports of renal dysfunction and increased mortality after CPB.[105,263,264] Some discussion of AP has been included in case the withdrawal is only temporary, as anticipated by the manufacturer.

ε-Aminocaproic Acid and Tranexamic Acid. EACA and TXA bind to produce a structural change in both plasminogen and plasmin. That structural change prevents the conversion of plasminogen to plasmin and also prevents plasmin from degrading fibrinogen and fibrin. The dual action of these agents results in two effects on the hemostatic mechanism. First, decreased conversion of plasminogen to plasmin results in reduced fibrinolysis. The second effect, the inactivation of plasmin, decreases the formation of degradation products of fibrinogen and fibrin. FDPs have anticoagulant effects, including the inhibition of platelet aggregation and the inhibition of the cross-linking of fibrin strands, which are thereby avoided. Their effectiveness in reducing blood loss in the wide variety of surgical situations previously mentioned is well confirmed.[261]

Aprotinin. AP produces its antifibrinolytic effect by a different mechanism. It is an inhibitor of numerous serine protease enzymes including plasmin and kallikrein. The latter participates in the process of contact activation of factor XII. As a consequence of its inhibition of plasmin, AP, like EACA and TXA, prevents degradation of fibrinogen and fibrin. As is the case with EACA and TXA, the reduction in FDPs should improve both platelet and coagulation function. However, AP is believed to have additional beneficial effects on the inflammatory response to CPB in general, and on platelets in particular.[265,266] The mechanism of these effects is not known with certainty. However, thrombin is a serine protease that can activate platelets via a "protease-activated receptor" on the platelet surface.[267] Better preservation of the GP1b receptor (which is necessary for initial platelet adhesion to vascular defects) has been reported during CPB in patients who received AP.[268] AP also appears to reduce neutrophil activation and transmigration across capillary endothelium, perhaps via an effect on an endothelial protease-activated receptor, and may therefore also blunt the neutrophil-mediated component of the response to endothelial injury.[266]

Use of Antifibrinolytics in Cardiac Surgery. Meta-analyses of the many studies performed in the context of CPB confirm that blood loss and the administration of allogeneic blood are diminished by the use of all three agents.[259,261,269,270] Concern has been expressed that antifibrinolysis might lead to an increased rate of graft occlusion, MI, and renal failure. While meta-analysis had not borne out any of those concerns,[261,269,270] as previously noted, increased renal dysfunction and mortality have recently been attributed to AP.[263,264,271] The mechanism of the renal dysfunction remains

a matter of speculation, and concern about selection bias in those investigations (i.e., "sicker" patients were more likely to receive AP) has been expressed.[266] As a result, at least three other retrospective reviews of existing databases, with attempts to control for covariates, have been performed. Two did not provide support for an adverse effect. Furnary et al.[272] reported no effect of AP on renal function, and Dietrich et al.[273] reported the absence of any dose-related effect of AP on renal function. However, Schneeweiss et al.[274] compared 33,517 patients who received AP with 44,682 who received EACA, and reported an adverse effect of AP on both mortality and renal function. AP is not currently available.

There is not a clear consensus as to which of the remaining two agents is most appropriate in the context of CPB. Meta-analysis has revealed both to be effective.[269] However, there is more evidence in support of TXA, and at least one study reported greater reduction of blood loss with TXA than EACA.[275]

The patterns of use of antifibrinolytic agents in cardiac surgery vary substantially among institutions. Few appear to use these agents for all CPB procedures. Most reserve them for situations more likely to be associated with post-CPB bleeding (e.g., repeat and circulatory arrest procedures). Still others appear to reserve antifibrinolytics for refractory bleeding post-CPB. The latter seems less logical because much of the activation of the hemostatic mechanism occurs during CPB.

Use of Antifibrinolytics in Liver Transplantation. Accelerated fibrinolysis occurs commonly during hepatic transplantation. This is probably, in part, the consequence of decreased clearance of activated clotting factors by the diseased liver. More importantly, hepatic clearance ceases entirely during the anhepatic phase. In addition, with reperfusion of the donor liver, there is a release of tPA into the systemic circulation. All three agents have all been used, and meta-analysis confirms reduced blood loss with AP and TXA, with too little information to draw conclusions about EACA.[262] Some advocate prophylactic administration to all patients, while others administer these agents only in response to the demonstration, typically by thromboelastography, of hyperfibrinolysis.

Use of Antifibrinolytics in Orthopaedic and Other Surgery. There have been numerous investigations of the effect of TXA and EACA on blood loss and transfusion requirement in scoliosis and joint replacement surgery. A meta-analysis confirmed the efficacy of TXA, but not EACA, in those circumstances.[260]

CONCLUSIONS

The approach to the bleeding patient requires a knowledge of the basic hemostatic mechanism and of common bleeding disorders, an ability to interpret coagulation tests, and an appreciation of the risks inherent to blood component therapy. The hemostatic balance is delicate and complex, and it is the responsibility of the anesthesiologist to anticipate, prevent, and treat disturbances of that balance. Preoperative evaluation must identify those patients whose inherited or acquired medical conditions or whose current medications may influence these processes. With respect to medications, there are a rapidly increasing number of agents that are administered specifically for the purpose of altering the hemostatic balance, such as clopidogrel, tPA, and LMWH. As the patient proceeds through the perioperative period, the anesthesiologist must determine whether bleeding is surgical in nature or is the result of a pre-existing or evolving hemostatic defect that will require the transfusion of hemostatic blood components—platelets, FFP, or cryoprecipitate—or the administration of pharmacologic agents.

ACKNOWLEDGMENT

The authors are grateful to Dzung Le, MD, Professor of Pathology, UCSD School of Medicine, for time spent in discussion of coagulation mechanisms and testing.

References

1. Whitaker BI, Sullivan M: The 2005 nationwide blood collection and utilization survey report. US Dept of Health and Human Services. http://www.hhs.gov/bloodsafety/2005NBCUS.pdf
2. Kleinman S, Chan P, Robillard P: Risks associated with transfusion of cellular blood components in Canada. Transfus Med Rev 2003; 17: 120.
3. Dodd RY: Current risk for transfusion transmitted infections. Curr Opin Hematol 2007; 14: 671.
4. Cable RG, Leiby DA: Risk and prevention of transfusion-transmitted babesiosis and other tick-borne diseases. Curr Opin Hematol 2003; 10: 405.
5. Busch MR: Evolving approaches to estimate risks of transfusion-transmitted viral infections: incidence-window period model after ten years. Dev Biol (Basel) 2007; 127: 87.
6. Busch MP, Glynn SA, Stramer SL, et al: A new strategy for estimating risks of transfusion-transmitted viral infections based on rates of detection of recently infected donors. Transfusion 2005; 45: 254.
7. Kleinman SH, Busch MP: Assessing the impact of HBV NAT on window period reduction and residual risk. J Clin Virol 2006; 36(Suppl 1): S23
8. Kuhns MC, Busch MP: New strategies for blood donor screening for hepatitis B virus: nucleic acid testing versus immunoassay methods. Mol Diagn Ther 2006; 10: 77
9. Satake M, Taira R, Yugi H, et al: Infectivity of blood components with low hepatitis B virus DNA levels identified in a lookback program. Transfusion 2007; 47: 1197
10. Conry-Cantilena C, VanRaden M, Gibble J, et al: Routes of infection, viremia, and liver disease in blood donors found to have hepatitis C virus infection. N Engl J Med 1996; 334: 1691
11. Tong MJ, el-Farra NS, Reikes AR, et al: Clinical outcomes after transfusion-associated hepatitis C. N Engl J Med 1995; 332: 1463
12. Goodnough LT, Brecher ME, Kanter MH, et al: Transfusion medicine. First of two parts—blood transfusion. N Engl J Med 1999; 340: 438
13. Shander A: Emerging risks and outcomes of blood transfusion in surgery. Semin Hematol 2004; 41: 117
14. Nichols WG, Price TH, Gooley T, et al: Transfusion-transmitted cytomegalovirus infection after receipt of leukoreduced blood products. Blood 2003; 101: 4195
15. Stephenson J: Investigation probes risk of contracting West Nile virus via blood transfusions. JAMA 2002; 288: 1573
16. Alter HJ: Emerging, re-emerging and submerging infectious threats to the blood supply. Vox Sang 2004; 87(Suppl 2): 56
17. Montgomery SP, Brown JA, Kuehnert M, et al: Transfusion-associated transmission of West Nile virus, United States 2003 through 2005. Transfusion 2006; 46: 2038
18. Brecher ME, Hay SN: Bacterial contamination of blood components. Clin Microbiol Rev 2005; 18: 195
19. Eder AF, Kennedy JM, Dy BA, et al: Bacterial screening of apheresis platelets and the residual risk of septic transfusion reactions: the American Red Cross experience (2004–2006). Transfusion 2007; 47: 1134
20. Stroncek DF, Rebulla P: Platelet transfusions. Lancet 2007; 370: 427
21. Stramer SL: Current risks of transfusion-transmitted agents: a review. Arch Pathol Lab Med 2007; 131: 702
22. Seitz R, von Auer F, Blumel J, et al: Impact of vCJD on blood supply. Biologicals 2007; 35: 79
23. Eder AF, Chambers LA: Noninfectious complications of blood transfusion. Arch Pathol Lab Med 2007; 131: 708
24. Heddle NM, Soutar RL, O'Hoski PL, et al: A prospective study to determine the frequency and clinical significance of alloimmunization post-transfusion. Br J Haematol 1995; 91: 1000
25. Slichter SJ: Platelet transfusion therapy. Hematol Oncol Clin North Am 2007; 21: 697
26. Eder AF, Herron R, Strupp A, et al: Transfusion-related acute lung injury surveillance (2003–2005) and the potential impact of the selective use of plasma from male donors in the American Red Cross. Transfusion 2007; 47: 599
27. Stainsby D, MacLennan S, Thomas D, et al: Guidelines on the management of massive blood loss. Br J Haematol 2006; 135: 634
28. Kleinman S: A perspective on transfusion-related acute lung injury two years after the Canadian Consensus Conference. Transfusion 2006; 46: 1465
29. Silliman CC, McLaughlin NJ: Transfusion-related acute lung injury. Blood Rev 2006; 20: 139
30. Wendel S, Biagini S, Trigo F, et al: Measures to prevent TRALI. Vox Sang 2007; 92: 258
31. Sheppard CA, Logdberg LE, Zimring JC, et al: Transfusion-related acute lung injury. Hematol Oncol Clin North Am 2007; 21: 163
32. Silliman CC, Boshkov LK, Mehdizadehkashi Z, et al: Transfusion-related acute lung injury: epidemiology and a prospective analysis of etiologic factors. Blood 2003; 101: 454
33. Kleinman S, Caulfield T, Chan P, et al: Toward an understanding of transfusion-related acute lung injury: statement of a consensus panel. Transfusion 2004; 44: 1774
34. Ventilation with lower tidal volumes as compared with traditional tidal volumes for acute lung injury and the acute respiratory distress syndrome. The Acute Respiratory Distress Syndrome Network. N Engl J Med 2000; 342: 1301
35. Insunza A, Romon I, Gonzalez-Ponte ML, et al: Implementation of a strategy to prevent TRALI in regional blood centre. Transfusion Medicine 2004; 157
36. Schroeder ML: Transfusion-associated graft-versus-host disease. Br J Haematol 2002; 117: 275
37. Lane TA: Leukocyte depletion of cellular blood components. Curr Opin Hematol 1994; 1: 443
38. Opelz G, Sengar DP, Mickey MR, et al: Effect of blood transfusions on subsequent kidney transplants. Transplantation Proceedings 1973; 5: 253
39. Vamvakas EC, Blajchman MA: Transfusion-related immunomodulation (TRIM): an update. Blood Rev 2007; 21: 327
40. Taylor RW, O'Brien J, Trottier SJ, et al: Red blood cell transfusions and nosocomial infections in critically ill patients. Crit Care Med 2006; 34: 2302
41. Malone DL, Dunne J, Tracy JK, et al: Blood transfusion, independent of shock severity, is associated with worse outcome in trauma. J Trauma 2003; 54: 898
42. Murphy GJ, Reeves BC, Rogers CA, et al: Increased mortality, postoperative morbidity, and cost after red blood cell transfusion in patients having cardiac surgery. Circulation 2007; 116: 2544
43. Netzer G, Shah CV, Iwashyna TJ, et al: Association of RBC transfusion with mortality in patients with acute lung injury. Chest 2007; 132: 1116
44. Vamvakas EC: Why have meta-analyses of randomized controlled trials of the association between non-white-blood-cell-reduced allogeneic blood transfusion and postoperative infection produced discordant results? Vox Sang 2007; 93: 196
45. Hebert PC, Wells G, Blajchman MA, et al: A multicenter, randomized, controlled clinical trial of transfusion requirements in critical care. Transfusion Requirements in Critical Care Investigators, Canadian Critical Care Trials Group. N Engl J Med 1999; 340: 409
46. Silliman CC, Moore EE, Johnson JL, et al: Transfusion of the injured patient: proceed with caution. Shock 2004; 21: 291
47. Hebert PC, Tinmouth A, Corwin HL: Controversies in RBC transfusion in the critically ill. Chest 2007; 131: 1583
48. Zallen G, Offner PJ, Moore EE, et al: Age of transfused blood is an independent risk factor for postinjury multiple organ failure. Am J Surg 1999; 178: 570
49. Hebert PC, Chin-Yee I, Fergusson D, et al: A pilot trial evaluating the clinical effects of prolonged storage of red cells. Anesth Analg 2005; 100: 1433
50. Basran S, Frumento RJ, Cohen A, et al: The association between duration of storage of transfused red blood cells and morbidity and mortality after reoperative cardiac surgery. Anesth Analg 2006; 103: 15
51. Koch CG, Li L, Sessler DI, et al: Duration of red-cell storage and complications after cardiac surgery. N Engl J Med 2008; 358: 1229
52. Spiess BD: Risks of transfusion: outcome focus. Transfusion 2004; 44: 4S
53. Vamvakas EC: White-blood-cell-containing allogeneic blood transfusion and postoperative infection or mortality: an updated meta-analysis. Vox Sang 2007; 92: 224
54. Collier AC, Kalish LA, Busch MP, et al: Leukocyte-reduced red blood cell transfusions in patients with anemia and human immunodeficiency virus infection: the Viral Activation Transfusion Study: a randomized controlled trial. JAMA 2001; 285: 1592
55. Hebert PC, Fergusson D, Blajchman MA, et al: Clinical outcomes following institution of the Canadian universal leukoreduction program for red blood cell transfusions. JAMA 2003; 289: 1941
56. Fergusson D, Hebert PC, Lee SK, et al: Clinical outcomes following institution of universal leukoreduction of blood transfusions for premature infants. JAMA 2003; 289: 1950
57. Nightingale S: Hypotension and bedside leukocyte reduction filters. JAMA 1999; 281: 1978
58. McLoughlin TM, Greilich PE: Preexisting hemostatic defects and bleeding disorders, Blood: Hemostasis, Transfusion, and Alternatives in the Perioperative Period. Edited by Lake CL MR. New York, Raven Press, 1995, pp 25.
59. Rajagopalan S, Mascha E, Na J, et al: The effects of mild perioperative hypothermia on blood loss and transfusion requirement. Anesthesiology 2008; 108: 71
60. Ferrara A, MacArthur JD, Wright HK, et al: Hypothermia and acidosis worsen coagulopathy in the patient requiring massive transfusion. Am J Surg 1990; 160: 515
61. Wang HE, Callaway CW, Peitzman AB, et al: Admission hypothermia and outcome after major trauma. Crit Care Med 2005; 33: 1296
62. Sessler DI: Mild perioperative hypothermia. N Engl J Med 1997; 336: 1730
63. Hiippala ST, Myllyla GJ, Vahtera EM: Hemostatic factors and replacement of major blood loss with plasma-poor red cell concentrates. Anesth Analg 1995; 81: 360

64. Yuan S, Ferrell C, Chandler WL: Comparing the prothrombin time INR versus the APTT to evaluate the coagulopathy of acute trauma. Thromb Res 2007; 120: 29

65. AuBuchon JP: Minimizing donor exposure in hemotherapy. Arch Pathol Lab Med 1994; 118: 380

66. Jameson LC, Popic PM, Harms BA: Hyperkalemic death during use of a high-capacity fluid warmer for massive transfusion. Anesthesiology 1990; 73: 1050

67. Rock G, Tittley P, Fuller V: Effect of citrate anticoagulants on factor VIII levels in plasma. Transfusion 1988; 28: 248

68. Crosby ET: Perioperative haemotherapy: I. Indications for blood component transfusion. Can J Anaesth 1992; 39: 695

69. Hebert PC, McDonald BJ, Tinmouth A: Overview of transfusion practices in perioperative and critical care. Vox Sang 2004; 87(Suppl 2): 209

70. Wu WC, Rathore SS, Wang Y, et al: Blood transfusion in elderly patients with acute myocardial infarction. N Engl J Med 2001; 345: 1230

71. Hebert PC, Wells G, Tweeddale M, et al: Does transfusion practice affect mortality in critically ill patients? Transfusion Requirements in Critical Care (TRICC) Investigators and the Canadian Critical Care Trials Group. Am J Respir Crit Care Med 1997; 155: 1618

72. Practice Guidelines for blood component therapy: A report by the American Society of Anesthesiologists Task Force on Blood Component Therapy. Anesthesiology 1996; 84: 732

73. Swerdlow PS: Red cell exchange in sickle cell disease. Hematology Am Soc Hematol Educ Program 2006; 48

74. Robertie PG, Gravlee GP: Safe limits of isovolemic hemodilution and recommendations for erythrocyte transfusion. Int Anesthesiol Clin 1990; 28: 197

75. Roth DM, Maruoka Y, Rogers J, et al: Development of coronary collateral circulation in left circumflex Ameroid-occluded swine myocardium. Am J Physiol 1987; 253: H1279

76. Weiskopf RB, Viele MK, Feiner J, et al: Human cardiovascular and metabolic response to acute, severe isovolemic anemia. JAMA 1998; 279: 217

77. Weiskopf RB, Kramer JH, Viele M, et al: Acute severe isovolemic anemia impairs cognitive function and memory in humans. Anesthesiology 2000; 92: 1646

78. Fluit CR, Kunst VA, Drenthe-Schonk AM: Incidence of red cell antibodies after multiple blood transfusion. Transfusion 1990; 30: 532

79. Tuman K: Tissue Oxygen Delivery- the Physiology of Anemia. Anesthesiol Clin North Am 1990; 8: 451

80. Practice guidelines for perioperative blood transfusion and adjuvant therapies: an updated report by the American Society of Anesthesiologists Task Force on Perioperative Blood Transfusion and Adjuvant Therapies. Anesthesiology 2006; 105: 198

81. Guidelines for the use of platelet transfusions. Br J Haematol 2003; 122: 10

82. Samama CM, Djoudi R, Lecompte T, et al: Perioperative platelet transfusion: recommendations of the Agence Francaise de Securite Sanitaire des Produits de Sante (AFSSaPS) 2003. Can J Anaesth 2005; 52: 30

83. Levi MM, Vink R, de Jonge E: Management of bleeding disorders by prohemostatic therapy. Int J Hematol 2002; 76(Suppl 2): 139

84. Shen YM, Frenkel EP: Acquired platelet dysfunction. Hematol Oncol Clin North Am 2007; 21: 647

85. Stanworth SJ, Brunskill SJ, Hyde CJ, et al: Is fresh frozen plasma clinically effective? A systematic review of randomized controlled trials. Br J Haematol 2004; 126: 139

86. O'Shaughnessy DF, Atterbury C, Bolton Maggs P, et al: Guidelines for the use of fresh-frozen plasma, cryoprecipitate and cryosupernatant. Br J Haematol 2004; 126: 11

87. Johansson PI, Hansen MB, Sorensen H: Transfusion practice in massively bleeding patients: Time for a change? Vox Sang 2005; 89: 92

88. Ho AM, Larmakar MK, Dion PW: Are we giving enough coagulation factors during major trauma resuscitation? Am J Surg 2005; 190: 479

89. Borgman MA, Spinella PC, Perkins JG, et al: The ratio of blood products transfused affects mortality in patients receiving massive transfusions at a combat support hospital. J Trauma 2007; 63: 805

90. Hess JR, Holcomb JB, Hoyt DB: Damage control resuscitation: the need for specific blood products to treat the coagulopathy of trauma. Transfusion 2006; 46: 685

91. Forestner JE: Massive transfusion protocol for trauma. American Society of Anesthesiologists Newsletter 2005; 69: 7

92. Lethagen S, Kyrle PA, Castaman G, et al: von Willebrand factor/factor VIII concentrate (Haemate P) dosing based on pharmacokinetics: a prospective multicenter trial in elective surgery. J Thromb Haemost 2007; 5: 1420

93. Carless P, Moxey A, O'Connell D, et al: Autologous transfusion techniques: a systematic review of their efficacy. Transfus Med 2004; 14: 123

94. Bern MM, Bierbaum BE, Katz JN, et al: Autologous blood donation and subsequent blood use in patients undergoing total knee arthroplasty. Transfus Med 2006; 16: 313

95. Boulton FE, James V: Guidelines for policies on alternatives to allogeneic blood transfusion. 1. Predeposit autologous blood donation and transfusion. Transfus Med 2007; 17: 354

96. Rock G, Berger R, Bormanis J, et al: A review of nearly two decades in an autologous blood programme: The rise and fall of activity. Transfus Med 2006; 16: 307

97. Goodnough LT, Shander A: Blood management. Arch Pathol Lab Med 2007; 131: 695

98. Goodnough LT: The use of erythropoietin in the enhancement of autologous transfusion therapy. Curr Opin Hematol 1995; 2: 214

99. Laupacis A, Fergusson D: Erythropoietin to minimize perioperative blood transfusion: a systematic review of randomized trials. The International Study of Peri-operative Transfusion (ISPOT) Investigators. Transfus Med 1998; 8: 309

100. Milbrink J, Birgegard G, Danersund A, et al: Preoperative autologous donation of 6 units of blood during rh-EPO treatment. Can J Anaesth 1997; 44: 1315

101. Monk TG, Goodnough LT, Brecher ME, et al: A prospective randomized comparison of three blood conservation strategies for radical prostatectomy. Anesthesiology 1999; 91: 24

102. Monk TG: Preoperative recombinant human erythropoietin in anemic surgical patients. Crit Care 2004; 8(Suppl 2): S45

103. Rosencher N, Poisson D, Albi A, et al: Two injections of erythropoietin correct moderate anemia in most patients awaiting orthopedic surgery. Can J Anaesth 2005; 52: 160

104. MacLaren R, Sullivan PW: Cost-effectiveness of recombinant human erythropoietin for reducing red blood cells transfusions in critically ill patients. Value Health 2005; 8: 105

105. Karkouti K, McCluskey SA, Evans L, et al: Erythropoietin is an effective clinical modality for reducing RBC transfusion in joint surgery. Can J Anaesth 2005; 52: 362

106. Pierson JL, Hannon TJ, Earles DR: A blood-conservation algorithm to reduce blood transfusions after total hip and knee arthroplasty. J Bone Joint Surg Am 2004; 86-A: 1512

107. Couvret C, Laffon M, Baud A, et al: A restrictive use of both autologous donation and recombinant human erythropoietin is an efficient policy for primary total hip or knee arthroplasty. Anesth Analg 2004; 99: 262

108. Marchetti M, Barosi G: Cost-effectiveness of epoetin and autologous blood donation in reducing allogeneic blood transfusions in coronary artery bypass graft surgery. Transfusion 2000; 40: 673

109. Avall A, Hyllner M, Bengtson JP, et al: Recombinant human erythropoietin in preoperative autologous blood donation did not influence the haemoglobin recovery after surgery. Acta Anaesthesiol Scand 2003; 47: 687

110. Rosengart TK, Helm RE, Klemperer J, et al: Combined aprotinin and erythropoietin use for blood conservation: results with Jehovah's Witnesses. Ann Thorac Surg 1994; 58: 1397

111. Price S, Pepper JR, Jaggar SI: Recombinant human erythropoietin use in a critically ill Jehovah's witness after cardiac surgery. Anesth Analg 2005; 101: 325

112. Corwin HL, Gettinger A, Pearl RG, et al: Efficacy of recombinant human erythropoietin in critically ill patients: a randomized controlled trial. JAMA 2002; 288: 2827

113. Egrie JC, Dwyer E, Browne JK, et al: Darbepoetin alfa has a longer circulating half-life and greater in vivo potency than recombinant human erythropoietin. Exp Hematol 2003; 31: 290

114. Segal JB, Blasco-Colmenares E, Norris EJ, et al: Preoperative acute normovolemic hemodilution: a meta-analysis. Transfusion 2004; 44: 632

115. Goodnough LT: Acute normovolemic hemodilution. Vox Sang 2002; 83(Suppl 1): 211

116. Weiskopf RB: Efficacy of acute normovolemic hemodilution assessed as a function of fraction of blood volume lost. Anesthesiology 2001; 94: 439

117. Matot I, Scheinin O, Jurim O, et al: Effectiveness of acute normovolemic hemodilution to minimize allogeneic blood transfusion in major liver resections. Anesthesiology 2002; 97: 794

118. Goodnough LT, Despotis GJ, Merkel K, et al: A randomized trial comparing acute normovolemic hemodilution and preoperative autologous blood donation in total hip arthroplasty. Transfusion 2000; 40: 1054

119. Wolowczyk L, Lewis DR, Nevin M, et al: The effect of acute normovolaemic haemodilution on blood transfusion requirements in abdominal aortic aneurysm repair. Eur J Vasc Endovasc Surg 2001; 22: 361

120. Bennett J, Haynes S, Torella F, et al: Acute normovolemic hemodilution in moderate blood loss surgery: a randomized controlled trial. Transfusion 2006; 46: 1097

121. Williamson KR, Taswell HF: Intraoperative blood salvage: A review. Transfusion 1991; 31: 662

122. Ereth MH, Oliver WC, Jr., Santrach PJ: Perioperative interventions to decrease transfusion of allogeneic blood products. Mayo Clin Proc 1994; 69: 575

123. Hughes LG, Thomas DW, Wareham K, et al: Intra-operative blood salvage in abdominal trauma: a review of 5 years' experience. Anaesthesia 2001; 56: 217

124. Desmond MJ, Thomas MJ, Gillon J, et al: Consensus conference on autologous transfusion. Perioperative red cell salvage. Transfusion 1996; 36: 644

125. Huet C, Salmi LR, Fergusson D, et al: A meta-analysis of the effectiveness of cell salvage to minimize perioperative allogeneic blood transfusion in cardiac and orthopedic surgery. International Study of Perioperative Transfusion (ISPOT) Investigators. Anesth Analg 1999; 89: 861

126. Hashimoto T, Kokudo N, Orii R, et al: Intraoperative blood salvage during liver resection: a randomized controlled trial. Ann Surg 2007; 245: 686

127. Fujimoto J, Okamoto E, Yamanaka N, et al: Efficacy of autotransfusion in hepatectomy for hepatocellular carcinoma. Arch Surg 1993; 128: 1065

128. Hart OJ, 3rd, Klimberg IW, Wajsman Z, et al: Intraoperative autotransfusion in radical cystectomy for carcinoma of the bladder. Surg Gynecol Obstet 1989; 168: 302

129. Bernstein HH, Rosenblatt MA, Gettes M, et al: The ability of the Haemonetics 4 Cell Saver System to remove tissue factor from blood contaminated with amniotic fluid. Anesth Analg 1997; 85: 831

130. Potter PS, Waters JH, Burger GA, et al: Application of cell-salvage during cesarean section. Anesthesiology 1999; 90: 619

131. Weiskopf RB: Erythrocyte salvage during cesarean section. Anesthesiology 2000; 92: 1519

132. Waters JH, Tuohy MJ, Hobson DF, et al: Bacterial reduction by cell salvage washing and leukocyte depletion filtration. Anesthesiology 2003; 99: 652

133. Biagini D, Filippucci E, Agnelli G, et al: Activation of blood coagulation in patients undergoing postoperative blood salvage and re-infusion of unwashed whole blood after total knee arthroplasty. Thromb Res 2004; 113: 211

134. Tawes RL, Jr., Sydorak GR, DuVall TB: Postoperative salvage: a technological advance in the 'washed' versus 'unwashed' blood controversy. Semin Vasc Surg 1994; 7: 98

135. Djaiani G, Fedorko L, Borger MA, et al: Continuous-flow cell saver reduces cognitive decline in elderly patients after coronary bypass surgery. Circulation 2007; 116: 1888

136. McKie JS, Herzenberg JE: Coagulopathy complicating intraoperative blood salvage in a patient who had idiopathic scoliosis. A case report. J Bone Joint Surg Am 1997; 79: 1391

137. Waters JH, Lee JS, Karafa MT: A mathematical model of cell salvage efficiency. Anesth Analg 2002; 95: 1312

138. Drummond JC, Petrovitch CT: Intraoperative blood salvage: Fluid replacement calculations. Anesth Analg 2005; 100(3): 645

139. Waters JH, Williams B, Yazer MH, et al: Modification of suction-induced hemolysis during cell salvage. Anesth Analg 2007; 104: 684

140. Waters JH, Dyga RM: Postoperative blood salvage: outside the controlled world of the blood bank. Transfusion 2007; 47: 362

141. Strumper D, Weber EW, Gielen-Wijffels S, et al: Clinical efficacy of postoperative autologous transfusion of filtered shed blood in hip and knee arthroplasty. Transfusion 2004; 44: 1567

142. Munoz M, Cobos A, Campos A, et al: Impact of postoperative shed blood transfusion, with or without leucocyte reduction, on acute-phase response to surgery for total knee replacement. Acta Anaesthesiol Scand 2005; 49: 1182

143. Moonen AF, Knoors NT, van Os JJ, et al: Retransfusion of filtered shed blood in primary total hip and knee arthroplasty: a prospective randomized clinical trial. Transfusion 2007; 47: 379

144. Griffith LD, Billman GF, Daily PO, et al: Apparent coagulopathy caused by infusion of shed mediastinal blood and its prevention by washing of the infusate. Ann Thorac Surg 1989; 47: 400

145. Winslow RM: Current status of oxygen carriers ('blood substitutes'): 2006. Vox Sang 2006; 91: 102

146. Spahn DR, Kocian R: The place of artificial oxygen carriers in reducing allogeneic blood transfusions and augmenting tissue oxygenation. Can J Anaesth 2003; 50: S41

147. The real value of blood (accessible at www.watchtower.org). Awake! August: 2006

148. Fung MK, Downes KA, Shulman IA: Transfusion of platelets containing ABO-incompatible plasma: a survey of 3156 North American laboratories. Arch Pathol Lab Med 2007; 131: 909

149. Kleinman SH, Glynn SA, Lee TH, et al: Prevalence and quantitation of parvovirus B19 DNA levels in blood donors with a sensitive polymerase chain reaction screening assay. Transfusion 2007; 47: 1756

150. Parsyan A, Candotti D: Human erythrovirus B19 and blood transfusion - an update. Transfus Med 2007; 17: 263

151. Reiner A: Massive Transfusion, Perioperative Transfusion Medicine. Edited by Spiess B, Counts R, Gould S. Philadelphia: Williams & Wilkins, 1998, pp 351.

152. Key NS, Negrier C: Coagulation factor concentrates: past, present, and future. Lancet 2007; 370: 439

153. Vinazzer H: Clinical use of antithrombin III concentrations. Vox Sang 1997; 53: 193

154. Avidan MS, Levy JH, Scholz J, et al: A phase III, double-blind, placebo-controlled, multicenter study on the efficacy of recombinant human antithrombin in heparin-resistant patients scheduled to undergo cardiac surgery necessitating cardiopulmonary bypass. Anesthesiology 2005; 102: 276

155. Wiedermann CJ, Kaneider NC: A systematic review of antithrombin concentrate use in patients with disseminated intravascular coagulation of severe sepsis. Blood Coagul Fibrinolysis 2006; 17: 521

156. Hoffman M, Monroe DM: Coagulation 2006: a modern view of hemostasis. Hematol Oncol Clin North Am 2007; 21: 1

157. Tilley R, Mackman N: Tissue factor in hemostasis and thrombosis. Semin Thromb Hemost 2006; 32: 5

158. Monroe D, MKey NS: The tissue factor-factor VIIa complex: procoagulant activity, regulation, and multitasking. J Thromb Haemost 2007; 5: 1097

159. Zarbock A, Polanowska-Grabowska R, KLey K: Platelet-neutrophil-interactions: linking hemostasis and inflammation. Blood Rev 2007; 21: 99

160. Ofosu FA: Protease activated receptors 1 and 4 govern the responses of human platelets to thrombin. Transfus Apher Sci 2003; 28: 265

161. Wettstein P, Haeberli A, Stutz M, et al: Decreased factor XIII availability for thrombin and early loss of clot firmness in patients with unexplained intraoperative bleeding. Anesth Analg 2004; 99: 1564

162. Wolberg AS: Thrombin generation and fibrin clot structure. Blood Rev 2007; 21: 131

163. Mosnier LO, Bouma BN: Regulation of fibrinolysis by thrombin activatable fibrinolysis inhibitor, an unstable carboxypeptidase B that unites the pathways of coagulation and fibrinolysis. Arterioscler Thromb Vasc Biol 2006; 26: 2445

164. Nilsson IM: Coagulation and fibrinolysis. Scand J Gastroenterol Suppl 1987; 137: 11

165. Hoffman M: A cell-based model of coagulation and the role of factor VIIa. Blood Rev 2003; 17(Suppl 1): S1

166. Buller HR, ten Cate JW: Acquired antithrombin III deficiency: laboratory diagnosis, incidence, clinical implications, and treatment with antithrombin III concentrate. Am J Med 1989; 87: 44S

167. Sniecinski RM, Chen EP, Levy JH, et al: Coagulopathy after cardiopulmonary bypass in Jehovah's Witness patients: management of two cases using fractionated components and factor VIIa. Anesth Analg 2007; 104: 763

168. Bucur SZ, Levy JH, Despotis GJ, et al: Uses of antithrombin III concentrate in congenital and acquired deficiency states. Transfusion 1998; 38: 481

169. Lemmer JH, Jr., Despotis GJ: Antithrombin III concentrate to treat heparin resistance in patients undergoing cardiac surgery. J Thorac Cardiovasc Surg 2002; 123: 213

170. Cardigan R, Turner C, Harrison P: Current methods of assessing platelet function: relevance to transfusion medicine. Vox Sang 2005; 88: 153

171. Rodgers RP, Levin J: A critical reappraisal of the bleeding time. Semin Thromb Hemost 1990; 16: 1

172. Agarwal S, Coakley M, Reddy K, et al: Quantifying the effect of antiplatelet therapy: a comparison of the platelet function analyzer (PFA-100) and modified thromboelastography (mTEG) with light transmission platelet aggregometry. Anesthesiology 2006; 105: 676

173. Dyszkiewicz-Korpanty A, Olteanu H, Frenkel EP, et al: Clopidogrel antiplatelet effect: an evaluation by optical aggregometry, impedance aggregometry, and the platelet function analyzer (PFA-100). Platelets 2007; 18: 491

174. Hayward CP: Further complexities in diagnosing acquired thrombocytopenia: unexpected parallels between antibody-mediated delayed thrombocytopenia with abciximab and heparin induced thrombocytopenia. Thromb Haemost 2004; 92: 674

175. Nemerson Y: The tissue factor pathway of blood coagulation. Semin Hematol 1992; 29: 170

176. Poller L: The British system for anticoagulant control. Thromb Diath Haemorrh 1975; 33: 157

177. Henriksen R: Instrumentation and quality control of hemostasis, Clinical Hematology. Edited by Lotspiech-Steininger C S-ME, Koepke J. Philadelphia, J.B. Lippincott, 1992, pp 695

178. Triplett DA: Overview of hemostasis, Hemostatic Disorders and the Blood Bank. Edited by Menitove JE ML. Arlington, Va, American Association of Blood Banks, 1984, pp 1

179. Casserly IP, Kereiakes DJ, Gray WA, et al: Point-of-care ecarin clotting time versus activated clotting time in correlation with bivalirudin concentration. Thromb Res 2004; 113: 115

180. Murphy GS, Marymont JH: Alternative anticoagulation management strategies for the patient with heparin-induced thrombocytopenia undergoing cardiac surgery. J Cardiothorac Vasc Anesth 2007; 21: 113

181. Carroll RC, Chavez JJ, Simmons JW, et al: Measurement of patients' bivalirudin plasma levels by a thrombelastograph ecarin clotting time assay: a comparison to a standard activated clotting time. Anesth Analg 2006; 102: 1316

182. Traverso CI, Caprini JA, Arcelus JI: The normal thromboelastogram and its interpretation. Semin Thromb Hemost 1995; 21(Suppl 4): 7

183. Tuman KJ, Spiess BD, McCarthy RJ, et al: Effects of progressive blood loss on coagulation as measured by thrombelastography. Anesth Analg 1987; 66: 856

184. Kang W: Blood coagulation during liver, kidney, and pancreas transplantation, Blood: Hemostasis, Transfusion, and Alternatives in the Perioperative Period. Edited by Lake CL MR. New York, Raven Press, 1995, pp 529

185. Zuckerman L, Cohen E, Vagher JP, et al: Comparison of thromboelastography with common coagulation tests. Thromb Haemost 1981; 46: 752

186. Levine JS, Branch DWRauch J: The antiphospholipid syndrome. N Engl J Med 2002; 346: 752

187. Neunert CE, Journeycake JM: Congenital platelet disorders. Hematol Oncol Clin North Am 2007; 21: 663

188. Ewenstein BM: Von Willebrand's disease. Annu Rev Med 1997; 48: 525

189. Vischer UM, de Moerloose P: von Willebrand factor: from cell biology to the clinical management of von Willebrand's disease. Crit Rev Oncol Hematol 1999; 30: 93

190. Federici AB, Mazurier C, Berntorp E, et al: Biologic response to desmopressin in patients with severe type 1 and type 2 von Willebrand disease: results of a multicenter European study. Blood 2004; 103: 2032

191. Rodeghiero F, Castaman G: Treatment of von Willebrand disease. Semin Hematol 2005; 42: 29

192. Franchini M: The use of desmopressin as a hemostatic agent: a concise review. Am J Hematol 2007; 82: 731

193. Mannucci PM: Treatment of von Willebrand's Disease. N Engl J Med 2004; 351: 683

194. Michiels JJ, Berneman ZN, van der Planken M, et al: Bleeding prophylaxis for major surgery in patients with type 2 von Willebrand disease with an

intermediate purity factor VIII-von Willebrand factor concentrate (Hae-mate-P). Blood Coagul Fibrinolysis 2004; 15: 323

195. Franchini M, Gandini G, Veneri D, et al: Safety and efficacy of subcuta-neous bolus injection of deferoxamine in adult patients with iron overload: an update. Blood 2004; 103: 747

196. Lee JW: von Willebrand disease, hemophilia A and B, and other factor defi-ciencies. Int Anesthesiol Clin 2004; 42: 59

197. Kaufmann JE, Vischer UM: Cellular mechanisms of the hemostatic effects of desmopressin (DDAVP). J Thromb Haemost 2003; 1: 682

198. Warrier AI, Lusher JM: DDAVP: a useful alternative to blood components in moderate hemophilia A and von Willebrand disease. J Pediatr 1983; 102: 228

199. Sohal AS, Gangji AS, Crowther MA, et al: Uremic bleeding: pathophysiol-ogy and clinical risk factors. Thromb Res 2006; 118: 417

200. Gangji AS, Sohal AS, Treleaven D, et al: Bleeding in patients with renal insuf-ficiency: a practical guide to clinical management. Thromb Res 2006; 118: 423

201. Moia M, Mannucci PM, Vizzotto L, et al: Improvement in the haemostatic defect of uraemia after treatment with recombinant human erythropoietin. Lancet 1987; 2: 1227

202. Tran HA, Anand SS, Hankey GJ, et al: Aspirin resistance. Thromb Res 2007; 120: 337

203. Steffel J, Luscher TF, Ruschitzka F, et al: Cyclooxygenase-2 inhibition and coagulation. J Cardiovasc Pharmacol 2006; 47(Suppl 1): S15

204. Kam PC, Egan MK: Platelet glycoprotein IIb/IIIa antagonists: pharmacol-ogy and clinical developments. Anesthesiology 2002; 96: 1237

205. Merlini PA, Rossi M, Menozzi A, et al: Thrombocytopenia caused by abciximab or tirofiban and its association with clinical outcome in patients undergoing coronary stenting. Circulation 2004; 109: 2203

206. Couris RR: Vitamins and minerals that affect hemostasis and antithrom-botic therapies. Thromb Res 2005; 117: 25

207. Szuwart T, Brzoska T, Luger TA, et al: Vitamin E reduces platelet adhesion to human endothelial cells in vitro. Am J Hematol 2000; 65: 1

208. Makris M, Watson HG: The management of coumarin-induced over-anti-coagulation Annotation. Br J Haematol 2001; 114: 271

209. Baglin TP, Keeling DM, Watson HG: Guidelines on oral anticoagulation (warfarin): third edition—2005 update. Br J Haematol 2006; 132: 277

210. Makris M: Optimisation of the prothrombin complex concentrate dose for warfarin reversal. Thromb Res 2005; 115: 451

211. Ghorashian S, Hunt BJ: "Off-license" use of recombinant activated factor VII. Blood Rev 2004; 18: 245

212. Dickneite G: Prothrombin complex concentrate versus recombinant factor VIIa for reversal of coumarin anticoagulation. Thromb Res 2007; 119: 643

213. O'Connell KA, Wood JJ, Wise RP, et al: Thromboembolic adverse events after use of recombinant human coagulation factor VIIa. JAMA 2006; 295: 293

214. Geerts WH, Pineo GF, Heit JA, et al: Prevention of venous thromboem-bolism: the Seventh ACCP Conference on Antithrombotic and Throm-bolytic Therapy. Chest 2004; 126: 338S

215. Bombeli T, Spahn DR: Updates in perioperative coagulation: physiology and management of thromboembolism and haemorrhage. Br J Anaesth 2004; 93: 275

216. Groce JB 3rd: Treatment of deep vein thrombosis using low-molecular-weight heparins. Am J Manag Care 2001; 7: S510

217. Boneu B, de Moerloose P: How and when to monitor a patient treated with low molecular weight heparin. Semin Thromb Hemost 2001; 27: 519

218. Walenga JM, Jeske WP, Prechel MM, et al: Decreased prevalence of heparin-induced thrombocytopenia with low-molecular-weight heparin and related drugs. Semin Thromb Hemost 2004; 30(Suppl 1): 69

219. Warkentin TE: Heparin-induced thrombocytopenia. Hematol Oncol Clin North Am 2007; 21: 589

220. Levy JH, Tanaka KA, Hursting MJ: Reducing thrombotic complications in the perioperative setting: an update on heparin-induced thrombocytopenia. Anesth Analg 2007; 105: 570

221. Gruel Y, Pouplard C, Nguyen P, et al: Biological and clinical features of low-molecular-weight heparin-induced thrombocytopenia. Br J Haematol 2003; 121: 786

222. Hirsh J, O'Donnell M, Eikelboom JW: Beyond unfractionated heparin and warfarin: current and future advances. Circulation 2007; 116: 552

223. Koster A, Kukucka M, Bach F, et al: Anticoagulation during cardiopul-monary bypass in patients with heparin-induced thrombocytopenia type II and renal impairment using heparin and the platelet glycoprotein IIb-IIIa antagonist tirofiban. Anesthesiology 2001; 94: 245

224. Despotis GJ, Joist JH: Anticoagulation and anticoagulation reversal with cardiac surgery involving cardiopulmonary bypass: an update. J Cardio-thorac Vasc Anesth 1999; 13: 18

225. Paparella D, Galeone A, Venneri MT, et al: Activation of the coagulation system during coronary artery bypass grafting: comparison between on-pump and off-pump techniques. J Thorac Cardiovasc Surg 2006; 131: 290

226. Paparella D, Al Radi OO, Meng QH, et al: The effects of high-dose heparin on inflammatory and coagulation parameters following cardiopulmonary bypass. Blood Coagul Fibrinolysis 2005; 16: 323

227. Body SC, Morse DS: Coagulation, transfusion and cardiac surgery, Perioperative Transfusion Medicine. Edited by Spiess BD, Counts RB, Gould SA. Baltimore, Williams & Wilkins, 1998, pp 419

228. White CM: Thrombin-directed inhibitors: pharmacology and clinical use. Am Heart J 2005; 149: S54

229. Wasowicz M, Vegas A, Borger MA, et al: Bivalirudin anticoagulation for cardiopulmonary bypass in a patient with heparin-induced thrombocy-topenia. Can J Anaesth 2005; 52: 1093

230. Dyke CM, Smedira NG, Koster A, et al: A comparison of bivalirudin to heparin with protamine reversal in patients undergoing cardiac surgery with cardiopulmonary bypass: the EVOLUTION-ON study. J Thorac Car-diovasc Surg 2006; 131: 533

231. Koster A, Chew D, Grundel M, et al: An assessment of different filter sys-tems for extracorporeal elimination of bivalirudin: an in vitro study. Anesth Analg 2003; 96: 1316

232. Bramlage P, Pittrow D, Kirch W: Current concepts for the prevention of venous thromboembolism. Eur J Clin Invest 2005; 35(Suppl 1): 4

233. Warkentin TE, Cook RJ, Marder VJ, et al: Anti-platelet factor 4/heparin antibodies in orthopedic surgery patients receiving antithrombotic prophy-laxis with fondaparinux or enoxaparin. Blood 2005; 106: 3791

234. Kahl B, Schwartz B, Mosher D: Profound imbalance of pro-fibrinolytic and anti-fibrinolytic factors (tissue plasminogen activator and plasminogen activator inhibitor type 1) and severe bleeding diathesis in a patient with cirrhosis: correction by liver transplantation. Blood Coagulation and Fibri-nolysis 2003; 14: 741

235. Staudinger T, Locker GJ, Frass M: Management of acquired coagulation disorders in emergency and intensive-care medicine. Semin Thromb Hemost 1996; 22: 93

236. Bick RL: Disseminated intravascular coagulation current concepts of etiol-ogy, pathophysiology, diagnosis, and treatment. Hematol Oncol Clin North Am 2003; 17: 149

237. Levi M: Current understanding of disseminated intravascular coagulation. Br J Haematol 2004; 124: 567

238. Zeerleder S, Hack CE, Wuillemin WA: Disseminated intravascular coagu-lation in sepsis. Chest 2005; 128: 2864

239. Carey MJ, Rodgers GM: Disseminated intravascular coagulation: clinical and laboratory aspects. Am J Hematol 1998; 59: 65

240. Dempfle CE: Coagulopathy of sepsis. Thromb Haemost 2004; 91: 213

241. Roberts HR, Monroe DM, White GC: The use of recombinant factor VIIa in the treatment of bleeding disorders. Blood 2004; 104: 3858

242. Welsby IJ, Monroe DM, Lawson JH, et al: Recombinant activated factor VII and the anaesthetist. Anaesthesia 2005; 60: 1203

243. Friederich PW, Henny CP, Messelink EJ, et al: Effect of recombinant acti-vated factor VII on perioperative blood loss in patients undergoing retrop-ubic prostatectomy: a double-blind placebo-controlled randomised trial. Lancet 2003; 361: 201

244. Boffard KD, Riou B, Warren B, et al: Recombinant factor VIIa as adjunc-tive therapy for bleeding control in severely injured trauma patients: two parallel randomized, placebo-controlled, double-blind clinical trials. J Trauma 2005; 59: 8

245. Diprose P, Herbertson MJ, O'Shaughnessy D, et al: Activated recombinant factor VII after cardiopulmonary bypass reduces allogeneic transfusion in complex non-coronary cardiac surgery: randomized double-blind placebo-controlled pilot study. Br J Anaesth 2005; 95: 596

246. Mayer SA, Brun NC, Begtrup K, et al: Recombinant activated factor VII for acute intracerebral hemorrhage. N Engl J Med 2005; 352: 777

247. Hedner U: Mechanism of action of factor VIIa in the treatment of coagu-lopathies. Semin Thromb Hemost 2006; 32(Suppl 1): 77

248. Martinowitz U, Michaelson M: Guidelines for the use of recombinant acti-vated factor VII (rFVIIa) in uncontrolled bleeding: a report by the Israeli Multidisciplinary rFVIIa Task Force. J Thromb Haemost 2005; 3: 640

249. Firozvi K, Deveras RA, Kessler CM: Reversal of low-molecular-weight heparin-induced bleeding in patients with pre-existing hypercoagulable states with human recombinant activated factor VII concentrate. Am J Hematol 2006; 81: 582

250. Khan AZ, Parry JM, Crowley WF, et al: Recombinant factor VIIa for the treatment of severe postoperative and traumatic hemorrhage. Am J Surg 2005; 189: 331

251. Shander A, Goodnough LT, Ratko T, et al: Consensus Recommendations for the Off-Label Use of Recombinant Human Factor VIIa (NovoSeven®) Therapy. P&T Journal 2005; 30: 644

252. Gordz S, Mrowietz C, Pindur G, et al: Effect of desmopressin (DDAVP) on platelet membrane glycoprotein expression in patients with von Wille-brand's disease. Clin Hemorheol Microcirc 2005; 32: 83

253. Cattaneo M, Harris AS, Stromberg U, et al: The effect of desmopressin on reducing blood loss in cardiac surgery—a meta-analysis of double-blind, placebo-controlled trials. Thromb Haemost 1995; 74: 1064

254. Salzman EW, Weinstein MJ, Weintraub RM, et al: Treatment with desmo-pressin acetate to reduce blood loss after cardiac surgery. A double-blind randomized trial. N Engl J Med 1986; 314: 1402

255. Czer LS, Bateman TM, Gray RJ, et al: Treatment of severe platelet dys-function and hemorrhage after cardiopulmonary bypass: reduction in blood product usage with desmopressin. J Am Coll Cardiol 1987; 9: 1139

256. Mongan PD, Hosking MP: The role of desmopressin acetate in patients undergoing coronary artery bypass surgery. A controlled clinical trial with thromboelastographic risk stratification. Anesthesiology 1992; 77: 38

257. Gratz I, Koehler J, Olsen D, et al: The effect of desmopressin acetate on postoperative hemorrhage in patients receiving aspirin therapy before coronary artery bypass operations. J Thorac Cardiovasc Surg 1992; 104: 1417

ANATOMY AND PHYSIOLOGY

258. Carless PA, Henry DA, Moxey AJ, et al: Desmopressin for minimising peri-operative allogeneic blood transfusion. Cochrane Database Syst Rev 2004; CD001884

259. Diprose P, Herbertson MJ, O'Shaughnessy D, et al: Reducing allogeneic transfusion in cardiac surgery: a randomized double-blind placebo-controlled trial of antifibrinolytic therapies used in addition to intra-opera-tive cell salvage. Br J Anaesth 2005; 94: 271

260. Zufferey P, Merquiol F, Laporte S, et al: Do antifibrinolytics reduce allo-geneic blood transfusion in orthopedic surgery? Anesthesiology 2006; 105: 1034

261. Henry DA, Carless PA, Moxey AJ, et al: Anti-fibrinolytic use for minimis-ing perioperative allogeneic blood transfusion. Cochrane Database Syst Rev 2007; CD001886

262. Molenaar IQ, Warnaar N, Groen H, et al: Efficacy and safety of antifibri-nolytic drugs in liver transplantation: a systematic review and meta-analy-sis. Am J Transplant 2007; 7: 185

263. Mangano DT, Tudor IC, Dietzel C: The risk associated with aprotinin in cardiac surgery. N Engl J Med 2006; 354: 353

264. Mangano DT, Miao Y, Vuylsteke A, et al: Mortality associated with apro-tinin during 5 years following coronary artery bypass graft surgery. JAMA 2007; 297: 471

265. Cirino G, Napoli C, Bucci M, et al: Inflammation-coagulation network: are serine protease receptors the knot? Trends Pharmacol Sci 2000; 21: 170

266. McEvoy MD, Reeves ST, Reves JG, et al: Aprotinin in cardiac surgery: a review of conventional and novel mechanisms of action. Anesth Analg 2007; 105: 949

267. Day JR, Taylor KM, Lidington EA, et al: Aprotinin inhibits proinflamma-tory activation of endothelial cells by thrombin through the protease-acti-vated receptor 1. J Thorac Cardiovasc Surg 2006; 131: 21

268. van Oeveren W, Harder MP, Roozendaal KJ, et al: Aprotinin protects platelets against the initial effect of cardiopulmonary bypass. J Thorac Cardiovasc Surg 1990; 99: 788

269. Levi M, Cromheecke ME, de Jonge E, et al: Pharmacological strategies to decrease excessive blood loss in cardiac surgery: a meta-analysis of clini-cally relevant endpoints. Lancet 1999; 354: 1940

270. Sedrakyan A, Treasure T, Elefteriades JA: Effect of aprotinin on clinical outcomes in coronary artery bypass graft surgery: a systematic review and meta-analysis of randomized clinical trials. J Thorac Cardiovasc Surg 2004; 128: 442

271. Karkouti K, Beattie WS, Dattilo KM, et al: A propensity score case-control comparison of aprotinin and tranexamic acid in high-transfusion-risk car-diac surgery. Transfusion 2006; 46: 327

272. Furnary AP, Wu Y, Hiratzka LF, et al: Aprotinin does not increase the risk of renal failure in cardiac surgery patients. Circulation 2007; 116: I127

273. Dietrich W, Busley R, Boulesteix AL: Effects of aprotinin dosage on renal function: an analysis of 8,548 cardiac surgical patients treated with differ-ent dosages of aprotinin. Anesthesiology 2008; 108: 189

274. Schneeweiss S, Seeger JD, Landon J, et al: Aprotinin during coronary-artery bypass grafting and risk of death. N Engl J Med 2008; 358: 771

275. Casati V, Guzzon D, Oppizzi M, et al: Hemostatic effects of aprotinin, tranexamic acid and epsilon-aminocaproic acid in primary cardiac surgery. Ann Thorac Surg 1999; 68: 2252

276. Bowden RA, Slichter SJ, Sayers MH, et al: Use of leukocyte-depleted platelets and cytomegalovirus-seronegative red blood cells for prevention of primary cytomegalovirus infection after marrow transplant. Blood 1991; 78: 246

277. Klein HG, Spahn DR, Carson JL: Red blood cell transfusion in clinical practice. Lancet 2007; 370: 415

278. Walker RH: Special report: transfusion risks. Am J Clin Pathol 1987; 88: 374

279. Kang Y, Lewis JH, Navalgund A, et al: Epsilon-aminocaproic acid for treat-ment of fibrinolysis during liver transplantation. Anesthesiology 1987; 66: 766

280. Kang Y: Monitoring and treatment of coagulation, Hepatic Transplanta-tion: Anesthetic and Periperative Management. Edited by Winter K, Kang Y. New York, Praeger, 1986, pp 151

CHAPTER 17 ■ INHALED ANESTHETICS

THOMAS J. EBERT AND PHILLIP G. SCHMID

ANESTHETIC AGENTS, ADJUVANTS, AND DRUG INTERACTION

KEY POINTS

1. At equilibrium, the CNS partial pressure of inhaled anesthetics equals their arterial partial pressure, which in turn equals their alveolar partial pressure if cardiopulmonary function is normal.

2. Isoflurane is the most potent of the volatile anesthetics in clinical use, desflurane is the least soluble, and sevoflurane is the least irritating to the airways.

3. The inspired concentration and the blood:gas solubility of an inhaled anesthetic are the major determinants of the speed of induction. Solubility alone determines the rate of elimination, provided there is normal cardiopulmonary function.

4. Nitrous oxide can expand a pneumothorax to double or triple its size in 10 to 30 minutes, and washout of nitrous oxide can lower alveolar concentrations of oxygen and carbon dioxide, a phenomenon called *diffusion hypoxia*.

5. Minimum alveolar concentration (MAC) is the alveolar concentration of an inhaled anesthetic at one atmosphere that prevents movement in response to a surgical stimulus in 50% of patients. Concentrations of inhaled anesthetics that provide loss of awareness and recall are about 0.4 to 0.5 MAC.

6. Excluding data in patients <1 year of age (where MAC is lower than in older children), MAC decreases approximately 6% per decade.

7. Volatile anesthetics depress cerebral metabolic rate and increase cerebral blood flow (CBF) in a dose-dependent manner. The latter effect may increase intracranial pressure in patients with a mass-occupying lesion of the brain.

8. Hypocapnia may blunt or abolish volatile anesthetic-induced increases in CBF depending on when the hypocapnia is produced and the nature of the cerebral disease process.

9. Volatile anesthetics produce dose-dependent depression of the electroencephalogram, sensory-evoked potentials, and motor-evoked potentials.

10. Volatile anesthetics in current use decrease arterial blood pressure, systemic vascular resistance, and myocardial function comparably and in a dose-dependent fashion.

11. Volatile anesthetics decrease tidal volume, decrease ventilatory response to hypercarbia and hypoxia, increase respiratory rate, and relax airway smooth muscle in a dose-dependent fashion.

12 Unlike halothane, volatile anesthetics in current use have minimal adverse effects on the liver and might afford some protection for hepatocytes from ischemic and/or hypoxic injury.

13 Volatile anesthetics are potent triggers for malignant hyperthermia in genetically susceptible patients, while nitrous oxide is only a weak trigger.

14 CO_2 absorbents degrade sevoflurane, desflurane, and isoflurane to carbon monoxide when the normal water content of the absorbent (13 to 15%) is markedly decreased (<5%).

Inhalation anesthetics are the most common drugs used for the provision of general anesthesia. Adding only a fraction of a volatile anesthetic to the inspired oxygen results in a state of unconsciousness and amnesia. When combined with intravenous adjuvants, such as opioids and benzodiazepines, a balanced technique is achieved that results in analgesia, further sedation/hypnosis, and amnesia. The popularity of the inhaled anesthetics for surgical procedures is because of their ease of administration and the ability to reliably monitor their effects with both clinical signs and end-tidal concentrations. In addition, the volatile anesthetic gases are relatively inexpensive in terms of the overall cost.

The most popular potent inhaled anesthetics used in adult surgical procedures are sevoflurane, desflurane, and isoflurane (Fig. 17-1). In pediatric cases, sevoflurane is most commonly employed. Although there are many similarities in terms of the overall effects of the volatile anesthetics (e.g., they all have a dose-dependent effect to decrease blood pressure), there are some unique differences that might influence the clinician's selection process depending on the patient's health and the surgical procedure. Discussion of the three most popular inhaled anesthetics provides the major emphasis of this chapter. For the sake of completeness and for historical perspective related to metabolism and toxicity, comments on halothane, enflurane, and methoxyflurane also are included.

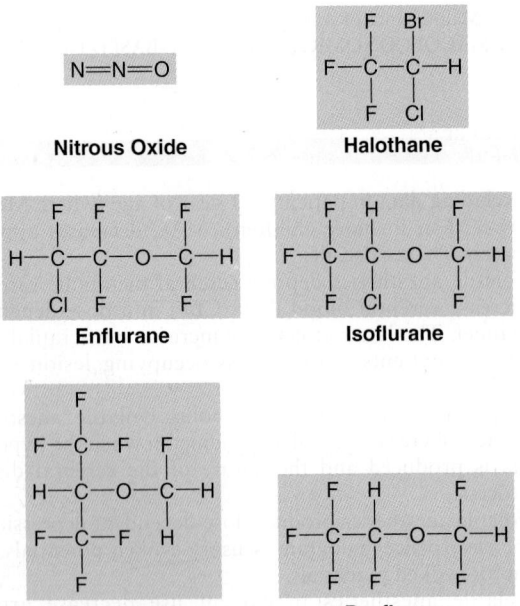

FIGURE 17-1. Chemical structure of inhaled anesthetics. Halothane is an alkane, a halogen-substituted ethane derivative. It is no longer available commercially. Isoflurane and enflurane are isomers that are methyl ethyl ethers. Desflurane differs from isoflurane in the substitution of a fluorine for a chlorine atom and sevoflurane is a methyl isopropyl ether.

PHARMACOKINETIC PRINCIPLES

Kety[1] in 1950 was the first to examine the pharmacokinetics of inhaled agents in a systematic fashion. Eger[2] accomplished much of the early research in the field, leading to his landmark text on the subject in 1974. The inhaled anesthetics differ substantially from nearly all other drugs because they are gases given via inhalation. This makes their pharmacokinetics unique as well, and thus discussion of pharmacokinetic principles of currently used agents is necessary for understanding and predicting their effects.

Drug pharmacology is classically divided into two disciplines, pharmacodynamics and pharmacokinetics. *Pharmacodynamics* can be defined as what drugs do to the body. It describes the desired and undesired effects of drugs, as well as the cellular and molecular changes leading to these effects. *Pharmacokinetics* can be defined as what the body does to drugs. It describes where drugs go, how they are transformed, and the cellular and molecular mechanisms underlying these processes.

Tissues are often grouped into hypothetical *compartments* based on perfusion. An important implication of different compartments and perfusion rates is the concept of redistribution. After a given amount of drug is administered, it reaches highly perfused tissue compartments first, where it can equilibrate rapidly and exert its effects. With time, however, compartments with lower perfusion rates receive the drug and additional equilibria are established between blood and these tissues. As the tissues with lower perfusion absorb drug, maintenance of equilibria throughout the body requires drug transfer from highly perfused compartments back into the bloodstream. This lowering of drug concentration in one compartment by delivery into another compartment is called *redistribution*.

In discussions of the inhaled anesthetics, the absorption phase is usually called *uptake*, the metabolic phase is usually called *biotransformation*, and the excretion phase is usually called *elimination*.

Unique Features of Inhaled Anesthetics

Speed, Gas State, and Route of Administration

The inhaled anesthetics are among the most rapidly acting drugs in existence, and when administering a general anesthetic, this speed provides a margin of safety. The ability to quickly increase or decrease anesthetic levels as necessary can mean the difference between an anesthetic state and an anesthetic misadventure. Speed also means efficiency. Rapid induction and recovery may lead to faster operating room turnover times, shorter recovery room stays, and earlier discharges to home.

Technically, of the inhaled anesthetics only nitrous oxide and xenon are true gases, while the so-called *potent agents* are the vapors of volatile liquids. But for simplicity, all of them are referred to as gases because they are all in the gas phase when administered via the lungs. As gases, none deviate significantly from ideal gas behavior. These agents are all non-ionized and have low molecular weights. This allows them to diffuse rapidly without the need for facilitated diffusion or active

TABLE 17-1

PHYSIOCHEMICAL PROPERTIES OF VOLATILE ANESTHETICS

PROPERTY	SEVOFLURANE	DESFLURANE	ISOFLURANE	ENFLURANE	HALOTHANE	N_2O
Boiling point (°C)	59	24	49	57	50	−88
Vapor pressure at 20°C (mm Hg)	157	669	238	172	243	38,770
Molecular weight (g)	200	168	184	184	197	44
Oil:gas partition coefficient	47	19	91	97	224	1.4
Blood:gas partition coefficient	0.65	0.42	1.46	1.9	2.50	0.46
Brain:blood solubility	1.7	1.3	1.6	1.4	1.9	1.1
Fat:blood solubility	47.5	27.2	44.9	36	51.1	2.3
Muscle:blood solubility	3.1	2.0	2.9	1.7	3.4	1.2
MAC in O_2 30–60 yr, at 37°C P_B760 (%)	1.8	6.6	1.17	1.63	0.75	104
MAC in 60–70% N_2O (%)	0.66	2.38	0.56	0.57	0.29	
MAC, >65 yr (%)	1.45	5.17	1.0	1.55	0.64	—
Preservative	No	No	No	No	Thymol	No
Stable in moist CO_2 absorber	No	Yes	Yes	Yes	No	Yes
Flammability (%) (in 70% N_2O/30% O_2)	10	17	7	5.8	4.8	
Recovered as metabolites (%)	2–5	0.02	0.2	2.4	20	

MAC, minimum alveolar concentration; N_2O, nitrous oxide.

transport from bloodstream to tissues. The other advantage of gases is that they can be delivered to the bloodstream via a unique route available in all patients: the lungs.

Speed, gaseous state, and the lung route of administration combine to form the major beneficial feature of the inhaled anesthetics: the ability to decrease plasma concentrations as easily and as rapidly as they are increased.

Physical Characteristics of Inhaled Anesthetics

The physical characteristics of inhaled anesthetics are shown in Table 17-1. The goal of delivering inhaled anesthetics is to produce the anesthetic state by establishing a specific concentration of anesthetic molecules in the central nervous system (CNS). This is done by establishing the specific partial pressure of the agent in the lungs, which ultimately equilibrates with the brain and spinal cord. At equilibrium, CNS partial pressure equals blood partial pressure, which in turn equals alveolar partial pressure:

$$P_{CNS} = P_{blood} = P_{alveoli} \qquad (17\text{-}1)$$

where P is partial pressure. Equilibration is a result of three factors:

1. Inhaled anesthetics are gases rapidly transferred bidirectionally via the lungs to and from the bloodstream and subsequently to and from CNS tissues as partial pressures equilibrate.
2. Plasma and tissues have a low capacity to absorb the inhaled anesthetics relative to the amount we can deliver to the lungs, allowing us to quickly establish or abolish anesthetizing concentrations of anesthetic in the bloodstream and ultimately the CNS.

3. Metabolism, excretion, and redistribution of the inhaled anesthetics are minimal relative to the rate at which they are delivered or removed from the lungs. This permits easy maintenance of blood and CNS concentrations.

The so-called *permanent gases*, such as oxygen and nitrogen, exist only as gases at ambient temperatures. Gases such as nitrous oxide can be compressed into liquids under high pressure at ambient temperature. Most *potent volatile anesthetics* are liquids at ambient temperature and pressure. If the system in which the volatile liquid resides is a closed container, molecules of the substance will equilibrate between the liquid and gas phases. At equilibrium, the pressure exerted by molecular collisions of the gas against the container walls is the *vapor pressure*. One important property of vapor pressure is that as long as *any* liquid remains in the container, the vapor pressure is independent of the volume of that liquid. As with any gas, however, vapor pressure is proportional to temperature.

For all of the potent agents, at 20°C the vapor pressure is below atmospheric pressure. If the temperature is raised, the vapor pressure increases. The *boiling point* of a liquid is the temperature at which its vapor pressure exceeds atmospheric pressure in an open container. Desflurane is bottled in a special container because its boiling point of 23.5°C makes it boil at typical room temperatures. Boiling does not occur within the bottle because it is countered by buildup of vapor pressure within the bottle, but once opened to air, the desflurane would quickly boil away. The bottle is designed to allow transfer of desflurane from bottle to vaporizer without exposure to the atmosphere.

Gases in Mixtures

For any mixture of gases in a closed container, each gas exerts a pressure proportional to its *fractional mass*. This is its *partial pressure*. The sum of the partial pressures of each gas in a mixture of gases equals the total pressure of the entire mixture (Dalton's law).

$$P_{total} = P_{gas1} + P_{gas2} + \cdots + P_{gasN} \qquad (17\text{-}2)$$

Another way to state this is that each gas in a mixture of gases at a given volume and temperature has a partial pressure that is the pressure it would have *if it alone* occupied the volume. The entire mixture behaves just as if it were a single gas according to the ideal gas law.

Gases in Solution

Partial pressure of a gas in solution is a bit complex because pressure can only be measured in the gas phase, while in solution the amount of gas is measured as a concentration. Partial pressure of a gas in solution refers to the pressure of the gas in the gas phase (if it were present) in equilibrium with the liquid. It is important to talk of partial pressures, however, because gases equilibrate based on partial pressures, not concentrations.

Gas molecules within a liquid interact with solvent molecules to a much larger extent than do molecules in the gas phase. *Solubility* is the term used to describe the tendency of a gas to equilibrate with a solution, hence determining its concentration in solution. Henry's law expresses the relationship of concentration of a gas in solution to the partial pressure of the gas with which the solution is in equilibrium:

$$C_g = kP_g \qquad (17\text{-}3)$$

where C_g is concentration of gas in solution, k is a solubility constant, and P_g is the partial pressure of the gas. From Equation 17-3 one can see that doubling the pressure of a gas doubles its concentration in solution. A more clinically useful expression of solubility is the solubility coefficient, λ:

$$\lambda = V_{dissolved\ gas}/V_{liquid} \text{ at } 37°C \qquad (17\text{-}4)$$

where V = volume. This equation states that for any gas in equilibrium with a liquid, a certain volume of that gas dissolves in a given volume of liquid.

The principles of partial pressures and solubility apply in mixtures of gases in solution. That is, the concentration of any one gas in a mixture of gases in solution depends on two factors: (1) its partial pressure in the gas phase in equilibrium with the solution, and (2) its solubility within that solution.

The implications of these properties are that anesthetic gases administered via the lungs diffuse into blood until the partial pressures in alveoli and blood are equal. The concentration of anesthetic in the blood depends on the partial pressure at equilibrium and the blood solubility. Likewise, transfer of anesthetic from blood to target tissues also proceeds toward equalizing partial pressures, but at this interface there is no gas phase. A partial pressure still exists to force anesthetic molecules out of solution and into a gas phase but there is no gas phase because blood (outside the lungs) and tissues are like closed, liquid-filled containers. Remember the principle: the partial pressure of a gas in solution represents the pressure that the gas in equilibrium with the liquid *would have* if a gas phase existed in contact with the liquid phase.

The concentration of anesthetic in target tissue depends on the partial pressure at equilibrium and the target tissue solubility. Because inhaled anesthetics are gases, and because partial pressures of gases equilibrate throughout a system, *monitoring the alveolar concentration of inhaled anesthetics provides an index of their effects in the brain*.

In summary:

1. Inhaled anesthetics equilibrate based on their partial pressures in each tissue (or tissue compartment), *not* based on their concentrations.
2. The partial pressure of a gas in solution is defined by the partial pressure in the gas phase with which it is in equilibrium. Where there is no gas phase the partial pressure reflects a force to escape out of solution.
3. The concentration of anesthetic in a tissue depends on its partial pressure and tissue solubility.

Finally, the particular terminology used when referring to gases in the gas phase or absorbed in plasma or tissues is important. Inspired concentrations or fractional volumes of inhaled anesthetic are typically used rather than partial pressure. Partial pressure is expressed in millimeters of mercury (mm Hg) or torr (1 torr = 1 mm Hg) or kilopascals (kPa). For most drugs, concentration is expressed as mass (milligram [mg]) per volume (milliliter [mL]), but it can also be expressed in percent by weight or volume. Because volume of a gas in the gas phase is directly proportional to mass according to the ideal gas law, it is easier to express this fractional concentration as a percent by volume. In the gas phase, fractional concentration is equal to the partial pressure divided by ambient pressure, usually atmospheric, or:

$$\text{Fractional Volume} = P_{anesthetic}/P_{barometric} \qquad (17\text{-}5)$$

Anesthetic Transfer: Machine to Central Nervous System

When the fresh gas flow and the vaporizer are turned on, fresh gas with a fixed fractional concentration of anesthetic leaves the fresh gas outlet and mixes with the gas in the circuit—the bag, tubing, absorbent canister, and piping. It is immediately diluted to a lower fractional concentration, then slowly rises as this compartment equilibrates with the fresh gas flow. With spontaneous patient ventilation by mask, the anesthetic gas passes from circuit to airways. The fractional concentration of anesthetic leaving the circuit is designated as F_I (fraction inspired). In the lungs the gas comprising the dead space in the airways (trachea, bronchi) and the alveoli further dilutes the circuit gas. The fractional concentration of anesthetic present in the alveoli is F_A (fraction alveolar). The anesthetic then passes across the alveolar–capillary membrane and dissolves in pulmonary blood according to the partial pressure of the gas and its blood solubility. It is further diluted and travels via bulk blood flow throughout the vascular tree. The anesthetic then passes via simple diffusion from blood to tissues as well as between tissues.

The vascular system delivers blood to three physiologic tissue groups; the vessel-rich group (VRG), the muscle group, and the fat group. The VRG includes the brain, heart, kidney, liver, digestive tract, and glandular tissues. The percent of body mass and perfusion of each group are shown in Table 17-2. The CNS tissues of the VRG are referred to as *tissues of desired effect*. The other tissues of the VRG that comprise the compartment are referred to as *tissues of undesired effects*. The tissues of the muscle and fat groups comprise the *tissues of accumulation*.

Anesthetic is delivered most rapidly to the VRG because of high blood flow. Here it diffuses according to partial pressure gradients. CNS tissue takes in the anesthetic according to the tissue solubility, and at a high enough tissue concentration, unconsciousness and anesthesia are achieved. Increasing CNS tissue concentrations cause progressively deeper stages of anesthesia. As this is occurring, anesthetic is also distributing to other VRG tissues. Also coincident with delivery to the

TABLE 17-2

DISTRIBUTION OF CARDIAC OUTPUT BY TISSUE GROUP

GROUP	% BODY MASS	% CARDIAC OUTPUT	PERFUSION (mL/min/100 g)
Vessel-rich	10	75	75
Muscle	50	19	3
Fat	20	6	3

CNS, anesthetic is being delivered—albeit more slowly because of lower perfusion—to muscle and fat, where it accumulates and may affect the speed of emergence from the anesthetic. In reality, the fat solubilities provide little influence on emergence in cases lasting <4 hours since the delivery of anesthetic to fat tissue is extremely slow as a result of low blood flow. The concentration of inhaled anesthetic in a given tissue at a particular time during the administration depends not only on tissue blood flow, but also on tissue solubility, which governs how the inhaled anesthetics partition themselves between blood and tissue. Partitioning depends on the relative solubilities of the anesthetic for each compartment. These relative solubilities are expressed by a partition coefficient, δ, which is the ratio of dissolved gas (by volume) in two-tissue compartments at equilibrium. Some of the partition coefficients for the inhaled anesthetics are shown in Table 17-1.

Uptake and Distribution

F_A/F_I

A simple, common way to assess anesthetic uptake is to follow the ratio of fractional concentration of alveolar anesthetic to inspired anesthetic (F_A/F_I) over time. Experimentally derived data for F_A/F_I versus time during induction are shown in Figure 17-2. The faster F_A rises relative to F_I, the faster the speed of induction since F_A is proportional to P_A ($F_A = P_A/P_{barometric}$) and $P_A = P_{blood} = P_{CNS}$; that is, the alveolar fraction is directly proportional to the partial pressure of anesthetic in the CNS.

As fresh gas carrying anesthetic begins to flow into the air-filled circuit (assuming complete mixing), the concentration in the circuit (F_I) will rise according to first-order kinetics:

$$F_I = F_{FGO}(1 - e^{-T/\tau}) \qquad (17\text{-}6)$$

F_{FGO} is the fraction of inspired anesthetic in the gas leaving the fresh gas outlet (i.e., the vaporizer setting), T is time, and τ is a time constant. The time constant is simply the volume or "capacity" of the circuit (V_C) divided by the fresh gas flow (FGF) or $\tau = V_C/FGF$. For example, if the bag, tubing, absorbent canister, and piping comprise 8 L, and the fresh gas flow is 2 L, the time constant $\tau = {}^8/_2 = 4$. One of the characteristics of first-order kinetics is that 95% of maximum is reached after three time constants—in this case, $3 \times 4 = 12$ minutes.

Because 12 minutes is relatively long, starting with a higher F_{FGO} can increase the rate of rise of F_I. Using the earlier example with $\tau = 4$, by first-order kinetics 63% of maximum is reached after one time constant, or 4 minutes. To attain an F_I of 2% at 4 instead of 12 minutes, the F_{FGO} can be set to 3.2% (2% divided by 0.63) and then lowered to 2% at the 4-minute mark.

Other ways to speed the increase in F_I include increasing the fresh gas flow, thus decreasing τ. Furthermore, the rebreathing bag can be collapsed prior to starting the fresh gas flow, such that the capacity in the circuit (V_C) is less, which also decreases τ. Finally, at high flows (>4 L/min) there is far

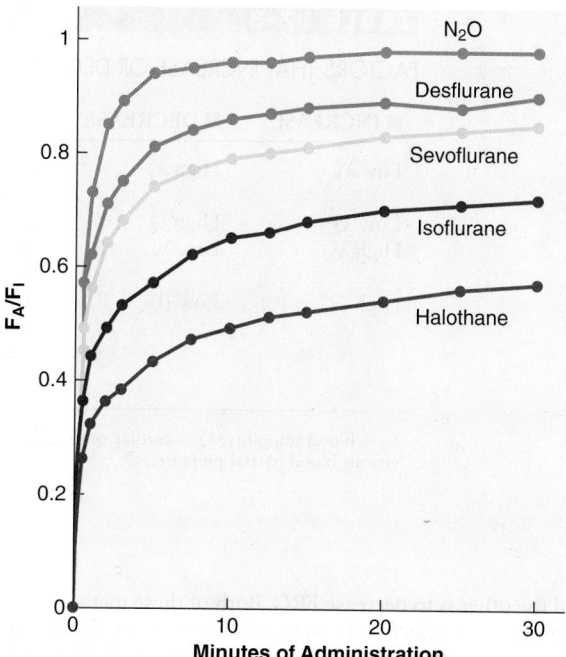

FIGURE 17-2. The rise in alveolar (F_A) anesthetic concentration toward the inspired (F_I) concentration is most rapid with the least soluble anesthetics, nitrous oxide (N_2O), desflurane, and sevoflurane. It rises most slowly with the more soluble anesthetics, such as halothane. All data are from human studies. (Adapted from Yasuda N, Lockhart SH, Eger EI II, et al: Comparison of kinetics of sevoflurane and isoflurane in humans. Anesth Analg 1991; 72: 316; and Yasuda N, Lockhart SH, Eger EI II, et al: Kinetics of desflurane, isoflurane, and halothane in humans. Anesthesiology 1991; 74: 489.)

less mixing because fresh gas pushes "old" gas out of the circuit via the pop-off valve before complete mixing occurs, causing F_I to increase at a greater rate; this is the most important factor in rapidly increasing F_I to the desired concentration.

One factor that delays the rate of rise of F_I is that CO_2 absorbent can adsorb and decompose the inhaled anesthetics. From a practical standpoint, this does not affect the rate of rise in F_I to a significant extent compared with other factors. Another factor that delays the rate of rise of F_I is solubility of the inhaled anesthetics in some of the plastic and rubber parts of the anesthesia circuit. This absorption has been quantified, but plays only a small role in decreasing the rate of rise of F_I.

Rise in F_A in the Absence of Uptake

The rate of rise in F_I discussed earlier assumes that no anesthetic is mixing with gas in the patient's lungs. In reality, circuit gas mixes with exhaled gases from the lung with each breath, thus lowering F_I within the circuit. If high fresh gas flows (>4 L/min), which produce a high volume of gas at the desired concentration, are used, little mixing with exhaled air occurs and F_I is relatively fixed. In this situation, circuit gas enters the lungs where it mixes with alveolar gas. If there were no blood flow to the lungs, F_A would rise in a fashion analogous to F_I; that is:

$$F_A = F_I(1 - e^{-T/\tau}) \qquad (17\text{-}7)$$

In this equation, τ is the time constant for alveolar rise in anesthetic concentration and equals the functional residual capacity (FRC) of the patient's lungs divided by minute ventilation, $\dot{V}_A$. There are two ways to speed the equilibration of F_A with F_I, that is, to decrease τ. One way is to increase minute ventilation,

TABLE 17-3

FACTORS THAT INCREASE OR DECREASE THE RATE OF RISE OF F_A/F_I

■ INCREASE	■ DECREASE	
Low λ_B	High λ_B	The lower the blood:gas solubility, the faster the rise in F_A/F_I
Low Q	High Q	The lower the cardiac output, the faster the rise in F_A/F_I
High $\dot{V}_A$	Low $\dot{V}_A$	The higher the minute ventilation, the faster the rise in F_A/F_I
High $(P_A - P_v)$	Low $(P_A - P_v)$	At the beginning of induction, P_v is zero but rises rapidly (thus $[P_A - P_v]$ falls rapidly) and F_A/F_I increases rapidly. Later during induction and maintenance P_v rises more slowly so F_A/F_I rises more slowly.

λ_B = blood solubility; Q = cardiac output; $\dot{V}$ = minute ventilation; P_A, P_V = pulmonary arterial and venous blood partial pressure.

and the other is to decrease FRC. Both of these methods can be used to speed induction by mask: the patient can exhale deeply before applying the mask (to decrease the initial FRC), and the patient can breathe deeply and rapidly (to increase) after the mask is applied. Importantly, high alveolar ventilation relative to uptake from the lungs to the bloodstream generates the initial high slope to the curves shown in Figure 17-2.

One of the reasons that pediatric inductions by spontaneous breathing of inhaled anesthetics are so much quicker than adult inductions is that the low FRC relative to $\dot{V}_A$ of children makes for a low time constant, and hence a more rapid increase in F_A/F_I. One important caveat about the relationship of F_A to FRC is that FRC includes airway dead space; thus, in reality, F_A by Equation 17-7 is not just the concentration of inhaled anesthetic in the alveoli but also the concentration in the entire lung. However, it is simply called the alveolar concentration because the dead space in the airways is relatively insignificant and only the alveolar gas is exchanging anesthetic with the blood.

Rise in F_A in the Presence of Uptake

Anesthetics *are* soluble in tissues, thus uptake of anesthetic from alveoli to blood is again characterized by first-order kinetics:

$$P_{bl} \text{ (blood)} = P_A \text{ (alveoli)} \times (1 - e^{-T/\tau}),$$
$$\text{where } P_A = F_A \times P_B \text{ (barometric)} \qquad (17\text{-}8)$$

Here, P_B is the barometric pressure and the time constant, τ, equals "capacity" (volume of anesthetic dissolved in blood at the desired alveolar partial pressure) divided by flow (volume of anesthetic delivered per unit time). For any given flow of anesthetic into the system, this capacity for the more soluble halothane is greater than the capacity for the less soluble desflurane; thus, τ for halothane is greater than that for desflurane. The more soluble the inhaled anesthetic, the larger the capacity of the blood and tissues for that anesthetic, and the longer it takes to saturate at any given delivery rate.

The most important factor in the rate of rise of F_A/F_I is uptake of anesthetic from the alveoli into the bloodstream. The rate of rise of F_A/F_I (especially the position of the "knees" in the curves of Figure 17-2) reflects the speed at which alveolar anesthetic (F_A) equilibrates with that being delivered to the lungs (F_I). Since there is uptake from alveoli to blood, F_A is not solely a function of F_I and time. The greater the uptake, the slower the rate of rise of F_A/F_I, and vice versa. Since uptake is proportional to tissue solubility, the less soluble the anesthetic (such as desflurane), the lesser its uptake and the faster it reaches equilibrium, $P_A = P_{blood} = P_{CNS}$.

Consider a hypothetical example. Suppose that halothane and desflurane are soluble in blood, but insoluble in all other tissues. Suppose further that total lung capacity and blood volume were both 5 L. If a fixed volume of anesthetic is delivered to the lungs (by asking the patient to take one deep breath and hold it), according to the blood:gas partition coefficients for halothane (2.5) and desflurane (0.42), 71.4% of the delivered halothane will be transferred to the blood while 28.6% remains in the alveoli (71.4/28.6 = 2.5). In contrast, 29.6% of the desflurane will be transferred to the blood while 70.4% remains in the alveoli (29.6/70.4 = 0.42). Therefore, 2.4 times (71.4/29.6) more halothane than desflurane (by volume or number of molecules) will be transferred from alveoli to bloodstream before partial pressures equilibrate. At equilibrium, the alveolar partial pressures of halothane and desflurane are 28.6% and 70.4% of their inhaled values, respectively. This means that F_A rises faster with desflurane than halothane, as does F_A/F_I.

Blood uptake of anesthetic is expressed by the equation:

$$\dot{V}_B = \delta_{b/g} * Q \times ((P_A - P_V)/P_B) \qquad (17\text{-}9)$$

where $\dot{V}_B$ is blood uptake, $\delta_{b/g}$ is the blood:gas partition coefficient, Q is cardiac output, P_A is alveolar partial pressure of anesthetic, P_v is mixed venous partial pressure of anesthetic, and P_B is barometric pressure. This is the Fick equation applied to blood uptake of inhaled anesthetics. *The greater the value of $\dot{V}_B$, the greater the uptake from alveoli to blood, and the slower the rise in F_A/F_I.*

From the preceding paragraphs, the parameters that increase or decrease the rate of rise in F_A/F_I during induction can now be clearly delineated and these important factors have been substantiated in experimental models (Table 17-3).

Distribution (Tissue Uptake)

The maximum F_A/F_I at a given inspired concentration of anesthetic, cardiac output, and minute ventilation depends entirely on the solubility of that drug in the blood as characterized by the blood:gas partition coefficient $\delta_{b/g}$. This can be seen in the time curves for the rise in F_A/F_I during induction for the various inhalation anesthetics shown in Figure 17-2. The first "knee" in each curve in Figure 17-2 represents the point at which the rapid rise in P_v begins to taper off; that is, when significant inhaled anesthetic concentrations begin to build up in the bloodstream because of distribution to and equilibration with the various tissue compartments.

As blood is equilibrating with alveolar gas, it also begins to equilibrate with the VRG, muscle, and, more gradually, the fat compartments based on perfusion. Muscle is not that different from the VRG, having partition coefficients that range from 1.2 (nitrous oxide) to 3.4 (halothane), just under a threefold difference; and for each anesthetic except nitrous oxide, the muscle partition coefficient is approximately double that for the VRG. Although both VRG and muscle are lean tissues, the muscle compartment equilibrates far more slowly than the VRG. The explanation comes in part due to the mass of the compartments relative to perfusion. The perfusion of the VRG is about 75 mL/min/100 g of tissue, whereas it is only 3 mL/min/100 g of tissue in the muscle (Table 17-2). This 25-fold difference in perfusion between VRG (especially brain) and muscle means that even if the partition coefficients were equal, the muscle would still take 25 times longer to equilibrate with blood.

Fat is perfused to a lesser extent than muscle and its time for equilibration with blood is considerably slower because the partition coefficients are so much greater. All of the potent agents are highly lipid-soluble. Partition coefficients range from 27 (desflurane) to 51 (halothane). On average, the solubility for these agents is about 25 times greater in fat than in the VRG group. Thus, fat equilibrates far more slowly with the blood and does not play a significant role in determining speed of induction. After long anesthetic exposures (>4 hours), the high saturation of fat tissue may play a role in delaying emergence.

Nitrous oxide represents an exception. Its partition coefficients are fairly similar in each tissue: it does not accumulate to any great extent and is not a very potent anesthetic. Its utility lies as an adjunct to the potent agents, and as a vehicle to speed induction.

Metabolism

Data suggest that enzymes responsible for biotransformation of inhaled anesthetics become saturated at less than anesthetizing doses of these drugs, such that metabolism plays little role in opposing induction. It may, however, have some significance to recovery from anesthesia, as discussed later.

Overpressurization and the Concentration Effect

There are several ways to speed uptake and induction of anesthesia with the inhaled anesthetics. The first is *overpressurization*, which is analogous to an intravenous bolus. This is the administration of a higher partial pressure of anesthetic than the alveolar concentration (F_A) actually desired for the patient. Inspired anesthetic concentration (F_I) can influence both F_A and the *rate of rise* of F_A/F_I. The greater the inspired concentration of an inhaled anesthetic, the greater the rate of rise. This concentration effect has two components: the concentrating effect and an augmented gas inflow effect.

For example, consider the administration of 10% anesthetic (10 parts anesthetic and 90 parts other gas) to a patient in whom 50% of the anesthetic in the alveoli is absorbed by the blood. In this case, five parts (0.5 × 10) anesthetic remain in the alveoli, five parts enter the blood, and 90 parts remain as other alveolar gas. The alveolar concentration is now 5/(90 + 5) = 5.3%. Consider next administering 50% anesthetic with the same 50% uptake. Now 25 parts anesthetic remain in alveoli, 25 parts pass into blood, and 50 parts remain as other alveolar gas. The alveolar concentration becomes 25/(50 + 25) = 33%. Giving 5 times as much anesthetic has led to a 33%/5.3% = 6.2 times greater alveolar concentration. The higher the F_I, the greater the effect. Thus nitrous oxide,

typically given in concentrations of 50 to 70%, has the greatest concentrating effect. This is why the F_A/F_I versus time curve in Figure 17-2 rises the most quickly with nitrous oxide, even though desflurane has a slightly lower blood:gas solubility.

This is not the complete picture; there is yet another factor to consider. As gas is leaving the alveoli for the blood, new gas at the original F_I is entering the lungs to replace that which is taken up by the blood. This other aspect of the concentration effect has been called *augmented gas inflow*. Again, take the example of 10% anesthetic delivered with 50% uptake into the bloodstream. The five parts anesthetic absorbed by the bloodstream are replaced by gas in the circuit that is still 10% anesthetic. The five parts anesthetic and 90 parts other gas left in the lungs mix with five parts replacement gas, or 5 × 0.10 = 0.5 parts anesthetic. Now the alveolar concentration is (5 + 0.5)/(100) = 5.5% (as compared to 5.3% without augmented inflow). For 50% anesthetic and 50% uptake, 25 parts of anesthetic removed from the alveoli are replaced with 25 parts of 50% anesthetic, giving a new alveolar concentration of (25 + 12.5)/(100) = 37.5% (as compared to 33% without augmented inflow). Thus, 5 times the F_I leads to 37.5/5.5 = 6.8 times greater F_A (compared to 6.2 times without augmented gas inflow). Of course, this cycle of absorbed gas being replaced by fresh gas inflow is continuous and has a finite rate, so our example is a simplification.

Second Gas Effect

A special case of concentration effect applies to administration of a potent anesthetic with nitrous oxide—that is, two gases simultaneously. Along with the concentration of potent agent in the alveoli via its uptake, there is further concentration via the uptake of nitrous oxide, a process called the *second gas effect*. The principle is simple (Figs. 17-3 and 17-4). Consider,

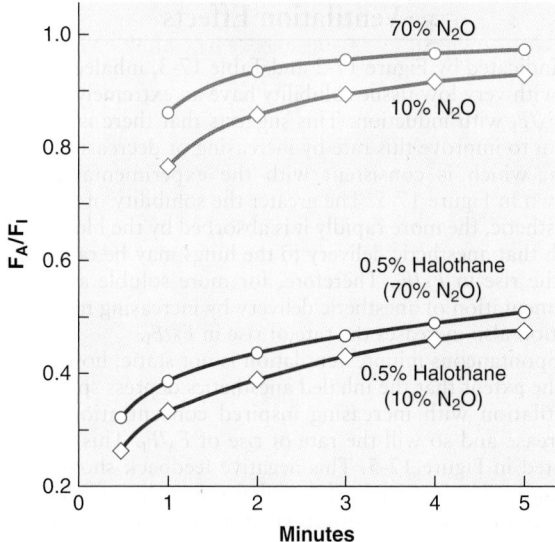

Concentration and Second-Gas Effects

FIGURE 17-3. The concentration effect is demonstrated in the top half of the graph from dogs receiving nitrous oxide (N_2O). Administration of 70% nitrous oxide produces a more rapid rise in the F_A/F_I ratio of nitrous oxide than administration of 10% nitrous oxide. The second gas effect is demonstrated in the lower graphs. The F_A/F_I ratio for 0.5% halothane rises more rapidly when given with 70% nitrous oxide than when given with 10% nitrous oxide. (Adapted from Epstein R, Rackow H, Salanitre E, et al: Influence of the concentration effect on the uptake of anesthetic mixtures: The second gas effect. Anesthesiology 1964; 25: 364.)

FIGURE 17-4. A graphic and relative equation to demonstrate the second-gas effect. In this hypothetical example, the second gas is set at 2% of a potent anesthetic and the model is set for 50% uptake of the first gas (nitrous oxide [N_2O]) in the first inspired breath. The second gas is concentrated because of the uptake of N_2O (**middle panel**). On replenishing the inspired second gas ($F_I = 2\%$) in the next breath, the second gas has been concentrated to be 2.7% because of the uptake of N_2O in the previous breath.

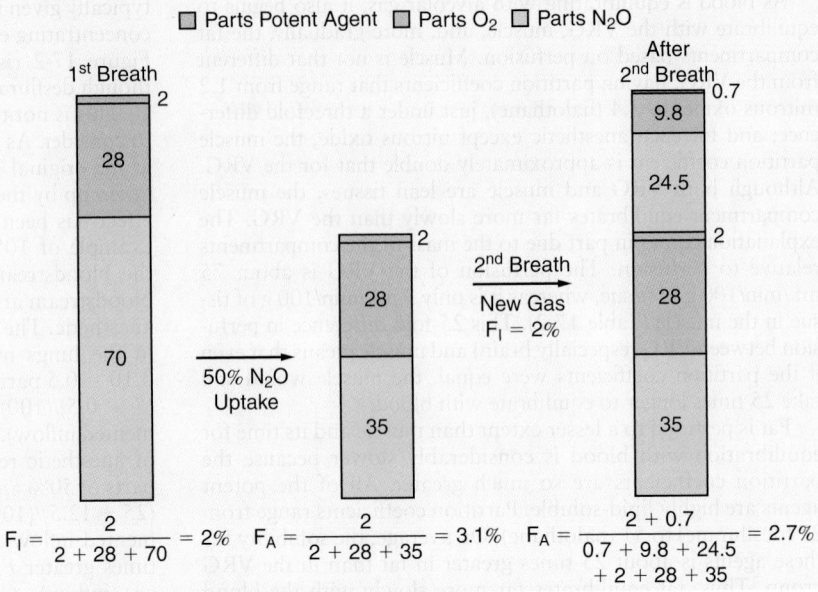

$$F_I = \frac{2}{2 + 28 + 70} = 2\% \quad F_A = \frac{2}{2 + 28 + 35} = 3.1\% \quad F_A = \frac{2 + 0.7}{0.7 + 9.8 + 24.5 + 2 + 28 + 35} = 2.7\%$$

for example, administering 2% of a potent anesthetic in 70% nitrous oxide and 28% oxygen. In this case, nitrous oxide, with its extremely high partial pressure (despite low solubility), partitions into the blood more rapidly than the potent anesthetic, decreasing the alveolar N_2O (nitrous oxide) concentration by some amount (e.g., by 50%). Ignoring uptake of the potent anesthetic, the uptake of N_2O is 35 parts, leaving 35 parts N_2O, 28 parts O_2, and two parts potent agent in the alveoli. The anesthetic gas is now present in the alveoli at a concentration of $2/(2 + 35 + 28) = 3.1\%$. The potent agent has been concentrated and F_A is increased.

Ventilation Effects

As indicated by Figure 17-2 and Table 17-3, inhaled anesthetics with very low tissue solubility have an extremely rapid rise in F_A/F_I with induction. This suggests that there is very little room to improve this rate by increasing or decreasing ventilation, which is consistent with the experimental evidence shown in Figure 17-5. The greater the solubility of an inhaled anesthetic, the more rapidly it is absorbed by the bloodstream, such that anesthetic delivery to the lungs may be rate limiting to the rise in F_A/F_I. Therefore, for more soluble anesthetics, augmentation of anesthetic delivery by increasing minute ventilation also increases the rate of rise in F_A/F_I.

Spontaneous minute ventilation is not static, however, and to the extent that the inhaled anesthetics depress spontaneous ventilation with increasing inspired concentration, $\dot{V}_A$ will decrease and so will the rate of rise of F_A/F_I. This is demonstrated in Figure 17-5. This negative feedback should not be considered a drawback of the inhaled anesthetics because the respiratory depression produced at high anesthetic concentrations essentially slows the rise in F_A/F_I. This might arguably add a margin of safety in preventing an overdose. Controlled ventilation does not offer this margin of safety.

Perfusion Effects

As with ventilation, cardiac output is not static during the course of induction. For the less soluble agents, changes in cardiac output do not affect the rate of rise of F_A/F_I to a great extent, but for the more soluble agents the effect is noticeable,

as seen in Figure 17-6. However, as inspired concentration increases, greater cardiovascular depression reduces anesthetic uptake and actually increases the rate of rise of F_A/F_I. This positive feedback can rapidly lead to profound cardiovascular depression. Figure 17-6 presents experimental data in which lower cardiac outputs lead to a much more rapid rise in F_A/F_I when $\dot{V}_A$ is held constant. This more rapid rise is greater than can be accounted for just by concentration effect.

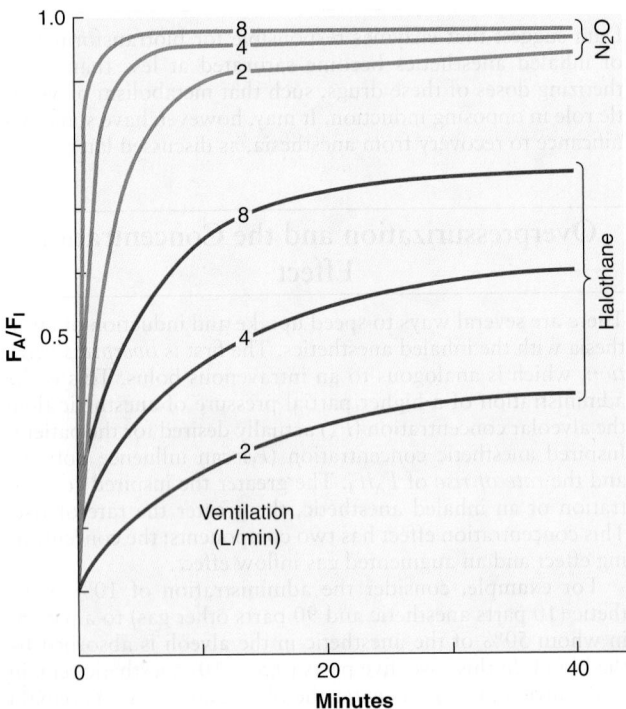

FIGURE 17-5. The F_A/F_I ratio rises more rapidly if ventilation is increased from 2 to 8 L/min. Solubility modifies this impact of ventilation; for example, the effect is greatest with the least-soluble anesthetic, nitrous oxide (N_2O; **top three lines**), and least with the more soluble anesthetic, halothane. (Adapted from Eger EI II: Ventilation, circulation and uptake, Anesthetic Uptake and Action. Baltimore, Williams & Wilkins, 1974, pp 122.)

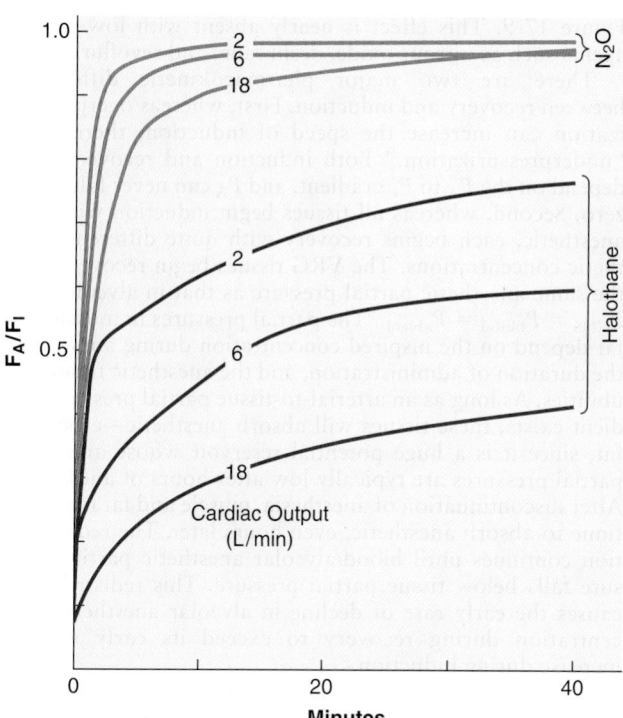

FIGURE 17-6.   If ventilation is fixed, an increase in cardiac output from 2 to 18 L/min will decrease the alveolar anesthetic concentration by augmenting uptake, thereby slowing the rise of the F_A/F_I ratio. This effect is most prominent with the more soluble anesthetics (halothane) than with the less soluble anesthetics (nitrous oxide [N_2O]). (Adapted from Eger EI II: Ventilation, circulation and uptake, Anesthetic Uptake and Action. Baltimore, Williams & Wilkins, 1974, p 131.)

Ventilation–Perfusion Mismatching

Ventilation and perfusion are normally fairly well matched in healthy patients such that P_A (alveolar partial pressure)/P_I and P_a (arterial partial pressure)/P_I are the same curve. However, if significant intrapulmonary shunt occurs, as in the case of inadvertent bronchial intubation, the rate of rise of alveolar and arterial anesthetic partial pressures can be affected. The effects, however, depend on the solubility of the anesthetic, as seen in Figure 17-7. Ventilation of the intubated lung is dramatically increased while perfusion increases slightly. The nonintubated lung receives no ventilation, while perfusion decreases slightly. For the less-soluble anesthetics, increased ventilation of the intubated lung cannot appreciably increase alveolar partial pressure relative to inspired concentration on that side, but alveolar partial pressure on the nonintubated side is essentially zero. Pulmonary mixed venous blood, therefore, comprises nearly equal parts blood containing normal amounts of anesthetic and blood containing no anesthetic; that is, diluted relative to normal. Thus the rate of rise in P_a relative to P_I is significantly reduced. There is less total anesthetic uptake, so the rate of rise of P_A relative to P_I increases even though induction of anesthesia is slowed because CNS partial pressure equilibrates with P_a. For the more soluble anesthetics, increased ventilation of the intubated lung *does* increase the alveolar partial pressure relative to inspired concentration on that side. Pulmonary venous blood from the intubated side contains a higher concentration of anesthetic that lessens the dilution by blood from the nonintubated side. Thus the rate of rise of P_a/P_I is not as depressed as that for the less soluble anesthetics, and induction of anesthesia is less delayed relative to normal.

Elimination

Percutaneous and Visceral Loss

Although the loss of inhaled anesthetics via the skin is very small, it does occur and the loss is the greatest for nitrous oxide. These anesthetics also pass across gastrointestinal viscera and the pleura. During open abdominal or thoracic surgery there is some anesthetic loss via these routes. Relative to losses by all other routes, losses via percutaneous and visceral routes are insignificant.

Diffusion Between Tissues

Using more elaborate mathematical modeling of inhaled anesthetic pharmacokinetics than presented here, several laboratories have derived a five-compartment model that best describes tissue compartments. These compartments are the alveoli, the VRG, the muscle, the fat, and one additional compartment. Current opinion is that this fifth compartment represents adipose tissue adjacent to lean tissue that receives anesthetic via intertissue diffusion. This transfer of anesthetic is not insignificant, and may account for up to one third of uptake during long administration.

Exhalation and Recovery

Recovery from anesthesia, like induction, depends on anesthetic solubility, cardiac output, and minute ventilation. Solubility is the primary determinant of the rate of fall of F_A

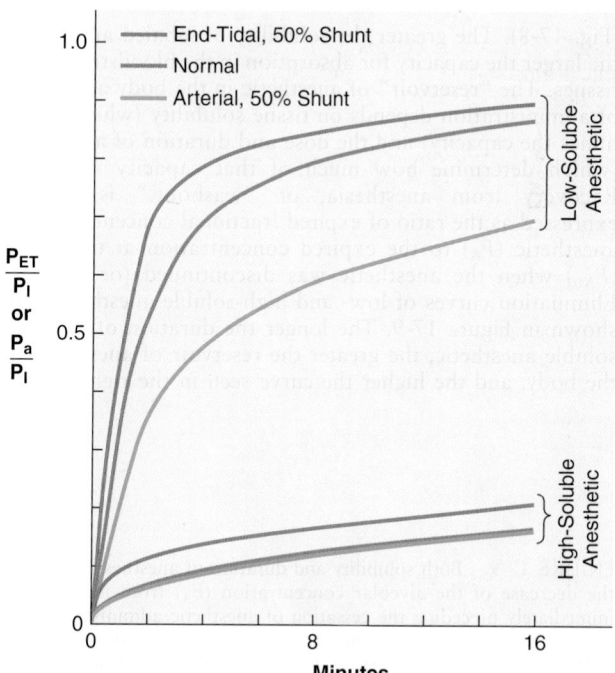

FIGURE 17-7.   When no ventilation/perfusion abnormalities exist, the alveolar (P_A) or end-tidal (P_{ET}) and arterial (P_a) anesthetic partial pressures rise together (*blue lines*) toward the inspired partial pressure (P_I). When 50% of the cardiac output is shunted through the lungs, the rate of rise of the end-tidal partial pressure (*orange lines*) is accelerated while the rate of rise of the arterial partial pressure (*green lines*) is slowed. The greatest effect of shunting is found with the least soluble anesthetics. (Adapted from Eger EI II, Severinghaus JW: Effect of uneven pulmonary distribution of blood and gas on induction with inhalation anesthetics. Anesthesiology 1964; 25: 620.)

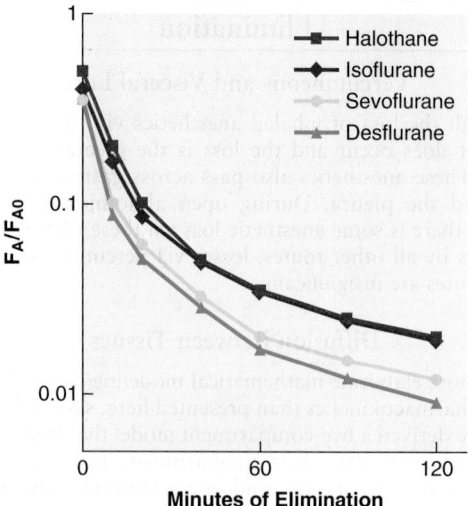

FIGURE 17-8. Elimination of anesthetic gases is defined as the ratio of end-tidal anesthetic concentration (F_A) to the last F_A during administration and immediately before the beginning of elimination (F_{A0}). During the 120-minute period after ending the anesthetic delivery, the elimination of sevoflurane and desflurane is 2 to 2.5 times faster than isoflurane or halothane (note logarithmic scale for the ordinate). (Adapted from Yasuda N, Lockhart SH, Eger EI II, et al: Comparison of kinetics of sevoflurane and isoflurane in humans. Anesth Analg 1991; 72: 316; and Yasuda N, Lockhart SH, Eger EI II, et al: Kinetics of desflurane, isoflurane, and halothane in humans. Anesthesiology 1991; 74: 489.)

(Fig. 17-8). The greater the solubility of inhaled anesthetic, the larger the capacity for absorption in the bloodstream and tissues. The "reservoir" of anesthetic in the body at the end of administration depends on tissue solubility (which determines the capacity) and the dose and duration of anesthetic (which determine how much of that capacity is filled). Recovery from anesthesia, or "washout," is usually expressed as the ratio of expired fractional concentration of anesthetic (F_A) to the expired concentration at time zero (F_{A0}) when the anesthetic was discontinued (or F_A/F_{A0}). Elimination curves of low- and high-soluble anesthetics are shown in Figure 17-9. The longer the duration of a highly soluble anesthetic, the greater the reservoir of anesthetic in the body, and the higher the curve seen in the right half of

Figure 17-9. This effect is nearly absent with low-soluble agents such as nitrous oxide, desflurane, and sevoflurane.[3]

There are two major pharmacokinetic differences between recovery and induction. First, whereas overpressurization can increase the speed of induction, there is no "underpressurization." Both induction and recovery rates depend on the P_A to P_v gradient, and P_A can never fall below zero. Second, whereas all tissues begin induction with zero anesthetic, each begins recovery with quite different anesthetic concentrations. The VRG tissues begin recovery with the same anesthetic partial pressure as that in alveoli, since $P_{CNS} = P_{blood} = P_{alveoli}$. The partial pressures in muscle and fat depend on the inspired concentration during anesthesia, the duration of administration, and the anesthetic tissue solubilities. As long as an arterial-to-tissue partial pressure gradient exists, these tissues will absorb anesthetic—especially fat, since it is a huge potential reservoir whose anesthetic partial pressures are typically low after hours of anesthesia. After discontinuation of anesthesia, muscle and fat may continue to absorb anesthetic, even hours later. The redistribution continues until blood/alveolar anesthetic partial pressure falls below tissue partial pressure. This redistribution causes the early rate of decline in alveolar anesthetic concentration during recovery to exceed its early rate of increase during induction.

Because VRG tissues are highly perfused and washout of anesthetic is mostly via elimination from these tissues early in recovery, all anesthetics, regardless of duration of administration, have approximately the same rate of elimination to 50% of F_{A0}. Unfortunately, halving the CNS concentration of anesthetic is rarely sufficient for waking the patient. More commonly, 80% to 90% of inhaled anesthetic must be eliminated before emergence. At these amounts of washout, the more soluble anesthetics are eliminated more slowly than less soluble agents.

Diffusion Hypoxia

During recovery from anesthesia, washout of high concentrations of nitrous oxide can lower alveolar concentrations of oxygen and carbon dioxide, a phenomenon called *diffusion hypoxia*. The resulting alveolar hypoxia can cause hypoxemia, and alveolar hypocarbia can depress respiratory drive, which may exacerbate hypoxemia. It is therefore appropriate to initiate recovery from nitrous oxide anesthesia with 100% oxygen rather than less concentrated O_2/air mixtures.

FIGURE 17-9. Both solubility and duration of anesthesia affect the decrease of the alveolar concentration (F_A) from its value immediately preceding the cessation of anesthetic administration (F_{A0}). A longer anesthetic time (from 15 minutes to 240 minutes) only slightly slows the decrease with low-soluble anesthetics (**left graph**). An agent with a higher blood and tissue solubility (**right graph**) slows the elimination of the anesthetic and enhances the effect of duration. (Adapted from Stoelting RK, Eger EI II: The effects of ventilation and anesthetic solubility on recovery from anesthesia: An in vivo and analog analysis before and after equilibrium. Anesthesiology 1969; 30: 290.)

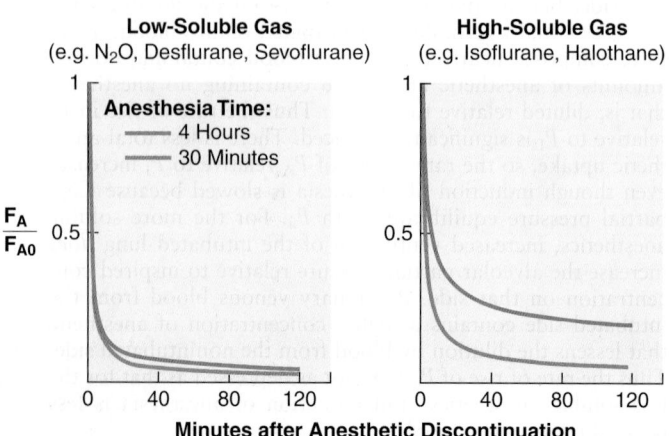

CLINICAL OVERVIEW OF CURRENT INHALED ANESTHETICS

Isoflurane

Isoflurane is a halogenated methyl ethyl ether that is a clear, nonflammable liquid at room temperature and has a high degree of pungency. It is the most potent of the volatile anesthetics in clinical use, has great physical stability, and undergoes essentially no deterioration during storage for up to 5 years or on exposure to sunlight. It has become the "gold standard" anesthetic since its introduction in the 1970s. There was a brief period of controversy concerning the use of isoflurane in patients with coronary disease because of the possibility for coronary "steal" arising from the potent effects of isoflurane on coronary vasodilation. In clinical use, however, this has been, at most, a rare occurrence.

Desflurane

Desflurane is a fluorinated methyl ethyl ether that differs from isoflurane by just one atom: a fluorine atom is substituted for a chlorine atom on the α-ethyl component of isoflurane (Fig. 17-1). The process of complete fluorination of the ether molecule has several effects. It decreases blood and tissue solubility (the blood:gas solubility of desflurane equals that of nitrous oxide), and it results in a loss of potency (the MAC of desflurane is 5 times higher than isoflurane). Moreover, fluorination of the methyl ether molecule results in a high vapor pressure owing to decreased intermolecular attraction. Thus, a new vaporizer technology was developed to deliver a regulated concentration of desflurane as a gas. It is a heated, pressurized vaporizer requiring electrical power and more frequent servicing. One of the advantages of desflurane is the near-absent metabolism to serum trifluoroacetate. This makes immune-mediated hepatitis a rare occurrence. Desflurane is the most pungent of the volatile anesthetics, and if administered via the face mask results in coughing, salivation, breath holding, and laryngospasm. In extremely dry CO_2 absorbers, desflurane (and to a lesser extent isoflurane, enflurane, and sevoflurane) degrades to form carbon monoxide. Desflurane has the lowest blood:gas solubility of the potent volatile anesthetics; moreover, its fat solubility is roughly half of that of the other volatile anesthetics. Thus, desflurane requires less downward titration in long surgical procedures to achieve a rapid emergence by virtue of decreased tissue saturation. Desflurane has been associated with tachycardia, hypertension, and, in select cases, myocardial ischemia when used in high concentrations or rapidly increasing the inspired concentration (without using opioid adjuvants to prevent such a response).

Sevoflurane

Sevoflurane is a sweet-smelling, completely fluorinated methyl isopropyl ether (Fig. 17-1). Its vapor pressure is roughly one-fourth that of desflurane and it can be used in a conventional vaporizer. The blood:gas solubility of sevoflurane is second only to desflurane in terms of potent volatile anesthetics. Sevoflurane is approximately half as potent as isoflurane, and some of the preservation of potency, despite fluorination, is because of the bulky propyl side chain on the ether molecule. Sevoflurane has minimal odor, no pungency, and is a potent bronchodilator. These attributes make sevoflurane an excellent candidate for administration via the face mask on induction of anesthesia in both children and adults. Sevoflurane is half as potent a coronary vasodilator as isoflurane, but is 10 to 20 times more vulnerable to metabolism than isoflurane. The metabolism of sevoflurane results in inorganic fluoride; the increase in plasma fluoride after sevoflurane administration has not been associated with renal-concentrating defects. Unlike other potent volatile anesthetics, sevoflurane is not metabolized to trifluoroacetate; rather, it is metabolized to an acyl halide (hexafluoroisopropanol). This does not stimulate formation of antibodies.

Sevoflurane can form carbon monoxide during exposure to dry CO_2 absorbents, and an exothermic reaction in dry absorbent has resulted in canister fires. New generic versions of sevoflurane have the potential to break down to hydrogen fluoride when exposed to metal compounds because of their lack of adequate water in the formulation. Sevoflurane also breaks down in the presence of the carbon dioxide absorber to form a vinyl halide called *compound A*. Compound A has been shown to be a dose-dependent nephrotoxin in rats, but has not been associated with renal injury in human volunteers or patients, with or without renal impairment, even when fresh gas flows are 1 L/min or less.

Xenon

Xenon is an inert gas. Difficult to obtain, and hence extremely expensive, it has received considerable interest in the last few years because it has many characteristics approaching those of an "ideal" inhaled anesthetic,[4,5] although it can trigger malignant hyperthermia. Its blood:gas partition coefficient is 0.14, and unlike the other potent volatile anesthetics (except methoxyflurane), xenon provides some degree of analgesia. The MAC of xenon in humans is 71%, which might prove to be a limitation. It is nonexplosive, nonpungent, and odorless, and thus can be inhaled with ease. In addition, it does not produce significant myocardial depression.[4] Because of its scarcity and high cost, new anesthetic systems need to be developed to provide for recycling of xenon. If this proves to be too difficult from either a technical or patient safety standpoint, it may be necessary to use it in a very low, or closed, fresh gas flow system to reduce wastage.

Nitrous Oxide

Nitrous oxide is a sweet-smelling, nonflammable gas of low potency (MAC = 104%) and is relatively insoluble in blood. It is most commonly administered as an anesthetic adjuvant in combination with opioids or volatile anesthetics during the conduct of general anesthesia. Although not flammable, nitrous oxide will support combustion. Unlike the potent volatile anesthetics in clinical use, nitrous oxide does not produce significant skeletal muscle relaxation, but it does have documented analgesic effects. Despite a long track record of use, controversy has surrounded nitrous oxide in four areas: its role in postoperative nausea and vomiting, its potential toxic effects on cell function via inactivation of vitamin B_{12}, its adverse effects related to absorption and expansion into air-filled structures and bubbles, and lastly, its effect on embryonic development. The one concern that seems most valid and most clinically relevant is the ability of nitrous oxide to expand air-filled spaces because of its greater solubility in blood compared to nitrogen. Several closed gas spaces, such as the bowel and middle ear, exist in the body and other spaces may occur as a result of disease or surgery, such as a pneumothorax. Because nitrogen in air-filled spaces cannot be removed readily via the bloodstream, nitrous oxide delivered to a patient diffuses from the blood into these closed gas spaces quite easily. Movement of nitrous oxide into these spaces continues until the partial pressure equals that of the blood and alveoli. Compliant spaces will continue to expand until sufficient pressure is generated to oppose further nitrous oxide flow into the space. The higher the inspired concentration of nitrous oxide, the higher the partial pressure required for equilibration.

Seventy-five percent nitrous oxide can expand a pneumothorax to double or triple its size in 10 and 30 minutes, respectively. Air-filled cuffs of pulmonary artery catheters and endotracheal tubes also expand with the use of nitrous oxide, possibly causing tissue damage via increased pressure in the pulmonary artery or trachea, respectively.[6,7] In a rabbit model, the volume of an air embolus resulting in cardiovascular compromise is less during coadministration of nitrous oxide.[8] Accumulation of nitrous oxide in the middle ear can diminish hearing postoperatively[9] and is relatively contraindicated for tympanoplasty because the increased pressure can dislodge a tympanic graft.

NEUROPHARMACOLOGY OF INHALED ANESTHETICS

Minimum Alveolar Concentration

The pharmacodynamic effects of inhaled anesthetics must be based on a dose, and this dose is the *minimum alveolar concentration* or MAC. MAC is the alveolar concentration of an anesthetic at one atmosphere that prevents movement in response to a surgical stimulus in 50% of patients. It is analogous to the ED_{50} expressed for intravenous drugs. A variety of surgical stimuli have been used to establish the MAC for each inhaled anesthetic, but the classic, defining, noxious stimulus is incision of the abdomen. Likewise, skeletal muscle movement is the defining patient response, but other responses have been used to establish MAC as well. Experimentally determined MAC values for humans for the inhaled anesthetics are shown in Table 17-1.

The 95% confidence ranges for MAC are approximately ±25% of the listed MAC values. Manufacturer's recommendations and clinical experience establish 1.2 to 1.3 times MAC as a dose that consistently prevents patient movement during surgical stimuli. Loss of consciousness typically precedes the absence of stimulus-induced movement by a wide margin. Although 1.2 to 1.3 MAC values do not *absolutely* ensure the defining criteria for brain anesthesia (the absence of self-awareness and recall), vast clinical experience suggests it is extremely unlikely for a patient to be aware of, or to recall, the surgical incision at these anesthetic concentrations unless other conditions exist such that MAC is increased in that patient (Table 17-4).

Concentrations of inhaled anesthetics that provide loss of self-awareness and recall are about 0.4 to 0.5 MAC. Several

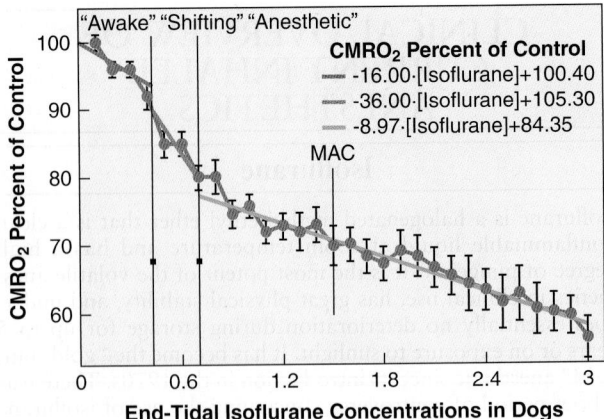

FIGURE 17-10. The effects of halothane on cerebral metabolic rate of oxygen consumption ($CMRO_2$) as a percentage of control ("awake"). $CMRO_2$ is plotted versus end-tidal isoflurane concentration. Regression lines for changes in $CMRO_2$ are drawn for each electroencephalogram-determined area. The pattern depicted here is characteristic of all of the anesthetics examined (enflurane, halothane, and isoflurane). MAC, minimum alveolar concentration. (Adapted from Stullken EH Jr, Milde JH, Michenfelder JD, et al: The nonlinear responses of cerebral metabolism to low concentrations of halothane, enflurane, isoflurane and thiopental. Anesthesiology 1977; 46: 28.)

lines of reasoning lead to this conclusion. First, most patients receiving only 50% nitrous oxide (approximately 0.4 to 0.5 MAC) as in a typical dentist's office will have no recall of their procedure during N_2O administration. Second, various studies have shown that a shift in electroencephalogram (EEG) dominance to the anterior leads, that is, the shift from self-aware to nonself-aware, accompanies loss of consciousness, and in primates, the EEG shift and loss of consciousness occur at 0.5 MAC.[10] Third, in dogs, loss of consciousness accompanies a sudden nonlinear fall in cerebral metabolic rate (CMR) at approximately 0.5 MAC (Fig. 17-10).

MAC values can be established for any measurable response. MAC-awake, or the alveolar concentration of anesthetic at which a patient opens his or her eyes to command, varies from 0.15 to 0.5 MAC.[11] Interestingly, transition from awake to unconscious and back typically shows some hysteresis in that it quite consistently takes 0.4 to 0.5 MAC to lose consciousness, but less than that (as low as 0.15 MAC) to regain consciousness. This may be because of the speed of alveolar wash-in versus wash-out.[12] MAC-BAR, or the alveolar concentration of anesthetic that blunts adrenergic responses to noxious stimuli, has likewise been established and is approximately 50% higher than standard MAC.[13] MAC also has been established for discreet levels of EEG activity, such as onset of burst suppression or isoelectricity.

Standard MAC values are roughly additive. Administering 0.5 MAC of a potent agent and 0.5 MAC of nitrous oxide is equivalent to 1 MAC of potent agent in terms of preventing *patient movement*, although this does not hold over the entire range of N_2O doses. MAC effects for other response parameters are not necessarily additive. Because MAC-movement probably differs from MAC for various secondary side effects (such hypothetical situations as "MAC-dysrhythmia," "MAC-hypotension," or "MAC-tachycardia"), combinations of a potent agent and nitrous oxide may decrease or increase these secondary effects relative to potent agent alone. For example, combining 0.6 MAC of nitrous oxide with 0.6 MAC of isoflurane produces less hypotension than 1.2 MAC of isoflurane alone because isoflurane is a more potent vasodilator and myocardial depressant at equivalent MAC than N_2O.

TABLE 17-4

FACTORS THAT INCREASE MINIMUM ALVEOLAR CONCENTRATION

- Increased central neurotransmitter levels (monoamine oxidase inhibitors, acute dextroamphetamine administration, cocaine, ephedrine, levodopa)
- Hyperthermia
- Chronic ethanol abuse (determined in humans)
- Hypernatremia

TABLE 17-5

FACTORS THAT DECREASE MINIMUM ALVEOLAR CONCENTRATION

- Increasing age
- Metabolic acidosis
- Hypoxia (PaO$_2$, 38 mm Hg)
- Induced hypotension (mean arterial pressure <50 mm Hg)
- Decreased central neurotransmitter levels (α-methyldopa, reserpine, chronic dextroamphetamine administration, levodopa)
- α_2-Agonists
- Hypothermia
- Hyponatremia
- Lithium
- Hypo-osmolality
- Pregnancy
- Acute ethanol administration[a]
- Ketamine
- Pancuronium[a]
- Physostigmine (10 times clinical doses)
- Neostigmine (10 times clinical doses)
- Lidocaine
- Opioids
- Opioid agonist-antagonist analgesics
- Barbiturates[a]
- Chlorpromazine[a]
- Diazepam[a]
- Hydroxyzine[a]
- Δ-9-Tetrahydrocannabinol
- Verapamil
- Anemia (<4.3 mL O$_2$/dL blood)

[a]Determined in humans.

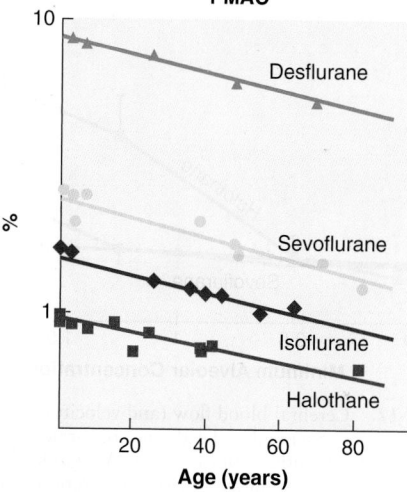

FIGURE 17-11. Effect of age on minimum alveolar concentration (MAC) is plotted. Regression lines are fitted to published values from separate studies. Data are from patients ages 1 to 80 years. (Adapted from Mapleson WW: Effect of age on MAC in humans: a meta-analysis. Br J Anaesth 1996; 76: 179.)

Various factors increase (Table 17-4) or decrease (Table 17-5) MAC. Unfortunately, no single mechanism explains these alterations in MAC, supporting the view that anesthesia is the net result of numerous and widely varying physiologic alterations. In general, those factors that increase CNS metabolic activity and neurotransmission, increase CNS neurotransmitter levels, and up-regulate of CNS responses to chronically depressed neurotransmitter levels (as in chronic alcoholism) also seem to increase MAC. Conversely, those factors that decrease CNS metabolic activity, neurotransmission, and CNS neurotransmitter levels, and down-regulate CNS responses to chronically elevated neurotransmitter levels seem to decrease MAC. Many notable factors do not alter MAC, including duration of inhaled anesthetic administration, gender, type of surgical stimulation, thyroid function, hypo- or hypercarbia, metabolic alkalosis, hyperkalemia, and magnesium levels. However, there may be a genetic component influencing MAC. Red-haired females have a 19% increase in MAC compared with dark-haired females.[14] These data suggest involvement of mutations of the *MCIR* allele. Variants of the *MCIR* allele also have been implicated in altering analgesic responses to a κ opioid.[15] MAC also can vary in relationship to genotype and chromosomal substitutions as shown in rats.[16]

The Effect of Age on MAC

The MAC for each of the potent anesthetic gases shows a clear, age-related change (Fig. 17-11). MAC decreases with age and there are similarities between agents in the decline in MAC and age. Excluding data in patients <1 year of age (where MAC can be lower[17]), there is a linear model that describes a change in MAC of approximately 6% per decade, a 22% decrease in MAC from age 40 to age 80, and a 27% decrease in MAC from age 1 to 40 years.[18]

Other Alterations in Neurophysiology

The three current, widely used, potent agents—isoflurane, desflurane, and sevoflurane—all have reasonably similar effects on a wide range of parameters including cerebral metabolic rate, the EEG, cerebral blood flow (CBF), and flow–metabolism coupling. There are notable differences in effects on ICP, cerebrospinal fluid (CSF) production and resorption, CO$_2$ vasoreactivity, CBF autoregulation, and cerebral protection. Nitrous oxide departs from the potent agents in several important respects, and is therefore discussed separately.

Cerebral Metabolic Rate and Electroencephalogram

All of the potent agents depress CMR to varying degrees in a nonlinear fashion. Once spontaneous cortical neuronal activity is absent (an isoelectric EEG), no further decreases in CMR are generated.

Isoflurane causes a larger MAC-dependent depression of CMR than halothane. Because of this greater depression in neuronal activity, isoflurane abolishes EEG activity at doses used clinically and can usually be tolerated from a hemodynamic standpoint.[19] Desflurane and sevoflurane both cause decreases in CMR similar to isoflurane.[20,21] Interestingly, while both desflurane and sevoflurane depress the EEG and abolish activity at clinically tolerated doses of approximately 2 MAC,[20,21] in *dogs* desflurane-induced isoelectric EEG reverts to continuous activity with time despite an unchanging MAC, a property unique to desflurane.[21]

At normal CO$_2$ and blood pressure, no evidence of sevoflurane cerebral toxicity exists.[22] With extreme hyperventilation to decrease cerebral blood flow by half, brain lactate levels increase, but significantly less than with halothane. There are conflicting data as to whether sevoflurane has a proconvulsant effect.[20,23] High, long-lasting concentrations of sevoflurane (1.5 to 2.0 MAC), a sudden increase in cerebral sevoflurane

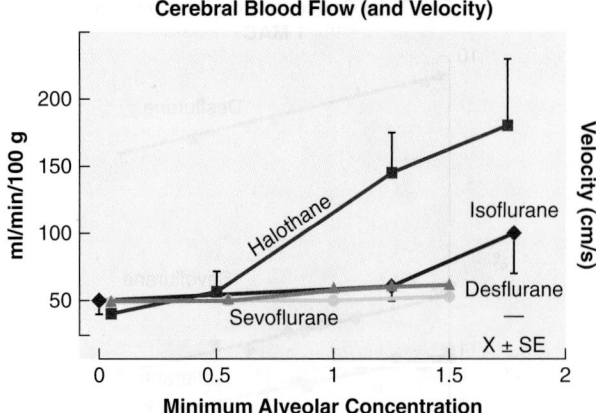

FIGURE 17-12. Cerebral blood flow (and velocity) measured in the presence of normocapnia and in the absence of surgical stimulation in volunteers receiving halothane or isoflurane. At light levels of anesthesia, halothane (but not isoflurane) increased cerebral blood flow. At 1.6 minimum alveolar concentration (MAC), isoflurane also increased cerebral blood flow. (Adapted from Eger EI II: Isoflurane (Forane): A compendium and reference. Madison, Ohio Medical Products, 1985.) Cerebral blood flow velocity measured before and during sevoflurane and desflurane anesthesia up to 1.5 MAC showed no change in cerebral blood flow and velocity. (Adapted from Bedforth NM, Hardman JG, Nathanson MH: Cerebral hemodynamic response to the introduction of desflurane: A comparison with sevoflurane. Anesth Analg 2000; 91: 152.)

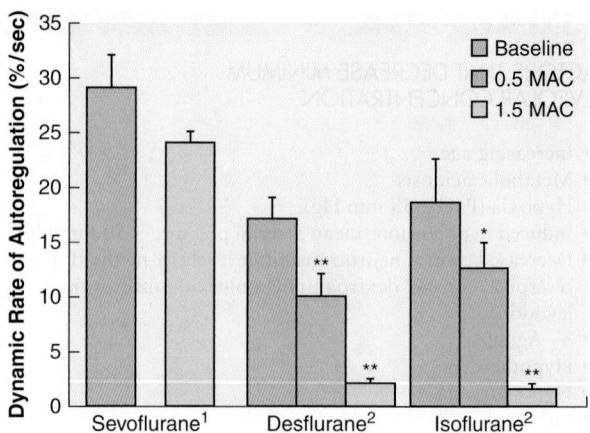

FIGURE 17-13. Dynamic rate of autoregulation (the change in middle cerebral artery blood flow after a rapid transient decrease in blood pressure) during awake (or fentanyl and N_2O baseline), 0.5, and 1.5 minimum alveolar anesthetic concentration (MAC) anesthesia. Values are mean ± SE (SD for sevoflurane). *$P < 0.05$ versus baseline, **$P < 0.001$ versus baseline and sevoflurane. (Adapted from Summors AC, Gupta AK, Matta BF: Dynamic cerebral autoregulation during sevoflurane anesthesia: A comparison with isoflurane. Anesth Analg 1999; 88: 341–345; and Strebel S, Lam A, Matta B, et al: Dynamic and static cerebral autoregulation during isoflurane, desflurane, and propofol anesthesia. Anesthesiology 1995; 83: 66–76.)

concentrations, and hypocapnia can trigger EEG abnormalities that often are associated with increases in heart rate in both adults and children.[24,25] This has raised the question as to the appropriateness of sevoflurane in patients with epilepsy.[26]

Cerebral Blood Flow, Flow–Metabolism Coupling, and Autoregulation

7 All of the potent agents increase CBF in a dose-dependent manner. Isoflurane, sevoflurane, and desflurane cause far less cerebral vasodilation per MAC-multiple than halothane (Fig. 17-12). In human studies, isoflurane produces insignificant or no changes in CBF.[27] Desflurane and sevoflurane both influence CBF in a fashion similar to isoflurane.[20,21] All of these inhaled anesthetic agents affect CBF in a time-dependent as well as dose-dependent manner. In animals, an initial dose-dependent increase in CBF with halothane and isoflurane administration recovers to preinduction levels approximately 2 to 5 hours after induction. The mechanism of this recovery is unclear.

The increase in CBF with increasing dose caused by the potent agents occurs despite decreases in CMR. This phenomenon has been called *uncoupling*, but from a mechanistic standpoint, true uncoupling of flow from metabolism may not occur. That is, as CMR is depressed by the volatile anesthetics, there still is a coupled decline in CBF opposed by a coincident direct vasodilatory effect on the cerebral blood vessels. The net effect on the cerebral vessels depends on the sum of indirect vasoconstricting and direct vasodilating influences.

Autoregulation is the intrinsic myogenic regulation of vascular tone. In normal brain, the mechanisms of autoregulation of CBF over a range of mean arterial pressures from 50 to 150 mm Hg are incompletely understood. Because the volatile anesthetics are direct vasodilators, all are considered to diminish autoregulation in a dose-dependent fashion such that at high anesthetic doses CBF is essentially pressure-passive. Sevoflurane preserves autoregulation up to approximately

1 MAC.[20] At 1.5 MAC, the dynamic rate of autoregulation (change in middle cerebral artery blood flow after a rapid transient decrease in blood pressure) is better preserved with sevoflurane than isoflurane (Fig. 17-13). This may be a result of less of a direct vasodilator effect of sevoflurane, preserving the ability of the vessel to respond to changes in blood pressure at 1.5 MAC. Based on a similar model but a separate study of dynamic autoregulation of cerebral blood flow, 0.5 MAC desflurane reduced autoregulation and isoflurane did not. At 1.5 MAC, both anesthetics substantially reduced autoregulation (Fig. 17-13).

Intracerebral Pressure

Probably the area of greatest clinical interest to the anesthesiologist is the effect of volatile anesthesia on intracerebral pressure (ICP). In general, ICP will increase or decrease in proportion to changes in CBF. Isoflurane increases ICP minimally in animals both with and without brain pathology, including those with an already elevated ICP.[28] In human studies there usually are mild increases in ICP with isoflurane administration that are blocked or blunted by hyperventilation or barbiturate coadministration.[29] There are some contradictory data, however. In one human study, hypocapnia did not prevent elevations in ICP with isoflurane administration in patients with space-occupying brain lesions.[30] However, isoflurane-induced increases in ICP tend to be of short duration, in one study only 30 minutes.[31]

Like isoflurane, both sevoflurane and desflurane >1 MAC produce mild increases in ICP, paralleling their mild increases in CBF.[20,21,32,33] One potential advantage of sevoflurane is that its lower pungency and airway irritation may lessen the risk of coughing and bucking and the associated rise in ICP as compared with desflurane or isoflurane. In fact, introduction of desflurane after propofol induction of anesthesia has led to significant increases in heart rate, mean arterial pressure, and middle cerebral artery blood flow velocity that were not noted in patients given sevoflurane.[34] This may relate to the airway irritant effects of desflurane rather than a specific alteration in neurophysiology. However, several studies in both children and adults suggest that increases in ICP from desflurane are slightly greater than from either isoflurane or sevoflurane.[35,36] The bottom line is that all three potent agents may be used at appropriate doses, especially with adjunctive and compensatory therapies, in just about any neurosurgical procedure.

Cerebrospinal Fluid Production and Resorption

Isoflurane does not appear to alter CSF production,[31] but may increase, decrease, or leave unchanged the resistance to resorption depending on dose. Sevoflurane at 1 MAC depresses CSF production up to 40%.[37] Desflurane at 1 MAC leaves CSF production unchanged or increased.[35,38] In general, anesthetic effects on ICP via changes in CSF dynamics are clinically far less important than anesthetic effects on CBF.

Cerebral Blood Flow Response to Hypercarbia and Hypocarbia

Significant hypercapnia is associated with dramatic increases in CBF whether or not volatile anesthetics are administered. As discussed earlier, hypocapnia can blunt or abolish volatile anesthetic-induced increases in CBF depending on when the hypocapnia is produced. This vasoreactivity to CO_2 may be somewhat altered by the volatile anesthetics as compared with normal. CO_2 vasoreactivity under desflurane anesthesia is normal up to 1.5 MAC,[28] and CO_2 vasoreactivity for sevoflurane is preserved at 1 MAC.[39]

Cerebral Protection

In one study, cerebral hypoperfusion secondary to hypotension from isoflurane was associated with better tissue oxygen content than during hypotension by other means, consistent with the profound decrease in cerebral metabolic rate of oxygen consumption ($CMRO_2$) seen with isoflurane.[40] Both sevoflurane and desflurane have been shown to improve neurologic outcome in comparison to N_2O-fentanyl after incomplete cerebral ischemia in a rat model.[41,42] In piglets undergoing low-flow cardiopulmonary bypass, desflurane improved neurologic outcome compared with a fentanyl/droperidol-based anesthetic.[43] In humans, desflurane has been shown to increase brain tissue PO_2 during administration, and to maintain PO_2 to a greater extent than thiopental during temporary cerebral artery occlusion during cerebrovascular surgery.[44] Human neuroprotection outcome studies for sevoflurane and desflurane have not been published.

Processed Electroencephalograms and Neuromonitoring

All of the volatile anesthetics produce dose-dependent effects on the EEG, sensory-evoked potentials (SEPs) and motor-evoked potentials (MEPs). EEGs recorded on the scalp can be processed to quantify the amount of activity in each of four frequency bands: delta (0 to 3 Hz), theta (4 to 7 Hz), alpha (8 to 13 Hz), and beta (>13 Hz). All three currently used agents at <1 MAC and N_2O at 30 to 70% can produce shifts to increasing frequencies. Between 1 and 2 MAC the potent agents produce shifts to decreasing frequencies and increases in amplitude. At >2 MAC, all of the potent agents can produce burst suppression or electrical silence. These are important factors to remember because EEG changes during administration of general anesthesia can also be caused by hypoxia, hypercarbia, and hypothermia. The EEG must always be interpreted within the appropriate clinical context.

All of the volatile agents cause a dose-dependent increase in latency and decrease in amplitude in all cortical SEP modalities. In subcortical modalities, such as brainstem auditory evoked potentials, these agents are associated with negligible effects. In general, visual evoked potentials are somewhat more sensitive to the effects of the volatile anesthetics than somatosensory evoked potentials. Like EEGs, these effects from anesthetics must be kept in mind when changes during SEPs occur, and appropriate doses of the volatile agents must be used. Sudden changes in the anesthetic regimen (>0.5 MAC) also seem to have greater effects on SEPs than more gradual changes.

MEPs evaluate the functional integrity of descending motor pathways. The evoked response is most commonly recorded as a muscle potential or a peripheral nerve signal. The trigger is typically transosseous activation via electrical or magnetic stimulation. MEPs are exquisitely sensitive to depression by volatile anesthetics, which are usually avoided in these cases.

Nitrous Oxide

The effects of nitrous oxide on cerebral physiology are not clear. Both the MAC for N_2O and its effects on CMR vary widely depending on species. The difference in CMR effects may in part be accounted for by differences in MAC, but MAC-equivalent effects on CMR also differ. Several studies in dogs, goats, and swine found that N_2O increases $CMRO_2$ and CBF, while in rodents no such increases or only slight increases occur. In human studies, N_2O administration preserved CBF but decreased $CMRO_2$.[19]

Another problem is the fact that N_2O is a coanesthetic used to supplement potent agents, not a complete anesthetic in itself, and CMR effects may differ depending on presence or absence of potent agent as well as the particular agent and dose. Addition of N_2O to 1 or 2.2 MAC isoflurane does not alter $CMRO_2$, but it does increase CBF at 1 MAC but not 2.2 MAC.

Barbiturates, narcotics, or a combination of the two appear to decrease or eliminate the increases in CMR and CBF produced by N_2O. The effect of pentobarbital/N_2O is dose-dependent, with preserved increases in CMR by N_2O at low-dose pentobarbital, and no changes in CMR at high-dose pentobarbital.[45] N_2O and benzodiazepine coadministration is particularly confusing. Midazolam/N_2O in dogs increased CBF but did not alter $CMRO_2$,[46] while the opposite was true in rats,[47] and both CBF and $CMRO_2$ declined in rats given diazepam/N_2O. N_2O administration increases ICP, but as is the case for CMR and CBF, changes in ICP are decreased or eliminated by a variety of coanesthetics and, more importantly, by hypocapnia.

N_2O appears to have an antineuroprotective effect, as addition of N_2O to isoflurane during temporary ischemia is associated with greater tissue damage and worsened neurologic outcome.[47] In a study in mice, survival time after a hypoxic event was decreased by addition of N_2O.[48] Given the conflicting data on the effects of N_2O on CMR, CBF, ICP, and the apparent antineuroprotective effect of this agent, avoidance or discontinuation of its use should be considered in surgical cases with a high likelihood of elevated ICP or significant cerebral ischemia.

THE CIRCULATORY SYSTEM

Hemodynamics

The cardiac, vascular, and autonomic effects of the volatile anesthetics have been carefully defined through a number of studies carried out in human volunteers not undergoing surgery.[49-54] In general, the information from these volunteer

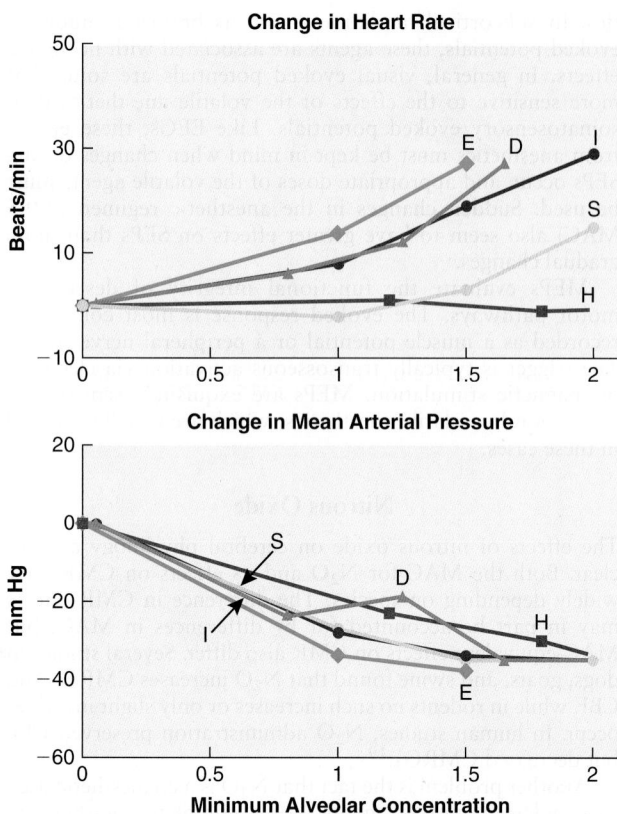

FIGURE 17-14. Heart rate and blood pressure changes (from awake baseline) in volunteers receiving general anesthesia with halothane (H), enflurane (E), isoflurane (I), desflurane (D), or sevoflurane (S). Halothane and sevoflurane produced little or no change in heart rate at <1.5 minimum alveolar concentration. All anesthetics caused similar decreases in blood pressure. (Adapted from Malan TP Jr, DiNardo JA, Isner RJ, et al: Cardiovascular effects of sevoflurane compared with those of isoflurane in volunteers. Anesthesiology 1995; 83: 918; Weiskopf RB, Cahalan MK, Eger EI II, et al: Cardiovascular actions of desflurane in normocarbic volunteers. Anesth Analg 1991; 73: 143; and Calverley RK, Smith NT, Prys-Roberts C, et al: Cardiovascular effects of enflurane anesthesia during controlled ventilation in man. Anesth Analg 1978; 57: 619.)

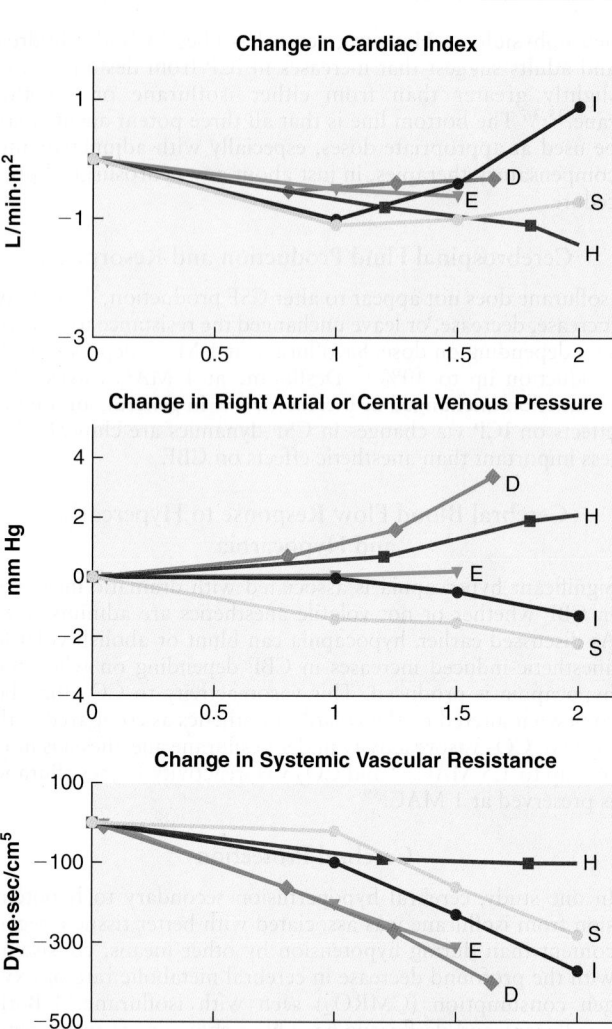

FIGURE 17-15. Cardiac index, central venous pressure (or right atrial pressure), and systemic vascular resistance changes (from awake baseline) in volunteers receiving general anesthesia with halothane (H), enflurane (E), isoflurane (I), desflurane (D), or sevoflurane (S). Increases in central venous pressure from halothane and desflurane might be due to different mechanisms. With halothane, the increase might be due to myocardial depression, whereas with desflurane, the increase is more likely due to venoconstriction. (Adapted from Malan TP Jr, DiNardo JA, Isner RJ, et al: Cardiovascular effects of sevoflurane compared with those of isoflurane in volunteers. Anesthesiology 1995; 83: 918; Weiskopf RB, Cahalan MK, Eger EI II, et al: Cardiovascular actions of desflurane in normocarbic volunteers. Anesth Analg 1991; 73: 143; and Calverley RK, Smith NT, Prys-Roberts C, et al: Cardiovascular effects of enflurane anesthesia during controlled ventilation in man. Anesth Analg 1978; 57: 619.)

studies has translated well to the patient population commonly exposed to these anesthetics during elective and emergent surgeries.

A common effect of the potent volatile anesthetics has been a dose-related decrease in arterial blood pressure, with essentially no differences noted between the volatile anesthetics at steady-state, equianesthetic concentrations (Fig. 17-14). Their primary mechanism to decrease blood pressure with increasing dose is related to their potent effects to lower regional and systemic vascular resistance (Fig. 17-15).

In volunteers, sevoflurane up to about 1 MAC results in minimal, if any, changes in steady-state heart rate while enflurane, isoflurane, and desflurane increase it 5 to 10% from baseline (Fig. 17-14). Both desflurane and, to a lesser extent, isoflurane have been associated with transient and significant increases in heart rate during rapid increases in the inspired concentration of either anesthetic.[55,56] The mechanism(s) underlying these transient heart rate surges is likely due to the relative pungency of these anesthetics, which stimulates airway receptors to elicit a reflex tachycardia.[57] The tachycardia can be lessened with fentanyl, alfentanil, or clonidine pretreatment.[58–60]

Myocardial Contractility

Myocardial contractility indices have been directly evaluated in animals and indirectly evaluated in humans during the administration of each of the volatile anesthetics. Human studies with isoflurane, sevoflurane, and desflurane have not demonstrated significant changes in echocardiographic-determined indices of myocardial function, including the more noteworthy measurement of the velocity of circumferential fiber shortening (Fig. 17-16). More precise indices of myocardial contractility have been obtained for sevoflurane, isoflurane, and desflurane in chronically instrumented dogs

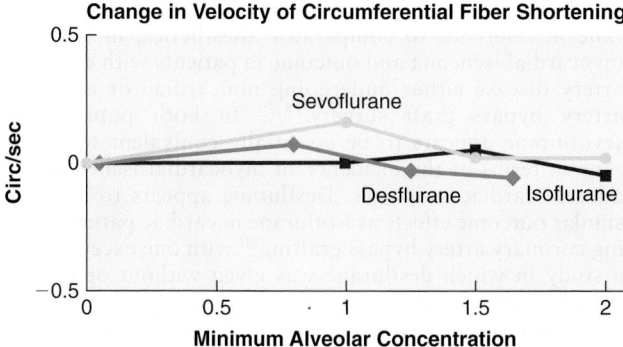

FIGURE 17-16. Noninvasive assessment of myocardial contractility with echocardiography during anesthesia in volunteers. Sevoflurane, desflurane, and isoflurane did not cause changes suggestive of myocardial depression. (Adapted from Malan TP Jr, DiNardo JA, Isner RJ, et al: Cardiovascular effects of sevoflurane compared with those of isoflurane in volunteers. Anesthesiology 1995; 83: 918; Weiskopf RB, Cahalan MK, Eger EI II, et al: Cardiovascular actions of desflurane in normocarbic volunteers. Anesth Analg 1991; 73: 143; and Calverley RK, Smith NT, Prys-Roberts C, et al: Cardiovascular effects of enflurane anesthesia during controlled ventilation in man. Anesth Analg 1978; 57: 619.)

after autonomic denervation of the heart. Isoflurane, desflurane, and sevoflurane resulted in a dose-dependent depression of myocardial function with no differences between the three anesthetics (Fig. 17-17).

Other Circulatory Effects

Most of the volatile anesthetics have been studied during both controlled and spontaneous ventilation.[51,61,62] The process of spontaneous ventilation reduces the high intrathoracic pressures from positive pressure ventilation. The negative intrathoracic pressure during the inspiratory phase of spontaneous ventilation augments venous return and cardiac filling and improves cardiac output and, hence, blood pressure. Spontaneous ventilation is associated with higher $PaCO_2$, causing cerebral and systemic vascular relaxation. This contributes to an improved cardiac output via afterload reduction. Thus, spontaneous ventilation decreases systemic vascular resistance and increases heart rate, cardiac output, and stroke volume as contrasted to positive pressure ventilation. It has been suggested that spontaneous ventilation might improve the safety of inhaled anesthetic administration because the concentration of a volatile anesthetic that produces cardiovascular collapse exceeds the concentration that results in apnea.[63]

A curious observation with the potent volatile anesthetics has been an alteration in the cardiovascular effects during prolonged anesthetic exposures, noted as a small increase in heart rate and cardiac index, a gradual decrease in systemic vascular resistance, and no change in myocardial indices.[51,52] The mechanism(s) of this effect are not clear.

Nitrous oxide is commonly combined with potent volatile anesthetics to maintain general anesthesia. Nitrous oxide has unique cardiovascular actions. It increases sympathetic nervous system activity and vascular resistance when given in a 40% concentration.[49,64] When nitrous oxide is combined with volatile anesthetics and compared with equipotent concentrations of the volatile anesthetic without nitrous oxide, there is an increased systemic vascular resistance and an improved arterial pressure with little effect on cardiac output.[51,65] These effects might not be due solely to sympathetic activation from nitrous oxide per se, but may be partially attributed to a

decrease in the concentration of the coadministered potent volatile anesthetic required to achieve a MAC equivalent when using nitrous oxide.

Oxygen consumption is decreased approximately 10 to 15% during general anesthesia.[66] The distribution of cardiac output also is altered by anesthesia. Blood flow to liver, kidneys, and gut is decreased, particularly at deep levels of anesthesia. In contrast, blood flow to the brain, muscle, and skin is increased or not changed during general anesthesia.[67] In humans, increases in muscle blood flow are noted with isoflurane, desflurane, and sevoflurane with very small differences between anesthetics at equipotent concentrations.[68]

Isoflurane, sevoflurane, and desflurane do not predispose patients to ventricular arrhythmias, nor sensitize the heart to the arrhythmogenic effects of epinephrine (Fig. 17-18). Some of the differences between volatile anesthetics in their ability to promote other arrhythmias can be attributed to their direct effects on cardiac pacemaker cells and conduction pathways.[69] Sinoatrial node discharge rate is slowed by the volatile anesthetics[70] and conduction in the His-Purkinje system and

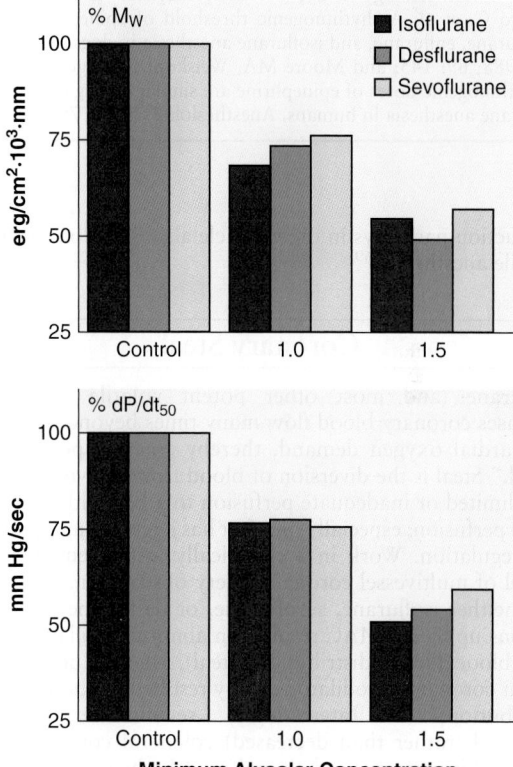

FIGURE 17-17. Myocardial contractility indices from chronically instrumented dogs. For these measurements, pharmacologic blockade of the autonomic nervous system was established to eliminate neural or circulating humoral influences on the inotropic state of the heart. The conscious control data were assigned 100%, and subsequent reductions in the inotropic state are depicted for both 1 and 1.5 minimum alveolar anesthetic concentrations of sevoflurane, desflurane, and isoflurane. There were no differences between these three volatile anesthetics. M_w, slope of the regional preload recruitable stroke work relationship; dP/dt_{50}, change in pressure per unit of time. (Adapted from Pagel PS, Kampine JP, Schmeling WT, et al: Influence of volatile anesthetics on myocardial contractility in vivo: Desflurane versus isoflurane. Anesthesiology 1991; 74: 900; and Harkin CP, Pagel PS, Kersten JR, et al: Direct negative inotropic and lusitropic effects of sevoflurane. Anesthesiology 1994; 81: 156.)

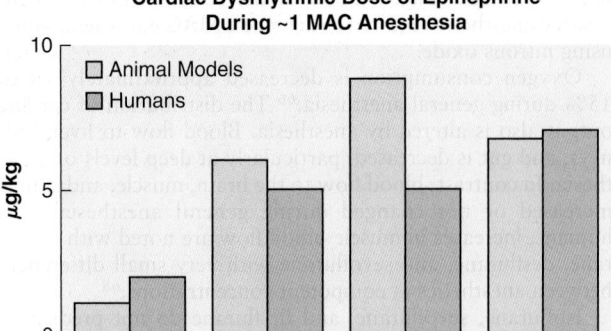

FIGURE 17-18. The dose of epinephrine associated with cardiac arrhythmias in animal and human models was least with halothane. The ether anesthetics—isoflurane, desflurane, and sevoflurane—required three- to sixfold greater doses of epinephrine to cause arrhythmias. (Adapted from Navarro R, Weiskopf RB, Moore MA, et al: Humans anesthetized with sevoflurane or isoflurane have similar arrhythmic response to epinephrine. Anesthesiology 1994; 80: 545; Weiskopf RB, Eger EI II, Holmes MA, et al: Epinephrine-induced premature ventricular contractions and changes in arterial blood pressure and heart rate during I-653, isoflurane, and halothane anesthesia in swine. Anesthesiology 1989; 70: 293; Hayashi Y, Sumikawa K, Tashiro C, et al: Arrhythmogenic threshold of epinephrine during sevoflurane, enflurane, and isoflurane anesthesia in dogs. Anesthesiology 1988; 69: 145; and Moore MA, Weiskopf RB, Eger EI II, et al: Arrhythmogenic doses of epinephrine are similar during desflurane or isoflurane anesthesia in humans. Anesthesiology 1993; 79: 943.)

conduction pathways in the ventricle also is prolonged by the volatile anesthetics.[69]

Coronary Steal

Isoflurane (and most other potent volatile anesthetics) increases coronary blood flow many times beyond that of the myocardial oxygen demand, thereby creating potential for "steal." Steal is the diversion of blood from a myocardial bed with limited or inadequate perfusion to a bed with more adequate perfusion; especially one that has a remaining element of autoregulation. Work in a chronically instrumented, canine model of multivessel coronary artery obstruction, has shown that neither isoflurane, sevoflurane, or desflurane at concentrations up to 1.5 MAC resulted in abnormal collateral coronary blood flow redistribution (steal), whereas adenosine, a potent coronary vasodilator, clearly resulted in abnormal flow distribution.[71–74] Interestingly, sevoflurane favorably increased (rather than decreased) collateral coronary blood flow in this instrumented animal model when aortic pressure was held constant by pharmacologic support of blood pressure.[73]

Myocardial Ischemia and Cardiac Outcome

Not surprisingly, the clinical relevance of coronary steal with isoflurane has been debated and is generally thought to be minimal.[75] Outcome studies have failed to associate the use of isoflurane in patients undergoing coronary artery bypass operations with an increased incidence of myocardial infarction or perioperative death.[75–77] Most studies would suggest that determinants of myocardial oxygen supply and demand, rather than the anesthetic, are of far greater importance to patient outcomes.

Several studies have evaluated sevoflurane and desflurane in reference to comparator anesthetics, in terms of myocardial ischemia and outcome in patients with coronary artery disease either undergoing noncardiac or coronary artery bypass graft surgery.[78,79] In both populations, sevoflurane appears to be essentially equivalent to isoflurane in terms of the incidence of myocardial ischemia and adverse cardiac outcomes. Desflurane appears to result in similar outcome effects as isoflurane in cardiac patients having coronary artery bypass grafting[80] with one exception. In a study in which desflurane was given without opioids to patients with coronary artery disease requiring coronary artery bypass graft surgery, significant ischemia mandating the use of beta-blockers was noted.[81] Desflurane has not been evaluated in terms of ischemia and outcome in a patient population with coronary disease undergoing noncardiac surgery.

Cardioprotection from Volatile Anesthetics

A preconditioning stimulus such as brief coronary occlusion and ischemia initiates a signaling cascade of intracellular events that reduces ischemia and reperfusion myocardial injury. There is a memory effect from an ischemic stimulus that offers 2 to 3 hours of protection. The volatile anesthetics mimic ischemic preconditioning and trigger a similar cascade of intracellular events resulting in myocardial protection that lasts beyond the elimination of the anesthetic.[82] Numerous factors may be involved in preconditioning, including the sodium:hydrogen exchanger, the adenosine receptor (particularly α_1 and α_2 subtypes), inhibitory G proteins, protein kinase C, tyrosine kinase, and potassium (K_{ATP}) channel opening. Pharmacologic blockade of these factors (e.g., with adenosine blockers, delta 1 opioids, pertussis toxin, or glibenclamide) reduces or eliminates the cardioprotective effect of ischemic or volatile anesthetic preconditioning.[82,83] Alternatively, administration of certain drugs can mimic ischemic or volatile anesthetic preconditioning. These include adenosine, opioid agonists, and K_{ATP} channel openers. In contrast to the inhalation of volatile anesthetics, these cardioprotective drugs must be delivered into a coronary artery because systemic administration can have serious side effects.

Lipophilic volatile anesthetics diffuse through myocardial cell membranes and alter mitochondrial electron transport, leading to reactive oxygen species formation.[83] This may be the trigger for preconditioning *via* protein kinase C activation of K_{ATP} channel opening.[84,85] Approximately 30 to 40% of the cardioprotection from the volatile anesthetics appears to be related to a reduced loading of calcium into the myocardial cells during ischemia. Preconditioned hearts may tolerate ischemia for 10 minutes longer than nonconditioned hearts.[86]

While these evolving data generally derive from animal models, there now is increasing evidence in cardiac patient populations that anesthetic cardioprotection lessens myocardial damage (based on troponin levels) during "on and off pump" cardiac surgery.[87,88] This effect seems to be common to all current potent volatile anesthetics, and may favorably influence intensive care unit length of stay after coronary surgery.[89] Sulfonylurea oral hyperglycemic drugs close K_{ATP} channels, abolishing anesthetic preconditioning. They should be discontinued 24 to 48 hours prior to elective surgery in high-risk patients.[82] But hyperglycemia also prevents preconditioning, so insulin therapy should be started when holding oral agents.[90] Recent evidence suggests that volatile anesthetics may protect other organs from ischemic injury including kidney, liver, and brain.[91–93]

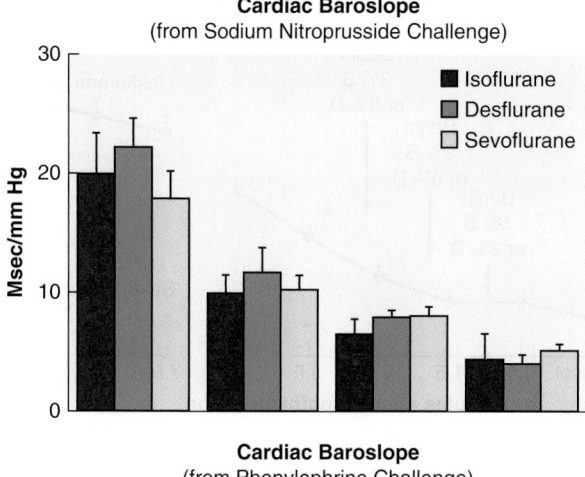

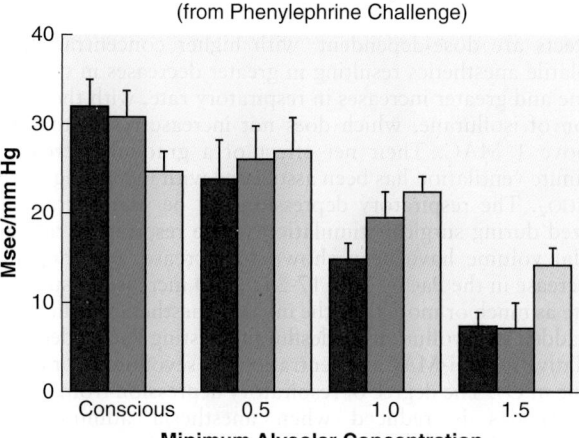

FIGURE 17-19. Summary data of the baroreflex regulation of heart rate (R-R interval) in response to a decreasing pressure stimulus (sodium nitroprusside) or in response to an increasing pressure stimulus (phenylephrine). These data were acquired in healthy volunteers who were randomized to receive isoflurane, desflurane, or sevoflurane. With increasing minimum alveolar anesthetic concentration, each of the volatile anesthetics led to a progressive reduction in the cardiac baroslope (an index of baroreflex sensitivity derived by relating changes in mean pressure to changes in R-R interval). There were no statistical differences between anesthetics. (Adapted from Ebert TJ, Harkin CP, Muzi M: Cardiovascular responses to sevoflurane: A review. Anesth Analg 1995; 81: S11.)

Autonomic Nervous System

10 Studies that have focused on the efferent activity of the parasympathetic and sympathetic nervous systems indicate that the volatile anesthetics depress their activity in a dose-dependent fashion.[94,95] However, because the autonomic nervous system is importantly modulated by baroreceptor reflex mechanisms, the effects of the anesthetic on the efferent system cannot be reported without taking into account their effects on different components of the baroreflex arc. Thus, although both limbs of the autonomic nervous system have been shown to be attenuated by the anesthetics, the afferent activity from the arterial baroreceptors has been found to be increased with some of the anesthetics, such as isoflurane.[96] This increased discharge of the baroreceptors actually contributes to the depression of the entire baroreflex arc by tonically lowering the overall level of outflow of the sympathetic nervous system. From the perspective of clinical relevance, studies have examined the behavior of the arterial baroreflex

system during a hypotensive or hypertensive stimulus by evaluating changes in heart rate and sympathetic nerve activity. The arterial baroreflex is the most rapidly responding system to blood pressure perturbations. Early investigations focused primarily on the regulation of heart rate, which reflects a primarily vagal-mediated end point. Isoflurane reduces, in a dose-dependent fashion, arterial baroreflex control of heart rate.[97] Similar effects on the reflex control of heart rate have recently been demonstrated with sevoflurane and desflurane (Fig. 17-19).[98–100]

There is greater difficulty in evaluating the sympathetic component of the baroreflex arc in humans, but a technique called *sympathetic microneurography* has been used to directly record vasoconstrictor impulses directed to blood vessels in humans.[50,55] There is a dose-dependent depression of the reflex control of sympathetic outflow that appears to be relatively equivalent for isoflurane, sevoflurane, and desflurane (Fig. 17-20). Importantly, at low levels of anesthesia (e.g., 0.5 MAC), there is little if any depression of reflex function and this might have important implications in the compromised patient population. Opioid and benzodiazepine adjuvants have only minimal effects on reflex function and combining these with low levels of potent anesthetics might preserve reflex function.[101,102] Another important observation has been the more rapid return of baroreflex function with the less soluble anesthetic sevoflurane versus isoflurane.[103] This might add to hemodynamic stability in the postoperative period when tissue concentrations of the volatile anesthetics are declining.

Desflurane has a unique and prominent effect on sympathetic outflow in humans, which is not apparent in animal models. With increasing steady-state concentrations of desflurane, there is a progressive increase in resting sympathetic nervous system activity and plasma norepinephrine levels.[50,55,104] Despite this increase in tonic sympathetic outflow, blood pressure decreases similarly to sevoflurane and isoflurane. This raises the question as to whether desflurane has the ability to uncouple neuroeffector responses. In addition, desflurane can cause marked activation of the sympathetic nervous system when the inspired concentration is increased, especially to

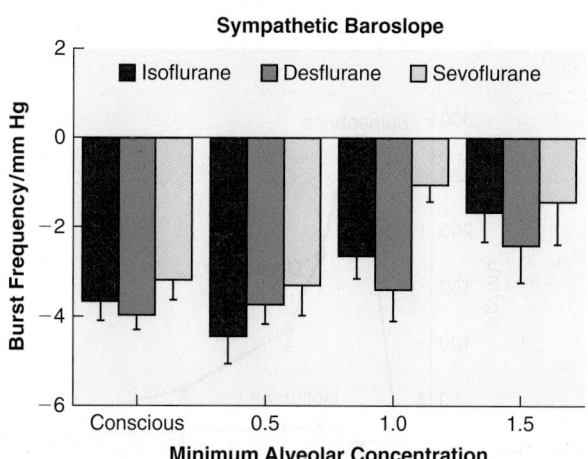

FIGURE 17-20. The sympathetic baroreflex function of healthy volunteers randomized to receive isoflurane, desflurane, or sevoflurane. The slope (sensitivity) is the relationship between decreasing diastolic pressure and increasing efferent sympathetic nerve activity. The reflex regulation of sympathetic outflow was fairly well preserved at 0.5 and 1.0 minimum alveolar anesthetic concentration (MAC) of anesthetic. At 1.5 MAC, there was a 50% decrease in the slope with all anesthetics. (Adapted from Ebert TJ, Harkin CP, Muzi M: Cardiovascular responses to sevoflurane: A review. Anesth Analg 1995; 81: S11.)

FIGURE 17-21. Consecutive measurements of sympathetic nerve activity (SNA; mean ± SE) from human volunteers during induction of anesthesia with propofol and the subsequent mask administration of sevoflurane or desflurane for a 10-minute period. The inspired concentration of these anesthetics was increased at 1-minute intervals beginning after propofol administration (0.41 MAC of sevoflurane and desflurane). In both groups, propofol reduced SNA and mean arterial pressure. Desflurane resulted in significant increases in SNA that persisted throughout the 10-minute mask administration period. (Adapted from Ebert TJ, Muzi M, Lopatka CW: Neurocirculatory responses to sevoflurane in humans. A comparison to desflurane. Anesthesiology 1995; 83: 88.)

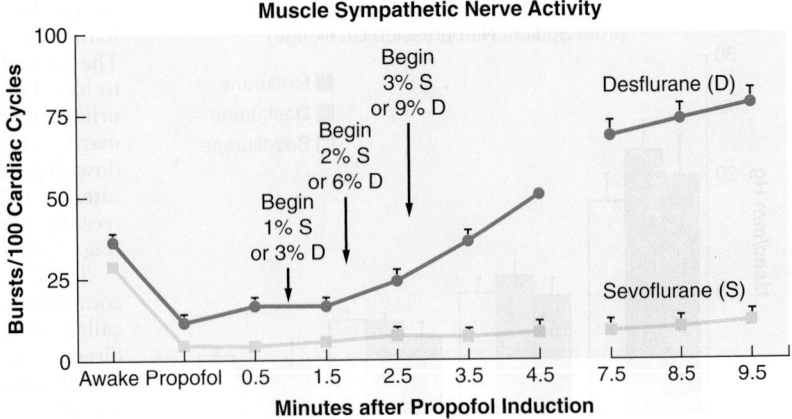

concentrations above 5 to 6% (Fig. 17-21).[50,55,104] There is a transient surge in sympathetic outflow leading to both hypertension and tachycardia. In addition, the endocrine axis is activated as evidenced by 15- to 20-fold increases in plasma antidiuretic hormone and epinephrine and norepinephrine (Fig. 17-22). The hemodynamic response persists for 4 to 5 minutes and the endocrine response persists for 15 to 25 minutes. Adequate concentrations of opioids or clonidine given prior to increasing the concentration of desflurane have been shown to attenuate these responses.[58–60] The source of the neuroendocrine activation has been actively sought, and it would appear that there are receptors in both the upper and the lower airways, and/or perhaps in a highly perfused tissue near the airways, that initiates the sympathetic activation.[57]

THE PULMONARY SYSTEM

General Ventilatory Effects

11 All volatile anesthetics decrease tidal volume and increase respiratory rate such that there are only minor effects on decreasing minute ventilation (Fig. 17-23). The ventilatory effects are dose-dependent, with higher concentrations of volatile anesthetics resulting in greater decreases in tidal volume and greater increases in respiratory rate, with the exception of isoflurane, which does not increase respiratory rate above 1 MAC. Their net effect of a gradual decrease in minute ventilation has been associated with increasing resting $PaCO_2$. The respiratory depression can be partially antagonized during surgical stimulation where respiratory rate and tidal volume have been shown to increase, resulting in a decrease in the $PaCO_2$ (Fig. 17-24). N_2O increases respiratory rate as much or more than the inhaled anesthetics. When N_2O is added to sevoflurane or desflurane, resting $PaCO_2$ decreases relative to equi-MAC concentrations of sevoflurane or desflurane in O_2. The degree of respiratory depression from inhaled anesthetics is reduced when anesthesia administration exceeds 5 hours.[105]

Ventilatory Mechanics

FRC is decreased during general anesthesia; this has been explained by a number of mechanisms including a decrease in the intercostal muscle tone, alteration in diaphragm position,

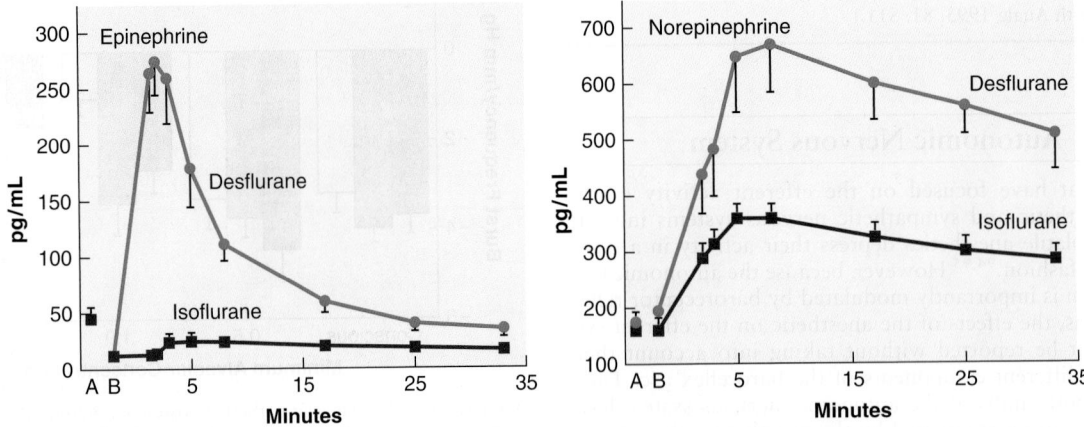

FIGURE 17-22. Stress hormone responses to a rapid increase in anesthetic concentration, from 4 to 12% inspired. Volunteers given desflurane showed a larger increase in plasma epinephrine and norepinephrine concentrations than when given isoflurane. Data are mean ± SE. A = awake value; B = value after 32 minutes of 0.55 minimum alveolar concentration; time represents minutes after the first breath of increased anesthetic concentration. (Adapted from Weiskopf RB, Moore MA, Eger EI II, et al: Rapid increase in desflurane concentration is associated with greater transient cardiovascular stimulation than with rapid increase in isoflurane concentration in humans. Anesthesiology 1994; 80: 1035.)

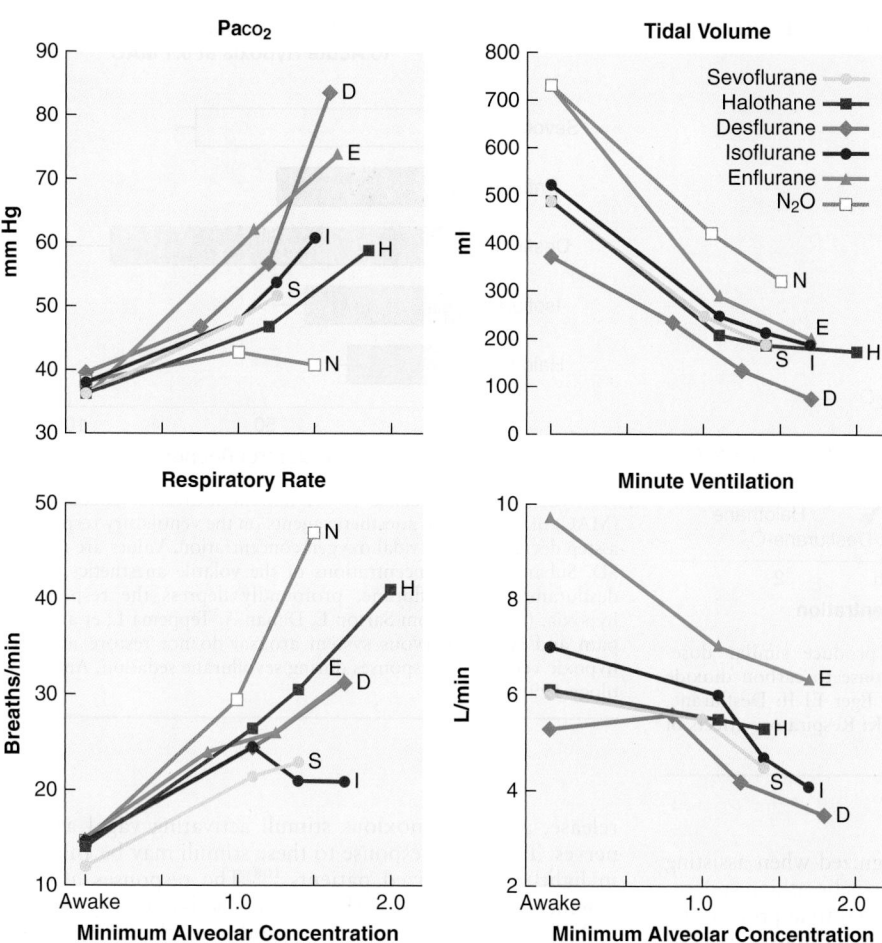

FIGURE 17-23. Comparison of mean changes in resting PaCO₂, tidal volume, respiratory rate, and minute ventilation in patients anesthetized with either halothane, isoflurane, enflurane, sevoflurane, desflurane, or nitrous oxide (N, N₂O). Anesthetic-induced tachypnea compensates in part for the ventilatory depression caused by all volatile anesthetics (decrease in minute ventilation and tidal volume, and concomitant increase in PaCO₂). Desflurane results in the greatest increase in PaCO₂ with corresponding reductions in tidal volume and minute ventilation. Isoflurane, like all other inhaled agents, increases respiratory rate, but does not result in dose-dependent tachypnea. (Adapted from Lockhart SH, Rampil IJ, Yasuda N, et al: Depression of ventilation by desflurane in humans. Anesthesiology 1991; 74: 484; Doi M, Ikeda K: Respiratory effects of sevoflurane. Anesth Analg 1987; 66: 241; Fourcade HE, Stevens WC, Larson CP Jr, et al: The ventilatory effects of Forane, a new inhaled anesthetic. Anesthesiology 1971; 35: 26; and Calverley RK, Smith NT, Jones CW, et al: Ventilatory and cardiovascular effects of enflurane anesthesia during spontaneous ventilation in man. Anesth Analg 1978; 57: 610.)

ANESTHETIC AGENTS, ADJUVANTS, AND DRUG INTERACTION

changes in thoracic blood volume, and the onset of phasic expiratory activity of respiratory muscles. About 40% of the muscular work of breathing is via intercostal muscles and about 60% is from the diaphragm. The diaphragmatic muscle function is relatively spared when contrasted to the parasternal intercostal muscles. However, inspiratory rib cage expansion is reasonably well maintained during anesthesia because of preserved activity of the scalene muscles. Expiration is generally considered a passive function mediated by the elastic recoil of the lung. The process of applying a resistance or load to expiration typically results in a slowing of respiration, but under anesthesia, additional responses include a substantial asynchrony of the thoracic movements with respiration. This suggests that in patients with pulmonary disease associated with increased expiratory resistance, the act of spontaneous ventilation during general anesthesia might be poorly tolerated.

Response to Carbon Dioxide and Hypoxemia

In awake humans, the central chemoreceptors respond vigorously to changes in arterial carbon dioxide tension such that minute ventilation increases 3 L/min per a 1-mm Hg increase in PaCO₂. All of the inhaled anesthetics produce a dose-dependent depression of the ventilatory response to hypercarbia (Fig. 17-25). The addition of nitrous oxide to a volatile anesthetic had been thought to diminish PaCO₂ responses less than an equi-MAC dose of the anesthetic alone, however, this does not appear to be the case for desflurane (Fig. 17-25). In patients with chronic obstructive pulmonary disease, there is an impaired response to increased PaCO₂ under anesthesia.

The threshold at which breathing stops, called the *apneic threshold*, can be determined during anesthesia with spontaneous ventilation. It is generally 4 to 5 mm Hg below the prevailing resting PaCO₂ and unrelated to the slope of the CO₂ response curves or to the level of the resting PaCO₂. The clinical

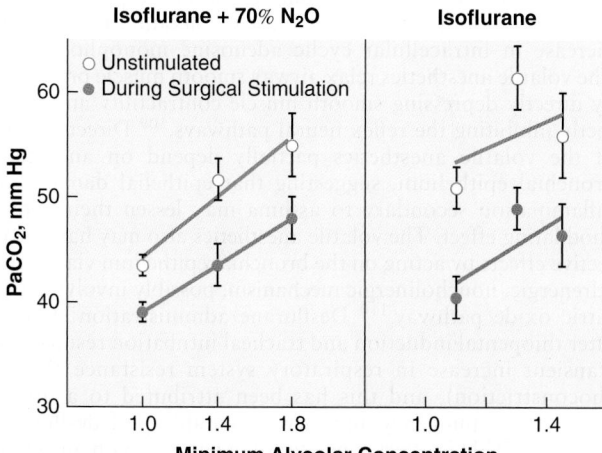

FIGURE 17-24. The effect of surgical stimulation on the ventilatory depression of inhaled anesthesia with isoflurane in the presence and absence of nitrous oxide (N₂O). Surgical stimulation increased alveolar ventilation and decreased PaCO₂ at all depths of anesthesia examined. (Adapted from Eger EI 2nd, Dolan WM, Stevens WC, et al: Surgical stimulation antagonizes the respiratory depression produced by Forane. Anesthesiology 1972; 36: 544.)

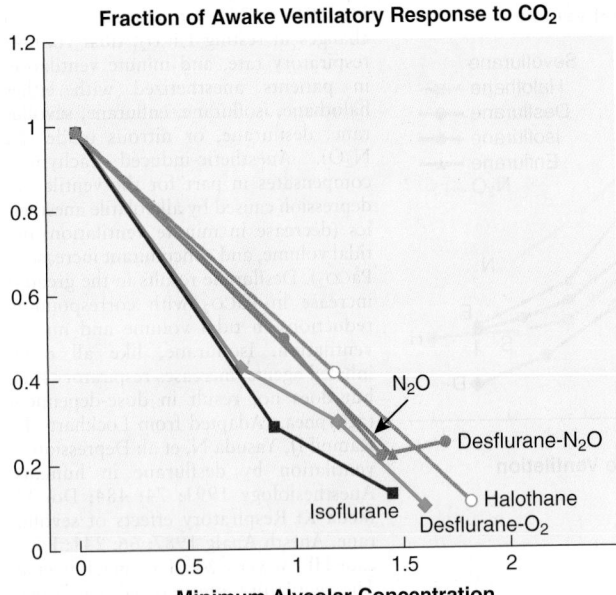

FIGURE 17-25. All inhaled anesthetics produce similar dose-dependent decreases in the ventilatory response to carbon dioxide (CO_2). N$_2$O, nitrous oxide. (Adapted from Eger EI II: Desflurane. Anesth Rev 1993; 20: 87; and Doi M, Ikeda K: Respiratory effects of sevoflurane. Anesth Analg 1987; 66: 241.)

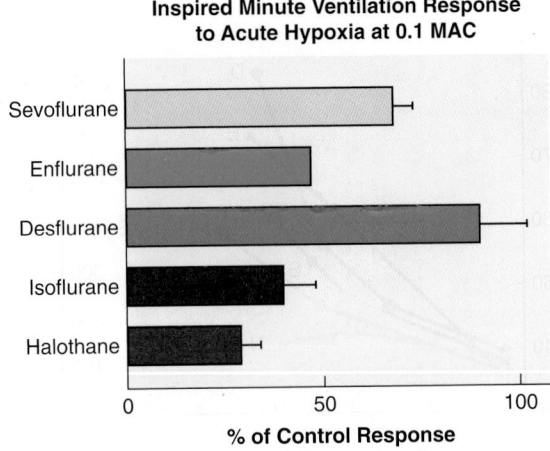

FIGURE 17-26. Influence of 0.1 minimum alveolar concentration (MAC) of five volatile anesthetic agents on the ventilatory response to a step decrease in end-tidal oxygen concentration. Values are mean ± SD. Subanesthetic concentrations of the volatile anesthetics, except desflurane and sevoflurane, profoundly depress the response to hypoxia. (Adapted from Sarton E, Dahan A, Teppema L, et al: Acute pain and central nervous system arousal do not restore impaired hypoxic ventilatory responses during sevoflurane sedation. Anesthesiology 1996; 85: 295.)

relevance of this threshold may be recognized when assisting ventilation in an anesthetized patient who is breathing spontaneously. This only serves to lower the PaCO$_2$ to approach that of the apneic threshold, therefore mandating more control of ventilation.

Inhaled anesthetics, including nitrous oxide, produce a dose-dependent attenuation of the ventilatory response to hypoxia. This action appears to depend on the peripheral chemoreceptors. In fact, even subanesthetic concentrations of volatile anesthetics (0.1 MAC) elicit anywhere from a 15 to 75% depression of the ventilatory drive to hypoxia (Fig. 17-26). The mechanism of this depression still remains poorly understood. Studies have suggested that hypoxia may decrease the probability that potassium channels are open, thus causing membrane depolarization, an influx of calcium ions, and a release of neurotransmitters.[106] One theory is that the potassium channels are responding to reactive oxygen species. One study found the administration of antioxidants prior to the administration of a volatile anesthetic prevented the depression of the hypoxic response.[107] The extreme sensitivity of the volatile anesthetics to inhibit ventilatory responses to hypoxia has important clinical implications. Residual effects of volatile anesthetics may impair the ventilatory drive of patients in the recovery room. In this regard, the short-acting anesthetics (sevoflurane and desflurane) may prove advantageous because of their more rapid washout and their minimal effect on hypoxic sensitivity at subanesthetic concentrations (Fig. 17-26). The effects of the volatile anesthetics on hypoxic drive may play an even more important role in patients who rely on hypoxic drive to set their level of ventilation, such as those with chronic respiratory failure or patients with obstructive sleep apnea.

Bronchiolar Smooth Muscle Tone

Bronchoconstriction under anesthesia occurs because of direct stimulation of the laryngeal and tracheal areas, from the administration of adjuvant drugs that cause histamine release, and from noxious stimuli activating vagal afferent nerves. The reflex response to these stimuli may be enhanced in lightly anesthetized patients.[108] The responses also are enhanced in patients with known reactive airway disease, including those requiring bronchodilator therapy or those with chronic smoking histories. Airway smooth muscle extends as far distally as the terminal bronchioles and is under the influence of both parasympathetic and sympathetic nerves. The parasympathetic nerves mediate baseline airway tone and reflex bronchoconstriction via M2 and M3 muscarinic receptors on the airway smooth muscle, which initiate increases in intracellular cyclic guanosine monophosphate. Adrenergic receptors also are located on bronchial smooth muscle, and the β_2-receptor subtype plays the predominant role in promoting bronchiolar muscle relaxation through an increase in intracellular cyclic adenosine monophosphate. The volatile anesthetics relax airway smooth muscle primarily by directly depressing smooth muscle contractility and indirectly inhibiting the reflex neural pathways.[109] Direct effects of the volatile anesthetics partially depend on an intact bronchial epithelium, suggesting that epithelial damage or inflammation secondary to asthma may lessen their bronchodilating effect. The volatile anesthetics also may have protective effects by acting on the bronchial epithelium via a nonadrenergic, noncholinergic mechanism, possibly involving the nitric oxide pathway.[110] Desflurane administration shortly after thiopental induction and tracheal intubation results in a transient increase in respiratory system resistance (bronchoconstriction), and this has been attributed to a direct effect of the pungency and airway irritability of desflurane (Fig. 17-27). This effect is worsened in patients with an active smoking history.[111] Volatile anesthetics have been used effectively to treat status asthmaticus when other conventional treatments have failed.[112,113] Although halothane has been historically used in these situations, it is no longer available commercially. Sevoflurane may be a better choice because of its quick onset, lack of pungency, lack of cardiovascular depression, and lower risk of cardiac arrhythmias compared with halothane.

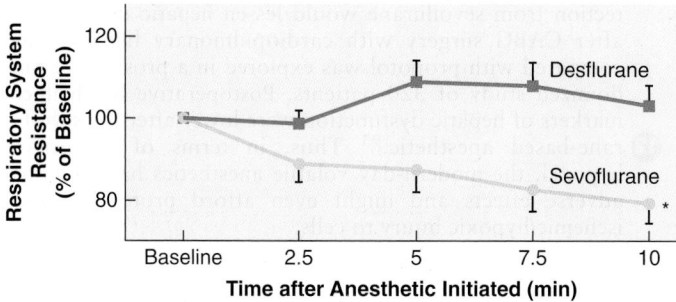

FIGURE 17-27. Changes in respiratory system resistance expressed as a percentage of the baseline recorded after tracheal intubation but prior to administration of sevoflurane or desflurane to the inspired gas mixture. Airway resistance responses to sevoflurane were significantly different from desflurane (*$p < 0.05$). (Adapted from Goff MJ, Arain SR, Ficke DJ, et al: Absence of bronchodilation during desflurane anesthesia: A comparison to sevoflurane and thiopental. Anesthesiology 2000; 93: 404.)

Mucociliary Function

Ciliated respiratory epithelium extends from the trachea to the terminal bronchioles. Cells and glands in the tracheobronchial tree secrete mucus that captures surface particles for transport via ciliary action. There are a number of factors involved in diminished mucociliary function, particularly in the mechanically ventilated patient in whom dried, inspired gases impair ciliary movement, thicken the protective mucus, and reduce the ability of mucociliary function to transport surface particles out of the airway. Volatile anesthetics and nitrous oxide reduce ciliary movement and alter the characteristics of mucus. It also is known that smokers have impaired mucociliary function compared with nonsmokers, and the combination of a volatile anesthetic in a smoker who is mechanically ventilated sets up a scenario for inadequate clearing of secretions, mucus plugging, atelectasis, and hypoxemia.

Pulmonary Vascular Resistance

Although vascular smooth muscle is clearly affected by the volatile anesthetics, the pulmonary vascular relaxation from clinically relevant concentrations of inhaled anesthetics is minimal. In addition, an anesthetic-related decrease in cardiac output tends to offset the direct vasodilator action of the anesthetic, resulting in little or no change in pulmonary artery pressures and pulmonary blood flow. Even nitrous oxide, which has little effect on cardiac output and pulmonary blood flow, has at best a small effect to increase pulmonary vascular resistance. However, the effect of nitrous oxide may be magnified in patients with resting pulmonary hypertension.[114]

Perhaps more important in terms of volatile anesthetics and pulmonary blood flow is their potential to attenuate hypoxic pulmonary vasoconstriction (HPV). During periods of hypoxemia, HPV reduces blood flow to underventilated areas of the lung, thereby diverting blood flow to areas of the lung with greater ventilation. The net effect is to improve the V/Q matching, resulting in a reduced amount of venous admixture and improved arterial oxygenation. Although all of the inhaled anesthetics in high concentrations have been shown to attenuate HPV in animal models, the situation is less clear in patient studies. This may reflect the multifactorial effects of the volatile anesthetics on factors involved in pulmonary blood flow, including their cardiovascular, autonomic, and humoral actions. Furthermore, nonpharmacologic variables impair HPV, including surgical trauma, temperature, pH, $PaCO_2$, size of the hypoxic segment, and intensity of the hypoxic stimulus. One-lung ventilation (OLV) serves as a model where HPV should lessen the expected decrease in PaO_2 and intrapulmonary shunt fraction (Qs/Qt). In patients undergoing OLV during thoracic surgery, volatile anesthetics have had minimal effects on PaO_2 and Qs/Qt when changing from two-lung to OLV (Fig. 17-28).[115,116] The efficacy of HPV to lessen shunt fraction varies inversely with pulmonary blood

flow (and cardiac output). Isoflurane, sevoflurane, and desflurane preserve cardiac output and have minimal-to-modest effects on shunt fraction during OLV. Propofol appears to be no more beneficial on shunt fraction during OLV compared with sevoflurane.[117]

HEPATIC EFFECTS

Postoperative liver dysfunction, to varying degrees, has been associated with all of the volatile anesthetics in current use. There are two distinct mechanisms by which anesthetics have caused hepatitis. One is more common and related to hepatocyte toxicity. It is relatively mild, does not require a previous exposure, and has a low morbidity. The second is associated with repeat exposure and probably represents an immune reaction to oxidatively derived metabolites of anesthetics. It has been associated with severe liver damage and fulminant hepatic failure and is discussed later in the chapter.

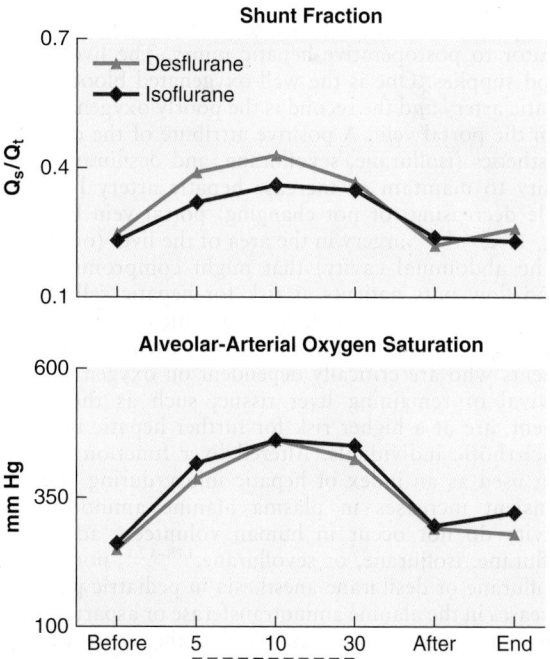

FIGURE 17-28. Shunt fraction (**top panel**) and the alveolar-arterial oxygen gradient (**bottom**) immediately before, during, and after one-lung ventilation (OLV) in patients anesthetized with desflurane or isoflurane. Data are means. (Adapted from Pagel PS, Fu JL, Damask MC, et al: Desflurane and isoflurane produce similar alterations in systemic and pulmonary hemodynamics and arterial oxygenation in patients undergoing one-lung ventilation during thoracotomy. Anesth Analg 1998; 87: 800.)

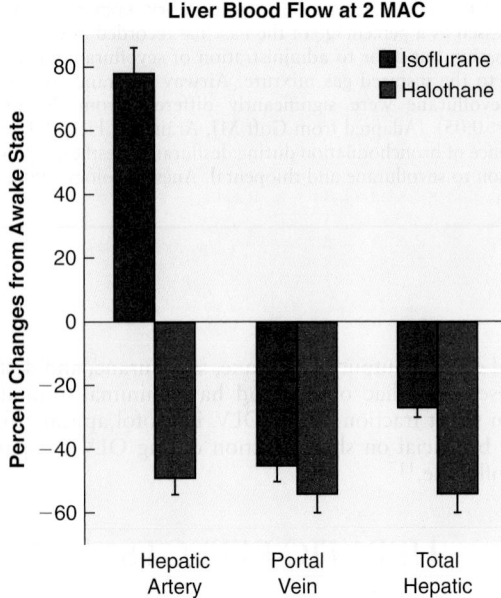

FIGURE 17-29. Changes (%, mean ± SE) in hepatic blood flow during administration of isoflurane or halothane. Decreases in portal vein blood flow produced by 2 minimum alveolar concentration (MAC) isoflurane are offset by increases in hepatic artery blood flow (autoregulation). Halothane resulted in decreases in both portal vein and hepatic artery blood flow, thereby significantly compromising total hepatic artery blood flow. (Adapted from Gelman S, Fowler KC, Smith LR: Liver circulation and function during isoflurane and halothane anesthesia. Anesthesiology 1984; 61: 726.)

Hypoxic injury to hepatocytes can be a significant contributor to postoperative hepatic injury. The liver has two blood supplies. One is the well-oxygenated blood from the hepatic artery and the second is the poorly oxygenated blood from the portal vein. A positive attribute of the ether-based anesthetics (isoflurane, sevoflurane, and desflurane) is their ability to maintain or increase hepatic artery blood flow while decreasing (or not changing) portal vein blood flow (Fig. 17-29).[118] Surgery in the area of the liver (or elsewhere in the abdominal cavity) that might compromise hepatic blood flow puts patients at risk for hepatic cell injury. In addition, hepatic enzyme induction, which increases oxygen demand, enhances the vulnerability of patients. Furthermore, patients who are critically dependent on oxygen supply for survival of remaining liver tissue, such as the cirrhotic patient, are at a higher risk for further hepatic injury than noncirrhotic individuals. Altered liver function tests have been used as an index of hepatic injury during anesthesia. Transient increases in plasma alanine aminotransferase activity do not occur in human volunteers administered desflurane, isoflurane, or sevoflurane,[118–120] nor following sevoflurane or desflurane anesthesia in pediatric patients.[121] Increases in the alanine aminotransferase or aspartate aminotransferase may not accurately reflect the extent of hepatic injury and are not uniquely specific to the liver. The centrilobular area of the liver is most susceptible to hypoxia. Therefore, a more sensitive measure of injury may be α-glutathione S-transferase (GST), since it is distributed primarily in the centrilobular hepatocytes. In patient studies, isoflurane did not increase GST.[122] In elderly patients with no pre-existing liver disease and having peripheral surgery under sevoflurane or desflurane, a brief impairment of splanchnic blood flow was demonstrated and this led to increases in GST that resolved in 24 hours.[123] The possibility that the organ pro-

tection from sevoflurane would lessen hepatic disturbances after CABG surgery with cardiopulmonary bypass when compared with propofol was explored in a prospective randomized study of 320 patients. Postoperative biochemical markers of hepatic dysfunction were lower after the sevoflurane-based anesthetic.[93] Thus, in terms of hepatocyte hypoxia, the modern-day volatile anesthetics have minimal adverse effects and might even afford protection from ischemic/hypoxic injury to cells.

NEUROMUSCULAR SYSTEM AND MALIGNANT HYPERTHERMIA

The inhaled anesthetics have two important actions on neuromuscular function. They directly relax skeletal muscle and they potentiate the action of neuromuscular blocking drugs.[124,125] In contrast, nitrous oxide does not relax skeletal muscles. The direct effects of volatile anesthetics to relax skeletal muscle are most prominent above 1 MAC and can be further enhanced, by 40%, in patients with myasthenia gravis.[126]

Volatile anesthetic potentiation of neuromuscular blockade has been well documented. For example, the infusion rate of rocuronium required to maintain neuromuscular blockade is 30 to 40% less during isoflurane, desflurane, and sevoflurane compared with propofol.[127] A similar left shift in the dose-response relationship has been observed with cisatracurium during volatile anesthetic administration versus during intravenous anesthesia.[125] While the mechanism of volatile anesthetic potentiation of the neuromuscular blocking drugs is not entirely clear, it appears to be largely because of a postsynaptic effect at the nicotinic acetylcholine receptor located at the neuromuscular junction. Specifically, at the receptor level, the volatile anesthetics act synergistically with the neuromuscular blocking drugs to enhance their action.[128] The degree of enhancement is related to their aqueous concentration so that at equi-MAC concentrations, the less potent anesthetics (e.g., desflurane and sevoflurane vs. isoflurane) should have a greater inhibitory effect on neuromuscular transmission. Support for this concept comes from a clinical study demonstrating 20% lower requirement for vecuronium to maintain a stable twitch depression during 1.25% desflurane compared with 1.25% isoflurane.[129] However, desflurane and isoflurane (and sevoflurane) at equipotent concentrations acted similarly to enhance the effect of cisatracurium on neuromuscular function.[125] This may relate to structural differences of the benzylisoquinolines versus aminosteroid neuromuscular blocking drugs.

All of the potent volatile anesthetics serve as triggers for malignant hyperthermia (MH) in genetically susceptible patients.[130,131] In contrast, nitrous oxide is only a weak trigger for MH.[132] The augmentation of caffeine-induced contractures by nitrous oxide is 1.3-fold, by isoflurane is 3-fold, and by halothane, 11-fold.[132] Although desflurane is a weak trigger for MH, it has been associated with an unusual delayed onset of symptoms of MH in animals and humans.[131,133]

GENETIC EFFECTS, OBSTETRIC USE, AND EFFECTS ON FETAL DEVELOPMENT

The potential for genetic toxicity from volatile anesthetics seems minimal. The Ames test identifies chemicals that act as mutagens and carcinogens and has been negative for isoflurane, desflurane, sevoflurane, and nitrous oxide.[134,135] A possible genotoxic effect of desflurane has been detected in female patients with a cytogenetic assay that detects sister chromatid exchanges (SCE) in lymphocytes from peripheral blood. Desflurane transiently increased the frequency of SCE, whereas in children, sevoflurane did not increase SCE.[136,137] The clinical implications of these findings are not clear in relation to the negative Ames test.

Volatile anesthetics can be teratogenic in animals,[138] but none have been shown to be teratogenic in humans. Animal studies have indicated that nitrous oxide exposure in the early periods of gestation may result in adverse effects, including an increased incidence of fetal resorption.[139] The same vulnerability does not exist during the administration of the potent volatile anesthetics.[139]

Nitrous oxide decreases the activity of vitamin B_{12}-dependent enzymes, methionine synthetase and thymidylate synthetase. The mechanism appears to be an irreversible oxidation of the cobalt atom of vitamin B_{12} by nitrous oxide. When 70% nitrous oxide is administered to patients, the time to 50% inactivation of methionine synthetase is 46 minutes. The concern that these changes might have an effect on a rapidly developing embryo/fetus seems appropriate because methionine synthetase and thymidylate synthetase are involved in the formation of myelin and the formation of DNA, respectively. Inhibition of these enzymes could manifest as depression of bone marrow function and neurologic disturbances. In fact, megaloblastic changes in bone marrow are consistently observed in patients exposed to nitrous oxide for 24 hours, and 4 days of exposure to nitrous oxide has resulted in agranulocytosis. Furthermore, animals exposed to 15% nitrous oxide for several weeks developed neurologic changes including spinal cord and peripheral nerve degeneration and ataxia. A sensory motor polyneuropathy that is often combined with signs of posterior lateral spinal cord degeneration has been described in humans who chronically inhale nitrous oxide for recreational use.[140] These effects have been attributed to reduced activity of the vitamin B_{12}-dependent enzymes.

Uterine smooth muscle tone is diminished by volatile anesthetics in similar fashion to the effects of volatile anesthetics on vascular smooth muscle. There is a dose-dependent decrease in spontaneous myometrial contractility that is consistent among the volatile anesthetics.[141,142] Desflurane and sevoflurane also inhibit the frequency and amplitude of myometrial contractions induced by oxytocin in a dose-dependent manner.[141] Uterine relaxation/atony can become problematic at concentrations of volatile anesthesia >1 MAC, and might delay the onset time of newborn respiration.[143] Consequently, a common technique used to provide general anesthesia for urgent cesarean sections is to administer low concentrations of the volatile anesthetic, such as 0.5 to 0.75 MAC, combined with nitrous oxide. This decreases the likelihood of uterine atony and blood loss, especially at a time after delivery when oxytocin responsiveness of the uterus is essential.[143] In some situations, uterine relaxation may be desirable, such as to remove a retained placenta. In this case, a brief, high concentration of a volatile anesthetic may be advantageous.

There has been an ongoing concern about the incidence of spontaneous abortions in operating room personnel chronically exposed to trace concentrations of inhaled anesthetics, especially nitrous oxide.[144] Early epidemiologic studies suggested that operating room personnel had an increased incidence of spontaneous abortions and congenital abnormalities in offspring. However, subsequent analysis of the data suggests inaccurate study design, confounding variables, and nonresponders might have led to flawed conclusions.[145] In prospective studies, no causal relationship has been shown between exposure to waste anesthetic gases, regardless of the presence or absence of scavenging systems, and adverse health effects.

Despite the unproven influence of trace concentrations of the volatile anesthetics on fetal development and spontaneous abortions, concerns for an adverse influence have resulted in the use of scavenging systems to remove anesthetic gases from the operating room and the establishment of standards for waste gas exposure. The National Institute for Occupational Safety and Health has recommended exposure levels for nitrous oxide is 25 parts per million (ppm) as a time-weighted average over 8 hours. The 1-hour exposure limit for halogenated anesthetics without nitrous oxide exposure is 2 ppm, and with nitrous oxide is 0.5 ppm.

In terms of neonatal effects from general anesthesia, Apgar scores and acid-base balance are not affected by anesthetic technique, such as spinal versus general.[146] More sensitive measures of neurologic and behavioral function, such as the Scanlon Early Neonatal Neurobehavioral Scale and the Neurologic and Adaptive Capacities Score (NACS) indicate some transient depression of scores following general anesthesia that resolves at 24 hours after delivery.[146,147]

ANESTHETIC DEGRADATION BY CARBON DIOXIDE ABSORBERS

Compound A

Sevoflurane undergoes base-catalyzed degradation in carbon dioxide absorbents to form a vinyl ether called *compound A*. The production of compound A is enhanced in low flow or closed circuit breathing systems and by warm or very dry CO_2 absorbents.[148,149] Barium hydroxide lime produces more compound A than soda lime and this can be attributed to slightly higher absorbent temperature during CO_2 extraction (Fig. 17-30).[150] Desiccated barium hydroxide lime also has been implicated in the heat and fires associated with sevoflurane, discussed later. This absorbent has been removed from the U.S. market.

There are well-defined species differences in the threshold for compound A-induced nephrotoxicity. The threshold is approximately 300 ppm·hr in 250-g rats, >612 ppm·hr in pigs, and between 600 and 800 ppm·hr in monkeys. In patients and volunteers receiving sevoflurane in closed circuit or low flow delivery systems, inspired compound A concentrations averaged 8 to 24 and 20 to 32 ppm with soda lime and barium hydroxide lime, respectively.[151–154] Total exposures as high as

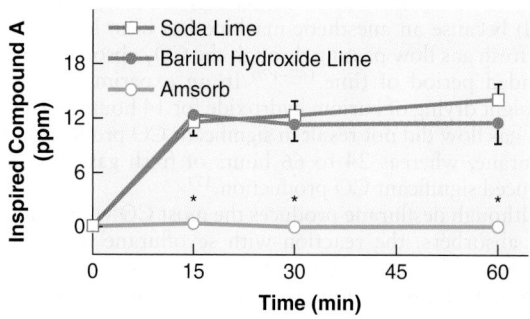

FIGURE 17-30. Compound A levels produced from three carbon dioxide absorbents during 1 minimum alveolar concentration sevoflurane anesthesia delivered to volunteers at 1 L/min fresh gas flow (mean ± SE). Gas samples were taken from the inspired limb of the anesthesia circuit. *Different from barium hydroxide lime or soda lime (p <0.05). (Adapted from Mchaourab A, Arain SR, Ebert TJ: Lack of degradation of sevoflurane by a new carbon dioxide absorbent in humans. Anesthesiology 2001; 94: 1007.)

320 to 400 ppm·hr have had no clear effect on clinical markers of renal function.[155–157] In randomized and prospective volunteer and patient studies, no adverse renal effects from low-flow (0.5 to 1.0 L/min) or closed circuit sevoflurane anesthesia were detected using both standard clinical markers of renal function (serum creatinine and blood urea nitrogen concentrations) and experimental markers of renal function and structural integrity (proteinuria, glucosuria and enzymuria).[152–154,158–161] In a prospective, multicenter, randomized study in patients with pre-existing renal disease, there were no adverse renal effects of long duration, low-flow sevoflurane.[162,163] In fact, transient proteinuria, glucosuria, and enzymuria have been noted after desflurane, isoflurane, and propofol anesthesia indicating these elevated markers of renal injury might represent common effects unrelated to the choice of anesthetic.[151,152] The majority of countries that have approved sevoflurane for clinical use have no flow restriction because of the proven safety of the anesthetic in scientific studies, where there has not been a single case report of renal injury from sevoflurane after a decade of use, despite a sensitized anesthesia community.

Carbon Monoxide and Heat

14 CO_2 absorbents degrade sevoflurane, desflurane, and isoflurane to carbon monoxide when the normal water content of the absorbent (13 to 15%) is markedly decreased <5%.[164–166] The degradation is the result of an exothermic reaction of the anesthetics with the absorbent. The anesthetic molecular structure and the presence of a strong base in the carbon dioxide absorbent are involved in the formation of carbon monoxide (CO).[165] Desflurane and isoflurane contain a difluoromethoxy moiety that is essential for the formation of CO. When studies are conducted with CO_2 absorbents maintained at or just above room temperature, desflurane given at just under 1 MAC produced up to 8,000 ppm of CO versus 79 ppm with nearly 2 MAC sevoflurane.[166] In desiccated barium hydroxide, CO production from desflurane was nearly threefold higher than with soda lime but was trivial with sevoflurane. In normal clinical use, CO_2 canister temperatures are 25 to 45°C, but can be higher when employing a very low fresh gas flow. In a laboratory setting, when CO_2 canister temperature is not controlled and sevoflurane is administered to desiccated barium hydroxide, the exothermic reaction can substantially increase canister temperatures. If the canister temperature exceeds 80°C, significant CO production is noted with sevoflurane.[164] Instances of CO poisoning of patients have been reported in situations where the CO_2 absorbent has been presumably dried (desiccated) because an anesthetic machine has been left on with a high fresh gas flow passing through the CO_2 absorbent over an extended period of time.[167–170] In an experimental setting, overnight drying of barium hydroxide for 14 hours at 10 L/min fresh gas flow did not result in significant CO production from desflurane, whereas 24 to 66 hours of fresh gas flow drying produced significant CO production.[171]

Although desflurane produces the most CO with desiccated CO_2 absorbers, the reaction with sevoflurane produces the most heat.[172] The strong exothermic reaction has caused significant heat production, fires, and patient injuries.[173–175] Although sevoflurane is not flammable at <11%, formaldehyde, methanol, and formate have been identified,[176] and these alone or in combination with oxygen might be flammable at high canister temperatures. In experimental settings, long exposure of 1 MAC sevoflurane to desiccated barium hydroxide resulted in canister temperatures in excess of 300°C, which can be associated with smoldering, melting of plastic components, explosions, and fires.[164] Barium hydroxide has been removed from the U.S. market.

There are newer CO_2 absorbents that do not degrade anesthetics (to either compound A or carbon monoxide), and they should reduce exothermic reactions. "From a patient safety perspective, widespread adoption of a nondestructive CO_2 absorbent should be axiomatic."[177] Although the cost of these new CO_2 absorbents Amsorb Plus (Armstrong Medical, Coleraine, UK) and DrägerSorb Free (Dräger, Lübek, Germany) is higher and the absorptive capacity may be lower than either barium hydroxide lime or soda lime, their benefit may be substantial. The use of a nondestructive absorbent eliminates all of the potential complications related to anesthetic breakdown and therefore minimizes the possibility of additional costs from those complications, including additional laboratory tests, hospital days, and medical/legal expenses. Adoption of these new absorbents into routine clinical practice is consistent with the patient safety goals of our anesthesia society.

Generic Sevoflurane Formulations

Generic formulations of sevoflurane were introduced into the clinical market in 2006. The methods for synthesizing sevoflurane differ between manufacturers.[178] Although the active ingredient of sevoflurane from different manufacturers is chemically equivalent, the water content in the formulations differs and this accounts for their different resistance to degradation to hydrogen fluoride when exposed to a Lewis acid (metal halides and metal oxides that are present in modern-day vaporizers). Adding water to the formulation inhibits the action of Lewis acids to degrade sevoflurane to hydrogen fluoride. The formulation of Abbott Labs was changed to contain 300 to 400 ppm of water, based on an early adverse experience with hydrogen fluoride formation from a low water formulation in 1996. The generic formulation marketed by Baxter Laboratories is low in water (~65 ppm) and has been shown in clinical and laboratory studies to degrade to toxic and corrosive hydrogen fluoride.[179] Recent reports indicate that the Penlon Sigma Delta sevoflurane vaporizer can degrade the Baxter low-water formulation of sevoflurane, resulting in etching of site glass and corrosion of the plastic on the vaporizer and discoloration of the anesthetic.[180] Whether these differences in formulation lead to patient safety issues remains to be seen.

ANESTHETIC METABOLISM

Fluoride-Induced Nephrotoxicity

The metabolism of enflurane may result in a well-described injury to renal collecting tubules.[181,182] The nephrotoxicity presents as a high-output renal insufficiency that is unresponsive to vasopressin and is characterized by dilute polyuria, dehydration, serum hypernatremia, hyperosmolality, elevated blood urea nitrogen, and creatinine. An association between increased plasma fluoride concentrations and metabolism led to a "fluoride hypothesis." This hypothesis has been re-examined recently in part because sevoflurane undergoes 5% metabolism that results in transient increases in serum fluoride concentrations, but it has not been associated with a renal-concentrating defect. The traditional hypothesis stated that both the duration of the high systemic fluoride concentrations (area under the fluoride-time curve) and the peak fluoride concentration (peaks above 50 μM appear to represent the toxic threshold) were related to nephrotoxicity (Fig. 17-31). The safety of sevoflurane with regard to fluoride concentrations may be the result of a rapid decline in plasma fluoride concentrations because of less availability of the anesthetic for metabolism from a faster washout compared with enflurane.[183] In addition, the site of metabolism is an important

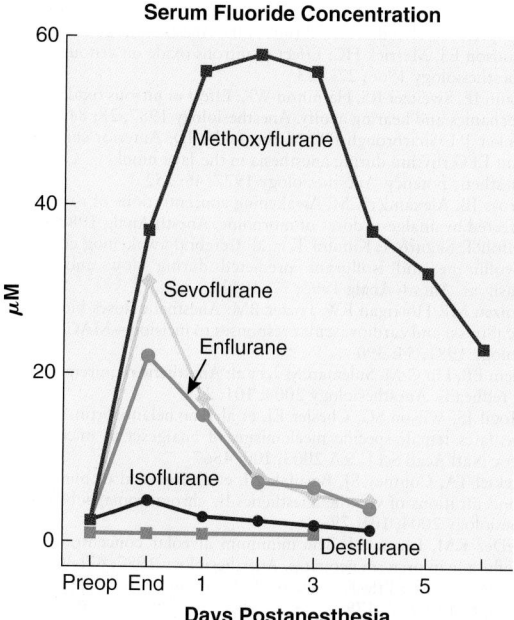

Serum Fluoride Concentration

FIGURE 17-31. Plasma inorganic fluoride concentrations (mean ± SE) before and after 2 to 4 hours of methoxyflurane, enflurane, sevoflurane, isoflurane, and desflurane anesthesia. (Adapted from Kharasch ED, Armstrong AS, Gunn K, et al: Clinical sevoflurane metabolism and disposition. II. The role of cytochrome P450 2E1 in fluoride and hexafluoroisopropanol formation. Anesthesiology 1995; 82: 1379; Mazze RI: Metabolism of the inhaled anaesthetics: Implications of enzyme induction. Br J Anaesth 1984; 56: 27S; and Sutton TS, Koblin DD, Gruenke LD, et al: Fluoride metabolites after prolonged exposure of volunteers and patients to desflurane. Anesth Analg 1991; 73: 180.)

factor in toxicity, that is, intrarenal metabolism contributes to nephrotoxicity. Therefore, the potential for toxicity from relatively high plasma levels of fluoride following long exposure to sevoflurane is offset by the minimal amount of renal defluorination and this may explain its relative absence of renal-concentrating defects.[184]

Factors such as total dose of anesthetic, liver enzyme induction, and obesity have been proven to enhance biotransformation. The activity of hepatic cytochrome P450 enzymes is increased by a variety of drugs, including phenobarbital, phenytoin, and isoniazid. Obesity causes increased metabolism (defluorination) of isoflurane.[185] However, the effects of obesity on the defluorination of sevoflurane are less clear.[186]

CLINICAL UTILITY OF VOLATILE ANESTHETICS

For Induction of Anesthesia

The appeal of mask induction in the adult population centers on the potential safety and utility of this technique.[187–190] Spontaneous ventilation is preserved with a gas induction since patients essentially regulate their own depth of anesthesia (too much sevoflurane would suppress ventilation). The availability of sevoflurane, which is potent, poorly soluble, and nonpungent, and therefore can be inhaled easily, has generated renewed interest in this technique.

Clinical studies indicate that stage two excitation is avoided with high concentrations of sevoflurane. The typical time to loss of consciousness is 60 seconds when delivering 8%

sevoflurane via the face mask. Sevoflurane also has been administered by mask as an approach to the difficult adult airway because it preserves spontaneous ventilation and does not cause salivation.[191] The traditional "awake look" in the suspected difficult airway (where intravenous drugs are titrated to a level that allows direct laryngoscopy in the awake patient) has been modified to consist of spontaneous ventilation of high concentrations of sevoflurane until laryngoscopic evaluation is tolerated. Laryngeal mask placement can be successfully achieved 2 minutes after administering 7% sevoflurane via the face mask.[189] The addition of nitrous oxide to the inspired gas mixture does not add significantly to the induction sequence. The gas induction technique is improved by pretreatment with benzodiazepines and worsened with opioid pretreatment because of apnea.[188] Importantly, patient acceptance of this technique has been relatively high, exceeding 90%.[187]

There are a number of techniques to administer sevoflurane via face mask. These include priming the circuit (emptying the rebreathing bag, opening the "pop-off" valve, dialing the vaporizer to 8% while using a fresh gas flow of 8 L/min, and maintaining this for 60 seconds prior to applying the face mask to the patient), a single-breath induction from end-expiratory volume to maximum inspired volume, or simply breathing while the vaporizer is set to 8%. All seem to have the successful end result of loss of consciousness, generally within 1 minute.

For Maintenance of Anesthesia

The volatile anesthetics are clearly the most popular drug used to maintain anesthesia. They are easily administered via inhalation, they are readily titrated, they have a high safety ratio in terms of preventing recall, and the depth of anesthesia can be quickly adjusted in a predictable way while monitoring tissue levels via end-tidal concentrations. They are effective regardless of age or body habitus. They have some properties that prove beneficial in the operating room, including relaxation of skeletal muscle, preservation of cardiac output and cerebral blood flow, relatively predictable recovery profiles, and organ protection from ischemic injury. Some of the drawbacks to the use of the current volatile anesthetics are their absence of analgesic effects, their association with postoperative nausea and vomiting, and their potential for carbon monoxide poisoning and hepatitis.

PHARMACOECONOMICS AND VALUE-BASED DECISIONS

In the current environment of cost containment, clinicians are constantly being pressured to use less expensive drugs, including antiemetics, neuromuscular blocking drugs, and volatile anesthetics. Factors involved in the value-based decision include the efficacy of the drug, the side effects, its direct costs, and its indirect effects. In terms of efficacy, all of the volatile anesthetics are reasonably similar; that is, they can be used to establish a state of anesthesia for surgical interventions and can be easily reversed. A common side effect of the volatile anesthetics is nausea and vomiting. The need for rescue medications to treat nausea and vomiting after volatile anesthesia needs to be considered in any legitimate cost analysis. Direct costs are not simply the cost per milliliter of liquid or cost per bottle of anesthetic. Rather, they reflect the combination of the potency of the drug to establish a MAC level, the fresh gas flow, and the cost of the anesthetic. Sevoflurane and isoflurane are generic products, whereas desflurane is still under patent protection. At 1 L/min fresh gas flow, delivering 1 MAC,

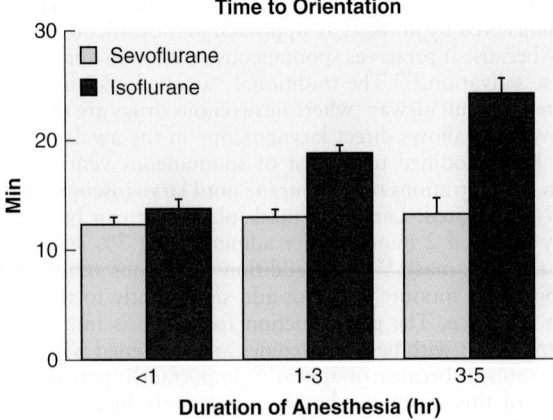

FIGURE 17-32. The recovery times to orientation after anesthesia of varying durations. With the less soluble anesthetic sevoflurane, the time to orientation was independent of the anesthetic duration. In contrast, long anesthetic durations with isoflurane were associated with delayed times to orientation. (Adapted from Ebert TJ, Robinson BJ, Uhrich TD, et al: Recovery from sevoflurane anesthesia: A comparison to isoflurane and propofol anesthesia. Anesthesiology 1998; 89: 1524.)

desflurane, sevoflurane, and isoflurane cost about US $11.00 per hour, US $5.00 per hour, and US $2.00 per hour, respectively, depending on the local cost of drug acquisition. The indirect costs are probably the most difficult to pinpoint, but may be the most important when evaluating the cost of using the new volatile anesthetics. Examples of indirect costs include costs associated with operating room time, time in the postanesthesia care unit versus bypassing the postanesthesia care unit to a step-down unit, labor costs, and outcome-related costs, such as litigation to defend a bad outcome from an anesthetic drug.

One of the arguments for using sevoflurane and desflurane has been their relative speed in terms of emergence from anesthesia. This argument has been tempered somewhat by the basic knowledge that titration of the volatile anesthetics can speed emergence times. Even the more soluble drug, isoflurane, can be titrated downward based on clinical experience or with the aid of processed EEG monitors, permitting fast wake-ups regardless of the choice of anesthetic agent. However, there is strong evidence to support the use of the less-soluble (but more expensive) drugs in the longest surgical cases (Fig. 17-32).[192] In these cases the high direct cost of the anesthetic is balanced by the much improved recovery profile including a more rapid time to emergence and a more rapid discharge from the recovery room. Curiously, the discharge advantage with the low-soluble anesthetics has been difficult to show after shorter surgical procedures.

References

1. Kety SS: The physiological and physical factors governing the uptake of anesthetic gases by the body. Anesthesiology 1950; 11: 517
2. Eger EI: Anesthetic Uptake and Action. Baltimore, Williams & Wilkins, 1974
3. Ebert TJ, Robinson BJ, Uhrich TD, et al: Recovery from sevoflurane anesthesia: A comparison to isoflurane and propofol anesthesia. Anesthesiology 1998; 89: 1524
4. Hettrick DA, Pagel PS, Kersten JR, et al: Cardiovascular effects of xenon in isoflurane-anesthetized dogs with dilated cardiomyopathy. Anesthesiology 1998; 89: 1166
5. Nakata Y, Goto T, Morita S: Comparison of inhalation inductions with xenon and sevoflurane. Acta Anaesthesiol Scand 1997; 41: 1157
6. Kaplan R, Abramowitz MD, Epstein BS: Nitrous oxide and air-filled balloon-tipped catheters. Anesthesiology 1981; 55: 71
7. Stanley TH, Kawamura R, Graves C: Effects of nitrous oxide on volume and pressure of endotracheal tube cuffs. Anesthesiology 1974; 41: 256
8. Munson ES, Merrick HC: Effect of nitrous oxide on venous air embolism. Anesthesiology 1966; 27: 783
9. Waun JE, Sweitzer RS, Hamilton WK: Effect of nitrous oxide on middle ear mechanics and hearing acuity. Anesthesiology 1987; 28: 846
10. Tinker JH, Sharbrough FW, Michenfelder JD: Anterior shift of the dominant EEG rhythm during anesthesia in the Java monkey: Correlation with anesthetic potency. Anesthesiology 1977; 46: 252
11. Gross JB, Alexander CM: Awakening concentrations of isoflurane are not affected by analgesic doses of morphine. Anesth Analg 1988; 67: 27
12. Katoh T, Suguro Y, Kimura T, et al: Cerebral awakening concentration of sevoflurane and isoflurane predicted during slow and fast alveolar washout. Anesth Analg 1993; 77: 1012
13. Roizen MF, Horrigan RW, Frazer BM: Anesthetic doses blocking adrenergic (Stress) and cardiovascular responses to incision—MAC BAR. Anesthesiology 1981; 54: 390
14. Liem EB, Lin C-M, Suleman M-I, et al: Anesthetic requirement is increased in redheads. Anesthesiology 2004; 101: 279
15. Mogil JS, Wilson SG, Chesler EJ, et al: The nelanocortin-1 receptor gene mediates female-specific mechanisms of analgesia in mice and humans. Proc Natl Acad Sci U S A 2003; 100: 4867
16. Stekiel TA, Contney SJ, Bosnjak ZJ, et al: Reversal of minimum alveolar concentrations of volatile anesthetics by chromosomal substitution. Anesthesiology 2004; 101: 796
17. LeDez KM, Lerman J: The minimum alveolar concentration (MAC) of isoflurane in preterm neonates. Anesthesiology 1987; 67: 301
18. Mapleson WW: Effect of age on MAC in humans: a meta-analysis. Br J Anaesth 1996; 76: 179
19. Smith AL, Wollman H: Cerebral blood flow and metabolism: Effects of anesthetic drugs and techniques. Anesthesiology 1972; 36: 378
20. Scheller MS, Nakakimura K, Fleischer JE, et al: Cerebral effects of sevoflurane in the dog: Comparison with isoflurane and enflurane. Br J Anaesth 1990; 65: 388
21. Lutz LJ, Milde JH, Milde LN: The cerebral functional, metabolic, and hemodynamic effects of desflurane in dogs. Anesthesiology 1990; 73: 125
22. Fujibayashi T, Sugiura Y, Yanagimoto M, et al: Brain energy metabolism and blood flow during sevoflurane and halothane anesthesia: effects of hypocapnia and blood pressure fluctuations. Acta Anaesthesiol Scand 1994; 38: 413
23. Yli-Hankala A, Vakkuri A, Särkelä M, et al: Epileptiform electroencephalogram during mask induction of anesthesia with sevoflurane. Anesthesiology 1999; 91: 1596
24. Jääskeläinen SK, Kaisti K, Suni L, et al: Sevoflurane is epileptogenic in healthy subjects at surgical levels of anesthesia. Neurology 2003; 61: 1073
25. Julliac B, Guehl D, Chopin F, et al: Sharp increase in cerebral sevoflurane concentration during mask induction in adults is a major risk factor of spike wave occurrence. Anesthesiology, 2004; A-132
26. Hisada K, Morioka T, Fukui K, et al: Effects of sevoflurane and isoflurane on electrocorticographic activities in patients with temporal lobe epilepsy. J Neurosurg Anesthesiol 2001; 13: 333
27. Algotsson L, Messeter K, Nordström CH, et al: Cerebral blood flow and oxygen consumption during isoflurane and halothane anesthesia in man. Acta Anaesthesiol Scand 1988; 32: 15
28. Lutz LJ, Milde JH, Milde LN: The response of the canine cerebral circulation to hyperventilation during anesthesia with desflurane. Anesthesiology 1991; 74: 504
29. Adams RW, Cucchiara RF, Gronert GA, et al: Isoflurane and cerebrospinal fluid pressure in neurosurgical patients. Anesthesiology 1981; 54: 97
30. Grosslight K, Foster R, Colohan AR, et al: Isoflurane for neuroanesthesia: risk factors for increases in intracranial pressure. Anesthesiology 1985; 63: 533
31. Artru AA: Isoflurane does not increase the rate of CSF production in the dog. Anesthesiology 1984; 60: 193
32. Talke P, Caldwell JE, Richardson CA: Sevoflurane increases lumbar cerebrospinal fluid pressure in normocapnic patients undergoing transsphenoidal hypophysectomy. Anesthesiology 1999; 91: 127
33. Talke P, Caldwell J, Dodsont B, et al: Desflurane and isoflurane increases lumbar cerebrospinal fluid pressure in normocapnic patients undergoing transsphenoidal hypophysectomy. Anesthesiology 1996; 85: 999
34. Michenfelder JD, Milde JH, Sundt JM Jr: Cerebral protection by barbiturate anesthesia. Use after middle cerebral artery occlusion in Java monkeys. Arch Neurol 1976; 33
35. Muzzi DA, Losasso TJ, Dietz NM, et al: The effect of desflurane and isoflurane on cerebrospinal fluid pressure in humans with supratentorial mass lesions. Anesthesiology 1992; 76: 720
36. Sponheim S, Skraastad Ø, Helseth E, et al: Effects of 0.5 and 1.0 MAC isoflurane, sevoflurane and desflurane on intracranial and cerebral perfusion pressures in children. Acta Anaesthesiol Scand 2003; 47: 932
37. Sugioka S: Effects of sevoflurane on intracranial pressure and formation and absorption of cerebrospinal fluid in cats. [Japanese]. Masui. Jpn J Anesthesiol 1992; 41: 1434
38. Artru AA: Rate of cerebrospinal fluid formation, resistance to reabsorption of cerebrospinal fluid, brain tissue water content, and electroencephalogram during desflurane anesthesia in dogs. J Neurosurg Anesthesiol 1993; 5: 178

39. Bundgaard H, von Oettingen G, Larsen KM, et al: Effects of sevoflurane on intracranial pressure, cerebral blood flow and cerebral metabolism. Acta Anaesthesiol Scand 1998; 42: 621

40. Seyde WC, Longnecker DE: Cerebral oxygen tension in rats during deliberate hypotension with sodium nitroprusside, 2-chloroadenosine, or deep isoflurane anesthesia. Anesthesiology 1986; 64: 480

41. Engelhard K, Werner C, Reeker W, et al: Desflurane and isoflurane improve neurological outcome after incomplete cerebral ischaemia in rats. Br J Anaesth 1999; 83: 415

42. Werner C, Möllenberg O, Kochs E, et al: Sevoflurane improves neurological outcome after incomplete cerebral ischaemia in rats. Br J Anaesth 1995; 75: 756

43. Loepke AW, Priestley MA, Schultz SEM, J. et al: Desflurane improves neurologic outcome after low-flow cardiopulmonary bypass in newborn pigs. Anesthesiology 2002; 97: 1521

44. Hoffman WE, Charbel FT, Edelman G, et al: Thiopental and desflurane treatment for brain protection. Neurosurgery 1998; 43: 1050

45. Sakabe T, Tsutsui T, Maekawa T, et al: Local cerebral glucose utilization during nitrous oxide and pentobarbital anesthesia in rats. Anesthesiology 1985; 63: 262

46. Fleischer JE, Milde JH, Moyer TP, et al: Cerebral effects of high-dose midazolam and subsequent reversal with Ro 15-1788 in dogs. Anesthesiology 1988; 68: 234

47. Hoffman WE, Miletich DJ, Albrecht RF: The effects of midazolam on cerebral blood flow and oxygen consumption and its interaction with nitrous oxide. Anesth Analg 1986; 65: 729

48. Hartung J, Cottrell JE: Nitrous oxide reduces thiopental-induced prolongation of survival in hypoxic and anoxic mice. Anesth Analg 1987; 66

49. Ebert TJ, Kampine JP: Nitrous oxide augments sympathetic outflow: Direct evidence from human peroneal nerve recordings. Anesth Analg 1989; 69: 444

50. Ebert TJ, Muzi M, Lopatka CW: Neurocirculatory responses to sevoflurane in humans. A comparison to desflurane. Anesthesiology 1995; 83: 88

51. Malan TP Jr, DiNardo JA, Isner RJ, et al: Cardiovascular effects of sevoflurane compared with those of isoflurane in volunteers. Anesthesiology 1995; 83: 918

52. Weiskopf RB, Cahalan MK, Eger EI II, et al: Cardiovascular actions of desflurane in normocarbic volunteers. Anesth Analg 1991; 73: 143

53. Stevens WC, Cromwell TH, Halsey MJ, et al: The cardiovascular effects of a new inhalation anesthetic, Forane, in human volunteers at a constant arterial carbon dioxide tension. Anesthesiology 1971; 35: 8

54. Calverley RK, Smith NT, Prys-Roberts C, et al: Cardiovascular effects of enflurane anesthesia during controlled ventilation in man. Anesth Analg 1978; 57: 619

55. Ebert TJ, Muzi M: Sympathetic hyperactivity during desflurane anesthesia in healthy volunteers. A comparison with isoflurane. Anesthesiology 1993; 79: 444

56. Weiskopf RB, Moore MA, Eger EI II, et al: Rapid increase in desflurane concentration is associated with greater transient cardiovascular stimulation than a rapid increase in isoflurane concentration in humans. Anesthesiology 1994; 80: 1035

57. Muzi M, Ebert TJ, Hope WG, et al: Site(s) mediating sympathetic activation with desflurane. Anesthesiology 1996; 85: 737

58. Weiskopf RB, Eger EI II, Noorani M, et al: Fentanyl, esmolol, and clonidine blunt the transient cardiovascular stimulation induced by desflurane in humans. Anesthesiology 1994; 81: 1350

59. Yonker-Sell AE, Muzi M, Hope WG, et al: Alfentanil modifies the neurocirculatory responses to desflurane. Anesth Analg 1996; 82: 162

60. Pacentine GG, Muzi M, Ebert TJ: Effects of fentanyl on sympathetic activation associated with the administration of desflurane. Anesthesiology 1995; 82: 823

61. Calverley RK, Smith NT, Jones CW, et al: Ventilatory and cardiovascular effects of enflurane anesthesia during spontaneous ventilation in man. Anesth Analg 1978 57: 610

62. Weiskopf RB, Cahalan MK, Ionescu P, et al: Cardiovascular actions of desflurane with and without nitrous oxide during spontaneous ventilation in humans. Anesth Analg 1991; 73: 165

63. Weiskopf RB, Holmes MA, Rampil IJ, et al: Cardiovascular safety and actions of high concentrations of I-653 and isoflurane in swine. Anesthesiology 1989; 70: 793

64. Ebert TJ: Differential effects of nitrous oxide on baroreflex control of heart rate and peripheral sympathetic nerve activity in humans. Anesthesiology 1990; 72: 16

65. Cahalan MK, Weiskopf RB, Eger EI II, et al: Hemodynamic effects of desflurane/nitrous oxide anesthesia in volunteers. Anesth Analg 1991; 73: 157

66. Theye RA, Michenfelder JD: Whole-body and organ VO2 changes with enflurane, isoflurane, and halothane. Br J Anaesth 1975; 47: 813

67. Crawford MW, Lerman J, Saldivia V, et al: Hemodynamic and organ blood flow responses to halothane and sevoflurane anesthesia during spontaneous ventilation. Anesth Analg 1992; 75: 1000

68. Ebert TJ, Harkin CP, Muzi M: Cardiovascular responses to sevoflurane: A review. Anesth Analg 1995; 81: S11

69. Atlee JL, III, Bosnjak ZJ: Mechanisms for cardiac dysrhythmias during anesthesia. Anesthesiology 1990; 72: 347

70. Bosnjak ZJ, Kampine JP: Effects of halothane, enflurane, and isoflurane on the SA node. Anesthesiology 1983; 58: 314

71. Hartman JC, Pagel PS, Kampine JP, et al: Influence of desflurane on regional distribution of coronary blood flow in a chronically instrumented canine model of multivessel coronary artery obstruction. Anesth Analg 1991; 72: 289

72. Hartman JC, Kampine JP, Schmeling WT, et al: Steal-prone coronary circulation in chronically instrumented dogs: isoflurane versus adenosine. Anesthesiology 1991; 74: 744

73. Kersten JR, Brayer AP, Pagel PS, et al: Perfusion of ischemic myocardium during anesthesia with sevoflurane. Anesthesiology 1994; 81: 995

74. Harkin CP, Pagel PS, Kersten JR, et al: Direct negative inotropic and lusitropic effects of sevoflurane. Anesthesiology 1994; 81: 156

75. Slogoff S, Keats AS, Dear WE, et al: Steal-prone coronary anatomy and myocardial ischemia associated with four primary anesthetic agents in humans. Anesth Analg 1991; 72: 22

76. O'Young J, Mastrocostopoulos G, Hilgenberg A, et al: Myocardial circulatory and metabolic effects of isoflurane and sufentanil during coronary artery surgery. Anesthesiology 1987; 66: 653

77. Tuman KJ, McCarthy RJ, Spiess BD, et al: Does choice of anesthetic agent significantly affect outcome after coronary artery surgery? Anesthesiology 1989; 70: 189

78. Ebert TJ, Kharasch ED, Rooke GA, et al: Myocardial ischemia and adverse cardiac outcomes in cardiac patients undergoing noncardiac surgery with sevoflurane and isoflurane. Anesth Analg 1997; 85: 993

79. Searle NR, Martineau RJ, Conzen P, et al: Comparison of sevoflurane/fentanyl and isoflurane/fentanyl during elective coronary artery bypass surgery. Can J Anaesth 1996; 43: 890

80. Thomson IR, Bowering JB, Hudson RJ, et al: A comparison of desflurane and isoflurane in patients undergoing coronary artery surgery. Anesthesiology 1991; 75: 776

81. Helman JD, Leung JM, Bellows WH, et al: The risk of myocardial ischemia in patients receiving desflurane versus sufentanil anesthesia for coronary artery bypass graft surgery. Anesthesiology 1992; 77: 47

82. Riess ML, Stowe DF, Warltier DC: Cardiac pharmacolocial preconditioning with volatile anesthetics: From bench to bedside? Am J Physiol 2004; 286: H1603

83. Stowe DF, Kevin LG: Cardiac preconditioning by volatile anesthetic agents: A defining role for altered mitochondrial bioenergetics. Antioxidants & Redox Signaling 2004; 6: 439

84. Novalija E, Kevin LG, Camara AK, et al: Reactive oxygen species precede the epsilon isoform of protein kinase C in the anesthetic preconditioning signaling cascade. Anesthesiology 2003; 99: 421

85. Kwok WM, Martinelli AT, Fujimoto K, et al: Differential modulation of the cardiac adenosine triphosphate-sensitive potassium channel by isoflurane and halothane. Anesthesiology 2002; 97: 50

86. Kevin LG, Katz P, Camara AK, et al: Anesthetic preconditioning: effects on latency to ischemic injury in isolated hearts. Anesthesiology 2003; 99: 385

87. De Hert SG, Turani F, Mathur S, et al: Cardioprotection with volatile anesthetics: mechanisms and clinical implications. Anesth Analg 2005; 100: 1584

88. Yu CH, Beattie WS: The effects of volatile anesthetics on cardiac ischemic complications and mortality in CABG: a meta-analysis. Can J Anaesth 2006; 53: 906

89. De Hert SG, Van der Linden PJ, Cromheecke S, et al: Choice of primary anesthetic regimen can influence intensive care unit length of stay after coronary surgery with cardiopulmonary bypass. Anesthesiology 2004; 101: 9

90. Gu W, Pagel PS, Warltier DC, et al: Modifying cardiovascular risk in diabetes mellitus. Anesthesiology 2003; 98: 774

91. Clarkson AN: Anesthetic-mediated protection/preconditioning during cerebral ischemia. Life Sci 2007; 80: 1157

92. Lee HT, Ota-Setlik A, Fu Y, et al: Differential protective effects of volatile anesthetics against renal ischemia-reperfusion injury in vivo. Anesthesiology 2004; 101: 1313

93. Lorsomradee S, Cromheecke S, Lorsomradee S, et al: Effects of sevoflurane on biomechanical markers of hepatic and renal dysfunction after coronary artery surgery. J Cardiothorac Vasc Anesth 2006; 20: 684

94. Seagard JL, Hopp FA, Bosnjak ZJ, et al: Sympathetic efferent nerve activity in conscious and isoflurane-anesthetized dogs. Anesthesiology 1984; 61: 266

95. Seagard JL, Hopp FA, Donegan JH, et al: Halothane and the carotid sinus reflex: evidence for multiple sites of action. Anesthesiology 1982; 57: 191

96. Seagard JL, Elegbe EO, Hopp FA, et al: Effects of isoflurane on the baroceptor reflex. Anesthesiology 1983; 59: 511

97. Muzi M, Ebert TJ: A randomized, prospective comparison of halothane, isoflurane and enflurane on baroreflex control of heart rate in humans, Advances in Pharmacology, Vol. 31: Anesthesia and Cardiovascular Disease. Edited by Bosnjak Z, Kampine JP. San Diego, Academic Press, 1994, pp. 379

98. Ebert TJ, Perez F, Uhrich TD, et al: Desflurane-mediated sympathetic activation occurs in humans despite preventing hypotension and baroreceptor unloading. Anesthesiology 1998; 88: 1227

99. Muzi M, Ebert TJ: A comparison of baroreflex sensitivity during isoflurane and desflurane anesthesia in humans. Anesthesiology 1995; 82: 919

100. Tanaka M, Nishikawa T: Arterial baroreflex function in humans anaesthetized with sevoflurane. Br J Anaesth 1999; 82: 350

101. Ebert TJ, Kotrly KJ, Madsen KS, et al: Fentanyl-diazepam anesthesia with or without N2O does not attenuate cardiopulmonary baroreflex-mediated vasoconstrictor responses to controlled hypovolemia in humans. Anesth Analg 1988; 67: 548

102. Kotrly KJ, Ebert TJ, Vucins EJ, et al: Effects of fentanyl-diazepam-nitrous oxide anaesthesia on arterial baroreflex control of heart rate in man. Br J Anaesth 1986; 58: 406

103. Tanaka M, Nishikawa T: Sevoflurane speeds recovery of baroreflex control of heart rate after minor surgical procedures compared with isoflurane. Anesth Analg 1999; 89: 284

104. Muzi M, Lopatka CW, Ebert TJ: Desflurane-mediated neurocirculatory activation in humans: Effects of concentration and rate of change on responses. Anesthesiology 1996; 84: 1035

105. Calverley RK, Smith NT, Jones CW, et al: Ventilatory and cardiovascular effects of enflurane anesthesia during spontaneous ventilation in man. Anesth Analg 1978; 57: 610

106. Lopez-Barneo J, Pardal R, Ortega-Saenz P: Cellular mechanisms of oxygen sensing. Ann Rev Physiol 2001; 63: 259

107. Dahan A, Teppema LJ: Influence of anaesthesia and analgesia on the control of breathing. Br J Anaesth 2003; 91: 40

108. Hirshman CA, Bergman NA: Factors influencing intrapulmonary airway calibre during anaesthesia. Br J Anaesth 1990; 65: 30

109. Hirshman CA, Edelstein G, Peetz S, et al: Mechanism of action of inhalational anesthesia on airways. Anesthesiology 1982; 56: 107

110. Lindeman KS, Baker SG, Hirshman CA: Interaction between halothane and the nonadrenergic, noncholinergic inhibitory system in porcine trachealis muscle. Anesthesiology 1994; 81: 641

111. Goff MJ, Arain SR, Ficke DJ, et al: Absence of bronchodilation during desflurane anesthesia: A comparison to sevoflurane and thiopental. Anesthesiology 2000; 93: 404

112. Mori N, Nagata H, Ohta S, et al: Prolonged sevoflurane inhalation was not nephrotoxic in two patients with refractory status asthmaticus. Anesth Analg 1996; 83: 189

113. Johnston RG, Noseworthy TW, Friesen EG, et al: Isoflurane therapy for status asthmaticus in children and adults. Chest 1990; 97: 698

114. Reiz S: Nitrous oxide augments the systemic and coronary haemodynamic effects of isoflurane in patients with ischaemic heart disease. Acta Anaesthesiol Scand 1983; 27: 464

115. Benumof JL, Augustine SD, Gibbons JA: Halothane and isoflurane only slightly impair arterial oxygenation during one-lung ventilation in patients undergoing thoracotomy. Anesthesiology 1987; 67: 910

116. Pagel PS, Fu JL, Damask MC, et al: Desflurane and isoflurane produce similar alterations in systemic and pulmonary hemodynamics and arterial oxygenation in patients undergoing one-lung ventilation during thoracotomy. Anesth Analg 1998; 87: 800

117. Beck DH, Doepfmer UR, Sinemus C, et al: Effects of sevoflurane and propofol on pulmonary shunt fraction during one-lung ventilation for thoracic surgery. Br J Anaesth 2001; 86: 38

118. Frink EJ Jr, Ghantous H, Malan TP, et al: Plasma inorganic fluoride with sevoflurane anesthesia: Correlation with indices of hepatic and renal function. Anesth Analg 1992; 74: 231

119. Eger EI II: Isoflurane (Forane): A compendium and reference. 2nd ed. Madison, Ohio Medical Products, 1985

120. Weiskopf RB, Eger EI II, Ionescu P, et al: Desflurane does not produce hepatic or renal injury in human volunteers. Anesth Analg 1992; 74: 570

121. Isik Y, Goksu S, Kocoglu H, et al: Low flow desflurane and sevoflurane anaesthesia in children. Eur J Anaesthesiol 2006; 23: 60

122. Hussey AJ, Aldridge LM, Paul D, et al: Plasma glutathione-S-transferase concentration as a measure of hepatocellular integrity following a single general anaesthetic with halothane, enflurane or isoflurane. Br J Anaesth 1988; 60: 130

123. Suttner SW, Schmidt CC, Boldt J, et al: Low-flow desflurane and sevoflurane anesthesia minimally affect hepatic integrity and function in elderly patients. Anesth Analg 2000; 91: 206

124. Kurahashi K, Maruta H: The effect of sevoflurane and isoflurane on the neuromuscular block produced by vecuronium continuous infusion. Anesth Analg 1996; 82: 942

125. Wulf H, Kahl M, Ledowski T: Augmentation of the neuromuscular blocking effects of cisatracurium during desflurane, sevoflurane, isoflurane or total i.v. anaesthesia. Br J Anaesth 1998; 80: 308

126. Nitahara K, Sugi Y, Higa K, et al: Neuromuscular effects of sevoflurane in myasthenia gravis patients. Br J Anaesth 2007; 98: 337

127. Bock M, Klippel K, Nitsche B, et al: Rocuronium potency and recovery characteristics during steady-state desflurane, sevoflurane, isoflurane or propofol anaesthesia. Br J Anaesth 2000; 84: 43

128. Paul M, Fokt RM, Kindler CH, et al: Characterization of the interactions between volatile anesthetics and neuromuscular blockers at the muscle nicotinic acetylcholine receptor. Anesth Analg 2002; 95: 362

129. Wright PMC, Hart P, Lau M, et al: The magnitude and time course of vecuronium potentiation by desflurane versus isoflurane. Anesthesiology 1995; 82: 404

130. Ducart A, Adnet P, Renaud B, et al: Malignant hyperthermia during sevoflurane administration. Anesth Analg 1995; 80: 609

131. Allen GC, Brubaker CL: Human malignant hyperthermia associated with desflurane anesthesia. Anesth Analg 1998; 86: 1328

132. Reed SB, Strobel GE: An in vitro model of malignant hyperthermia: differential effects of inhalation anesthetics on caffeine-induced muscle contractures. Anesthesiology 1978; 48: 254

133. Papadimos TJ, Almasri M, Padgett JS, et al: A suspected case of delayed onset malignant hyperthermia with desflurane anesthesia. Anesth Analg 2004; 98: 548

134. Hobbhahn J, Wiesner G, Taeger K: [Occupational exposure and environmental pollution: the role of inhalation anesthetics with special consideration of sevoflurane.]. Anaesthesist 1998; 47: S77

135. Baden J, Kelley M, Mazze R: Mutagenicity of experimental inhalational anesthetic agents: sevoflurane, synthane, diozychlorane, and dioxyflurane. Anesthesiology 1982; 56: 462

136. Krause T, Scholz J, Jansen L, et al: Sevoflurane anaesthesia does not induce the formation of sister chromatid exchanges in peripheral blood lymphocytes of children. Br J Anaesth 2003; 90: 233

137. Akin A, Ugur F, Ozkul Y, et al: Desflurane anaesthesia increases sister chromatid exchanges in human lymphocytes. Acta Anaesthesiol Scand 2005; 49: 1559

138. Mazze RI, Wilson AI, Rice SA, et al: Fetal development in mice exposed to isoflurane. Teratology 1985; 32: 339

139. Mazze RI, Fujinaga M, Rice SA, et al: Reproductive and teratogenic effects of nitrous oxide, halothane, isoflurane, and enflurane in Sprague-Dawley rats. Anesthesiology 1986; 64: 339

140. Layzer RB, Fishman RA, Schafer JA: Neuropathy following use of nitrous oxide. Neurology 1978; 28: 504

141. Yildiz K, Dogru K, Dalgic H, et al: Inhibitory effects of desflurane and sevoflurane on oxytocin-induced contractions of isolated pregnant human myometrium. Acta Anaesthesiol Scand 2005; 49: 1355

142. Munson ES, Embro WJ: Enflurane, isoflurane and halothane and isolated human uterine muscle. Anesthesiology 1977; 46: 11

143. Abboud TK, Zhu J, Richardson M, et al: Desflurane: a new volatile anesthetic for cesarean section. Maternal and neonatal effects. Acta Anaesthesiol Scand 1995; 39: 723

144. Lane GA, Nahrwold ML, Tait AR: Anesthetics as teratogens: Nitrous oxide is fetotoxic, xenon is not. Science 1980; 210: 899

145. McGregor DG: Occupational exposure to trace concentrations of waste anesthetic gases. Mayo Clin Proc 2000; 75: 273

146. Abboud TK, Nagappala S, Murakawa K, et al: Comparison of the effects of general and regional anesthesia for cesarean section on neonatal neurologic and adaptive capacity scores. Anesth Analg 1985; 64: 996

147. Warren TM, Datta S, Ostheimer GW, et al: Comparisons of the maternal and neonatal effects of halothane, enflurane and isoflurane for cesarean delivery. Anesth Analg 1983; 62: 516

148. Ruzicka JA, Hidalgo JC, Tinker JH, et al: Inhibition of volatile sevoflurane degradation product formation in an anesthesia circuit by a reduction in soda lime temperature. Anesthesiology 1994; 81: 238

149. Fang ZX, Kandel L, Laster MJ, et al: Factors affecting production of compound A from the interaction of sevoflurane with Baralyme and soda lime. Anesth Analg 1996; 82: 775

150. Frink EJ Jr, Malan TP, Morgan SE, et al: Quantification of the degradation products of sevoflurane in two CO2 absorbents during low-flow anesthesia in surgical patients. Anesthesiology 1992; 77: 1064

151. Ebert TJ, Arain SR: Renal effects of low-flow anesthesia with desflurane and sevoflurane in patients. Anesthesiology, 1999: A404

152. Kharasch ED, Frink EJ Jr, Zager R, et al: Assessment of low-flow sevoflurane and isoflurane effects on renal function using sensitive markers of tubular toxicity. Anesthesiology 1997; 86: 1238

153. Bito H, Ikeuchi Y, Ikeda K: Effects of low-flow sevoflurane anesthesia on renal function. Comparison with high-flow sevoflurane anesthesia and low-flow isoflurane anesthesia. Anesthesiology 1997; 86: 1231

154. Bito H, Ikeda K: Closed-circuit anesthesia with sevoflurane in humans. Effects on renal and hepatic function and concentrations of breakdown products with soda lime in the circuit. Anesthesiology 1994; 80: 71

155. Eger EI II, Koblin DD, Bowland T, et al: Nephrotoxicity of sevoflurane versus desflurane anesthesia in volunteers. Anesth Analg 1997; 84: 160

156. Ebert TJ, Frink EJ Jr, Kharasch ED: Absence of biochemical evidence for renal and hepatic dysfunction after 8 hours of 1.25 minimum alveolar concentration sevoflurane anesthesia in volunteers. Anesthesiology 1998; 88: 601

157. Eger EI II, Gong D, Koblin DD, et al: Dose-related biochemical markers of renal injury after sevoflurane versus desflurane anesthesia in volunteers. Anesth Analg 1997; 85: 1154

158. Groudine SB, Fragen RJ, Kharasch ED, et al: Comparison of renal function following anesthesia with low-flow sevoflurane and isoflurane. J Clin Anesth 1999; 11: 201

159. Bito H, Ikeda K: Renal and hepatic function in surgical patients after low-flow sevoflurane or isoflurane anesthesia. Anesth Analg 1996; 82: 173

160. Ebert TJ, Messana LD, Uhrich TD, et al: Absence of renal and hepatic toxicity after four hours of 1.25 minimum alveolar concentration sevoflurane anesthesia in volunteers. Anesth Analg 1998; 86: 662

161. Ebert TJ, Frink EJ Jr, Kharasch ED: Absence of biochemical evidence for renal and hepatic dysfunction after 8 hours of 1.25 minimum alveolar concentration sevoflurane anesthesia in volunteers. Anesthesiology 1998; 88: 601

162. Conzen PF, Kharasch ED, Czerner SFA, et al: Low-flow sevoflurane compared with low-flow isoflurane anesthesia in patients with stable renal insufficiency. Anesthesiology 2002; 97: 578

163. Litz RJ, Hübler M, Lorenz W, et al: Renal responses to desflurane and isoflurane in patients with renal insufficiency. Anesthesiology 2002; 97: 1133

164. Holak EJ, Mei DA, Dunning MB, III, et al: Carbon monoxide production from sevoflurane breakdown: Modeling of exposures under clinical conditions. Anesth Analg 2003; 96: 757

165. Baxter PJ, Garton K, Kharasch ED: Mechanistic aspects of carbon monoxide formation from volatile anesthetics. Anesthesiology 1998; 89: 929

166. Fang ZX, Eger EI II, Laster MJ, et al: Carbon monoxide production from degradation of desflurane, enflurane, isoflurane, halothane, and sevoflurane by soda lime and baralyme. Anesth Analg 1995; 80: 1187

167. Berry PD, Sessler DI, Larson MD: Severe carbon monoxide poisoning during desflurane anesthesia. Anesthesiology 1999; 90: 613

168. Woehlck HJ: Severe intraoperative CO poisoning. Anesthesiology 1999; 90: 353

169. Woehlck HJ, Dunning M, III, Gandhi S, et al: Indirect detection of intraoperative carbon monoxide exposure by mass spectrometry during isoflurane anesthesia. Anesthesiology 1995; 83: 213

170. Woehlck HJ, Dunning M, Connolly LA: Reduction in the incidence of carbon monoxide exposures in humans undergoing general anesthesia. Anesthesiology 1997; 87: 228

171. Woehlck HJ, Dunning M, III, Raza T, et al: Physical factors affecting the production of carbon monoxide from anesthetic breakdown. Anesthesiology 2001; 94: 453

172. Wissing H, Kuhn I, Warnken U, et al: Carbon monoxide production from desflurane, enflurane, halothane, isoflurane and sevoflurane with dry soda lime. Anesthesiology 2001; 95: 1205

173. Castro BA, Freedman LA, Craig WL, et al: Explosion within an anesthesia machine: Baralyme®, high fresh gas flows and sevoflurane concentration. Anesthesiology 2004; 101: 537

174. Wu J, Previte JP, Adler E, et al: Spontaneous ignition, explosion, and fire with sevoflurane and barium hydroxide lime. Anesthesiology 2004; 101: 534

175. Fatheree RS, Leighton BL: Acute respiratory distress syndrome after an exothermic Baralyme®-sevoflurane reaction. Anesthesiology 2004; 101: 531

176. Hanaki C, Fujii K, Morio M, et al: Decomposition of sevoflurane by sodalime. Hiroshima J Med Sci 1987; 36: 61

177. Kharasch ED: Putting the brakes on anesthetic breakdown. Anesthesiology 1999; 91: 1192

178. Baker MT: Sevoflurane: are there differences in products? Anesth Analg 2007; 104: 1447

179. Kharasch ED, Subbarao GN, Stephens DA, et al: Influence of sevoflurane formulation water content on degradation to hydrogen fluoride in vaporizers. Anesthesiology 2007; 107: A1591

180. O'Neill B, Hafiz MA, De Beer DA: Corrosion of Penlon sevoflurane vaporisers. Anaesthesia 2007; 62: 421

181. Frink EJ Jr, Malan TP Jr, Isner RJ, et al: Renal concentrating function with prolonged sevoflurane or enflurane anesthesia in volunteers. Anesthesiology 1994; 80: 1019

182. Mazze RI, Calverley RK, Smith NT: Inorganic fluoride nephrotoxicity: Prolonged enflurane and halothane anesthesia in volunteers. Anesthesiology 1977; 46: 265

183. Mazze RI: The safety of sevoflurane in humans. Anesthesiology 1992; 77: 1062

184. Kharasch ED, Hankins DC, Thummel KE: Human kidney methoxyflurane and sevoflurane metabolism. Intrarenal fluoride production as a possible mechanism of methoxyflurane nephrotoxicity. Anesthesiology 1995; 82: 689

185. Strube PJ, Hulands GH, Halsey MJ: Serum fluoride levels in morbidly obese patients: enflurane compared with isoflurane anaesthesia. Anaesthesia 1987; 42: 685

186. Frink EJ Jr, Malan TP Jr, Brown EA, et al: Plasma inorganic fluoride levels with sevoflurane anesthesia in morbidly obese and nonobese patients. Anesth Analg 1993; 76: 1333

187. Thwaites A, Edmends S, Smith I: Inhalation induction with sevoflurane: A double-blind comparison with propofol. Br J Anaesth 1997; 78: 356

188. Muzi M, Colinco MD, Robinson BJ, et al: The effects of premedication on inhaled induction of anesthesia with sevoflurane. Anesth Analg 1997; 85: 1143

189. Muzi M, Robinson BJ, Ebert TJ, et al: Induction of anesthesia and tracheal intubation with sevoflurane in adults. Anesthesiology 1996; 85: 536

190. Tanaka S, Tsuchida H, Nakabayashi K, et al: The effects of sevoflurane, isoflurane, halothane, and enflurane on hemodynamic responses during an inhaled induction of anesthesia via a mask in humans. Anesth Analg 1996; 82: 821

191. Mostafa SM, Atherton AMJ: Sevoflurane for difficult tracheal intubation. Br J Anaesth 1997; 79: 392

192. Eger EI II, Johnson BH: Rates of awakening from anesthesia with I-653, halothane, isoflurane, and sevoflurane: A test of the effect of anesthetic concentration and duration in rats. Anesth Analg 1987; 66: 977

ANESTHETIC AGENTS, ADJUVANTS, AND DRUG INTERACTION

CHAPTER 18 ■ INTRAVENOUS ANESTHETICS

PAUL F. WHITE AND MATTHEW R. ENG

KEY POINTS

1 With the exception of ketamine, intravenous (IV) anesthetics lack intrinsic analgesic properties.

2 Dexmedetomidine is an α_2-agonist with sedative and opioid-sparing effects that is used as an anesthetic adjuvant in the operating room and intensive care unit.

3 Low doses of IV anesthetics produce sedation, and high doses produce hypnosis (or unconsciousness).

4 All IV anesthetics are sedative-hypnotics and produce dose-dependent central nervous system (CNS) depression.

5 Compared to thiopental and propofol, methohexital produces less CNS depression.

6 Propofol possesses unique antiemetic and appetite-stimulating properties.

7 Etomidate produces less cardiovascular depression than the barbiturates and propofol.

8 Ketamine possesses analgesic and psychomimetic properties.

9 Midazolam possesses amnestic and anxiolytic properties.

10 IV anesthetics in combination with potent opioid analgesics and/or local anesthetics can be used to produce total intravenous anesthesia.

The concept of intravenous (IV) anesthesia has evolved from primarily induction of general anesthesia to total IV anesthesia (TIVA). TIVA has assumed increasing importance for therapeutic, as well as diagnostic, procedures in both adults and children. IV anesthetic techniques are used for procedures in the operating room (OR) and remote from the OR. In many centers in Europe and South America, TIVA has become more popular for general anesthesia than classic "balanced anesthesia" or volatile anesthetic-based techniques. This change has been a result of (1) the development of rapid, short-acting IV hypnotic, analgesic, and muscle relaxant drugs; (2) the availability of pharmacokinetic and dynamic-based IV delivery systems; and (3) the development of the electroencephalogram (EEG)-based cerebral monitoring devices, which measure the hypnotic component of the anesthetic state. This chapter focuses on the pharmacologic properties and clinical uses of the currently available IV anesthetics.

Following its introduction into clinical practice, thiopental quickly became the gold standard of IV anesthetics against which all the newer IV drugs were compared. Many different hypnotic drugs are currently available for use during IV anesthesia (Fig. 18-1). However, it is clear that the "ideal" IV anesthetic is yet to be developed. The physical and pharmacologic properties that an ideal IV anesthetic would possess include the following:

1. Drug compatibility (water-solubility) and stability in solution.

2. Lack of pain on injection, veno-irritation, and local tissue damage following extravasation.
3. Low potential to release histamine or precipitate hypersensitivity reactions.
4. Rapid and smooth onset of hypnotic action without excitatory activity.
5. Rapid metabolism to pharmacologically inactive metabolites.
6. A steep dose-response relationship to enhance titratability and minimize tissue accumulation.
7. Lack of acute cardiovascular and respiratory depression.
8. Decreases in cerebral metabolism and intracranial pressure.
9. Rapid and smooth return of consciousness and cognitive skills with residual analgesia.
10. Absence of postoperative nausea and vomiting, amnesia, psychomimetic reactions, dizziness, headache, or prolonged sedation (hangover effects).

Despite thiopental's proven clinical usefulness, safety, and widespread acceptance over many decades of use, it has been supplanted by a variety of agents from different drug groups. The sedative-hypnotic drugs that have been more recently introduced into clinical practice (e.g., midazolam, ketamine, etomidate, propofol) have proven to be extremely valuable in specific clinical situations. These newer compounds combine many of the characteristics of the ideal IV anesthetic, but fail in aspects where the other drugs succeed. For some of these IV

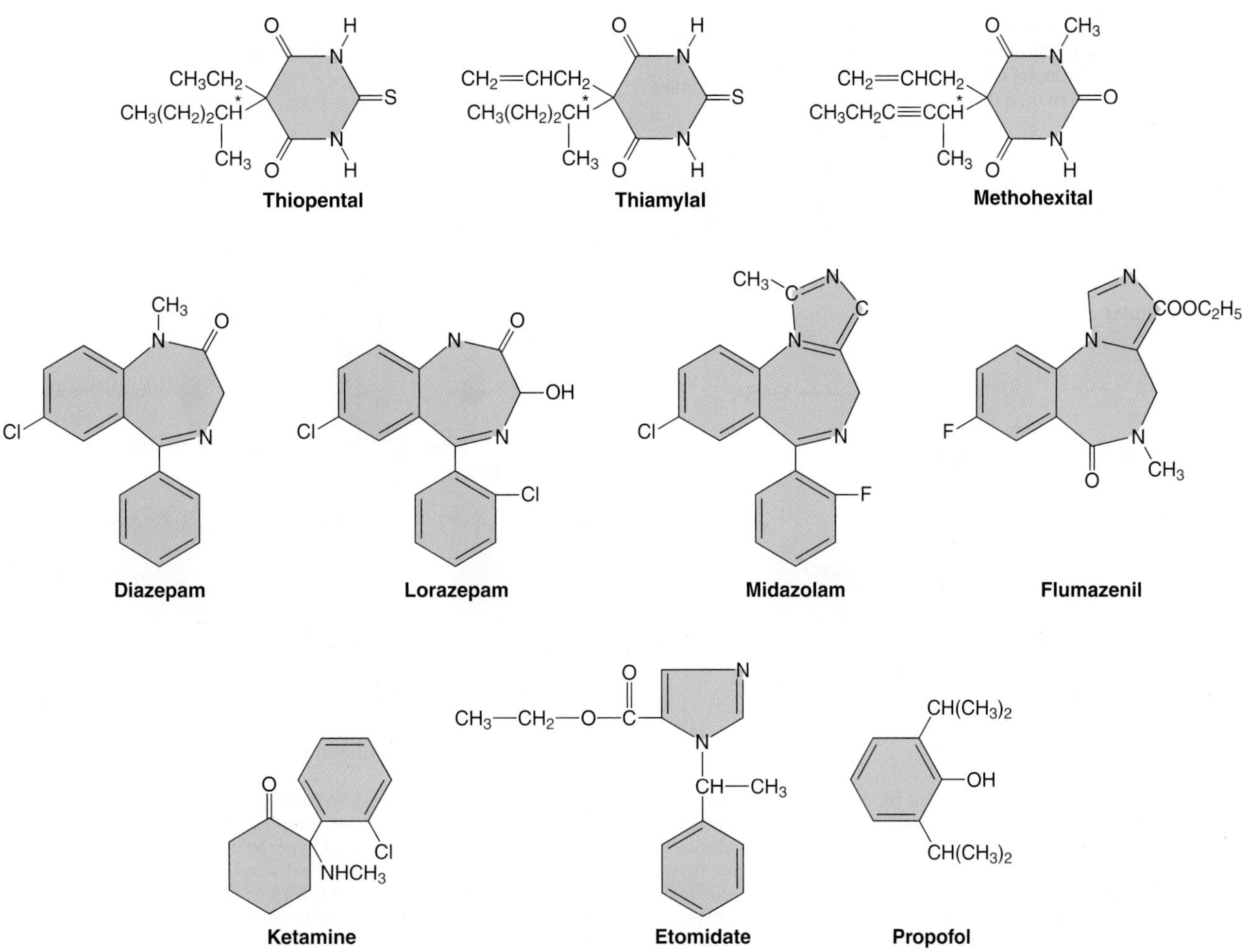

FIGURE 18-1. Chemical structures of currently available nonopioid intravenous anesthetics.

sedative-hypnotics, disadvantages have led to "restricted" indications (e.g., ketamine, etomidate). Because the optimal pharmacologic properties are not equally important in every clinical situation, the anesthesiologist must make the choice of the IV anesthetic drug that best fits the needs of the individual patient and the operative (or diagnostic) procedure.

GENERAL PHARMACOLOGY OF INTRAVENOUS HYPNOTICS

Mechanism of Action

A widely accepted theory of anesthetic action is that both IV and inhalational anesthetics exert their primary sedative and hypnotic effects through an interaction with the inhibitory γ-aminobutyric acid (GABA) neurotransmitter system.[1] GABA is the principal inhibitory neurotransmitter within the CNS. The GABA and adrenergic neurotransmitter systems counterbalance the action of excitatory neurotransmitters. The GABA type A ($GABA_A$) receptor is a receptor complex consisting of up to five glycoprotein subunits. When the $GABA_A$ receptor is activated, transmembrane chloride conductance increases, resulting in hyperpolarization of the postsynaptic cell membrane and functional inhibition of the postsynaptic neuron. Sedative-hypnotic drugs interact with different components of the GABA-receptor complex (Fig. 18-2). However, the allosteric (structural) requirements for

activation of the receptor are different for IV and volatile anesthetics.

Benzodiazepines bind to specific receptor sites that are part of the $GABA_A$-receptor complex. The binding of benzodiazepines to their receptor site increases the efficiency of the coupling between the GABA receptor and the chloride ion channel. The degree of modulation of the GABA-receptor function is limited, which explains the maximal "ceiling effect" produced by benzodiazepines with respect to CNS depression. The dose-dependent CNS depressant effect of benzodiazepines produce hypnosis, sedation, anxiolysis, amnesia, and anticonvulsant effects.[2] These CNS effects are presumed to be associated with stimulation of different receptor subtypes and/or concentration-dependent receptor occupancy.[1] For example, it has been suggested that benzodiazepine receptor occupancy of 20% provides anxiolysis, while 30 to 50% receptor occupancy is associated with amnesia to sedation, and 60% receptor occupancy is required for hypnosis (or unconsciousness).[2]

The interaction of barbiturates and propofol with specific membrane structures appears to decrease the rate of dissociation of GABA from its receptor, thereby increasing the duration of the GABA-activated opening of the chloride ion channel (Fig. 18-2). Barbiturates can also mimic the action of GABA by directly activating the chloride channels. The proposed mechanism of action of thiopental relates to its ability to function as a competitive inhibitor at the nicotinic acetylcholine receptors in the CNS.[3] Etomidate augments GABA-gated chloride currents (i.e., indirect modulation) and at

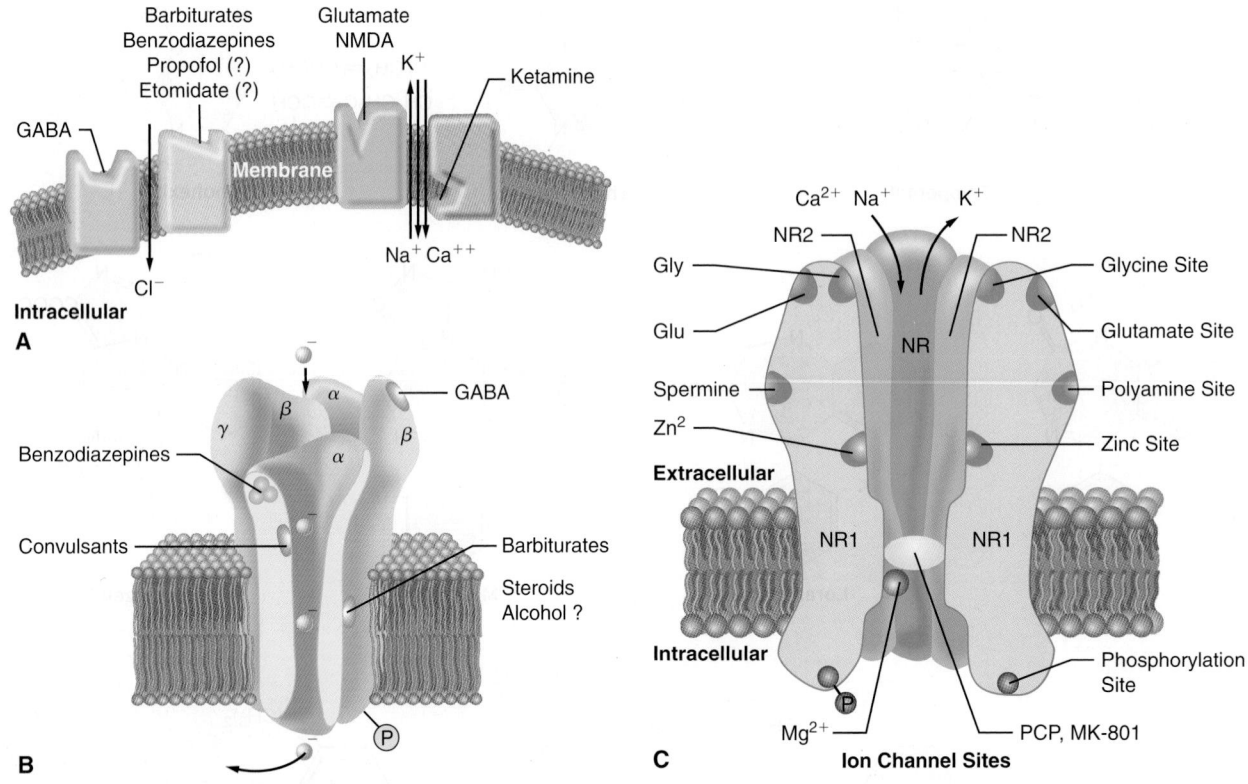

FIGURE 18-2.   A. This model depicts the postsynaptic site of γ-aminobutyric acid (GABA) and glutamate within the CNS. GABA decreases the excitability of neurons by its action at the $GABA_A$-receptor complex. When GABA occupies the binding site of this complex, it allows inward flux of chloride ion, resulting in hyperpolarizing of the cell and subsequent resistance of the neuron to stimulation by excitatory transmitters. Barbiturates, benzodiazepines, propofol, and etomidate decrease neuronal excitability by enhancing the effect of GABA at this complex, facilitating this inhibitory effect on the postsynaptic cell. Glutamate and its analog N-methyl-D-aspartate (NMDA) are excitatory amino acids. When glutamate occupies the binding site on the NMDA subtype of the glutamate receptor, the channel opens and allows Na^+, K^+, and Ca^{2+} to either enter or leave the cell. Flux of these ions leads to depolarization of the postsynaptic neuron and initiation of an action potential and activation of other pathways. Ketamine blocks this open channel and prevents further ion flux, thus inhibiting the excitatory response to gluta-mate. (Reprinted with permission from Van Hemelrijck J, Gonzales JM, White PF: Use of intravenous sedative agents, Principles and Practice of Anesthesiology. Edited by Rogers MC, Tinker JH, Covino BG, Longnecker DE. St. Louis, Mosby, 1992, p 1131.) **B.** Schematic model of the $GABA_A$-receptor complex illustrating recognition sites for many of the substances that bind to the receptor. **C.** Model of the NMDA receptor showing sites for antagonist action. Ketamine binds to the site labeled PCP (phencyclidine). The pentameric structure of the receptor, composed of a combination of the subunits NR 1 and NR 2, is illustrated. (Altered with permission from Leeson TD, Iversen LL: The glycine site on the NMDA receptor: Structure-activity relationships and therapeutic potential. J Med Chem 1994; 37: 4053.)

higher concentrations evokes chloride currents in the absence of GABA (i.e., direct activation). Although the mechanism of action of propofol is similar to that of the barbiturates (i.e., enhancing the activity of the GABA-activated chloride chan-nel), it also possesses ion channel-blocking effects in cerebral cortex tissue and nicotinic acetylcholine receptors, as well as an inhibitory effect on lysophosphatidate signaling in lipid mediator receptors.[4]

Ketamine produces a functional dissociation between the thalamocortical and limbic systems, a state that has been termed *dissociative* anesthesia. Ketamine depresses neuronal function in the cerebral cortex and thalamus, while simultane-ously activating the limbic system. Ketamine's effect on the medial medullary reticular formation may be involved in the affective component of its nociceptive activity. The CNS effects of ketamine appear to be primarily related to its antagonistic activity at the N-methyl-D-aspartate (NMDA) receptor (Fig. 18-2). Unlike the other IV anesthetics, ketamine does not inter-

act with GABA receptors; however, it binds to non-NMDA glu-tamate receptors and nicotinic, muscarinic, monoaminergic, and opioid receptors. In addition, it also inhibits neuronal sodium channels (producing a modest local anesthetic action) and calcium channels (causing cerebral vasodilatation).

The centrally-active α_2-adrenergic receptor agonists, clonidine and dexmedetomidine, have potent sedative and opioid analgesic-sparing properties. These drugs also have significant effects on the peripheral α_2 receptors involved in regulating the cardiovascular system by inhibiting norepi-nephrine release. This class of anesthetic adjuncts can also reduce blood pressure and heart rate by decreasing the tonic levels of sympathetic outflow from the CNS and augment-ing cardiac vagal activity, respectively.[5,6] However, dexme-detomidine failed to block the acute hyperdynamic response to electroconvulsive therapy when administered as an adju-vant to methohexital anesthesia.[7] Earlier studies with cloni-dine demonstrated that this α_2 agonist-antagonist could also reduce the IV[8] and volatile[9] anesthetic requirements, as well as the postoperative opioid analgesic requirement.

Pharmacokinetics and Metabolism

An understanding of basic pharmacokinetic principles is integral to the understanding the pharmacologic actions and interactions of IV anesthetic and adjunctive drugs, and will allow the anesthesiologist to develop more optimal dosing strategies when using IV techniques. Although lipid solubility facilitates diffusion of IV anesthetics across cellular membranes, including the blood–brain barrier, only the nonionized form is able to readily cross neuronal membranes. The ratio of the unionized-to-ionized fraction depends on the pKa of the drug and the pH of the body fluids.

The rapid onset of the CNS effect of most IV anesthetics can be explained by their high lipid solubility and the relatively high proportion of the cardiac output (20%) perfusing the brain. However, a variable degree of hysteresis exists between the blood concentration of the hypnotic drug and its onset of action on the CNS. The hysteresis is related in part to diffusion of these drugs into brain tissue and nonspecific CNS receptor binding. However, the number of CNS binding sites is usually saturable and only a small fraction of the available binding sites needs to be occupied to produce clinical effects. Although the total amount of drug in the blood is available for diffusion, the diffusion rate will be more limited for IV anesthetics with a high degree of plasma protein binding (90%) because only the "free" unbound drug can diffuse across membranes and exert central effects. When several drugs compete for the same binding sites, or when the protein concentration in the blood is decreased by preexisting disease (e.g., hepatic failure, malnutrition), a higher fraction of the unbound drug will be available to exert an effect on the CNS. Since only unbound drug is available for uptake and metabolism in the liver, highly protein-bound drugs may have a lower rate of hepatic metabolism as a result of their decreased hepatic extraction ratio (i.e., the fraction of the hepatic blood flow that is cleared of the drug).

The pharmacokinetics of IV hypnotics are characterized by rapid distribution and subsequent redistribution into several hypothetical compartments (determined by their effect on blood flow to various tissues), followed by elimination (Table 18-1). The initial pharmacologic effects are related to the activity of the drug in the central compartment. The primary mechanism for terminating the central effects of IV anesthetics

administered for induction of anesthesia is redistribution from the central highly perfused compartment (brain) to the larger, but less well perfused "peripheral" compartments (muscle, fat). Even for drugs with a high hepatic extraction ratio, elimination does not usually play a major role in terminating the drug's CNS effects because elimination of the drug can occur only from the central compartment. The rate of elimination from the central compartment, the amount of drug present in the peripheral compartments, and the rate of redistribution from the peripheral compartments "back" into the central compartment determine the time necessary to eliminate the drug from the body and directly influence recovery times.

Most IV anesthetic agents are eliminated via hepatic metabolism followed by renal excretion of more water-soluble metabolites. Some metabolites have pharmacologic activity and can produce prolonged drug effects (e.g., oxazepam, desmethyldiazepam, norketamine). Moreover, there is considerable interpatient variability in the clearance rates for commonly used IV anesthetic drugs. The elimination clearance is the distribution volume cleared of drug over time and is a measure of the efficacy of the elimination process. The slow elimination of some anesthetics is partly due to their high degree of protein binding that reduces their hepatic extraction ratio. Other drugs may have a high hepatic extraction ratio and elimination clearance despite extensive plasma protein binding (e.g., propofol), indicating that protein binding is not always a rate-limiting factor.

For most drugs, the hepatic enzyme systems are not saturated at clinically relevant drug concentrations, and the rate of drug elimination will decrease as an exponential function of the drug's plasma concentration (first-order kinetics). However, when high steady-state plasma concentrations are achieved with prolonged infusions, hepatic enzyme systems can become saturated and the elimination rate becomes independent of the drug concentration (zero-order kinetics). The elimination half-life ($t_{1/2}\beta$) is the time required for the anesthetic concentration to decrease by 50% during the terminal phase of the plasma decay curve. The $t_{1/2}\beta$ depends on the volume to be cleared (the distribution volume) and the efficiency of the metabolic clearance system. Because their volumes of distribution are similar, the wide variation in elimination half-life values for the IV anesthetics is a reflection of differences in their clearance values.

When a drug infusion is administered without a loading dose, at least 3 times the $t_{1/2}\beta$ value may be required to achieve a true "steady-state" plasma concentration. The steady-state concentration obtained during an anesthetic infusion depends on the rate of drug administration and its clearance rate. When an infusion is discontinued, the rate at which the plasma concentration

TABLE 18-1

PHARMACOKINETIC VALUES FOR THE CURRENTLY AVAILABLE INTRAVENOUS SEDATIVE-HYPNOTIC DRUGS

■ DRUG NAME	■ DISTRIBUTION HALF-LIFE (min)	■ PROTEIN BINDING (%)	■ DISTRIBUTION VOLUME AT STEADY STATE (L/kg)	■ CLEARANCE (mL/kg/min)	■ ELIMINATION HALF-LIFE (hr)
Thiopental	2–4	85	2.5	3.4	11
Methohexital	5–6	85	2.2	11	4
Propofol	2–4	98	2–10	20–30	4–23
Midazolam	7–15	94	1.1–1.7	6.4–11	1.7–2.6
Diazepam	10–15	98	0.7–1.7	0.2–0.5	20–50
Lorazepam	3–10	98	0.8–1.3	0.8–1.8	11–22
Etomidate	2–4	75	2.5–4.5	18–25	2.9–5.3
Ketamine	11–16	12	2.5–3.5	12–17	2–4

From White PF. Textbook of Intravenous Anesthesia. Baltimore, Williams & Wilkins, 1997, pp. 27 and 77.

decreases largely depends on the clearance rate (as reflected by the terminal $t_{1/2}\beta$ value). For drugs with shorter elimination half-lives, plasma concentration will decrease at a rate that allows for a more rapid recovery (e.g., propofol). Drugs with long $t_{1/2}\beta$ values (e.g., thiopental and diazepam) are usually only administered by continuous IV infusion when the medical condition requires long-term treatment (e.g., elevated intracranial pressure [ICP] as a result of brain injury or prolonged sedation in the intensive care unit [ICU] because of respiratory failure).

3 Careful titration of an anesthetic drug to achieve the desired clinical effect is necessary to avoid drug accumulation and the resultant prolonged CNS effects after the infusion has been discontinued. Although the value of the $t_{1/2}\beta$ indicates how fast a drug is eliminated from the body, a more useful indicator of the acceptability of a hypnotic infusion for maintenance of anesthesia or sedation is the context-sensitive half-time, a value derived from computer simulations of drug infusions.[10] The context-sensitive half-time is defined as the time necessary for the effect-compartment (i.e., effect site) concentration to decrease by 50% in relation to the duration of the infusion. The context-sensitive half-time becomes particularly important in determining recovery after prolonged infusions of sedative-hypnotic drugs. Drugs (e.g., propofol) may have a relatively short context-sensitive half-time despite the fact that a large amount of drug remains present in the "deep" (less well-perfused) compartment. The slow return of the anesthetic from the deep compartment contributes little to the concentration of drug in the central compartment from which it is rapidly cleared. Therefore, the concentration in the central compartment rapidly declines below the hypnotic threshold after discontinuation of the infusion, contributing to short emergence times despite the fact that a substantial quantity of anesthetic drug may remain in the body.

Marked interpatient variability exists in the pharmacokinetics of IV sedative-hypnotic drugs. Factors that can influence anesthetic drug disposition include the degree of protein binding, the efficiency of hepatic and renal elimination processes, physiologic changes with aging, pre-existing disease states, the operative site, body temperature, and drug interactions (e.g., coadministration of volatile anesthetics). For example, increased age, lean body (muscle) mass, and total body water decrease result in an increase in the steady-state volume of distribution of most IV anesthetics. The increased distribution volume and decreased hepatic clearance leads to a prolongation of their $t_{1/2}\beta$ values. Moreover, a decrease of the volume of the central compartment may result in higher initial drug concentrations and can at least partially explain the decreased induction requirement in the elderly. Additionally, the slower redistribution from the vessel-rich tissues to intermediate compartments (muscles) also contributes to the age-related decrease in the induction dose requirements.[10] Although prolongation of the elimination half-time does not provide an explanation for the decreased induction dose requirement, it is responsible for producing higher steady-state plasma concentrations at any given infusion rate, contributing to a slower recovery from the subhypnotes (residual effects).

The hepatic clearance of IV anesthetics with a high (e.g., etomidate, propofol, ketamine) or intermediate (e.g., methohexital, midazolam) extraction ratio largely depends on hepatic blood flow, with most of the drug being removed from the blood as it flows through the liver (so-called perfusion-limited clearance). The elimination rate of drugs with low hepatic extraction ratios (e.g., thiopental, diazepam, lorazepam) depends on the enzymatic activity of the liver and is less dependent of hepatic blood flow (so-called capacity-limited clearance). Hepatic blood flow decreases during upper abdominal and laparoscopic surgery and, as a result, higher blood levels of drugs with perfusion-limited clearance are achieved at any given infusion rate. With aging, a decreased cardiac output and a redistribution of blood flow can partly explain the lower clearance rate for drugs with perfusion-limited clearance. Although concomitant administra-

tion of volatile anesthetics (which are known to decrease liver blood flow) has little influence on the elimination of thiopental, they can decrease the clearance of etomidate, ketamine, methohexital, and propofol. Other factors that decrease hepatic blood flow include hypocapnia, congestive heart failure, intravascular volume depletion, acute alcohol intoxication, circulatory collapse, increase intra-abdominal pressure, β-adrenergic blockade, and norepinephrine administration.

Hepatic disease can influence the pharmacokinetics of drugs by (1) altering the plasma protein content and changing the degree of protein binding, (2) decreasing hepatic blood flow and producing intrahepatic shunting, and (3) depressing the metabolic enzymatic activity of the liver. Therefore, the influence of hepatic disease on pharmacokinetics and dynamics of IV anesthetics is difficult to predict. Renal disease can also alter the concentration of plasma and tissue proteins, as well as the degree of protein binding, thereby producing changes in free drug concentrations. Because IV anesthetic agents are primarily metabolized by the liver, renal insufficiency has little influence on their rate of metabolic inactivation or elimination of the primary compound.

Pharmacodynamic Effects

4 The principal pharmacologic effect of IV anesthetics is to produce progressively increasing sedation and ultimately hypnosis as a result of dose-dependent CNS depression. However, all sedative-hypnotics also directly or indirectly affect other major organ systems. The relationship between the dose of a sedative-hypnotic and its CNS effects can be defined by dose-response curves. Although most IV anesthetics are characterized by steep dose-response curves, they are not always parallel (Fig. 18-3). However, the characteristics of a dose-

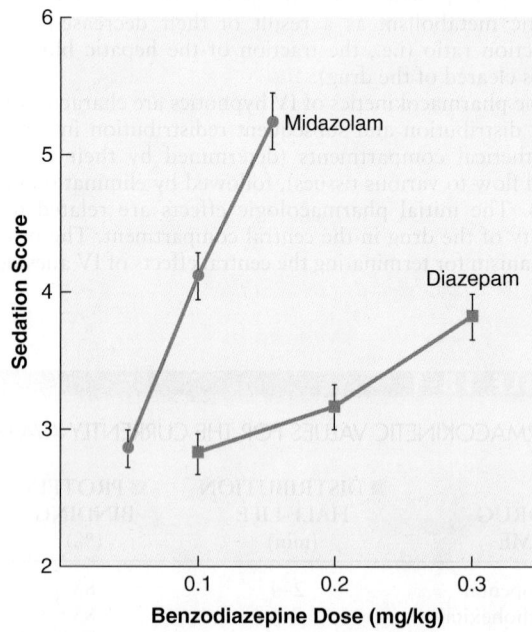

FIGURE 18-3. Dose-response relationships for sedation with midazolam (•) and diazepam (□). The level of sedation (2 = awake and alert to 6 = asleep and unarousable) was assessed 5 minutes after bolus doses of midazolam (0.05, 0.1, or 0.15 mg/kg) or diazepam (0.1, 0.2, or 0.3 mg/kg). Values represent mean values ± SEM. (Reprinted with permission from White PF, Vascones LO, Mathes SA, et al: Comparison of midazolam and diazepam for sedation during plastic surgery. J Plast Reconstruct Surg 1988; 81: 703.)

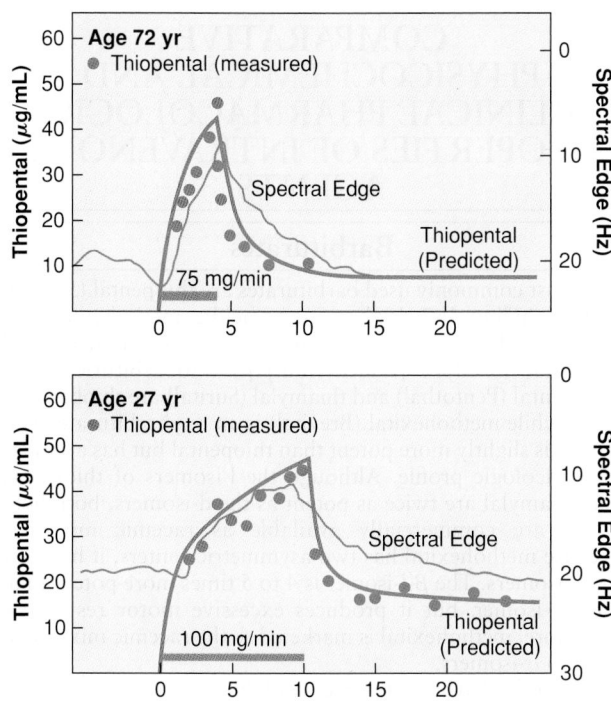

FIGURE 18-4. The concentration of thiopental versus time and spectral edge in an elderly patient (**top**) and in a younger patient (**bottom**). *Solid horizontal bars* represent the length of thiopental infusion. *Filled circles* represent the measured thiopental concentration (linear scale), and the *solid line* next to them represents the fitted data from the pharmacokinetic model. The axis for spectral edge has been inverted for visual clarity. (Reprinted with permission from Homer TD, Stanski DR: The effect of increasing age on thiopental disposition and anesthetic requirement. Anesthesiology 1985; 62: 714.)

response curve can only be interpreted in relation to the specific response for which it was constructed.

When steady-state plasma concentrations are achieved, one can assume that the plasma concentration is in quasiequilibrium with the effect-site concentration. Under these circumstances, it is possible to describe the relationship between drug and effect using a concentration-effect curve (Fig. 18-4). Because of the pharmacodynamic variability that exists among individuals, the plasma drug concentration necessary to obtain a particular effect is often described in terms of an effective concentration range, the so-called therapeutic window. Efficacy of an IV anesthetic relates to the maximum effect that can be achieved with respect to some measure of CNS function. Depending on the drug effect under consideration, the efficacy of sedative-hypnotics may appear to be <100%. For example, it is virtually impossible to produce a burst-suppressive EEG pattern with a benzodiazepine. Potency, on the other hand, relates to the quantity of drug necessary to obtain the maximum CNS effect. The relative potency of sedative-hypnotics also varies depending on the end point chosen. In the presence of an antagonist drug (e.g., flumazenil), the maximal response that can be obtained with a benzodiazepine agonist is further reduced because of competition for the same CNS receptor binding sites.

The influence of sedative-hypnotics on cerebral metabolism, cerebral hemodynamics, and ICP is of particular importance during neuroanesthesia. In patients with reduced cerebral compliance, a small increase in cerebral blood volume can cause a life-threatening increase in ICP. Most sedative-hypnotic drugs cause a proportional reduction in cerebral

metabolism ($CMRO_2$) and cerebral blood flow (CBF), resulting in a decrease in ICP. Although a decrease in $CMRO_2$ probably provides only a modest degree of protection against CNS ischemia or hypoxia, some hypnotics appear to possess cerebroprotective potential (e.g., thiopental, propofol). Explanations for the alleged neuroprotective effects of these compounds include a biochemical role as free-radical scavengers and membrane stabilizers (barbiturates and propofol) or NMDA-receptor antagonists (ketamine). With the exception of ketamine, all sedative-hypnotics also lower intraocular pressure. The changes in intraocular pressure generally reflect the effects of the IV agent on systemic arterial pressure and intracranial hemodynamics. However, none of the available sedative-hypnotic drugs protect against the transient increase in intraocular pressure that occurs with laryngoscopy and tracheal intubation.

Most IV hypnotics have similar EEG effects. Activation of high-frequency EEG activity (15 to 30 Hz) is characteristic of low concentrations (so-called sedative doses) of IV anesthetics. At higher concentrations, an increase in the relative contribution of the lower frequency higher amplitude waves is observed. At high concentrations, a burst-suppressive pattern develops with an increase in the isoelectric periods. Most sedative-hypnotic drugs have been reported to cause occasional EEG seizurelike activity. Interestingly, these same drugs also possess anticonvulsant properties.[11,12] When considering possible epileptogenic properties of CNS-depressant drugs, it is important to differentiate between true epileptogenic activity (e.g., methohexital) and myoclonic-like phenomena (e.g., etomidate, ketamine, propofol). Myoclonic activity is generally considered to be the result of an imbalance between excitatory and inhibitory subcortical centers, produced by an unequal degree of suppression of these brain centers by low concentrations of hypnotic drugs. Epileptic activity refers to a sudden alteration in CNS seizurelike activity resulting from a high-voltage electrical discharge at either cortical or subcortical sites, with subsequent spreading to the thalamic and brainstem centers. As a result of its vasoconstrictive effects on the cerebral vasculature, propofol may be useful for treatment of intractable migraine headaches.[13]

Although some induction drugs can increase airway sensitivity, coughing and airway irritation (e.g., bronchospasm) are usually a result of manipulation of the airway during "light" (inadequate) levels of IV anesthesia rather than to a direct drug effect. With the exception of ketamine (and to a lesser extent, etomidate), IV anesthetics produce dose-dependent respiratory depression, which is enhanced in patients with chronic obstructive pulmonary disease. The respiratory depression is characterized by a decrease in tidal volume and minute ventilation, as well as a transient rightward shift in the CO_2 response curve. Following the rapid injection of a large bolus dose of an IV anesthetic, transient apnea lasting 30 to 90 seconds is usually produced. Ketamine causes minimal respiratory depression when administered in the usual induction doses, while etomidate is associated with less respiratory depressant effects than the barbiturate compounds or propofol. The α_2-agonist dexmedetomidine has minimal depressant effects on respiratory function.[14] The sympatholytic effects of dexmedetomidine when administered for premedication may increase the incidence of intraoperative hypotension and bradycardia.[15]

Many different factors contribute to the hemodynamic changes associated with IV induction of anesthesia, including the patient's pre-existing cardiovascular and fluid status, resting sympathetic nervous system tone, chronic cardiovascular drugs, preanesthetic medication, the speed of drug injection, and the onset of unconsciousness. In addition, cardiovascular changes can be attributed to the direct pharmacologic actions of anesthetic and analgesic drugs on the heart and peripheral vasculature. IV anesthetics can depress the CNS and peripheral nervous system responses, blunt the compensatory baroreceptor reflex mechanisms, produce direct myocardial depression, and lower peripheral vascular resistance (and/or dilate venous capacitance vessels), thereby decreasing venous return. Profound hemodynamic effects occur at induction of anesthesia in the presence of hypovolemia because a higher than expected drug concentration is achieved in the central compartment. Not surprisingly, the acute cardiocirculatory depressant effects of all IV anesthetics are accentuated in the elderly, as well as in the presence of pre-existing cardiovascular disease (e.g., coronary artery disease, hypertension).

The effects of IV anesthetics on neuroendocrine function are also influenced by the surgical stimuli. Surgery-induced increases in stress hormones (e.g., vasopressin, catecholamines) can result in increased peripheral vascular resistance, and a reduction of urine output. Similarly, glucose tolerance appears to be decreased by surgical stress, resulting in elevations in the glucose concentration. Unlike ketamine and dexmedetomidine, most IV sedative-hypnotic drugs lack intrinsic analgesic activity. In fact, thiopental has been alleged to possess so-called antianalgesic activity (i.e., appearing to lower the pain threshold). Although propofol possesses dose-dependent effects on thalamocortical transfer of nociceptive information, pain-evoked cortical activity remains intact after loss of consciousness.[16]

Hypersensitivity (Allergic) Reactions

Allergic or hypersensitivity-type reactions to IV anesthetics are rare but can be severe and even life-threatening. IV drug administration bypasses the normal "protective barriers" against entrance of foreign molecules into the body. With the exception of etomidate, all IV induction agents have been alleged to cause some histamine release. However, the incidence of severe anaphylactic reactions is extremely low with the currently available IV induction agents. The high frequency of allergic reactions to the Cremophor EL–containing formulations led to the early withdrawal of IV anesthetics containing this solubilizing agent (e.g., propofol EL, propanidid, Alphadione [Althesin]). The possible mechanisms for immunologic reactions include (1) direct action on mast cells, (2) classic complement activation after previous exposure and antibody formation, (3) complement activation through the alternative pathway without previous antigen exposure, (4) antigen-antibody reactions, and (5) the "mixed type" of anaphylactoid reactions.

Severe anaphylactic reactions to IV anesthetics are extremely uncommon; however, profound hypotension attributed to nonimmunologically mediated histamine release has been reported with thiopental use. Although anaphylactic reactions to etomidate have been reported, it does not appear to release histamine, and is considered to be the most "immunologically safe" IV anesthetic. Propofol does not normally trigger histamine release, but life-threatening anaphylactoid reactions have been reported in patients with a previous history of multiple-drug allergies. Barbiturates can also precipitate episodes of acute intermittent porphyria and their use is contraindicated in patients who are predisposed to acute intermittent porphyria. Although benzodiazepines, ketamine, and etomidate are reported to be safe in humans, these drugs have been shown to be porphyrogenic in animal models. The most common cause of profound hypotension following IV induction of anesthesia is that of drug interactions and/or unrecognized hypovolemia.

COMPARATIVE PHYSICOCHEMICAL AND CLINICAL PHARMACOLOGIC PROPERTIES OF INTRAVENOUS AGENTS

Barbiturates

The most commonly used barbiturates are thiopental (5-ethyl-5-[1-methylbutyl]-2-thiobarbituric acid), methohexital (1-methyl-5-allyl-5-[1-methyl-2-pentanyl] barbituric acid), and thiamylal (5-allyl-5-[1-methylbutyl]-2-thiobarbituric acid). Thiopental (Pentothal) and thiamylal (Surital) are thiobarbiturates, while methohexital (Brevital) is an oxybarbiturate. Thiamylal is slightly more potent than thiopental but has a similar pharmacologic profile. Although the l-isomers of thiopental and thiamylal are twice as potent as the d-isomers, both hypnotics are commercially available as racemic mixtures. Because methohexital has two asymmetric centers, it has four stereoisomers. The β-l-isomer is 4 to 5 times more potent than the α-l-isomer, but it produces excessive motor responses. Therefore, methohexital is marketed as the racemic mixture of the two α-isomers.

All three barbiturates are available as sodium salts and must be dissolved in isotonic sodium chloride (0.9%) or water to prepare solutions of 2.5% thiopental, 1 to 2% methohexital, and 2% thiamylal. If refrigerated, solutions of the thiobarbiturates are stable for up to 2 weeks. Solutions of methohexital are stable for up to 6 weeks. When barbiturates are added to Ringer lactate or an acidic solution containing other water-soluble drugs, precipitation will occur and can occlude the IV catheter. Although the typical solution of thiopental (2.5%) is highly alkaline (pH 9) and can be irritating to the tissues if injected extravenously, it does not cause pain on injection and venoirritation is rare. In contrast, a 1% methohexital solution frequently causes discomfort when injected into small veins. Intra-arterial injection of thiobarbiturates is a serious complication as crystals can form in the arterioles and capillaries, causing intense vasoconstriction, thrombosis, and even tissue necrosis. Accidental intra-arterial injections should be treated promptly with intra-arterial administration of papaverine and lidocaine (or procaine), as well as a regional anesthesia-induced sympathectomy (stellate ganglion block, brachial plexus block) and heparinization.

Thiopental is metabolized in the liver to hydroxythiopental and the carboxylic acid derivative, which are more water soluble and have little CNS activity. When high doses of thiopental are administered, a desulfuration reaction can occur with the production of pentobarbital, which has long-lasting CNS-depressant activity. The low elimination clearance of thiopental (3.4 mL/kg/min) contributes to a long elimination half-life ($t_{1/2}\beta$ of 11 hours). Pre-existing hepatic and renal disease result in decreased plasma protein binding, thereby increasing the free fraction of thiopental and enhancing its CNS and cardiovascular-depressant properties. During prolonged continuous administration of thiopental, the concentration in the tissues approaches the concentration in the central compartment, with termination of its CNS effects becoming solely dependent on elimination by nonlinear hepatic metabolism. Methohexital is metabolized in the liver to inactive hydroxyderivatives. The clearance of methohexital (11 mL/kg/min) is higher and more dependent on hepatic blood flow than thiopental, resulting in a shorter elimination half-life ($t_{1/2}\beta$ 4 hours).

The usual induction dose of thiopental is 3 to 5 mg/kg in adults, 5 to 6 mg/kg in children, and 6 to 8 mg/kg in infants. Because methohexital is approximately 2.7 times more potent than thiopental, a dose of 1.5 mg/kg is equivalent to 4 mg/kg of thiopental in adults. The dose of barbiturates necessary to induce anesthesia is reduced in premedicated patients, patients in early pregnancy (7 to 13 weeks' gestation), and those of more advanced American Society of Anesthesiologists physical status (III or IV). Geriatric patients require a 30 to 40% reduction in the usual adult dose because of a decrease of the volume of the central compartment and slowed redistribution of thiopental from the vessel-rich tissues to lean muscle.[17] When the calculation of the induction dose is based on the lean body mass rather than total body weight, dosage adjustments for age, sex, or obesity are not necessary. Thiopental infusion is seldom used to maintain anesthesia because of the long context-sensitive half-time and prolonged recovery period. Plasma thiopental levels necessary to maintain a hypnotic state range between 10 and 20 mg/mL. A typical infusion rate necessary to treat intracranial hypertension or intractable convulsions is 2 to 4 mg/kg/hr. The plasma concentration of methohexital needed to maintain hypnosis during anesthesia ranges between 3 and 5 mg/mL and can be achieved with an infusion rate of methohexital 50–120 μg/kg/min.

Barbiturates produce a proportional decrease in $CMRO_2$ and CBF, thereby lowering ICP. The maximal decrease in $CMRO_2$ (55%) occurs when the EEG becomes isoelectric (burst-suppressive pattern). An isoelectric EEG can be maintained with a thiopental infusion rate of 4 to 6 mg/kg/hr (resulting in plasma concentrations of 30 to 50 μg/mL). Because the decrease in systemic arterial pressure is usually less than the reduction in ICP, thiopental should improve cerebral perfusion and compliance. Therefore, thiopental is widely used to improve brain relaxation during neurosurgery and to improve cerebral perfusion pressure (CPP) after acute brain injury. Although barbiturate therapy is widely used to control ICP after brain injury, the results of outcome studies are no better than with other aggressive forms of cerebral antihypertensive therapy.

It has been suggested that barbiturates also possess "neuroprotective" properties secondary to their ability to decrease oxygen demand. Alternative explanations have been suggested, including a reverse steal ("Robin Hood effect") on CBF, free-radical scavenging, stabilization of liposomal membranes, as well as excitatory amino acid receptor blockade. Based on evidence from experimental studies and a large randomized prospective multi-institutional study,[18] experts have concluded that barbiturates have no place in the therapy following resuscitation of a cardiac arrest patient. In contrast, barbiturates are frequently used for cerebroprotection during incomplete brain ischemia (e.g., carotid endarterectomy, temporary occlusion of cerebral arteries, profound hypotension, and cardiopulmonary bypass). By improving the brain's tolerance of incomplete ischemia in patients undergoing open heart surgery with cardiopulmonary bypass, barbiturates were alleged to decrease the incidence of postbypass neuropsychiatric disorders.[19] However, during valvular open heart cardiac surgery, a protective effect of barbiturate loading could not be demonstrated.[20] Given the lack a demonstrable neuroprotective effect, use of barbiturates during cardiac surgery is not recommended. Use of moderate degrees of hypothermia (33 to 34°C) might provide superior neuroprotection to the barbiturates without prolonging recovery.

Barbiturates cause predictable, dose-dependent EEG changes and possess potent anticonvulsant activity. Continuous infusions of thiopental have been used to treat refractory status epilepticus. However, low doses of thiopental may induce spike wave activity in epileptic patients. Methohexital has well-established epileptogenic effects in patients with psychomotor epilepsy. Low-dose methohexital infusions are frequently used to activate cortical EEG seizure discharges in patients with temporal lobe epilepsy. It is also the IV anesthetic of choice for electroconvulsive therapy.[21] Since the frequency of epileptiform EEG activity during induction of anesthesia with methohexital is significantly less than that which occurs during normal periods of sleep in epileptic patients, this suggests that higher doses of methohexital produces anticonvulsant activity. Methohexital also causes myoclonic-like muscle tremors and other signs of excitatory activity (e.g., hiccoughing).

Barbiturates cause dose-dependent respiratory depression.[22] However, bronchospasm or laryngospasm following induction with thiopental is usually the result of airway manipulation in "lightly" anesthetized patients. Laryngeal reflexes appear to be more active after induction with thiopental than with propofol. The cardiovascular effects of thiopental and methohexital include decreases in cardiac output, systemic arterial pressure, and peripheral vascular resistance. The depressant effects of thiopental on cardiac output are primarily a result of a decrease in venous return caused by peripheral pooling, as well as a result of a direct myocardial depressant effect, which assumes increasing importance in the presence of hypovolemia and myocardial disease.[23] Use of appropriate doses can minimize the cardiodepressant effects of thiopental, even in infants. Bhutada et al.[24] demonstrated that thiopental could be used for induction in infants without important changes in heart rate and blood pressure during the intubation period. An equipotent dose of methohexital produces even less hypotension than thiopental because of a greater tachycardic response to the blood pressure-lowering effects of the drug. If the blood pressure remains stable, the myocardial oxygen demand/supply ratio remains normal despite the increase in heart rate because of a concurrent decrease in coronary vascular resistance.

Propofol

Propofol (2,6-disopropylphenol), an alkylphenol compound, is virtually insoluble in aqueous solution. The initial Cremophor EL formulation of propofol was withdrawn from clinical testing because of the high incidence of anaphylactic reactions. Subsequently, propofol (10 mg/mL) was reintroduced as an egg lecithin emulsion formulation (Diprivan), consisting of 10% soybean oil, 2.25% glycerol, and 1.2% egg phosphatide. Pain on injection occurs in 32 to 67% of patients when injected into small hand veins but can be minimized by injection into larger veins and by prior administration of either lidocaine or a potent opioid analgesic (e.g., fentanyl or remifentanil). A wide variety of drugs have been alleged to reduce pain on injection of propofol (e.g., metoprolol,[25] granisetron,[26] dolasetron,[27] and even thiopental[28]). Diluting the formulation with additional solvent (Intralipid) or changing the lipid carrier (Lipofundin) also reduced propofol-induced injection pain, probably because of a decrease in the concentration of free propofol in the aqueous phase of the emulsion. A new propofol formulation with sodium metabisulphite (instead of disodium edentate) as an antimicrobial has been shown to be associated with less severe pain on injection.[29] Although the presence of the metabisulphite has raised concerns regarding its use in sulphite-allergic patients, this does not appear to be a clinically important problem. Of interest, a 2% formulation is available for long-term sedation to decrease the fluid volume infused as well as the lipid load.

More recently, a lower-lipid formulation of propofol (Ampofol) has been introduced into clinical practice for both general anesthesia[30] and sedation.[31] The increased "free" fraction of propofol leads to increased pain when it is injected into small veins. Therefore, it is important to add lidocaine to the Ampofol formulation to minimize the pain on injection. A new water-soluble prodrug of propofol (Aquavan) is in clinical development. This prodrug is rapidly hydrolyzed by plasma alkaline phosphatases in the circulation to release free propofol.[32] It has a slower onset than propofol but a similar recovery profile.[33] Although Aquavan does not produce injection site discomfort, a transient burning sensation has been reported in the perineal region following IV injection.

Propofol's pharmacokinetics has been studied using single-bolus dosing and continuous infusions.[34] In studies using a two-compartment kinetic model, the initial distribution half-life is 2 to 4 minutes and the elimination half-life is 1 to 3 hours. Using a three-compartment model, the initial and slow distribution half-life values are 1 to 8 minutes and 30 to 70 minutes, respectively. The elimination half-life depends largely on the sampling time after discontinuing the administration of propofol and ranges from 2 to 24 hours. This long elimination half-life is indicative of the existence of a poorly perfused compartment from which propofol slowly diffuses back into the central compartment. Propofol is rapidly cleared from the central compartment by hepatic metabolism and the context-sensitive half-life for propofol infusions up to 8 hours is <40 minutes. Propofol is rapidly and extensively metabolized to inactive, water-soluble sulphate and glucuronic acid metabolites, which are eliminated by the kidneys. Propofol's clearance rate (20–30 mL/kg/min) exceeds hepatic blood flow, suggesting that an extrahepatic route of elimination (lungs) also contributes to its clearance. Nevertheless, changes in liver blood flow would be expected to produce marked alterations in propofol's clearance rate. Surprisingly, few changes in propofol's pharmacokinetics have been reported in the presence of hepatic or renal disease.

The induction dose of propofol in healthy adults is 1.5 to 2.5 mg/kg, with blood levels of 2 to 6 μg/mL producing unconsciousness depending on the concomitant medications (e.g., opioid analgesics), the patient's age and physical status, and the extent of the surgical stimulation.[35] In one of the first reports describing the use of propofol for induction and maintenance of anesthesia with nitrous oxide, an average infusion rate of 120 μg/kg/min was required.[36] The recommended maintenance infusion rate of propofol varies between 100 and 200 μg/kg/min for hypnosis and 25 to 75 μg/kg/min for sedation. Awakening typically occurs at plasma propofol concentrations of 1 to 1.5 μg/mL.[37] Because a 50% decrease in the plasma propofol concentration is usually required for awakening, emergence following anesthesia is usually rapid even following prolonged infusions.

Analogous to the barbiturates, children require higher induction and maintenance doses of propofol on a milligram per kilogram basis as a result of their larger central distribution volume and higher clearance rate. Elderly patients and those in poor health require lower induction and maintenance doses of propofol as a result of their smaller central distribution volume and decreased clearance rate. Although subhypnotic doses of propofol produce sedation and amnesia,[37] awareness has been reported even at higher infusion rates when propofol is used as the sole anesthetic.[38] Propofol often produces a subjective feeling of well-being (and even euphoria) on emergence, and has been abused by health care professionals as a result of this CNS action.[39]

Propofol decreases $CMRO_2$ and CBF, as well as ICP.[40] However, when larger doses are administered, the marked depressant effect on systemic arterial pressure can significantly decrease CPP. Cerebrovascular autoregulation in response to changes in systemic arterial pressure and reactivity of the cerebral blood flow to changes in carbon dioxide tension are not affected by propofol. Evidence for a possible neuroprotective effect has been reported with in vitro preparations, and the use of propofol to produce EEG burst suppression has been proposed as a method for providing neuroprotection during aneurysm surgery. Its neuroprotective effect may at least partially be related to the antioxidant potential of propofol's phenol ring structure, which may act as a free-radical scavenger, decreasing free-radical–induced lipid peroxidation. A recent study reported that this antioxidant activity may offer many advantages in preventing the hypoperfusion-reperfusion phenomenon that can occur during major laparoscopic surgery.[41] Although TIVA with propofol and an opioid analgesic is a safe and effective alternative to standard inhalation techniques (i.e., volatile anesthetic with nitrous oxide) for maintenance of anesthesia, concerns have been raised regarding the cost-effectiveness of this technique.[42]

Propofol produces cortical EEG changes that are similar to those of thiopental. However, sedative doses of propofol increase β-wave activity analogous to the benzodiazepines. Induction of anesthesia with propofol is occasionally accompanied by excitatory motor activity (so-called nonepileptic myoclonia). In a study involving patients without a history of seizure disorders, excitatory movements following propofol were not associated with EEG seizure activity.[43] Propofol appears to possess profound anticonvulsant properties.[44] Propofol has been reported to decrease spike activity in patients with cortical electrodes implanted for resection of epileptogenic foci and has been used successfully to terminate status epilepticus. The duration of motor and EEG seizure activity following electroconvulsive therapy is significantly shorter with propofol than with other IV anesthetics. Propofol produces a decrease in the early components of somatosensory and motor-evoked potentials but does not influence the early components of the auditory-evoked potentials.

Propofol produces dose-dependent respiratory depression, with apnea occurring in 25 to 35% of patients after a typical induction dose. A maintenance infusion of propofol decreases tidal volume and increases respiratory rate. The ventilatory response to carbon dioxide and hypoxia is also significantly decreased by propofol. Propofol can produce bronchodilation in patients with chronic obstructive pulmonary disease and does not inhibit hypoxic pulmonary vasoconstriction.

Propofol's cardiovascular depressant effects are generally considered to be more profound than those of thiopental. Both direct myocardial depressant effects and decreased systemic vascular resistance have been implemented as important factors in producing cardiovascular depression. Direct myocardial depression and peripheral vasodilation are dose- and concentration-dependent. In addition to arterial vasodilation, propofol produces venodilation (caused both to a reduction in sympathetic activity and by a direct effect on the vascular smooth muscle), which further contributes to its hypotensive effect. The relaxation of the vascular smooth muscle may be because of an effect on intracellular calcium mobilization or because of an increase in the production of nitric oxide. Experiments in isolated myocardium suggest that the negative inotropic effect of propofol results from a decrease in intracellular calcium availability secondary to inhibition of transsarcolemmal calcium influx.

Propofol also alters the baroreflex mechanism, resulting in a smaller increase in heart rate for a given decrease in arterial pressure.[45] The smaller increase in heart rate with propofol may account for the larger decrease in arterial pressure than with an equipotent dose of thiopental. Recent studies suggest that induction of anesthesia with propofol attenuates desflurane-mediated sympathetic activation.[46] Age enhances the cardiodepressant response to propofol and a reduced dosage is required in the elderly. Patients with limited cardiac reserve seem to tolerate the cardiac depression and systemic vasodilation produced by carefully titrated doses of propofol, and maintenance infusions are increasingly used at the end of cardiac surgery when early extubation is desired.

Propofol appears to possess antiemetic properties that contribute to a lower incidence of emetic sequelae after general anesthesia.[36] In fact, subanesthetic doses of propofol (10 to

20 mg) have also been successfully used to treat nausea and emesis in the early postoperative period.[47] The postulated mechanisms include antidopaminergic activity, depressant effect on the chemoreceptor trigger zone and vagal nuclei, decreased release of glutamate and aspartate in the olfactory cortex, and reduction of serotonin concentrations in the area postrema. However, the ability of propofol to produce a sense of well-being may also contribute to its antiemetic action. Interestingly, propofol also decreases the pruritus produced by spinal opioids.

Propofol does not trigger malignant hyperthermia and may be considered the induction agent of choice in malignant hyperthermia-susceptible patients. The use of propofol infusions for sedation in the pediatric ICU has been linked to several deaths following prolonged administration because of lipid accumulation and hypotension. Although clinical doses of propofol do not affect cortisol synthesis or the response to adrenocorticotropic hormone stimulation, propofol has been reported to inhibit phagocytosis and killing of bacteria in vitro and to reduce proliferative responses when added to lymphocytes from critically ill patients.[48] Because fat emulsions are known to support the growth of micro-organisms, contamination can occur as a result of dilution or fractionated use.[49]

In critically-ill children and adults receiving high-dose infusions of propofol, some patients have been reported to experience "propofol syndrome," which is characterized by myocardial failure, metabolic acidosis, and rhabdomyolysis. The etiology of this syndrome may be related to the large lipid load associated with prolonged infusions of the current formulations of propofol.

Benzodiazepines

The parenteral benzodiazepines include diazepam (Valium), lorazepam (Ativan), and midazolam (Versed), as well as the antagonist flumazenil (Romazicon). Diazepam and lorazepam are insoluble in water and their formulation contains propylene glycol, a tissue irritant that causes pain on injection and venous irritation. Diazepam is available in a lipid emulsion formulation, which does not cause pain or thrombophlebitis but is associated with a slightly lower bioavailability. Midazolam is a water-soluble benzodiazepine that is available in an acidified (pH 3.5) aqueous formulation that produces minimal local irritation after IV or intramuscular (IM) injection.[50] At physiologic pH, an intramolecular rearrangement occurs that changes the physicochemical properties of midazolam such that it becomes more lipid soluble.

Benzodiazepines undergo hepatic metabolism via oxidation and glucuronide conjugation. Oxidation reactions are susceptible to hepatic dysfunction and coadministration of other anesthetic drugs. Diazepam is metabolized to active metabolites (desmethyldiazepam, 3-hydroxydiazepam), which can prolong diazepam's residual sedative effects because of their long $t_{1/2}\beta$ values. These metabolites undergo secondary conjugation to form inactive water-soluble glucuronide conjugates. Drugs that inhibit the oxidative metabolism of diazepam include the H_2-receptor blocking drug cimetidine. Severe liver disease reduces diazepam's protein-binding and hepatic-clearance rate, increases its volume of distribution, and thereby further prolongs the $t_{1/2}\beta$ value. Chronic renal disease decreases protein binding and increases the free drug fraction, resulting in enhanced hepatic metabolism and a shorter $t_{1/2}\beta$ value. In elderly patients, the clearance rate of diazepam is significantly decreased, prolonging its $t_{1/2}\beta$ to 75 to 150 hours.

Lorazepam is directly conjugated to glucuronic acid to form pharmacologically inactive metabolites. Age and renal disease have little influence on the kinetics of lorazepam; however, severe hepatic disease decreases its clearance rate. Midazolam undergoes extensive oxidation by hepatic enzymes to form water-soluble hydroxylated metabolites, which are excreted in the urine. However, the primary metabolite, 1-hydroxymethylmidazolam, has mild CNS-depressant activity. The hepatic clearance rate of midazolam is 5 times greater than lorazepam and 10 times greater than diazepam. Although changes in liver blood flow can affect the clearance of midazolam, age has relatively little influence on midazolam's elimination half-life.

The benzodiazepines used in anesthesia are classified as either short- (midazolam, flumazenil), intermediate- (diazepam), or long-acting (lorazepam). Because the distribution volumes are similar, the large difference in the elimination half-times is because of differences in their differing clearance rates (Table 18-1). The context-sensitive half-times for diazepam and lorazepam are very long; therefore, only midazolam should be used by continuous infusion to avoid excessive accumulation.

All benzodiazepines produce dose-dependent anxiolytic, anterograde amnestic, sedative, hypnotic, anticonvulsant, and spinally mediated muscle relaxant properties. Benzodiazepines differ in potency and efficacy with regard to their distinctive pharmacologic properties.[50] The dose-dependent pharmacologic activity implies that the CNS effects of various benzodiazepine compounds depend on the affinity for receptor subtypes and their degree of receptor binding. Although benzodiazepines can be used as hypnotics, they are primarily used as premedicants and adjuvant drugs because of their anxiolytic, sedative, and amnestic properties. For example, midazolam (0.04 to 0.08 mg/kg IV/IM) is the most commonly used premedicant. In addition, midazolam, 0.4 to 0.8 mg/kg administered orally 10 to 15 minutes before parental separation, is an excellent premedicant in children. In contrast to lorazepam, both diazepam and midazolam can be used to induce anesthesia because they have a relatively short onset time after IV administration. The half-life of equilibration between the plasma concentration of midazolam and its maximal EEG effect is only 2 to 3 minutes. The therapeutic window to maintain unconsciousness with midazolam is reported to be 100 to 200 ng/mL, with awakening occurring at plasma concentrations below 50 ng/mL. However, significant hypnotic synergism occurs when midazolam and opioid analgesics are administered in combination.

The usual induction dose of midazolam in premedicated patients is 0.1 to 0.2 mg/kg IV, with infusion rates of 0.25–1.0 µg/kg/min required to maintain hypnosis and amnesia in combination with inhalational agents and/or opioid analgesics. Higher maintenance infusion rates and prolonged administration will result in accumulation and prolonged recovery times. Lower infusion rates are sufficient to provide sedation and amnesia during local and regional anesthesia.[51] Patient-controlled administration of midazolam during procedures under local anesthesia is well accepted by patients and associated with few perioperative complications.[52]

Benzodiazepines decrease both $CMRO_2$ and CBF analogous to the barbiturates and propofol. However, in contrast to these compounds, midazolam is unable to produce a burst-suppressive (isoelectric) pattern on the EEG. Accordingly, there is a "ceiling" effect with respect to the decrease in $CMRO_2$ produced by increasing doses of midazolam. Midazolam produces a dose-related decrease in regional cerebral perfusion in the parts of the brain that subserve arousal, attention, and memory. Cerebral vasomotor responsiveness to carbon dioxide is preserved during midazolam anesthesia. In patients with severe head injury, a bolus dose of midazolam may decrease CPP with little effect on ICP. Although midazolam may improve neurologic outcome after incomplete ischemia in animal experiments, benzodiazepines have not been shown to possess neuroprotective activity in humans. Like the other sedative-hypnotic drugs, the benzodiazepines are potent anticonvulsants that are commonly used to treat status epilepticus.

Benzodiazepines produce dose-dependent respiratory depression. In healthy patients, the respiratory depression associated with benzodiazepine premedication is insignificant. However, the depressant effect is enhanced in patients with chronic respiratory disease, and synergistic depressant effects occur when benzodiazepines are coadministered with opioid analgesics. Benzodiazepines also depress the swallowing reflex and decrease upper airway reflex activity.

Both midazolam and diazepam produce decreases in systemic vascular resistance and blood pressure when large doses are administered for induction of anesthesia. However, the cardiovascular depressant effects of benzodiazepines are frequently "masked" by the stimulus of laryngoscopy and intubation. The cardiovascular depressant effects are directly related to the plasma concentration; however, a plateau plasma concentration appears to exist above which little further change in arterial blood pressure occurs. In the presence of heart failure, the decrease in preload and afterload produced by benzodiazepines may be beneficial in improving cardiac output. However, the cardiodepressant effect of benzodiazepines may be more marked in hypovolemic patients.

A short-acting intravenous sedative, Ro 48-6791, is a water-soluble benzodiazepine that has full agonistic activity at CNS benzodiazepine receptors. Compared with midazolam, it is 2- to 2.5-fold more potent, has a higher plasma clearance rate, and has a similar onset and duration of action.[53] In a study involving outpatients undergoing endoscopy procedures, the times to ambulation and to recovery from psychomotor impairment were decreased compared to midazolam, although the later recovery end points (e.g., "fitness-for-discharge") were similar.[54]

In contrast to all other sedative-hypnotic drugs, there is a specific antagonist for benzodiazepines. Flumazenil, a 1,4-imidazobenzodiazepine derivative, has a high affinity for the benzodiazepine receptor but minimal intrinsic activity.[55] Flumazenil's molecular structure is similar to other benzodiazepines except for the absence of a phenyl group, which is replaced by a carbonyl group. It is water soluble and possesses moderate lipid solubility at physiologic pH. Flumazenil is rapidly metabolized in the liver, and its metabolites are excreted in the urine as glucuronide conjugates. Flumazenil acts as a competitive antagonist in the presence of benzodiazepine agonist compounds. The residual activity of the benzodiazepines in the presence of flumazenil depends on the relative concentrations of the agonist and antagonist drugs. As a result, it is possible to reverse benzodiazepine-induced anesthesia (or deep sedation) either completely or partially, depending on the dose of flumazenil. Flumazenil is short acting, with an elimination half-life of ~1 hour.

Recurrence of the central effects of benzodiazepines (resedation) may occur after a single dose of flumazenil because of residual effects of the more slowly eliminated agonist drug.[56] If sustained antagonism is desired, it may be necessary to administer flumazenil as repeated bolus doses or a continuous infusion. In general, 45 to 90 minutes of antagonism can be expected following flumazenil 1 to 3 mg IV. However, the respiratory depression produced by benzodiazepines is not completely reversed by flumazenil.[57] Reversal of benzodiazepine sedation with flumazenil is not associated with adverse cardiovascular effects or evidence of an acute stress response.[58] Although flumazenil does not appear to change CBF or $CMRO_2$ following midazolam anesthesia for craniotomy, acute increases in ICP have been reported in head-injured patients receiving flumazenil.

Etomidate

Etomidate is a carboxylated imidazole-containing anesthetic compound (R-1-ethyl-1-[a-methylbenzyl] imidazole-5-carboxylate) that is structurally unrelated to any other IV anesthetic. Only the d-isomer of etomidate possesses anesthetic activity. Analogous to midazolam (which also contains an imidazole nucleus), etomidate undergoes an intramolecular rearrangement at physiologic pH, resulting in a closed-ring structure with enhanced lipid solubility. The aqueous solution of etomidate (Amidate) is unstable at physiologic pH and is formulated in a 0.2% solution with 35% propylene glycol (pH 6.9), contributing to a high incidence of pain on injection, venoirritation, and hemolysis. A new lipid emulsion formulation (Etomidate-Lipuro) has recently been introduced in Europe and appears to be associated with a lower incidence of side effects compared with the original propylene glycol formulation.

The standard induction dose of etomidate (0.2–0.3 mg/kg IV) produces a rapid onset of anesthesia. Involuntary myoclonic movements are common during the induction period as a result of subcortical disinhibition and are unrelated to cortical seizure activity. The frequency of this myocloniclike activity can be attenuated by prior administration of opioid analgesics, benzodiazepines, or small sedative doses (0.03 to 0.05 mg/kg) prior to induction of anesthesia.[59] Recently, remifentanil reduced etomidate-induced myoclonic activity without increasing side effects like apnea, emesis, or pruritus.[60] Emergence time after etomidate anesthesia is dose-dependent but remains short even after administration of repeated bolus doses or continuous infusions. For maintenance of hypnosis, the target concentration is 300 to 500 ng/mL and can be rapidly achieved by administering a two- or three-stage infusion (e.g., 100 mg/kg/min for 10 minutes followed by 10 mg/kg/min or 100 mg/kg/min for 3 to 5 minutes, followed by 20 mg/kg/min for 20 to 30 minutes, and then 10 mg/kg/min). The pharmacokinetics of etomidate are optimally described by a three-compartment open model.[61] The high clearance rate of etomidate (18 to 25 mL/kg/min) is a result of extensive ester hydrolysis in the liver (forming inactive water-soluble metabolites). A significant decrease in plasma protein binding has been reported in the presence of uremia and hepatic cirrhosis. Severe hepatic disease causes a prolongation of the elimination half-life secondary to an increased volume of distribution and a decreased plasma clearance rate.

Analogous to the barbiturates, etomidate decreases $CMRO_2$, CBF, and ICP. However, the hemodynamic stability associated with etomidate will maintain adequate CPP. Etomidate has been used successfully for both induction and maintenance of anesthesia for neurosurgery. Etomidate's well-known inhibitory effect on adrenocortical synthetic function[62] limits its clinical usefulness for long-term treatment of elevated ICP. Although clear evidence for a neuroprotective effect in humans is lacking, etomidate is frequently used during temporary arterial occlusion and intraoperative angiography (for the treatment of cerebral aneurysms). Etomidate produces an EEG pattern that is similar to thiopental except for the absence of increased β activity at lower doses. Etomidate has been alleged to produce convulsionlike EEG potentials in epileptic patients without the appearance of myoclonic or convulsant-like motor activity, a property that has been proven useful for intraoperative mapping of seizure foci. Analogous to methohexital, etomidate possesses anticonvulsant properties and has been used to terminate status epilepticus. Etomidate also produces a significant increase of the amplitude of somatosensory-evoked potentials while only minimally increasing their latency. Consequently, etomidate can be used to facilitate the interpretation of somatosensory-evoked potentials when the signal quality is poor.

(7) Etomidate causes minimal cardiorespiratory depression even in the presence of cardiovascular and pulmonary disease.[63] The drug does not induce histamine release and can be safely used in patients with reactive airway disease. Consequently, etomidate is considered to be the induction agent of choice for poor-risk patients with cardiorespiratory disease, as well as in those situations in which preservation of a normal blood pressure is crucial (e.g., cerebrovascular disease). However, etomidate does not effectively blunt the sympathetic response to laryngoscopy and intubation unless combined with a potent opioid analgesic.

Etomidate is associated with a high incidence of postoperative nausea and emesis when used in combination with opioids for brief outpatient procedures. In addition, the increased mortality in critically ill patients sedated with an etomidate infusion has been attributed to its inhibitory effect on cortisol synthesis.[64] Etomidate inhibits the activity of 11-β-hydroxylase, an enzyme necessary for the synthesis of cortisol, aldosterone, 17-hydroxyprogesterone, and corticosterone. Even after a single induction dose of etomidate,[64] adrenal suppression persists for 5 to 8 hours. Although the clinical significance of short-term blockade of cortisol synthesis is not known, the use of etomidate for maintenance of anesthesia has been questioned. Recently, etomidate has been reported to inhibit platelet function, resulting in prolongation of the bleeding time.[65] In spite of its side effect profile, etomidate remains a valuable induction drug for specific indications (e.g., in patients with severe cardiovascular and cerebrovascular disease).

Ketamine

Ketamine (Ketalar or Ketaject) is an arylcyclohexylamine that is structurally related to phencyclidine.[66] Ketamine is a water-soluble compound with a pKa of 7.5 and is available in 1%, 5%, and 10% aqueous solutions. The ketamine molecule contains a chiral center producing two optical isomers. The S(+) isomer of ketamine possesses more potent anesthetic and analgesic properties despite having a similar pharmacokinetic and pharmacodynamic profile as the racemic mixture (or the R[−] isomer).[67,68] Although the S(+)-ketamine is approved for clinical use in Europe, the commonly used solution is a racemic mixture of the two isomers. Ketamine is extensively metabolized by hepatic microsomal cytochrome P450 enzymes and its primary metabolite, norketamine, is one third to one fifth as potent as the parent compound. The metabolites of norketamine are excreted by the kidney as water-soluble hydroxylated and glucuronidated conjugates. Analogous to the barbiturates and propofol, ketamine has relatively short distribution and redistribution half-life values. Ketamine also has a high hepatic clearance rate (1 L/min) and a large distribution volume (3 L/kg), resulting in an elimination half-life of 2–4 hours. The high hepatic extraction ratio suggests that alterations in hepatic blood flow can significantly influence ketamine's clearance rate.

(8) Ketamine produces dose-dependent CNS depression leading to a so-called dissociative anesthetic state characterized by profound analgesia and amnesia, even though patients may be conscious and maintain protective reflexes. The proposed mechanism for this cataleptic state includes electrophysiologic inhibition of thalamocortical pathways and stimulation of the limbic system. Although it is most commonly administered parenterally, oral and intranasal administration of ketamine (6 mg/kg) has been used for premedication of pediatric patients. Following benzodiazepine premedication, ketamine 1 to 2 mg/kg IV (or 4 to 8 mg/kg IM) can be used for induction of anesthesia. The duration of ketamine-induced anesthesia is in the range of 10 to 20 minutes after a single induction dose; however, recovery to full orientation may require an additional 60 to 90 minutes. Emergence times are even longer following repeated bolus injections or a continuous infusion. S(+)-ketamine has a shorter recovery time compared with the racemic mixture. The therapeutic window for maintenance of unconsciousness with ketamine is between 0.6 and 2 μg/mL in adults and between 0.8 and 4 μg/mL in children. Analgesic effects are evident at subanesthetic doses of 0.1 to 0.5 mg/kg IV and plasma concentrations of between 85 and 160 ng/mL. A low-dose infusion of 4 μg/kg/min IV was reported to result in equivalent postoperative analgesia as an IV morphine infusion at 2 mg/hr.

As a result of its NMDA-receptor blocking activity, ketamine should be highly effective for "pre-emptive" analgesia and opioid-resistant chronic pain states.[69] Unfortunately, a well-controlled study failed to demonstrate a pre-emptive effect when ketamine was administered prior to the surgical incision (vs. intraoperatively).[70] Nevertheless, other studies[71,72] described a beneficial opioid-sparing effect of small doses of ketamine (75 to 150 μg/kg IV) when administered as an adjuvant during surgery.

An important consideration in the use of ketamine anesthesia relates to the high incidence of psychomimetic reactions (namely, hallucinations, nightmares, altered short-term memory, and cognition) during the early recovery period. The incidence of these reactions is dose-dependent and can be reduced by coadministration of benzodiazepines, barbiturates, or propofol. Ketamine has been traditionally contraindicated for patients with increased ICP or reduced cerebral compliance because it increases $CMRO_2$, CBF, and ICP. However, there is recent evidence that IV induction doses of ketamine actually decrease ICP in traumatic–brain-injury patients during controlled ventilation with propofol sedation.[73] Prior administration of thiopental or benzodiazepines can blunt ketamine-induced increases in CBF. Because ketamine has antagonistic activity at the NMDA receptor, it may possess some inherent protective effects against brain ischemia. However, ketamine can adversely affect neurologic outcome in the presence of brain ischemia despite its NMDA-receptor blocking activity. Cortical EEG recordings following ketamine induction are characterized by the appearance of fast β activity (30 to 40 Hz) followed by moderate-voltage θ activity, mixed with high-voltage δ waves recurring at 3- to 4-second intervals. At higher dosages, ketamine produces a unique EEG burst-suppression pattern (Fig. 18-5).

Although ketamine-induced myoclonic and seizurelike activity has been observed in normal (nonepileptic) patients, ketamine appears to possess anticonvulsant activity.[11,12] Two studies have demonstrated the opioid-sparing effects of low-

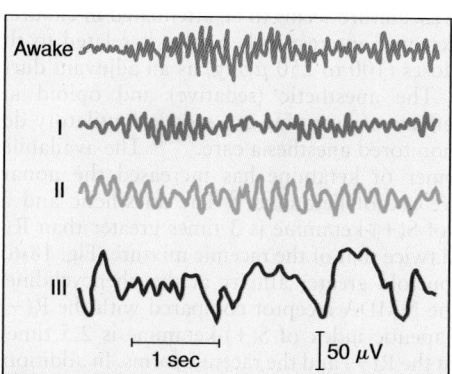

FIGURE 18-5. Progressive changes in the electroencephalogram (EEG) produced by ketamine. Stages I through III are achieved with racemic ketamine and its S(+)isomer. With R(−)ketamine, Stage II was the maximal EEG depression produced. (Reprinted with permission from Shüttler J, Stanski DR, White PF, et al: Pharmacodynamic modeling of the EEG effect of ketamine and its enantiomers in man. J Pharmacokinet Biopharm 1987; 15: 241.)

dose ketamine (75 to 200 μg/kg) when administered as an adjuvant during anesthesia.[71,72] Interestingly, small doses of ketamine have also been used in the treatment of severe depression in patients with chronic pain syndromes.[74,75] However, ketamine can produce adverse effects when administered in the presence of tricyclic antidepressants because both drugs inhibit norepinephrine reuptake and could produce severe hypotension, heart failure, and/or myocardial ischemia.[75,76]

Ketamine has well-characterized bronchodilatory activity. In the presence of active bronchospasm, ketamine is considered to be the IV induction agent of choice. Ketamine has been used in subanesthetic dosages to treat persistent bronchospasm in the OR and ICU. It is also used in combination with midazolam to provide sedation and analgesia for asthmatic patients. In contrast to the other IV anesthetics, protective airway reflexes are more likely to be preserved with ketamine. However, it must be emphasized that the use of ketamine does not obviate the need for tracheal intubation in the patient with a full stomach (because tracheal soiling has been reported in this situation). Ketamine causes minimal respiratory depression in clinically relevant doses and can facilitate the transition from mechanical to spontaneous ventilation after anesthesia. However, its ability to increase oral secretions can lead to laryngospasm during "light" anesthesia.

Ketamine has prominent cardiovascular-stimulating effects secondary to direct stimulation of the sympathetic nervous system. Ketamine is the only anesthetic that actually increases peripheral arteriolar resistance. As a result of its vasoconstrictive properties, ketamine can reduce the magnitude of redistribution hypothermia.[77] Induction of anesthesia with ketamine often produces significant increases in arterial blood pressure and heart rate. Although the mechanism of the cardiovascular stimulation is not entirely clear, it appears to be centrally mediated. There is evidence to suggest that ketamine attenuates baroreceptor activity via an effect on NMDA receptors in the nucleus tractus solitarius. Because of the increased cardiac work and myocardial oxygen consumption, ketamine negatively affects the balance between myocardial oxygen supply and demand. Consequently, its use is not recommended in patients with severe coronary artery disease. In contrast to the secondary cardiovascular stimulation, ketamine has intrinsic myocardial depressant properties that only become apparent in the seriously ill patient with depleted catecholamine reserves. Because ketamine can also increase pulmonary artery pressure, its use is contraindicated in adult patients with poor right ventricular reserve. Interestingly, the effect on the pulmonary vasculature seems to be attenuated in children.

The renewed interest in ketamine is related to the use of smaller doses (100 to 250 μg/kg) as an adjuvant during anesthesia.[78] The anesthetic (sedative) and opioid analgesic-sparing effects of ketamine can reduce ventilatory depression during monitored anesthesia care.[79–81] The availability of the stereoisomer of ketamine has increased the nonanesthetic adjunctive use of ketamine.[82] The anesthetic and analgesic potency of S(+)-ketamine is 3 times greater than R(−)-ketamine and twice that of the racemic mixture (Fig. 18-6), reflecting its fourfold greater affinity at the phencyclidine binding site on the NMDA receptor compared with the R(−) isomer. The therapeutic index of S(+)-ketamine is 2.5 times greater than both the R(−) and the racemic forms. In addition, hepatic biotransformation of S(+)-ketamine occurs 20% faster than that of the R(−) enantiomer, contributing to shorter emergence times and faster return of cognitive function. Both isomers produce similar cardiovascular-stimulating effects and hormonal responses during surgery. Although the incidence of dreaming is similar with S(+)-ketamine and the racemic mixture, subjective mood and patient acceptance are higher with the S(+) isomer.[67,68]

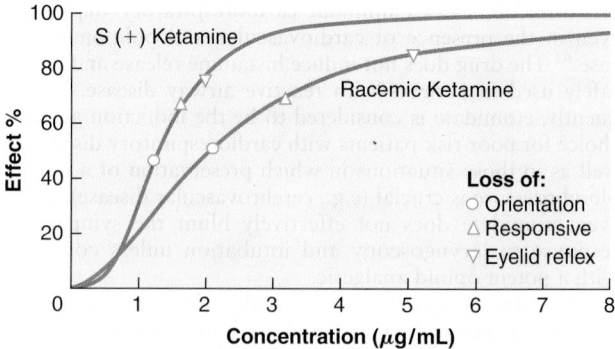

FIGURE 18-6.   Concentration-response relationship for racemic ketamine and S(+)ketamine in relation to specific clinical end points. The slowing of the median electroencephalogram frequency was used as the effect (end point) and was related to the arterial blood concentrations of ketamine. (Reprinted with permission from Schüttler J, Kloos S, Ihmsen H, et al: Pharmacokinetic-pharmacodynamic properties of S(+) ketamine versus racemic ketamine: A randomized double-blind study in volunteers. Anesthesiology 1992; 77: A330.)

Dexmedetomidine

Dexmedetomidine is a highly selective α_2-adrenoceptor agonist that has been approved by the Food and Drug Administration for the short-term (<24 hours) sedation of mechanically ventilated patients in the ICU setting. In this setting it appears to offer some clinical advantages because it produces a unique type of sedation-analgesia with less ventilatory depression than the commonly used sedative-hypnotic and opioid analgesic drugs.[14] Although dexmedetomidine is being used for sedating patients undergoing diagnostic and therapeutic procedures outside the operating and ICU environments, these represent "off label" uses of this drug.

When used for premedication prior to general anesthesia, dexmedetomidine produced preoperative sedation and anxiolysis comparable to midazolam.[15] However, its use led to an increased incidence of intraoperative hypotension and bradycardia compared with the commonly used benzodiazepine compound. When used for premedication prior to regional anesthesia, dexmedetomidine reduced patient anxiety, sympathoadrenal (stress) responses, and perioperative opioid analgesic requirements.[83] Hall et al.[84] also demonstrated the sedative, amnestic, and analgesic effects of low-dose infusions of dexmedetomidine (0.2 to 0.6 μg/kg/hr).

As an IV adjuvant during induction and/or maintenance of general anesthesia, dexmedetomidine will blunt the acute hemodynamic response to laryngoscopy and intubation.[85] It has also been used to facilitate awake fiberoptic intubation.[86,87] When used as an anesthetic adjuvant during general anesthesia, dexmedetomidine has been reported to improve perioperative hemodynamic stability in neurosurgical patients,[88] and improve postoperative pain control after major surgery.[89,90] However, a recent study[91] failed to demonstrate any clinically significant improvements in patient outcomes after bariatric surgery despite producing both anesthetic and analgesic-sparing effects.

In summary, dexmedetomidine appears to be a potentially useful adjuvant during local and regional anesthesia. It provides comparable sedation to midazolam[92] but has a slower onset and offset of sedation than propofol.[93] When administered as an adjuvant during IV regional anesthesia[94] it improved the quality of both intra- and postoperative analgesia. Because of its high cost, dexmedetomidine's cost-benefit ratio as an IV adjuvant during general anesthesia clearly requires further investigation.

CLINICAL USES OF INTRAVENOUS ANESTHETICS

Induction Agents

The induction characteristics and recommended dosages of the available IV anesthetic agents are summarized in Table 18-2. As a result of differences in pharmacokinetic (e.g., altered clearance and distribution volumes) and pharmacodynamic (altered brain sensitivity) variables, the induction dosages of all IV anesthetics need to be adjusted to meet the needs of individual patients. For example, advanced age, preexisting diseases (e.g., hypothyroidism, hypovolemia), premedication (e.g., benzodiazepines), and coadministration of adjuvant drugs (e.g., opioids, α_2-agonists) decrease the induction dose requirements. When there is concern regarding a possible abnormal response, assessing the effect of a small "test dose" (equal to 10 to 20% of the usual induction dose) will often identify those patients for whom a dosage adjustment is required. Before administering additional medication, adequate time should be allowed for the anesthetic to exert its effect, especially when using drugs with a slow onset of action (midazolam) or in the presence of a "slow" circulation time in elderly patients and those with congestive heart failure.

The clinical uses of propofol have expanded greatly since its introduction into clinical practice in 1989.[95] IV administration of propofol results in a rapid loss of consciousness (usually within one arm-to-brain circulation) that is comparable to that of the barbiturates. Although an induction dose of 2.5 mg/kg was initially recommended, the use of smaller induction doses of propofol (1 to 2 mg/kg) has minimized its acute cardiovascular and respiratory depressant effects. Recovery from propofol's sedative-hypnotic effects is rapid with less residual sedation, fatigue ("hangover"), and cognitive impairment than with other available sedative-hypnotic drugs after short surgical procedures. Consequently, propofol has become the IV drug of choice for outpatients undergoing ambulatory surgery.

With benzodiazepines, there is wide variation in the dose-response relationships in unpremedicated elective surgery patients. Compared with midazolam, diazepam and lorazepam have slower onset times to achieve a peak effect and their dose-effect relationship is less predictable. As a result, diazepam and lorazepam are rarely used for induction of general anesthesia. In addition, the slow hepatic clearance of diazepam and lorazepam may contribute to prolonged residual effects (e.g., sedation, amnesia, fatigue) when they are used for premedication. Midazolam has a slightly more rapid onset and may be a useful induction agent for special indications (e.g., when nitrous oxide is contraindicated, or as part of a total IV anesthetic technique). However, when midazolam is used for induction and/or maintenance of anesthesia, return of consciousness takes substantially longer than with other sedative-hypnotic drugs. In spite of its extensive hepatic metabolism, recovery of cognitive function is still slower after midazolam compared with thiopental, methohexital, etomidate, or propofol.

In an effort to optimize the clinical use of midazolam during the induction period, it is used increasingly as a coinduction agent with other sedative-hypnotic drugs (propofol, ketamine). Midazolam 2 to 5 mg IV can provide for increased sedation, amnesia, and anxiolysis during the preinduction period. When midazolam is used in combination with propofol, 1.5 to 2 mg/kg IV,[112] or ketamine, 0.75 to 1 mg/kg IV,[96] it facilitates the onset of anesthesia and decreases the possibility of intraoperative recall without delaying emergence times. Midazolam also attenuates the cardiostimulatory response to ketamine, as well as its psychomimetic emergence reactions. Use of midazolam, 2 to 3 mg IV, with propofol reduces recall during the induction period; however, larger doses of midazolam (5 mg IV) will delay emergence after brief surgical procedures.

As a result of their side effect profiles, the clinical use of etomidate and ketamine for induction of anesthesia is restricted to specific situations in which their unique pharmacologic profiles offer advantages over other available IV anesthetics. For example, etomidate can facilitate maintenance of a stable blood pressure in high-risk patients with critical stenosis of the cerebral vasculature and in patients with severe cardiac impairment or unstable angina. Ketamine is a useful induction agent for patients with reactive airway disease, as well as for those situations where continued spontaneous ventilation is desirable during surgery.

ANESTHETIC AGENTS, ADJUVANTS, AND DRUG INTERACTION

TABLE 18-2

INDUCTION CHARACTERISTICS AND DOSAGE REQUIREMENTS FOR THE CURRENTLY AVAILABLE SEDATIVE-HYPNOTIC DRUGS

DRUG NAME	INDUCTION DOSE (mg/kg)	ONSET (sec)	DURATION (min)	EXCITATORY ACTIVITY	PAIN ON INJECTION	HEART RATE	BLOOD PRESSURE
Thiopental	3–6	<30	5–10	+	0–+	↑	↓
Methohexital	1–3	<30	5–10	++	+	↑↑	↓
Propofol	1.5–2.5	15–45	5–10	+	++	0–↓	↓↓
Midazolam	0.2–0.4	30–90	10–30	0	0	0	0/↓
Diazepam	0.3–0.6	45–90	15–30	0	+/+++	0	0/↓
Lorazepam	0.03–0.06	60–120	60–120	0	++	0	0/↓
Etomidate	0.2–0.3	15–45	3–12	+++	+++	0	0
Ketamine	1–2	45–60	10–20	+	0	↑↑	↑↑

0, none; +, minimal; ++, moderate; +++, severe; ↓, decrease; ↑, increase.
From White PF. Textbook of Intravenous Anesthesia. Baltimore, Williams & Wilkins, 1997, pp. 27–46 and 77–92.

Maintenance of Anesthesia

The continued popularity of volatile anesthetics for maintenance of anesthesia is primarily related to their rapid reversibility and ease of administration when using a conventional vaporizer delivery system. The availability of IV drugs with more rapid onset and shorter recovery profiles, as well as user-friendly infusion delivery systems, has facilitated the maintenance of anesthesia with continuous infusions of IV drugs, producing an anesthetic state (namely, TIVA) that compares favorably with the volatile anesthetics. In a comparison of the requirement of postoperative analgesics after inhalation and TIVA techniques, not surprisingly, the postoperative pain was reduced after TIVA.[97] For example, in morbidly obese patients undergoing bariatric surgery, the use of TIVA technique was associated with a superior recovery profile compared with a sevoflurane-based inhalation technique.[98] However, TIVA techniques are more expensive than inhalation or "balanced" anesthetic techniques.[42]

The traditional intermittent bolus administration of IV drugs results in depth of anesthesia (and analgesia) that oscillates above and below the desired level.[99] Because of rapid distribution and redistribution of the IV anesthetics, the high peak blood concentration after each bolus is followed by a rapid decrease, producing fluctuating drug levels in the blood and hence the brain. The magnitude of the drug level fluctuation depends on the size of the bolus dose and the frequency of its administration. Wide variation in the plasma drug concentrations can result in hemodynamic and respiratory instability as a result of changes in the depth of anesthesia or sedation. By providing more stable blood (and brain) concentrations with a continuous IV infusion, it might be possible to improve anesthetic conditions and hemodynamic stability, as well as decreasing side effects and recovery times with IV anesthetics.[100] Administration of IV anesthetics by a variable-rate infusion is a logical extension of the incremental bolus method of drug titration, as a continuous infusion is equivalent to the sequential administration of infinitely small bolus doses.

Although an IV anesthetic can be titrated to achieve and maintain the desired clinical effect, a knowledge of basic pharmacokinetic principles is helpful in more accurately predicting the optimal dosage requirements. The required plasma concentration depends on the desired pharmacologic effect (hypnosis, sedation), the concomitant use of other adjunctive drugs (opioid analgesics, muscle relaxants, cardiovascular drugs), the type of operation (superficial, intraabdominal, intracranial), and the patient's sensitivity to the drug (age, drug history, preexisting diseases). Preexisting diseases (cirrhosis, congestive heart failure, renal failure) can markedly alter the pharmacokinetic variables of the highly protein-bound, lipophilic IV anesthetic drugs. In general, children have higher clearance rates, while the elderly have reduced clearance values. Various intraoperative interventions (e.g., laryngoscopy, tracheal intubation, skin incision, entry into body cavities) transiently increase the anesthetic and/or analgesic requirements. Therefore, the infusion scheme should be tailored to provide peak drug concentrations during the periods of most intense stimulation. For specific surgical interventions, the so-called therapeutic window of an IV anesthetic is defined as the blood concentration range required to produce a given effect (Table 18-3). It must be emphasized that the therapeutic window for sedative-hypnotics is markedly influenced by the presence of adjunctive drugs (e.g., opioids, α_2-agonists, nitrous oxide).

The use of IV anesthetic techniques requires continuous titration of the drug infusion rate to the desired pharmacodynamic end-point.[96] Most anesthesiologists rely on somatic and autonomic signs for assessing depth of IV anesthesia, analogous to the manner in which they titrate the volatile anesthetics. The most sensitive clinical signs of depth of anesthesia appear to be changes in muscle tone (i.e., electromyography [EMG]) and ventilatory rate and pattern.[101] However, if the patient has been given muscle relaxants, the anesthesiologist must rely on signs of autonomic hyperactivity (e.g., tachycardia, hypertension, lacrimation, diaphoresis). Unfortunately, the anesthetic drugs (ketamine), as well as adjunctive agents (α_2-agonists, beta-blockers, adenosine, calcium channel blockers), can directly influence the cardiovascular response to surgical stimulation. Although the cardiovascular signs of autonomic nervous system hyperactivity may be masked, other autonomic signs (e.g., diaphoresis) and purposeful movements may be more reliable indicators of depth of anesthesia than blood pressure because the latter depends on the ability of the heart to maintain the cardiac output in the face of acute changes in afterload. The heart rate response to surgical stimulation appears to be more useful than the blood pressure response in determining the need for additional analgesic medication. Moreover, it would appear that blood pressure and heart rate responses to surgical stimulation are a less useful guide with IV techniques than with volatile anesthetics. Interestingly, supplementation with a sedative-hypnotic (propofol) was as effective as a potent opioid analgesic in controlling acute autonomic responses during TIVA.[102]

The clinical assessment of anesthetic depth has become more challenging because IV anesthetic techniques involve a combination of hypnotics, opioids, muscle relaxants, and adjuvant drugs. The interactions between these drugs can result in additive, supra-additive, infra-additive, or even antagonistic effects. An ideal "depth of anesthesia" indicator would integrate the physiologic and neurologic information from all

TABLE 18-3

THERAPEUTIC BLOOD CONCENTRATIONS WHEN INTRAVENOUS ANESTHETICS ARE INFUSED FOR HYPNOSIS OR SEDATION

■ DRUG NAME	■ MAJOR SURGERY PROCEDURES	■ MINOR SURGERY PROCEDURES	■ SEDATIVE CONCENTRATION	■ AWAKENING CONCENTRATION
Thiopental	10–20 µg/mL	10–20 µg/mL	4–8 µg/mL	4–8 µg/mL
Methohexital	6–15 µg/mL	5–10 µg/mL	1–3 µg/mL	1–3 µg/mL
Propofol	4–6 µg/mL	2–4 µg/mL	1–2 µg/mL	1–1.5 µg/mL
Midazolam	100–200 ng/mL	50–200 ng/mL	40–100 ng/mL	50–150 ng/mL
Etomidate	500–1000 ng/mL	300–600 ng/mL	100–300 ng/mL	200–350 ng/mL
Ketamine	1–4 µg/mL	0.6–2 µg/mL	0.1–1 µg/mL	NA

NA, not available.
From White PF. Textbook of Intravenous Anesthesia. Baltimore, Williams & Wilkins, 1997, pp. 27 and 77.

aspects of the anesthetic state. In the absence of a global cerebral function monitor, the depth of anesthesia device should provide an indication of one or more of the key components of general anesthesia (e.g., hypnosis, analgesia, amnesia, suppression of the stress response, or muscle relaxation). A simple, noninvasive monitor of the depth of anesthesia, which would reliably predict a patient's response to surgical stimulation, would be extremely valuable when using IV anesthetic techniques.

The EMG activity of the frontalis muscles increases significantly in patients who move in response to specific surgical stimuli.[101] However, EMG changes occur late and their interpretation is obscured by muscle relaxant drugs. The EEG changes depend largely on the type of anesthetic drugs used. Although a common EEG pattern can be recognized with increasing depression of CNS function by sedative-hypnotics and opioid analgesics, there is no characteristic EEG pattern associated with unconscious and amnestic states.[103] Univariate descriptors of EEG activity appear to be of limited clinical usefulness, and no meaningful correlation could be found between EEG spectral edge frequency and hemodynamic response to surgical stimuli during propofol anesthesia.[104] Although EEG variables (spectral edge frequency, median frequency) appear to be useful indicators of the CNS effects of anesthetic and analgesic drugs in the experimental setting, their usefulness in clinical practice is limited because the many confounding factors during the operation (changing drug levels and surgical stimulation). The EEG-based bispectral index (BIS), patient state index, state entropy and response entropy, and cerebral state index represent monitoring approaches that reply on sophisticated computerized algorithms to analyze the spontaneous EEG. All of these cerebral monitoring devices have proved to be a useful indicator of anesthetic (hypnotic) depth. Several recent studies have demonstrated that the use of these indices can improve titration of both IV and volatile anesthetics during surgery, thereby facilitating the recovery process.[105] Using EEG-based monitoring can reduce the time required to achieve fast-track eligibility and facilitate earlier discharge home after ambulatory surgery.[106,107]

An alternative to the spontaneous EEG involves the use of the evoked response of the EEG to sensory stimuli (e.g., auditory-evoked potential monitors). The ability to quantitatively assess the response of the body to varying levels of stimulation (sensory- or auditory-evoked responses) may be useful in improving the assessment of depth of anesthesia.[108] Although all sedative-hypnotic drugs affect the brainstem evoked potentials, uncertainty still exists regarding the most useful evoked response(s) to measure. The complexity associated with recording evoked responses is much greater than recording the spontaneous EEG because the value is critically dependent on technical factors (e.g., stimulus intensity, stimulus rate, electrode position), body temperature, as well as the anesthetic drugs. Although most IV anesthetics produce dose-dependent changes in the somatosensory-evoked potentials, the correlation between the acute hemodynamic changes to surgical stimuli and the early auditory-evoked responses is poor. However, the early cortical (midlatency) auditory-evoked response might be useful in detecting awareness under anesthesia. Furthermore, the auditory-evoked potential index may be more discriminating than the spontaneous EEG-based devices in characterizing the transition from wakefulness to unresponsiveness.[109]

As a result of the availability of more rapid and shorter acting sedative-hypnotics, sophisticated computer technology, and new insights into pharmacokinetic-dynamic interactions, use of TIVA techniques has been steadily increasing throughout the world during the last decade. When using constant rate IV infusions, 4 to 5 half-lives may be required to achieve a steady-state anesthetic concentration (Fig. 18-7).

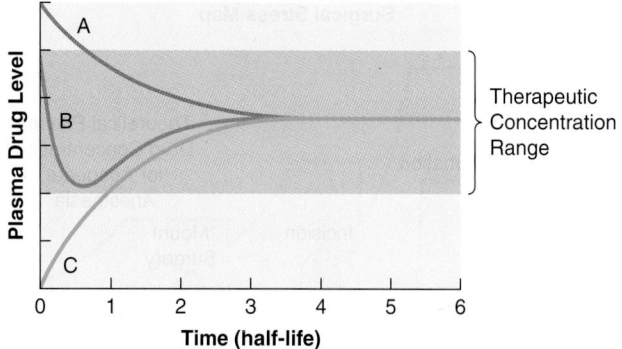

FIGURE 18-7.   Simulated drug level curves when a constant infusion is administered following a "full" loading dose equal to [Cp] × Vd_ss (*Curve A*), a smaller loading dose equal to [Cp] × Vc (*Curve B*), or in the absence of a loading (*Curve C*). See text for details. (Reprinted with permission from White PF: Clinical uses of intravenous anesthetic and analgesic infusions. Anesth Analg 1989; 68: 161.)

To more rapidly achieve a therapeutic blood concentration, it is necessary to administer a loading (priming) dose and to maintain the desired drug concentration using a maintenance infusion. The loading dose (LD) and initial maintenance infusion rate (MIR) can be calculated from previously determined population kinetic values using the following equations:

$$LD = Cp \ (mg/mL) \cdot Vd \ (mL/kg)$$
$$MIR = Cp \ (mL/kg) \cdot Cl \ (mL/kg/min)$$

where Cp = plasma drug concentration, Vd = distribution volume, and Cl = drug clearance.

The use of the smaller central volume of distribution (Vc) for the Vd component of the LD equation will underestimate the LD, whereas use of the larger steady-state volume of distribution (Vd_ss) will result in drug levels that transiently exceed those that are desired. If a smaller LD is administered, a higher initial MIR will be required to compensate for the drug that is removed from the brain by both redistribution and elimination processes. As the redistribution phase assumes less importance, the MIR will decrease because it becomes solely dependent on the drug's elimination and the desired plasma concentration.

An alternative approach is to begin with a rapid loading infusion with a bolus-elimination transfer scheme that combines three functions, as shown in the following equation:

$$Input = V1 \cdot C_{ss} + Cl \cdot C_{ss} + V1 \cdot C_{ss} \ (k_{21} \cdot e^{-k21t})$$

where V1 = distribution volume of the central compartment, C_{ss} = steady-state plasma concentration, Cl = drug clearance; k_{21} = redistribution constant from the central to the peripheral compartment, and k_{21} = redistribution constant from the peripheral to the central compartment. Implementation of the bolus-elimination transfer infusion scheme requires the use of a microprocessor-controlled pump. If a continuous infusion is to be used in an optimal manner to suppress responses to surgical stimuli, the MIR should be varied according to the individual patient responses (Fig. 18-8). Using an MIR large enough to suppress responses to the most intense surgical stimuli will lead to excessive drug accumulation, postoperative side effects, and delayed recovery. More gradual signs of inadequate or excessive anesthesia can be treated by making 50 to 100% changes in the MIR. Abrupt increases in autonomic activity can be treated by giving a small bolus dose equal to 10 to 25% of the initial loading dose and increasing the MIR.

Surgical Stress Map

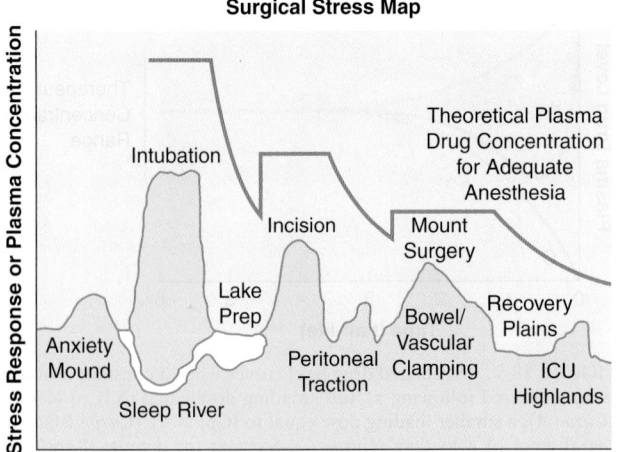

FIGURE 18-8.   The "landscape" of surgical anesthesia. The surgical stimuli are not constant during an operation; therefore, the plasma concentration of an intravenous anesthetic should be titrated to match the needs of the individual patient. ICU, intensive care unit. (Reprinted with permission from Glass PSA, Shafer SL, Jacobs JR, et al: Intravenous drug delivery systems, Miller's Anesthesia, 4th ed. New York, Churchill Livingstone, 1994, p. 391.)

Despite the marked pharmacokinetic and pharmacodynamic variability that exists among surgical patients, computer programs have been developed that allow reasonable predictions of concentration-time profiles for IV anesthetics and analgesics. This new technology has led to the development of target-controlled infusions (TCI), whereby the anesthesiologist chooses a "target" blood or brain (effective site) drug concentration and the micropressor-controlled infusion pump infuses the drug at the rate needed to rapidly achieve and maintain the desired concentration based on population pharmacokinetic-dynamic data.[109] It is obvious that the target concentration must be altered depending on the observed pharmacodynamic effect and the anticipated changes in surgical stimulation.

Closed-loop control based on plasma drug concentrations is not possible because there is no available method to obtain frequent measurements of drug concentrations in real time. A more advanced form of TCI uses a feedback signal generated by simulating a mathematical model of the control process. Clearly, the precision of control achievable with a model-based system is only as accurate as the model. An example of a model-based drug delivery system is the computer-assisted continuous infusion system. An ideal automatic anesthesia delivery device would titrate anesthetic to meet the needs of the individual patient using an acquired feedback signal that accurately reflects the effect site concentration of the drug. The most successful efforts at feedback control of anesthesia have used the BIS and cortical auditory-evoked responses to assess the pharmacodynamic end point.[108]

The rapid, short-acting sedative-hypnotics (e.g., methohexital, propofol) and opioids (e.g., alfentanil, remifentanil) are better suited for continuous administration techniques than the more traditional anesthetic and analgesic agents because they can be more precisely titrated to meet the unique and changing needs of the individual patient. Traditionally, the elimination half-life of a particular drug has been used in attempting to predict the duration of drug action and the time to awakening after discontinuation of the anesthetic infusion. Using conceptual modeling techniques, it has been shown that the concept of context-sensitive half-time is more appropriate in choosing drugs for continuous IV administration (Fig. 18-9). Because none of the currently available IV drugs can

provide for a complete anesthetic state without producing prolonged recovery times and undesirable side effects, it is necessary to administer a combination of IV drugs that provide for hypnosis, amnesia, hemodynamic stability, analgesia, and muscle relaxation. Selecting a combination of drugs with similar pharmacokinetics and compatible pharmacodynamic profiles should improve the anesthetic and surgical conditions. Sedative-hypnotics, opioids, sympatholytics, and muscle relaxants can be successfully administered using continuous infusion TIVA techniques as alternatives to the volatile anesthetics and nitrous oxide.

Sedation in the Operating Room and Intensive Care Unit

The use of sedative-hypnotic drugs as part of a monitored anesthesia care technique in combination with local anesthetics is becoming increasingly popular.[110–112] During local or regional anesthesia, subhypnotic dosages of IV anesthetics can be infused to produce sedation, anxiolysis, and amnesia and enhance patient comfort. The optimum sedation technique achieves the desired clinical end points without producing perioperative side effects (e.g., respiratory depression, nausea, and vomiting).[113] In addition, it should provide for ease of titration to the desired level of sedation while providing for a rapid return to a "clear-headed" state on completion of the surgical procedure.

Sedation also constitutes an essential element in the management of patients in the ICU. The ideal sedative agent for critically ill patients would have minimal depressant effects on the respiratory and cardiovascular systems, would not influence biodegradation of other drugs, and would be independent of renal and hepatic function for its elimination. Recently, the BIS monitor has been used to monitor the depth of sedation in the ICU. For patients undergoing cardiac surgery, rapid reversibility of the sedative state may result in earlier extubation and lead to a shorter stay in the ICU. Although intermittent bolus injections of sedative-hypnotic drugs (e.g., diazepam 2.5 to 5 mg, lorazepam 0.5 to 1 mg, midazolam 1.25

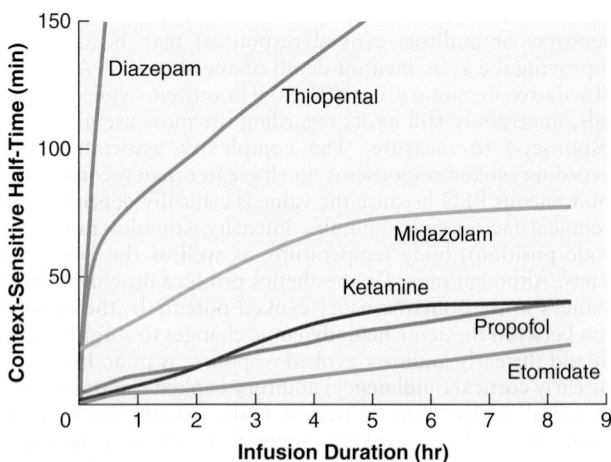

FIGURE 18-9.   Context-sensitive half-time values as a function of infusion duration for intravenous anesthetics, including thiopental, midazolam, diazepam, ketamine, etomidate, and propofol. The context-sensitive half-time for thiopental and diazepam is significantly longer compared with etomidate, propofol, and midazolam, with an increasing infusion duration increase. (Reprinted with permission from Hughes MA, Glass PSA, Jacobs JR: Context-sensitive half-time in multicompartment pharmacokinetic models for intravenous anesthesia. Anesthesiology 1992; 76: 334.)

to 2.5 mg) have been administered during local anesthesia, continuous infusion techniques with propofol are becoming increasingly popular for maintaining a stable level of sedation in the OR and ICU settings.

Benzodiazepines, particularly midazolam, are still the most widely used for sedation in the ICU and for relief of acute situational anxiety during local and regional anesthesia. Midazolam has a steeper dose-response curve than diazepam (Fig. 18-3),[111] and therefore careful titration is necessary to avoid oversedation and respiratory depression. Midazolam infusion, 0.05–5.0 μg/kg/min, can be highly effective in providing sedation for hemodynamically unstable patients in the ICU.[114] Use of a midazolam infusion has been shown to control agitation and decrease analgesic requirements without producing cardiovascular or respiratory instability. However, marked variability exists for midazolam in the individual patient dose-effect relationships. In addition, marked tolerance may develop to the CNS effects of midazolam with prolonged administration.

Propofol sedation offers advantages over the other sedative-hypnotics (including midazolam) because of its rapid recovery and favorable side effect profile. In addition, the degree of sedation is readily changeable from "light" to "deep" levels by varying the MIR. Following a propofol loading dose of 0.25 to 0.5 mg/kg, a carefully titrated subhypnotic infusion of 25 to 75 μg/kg/min produces a stable level of sedation with minimal cardiorespiratory depression and a short recovery period. Because even low concentrations of propofol can depress the ventilatory response to hypoxia, supplemental oxygen should always be provided. Sedative infusions of propofol produce less perioperative amnesia than midazolam, and propofol-induced amnesia appears to be directly related to the infusion rate.

A small dose of midazolam (2 mg IV) administered immediately before a variable-rate infusion of propofol has also been shown to significantly decrease intraoperative anxiety and recall of uncomfortable events without compromising the rapid recovery from propofol sedation.[112] Propofol sedation can also be supplemented with potent opioid and nonopioid analgesics to provide sedation analgesia. In comparing propofol and midazolam for patient-controlled sedation,[115] midazolam was associated with less intraoperative recall and pain on injection than propofol, while propofol was associated with less residual impairment of cognitive function. Compared with anesthesiologist-controlled sedation, patient-controlled sedation was associated with fewer propofol dosages, "lighter" levels of sedation, and reduced patient comfort.[116] Computer "target-controlled" sedation was also associated with more frequent "oversedation."[117] Finally, music can reduce the propofol dosage requirement during local and regional anesthesia.[118]

Compared with midazolam in the ICU setting, use of propofol sedation allowed for more rapid weaning of critically ill patients from artificial ventilation.[119] It has been suggested that the more rapid weaning after propofol sedation may be cost-saving compared with midazolam when only a limited period of sedation (<48 hours) is required.[120] Although a pharmacokinetic study yielded no evidence of a change in receptor sensitivity or drug accumulation over a 4-day study period, preliminary data suggest that tolerance to the CNS effects of propofol may develop with more prolonged administration (>1 week). Increasingly, dexmedetomidine infusions are being used in critically ill patients who require both sedation and analgesia.

Concerns have been raised about elevated lipid plasma levels in patients sedated with standard formulations of propofol over a period of several days, especially when high infusion rates (>6 mg/kg/hr) are used. However, the availability of a propofol formulation with reduced lipid content (Ampofol)

should decrease the risk of this problem in the future. Because of conflicting evidence regarding increased mortality as a result of myocardial failure when propofol was used for sedation in the neonatal ICU,[121–124] more safety data are needed to define the indications for the use of prolonged propofol infusions, especially in this patient population. Low-dose ketamine infusions (5 to 25 μg/kg/min) can also be used for sedation and analgesia during local or regional anesthetic procedures, as well as in the ICU setting.[67] Midazolam, 0.07 to 0.15 mg/kg infused over 3 to 5 minutes, followed by ketamine, 0.25 to 0.5 mg/kg IV over 1 to 3 minutes, produced excellent sedation, amnesia, and analgesia without significant cardiorespiratory depression.

Another alternative to propofol for sedation outside the OR is dexmedetomidine. The α_2-agonist can be infused at rates of 0.25 to 0.75 μg/kg/hr to produce sedation during gynecologic procedures[90] and in the ICU. Although the onset of sedation is slower than that of propofol, its opioid-sparing effects reduce the risk of ventilatory depression during procedures outside the OR and may facilitate weaning from mechanical ventilation in the ICU. In the ambulatory setting, recovery from dexmedetomidine's sedative effects is slower than with propofol.

CONCLUSIONS

Despite the introduction of new anesthetic agents, it is obvious that many of the goals desirable in an ideal IV anesthetic have not been achieved with any of the currently available drugs. Nevertheless, each of these sedative-hypnotic drugs possesses characteristics that may be useful in specific clinical situations and when combined with an appropriate multimodal analgesic technique (e.g., opioids, nonsteroidal anti-inflammatory drugs, local anesthetics) can provide excellent anesthetic conditions. In situations in which a rapid recovery is not essential (e.g., inpatient procedures), the barbiturates thiopental and methohexital may be the most cost-effective IV anesthetics. Although recovery from anesthesia with methohexital is more rapid than with thiopental (and compares favorably with propofol), excitatory side effects (e.g., myoclonus, hiccoughing) are more prominent than with thiopental or propofol. Methohexital remains the anesthetic of choice for electroconvulsive therapy procedures.

Propofol is the IV drug of choice when a rapid and smooth recovery is essential (e.g., outpatient [ambulatory] anesthesia); increasingly, propofol has been used for all inpatient procedures because of the availability of less costly generic formulations. Recovery from propofol anesthesia is characterized by the absence of a "hangover effect" and reduced postoperative nausea and vomiting symptoms. The cardiovascular-depressant effects produced by propofol appear to be more pronounced than those of thiopental, but can be minimized by careful titration and the use of a variable-rate infusion during the maintenance period. The ability to combine propofol with potent, rapid, and short-acting opioid analgesics (e.g., remifentanil) has facilitated the use of TIVA techniques. Improvements in the TCI delivery systems for IV anesthetics (propofol) and analgesics (remifentanil) will lead to an ever greater acceptance of TIVA techniques in the future.[125]

When administered alone for induction of anesthesia, benzodiazepines are associated with a slower onset and more prolonged recovery profile. In the usual induction doses, benzodiazepines are associated with minimal cardiorespiratory depression and the reliable amnestic effect may be valuable during TIVA (e.g., for acute sedation prior to induction of anesthesia, for maintenance in the absence of nitrous oxide). When administered in smaller doses, midazolam can also be a valuable adjunct as part of a coinduction and/or maintenance technique. Other shorter-acting benzodiazepines may be developed in the future (e.g., Ro 48-6791).

Etomidate has minimal cardiovascular and respiratory depressant effects and is therefore an extremely useful induction agent in high-risk patients. It is also occasionally used as an alternative to methohexital for electroconvulsive therapy procedures. The occurrence of pain on injection, excitatory phenomena, adrenocortical suppression, and a high incidence of postoperative nausea and vomiting have limited the use of etomidate to special situations in which its cardiovascular profile offers significant advantages over other available IV anesthetics. A new lipid formulation of etomidate is apparently associated with its fewer side effects and may allow this IV anesthetic to gain wider clinical acceptance in the future.

Ketamine is a unique IV anesthetic that produces a wide spectrum of pharmacologic effects including sedation, hypnosis, somatic analgesia, bronchodilation, and sympathetic nervous system stimulation. Induction of anesthesia can be rapidly achieved following IM injection, making ketamine a valuable alternative to an inhalation induction when IV access is difficult to establish. Ketamine is also indicated for induction of anesthesia in the presence of severe hypovolemic shock, acute bronchospastic states, right-to-left intracardiac shunts, and cardiac tamponade. The adverse hyperdynamic cardiovascular, cerebrodynamic, and psychomimetic effects of ketamine can be minimized by prior administration of a benzodiazepine (e.g., midazolam) or a sedative-hypnotic drug (e.g., thiopental, propofol). Ketamine is also useful as part of coinduction and maintenance anesthetic techniques when avoiding opioid analgesics is desirable. The introduction of the more potent S(+)-ketamine may increase use of ketamine in small doses or by continuous infusion as an IV adjuvant during general anesthesia because of its anesthetic and analgesic-sparing activity.

In summary, IV anesthesia has evolved from being used mainly for induction of anesthesia to providing unconsciousness and amnesia for surgical procedures performed under local, regional, and general anesthesia. New insights into the pharmacokinetics and dynamics of IV anesthetics, as well as the development of computer technology to facilitate IV drug delivery (e.g., TCIs), have greatly enhanced the use of TIVA techniques. The shorter context-sensitive half-life values of the newer sedative-hypnotic drugs make these compounds more useful as continuous infusions for maintenance of anesthesia and sedation. While the search for the ideal IV anesthetic continues, the major challenge for anesthesiologists is to choose the sedative-hypnotic drug that most closely matches the patient's needs in specific clinical situations.

References

1. Franks NP, Lieb WR: Molecular and cellular mechanisms of general anaesthesia. Nature 1994; 367: 607
2. White PF: Textbook of Intravenous Anesthesia. Baltimore, Williams & Wilkins, 1997, pp 27 and 77
3. Coates KM, Mather LE, Johnson R, et al: Thiopental is a competitive inhibitor at the human alpha-7 nicotinic acet ylcholine receptor. Anesth Anal 2001; 92: 930
4. Rossi MA, Chan CK, Christensen JD, et al: Interactions between propofol and lipid mediator receptors: inhibition of lysophosphatidate signaling. Anesth Analg 1996; 83: 1090
5. Shelly MP: Dexmedetomidine: A real innovation or more of the same? Br J Anaesth 2001; 87: 677
6. Thomas JE, Judith E, Hall, MA et al: The effects of increasing plasma concentrations of Dexmedetomidine in humans. Anesthesiology 2000; 93: 382
7. Fu W, White PF: Dexmedetomidine failed to block the acute hyperdynamic response to electroconvulsive therapy. Anesthesiology 1999; 90: 422
8. Higuchi H, Adachi Y, Dahan A, et al: The interaction between propofol and clonidine for loss of consciousness. Anesth Analg 2002; 94: 886
9. Segal IS, Jarvis DJ, Duncan SR, et al: Clinical efficacy of oral-transdermal clonidine combinations during the perioperative period. Anesthesiology 1991; 74: 220
10. Hughes MA, Jacobs JR, Glass PSA: Context-sensitive half-time in multi-compartment pharmacokinetic models for intravenous anesthesia. Anesthesiology 1992; 76: 334
11. Modica PA, Tempelhoff R, White PF: Pro- and anticonvulsant effects of anesthetics (Part I). Anesth Analg. 1990; 70: 303
12. Modica PA, Tempelhoff R, White PF: Pro- and anticonvulsant effects of anesthetics (Part II). Anesth Analg 1990; 70: 433
13. Drummond-Lewis J, Scher C: Propofol: A new treatment strategy for refractory migraine headache. Pain Med 2002; 3: 366
14. Hsu YW, Cortinez LI, Robertson KM, et al: Dexmedetomidine pharmacodynamics: part I: crossover comparison of the respiratory effects of dexmedetomidine and remifentanil in healthy volunteers. Anesthesiology 2004; 101: 1066
15. Scheinin H, Jaakola ML, Sjovall S, et al: Intramuscular dexmedetomidine as premedication for general anesthesia. A comparative multicenter study. Anesthesiology 1993; 78: 1065
16. Hofbauer RK, Fiset P, Plourde G, et al: Dose-dependent effects of propofol on the central processing of thermal pain. Anesthesiology 2004; 100: 386
17. Avram J, Krejcie TC, Henthorn TK: The relationship of age to pharmacokinetics of early drug distribution: The concurrent disposition of thiopental and indocyanine green. Anesthesiology 1990; 72: 403
18. (No authors listed): Randomized clinical study of thiopental loading in comatose survivors of cardiac arrest. Am J Emerg Med 1986; 4: 72
19. Gunaydin B, Babacan A: Cerebral hypoperfusion after cardiac surgery and anesthetic strategies: A comparative study with high-dose fentanyl and barbiturate anesthesia. Ann Thorac Cardiovasc Surg 1998; 4: 12
20. Newman MF, Croughwell ND, White WD, et al: Pharmacologic electroencephalograhic suppression during cardiopulmonary bypass: A comparison of thiopental and isoflurane. Anesth Analg 1998; 86: 246
21. Ding Z, White PF: Anesthesia for electroconvulsive therapy. Anesth Analg 2002; 94: 1351
22. Blouin RT, Conard PF, Gross JB: Time course of ventilatory depression following induction doses of propofol and thiopental. Anesthesiology 1991; 75: 940
23. Vohra A, Thomas AN, Harper NJN, et al: Non-invasive measurement of cardiac output during induction of anaesthesia and tracheal intubation: Thiopentone and propofol compared. Br J Anaesth 1991; 67: 64
24. Bhutada A, Shani R, Rastogi S, et al: Randomised controlled trial of thiopental for intubation in neonates. Arch Dis Child Fetal Neonatal Ed 2000; 82: F34
25. Asik I, Yorukoglu D, Gulay I, et al: Pain on injection of propofol: Comparison of metoprolol with lidocaine. Eur J Anaesthesiol 2003; 20: 487
26. Dubey PK, Prasad SS: Pain on injection of propofol: The effect of granisetron pretreatment. Clini J Pain 2003; 19: 121
27. Piper SN, Rohm KD, Papsdorf M, et al: Dolasetron reduces pain on injection of propofol. Anaesthesiol Intensivmed Notfallmed Schmerzther 2002; 37: 528
28. Agarwal A, Ansari MF, Gupta D, et al: Pretreatment with thiopental for prevention of pain associated with propofol injection. Anaesth Analg 2004; 98: 683
29. Shao X, Li H, White PF, et al: Bisulfite-containing propofol: is it a cost-effective alternative to Diprivan for induction of anesthesia? Anesth Analg 2000; 91: 871
30. Song D, Hamza M, White PF, et al: The pharmacodynamic effects of a lower-lipid emulsion of propofol: A comparison with the standard propofol emulsion. Anesth Analg 2004; 98: 687
31. Song D, Hamza M, White PF, et al: Comparison of a lower-lipid propofol emulsion with the standard emulsion for sedation during monitored anesthesia care. Anesthesiology, 2004; 100: 1072
32. Gibiansky E, Struys MM, Gibiansky L, et al: AQUAVAN injection, a water-soluble prodrug of propofol, as a bolus injection: a phase I dose-escalation comparison with DIPRIVAN (part 1): pharmacokinetics. Anesthesiology 2005; 103: 718
33. Struys MM, Vanluchene AL, Gibiansky E, et al: AQUAVAN injection, a water-soluble prodrug of propofol, as a bolus injection: a phase I dose-escalation comparison with DIPRIVAN (part 2): pharmacodynamics and safety. Anesthesiology 2005; 103: 730
34. Shafer A, Doze VA, Shafer SL, et al: Pharmacokinetics and pharmacodynamics of propofol infusions during general anesthesia. Anesthesiology 1988; 69: 348
35. Sebel PS, Lowdon JD: Propofol: A new intravenous anesthetic. Anesthesiology 1989; 71: 260
36. Doze VA, Westphal LM, White PF: Comparison of propofol with methohexital for outpatient anesthesia. Anesth Analg 1986; 65: 1189
37. Smith I, White PF, Nathanson M, et al: Propofol: An update on its clinical use. Anesthesiology 1994; 81: 1005
38. Glass PSA: Prevention of awareness during total intravenous anesthesia. Anesthesiology 1993; 78: 399
39. Oxorn D, Orser B, Ferris LE, et al: Propofol and thiopental anesthesia: A comparison of the incidence of dreams and perioperative mood alterations. Anesth Analg 1994; 79: 553
40. Pinaud M, Lelausque JN, Chetanneau A, et al: Effects of propofol on cerebral hemodynamics and metabolism in patients with brain trauma. Anesthesiology 1990; 73: 404
41. Yagmurdur H, Cakan T, Bayrak A, et al: The effects of etomidate, thiopental, and propofol in induction on hypoperfusion-reperfusion phenomenon

during laparoscopic cholecystectomy. Acta Anaesthesiol Scand 2004; 48: 772

42. Dolk A, Cannerfelt R, Anderson RE, et al: Inhalation anaesthesia is cost-effective for ambulatory surgery clinical comparison with propofol during elective knee arthroscopy. Eur J Anaesthesiol 2002; 19: 88

43. Reddy RV, Moorthy SS, Dierdorf SF, et al: Excitatory effects and electroencephalographic correlation of etomidate, thiopental, methohexital, and propofol. Anesth Analg 1993; 77: 1008

44. Ebrahim ZY, Schubert A, Van Ness P, et al: The effect of propofol on the electroencephalogram of patients with epilepsy. Anesth Analg 1994; 78: 275

45. Sellgren J, Ejnell H, Elam M, et al: Sympathetic muscle nerve activity, peripheral blood flows, and baroreceptor reflexes in humans during propofol anesthesia and surgery. Anesthesiology 1994; 80: 534

46. Lopatka CW, Muzi M, Ebert TJ: Propofol, but not etomidate, reduces desflurane-mediated sympathetic activation in humans. Can J Anaesth 1999; 46: 342

47. Gan TJ, Glass PSA, Howell ST, et al: Determination of plasma concentrations associated with 50% reduction in postoperative nausea. Anesthesiology 1997; 87: 779

48. Krumholz W, Endrass J, Hempelmann G: Propofol inhibits phagocytosis and killing of Staphylococcus aureus and Escherichia coli by polymorphonuclear leukocytes in vitro. Can J Anaesth 1994; 41: 446

49. Crowther J, Hrazdil J, Jolly DT, et al: Growth of microorganisms in propofol, thiopental, and a 1: 1 mixture of propofol and thiopental. Anesth Analg 1996; 82: 475

50. Reves JG, Fragen RJ, Vinik HR, et al: Midazolam—Pharmacology and uses. Anesthesiology 1985; 62: 310

51. Urquhart ML, White PF: Comparison of sedative infusions during regional anesthesia: Methohexital, etomidate, and midazolam. Anesth Analg 1988; 68: 249

52. Ghouri A, Taylor E, White PF: Patient-controlled drug administration during local anesthesia: A comparison of midazolam, propofol, and alfentanil. J Clin Anesth 1992; 4: 476

53. Dingemanse J, van Gerven JMA, Schoemaker RC, et al: Integrated pharmacokinetics and pharmacodynamics of Ro 48-6791, a new benzodiazepine, in comparison with midazolam during first administration to healthy male subjects. Br J Clin Pharmacol 1997; 44: 477

54. Tang J, Wang B, White PF, et al: Comparison of the sedation and recovery profiles of Ro 48-6791, a new benzodiazepine, and midazolam in combination with meperidine for outpatient endoscopic procedures. Anesth Analg 1999; 89: 893

55. Brodgen RN, Goa KL: Flumazenil. Drugs 1991; 42: 1061

56. Ghouri AF, Ramirez Ruiz MA, et al: Effect of flumazenil on recovery after midazolam and propofol sedation. Anesthesiology 1994; 81: 333

57. Flogel CM, Ward DS, Wada DR, et al: The effects of large-dose flumazenil on midazolam-induced ventilatory depression. Anesth Analg 1993; 77: 1207

58. White PF, Shafer A, Boyle WA, et al: Benzodiazepine antagonism does not provoke a stress response. Anesthesiology 1989; 70: 636

59. Doenicke AW, Roizen MF, Kugler J, et al: Reducing myoclonus after etomidate. Anesthesiology 1999; 90: 113

60. Kelsaka E, Karakaya D, Sarihasan B, et al: Remifentanil pretreatment reduces myoclonus after etomidate. J Clin Anesth 2006; 18: 83

61. Van Hamme MJ, Ghoneim MM, Amber JJ: Pharmacokinetics of etomidate, a new intravenous anesthetic. Anesthesiology 1978; 49: 274

62. Wagner RL, White PF, Kan PB, et al: Inhibition of adrenal steroidogenesis by the anesthetic etomidate. N Engl J Med 1984; 310: 1415

63. Gooding JM, Weng JT, Smith RA: Cardiovascular and pulmonary response following etomidate induction of anesthesia in patients with demonstrated cardiac disease. Anesth Analg 1979; 50: 40

64. Wagner RL, White PF: Etomidate inhibits adrenocortical function in surgical patients. Anesthesiology 1984; 61: 647

65. Gries A, Weis S, Herr A, et al: Etomidate and thiopental inhibit platelet function in patients undergoing infrainguinal vascular surgery. Acta Anaesthesiol Scand 2001; 45: 449

66. White PF, Way WL, Trevor AJ: Ketamine—Its pharmacology and therapeutic uses. Anesthesiology 1982; 56: 119

67. White PF, Ham J, Way WL, et al: Pharmacology of ketamine isomers in surgical patients. Anesthesiology 1980; 52: 231

68. White PF, Schuttler J, Shafer A, et al: Comparative pharmacology of the ketamine isomers. Studies in volunteers. Br J Anaesth 1985; 57: 197

69. Rabben T, Skjelbred P, Oye I: Prolonged analgesia effect of ketamine, an N-methyl-D-aspartate receptor inhibitor, in patients with chronic pain. J Pharmacol Ther 1999; 289: 1060

70. Dahl V, Ernoe PE, Steen T, et al: Does ketamine have preemptive effects in women undergoing abdominal hysterectomy procedures? Anesth Analg 2000; 90: 1419

71. Susuki M, Tsueda K, Lansing PS, et al: Small-dose ketamine enhances morphine-induced analgesia after outpatient surgery. Anesth Analg 1999; 89: 98

72. Menigaux C, Fletcher D, Dupont X, et al: The benefits of intraoperative small-dose ketamine on postoperative pain after anterior cruciate ligament repair. Anesth Analg 2000; 90: 129

73. Albanese J, Arnaud S, Rey M, et al: Ketamine decreases intracranial pressure and electroencephalographic activity in traumatic brain injury patients during propofol sedation. Anesthesiology 1997; 87: 1328

74. Berman RM, Capiello A, Anand A, et al: Antidepressant effects of ketamine in depressed patients. Biol Psychiatry 2000; 47: 351

75. Kudoh A, Takahira Y, Katagai H, et al: Small-dose ketamine improves the postoperative state of depressed patients. Anesth Analg 2002; 95: 114

76. Mortero RF, Clark LD, Tolan MM, et al: The effects of small-dose ketamine on propofol sedation: Respiration, postoperative mood, perception, cognition and pain. Anesth Analg 2001; 92: 1465

77. Ikeda T, Kazama T, Sessler DI, et al: Induction of anesthesia with ketamine reduces the magnitude of redistribution hypothermia. Anesth Analg 2001; 93: 934

78. Khos R, Duriex ME: Ketamine: Teaching an old drug new tricks. Anesth Analg 1998; 87: 1186

79. Badrinath S, Avramov MN, Shadrick M, et al: The use of a ketamine-propofol combination during monitored anesthesia care. Anesth Analg 2000; 90: 858

80. Deng XM, Xiao WJ, Luo MP, et al: The use of midazolam and small-dose ketamine for sedation and analgesia during local anesthesia. Anesth Analg 2001; 93: 1174

81. Mortero RF, Clark LD, Tolan MM, et al: The effects of small-dose ketamine on propofol sedation: respiration, postoperative mood, perception, cognition, and pain. Anesth Analg 2001; 92: 1465

82. Sneyd JR: Recent advances in intravenous anaesthesia. Br J Anaesth 2004; 93: 725

83. Jaakola ML: Dexmedetomidine premedication before intravenous regional anesthesia in minor outpatient hand surgery. J Clin Anesth 1994; 6: 204

84. Hall JE, Uhrich TD, Barney JA, et al: Sedative, amnestic, and analgesic properties of small-dose dexmedetomidine infusions. Anesth Analg 1995; 90: 699

85. Yildiz M, Tavlan A, Tuncer S, et al: Effect of dexmedetomidine on haemodynamic responses to laryngoscopy and intubation: perioperative haemodynamics and anaesthetic requirements. Drugs R D 2006; 7: 43

86. Scher CS, Gitlin MC: Dexmedetomidine and low-dose ketamine provide adequate sedation for awake fibreoptic intubation. Can J Anaesth 2003; 50: 607

87. Bergese SD, Khabiri B, Roberts WD, et al: Dexmedetomidine for conscious sedation in difficult awake fiberoptic intubation cases. J Clin Anesth 2007; 19: 141

88. Tanskanen PE, Kyttä JV, Randell TT, et al: Dexmedetomidine as an anaesthetic adjuvant in patients undergoing intracranial tumour surgery: a double-blind, randomized and placebo-controlled study. Br J Anaesth. 2006; 97: 658

89. Arain SR, Ruehlow RM, Uhrich TD, et al: The efficacy of dexmedetomidine versus morphine for postoperative analgesia after major inpatient surgery. Anesth Analg 2004; 98: 153

90. Gurbet A, Basagan-Mogol E, Turker G, et al: Intraoperative infusion of dexmedetomidine reduces perioperative analgesic requirements. Can J Anaesth 2006; 53: 646

91. Tufanogullari B, White PF, Peixoto MP, et al: Dexmedetomidine infusion during laparoscopic bariatric surgery: Effect on recovery outcome variables. Anesth Analg 2008 (in press)

92. Alhashemi JA: Dexmedetomidine vs midazolam for monitored anaesthesia care during cataract surgery. Br J Anaesth 2006; 96: 722

93. Arain SR, Ebert TJ: The efficacy, side effects, and recovery characteristics of dexmedetomidine versus propofol when used for intraoperative sedation. Anesth Analg 2002; 95: 461

94. Memis D, Turan A, Karamanlioglu B, et al: Adding dexmedetomidine to lidocaine for intravenous regional anesthesia. Anesth Analg 2004; 98: 835

95. Smith I, White PF, Nathanson M, et al: Propofol: An update on its clinical use. Anesthesiology 1994; 81: 1005

96. White PF: Comparative evaluation of intravenous agents for rapid sequence induction: Thiopental, ketamine, and midazolam. Anesthesiology 1982; 57: 279

97. Kamata K, Nagata O, Iwakiri H, et al: Comparison of requirement for postoperative analgesics after inhalation and total intravenous anesthesia. Masui 2003; 52: 1200

98. Salihoglu Z, Karaca S, Kose Y, et al: Total intravenous anesthesia versus single breath technique and anesthesia maintenance with sevoflurane for bariatric operations. Obes Surg 2001; 11: 496

99. White PF: Use of continuous infusion versus intermittent bolus administration of fentanyl or ketamine during outpatient anesthesia. Anesthesiology 1983; 59: 294

100. White PF: Clinical uses of intravenous anesthetic and analgesic infusions. Anesth Analg 1989; 68: 161

101. Chang T, Dworsky WA, White PF: Continuous electromyography for monitoring depth of anesthesia. Anesth Analg 1988; 53: 315

102. Monk TG, Ding Y, White PF: Total intravenous anesthesia: effects of opioid versus hypnotic supplementation on autonomic responses and recovery. Anesth Analg 1992; 75: 798

103. Plourde G: Depth of anaesthesia. Can J Anaesth 1991; 31: 270

104. White PF, Boyle WA: Relationship between hemodynamic and electroencephalographic changes during general anesthesia. Anesth Analg 1989; 68: 177

105. White PF: Use of cerebral monitoring during anesthesia: Effect on recovery profile. Best Prac Res Clin Anaesth 2006; 20: 181

106. Song D, van Vlymen J, White PF: Is the bispectral index useful in predicting fast-track eligibility after ambulatory anesthesia with propofol and desflurane? Anesth Analg 1998; 87: 1245

107. White PF, Ma H, Tang J, et al: Does the use of electroencephalographic bispectral index or auditory evoked potential index monitoring facilitate

recovery after desflurane anesthesia in the ambulatory setting? Anesthesiology 2004; 100: 811

108. Struys M, Versichelen L, Mortier E, et al: Comparison of spontaneous frontal EMG, EEG power spectrum and bispectral index to monitor propofol drug effect and emergence. Acta Anaesthesiol Scand 1998; 42: 628

109. Schraag S, Bothner U, Gajraj R, et al: The performance of electroencephalogram bispectral index and auditory evoked potential index to predict loss of consciousness during propofol infusion. Anesth Analg 1999; 89: 1311

110. Milne SE, Kenny GN: Future applications for TCI systems. Anaesthesia 1998; 53: 56

111. White PF, Vascones LO, Mathes SA, et al: Comparison of midazolam and diazepam for sedation during plastic surgery. J Plast Reconstruct Surg 1998; 81: 703

112. Taylor E, Ghouri AF, White PF: Midazolam in combination with propofol for sedation during local anesthesia. J Clin Anesth 1992; 4: 213

113. Sä Règo MM, Watcha, MF, White PF: The changing role of monitored anesthesia care in the ambulatory setting. Anesth Analg 1997; 85: 1020

114. Shafer A, Doze VA, White PF: Pharmacokinetic variability of midazolam infusions in critically ill patients. Crit Care Med 1990; 18: 1039

115. Ghouri AF, Taylor E, White PF: Patient-controlled drug administration during local anesthesia: a comparison of midazolam, propofol, and alfentanil. J Clin Anesth 1992; 4: 476

116. Alhashemi JA, Kaki AM: Anesthesiologist-controlled versus patient-controlled propofol sedation for shockwave lithotripsy. Can J Anaesth 2006; 53: 449

117. Burns R, McCrae AF, Tiplady B: A comparison of target-controlled therapy with patient-controlled administration of propofol combined with midazolam for sedation during dental surgery. Anaesthesia 2003; 58: 170

118. Ayoub CM, Rizk LB, Yaacoub CI, et al: Music and ambient operating room noise in patients undergoing spinal anesthesia. Anesth Analg 2005; 100: 1316

119. White PF, Negus JB: Sedative infusions during local or regional anesthesia: A comparison of midazolam and propofol. J Clin Anesth 1991; 3: 32

120. Aitkenhead AR, Pepperman ML, Willatts SM, et al: Comparison of propofol and midazolam for long-term sedation in critically ill patients. Lancet 1989; 2: 704

121. Carrasco G, Molina R, Costa J, et al: Propofol vs. midazolam in short-, medium-, and long-term sedation of critically ill patients: A cost-benefit analysis. Chest 1993; 103: 557

122. McFarlan CS, Anderson BJ, Short TG: The use of propofol infusions in paediatric anaesthesia: A practical guide. Paediatr Anaesth 1999; 9: 209

123. Parke TJ, Steven JE, Rice ASC, et al: Metabolic acidosis and fatal myocardial failure after propofol infusion in children: five case reports. BMJ 1992; 305: 613

124. Martin PH, Murphy BVS, Petros AJ: Metabolic, biochemical and haemodynamic effects of infusion of propofol for long-term sedation of children undergoing intensive care. Br J Anaesth 1997; 79: 276

125. Egan TD, Shafer SL: Target-controlled infusions for intravenous anesthetics. Anesthesiology 2003; 99: 1039

CHAPTER 19 ■ OPIOIDS

BARBARA A. CODA

KEY POINTS

1 The term *opioid* designates all drugs, both natural and synthetic, including endogenous peptides, which have morphinelike properties. In its broadest sense, it refers to agonists, partial agonists, and mixed agonist–antagonists at one or more of the opioid receptors.

2 Opioid receptor classification is based on binding activity of specific ligands: morphine at mu (μ), ketocyclazocine at kappa (κ), enkephalins at delta (δ), and endorphin at epsilon (ε) receptors, and specific opioid receptors are responsible for different opioid effects. Most opioids used in clinical anesthesia today (e.g., fentanyl, morphine, and their derivatives) are highly selective for μ-opioid receptors. Naloxone, the most commonly used opioid antagonist, is not selective for opioid receptor type. Very few endogenous opioids exhibit great selectivity for a single receptor type.

3 Opioids are administered primarily for their analgesic effect, which results from complex interactions at discrete sites in the brain, spinal cord, and under certain conditions, peripheral tissues, and involves both μ_1 and μ_2 opioid effects. Morphine also appears to exert anti-inflammatory effects at μ_3-opioid receptors. For the mixed agonist–antagonist opioids, analgesic effects are also mediated at κ receptors. Opioids act selectively on neurons that transmit and modulate nociception, leaving other sensory modalities and motor functions intact.

4 Opioids are used in combination with inhaled anesthetics to produce balanced anesthesia. Fentanyl and its derivatives reduce the minimum alveolar concentration (MAC) of volatile agents in a dose-dependent fashion. An apparent ceiling effect is seen at 70% MAC reduction, although reduction of up to 90% has been reported for sufentanil and remifentanil.

5 Fentanyl and its derivatives can be combined with a sedative-hypnotic agent to provide total intravenous anesthesia (TIVA). Alfentanil and remifentanil are particularly suited for TIVA because of their rapid onset and short duration of action.

6 Fentanyl and its derivatives can be given in very high doses for "opioid anesthesia," but even at extremely high doses, that is, those that produce profound analgesia as well as apnea, unconsciousness is not assured.

7 Muscle hypertonus occurs with high-dose opioid administration, and severe chest wall rigidity can interfere with ventilation. It is seen most often on induction with rapid-acting opioids. Opioid-induced muscle rigidity is increased in the presence of nitrous oxide and can be prevented or treated with sedative-hypnotics or low-dose muscle relaxants.

8 All opioids depress respiratory drive in a dose-dependent manner, and ventilatory depression is seen even at doses associated with mild analgesia. Equianalgesic opioid doses produce equivalent magnitudes of respiratory depression. When given in combination with benzodiazepines, opioids can blunt hypoxic drive to a greater extent than the hypercarbic drive and produce profound respiratory depression.

9 Fentanyl or one of its derivatives is often used as a component of anesthetic induction. Small opioid doses reduce the dosage requirements of sedative-hypnotics, and blunt airway reflexes (sympathetic activity in response to laryngoscopy).

10 In low doses, opioids have minimal cardiovascular effects, but bradycardia and hypotension are seen with higher doses. A prominent feature of fentanyl and its derivatives is their remarkable hemodynamic stability. Morphine and meperidine cause histamine release, and high doses of these opioids can produce hypotension.

11 All opioids can produce nausea and vomiting through complex interactions at nausea and vomiting centers in the medulla. In general, equianalgesic doses of opioids produce similar magnitude of nausea. Opioid-induced nausea can be exacerbated by vestibular input, and is particularly problematic in ambulatory patients.

12 Opioids produce smooth muscle spasm throughout the gastrointestinal tract. They decrease gastric secretions and delay gastric emptying. Opioids increase the tone of the common bile duct and sphincter of Oddi, although meperidine and the mixed agonist–antagonists cause less biliary spasm than morphine and fentanyl.

HISTORY

Opioids have been used in the treatment of pain for thousands of years. The drug opium, which contains more than 20 alkaloids, is obtained from the exudate of *Papaver somniferum* seed pods, and the word *opium* is derived from *opos*, the Greek word for juice. The first undisputed reference to poppy juice is found in the third century (BCE) writings of Theophrastus.[1] The German pharmacist Sertuener isolated what he called the "soporific principle" in opium in 1806, and in 1817 named it morphine, after the Greek god of dreams, Morpheus.[2] Isolation of other opium alkaloids followed, and by the mid-1800s, the medical use of pure alkaloids rather than crude opium preparations began to spread.[1] Morphine was used widely to treat wounded soldiers during the American Civil War, and in 1869 its use as a premedication was described by Claude Bernard. However, in the absence of muscle relaxants and controlled ventilation, opioids were associated with a significant risk of severe respiratory depression and death. Thus their use in anesthesia was limited at that time.

With the advent of cardiac surgery in the late 1950s came the development of "opioid anesthesia." A decade later, Lowenstein[3] reported the use of progressively higher doses of morphine (0.5 to 3 mg/kg), but found limitations including incomplete suppression of the stress response, hypotension, awareness during anesthesia, and increased fluid and blood requirements.

Fentanyl, a 4-anilinopiperidine derivative of phenoperidine, was synthesized in 1960. The completely synthetic opioids were more potent and had a better safety margin (ratio of median lethal dose to lowest effective dose for surgery) than meperidine. Advances in surgical techniques created the need for potent opioids with a rapid onset, a brief, predictable duration, and a maximal safety margin for use in clinical anesthesia, and led to development of sufentanil, alfentanil, and other fentanyl derivatives between 1974 and 1976. The newest potent opioid, remifentanil, has an ultrashort duration of action because of rapid metabolism by ester hydrolysis and offers an advantage in specific clinical settings.

The search for opioid analgesics without potential for dependence was stimulated by concerns about opioid addiction and led to the identification of multiple opioid receptor types. In the mid-1960s, nalorphine, a morphine antagonist, was also found to have analgesic properties. Two other compounds, pentazocine and cyclazocine, antagonized some of morphine's effects. Pentazocine also produced analgesia, and both produced some psychotropic effects that morphine did not. These and other observations led Martin[4] to propose the theory of receptor dualism. Intrinsic to this theory were two key concepts: (1) the existence of multiple opioid receptors (originally only two were proposed) and (2) the idea of pharmacologic redundancy (i.e., more than one receptor could mediate a physiologic function, such as analgesia). Thus, a drug could be a strong agonist, a partial agonist, or a competitive antagonist at one or more of the different receptor types. Subsequent research has revealed three distinct families of opioid peptides and multiple categories of opioid receptors.

TERMINOLOGY

The term *opiate* was originally used to refer to drugs derived from opium, including morphine, its semisynthetic derivatives, and codeine. The more general term *opioid* was introduced to designate all drugs, both natural and synthetic, with morphinelike properties, including endogenous peptides. The nonspecific term *narcotic* has been used to refer to morphine and morphinelike analgesics. However, because of its use in a legal

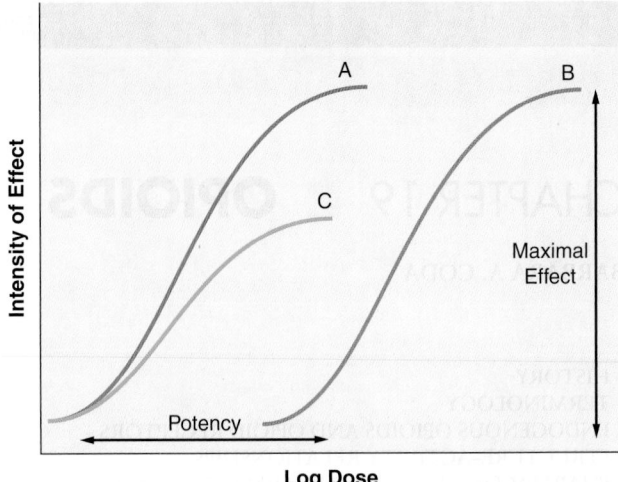

FIGURE 19-1. Log dose-effect curves for two agonists (A and B) with equal efficacy but different potency, and a partial agonist (C). Note that the potencies of A and C are similar, but the efficacy is less and the slope of the dose-response curve is shallower for the partial agonist. Note also that at lower doses, the partial agonist C is more potent than the full agonist B.

context, referring to any drug (including nonopioids such as cocaine) that can produce dependence, the term narcotic is not useful in a pharmacologic or clinical context.

In its broadest sense, the term *opioid* can refer to agonists, partial agonists, mixed agonist–antagonists, and competitive antagonists. Differentiation of these terms requires understanding of receptor-ligand interactions. Receptor theory states that drugs have two independent characteristics at receptor sites: *affinity*, the ability to bind a receptor to produce a stable complex, and intrinsic activity or *efficacy*, which is described by the dose-effect curve resulting from the drug–receptor combination. Efficacy can range from zero (i.e., no effect) to the maximum possible effect, depicted graphically as the plateau of the dose-effect curve (Fig. 19-1). Given a high enough dose, an *agonist* will produce the maximum possible effect of binding with the receptor, whereas an *antagonist* produces no direct effect when it binds the receptor. A *partial agonist* has a dose-effect ceiling that is lower than the maximum possible effect produced by a full agonist, as well as a dose-effect curve that is less steep than that of a full agonist. A *mixed agonist–antagonist* acts as an agonist (or partial agonist) at one receptor and an antagonist at another. It is important to differentiate the term *potency* from efficacy. Whereas efficacy defines the range in magnitude of an effect produced by a drug-receptor combination relative to the maximum possible effect, potency refers to the relative dose required to achieve an effect, and is related to receptor affinity. Thus, at the lower end of the effect range, a partial agonist may be more potent than a full agonist (Fig. 19-1). However, even at very large doses the efficacy, or maximum effect achieved by the partial agonist, will be less than the maximum possible effect of a full agonist.

ENDOGENOUS OPIOIDS AND OPIOID RECEPTORS

All of the endogenous opioids are derived from three prohormones: proenkephalin, prodynorphin, and pro-opiomelanocortin (POMC). Each of these precursors is encoded by a separate gene. The three families of peptides differ in their distribution, receptor selectivity, and neurochemical role,[5] but share some features. For example, all begin with the pentapeptide sequences of [Leu]- or [Met]-enkephalin. Proenkephalin includes the pentapeptide sequences for [Met]- and [Leu]-enkephalin, and cells that synthesize proenkephalin are widely distributed throughout the brain, spinal cord, and peripheral sites, particularly the adrenal medulla.[6] Pro-opiomelanocortin is the common precursor of β-endorphin, adrenocorticotropic hormone (ACTH), and melanocyte-stimulating hormone. The term *endorphin* is reserved for peptides of the POMC family. The major site of POMC synthesis is the pituitary, but it is also found in the pancreas and placenta. The dynorphin peptides all begin with the [Leu]-enkephalin sequence and are widely distributed throughout the brain, spinal cord, and peripheral sites.

Endogenous opioids bind to a number of opioid receptors to produce their effects. The initial classification by Martin[4] of opioid receptors into the three types was based on binding activity of the exogenous ligands morphine, ketocyclazocine, and SKF10,047 at mu (μ), kappa (κ), and sigma (σ) receptors, respectively. Other opioid receptors identified since that time are delta (δ) receptors, bound by enkephalins, and epsilon (ε) receptors, bound by endorphin.[5,6] There is also evidence supporting the existence of two μ, two δ, and three κ receptor subtypes.[7] Increasing evidence supports a third μ receptor subtype, present on human vascular tissues and leukocytes.[8] While it appears that specific opioid receptors are responsible for different opioid effects and that synthetic opioids may be highly selective for a receptor type or subtype, it is important to note that very few endogenous opioids exhibit great selectivity for a single receptor type.[9]

Remember also, that the theory of receptor dualism includes the concept of pharmacologic redundancy of receptor function. Thus, observed opioid effects typically involve complex interactions among the different receptor systems at supraspinal, spinal, and peripheral sites. The expression of endogenous opioids and opioid receptors is not a static phenomenon. For example, acute inflammation has been shown to up-regulate the expression of both β-endorphin and met-enkephalin as well as peripheral μ- and δ-opioid receptors.[10,11] Conversely, chronic inflammation is associated with down-regulation of μ-opioid receptors.[12] μ-opioid receptor expression was also decreased in the dorsal root ganglia in a nerve injury model of neuropathic pain.[13] Table 19-1 summarizes our current understanding of which opioid receptors are responsible for mediating opioid analgesic and side effects. One caveat in interpreting this summary is that species differences in opioid receptor systems exist, so the results of animal studies, from which most of this information is derived, may not always be directly applicable to humans. Most opioids used in clinical anesthesia today (e.g., fentanyl, morphine, and their derivatives) are highly selective for μ-opioid receptors. Naloxone, the most commonly used opioid antagonist, is not selective for opioid receptor type. In fact, current identification of an opioid-receptor–mediated drug effect requires demonstration of naloxone reversibility. Development of selective

TABLE 19-1

TENTATIVE CLASSIFICATION OF OPIOID RECEPTOR SUBTYPES AND THEIR ACTIONS

■ RECEPTOR	■ ANALGESIA	■ RESPIRATORY	■ GASTROINTESTINAL	■ ENDOCRINE	■ OTHER
μ	Peripheral	—	↓ Gastric secretion ↓ GI transit—supraspinal and peripheral Antidiarrheal	—	Pruritus Skeletal muscle rigidity ?Urinary retention (and/or δ) Biliary spasm (probably >1 receptor type)
μ_1	Supraspinal	—	—	Prolactin release	Acetylcholine turnover Catalepsy
μ_2	Spinal and supraspinal (synergism with spinal)	Respiratory depression	↓ GI transit—spinal and supraspinal	—	Most cardiovascular effects
μ_3	—	—	—	—	Anti-inflammatory
κ	Peripheral	—	—	↓ ADH release	Sedation
κ_1	Spinal	—	—	—	Antipruritic
κ_2	?	—	—	—	(Pharmacology unknown)
κ_3	Supraspinal	—	—	—	
δ	Peripheral	?Respiratory depression	↓ GI transit—spinal Antidiarrheal—spinal and supraspinal	?Growth hormone release	?Urinary retention (and/or μ)
δ_1	Spinal	—	—	—	Dopamine turnover
δ_2	Supraspinal	—	—	—	
Unknown (receptor type not identified)	Supraspinal	—	—	—	Pupillary constriction Nausea and vomiting

GI, gastrointestinal; ADH, antidiuretic hormone.
Adapted from Pasternak GW: Pharmacological mechanisms of opioid analgesics. Clin Neuropharmacol 1993; 16: 1.

opioid receptor subtype antagonists, such as naltrindole (a δ-opioid receptor antagonist) and nor-binaltorphimine (a κ-opioid receptor antagonist) are currently improving our understanding of which receptor subtypes mediate specific opioid effects.

At the cellular level, endogenous and exogenous opioids produce their effects by altering patterns of interneuronal communication. Receptor binding initiates a series of physiologic functions resulting in cellular hyperpolarization and inhibition of neurotransmitter release, effects that are mediated by second messengers. All opioid receptors appear to be coupled to G proteins,[5] which regulate the activity of adenylate cyclase among other functions. G protein interactions, in turn, affect ion channels; different ion conductances may be involved at different opioid receptor types.[9]

STRUCTURE–ACTIVITY RELATIONSHIPS

The wide array of different molecules that produce morphine-like analgesia and side effects, including endogenous opioids, all share some common structural characteristics. Horn and Rodgers[7] suggested that the tyrosine moiety at the amino terminal of the enkephalins formed the basis of a significant conformational relationship between the enkephalins and opiates. The structure of the phenanthrene class of opium alkaloids is complex and consists of five or six fused rings. Morphine, one of three phenanthrenes, has a rigid five-ring structure that conforms to a "T" shape (Fig. 19-2).[14] The other phenanthrenes are codeine, a derivative of morphine, and thebaine, a precursor of oxycodone and naloxone. Progressively reducing the number of fused rings from the phenanthrenes yields the morphinans, with four rings; the benzomorphans, with three rings; the phenylpiperidines, with two rings; and finally, the tyramine moiety of the endogenous opioid peptides, with a single hydroxylated ring. All of these distinct classes of drugs possess morphinelike activity. The opiate receptor model of Thorpe[14] is based on these structural similarities with two aromatic binding sites and one anionic site responsible for binding the positively charged nitrogen. In this model, differences in binding at the aromatic or anionic sites could account for receptor specificity or for agonist versus antagonist activity. Structural modifications alter such important properties as opioid receptor affinity, agonist versus antagonist activity, resistance to metabolic breakdown, lipid solubility, and pharmacokinetics.[1]

PHARMACOKINETICS AND PHARMACODYNAMICS

Opioid effects are initiated by the combination of an opioid with one or more receptors at specific tissue sites. The relationship between opioid dose and effects depends on both pharmacokinetic and pharmacodynamic variables. *Pharmacokinetics* determines the relationship between drug dose and its concentration at the effect site(s). *Pharmacodynamic* variables relate the concentration of a drug at its site of action, in this case opioid receptors in the brain and other tissues, and the intensity of its effects. Pharmacokinetics generally refers to the study of blood or plasma drug concentration versus time because blood is easy to sample, bears a definable relationship to tissue concentration, and is the medium by which drugs are distributed throughout the body. Changes in drug concentration over time in the blood, at the effect site and at other sites, are determined by physicochemical properties of the drug as well as the processes of absorption, redistribution, biotransformation, and elimination.

In clinical anesthesia practice, opioids are typically administered intravenously. After an intravenous (IV) bolus dose or brief infusion, peak plasma opioid concentrations occur within minutes. Plasma drug concentrations then fall rapidly as the drug is distributed to extravascular sites, including sites of action, noneliminating tissues, and eliminating organs. Compartmental models describe the time course of change in plasma concentration; typically, opioids used in anesthesia are characterized by two- or three-compartment models (see Chapter 7). The early rapid decline in plasma concentration after the peak is called the *distribution phase*, and the subsequent slower decline is the *elimination phase*. From a mathematical curve fitted to measured plasma concentration versus time data, distribution and elimination half-lives, systemic

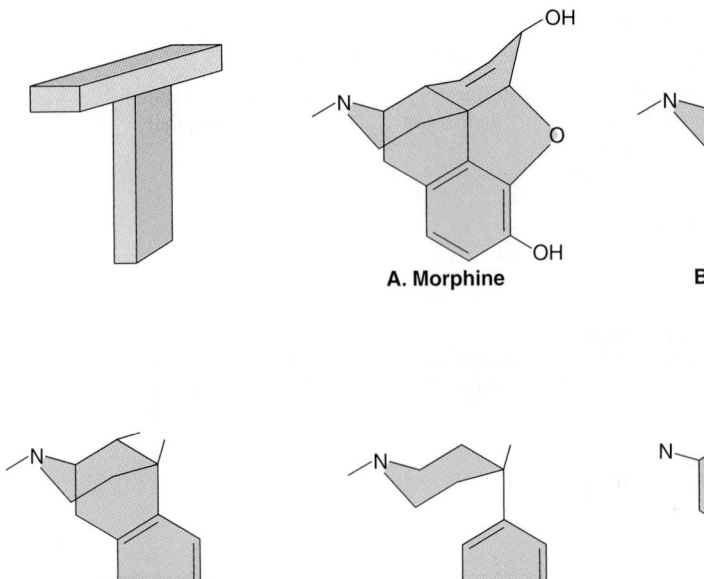

FIGURE 19-2. "T"-shape conformation of opioid molecules. **A.** Morphine, one of the phenanthrene alkaloids, has a rigid five-ring structure, with a phenylpiperidine ring forming a crossbar and a hydroxylated aromatic ring in the vertical axis. **B.** Reducing the number of fused rings to four yields the morphinan class of opium alkaloids. **C.** Benzomorphans have three fused rings. **D.** Phenylpiperidines and the 4-anilinopiperidines such as fentanyl have a flexible two-ring structure. **E.** Finally, the tyramine moiety, which is the amino terminal peptide of both [Leu]- and [Met]-enkephalin, is shown, with a single aromatic ring. Another key feature is the positively charged basic nitrogen equidistant (4.55 Å) from the aromatic ring. (Adapted with permission from Thorpe DH: Opiate structures and activity: A guide to understanding the receptor. Anesth Analg 1984; 63: 143.)

A. Morphine

B. Morphinans

C. Benzomorphans

D. Phenylpiperidines

E. Tyramine Moiety

TABLE 19-2

PHYSICOCHEMICAL CHARACTERISTICS AND PHARMACOKINETICS OF COMMONLY USED OPIOID AGONISTS IN ADULTS

PARAMETER	MORPHINE	MEPERIDINE	FENTANYL	SUFENTANIL	ALFENTANIL	REMIFENTANIL
pKa	7.9	8.5	8.4	8.0	6.5	7.26[a]
% Nonionized (pH 7.4)	23	7	8.5	20	89	58[a]
λ_{ow}	1.4	39	816	1,757	128	17.9[b]
Protein binding (%)	35	70	84	93	92	66–93[a]
Clearance (mL/min)	1,050	1,020	1,530	900	238	4,000
Vd_{ss} (L)	224	305	335	123	27	30
Rapid distribution half-life ($T_{1/2}\pi$, min)	—	—	1.2–1.9	1.4	1.0–3.5	0.4–0.5
Slow redistribution half-life ($T_{1/2}\pi$, min)	1.5–4.4	4–16	9.2–19	17.7	9.5–17	2.0–3.7
Elimination half-life ($T_{1/2}\beta$, h)	1.7–3.3	3–5	3.1–6.6	2.2–4.6	1.4–1.5	0.17–0.33

λ_{ow}, octanol: water partition coefficient; Vd_{ss}, steady-state volume of distribution.
[a]Unpublished information from Glaxo. J. G. Bovill, personal communication, 1995.
[b]Glass PSA, et al: Anesth Analg 1999; 89: S7.
Adapted from Bovill JG: Pharmacokinetics and pharmacodynamics of opioid agonists. Anaesth Pharmacol Rev 1993; 1: 122.

ANESTHETIC AGENTS, ADJUVANTS, AND DRUG INTERACTION

clearance, compartment volumes, and intercompartmental transfer rate constants can be calculated. Table 19-2 summarizes the estimates of key pharmacokinetic parameters and physicochemical characteristics for the most commonly used opioids in clinical anesthesia.

It is important to note that there is tremendous variability in the values published for opioid pharmacokinetic parameters. This is partly because of real population differences (e.g., age, diseases) and partly because of differences in study design (e.g., sampling site, duration, concomitant events such as surgery, or other drugs that may affect differential flow to sites of metabolism or elimination). In addition, the distributional and elimination half-lives are of limited use in predicting the onset and duration of opioid action in clinical anesthesia. Contributions of distribution processes between physiologic compartments vary with time. In an effort to relate pharmacokinetics to the time of onset and duration of action, concepts such as *effect compartment* in pharmacodynamic modeling[15] and *context-sensitive half-times*[16] have been developed. The application of these concepts is considered later in this chapter.

Physicochemical properties of opioids influence both pharmacokinetics and pharmacodynamics. To reach its effector sites in the central nervous system (CNS), an opioid must cross biologic membranes from the blood to receptors on neuronal cell membranes. The ability of opioids to cross this blood–brain barrier depends on such properties as molecular size, ionization, lipid solubility, and protein binding (Table 19-2). Of these characteristics, lipid solubility and ionization assume major importance in determining the rate of penetration to the CNS. In the laboratory, lipid solubility is measured as an octanol: water or octanol: buffer partition coefficient. Drug ionization is also an important determinant of lipid solubility; nonionized drugs are 1,000 to 10,000 times more lipid-soluble than the ionized form.[17] The degree of ionization depends on the pKa of the opioid and the pH of the environment. An opioid with a pKa much lower than 7.4 will have a much greater

nonionized fraction in plasma than one with a pKa close to or greater than physiologic pH. While greater lipid solubility correlates with membrane permeability, the relationship is not simply a linear one. Hansch and Dunn[18] have shown that there is an optimal hydrophobicity for blood–brain barrier penetration, and Bernards and Hill[19] have demonstrated a similar biphasic relationship between the octanol: buffer distribution coefficient and spinal meningeal permeability. Plasma protein binding also affects opioid redistribution because only the unbound fraction is free to diffuse across cell membranes. The major plasma proteins to which opioids bind are albumin and α_1-acid glycoprotein. Alterations in α_1-acid glycoprotein concentration occur in a variety of conditions and disease states and result in acute or chronic changes in opioid requirements.

Two main mechanisms are responsible for drug elimination: *biotransformation* and *excretion*. Opioids are biotransformed in the liver by two types of metabolic processes. Phase I reactions include oxidative and reductive reactions, such as those catalyzed by cytochrome P450 system, and hydrolytic reactions. Phase II reactions involve conjugation of a drug or its metabolite to an endogenous substrate, such as D-glucuronic acid.[17] Remifentanil is metabolized via ester hydrolysis, which is unique for an opioid. With the exceptions of the *N*-dealkylated metabolite of meperidine and the 6- and possibly 3-glucuronides of morphine, opioid metabolites are generally inactive. Opioid metabolites and, to a lesser extent, their parent compounds are excreted primarily by the kidneys. The biliary system and gut are other routes of opioid excretion.

MORPHINE

Morphine produces its major effects in the CNS and the gastrointestinal system, but other systems are also affected. CNS effects include analgesia, sedation, changes in affect, respiratory depression, nausea and vomiting, pruritus, and changes in pupil size. Morphine also affects gastric secretions and gut motility, and has endocrine, urinary, and autonomic effects. It mimics the effects of endogenous opioids by acting as an agonist at μ_1- and μ_2-opioid receptors throughout the body and is considered the standard agonist to which other μ-agonists are compared.

Analgesia

Morphine analgesia results from complex interactions at a number of discrete sites in the brain, spinal cord, and under certain conditions, peripheral tissues, and involves both μ_1 and μ_2 opioid effects. Morphine and related opioids act selectively on neurons that transmit and modulate nociception, leaving other sensory modalities and motor functions intact. At the spinal cord level, morphine acts presynaptically on primary afferent nociceptors to decrease the release of substance P and also hyperpolarizes postsynaptic neurons in the substantia gelatinosa of the dorsal spinal cord to decrease afferent transmission of nociceptive impulses.[20] Spinal morphine analgesia is mediated by μ_2-opioid receptors. Supraspinal opioid analgesia originates in the periaqueductal gray matter, the locus ceruleus, and nuclei within the medulla, notably the nucleus raphe magnus, and primarily involves μ_1-opioid receptors. Microinjections of morphine into any of these regions activate the respective descending modulatory systems to produce profound analgesia.[6,20] Endogenous pain transmission and modulation pathways are discussed in Chapter 58. Morphine can act at a number of these discrete regions in the CNS to produce synergistic analgesic effects. For example, coadministration at the level of the brain and spinal cord increases morphine's analgesic potency nearly tenfold,[21] an effect mediated by μ_2-opioid receptors.[6] There are also synergistic interactions between supraspinal sites of opioid action (e.g., between the periaqueductal gray matter and the nucleus raphe magnus).[6] When acute inflammation is present, morphine may also produce analgesia by activating peripheral opioid receptors.[11,22] In chronic pain conditions such as neuropathic pain or chronic arthritis, spinal and peripheral receptors may be down-regulated, a state that can decrease morphine analgesia.[12,13]

Although rapidly changing plasma morphine concentrations, such as those that follow bolus dosing, do not correlate well with analgesic effects, constant or very slowly changing (i.e., steady-state) plasma concentrations do correlate with effect intensities. The minimum effective analgesic concentration (MEAC) of morphine for postoperative pain relief is 10 to 15 ng/mL.[23] For more severe pain, plasma morphine concentrations of 30 to 50 ng/mL are needed to achieve adequate analgesia.[24]

Effect on Minimum Alveolar Concentration of Volatile Anesthetics

μ-agonists are used extensively in conjunction with inhaled anesthetics to provide "balanced anesthesia." In animals, morphine decreases the minimum alveolar concentration (MAC) of volatile anesthetics in a dose-dependent manner,[25,26] but there appears to be a ceiling effect to the anesthetic-sparing ability of morphine, with a plateau at 65% MAC.[25] Morphine 1 mg/kg administered with 60% nitrous oxide (N_2O) blocks the adrenergic response to skin incision in 50% of patients, a characteristic called *MAC-BAR*.[27] Neuraxial morphine may also reduce MAC. Epidural morphine 4 mg given 90 minutes prior to incision reduces halothane MAC by nearly 30%.[28] The effect of intrathecal morphine on MAC is unclear. In one study, a relatively large dose of intrathecal morphine (750 μg) reduced halothane MAC approximately 40%,[29] but an equally large dose (15 μg/kg) failed to reduce halothane MAC in another.[30]

Other Central Nervous System Effects

Morphine can produce sedation, as well as cognitive and fine motor impairment, even at plasma concentrations commonly achieved during management of moderate to severe pain.[31] Other subjective side effects include euphoria, dysphoria, and sleep disturbances. High doses of morphine and similar opioids produce a slowing of electroencephalogram (EEG) activity associated with a marked shift toward increased voltage and decreased frequency.[1,32] In routine analgesic doses, morphine can produce sleep disturbances, including reduction in rapid eye movement and slow-wave sleep,[1] as well as vivid dreams.

Morphine produces dose-dependent pupillary constriction (miosis).[33] In the absence of other drugs, miosis appears to correlate with opioid-induced ventilatory depression. However, hypoxemia from severe opioid-induced respiratory depression will cause pupillary dilation.

Systemic and neuraxial administration of morphine can produce pruritus, although this symptom is more common with spinal administration.[1] Pruritus appears to be a μ receptor-mediated effect produced at the level of the medullary dorsal horn,[34] although there may also be a direct antipruritic effect mediated by κ receptors.[35] Antihistamines are often used to treat this side effect, but pruritus induced by morphine microinjection into the medullary dorsal horn is not histamine-mediated.[34] Thus, their effectiveness is probably related to nonspecific sedative effects.

Morphine can also affect the release of several pituitary hormones, both directly and indirectly. Inhibition of corticotropin-releasing factor and gonadotropin-releasing hormone decreases circulating concentrations of ACTH, β-endorphin, follicle-stimulating hormone, and luteinizing hormone. Prolactin and growth hormone concentrations may be increased by opioids, and antidiuretic hormone release is inhibited by opioids.[1]

Respiratory Depression

Morphine and other μ agonists produce dose-dependent ventilatory depression primarily by decreasing the responsivity of the medullary respiratory center to CO_2.[33] Standard therapeutic doses of morphine produce a shift to the right and a decrease in slope of the ventilatory response to CO_2 curve, as well as abnormal breathing patterns.[36,37] The respiratory depressant effects of morphine are similar for young and elderly patients,[36,37] but normal sleep markedly potentiates morphine-induced ventilatory depression.[38] Frequent periods of oxygen desaturation associated with obstructive apnea, paradoxic breathing, and slow respiratory rate have been reported in patients receiving morphine infusions for postoperative analgesia, but occurred only when the patients were asleep.[39] Such reports emphasize the need to consider both the expected severity of postoperative pain as well as diurnal variations in pain and opioid sensitivity when including long-acting opioids such as morphine in an anesthetic. Sleep apnea, often seen in association with obesity, increases the risk of morphine-induced respiratory depression. With increasing morphine doses, periodic breathing resembling Cheyne-Stokes breathing, decreased hypoxic ventilatory drive, and apnea can occur.[40] However, even with severe ventilatory depression, patients are usually arousable and will breathe on command.

Cough Reflex

Morphine and related opioids depress the cough reflex, at least in part by a direct effect on the medullary cough center. Doses required to attenuate the cough reflex are smaller than the usual analgesic dosage, and receptors mediating this effect appear to be less stereospecific and less sensitive to naloxone than those responsible for analgesia.[1] Dextroisomers of opioids, which do not produce analgesia, are also effective cough suppressants.[1]

Muscle Rigidity

Large doses of IV morphine (2 mg/kg infused at 10 mg/min) can produce abdominal muscle rigidity and decrease thoracic compliance; this effect plateaus 10 minutes after morphine administration is complete.[41] Subjects receiving smaller doses of IV morphine (10 to 15 mg) also report feelings of muscle tension, most frequently in the neck or legs, but occasionally in the chest wall (unpublished observations). Muscle rigidity is drastically increased by the addition of 70% N_2O.[41] Opioid-induced muscle rigidity appears to be mediated by μ receptors at supraspinal sites.[42] Myoclonus, sometimes resembling seizures, but without EEG evidence of seizure activity, has also been observed with high-dose opioids.[43] In clinical practice, opioid-induced muscle rigidity and myoclonus are most often observed on induction of anesthesia, but have been observed postoperatively[44] and can be severe enough to interfere with manual or mechanical ventilation. These effects are reduced or eliminated by naloxone,[44] drugs that facilitate γ-aminobutyric acid agonist activity (such as thiopental[41] and diazepam), and muscle relaxants.[44]

Nausea and Vomiting

Nausea and vomiting are among the most distressing side effects of morphine and its derivatives. Increased postoperative vomiting is seen with morphine premedication as well as with the use of intraoperative opioids.[45] The incidence of opioid-induced nausea appears to be similar irrespective of the route of administration, including oral, IV, intramuscular, subcutaneous, transmucosal, transdermal, intrathecal, and epidural.[45] Furthermore, laboratory and clinical studies comparing the incidence or severity of nausea and vomiting have found no differences among opioids in equianalgesic doses, including morphine, hydromorphone, meperidine, fentanyl, sufentanil, alfentanil, and remifentanil.[45–48] The physiology and neuropharmacology of opioid-induced nausea and vomiting are complex (Fig. 19-3). The vomiting center receives input from the chemotactic trigger zone (CTZ) in the area postrema of the medulla, the pharynx, gastrointestinal tract, mediastinum, and visual center.[45,49] The CTZ is rich in opioid, dopamine, serotonin, histamine, and (muscarinic) acetylcholine receptors, and also receives input from the vestibular portion of the eighth cranial nerve. Morphine and related opioids induce nausea by direct stimulation of the CTZ and can also produce increased vestibular sensitivity.[1] Therefore, vestibular stimulation such as ambulation markedly increases the nauseant and emetic effects of morphine. This can be especially problematic in outpatient surgery, when early ambulation is a clinical priority. High doses of morphine and other opioids also have naloxone-reversible antiemetic effects at the level of the vomiting center.[50] In volunteer studies, morphine-induced nausea and vomiting increase after a morphine infusion is stopped,[51] which suggests that antiemetic effects are more short-lived than emetic effects. Another possible explanation for this observation is that the active metabolite morphine-6-glucuronide accumulates and worsens nausea. Prophylaxis and treatment of opioid-induced nausea and vomiting includes the use of drugs that act as antagonists at the various receptor sites in the CTZ as well agents such as propofol and benzodiazepines, whose antiemetic mechanisms are unknown.[45]

Gastrointestinal Motility and Secretion

Morphine and other opioids affect gastrointestinal motility and propulsion, as well as gastric and pancreatic secretions via stimulation of opioid receptors in the brain, spinal cord, enteric muscle, and smooth muscle,[40,52] and are mediated by μ-, κ-, and δ-opioid receptors at different anatomic sites.[52] In rodents, μ agonists inhibit gastric secretion, decrease gastrointestinal motility and propulsion, and suppress diarrhea when administered by intracerebroventricular, intrathecal, and peripheral injection.[52] Animal and human studies demonstrate that methylnaltrexone and alvimopan, opioid antagonists that do not cross the blood–brain barrier, attenuate morphine-induced gastrointestinal dysfunction.[53,54] Such studies also suggest that effects such as delayed gastric emptying, ileus, and constipation are mediated primarily by a peripheral opioid mechanism. Morphine decreases lower esophageal sphincter

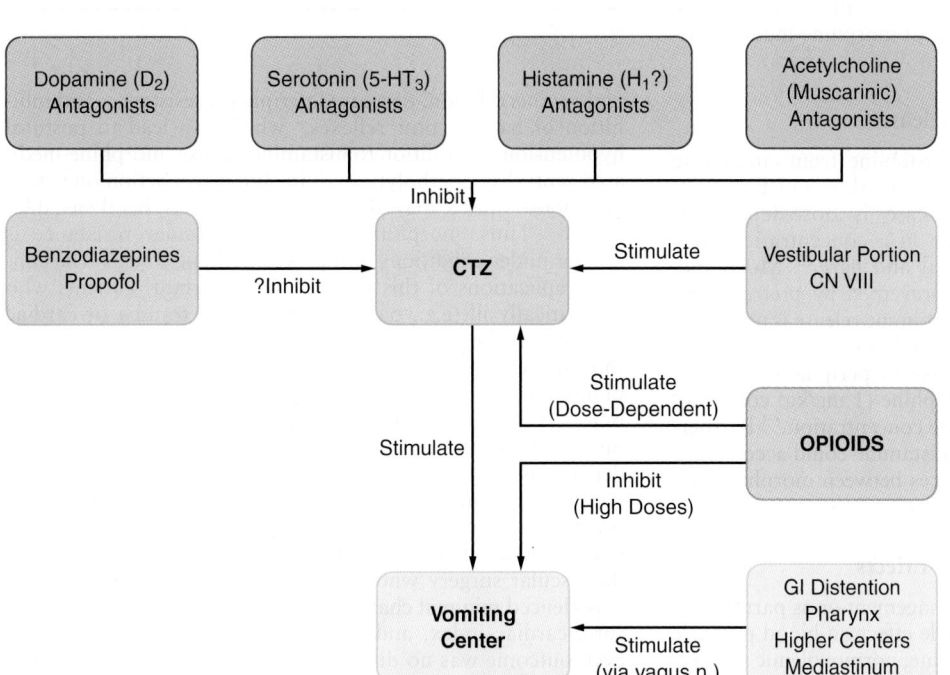

FIGURE 19-3. Pharmacology of nausea and vomiting. The chemotactic trigger zone (CTZ), located in the area postrema of the brainstem, contains dopamine, serotonin, histamine, and muscarinic acetylcholine as well as opioid receptors. The vomiting center receives input from the CTZ as well as peripheral sites via the vagus nerve. As illustrated, the role of opioids is complex, and they appear to have both emetic and antiemetic effects. CN, cranial nerve; GI, gastrointestinal; n., nerve.

ANESTHETIC AGENTS, ADJUVANTS, AND DRUG INTERACTION

tone and produces symptoms of gastroesophageal reflux,[40] and diamorphine significantly slows gastric emptying. Thus, preoperative opioid administration should be considered when evaluating the risk of regurgitation and aspiration of gastric contents in patients who will be anesthetized or sedated. Like other opioid effects, gastrointestinal effects are probably dose-related. Tone in both the small and large bowel is increased, but propulsive activity is decreased, leading to constipation. Epidurally administered morphine can also delay gastric emptying.[55]

Biliary Tract

Morphine and other opioids increase the tone of the common bile duct and sphincter of Oddi. Symptoms accompanying increases in biliary pressure can vary from epigastric distress to typical biliary colic, and may even mimic angina. When produced, biliary spasm can elevate plasma amylase and lipase for up to 24 hours.[1] Morphine and other μ agonists such as fentanyl are used in provocative tests to evaluate sphincter of Oddi dysfunction and biliary-type pain. In volunteers, morphine caused a greater delay in gallbladder emptying[56] and an increase in contractions of the sphincter of Oddi[57] than meperidine. Nitroglycerine, atropine, and naloxone can reverse opioid-induced increases in biliary pressure.[1] It has been suggested that morphine causes biliary tract contraction via histamine release, and antagonism of morphine's biliary effects by diphenhydramine supports this hypothesis.[58]

Genitourinary Effects

Urinary retention, seen after both systemic and spinal morphine administration, is caused by complex effects on central and peripheral neurogenic mechanisms. It results in dyssynergia between the bladder detrusor muscle and the urethral sphincter because of a failure of sphincter relaxation.[1,59] Estimates of the incidence of this bothersome side effect vary widely and are confounded by the effects of anesthesia and surgery on urinary retention, but it is probably more common after spinal administration. Spinal morphine appears to cause naloxone-reversible urinary retention via μ- and/or δ-, but not κ-opioid receptors.[59] In an animal study, cholinomimetic agents and α-adrenergic agonists aggravated morphine-induced high intravesical pressures, and therefore may be harmful agents to use for treatment of morphine-induced urinary retention.[60]

Histamine Release

Opioids stimulate the release of histamine from circulating basophils and from tissue mast cells in skin and lung.[61,62] Morphine-mediated histamine release is dose-dependent; intradermal injection of morphine in a concentration of 1 mg/mL induces an urticarial wheal and flare.[62] Morphine-induced histamine release is not prevented by pretreatment with naloxone,[62] suggesting that histamine release is not mediated by opioid receptors. Morphine-induced histamine release has clinical relevance. The decrease in peripheral vascular resistance seen with high-dose morphine (1 mg/kg) correlates well with elevated plasma histamine concentration.[63] Furthermore, differences in the release of histamine could account for most of the hemodynamic differences between morphine and fentanyl (Fig. 19-4).[63]

Cardiovascular Effects

In doses typically used for pain management or as part of balanced anesthesia, morphine has little effect on blood pressure or heart rate and rhythm in the supine, normovolemic patient. However, higher doses of morphine can produce arteriolar

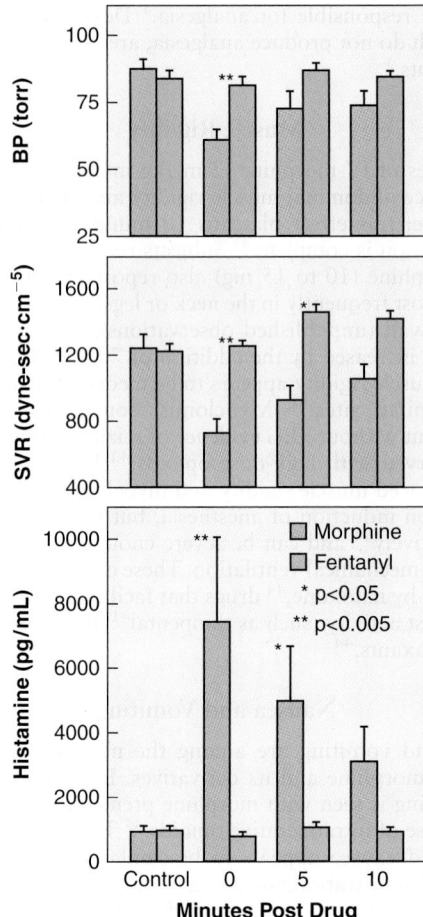

FIGURE 19-4.   Mean arterial pressure (BP), systemic vascular resistance (SVR), and plasma histamine concentration (mean ± SE) before and after morphine 1 mg/kg and fentanyl 50 μg/kg (both infused over 10 minutes). Morphine, but not fentanyl, causes significant decrements in BP and SVR, which parallel the increase in plasma histamine concentration. (Reprinted with permission from Rosow CE, Moss J, Philbin DM, et al: Histamine release during morphine and fentanyl anesthesia. Anesthesiology 1982; 56: 93.)

and venous dilation, decreased peripheral resistance, and inhibition of baroreceptor reflexes,[1] which can lead to postural hypotension. In addition to histamine release, morphine-mediated central sympatholytic activity and direct action on vascular smooth muscle may also contribute to peripheral vasodilation.[64] Thus, morphine's effect on vascular resistance is greater under conditions of high sympathetic tone.[57] The clinical implications of this finding are important. Patients who are critically ill (e.g., patients with severe trauma or cardiac disease) can be expected to have high sympathetic tone, and thus may experience hypotension in response to doses of morphine that would not normally produce hemodynamic instability. At clinically relevant doses, morphine does not suppress myocardial contractility.[1] However, opioids do produce dose-dependent bradycardia, probably by both sympatholytic and parasympathomimetic mechanisms.[65] In clinical anesthesia practice, opioids are often used to prevent tachycardia and reduce myocardial oxygen demand. Patients undergoing cardiovascular surgery who received 1 to 2 mg/kg of morphine experienced minimal changes in heart rate, mean arterial pressure, cardiac index, and systemic vascular resistance. However, outcome was no different from that achieved with carefully administered inhalation-based anesthesia.[65] Morphine's specific ability to reduce systemic inflammation by its action at the μ_3-opioid receptor may benefit patients undergoing cardiopulmonary bypass.[66] Murphy et al.[67] demonstrated that morphine suppresses several components of the inflammatory response to cardiopulmonary bypass. Clinical benefits of morphine 40 mg, given prior to cardioplegia, include better recovery of global ventricular function and prevention of postoperative hypothermia.[68]

Morphine does not directly affect cerebral circulation, but with morphine-induced respiratory depression, CO_2 retention causes cerebral vasodilation and an elevation in cerebrospinal fluid pressure. This effect is not seen when mechanical ventilation is used to prevent hypercarbia.[1] Thus, morphine and other μ agonists must be used cautiously in spontaneously breathing patients with head injury or other conditions associated with elevated intracranial pressure.

Disposition Kinetics

Morphine is rapidly absorbed after intramuscular, subcutaneous, and oral administration. Following intramuscular administration, peak plasma concentration is seen at 20 minutes and absorption half-life is estimated at 7.7 minutes (range, 2 to 15 minutes).[69] After IV administration morphine undergoes rapid redistribution, with a mean redistribution half-time between 1.5 and 4.4 minutes in awake and anesthetized adults.[69–71] Morphine has a terminal elimination half-life between 1.7 and 3.3 hours.[70–72] Age affects morphine pharmacokinetics. The average elimination half-life of morphine is 7 to 8 hours in neonates <1 week of age and 3 to 5 hours in older infants.[73] In patients between 61 and 80 years old, morphine's terminal elimination half-life was 4.5 hours compared with 2.9 hours in younger patients.[72]

Morphine is about 35% protein bound, mostly to albumin.[17] Its steady-state volume of distribution is large, with estimates in the range of 3 to 4 L/kg in normal adults.[69–71] Morphine's major metabolic pathway is hepatic phase II conjugation, to form morphine-3-glucuronide (M3G) and morphine-6β-glucuronide (M6G). 3-Glucuronidation is the predominant pathway, and following a single IV dose, 40% and 10% of the dose are excreted in the urine as M3G and M6G, respectively.[74] Unchanged morphine in the urine accounts for only about 10% of the dose. The rate of hepatic clearance of morphine is high, with a hepatic extraction ratio of 0.7.[69] Thus, morphine elimination may be slowed by processes that decrease hepatic blood flow.[71] Extrahepatic sites such as kidney, intestine, and lung have been suggested for morphine glucuronidation, but their importance in humans is unknown.

Active Metabolites

M6G possesses significant μ receptor affinity and potent antinociceptive activity. Appreciable plasma concentrations of M6G and M3G have been measured in cancer patients receiving high doses of oral morphine. During chronic oral morphine therapy, plasma M6G concentrations can be higher than those of the parent morphine compound.[75] Because morphine glucuronides are eliminated by the kidney, it is not surprising that very high M6G-to-morphine ratios have been reported in patients with renal dysfunction. This accumulation of the active metabolite is thought to be responsible for the unusual sensitivity of renal failure patients to morphine. While common wisdom suggests that glucuronide conjugates do not penetrate the blood–brain barrier, M6G concentration in cerebrospinal fluid is 20 to 80% that of morphine.[76] Despite animal literature demonstrating the analgesic potency of M6G, there is little information in humans concerning the magnitude of analgesia and side effects of M6G relative to morphine. Portenoy et al.[76] demonstrated that in cancer patients receiving chronic mor-

phine therapy, pain relief correlated positively with the M6G-to-morphine ratio, suggesting a contributing role of M6G to overall morphine analgesia. In a study of cancer patients who received synthetic M6G (up to 60 μg/kg), 17 of 19 patients experienced effective analgesia and no adverse effects.[77] In contrast, dizziness, nausea, sedation, muscle aches, and respiratory depression have been reported in volunteers who received M6G.[75] However, the role of M6G in acute dosing is unclear because there is a long delay (6 to 8 hours) between the time course of plasma concentration and CNS effects.[78] While the contribution of M6G to morphine-induced analgesia and side effects remains to be determined, morphine should be administered cautiously to patients with renal failure.

Dosage and Administration of Morphine

In current clinical practice morphine is used mainly as a premedicant and for postoperative analgesia, and less often as a component of balanced or high-dose opioid anesthesia. Intravenous analgesic doses of morphine for adults typically range from 0.01 to 0.20 mg/kg. When used in a balanced anesthetic technique with N_2O, morphine can be given in total doses of up to 3 mg/kg with remarkable hemodynamic stability, but awareness under anesthesia is a risk. When combined with other inhalation agents, it is unlikely that more than 1 to 2 mg/kg of morphine is necessary. The morphine dose associated with apparent cardioprotective effect is a single dose of 40 mg, given before cardioplegia and cardiopulmonary bypass.[68] Because of its hydrophilicity, morphine crosses the blood–brain barrier relatively slowly; and while its onset can be observed within 5 minutes, peak effects may be delayed for 10 to 40 minutes. This delay makes morphine more difficult to titrate as an anesthetic supplement than the more rapidly acting opioids.

MEPERIDINE

Meperidine, a phenylpiperidine derivative (Fig. 19-5), was the first totally synthetic opioid. It was initially studied as an anticholinergic agent, but was found to have significant analgesic activity.[1]

Analgesia and Effect on Minimum Alveolar Concentration of Volatile Anesthetics

Meperidine's analgesic potency is about one-tenth that of morphine's and is most likely mediated by μ-opioid receptor activation. However, meperidine also has moderate affinity for κ- and δ-opioid receptors.[1,79] Unlike morphine, meperidine plasma concentrations correlate reasonably well with analgesic effects.[80] Although there is considerable interpatient variability, the MEAC of meperidine is approximately 200 ng/mL. There is very little information available on the effect of meperidine on the MAC of inhaled anesthetics, but a study in dogs demonstrated a dose-dependent reduction in the MAC of halothane.[81]

Meperidine also has well-recognized weak local anesthetic properties. Compared with morphine, fentanyl, and buprenorphine injected perineurally, only meperidine alters nerve conduction and produces analgesia.[82] This has led to some popularity for epidural and subarachnoid administration, particularly in obstetric anesthesia. But because of its local anesthetic effects, neuraxial meperidine may also produce sensory and motor blockade as well as sympatholytic effects that are not seen with other opioids.

Side Effects

Like morphine, therapeutic doses of meperidine can produce sedation, pupillary constriction, and euphoria, and very high

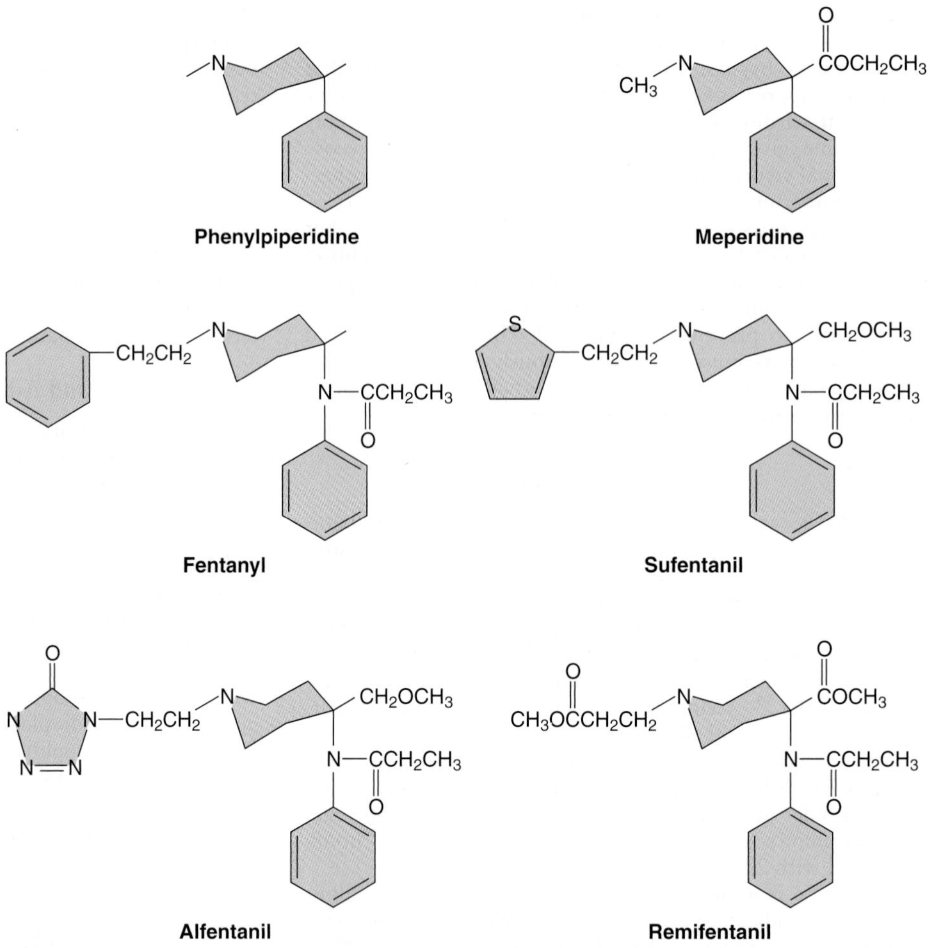

FIGURE 19-5. Chemical structures of phenylpiperidine, meperidine, and the 4-anilinopiperidine derivatives fentanyl, sufentanil, alfentanil, and remifentanil.

Phenylpiperidine

Meperidine

Fentanyl

Sufentanil

Alfentanil

Remifentanil

doses are associated with CNS excitement and seizures (see later discussion). In equianalgesic doses, meperidine produces respiratory depression equal to that of morphine, as well as nausea, vomiting, and dizziness, particularly in ambulatory patients.[1]

Like other opioids, meperidine causes significant delay in gastric emptying. While meperidine does increase common bile duct pressure, this occurs to a lesser extent than with equianalgesic doses of morphine and fentanyl (Fig. 19-6).[56,83]

Analgesic doses of meperidine in awake patients are not associated with hemodynamic instability, but 1 mg/kg in patients with cardiac disease decreased heart rate, cardiac index, and rate–pressure product.[84] In an isolated papillary muscle preparation, high concentrations of meperidine depressed contractility. This effect was not naloxone-reversible and is consistent with a nonspecific, local anesthetic effect.[85] In higher doses, meperidine causes significantly more hemodynamic instability than morphine or fentanyl and its derivatives,[86] an effect at least partially related to histamine release. In a comparison of opioids administered as part of balanced anesthesia, Flacke et al.[86] found that 25% patients in the meperidine group experienced severe hypotension and had abnormally elevated plasma histamine concentrations. Interestingly, only one patient in the morphine group (0.6 mg/kg morphine given) had a similar histamine plasma concentration. Thus, meperidine is not recommended in high doses for clinical anesthesia.

Shivering

Meperidine is effective in reducing shivering from diverse causes, including general and epidural anesthesia, fever,

hypothermia, transfusion reactions, and administration of amphotericin B. Meperidine reduces or eliminates visible shivering as well as the accompanying increase in oxygen consumption[87] following general and epidural anesthesia. Equianalgesic doses of fentanyl (25 μg) and morphine (2.5 mg) did not reduce postoperative shivering, suggesting that the antishivering effect of meperidine is not mediated by μ-opioid receptors. This effect may be mediated by κ-opioid receptors. Butorphanol, a drug with significant κ agonist activity, effectively reduces postoperative shivering in a dose of 1 mg.[88] Furthermore, low doses of naloxone, sufficient to block μ receptors, did not reverse the antishivering effect of meperidine, but high-dose naloxone, designed to block both μ and κ receptors, did reverse the antishivering effect.[79] The observation that other types of drugs, such as α_1-adrenergic agonists (clonidine 1.5 μg/kg), serotonin antagonists,[89] and propofol,[90] can reduce postoperative shivering suggests that a nonopioid mechanism may be involved. Physostigmine 0.04 mg/kg can also prevent postoperative shivering, suggesting a role for the cholinergic system.[91]

Disposition Kinetics

Following IV administration, meperidine plasma concentration falls rapidly. Meperidine's redistribution half-life is 4 to 16 minutes, and its terminal elimination half-life is between 3 and 5 hours.[92,93] The elimination half-life is not prolonged in elderly patients; however, in neonates and infants, the median elimination half-life is 8 to 10 hours, with greater individual variability (three- to fivefold) compared with adults.

Meperidine is moderately lipid soluble, and is 40 to 70% protein bound, mostly to albumin and α_1-acid glycoprotein

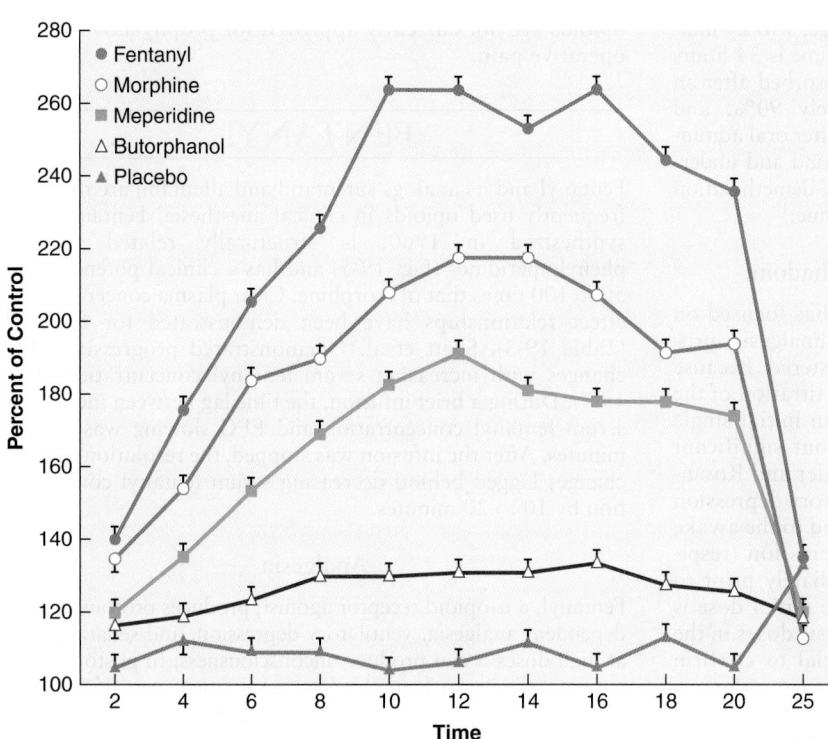

FIGURE 19-6. The effect of several opioids on common bile duct pressures in patients anesthetized with enflurane and N_2O-O_2. Patients received either fentanyl 100 μg/70 kg, morphine 10 mg/70 kg, meperidine 75 mg/70 kg, or butorphanol 2 mg/70 kg. After 20 minutes, the effects were reversed with naloxone. (Reprinted with permission from Radnay PA, Duncalf D, Novakovik M, et al: Common bile duct pressure changes after fentanyl, morphine, meperidine, butorphanol, and naloxone. Anesth Analg 1984; 63: 441.)

(Table 19-2).[94] Meperidine has a large steady-state volume of distribution, with estimates in the range of 3.5 to 5 L/kg in adults.[92,93] The high clearance rate (10 mL/kg/min) reflects a high hepatic extraction ratio; it is N-demethylated in the liver to form normeperidine, the principal metabolite, and also hydrolyzed to meperidinic acid. Both metabolites may then be conjugated[1] and excreted renally. Normeperidine is pharmacologically active and potentially toxic (see later discussion).

Active Metabolites

Normeperidine has appreciable pharmacologic activity and can produce signs of CNS excitation. Mood alterations such as apprehension and restlessness, as well as neurotoxic effects such as tremors, myoclonus, and seizures, have been reported.[95] The elimination half-life of the metabolite normeperidine (14 to 21 hours) is considerably longer than the parent compound, and therefore is likely to accumulate with repeated or prolonged administration, particularly in patients with renal dysfunction.[95] Myoclonus and seizures have been reported in patients receiving meperidine for postoperative or chronic pain. Patients who developed seizures had a mean plasma normeperidine concentration of 0.81 μg/mL.[95] It appears that a total daily meperidine dosage of 1,000 mg is associated with an increased risk of seizures, even in patients without renal dysfunction.

Dosage and Administration of Meperidine

A single dose of meperidine is approximately one-tenth as potent as morphine when given parenterally, but has a shorter duration of action. Intravenous analgesic doses of meperidine for adults typically range from 0.1 to 1 mg/kg. Intravenous doses of 12.5 to 50 mg are effective in reducing postoperative shivering. As discussed earlier, high doses of meperidine for intraoperative use are not recommended because of hemodynamic instability. In addition, large single doses or prolonged administration may produce seizures because of the metabolite normeperidine; the total daily dose should not exceed 1,000 mg in 24 hours.

METHADONE

Methadone, a synthetic opioid introduced in the 1940s, is primarily a μ agonist with pharmacologic properties that are similar to morphine. Although its chemical structure is very different from that of morphine, steric factors force the molecule to simulate the pseudopiperidine ring conformation that appears to be required for opioid activity.[1] Because of its long elimination half-life, methadone is most often used for long-term pain management and for treatment of opioid abstinence syndromes.

Analgesia and Use in Anesthesia

Following parenteral administration, the onset of analgesia is rapid, within 10 to 20 minutes. After single doses of up to 10 mg, the duration of analgesia is similar to morphine,[1] but with large or repeated parenteral doses, prolonged analgesia can be obtained. Several investigators have administered methadone intra- and postoperatively with the aim of providing prolonged postoperative analgesia. Patients who received 20 mg methadone intraoperatively and up to 20 mg additional methadone in the immediate postoperative period had a median duration of postoperative analgesia of over 20 hours.[96,97]

Side Effects

Side effects of methadone are similar in magnitude and frequency to those of morphine.[1,96] Patients who received 20 mg methadone at the beginning of surgery were sedated in the immediate postoperative period but did not appear to have clinically significant respiratory depression. About 50% experienced nausea or vomiting, which was easily treated with standard antiemetic therapy.[96] Methadone produces typical opioid effects on smooth muscle. Like morphine, it markedly decreases intestinal propulsive activity and can cause constipation as well as biliary spasm.[1]

Disposition Kinetics

Following an IV dose, the plasma concentration–time data for methadone are described by a biexponential equation. The mean redistribution half-time is 6 minutes (range, 1 to 24 minutes), and the mean terminal elimination half-time is 34 hours (range, 9 to 87 hours).[97] Methadone is well absorbed after an oral dose, with bioavailability approximately 90%, and reaches peak plasma concentration at 4 hours after oral administration.[1] It is nearly 90% plasma protein bound and undergoes extensive metabolism in the liver, mostly N-demethylation and cyclization to form pyrrolidines and pyrroline.[1]

Dosage and Administration of Methadone

The use of methadone in clinical anesthesia has focused on attempts to achieve prolonged postoperative analgesia, providing that an adequate initial dose is administered. Because adverse effects can also be prolonged, careful titration of the dose is necessary. In opioid-naïve patients, an initial single dose of 20 mg can provide analgesia without significant postoperative respiratory depression.[96] Wangler and Rosenblatt[98] described a technique to avoid respiratory depression in which 8 to 12 mg methadone is administered to the awake patient until the threshold of respiratory depression (respiratory rate of 6 to 8/min) is reached. Immediately prior to incision, an additional dose equal to half the initial dose is given. For administering supplemental analgesic doses in the immediate postoperative period, it is essential to confirm that patients with ongoing significant pain have no depression of respiration or level of consciousness, and that a 30- to 40-minute interval should elapse between 5-mg doses to allow full assessment of adverse effects. It may be easier and safer to use a sustained-release opioid preparation (containing oxycodone or morphine) with a shorter time to peak effect if a long-acting analgesic is desired. This is most easily accomplished by administering the oral medication preoperatively, but it is also important to note that these long-acting opioids are not currently approved for prophylaxis of postoperative pain.

FENTANYL

Fentanyl and its analogs sufentanil and alfentanil are the most frequently used opioids in clinical anesthesia. Fentanyl, first synthesized in 1960, is structurally related to the phenylpiperidines (Fig. 19-5) and has a clinical potency ratio 50 to 100 times that of morphine. Clear plasma concentration-effect relationships have been demonstrated for fentanyl (Table 19-3). Scott et al.[99] demonstrated progressive EEG changes with increasing serum fentanyl concentration (Fig. 19-7). During a brief infusion, the time lag between increasing serum fentanyl concentration and EEG slowing was 3 to 5 minutes. After the infusion was stopped, the resolution of EEG changes lagged behind decreasing serum fentanyl concentration by 10 to 20 minutes.

Analgesia

Fentanyl, a μ-opioid receptor agonist, produces profound dose-dependent analgesia, ventilatory depression, and sedation, and at high doses it can produce unconsciousness. In postoperative patients, the mean fentanyl dose requirement was 55.8 μg/hr, and mean MEAC in blood was 0.63 ng/mL.[100] A large interpatient variability in MEAC (0.23 to 1.18 ng/mL) typical of opioids was observed, but over the 2-day study period, the MEAC for any individual patient remained relatively constant. In volunteers, a mean plasma fentanyl concentration of 1.3 ng/mL reduced experimental pain intensity ratings by 50%,[46] consistent with other estimates of plasma fentanyl concentrations producing moderate-to-strong analgesia.[101]

TABLE 19-3

PLASMA CONCENTRATION RANGES (ng/ml) FOR VARIOUS THERAPEUTIC AND NONTHERAPEUTIC OPIOID EFFECTS[a]

EFFECT	MORPHINE	MEPERIDINE	FENTANYL	SUFENTANIL	ALFENTANIL	REMIFENTANIL
MEAC	10–15	200	0.6	0.03	15	—
Moderate-to-strong analgesia	20–50	400–600	1.5–5	0.05–0.10	40–80	—
50% MAC reduction	NA	>500	0.5–2	0.145	200	1.3
Surgical analgesia with ~70% N₂O	NA	NA	15–25	NA	300–500	4–7.5
Respiratory depression threshold	25	200	1	0.02–0.04	50–100	—
50% ↓ ventilatory response to CO₂	50	NA	1.5–3	0.04	120–350	0.9–1.2
Apnea	NA	NA	7–22	NA	300–600	—
Unconsciousness (not reliably achieved with opioids alone)	—	(Seizures)	15–20	NA	500–1500	—

[a]Effects were generally achieved during continuous infusions or patient-controlled analgesia systems. Note that plasma concentrations associated with measurable depression of ventilatory drive are similar to those associated with analgesia for all opioids.
MEAC, minimum effective analgesic concentration, defined in most studies as the plasma opioid concentration associated with just perceptible analgesia; MAC, minimum alveolar concentration; NA, information not available.

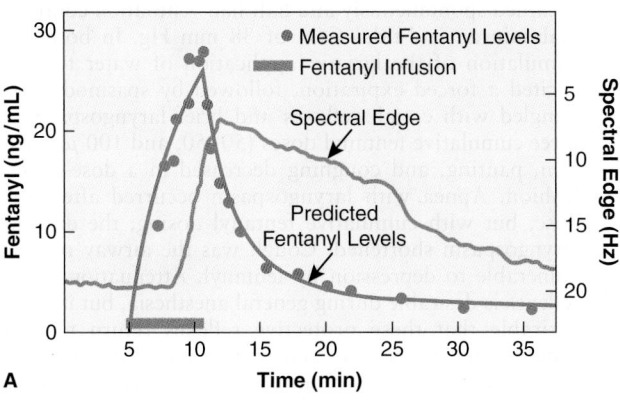
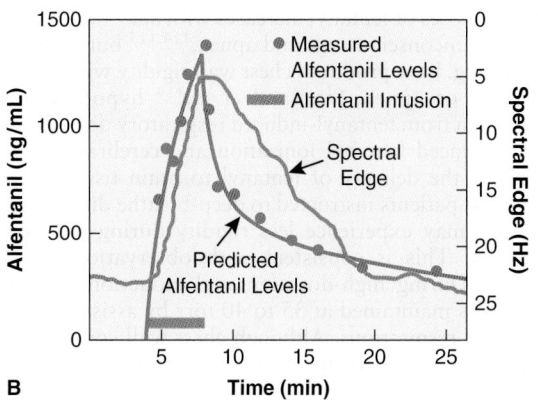

FIGURE 19-7. The time course of electroencephalogram (EEG) spectral edge and serum concentrations of fentanyl (**A**) and alfentanil (**B**). Infusion rates were 150 μg/min fentanyl and 1,500 μg/min alfentanil. Increasing opioid effect is seen as a decrease in spectral edge. Changes in spectral edge follow serum concentrations more closely with alfentanil than with fentanyl. (Reprinted with permission from Scott JC, Ponganis KV, Stanski DR: EEG quantitation of narcotic effect: The comparative pharmacodynamics of fentanyl and alfentanil. Anesthesiology 1985; 62: 234.)

Use in Anesthesia

Fentanyl reduces the MAC of volatile anesthetics in a concentration- or dose-dependent fashion. A single IV bolus dose of fentanyl 3 μg/kg, given 25 to 30 minutes prior to incision, reduced both isoflurane and desflurane MAC by approximately 50%.[102] Fentanyl 1.5 μg/kg administered 5 minutes prior to skin incision reduces the minimum alveolar concentration that blocks adrenergic responses to stimuli (MAC-BAR) of isoflurane or desflurane in 60% N_2O by 60 to 70%.[103] No further drop is seen with an increase in fentanyl dose to 3 μg/kg. During constant plasma concentration of 0.5 to 1.7 ng/mL, fentanyl reduced isoflurane MAC by 50%.[104] Fentanyl produces a steep plasma concentration-related reduction in sevoflurane MAC[105]; 3 ng/mL provides a 59% reduction, but a ceiling effect is reached, such that a threefold increase to 10 ng/mL reduced MAC by only an additional 17%.

Epidural fentanyl also reduces inhaled anesthetic requirements.[106] Epidural fentanyl 1, 2, and 4 μg/kg reduced halothane MAC by 45, 58, and 71%, respectively, while the same doses of fentanyl given IV reduced halothane MAC to a lesser extent, by 8, 40, and 49%, respectively.

Combining opioids with propofol rather than an inhalation agent is a technique for providing general anesthesia, referred to as *total intravenous anesthesia* or TIVA. For an IV anesthetic, the potency index is described as the plasma concentration required to prevent a response in 50% (CP$_{50}$) or 95% (CP$_{95}$) of patients to various surgical stimuli. Plasma concentrations of fentanyl and propofol that reduce hemodynamic or somatic responses to various surgical stimuli in 50% of patients have been determined using computer-assisted infusion.[107] Fentanyl plasma concentrations of 1.2, 1.8, and 2.8 ng/mL were required for 50% reductions in propofol's CP$_{50}$s for skin incision, peritoneal incision, and abdominal retraction, respectively. Greater fentanyl concentrations were required to suppress hemodynamic responses to these same stimuli. Thus, fentanyl reduces requirements for both volatile agents and propofol by a similar proportion.

Computer-assisted infusion of fentanyl has been included as a component of a balanced anesthetic technique.[108,109] In combination with 50 to 70% N_2O in oxygen, loss of consciousness, and absence of response to skin incision are achieved at plasma fentanyl concentrations of 15 to 25 ng/mL and >3.7 ng/mL, respectively. Intraoperative concentration requirements varied between 1 and 9 ng/mL. Spontaneous

ventilation returned when the fentanyl concentration dropped to 1.5 to 2 ng/mL.[108,109]

Fentanyl has been used as the sole agent for anesthesia, a technique that requires a large initial dose of 50 to 150 μg/kg or stable plasma fentanyl concentrations in the range of 20 to 30 ng/mL.[101] The major advantage of this technique is reliable hemodynamic stability. High doses of fentanyl significantly blunt the "stress response"—that is, hemodynamic and hormonal responses to surgical stimuli—while producing only minimal cardiovascular depression. Thus, the technique is sometimes referred to as *stress-free anesthesia*. There are also disadvantages to using high-dose fentanyl as the sole anesthetic agent. It precludes early extubation and "fast-track" techniques because of prolonged respiratory depression accompanying high-dose fentanyl. Furthermore, it appears that no dose of fentanyl will completely block hemodynamic or hormonal responses in all patients.[110] Finally, there have been reports of intraoperative awareness and recall in patients who received very high doses (>50 μg/kg) of fentanyl. Because opioids do not produce muscle relaxation, and high-dose fentanyl can produce muscle rigidity, a muscle relaxant is generally required to achieve adequate surgical conditions. This can potentially increase the difficulty in detecting signs of intraoperative awareness.

Other Central Nervous System Effects

The effects of fentanyl on cerebral blood flow and intracranial pressure (ICP) have been studied in patients with and without neurologic disease. An induction dose of 16 μg/kg increased middle cerebral artery flow by 25% in normal patients having noncranial neurosurgery.[111] A smaller dose (3 μg/kg) resulted in an elevation in ICP in ventilated patients with head trauma,[112] but in brain tumor patients, a dose of 5 μg/kg of fentanyl with N_2O–O_2 did not result in elevated ICP.[113] In all cases of elevation in ICP and cerebral blood flow, there were decreases in mean arterial pressure, which may have contributed to these changes.

The muscle rigidity often seen on induction with high-dose fentanyl and its derivatives may make it difficult or impossible to ventilate the patient. In a study in normal volunteers, 1,500 μg fentanyl infused over 10 minutes produced rigidity in 50% of subjects.[114] A similar incidence, 35%, was seen in patients receiving 750 to 1,000 μg fentanyl during induction of general anesthesia, and up to 80% of patients receiving 30 μg/kg developed moderate-to-severe rigidity.[115] Muscle rigidity seen with high doses of fentanyl increases with age[115] and is accompanied by unconsciousness and apnea,[114,115] but lower doses, 7 to 8 μg/kg, have produced chest wall rigidity without unconsciousness or apnea. Streisand et al.[114] hypothesized that hypercarbia from fentanyl-induced respiratory depression may have influenced fentanyl ionization and cerebral blood flow and hence the delivery of fentanyl to brain tissue. It would follow that patients instructed to deep-breathe during fentanyl induction may experience less rigidity during induction of anesthesia. This is consistent with observations by Lunn et al.[116] During high-dose fentanyl induction (75 μg/kg), $PaCO_2$ was maintained at 35 to 40 torr by assisting and then controlling respirations. Although chest wall compliance was reduced in 4 of 18 patients, no patient developed rigidity sufficient to impair ventilation.

Fentanyl has been associated with seizurelike movements during anesthetic induction, which are not associated with seizure activity on the EEG.[117] Such activity may represent myoclonus, a result of opioid-mediated blockade of inhibitory motor pathways of cortical origin, or may represent exaggerations of opioid-induced muscle rigidity.[117] However, fentanyl can activate epileptiform EEG activity in patients having surgery for intractable temporal lobe epilepsy.[118]

Fentanyl-induced pruritus typically presents as facial itching, but can be generalized. Equianalgesic plasma concentrations of fentanyl, morphine, and alfentanil produce equivalent intensity of pruritus.[46] Fentanyl has also been reported to have a tussive effect. The mechanism is unclear, and it is not attenuated by pretreatment with atropine or midazolam.[119]

Respiratory Depression

Fentanyl produces approximately the same degree of ventilatory depression as equianalgesic doses of morphine.[46] Respiratory depression—expressed as an elevation in end-tidal CO_2, a decrease in the slope of the CO_2 response curve, or the minute ventilation at an end-tidal CO_2 of 50 mm Hg (V_E50)—develops rapidly, reaching a peak in ~5 minutes,[99,120,121] and the time course closely follows plasma fentanyl concentration.[120,122] Even at plasma concentrations associated with mild analgesia, ventilatory depression can be detected, and the magnitude of respiratory depression is linearly related to intensity of analgesia (Table 19-3).[46,123] In postoperative patients, plasma fentanyl concentrations of 1.5 to 3.0 ng/mL were associated with a 50% reduction in CO_2 responsiveness.[124]

Fentanyl's respiratory depression is greatly increased when it is given in combination with another respiratory depressant such as midazolam. Bailey et al.[121] determined that midazolam alone (0.05 mg/kg) did not depress ventilation or cause hypoxemia. Fentanyl alone (2 μg/kg) reduced the slope of the CO_2 response curve and the V_E50 by 50%, and 6 of 12 subjects became hypoxemic. Fentanyl and midazolam produced no greater depression of the ventilatory response to CO_2 than fentanyl alone, but 11 of 12 subjects became hypoxemic and 6 of 12 became apneic within 5 minutes. These observations suggest that this frequently used combination blunts the hypoxic ventilatory drive to a greater extent than the hypercarbic ventilatory drive. Precautions such as supplemental oxygen and pulse oximetry monitoring are recommended when such drug combinations are used.

Airway Reflexes

Although obtundation of airway reflexes by general inhalation anesthetics is well described, little is known about the direct effects of opioids on these protective reflexes. Tagaito et al.[125] examined the dose-related effects of fentanyl on airway responses to laryngeal irritation during propofol anesthesia in humans. All patients had laryngeal mask airways; half

breathed spontaneously and half had ventilation controlled to maintain an end-tidal CO_2 of 38 mm Hg. In both groups, stimulation of the larynx (application of water to mucosa) elicited a forced expiration, followed by spasmodic panting mingled with cough reflexes and brief laryngospasm. With three cumulative fentanyl doses (50, 50, and 100 μg), expiration, panting, and coughing decreased in a dose-dependent fashion. Apnea with laryngospasm occurred after the first dose, but with cumulative fentanyl dosing, the duration of laryngospasm shortened. Cough was the airway reflex most vulnerable to depression by fentanyl. Attenuation of airway reflexes is desirable during general anesthesia, but it is equally desirable that these protective reflexes return to baseline rapidly after emergence, and remain intact throughout conscious sedation. Doses required to suppress cough and other reflexes in awake or sedated individuals have not been characterized.

Cardiovascular and Endocrine Effects

Isolated heart muscle models demonstrate concentration-dependent negative inotropic effects of opioids, including morphine, meperidine, and fentanyl.[65] A very high fentanyl concentration (10 μg/mL) reduced contractility by 50%, but 1 μg/mL had no significant effects on papillary muscle mechanics. In clinical practice, even high-dose fentanyl administration (up to 75 μg/kg) produces much lower plasma concentrations, in the range of 50 ng/mL,[116] and is associated with remarkable hemodynamic stability. Patients who received 7 μg/kg fentanyl at induction of anesthesia had a slight decrease in heart rate, but no change in mean arterial pressure compared with control.[86] Fentanyl-induced bradycardia is more marked in anesthetized than conscious subjects, and usually resolves with atropine. With higher fentanyl doses, in the range of 20 to 25 μg/kg, decreases in heart rate, mean arterial pressure, systemic and pulmonary vascular resistance, and pulmonary capillary wedge pressure of approximately 15% were seen in patients with coronary artery disease.[116,126] Very high fentanyl doses, up to 75 μg/kg, produced no further hemodynamic changes. All of these patients had been premedicated with diazepam, pentobarbital, scopolamine, and/or atropine. In unpremedicated patients undergoing noncardiac surgery, induction with fentanyl 30 μg/kg produced no changes in heart rate or systolic blood pressure.[115] Hypertension in response to sternotomy is the most common hemodynamic disturbance during high-dose fentanyl anesthesia and occurs in 40 and 100% in patients receiving 50 to 100 μg/kg.[127] Unlike morphine and meperidine, which induce hypotension, at least in part because of histamine release,[64,128] high-dose fentanyl (50 μg/kg) is not associated with significant histamine release (Fig. 19-4).

Although high doses of fentanyl are associated with minimal cardiovascular changes, combining fentanyl with other drugs can compromise hemodynamic stability. The combination of fentanyl and diazepam produces significant cardiovascular depression.[115,126] Diazepam 10 mg given after 20 to 50 μg/kg of fentanyl decreased stroke volume, cardiac output, systemic vascular resistance, and mean arterial pressure, and increased central venous pressure significantly.[126] Adding 60% N_2O to high-dose fentanyl produced a significant decrease in cardiac output and increases in systemic and pulmonary vascular resistance.[116]

High-dose fentanyl (100 μg/kg) prevented increases in plasma epinephrine, cortisol, glucose, free fatty acids, and growth hormone (the "stress response") during surgery, but a lower dose of fentanyl (5 μg/kg followed by an infusion of 3 μg/kg/h) did not.[129] Unlike morphine, fentanyl does not prevent the inflammatory effects associated with cardiopulmonary bypass, nor does it produce the apparent cardioprotective effects seen with morphine.[67,68]

Smooth Muscle and Gastrointestinal Effects

⓫ Fentanyl, like morphine and meperidine, significantly increases common bile duct pressure (Fig. 19-6).[83] Like other ⓬ opioids, fentanyl can cause nausea and vomiting, particularly in ambulatory patients, and can delay gastric emptying and intestinal transit.

Disposition Kinetics

Fentanyl's extreme lipid solubility (Table 19-2) allows rapid crossing of biologic membranes and uptake by highly perfused tissue groups, including the brain, heart, and lung. Thus, after a single bolus dose, the onset of effects is rapid and the duration brief. Hug and Murphy[130] determined the relationships between fentanyl effects and its concentration over time in plasma and various tissues in rats given fentanyl 50 μg/kg (Fig. 19-8). The onset of opioid effects occurred within 10 seconds and correlated with a rapid increase in brain tissue fentanyl concentration, which equilibrated with plasma by 1.5 minutes. Recovery from fentanyl effects started within 5 minutes and was complete by 60 minutes. Elimination from the "central tissues" (brain, heart, and lung) was also rapid, as fentanyl was redistributed to other tissues, particularly muscle and fat. Peak muscle concentration was seen at 5 minutes, while fat concentration reached a maximum approximately 30 minutes after the dose. The delay in fat uptake despite fentanyl's high lipid solubility is because of the limited blood supply to that tissue. Thus, redistribution to muscle and fat limits the duration of a bolus dose of fentanyl, and accumulation in peripheral tissue compartments can be extensive because of the large mass of muscle and high affinity of fentanyl for fat. With prolonged administration of fentanyl, fat can act as a reservoir of drug.

Fentanyl pharmacokinetics has been studied in awake and anesthetized individuals. After an IV dose, plasma fentanyl concentration falls rapidly, and the concentration-time curve has been described by both two- and three-compartment models.[130] McClain and Hug[120] administered fentanyl 3.2 or 6.4 μg/kg to healthy male volunteers and found that nearly 99% of the dose was eliminated from plasma by 60 minutes. These investigators found both rapid and slower distribution phases,

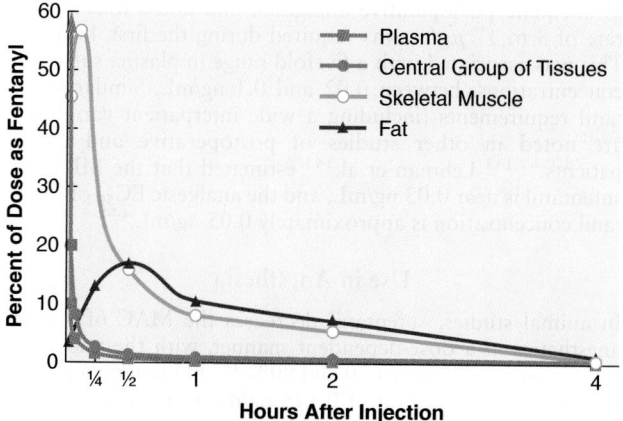

FIGURE 19-8.　Fentanyl uptake and elimination in various tissues of the rat following intravenous injection. Unchanged fentanyl tissue concentrations (means for six rats) are expressed as percentage of dose. "Central" represents the combined content of brain, heart, and lung tissues. The large mass of muscle (50% body weight of the rat) and high affinity of fat for fentanyl (despite slow equilibration) serve as a drain on the central compartment. (Reprinted with permission from Hug CC, Murphy MR: Tissue redistribution of fentanyl in terms of its effects in rats. Anesthesiology 1981; 55: 369.)

with half-times of 1.2 to 1.9 minutes and 9.2 to 19 minutes, respectively. The terminal elimination half-time ranged from 3.1 to 6.6 hours, somewhat longer than that for morphine. Similar values were noted in surgical patients <50 years old,[113,131] including morbidly obese patients.[113] Reports of age effects on fentanyl kinetics are conflicting. The fentanyl requirement decreases with increasing age (20 to 89 years), but pharmacokinetic parameters do not change.[132] In contrast, Bentley et al.[131] observed a marked decrease in clearance and an increase in terminal elimination half-time to approximately 15 hours in patients >60 years old compared with 4.4 hours in patients <50 years old.

Unlike its derivatives, fentanyl is significantly bound to red blood cells, approximately 40%, and has a blood: plasma partition coefficient of approximately 1.[133] Plasma fentanyl is highly protein bound, with estimates in the range of 79 to 87%. It binds avidly to α_1-acid glycoprotein but also binds to albumin.[133,134] Fentanyl protein binding is pH-dependent, such that a decrease in pH will increase the proportion of fentanyl that is unbound.[133] Thus, a patient with respiratory acidosis will have a higher proportion of unbound (active) fentanyl, which could exacerbate respiratory depression. Clearance of fentanyl is primarily by rapid and extensive metabolism in the liver. Clearance estimates of 8 to 21 mL/kg/min approach liver blood flow and indicate a high hepatic extraction ratio.[120,132] Thus, hepatic metabolism of fentanyl is expected to be dependent on liver blood flow. Metabolism is primarily by N-dealkylation to norfentanyl and by hydroxylation of both the parent and norfentanyl.[133] Only about 6% of the dose of fentanyl is excreted unchanged in the urine.[120]

Dosage and Administration of Fentanyl

From administration as a single bolus dose, fentanyl developed an early reputation as a short-acting opioid, but experience with very large doses and multiple doses revealed that prolonged respiratory depression and delayed recovery could occur (Table 19-4). These observations demonstrate that fentanyl's clinical duration is limited by redistribution, and that with prolonged administration, accumulation can occur, as discussed later in this chapter.

Fentanyl can be useful as a sedative/analgesic premedication when given a short time prior to induction. For this use, incremental doses of 25 to 50 μg IV are titrated until the desired effect is achieved. It is important to note that although the onset of fentanyl's effects is rapid, peak effect lags behind peak plasma concentration by up to 5 minutes.[99] A transmucosal delivery system for fentanyl is also available and has been shown to be an effective premedicant for pediatric and adult patients as well as an effective treatment for "breakthrough" pain in chronic pain patients. Doses of 10 to 20 μg/kg in children and 400 to 800 μg in adults, administered 30 minutes prior to induction or a painful procedure, are safe and effective, but dose-dependent side effects typical of opioids are reported.[135,136] Because respiratory depression and hypoxemia can occur, transmucosal fentanyl usually should be administered in a monitored environment.

Fentanyl is used frequently as an adjunct to induction agents to blunt the hemodynamic response to laryngoscopy and tracheal intubation, which can be particularly severe in patients with hypertension or cardiovascular disease. Common clinical practice involves titration of fentanyl in doses of 1.5 to 5 μg/kg prior to administration of the induction agent. Because its peak effect lags behind peak plasma concentration by 3 to 5 minutes, fentanyl titration should be complete approximately 3 minutes prior to laryngoscopy to maximally blunt hemodynamic responses to tracheal intubation. Perhaps the most common clinical use of fentanyl and its derivatives is

TABLE 19-4

DOSAGE FOR FENTANYL, SUFENTANIL, ALFENTANIL, AND REMIFENTANIL DURING ELECTIVE SURGERY IN ADULTS[a]

■ ANESTHETIC PHASE	■ FENTANYL	■ SUFENTANIL	■ ALFENTANIL	■ REMIFENTANIL
Premedication (μg)	25–50	2–5	250–500	—
Induction				—
With hypnotic (μg/kg)	1.5–5	0.1–1	10–50	0.5–1.0 and/or 0.25–0.5 μg/kg/min
With 60–70% N_2O (μg/kg)	8–23	1.3–2.8		—
High-dose opioid (μg/kg)	50	10–30	120	2–5 +/or 2 μg/kg/min
Maintenance				
Balanced anesthesia				
Intermittent bolus (μg)	25–100	5–20	250–500	25–50
Infusion (μg/kg/min)	0.033	0.005–0.015	0.5–1.5	0.25–0.05
High dose opioid (μg/kg/min)	0.5	—	2.5–10	1.0–3.0
Transition to PACU (μg/kg/min)				0.05–0.15
Monitored Anesthesia Care				
Intermittent bolus (μg)	12.5–50	2.5–10	125–250	12.5–25
Infusion (μg/kg/min)	—	—	—	0.01–0.2

PACU, postanesthesia care unit.
[a]Doses are guidelines for hemodynamically stable adults. They should be adjusted downward for elderly patients and those with cardiac dysfunction and hemodynamic instability.

as an analgesic component of balanced general anesthesia. With this technique, incremental doses of fentanyl 0.5 to 2.5 μg/kg are administered intermittently as dictated by the intensity of the surgical stimulus and may be repeated approximately every 30 minutes. Generally, administration of up to 3 to 5 μg/kg/hr will allow recovery of spontaneous ventilation at the end of surgery. As an alternative to intermittent dosing, a loading dose of 5 to 10 μg/kg and continuous fentanyl infusion at a rate between 2 and 10 μg/kg/hr are recommended.[109] It is important to remember, however, that anesthetic requirements vary with age, concurrent diseases, and the surgical procedure. For example, fentanyl requirements decrease by 50% as age increases from 20 to 89 years.[132] Fentanyl requirements can also be expected to decrease with the duration of infusion (see "Context-Sensitive Half-Time").

Fentanyl combined with high-dose droperidol and nitrous oxide, a technique called *neuroleptanesthesia*,[137] is rarely used today because of concerns about prolongation of the QT interval of the electrocardiogram by high-dose droperidol.[138] High-dose (e.g., 50 to 150 μg/kg) fentanyl "anesthesia" has been used extensively for cardiac surgery. With this technique, a mean plasma fentanyl concentration of 15 ng/mL, which prevents hemodynamic changes in response to noxious stimuli,[139] can be achieved with a loading dose of 50 μg/kg, followed by a continuous infusion of 30 μg/kg/hr. With high-dose fentanyl, muscle relaxants and mechanical ventilation are required.

The use of fentanyl in the management of acute and chronic pain is discussed in Chapters 57 and 58).

SUFENTANIL

Sufentanil, a thienyl derivative of fentanyl (Fig. 19-5) first described in the mid-1970s, has a clinical potency ratio 2,000 to 4,000 times that of morphine and 10 to 15 times that of fentanyl.[140,141] Like fentanyl, sufentanil equilibrates rapidly between blood and brain, and demonstrates clear plasma concentration-effect relationships. In a study comparing effects of sufentanil and fentanyl on the EEG, Scott et al.[141] noted simi-

lar pharmacodynamic profiles. During a 4-minute sufentanil infusion, the change in spectral edge lagged behind the rising sufentanil concentration by approximately 2 to 3 minutes, while resolution of the EEG changes lagged behind plasma concentration changes by 20 to 30 minutes.

Analgesia

Sufentanil is a highly selective μ-opioid receptor agonist and exerts potent analgesic effects in animals when given by either systemic or spinal routes. While the literature describing clinical experience with sufentanil as a component of general anesthesia is extensive, available information regarding the analgesic potency of systemically administered sufentanil in humans is limited. Geller et al.[142] titrated an IV infusion rate to adequate postoperative analgesia, and noted that a mean rate of 8 to 17 μg/hr was required during the first 48 hours. This was associated with a fivefold range in plasma sufentanil concentrations, between 0.02 and 0.1 ng/mL. Similar sufentanil requirements (including a wide interpatient variability) are noted in other studies of postoperative and cancer patients.[47,143] Lehman et al.[143] estimated that the MEAC of sufentanil is near 0.03 ng/mL, and the analgesic EC_{50} of sufentanil concentration is approximately 0.05 ng/mL.[144]

Use in Anesthesia

In animal studies, sufentanil decreases the MAC of volatile anesthetics in a dose-dependent manner, with the maximum MAC reduction between 70 and 90%.[145] In humans, a plasma sufentanil concentration of 0.145 ng/mL is associated with a 50% reduction in isoflurane MAC.[146] Increasing the plasma sufentanil concentration to 0.5 ng/mL reduced isoflurane MAC by 78%, and a ceiling effect was approached with greater plasma sufentanil concentrations. The maximum MAC reduction seen in humans was 89% at a sufentanil concentration of 1.4 ng/mL.

In clinical anesthesia practice, sufentanil is used as a component of balanced anesthesia and has been employed extensively in high doses (10 to 30 μg/kg) with oxygen and muscle relaxants for cardiac surgery. In this dose range, sufentanil is at least as effective as fentanyl in its ability to produce and maintain hypnosis. In addition, hemodynamic stability appears to be as good as or better than that achieved with fentanyl.[86,140] Bailey et al.[147] used a computer-assisted continuous infusion system to determine the sufentanil plasma concentration response to various noxious stimuli during high-dose sufentanil anesthesia for cardiac surgery. They estimated the plasma concentration associated with a 50% probability of no response (movement, hemodynamic, or sympathetic) to intubation, incision, sternotomy, and mediastinal dissection (CP_{50}). The CP_{50} for intubation, incision, and sternotomy (pooled data) was 7.06 ng/mL, and for mediastinal dissection CP_{50} was 12.1 ng/mL. As is typical of opioids, a wide intersubject variability (three- to tenfold) was noted in sufentanil concentration requirements. However, when used as the sole anesthetic agent, even high doses may not completely block the hemodynamic responses to noxious stimuli.[110]

Other Central Nervous System Effects

Equianalgesic doses of sufentanil and fentanyl produce similar changes in the EEG.[140,141] In patients who received sufentanil 15 μg/kg, α activity became prominent within a few seconds, and within 3 minutes, the EEG consisted almost entirely of slow δ activity.[140] Rigidity and myoclonic activity resembling seizures have been reported during induction of, and on emergence from, anesthesia with sufentanil in doses of approximately 1 to 2 μg/kg.[43,44]

In patients with intracranial tumors, sufentanil 1 μg/kg was associated with an elevation in spinal cerebrospinal pressure and a decrease in cerebral perfusion pressure.[148] As seen with fentanyl, mean arterial pressure had dropped significantly in these patients. In normal volunteers, a smaller dose of sufentanil (0.5 μg/kg) was not associated with changes in cerebral blood flow.[149] Very large doses of sufentanil (20 μg/kg) in dogs decreased cerebral blood flow in proportion to cerebral metabolism, and intracranial pressure did not change.[150]

Respiratory Depression

Like other μ opioid agonists, sufentanil causes respiratory depression in doses associated with clinical analgesia.[122,123] Respiratory depression can be especially marked in the presence of inhalation anesthetics. In spontaneously breathing patients anesthetized with 1.5% halothane and N_2O, a small dose of sufentanil (approximately 2.5 μg) reduced mean minute ventilation by 50%, and 4 μg reduced mean respiratory rate by 50%.[151] Postoperative respiratory depression after apparent recovery from anesthesia has been reported for both fentanyl and sufentanil.[152] The lack of exogenous stimulation in the early postoperative period may be an important factor during early recovery from anesthesia.

In normal volunteers who received bolus doses of fentanyl and sufentanil, changes in end-tidal CO_2 were the same for fentanyl and sufentanil, but the slope of the ventilatory response to CO_2 was depressed to a greater extent by fentanyl.[122] In another volunteer study, a fourfold range of equianalgesic plasma concentrations of morphine and sufentanil produced equivalent respiratory depression, measured as both increased end-tidal CO_2 and a decreased ventilatory response to CO_2.[144]

Cardiovascular and Endocrine Effects

In animal studies, sufentanil produces vasodilation by a sympatholytic mechanism but may also have a direct smooth muscle effect.[153] Clinically, a prominent feature of many trials involving sufentanil is the remarkable hemodynamic stability achieved during balanced and high-dose (up to 30 μg/kg) opioid anesthesia. Only a modest decrease in mean arterial pressure is observed when sufentanil (approximately 15 μg/kg) is used for induction of anesthesia.[86,154]

In general, sufentanil and fentanyl have been found to be equivalent for use in balanced and high-dose opioid anesthesia,[110,155] but one clinical comparison noted better analgesia and respiratory function with sufentanil in the immediate postoperative period.[156] The choice of premedication and muscle relaxant may significantly affect hemodynamics during induction and maintenance of anesthesia with sufentanil. Combining vecuronium and sufentanil can cause a decrease in mean arterial pressure during induction,[157] and significant bradycardia and sinus arrest[158] have been reported. Bradycardia is not seen when pancuronium is used during anesthesia with sufentanil.

Sufentanil, like fentanyl, reduces the endocrine and metabolic responses to surgery.[140] However, even a large induction dose (20 μg/kg) did not prevent increases in cortisol, catecholamines, glucose, and free fatty acids during and after cardiopulmonary bypass.[159]

Disposition Kinetics

Sufentanil is extremely lipophilic and has pharmacokinetic properties similar to that of fentanyl. Because of a smaller degree of ionization at physiologic pH and higher degree of plasma protein binding, its volume of distribution is somewhat smaller and its elimination half-life shorter than that of fentanyl (Table 19-2). Sufentanil pharmacokinetics has been studied in anesthetized patients who had received methohexital for anesthetic induction, followed by the sufentanil dose of 5 μg/kg, and N_2O in oxygen 33%.[160] Plasma sufentanil concentration drops very rapidly after an IV bolus dose, and 98% of the drug is cleared from plasma within 30 minutes. Plasma concentration–time data in this study were best fitted to a three-compartment model, with rapid and slower distribution half-times of 1.4 and 17.7 minutes, respectively, and an elimination half-life of 2.7 hours. In other pharmacokinetic studies with anesthetized patients, reported mean elimination half-lives were in the range of 2.2 to 4.6 hours.[161,163] Obese patients have a larger total volume of distribution and a longer elimination half-life (3.5 vs. 2.2 hours) compared with nonobese patients.[161]

Sufentanil is less red cell bound than fentanyl (22 compared with 40%).[133] Plasma sufentanil is approximately 92% protein bound at pH 7.4, mostly to α_1-acid glycoprotein. Clearance of sufentanil is rapid, and like fentanyl, it has a high hepatic extraction ratio.[133] Metabolism in the liver is by N-dealkylation and O-demethylation, but sufentanil clearance and elimination half-life in patients with cirrhosis are similar to controls.[162]

Dosage and Administration of Sufentanil

Sufentanil is most often used as a component of balanced anesthesia, or as a single agent in high doses, particularly for cardiac surgery (Table 19-4). Several investigations have found similar sufentanil dose requirements for induction of anesthesia.[86,147,163] When sufentanil is titrated during induction, loss of consciousness is seen with total doses between 1.3 and 2.8 μg/kg. Doses in the range of 0.3 to 1.0 μg/kg given 1 to 3 minutes prior to laryngoscopy can be expected to blunt hemodynamic responses to intubation, but muscle rigidity can occur even at these lower doses, particularly in the elderly.

Balanced anesthesia is maintained with intermittent bolus doses or a continuous infusion. With bolus doses of 0.1 to 0.5 μg/kg, mean maintenance requirements of 0.35 μg/kg/hr have been reported.[86] Cork et al.[164] administered an initial bolus of 0.5 μg/kg followed by an infusion of 0.5 μg/kg/hr, titrated to patient need. This regimen of sufentanil in combination with

N_2O 70% in oxygen, with or without isoflurane, provided satisfactory anesthesia with good hemodynamic stability. Thus, for balanced anesthesia, dose requirements for bolus administration and continuous infusion are similar, in the range of 0.3 to 1 $\mu g/kg/hr$. Much higher bolus doses (10 $\mu g/kg$) and/or infusion rates (0.15 $\mu g/kg/min$) are required to achieve the plasma sufentanil concentration range of 6 to 60 ng/mL required during cardiac anesthesia using sufentanil as the sole agent.

ALFENTANIL

Alfentanil, a tetrazole derivative of fentanyl (Fig. 19-5), was synthesized 2 years after sufentanil and introduced into clinical practice in the early 1980s. On a milligram basis, its clinical potency is approximately 10 times that of morphine and one-fourth to one-tenth that of fentanyl when given in single doses. Alfentanil differs from fentanyl in its pharmacokinetics as well as in its speed of equilibration between plasma and effect site in the brain. In a comparison using EEG spectral-edge effects to quantify fentanyl and alfentanil pharmacodynamics, Scott et al.[99] demonstrated that alfentanil's effect followed serum drug concentration more closely than fentanyl (Fig. 19-8). Peak effect lagged behind peak plasma concentration by <1 minute, and resolution of effect followed decreasing serum alfentanil concentration by no more than 10 minutes. Alfentanil is a μ-opioid receptor agonist and produces typical naloxone-reversible analgesia and side effects such as sedation, nausea, and respiratory depression.

Analgesia

Clear concentration and dose-related analgesic effects have been demonstrated for alfentanil, but, as is typical for opioids, individual requirements vary widely. For postoperative analgesia, the MEAC is approximately 10 ng/mL, with a range of 2 to >40 ng/mL.[165] In a laboratory investigation, 80 ng/mL was associated with a 50% reduction in pain intensity.[46] Similar results are seen in clinical studies, in which mean alfentanil plasma concentrations required for relief of moderate-to-severe pain are approximately 40 to 80 ng/mL (Table 19-3).[166] Following an adequate loading dose, average alfentanil requirements for postoperative analgesia are approximately 10 to 20 $\mu g/kg/hr$.[167,168]

Use in Anesthesia

Like other opioids, alfentanil decreases the MAC of enflurane in a curvilinear fashion up to a plateau.[26,169] In dogs, an infusion rate of 8 $\mu g/kg/min$ (plasma concentration, 223 ng/mL) reduced enflurane MAC by 69%, but increasing the infusion rate fourfold did not reduce enflurane MAC further.[158]

Alfentanil plasma concentrations required to supplement N_2O anesthesia have been determined.[170] Patients received a loading dose of 150 $\mu g/kg$, followed by an infusion titrated between 25 and 150 $\mu g/kg/hr$ according to responses to surgical stimuli. Plasma concentrations required along with 66% N_2O to obtund somatic, autonomic, and hemodynamic responses to stimuli in 50% of patients were 475, 279, and 150 ng/mL for tracheal intubation, skin incision, and skin closure, respectively. The plasma alfentanil concentration associated with spontaneous ventilation after discontinuation of N_2O was 223 ng/mL. Nearly identical results were obtained in a similar study using computer-controlled infusions to deliver alfentanil (Fig. 19-9).[171] Plasma alfentanil concentrations required in combination with propofol to obtund responses to intubation and surgical stimuli have also been determined.[172] In contrast to combining alfentanil and N_2O, much lower alfentanil plasma concentrations (55 to 92 ng/mL) were

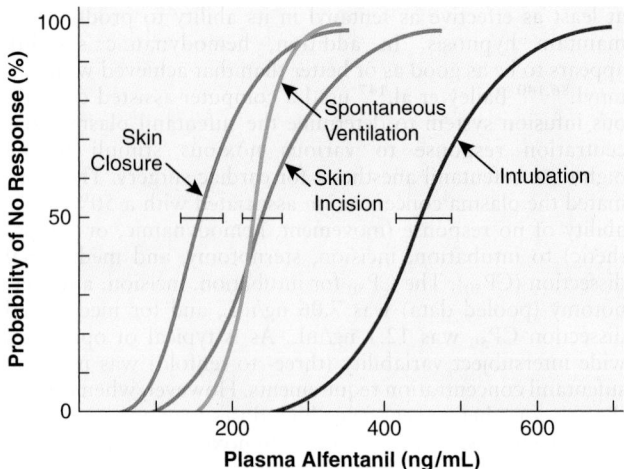

FIGURE 19-9. The relationship between alfentanil plasma concentration (with 66% N_2O) and the probability of no response for intubation, skin incision, and skin closure; and the relationship of plasma alfentanil concentration (without N_2O) and the recovery of adequate spontaneous ventilation. (Reprinted with permission from Ausems ME, Vuyk J, Hug CC, et al: Comparison of a computer-assisted infusion vs. intermittent bolus administration of alfentanil as a supplement to nitrous oxide for lower abdominal surgery. Anesthesiology 1988; 68: 851.)

required to prevent responses in 50% of patients when alfentanil was combined with propofol at a plasma concentration of 3 $\mu g/mL$ (Fig. 19-10).

High-dose alfentanil has been used as an induction agent for patients with and without cardiac disease[173] and for induction and maintenance of cardiac anesthesia.[127,174] Patients with cardiac valvular or coronary artery disease required half as much alfentanil to induce unconsciousness.[173] When used as the sole anesthetic agent, mean plasma alfentanil concentrations required to significantly blunt hemodynamic responses to intubation and sternotomy were 700 to 830 ng/mL and 1,200 to 1,800 ng/mL, respectively.[175] These values are approximately twice those reported for alfentanil in combination with 66% nitrous oxide.[170,171] However, even doses that produced very high plasma alfentanil concentrations (1,200 to >2,000 ng/mL) did not eliminate responses to intubation and intraoperative stimuli in all patients.[170] In contrast to fentanyl and sufentanil, the duration of even very large doses of alfentanil is short, so repeated doses or a continuous infusion of alfentanil is required.

Other Central Nervous System Effects

Alfentanil produces the typical generalized slowing of the EEG.[99,176] Like fentanyl, alfentanil can increase epileptiform EEG activity in patients with intractable temporal lope epilepsy having surgery under general anesthesia.[143] Like fentanyl and sufentanil, alfentanil can produce intense muscle rigidity accompanied by loss of consciousness. In 90 to 100% of patients, induction doses of 150 to 175 $\mu g/kg$ were associated with muscle rigidity, which was not limited to the chest wall or trunk. Rather, electromyography has shown increased activity of comparable magnitude in muscles of the neck, extremities, chest wall, and abdomen.[148,177]

Alfentanil has been reported to increase cerebrospinal fluid pressure in patients with brain tumors, whereas fentanyl does not.[113] However, when normocapnia and blood pressure were maintained at baseline, no clinically significant changes in ICP and no evidence of cerebral vasodilation or vasoconstriction were seen in neurosurgical patients who received 25 and

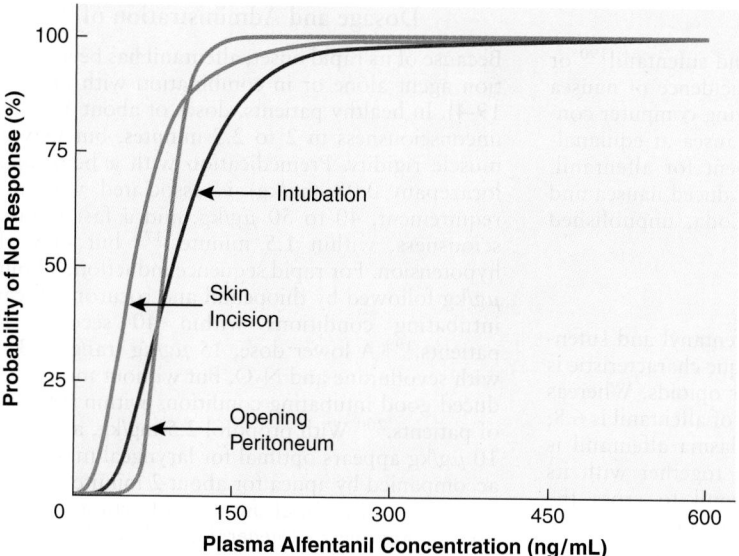

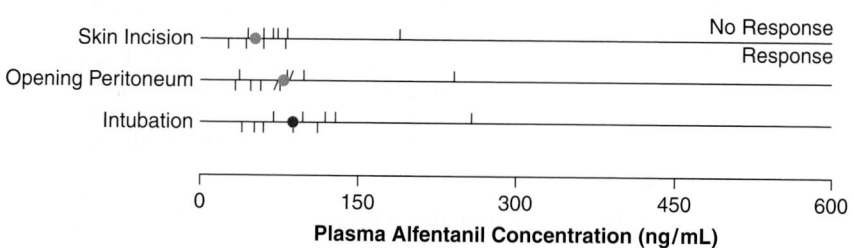

FIGURE 19-10. The alfentanil plasma concentration-effect relationships for intubation, skin incision, and the opening of the peritoneum when given as a supplement to propofol. (Reprinted with permission from Vuyk J, Lim T, Engbers FHM, et al: Pharmacodynamics of alfentanil as a supplement to propofol or nitrous oxide for lower abdominal surgery in female patients. Anesthesiology 1993; 78: 1036.)

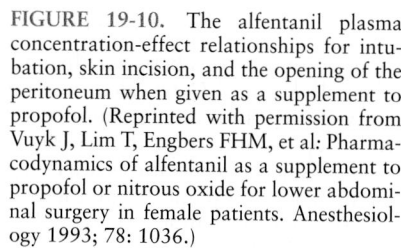

50 μg/kg of alfentanil with N_2O.[178] When the effects of three-dose regimens of alfentanil, 10, 20, and 30 μg/kg, followed by 10, 20 and 30 μg/kg/hr, were compared with placebo in brain tumor patients anesthetized with propofol and fentanyl, mean arterial pressure and cerebral perfusion pressure decreased in a dose-dependent fashion, but there were no changes in subdural ICP or arteriovenous O_2 content difference.[179]

Respiratory Depression

In animal and human studies, antinociceptive effects could not be separated from respiratory depression in volunteers; mild ventilatory depression (increased end-tidal CO_2; decreased slope of the CO_2 response curve) was seen at plasma concentrations as low as 20 ng/mL. At plasma concentrations associated with 50% reduction in pain intensity, respiratory depression was equivalent for alfentanil, fentanyl, and morphine.[15] A clinical study examined postoperative analgesia and respiratory effects of alfentanil administered by a patient-controlled analgesia system.[180] In patients who received a continuous alfentanil infusion at 900 μg/hr plus 100- to 200-μg doses as needed, three of ten patients developed respiratory depression (respiratory rate <8/min). Mean alfentanil blood concentration in this group of patients was 80 ng/mL.

Two clinical studies examined the intensity and duration of respiratory depressant effects of alfentanil in the immediate postoperative period.[181,182] Patients received balanced anesthesia 67% N_2O with or without 0.5% halothane and alfentanil 20 to 100 μg/kg/hr. At the end of surgery the infusion was decreased to 20 μg/kg/hr, which produced plasma alfentanil concentrations between 106 and 120 ng/mL, and good analgesia. Ventilatory response to CO_2 was decreased to 50% of the baseline value, but $PaCO_2$ was only moderately elevated (42 to 48 torr). By 2 hours after alfentanil was discontinued, respiratory function was near baseline. Recovery of ventila-

tory function was faster with alfentanil compared with fentanyl.[182] Another comparison found that for anesthetics of 1.5 to 2 hours' duration, recovery of respiratory function was similar with alfentanil and fentanyl.[183] Like its congeners, alfentanil has been associated with apnea and unconsciousness after apparent recovery from anesthesia.[184]

Cardiovascular Effects

The cardiovascular effects of alfentanil are influenced by preoperative medication, muscle relaxant used, method of administration, and the degree of surgical stimulation. In general, heart rate and mean arterial pressure are unchanged or slightly decreased during induction with alfentanil 40 to 120 μg/kg,[173] but rapid induction with 150 to 175 μg/kg alfentanil can decrease mean arterial pressure by 15 to 20 torr. After induction with etomidate, alfentanil 120 μg/kg decreased mean arterial pressure by approximately 30 torr,[185] and following thiopental (3 to 5 mg/kg) induction, a smaller dose of alfentanil (40 μg/kg) decreased mean arterial pressure by approximately 40 torr.[186] Alfentanil does not appear to have negative inotropic effects,[185] but severe hypotension has been observed when alfentanil is given after 0.125 mg/kg diazepam.[187] In combination with lorazepam premedication or thiopental induction, moderate doses (10 to 50 μg/kg) of alfentanil blunt the cardiovascular and catecholamine responses to laryngoscopy and intubation,[175,186] but for patients >70 years old, doses in this range given with thiopental can produce significant hypotension after induction.[188] Alfentanil can also cause bradycardia, but this effect is minimized by premedication with atropine and by the vagolytic effect of pancuronium. Alfentanil 50 μg/kg combined with propofol 1 mg/kg for induction of anesthesia can produce significant bradycardia and hypotension after intubation, but premedication with glycopyrrolate prevents these effects.[189]

Nausea and Vomiting

Clinical comparisons between alfentanil and sufentanil[190] or fentanyl[191] and N_2O revealed the same incidence of nausea and vomiting. In normal volunteers receiving computer-controlled opioid infusions, the severity of nausea at equianalgesic plasma concentrations was equivalent for alfentanil, fentanyl, and morphine,[46] but alfentanil-induced nausea and vomiting resolved more quickly (B.A. Coda, unpublished observations, 1988–90).

Disposition Kinetics

Alfentanil pharmacokinetics differs from fentanyl and sufentanil in several respects (Table 19-3). A unique characteristic is that alfentanil is a weaker base than other opioids. Whereas other opioids have pKa above 7.4, the pKa of alfentanil is 6.8; consequently, nearly 90% of unbound plasma alfentanil is nonionized at pH 7.4.[131] This property, together with its moderate lipid solubility, enables alfentanil to cross the blood–brain barrier rapidly and accounts for its rapid onset of action. Compared with fentanyl and sufentanil, which have mean plasma-brain equilibration half-times of 6.4 and 6.2 minutes, respectively,[99,141] alfentanil has a blood–brain equilibration half-time of 1.1 minutes.[121] Alfentanil also has a smaller volume of distribution than fentanyl, which is a result of lower lipid solubility and high protein binding.[192] Approximately 92% of alfentanil is protein bound, mostly to α_1-acid glycoprotein.[131,134]

After IV administration, plasma alfentanil concentration falls rapidly; 90% of the administered dose has left the plasma by 30 minutes,[193] mostly because of distribution to highly perfused tissues. Plasma concentration decay curves in patients most often fit a three-compartment model.[24,193] Like fentanyl, alfentanil is quickly distributed, with rapid and slow distribution half-times of 1.0 to 3.5 minutes and 9.5 to 17 minutes, respectively. However, alfentanil has a terminal elimination half-life of 84 to 90 minutes, which is considerably shorter than those of fentanyl and sufentanil. Clearance of alfentanil, 6.4 mL/kg/min, is just half that of fentanyl, but because alfentanil's volume of distribution is 4 times smaller than fentanyl's, relatively more of the dose is available to the liver for metabolism.[194] Chauvin et al.[195] found that alfentanil has an intermediate hepatic extraction coefficient (32 to 53%) in humans, and that its elimination depends on hepatic plasma flow.

In animals, alfentanil undergoes N-dealkylation and O-demethylation in the liver to form inactive metabolites.[131] Liver disease can significantly prolong the elimination half-life of alfentanil. Patients with moderate hepatic insufficiency as a result of cirrhosis have reduced binding to α_1-acid glycoprotein and a plasma clearance one-half that of control patients. These changes result in a marked increase in the elimination half-life, 219 minutes versus 90 minutes in controls.[196] Renal disease also decreases alfentanil protein binding, but does not result in decreased plasma clearance or a prolonged terminal elimination half-life.[197] Alfentanil's elimination half-life is prolonged by about 30% in the elderly and appears to be much shorter (about 40 minutes) in children 5 to 8 years old.[198] Obesity is also associated with a 50% decrease in alfentanil clearance and a prolonged (172 minutes) elimination half-life.[198]

The combination of moderate lipid solubility and short elimination half-life suggests that both redistribution and elimination are important in the termination of alfentanil's effects.[182] After a single bolus dose, redistribution will be the most important mechanism, but after a very large dose, repeated small doses, or a continuous infusion, elimination will be a more important determinant of the duration of alfentanil's effects.

Dosage and Administration of Alfentanil

Because of its rapid onset, alfentanil has been used as an induction agent alone or in combination with other drugs (Table 19-4). In healthy patients, doses of about 120 μg/kg produce unconsciousness in 2 to 2.5 minutes, but may also produce muscle rigidity. Premedication with a benzodiazepine (e.g., lorazepam 0.08 mg/kg) is associated with a lower dose requirement, 40 to 50 μg/kg, and a faster onset of unconsciousness, within 1.5 minutes,[173] but may also produce hypotension. For rapid sequence induction, a bolus dose of 36 μg/kg followed by thiopental and rocuronium can yield ideal intubating conditions within 40 seconds in 95% of patients.[199] A lower dose, 15 μg/kg (range, 13 to 31 μg/kg) with sevoflurane and N_2O, but without muscle relaxants produced good intubating conditions within 90 seconds in 95% of patients.[200] With propofol 2.5 mg/kg, an alfentanil dose of 10 μg/kg appears optimal for laryngeal mask insertion, but is accompanied by apnea for about 2 minutes.[201]

Because of its brief duration of action, alfentanil can be a useful component of general anesthesia in short surgical procedures, especially those associated with minimal postoperative pain, particularly in the outpatient surgery. In this setting, loading doses of 5 to 10 μg/kg provide good analgesia with rapid recovery.[192] For longer procedures, alfentanil can be administered as needed in repeated small bolus doses, but its pharmacokinetic properties make it ideal for administration as a continuous infusion. After induction of anesthesia, a loading dose of alfentanil 10 to 50 μg/kg is followed with supplemental bolus doses of 3 to 5 μg/kg as needed or a continuous infusion starting at 0.4 to 1.7 μg/kg/min with 60 to 70% N_2O or a propofol infusion.[170,171,192,200–203] A pediatric study reported use of similar doses of alfentanil and propofol,[204] while another used higher alfentanil doses (100 μg/kg loading dose followed by 2.5 μg/kg/min) combined with 70% N_2O without propofol.[205]

When high-dose alfentanil is used as the sole anesthetic agent, a continuous infusion of up to 150 to 600 μg/kg/hr is adjusted according to the patient's responses to stimuli, but much lower doses can be effective for cardiac surgery if adequate premedication is given.[174]

REMIFENTANIL

Remifentanil, a 4-anilidopiperidine with a methyl ester side chain (Fig. 19-5) that was first described in 1990 and approved for clinical use in 1996, was developed to meet the need for an ultrashort-acting opioid. Because its ester side chain is susceptible to metabolism by blood and tissue esterases, remifentanil is rapidly metabolized to a substantially less active compound. Thus, because its ultrashort action is due to metabolism rather than to redistribution, it does not accumulate with repeated dosing or prolonged infusion. Remifentanil demonstrates potent, naloxone-reversible μ-selective opioid agonist activity in animal assays.[206]

Analgesia

In animals and humans, remifentanil produces dose-dependent analgesic effects. Human laboratory studies have examined analgesic effects of bolus IV doses (0.0625 to 2.0 μg/kg)[207] as well as computer-controlled infusions with targeted plasma concentrations (0.75 to 3.0 ng/mL).[208] Bolus doses produced a peak analgesic effect between 1 and 3 minutes and a duration of approximately 10 minutes. In volunteers, MEAC is approximately 0.75 ng/mL and analgesic EC_{50} is approximately 3 ng/mL.[208] Both studies found remifentanil to be about 40 times as potent as alfentanil.

Clinical investigations have evaluated early postoperative analgesia. One study reported that after remifentanil–propofol anesthesia, nearly 80% of patients were titrated to satisfactory analgesia with remifentanil infusion of 0.05 to 0.15 μg/kg/min.[209] Another early postoperative evaluation demonstrated effective analgesia with patient-controlled infusion of remifentanil to a mean target blood concentration of 2 ng/mL, but noted a fairly high incidence of nausea (26%) with this regimen.[210] Clinical evaluations of remifentanil for labor analgesia have produced conflicting results, and some have found prohibitive rates of unacceptable side effects such as nausea and respiratory depression. However, a dose-ranging study that used remifentanil via patient-controlled analgesia reported a median effective bolus dose of 0.4 μg/kg (range, 0.2 to 0.8 μg/kg) and consumption of 0.066 μg/kg/min (range, 0.027 to 0.207 μg/kg/min).[211] Although these results are preliminary, remifentanil may offer an alternative for laboring patients in whom regional anesthesia is absolutely contraindicated.

Use in Anesthesia

The effect of remifentanil on the MAC of volatile anesthetics is characterized by steep dose-effect or concentration-effect curves typical of other μ opioid agonists. In animals, remifentanil decreases enflurane and isoflurane MAC in a dose-dependent fashion up to a maximum near 65%, similar to fentanyl.[212,213] In humans, remifentanil reduces isoflurane MAC logarithmically in a blood concentration-dependent fashion.[214] A whole blood remifentanil concentration of 1.3 ng/mL reduced isoflurane MAC by 50%, with a maximum MAC reduction (91%) at 32 ng/mL. Remifentanil's effects on the MAC-BAR (requirement for blunting the sympathetic response to skin incision) of sevoflurane[215] and desflurane[216] in 60% N_2O are similar. A remifentanil plasma concentration of 1 ng/mL reduced MAC-BAR of the inhalation agents by 60%, while 3 ng/mL decreased MAC-BAR another 30%.

The rapid onset and brief duration of remifentanil suggest that it is suitable for induction of anesthesia. Although a median ED_{50} of 12 μg/kg for loss of consciousness has been reported, clinical investigations have also found that, as with other opioids, loss of consciousness is not reliably achieved with remifentanil alone, even in doses of 20 μg/kg or more.[217,218] Furthermore, a high incidence of muscle rigidity and purposeless movement was seen. Even at 2 μg/kg remifentanil, moderate muscle rigidity was seen in 40% of patients, and at 20 μg/kg, 60% of patients had severe muscle rigidity.[217]

Drover and Lemmens[219] used computer-assisted infusions to determine the blood concentrations of remifentanil required to supplement 66% N_2O in patients having abdominal surgery. Other than premedication with 1 to 2 mg midazolam, no sedatives or hypnotics were given. During surgery, the remifentanil EC_{50} for adequate anesthesia was 4.1 ng/mL for men and 7.5 ng/mL for women. The reason for gender differences in these results was not clear, but could have been related to different types of surgeries. Pediatric patients require twice as much remifentanil as adults (0.15 μg/kg/min vs. 0.08 μg/kg/min) when it is used with propofol for TIVA.[220]

Investigations of remifentanil for balanced anesthesia, including combination with isoflurane,[221,222] sevoflurane,[223] and desflurane,[224] report similar findings of hemodynamic stability and easy titratability. A clinical trial of remifentanil and desflurane–N_2O identified blood remifentanil concentrations that provide an optimal balance between hemodynamic stability and blunting responses to noxious stimulation while permitting rapid recovery.[224] In the presence of 2.2 to 2.7% end-tidal desflurane and N_2O, optimal remifentanil plasma concentrations were 5 to 7 ng/mL for laryngoscopy and skin closure and 10 ng/mL during abdominal surgery. It is interesting to note that adjustments in remifentanil blunted the sympathetic response to noxious stimulation but did not alter desflurane's effect on the bispectral index analysis of the EEG.

Remifentanil is infused as a component of TIVA more frequently than other opioids. Both remifentanil and propofol can be administered at fixed infusion rates or by computer-controlled systems that provide target plasma concentrations, commonly referred to as target-controlled infusions or TCI. The combination of remifentanil and propofol for TIVA has been used successfully for a variety of inpatient procedures, including coronary artery bypass graft; other major thoracic, neurosurgical, abdominal, and orthopaedic procedures; as well as ambulatory surgery and other painful procedures in adults and children. Two studies demonstrated that a fairly low plasma concentration of remifentanil, TCI at 3.4 to 4 ng/mL, reduces propofol EC_{50} for intubation by 66%, from approximately 6 to 2 ng/mL,[218,225] but further increases in remifentanil dosage only modestly reduced propofol dose requirements, an apparent ceiling effect.[225] A clinical dose ranging study found that remifentanil EC_{50} for laryngoscopy was 14.3 and 1.4 ng/mL with propofol infusions of 44 and 200 μg/kg/min, respectively.[226] Response to intubation was prevented in 80% of patients by approximately doubling the remifentanil. A small bolus dose of remifentanil (20 μg) given 30 seconds before induction, can reduce the pain of propofol injection.[227]

As previously noted, pediatric patients receiving propofol infusion require higher remifentanil doses than adults.

While high-dose remifentanil (1 to 2 μg/kg/min) has been used as a single agent for cardiac anesthesia,[228] it is more commonly administered with propofol or isoflurane for "fast-track cardiac anesthesia." Target remifentanil and propofol concentrations for cardiac surgery[228,229] are very similar to those for other procedures with low-dose propofol. In a study comparing remifentanil, sufentanil, and fentanyl for fast-track cardiac anesthesia, Engoren et al.[230] found that remifentanil patients were more likely to require treatment for blood pressure fluctuations during and after surgery, but otherwise, the three regimens produced similar outcomes with respect to extubation, intensive care unit stay, and cost.

One drawback of remifentanil use for general anesthesia is that patients require analgesics very soon after an infusion is stopped. A continuation of remifentanil to transition to postoperative analgesia can avoid early pain and accompanying detrimental sympathoadrenal stimulation and is essential for patients undergoing cardiac or other major surgery.

Remifentanil administered by infusion also appears to be useful during monitored anesthesia care for conscious sedation in procedures such as extracorporeal shock wave lithotripsy and colonoscopy,[231,232] or in conjunction with regional anesthesia.[233–235] When compared with propofol, remifentanil provides better analgesia, but results in more nausea and respiratory depression, whereas propofol causes more oversedation. Times required for readiness for discharge are clinically similar. For monitored anesthesia care, the ideal administration regimen appears to be small bolus doses of remifentanil with a continuous infusion combined with low-dose propofol or midazolam.

Other Central Nervous System Effects

Remifentanil produces classic μ opioid agonist effects on the EEG, that is, a concentration-dependent slowing. The plasma concentration associated with 50% maximal EEG changes (EC_{50}) is 15 to 20 ng/mL.[236,237] Remifentanil's rapid onset and very short duration results in extremely close tracking of changes in EEG spectral edge with plasma remifentanil concentration.[236,237] Like other opioids, remifentanil can produce muscle rigidity, especially with bolus doses. This can be avoided with using smaller doses and injecting over 60 seconds or more.

Neither remifentanil (0.5 or 1.0 μg/kg) nor alfentanil (10 or 20 μg/kg) given during isoflurane/N_2O anesthesia with controlled ventilation affect intracranial pressure, and both produce modest, dose-dependent decreases in mean arterial pressure.[238] A multicenter clinical trial comparing remifentanil/N_2O with fentanyl/N_2O anesthesia found that intracranial pressure and cerebral perfusion pressure were similar with the two regimens.[239] In a study comparing cerebrovascular autoregulation in the awake and anesthetized states, remifentanil 0.5μg/kg/min plus propofol preserved cerebral autoregulation, whereas isoflurane 1.8% did not.[240]

In many cranial and spinal neurosurgical procedures, the ability to monitor motor-evoked potentials (MEPs) is important; opioids, sedative hypnotic drugs, and inhalation agents used in general anesthesia are known to suppress MEPs. A human and animal study compared the effects of phenylpiperidine opioids and hypnotics including thiopental, midazolam, and propofol on MEPs.[241] While all opioids and propofol suppressed MEPs in a dose-dependent fashion, remifentanil exerted less suppression than the other opioids and propofol. A target plasma concentration of 9 ng/mL reduced amplitude by 50%, but the quality and reproducibility of MEPs was preserved even at plasma concentration of 15 ng/mL, well within the plasma concentration range that provides surgical anesthesia.

Although remifentanil has not been shown to produce seizure activity, it can be used to reduce methohexital requirement in patients having electroconvulsive therapy. Remifentanil 1 μg/kg allowed a 50% reduction in methohexital dose, which results in seizure prolongation by 50%.[242]

Respiratory Depression

Remifentanil produces dose-dependent respiratory depression as measured by increases in end-tidal CO_2 and decreased oxygen saturation. In a dose-escalation study in normal volunteers, the respiratory depressant effects of remifentanil and alfentanil were compared.[207] Peak respiratory depression occurred at 5 minutes after each dose of remifentanil and alfentanil, and the maximal respiratory depressant effect seen after 2 μg/kg remifentanil was similar to that caused by 32 μg/kg alfentanil. The duration of respiratory depression, measured as time to return of blood gases to within 10% of baseline values, was 10 minutes after 1.5 μg/kg and 20 minutes after 2 μg/kg remifentanil compared with 30 minutes after 32 μg/kg alfentanil. During continuous opioid infusion, the ventilatory response to CO_2 decreased by approximately 30, 45, and 60% in response to 4-hour remifentanil infusions of 0.025, 0.050, and 0.075 μg/kg/min, respectively.[243] Recovery from remifentanil-induced respiratory depression was rapid, and minute ventilation returned to baseline by 8 minutes (range, 5 to 15 minutes) after the infusion was stopped for all infusion rates. In contrast, a 50% decrease in minute ventilation produced by a 4-hour infusion of alfentanil at 0.5 μg/kg/min required 61 minutes (range, 5 to 90 minutes) to return to baseline.[243] In a volunteer study, Glass et al.[244] reported that the blood remifentanil concentration needed to depress ventilatory response to inspired 8% CO_2 by 50% (EC_{50}) was 1.17 ng/mL. Bouillon et al.[245] reported a similar EC_{50} (0.92 ng/mL) and also noted that remifentanil concentrations that are well tolerated at steady state will produce clinically significant respiratory depression when achieved with bolus dosing. In general, clinical comparisons report that respiratory parameters (respiratory rate, O_2 saturation, and end-tidal CO_2) recover more rapidly after remifentanil compared with other opioids given in equipotent dosage.

Maintenance of spontaneous respiration during general anesthesia with remifentanil and volatile agents or propofol may not be feasible unless low doses of remifentanil are used.[246] Clinical experience in spontaneously breathing humans receiving remifentanil combined with either isoflurane or propofol demonstrates respiratory depression in 10 to 35% of patients receiving remifentanil at 0.025 μg/kg/min. It increases to nearly 50% in patients receiving 0.05 μg/kg/min and to >90% with remifentanil 0.075 μg/kg/min.[247,248] A similar rate of respiratory depression (20%) with need for assisted ventilation is seen in pediatric patients receiving remifentanil/propofol infusions for general anesthesia during bone marrow aspiration.[249] As discussed earlier, remifentanil alone or combined with low-dose propofol or midazolam can be used for conscious sedation and to supplement regional or local anesthesia during monitored anesthesia care. Clinical reports describing these regimens report respiratory depression (respiratory rate <8 or SpO_2 <90%) in 2 to 30% of patients, but in all cases, recovery from respiratory depression with remifentanil is more rapid than other agents.[231–234] As with other opioids, higher rates of respiratory depression are seen when propofol is combined with remifentanil (15 to 50% of patients), and careful monitoring and titration are required to minimize this side effect.

Hemodynamic Effects

In healthy volunteers, remifentanil in bolus doses >1.0 μg/kg produce brief increases in systolic blood pressure (5 to 20 torr) and heart rate (10 to 25 beats/min).[207] In patients anesthetized with isoflurane and 66% N_2O in oxygen, remifentanil (up to 5 μg/kg) produces dose-dependent decreases in systolic blood pressure and heart rate. These effects are attenuated by premedication with glycopyrrolate 0.3 to 0.4 mg and are readily reversed with ephedrine or phenylephrine.[248] Sebel et al.[250] evaluated hemodynamic responses in patients receiving remifentanil 2 to 30 μg/kg (escalating doses) given during general anesthesia and found that systolic heart rate decreased more than 20% for doses >2 μg/kg. These hemodynamic effects were not mediated by histamine release. Clinical reports of experience with patients receiving opioid-based anesthetics have characterized hemodynamic changes during balanced anesthesia with remifentanil combined with isoflurane $\pm$ N_2O/O_2 or propofol. During a comparison of remifentanil versus alfentanil-based TIVA, a 20% drop in mean arterial pressure, with minimal change in heart rate, was noted after induction, with 35 to 50% of patients experiencing at least one episode of mean arterial pressure <70 mm Hg.[203] Decreases in blood pressure were transient and easily treated with fluids and downward titration of propofol. In a comparison of remifentanil- and fentanyl-based general anesthetics in >2,400 patients (80% American Society of Anesthesiology grade I and II), hypotension (systolic blood pressure <80 or treated pharmacologically) occurred in 12% of patients receiving remifentanil compared with 4% with fentanyl.[221] Bradycardia was less common, with 2% and 1% of patients in the remifentanil and fentanyl groups, respectively.

Greater hemodynamic changes can be seen in patients with coronary disease. In a comparison of high-dose remifentanil (2 μg/kg/min) and remifentanil 0.5 μg/kg/min plus propofol targeted to 2 μg/mL plasma concentration, both techniques produced similar changes: 30% drop in mean arterial pressure and 25% drop in cardiac index. Myocardial blood flow and oxygen consumption decreased by about 30 and 40%, respectively. More moderate hemodynamic changes were reported with lower doses (remifentanil TCI 4 to 8 ng/mL and propofol 1.2 ng/mL).[229] Heart rate and cardiac index dropped 20 and 6%, respectively, and no hypotension was seen. In an early clinical report, DeSouza et al.[251] reported a series of severe bradycardia (heart rate <30 beats/min) and hypotension (systolic blood pressure <80 mm Hg) in six patients who received a rapid injection of remifentanil 1 μg/kg followed by a continuous infusion at 0.1 to 0.2 μg/kg/min on induction for cardiac surgery. Hypotension was effectively treated by ephedrine and temporary discontinuation of remifentanil. These severe effects can often be avoided by slower administration (>60 seconds or longer) of the loading dose, as smaller bolus doses of remifentanil (0.3 to 0.5 μg/kg) are apparently not associated with severe bradycardia and hypotension.

Gastrointestinal Effects

Like other μ agonists, remifentanil can cause nausea and vomiting, but the occurrence of these adverse effects is influenced to a large extent by surgery, adjuvant anesthetic agents, and antiemetic prophylaxis. In a volunteer study, high infusion rates (1 to 8 μg/kg/min) produced nausea in 70% of subjects,[236] but much lower doses are typically used for general anesthesia. Philip et al.[202] compared nausea and vomiting at multiple time points in outpatient adults for laparoscopic surgery who received remifentanil or alfentanil combined with N_2O and propofol. Overall, the incidence of nausea was 44 and 53% for remifentanil and alfentanil, respectively; the incidence of vomiting was 21 and 29% for remifentanil and alfentanil, respectively. In outpatients with similar opioid infusions combined with 0.8% isoflurane, nausea occurred in 18 and 20% of patients with remifentanil and alfentanil, respectively.[252] In contrast, a report summarizing adverse events in >2,400 patients who received remifentanil (range, 0.25 to 2 μg/kg/min) or fentanyl with isoflurane or propofol for a variety of surgeries, nausea and vomiting were rare.[221] Other clinical comparisons of remifentanil plus propofol to alfentanil plus propofol reported very low incidence of nausea and vomiting (6 to 22%).[42,253] In a pediatric study, the addition of remifentanil 0.2 μg/kg/min to desflurane anesthesia produced no increase in nausea or vomiting after dental surgery; nausea and vomiting occurred in <5% of patients who received remifentanil. For strabismus surgery in children, vomiting occurred with equal frequency (26 to 31%) with remifentanil, alfentanil, isoflurane, and propofol.[254] Thus, remifentanil appears to produce dose-dependent nausea and vomiting similar to other short-acting μ-agonist opioids that can be attenuated by propofol. Taken together, remifentanil studies confirm the wide variability in occurrence of nausea and vomiting in the clinical setting.

Like other opioids, remifentanil delays gastric emptying[255] and biliary drainage.[256] As expected, biliary effects resolve more quickly than biliary drainage delay from morphine of meperidine.

Other Side Effects

Postoperative shivering occurred in about 40% of patients undergoing otorhinolaryngeal surgery despite active warming and independent of temperature,[48] while another study noted shivering in only 10% of outpatients.[252] In both of these studies, shivering was less common with alfentanil. One pediatric investigation reported pruritus in 12% of patients.[254]

In volunteers, remifentanil produced concentration-related subjective and psychomotor side effects typical of μ opioids.[208] Subjective side effects induced by remifentanil included dry mouth, itching, flushing, sweating, and "turning of the stomach." Remifentanil also impaired performance of psychomotor tests and caused miosis and respiratory depression. Some of these effects lasted an hour or more after remifentanil administration was stopped.

Disposition Kinetics

The key structural feature of remifentanil is an ester functional group that is susceptible to hydrolysis by blood and tissue nonspecific esterases and results in very rapid metabolism. Because butyrocholinesterase (pseudocholinesterase) does not appear to metabolize remifentanil, plasma cholinesterase deficiency and anticholinergic administration do not affect remifentanil clearance.[255] Unlike other opioids, redistribution plays only a minor role in remifentanil clearance. This property reduces its pharmacokinetic variability compared with other opioids. Remifentanil has a small volume of distribution, approximately 0.3 to 0.5 L/kg,[257,258] or about 25 L in an average adult.[259] Remifentanil's clearance, 3 to 5 L /min, is approximately 3 to 4 times normal hepatic blood flow.[192,240,241] Both two- and three-compartment models have been used to describe the plasma concentration decay curve of remifentanil. A rapid distribution phase of 0.9 minutes and a very short terminal elimination half-life of 9.5 minutes characterized a two-compartment model in adults.[207] In pediatrics, elimination half-life is about 3.5 to 6 minutes.[260] In the three-compartment model, rapid and slow distribution half-times were 0.4 to 0.9 and 2 to 6 minutes, respectively, and the elimination half-time was about 10 to 30 minutes.[237,258]

As for other fentanyl congeners, gender does not affect remifentanil pharmacokinetics, but advanced age is associated with a decrease in clearance and volume of distribution, as well as an apparent increase in potency.[261] Remifentanil pharmacokinetics are similar in lean (within 20% ideal body weight) and obese (at least 80% over ideal body weight) patients, indicating that remifentanil dosing should be based on lean body mass.[262] Although pharmacokinetic parameters of remifentanil are unchanged in patients with severe liver disease[263] or renal failure,[264] patients with hepatic disease appear to be more sensitive to remifentanil-induced respiratory depression.

Dosage and Administration of Remifentanil

Because of its extremely short duration of action, remifentanil is best administered as a continuous infusion, although administration as repeated bolus doses can also be effective (Table 19-4). Outside the United States, remifentanil is often administered by TCI, a pump system designed to infuse the drug based on population kinetics to achieve desired target plasma concentrations. Theoretically, this makes sense especially for remifentanil because its pharmacodynamic effects track plasma concentrations very closely. However, two studies have found that simple manually controlled infusion is as effective[265,266] and is more economical than computer-controlled infusions.

Numerous reports have described dosing regimens for remifentanil alone or in combination with IV and inhaled agents for induction and maintenance of general anesthesia, and as a component of sedation and monitored anesthesia care.

Induction Dosage, Intubation, Laryngeal Mask Airway Placement. As described earlier, remifentanil alone has not been found to be a satisfactory single agent for induction of anesthesia because of unreliability in loss of consciousness and significant muscle rigidity.[217] However, induction of anesthesia with high-dose remifentanil, 4 to 5 μg/kg, or an infusion of 2 μg/kg/min has been reported.[228] It is important to note that bolus doses of >2 μg/kg can drop arterial pressure 20 to 30%, while hemodynamic changes in cardiac patients receiving high-dose infusion are similar to remifentanil plus propofol.[267] Combined with a potent inhalation agent, a loading dose of 1 μg/kg given slowly (over 60 seconds) can provide adequate intubating conditions with hemodynamic stability. By far the most commonly reported remifentanil-based regimen for anesthetic induction and laryngoscopy consists of remifentanil 0.5 to 1 μg/kg given over 60 seconds plus propofol 1 to 2 mg/kg, followed by remifentanil infusion of 0.25 to 0.5 μg/kg/min.[221,222,268,269] This may be given with or without a midazolam 1- to 2-mg IV premedication. Similar regimens are recommended for pediatric patients, with substitution of oral midazolam premedication 0.5 mg/kg. In the elderly, dose reduction is indicated, with remifentanil 0.05 μg/kg over 60 seconds plus propofol titrated to loss of consciousness in 10-mg increments, followed by remifentanil infusion of 0.1 μg/kg/min. If TCI is used for induction of anesthesia, an initial remifentanil target of 5 to 7 ng/mL accompanied by 0.5 to 1 MAC inhaled anesthetic or propofol TCI of 2 ng/mL is recommended.[219,259]

Maintenance of General Anesthesia. In combination with 70% N_2O in O_2, remifentanil 0.6 μg/kg/min is generally adequate, but at least one study reported a wide range of infusion rates (0.025 to 2 μg/kg/min).[270] A similar infusion rate for remifentanil with N_2O is recommended for pediatric patients. A lower infusion rate (0.2 to 0.25 μg/kg/min) is needed when remifentanil is combined with sevoflurane (1 to 2%),[223] desflurane (3 to 3.6%),[224,271] or isoflurane (0.2 to 0.8%).[221,222,252] For TIVA, maintenance infusion rates for remifentanil and propofol are 0.25 to 0.5 μg/kg/min and 75 to 100 μg/kg/min, respectively.[203,221,268,272,273] If N_2O is added, remifentanil infusion rates as low as 0.125 μg/kg/min and propofol infusion of 50 to 75 μg/kg/min can be used.[272] For elderly patients or those with cardiac disease, a reduction in propofol by about 25% is recommended. Although children require higher remifentanil doses to block responses to skin incision, effective infusion rates for anesthetic maintenance are similar to those of adults, with remifentanil at 0.25 μg/kg/min and propofol about 100 μg/kg/min. For high-dose opioid anesthesia for cardiac surgery, the remifentanil infusion is maintained at 1 to 3 μg/kg/min and should be adjusted downward for hypothermia, as discussed earlier.[228] Adding a low-dose propofol infusion of 50 μg/kg/min to this high infusion rate effectively suppressed responses to skin incision, sternotomy, and aortic cannulation.[274]

If TCI is used, a target range for remifentanil is 4 to 10 ng/mL for balanced anesthesia and TIVA, and a starting rate of 25 to 30 ng/mL is recommended for high-dose opioid anesthesia.[228,259]

A disadvantage of remifentanil, related to its short duration of action, is that patients may experience substantial pain on emergence from anesthesia. Thus, if moderate-to-severe postoperative pain is anticipated, continuing the remifentanil infusion between 0.05 and 0.15 μg/kg/min ensures adequate analgesia in most patients.[209] The use of local and regional anesthetic techniques is also effective. When only mild postoperative pain is anticipated, intraoperative administration of a nonsteroidal anti-inflammatory drug 30 to 60 minutes before the end of surgery may provide effective analgesia without additional opioids.

Monitored Anesthesia Care. Remifentanil can also be used for conscious sedation/analgesia and as an adjunct for sedation or analgesia during regional anesthesia, or for block placement, as part of monitored anesthesia care. When local or regional anesthesia is not used and the procedure is expected to be painful, remifentanil and propofol can be beneficial. During colonoscopy, a continuous remifentanil infusion of 0.2 to 0.25 μg/kg/min, supplemented with small (10-mg) doses of propofol provided good analgesia but mild respiratory depression was common.[232] In another clinical evaluation, patients having extracorporeal shock wave lithotripsy received low-dose

propofol (50 μg/kg/min) as well as remifentanil. Patients who received low-dose (12.5 to 25 μg) intermittent bolus injection of remifentanil with or without infusion at 0.05 μg/kg/min reported better analgesia than continuous infusion of 0.1 μg/kg/min alone.[231] Remifentanil 1 μg/kg with or without a subsequent infusion of 0.2 μg/kg/min administered 90 seconds prior to placement of ophthalmologic block resulted in excellent analgesia,[275] but 14% of patients who received an infusion experienced respiratory depression.

When used as an adjunct to local or regional anesthesia, a much lower maintenance infusion rate, 0.05 to 0.1 μg/kg/min, provides adequate sedation and analgesia.[234,235] Finally, the dose requirement of remifentanil for sedation/analgesia is reduced approximately 50% when combined with midazolam or propofol. When 1 to 2 mg of midazolam premedication is given, 0.01 to 0.07 μg/kg/min remifentanil provides good sedation/analgesia for procedures performed under local or regional anesthesia.[233,234]

PARTIAL AGONISTS AND MIXED AGONIST–ANTAGONISTS

The partial agonist and mixed agonist–antagonist opioids are synthetic or semisynthetic compounds that are structurally related to morphine. They are characterized by binding activity at multiple opioid receptors and their differential effects (agonist, partial agonist, or antagonist) at each receptor type. The clinical effect of a partial agonist at the μ-opioid receptor is complex (Fig. 19-11). Administered alone, a partial agonist has a flatter dose-response curve and a lower maximal effect than a full agonist (see Fig. 19-1 and the lowermost curve in Fig. 19-11). Combined with a low concentration (compare the curve indicated by [A] = 0.25 in Fig. 19-11) of a full agonist,

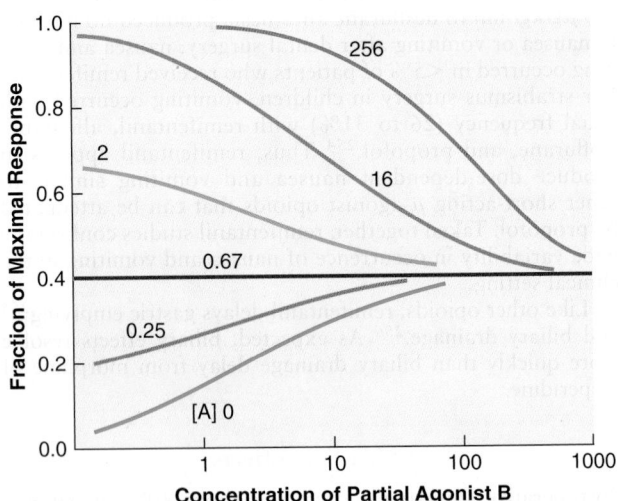

FIGURE 19-11. Hypothetical log dose-effect curves for the combination of a partial agonist, B (intrinsic efficacy of 0.4), with a range of concentrations of a full agonist, A. The observed effect of the combination of A and B is expressed as a fraction of the maximal effect of the full agonist. As the concentration of the partial agonist increases, the effect of the combination converges on the maximum effect of the partial agonist. When added to a low concentration (e.g., [A] = 0.25) of agonist, the partial agonist increases the response; but when added to a large concentration of the agonist, the response decreases—that is, B acts like an antagonist. (Modified with permission from Bowdle TA: Partial agonist and agonist–antagonist opioids: Basic pharmacology and clinical applications. Anaesth Pharmacol Rev 1993; 1: 135.)

TABLE 19-5

ACTIONS OF NALBUPHINE, BUTORPHANOL, AND BUPRENORPHINE AT OPIOID RECEPTORS[a]

■ DRUG	■ μ RECEPTOR	■ κ RECEPTOR
Nalbuphine	Partial agonist	Partial agonist
Butorphanol	Partial agonist	Partial agonist
Buprenorphine	Partial agonist	—

[a]Although nalbuphine and butorphanol have been reported to be antagonists at the μ opioid receptor, they do cause respiratory depression, which is not a function of κ agonists. Thus, they appear to have at least partial agonist activity at the μ-opioid receptor.
Adapted from Bowdle TA: Partial agonist and agonist–antagonist opioids: Basic pharmacology and clinical applications. Anesth Pharmacol Rev 1993; 1: 135.

the effects of the partial agonist are additive up to the maximum effect of the partial agonist. Combined with increasing concentrations ([A] = 0.67 to 256) of full agonist, the partial agonist will act as an antagonist. These drugs mediate their clinical effects via μ and κ-opioid receptors, as summarized in Table 19-5. The classification scheme presented may change as our understanding of these drugs and of opioid receptors continues to grow. Bowdle[276] extensively reviewed the pharmacology and clinical uses of these and other drugs in this class. Only nalbuphine, butorphanol, and buprenorphine are considered in this chapter.

The major role of the opioid agonist–antagonist and partial agonist drugs continues to be in the provision of postoperative analgesia, but they have also been used for intraoperative sedation, as adjuncts during general anesthesia, and to antagonize some effects of full μ opioid agonists.

Nalbuphine

Nalbuphine is a phenanthrene opioid derivative. Although often classified as a κ agonist and μ antagonist, it is more accurately described as a partial agonist at both κ and μ receptors.[276] While studies have not been done in humans, Murphy and Hug[25] reported that a 0.5 mg/kg dose reduced enflurane MAC by 8% in dogs. However, increasing the dose eightfold produced no further reduction in enflurane MAC. This modest MAC reduction, compared with 65% for morphine, suggests nalbuphine may not be a useful adjunct for general anesthesia. However, several investigators have examined its effectiveness as a component of balanced anesthesia for cardiac[277] and lower abdominal surgery.[25,278] Combined with diazepam 0.4 mg/kg and 50% N_2O in oxygen, a loading dose of 3 mg/kg was followed by additional doses of 0.25 mg/kg as needed throughout surgery. No significant increases in blood pressure, stress hormones, or histamine were seen, and emergence from anesthesia was uncomplicated.[277] Nalbuphine 0.2 mg/kg was compared with meperidine 0.5 mg/kg as an adjuvant to general anesthesia with 1% halothane and 70% N_2O in oxygen in spontaneously breathing patients undergoing inguinal hernia repair.[279] Both drugs produced a similar degree of respiratory depression, postoperative analgesia, and side effects. The most common side effect was drowsiness. In a double-blind comparison with fentanyl for gynecologic surgery, fentanyl was found to better attenuate hypertensive responses to intubation and surgical stimulation.[278] However, significant respiratory depression was seen in 8 of 30 patients who received fentanyl; 4 required naloxone, compared with no respiratory depression in the nalbuphine group. Analgesia was similar and, as in other studies, postoperative sedation was common in the nalbuphine group.

The respiratory depression produced by nalbuphine, most likely mediated by μ-opioid receptors, has a ceiling effect equivalent to that produced by ~0.4 mg/kg morphine.[276] Analgesia is mediated by both κ and μ receptors. Because of these effects, nalbuphine has been used to antagonize the respiratory depressant effects of full agonists while still providing analgesic effects. In a double-blind comparison, both nalbuphine and naloxone antagonized fentanyl-induced postoperative respiratory depression, but patients who received nalbuphine had less reversal of analgesia.[280] Nalbuphine can also antagonize respiratory depression following high-dose (100 to 120 μg/kg) fentanyl for cardiac surgery.[281] Only 3 of 21 patients experienced pain after nalbuphine administration, and this was adequately treated with additional nalbuphine. However, in a volunteer study, nalbuphine 0.21 mg/kg did not antagonize the respiratory depressant effects of 0.21 mg/kg morphine.[282] While nalbuphine and other agonist–antagonists have ceiling analgesic and respiratory depressant effects, they can be as effective as full μ agonists in providing postoperative analgesia. Nalbuphine 5 to 10 mg has also been used to antagonize pruritus induced by epidural and intrathecal morphine. The usual adult dose of nalbuphine is 10 mg as often as every 3 hours. It is important to be aware that nalbuphine can precipitate withdrawal symptoms in patients who are physically dependent on opioids.

Butorphanol

Butorphanol, a morphinan congener, has partial agonist activity at κ- and μ-opioid receptors, similar to those of nalbuphine. Compared with nalbuphine and similar drugs, however, butorphanol has a pronounced sedative effect, which is probably mediated by κ receptors. In a laboratory study as well as in clinical use as a premedicant, butorphanol produced dose-dependent sedation comparable to that of midazolam.[283] Like nalbuphine, butorphanol decreases enflurane MAC, in dogs, by a modest amount, 11%, at 0.1 mg/kg.[30] Increasing the butorphanol dose 40-fold does not produce a further reduction. However, like nalbuphine, butorphanol has also been reported to be an effective component of balanced general anesthesia. Combined with diazepam and nitrous oxide, butorphanol and morphine provided equally satisfactory anesthesia.[276]

Given alone, butorphanol produces respiratory depression with a ceiling effect below that of full μ agonists. In postoperative patients a parenteral dose of 3 mg produces respiratory depression approximately equal to that of 10 mg morphine. In a clinical study examining its effectiveness in reversing fentanyl-induced respiratory depression,[284] patients anesthetized with isoflurane, nitrous oxide, and fentanyl 5 μg/kg followed by an infusion of 3 μg/kg/hr received three sequential doses of butorphanol 1 mg at 10- to 15-minute intervals. After the first 1-mg dose, respiratory rate and ventilatory response to CO_2 increased, while end-tidal CO_2 decreased significantly. Further progressive changes were not significantly different from the initial response to butorphanol and analgesia was not significantly affected in 21 of 22 patients.

In contrast to morphine, fentanyl, and even meperidine, butorphanol does not produce significant elevation in intrabiliary pressure[83] (Fig. 19-6). Butorphanol has also been effective in the treatment of postoperative shivering,[88] but the mechanism for this effect is unknown. Butorphanol's agonist activity at the κ receptor produces an antipruritic effect that is blocked by a selective κ antagonist.[35] Thus, butorphanol may be able to reduce morphine-induced pruritus without completely blocking its analgesic effect. On the other hand, it is unknown whether increased sedation, which is possible with such coadministration, would outweigh an antipruritic benefit.

Butorphanol is indicated for use as a sedative and in treatment of moderate postoperative pain. Preliminary clinical experience suggests that butorphanol administered as patient-controlled analgesia is associated with a lower incidence of opioid-induced ileus compared with μ-selective opioids (P. J. Dunbar, personal communication, 1996). A dose as low as 0.5 mg can provide clinically useful sedation, while single analgesic doses range from 0.5 to 2 mg. Butorphanol has also been administered epidurally and transnasally.

Buprenorphine

Buprenorphine is a highly lipophilic thebaine derivative, and is a partial μ opioid agonist. At small-to-moderate doses it is 25 to 50 times more potent than morphine.[1] Unlike nalbuphine and butorphanol, buprenorphine does not appear to have agonist activity at the κ-opioid receptor (Table 19-5).[276] Another unique characteristic of buprenorphine is its slow dissociation from μ receptors, which can lead to prolonged effects not easily antagonized by naloxone. Buprenorphine also appears to have an unusual bell-shaped dose-response curve such that, at very high doses, it produces progressively less analgesia.[276] In a clinical study, patients who received 10 or 20 μg/kg buprenorphine during surgery were pain-free postoperatively, but half of the patients who received 30 or 40 μg/kg had significant postoperative pain.[285] This observation is consistent with buprenorphine's bell-shaped dose-effect curve, and patients who received very high buprenorphine doses probably had plasma drug concentrations in the range at which declining analgesia is seen.

Buprenorphine also appears to have a ceiling effect to its respiratory depressant dose-response curve. However, although buprenorphine-induced respiratory depression can be prevented by prior naloxone administration, it is not easily reversed by naloxone once the effects have been produced.[1] A dose of 0.3 mg buprenorphine reduces CO_2 responsiveness to about 50% of control values.[286] Large doses of naloxone (5 to 10 mg) were required to antagonize buprenorphine respiratory depression in volunteers, while 1-mg doses were not effective. In addition, the maximum antagonist effect did not occur until 3 hours after naloxone administration, an observation consistent with buprenorphine's slow dissociation from μ receptors. Buprenorphine has been compared with naloxone in its ability to antagonize fentanyl-induced respiratory depression, and appears to increase respiratory rate without antagonizing analgesic effects in slowly administered doses up to 0.5 mg.[287]

Buprenorphine can be effective in treatment of moderate-to-severe pain. Its onset can be slow, but analgesic duration can be >6 hours. A single dose of 0.3 to 0.4 mg appears to produce analgesia equivalent to 10 mg morphine.[1]

OPIOID ANTAGONISTS (NALOXONE AND NALTREXONE)

Under normal conditions, opioid antagonists produce few effects. They are competitive inhibitors of the opioid agonists, so the effect profile depends on the type and dose of agonist administered as well as the degree to which physical dependence on the opioid agonist has developed. The most widely used opioid antagonist is *naloxone*, which is structurally related to morphine and oxymorphone, and is a pure antagonist at μ-, κ-, and δ-opioid receptors.[1] *Naltrexone* is a long-acting oral agent, which also has relatively pure antagonist activity. In some circumstances, naloxone can antagonize effects that appear to be mediated by endogenous opioids. For example, naloxone can reverse "stress analgesia" in animals and man, it can antagonize analgesia produced by low-frequency stimulation with acupuncture needles, and it can also reverse analgesia produced by placebo medications.[1]

In clinical anesthesia practice, naloxone is administered to antagonize opioid-induced respiratory depression and sedation. Because opioid antagonists will reverse all opioid effects, including analgesia, naloxone should be carefully titrated to avoid producing sudden, severe pain in postoperative patients. Sudden, complete antagonism of opioid effects with naloxone has been reported to cause severe hypertension, tachycardia, ventricular dysrhythmias, and acute, sometimes fatal, pulmonary edema.[288] Naloxone-induced pulmonary edema can occur even in healthy young patients who have received relatively small doses (80 to 500 μg) of naloxone.[289,290] The mechanism for this phenomenon is thought to be centrally mediated catecholamine release, which causes acute pulmonary hypertension. Because most patients with opioid-induced respiratory depression will often breathe on command, it is important to stimulate them in addition to administering carefully titrated naloxone doses in the immediate postoperative period. It is also essential to monitor vital signs and oxygenation closely after naloxone is administered to detect occurrence of any of these potentially serious complications.

Naloxone will precipitate opioid withdrawal symptoms in opioid-dependent individuals. Clinicians tend to be aware of this risk when treating patients with known opioid addiction, but it is important to consider the potential for opioid withdrawal syndrome when treating nonaddicts who use opioids chronically, such as cancer patients and severe burn and trauma patients with protracted recovery courses.

Naloxone has a very fast onset of action, and thus is easily titrated. Peak effects occur within 1 to 2 minutes, and duration is dose-dependent, but total doses of 0.4 to 0.8 mg generally last 1 to 4 hours.[1] Suggested incremental doses for IV titration are 20 to 40 μg given every few minutes until the patient's ventilation improves, but analgesia is not completely reversed. Because naloxone has a short duration of action, respiratory depression may recur if large doses and/or long-acting opioid agonists have been administered. When prolonged ventilatory depression is anticipated, an initial loading dose followed by a naloxone infusion can be used. Infusion rates between 3 and 10 μg/hr have been effective in antagonizing respiratory depression from systemic as well as epidural opioids.[291]

While peripherally acting μ antagonists are undergoing preliminary trials in prevention of treatment of opioid-mediated gastrointestinal dysfunction,[54] they are not yet available for clinical use.

USE OF OPIOIDS IN CLINICAL ANESTHESIA

Opioids are used alone or in combination with other agents, such as sedatives or anticholinergic agents, as "premedications." For this purpose, longer-acting opioids such as morphine are administered as single doses that are generally within the "analgesic" range. The goal of opioid premedication is to provide moderate sedation, anxiolysis, and analgesia while maintaining hemodynamic stability. Potential risks of opioid premedication include oversedation, respiratory depression, and nausea and vomiting. For induction of anesthesia, opioids are often used to blunt or prevent the hemodynamic responses to tracheal intubation. Opioids with rapid onset of action, such as fentanyl and its derivatives, are appropriate for this use.

Intraoperatively, opioids are administered as components of balanced anesthesia, or alone in high-dose opioid anesthesia. During maintenance of general anesthesia, opioid dosage is titrated to the desired effect based on the surgical stimulus as well as individual patient characteristics, such as age, volume status, neurologic status, liver dysfunction, or other systemic disease states. Plasma opioid concentrations required to blunt hemodynamic responses to laryngoscopy, tracheal intubation, and various surgical stimuli, as well as plasma opioid concentration associated with awakening from anesthesia, have been determined for several opioids. Titration to achieve these plasma concentrations (Table 19-3), which reflect brain (effect site) concentrations, can be accomplished by administering repeated small bolus doses or by manual- or target-controlled infusion. Fentanyl and its derivatives sufentanil and alfentanil are the opioids most widely used as supplements to general anesthesia; remifentanil is a useful alternative when ultrashort duration is desirable. All of these opioids are more easily titrated than morphine because of their rapid onset of action. However, Shafer and Varvel[15] have emphasized that making a rational choice among these opioids requires an understanding of the relationships between their pharmacokinetics and pharmacodynamics. They have used elegant computer models to simulate the rate of decrease in plasma and effect site (brain) concentrations after various administration methods, including bolus doses, brief infusion, and prolonged infusion. Decreases in effect site concentration will determine time to recovery from various opioid effects. Comparable simulations have also been done for the newer opioid remifentanil.[218] Important pharmacokinetic differences among these opioids include volumes of distribution and intercompartmental (distributional) and central (elimination) clearances. A smaller distribution volume tends to shorten recovery time, and a reduction in clearance tends to increase recovery time.[15] The major pharmacodynamic differences among these opioids are potency and the equilibration times between the plasma and the site of drug effect. Equilibration half-times between plasma and effect site are 5 to 6 minutes for fentanyl and sufentanil and 1.3 to 1.5 minutes for alfentanil and remifentanil.[15,207] Computer simulations demonstrate that simply comparing elimination half-lives will not predict the relative rate of decline in drug concentration at the effect site after either bolus doses or continuous infusion of fentanyl, sufentanil, and alfentanil. The rate of recovery after a continuous infusion will depend on the duration of the infusion as well as the magnitude of decline that is required. Figure 19-12 demonstrates

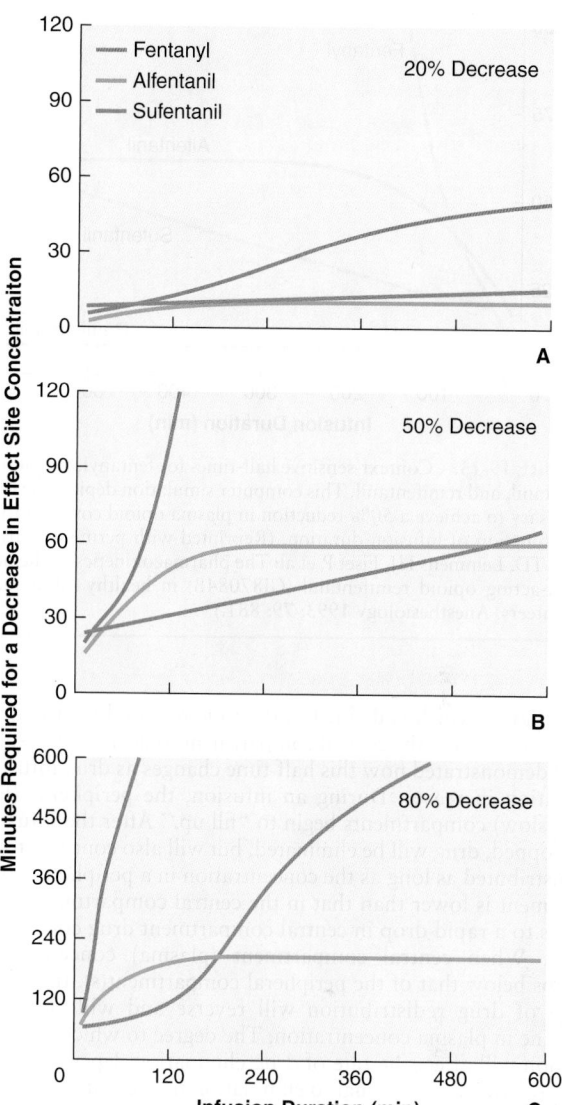

FIGURE 19-12. Recovery curves for fentanyl, sufentanil, and alfentanil showing the time required for decreases of 20% (**A**), 50% (**B**), and 80% (**C**) from maintained intraoperative effect site (brain) concentrations after termination of the infusion. (Reprinted with permission from Shafer SL, Varvel JR: Pharmacokinetics, pharmacodynamics, and rational opioid selection. Anesthesiology 1991; 74: 53.)

how the times required for 20, 50, and 80% decrements in effect site (i.e., brain) concentrations vary with each opioid depending on infusion duration. If only a 20% drop in effect site concentration is required (upper panel), recovery from all three opioids will be rapid, although recovery time increases for fentanyl after 3 hours of drug infusion. However, if a 50% decrease is required, recovery from sufentanil will be fastest for infusions <6 to 8 hours in duration, but more rapid for alfentanil if infusions are continued for >8 hours.

Context-Sensitive Half-Time

Hughes et al.[16] expanded the concepts of Shafer and Varvel[15] to define the relative contributions of distribution compartments to central compartment (plasma) drug distribution. These relative contributions vary according to infusion duration. Hughes et al. devised the concept of "context-sensitive

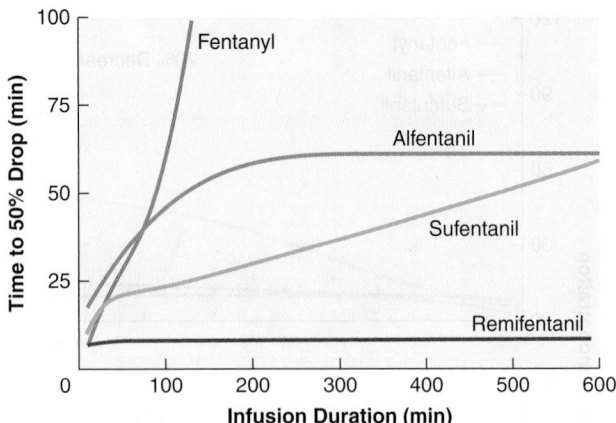

FIGURE 19-13. Context-sensitive half-times for fentanyl, sufentanil, alfentanil, and remifentanil. This computer simulation depicts the time necessary to achieve a 50% reduction in plasma opioid concentration as a function of infusion duration. (Reprinted with permission from Egan TD, Lemmens HJ, Fiset P, et al: The pharmacokinetics of the new short-acting opioid remifentanil (GI87084B) in healthy adult male volunteers. Anesthesiology 1993; 79: 881.)

half-time," which is defined as the time required for the drug concentration in the central compartment to decrease by 50%, and demonstrated how this half-time changes as drug infusion duration increases. During an infusion, the peripheral (fast and slow) compartments begin to "fill up." After the infusion is stopped, drug will be eliminated, but will also continue to be redistributed as long as the concentration in a peripheral compartment is lower than that in the central compartment. This leads to a rapid drop in central compartment drug concentration. When central compartment (plasma) concentration drops below that of the peripheral compartment(s), the direction of drug redistribution will reverse and will slow the decline in plasma concentration. The degree to which redistribution will affect the rate of drug elimination depends on the ratio of the distributional to elimination time constants. Thus, a drug that can rapidly redistribute will have a correspondingly larger contribution from the peripheral compartment(s), and plasma concentration will drop progressively more slowly as infusion duration continues. Figure 19-13 illustrates the context-sensitive half-times for fentanyl, alfentanil, sufentanil, and remifentanil. This model predicts the time to a 50% concentration decrease in the plasma, which will reflect, but not be equal to, effect site concentrations depicted in Figure 19-12.

Some testing of these computer models in humans has been done. Kapila et al.[292] compared modeled context-sensitive half-times with measured decreases in drug concentration and drug effect (respiratory depression) in volunteers receiving remifentanil and alfentanil. After 3-hour opioid infusions, measured whole blood opioid concentrations and recovery of ventilatory drive corresponded closely to modeled values for both drugs. Although the concept of a context-sensitive half-time appears to be useful, Hughes et al.[16] noted that it is unknown whether a decrement of 50% provides the most clinically useful description of the rate of offset of opioid effects. If one closely titrates infusions so that minimum effective concentrations are achieved, perhaps much smaller decrements will be necessary. For example, it can be seen in the upper panel of Figure 19-12 that if only a 20% decline in effect site concentration is needed, fentanyl, sufentanil, and alfentanil concentrations all drop rapidly if the infusion duration is 2 hours or less. This rapid resolution is seen for sufentanil and alfentanil even with prolonged (5- to 10-hour) administration if only a 20% decrement is required. In practice, it is relatively

easy to administer higher than necessary doses of opioids, particularly to mechanically ventilated patients, because hemodynamic consequences are minimal. Titrating against a quantifiable parameter, such as minute ventilation in a spontaneously breathing patient, may allow a tighter dose titration, but this may not be practical for many surgeries—for example, those requiring the use of muscle relaxants. It does seem clear, however, that some context-sensitive index is more useful than the elimination half-life. Understanding these concepts can be useful when deciding which opioid to use, as well as in adapting guidelines for opioid dosage and infusion rates depending on the duration of anesthesia.

References

1. Jaffe JH, Martin WR: Opioid analgesics and antagonists, The Pharmacological Basis of Therapeutics. Edited by Gilman AG, Goodman LS, Rall TW, et al. New York, Macmillan, 1985, p 49
2. Rey A: L'Examen Clinique en Psychologie. Paris, Presses Universitaires de France, 1964
3. Lowenstein E: Morphine anesthesia: A perspective. Anesthesiology 1971; 35: 563
4. Martin WR: Multiple opioid receptors. Life Sci 1981; 128: 1547
5. Pleuvry BJ: The endogenous opioid system. Anaesth Pharmacol Rev 1993; 1: 114
6. Pasternak GW: Pharmacologic mechanisms of opioid analgesics. Clin Neuropharmacol 1993; 16: 1
7. Horn AS, Rodgers JR: Structural and conformational relationships between the enkephalins and the opiates. Nature 1976; 260: 795
8. Stefano GB, Zhu W, Cadet P, et al: Morphine enhances nitric oxide release in the mammalian gastrointestinal tract via the micro(3) opioate receptor subtype: a hormonal role for endogenous morphine. J Physiol Pharmacol 2004; 55: 279
9. McFadzean I: The ionic mechanisms underlying opioid mechanisms. Neuropeptides 1988; 11: 173
10. Mousa SA, Straub RH, Shäfer M, et al: Beta-endorphin, Met-enkephalin and corresponding opioid receptors within synovium of patients with joint trauma, osteoarthritis and rheumatoid arthritis. Ann Rheum Dis 2007; 66: 871
11. Nuñéz S, Lee JS, Zhang Y, et al: Role of peripheral μ-opioid receptors in inflammatory orofacial muscle pain. Neuroscience 2007; 146: 1346
12. Li Z, Proud D, Zhang C, et al: Chronic arthritis down-regulates peripheral μ-opioid receptor expression with concomitant loss of endomorphin 1 antinociception. Arthritis Rheum 2005; 52: 3210
13. Rashid MH, Inoue M, Toda K, et al: Loss of peripheral morphine analgesia contributes to the reduced effectiveness of systemic morphine in neuropathic pain. J Pharmacol Ther 2004; 309: 380
14. Thorpe DH: Opiate structures and activity: A guide to underlying opioid actions. Anesth Analg 1984; 63: 143
15. Shafer SL, Varvel JR: Pharmacokinetics, pharmacodynamics, and rational opioid selection. Anesthesiology 1991; 74: 53
16. Hughes MA, Glass PSA, Jacobs JR: Context-sensitive half-time in multicompartment pharmacokinetic models for intravenous anesthetic drugs. Anesthesiology 1992; 76: 334
17. Bovill JG: Pharmacokinetics and pharmacodynamics of opioid agonists. Anaesth Pharmacol Rev 1993; 1: 122
18. Hansch C, Dunn WJ: Linear relationships between lipophilic character and biological activity of drugs. J Pharm Sci 1972; 61: 1
19. Bernards CM, Hill HF: Physical and chemical properties of drug molecules governing their diffusion through the spinal meninges. Anesthesiology 1992; 77: 750
20. Lipp J: Possible mechanisms of morphine analgesia. Clin Neuropharmacol 1991; 14: 31
21. Yeung JC, Rudy TA: Multiplicative interaction between narcotic agonisms expressed at spinal and supraspinal sites of antinociceptive action as revealed by concurrent intrathecal and intracerebroventricular injections of morphine. J Pharmacol Exp Ther 1980; 215: 633
22. Stein C, Millan MJ, Shippenberg TS, et al: Peripheral opioid receptors mediating antinociception in inflammation: Evidence for involvement of μ, δ and κ receptors. J Pharmacol Exp Ther 1989; 248: 1269
23. Dahlstrom B, Tamsen A, Psalzow I, et al: Patient-controlled analgesia therapy. Part IV: Pharmacokinetics and analgesic plasma concentrations of morphine. Clin Pharmacokinetics 1982; 7: 266
24. Hill HF, Coda BA, Mackie AM, et al: Patient-controlled analgesic infusions: Alfentanil versus morphine. Pain 1992; 49: 301
25. Murphy MR, Hug CC: The enflurane-sparing effect of morphine, butorphanol, and nalbuphine. Anesthesiology 1982; 57: 489
26. Lake CL, DiFazio CA, Moscicki JC, et al: Reduction in halothane MAC: Comparison of morphine and alfentanil. Anesth Analg 1985; 64: 807
27. Roizen MF, Horrigan RW, Frazer BM: Anesthetic doses blocking adrenergic (stress) and cardiovascular responses to incision-MAC BAR. Anesthesiology 1981; 54: 390

28. Schweiger IM, Klopfenstein CE, Forster A: Epidural morphine reduces halothane MAC in humans. Can J Anaesth 1992; 39: 911

29. Drasner K, Bernards CM, Ozanne GM: Intrathecal morphine reduces the minimum alveolar concentration of halothane in humans. Anesthesiology 1988; 69: 310

30. Licina MG, Schubert A, Tobin JE, et al: Intrathecal morphine dose not reduce minimum alveolar concentration of halothane in humans: Results of a double-blind study. Anesthesiology 1991; 74: 660

31. Coda BA, Hill HF, Hunt EB, et al: Cognitive and motor function impairments during continuous opioid analgesic infusions. Hum Psychopharmacol 1993; 8: 383

32. Smith NT, Dee-Silver H, Sanford TJ, et al: EEGs during high-dose fentanyl–, sufentanil–, or morphine–oxygen anesthesia. Anesth Analg 1984; 63: 386

33. Martin WR: Pharmacology of opioids. Pharmacol Rev 1984; 35: 283

34. Thomas DA, Williams GM, Iwata K, et al: The medullary dorsal horn: A site of action of morphine in producing facial scratching in monkeys. Anesthesiology 1993; 79: 548

35. Lee H, Naughton NN, Woods JH, et al: Effects of Butorphanol on morphine-induced itch and analgesia in primates. Anesthesiology 2007; 107: 478

36. Arunasalam K, Davenport HT, Painter S, et al: Ventilatory response to morphine in young and old subjects. Anaesthesia 1983; 38: 529

37. Daykin AP, Bowen DJ, Saunders DA, et al: Respiratory depression after morphine in the elderly. Anaesthesia 1986; 41: 910

38. Forrest WH, Bellville JW: The effect of sleep plus morphine on the respiratory response to carbon dioxide. Anesthesiology 1964; 25: 137

39. Catley DM, Thornton C, Jordan C, et al: Pronounced episodes of oxygen desaturation on the postoperative period: Its association with ventilatory pattern and analgesic regimen. Anesthesiology 1985; 63: 20

40. Duthie DJR, Nimmo WS: Adverse effects of opioid analgesic drugs. Br J Anaesth 1987; 59: 61

41. Freund FG, Martin WE, Wong KC, et al: Abdominal-muscle rigidity induced by morphine and nitrous oxide. Anesthesiology 1973; 38: 358

42. Weinger MB, Cline EJ, Smith NT, et al: Localization of brainstem sites which mediate alfentanil-induced muscle rigidity in the rat. Pharmacol Biochem Behav 1988; 29: 573

43. Smith NT, Benthuysen JL, Bickford RG, et al: Seizures during opioid anesthetic induction: Are they opioid-induced rigidity? Anesthesiology 1989; 71: 852

44. Bowdle TA, Rooke GA: Postoperative myoclonus and rigidity after anesthesia with opioids. Anesth Analg 1994; 78: 783

45. Watcha MF, White PF: Postoperative nausea and vomiting. Anesthesiology 1992; 77: 162

46. Hill HF, Chapman CR, Saeger LS, et al: Steady-state infusions of opioids in human. II. Concentration–effect relationships and therapeutic margins. Pain 1990; 43: 69

47. Coda BA, O'Sullivan B, Donaldson G, et al: Comparative efficacy of patient-controlled administration of morphine, hydromorphone, or sufentanil for the treatment of oral mucositis pain following bone marrow transplantation. Pain 1997; 72: 333

48. Crozier TA, Kietzmann D, Dobermeier B: Mood change after anaesthesia with remifentanil or alfentanil. Eur J Anaesthesiol 2004; 21: 20

49. Peroutka SJ, Snyder SH: Antiemetics: Neurotransmitter receptor binding predicts therapeutic actions. Lancet 1982; 20: 659

50. Costello DJ, Borison HL: Naloxone antagonizes narcotic self blockade of emesis in the cat (abs). J Pharmacol Exp Ther 1977; 203: 222

51. Coda BA, Mackie A, Hill HF: Influence of alprazolam on opioid analgesia and side effects during steady-state morphine infusions. Pain 1992; 50: 309

52. Burks TF, Fox DA, Hirning LD, et al: Regulation of gastrointestinal function by multiple opioid receptors. Life Sci 1988; 43: 2177

53. Murphy DB, Sutton JA, Prescott LF, et al: Opioid-induced delay in gastric emptying: A peripheral mechanism in humans. Anesthesiology 1997; 87: 765

54. Holzer P: Treatment of opioid-induced gut dysfunction. Expert Opin Investig Drugs 2007; 16: 181

55. Thorén T, Wattwil M: Effects on gastric emptying of thoracic epidural analgesia with morphine or bupivicaine. Anesth Analg 1988; 67: 687

56. Hahn M, Baker R, Sullivan S: The effect of four narcotics on cholecystokinin octapeptide stimulated gallbladder contraction. Aliment Pharmacol Ther 1988; 2: 129

57. Thune A, Baker RA, Saccone GT, et al: Differing effects of pethidine and morphine on human sphincter of Oddi motility. Br J Surg 1990; 77: 992

58. Ehrenpreis S, Kimura I, Kobayashi T, et al: Histamine release as the basis for morphine action on bile duct and sphincter of Oddi. Life Sci 1987; 40: 1695

59. Dray A: Epidural opiates and urinary retention: New models provide new insights. Anesthesiology 1988; 68: 323

60. Durant PAC, Yaksh TL: Drug effects on urinary bladder tone during spinal morphine-induced inhibition of the micturition reflex in unanesthetized rats. Anesthesiology 1988; 68: 325

61. Stellato C, Cirillo R, de Paulis A, et al: Human basophil/mast cell releasability: IX. Heterogeneity of the effects of opioids on mediator release. Anesthesiology 1992; 77: 32

62. Hermens JM, Ebertz JM, Hanifin JM, et al: Comparison of histamine release in human skin mast cells induced by morphine, fentanyl, and oxymorphone. Anesthesiology 1985; 62: 124

63. Rosow CE, Moss J, Philbin DM, et al: Histamine release during morphine and fentanyl anesthesia. Anesthesiology 1982; 56: 93

64. Lowenstein E, Whiting RB, Bittar DA, et al: Local and neurally mediated effects of morphine on skeletal muscle vascular resistance. J Pharmacol Exp Ther 1972; 180: 359

65. Roizen MF: Does the choice of anesthetic (narcotic versus inhalational) significantly affect cardiovascular outcome after cardiovascular surgery?, Opioids in Anesthesia. Edited by Estafanous FG. Boston, Butterworth, 1984, pp 180

66. Bilfinger TV, Fimiani C, Stefano GB: Morphine's immunoregulatory actions are not shared by fentanyl. Int J Cardiol 1998; 64(Suppl 1): S61

67. Murphy GS, Szokol JW, Marymount JH, et al: The effects of morphine and fentanyl on the inflammatory response to cardiopulmonary bypass in patients undergoing elective coronary artery bypass graft surgery. Anesth Analg 2007; 104: 1334

68. Murphy GS, Szokol JW, Marymount JH, et al: Opioids and cardioprotection: the impact of morphine and fentanyl on recovery of ventricular function after cardiopulmonary bypass. J Cardiothorac Vasc Anesth 2006; 20: 493

69. Stanski DR, Greenblatt DJ, Lowenstein E: Kinetics of intravenous and intramuscular morphine. Clin Pharmacol Ther 1978; 24: 52

70. Murphy MR, Hug CC: Pharmacokinetics of intravenous morphine in patients anesthetized with enflurane–nitrous oxide. Anesthesiology 1981; 54: 187

71. Mazoit JX, Sandouk P, Zetlaoui P: Pharmacokinetics of unchanged morphine in normal volunteers. Anesth Analg 1987; 66: 293

72. Sear JW, Hand CW, Moore RA, et al: Studies on morphine disposition: influence of general anesthesia on plasma concentrations of morphine and its metabolites. Br J Aneasth 1989; 662: 22

73. Lynn AM, Slattery JT: Morphine pharmacokinetics in early infancy. Anesthesiology 1987; 66: 136

74. Osborne R, Joel S, Trew D, et al: Morphine and metabolite behavior after different routes of morphine administration: Demonstration of the importance of the active metabolite morphine-6-glucuronide. Clin Pharmacol Ther 1990; 47: 12

75. Lehmann KA, Zech D: Morphine-6-glucuronide, a pharmacologically active morphine metabolite: A review of the literature. Eur J Pain 1993; 14: 28

76. Portenoy RK, Thaler HT, Inturrisi CE, et al: The metabolite morphine-6-glucuronide contributes to the analgesia produced by morphine infusion in patients with pain and normal renal function. Clin Pharmacol Ther 1992; 51: 422

77. Osborne R, Thompson P, Joel S, et al: The analgesic activity of morphine-6-glucuronide. Br J Clin Pharmacol 1992; 34: 130

78. Lötsch J: Morphine metabolites as novel analgesic drugs? Curr Opin Anaesthesiol 2004; 17: 449

79. Kurz M, Belani KG, Sessler DI, et al: Naloxone, meperidine, and shivering. Anesthesiology 1993; 79: 1193

80. Tamsen A, Hartvig P, Fagerlund C, et al: Patient-controlled analgesic therapy, part II: Individual analgesic demand and analgesic plasma concentrations of pethidine in postoperative pain. Clin Pharmacokinet 1982; 7: 164

81. Steffey EP, Martucci R, Howland D, et al: Meperidine–halothane interaction in dogs. Can Anaesth Soc J 1977; 24: 459

82. Kaya K, Babacan A, Beyazova M, et al: Effects of perineural opioids on nerve conduction of N. suralis in man. Acta Neurol Scand 1992; 85: 337

83. Radnay PA, Duncalf D, Novakovic M, et al: Common bile duct pressure changes after fentanyl, morphine, meperidine, butorphanol, and naloxone. Anesth Analg 1984; 63: 441

84. Yrjola H, Heinonen J, Tuominen M, et al: Comparison of haemodynamic effects of pethidine and anileridine in anaesthetised patients. Acta Anaesthesiol Scand 1981; 25: 412

85. Rendig SV, Amsterdam EA, Henderson GL, et al: Comparative cardiac contractile actions of six narcotic analgesics: Morphine, meperidine, pentazocine, fentanyl, methadone and L-α-acetylmethadol (LAAM). J Pharmacol Exp Ther 1980; 215: 259

86. Flacke JW, Bloor BC, Kripke BJ, et al: Comparison of morphine, meperidine, fentanyl, and sufentanil in balanced anesthesia: A double-blind study. Anesth Analg 1985; 64: 897

87. Macintyre PE, Pavlin EG, Dwersteg JF: Effect of meperidine on oxygen consumption, carbon dioxide production, and respiratory gas exchange in postanesthesia shivering. Anesth Analg 1987; 66: 751

88. Vogelsang J, Hayes SR: Butorphanol tartrate (Stadol) relieves postanesthesia shaking more effectively than meperidine (Demerol) or morphine. J Post Anesth Nurs 1992; 7: 94

89. Joris J, Banache M, Bonnet F, et al: Clonidine and ketanserin both are effective treatment for postanesthetic shivering. Anesthesiology 1993; 79: 532

90. Matsukawa T, Kurz A, Sessler DI, et al: Propofol linearly reduces the vasoconstriction and shivering thresholds. Anesthesiology 1995; 82: 1169

91. Horn E-P, Standl T, Sessler DI, et al: Physostigmine prevents postanesthetic shivering as does meperidine or clonidine. Anesthesiology 1998; 88: 108

92. Mather LE, Tucker GT, Pflug AE, et al: Meperidine kinetics in man: Intravenous injection in surgical patients and volunteers. Clin Pharmacol Ther 1975; 17: 27

93. Koska AJ, Kramer WG, Romagnoli A, et al: Pharmacokinetics of high-dose meperidine in surgical patients. Anesth Analg 1981; 60: 8

94. Wong YC, Chan K, Lau OW, et al: Protein binding characterization of pethidine and norpethidine and lack of interethnic variability. Methods Find Exp Clin Pharmacol 1991; 13: 273

95. Kaiko RF, Foley KM, Grabinski PY, et al: Central nervous system excitatory effects of meperidine in cancer patients. Ann Neurol 1983; 13: 180

96. Gourlay GK, Wilson PR, Glynn CJ: Pharmacodynamics and pharmacokinetics of methadone during the perioperative period. Anesthesiology 1982; 57: 458

97. Gourlay GK, Willis RJ, Wilson PR: Postoperative pain control with methadone: Influence of supplementary methadone doses and blood concentration–response relationships. Anesthesiology 1984; 61: 19

98. Wangler MA, Rosenblatt RM: Methadone titration to avoid excessive respiratory depression. Anesthesiology 1983; 59: 363

99. Scott JC, Ponganis KV, Stanski DR: EEG quantitation of narcotic effect: The comparative pharmacodynamics of fentanyl and alfentanil. Anesthesiology 1985; 62: 234

100. Gourlay GK, Kowalski SR, Plummer JL, et al: Fentanyl blood concentration–analgesic response relationship in the treatment of postoperative pain. Anesth Analg 1988; 67: 329

101. Hug CC: Pharmacokinetics of new synthetic narcotic analgesics, Opioids in Anesthesia. Edited by Estafanous FG. Boston, Butterworth, 1984, p 50

102. Sebel PS, Glass PSA, Fletcher JE, et al: Reduction of the MAC of desflurane with fentanyl. Anesthesiology 1992; 76: 52

103. Daniel M, Weiskopf RB, Noorani M, et al: Fentanyl augments the blockade of the sympathetic response to incision (MAC-BAR) produced by desflurane and isoflurane. Anesthesiology 1998; 88: 43

104. Westmoreland CL, Sebel PS, Gropper A: Fentanyl or alfentanil decreases the minimum alveolar anesthetic concentration of isoflurane in surgical patients. Anesth Analg 1994; 78: 23

105. Katoh T, Ikeda K: The effects of fentanyl on sevoflurane requirements for loss of consciousness and skin incision. Anesthesiology 1998; 88: 18

106. Inagaki Y, Mashimo T, Yoshiya I: Segmental analgesic effect and reduction of halothane MAC from epidural fentanyl in humans. Anesth Analg 1992; 74: 856

107. Kazama T, Ikeda K, Morita K: The pharmacodynamic interaction between propofol and fentanyl with respect to the suppression of somatic or hemodynamic responses to skin incision, peritoneum incision, and abdominal wall retraction. Anesthesiology 1998; 89: 894

108. Shafer SL, Varvel JR, Aziz N, et al: Pharmacokinetics of fentanyl administered by computer-controlled infusion pump. Anesthesiology 1990; 73: 1091

109. Glass PSA, Jacobs JR, Smith LR, et al: Pharmacokinetic model-driven infusion of fentanyl: Assessment of accuracy. Anesthesiology 1990; 73: 1082

110. Philbin DM, Rosow CE, Schneider RC, et al: Fentanyl and sufentanil anesthesia revisited: How much is enough? Anesthesiology 1990; 73: 5

111. Trindle MR, Dodson BA, Rampil IJ: Effects of fentanyl versus sufentanil in equianesthetic doses on middle cerebral artery blood flow volume. Anesthesiology 1993; 78: 454

112. Sperry RJ, Bailey PL, Reichman MV, et al: Fentanyl and sufentanil increase intracranial pressure in head trauma patients. Anesthesiology 1992; 77: 416

113. Jung R, Shah N, Reinsel R, et al: Cerebrospinal fluid pressure in patients with brain tumors: Impact of fentanyl versus alfentanil during nitrous oxide–oxygen anesthesia. Anesth Analg 1990; 71: 419

114. Streisand JB, Bailey PL, LeMaire L, et al: Fentanyl-induced rigidity and unconsciousness in human volunteers. Anesthesiology 1993; 78: 629

115. Bailey PL, Wilbrink J, Zwanikken P, et al: Anesthetic induction with fentanyl. Anesth Analg 1985; 64: 48

116. Lunn JK, Stanley TH, Eisele J, et al: High dose fentanyl anesthesia for coronary artery surgery: Plasma fentanyl concentrations and influence of nitrous oxide on cardiovascular responses. Anesth Analg 1979; 58: 390

117. Scott JC, Sarnquist FH: Seizure-like movements during a fentanyl infusion with absence of seizure activity in a simultaneous EEG recording. Anesthesiology 1985; 62: 812

118. Manninen PH, Burke SJ, Wennberg R, et al: Intraoperative localization of epileptogenic focus with alfentanil and fentanyl. Anesth Analg 1999; 88: 1101

119. Phua WT, Teh BT, Jong W, et al: Tussive effect of a fentanyl bolus. Can J Anaesth 1991; 38: 330

120. McClain DA, Hug CC: Intravenous fentanyl kinetics. Clin Pharmacol Ther 1980; 28: 106

121. Bailey PL, Pace NL, Ashburn MA, et al: Frequent hypoxemia and apnea after sedation with midazolam and fentanyl. Anesthesiology 1990; 73: 826

122. Bailey PL, Streisand JB, East KA, et al: Differences in magnitude and duration of opioid-induced respiratory depression and analgesia with fentanyl and sufentanil. Anesth Analg 1990; 70: 8

123. Knill RL: Does sufentanil produce less ventilatory depression than fentanyl? Anesth Analg 1990; 71: 564

124. Cartwright P, Prys-Roberts C, Gill K, et al: Ventilatory depression related to plasma fentanyl concentrations during and after anesthesia in humans. Anesth Analg 1983; 62: 966

125. Tagaito Y, Isono S, Nishino T: Upper airway reflexes during a combination of propofol and fentanyl anesthesia. Anesthesiology 1998; 88: 1459

126. Stanley TH, Webster LR: Anesthetic requirements and cardiovascular effects of fentanyl–oxygen and fentanyl–diazepam–oxygen anesthesia in man. Anesth Analg 1978; 57: 411

127. Bovill JG, Sebel PS, Stanley TH: Opioid analgesics in anesthesia: With special reference to their use in cardiovascular anesthesia. Anesthesiology 1984; 61: 731

128. Flacke JW, Flacke WE, Bloor BC, et al: Histamine release by four narcotics: A double-blind study in humans. Anesth Analg 1987; 66: 723

129. Giesecke K, Hamberger B, Järnberg PO, et al: High- and low-dose fentanyl anaesthesia: Hormonal and metabolic responses during cholecystectomy. Br J Anaesth 1988; 61: 575

130. Hug CC, Murphy MR: Tissue redistribution of fentanyl and termination of its effects in rats. Anesthesiology 1981; 55: 369

131. Bentley JB, Borel JD, Nenad RE, et al: Age and fentanyl pharmacokinetics. Anesth Analg 1982; 61: 968

132. Scott JC, Stanski DR: Decreased fentanyl and alfentanil dose requirements with age: A simultaneous pharmacokinetic and pharmacodynamic evaluation. J Pharmacol Exp Ther 1987; 240: 159

133. Mather LE: Clinical pharmacokinetics of fentanyl and its newer derivatives. Clin Pharmacokinetics 1983; 8: 422

134. Meuldermans WEG, Hurkmans RMA, Heykants JJP: Plasma protein binding and distribution of fentanyl, sufentanil, alfentanil and lofentanil in blood. Arch Int Pharmacodyn 1982; 257: 4

135. Streisand JB, Stanski DR, Hague B, et al: Oral transmucosal fentanyl citrate premedication in children. Anesth Analg 1989; 69: 28

136. Gerwels JW, Bezzant JL, Le Maire L, et al: Oral transmucosal fentanyl citrate for painful procedures in patients undergoing outpatient dermatologic procedures. J Dermatol Surg Oncol 1994; 20: 823

137. Foldes FF: Neuroleptanesthesia for general surgery, International Anesthesiology Clinics. Edited by Oyama T. Boston, Little, Brown, 1973, pp 1

138. White P: Droperidol: A cost-effective antiemetic for over thirty years. Anesth Analg 2002; 95: 789

139. Sprigge JS, Wynands JE, Whalley DG, et al: Fentanyl infusion anesthesia for aortocoronary bypass surgery: Plasma levels and hemodynamic response. Anesth Analg 1982; 61: 972

140. Monk JP, Beresford R, Ward A: Sufentanil: A review of its pharmacological properties and therapeutic use. Drugs 1988; 36: 286

141. Scott JC, Cooke JE, Stanski DR: Electroencephalographic quantitation of opioid effect: Comparative pharmacodynamics of fentanyl and sufentanil. Anesthesiology 1991; 74: 34

142. Geller E, Chrubasik J, Graf R, et al: A randomized double-blind comparison of epidural sufentanil versus intravenous sufentanil or epidural fentanyl analgesia after major abdominal surgery. Anesth Analg 1993; 76: 1243

143. Lehmann KA, Gerhard A, Horrichs-Haermeyer G, et al: Postoperative patient-controlled analgesia with sufentanil: Analgesic efficacy and minimum effective concentrations. Acta Anaesthesiol Scand 1991; 35: 221

144. Coda BA, Hill HF, Bernards C, et al: Comparison of therapeutic margins of sufentanil and morphine during steady-state infusions in volunteers. Anesthesiology 1991; 75: A673

145. Hall RI, Murphy MR, Hug CC: The enflurane sparing effect of sufentanil in dogs. Anesthesiology 1987; 67: 518

146. Brunner MD, Braithwaite P, Jhaveri R, et al: MAC reduction of isoflurane by sufentanil. Br J Anaesth 1994; 72: 42

147. Bailey JM, Schweiger IM, Hug CC: Evaluation of sufentanil anesthesia obtained by a computer-controlled infusion for cardiac surgery. Anesth Analg 1993; 76: 247

148. Marx W, Shah N, Long C, et al: Sufentanil, alfentanil, and fentanyl: Impact on cerebrospinal fluid pressure in patients with brain tumors. J Neurosurg Anesth 1989; 1: 3

149. Mayer N, Weinstabl C, Podreka I, et al: Sufentanil does not increase cerebral blood flow in healthy human volunteers. Anesthesiology 1990; 73: 240

150. Werner C, Hoffman WE, Baughman VL, et al: Effects of sufentanil on cerebral blood flow, cerebral blood flow velocity, and metabolism in dogs. Anesth Analg 1991; 72: 177

151. Welchew EA, Herbert P: Effects of sufentanil on respiration and heart rate during nitrous oxide and halothane anaesthesia. Br J Anaesth 1986; 58: 120P

152. Robinson D: Respiratory arrest after recovery from anaesthesia supplemented with sufentanil. Can J Anaesth 1988; 35: 101

153. Karasawa F, Iwanov V, Moulds RF: Sufentanil and alfentanil cause vasorelaxation by mechanisms independent of the endothelium. Clin Exp Pharmacol Physiol 1993; 20: 705

154. Sebel PS, Bovil JG: Cardiovascular effects of sufentanil. Anesth Analg 1982; 61: 115

155. Rosow CE: Cardiovascular effects of opioid analgesia. Mt Sinai J Med 1987; 54: 273

156. Clark NJ, Meuleman T, Liu W, et al: Comparison of sufentanil–N_2O and fentanyl–N_2O in patients without cardiac disease undergoing general surgery. Anesthesiology 1987; 66: 130

157. Thomson IR, MacAdams CL, Hudson RJ, et al: Drug interactions with sufentanil. Anesthesiology 1992; 76: 922

158. Schmeling WT, Bernstein JS, Vucins EJ, et al: Persistent bradycardia with episodic sinus arrest after sufentanil and vecuronium administration: Successful treatment with isoproterenol. J Cardiothorac Anesth 1990; 4: 89

159. Bovill JG, Sebel PS, Fiolet JWT, et al: The influence of sufentanil on endocrine and metabolic responses to cardiac surgery. Anesth Analg 1983; 62: 391

160. Bovill JG, Sebel PS, Blackburn CL, et al: The pharmacokinetics of sufentanil in surgical patients. Anesthesiology 1984; 61: 502

161. Schwartz AE, Matteo RS, Ornstein E, et al: Pharmacokinetics of sufentanil in obese patients. Anesth Analg 1991; 73: 790

162. Chauvin M, Ferrier C, Haberer JP, et al: Sufentanil pharmacokinetics in patients with cirrhosis. Anesth Analg 1989; 68: 1

163. Bowdle TA, Ward RJ: Induction of anesthesia with small doses of sufentanil or fentanyl: Dose versus EEG response, speed of onset, and thiopental requirement. Anesthesiology 1989; 70: 26

164. Cork RC, Gallo JA, Weiss LB, et al: Sufentanil infusion: Pharmacokinetics compared to bolus. Anesth Analg 1988; 67: S1

165. Lehmann KA: The pharmacokinetics of opioid analgesics with special reference to patient-controlled administration, Patient-Controlled Analgesia. Edited by Harmer M, Rosen M, Vickers MD. Oxford, Blackwell Scientific, 1985, pp 18

166. van den Nieuwenhuyzen MCO, Engbers FHM, Burm AGL, et al: Computer-controlled infusion of alfentanil for postoperative analgesia: A pharmacokinetic and pharmacodynamic evaluation. Anesthesiology 1993; 79: 481

167. Welchew EA, Hosking J: Patient-controlled postoperative analgesia with alfentanil. Anaesthesia 1985; 40: 1172

168. Chauvin M, Hongnat JM, Mourgeon E, et al: Equivalence of postoperative analgesia with patient-controlled intravenous or epidural alfentanil. Anesth Analg 1993; 76: 1251

169. Hall RI, Szlam F, Hug CC: The enflurane-sparing effect of alfentanil in dogs. Anesth Analg 1987; 66: 1287

170. Ausems ME, Hug CC, Stanski DR, et al: Plasma concentrations of alfentanil required to supplement nitrous oxide anesthesia for general surgery. Anesthesiology 1986; 65: 362

171. Ausems ME, Vuyk J, Hug CC, et al: Comparison of a computer-assisted infusion versus intermittent bolus administration of alfentanil as a supplement to nitrous oxide for lower abdominal surgery. Anesthesiology 1988; 68: 851

172. Vuyk J, Lim T, Engbers FHM, et al: Pharmacodynamics of alfentanil as a supplement to propofol or nitrous oxide for lower abdominal surgery in female patients. Anesthesiology 1993; 78: 1036

173. Nauta J, de Lange S, Koopman D, et al: Anesthetic induction with alfentanil: A new short-acting narcotic analgesic. Anesth Analg 1982; 61: 267

174. Hug CC, Hall RI, Angert KC, et al: Alfentanil plasma concentration vs. effect relationships in cardiac surgical patients. Br J Anaesth 1988; 61: 435

175. Hynynen M, Takkunen O, Salmenperä M, et al: Continuous infusion of fentanyl or alfentanil for coronary artery surgery. Br J Anaesth 1986; 58: 1252

176. Bovill JG, Sebel PS, Wauquier A, et al: Influence of high-dose alfentanil anaesthesia on the electroencephalogram: Correlation with plasma concentrations. Br J Anaesth 1983; 55: 199

177. Benthuysen JL, Smith NT, Sanford TJ, et al: Physiology of alfentanil-induced rigidity. Anesthesiology 1986; 64: 440

178. Mayberg TS, Lam AM, Eng CC, et al: The effect of alfentanil on cerebral blood flow velocity and intracranial pressure during isoflurane–nitrous oxide anesthesia in humans. Anesthesiology 1993; 78: 288

179. Olsen KS, Juul N, Cold GE: Effect of alfentanil on intracranial pressure during propofol-fentanyl anesthesia for craniotomy. A randomized prospective dose-response study. Acta Anaesthesiol Scand 2005; 49: 445

180. Owen H, Currie JC, Plummer JL: Variation in the blood concentration/analgesic response relationship during patient-controlled analgesia with alfentanil. Anaesth Intens Care 1991; 19: 555

181. O'Connor M, Escarpa A, Prys-Roberts C: Ventilatory depression during and after infusion of alfentanil in man. Br J Anaesth 1983; 55: 217S

182. Andrews CJH, Sinclair M, Prys-Roberts C, et al: Ventilatory effects during and after continuous infusion of fentanyl or alfentanil. Br J Anaesth 1983; 55: 211S

183. Stanley TH, Pace NL, Liu WS, et al: Alfentanil–N2O vs fentanyl–N2O balanced anaesthesia: Comparison of plasma hormonal changes, early postoperative respiratory function, and speed of postoperative recovery. Anesth Analg 1983; 62: 245

184. Hudson RJ: Apnoea and unconsciousness after apparent recovery from alfentanil-supplemented anaesthesia. Can J Anaesth 1990; 37: 255

185. Rucquoi M, Camu F: Cardiovascular responses to large doses of alfentanil and fentanyl. Br J Anaesth 1983; 55: 223S

186. Crawford DC, Fell D, Achola KJ, et al: Effects of alfentanil on the pressor and catecholamine responses to tracheal intubation. Br J Anaesth 1987; 59: 707

187. Silbert BS, Rosow CE, Keegan CR, et al: The effect of diazepam on induction of anesthesia with alfentanil. Anesth Analg 1986; 65: 71

188. Kirby IJ, Northwood D, Dodson ME: Modification by alfentanil of the haemodynamic response to tracheal intubation in elderly patients. Br J Anaesth 1988; 60: 384

189. Skues MA, Richards MJ, Jarvis A, Prys-Roberts C: Preinduction atropine or glycopyrrolate and hemodynamic changes associated with induction and maintenance of anesthesia with propofol and alfentanil. Anesth Analg 1989; 69: 386

190. Bloomfield EL: The incidence of postoperative nausea and vomiting: A retrospective comparison of alfentanil versus sufentanil. Mil Med 1992; 157: 59

191. Sfez M, Mapihan YL, Gaillard JL, et al: Analgesia for appendectomy: A comparison of fentanyl and alfentanil in children. Acta Anaesthesiol Scand 1990; 34: 30

192. Bovill JG: Which potent opioid? Important criteria for selection. Drugs 1987; 33: 520

193. Bovill JG, Sebel PS, Blackburn CL, et al: The pharmacokinetics of alfentanil (R39209): A new opioid analgesic. Anesthesiology 1982; 57: 439

194. Stanski DR, Hug CC: Alfentanil: A kinetically predictable narcotic analgesic. Anesthesiology 1982; 57: 435

195. Chauvin M, Bonnet F, Montembault C, et al: The influence of hepatic plasma flow on alfentanil plasma concentration plateaus achieved with an infusion model in humans: Measurement of alfentanil hepatic extraction coefficient. Anesth Analg 1986; 65: 999

196. Ferrier C, Marty J, Bouffard Y, et al: Alfentanil pharmacokinetics in patients with cirrhosis. Anesthesiology 1985; 62: 480

197. Chauvin M, Lebrault C, Levron JC, et al: Pharmacokinetics of alfentanil in chronic renal failure. Anesth Analg 1987; 66: 53

198. Larijani GE, Goldberg ME: Alfentanil hydrochloride: A new short-acting narcotic analgesic for surgical procedures. Clin Pharm 1987; 6: 275

199. Abou-Arab MH, Heiser T, Caldwell JE: Dose of alfentanil needed to obtain optimal intubation conditions during rapid-sequence induction of anaesthesia with thiopentone and rocuronium. Br J Anaesth 2007; 98: 604

200. Kim JY, Kwak YL, Lee KC, et al: The optimal bolus dose of alfentanil for trachea intubation during sevoflurane induction without neuromuscular blockade in day-case anaesthesia. Acta Anaesthesiol Scand 2008; 52: 106

201. Yu AL, Critchey LA, Lee A, et al: Alfentanil dosage when inserting the classic laryngeal mask airway. Anesthesiology 2006; 105: 684

202. Philip BK, Scuderi PE, Chung F, et al: Remifentanil compared with alfentanil for ambulatory surgery using total intravenous anesthesia. The Remifentanil/Alfentanil Outpatient TIVA Group. Anesth Analg 1997; 84: 515

203. Ozkose Z, Cok OY, Tuncer B, et al: Comparison of hemodynamics, recovery profile, early postoperative pain, and costs of remifentnail versus alfentanil-based total intravenous anesthesia (TIVA). J Clin Anesthesia 2002; 14: 161

204. Ganidagli S, Cengiz M, Baysal Z: Remifentanil vs. alfentanil in the total intravenous anaesthesia for pediatric surgery. Paediatric Anaesthesia 2003; 13: 695

205. Davis PJ, Lerman J, Suresh S, et al: A randomized multicenter study of remifentanil compared with alfentanil, isoflurane, or propofol in anesthetized pediatric patients undergoing elective strabismus surgery. Anesth Analg 1997; 84: 282

206. James MK, Feldman PL, Schuster SV, et al: Opioid receptor activity of GI87084B, a novel ultra-short acting analgesic, in isolated tissues. J Pharmacol Exp Ther 1991; 259: 712

207. Glass PSA, Hardman D, Kamiyama Y, et al: Preliminary pharmacokinetics and pharmacodynamics of an ultra-short-acting opioid: Remifentanil (GI87084B). Anesth Analg 1993; 77: 1031

208. Black ML, Hill JL, Zacny JP: Behavioral and physiological effects of remifentanil and alfentanil in human volunteers. Anesthesiology 1999; 90: 718

209. Bowdle TA, Camporesi EM, Maysick L, et al: A multicenter evaluation of remifentanil for early postoperative analgesia. Anesth Analg 1996; 83: 1292

210. Schraag S, Kenny GN, Mohl U, et al: Patient-maintained remifentanil target-controlled infusion for the transition to early postoperative analgesia. Br J Anaesth 1998; 81: 365

211. Volmanen P, Akural EI, Raudaskoski T, et al: Remifentanil in obstetric analgesia: A dose-finding study. Anesth Analg 2002; 94: 913

212. Michlesen LG, Salmenpera M, Hug CC, et al: Anesthetic potency of remifentanil in dogs. Anesthesiology 1996; 84: 865

213. Criado AB, Gómez de Segura IA: Reduction in isoflurane MAC by fentanyl or remifentanil in rats. Veterinary Anesthesia and Analgesia 2003; 30: 250

214. Lang E, Kapila A, Shlugman D, et al: Reduction of isoflurane minimal alveolar concentration by remifentanil. Anesthesiology 1996; 85: 721

215. Albertin A, Casati A, Bergonzi P, et al: Effects of two target-controlled concentrations (1 and 3 ng/ml) of remifentanil on MAC(BAR) of sevoflurane. Anesthesiology 2004; 100: 255

216. Albertin A, Dedola E, Bergonzi PC, et al: The effect of adding two target-controlled concentrations (1–3 ng/ml) of remifenatnil on MAC BAR of desflurane. Eur J Anaesthesiol 2006; 23: 510

217. Jhaveri R, Joshi P, Batenhorst R, et al: Dose comparison of remifentanil and alfentanil for loss of consciousness. Anesthesiology 1997; 87: 253

218. Bouillon TW, Bruhn J, Radulescu L, et al: Pharmacodynamic interaction between remifentanil and propofol regarding hypnosis, tolerance of laryngoscopy, bispectral index, and electroencephalographic approximate entropy. Anesthesiology 2004; 100: 1353

219. Drover DR, Lemmens HJ: Population pharmacodynamics and pharmacokinetics of remifentanil as a supplement to nitrous oxide anesthesia for elective abdominal surgery. Anesthesiology 1998; 89: 869

220. Muñoz HR, Cortinez LI, Ibacache ME, et al: Remifentanil requirements during propofol administration to block the somatic response to skin incision in children and adults. Anesth Analg 2007; 104: 77

221. Joshi GP, Warner DS, Twersky RS, et al: A comparison of the remifentanil and fentanyl adverse effect profile in a multicenter phase IV study. J Clin Anesth 2002; 14: 494

222. Snyed JR, Camu F, Doenicke A, et al: Remifentanil during anaesthesia for major abdominal and gynaecological surgery. An open, comparative study of safety and efficacy. Eur J Anaesthesiol 2001; 18: 605, 2110

223. Van Delden PG, Houweling PL, Bencini AF, et al: Remifentanil-sevoflurane anaesthesia for laparoscopic cholecystectomy: comparison of three dose regimens. Anaesthesia 2002; 57: 212

224. Billard V, Servin F, Guignard B, et al: Desflurane-remifantnail-nitrous oxide anesthesia for abdominal surgery: Optimal concentrations and recovery features. Acta Anaesthesiol Scand 2004; 48: 355

225. Mertens MJ, Olofsen E, Engbers FH, et al: Propofol reduces perioperative remifentanil requirements in a synergistic manner. Response surface modeling of perioperative remifentanil-propofol interactions. Anesthesiology 2003; 99: 347

226. Fragen RJ, Randel GI, Librojo ES, et al: The interaction of remifentanil and propofol to prevent response to tracheal intubation and the start of surgery for outpatient knee arthroscopy. Anesthesiology 1994; 81: A376

227. Ivilicki L, Balkan BK, Gökel BK, et al; The effects of alfentnail or remifentanil pretreatment on propofol injection pain. J Clin Anesth 2004; 16: 499

228. Barvais L, Sutcliffe N: Remifentanil for cardiac anesthesia. Adv Exp Med Biol 2003; 523: 171

229. Guarracino F, Penzo D, De Cosmo D, et al: Pharmacokinetic-based total intravenous anaesthesia using remifentanil and propofol for surgical myocardial revascularization. Eur J Anaesthesiol 2003; 20: 385

230. Engoren M, Luther G, Fenn-Buderer N: A comparison of fentanyl, sufentanil, and remifentanil for fast-track cardiac anesthesia. Anesth Analg 2001; 93: 859

231. Sá Rêgo MM, Inagaki Y, White PF: Remifentanil administration during monitored anesthesia care: Are intermittent boluses an effective alternative to a continuous infusion? Anesth Analg 1999; 88: 518

232. Rudner R, Przemyslaw J, Kawecki P, et al: Conscious analgesia/sedation with remifentanil and propofol versus total intravenous anesthesia with fentanyl, midazolam, and propofol for outpatient colonoscopy, Gastrointest Endosc 2003; 57: 657

233. Gold MI, Watkins WD, Sung YF, et al: Remifentanil vs. remifentanil/midazolam for ambulatory surgery during monitored anesthesia care. Anesthesiology 1997; 87: 51

234. Lauwers M, Camu F, Breivik H, et al: The safety and effectiveness of remifentanil as an adjunct sedative for regional anesthesia. Anesth Analg 1999; 88: 134

235. Servin FS, Raeder JC, Merle JC, et al: Remifentanil sedation compared with propofol during regional anaesthesia. Acta Anaesthesiol Scand 2002; 46: 309

236. Egan TD, Lemmens HJM, Fiset P, et al: The pharmacokinetics of the new short-acting opioid remifentanil (GI87084B) in healthy adult male volunteers. Anesthesiology 1993; 79: 881

237. Egan TD, Minto CF, Hermann DJ, et al: Remifentanil vs. alfentanil: Comparative pharmacokinetics and pharmacodynamics in healthy adult male volunteers [published erratum appears in Anesthesiology 85(3): 695, 1996]. Anesthesiology 1996; 84: 821

238. Warner DS, Hindman BJ, Todd MM, et al: Intracranial pressure and hemodynamic effects of remifentanil vs. alfentanil in patients undergoing supratentorial craniotomy. Anesth Analg 1996; 83: 348

239. Guy J, Hindman BJ, Baker KZ, et al: Comparison of remifentanil and fentanyl in patients undergoing craniotomy for supratentorial space-occupying lesions [see comments]. Anesthesiology 1997; 86(3): 514

240. Engelhard K, Waser C, Mollenaz O, et al: Effects of remifentanil/propofol in comparison with isoflurane on dynamic cerebrovascular autoregulation in humans. Acta Anaesthesiol Scand 2001; 45: 971

241. Scheufler KM, Zentner J: Total intravenous anesthesia for intraoperative monitoring of the motor pathways: An integral view combining clinical and experimental data. J Neurosurg 2002; 96: 571

242. Smith DL, Angst MS, Brock-Utne JG, et al: Seizure duration with remifentanil/methohexital vs. methohexital alone in middle-aged patients undergoing electroconvulsive therapy. Acta Anaesthesiol Scand 2003; 47: 1064

243. Glass PSA, Hardman HD, Kamiyama Y, et al: Pharmacodynamic comparison of GI87084B (GI), a novel ultra-short acting opioid, and alfentanil. Anesth Analg 1992; 74: S113

244. Glass PS, Iselin Chaves IA, Goodman D, et al: Determination of the potency of remifentanil compared with alfentanil using ventilatory depression as the measure of opioid effect. Anesthesiology 1999; 90: 1556

245. Bouillon T, Bruhn J, Radu-Radulescu L, et al: Model of the ventilatory depressant potency of remifentanil in the non-steady state. Anesthesiology 2003; 99: 779

246. Ma D, Chakrabarti MK, Whitwam JG: The combined effects of sevoflurane and remifentanil on central respiratory activity and nociceptive cardiovascular responses in anesthetized rabbits. Anesth Analg 1999; 89: 453

247. Peacock JE, Phillip BK: Ambulatory anesthesia experience with remifentanil. Anesth Analg 1999; 89: S22

248. Pitts MC, Palmore MM, Salmenpera MT, et al: Pilot study: Hemodynamic effects of intravenous GI87084B (GI) in patients undergoing elective surgery. Anesthesiology 1992; 77: A101

249. Keidan I, Berkenstadt H, Sidi A, et al: Propofol/remifentanil versus propofol alone for bone marrow aspiration in paediatric haemato-oncological patients. Paediatric Anaesthesia 2001; 11: 297

250. Sebel PS, Hoke JF, Westmoreland C, et al: Histamine concentrations and hemodynamic responses after remifentanil. Anesth Analg 1995; 80: 990

251. DeSouza G, Lewis MC, TerRiet MF: Severe bradycardia after remifentanil [letter]. Anesthesiology 1997; 87: 1019

252. Cartwright DP, Kvalsvik O, Cassuto J, et al: A randomized, blind comparison of remifentanil and alfentanil during anesthesia for outpatient surgery. Anesth Analg 1997; 85: 1014

253. Dershwitz M, Michalowski P, Chang Y, et al: Postoperative nausea and vomiting after total intravenous anesthesia with propofol and remifentanil or alfentanil: How important is the opioid? J Clin Anesth 2002; 14: 275

254. Davis PJ, Lerman J, Suresh S, et al: A randomized multicenter study of remifentanil compared with alfentanil. Isoflurane or propofol; in anesthetized pediatric patients undergoing elective strabismus surgery. Anesth Analg 1997; 84: 982

255. Walldén J, Thörn SE, Wattwil M: The delay of gastric emptying induced by remifentanil is not influenced by posture. Anesth Analg 2004; 99: 429

256. Fragen RJ, Vilich F, Spies SM, et al: The effect of remifentanil on biliary tract drainage into the duodenum. Anesth Analg 1999; 89: 1561

257. Manullang J, Egan TD: Remifentanil's effect is not prolonged in a patient with pseudocholinesterase deficiency. Anesth Analg 1999; 89: 529

258. Westmoreland CL, Hoke JF, Sebel PS, et al: Pharmacokinetics of remifentanil (GI87084B) and its major metabolite (GI90291) in patients undergoing elective inpatient surgery. Anesthesiology 1993; 79: 893

259. Servin F: Remifentanil; from pharmacological properties to clinical practice. Adv Exp Med Biol 2003; 523: 245

260. Ross AK, Davis PJ, Dear G deL, et al: Pharmacokinetics of remifentanil in aesthetized pediatric patients undergoing elective surgery or diagnostic procedures. Anesth Analg 2001; 93: 1393

261. Minto CF, Schnider TW, Egan TD, et al: Influence of age and gender on the pharmacokinetics and pharmacodynamics of remifentanil. I. Model development. Anesthesiology 1997; 86: 10

262. Egan TD, Huizinga B, Gupta SK, et al: Remifentanil pharmacokinetics in obese vs. lean patients [see comments]. Anesthesiology 1998; 89: 562

263. Dershwitz M, Hoke JF, Rosow CE, et al: Pharmacokinetics and pharmacodynamics of remifentanil in volunteer subjects with severe liver disease. Anesthesiology 1996; 84: 812

264. Hoke JF, Shlugman D, Dershwitz M, et al: Pharmacokinetics and pharmacodynamics of remifentanil in persons with renal failure compared with healthy volunteers. Anesthesiology 1997; 87: 533

265. Lehmann A, Boldt J, Rompert R, et al: Target-controlled or manually controlled infusion of propofol in high-risk patients with severely reduced left ventricular function. J Cardiothorac Vasc Anesth 2001; 15: 445

266. Fragen RJ, Fitzgerald PC: Is an infusion pump necessary to safely administer remfentanil? Anesth Analg 2000; 90: 713

267. Kazmaier S, Hanekop GG, Buhre W, et al: Myocardial consequences of remifentanil in patients with coronary artery disease. Br J Anaesth 2000; 84: 578

268. Hogue CW Jr, Bowdle TA, O'Leary C, et al: A multicenter evaluation of total intravenous anesthesia with remifentanil and propofol for elective inpatient surgery. Anesth Analg 1996; 83: 279

269. Song D, Whitten CW, White PF: Use of remifentanil during anesthetic induction: A comparison with fentanyl in the ambulatory setting. Anesth Analg 1999; 88: 734

270. Dershwitz M, Randel GI, Rosow CE, et al: Initial clinical experience with remifentanil, a new opioid metabolized by esterases. Anesth Analg 1995; 81: 619

271. Pinsker MC, Carroll NV: Quality of emergence from anesthesia and incidence of vomiting with remifentanil in a pediatric population. Anesth Analg 1999; 89: 71

272 Jellish WS, Sheikh T, Baker W, et al: Hemodynamic stability, myocardial ischemia, and perioperative outcome after carotid surgery with remifentanil/propofol or isoflurane/fentanyl anesthesia. J Neurosurgical Anesthesiology 2003; 3: 176

273. Phillip BK, Scuderi PE, Chung F, et al: Remifentanil compared to alfentanil for ambulatory surgery using total intravenous anesthesia. Anesth Analg 1997; 84: 515

274. Randel GI, Fragen RJ, Librojo ES, et al: Remifentanil blood concentration effect relationship at intubation and skin incision in surgical patients compared to alfentanil. Anesthesiology 1994; 81: A375

275. Ahmad S, Leavell ME, Fragen RJ, et al: Remifentanil vs. alfentanil as analgesic adjuncts during placement of ophthalmologic nerve blocks. Reg Anesth Pain Med 1999; 24: 331

276. Bowdle TA: Partial agonist and agonist–antagonist opioids: Basic pharmacology and clinical applications. Anaesth Pharmacol Rev 1993; 1: 135

277. Zsigmond EK, Winnie AP, Raza SMA, et al: Nalbuphine as an analgesic component in balanced anesthesia for cardiac surgery. Anesth Analg 1987; 66: 1155

278. Rawal N, Wennhager M: Influence of perioperative nalbuphine and fentanyl on postoperative respiration and analgesia. Acta Anaesthesiol Scand 1990; 34: 197

279. O'Connor SA, Wilkinson DJ: A double-blind study of the respiratory effects of nalbuphine hydrochloride in spontaneously breathing anesthetized patients. Anesthesiology 1988; 67: 324.

280. Bailey PL, Clark NJ, Pace NL, et al: Antagonism of postoperative opioid-induced respiratory depression: Nalbuphine vs. naloxone. Anesth Analg 1987; 66: 1109

281. Moldenhauer CC, Roach GW, Finlayson DC, et al: Nalbuphine antagonism of ventilatory depression following high-dose fentanyl anesthesia. Anesthesiology 1985; 62: 647

282. Bailey PL, Clark NJ, Pace NL, et al: Failure of nalbuphine to antagonize morphine: A double-blind comparison with naloxone. Anesth Analg 1986; 65: 605

283. Dershwitz M, Rosow CE, DiBiase PM, et al: Comparison of the sedative effects of butorphanol and midazolam. Anesthesiology 1991; 74: 717

284. Bowdle TA, Greichen SL, Bjurstrom RI, et al: Butorphanol improves CO_2 response and ventilation after fentanyl anesthesia. Anesth Analg 1987; 66: 517

285. Pedersen JE: Perioperative buprenorphine: Do high doses shorten analgesia postoperatively? Acta Anaesthesiol Scand 1986; 30: 660

286. Gal TL: Naloxone reversal of buprenorphine-induced respiratory depression. Clin Pharmacol Ther 1989; 45: 66

287. Boysen K, Hertel S, Chraemmer-Jorgansen B, et al: Buprenorphine antagonism of ventilatory depression following fentanyl anaesthesia. Acta Anesthesiol Scand 1988; 32: 490

288. Pallasch TJ, Gill CJ: Naloxone-associated morbidity and mortality. Oral Surg Oral Med Oral Pathol 1981; 52: 602

289. Partridge BL, Ward CF: Pulmonary edema following low-dose naloxone administration. Anesthesiology 1986; 65: 709

290. Prough DS, Roy R, Bumgarner J, et al: Acute pulmonary edema in healthy teenagers following conservative doses of intravenous naloxone. Anesthesiology 1984; 60: 485

291. Rawal N, Schött U, Dahlström B, et al: Influence of naloxone infusion on analgesia and respiratory depression following epidural morphine. Anesthesiology 1986; 64: 194

292. Kapila A, Glass PSA, Jacobs JR, et al: Measured context-sensitive half-times of remifentanil and alfentanil. Anesthesiology 1995; 83: 968

ANESTHETIC AGENTS, ADJUVANTS, AND DRUG INTERACTION

CHAPTER 20 ■ NEUROMUSCULAR BLOCKING AGENTS

FRANÇOIS DONATI AND DAVID R. BEVAN

KEY POINTS

1. Neuromuscular blocking agents are used to improve conditions for tracheal intubation, to provide immobility during surgery, and to facilitate mechanical ventilation.

2. The main site of action of neuromuscular blocking agents (muscle relaxants) is on the nicotinic cholinergic receptor at the endplate of muscle. They also have effects at presynaptic receptors located on the nerve terminal.

3. Succinylcholine is a blocking agent that produces depolarization at the endplate and binds to extrajunctional receptors. In spite of many side effects, such as hyperkalemia, its rapid offset makes it the drug of choice for rapid sequence induction.

4. All other drugs available are nondepolarizing. They compete with acetylcholine for the same binding sites.

5. Fade in response to high-frequency stimulation (e.g. train-of-four, 2 Hz for 2 seconds) is a characteristic of nonde-polarizing blockade. Train-of-four fade is difficult to evaluate manually or visually during recovery when ratio is >0.4.

6. The upper airway is particularly sensitive to the effects of nondepolarizing blockade. Complete recovery does not occur until train-of-four ratio at the adductor pollicis is >0.9.

7. Residual paralysis is more frequent with long-duration than intermediate-duration agents.

8. Reversal with anticholinesterases should be attempted when a certain degree of spontaneous recovery is manifest. Ideally, all four twitches in response to train-of-four stimulation should be visible before reversal is given.

9. After injection of the selective binding agent sugammadex, neuromuscular transmission is restored because of 1:1 binding of sugammadex to rocuronium.

It appears paradoxical that drugs having peripheral effects on neuromuscular transmission might have a role in anesthesia. If the patient is anesthetized, why provide agents to prevent movement? Yet, the introduction of muscle relaxants, more appropriately called *neuromuscular blocking agents*, into clinical practice in 1942 was an important mile-stone in the history of anesthesia.[1] While the usefulness of the new drugs became apparent, there were doubts regarding patient safety. In 1954, Beecher and Todd[2] claimed that anesthetic mortality increased sixfold when muscle relaxants were used. This situation was probably because of the sub-optimal use of mechanical ventilation and reversal drugs,

498

but other controversies have arisen in recent years for a variety of reasons.

For example, the incidence of awareness appears to be greater when neuromuscular blocking agents are used,[3] and some authors recommend restricting the use of these drugs whenever possible, as patient movement might be an indicator of consciousness. However, anesthetics act at the spinal cord level to produce immobility; thus, movement in response to a noxious stimulus indicates inadequate analgesia and does not necessarily mean the patient is conscious.[4] Therefore, awareness does not occur because too much neuromuscular blocking agent has been given, but because too little anesthetic is administered. The controversy regarding neuromuscular blocking agents and awareness is complicated by the fact that neuromuscular blockade seems to affect the bispectral index (BIS), which is the most widely used measure of unconsciousness.[5] Reductions in BIS have been reported in awake individuals receiving succinylcholine and in mildly sedated patients given mivacurium.

Complete paralysis is not required for the duration of all surgical procedures. However, neuromuscular blocking agents were found to make a difference in lower abdominal surgery, where surgical conditions were better in patients receiving vecuronium (Fig. 20-1).[6] In addition to providing immobility and better surgical conditions, neuromuscular blocking agents improve intubating conditions. The doses of opioids required for acceptable intubating conditions in the absence of muscle paralysis produce significant hypotension (Fig. 20-2).[7] Providing optimal intubating conditions is not a trivial objective. Poor intubating conditions may increase the incidence of laryngeal injury, as manifested by voice hoarseness and vocal cord damage (Fig. 20-3), and the best way to improve intubating conditions is to administer neuromuscular blocking agents.[8]

It is also essential to make sure that the effects of neuromuscular blocking drugs have worn off or are reversed before the patient regains consciousness. With the introduction of shorter-acting neuromuscular blocking agents, many thought that reversal of blockade could be omitted. However, residual paralysis is still a problem, nearly 30 years after if was first

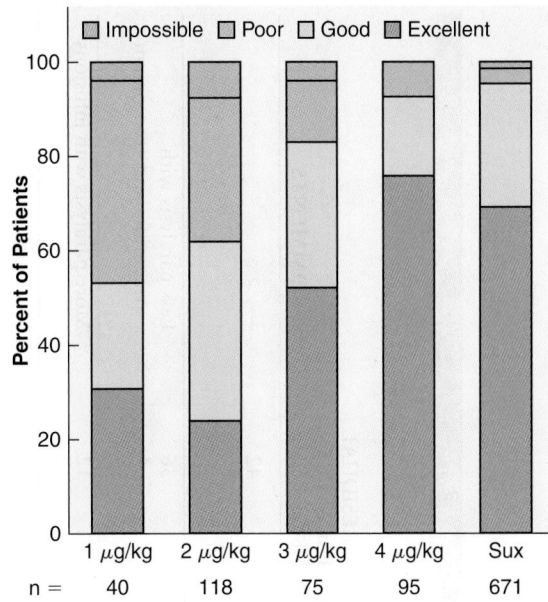

FIGURE 20-2. Neuromuscular blocking agents provide better intubating conditions than high doses of opioids, without hypotension. Hypnotic agent was propofol or thiopental. Intubating conditions are plotted against dose of remifentanil (in micrograms per kilogram). Results for succinylcholine (Sux), 1 mg/kg (with little opioid) are given for comparison. Hypotension was seen with remifentanil, 4 μg/kg.[7] (Data obtained from several different studies; references 7, 37, 38, 69, 72, 159, and 160.)

described (Table 20-1), and in spite of the availability of shorter-acting neuromuscular blocking drugs and widespread use of neuromuscular monitoring.[9] Part of this might be related to the recognition that the threshold for complete neuromuscular recovery is a train-of-four ratio of 0.9, instead of the traditional 0.7 (Fig. 20-4).[132] Thus, an understanding of the pharmacology of neuromuscular blocking agents and reversal drugs is essential.

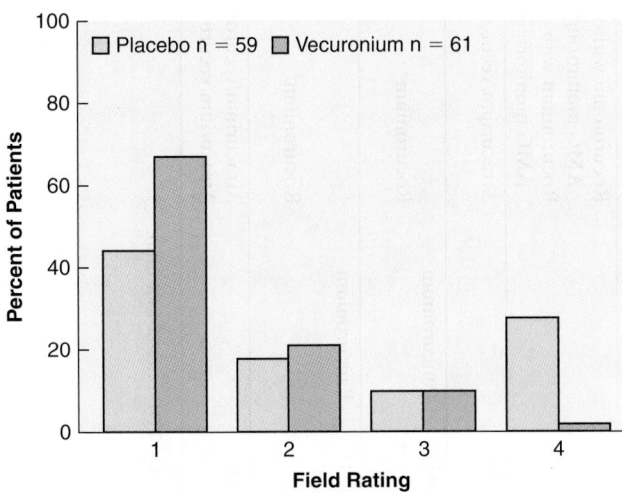

FIGURE 20-1. Surgeon's assessment of muscle relaxation during lower abdominal surgery. Rating goes from 1 (excellent) to 4 (poor). The incidence of poor rating was greater in patients not given vecuronium (29%) compared with those who received the drug (2%). (Redrawn from King M, Sujirattanawimol N, Danielson DR, et al: Requirements for muscle relaxants during radical retropubic prostatectomy. Anesthesiology 2000; 93: 1392.)

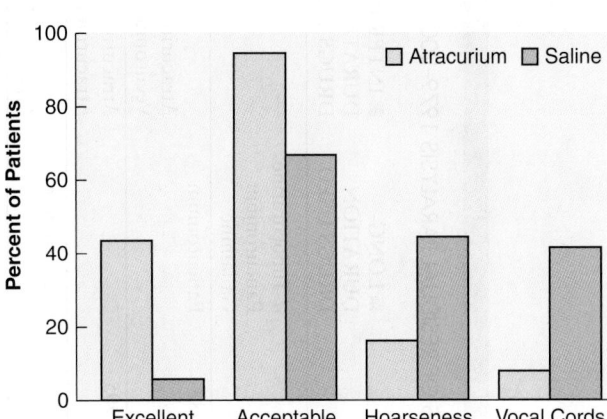

FIGURE 20-3. Neuromuscular blocking agents improve intubating conditions and reduce vocal cord sequelae. The graph depicts the incidence of excellent and acceptable (defined as good or excellent) intubating conditions after atracurium or saline. The percentage of patients who reported hoarseness and those with vocal cord lesions documented by stroboscopy is also shown. (Data from Mencke et al.[8])

TABLE 20-1

SELECTED REPORTS OF RESIDUAL PARALYSIS 1979–2007

STUDY	LONG-DURATION DRUGS USED	INTERMEDIATE-DURATION DRUGS USED	REVERSAL	TOF THRESHOLD	RESIDUAL PARALYSIS (% OF PATIENTS)	COMMENTS
Viby-Mogensen et al.,[138] 1979	*d*-Tubocurarine Pancuronium Gallamine	—	Yes	0.7	42	—
Bevan et al.,[163] 1988	Pancuronium	Atracurium Vecuronium	Yes Yes Yes	0.7 0.7 0.7	36 4 9	Less paralysis with atracurium and vecuronium
Fawcett et al.,[90] 1995		Atracurium/vecuronium bolus Atracurium/vecuronium infusion	Yes Yes	0.7 0.7	12 24	More paralysis with infusions
Berg et al., 1997[140]	Pancuronium	Atracurium/vecuronium	Yes Yes	0.7 0.7	26 5	More atelectasis when residual paralysis present
Bissinger et al.,[164] 2000	Pancuronium	Vecuronium	Yes Yes	0.7 0.7	20 8	More hypoxia with TOF < 0.7
Gatke et al.,[121] 2002		Rocuronium without AMG monitoring Rocuronium with AMG monitoring	Yes Yes	0.8 0.8	17 3	Less paralysis when AMG used
Debaene et al.,[120] 2003		Atracurium/vecuronium/rocuronium	No	0.7 0.9	16 45	Paralysis could be present even 4 hr after injection
Murphy et al.,[66] 2003	Pancuronium	Rocuronium	No No	0.8 0.8	82 0	After cardiac surgery when ready to wean from ventilatory support
Murphy et al.,[67] 2004	Pancuronium	Rocuronium	Yes Yes	0.7 0.9 0.7 0.9	47 97 7 33	More hypoxia and discharge delayed with pancuronium
Baillard et al.,[141] 2005		Atracurium/vecuronium/rocuronium Atracurium/vecuronium/rocuronium	No (94%) No (58%)	0.9 0.9	63 3	Less paralysis when reversal and monitoring used

AMG, acceleromyography; TOF, train-of-four ratio.

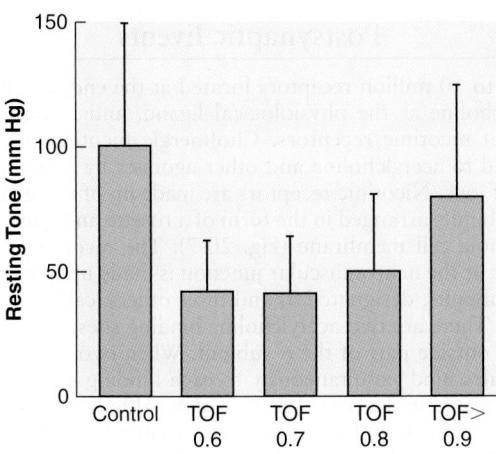

FIGURE 20-4. Upper esophageal resting tone in volunteers given vecuronium. Train-of-four ratio (TOF) was measured at the adductor pollicis muscle. Statistically significant decreases compared with control were found at all levels of paralysis until TOF >0.9. (Redrawn from Eriksson LI, Sundman E, Olsson R, et al: Functional assessment of the pharynx at rest and during swallowing in partially paralyzed humans: simultaneous videomanometry and mechanomyography of awake human volunteers. Anesthesiology 1997; 87: 1035.)

PHYSIOLOGY AND PHARMACOLOGY

Structure

The cell bodies of motor neurons supplying skeletal muscle lie in the spinal cord. They receive and integrate information from the central nervous system. This information is carried via an elongated structure, the axon, to distant parts of the body. Each nerve cell supplies many muscle cells (or fibers) a short distance after branching into nerve terminals. The terminal portion of the axon is a specialized structure, the synapse, designed for the production and release of acetylcholine. The synapse is separated from the endplate of the muscle fiber by a narrow gap, called the *synaptic cleft*, which is approximately 50 nm in width (0.05 μm) (Fig. 20-5).[11] The nerve terminal is surrounded by a Schwann cell, and the synaptic cleft has a basement membrane and contains filaments that anchor the nerve terminal to the muscle.

The endplate is a specialized portion of the membrane of the muscle fiber where nicotinic acetylcholine receptors are concentrated. During development, multiple connections are made between nerve terminals and a single muscle fiber. However, as maturation continues, most of these connections atrophy and disappear, usually leaving only one connection per muscle fiber. This endplate continues to differentiate from the rest of the muscle fiber. The nerve terminal enlarges, and folds appear. The acetylcholine receptors cluster at the endplate, especially at the crests of the folds, and their density decreases to almost zero in extrajunctional areas.[12] Mammalian endplates usually have an oval shape with the short axis perpendicular to the fiber. The width of the endplate is sometimes as large as the diameter of the fiber, but is usually smaller. However, its length is only a small fraction of that of the fiber.

Nerve Stimulation

Under resting conditions, the electrical potential of the inside of a nerve cell is negative with respect to the outside (typically –90 mV). If this potential is made less negative (depolarization), sodium channels open and allow sodium ions to enter the cell. This influx of positive ions makes the potential inside the membrane positive with respect to the outside. This potential change, in turn, causes depolarization of the next segment of membrane, causing more sodium channels to open, and an electrical impulse, or action potential, propagates. The duration of the action potential is brief (<1 msec) because of rapid inactivation of sodium channels and activation of potassium channels. An action potential also triggers the opening of calcium channels, allowing calcium ions to penetrate the cell. This entry of calcium facilitates release of the neurotransmitter at the nerve terminal.

The sodium channels in the axon may be activated in response to electrical depolarization provided by a nerve stimulator. A peripheral nerve is made up of a large number of axons, each of which responds in an all-or-none fashion to the stimulus applied. Thus, in the absence of neuromuscular blocking agents, the relationship between the amplitude of the muscle contraction and current applied is sigmoid. At low currents, the depolarization is insufficient in all axons. As current increases, more and more axons are depolarized to threshold and the strength of the muscle contraction increases. When the stimulating current reaches a certain level, all axons are depolarized to threshold and

FIGURE 20-5. Schematic representation of the neuromuscular junction (not drawn to scale).

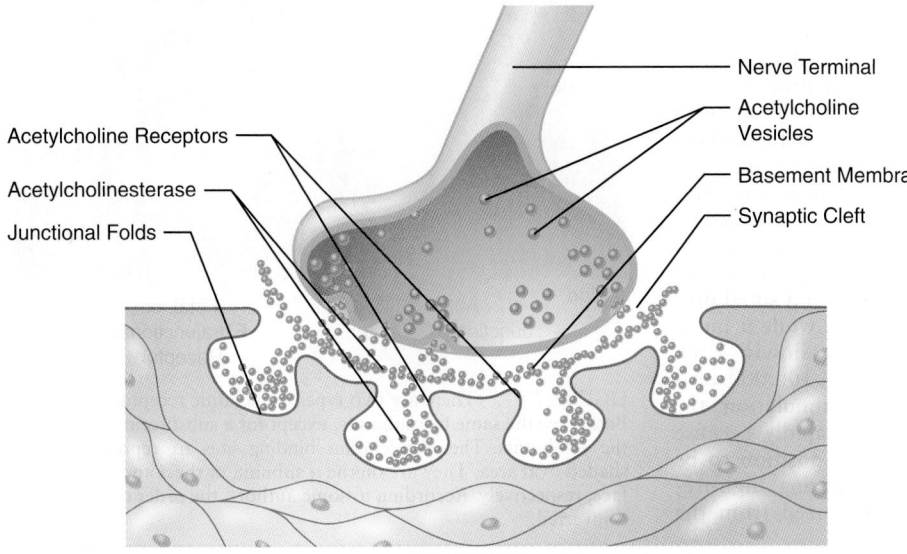

Nerve Terminal

Acetylcholine Vesicles

Basement Membrane

Synaptic Cleft

Acetylcholine Receptors

Acetylcholinesterase

Junctional Folds

Muscle Cell

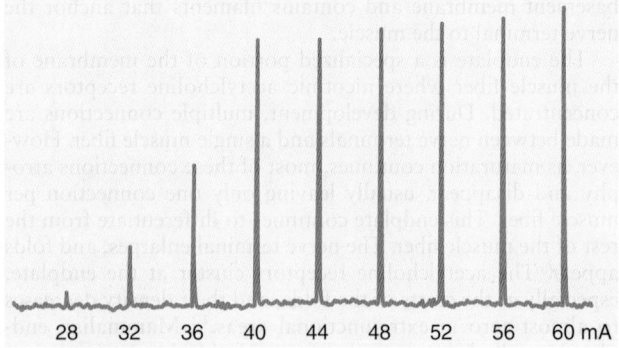

FIGURE 20-6. Example of increasing stimulating current in one patient. Current pulses, 0.2-msec duration, were delivered to the ulnar nerve at the wrist every 10 seconds. The force of contraction of the adductor pollicis muscle was measured and appears as spikes. No twitch was seen if the current was <28 mA. At current strengths of ≥40 mA, the current became supramaximal; increasing the current produced little change in force.

propagate an action potential. Increasing current beyond this point does not increase the amplitude of muscle contraction: the stimulation is supramaximal (Fig. 20-6). Most commercially available stimulators deliver impulses lasting 0.1 to 0.2 msec.

Release of Acetylcholine

Acetylcholine is synthesized from choline and acetate and packaged into 45-nm vesicles. Each vesicle contains 5,000 to 10,000 acetylcholine molecules. Some of these vesicles cluster near the cell membrane opposite the crests of the junctional folds of the endplate, in areas called *active zones* (Fig. 20-5).[12]

It is now widely accepted that acetylcholine is released in packets, or quanta, and that a quantum represents the contents of one vesicle. In the absence of nerve stimulation, quanta are released spontaneously, at random, and this is seen as small depolarizations of the endplate (miniature endplate potential). When an action potential invades the nerve terminal, approximately 200 to 400 quanta are released simultaneously, unloading approximately 1 to 4 million acetylcholine molecules into the synaptic cleft.[11] Calcium, which enters the nerve terminal through channels that open in response to depolarization, is required for vesicle fusion and release. Calcium channels are located near docking proteins, and this special geometric arrangement provides high intracellular concentrations of calcium to allow binding of specialized proteins on the vesicle membrane with docking proteins.[12] Binding produces fusion of the membranes and release of acetylcholine ensues. When the calcium concentration is decreased, or if the action of calcium is antagonized by magnesium, the release process is inhibited and transmission failure may occur. Other proteins regulate storage and mobilization of acetylcholine vesicles. It appears that a small proportion of vesicles is immediately releasable, while a much larger reserve pool can be mobilized more slowly. Each impulse releases 0.2 to 0.5% of the 75,000 to 100,000 vesicles in the nerve terminal. With repetitive stimulation, the amount of acetylcholine released decreases rapidly because only a small fraction of the vesicles is in a position to be released immediately. To sustain release during high-frequency stimulation, vesicles must be mobilized from the reserve pool.

Postsynaptic Events

The 1 to 10 million receptors located at the endplate bind to acetylcholine as the physiological ligand, and belong to the class of nicotinic receptors. Cholinergic nicotinic receptors respond to acetylcholine and other agonists by allowing passage of ions. Nicotinic receptors are made up of five glycoprotein subunits arranged in the form of a rosette and lying across the whole cell membrane (Fig. 20-7). The nicotinic subtype present at the neuromuscular junction is made up of two identical subunits, designated α, and three others, called β, δ, and γ or ε. There are two acetylcholine binding sites, each located on the outside part of the α subunit. When two acetylcholine molecules bind simultaneously to each binding site, an opening is created in the center of the rosette, allowing sodium ions to enter the cell and potassium ions to exit.[11,12] The inward movement of sodium is predominant because it is attracted by the negative voltage of the inside of the cell. This movement of sodium depolarizes the endplate; that is, its inside becomes less negative. There is a high density of sodium channels in the folds of synaptic clefts and in the perijunctional area.[12,13] These channels open when the membrane is depolarized beyond a critical point, allowing more sodium to enter the cell and producing further depolarization. This depolarization generates an action potential, which propagates by activation of sodium channels along the whole length of the muscle fiber. The muscle action potential has a duration of 5 to 15 msec and can be recorded as an electromyogram (EMG). It precedes the onset of contraction, or twitch, which lasts 100 to 200 msec. With high-frequency (>10 Hz) stimulation, the muscle fiber does not have time to relax before the next impulse, so contractions fuse and add up, and a tetanus is obtained.

There are two types of nicotinic acetylcholine receptors. Early in development, receptors are evenly distributed along the whole length of the muscle fiber. These receptors, called *fetal* receptors, have a γ subunit (Fig. 20-7). When the endplate develops, receptors tend to cluster at the neuromuscular junction and leave only few receptors in the extrajunctional areas. As maturation continues, the γ subunit is substituted by an ε subunit, which is characteristic of the *adult* type, junctional receptor.[12] In humans, the switch occurs in the third trimester of pregnancy. Maintenance of adult receptors at the endplate depends on the integrity of nerve supply. A few γ-type, extrajunctional receptors still persist in adults and can proliferate in cases of denervation. Both types of receptor have

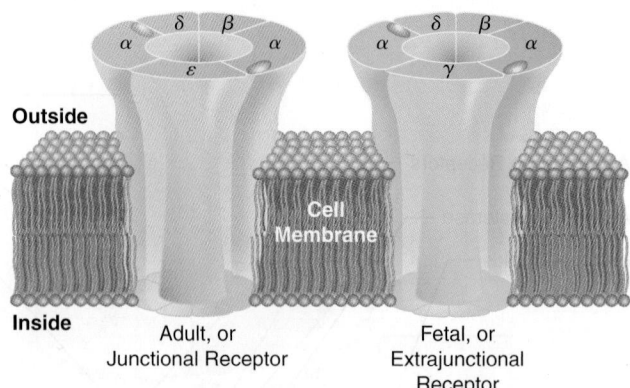

FIGURE 20-7. There are two types of nicotinic receptors in muscle. Both have the same five subunits, except for a substitution of the ε for the γ subunits. The acetylcholine binding sites are represented by a shaded oval area. They are on the α subunit, at the δ and ε or γ interface, respectively. According to some authors, the order of the β and δ is inverted.

two binding sites for acetylcholine, located on each of the α subunits, but they have slightly different sensitivities to agonist and antagonist drugs.[12]

2 The main action of nondepolarizing neuromuscular blocking drugs is to bind to at least one of the two α subunits of the postsynaptic receptor. This prevents access to the receptor by acetylcholine and does not produce opening of the receptor. Under normal circumstances, only a small fraction of available receptors must bind to acetylcholine to produce sufficient depolarization to trigger a muscle contraction. In other words, there is a wide "margin of safety."[13] This redundancy implies that neuromuscular blocking drugs must be bound to a large number of receptors before any blockade is detectable. Animal studies suggest that 75% of receptors must be occupied before twitch height decreases in the presence of d-tubocurarine, and blockade is complete when 92% of receptors are occupied.[14] The actual number depends on species and type of muscle, and humans might have a reduced margin of safety compared with other species.[13] So it is futile to correlate receptor occupancy data obtained in cats with certain clinical tests in humans, such as hand grip and head lift, which involve different muscle groups. However, the general concept that a large proportion of receptors must be occupied before blockade becomes detectable, and that measurable blockade occurs over a narrow range of receptor occupancy, remains applicable to clinical practice. Because it must overcome the margin of safety, the initial dose of neuromuscular blocking agent is greater than maintenance doses.

Acetylcholine is hydrolyzed rapidly by the enzyme acetyl cholinesterase, which is present in the folds of the endplate as well as embedded in the basement membrane of the synaptic cleft. The presence of the enzyme in the synaptic cleft suggests that not all the acetylcholine released reaches the endplate; some is hydrolyzed en route.[12,15]

Presynaptic Events

The release of acetylcholine normally decreases during high-frequency stimulation because the pool of readily releasable acetylcholine becomes depleted faster than it can be replenished. Under normal circumstances, the reduced amount released is well above what is required to produce muscle contraction because of the high margin of safety at the neuromuscular junction. In addition, a positive feedback system involving activation of presynaptic receptors helps in the mobilization of acetylcholine vesicles. Although studies aimed at identifying these receptors are extremely difficult to perform, there is some evidence that there the presynaptic and postsynaptic receptors are of different subtypes. Presynaptic receptors are most likely of the $\alpha_3\beta_2$ subtype, that is they are made up of only α and β subunits.[16,17] Both the α subunits are slightly different from those found in postsynaptic receptors (thus the designation as α_3, instead of the α_1 given to postsynaptic receptors). The other three subunits are all identical (β_2), and slightly different from the β_1 subunit found in postsynaptic receptors.

The physiologic role of the presynaptic receptors is to maintain the number of vesicles ready to be released. Nondepolarizing neuromuscular blocking drugs produce characteristic TOF and tetanic fade, probably by blocking presynaptic nicotinic receptors,[16] thus preventing mobilization of acetylcholine vesicles and leading to reduced acetylcholine release during high-frequency stimulation. Succinylcholine has virtually no effect on these presynaptic receptors, which would explain the lack of fade observed with this drug.[17] Fade constitutes a key property of nondepolarizing

neuromuscular blocking drugs and is useful for monitoring purposes.

NEUROMUSCULAR BLOCKING AGENTS

Neuromuscular blocking drugs interact with the acetylcholine receptor either by depolarizing the endplate (depolarizing agents) or by competing with acetylcholine for binding sites (nondepolarizing agents). The only depolarizing agent still in use is succinylcholine. All others are of the nondepolarizing type.

Pharmacologic Characteristics of Neuromuscular Blocking Agents

The effect of neuromuscular blocking drugs is measured as the depression of adductor muscle contraction (twitch) following electrical stimulation of the ulnar nerve. The value is compared with a control value, obtained before injection of the drug. Each drug has characteristic onset, potency, duration of action, and recovery index.

Potency of each drug is determined by constructing dose-response curves, which describe the relationship between twitch depression and dose (Fig. 20-8).[18] Then, the effective dose 50, or ED_{50}, which is the median dose corresponding to 50% twitch depression, is obtained. Because clinically useful relaxation is attained when twitch is abolished almost completely, the ED_{95}, corresponding to 95% block, is more commonly used. For example, the ED_{95} for vecuronium is 0.05 mg/kg, which means that half the patients will achieve at least 95% block of single twitch (compared with the prevecuronium value) with that dose, and half the subjects will reach <95% block. Rocuronium has an ED_{95} of 0.3 mg/kg. Therefore, it has one-sixth the potency of vecuronium. In other words, compared with vecuronium, 6 times as much rocuronium has to be given to produce the same effect. The ED_{95} of known neuromuscular blocking agents vary over two orders of magnitude (Table 20-2).

Onset time, or time to maximum blockade, can be shortened if the dose is increased. When two or more drugs are

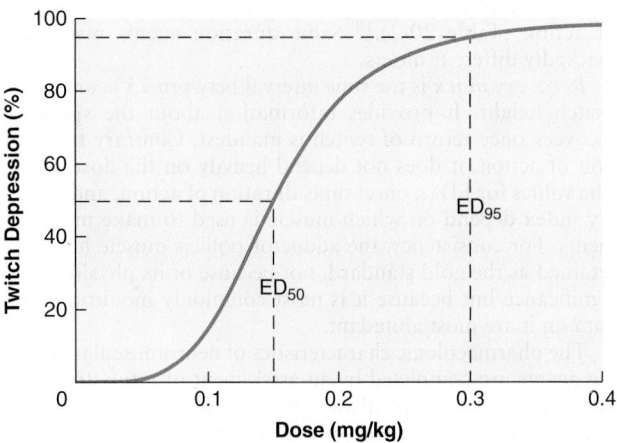

FIGURE 20-8.   Example of a dose-response relationship. The actual numbers are approximately those for rocuronium. The ED_{50} is the dose corresponding to 50% blockade and ED_{95} is the dose corresponding to 95% blockade.

TABLE 20-2

POTENCY, ONSET TIME, DURATION, AND RECOVERY INDEX OF NEUROMUSCULAR BLOCKING AGENTS[a]

■ AGENT	■ ED$_{95}$ (mg/kg)	■ ONSET TIME (min)	■ DURATION TO 25% RECOVERY (min)	■ RECOVERY INDEX (25–75% RECOVERY) (min)
■ ULTRASHORT-DURATION AGENTS				
Succinylcholine	0.3	1–1.5	6–8	2–4
Gantacurium[b]	0.19	1.7	6–8	2.5
■ SHORT-DURATION AGENTS				
Mivacurium[c]	0.08	3–4	15–20	7–10
Rapacuronium[c]	0.75	1–1.5	15–25	5–7
■ INTERMEDIATE-DURATION AGENTS				
Atracurium	0.2–0.25	3–4	35–45	10–15
Cisatracurium	0.05	5–7	35–45	12–15
Rocuronium	0.3	1.5–3	30–40	8–12
Vecuronium	0.05	3–4	35–45	10–15
■ LONG-DURATION AGENTS				
Alcuronium[c]	0.25	3–5	60–90	30–40
Doxacurium	0.025	5–10	40–120	30–40
d-Tubocurarine[c]	0.5	2–4	60–120	30–45
Gallamine[c]	2	1.5–3	60–120	30–60
Metocurine[c]	0.3	3–5	60–150	40–60
Pancuronium	0.07	2–4	60–120	30–40
Pipecuronium[c]	0.05	3–5	90–130	35–45

[a]Typical values for the average young adult patient. Onset and duration data depend on dose. The values presented are the best estimates available for twice the ED$_{95}$ and are measured at the adductor pollicis muscle with nitrous oxide and no volatile agent. Actual values may vary markedly from one individual to the next, and may be affected by age, other medications, and/or disease states. The categories under which the drugs are classified are somewhat arbitrary.
[b]Being investigated at the time of writing.
[c]No longer used or very limited use in North America.

compared, it is meaningful to compare only equipotent doses and usually clinically relevant doses (2 × ED$_{95}$) are considered.[18]

Duration of action is the time from injection of the neuromuscular blocking agent to return of 25% twitch height (compared with control). Duration increases with dose, so comparisons are normally made with 2 × ED$_{95}$ doses. The 25% twitch height figure was chosen because rapid reversal can normally be achieved at that level. Categories were proposed for neuromuscular blocking drugs according to their duration of action (Table 20-2).[18] Same duration agents may have markedly different onsets.

Recovery index is the time interval between 25% and 75% twitch height. It provides information about the speed of recovery once return of twitch is manifest. Contrary to duration of action, it does not depend heavily on the dose given. The values for ED$_{95}$, onset time, duration of action, and recovery index depend on which muscle is used to make measurements. For consistency, the adductor pollicis muscle has been retained as the gold standard, not because of its physiological significance but because it is most commonly monitored and data on it are most abundant.

The pharmacologic characteristics of neuromuscular blocking agents are completed by an assessment of *intubating conditions*, which do not always parallel twitch height at the adductor pollicis muscle. Intubating conditions depend on paralysis of centrally located muscles, but also on the type and quantity of opioid and hypnotic drugs given for induction of anesthesia. To decrease variability between studies, criteria to grade intubating conditions as excellent, good, poor, or impossible in a scoring system were adopted by a group of experts who met in Copenhagen in 1994.[19]

DEPOLARIZING DRUGS: SUCCINYLCHOLINE

Among drugs that depolarize the endplate, only succinylcholine is still used clinically. In spite of a long list of undesired effects, succinylcholine remains popular because it is the only ultrarapid onset/ultrashort duration neuromuscular blocking drug currently available.

Neuromuscular Effects

The effects of succinylcholine at the neuromuscular junction are not completely understood. The drug depolarizes postsynaptic and extrajunctional receptors. However, when the receptor is in contact with any agonist, including acetylcholine, for a prolonged time it ceases to respond to the agonist. Normally, this desensitization process does not occur with acetylcholine because of its rapid breakdown (<1 msec). However, succinylcholine remains at the endplate for much longer, so desensitization develops after a brief period of activation.[17] Another possible mechanism is the inactivation of sodium channels in the junctional and perijunctional areas, which occurs when the membrane remains depolarized.[17] This inactivation prevents the propagation of the action potential. Both desensitization of the receptor and inactivation of sodium channels might be present together.

Within 1 minute after succinylcholine injection and before paralysis is manifest, some disorganized muscular activity is frequently observed. This phenomenon is called *fasciculation*.

This activity probably reflects the agonist effect of succinylcholine, before desensitization takes place. Small doses of nondepolarizing drugs are effective in reducing the incidence of fasciculations.[20]

Succinylcholine has yet another neuromuscular effect. In some muscles, like the masseter and to a lesser extent the adductor pollicis, a sustained increase in tension that may last for several minutes can be observed. The mechanism of action of this tension change is uncertain but is most likely mediated by acetylcholine receptors because it is blocked by large amounts of nondepolarizing drugs.[21] The increase in masseteric tone, which is probably always present to some degree but greater in some susceptible individuals, may lead to imperfect intubating conditions in a small proportion of patients. Masseter muscle spasm may be an exaggerated form of this response.

Characteristics of Depolarizing Blockade

After injection of succinylcholine, single-twitch height is decreased. However, the response to high-frequency stimulation is sustained: minimal train-of-four and tetanic fade is observed. The block is antagonized by nondepolarizing agents so that the ED$_{95}$ is increased by a factor two if a small dose of nondepolarizing drug is given before.[22] Succinylcholine blockade is potentiated by inhibitors of acetyl cholinesterase, such as neostigmine and edrophonium.[23]

Phase II Block

After administration of 7 to 10 mg/kg, or 30 to 60 minutes of exposure to succinylcholine, train-of-four and tetanic fade become apparent. Neostigmine or edrophonium can antagonize this block, which has been termed *nondepolarizing, dual,* or *phase II* block. The onset of phase II block coincides with tachyphylaxis, as more succinylcholine is required for the same effect.

Pharmacology of Succinylcholine

Succinylcholine is rapidly hydrolyzed by plasma cholinesterase (also called *pseudocholinesterase*), with an elimination half-life of <1 minute in patients.[24] Because of the rapid disappearance of succinylcholine from plasma, the maximum effect is reached quickly. Subparalyzing doses (up to 0.3 to 0.5 mg/kg) reach their maximal effect within approximately 1.5 to 2 minutes at the adductor pollicis muscle,[22] and within 1 minute at more central muscles, such as the masseter, the diaphragm, and the laryngeal muscles. With larger doses (1 to 2 mg/kg), abolition of twitch response can be reached even more rapidly.

The mean dose producing 95% blockade (ED$_{95}$) at the adductor pollicis muscle is 0.30 to 0.35 mg/kg with opioid–nitrous oxide anesthesia.[22] In the absence of nitrous oxide, the ED$_{95}$ is increased to 0.5 mg/kg.[25] These values are doubled if *d*-tubocurarine, 0.05 mg/kg, is given as a defasciculating agent.[22] The time until full recovery is dose-dependent and reaches 10 to 12 minutes after a dose of 1 mg/kg.

Side Effects

Cardiovascular

Sinus bradycardia with nodal or ventricular escape beats (or both) may occur, especially in children, and asystole has been described after a second dose of succinylcholine in both pediatric and adult patients. These effects can be attenuated with atropine or glycopyrrolate.[26] The mechanisms for the cardiovascular side effects of succinylcholine are not known because

succinylcholine appears to have little effect of autonomic cholinergic receptors.[17] Succinylcholine increases catecholamine release, and tachycardia is seen frequently.

Anaphylaxis

Succinylcholine has been incriminated as the trigger of allergic reactions more often than any other drug used in anesthesia. Successive studies conducted in France indicate that the number of reported events is decreasing, corresponding to the gradual replacement of succinylcholine by nondepolarizing drugs.[27] The incidence of anaphylactic reactions to succinylcholine is difficult to establish, but is probably of the order of 1:5,000 to 1:10,000.

Fasciculations

The prevalence of fasciculations is high (60 to 90%) after the rapid injection of succinylcholine, especially in muscular adults. Fasciculations are a benign side effect of the drug, but many clinicians prefer to prevent fasciculations. In this respect, a small dose of a nondepolarizing neuromuscular blocking drug is given 3 to 5 minutes before succinylcholine is effective.[20] When the drug was available, *d*-tubocurarine 0.05 mg/kg was used for this purpose. Rocuronium is an acceptable alternative, as long as appropriate doses (0.03 to 0.04 mg/kg, or 10% of the ED$_{95}$) are given.[28] In one study, rocuronium, 0.03 mg/kg, decreased the incidence of fasciculations from 90 to 10%.[29] A dose of 0.06 mg/kg leads to an unacceptably high incidence of symptoms of neuromuscular weakness, such as blurred vision, heavy eyelids, voice changes, difficulty swallowing, or even dyspnea, in the awake patient.[30] A recent meta-analysis shows that these side effects have been observed frequently in studies of defasciculating doses of neuromuscular blocking agents,[20] but these side effects are most likely related to the high dose given.[28] Atracurium, 0.02 mg/kg, is also effective. Pancuronium, vecuronium, cisatracurium, and mivacurium are not as effective as defasciculants. After these nondepolarizing drugs, the dose of succinylcholine must be increased from 1 mg/kg to 1.5 or even 2 mg/kg because of the antagonism between depolarizing and nondepolarizing drugs.[22] Other drugs, such as diazepam, lidocaine, fentanyl, calcium, vitamin C, magnesium, and dantrolene, have all been used to prevent fasciculations. The results are no better than with nondepolarizing relaxants and they may have undesirable effects of their own. The administration of small (10-mg) doses of succinylcholine 1 minute before the intubating dose, does not appear to be effective[29] and has largely been abandoned.

Muscle Pains

Generalized aches and pains, similar to the myalgia that follows violent exercise, are common 24 to 48 hours after succinylcholine administration. Their incidence is variable (1.5 to 89% of patients receiving succinylcholine) and are more common in young, ambulatory patients.[31] The intensity of muscle pains is not always correlated with the intensity of fasciculations, but the methods that have been shown effective to prevent fasciculations usually prevent muscle pains. For example, a precurarization dose of a nondepolarizing neuromuscular blocking agent is effective. Lidocaine (1 to 1.5 mg/kg), especially in conjunction with precurarization, has also been shown to be of value.[31] Calcium, vitamin C, benzodiazepines, magnesium, and dantrolene have been tried with inconclusive results.[31]

Intragastric Pressure

Succinylcholine increases intragastric pressure, and this effect is blocked by precurarization. However, succinylcholine causes even greater increases in lower esophageal sphincter pressure. Thus, succinylcholine does not appear to increase the risk of aspiration of gastric contents unless the lower esophageal sphincter is incompetent.

Intraocular Pressure

Intraocular pressure increases by 5 to 15 mm Hg after injection of succinylcholine. The mechanism is unknown but occurs after detachment of extraocular muscle, suggesting an intraocular etiology. Precurarization with a nondepolarizing blocker has little or no effect on this increase. This information has led to the widespread recommendation to avoid succinylcholine in open-eye injuries. However, it must be appreciated that inadequate anesthesia, elevated systemic blood pressure, and insufficient neuromuscular blockade during laryngoscopy and tracheal intubation might increase intraocular pressure more than succinylcholine. In addition, there is little evidence that the use of succinylcholine has led to blindness or extrusion of eye content.[32]

Intracranial Pressure

Succinylcholine may increase intracranial pressure, and this response is probably diminished by precurarization.[33] Again, laryngoscopy and tracheal intubation with inadequate anesthesia or muscle relaxation are likely to increase intracranial pressure even more than succinylcholine.

Hyperkalemia

Serum potassium increases by approximately 0.5 mEq/L after injection of succinylcholine. This increase is not prevented completely by precurarization. In fact, only large doses of nondepolarizing blockers reliably abolish this effect.[34] Subjects with pre-existing hyperkalemia, such as patients in renal failure, do not have a greater increase in potassium levels, but the absolute level might reach the toxic range. Succinylcholine is safe in normokalemic renal-failure patients.[35] Severe hyperkalemia, occasionally leading to cardiac arrest, has been described in patients after major denervation injuries, spinal cord transection, peripheral denervation, stroke, trauma, extensive burns, and prolonged immobility with disease, and may be related to potassium loss via a proliferation of extrajunctional receptors.[34] Hyperkalemia has been reported with myotonia and muscle dystrophies, and cardiac arrests have been reported in children before the diagnosis of the disease was made.[34] Severe hyperkalemia after succinylcholine resulting in cardiac arrest has also been observed in acidotic hypovolemic patients.

Abnormal Plasma Cholinesterase

Plasma cholinesterase activity can be reduced by a number of endogenous and exogenous causes, such as pregnancy, liver disease, uremia, malnutrition, burns, plasmapheresis, and oral contraceptives. These conditions usually lead to a slight, clinically unimportant increase in the duration of action of succinylcholine.[36] Plasma cholinesterase activity is reduced by some anticholinesterases (e.g., neostigmine) so that the duration of succinylcholine given after neostigmine, but not after edrophonium, is increased.[23]

A small proportion of patients have a genetically determined inability to metabolize succinylcholine. Either plasma cholinesterase is absent or an abnormal form of the enzyme is present. Only patients homozygous for the condition (approximately 1:2,000 individuals) have prolonged paralysis (3 to 6 hours) after usual doses of succinylcholine (1 to 1.5 mg/kg). In heterozygous patients (1:30 cases), the duration of action is only slightly prolonged compared with normal individuals.

Traditional methods for identifying plasma cholinesterase phenotype involve measurement of enzyme activity with a substrate and inhibition with dibucaine, fluoride, and chloride. These tests are only capable of identifying some enzyme variants. The complete amino acid sequence of plasma cholinesterase has now been determined using molecular genetics techniques. The cholinesterase gene is located on chromosome 3 at q26,[36] and over 20 mutations in the coding region of the plasma cholinergic gene have been identified. Whole blood or fresh-frozen plasma can accelerate succinylcholine metabolism in patients with low or absent plasma cholinesterase, but the best course of action is probably mechanical ventilation of the lungs until full recovery of neuromuscular function can be demonstrated. Neostigmine and edrophonium are unpredictable in the reversal of abnormally prolonged succinylcholine blockade and are best avoided.

Clinical Uses

The main indication for succinylcholine is to facilitate tracheal intubation. In adults, a dose of 1.0 mg/kg yields 75 to 80% excellent intubation conditions within 1 to 1.5 minutes after an induction sequence that includes a hypnotic (propofol or thiopental) and a moderate opioid dose.[37,38] The dose must be increased to 1.5 to 2.0 mg/kg if a precurarizing dose of nondepolarizing blocker has been used.[22] Intubating conditions without precurarization are only marginally improved by increasing the dose to 2 mg/kg.[38]

Succinylcholine is especially indicated for "rapid sequence induction," when a patient presents with a full stomach and the possibility of aspiration of gastric contents. In this situation, manual ventilation of the lungs is avoided, if possible, to reduce the probability of aspiration because of excessive intragastric pressure caused by gas forced via face mask. Thus, the ideal neuromuscular blocking agent has both a fast onset, to reduce the time between induction and intubation of the airway, and a rapid recovery, to allow return of normal breathing before the patient becomes hypoxic. The duration of action of succinylcholine, given at a dose of 1 mg/kg, is short enough so that in the majority of properly preoxygenated patients resume respiratory efforts (5 to 6 minutes) before hypoxia can be detected.[39] It has been argued that this is valid only in relatively healthy subjects and not in all cases. As a result, a lower dose has been suggested. However, a dose of 0.5 to 0.6 mg/kg results in substantially fewer patients with excellent intubating conditions, and the decrease in duration is modest.[37,38] For maintenance of relaxation, typical infusion rates are approximately 50 to 100 μg/kg/min. However, the availability of short and intermediate nondepolarizing drugs makes succinylcholine infusions obsolete.

Children are slightly more resistant to succinylcholine than adults,[40] and doses of 1 to 2 mg/kg are required to facilitate intubation. In infants, 2 to 3 mg/kg may be required. Precurarization is not necessary in patients younger than 10 years because fasciculations are uncommon in this age group. Bradycardia is common in children unless atropine or glycopyrrolate is given.[26] Succinylcholine, at a dose of 4 mg/kg, is the only effective intramuscular neuromuscular blocking agent in children with difficult intravenous access and provides adequate intubating conditions in about 4 minutes. However, this route of administration should not be the method of choice.[41]

In obese individuals, the dose of succinylcholine, in milligrams per kilogram of actual body weight, is the same as in leaner patients. Calculating the dose per kilogram ideal body weight might lead to underdosing and inadequate intubating conditions.[42] The volume of distribution, expressed per kilogram of actual body weight, of succinylcholine is probably decreased in obese individuals, but this is compensated by an increase in plasma cholinesterase activity.

NONDEPOLARIZING DRUGS

4 Nondepolarizing neuromuscular blocking drugs bind to the postsynaptic receptor in a competitive fashion, by binding to one of the α subunits of the receptor (Fig. 20-7).[12]

Characteristics of Nondepolarizing Blockade

5 The fade observed in response to high-frequency stimulation (>0.1 Hz) is characteristic of nondepolarizing blockade.[16] With EMG recordings, fade is relatively constant in the range 2 to 50 Hz.[43] Mechanical fade is greater with 100 Hz than with 50 Hz.[44] Tetanic stimulation is followed by posttetanic facilitation, which is an increased response to any stimulation applied soon after the tetanus. The intensity and duration of this effect depend on the frequency and duration of the tetanic stimulation. With a 50-Hz tetanus of 5-second duration, twitch responses have been found to fall within 10% of their pretetanic values in 1 to 2 minutes[45] (Fig. 20-9).

Finally, nondepolarizing blockade can be antagonized with anticholinesterase agents such as edrophonium, neostigmine, or pyridostigmine. It is also antagonized by depolarizing agents such as succinylcholine provided that the nondepolarizing blockade is intense and that the succinylcholine dose is too small to produce a block of its own.

Pharmacokinetics

As is the case for other drugs used in anesthesia, the *elimination half-life* of neuromuscular blocking agents does not always correlate with duration of action because termination of action sometimes depends on redistribution instead of elimination. However, knowledge of the kinetics of the drug helps us understand the behavior of the drug in special situations (prolonged administration, disease of the organs of elimination, and so on).

Several mechanisms can explain the various categories of durations of action listed in Table 20-3:

1. All *long-duration* drugs all have a long (1 to 2 hours) elimination half-life and depend on liver and/or kidney function for termination of action.

2. *Intermediate-duration* drugs either have an intermediate elimination half-life (atracurium and cisatracurium) or they have long elimination half-lives (1 to 2 hours) but depend on redistribution rather than elimination for termination of effect (vecuronium and rocuronium; Fig. 20-10).

3. *Short-duration* drugs have either short elimination half-lives (the active isomers of mivacurium) or long elimination half-life but extensive redistribution (rapacuronium).

4. *Ultrashort-duration* drugs have a very short elimination half-life (succinylcholine).

The *volume of distribution* of all these agents is approximately equal to extracellular fluid (ECF) volume (0.2 to 0.4 L/kg; Table 20-3). In infants, in whom the ECF volume as a proportion of body weight, is increased, the volume of distribution of neuromuscular blocking drugs parallels ECF volume closely.

Onset and Duration of Action

Onset time of neuromuscular blocking drugs is determined by the time required for drug concentrations at the site of action to reach a critical level, usually that corresponding to 100% block. Onset time (2 to 7 minutes) is longer than time to peak plasma concentrations (<1 minute). This delay reflects the time required for drug transfer between plasma and neuromuscular junction and is represented quantitatively by a rate constant (k_{eo}). This rate constant corresponds to half-times of 5 to 10 minutes for most nondepolarizing drugs and is determined by all the factors that modify access of the drug to, and its removal from, the neuromuscular junction. These include cardiac output, distance of the muscle from the heart, and muscle blood flow. Thus, onset times are not the same in all muscles because of different blood flows. Also, if metabolism or redistribution is very rapid, for example, in the case of succinylcholine, the onset time is accelerated. Finally, potent drugs have a slower onset of action than less potent agents (Fig. 20-11).[46] This is because a large proportion of receptors must be occupied before blockade can be observed. Blockade of these receptors will occur faster, and onset will be more rapid, if more drug molecules are available, that is, if potency is low. Table 20-2 shows that onset tends to be slower if a drug is potent, that is, if ED_{95} is small.

Duration of action is determined by the time required for drug concentrations at the site of action to decrease below a certain level, usually corresponding to 25% first twitch blockade. Duration is determined chiefly by plasma concentrations, at least for intermediate- and long-duration drugs.

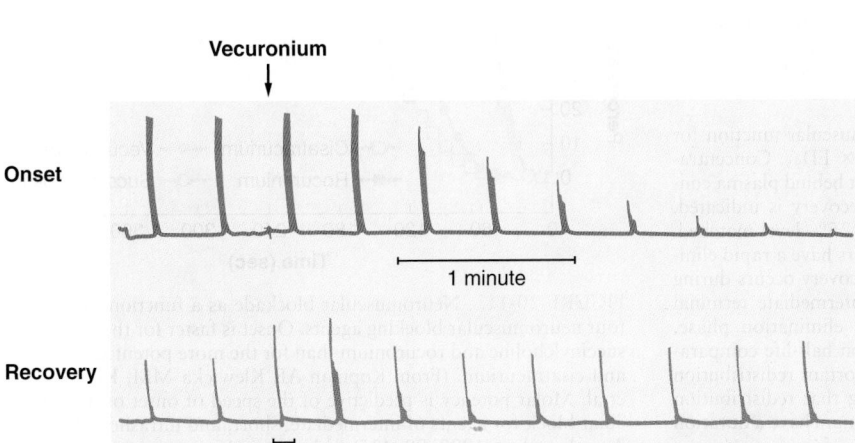

Onset

Recovery

Vecuronium

1 minute

Tetanus

FIGURE 20-9. Characteristics of nondepolarizing blockade. Train-of-four responses are equal before administration of vecuronium (*arrow*). For a given twitch depression, fade is less during onset (*top trace*) than recovery (*bottom trace*). A 50-Hz tetanus was applied during recovery. Tetanic fade is seen with posttetanic facilitation, that is a greater train-of-four response after than before the train.

ANESTHETIC AGENTS, ADJUVANTS, AND DRUG INTERACTION

TABLE 20-3

TYPICAL PHARMACOKINETIC DATA FOR NEUROMUSCULAR BLOCKING AGENTS IN ADULTS, EXCEPT WHERE STATED

■ DRUG	■ VOLUME OF DISTRIBUTION (L/kg)	■ CLEARANCE (mL/kg/min)	■ ELIMINATION HALF-LIFE (min)
■ ULTRASHORT-DURATION AGENTS			
Succinylcholine	0.04	37	0.65
■ SHORT-DURATION AGENTS			
Mivacurium			
Trans–trans	0.05	29	2.4
Cis–trans	0.05	46	2.0
Cis–cis	0.18	7	30
Rapacuronium	0.2	7	100
■ INTERMEDIATE-DURATION AGENTS			
Atracurium	0.14	5.5	20
Cisatracurium			
Adults	0.12	5	23
Intensive care	0.26	6.5	25
Rocuronium			
Adults	0.3	3	90
Intensive care	0.7	3	330
Vecuronium	0.4	5	70
■ LONG-DURATION AGENTS			
Doxacurium	0.2	2.5	95
d-Tubocurarine			
Adults	0.3	1–3	90
Elderly	0.3	0.8	270
Neonates	0.7	1.1	300
Infants	0.5	1.0	300
Children	0.3	1.5	90
Pancuronium	0.3	1.8	140

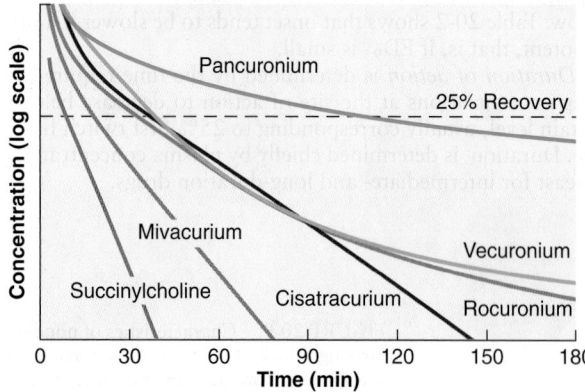

FIGURE 20-10. Concentrations at the neuromuscular junction for six representative drugs, after bolus doses of 2 × ED$_{95}$. Concentrations at the neuromuscular junction lag somewhat behind plasma concentrations. The level corresponding to 25% recovery is indicated. The curves were moved up or down so that the 25% level matched. Succinylcholine and the active mivacurium isomers have a rapid elimination. Pancuronium has a long half-life and recovery occurs during the elimination phase. Cisatracurium has an intermediate terminal half-life, and recovery also occurs during the elimination phase. Rocuronium and vecuronium have an elimination half-life comparable with that of pancuronium. However, an important redistribution occurs before, and 25% recovery occurs during that redistribution process. As a result, both rocuronium and vecuronium have a duration of action comparable with that of cisatracurium.

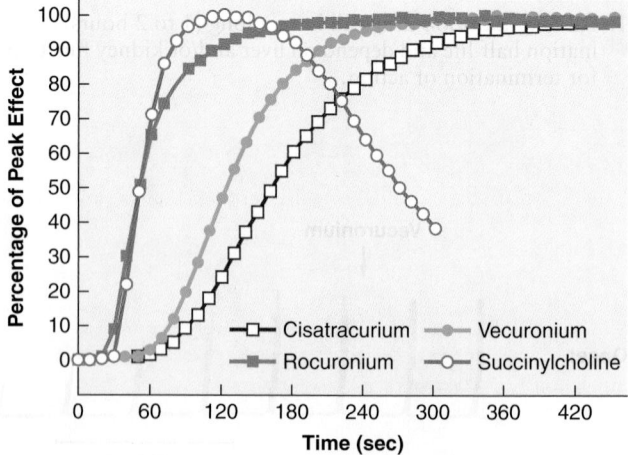

FIGURE 20-11. Neuromuscular blockade as a function of time for four neuromuscular blocking agents. Onset is faster for the less potent succinylcholine and rocuronium than for the more potent vecuronium and cisatracurium. (From Kopman AF, Klewicka MM, Kopman DJ, et al: Molar potency is predictive of the speed of onset of neuromuscular block for agents of intermediate, short, and ultrashort duration. Anesthesiology 1999; 90: 425, with permission.)

Individual Nondepolarizing Agents

Since 1942, nearly 50 nondepolarizing neuromuscular blocking agents have been introduced into clinical anesthesia. This section covers only those drugs currently available in North America and Europe, plus a few others of historical interest. The first agent to undergo clinical investigation was Intocostrin, or d-tubocurarine, the purified and standardized product of curare obtained from the plant *Chondodendrom tomentosum*.[1] d-Tubocurarine has been completely replaced by more modern synthetic analogues.

d-Tubocurarine

The dose of d-tubocurarine required to produce 95% twitch block of at the adductor pollicis muscle, or ED_{95}, is 0.5 mg/kg. At that dose, the duration of action is typical of a long-duration agent (Table 20-2).[47]

Pharmacology. The molecule undergoes minimal metabolism so that 24 hours after its administration about 10% of the compound is found in the urine and 45% in the bile. Like most other neuromuscular blocking drugs, it is not extensively (30 to 50%) protein bound. Excretion is impaired in renal failure.

Cardiovascular Effects. Hypotension frequently accompanies the administration of d-tubocurarine even at doses <ED_{95}. The mechanism involved is mainly histamine release, and skin flushing is frequently observed. Autonomic ganglionic blockade may also play a minor role.

Age. Pharmacokinetic studies have been performed in all age groups, and the results are helpful in understanding the behavior of all nondepolarizing agents in patients at the extremes of age. The potency of d-tubocurarine on a milligram per kilogram basis does not vary greatly with age. Infants demonstrate greater blockade than older children or adults if the same concentration of d-tubocurarine is applied. However, infants have an increased volume of distribution, when expressed in milliliters per kilogram of body weight, so that the same milligram per kilogram dose produces a reduced concentration. The net effect is similar blockade after a given milligram per kilogram dose in infants, older children, and adults (Table 20-3).[48] This phenomenon has also been observed with other neuromuscular blocking agents. However, the decreased glomerular filtration rate in the very young and the very old results in an increased elimination half-life and prolonged duration of action.[48] The onset of action is more rapid in the young as a result of a more rapid circulation time.

Burns. Patients with massive burns demonstrate resistance to d-tubocurarine and other nondepolarizing drugs that depends on the size of the burn and the time since injury.[49] Higher concentrations of the free drug are required to produce a given degree of twitch depression compared with nonthermally injured patients. Compared with normal subjects, the number of acetylcholine receptors is increased in muscles close to the site of burn injury, but also, to a lesser extent, in more distant muscles.[50]

Clinical Use. The long duration and cardiovascular effects of d-tubocurarine have restricted its use and constituted a stimulus for the production of alternative agents. Initially, this led to the introduction of pancuronium, which replaced the hypotension of d-tubocurarine with hypertension and tachycardia. More recently, drugs of intermediate duration (atracurium, cisatracurium, vecuronium, and rocuronium) with virtually no cardiovascular effects have almost eliminated the use of d-tubocurarine. When available, d-tubocurarine has been mainly confined to be used as a "precurarization" (3 mg/70 kg) before succinylcholine to reduce fasciculations and muscle pains. Rocuronium has largely replaced d-tubocurarine for this indication.

Alcuronium

Although it has never been available in North America, alcuronium still enjoys limited use in some countries. The ED_{95} is approximately 0.2 to 0.25 mg/kg. Intubating doses are usually limited to 0.3 mg/kg because of the long duration of action. Although it was introduced as an intermediate-duration drug, its recovery index (37 minutes) makes it a long-acting neuromuscular blocking agent.[51]

Atracurium

Atracurium is a bisquaternary ammonium benzylisoquinoline compound of intermediate duration of action. It is degraded via two metabolic pathways. One of these pathways is the Hofmann reaction, a nonenzymatic degradation with a rate that increases as temperature and/or pH increases. The second pathway is nonspecific ester hydrolysis. The enzymes involved in this metabolic pathway are a group of tissue esterases, which are distinct from plasma or acetyl cholinesterases.[52] The same group of enzymes is involved in the degradation of esmolol and remifentanil. It has been estimated that two thirds of atracurium is degraded by ester hydrolysis and one third by Hofmann reaction. Subjects with abnormal plasma cholinesterase have a normal response to atracurium.

The end products of the degradation of atracurium are laudanosine and acrylate fragments. Laudanosine has been reported as causing seizures in animals, but at doses largely exceeding the clinical range. No deleterious effect of laudanosine has been demonstrated conclusively in humans.[52] Laudanosine is excreted by the kidney. Acrylates have been shown to inhibit human cell proliferation in vitro.[53] However, the concentrations and exposure times required to obtain this effect are much greater than what is obtained normally in clinical practice.

Pharmacology. Atracurium is an intermediate-duration drug, with a terminal half-life of approximately 20 minutes. Termination of effect occurs during the elimination phase of the drug. Duration of action does not depend on age, renal function, or hepatic function.

The ED_{95} of atracurium is 0.2 to 0.25 mg/kg. The onset of action (3 to 5 minutes at 2 × ED_{95}) of equipotent doses is similar for atracurium, pancuronium, d-tubocurarine, and vecuronium. It is slower than succinylcholine. As with any neuromuscular blocking agent, onset of atracurium can be shortened if the dose is increased, but it is not recommended to exceed 0.5 mg/kg because of hypotension and histamine release. The duration of action is also dose-related. The time to 25% first twitch recovery after 0.5 mg/kg is approximately 30 to 40 minutes.

Cardiovascular Effects. Like d-tubocurarine, atracurium releases histamine in a dose-related manner. If large doses (≥0.5 mg/kg) are administered, hypotension, tachycardia, and skin flushing are frequent manifestations. Bronchospasm may also occur. These responses can be avoided by slow injection of atracurium over 1 to 3 minutes or by pretreatment with H_1 and H_2 receptor blockade. This histamine release, which occurs in virtually every subject given a large enough dose, should not be confused with an anaphylactic reaction, which is observed irrespective of dose in a small number of individuals. Anaphylactic reactions to atracurium have been described, but they do not appear to be more frequent than after other neuromuscular blocking drugs.[27]

Special Situations. Dosage requirements are similar in the elderly, younger adults, and children, presumably reflecting the organ independence of atracurium's elimination. Similarly, no dosage adjustment is required in individuals with renal or hepatic failure. As with other nondepolarizing agents, the dose must be increased in burn patients, partly because of increased protein binding and partly because of up-regulation of receptors, causing resistance at the endplate. In the obese patient, the dose of atracurium, as for all neuromuscular blocking agents, should be calculated based on lean body mass.

Clinical Uses. To obtain adequate intubating conditions, relatively large doses must be used (0.5 mg/kg), and laryngoscopy should be attempted only after 2 to 3 minutes. Cardiovascular manifestations of histamine release are often seen at that dose, and perfect intubating conditions are seen in only half the patients (Fig. 20-3).[8] Increasing the dose may improve intubating conditions, but at the expense of greater cardiovascular effects. For intubation, there has been a tendency to replace atracurium by agents with a shorter onset time and more cardiovascular stability, such as rocuronium. However, atracurium is convenient and versatile for maintenance of relaxation, either as a continuous infusion (5 to 10 μg/kg/min) or as intermittent injections (0.05 to 0.1 mg/kg every 10 to 15 minutes).

Cisatracurium

In an attempt to increase the margin of safety between the neuromuscular blocking dose and the histamine-releasing dose, a potent isomer of atracurium, cisatracurium, was identified. Like atracurium, its cardiovascular effects are manifest only at doses exceeding 0.4 mg/kg, but its ED_{95} (0.05 mg/kg) is much lower. As a result, manifestations of histamine release are not seen in practice. The metabolism of cisatracurium is similar to that of atracurium, with Hofmann and ester hydrolysis both playing a role.[52]

Pharmacology. Because cisatracurium is a potent drug, its onset time is longer than that of atracurium and longer still than that of rocuronium. For example, equipotent doses of cisatracurium (0.092 mg/kg) and rocuronium (0.72 mg/kg) had onset times of 4 minutes and 1.7 minutes, respectively.[54] The elimination half-life (22 to 25 minutes) is similar to that of atracurium,[55] so the duration of action for 2 × ED_{95} doses (0.1 mg/kg) is 30 to 45 minutes. However, in an attempt to accelerate onset, the recommended intubating dose is increased to 0.15 mg/kg. This dose is well below the threshold for histamine release, but the duration of action is prolonged to 45 to 60 minutes.

Because the doses required to obtain paralysis are considerably less for cisatracurium than for atracurium, less laudanosine and less acrylate byproducts are produced.[52,53] Thus, the concerns raised by the potential toxic effects of these metabolites are virtually eliminated.

Special Situations. Like atracurium, there is no need to adjust dosage in the elderly, children, or infants, when compared with young adults. The experience in burn patients is limited, but the same principles that are valid for atracurium are expected to apply. In obese individuals, the dose of cisatracurium should be calculated on the basis of ideal body weight.[56]

Side Effects. In contrast to atracurium, cisatracurium is devoid of histamine-releasing properties even at high doses (8 × ED_{95}). It is also devoid of cardiovascular effects. However, anaphylactic reactions have been described.[27]

Clinical Use. Cisatracurium may be used to facilitate tracheal intubation at doses equivalent to 3 to 4 times the ED_{95} (0.15 to 0.2 mg/kg) when manual ventilation is possible after induction of anesthesia and when the duration of the procedure is expected to exceed 1 hour. Duration is shorter with lower doses, but onset time is prolonged and intubating conditions are less ideal. Neuromuscular blockade is easily maintained at a stable level by continuous intravenous infusion of cisatracurium (1 to 2 μg/kg/min) at a constant rate and does not change with time, suggesting the lack of a significant cumulative drug effect and lack of dependence on renal and/or hepatic clearance mechanisms.[57] The rate of recovery is independent of the dose of cisatracurium and the duration of the administration.

Because cisatracurium does not depend on end-organ function for its elimination, the drug appears suitable for administration in the intensive care unit (ICU). The infusion rates to keep patients paralyzed are greater than in the operating room (typically 5 μg/kg/min), with wide interindividual variability.[58] It is likely that prolonged exposure of the receptors to a neuromuscular blocking agent causes some up-regulation, with a corresponding requirement for a higher dose.[49]

Doxacurium

Doxacurium is a potent, long-acting benzylisoquinoline compound that is not degraded by Hofmann elimination or ester hydrolysis. It has a prolonged elimination half-life (1 to 2 hours) and depends on the kidney and the liver for its disposition. Thus, duration of action is prolonged in the elderly and in subjects with impaired renal or hepatic function. The ED_{95} for doxacurium is 25 μg/kg (Table 20-2).[59] Doxacurium has a limited place in clinical practice because of its very slow onset and long duration of action. Nevertheless, its cardiovascular stability may be useful in patients with ischemic heart disease who are undergoing prolonged anesthesia or long-term mechanical ventilation of the lungs. It is unsuitable for facilitating tracheal intubation or for providing skeletal muscle relaxation during brief surgical procedures. When infused for several days to patients in the ICU, recovery after stopping the infusion exceeded 10 hours.

Gallamine

Gallamine was introduced in 1948 and has only historical interest. It is a low potency nondepolarizing drug (ED_{95} = 2 mg/kg) with a long duration of action. Gallamine produces significant tachycardia because of a vagolytic effect, even at doses associated with incomplete blockade at the adductor pollicis muscle. It is effective when used to prevent succinylcholine-induced fasciculations.[20]

Gantacurium

Gantacurium is a new compound, still under investigation. It is a nondepolarizing drug and belongs to the class of asymmetric mixed-onium chlorofumarates. Its main degradation pathway involves cysteine in the plasma and is independent of plasma cholinesterase. The ED_{95} in humans is approximately 0.19 mg/kg.[60] Cardiovascular effects are observed at doses exceeding 3 × ED_{95}, and are most probably related to histamine release. At doses anticipated to be required for tracheal intubation (0.4 to 0.6 mg/kg), onset at the adductor pollicis muscle is 1.5 minutes and duration to 25% T_1 recovery is 8 to 10 minutes, comparable with that of succinylcholine.

Metocurine

Metocurine, produced by methylation of two hydroxy groups of *d*-tubocurarine, is twice as potent as the parent compound and produces less histamine release. Its ED$_{95}$ is approximately 0.3 mg/kg.[47] Its duration of action is comparable with that of *d*-tubocurarine, making it a long-acting agent. Metocurine enjoyed a brief period of popularity before the introduction of atracurium and vecuronium. Metocurine and pancuronium combined were found to be synergistic with opposing cardiovascular effects, and the mixture was recommended for use in patients with severe cardiovascular disease. However, the introduction of shorter-duration alternatives without cardiovascular effects has made metocurine obsolete.

Mivacurium

Mivacurium is a benzylisoquinoline derivative with a short duration of action that is hydrolyzed by plasma cholinesterase, like succinylcholine.[61] Contrary to succinylcholine, however, mivacurium produces nondepolarizing blockade. The drug is presented as a mixture of three isomers. Two, the cis–trans and trans–trans, have short half-lives, but the cis–cis isomer has a much longer half-life (Table 20-3). The pharmacology of mivacurium is governed largely by the behavior of the trans–trans and cis–trans isomers, because the cis-cis isomer accounts for only 6% of the mixture and has less potent that the other two isomers.

Pharmacology. The ED$_{95}$ of mivacurium has been estimated in the range 0.08 to 0.15 mg/kg (Table 20-2). Intubating doses are 0.2 or 0.25 mg/kg but intubating conditions are not as good as with succinylcholine.[62] Onset time is surprisingly long for a drug whose active isomers have a terminal half-life of <2 minutes. At 2 to 3 × ED$_{95}$, twitch disappears in 2.5 to 4 minutes.[61] This long onset time is probably the result of the high potency of mivacurium.[46] Recovery to 25% does not depend heavily on dose, being in the range of 15 to 25 minutes for doses of 0.15 to 0.25 mg/kg. The infusion rate to maintain blockade constant does not vary with time, and recovery is as rapid after many hours of infusion than after a bolus dose.[61]

Side Effects. Like atracurium, mivacurium releases histamine in a dose-related fashion. Hypotension, tachycardia, and cutaneous signs, such as erythema and flushing, are seen frequently when doses are increased to 0.2 mg/kg or more. These histamine-related effects are short-lived (2 to 3 minutes) and should not normally be considered a manifestation of anaphylaxis, which is a rare event. Bronchospasm is rare. Manifestations of histamine release may be decreased if the drug is either given slowly (in >30 seconds) or in divided doses (0.15 mg/kg followed 30 seconds later by 0.1 mg/kg).

Special Situations. In infants and children the ED$_{95}$ is approximately the same as in adults, but onset of block and recovery are more rapid.[63] Cardiovascular effects are not as important as in adults, so doses up to 0.3 mg/kg have been used. The infusion rate required to maintain blockade is greater in children than in adults, and less in the elderly than in younger adults.

Burns. In burn patients, up-regulation of the receptors, and to a lesser extent increased protein binding, causes a resistance to all nondepolarizing neuromuscular blocking agents. However, for mivacurium, the situation is different because plasma cholinesterase activity is decreased in burn patients. The net effect is either a normal or even an enhanced effect of usual doses.[64]

Reversal. Administration of anticholinesterase agents after mivacurium has been controversial. Neostigmine has two opposing effects on mivacurium: it inhibits plasma cholinesterase, thus interfering with the breakdown of mivac-

urium, but it also reverses nondepolarizing blockade. In fact, neostigmine has been shown to delay recovery if given during intense mivacurium neuromuscular block,[65] but to accelerate recovery if signs of spontaneous recovery are present (two twitches or more present). Edrophonium does not interfere with plasma cholinesterase activity and was found to accelerate recovery, even when given when blockade is profound (one twitch in the train-of-four).[65] Mivacurium reversal has been suggested to be unnecessary because spontaneous recovery is rapid. However, residual block may be seen, particularly if large doses of mivacurium are used up to the end of anesthesia.

Plasma Cholinesterase. Mivacurium is metabolized by plasma cholinesterase somewhat more slowly than succinylcholine. The conditions associated with a decrease plasma cholinesterase activity known to affect succinylcholine metabolism also alter mivacurium duration of action.

Clinical Use. Mivacurium is no longer available in North America, but it is used in other parts of the world. It is well suited to surgical procedures requiring brief muscle relaxation, particularly those in which rapid recovery is required, such as ambulatory and laparoscopic surgery. However, it is not recommended for rapid-sequence induction. Cardiovascular effects may be avoided by administering the drug slowly or by splitting the dose into two injections 30 seconds apart. Small doses of mivacurium (0.04 to 0.08 mg/kg) have been suggested to facilitate insertion of a laryngeal mask airway. Conditions and success rate are usually better than in the absence of neuromuscular blocking agent. Maintenance of relaxation is accomplished more easily by constant infusion (5 to 7 μg/kg/min in young and middle-aged adults) than by intermittent bolus injection. This infusion rate has to be increased in children and reduced in the elderly. In children, mivacurium has a faster onset of action and more rapid recovery than in adults, so the drug can be used for intubation and maintenance of relaxation for short procedures.[63]

Pancuronium

Pancuronium belongs to a series of bisquaternary aminosteroid compounds. It is metabolized to a 3-OH compound, which has one-half the neuromuscular blocking activity of the parent compound. The ED$_{95}$ of pancuronium is 0.07 mg/kg. The duration of action is long, being 1.5 to 2 hours after a 0.15 mg/kg dose. Clearance is decreased in renal and hepatic failure, demonstrating that excretion depends on both organs. The onset of action is more rapid in infants and children than in adults, and recovery is slower in the elderly.

Cardiovascular Effects. Pancuronium is associated with increases in heart rate, blood pressure, and cardiac output, particularly after large doses (2 × ED$_{95}$). The cause is uncertain but includes a vagolytic effect at the postganglionic nerve terminal, a sympathomimetic effect as a result of blocking of muscarinic receptors that normally exert some braking on ganglionic transmission, and an increase in catecholamine release. Pancuronium does not release histamine.

Clinical Use. The slow onset of action of pancuronium limits its usefulness in facilitating tracheal intubation. Administration in divided doses, with a small dose given 3 minutes before induction of anesthesia (priming principle), produces a small but measurable acceleration. However, the intermediate-acting compounds are more suitable when succinylcholine is contraindicated. In cardiac anesthesia, pancuronium has enjoyed popularity because it counteracts the bradycardic effect of high doses of opioids. With the increased tendency toward early extubation in cardiac surgery, the appropriateness of pancuronium in this setting must be re-evaluated. The use of pancuronium instead of rocuronium is associated with a greater incidence of muscular weakness after cardiac surgery,[66] and reversal in this setting should be considered seriously. The continued popularity of pancuronium relates to cost: generic pancuronium is cheaper than other nondepolarizing relaxants. In noncardiac patients, its use is associated with a high incidence of residual block in the postanesthesia care unit, even when reversal is given (Table 20-1).[9,67] Pancuronium neuromuscular block is more difficult to reverse than that of the intermediate duration agents.[68]

Pipecuronium

Pipecuronium was developed in an effort to obtain a pancuronium without cardiovascular side effects. Its ED_{95} is slightly less (0.05 mg/kg) than that of pancuronium, and it is virtually without any cardiovascular effects. However, pipecuronium soon became obsolete because it had the drawbacks of long-acting agents (difficulty to reverse, residual paralysis, lack of versatility), and the absence of cardiovascular effects was also seen with the shorter-acting vecuronium and rocuronium.

Rapacuronium

Rapacuronium is also an aminosteroid compound that was introduced for clinical use in 1999. It was withdrawn in 2001 because of rare, but severe, cases of bronchospasm after intubation. Being less potent than rocuronium, it had a more rapid onset of action. Following 1.5 mg/kg, good-to-excellent intubation conditions were produced at 60 seconds, mean clinical duration was 17 minutes, and spontaneous recovery to train-of-four ratio of 0.7 occurred in 35 minutes.[69] The intubating conditions were not as good as with succinylcholine and the duration of action was longer. Rapacuronium is metabolized to an active 17-OH derivative (ORG 9488) that has twice the neuromuscular blocking activity of the parent compound and is excreted slowly via the kidneys.

Rapacuronium produced mild dose-related tachycardia and hypotension. Increases in airway pressure and bronchospasm were observed in more patients given rapacuronium than succinylcholine.[69] The mechanism for this effect is not an allergic or histamine-related reaction, but is most likely related to the effect of rapacuronium on M2 and M3 muscarinic receptors in the lung. Activation of the postsynaptic M3 receptors by acetylcholine produces bronchosconstriction in the lungs, and the effect is terminated by presynaptic M2 receptors that counteract this effect. Rapacuronium has the potential to block both receptors, but it has a greater affinity for the M2 receptor. The concentrations required for M2 blockade are well within the clinical range, while much more is required for M3 inhibition. The net effect is that if M2 receptors are blocked selectively, for example, in susceptible individuals, bronchoconstriction by activation of the M3 receptors is unopposed.[70] Other neuromuscular blocking agents, such as vecuronium and cisatracurium, have similar differential effects on the M2 and M3 receptors, but at concentrations higher than encountered clinically.[70]

Rocuronium

Rocuronium is an aminosteroid compound with structural similarity with vecuronium and pancuronium. Its duration of action is comparable with that of vecuronium, but its onset is shorter.

Pharmacology. Plasma concentrations of rocuronium decrease rapidly after bolus injection because of hepatic uptake.[71] Thus, the duration of action of the drug is determined chiefly by redistribution, rather than by its rather long terminal elimination half-life (1 to 2 hours; Fig. 20-10). Metabolism to 17-deacetylrocuronium is a very minor elimination pathway. Most of the drug is excreted unchanged in the urine, bile, or feces.[71]

With an ED_{95} of 0.3 mg/kg, rocuronium has one-sixth the potency of vecuronium, a more rapid onset, but a similar duration of action and similar pharmacokinetic behavior. With equipotent doses, rocuronium onset at the adductor pollicis muscle is much faster than that of cisatracurium, atracurium, and vecuronium (Fig. 20-11).[46] After doses of 0.6 mg/kg (2 × ED_{95}) maximal block occurs in 1.5 to 2 minutes. In a multicenter study of 349 patients, intubating conditions at 60 seconds after 0.6 mg/kg rocuronium were good to excellent in 77% of cases. To obtain results similar to those after 1 mg/kg succinylcholine, the dose of rocuronium had to be increased to 1.0 mg/kg, which provided 92% good or excellent conditions.[72] However, the duration of action is longer than for succinylcholine, ranging between 30 and 40 minutes for a 0.6-mg/kg dose to approximately 60 minutes after 1 mg/kg in adults. Thus, rocuronium is an intermediate-duration drug.

As for other nondepolarizing agents, the onset of action of rocuronium is more rapid at the diaphragm and adductor laryngeal muscles than at the adductor pollicis muscle,[73] probably a result of a greater blood flow to centrally located muscles. Laryngeal adductor muscles are important in anesthesia because they close the vocal cords and insufficient relaxation prevents easy passage of the tracheal tube. Laryngeal adductor muscles are resistant to the effect of rocuronium, and the plasma concentration required for equivalent blockade is greater at the larynx than at the adductor pollicis muscle.[74] The same is true of the diaphragm, which is resistant to the effect of rocuronium and other neuromuscular blocking agents. Recovery is faster at the diaphragm and larynx than at the adductor pollicis muscle.[75]

Cardiovascular Effects. No hemodynamic changes (blood pressure, heart rate, or ECG) were seen in humans, and there were no increases in plasma histamine concentrations after doses of up to 4 × ED_{95} (1.2 mg/kg).[76] Only slight hemodynamic changes are observed during coronary artery bypass surgery. Anaphylactic reactions have been described, and a French study indicated that these events occurred more frequently with rocuronium than with other neuromuscular blocking agents,[27] contrary to the findings of an Australian study.[77] However, it now appears that many of these reports might not be a true anaphylactic reaction to rocuronium because up to 50% of the general population show a positive intradermal or pick test to the drug.[78] Clearly, many patients who were investigated for a possible anaphylactic reaction were falsely labeled allergic to the drug because of the high rate of false-positive tests. It is possible that overdiagnosis has played a role in the relatively high incidence of rocuronium anaphylaxis reported in Norway (29 cases in 150,000 administrations, or 1:5,000)[79] or in France,[27] while reports from other Nordic countries suggest a much lower incidence (7 cases in 800,000 administrations, or <1:100,000).[79]

Another hypothesis that was put forward recently is sensitization of patients by over-the-counter cough medication containing pholcodine. In a study comparing subjects from Norway, where the number of reported anaphylactic cases is high, and Sweden, where those reports are virtually nonexistent, it was found that a large proportion of Norwegians was sensitized to pholcodine, but this sensitization did not occur in Swedes.[80] Pholcodine is available as an antitussive in cough syrups in certain countries like Norway, France, Ireland, the United Kingdom, and Australia. It is not available in Sweden, Denmark, Germany, the United States, and Canada. In the United States, the incidence of anaphylactic reactions to rocuronium and vecuronium may be as low as 1:1,000,000.[81] It is hypothesized that cross-sensitization may occur between pholcodine and neuromuscular blocking agents such as rocuronium and succinylcholine. However, its should be remembered that the role of pholcodine in the context remains a hypothesis, and the incidence of anaphylactic reactions to rocuronium remains very low, even in countries where pholcodine is available. Thus, current evidence suggests that withholding rocuronium because of the fear of anaphylactic reactions is unjustified.

Special Situations. The potency of rocuronium has been reported to be slightly greater in women than in men, the ED_{95} being 0.27 and 0.39 mg/kg, respectively, with an increased duration in women.[82] Some ethnic groups are more sensitive to the drug. Chinese subjects living in Vancouver were found to be more sensitive than whites.[83] As with other nondepolarizing drugs, potency has been reported to vary according to geographical distribution. Most studies reported a greater potency in North America compared with Europe,[84] with one report showing a potency of rocuronium in mainland China as intermediate between European and American values.[84] Children (2 to 12 years old) require more rocuronium and duration of action is less. Onset of action is shorter in the pediatric than in the adult population. For example, a dose of 1.2 mg/kg provides an onset time (39 seconds) comparable with that of succinylcholine, 2 mg/kg, and mean duration of action is 41 minutes.[85] Thus, the recommended doses are 0.9 to 1.2 mg/kg in this age group. Rocuronium is more potent in infants than in older children. Doses of 0.6 mg/kg have a longer duration in neonates (<1 month) than in infants (5 to 12 months), so a reduced dosage (0.45 mg/kg) is recommended.[86] Rocuronium may be used for rapid-sequence induction as succinylcholine is relatively contraindicated because of the possible presence of undiagnosed muscle dystrophy in pediatric patients, especially in boys.[34] The use of rocuronium in large doses (1.2 mg/kg) might become widespread in all age groups for rapid-sequence induction if and when the selective binding agent sugammadex becomes available (see "Sugammadex").

In elderly patients, the ED_{95} is similar to that found in younger adults, but the duration of action is prolonged slightly.[87] Rocuronium has an increased terminal half-life in renal-failure patients, probably because of its partial renal elimination, but this translates into very minor, if any, prolongation of block.[88] In hepatic disease, the slower uptake and elimination of rocuronium by the liver tends to prolong the duration of action of the drug, but this is compensated to some extent by the larger volume of distribution.[89]

Clinical Use. The rapid onset and intermediate duration of action makes this agent a potential replacement for succinylcholine in conditions where rapid tracheal intubation is indicated. However, large doses (>1 mg/kg) are required, with the drawback being a prolonged duration of action. Contrary to succinylcholine, the option to wait for spontaneous breathing to resume before hypoxia is manifest does not exist with rocuronium. To shorten the onset time, the "priming principle," which involves the administration of a small dose of rocuronium usually 3 minutes before induction, has been advocated. Unfortunately, the optimal priming dose, that is the largest dose that will not produce symptoms of weakness in the awake patient, is rather small. As with defasciculating doses before succinylcholine, it is not recommended to administer more than $0.1 \times ED_{95}$,[28] which, in the case of rocuronium, amounts to 0.03 mg/kg. Such a small dose has minimal effects on onset times provided by much larger doses (0.6 to 1.0 mg/kg). However, priming might have an effect if the intubating dose is small (0.45 mg/kg). A "timing principle" has been described in which 0.6 mg/kg rocuronium is given *before*

the induction agent, which is administered at the onset of ptosis. Considering that loss of consciousness does not occur immediately after injection of the induction agent, this technique is not recommended. Rocuronium and thiopental do not mix. They form a precipitate when they are in the same intravenous line. If thiopental is used for induction of anesthesia, the line must be flushed carefully before rocuronium is given.

Rocuronium has gradually replaced vecuronium as an intermediate-duration relaxant because of its more rapid onset. Initial doses of 0.6 mg/kg intravenously will usually produce good intubating conditions within 90 seconds. Duration of action is 30 to 40 minutes. Smaller doses (typically, 0.45 mg/kg) have a shorter duration of action, but time to intubation must be increased. Subsequent doses of 0.1 to 0.2 mg/kg will provide clinical relaxation for 10 to 20 minutes. Alternatively, rocuronium might be given by continued infusion, titrated with the help of a nerve stimulator. Infusion rates are in the range 5 to 10 $\mu g/kg/min$.[57] Recovery after infusions is slower than after bolus doses.

Vecuronium

Vecuronium is an intermediate-duration aminosteroid neuromuscular relaxant without cardiovascular effects. Its ED_{95} is 0.04 to 0.05 mg/kg. Its duration and recovery characteristics are comparable with those of rocuronium. However, its onset of action is slower.

Pharmacology. Vecuronium is a monoquaternary ammonium compound produced by demethylation of the pancuronium molecule. Vecuronium undergoes spontaneous deacetylation to produce 3-OH, 17-OH, and 3,17-$(OH)_2$ metabolites. The most potent of these metabolites, 3-OH vecuronium, about 60% of the activity of vecuronium, is excreted by the kidney and may be responsible, in part, for prolonged paralysis in patients in the ICU. Like rocuronium, vecuronium has been found less potent and with a shorter duration of action in men than in women, probably because of a greater volume of distribution in men.

Duration of action of vecuronium, like that of rocuronium, is governed by redistribution, not by elimination (Fig. 20-10). Attempts have been made to speed the onset of action by using the priming principle, that is, by administering a small, subparalyzing dose several minutes before the principal dose is given. With the availability of rocuronium, which has a more rapid onset of action than that of vecuronium, "priming" becomes an obsolete practice.

Cardiovascular Effects. Vecuronium usually produces no cardiovascular effects with clinical doses. It does not induce histamine release. Bradycardia has been described with high-dose opioid anesthesia, and this might be the reflection of the opioid effect. Allergic reactions have been described, but no more frequently than after the use of other neuromuscular blocking drugs.[27,81]

Clinical Use. The cardiovascular neutrality and intermediate duration of action make vecuronium a suitable agent for use in patients with ischemic heart disease or those undergoing short, ambulatory surgery. As with rocuronium, care should be taken when vecuronium is administered immediately after thiopental because a precipitate of barbituric acid may be formed that may obstruct the intravenous cannula.

Large doses (0.1 to 0.2 mg/kg) can be used to facilitate tracheal intubation instead of succinylcholine. For maintenance of relaxation, vecuronium may be given using intermittent boluses, 0.01 to 0.02 mg/kg, or by continuous infusion at a rate of 1 to 2 $\mu g/kg/min$. However, the rate of spontaneous recovery of neuromuscular function is slower after administration by infusion than by intermittent boluses.[90] Vecuronium has now largely been replaced by the more rapid rocuronium.

DRUG INTERACTIONS

Interactions between neuromuscular blocking drugs and several anesthetic and nonanesthetic drugs have been suggested. Although some interactions have been confirmed, many remain as isolated case reports or theoretical possibilities. Only some of the most clinically relevant interactions will be discussed here.

Anesthetic Agents

Inhalational Agents

The anesthetic vapors potentiate neuromuscular blockade in a dose-related fashion. Studies attempting to quantify the magnitude of this effect have led to conflicting results because the time factor is also important. The older halogenated agents halothane, enflurane, and isoflurane may take 2 hours or more to equilibrate with muscle, so in practice the potentiating effect of these vapors might not be immediately apparent. At similar minimum alveolar concentration (MAC), enflurane appears to potentiate nondepolarizing blockade more than does isoflurane, which in turn potentiates to a greater extent than halothane. The newer agents sevoflurane and desflurane equilibrate more rapidly with muscle, but the effect may be measurable only after 30 minutes or more. For example, the duration of action of a bolus dose of mivacurium given at induction of anesthesia is not altered by the presence of sevoflurane (1 MAC). However, the infusion rate required to maintain block decreases by 75% over the next 1.5 hours, compared with no change under propofol anesthesia.[91] The degree of potentiation increases with the concentration of sevoflurane. Recovery rate is longer in the presence of sevoflurane, even if the infusion rate of mivacurium was less. There is evidence that desflurane might have a greater potentiating effect on the neuromuscular junction than sevoflurane.[92]

Nitrous oxide (70% inspired) has been considered as having no effect on neuromuscular blockade. Recent evidence suggests that the presence of nitrous oxide has a slight potentiating effect on neuromuscular block, decreasing the ED_{50} of rocuronium by approximately 20%.[93]

The mechanism of action of potentiation by halogenated agents is uncertain, but it appears that they produce their effects at the neuromuscular junction. Isoflurane and sevoflurane inhibit current through the nicotinic receptor at the neuromuscular junction, and this inhibition is dose-dependent.[94]

Intravenous Anesthetics

Although some slight potentiation of neuromuscular blockade has been demonstrated with high doses of most intravenous induction agents in animals, clinical doses of drugs such as midazolam, thiopental, propofol, fentanyl, and ketamine have little or no neuromuscular effect in humans.

Local Anesthetics

Lidocaine, procaine, and other local anesthetic agents produce neuromuscular blockade in their own right as well as potentiating the effects of depolarizing and nondepolarizing neuromuscular blocking drugs. Contrary to the findings of other studies, a longer duration of action of vecuronium was found in patients under general anesthesia with an epidural catheter injected with mepivacaine.[95] The exact mechanisms for this interaction are uncertain, but it is unlikely that the systemic levels of local anesthetic are sufficient to produce this effect at the neuromuscular junction.

Interactions Between Nondepolarizing Blocking Drugs

Combinations of two nondepolarizing neuromuscular blocking drugs are either additive or synergistic, depending on which two drugs are involved. Addition occurs when the total effect equals that of equipotent doses of each drug. For instance, pancuronium and vecuronium have an additive interaction.[96] An ED_{95} of either pancuronium (0.07 mg/kg) or vecuronium (0.05 mg/kg) yields 95% blockade. Half the ED_{95} of pancuronium (0.035 mg/kg) administered with half the ED_{95} of vecuronium (0.025 mg/kg) will also produce 95% block. However, some combinations are synergistic; that is, their combined effect is greater than if an equipotent dose of either one of the constituents is given alone. For example, cisatracurium (ED_{95} = 0.05 mg/kg) and rocuronium (ED_{95} = 0.3 mg/kg) will produce a greater blockade than equipotent amounts of each drug given alone. If half the ED_{95} of cisatracurium (0.025 mg/kg) is administered with half the ED_{95} of rocuronium (0.15 mg/kg), the effect will be >95% twitch depression. To get 95% block, only approximately one-fourth the ED_{95} of each drug needs to be given together; that is, cisatracurium, 0.0125 mg/kg with rocuronium, 0.075 mg/kg.[97] Generally, combinations of chemically similar drugs—for example, pancuronium–vecuronium, *d*-tubocurarine–metocurine, and atracurium–mivacurium—have additive effects. Combinations of dissimilar agents tend to show potentiation, but the rule is not always followed. The first such synergism was demonstrated for pancuronium–metocurine combinations, and the mixture was advocated for its lack of cardiovascular effects. The use of combinations may be recommended to reduce cost or to take advantage of the properties of two drugs. For example, synergism occurs between mivacurium and rocuronium, and the mixture retains the fast onset of rocuronium, while having the short duration of action of mivacurium.

The mechanism by which two drugs produce a greater effect than either one alone is uncertain. Synergism is expected between mivacurium and pancuronium because of the inhibition of plasma cholinesterase that pancuronium produces, thus accentuating the effect of mivacurium. However, such a simple mechanism is absent in most cases. Surprisingly, when drug mixtures are applied to receptors in vitro, no potentiation is observed.[98]

Interactions of a different nature occur when administration of a nondepolarizing agent is followed by injection of another nondepolarizing agent. Usually, the duration of action of the second agent is that of the first drug given. For example, if vecuronium, an intermediate-acting agent, is given after the long-acting pancuronium, it has a long duration of action.[99] On the contrary, if vecuronium is the first drug, pancuronium given as a top-up dose has an intermediate duration of action. Thus, switching from a long-duration agent to an intermediate-duration drug to obtain paralysis of intermediate duration at the end of a case will not provide paralysis of intermediate duration. The reason why the characteristics of the first agent given are determinant is that the size of the loading dose is greater than that of the maintenance dose, so that even when the second dose is given, the majority of receptors is still occupied by the first drug.

Nondepolarizing–Depolarizing Interactions

Depolarizing and nondepolarizing relaxants are mutually antagonistic. When *d*-tubocurarine or other nondepolarizing agents are given before succinylcholine to prevent fasciculations and muscle pain, the succinylcholine is less potent and has a shorter duration of action.[22] The exception is with pancuronium because it inhibits plasma cholinesterase. However, nondepolarizing drugs are somewhat more effective when administered after the effect of succinylcholine has worn off, compared with no prior succinylcholine.[17] Finally, the response to a small dose of succinylcholine at the end of an anesthetic in which a nondepolarizing agent has been used is difficult to predict. It may either antagonize or potentiate the blockade, depending on the degree of nondepolarizing block. Antagonism is more likely if blockade is deep and potentiation if blockade is shallow. If an anticholinesterase agent has been given, then the effect of the succinylcholine is potentiated because of inhibition of plasma cholinesterase.

Antibiotics

Neomycin and streptomycin are the most potent of the aminoglycosides in depressing neuromuscular function.[100] The polymyxins also depress neuromuscular transmission.[100] These antibiotics are no longer used frequently. Other aminoglycosides (e.g., gentamicin, netilmicin, tobramycin) also potentiate nondepolarizing neuromuscular blockade. They prolong the action of steroidal neuromuscular agents, but their effect on benzylisoquinoline compounds is less apparent.[101] The lincosamides clindamycin and lincomycin have prejunctional and postjunctional effects, but prolongation of blockade by clindamycin is unlikely to occur clinically unless large doses are used. The penicillins, cephalosporins, tetracyclines, and erythromycin are devoid of neuromuscular effects at clinically relevant doses. Metronidazole does not appear to have clinically significant effects at the neuromuscular junction.

Anticonvulsants

Acute administration of phenytoin produces augmentation of neuromuscular block.[102] Resistance to pancuronium, metocurine, vecuronium, and rocuronium has been demonstrated in patients receiving chronic anticonvulsant therapy with carbamazepine or phenytoin.[103,104] The requirements for atracurium, mivacurium, and cisatracurium are the same or increased slightly by chronic administration of anticonvulsant drugs.[105] A least part of the phenomenon has a pharmacokinetic origin. In patients with chronic carbamazepine therapy, the clearance of vecuronium was found to be increased and its terminal half-life decreased.[103]

Cardiovascular Drugs

Beta-blocking drugs and calcium channel antagonists have been found to have neuromuscular effects in vitro, but in practice, the duration of action of neuromuscular blocking agents is not altered in patients taking these drugs chronically.[104] Ephedrine given at induction of anesthesia has been found to accelerate onset of action of rocuronium while esmolol prolongs onset time.[106] The mechanism for this effect is probably by alteration of drug delivery to the site of action by changes in cardiac output. It is possible to take advantage of this phenomenon to improve intubating conditions. Use of ephedrine, 5 to 10 mg in the average adult, at induction has been shown to improve intubating conditions provided by rocuronium.[107]

Magnesium

Calcium is required for the release of acetylcholine,[12] and magnesium antagonizes this effect. In doses of 30 mg/kg at induction followed by 10 mg/kg/hr, magnesium was found to reduce maintenance rocuronium requirements by 50% and to increase recovery times.[108] Similar effects have been reported with other nondepolarizing agents. Previous administration of magnesium abolishes succinylcholine-induced fasciculations, but it does not prolong the duration of neuromuscular blockade.[109]

Miscellaneous

Metoclopramide inhibits plasma cholinesterase and thus prolongs the action of succinylcholine and mivacurium. Inconsistent interactions have been described for diuretics, digoxin, and corticosteroids, probably because these drugs induce chronic fluid and electrolyte shifts, the magnitude of which depends on the condition being treated.

ALTERED RESPONSES TO NEUROMUSCULAR BLOCKING AGENTS

Intensive Care Unit

Neuromuscular blocking agents are useful in the ICU to facilitate mechanical ventilation, and their use is frequent in patients requiring ventilation in the prone position, permissive hypercapnia, high positive end-expiratory pressure, and elevated airways pressure.[110] It is essential to provide sedation to patients who receive paralyzing agents, to prevent discomfort associated with the inability to move. Enthusiasm for the liberal use of neuromuscular blocking agents in the ICU has waned considerably over the past 10 to 20 years because of several reports of critically ill patients who demonstrated residual weakness for unexpectedly long periods after discontinuation of a neuromuscular blocking agent. In some, recovery took several months.[111] Pancuronium and vecuronium have been used most frequently, but recent descriptions of similar syndromes after atracurium and cisatracurium suggest that the frequency of reports of weakness reflects the popularity of the drugs rather than a particular association with steroid-based compounds. Electromyographic studies have shown variable lesions from myopathy to axonal degeneration of motor and sensory fibers. The picture is complicated by the syndrome of "critical illness neuropathy," which occurs in patients with sepsis and multiorgan failure, even in individuals not given neuromuscular blocking agents. Administration of corticosteroids is also considered a risk factor.[110] Symptoms include failure to wean from mechanical ventilation, limb weakness, and impaired deep tendon reflexes, but sensory function is usually not affected. There are no controlled clinical studies to allow the several initiating factors to be identified and matched with particular syndromes. In the absence of more definitive studies, it is recommended to administer neuromuscular blocking agents only to patients who cannot be managed otherwise, to limit the duration of administration to a few days or less, to use only the dose that is necessary, and to interrupt temporarily the administration of the neuromuscular blocking agent every day or so.[110]

Studies in ICU patients in whom the administration of relaxant was adjusted according to strict neuromuscular monitoring criteria have shown considerable variation in the requirement for neuromuscular blocking agent to maintain the same effect among patients and a wide within-patient pharmacokinetic variability.[58] Vecuronium and rocuronium have been associated with prolonged recovery times. For example, a mean of 3 hours was found between the end of rocuronium infusion and a train-of-four ratio of 0.7.[112] With cisatracurium, this interval was shorter (approximately 1 hour) and less variable.[58] Drug requirement is variable from patient to patient, is usually greater than in the operating room, and tends to increase with time. These reports suggest the need for more careful monitoring of neuromuscular block in ICU patients, although the optimal method and level of block to be achieved are uncertain. It is suggested to titrate neuromuscular blocking agents to the minimum infusion rate that will optimize oxygenation.

Myasthenia Gravis

Myasthenia gravis is an autoimmune disease in which circulating antibodies produce a functional reduction in the number of postsynaptic acetylcholine receptors.[113]

Diagnosis and Management

The hallmark of myasthenia gravis is fatigue. Presentation is extremely varied but typically, ocular symptoms, such as diplopia and ptosis, occur first. Bulbar involvement is usually seen next. Patients may proceed to have extremity weakness and respiratory difficulties.[113] The characteristic EMG finding in myasthenia gravis is a voltage decrement to repeated stimulation at 2 to 5 Hz. This finding is also characteristic of nondepolarizing blockade in nonmyasthenic individuals. Edrophonium, 2 to 8 mg, produces brief recovery from myasthenia gravis and can be used as a diagnostic test. Finally, up to 80% of patients have an increased titer of the acetylcholine receptor antibody.

Treatment is largely symptomatic. Anticholinesterase agents such as pyridostigmine are used to increase neurotransmission at the neuromuscular junction. Corticosteroids and immunotherapy with azathioprine might produce long-term improvement. Plasmapheresis might be effective by eliminating the circulating antibody. Finally, many myasthenic patients have an associated thymoma, and surgical removal of the thymus may be indicated.[113]

Response to Neuromuscular Blocking Agents

Patients with myasthenia gravis are usually resistant to succinylcholine, with larger than usual doses required to produce complete blockade. This effect might be offset by the inhibition of plasma cholinesterase activity provided by pyridostigmine. Sensitivity to nondepolarizing neuromuscular blocking drugs is increased to a variable extent, depending on the severity of the disease. The ED$_{95}$ of vecuronium was found to be decreased by more than half in myasthenic patients, and the response of the orbicularis oculi muscle is depressed even more than that of the adductor pollicis muscle, reflecting some degree of ocular involvement.[114]

Management of Anesthesia

Traditionally, neuromuscular blocking drugs have been avoided in the patient with myasthenia gravis by the use of inhalational vapors with or without local anesthesia. More recently, there have been several reports of the successful use of small, titrated doses of atracurium, mivacurium, vecuronium, or rocuronium, administered under careful neuromuscular monitoring.[113] The effect of reversal drugs might be less than expected because myasthenic patients already receive drugs that produce cholinesterase inhibition. Thus, it is preferable to continue mechanical ventilation until spontaneous recovery is manifest.

After thymectomy, the need for mechanical support of ventilation can usually be predicted from preoperative lung function tests. The dose of anticholinesterases should be adjusted and is usually is reduced for 1 to 2 days after surgery.

Myotonia

Myotonia is characterized by an abnormal delay in muscle relaxation after contraction. Several forms have been described: myotonic dystrophy (dystrophia myotonica, myotonia atrophica, Steinert disease), myotonia congenita (Thomsen disease), hyperkalemic periodic paralysis, and paramyotonia congenita.

Diagnosis

Repeated nerve stimulation leads to a gradual but persistent increase in muscle tension. The EMG is pathognomonic; myotonic after-discharges are seen in peripheral muscle, consisting of rapid bursts of potential produced by tapping the muscle or moving the needle. They produce typical "dive-bomber" sounds on the loudspeaker.

Response to Neuromuscular Blocking Agents

The characteristic response to succinylcholine is a sustained, dose-related contracture that may make ventilation difficult for several minutes. Muscle membrane fragility may be responsible for the exaggerated hyperkalemia that is produced after succinylcholine.[34] Most case reports suggest that the response to nondepolarizing drugs is normal. However, myotonic responses have been observed after reversal with neostigmine.

Anesthesia

Succinylcholine is best avoided. Short- or intermediate-duration nondepolarizing agents may be used in usual doses with careful neuromuscular monitoring. Reversal agents are best avoided. Thus, mechanical ventilation should be maintained until the effects of nondepolarizing agents have worn off completely.

Muscular Dystrophy

The muscular dystrophies are a group of many diseases, with variability in presentation and typical age at onset of symptoms. The most common of these is the Duchenne-type muscular dystrophy (DMD), an X-linked hereditary disease that usually becomes apparent in childhood. Other types of muscular dystrophy include Becker, limb-girdle, fasciohumeral, Emery-Dreifuss, nemaline rod, and oculopharyngeal dystrophy. There have been several reports of cardiac arrest after administration of succinylcholine in children, often associated with hyperkalemia. Resuscitation was found to be difficult, and several of these cases were fatal.[34] The most likely explanation for these adverse events is previously undiagnosed, latent, muscular dystrophy.

Response to Neuromuscular Blocking Agents

In most case reports, the response to nondepolarizing agents, such as vecuronium, atracurium, and mivacurium, has been described as normal, although there have been sporadic instances of increased sensitivity. There are little data on the response to anticholinesterases. There is considerable controversy over whether DMD patients are susceptible to malignant hyperthermia.

Anesthesia

Succinylcholine should be avoided in patients with muscular dystrophy, especially if onset of symptoms occurred in childhood or adolescence. The possibility of latent or unrecognized DMD in young males (<10 years old) may be a reason to avoid succinylcholine in this patient population. Careful titration of short- or intermediate-duration nondepolarizing agents should be done. Reversal agents do not appear to be contraindicated.

Upper Motor Neuron Lesions

Patients with hemiplegia or quadriplegia as a result of central nervous system lesions show an abnormal response to both depolarizing and nondepolarizing agents. Hyperkalemia and cardiac arrest have been described after succinylcholine, probably as a result of extrajunctional receptor proliferation. Hyperkalemia is typically seen if the drug is given between from 1 week to 6 months after the lesion, but may be seen before and after that period.[34] There is resistance to nondepolarizing neuromuscular blocking drugs below the level of the lesion. In hemiplegic patients, monitoring of the affected side shows that the block is less intense and recovery is more rapid than on the unaffected side. However, the apparently normal side also demonstrates some resistance to nondepolarizing drugs. Similar findings have been reported after a stroke, with a greater resistance on the affected side.

Burns

As a result of the proliferation of extrajunctional receptors, succinylcholine produces severe hyperkalemia in patients with burns, and this may lead to cardiac arrest. The magnitude of the problem depends on the extent of the injury. It may appear as early as 24 to 48 hours after the burn injury and usually ends with healing.[34] Resistance to the effects of nondepolarizing neuromuscular blocking agents is manifest, even in muscles that are apparently not affected by the burn.[49,50]

Miscellaneous

Denervated muscle demonstrates potassium release after succinylcholine and resistance to nondepolarizing relaxants. Contractures in response to succinylcholine have also been observed in amyotrophic lateral sclerosis and multiple sclerosis. There have been isolated reports of hyperkalemia after succinylcholine in several neurologic diseases, including Friedrich's ataxia, polyneuritis, and Parkinson disease.

MONITORING NEUROMUSCULAR BLOCKADE

Why Monitor?

Deep levels of paralysis are usually desired during anesthesia to facilitate tracheal intubation and to obtain an immobile surgical field. However, complete return of respiratory function must be attained before the trachea is extubated. Administration of neuromuscular blocking drug must be individualized because blockade occurs over a narrow range of receptor occupancy, and because there is considerable interindividual variability in response. Thus, it is important for the clinician to assess the effect of neuromuscular blocking drugs without the confounding influence of volatile agents, intravenous anesthetics, and opioids. One should remember, however, that monitoring is a tool, not a cure. Neuromuscular blocking agents have the same effects, whether or not monitoring is used. Most studies found that monitoring is not associated with a decrease in the incidence of residual paralysis.[9] To test the function of the neuromuscular junction, a peripheral nerve is stimulated electrically, and the response of the muscle is assessed.

Stimulator Characteristics

The response of the nerve to electrical stimulation depends on three factors: the current applied, the duration of the current, and the position of the electrodes. Stimulators should deliver a maximum current in the range of 60 to 80 mA. Most stimulators are designed to provide constant current, irrespective of impedance changes because of drying of the electrode gel, cooling, decreased sweat gland function, and so forth. However, this constant current feature does not hold for high impedances (>5 kΩ). Thus, electrodes should be firmly applied to the skin. A current display monitor on the stimulator is an asset because accidental disconnection can be identified easily by a current approaching 0 mA. The duration of the current pulse should be long enough for all axons in the nerve to depolarize but short enough to avoid the possibility of exceeding the refractory period of the nerve. In practice, pulse durations of 0.1 to 0.2 msec are acceptable. At least one electrode should be on the skin overlying the nerve to be stimulated. If the negative electrode is used for this purpose, the threshold to supramaximal stimulation is less than for the positive electrode. However, the difference is not large in practice. The position of the other electrode is not critical, but it should not be placed in the vicinity of other nerves. There is no need to use needle electrodes. Silver–silver chloride surface electrodes, used to monitor the electrocardiogram, are adequate for peripheral nerve stimulation, without the risk of bleeding, infection, and burns. In practice, applying these electrodes along the course of a nerve gives the best results (Fig. 20-12).

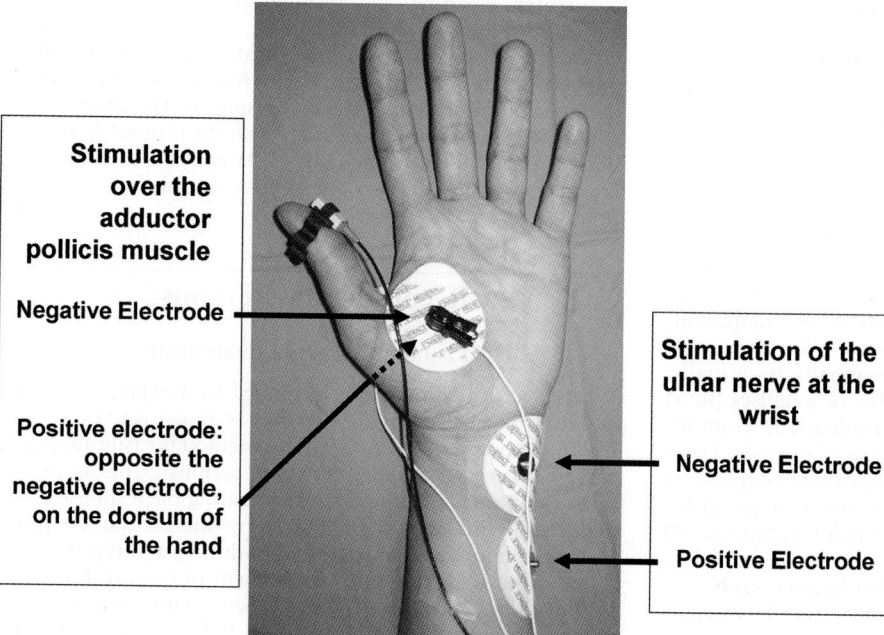

FIGURE 20-12. Electrode placement to obtain contraction of the adductor pollicis muscle. The traditional method is to apply the electrodes over the course of the ulnar nerve at the wrist, with the negative electrode distal (*right*). An alternate method is to position the electrodes over the adductor pollicis muscle (*left*), the negative electrode on the palm of the hand, the positive in the same location, but on the dorsum of the hand. The device fixed to the thumb is an accelerometer.

Stimulation over the adductor pollicis muscle

Negative Electrode

Positive electrode: opposite the negative electrode, on the dorsum of the hand

Stimulation of the ulnar nerve at the wrist

Negative Electrode

Positive Electrode

Monitoring Modalities

Different stimulation modalities were introduced into clinical practice to take advantage of the characteristic features of nondepolarizing neuromuscular blockade: fade and post-tetanic facilitation with high-frequency stimulation. Thus, the following discussion refers mostly to nondepolarizing block.

Single Twitch

The simplest way to stimulate a nerve is to apply a single stimulus, at intervals of >10 seconds (frequency, <0.1 Hz). This interval is needed to allow the neuromuscular junction to recover if nondepolarizing agents are used. With shorter intervals, fade might be present. With depolarizing agents like succinylcholine, little fade occurs and a higher frequency, such as 1 Hz, may be used without concern for fade. The amplitude of response is compared with a control, preblockade twitch height. The single-twitch modality is useful to construct dose-response curves and to evaluate onset time. However, because a control value is required, the clinical usefulness of this mode of stimulation is limited.

Tetanus

When stimulation is applied at a frequency of ≥30 Hz, the mechanical response of the muscle is fusion of individual twitch responses. In the absence of neuromuscular blocking drugs, no fade is present and the response is sustained. During nondepolarizing blockade, the mechanical response appears as a peak, followed by a fade (Fig. 20-9). The sensitivity of tetanic stimulation in the detection of residual neuromuscular blockade is greater than that of single twitch; that is, tetanic fade might be present while twitch height is normal. Most nerve stimulators provide a 5-second train at a frequency of 50 Hz. This frequency was adopted because at >100 Hz, some fade may be seen even in the absence of neuromuscular blocking drugs. However, more fade is seen with 100-Hz than 50-Hz frequencies, and 100-Hz, 5-second trains are most useful in the detection of residual block.[44,115] With tetanic stimulation, no control prerelaxant response is required, as the degree of muscle paralysis can be assessed by the degree of fade following tetanic stimulation. However, the main disadvantage of this mode of stimulation is posttetanic facilitation (Fig. 20-9), the extent of which depends on the frequency and duration of the tetanic stimulation. For a 50-Hz tetanus applied for 5 seconds, the duration of this interval appears to be at least 1 to 2 minutes.[45] If single-twitch stimulation is performed during that time, the response is spuriously exaggerated.

Train-of-Four

With 2-Hz stimulation, the mechanical or electrical response decreases little after the fourth stimulus, and the degree of fade is similar to that found at 50 Hz.[43] Thus, applying train-of-four stimulation at 2 Hz provides more sensitivity than single twitch and approximately the same sensitivity as tetanic stimulation at 50 Hz. In addition, this relatively low frequency allows the response to be evaluated manually or visually. Moreover, the presence of a small number of impulses (four) eliminates the problem of posttetanic facilitation. Train-of-four stimulation can be repeated every 12 to 15 seconds. There is a fairly close relationship between single-twitch depression and train-of-four response,[116] and no control is required for the latter. During recovery, the second twitch reappears at 80 to 90% single-twitch block, the third at 70 to 80%, and when blockade is 65 to 75%, all four twitches become visible.[117] Then, the train-of-four ratio, the height of the fourth twitch to that of the first twitch, is linearly related to first twitch height

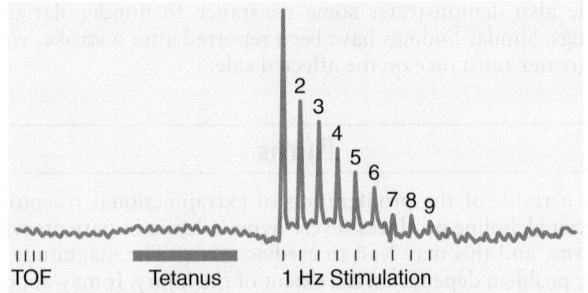

FIGURE 20-13. Posttetanic count (PTC). During profound blockade, no response is seen to train-of-four (TOF) or tetanus. However, because there is posttetanic facilitation, some twitches can be seen after tetanic stimulation. In this example, the PTC is 9.

when blockade is <70%. When single-twitch height has recovered to 100%, the train-of-four ratio is approximately 70%.

Posttetanic Count

During profound neuromuscular blockade, there is no response to single-twitch, tetanic, or train-of-four stimulation. To estimate the time required before the return of a response, one may use a technique that depends on the principle of posttetanic facilitation. A 50-Hz tetanus is applied for 5 seconds, followed by a 3-second pause and by stimulation at 1 Hz. The train-of-four and tetanic responses are undetectable, but facilitation produces a certain number of visible posttetanic twitches (Fig. 20-13). The number of visible twitches correlates inversely with the time required for a return of single-twitch or train-of-four responses.[118] For intermediate-duration drugs, the time from a posttetanic count (PTC) of 1 to reappearance of twitch is 15 to 20 minutes.

Double-Burst Stimulation

Train-of-four fade may be difficult to evaluate by visual or tactile means during recovery from neuromuscular blockade. Irrespective of experience, it is difficult for anesthesiologists to detect train-of-four fade when actual train-of-four ratio is 0.4 or greater, meaning that residual paralysis can go undetected.[115] This shortcoming can be overcome, to a certain extent, by applying two short tetanic stimulations (three impulses at 50 Hz, separated by 750 msec), and by evaluating the ratio of the second to the first response. The double-burst stimulation ratio correlates closely with the train-of-four ratio, but is easier to detect manually.[115] At least 12 to 15 seconds must elapse between two consecutive double-burst stimulations.

Recording the Response

Visual and Tactile Evaluation

When electrical stimulation is applied to a nerve, the easiest and least expensive way to assess the response is to observe or feel the response of the muscle. This method is easily adaptable to any superficial muscle. However, serious errors in assessment can be made. In the case of evaluating the response of the adductor pollicis muscle to ulnar nerve stimulation, the train-of-four count can be made reliably during a surgical procedure,[117] but the quantitative assessment of train-of-four ratio is difficult to make during recovery. Several investigations suggest that train-of-four ratios as low as 0.3[115] can remain undetected. The detection rate for tetanic fade (50 Hz) is no better.[115] With double-burst stimulation, fade can be detected reliably up to train-of-four ratios in the range of 0.6 to 0.7.[115] With 100-Hz tetanic stimulation, fade might be detected at train-of-four ratios of 0.8 to 1.0[44,115] and may be seen in individuals with no neuromuscular block.

Measurement of Force

A force transducer can overcome the shortcomings of one's senses. If applied correctly, the device provides accurate and reliable responses, displayed as either a digital or an analog signal on a monitor. Force measurement can be measured after single-twitch, tetanus, train-of-four, double-burst, or post-tetanic stimulation. However, the availability of tetanus and double-burst stimulation is superfluous if accurate measurement of the train-of-four response can be made. Unfortunately, transducers are expensive, bulky, cumbersome, and can be applied to only one muscle, usually the adductor pollicis.

Electromyography

It is possible to measure the electrical instead of the mechanical response of the muscle. One electrode should be positioned over the neuromuscular junction, which is usually close to the midportion of the muscle, and the other near the insertion of the muscle. A third, neutral electrode can be located anywhere else. Theoretically, any superficial muscle can be used for EMG recordings. In practice, such recordings are limited to the hypothenar eminence, the first dorsal interosseous, and the adductor pollicis muscles, which are supplied by the ulnar nerve. Most EMG recording devices compute the area under the EMG curve during a specified time window after the stimulus is applied. There is usually good correlation between EMG and force of the adductor pollicis muscle if the EMG signal is taken from the thenar eminence. The signal obtained from the hypothenar eminence is larger and less subject to movement artifacts, but it can underestimate the degree of paralysis when compared with the adductor pollicis muscle.[119]

Accelerometry

According to Newton's law, acceleration is proportional to force if mass remains unchanged. The device is usually attached to the tip of the thumb (Fig. 20-12) and a digital readout is obtained. The setup is sensitive to inadvertent displacement of the thumb and, in the absence of neuromuscular blocking drugs, train-of-four ratios >100% can be obtained.[116] In spite of these shortcomings, accelerometers have become increasingly popular because they are easy to use, are less cumbersome, can be used on muscles other than the adductor pollicis, and are relatively inexpensive. The use of accelerometry is helpful in the diagnosis of residual paralysis[120] and, in certain circumstances,[121] but not all,[9] it can reduce the incidence of the condition.

Displacement

A variety of devices have been proposed that respond to motion or displacement. They are designed for the adductor pollicis muscle. A thorough evaluation of these devices has not been made, but data indicate that there are slight but clinically insignificant differences between the results such displacement transducers and mechanomyography provide.[122]

Phonomyography

A contracting muscle emits low frequency sounds. Train-of-four response and fade can be heard with a stethoscope placed over the adductor pollicis muscle. A quantitative response can be obtained with special microphones sensitive to frequencies (2 Hz) below the threshold of the human ear. An excellent correlation between phonomyography and force measurement has been found at several muscles, including the adductor pollicis and the corrugator supercilii.[123] At the time of writing, no commercial devices using phonomyography were available.

Choice of Muscle

Muscles do not respond in a uniform fashion to neuromuscular blocking drugs. After administration of a neuromuscular blocking agent, differences can be measured with respect to onset time, maximum blockade, and duration of action. It is not practical to monitor the muscles of physiological importance, for example, the abdominal muscles during surgery, or the respiratory and upper airway muscles postoperatively. A better approach is to choose a monitoring site that has a response similar to the muscle of interest. For example, monitoring the response of the facial nerve around the eye is a good indicator of intubating conditions, and the use of the adductor pollicis muscle during recovery reflects upper airway muscle function. Another strategy is to stick to one monitoring site, such as the adductor pollicis muscle, and interpret the information provided from knowledge of the different responses between muscles (Fig. 20-14).

Adductor Pollicis Muscle

The adductor pollicis muscle is accessible during most surgical procedures. It is supplied by the ulnar nerve, which becomes superficial at the wrist where a negative electrode can be positioned. The positive electrode is applied a few centimeters proximally (Fig. 20-12). The force of contraction of the adductor pollicis muscle can be measured easily, and it has become a standard in research. After injection of a dose that produces less than 100% blockade, the time to maximal blockade is longer than in centrally located muscles.[124,125] The adductor pollicis muscle is relatively sensitive to nondepolarizing neuromuscular blocking drugs, and during recovery it is blocked more than some respiratory muscles such as the diaphragm,[124] laryngeal adductors,[125] and abdominal muscles (Fig. 20-14).[126] There is evidence that recovery of the adductor pollicis and of upper airway muscles occurs more or less simultaneously (Fig. 20-14).[127]

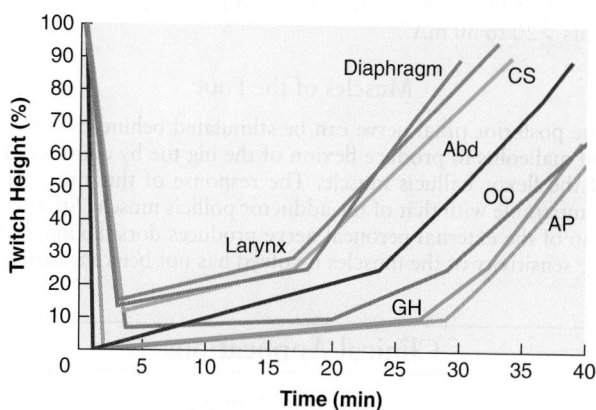

FIGURE 20-14. Approximate time course of twitch height after rocuronium, 0.6 mg/kg, at different muscles. Diaphragm, diaphragm; larynx, laryngeal adductors (vocal cords); CS, corrugator supercilii muscle (eyebrow); Abd, abdominal muscles; OO, orbicularis oculi muscle (eyelid); GH, geniohyoid muscle (upper airway); AP, adductor pollicis muscle (thumb). (Data are taken or inferred from references 75, 126, 127, and 129.)

The adductor pollicis muscle can also be stimulated by applying electrodes directly over it. This can be accomplished by placing the two electrodes in the space lying between the base of the first and second metacarpals, on the palmar and dorsal aspects on the hand, respectively (Fig. 20-12). Such a stimulation avoids the confounding movement of hypothenar muscles. Direct muscle stimulation with this electrode position does not normally occur because neuromuscular blocking agents abolish the response completely.[128] The ability to detect fade by visual or tactile means is the same, whether the stimulating electrodes are applied at the wrist or the hand.[115]

Other Muscles of the Hand

Ulnar nerve stimulation also produces flexion and abduction of the fifth finger, which usually recovers before the adductor pollicis muscle, the discrepancy in first twitch or train-of-four ratio being of the order of 15 to 20%.[119] Relying on the response of the fifth finger might overestimate recovery from blockade. Abduction of the index finger also results from stimulation of the ulnar nerve because of contraction of the first dorsal interosseous, the sensitivity of which is comparable with that of the adductor pollicis muscle. The hypothenar eminence (near the fifth finger) and the first dorsal interosseous are particularly well suited for EMG recordings.[119] Stimulation in the hand (Fig. 20-12) eliminates contraction of the hypothenar muscles, but may evoke movement of the first dorsal interosseous.

Muscles Surrounding the Eye

There seem to be major differences in the response of muscles innervated by the facial nerve and located around the eye, and these differences have introduced some confusion in the literature. The orbicularis oculi muscle essentially covers the eyelid, and its response to neuromuscular blocking agents is similar to that of the adductor pollicis muscle.[129] However, it is customary to observe the movement of the eyebrow, and recordings at that site are similar to that of the laryngeal adductors (Fig. 20-14).[129] Onset of blockade is more rapid and recovery occurs sooner than at the adductor pollicis. Thus, facial nerve stimulation with inspection of the response of the eyebrow (which most likely represents the effect of the corrugator supercilii, not the orbicularis oculi muscle) is indicated to predict intubating conditions and to monitor profound blockade. The facial nerve can be stimulated 2 to 3 cm posterior to the lateral border of the orbit. There is no need to use stimulating currents >20 to 30 mA.

Muscles of the Foot

The posterior tibial nerve can be stimulated behind the internal malleolus to produce flexion of the big toe by contraction of the flexor hallucis muscle. The response of this muscle is comparable with that of the adductor pollicis muscle. Stimulation of the external peroneal nerve produces dorsiflexion, but the sensitivity of the muscles involved has not been measured.

Clinical Applications

Monitoring Onset

The quality of intubating conditions depends chiefly on the state of relaxation of muscles of the jaw, pharynx, larynx, and respiratory system. Onset of action is faster in all these muscles than in the hand or foot because they are closer to the central circulation and they receive a greater blood flow. Among these central muscles, the diaphragm and especially the laryngeal adductors are the most resistant to nondepolarizing agents.

The diaphragm is an important muscle because its blockade prevents coughing, and if laryngeal muscles are paralyzed, vocal cords are relaxed, allowing easy passage of a tracheal tube. The relationship between onset time in laryngeal and hand muscles depends on dose. At relatively low doses (e.g., rocuronium, 0.3 to 0.4 mg/kg), onset time is slower at the adductor pollicis than at the laryngeal muscles. If the dose is increased (e.g., rocuronium, 0.6 to 1.0 mg/kg), onset is faster at the adductor pollicis muscle because these doses produce 100% blockade at the adductor pollicis without blocking laryngeal muscles completely (Fig. 20-14).[73] Onset time decreases considerably in any muscle if the dose given is sufficient to reach 100%. Finally, if the dose is large enough to block the laryngeal muscles completely, onset time again becomes shorter at the larynx. It is not surprising that monitoring the adductor pollicis muscle predicts intubating conditions poorly. Facial nerve stimulation with visual observation of the response over the eyebrow gives better results because the response of the corrugator supercilii is close to that of the vocal cords. Train-of-four fade takes longer to develop than single-twitch depression (Fig. 20-9), and during onset, train-of-four stimulation does not have any advantages over single-twitch stimulation at 0.1 Hz.

Monitoring Surgical Relaxation

Adequate surgical relaxation is usually obtained when fewer than two or three visible twitches are observed at the adductor pollicis muscle. However, this criterion might prove inadequate in certain circumstances when profound relaxation is required owing to the discrepancy between the adductor pollicis and other muscles. In this case, the PTC can be used at the adductor pollicis muscle,[118] provided that this type of stimulation is not repeated more often than every 2 to 3 minutes. A suitable alternative is stimulation of the facial nerve with observation of the response over the eyebrow, which recovers at the same rate as such resistant muscles as the diaphragm.[124,129]

Monitoring Recovery

Complete return of neuromuscular function should be achieved at the conclusion of surgery unless mechanical ventilation is planned. Thus, monitoring is useful in determining whether spontaneous recovery has progressed to a degree that allows reversal agents to be given and to assess the effect of these agents.

The effectiveness of anticholinesterase agents depends directly on the degree of recovery present when they are administered. Preferably, reversal agents should be given only when four twitches are visible at the adductor pollicis muscle,[130] which corresponds to a first-twitch recovery of >25%. The presence of spontaneous breathing is not a sign of adequate neuromuscular recovery. The diaphragm recovers earlier than the much more sensitive upper airway muscles, such as the geniohyoid, which recovers, on average, at the same time as the adductor pollicis muscle.[127] To prevent upper airway obstruction after extubation, it is preferable to use the adductor pollicis muscle to monitor recovery, instead of the more resistant muscles of the hypothenar eminence or those around the eye.

Finally, the adequacy of recovery should be assessed. Traditionally, a train-of-four ratio of 0.7 was considered to be the threshold below which residual weakness of the respiratory muscles could be present. There is abundant evidence that significant weakness may occur up to train-of-four ratio values of 0.9.[10,123] Awake volunteers given mivacurium failed to perform the head-lift test when the train-of-four ratio at the adductor pollicis muscle decreased below 0.62, but needed a train-of-four ratio of at least 0.86 to hold a tongue depressor

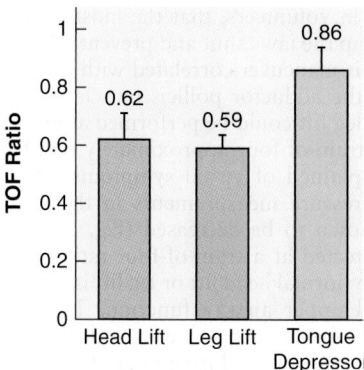

FIGURE 20-15.   Correlation between train-of-four (TOF) responses at the adductor pollicis muscle and certain clinical tests of neuromuscular recovery. Volunteers were given mivacurium and were asked to lift their heads for 5 seconds (head lift), lift their legs for 5 seconds (leg lift), or hold a tongue depressor between their teeth against force (tongue depressor). The minimum TOF ratio (and SD) when each of these tests was passed is indicated. (Data from Kopman et al.[131])

between their teeth (Fig. 20-15).[131] This suggests that the head-lift test does not guarantee full recovery, and that the upper airway muscles used to retain a tongue depressor are very sensitive to the residual effects of neuromuscular blocking drugs. Furthermore, impairment in swallowing and laryngeal aspiration of a pharyngeal fluid was observed at train-of-four ratios as high as 0.9 in volunteers given vecuronium (Fig. 20-4).[132]

Anesthetized patients appear considerably more sensitive to the ventilatory effects of neuromuscular blocking drugs than are awake patients. Whereas tidal volume and end-tidal CO_2 are preserved in awake patients receiving relatively high doses of neuromuscular blocking drugs,[133] anesthetized adults have a decreased tidal volume and increased PCO_2 with doses of pancuronium as low as 0.5 mg.[134] In conscious volunteers, administration of small doses of vecuronium to maintain train-of-four at <0.9 leads to severe impairment of the ventilatory response to hypoxia (Fig. 20-16).[135] The response to hypercapnia is maintained, and this indicates that the response to hypoxia is not a result of respiratory muscle weakness.[135]

Taken together, the results of these investigations indicate that normal respiratory and upper airway function does not return to normal unless the train-of-four ratio at the adductor

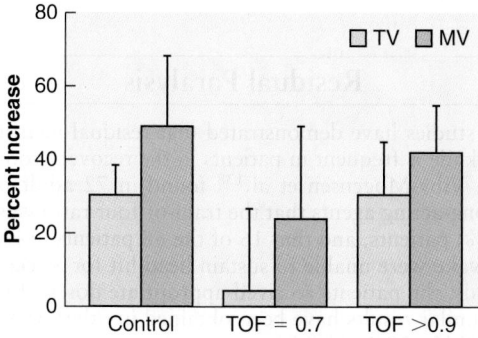

FIGURE 20-16.   Response to hypoxia is impaired during recovery from vecuronium blockade. Normal response is an increase in minute volume (MV) or tidal volume (TV; control). These increases are decreased significantly when vecuronium produces a train-of-four ratio (TOF) of 0.7 at the adductor pollicis muscle. They return to near-normal values at a TOF >0.9. (Data from Eriksson et al.[135])

pollicis muscle is 0.9 or more. However, it has become apparent that human senses fail to detect either a train-of-four or 50-Hz tetanic fade when the train-of-four ratio is as low as 0.3.[115] With double-burst stimulation, detection failures may occur at train-of-four ratios of 0.6 to 0.7.[115] Compared with the train-of-four, the ability to detect fade is not improved by using tetanic stimulation at 50 Hz for 5 seconds. However, fade can be detected visually at train-of-four ratios of 0.8 to 0.9 by using 100-Hz tetanic stimulation,[46,115] although this threshold may vary from patient to patient.[115] Because of the presence of posttetanic facilitation, 50- or 100-Hz stimuli should not be applied more often than every 2 minutes. Because of the limitations of one's senses, it has been advocated that quantitative assessment of the train-of-four ratio be made routinely.[10] Mechanographic and EMG equipment give reliable values of train-of-four ratio, but the use of this equipment is limited by size, cost, and convenience. Accelerometers are less bulky and cheaper, but they can overestimate the value of train-of-four ratio during recovery.[116] It has been suggested that a train-of-four ratio of 1.0 obtained by accelerometry must be obtained before neuromuscular function can be considered complete.[115] Monitoring devices based on the measurement of displacement or sound may prove to have more reliable train-of-four ratios than accelerometry. In one study, a transmission module sensitive to bending and deformation was found to yield train-of-four ratio values comparable to mechanomyography during the recovery period.[122]

In response to the shortcomings of visual or tactile evaluations, another approach to recovery is to wait until sufficient spontaneous recovery is present and give reversal agents systematically. If given at a train-of-four count of 2 during cisatracurium or rocuronium blockade, complete recovery is not achieved until 15 minutes or so later, with some patients still having train-of-four ratios <0.9 after 30 minutes.[136] Thus, the recommendation is to wait until all four twitches have reappeared. In any event, clinicians must be aware of the limitations of the tests they are using and complete their evaluations with clinical tests.

Factors Affecting the Monitoring of Neuromuscular Blockade

Many drugs interfere with neuromuscular function and these are dealt with elsewhere (see "Drug Interactions"). However, certain situations make the interpretation of data on neuromuscular function difficult. Central hypothermia may slow the metabolism of neuromuscular blocking agents and prolong blockade in all muscles of the body.[137] If the extremity where monitoring is performed is cold, the degree of block will be accentuated. Thus, if only the monitored hand is cold, without central hypothermia, the degree of paralysis will appear to be increased.[137] Resistance to nondepolarizing neuromuscular blocking drugs occurs with nerve damage, including peripheral nerve trauma, cord transection, and stroke. In this case, monitoring of the involved limb would tend to underestimate the degree of muscle paralysis. The level of paralysis should also be adjusted for the type of patient, as well as the type of surgery. For example, it is not necessary to paralyze frail individuals or patients at the extremes of age to the same extent as young muscular adults. The same applies to patients with debilitating muscular diseases.

Neuromuscular monitoring by itself does not guarantee adequate relaxation during surgery and complete recovery postoperatively. The surgical field may be poor in spite of full paralysis of the hand because of difference in response between muscles. For example, evidence of breathing efforts can be manifest on the expired CO_2 curve when no twitch is present at the adductor pollicis muscle following ulnar nerve stimulation, reflecting the earlier recovery of the diaphragm.[124,126] Residual paralysis might occur because of excess neuromuscular blocking agents given, early administration of reversal, or an abnormal response of the patient. The effect of the neuromuscular blocking drug is the same whether or not monitoring is used. Neuromuscular monitoring can help in the diagnosis of inadequate skeletal muscle relaxation during surgery or insufficient recovery after surgery, but does not, in itself, treat these conditions.[9]

ANTAGONISM OF NEUROMUSCULAR BLOCK

In most circumstances, all efforts should be made to ensure that the patient leaves the operating room with unimpaired muscle strength. Specifically, respiratory and upper airway muscles must function normally so the patient can breathe, cough, swallow secretions, and keep his or her airway patent. Two strategies can be adopted to achieve this goal. The first is to titrate neuromuscular blocking agents carefully so that no residual effect is manifest at the end of surgery. The second is to accelerate recovery by giving a reversal drug. This second option is probably safer, but both strategies require careful assessment of blockade. A third possibility that might be available in the near future is selective binding of neuromuscular blocking agents with a cyclodextrin molecule to restore neuromuscular function.

Assessment of Neuromuscular Blockade

Spontaneous breathing can resume even if relatively deep degrees of paralysis are still present because of the relative diaphragm-sparing effect of neuromuscular blocking agents. Spontaneous ventilation, adequate to prevent hypercapnia, can be maintained despite considerable measurable skeletal muscle weakness if a patent airway is ensured. The ability to perform maneuvers such as vital capacity, maximum voluntary ventilation, and forced expiratory flow rate recovers at less intense levels of paralysis because it requires a greater strength.[133] However, such tests are difficult to perform in everyday practice, particularly when the patient is recovering from general anesthesia. Moreover, the weakest point in the respiratory system is the upper airway. When given vecuronium, swallowing was impaired and laryngeal aspiration occurred when the train-of-four ratio was ≤0.9.[132] These problems are difficult to diagnose when a tracheal tube is in place. Consequently, several indirect indices, which are easier to measure, have been correlated with the more specific tests of lung and upper airway function.

Clinical Evaluation

Several crude tests have been suggested, including head lift for 5 seconds, tongue protrusion, and the ability to lift the legs off the bed to determine recovery of neuromuscular function. Pavlin et al.[133] correlated the maximum inspiratory pressure with tests of skeletal muscle strength and of airway musculature in conscious volunteers receiving d-tubocurarine. As the dose was increased, head lift and leg raising were affected first. Then, the ability to swallow, touch teeth, and maintain a patent airway was impaired. At that time, hand grip strength was decreased markedly. Nevertheless, as long as the mandible was elevated by an observer, end-tidal CO_2 was normal even when the subject failed all other tests. From these data, Eriksson et al.[132] concluded that ability to maintain head lift for 5 seconds usually indicates sufficient strength to protect the airway and support ventilation. However, Kopman et al.[131]

have shown, in volunteers, that the most sensitive test is the ability to clamp the jaws shut and prevent removal of a tongue depressor. This maneuver correlated with a train-of-four ratio measured at the adductor pollicis muscle of >0.86, whereas head lift and leg lift could be performed at more intense levels of paralysis (train-of-four approximately 0.6; Fig. 20-15). All subjects complained of visual symptoms until train-of-four was >0.9. Pressure measurements in the upper esophagus have been shown to be decreased (Fig. 20-4) and laryngeal aspiration detected at a train-of-four ratio <0.9.[132] Thus, it appears that a normal head lift or leg lift is insufficient to guarantee normal upper airway function. The ability to resist removal of an object (such as a tongue depressor or a tracheal tube) from the mouth by closing the teeth probably correlates better with adequate upper airway function.

Evoked Responses to Nerve Stimulation

The clinical tests previously described are usually unobtainable in the patient recovering from anesthesia. Furthermore, it is preferable to assess the degree of recovery before emergence. Evoked responses to nerve stimulation are then appropriate. The target is a train-of-four >0.9, considering that upper airway function does not recover completely until the train-of-four ratio at the adductor pollicis muscle is at least 0.9.

With the introduction of short- and intermediate-duration nondepolarizing agents into clinical practice, the use of reversal agents has been considered by some as optional. The decision to omit pharmacologic reversal of neuromuscular blockade must be made carefully because the presence of residual paralysis may be missed. As mentioned earlier, manual and tactile evaluation of neuromuscular blockade by train-of-four or 50-Hz tetanic stimulation may fail to detect fade.[115] Double-burst stimulation is more sensitive, but becomes unreliable at train-of-four ratios in the range of 0.6 to 0.9.[115] The most sensitive test is the ability to maintain sustained contraction to 100-Hz tetanus for 5 seconds. Fade may be detected when train-of-four ratio is as high as 0.8 to 0.9.[46,115] Tetanic stimulation at 100 Hz is painful and must be performed only in adequately anesthetized patients.

Because of the limitations of the visual and tactile estimate of the train-of-four response during recovery, objective measurement has been advocated.[10] Acceleromyographic recordings might be the most practical because accelerometers are cheap and easy to use. However, it must be appreciated that the train-of-four ratio obtained with accelerometry is greater than that measured with mechanomyography and may exceed 1.0. An accelerographic train-of-four ratio of 1.0 has been proposed as the equivalent of a mechanomyographic train-of-four of 0.9.[115]

Residual Paralysis

Several studies have demonstrated that residual neuromuscular blockade is frequent in patients in the recovery room after surgery. Viby-Mogensen et al.[138] found in 72 adult patients given long-acting agents that the train-of-four ratio was 0.7 in 30 (42%) patients, and that 16 of the 68 patients (24%) who were awake were unable to sustain head lift for 5 seconds. In that study, the patients received appropriate doses of neostigmine. Similar results have been obtained in other parts of the world (Table 20-1).[9,139] The incidence of train-of-four ratio 0.7 is reduced from about 30% to <10% if the intermediate agents atracurium or vecuronium are substituted for the long-acting drugs and if reversal is given.[9,139,140] However, the actual incidence of residual paralysis was certainly underestimated in the earlier studies because of the criterion used (train-of-four ratio of 0.7).

Recently, there has been a trend for a greater incidence of residual paralysis, even with intermediate-duration drugs. This can be explained by two factors. The threshold for residual paralysis has been raised from a train-of-four ratio of 0.7 to 0.8 and then to 0.9.[9] However, the most important reason for high incidence of residual paralysis seems to be omission of reversal. In one study, more systematic institution of pharmacologic reversal was associated with a decrease in the incidence of residual paralysis (train-of-four >0.9) from 62% to 3%.[141]

Clinical Importance

Residual paralysis in the recovery room has been shown to be associated with significant morbidity. In 1997, Berg et al.[140] studied nearly 700 general surgical patients who randomly received pancuronium, vecuronium, or atracurium to produce surgical relaxation. In patients who had received pancuronium, the incidence of postoperative partial paralysis, defined by the then-accepted criterion of a train-of-four ratio <0.7, was 5 times that in patients receiving either of the two intermediate-acting drugs (26 vs. 5%). In addition, the incidence of atelectasis demonstrated on chest radiographs taken 2 days later was greater in patients who had received pancuronium and who had not attained a train-of-four ratio of 0.7 (16%) than in those who exceeded this threshold (4.8%).[140] Intense residual block has been demonstrated in patients after cardiac surgery, especially if pancuronium was chosen over rocuronium.[66]

Reversal Agents

So far, the only compounds that have been widely used to reverse the effect of neuromuscular blocking agents are the anticholinesterase drugs. The pharmacologic principle involved is inhibition of acetylcholine breakdown to increase its concentration of acetylcholine at the neuromuscular junction, thus tilting the competition for receptors in favor of the neurotransmitter.[139] Other drugs such as suramin and 3-4 aminopyridine are not as effective, or more toxic, or both. The monopoly occupied by anticholinesterase agents might be challenged soon with the introduction of a selective binding agent, sugammadex, which is now undergoing clinical trials in North America and Europe.

Anticholinesterases: Mechanism of Action

Neostigmine, edrophonium, and pyridostigmine inhibit acetylcholinesterase, but this may not be the only mechanism by which blockade is antagonized. This inhibition is present at all cholinergic synapses in the peripheral nervous system. Thus, the anticholinesterases have potent parasympathomimetic activity, which is attenuated or abolished by the administration of an antimuscarinic agent, atropine or glycopyrrolate. Neostigmine, edrophonium, and pyridostigmine are quaternary ammonium compounds, which do not penetrate the blood-brain barrier well. Thus, although these agents have the ability to affect cholinergic function in the central nervous system, the concentrations in the brain are usually too small for such an effect. Physostigmine is an anticholinesterase that can cross the blood-brain barrier easily. For this reason, it is not used to reverse neuromuscular blockade.

Neostigmine and pyridostigmine are attached to the anionic and esteratic sites of the acetylcholinesterase molecule and produce longer lasting inhibition than edrophonium. Neostigmine and pyridostigmine are inactivated by the interaction with the enzyme, whereas edrophonium is unaffected.[139]

Inhibition of acetylcholinesterase results in an increased amount of acetylcholine reaching the receptor and in a longer time for acetylcholine to remain in the synaptic cleft. This causes an increase in the size and duration of the end plate potentials.[142] There is evidence that some of the effects of neostigmine are not the result of cholinesterase inhibition.[142]

Anticholinesterases also have presynaptic effects. In the absence of neuromuscular blocking drugs, they potentiate the normal twitch response in a way similar to succinylcholine, probably as a result of the generation of action potentials that spread antidromically. A ceiling effect, that is, the inability for large doses to produce an increasing effect, has been demonstrated in vitro[143] and can be observed in patients.[144]

Neostigmine Block

Large doses of anticholinesterases, especially if given when neuromuscular block is absent, may produce evidence of neuromuscular dysfunction. For example, dose-dependent decreases in the EMG activity of the genioglossus and the diaphragm have been measured following neostigmine administration in rats.[145] The problem might be less when some degree of neuromuscular blockade is present before neostigmine is given. The mechanism involved is uncertain. There are no clinical reports of postoperative weakness attributed to reversal agents. Still, it appears prudent to reduce the dose of anticholinesterase agent if recovery from neuromuscular block is almost complete.

Potency

Dose-response curves have been constructed for edrophonium, neostigmine, and pyridostigmine. During a constant infusion of neuromuscular blocking drugs, the curves are obtained by plotting the peak effect versus the dose of reversal agent. In this situation, neostigmine was found to be approximately 12 times as potent as edrophonium.[146] However, the curves are not parallel, that of edrophonium being flatter. This indicates that edrophonium is effective over a narrower range of blockade and less effective against deep blockade. This was verified when neostigmine and edrophonium were used to reverse atracurium blockade. More neostigmine and edrophonium were required to reverse deep (99%) than moderate (90%) block, but the difference was greater for edrophonium.[147] There is no difference in the dose-response relationship of anticholinesterases if vecuronium is infused instead of pancuronium, but there is a marked shift to the left for the curves obtained during vecuronium block if the reversal agent is given during spontaneous recovery.[148] This indicates that anticholinesterase-assisted recovery is the sum of two components: (1) spontaneous recovery from the neuromuscular blocking agent itself, which depends on the pharmacokinetic characteristics of the drug, and (2) assisted recovery, which is a function of the dose and type of anticholinesterase agent given.

Pharmacokinetics

Following bolus intravenous injection, the plasma concentration of the anticholinesterases decreases rapidly during the first 5 to 10 minutes and then more slowly.[139] Volumes of distribution are in the range of 0.7 to 1.4 L/kg and the elimination half-life is 60 to 120 minutes. The drugs are water-soluble, ionized compounds so that their principal route of excretion is the kidney. Their clearances are in the range of 8 to 16 mL/kg/min, which is much greater than the glomerular filtration rate because they are actively secreted into the tubular lumen. Their clearance is reduced markedly in patients in renal failure.

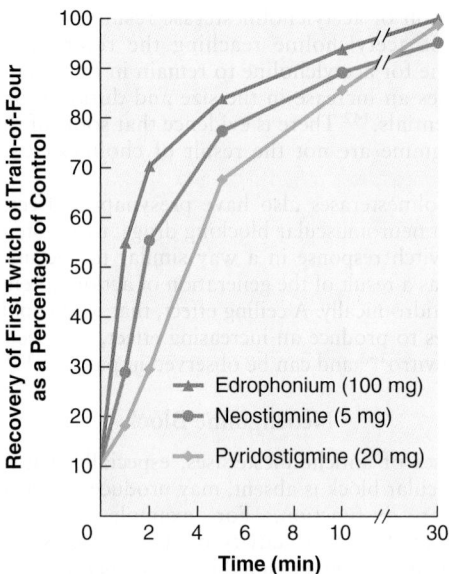

FIGURE 20-17. Reversal of pancuronium blockade at 10% twitch recovery. Reversal is given at time zero. Edrophonium is faster than neostigmine, which is faster than pyridostigmine. (Redrawn from Ferguson A, Egerszegi P, Bevan DR: Neostigmine, pyridostigmine, and edrophonium as antagonists of pancuronium. Anesthesiology 1980; 53: 390.)

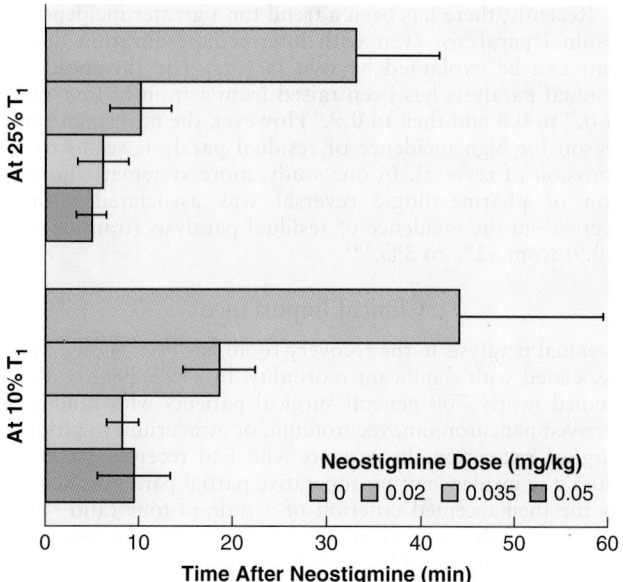

FIGURE 20-18. Neostigmine is more effective at greater degree of recovery from rocuronium blockade. Time to reach a train-of-four ratio of 0.8 after various doses of neostigmine. This time is less if neostigmine is given at 25% than at 10% first-twitch recovery. Notice a ceiling effect for neostigmine at doses >0.035 mg/kg. A dose of 0 indicates no reversal given. (Data from McCourt et al.[144])

Pharmacodynamics

The onset of action of edrophonium (1 to 2 minutes) to peak effect is much more rapid than that of neostigmine (7 to 11 minutes) or pyridostigmine (15 to 20 minutes; Fig. 20-17).[162] The reason for the differences is uncertain, but may be related to the different rates of binding to the enzyme. The duration of action (1 to 2 hours) is similar to their elimination half-life. Even when used to reverse blockade produced by long-acting agents, duration of action of anticholinesterase agents is comparable with or most often exceeds that of the neuromuscular blocking drug. Well-documented recurarization has not been reported. In practice, cases of apparent reparalysis in the recovery room are incomplete reversal that was initially thought to be complete. Either manual or visual assessment is performed using the train-of-four or tetanus mode, which can yield to gross underevaluation of residual paralysis, or respiratory function appeared adequate when the tracheal tube is in place, but once extubated, the patient cannot maintain a patent airway.

Factors Affecting Reversal

Several factors modify the rate of recovery of neuromuscular activity after reversal.

Intensity of Block

The more intense the block at the time of reversal, the longer the recovery of neuromuscular activity (Fig. 20-18).[144] In addition, neostigmine is more effective than edrophonium or pyridostigmine in antagonizing intense (90%) blockade. When reversal is administered after spontaneous recovery to ≥25% T_1 has occurred, recovery is rapid and the time from reversal to train-of-four >0.9 is usually only a few minutes, although recovery after pancuronium may not be complete.[68] Thus, Kopman et al.[136] recommended that reversal should not be attempted until T_1 ≥25% when four twitches to train-of-four stimulation are visible. Attempted reversal at only two twitches may take 30 minutes or more to reach train-of-four of 0.9.

One might argue that reversal can be attempted earlier, for instance when there is only one or no twitch visible following train-of-four stimulation, because one would otherwise spend time waiting for all four twitches to reappear. Several studies dealt with the problem of total time between injection of the neuromuscular blocking agent until complete recovery, with the reversal agent given at different levels of spontaneous recovery. Bevan et al.[148] administered large doses of neostigmine (0.07 mg/kg) after rocuronium and vecuronium and measured time until train-of-four ratio was 0.9. Neostigmine decreased the time to recovery, no matter when it was given. However, time from injection to full reversal was not less when neostigmine was given 5 minutes after rocuronium (42.1 minutes) than at 25% recovery (28.2 minutes; Fig. 20-19).[148] In addition, giving the reversal agent too early leads to a period of "blind paralysis" because neostigmine-assisted recovery is characterized by an early, rapid phase, followed by slower recovery. As a result, the interval between a train-of-four ratio of 0.4 to 0.9, that is, the time when fade is difficult to detect, is likely to be much longer with early neostigmine administration. Thus, there is little advantage in attempting early reversal.

Dose

Over a certain dose range, the degree and rate of reversal depends directly on dose.[144,147] However, all anticholinesterase agents demonstrate a ceiling effect (Fig. 20-18). Usually, there is no added benefit in giving doses exceeding 0.07 mg/kg neostigmine, or 1.0 mg/kg edrophonium.

Choice of Neuromuscular Blocking Agent

Recovery of neuromuscular activity after reversal depends on the rate of spontaneous recovery as well as the acceleration induced by the reversal agent. Consequently, the overall recovery of intermediate-acting agents (atracurium, vecuronium, mivacurium, rocuronium) following the same dose of anticholinesterase is more rapid and more complete than after pancuronium,

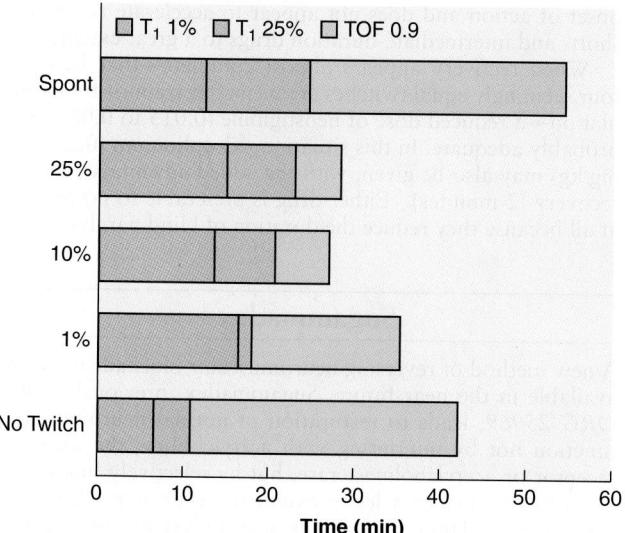

FIGURE 20-19.   Time from injection of rocuronium until recovery to train-of-four ratio (TOF) of 0.9 in adults. Reversal with neostigmine was either not given (Spont) or given at 25%, 10%, or 1% twitch recovery, or given 5 minutes after rocuronium, when there was no twitch. Times from rocuronium injection to 1% first twitch, 25% first twitch, and TOF of 0.9 are indicated. Neostigmine was optimal when given at 10 to 25%. Giving it early had no advantage. (Data from Bevan et al.[148])

d-tubocurarine, or gallamine.[68] This difference is probably why residual paralysis is more frequent with longer-acting neuromuscular blocking agents. After prolonged infusions, recovery is slower than after intermittent bolus administration.

Age

Recovery of neuromuscular activity occurs more rapidly with smaller doses of anticholinesterases in infants and children than in adults (Fig. 20-20).[148] Residual weakness in the recovery room is found less frequently in children than in adults.

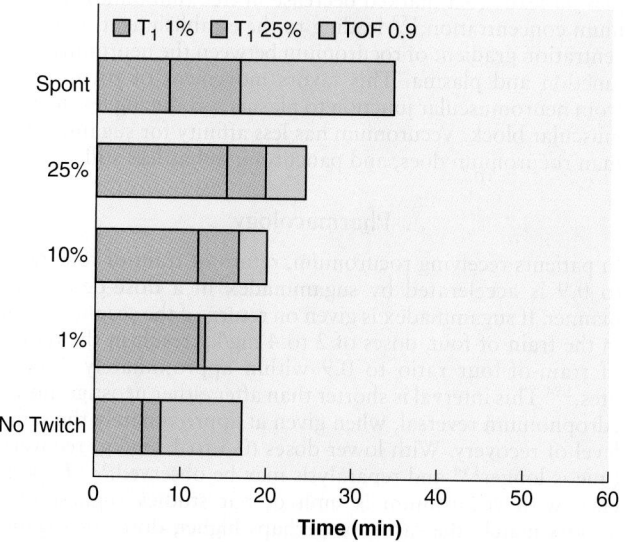

FIGURE 20-20.   Same graph as in Figure 20-19, but in children 2 to 12 years old. Spontaneous recovery from rocuronium blockade (Spont) is more rapid, as well as neostigmine-assisted recovery. (Data from Bevan et al.[148])

The effectiveness of reversal has not been studied extensively in the elderly. Although the elimination of anticholinesterases is reduced in this age group, this reduction is counterbalanced by the tendency for neuromuscular blockade to wear off more slowly. This is especially true of steroidal neuromuscular blocking agents, such as vecuronium and rocuronium, which have a slower recovery index in the elderly.

Drug Interactions

Drugs that potentiate neuromuscular blockade can slow reversal or produce recurarization if given after anticholinesterase administration. Halogenated agents, when continued after neostigmine administration, prolong time to full reversal. Even when they are discontinued at the time of anticholinesterase drug administration, reversal time is not reduced significantly, probably because washout of the vapor from muscle tissue takes time. Care must be taken if aminoglycoside antibiotics or magnesium must be given shortly after reversal agents.

Renal Failure

Anticholinesterases are actively secreted into the tubular lumen so that their clearance is reduced in renal failure.[139] Thus, duration of action of neostigmine and edrophonium is increased in renal failure, at least to a comparable extent as duration of action of the neuromuscular blocking agent. No cases of recurarization have been reported.

Anticholinesterases: Other Effects

Cardiovascular

Anticholinesterases provoke profound vagal stimulation. The time course of the vagal effects parallels the reversal of block, which is rapid for edrophonium and slower for neostigmine. However, the bradycardia and bradyarrhythmias can be prevented with anticholinergic agents. Atropine has a rapid onset of action (1 minute), duration of 30 to 60 minutes, and crosses the blood–brain barrier. Its time course makes it appropriate for use in combination with edrophonium,[146] whereas glycopyrrolate (onset 2 to 3 minutes) is more suitable with neostigmine or pyridostigmine. Because glycopyrrolate does not cross the blood–brain barrier, it is believed that the incidence of memory deficits after anesthesia is less than that after atropine. If atropine is given with neostigmine, the dose is approximately half that of neostigmine (atropine 20 μg/kg for neostigmine 40 μg/kg). Such a combination leads to an initial tachycardia followed by a slight bradycardia. With glycopyrrolate, the dose is one-fourth to one-fifth that of neostigmine. Atropine requirements are less with edrophonium than with neostigmine (atropine 7 to 10 μg/kg with edrophonium 0.5 mg/kg).

Other Cholinergic Effects

Anticholinesterases produce increased salivation and bowel motility. Although atropine blocks the former, it appears to have little effect on peristalsis. Some reports claim an increase in bowel anastomotic leakage after the reversal of neuromuscular blockade. There has been concern over the possible impact of anticholinesterase agents on postoperative nausea and vomiting (PONV). A meta-analysis, published in 1999, concluded that neostigmine had no effect on the overall incidence of PONV, but large doses (2.5 mg or more in adults) was associated with a higher incidence of PONV than no reversal, while lower doses led to less PONV.[149] A more recent meta-analysis reanalyzed the data and incorporated additional studies. It concluded that there was no relation between administration of neostigmine and PONV.[150] At any rate, possible nausea and vomiting is preferable to signs and symptoms of respiratory paralysis.

Respiratory Effects

Anticholinesterases may cause an increase in airway resistance, but anticholinergics reduce this effect. Several other factors, such as pain, the presence of an endotracheal tube, or light anesthesia, may predispose to bronchoconstriction at the end of surgery so that it is difficult to incriminate the reversal agents.

Clinical Use

Several strategies have been proposed to restore neuromuscular function at the end of surgery and anesthesia. One of them involves restricting the dose of nondepolarizing blocking agent at induction of anesthesia to what is necessary for the duration of the procedure, minimal additional doses and reliance of complete spontaneous recovery in an attempt to avoid reversal with anticholinesterase agents. This approach is not without dangers. Even relatively modest doses ($2 \times ED_{95}$) of atracurium, vecuronium, or rocuronium are associated with residual paralysis (train-of-four ratio <0.9) after as long as 4 hours after injection.[120] Visual or tactile monitoring with train-of-four, 50 Hz-tetanus, or double-burst stimulation stimulation cannot rule out some degree of residual paralysis.[115] Only a sustained response to a 100-Hz tetanus may rule out the presence of residual paralysis by tactile or visual means.[44,115] The use of objective monitoring, such as acceleromyography, is even better.[115] Still, pharmacologically assisted recovery is expected in most cases, as it is illusory to aim for complete recovery only by careful titration of neuromuscular blocking agents. In a study examining anesthetic outcomes in The Netherlands, the use of reversal agents was found to be associated with a tenfold reduction in mortality.[151] Not surprisingly, the more systematic use of reversal agents in one institution led to a substantial decrease in residual paralysis.[141]

Administration of anticholinesterase agents will accelerate recovery, no matter when they are given in the course of recovery (Fig. 20-19). However, there are advantages in giving ❽ reversal agents when spontaneous recovery is well under way, preferably when four twitches are present after train-of-four stimulation. If neostigmine is given when deep blockade is present (no twitch or only one twitch present; Figs. 20-18 and 20-19), reversal takes longer than if four twitches are present. As a result, time from injection of rocuronium until full recovery (train-of-four >0.9) is not reduced, and my in fact be increased, if neostigmine is given too early (Fig. 20-19). Furthermore, the patient might be more difficult to manage with early reversal: duration of blind paralysis (from train-of-four of 0.4, when train-of-four fade becomes undetectable, until train-of-four is 0.9) is longer with early reversal. This means that missing residual paralysis is more likely with hasty administration of anticholinesterase agents. Therefore, if four twitches are not visible after train-of-four stimulation, it is recommended to keep the patient anesthetized and mechanically ventilated until four twitches reappear and then administer anticholinesterases.

Intense blockade is not expected to be reversed effectively by increasing the dose of anticholinesterase (Fig. 20-18). In general, neostigmine doses of 0.04 to 0.05 mg/kg should be sufficient, and there is no advantage in exceeding 0.07 mg/kg because of the ceiling effect of the drug. Edrophonium is not recommended for intense block. Pyridostigmine has a slow

onset of action and does not appear to accelerate reversal of short- and intermediate-duration drugs to a great extent.

When recovery appears almost complete—that is, when four seemingly equal twitches are seen after train-of-four stimulation—a reduced dose of neostigmine (0.015 to 0.02 mg) is probably adequate. In this situation, edrophonium (0.2 to 0.5 mg/kg) may also be given, with the added advantage of rapid recovery (2 minutes). Either drug is preferable to no reversal at all because they reduce the duration of blind paralysis.

Sugammadex

A new method of reversing neuromuscular blockade might be available in the near future. Sugammadex, previously called ORG 25969, leads to restoration of normal neuromuscular function not by interfering with acetylcholine, the nicotinic receptor or acetylcholinesterase, but by selectively binding to rocuronium, and to a lesser extent to vecuronium and pancuronium.[152] The compound is a cyclodextrin, made up of eight sugars arranged in a ring to make a center to accommodate the rocuronium molecule. Once bound, rocuronium is held in place by polar side chains attached to the ring. Because sugammadex does not bind to any known receptor, it is devoid of major cardiovascular or other side effects. It does not bind neuromuscular blocking drugs that do not have a steroid nucleus. The benzylisoquinolines, such as atracurium, cisatracurium and mivacurium, and succinylcholine are unaffected by sugammadex.

Mechanism of Action

❾ Sugammadex has a molecular weight of 2,178 Daltons[152] and binds with rocuronium in a 1:1 molar ratio. The rocuronium molecule is less bulky (610 Daltons), so 3.6 mg (or mg/kg) of sugammadex is required to bind 1.0 mg (or mg/kg) of rocuronium. Binding is tight, but not irreversible. This means that rocuronium–sugammadex complexes form while some others break up into their two constituents. The dissociation constant has been estimated to be 0.1 μM,[152] and it is not known whether it is affected by pH, temperature, type of fluid or tissue, or other factors. After injection of sugammadex, evidence suggests that binding of rocuronium to sugammadex in plasma leads to a marked decrease in free (unbound) rocuronium concentration,[153] leading to the establishment of a concentration gradient of rocuronium between the neuromuscular junction and plasma. This favors movement of rocuronium from neuromuscular junction to plasma, producing less neuromuscular block. Vecuronium has less affinity for sugammadex than rocuronium does, and pancuronium has less still.

Pharmacology

In patients receiving rocuronium, return of train-of-four ratio to 0.9 is accelerated by sugammadex in a dose-dependent manner. If sugammadex is given on return of the second twitch in the train-of-four, doses of 2 to 4 mg/kg result in the return of train-of-four ratio to 0.9 within approximately 2 minutes.[154] This interval is shorter than after either neostigmine or edrophonium reversal, when given at approximately the same level of recovery. With lower doses (0.5 to 1 mg/kg) recovery time is longer[154] and reparalysis may be observed.[155] Experience with vecuronium is limited, but studies suggest that approximately the same, or perhaps higher, doses of sugammadex are required for the same effect.[154]

Sugammadex is also effective when blockade is deep, but larger doses are required (Fig. 20-21). When a PTC of 2 is present, which for rocuronium occurs 15 to 20 minutes before return of twitch, the required dose is probably 4 to 8 mg/kg.[156]

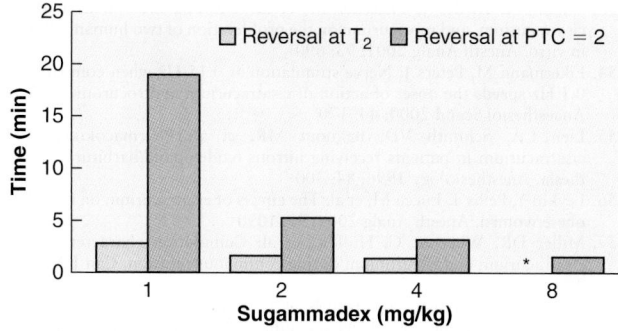

FIGURE 20-21. Relationship between time to achieve a train-of-four ratio of 0.9 and dose of sugammadex at moderate (spontaneous recovery to T_2 or two visible twitches) or profound (posttetanic count [PTC] of 2). Dose of sugammadex required is greater with profound blockade. *No data available for moderate blockade. (Data from references 153, 154, and 156.)

Sugammadex could also be used in the case of a failed intubation. If rocuronium 0.6 mg/kg was given, sugammadex 8 mg/kg might be effective as early as 3 minutes after rocuronium injection, and if the dose of rocuronium is doubled to 1.2 mg/kg, one might need 16 mg/kg of sugammadex.[157] The availability of sugammadex might make succinylcholine obsolete for intubation.[152]

Pharmacokinetics

Sugammadex has a volume of distribution that is similar to ECF (13 L). Its terminal half-life is approximately 2 hours.[158] Both sugammadex and sugammadex–rocuronium complexes are excreted unchanged via the kidney. No data are available in renal-failure patients. In patients receiving rocuronium, injection of sugammadex increases the total (free plus bound) plasma concentrations of rocuronium, which suggests that it causes sequestration of rocuronium in the plasma by drawing it from peripheral tissues.

Clinical Use

At the time of writing (end of 2007), sugammadex had not been approved for clinical use anywhere in the world. Not all clinical data had been published, so the following comments should be taken with caution. Although administration of doses as high as 40 mg/kg have been reported as safe, it appears prudent to use the lowest effective dose, to keep costs down and because safety of high doses will be established only after use is widespread. Because the effective dose depends on the depth of blockade, monitoring is recommended, if not essential. For reversal of rocuronium blockade when spontaneous recovery has already started (two to four twitches present), sugammadex 2 to 4 mg/kg will produce faster recovery than neostigmine would, without cardiovascular side effects.[154] When recovery is even greater (four apparently equal twitches), 0.5 to 1 mg/kg might be sufficient, but more data are needed on this.

The usefulness of sugammadex might be even greater in cases of deep blockade, when no twitch is seen after train-of-four stimulation. The use of the PTC mode of stimulation will probably be useful in establishing the dose, but if any PTC count is present, it is expected that 4 to 8 mg/kg will be required.[156] The dose will be doubled in cases of deeper blockade (no PTC count) or rescue after failed intubation. It is expected that as confidence in the efficacy of sugammadex in the context of profound blockade builds up, clinicians

might have a tendency to give larger doses of rocuronium. This change in practice could yield some benefits. More profound relaxation provides better and faster intubating conditions, better surgical conditions, and less damage to the laryngeal structures. Faster and more predictable recovery could diminish the incidence of residual paralysis and reduce turn-around time. But these benefits will come at a cost. Of course, it will be more expensive to establish muscle relaxation if the dose of rocuronium is increased, and the cost of reversal will undoubtedly be substantial, especially if large doses are given consistently. In addition, however, all movement will be abolished during surgery, so an important sign of inadequate analgesia and anesthesia will be lost. It is unclear whether awareness can be totally avoided by the use of BIS monitoring, as large doses of neuromuscular blocking agents can depress BIS in certain circumstances.[5] Finally, many foreseeable problems regarding sugammadex have not been addressed, such as its use in renal-failure patients, the management of a patient who has recently received sugammadex who needs surgery (for re-exploration for instance), the interaction with steroid-type drugs or naturally occurring molecules, and the potential for bypassing the postanesthesia care unit. Future experience with this new agent will be critical.

References

1. Griffith HR, Johnson GE: The use of curare in general anesthesia. Anesthesiology 1942; 3: 418
2. Beecher HK, Todd DP: A study of the deaths associated with anesthesia and surgery: Based on a study of 599, 548 anesthesias in ten institutions 1948–1952, inclusive. Ann Surg 1954; 140: 2
3. Sandin RH, Enlund G, Samuelsson P, et al: Awareness during anaesthesia: A prospective case study. Lancet 2000; 355: 707
4. Sonner JM, Antognini JF, Dutton RC, et al: Inhaled anesthetics and immobility: Mechanisms, mysteries, and minimum alveolar anesthetic concentration. Anesth Analg 2003; 97: 718
5. Ekman A, Stalberg E, Sundman E, et al: The effect of neuromuscular block and noxious stimulation on hypnosis monitoring during sevoflurane anesthesia. Anesth Analg 2007; 105: 688
6. King M, Sujirattanawimol N, Danielson DR, et al: Requirements for muscle relaxants during radical retropubic prostatectomy. Anesthesiology 2000; 93: 1392
7. McNeil IA, Culbert B, Russell I: Comparison of intubating conditions following propofol and succinylcholine with propofol and remifentanil 2 micrograms kg-1 or 4 micrograms kg-1. Br J Anaesth 2000; 85: 623
8. Mencke T, Echternach M, Kleinschmidt S, et al: Laryngeal morbidity and quality of tracheal intubation: a randomized controlled trial. Anesthesiology 2003; 98: 1049
9. Naguib M, Kopman AF, Ensor JE: Neuromuscular monitoring and postoperative residual curarisation: a meta-analysis. Br J Anaesth 2007; 98: 302
10. Eriksson LI: Evidence-based practice and neuromuscular monitoring: it's time for routine quantitative assessment. Anesthesiology 2003; 98: 1037
11. Boonyapisit K, Kaminski HJ, Ruff RL: Disorders of neuromuscular junction ion channels. Am J Med. 1999; 106: 97
12. Naguib M, Flood P, McArdle JJ, et al: Advances in neurobiology of the neuromuscular junction: implications for the anesthesiologist. Anesthesiology 2002; 96: 202
13. Wood SJ, Slater CR: Safety factor at the neuromuscular junction. Prog. Neurobiol. 2001; 64: 393
14. Waud BE, Waud DR: The relation between the response to "train-of-four" stimulation and receptor occlusion during competitive neuromuscular block. Anesthesiology 1972; 37: 413
15. Rotundo RL: Expression and localization of acetylcholinesterase at the neuromuscular junction. J Neurocytol. 2003; 32: 743
16. Jonsson M, Gurley D, Dabrowski M, et al: Distinct pharmacologic properties of neuromuscular blocking agents on human neuronal nicotinic acetylcholine receptors: a possible explanation for the train-of-four fade. Anesthesiology 2006; 105: 521
17. Jonsson M, Dabrowski M, Gurley DA, et al: Activation and inhibition of human muscular and neuronal nicotinic acetylcholine receptors by succinylcholine. Anesthesiology 2006; 104: 724
18. Donati F: Neuromuscular blocking drugs for the new millennium: current practice, future trends—comparative pharmacology of neuromuscular blocking drugs. Anesth Analg 2000; 90: S2
19. Viby-Mogensen J, Engbaek J, Eriksson LI, et al: Good clinical research practice (GCRP) in pharmacodynamic studies of neuromuscular blocking agents. Acta Anaesthesiol Scand 1996; 40: 59

20. Schreiber JU, Lysakowski C, Fuchs-Buder T, et al: Prevention of succinyl-choline-induced fasciculation and myalgia: a meta-analysis of randomized trials. Anesthesiology 2005; 103: 877

21. Smith CE, Saddler JM, Bevan JC, et al: Pretreatment with non-depolarizing neuromuscular blocking agents and suxamethonium-induced increases in resting jaw tension in children. Br J Anaesth 1990; 64: 577

22. Szalados JE, Donati F, Bevan DR: Effect of d-tubocurarine pretreatment on succinylcholine twitch augmentation and neuromuscular blockade. Anesth Analg 1990; 71: 55

23. McCoy EP, Mirakhur RK: Comparison of the effects of neostigmine and edrophonium on the duration of action of suxamethonium. Acta Anaesthesiol Scand 1995; 39: 744

24. Roy JJ, Donati F, Boismenu D, Varin F: Concentration-effect relation of succinylcholine chloride during propofol anesthesia. Anesthesiology 2002; 97: 1082

25. Szalados JE, Donati F, Bevan DR: Nitrous oxide potentiates succinyl-choline neuromuscular blockade in humans. Anesth Analg 1991; 72: 18

26. Lerman J, Chinyanga HM: The heart rate response to succinylcholine in children: a comparison of atropine and glycopyrrolate. Can Anaesth. Soc. J 1983; 30: 377

27. Mertes PM, Laxenaire MC, Alla F: Anaphylactic and anaphylactoid reactions occurring during anesthesia in France in 1999–2000. Anesthesiology 2003; 99: 536

28. Donati F: Dose inflation when using precurarization. Anesthesiology 2006; 105: 222

29. Harvey SC, Roland P, Bailey MK, et al: A randomized, double-blind comparison of rocuronium, d-tubocurarine, and "mini-dose" succinylcholine for preventing succinylcholine-induced muscle fasciculations. Anesth Analg 1998; 87: 719

30. Mencke T, Schreiber JU, Becker C, et al: Pretreatment before succinyl-choline for outpatient anesthesia? Anesth Analg 2002; 94: 573

31. Wong SF, Chung F: Succinylcholine-associated postoperative myalgia. Anaesthesia 2000; 55: 144

32. Vachon CA, Warner DO, Bacon DR: Succinylcholine and the open globe. Tracing the teaching. Anesthesiology 2003; 99: 220

33. Minton MD, Grosslight K, Stirt JA, Bedford RF: Increases in intracranial pressure from succinylcholine: prevention by prior nondepolarizing blockade. Anesthesiology 1986; 65: 165

34. Gronert GA: Cardiac arrest after succinylcholine: mortality greater with rhabdomyolysis than receptor upregulation. Anesthesiology 2001; 94: 523

35. Thapa S, Brull SJ: Succinylcholine-induced hyperkalemia in patients with renal failure: an old question revisited. Anesth Analg 2000; 91: 237

36. Davis L, Britten JJ, Morgan M: Cholinesterase. Its significance in anaesthetic practice. Anaesthesia 1997; 52: 244

37. Donati F: The right dose of succinylcholine. Anesthesiology 2003; 99: 1037

38. Naguib M, Samarkandi AH, El Din ME, et al: The dose of succinylcholine required for excellent endotracheal intubating conditions. Anesth Analg 2006; 102: 151

39. Hayes AH, Breslin DS, Mirakhur RK, et al: Frequency of haemoglobin desaturation with the use of succinylcholine during rapid sequence induction of anaesthesia. Acta Anaesthesiol Scand 2001; 45: 746

40. Meakin G, McKiernan EP, Morris P, et al: Dose-response curves for suxamethonium in neonates, infants and children. Br J Anaesth 1989; 62: 655

41. Donati F, Guay J: No substitute for the intravenous route. Anesthesiology 2001; 94: 1

42. Lemmens HJ, Brodsky JB: The dose of succinylcholine in morbid obesity. Anesth Analg 2006; 102: 438

43. Lee C, Katz RL: Fade of neurally evoked compound electromyogram during neuromuscular block by d-tubocurarine. Anesth Analg 1977; 56: 271

44. Baurain MJ, Hennart DA, Godschalx A, et al: Visual evaluation of residual curarization in anesthetized patients using one hundred-hertz, five-second tetanic stimulation at the adductor pollicis muscle. Anesth Analg 1998; 87: 185

45. Brull SJ, Connelly NR, O'Connor TZ, et al: Effect of tetanus on subsequent neuromuscular monitoring in patients receiving vecuronium. Anesthesiology 1991; 74: 64

46. Kopman AF, Klewicka MM, Kopman DJ, et al: Molar potency is predictive of the speed of onset of neuromuscular block for agents of intermediate, short, and ultrashort duration. Anesthesiology 1999; 90: 425

47. Savarese JJ, Ali HH, Antonio RP: The clinical pharmacology of metocurine: dimethyltubocurarine revisited. Anesthesiology 1977; 47: 277

48. Fisher DM, O'Keeffe C, Stanski DR, et al: Pharmacokinetics and pharmacodynamics of d-tubocurarine in infants, children, and adults. Anesthesiology 1982; 57: 203

49. Martyn JA, White DA, Gronert GA, et al: Up-and-down regulation of skeletal muscle acetylcholine receptors. Effects on neuromuscular blockers. Anesthesiology 1992; 76: 822

50. Ibebunjo C, Martyn JA: Thermal injury induces greater resistance to d-tubocurarine in local rather than in distant muscles in the rat. Anesth Analg 2000; 91: 1243

51. Diefenbach C, Kunzer T, Buzello W, et al: Alcuronium: a pharmacodynamic and pharmacokinetic update. Anesth Analg 1995; 80: 373

52. Fodale V, Santamaria LB: Laudanosine, an atracurium and cisatracurium metabolite. Eur. J Anaesthesiol. 2002; 19: 466

53. Amann A, Rieder J, Fleischer M, et al: The influence of atracurium, cisatracurium, and mivacurium on the proliferation of two human cell lines in vitro. Anesth Analg 2001; 93: 690

54. Eikermann M, Peters J: Nerve stimulation at 0.15 Hz when compared to 0.1 Hz speeds the onset of action of cisatracurium and rocuronium. Acta Anaesthesiol Scand 2000; 44: 170

55. Lien CA, Schmith VD, Belmont MR, et al: Pharmacokinetics of cisatracurium in patients receiving nitrous oxide/opioid/barbiturate anesthesia. Anesthesiology 1996; 84: 300

56. Leykin Y, Pellis T, Lucca M, et al: The effects of cisatracurium on morbidly obese women. Anesth Analg 2004; 99: 1090

57. Miller DR, Wherrett C, Hull K, et al: Cumulation characteristics of cisatracurium and rocuronium during continuous infusion. Can J Anaesth 2000; 47: 943

58. Lagneau F, D'Honneur G, Plaud B, et al: A comparison of two depths of prolonged neuromuscular blockade induced by cisatracurium in mechanically ventilated critically ill patients. Intensive Care Med. 2002; 28: 1735

59. Basta SJ, Savarese JJ, Ali HH, et al: Clinical pharmacology of doxacurium chloride. A new long-acting nondepolarizing muscle relaxant. Anesthesiology 1988; 69: 478

60. Belmont MR, Lien CA, Tjan J, et al: Clinical pharmacology of GW280430A in humans. Anesthesiology 2004; 100: 768

61. Savarese JJ, Ali HH, Basta SJ, et al: The clinical neuromuscular pharmacology of mivacurium chloride (BW B1090U). A short-acting nondepolarizing ester neuromuscular blocking drug. Anesthesiology 1988; 68: 723

62. Maddineni VR, Mirakhur RK, McCoy EP, et al: Neuromuscular effects and intubating conditions following mivacurium: a comparison with suxamethonium. Anaesthesia 1993; 48: 940

63. Brandom BW, Meretoja OA, Simhi E, et al: Age related variability in the effects of mivacurium in paediatric surgical patients. Can J Anaesth 1998; 45: 410

64. Martyn JA, Goudsouzian NG, Chang Y, et al: Neuromuscular effects of mivacurium in 2- to 12-yr-old children with burn injury. Anesthesiology 2000; 92: 31

65. Kao YJ, Le ND: The reversal of profound mivacurium-induced neuromuscular blockade. Can J Anaesth 1996; 43: 1128

66. Murphy GS, Szokol JW, Marymont JH, et al: Recovery of neuromuscular function after cardiac surgery: pancuronium versus rocuronium. Anesth Analg 2003; 96: 1301

67. Murphy GS, Szokol JW, Franklin M, et al: Postanesthesia care unit recovery times and neuromuscular blocking drugs: a prospective study of orthopedic surgical patients randomized to receive pancuronium or rocuronium. Anesth Analg 2004; 98: 193

68. Baurain MJ, Hoton F, d'Hollander AA, et al: Is recovery of neuromuscular transmission complete after the use of neostigmine to antagonize block produced by rocuronium, vecuronium, atracurium and pancuronium? Br J Anaesth 1996; 77: 496

69. Sparr HJ, Mellinghoff H, Blobner M, et al: Comparison of intubating conditions after rapacuronium (Org 9487) and succinylcholine following rapid sequence induction in adult patients. Br J Anaesth 1999; 82: 537

70. Jooste E, Klafter F, Hirshman CA, et al: A mechanism for rapacuronium-induced bronchospasm: M2 muscarinic receptor antagonism. Anesthesiology 2003; 98: 906

71. Proost JH, Eriksson LI, Mirakhur RK, et al: Urinary, biliary and faecal excretion of rocuronium in humans. Br J Anaesth 2000; 85: 717

72. Andrews JI, Kumar N, van den Brom RH, et al: A large simple randomized trial of rocuronium versus succinylcholine in rapid-sequence induction of anaesthesia along with propofol. Acta Anaesthesiol Scand 1999; 43: 4

73. Wright PM, Caldwell JE, Miller RD: Onset and duration of rocuronium and succinylcholine at the adductor pollicis and laryngeal adductor muscles in anesthetized humans. Anesthesiology 1994; 81: 1110

74. Plaud B, Proost JH, Wierda JM, et al: Pharmacokinetics and pharmacodynamics of rocuronium at the vocal cords and the adductor pollicis in humans. Clin Pharmacol Ther 1995; 58: 185

75. Dhonneur G, Kirov K, Slavov V, et al: Effects of an intubating dose of succinylcholine and rocuronium on the larynx and diaphragm: an electromyographic study in humans. Anesthesiology 1999; 90: 951

76. Levy JH, Davis GK, Duggan J, et al: Determination of the hemodynamics and histamine release of rocuronium (Org 9426) when administered in increased doses under N2O/O2-sufentanil anesthesia. Anesth Analg 1994; 78: 318

77. Rose M, Fisher M: Rocuronium: high risk for anaphylaxis? Br J Anaesth 2001; 86: 678

78. Dhonneur G, Combes X, Chassard D, et al: Skin sensitivity to rocuronium and vecuronium: a randomized controlled prick-testing study in healthy volunteers. Anesth Analg 2004; 98: 986

79. Laake JH, Rottingen JA: Rocuronium and anaphylaxis—a statistical challenge. Acta Anaesthesiol Scand 2001; 45: 1196

80. Florvaag E, Johansson SG, Oman H, et al: Prevalence of IgE antibodies to morphine. Relation to the high and low incidences of NMBA anaphylaxis in Norway and Sweden, respectively. Acta Anaesthesiol Scand 2005; 49: 437

81. Bhananker SM, O'Donnell JT, Salemi JR, et al: The risk of anaphylactic reactions to rocuronium in the United States is comparable to that of vecuronium: an analysis of food and drug administration reporting of adverse events. Anesth Analg 2005; 101: 819

82. Xue FS, Tong SY, Liao X, et al: Dose-response and time course of effect of rocuronium in male and female anesthetized patients. Anesth Analg 1997; 85: 667

83. Collins LM, Bevan JC, Bevan DR, et al: The prolonged duration of rocuronium in Chinese patients. Anesth Analg 2000; 91: 1526

84. Dahaba AA, Perelman SI, Moskowitz DM, et al: Geographic regional differences in rocuronium bromide dose-response relation and time course of action: an overlooked factor in determining recommended dosage. Anesthesiology 2006; 104: 950

85. Woolf RL, Crawford MW, Choo SM: Dose-response of rocuronium bromide in children anesthetized with propofol: a comparison with succinylcholine. Anesthesiology 1997; 87: 1368

86. Rapp HJ, Altenmueller CA, Waschke C: Neuromuscular recovery following rocuronium bromide single dose in infants. Paediatr Anaesth 2004; 14: 329

87. Bevan DR, Fiset P, Balendran P, et al: Pharmacodynamic behaviour of rocuronium in the elderly. Can J Anaesth 1993; 40: 127

88. Szenohradszky J, Fisher DM, Segredo V, et al: Pharmacokinetics of rocuronium bromide (ORG 9426) in patients with normal renal function or patients undergoing cadaver renal transplantation. Anesthesiology 1992; 77: 899

89. Khalil M, D'Honneur G, Duvaldestin P, et al: Pharmacokinetics and pharmacodynamics of rocuronium in patients with cirrhosis. Anesthesiology 1994; 80: 1241

90. Fawcett WJ, Dash A, Francis GA, et al: Recovery from neuromuscular blockade: residual curarisation following atracurium or vecuronium by bolus dosing or infusions. Acta Anaesthesiol Scand 1995; 39: 288

91. Motamed C, Donati F: Sevoflurane and isoflurane, but not propofol, decrease mivacurium requirements over time. Can J Anaesth 2002; 49: 907

92. Hemmerling TM, Schuettler J, Schwilden H: Desflurane reduces the effective therapeutic infusion rate (ETI) of cisatracurium more than isoflurane, sevoflurane, or propofol. Can J Anaesth 2001; 48: 532

93. Kopman AF, Chin WA, Moe J, et al: The effect of nitrous oxide on the dose-response relationship of rocuronium. Anesth Analg 2005; 100: 1343

94. Paul M, Fokt RM, Kindler CH, et al: Characterization of the interactions between volatile anesthetics and neuromuscular blockers at the muscle nicotinic acetylcholine receptor. Anesth Analg 2002; 95: 362

95. Suzuki T, Mizutani H, Ishikawa K, et al: Epidurally administered mepivacaine delays recovery of train-of-four ratio from vecuronium-induced neuromuscular block. Br J Anaesth 2007; 99: 721

96. Ferres CJ, Mirakhur RK, Pandit SK, et al: Dose-response studies with pancuronium, vecuronium and their combination. Br J Clin Pharmacol 1984; 18: 947

97. Kim KS, Chun YS, Chon SU, et al: Neuromuscular interaction between cisatracurium and mivacurium, atracurium, vecuronium or rocuronium administered in combination. Anaesthesia 1998; 53: 872

98. Paul M, Kindler CH, Fokt RM, et al: Isobolographic analysis of non-depolarising muscle relaxant interactions at their receptor site. Eur J Pharmacol 2002; 438: 35

99. Kay B, Chestnut RJ, Sum Ping JS, et al: Economy in the use of muscle relaxants. Vecuronium after pancuronium. Anaesthesia 1987; 42: 277

100. Sokoll MD, Gergis SD: Antibiotics and neuromuscular function. Anesthesiology 1981; 55: 148

101. Dupuis JY, Martin R, Tetrault JP: Atracurium and vecuronium interaction with gentamicin and tobramycin. Can J Anaesth. 1989; 36: 407

102. Spacek A, Nickl S, Neiger FX, et al: Augmentation of the rocuronium-induced neuromuscular block by the acutely administered phenytoin. Anesthesiology 1999; 90: 1551

103. Alloul K, Whalley DG, Shutway F, et al: Pharmacokinetic origin of carbamazepine-induced resistance to vecuronium neuromuscular blockade in anesthetized patients. Anesthesiology 1996; 84: 330

104. Loan PB, Connolly FM, Mirakhur RK, et al: Neuromuscular effects of rocuronium in patients receiving beta-adrenoreceptor blocking, calcium entry blocking and anticonvulsant drugs. Br J Anaesth 1997; 78: 90

105. Richard A, Girard F, Girard DC, et al: Cisatracurium-induced neuromuscular blockade is affected by chronic phenytoin or carbamazepine treatment in neurosurgical patients. Anesth Analg 2005; 100: 538

106. Szmuk P, Ezri T, Chelly JE, et al: The onset time of rocuronium is slowed by esmolol and accelerated by ephedrine. Anesth Analg 2000; 90: 1217

107. Gopalakrishna MD, Krishna HM, Shenoy UK: The effect of ephedrine on intubating conditions and haemodynamics during rapid tracheal intubation using propofol and rocuronium. Br J Anaesth 2007; 99: 191

108. Gupta K, Vohra V, Sood J: The role of magnesium as an adjuvant during general anaesthesia. Anaesthesia 2006; 61: 1058

109. Stacey MR, Barclay K, Asai T, et al: Effects of magnesium sulphate on suxamethonium-induced complications during rapid-sequence induction of anaesthesia. Anaesthesia 1995; 50: 933

110. Arroliga A, Frutos-Vivar F, Hall J, et al: Use of sedatives and neuromuscular blockers in a cohort of patients receiving mechanical ventilation. Chest 2005; 128: 496

111. Fletcher SN, Kennedy DD, Ghosh IR, et al: Persistent neuromuscular and neurophysiologic abnormalities in long-term survivors of prolonged critical illness. Crit Care Med 2003; 31: 1012

112. Sparr HJ, Wierda JM, Proost JH, et al: Pharmacodynamics and pharmacokinetics of rocuronium in intensive care patients. Br J Anaesth 1997; 78: 267

113. Hirsch NP: Neuromuscular junction in health and disease. Br J Anaesth 2007; 99: 132

114. Itoh H, Shibata K, Yoshida M, et al: Neuromuscular monitoring at the orbicularis oculi may overestimate the blockade in myasthenic patients. Anesthesiology 2000; 93: 1194

115. Capron F, Fortier LP, Racine S, et al: Tactile fade detection with hand or wrist stimulation using train-of-four, double-burst stimulation, 50-hertz tetanus, 100-hertz tetanus, and acceleromyography. Anesth Analg 2006; 102: 1578

116. Kopman AF, Klewicka MM, Neuman GG: The relationship between acceleromyographic train-of-four fade and single twitch depression. Anesthesiology 2002; 96: 583

117. O'Hara DA, Fragen RJ, Shanks CA: Comparison of visual and measured train-of-four recovery after vecuronium-induced neuromuscular blockade using two anaesthetic techniques. Br J Anaesth 1986; 58: 1300

118. Viby-Mogensen J, Howardy-Hansen P, Chraemmer-Jorgensen B, et al: Posttetanic count (PTC): a new method of evaluating an intense nondepolarizing neuromuscular blockade. Anesthesiology 1981; 55: 458

119. Kopman AF: The relationship of evoked electromyographic and mechanical responses following atracurium in humans. Anesthesiology 1985; 63: 208

120. Debaene B, Plaud B, Dilly MP, et al: Residual paralysis in the PACU after a single intubating dose of nondepolarizing muscle relaxant with an intermediate duration of action. Anesthesiology 2003; 98: 1042

121. Gatke MR, Viby-Mogensen J, Rosenstock C, et al: Postoperative muscle paralysis after rocuronium: less residual block when acceleromyography is used. Acta Anaesthesiol Scand 2002; 46: 207

122. Dahaba AA, von Klobucar F, Rehak PH, et al: The neuromuscular transmission module versus the relaxometer mechanomyograph for neuromuscular block monitoring. Anesth Analg 2002; 94: 591

123. Hemmerling TM, Le N: Brief review: Neuromuscular monitoring: an update for the clinician. Can J Anaesth. 2007; 54: 58

124. Donati F, Meistelman C, Plaud B: Vecuronium neuromuscular blockade at the diaphragm, the orbicularis oculi, and adductor pollicis muscles. Anesthesiology 1990; 73: 870

125. Donati F, Meistelman C, Plaud B: Vecuronium neuromuscular blockade at the adductor muscles of the larynx and adductor pollicis. Anesthesiology 1991; 74: 833

126. Kirov K, Motamed C, Dhonneur G: Differential sensitivity of abdominal muscles and the diaphragm to mivacurium: an electromyographic study. Anesthesiology 2001; 95: 1323

127. D'Honneur G, Guignard B, Slavov V, et al: Comparison of the neuromuscular blocking effect of atracurium and vecuronium on the adductor pollicis and the geniohyoid muscle in humans. Anesthesiology 1995; 82: 649

128. Nepveu ME, Donati F, Fortier LP: Train-of-four stimulation for adductor pollicis neuromuscular monitoring can be applied at the wrist or over the hand. Anesth Analg 2005; 100: 149

129. Plaud B, Debaene B, Donati F: The corrugator supercilii, not the orbicularis oculi, reflects rocuronium neuromuscular blockade at the laryngeal adductor muscles. Anesthesiology 2001; 95: 96

130. Kirkegaard H, Heier T, Caldwell JE: Efficacy of tactile-guided reversal from cisatracurium-induced neuromuscular blockade. Anesthesiology 2002; 96: 45

131. Kopman AF, Yee PS, Neuman GG: Relationship of the train-of-four fade ratio to clinical signs and symptoms of residual paralysis in awake volunteers. Anesthesiology 1997; 86: 765

132. Eriksson LI, Sundman E, Olsson R, et al: Functional assessment of the pharynx at rest and during swallowing in partially paralyzed humans: simultaneous videomanometry and mechanomyography of awake human volunteers. Anesthesiology 1997; 87: 1035

133. Pavlin EG, Holle RH, Schoene RB: Recovery of airway protection compared with ventilation in humans after paralysis with curare. Anesthesiology 1989; 70: 381

134. Nishino T, Yokokawa N, Hiraga K, et al: Breathing pattern of anesthetized humans during pancuronium-induced partial paralysis. J Appl.Physiol 1988; 64: 78

135. Eriksson LI, Lennmarken C, Wyon N, et al: Attenuated ventilatory response to hypoxaemia at vecuronium-induced partial neuromuscular block. Acta Anaesthesiol Scand 1992; 36: 710

136. Kopman AF, Zank LM, Ng J, et al: Antagonism of cisatracurium and rocuronium block at a tactile train-of-four count of 2: should quantitative assessment of neuromuscular function be mandatory? Anesth Analg 2004; 98: 102

137. Heier T, Caldwell JE: Impact of hypothermia on the response to neuromuscular blocking drugs. Anesthesiology 2006; 104: 1070

138. Viby-Mogensen J, Jorgensen BC, Ording H: Residual curarization in the recovery room. Anesthesiology 1979; 50: 539

139. Bevan DR, Donati F, Kopman AF: Reversal of neuromuscular blockade. Anesthesiology 1992; 77: 785

140. Berg H, Roed J, Viby-Mogensen J, et al: Residual neuromuscular block is a risk factor for postoperative pulmonary complications. A prospective, randomised, and blinded study of postoperative pulmonary complications after atracurium, vecuronium and pancuronium. Acta Anaesthesiol Scand 1997; 41: 1095

141. Baillard C, Clec'h C, Catineau J, et al: Postoperative residual neuromuscular block: a survey of management. Br J Anaesth 2005; 95: 622

142. Fiekers JF: Concentration-dependent effects of neostigmine on the endplate acetylcholine receptor channel complex. J Neurosci 1985; 5: 502

143. Bartkowski RR: Incomplete reversal of pancuronium neuromuscular blockade by neostigmine, pyridostigmine, and edrophonium. Anesth Analg 1987; 66: 594

144. McCourt KC, Mirakhur RK, Kerr CM: Dosage of neostigmine for reversal of rocuronium block from two levels of spontaneous recovery. Anaesthesia 1999; 54: 651

145. Eikermann M, Fassbender P, Malhotra A, et al: Unwarranted administration of acetylcholinesterase inhibitors can impair genioglossus and diaphragm muscle function. Anesthesiology 2007; 107: 621

146. Cronnelly R, Morris RB, Miller RD: Edrophonium: duration of action and atropine requirement in humans during halothane anesthesia. Anesthesiology 1982; 57: 261

147. Donati F, Smith CE, Bevan DR: Dose-response relationships for edrophonium and neostigmine as antagonists of moderate and profound atracurium blockade. Anesth Analg 1989; 68: 13

148. Bevan JC, Collins L, Fowler C, et al: Early and late reversal of rocuronium and vecuronium with neostigmine in adults and children. Anesth Analg 1999; 89: 333

149. Tramer MR, Fuchs-Buder T: Omitting antagonism of neuromuscular block: effect on postoperative nausea and vomiting and risk of residual paralysis. A systematic review. Br J Anaesth 1999; 82: 379

150. Cheng CR, Sessler DI, Apfel CC: Does neostigmine administration produce a clinically important increase in postoperative nausea and vomiting? Anesth Analg 2005; 101: 1349

151. Arbous MS, Meursing AE, van Kleef JW, et al: Impact of anesthesia management characteristics on severe morbidity and mortality. Anesthesiology 2005; 102: 257

152. Naguib M: Sugammadex: another milestone in clinical neuromuscular pharmacology. Anesth Analg 2007; 104: 575

153. Gijsenbergh F, Ramael S, Houwing N, et al: First human exposure of Org 25969, a novel agent to reverse the action of rocuronium bromide. Anesthesiology 2005; 103: 695

154. Suy K, Morias K, Cammu G, et al: Effective reversal of moderate rocuronium- or vecuronium-induced neuromuscular block with sugammadex, a selective relaxant binding agent. Anesthesiology 2007; 106: 283

155. Eleveld DJ, Kuizenga K, Proost JH, et al: A temporary decrease in twitch response during reversal of rocuronium-induced muscle relaxation with a small dose of sugammadex. Anesth Analg 2007; 104: 582

156. Groudine SB, Soto R, Lien C, et al: A randomized, dose-finding, phase II study of the selective relaxant binding drug, Sugammadex, capable of safely reversing profound rocuronium-induced neuromuscular block. Anesth Analg 2007; 104: 555

157. de Boer HD, Driessen JJ, Marcus MA, et al: Reversal of rocuronium-induced (1.2 mg/kg) profound neuromuscular block by sugammadex: a multicenter, dose-finding and safety study. Anesthesiology 2007; 107: 239

158. Sparr HJ, Vermeyen KM, Beaufort AM, et al: Early reversal of profound rocuronium-induced neuromuscular blockade by sugammadex in a randomized multicenter study: efficacy, safety, and pharmacokinetics. Anesthesiology 2007; 106: 935

159. Durmus M, Ender G, Kadir BA, et al: Remifentanil with thiopental for tracheal intubation without muscle relaxants. Anesth Analg 2003; 96: 1336

160. Klemola UM, Mennander S, Saarnivaara L: Tracheal intubation without the use of muscle relaxants: remifentanil or alfentanil in combination with propofol. Acta Anaesthesiol Scand 2000; 44: 465

161. Eriksson LI, Lennmarken C, Wyon N, et al: Attenuated ventilatory response to hypoxaemia at vecuronium-induced partial neuromuscular block. Acta Anaesthesiol Scand 1992; 36: 710

162. Ferguson A, Egerszegi P, Bevan DR: Neostigmine, pyridostigmine, and edrophonium as antagonists of pancuronium. Anesthesiology 1980; 53: 390

163. Bevan DR, Smith CE, Donati F: Postoperative neuromuscular blockade: a comparison between atracurium, vecuronium, and pancuronium. Anesthesiology 1988; 69: 272

164. Bissinger U, Schimek F, Lenz G: Postoperative residual paralysis and respiratory status: a comparative study of pancuronium and vecuronium. Physiol Res. 2000; 49: 455

CHAPTER 21 ■ LOCAL ANESTHETICS

SPENCER S. LIU AND YI LIN

KEY POINTS

1. Local anesthetics provide anesthesia and analgesia by blocking the transmission of pain sensation along nerve fibers

2. The key target of local anesthetics is the voltage-gated sodium channel. The binding is intracellular and is mediated by hydrophobic interactions.

3. The degree of nerve blockade depends on both drug concentration and volume.

4. Most clinically relevant agents contain a lipid-soluble benzene ring connected to an amide group and are categorized as either aminoesters or aminoamides, based on their chemical linkage.

5. Potency is related to hydrophobicity and physiochemical properties of the agent. In general, more potent agents are more lipid soluble.

6. Efficacy for clinical use of local anesthetics may be increased by addition of epinephrine, opioids, and α_2-adrenergic agonists. The value of alkalinization of local anesthetics appears to be debatable as a clinically useful tool to improve anesthesia.

7. Systemic toxicity from the clinical use of local anesthetics is an uncommon occurrence. Patients with cardiovascular collapse from bupivacaine, ropivacaine, and levobupivacaine may be especially difficult to resuscitate; however intravenous lipid infusion is a promising new therapy.

---

1. Local anesthetics block the conduction of impulses in electrically excitable tissues. One of the important uses is to provide anesthesia and analgesia by blocking the transmission of pain sensation along nerve fibers. The molecular target of these agents is specific and the interaction has been extensively studied. Existing clinical applications are numerous and continue to expand. A comprehensive understanding of the mechanisms and the physiochemical properties of these agents would enable optimization of the therapeutic potential and avoid complications associated with inadvertent systemic toxicity.

MECHANISMS OF ACTION OF LOCAL ANESTHETICS

Anatomy of Nerves

Local anesthetics are used to block nerves in the peripheral nervous system (PNS) and central nervous system (CNS). In the peripheral nervous system, nerves contain both afferent and efferent fibers, which are bundled into one or more fascicles and organized within three tissue layers.[1] Individual nerve fibers within each fascicle are surrounded by the endoneurium, a loose connective tissue containing glial cells, fibroblasts, and blood capillaries. A dense layer of collagenous connective tissue called the *perineurium* surrounds each fascicle. A final layer of dense connective tissue, the epineurium, encases groups of fascicles into a cylindrical sheath (Fig. 21-1). These layers of tissue offer protection to the surrounded nerve fibers and act as barriers to passive diffusion of local anesthetics.[2]

Nerves in both the central and peripheral nervous system are differentiated by the presence or the absence of myelin sheath. Myelinated nerve fibers are surrounded by Schwann cells in the PNS and by oligodendrocytes in the CNS. The cells form a concentrically wrapped lipid bilayer sheath around the axons that cover the length of the nerve.[3] The myelin sheath is interrupted at short, regular intervals by specialized regions called *nodes of Ranvier*, which contain densely clustered protein elements essential for transmission of neuronal signals[4] (Fig. 21-2). As electrical signals are renewed at each node, nerve impulses move in myelinated fibers by saltatory conduction. In contrast, there are no nodes of Ranvier in nonmyelinated nerve fibers. Although these nerve fibers are similarly encased in Schwann cells, the plasma membrane does not wrap around the axons concentrically. Several nerve fibers may be simultaneously embedded within a single Schwann cell[1] (Fig. 21-3).

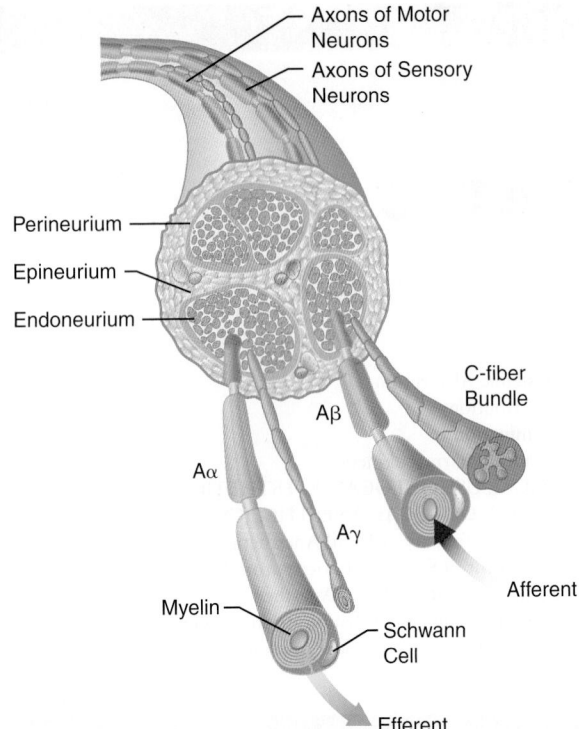

FIGURE 21-1. Schematic cross section of typical peripheral nerve. The epineurium, consisting of collagen fibers, is oriented along the long axis of the nerve. The perineurium is a discrete cell layer, whereas the endoneurium is a matrix of connective tissue. Both afferent and efferent axons are shown. Sympathetic axons (not shown) are also present in mixed peripheral nerves. (Adapted from Strichartz GR: Neural physiology and local anesthetic action, Neural Blockade in Clinical Anesthesia and Management of Pain. Edited by Cousins MJ, Bridenbaugh PO. Philadelphia, Lippincott–Raven, 1998, p 35, with permission.)

Nerve fibers are commonly classified according to their size, conduction velocity, and function (Table 21-1). In general, nerve fibers with cross-sectional diameter greater than 1 micron are myelinated. Both a larger nerve size and the presence of myelin sheath are associated with faster conduction velocity.[5] Nerve fibers with large diameters have better intrinsic electric conductance. Myelin improves the electrical insulation of nerve fibers and permits more rapid impulse transmission via saltatory con-

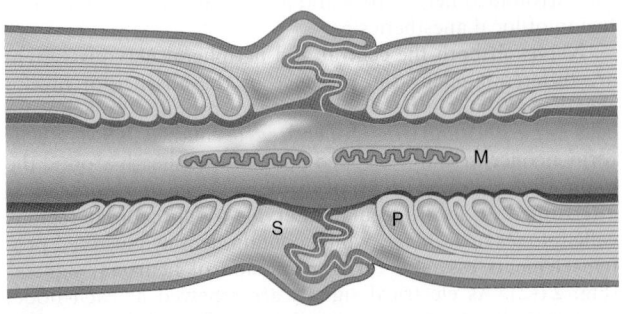

FIGURE 21-2. Diagram of node of Ranvier displaying mitochondria (M), tight junctions in paranodal area (P), and Schwann cell (S) surrounding node. (Adapted from Strichartz GR: Mechanisms of action of local anesthetic agents, Principles and Practice of Anesthesiology. Edited by Rogers MC, Tinker JH, Covino BG, et al. St. Louis, Mosby Year Book, 1993, p 1197, with permission.)

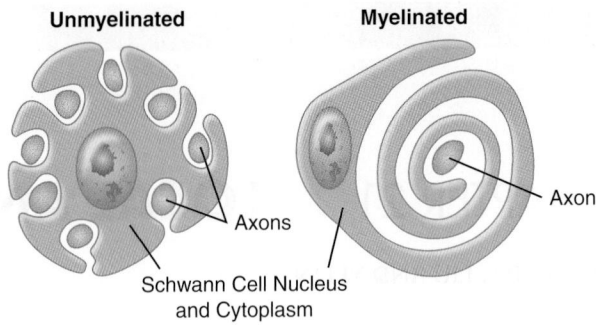

FIGURE 21-3. Schwann cells form myelin around one myelinated axon or encompass several unmyelinated axons. (Adapted from Carpenter RL, Mackey DC: Local anesthetics, Clinical Anesthesia 3e. Edited by Barash PG, Cullen BF, Stoelting RF. Philadelphia, Lippincott–Raven, 1996, p 413, with permission.)

duction. Large-diameter, myelinated fibers, many of which are classified as A fibers, are typically involved in motor and sensory functions in which speed of nerve transmission is critical. In contrast, the small-diameter, nonmyelinated C fibers have slower conduction velocity and relay sensory information such as pain, temperature, and autonomic functions.

Electrophysiology of Neural Conduction and Voltage-Gated Sodium Channels

Transmission of electrical impulses along the cell membrane forms the basis of signal transduction along nerve fibers. Energy necessary for the propagation and maintenance of the electric potential is maintained on the cell surface by ionic disequilibria across the semipermeable cell membrane.[6] The resting membrane potential, approximately −60 to −70 mV in neurons (the extracellular electric potential is by convention defined as zero, and the intracellular potential is thus negative to it), is derived predominantly from a difference in the intracellular and extracellular concentrations of potassium and sodium ions. Neurons at rest are more permeable to potassium ions than sodium ions because of potassium leak channels; therefore membrane potential is closer to the equilibrium potential of potassium (E_K − 80 mV) than that of sodium (E_{Na} + 60 mV). The ion gradient is continuously regenerated by protein pumps, cotransporters, and channels via adenosine triphosphate-dependent process.

Electrical impulses are conducted along nerve fibers as action potentials. They are brief, localized spikes of positive charge, or depolarizations, on the cell membrane caused by rapid influx of sodium ions down its electrochemical gradient.[7] An action potential is initiated by local membrane depolarization, such as at the cell body or nerve terminal by ligand-receptor complex. When a certain charge threshold is reached, an action potential is triggered and further depolarization occurs in an "all-or-none" fashion.[8] The spike in membrane potential peaks around +50 mV, at which point the influx of sodium is replaced with an efflux of potassium, causing a reversal of membrane potential, or repolarization. The passive diffusion of membrane depolarization triggers other action potentials in either adjacent cell membrane in *nonmyelinated* nerve fibers or adjacent nodes of Ranvier in *myelinated* nerve fibers, resulting in a wave of action potential being propagated along the nerve. A short refractory period that ensues after each action potential prevents the retrograde spread of action potential on previously activated membranes.[7]

The flow of ions responsible for action potentials is mediated by a variety of channels and pumps, the most important

TABLE 21-1

CLASSIFICATION OF NERVE FIBERS

■ CLASSIFICATION	■ DIAMETER (μ)	■ MYELIN	■ CONDUCTION (m/sec)	■ LOCATION	■ FUNCTION
A-alpha, A-beta	6–22	+	30–120	Afferents/efferents for muscles and joints	Motor and proprioception
A-gamma	3–6	+	15–35	Efferent to muscle spindle	Muscle tone
A-delta	1–4	+	5–25	Afferent sensory nerve	Pain Touch Temperature
B	<3	+	3–15	Preganglionic sympathetic	Autonomic function
C	0.3–1.3	−	0.7–1.3	Postganglionic sympathetic Afferent sensory nerve	Autonomic function Pain Temperature

of which are the voltage-gated sodium channels. They are essential for the influx of sodium ions during the rapid depolarization phase of action potential and belong to a family of channel proteins that also includes voltage-gated potassium and voltage-gated calcium channels. Each voltage-gated sodium channel is a complex made up of one principal alpha subunit and one or more auxiliary beta subunits.[9] The alpha subunit is a single-polypeptide transmembrane protein that contains most of the key components of the channel function. They include four homologous alpha-helical domains (D1 to D4) that form the channel pore and control ion selectivity, voltage-sensing regions that regulate gating function and inactivation, and phosphorylation sites for modulation by protein kinases. Beta subunits are short polypeptide proteins with a single transmembrane domain. They are linked to alpha subunits by either noncovalent or disulfide bonds; although they are dispensable for channel activity, evidence suggests that they perhaps play a role in modulation of channel expression, localization and function.

In the absence of a stimulus, voltage-gated sodium channels exist predominantly in the resting or closed state (Fig. 21-4). On membrane depolarization, positive charges on the membrane interact with charged amino acid residues in the voltage-sensing regions (S4).[10] This induces a conformational change in the channel, converting it to the open state. Sodium ions rush through the opened pore, which is lined with negatively charged residues. Ion selectivity is determined by these amino acid residues; changes in their composition can lead to increased permeability for other cations, such as potassium and calcium.[11] Within milliseconds after opening, channels undergo a transition to the inactivated state. Depending on the frequency and the voltage of the initial depolarizing stimulus, the channel may undergo either a fast or slow inactivation. Slow or fast inactivation refers to the duration in which the channel remains refractory to repeat depolarization before resetting to the closed state. Fast inactivation completes within a millisecond and is sensitive to the action of local anesthetics. It is mediated by a short mobile intracellular polypeptide loop connecting domains D3 and D4 that closes the channel from inside the cell via a hinge-lid mechanism.[12] A triad of highly hydrophobic amino acids (isoleucine, phenylalanine, and methionine, or IFM) appears to be an important structural determinant of fast activation; disrupting the loop or changing the hydrophobicity of the amino acids abrogates fast inactivation.[13,14] Slow activation, lasting seconds to minutes, is distinct from fast activation. It is resistant to the action of local anesthetics and its mechanism is less well understood. It often occurs after prolonged depolarization and is believed to be important in regulating membrane excitability.

Nine isoforms of voltage-gated sodium channels (Na_V 1.1 to Na_V 1.9) have been identified, each relates to a unique alpha subunit subtype (Table 21-2). Each isoform varies slightly in its channel kinetics, such as threshold of activation and mode of inactivation, and its sensitivity to blocking agents like tetrodotoxins and local anesthetics. Cell and tissue expression of individual isoforms may be quite specific; for instance, Na_V 1.2 is found almost exclusively in the CNS, whereas Na_V 1.6 is restricted to nodes of Ranvier in both CNS and PNS.[15] Likewise, several isoforms could be present on a single cell type; both Na_V 1.8 and Na_V 1.9 have been found in small to medium-sized neurons in dorsal root ganglions that are connected to A delta and C fibers. Whether individual isoforms each has a separate and defined role remains to be seen;

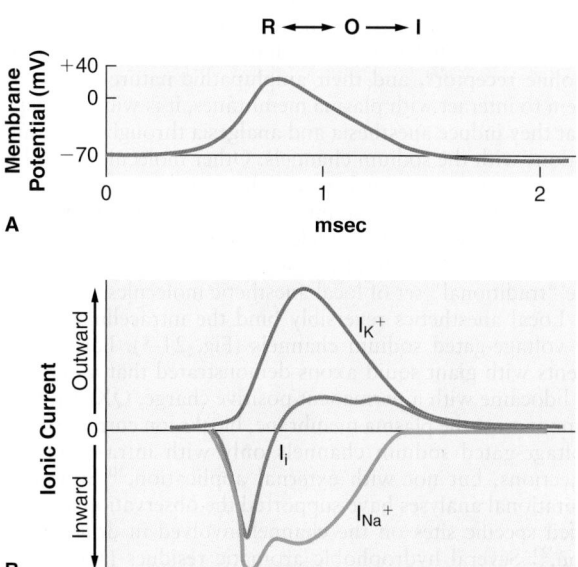

FIGURE 21-4.   Illustration of dominant form of sodium channel during generation of an action potential. R, resting form; O, open form; I, inactive form. **A.** The concurrent generation of an action potential as the membrane depolarizes from resting potential. **B.** The concurrent changes in ion flux, as inward sodium current (I_{NA+}) and outward potassium current (I_{K+}) together yield the net ionic current across the membrane (I_i). (Adapted from Strichartz GR: Neural physiology and local anesthetic action, Neural Blockade in Clinical Anesthesia and Management of Pain. Edited by Cousins MJ, Bridenbaugh PO. Philadelphia, Lippincott–Raven, 1998, p 35, with permission.)

TABLE 21-2

VOLTAGE-GATED SODIUM CHANNELS

■ NAME	■ TISSUE EXPRESSION	■ TETRODOTOXIN	■ ASSOCIATED CHANNELOPATHIES
Na$_V$ 1.1	CNS, heart	Sensitive	Inherited febrile epilepsy
Na$_V$ 1.2	CNS nonmyelinated axons	Sensitive	Inherited febrile epilepsy
Na$_V$ 1.3	Fetal DRG	Sensitive	None known
Na$_V$ 1.4	Skeletal muscle	Sensitive	Hyperkalemic periodic paralysis, paramyotonia congenita
Na$_V$ 1.5	Heart, embryonic neurons	Insensitive	Brugada syndrome, long QT syndrome
Na$_V$ 1.6	Nodes of Ranvier	Sensitive	None known
Na$_V$ 1.7	CNS, DRG, sympathetic neurons	Sensitive	Erythromelalgia, paroxysmal extreme pain disorder, congenital insensitivity to pain
Na$_V$ 1.8	Small DRG neurons	Insensitive	None known
Na$_V$ 1.9	Small DRG neurons	Insensitive	None known

Data adapted from Benarroch EE: Sodium channels and pain. Neurology 2007: 68: 233, and Koopmann TT, Bezzina CR, Wilde AA: Voltage-gated sodium channels: Action players with many faces. Ann Med 2006: 38: 472.

however, clues of their function may be inferred from studies of several inherited diseases that have been associated with sodium channelopathies. Hyperexcitability of Na$_V$ 1.7 has been implicated in several painful disease states, such as primary erythromelalgia and paroxysmal extreme pain disorder.[16,17] Conversely, null mutation of Na$_V$ 1.7 is linked to a rare genetic condition in which otherwise normal individuals have severely impaired perception to pain.[18,19]

Molecular Mechanisms of Local Anesthetics

Local anesthetics block the transmission of nerve impulses by targeting the function of voltage-gated sodium channels. Although several local anesthetics can bind to other receptors like voltage-gated potassium channels and nicotinic acetylcholine receptors, and their amphipathic nature may enable them to interact with plasma membranes, it is widely accepted that they induce anesthesia and analgesia through direct interactions with the sodium channels. Other molecules with local anesthetic properties such as tricyclic antidepressants and anticonvulsants may likewise interact with voltage-gated sodium channels; however, it is unclear if they act through similar mechanisms. Therefore, the following discussion is limited to the "traditional" set of local anesthetic molecules.

2 Local anesthetics reversibly bind the intracellular portion of voltage-gated sodium channels (Fig. 21-5). Early experiments with giant squid axons demonstrated that a derivative of lidocaine with a permanent positive charge, QX314, which cannot cross the plasma membrane, blocks ion current through voltage-gated sodium channels only with intra-axoplasmic injections, but not with external application.[20] Subsequent mutational analyses have supported the observation and identified specific sites on the channel involved in drug recognition.[21] Several hydrophobic aromatic residues (a phenylalanine at position 1764 and a tyrosine at position 1771 in Na$_V$ 1.2) located within an alpha helix (S6) of domains 1, 3, and 4 are essential for drug binding (Fig. 21-6). They line an inner cavity within the intracellular portion of the channel pore and span a region about 11 Å apart, roughly the size of a local anesthetic molecule. Changes in either residue severely reduce the binding affinity. Another hydrophobic amino acid (an isoleucine at position 1760), located near the outer pore opening, has similarly been found to influence the dissociation of local anesthetics from the channel by antagonizing the release of drugs through the channel pore.

Application of local anesthetics typically produces a concentration-dependent decrease in the peak sodium current.[22,23] Known as "tonic blockade," it reflects the reduction of the number of sodium channels for a given drug concentration present in the open state at equilibrium. In contrast, repetitive stimulation of the sodium channels often leads to a shift in the steady-state equilibrium, resulting in a greater number of channels being blocked at the same drug concentration. Termed *use-dependent blockade*, the exact mechanism is incompletely understood and has been the subject of many competing hypotheses. One popular theory, the *modulated-receptor*

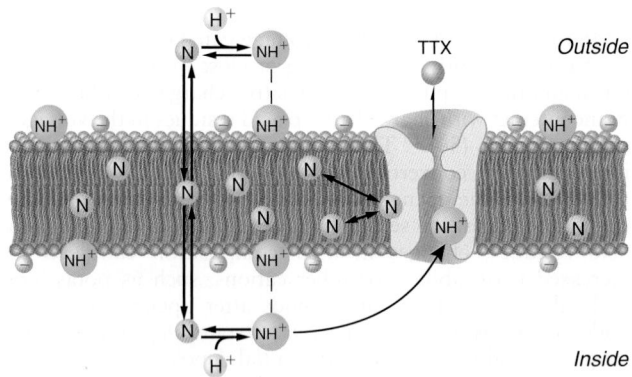

FIGURE 21-5. Diagram of bilayer lipid membrane of conductive tissue with sodium channel spanning the membrane. Tertiary amine local anesthetics exist as neutral base (N) and protonated, charged form (NH+) in equilibrium. The neutral base (N) is more lipid soluble, preferentially partitions into the lipophilic membrane interior, and easily passes through the membrane. The charged form (NH+) is more water soluble and binds to the sodium channel at the negatively charged membrane surface. Both forms can affect function of the sodium channel. The N form can cause membrane expansion and closure of the sodium channel. The NH+ form will directly inhibit the sodium channel by binding with a local anesthetic receptor. The natural "local anesthetic" tetrodotoxin (TTX) binds at the external surface of the sodium channel and has no interaction with clinically used local anesthetics. (Adapted from Strichartz GR: Neural physiology and local anesthetic action, Neural Blockade in Clinical Anesthesia and Management of Pain. Edited by Cousins MJ, Bridenbaugh PO. Philadelphia, Lippincott–Raven, 1998, p 35, with permission.)

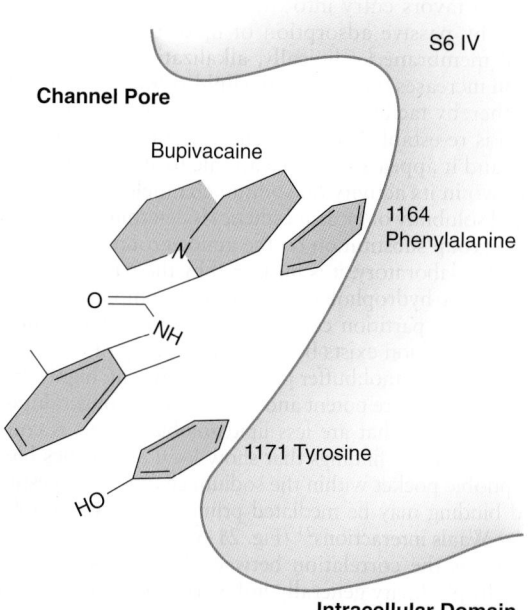

FIGURE 21-6. Diagram of local anesthetic binding site, depicting a hydrophobic pocket within the channel pore. (Adapted from Ragsdale DS, McPhee JC, Scheuer T, et al: Molecular determinants of state-dependent block of Na+ channels by local anesthetics. Science 1994; 265: 1724, with permission.)

theory, proposes that local anesthetics bind to the open or the inactivated channels more avidly than the resting channels, suggesting that drug affinity is a function of a channel's conformational state. An alternate theory, the *guarded-receptor theory*, assumes that the intrinsic binding affinity remains essentially constant regardless of a channel's conformation; rather, the apparent affinity is associated with increased access to the recognition site resulting from channel gating. Experimental evidence so far has been inconclusive.

Mechanism of Nerve Blockade

Local anesthetics block peripheral nerves by disrupting the transmission of action potentials along nerve fibers. To get to its site of action, principally the voltage-gated sodium channels, local anesthetics have to reach the targeted nerve membrane. This entails the diffusion of drugs through tissues and the generation of a concentration gradient. Even with close proximity of deposition, only about 1 to 2% of the injected local anesthetics ultimately penetrate into the nerve.[24] As discussed earlier, the perineural sheath encasing nerve fibers appears to be an important determinant; nerves that have been desheathed in vitro require about a hundred-fold lower local anesthetic concentration (in the 0.7- to 0.9-mM range for lidocaine) than nerves in vivo (the typical 2% lidocaine used clinically is equivalent to 75 mM concentration). Although it may vary with anatomic location and nerve physiology, functional block typically occurs within 5 minutes of injection in rat sciatic nerves, and this time course corresponds to the peak in the intraneural drug absorption.

The degree of nerve blockade depends on the local anesthetic concentration and volume. For a given drug, a minimal concentration is necessary to effect complete nerve blockade. It reflects the potency of the local anesthetics and the intrinsic conduction properties of nerve fibers, which in turn likely depend on the drug's binding affinity to the ion channels and the degree of drug saturation necessary to halt the transmission of action potentials. Accordingly, individual types of nerve fibers differ in their minimal blocking concentration, such that some A fibers are blocked by lower drug concentrations than C fibers.[25] Likewise, the pattern of stimulation (tonic vs. use-dependent blockade) influences the degree of conduction failure; repetitive stimulations, which can lead to a shift in steady-state equilibrium of blocked sodium channels, are associated with higher conduction failure than tonic stimulation at a given drug concentration.[26]

Of equal importance as drug concentration is the local anesthetics volume. A sufficient volume is needed to suppress the regeneration of nerve impulse over a critical length of nerve fiber. According to the model of decremental conduction (Fig. 21-7), as membrane depolarization from an action potential passively decays with distance along nerve fibers, the presence of local anesthetics decreases the ability of adjacent membrane or successive nodes of Ranvier to regenerate the impulse.[27] Transmission stops once the membrane depolarization falls below the threshold for action potential activation. Too short an exposure length allows impulses to "skip" over membranes or nodes that are blocked by even the highest drug concentration, whereas exposure of a long nerve segment to a relatively low drug concentration can still result in gradual extinction of impulses by decremental decay.

Not all sensory and motor modalities are blocked by local anesthetics equally. It has been long observed that application of local anesthetics produced an ordered progression of sensory and motor deficits, starting commonly with the disappearance of temperature sensation, followed by proprioception, motor function, sharp pain, and then light touch. Termed *differential blockade*, historically this had been thought to be related simply to the diameter of the nerve fibers, with the smaller fibers inherently more susceptible to drug blockade than larger fibers.[28] However, while the "size principle" of differential blockade is consistent with many experimental findings, it does not appear to be universally true. Larger, myelinated A delta fibers (believed to mediate sharp pain) have been found to be blocked preferentially over small, nonmyelinated

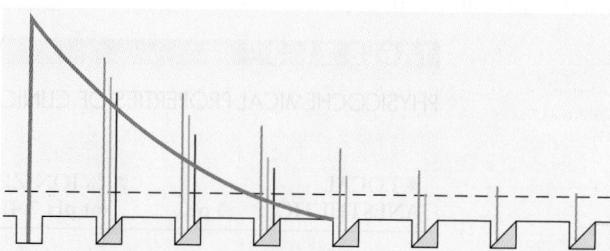

FIGURE 21-7. Diagram illustrating the principle of decremental conduction block by local anesthetic at a myelinated axon. The first node of Ranvier at left contains no local anesthetic and gives rise to a normal action potential (*solid curve*). If the nodes succeeding the first are occupied by a concentration of local anesthetic high enough to block 74 to 84% of the sodium conductance, then the action potential amplitudes decrease at successive nodes (amplitudes are indicated by interrupted bars representing three increasing concentration of local anesthetic). Eventually, the impulse decays to below-threshold amplitude if the series of local anesthetic containing nodes is long enough. Propagation of the impulse is then blocked by decremental conduction, even though none of the nodes are completely blocked. Concentrations of local anesthetic that block more than 84% of the sodium conductance at three successive nodes prevent any impulse propagation at all. (Adapted from Fink BR: Mechanisms of differential axial blockade in epidural and spinal anesthesia. Anesthesiology 1989; 70: 851, with permission.)

C fibers (dull pain). Furthermore, within the C fibers are fast and slow components of impulse transmission, each with distinct susceptibility to drug blockade.[29] These observations argue against a purely pharmacokinetic mechanism as the sole basis for explaining differential blockade. Instead, it may also likely depend on the intrinsic excitatory properties of the nerve fibers, namely, the patterned expression of voltage-gated sodium channels. Indeed, two channel isoforms, $Na_V 1.7$ and $Na_V 1.8$, both present on dorsal root ganglions, have been shown to possess different sensitivities to lidocaine blockade.[30] It remains to be seen how differential blockade of certain channels might translate into selective inhibition of pain and other sensory modalities.

PHARMACOLOGY AND PHARMACODYNAMICS

Chemical Properties and Relationship to Activity and Potency

Most clinically relevant local anesthetics are made up of a lipid-soluble, aromatic benzene ring connected to an amide group via either an amide or ester moiety. The type of linkage divides them broadly into two categories, the *aminoesters* and the *aminoamides*. Aside from a difference in their metabolic pathways (aminoesters are hydrolyzed by plasma cholinesterases and aminoamides are degraded by hepatic carboxylesterase) and the incidence of allergic reactions attributed, their membership in either category offers little in distinction of their biophysical properties. Rather, the distinguishing physiochemical characteristics are associated with the alkalinity of the amide group, the lipophilicity conferred by the alkyl substitution on the amide group and the benzene ring, and the stereochemistry of related isomers.

The tertiary amide found in local anesthetics is capable of accepting a proton, albeit with low affinity; thus, these compounds are classified as weak bases. At physiological pH, local anesthetics in solution are in equilibrium between the protonated, cationic form and the lipid-soluble, neutral forms. The ratio of the two forms depends on the pK_a or the dissociation constant, of the local anesthetics and the surrounding pH

(Table 21-3). A ratio with high concentration of the lipid-soluble form favors entry into the cell as the main pathway for entry is by passive adsorption of lipid-soluble form through the cell membrane.[2] Clinically, alkalization of the anesthetic solution increases the ratio of the lipid-soluble form to cationic form, thereby facilitating cell entry. Once inside the cell, equilibrium is re-established between the cationic and the neutral forms, and it appears that the cationic form is the more potent of the two in its activity on sodium channels.[31]

Lipid solubility of local anesthetics is determined by the degree of alkyl group substitution on the amide group and the benzene ring. In the laboratory, it is measured by the partition coefficient in octanol, a hydrophobic solvent, and compounds with high octanol:buffer partition coefficients are more lipid soluble.[32] A positive correlation exists between the potency of the local anesthetics and its octanol:buffer partition coefficient; highly lipid-soluble agents are more potent and tend to have a longer duration of action than ones that are less lipid soluble.[33] This is consistent with experimental findings that show local anesthetics bind to a hydrophobic pocket within the sodium channels, suggesting that ligand binding may be mediated primarily by hydrophobic and van der Waals interactions[21] (Fig. 21-6).

Whereas the correlation between local anesthetic potency and hydrophobicity generally holds true in vitro, it may not be as exact in vivo. As opposed to setups with isolated nerves, other factors may influence the potency of local anesthetics on nerves in situ.[34] For example, highly lipid-soluble agents may be sequestered into surrounding adipose cells. Vasodilatory properties of local anesthetics may likewise alter drug redistribution into the neighboring tissues.[35,36] Relative potency of local anesthetics has been determined for different clinical applications and these values are listed in Table 21-4.

Finally, anesthetic activity and potency are affected by the stereochemistry of local anesthetics. Many older drugs exist as racemic mixtures; that is, enantiomeric stereoisomers differing in the arrangement at the asymmetric or chiral carbon atom are in equal proportion. Newer agents, namely ropivacaine and levobupivacaine, are available as purely single enantiomers. They were initially developed as less cardiotoxic alternatives to bupivacaine. While the desired improvement in the safety index has been generally supported by clinical studies, it appears that overall, this is at the expense of a slight decrease in potency and shorter duration of action compared with the racemic

TABLE 21-3

PHYSICOCHEMICAL PROPERTIES OF CLINICALLY USED LOCAL ANESTHETICS

■ LOCAL ANESTHETIC	■ pK_a	■ % IONIZED (at pH 7.4)	■ PARTITION COEFFICIENT (LIPID SOLUBILITY)	■ % PROTEIN BINDING
■ AMIDES				
Bupivacaine[a]	8.1	83	3,420	95
Etidocaine	7.7	66	7,317	94
Lidocaine	7.9	76	366	64
Mepivacaine	7.6	61	130	77
Prilocaine	7.9	76	129	55
Ropivacaine	8.1	83	775	94
■ ESTERS				
Chloroprocaine	8.7	95	810	N/A
Procaine	8.9	97	100	6
Tetracaine	8.5	93	5,822	94

N/A, not available.
[a]Levobupivacaine has same physicochemical properties as racemate.
Data from Liu SS: Local anesthetics and analgesia, The Management of Pain. Edited by Ashburn MA, Rice LJ. New York, Churchill Livingstone, 1997, pp 141.

TABLE 21-4

RELATIVE POTENCY OF LOCAL ANESTHETICS FOR DIFFERENT CLINICAL APPLICATIONS

	■ BUPIVACAINE	■ CHLORO-PROCAINE	■ LIDOCAINE	■ MEPIVACAINE	■ PRILOCAINE	■ ROPIVACAINE
Peripheral nerve	3.6	N/A	1	2.6	0.8	3.6
Spinal	9.6	1	1	1	1	N/A
Epidural	4	0.5	1	1	1	4

N/A, not available.
Data from Camorcia M: Minimum local analgesic doses of ropivacaine, levobupivacaine, and bupivacaine for intrathecal labor analgesia. Anesthesiology 2005; 102: 646. Faccenda KA: A comparison of levobupivacaine 0.5% and racemic bupivacaine 0.5% for extradural anesthesia for caesarean section. Reg Anesth Pain Med 2003; 28: 394. McDonald SB. Hyperbaric spinal ropivacaine: A comparison to bupivacaine in volunteers. Anesthesiology 1999; 90: 971. Marsan A: Prilocaine or mepivacaine for combined sciatic-femoral nerve block in patients receiving elective knee arthroscopy. Minerva Anestesiol 2004; 70: 763. Casati A: Lidocaine versus ropivacaine for continuous interscalene brachial plexus block after open shoulder surgery. Acta Anaesthesiol Scand 2003; 47: 35. Casati A: A double-blind study of axillary brachial plexus block by 0.75% ropivacaine or 2% mepivacaine. Eur J Anaesthesiol 1998; 15: 549. Fanelli G: A double-blind comparison of ropivacaine, bupivacaine, and mepivacaine during sciatic and femoral nerve blockade. Anesth Analg, 1998; 87: 597. Yoos JR: Spinal 2-chloroprocaine: a comparison with small-dose bupivacaine in volunteers. Anesth Analg 2005; 100: 566. Kouri ME: Spinal 2-chloroprocaine: A comparison with lidocaine in volunteers. Anesth Analg 2004; 98: 75.

mixtures.[37,38] A theoretical basis for the difference between the enantiomeric stereoisomers can be readily hypothesized; however, little is known of the exact mechanisms involved. Likely, it may include subtle stereoselective preference in local anesthetic binding among the individual sodium channel isoforms.

Additives to Increase Local Anesthetic Activity

Epinephrine

Reported benefits of epinephrine include prolongation of local anesthetic block, increased intensity of block, and decreased systemic absorption of local anesthetic.[39] Epinephrine's vasoconstrictive effects augment local anesthetics by antagonizing inherent vasodilating effects of local anesthetics, decreasing systemic absorption and intraneural clearance, and perhaps by redistributing intraneural local anesthetic.[39,40]

Direct analgesic effects from epinephrine may also occur via interaction with α_2-adrenergic receptors in the brain and spinal cord,[41] especially because local anesthetics increase the vascular uptake of epinephrine.[42] Clinical use of epinephrine is listed in Table 21-5. The smallest dose is suggested because epinephrine combined with local anesthetics may have toxic effects on tissue,[43] the cardiovascular system,[44] peripheral nerves, and the spinal cord.[39]

Alkalinization of Local Anesthetic Solution

Local anesthetic solutions are alkalinized in order to hasten onset of neural block.[45] The pH of commercial preparations of

TABLE 21-5

EFFECTS OF ADDITION OF EPINEPHRINE TO LOCAL ANESTHETICS

	■ INCREASE DURATION	■ DECREASE BLOOD LEVELS (%)	■ DOSE/CONCENTRATION OF EPINEPHRINE
■ NERVE BLOCK			
Bupivacaine	+/−	10–20	1:200,000
Lidocaine	++	20–30	1:200,000
Mepivacaine	++	20–30	1:200,000
Ropivacaine	−−	0	1:200,000
■ EPIDURAL			
Bupivacaine	+/−	10–20	1:300,000–1:200,000
Levobupivacaine	+/−	10	1:200,000–1:400,000
Chloroprocaine	++		1:200,000
Lidocaine	++	20–30	1:600,000–1:200,000
Mepivacaine	++	20–30	1:200,000
Ropivacaine	−−	0	1:200,000
■ SPINAL			
Bupivacaine	+/−		0.2 mg
Lidocaine	++		0.2 mg
Tetracaine	++		0.2 mg

++, overall supported; −−, overall not supported; +/−, inconsistent.
Data from Liu SS: Local anesthetics and analgesia, The Management of Pain. Edited by Ashburn MA, Rice LJ. New York, Churchill Livingstone, 1997, pp 141; and Kopacz DJ: A comparison of epidural levobupivacaine 0.5% with or without epinephrine for lumbar spine surgery. Anesth Analg 2001; 93: 755.

local anesthetics ranges from 3.9 to 6.47 and is especially acidic if prepackaged with epinephrine.[46] As the pK_a of commonly used local anesthetics ranges from 7.6 to 8.9 (Table 21-3), <3% of the commercially prepared local anesthetic exists as the lipid-soluble neutral form. The neutral form is believed to be the most important for penetration into the neural cytoplasm, whereas the charged form primarily interacts with the local anesthetic receptor within the sodium channel. Therefore, the rationale for alkalinization was to increase the percentage of local anesthetic existing as the lipid-soluble neutral form. However, clinically used local anesthetics cannot be alkalinized beyond a pH of 6.05 to 8 before precipitation occurs,[46] and such pHs will only increase the neutral form to about 10%.

Clinical studies that have shown an association between alkalinization of local anesthetics and hastening of block onset have shown a decrease of <5 minutes when compared with commercial preparations.[45,47] In addition, a study in rats suggests that alkalinization of lidocaine decreases the duration of peripheral nerve blocks if the solution does not also contain epinephrine.[48] Overall, the value of alkalinization of local anesthetics appears debatable as a clinically useful tool to improve anesthesia.

Opioids

Opioids have multiple central neuraxial and peripheral mechanisms of analgesic action. Spinal administration of opioids provides analgesia primarily by attenuating C fiber nociception[49] and is independent of supraspinal mechanisms.[50] Coadministration of opioids with central neuraxial local anesthetics results in synergistic analgesia.[51] An exception to this analgesic synergy is 2-chloroprocaine, which appears to decrease the effectiveness of epidural opioids when used for epidural anesthesia.[52] The mechanism for this action is unclear but does not appear to involve direct antagonism of opioid receptors.[53] Overall, clinical studies support the practice of central neuraxial coadministration of local anesthetics and opioids in humans for prolongation and intensification of analgesia and anesthesia.[51]

The discovery of peripheral opioid receptors initially offered another circumstance in which the coadministration of local anesthetics and opioids may be useful.[54] However, cumulative evidence now suggests that neither intra-articular administration of local anesthetic and opioid for postoperative analgesia[55] nor combining local anesthetics and opioids for nerve blocks increases efficacy.[56]

α_2-Adrenergic Agonists

α_2-Adrenergic agonists can be a useful adjuvant to local anesthetics. α_2-Agonists, such as clonidine, produce analgesia via supraspinal and spinal adrenergic receptors.[57] Clonidine also has direct inhibitory effects on peripheral nerve conduction (A and C nerve fibers).[58] Thus, addition of clonidine may have multiple routes of action depending on type of application. Preliminary evidence suggests that coadministration of an α_2-agonist and local anesthetic results in central neuraxial and peripheral nerve analgesic synergy,[59] whereas systemic (supraspinal) effects are additive.[60] Overall, clinical trials indicate that clonidine enhances intrathecal and epidural anesthesia, peripheral nerve blocks,[61] and intravenous regional anesthesia.[62]

PHARMACOKINETICS OF LOCAL ANESTHETICS

Plasma concentration of local anesthetics is a function of the dose administered and the rates of systemic absorption, tissue distribution, and drug elimination. Elevated levels may pro-duce unintended effects in other electric-sensitive systems, most importantly, the cardiovascular and the central nervous systems. Having a thorough understanding of the factors involved would enable one to maximize the local anesthetic potential while avoiding possible complications arising from systemic local anesthetic toxicity.

Systemic Absorption

Decreasing systemic absorption of local anesthetics increases their safety margin in clinical uses. The rate and extent of systemic absorption depends on the site of injection, the dose, the drug's intrinsic pharmacokinetic properties, and the addition of a vasoactive agent. The vascularity of the tissue markedly influences the rate of drug absorption, such that deposition of local anesthetics in vessel-rich tissues results in higher peak plasma levels in a shorter period of time. Accordingly, the rate of systemic absorption is greatest with intercostal nerve blocks, and followed in decreasing order, by caudal and epidural injections, brachial plexus block, and femoral and sciatic nerve blocks (Table 21-6). Thus, the same amount of local anesthetics injected would result in unequal peak plasma levels, depending on the site of drug delivery.

For a given site of injection, the rate of systemic absorption and the peak plasma level are directly proportional to the dose of local anesthetic deposited. This relationship is nearly linear (Fig. 21-8) and independent of the drug concentration and the speed of injection.[63]

The rate of systemic absorption differs with individual local anesthetics. In general, more potent, lipid-soluble agents are associated with a slower rate of absorption than less lipid-soluble compounds (Fig. 21-9). Sequestration into lipid-rich compartments may not be the only explanation. Local anesthetics exert direct effects on vascular smooth muscles in a concentration-dependent manner. At low concentrations, more potent agents appear to cause more vasoconstriction than less potent agents, thereby decreasing the rate of vascular absorption.[36] At high concentrations, vasodilatory effects seem to predominate for most local anesthetics.

Distribution

Systemic absorption of local anesthetics leads to rapid distribution throughout the body. While the apparent volume of distribution (VD_{ss}) adequately describes the steady-state concentration of local anesthetics in plasma (Table 21-7), it offers little information regarding the pattern of distribution. Regional dif-

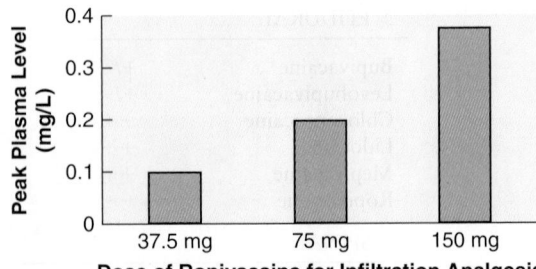

FIGURE 21-8. Increasing doses of ropivacaine used for wound infiltration result in linearly increasing maximal plasma concentrations (C_{max}). (Data from Mulroy MF, Burgess FW, Emanuelsson B-M: Ropivacaine 0.25% and 0.5%, but not 0.125%, provide effective wound infiltration analgesia after outpatient hernia repair, but with sustained plasma drug levels. Reg Anesth Pain Med 1999; 24: 136.)

TABLE 21-6

TYPICAL C_{max} AFTER REGIONAL ANESTHETICS WITH COMMONLY USED LOCAL ANESTHETICS

LOCAL ANESTHETIC	TECHNIQUE	DOSE (mg)	C_{max} (μg/mL)	T_{max} (min)	TOXIC PLASMA CONCENTRATION (μg/mL)
Bupivacaine	Brachial plexus	150	1.0	20	3
	Celiac plexus	100	1.50	17	
	Epidural	150	1.26	20	
	Intercostal	140	0.90	30	
	Lumbar sympathetic	52.5	0.49	24	
	Sciatic femoral	400	1.89	15	
Levobupivacaine	Epidural	75	0.36	50	4
	Brachial plexus	250	1.2	55	
Lidocaine	Brachial plexus	400	4.00	25	5
	Epidural	400	4.27	20	
	Intercostal	400	6.8	15	
Mepivacaine	Brachial plexus	500	3.68	24	5
	Epidural	500	4.95	16	
	Intercostal	500	8.06	9	
	Sciatic/femoral	500	3.59	31	
Ropivacaine	Brachial plexus	190	1.3	53	4
	Epidural	150	1.07	40	
	Intercostal	140	1.10	21	

C_{max}, peak plasma levels; T_{max}, time until C_{max}.
Data from Liu SS: Local anesthetics and analgesia, The Management of Pain. Edited by Ashburn MA, Rice LJ. New York, Churchill Livingstone, 1997, pp 141. Berrisford RG: Plasma concentrations of bupivacaine and its enantiomers during continuous extrapleural intercostal nerve block. Br J Anaesth 1993; 70: 201. Kopacz DJ: A comparison of epidural levobupivacaine 0.5% with or without epinephrine for lumbar spine surgery. Anesth Analg 2001; 93: 755. Crews JC: Levobupivacaine for axillary brachial plexus block: A pharmacokinetic and clinical comparison in patients with normal renal function or renal disease. Anesth Analg 2002; 95: 219.

ferences in local anesthetic concentrations are seen among individual organ systems and the pattern of distribution largely depends on organ perfusion, the partition coefficient between compartments, and plasma protein binding.[64] Organs that are well perfused, such as the heart and the brain, have higher drug

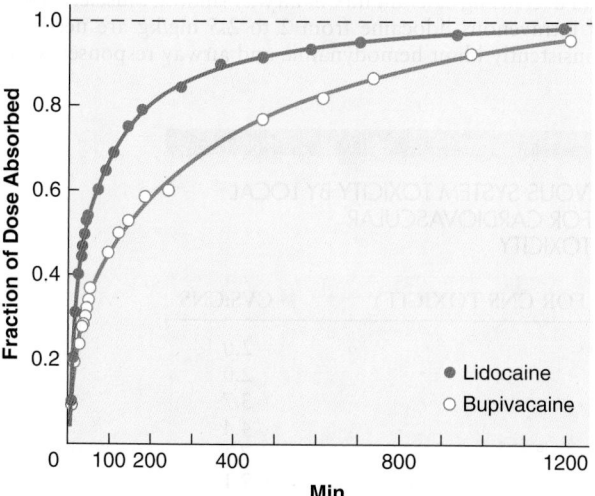

FIGURE 21-9. Fraction of dose absorbed into the systemic circulation over time from epidural injection of lidocaine or bupivacaine. Bupivacaine is a more lipid soluble, more potent agent with less systemic absorption over time. (Adapted from Tucker GT, Mather LE: Properties, absorption, and disposition of local anesthetic agents, Neural Blockade in Clinical Anesthesia and Management of Pain. Edited by Cousins MJ, Bridenbaugh PO. Philadelphia, Lippincott–Raven, 1998, p 55, with permission.)

concentrations. Unfortunately, they are also the organs most seriously affected by local anesthetic toxicity.

Elimination

The metabolic pathway for clearance of local anesthetics is primarily determined by their chemical linkage. Aminoesters are hydrolyzed by plasma cholinesterases and aminoamides are transformed by hepatic carboxylesterases and cytochrome P450 enzymes. Severe liver disease may slow the clearance of aminoamide local anesthetics and significant drug levels may therefore accumulate.[65]

Clinical Pharmacokinetics

The primary benefit of knowledge of the systemic pharmacokinetics of local anesthetics is the ability to predict the peak plasma level (C_{max}) after the agents are administered, thereby avoiding the administration of toxic doses (Tables 21-6, 21-8, and 21-9). However, pharmacokinetics are difficult to predict in any given circumstance as both physical and pathophysiologic characteristics will affect the individual pharmacokinetics. There is some evidence for increased systemic levels of local anesthetics in the very young and in the elderly owing to decreased clearance and increased absorption,[66] whereas correlation of resultant systemic blood levels between dose of local anesthetic and patient weight is often inconsistent (Fig. 21-10).[67] Effects of gender on clinical pharmacokinetics of local anesthetics have not been well defined,[68] although pregnancy may decrease clearance.[69] Pathophysiologic states such as cardiac and hepatic disease will alter expected pharmacokinetic parameters (Table 21-10), and lower doses of local anesthetics should be used for these patients. As expected, renal

TABLE 21-7

PHARMACOKINETIC PARAMETERS OF CLINICALLY USED LOCAL ANESTHETICS

LOCAL ANESTHETIC	VDss (L/kg)	CL (L/kg/hr)	$T_{1/2}$ (hr)
Bupivacaine	1.02	0.41	3.5
Levobupivacaine	0.78	0.32	2.6
Chloroprocaine	0.50	2.96	0.11
Etidocaine	1.9	1.05	2.6
Lidocaine	1.3	0.85	1.6
Mepivacaine	1.2	0.67	1.9
Prilocaine	2.73	2.03	1.6
Procaine	0.93	5.62	0.14
Ropivacaine	0.84	0.63	1.9

VDss, volume of distribution at steady state; CL, total body clearance; $T_{1/2}$, terminal elimination half-life. Data from Denson DD: Physiology and pharmacology of local anesthetics, Acute Pain. Mechanisms and Management. Edited by Sinatra RS, Hord AH, Ginsberg B, et al. St. Louis, Mosby Year Book, 1992. p 124; and Burm AG, van der Meer AD, van Kleef JW et al: Pharmacokinetics of the enantiomers of bupivacaine following intravenous administration of the racemate. Br J Clin Pharmacol 1994; 38: 125.

disease has little effect on pharmacokinetic parameters of local anesthetics (Table 21-10). All of these factors should be considered when using local anesthetics and minimizing systemic toxicity, the commonly accepted maximal dosages (Table 21-9) notwithstanding.

CLINICAL USE OF LOCAL ANESTHETICS

Local anesthetics are used in a variety of ways in clinical anesthesia practice. Probably the most common clinical use of local anesthetics for anesthesiologists is for regional anesthesia and analgesia. Central neuraxial anesthesia and analgesia can be accomplished by epidural or spinal injections of local anesthetics. Placement of epidural and spinal catheters can allow continuous infusion of local anesthetics and other analgesics for extended durations. Intravenous regional anesthesia and peripheral nerve blocks allow for anesthesia of the head and neck, including the airway, upper extremities, trunk, and lower extremities. Catheters for continuous peripheral nerve blocks and continuous

surgical wound infusions can also be placed to allow continuous infusions of local anesthetics for prolonged analgesia.[70]

Topical application of local anesthetics to the airway, eye, and skin provides sufficient anesthesia for painless performance of minor anesthetic and surgical procedures such as tracheal intubation, intravenous catheter placement, or dural puncture.[71] Typical applications for each local anesthetic are listed in Table 21-9.[72]

Other common clinical uses for local anesthetics include administration of lidocaine to blunt responses to tracheal instrumentation and to suppress cardiac dysrhythmias. Intravenous or topical administrations of lidocaine have been used with variable success to blunt hemodynamic response to tracheal intubation and extubation.[73] In addition to hemodynamic responses, instrumentation of the airway can result in coughing, bronchoconstriction, and other airway responses. Intravenous lidocaine can be effective for decreasing airway sensitivity to instrumentation by depressing airway reflexes and decreasing calcium flux in airway smooth muscle.[74] Doses of intravenous lidocaine from 2 to 2.5 mg/kg are needed to consistently blunt hemodynamic and airway responses to tra-

TABLE 21-8

RELATIVE POTENCY FOR SYSTEMIC CENTRAL NERVOUS SYSTEM TOXICITY BY LOCAL ANESTHETICS AND RATIO OF DOSAGE NEEDED FOR CARDIOVASCULAR SYSTEM:CENTRAL NERVOUS SYSTEM (CVS:CNS) TOXICITY

AGENT	RELATIVE POTENCY FOR CNS TOXICITY	CVS:CNS
Bupivacaine	4.0	2.0
Levobupivacaine	2.9	2.0
Chloroprocaine	0.3	3.7
Etidocaine	2.0	4.4
Lidocaine	1.0	7.1
Mepivacaine	1.4	7.1
Prilocaine	1.2	3.1
Procaine	0.3	3.7
Ropivacaine	2.9	2.0
Tetracaine	2.0	

Data from Liu SS: Local Anesthetics and Analgesia, The Management of Pain. Edited by Ashburn MA, Rice LJ. New York, Churchill Livingstone, 1997, pp 141; and Groban L: Central nervous system and cardiac effects from long-acting amide local anesthetic toxicity in the intact animal model. Reg Anesth Pain Med 2003; 28: 3.

TABLE 21-9

CLINICAL PROFILE OF LOCAL ANESTHETICS

▪ LOCAL ANESTHETIC	▪ CONCENTRATION (%)	▪ CLINICAL USE	▪ ONSET	▪ DURATION (hr)	▪ RECOMMENDED MAXIMUM SINGLE DOSE (mg)
▪ AMIDES					
Bupivacaine	0.25	Infiltration	Fast	2–8	175/225 + epinephrine
Levobupivacaine	0.25–0.5	Peripheral nerve block	Slow	4–12	150
	0.5–0.75	Epidural anesthesia	Moderate	2–5	150
	0.03–0.25	Epidural analgesia	NA	NA	NA
	0.5–0.75	Spinal anesthesia	Fast	1–4	20
Etidocaine	0.5%	Infiltration	Fast	2–8	300/400 + epinephrine
	0.5–1	Peripheral nerve block	Fast	3–12	300/400 + epinephrine
	1–1.5	Epidural anesthesia	Fast	2–4	300/400 + epinephrine
Lidocaine	0.5–1	Infiltration	Fast	1–4	300/500 + epinephrine
	0.25–0.5	IV regional anesthesia	Fast	0.5–1	300
	1–1.5	Peripheral nerve block	Fast	1–3	300/500 + epinephrine
	1.5–2	Epidural anesthesia	Fast	1–2	300/500 + epinephrine
	1.5–5	Spinal anesthesia	Fast	0.5–1	100
	4	Topical	Fast	0.5–1	300
Mepivacaine	0.5–1	Infiltration	Fast	1–4	400/500 + epinephrine
	1–1.5	Peripheral nerve block	Fast	2–4	400/500 + epinephrine
	1.5–2	Epidural anesthesia	Fast	1–3	400/500 + epinephrine
	2–4	Spinal anesthesia	Fast	1–2	100
Prilocaine	0.5–1	Infiltration	Fast	1–2	600
	0.25–0.5	IV regional anesthesia	Fast	0.5–1	600
	1.5–2	Peripheral nerve block	Fast	1.5–3	600
	2–3	Epidural	Fast	1–3	600
Ropivacaine	0.2–0.5	Infiltration	Fast	2–6	200
	0.5–1	Peripheral nerve block	Slow	5–8	250
	0.5–1	Epidural anesthesia	Moderate	2–6	200
	0.05–0.2	Epidural analgesia	NA	NA	NA
▪ MIXTURE					
Lidocaine + prilocaine	2.5/2.5	Skin topical	Slow	3–5	20 gm
▪ ESTERS					
Benzocaine	Up to 20%	Topical	Fast	0.5–1	200
Chloroprocaine	1	Infiltration	Fast	0.5–1	800/1000 + epinephrine
	2	Peripheral nerve block	Fast	0.5–1	800/1000 + epinephrine
	2–3	Epidural anesthesia	Fast	0.5–1	800/1000 + epinephrine
Cocaine	4–10	Topical	Fast	0.5–1	150
Procaine	10	Spinal anesthesia	Fast	0.5–1	1,000
Tetracaine	2	Topical	Fast	0.5–1	20
	0.5	Spinal anesthesia	Fast	2–6	20

IV, intravenous.
Adapted from Covino BG, Wildsmith JAW: Clinical pharmacology of local anesthetic agents.
Neural Blockade in Clinical Anesthesia and Management of Pain. Edited by Cousins MJ, Bridenbaugh PO. Philadelphia, Lippincott–Raven, 1998, pp 97, with permission.

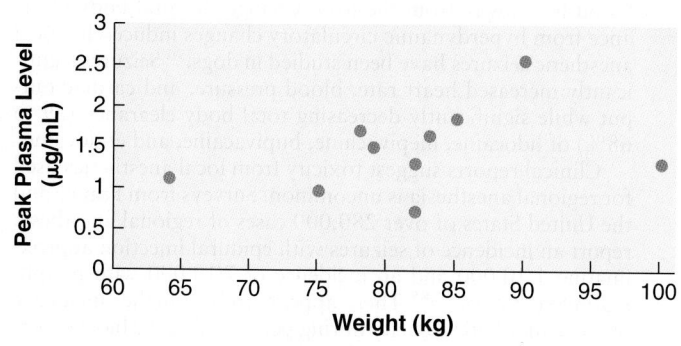

FIGURE 21-10.   Lack of correlation between patient weight and peak plasma concentration after epidural administration of 150 mg of bupivacaine. (Data from Sharrock NE, Mather LE, Go G, et al: Arterial and pulmonary concentrations of the enantiomers of bupivacaine after epidural injection in elderly patients. Anesth Analg 1998; 86: 812.)

TABLE 21-10

EFFECTS OF CARDIAC, HEPATIC, AND RENAL DISEASE ON
LIDOCAINE PHARMACOKINETICS

	■ VD_{ss} (L/Kg)	■ CL (mL/kg/min)	■ $T_{1/2}$ (hr)
Normal	1.32	10.0	1.8
Cardiac failure	0.88	6.3	1.9
Hepatic disease	2.31	6.0	4.9
Renal disease	1.2	13.7	1.3

VDss, volume of distribution at steady state; CL, total body clearance; $T_{1/2}$, terminal elimination half-life.
Data from Thomson PD: Lidocaine pharmacokinetics in advanced heart failure, liver disease, and renal
failure in humans. Ann Intern Med 1973; 78: 499.

cheal instrumentation.[74,75] Intravenous lidocaine is also effective for attenuating increases in intraocular pressure, intracranial pressure, and intra-abdominal pressure during airway instrumentation.[76] Attenuation of all these responses may be beneficial in selected clinical situations (e.g., corneal laceration or increased intracranial pressure). Intravenous lidocaine has well-recognized cardiac antidysrhythmic effects.[77]

Finally, intravenous lidocaine (1 to 5 mg/kg) is an effective analgesic and has been used to treat postoperative[78] and chronic neuropathic pain.[79] Peripheral and central inhibition of generation and propagation of spontaneous electrical activity in injured C nerve fibers and Aδ nerve fibers are thought to be primary mechanisms as opposed to typical conduction block.[80] Positron emission tomography in patients with neuropathic pain suggests that altered activity in cerebral blood flow to the thalamus[81] may also contribute to systemic analgesic effects of local anesthetics. The ability of local anesthetics to provide systemic analgesic effects at central and peripheral sites may partly explain the ability of a single neural block to provide long-lasting analgesia from neuropathic pain.

TOXICITY OF LOCAL ANESTHETICS

❼ Systemic Toxicity of Local Anesthetics

Central Nervous System Toxicity

Local anesthetics readily cross the blood–brain barrier, and generalized CNS toxicity may occur from systemic absorption or direct vascular injection. Signs of generalized CNS toxicity because of local anesthetics are dose-dependent (Table 21-11).

TABLE 21-11

DOSE-DEPENDENT SYSTEMIC EFFECTS OF LIDOCAINE

■ PLASMA CONCENTRATION (μg/mL)	■ EFFECT
1–5	Analgesia
5–10	Lightheadedness
	Tinnitus
	Numbness of tongue
10–15	Seizures
	Unconsciousness
15–25	Coma
	Respiratory arrest
>25	Cardiovascular depression

Low doses produce CNS depression, and higher doses result in CNS excitation and seizures.[82] The rate of intravenous administration of local anesthetic will also affect signs of CNS toxicity, as higher rates of infusion of the same dose will lessen the appearance of CNS depression while leaving excitation intact.[83] This dichotomous reaction to local anesthetics may be a result of a greater sensitivity of cortical inhibitory neurons to the impulse blocking effects of local anesthetics.[82,84,85]

Local anesthetic potency for generalized CNS toxicity approximately parallels action potential blocking potency (Tables 21-4 and 21-8).[82] In general, decreased local anesthetic protein binding and clearance will increase potential CNS toxicity. External factors can increase potency for CNS toxicity, such as acidosis and increased PCO_2, perhaps via increased cerebral perfusion or decreased protein binding of local anesthetic.[82] There are also external factors that can decrease local anesthetic potency for generalized CNS toxicity. For example, seizure thresholds of local anesthetics are increased by administration of barbiturates and benzodiazepines.[86]

Addition of vasoconstrictors such as epinephrine may reduce or promote the potential for generalized local anesthetic CNS toxicity. Addition of epinephrine to local anesthetics will decrease systemic absorption and peak blood levels and increase the safety margin. On the other hand, the convulsive threshold for intravenous administration of lidocaine in the rat is decreased by about 42% when epinephrine (1:100,000), norepinephrine, or phenylephrine is added to the plain solution.[87] The mechanisms of increased toxicity with addition of epinephrine are unclear but appear to depend on the development of hypertension from vasoconstriction. A hyperdynamic circulatory system may enhance the toxic effects of local anesthetics by causing increased cerebral blood flow and delivery of lidocaine to the brain[88] or through disruption of the blood–brain barrier.[89] In addition to enhancing distribution of local anesthetic to the brain, hyperdynamic circulatory changes can also decrease clearance of local anesthetic from the body because of changes in distribution of blood flow away from the liver. Changes in total body clearance from hyperdynamic circulatory changes induced by local anesthetic seizures have been studied in dogs.[90] Seizures significantly increased heart rate, blood pressure, and cardiac output while significantly decreasing total body clearance (29 to 68%) of lidocaine, mepivacaine, bupivacaine, and etidocaine.

Clinical reports suggest toxicity from local anesthetics used for regional anesthesia is uncommon. Surveys from France and the United States of over 280,000 cases of regional anesthesia report an incidence of seizures with epidural injection approximating 1/10,000 and an incidence of 7/10,000 with peripheral nerve blocks.[84,85] There appears to be a higher incidence of local anesthetic toxicity during peripheral nerve blocks, perhaps because of differences in practice or less clinical awareness. Nonetheless, in an analysis of closed malpractice claims in the United States from 1980 to 1999, epidural anesthesia (primarily obstetrical) constituted all of the cases of death or brain damage resulting from unintentional intravenous injection of local anesthetic.[91]

Cardiovascular Toxicity of Local Anesthetics

In general, much greater doses of local anesthetics are required to produce cardiovascular toxicity than CNS toxicity. Similar to CNS toxicity, potency for cardiovascular toxicity reflects the anesthetic potency of the agent (Tables 21-4 and 21-8). Attention has focused on the increased cardiotoxicity of the more potent, more lipid-soluble agents (bupivacaine, levobupivacaine, ropivacaine). These agents appear to have a different sequence of cardiovascular toxicity than less potent agents, with bupivacaine being the most cardiotoxic. For example, increasingly toxic doses of lidocaine leads to hypotension, bradycardia, and hypoxia, whereas toxic doses of bupivacaine, levobupivacaine, and ropivacaine often result in sudden cardiovascular collapse as a result of ventricular dysrhythmias that are resistant to resuscitation (Fig. 21-11).[82,86,92]

Use of the single–optical isomer preparations of ropivacaine and levo-bupivacaine may improve the safety profile for long-lasting regional anesthesia. Both ropivacaine and levobupivacaine appear to be approximately equipotent to racemic bupivacaine for epidural and plexus anesthesia (Table 21-4).[93,94] Both ropivacaine and levobupivacaine have approximately 30 to 40% less systemic toxicity than bupivacaine on a milligram to milligram basis in animal studies[82,92,95] (Fig. 21-12), although human studies are less dramatic (Fig. 21-13).[96,97] Reduced potential for cardiotoxicity is likely because of reduced affinity for brain and myocardial tissue from their single isomer preparation.[18,82,98] In addition to stereoselectivity, the larger butyl side chain in bupivacaine may also have more of a cardiodepressant effect as opposed to the propyl-side chain of ropivacaine.[99]

Cardiovascular Toxicity Mediated at the CNS. It has been demonstrated that the central and peripheral nervous systems

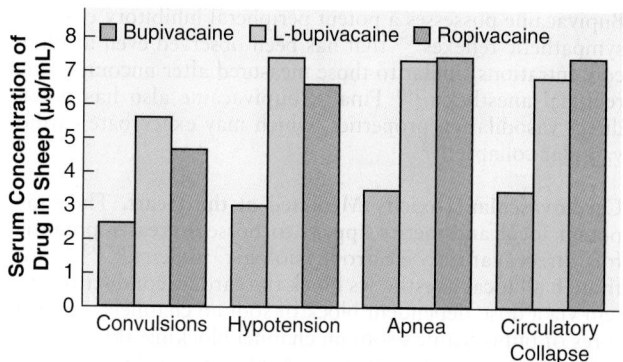

FIGURE 21-12. Serum concentrations in sheep at each toxic manifestation for bupivacaine, levo (L)-bupivacaine, and ropivacaine in sheep. Both levobupivacaine and ropivacaine required significantly greater serum concentrations than bupivacaine. (Data from Santos AC, DeArmas PI: Systemic toxicity of levobupivacaine, bupivacaine, and ropivacaine during continuous intravenous infusion to nonpregnant and pregnant ewes. Anesthesiology 2001; 95: 1256.)

may be involved in the increased cardiotoxicity with bupivacaine. The nucleus tractus solitarii in the medulla is an important region for autonomic control of the cardiovascular system. Neural activity in the nucleus tractus solitarii of rats is markedly diminished by intravenous doses of bupivacaine immediately prior to development of hypotension. Furthermore, direct intracerebral injection of bupivacaine can elicit sudden dysrhythmias and cardiovascular collapse.[100]

Peripheral effects of bupivacaine on the autonomic and vasomotor systems may also augment its cardiovascular toxicity.

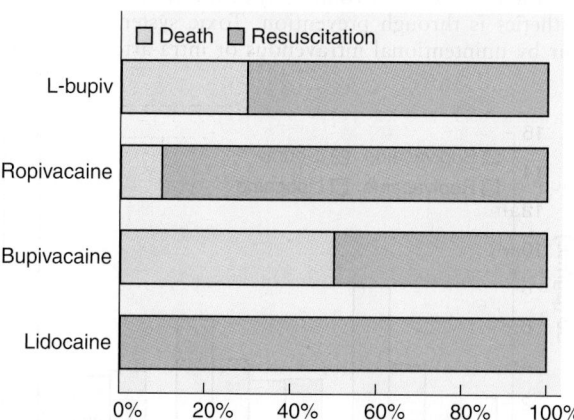

FIGURE 21-11. Success of resuscitation of dogs after cardiovascular collapse from intravenous infusions of lidocaine, bupivacaine, levobupivacaine (L-bupiv), and ropivacaine. Success rates were greater for lidocaine (100%), than ropivacaine (90%), than levobupivacaine (70%), and than bupivacaine (50%). Required doses to induce cardiovascular collapse were greater for lidocaine (127 mg/kg), than ropivacaine (42 mg/kg), than levobupivacaine (27 mg/kg), and than bupivacaine (22 mg/kg). (Data from Groban L, Deal DD, Vernon JC, et al: Cardiac resuscitation after incremental overdosage with lidocaine, bupivacaine, levobupivacaine, and ropivacaine in anesthetized dogs. Anesth Analg 2001; 92: 37.)

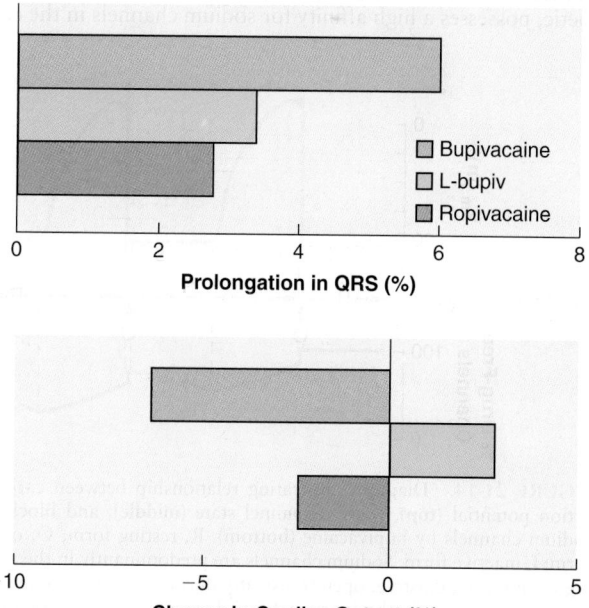

FIGURE 21-13. Mild prolongation in QRS interval and change in cardiac output after intravenous infusions of bupivacaine (103 mg), levobupivacaine (L-bupiv; 37 mg), and ropivacaine (115 mg) in healthy volunteers. (Data from Knudsen K, Beckman Suurkula M, et al: Central nervous and cardiovascular effects of i.v. infusions of ropivacaine, bupivacaine and placebo in volunteers. Br Anaesth 1997; 78: 507; and Stewart J, Kellett N, Castro D: The central nervous system and cardiovascular effects of levobupivacaine and ropivacaine in healthy volunteers. Anesth Analg 2003; 97: 412.)

Bupivacaine possesses a potent peripheral inhibitory effect on sympathetic reflexes[100] that has been observed even at blood concentrations similar to those measured after uncomplicated regional anesthesia.[101] Finally, bupivacaine also has potent direct vasodilating properties, which may exacerbate cardiovascular collapse.[102]

Cardiovascular Toxicity Mediated at the Heart. The more potent local anesthetics appear to possess greater potential for direct cardiac electrophysiologic toxicity.[82,92,98] Although all local anesthetics block the cardiac conduction system via a dose-dependent block of sodium channels, two features of bupivacaine's sodium channel blocking abilities may enhance its cardiotoxicity. First, bupivacaine exhibits a much stronger binding affinity to resting and inactivated sodium channels than lidocaine.[103] Second, local anesthetics bind to sodium channels during systole and dissociate during diastole (Fig. 21-14). Bupivacaine dissociates from sodium channels during cardiac diastole much more slowly than lidocaine. Indeed, bupivacaine dissociates so slowly that the duration of diastole at physiologic heart rates (60 to 180 beats/min) does not allow enough time for complete recovery of sodium channels and bupivacaine conduction block accumulates. In contrast, lidocaine fully dissociates from sodium channels during diastole and little accumulation of conduction block occurs (Fig. 21-15).[103,104] Thus, enhanced electrophysiologic effects of more potent local anesthetics on the cardiac conduction system may explain their increased potential to produce sudden cardiovascular collapse via cardiac dysrhythmias.

Increased potency for direct myocardial depression from the more potent local anesthetics is another contributing factor to increased cardiotoxicity (Fig. 21-16).[82,99] Again, multiple mechanisms may account for the increased potency for myocardial depression from more potent local anesthetics. Bupivacaine, the most completely studied potent local anesthetic, possesses a high affinity for sodium channels in the car-

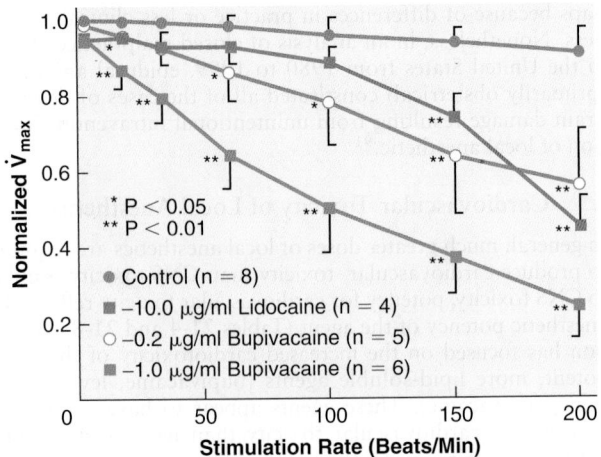

FIGURE 21-15. Heart rate-dependent effects of lidocaine and bupivacaine on velocity of the cardiac action potential ($\dot{V}_{max}$). Bupivacaine progressively decreases $\dot{V}_{max}$ at heart rates above 10 beats/min because of accumulation of sodium channel block, whereas lidocaine does not decrease $\dot{V}_{max}$ until heart rate exceeds 150 beats/min. (Adapted from Clarkson CW, Hondegham LM: Mechanisms for bupivacaine depression of cardiac conduction: Fast block of sodium channels during the action potential with slow recovery from block during diastole. Anesthesiology 1985; 62: 396 with permission.)

diac myocyte.[82,98] Furthermore, bupivacaine inhibits myocyte release and utilization of calcium[105] and reduces mitochondrial energy metabolism, especially during hypoxia.[106] Thus, multiple direct effects of bupivacaine on activity of the cardiac myocyte may explain the cardiotoxicity of bupivacaine and other potent local anesthetics.

Treatment of Systemic Toxicity from Local Anesthetics

The best method for avoiding systemic toxicity from local anesthetics is through prevention. Toxic systemic levels can occur by unintentional intravenous or intra-arterial injection

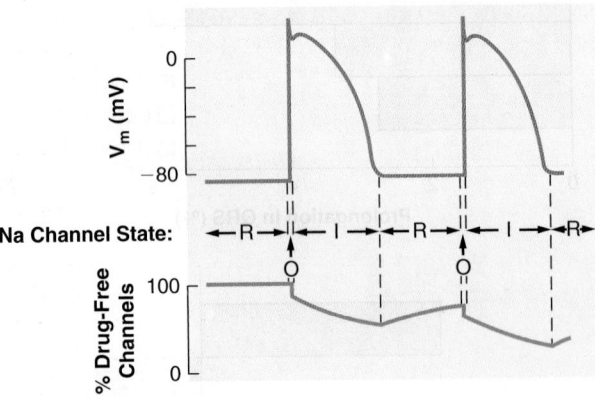

FIGURE 21-14. Diagram illustrating relationship between cardiac action potential (**top**), sodium channel state (**middle**), and block of sodium channels by bupivacaine (**bottom**). R, resting form; O, open form; I, inactive form. Sodium channels are predominantly in the resting form during diastole, open transiently during the action potential upstroke, and are in the inactive form during the action potential plateau. Block of sodium channels by bupivacaine accumulates during the action potential (systole) with recovery occurring during diastole. Recovery of sodium channels is from dissociation of bupivacaine and is time-dependent. Recovery during each diastolic interval is incomplete and results in accumulation of sodium channel block with successive heartbeats. (Adapted from Clarkson CW, Hondegham LM: Mechanisms for bupivacaine depression of cardiac conduction: Fast block of sodium channels during the action potential with slow recovery from block during diastole. Anesthesiology 1985; 62: 396, with permission.)

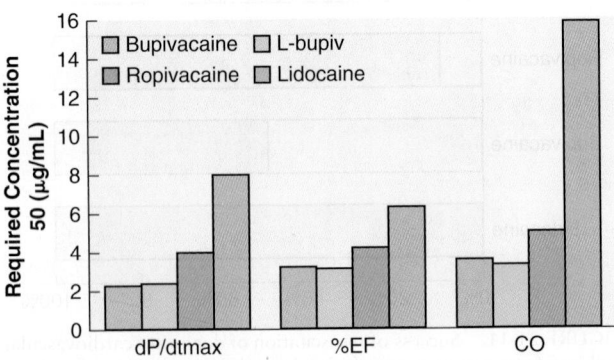

FIGURE 21-16. Plasma concentrations required to induce myocardial depression in dogs administered bupivacaine, levo (L)-bupivacaine, ropivacaine, and lidocaine. dP/dtmax, 35% reduction of inotropy from baseline measure; %EF, 35% reduction in ejection fraction from baseline measure; CO, 25% reduction in cardiac output from baseline measure. (Data from Groban L, Deal DD, Vernon JC, et al: Does local anesthetic stereoselectivity or structure predict myocardial depression in anesthetized canines? Reg Anesth Pain Med 2002; 27: 460.)

or by systemic absorption of excessive doses placed in the correct area. Unintentional intravascular and intra-arterial injections can be minimized by frequent syringe aspiration for blood, use of a small test dose of local anesthetic (approximately 3 mL) to test for subjective systemic effects from the patient (e.g., tinnitus, circumoral numbness), and either slow injection or fractionation of the rest of the dose of local anesthetic.[86] Detailed knowledge of local anesthetic pharmacokinetics will also aid in reducing the administration of excessive doses of local anesthetics. Ideally, heart rate, blood pressure, and the electrocardiogram should be monitored during administration of large doses of local anesthetics. Pretreatment with a benzodiazepine, such as midazolam, may also lower the probability of seizure by raising the seizure threshold.

Treatment of systemic toxicity is primarily supportive. Injection of local anesthetic should be stopped. Oxygenation and ventilation should be maintained, as systemic toxicity of local anesthetics is enhanced by hypoxemia, hypercarbia, and acidosis.[86] If needed, the patient's trachea should be intubated and positive pressure ventilation instituted. As previously discussed, signs of CNS toxicity will typically occur prior to cardiovascular events. Seizures can increase body metabolism and cause hypoxemia, hypercarbia, and acidosis. Pharmacologic treatment to terminate seizures may be needed if oxygenation and ventilation cannot be maintained. Intravenous administration of thiopental (50 to 100 mg), midazolam (2 to 5 mg), and propofol (1 mg/kg) can terminate seizures from systemic local anesthetic toxicity. Succinylcholine (50 mg) can terminate muscular activity from seizures and facilitate ventilation and oxygenation. However, succinylcholine will not terminate seizure activity in the CNS, and increased cerebral metabolic demands will continue unabated.

Cardiovascular depression from less potent local anesthetics (e.g., lidocaine) is usually mild and caused by mild myocardial depression and vasodilation. Hypotension and bradycardia can usually be treated with ephedrine (10 to 30 mg) and atropine (0.4 mg). As previously discussed, potent local anesthetics (e.g., bupivacaine) can produce profound cardiovascular depression and malignant dysrhythmias that should be promptly treated. Oxygenation and ventilation must be immediately instituted, with cardiopulmonary resuscitation if needed. Ventricular dysrhythmias may be difficult to treat and may need large and multiple doses of electrical cardioversion, epinephrine, vasopressin, and amiodarone. The use of calcium channel blockers in this setting is not recommended, as its cardiodepressant effect is exaggerated.[86]

A novel and promising treatment for cardiac toxicity is the administration of intravenous lipid to theoretically remove bupivacaine from sites of action. Administration of 100 mL of 20% lipid solution has been reported to allow successful resuscitation of a patient from bupivacaine-induced dysrhythmias refractory to conventional therapy.[107] These findings raise the question of whether standard propofol in a 10% lipid solution would be a preferred treatment for cardiac toxicity. However, the dose of lipid in a standard induction dose of propofol would be too small and the dose of propofol would lead to unacceptable cardiac depression.[107]

Neural Toxicity of Local Anesthetics

In addition to systemic toxicity, local anesthetics can cause injury to the central and peripheral nervous systems from direct exposure. Mechanisms for local anesthetic neurotoxicity remain speculative, but previous studies have demonstrated local anesthetic–induced injury to Schwann cells, inhibition of fast axonal transport, disruption of the blood-nerve barrier, decreased neural blood flow with associated ischemia, and disruption of cell membrane integrity via a detergent property of

local anesthetics.[108,109] Although all clinically used local anesthetics can cause concentration-dependent nerve fiber damage in peripheral nerves when used in high enough concentrations, previous studies have demonstrated that local anesthetics in clinically used concentrations are generally safe for peripheral nerves.[110] The spinal cord and the nerve roots, on the other hand, are more prone to injury.

Concentration-dependent spinal cord toxicity of local anesthetics has been assessed by administration of local anesthetics to rabbits via intrathecal catheters. These studies suggest that bupivacaine (2%), lidocaine (8%), and tetracaine (1%) cause histopathologic changes and neurologic deficits. On the other hand, clinically relevant concentrations of ropivacaine (2%) did not disrupt spinal cord histology or cause neurologic deficits.[111] Desheathed peripheral nerve models, designed to mimic unprotected nerve roots in the cauda equina, have been used to further assess electrophysiologic neurotoxicity of local anesthetics.[112,113] Lidocaine 5% and tetracaine 0.5% caused irreversible conduction block in these models, whereas lidocaine 1.5%, bupivacaine 0.75%, and tetracaine 0.06% did not. Although such studies do not reflect in vivo conditions, they suggest that lidocaine and tetracaine may be especially neurotoxic in a concentration-dependent fashion and that neurotoxicity could theoretically occur with clinically used solutions.

Nonetheless, clinical injury is rare. A systematic review of approximately 2.7 million central neuraxial blocks determined rates of occurrence of radiculopathy to be approximately 0.03% and of paraplegia to be approximately 0.0008%.[114]

Transient Neurologic Symptoms After Spinal Anesthesia

Prospective, randomized studies reveal a 4 to 40% incidence of transient neurologic symptoms (TNS), including pain or sensory abnormalities in the lower back, buttocks, or lower extremities, after lidocaine spinal anesthesia[115,116] (see also Chapter 34). These symptoms have been reported with other local anesthetics as well (Table 21-12) but have not resulted in permanent neurologic injury.[116] Increased risk of TNS is associated with lidocaine, the lithotomy position, and ambulatory anesthesia, but not with baricity of solution or dose of local anesthetic.[115,116] The potential neurologic etiology of this syndrome coupled with known concentration-dependent toxicity of lidocaine led to concerns over a neurotoxic etiology for TNS from spinal lidocaine.

As previously discussed, laboratory work in both intrathecal and desheathed peripheral nerve models has proved that the concentration of lidocaine is a critical factor in neurotoxicity. However, TNS does not display a dose-dependent response, as 0.5% lidocaine results in similar incidences of TNS as 5% spinal lidocaine.[117] Furthermore, a volunteer study comparing individuals with and without TNS symptoms after lidocaine spinal anesthesia showed no difference detected by electromyography, nerve conduction studies, or somatosensory-evoked potentials. Finally, effective treatment for TNS includes nonsteroidal anti-inflammatory agents and trigger point injections. These are typically effective treatments for myofascial pain and not for neuropathic pain.[115] Overall, there is little evidence to support a neurotoxic etiology for TNS.[115] Other potential etiologies for TNS include patient positioning, sciatic nerve stretch, muscle spasm, and myofascial strain.[115]

Myotoxicity of Local Anesthetics

Toxicity to skeletal muscle is an uncommon side effect of local anesthetic injection. Experimental data suggest, however, that local anesthetics have the potential for myotoxicity in clini-

TABLE 21-12

THE INCIDENCE OF TRANSIENT NEUROLOGIC SYMPTOMS (TNS) VARY WITH TYPE OF SPINAL LOCAL ANESTHETIC AND SURGERY

■ LOCAL ANESTHETIC	■ CONCENTRATION (%)	■ TYPE OF SURGERY	■ APPROXIMATE INCIDENCE OF TNS (%)
Lidocaine	2–5	Lithotomy position	30–36
	2–5	Knee arthroscopy	18–22
	0.5	Knee arthroscopy	17
	2–5	Mixed supine position	4–8
Mepivacaine	1.5–4	Mixed	23
Procaine	10	Knee arthroscopy	6
Bupivacaine	0.5–0.75	Mixed	1
Levobupivacaine	0.5	Mixed	1
Prilocaine	2–5	Mixed	1
Ropivacaine	0.5–0.75	Mixed	1

Data from Pollock JE: Transient neurologic symptoms: Etiology, risk factors, and management. Reg Anesth Pain Med 2002; 27: 581; and Breebaart MB: Urinary bladder scanning after day-case arthroscopy under spinal anaesthesia: Comparison between lidocaine, ropivacaine, and levobupivacaine. Br J Anaesth 2003; 90: 309.

cally applicable concentrations (Fig. 21-17). Histopathologic evidence shows that the injection of these agents causes diffuse myonecrosis, which is typically both reversible and clinically imperceptible.[118] The reversible nature of this injury is possibly because of the relative resilience of myoblasts, which regenerate damaged tissue. Theoretical mechanisms of injury are numerous but dysregulation of intracellular calcium concentrations is the most likely culprit. Laboratory studies demonstrate that ropivacaine is less myotoxic than bupivacaine, primarily because of the latter causing apoptosis (programmed cell death).[118] Further investigation is needed to determine the clinical relevance of local or systemic myotoxicity following single injection or continuous infusion of local anesthetics.

Allergic Reactions to Local Anesthetics (see also Chapter 12)

True allergic reactions to local anesthetics are rare and usually involve type I (immunoglobulin E) or type IV (cellular immunity) reactions.[119,120] Type I reactions are worrisome, as anaphylaxis may occur, and are more common with ester than amide local anesthetics. True type I allergy to aminoamide agents is extremely rare.[120] Increased allergenic potential with esters may be a result of hydrolytic metabolism to para-aminobenzoic acid, which is a documented allergen. Added preservatives such as methylparaben and metabisulfite can also provoke an allergic response. Skin testing with intradermal injections of preservative-free local anesthetics has been advocated as a means to determine tolerance to local anesthetic. These tests should be undertaken with caution because potentially severe and even fatal reactions can occur in truly allergic patients.[120]

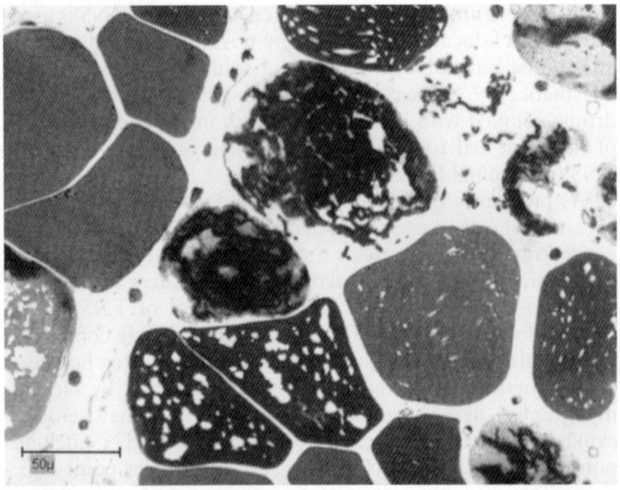

FIGURE 21-17.   Skeletal muscle cross section with characteristic histologic changes after continuous exposure to bupivacaine for 6 hours. A whole spectrum of necrobiotic changes can be encountered, ranging from slightly damaged vacuolated fibers and fibers with condensed myofibrils to entirely disintegrated and necrotic cells. The majority of the myocytes are morphologically affected. Additionally, a marked interstitial and myoseptal edema appears within the sections. However, scattered fibers remain intact. (Reprinted from Zink W, Graf B: Local anesthetic myotoxicity. Reg Anesth Pain Med 2004; 29: 333–340, with permission.)

References

1. Wheater PR, Burkitt HG, Daniels VG: Functional Histology, 2nd edition. New York, Churchill Livingstone, 1987, p 95
2. Ritchie JM, Ritchie B, Greengard P: The effect of the nerve sheath on the action of local anesthetics. J Pharmacol Exp Ther 1965; 150: 160
3. Coggeshall RE: A fine structural analysis of the myelin sheath in rat spinal roots. Anat Rec 1979; 194: 201
4. Waxman SG, Ritchie JM: Organization of ion channels in the myelinated nerve fiber. Science 1985; 228: 1502
5. Koester J: Passive Membrane Properties of the Neuron, Principles of Neuroscience, 3rd edition. Edited by Kandel ER, Schwartz JH, Jessell TM. New York, Elsevier Science, 1991
6. Hodgkin AL, Katz B: The effect of sodium ions on the electrical activity of the giant axon of the squid. J Physiol 1949; 108: 37
7. Hodgkin AL, Huxley AF: A quantitative description of membrane current and its application to conduction and excitation in nerve. J Physiol 1952; 117: 500
8. Sigworth FJ, Neher E: Single Na+ channel currents observed in cultured rat muscle cells. Nature 1980; 287: 447

9. Catterall WA: From ionic currents to molecular mechanisms: the structure and function of voltage-gated sodium channels. Neuron 2000; 26: 13

10. Hirschberg B, Rovner A, Lieberman M, et al: Transfer of twelve charges is needed to open skeletal muscle Na+ channels. J Gen Physiol 1995; 106: 1053

11. Heinemann SH, Terlau H, Stühmer W, et al: Calcium channel characteristics conferred on the sodium channel by single mutations. Nature 1992; 356: 441

12. Armstrong CM: Sodium channels and gating currents. Physiol Rev 1981; 61: 644

13. Stühmer W, Conti F, Suzuki H, et al: Structural parts involved in activation and inactivation of the sodium channel. Nature 1989; 339: 597

14. West JW, Patton DE, Scheuer T, et al: A cluster of hydrophobic amino acid residues required for fast Na(+)-channel inactivation. Proc Natl Acad Sci USA 1992; 89: 10910

15. Woods JN, Boorman JP, Okuse K, et al: Voltage-Gated Sodium Channels and Pain Pathways. J Neurobiol 2004; 61: 55

16. Drenth JP, te Morsche RH, Guillet G, et al: SCN9A mutations define primary erythermalgia as a neuropathic disorder of voltage gated sodium channels. J Invest Dermatol 2005; 124: 1333

17. Fertleman CR, Baker MD, Parker KA, et al: SCN9A mutations in paroxysmal extreme pain disorder: allelic variants underlie distinct channel defects and phenotypes. Neuron 2006; 52: 767

18. Cox JJ, Reimann F, Nicholas AK, et al: An SCN9A channelopathy causes congenital inability to experience pain. Nature 2006; 444: 894

19. Goldberg Y, Macfarlane J, Macdonald M, et al: Loss-of-function mutations in the Na(v) 1.7 gene underlie congenital indifference to pain in multiple human populations. Clin Genet 2007; 71: 311

20. Frazier DT, Narahashi T, Yamada M: The site of action and active form of local anesthetics. II. Experiments with quaternary compounds. J Pharmacol Exp Ther 1970; 171: 45

21. Ragsdale DS, McPhee JC, Scheuer T, et al: Molecular determinants of state-dependent block of Na+ channels by local anesthetics. Science 1994; 265: 1724

22. Scholz A: Mechanisms of (local) anaesthetics on voltage-gated sodium and other ion channels. Br J Anaesth 2002; 89: 52

23. Ulbricht W: Sodium channel inactivation: molecular determinants and modulation. Physiol Rev 2005; 85: 1271

24. Popitz-Bergez FA, Leeson S, Strichartz GR, et al: Relation between functional deficit and intraneural local anesthetic during peripheral nerve block. A study in the rat sciatic nerve. Anesthesiology 1995; 83: 583

25. Fink BR, Cairns AM: Differential slowing and block of conduction by lidocaine in individual afferent myelinated and unmyelinated axons. Anesthesiology 1984; 60: 111

26. Fink BR, Cairns AM: Differential use-dependent (frequency-dependent) effects in single mammalian axons: Data and clinical considerations. Anesthesiology 1987; 67: 477

27. Fink BR: Mechanisms of differential axial blockade in epidural and subarachnoid anesthesia. Anesthesiology 1989; 70: 851

28. Gasser HS, Erlanger J: The role of fiber size in the establishment of a nerve block by pressure or cocaine. Am J Physiol 1929; 88: 581

29. Gokin AP, Philip B, Strichartz GR: Preferential block of small myelinated sensory and motor fibers by lidocaine: in vivo electrophysiology in the rat sciatic nerve. Anesthesiology 2001; 95: 1441

30. Chevrier P, Vijayaragavan K, Chahine M: Differential modulation of Nav 1.7 and Nav 1.8 peripheral nerve sodium channels by the local anesthetic lidocaine. Br J Pharmacol 2004; 142: 576

31. Chernoff DM, Strichartz GR: Tonic and phasic block of neuronal sodium currents by 5-hydroxyhexano-2′,6′-xylide, a neutral lidocaine homologue. J Gen Physiol 1989: 93: 1075

32. Strichartz GR, Sanchez V, Arthur GR et al: Fundamental properties of local anesthetics. II. Measured octanol:buffer partition coefficients and pKa values of clinically used drugs. Anesth Analg 1990; 71: 158

33. Bokesch PM, Post C, Strichartz G: Structure-activity relationship of lidocaine homologs producing tonic and frequency-dependent impulse blockade in nerve. J Pharmacol Exp Ther 1986; 237: 773

34. Gissen AJ, Covino BG, Gregus J: Differential sensitivity of fast and slow fibers in mammalian nerve. III. Effect of etidocaine and bupivacaine on fast/slow fibers. Anesth Analg 1982; 61: 570

35. Johns RA, DiFazio CA, Longnecker DE: Lidocaine constricts or dilates rat arterioles in a dose-dependent manner. Anesthesiology 1985; 62: 141

36. Johns RA, Seyde WC, DiFazio CA, et al: Dose-dependent effects of bupivacaine on rat muscle arterioles. Anesthesiology 1986; 65: 186

37. Foster RH, Markham A: Levobupivacaine: A review of its pharmacology and use as a local anaesthetic. Drugs 2000; 59: 551

38. McClellan KJ, Faulds D: Ropivacaine: an update of its use in regional anaesthesia. Drugs 2000; 60: 1065

39. Neal JM: Effects of epinephrine in local anesthetics on the central and peripheral nervous systems: Neurotoxicity and neural blood flow. Reg Anesth Pain Med 2003; 28: 124

40. Sinnott CJ, Cogswell III LP, Johnson A, et al: On the mechanism by which epinephrine potentiates lidocaine's peripheral nerve block. Anesthesiology 2003; 98: 181

41. Curatolo M, Petersen-Felix S, Arendt-Nielsen L, et al: Epidural epinephrine and clonidine: Segmental analgesia and effects on different pain modalities. Anesthesiology 1997; 87: 785

42. Ueda W, Hirakawa M, Mori K: Acceleration of epinephrine absorption by lidocaine. Anesthesiology 1985; 63: 717

43. Magee C, Rodeheaver GT, Edgerton MT, et al: Studies of the mechanisms by which epinephrine damages tissue defenses. J Surg Res 1977; 23: 126

44. Hall JA, Ferro A: Myocardial ischaemia and ventricular arrhythmias precipitated by physiological concentrations of adrenaline in patients with coronary artery disease. Br Heart J 1992; 67: 419

45. Lambert DH: Clinical value of adding sodium bicarbonate to local anesthetics. Reg Anesth Pain Med 2002; 27: 328

46. Ikuta PT, Raza SM, Durrani Z: pH adjustment schedule for the amide local anesthetics. Reg Anesth 1989; 14: 229

47. Neal JM, Hebl JR, Gerancher JC, et al: Brachial plexus anesthesia: essentials of our current understanding. Reg Anesth Pain Med 2002; 27: 402

48. Sinnott CJ, Garfield JM, Thalhammer JG: Addition of sodium bicarbonate to lidocaine decreases the duration of peripheral nerve block in the rat. Anesthesiology 2000; 93: 1045

49. Wang C, Chakrabarti MK, Galletly DC, et al: Relative effects of intrathecal administration of fentanyl and midazolam on A delta and C fibre reflexes. Neuropharmacology 1992; 31: 439

50. Niv D, Nemirovsky A, Rudick V: Antinociception induced by simultaneous intrathecal and intraperitoneal administration of low doses of morphine. Anesth Analg 1995; 80: 886

51. Walker SM, Goudas LC, Cousins MJ, et al: Combination spinal analgesic chemotherapy: a systematic review. Anesth Analg 2002; 95: 674

52. Karambelkar DJ, Ramanathan S: 2-Chloroprocaine antagonism of epidural morphine analgesia. Acta Anaesth Scand 1997; 41: 774

53. Coda B, Bausch S, Haas M, et al: The hypothesis that antagonism of fentanyl analgesia by 2-chloroprocaine is mediated by direct action on opioid receptors. Reg Anesth 1997; 22: 43

54. Janson W, Stein C: Peripheral opioid analgesia. Curr Pharm Biotechnol 2003; 4: 270

55. Rosseland LA: No evidence for analgesic effect of intra-articular morphine after knee arthroscopy: A qualitative systematic review. Reg Anesth Pain Med 2005; 30: 83

56. Picard PR, Tramer MR, McQuay HJ, et al: Analgesic efficacy of peripheral opioids (all except intra-articular): A qualitative systematic review of randomised controlled trials. Pain 1997; 72: 309

57. Eisenach JC, De Kock M, Klimscha W: Alpha(2)-adrenergic agonists for regional anesthesia: A clinical review of clonidine (1984–1995). Anesthesiology 1996; 85: 655

58. Butterworth JF, Strichartz GR: The $α_2$-adrenergic agonists clonidine and guanfacine produce tonic and phasic block of conduction in rat sciatic nerve fibers. Anesth Analg 1993; 76: 295

59. Gaumann DM, Brunet PC, Jirounek P: Clonidine enhances the effects of lidocaine on C fiber action potential. Anesth Analg 1992; 74: 719

60. Pertovaara A, Hamalainen MM: Spinal potentiation and supraspinal additivity in the antinociceptive interaction between systemically administered $α_2$-adrenoreceptor agonist and cocaine in the rat. Anesth Analg 1994; 79: 261

61. Colin JL, McCartney ED, Apatu E: Should we add clonidine to local anesthetic for peripheral nerve blockade? A qualitative systematic review of the literature. Reg Anesth Pain Med 2007; 32: 330

62. Reuben SS, Steinberg RB, Klatt JL, et al: Intravenous regional anesthesia using lidocaine and clonidine. Anesthesiology 1999; 91:654

63. Morrison LM, Emanuelsson BM, McClure JH, et al: Efficacy and kinetics of extradural ropivacaine: Comparison with bupivacaine. Br J Anaesth 1994; 72: 164

64. Tucker GT, Mather LE: Pharmacology of local anaesthetic agents. Pharmacokinetics of local anaesthetic agents. Br J Anaesth 1975; 47(Suppl): 213

65. Thomson PD, Melmon KL, Richardson JA, et al: Lidocaine pharmacokinetics in advanced heart failure, liver disease, and renal failure in humans. Ann Intern Med 1973; 78: 499

66. Rosenberg PR, Veering BT, Urmey WF: Maximum recommended doses of local anesthetics: A multifactorial concept. Reg Anesth Pain Med 2004; 29: 564

67. Braid DP, Scott DB: Dosage of lignocaine in epidural block in relation to toxicity. Br J Anaesth 1996; 38: 596

68. Adinoff B, Devous MD Sr, Best SE, et al: Gender differences in limbic responsiveness, by SPECT, following pharmacologic challenge in healthy subjects. Neuroimage 2003; 18: 697

69. Tucker GT, Mather LE: Properties, absorption, and disposition of local anesthetic agents, Neural Blockade in Clinical Anesthesia and Management of Pain, 3rd edition. Edited by Cousins MJ, Bridenbaugh PO. Philadelphia, Lippincott–Raven Publishers, 1998, p 55

70. Liu SS, Richman JM, Thirlby RC, et al: Efficacy of continuous wound catheters delivering local anesthetic for postoperative analgesia: A quantitative and qualitative systematic review of randomized controlled trials. J Am Coll Surg. 2006; 203; 914

71. Lander JA, Weltman BJ, So SS: EMLA and amethocaine for reduction of children's pain associated with needle insertion. Cochrane Database Syst Rev 2006; 3: CD004236

72. Covino BG, Wildsmith JAW: Clinical pharmacology of local anesthetic agents, Neural Blockade in Clinical Anesthesia and Management of Pain, 3rd edition. Edited by Cousins MJ, Bridenbaugh PO. Philadelphia, Lippincott–Raven Publishers, 1998, p 97

ANESTHETIC AGENTS, ADJUVANTS, AND DRUG INTERACTION

73. Ugur B, Ogurlu M, Gezer E, et al: Effects of esmolol, lidocaine and fentanyl on haemodynamic responses to endotracheal intubation: A comparative study. Clin Drug Investig. 2007; 27: 269

74. Adamzik M, Groeben H, Farahani R, et al: Intravenous lidocaine after tracheal intubation mitigates bronchoconstriction in patients with asthma. Anesth Analg 2007; 104 :168

75. Yukioka H, Hayashi M, Terai T, et al: Intravenous lidocaine as a suppressant of coughing during tracheal intubation in elderly patients. Anesth Analg 1993; 77: 309

76. Nakayama M, Fujita S, Kanaya N, et al: Effect of intravenous lidocaine on intraabdominal pressure response to airway stimulation. Anesth Analg 1994; 78: 1149

77. Spöhr F, Wenzel V, Böttiger BW: Drug treatment and thrombolytics during cardiopulmonary resuscitation. Curr Opin Anaesthesiol 2006; 19: 157

78. Kaba A, Laurent SR, Detroz BJ, et al: Intravenous lidocaine infusion facilitates acute rehabilitation after laparoscopic colectomy. Anesthesiology 2007; 106: 11

79. Tremont-Lukats IW, Challapalli V, McNicol ED, et al: Systemic administration of local anesthetics to relieve neuropathic pain: a systematic review and meta-analysis. Anesth Analg 2005; 101: 1738

80. Yanagidate F, Strichartz GR: Local anesthetics. Handb Exp Pharmacol 2007; 177: 95

81. Cahana A, Carota A, Montadon ML et al: The long-term effect of repeated intravenous lidocaine on central pain and possible correlation in positron emission tomography measurements. Anesth Analg 2004; 98: 1581

82. Groban L: Central nervous system and cardiac effects from long-acting amide local anesthetic toxicity in the intact animal model. Reg Anesth Pain Med 2003; 28: 3

83. Shibata M, Shingu K, Murakawa M: Tetraphasic actions of local anesthetics on central nervous system electrical activity in cats. Reg Anesth 1994; 19: 255

84. Brown DL, Ransom DM, Hall JA, et al: Regional anesthesia and local anesthetic-induced systemic toxicity: Seizure frequency and accompanying cardiovascular changes. Anesth Analg 1995; 81: 321

85. Auroy Y, Benhamou D, Bargues L, et al: Major complications of regional anesthesia in France: The SOS Regional Anesthesia Hotline Service. Anesthesiology 2002; 97: 1274

86. Weinberg GL: Current concepts in resuscitation of patients with local anesthetic cardiac toxicity. Reg Anesth Pain Med 2002; 27: 568

87. Yokoyama M, Hirakawa M, Goto H: Effect of vasoconstrictive agents added to lidocaine on intravenous lidocaine-induced convulsions in rats. Anesthesiology 1995; 82: 574

88. Yamauchi Y, Kotani J, Ueda Y: The effects of exogenous epinephrine on a convulsive dose of lidocaine: Relationship with cerebral circulation. J Neurosurg Anesth 1998; 10: 178

89. Mayhan WG, Faraci FM, Siems JL: Role of molecular charge in disruption of the blood–brain barrier during acute hypertension. Circ Res 1989; 64: 658

90. Arthur GR, Feldman HS, Covino BG: Alterations in the pharmacokinetic properties of amide local anaesthetics following local anaesthetic induced convulsions. Acta Anaesthesiol Scand 1988; 32: 522

91. Lee LA, Posner KL, Domino KB, et al: Injuries associated with regional anesthesia in the 1980s and 1990s: A closed claim analysis. Anesthesiology 2004; 101: 143

92. Mather LE, Copeland SE, Ladd LA: Acute toxicity of local anesthetics: Underlying pharmacokinetic and pharmacodynamic concepts. Reg Anesth Pain Med 2005; 30: 553

93. Simpson D, Curran MP, Oldfield V, et al: Ropivacaine: a review of its use in regional anaesthesia and acute pain management. Drugs 2005; 65: 2675

94. Casati A, Putzu M: Bupivacaine, levobupivacaine and ropivacaine: are they clinically different? Best Pract Res Clin Anaesthesiol 2005; 19: 247

95. Strichartz GR, Sanchez V, Arthur GR: Fundamental properties of local anesthetics. II. Measured octanol:buffer partition coefficients and pK_a values of clinically used drugs. Anesth Analg 1990; 71: 158

96. Knudsen K, Beckman Suurkula M, Blomberg S, et al: Central nervous and cardiovascular effects of i.v. infusions of ropivacaine, bupivacaine and placebo in volunteers. Br J Anaesth 1997; 78: 507

97. Stewart J, Kellett N, Castro D: The central nervous system and cardiovascular effects of levobupivacaine and ropivacaine in healthy volunteers. Anesth Analg 2002; 97: 412

98. Heavner JE: Cardiac toxicity of local anesthetics in the intact isolated heart model: A review. Reg Anesth Pain Med 2002; 27: 545

99. Groban L, Deal DD, Vernon JC, et al: Does local anesthetic stereoselectivity or structure predict myocardial depression in anesthetized canines? Reg Anesth Pain Med 2002; 27: 460

100. Pickering AE, Waki H, Headley PM, et al: Investigation of systemic bupivacaine toxicity using the in situ perfused working heart-brainstem preparation of the rat. Anesthesiology 2002; 97: 1550

101. Chang KSK, Yang M, Andresen MC: Clinically relevant concentrations of bupivacaine inhibit rat aortic baroreceptors. Anesth Analg 1994; 78: 501

102. Hogan QH, Stadnicka A, Bosnjak ZJ, et al: Effects of lidocaine and bupivacaine on isolated rabbit mesenteric capacitance veins. Reg Anesth Pain Med 1998; 23: 409

103. Guo XT, Castle NA, Chernoff DM, et al: Comparative inhibition of voltage-gated cation channels by local anesthetics. Ann N Y Acad Sci 1991; 625: 181

104. Clarkson CW, Hondeghem LM: Mechanisms for bupivacaine depression of cardiac conduction: Fast block of sodium channels during the action potential with slow recovery from block during diastole. Anesthesiology 1985; 62: 396

105. Mio Y, Fukuda N, Kusakari Y, et al: Bupivacaine attenuates contractility by decreasing sensitivity of myofilaments to Ca2+ in rat ventricular muscle. Anesthesiology 2002; 97: 1168

106. Nouette-Gaulain K, Forestier F, Malgat M, et al: Effects of bupivacaine on mitochondrial energy metabolism in heart of rats following exposure to chronic hypoxia. Anesthesiology 2002; 97: 1507

107. Weinberg G: Lipid infusion resuscitation for local anesthetic toxicity: Proof of clinical efficacy. Anesthesiology 2006; 105: 7

108. Kitagawa N, Oda M, Totoki T: Possible mechanism of irreversible nerve injury caused by local anesthetics and membrane disruption. Anesthesiology 2004; 100: 962

109. Kalichman MW: Physiologic mechanisms by which local anesthetics may cause injury to nerve and spinal cord. Reg Anesth 1993; 18: 448

110. Selander D: Neurotoxicity of local anesthetics: Animal data. Reg Anesth 1993; 18: 461

111. Yamashita A, Matsumoto M, Matsumoto S, et al: A comparison of the neurotoxic effects on the spinal cord of tetracaine, lidocaine, bupivacaine, and ropivacaine administered intrathecally in rabbits. Anesth Analg 2003; 97: 512

112. Bainton C, Strichartz G: Concentration dependence of lidocaine-induced irreversible conduction loss in frog nerve. Anesthesiology 1994; 81: 657

113. Lambert L, Lambert D, Strichartz G: Irreversible conduction block in isolated nerve by high concentrations of local anesthetics. Anesthesiology 1994; 80: 1082

114. Brull R, McCartney CJL, Chan VWS, et al: Neurological complications after regional anesthesia: contemporary estimates of risk. Anesth Analg 2007; 104: 965

115. Pollock JE: Transient neurologic symptoms: Etiology, risk factors, and management. Reg Anesth Pain Med 2002; 27: 581

116. Zaric D, Christiansen C, Pace NL, et al: Transient neurologic symptoms after spinal anesthesia with lidocaine versus other local anesthetics: A systematic review of randomized, controlled trials. Anesth Analg 2005; 100: 1811

117. Pollock JE, Liu SS, Neal JM, et al: Dilution of lidocaine does not reduce the incidence of transient neurologic symptoms. Anesthesiology 1999; 90: 445

118. Zink W, Bohl JRE, Hacke N, et al: The long term myotoxic effects of bupivacaine and ropivacaine after continuous peripheral nerve blocks. Anesth Analg 2005; 101: 548

119. Boren E, Teuber SS, Naguwa SM, et al: A critical review of local anesthetic sensitivity. Clin Rev Allergy Immunol. 2007; 32: 119

120. Finder RL, Moore PA: Adverse drug reactions to local anesthesia. Dent Clin North Am 2002; 46: 747

CHAPTER 22 ■ DRUG INTERACTIONS

CARL E. ROSOW AND WILTON C. LEVINE

KEY POINTS

1 Drug combinations are a useful and necessary part of anesthesia practice, but they are occasionally a source of morbidity. The qualitative nature of most anesthetic interactions is predictable even though the magnitude of the response might not be known with certainty. Drugs that interact to produce a totally unexpected or dangerous effect stand out because of their rarity.

2 A *pharmaceutical* interaction is a chemical or physical interaction that occurs before a drug is administered or absorbed systemically.

3 A *pharmacokinetic* interaction occurs when one drug alters the absorption, distribution, metabolism, or elimination of another.

4 A *pharmacodynamic* interaction occurs when one drug alters the sensitivity of a target receptor or tissue to the effects of a second drug. We commonly classify these interactions by their direction and intensity, that is, additive, antagonistic, or supra-additive (synergistic).

5 *Additive interactions* are most likely to occur when drugs with identical mechanisms are combined.

6 The most common *antagonistic interactions* are those involving deliberate reversal with competitive antagonists. Antagonism that is unintended is a much less common event.

7 *Synergistic interaction* is most likely to occur when drugs with different mechanisms are combined.

8 Most cardiovascular drug–drug interactions are simply extensions of the known pharmacology of the agents. With few exceptions, there is little reason to withhold most vasoactive medications before surgery.

9 Combinations of central nervous system (CNS) depressants almost always produce additive or synergistic increases in CNS effect. These interactions are usually useful and predictable.

10 Among the thousands of herbal preparations available, only a few have been documented to cause problems either through intrinsic toxicity or pharmacokinetic and pharmacodynamic interactions. There are no studies demonstrating specific adverse interactions between herbals and anesthetic drugs.

Modern drug regimens for medical ailments such as hypertension, angina, bronchospasm, or malignancy nearly always involve the use of multiple agents. This strategy is frequently successful because many medical conditions are responsive to groups of drugs that act by different mechanisms and have different dose-limiting toxicities. The goal in each case is to produce an increased therapeutic effect with decreased toxicity compared with treatment with individual agents. Unfortunately, the mixing of drugs is not without risk, and hundreds of research articles on the benefits and drawbacks of drug interactions appear every year. A sizable industry has now evolved to provide clinicians with reference books and computer databases on the subject.

Anesthesiologists face the same dilemma as all other physicians: drug combinations are a useful and necessary part of practice, but they are occasionally a source of morbidity. This

chapter reviews the reasons that drugs are combined and the ways in which the combinations can alter either pharmacokinetics or pharmacodynamics. This is *not* a comprehensive list of anesthetic drug interactions—entire books have been devoted to the subject.[1] The examples included have been chosen largely on the basis of proven or likely clinical relevance and the strength of their documentation. When possible, prototypical interactions are illustrated with examples that have direct relevance to anesthesia, although in some cases no such examples are available. The emphasis throughout is on mechanism, but it will quickly be apparent that our understanding of mechanism is incomplete for many pharmacodynamic interactions. Finally, it is important to know how to read the relevant literature, and a short section is devoted to some of the common ways interactions can be studied.

HISTORICAL PERSPECTIVE

Historically, anesthesiologists were trained to regard drug interactions as a danger and something to be avoided. The generations of clinicians who administered open-drop diethyl ether probably had good reason to limit the number of anesthetic drugs administered: ether by itself could produce hypnosis, reasonable levels of analgesia, and muscle relaxation. Ventilation and blood pressure were usually well maintained because ether has respiratory stimulant and sympathomimetic properties. Clinicians could adjust the dose of this single agent fairly accurately using Guedel's criteria for pupil size, respiratory pattern, muscle tone, and so forth. This meant that a patient requiring even major abdominal surgery could be anesthetized using nothing more than a can of ether and a simple mask.

Before World War II, endotracheal intubation and controlled ventilation were usually not options, and muscle relaxants had not been introduced. Clinicians in this era were well served to keep things simple: if an anesthesiologist chose to add morphine to an ether anesthetic, the pupil and respiratory signs would no longer be reliable, muscle relaxation would probably decrease, and ventilatory depression (if it occurred) could not be treated easily.

The introduction of muscle relaxants, opioid-based anesthesia, and modern intravenous (IV) and inhaled anesthetics completely changed these considerations. The signs and stages of ether anesthesia are no longer applicable, and controlled or assisted ventilation is often necessary because most of these drugs have profound effects on respiration. Most importantly, clinicians now realize that anesthetics are highly specific drugs, and no single agent can produce all the "desirable" components of anesthesia. There is good evidence that even the potent volatile anesthetics are not sufficient to produce optimal anesthetic conditions when given alone. Zbinden, et al.[2] showed that even moderately high concentrations of isoflurane in oxygen cannot suppress many cardiovascular responses to surgical stimuli. This finding is reflected in common clinical practice because isoflurane is routinely supplemented with opioids and other drugs to control blood pressure and heart rate.

Our views of what is desirable in anesthesia have also changed markedly. For example, most patients now expect and prefer an IV hypnotic, rather than a mask, for anesthetic induction. Similarly, the long emergence after ether is no longer expected or acceptable. A smooth recovery, free of pain or delirium, is now common within minutes after major surgical interventions. These goals are difficult to accomplish without using multiple drugs.

PROBLEMS CREATED BY DRUG–DRUG INTERACTIONS

❶ There are almost no data on the true incidence of perioperative drug interaction, although there are data on general inpatient populations. It is logical that the probability of drug–drug interaction increases with the number of drugs administered.[3] Many patients are routinely taking three or four antihypertensives, antidepressants, or gastrointestinal drugs in the preoperative period. Most also receive five to ten drugs during general anesthesia, but we do not normally hear about significant complications attributable to drug interaction. There are a number of possible explanations for this:

1. Interactions may occur, but they usually do not present a problem. Toxicity from a drug interaction is likely to become a source of morbidity primarily when it occurs in a setting where it is not rapidly recognized and treated. For example, this can happen when opioid and midazolam combinations are used by untrained personnel for endoscopic, radiologic, and outpatient procedures performed under "conscious sedation". The unexpectedly large sedative and ventilatory effects can lead to death.[4]
2. Many of the effects introduced by mixing drugs are hard to distinguish from clinical "noise." Variability in response to anesthetic drugs is the rule: the data on IV opioids[5] and hypnotics,[6] for example, show that different patients may have a three- to fivefold difference in the therapeutic and toxic effects of a given dose—even when the drug is given alone.
3. The qualitative nature of most anesthetic interactions is predictable even though the magnitude of the responses might not be known with certainty. Combining two cardiovascular depressants will produce more hypotension; two CNS depressants will produce more sedation, and so forth. Drugs that interact to produce a totally unexpected or dangerous effect stand out because of their rarity. A notorious example of such an idiosyncratic interaction is the CNS excitation that may occur when meperidine is administered to patients taking monoamine oxidase inhibitors (MAOIs).
4. Many IV anesthetic drugs (diazepam, fentanyl) have large safety margins—especially when respiration is supported—so changes in drug effect have few consequences. The mere fact that a measurable interaction exists does not mean it will cause a difference in outcome or the need for intervention. Dangerous interactions most often involve drugs such as warfarin, digoxin, and theophylline, agents with only small differences between therapeutic and toxic concentrations.
5. Finally, it is likely that many instances of anesthetic drug interaction go unrecognized. Excessive drug effects are often attributed to some ill-defined patient "sensitivity." When a drug *fails* to produce an effect, it is because the patient is "tolerant" or "resistant." It is almost never considered a drug reaction or interaction.

WHY COMBINE DRUGS?

The goal of combining drugs is to decrease toxicity while maintaining or increasing efficacy. It is instructive to see how this principle has been applied in other areas of medicine:

1. Combination therapy can reduce toxicity. For example, a β-adrenergic antagonist and a vasodilator have at least additive effects on blood pressure, but their side effects are different and (presumably) nonadditive. Lower doses of each drug may be used in combination so dose-related side effects are decreased.
2. Combination chemotherapy for malignancy can increase efficacy. To produce the maximum decrease in tumor burden, each chemotherapeutic drug is given at its maximally tolerated dose, an end point determined by its toxic effects on some normal cell population. Drugs such as alkylating agents and vinca alkaloids are combined because they have different dose-limiting organ toxicities (bone marrow and nerve, respectively), so each drug can be given at a full tumor-suppressing dose.
3. Single-drug therapy is sometimes preferable. The mainstay drugs for prophylaxis of seizures (phenytoin, carbamazepine) have similar dose-limiting side effects such as ataxia and drowsiness, so there is little to be gained by combining them.

PHARMACEUTICAL INTERACTIONS

❷ A *pharmaceutical* interaction is a chemical or physical interaction that occurs before a drug is administered or absorbed systemically. The most obvious pharmaceutical interactions are the incompatibilities that can occur between drugs in solution:

- Precipitation of thiopental may occur when it is injected together with succinylcholine into the IV catheter line.
- Bicarbonate can decrease the solubility of bupivacaine and cause it to precipitate.
- Catecholamine solutions (norepinephrine, epinephrine) can be inactivated if they are alkalinized by the addition of sodium bicarbonate, a circumstance that could occur during cardiopulmonary resuscitation.

The number of these incompatibilities is large, and the anesthesiologist should avoid mixing drugs unless they are known to be compatible. Information on specific IV drug incompatibilities is readily available from most hospital pharmacists.

Occasionally, two drugs may interact chemically to form a toxic compound:

- The halogenated anesthetics—desflurane, enflurane, and isoflurane—have been shown to interact with dry soda lime or Baralyme to produce carbon monoxide[7] and heat.[8] Desiccation of soda lime is most likely to occur when oxygen has been left flowing through the canister overnight. Older anesthesiologists recall that trichloroethylene interacted with soda lime to produce the neurotoxin, dichloroacetylene.
- Nitric oxide (NO) is a selective pulmonary vasodilator that has been approved in the United States for treatment of primary pulmonary hypertension in the newborn. If NO is allowed more than fleeting contact with oxygen, it forms nitrogen dioxide (NO_2). The latter compound can be quite toxic, and concentrations >10 ppm can produce pulmonary edema and alveolar hemorrhage. The problem is circumvented by allowing oxygen and NO to mix in the breathing circuit just before administration.

PHARMACOKINETIC INTERACTIONS

❸ A *pharmacokinetic* interaction occurs when one drug alters the absorption, distribution, metabolism, or elimination of another. Many of the basic pharmacokinetic principles underlying these interactions are reviewed in Chapter 7.

Absorption

Alteration of absorption may occur because of direct chemical or physical interaction between drugs in the body or because one drug alters the physiologic mechanisms governing absorption of the second:

- Orally administered tetracycline can be inactivated by chelation if it is given together with antacids containing polyvalent cations such as Mg^{2+}, Ca^{2+}, or Al^{3+}.
- Oral antidiarrheal drugs such as kaolin and pectin can physically adsorb digoxin and prevent it from being absorbed.
- The bile acid-binding resin, cholestyramine, can bind to warfarin and prevent its absorption. It can also reduce the absorption of vitamin K and other fat-soluble compounds.

Another interaction of significance to anesthesiologists is the delay of gastric emptying produced by medications such as opioids and anticholinergics. Opioids produce hypertonus of smooth muscle, reduction of peristalsis, and contraction of sphincters throughout the gastrointestinal tract, and it appears that both central and peripheral mechanisms play a role in this

effect. Murphy, et al.[9] gave volunteers 500 mL of distilled water to drink and showed that 0.09 mg/kg of morphine increased the half-time for gastric emptying from 5.5 to 21 minutes. Morphine can also reduce the absorption of orally administered drugs because the primary site for absorption is the small intestine, and gastric emptying is rate-limiting. Asai, et al.[10] demonstrated that morphine significantly reduces the absorption of oral acetaminophen in patients.

Changes in regional blood flow (vasodilators, vasoconstrictors) can affect the absorption of parenterally administered drugs. Shock or congestive heart failure decreases perfusion of peripheral tissues such as skin and muscle, so the onset and intensity of effect may become unpredictable for drugs given by intramuscular or subcutaneous injection:

- Local administration of epinephrine and other vasoconstrictors retard absorption of infiltrated local anesthetics and therefore prolong their effects.
- Drugs that decrease effective pulmonary ventilation have the potential to reduce the uptake of volatile anesthetics. Drugs that increase minute ventilation, reduce intrapulmonary shunting, or relieve bronchospasm can increase the uptake of volatile anesthetics even though the inspired concentration remains constant.
- The rapid uptake of nitrous oxide can increase the alveolar concentration of concomitantly administered volatile anesthetics (the "second gas effect").

Distribution

Many drug–drug interactions occur when one drug alters the distribution of a second. This may occur because of alterations in hemodynamics, drug ionization, or binding to plasma and tissue proteins. Much has been written about the involvement of these mechanisms in drug interactions (particularly the last two), but there are few examples of proven relevance to anesthesia.

Drugs such as volatile anesthetics, beta-blockers, calcium channel blockers, and vasodilators can decrease cardiac output and produce significant changes in drug distribution. A decrease in cardiac output increases the arterial concentrations of other drugs in highly perfused tissues such as the brain and myocardium[11]:

- In a patient with depressed cardiac function, normal doses of IV agents such as propofol, thiopental, and remifentanil can produce substantially greater cardiovascular and CNS effects. This can be due to an increase in tissue drug concentrations or an increase in tissue sensitivity to the effects of the drug.[12–14]
- The same effect is seen with volatile anesthetics. Low cardiac output increases end-tidal concentrations and intensifies cardiovascular and CNS effects.

Drug-induced changes in pH in a particular body region or fluid compartment can alter the distribution of other drugs by so-called "ion trapping." Most of our therapeutic agents are weak acids or bases that are partially ionized at normal body pH. It is only the nonionized fraction that can cross lipid membranes and come to equilibrium. The amount ionized can be determined for acids or bases from the general form of the Henderson-Hasselbalch equation:

$$\frac{[\text{Protonated}]}{[\text{Unprotonated}]} = 10^{(pk_a - pH)}$$

Recall that an unprotonated acid is ionized, whereas an unprotonated base is nonionized. It is apparent from this relationship that a weak base (fentanyl, lidocaine) will be progressively ionized as the pH decreases, whereas a weak acid (aspirin, phenobarbital) will be more nonionized.

For certain membrane barriers, such as those in the stomach, placenta, or renal tubules, the pH on either side is very different, and this creates the necessary conditions for ion trapping. Consider the case of a weak acid (ionization constant $[pK_a] = 3.4$) that is distributing between stomach and blood. In stomach acid (pH 2.4), the ratio of uncharged to charge drug is:

$$\frac{[\text{Nonionized}]}{[\text{Ionized}]} = 10^{(3.4 - 2.4)} = 10$$

In blood (pH 7.4),

$$\frac{[\text{Nonionized}]}{[\text{Ionized}]} = 10^{(3.4 - 2.4)} = 0.0001$$

At equilibrium, the concentrations of nonionized (uncharged) drug must be the same on either side of the gastric membrane barrier. This means that a 10,000-fold concentration gradient is established for total drug (nonionized + ionized):

	■ STOMACH (pH 2.4)	■ BLOOD (pH 7.4)
Nonionized drug	1	1
Ionized drug	0.1	10,000
Total drug	1.1	10,001

It is easy to see why weak acids such as aspirin are well absorbed from the stomach. The potential for drug interaction is great. Even moderate changes in pH can have large effects on this equilibrium—raising intragastric pH to 5.4 decreases the concentration gradient by 100-fold:

- Administration of antacids, histamine type 2 receptor antagonists, or proton pump inhibitors such as omeprazole can reduce the gastric absorption of some acidic drugs. Alteration of pH has been shown to change the oral bioavailability of ketoconazole[15] and midazolam.[16]
- Lipid-soluble basic drugs such as fentanyl and meperidine can diffuse *into* the stomach from the bloodstream. They become ionized and trapped in gastric acid only to be reabsorbed when they enter the more alkaline environment of the proximal jejunum. This gastric "recycling" is believed to be the basis for secondary increases in plasma concentrations of these opioids.[17]
- Alteration of urine pH can markedly affect the renal clearance of certain drugs (described in "Drug Elimination").

Much has been written about the role of plasma protein binding in drug–drug interaction. The fraction of a dose that remains intravascular is either free or bound to circulating proteins. Acidic drugs usually bind to albumin and various globulin fractions. Many basic drugs such as meperidine, lidocaine, bupivacaine, and propranolol bind to α_1-acid glycoprotein, an acute-phase reactant. Drug binding by α_1-acid glycoprotein can increase after surgery and in certain other conditions such as burns, myocardial infarction, trauma, and malignancies. Conversely, hepatic cirrhosis and the nephrotic syndrome are often accompanied by hypoproteinemia and decreases in both albumin and globulin binding.

The extent to which drug is bound versus free is important because it is only the unbound fraction that is available for crossing membranes, entering tissues, and binding to receptors to produce the pharmacologic effect. Protein-bound drug is not filtered by a normal glomerulus and (for some drugs) is not acted on by drug-metabolizing enzymes. A drug that is highly bound to plasma protein effectively exists in a "depot," not unlike a drug given by deep intramuscular injection. The potential therefore exists that one drug could alter the disposition, clearance, or biological effect of another by affecting its binding:

- The classic example of such an interaction is drug displacement of bilirubin in infants. Premature infants have immature glucuronyl transferase and are unable to conjugate bilirubin formed by destruction of erythrocytes. Much of the load of unconjugated bilirubin is bound to albumin and thus prevented from entering tissues. Sulfonamides and other drugs can compete for albumin-binding sites, and the bilirubin they displace can enter tissues. Excessive levels of bilirubin in the brain can lead to kernicterus, a potentially fatal problem. This effect was discovered accidentally in 1956 during a clinical drug trial. When premature infants were given a penicillin-sulfonamide mixture, the mortality rate increased, and many were found to have kernicterus at autopsy.[18]
- The same mechanism has been postulated for numerous drug–drug interactions. Highly bound, potentially toxic drugs such as warfarin and phenytoin may be displaced by other highly bound drugs. Warfarin is >98% bound to albumin, meaning that only 1 to 2% of the circulating drug accounts for the entire biological effect. Phenylbutazone is a nonsteroidal anti-inflammatory drug (NSAID) that competes effectively for the same binding sites. If phenylbutazone displaces only 2% of warfarin, this theoretically doubles the free (active) fraction and greatly increases the warfarin effect.

This type of drug–drug interaction has been dogma for years, but it is nearly impossible to find documented evidence that it causes harm[19]:

1. Most drugs are widely distributed in the body, so most of the administered dose is *extravascular*—two thirds of the total dose in the case of warfarin. Even a large change in plasma unbound fraction (e.g., 10%) will therefore release only 3 to 4% of total warfarin in the body.
2. The body acts as a sink or buffer against large changes in unbound fraction (any unbound drug in plasma is rapidly distributed into peripheral tissues).

Some caution is still warranted for anesthesiologists and other clinicians who use IV drug regimens with doses often in the toxic range (e.g., high doses of opioids, hypnotics, and muscle relaxants). In these circumstances, it is possible that even a temporary change in free drug concentration can have clinical consequences.

Metabolism

There are numerous examples in anesthesia of drugs that increase or decrease the metabolism of others. Interactions may occur in extrahepatic or hepatic sites of metabolism.

Many drugs—especially those with ester linkages—undergo hydrolysis by specific or nonspecific esterases found in blood and peripheral tissues:

- Drugs given to inhibit acetylcholinesterase at the motor end plate usually inhibit butyrylcholinesterase (pseudocholinesterase) in plasma. Thus, administration of neostigmine or pyridostigmine intensifies and prolongs the effects of succinylcholine and can also theoretically affect ester local anesthetics (procaine, chloroprocaine, tetracaine, cocaine). Enzyme inhibition needs to be substantial (<20% of normal activity remaining) before the clinical effects of these local anesthetics become prolonged.[20,21] The prolongation of effect depends on the specific inhibitor. Neostigmine, for example, can prolong the effect of succinylcholine by several hours. The organophosphate, echothiophate, is a powerful miotic used topically for refractory glaucoma. This compound irreversibly inhibits pseudocholinesterase,[20,22] and the effect persists for weeks, so the risk for interaction is prolonged.

- Drugs such as esmolol and remifentanil are hydrolyzed by so-called nonspecific esterases in blood and peripheral tissues. These drugs are not good substrates for cholinesterases, so they are not subject to this interaction.[23] The nonspecific esterases constitute a large group of isozymes with extremely high capacity and low substrate specificity. This enzyme system is not likely to be involved in drug–drug interactions because inhibition of any one isozyme usually does not affect overall drug clearance.

Monamide Oxidase Interactions

The enzyme, monamide oxidase (MAO), is distributed throughout the body, with the largest amounts found in the liver, kidney, and brain. MAO is located on the outer surface of mitochondria in the presynaptic terminals of noradrenergic, dopaminergic, and serotonergic neurons in the CNS and periphery. It acts to regulate the presynaptic pool of norepinephrine, dopamine, epinephrine, and serotonin available for synaptic transmission (see Chapter 15). MAO exists in two isoforms: MAO-A predominates in the gut wall, whereas MAO-B is the major isoform in the CNS.

The MAOIs are used mainly for the treatment of refractory endogenous depression and certain other mood disorders. They have gained some notoriety in medicine because they are the cause of more clinically important drug–drug interactions than almost any other class of drugs. Many of the purported interactions are poorly documented, although they cannot be discounted completely.

There are currently only three MAOIs marketed in the United States. Phenelzine (Nardil) is an older, nonselective MAOI derived from hydrazine. It irreversibly inhibits the enzyme, and synthesis of new enzyme can take 10 to 14 days. Tranylcypromine (Parnate) is a slightly shorter-acting MAOI derived from amphetamine. The newest member of this class is selegiline (deprenyl, Eldepryl), which is used as an adjunct in the treatment of Parkinson disease. In lower doses, selegiline is relatively selective for MAO-B. The antibiotics, furazolidone and linezolid, and the chemotherapeutic drug, procarbazine, also cause substantial inhibition of MAO and can potentially cause many of the same interactions.

Reported MAOI interactions are broadly of two types: the first group involves drugs that affect sympathetic neurotransmission:

- The well-known interaction with indirect-acting sympathomimetic drugs (ephedrine, amphetamine) occurs because MAOI treatment increases the amount of presynaptic transmitter that can be released by these drugs. Normal doses of ephedrine have produced severe hypertensive crises, occasionally leading to cerebral hemorrhage and death.
- The "wine and cheese" reaction is essentially the same interaction. Many foods such as aged cheese contain tyramine, a phenylethylamine that has ephedrinelike actions at sympathetic nerve endings. Normally, exogenous tyramine is degraded by MAO-A in the gut wall and liver, but patients taking an MAOI may achieve high systemic concentrations and consequently have hypertensive crises. Selegiline is now being marketed in a transdermal patch formulation (Emsam) that may reduce the exposure of gut and liver MAO to the inhibitor. This would not be expected to reduce the interactions with IV agents, however.
- Paradoxically, a patient who has been taking an MAOI for some time may actually have *decreased* adrenergic responsiveness (some of the older MAOIs were marketed as treatments for hypertension). Even with good dietary compliance, these patients absorb some tyramine. Chronic exposure to low levels of tyramine allows this compound to be taken up by adrenergic terminals (in place of tyrosine), where it is metabolized to octopamine (rather than norepinephrine). Octopamine is a "false transmitter" with little activity, so sympathetic nerve function may eventually be impaired.
- Because MAO plays only a small role in the metabolism of compounds in the synaptic cleft, the response to sympathomimetics that act directly on postsynaptic receptor sites (phenylephrine, norepinephrine, epinephrine) should be affected less by such interactions. In a small study of four healthy volunteers (two receiving tranylcypromine and two receiving phenelzine), there was a moderate (twofold) increase in the response to phenylephrine, but the responses to norepinephrine and epinephrine were not exaggerated.[24] This is reassuring, but any sympathomimetic drug should still be administered with caution to patients taking an MAOI.
- Adverse interactions have been described with older MAOIs and levodopa, possibly because both drugs increase dopamine concentrations. Nevertheless, there is some experience that levodopa and selegiline may be combined safely in patients with Parkinson disease. The MAOI is given in this case to decrease the clearance of levodopa from brain tissue and to prevent free radical formation believed to be involved in neuronal degeneration.[25]
- Inhibition of norepinephrine reuptake by tricyclic antidepressants (TCAs) increases the amount of neurotransmitter in the synaptic cleft. This would seem to be a recipe for adverse interaction with MAOIs, but with careful monitoring, this combination has been used successfully for therapy.

The second group of MAOI interactions involves CNS depressants. As stated previously, some of these are poorly documented, and the mechanisms are unknown:

- The most important interaction is unquestionably with meperidine and other drugs that inhibit serotonin reuptake. When meperidine is given to a patient taking an MAOI, a life-threatening "serotonin syndrome" may occur, accompanied by excitation, hyperpyrexia, hypertension, profuse sweating, and rigidity.[26] This may progress to seizures, coma, and death. The reaction does not occur in every instance. It has also been described with selegiline,[27] and case reports suggest that toxic interactions may occur with the antitussive, dextromethorphan,[28] and the analgesics, propoxyphene,[29] and tramadol.[26] Other than some poorly documented case reports, the evidence suggests that morphine and fentanyl do not produce this interaction.[30]
- Anecdotal reports have appeared regarding adverse MAOI interactions with other psychotropic drugs, including alcohol, phenothiazine, benzodiazepines, and barbiturates,[31] but the evidence is weak. Some wines, such as Chianti, could be dangerous because they contain tyramine. It is possible (but probably not advisable) to use ketamine for induction of anesthesia in patients taking an MAOI.[32]

Should MAOIs be discontinued before elective surgery? The issue is still a matter of debate,[33,34] although drug package inserts usually advise an extremely conservative position (i.e., waiting 2 weeks for the enzyme to regenerate). Current clinical opinion probably favors continuing MAOI therapy up to the time of surgery, and our own experience supports this view. Most patients are receiving these drugs for moderate-to-severe psychiatric disorders that have not responded to other treatments. It is unpleasant and possibly risky for a patient

FIGURE 22-1.   The effects of increasing or decreasing hepatic blood flow with isoproterenol (**A**) and norepinephrine (NE) (**B**) on steady-state arterial lidocaine concentrations in the rhesus monkey. The pressors were administered during the period indicated by the *shaded bar*. The *dashed lines* show the steady-state concentration expected in the absence of pressors. (Reprinted from Benowitz NL, Forsyth RP, Melmon KL, et al: Lidocaine disposition kinetics in monkey and man: II. Effects of hemorrhage and sympathomimetic drug administration. Clin Pharmacol Ther 1974; 16: 99, with permission.)

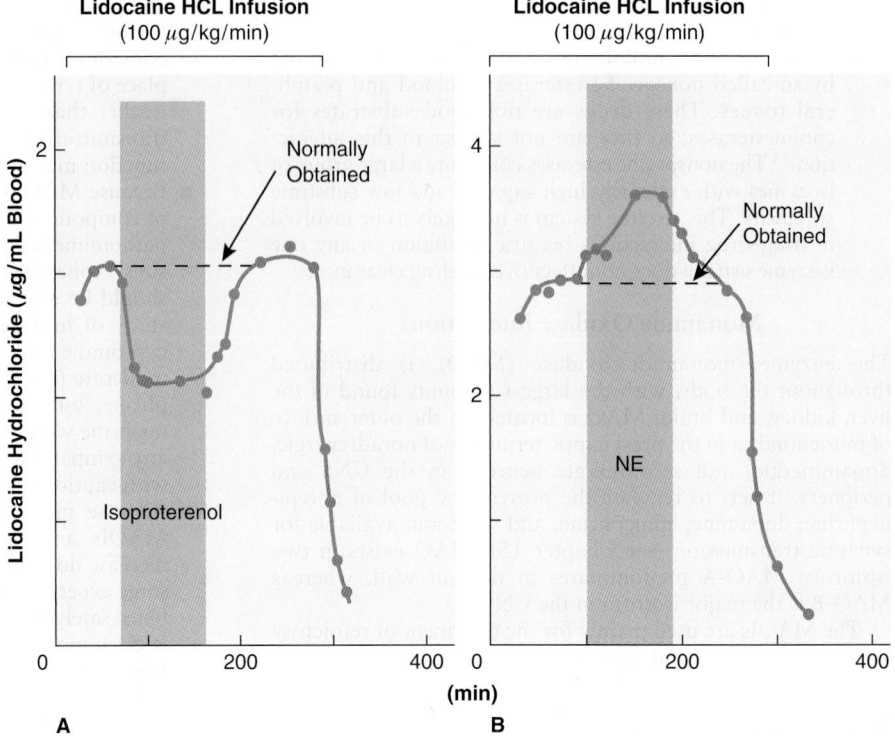

Hepatic Biotransformation

Many anesthetic drugs undergo oxidative metabolism by one of the isoforms of cytochrome P450 found in liver microsomes. The P450 isoforms have low substrate specificity, which means that drugs of diverse structures, such as general inhalation anesthetics, meperidine, barbiturates, and benzodiazepines, can be biotransformed by a single group of enzymes. It is not surprising that inhibitors or inducers of these enzymes can also affect the clearance of broad groups of drugs.

The removal of drug from the blood by hepatic biotransformation (hepatic clearance) is a function of two independent variables, the hepatic blood flow and the intrinsic clearance (the maximal ability of the liver to metabolize that drug). The intrinsic clearance is often expressed as the *extraction ratio* (ER)—the fraction of drug that can be metabolized in a single pass through the liver (see Chapter 7).

$$ER = \frac{C_a - C_v}{C_a}$$

with refractory depression to endure 2 to 3 weeks without effective therapy. If a general anesthetic is planned, it seems prudent to use the fewest possible drugs. Avoiding drugs with substantial sympathetic effects (e.g., pancuronium, cocaine, ketamine) probably makes sense.

There is little doubt that patients taking MAOIs have the potential for perioperative hemodynamic instability, yet beta-blockers, direct vasodilators, and direct-acting pressors appear to be safe and effective treatments in most circumstances. Roizen[35] concluded, "The major problem with continuing MAO inhibitors preoperatively is not the hemodynamic fluctuations that might occur . . . but rather the rare instance of hyperpyrexic coma following narcotic administration. . . ." Because opioids such as fentanyl appear safe and there are no major interactions with local anesthetics or NSAIDs, providing analgesia without meperidine should not be a hardship.

where C_a is the drug concentration coming to the liver (mixed portal vein + hepatic artery) and C_v is the drug concentration leaving (hepatic vein). So,

$$\text{Hepatic clearance} = ER \times \text{hepatic blood flow}$$

Drugs may be classed broadly as "high extraction" and "low extraction," a distinction with important implications for drug interaction:

A high-extraction drug (e.g., lidocaine, propranolol) may have an ER of 0.7 to 0.8 or more (70 to 80% is cleared in one pass through the liver). For these drugs, hepatic blood flow is the rate-limiting factor in overall hepatic clearance, that is, the delivery of drug to the liver determines the amount cleared. Clearance is decreased by drugs or maneuvers that lower hepatic blood flow, such as beta-blockade, cimetidine, halothane, hypotension, and upper abdominal surgery. The clearance of these rapidly metabolized drugs is much less sensitive to changes in enzyme activity. Nor does plasma protein binding have a large effect; the enzymes are so active that a drug such as lidocaine is simply stripped off its binding proteins as it traverses the liver:

- Decreases in hepatic blood flow secondary to decreased cardiac output elevate lidocaine concentrations in humans.[36]
- Pressor administration can also accomplish the same thing. This effect was elegantly demonstrated by Benowitz, et al.[37] in rhesus monkeys (Fig. 22-1). Steady-state infusions of lidocaine were established, then hepatic blood flow was increased or decreased by infusions of isoproterenol or norepinephrine, respectively. During isoproterenol infusion, the concentration of lidocaine decreased, indicating increased clearance. During norepinephrine infusion, lidocaine concentrations increased.
- Lidocaine clearance is decreased and toxicity is increased when patients are treated chronically with cimetidine.[38] It is not clear whether single-dose premedication with cimetidine produces the same effect.

- Other high-extraction drugs, such as morphine and sufentanil, are affected the same way. The clearance of morphine may be very slow in a patient with decreased hepatic blood flow.

Low-extraction drugs such as diazepam, alfentanil, or mepivacaine have ERs of 0.3 or less. These drugs behave quite differently because hepatic enzyme activity is rate-limiting (hepatic clearance is limited by intrinsic clearance). Stimulation or inhibition of enzyme activity can have a large effect on overall pharmacokinetics. Protein binding is also more likely to affect clearance because the bound forms of these drugs are protected from hepatic metabolism. The most common reason for increased intrinsic clearance is enzyme induction. Many drugs of importance in anesthesiology are metabolized by the cytochrome P450 enzymes (so-called microsomal or CYP enzymes). Several families and numerous subfamilies of these enzymes have been identified based on the homology of their amino acid sequences. The most important subfamily appears to be CYP3A, which is found in greatest abundance in human liver and is responsible for the metabolism of a huge number of drugs. Other subfamilies play important roles in drug metabolism, such as CYP2C19 (diazepam) or CYP2E1 (defluorination of volatile anesthetics). There are hundreds of drugs and environmental toxins that can stimulate or "induce" microsomal enzymes. Typically, a single inducer can affect the products of several gene families. For example, phenobarbital can increase the amount of the P450 enzymes CYP2B, 2C, 2E, 3A, and 4B.[39] An increase in the quantity of enzyme protein can therefore increase the clearance of many drugs simultaneously. However, not all inducers affect the same enzymes.

Treatment with an enzyme inducer (Table 22-1) can make an otherwise stable drug regimen ineffective or inconsistently effective:

- A classic example is the interaction between phenobarbital and coumarin-type anticoagulants (Fig. 22-2). Increased metabolism may also result in the production of an active or toxic metabolite.
- In rat microsomal preparations, the liberation of inorganic fluoride by isoflurane, methoxyflurane, and enflurane can be increased by pretreatment with barbiturates,[40] but this interaction appears to be clinically important only for methoxyflurane.[41] In humans, phenobarbital does not induce defluorination of enflurane.
- Reductive pathways also involve P450 enzymes, and the production of toxic reduced intermediates has been postulated as a mechanism for "halothane hepatitis." In animal models, administration of halothane after enzyme inducers can lead to centrilobular necrosis.[42] The clinical relevance of this finding is unknown.

There are many examples of drugs that inhibit the hepatic biotransformation of other drugs (Table 22-1):

TABLE 22-1

DRUGS THAT INDUCE OR INHIBIT HEPATIC DRUG METABOLISM IN HUMANS

INDUCERS	INHIBITORS
Phenobarbital	Cimetidine
Phenytoin	Ketoconazole
Rifampicin	Erythromycin
Carbamazepine	Disulfiram
Ethanol	Ritonavir

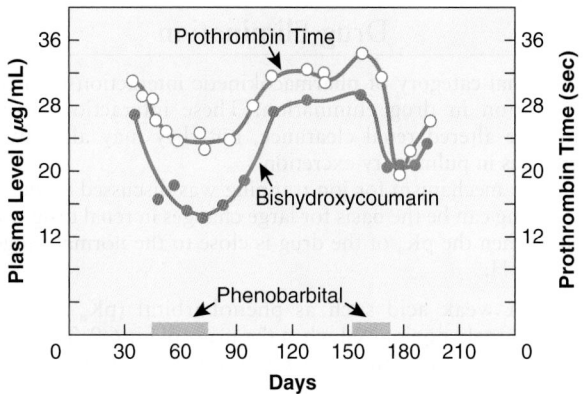

FIGURE 22-2. Effect of phenobarbital on plasma levels of bishydroxycoumarin. The anticoagulant was given at a dose of 75 mg/day. Phenobarbital, 65 mg/day, was given during the periods indicated on the x-axis. Induction of hepatic enzymes decreased anticoagulant concentrations and reduced the effect. (Reprinted from Cucinell SA, Conney AH, Sansur M, et al: Drug interactions in man: I. Lowering effect of phenobarbital on plasma levels of bishydroxy coumarin [dicumarol] and diphenylhydantoin [Dilantin]. Clin Pharmacol Ther 1965; 6: 420, with permission.)

- When two drugs are substrates for the same P450 enzymes, they can interact competitively and reduce the clearance of both. For example, it has been demonstrated that midazolam and fentanyl are competitive inhibitors in vitro of metabolism by CYP3A4.[43] This pharmacokinetic interaction is probably far less important than the pharmacodynamic interaction between these drugs (described later).
- Another study concluded that propofol competitively inhibits CYP3A4, and it can reduce the clearance of midazolam by 37%.[44] Propofol itself appears to be metabolized by a different isoform, CYP2B6.[45]
- Alfentanil and erythromycin are both metabolized by CYP3A4,[46] and the antibiotic greatly prolongs the effect of the opioid.[46] Sufentanil and fentanyl are also metabolized by CYP3A4,[47] but the clearance of sufentanil is not changed by erythromycin.[48] Perhaps this is because it is a high-clearance opioid.
- Cimetidine has an imidazole group that binds to the heme iron of cytochrome P450 and forms an inactive complex. Cimetidine inhibits the metabolism of many drugs, including warfarin, diazepam, phenytoin, and morphine. Several studies have demonstrated that coadministration of cimetidine and diazepam causes clinically significant elevations in the concentration of both diazepam and its active metabolite.[49] As stated previously, cimetidine can decrease hepatic blood flow, so it can also decrease the clearance of high-extraction drugs.[38]
- Protease inhibitors such as saquinavir[50] and ritonavir[51] can inhibit the metabolism of midazolam and fentanyl, respectively, by inhibiting CYP3A4.
- Other imidazole drugs such as the antifungals, ketoconazole and itraconazole, can inhibit a wide variety of microsomal enzymes. They have been shown to decrease the clearance (and increase the toxicity) of glyburide, terfenadine, digoxin, midazolam, theophylline, and warfarin.
- The related benzimidazole, etomidate, blocks the synthesis of cortisol and aldosterone by inhibiting the P450-dependent mitochondrial enzymes, 17α-hydroxylase and 11β-hydroxylase.[52] Etomidate can inhibit the metabolism of other drugs, but the effects do not appear to be clinically important.

Drug Elimination

The final category of pharmacokinetic interaction is through alteration in drug elimination. These interactions usually involve altered renal clearance, but they may also involve changes in pulmonary excretion.

The mechanism for ion trapping was discussed earlier. Ion trapping can be the basis for large changes in renal drug excretion when the pK_a of the drug is close to the normal range of urine pH:

■ A weak acid such as phenobarbital ($pK_a = 7.4$) is largely nonionized when the urine pH is 6.0. This means that much of the filtered drug is in a relatively lipid-soluble form and available for tubular reabsorption. If the urine pH is raised to 8 or 9 (e.g., with sodium bicarbonate), most of the phenobarbital becomes ionized, reabsorption decreases, and clearance increases. For a weak base, the reverse situation is true—excretion can be promoted when the urine is acidified. This type of interaction has been used therapeutically in certain cases of drug overdose.

Organic anions and cations are actively secreted by separate transporters in the renal tubule. The cation system handles the elimination of atropine, isoproterenol, neostigmine, and meperidine. The anion system is involved in the excretion of salicylate, penicillins, cephalosporins, and most of the potent diuretics. The various anions and cations can compete for their respective transport sites:

■ Probenecid inhibits the secretion of penicillin, increasing plasma concentrations and prolonging the duration of action.
■ Quinidine has been shown to decrease both the volume of distribution and the renal clearance of digoxin, and plasma digoxin concentrations may increase by two- to fivefold.[53] The renal effect is believed to be due to a reduction in tubular secretion of digoxin.

PHARMACODYNAMIC INTERACTIONS

Up to this point, we have been discussing pharmacokinetic interactions that change the amount of active drug reaching receptor sites. A *pharmacodynamic* interaction occurs when one drug alters the sensitivity of a target receptor or tissue to the effects of a second drug. This means that the dose-response or concentration-response curve for one drug is shifted by another (Fig. 22-3). It is often difficult to assign a specific mechanism to these interactions. We commonly classify them by their direction and intensity, that is, additive, antagonistic, or supra-additive (synergistic).

Additive interactions are most likely to occur when drugs with identical mechanisms are combined. The clinician normally expects additivity when combining two benzodiazepines, two fentanyl analogs, or two volatile anesthetics. Most additive interactions tend not to be particularly surprising, although some are clinically useful:

■ The administration of two aminosteroid nondepolarizing muscle relaxants, such as rocuronium and vecuronium, gives an additive effect[54] (Fig. 22-4). Notably, the interactions between nondepolarizing relaxants of different chemical classes are often synergistic (see later discussion).
■ The interaction of two volatile anesthetics or nitrous oxide with volatile anesthetics is additive.[55–57]
■ In animals, mixtures of lidocaine-tetracaine or lidocaine-etidocaine produce approximately additive CNS toxicity when given intravenously.[58]

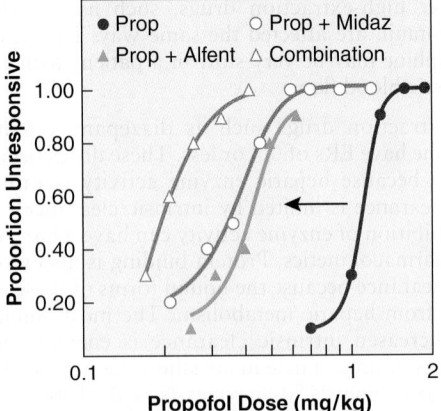

FIGURE 22-3. Dose-response curves for loss of consciousness after an intravenous bolus dose of propofol (Prop) alone, propofol plus midazolam (Midaz), propofol plus alfentanil (Alfent), or all three drugs. Drug combinations were given as constant ratios, based on the measured ED_{50}s of the individual drugs. Both the benzodiazepine and the opioid shifted the dose-response curve for propofol significantly to the left. (Redrawn from data in Short TG, Plummer JL, Chui PT: Hypnotic and anaesthetic interactions between midazolam, propofol and alfentanil. Br J Anaesth 1992; 69: 162, with permission.)

The most common *antagonistic drug interactions* in anesthesia are those involving deliberate reversal of effect with competitive antagonists such as neostigmine, naloxone, or flumazenil. Pharmacodynamic antagonism that is *unintended* is a much less common event:

■ An antagonistic interaction occurs between succinylcholine and the nondepolarizing relaxants.[59]
■ When epidural morphine or fentanyl is administered after establishing a block with 2-chloroprocaine, both the duration and the intensity of opioid analgesia are decreased.[60] The mechanism for this interaction is unclear.
■ When butorphanol is combined with midazolam, the mixture increases sedation but has less anterograde amnestic effect than midazolam alone (Fig. 22-5). This illustrates the important concept that a drug combination

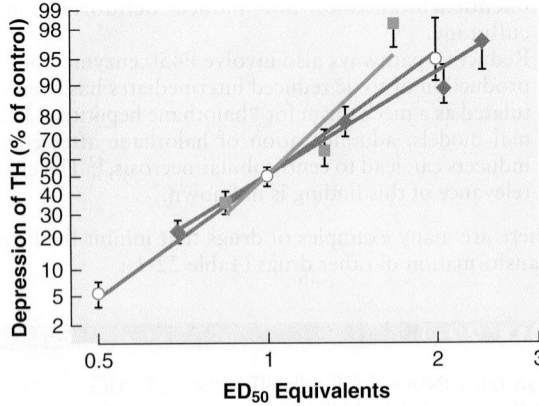

FIGURE 22-4. The interaction of rocuronium and vecuronium is additive in man. Log dose-probit graph plots twitch height (TH) as percentage of control value. Dose is given in terms of ED_{50} multiples. Diamonds (blue), squares (green), and circles (red) represent rocuronium, vecuronium, and the combination, respectively. The dose-response curve for the combination cannot be distinguished from those of the individual drugs. (Reprinted from Naguib M, Samarkandi AH, Bakhamees HS, et al: Comparative potency of steroidal neuromuscular blocking drugs and isobolographic analysis of the interaction. Br J Anaesth 1995; 75: 37, with permission.)

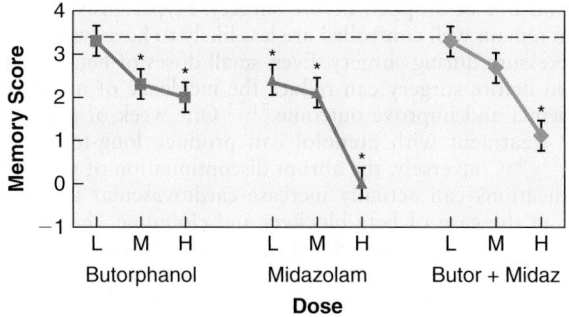

FIGURE 22-5. Memory scores of patients 5 minutes after receiving butorphanol, midazolam, or the combination. L, M, and H signify low, medium, and high doses (7.1, 22.5, and 71.4 μg/kg butorphanol; 4.3, 13.6, and 42.9 μg/kg midazolam; or 3.6 + 2.2, 11.3 + 6.8, and 35.7 + 21.5 μg/kg butorphanol and midazolam in combination). The *dashed line* indicates mean pretreatment value. Midazolam, but not butorphanol, produced a profound anterograde amnestic effect. Giving one-half the dose of each drug in combination produced an effect that was less than that after midazolam alone. (Reprinted from Dershwitz M, Rosow CE, DiBiase PM, et al: A comparison of the sedative effects of butorphanol and midazolam. Anesthesiology 1991; 74: 717, with permission.)

may simultaneously be synergistic and antagonistic for different effects. In the case of the amnestic effect, butorphanol may simply be diluting the effects of midazolam.[61]

7 The most interesting and clinically important interactions tend to be the *synergistic interactions,* in which small doses of two or more drugs can sometimes produce large effects. Synergy is most likely to occur when drugs of different classes, or even those with slightly different mechanisms, are used to produce the same effects:

- The potentiation of opioids by NSAIDs is a classic and useful interaction between analgesic drugs with completely different mechanisms.[62]
- The potentiation of nondepolarizing relaxants by the various volatile anesthetics is a useful interaction on a daily basis. The exact mechanism is unknown, but several theories have been proposed, including increased blood flow to muscle, depression of centrally mediated muscle tone, decreased neurotransmitter release, and decreased sensitivity of postjunctional or muscle membranes.
- A much more subtle supra-additive interaction occurs between aminosteroid and benzylisoquinolines. Pancuronium and *d*-tubocurarine were shown to produce a synergistic relaxant effect in combination,[63] and this is also seen with similar combinations across these two chemical classes (atracurium and vecuronium, *d*-tubocurarine and vecuronium, mivacurium and rocuronium). Various mechanisms have been proposed, including multiple binding sites[64] (presynaptic for aminosteroid versus postsynaptic for benzylisoquinolines) and allosteric interactions between separate agonist and antagonist binding sites.[65]
- Sedatives and hypnotics with related (but not identical) mechanisms of action usually interact synergistically to produce greater CNS depression. This is discussed in more detail later in this chapter.

STUDYING DRUG INTERACTIONS

As already discussed, a study that demonstrates that a drug–drug interaction exists does not necessarily establish its mechanism, its magnitude, or its clinical relevance. What information is needed to conclude that an interaction is pharmacodynamic rather than pharmacokinetic? How do we know it is really synergistic? Let us consider four clinical

experiments to study the interaction of midazolam and thiopental. Given the different mechanisms for these two drugs, we might predict a synergistic interaction: benzodiazepines increase neuronal chloride conductance by facilitating γ-aminobutyric acid (GABA) binding, whereas barbiturates bind to a separate site and increase GABA efficacy:

1. In the simplest study design, two groups of patients are randomly assigned to receive midazolam-thiopental or placebo-thiopental. The percentage that becomes unresponsive in each group is assessed at a standard time after thiopental administration. The data show that midazolam increases the percentage unresponsive.

   Such a study is severely limited: it tells us that an interaction has occurred, but the results cannot be generalized beyond the conditions examined (a single dose of midazolam, a single dose of thiopental). Nothing may be inferred about mechanism.

2. A more complex (but more useful) experiment would be to study a thiopental dose-response curve in the presence and absence of midazolam. This would show that the dose of thiopental required to produce hypnosis in half the patients (ED_{50}) is decreased by midazolam.

   These results allow us to conclude that the interaction occurs over a range of thiopental doses relevant to clinical practice. The data still apply only to a single dose of midazolam, and they tell us nothing about the mechanism of the interaction.

3. A useful modification of this experiment is to administer the thiopental by a constant-rate infusion (with or without midazolam) and measure its concentration over time. The data show that concentrations of thiopental rise at the same rate in both groups, but midazolam decreases the concentration needed to produce hypnosis in 50% of the patients (the EC_{50}).

   This tells us that midazolam has not changed the pharmacokinetics of thiopental, so the interaction must have a pharmacodynamic mechanism.

4. Finally, there are a number of experimental designs for demonstrating synergy, and these have been reviewed in the clinical literature.[66] Two of the most common techniques used by experimental pharmacologists are algebraic (fractional)[67] and isobolographic[68,69] analysis, and clinical anesthesia studies using these methods have been appearing frequently. The interaction of thiopental and midazolam was studied with an isobolographic technique, and the results are shown in Figure 22-6.[70] In general, this analysis

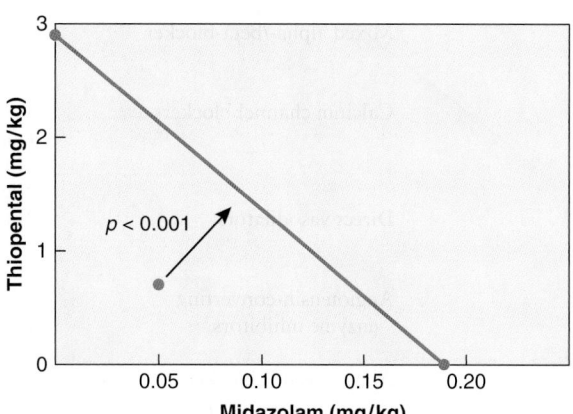

FIGURE 22-6. Isobolographic analysis of the interaction between midazolam and thiopental in humans (see text for details). The ED_{50} of the combination was significantly less than predicted by the red "line of additivity." (Redrawn from data of Tverskoy M, Fleyshman G, Bradley EL Jr et al: Midazolam-thiopental anesthetic interaction in patients. Anesth Analg 1988; 67: 342, with permission.)

requires a minimum of *three* dose-response experiments, one with each drug alone and one with the drugs in combination. The drug combination can be studied as a fixed ratio, or one of the drugs can be given at a fixed dose and the dose of the second drug varied. From these experiments, three estimates of ED_{50} are made, and an isobologram is constructed as shown in Figure 22-6. The ED_{50}s for thiopental and midazolam alone are graphed on the two axes, and these points are connected by the theoretic "line of additivity." If the two drugs are simply additive when combined, we would expect the ED_{50} of the mixture to fall somewhere along this line. Because the actual ED_{50} of the mixture is significantly less than predicted by this line, the interaction is synergistic (an ED_{50} greater than predicted would signify antagonism).

PHARMACODYNAMIC INTERACTIONS AFFECTING HEMODYNAMICS

The treatment of hypertension, angina, dysrhythmias, and congestive heart failure involves the use of drugs with powerful effects on autonomic function and cardiovascular homeostasis. Until the 1970s, the teaching was generally that cardiovascular depressant or stimulant medications should be discontinued before surgery because they interfered with protective responses to the trauma of anesthesia and surgery. Some older antihypertensives like reserpine and α-methyl dopa altered the depth of anesthesia, and this was believed to be undesirable. There is now a substantial body of evidence showing that most cardiovascular medications need not and

should not be stopped before surgery. Hypertensive patients who remain well controlled are less likely to have wide swings in pressure during surgery. Even small doses of beta-blockers given before surgery can reduce the incidence of myocardial ischemia and improve outcome.[71,72] One week of perioperative treatment with atenolol can produce long-term benefits.[73,74] Conversely, the abrupt discontinuation of vasoactive medications can actually increase cardiovascular instability, and in the case of beta-blockers and clonidine, the rebound hypertension and dysrhythmias may be dangerous.

Given the foregoing observations, it is fortunate that most cardiovascular drug–drug interactions are simply extensions of the known pharmacology of the agents (Table 22-2). In short, the hypotensive effects of general or regional anesthesia may be increased by all antihypertensive medications. Using similar logic, antidysrhythmic drugs such as amiodarone or procainamide increase the possibility of bradycardia, hypotension, and decreased cardiac output.

8 With the possible exception of angiotensin-converting enzyme inhibitors (ACEIs) and angiotensin receptor blockers (ARBs), there is little reason to withhold most vasoactive medications before surgery. It may be prudent to stop diuretic treatment before procedures with large anticipated fluid requirements or significant use of nephrotoxic antibiotics. Several studies suggest that continuation of the ACEIs and ARBs leads to a high incidence of severe, sometimes refractory, hypotension during induction of general anesthesia.[75,76] These drugs decrease afterload, and they also potentiate anesthetic-induced reduction in preload. The effect on preload may be quite important in hypertensive patients who have pre-existing diastolic dysfunction.

Like the baroreceptor reflexes, the renin-angiotensin system is an important way the body can respond to hypovolemia or hypotension. Within minutes after a pressure decrease is

TABLE 22-2

EFFECTS OF ANTIHYPERTENSIVE DRUGS DURING ANESTHESIA

CLASS	DRUGS	CLASS EFFECTS
Alpha-blockers	Phenoxybenzamine Phentolamine Prazosin	Hypotension/vasodilation Reflex tachycardia
Beta-blockers	Propranolol Metoprolol Atenolol	Hypotension Decreased contractility Bradycardia AV block
Mixed alpha-/beta-blocker	Labetalol	Hypotension/vasodilation Bradycardia AV block
Calcium channel blockers	Verapamil Diltiazem Nifedipine Nicardipine	Hypotension/vasodilation Decreased contractility Bradycardia AV block
Direct vasodilators	Nitroglycerin Isosorbide Hydralazine	Hypotension/vasodilation Reflex tachycardia
Angiotensin-converting enzyme inhibitors	Captopril Enalapril Lisinopril	Hypotension/vasodilation Hyperkalemia
Angiotensin II blocker	Losartan Valsartan	Hypotension/vasodilation Hyperkalemia
Diuretics	Thiazides Furosemide Bumetanide	Hypovolemia Hypokalemia Possible vasodilation

AV, atrioventricular.

sensed by the juxtaglomerular apparatus, angiotensin II causes vasoconstriction by both central and peripheral actions. Chronic blockade of this system not only inhibits the angiotensin response, but it also reduces the vasoconstrictor response to norepinephrine.[77] This may explain why ACEI-induced and ARB-induced hypotension can be so resistant to sympathetic drugs such as phenylephrine, ephedrine, and norepinephrine.[78] Vasopressin and various vasopressin analogs can restore sympathetic response[79,80] and may be useful pressors in cases of refractory hypotension.

There is currently no consensus on the preoperative management of patients taking ACEIs or ARBs. Withholding them for 24 hours may decrease hypotension but also make blood pressure extremely labile during surgery. Some have found them to be beneficial during surgery.[81,82] In addition, ACEIs do not appear to significantly impact the hemodynamic management of neuraxial anesthesia.[83] The considerations are probably different for patients receiving ACEIs for chronic congestive heart failure. ACEIs are given to these patients for afterload reduction; they improve baroreceptor sensitivity, reduce ventricular remodeling, and decrease the mortality rate. Perioperative use of ACEIs in this population may not increase the already high incidence of hypotension during induction.[84]

Most perioperative hemodynamic interactions involve the use of cardiovascular depressants. It is also useful to consider several groups of patients who are treated (or who "self-treat") before surgery with cardiovascular *stimulants*:

1. Patients with bronchospasm may require treatment with rapid-acting β_2 agonists (albuterol, terbutaline), anticholinergics (ipratropium), or phosphodiesterase inhibitors (theophylline). These patients are at increased risk for tachydysrhythmias and ectopic rhythms. Similar considerations apply to the patient receiving the IV β_2 agonist, ritodrine, for premature labor.

2. Patients who receive TCAs such as imipramine, desipramine, amitriptyline, and nortriptyline present several possible scenarios for adverse drug interaction. These drugs work by blocking presynaptic reuptake of norepinephrine or serotonin, so they can theoretically increase the effects of direct-acting or indirect-acting agonists at these synapses. Most TCAs also have prominent anticholinergic effects. In overdose situations, TCAs can create the entire range of cardiovascular toxicity, including myocardial infarction and sudden death. In spite of this, hypotension and tachydysrhythmias are not common intraoperative problems for patients taking these older antidepressants. It is still reasonable to minimize the use of pancuronium, halothane, ketamine, and other agents with the potential to increase the incidence of dysrhythmias. If TCA-induced hypotension occurs, there is disagreement about the best way to treat it.[85] One case report describes a patient on chronic nifedipine and nortriptyline therapy who had hypotension that was resistant to ephedrine, phenylephrine, and dopamine (norepinephrine was eventually successful).[86]

3. Finally, we must all be prepared to treat patients who are acutely or chronically intoxicated with cocaine. In addition to its local anesthetic properties, cocaine decreases norepinephrine reuptake, like TCAs. Acute intoxication presents a particular challenge. Young, otherwise healthy people may present with fulminant hypertension, tachycardia, and myocardial ischemia (the latter may be severe because cocaine can also induce a thrombotic diathesis). Management of the acute cardiovascular effects is similar to that for pheochromocytoma: these patients need both vasodilators and beta-blockers. A beta-blocker should not be given alone because unopposed α-adrenergic stimulation can cause a further increase in systemic vascular resistance. Patients with chronic cocaine intoxication are less of a problem, but they

are still at risk for dysrhythmias (avoiding halothane, pancuronium, atropine, and sympathomimetics still seems like a good idea). Chronic cocaine exposure increases halothane minimum alveolar concentration (MAC) in dogs[87] and isoflurane MAC in sheep,[88] and acute ingestion may antagonize the sedative effects of benzodiazepines in humans.[89] This is an interesting contrast to chronic treatment with amphetamine, which appears to decrease MAC in dogs.[90] It might be believed that the adrenergic overactivity induced by cocaine would produce receptor down-regulation over time, but several animal studies suggest that chronic cocaine treatment does not decrease brain catecholamine content or sympathetic responsiveness.[91,92] The relevance of these data to human cardiovascular responses remains to be proven.

PHARMACODYNAMIC INTERACTIONS AFFECTING ANALGESIA OR HYPNOSIS

9 Combinations of CNS depressants almost always produce additive or synergistic increases in CNS effect. These interactions are usually useful and predictable. All the common IV and inhaled anesthetic agents have been tested in combination in humans. The following sections highlight some of the most important interactions.

Opioid–Hypnotic Interactions

This is arguably the most commonly used synergistic combination in IV anesthesia:

- Fentanyl and alfentanil have been shown to reduce the requirement for barbiturates, and there is some evidence that the interaction is beneficial. Reducing the total dose of thiopental[93] or thiamylal[94] during short procedures decreases the time to awakening and orientation.
- Opioids also potentiate propofol, but it has been much more difficult to show that the combination improves recovery compared with propofol alone. Short, et al.[95] found that a small dose of alfentanil can reduce the induction dose of propofol by 50% (Fig. 22-3). During total IV anesthesia, infusions of remifentanil or alfentanil tremendously reduce the infusion rate of propofol needed to suppress response to voice and movement responses to surgical stimuli.[96,97] Target effect-site concentrations of only 1 to 2 μg/mL of propofol produce adequate anesthesia in many cases. These are routinely achieved with propofol doses used for conscious sedation (25 to 50 μg/kg per minute).

Opioid–Benzodiazepine Interactions

This important interaction was alluded to earlier, and it illustrates why opioids are so commonly used in combination with diazepam or midazolam. Opioids are highly selective CNS depressants; they can produce sedation, but they are relatively weak hypnotics. Even huge doses of fentanyl and its congeners do not dependably produce sleep by themselves.[98] For example, alfentanil doses as high as 100 to 200 μg/kg cannot always induce unconsciousness in unpremedicated patients.[99] Such opioid doses uniformly produce apnea, rigidity, and profound analgesia.

Kissin et al.[100] found, however, that a tiny dose of alfentanil (3 μg/kg) is sufficient to reduce the hypnotic ED_{50} of midazolam by 50%. This dose is subanalgesic and subhypnotic when given alone. This means that a small dose of opioid

ANESTHETIC AGENTS, ADJUVANTS, AND DRUG INTERACTION

(50 μg fentanyl, 500 μg alfentanil) may have almost no hypnotic effect by itself, but can still be an extremely effective potentiator of other hypnotics. It also means that when fentanyl and midazolam are combined for conscious sedation, the opioid is producing sleep as well as analgesia.

Benzodiazepine–Hypnotic Interactions

The theoretical basis for the interaction between barbiturates and benzodiazepines was discussed earlier, and the thiopental–midazolam interaction is shown in Figure 22-6.

- Thiopental–midazolam interaction has been studied in humans, and the combination was found to have 1.8 times the expected potency of the individual agents.[70,101] Similar results have been described with the combination of midazolam and methohexital.[102]
- Propofol also acts by modulation of GABA neurotransmission, and its hypnotic effects are potentiated when it is combined with midazolam.[95]

The clinical benefits of benzodiazepine premedication are most obvious during the preoperative period. Intraoperative benefits (i.e., increased efficacy or reduced toxicity) of benzodiazepine–hypnotic combinations have not been demonstrated. The patient premedicated with midazolam needs less thiopental or propofol for induction (or maintenance), but it has not been established that this results in a smoother anesthetic or more rapid awakening.

Volatile Anesthetic–Opioid Interactions

Opioids produce dose-dependent and concentration-dependent decreases in MAC for all the inhalation anesthetics:

- A steady-state plasma fentanyl concentration of 1.67 ng/mL decreases human isoflurane MAC by 50%[103] (Fig. 22-7).

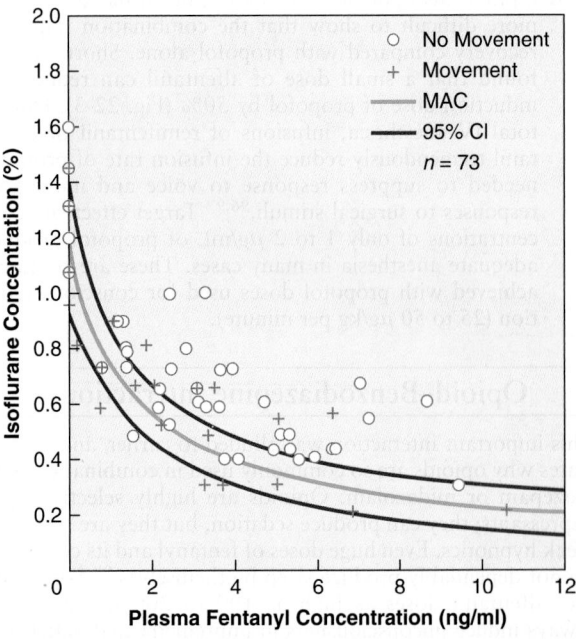

FIGURE 22-7. The interaction between fentanyl and isoflurane. The *green line* represents the concentration of the two drugs that prevents movement in 50% of patients. MAC, minimum alveolar concentration; CI, confidence interval. (Reprinted from McEwan AI, Smith C, Dyar O, et al: Isoflurane minimum alveolar concentration reduction by fentanyl. Anesthesiology 1993; 78: 864, with permission.)

- Opioid partial agonists such as nalbuphine and butorphanol produce smaller reductions in MAC.[104]
- Animal data consistently show that an approximately 70% reduction in MAC is the maximum effect obtainable with a full agonist like fentanyl.[105] The mechanism for this interaction is unknown, but Licina, et al.[106] showed that administration of lumbar intrathecal morphine (15 μg/kg) does not alter halothane MAC in humans. This suggests that the effect may be due to supraspinal opioid actions. Rampil, et al.[107] showed that MAC in the rat is not altered when the cerebral cortex and all other precollicular brain structures are removed. MAC therefore appears to reflect an action of the volatile anesthetics on the spinal cord, whereas MAC reduction by opioids is most likely to be mediated by structures in the brainstem or higher. One possible site for interaction is the locus coeruleus (LC).

Opioids and volatile agents are often combined to smooth the intraoperative and postoperative course. In some patients, the combination of opioid and volatile agent is hemodynamically better tolerated than the volatile agent alone. Addition of an opioid may also reduce the incidence of emergence delirium.

Is there any evidence that decreasing the dose of the inhaled agent in this manner speeds awakening? Two studies indicate that "MAC awake" (the concentration at which 50% of subjects respond to voice) is much less affected by opioids than MAC.[108,109] This suggests that the combination might speed emergence, but there have been no studies specifically designed to test this hypothesis.

Other IV agents such as lidocaine,[110] midazolam,[111] and α_2 agonists have been shown to decrease MAC in experimental animals. For lidocaine and midazolam, the plasma concentrations required to produce a meaningful decrease in MAC are so high that the interaction is unlikely to have clinical utility. There is some evidence that the simultaneous use of volatile anesthetics and benzodiazepines causes increased cortical binding of the latter.[112]

α_2-Agonist Interactions

It has long been known that drugs that depress CNS sympathetic function can produce sedation and potentiate anesthesia. Older antihypertensives such as reserpine and α-methyldopa can produce drowsiness and reduce halothane MAC.[113] The newer autonomic modulators—α_2 agonists such as clonidine or dexmedetomidine—are powerful sedatives and analgesics in humans.

- In animals, dexmedetomidine produces marked potentiation of opioid analgesia and benzodiazepine-induced hypnosis.[114]
- Dexmedetomidine also lowers halothane MAC by nearly 100% through a specific postsynaptic α_2 mechanism.[115]

Dexmedetomidine interacts with both presynaptic and postsynaptic α_2-adrenergic receptors to decrease central sympathetic tone. Its hypnotic effect is largely the result of depression of function in the LC in the pons.[116] This is the main adrenergic nucleus in the brain and an important input for endogenous sleep pathways through the ventrolateral preoptic nucleus. There is evidence to suggest that the LC is an important site for control of sleep, attention, memory, analgesia, and autonomic function.[117] The LC contains receptors for glutamate, GABA, acetylcholine, opioids, and benzodiazepines, and experimental evidence suggests that it may be the site for some important anesthetic drug effects and interactions:

1. The LC is the rostral portion of an important descending inhibitory pathway, which plays a part in the production of opioid analgesia.[118]

2. In the rat, destroying the LC produces a state of narcolepsy and decreases halothane MAC by 30 to 40%.[119]

3. Agonists at GABA, opioid, and α_2 receptors are all inhibitory when microinjected into the LC. These drugs all have sedative-hypnotic properties, and all of them lower the requirement for volatile anesthetics.

4. Acetylcholine and glutamate receptor agonists are excitatory in the LC, and antagonists at these receptors (e.g., scopolamine, ketamine) are hypnotics. Some glutamate effects are mediated by NO, and inhibitors of neuronal NO synthase can decrease the requirement for halothane[120] and isoflurane.[121]

Three-Way Interactions

In clinical practice, it is common to combine more than two drugs with sedative-hypnotic effects. We have relatively little information on what happens when a third drug is added to two that already have synergistic effects:

- Short, et al.[95] performed a clinical study of hypnotic interactions among propofol, midazolam, and alfentanil (Fig. 22-3). Propofol requirement was reduced by 82% with the three-way combination, but it produced less potentiation than would have been predicted by adding the effects of the two-way combinations.

- Vinik, et al.[122] studied the same combination and also found profound hypnotic synergism: the dose of propofol could be decreased by 86% in the presence of alfentanil and midazolam. The data also suggested that the interaction between midazolam and alfentanil was a marked potentiation, but the addition of propofol did not produce significant additional change. Figure 22-8 shows the data from this experiment analyzed with a three-way isobologram.

- A three-way interaction involving enflurane, dexmedetomidine, and fentanyl was investigated in dogs. Salmenpera, et al.[123] found that each of the two IV agents lowered enflurane MAC, and combining the three drugs produced a MAC reduction that was probably greater than predicted by simple additivity. In this case, the three-way combination produced more bradycardia than enflurane alone.

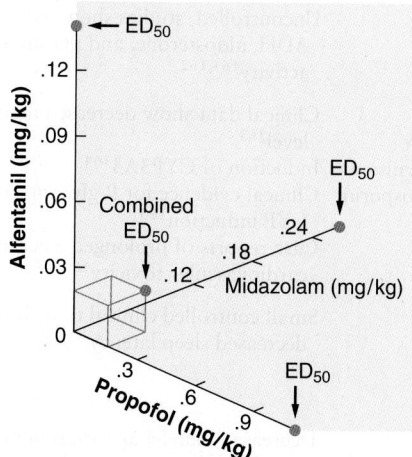

FIGURE 22-8. ED_{50} isobolograms for the three-way hypnotic interactions among midazolam, alfentanil, and propofol. The reader can imagine a triangular "plane of additivity" with its corners at the individual ED_{50} values. The ED_{50} for the triple combination was significantly lower than predicted by additivity. (Reprinted from Vinik HR, Bradley EL Jr, Kissin I: Triple anesthetic combination: Propofol-midazolam-alfentanil. Anesth Analg 1994; 78: 354, with permission.)

Herbal Preparations and Drug Interactions

American have increasingly used herbal, vitamin, and over-the-counter preparations in an attempt to treat various ailments. While the use of these preparations increased significantly during the 1990s, over recent years the use seems to have slowed.[1] In 2003, over-the-counter sales of herbals and vitamins were approximately $62.9 billion, an 8% growth from 2002.[124] A survey of 3,842 patients during preoperative evaluations found that 22% used herbal medications and 51% used vitamins. The most likely patients to use these products were women ages 40 to 60 years.[125] Another survey of 1,017 patients found 32% used one or more herb-related compounds, and 70% did not report this information when asked during routine preanesthetic assessment.[126]

Herbal preparations are classified as dietary supplements in the Dietary Supplement Heath and Education Act of 1994.[127] By this act, herbal preparations are exempt from the safety and efficacy requirements and regulations that prescription and over-the-counter drugs must fulfill. Instead, the U.S. Food and Drug Administration must prove lack of safety.[128] There is no regulatory oversight of the specific contents of the herbal preparations, and different batches or brands of the same herbal often do not contain equal amounts of the active compound.

The *Physicians' Desk Reference for Herbal Medicines* is now in its fourth edition,[129] but there is still relatively little peer-reviewed literature addressing herbals and dietary supplements with specific reference to perioperative care. Among the thousands of herbal preparations available, only a few have been documented to cause problems either through intrinsic toxicity or through pharmacokinetic and pharmacodynamic interactions.[130–132] The herbals most commonly cited are echinacea, ephedra (ma huang), garlic, gingko, ginseng, kava, and St. John's wort. As Fugh-Berman[133] noted, many of the articles on herbals contain significant errors and unsubstantiated conclusions. Some commonly mentioned herbal-based interactions are listed in Table 22-3, along with an assessment of the strength of the evidence. We were unable to find clinical trials proving that there are specific adverse interactions between herbals and anesthetic drugs.

MODELS FOR THE FUTURE: DRUG INTERACTION DURING TOTAL INTRAVENOUS ANESTHESIA

Anesthesia must always be titrated to effect, but the clinician usually begins dosing each drug with some notion of a "normal" dose range and a reasonable incremental dose. As additional drugs are added to the anesthetic, these doses need to be modified. Are there any reliable data to guide the administration of anesthetic drugs in combination? The answer for most routine balanced anesthetics is probably "no." As we have seen, almost all anesthetic drugs interact in a nonlinear, synergistic fashion, and the magnitude of the interaction depends on the specific doses of each agent. If the drugs are given by bolus injection or variable-rate infusion, the interaction changes constantly with time. Predicting anesthetic interaction, then, is like aiming at a moving target. Even a relatively simple anesthetic seems to require the analysis of an impossibly large number of potential variables.

In spite of the obstacles, there have been some attempts to apply quantitative models to total intravenous anesthesia (TIVA). The TIVA technique offers several advantages in this regard:

1. Anesthesia is often induced and maintained with only two drugs, a rapid-acting hypnotic (e.g., propofol) and a rapid-acting opioid (e.g., alfentanil, remifentanil). The

TABLE 22-3

PUBLISHED EVIDENCE FOR HERBAL TOXICITY

■ NAME(S)	■ COMMON USE	■ CLAIMED TOXICITY[130,132,133,135]	■ PUBLISHED EVIDENCE[a]
Ephedra Ma huang Ephedrine Chinese joint fir	Weight loss Antitussive Bacteriostatic	Halothane: arrhythmias MAOI: enhanced sympathetic effects Oxytocin: hypertension Stroke, hypertension, cardiac arrest	IV ephedrine well characterized Inadequate data on specific interactions with oral ephedra Oral ephedra known to cause adverse CNS and cardiac events[136]
Echinacea	Common cold prevention	Hepatotoxicity	No evidence of hepatotoxicity[133] Inhibitor of CYP1A2 and intestinal CYP3A activity[137] Inducer of hepatic CYP3A[137]
Purple cone flower	Wounds and burns Urinary tract infections Coughs and bronchitis	Decrease corticosteroid effect	Laboratory evidence of macrophage activation and enhanced natural killer cell activation[138,139]
Garlic Ajo	Lipid lowering Hypertension Antiplatelet, antioxidant	Potentiate warfarin	No controlled trials demonstrating interaction with warfarin[140] Decreased platelet aggregation in vitro[141-146]
Ginger	Nausea Antispasmodic	Inhibit thromboxane synthetase	In vitro evidence of thromboxane synthetase inhibition[147-150] No effect on platelet function with 2 g, but inhibition with 5 g[151,152]
Ginkgo Maidenhair tree Fossil tree	Circulatory stimulant	Inhibit PAF	Case reports of increased bleeding in humans[153] In vitro evidence of PAF inhibition[154,155]
Goldenseal Orange root Yellow root Ground raspberry Tumeric root Eye root	Diuretic Anti-inflammatory Laxative Hemostatic	Oxytocic Paralysis in overdose Edema Hypertension	No evidence
Kava Ava/ava pepper Kawa	Anxiolytic	Hepatotoxicity Potentiate barbiturates, benzodiazepines	Case reports of hepatotoxicity[156,157] May interact to increase sedation via GABA receptor activation[158] Clinical and animal studies demonstrating sedation and anxiolysis[159,160]
Licorice Sweet root	Gastric/duodenal ulcer Gastritis Cough and bronchitis	Hypertension Hypokalemia Edema	Licorice abuse can cause hypokalemia Uncontrolled, studies show reductions in ADH, aldosterone, and plasma renin activity[161,162]
St. John's wort Hardhay Amber Goat weed	Depression	Decreased efficacy of digoxin Decreased efficacy of warfarin Decreased efficacy of anticonvulsants Decreased serum level of cyclosporin Enzyme induction Prolonged anesthesia	Clinical data show decreased digoxin level[163] Induction of CYP3A4[164] Clinical evidence for P-glycoprotein and CYP induction[163] Case reports of prolonged emergence, cardiovascular toxicity[165,166]
Valerian All-heal Setwall Vandal root	Sedative Anxiolytic	Potentiate barbiturates	Small controlled clinical trial showed decreased sleep latency[167,168]
Vitamin E	Antiaging Prevent stroke, pulmonary emboli Prevent atherosclerosis Promote wound healing	Increased bleeding Increased hypertension	Decreased platelet aggregation in vitro[169-171] Small clinical trial shows reduction in platelet aggregation[80] No evidence for hypertension

IV, intravenous; MAOI, monamide oxidase inhibitor; CNS, central nervous system; PAF, platelet activating factor; GABA, γ-aminobutyric acid; ADH, antidiuretic hormone.
[a]Based on search of Medline and Cochrane databases, January 1, 1966, to November 1, 2007.

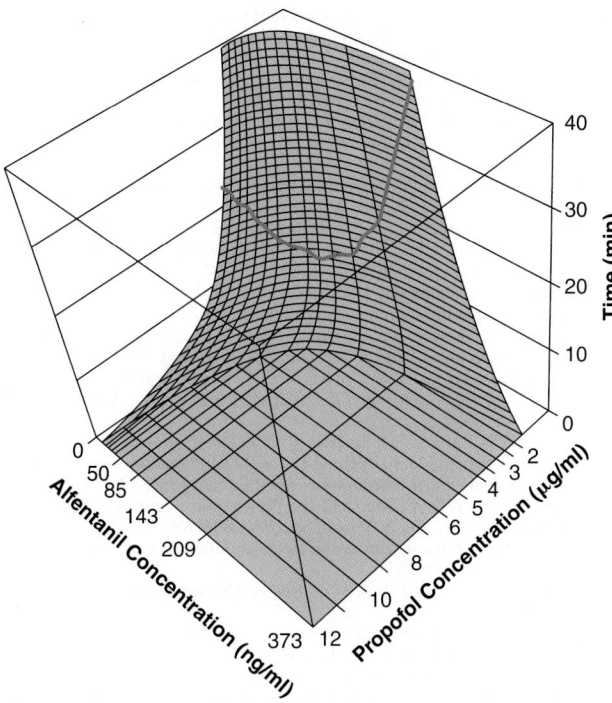

FIGURE 22-9. Computer simulation of the decay in blood propofol and plasma alfentanil concentrations during the first 40 minutes after the termination of a computer-controlled infusion (see text for details). (Reprinted from Vuyk J, Lim T, Engbers FHM, et al: The pharmacodynamic interaction of propofol and alfentanil during lower abdominal surgery in women. Anesthesiology 1995; 83: 8, with permission.)

pharmacokinetics and pharmacodynamics of these drugs are exceptionally well studied.
2. The drugs have pharmacokinetics well suited to administration by continuous infusion with microprocessor-driven pumps. During anesthesia, plasma concentrations of the drugs may be held relatively constant, so blood and brain attain pseudoequilibrium. The researcher may vary the infusion of each drug independently and relate stable plasma concentrations to clinical effects.

In one of the first quantitative studies of drug interaction during TIVA, Vuyk and colleagues[96] gave computer-controlled infusions of propofol and alfentanil to women undergoing lower abdominal surgery. First, the target concentration of alfentanil was held constant and propofol was varied; then, the reverse experiment was done. The onset of sleep and the time to awakening were measured, as was presence or absence of somatic and hemodynamic responses to laryngoscopy, intubation, incision, and opening of peritoneum. Arterial blood samples were collected, and the EC_{50} of alfentanil for each clinical end point was related to blood propofol concentration. As expected, the data showed that propofol potentiated the analgesic effects of alfentanil, and alfentanil potentiated the hypnotic effects of propofol. More importantly, the authors were able to relate various concentrations of each agent to a given end point.

The interest in these data lie in the way they can be used to model drug interactions.[134] In Figure 22-9, Vuyk, et al.[96] simulated the time to regain consciousness at different ratios of propofol and alfentanil. The graph is somewhat complex, but it is worth considering for a few moments. Vuyk and colleagues assume that a 180-minute anesthetic has been given with propofol and alfentanil targeted at various concentrations. Regardless of the ratio of the two drugs, the resulting anes-

thetic is sufficient to prevent the response to intra-abdominal surgery in 50% of patients. The three-axis graph relates the concentrations of each drug to the time after discontinuation of the infusions. At time 0 (the floor of the graph), we see the steady-state concentrations just when the infusions are stopped. The disappearance of both drugs is shown, and the family of plasma decay curves (all possible combinations of propofol and alfentanil) is depicted on the graph surface. The curved line that crosses the time-versus-concentration surface identifies the time at which a patient has a 50% probability of awakening. The fastest emergence (10 minutes) occurs when propofol and alfentanil are targeted at concentrations of 3.5 μg/mL and 85 ng/mL, respectively. Emergence is significantly longer if the anesthetic is mostly propofol or mostly alfentanil.

How will these data help anyone give an anesthetic? What if the infusion is much shorter or longer than 180 minutes? What if the patients are old and sick? What if the anesthesiologist does not have a computer or an infusion pump? The answer could be another set of questions: "What is the value of knowing that the MAC of halothane is 0.74 vol%, the induction dose of propofol is 2.5 mg/kg, or the analgesic dose of morphine is 0.1 mg/kg?" We all understand that the value of such numbers is to give us a frame of reference for titrating the agents. The value of the model created by Vuyk and colleagues[96] is not as a "recipe" for a good IV anesthetic, it is a way to think about dosing guidelines for two or more drugs simultaneously. It is not far-fetched to imagine that the Food and Drug Administration will someday require information on "optimal combinations" for each new pharmacologic agent.

References

1. Smith NT, Corbascio AN: Drug Interactions in Anesthesia, 2nd edition. Philadelphia, Lea and Febiger, 1986
2. Zbinden AM, Petersen-Felix S, Thomson DA: Anesthetic depth defined using multiple noxious stimuli during isoflurane/oxygen anesthesia: II. Hemodynamic responses. Anesthesiology 1994; 80: 261
3. Smith JW, Seidl LG, Cluff LG: Studies on the epidemiology of adverse drug reactions: V. Clinical factors influencing susceptibility. Ann Intern Med 1966; 65: 629
4. Bailey PL, Pace NL, Ashburn MA, et al: Frequent hypoxemia and apnea after sedation with midazolam and fentanyl. Anesthesiology 1990; 73: 826
5. Ausems ME, Hug CC Jr, Stanski DR, et al: Plasma concentrations of alfentanil required to supplement nitrous oxide anesthesia for general surgery. Anesthesiology 1986; 65: 362
6. Dundee JW, Robinson FP, McCullum JS, et al: Sensitivity to propofol in the elderly. Anaesthesia 1986; 41: 482
7. Baxter PJ, Garton K, Kharasch ED: Mechanistic aspects of carbon monoxide formation from volatile anesthetics. Anesthesiology 1998; 89: 929
8. Laster MJ, Eger EI: Temperature in soda lime during degradation of desflurane, isoflurane, and sevoflurane by dessicated soda lime. Anesth Analg 2005; 101: 753
9. Murphy DB, Sutton JA, Prescott LF, et al: Opioid-induced delay in gastric emptying: A peripheral mechanism in humans. Anesthesiology 1997; 87: 765
10. Asai T, McBeth C, Stewart JIM, et al: Effect of clonidine on gastric emptying of liquids. Br J Anaesth 1997; 78: 28
11. Avram MJ, Krejcie TC, Henthorn TK, et al: Beta-adrenergic blockade affects initial drug distribution due to decreased cardiac output and altered blood flow distribution. J Pharmacol Exp Ther 2004; 311: 617
12. Johnson KB, Kern SE, Hamber EA, et al: The influence of hemorrhagic shock on remifentanil: A pharmacokinetic and pharmacodynamic analysis. Anesthesiology 2001; 94: 322
13. Adams P, Gelman S, Reves JG, et al: Midazolam pharmacodynamics and pharmacokinetics during acute hypovolemia. Anesthesiology 1985; 63: 140
14. Klockowski PM, Levy G: Kinetics of drug action in disease states: XXV. Effect of experimental hypovolemia on the pharmacodynamics and pharmacokinetics of desmethyldiazepam. J Pharmacol Exp Ther 1988; 245: 508
15. van der Meer JWM, Keuning JJ, et al: The influence of gastric acidity on the bioavailability of ketoconazole. J Antimicrob Chemother 1980; 6: 552
16. Elwood RJ, Hildebrand PJ, et al: Influence of ranitidine on uptake of oral midazolam. Br J Anaesth 1983; 55: 241
17. Trudnowski RJ, Gessner T: Gastric excretion of intravenously administered meperidine in surgical patients. Anesth Analg 1979; 58: 88
18. Silverman WA, Andersen DH, Blanc WA, et al: A difference in mortality rate and incidence of kernicterus among premature infants allotted to two prophylactic antibacterial regimens. Pediatrics 1956; 18: 614

19. Holford NHG: Pharmacokinetics and pharmacodynamics: Rational dosing and the time course of drug action, Basic and Clinical Pharmacology, 9th ed. Edited by Katzung B. New York, McGraw-Hill, 2004, pp 48

20. Brodsky JB, Campos FA: Chloroprocaine analgesia in a patient receiving echothiophate eye drops. Anesthesiology 1978; 48: 288

21. Kuhnert BR, Philipson EH, Pimental R, et al: A prolonged chloroprocaine epidural block in a postpartum patient with abnormal pseudocholinesterase. Anesthesiology 1982; 56: 477

22. Lanks WK, Sklar GS: Pseudocholinesterase levels and rates of chloroprocaine hydrolysis in patients receiving adequate doses of phospholine iodide. Anesthesiology 1980; 52: 434

23. Davis PJ, Stiller RL, Wilson AS, et al: In vitro remifentanil metabolism: The effects of whole blood constituents and plasma butyrylcholinesterase. Anesth Analg 2002; 95: 1305

24. Boakes AJ, Laurence DR, Teoh PC, et al: Interactions between sympathomimetic amines and antidepressant agents in man. Br Med J 1973; 311

25. Parkinson's Study Group: Effects of tocopherol and deprenyl on the progression of disability in early Parkinson's disease. N Engl J Med 1993; 328: 176

26. Gillman PK: Monoamine oxidase inhibitors, opioid analgesics and serotonin toxicity, Br J Anaesth 2005; 95: 434

27. Zornberg GL, Bodkin JA, Cohen BM: Severe adverse interaction between pethidine and selegiline. Lancet 1991; 337: 246

28. Rivers N, Horner B: Possible lethal reaction between nardil and dextromethorphan [Letter]. CMAJ 1970; 103: 85

29. Zornberg GL, Hegarty JD: Adverse interaction between propoxyphene and phenelzine. Am J Psychiatry 1993; 150: 1270

30. Michaels I, Serrins M, Shier NQ, et al: Anesthesia for cardiac surgery in patients receiving monoamine oxidase inhibitors. Anesth Analg 1984; 63: 1041

31. Sjoqvist F: Psychotropic drugs (2): Interaction between monoamine oxidase (MAO) inhibitors and other substances. Proc R Soc Med 1965; 58: 967

32. Doyle DJ: Ketamine induction and monoamine oxidase inhibitors. J Clin Anesth 1990; 2: 324

33. El-Ganzouri AR, Ivankovich AD, Braverman B, et al: Monoamine oxidase inhibitors: Should they be discontinued preoperatively? Anesth Analg 1985; 64: 592

34. Dolenc TJ, Habl SS, Barnes RD, Rasmussen KG. Electroconvulsive therapy in patients taking monoamine oxidase inhibitors. J ECT 2004; 20: 258

35. Roizen MF: Monoamine oxidase inhibitors: Are we condemned to relive history or is history no longer relevant? J Clin Anesth 1990; 2: 293

36. Stenson RE, Constantino RT, Harrison DC: Interrelationship of hepatic blood flow, cardiac output and blood levels of lidocaine in man. Circulation 1971; 18: 205

37. Benowitz NL, Forsyth RP, Melmon KL, et al: Lidocaine disposition kinetics in monkey and man: II. Effects of hemorrhage and sympathomimetic drug administration. Clin Pharmacol Ther 1974; 16: 99

38. Feely J, Wilkinson GR, McAllister CB, et al: Increased toxicity and reduced clearance of lidocaine by cimetidine. Ann Intern Med 1982; 96: 592

39. Tukey RH, Johnson EF: Molecular aspects of regulation and structure of the drug-metabolizing enzymes, Principles of Drug Action: The Basis of Pharmacology, 3rd ed. Edited by Pratt WB, Taylor P., New York, Churchill Livingstone, 1990, pp 435

40. Greenstein LR, Hitt BA, Mazze RI: Metabolism in vitro of enflurane, isoflurane, and methoxyflurane. Anesthesiology 1975; 42: 420

41. Mazze RI, Trudell JR, Cousins MJ: Methoxyflurane metabolism and renal dysfunction: Clinical correlation in man. Anesthesiology 1971; 35: 247

42. Sipes JG, Brown BR Jr: An animal model of hepatotoxicity associated with halothane anesthesia. Anesthesiology 1976; 45: 622

43. Oda Y, Mizutani K, Hase I, et al: Fentanyl inhibits metabolism of midazolam: Competitive inhibition of CYP3A4 in vitro. Br J Anaesth 1999; 82: 900

44. Hamaoka N, Oda Y, Hase I, et al: Propofol decreases the clearance of midazolam by inhibiting CYP3A4: In vivo and in-vitro study. Clin Pharmacol Ther 1999; 66: 110

45. Oda Y, Hamaoka N, Hiroi T, et al: Involvement of human liver cytochrome P4502B6 in the metabolism of propofol. Br J Clin Pharmacol 2001; 51: 281

46. Bartkowski RR, Goldberg ME, Larijani GE, et al: Inhibition of alfentanil metabolism by erythromycin. Clin Pharmacol Ther 1989; 46: 99

47. Tateishi T, Krivoruk Y, Ueng Y, et al: Identification of human liver cytochrome P-450 3A4 as the enzyme responsible for fentanyl and sufentanil N-dealkylation. Anesth Analg 1996; 82: 167

48. Bartkowski RR, Goldberg ME, Huffnagle S, et al: Sufentanil disposition. Anesthesiology 1993; 78: 260

49. Klotz U, Reimann I: Delayed clearance of diazepam due to cimetidine. N Engl J Med 1980; 302: 1012

50. Palkama VJ, Ahonen J, Neuvonen J, et al: Effect of saquinavir on the pharmacokinetics and dynamics of oral and intravenous midazolam. Clin Pharmacol Ther 1999; 66: 33

51. Olkkola KT, Palkama VJ, Neuvonen PJ: Ritonavir's role in reducing fentanyl clearance and prolonging its half life. Anesthesiology 1999; 91: 681

52. Wagner RL, White PF, Kan PB, et al: Inhibition of adrenal steroidogenesis by the anesthetic etomidate. N Engl J Med 1984; 310: 1415

53. Leahey EB Jr, Reiffel JA, Drusin RE, et al: Interaction between quinidine and digoxin. JAMA 1978; 240: 533

54. Naguib M, Samarkandi AH, Bakhamees HS, et al: Comparative potency of steroidal neuromuscular blocking drugs and isobolographic analysis of the interaction. Br J Anaesth 1995; 75: 37

55. Quasha AL, Eger EI II, Tinker JH: Determination and applications of MAC. Anesthesiology 1980; 53: 315

56. Murray TJ, Mehta MP, Forbes RB, et al: Additive contribution of nitrous oxide to halothane MAC in infants and children. Anesth Analg 1990; 71: 120

57. Eger EI II. Does 1 + 1 = 2? Anesth Analg 1989; 41: 482

58. Munson ES, Paul WL, Embro WJ: Central nervous system toxicity of local anesthetic mixtures in monkeys. Anesthesiology 1977; 46: 179

59. Kim KS, Na DJ, Chon SU: Interactions between suxamethonium and mivacurium or atracurium. Br J Anaesth 1996; 77: 612

60. Eisenach JC, Schlairet TJ, Dobson CE II, et al: Effect of prior anesthetic solution on epidural morphine analgesia. Anesth Analg 1991; 73: 119

61. Dershwitz M, Rosow CE, DiBiase PM, et al: A comparison of the sedative effects of butorphanol and midazolam. Anesthesiology 1991; 74: 717

62. Maves TJ, Pechman PS, Meller ST, et al: Ketorolac potentiates morphine antinociception during visceral nociception in the rat. Anesthesiology 1994; 80: 1094

63. Lebowitz PW, Ramsey FM, Savarese JJ, et al: Potentiation of neuromuscular blockade in man produced by combinations of pancuronium and metocurine or pancuronium and d-tubocurarine. Anesth Analg 1980; 59: 604

64. Bowman WC, Prior C, Marshall IG: Presynaptic receptors in the neuromuscular junction. Ann N Y Acad Sci 1990; 604: 69

65. Standaert FG: Basic chemistry of acetylcholine receptors. Anesth Clin North Am 1993; 11: 205

66. Tallarida RJ: Statistical analysis of drug combinations for synergism. Pain 1992; 49: 93

67. Berenbaum MC: Synergy, additivism and antagonism in immunosuppression. J Clin Exp Immunol 1977; 28: 1

68. Berenbaum MC: What is synergy? Pharm Rev 1989; 41: 93

69. Tallarida RJ, Porreca F, Cowan A: Statistical analysis of drug-drug and site-site interactions with isobolograms. Life Sci 1989; 45: 947

70. Tverskoy M, Fleyshman G, Bradley EL Jr, et al: Midazolam-thiopental anesthetic interaction in patients. Anesth Analg 1988; 67: 342

71. Stone JG, Foex P, Sear JW: Myocardial ischemia in untreated hypertensive patients: Effect of a single small oral dose of a beta-adrenergic blocking agent. Anesthesiology 1988; 68: 495

72. Pasternack PF, Grossi EA, Baumann FG, et al: Beta blockade to decrease silent myocardial ischemia during peripheral vascular surgery. Am J Surg 1989; 158: 113

73. Wallace A, Layug B, Tateo I, et al: Prophylactic atenolol reduces postoperative myocardial ischemia. Anesthesiology 1998; 88: 7

74. Warltier DC: β-Adrenergic-blocking drugs: Incredibly useful, incredibly underutilized. Anesthesiology 1998; 88: 2

75. Colson P, Saussine M, Séguin JR, et al: Hemodynamic effects of anesthesia in patients chronically treated with angiotensin converting enzyme inhibitors. Anesth Analg 1992; 74: 805

76. Coriat P, Richer C, Douraki T, et al: Influence of chronic angiotensin-converting enzyme inhibition on anesthetic induction. Anesthesiology 1994; 81: 299

77. Fruncillo RJ, Rotmensch HH, Vlasses PH, et al: Effect of captopril and hydrochlorothiazide on the response to pressor agents in hypertensives. Eur J Clin Pharmacol 1985; 28: 5

78. Boccara G, Ouattara A, Godet G, et al: Terlipressin versus norepinephrine to correct refractory arterial hypotension after general anesthesia in patients chronically treated with renin-angiotensin system inhibitors. Anesthesiology 2003; 98: 1338

79. Noguera I, Medina P, Segarra G, et al: Potentiation by vasopressin of adrenergic vasoconstriction in the rat isolated mesenteric artery. Br J Pharmacol 1997; 122: 431

80. Meersschaert K, Brun L, Gourdin M, et al: Terlipressin-ephedrine versus ephedrine to treat hypotension at the induction of anesthesia in patients chronically treated with angiotensin converting-enzyme inhibitors: A prospective, randomized, double-blinded, crossover study. Anesth Analg 2002; 94: 835

81. Licker M, Bednarkiewicz M, Neidhart P, et al: Preoperative inhibition of angiotensin-converting enzyme improves systemic and renal haemodynamic changes during aortic abdominal surgery. Br J Anaesth 1996; 76: 632

82. Comfere T, Sprung J, Kumar MM, et al: Angiotensin system inhibitors in a general surgical population. Anesth Analg 2005; 100: 636

83. Hohne C, Meier L, Boemke W, et al: ACE inhibition does not exaggerate the blood pressure decrease in the early phase of spinal anaesthesia. Acta Anaesth Scand 2003; 47: 891

84. Ryckwaert F, Colson P: Hemodynamic effects of anesthesia in patients with ischemic heart failure chronically treated with angiotensin-converting enzyme inhibitors. Anesth Analg 1997; 84: 945

85. Rosenthal JA: American Heart Association recommendations for treating tricyclic antidepressant-induced hypotension [Letter]. Anesthesiology 1997; 87: 1259

86. Sprung J, Schoenwald P, Levy P, et al: Treating intraoperative hypotension in a patient on long-term tricyclic antidepressants: A case of aborted aortic surgery. Anesthesiology 1997; 86: 990

87. Stoelting RK, Creasser CW, Martz RC: Effect of cocaine administration on halothane MAC in dogs. Anesth Analg 1975; 54: 422

88. Bernards C, Kern C, Cullen BF: Chronic cocaine administration reversibly increases isoflurane minimum alveolar concentration in sheep. Anesthesiology 1996; 85: 91

89. Bernards C, Teijeiro A: Illicit cocaine ingestion during anesthesia. Anesthesiology 1995; 84: 218

90. Johnston R, Way W, Miller R: Alteration of anesthetic requirement by amphetamine. Anesthesiology 1972; 36: 357

91. Seidler F, Slotkin T: Fetal cocaine exposure causes persistent noradrenergic hyperactivity in rat brain regions: Effects on neurotransmitter turnover and receptors. J Pharmacol Exp Ther 1992; 263: 413

92. Kelley K, Han D, Fellingham G, et al: Cocaine and exercise: Physiological responses of cocaine-conditioned rats. Med Sci Sports Exerc 1995; 27: 65

93. Epstein B, Levy M-L, Thein M, et al: Evaluation of fentanyl as an adjunct to thiopental-nitrous oxide-oxygen anesthesia for short procedures. Anesth Rev 1985; 2: 24

94. Rosow CE, Latta WB, Keegan CR, et al: Alfentanil for use in short surgical procedures, Opioids in Anesthesia. Edited by Estafanous FG. Boston, Butterworth, 1984, pp 93

95. Short TG, Plummer JL, Chui PT: Hypnotic and anaesthetic interactions between midazolam, propofol and alfentanil. Br J Anaesth 1992; 69: 162

96. Vuyk J, Lim T, Engbers FHM, et al: The pharmacodynamic interaction of propofol and alfentanil during lower abdominal surgery in women. Anesthesiology 1995; 83: 8

97. Smith C, McEwan AI, Jhaveri R, et al: The interaction of fentanyl on the Cp50 of propofol for loss of consciousness and skin incision. Anesthesiology 1994; 81: 820

98. Bailey PL, Wilbrink J, Zwanikken P, et al: Anesthetic induction with fentanyl. Anesth Analg 1985; 64: 48

99. Silbert BS, Rosow CE, Keegan CR, et al: The effect of diazepam on induction of anesthesia with alfentanil. Anesth Analg 1986; 65: 71

100. Kissin I, Vinik HR, Castillo R, et al: Alfentanil potentiates midazolam-induced unconsciousness in subanalgesic doses. Anesth Analg 1990; 71: 65

101. Short TG, Galletly DC, Plummer JL: Hypnotic and anaesthetic action of thiopentone and midazolam alone and in combination. Br J Anaesth 1991; 66: 13

102. Tverskoy M, Ben-Shlomo I, Finger EJ, et al: Midazolam acts synergistically with methohexitone for induction of anaesthesia. Br J Anaesth 1989; 63: 109

103. McEwan AI, Smith C, Dyar O, et al: Isoflurane minimum alveolar concentration reduction by fentanyl. Anesthesiology 1993; 78: 864

104. Murphy MR, Hug CC Jr: The enflurane sparing effect of morphine, butorphanol and nalbuphine. Anesthesiology 1982; 57: 489

105. Murphy RM, Hug CC Jr: The anesthetic potency of fentanyl in terms of its reduction of enflurane MAC. Anesthesiology 1982; 57: 485

106. Licina MG, Schubert A, Tobin JE, et al: Intrathecal morphine does not reduce minimum alveolar concentration of halothane in humans: Results of a double-blind study. Anesthesiology 1991; 74: 660

107. Rampil IJ, Mason P, Singh H: Anesthetic potency (MAC) is independent of forebrain structures in the rat. Anesthesiology 1993; 78: 707

108. Gross JB, Alexander CM: Awakening concentrations of isoflurane are not affected by analgesic doses of morphine. Anesth Analg 1988; 67: 27

109. Katoh T, Ikeda K: The effects of fentanyl on sevoflurane requirements for loss of consciousness and skin incision. Anesthesiology 1998; 88: 18

110. Himes RS, DiFazio CA, Burney RG: Effects of lidocaine on the anesthetic requirements for nitrous oxide and halothane. Anesthesiology 1977; 47: 437

111. Hall RI, Schwieger IM, Hug CC: The anesthetic efficacy of midazolam in the enflurane-anesthetized dog. Anesthesiology 1988; 68: 862

112. Hansen TD, Warner DS, Todd MM, et al: The influence of inhalational anesthetics on in vivo and in vitro benzodiazepine receptor binding in the rat cerebral cortex. Anesthesiology 1991; 74: 97

113. Miller RD, Way WL, Eger EI II: The effects of alpha-methyldopa, reserpine, guanethidine and ipronazide on minimum alveolar anesthetic concentration (MAC). Anesthesiology 1968; 29: 1156

114. Salonen M, Reid K, Maze M: Synergistic interaction between α-2-adrenergic agonists and benzodiazepines in rats. Anesthesiology 1992; 76: 1004

115. Segal IS, Vickery RG, Walton JK, et al: Dexmedetomidine diminishes halothane anesthetic requirements in rats through a postsynaptic α-2-adrenergic receptor. Anesthesiology 1988; 69: 818

116. Correa-Sales C, Rabin BC, Maze M: A hypnotic response to dexmedetomidine, an α-2-agonist, is mediated in the locus coeruleus in rats. Anesthesiology 1992; 76: 948

117. Scheinin M, Schwinn DA: The locus coeruleus: Site of hypnotic actions of α-2-adrenoceptor agonists? [Editorial]. Anesthesiology 1992; 76: 873

118. Advokat C: The role of descending inhibition in morphine-induced analgesia. Trends Pharmacol Sci 1988; 9: 330

119. Roizen MF, White PF, Eger EI II, et al: Effects of ablation of serotonin or norepinephrine brain-stem areas on halothane and cyclopropane MACs in rats. Anesthesiology 1978; 49: 252

120. Johns RA, Moscicki JC, DiFazio CA: Nitric oxide synthase inhibitor dose-dependently and reversibly reduces the threshold for halothane anesthesia: A role for nitric oxide in mediating consciousness? Anesthesiology 1992; 77: 779

121. Pajewski TN, DiFazio CA, Moscicki JC, et al: Nitric oxide synthase inhibitors, 7-nitro-indazole and nitroG-L-arginine-methyl ester, dose-dependently reduce the threshold for isoflurane anesthesia. Anesthesiology 1996; 85: 1111

122. Vinik HR, Bradley EL Jr, Kissin I: Triple anesthetic combination: Propofol-midazolam-alfentanil. Anesth Analg 1994; 78: 354

123. Salmenpera M, Szlam F, Hug CC Jr: Anesthetic and hemodynamic interactions of dexmedetomidine and fentanyl in dogs. Anesthesiology 1994; 80: 837

124. Nutrition Business Journal. Available at: www.nutritionbusiness.com. Accessed March 15, 2005

125. Tsen LC, Segal S, Pothier M, et al: Alternative medicine use in presurgical patients. Anesthesiology 2000; 93: 148

126. Kaye AD, Clarke RC, Sabar R, et al: Herbal medicines: Current trends in anesthesiology practice—a hospital survey. J Clin Anesth 2000; 12: 468

127. Dietary Supplement Health and Education Act, 1994, PL 103-417(180 Stat 2126)

128. Marwick C: Growing use of medicinal botanicals forces assessment by drug regulators. JAMA 1995; 273: 607

129. Kush RD, Bleicher P, Raymond S, Kubich W, Marks R, Tardiff B. Physicians' Desk Reference (PDR) for Herbal Medicines, 4th ed. Montvale, NJ, Thomson Healthcare, 2004

130. Ang-Lee MK, Moss J, Yuan CS: Herbal medicines and perioperative care. JAMA 2001; 286: 208

131. Fugh-Berman A: Herb-drug interactions. Lancet 2000; 355: 134

132. Miller LG: Herbal medicinals: Selected clinical considerations focusing on known or potential drug-herb interactions. Arch Intern Med 1998; 158: 2200

133. Fugh-Berman A: Herbal medicinals: Selected clinical considerations, focusing on known or potential drug-herb interactions. Arch Intern Med 1999; 159: 1957

134. Stanski DR, Shafer SL: Quantifying anesthetic drug interaction. Implications for drug dosing [Editorial]. Anesthesiology 1995; 83: 1

135. American Society of Anesthesiologists: Considerations for anesthesiologists: What you should know about your patients' use of herbal medicines and other dietary supplements. ASA pamphlet. American Society of Anesthesiologists, 2003

136. Haller CA, Benowitz NL: Adverse cardiovascular and central nervous system events associated with dietary supplements containing ephedra alkaloids. N Engl J Med 2000; 343: 1833

137. Gorski JC, Huang SM, Pinto A, et al: The effect of echinacea (Echinacea purpurea root) on cytochrome P450 activity in vivo. Clin Pharmacol Ther 2004; 75: 89–100

138. See DM, Broumand N, Sahl L, et al: In vitro effects of echinacea and ginseng on natural killer and antibody-dependent cell cytotoxicity in healthy subjects and chronic fatigue syndrome or acquired immunodeficiency syndrome patients. Immunopharmacology 1997; 35: 229

139. Luettig B, Steinmuller C, Gifford GE, et al: Macrophage activation by the polysaccharide arabinogalactan isolated from plant cell cultures of Echinacea purpurea. J Natl Cancer Inst 1989; 81: 669

140. Vaes LP, Chyka PA: Interactions of warfarin with garlic, ginger, ginkgo, or ginseng: Nature of the evidence. Ann Pharmacother 2000; 34: 1478

141. Bordia A: Effect of garlic on human platelet aggregation in vitro. Atherosclerosis 1978; 30: 355

142. Bordia A, Verma SK, Srivastava KC: Effect of garlic (Allium sativum) on blood lipids, blood sugar, fibrinogen and fibrinolytic activity in patients with coronary artery disease. Prostaglandins Leukot Essent Fatty Acids 1998; 58: 257

143. Ali M, Bordia T, Mustafa T: Effect of raw versus boiled aqueous extract of garlic and onion on platelet aggregation. Prostaglandins Leukot Essent Fatty Acids 1999; 60: 43

144. Kiesewetter H, Jung F, Jung EM, et al: Effect of garlic on platelet aggregation in patients with increased risk of juvenile ischaemic attack. Eur J Clin Pharmacol 1993; 45: 333

145. Kiesewetter H, Jung C, Mrowietz G, et al: Effects of garlic on blood fluidity and fibrinolytic activity: A randomised, placebo-controlled, double-blind study. Br J Clin Pract 1990; 69(Suppl): 24

146. Das IKN, Sooranna SR: Potent activation of nitric oxide synthase by garlic: A basis for its therapeutic applications. Curr Med Res Opin 1995; 13: 257

147. Bordia A, Verma SK, Srivastava KC: Effect of ginger (Zingiber officinale Rosc.) and fenugreek (Trigonella foenumgraecum L.) on blood lipids, blood sugar and platelet aggregation in patients with coronary artery disease. Prostaglandins Leukot Essent Fatty Acids 1997; 56: 379

148. Srivastava KC: Effect of onion and ginger consumption on platelet thromboxane production in humans. Prostaglandins Leukot Essent Fatty Acids 1989; 35: 183

149. Thomson M, Al-Qattan KK, Al-Sawan SM, et al: The use of ginger (Zingiber officinale Rosc.) as a potential anti-inflammatory and antithrombotic agent. Prostaglandins Leukot Essent Fatty Acids 2002; 67: 475

150. Lumb AB: Effect of dried ginger on human platelet function. Thromb Haemost 1994; 71: 110

151. Janssen PL, Meyboom S, van Staveren WA, et al: Consumption of ginger (Zingiber officinale roscoe) does not affect ex vivo platelet thromboxane production in humans. Eur J Clin Nutr 1996; 50: 772

152. Meisel C, Johne A, Roots I: Fatal intracerebral mass bleeding associated with ginkgo biloba and ibuprofen. Atherosclerosis 2003; 167: 367

153. Chung KF, Dent G, McCusker M, et al: Effect of a ginkgolide mixture (BN 52063) in antagonising skin and platelet responses to platelet activating factor in man. Lancet 1987; 1: 248

154. Bal Dit Sollier C, Caplain H, Drouet L: No alteration in platelet function or coagulation induced by EGb761 in a controlled study. Clin Lab Haematol 2003; 25: 251

155. Russmann S, Lauterburg BH, Helbling A: Kava hepatotoxicity. Ann Intern Med 2001; 135: 68

156. Stickel F, Baumuller HM, Seitz K, et al: Hepatitis induced by Kava (*Piper methysticum rhizoma*). J Hepatol 2003; 39: 62

157. Lehrl S: Clinical efficacy of kava extract WS 1490 in sleep disturbances associated with anxiety disorders. Results of a multicenter, randomized, placebo-controlled, double-blind clinical trial. J Affect Disord 2004; 78: 101

158. Pittler MH, Ernst E: Efficacy of kava extract for treating anxiety: systemic review and meta-analysis. J Psychopharmacol 2000; 20: 84

159. Garrett KM, Basmadjian G, Khan IA, et al: Extracts of kava (*Piper methysticum*) induce acute anxiolytic-like behavioral changes in mice. Psychopharmacology (Berl) 2003; 170: 33

160. Forslund T, Fyhrquist F, Froseth B, et al: Effects of licorice on plasma atrial natriuretic peptide in healthy volunteers. J Intern Med 1989; 225: 95

161. Bernardi M, D'Intino PE, Trevisani F, et al: Effects of prolonged ingestion of graded doses of licorice by healthy volunteers. Life Sci 1994; 55: 863

162. Durr D, Stieger B, Kullak-Ublick GA, et al: St John's wort induces intestinal P-glycoprotein/MDR1 and intestinal and hepatic CYP3A4. Clin Pharmacol Ther 2000; 68: 598

163. Crowe S, McKeating K: Delayed emergence and St. John's wort. Anesthesiology 2002; 96: 1025

164. Markowitz JS, Donovan JL, DeVane C, et al: Effect of St John's wort on drug metabolism by induction of cytochrome P450 3A4 enzyme. JAMA 2003; 290(11): 1500

165. Irefin S, Sprung J: A possible cause of cardiovascular collapse during anesthesia: Long-term use of St. John's wort. J Clin Anesth 2000; 12: 498

166. Balderer G, Borbely AA: Effect of valerian on human sleep. Psychopharmacology (Berl) 1985; 87: 406

167. Donath F, Quispe K, Diefenbach A, et al: Critical evaluation of the effect of valerian extract on sleep structure and sleep quality. Pharmacopsychiatry 2000; 33: 47

168. Celestini A, Pulcinelli FM, Pignatelli P, et al: Vitamin E potentiates the antiplatelet activity of aspirin in collagen-stimulated platelets. Haematologica 2002; 87: 420

169. Szuwart T, Brzoska T, Luger TA, et al: Vitamin E reduces platelet adhesion to human endothelial cells in vitro. Am J Hematol 2000; 65: 1

170. Pignatelli P, Pulcinelli FM, Lenti L, et al: Vitamin E inhibits collagen-induced platelet activation by blunting hydrogen peroxide. Arterioscler Thromb Vasc Biol 1999; 19: 2542

171. Steiner M: Vitamin E, a modifier of platelet function: Rationale and use in cardiovascular and cerebrovascular disease. Nutr Rev 1999; 57: 306

SECTION V ■ PREANESTHETIC EVALUATION AND PREPARATION

CHAPTER 23 ■ PREOPERATIVE PATIENT ASSESSMENT AND MANAGEMENT

TARA M. HATA AND JOHN R. MOYERS

KEY POINTS

1 The Joint Commission requires that all patients receive a preoperative anesthetic evaluation, and the American Society of Anesthesiologists (ASA) published a Practice Advisory for Preanesthesia Evaluation in 2002 and Approved Basic Standards for Preoperative Care.

2 The goals of a preoperative evaluation are to reduce patient risk and morbidity associated with surgery and coexisting diseases, promote efficiency and reduce costs, as well as to prepare the patient medically and psychologically for surgery and anesthesia.

3 It is important for the evaluation to be complete, accurate, and clear, not only to allow the information to be relayed to others who may care for the patient perioperatively, but also for medicolegal purposes.

4 The preoperative evaluation serves as a screening tool to anticipate and avoid airway difficulties or problems with anesthetic drugs. In addition to the history and physical, previous anesthesia records should be reviewed. Contraindications to specific drugs, such as succinylcholine, nitrous oxide, or volatile agents, should be sought.

5 Review of the patient's allergies and medication list, including over-the-counter and herbal medications, should specifically screen for latex allergy and potential drug interactions. It should also alert the anesthesiologist to the need for steroid coverage.

6 When evaluating the patient with hypertension, diabetes, or obesity it is important to determine the presence of end-organ damage such as heart, lung, renal, and cerebrovascular dysfunction.

7 Exercise tolerance is the most important determinant of cardiac risk. The algorithm for preoperative evaluation of cardiac patients undergoing noncardiac surgery is a useful guide to determine the need for further testing and evaluation.

8 Preoperative laboratory tests should be ordered on the basis of positive findings from the history and physical examination, or anticipated physiological disturbances during surgery such as blood loss.

9 Optimization of the patient's health status prior to surgery includes clear instruction regarding nothing by mouth times as well as which medications to administer immediately before surgery. In general, most medications for hypertension or cardiac disease should be considered, and consideration should be given to initiating a beta-blocker in patients at risk. The need for subacute bacterial endocarditis prophylaxis should be anticipated. Likewise, drugs for asthma or chronic obstructive pulmonary disease should be continued or administered prophylactically. Medications taken for the treatment of reflux should be continued, or initiated for those patients with untreated symptoms. For diabetic patients, oral hypoglycemic agents should often be held, but patients requiring insulin will need to continue to take adjusted doses.

10 Although preoperative sedation is generally limited to drugs given immediately prior to anesthesia, the timing of administration must be planned when oral sedation is needed in children to allow optimal effect and avoid operating room delays.

The goals of preoperative evaluation are to reduce patient risk and the morbidity of surgery, as well as to promote efficiency and reduce costs. The Joint Commission requires that all patients receive a preoperative anesthetic evaluation. The American Society of Anesthesiologists (ASA) approved Basic Standards for Preanesthetic Care, which outlines the minimum requirements for a preoperative evaluation. Conducting a preoperative evaluation is based on the premise that it will modify patient care and improve outcome. There is evidence, although not entirely convincing in all instances, that the preoperative evaluation will increase patient safety. That is, armed with knowledge preoperatively, the anesthesiologist can formulate and conduct an anesthetic plan that avoids dangers inherent in patient disease states. Furthermore, preoperative evaluations may reduce costs and cancellation rates, increasing resource utilization in the operating room. This notion assumes that evaluations are done by anesthesiologists and others familiar with anesthetics, surgery, and perioperative events.

The preoperative evaluation has several components and goals. One should obtain a history and perform a physical examination pertinent to the patient and contemplated surgery. Based on the history and physical examination, the appropriate laboratory tests and preoperative consultations should be obtained. Through these, one needs to determine whether the patient's preoperative condition may be improved prior to surgery. Guided by these factors, the anesthesiologist should choose the appropriate anesthetic and care plan. Finally, the process should be used to educate the patient about anesthesia and the perioperative period, answer all questions, and obtain informed consent.

The first part of this chapter outlines clinical risk factors pertinent to patients scheduled for anesthesia and surgery and the use of tests to confirm diagnoses. The second part discusses preoperative medication. The chapter provides only an overview of the preoperative management process; for more details, the reader is referred to chapters focusing on specific organ systems.

CHANGING CONCEPTS IN PREOPERATIVE EVALUATION

In the past, patients were admitted to the hospital at least a day prior to surgery. Currently, more and more patients are admitted to the hospital from the postanesthesia care unit. Older patients are scheduled for more complex procedures, and there is more pressure on the anesthesiologist to reduce the time between cases. The first time the anesthesiologist performing the anesthetic sees the patient may be just prior to anesthesia and surgery. Others may have seen the patient previously in a preoperative evaluation clinic. Only a short time exists to engender trust and answer last-minute questions. It is often impossible to alter medical therapy at this juncture immediately preoperatively. However, preoperative screening clinics are becoming more effective and clinical practice guidelines are becoming more prevalent. Information technology has helped the anesthesiologist in previewing the upcoming patients who will be anesthetized. Preoperative questionnaires and computer-driven programs have become alternatives to traditional information gathering. Finally, when anesthesiologists are responsible for ordering preoperative laboratory tests, cost saving occurs and cancellations of planned surgical procedures become less likely. In this setting it is important that there is communication between the preoperative evaluation clinic and the anesthesiologist performing the anesthetic.

APPROACH TO THE HEALTHY PATIENT

The preoperative evaluation form is the basis for formulating the best anesthetic plan tailored to the patient. It should aid the anesthesiologist in identifying potential complications, as well as serve as a medicolegal document. The importance of the design has increased because it is more common today for the evaluation to be completed in a preoperation clinic by another physician or health professional who will not personally be performing the anesthetic, but also because regulatory agencies such as JCAHO demand better documentation. Therefore, the information obtained needs to be complete, concise, and legible. In those hospitals that have electronic medical records, legibility is no longer an issue. A group from University of California, San Diego studied the quality of preoperative evaluation forms across the United States and rated them in three categories: informational content, ease of use, and ease of reading.[1] Their results revealed that a surprisingly high percentage of forms are missing important information. Figure 23-1 is an example of the preoperative evaluation form in use at the University of Iowa Hospitals, which attempts to document all pertinent information.

The approach to the patient should always begin with a thorough history and physical examination. These two evaluations alone may be sufficient (without additional routine laboratory tests).

The indication for the surgical procedure is part of the preoperative history because it will help determine the urgency of the surgery. True emergency procedures, which are associated with a recognized higher anesthetic morbidity and mortality, require a more abbreviated evaluation. A less-defined area is the approach to urgent procedures. For example, ischemic limbs require surgery soon after presentation, but can usually be delayed for 24 hours for further evaluation. The indication for the surgical procedure may also have implications on other aspects of perioperative management. For example, the presence of a small bowel obstruction has implications regarding the risk of aspiration and the need for a rapid sequence induction. The extent of a lung resection will dictate the need for further pulmonary testing and perioperative monitoring. Patients undergoing carotid endarterectomy may require a more extensive neurologic examination, as well as testing to rule out coronary artery disease (CAD). Frequently, further information will be required that necessitates contacting the surgeon. Perioperative care of the patient, as well as efficiency in the operating room, is always enhanced by close communication with the surgeons.

The ability to review previous anesthetic records is helpful in detecting the presence of a difficult airway, a history of malignant hyperthermia, and the individual's response to surgical stress and specific anesthetics. The patient should be questioned regarding any previous difficulty with anesthesia or other family members having difficulty with anesthesia. A patient history relating an "allergy" to anesthesia should make one suspicious for malignant hyperthermia.

The history should include a complete list of medications, including over-the-counter and herbal products, to define a preoperative medication regimen, anticipate potential drug interactions, and provide clues to underlying disease. A complete list of drug allergies, including previous reactions, should be obtained, as well as an inquiry concerning reaction to latex.

The anesthesiologist should determine when the patient last ate, as well as note the sites of pre-existing intravenous cannulae and invasive monitors. Once the general issues are completed, the preoperative history and physical examination can focus on specific systems.

PRE-ANESTHETIC EVALUATION Patient Name _____ Hospital Number _____

Operation Proposed _____

Surgical Diagnosis _____

Age _____ Gender _____ Wt _____ Ht _____

BP ___ P ___ rr ___ T ___

Allergies ☐ Latex allergy

Medications (Include Drugs, OTC and Herbals):

Anesthetic History ☐ Malignant hyperthermia

HEENT ☐ Hx of difficult airway
Teeth:
Class: I II III IV
Chin:
Neck:

Respiratory System ☐ WNL
☐ Asthma ☐ Bronchitis ☐ COPD ☐ Pneumonia
☐ TB ☐ Penumothorax ☐ Recent URI ☐ Dyspnea
☐ Cough ☐ RequiresO2 ☐ Steroids ☐ Snoring/Sleep Apnea
Tobacco: ___ ppd ___ YR
Chest Exam:
CxR:

Anesthetic options / risks discussed _____

☐ Risks discussed and patient/guardian understands.

Print Name/Signature   Time   Date

Cardiovascular System ☐ WNL
☐ CHD ☐ HTN ☐ CAD ☐ MI ☐ Valve disease
☐ Cardiomyopathy ☐ CHF ☐ RF ☐ Pacer ☐ Dysrrhythmia
☐ PVD ☐ Angina ☐ DOE ☐ Orthopnea ☐ Murmur
Exercise tolerance:
CV Exam:
EKG:
Echo/Cath:

Central Nervous System ☐ WNL
☐ CVA ☐ TIA ☐ LOC ☐ Seizures ☐ ↑ICP
☐ HA ☐ NM disease ☐ Weakness ☐ Parethesias ☐ Psych disorder
☐ Altered MS/GCS ☐ Spinal cord injury

Renal ☐ WNL
☐ Insufficiency ☐ Failure ☐ Dialysis: last date _____

GI, Hepatic ☐ WNL
☐ Liver disease ☐ Hepatitis ☐ Bowel obstruction ☐ N/V ☐ Reflux
ETOH_drinks / _____

Endocrine, Metabolic, Infections, Other ☐ WNL
☐ Diabetes ☐ Thyroid disease ☐ RA ☐ Steroids
☐ Coagulopathy ☐ Chemotherapy ☐ Sickle Cell ☐ Pregnant
☐ Anemia ☐ HIV ☐ MRSA ☐ VRE

Additional Information / Interval History
☐ Advance directive(s) documented elsewhere

NPO Status:
Invasive monitors:
IV Access:

Pt Instructions:

Print Staff Name/Signature   Time   Date

Lab Data

☐ Patient examined and chart reviewed.
   Patient approved for anesthesia.
☐ Potential post-op ICU admission
A/P:

Attending Signature   Time   Date
POSTANESTHETIC EVALUATION
   PACU / ICU / Ward
☐ Extubated O₂ sat _____
☐ Satisfactory spont vent P _____
☐ Protective reflexes BP _____
☐ Follows commands IT _____
☐ Report given T _____

Signature   Time   Date
POSTANESTHETIC PROGRESS NOTE
☐ No anesthesia related adverse events

Signature   Time   Date

FIGURE 23-1.   Example of preanesthetic evaluation form.

Systems Approach

Airway

A basic concern of the anesthesiologist is always the patient's airway. The ability to review previous anesthetic records is especially useful in uncovering unsuspected "difficult airways" or to confirm previous uneventful intubations, assuming the patient's body habitus has not changed in the interim. Evaluation of the airway involves determination of the thyromental distance, the ability to flex the base of the neck and extend the head, and examination of the oral cavity, including dentition. The Mallampati classification has become the standard for assessing the relationship of the tongue size relative to the oral cavity (Table 23-1),[2] although by itself the Mallampati classification has a low positive predictive value in identifying patients who are difficult to intubate.[3,4] Most anesthesiologists find a multifactorial approach very helpful (Table 23-2). In trauma patients, as well as those with severe rheumatoid arthritis or Down syndrome, assessment of the cervical spine is critical. In appropriate patients, the presence of pain or symptoms of cervical cord compression on movement should be assessed. In other instances, radiographic examination may be required.

Pulmonary

A screening evaluation should include questions regarding the history of tobacco use, shortness of breath, cough, wheezing, stridor, and snoring or sleep apnea. The patient should also be questioned regarding the presence or recent history of an upper respiratory tract infection. Physical examination should assess the respiratory rate as well as the chest excursion, use of accessory muscles, nail color, and the patient's ability to carry on a conversation or to walk without dyspnea. Auscultation should be used to detect decreased breath sounds, wheezing,

TABLE 23-1

AIRWAY CLASSIFICATION SYSTEM

■ CLASS	■ DIRECT VISUALIZATION, PATIENT SEATED	■ LARYNGOSCOPIC VIEW
I	Soft palate, fauces, uvula, pillars	Entire glottic
II	Soft palate, fauces, uvula	Posterior commissure
III	Soft palate, uvular base	Tip of epiglottis
IV	Hard palate only	No glottal structures

Modified from Mallampati RS, Gatt SP, Gugino LD, et al: A clinical sign to predict difficult tracheal intubation: A prospective study. Can Anaesth Soc J 1985; 32: 429, with permission.

TABLE 23-2

COMPONENTS OF THE AIRWAY PHYSICAL EXAMINATION[a]

■ AIRWAY EXAMINATION COMPONENT	■ SUGGESTIVE OF DIFFICULTY WITH INTUBATION
1. Length of upper incisors	Long compared to the rest of dentition
2. Relation of maxillary and mandibular incisors during normal jaw closure	Prominent "overbite"
3. Relation of maxillary and mandibular incisors during voluntary protrusion of mandible	Patient cannot bring mandibular incisors anterior to maxillary incisors
4. Interincisor distance	Less than 3 cm
5. Visibility of uvula	Not visible when tongue is protruded with patient in sitting position
6. Shape of palate	Highly arched or very narrow
7. Compliance of mandibular space	Stiff, indurated, occupied by mass, or nonresilient
8. Thyromental distance	Less than three fingerbreadths
9. Length of neck	Short neck
10. Thickness of neck	Thick neck
11. Range of motion of head and neck	Patient cannot touch tip of chin to chest or is unable to extend neck

[a]This table displays some findings of the airway physical examination that may suggest difficulty with intubation. Clinical context and judgment determine which of the components apply to a particular patient. The order of presentation in this table follows the "line of sight" that occurs during conventional oral laryngoscopy.
Modified from the Task Force on Difficult Airway Management: Practice guidelines for management of the difficult airway: An updated report by the American Society of Anesthesiologist Task Force on Management of the Difficult Airway. *Anesthesiology* 2003; 98: 1269.

stridor, or rales. For the patient with positive findings, see the section on the preoperative evaluation of the patient with Pulmonary Disease.

Cardiovascular System

When screening a patient for cardiovascular disease prior to surgery, the anesthesiologist is most interested in recognizing signs and symptoms of uncontrolled hypertension and unstable cardiac disease such as myocardial ischemia, congestive heart failure, valvular heart disease, and significant cardiac dysrhythmias. Symptoms of cardiovascular disease should be carefully determined, especially the characteristics of chest pain, if present. Certain populations of patients, such as the elderly, women, or diabetics, may present with more atypical features. The presence of unstable angina has been associated with a high perioperative risk of myocardial infarction (MI).[5] The perioperative period is associated with a hypercoagulable state and surges in endogenous catecholamines, both of which may exacerbate the underlying process in unstable angina, increasing the risk of acute infarction.[6] The preoperative evaluation can affect both a patient's short- and long-term health by instituting treatment of unstable angina. Symptoms of clinically important valvular disease should be sought, such as angina, syncope, or congestive heart failure from aortic stenosis that would require further evaluation. A history of other valvular disease such as mitral valve prolapse may simply dictate the need for subacute bacterial endocarditis prophylaxis.

The examination of the cardiovascular system should include blood pressure, measuring both arms when appropriate. The anesthesiologist should take into account the effects of preoperative anxiety and may want a record of resting blood pressure measurements. However, Bedford and Feinstein[7] reported that the admission blood pressure was the best predictor of HR and BP response to laryngoscopy. Auscultation of the heart is performed, specifically listening for a murmur radiating to the carotids suggestive of aortic stenosis, abnormal rhythms, or a

gallop suggestive of heart failure. The presence of bruits over the carotid arteries would warrant further workup to determine the risk of stroke. The extremities should also be examined for the presence of peripheral pulses to exclude peripheral vascular disease or congenital cardiovascular disease.

Neurologic System

A screening of the neurologic system in the apparently healthy patient mostly can be accomplished through simple observation. The patient's ability to answer health history questions practically ensures a normal mental status. Questions can be directed to exclude the presence of increased intracranial pressure, cerebrovascular disease, seizure history, pre-existing neuromuscular disease, or nerve injuries. The neurologic examination may be cursory in healthy patients, or extensive in patients with coexisting disease. Testing of strength, reflexes, and sensation may be important in patients if the anesthetic plan or surgical procedure may result in a change in the condition.

Endocrine System

Each patient should be screened for endocrine diseases that may affect the perioperative course: diabetes, thyroid disease, parathyroid disease, endocrine-secreting tumors, and adrenal cortical suppression.

EVALUATION OF THE PATIENT WITH KNOWN SYSTEMIC DISEASE

Cardiovascular Disease

The preoperative evaluation of the patient with suspected cardiovascular disease has been approached in two ways: clinical

TABLE 23-3

AMERICAN SOCIETY OF ANESTHESIOLOGISTS (ASA) PHYSICAL STATUS CLASSIFICATION

■ DISEASE	■ STATE
ASA Class 1	No organic, physiologic, biochemical, or psychiatric disturbance
ASA Class 2	Mild-to-moderate systemic disturbance that may not be related to the reason for surgery
ASA Class 3	Severe systemic disturbance that may or may not be related to the reason for surgery
ASA Class 4	Severe systemic disturbance that is life-threatening with or without surgery
ASA Class 5	Moribund patient who has little chance of survival but is submitted to surgery as a last resort (resuscitative effort)
Emergency operation (E)	Any patient in whom an emergency operation is required

From information derived from American Society of Anesthesiologists: New classification of physical status. Anesthesiology 1963; 24: 111.

risk indices and preoperative cardiac testing. The goals are to define risk, determine which patients will benefit from further testing, form an appropriate anesthetic plan, and identify patients who will benefit from perioperative beta-blockade, intervention therapy, or even surgery. Clinical risk indices range from the physical status index of the American Society of Anesthesiologists (Table 23-3) to the Goldman Cardiac Risk Index, which has recently been updated.

In an update of the Goldman Cardiac Risk Index, the investigators studied 4,315 patients aged 50 years and older who were undergoing elective, major noncardiac procedures.[8] Six independent predictors of complications were identified and included in a revised risk index: high-risk type of surgery, history of ischemic heart disease, history of congestive heart failure, history of cerebrovascular disease, preoperative treatment with insulin, and preoperative serum creatinine >2.0 mg/dL. Cardiac complications rose with an increase in the number of risk factors present. Rates of major cardiac complications with 0, 1, 2, or 3 of these factors were 0.5, 1.3, 4, and 9%, respectively, in the derivation cohort and 0.4, 0.9, 7, and 11%, respectively, among 1,422 patients in the validation cohort (Fig. 23-2).

While all of these indices provide information to assess the probability of complications and provide an estimate of risk, they do not prescribe perioperative management. In contrast, the anesthesiologist is most concerned with forming an anesthetic plan after defining the cardiovascular risk factors.

In patients with symptomatic coronary disease, the preoperative evaluation may lead to the recognition of a change in the frequency or pattern of anginal symptoms. Certain populations of patients—for example, the elderly, women, or diabetics—may present with more atypical features. The presence of unstable angina has been associated with a high perioperative risk of MI.[5]

In virtually all studies, the presence of active congestive heart failure preoperatively has been associated with an increased incidence of perioperative cardiac morbidity.[9,10] Stabilization of ventricular function and treatment for pulmonary congestion are important prior to elective surgery. Because the type of perioperative monitoring and treatments would be different, clarifying the cause of heart failure is important. Congestive symptoms may be a result of nonischemic cardiomyopathy or cardiac valvular insufficiency and/or stenosis.

Adults with a prior MI almost always have coronary artery disease, (CAD). Traditionally, risk assessment for noncardiac surgery was based on the time interval between the MI and surgery. Multiple older studies have demonstrated an increased incidence of reinfarction if the MI was within 6 months of surgery.[11–13] With improvements in perioperative care, this difference has decreased. Therefore, the importance of the intervening time interval may no longer be valid in the current era of interventional therapy and risk stratification after an acute MI. Although many patients with an MI may continue to have myocardium at risk for subsequent ischemia and infarction, other patients may have their critical coronary stenoses either totally occluded or widely patent. For example, the use of percutaneous transluminal coronary angioplasty, thrombolysis, and early coronary artery bypass grafting (CABG) has changed the natural history of the disease.[14,15] Therefore, patients should be evaluated from the perspective of their risk for ongoing ischemia. The American Heart Association/American College of Cardiology Task Force on Perioperative Evaluation of the Cardiac Patient Undergoing Noncardiac Surgery has defined three risk groups—major, intermediate, and minor (Table 23-4). They indicate that recent MI (<30 days) places patients in the group at highest risk; after that period, a prior MI places the patient at intermediate risk.[16]

Patients with Coronary Artery Disease

For those patients without overt symptoms or history, the probability of CAD varies with the type and number of

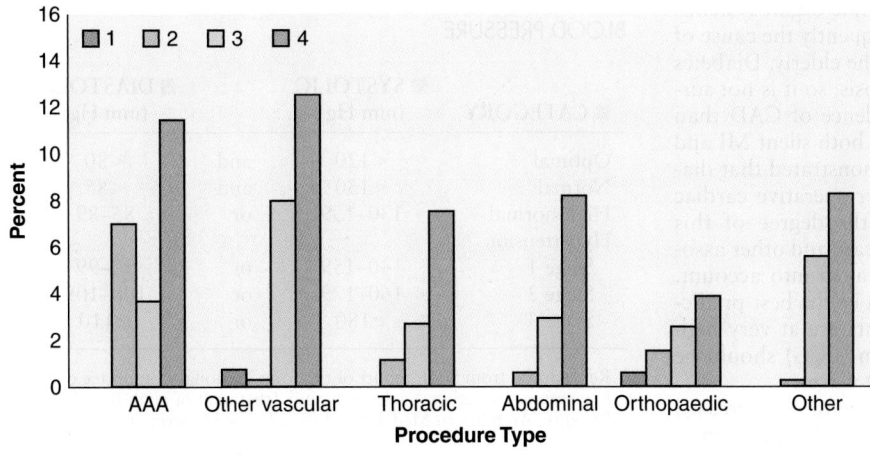

FIGURE 23-2. Cardiac risk index (CRI). Bars represent rate of major cardiac complications in entire patient population (both derivation and validation cohorts combined) for patients in revised CRI classes according to type of procedure performed. Note that, by definition, patients undergoing abdominal aortic aneurysm (AAA), thoracic, and abdominal procedures were excluded from Class I. In all subsets except patients undergoing AAA, there was a statistically significant trend toward greater risk with higher-risk class. See text for details. (Reproduced from Lee TH, Marcantonio ER, Mangione CM, et al: Derivation and prospective validation of a simple index for prediction of cardiac risk of major noncardiac surgery. Circulation 1999; 100: 1043, with permission.)

TABLE 23-4

CLINICAL PREDICTORS OF INCREASED PERIOPERATIVE CARDIOVASCULAR RISK (MYOCARDIAL INFARCTION, CONGESTIVE HEART FAILURE, DEATH)

MAJOR

Unstable coronary syndromes
- Recent myocardial infarction[a] with evidence of important ischemic risk by clinical symptoms or noninvasive study
- Unstable or severe[b] angina (Canadian Class III or IV)[c]

Decompensated congestive heart failure

Significant dysrhythmias
- High-grade atrioventricular block
- Symptomatic ventricular arrhythmias in the presence of underlying heart disease
- Supraventricular arrhythmias with uncontrolled ventricular rate

Severe valvular disease

INTERMEDIATE

Mild angina pectoris (Canadian Class I or II)

Prior myocardial infarction by history or pathologic Q waves

Compensated or prior congestive heart failure

Diabetes mellitus

MINOR

Advanced age

Abnormal ECG (left ventricular hypertrophy, left bundle-branch block, ST-T abnormalities)

Rhythm other than sinus (e.g., atrial fibrillation)

Low functional capacity (e.g., inability to climb one flight of stairs with a bag of groceries)

History of stroke

Uncontrolled systemic hypertension

ECG, electrocardiogram.

[a]The American College of Cardiology National Database Library defines recent myocardial infarction as >7 days but ≤1 month (30 days).

[b]May include "stable" angina in patients who are unusually sedentary.

[c]Campeau L: Grading of angina pectoris. Circulation 1976; 54: 522. Reproduced from Eagle K, Brundage B, Chaitman B, et al: Guidelines for perioperative cardiovascular evaluation of the noncardiac surgery. A report of the American Heart Association/American College of Cardiology Task Force on Assessment of Diagnostic and Therapeutic Cardiovascular Procedures. Circulation 1996; 93: 1278, with permission.

---

atherosclerotic risk factors present. Peripheral arterial disease has been shown to be associated with CAD in multiple studies.[17]. Diabetes mellitus is a common disease in the elderly and represents a process that affects multiple organ systems. Complications of diabetes mellitus are frequently the cause of urgent or emergent surgery, especially in the elderly. Diabetes accelerates the progression of atherosclerosis, so it is not surprising that diabetics have a higher incidence of CAD than nondiabetics. There is a high incidence of both silent MI and myocardial ischemia.[18] Eagle, et al.[19] demonstrated that diabetes is an independent risk factor for perioperative cardiac morbidity. In attempting to determine the degree of this increased probability, the length of the disease and other associated end-organ dysfunction should be taken into account. Autonomic neuropathy has been found to be the best predictor of silent CAD.[20] Because these patients are at very high risk for a silent MI, an electrocardiogram (ECG) should be obtained to examine for the presence of Q waves.

Hypertension has also been associated with an increased incidence of silent myocardial ischemia and infarction.[18]

Hypertensive patients who have left ventricular hypertrophy and are undergoing noncardiac surgery are at a higher perioperative risk than nonhypertensive patients.[21]

Investigators have suggested that the presence of a strain pattern on ECG suggests a chronic ischemic state.[22] Therefore, these patients should also be considered to have an increased probability of CAD and for perioperative morbidity.

There is controversy regarding a trigger to delay or cancel a surgical procedure in a patient with untreated or inadequately treated hypertension. Hypertension has been divided into three stages, with stage 3 denoting that which might be used as a cutoff (Table 23-5).[23] Aggressive treatment of blood pressure is associated with increased reduction in long-term risk, although the effect diminishes in all but diabetic patients as diastolic blood pressure is reduced below 90 mm Hg. Although there has been a suggestion in the literature that a case should be delayed if the diastolic pressure is >110 mm Hg, the study often quoted as the basis for this determination demonstrated no major morbidity in that small group of patients.[24] Other authors state that there is little association between blood pressures of <180 mm Hg systolic or 110 mm Hg diastolic and postoperative outcomes. However, such patients are prone to perioperative myocardial ischemia, ventricular dysrhythmias, and lability in blood pressure. It is less clear in patients with blood pressures above 180/100 mm Hg, although no absolute evidence exists that postponing surgery will reduce risk.[25,26] In the absence of end-organ changes, such as renal insufficiency or left ventricular hypertrophy with strain, the benefits of optimizing blood pressure must be weighed against the risks of delaying surgery.

Several other risk factors have been used to suggest an increased probability of CAD. These include the atherosclerotic processes associated with tobacco use and hypercholesterolemia. Although these risk factors increase the probability of developing CAD, they have not been shown to increase perioperative risk. When attempting to determine the overall probability of disease, the number of risk factors and severity of each are important.

Importance of Surgical Procedure

The surgical procedure influences the scope of preoperative evaluation required by determining the potential range of physiologic flux during the perioperative period. Few hard data exist defining the surgery-specific incidence of complications. It is known that peripheral procedures, such as those included in a study of ambulatory surgery completed at the Mayo Clinic, are associated with an extremely low incidence of morbidity and mortality,[27] while major vascular procedures

TABLE 23-5

BLOOD PRESSURE

CATEGORY	SYSTOLIC (mm Hg)		DIASTOLIC (mm Hg)
Optimal	<120	and	<80
Normal	<130	and	<85
High-normal	130–139	or	85–89
Hypertension			
Stage 1	140–159	or	90–99
Stage 2	160–179	or	100–109
Stage 3	≥180	or	≥110

Reproduced from Sixth report of the Joint National Committee on Prevention, Detection, Evaluation, and Treatment of High Blood Pressure. Arch Intern Med 1997; 157: 2413, with permission.

PREANESTHETIC EVALUATION
AND PREPARATION

TABLE 23-6

CARDIAC RISKᵃ STRATIFICATION FOR NONCARDIAC SURGICAL PROCEDURES IN PATIENTS WITH KNOWN CORONARY ARTERY DISEASE

HIGH	(Reported cardiac risk often >5%) • Emergent major operations, particularly in the elderly • Aortic and other major vascular • Peripheral vascular • Anticipated prolonged surgical procedures associated with large fluid shifts and/or blood loss
INTERMEDIATE	(Reported cardiac risk generally <5%) • Renal insufficiency • Carotid endarterectomy • Head and neck • Intraperitoneal and intrathoracic • Orthopaedic • Prostate
LOWᵇ	(Reported cardiac risk generally <1%) • Endoscopic procedures • Superficial procedures • Cataract • Breast

ᵃCombined incidence of cardiac death and nonfatal myocardial infarction.
ᵇDo not generally require further preoperative cardiac testing.
Reproduced from Eagle K, Brundage B, Chaitman B, et al: Guidelines for perioperative cardiovascular evaluation of the noncardiac surgery. A report of the American Heart Association/American College of Cardiology Task Force on Assessment of Diagnostic and Therapeutic Cardiovascular Procedures. Circulation 1996; 93: 1278, with permission.

are associated with the highest incidence of complications. Eagle, et al.[28] published data on the incidence of perioperative MI and mortality by procedure for patients enrolled in the Coronary Artery Surgery Study. They determined the overall risk of perioperative morbidity in patients with known CAD treated either medically or with prior CABG. They found that high-risk procedures include major vascular, abdominal, thoracic, and orthopaedic surgery. The American Heart Association/American College of Cardiology Guidelines described risk stratification for noncardiac surgery that is shown in Table 23-6.[16]

Importance of Exercise Tolerance

❼ Exercise tolerance is one of the most important determinants of perioperative risk and the need for further testing and invasive monitoring. An excellent exercise tolerance, even in patients with stable angina, suggests that the myocardium can be stressed without failing. If a patient can walk a mile without becoming short of breath, the probability of extensive CAD is small. Alternatively, if patients experience dyspnea associated with chest pain during minimal exertion, the probability of extensive CAD is high, which has been associated with greater perioperative risk. Additionally, these patients are at risk for developing hypotension with ischemia, and therefore may benefit from more extensive monitoring, coronary intervention therapy, or revascularization. Exercise tolerance can be assessed with formal treadmill testing or with a questionnaire that assesses activities of daily living (Table 23-7).[16]

Reilly, et al.[29] have evaluated the predictive value of self-reported exercise tolerance for serious perioperative complications and demonstrated that a poor exercise tolerance (could not walk four blocks and climb two flights of stairs) independently predicted a complication with an odds ratio of 1.94. The likelihood of a serious adverse event was inversely related to the number of blocks that could be walked. Therefore, there is good evidence to suggest that minimal additional testing is necessary if the patient is able to describe a good exercise tolerance.

Indications for Further Cardiac Testing

Multiple algorithms have been proposed to determine which patients require further testing. As described previously, the risk associated with the proposed surgical procedure influences the decision to perform further diagnostic testing and interventions. Guidelines must be tempered by recent studies in which perioperative cardiac morbidity was greatly reduced by perioperative β-adrenergic blockade administration.[30]

TABLE 23-7

ESTIMATED ENERGY REQUIREMENT FOR VARIOUS ACTIVITIESᵃ

1 MET	Can you take care of yourself? Eat, dress, or use the toilet? Walk indoors around the house? Walk a block or two on level ground at 2–3 mph or 3.2–4.8 km/hr? Do light work around the house, like dusting or washing dishes?	4 METs	Walk on level ground at 4 mph or 6.4 km/hr? Run a short distance? Do heavy work around the house, like scrubbing floors or lifting or moving heavy furniture? Participate in moderate recreational activities like golf, bowling, dancing, doubles tennis, or throwing a baseball or football?
4 METs	Climb a flight of stairs or walk up a hill?	>10 METs	Participate in strenuous sports like swimming, singles tennis, football, basketball, or skiing

MET, metabolic equivalent.
ᵃAdapted from the Duke Activity Status Index and American Heart Association Exercise Standards. Reproduced from Eagle K, Brundage B, Chaitman B, et al: Guidelines for perioperative cardiovascular evaluation of the noncardiac surgery. A report of the American Heart Association/American College of Cardiology Task Force on Assessment of Diagnostic and Therapeutic Cardiovascular Procedures. Circulation 1996; 93: 1278, with permission.

With the reduction in perioperative morbidity, it has been suggested that extensive cardiovascular testing is not necessary. However, until these findings can be confirmed, further testing may be warranted.

The algorithm to determine the need for testing proposed by the American College of Cardiology/American Heart Association Task Force updated in 2002,[31] and again in 2007[32] is based on the available evidence and expert opinion that integrates clinical history, surgery-specific risk, and exercise tolerance (See Fig. 42-6 on p. 1113). In step one, the clinician evaluates the urgency of the surgery and the appropriateness of a formal preoperative assessment. Next, one should determine if the patient has undergone a recent revascularization procedure or coronary evaluation. Those patients with unstable coronary syndromes should be identified, and appropriate treatment instituted. Finally, the decision to undergo further testing depends on the interaction of the clinical risk factors, surgery-specific risk, and functional capacity. For patients at intermediate clinical risk, both exercise tolerance and the extent of the surgery are taken into account to determine the need for further testing. Importantly, no preoperative cardiovascular testing should be performed if the results will not change perioperative management.

Cardiovascular Tests

Electrocardiogram.   Preoperative 12-lead electrocardiogram can provide important information on the state of the patient's myocardium and coronary circulation. Abnormal Q waves in high-risk patients are highly suggestive of a past MI. Confirmation of active ischemia usually requires changes in at least two leads. It has been estimated that approximately 30% of MIs occur without symptoms ("silent infarctions") and can only be detected on routine ECGs, with the highest incidence occurring in patients with either diabetes or hypertension. The Framingham study showed that long-term prognosis is not improved by lack of symptoms.[18] The absence of Q waves on the ECG does not exclude the occurrence of a Q-wave MI in the past. Between 5 and 27% of Q waves disappear over the 10-year period following an infarction during the 1970s.[33] Those patients in whom the ECG reverts to normal have improved survival compared with those with consistent abnormalities, with or without Q waves. The presence of Q waves on a preoperative ECG in a high-risk patient, regardless of symptoms, should alert the anesthesiologist to the increased perioperative risk and the possibility of active ischemia.

It has not been established that information obtained from the preoperative ECG affects clinical care. A review of clinical studies on the matter is inconclusive. In one retrospective review of adult patients undergoing ambulatory surgery, the preoperative ECG was not predictive of perioperative risk.[34] Although controversy exists, there are current recommendations for the need for a preoperative ECG. A preoperative resting 12-lead ECG is recommended for patients with at least one clinical risk factor who are undergoing vascular surgical procedures and for patients with known CAD, peripheral arterial disease, or cerebrovascular disease who are undergoing intermediate-risk surgical procedures. A perioperative ECG is reasonable in persons with no clinical risk factors who are about to undergo vascular surgical procedures and may be reasonable in patients with at least one clinical risk factor who are undergoing intermediate-risk operative procedures.[32]

Noninvasive Cardiovascular Testing.   The exercise ECG has been the traditional method in the past for evaluating patients with suspected CAD. It represents the most cost-effective and least invasive method for detecting ischemia, with a sensitivity of 70 to 80% and a specificity of 60 to 75% for identifying CAD. A positive exercise stress test alerts the anesthesiologist that the patient is at risk for ischemia over a wide range of heart rates, with the greatest risk in those who develop ischemia only after mild exercise. However, as discussed previously, the ability to exercise suggests that no further testing is necessary, and therefore stress electrocardiography is infrequently indicated.

A number of high-risk patients are either unable to exercise or have contraindications to exercise, for example, those with claudication. Therefore, pharmacologic stress testing and ambulatory electrocardiography have come into vogue, particularly as preoperative cardiovascular tests in patients scheduled for vascular surgery. Pharmacologic stress thallium imaging is useful in those patients who are unable to exercise. Dipyridamole or adenosine is administered as a coronary vasodilator to assess flow heterogeneity. The presence of a redistribution defect is predictive of postoperative cardiac events, especially in patients undergoing peripheral vascular surgery. Similarly, dobutamine can be used to increase myocardial oxygen demand, by increasing heart rate and blood pressure, in those patients who cannot exercise.

The ambulatory ECG (Holter monitoring) provides a means of continuously monitoring the ECG for significant ST segment changes preoperatively. One study demonstrated that the presence of silent ischemia is a strong predictor of outcome, while its absence is associated with a favorable outcome in 99% of the patients studied.[35] Other investigators have demonstrated the value of ambulatory ECG monitoring, although the negative predictive values have not been as high as reported by some.

Stress echocardiography is another preoperative test that may be of value in evaluating patients with suspected CAD. The appearance of either new or more severe regional wall motion abnormalities with exercise is considered a positive test. Either represents areas at risk for myocardial ischemia. The advantage of the stress echocardiogram is that it is a dynamic assessment of ventricular function. Dobutamine echocardiography has also been studied and found to have among the best predictive values. It is generally accepted that the group at risk is composed of those who demonstrate regional wall motion abnormalities at low heart rates.

Several groups have published meta-analyses of preoperative diagnostic tests. One group of investigators demonstrated good predictive values using ambulatory ECG monitoring, radionuclide angiography, dipyridamole thallium imaging, or dobutamine stress echocardiography.[36] Shaw, et al.[37] also demonstrated good predictive values of dipyridamole thallium imaging and dobutamine stress echocardiography. Both of these studies demonstrated the superior value of dobutamine stress echocardiography; however, there was significant overlap of the confidence intervals with other tests. The most important determinant with respect to the choice of preoperative testing is the expertise of the local institution.

Current recommendations are that patients with active cardiac conditions such as unstable angina, congestive heart failure, significant dysrhythmias and severe valvular disease should undergo noninvasive stress testing before noncardiac surgery. Noninvasive stress testing for patients with multiple clinical risk factors and poor functional capacity (less than four metabolic equivalents) who require vascular surgery is reasonable if it will change management. Noninvasive testing in other patients about to go under intermediate-risk noncardiac surgery or vascular surgery is less clear.[32]

Assessment of Ventricular and Valvular Function.   Both echo and radionuclide angiography can assess cardiac ejection fraction at rest and under stress, but echo is less invasive and is also able to assess regional wall motion abnormalities, wall thickness, valvular function, and valve area. Pulse-wave Doppler can be used to determine the velocity time integral. Ejection fraction can then be calculated by determining the cross-sectional area of the ventricle. Conflicting results exist with regard to the predictive value of ejection fraction using either echocardiographic or radionuclide measurements. It is reasonable for those with dyspnea of unknown origin and for those with current or prior heart failure with worsening dyspnea or other change in clinical status to have preoperative evaluations of left ventricular function. The wisdom of reassessment of left ventricular function in clinically stable patients with previous cardiomyopathy is unknown.[32] Echocardiography can provide important information regarding valvular function, which may have important implications for either cardiac or noncardiac surgery, and is discussed more fully later in this text. Aortic stenosis has been associated with a poor prognosis in noncardiac surgical patients, and knowledge of valvular lesions may modify perioperative hemodynamic therapy.[9]

Coronary Angiography.   Coronary angiography is currently the best method for defining coronary anatomy. In addition, information regarding ventricular and valvular function can also be assessed. Hemodynamic indices can be determined such as ventricular pressures and pressure gradients across valves. This information is routinely available in patients scheduled for CABG. Narrowing of the left main coronary artery and certain other lesions may be associated with a greater perioperative risk. Diffuse atherosclerosis in small vessels, as seen in diabetics, may lead to incomplete revascularization and a risk of developing ischemia despite CABG. Coronary angiography is used by cardiologists to determine whether coronary vascularization is an option.

Unlike the exercise or pharmacologic stress tests discussed earlier, coronary angiography provides anatomic, not functional, information. Although a critical coronary stenosis delineates an area of risk for developing myocardial ischemia, the functional response of that ischemia cannot be assessed by angiography alone. A critical stenosis may or may not be the underlying cause for a perioperative MI that occurs. In the ambulatory population, many infarctions are the result of acute thrombosis of a noncritical stenosis. Therefore, the value of routine angiography prior to noncardiac surgery depends on the identification of lesions that will cause morbidity and mortality.

Patients with restricted physical activity in whom functional capacity is difficult to determine may benefit from sophisticated imaging techniques such as cardiac computed tomography.[38]

Perioperative Coronary Interventions

The strategies to reduce the perioperative risk of noncardiac surgery have recently been studied. There are several large studies that suggest that in patients who survive CABG, the risk of subsequent noncardiac surgery is low.[5,8] Although there are little data to support the notion of coronary revascularization solely for the purpose of improving perioperative outcome, it is true that for some patients scheduled for high-risk surgery, long-term survival may be enhanced by revascularization. Two studies used the Coronary Artery Surgery Study database and found that CABG significantly improved survival in those patients with both peripheral vascular disease and triple-vessel coronary disease, especially the group with depressed ventricular function.[6] After reviewing all available data, most clinicians believe the indication for CABG prior to noncardiac surgery remains the same as in other settings and is independent of the proposed noncardiac surgery.

The value of percutaneous transluminal coronary angioplasty is less well established. The current evidence does not support the use of percutaneous transluminal coronary angioplasty beyond established indications for nonoperative patients.

Early surgery after coronary stent placement has been associated with adverse cardiac events. A significant incidence of perioperative death and of hemorrhage in patients after stent placement has been reported. The waiting period for surgery after bare metal stent placement is generally recognized one month as a minimum, while the waiting period for drug eluting stents is 12 months. This difference is because the incidence of stent thrombosis for the drug-eluting stents has been found to be similar to the bare metal stents in the early phase after placement, but less well defined over a longer period of time. Currently, patients are invariably taking aspirin and clopidogrel as antiplatelet therapy after stent placement. A thienopyridine (ticlopidine or clopidogrel) is generally continued with aspirin for 1 month after bare-metal stenting and for 12 months after drug-eluting stent placement (Fig. 23-3). Perioperative management weighs the risk of bleeding versus a stent thrombosis. The decision must involve anesthesiologist, surgeons, cardiologists, and intensivists. In those patients who have a high risk for stent thrombosis many advocate that at least aspirin be continued in the perioperative period. Also, the anesthesiologist must weigh the risk of regional versus general anesthesia when these patients are taking antiplatelet therapy. Surgery in patients with recent stent placement should probably only be considered in centers where 24 hour interventional cardiologists are available.[39–41]

Pulmonary Disease

Pulmonary complications remain a major cause of morbidity and mortality for patients undergoing surgery and anesthesia. They occur more frequently than cardiac complications, with an incidence of 5 to 10% in those having major noncardiac procedures. Perioperative pulmonary complications include atelectasis, pneumonia, bronchitis, bronchospasm, hypoxemia, exacerbation of chronic obstructive pulmonary disease, and respiratory failure requiring mechanical ventilation.[42]

The site and type of surgery are the strongest predictors of complications. With regard to the surgical *site*, thoracic, aortic, or upper abdominal surgery is associated with the highest risk for postoperative pulmonary problems. Risk increases as the incision approaches the diaphragm.[42–45] Decreases in postoperative vital capacity and functional residual capacity, as well as diaphragmatic dysfunction, contribute to hypoxemia and atelectasis.[46] Functional residual capacity may take up to 2 weeks to return to baseline. Diaphragmatic dysfunction occurs despite adequate analgesia and is theorized to be because of phrenic nerve inhibition.[47] The *types* of surgery carrying the highest risks were abdominal aortic aneurysm repair, thoracic, and upper abdominal surgery, followed by neck, peripheral vascular, and neurosurgery. Neurosurgery and neck surgery may be associated with perioperative aspiration pneumonia.

The need for emergency surgery and the need for general anesthesia are also associated with a slightly increased risk. Not only can the surgery affect pulmonary function, but general anesthesia also results in mechanical changes such as a decrease in the functional residual capacity and altered diaphragmatic motion leading to $\dot{V}/\dot{Q}$ mismatch with shunting and dead-space ventilation. General anesthesia also aggravates these changes by its effects at the microscopic level: inhibition of mucociliary clearance, increased alveolar-capillary permeability, inhibition of surfactant release, increased nitric oxide synthetase, and increased sensitivity of the pulmonary vasculature to neurohumoral mediators. Subanesthetic levels of intravenous or volatile agents have the ability to blunt the ventilatory response to hypoxemia and hypercarbia. Duration of anesthesia is a well-established risk factor for postoperative pulmonary complications, with morbidity rates increasing after 2 to 3 hours.[48] However, although laparoscopic surgery is often longer in duration, the decreased pulmonary complications postoperatively compared with an

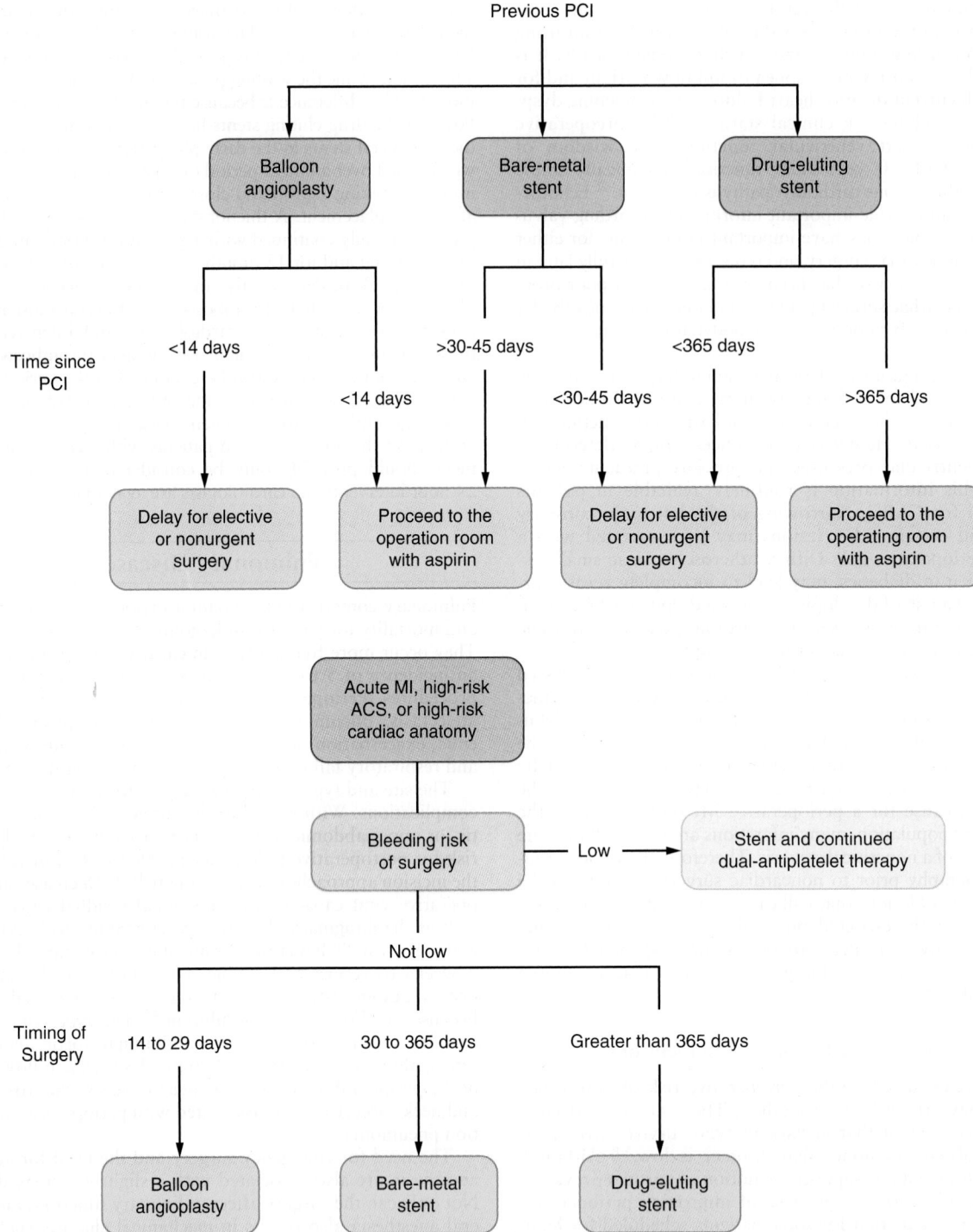

FIGURE 23-3. **A.** Proposed approach to the management of patients with previous percutaneous coronary intervention (PCI) who require noncardiac surgery, based on expert opinion. **B.** Proposed treatment for patients requiring percutaneous coronary intervention who need subsequent surgery. ACS indicates acute coronary syndrome; COR, class of recommendation; LOE, level of evidence; and MI, myocardial infarction. (Reused with permission from ACC/AHA 2007 Guidelines on Perioperative Cardiovascular Evaluation and Care for Noncardiac Surgery. Circulation 2007;116:e418–e500.

TABLE 23-8

POTENTIAL PATIENT-RELATED RISK FACTORS FOR POSTOPERATIVE PULMONARY COMPLICATIONS

■ POTENTIAL RISK FACTOR	■ TYPE OF SURGERY	■ UNADJUSTED RELATIVE RISK ASSOCIATED WITH FACTOR
Smoking	Coronary bypass	3.4
	Abdominal	1.4–4.3
ASA Class >II	Unselected	1.7
	Thoracic or abdominal	1.5–3.2
Age >70 yr	Unselected	1.9–2.4
	Thoracic or abdominal	0.9–1.9
Obesity	Unselected	1.3
	Thoracic or abdominal	0.8–1.7
COPD	Unselected	2.7–3.6
	Thoracic or abdominal	4.7

ASA, American Society of Anesthesiologists; COPD, chronic obstructive pulmonary disease.
Adapted from Smetana GW: Preoperative pulmonary evaluation. N Engl J Med 1999; 340: 942.

open procedure usually outweigh the risks of increased anesthesia time.[49]

Patient-Related Factors

Preoperative evaluation of patients with pre-existing pulmonary disease should include assessment of the type and severity of disease, as well as its reversibility (Table 23-8). Because clinical observations are often the best predictors for the development of postoperative pulmonary complications, a careful history and physical examination is imperative. The anesthesiologist should inquire about exercise intolerance, chronic cough, or unexplained dyspnea. On physical examination, findings of wheezing, rhonchi, decreased breath sounds, dullness to percussion, and a prolonged expiratory phase are important. Preoperative pulmonary function testing is usually reserved for those scheduled for lung resection, or for those scheduled for major surgery who have unexplained pulmonary signs and symptoms after a careful history and physical examination. Early intervention helps to ensure that the patient's medical status is optimal prior to surgery.

Tobacco

The use of tobacco is an important risk factor, but one that usually cannot be influenced. Even among smokers who have not developed chronic lung disease, smoking is known to increase carboxyhemoglobin levels, decrease ciliary function, and increase sputum production, as well as cause stimulation of the cardiovascular system secondary to the nicotine. While cessation of smoking for 2 days can decrease carboxyhemoglobin levels, abolish the nicotine effects, and improve mucous clearance, prospective studies show that smoking cessation for at least 4 to 8 weeks was necessary to reduce the rate of postoperative pulmonary complications.[50,51] Because smokers often show increased airway reactivity under general anesthesia, it is useful to administer a bronchodilator such as albuterol preoperatively.

Asthma

Asthma is one of the most common coexisting diseases that confronts the anesthesiologist. In general, the preoperative management of asthma is the same as for patients with asthma not undergoing surgery. During the patient interview it is important to elicit information regarding inciting factors, severity, reversibility, and current status. Frequent use of bronchodilators, hospitalizations for asthma, and the requirement for systemic steroids are all indicators of the severity of the disease. After an episode of asthma, airway hyperreactivity may persist for several weeks.[52] In addition to bronchodilators, perioperative steroids are worth considering as prophylaxis for the severe asthmatic; for example, hydrocortisone 100 mg intravenously every 8 hours on the day of surgery. The possibility of adrenal insufficiency is also a concern in those patients who have received more than a "burst and taper" of steroids in the previous 6 months. This group of patients should be administered "stress doses" of steroids perioperatively. Kabalin, et al.[53] found there was a low complication rate for asthmatics treated with short-term steroids undergoing surgery. Significantly, they found no association with impaired wound healing or infections. For patients using inhaled steroids, they should be administered regularly, starting at least 48 hours prior to surgery for optimal effectiveness.

Obstructive Sleep Apnea

Obstructive sleep apnea (OSA) is a syndrome defined by periodic obstruction of the upper airway during sleep, leading to episodic oxygen desaturation and hypercarbia. This episodic desaturation in turn causes episodic arousal, leading to chronic sleep deprivation with daytime hypersomnolence and even behavioral changes in children. Depending on the frequency and severity of events, it may lead to other changes such as chronic pulmonary hypertension and right heart failure. It is estimated to be present in 9% of women and 24% of men, with the great majority of these being undiagnosed. Factors commonly associated with an increased risk of sleep apnea include obesity (body mass index >35 kg/m^2 or 95th percentile for age), increased neck circumference, severe tonsillar hypertrophy, and anatomic abnormalities of the upper airway.

Because of their propensity for airway collapse and sleep deprivation, patients with OSA are especially susceptible to the respiratory depressant and airway effects of sedatives, narcotics, and inhaled anesthetics both intraoperatively and postoperatively. Preoperative identification of those patients at risk allows them to undergo a formal sleep study to determine the presence and severity of symptoms, and also allows preoperative initiation of continuous positive airway pressure (CPAP). The ASA in 2006 published practice guidelines for the perioperative management of patients with OSA, and the following will attempt to summarize those guidelines.[54] During the preoperative evaluation, specific questions should be directed toward the patient and family regarding the presence of symptoms and signs of OSA:

- Does the patient snore loudly enough to be heard through a door, or snore frequently?
- Are there observed pauses in breathing during sleep?
- Are there frequent arousals during sleep, or awakenings with a choking sensation?
- Is frequent daytime somnolence, fatigue, or falling asleep easily in a nonstimulating environment noted?
- Do the child's parents notice restless sleep or difficulty with breathing?
- Is the child overly aggressive or have trouble concentrating?

If a patient has predisposing anatomy and/or signs or symptoms in two or more areas, he or she should be referred for a sleep study. If this is not possible, the patient should be managed as having OSA. The risk of perioperative complications in patients with OSA increases with the severity of sleep apnea, the invasiveness of surgery and anesthesia, and the amount of postoperative opioids required. There is a general consensus that preoperative initiation of airway support such as CPAP reduces perioperative risk, perhaps by decreasing the sleep deprivation and secondary hypersomnolence.[54] Importantly, OSA is also associated with difficult airway management, making it prudent to examine previous anesthesia records as well as to perform a thorough airway examination. The difficult airway algorithm[54] should be followed and emergency airway equipment should be readily available at the surgical center.

There are multiple management decisions to make in coordination with the surgeon with respect to the OSA patient:

- Determine whether there are noninvasive ways of performing the surgery that would decrease the need for narcotics postoperatively.
- Discuss whether it is feasible to perform surgery under neuraxial, regional, or local anesthesia, decreasing the total amount of anesthesia or opioids needed.
- Determine whether nonsteroidal anti-inflammatory agents are acceptable for postoperative analgesia.
- Discuss whether outpatient surgery a safe option.
- Determine whether the patient will be able to use CPAP postoperatively.
- Determine whether postoperative admission to an intensive care unit is required for the patient who is a first-time user of CPAP.

The ASA practice guidelines recommend hospitalization after uvulopalatoplasty surgery and after tonsillectomy for OSA in children younger than 3 years. Postoperative hospitalization is also recommended for those OSA patients with other coexisting diseases. When procedures are performed on an outpatient basis, prolonged postoperative monitoring should be continued to ensure that the patient is able to maintain room air saturation without obstruction when left undisturbed in recovery. Recovery in the nonsupine position (elevation of the head and thorax) is also recommended to optimize airway patency. The task force recommends continuous pulse oximetry during hospitalization, as well as supplemental oxygen until the patient can maintain their baseline saturation on room air.

Endocrine Disease

Diabetes Mellitus

Diabetes mellitus is the most common endocrinopathy, with the incidence of type 1 diabetes at 0.4% of the population, and type 2 diabetes affecting approximately 8 to 10% of Americans, but projected to develop in >30% of Americans born after 2000, largely because of the rise in obesity.[55] Critical illness-induced hyperglycemia, defined as a blood glucose >200 mg/dL in the absence of known diabetes, occurs frequently, particularly in the elderly.[56] Diabetes has acute and chronic disease manifestations, making it more likely for diabetics to require surgery. The majority of diabetics develop secondary disease in one or more organ systems, which must be identified preoperatively so that an appropriate plan can be developed for perioperative management. While long-term, close control of glucose may limit some of the microvascular effects of diabetes (retinopathy, neuropathy, and nephropathy), macrovascular events such as MIs or stroke may not be decreased. Diabetics have an increased risk of CAD, hypertension, congestive heart failure, and perioperative MI. The 2002 American College of Cardiology/American Heart Association guidelines on perioperative cardiac assessment of patients undergoing noncardiac surgery place diabetics, especially those receiving insulin, at a minimum of intermediate risk.[57] They also state that most diabetic patients >65 years of age have significant CAD, with the incidence of silent ischemia increased by associated diabetic autonomic neuropathy.

Diabetics are also more likely than the general population to have cerebral vascular, peripheral vascular, and renal vascular disease. Diabetes is the leading cause of renal failure requiring dialysis. Peripheral neuropathies and vascular disease make these patients more susceptible to positioning injuries during surgery as well as postoperatively. Autonomic neuropathy is also common in diabetics, and may predispose the patient to hemodynamic instability during anesthesia, and theoretically increase the risk of pulmonary aspiration because of the associated gastroparesis. These deficits should be documented prior to anesthesia and the anesthetic plan adjusted accordingly. Stiff joint syndrome due to glycosylation of proteins and abnormal collagen cross-linking, may significantly affect the temporomandibular, atlantooccipital, and cervical spine joints in patients with long-standing type 1 diabetes, resulting in difficulty with intubation. A thorough airway examination should be performed prior to anesthesia and a high index of suspicion maintained for a potentially difficult airway. Some suggest using the "prayer sign" as an evaluation tool: patients who are unable to completely oppose their hands (with no space between) should be suspected of also having changes in other joints potentially impacting airway manipulation.

Regimens for perioperative glycemic control vary enormously, not only between type 1 and type 2 diabetics, but also within each group. Patients with type 1 diabetes have an absolute insulin deficiency usually due to destruction of pancreatic beta cells. These patients must receive insulin to prevent diabetic ketoacidosis. Home glucose management most often relies on a combination of short- and intermediate- or long-acting insulin regimens. Insulin pumps are increasingly common and are used to administer a continuous subcutaneous infusion of a short-acting insulin, supplemented by boluses dictated by glucose levels, diet, and exercise. Type 2 diabetes accounts for the great majority of diabetics and is defined by variable degrees of insulin deficiency and resistance. Although most commonly associated with obesity, it may also be induced by corticosteroids or pregnancy. Ketoacidosis is uncommon in type 2 diabetes, and the stress of severe infection or illness is more likely to provoke a nonketotic hyperosmolar state, which is characterized by severe dehydration, hyperglycemia, and hyperosmolarity. In type 2 diabetics, glucose control is most commonly achieved with diet, exercise, and/or oral hypoglycemic drugs. These agents primarily work by increasing endogenous insulin release, increasing insulin sensitivity, and/or decreasing hepatic gluconeogenesis. These drugs fall under the main categories of sulfonylureas, biguanides, thiazolidinediones, and meglitinides. If glycemic control is unsuccessful, then insulin is generally added to the regimen.

Ideally, both type 1 and 2 diabetic patients should be evaluated by the preoperative clinic as well as the patient's endocrinologist 1 to 2 weeks before elective surgery. In addition to a thorough history and physical, a judicious laboratory investigation should include a blood glucose, hemoglobin-A1c, serum electrolytes, creatinine, and an ECG. If the patient's glycemic control is inadequate based on a hemoglobin A1c out of the target range (7 to 9% for <5 years old; 6 to 8% for >5 years old), abnormal electrolytes, or ketonuria, then elective surgery should be delayed to allow optimization of preoperative glycemic control. Administration of perioperative beta-blockers should be considered in diabetic patients with CAD in an attempt to limit perioperative myocardial ischemia, as there is no evidence of worsened glucose intolerance or masking of hypoglycemic symptoms. However, the physician should be attentive to the possibility of precipitating heart failure.

Preoperative Glucose Management.

Anesthesia and surgery interrupt the regular meal schedule and insulin administration of diabetics. Perioperative stress may increase serum glucose concentrations secondary to the release of cortisol and catecholamines. The majority of available literature suggests that better glycemic control may limit morbidity (length of hospital/intensive care unit stay, infection rate, wound healing, outcomes after strokes/MIs) and mortality particularly in cardiac surgery patients, carotid endarterectomy patients, and the critically ill,[56,58-60] although a recent randomized trial found an increase in the incidence of death and perioperative stroke in cardiac surgery patients where an attempt was made to maintain the glucose between 80 and 100 mg/dL.[61] More studies are needed to determine whether strict glycemic control will improve outcome in all diabetics undergoing surgery.

Because good evidence is lacking to be able to set standards for the perioperative glucose management of diabetic patients, at a minimum, an attempt should be made to control the glucose within a range of 100 to 200 mg/dL, although some will argue that tighter control with a top limit of 150 mg/dL is warranted. The following recommendations can serve as a general guide:

- Plan with the surgeon to schedule the surgery as the first case of the day to prevent prolonged fasting.
- As a general rule, oral hypoglycemic agents are held on the day of surgery to avoid reactive hypoglycemia. The exception is metformin, which should be held for at least 24 hours preoperatively to avoid the risk drug-induced lactic acidosis.
- Insulin should be continued through the evening before surgery, including the usual dose of insulin glargine (Lantus).
- Patients should be counseled to take a glucose tablet or clear juice if hypoglycemia occurs prior to arrival at the hospital, in order to prevent delay of the surgery.
- Schedule the patient to arrive without having ingested anything by mouth in early morning and check blood glucose, electrolytes, and ketones.
- Type 1 diabetics should be continued on basal insulin replacement even while nothing by mouth status to prevent ketoacidosis. Administer half the usual morning dose of

intermediate- or long-acting insulin after arrival to the surgery center, but hold the usual dose of rapid- or short-acting insulin.
- Patients on insulin pumps may be managed by continuing the pump for short surgeries, or changing over to an intravenous insulin infusion for moderate or major surgeries.
- Use the patient's own sliding scale to administer a short-acting insulin subcutaneously to maintain the glucose between 100 and 200 mg/dL prior to the scheduled surgery.

This strategy, along with blood glucose determinations every 1 to 2 hours, may be all that is necessary for well-controlled diabetics undergoing short, noninvasive outpatient surgeries. Additionally, it is important to prevent postoperative nausea and vomiting and to encourage the early resumption of diet, allowing return to their previous insulin regimen. For type 1 or 2 diabetics undergoing moderate or major surgery, insulin is generally administered in the form of an infusion of regular insulin. Discontinuing the patient's own insulin pump to avoid problems with insulin preparations and pump technology is often advised.

There are several methods of administering an insulin infusion, none of which has proved superior to the others. Some recommend a combined infusion of glucose, insulin, and potassium because of the inherent safety of avoiding the possibility of having a glucose infusion inadvertently stopped while an insulin infusion continues. However, concurrent separate infusions of insulin and glucose are more easily adjusted and may provide better glycemic control. To increase the safety, the insulin infusion (which is on a separate pump) is added via a side port to the same line delivering the glucose infusion. A separate nonglucose isotonic solution should be used to replace deficits and intraoperative fluid losses. All protocols rely on the frequent determination of a plasma glucose level at least every 1 to 2 hours to allow titration of insulin.[62-64]

Thyroid and Parathyroid Disease

Thyroid and parathyroid disease have clinical manifestations that are important to the preoperative evaluation (Table 23-9). Thyroid disease is usually adequately evaluated by clinical history, although of course the thyroid function tests are more sensitive. The preoperative evaluation should focus on evaluating the signs and symptoms of hyperthyroidism and hypothyroidism. Hypothyroidism can lead to the development of hypothermia, hypoglycemia, hypoventilation and hyponatremia, as well as a susceptibility to depressant drugs. Anesthesiologists should be alerted to the possibility of the hypermetabolic state of thyroid storm in patients with hyperthyroidism. A large thyroid mass may distort the upper airway, producing inspiratory stridor or wheezing, especially evident in the supine position. In these cases, a chest x-ray should be obtained looking for evidence of tracheal deviation or narrowing. A computed tomography scan of the upper airway and trachea will provide better detail of any airway compromise. Patients with hyperparathyroidism often have hypercalcemia, indicating the need for preoperative determination of a serum calcium level.

Adrenal Disorders

The classic findings for pheochromocytoma include intermittent hypertension, headache, diaphoresis, and tachycardia. In patients with other endocrine tumors, a pheochromocytoma should be ruled out as the cause of unexplained hypertension as part of a multiple endocrine neoplasia syndrome. Over time the mortality for surgical resection of a pheochromocytoma has decreased because of improvements

TABLE 23-9

CLINICAL MANIFESTATIONS OF THYROID AND PARATHYROID DISEASES

	■ HYPERTHYROIDISM	■ HYPOTHYROIDISM	■ HYPERPARATHYROIDISM
General	Weight loss; heat intolerance; warm, moist skin	Cold intolerance	Weight loss, polydipsia
Cardiovascular	Tachycardia, atrial fibrillation, congestive heart failure	Bradycardia, congestive heart failure, cardiomegaly, pericardial or pleural effusion	Hypertension, heart block
Neurologic	Nervousness, tremor, hyperactive reflexes	Slow mental function, minimal reflexes	Weakness, lethargy, headache, insomnia, apathy, depression
Musculoskeletal	Muscle weakness, bone resorption	Large tongue, amyloidosis	Bone pains, arthritis, pathologic fractures
Gastrointestinal	Diarrhea	Delayed gastric emptying	Anorexia, nausea, vomiting, constipation, epigastric pain
Hematologic	Anemia, thrombocytopenia		
Renal		Impaired free water clearance	Polyuria, hematuria

Adapted from Roizen MF: Anesthesia for the patient with endocrine disease, Part 1. Curr Rev Clin Anesth 1987; 6: 43.

in perioperative therapy for patients with the syndrome. The important issue is to identify patients with a pheochromocytoma preoperatively before they are scheduled for other types of surgery.

In patients taking long-term corticosteroids, one should have a high index of suspicion for adrenal-cortical suppression and Cushing syndrome. The hallmark symptoms found in Cushing syndrome include moon facies, striations of the skin, trunk obesity, hypertension, easy bruisability, and hypovolemia. The preoperative preparation includes correction of the fluid and electrolyte abnormalities. There is consensus that for patients taking corticosteroids for long periods, perioperative steroid supplementation is indicated to cover the stresses of anesthesia and surgery. However, in patients who have had only a short course of steroids within the 12 months prior to surgery, the use of steroid supplementation is controversial, although most clinicians would favor their use preoperatively (Table 23-10).

Other Organ Systems

Renal disease has important implications for fluid and electrolyte management, as well as metabolism of drugs. Liver disease is associated with altered protein binding and volume of distribution of drugs, as well as coagulation abnormalities. Coagulation disorders may influence the choice of regional anesthesia. The anesthesiologist should inquire about bruising, bleeding, and the use of medications that influence platelet function such as aspirin, other nonsteroidal anti-inflammatory drugs, and anticoagulants. Musculoskeletal disorders have been associated with an increased risk of malignant hyperthermia. Osteoarthritis may result in difficulty exposing the glottic opening for tracheal intubation or difficulty in positioning for regional anesthetic. Because rheumatoid arthritis is a multisystem disease, it is important in such patients to perform a thorough review of systems. These patients may have restrictive lung disease, pleural effusions, pericarditis, anemia, and atlanto-occipital instability. Finally, the anesthesiologist should inquire about infectious diseases such as human immunodeficiency virus or antibiotic-resistant infections.

TABLE 23-10

PERIOPERATIVE CORTICOSTEROID COVERAGE

For minor surgery	The patient should take 1.5–2 times his or her usual prednisone dosage on the morning of surgery. The following day the patient should take his or her normal prednisone dose (or parenteral equivalent if gut cannot be used). The surgeon and anesthesiologist should be aware that the patient is glucocorticoid-dependent and should be prepared to administer more "steroids" if the surgery becomes prolonged or more extensive.
For moderate surgery	The patient should be given 2 times his or her usual glucocorticoid dosage orally (if possible) on the morning of surgery and/or 25 mg hydrocortisone IV before the operation, then 75 mg hydrocortisone IV during the operation, and 50 mg hydrocortisone IV after the operation; then the dose should be rapidly tapered over 48 hr to the usual dose—if the postoperative course is uncomplicated.
For major surgery	The patient should be given 2 times his or her usual glucocorticoid dosage orally (if possible) on the morning of surgery and/or 50 mg hydrocortisone IV before the operation, then 100 mg hydrocortisone IV during the operation. After the operation, 100 mg IV q 8 hr × 24 hr should be administered and then rapidly tapered (over 48–72 hr) to the patient's usual glucocorticoid dosage—if the postoperative course is uncomplicated.

IV, intravenously.
Adapted from Brussel T, Chernow B: Perioperative management of endocrine problems: Thyroid, adrenal cortex, pituitary. Am Soc Anesthesiol 1990; 3: 48.

PREOPERATIVE LABORATORY TESTING

The Value of Preoperative Testing: Normal Values

8 In attempting to determine the optimal choice of preoperative tests, it is important to understand the interpretation of the results. Ideally, tests would either confirm or exclude the presence of a disease; however, most tests only increase or decrease the probability of disease. In determining reference ranges for diagnostic tests, values that fall outside the 95% confidence intervals for normal individuals are considered abnormal. Therefore, up to 5% of normal individuals can have "abnormal" test results. To determine its clinical relevance, a test must be interpreted within the context of the clinical situation. Performing tests in patients with no risk for having the pathophysiologic process of interest can yield a high number of false-positive results. For example, a low potassium value (3.0 mg/dL) in an otherwise healthy individual is most likely a normal result. Interpreting this test as abnormal, and initiating treatment, could lead to harm without any benefit.

Risks and Costs Versus Benefits

The use of medical testing is associated with significant cost, both in real dollars and in potential harm. Routine preoperative testing has been estimated to cost $3 billion annually. An "abnormal" test that is later determined to be a false result can lead to significant cost and real harm. For example, a positive exercise electrocardiographic stress test in a healthy 40-year-old woman may lead to coronary angiography. Coronary angiography is not a benign procedure, and can lead to vascular injuries. Based on Bayesian analysis, a positive test result in this patient is most likely a false-positive, and the test was inappropriately used. Therefore, the woman and her physician would gain no additional information, thousands of dollars in medical costs would accrue, and she would sustain morbidity.

Several studies have evaluated the implications of reduced testing. Golub, et al.[65] retrospectively reviewed the records of 325 patients who had undergone preadmission testing prior to ambulatory surgery. Of these, 272 (84%) had at least one abnormal screening test result, while only 28 surgeries were delayed or canceled. The authors estimated that only three patients potentially benefited from preadmission testing, including a new diagnosis of diabetes in one and nonspecific ECG changes in two, one of which had known ischemic heart disease.

In a study published in 1991, Narr et al.[66] at the Mayo Clinic demonstrated minimal benefits from routine testing and proposed that routine laboratory screening tests were not required in healthy patients. In a follow-up study published in 1997, a cohort of patients who had no preoperative testing during 1994 was reviewed and found to include no deaths or major perioperative morbidity.[67] The authors concluded that current anesthetic and medical practices rapidly identify indications for laboratory evaluation when necessary, and therefore routine testing was not indicated in this healthy cohort.

Even if testing better defines a disease state, the risks of any intervention based on the results may outweigh the benefit. Cardiovascular testing is a classic example (Fig. 23-4). If a noninvasive test is positive, coronary angiography may be performed. A positive angiogram may then result in CABG prior to the planned noncardiac surgery. Although cardiovascular morbidity and mortality may be reduced in patients with significant CAD who have undergone coronary revascularization, the morbidity associated with both the testing and revascularization procedure may be greater than any potential benefit. Roizen and Cohn[68] have suggested a protocol for screening tests based on the preoperative evaluation using a risk-benefit analysis. The following is modified from those recommendations and the "Practice Advisory for Preanesthetic Evaluation" from the ASA (*Class C procedures* are highly invasive and commonly necessitate blood administration, invasive monitoring and postoperative care in a critical care unit).

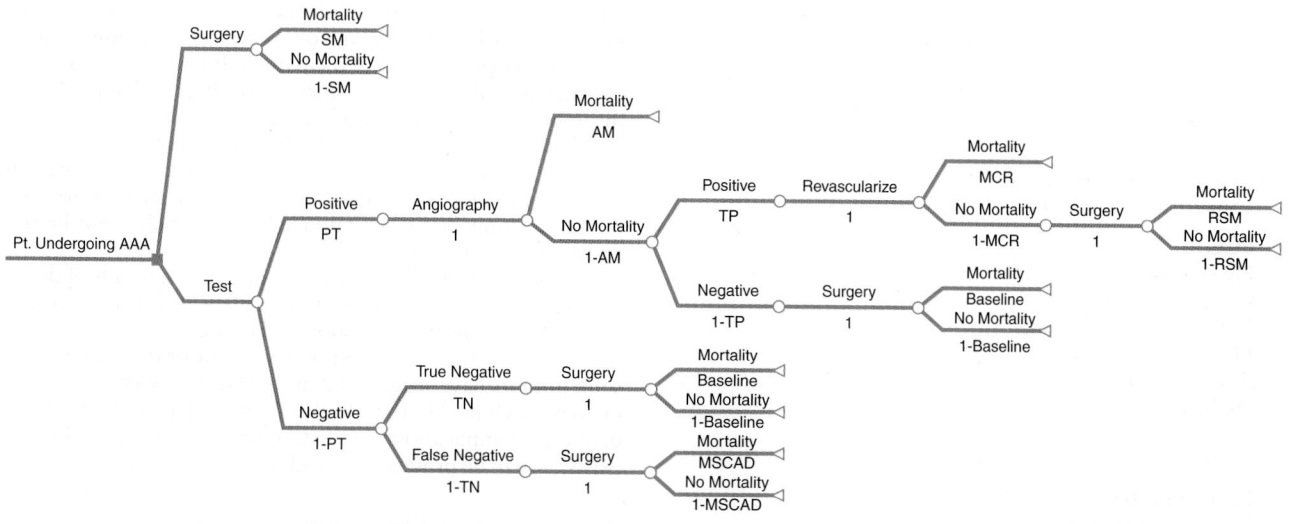

FIGURE 23-4. A decision algorithm evaluating the decision between vascular surgery alone or coronary artery revascularization before vascular surgery. There are currently no randomized trials to address the optimal strategy. By outlining the multiple decision points at which a patient can sustain mortality by choosing to undergo coronary revascularization first, the optimal strategy for preoperative evaluation can be demonstrated. Specifically, variation in mortalities at each decision point can change the optimal strategy. (Reproduced from Fleisher LA, Skolnick ED, Holroyd KJ, et al: Coronary artery revascularization before abdominal aortic aneurysm surgery: A decision analytic approach. Anesth Analg 1994; 79: 661, with permission.)

Recommended Laboratory Testing

Blood Count
Neonates
Physiologic age ≥75 years
Class C procedure
Malignancy
Renal disease
Tobacco use
Anticoagulant use
Bleeding disorder

Coagulation Studies
Chemotherapy
Hepatic disease
Bleeding disorder
Anticoagulants

Electrolytes
Renal disease
Diabetes
Diuretic, digoxin, or steroid use
CNS disease
Endocrine disorders

Blood Urea Nitrogen/Creatinine
Physiologic age ≥75 years
Class C procedure
Cardiovascular disease
Renal disease
Diabetes
Diuretic or digoxin use
CNS disease

Blood Glucose
Physiologic age ≥75 years
Class C procedure
Diabetes
Steroid use
CNS disease

Liver Function Tests
Hepatic disease
Hepatitis exposure
Malnutrition

Chest X-Ray
Recent upper respiratory infection
Physiologic age ≥75 years
Cardiovascular disease
Pulmonary disease
Malignancy
Radiation Therapy
Tobacco ≥20 pack-years

ECG
Physiologic age ≥75 years
Class C procedure
Cardiovascular disease
Pulmonary disease
Radiation therapy
Diabetes
Digoxin use
CNS disease

Pregnancy Test
Possible pregnancy

Albumin
Physiologic age ≥75 years
Class C procedure
Malnutrition

Type and Screen
Physiologic age ≥75 years
Class C procedure

Complete Blood Count and Hemoglobin Concentration

The use of a preoperative hemoglobin has been suggested as the only test necessary in many patients prior to elective surgery; however, even this minimal standard has been questioned. Baron, et al.[69] reviewed the records of 1,863 pediatric patients scheduled for elective outpatient procedures. In only 1.1% of patients was the hematocrit abnormal, and in none of these patients was the procedure canceled or the anesthetic plan modified. However, a baseline hematocrit is still indicated in any procedure with a risk of blood loss.

The standard regarding the lowest acceptable perioperative hematocrit and indication for a preoperative transfusion has changed during the past decade. The current recommendations of the National Blood Resource Education Committee are that a hemoglobin level of 7 g/dL is acceptable in patients without systemic disease. In patients with systemic disease, signs of inadequate systemic oxygen delivery (tachycardia, tachypnea) are an indication for transfusion.

Electrolytes

In the past, patients routinely received a chemistry panel prior to surgery. Because of technology issues, it may be cheaper to obtain a standard battery than to determine one particular test. However, testing rarely leads to any change in perioperative management.

There are numerous guidelines regarding the need for preoperative electrolytes. The only consensus is the lack of routine testing in asymptomatic adults, although a creatinine and glucose has been recommended in older patients. In patients with systemic diseases or on medications that affect the kidneys, a blood urea nitrogen and creatinine evaluation are indicated.

Coagulation Studies

Coagulation disorders can have significant impact on the surgical procedure and perioperative management. However, abnormal laboratory studies in the absence of clinical abnormalities with hemophilia or von Willebrand disease, require preoperative preparation of the patient. It is important to identify such disorders from a history of bleeding problems. A prothrombin and partial thromboplastin time analysis are indicated with a past history of bleeding disorders following injuries, tooth extraction, or surgical procedures; and in patients with known or suspected liver disease, malabsorption, or malnutrition, and on certain medications such as antibiotics and chemotherapeutic agents.

Bleeding time previously was advocated as a means of determining the presence of a qualitative platelet defect. However, recently clinicians have questioned the value of this test in clinical practice. The test is extremely operator-dependent, and some authors have suggested that the test should be abandoned in favor of clinical history. In the absence of a clinical bleeding diathesis, complications are extremely rare. If such a history exists, it may be prudent to avoid regional anesthesia.

Pregnancy Testing

Routine pregnancy testing in women of childbearing potential is a subject of considerable debate. The rationale is that specific agents may be avoided, or surgery may be delayed. Information regarding the last menstrual period can help define the potential, but does not eliminate the possibility. Roizen and Cohn[68] suggest that pregnancy testing should be limited to female patients who believe they are pregnant or cannot tell if they are pregnant. However, a number of studies have evaluated the validity of history as a means of assessing pregnancy status in adolescents with conflicting results. Current practice varies dramatically among centers, and anesthesiologists and may be a function of the population served with regard to the need to routinely test those women with a negative pregnancy history.

Chest X-Rays

A preoperative chest x-ray can identify abnormalities that may lead to either delay or cancellation of the planned surgical procedure or modification of perioperative care. For example, identification of pneumonia, pulmonary edema, pulmonary nodules, or a mediastinal mass could all lead to modification of care. However, routine testing in the population without risk factors can lead to more harm than benefit. Roizen and Cohn[68] have demonstrated substantial harm from additional procedures based on shadows performed solely as a routine preoperative chest x-ray.

The American College of Physicians suggests that a chest x-ray is indicated in the presence of active chest disease or an intrathoracic procedure, but not on the basis of advanced age alone.[70] Other guidelines suggest that a preoperative chest x-ray is reasonable in patients over the age of 60 years. In a meta-analysis, Archer, et al.[71] reviewed the published reports from 1966 to 1992 in the English, French, and Spanish literature. Twenty-one reports were identified with sufficient data to evaluate the use of testing. On average, abnormalities were reported in 10% of routine preoperative chest x-rays, of which only 1.3% were unexpected. These findings result in modification in management in only 0.1% of patients, with unknown influence on outcome. The authors estimated that each finding that influenced management would cost $23,000, concluding that routine chest x-rays without a clinical indication were not justified. Therefore, a preoperative chest x-ray is indicated in patients with a history or clinical evidence of active pulmonary disease, and *may* be indicated routinely only in patients with advanced age.

Pulmonary Function Tests

Pulmonary function tests can be generally divided into two categories, spirometry and an arterial blood gas. Spirometry can provide information on forced vital capacity (FVC), forced expiratory volume in 1 second (FEV_1), ratio of FEV_1/FVC, and average forced expiratory flow from 25 to 75% (FEF 25–75%). Although each of these measures has a sound physiologic basis, their practical assessment can vary greatly among healthy persons. Objective measures defining high risk for pulmonary resection have been proposed. For nonpulmonary surgery, they rarely provide additional information beyond that obtained from history. Possible indications are the use of pulmonary function testing with bronchodilator therapy to assess responsiveness in a patient who is wheezing and when the history and physical leave the degree of perioperative risk uncertain.

With the advent of the pulse oximeter, the use of preoperative arterial blood gas sampling has become less important. It may still be indicated, since determining the baseline CO_2 is useful in managing postoperative ventilation settings and resting hypercapnia is associated with increased perioperative risk. However, the physical act of obtaining an arterial blood gas can lead to hyperventilation and change the $PaCO_2$. One method of assessing the probability of CO_2 retention is evaluation of the serum bicarbonate. A normal serum bicarbonate will virtually exclude the diagnosis of CO_2 retention. If the serum bicarbonate is elevated, then an arterial blood gas test either preoperatively or immediately prior to induction may be indicated.

Another indication for an arterial blood gas has been determination of oxygen concentration. With the advent and availability of pulse oximetry in the preoperative screening clinic, this is rarely an indication.

SUMMARY OF THE PREOPERATIVE EVALUATION

9 The preoperative evaluation of the surgical patient continues to be an important component of the anesthesiologist's role. A thorough history and physical examination can be used to identify those medical conditions that might affect perioperative management and direct further laboratory testing. In the current era of capitated care and the desire to reduce inappropriate utilization of medical technology, the anesthesiologist can have a significant impact on health resource utilization by performing appropriate laboratory tests. By combining data from the history, physical examination, exercise tolerance, and the stress of the surgical procedure, inappropriate testing can be reduced; but more importantly, appropriate screening tests will be performed.

PREOPERATIVE MEDICATION

Anesthetic management for patients begins with preoperative psychological preparation and, if necessary, preoperative medication. Specific pharmacologic actions should be kept in mind when these drugs are administered before operation, and they should be tailored to the needs of each patient. The anesthesiologist should assess the patient's mental and physical condition during the preoperative visit. Because it is actually the beginning of the anesthetic, choice of preoperative medication should be based on the same considerations as the choice of anesthesia, including considerations of the patient's medical problems, requirements of the surgery, and the anesthesiologist's skills. Satisfactory preoperative preparation and medication facilitate an uneventful perioperative course. Poor preparation may begin a series of problems and misadventures.

10 No consensus exists on the choice of preoperative medications. Their use has been dominated by tradition, which has been modified somewhat by the change in anesthetic agents and techniques over the years. Beecher[72] stated that "empirical procedures firmly established in the habits of good doctors have a life, not to say, immortality of their own." Similarly, "the emotional attachment of an anesthesiologist to his own regimen is often more obvious than his objective assessment of its effects."[73] Another reason for lack of consensus may be that several different drugs or combinations of drugs can accomplish the same goals. However, there is general agreement that most patients should enter the operating room after anxiety has been relieved and other specific goals have been met through preoperative preparation and medication. Anxiolysis should be accomplished without undue sedation, which can interfere with patient safety or, given the dramatic increase in the number of outpatient surgical procedures, prolong length of stay in the operating room.

Psychological Preparation

Psychological preparation of the patient involves the preoperative visit and interview with the patient and family members. The anesthesiologist should explain anticipated events and the proposed anesthetic management in an effort to reduce anxiety and allay apprehension. Patients may perceive the day of surgery as the biggest, most threatening day in their lives; they do not wish to be treated impersonally in the operating room. The anesthesiologist's first direct encounter with the patient may be in the immediate preoperative period. A growing

TABLE 23-11

COMPARISON OF PREOPERATIVE VISIT (PERCENTAGE OF PATIENTS) AND PENTOBARBITAL (2 mg/kg IM)

	▪ FELT DROWSY	▪ FELT NERVOUS	▪ ADEQUATE PREPARATION
Control group	18	58	35
Pentobarbital group	30	61	48
Preoperative visit	26	40	65
Preoperative visit and pentobarbital	38	38	71

IM, intramuscularly.
Data from Egbert LD, Battit GE, Turndorf H, et al: The value of the preoperative visit by the anesthetist. JAMA 1963; 185: 553.

TABLE 23-12

VARIOUS GOALS FOR PREOPERATIVE MEDICINE

1. Relief of anxiety
2. Sedation
3. Amnesia
4. Analgesia
5. Drying of airway secretions
6. Prevention of autonomic reflex responses
7. Reduction of gastric fluid volume and increased pH
8. Antiemetic effects
9. Reduction of anesthetic requirements
10. Facilitation of smooth induction of anesthesia
11. Prophylaxis against allergic reactions

Modified from Stoelting RK: Psychological preparation and preoperative medication. Anesthesia. Edited by Miller RD. New York, Churchill Livingstone, 1981.

number of patients receive their preanesthetic evaluations by others in preoperative evaluation clinics or just prior to surgery. Preoperative visits must be conducted efficiently, but they must also be informative and reassuring, answering all questions. Most of the anesthesiologist's time is spent with an unconscious or sedated patient; therefore, he or she must take time before the operation to earn the trust and confidence of that patient.

Most patients are anxious before surgery. Studies show that, depending on the intensity of inquiry, 40 to 85% of patients are apprehensive before surgery. Preoperative anxiety states are at a high level, and most patients expect apprehension to be relieved before they arrive in the operating room. The classic study by Egbert, et al.[74] showed that an average of 57% of patients felt anxious before operation. An informative and comforting preoperative visit may replace many milligrams of depressant medication. For example, the study by Egbert et al. showed that more patients were adequately prepared for surgery after a preoperative interview than after 2 mg/kg of pentobarbital given intramuscularly 1 hour before surgery (Table 23-11).[74] However, psychological preparation cannot accomplish everything and will not relieve all anxiety.

Besides psychological preparation, there are other goals of preoperative medication. Control of pain and satisfactory levels of amnesia or sedation cannot be achieved with consistent success at the preoperative visit alone. In addition, emergency situations may provide little or no time for a preoperative interview. More seriously ill or elderly patients, conversely, may not tolerate the physiologic effects of sedative medications. Always remember that the substitution of preoperative depressant drugs for a comforting and tactful preoperative visit may compromise patient safety.

Pharmacologic Preparation

The ideal drug or combination of drugs for preoperative pharmacologic preparation is as elusive as is the ideal anesthetic technique and is not based on a large body of data that is either definitive or persuasive. Routine administration of the same drugs to all patients has fallen into disfavor as a selective approach has emerged. In selecting the appropriate drugs for preoperative medication, the patient's psychological condition, physical status, and age must be considered. The surgical procedure and its duration are important factors, as well. Is this an outpatient procedure? Is it elective surgery or emergency surgery? The anesthesiologist must know the patient's weight, prior response to depressant drugs, including

unwanted side effects, and allergies. Finally, the anesthesiologist's experience and familiarity with certain preoperative medications more than others are determinants.

The goals to be achieved for each patient with preoperative medication are intimately involved in the selection process (Table 23-12). The desired goals may be multiple and should be tailored to the needs of each patient. Some of the goals, such as relief of anxiety and production of sedation, apply to almost every patient, whereas others are important only occasionally. Prophylaxis against allergic reactions applies in only a few instances. Prevention of autonomic reflexes mediated through the vagus nerve or an antiemetic effect may be better attempted immediately before the anticipated need rather than achieved at the time of preoperative medication. Preoperative medication regimens should not produce sufficient obtundation to be clinically significant in reducing anesthetic requirement.

Some patients should not receive depressant drugs before surgery. Patients with little physiologic reserve, at the extremes of age, with a head injury, or with hypovolemia may be harmed more than helped by many of the medications normally used before operation. In contrast, the conditions of others demand that attempts be made pharmacologically to reduce anxiety, provide analgesia, or dry secretions in the airway to produce a safer perioperative course. For elective surgery, the anesthesiologist will, in most instances, want the patient to enter the operating room free of anxiety and sedated, yet easily aroused and cooperative. The patient should not be overly obtunded or display other unwanted side effects of the preoperative drugs. The patient who asks to be "asleep" before leaving the hospital room should be told that apprehension and sedation may be reduced but it would be unsafe to produce a comatose state. The time and route of administration of the preoperative medications are important. As a general rule, oral medications should be given to the patient 60 to 90 minutes before arrival in the operating room. It is acceptable to administer oral drugs with up to 150 mL of water.[75] Intravenous agents produce effects after a few circulation times, while for full effect, intramuscular medications should be given at least 20 minutes and preferably 30 to 60 minutes before the patient's arrival in the operating room. Every attempt should be made to have the preoperative medications achieve their full effect before the patient's arrival in the operating room rather than after induction of anesthesia. The drug(s), doses, route of administration, and effects should be recorded on the anesthetic record. A list of common preoperative medications is presented in Table 23-13.

TABLE 23-13

COMMON PREOPERATIVE MEDICATIONS, DOSES, AND ADMINISTRATION ROUTES

■ MEDICATION	■ ADMINISTRATION ROUTE	■ DOSE (mg)
Lorazepam	Oral, IV	0.5–4
Midazolam	IV	Titration of 1.0–2.5-mg doses
Fentanyl	IV	Titration of 25–100-µg doses
Morphine	IV	Titration of 1.0–2.5-mg doses
Meperidine	IV	Titration of 10–25-mg doses
Cimetidine	Oral, IV	150–300
Ranitidine	Oral	50–200
Metoclopramide	IV	5–10
Atropine	IV	0.3–0.4
Glycopyrrolate	IV	0.1–0.2
Scopolamine	IV	0.1–0.4

IV, intravenous.
Modified from Stoelting RK, Miller RD, eds: Basics of Anesthesia. New York, Churchill Livingstone, 1984.

PREANESTHETIC EVALUATION AND PREPARATION

Sedative–Hypnotics and Tranquilizers

Benzodiazepines. Benzodiazepines are among the most popular drugs used for preoperative medication (Table 23-14). They are used to produce anxiolysis, amnesia, and sedation. Because the site of action of benzodiazepines is on specific receptors in the central nervous system (Fig. 23-5) there is relatively little depression of ventilation or of the cardiovascular system with premedicant doses. Benzodiazepines have a wide therapeutic index and a low incidence of toxicity. Other than central nervous system depression, there are few side effects of this group of drugs. Specifically, nausea and vomiting are not usually associated with administration of benzodiazepines for preoperative medication.

There are some hazards and unwanted side effects of benzodiazepines. The central nervous system depression these drugs cause is sometimes long and excessive, especially with use of lorazepam. These drugs are not analgesic agents. Benzodiazepines may not always produce a calming effect but may cause agitation, as evidenced by restlessness and delirium.

Lorazepam. Lorazepam resembles oxazepam structurally and is 5 to 10 times as potent as diazepam. Lorazepam can produce profound amnesia, relief of anxiety, and sedation (Fig. 23-6).[76] When lorazepam is compared with diazepam, their effects are very similar. Although it is insoluble in water and requires a solvent such as polyethylene glycol or propylene glycol, administration of lorazepam, unlike diazepam, is not associated with pain on injection or phlebitis. Prolonged sedation is more likely after lorazepam administration. Even though the elimination half-life of diazepam is longer than that of lorazepam (20 to 40 hours vs. 10 to 20 hours), the effect of diazepam may be shorter because it more rapidly dissociates from the benzodiazepine receptor.[77]

In addition to the intravenous route, lorazepam is reliably absorbed orally. Bradshaw, et al.[78] demonstrated clinical effects 30 to 60 minutes after oral administration of lorazepam. Peak plasma concentrations may not occur until 2 to 4 hours after oral administration. Therefore, lorazepam must be ordered well before surgery so that the drug has time to be effective before the patient arrives in the operating room. Lorazepam also may be given sublingually. As stated previously, the elimination half-life is 10 to 20 hours. The usual dose is about 25 to 50 µg/kg. The dose for an adult should usually not exceed 4.0 mg.[76,77] With recommended doses, anterograde amnesia may be produced for as long as 4 to 6 hours without excessive sedation. Higher doses lead to prolonged and excessive sedation without more amnesia. Because of its slow onset and length of action, lorazepam is not useful in instances in which rapid awakening is necessary, such as with outpatient anesthesia. There are no active metabolites of lorazepam; because its metabolism is not dependent on microsomal enzymes, there is less influence on its effect from age or liver disease. As with diazepam, little cardiorespiratory depression occurs with lorazepam. However, there is the danger of unwanted respiratory depression in those with lung disease.

TABLE 23-14

COMPARISON OF PHARMACOLOGIC VARIABLES OF BENZODIAZEPINES

	■ DIAZEPAM	■ LORAZEPAM	■ MIDAZOLAM
Dose equivalent (mg)	10	1–2	3–5
Time to peak effect after oral dose (hr)	1–1.5	2–4	0.5–1
Elimination half-time (hr)	20–40	10–20	1–4
Clearance (mL/kg/min)	0.2–0.5	0.7–1.0	6.4–11.1
Volume of distribution (L/kg)	0.7–1.7	0.8–1.3	1.1–1.7

Adapted from Reves JG, Fragen RJ, Vinick HR, et al: Midazolam: Pharmacology and uses. Anesthesiology 1985; 62: 310; and Stoelting RK: Pharmacology and Physiology in Anesthetic Practice. Philadelphia, JB Lippincott, 1987.

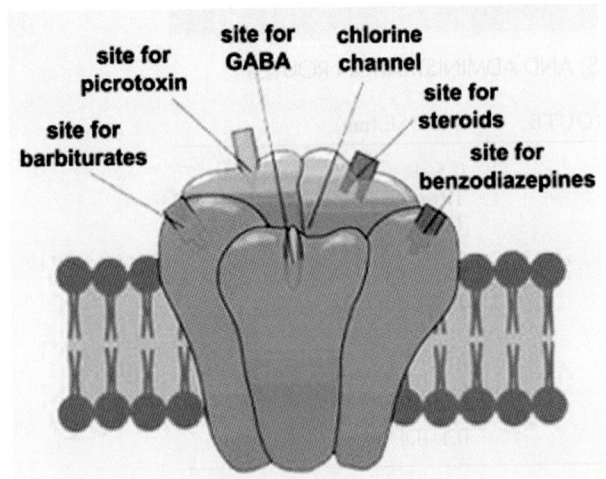

FIGURE 23-5. Schematic diagram of the benzodiazepine site on the GABA (γ-aminobutyric acid) receptor. [Reproduced with permission from Carlson N: Foundations of Physiological Psychology (7th edition). Boston, Pearson Education, Inc, 2007, p 115)]

Midazolam. Midazolam has predominantly replaced the use of diazepam for preoperative medication and conscious sedation. It is common to administer sedative doses intravenously just prior to the trip to the operating room. The physicochemical properties of the drug allow for its water solubility and rapid metabolism. As with other benzodiazepines, midazolam produces anxiolysis, sedation, and amnesia. It is 2 to 3 times as potent as diazepam because of its increased affinity for the benzodiazepine receptor. The usual intramuscular dose is 0.05 to 0.1 mg/kg and titration of 1.0 to 2.5 mg at a time intravenously. There is no irritation or phlebitis with injection of midazolam. The incidence of side effects after administration is low, although depression of ventilation and sedation may be greater than expected, especially in elderly patients or when the drug is combined with other central nervous system depressants. There is more rapid onset of action and predictable absorption after intramuscular injection of midazolam than after diazepam. The time of onset after intramuscular injection is 5 to 10 minutes, with peak effect occurring after 30 to 60 minutes. The onset after intravenous administration of 5 mg would be expected to occur after 1 to 2 minutes. In addition to quicker onset, more rapid recovery occurs after midazolam administration compared with diazepam. This is probably the result of the lipid solubility of midazolam and its rapid distribution in the peripheral tissues and metabolic biotransformation. For these reasons, midazolam usually should be given within an hour of induction.[63] Midazolam is metabolized by hepatic microsomal enzymes to essentially inactive hydroxylated metabolites. H_2 receptor antagonists do not interfere with its metabolism. The elimination half-life of midazolam is approximately 1 to 4 hours and may be extended in the elderly. Tests show that mental function usually returns to normal within 4 hours of administration.[79] After administration of 5 mg, amnesia lasts from 20 to 30 minutes. Intramuscular administration may produce longer periods of amnesia. The lack of recall may be augmented by concomitant administration of scopolamine. The properties of midazolam make it ideal for shorter procedures.

Other Benzodiazepines. Oxazepam, another benzodiazepine that has been used for preoperative medication, is one of the pharmacologically active metabolites of diazepam. It is absorbed slowly after oral administration and has an elimination half-life of 5 to 15 hours. Temazepam has been given in oral doses of 20 to 30 mg before surgery. It must be given well before surgery because peak plasma levels do not occur until approximately 2 to 2.5 hours after administration. Triazolam is a short-acting benzodiazepine. The adult oral dose of the drug is 0.25 to 0.5 mg. Peak plasma concentrations occur in about 1 hour and its elimination half-life is 1.7 to 5.2 hours. The drug may become long-acting in the elderly. Similarly, a study by Pinnock, et al. did not show triazolam to be of short duration when compared with diazepam for premedication for minor gynecologic surgery.[80] Alprazolam (1 mg) given to adults has been shown to produce a modest reduction in anxiety before surgery.

Other Sedative Drugs

Diphenhydramine. Diphenhydramine is a histamine receptor antagonist with sedative and anticholinergic activity. It is also an antiemetic. A dose of 50 mg will last 3 to 6 hours in an adult. Diphenhydramine has been used recently in combination with cimetidine, steroids, and other drugs for prophylaxis in patients with chronic atopy, latex allergy, and for prophylaxis before chemonucleolysis and dye studies. Diphenhydramine blocks the histamine-1 receptor to prevent effects of histamine peripherally.

FIGURE 23-6. Percentage of patients in each group failing to recall specific events of the operative day. Medications were administered intramuscularly. O.R., operating room; I.V., intravenous. (Reprinted from Fragen RJ, Caldwell N: Lorazepam premedication: Lack of recall and relief of anxiety. Anesth Analg 1976; 55: 792, with permission.)

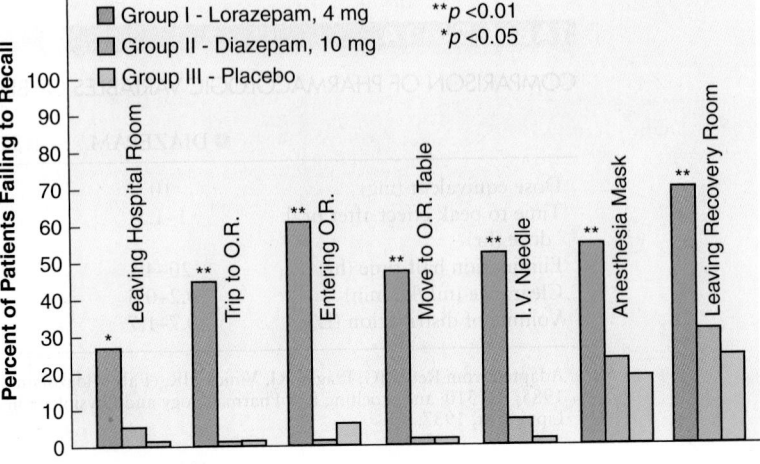

Opioids

Morphine and meperidine were historically the most frequently used opioids for intramuscular preoperative medication. Recently, the use of intravenous fentanyl just before surgery has become much more popular. Opioids are used when analgesia is needed before operation. Cohen and Beecher[81] opined that "unless there is pain, there is no need for narcotic in preanesthetic medication." For the patient experiencing pain before operation, the opioids can produce good analgesia and even euphoria. Opioids have been ordered for patients before operation to ameliorate the discomfort that may occur during regional anesthesia or the insertion of invasive monitoring catheters or large intravenous lines. The dose of opioid may need to be reduced in the debilitated or elderly patient. The elderly patient often exhibits a reduced sensitivity to pain. Furthermore, elderly patients can have an increased analgesic response to opioids. Opioids also have been used before operation in the opioid-dependent patient.

Preoperative administration of opioids in other settings has been controversial. Preoperative opioids prior to a nitrous oxide–opioid anesthetic may help to establish a basal state of anesthesia when the patient arrives in the operating room and to get a preview of the patient's response to opioids. Opioids have been given to patients before operation to provide analgesia on their awakening in the recovery room. The other approach is to titrate the opioid intravenously during emergence or on the patient's arrival in the recovery room. Preoperative administration of opioids can lower anesthetic requirements. Some anesthesiologists use opioids in combination with other drugs before operation to facilitate anesthetic induction by mask, although opioids do decrease ventilatory response and therefore decrease uptake of inhalation drugs. If necessary, the anesthesiologist may want to use assisted or controlled ventilation of the lungs to overcome the respiratory depressant effects of the opioids. Finally, opioids do not relieve apprehension, produce sedation, or prevent recall.

Opioids administration has the potential to cause several side effects. Preoperatively, opioids usually exhibit no direct myocardial effects. However, some opioids do interfere with the compensatory constriction of smooth muscles of the peripheral vasculature. This venodilation may lead to orthostatic hypotension. Histamine release after injection of morphine may compound these circulatory effects. As with most preoperative medications, it is probably safest to have the patient remain at bed rest after opioid premedication. The analgesic properties and respiratory depressant effects of opioids usually go hand in hand. The decrease in the carbon dioxide drive at the medullary respiratory center may be prolonged. Furthermore, there is a decrease in the responsiveness to hypoxia at the carotid body after injection of only low doses of opioids.[82] The anesthesiologist may wish to consider supplemental oxygen for the patient receiving opioid premedication.

In general, the opioid agonist–antagonists produce less respiratory depression, but they also produce less analgesia. Rather than euphoria, the opioids may produce dysphoria. When this side effect does occur, it is most commonly seen in a patient who does not have pain before operation and has received the opioid premedication. Nausea and vomiting may result from opioid administration. The effect of opioids on the vestibular apparatus leading to motion sickness or stimulation of the medullary chemoreceptor trigger zone is a postulated reason for nausea and vomiting. Choledochoduodenal sphincter (sphincter of Oddi) spasm has occasionally been noted subsequent to injection of opioids. The opioid produces smooth muscle constriction, which leads to right upper quadrant pain. Pain relief may be achieved with naloxone or possibly glucagon. Occasionally, the pain from biliary tract spasm is difficult to differentiate from the pain of angina pectoris. The administration of nitroglycerin should relieve angina pectoris and pain resulting from biliary tract spasm; an opioid antagonist should relieve only pain resulting from biliary tract spasm. Some question the use of opioid premedication in patients with biliary tract disease. All opioids have the potential to induce choledochoduodenal sphincter spasm. Fentanyl and meperidine are less likely than morphine to produce this side effect. Opioids may produce pruritus. Morphine, possibly through histamine release, often produces itching, especially around the nose. Opioids also may cause flushing, dizziness, and miosis.

Other drugs are often combined with opioids for their additive effects or to overcome the disadvantages of opioid side effects. A sedative-hypnotic is often used with opioids to produce sedation, anxiolysis, and amnesia in addition to analgesia.

Morphine. Morphine is well absorbed after intramuscular injection. The onset of effect should occur within 15 to 30 minutes. The peak effect occurs in 45 to 90 minutes and lasts as long as 4 hours. After intravenous administration, the peak effect usually occurs within 20 minutes. Morphine is not reliably absorbed after oral administration. As with the other opioids, depression of ventilation and orthostatic hypotension may occur after injection of morphine. The effect of morphine on the chemoreceptive trigger zone may produce nausea and vomiting. Nausea and vomiting may also occur owing to a vestibular component.

Meperidine. Meperidine is about one-tenth as potent as morphine. It may be given orally or parenterally. A single dose of meperidine usually lasts 2 to 4 hours. The onset after intramuscular injection is unpredictable, and a great deal of variability in time to peak effect exists.

Fentanyl. Fentanyl is a synthetic opioid agonist structurally similar to meperidine. It is 75 to 125 times more potent than morphine in its analgesic characteristics. The lipid solubility of fentanyl is greater than that of morphine, which contributes to its rapid onset of action. Peak plasma concentrations occur within 6 to 7 minutes following intravenous administration and its elimination half-time is 3 to 6 hours. The drug's short duration of action is attributed to redistribution to inactive tissues, such as the lungs, fat, and skeletal muscle. Metabolism occurs primarily by N-demethylation to norfentanyl, which is a less potent analgesic. A decreased clearance rate in the elderly may prolong elimination.

In doses of 1 to 2 μg/kg intravenously, fentanyl may be used to provide preoperative analgesia. Oral transmucosal fentanyl preparations of fentanyl are available, delivering 5 to 20 μg/kg of the drug. This form has been examined as a premedicant in both adults and children to relieve anxiety and pain. Fentanyl causes neither myocardial depression nor histamine release, but may be associated with ventilatory depression and profound bradycardia. Synergistic effects with benzodiazepines warrant close observation when this combination is given in the preoperative period.

Gastric Fluid pH and Volume

Many patients who come to the operating room are at risk for aspiration pneumonitis. The classic example is the patient with acute pain and a "full stomach" who must have emergency surgery. The pregnant patient, the obese patient, the diabetic, the patient with hiatal hernia or gastroesophageal reflux, all may be at risk for aspiration of gastric contents and subsequent chemical pneumonitis. Although uncertain it is believed, if adults aspirate more than 25 mL of gastric fluid with a pH lower than 2.5, pulmonary sequelae will result. This "fact" has not been, and probably never will be, proved in humans.

TABLE 23-15

SUMMARY OF FASTING RECOMMENDATIONS TO REDUCE THE RISK OF PULMONARY ASPIRATION[a]

■ INGESTED MATERIAL	■ MINIMUM FASTING PERIOD, APPLIED TO ALL AGES (hr)
Clear liquids[b]	2
Breast milk	4
Infant formula	6
Nonhuman milk	6
Light meal (toast and clear liquids)	6

[a]Applies only to healthy patients who are undergoing elective procedures and are not intended for women in labor. Following the guidelines does not guarantee complete gastric emptying.
[b]Examples of clear liquids include water, fruit juices without pulp, carbonated beverages, clear tea, and black coffee.
Adapted from Practice Guidelines for Preoperative Fasting and the Use of Pharmacologic Agents to Reduce the Risk of Pulmonary Aspiration: Application to Healthy Patients Undergoing Elective Procedures. A Report by the American Society of Anesthesiologists Task Force on Preoperative Fasting. Anesthesiology 1999; 90: 896.

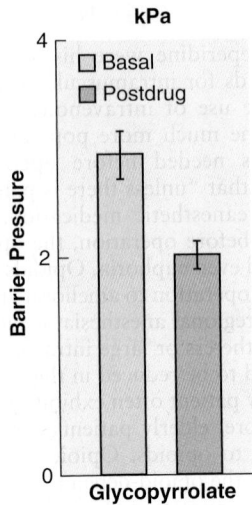

FIGURE 23-7. Barrier pressure (esophageal sphincter pressure minus gastric pressure) before and after intravenous administration of glycopyrrolate, 0.3 mg, to adult patients. Mean ± SE. (Reprinted from Brock-Utne JG, Welman RS, Moshal MG, et al: The effect of glycopyrrolate [Robinul] on the lower esophageal sphincter. Can Anaesth Soc J 1978; 25: 144, with permission.)

However, using these guidelines, some have estimated that 40 to 80% of patients scheduled for elective surgery may be at risk.[83,84] However, clinically significant pulmonary aspiration of gastric contents is very rare in healthy patients having elective surgical procedures, and few anesthesiologists advocate routine prophylaxis.[85]

Many anesthesiologists follow the American Society of Anesthesiologists practice recommendations,[85] however the necessity of prolonged fasting (nothing by mouth after midnight) before induction of anesthesia for elective surgery has been challenged.[86] Some institutions allow ingestion of clear liquids until 3 or even 2 hours before surgery in selected patients. Indeed, gastric fluid volume may not be increased by ingestion of 150 mL of water, coffee, or orange juice 2 to 3 hours prior to the induction of anesthesia. For example, a study by Shevde and Trivedi described the administration of 240 mL of water, coffee, or pulp-free orange juice to healthy volunteers. All had gastric volumes of less than 25 mL with a slight decrease in pH within 2 hours of taking one of the three liquids.[87] There is concern about comfort, hypovolemia, and hypoglycemia in the pediatric age group perioperatively after prolonged fasting. Studies in infants, children, and healthy adults scheduled for elective surgery have found that drinking clear fluid up to 3 hours before scheduled surgery does not have a measurable effect on gastric volume and pH. It must be appreciated, however, that these data are from healthy patients not "at risk" for aspiration and apply only to ingestion of clear liquids. As stated before, most clinicians adhere to The American Society of Anesthesiologists' preoperative fasting guidelines, which were adapted in 1998 (Table 23-15).[85]

Many different kinds of drugs have been used to alter gastric fluid volume and increase the pH of gastric fluid. Anticholinergics, H_2 receptor antagonists, antacids, and gastrokinetic agents have all been used to reduce the possibility of aspiration pneumonitis.

Anticholinergics. Neither atropine nor glycopyrrolate has been shown to be very effective in increasing gastric fluid pH or reducing gastric fluid volume.[83,84] Furthermore, intravenous doses of anticholinergics may cause relaxation of the gastroesophageal junction (Fig. 23-7). Therefore, the risk of aspiration pneumonitis may be increased, but this specific effect of intramuscular administration of anticholinergics for preoperative use has not been proved.

Histamine Receptor Antagonists. The H_2 receptor antagonists cimetidine, ranitidine, famotidine, and nizatidine reduce gastric acid secretion. They block the ability of histamine to induce secretion of gastric fluid with a high hydrogen ion concentration. Therefore, the H_2 receptor antagonists increase gastric fluid pH. Their antagonism of the histamine receptor occurs in a selective and competitive manner. It is important to remember that these drugs cannot be expected reliably to affect gastric fluid volume or gastric emptying time. Compared with other premedicants, they have relatively few side effects. Because there are few side effects, many anesthesiologists have advocated the liberal preoperative use of H_2 receptor antagonists. Multiple-dose regimens may be more effective in increasing gastric pH than a single dose before operation on the day of surgery. An H_2 antagonist also may be used for the allergic patient or in preparing a patient for exposure to a trigger of the allergic response, such as radiologic dye.

Cimetidine. Cimetidine usually is administered in 150 to 300 mg doses orally or parenterally. Administration of 300 mg of cimetidine orally 1 to 1.5 hours before surgery has been shown to increase the gastric fluid pH above 2.5 in 80% of patients.[88,89] Cimetidine can be given intravenously for those unable to take oral medications. Cimetidine can cross the placenta, but adverse fetal effects are unproved. The gastric effects of cimetidine last as long as 3 or 4 hours, and therefore this drug is suitable for operations of that duration.

Cimetidine has few side effects, but there are some of note. It inhibits the hepatic mixed-function oxidase enzyme system; therefore, it can prolong the half-life of many drugs, including diazepam, chlordiazepoxide, theophylline, propranolol, and lidocaine. The clinical significance of this after one or two preoperative doses of cimetidine is uncertain. Life-threatening cardiac dysrhythmias, hypotension, cardiac arrest, and central nervous system depression have been reported after cimetidine administration. These side effects may be especially likely to occur in critically ill patients after rapid intravenous administration. As discussed previously, cimetidine does not affect gastric fluid already present.

Ranitidine. Ranitidine is more potent, specific, and longer acting than cimetidine. The usual oral dose is 50 to 200 mg. Ranitidine, 50 to 100 mg, given parenterally will decrease gastric fluid pH within 1 hour. It is as effective in reducing the number of patients at risk for gastric aspiration as cimetidine and produces fewer cardiovascular or central nervous system side effects. The effects of ranitidine last up to 9 hours. Thus, it may be superior to cimetidine at the conclusion of lengthy procedures in reducing the risk of aspiration pneumonitis during emergence from anesthesia and extubation of the trachea.

Other Histamine Receptor Antagonists. Famotidine is a third H_2 receptor blocker that has been given preoperatively to raise gastric fluid pH. Its pharmacokinetics are similar to those of cimetidine and ranitidine, with the exception of having a longer serum elimination half-life than the other two drugs. Famotidine in a dose of 40 mg orally 1.5 to 3 hours preoperatively has been shown to be effective in increasing gastric pH. Nizatidine 150 to 300 mg orally 2 hours before surgery will similarly decrease preoperative gastric acidity.[90–92]

Antacids. Antacids are used to neutralize the acid in gastric contents. A single dose of antacid given 15 to 30 minutes before induction of anesthesia is almost 100% effective in increasing gastric fluid pH above 2.5. The nonparticulate antacid, 0.3 M sodium citrate, is commonly given before operation when an increase in gastric fluid pH is desired. The nonparticulate antacids do not produce pulmonary damage themselves if aspiration of gastric fluid containing these antacids should occur. Colloid antacid suspension may be more effective than the nonparticulate antacids in increasing gastric fluid pH. However, aspiration of gastric fluid containing particulate antacids may cause significant and persistent pulmonary damage, despite the increase in gastric fluid pH. The serious pulmonary sequelae have been manifested in the form of pulmonary edema and arterial hypoxemia.

Antacids work at the time given. There is no "lag time," as with the H_2 receptor blockers. Antacids are effective on the fluid already present in the stomach. This makes them especially attractive in emergency situations for those patients who are able to take medications orally.

However, antacids do increase gastric fluid volume, unlike H_2 receptor blockers.[88] The risk of aspiration depends on both the pH and the volume of gastric content. The increase in gastric fluid volume from antacid administration may become readily apparent after repeated doses, such as during labor, during which opioid administration may also contribute to delayed gastric emptying. Withholding antacids because of concern about increasing gastric volume is not warranted, considering animal evidence documenting increased mortality after aspiration of low volumes of acidic gastric fluid (0.3 mL/kg, pH 1) compared with aspiration of large volumes of buffered gastric fluid (1 to 2 mL/kg, pH 1.8).[93] Antacids may slow gastric emptying, and complete mixing with all gastric contents may be questionable in the immobile patient. The effect of antacids on food particles within the stomach is unknown.

Omeprazole. Omeprazole suppresses gastric acid secretion in a dose-dependent manner by binding to the proton pump of the parietal cell. For an adult patient, intravenous doses of 40 mg 30 minutes before induction have been used. Oral doses of 40 to 80 mg must be given 2 to 4 hours before surgery to be effective. Effect on gastric pH may last as long as 24 hours. Much like the other H_2 receptor antagonists, investigators have found increases in gastric pH and inconsistent effects on gastric volume with administration of omeprazole.[94–96]

Gastrokinetic Agents. Gastrokinetic agents are useful because of their effectiveness in reducing gastric fluid volume.

Metoclopramide. Metoclopramide is a dopamine antagonist that stimulates upper gastrointestinal motility, increases gastroesophageal sphincter tone, and relaxes the pylorus and duodenum. It also has antiemetic properties. Metoclopramide speeds gastric emptying but has no known effect on acid secretion and gastric fluid pH. It may be administered orally or parenterally. A parenteral dose of 5 to 10 mg is usually given 15 to 30 minutes before induction. When the drug is administered intravenously over 3 to 5 minutes, it usually prevents the abdominal cramping that can occur from more rapid administration. An oral dose of 10 mg achieves onset within 30 to 60 minutes. The elimination half-life of metoclopramide is approximately 2 to 4 hours.

The clinical usefulness of the gastrokinetic agents is found in those patients who are likely to have large gastric fluid volumes, such as parturients, patients scheduled for emergency surgery who have just eaten, obese patients, patients with trauma, outpatients, and those with gastroparesis secondary to diabetes mellitus. However, it is not recommended in those patients with bowel obstruction.

However, the administration of metoclopramide does not guarantee gastric emptying. Significant gastric fluid volume may still be present despite its administration. The effect of metoclopramide on the upper gastrointestinal tract may be offset by concomitant atropine administration or prior injection of opioids. It will not further reduce gastric volume in patients undergoing elective surgery with already small gastric volumes. It may not be effective after administration of sodium citrate. In contrast, metoclopramide may be especially effective in reducing the risk of aspiration pneumonitis when combined with an H_2 receptor antagonist (e.g., ranitidine) before elective surgery.

As mentioned previously, the drugs used to alter gastric fluid pH and volume are relatively free of side effects. The risk–benefit ratio for these drugs in reducing the risk of pulmonary sequelae from aspiration is often very favorable. Indeed, the drugs do decrease the number of patients at risk. However, none of the drugs or combinations of drugs is absolutely reliable in preventing the risk of aspiration pneumonitis in all patients all of the time. Therefore, their use does not eliminate the need for careful anesthetic techniques to protect the airway during induction, maintenance, and emergence from anesthesia.

Antiemetics

There are several groups of patients in whom the antiemetic effects of drugs may be helpful in reducing nausea and vomiting. These are patients scheduled for ophthalmologic surgery, patients with a prior history of nausea and vomiting or motion sickness, patients scheduled for laparoscopic surgery or gynecologic procedures, and patients who are obese. A risk score for predicting postoperative nausea and vomiting after inhalation anesthesia identified four risk factors: female gender, prior history of motion sickness or postoperative nausea, nonsmoking, and the use of postoperative opioids. The investigators suggested prophylactic antiemetic therapy when two or more of the risk factors were present when using volatile anesthetics. Droperidol, metoclopramide, ondansetron, and dexamethasone, singly or in combination, are agents in common usage.[97,98] Many anesthesiologists prefer not to administer antiemetics as part of a preoperative regimen, but believe that antiemetics should be administered intravenously just before they are needed at the conclusion of surgery.

Anticholinergics

Previously, anticholinergic drugs were widely used when inhalation anesthetics produced copious respiratory tract

TABLE 23-16

COMPARISON OF SOME OF THE EFFECTS OF ANTICHOLINERGIC DRUGS

	■ ATROPINE	■ GLYCOPYRROLATE	■ SCOPOLAMINE
Increased heart rate	+++	++	+
Antisialagogue	+	++	+
Sedation	+	0	+++

0, no effect; +, small effect; ++, moderate effect; +++, large effect.
Adapted from Stoelting RK: Pharmacology and Physiology in Anesthetic Practice. Philadelphia, JB Lippincott, 1991.

secretions, and intraoperative bradycardia was a frequent danger. The advent of newer inhalation agents has almost completely dispelled the routine use of anticholinergic drugs for preoperative medication. Their routine use has been questioned by several authors who believe that the same care in selection of anticholinergics should be exhibited as in the choice of other drugs. Specific indications for an anticholinergic before surgery are (1) antisialagogue effect and (2) sedation and amnesia (Table 23-16). Uses that are less firmly established and not universally agreed on include the preoperative prescription of anticholinergics for their vagolytic action or in an attempt to decrease gastric acid secretion.

Antisialagogue Effect. Anticholinergics have been prescribed in a selective fashion when drying of the upper airway is desirable. For example, when endotracheal intubation is contemplated, an anesthesiologist may want to reduce secretions. In the study by Falick and Smiler,[99] conditions were more often rated as satisfactory after endotracheal intubation when an anticholinergic drug had been administered.

The antisialagogue effect may be important for intraoral operations and instrumentations of the airway such as bronchoscopic examination. Administration of anticholinergics may be desirable before the use of topical anesthesia for the airway to prevent a dilutional effect of secretions and to allow contact of the local anesthetic with the mucosa.

Scopolamine is a more potent drying agent than atropine. It is less likely to increase heart rate and more likely to produce sedation and amnesia. Glycopyrrolate is a more potent and longer acting antisialagogue than atropine, with less likelihood of increasing heart rate. Because glycopyrrolate is a quaternary amine, it does not easily cross the blood–brain barrier and does not produce sedation. Anticholinergics are not the only drugs that can dry secretions. As demonstrated by the study of Forrest, et al.,[100] several other drugs and placebo (presumably a reflection of apprehension) can cause a patient to have a dry mouth before operation.

Sedation and Amnesia. When sedation and amnesia are desired before operation, scopolamine is frequently the anticholinergic chosen, especially in combination with morphine. Scopolamine and atropine both cross the blood–brain barrier. Scopolamine is a much more potent sedative and amnestic drug than atropine. In a study of patient acceptance of preoperative medication, the combination of morphine and scopolamine was superior to that of morphine and atropine.[101] Scopolamine does not produce amnesia in all patients. It may not be as effective as lorazepam or diazepam in preventing recall. Scopolamine has an additive amnestic effect when combined with benzodiazepines. The study by Frumin, et al.[102] showed that the combination of diazepam and scopolamine produced amnesia more often than did diazepam alone.

Vagolytic Action. Vagolytic action of the anticholinergic drugs is produced through the blockade of effects of acetylcholine on the sinoatrial node. Atropine given intravenously is more potent than glycopyrrolate and scopolamine in increasing heart rate. The vagolytic action of the anticholinergic drugs is useful in the prevention of reflex bradycardia during surgery. Bradycardia may result from traction on extraocular muscles or abdominal viscera, from carotid sinus stimulation, or after the administration of repeated doses of intravenous succinylcholine. The prevention of reflex bradycardia with intramuscular doses of the anticholinergics is unreliable, given the drug dosages and timing usually involved with preoperative medication administered on the ward. Many anesthesiologists prefer to give atropine or glycopyrrolate intravenously just before surgery and the anticipated bradycardic stimulus. Atropine and glycopyrrolate given intravenously immediately before surgery have been equally effective in preventing bradycardia resulting from repeated doses of succinylcholine.

Side Effects of Anticholinergic Drugs. Scopolamine and atropine may cause central nervous system toxicity, the so-called central anticholinergic syndrome. This syndrome is most likely to occur after the administration of scopolamine, but can be seen after high doses of atropine. The symptoms of central nervous system toxicity resulting from anticholinergic drugs include delirium, restlessness, confusion, and obtundation. Elderly patients and patients with pain appear to be particularly susceptible. The central nervous system toxic effect of anticholinergics has been noted to be potentiated by inhalation anesthetics. The administration of 1 to 2 mg of physostigmine intravenously can successfully treat the syndrome.

Mydriasis and cycloplegia from anticholinergic drugs is unwanted in patients with glaucoma because of resulting increased intraocular pressure, which seems unlikely with the small doses used for preoperative medication. Atropine and glycopyrrolate may be less likely to increase intraocular pressure than scopolamine. In patients with glaucoma, most anesthesiologists feel safe in continuing medications for glaucoma up until the time of surgery and using atropine or glycopyrrolate when necessary.

Because anticholinergic drugs block vagal activity, relaxation of bronchial smooth muscle occurs and respiratory dead space increases. The magnitude of the increase in dead space depends on prior bronchomotor tone, but increases as large as 25 to 33% have been reported. Anticholinergic drugs cause secretions to dry and thicken. In theory, a dose of anticholinergic drug given before operation could lead to inspissation of secretions and an increase in airway resistance. The threat of inspissated secretions may develop into more than a theoretical issue for patients with diseases such as cystic fibrosis.

Sweat glands of the body are innervated by the sympathetic nervous system and use cholinergic transmission. Therefore, administration of anticholinergic agents interferes with the sweating mechanism, which may cause body temperature to increase. This side effect of anticholinergic medication must be considered carefully in a child with a fever.

Atropine is more likely than glycopyrrolate or scopolamine to cause an increase in heart rate. Unwanted increases in heart rate are much more likely after intravenous administration than after intramuscular administration. In fact, heart rate may transiently decrease after intramuscular administration as a result of a peripheral agonist effect of the anticholinergic agent.

Adrenergic Agonists

α_2 Adrenergic agonists have been used as premedicants.[103,104] Clonidine in doses of 2.5 to 5 μg/kg has been administered preoperatively to produce sedation, reduce maximum allowable concentration, and prevent hypertension and tachycardia from endotracheal intubation and surgical stimulation. It has even been used as part of anesthetic technique to produce induced hypotension. Dexmedetomidine is another α_2 adrenergic agonist studied for preoperative use to attenuate intraoperative sympathoadrenal responses.[103] After the administration of clonidine preoperatively, one is more likely to see episodes of hypotension and bradycardia during anesthesia when there are periods of little surgical stimulation. Furthermore, some anesthesiologists ask if preoperative α_2-adrenergic agonists are a substitute for a properly conducted anesthetic if appropriate attention is given to depth of anesthesia.

Other Drugs Given with Preoperative Medications

Although they are not preoperative medications in the strict sense, other drugs are often given at the time of preoperative medication. Examples of such drugs are insulin, steroids, antibiotics, and methadone for patients who are addicted to opioids. They may be prescribed by either the anesthesiologist or the surgeon to be given on the ward or in the operating room immediately prior to surgery. Regardless of these factors, their actions may affect the anesthetic, and the anesthesiologist must be knowledgeable about their administration and actions.

Beta-Blockers. For patients with known or suspected CAD, preoperative beta-blockers may add to safety in the perioperative period. Clinical studies have shown that beta-blockers in this setting have reduced mortality and the incidence of nonfatal MI after surgery.[104] Because benefit has been shown with several different beta-blockers, it is probably a drug class effect or hemodynamic effect rather than the result of employing a specific beta-blocker. Contraindications to preoperative beta-blocker therapy include known allergy to beta-blockers, second- or third-degree heart block, congestive heart failure, acute bronchospasm, low systolic blood pressure (<100 mm Hg), slow heart rate (<60 beats per minute), and other hemodynamic instability. Many clinicians use either atenolol (50 to 100 mg orally daily) or metoprolol (25 to 50 mg orally twice daily). They are chosen because of their long action and relative β_1 selectivity.

Although shown to be effective in patients with ischemic heart disease perioperatively, the best beta-blocker to administer, the dose, and target heart rate are unknown. Attention to perioperative heart rate may be the most important factor. Current guidelines recommend that beta-blockers be continued in those receiving beta-blockers to treat such maladies as angina, symptomatic arrhythmias, hypertension or for other indications. Perioperative beta-blocker therapy should be initiated for patients about to undergo vascular surgery at high cardiac risk due to signs of ischemia on preoperative testing. Beta-blockers should probably be started in patients about to undergo vascular surgery who have evidence of CAD.[105]

In the ambulatory surgery population, current evidence does not support beta-blockade for those not currently taking beta-blockers and for whom long-term therapy is unwarranted.[106]

Although unproven, many strive for heart rate near 60 to 70 beats per minute, while maintaining a systolic blood pressure >110 mm Hg. The beta-blockade is usually maintained throughout the perioperative period to achieve maximum effect. Intravenous metoprolol may be given just prior to surgery if inadequate blockade has been achieved with the oral medications. The oral beta-blockers may be started several days prior to surgery.

Statins. Like beta-blockers, statin drugs have been recommended preoperatively in patients with cardiovascular disease. Studies have shown that statins can reduce cardiovascular morbidity and mortality, have a lipid lowering effect, enhance nitric-oxide–mediated pathways, reduce vascular inflammation, and have direct cardioprotective effects. There is a small risk of rhabdomyolysis with statin therapy.

Some have recommended these medications be given in the perioperative period for those with CAD. Current guidelines recommend continuing statin therapy in the perioperative period for those already taking the medication. More studies are needed in regard to initiating statin therapy preoperatively in others. There is some evidence that this class of drugs may have benefit in those undergoing vascular surgery and in those with one clinical risk factor for myocardial ischemia about to undergo an intermediate risk surgical procedure. If indeed statin therapy is effective preoperatively, the dose, timing of initiation of therapy, and the length of therapy are yet to be determined.[107,108]

Antibiotics. Antibiotics are often administered 1 hour, 15 minutes before operation for contaminated, potentially contaminated, or dirty surgical wounds. Prophylactic antibiotics may be warranted for "clean" surgical procedures when infection would be catastrophic. Other instances for the use of prophylactic antibiotics include in the immunosuppressed patient, in the aged, or in patients taking steroids. Antibiotics given immediately before surgery are also used for the prevention of endocarditis.[109] It has been estimated that 60 to 70% of surgical patients receive antibiotics just before surgery or intraoperatively. Antibiotic administration comes under the anesthesiologist's purview because of the desire to have such agents given immediately before exposure to pathogens, which is just before the beginning of surgery.

Cephalosporins are the most popular antibiotics because they cover the microbes on the skin. For intestinal surgery anaerobic and Gram-negative coverage is needed. The National Surgical Infection Project recommends that antibiotics be administered 1 hour prior to incision.[110,111] There are two exceptions to this policy: (1) vancomycin should be given 2 hours prior to incision, and (2) when a tourniquet is used, the antibiotics should be administered prior to its inflation.

Those allergic to penicillin, cephalosporins, and related compounds (beta lactam allergy) may receive either vancomycin or clindamycin. The optimal dose of antibiotics in obese patients is under review. There is some question as to the dose needed to achieve adequate tissue levels in morbidly obese patients. Furthermore, obese patients may have other factors that predispose them to infections, such as diabetes mellitus.

Steroids. Steroid administration may be necessary immediately before surgery in the patient treated for hypoadrenocorticism or in the patient with suppression of the pituitary-adrenal axis owing to present or previous administration of corticosteroids. It is impossible to identify the specific duration of therapy or dose of steroids that produces pituitary and adrenal suppression. Marked variability among patients exists. Certainly, more suppression may be expected with a higher dose and a longer duration of therapy. A conservative estimate is to consider treatment in any patient who has received corticosteroid therapy for at least 1 month in the past 6 to 12 months.

Because of disease states of the pituitary-adrenal axis or its suppression from steroid therapy, patients may not be able to respond to the stress of surgery. The dose and duration of supplemental steroid administration depend on an estimate of the stress of the surgical procedure in the perioperative period. One regimen is to administer 25 mg of cortisol preoperatively and then give an intravenous infusion of 100 mg of cortisol over the next 12 to 24 hours for adult patients. Another method is to administer 100 mg of hydrocortisone intravenously before, during, and after surgery. This dose is meant to equal the estimated maximum amount of steroid that stress could produce in patients perioperatively. When considering whether to administer steroids or a higher dose of steroids, the anesthesiologist should keep in mind that the risk–benefit ratio is usually very small.

Insulin.   See "Diabetes Mellitus."

Opioid Dependency

Withdrawal produced by drug cessation is a preoperative issue in the patient who is taking methadone or is dependent on other opioids. There should be an attempt to maintain opioid use at the usual level by continuing methadone or substituting other appropriate agents for methadone. The anesthesiologist should be cautioned about using agonist-antagonist drugs in these patients in the preoperative period for fear of producing withdrawal.

DIFFERENCES IN PREOPERATIVE MEDICATION BETWEEN PEDIATRIC AND ADULT PATIENTS

Compared with adults, preoperative medications for children include aspects of psychological preparation, the emphasis on oral medications when pharmacologic preparation is desired, and more frequent use of anticholinergics for their vagolytic activity. What remains the same is the need to assess the needs of each child individually and to tailor the psychological preparation and preoperative medication accordingly.

Psychological Factors in Pediatric Patients

Hospital admission and major surgery can produce long-lasting psychological effects in some children. The hospital stay is stressful and full of apprehension over the short term for almost all children. The demeanor and communicative efforts of the anesthesiologist can make a difference to the child and family who are getting ready for a trip to the operating room, anesthesia, and surgery.

Age is probably the most important aspect when psychological preparation of the pediatric patient is considered. A baby younger than 6 to 8 months of age is not emotionally upset when separated from his or her mother. Others in the health care team can substitute very easily. Preoperative preparation in this age group is often directed toward other goals, for example, obtundation of vagal reflex responses. However, preschool children are at an age when hospitalization may be the most upsetting and will become upset when

separated from their parents and they fear the operating room. It is difficult to explain the forthcoming events to children in this age group. It is easier to communicate with patients from age 5 years to adolescence. The anesthesiologist can explain and offer reassurance about such issues as separation from parents and the home, operating room events, and any of the patient's perceived fears of surgery and anesthesia. Adolescent patients may already be anxious and apprehensive. They may also be worried about loss of consciousness, have a fear of death, or be apprehensive about what they will do or say after preoperative sedation or during anesthesia. The more fearful child may be difficult to identify, but is usually the child who is quiet during the preoperative interview and appears nonchalant or even detached. If these patients can be identified before operation, they are often candidates for heavy pharmacologic preparation.

Psychological Preparation

For the previously mentioned reasons, a good preoperative visit and proper psychological preparation may be even more important in children than adults. The art of psychological preparation that is acquired by the anesthesiologist makes the preoperative visit a time of reassurance and explanation. It is an opportunity to gain the child's trust. Most anesthesiologists will want to involve the parents when possible. Some hospitals have found brochures, motion pictures, and slide shows to be helpful in preparing pediatric patients for the operating room but are not uniformly satisfactory. The child may want to bring a personal belonging, such as a stuffed animal or blanket, to the operating room for security. Some children wish to take an active role by doing such things as holding the face mask during inhalation induction of anesthesia. It may be helpful in a case with supportive parents to have them accompany the child to the operating room suite after an explanation of events that may occur during induction. The emphasis is on support from the parent rather than simply their presence.[112] It is common in many hospitals for a parent to go into the operating room and stay until induction is complete.

Differences in Pharmacologic Preparation

The discussion of pharmacologic preparation for the pediatric patient presumes proper psychological preparation, a satisfactory operating room environment, and preparation for an efficient and timely induction of anesthesia.

Sedative–Hypnotics

As in adults, the sedative–hypnotic medications are used to reduce apprehension, produce sedation and amnesia, and to facilitate smooth induction of anesthesia when an inhalation method is to be used. The use of preoperative medication is controversial in pediatric patients and may not be completely successful in as many as 20% of instances.[113] It has not been proved to reduce unwanted psychological outcome after surgery and anesthesia. Neither has it been shown that the uneventful induction of anesthesia is less likely to produce long-lasting psychological problems in children. After 6 months to 1 year of age, the child scheduled for a surgical procedure may benefit from a sedative–hypnotic drug before surgery. There is emphasis on avoiding intramuscular injections in children. The oral route is often preferred for preoperative medication in the older child, whereas in preschool children drugs may also be given rectally. Many different sedative–hypnotic drugs via different routes (oral, intranasal, and rectal) have been prescribed for children before operation. Midazolam

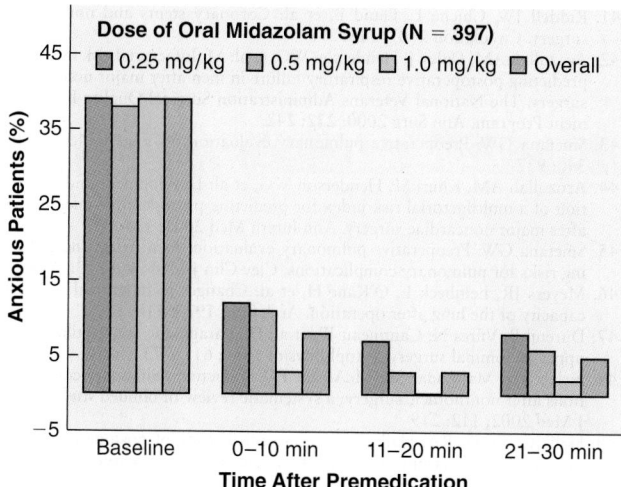

FIGURE 23-8. Percentage of patients exhibiting anxiety from baseline to time after oral midazolam. There was a positive association between dose and onset of anxiolysis ($p = 0.01$); a larger proportion of children achieved satisfactory anxiolysis within 10 minutes at the higher doses. (Reprinted from Coté CJ, Cohen IT, Suresh S, et al: A comparison of three doses of a commercially prepared oral midazolam syrup in children. Anesth Analg 2002; 94: 37, with permission.)

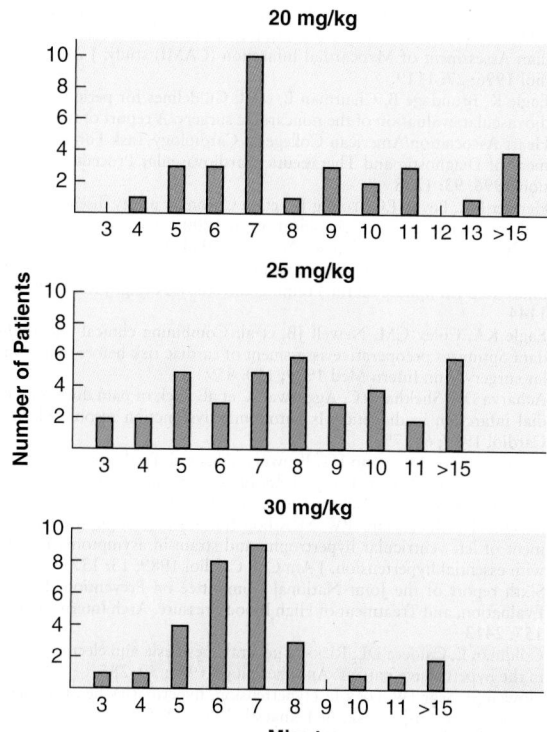

FIGURE 23-9. Frequency distribution of sleep induction times after rectal instillation of methohexital. Patients averaged 3.3 years in age and 15 kg in body weight. (Reprinted from Liu LMP, Goudsouzian NG, Liu PL: Rectal methohexital premedication in children, a dose-comparison study. Anesthesiology 1980; 53: 343, with permission.)

can be given intramuscularly (0.05 to 0.2 mg/kg). However, the most common, effective and acceptable route for midazolam is the oral route at a dose of 0.5 to 0.75 mg/kg (Fig. 23-8).[114,115] The cherry-flavored oral preparation is acceptable to most children. It is effective in producing sedation and compliance, but not usually sleep, in about 15 minutes and lasts for 30 to 60 minutes. Oral ketamine (5 to 10 mg) has been prescribed 20 to 30 minutes before induction. Although often allowing smooth separation from parents, oral secretions and preoperative or postoperative delirium can be problems. Intramuscular ketamine (5 to 10 mg/kg) can be particularly helpful in the extremely recalcitrant or combative child. Both ketamine (3 to 8 mg/kg) and midazolam (0.2 mg/kg) can be given using a nasal atomizer, with the caveat that irritation of the nasal cavity and bitter aftertaste are disadvantageous. Ketamine (5 mg/kg) and midazolam (0.3 to 1.0 mg/kg) have also been given rectally before induction of anesthesia. A further option in the pharmacologic preparation of children is the rectal administration of methohexital (Fig. 23-9). Methohexital (20 to 30 mg/kg) may be given immediately before operation, using pulse oximetry and while the child is still in the parent's arms. The intramuscular route is also possible.

Opioids

There is the occasional need for opioid premedication in children. Methadone has the advantage of oral administration, usually prescribed in the 0.1 to 0.2 mg/kg dose range. Transmucosal administration of fentanyl (5 to 20 µg/kg) appears to be effective in producing sedation preoperatively. However, transmucosal fentanyl may increase gastric fluid volume and also increase the incidence of rigidity, respiratory depression, pruritus, nausea, and vomiting.[68] Fentanyl (2 µg/kg) and sufentanil (3.0 µg/kg) given by the intranasal route have been shown to calm pediatric patients preoperatively. Again, postoperative nausea and vomiting, in addition to respiratory complications, have resulted in lack of enthusiasm for this technique.

For information on anesthesia for ambulatory surgery, see Chapter 32.

References

1. Takata MN, Benumof JL, Mazzei WJ: The preoperative evaluation form: Assessment of quality from one hundred thirty-eight institutions and recommendations for a high-quality form. J Clin Anes 2001; 13: 345
2. Mallampati RS, Gatt SP, Gugino LD, et al: A clinical sign to predict difficult tracheal intubation: A prospective study. Can Anaesth Soc J 1985; 32: 429
3. Frerk CM: Predicting difficult intubation. Anaesthesia 1991; 46: 1005
4. Savva D: Prediction of difficult tracheal intubation. Br J Anaesth 1994; 73: 149
5. Shah KB, Kleinman BS, Rao T, et al: Angina and other risk factors in patients with cardiac diseases undergoing noncardiac operations. Anesth Analg 1990; 70: 240
6. Tuman KJ, McCarthy RJ, March RJ, et al: Effects of epidural anesthesia and analgesia on coagulation and outcome after major vascular surgery. Anesth Analg 1991; 73: 696
7. Bedford R, Feinstein B: Hospital admission blood pressure, a predictor for hypertension following endotracheal intubation. Anesth Analg 1980; 59: 367
8. Lee TH, Marcantonio ER, Mangione CM, et al: Derivation and prospective validation of a simple index for prediction of cardiac risk of major noncardiac surgery. Circulation 1999; 100: 1043
9. Goldman L, Caldera DL, Nussbaum SR, et al: Multifactorial index of cardiac risk in noncardiac surgical procedures. N Engl J Med 1977; 297: 845
10. Detsky A, Abrams H, McLaughlin J, et al: Predicting cardiac complications in patients undergoing non-cardiac surgery. J Gen Intern Med 1986; 1: 211
11. Tarhan S, Moffitt EA, Taylor WF, et al: Myocardial infarction after general anesthesia. JAMA 1972; 220: 1451
12. Rao TL, Jacobs KH, El-Etr AA: Reinfarction following anesthesia in patients with myocardial infarction. Anesthesiology 1983; 59: 499
13. Shah KB, Kleinman BS, Sami H, et al: Reevaluation of perioperative myocardial infarction in patients with prior myocardial infarction undergoing noncardiac operations. Anesth Analg 1990; 71: 231
14. Califf RM, Topol EJ, George BS, et al: One-year outcome after therapy with tissue plasminogen activator: Report from the Thrombolysis and Angioplasty in Myocardial Infarction trial. Am Heart J 1990; 119: 777

15. Rouleau JL, Talajic M, Sussex B, et al: Myocardial infarction patients in the 1990s—their risk factors, stratification and survival in Canada: The Canadian Assessment of Myocardial Infarction (CAMI) study. J Am Coll Cardiol 1996; 27: 1119

16. Eagle K, Brundage B, Chaitman B, et al: Guidelines for perioperative cardiovascular evaluation of the noncardiac surgery. A report of the American Heart Association/American College of Cardiology Task Force on Assessment of Diagnostic and Therapeutic Cardiovascular Procedures. Circulation 1996; 93: 1278

17. Hertzer NR, Bevan EG, Young JR, et al: Coronary artery disease in peripheral vascular patients: A classification of 1000 coronary angiograms and results of surgical management. Ann Surg 1984; 199: 223

18. Kannel W, Abbott R: Incidence and prognosis of unrecognized myocardial infarction: An update on the Framingham study. N Engl J Med 1984; 311: 1144

19. Eagle KA, Coley CM, Newell JB, et al: Combining clinical and thallium data optimizes preoperative assessment of cardiac risk before major vascular surgery. Ann Intern Med 1989; 110: 859

20. Acharya DU, Shekhar YC, Aggarwal A, et al: Lack of pain during myocardial infarction in diabetics: Is autonomic dysfunction responsible? Am J Cardiol 1991; 68: 793

21. Hollenberg M, Mangano DT, Browner WS, et al: Predictors of postoperative myocardial ischemia in patients undergoing noncardiac surgery. The Study of Perioperative Ischemia Research. JAMA 1992; 268: 205

22. Pringle SD, MacFarlane PW, McKillop JH, et al: Pathophysiologic assessment of left ventricular hypertrophy and strain in asymptomatic patients with essential hypertension. J Am Coll Cardiol 1989; 13: 1377

23. Sixth report of the Joint National Committee on Prevention, Detection, Evaluation, and Treatment of High Blood Pressure. Arch Intern Med 1997; 157: 2413

24. Goldman L, Caldera DL: Risks of general anesthesia and elective operation in the hypertensive patient. Anesthesiology 1979; 50: 285

25. Howell SJ, Sear JW, Foex P: Hypertension, hypertensive heart disease and perioperative cardiac risk. Br J Anaesth 2004; 92: 570

26. Wesker N, Klien M, Szendro G: The dilemma of immediate preoperative hypertension. J Clin Anesth 2003; 15: 179

27. Warner MA, Shields SE, Chute CG: Major morbidity and mortality within 1 month of ambulatory surgery and anesthesia. JAMA 1993; 270: 1437

28. Eagle KA, Rihal CS, Mickel MC, et al: Cardiac risk of noncardiac surgery: Influence of coronary disease and type of surgery in 3368 operations. CASS Investigators and University of Michigan Heart Care Program. Circulation 1997; 96: 1882

29. Reilly DF, McNeely MJ, Doerner D, et al: Self-reported exercise tolerance and the risk of serious perioperative complications. Arch Intern Med 1999; 159: 2185

30. Poldermans D, Boersma E, Bax JJ, et al: The effect of bisoprolol on perioperative mortality and myocardial infarction in high-risk patients undergoing vascular surgery. N Engl J Med 1999; 341: 1789

31. American College of Cardiology and the American Heart Association: ACC/AHA Guideline Update on Perioperative Cardiovascular Evaluation for Noncardiac Surgery. ACC/AHA Practice Guidelines 2002

32. American College of Cardiology/American Heart Association Task Force on Practice Guidelines (Writing Committee to Revise the 2002 Guidelines on Perioperative Cardiovascular Evaluation for Noncardiac Surgery); American Society of Echocardiography; American Society of Nuclear Cardiology; Heart Rhythm Society; Society of Cardiovascular Anesthesiologists; Society for Cardiovascular Angiography and Interventions; Society for Vascular Medicine and Biology; Society for Vascular Surgery, Fleisher LA, et al. ACC/AHA 2007 guidelines on perioperative cardiovascular evaluation and care for noncardiac surgery. Executive summary: A report of the American College of Cardiology/American Heart Association Task Force on Practice Guidelines (Writing Committee to Revise the 2002 Guidelines on Perioperative Cardiovascular Evaluation for Noncardiac Surgery). Anesth Analg 2008; 106: 685

33. Kalbfleisch JM, Shudaksharappa KS, Conrad LL, et al: Disappearance of the Q deflection following myocardial infarction. Am Heart J 1968; 76: 193

34. Gold BS, Young ML, Kinman JL, et al: The utility of preoperative electrocardiograms in the ambulatory surgical patient. Arch Intern Med 1992; 152: 301

35. Raby KE, Goldman L, Creager MA, et al: Correlation between perioperative ischemia and major cardiac events after peripheral vascular surgery. N Engl J Med 1989; 321: 1296

36. Mantha S, Roizen MF, Barnard J, et al: Relative effectiveness of four preoperative tests for predicting adverse cardiac outcomes after vascular surgery: A meta-analysis. Anesth Analg 1994; 79: 422

37. Shaw LJ, Eagle KA, Gersh BJ, et al: Meta-analysis of intravenous dipyridamole–thallium-201 imaging (1985 to 1994) and dobutamine echocardiography (1991 to 1994) for risk stratification before vascular surgery. J Am Coll Cardiol 1996; 27: 787

38. Lavi R, Lavi S, Daghini E, et al: New frontiers in the evaluation of cardiac patients for noncardiac surgery. Anesthesiology 2007; 107: 1018

39. Dupuis JY, Labinaz M: Noncardiac surgery in patients with coronary artery stent: what should the anesthesiologist know? Can J Anesth 2005; 52: 356

40. Schouten O, Jeroen JB, Poldermans D: Management of patients with cardiac stents undergoing noncardiac surgery. Curr Opin Anaesthesiol 2007; 20: 274–278

41. Riddell JW, Chiche L, Plaud B, et al: Coronary stents and noncardiac surgery. Circulation 2007; 116: 378

42. Arozullah AM, Daley J, Henderson WG, et al: Multifactorial risk index for predicting postoperative respiratory failure in men after major noncardiac surgery. The National Veterans Administration Surgical Quality Improvement Program. Ann Surg 2000; 232: 242

43. Smetana GW: Preoperative pulmonary evaluation. N Engl J Med 1999; 340: 937

44. Arozullah AM, Khuri SF, Henderson WG, et al: Development and validation of a multifactorial risk index for predicting postoperative pneumonia after major noncardiac surgery. Ann Intern Med 2001; 135: 847

45. Smetana GW: Preoperative pulmonary evaluation: Identifying and reducing risks for pulmonary complications. Clev Clin J Med 2006; 73: 3646.

46. Meyers JR, Lembeck L, O'Kane H, et al: Changes in functional residual capacity of the lung after operation. Arch Surg 1975; 110: 576

47. Dureuil B, Viires N, Cantineau JP, et al: Diaphragmatic contractility after upper abdominal surgery. J Appl Physiol 1986; 61: 1775

48. Fisher BW, Majumdar SR, McAlistar FA: Predicting pulmonary complications after nonthoracic surgery: a systematic review of blinded studies. Am J Med 2002; 112: 219

49. Hall JC, Tarala RA, Hall JL: A case-control study of postoperative pulmonary complications after laparoscopic and open cholecystectomy. J Laparoendosc Surg 1996; 6: 87

50. Warner MA, Divertie MB, Tinker JH: Preoperative cessation of smoking and pulmonary complications in coronary artery bypass patients. Anesthesiology 1984; 60: 609

51. Rock P, Passannante A: Preoperative assessment: pulmonary. Anesthesiol Clin N Am 2002; 22: 77

52. Whyte MK, Choudry NB, Ind PW: Bronchial hyperresponsiveness in patients recovering from acute severe asthma. Respir Med 1993; 87: 29

53. Kabalin CS, Yarnold PR, Grammer LC: Low complication rate of corticosteroid-treated asthmatics undergoing surgical procedures. Arch Intern Med 1995; 155: 1379

54. Practice guidelines for the perioperative management of patients with obstructive sleep apnea: (OSA) A report by the ASA Task Force. Anesthesiology 2006; 104: 1081

55. Narayan KM, Boyle JP, Thompson TJ, et al: Lifetime risk for diabetes mellitus in the United States. JAMA 2003; 290: 1884

56. Coursin DB, Connery LE, Ketzler JT: Perioperative diabetic and hyperglycemic management issues. Crit Care Med 2004; 32(4 Suppl): S116

57. Eagle KA, Berger PB, Calkins H, et al: ACC/AHA guideline update for perioperative cardiovascular evaluation for noncardiac surgery—executive summary a report of the American College of Cardiology/American Heart Association Task Force on Practice Guidelines (Committee to Update the 1996 Guidelines on Perioperative Cardiovascular Evaluation for Noncardiac Surgery). Circulation 2002; 105: 1257

58. Furnary AP, Wu Y: Clinical effects of hyperglycemia in the cardiac surgery population: The Portland Diabetic Project. Endocr Pract 2006; 12(Suppl 3): 22

59. McGirt MJ, Woodworth GF, Brooke BS, et al: Hyperglycemia independently increases the risk of perioperative stroke, myocardial infarction, and death after carotid endarterectomy. Neurosurgery 2006; 58: 1066

60. Blondet JJ, Beilman GJ: Glycemic control and prevention of perioperative infection. Curr Opin Crit Care 2007; 13: 421

61. Gandhi GY, Nuttall GA, Abel MD, et al: Intensive intraoperative insulin therapy versus conventional glucose management during cardiac surgery: A randomized trial. Ann Intern Med 2007; 146: 233

62. Furnary AP, Cheek DB, Holmes SC, et al: Achieving tight glycemic control in the operating room: Lessons learned from 12 years in the trenches of a paradigm shift in anesthetic care. Semin Thorac Cardiovasc Surg 2006; 18: 339

63. Robertshaw HJ, Hall GM: Diabetes mellitus: anaesthetic management. Anaesthesia 2006; 61: 1187

64. Rhodes ET, Ferrari LR, Wolfsdorf JI, et al: Perioperative management of pediatric surgical patients with diabetes mellitus. Anesth Analg 2005; 101: 986

65. Golub R, Cantu R, Sorrento JJ, et al: Efficacy of preadmission testing in ambulatory surgical patients. Am J Surg 1992; 163: 565

66. Narr BJ, Hansen TR, Warner MA: Preoperative laboratory screening in healthy Mayo patients: Cost-effective elimination of tests and unchanged outcomes. Mayo Clin Proc 1991; 66: 155

67. Narr BJ, Warner ME, Schroeder DR, et al: Outcomes of patients with no laboratory assessment before anesthesia and a surgical procedure. Mayo Clin Proc 1997; 72: 505

68. Roizen MF, Cohn S: Preoperative evaluation for elective surgery: What laboratory tests are needed?, Advances in Anesthesia. St Louis, Mosby–Year Book, 1993, p 25

69. Baron MJ, Gunter J, White P: Is the pediatric preoperative hematocrit determination necessary? South Med J 1992; 85: 1187

70. Sox HCJ: Common Diagnostic Tests: Use and Interpretation. Philadelphia, American College of Physicians, 1990

71. Archer C, Levy AR, McGregor M: Value of routine preoperative chest x-rays: A meta-analysis. Can J Anaesth 1993; 40: 1022

72. Beecher HK: Preanesthetic medication. JAMA 1955; 157: 242

73. Lyons SM, Clarke RSJ, Vulgaraki K: The premedication of cardiac surgical patients. Anaesthesia 1975; 30: 459

74. Egbert LD, Battit GE, Turndorf H, et al: The value of the preoperative visit by the anesthetist. JAMA 1963; 185: 553

75. Soreide E, Holst-Larsen K, Reite K, et al: Effects of giving water 20–450 ml with oral diazepam premedication 1–2 h before operation. Br J Anaesth 1993; 71: 503

76. Fragen RJ, Caldwell N: Lorazepam premedication: Lack of recall and relief of anxiety. Anesth Analg 1976; 55: 792

77. White PF: Pharmacologic and clinical aspects of preoperative medication. Anesth Analg 1986; 65: 963

78. Bradshaw EG, Ali AA, Mulley BA, et al: Plasma concentrations and clinical effects of lorazepam after oral administration. Br J Anaesth 1981; 53: 517

79. Reves JG, Fragen RJ, Vinick HR, et al: Midazolam: Pharmacology and uses. Anesthesiology 1985; 62: 310

80. Pinnock CA, Fell D, Hunt PCW, et al: A comparison of triazolam and diazepam as premedication for minor gynaecologic surgery. Anaesthesia 1985; 40: 324

81. Cohen EN, Beecher HK: Narcotics in preanesthetic medication: A controlled study. JAMA 1951; 147: 1664

82. Weil JV, McCullough RE, Kline JS: Diminished ventilatory response to hypoxia and hypercapnia after morphine in man. N Engl J Med 1975; 292: 1103

83. Stoelting RK: Responses to atropine, glycopyrrolate and Riopan on gastric fluid pH and volume in adult patients. Anesthesiology 1978; 48: 367

84. Manchikanti L, Roush JR: The effect of preanesthetic glycopyrrolate and cimetidine in gastric fluid pH and volume in outpatients. Anesth Analg 1984; 63: 40

85. A Report by the American Society of Anesthesiologists Task Force on Preoperative Fasting: Practice guidelines for preoperative fasting and the use of pharmacologic agents to reduce the risk of pulmonary aspiration: Application to healthy patients undergoing elective procedures. Anesthesiology 1999; 90: 896

86. Kallar SK, Everett LL: Potential risks and preventive measures for pulmonary aspiration: New concepts in preoperative fasting guidelines. Anesth Analg 1993; 77: 171

87. Shevde K, Trivedi N: Effects of clear liquids on gastric volume and pH in healthy volunteers. Anesth Analg 1991; 72: 528

88. Stoelting RK: Gastric fluid pH in patients receiving cimetidine. Anesth Analg 1978; 57: 675

89. Maliniak K, Vahil AH: Pre-anesthetic cimetidine and gastric pH. Anesth Analg 1979; 58: 309

90. Feldman M, Burton ME: Histamine-2 receptor antagonists. N Engl J Med 1990; 323: 1672

91. Escolano F, Castaño J, Lopez R, et al: Effects of omeprazole, ranitidine, famotidine and placebo on gastric secretion in patients undergoing elective surgery. Br J Anaesth 1992; 69: 404

92. Mikawa K, Nishina K, Maekawa N, et al: Gastric fluid volume and pH after nizatidine in adults undergoing elective surgery: Influence of timing and dose. Can J Anaesth 1995; 42: 730

93. James CF, Modell JH, Gibbs CP, et al: Pulmonary aspiration: Effects of volume and pH in the rat. Anesth Analg 1984; 63: 665

94. Rocke DA, Rout CC, Gouws E: Intravenous administration of the proton pump inhibitor omeprazole reduces the risk of acid aspiration at emergency cesarean section. Anesth Analg 1994; 78: 1093

95. Haskins DA, Jahr JS, Texidor M, et al: Single-dose oral omeprazole for reduction of gastric residual acidity in adults for outpatient surgery. Acta Anaesthesiol Scand 1992; 36: 513

96. Atanassoff PG, Alon E, Pasch T: Effects of single-dose intravenous omeprazole and ranitidine on gastric pH during general anesthesia. Anesth Analg 1992; 75: 95

97. Apfel CC, Korttila K, Abdalla M, et al: A factorial trial of six interventions for the prevention of postoperative nausea and vomiting. N Engl J Med 2004; 350: 2441

98. Apfel CC, Läärä E, Koivuranta M, et al: A simplified risk score for predicting postoperative nausea and vomiting. Anesthesiology 1999; 91: 693

99. Falick YS, Smiler BG: Is anticholinergic premedication necessary? Anesthesiology 1975; 43: 472

100. Forrest WH, Brown CR, Brown BW: Subjective responses to six common preoperative medications. Anesthesiology 1977; 47: 241

101. Conner JT, Bellville JW, Wender R, et al: Morphine, scopolamine and atropine as intravenous surgical premedicants. Anesth Analg 1977; 56: 606

102. Frumin MJ, Herekar VR, Jarvik ME: Amnesic actions of diazepam and scopolamine in man. Anesthesiology 1976; 45: 406

103. Abi-Jaoude F, Brusset A, Ceddaha A, et al: Clonidine premedication for coronary artery bypass grafting under high-dose alfentanil anesthesia: Intraoperative and postoperative hemodynamic study. J Cardiothorac Vasc Anesth 1993; 7: 35

104. Feringa HH, Bax JJ, Poldermans D: Perioperative medical management of ischemic heart disease in patients undergoing noncardiac surgery. Curr Opin Anaesth 2007; 20: 254

105. Guideline Update on Perioperative Cardiovascular Evaluation for Noncardiac Surgery: Focused Update on Perioperative Beat-Blocker Therapy: A Report of the American College of Cardiology/American Heart Association Task Force on Practice Guidelines. Circulation 2006; 113: 2662

106. Fleisher LA: Should my outpatient center have a (beta)-blocker protocol? Curr Opin Anaesth 2007; 20: 526

107. Kersten JR, Fleisher LA: Statins: The next adavance in cardioprotection? Anesthesiology 2006; 105: 1079

108. Hindler K, Shaw A, Samuels J, et al: Improved postoperative outcomes associated with preoperative statin therapy. Anesthesiology 2006; 105: 1260

109. Dajani AS, Taubert KA, Wilson W, et al: Prevention of bacterial endocarditis. Recommendations by the American Heart Association. JAMA 1997; 277: 1794

110. Bratzler DW, Houck PM: Antimicrobial prophylaxis for surgery: an advisory statement from the National Surgical Infection Prevention Project. Am J Surg 2005; 189: 395

111. Pold HC Jr., Lopez-Mayor JF: Postoperative wound infection: A prospective study of determinant factors and prevention. Surgery 1969; 66: 97

112. Vetter TR: The epidemiology and selective identification of children at risk for preoperative anxiety reactions. Anesth Analg 1993; 77: 96

113. Kain ZN, MacLaren J, McClain BC, et al: Effects of age and emotionality on the effectiveness of midazolam administered preoperatively to children. Anesthesiology 2007; 107: 545

114. Weldon BC, Watcha MF, White PF: Oral midazolam in children: Effect of time and adjunctive therapy. Anesth Analg 1992; 75: 51

115. Coté CJ, Cohen IT, Suresh S, Rabb M, et al: A comparison of three doses of a commercially prepared oral midazolam syrup in children. Anesth Analg 2002; 94: 37

PREANESTHETIC EVALUATION AND PREPARATION

CHAPTER 24 ■ MALIGNANT HYPERTHERMIA AND OTHER INHERITED DISORDERS

HENRY ROSENBERG, BARBARA W. BRANDOM, AND NYAMKHISHIG SAMBUUGHIN

KEY POINTS

1 Malignant hyperthermia syndrome (MH) is an uncommon pharmacogenetic disorder of skeletal muscle. MH susceptibility is inherited. MH is induced by pharmacologic agents in almost all cases. A few well-documented cases have resulted from exercise and heat exposure. The increase in metabolism that is pathognomonic of MH is due to the biochemical effect of uncontrolled, increased calcium in muscle sarcoplasm.

2 Unexpected elevation of end-tidal carbon dioxide in the absence of equipment malfunction is the most sensitive and specific sign of MH. Other signs include tachycardia, tachypnea, acidosis, muscle rigidity, and sometimes rhabdomyolysis. MH may occur at any time in the course of an anesthetic from induction to emergence.

3 Masseter muscle rigidity after succinylcholine is more common in children than adults. It is predictive of MH susceptibility in up to 25% of cases and is associated with myoglobinuria. Trigger agents should be discontinued after masseter muscle rigidity. With generalized rigidity the likelihood of MH is very high.

4 Sudden cardiac arrest in a young male during general anesthesia, with or without succinylcholine, is likely a result of hyperkalemia in a patient with an occult myopathy, most often Duchenne muscular dystrophy.

5 Disorders that predispose patients to MH include central core disease, multiminicore disease, and rarer forms of myotonia.

6 Trigger agents for MH include all potent inhalation agents and succinylcholine.

7 The gold standard test for diagnosis of MH susceptibility is the caffeine-halothane contracture test (of freshly biopsied

muscle) wherein muscle is exposed to incremental doses of caffeine or to halothane. See www.mhaus.org for the addresses of MH diagnostic centers.

8 The essential points in treatment of MH are the immediate discontinuation of trigger agents, hyperventilation, administration of dantrolene in doses of 2.5 mg/kg, repeated as needed to control signs of MH, and cooling by all routes available (especially nasogastric lavage), treatment of hyperkalemia in a standard fashion. Following an MH episode the patient should be observed in a hospital and treated with dantrolene for at least 36 hours.

9 To minimize injury from MH it is necessary to monitor core body temperature and end-tidal CO_2 along with minute ventilation during general anesthesia, have dantrolene immediately available, obtain a thorough personal and family history related to anesthetic complications, and avoid MH trigger agents in susceptible patients and their relatives.

10 MH susceptibility is inherited in an autosomal dominant pattern in humans. MH has been associated with mutations in three genes, most frequently the ryanodine receptor gene (*RYR1*), rarely the dihydropyridine receptor gene, and the gene that elaborates the sodium channel of muscle. In humans, over 28 mutations in *RYR1* have been found to be causal for MH. These *RYR1* mutations increase the sensitivity of the ryanodine receptor calcium channel to agonists, leading to increased calcium release from the sarcoplasmic reticulum. There are over 150 DNA variants in *RYR1* whose significance in regard to MH susceptibility is yet to be determined.

11 Molecular genetic testing for MH susceptibility, using examination of part of *RYR1*, is available in the United

States, Europe, and several other countries. Genetic testing may be recommended for those with positive caffeine halothane contracture test results and a confirmed MH episode in a family member. Despite low sensitivity,

approximately 25%, many patients were able to be diagnosed as being MH-susceptible without resorting to the muscle contracture test.

Many inherited disorders have significant implications for anesthetic management. In this chapter we discuss those disorders that are precipitated by drugs often administered by anesthesiologists. In some cases, such as the porphyrias, the illness may be induced by agents other than anesthetics. In other enzymatic disorders, such as pseudocholinesterase abnormalities, it would be unlikely for a patient to have any problem until exposed to the depolarizing neuromuscular blocking agent succinylcholine. Malignant hyperthermia (MH) or malignant hyperpyrexia is perhaps the most significant inherited disorder triggered by exposure to anesthetic drugs.

MALIGNANT HYPERTHERMIA

Historical Aspects

MH was first formally described in 1960 in *Lancet* by Denborough and Lovell.[1] That first case described well the clinical presentation of MH. The young patient claimed that several of his relatives died without apparent cause during anesthesia. He was anesthetized with halothane and developed tachycardia, hot sweaty skin, peripheral mottling, and cyanosis. Early recognition and symptomatic treatment saved him. This new syndrome was unique: patients were healthy unless exposed to anesthesia, temperature elevation was a hallmark, a heritable component was present, and death was common. It was soon realized that it was possible to abort the malignant effects of the syndrome with early recognition and treatment.

The association between porcine stress syndrome (PSS) or "pale soft exudative pork syndrome" and MH was described in the early 1970s, thus providing an animal model for MH.[2] Porcine breeds such as the Landrace, Poland China, and Pietrain show the classic presentations of MH when potent inhalation agents and/or succinylcholine are administered. The development of an in vitro diagnostic bioassay of muscle was suggested by Kalow et al.[3] In 1975, Harrison[4] reported that dantrolene could be effective in treating and preventing MH in pigs. In 1979 intravenous dantrolene was approved by the U.S. Food and Drug Administration for treatment of the human form of MH. In the 1980s, lay organizations in the United States, Canada, and Great Britain were formed to disseminate information to patients affected by MH as well as to increase awareness of the syndrome among physicians. The muscle bioassay, the diagnostic halothane-caffeine contracture test, was standardized by work from the North America MH Registry, created in the United States in the late 1980s. A variety of other tests for diagnosing MH susceptibility were introduced, which subsequently were found to have little validity.

A major step forward in the understanding of the pathophysiology of MH occurred in 1985, when Lopez and colleagues[5] demonstrated increased intracellular concentration of calcium ion in muscle from MH-susceptible pigs and humans. The intracellular calcium concentration dramatically increased during an MH crisis and was reversed by the administration of dantrolene.

In the 1990s molecular biologic techniques identified genes associated with MH susceptibility. This allowed, in 2003, the introduction of a clinically useful genetic test for MH, although with limited sensitivity. Later, MH causative mutations were introduced in mice who then displayed clinical signs of MH on exposure to trigger agents and heat.[6,7]

Analysis of epidemiologic data gathered by the Malignant Hyperthermia Association of the United States (MHAUS) in the North American MH Registry led to differentiation between MH and some other life-threatening anesthetic complications. In particular, some deaths in children formerly attributed to MH were really the result of destruction of muscle cells that occurred during anesthesia with volatile agents and succinylcholine in patients with unrecognized myopathies, specifically the dystrophinopathies and Duchenne and Becker muscular dystrophy.[8]

Clinical Presentations

As understanding of MH grew, the definition of MH changed. At first, MH was thought in all cases to be a heritable syndrome consisting of an extremely elevated body temperature, skeletal muscle rigidity, and acidosis associated with a high mortality rate. However, it is more useful to think of MH in terms of its underlying pathophysiologic characteristics because recognition of MH prior to hyperthermia will facilitate treatment. MH is a hypermetabolic disorder of skeletal muscle with varied presentations, depending on species, breed, exposure to triggering agents, and genetic makeup of the individual. The pathophysiologic process in this disorder is intracellular hypercalcemia in skeletal muscle, which activates metabolic pathways resulting in adenosine triphosphate (ATP) depletion, acidosis, membrane destruction, and cell death. The heritable component is not always apparent from family history unless there is a history of anesthetic problems suggestive of the syndrome. Disorders that may have symptoms and signs similar to those of MH, such as neuroleptic malignant syndrome (NMS), and heat stroke do not appear to have an inherited basis.

Classic Malignant Hyperthermia

In the classic case, the initial signs of tachycardia and tachypnea result from sympathetic nervous system stimulation secondary to underlying hypermetabolism derived primarily from the skeletal muscle. Because many patients receive neuromuscular blockers and controlled ventilation during general anesthesia, tachypnea usually is not recognized. Shortly after the increase in heart rate, an increase in blood pressure occurs, often associated with ventricular dysrhythmias induced by sympathetic nervous system stimulation resulting from hypercarbia, hyperkalemia, and or catecholamine release. An increase in muscle tone may (or may not) become apparent. Increase in body temperature, at a rate of 1 to 2°C every 5 minutes, follows. CO_2 absorbent becomes warm to the touch (because the reaction with CO_2 is exothermic). The patient may display peripheral mottling, sweating, and cyanosis. Blood gas analysis reveals respiratory and/or metabolic acidosis without marked oxygen desaturation.

Elevation of end-tidal CO_2 is one of the earliest, most sensitive and specific signs of MH. However, vigorous hyperventilation may mask such hypercarbia and delay the diagnosis.[9] A mixed venous blood sample will show even more dramatic evidence of CO_2 retention and metabolic acidosis.[10] Hyperkalemia, hypercalcemia, lactacidemia, and myoglobinuria are characteristic. An increase in creatine kinase (CK) levels is dramatic, often exceeding 20,000 units in the first 12 to 24 hours. But increased CK is not a constant feature, particularly if the syndrome is detected promptly and treatment begun rapidly.[11] Death results unless the syndrome is recognized and treated promptly. Even with treatment, the patient is at risk for myoglobinuric renal failure and disseminated intravascular coagulation. Another significant clinical problem is a 25% recrudescence rate of the syndrome within the first 24 to 36 hours.[12,13] If succinylcholine is used during induction of anesthesia, an acceleration of the manifestations of MH may occur with tachycardia, hypertension, marked temperature elevation, and dysrhythmias over the course of 5 to 10 minutes. However, a completely normal response to succinylcholine does not rule out the subsequent development of MH when potent volatile agents are used.

Masseter Muscle Rigidity

3 Rigidity of the jaw muscles after administration of succinylcholine is referred to as *masseter muscle rigidity* (MMR) or *masseter spasm*. This phenomenon was associated with MH from case reports of MMR preceding MH. Although MMR probably occurs in patients of all ages, it is more common in children and young adults. A retrospective study from the Danish Malignant Hyperthermia Registry found that the incidence of MMR was 1 in 12,000 (including adults and children).[14] A prospective study found MMR in 1 of 500 apparently normal children who received halothane and then intravenous succinylcholine.[15] In most cases of MMR, anesthesia was induced by inhalation of halothane or sevoflurane, after which succinylcholine was administered. Although less common, MMR may follow succinylcholine administration after intravenous induction.[16] MMR may even occur after induction with any anesthetic agent, intravenous or inhalation, before succinylcholine administration.[17] Repeat doses of succinylcholine do not relieve MMR nor do nondepolarizing relaxants. A peripheral nerve stimulator usually reveals flaccid paralysis. If generalized rigidity is noted, the likelihood of MH susceptibility is very high. Tachycardia and dysrhythmias are not infrequent. Only in about 30% of cases does frank MH supervene immediately after MMR. More commonly (if the anesthetic is continued with a triggering agent), the initial signs of MH appear in 20 minutes or more. However, a study by Littleford et al.[18] has shown that although acidosis and rhabdomyolysis may be present when anesthesia is continued with a volatile inhalation agent in children after MMR, fulminant MH may not occur. If the anesthetic is discontinued, the patient usually appears to recover uneventfully. However, within 12 hours, myoglobinuria often occurs and CK elevation is detectable. Therefore, if MMR occurs, urine should be examined for myoglobin. Patients experiencing MMR should be hospitalized for at least 24 hours.

Muscle biopsy with caffeine-halothane contracture testing has shown that many patients who experience MMR are also susceptible to MH.[19,20] But reports have also shown that succinylcholine increases jaw muscle tone in patients with normal muscle.[21–23] This normal agonistic effect of succinylcholine, further increased by temperature[24] and epinephrine in the presence of halothane, accounts for some cases of MMR. When MMR is accompanied by rigidity of chest or limb muscles, MH is more likely to follow than after isolated jaw rigidity.[25,26]

The differential diagnosis of MMR consists of the following: (1) myotonic syndrome, (2) temporomandibular joint dysfunction, (3) underdosing with succinylcholine, (4) not allowing sufficient time for succinylcholine to act before intubation, (5) increased resting tension after succinylcholine in the presence of fever or elevated plasma epinephrine, and (6) MH. Signs of temporomandibular dysfunction as well as myotonia should be sought following the MMR episode. If rigidity precluding laryngoscopy occurred without temporomandibular joint dysfunction, the patient should be evaluated by a neurologist for the presence of occult myopathy and counseled regarding the need for a muscle biopsy with diagnostic contracture test to evaluate MH susceptibility. It is incumbent on the anesthesiologist to alert the patient to the possibility that MH may follow in subsequent procedures.

Our advice regarding MMR is as follows:

1. When it occurs, the anesthesiologist should, if at all possible, discontinue the anesthetic and postpone surgery. If end-tidal CO_2 monitoring and dantrolene are available and the anesthesiologist is experienced in managing MH, he or she may elect to continue with a nontriggering anesthetic.
2. Dantrolene administration is advised only if there is generalized rigidity and/or signs of hypermetabolism.
3. After MMR, the patient should be admitted to the hospital for a period of 12 to 24 hours with monitoring for myoglobinuria and signs of MH. Administration of 1 to 2 mg/kg of dantrolene should be considered.
3. The family should be informed of the episode of MMR and its implications.
4. CK levels should be checked 6, 12, and 24 hours after the episode. If the CK level is still grossly elevated at 12 hours, additional samples should be drawn until CK returns to normal.
5. If the CK level is >20,000 IU in the perioperative period and a concomitant myopathy is not present, the diagnosis of MH is very likely.[25,27] If contracture test results are within normal limits after an episode of MMR, we currently do not recommend that other family members undergo testing, but advise that succinylcholine be avoided in future anesthetics for that patient.

Variations in Presentation of Malignant Hyperthermia

There are a large number of variations in the presentation of MH. Some patients may undergo multiple anesthetics before experiencing MH. Similarly, MH may present after several hours of anesthesia or rarely in the early postoperative period, within 1 hour of discontinuing anesthesia. In some cases rigidity is not found at all, and in others temperature elevation is unimpressive. Interestingly, postoperative myoglobinuria may be the only sign of MH and may occur without an obvious increase in metabolism.[28] However the differential diagnosis of postoperative myoglobinuria is large. Succinylcholine may cause rhabdomyolysis in patients who have other muscle disorders that may not be clinically obvious on cursory examination.[8,29] Myoglobinuria may follow succinylcholine in patients who are taking inhibitors of cholesterol formation in patients with apparently normal muscle.[30]

Gross myoglobinuria (dark or cola-colored urine) is serious, as renal failure is likely. The patient should be evaluated and treatment begun with intravenous fluids and possibly mannitol and bicarbonate to avoid renal injury. Urine dipstick can be used to screen for myoglobinuria. If the dipstick is negative for blood, then there is no myoglobin present. If there is a strong positive reaction for blood and no red blood cells are seen microscopically, then myoglobinuria is likely and confirmatory tests indicated.

Myodystrophies Exacerbated by Anesthesia

Duchenne muscular dystrophy (DMD) occurs in 1 in 3,000 males. Boys are usually asymptomatic until the age of 4 or 5 years, but elevated CK is a constant finding from birth. Dystrophin is a major element in the dystroglycan complex that provides stability to the muscle cell membrane. *Becker dystrophy*, an order of magnitude less common than Duchenne muscular dystrophy is due to lower than normal levels of dystrophin and often does not produce symptoms until adolescence. Any patient with *dystrophinopathy* may experience hyperkalemic cardiac arrest after administration of succinylcholine.

The same may occur following administration of volatile anesthetic agents only.[31] These adverse events were first believed to represent a form of MH.[32,33] It now appears that the pathophysiology of the hyperkalemic episodes and MH is different. Case reports collected by the MHAUS and the North American MH Registry indicate that when an apparently healthy child experiences a sudden unexpected cardiac arrest on induction of anesthesia, once hypoxemia and ventilatory problems are ruled out, hyperkalemia should be considered. Of 29 patients with such a presentation, 60% died. In 50% there was evidence of undiagnosed myopathy (usually muscular dystrophy).[8] The treatment of the hyperkalemic arrest includes administration of calcium chloride, glucose, insulin, bicarbonate, and hyperventilation, but not dantrolene.

Because of the potentially fatal hyperkalemic event in patients with undiagnosed myopathy, succinylcholine should not be used routinely in children and young adolescents. Of course, in special circumstances, such as airway emergencies and the presence of a "full stomach," succinylcholine may still be appropriate in children without signs of a myopathy. However, administration of rapid-acting nondepolarizing neuromuscular blockers in these situations may be an appropriate alternative to use of succinylcholine.

In contrast to dystrophinopathies, congenital myopathies are a heterogeneous group of diseases defined histopathologically, with incidence of approximately 1 in 16,500 births.[34] There is marked phenotypic variability as well as genetic and histologic overlap between these conditions; *central core disease* (CCD), *nemaline myopathy*, *multiminicore disease*,[35] and *centronuclear myopathy*. CCD, the most common congenital myopathy, is defined by muscle weakness that has a variable onset and progression. The syndrome derives its name from the histologic appearance of reduced oxidative activity in areas along the longitudinal axis of the fiber. These are the histologic central cores, which may not be present at a young age. Among CCD patients there is significant variability in muscle weakness, even within affected families, but weakness usually involves the spine and pelvis. Foot deformities and patellar instability are common. CCD is generally inherited in an autosomal dominant manner linked with *RYR1* mutations. Many cases of MH have been reported in patients with CCD. Therefore, precautions regarding MH must be taken for all patients with CCD.[34] Recessive inheritance of *RYR1* mutations has been reported in a few patients with congenital myopathy[36] and mulitminicores[35] or central nuclei. MH episodes were reported in only 4 of 28 such patients, but exposure to anesthetic MH triggers was not described.[37]

Myotonias and *periodic paralyses* are a varied set of inherited disorders due to point mutations in an ion channel. Mutations in the human skeletal muscle sodium channel produce hyperkalemic periodic paralysis, potassium-aggravated myotonia, paramyotonia congenital, and hypokalemic periodic paralysis type 2. Hypokalemic periodic paralysis is due to point mutations in the calcium channel. Myotonia congenita is caused by mutations in the chloride channel.[38] The common pathophysiologic process is prolonged depolarization of the muscle membrane following activation. Patients with any form of myotonia will display muscle contractures after succinylcholine. Hypokalemic periodic paralysis and a rare form of myotonia, myotonia fluctuans, have been linked to MH susceptibility by the halothane-caffeine contracture test.[39,40] Periodic paralyses are characterized by marked muscle weakness resulting from small deviations in potassium concentrations. *King* or *King-Denborough* syndrome is a rare myopathy characterized by cryptorchidism, markedly slanted eyes, low-set ears, pectus deformity, scoliosis, small stature, and hypotonia. This syndrome was associated with MH soon after the original description of MH. Several patients with this disorder have been diagnosed as MH-susceptible both clinically and by muscle biopsy.[41,42]

Skeletal abnormalities such as osteogenesis imperfecta[43] and the Schwartz-Jampel[44] syndrome have been associated with signs of MH. Metabolism is increased in osteogenesis imperfecta because of the bone disease without exposure to drugs. Fever during anesthesia is common in these patients.[45] The Schwartz-Jampel syndrome is an autosomal recessive myotonic-like condition with osteoarticular deformities. In some patients there is an abnormality of muscle; in others, a neurologic abnormality is present and the symptoms can be blocked by nondepolarizing neuromuscular blockers. Fever is common in these patients because of continuous muscle activity. In both these conditions, association with MH is unlikely. Despite a few well-documented cases of MH in patients with osteogenesis imperfecta, we (and others[46]) have not confirmed MH susceptibility in three cases of osteogenesis imperfecta tested with the halothane-caffeine contracture test. Inhalation anesthetics have been administered without complication to many patients with osteogenesis imperfecta.

Syndromes with a Clinical Resemblance to Malignant Hyperthermia

Pheochromocytoma may be mistaken for MH because it presents with tachycardia, hypertension, and fever during anesthesia. However, pheochromocytoma does not predispose to MH.[47] *Thyrotoxicosis* could also be mistaken for MH. Carbon dioxide production is lower in these endocrine disorders than in MH. Hypertension is usually greater in pheochromocytoma than in thyrotoxicosis, and even less in MH. Neither endocrine crisis is associated with muscle rigidity, as is MH. Metabolic acidosis is generally not present during thyrotoxicosis and not as great during pheochromocytoma as during MH. Thyroid crisis did not trigger MH, without exposure to anesthetic triggers, even in susceptible pigs.[48]

Sepsis is often confused with MH. Patients most at risk are those undergoing urinary tract surgery, oral surgery, or appendectomy. They are afebrile intraoperatively but develop fever, rigors (which may be mistaken for MH-related rigidity), and sometimes acidosis in the postanesthesia care unit. Hyperkalemia may also appear during episodes of sepsis. Unlike MH, however, persistent muscle rigidity is rare. In addition, signs of sepsis may be treated effectively with nonsteroidal anti-inflammatory agents, antibiotics, and cardiovascular support. MH will not respond to such nonspecific therapy. Dantrolene administration in the presence of sepsis may be followed by acute reduction of fever because dantrolene reduces the metabolism of normal muscle.

Hypoxic encephalopathy is characterized by failure to awaken from anesthesia, posturing, opisthotonus, and hyperthermia. It has been mistaken for MH. A marked hypoxic episode with or without outright cardiac arrest precedes such clinical signs.

Mitochondrial myopathies resemble MH in that weakness and acidosis may be observed in both syndromes. Defects within the mitochondrial genome affect oxidative phosphorylation and result in impaired production of ATP. Mitochondrial disease has many manifestations, usually presenting at an early age with central nervous system, gastrointestinal, and muscle pathology. Failure to thrive, developmental delays, muscle weakness, cardiomyopathy, and intolerance to heat may be present. Elevated serum lactate and pyruvate are found on laboratory examination. CK may be elevated. Anesthesia for patients with mitochondrial disease should be designed to be "stress-free". Succinylcholine is best avoided in these patients because of the potential for hyperkalemia. The general consensus is that mitochondrial myopathies do not predispose to MH.

Malignant Hyperthermia Outside the Operating Room

The often-repeated observation that an MH-like syndrome can occur in certain pig breeds in response to stressful situations supports the suggestion that MH may occur outside the operating room in humans. However, such events are exceedingly rare. Gronert et al.[49] have described a patient who had episodic fevers and whose muscle produced a contracture consistent with MH susceptibility. The fevers were controlled by dantrolene. A mutation in *RYR1*, known to be causative of MH, was found in a patient who survived anesthesia-induced MH and then died after soccer practice. Other family members also had the same mutation.[50] A few patients with exercise-induced rhabdomyolysis have been found to harbor one of the MH-related mutations.[51] Exercise-induced rhabdomyolysis may occur in patients with other myopathies with or without exposure to myotoxic drugs such as those that lower serum cholesterol.[52] But most cases of heat stroke, even with marked rhabdomyolysis, are not associated with MH susceptibility.[53]

Neuroleptic Malignant Syndrome and Other Drug-Induced Hyperthermic Reactions

The symptoms and signs of the NMS include fever, rhabdomyolysis, tachycardia, hypertension, agitation, muscle rigidity, and acidosis.[54] NMS results from treatment with a variety of antipsychotic agents, including the atypical antipsychotics and haloperidol. NMS complicates such treatment in <0.1% of patients taking such medications. Death is uncommon if diagnosed rapidly and treated promptly. Nevertheless hundreds of people die from NMS each year. A variety of drugs have been found useful in the treatment of NMS including benzodiazepines, bromocriptine, and dantrolene. Because of the clinical resemblance to MH, it is not unusual for an anesthesiologist to be consulted in the management of patients with this disorder. A 24/7 Helpline staffed by psychiatrists experienced in the treatment of NMS and serotonin syndrome is available at 1-888-667-8367. The Neurolept Malignant Syndrome Information Service is available at www.nmsis.org.

Although the resemblance of NMS to MH is striking, there are significant differences between the two. MH is acute, whereas NMS often occurs after longer-term drug exposure. Phenothiazines, haloperidol, or any of the newer potent antipsychotics are usually triggering agents for NMS. Sudden withdrawal of drugs used to treat Parkinson disease may also trigger NMS. Electroconvulsive therapy with succinylcholine does not appear to trigger the syndrome.[55] Also, NMS does not seem to be inherited, and there are no case reports of it in family members who have had an episode of MH.

NMS is related to dopamine depletion in the central nervous system by psychoactive agents. In support of this theory, therapy with bromocriptine, a dopamine agonist, is often useful in treatment of NMS. Although there appear to be similarities between MH and NMS,[54] a common pathophysiology is not readily apparent. From an anesthesiologist's viewpoint, it is best to monitor patients with NMS as though they were susceptible to MH. However, drugs such as succinylcholine have been used for electroconvulsive therapy without problems in MH patients.

A similar set of signs may be observed in some patients taking serotonin uptake inhibitors(so-called serotonin syndrome).[56]

Other drugs known to induce a hypermetabolic syndrome and rhabdomyolysis, probably by stimulation of the sympathetic nervous system and uncoupling proteins, mechanisms not related to those of MH, are cocaine, amphetamines, and MDMA (i.e., the street drug Ecstasy). Dantrolene has been used

TABLE 24-1

SAFE VERSUS UNSAFE DRUGS IN MALIGNANT HYPERTHERMIA

■ SAFE DRUGS	■ UNSAFE DRUGS
Antibiotics	All inhalation agents
Antihistamines	(except nitrous oxide)
Barbiturates	Succinylcholine
Benzodiazepines	
Droperidol	
Ketamine	
Local anesthetics	
Nitrous oxide	
Nondepolarizing	
neuromuscular blockers	
Opioids	
Propofol	
Propranolol	
Vasoactive drugs	

sporadically as an adjunct to treatment of marked hyperthermia in these cases and in NMS.[57] Experimental evidence in animals supports treatment with β_3 blocker such as carvedilol.[58]

Drugs That Trigger Malignant Hyperthermia

6 It is clearly established that the potent inhalation agents, including sevoflurane, desflurane, isoflurane, halothane, methoxyflurane, and cyclopropane, may trigger MH. Succinylcholine is also a trigger. Other anesthetic drugs and adjuvants are not MH triggers (Table 24-1). All local anesthetics are safe for MH-susceptible patients.[59] Amide local anesthetics given during an MH crisis (e.g., for dysrhythmia control) do not worsen the episode.

Although plasma catecholamines increase during an MH crisis, such an elevation is usually secondary to metabolic and cardiovascular changes. Vasopressors and other catecholamines are not involved in triggering MH.[60] Therefore, these drugs should be given as necessary, but only with simultaneous treatment of the MH crisis.

Vecuronium, rocuronium, cisatracurium, pancuronium, and all other nondepolarizing drugs are considered safe to use in patients with MH. Clinical studies have shown that anticholinesterase–anticholinergic combinations are safe for reversal of nondepolarizing relaxants in MH-susceptible patients.[61]

Digoxin, quinidine, and calcium salts do not induce MH in swine.[62] Therefore, it is reasonable to assume that they are safe to use in clinical situations. Neither ketamine nor propofol are MH triggers. Although a wide variety of drugs may precipitate NMS, these do not produce MH crises. The two syndromes are not related in this manner.

Incidence and Epidemiology

The incidence of MH varies from country to country, based on differences in gene pools, exposure to triggers, and reporting mechanisms. In the upper midwest of the United States there are many large families of MH-susceptible people. In contrast, other areas of this country and the world have rarely reported MH. Bachand and colleagues[63] examined the incidence of MH in a province of Quebec, Canada, where many families had undergone biopsy. They traced the pedigrees of patients to the original immigrants from France and found an incidence of MH susceptibility of 0.2% in this province. However, that represented only five extended families. The best epidemiologic study of MH was done in the mid 1980s by Ording[14] based on the Danish Malignant Hyperthermia Registry. She found that fulminant MH occurred once in 250,000 administered anesthetics. However, if the definition of MH was expanded to include abortive cases of MH, the incidence increased to 1 in 4,000 exposures to inhalation anesthetics and succinylcholine!

A better understanding of the prevalence of MH susceptibility may emerge from the use of molecular genetics. For example, Monnier and colleagues[64] estimate that one in 2,000 to 3,000 persons in France harbor one of the known MH causative mutations. A similar prevalence has been reported in the Japanese population, although associated with different mutations than found in Europe.[65] Currently, the consensus is that mortality from MH is under 5% in Western countries. However, the epidemiologic characteristics of MH are very difficult to define for the following reasons:

1. Widespread diagnostic testing for MH is difficult to apply.
2. The clinical diagnosis of MH is often questionable.
3. Triggering of MH may not occur on each anesthetic exposure. Susceptible patients have received triggering agents for more than ten anesthetics without any problems, only to have MH triggered on the subsequent anesthetic. Investigation of the Danish Malignant Hyperthermia Registry found the MH genotype to be expressed in only 34 to 54% of anesthetic exposures.[66]
4. Registries of MH cases do not capture all relevant data. There is a paucity of data concerning the frequency of use of anesthesia in the general population.

Diagnostic Tests for Malignant Hyperthermia

❼ The gold standard muscle bioassay for MH susceptibility derives from the observation that viable muscle biopsied from MH patients responds with marked rigidity to halothane, caffeine, chlorocresol, and a variety of other agents known to release calcium from the sarcoplasmic reticulum. Although the test is conducted somewhat differently in Europe[67,68] than in North America,[69–71] the principles of the test are similar.

Halothane-Caffeine Contracture Test

Although some procedures and interpretations differ between the European Malignant Hyperthermia Group (EMHG) and North American Malignant Hyperthermia Group (NAMHG) protocols, the following steps are similar. Skeletal muscle (1 to 3 g) is usually biopsied from a thigh muscle, usually the vastus lateralis muscle. Strips of muscle weighing 100 to 200 mg and measuring 15 to 30 mm ($\geq$25 mm preferred) in length by 2 to 3 mm in width by 2 to 3 mm in thickness are carefully isolated and mounted in a standard muscle bath apparatus (Fig. 24-1). The tissue bath contains a modified Krebs solution at 37°C bubbled with O_2 and CO_2 (95%/5%), and the resting tension is adjusted to the optimum length for maximal twitch tension (usually about 2 g). The bundles are stimulated supramaximally with pulses of frequency 0.1 to 0.2 Hz with 2-msec pulses to verify viability. After a 15- to 60-minute equilibration with O_2/CO_2 (95%/5%), halothane is added to the gas phase, either as a bolus dose or in incrementally increasing concentrations (Fig. 24-2). The concentration of halothane is verified by gas chromatography. A second set of muscle strips is equilibrated and subsequently exposed to incrementally increasing concentrations of caffeine-free base (Fig. 24-2). It is recommended that the caffeine strips be tested early in the procedure because they tend to be more sensitive to instability over time.

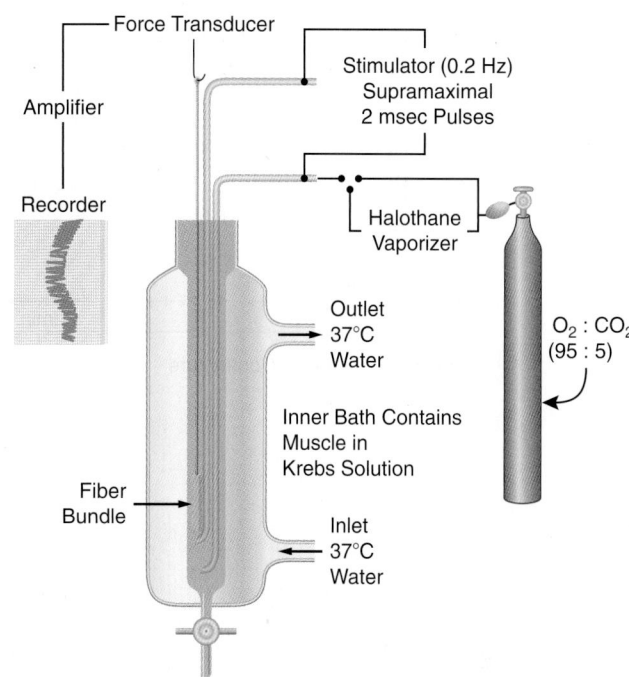

FIGURE 24-1. Diagram of the muscle bath apparatus used for contracture testing for diagnosing MH susceptibility.

Testing is usually completed within about 5 hours of biopsy to ensure adequate viability of the muscle preparations. Therefore, it is essential that the biopsy be performed $\leq$1 hour away from the testing laboratory. Usually, histologic and biochemical evaluation accompanies the contracture test to characterize potential muscle disorders.

Sensitivity and Specificity of the Halothane-Caffeine Contracture Test. The sensitivity of the NAMHG protocol caffeine-halothane contracture test is 100% with specificity 78% (false-negatives are to be avoided).[70,71] The EMHG test in vitro contracture test has sensitivity of 98% with specificity of 93%. It is difficult to be certain of the sensitivity and specificity of the contracture test because although one can be fairly certain of the clinical phenotype of MHS based on anesthetic exposures, it is almost impossible to be assured that control subjects do not harbor a causative mutation. Determination of the sensitivity and specificity is based on contracture studies of patients with no known MH history undergoing routine surgery (controls) compared with contracture studies from patients who experienced an unequivocal clinical episode of MH.

Other Agents used in the Contracture Tests

In attempts to further improve the specificity and sensitivity of the contracture test, other agents have been tested for their effect on skeletal muscle.

Ryanodine. An additional contracture test using the plant alkaloid ryanodine was proposed for inclusion in the EMHG protocol. Ryanodine binds to and activates the calcium release channel of the sarcoplasmic reticulum. It was reasoned that this test would afford maximum specificity for MH, and early studies supported this concept.[72–75]

The basic testing conditions for ryanodine are similar to those described for halothane and caffeine testing. High-purity ryanodine is employed. A bolus of ryanodine to produce one $\mu M/L$ is added to the bath and the time to onset of contracture, time to

PREANESTHETIC EVALUATION AND PREPARATION

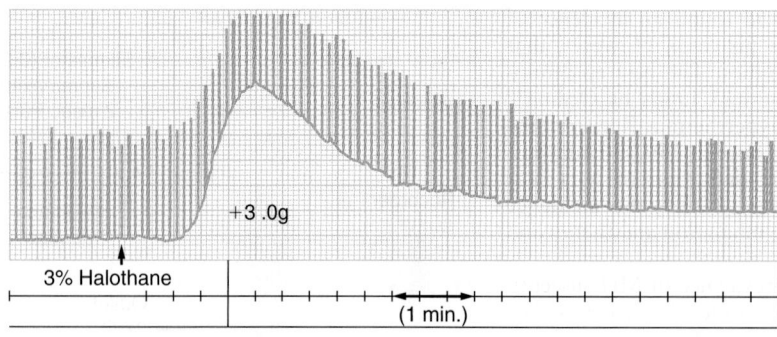

Abnormal Halothane Contracture

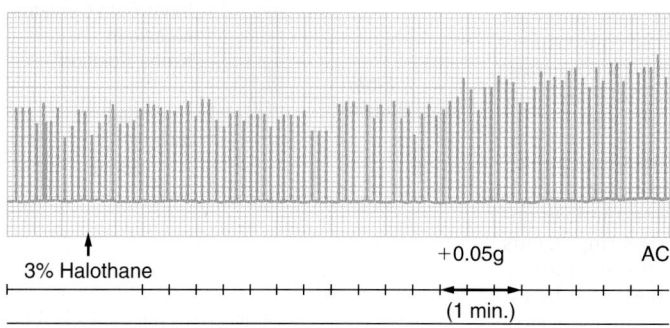

A Normal Halothane Contracture

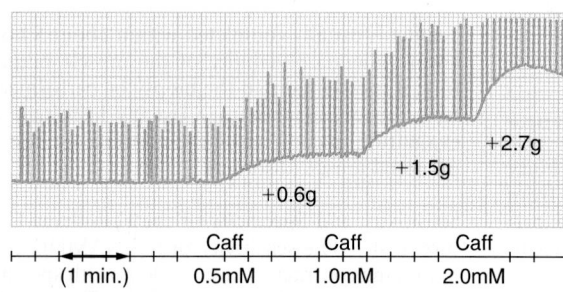

Abnormal Caffeine Dose Response

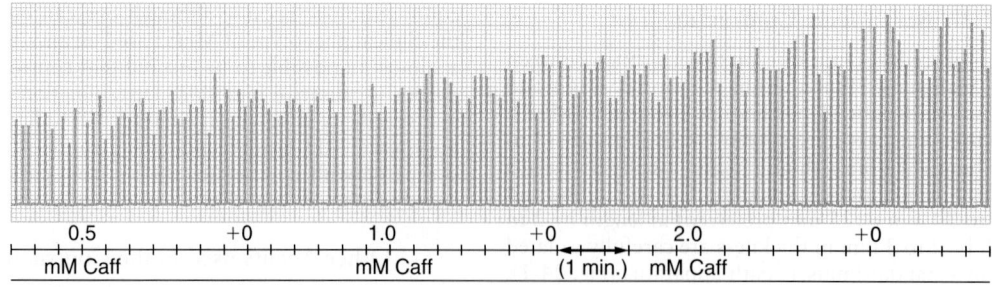

B Normal Caffeine Dose Response

FIGURE 24-2.   Muscle strips weighing approximately 150 mg and stimulated supramaximally are exposed to 3% halothane or incremental doses of caffeine. **A.** A 3-g contracture is recorded from this strip from a patient with malignant hyperthermia syndrome (MHS) after exposure of the muscle to 3% halothane (*top*); a normal response to 3% halothane (*bottom*). **B.** Contractures noted after exposure to 0.5, 1, and 2 m*M* caffeine (Caff) in MHS muscle (*top*); no contracture response to the same caffeine concentrations. Twitch height augmentation is normal following caffeine addition (*bottom*).

0.2-g contracture, time to 1-g contracture, and the time and amplitude of maximum contracture are recorded. Discrimination was improved by using the time to initial contracture and time to development of a 10-mN (1 g) contracture.[76]

4-Chloro-*m*-Cresol.

4-Chloro-*m*-cresol (4-CmC) is a potent activator of ryanodine receptor–mediated Ca^{2+} release. Cumulative administration of 25, 50, 75, 100, 150, and 200 μmol/L of 4-CmC produced concentration-dependent contractures. Contractures developed earlier and to a greater magnitude in muscle from patients identified as MHS by the EMHG protocol than in normal muscle.[77] The EMHG-approved bioassay includes administration of a single bolus of 4-CmC so that the bathed muscle is exposed to a concentration of 75 μmol/L.

Pitfalls in the Contracture Test

Ideally, each laboratory should derive specimens from patients who are clearly and unequivocally normal and those who are clearly and unequivocally MH-susceptible to verify that cutpoints for MH susceptibility are diagnostic within the laboratory. Unfortunately, because of the variation in presentation of MH, it is not always possible to have complete agreement on the MH status of a patient based on a clinical history, even among experts in the field.

There have been a few reports describing patients who were diagnosed as nonsusceptible by contracture testing subsequently experiencing clinical episodes highly suggestive of MH; and in one case, the estimated false-negative rate was 4 of 171 subjects (2%).[78,79] MH experts are not convinced that these were valid cases of MH. A mimic of MH such as sepsis may explain the clinical problem.[79] In contrast, studies have reported patients with negative results for MH receiving triggering agents on multiple occasions,[80,81] all without complications. Unfortunately, studies like these are difficult to conduct because they require large patient populations and tracking of subjects diagnosed several years before the actual study.

Tests with More Limited Usefulness in Malignant Hyperthermia Diagnosis

Alternative tests that have not gained acceptance within the EMHG or NAMHG have been reviewed elsewhere.[82,83]

Elevated resting CK values are associated with MH susceptibility in a few families. However, many subjects susceptible to MH do not have elevated CK values, making this method of diagnosis relatively insensitive.[83] Also, several muscle disorders are associated with elevated resting CK values, making this test nonspecific.[83] Elevated CK values may be useful in preliminarily identifying key family members to be referred for contracture testing and in identifying muscle disease in children too young to undergo contracture testing.

Although the use of resting CK values for general screening of MH susceptibility is neither sensitive nor specific, there is a relationship between high postoperative CK values associated with MMR and the probability of diagnosis as MH-susceptible by the contracture test.[20,27] Although it is not a perfect indicator of MH susceptibility,[84] the chances are about 80% that a CK value >20,000 after MMR will yield a positive diagnosis by contracture testing.[20,27] A relatively normal CK level postoperatively does not rule out the possibility of an acute MH reaction during that anesthetic.[11,85]

A variety of minimally invasive diagnostic tests have been presented. One uses nuclear magnetic resonance spectroscopy to evaluate ATP depletion during graded exercise in vivo. MH patients have a greater breakdown of ATP and creatine phosphate as well as an increase in acid content compared with normal patients.[86] Using cultured muscle cells[87] or B lymphocytes,[88] it has been shown that agents such as caffeine and

chlorocresol will raise intracellular calcium ion concentrations to a greater extent in tissue derived from MHS individuals than normal patients.

By fine dissection of muscle to separate single muscle fibers it has been shown that specially prepared fibers will demonstrate accentuated contractures, as with the muscle bundles. One advantage is that the muscle may be preserved for repeated studies. On the other hand, even in MH muscle, some fibers may behave normally. This test is used routinely in Japan.

A rather novel approach entails injection of a small amount of caffeine or inhalation anesthetic through a microdialysis catheter inserted into the thigh muscle and sampling local CO_2 and/or lactate levels.[89] This method is being studied further.[90–92]

Clinical Diagnosis of Malignant Hyperthermia: The Grading Scale

A clinical grading scale has been developed to address concerns for objectively evaluating the clinical episode.[93] This scale lacks sensitivity because incomplete recording of necessary data or early termination of the crisis would not yield scores indicative of MH, even in the presence of a true MH episode. The value of the grading scale is mainly in identifying those subjects with the most convincing episodes of MH for subsequent evaluation of the sensitivity of the diagnostic tests. The clinical grading scale (Table 24-2) is useful for documentation of clinical episodes in those cases in which the subject is rated a D6 (Diagnostic rank 6, almost certainly MH), but lower scores should not be used for diagnosis. We encourage the practice of sending patients rated D6 for diagnostic muscle contracture testing because these individuals are rare and essential for the continuing

TABLE 24-2

CRITERIA USED IN THE MALIGNANT HYPERTHERMIA CLINICAL GRADING SCALE

Process I: Muscle rigidity	
Generalized rigidity	15
Masseter rigidity	15
Process II: Myonecrosis	
Elevated CK >20,000 (after succinylcholine administration)	15
Elevated CK >10,000 (without exposure to succinylcholine)	15
Cola-colored urine	10
Myoglobin in urine >60 μg/L	5
Blood/plasma/serum K^+ >6 mEg/L	3
Process III: Respiratory acidosis	
$PetCO_2$ >55 with controlled ventilation	15
$PaCO_2$ >60 with controlled ventilation	15
$PetCO_2$ >60 with spontaneous ventilation	15
Inappropriate hypercarbia	15
Inappropriate tachypnea	10
Process IV: Temperature increase	
Rapid increase in temperature	15
Inappropriate temperature >38.8°C in perioperative period	10
Process V: Cardiac involvement	
Inappropriate tachycardia	3
Ventricular tachycardia or fibrillation	3

CK, creatine kinase.
See Larach, et al.[93] for full details of this scoring system. Briefly, a case may receive 15 points for the worst presentation in five of the first six categories. A sum of more than 50 points is termed *D6*, almost certainly a case of malignant hyperthermia (MH). A sum of 35 to 49 points is *D5*, very likely to be a case of MH.

evaluation of the sensitivity and specificity of the contracture test and for study of the genetics of MH.

Molecular Genetic Testing for Malignant Hyperthermia Susceptibility

The discovery of multiple MH causing mutations in the *RYR1*[94] has led to the introduction of genetic testing of MH susceptibility on a limited basis in Europe and the United States. The guidelines published by the European Malignant Hyperthermia Group (www.emhg.org) suggest that for clinical diagnosis, a panel of 28 *RYR1* mutations should be examined. A limitation of genetic testing in the United States has been sensitivity of about 23% when testing for 21 mutations.[95] Screening of the entire coding region of the *RYR1* identifies sequence variants in 70%[65,96] to 86%[97] of patients. Therefore, sensitivity of genetic tests will improve as more mutations are identified as causative of MH.

Patients should consider genetic testing if:

1. They have had a positive contracture test.
2. A family member has had a positive contracture test.
3. They have suffered a very likely MH episode, but have not had a contracture test.
4. A family member has been found to have a causal mutation.

When a mutation known to be causative for MH is identified in a family member who has had an abnormal contracture response to halothane or caffeine, it is possible to determine MH susceptibility in other members of that family by examination of their *RYR1* DNA for that mutation. Those with the mutation are MH-susceptible (with high specificity) but those without the mutation cannot be considered MH-negative as they may harbor another mutation. The patient cannot be presumed to be MH-negative without negative results on muscle contracture testing.[98] The decision to undergo genetic testing is complex. The pros and cons of testing should be discussed with either an MH expert or a genetic counselor. At the current time, there are two clinical laboratories offering molecular genetic testing for MH:

■ LABORATORY	■ CONTACT
PreventionGenetics, LLC Eric W. Johnson, PhD 3700 Downwind Drive Marshfield, WI 54449 www.preventiongenetics.com A College of American Pathology diagnostic laboratory	715-387-0484 clinicaltesting@ preventiongenetics.com

Center for Medical Genetics
University of Pittsburgh
   Medical Center
J. Kant, MD, PhD
S701 Scaife Hall
3550 Terrace Street
Pittsburgh, PA 15213
http://path.upmc.edu/
   divisions/mdx/diagnostics.html
	Deanna Steele, CGC
	800-454-8155
	or
	412-648-8519
	(laboratory)

See the section on pathogenesis and etiology of MH for more details.

Treatment of Malignant Hyperthermia

MH is a treatable disorder. All institutions in which anesthetic agents known to trigger MH are administered should have dantrolene available (36 ampules [720 mg] is recommended) and a management plan.

The Acute Episode

8 The following steps should be taken immediately when MH is diagnosed:

1. Administration of all inhalation agents and succinylcholine should be discontinued and assistance should be secured. (It is helpful to have a dedicated cart available containing the agents for treatment of MH.)
2. Hyperventilation with 100% oxygen should be instituted at >10 L/min. Oxygen flow should be 10 L/min to hasten purging of residual anesthetic gases. Time should not be wasted in securing another anesthetic machine, but an Ambu bag and E-cylinder of oxygen may be used.
3. Assistance should be obtained in mixing dantrolene. The present preparation of dantrolene is poorly soluble. Each vial containing 20 mg should be mixed with 50 mL of bacteriostatic sterile distilled water (not saline solution). It is important to store sterile water in clearly labeled containers of a different size from that used for routine intravenous solutions. It may be helpful to keep a mixing system adjacent. Dantrolene will dissolve faster as temperature of the diluent increases from 20 to 40°C[99] or 41°C.[100] Intravenous therapy should be started with 2.5 mg/kg with repeat doses as needed. More than 10 mg/kg of dantrolene may be given as dictated by clinical circumstances; however, many acute episodes are controlled with 2 to 3 mg/kg. There are 3 g of mannitol with each 20 mg of dantrolene. Therefore, a bladder catheter should be inserted to facilitate monitoring urine output.
4. Titration of dantrolene to heart rate, body temperature, and $PaCO_2$ is the best clinical guideline of therapy.
5. In fulminant cases in which significant metabolic acidosis is present, 2 to 4 mEq/kg bicarbonate should be given. Large volumes of fluid may be needed to replace loss into edematous tissues and into the urine.
6. If it is not already available, a capnometer should be obtained so that CO_2 excretion can be documented.
7. Dysrhythmia control usually follows hyperventilation, dantrolene therapy, and correction of acidosis. Calcium channel blockers should not be used in the acute treatment of MH. Verapamil can interact with dantrolene to produce hyperkalemia and myocardial depression.[101,102] Lidocaine can be given safely during an MH crisis.
8. Body temperature elevation should be managed by giving cool fluid intravenously, placing ice packs on the groin and in the axillae, and by use of gastric, wound, and rectal lavage. Some have recommended peritoneal dialysis and others recommend cardiopulmonary bypass. Cooling should be stopped when core temperature reaches 38°C to avoid hypothermia.
9. Although arterial blood is useful for assessing acidosis, central mixed venous blood gas determinations (or, if not available, femoral venous blood gas readings) serve as a better guideline for therapy. Serum potassium should be measured early.
10. Hyperkalemia should be managed in the usual fashion with glucose, insulin, bicarbonate, and hyperventilation (see Chapter 14). If hyperkalemia is associated with significant cardiac effects, calcium chloride, 1 gram or 10 mg/kg, should be given. Hypokalemia frequently results during therapy of MH. However, potassium replacement should be undertaken very cautiously, if at all, because potassium may retrigger an MH episode.
11. Baseline laboratory tests should include creatinine, coagulation profile, CK as well as liver function tests. CK elevations may not occur for 6 to 12 hours after an MH episode

and should be followed as a rough guide to therapy. Myoglobin levels in blood and urine should be obtained early in the episode.

Management After the Acute Episode

After the acute episode, the clinician should be concerned about three complications of MH:

1. Recrudescence of MH. As many as 25% of patients may experience acute recrudescence, a relapse, within hours of the first episode.[13]
2. Disseminated intravascular coagulation (DIC)[103] (see Chapter 16). DIC has often been described in cases of MH, probably resulting from release of thromboplastins secondary to shock and core temperature >41°C[104] and/or release of cellular contents on membrane destruction. The usual regimen for treatment of DIC should be followed.
3. Myoglobinuric renal failure (see Chapter 52). Myoglobinuria may occur within hours after the episode begins. If the urine is acid, bicarbonate should be given to decrease the chance that myoglobin will injure renal tubules. Mannitol should be given to produce >1 ml/kg/hr urine output.

The guidelines for the dose and duration of dantrolene therapy after resolution of acute MH are empirical. It would seem prudent to continue dantrolene, 1 mg/kg every 6 hours intravenously, for at least 24 to 36 hours, but more may be given if signs of MH reappear. Some recommend conversion of dantrolene therapy from intravenous to oral form (4 mg/kg per day or more) with continuation for several days.

Significant muscle weakness and pain may follow MH, resulting from muscle destruction along with dantrolene administration; this should be managed symptomatically. Recovery of strength may require weeks to months.

A variety of other electrolyte changes may occur, such as hypocalcemia and hyperphosphatemia. Sodium and chloride changes may occur secondary to fluid shifts during the acute episode. All these changes usually respond to control of the acute episode.

Dantrolene

Dantrolene sodium is a hydantoin derivative (1-[[[5-(4-nitrophenyl)-2-furanyl]methylene]amino]-2,4-imidazolidinedione). In 1979, intravenous dantrolene was approved for treatment of MH. Until that time, the primary use of dantrolene was in the management of spasticity. Dantrolene is a unique muscle relaxant. Unlike neuromuscular blocking agents (whose site of action is at the nicotinic receptor of the neuromuscular junction) or the nonspecific relaxants (which modulate spinal cord synaptic reflexes), dantrolene acts within the muscle cell itself by reducing calcium release by the sarcoplasmic reticulum. [^{3}H]Azidodantrolene, a pharmacologically active, photoaffinity analog of dantrolene, specifically binds to a site on the ryanodine receptor.[105,106] During an MH episode, dantrolene reduces intracellular calcium levels. Therefore, dantrolene is a specific and effective agent in the treatment of MH. In the usual clinical doses, dantrolene has little effect on myocardial contractility.[107]

Studies have also indicated that doses of neuromuscular blocking agents need not be changed significantly after dantrolene administration. However, the drug should be used cautiously in patients with neuromuscular disease.[108]

The serum level of dantrolene required for prophylaxis against MH is about 2.5 μg/mL. The half-life of intravenous dantrolene, the only form recommended, is approximately 12 hours. However, the therapeutic level of dantrolene usually persists for 4 to 6 hours after a usual intravenous dose of 2.5 mg/kg.[109,110] Therefore, dantrolene should be supplemented at least every 6 hours after a clinical episode. Muscle weakness

may persist for 24 hours after dantrolene therapy is discontinued. Nausea and phlebitis are other complications of acute dantrolene administration. Hepatotoxicity has been demonstrated only with long-term use of oral dantrolene. Prophylaxis for MH should be carried out with intravenous or oral dantrolene[111] (5 mg/kg per 24 hours) in those *rare* situations in which prophylaxis is desired.

Management of the Patient Susceptible to Malignant Hyperthermia

Because of an increasing awareness of MH and more widespread use of diagnostic tests, it is not unusual for an anesthesiologist to be confronted with a MH-susceptible patient or a patient who has a family history of MH. The management of such patients should be carefully planned.

In the preoperative interview, the anesthesiologist should try to obtain sufficient information regarding previous episodes of MH and their documentation. If the family has participated in the North American Malignant Hyperthermia Registry, the Registry may be able to give details to the anesthesia provider. The anesthesiologist should allow adequate time to reassure patients and their families that he or she is familiar with MH and its implications and that appropriate monitoring and therapy will be instituted as necessary. It may be worth mentioning that there have been no deaths from MH in previously diagnosed MH-susceptible patients when the anesthesia team was aware of the problem. Anesthesia and premedication should be designed to produce a low normal heart rate. Standard premedicant drugs such as opioids, benzodiazepines, ataractics, barbiturates, antihistamines, and anticholinergics do not cause problems in MH-susceptible patients when administered in appropriate doses; however, phenothiazines are not recommended. Dantrolene need not be given preoperatively because nontriggering agents are used and end-tidal CO_2 and core temperature are monitored. Dantrolene must be immediately available in the operating room, and equipment for rapid measurement of blood gases and electrolytes should be available.

The anesthesia machine is prepared by draining, removing, or disabling anesthetic vaporizers, and changing tubing and CO_2 absorbent and flowing oxygen at 10 L/min for 10 minutes or longer. The modern anesthesia workstation is larger than older anesthesia machines and can require >10 minutes to purge of inhalation agents unless many components have been replaced.[112,113] Obviously, iced solutions and adequate supplies of dantrolene must be available in the vicinity of the operating room when MH-susceptible patients are anesthetized.

Exhaled CO_2 should be monitored because the earliest sign of MH is an increase in CO_2 production and excretion. Arterial and central venous monitoring is recommended for MH-susceptible patients, only as dictated by the surgical procedure. Body core temperature should be monitored by nasopharyngeal, rectal, or esophageal routes in all patients for all surgical procedures. Skin temperature, although acceptable, is not as desirable because it may not reflect core temperature.[114]

If possible, a regional, local, or major conduction anesthetic should be used. If not possible, intravenous induction of anesthesia followed by nitrous oxide, oxygen, and a nondepolarizing relaxant with opioid supplementation is recommended. Agents that have not been implicated in MH are midazolam, dexmedetomidine, diazepam, droperidol, and propofol.

Neuromuscular blocking agents such as pancuronium, vecuronium, atracurium, cisatracurium, and rocuronium are safe. Routine reversal of nondepolarizing relaxants with anticholinesterase and anticholinergic agents is recommended.

Many thousands of safe anesthetics have been administered with nitrous oxide in MH-susceptible patients. Two cases have been reported in which early signs of MH have been documented despite the use of a safe anesthetic technique.[115] Therefore, even under the most controlled circumstances, the anesthesiologist should be alert to the early signs of MH.

Administration of dantrolene after surgery is not recommended if there are no signs of MH. If there is no sign of MH in the first hour postoperatively after safe anesthetic techniques were used, it is very unlikely that MH will occur later. The patient may be discharged on the same day as surgery.[116,117] Complete rehydration with intravenous fluid and adequate oral intake decreases the chance that fever will occur postdischarge as a result of dehydration.

The same precautions should be taken for the obstetric patient as for the routine surgical patient. Evidence that the stress of labor may precipitate MH is not convincing, and well-conducted epidural anesthesia for labor and delivery without dantrolene pretreatment but with careful monitoring of vital signs is recommended. If an emergency cesarean section with general anesthesia is necessary, alternatives to succinylcholine should be used. The maternal:fetal partition ratio for dantrolene is probably 0.4.[118] Dantrolene has not been reported to produce significant problems for the fetus or newborn, but existing data are very scanty.

Malignant Hyperthermia in Species Other Than Pigs and People

MH has been reported sporadically in many species. Clinical episodes have been documented in cats, dogs, and horses.[119] *Capture myopathy* is a syndrome characterized by temperature elevation, rhabdomyolysis, acidosis, and death in wild animals (e.g., zebra, elk). This also has been suggested to be an MH variant.

Medicolegal Aspects

It is not surprising that MH cases have been the subject of malpractice suits. Because MH may be considered an inborn genetic problem with a relatively fixed associated mortality that may go unrecognized before a patient's exposure to triggering agents, it may be used as a "cover" for other problems.

Fever, opisthotonic posturing, and neurologic abnormalities may accompany hypoxic brain injury, and because of their similarity to MH, MH may be incorrectly implicated in the differential diagnosis. Furthermore, after cardiac arrest from any cause, CK and potassium levels may be significantly elevated.

Some have stated that, with the advent of dantrolene, there should be no deaths from MH. This is unrealistic because the syndrome may be truly explosive in some cases and impossible to control with current therapy. When muscle is rigid, perfusion will decrease; delivery of dantrolene to muscle may be impaired, and increasing muscle acidosis and temperature will produce resistance to the effects of dantrolene. The dose of dantrolene needed to prevent recrudescence cannot be determined with certainty. Nevertheless, certain common themes underlie the basis for litigation in MH:

1. Failure to obtain a thorough personal history in regard to anesthetic problems and a family history of any unexplained perioperative problems.
2. Failure to monitor core temperature continuously with an electronic temperature monitoring device. Intraoperative temperature monitoring is now considered a "standard of care" in the United States.
3. Failure to have adequate supplies of dantrolene on hand with a plan of management of MH.

4. Failure to investigate unexplained increases in body temperature and increased skeletal muscle tone (especially after succinylcholine administration) when associated with increased heart rate and dysrhythmias.

Several examples of medicolegal cases involving these principles are described:

1. A young female patient had shoulder surgery with isoflurane–nitrous oxide–oxygen. Temperature was not monitored continuously. At the end of the procedure, premature ventricular beats and increasing end-tidal CO_2 were noted. The patient had a cardiac arrest as the dysrhythmia was being treated. As the drapes were being removed, the patient felt warm. A temperature probe revealed a reading of nearly 42°C. The patient was diagnosed as having an acute episode of MH. Dantrolene was administered an hour later. The patient developed DIC over the next day and died. The case was settled out of court.
2. A 26-year-old woman was undergoing a breast augmentation in a plastic surgeon's office using general anesthesia with isoflurane. Toward the end of the procedure, her heart rate increased as did end-tidal CO_2 and skin temperature. Dantrolene was not available and the patient was sent to a nearby emergency department. By the time dantrolene was given, her temperature was about 43°C. She developed DIC and died. The case was settled without jury trial. The company providing insurance for the physician now mandates that dantrolene be immediately available wherever general anesthesia is administered.
3. Symptoms of bowel obstruction developed in a middle-aged man. He was taken to a local hospital, and anesthesia was administered with nitrous oxide–oxygen–halothane and succinylcholine. His temperature was not monitored, but an unexplained tachycardia (140 to 160 beats/min) was present throughout the 2-hour procedure. On arrival in the intensive care unit after the operation, the patient was slightly hypotensive. Invasive monitoring was started. Despite marked metabolic and respiratory acidosis, a $PaCO_2$ of 100 mm Hg, and a recorded temperature of nearly 42°C, MH was not diagnosed. A cooling blanket and antibiotics failed to arrest the decrease in the patient's blood pressure, which eventually led to cardiac arrest. A judgment against the physicians and hospital of $4.5 million was reached.

There have been several malpractice cases filed against anesthesiologists in which cardiac arrest and death occurred after succinylcholine was used in patients with an undiagnosed myopathy. The usual outcome is an out-of-court settlement.

The message is clear. All facilities where general anesthesia is administered (including hospitals, outpatient surgery centers, physician offices, and dental offices) should have a full supply of dantrolene available. All patients undergoing general anesthesia should have standard monitoring, including end-tidal CO_2 and, except for brief cases, body temperature.

Patient Support Services

To answer the needs of patients and families who wished to learn more about MH and of those families whose relatives have died from MH, support groups were founded in several countries. The MHAUS provides a variety of services, such as a quarterly newsletter, *The Communicator,* with excerpts from the medical literature, explanatory articles, questions and answers, and related information, much of which is available on the Web site (www.mhaus.org). In addition MHAUS organized two hotlines so that a health care provider with an urgent question about MH or NMS can be placed in contact with a knowledgeable volunteer specialist. Approximately 30 to 40 calls a month are handled by the MH Hotline, 1-800-644-9737, and a smaller number by the Neurolept Malignant Syndrome Information Service, 1-888-667-8367.

The address of the Malignant Hyperthermia Association of the United States is 11E State Street, Box 1069, Sherburne, NY 13460-1069; FAX, 607-674-7910; phone, 1-607-674-7901. The hotline number is 1-800-MHHyper, (644-9737).

In 1989, the North American MH Registry was formed. Now based in Pittsburgh, Pennsylvania (Children's Hospital of Pittsburgh, 412-692-5464), the Registry is the repository for patient and family specific information for MH-susceptible patients. MH-susceptible patients are invited to contact the Registry. If an MHS individual wishes to join the Registry, he or she must complete a questionnaire and sign a consent form. A description of the Registry is available at www.anesth.upmc.edu. The forms used in the Registry can be reviewed at www.mhaus.org.

Pathogenesis and Etiology

Within 10 years of the first description of MH it became clear that the root cause was an abnormality (or abnormalities) in skeletal muscle biochemistry. This was first demonstrated by the observation that isolated skeletal muscle in vitro displayed enhanced contracture responses to halothane and to calcium-releasing compounds in MH-susceptible people and swine. Several other major developments contributed to the present understanding of the complex pathophysiology of MH. One was the recognition that the syndrome is genetically transmitted. This finding is significant because it suggests that a rigorous application of modern molecular genetics will lead to the identification of mutations in specific proteins causing the disorder (see Chapter 6). Another was the recognition of similarities between human MH and porcine stress syndrome. This animal model was used to evaluate drugs that caused the syndrome and elucidate the role of altered Ca^{2+} regulation in MH. This led to the finding that a mutation in the ryanodine receptor gene was associated with MH in swine[120] and in many humans. Yet another was that MH is a heterogenetic (more than one gene) disorder. Heterogeneity may account for some variability in presentation and forces investigators to consider the role of a final common pathway resulting from a mutation in any one of several different proteins. Finally, the observation that pigs or human subjects with MH susceptibility do not always experience MH when exposed to adequate triggering agents has suggested that modulators influence the expression of the syndrome.[121,122]

It has been observed that mutations (DNA variants) in the ryanodine receptor gene are associated with 80% of all cases of MH.[97] But other genetic loci may also less often be associated with MHS (Table 24-3). *RYR1* variants have also been associated with CCD,[34,123] a disorder known to predispose to MH.

Altered Calcium Regulation: The Common Final Pathway

Ultimately, the main problem in skeletal muscle leading to the signs of MH is a lack of control of myoplasmic Ca^{2+} concentration during anesthesia.[5,124] Ca^{2+} levels are controlled by a complex interaction of Ca^{2+} release from the terminal cisternae, the ATP–driven Ca^{2+} pumps at the sarcoplasmic reticulum and sarcolemma, which resequester released calcium, Na^+/Ca^{2+} exchange, several Ca^{2+} buffering proteins (calsequestrin, parvalbumin), and mitochondrial Ca^{2+} regulation (Fig. 24-3). Although several of these systems may become involved as the MHS progresses, the difficulty in Ca^{2+} regulation appears to originate in the Ca^{2+} release mechanism in the terminal cisternae, that is, the calcium channel known as the ryanodine receptor. The Ca^{2+} release mechanism could be made sensitive to anesthetics by any of several possibilities, including a mutation in the skeletal muscle calcium release channel (the ryanodine receptor, *RYR1*), a protein directly coupled to *RYR1* (e.g., dihydropyridine receptor), or an altered modulator of *RYR1* function (e.g., fatty acids). Succinylcholine opens the acetylcholine receptor and depolarizes the muscle membrane by opening the voltage-dependent sodium channels, which may have altered function in MH. Depolarization leads to Ca^{2+} release from the sarcoplasmic reticulum. Dantrolene antagonizes Ca^{2+} release from the sarcoplasmic reticulum, lowers elevated intracellular Ca^{2+} levels, and reverses an episode of MH.[5]

Understanding the Malignant Hyperthermia Defect: Necessary Concepts

A hypothesis explaining MH must account for the puzzling clinical observations surrounding this disorder. Most importantly, the large majority of these patients function normally in the absence of anesthetics. Therefore, the defect should not significantly interfere with normal muscle physiology. The defect, at least in humans, appears to be expressed significantly only in skeletal muscle. The expression of the syndrome shows a large variability among individuals. For example, 30% of patients have had up to three uneventful anesthetics before experiencing MH.[66,125] A spectrum of presentations can occur, ranging from relatively minor intraoperative complications to rapid temperature rise, muscle rigidity, acidosis, dysrhythmias, and death. Some cases have a greater latency to onset and are not made manifest until several hours postoperatively. MH does not always occur in response to triggering agents. The large variability among individuals may be explained by different genes causing MH in different families or by other predisposing factors being expressed differently in different patients or families.[126] The function of many different proteins has been reported to be altered in MH skeletal muscle. Thus, it is reasonable to assume that systems other than those directly involved in Ca^{2+} regulation are secondarily altered in MH and these may play a crucial role in modifying

TABLE 24-3

MOLECULAR GENETICS OF MALIGNANT HYPERTHERMIA

■ LOCUS NAME	■ GENE SYMBOL	■ CHROMOSOMAL LOCUS	■ PROTEIN NAME
MHS1	*RYR1*	19q13.1	Ryanodine receptor type 1
MHS5	*CACNA1S*	1q32	Voltage-dependent L-type calcium channel subunit alpha-1S

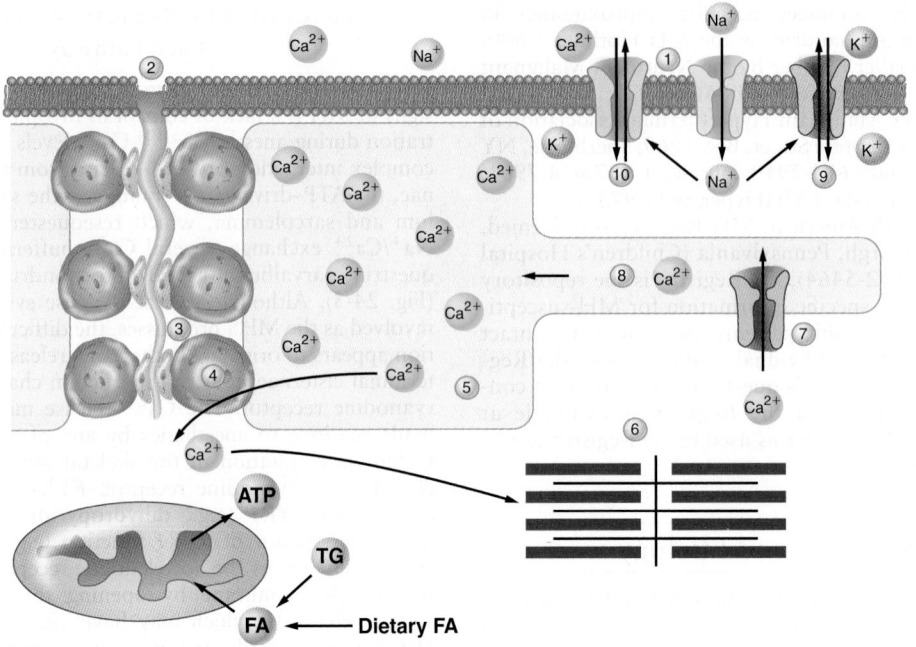

FIGURE 24-3. Excitation-contraction coupling and malignant hyperthermia. The action potential generated at the endplate region of the neuromuscular junction is propagated down the sarcolemma (muscle plasma membrane) by the opening of voltage-dependent Na^+ channels (*1*). The action potential continues down into the t-tubules (*2*) to the dihydropyridine receptors (*3*). The dihydropyridine receptors in skeletal muscle function as voltage sensors and are coupled to the Ca^{2+} release channels (*4*). Through this coupled signaling process, the Ca^{2+} release channels are opened, some of the available terminal cisternae Ca^{2+} stores (*5*) are released, and the levels of myoplasmic Ca^{2+} are elevated. The Ca^{2+} then diffuses to the myofibrils (*6*) and interacts with the troponin/tropomyosin complex associated with actin (*thin lines*) and allows interaction of actin with myosin (*thick lines*) for mechanical movement. The Ca^{2+} diffuses away from the myofibrils and this Ca^{2+} signal is terminated by an adenosine triphosphate (ATP)-driven Ca^{2+} pump (*7*), which pumps Ca^{2+} into the longitudinal sarcoplasmic reticulum (*8*). The Ca^{2+} diffuses from the longitudinal sarcoplasmic reticulum to the terminal cisternae, where it is concentrated for release by Ca^{2+} binding proteins. Na^+ entering during the action potential is subsequently extruded from the cell by the Na^+/K^+-ATPase (*9*) and possibly through Na^+/Ca^{2+} exchange (*10*). This latter process would elevate intracellular Ca^{2+} and could result from delayed inactivation of Na^+ currents. A major form of energy for supplying cellular ATP for the ion pumps and numerous other energy consuming processes is fatty acids (FA) derived from the serum (dietary FA), or from intramuscular triglyceride (TG) stores. Therefore, a defect in the intracellular Ca^{2+} regulating processes (increased Ca^{2+} release or decreased Ca^{2+} uptake), or a defect in the sarcolemma could account for an increase in myoplasmic Ca^{2+}.

the response to triggering agents. The involvement of secondary systems would explain the high variability in the phenotype. Such modifying proteins, genes, or other chemical compounds are yet to be clearly defined.

The Sarcolemma and MH

The sarcolemma (Fig. 24-3) maintains the membrane potential of the muscle cell and acts as a permeability barrier to ions, including Na^+, K^+, Cl^-, and Ca^{2+}. Skeletal muscle, in most cases, does not require extracellular Ca^{2+} for nerve or electrically evoked contractility. In contrast, halothane-induced contractures[124,127] and, to a lesser extent (depending on the species), caffeine-induced contractures[124] require extracellular Ca^{2+}. However, the sarcolemma per se has not been implicated directly in the pathophysiology of MH.

Terminal Cisternae: Ca^{2+} Release. The terminal cisternae of the sarcoplasmic reticulum are the sites of Ca^{2+} sequestration. They are coupled to the t-tubules through the ryanodine receptor and the dihydropyridine receptor (Fig. 24-4; also see Fig. 24-3). Several investigators have reported a hypersensitive Ca^{2+}-induced Ca^{2+} release in terminal cisternae preparations from porcine MH muscle.[128–130]

In muscle preparations containing triads and sarcoplasmic reticulum, halothane at clinically relevant concentrations cannot induce a sustained net Ca^{2+} release if physiologic levels of ATP and Mg^{2+} are included. This ability to overcome the effects of halothane under approximate physiologic conditions is because of the enormous capacity of the Ca^{2+} pumping system. The addition of fatty acids, even to vesicles isolated from normal muscle, markedly (approximately 20- to 30-fold) decreases the concentration of halothane required for the sustained opening of the Ca^{2+} release channel in the presence of ATP and Mg^{2+}. Under these conditions, fatty acids can cause a sustained Ca^{2+} release at clinical concentrations of halothane. Unlike studies of Ca^{2+} release in the absence of fatty acids, there is an absolute temperature dependence (occurs at 37°C, not at 25°C) of the fatty acid enhancement of halothane-induced Ca^{2+} release, which is consistent with the temperature dependence of halothane-induced contractures of MH muscle.[131] Hence, the type and concentration of fatty acids may modulate the expression of MH.

Mitochondria. Mitochondria oxidize a variety of substrates to generate the form of energy (ATP) most useful for driving cellular reactions. Defects in mitochondrial function do not appear to initiate the MHS, although they may produce increased temperature, acidosis, and cardiovascular failure.

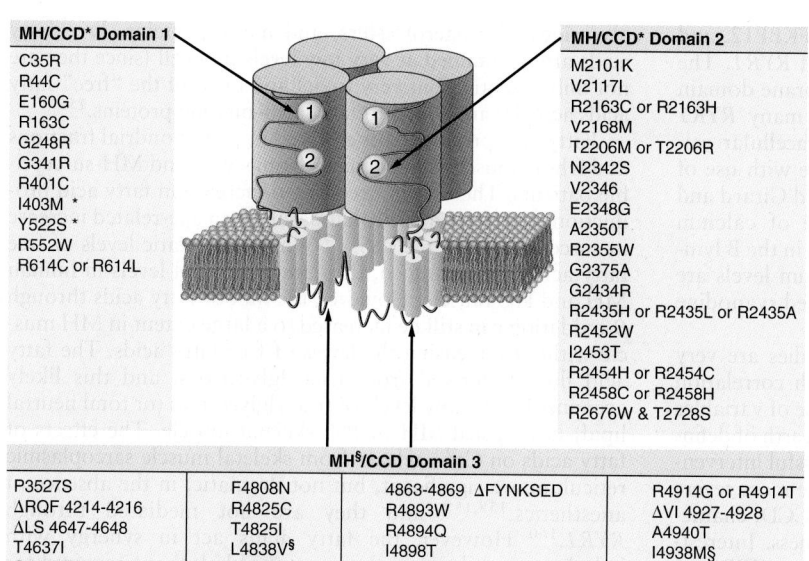

MH/CCD* Domain 1
C35R
R44C
E160G
R163C
G248R
G341R
R401C
I403M *
Y522S *
R552W
R614C or R614L

MH/CCD* Domain 2
M2101K
V2117L
R2163C or R2163H
V2168M
T2206M or T2206R
N2342S
V2346
E2348G
A2350T
R2355W
G2375A
G2434R
R2435H or R2435L or R2435A
R2452W
I2453T
R2454H or R2454C
R2458C or R2458H
R2676W & T2728S

FIGURE 24-4. Schematic illustration of the homotetrameric ryanodine receptor, the calcium release channel situated in the membrane of the sarcoplasmic reticulum. The cytosolic part of the protein complex, the so-called foot, bridges the gap between the transverse tubular system and the sarcoplasmic reticulum. Mutations have been described for the skeletal muscle ryanodine receptor (RYR1), which cause susceptibility to malignant hyperthermia (MH) and central core disease (CCD). (Reprinted from Treves S, Anderson AA, Ducreux S, et al: Ryanodine receptor 1 mutations, dysregulation of calcium homeostasis and neuromuscular disorders. Neuromusc Disord 1:2005; 5: 577, with permission.)

MH§/CCD Domain 3			
P3527S	F4808N	4863-4869 ΔFYNKSED	R4914G or R4914T
ΔRQF 4214-4216	R4825C	R4893W	ΔVI 4927-4928
ΔLS 4647-4648	T4825I	R4894Q	A4940T
T4637I	L4838V§	I4898T	I4938M§
G4638D	V4849I	G4891R	A14646+2.9kb
H4651P	Δ4860	G4899R	
L4796C	R4861H	A4906V	

Longitudinal Sarcoplasmic Reticulum: Ca^{2+} Uptake. The longitudinal sarcoplasmic reticulum (Fig. 24-3) is primarily involved in removing Ca^{2+} from the myoplasm through the ATP–driven Ca^{2+} pump. While earlier studies had suggested a defect in Ca^{2+} uptake might cause the loss of Ca^{2+} regulation associated with MH, subsequent studies have ruled out a role for the Ca^{2+} pump in causing MH.

Myofibrils. No defect in the Ca^{2+} sensitivity of the fast or slow fibers of the contractile system from MH skeletal muscle has been observed.

Calcium Release Channel of Skeletal Muscle and its role in MH

The human skeletal muscle calcium release channel is encoded by a ryanodine receptor type 1 (RYR1) gene located on chromosome 19q13.1.[132] (Fig. 24-4). There are other types of RYR that exist in cardiac muscle (type 2) and brain (type 3) tissues, respectively. However, those organs do not appear to be involved primarily in the pathophysiology of MH. RYR1 is the primary conduit through which the sarcoplasmic reticulum stores of Ca^{2+} are released to the sarcoplasm. RYR1 is an extremely large homotetramer, having subunits of about 560,000 MW each. RYR1 has binding sites for the contracture-inducing plant alkaloid ryanodine[133] and the preservative 4-CmC.[134]

🔟 Susceptibility to MH is associated with mutations in RYR1.[94,135,136] The hypothesis that mutation in RYR1 causes MH susceptibility is supported by physiologic studies showing subtle effects of halothane on isolated RYR1 currents in human MH muscle.[137] Halothane can open a hypersensitive RYR1, leading to an uncontrolled release of Ca^{2+} into the myoplasm and the MHS. However, the buffering capacity of the Ca^{2+} pump in the presence of ATP is able to sustain normal Ca^{2+} regulation in the presence of halothane in terminal cisternae preparations isolated from MH muscle. These observations are consistent with the observed interindividual variability in human MH and the occurrence of nonrigid MH. When ATP is low, the syndrome occurs, and the lower the energy stores, the worse the MH syndrome is.

Consistent with the altered function of RYR1, there has been a specific mutation identified (Arg^{615} to Cys^{615}) in RYR1 in susceptible swine.[138] The mutation is on the cytoplasmic surface of RYR1.[139] It accounts for the altered functional states of RYR1 and ryanodine binding in these animals. The human equivalent

(Arg^{614} to Cys^{614}) to the swine RYR1 mutation has been identified in 2 to 11% of MH families, depending on population studied. However, in some cases there is a discordance between the presence of this mutation and the outcome of the diagnostic contracture test.[140–142] A major reason for the attenuated effects of the RYR1 mutation in human muscle is likely the dominant mode of inheritance with reduced penetrance and genetic heterogeneity of MH versus recessive mutation in the pig. Thus, normal copies of RYR1 are expressed in human MH muscle, but not susceptible animal muscle. The number of sequence variants in RYR1 associated with MH to date is >150, including Arg614Cys, and this number is constantly rising. Many of these are found in only a few families.

In summary, there are physiologic, biochemical, pharmacologic, and molecular genetic data supporting a mutation in RYR1 as an important factor, and perhaps an initiating factor, in >70% of the families with MH. The effects of the altered RYR1 function on Ca^{2+} regulation determined in vitro are not as pronounced in humans as in swine, possibly owing to the dominant mode of inheritance and genetic heterogeneity of MH in humans. It is highly probable that other systems come into play as modulators of the MH response. This may better explain the extreme intra- and interindividual variability in the human MH syndrome, which is in contrast to the more consistent response in MH swine.

Molecular Biology of Malignant Hyperthermia

The identification of the porcine mutation causing porcine stress syndrome, and the location of the human RYR1 gene on chromosome 19q13.1, has helped to establish a direct link of this gene to MH.[132,143] About 70% of MH families have a RYR1 variant.

RYR1 is one of the largest human genes. It contains 106 exons that are transcribed into a 15,364 nucleotide mRNA. Transcription occurs mainly in skeletal muscle. More than 200 different sequence variants have been identified in RYR1. The majority are clustered in three regions: the N-terminal region between codons 34 and 614, the central region between codons 2163 and 2458, and the C-terminal region between codons 4136 and 4973.[94,96, 123,135, 144] This preferential localization raised speculations concerning the specific role of these regions. The central region is close to the region where the protein would interact with the regulatory protein, FKBP12, and the dihydropyridine receptor, a voltage sensor of *RYR1*. The C-terminal region corresponds to the transmembrane domain of the protein.[123] The pathogenic character of many *RYR1* mutations has been studied by measures of intracellular calcium release in response to caffeine or halothane with use of different cell lines.[145,146] Sei and colleagues[147] and Girard and colleagues[148] have demonstrated the presence of calcium channels similar to those found in skeletal muscle in the B lymphocyte along with enhanced intracellular calcium levels are found in lymphocytes from cell lines with mutated ryanodine genes on exposure to caffeine or chlorocresol.

The phenotype and genotype correlation studies are very limited in MH because it is difficult to establish correlation between the mutation and contractile data because of variables among diagnostic laboratories and because of a dearth of definitive clinical episodes of MHS as a result of successful intervention during onset of an episode. Nevertheless, the most severe phenotype associated with *RYR1* mutation(s) is CCD, characterized by marked hypotonia and muscle weakness. Interestingly, the majority of *RYR1* mutations causing CCD are located in the transmembrane region of the protein, suggesting a critical role of this region in Ca^{2+} regulation. In addition, the mutations causing both MH and CCD (R163C, R2163H, and R2435H) exhibit more severe caffeine and halothane responses than those associated with MH alone.[149]

Genetic studies have identified linkage of four other chromosomal regions to MH, suggesting genetic heterogeneity of the disorder, including MHS2 at 17q11.2-q24, MHS3 at 7q21-q22, and MHS6 at 5p. However, only one gene other than *RYR1* has been identified (Table 24-3). The Arg1086His mutation was identified in the *CACNL1A3*, also referred to as the *CACNA1S* gene, of a large French MH family. *CACNL1A3* codes for the α_1 subunit of the dihydropyridine receptor (*DHPR*) the voltage sensor for *RYR1*.[150] Mutational screening studies, however, indicate that only 1% of MHS families exhibit mutations in the *DHPR*. No mutation has been found in the MHS 3 locus in a MHS family.

As mentioned already, discordance between segregation of mutations identified in *RYR1* and the outcome of the in vitro contracture test for MH[140,141,151,152] has been reported. This discordance is uncommon and the reasons for it range from specimen mix-up or false-positive contracture test to silencing of the expression of the abnormal gene. In contrast, a study in swine has demonstrated that there is an excellent correlation between the contracture test outcome and the genetic susceptibility for MH. In human families, specific ryanodine mutations usually correlate extremely well with the in vitro contracture test result. Hence, in a particular family the presence of the familial MH mutation predicts MH susceptibility with an extremely high specificity.[153]

Do Fatty Acids Contribute to the Pathophysiology of Malignant Hyperthermia?

One theory accounting for the observed clinical variability of the MHS postulates a role for free fatty acids in the pathophysiology of the syndrome.

Lipids are an important component of a cell, as they provide energy and structure (e.g., membranes) and participate in function. Several lipid metabolites, including fatty acids, serve second-messenger functions.[154] Fatty acids are the major source of energy in the resting state of skeletal muscle and can also contribute up to 65% of the energy during exercise.[155] Fatty acids provide about 70% of the energy in resting muscle. Therefore, fatty acid utilization is likely up-regulated in MH muscle to compensate for the energy consumed by the adenosine triphosphatases to maintain Na^+ and Ca^{2+} homeostasis.

In addition to existing in a free form, fatty acids are esterified to phospholipids, triacylglycerides, diacylglycerides, monoacyl-

glycerides, cholesterol esters, and many proteins. Free fatty acids are maintained at very low levels in a cell (since they are not only essential, but very toxic) and most of the "free" fatty acids actually are bound to fatty acid–binding proteins.[156]

Fatty acid production is elevated in mitochondrial fractions and whole-muscle homogenates from swine and MH-susceptible patients. There is an age-related increase in fatty acid production in skeletal muscle that parallels an age-related increase in susceptibility to the PSS.[157] When only static levels of free fatty acids are examined, they are at normal levels in human MH and PSS muscle. However, the flux of fatty acids through β-oxidation can still be increased to a large extent in MH muscle without increasing the levels of free fatty acids. The fatty acid flux is derived from triacylglycerides, and this likely accounts for the low levels of triacylglycerides (or total neutral lipid) in biopsied MH or PSS skeletal muscle. The effects of fatty acids on Ca^{2+} release from skeletal muscle sarcoplasmic reticulum are significant, but not dramatic, in the absence of anesthetics,[158,159] and they are not mediated through *RYR1*.[160] However, the fatty acids act in synergy with halothane and decrease the amount of halothane required for sustained Ca^{2+} release by 20- to 30-fold![122,129] This fatty acid enhancement of halothane-induced Ca^{2+} release, in contrast with all other studies of Ca^{2+} release, exhibits the same temperature dependence (i.e., it occurs only at 37°C, not at 25°C) as halothane-induced contractures of skeletal muscle and is mediated through *RYR1*.[122] While the concentration of fatty acid required for this effect exceeds that of the normal unbound form, halothane can displace fatty acids from fatty acid–binding proteins.[161] Therefore, it is highly likely that sufficient concentrations of fatty acids could be achieved at the site of halothane action. If the production of free fatty acids is sustained by accelerated triacylglyceride breakdown and the fatty acids are shunted toward acylation of *RYR1* and the sodium channel, then this could lead to greatly elevated myoplasmic Ca^{2+} levels. In the case of *RYR1*, this would lead to a greater sensitivity to halothane.

The Future of Research in Malignant Hyperthermia

While molecular genetics has dominated the research in MH in recent years, a deeper understanding of the physiology and biochemistry of the interplay among *RYR1*, the Na^+ channel, and fatty acid metabolism still is needed. DNA-based linkage analyses are no longer pursued to the same extent as in the early 1990s. Instead, the focus of recent molecular genetic studies has been on identifying new mutations in *RYR1* and the phenotypic effects associated with such mutations.[162] Further linkage studies are necessary to identify other genes linked to MH.

⓫   It seems clear that the accuracy of molecular genetic testing for MH susceptibility will improve as additional mutations are found to be causal for MH. As such, genetic testing will increasingly replace the contracture test despite the numerous DNA changes that are likely to be causal. With advances in molecular genetics technology, it is likely that it will be possible to screen for all mutations in a cost-effective manner.

One of the major clinical concerns of MH-susceptible patients is their possible risk for heat stroke, exercise-induced rhabdomyolysis, and other environmental stressors that might affect muscle function. DNA testing facilitates evaluation of those who have experienced one of these nonanesthetic-associated problems. But to rule out the diagnosis of MHS, it is still necessary to undergo muscle biopsy and contracture testing. Genes other than *RYR1* influence the response of muscle to exercise.[163] Creation of the "knock-in" mouse model for MH, whereby one of the causal mutations is incorporated into the mouse genome, has shown that indeed high environmental temperature[6,7] is fatal in these animals. Such artificial constructs will likely reveal more information concerning genotype and phenotype.

Summary

Mutations associated with skeletal muscle control of intracellular calcium by the *RYR1* channel are causal for most cases of classic MH. Any one of three different genes may cause MH, although the exact proteins that are abnormal in MH remain to be identified in some cases. Mutations have been identified in *RYR1* and in the dihydropyridine receptor gene. A variety of poorly understood biochemical and/or gene expression factors influence the clinical manifestations of MH. For example, mutations in a sodium channel subunit may be associated with some signs of MH, but this clinical MH requires the expression of other factors also. A disturbance in fatty acid metabolism, as a secondary effect, alters the function of several organelles and can lead to a hypersensitive *RYR1* response to halothane and altered Na⁺ channel subunit expression in skeletal muscle. The MHS is the result of a complex and poorly understood interaction among several systems in skeletal muscle.

OTHER INHERITED DISORDERS

Inherited diseases affect every bodily organ and every physiologic and biochemical process. Some are mild and allow a relatively normal life span, whereas others are incompatible with extrauterine existence even for a few days. Adding to the complexity is a natural variability of genetic penetrance and expressivity even in a single family. All of these disorders have as a common feature an abnormality in one or more genes that affects the function of one or more enzymes. The metabolic basis of inherited diseases is the subject of several well-known books, which may be consulted for an in-depth appreciation of our state of knowledge of many of these disorders.

DISORDERS OF PLASMA CHOLINESTERASE

Plasma cholinesterase, pseudocholinesterase, or butyrylcholinesterase (BChE) is an enzyme with a molecular weight of 320,000 and a tetrahedral structure. The four exons that code for this protein are located on chromosome 3q26. BChE is found in plasma and most tissue but not in red blood cells. BChE degrades acetylcholine released at the neuromuscular junction, as well as other choline and aliphatic esters.[164] The half-life of BChE has been estimated to be 8 to 16 hours. It is very stable in serum samples and can be stored for long periods of time at –20°C with little or no activity loss. BChE is synthesized in the liver. Therefore, BChE activity is decreased in advanced cases of hepatocellular dysfunction from any cause.

Inherited variants of BChE are of interest to the anesthesiologist because the duration of action of succinylcholine and (in some cases) ester-linked local anesthetics, as well as the toxicity of cocaine,[165] is a function of the activity of this enzyme (see Chapter 20). Prolonged apnea after succinylcholine administration occurs in patients who have low absolute activity of BChE or enzyme variants.[166,167] Low BChE activity predisposes patients to toxicity from standard doses of anti-Alzheimer drugs.[168] Otherwise, BChE-deficient patients have no symptoms.

Many physiologic, pharmacologic, and pathologic factors can either increase or decrease the activity of this enzyme to a significant extent (Table 24-4). Only when there is a >75% decrease in the levels of the normal BChE is there clinically evident prolongation of succinylcholine activity.

TABLE 24-4

SOME CAUSES OF CHANGES IN CHOLINESTERASE ACTIVITY[a]

■ INHERITED

Cholinesterase variants that may lead to decreased or increased activity (e.g., silent gene or C5 variant)

■ PHYSIOLOGIC

Decreases in last trimester of pregnancy
Reduced activity of the newborn

■ ACQUIRED DECREASES

Liver diseases
Carcinoma
Debilitating diseases
Collagen diseases
Uremia
Malnutrition
Myxedema

■ ACQUIRED INCREASES

Obesity
Alcoholism
Thyrotoxicosis
Nephrosis
Psoriasis
Electroshock therapy

■ DRUGS RELATED TO DISEASES

Neostigmine
Pyridostigmine
Chlorpromazine
Echothiophate iodide
Cyclophosphamide
Monoamine oxidase inhibitors
Pancuronium
Contraceptives
Organophosphorus insecticides
Hexafluorenium

■ OTHER CAUSES OF DECREASED ACTIVITY

Plasmapheresis
Extracorporeal circulation
Tetanus
Radiation therapy
Burns

[a]The significance of these factors depends on the severity of disease, drug dosage, and individual variation.
Adapted from Whittaker M: Plasma cholinesterase variants and the anesthetist. Anaesthesia 1980; 35: 174.

Succinylcholine-Related Apnea

Succinylcholine is hydrolyzed by a two-step process, first to succinylmonocholine and then to succinic acid. It has been estimated that only about 5% of the injected drug reaches the endplate region because of a combination of both hydrolysis and diffusion from the plasma. Urinary excretion and protein binding play unimportant roles in the disposition of the drug when BChE activity is normal. The rate of metabolism determines the duration of action of succinylcholine.

A variety of assay procedures are available for BChE. However, most involve the reaction of a thiocholine (e.g.,

TABLE 24-5

BIOCHEMICAL CHARACTERISTICS OF SOME CHOLINESTERASE VARIANTS

■ GENOTYPE	■ ACTIVITY	■ DIBUCAINE NUMBER	■ FLUORIDE NUMBER	■ CHLORIDE NUMBER	■ SUCCINYLCHO-LINE NUMBER
EuEu	677–1,860	78–86	55–65	1–12	89–98
EaEa	140–525	18–26	16–32	46–58	4–19
EuEa	285–1008	51–70	38–55	15–34	51–78
EuEf	579–900	74–80	47–48	14–30	87–91
EfEa	475–661	49–59	25–33	31–36	56–59
EfEs	351	63	26	25	81

Eu, normal enzyme gene; Ea, atypical enzyme gene; Ef, fluoride-resistant gene; Es, silent gene.
Reproduced from Viby-Mogensen J: Succinylcholine neuromuscular blockade in subjects homozygous for atypical plasma cholinesterase. Anesthesiology 1981; 55: 429, with permission.

butyrylthiocholine) with serum- or plasma-containing cholinesterase. The reaction product is coupled with 5,5′-dithiobis(2-nitrobenzoic acid) and forms a colored product that can be followed spectrophotometrically. The use of benzoylcholine, a specific substrate for BChE, avoids contamination of the assay for BChE by the esterase in red blood cells that is released when hemolysis occurs.

Kalow and Genest[169] were the first to show that qualitative as well as quantitative differences in BChE determine the duration of succinylcholine apnea. They found that in certain persons displaying succinylcholine sensitivity, the local anesthetic dibucaine (Nupercaine) inhibited the hydrolysis of a benzoylcholine substrate less than it inhibited the reaction in those displaying a normal response to succinylcholine. Thus, this atypical phenotype may be referred to as *dibucaine-resistant*. The percentage inhibition of the reaction was termed the *dibucaine number*. It was found to be constant for a person and did not depend on the concentration of the enzyme.

A discontinuous distribution of dibucaine numbers suggested an inheritance pattern based on alteration at a single gene locus (Table 24-5). Those with dibucaine numbers in the range of 80 would be homozygous normal with a normal response to succinylcholine; those with dibucaine numbers of 20 would be homozygous atypical with a marked prolongation of succinylcholine activity; and those with dibucaine numbers in the 60 range would be heterozygous and, in general, have a normal response to succinylcholine.

Many point mutations have been discovered. Nevertheless, the effects of these mutations are still described by a few categories of functional change. In one case, the silent type, enzyme is not produced. In the other, there is a differential inhibition of BChE by fluoride.[170] In those with prolonged duration of succinylcholine activity with this genotype, fluoride ion inhibits the in vitro hydrolysis of substrate by the enzyme less than it does in normal patients. Thus, the phenotype may be referred to as *fluoride-resistant*. A *fluoride number,* similar to a dibucaine number, is thereby created. Other variants exist, including the K variant, which can be identified only by genetic analysis, not by the current tests of substrate degradation.

When there is a question of succinylcholine sensitivity, the absolute activity of BChE should be determined as well as the dibucaine and fluoride numbers. In some cases, because of biologic variability or unusual combinations of genotype (e.g., combination of atypical and fluoride genes), it is helpful to use other inhibitors of the cholinesterase reaction in genotyping the patient. Bromide, urea, sodium chloride, and succinylcholine have been used to distinguish the various genotypes (Table 24-5).

Molecular genetic techniques have been successfully applied to BChE variants. Primo-Parma et al.[171] and McGuire et al.[172]

identified a point mutation in the gene for human BChE in which a nucleotide change leads to an alteration of a single amino acid (adenine to guanine) in the protein. This change apparently alters the affinity of atypical BChE for choline esters. Other base pair alterations account for other atypical variants, including the K and J silent gene variants, which, although common, produce little to no clinical prolongation of succinylcholine action (Table 24-6).

In European studies, the approximate percentages in the population of the genotypes are as follows: EuEu (96%), EuEa (2.5%), EuEf or EuEs (0.3%), EaEf (0.005%), EaEa (0.05%), and EfEf or EfEs (0.006%).[173] Patients homozygous for atypical, fluoride, or silent genes as well as those with the combination of atypical with fluoride, atypical with silent genes, or fluoride with silent genes should wear safety identification bracelets indicating that succinylcholine administration will lead to prolonged apnea. Relatives should be tested as well.

Clinical Implications of Pseudocholinesterase Abnormalities

Important questions for the anesthesiologist are: Which patients are at risk for development of an abnormal response to succinylcholine? What are the clinical characteristics of this response? What are the treatment options?

Significant prolongation of succinylcholine's effects occurs in the following genotypes: EaEa, EfEf, EaEs, EfEa, and EsEs. The more common situations in which homozygote normal patients and heterozygotes are at risk are as follows: patients who have been receiving echothiophate eyedrops (up to 2 weeks after therapy is discontinued), patients who are undergoing plasmapheresis, patients with severe liver disease, and patients (particularly heterozygotes) who have received succinylcholine after reversal of nondepolarizing blockade with neostigmine.

TABLE 24-6

STRUCTURAL CHANGES OF BChE VARIANTS

Fluoride-2	117 GLY → Frame shift
Atypical	70ASP → GLY
Silent	117 GLY → Frame shift
Fluoride-1	243 THR → MET
Fluoride-2	390 GLY → VAL
K Variant	539 ALA → THR
H Variant	142 VAL → MET
J Variant	497 GLU → VAL

Viby-Mogensen[166,167] has studied the question of BChE apnea in detail. His cholinesterase unit found that 6.2% of patients who displayed apnea for 50 to 250 minutes after a "usual" dose of succinylcholine had an acquired deficiency of BChE. He then studied 70 patients who were genotypically normal for BChE and administered 1.0 mg/kg of succinylcholine during a 50% nitrous oxide–oxygen–1% halothane anesthetic and followed the depression and return of thumb twitch. He found that there was indeed a relationship between the duration of apnea, the return of a full twitch response, and BChE activity. However, only moderate prolongation of apnea was found when BChE was depressed by as much as 70%. Apnea is significantly prolonged only with extreme depression of BChE activity.

In a second study with a similar protocol, he found that heterozygotes having one normal gene (e.g., EuEa, EuEf) had a normal response to succinylcholine, including typical fasciculations and a depolarizing type of block with train-of-four stimulations.[167] However, heterozygotes without the usual gene (e.g., EaEf) had a prolonged response to succinylcholine, with apnea lasting as long as 24 minutes. Apnea lasts from 120 minutes to >300 minutes in homozygous atypical patients (EaEa) when they are given succinylcholine.[167] The other class of patients who regularly display prolonged apnea after succinylcholine administration comprises patients who are homozygous for the silent gene.

Treatment of Succinylcholine Apnea

The safest course of treatment when the patient fails to breathe 10 to 15 minutes after succinylcholine administration is to continue mechanical ventilation until adequate muscle tone has returned. Two units of fresh-frozen plasma may contain adequate amounts of BChE to hydrolyze the succinylcholine,[174] although blood transfusion is not recommended for routine treatment of succinylcholine-induced apnea.

The use of cholinesterase inhibitors in treating succinylcholine apnea is controversial. If they are administered before there is evidence of fade with train-of-four stimulation, there may be a transient improvement followed by intensification of the neuromuscular block. Remember that neostigmine inhibits the degradation of succinylcholine by BChE. The best chance for reversal of succinylcholine-related apnea in these situations occurs when no more than 0.03 mg/kg of neostigmine is given 90 to 120 minutes after succinylcholine when a nondepolarizing type of blockade is present.

C5 Variant

An isoenzyme of BChE has been demonstrated whereby the hydrolysis of succinylcholine is increased, and therefore the duration of apnea is decreased after succinylcholine administration. The gene does not appear to be an allele of the Eu and Ea gene and is found infrequently in the population.[175]

Plasma Cholinesterase Abnormalities and the Metabolism of Local Anesthetics

Although the ester-linked local anesthetics (e.g., procaine, tetracaine, 2-chloroprocaine) are metabolized by BChE, prolongation of block and/or clinical toxicity of these local anesthetics in homozygous atypical patients has rarely been documented.[176,177] Jatlow et al.[178] have shown delayed hydrolysis of cocaine in vitro with plasma from homozygote atypical patients. They theorized that such persons may be at risk for toxic reaction from normal doses of cocaine.

THE PORPHYRIAS

All the porphyrias result from a defect in heme synthesis. The heme pigments are tetrapyrroles that are the essential elements in hemoglobin, myoglobin, and the cytochromes. That is, compounds that are involved in the transport of oxygen, activation of oxygen, and the electron transport chain. Cytochrome P450 is a hemoprotein intimately involved in the conversion of lipid-soluble nonpolar drugs to soluble polar compounds that may be excreted in the urine.

A complete deficiency of enzymes that are involved in heme synthesis is incompatible with life. However, a partial deficiency may lead to the accumulation of one or more of the molecular intermediates in heme production. Such an accumulation of precursors is responsible for the clinical manifestations of the porphyrias in an as-yet unexplained manner.

The rate-limiting step in heme synthesis is the conjugation of succinyl-CoA with glycine to form D-aminolevulinic acid (the enzyme is aminolevulinic acid synthetase). In the porphyrias, there is a partial deficiency of enzymes subsequent to this initial step, which results in a stimulation of this reaction to form aminolevulinic acid. The result is overproduction of intermediate products before the deficient step (Fig. 24-5).

The porphyrias generally manifest after puberty. Inheritance is autosomal dominant, except for the autosomal recessive congenital erythropoietic porphyria.

A functional classification for the anesthesiologist is based on a division of the porphyrias into inducible and noninducible. The inducible porphyrias are those in which the acute symptoms are precipitated on drug exposure (Table 24-6).[179] Acute intermittent porphyria, variegate porphyria, and hereditary coproporphyria are inducible. These porphyrias cause an acute neurologic syndrome with a variety of presentations. Cutaneous manifestations, with particular sensitivity

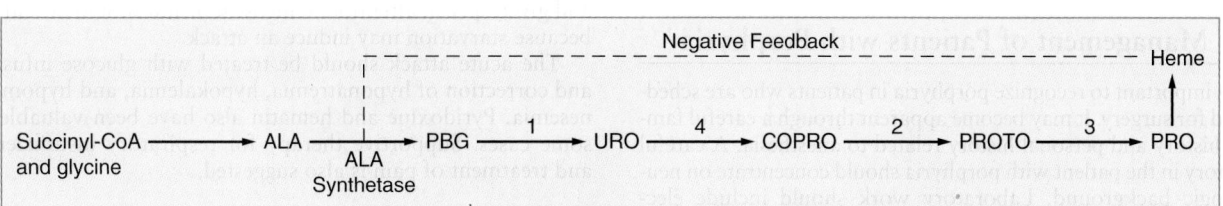

FIGURE 24-5. Biosynthesis of heme and sites of defects in certain porphyrias. In intermittent acute porphyria, there is a partial deficiency of the enzyme at site 1. In hereditary coproporphyria, there is an enzyme deficiency at site 2. In variegate porphyria, the enzyme problem is at site 3. In porphyria cutanea tarda, there is a deficiency at site 4. ALA, aminolevulinic acid; PBG, porphobilinogen; URO, uroporphyrinogen; COPRO, coproporphyrinogen; PROTO, protoporphyrinogen; PRO, protoporphyrin. (Reprinted from Mees DL, Frederickson EL: Anesthesia and the porphyrias. South Med J 1975; 68: 29, with permission.)

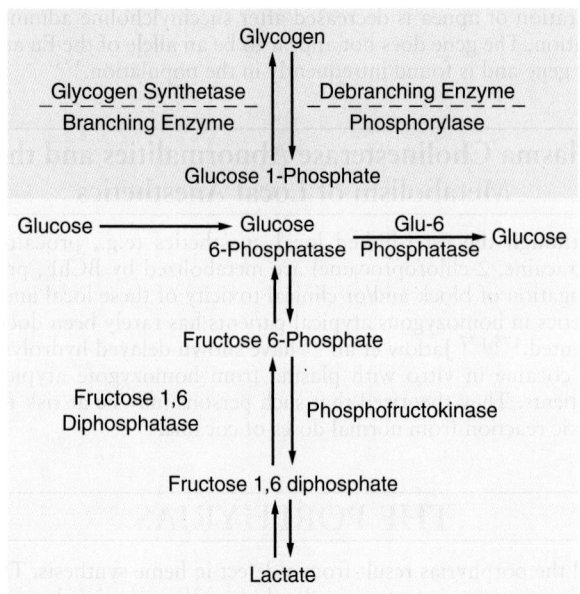

FIGURE 24-6.   The glycogen–glucose–lactate pathway. GLU-6, glucose 6-phosphatase.

to ultraviolet light exhibited by skin fragility and bleeding, are other chief features of the porphyrias. About 80% of patients with variegate porphyria are photosensitive. Some patients with hereditary coproporphyria also may have skin lesions. The porphyrias are very difficult to diagnose in the latent phase of the disorder. Direct assay of the intermediates themselves may be used in the acute state to measure the elevated levels of the heme intermediates.

The central, peripheral, and autonomic nervous systems may be involved in the porphyrias. A frequent manifestation is colicky abdominal pain, often with nausea and vomiting, which may suggest the diagnosis of acute abdomen, leading to exploratory laparotomy. Other symptoms are psychiatric disturbance, quadriplegia, hemiplegia, alterations of consciousness, and pain. Hyponatremia and hypokalemia may result from vomiting during the acute attack or may be related to hypothalamic disturbance. Death may result from paralysis of the respiratory muscles. The cause of these changes is unknown; they may be related to metabolites of the intermediates or result from deficiency of the heme pigment in the nerve cell itself.

Because the porphyrias are unusual disorders, there is limited experience with the clinical use of many anesthetic drugs. In vitro studies suggest that certain anesthetics or anesthetic adjuvants may be contraindicated, but sufficient clinical experience is lacking.[180]

Management of Patients with Porphyria

It is important to recognize porphyria in patients who are scheduled for surgery. It may become apparent through a careful family history and personal history related to anesthesia. A careful history in the patient with porphyria should concentrate on neurologic background. Laboratory work should include electrolyte and blood urea nitrogen levels. Physical examination includes inspection of cutaneous lesions over the body.

In the anesthetic management of patients with porphyria, the chief concern is to avoid the administration of drugs that can induce a crisis; the drugs that induce cytochrome enzyme production can trigger the syndrome. Chief among those are the barbiturates; therefore, all barbiturates are contraindicated

TABLE 24-7

DRUGS KNOWN TO PRECIPITATE PORPHYRIA

■ SEDATIVES

Barbiturates
Hypnotics such as chlordiazepoxide, glutethimide, diazepam

■ ANALGESICS

Pentazocine, antipyrine, aminopyridine
Lidocaine

■ ANTICONVULSANTS

Phenytoin, methsuximide

■ ANTIBIOTICS

Sulfonamides, chloramphenicol

■ STEROIDS

Estrogens, progesterones

■ HYPOGLYCEMIC SULFONYLUREAS

Tolbutamide, chlorpropamide

■ TOXINS

Lead, ethanol

■ MISCELLANEOUS

Ergot preparations
Amphetamines
Methyldopa

in porphyria. Ethyl alcohol, nonbarbiturate sedatives, hydantoin anticonvulsants, and a variety of other drugs also can induce a crisis (Table 24-7). Other factors, such as fasting, infection, and estrogens, may also precipitate porphyria. Diagnosis can be especially difficult because attacks may occur at a variable time after drug administration or they may not occur at all despite administration of inducing drugs.

Propofol appears to be a safe induction agent.[181] Nitrous oxide, muscle relaxants, and opioids are unequivocally safe drugs. Experience with other inhalation agents[182] and reversal agents has been favorable, but in vitro studies suggest that they might exacerbate a crisis.

Most experts have advised that regional techniques be avoided to prevent confusion should neurologic signs develop after operation. However, reports of uneventful epidural anesthesia in the parturient with acute intermittent porphyria may indicate that this technique can be safely performed in these patients.[183] Blistered or fragile skin areas should be padded and given special attention. Glucose infusion should be started because starvation may induce an attack.

The acute attack should be treated with glucose infusion and correction of hyponatremia, hypokalemia, and hypomagnesemia. Pyridoxine and hematin also have been valuable in some cases. Supportive therapy for respiratory insufficiency and treatment of pain is also suggested.

GLYCOGEN STORAGE DISEASES

The metabolic pathways involving glucose degradation to lactate, glucose conversion to glycogen, and the breakdown of glycogen to glucose are important to the whole-body biochemistry as well as to cellular physiology. Glucose metabolism has been studied intensively since the earliest days of modern biochemistry. The inherited glycogen storage diseases are characterized by dysfunction of one of the many enzymes involved in glucose metabolism. Some of the glycogen storage diseases are incompatible with life past infancy, whereas others are not. Anesthetic experience with these diseases is limited, but several significant problems have been identified.[184,185]

Hypoglycemia. Hypoglycemia is a constant risk in these patients. It results from failure to metabolize stored glycogen to glucose.

Acidosis. This is related to fat and protein metabolism because glycogen stores are not metabolically available.

Cardiac and Hepatic Dysfunction. This is secondary to destruction and displacement of normal tissue by the accumulated glycogen.

Detailed descriptions of glucose metabolism are given elsewhere. Figure 24-6 outlines the glycogen–glucose–lactate pathway. There are, of course, multiple enzymatic steps to reach each of the endpoints.

Defects in Glucose Metabolism

Type I (Von Gierke Disease; Glucose-6-Phosphate Deficiency)

Inheritance is autosomal recessive. The prognosis is moderately good, with many patients surviving into adulthood. Short stature and liver enlargement are characteristic. These patients tolerate fasting very poorly. Hypoglycemia, acidosis, and convulsions may be a problem. Prolonged bleeding has been described. Often, preoperative hyperalimentation is used to reduce liver glycogen stores. Portacaval shunt has been performed with limited success in these patients.

Type II (Pompe Disease)

Inheritance is considered autosomal recessive. This is a devastating disease with a very poor prognosis. There is a deficiency of lysosomal acid maltase with an accumulation of glycogen in the lysosomes, especially in the heart, liver, muscle, and central nervous system. Cardiac compromise resulting from outflow obstruction of hypertrophied muscle occurs, as does congestive heart failure secondary to myocardial disruption by glycogen stores. A late-onset form with a better prognosis has also been described. Enzyme replacement therapy may improve clinical outcome.[186]

Type III (Forbes Disease; Debranching Enzyme Deficiency)

Inheritance of this disease is autosomal recessive.

Type IV (Andersen Disease; Branching Enzyme Deficiency)

This is a very rare disorder, characterized by a defect in the synthesis of normal glycogen. Cirrhosis of the liver and death are characteristic before 2 years of age.

Type V (McArdle Disease; Muscle Phosphorylase Deficiency)

An autosomal recessive inheritance pattern and cramping with exercise are characteristic of this disorder. Skeletal muscle is not able to mobilize glycogen stores, the usual fuel in muscle, for sustained exercise. Myoglobinuria occurs with overexertion in these patients and may occur after succinylcholine administration as well. Muscle atrophy occurs in adulthood. Tourniquets should not be used in these patients, and frequent

automated blood pressure readings should be done with caution. Severe rhabdomyolysis has been observed after bypass for cardiac surgery.[187]

Type VI (Hers Disease; Reduced Hepatic Phosphorylase)

A decreased ability to mobilize hepatic glycogen occurs in this disorder, with normal muscle and cardiac physiology.

Type VII (Muscle Phosphofructokinase Deficiency)

This disorder is similar to McArdle disease and is characterized by muscle cramping. The same enzymatic defect in erythrocytes leads to chronic hemolysis.

Type VIII (Deficient Hepatic Phosphorylase Kinase)

Type VIII results from a deficiency in the regulatory enzyme controlling the phosphorylase enzyme. A case report has described fever and acidosis during succinylcholine, halothane, and ketamine anesthesia.[188] Liver transplantation has been used with success in the more severe forms of the glycogen storage diseases.

THE MUCOPOLYSACCHARIDOSES

The mucopolysaccharides are polysaccharides that yield mixtures of monosaccharides and derived products after hydrolysis. The mucopolysaccharides contain *N*-acetylated hexosamine in a characteristic repeating unit. For example, chondroitin sulfate A is a monosaccharide of *d*-glucuronic acid and *N*-acetyl *d*-galactosamine 4-sulfate. Mucopolysaccharides are found in all cells.

The mucopolysaccharidoses are genetically determined diseases in which mucopolysaccharides are stored in tissues in abnormal quantities and excreted in large amounts in the urine. The disorders result from a deficiency of a specific lysosomal enzyme that is required to break down these compounds. As a result, mucopolysaccharides accumulate in tissues, producing specific clinical manifestations. There are seven basic forms of mucopolysaccharidoses and several subgroups. Most of the mucopolysaccharidoses are inherited as autosomal recessive traits. All the mucopolysaccharidoses are progressive, and patients characteristically are marked by coarse facial features (gargoylism); associated skeletal abnormalities such as lumbar lordosis, stiff joints, chest deformity, dwarfing, and hypoplasia of the odontoid process (Morquio syndrome); corneal opacities; limitation of joint motion; and heart, liver, and spleen enlargement resulting from mucopolysaccharide accumulation. Mental deterioration also occurs frequently. Some cases have been successfully treated by bone marrow transplantation at a young age.

The Hunter and Hurler syndromes are the best-known variants of the mucopolysaccharidoses. The Hunter syndrome is an X-linked recessive disease.[189] Respiratory infection and heart disease, both valvular and ischemic, often lead to death at a young age. The thick, soft tissues and the copious, thick secretions make perioperative and intraoperative airway management a particular problem. In the series of Leroy and Crocker,[189] minor difficulties occurred with anesthesia in patients in more than one third of 60 operations. The use of a laryngeal mask airway may not be successful.[190] Postoperative respiratory obstruction was noted in several cases.[191] Because of the underlying heart disease, these patients should have electrocardiograms and echocardiographic tests performed before surgery. The same considerations apply in other even less frequent lysosomal storage diseases.[192]

Mucopolysaccharidosis IV (Morquio syndrome) is associated with perhaps the most significant skeletal deformities. In addition to cardiovascular disorders and respiratory insufficiency from marked chest wall deformity, acute, subacute, or chronic myelopathy is extremely common. This is secondary to severe hypoplasia or absence of the odontoid process of the second cervical vertebra. In anesthesia care, the head should be positioned carefully, and precautions such as avoidance of succinylcholine should be taken with patients with spinal cord compromise.

OSTEOGENESIS IMPERFECTA

Osteogenesis imperfecta is seen in approximately 1 of 50,000 births. Most cases are autosomal dominant; some are autosomal recessive. The pathophysiologic characteristics include decreased collagen synthesis, which leads to osteoporosis, joint laxity, and tendon weakness. The manifestations of osteogenesis imperfecta are small bowed limbs, large head, short neck, blue sclerae, otosclerosis, joint laxity, brittle teeth, and a tendency to fractures. Abnormal platelet function produces increased surgical blood loss, and dilation of the valve rings may cause aortic and mitral valve dysfunction. Kyphoscoliosis may produce pulmonary compromise. Temperature elevation is common, possibly because of elevated basal metabolic rate.

The patient should be handled carefully because minor trauma may lead to fractures. Airway management may also be difficult because of cervical spine involvement. Patients have short necks, and mandibular fractures frequently occur. Particular care should be taken to pad the areas that will receive pressure. Platelet transfusion may be needed. Core temperature should be monitored because hyperthermia has been reported.[193] Signs consistent with MH have been observed, but contracture tests for MH susceptibility have not confirmed a constant association between osteogenesis imperfecta and MH.[46] Lactic acidosis has also been observed with no increase in temperature.[194]

SUMMARY NOTE

Many other inherited disorders impact drug disposition, metabolism, and other aspects of anesthesia care ranging from altered airway anatomy in Treacher Collins syndrome to abnormal physiologic responses to anesthetic agents in familial dysautonomia. The readers should consult the literature when confronted with one of the numerous disorders affecting drug metabolism and disposition. At present, assessment of previous anesthetic experience of the patient and family is still the most efficient way to anticipate variable response to analgesics and anesthetic drugs.

References

1. Denborough MA, Lovell RRH: Anaesthetic deaths in a family. Lancet 1960; 2: 45
2. Nelson TE: Porcine stress syndromes, International Symposium on Malignant Hyperthermia. Edited by Gordon RA, Britt BA, Kalow W. Springfield, IL, Charles C Thomas, 1973, p 191
3. Kalow W, Britt BA, Terreau ME, Haist C: Metabolic error of muscle metabolism after recovery from malignant hyperthermia. Lancet 1970; 2: 895
4. Harrison GG: Control of the malignant hyperpyrexic syndrome in MHS swine by dantrolene sodium. Br J Anaesth 1975; 47: 62
5. Lopez JR, Allen PD, Alamo L, et al: Myoplasmic free [Ca^{2+}] during a malignant hyperthermia episode in swine. Muscle Nerve 1988; 11: 82
6. Chelu MG, Goonasekera SA, Durham WJ, et al: Heat- and anesthesia-induced malignant hyperthermia in an RyR1 knock-in mouse. FASEB J 2005; 10.1096/fj.05-4497fje
7. Yang T, Riehl J, Esteve E, et al: Pharmacologic and functional characterization of malignant hyperthermia in the R163C RyR1 knock-in mouse. Anesthesiology 2006; 105: 1164
8. Larach MG, Rosenberg H, Gronert GA, et al: Hyperkalemic cardiac arrest during anesthesia in infants and children with occult myopathies. Clin Pediatr 1997; 36: 9
9. Karan SM, Crowl F, Muldoon SM: Malignant hyperthermia masked by capnographic monitoring. Anesth Analg 1994; 78: 590
10. Gronert GA, Ahern CP, Milde JH: Treatment of porcine malignant hyperthermia: Lactate gradient from muscle to blood. Can Anaesth Soc J 1986; 33: 729
11. Newmark JL, Voelkel M, Brandom BW, Wu J: Delayed onset of malignant hyperthermia without creatine kinase elevation in a geriatric, ryanodine receptor type 1 gene compound heterozygous patient. Anesthesiology 2007; 107: 350
12. Short JA, Cooper CM: Suspected recurrence of malignant hyperthermia after post-extubation shivering in the intensive care unit, 18 h after tonsillectomy. Br J Anaesth 1999; 82: 945
13. Burkman JM, Posner KL, Domino KB. Analysis of the clinical variables associated with recrudescence after malignant hyperthermia reactions. Anesthesiology 2007; 106: 901
14. Ording H: Incidence of malignant hyperthermia in Denmark. Anesth Analg 1985; 64: 700
15. Hannallah RS, Kaplan RF: Jaw relaxation after a halothane/succinylcholine sequence in children. Anesthesiology 1994; 81: 99
16. Roman CS, Rosin A: Succinylcholine-induced masseter muscle rigidity associated with rapid sequence intubation. Am J Emerg Med 2007; 25: 102
17. Albrecht A, Wedel DJ, Gronert GA: Masseter muscle rigidity and nondepolarizing neuromuscular blocking agents. Mayo Clin Proc 1997; 72: 329
18. Littleford JA, Patel LR, Bose D et al: Masseter muscle spasm in children: Implications of continuing the triggering anesthetic. Anesth Analg 1991; 72: 151
19. Ellis FR, Halsall PJ: Suxamethonium spasm. A differential diagnostic conundrum. Br J Anaesth 1984; 56: 381
20. O'Flynn RP, Shutack JG, Rosenberg H, Fletcher JE: Masseter muscle rigidity and malignant hyperthermia susceptibility in pediatric patients: An update on management and diagnosis. Anesthesiology 1994; 80: 1228
21. Van Der Speck AF, Fang WB, Ashton-Miller JA et al: The effects of succinylcholine on mouth opening. Anesthesiology 1987; 67: 459
22. Van Der Spek AF, Fang WB, Ashton-Miller JA et al: Increased masticatory muscle stiffness during limb muscle flaccidity associated with succinylcholine administration. Anesthesiology 1988; 69: 11
23. Van Der Spek AF, Reynolds PI, Fang WB et al. Changes in resistance to mouth opening induced by depolarizing and non-depolarizing neuromuscular relaxants. Br J Anaesth 1990; 64: 21
24. Storella RJ, Keykhah MM, Rosenberg H: Halothane and temperature interact to increase succinylcholine-induced jaw contracture in the rat. Anesthesiology 1993; 79: 1261
25. Larach MG, Rosenberg H, Larach DG, Broennle AM: Prediction of malignant hyperthermia susceptibility by clinical signs. Anesthesiology 1987; 66: 57
26. Hackl W, Mauritz W, Schemper M, et al: Prediction of malignant hyperthermia susceptibility: Statistical evaluation of clinical signs. Br J Anaesth 1990; 64: 425
27. Rosenberg H, Fletcher JE: Masseter muscle rigidity and malignant hyperthermia susceptibility. Anesth Analg 1986; 65: 161
28. Friedman S, Baker T, Gatti M et al: Probable succinylcholine-induced rhabdomyolysis in a male athlete. Anesth Analg 1995; 81: 422
29. Sullivan M, Thompson WK, Gill GD: Succinylcholine-induced cardiac arrest in children with undiagnosed myopathy. Can J Anaesth 1994; 41: 497
30. Rosenberg AD, Neuwirth MG, Kagen LJ, et al: Intraoperative rhabdomyolysis in a patient receiving pravastatin, a 3-hydroxy-3-methylglutaryl coenzyme A (HMG CoA) reductase inhibitor. Anesth Analg 1995; 81: 1089
31. Girshin M, Mukherjee J, Clowney R et al: The post-operative cardiovascular arrest of a 5-year-old male: an initial presentation of Duchenne's muscular dystrophy. Pediatr Anesth 2006; 16: 170
32. Kelfer HM, Singer WD, Reynolds RN: Malignant hyperthermia in a child with Duchenne muscular dystrophy. Pediatrics 1983; 71: 118
33. Smith CL, Bush GH: Anaesthesia and progressive muscular dystrophy. Br J Anaesth 1985; 57: 1113
34. Jungbluth H: Central core disease. Orphanet J Rare Dis 2007; 2: 25
35. Jungbluth H: Multi-minicore disease. Orphanet J Rare Dis 2007; 2: 31
36. Treves S, Anderson AA, Ducreux S, et al: Ryanodne receptor 1 mutations, dysregulation of calcium homeostasis and neuromuscular disorders. Neuromusc Disord 2005; 15: 577
37. Zhou H, Jungbluth H, Sewry CA, et al: Molecular mechanisms and phenotypic variation in RYR1-related congential myopathies. Brain 2007; 103: 2024
38. Meola G, Sansone V, Rotondo G, Mancinelli E. Muscle biopsy and cell cultures: potential diagnostic tools in hereditary skeletal muscle channelopathies. Eur J Histochem 2003; 47: 17
39. Lambert C, Blanloeil Y, Krivosic-Horber R, et al: Malignant hyperthermia in a patient with hypokalemic periodic paralysis. Anesth Analg 1994; 79: 1012
40. Vita GM, Olckers A, Jedlicka AE, et al: Masseter muscle rigidity associated with glycine 1306-to-alanine mutation in the adult muscle sodium channel α-subunit gene. Anesthesiology 1995; 82: 1097
41. McPherson EW, Taylor CA Jr: The King syndrome: Malignant hyperthermia, myopathy, and multiple anomalies. Am J Med Genet 1981; 8: 159
42. Isaacs H, Badenhorst ME: Dominantly inherited malignant hyperthermia (MH) in the King-Denborough syndrome. Muscle Nerve 1992; 15: 740

43. Rampton AJ, Kelly DA, Shanahan EC, Ingram GS: Occurrence of malignant hyperpyrexia in a patient with osteogenesis imperfecta. Br J Anaesth 1984; 56: 1443

44. Viljoen D, Beighton P: Schwartz-Jampel syndrome (chondrodystrophic myotonia). J Med Gen 1992; 29: 58

45. Ghert M, Allen B, Davids J, et al: Increased postoperative febrile response in children with osteogenesis imperfecta. J Pediatr Orthop 2003; 23: 261

46. Porsborg P, Astrup G, Bendixen D et al: Osteogenesis imperfecta and malignant hyperthermia. Is there a relationship? Anaesthesia 1996; 61: 863

47. Allen GC, Rosenberg H: Phaeochromocytoma presenting as acute malignant hyperthermia—a diagnostic challenge. Can J Anaesth 1990; 37: 593

48. Kumar MV, Carr RJ, Komanduri V et al: Differential diagnosis of thyroid crisis and malignant hyperthermia in an anesthetized porcine model. Endocr Res 1999; 25: 87

49. Gronert GA, Thompson RL, Onofrio BM: Human malignant hyperthermia: Awake episodes and correction by dantrolene. Anesth Analg 1980; 59: 377

50. Tobin JR, Jason DR, Challa VR, Nelson TE, Sambuughin N: Malignant hyperthermia and apparent heat stroke. JAMA 2001; 286: 168

51. Wappler F, Fiege M, Steinfath M et al: Evidence for susceptibility to malignant hyperthermia in patients with exercise-induced rhabdomyolysis. Anesthesiology 2001; 94: 95

52. Lorenzoni PJ, Silvado CE, Scola RH, et al: McArdle disease with rhabdomyolysis induced by rosuvastatin. Arq Neuropsiquiatr 2007; 65: 834

53. Fink E, Brandom BW, Torp KD: Heatstroke in the super-sized athlete. Pediatric Emergency Care 2006; 22: 510

54. Mann SC, Caroff SN, Keck PE, Lazarus A: The Neuroleptic Malignant Syndrome and Related Conditions, 2nd edition. Washington, DC, American Psychiatric Publishing, Inc., 2003

55. Addonizio G, Susman VL: ECT as a treatment alternative for patients with symptoms of neuroleptic malignant syndrome. J Clin Psych 1987; 48: 102

56. Nisijima K, Shioda K, Iwamura T: Neuroleptic malignant syndrome and serotonin syndrome. Prog Brain Res 2007; 162; 81

57. Brvar M, Bunc M: Video of dantrolene effectiveness on neuroleptic malignant syndrome associated muscular rigidity and tremor. Crit Care 2007; 11: 415

58. Sprague JE, Moze P, Caden D, Rusyniak DE, Holmes C, Goldstein DS, Mills EM. Carvediol reverses hyperthermia and attenuates rhabdomyolysis induced by 3,4-methlenedioxymethamphetamine (MDMA, Ecstasy) in an animal model. Crit Care Med 2005; 33: 1311

59. Berkowitz A, Rosenberg H: Femoral block with mepivacaine for muscle biopsy in malignant hyperthermia patients. Anesthesiology 1985; 62: 651

60. Gronert GA, Milde JH, Taylor SR: Porcine muscle responses to carbachol, α and α adrenoreceptor agonist, halothane or hyperthermia. J Physiol 1980; 307: 319

61. Ording H, Nielsen VG: Atracurium and its antagonism by neostigmine (plus glycopyrrolate) in patients susceptible to malignant hyperthermia. Br J Anaesth 1986; 58: 1001

62. Gronert GA, Ahern CP, Milde JH et al: Effect of CO_2, calcium, digoxin, and potassium on cardiac and skeletal muscle metabolism in malignant hyperthermia susceptible swine. Anesthesiology 1986; 64: 24

63. Bachand M, Vachond N, Boisvert M et al: Clinical reassessment of malignant hyperthermia in Abitibi-Temiscamingue. Can J Anaesth 1997; 44: 696

64. Monnier N, Krivosic-Horber R, Payen J-F et al: Presence of two different genetic traits in malignant hyperthermia families: implications for genetics analysis, diagnosis, and incidence of malignant hyperthermia susceptibility. Anesthesiology 2002; 97: 1067

65. Ibarra MCA, Wu S, Murayama K, et al: Malignant hyperthermia in Japan: mutation screening of the entire ryanodine receptor type 1 gene coding region by direct sequencing. Anesthesiology 2006; 104: 1146

66. Bendixen D, Skovgaard LT, Ording H: Analysis of anaesthesia in patients suspected to be susceptible to malignant hyperthermia before diagnostic in vitro contracture test. Acta Anaesthesiol Scand 1997; 41: 480

67. European Malignant Hyperpyrexia Group: A protocol for the investigation of malignant hyperpyrexia. Br J Anaesth 1984; 56: 1267

68. European MH Group: Laboratory diagnosis of malignant hyperpyrexia susceptibility (MHS). Br J Anaesth 1985; 57: 1038

69. Larach MG: Standardization of the caffeine–halothane muscle contracture test. Anesth Analg 1989; 69: 511

70. Allen GC, Larach MG, Kunselman AR: The sensitivity and specificity of the caffeine–halothane contracture test: A report from the North American Malignant Hyperthermia Registry. The North American Malignant Hyperthermia Registry of MHAUS. Anesthesiology 1998; 88: 570

71. Larach MG, Landis JR, Bunn JS, et al: Prediction of malignant hyperthermia susceptibility in low-risk subjects. An epidemiologic investigation of caffeine–halothane contracture responses. Anesthesiology 1992; 76: 16

72. Lenzen C, Roewer N, Wappler F, et al: Accelerated contractures after administration of ryanodine to skeletal muscle of malignant hyperthermia susceptible patients. Br J Anaesth 1993; 71: 242

73. Wappler F, Roewer N, Lenzen C, et al: High-purity ryanodine and 9,21-dehydroryanodine for in vitro diagnosis of malignant hyperthermia in man. Br J Anaesth 1994; 72: 240

74. Hopkins PM, Ellis FR, Halsall PJ: Comparison of in vitro contracture testing with ryanodine, halothane and caffeine in malignant hyperthermia and other neuromuscular disorders. Br J Anaesth 1993; 70: 397

75. Bendahan D, Guis S, Monnier N, et al: Comparative analysis of in vitro contracture tests with ryanodine and a combination of ryanodine with

76. Hopkins PM, Hartung E, Wappler F: Multicentre evaluation of ryanodine contracture testing in malignant hyperthermia. The European Malignant Hyperthermia Group. Br J Anaesth 1998; 80: 389

77. Wappler F, Scholz J, von Richthofen, et al: 4-Chloro-m-cresol-induced contractures of skeletal muscle specimen from patients at risk for malignant hyperthermia. Anaesthesiol Intensivmed Notfallmed Schmerzther 1997; 32: 541

78. Isaacs H, Badenhorst M: False-negative results with muscle caffeine–halothane contracture testing for malignant hyperthermia. Anesthesiology 1993; 79: 5

79. Wedel DJ, Nelson TE: Malignant hyperthermia—diagnostic dilemma: False-negative contracture responses with halothane and caffeine alone. Anesth Analg 1994; 78: 787

80. Allen GC, Rosenberg P, Fletcher JE: Safety of general anesthesia in patients previously tested negative for malignant hyperthermia susceptibility. Anesthesiology 1990; 72: 619

81. Ording H, Hedengran AM, Skovgaard LT: Evaluation of 119 anaesthetics received after investigation for susceptibility to malignant hyperthermia. Acta Anaesthesiol Scand 1991; 35: 711

82. Fletcher JE: Current laboratory methods for the diagnosis of malignant hyperthermia susceptibility, Anesthesia Clinics of North America, Temperature Regulation in Anesthesia. Edited by Levitt RC. Philadelphia, WB Saunders, 1994, p 553

83. Ording H: Diagnosis of susceptibility to malignant hyperthermia in man. Br J Anaesth 1988; 60: 287

84. Kaplan RF, Rushing E: Isolated masseter muscle spasm and increased creatine kinase without malignant hyperthermia susceptibility or other myopathies. Anesthesiology 1992; 77: 820

85. Antognini JF: Creatine kinase alterations after acute malignant hyperthermia episodes and common surgical procedures. Anesth Analg 1995; 81: 1039

86. Bendahan D, Kozak-Ribbens G, Rodet L, et al: ^{31}Phosphorus magnetic resonance spectroscopy characterization of muscular metabolic anomalies in patients with malignant hyperthermia: application to diagnosis. Anesthesiology 1998; 88: 96

87. Treves S, Larini F, Menegazzi P, et al: Alteration of intracellular Ca^{2+} transients in COS-7 cells transfected with the cDNA encoding skeletal-muscle ryanodine receptor carrying a mutation associated with malignant hyperthermia. Biochem J 1994; 301: 661

88. Sei Y, Brandom BW, Bina S, Hosoi E, et al: Patients with malignant hyperthermia demonstrate an altered calcium control mechanism in B lymphocytes. Anesthesiology 2002; 97: 1052

89. Anetseder M, Hager M, Muller-Reible C, Roewer N. Diagnosis of susceptibility to malignant hyperthermia by use of a metabolic test. Lancet 2003; 362: 494

90. Schuster F, Metterlein T, Negele S, et al: Intramuscular injection of sevoflurane detects malignant hyperthermia predisposition in susceptible pigs. Anesthesiology 2007; 107: 616

91. Schuster F, Scholl H, Hager M, et al: The dose-response relationship and regional distribution of lactate after intramuscular injection of halothane and caffeine in malignant hyperthermia-susceptible pigs. Anesth Analg 2006; 102: 468

92. Bina S, Cowan G, Karaian J, et al: Effects of caffeine, halothane, and 4-chloro-m-cresol on skeletal muscle lactate and pyruvate in malignant hyperthermia-susceptible and normal swine as assessed by microdialysis. Anesthesiology 2006; 104: 90

93. Larach MG, Localio AR, Allen GC, et al: A clinical grading scale to predict malignant hyperthermia susceptibility. Anesthesiology 1994; 80: 771

94. Jurkat-Rott K, McCarthy T, Lehmann-Horn F: Genetics and pathogenesis of malignant hyperthermia. Muscle Nerve 2000; 23: 4

95. Sei Y, Sambuughin NN, Davis EJ, et al: Malignant hyperthermia in North America genetic screening of the three hot spots in the type 1 ryanodine receptor gene. Anesthesiology 2004; 101: 824

96. Sambuughin N, Holley H, Muldoon S, et al: Screening of the entire ryanodine receptor type 1 coding region for sequence variants associated with malignant hyperthermia susceptibility in the North American population. Anesthesiology 2005; 102: 515

97. Galli L, Orrico A, Lorenzini S, et al: Frequency and localization of mutations in the 106 exons of the RYR1 gene in 50 individuals with malignant hyperthermia. Human Mutation, Mutation in Brief #913, Online 2006

98. Urwyler A, Deufel T, McCarthy T, West S: Guidelines for molecular genetic detection of susceptibility to malignant hyperthermia. Br J Anaesth 2001; 86: 283

99. Mitchell LW, Leighton BL: Warmed diluent speeds dantrolene reconstitution. Can J Anaesth 2003; 50: 127

100. Quraishi SA, Orkin FK, Murray WB. Dantrolene reconstitution: can warmed diluent make a difference? J Clin Anesh 2006; 18: 339

101. Rubin AS, Zablocki AD: Hyperkalemia, verapamil, and dantrolene. Anesthesiology 1987; 66: 246

102. Saltzman LS, Kates RA, Corke BC, et al: Hyperkalemia and cardiovascular collapse after verapamil and dantrolene administration in swine. Anesth Analg 1984; 63: 473

103. Jensen AG, Bach V, Werner MU, et al: A fatal case of malignant hyperthermia following isoflurane anaesthesia. Acta Anaesthesiol Scand 1986; 30: 293

104. Bouchama A, Knochel JP: Heat stroke. N Engl J Med 2002; 346: 1978

105. Paul-Pletzer K, Palnitkar SS, Jimenez LS, et al: The skeletal muscle ryanodine receptor identified as a molecular target of [³H]azidodantrolene by photoaffinity labeling. Biochemistry 2001; 40: 531

106. Paul-Pletzer K, Yamamoto T, Bhat MB, et al: Identification of a dantrolene-binding sequence on the skeletal muscle ryanodine receptor. J Biol Chem 2002; 277: 34918

107. Britt BA: Dantrolene. Can Anaesth Soc J 1984; 31: 61

108. Watson CB, Reierson N, Norfleet EA: Clinically significant muscle weakness induced by oral dantrolene sodium prophylaxis for malignant hyperthermia. Anesthesiology 1986; 65: 312

109. Flewellen EH, Nelson TE, Jones WP, et al: Dantrolene dose response in awake man: implications for management of malignant hyperthermia. Anesthesiology 1983; 59: 275

110. Lerman J, McLeod ME, Strong HA: Pharmacokinetics of intravenous dantrolene in children. Anesthesiology 1989; 70: 625

111. Allen GC, Cattran CB, Peterson RG, Lalande M: Plasma levels of dantrolene following oral administration in malignant hyperthermia-susceptible patients. Anesthesiology 1988; 69: 900

112. Crawford MW, Prinhazen H, Petroz GC: Accelerating the washout of inhalational anesthetics from the Drager Primus anesthetic workstation: effect of exchangeable internal components. Anesthesiology 2007; 106: 289

113. Schonell LH, Sims C, Bulsara M: Preparing a new generation anaesthetic machine for patients susceptible to malignant hyperthermia. Anaesth Intensive Care 2003; 31: 58

114. Vaughan MS, Cork RC, Vaughan RW: Inaccuracy of liquid crystal thermometry to identify core temperature trends in postoperative adults. Anesth Analg 1982; 61: 284

115. Ruhland G, Hinkle AJ: Malignant hyperthermia after oral and intravenous pretreatment with dantrolene in a patient susceptible to malignant hyperthermia. Anesthesiology 1984; 60: 159

116. Pollock N, Langton E, Stowell K, Simpson C, McDonnell N: Safe Duration of Postoperative Monitoring for Malignant Hyperthermia Susceptible Patients. Anaesthesia Intensive Care 2004; 32: 502

117. Yentis SM, Levine MF, Hartley EJ: Should all children with suspected or confirmed malignant hyperthermia susceptibility be admitted after surgery? A 10-year review. Anesth Analg 1992; 75: 345

118. Shime J, Gare D, Andrews J, Britt B: Dantrolene in pregnancy: Lack of adverse effects on the fetus and newborn infant. Am J Obstet Gynecol 1988; 159: 831

119. Aleman M, Riehl J, Aldridge BM, Lecouteur RA, Stot JL, Pessah IN: Association of a mutation in the ryanodine receptor 1 gene with equine malignant hyperthermia. Muscle Nerve 2004; 30: 356

120. MacLennan DH, Phillips MS: Malignant hyperthermia. Science 1992; 256: 789

121. Fletcher JE, Calvo PA, Rosenberg H: Phenotypes associated with malignant hyperthermia susceptibility in swine genotyped as homozygous or heterozygous for the ryanodine receptor mutation. Br J Anaesth 1993; 71: 410

122. Fletcher JE, Tripolitis L, Rosenberg H, Beech J: Malignant hyperthermia: Halothane- and calcium-induced calcium release in skeletal muscle. Biochem Mol Biol Int 1993; 29: 763

123. Nelson TE: A pharmacogenetic disease of Ca⁺⁺-regulating proteins. Curr Mol Med 2002; 2: 347

124. Iaizzo PA, Klein W, Lehmann-Horn F: Fura-2 detected myoplasmic calcium and its correlation with contracture force in skeletal muscle from normal and malignant hyperthermia susceptible pigs. Pflugers Arch 1988; 411: 648

125. Halsall PJ, Cain PA, Ellis FR: Retrospective analysis of anaesthetics received by patients before susceptibility to malignant hyperpyrexia was recognized. Br J Anaesth 1979; 51: 949

126. Urwyler A, Censier K, Kaufmann MA, Drewe J: Genetic effects on the variability of the halothane and caffeine muscle contracture tests. Anesthesiology 1994; 80: 1287

127. Fletcher JE, Huggins FJ, Rosenberg H: The importance of calcium ions for in vitro malignant hyperthermia testing. Can J Anaesth 1990; 37: 695

128. Nelson TE: Abnormality in calcium release from skeletal sarcoplasmic reticulum of pigs susceptible to malignant hyperthermia. J Clin Invest 1983; 72: 862

129. Fletcher JE, Mayerberger S, Tripolitis L, et al: Fatty acids markedly lower the threshold for halothane-induced calcium release from the terminal cisternae in human and porcine normal and malignant hyperthermia susceptible skeletal muscle. Life Sci 1991; 49: 1651

130. Mickelson JR, Ross JA, Reed BK, Louis CF: Enhanced Ca²⁺-induced calcium release by isolated sarcoplasmic reticulum vesicles from malignant hyperthermia susceptible pig muscle. Biochim Biophys Acta 1986; 862: 318

131. Sullivan JS, Denborough MA: Temperature dependence of muscle function in malignant hyperpyrexia-susceptible swine. Br J Anaesth 1981; 53: 1217

132. McCarthy TV, Healy JM, Heffron JJ, et al: Localization of the malignant hyperthermia susceptibility locus to human chromosome 19q12-13.2. Nature 1990; 343: 562

133. Hawkes MJ, Nelson TE, Hamilton SL: [3H]ryanodine as a probe of changes in the functional state of the Ca²⁺-release channel in malignant hyperthermia. J Biol Chem 1992; 267: 6702, 1992

134. Herrmann-Frank A, Richter M, Sarkozi S, et al: 4-Chloro-m-cresol, a potent and specific activator of the skeletal muscle ryanodine receptor. Biochim Biophys Acta 1996; 1289: 31

135. McCarthy TV, Quane KA, Lynch PJ: Ryanodine receptor mutations in malignant hyperthermia and central core disease. Hum Mut 2000; 15: 410

136. Robinson R, Curran JL, Hall WJ, et al: Genetic heterogeneity and HOMOG analysis in British malignant hyperthermia families. J Med Genet 1998; 35: 196

137. Nelson TE: Halothane effects on human malignant hyperthermia skeletal muscle single calcium-release channels in planar lipid bilayers. Anesthesiology 1992; 76: 588

138. Fujii J, Otsu K, Zorzato F, et al: Identification of a mutation in porcine ryanodine receptor associated with malignant hyperthermia. Science 1991; 253: 448

139. Mickelson JR, Knudson CM, Kennedy CF, et al: Structural and functional correlates of a mutation in the malignant hyperthermia-susceptible pig ryanodine receptor. FEBS Lett 1992; 301: 49

140. Deufel T, Sudbrak R, Feist Y, et al: Discordance, in a malignant hyperthermia pedigree, between in vitro contracture-test phenotypes and haplotypes for the MHS1 region on chromosome 19q12-13.2, comprising the C1840T transition in the RYR1 gene. Am J Hum Genet 1995; 56: 1334 [erratum: Am J Hum Genet 1995; 57(2): 520]

141. Fagerlund TH, Ording H, Bendixen D, et al: Discordance between malignant hyperthermia susceptibility and RYR1 mutation C1840T in two Scandinavian MH families exhibiting this mutation. Clin Genet 1997; 52: 416

142. Robinson RL, Anetseder MJ, Brancadoro V, et al: Recent advances in the diagnosis of malignant hyperthermia susceptibility: how confident can we be of genetic testing? Eur J Hum Genet 2003; 11: 342

143. MacLennan DH, Duff C, Zorzato F, et al: Ryanodine receptor gene is a candidate for predisposition to malignant hyperthermia. Nature 1990; 343: 559

144. Davis MR, Haan E, Jungbluth H, et al: Principal mutation hotspot for central core disease and related myopathies in the C-terminal transmembrane region of the RYR1 gene. Neuromuscul Disord 2003; 13: 151

145. Tilgen N, Zorzato F, Halliger-Keller B, et al: Identification of four novel mutations in the C-terminal membrane spanning domain of the ryanodine receptor 1: association with central core disease and alteration of calcium homeostasis. Hum Mol Genet 2001; 10: 2879

146. Wehner M, Rueffert H, Koenig F, Olthoff D: Functional characterization of malignant hyperthermia-associated RyR1 mutations in exon 44, using the human myotube model. Neuromuscul Disord 2004; 14: 429

147. Sei Y, Gallagher KL, Basile AS: Skeletal muscle type ryanodine receptor is involved in calcium signaling in human B lymphocytes. J Biol Chem 1999; 274: 5995

148. Girard T, Cavagna D, Padocan E, et al: B-lymphocytes from malignant hyperthermia susceptible patients have an increased sensitivity to skeletal muscle ryanodine receptor activators. J Biol Chem 2001; 276: 48077

149. Robinson RL, Brooks C, Brown SL, et al: RYR1 mutations causing central core disease are associated with more severe malignant hyperthermia in vitro contracture test phenotypes. Hum Mutat 2002; 20: 88

150. Monnier N, Procaccio V, Stieglitz P, Lunardi J: Malignant-hyperthermia susceptibility is associated with a mutation of the alpha 1-subunit of the human dihydropyridine-sensitive L-type voltage-dependent calcium-channel receptor in skeletal muscle. Am J Hum Genet 1997; 60: 1316

151. Serfas KD, Bose D, Patel L, et al: Comparison of the segregation of the RYR1 C1840T mutation with segregation of the caffeine/halothane contracture test results for malignant hyperthermia susceptibility in a large Manitoba Mennonite family. Anesthesiology 1996; 84: 322

152. Heytens L: Molecular genetic detection of susceptibility to malignant hyperthermia in Belgian families. Acta Anaesthesiol Belg 2007; 58: 113

153. Girard T, Treves S, Voronkov E, Siegemund M, Urwyler A: Molecular genetic testing for malignant hyperthermia susceptibility. Anesthesiology 2004; 100: 1076

154. Graber R, Sumida C, Nunez EA: Fatty acids and cell signal transduction. J Lipid Mediat Cell Signal 1994; 9: 91

155. Carroll JE: Myopathies caused by disorders of lipid metabolism. Neurol Clin 1988; 6: 563

156. Glatz JF, Vork MM, Cistola DP, van der Vusse GJ: Cytoplasmic fatty acid binding protein: Significance for intracellular transport of fatty acids and putative role on signal transduction pathways. Prostaglandins Leukot Essent Fatty Acids 1993; 48: 33

157. Cheah KS, Cheah AM, Waring JC: Phospholipase A2 activity, calmodulin, Ca²⁺ and meat quality in young and adult halothane sensitive and halothane insensitive British Landrace pigs. Meat Sci 1986; 17: 37

158. Cheah AM: Effect of long chain unsaturated fatty acids on the calcium transport of sarcoplasmic reticulum. Biochim Biophys Acta 1981; 648: 113

159. Messineo FC, Rathier M, Favreau C, et al: Mechanisms of fatty acid effects on sarcoplasmic reticulum. III. The effects of palmitic and oleic acids on sarcoplasmic reticulum function—a model for fatty acid membrane interactions. J Biol Chem 1984; 259: 1336

160. Dettbarn C, Palade P: Arachidonic acid-induced Ca²⁺ release from isolated sarcoplasmic reticulum. Biochem Pharmacol 1993; 45: 1301

161. Dubois BW, Evers AS: ⁹F-NMR spin-spin relaxation (T2) method for characterizing volatile anesthetic binding to proteins. Analysis of isoflurane binding to serum albumin. Biochemistry 1992; 31: 7069

162. Jurkat-Rott K, Lehmann-Horn F: Muscle channelopathies and critical points in functional and genetic studies. J Clin Inv 2005; 115: 2000

163. Clarkson PM, Hoffman EP, Zambraski E, et al: ACTN3 and MLCK genotype associations with exertional muscle damage. J Appl Physiol 2005; 99: 564

164. Whittaker M: Chemical and Biochemical Properties In Monographs in Human Genetics, Vol. 11. New York, Karger, 1986

165. Xie W, Altamirano CV, Bartels CF, et al: An improved cocaine hydrolase: The A328Y mutant of human butyrylcholinesterase is 4-fold more efficient. Mol Pharmacol 1999; 55: 83

166. Viby-Mogensen J: Correlation of succinylcholine duration of action with plasma cholinesterase activity in subjects with normal enzyme. Anesthesiology 1980; 53: 517

167. Viby-Mogensen J: Succinylcholine neuromuscular blockade in subjects heterozygous for abnormal plasma cholinesterase. Anesthesiology 1981; 55: 231

168. Duysen EG, Li B, Darvesh S, Lockridge O: Sensitivity of butyrylcholinesterase knockout mice to (—)-huperizine A and donepizil suggests humans with butyrylcholinesterase deficiency may not tolerate these Alzheimer's disease drugs and indicates butyrylcholinesterase function in neurotransmission. Toxicology 2007; 233: 60

169. Kalow W, Genest K: A method for the detection of atypical forms of human serum cholinesterase: Determination of dibucaine numbers. Can J Biochem 1957; 35: 339

170. Harris H, Whittaker M: Differential inhibition of serum cholinesterase with fluoride: Recognition of two new phenotypes. Nature (Lond) 1961; 191: 496

171. Primo-Parma SL, Bartels CF, Wiersema B, et al: Characterization of 12 silent alleles of the human butyrylcholinesterase (BCHE) gene. Am J Hum Genet 1996; 58: 52

172. McGuire M, Noguiera CG, Bartels CF, et al: Identification of the structured mutation responsible for the dibucaine-resistant (atypical) variant form of human cholinesterase. Proc Natl Acad Sci USA 1989; 86: 953

173. Hanel HK, Viby-Mogensen J, Schaffalitzky de Muckadell OB: Serum cholinesterase variants in the Danish population. Acta Anaesthesiol Scand 1978; 22: 505

174. Lovely MJ, Patteson SK, Beuerlein FJ, Chesney JT: Perioperative blood transfusion may conceal atypical pseudocholinesterase. Anesth Analg 1990; 70: 326

175. Harris H, Hopkinson DA, Robson EB, et al: Genetic studies on a new variant of serum cholinesterase detected by electrophoresis. Ann Hum Genet 1963; 26: 359

176. Brodsky JB, Campos FA: Chloroprocaine analgesia in a patient receiving echothiophate iodide eye drops. Anesthesiology 1978; 48: 288

177. Raj PP, Rosenblatt R, Miller J, et al: Dynamics of local anesthetic compounds in regional anesthesia. Anesth Analg 1977; 56: 110

178. Jatlow P, Barash PG, Van Dyke C, et al: Cocaine and succinylcholine sensitivity: A new caution. Anesth Analg 1979; 58: 235

179. Murphy PC: Acute intermittent porphyria: The anaesthetic problem and its background. Br J Anaesth 1964; 36: 801

180. James MFM, Hift RJ: Porphyrias. Br J Anaesth 2000; 85: 143

181. McLoughlin C: Use of propofol in a patient with porphyria. Br J Anaesth 1989; 62: 114

182. Sheppard L, Dorman T: Anesthesia in a child with homozygous porphobilinogen deaminase deficiency: a severe form of acute intermittent porphyria. Pediatric Anaesth 2005; 15: 426

183. McNeill MJ, Bennet A: Use of regional anaesthesia in a patient with acute porphyria. Br J Anaesth 1990; 64: 371

184. Cox JM: Anesthesia and glycogen storage disease. Anesthesiology 1963; 29: 1221

185. Bustamante SE, Appachi E: Acute pancreatitis after anesthesia with propofol in a child with glycogen storae disease type IA. Paediatric Anaesthesia 2006; 16: 680

186. Ing RJ, Cook DR, Bengur RA, et al: Anaesthetic management of infants with glycogen storage disease type II: a physiologic approach. Paediatric Anaesthesia 2004; 14: 514

187. Lobato EB, Janelle GM, Urdaneta F, Malias MA: Noncardiogenic pulmonary edema and rhabdomyolysis after protamine administration in a patient with unrecognized McArdle's disease. Anesthesiology 1999; 91: 303

188. Edelstein G, Hirshman CA: Hyperthermia and ketoacidosis during anesthesia in a child with glycogen-storage disease. Anesthesiology 1980; 52: 90

189. Leroy JG, Crocker AC: Clinical definition of the Hurler-Hunter phenotypes. Am J Dis Child 1966; 112: 518

190. Busoni P, Cognani G: Failure of laryngeal mask to secure the airway in a patient with Hunter's syndrome (mucopolysaccharidosis type II). Paediatr Anaesth 1999; 9: 153

191. Walker RW, Colovic V, Robinson DN, Dearlove OR. Postobstructive pulmonary oedema during anaesthesia in children with mucopolysaccharidoses. Paediatr Anaesth 2003; 13: 441

192. Friedhoff RJ, Rose SH, Brown MJ, et al: Galactosialidosis: a unique disease with significant clinical implications during perioperative anesthesia management. Anesth Analg 2003; 97: 53

193. Oliverio RM: Anesthetic management of intramedullary nailing in osteogenesis imperfecta: Report of a case. Anesth Analg 1973; 52: 232

194. Kill C, Leonhardt A, Wulf H: Lacticacidosis after short-term infusion of propofol for anaesthesia in a child with osteogenesis imperfecta. Paediatric Anaesth 2003; 13: 823

STEPHEN F. DIERDORF. AND J. SCOTT WALTON

MUSCULOSKELETAL DISEASES
  Muscular Dystrophy
  The Myotonias
  Familial Periodic Paralysis
  Myasthenia Gravis
  Myasthenic Syndrome (Lambert-Eaton)
  Guillain-Barré Syndrome (Polyradiculoneuritis)
CENTRAL NERVOUS SYSTEM DISEASES
  Multiple Sclerosis
  Epilepsy
  Parkinson Disease
  Huntington Disease
  Alzheimer Disease
  Amyotrophic Lateral Sclerosis

  Creutzfeldt-Jakob Disease
ANEMIAS
  Nutritional Deficiency Anemias
  Hemolytic Anemias
  Hemoglobinopathies
COLLAGEN VASCULAR DISEASES
  Rheumatoid Arthritis
  Systemic Lupus Erythematosus
  Scleroderma
  Polymyositis/Dermatomyositis (Inflammatory Myopathies)
SKIN DISORDERS
  Epidermolysis Bullosa
  Pemphigus

KEY POINTS

1 The cytoskeleton of the muscle membrane in patients with muscular dystrophy is abnormal and is susceptible to damage from succinylcholine. Massive release of intracellular contents, including potassium, may occur.

2 Myotonic dystrophy produces cardiac conduction delay that can manifest as high-grade atrioventricular block.

3 Patients with myasthenia gravis are exquisitely sensitive to nondepolarizing muscle relaxants. Short-acting muscle relaxants and objective monitoring of neuromuscular function are indicated.

4 Many types of cancer, in addition to small cell lung carcinoma, can produce myasthenic syndrome.

5 Patients with multiple sclerosis should be advised that an exacerbation of their neurologic symptoms may occur during the perioperative period.

6 Repeated episodes of sickling in patients with sickle cell disease cause pulmonary hypertension. Pulmonary hypertension in sickle cell patients is associated with increased mortality.

7 Rheumatoid arthritis is a multisystem disease that causes subclinical cardiac and pulmonary dysfunction.

8 Many patients with rheumatoid arthritis have significant degeneration of the cervical spine with few neurologic symptoms. Cervical manipulation during laryngoscopy and intubation requires special precautions.

9 Esophageal dysfunction in patients with scleroderma or dermatomyositis increases the risk of aspiration pneumonitis.

10 Patients with epidermolysis bullosa can have undiagnosed dilated cardiomyopathy.

A variety of rare disorders may influence the selection and conduct of anesthesia. Recent advances in molecular genetics and biology have clarified the disease mechanisms and inheritance of many uncommon diseases. These discoveries have radically altered the treatment of some disorders. Anesthesiologists must periodically update their diagnostic skills and clinical knowledge to recognize when additional evaluation or treatment may be required and how these diseases influence the management of anesthesia.

MUSCULOSKELETAL DISEASES

The cytoskeleton of the muscle cell is composed of proteins such as dystrophin, merosin, utrophin, syntrophin, dystrobrevin, and sarcoglycans (Fig. 25-1). Abnormal proteins or insufficient quantities of normal proteins may diminish the

integrity of the muscle membrane, making it more susceptible to damage. The muscular dystrophies are diseases associated with abnormalities of the muscle membrane (Table 25-1).[1]

Muscular dystrophies are characterized by a progressive loss of skeletal muscle function (Fig. 25-2). Although less evident, cardiac and smooth muscle are also affected.

Muscular Dystrophy

Duchenne Muscular Dystrophy

Duchenne muscular dystrophy is caused by a lack of production of dystrophin, a major component of the skeleton of the muscle membrane. Duchenne dystrophy is characterized by painless degeneration and atrophy of skeletal muscle. This disorder is a sex-linked recessive trait clinically evident in boys.

PREANESTHETIC EVALUATION AND PREPARATION

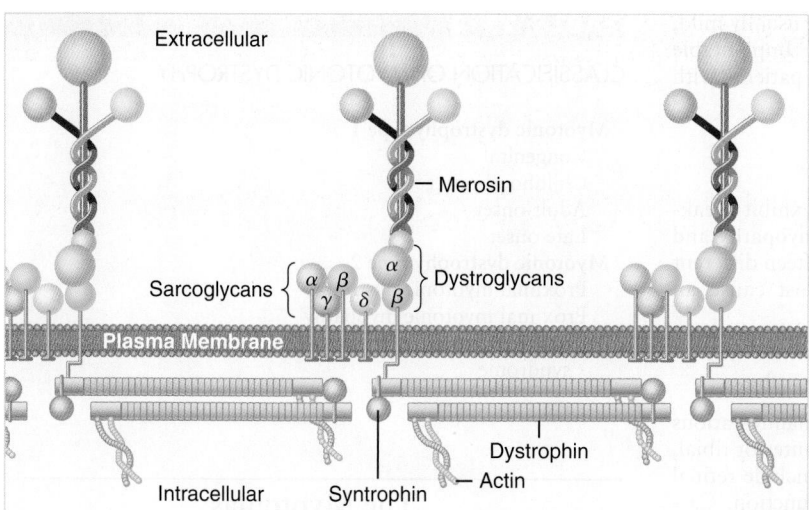

FIGURE 25-1.   Muscle cell cytoskeleton. (Reprinted from Duggan DJ, Gorospe JR, Fanin M, et al: Mutations in the sarcoglycan genes in patients with myopathy. N Engl J Med 1997; 336: 618–624, with permission.)

Progressive muscle weakness produces symptoms between the ages of 2 and 5 years and significant limitation by age 12 years. Axial muscle imbalance produces kyphoscoliosis that may require operative instrumentation for stabilization. Death is usually secondary to congestive heart failure or pneumonia. Aggressive treatment of cardiopulmonary dysfunction has improved survival for many patients until the age of 30 years. Serum creatine kinase levels reflect the progression of the disease. Early in the patient's life the creative kinase level is increased. Later, as significant amounts of muscle have degenerated, the creatine kinase level decreases.

As the patient ages, loss of cardiac muscle is reflected by a progressive decrease in R-wave amplitude in the lateral precordial leads of the electrocardiogram (ECG). Serial echocardiography can provide important information about cardiac function. Progressive loss of myocardial tissue results in cardiomyopathy, ventricular dysrhythmias, and mitral regurgitation. Treatment of cardiac dysfunction includes angiotensin-converting enzyme (ACE) inhibitors, β-adrenergic blockers, and dysrhythmia surveillance.[2]

Diminished muscle strength produces an ineffective cough, resulting in retention of pulmonary secretions, pneumonia, and death. Smooth muscle involvement causes intestinal hypomotility, delayed gastric emptying, and gastroparesis.

Although the genetic defect that causes Duchenne dystrophy is known, specific genetic therapy remains elusive. Current treatment is supportive and directed at better nutrition and improvement of cardiorespiratory function. Prolonged therapy with corticosteroids may improve skeletal muscle function.

Emery-Dreifuss Muscular Dystrophy

Emery-Dreifuss muscular dystrophy is characterized by contractures of the elbows, ankles, spine, and humeropectoral

TABLE 25-1

TYPES OF MUSCULAR DYSTROPHY

Duchenne
Becker
Emery-Dreifuss
Limb-girdle
Oculopharyngeal
Fascioscapulohumeral
Congenital muscular dystrophy

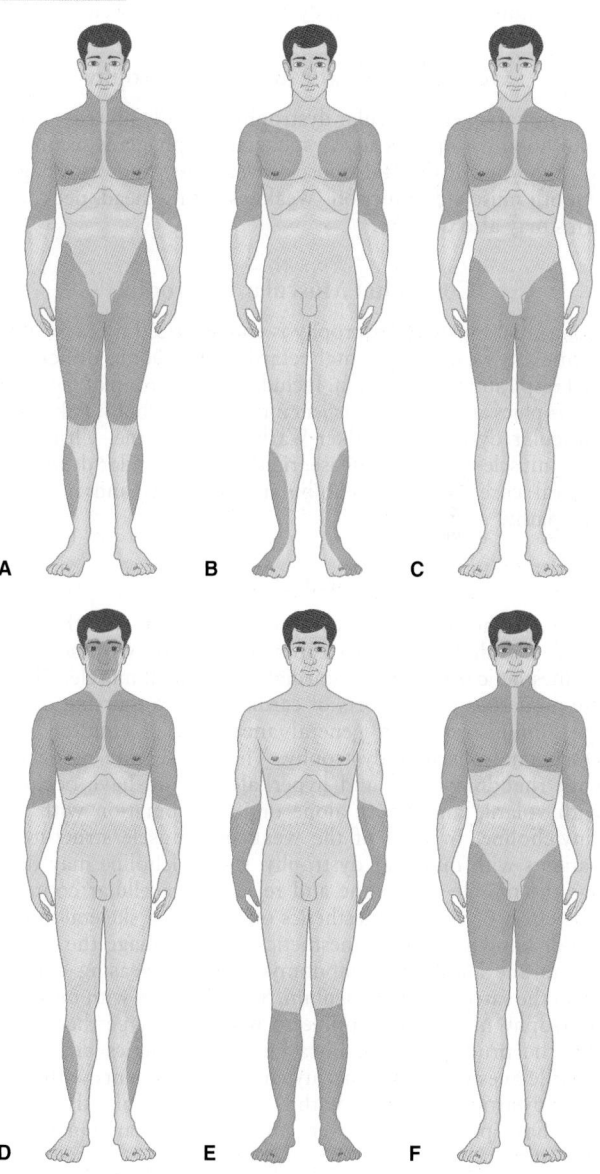

FIGURE 25-2.   Distribution of predominant muscle weakness in different types of muscular dystrophy. A. Duchenne-type and Becker-type. B. Emery-Dreifuss. C. Limb-girdle. D. Fascioscapulohumeral. E. Distal. F. Oculopharyngeal. (Reproduced from BMJ Publishing Group. Emery AEH: The muscular dystrophies. BMJ 1998; 317: 991–995, with permission.)

weakness. The skeletal muscle manifestations are usually mild, whereas cardiac conduction defects can be fatal.[3] Implantable defibrillating pacemakers are often indicated for patients with Emery-Dreifuss muscular dystrophy.

Limb-Girdle Muscular Dystrophy

Patients with limb-girdle muscular dystrophy exhibit weakness of the shoulder and pelvic girdles. Cardiomyopathy and atrioventricular conduction defects can occur. Fifteen different genetic defects have been discovered, and most cause an abnormality in the sarcoglycan proteins.

Facioscapulohumeral Muscular Dystrophy

Patients with this disease have diverse clinical manifestations such as weakness of the facial, scapulohumeral, anterior tibial, and pelvic girdle muscles. Other abnormalities include retinal vascular disease, deafness, and neurologic dysfunction. Cardiac conduction defects and dysrhythmias may occur.

Oculopharyngeal Muscular Dystrophy

Oculopharyngeal muscular dystrophy typically presents in late adulthood with ptosis and dysphagia. Dysphagia is secondary to pharyngeal skeletal muscle weakness and esophageal smooth muscle dysfunction. Weakness of the head, neck, and arms may also develop.

Congenital Muscular Dystrophy

Congenital muscular dystrophy is characterized by early onset of muscle weakness, mental retardation, feeding difficulties, and respiratory dysfunction. Included in this group of muscular dystrophies are merosin-deficient muscular dystrophy, Fukuyama muscular dystrophy, Walker-Warburg syndrome, Ulrich disease, muscle-eye-brain disease, rigid spine muscular dystrophy, central core disease, myotubular myopathy, and nemaline myopathy.[4]

Management of Anesthesia

Most of the significant complications from anesthesia in patients with muscular dystrophy are secondary to the effects of anesthetic drugs on myocardial and skeletal muscle.[5] There are numerous case reports of cardiac arrest occurring during the administration of general anesthesia in children with Duchenne muscular dystrophy. These cases are associated with rhabdomyolysis and hyperkalemia and have occurred with volatile anesthetics alone or in combination with succinylcholine. In view of the weakened muscle structure of patients with muscular dystrophy, succinylcholine may damage the muscle membrane and release intracellular contents. The effect of volatile anesthetics on abnormal skeletal muscle is not known. Volatile anesthetics could damage the muscle membrane and cause rhabdomyolysis by releasing calcium from the sarcoplasmic reticulum. Some patients with muscular dystrophy may be susceptible to malignant hyperthermia. It may be prudent to use intravenous anesthetics and avoid volatile anesthetics and succinylcholine for patients with muscular dystrophy.[6] Patients with Duchenne muscular dystrophy may have prolonged recovery from nondepolarizing muscle relaxants.

Degeneration of gastrointestinal smooth muscle with hypomotility of the intestinal tract and delayed gastric emptying in conjunction with impaired swallowing increases the risk of perioperative aspiration of gastric contents. Vigorous respiratory therapy and mechanical ventilation may be required during the early postoperative period.

TABLE 25-2

CLASSIFICATION OF MYOTONIC DYSTROPHY

Myotonic dystrophy type 1
  Congenital
  Childhood-onset
  Adult-onset
  Late onset
Myotonic dystrophy type 2
  Proximal myotonic dystrophy
  Proximal myotonic myopathy
  Proximal myotonic myopathy
    syndrome

The Myotonias

Myotonia is the delayed relaxation of skeletal muscle after voluntary contraction. Electromyography demonstrates repetitive muscle fiber discharges that fluctuate. These abnormalities are secondary to dysfunction of ion channels in the muscle membrane. There are two types of myotonic dystrophy caused by abnormalities in two distinct gene loci: myotonic dystrophy type 1 and myotonic dystrophy type 2 (Table 25-2). The genetic alteration in type 1 is an unstable trinucleotide expansion on chromosome 19q; type 2 is caused by a quadnucleotide expansion on chromosome 3q. Myotonic dystrophy type 1 is the more common form and is further subdivided by age of onset into congenital, childhood-onset, adult-onset (most prevalent), and late onset.[7]

Adult-onset myotonic dystrophy is an autosomally dominant inherited disorder with symptoms occurring during the second and third decades of life. Other clinical features include muscle degeneration, cataracts, premature balding, diabetes mellitus, thyroid dysfunction, adrenal insufficiency, gonadal atrophy, and cardiac abnormalities. Cardiac manifestations include atrioventricular conduction delay, atrial tachydysrhythmias, diastolic dysfunction, cardiomyopathy, and mitral valve prolapse. First-degree atrioventricular block may precede the onset of skeletal muscle symptoms. Sudden death may be secondary to third-degree atrioventricular block or ventricular dysrhythmias. Echocardiography may reveal subclinical evidence of left ventricular systolic and diastolic dysfunction.[8] Although cardiac abnormalities are less commonly reported in patients with myotonic dystrophy type 2, fatal dysrhythmias can occur.

Pulmonary function studies demonstrate a restrictive lung disease pattern, mild arterial hypoxemia, and diminished ventilatory responses to hypoxia and hypercapnia. Brainstem respiratory control mechanisms may also be defective. Weakness of the respiratory muscles diminishes the effectiveness of cough and may lead to pneumonia. Myotonia of the respiratory muscles can produce intense dyspnea requiring treatment with procainamide. Alteration of smooth muscle function produces gastric atony and intestinal hypomotility. Pharyngeal muscle weakness in conjunction with delayed gastric emptying increases the risk of aspiration of gastric contents.

Pregnancy may produce an exacerbation of myotonic dystrophy, and congestive heart failure is more likely to occur during pregnancy. Cesarean section is often required because of uterine smooth muscle dysfunction. Some infants of mothers with myotonic dystrophy may develop congenital myotonic dystrophy. Congenital myotonic dystrophy is characterized by hypotonia, respiratory insufficiency, and difficulty with feeding.

Therapy for myotonic dystrophy is directed at treatment of cardiac dysrhythmias (pacemaker implantation) and surgical therapy for cataracts and gallbladder disease. Sodium channel blockers, including mexiletine, phenytoin, procainamide,

Succinylcholine (mg/kg)

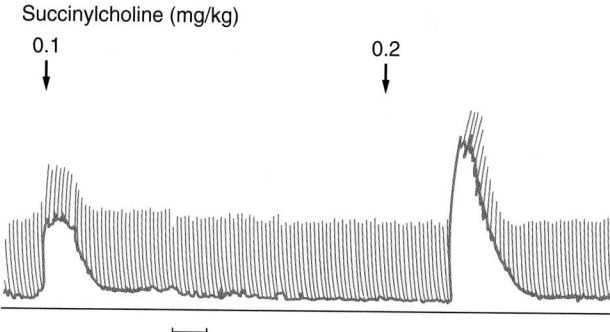

FIGURE 25-3. Administration of low doses of succinylcholine to a patient with myotonic dystrophy produces an exaggerated contraction of skeletal muscle. (Reprinted from Mitchell MM, Ali HH, Savarese JJ: Myotonia and neuromuscular blocking drugs. Anesthesiology 1978; 49: 44–48, with permission.)

taurine, clomipramine, and imipramine have been used for the treatment of myotonia with less than conclusive results.

Management of Anesthesia

Considerations for anesthesia for patients with myotonic dystrophy include the presence of cardiac and respiratory muscle disease and the abnormal responses to drugs used during anesthesia. Succinylcholine produces an exaggerated contracture and its use should be avoided (Fig. 25-3). The myotonic response to succinylcholine can be so severe that ventilation and tracheal intubation are difficult or impossible. Most patients with myotonic dystrophy develop a chronic myopathy and the response to nondepolarizing muscle relaxants may be enhanced. Reversal with neostigmine may provoke myotonia. The response to the peripheral nerve stimulator must be carefully interpreted because muscle stimulation may produce myotonia. The myotonic response may be misinterpreted as sustained tetanus when significant neuromuscular blockade still exists.

Patients with myotonic dystrophy are sensitive to the respiratory depressant effects of opioids, barbiturates, benzodiazepines, and inhaled anesthetics. Respiratory complications are more likely to occur in the early postoperative period after upper abdominal surgery or in those patients in whom preoperative upper extremity weakness was evident.[9]

No specific anesthetic technique has been shown to be superior for patients with myotonic dystrophy. Carefully controlled propofol infusions have been used successfully. Inhaled anesthetics may be used but close monitoring of cardiac rhythm and cardiovascular function is indicated. Postoperative mechanical ventilation should be employed until muscle strength and function return.[10] Regional anesthesia has been described for both children and adults with myotonic dystrophy.[11]

Skeletal muscle weakness and myotonia are exacerbated during pregnancy. Labor is typically prolonged and there is an increased incidence of postpartum hemorrhage (placenta accreta). Spinal and epidural anesthesia have been successfully used for pregnant patients.

Familial Periodic Paralysis

The familial periodic paralyses are a subgroup of diseases referred to as the *skeletal muscle channelopathies*. This group of diseases include hyperkalemic and hypokalemic periodic paralysis, paramyotonia congenita, potassium-aggravated myotonia, normokalemic periodic paralysis, and Andersen syndrome. The common mechanism for these diseases appears to be a persistent

TABLE 25-3

CLINICAL FEATURES OF FAMILIAL PERIODIC PARALYSIS

Hypokalemic
Calcium channel defect
Potassium level <3 mEq/L during symptoms
Precipitating factors
    High glucose meals
    Strenuous exercise
    Glucose-insulin infusions
    Stress
    Hypothermia
Chronic myopathy with aging
Hyperkalemic
Sodium channel defect
Potassium level >5.5 mEq/L during symptoms
Precipitating factors
    Rest after exercise
    Potassium infusions
    Metabolic acidosis
    Hypothermia
Skeletal muscle weakness may be localized to tongue and eyelids

sodium inward current depolarization causing muscle membrane inexcitability and subsequent muscle weakness.[12]

Hyperkalemic Periodic Paralysis

Hyperkalemic periodic paralysis is characterized by episodes of myotonia and muscle weakness that may last for several hours after exposure to a trigger. Weakness can occur during rest after strenuous exercise, infusion of potassium, metabolic acidosis, or hypothermia (Table 25-3). The weakness may be so severe that ventilatory support is required. The hyperkalemia is often transient and occurs only at the time of weakness, and potassium levels measured during the attack may be normal or decreased. Treatment consists of a low-potassium diet and the administration of thiazide diuretics.

Hypokalemic Periodic Paralysis

Hypokalemic periodic paralysis is caused by a defect in the calcium ion channel. Paralysis may be produced by a decrease in serum potassium levels, ingestion of carbohydrates, strenuous exercise, and infusion of glucose and insulin (Table 25-3). Paralysis is usually incomplete, affecting the limbs and trunk, but sparing the diaphragm. Low potassium levels during acute episodes can cause cardiac dysrhythmias. Chronic muscle weakness occurs in most patients with hypokalemic periodic paralysis as they age.[13]

Treatment consists of potassium infusion and the administration of acetazolamide and dichlorphenamide. Potassium-sparing diuretics such as triamterene and spironolactone may be beneficial.

Management of Anesthesia

The primary goal with both forms of periodic paralysis is maintenance of normal potassium levels and avoidance of events that precipitate weakness. Any electrolyte abnormality should be corrected prior to surgery. These patients may be sensitive to nondepolarizing muscle relaxants, and short-acting muscle relaxants are preferred. Succinylcholine is best avoided as its administration may alter potassium levels. Metabolic changes (acidosis and alkalosis) or medications (glucose and insulin, diuretics) that reduce potassium levels may initiate an episode of paralysis. Because changes in

TABLE 24-4

DIFFERENT PRESENTATIONS OF MYASTHENIA GRAVIS

■ TYPE	■ ETIOLOGY	■ ONSET	■ SEX	■ THYMUS	■ COURSE
Neonatal myasthenia	Passage of antibodies from myasthenic mothers across the placenta	Neonatal	Both sexes	Normal	Transient
Congenital myasthenia	Congenital end-plate pathology, genetic autosomal recessive pattern of inheritance	0–2 yr	Male > female	Normal	Nonfluctuating compatible with long survival
Juvenile myasthenia	Autoimmune disorder	2–20 yr	Female > male (4:1)	Hyperplasia	Slowly progressive, tendency to relapse and remission
Adult myasthenia	Autoimmune disorder	20–40 yr	Female > male thymoma	Hyperplasia > within 3–5 yr	Maximum severity
Elderly myasthenia	Autoimmune disorder	>40 yr	Male > female	Thymoma (benign or locally invasive)	Rapid progress, higher mortality

Reproduced from Baraka A: Anesthesia and myasthenia gravis. Can J Anaesth 1992; 39: 476, with permission.

potassium levels may precede the onset of weakness, serial measurement of potassium levels during prolonged surgical procedures and the early postoperative period should be considered. The ECG should be monitored for evidence of potassium-related dysrhythmias. Other recommendations include the avoidance of carbohydrate loads, hypothermia, and excessive hyperventilation. Any cause of potassium depletion can produce muscle weakness. Halogenated inhaled anesthetics have been administered without complication and regional anesthesia has been used.[14] Malignant hyperthermia has been associated with both forms of periodic paralysis.

Myasthenia Gravis

Myasthenia gravis is an autoimmune disease with antibodies directed against the nicotinic acetylcholine receptor or other muscle membrane proteins. Eighty-five percent of patients with myasthenia gravis have identifiable antiacetylcholine receptor antibodies and are considered seropositive. The majority of seronegative patients have antibodies to other muscle membrane proteins such as muscle-specific receptor tyrosine kinase, rapsyn, or agrin. These autoantibodies damage muscle membranes by activation of complement, degradation of acetylcholine receptor molecules, or blockade of the acetylcholine receptor. The different pathophysiologic mechanisms explain the heterogeneity of the clinical manifestations of myasthenia gravis.[15] The thymus may play a central role in the pathogenesis of myasthenia gravis as 90% of patients have histologic abnormalities such as thymoma, thymic hyperplasia, or thymic atrophy.

The clinical hallmark of myasthenia gravis is skeletal muscle weakness. The weakness is aggravated by repetitive muscle use and there are periods of exacerbation alternating with remission. Any skeletal muscle may be affected, although there is a predilection for muscles innervated by cranial nerves. Initial symptoms include diplopia, dysarthria, dysphagia, or limb muscle weakness. Myasthenic crises occur in 15 to 50% of patients and are often precipitated by pulmonary infections and result in respiratory failure requiring mechanical ventilation. Cardiac manifestations of myasthenia gravis include

focal myocarditis, atrial fibrillation, atrioventricular conduction delay, and left ventricular diastolic dysfunction.

Viral infection, pregnancy, extreme heat, stress, and surgery may initiate or exacerbate the symptoms of myasthenia, but the response to stressors is unpredictable. Some pregnant patients have a remission during pregnancy while others (20 to 40%) have increased symptoms during gestation. Postpartum respiratory failure can occur. Fifteen to 20% of neonates born to myasthenic mothers have transient myasthenia from passive transfer of acetylcholine receptor antibodies. Signs and symptoms of neonatal myasthenia begin 12 to 48 hours after birth and may persist for several weeks.[16]

Disease classification is based on skeletal muscle groups affected as well as age of onset (Table 25-4). The Osserman staging system is based on the severity of the disease: type I, ocular signs and symptoms only; type IIA, generalized muscle weakness; type IIB, generalized moderate weakness and/or bulbar dysfunction; type III, acute fulminant presentation and/or respiratory dysfunction; and type IV, severe generalized myasthenia.

The diagnosis of myasthenia is based on the clinical history, the edrophonium test, electromyography, and the detection of circulating acetylcholine receptor antibodies. No single test is definitive.

Treatment includes the administration of cholinesterase inhibitors, corticosteroids, immunosuppressants, plasmapheresis, and intravenous immunoglobulin. Cholinesterase inhibitors function by increasing the concentration of acetylcholine at the postsynaptic membrane. Consistent control of myasthenia with cholinesterase inhibitors can be quite challenging. Underdosing will result in increased muscle weakness, whereas overdosing will produce a "cholinergic crisis" characterized by abdominal pain, salivation, bradycardia, and skeletal muscle weakness.

Corticosteroids produce an improvement in muscle strength in myasthenic patients, although the precise mechanism is unknown. Immunosuppressants used for the treatment of myasthenic include azathioprine, cyclosporine, cyclophosphamide, tacrolimus, rituximab, and mycophenolate mofetil. Plasmapheresis removes acetylcholine receptor antibodies from the circulation and is effective during a myasthenic crisis. Intravenous immunoglobulin may also be effective.

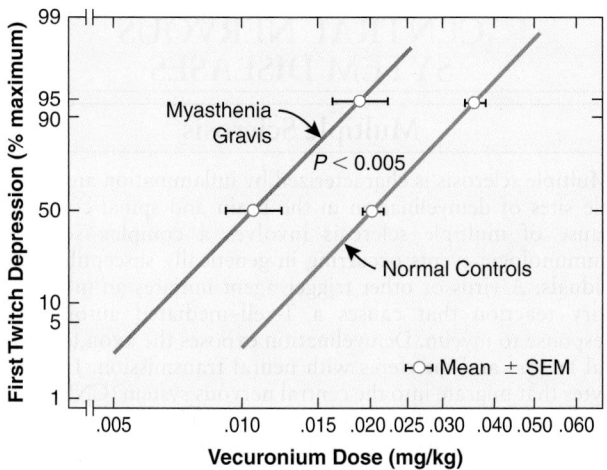

FIGURE 25-4. Dose-response for vecuronium in normal patients and patients with myasthenia gravis. (Reprinted from Eisenkraft JB, Book WJ, Papatestas AE: Sensitivity to vecuronium in myasthenia gravis: A dose-response study. Can J Anaesth 1990: 37: 301–306, with permission.)

The role of thymectomy for the treatment of myasthenia is not clearly established. Although a thymoma is a clear indication for thymectomy, the operation for other myasthenic patients is controversial. Different surgical techniques include sternal splitting with extended thymectomy, transcervical, video-assisted thoracoscopy, and robotic surgery.[17] Less invasive approaches offer fewer postoperative complications, but may result in incomplete resection of the thymus.

Management of Anesthesia

The primary concern for anesthesia is the potential interaction between the disease, treatment of the disease, and neuromuscular blocking drugs. The uncontrolled or poorly controlled myasthenic patient is exquisitely sensitive to nondepolarizing muscle relaxants (Fig. 25-4). Small defasciculating doses of nondepolarizing drugs can produce significant respiratory muscle weakness and respiratory distress. An anesthetic technique that avoids the use of a muscle relaxant may be preferred.[18] Isoflurane, sevoflurane, and desflurane depress neuromuscular transmission and may provide adequate muscle relaxation for tracheal intubation.

Cholinesterase inhibitor drugs used to treat myasthenia will influence the response to both depolarizing and nondepolarizing muscle relaxants. If muscle relaxation is required, small doses of short-acting nondepolarizing muscle relaxants should be administered. Close, objective monitoring of neuromuscular transmission and clinical effect is necessary. Although patients with myasthenia have a resistance to succinylcholine, a dose of 1.5 to 2 mg/kg will be adequate for rapid tracheal intubation. Preoperative administration of pyridostigmine, however, may prolong the duration of action of succinylcholine.[19]

Adjuvant drugs that may exacerbate muscle weakness in myasthenic patients include aminoglycoside antibiotics, polymyxins, β-adrenergic blockers, procainamide, corticosteroids, and phenytoin. Patients with myasthenia have central respiratory depression, and the respiratory depressant effects of barbiturates, benzodiazepines, opioids, and propofol may be accentuated.

Most anesthetic techniques permit weaning form mechanical ventilation and tracheal extubation of myasthenic patients soon after surgery; however, these patients can be quite challenging to wean from ventilatory support.[20]

Epidural analgesia can be used during labor and delivery. Muscle relaxation induced by regional anesthesia may compound the weakness caused by myasthenia. Amide local anesthetics may be better than ester local anesthetics as the metabolism of amides is not affected by cholinesterase activity. Exacerbations of myasthenia must be anticipated during pregnancy.

Myasthenic Syndrome (Lambert-Eaton)

The Lambert-Eaton myasthenic syndrome is a disorder of neuromuscular transmission associated with carcinomas, particularly small cell carcinoma of the lung and lymphoproliferative diseases (Table 25-5). Lambert-Eaton myasthenic syndrome is an autoimmune disease in which antibodies against voltage-gated calcium ion channels (presynaptic) are produced. The result is a decreased release of acetylcholine in response to nerve stimulation. The typical patient is a man older than 40 years of age with proximal extremity weakness (hip, shoulder) that affects gait and the ability to stand and climb stairs. Autonomic dysfunction, such as xerostomia, impotence, orthostatic hypotension, constipation, and altered sweating responses may develop.[21]

Treatment of the underlying neoplasm may improve the neurologic condition. The most effective drug for treatment of

---

TABLE 25-5

COMPARISON OF MYASTHENIC SYNDROME AND MYASTHENIA GRAVIS

	■ MYASTHENIC SYNDROME	■ MYASTHENIA GRAVIS
Manifestations	Proximal limb weakness (arms > legs)	Extraocular, bulbar, and facial muscle weakness
	Strength improves with exercise	Fatigue with exercise
	Muscle pain common	Muscle pain uncommon
	Reflexes absent or decreased	Reflexes normal
Gender	Male > female	Female > male
Coexisting pathology	Small cell carcinoma of lung	Thymoma
Response to muscle relaxants	Sensitive to succinylcholine and nondepolarizing muscle relaxants	Resistant to succinylcholine
		Sensitive to nondepolarizing muscle relaxants
	Poor response to anticholinesterases	Poor response to anticholinesterases

Reprinted from Stoelting RK, Dierdorf SF, eds: Anesthesia and Co-Existing Disease, 3rd ed. New York, Churchill Livingstone, 1993, with permission.

myasthenic syndrome is 3,4-diaminopyridine, which prolongs the action potential and increases release of acetylcholine. Immunosuppression with corticosteroids, azathioprine and cyclosporine may be effective. Plasmapheresis and intravenous immunoglobulin may produce short-term improvement.[22]

Management of Anesthesia

Patients with myasthenic syndrome are sensitive to the effects of both depolarizing and nondepolarizing muscle relaxants. The administration of 3,4-diaminopyridine should be continued to the time of surgery.

Guillain-Barré Syndrome (Polyradiculoneuritis)

Guillain-Barré syndrome is the acute form of a group of disorders classified as inflammatory neuropathies. Other inflammatory neuropathies include acute inflammatory polyneuropathy, acute motor axonal neuropathy, acute motor-sensory axonal neuropathy, Miller-Fisher syndrome, and chronic inflammatory demyelinating neuropathy. Guillain-Barré syndrome is an autoimmune disease caused by a bacterial or viral infection that triggers an immune response that produces antibodies that damage the myelin sheath and cause axonal degeneration.[23]

Most patients have a history of a respiratory or gastrointestinal infection within 4 weeks of the onset of neurologic symptoms. Guillain-Barré syndrome is characterized by the acute or subacute onset of skeletal muscle weakness or paralysis of the legs. Paresthesias may precede the onset of paralysis. The paralysis progresses cephalad to include the muscles of the trunk and arms. Difficulty swallowing and impaired ventilation secondary to intercostal muscle paralysis can occur. Progression occurs over 10 to 12 days, followed by gradual recovery. The most serious immediate problem is ventilatory insufficiency. If the vital capacity decreases to <15 to 20 mL/kg, mechanical ventilation of the lungs is indicated. The more rapid the onset of quadriplegia, the more likely is the need for mechanical ventilation. Although 85% of patients with this syndrome achieve a good recovery, chronic recurrent neuropathy develops in 3 to 5% of patients.

Intensive respiratory care and management of autonomic dysfunction have reduced mortality to <5%. Plasmapheresis and the administration of intravenous immunoglobulin may modulate the disordered immune response.

Autonomic nervous system dysfunction can produce wide fluctuations in cardiovascular parameters. In a manner similar to autonomic hyperreflexia, physical stimulation can precipitate hypertension, tachycardia, and cardiac dysrhythmias.

Management of Anesthesia

Autonomic nervous system dysfunction may cause hypotension secondary to postural changes, blood loss, or positive airway pressure. Noxious stimuli such as laryngoscopy and tracheal intubation may produce exaggerated increases in heart rate and blood pressure.

The administration of succinylcholine should be avoided because of the danger of potassium release and hyperkalemia. This risk may persist after clinical recovery from the disease.[24] A short-acting, nondepolarizing muscle relaxant with minimal cardiovascular effects such as cisatracurium or rocuronium would be a useful choice. The sensitivity to nondepolarizing muscle relaxants may vary from extreme sensitivity to resistance, depending on the phase of the disease.[25] It is likely that mechanical ventilation will be required during the immediate postoperative period. Patients with Guillain-Barré syndrome who have pronounced sensory disturbances may benefit form the administration of neuraxial opioids.

CENTRAL NERVOUS SYTEM DISEASES

Multiple Sclerosis

Multiple sclerosis is characterized by inflammation and multiple sites of demyelination in the brain and spinal cord. The cause of multiple sclerosis involves a complex series of immunologic events occurring in genetically susceptible individuals. A virus or other trigger agent initiates an inflammatory reaction that causes a T-cell–mediated autoimmune response to myelin. Demyelination exposes the axon to harmful factors and interferes with neural transmission. Lymphocytes that migrate into the central nervous system (CNS) mediate much of the inflammatory reaction. The ability of neural tissue to repair itself during the early phases of the process explains the relapsing nature of the disease.[26]

The symptoms of multiple sclerosis depend on the sites of injury in the brain and spinal cord. Demyelination of the optic tracts produces visual disturbances, whereas demyelination of the oculomotor pathways results in nystagmus. Lesions of the spinal cord produce limb weakness and paresthesias. The legs are affected more than the arms. Bowel retention and urinary incontinence are frequent complaints. Brainstem involvement can produce diplopia, trigeminal neuralgia, cardiac dysrhythmias, and autonomic dysfunction, while alterations in ventilation can lead to hypoxemia, apnea, and respiratory failure. The course of multiple sclerosis is characterized by exacerbation of symptoms at unpredictable intervals over a period of years. During the early phase of the disease patients are classified as either relapsing-remitting multiple sclerosis (85%) or primary-progressive multiple sclerosis. Over time, many patients with relapsing-remitting multiple sclerosis develop neurodegeneration and are categorized as secondary-progressive multiple sclerosis. Patients with primary-progressive multiple sclerosis are generally devoid of acute episodes, but develop progressive degeneration. Pregnancy is associated with an improvement in symptoms, but relapse frequently occurs in the first 3 postpartum months.

Clinical criteria for diagnosis include age of onset between 10 and 50 years, neurologic signs and symptoms of CNS white matter disease, two or more attacks separated by a month or more, and involvement of two or more noncontiguous anatomic areas. Elevated levels of immunoglobulin (Ig) G and albumin in the cerebrospinal fluid are characteristic of multiple sclerosis. Magnetic resonance imaging (MRI) is a sensitive diagnostic tool for multiple sclerosis and provides direct evidence of the location of demyelinated plaques in the CNS.

Therapy for multiple sclerosis is directed at modulating the immunologic and inflammatory responses that damage the CNS. Corticosteroids are the primary agents for treatment of acute exacerbations of multiple sclerosis. Corticosteroids have diverse effects that suppress cellular immune responses and inflammatory edema. Interferon alters the inflammatory response and augments natural disease suppression and has been shown to reduce the relapse rate. Glatiramer is a mixture of polypeptides that mimic the structure of myelin and serves as a decoy for autoantibodies. Patient response to immunosuppressants has been variable. Mitoxantrone, which can be cardiotoxic, can be used to treat aggressive multiple sclerosis.[27] Symptomatic therapy includes diazepam, dantrolene, and baclofen for spasticity. Painful dysesthesia, tonic seizures, dysarthria, and ataxia can be treated with carbamazepine. Nonspecific measures include the avoidance of excessive fatigue, emotional stress, and hyperthermia. Demyelinated nerve fibers are extremely sensitive to increases in temperature. A temperature increase of 0.5°C can block impulse conduction in demyelinated fibers.

Management of Anesthesia

The effect of surgery and anesthesia on the course of multiple sclerosis is controversial. Regional anesthesia and general anesthesia have been reported to exacerbate multiple sclerosis, while other reports have found no correlation between anesthesia and the course of the disease. Factors other than anesthesia such as infection, emotional stress, and hyperpyrexia may contribute to an increased risk of a perioperative exacerbation. Preoperatively, the patient should be advised that surgery and anesthesia could produce a relapse despite a well-managed anesthetic.

Although the mechanism is not known, spinal anesthesia has been associated with an exacerbation of the disease. It could be speculated that demyelinated areas of the spinal cord are more sensitive to the effects of the local anesthetic, causing a relative neurotoxicity. Evidence for this theory is found by the observation that higher concentrations of bupivacaine (0.25%) used for labor epidural analgesia were more likely to cause relapse than lower concentrations.[28] With such a precaution, epidural analgesia can be safely provided for women during labor.

Patients being treated with corticosteroids may require intravenous corticosteroid supplementation during the perioperative period. Immunosuppressants can produce cardiotoxicity and subclinical cardiac dysfunction. Baclofen can produce an increased sensitivity to nondepolarizing muscle relaxants, while anticonvulsants produce resistance to nondepolarizing muscle relaxants. In theory, succinylcholine could produce an exaggerated release of potassium, although this has not been reported. Autonomic dysfunction may exaggerate the hypotensive effects of volatile anesthetics. Respiratory muscle weakness and respiratory control dysfunction increase the likelihood of the need for supplemental oxygen and/or mechanical ventilation during the immediate postoperative period.[29]

Epilepsy

A seizure is a common manifestation of many types of CNS diseases and is the external manifestation of epilepsy. A seizure results from an excessive discharge of large numbers of neurons that become depolarized in a synchronous fashion. Idiopathic seizures usually begin during childhood. The sudden onset of seizures in a young or middle-aged adult may indicate focal brain disease, particularly a tumor. The onset of seizures after 60 years of age can be a result of cerebrovascular disease, head injury, tumor, infection, or metabolic disturbances. Some rare forms of epilepsy are caused by mutations in ion channels. The availability of new antiseizure drugs has increased the therapeutic options for patients with epilepsy (Table 25-6).[30]

TABLE 25-6

ANTICONVULSANT DRUGS

■ DRUG	■ SEIZURE TYPE	■ THERAPEUTIC BLOOD LEVELS (μg/mL)	■ SIDE EFFECTS*
Phenobarbital	Generalized	15–35	Sedation, increased drug metabolism
Valproate	Generalized Absence	50–100	Pancreatitis, hepatic dysfunction
Felbamate	Generalized Partial	20–140	Insomnia, ataxia, nausea
Phenytoin	Generalized Partial	10–20	Gingival hyperplasia Dermatitis Resistance to NM blockers
Fosphenytoin	Generalized Partial		Paresthesias Hypotension
Carbamazepine	Generalized Partial	6–12	Cardiotoxic, hepatitis Resistance to NM blockers
Lamotrigine	Generalized Partial	2–16	Rash Stevens-Johnson syndrome
Topiramate	Generalized Partial	4–10	Severe metabolic acidosis Hyperthermia
Gabapentin	Generalized Partial	4–16	Fatigue, somnolence
Primidone	Generalized Partial	6–12	Nausea, ataxia
Clonazepam	Absence	0.01–0.07	Ataxia
Ethosuximide	Absence	40–100	Leukopenia, Erythema multiforme
Levetiracetam	Generalized Partial	5–45	Dizziness, headache Somnolence
Oxcarbazepine	Partial	10–35	Hyponatremia, diplopia Somnolence
Tiagabine	Partial		Tremor, depression
Zonisamide	Generalized	10–40	Anorexia Decreased cognition

Partial listing NM, neuromuscular.

The most frequently encountered types of seizures are:

1. *Grand mal seizure*: A grand mal seizure is characterized by generalized tonic-clonic activity. All respiratory activity is arrested and a period of arterial hypoxemia ensues. The tonic phase lasts for 20 to 40 seconds and is followed by the clonic phase. In the postictal period, the patient is lethargic and confused. Diazepam and thiopental are effective for treatment of acute, generalized seizures. Epileptic patients resistant to drug therapy may benefit from surgical resection of a seizure focus or vagal nerve stimulator implantation.

2. *Focal cortical seizure*: Focal cortical seizures may be sensory or motor, depending on the site of neuronal discharge. There is usually no loss of consciousness, although the seizure activity may spread to produce a grand mal seizure.

3. *Absence seizure (petit mal)*: Absence seizures are characterized by a brief loss of awareness lasting 30 seconds. Additional manifestations include staring, blinking, and rolling of the eyes. Absence seizures typically occur in children and young adults.

4. *Akinetic seizure*: Akinetic seizures are characterized by a sudden, brief loss of consciousness and postural tone. These types of seizures usually occur in children and can result in severe head injury from a fall.

5. *Status epilepticus*: Status epilepticus is defined as two consecutive tonic-clonic seizures without regaining consciousness, or seizure activity that is unabated for 30 minutes or more. Grand mal status epilepticus typically lasts for 48 hours with a seizure frequency of four to five per hour; mortality can be as high as 20%. As the seizure progresses, skeletal muscle activity diminishes and seizure activity may be evident only on the electroencephalogram (EEG). Respiratory effects of status epilepticus include inhibition of the respiratory centers, uncoordinated skeletal muscle activity that impairs ventilation, and abnormal autonomic activity that produces bronchoconstriction. There is a high likelihood of permanent neuronal damage from continued seizures. Diazepam and lorazepam are considered the drugs of choice for the treatment of status epilepticus. Because the effects of benzodiazepines are transient, a longer-acting anticonvulsant such as phenytoin or phenobarbital must also be administered. Thiopental is quite effective for the initial treatment of status epilepticus, but the effect is brief. On rare occasions, general anesthesia with isoflurane or barbiturates may be required.

Management of Anesthesia

Patients receiving antiseizure medications should be maintained on their normal medication regimen until the time of surgery and administration resumed as soon as possible after surgery. A decline in blood levels of anticonvulsant drugs increases the likelihood of postoperative seizures. An anesthesia technique should be used that minimizes the risk of seizure activity. Stimulation of the hepatic microsomal enzymes by anticonvulsants may increase the rate of biotransformation of volatile halogenated anesthetics and increase the risk of organ toxicity. Side effects of anticonvulsants include leukopenia, anemia, hepatitis, pancreatitis, hepatic failure, coagulopathy, aplastic anemia, cardiotoxicity, hypothyroidism, rash, and hypersensitivity.[31]

Although most inhaled anesthetics, including nitrous oxide, have been reported to produce seizure activity, such activity during the administration of isoflurane and desflurane is extremely rare. These drugs generally produce a dose-dependent depression of EEG activity. However, sevoflurane may be epileptogenic, although the clinical significance of this finding is uncertain.[32] Ketamine and methohexital may produce seizure activity in patients with known seizure disorders. It would seem to be reasonable to avoid the use of ketamine and

methohexital in patients with seizure disorders when alternative drugs such as thiopental, propofol, and benzodiazepines are available. Potent opioids such as fentanyl, sufentanil, alfentanil, and remifentanil may produce myoclonic activity or chest wall rigidity that can be confused with seizure activity. Patients receiving phenytoin or carbamazepine exhibit resistance to nondepolarizing muscle relaxants.

Parkinson Disease

Parkinson disease is a degenerative disease of the CNS caused by loss of dopaminergic fibers in the basal ganglia of the brain. The characteristic pathologic feature is destruction of dopamine-containing nerve cells in the substantia nigra of the basal ganglia. Lewy bodies, a hallmark of the pathology of Parkinson disease, are cytoplasmic aggregates of α-synuclein. α-Synuclein inclusions occur in other areas of the brain and peripheral nerves. The cause of Parkinson disease is multifactorial, with genetic and environmental factors. Other than the well-known postencephalitic Parkinson disease, however, there is little evidence that Parkinson disease is caused by a virus.[33]

The clinical effects of Parkinson disease are caused by dopamine deficiency. Dopamine deficiency increases activity of γ-aminobutyric acid, which inhibits thalamic and brainstem nuclei, which suppresses cortical motor activity, thereby causing tremor, akinesia, and gait and posture abnormalities. The most characteristic clinical features of Parkinson disease are resting tremor, cogwheel rigidity of the extremities, bradykinesia, shuffling gait, stooped posture, and facial immobility. These features are secondary to diminished inhibition of the extrapyramidal motor system as a result of dopamine depletion in the basal ganglia. Other clinical features are seborrhea, sialorrhea, orthostatic hypotension, bladder dysfunction, papillary abnormalities, diaphragmatic spasm, oculogyric crises, dementia, and mental depression.

Treatment is directed toward increasing dopamine levels in the brain, but preventing the adverse peripheral effects of dopamine. Levodopa is the single most effective therapy for patients with Parkinson disease. When administered orally, levodopa is converted to dopamine and causes side effects such as nausea, vomiting, and hypotension. To avoid such side effects, levodopa is administered with a peripheral decarboxylase inhibitor (carbidopa). Cardiovascular effects of levodopa include depletion of myocardial norepinephrine stores, peripheral vasoconstriction, hypovolemia, and hypotension. More recently, entacapone, a catechol-O-methyltransferase inhibitor has been added to the combination of levodopa and carbidopa. Entacapone blocks the peripheral metabolism of levodopa and increases the bioavailability of levodopa. Other drugs that improve function in patients with Parkinson disease include the monoamine oxidase-B inhibitors selegiline and rasagiline. Dopamine receptor agonists, such as bromocriptine, pergolide, cabergoline, pramipexole, ropinirole, exert their effect on dopamine receptors in the brain. The ergot-related dopamine agonists (pergolide and cabergoline) have been associated with the development of cardiac valvular fibrosis. Pallidotomy and implantation of deep-brain stimulators may be a good option for selected patients. The therapeutic regimen for patients with Parkinson disease is complex and requires a skilled neurologist to individualize therapy.[34]

Management of Anesthesia

The patient's medications should be administered on the morning of surgery. The half-life of levodopa is short, and interruption of therapy for more than 6 to 12 hours can result in severe skeletal muscle rigidity that interferes with ventilation. Apomorphine is a dopamine agonist that can be administered subcutaneously or intravenously if oral levodopa cannot be administered. Dopamine antagonists such as phenothiazines, droperidol, and metoclopramide should be avoided. Alfentanil and fentanyl may produce acute dystonic reactions in patients with Parkinson disease. Although ketamine could produce an exaggerated sympathetic nervous system response with resultant tachycardia and hypertension, it has been used without difficulty in patients with Parkinson disease. There are no reports of adverse responses to isoflurane, sevoflurane, or desflurane. The likelihood of coexisting heart disease in elderly patients with Parkinson disease may influence the selection of anesthetics and monitoring techniques. Although definitive studies of anesthesia for patients receiving monoamine oxidase-B inhibitors (selegiline, rasagiline) have not been performed, clinical experience indicates that anesthesia is usually uneventful. There have been reports of agitation, muscle rigidity, and hyperthermia in patients receiving meperidine and selegiline. Patients being treated with dopamine agonists may be at risk for neuroleptic malignant syndrome.

Autonomic dysfunction is common. The most consistent cardiovascular abnormality is orthostatic hypotension that may be compounded by the vasodilatory effects of anti-Parkinson drugs. Patients with Parkinson disease would be more likely to develop exaggerated responses in blood pressure in response to inhaled halogenated anesthetics. Gastrointestinal dysfunction is manifested be excessive salivation and esophageal dysfunction. The patient with Parkinson disease should be considered to be at risk for aspiration pneumonitis.

Perioperative respiratory complications are common.[35] Upper airway obstruction may occur as a result of poor coordination of upper airway muscles secondary to neurotransmitter imbalance caused the disease process or induced by the administration of antidopaminergic drugs. Some patients with upper airway obstruction may respond to anti-Parkinson drugs.

In the postoperative period, patients with Parkinson disease are susceptible to mental confusion and hallucinations. Such alterations in mental function may not appear until the day after surgery.

Huntington Disease

Huntington disease is an autosomal dominant inherited disease characterized by progressive neurodegeneration. Huntington disease is one of the trinucleotide repeat disorders. An increase in cytosine, adenine, and guanine (CAG) repeat sequences on chromosome 4 is the genetic defect that produces a mutant huntingtin protein that causes Huntington disease. Huntingtin is found in all human cells, but most notably brain cells. The precise function of this protein is unknown. Neurons from patients with Huntington disease show abnormal inclusions containing mutant huntingtin and polyglutamine. It has been speculated that degradation of the mutant huntingtin by caspase-6 produces a cytotoxic metabolite. Brain specimens show marked atrophy and cell loss in the caudate and putamen. Identification of the Huntington gene provides a reliable predictive test; however, the delayed nature of the clinical manifestations of the disease presents legal and ethical concerns about predictive testing.[36]

Clinical features are choreiform movements and dementia. Onset is typically between the ages of 35 and 40 years, but onset has been reported as early as age 2 and as late as age 80. The disease progresses for several years and depression makes suicide a frequent occurrence. Death usually results from malnutrition and aspiration pneumonitis. Hypothalamic atrophy can cause endocrine changes such as elevated cortisol levels, reduced testosterone levels, and diabetes. The duration of Huntington disease averages 17 years from the time of diagnosis to death.

There is no specific therapy for Huntington disease. Drugs used for the treatment of chorea include haloperidol, fluphenazine, olanzapine, amantadine, riluzole, and tetrabenazine. Antidepressants are commonly used to alleviate depression. Coenzyme Q10 and minocycline are under investigation as neuroprotectants.

Management of Anesthesia

The medical literature is sparse with regard to the anesthetic management of patients with Huntington disease.[37] Many of the manifestations of Huntington disease are typical of patients with neurodegenerative disorders. As the disease progresses, the pharyngeal muscles become dysfunctional and the risk of aspiration pneumonitis increases. Although there are no specific contraindications to the use of inhaled or intravenous anesthetics, recovery from propofol may be faster than from other intravenous hypnotics. Short-acting muscle relaxants would be preferable to longer-acting relaxants. Decreased plasma cholinesterase may prolong the effect of succinylcholine. Spinal anesthesia has been successfully used.

As for any patient with a progressive neurologic disease, delayed emergence and an increased likelihood of respiratory complications must be anticipated in the immediate postoperative period.

Alzheimer Disease

Alzheimer disease is the major cause of dementia in the United States. The incidence of Alzheimer disease is 1% in 60-year-old patients and 30% in 85-year-old patients. Although dementia is caused by >60 disorders, Alzheimer disease is responsible for 50 to 60% of the cases. Memory impairment and language deterioration occur early in the disease process. Motor and sensory abnormalities, gait disturbances, seizures, agitation, and psychosis are later features of the disease. Computed tomography (CT), MRI, and positron emission tomography are helpful in differentiating Alzheimer disease from other causes of dementia. Evidence of hippocampal atrophy may precede the onset of clinical symptoms.

The deposition of amyloid beta peptide oligomers appears to be central to the process of degeneration and death of neurons. Deposition of this peptide produces neuritic plaques and neurofibrillary tangles and activates the apoptotic cell death cascade that causes neurotransmitter dysfunction. Therapy is currently limited but ongoing research is directed at three areas: (1) antiamyloid deposition: statins, metal chelation (copper, zinc), antifibrillation, beta and gamma secretase inhibition; (2) neuroprotection: antioxidants, nerve growth factor, anti-inflammation, caspase inhibition, monoamine oxidase inhibition, cholinesterase inhibition; and (3) neurorestoration: nerve growth factor, cell transplantation, and stem cell therapy.[38] The administration of cholinesterase inhibitors is considered standard of care for patients with early Alzheimer disease. The three most commonly used cholinesterase inhibitors are donepezil, rivastigmine, and galantamine. Cholinesterase inhibitors improve the patient's ability to perform daily living activities and may improve cognition. Side effects of cholinesterase inhibitors include nausea, vomiting, bradycardia, syncope, and fatigue.

Management of Anesthesia

Selection of anesthetic drugs and techniques for patients with Alzheimer disease is guided by the patient's general physiologic condition, the degree of neurologic impairment, and the potential for interaction between anesthetics and medications the patient is receiving. The patient's preoperative drug list should be reviewed for the possibility of interactions with anesthetics. Patients are likely to be disoriented and uncooperative because of dementia. Sedative premedications are rarely indicated as further mental confusion could result. Anesthetics known to result in rapid recovery, such as propofol, desflurane, and sevoflurane, are advantageous. Although isoflurane may increase amyloid beta protein generation and aggregation in isolated human neurons, the clinical significance is unknown.[39] If an anticholinergic is required, glycopyrrolate, which does not cross the blood–brain barrier, is preferable to atropine or scopolamine. An anticholinergic that crosses the blood–brain barrier could exacerbate dementia. Patients receiving cholinesterase inhibitors may have a prolonged response to succinylcholine.

Amyotrophic Lateral Sclerosis

Amyotrophic lateral sclerosis (ALS, Lou Gehrig disease, motor neuron disease) is a degenerative disease of motor cells throughout the CNS. Upper and lower motor neurons are involved. Progression of the disease is relentless and death usually follows within 3 to 5 years of diagnosis, although 10% of ALS patients survive for 10 years. The cause of ALS is unknown and many hypotheses have been proposed, including heavy metal exposure and environmental causes. Current research has centered on glutamate excitotoxicity and oxidant stress. Five to 10 % of ALS cases are hereditary and patients exhibit a mutation of superoxide dismutase.[40]

The signs and symptoms of ALS reflect the upper and lower motor neuron dysfunction. Onset patterns such as bulbar, cervical, and lumbar are determined by the area of the CNS first affected. Initial symptoms are weakness, atrophy, and skeletal muscle fasciculation. As the disease progresses, the atrophy and weakness involve most skeletal muscles, including those of the tongue, pharynx, larynx, and chest. Dysarthria and dysphagia are a result of bulbar involvement. Pulmonary function tests demonstrate a decrease in vital capacity, maximal voluntary ventilation, and diminished expiratory muscle reserve. Respiratory failure eventually develops and ventilatory support is required. Patients with ALS have autonomic dysfunction as evidenced by an increased resting heart rate, orthostatic hypotension, and elevated levels of epinephrine and norepinephrine. There may be decreased R-R interval variation on the ECG and a decreased heart rate response to atropine. The cause of death for patients with ALS is usually respiratory failure. Sudden death from circulatory collapse may occur in ventilator-dependent patients with ALS.

Riluzole, a glutamate release inhibitor, is the only drug currently approved for the treatment of ALS. Although not curative, riluzole may modestly prolong survival (4 to 18 months) and delay the need for tracheostomy. Therapeutic agents under investigation include antioxidants, mitochondrial enhancers, antiapoptotics, immunomodulators, anti-inflammatories, and proteasome inhibitors.

Management of Anesthesia

Neuromuscular transmission is markedly abnormal in patients with ALS, and these patients can be very sensitive to nondepolarizing muscle relaxants. As with other patients with motor neuron disease, ALS patients should be considered to be vulnerable to hyperkalemia in response to succinylcholine. Dysfunction of pharyngeal and laryngeal muscles predisposes patients with ALS to pulmonary aspiration. The need for postoperative ventilatory support is likely for these patients. There is no evidence that a specific anesthetic drug or combination of drugs is best for patients with ALS. Subclinical autonomic dysfunction can produce exaggerated decreases in cardiovascular function in response to anesthesia.[41]

Creutzfeldt-Jakob Disease

Creutzfeldt-Jakob disease (CJD) is one of a group of diseases termed the *transmissible spongiform encephalopathies*. Pathologically, these diseases are characterized by vacuolation of brain tissue and neuronal death. There are four types of CJD: familial (fCJD, sporadic (sCJD), iatrogenic (iCJD), and variant (vCJD). CJD is most likely an infection caused by a prion (PrP), a small proteinaceous substance devoid of nucleic acids. Presumably, the pathologic prion (PrP^{Sc}) converts naturally occurring prion material (PcP^C) to PrP^{Sc}. PrP^{Sc} initially invades peripheral nerves and then spreads centrally. Hematogenous and lymphoid reticular system (tonsils, spleen) spread may also occur. sCJD is a rare cause of dementia, but the discovery of transmission of a prion disease (bovine spongiform encephalopathy, mad cow disease) from cows to humans in the mid-1990s catapulted CJD to prominence. This disease is vCJD.[42]

The clinical characteristics of sCJD are subacute dementia, myoclonus, and EEG changes. The EEG pattern is relatively characteristic, with diffuse slow activity and periodic complexes. Progressive loss of cognitive and neurologic function occurs. Patients with vCJD present at an earlier age with psychiatric features such as dysphoria, withdrawal, anxiety, and insomnia. Neurologic features develop 1 to 2 months after the psychiatric changes commence. Transmission of vCJD is by ingestion of contaminated animal products. Iatrogenic transmission of iCJD has been linked to contaminated dural graft material, corneal transplants, contaminated surgical instruments, pooled human growth hormone, and blood.[43] There is no treatment for CJD. Investigational therapies are aimed at preventing prion transport from the periphery to the CNS and at neuron regeneration.

Management of Anesthesia

CJD is a transmissible disease and appropriate precautions must be observed when administering anesthesia. High-risk patient tissues include brain, spinal cord, cerebrospinal fluid, lymphoid tissue, and blood. Single-use anesthesia supplies, including face masks, breathing circuits, laryngoscopes, and tracheal tubes, should be employed.[44]

Patients with degenerative neurologic diseases are prone to aspirate gastric contents because they have impaired swallowing function and decreased laryngeal reflexes. Because lower motor neuron dysfunction occurs in CJD patients, succinylcholine should be avoided. The autonomic and peripheral nervous systems may be adversely affected and abnormal cardiovascular responses to anesthesia and vasoactive drugs may occur.

ANEMIAS

Anemia is an absolute or relative deficiency in the concentration of circulating red blood cells. Anemias can be classified as nutritional, hemolytic, and genetic (hemoglobinopathies, thalassemias; Table 25-7). Compensatory mechanisms develop to offset the decreased oxygen-carrying capacity of the blood (Table 25-8). In a healthy person, symptoms do not develop until the hemoglobin level decreases below 7 g/dL. Symptoms are variable and depend on concurrent disease processes. There is no universally accepted hematocrit level that demands transfusion. The patient's physiologic condition and coexisting diseases must be factored into a subjective decision.

Nutritional Deficiency Anemias

The three primary causes of nutritional deficiency anemia are iron deficiency, vitamin B$_{12}$ deficiency, and folic acid deficiency.

TABLE 25-7

TYPES OF ANEMIAS

Nutritional
  Iron deficiency
  Vitamin B_{12} deficiency
  Folic acid deficiency
  Chronic illness
Hemolytic
  Spherocytosis
  Glucose-6-phosphate dehydrogenase deficiency
  Immune-mediated
  Drug-induced ABO incompatibility
Genetic
  Hemoglobin S (sickle cell)
  Thalassemia major (Cooley's anemia)
  Thalassemia intermedia
  Thalassemia minor

Chronic illness, cancer, and poor dietary intake can result in nutritional deficiency anemia.

Iron deficiency anemia produces a microcytic, hypochromic red blood cell. Iron deficiency anemia may be an absolute deficiency secondary to decreased oral intake or a relative deficiency caused by a rapid turnover of red blood cells (e.g., chronic blood loss, hemolysis).

Megaloblastic anemia can be caused by vitamin B_{12} (cobalamin) deficiency, folate deficiency, or refractory bone marrow disease. Absorption of vitamin B_{12} by the gastrointestinal tract depends on release of intrinsic factor, a glycoprotein produced by gastric parietal cells. Atrophy of the gastric mucosa causes vitamin B_{12} deficiency and megaloblastic anemia. Chronic gastritis and gastric atrophy may be caused by autoantibodies to gastric parietal cells. In addition to anemia, vitamin B_{12} deficiency can interfere with myelination and cause nervous system dysfunction. This is manifested by a peripheral neuropathy secondary to degeneration of the lateral and posterior spinal cord columns. Symmetric loss of proprioception and vibratory sensation in the lower extremities occur. Administration of parenteral vitamin B_{12} reverses both the hematologic and neurologic changes in adults. The coexisting neuropathy of vitamin B_{12} deficiency must be considered when regional or peripheral nerve blocks might be used. The clinical significance of the effects of nitrous oxide on vitamin B_{12} metabolism is controversial. Nitrous oxide inactivates the vitamin B_{12} component of methionine synthetase and prolonged exposure to nitrous oxide produces megaloblastic anemia and neurologic changes similar to those that occur with pernicious anemia. In susceptible patients (those with chronic illness, the elderly) there is also evidence that short-term exposure to nitrous oxide can cause megaloblastic red blood cell changes.[45] The issue of nitrous oxide causing postoperative neurologic dysfunction is also controversial and case reports of neuropathy linked to intraoperative nitrous oxide exposure have increased.

TABLE 25-8

COMPENSATORY MECHANISMS TO INCREASE OXYGEN DELIVERY WITH CHRONIC ANEMIA

Increased cardiac output
Increased red blood cell 2,3-diphosphoglycerate
Increased P-50
Increased plasma volume
Decreased blood viscosity

Folic acid deficiency also produces megaloblastic anemia. Although peripheral neuropathy may occur, it is not as common as with vitamin B_{12} deficiency. Causes of folic acid deficiency include alcoholism, pregnancy, and malabsorption syndromes. Methotrexate, phenytoin, and ethanol are among the drugs known to interfere with folic acid absorption.

Hemolytic Anemias

The normal life span of an erythrocyte is 120 days. Abnormalities in the erythrocyte may result in premature destruction of the cell (hemolysis). Causes of hemolytic anemia include structural erythrocyte abnormalities, enzyme deficiencies, and immune hemolytic anemias.

Hereditary Spherocytosis

Spherocytosis, elliptocytosis, pyropoikilocytosis, and stomatocytosis are the four types of hereditary membrane defects resulting in abnormally shaped red blood cells.

Spherocytosis is the most common of the red cell membrane defects producing hemolysis. This defect is caused by an abnormality in the proteins that comprise the skeleton of the red blood cell membrane. The red blood cell is rounded, fragile, and more susceptible to hemolysis than the normal biconcave red blood cell. The spleen destroys the abnormal red blood cells and chronic anemia ensues. Cholelithiasis from chronic hemolysis and elevation of the serum bilirubin occur in patients with hereditary spherocytosis. Patients with hereditary spherocytosis may have hemolytic crises accompanied by anemia, vomiting, and abdominal pain. These crises may be triggered by infection or folic acid deficiency.

Hereditary spherocytosis is treated by splenectomy that is usually delayed until the patient is age 6 years or older. Splenectomy before that age is associated with a high incidence of bacterial infections, especially pneumococcal type. Transfusion is rarely necessary because adequate compensatory mechanisms for chronic anemia have developed.

Glucose-6-Phosphate Dehydrogenase Deficiency

Glucose-6-phosphate dehydrogenase (G6PD) deficiency is the most common enzymopathy in humans and afflicts 400 million people worldwide. G6PD deficiency may confer malarial resistance and the distribution of this variant parallels the geographic distribution of malaria. African Americans, Africans, Asians, Indians, and Mediterranean populations are susceptible to the abnormality. G6PD initiates the hexose monophosphate shunt that begins the metabolism of glucose in the red blood cell. This pathway produces nicotinamide-adenine dinucleotide phosphate (NADPH). Without NADPH, the red blood cell is vulnerable to damage by oxidation. A deficiency of G6PD results in decreased levels of glutathione when the erythrocyte is exposed to oxidants. This increases the rigidity of the red blood cell membrane and accelerates clearance of the cell from the circulation. In severe forms of G6PD deficiency, oxidation produces denaturation of globin chains and causes intravascular hemolysis. NADPH contributes to the synthesis of endogenous nitric oxide and a deficiency of NADPH caused by G6PD deficiency may adversely affect neutrophil function, thereby increasing the risk of sepsis in critically ill patients.

There are a number of drugs that enhance the destruction of erythrocytes in patients with G6PD deficiency (Table 25-9). There is considerable variability in the hemolytic response to drugs; many drugs (e.g., aspirin) cause hemolysis only in very high doses. Patients with G6PD deficiency are unable to reduce methemoglobin produced by sodium nitrate; therefore, sodium nitroprusside and prilocaine should not be administered.

TABLE 25-9

DRUGS THAT PRODUCE HEMOLYSIS IN PATIENTS WITH GLUCOSE-6-PHOSPHATE DEHYDROGENASE DEFICIENCY

Phenacetin	Nalidixic acid
Aspirin (high doses)	Isoniazid
Penicillin	Primaquine
Streptomycin	Quinine
Chloramphenicol	Quinidine
Sulfacetamide	Doxorubicin
Sulfanilamide	Methylene blue
Sulfapyridine	Nitrofurantoin

Characteristically, the crisis begins 2 to 5 days after drug administration. The hemolytic episode is usually self-limited as only the older red blood cells are affected. Bacterial infections can trigger hemolytic episodes and oxidants produced by active white blood cells may hemolyze susceptible red blood cells. Anesthetic drugs have not been implicated as hemolytic agents; however, early postoperative evidence of hemolysis might suggest a G6PD deficiency.

Pyruvate Kinase Deficiency

Pyruvate kinase is a glycolytic enzyme of the Embden-Meyerhof pathway. This pathway converts glucose to lactate and is the primary pathway for adenosine triphosphate synthesis in the red blood cell. A deficiency of pyruvate kinase results in a potassium leak from the red blood cell, increasing their rigidity and accelerating destruction in the spleen.

Clinically, these patients exhibit anemia, premature cholelithiasis, and splenomegaly. The degree of anemia varies from very mild to a severe, transfusion-dependent anemia. The clinical features resemble those for patients with spherocytosis. There are no special considerations for anesthesia other than those for any patient with chronic anemia.

Immune Hemolytic Anemia

The immune hemolytic anemias are characterized by immunologic alterations in the red blood cell membrane and are caused by drugs, disease, or erythrocyte sensitization. There are three types of immune hemolytic anemia: autoimmune hemolysis, drug-induced immune hemolysis, and alloimmune hemolysis (erythrocyte sensitization).[46] Autoimmune hemolytic anemia includes both warm and cold antibody hemolytic anemia. Cold autoimmune hemolytic anemia is of special concern to the anesthesiologist because of the likelihood that the cold operating room environment and hypothermia during cardiopulmonary bypass may initiate a hemolytic crisis. Cold hemagglutinin disease is caused by IgM autoantibodies that react with I antigens of red blood cells. Maintaining a warm environment is essential for prevention of hemolysis. Plasmapheresis to reduce the titer of cold antibody is recommended before hypothermic procedures such as cardiopulmonary bypass. Collagen vascular diseases, solid organ transplant, blood transfusion, neoplasia, and infections can produce immune hemolytic anemia by a variety of mechanisms including warm and cold antibody-mediated hemolysis.

There are three types of drug-induced immune hemolysis: autoantibody type, hapten-induced type, and immune complex type. Hemolysis induced by α-methyldopa is of the autoimmune type mediated by an IgG antibody that does not fix complement. The hapten-induced type is characteristic of the response to penicillin. The immune type of reaction can occur after the administration of quinidine, quinine, sulfonamides,

isoniazid, phenacetin, acetaminophen, cephalosporins, tetracyclines, hydralazine, and hydrochlorothiazide.

The classic example of alloimmune hemolysis (erythrocyte sensitization) is hemolytic disease of the newborn produced by Rh sensitization. An Rh-negative mother with Rh antibodies produces hemolysis in an Rh-positive fetus. Differences in fetal and maternal ABO groups may also cause hemolysis. However, this is unusual because A and B antibodies are of the IgM class and do not readily cross the placenta.

Treatment of immune hemolytic anemias is with corticosteroids and immunosuppressants. Splenectomy may be beneficial in some patients.

Hemoglobinopathies

Hemoglobinopathies are diseases caused by genetic errors in hemoglobin synthesis and production. Illness is caused by anemia, accumulation of inappropriate hemoglobin precursors, immunocompromise, tissue infarction, inflammation and other factors.

The hemoglobinopathies convey survival protection in malarial endemic areas by decreasing erythrocyte life span and promoting erythrocyte turnover. In the case of sickle cell disease, survival advantage is conveyed only to heterozygous carriers of the disease. The hemoglobinopathies most likely to be encountered are sickle cell disease, hemoglobin C, and the thalassemias.

Sickle Cell Disease

Sickle cell disease (SCD) was one of the first diseases determined to be caused by a single molecular abnormality. SCD results from mutation of chromosome 11 that causes substitution of valine for glutamic acid at the sixth position of the β-globin protein. Persons heterozygous for the sickle cell gene (*HbSA*) are usually asymptomatic and live a normal life while homozygous individuals suffer SCD (*HbSS*).[47]

Normal hemoglobin molecules are composed of four globin proteins bound to a single iron-containing heme structure. The normal adult globin arrangement is two α-globins and two β-globins. This structure is hemoglobin A (HbA) and comprises 95 to 98% of hemoglobin in the normal adult. In SCD the β-globins are abnormal, causing instability and decreased solubility of the β^{Sickle} (β^S)-globin. The hemoglobin of SCD is termed *hemoglobin S* (HbS). When sickle cell hemoglobin (HbS) is exposed to low oxygen concentrations, a conformational change of β^S causes polymerization and precipitation of HbS with deformation of the erythrocyte, hemolysis, and premature red blood cell destruction. Red blood cell life span in SCD is only 12 to 17 days versus a normal life span of 120 days. Hemoglobin electrophoresis can be performed to diagnose SCD and determine the relative concentrations of HbA, HbF, and HbS. Sickle cell trait may also be combined with hemoglobin C (HbC) or thalassemia. Hemoglobin C is produced by a mutation affecting the same amino acid on the β-globin as HbS. The number 6 glutamic acid is replaced by lysine in HbC. HbC is mildly unstable and even those homozygous for HBC have few symptoms. Individuals with HbSC suffer symptoms approaching the severity of SCD.

Linking the molecular basis of SCD to its many varied clinical manifestations has proven difficult. The traditional explanation has been the "vicious cycle" theory. Erythrocytes in a deoxygenated capillary deform to the sickle shape and create a mechanical obstruction to blood flow. The slowing of blood flow creates stasis and further reductions in oxygenation. The sickling of additional erythrocytes causes a vicious cycle that manifests as pain, tissue ischemia, and infarction. At best, this theory is incomplete and many other mechanisms are operable (Table 25-10).[48]

TABLE 25-10

MECHANISMS OF CELLULAR AND TISSUE INJURY IN SICKLE CELL DISEASE

Erythrocyte and platelet adhesion to endothelium
Activation of coagulation system with thrombosis and ischemia
Reperfusion injury
Leukocytosis and immune system activation
Free radical injury due to leukocyte superoxide release
Decreased nitric oxide due to leukocyte superoxide release
Activation of cytokine and inflammatory mediators
Hemolysis and release of free hemoglobin
Free radical injury secondary to free hemoglobin
Decreased nitric oxide due to uptake by free hemoglobin
Endothelial dysfunction secondary to inflammation and depletion of nitric oxide
Excessive iron stores secondary to repeated erythrocyte transfusion

The clinical manifestations of SCD are diverse and involve all organ systems (Table 25-11). The most common problem is pain that may be poorly localized, bilateral, and described as aching. When the pain becomes severe, the patient may be experiencing a painful crisis. The pain can be treated with non-steroidal anti-inflammatory drugs (NSAIDs) and narcotics. Hydration and supplemental oxygen are often administered to improve tissue oxygen delivery. Blood transfusion is required when routine measures fail to relieve the symptoms. Splenic

TABLE 25-11

CLINICAL MANIFESTATIONS OF SICKLE CELL DISEASE

Hematologic	**Pulmonary**
Hemolytic anemia	Acute chest syndrome
Aplastic anemia	Hypoxemia
Leukocytosis	Pulmonary infarction
Spleen	Fibrosis
Infarction	Asthma
Hyposplenism	Sleep apnea
Splenic sequestration	Thromboembolism
Central Nervous System	Pneumonia
Stroke	**Genitourinary**
Hemorrhage	Priapism
Aneurysm	Infection
Meningitis	**Hepatobiliary**
Musculoskeletal	Jaundice
Painful crises	Hepatitis
Bone marrow hyperplasia	Cirrhosis
Avascular necrosis	Cholelithiasis
Osteomyelitis	Cholestasis
Bone infarcts	**Eye**
Skeletal deformity	Retinopathy
Growth retardation	Hemorrhage
Cutaneous ulceration	Visual loss
Cardiac	**Immune System**
Cardiomegaly	Immunosuppression
Pulmonary hypertension	Leukocytosis
Cor pulmonale	**Psychosocial**
Diastolic dysfunction	Depression
Cardiomyopathy	Anxiety
Renal	Substance abuse
Papillary necrosis	Narcotic dependence
Glomerular sclerosis	
Renal failure	

autoinfarction is a universal feature of SCD, and lifelong penicillin therapy and an aggressive immunization program are required to compensate for functional asplenia. Sepsis, aplastic crisis, splenic sequestration crisis, and acute chest syndrome (ACS) are four life-threatening events that must be recognized and promptly treated. Aplastic crisis occurs when bone marrow suppression prevents the timely replacement of erythrocytes. Transfusion of red blood cells must be performed until normal marrow function is re-established. A viral infection is a frequent precipitant of aplastic crisis. Splenic sequestration crisis occurs when large numbers of erythrocytes are trapped by an enlarged spleen. The ensuing anemia and hypovolemia require volume resuscitation and red blood cell transfusions. Splenectomy is performed after resolution of the crisis.

ACS represents the single greatest threat to the patient with SCD. The mortality of ACS is 1 to 20%. Signs and symptoms of ACS include dyspnea, wheezing, chest pain, hypoxemia, and pulmonary infiltrates. ACS may progress to adult respiratory distress syndrome, respiratory failure, and pneumonia. Treatment includes supplemental oxygen, erythrocyte transfusion, inhaled bronchodilators, antibiotics, and in some cases steroids. Mechanical ventilation may be necessary. Precipitants of ACS include pulmonary infection, fat embolism from bony infarcts, worsening of asthma, and perioperative respiratory dysfunction.[49]

Most treatment of SCD is supportive and directed at early treatment of complications. Many SCD patients are treated with hydroxyurea to increase circulating levels of fetal hemoglobin. All SCD patients should be enrolled in a multidisciplinary clinical care program. Advances in preventive and acute care have improved the mean age of survival for SCD patients to >50 years. Curative treatment for some patients is possible with bone marrow transplantation from a matched sibling. Bone marrow transplantation is typically reserved for SCD patients with severe symptoms at an early age.

Management of Anesthesia. Preparation of the SCD patient for surgery should be done in close collaboration with the sickle cell specialty service that provides the patient's routine care. The underlying condition of the patient and the extent of the surgery will determine the need for preoperative testing and erythrocyte transfusion. Age >30 years, history of ACS, asthma, resting hypoxemia, pulmonary hypertension, previous stroke, and frequent painful crises increase the risk of perioperative complications. Minor procedures such as myringotomy, tonsillectomy and adenoidectomy, and vascular access procedures have mild perioperative risk and generally do not require transfusion. However, patients with severe disease may require transfusion for even minor procedures. Intra-abdominal and orthopaedic procedures pose moderate risk and transfusion is usually indicated. Thoracic, cardiac, and intracranial operations should be considered high risk with transfusion required. Transfusion of erythrocytes to raise the hematocrit to 30 to 35% is desired. Routine preoperative testing should include a hematocrit before and after transfusion, creatinine, blood urea nitrogen, electrolytes, room air oximetry, and prothrombin time/partial thromboplastin time with international normalized ratio. ECG, echocardiography, chest radiography, and arterial blood gas analysis should be considered for patients with symptoms suggestive of cardiac disease, pulmonary hypertension, a history of ACS, exertional dyspnea, or chronic hypoxemia. Pulmonary hypertension and diastolic dysfunction are relatively common and are associated with increased morbidity and mortality.[50]

Prevention of conditions that favor sickling is the basis of perioperative management. Adequate oxygenation, avoidance of increased oxygen consumption, and prevention of vascular stasis are imperative. Normothermia should be achieved to avoid problems associated with hyperthermia and hypothermia. Hyperthermia increases oxygen consumption and hypothermia causes vascular constriction that promotes blood stasis. Perioperative shivering increases oxygen consumption and is undesirable. The use of tourniquets may be considered if essential to the success of the operation.

Drugs used for anesthesia are not known to have direct effects on the sickling process. General anesthesia is usually employed, but regional anesthesia can be used if indicated (e.g., labor and delivery, cesarean section). The presence of pulmonary hypertension or cardiac dysfunction may require more aggressive perioperative monitoring and postoperative management to avoid decompensation. Ten percent of SCD patients may experience ACS in the perioperative period. Supplemental oxygen, chest physiotherapy, good pain control, and maintenance of the hematocrit between 30 and 35% may reduce the risk of postoperative ACS. Anecdotally, mainstem bronchial intubation may precipitate ACS and inadvertent one-lung ventilation is to be avoided.[47,48,50]

Thalassemia

Thalassemia is a hemoglobinopathy in which there is inadequate synthesis of either the α- or β-globin proteins. Thalassemia is more common in the Mediterranean, Middle Eastern, and Southeast Asian regions. If β-globin synthesis is inadequate, the excess α globin is reactive and causes premature destruction of erythrocytes. If β-globin synthesis is inadequate, the excess β-globin forms nonfunctional tetramers called *hemoglobin H*.

Erythrocyte life is shortened with resultant hemolytic anemia, splenomegaly, hepatomegaly, cholelithiasis, and jaundice. Bone marrow hyperplasia causes skeletal abnormalities such as growth retardation, facial dysmorphism, and pathologic fractures. Extramedullary bone marrow that is susceptible to spontaneous hemorrhage may form in the pleura, paranasal sinuses, and epidural space.

The expression of thalassemia is variable, ranging from asymptomatic mild anemia to death at an early age. The terms *thalassemia major, intermedia*, and *minor* refer to the clinical severity. Patients with thalassemia major require lifelong transfusions. Hypertransfusion is used to maintain the patient's hemoglobin at 9 to 10 g/dL in order to suppress thalassemic erythropoiesis. This suppresses extramedullary bone marrow formation and reduces the likelihood of skeletal deformity, causes less hemolysis, and decreased production of toxic hemoglobin precursors. Chelation therapy must be instituted early to prevent the complications of iron overload. The pathophysiology of thalassemia is very similar to that of SCD. Chronic hemolysis, globin excess, and iron overload result in chronic inflammation, depletion of nitric oxide, endothelial dysfunction, and activation of the coagulation system. These result in pulmonary hypertension, cardiomyopathy, cirrhosis, and splenomegaly.[51]

Management of Anesthesia. Anesthetic considerations are related to the degree of anemia, skeletal deformity, and secondary organ damage. The craniofacial deformities common in patients with thalassemia may make direct laryngoscopy and tracheal intubation difficult. Neuraxial anesthesia may be complicated by skeletal abnormalities and extramedullary bone marrow deposits. Spinal anesthesia, however, has been used for cesarean section. In general, many of the assessment and management recommendations for SCD are also applicable for patients with thalassemia.[52]

COLLAGEN VASCULAR DISEASES

The four most common collagen vascular diseases are rheumatoid arthritis, systemic lupus erythematosus, scleroderma, and dermatomyositis/polymyositis. Although many patients can be categorized as having discrete disease syndromes, many others with collagen vascular diseases are considered to have overlap syndromes (mixed connective tissue diseases) with features of different collagen vascular diseases and cannot be conveniently classified. The etiology of the collagen vascular diseases is unknown, although the immune system is clearly involved in the cascade of pathologic events that cause clinical manifestations of the diseases. Although all of these diseases have effects on joints, each has diffuse systemic effects as well. The alterations in joint function and systemic effects will both have significant impact on the management of anesthesia.

Rheumatoid Arthritis

Rheumatoid arthritis is a chronic inflammatory disease characterized by symmetric polyarthropathy and a variety of systemic effects. Although the etiology of rheumatoid arthritis is unknown, extensive research has revealed the pathogenesis. Activated endothelial cells attract adhesion molecules that bind to proteins and initiate a sequence of events that stimulate T cells and B lymphocytes. Cytokines (tumor necrosis factor, interleukin-1, interleukin-6) are released that accelerate the inflammatory cascade. B lymphocytes produce autoantibodies (rheumatoid factor) that enhance cytokine production and can be found in 75% of patients with rheumatoid arthritis. The pathologic changes of rheumatoid arthritis begin with cellular hyperplasia of the synovium followed by invasion of the synovium by lymphocytes, plasma cells, and fibroblasts. Cartilage and articular surfaces are ultimately destroyed.[53]

The hands and wrists are involved first, particularly the metacarpophalangeal and interphalangeal joints. The knee is involved most frequently in the lower extremity. The upper cervical spine is affected in nearly 80% of patients with rheumatoid arthritis. Instability of the upper cervical spine can manifest as atlantoaxial instability, cranial settling, and subaxial instability. Plain radiography and CT of the cervical spine will demonstrate the bony changes caused by rheumatoid arthritis. MRI is better suited to study the effects of the bony and soft tissues changes on the spinal cord. However, the degree of cord compression may not correlate with the patient's symptoms. Although a very rare event, spinal cord damage after laryngoscopy and tracheal intubation has been reported.[54] Intradural cord compression secondary to rheumatoid nodules or pannus formation can also occur. Rheumatoid arthritis commonly affects the joints of the larynx, resulting in limitation of vocal cord movement and generalized erythema and edema of the laryngeal mucosa that may progress to airway obstruction. Arthritic changes in the temporomandibular joints also occur. All of these abnormalities can complicate laryngoscopy and tracheal intubation.

Extra-articular and systemic manifestations of rheumatoid arthritis are diverse (Table 25-12). Cardiovascular disease is a common cause of mortality in patients with rheumatoid arthritis and there is a high incidence of subclinical cardiac dysfunction.[55] Pericarditis occurs in one third of patients with rheumatoid arthritis and can produce constrictive pericarditis or cardiac tamponade. Other cardiovascular manifestations include coronary artery disease, myocarditis, pulmonary hypertension, diastolic dysfunction, dysrhythmias, and aortitis (aortic root dilation, aortic valve regurgitation). Pulmonary changes include pleural effusions, pulmonary nodules, interstitial lung disease, reduced diffusion capacity, obstructive lung disease, and restrictive lung disease. Several of the antirheumatic drugs can cause or accentuate pulmonary dysfunction. Renal failure is a common cause of death in patients with rheumatoid arthritis and may be secondary to vasculitis, amyloidosis, and antirheumatic drugs.

Mild anemia is present in almost all patients with rheumatoid arthritis. The anemia may be secondary to a decrease in erythropoiesis or may be a side effect of drug therapy.

TABLE 25-12

EXTRA-ARTICULAR MANIFESTATIONS OF RHEUMATOID ARTHRITIS

Skin
  Raynaud phenomenon
  Digital necrosis
Eyes
  Scleritis
  Corneal ulceration
Lung
  Pleural effusion
  Pulmonary fibrosis
Heart
  Pericarditis
  Cardiac tamponade
  Coronary arteritis
  Aortic insufficiency
Kidney
  Interstitial fibrosis
  Glomerulonephritis
  Amyloid deposition

Peripheral Nervous System
  Compression syndromes
  Mononeuritis
Central Nervous System
  Dural nodules
  Necrotizing vasculitis
Liver
  Hepatitis
Blood
  Anemia
  Leukopenia

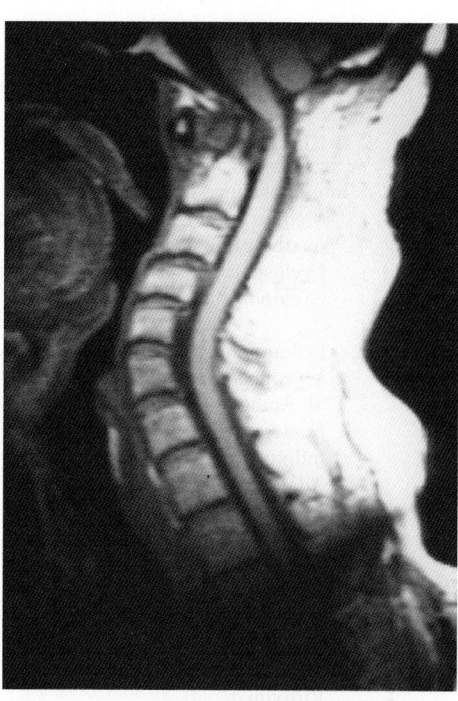

FIGURE 25-5. Magnetic resonance imaging of a cervical spine in a patient with rheumatoid arthritis. Although the patient had no neurologic symptoms, there is severe spinal stenosis in the upper cervical spine.

Neurologic complications of rheumatoid arthritis include peripheral nerve compression (carpal tunnel syndrome) and cervical nerve root compression. Mononeuritis multiplex is presumed to be caused by deposition of immune complexes in blood vessels supplying the affected nerves. Rheumatoid vasculitis may affect cerebral blood vessels, producing a cerebral necrotizing vasculitis.

There is no cure for rheumatoid arthritis. The disease process of immunoinflammation that causes rheumatoid arthritis is extremely complex and monotherapy is unlikely to be completely successful. The goals of therapy are induction of a remission, improved function, and maintenance of a remission. There are three groups of drugs used for treatment: NSAIDs, corticosteroids, and disease modifying antirheumatic drugs (DMARDs). Because NSAIDs do not affect the course of the disease, they are used in conjunction with DMARDs. Corticosteroids are effective but the side effects associated with long-term treatment limit their usefulness. DMARDs are now the first line of therapy for the early treatment of rheumatoid arthritis. Methotrexate has proven to be very effective and is often the initial drug of choice. Other less commonly used synthetic DMARDs include leflunomide, cyclosporine, azathioprine, gold, sulfasalazine, minocycline, and hydroxychloroquine. Biologic DMARDs that inhibit tumor necrosis factor-α include infliximab, etanercept, and adalimumab. Anakinra inhibits interleukin-1 and tocilizumab inhibits interleukin-6. Abatacept is a cytotoxic T-lymphocyte immunoglobulin and rituximab is a monoclonal antibody directed at antigens on B lymphocytes. The primary side effect of biologic DMARDs is an increased susceptibility to infection.[56] Most of the drugs used for the treatment of rheumatoid arthritis have significant side effects that may limit their usefulness (Table 25-13). Surgical procedures such as synovectomy, tenolysis, and joint replacement are performed to relieve pain and restore joint function.

Management of Anesthesia

Because rheumatoid arthritis is a multisystem disease and the clinical manifestations are so diverse, individualized preoperative evaluation is important in the identification of systemic effects.

The joint effects including arthritic changes in the temporomandibular joints, cricoarytenoid joints, and cervical spine can render rigid, direct laryngoscopy and tracheal intubation difficult. The mobility of these joints should be evaluated before surgery so that a plan for airway management can be formulated. If atlantoaxial instability exists, flexion of the neck may compress the spinal cord. Neck pain radiating to the occiput may be the first sign of cervical spine involvement. Patients with symptoms or evidence of cervical cord compression can be fitted with a cervical collar preoperatively to minimize the risk of overmanipulation of the neck during surgery. Many patients with rheumatoid arthritis, however, are asymptomatic with respect to cervical spine disease (Fig. 25-5). Preoperative imaging (radiography, CT, MRI) may be indicated if the degree of cervical involvement is unknown. Although there have been no documented reports of spinal cord damage in patients with rheumatoid arthritis undergoing tracheal intubation for elective surgery, alleged neurologic damage after laryngoscopy has been the source of litigation against anesthesiologists. If tracheal intubation is required, awake, fiberoptic-assisted tracheal intubation may be the best way to minimize the risk of neurologic damage in patients with significant cervical spine involvement. Cricoarytenoid arthritis produces erythema and edema of the vocal cords and may reduce the size of the glottic inlet, necessitating the use of a smaller than predicted tracheal tube.

The degree of cardiopulmonary involvement by the rheumatoid process influences the selection of the type of anesthesia. Preoperative evaluation of the heart and lungs is necessary if the clinical history suggests dysfunction. The need for postoperative ventilatory support should be anticipated if severe pulmonary disease is present.

Medications that the patient is receiving can influence the management of anesthesia. Corticosteroid supplementation may be necessary during the perioperative period. Aspirin and other anti-inflammatory drugs interfere with platelet function and clotting may be abnormal. Many rheumatoid medications suppress red blood cell formation, and anemia is common. Drug-induced hepatic and renal dysfunction may be present.

TABLE 25-13

ADVERSE EFFECTS OF DRUGS USED TO TREAT COLLAGEN VASCULAR DISEASES

■ CLASS OF DRUGS	■ EFFECTS
Immunosuppressants	
Methotrexate	Hepatotoxicity, anemia, leucopenia
Azathioprine	Biliary stasis, leucopenia
Cyclosporine	Renal dysfunction, hypertension hypomagnesemia
Cyclophosphamide	Leukopenia, hemorrhagic cystitis, inhibition of pseudocholinesterase
Leflunomide	Hepatotoxicity, weight loss, hypertension
Mycophenolate mofetil	Nausea, vomiting, diarrhea
TNF Antagonists	
Etanercept	Infections, tuberculosis
Infliximab	Lymphoma, heart failure
Adalimumab	
Interleukin-1 Antagonists	
Anakinra	Infection, skin irritation
T-Cell Inhibitors	
Abatacept	Infection
Interleukin-6 Antagonists	
Tocilizumab	Infection, headache, stomatitis, fever
CD20 Monoclonal Antibody	
Rituximab	Infection, infusion reaction
Corticosteroids	Hypertension, fluid retention, osteoporosis, infection, glucose intolerance
Aspirin	Platelet dysfunction, peptic ulcer, hypersensitivity
NSAIDs	Peptic ulcer, leukopenia, coronary artery disease
COX-2 Inhibitors	Renal dysfunction
	Adverse cardiovascular events
Gold	Aplastic anemia, dermatitis, nephritis
Antimalarials	Myopathy, retinopathy
Penicillamine	Glomerulonephritis, myasthenia, aplastic anemia

TNF, tumor necrosis factor; NSAIDs, nonsteroidal anti-inflammatory drugs; COX-2, cyclooxygenase-2.

Restriction of joint mobility necessitates careful positioning of the patient during the operation. The extremities should be positioned to minimize the risk of neurovascular compression and further joint injury. Preoperative examination of joint motion will help determine how the extremities should be positioned.

Rheumatoid arthritis is a multisystem disease. Joint disabilities have been well documented in the medical literature and are often obvious. More significant and less evident are the effects of the spinal cord, heart, lungs, kidneys, and liver. The type and severity of systemic dysfunction must be considered when planning an anesthetic for patients with rheumatoid arthritis.[57,58]

Systemic Lupus Erythematosus

Systemic lupus erythematosus (SLE) is an autoimmune disorder with diverse clinical and immunologic manifestations. The etiology of SLE is unknown, but appears to be a complex interaction between genetic susceptibility and hormonal and environmental factors. Patients with SLE are predominantly female of child-bearing age and of African and Asian ethnicity. Patients with SLE produce autoantibodies primarily to DNA, but also RNA polymerase, cardiolipin, and ribosomal phosphoproteins. It has been speculated that cell apoptosis releases intracellular proteins that generate an antibody response in susceptible patients. Some of the clinical manifestations of SLE may be the result of the production of an autoantibody highly specific for a single protein within an organ. Many patients with SLE have detectable anti-DNA antibodies 2 to 9 years before diagnosis.[59]

The clinical manifestations of SLE are diverse. The most common presenting features are polyarthritis and dermatitis. The arthritis is migratory and any joint can be involved, including the cervical spine. The classic malar rash is present in only one third of SLE patients. Renal disease is present in 50 to 60% of the patients and is a common cause of morbidity and mortality. Dialysis or renal transplantation is required in 10 to 20% of SLE patients. Proteinuria, hypertension, and decreased creatinine clearance are the usual manifestations of lupus nephritis. CNS involvement occurs in 50% of the patients and is secondary to vasculitis. CNS manifestations include seizures, stroke, dementia, psychosis, myelitis, and peripheral neuropathy.

SLE produces a diffuse serositis that manifests as pleuritis and pericarditis. Although 60% of SLE patients have pericardial effusions, cardiac tamponade is uncommon. In rare cases, however, tamponade may be the presenting sign of SLE. Accelerated arteriosclerosis, cardiac conduction abnormalities, and ventricular dysfunction are other cardiac features of SLE. A noninfectious endocarditis (Libman-Sachs endocarditis) may cause mitral regurgitation. Pulmonary manifestations of SLE include pleural effusion, pneumonitis, pulmonary hypertension, and alveolar hemorrhage. Pulmonary function studies typically demonstrate a restrictive disease pattern and a decreased diffusing capacity. There is a high incidence of pulmonary hypertension in SLE patients who have Raynaud syndrome. Patients with SLE are susceptible to infection that may present as pneumonia or adult respiratory distress syndrome. Cricoarytenoid arthritis can manifest as hoarseness, stridor, or airway obstruction.

Nearly one third of SLE patients has detectable antiphospholipid antibodies and may have thromboembolic complications. Gastrointestinal manifestations of lupus include peritonitis, pancreatitis, and bowel ischemia. Lupoid hepatitis is an autoimmune hepatitis that occurs in <10% of patients with SLE.

Despite the diverse effects of SLE and the lack of specific therapy, current treatment regimens have improved survival. NSAIDs are used for mild arthritis. Antimalarials (hydroxychloroquine) control arthritis and dermatitis and exert antithrombotic effects. Corticosteroids are effective for moderate and severe SLE. Immunosuppressants such as cyclophosphamide, azathioprine, methotrexate, cyclosporine, and mycophenolate mofetil are effective and permit lower dosages of corticosteroids. The potential for side effects from any of the drugs is significant and can cause morbidity.[60]

More than 80 drugs have been reported to cause drug-induced lupus, with the most common agents being procainamide, quinidine, hydralazine, methyldopa, enalapril, captopril, clonidine, isoniazid, and minocycline. Drug-induced lupus may be caused by drug metabolites that stimulate T cells. The clinical manifestations of drug-induced lupus are generally mild and include arthralgia, fever, anemia, and leukopenia. These effects typically resolve within weeks to months after discontinuation of the drug.

Management of Anesthesia

Careful preoperative evaluation of the patient with SLE is necessary because of the diverse systemic effects of the disease. Preoperative chest radiography, echocardiography, or pulmonary function testing may be necessary if the clinical history suggests cardiopulmonary dysfunction. Although there are no specific contraindications to a particular type of anesthetic, myocardial dysfunction will certainly influence the choice of anesthetic and the type of intraoperative monitors. Because renal dysfunction is so common, renal function should be quantified if there is a suggestion of a recent change in renal function. Although minor abnormalities in hepatic function are often present, these changes are usually not significant. Patients with SLE are at increased risk for postoperative infections.

Arthritic involvement of the cervical spine is unusual in patients with SLE and tracheal intubation is generally not difficult. However, the potential for laryngeal involvement and upper airway obstruction does require clinical evaluation of laryngeal function. Should postextubation laryngeal edema or stridor occur, intravenous administration of corticosteroids is effective for alleviation of symptoms.

Drugs used for the treatment of SLE may influence the choice of drugs. Patients receiving corticosteroids will usually require corticosteroid replacement during the perioperative period. Cyclophosphamide inhibits plasma cholinesterase and may prolong the response to succinylcholine.

Scleroderma

Scleroderma results in excessive fibrosis in the skin and internal organs. Endothelial cell activation gives rise to inflammation and increased immune cell activity with activation of T cells and B lymphocytes. The endothelial cells appear to be deficient in intrinsic vasodilators while having increased levels of the potent vasoconstrictor endothelin-1. This process causes inflammation and obliteration of small arteries and arterioles

and ultimately fibrosis and atrophy of organs. Autoantibodies are frequently present and may correlate with disease activity.[61]

The manifestations of scleroderma are most evident in the skin, which becomes thickened and swollen. Eventually the skin becomes atrophic and small arteries are obliterated. The skin becomes fibrotic and taut and produces severe restriction of joint mobility. Raynaud phenomenon is present in 85% of patients with scleroderma and is often the presenting symptom.

The same pathologic process that affects the vascular system of the skin affects small blood vessels in other organs. Lung involvement occurs in 80 to 90% of patients with scleroderma and is characterized by interstitial fibrosis, pulmonary hypertension, and an impaired diffusing capacity. These changes in conjunction with the effects of chronic aspiration pneumonitis produce a restrictive lung disease. Myocardial fibrosis occurs in 70 to 80% of patients with scleroderma, although only 25% have clinical symptoms. Echocardiography may reveal a decreased ejection fraction and impaired left ventricular filling. Degeneration of the cardiac conduction tissue may cause conduction defects and cardiac dysrhythmias. Pericarditis with effusion is very common.

Renal dysfunction is relatively common and is secondary to pathologic changes in the renal vasculature similar to the changes in the digital arteries that produce Raynaud phenomenon. Renal dysfunction can be so severe that a scleroderma renal crisis develops with hypertension, retinopathy, and a rapid deterioration in renal function.

Gastrointestinal motility is decreased and is very pronounced in the esophagus. The frequent episodes of gastroesophageal reflux and aspiration pneumonitis exacerbate pulmonary dysfunction. Involvement of the colon and small intestine may result in pseudo-obstruction.

Therapy has been directed at a number of pathways. Corticosteroids are beneficial, but the likelihood of side effects is great. Cyclophosphamide is the immunosuppressant with the greatest effect. Vasodilators such as calcium channel blockers, ACE inhibitors, and prostacyclins are often used for the treatment of cardiac dysfunction, pulmonary hypertension, and Raynaud phenomenon. Statins may be effective by virtue of their endothelial protective effects and anti-inflammatory effects. The endothelin A receptor antagonists ambrisentan and sitaxsentan are currently under investigation.

Management of Anesthesia

Scleroderma, like other collagen vascular diseases, is a multisystem disease with many systemic manifestations. There are no specific contraindications to the use of any type of anesthesia, although the selection must be guided by identification of organ dysfunction.

Tracheal intubation can be quite difficult. Fibrotic and taut facial skin can markedly hinder active and passive motion of the temporomandibular joint. Awake, fiberoptic-assisted laryngoscopy may be required; tracheostomy may be necessary in severely affected patients. Orotracheal intubation is preferred as the fragility of the nasal mucosa increases the risk of severe nasal hemorrhage form nasotracheal intubation.

The patient with scleroderma is at risk for aspiration pneumonitis during the induction of anesthesia because of the high incidence of esophageal dysmotility and gastroesophageal reflux.

Chronic arterial hypoxemia is often present because of restriction of lung expansion and impaired oxygen diffusion. Compromised myocardial function and decreased coronary vascular reserve often necessitate the use of invasive cardiovascular monitors because the response to inhaled anesthetics may be exaggerated. Transesophageal echocardiography can provide valuable information about cardiac function, although passage of the probe may be difficult because of esophageal stricture. Venous access can be difficult and a venous cutdown or central venous catheterization may be required. Myopathy with subsequent muscle weakness is present in most patients with scleroderma and increased sensitivity to muscle relaxants should be anticipated.

Regional anesthesia may be administered to patients with scleroderma, although the response to local anesthetics may be prolonged. The anesthesiologist is often consulted as to the efficacy of sympathetic blockade for the treatment of vasospasm secondary to Raynaud phenomenon.

Polymyositis/Dermatomyositis (Inflammatory Myopathies)

Three diseases comprise the inflammatory myopathies: polymyositis, dermatomyositis, and inclusion-body myositis. Although the clinical features of the three diseases are diverse, severe muscle weakness and noninfectious muscle inflammation are present in all three. Dermatomyositis is the result of an antibody-induced complement activation that lyses muscle capillaries and causes muscle necrosis. Muscle fiber necrosis in polymyositis and inclusion-body myositis is caused by cytotoxic T cells.[62]

Common presenting symptoms of polymyositis are muscle pain, tenderness, and proximal muscle weakness. Patients with dermatomyositis have a characteristic skin rash that often precedes the onset of weakness. The skin rash is characterized by a purplish discoloration of the eyelids (heliotrope rash), periorbital edema, erythematous lesions on the knuckles, and a photosensitive rash on the face, neck, and chest. Inclusion-body myositis presents with weakness of the quadriceps and ankle dorsiflexors in men >50 years of age. Fifty percent of patients with polymyositis and dermatomyositis have evidence of pulmonary disease. Pulmonary manifestations include interstitial pneumonitis, alveolitis, and bronchopneumonia. Aspiration pneumonitis is very common in patients with polymyositis. Intrinsic lung disease and thoracic muscle weakness produce a restrictive pulmonary pattern and a decreased diffusion capacity. Myocardial fibrosis can result in congestive heart failure and cardiac dysrhythmias. Patients with polymyositis and dermatomyositis are at increased risk to develop cancer and careful screening is indicated.

The most effective treatment for the inflammatory myopathies is corticosteroids (prednisone). Immunosuppressants such as methotrexate, azathioprine, cyclophosphamide, cyclosporine, and mycophenolate mofetil are also effective. Intravenous immunoglobulin has been shown to be effective in patients resistant to corticosteroids. Monoclonal antibodies such as infliximab, etanercept, and rituximab are currently under investigation.[63]

Management of Anesthesia

Mobility of the temporomandibular joints and cervical spine is usually adequate in patients with polymyositis. Some patients, however, have restricted mobility that can make direct laryngoscopy difficult. Awake, fiberoptic-assisted tracheal intubation may be required for those patients with restricted neck mobility and inadequate mouth opening.

Dysphagia and gastroesophageal reflux are very common and there is an increased likelihood of aspiration pneumonitis. Gastrointestinal perforations that necessitate surgical intervention are relatively common in patients with polymyositis.

Although the electromyographic changes of polymyositis suggest the potential for hyperkalemia after succinylcholine, it has been administered to patients with polymyositis without complication.[64] Prolonged neuromuscular blockade may occur after the administration of nondepolarizing muscle relaxants. This prolonged response may be secondary to the myopathy or an interaction between the muscle relaxant and immunosuppressants. The reported experience with anesthesia for patients with inflammatory myopathies is very limited and generalizations from a few case reports must be interpreted with caution. It should be anticipated that considerable variation in response to muscle relaxants will occur. It may be prudent to avoid the administration of succinylcholine and to use short-acting muscle relaxants. Because of the preoperative muscle weakness, postoperative mechanical ventilation may be necessary.

The degree of cardiopulmonary dysfunction influences the choice of anesthetics and intraoperative monitors. The cardiac dysfunction may be subclinical and preoperative echocardiography may be necessary to quantify cardiac function.

SKIN DISORDERS

Most primary diseases of the skin are localized and cause few systemic effects or complications during the administration of anesthesia. Two blistering skin disorders can result in complications during the perioperative period: epidermolysis bullosa and pemphigus.

Epidermolysis Bullosa

Epidermolysis bullosa is a rare skin disease that can be inherited or acquired. Patients with heritable forms have abnormalities in the anchoring systems of skin layers. The acquired forms are autoimmune disorders in which autoantibodies are produced that destroy the basement membrane of the skin and mucosa. The end result is the loss or absence of normal intercellular bridges and separation of skin layers, intradermal fluid accumulation, and bullae formation (Fig. 25-6). Lateral shearing forces applied to the skin are especially damaging. Pressure applied perpendicular to the skin is not as hazardous. Although defects in 10 different genes have been discovered and there are over 30 subtypes of epidermolysis bullosa, these disorders can be categorized into 3 groups depending on where the actual skin separation occurs: epidermolysis simplex, junctional epidermolysis, and epidermolysis bullosa dystrophica. Although serious complications from skin and mucosal loss can occur with any form of epidermolysis, the simplex form is generally benign. There are two forms of junctional epidermolysis (JEB): Herlitz type (H-JEB) and non-Herlitz (NH-JEB). H-JEB is lethal by 1 year of age and often has laryngeal involvement.[65]

Epidermolysis bullosa dystrophica (DEB) is caused by a defect in type VII collagen. DEB produces severe scarring of the fingers and toes with pseudosyndactyly formation and ankylosis of the interphalangeal joints and resorption of the metacarpals and metatarsals (Fig. 25-7). Secondary infection of bullae and malignant degeneration of the skin are common. Involvement of the esophagus is present in most patients, resulting in dysphagia and esophageal strictures that contribute to poor nutrition. Dilated cardiomyopathy with a markedly decreased ejection fraction and formation of intracardiac thrombi can develop in patients with DEB and serial echocardiography may be indicated.[66] Glomerulonephritis may be secondary to streptococcal infection. Hypoalbuminemia, secondary to nephritis, protein loss into bullae, and poor nutrition is usual. Anemia is usually present as a result of poor nutrition and repeated infections. Hypoplasia of tooth enamel results in carious degeneration of the teeth and the need for extensive dental restorations. Patients with DEB rarely survive beyond the third decade.

Medical therapy for DEB has not been very successful. Corticosteroids are not effective. Phenytoin, a collagenase inhibitor, may produce short-term improvement. Skin transplantation with genetically modified sheets of epidermal cells

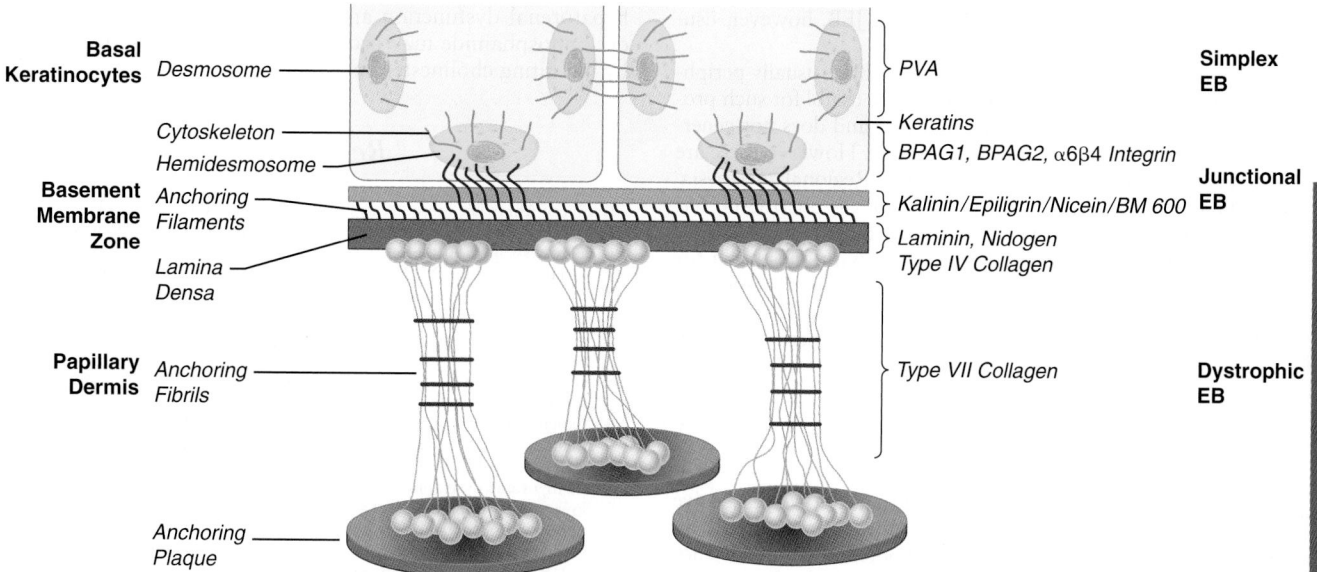

Basal Keratinocytes
Desmosome
Cytoskeleton
Hemidesmosome

Basement Membrane Zone
Anchoring Filaments
Lamina Densa

Papillary Dermis
Anchoring Fibrils

Anchoring Plaque

PVA — **Simplex EB**

Keratins
BPAG1, BPAG2, α6β4 Integrin — **Junctional EB**

Kalinin/Epiligrin/Nicein/BM 600

Laminin, Nidogen
Type IV Collagen

Type VII Collagen — **Dystrophic EB**

FIGURE 25-6. The ultrastructure of the zones of the skin. The diagram demonstrates where skin separation occurs in different types of epidermolysis bullosa (EB). (Reproduced from Uitto J, Christiano AM: Molecular genetics of the cutaneous basement membrane zone. J Clin Invest 1992; 90: 687–692, with permission.)

is under investigation and may be effective for some forms of epidermolysis. Surgical therapy is directed at preservation and improvement of hand function.

Management of Anesthesia

It is critical that trauma to the skin and mucous membranes be avoided or minimized during the intraoperative period. Gel pads can be used for ECG electrodes. The blood pressure cuff should be well padded with loose cotton dressing, and intravascular catheters should be anchored with sutures or a gauze dressing rather than tape. Trauma from a face mask can be minimized by lubrication of the mask and the patient's face. The use of upper airway instruments, including oropharyngeal and nasopharyngeal airways, should be kept to a minimum because

the squamous cell epithelial lining of the oropharynx and esophagus is susceptible to bullous formation. Frictional trauma to the oropharynx can result in the formation of large intraoral bullae, airway obstruction, and extensive hemorrhage from denuded mucosa. For similar reasons, insertion of an esophageal stethoscope should be avoided. Laryngeal involvement is rare in patients with DEB. If tracheal intubation is required, the laryngoscope and tracheal tube should be well lubricated to reduce friction against the oropharyngeal mucosa. Scarring of the oral cavity can cause microstomia and immobility of the tongue that increases the difficulty of tracheal intubation. Fiberoptic-assisted tracheal intubation may be required. Although tracheal intubation is generally safe for patients with DEB, similar safety has not been established for patients with JEB. JEB affects all mucosa, including the respiratory epithelium. The types of surgical procedures

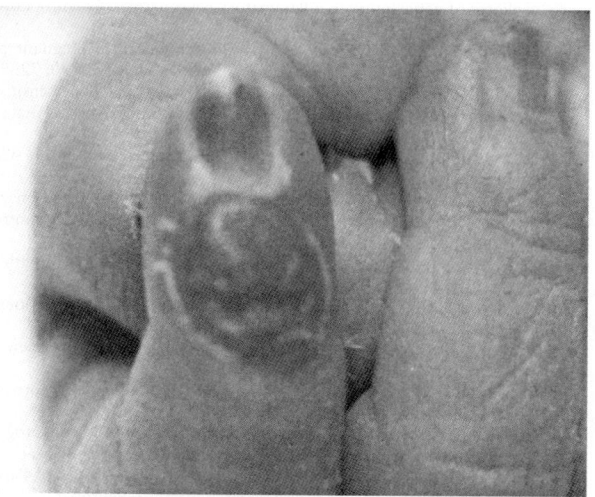

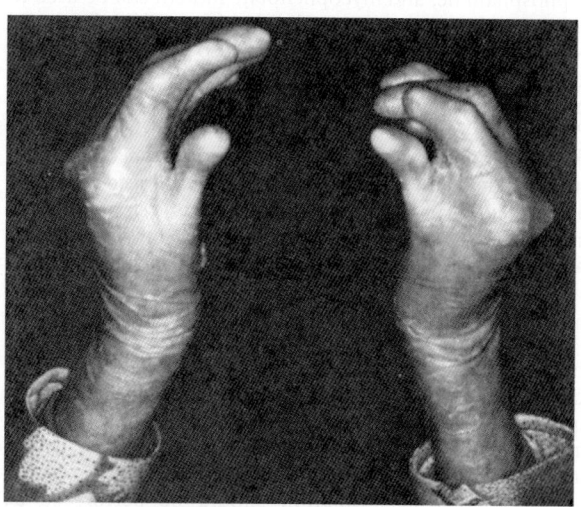

A   **B**

FIGURE 25-7. Epidermolysis bullosa. **A.** Bullous lesion of the finger in a neonate with epidermolysis. **B.** Hands of an older child with epidermolysis progression to produce severe scarring and pseudosyndactyly. (Courtesy of James E. Bennett, MD, Division of Plastic Surgery, Indiana University School of Medicine, Indianapolis, IN.)

(intra-abdominal) required in infants with JEB, however, usually mandate tracheal intubation.

Surgical procedures for patients with DEB are usually peripheral and involve the hands. Ketamine is very useful for such procedures because it provides good analgesia and does not generally require supplemental inhaled anesthesia. However, there are no contraindications to inhaled anesthetics. Regional anesthesia, including spinal, epidural, and brachial plexus anesthesia, has been used successfully for patients with DEB.

Despite all the potential complications with anesthesia for patients with epidermolysis, intraoperative management is associated with surprisingly few adverse effects. This is especially true when care is provided at a center experienced with the management of patients with epidermolysis bullosa.[67,68]

Pemphigus

Pemphigus is a vesiculobullous disease that involves extensive areas of the skin and mucous membranes. Pemphigus is an autoimmune disease in which IgG antibodies attack the desmosomal proteins desmoglein 3 and desmoglein 1, leading to loss of cell adhesion and separation of epithelial layers. A number of drugs have been implicated as the cause of pemphigus, including penicillamine, cephalosporins, ACE inhibitors, phenobarbital, propranolol, levodopa, nifedipine, and NSAIDs.[69]

Although there are several types of pemphigus, pemphigus vulgaris is the most common type and the most significant for the anesthesiologist because of the occurrence of oral lesions. Oral lesions develop in 50 to 70% of patients with pemphigus vulgaris and may precede the cutaneous lesions.[70] Lesions of the pharynx, larynx, esophagus, conjunctiva, urethra, cervix, and anus can develop. Extensive oropharyngeal lesions may make eating painful to the extent that malnutrition occurs. Skin denudation and bullae formation can cause significant fluid and protein losses and the risk of secondary bacterial infection is great. As with epidermolysis bullosa, lateral shearing force is more likely to produce bullae than pressure exerted perpendicular to the skin surface. Systemic corticosteroids are the most effective therapy for pemphigus vulgaris. Improvement may be seen within days of corticosteroid therapy, with full healing in 6 to 8 weeks. Dapsone, an anti-inflammatory agent, can be used in conjunction with corticosteroids or as monotherapy. Immunosuppressants such as methotrexate, cyclophosphamide, and mycophenolate mofetil can be used to reduce corticosteroid doses and side effects. Rituximab, an anti-CD20 monoclonal antibody, has also been shown to be effective. Severe progressive pemphigus has also been treated with intravenous immune globulin.[71]

Paraneoplastic pemphigus is an autoimmune disease associated with a number of malignant tumors, especially lymphomas and leukemias. IgG antibodies are produced that react to desmoglein 3 and 1. Oral and cutaneous lesions occur in most patients. Obstructive respiratory failure may result form inflammation and sloughing of the tracheobronchial tree.

Management of Anesthesia

Preoperative drug therapy and the extreme fragility of the mucous membranes are the primary concerns for management of anesthesia for patients with pemphigus. Corticosteroid supplementation will be necessary during the perioperative period if the patient's therapy includes steroids. Management of the airway and tracheal intubation should be performed as described for patients with epidermolysis bullosa. Ketamine and regional anesthesia have been used successfully for patients with pemphigus.[72]

There are no specific contraindications to the use of any inhaled or intravenous anesthetic. Methotrexate produces

hepatorenal dysfunction and bone marrow suppression, and cyclophosphamide may prolong the action of succinylcholine by inhibiting cholinesterase activity.

References

1. Emery AEH: The muscular dystrophies. Lancet 2002; 359: 687
2. McNally EM: New approaches in the therapy of cardiomyopathy in muscular dystrophy. Annu Rev Med 2007; 58: 75
3. Boriani G, Gallina M, Merlini L, et al: Clinical relevance of atrial fibrillation/flutter, stroke, pacemaker implant, and heart failure in Emery-Dreifuss muscular dystrophy: A long term longitudinal study. Stroke 2003; 34: 901
4. Wagner KR: Genetic diseases of muscle. Neurol Clin North Am 2002; 20: 645
5. Klingler W, Lehmann-Horn F, Jurkat-Rott K: Complications of anaesthesia in neuromuscular disorders. Neuromusc Dis 2005; 15: 195
6. Yemen TA, McClain: Muscular dystrophy, anesthesia and the safety of inhalational agents revisited; again. Pediatr Anes 2006; 16: 105
7. Machuca-Tzili L, Brook D, Hilton-Jones: Clinical and molecular aspects of the myotonic dystrophies: A review. Muscle Nerve 2005; 32: 1
8. Sovari AA, Bodine CK, Farokhi F: Cardiovascular manifestations of myotonic dystrophy-1. Cardiol Rev 2007; 15: 191
9. Mathieu J, Allard P, Gobeil G, et al: Anesthetic and surgical complications in 219 cases of myotonic dystrophy. Neurology 1997; 49: 1646
10. Rosenbaum HK, Miller JD: Malignant hyperthermia and myotonic disorders. Anes Clin N Am 2002; 20: 623
11. White RJ, Bass SP: Myotonic dystrophy and paediatric anaesthesia. Pediatr Anaesth 2003; 13: 94
12. Jurkat-Rott K, Lerche H, Lehmann-Horn F: Skeletal muscle channelopathies. J Neurol 2002; 249: 1493
13. Jurkat-Rott K, Lehmann-Horn F: Paroxysmal muscle weakness—the familial periodic paralyses. J Neurol 2006; 253: 1391
14. Weller JF, Elliott RA, Pronovost PJ: Spinal anesthesia for a patient with familial hyperkalemic periodic paralysis. Anesthesiology 2002; 97: 259
15. Conti-Fine BM, Milani M, Kaminski HJ: Myasthenia gravis: past, present, and future. J Clin Invest 2006; 116: 2843
16. Sax TW, Rosenbaum RB: Neuromuscular disorders in pregnancy. Muscle Nerve 2006; 34: 559
17. Cakar F, Werner P, Augustin F, et al: A comparison of outcomes after robotic extended thymectomy for myasthenia gravis. Eur J Card-Thor Surg 2007; 31: 501
18. Della Rocca G, Coccia C, Diana L, et al: Propofol or sevoflurane anesthesia without muscle relaxants allow early extubation of myasthenic patients. Can J Anaesth 2003; 50: 547
19. Abel M, Eisenkraft JB: Anesthetic implications of myasthenia gravis. Mount Sinai J Med 2002; 69: 31
20. Dillon FX: Anesthesia issues in the perioperative management of myasthenia gravis. Semin Neurol 2004; 24: 83
21. Mareska M, Gutmann L: Lambert-Eaton myasthenic syndrome. Semin Neurol 2004; 24: 149
22. Maddison P, Newsom-Davis: Treatment for Lambert-Eaton myasthenic syndrome. Cochrane Database of Systemic Diseases 2005; (2): CD003279
23. Lehmann HC, Kohne A, Meyer zu Horste G, et al: Role of nitric oxide as mediator of nerve injury in inflammatory neuropathies. J Neuropathol Exp Neurol 2007; 66: 305
24. Feldman JM: Cardiac arrest after succinylcholine in a pregnant patient recovered from Guillain-Barré syndrome. Anesthesiology 1990; 72: 942
25. Fiacchino F, Gemma M, Bricchi M, et al: Hypo- and hypersensitivity to vecuronium in a patient with Guillain-Barre syndrome. Anesth Analg 1994; 78: 187
26. DeJager PL, Hafler DA: New therapeutic approaches for multiple sclerosis. Annu Rev Med 2007; 58: 417
27. Neuhaus O, Kieseier BC, Hartung H-P: Pharmacokinetics and pharmacodynamics of the interferon-betas, glatiramer acetate, and mitoxantrone in multiple sclerosis. J Neurol Sci 2007; 259: 27
28. Bader AM, Hunt CO, Datta S, et al: Anesthesia for the patient with multiple sclerosis J Clin Anesth 1988; 1: 21
29. Dorotta IR, Schubert A: Multiple sclerosis and anesthetic implications. Curr Opin Anaesthesiol 2002; 15: 365
30. Vajda FJE: Pharmacotherapy of epilepsy: New armamentarium, new issues. J Clin Neurosci 2007; 14: 813
31. Bazil CW, Pedley TA: Clinical pharmacology of antiepileptic drugs. Clin Neuropharm 2003; 26: 38
32. Jaaskelainen SK, Kaisti K, Suni L, et al: Sevoflurane is epileptogenic in healthy subjects at surgical levels of anesthesia. Neurology 2003; 61: 1073.
33. Litvan I, Halliday G, Hallett M, et al: The etiopathogenesis of Parkinson disease and suggestions for future research. Part I. J Neuropathol Exp Neurol 2007; 66: 251
34. Schapira AHV: Treatment options in the modern management of Parkinson disease. Arch Neurol 2007; 64: 1083
35. Galvez-Jimenez N, Lang AE: The perioperative management of Parkinson's disease revisited. Neurol Clin N Am 2004; 22: 367
36. Walker FO: Huntington's disease. Lancet 2007; 369: 218

37. Gilli E, Bartoloni A, Fiocca F, et al: Anaesthetic management in a case of Huntington's chorea. Minerva Anesthsiol 2006; 72: 757

38. Cummings JL, Doody R, Clark C: Disease-modifying therapies for Alzheimer disease. Neurology 2007; 69: 1622

39. Xie Z, Dong Y, Maeda U, et al: Isoflurane-induced apoptosis: A potential pathogenic link between delirium and dementia. J Neurosci 2007; 27: 1247.

40. Mitchell JD, Borasio GD: Amyotrophic lateral sclerosis. Lancet 2007; 369: 2031

41. Jacka MJ, Sanderson F: Amyotrophic lateral sclerosis presenting during pregnancy. Anesth Analg 1998; 86: 542

42. Aguzzi A: Prion diseases of humans and farm animals: Epidemiology, genetics, and pathogenesis. J Neurochem 2006; 97: 1726

43. Sutton JM, Dickinson J, Walker JT, et al: methods to minimize the risks of Creutzfeldt-Jakob disease transmission by surgical procedures: Where to set the standard. Clin Infect Dis 2006; 43: 757

44. Farling P, Smith G: Anaesthesia for patients with Creutzfeld-Jakob disease. A practical guide. Anaesthesia 2003; 58: 627

45. Myles PS, Leslie K, Sibert B, et al: A review of the risks and benefits of nitrous oxide in current anaesthetic practice. Anaesth Intens Care 2004; 32: 165

46. Gehrs BC, Friedberg RC: Autoimmune hemolytic anemia. Am J Hematol 2002; 69: 258

47. Firth PG: Anaesthesia for peculiar cells—a century of sickle cell disease. Br J Anesth 2005; 95: 287

48. Firth PG, Head CA: Sickle cell disease and anesthesia. Anesthesiology 2004; 101: 766

49. Vichinsky EP, Neumayr LD, Earles AN, et al: Causes and outcomes of the acute chest syndrome in sickle cell disease. N Engl J Med 2000; 342: 1855

50. Frietsch T, Ewen I, Waschke KF: Anaesthetic care for sickle cell disease. Eur J Anaesthesiol 2001; 18: 137

51. Kato GJ, Onyekwere OC, Gladwin MT: Pulmonary hypertension in sickle cell disease. Relevance to children. Pediatr Hematol Oncol 2007; 24: 159

52. Butwick A, Findley I, Wonke B: Management of pregnancy in a patient with β thalassemia. Int J Obstet Anes 2005; 14: 351

53. Scrivo R, Di Franco M, Spadaro A, et al: The immunology of rheumatoid arthritis. Ann NY Acad Sci 2007; 1108: 312

54. Yaszemski MJ, Shepler TR: Sudden death from cord compression associated with atlantoaxial instability in rheumatoid arthritis. Spine 1990; 15: 338

55. Gonzalez-Juanatey C, Testa A, Garcia-Castelo A, et al: Echocardiographic and Doppler findings in long term treated rheumatoid arthritis patients without clinically evident cardiovascular disease. Semin Arthritis Rheum 2004; 33: 231

56. Siddiqui MAA: The efficacy and tolerability of newer biologics in rheumatoid arthritis: best current evidence. Curr Opin Rheumatol 2007; 19: 308

57. Petrozza PH: Major spine surgery. Anes Clin N Am 2002; 20: 405

58. Takenaka I, Urakami Y, Aoyama K, et al: Severe subluxation in the sniffing position in a rheumatoid patient with anterior atlantoaxial subluxation. Anesthesiology 2004; 101: 1235

59. D'Cruz DP, Khamashta MA, Hughes GRV: Systemic lupus erythematosus. Lancet 2007; 369: 587.

60. Moldovan I: Systemic lupus erythematosus. Comp Ther 2006; 32: 158

61. Varga J, Abraham D: Systemic sclerosis: A prototypic multisystem fibrotic disorder. J Clin Invest 2007; 117: 557

62. Dalakas MC: Inflammatory disorders of muscle: progress in polymyositis, dermatomyositis and inclusion body myositis. Curr Opin Neurol 2004; 17: 561

63. Briani C, Doria A, Sarzi-Puttini P, et al: Update on idiopathic myopathies. Autoimmunity 2006; 39: 161

64. Brown S, Shupak RC, Patel C, et al: Neuromuscular blockade in a patient with active dermatomyositis. Anesthesiology 1992; 77: 1031

65. Uitto J, Richard G: Progress in epidermolysis bullosa: From eponyms to molecular genetic classification. Clin Dermatol 2005; 23: 33

66. Sidwell RU, Yates R, Atherton D: Dilated cardiomyopathy in dystrophic epidermolysis bullosa. Arch Dis Child 2000; 83: 59

67. Hore I, Bajaj Y, Denyer J, et al: The management of general and specific ENT problems in children with epidermolysis bullosa—a retrospective case note review. Int J Paediatr Otolaryngol 2007; 71: 385

68. Herod J, Denyer J, Goldman A, et al: Epidermolysis bullosa in children: pathophysiology, anesthesia and pain management. Pediatr Anaesth 1994; 12: 388

69. Bystryn J-C, Rudolph JL: Pemphigus. Lancet 2005; 366: 61

70. Espana A, Fernandez S, del Olmo J, et al: Ear, nose and throat manifestations in pemphigus vulgaris. Br J Dermatol 2007; 156: 733

71. Yeh SW, Sami N, Ahmed RA: Treatment of pemphigus vulgaris. Am J Clin Dermatol 2005; 6: 327

72. Mahalingam TG, Karthivel S, Sodhi P: Anaesthetic management of a patient with pemphigus vulgaris for emergency laparotomy. Anaesthesia 2000; 55: 160

PREANESTHETIC EVALUATION AND PREPARATION

CHAPTER 26 ■ THE ANESTHESIA WORKSTATION AND DELIVERY SYSTEMS

KEVIN T. RIUTORT, RUSSELL C. BROCKWELL, SORIN J. BRULL, AND J. JEFFREY ANDREWS

KEY POINTS

1 The low-pressure circuit (LPC) is the "vulnerable area" of the anesthesia workstation because it is most subject to breakage and leaks. The LPC is located downstream from all anesthesia machine safety features except the oxygen analyzer (or, in some cases, the ratio controller), and it is the portion of the machine where a leak is most likely to go unrecognized if an inappropriate LPC leak test is performed. Leaks in the LPC can cause delivery of a hypoxic or subanesthetic mixture, leading to patient hypoxic injury or awareness during anesthesia. Hypoxic delivery is typically caused by a cracked oxygen flow tube that is located downstream to the nitrous/air/helium tubes. Hypoxic mixtures would not likely occur in the workstations that have electronically metered fresh gas. Even with these workstations, however, hypoxic mixtures could be delivered as the oxygen is consumed from the rest of the breathing circuit.

2 Because most General Electric (GE) Healthcare/Datex-Ohmeda anesthesia machines have a one-way check valve in the LPC, a negative leak test is required to detect leaks in the LPC. A positive pressure leak test will not detect leaks in the LPC of most GE Healthcare/Datex-Ohmeda products.

3 Internal vaporizer leaks can be detected only with the vaporizer turned to the "on" position.

4 Prior to an anesthetic, the circle system must be checked for leaks and for flow. To test for leaks, the circle system is pressurized to 30-cm water pressure and the circle system airway pressure gauge is observed (static test). To check for appropriate flow to rule out obstructions and faulty valves, the ventilator and a test lung (breathing bag) are used (dynamic test). Additionally, the manual circuit must be actuated by compressing the reservoir bag in order to rule out obstructions to flow in the manual mode.

5 Many new anesthesia workstation self-tests do not detect internal vaporizer leaks unless each vaporizer is individually turned on during repeated self-tests.

6 In the event of a pipeline crossover, two actions must be taken. The backup oxygen cylinder must be turned on (because the yoke valve should always be turned off during normal operation) and the wall supply sources must be disconnected.

7 The oxygen failure cutoff valves (also known previously as fail-safe valves, hypoxic guards, or proportioning systems) help minimize delivery of a hypoxic mixture, but they are not foolproof. Delivery of a hypoxic mixture may still result from: (1) the wrong supply gas, either in the cylinder or in the main pipeline; (2) a defective or broken safety device; (3) leaks downstream from the safety devices; (4) inert gas administration (for instance, helium may not be subject to the oxygen failure cutoff valve); and (5) dilution of the inspired oxygen concentration by high concentrations of inhaled anesthetics.

8 Because of its low boiling point and high vapor pressure, controlled vaporization of desflurane requires specially designed vaporizers, such as the GE Healthcare/Datex-Ohmeda Tec 6 and the Aladin Cassette vaporizer.

9 Misfilling an empty variable bypass vaporizer with desflurane could theoretically be catastrophic, resulting in delivery of a hypoxic mixture and a massive overdose of inhaled desflurane anesthetic.

10 Inhaled anesthetics can interact with CO_2 absorbents and produce toxic compounds. During sevoflurane (only) anesthesia, compound A can be formed, particularly at low fresh gas flow rates, and during desflurane, and to a lesser extent sevoflurane anesthesia, carbon monoxide can be produced, particularly with desiccated absorbents.

11 Desiccated strong base absorbents (particularly barium hydroxide lime, Baralyme) can react with sevoflurane, producing extremely high absorber temperatures and combustible decomposition products. These in combination with the oxygen or nitrous oxide-enriched environment of the circle system can produce high temperatures and fires within the breathing system.

12 Anesthesia ventilators with ascending bellows (bellows that ascend during the expiratory phase) were initially thought to be safer than descending bellows because disconnections would readily manifest with ascending bellows. The descending bellows machines, however, have been carefully redesigned to address these initial limitations. Current ventilators have featherlight bellows, they have an electric eye at the bottom to detect bellows movement, and the canister is subjected to positive end-expiratory pressure (PEEP), such that in case of disconnection, the bellows would actually rise and stay up.

13 With older-design machines, use of the oxygen flush valve during the inspiratory phase of mechanical ventilation could cause barotrauma, particularly in pediatric patients. The newer workstations have fresh gas decouplers or peak-inspiratory pressure limiters that were designed to prevent these complications. Ventilators that use fresh gas decoupling technology virtually eliminate the possibility of barotrauma by oxygen flushing during the inspiratory phase because fresh gas flow and oxygen flush flow are diverted to the reservoir breathing bag. However, if the breathing bag has a large leak or is absent altogether, patient awareness under anesthesia and delivery of a lower than expected oxygen concentration could occur because of entrainment of room air.

14 Modern ventilators compensate for the fresh gas flow as the tidal volume is delivered. Thus, the delivered tidal volume does not change as a function of the fresh gas flow. This compensation is achieved either by "fresh gas decoupling" (in Dräger Narkomed 6000 series, Apollo and Fabius machines) or by "fresh gas compensation" in GE Healthcare/Datex-Ohmeda machines.

15 With newer GE Healthcare/Datex-Ohmeda anesthetic ventilators such as the 7100 and 7900 SmartVent, both the patient gas and the drive gas are scavenged, resulting in substantially increased volumes of scavenged gas. Thus, the scavenging systems must be set appropriately high to accommodate the increased volume; otherwise, undesired PEEP and pollution of the operating room environment could result.

The function of the anesthesia machine is to (1) extract gases from the central supply and cylinders, (2) meter them and load them with anesthetic vapors, and (3) deliver them to the patient for breathing.[1] The anesthesia machine is, conceptually, a pump for delivering medical gases and inhalation agents to the patient's lungs. This machine has evolved over the past 160 years from a rather simple ether inhaler to a complex device of valves, pistons, vaporizers, monitors, and electronic circuitry.

The "pump" in the modern anesthesia machine is either a mechanical ventilator or the lungs of the spontaneously breathing patient, or perhaps, a combination of the two. The anesthesia pump has a supply system: medical gases from either a pipeline supply or a gas canister, alongside vaporizes delivering inhalation agents that are mixed with the medical gases. The anesthesia pump also has an exhaust system, the waste gas scavenging system, which removes excess gases from the machine's circuit. The breathing circuit is a series of hoses, valves, filters, switches, and regulators that interconnect the supply system, the patient, and the exhaust system.

Modern anesthesia machines (Figs. 26-1 and 26-2) are now more properly referred to as *anesthesia workstations*. The anesthesia workstation, as defined by ASTM International (originally known as the American Society for Testing and Materials), is a system for administering anesthetics to patients consisting of the *anesthesia gas supply device*, *the anesthesia ventilator*, *monitoring devices*, and *protection devices*.[2] The protection device is designed to prevent the patient from hazardous output due to incorrect delivery of energy or substances, for example, the adjustable pressure-limiting valve prevents barotrauma.

In this chapter, the anesthesia workstation is examined piece by piece. The normal operation, function, and integration of major anesthesia workstation subsystems are described. More importantly, the potential problems and hazards associated with the various components of the anesthesia delivery system, and the appropriate preoperative checks that may help to detect and prevent such problems, are illustrated.

ANESTHESIA WORKSTATION STANDARDS AND PRE-USE PROCEDURES

A few years ago, a fundamental knowledge of the basic anesthesia machine pneumatics would have sufficed for most anesthesia providers. Today, a detailed understanding of pneumatics, electronics, and even computer science is necessary to fully

FIGURE 26-1. Dräger Medical Fabius GS anesthesia workstation. (Courtesy of Dräger Medical AG.)

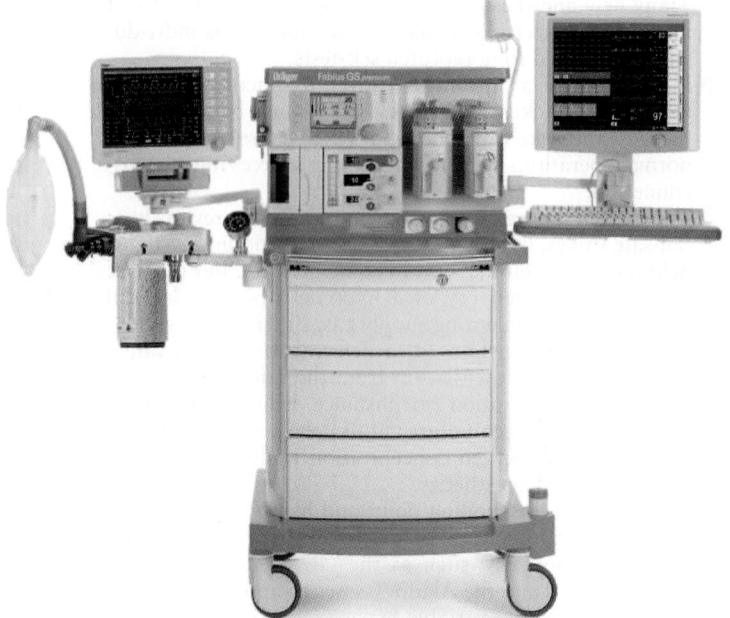

understand the capabilities and complexities of the anesthesia workstation. Along with the changes in the composition of the anesthesia workstation to include more complex ventilation systems and integrated monitoring, recently there has also been increasing divergence between anesthesia workstation designs from different manufacturers. In 1993, a joint effort between the American Society of Anesthesiologists (ASA) and the U.S. Food and Drug Administration (FDA) produced the 1993 FDA Anesthesia Apparatus Pre-Use Checkout Recommendations (Appendix A). This pre-use checklist was versatile and could be applied to most commonly available anesthesia

machines equally well and did not require users to vary the pre-use procedure significantly from machine to machine.

Today, because of increasing fundamental anesthesia workstation design variations, the 1993 FDA pre-use checklist may no longer be applicable to many anesthesia workstations. Anesthesia providers must be aware of this limitation, and the original equipment manufacturer's recommended pre-use checklist should be followed. Some of the newer workstations even have computer-assisted self-tests that automatically perform all or a part of the pre-use machine checkout procedure. The availability of such automated checkout features further adds to the complexity of constructing a standardized pre-use anesthesia machine checklist such as the one used in the recent past. Ultimately, the responsibility of performing adequate pre-use testing of the anesthesia workstation falls to the individual user: regardless of the level of training and the quality of technical support, the anesthesia care provider has the ultimate responsibility for proper function of all anesthesia equipment. The anesthesia provider of record must be aware of which anesthesia workstation components are tested by the automated self-tests and which ones are not. Because of the number of machines available and the variability among their self-testing procedures, the following discussion will be limited to general topics related to these systems.

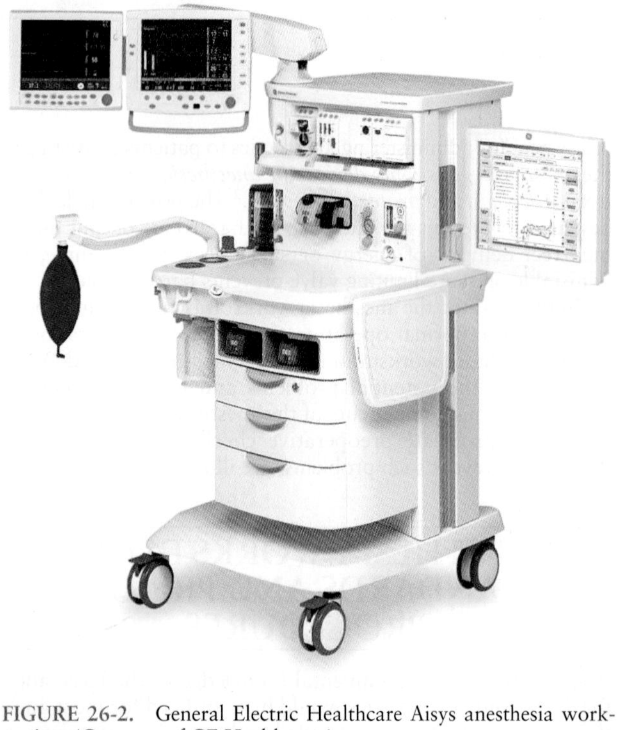

STANDARDS FOR ANESTHESIA MACHINES AND WORKSTATIONS

Standards for anesthesia machines and workstations provide guidelines to manufacturers regarding their minimum performance, design characteristics, and safety requirements. During the past 2 decades, the progression of anesthesia machine standards has been as follows:

1979: American National Standards Institute, Z79.8-1979[3]

1988: American Society for Testing and Materials, F1161-88[4]

1994: ASTM F1161-94 (reapproved in 1994 and discontinued in 2000)[5]

2005: International Electrical Commission (IEC), 60601-1[6]

2005: ASTM F1850-00 (reapproved)[2]

FIGURE 26-2. General Electric Healthcare Aisys anesthesia workstation. (Courtesy of GE Healthcare.)

The ASTM F1850-00 specification applies to workstation design in conjunction with the IEC publication 60601-1. IEC publication 60601-1 is an umbrella specification that describes general requirements for basic safety and essential performance of medical electrical equipment. To comply with the 2005 ASTM F1850-00 standard, newly manufactured workstations must have monitors that measure the following parameters: continuous breathing system pressure, exhaled tidal volume, ventilatory CO_2 concentration, anesthetic vapor concentration, inspired oxygen concentration, oxygen supply pressure, arterial hemoglobin oxygen saturation, arterial blood pressure, and continuous electrocardiogram. The anesthesia workstation must have a prioritized alarm system that groups the alarms into three categories: high, medium, and low. These monitors and alarms may be enabled automatically and made to function by turning on the anesthesia workstation, or the monitors and alarms can be enabled manually and made functional by following a pre-use checklist.[2]

Perhaps just as important as the specifications for new anesthesia machines and workstations that are introduced into clinical care are the characteristics that render older machines obsolete. This is not an inconsequential issue because on the one hand, the financial investment for replacing older machines is significant, while on the other hand, the implications for patient safety are huge. The "Guidelines for Determining Anesthesia Machine Obsolescence" document addresses some of the absolute as well as relative criteria that can help institutions make a decision on when even otherwise functioning equipment should be replaced.[7]

FAILURE OF ANESTHESIA EQUIPMENT

An 11-year study of 1,000 anesthesia incidents in the United Kingdom revealed that the most common failure was due to an equipment leak (61/1,000).[8] The authors stated the most likely underlying cause of system leaks was due to "design weakness"; for example, push-on tapers in breathing circuits that can easily become disconnected. Poor equipment maintenance and setup were the second most common underlying causes of equipment failure. Equipment failure from entrapped cables may result in the inability to ventilate the patient (thus warranting careful attention to organization and tidiness of the anesthesia workstation environment by the anesthesia provider).[9] The authors found that pulse oximetry alarm was the most common principal monitor alerting the anesthesiologist to an equipment problem.

In a review of the ASA "Closed Claims" database, Caplan et al.[10] found that although claims related to the medical gas-delivery system were rare, when they occurred, they were usually severe, often resulting in death or permanent brain injury. The most common malfunction, in the authors' review, was the breathing circuit (39%), followed by vaporizers (21%), ventilators (17%), gas tanks or gas lines (11%), and the anesthesia machine itself (7%).

SAFETY FEATURES OF NEWER ANESTHESIA WORKSTATIONS

Older or conventional anesthesia machines have design limitations that limit their safety. For example, machines such as the Dräger Narkomed series and the Narkomed G (Dräger Medical, Inc., Telford, PA) may lack features to prevent barotraumas during oxygen flush, lack automated checkout, often have multiple external connections, may have gas-driven ventilator bellows that do not fully empty, and allow breath stacking as well as inaccurate tidal volume delivery.[11]

Newer workstations—including the General Electric (GE) Healthcare/Datex-Ohmeda Aestiva/5 with 7900 ventilator (GE Healthcare, Madison, WI), the Anesthesia Delivery Unit (ADU), and the Dräger Medical Fabius GS v1.3, Julian, and Narkomed 6400—have designs that incorporate additional safety features such as fresh gas flow decoupling to prevent barotrauma during oxygen flush; integrated, software-driven self checkout routines; limited external connections; and electronic, piston-driven ventilators that deliver accurate tidal volumes.[11] Table 26-1 summarizes relevant safety features of newer anesthesia workstations.

CHECKOUT OF THE ANESTHESIA WORKSTATION

A complete anesthesia apparatus checkout procedure must be performed each day prior to the first use of the anesthesia workstation. An abbreviated checkout procedure should be performed before each subsequent case. The 1993 FDA Anesthesia Apparatus Checkout Recommendations reproduced in Appendix A remain applicable to the majority of older anesthesia machines in use worldwide.[12–16]

In 2007 the ASA published recommendations for preanesthesia checkout machines, taking into consideration newer workstations that perform automated checkout.[17] Because the design of newer workstations varies considerably, no single pre-use procedure is applicable. Hence, the Subcommittee of ASA Committee on Equipment and Facilities developed in 2007 the "Recommendations for Preanesthesia Checkout Procedures." These guidelines present a template for individual departments and practitioners to design preanesthesia checkout procedures specific to their needs and equipment (Appendix B). Sample checkout procedures are published on the ASA Web site[a] and they encompass adult as well as pediatric equipment from both major equipment manufacturers in the United States.

The three most important preoperative checks are: (1) oxygen analyzer calibration, (2) the low-pressure circuit leak test, and (3) the circle system test. Each is discussed in the following sections. Additional details regarding these systems will be presented briefly in subsequent sections describing the anatomy of the anesthesia workstation; for a more comprehensive review, the reader is encouraged to consult his or her own equipment manufacturer's user manual. For a simplified diagram of a two-gas anesthesia machine and the components described in the following discussion, please refer to Figure 26-3. A comprehensive discussion of Figure 26-3 can also be found in "Anesthesia Workstation Pneumatics."

Oxygen Analyzer Calibration

The oxygen analyzer is one of the most important monitors on the anesthesia workstation. It is the only machine safety device that evaluates the integrity of the low-pressure circuit in an ongoing fashion. Other machine safety devices, such as the oxygen failure cutoff ("failsafe") valve, the oxygen supply failure alarm, and the proportioning system, are all upstream from the flow control valves. The only machine monitor that detects problems downstream from the flow control valves is the oxygen analyzer. Calibration of this monitor is described in Appendix A (Anesthesia Apparatus Checkout Recommendations, 1993, Step 9). The actual procedure for calibrating the oxygen analyzer has remained reasonably similar over the recent generations of the anesthesia workstations (Guideline for Designing Preanesthesia Checkout Procedures, 2007, Item 10 in Appendix B). Generally, the oxygen concentration sensing

---

[a]http://www.asahq.org.

TABLE 26-1

COMPARISON OF ANESTHESIA WORKSTATION FUNCTIONS

ANESTHESIA WORKSTATION FUNCTION	OHMEDA 7800	DRÄGER NARKOMED AV2+	DRÄGER-NARKOMED 6400	DRÄGER JULIAN	DRÄGER FABIUS GS 1.3	GE/DATEX-OHMEDA AESTIVA/5	GE/DATEX-OHMEDA ADU	GE AISYS	DRÄGER APOLLO
Increase in FGF increases V_T	Yes	Yes	No	No	No	Initially	No	No	No
Pre-use system leakage is measured	No	No	Yes	Yes	Yes	No	Yes	Yes	Yes
Proximal leak compensation	No	No	No	No	No	Yes	No	Yes	Yes
Leakage measurement during operation	No	No	Yes	No	No	No	No	Yes	Yes
Hose compliance compensation	No	No	Yes	Yes	Yes	No	Yes	Yes	Yes
System compliance compensation	No	No	Yes	Yes	Yes	Yes	Yes	Yes	Yes
The reported exhaled V_T is adjusted for hose compliance	No	No	Yes	No	Yes	No	No	Yes	Yes
The fresh gas inflow is distal to:	Absorber	Absorber	Absorber	Midabsorber	Absorber	Absorber	Inspiratory valve	Absorber	Absorber
The fresh gas inflow is proximal to:	Inspiratory valve	Inspiratory valve	Decoupling valve	Midabsorber	Decoupling valve	Inspiratory valve	Y-piece	Inspiratory valve	Decoupling valve
At low FGF, what gas fills the reservoir bag?	Exhaled	Exhaled	Scrubbed	Exhaled	Scrubbed	Exhaled	Exhaled	Exhaled	Exhaled
Mechanism of VCV	Mechanical limit	Mechanical limit	Displacement	Metered	Displacement	Metered/servo	Metered/calculated	Metered, calculated	Metered
Limiting of pressure control ventilation	Pressure limited	Pressure limited	Flow/pressure limited	Flow/pressure limited	Flow/pressure limited	Pressure limited	Flow/pressure limited	Flow/pressure limited	Flow/pressure limited
FiO_2 compensated for volatile agent	No	No	No	No	No	No	Yes	Yes	Yes
Synchronized intermittent mechanical ventilation	No	No	Yes	No	No	Yes	Yes	Yes	Yes
The manufacturer specified minimum V_T (mL)	18	N/A	10	50	20	20	20	20	20
FGF control	Needle valve	Needle valve	Needle valve	Digital control	Needle valve	Needle valve	Needle valve	Digital control	Needle valve

(continued)

TABLE 26-1

(Continued)

ANESTHESIA WORKSTATION FUNCTION	DRÄGER NARKOMED AV2+	OHMEDA 7800	DRÄGER NARKOMED 6400	DRÄGER JULIAN	DRÄGER FABIUS GS 1.3	GE/DATEX-OHMEDA AESTIVA/5	GE/DATEX-OHMEDA ADU	GE AISYS	DRÄGER APOLLO
FGF measurement	Flow tubes	Flow tubes	Flow tubes	Electronic	Electronic	Flow tubes	Electronic	Electronic	Electronic
Backup flow tube	N/A	N/A	N/A	No	Yes	N/A	Yes	Yes (failsafe mode)	Yes
Integrated capnography	No	No	Yes	Yes	No	No	Yes	Yes	Yes
Integrated anesthetic gas monitoring	No	No	Yes	Yes	No	No	Yes	Yes	Yes
Effect of lost oxygen pressure on FGF	No FGF	No FGF	No FGF	Auto air on	Air available	Air available	Air available	Air available	Air available
Sampled gas returned to circuit	No	No	No	No	No	No	Yes	No	Yes
Mechanical airway pressure gauge	Yes	Yes	No	No	Yes	Yes	No	No	Yes
Absorber removable during VCV	No	No	No	No	Yes	No	Yes	Yes (optional)	Yes (optional)
Room air entrained during a circuit leak	No	No	Yes	Yes	Yes	No	No	No	Yes
Room air entrained with inadequate FGF	No	No	No	No	Yes	No	No	No	No
Effect of O2 flush during VCV inspiration	>VT, held at pressure limit	>VT, end at pressure limit	None	>VT, held at pressure limit	None	>VT, end at pressure limit	>VT, end at pressure release	>VT, end at pressure release	None
Failsafe integrated with the ratio controller	No	No	No	Yes, electronic	Yes, pneumatic	No	Yes, electronic	Yes, electronic	Yes, electronic
Method to find a low pressure/vaporizer leak	Positive pressure	Negative pressure	Automatic, vaporizer open	Automatic, vaporizer open	Automatic, vaporizer open	Negative pressure	Automatic	Automatic	Automatic, vaporizer open
Ventilator drive gas scavenging	No	No	N/A	Yes	N/A	Yes	No	Yes	N/A

FGF, fresh gas flow; VT, tidal volume; VCV, volume control ventilation; N/A, not available. Modern anesthesia machines offer new safety features. APSF Newsletter 2003; 18: 17.
Adapted from Olympio MA:

FIGURE 26-3. Diagram of a generic two-gas anesthesia machine. (Modified from Check-Out, A Guide for Preoperative Inspection of an Anesthesia Machine. Park Ridge, IL, American Society of Anesthesiologists, 1987, with permission.)

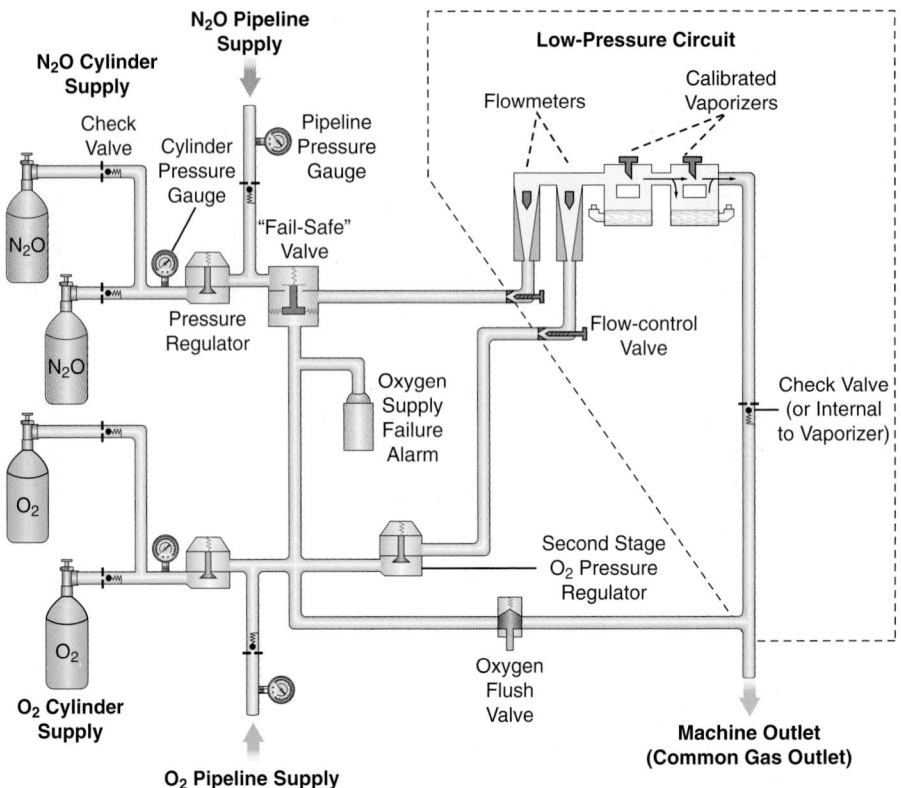

element must be exposed to room air for calibration to 21%. This may require manually setting a dial on older machines, but on newer ones, it usually involves only temporary removal of the sensor, selecting and then confirming that the oxygen calibration is to be performed from a set of menus on the workstation's display screen, and finally reinstalling the sensor. The function of the low-oxygen alarm should be verified by setting the alarm to trigger above the current oxygen reading. Newer workstations have automatic oxygen sensor calibration.

Low-Pressure Circuit Leak Test

❶ The low-pressure leak test checks the integrity of the anesthesia machine from the flow control valves to the common outlet. It evaluates the portion of the machine that is downstream from all safety devices except the oxygen analyzer. The components located within this area are *precisely* the ones most subject to breakage and leaks. Leaks in the low-pressure circuit can cause hypoxia or patient awareness.[18,19] Flow tubes, the most delicate pneumatic component of the machine, can crack or break. A typical three-gas anesthesia machine has 16 O-rings in the low-pressure circuit. Leaks can occur at the interface between the glass flow tubes and the manifold, and at the O-ring junctions between the vaporizer and its manifold. Loose filler caps on vaporizers are a common source of leaks, and these leaks can lead to delivery of subanesthetic doses of inhaled agents, causing patient awareness during general anesthesia.[18,20]

Several different methods have been used to check the low-pressure circuit for leaks. They include the oxygen flush test, the common gas outlet occlusion test, the traditional positive pressure leak test, the North American Dräger positive pressure leak test, the Ohmeda 8000 internal positive pressure leak test, the Ohmeda negative pressure leak test, the 1993 FDA universal negative pressure leak test, and others. One reason for the large number of methods is that the internal

design of various machines differs considerably. The most notable example is that most GE Healthcare/Datex-Ohmeda (hereafter referred to as Datex-Ohmeda) workstations have a check valve near the common gas outlet, whereas Dräger Medical workstations do not. The presence or absence of the check valve profoundly influences which preoperative check is indicated.

Several mishaps have resulted from application of the wrong leak test to the wrong machine.[21–24] Therefore, it is mandatory to perform the appropriate low-pressure leak test each day. To do this, it is essential to understand the exact location and operating principles of the Datex-Ohmeda check valve. Many Datex-Ohmeda anesthesia workstations have a machine outlet check valve located in the low-pressure

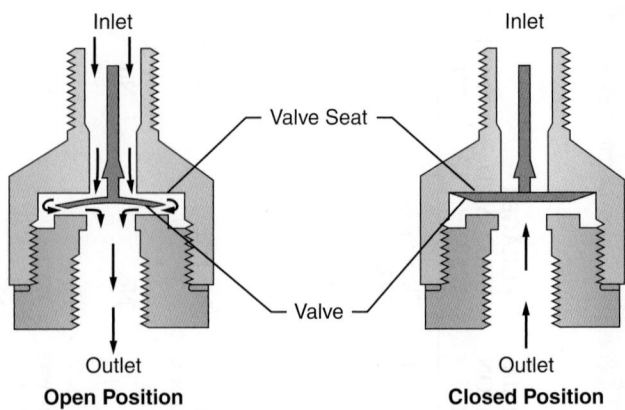

FIGURE 26-4. Machine outlet check valve. See text for details. (Reproduced from Bowie E, Huffman LM: The Anesthesia Machine: Essentials for Understanding. Madison, Ohmeda, Inc., a Division of BOC Health Care, 1985, with permission.)

circuit (Table 26-1). The check valve is located downstream from the vaporizers and upstream from the oxygen flush valve (Fig. 26-3). It is open (Fig. 26-4, *left*) in the absence of back pressure. Gas flow from the manifold moves the rubber flapper valve off its seat and allows gas to proceed freely to the common outlet. The valve closes (Fig. 26-4, *right*) when back pressure is exerted on it.[13] Back pressure sufficient to close the check valve may occur with the following conditions: oxygen flushing, peak breathing circuit pressures generated during positive pressure ventilation, or use of a positive pressure leak test.

Generally speaking, the low-pressure circuit of anesthesia workstations without an outlet check valve can be tested using a positive pressure leak test, and machines with check valves must be tested using a negative pressure leak test. When performing a positive pressure leak test, the operator generates positive pressure in the low-pressure circuit using flow from the anesthesia machine or from a positive pressure bulb to detect a leak. When performing a negative pressure leak test, the operator creates negative pressure in the low-pressure circuit using a suction bulb to detect leaks. Two different low-pressure circuit leak tests are described here.

Oxygen Flush Positive-Pressure Leak Test

❷ Historically, older anesthesia machines did not have check valves in the low-pressure circuit. Therefore, it was common practice to pressurize the breathing circuit and the low-pressure circuit with the oxygen flush valve to test for internal anesthesia machine leaks. Because many modern Datex-Ohmeda machines now have check valves in the low-pressure circuit, application of a positive-pressure leak test to these machines can be misleading or even dangerous (Fig. 26-5).

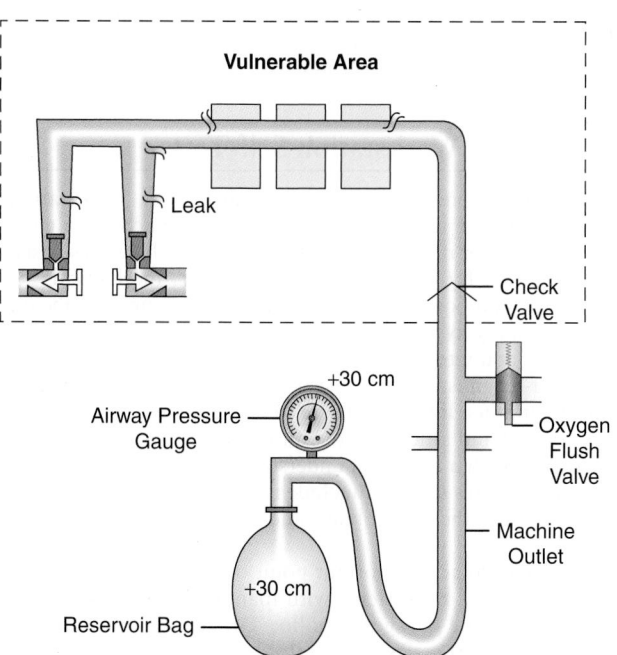

FIGURE 26-5. Inappropriate use of the oxygen flush valve to check the low-pressure circuit of an Ohmeda machine equipped with a check valve. The area within the rectangle is not checked by the inappropriate use of the oxygen flush valve. The components located within this area are *precisely* the ones most subject to breakage and leaks. Positive pressure within the patient circuit closes the check valve, and the value on the airway pressure gauge does not decline, despite leaks in the low-pressure circuit.

Inappropriate use of the oxygen flush valve or the presence of a leaking flush valve may lead to inadequate evaluation of the low-pressure circuit for leaks. In turn, this can lead the workstation user into a false sense of security despite the presence of large leaks.[21–23,25,26] Positive pressure from the breathing circuit results in closure of the outlet check valve, and the value on the airway pressure gauge will fail to decline. The system appears to be tight, but in actuality, only the circuitry downstream from the check valve is leak free.[27] Thus, a vulnerable area exists from the check valve back to the flow control valves because this area is not tested by a positive pressure leak test.

Verifying the Integrity of the Gas Supply Lines Between the Flowmeters and the Common Gas Outlet. The 1993 FDA universal negative pressure leak test (Appendix A, Step 5) was named "universal" because at that time it could be used to check all contemporary anesthesia machines regardless of the presence or absence of check valves in the low-pressure circuit.[14] It remains effective for many older anesthesia workstations, but many newer machines are no longer compatible with this universal test. Table 26-1 describes how newer workstations test for low-pressure circuit and vaporizer leaks. Leaks in the gas supply lines between the flowmeters and the common gas outlet should be checked daily or whenever a vaporizer is changed (Appendix B, Item 8). The most thorough technique is to check each vaporizer individually by turning it on and then evaluating for leaks. It is important to note that automated checkout procedures may not necessarily evaluate leaks at the vaporizer, if the vaporizer is not turned on during testing. Additionally, vaporizers should be adequately filled and filler ports should be tightly closed (Appendix B, Item 7). As mentioned previously, the ASA now recommends that individual institutions develop internal guidelines specific to their own equipment and needs.

The 1993 FDA check is based on the Datex-Ohmeda negative-pressure leak test (Fig. 26-6). It is performed using a negative-pressure leak testing device, which is a simple suction bulb. The machine master switch, the flow control **❸** valves, and vaporizers are turned off. The suction bulb is attached to the common fresh gas outlet and squeezed repeatedly until it is fully collapsed. This action creates a vacuum in the low-pressure circuitry. The machine is leak-free if the hand bulb remains collapsed for at least 10 seconds. A leak is present if the bulb reinflates during this period. The test is repeated with each vaporizer individually turned to the on position because internal vaporizer leaks can be detected only with the vaporizer turned on. If the bulb reinflates in <10 seconds, a leak is present somewhere in the low-pressure circuit.

Evaluation of the Circle System

The circle system tests (Appendix B, Items 12 and 13) evaluate the integrity of the circle breathing system, which spans from the common gas outlet to the Y-piece (Fig. 26-7). It has two components: (1) *breathing system pressure and leak testing* and (2) *verification that gas flows properly through the breathing circuit during both inspiration and exhalation*. To thoroughly check the circle system for leaks, valve integrity, and obstruction, both tests must be performed preoperatively. The 2008 recommendations call for performing the breathing system test and leak test prior to each case, such that pressure can be developed in the system during manual and mechanical ventilation. Automated leak-testing routines are implemented in modern workstations; system compliance is also calculated and used to adjust volume delivery during mechanical ventilation (Appendix B, Item 12). Because pressure and leak testing cannot identify all obstructions in the breathing circuit or confirm the function of the inspiratory and expiratory unidirectional valves, a test lung or second reservoir bag can be used to confirm circuit

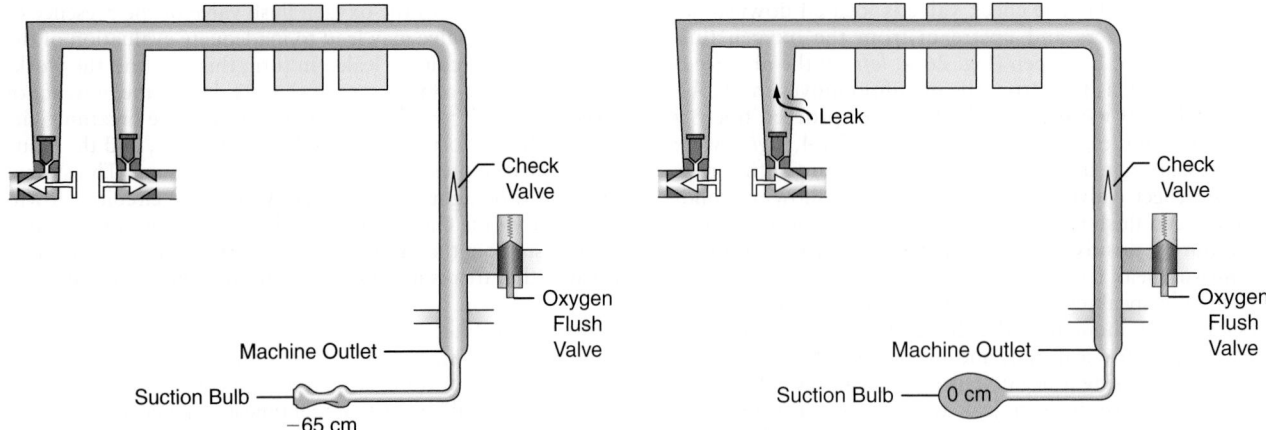

FIGURE 26-6.   Food and Drug Administration negative-pressure leak test. *Left.* A negative-pressure leak testing device is attached directly to the machine outlet. Squeezing the bulb creates a vacuum in the low-pressure circuit and opens the check valve. *Right.* When a leak is present in the low-pressure circuit, room air is entrained through the leak and the suction bulb inflates. (Reprinted from Andrews JJ: Understanding anesthesia machines, 1988 Review Course Lectures. Cleveland, International Anesthesia Research Society, 1988, p. 78, with permission.)

integrity. However, visual inspection of the unidirectional valves should be performed daily because subtle damage to these valves is very difficult to determine. Older 1993 FDA checkout procedures to identify valve incompetence that may not be visually obvious can be implemented, but are typically too complex for daily testing (Appendix B, Item 13).

In the 1993 FDA Anesthesia Apparatus Checkout Recommendations, a *leak test* is performed by closing the pop-off valve, occluding the Y-piece, and pressurizing the circuit to 30 cm water pressure using the oxygen flush valve. The value on the pressure gauge will not decline if the circle system is leak-free, but this does not assure valve integrity. The value on the gauge will read a pressure of 30 cm H_2O even if the unidirectional valves are stuck shut or if the valves are incompetent. Additionally, a *flow test* checks the integrity of the unidirec-

tional valves, and it detects obstruction in the circle system. It can be performed by removing the Y-piece from the circle system and breathing through the two corrugated hoses individually. The valves should be present, and they should move appropriately. The operator should be able to inhale but not be able to exhale through the inspiratory limb. The operator should be able to exhale but not inhale through the expiratory limb. The flow test can also be performed by using the ventilator and a breathing bag attached to the Y-piece as described in the 1993 FDA Anesthesia Apparatus Checkout Recommendations (Appendix A, Steps 11 and 12).[14]

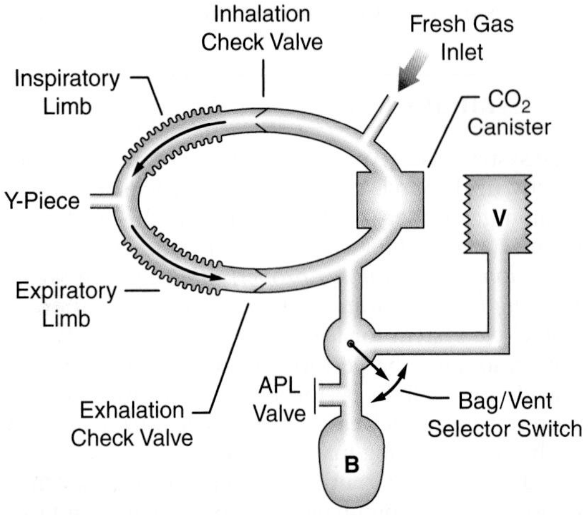

Workstation Self-Tests

As mentioned previously, many new anesthesia workstations now incorporate technology that allows the machine to either automatically or manually walk the user through a series of self-tests to check for functionality of electronic, mechanical, and pneumatic components. Tested components commonly include the gas supply system, flow control valves, the circle system, ventilator, and integrated vaporizers. The comprehensiveness of these self-diagnostic tests varies from one model and manufacturer to another. If these tests are to be employed, users must be sure to read and strictly follow all manufacturer recommendations. Although a thorough understanding of what the particular workstation's self-tests include is very helpful, this information is often difficult to obtain and may vary greatly between devices.

One particularly important point of caution with self-tests should be noted on systems with manifold-mounted vaporizers such as the Dräger Apollo, Dräger Fabius GS, and Narkomed 6000 series. A manifold-mounted vaporizer does not become a part of an anesthesia workstation's gas flow stream until its concentration control dial is turned to the on position. Therefore, to detect internal vaporizer leaks on this type of a system, the "leak test" portion of the self-diagnostic must be repeated separately with each individual vaporizer turned to the on position. If this precaution is not taken, large leaks that could potentially result in patient awareness, such those from a loose filler cap or cracked fill indicator, could go undetected.

FIGURE 26-7.   Components of the circle system. APL, adjustable pressure limiting; B, reservoir bag; V, ventilator. (Reproduced from Brockwell RC: Inhaled anesthetic delivery systems, Anesthesia, 6th editiion. Edited by Miller: Philadelphia, Churchill Livingstone, 2004, p. 295, with permission.)

ANESTHESIA WORKSTATION PNEUMATICS

Anatomy of an Anesthesia Workstation

A simplified diagram of a generic two-gas anesthesia machine is shown in Figure 26-3. The pressures within the anesthesia workstation can be divided into three circuits: a high-pressure, an intermediate-pressure, and a low-pressure circuit. The *high-pressure circuit* is confined to the cylinders and the cylinder primary pressure regulators. For oxygen, the pressure range of the high-pressure circuit extends from a high of 2,200 pounds per square inch gauge (psig) to 45 psig, which is the regulated cylinder pressure. For nitrous oxide in the high-pressure circuit, pressures range from a high of 750 psig in the cylinder to a low of 45 psig. The *intermediate-pressure circuit* begins at the regulated cylinder supply sources at a pressure of 45 psig and it includes the pipeline sources at 50 to 55 psig and extends to the flow control valves. Depending on the manufacturer and specific machine design, second-stage pressure regulators may be used to decrease the pipeline supply pressures to the flow control valves to even lower pressures such as 14 psig or 26 psig within the intermediate pressure circuit.[28,29] Finally, the *low-pressure circuit* extends from the flow control valves to the common gas outlet. Therefore, the low-pressure circuit includes the flow tubes, vaporizer manifold, vaporizers, and the one-way check valve on most GE Healthcare/Datex-Ohmeda machines.[29]

Both oxygen and nitrous oxide have two supply sources. These consist of a pipeline supply source and a cylinder supply source. The pipeline supply source is the primary gas source for the anesthesia machine. The hospital pipeline supply system provides gases to the machine at approximately 50 psig, which is the normal working pressure of most machines. The cylinder supply source serves as a backup if the pipeline supply fails, or acts as the primary supply if the anesthesia workstation is being used in a location without the availability of pipeline-supplied gases. As previously described, the oxygen cylinder source is regulated from 2,200 to approximately 45 psig, and the nitrous oxide cylinder source is regulated from 745 to approximately 45 psig.[28–30]

A safety device traditionally referred to as the *failsafe* valve (and currently more appropriately termed the *oxygen failure cutoff valve*) is located downstream from the nitrous oxide supply source. It serves as an interface between the oxygen and nitrous oxide supply sources. This valve shuts off, or proportionally decreases, the supply of nitrous oxide (and other gases) if the oxygen supply pressure decreases. To meet ASTM standards, contemporary machines have an alarm device to monitor the oxygen supply pressure. A high-priority alarm is actuated as declining oxygen supply pressure reaches a predetermined threshold, such as 30 psig.[28–30]

Many GE Healthcare/Datex-Ohmeda machines have a second-stage oxygen regulator located downstream from the oxygen supply source in the intermediate pressure circuit. It is adjusted to a precise pressure level, such as 14 psig.[28] This regulator supplies a constant pressure to the oxygen flow control valve regardless of fluctuating oxygen pipeline pressures. For example, the flow from the oxygen flow control valve will be constant if the oxygen supply pressure is >14 psig.

The flow control valves represent an important anatomic landmark within the anesthesia workstation because they separate the intermediate-pressure circuit from the low-pressure circuit. The low-pressure circuit is that part of the machine that lies downstream from the flow control valves. The operator regulates flow entering the low-pressure circuit by adjusting the flow control valves. The oxygen and nitrous oxide flow control valves are linked mechanically or pneumatically by a proportioning system to help prevent inadvertent delivery of a hypoxic mixture. After leaving the flow tubes, the mixture of gases travels through a common manifold and may be directed to a calibrated vaporizer. Precise amounts of inhaled anesthetic can be added, depending on vaporizer control dial setting. The total fresh gas flow plus the anesthetic vapor then travel toward the common gas outlet.[28,29]

Many Datex-Ohmeda anesthesia machines have a one-way check valve located between the vaporizers and the common gas outlet in the mixed-gas pipeline. Its purpose is to prevent back flow into the vaporizer during positive pressure ventilation, therefore minimizing the effects of downstream intermittent pressure fluctuations on inhaled anesthetic concentration (see "Vaporizers: Intermittent Back Pressure"). The presence or absence of this check valve *profoundly* influences which preoperative leak test is indicated (see "Checkout of the Anesthesia Workstation"). The oxygen flush connection joins the mixed-gas pipeline between the one-way check valve (when present) and the machine outlet. Thus, when oxygen flush valve is activated the pipeline oxygen pressure has a "straight shot" to the common gas outlet in machines that do not use fresh gas decoupling technology.[28,29]

Pipeline Supply Source

Under normal conditions, the pipeline supply serves as the primary gas source for the anesthesia machine. Most hospitals today have a central piping system to deliver medical gases such as oxygen, nitrous oxide, and air to the operating room. The central piping system must supply the correct gases at the appropriate pressure for the anesthesia workstation to function properly. Unfortunately, this does not always occur. Even as recently as 2002, large medical centers with huge cryogenic bulk oxygen storage systems are not immune to component failures that may contribute to critical oxygen pipeline supply failures.[31] In the 2002 case, a faulty joint ruptured at the bottom of the primary cryogenic oxygen storage tank, releasing 8,000 gallons of liquid oxygen to flood the streets in the surrounding area. This mishap suddenly compromised the oxygen delivery to a major medical center.

In a survey of approximately 200 hospitals in 1976, 31% reported difficulties with pipeline systems.[32] The most common problem was inadequate oxygen pressure, followed by excessive pipeline pressures. The most devastating reported hazard, however, was accidental crossing of oxygen and nitrous oxide pipelines, which has led to many deaths. This problem caused 23 deaths in a newly constructed wing of a general hospital in Sudbury, Ontario, during a 5-month period.[32,33] More recently, in 2002, two additional hypoxic deaths were reported in New Haven, Connecticut. These resulted from a medical gas system failure in which an altered oxygen flowmeter was inadvertently connected to a wall supply source for nitrous oxide.[34]

In the event that a pipeline crossover is suspected, the workstation user must immediately make *two* corrective actions. First, the backup oxygen cylinder should be turned on. Then the pipeline supply must be disconnected. This second step is mandatory because the machine will preferentially use the (potentially) inappropriate 50 psig pipeline supply source instead of the lower-pressure (45 psig) oxygen cylinder source if the wall supply is not disconnected.

Gas enters the anesthesia machine through the pipeline inlet connections (Fig. 26-3, arrows). The pipeline inlet fittings are gas-specific Diameter Index Safety System threaded body fittings. The Diameter Index Safety System provides threaded, noninterchangeable connections for medical gas lines, which minimize the risk of misconnection. A check valve is located downstream from the inlet. It prevents reverse flow of gases from the machine to the pipeline or the atmosphere.

Cylinder Supply Source

Anesthesia workstations have E-cylinders for use when a pipeline supply source is not available or if the pipeline system fails. Anesthesia providers can easily become complacent and falsely assume that backup gas cylinders are in fact present on the back of the anesthesia workstation, and further, if they are present, that they contain an adequate supply of compressed gas. The pre-use checklist should contain steps that confirm both.

Medical gases supplied in E-cylinders are attached to the anesthesia machine via the hanger yoke assembly. The hanger yoke assembly orients and supports the cylinder, provides a gas-tight seal, and ensures a unidirectional flow of gases into the machine.[29] Each hanger yoke is equipped with the Pin Index Safety System. This system is a safeguard introduced to eliminate cylinder interchanging and the possibility of accidentally placing the incorrect gas on a yoke designed to accommodate another gas. Two metal pins on the yoke assembly are arranged so that that they project into corresponding holes on the cylinder valve. Each gas or combination of gases has a specific and unique pin arrangement.[35]

Once the cylinders are turned on, compressed gases may pass from their respective high-pressure cylinder sources into the anesthesia machine (Fig. 26-3). A check valve is located downstream from each cylinder if a double-yoke assembly is used. This check valve serves several functions. First, it minimizes gas transfer from a cylinder at high pressure to one with lower pressure. Second, it allows an empty cylinder to be exchanged for a full one while gas flow continues from the other cylinder into the machine with minimal loss of gas or supply pressure. Third, it minimizes leakage from an open cylinder to the atmosphere if one cylinder is absent.[28,29] A cylinder supply pressure gauge is located downstream from the check valves. The gauge will indicate the pressure in the cylinder having the higher pressure when two reserve cylinders of the same gas are opened at the same time.

Each cylinder supply source has a pressure-reducing valve known as the *cylinder pressure regulator*. It reduces the high and variable storage pressure present in a cylinder to a lower, more constant pressure suitable for use in the anesthesia machine. The oxygen cylinder pressure regulator reduces the oxygen cylinder pressure from a high of 2,200 psig to approximately 45 psig. The nitrous oxide cylinder pressure regulator receives pressure of up to 745 psig and reduces it to approximately 45 psig.[28,29]

The gas supply cylinder valves should be turned off when not in use, except during the preoperative machine checking period. If the cylinder supply valves are left on, the reserve cylinder supply can be silently depleted whenever the pressure inside the machine decreases to a value lower than the regulated cylinder pressure. For example, oxygen pressure within the machine can decrease below 45 psig with oxygen flushing or possibly even during the use of a pneumatically driven ventilator, particularly at high inspiratory flow rates. Additionally, the pipeline supply pressures of all gases can fall to <45 psig if problems exist in the central piping system. If the cylinders are left on when this occurs, they will eventually become depleted and no reserve supply may be available if a complete central pipeline failure occurred.[27,28]

The amount of time that an anesthesia machine can operate from the E-cylinder supply is important knowledge, and is particularly important now that anesthesia is being provided more frequently in office-based and in remote (outside the operating room) hospital settings. For oxygen, the volume of gas remaining in the cylinder is proportional to the cylinder pressure. One author has proposed the following equation to help estimate the remaining time.[36]

$$\text{Approx. remaining time (Hr)} \approx \frac{\text{Oxygen cylinder pressure (psig)}}{200 \times \text{oxygen flow rate (L/min)}}$$

It should be noted that this calculation will provide only a gross estimate of remaining time and may not be exact. Furthermore, users should be cautioned that use of a pneumatically driven mechanical ventilator will dramatically increase oxygen utilization rates and decrease the remaining time until cylinder depletion. Hand ventilating with low fresh gas flow rates may consume <5% the amount of oxygen, as compared with intermediate flowmeter settings coupled with the use of pneumatically powered mechanical ventilation.[31] Because piston-type anesthesia ventilators such as found in the Dräger Medical Fabius GS and Narkomed 6000 series do not affect oxygen consumption rates, they may be preferable to conventional gas-driven ventilators in practice settings that depend on the use of compressed gas cylinders as the primary gas sources.

Oxygen Supply Pressure Failure Safety Devices

Oxygen and nitrous oxide supply sources existed as independent entities in older models of anesthesia machines, and they were not pneumatically or mechanically interfaced. Therefore, abrupt or insidious oxygen pressure failure had the potential to lead to the delivery of a hypoxic mixture. The 2000 ASTM F1850-00 standard states that, "The anesthesia gas supply device shall be designed so that whenever oxygen supply pressure is reduced to below the manufacturer specified minimum, the delivered oxygen concentration shall not decrease below 19% at the common gas outlet."[37] Contemporary anesthesia machines have a number of safety devices that act together in a cascade manner to minimize the risk of delivery of a hypoxic gas mixture as oxygen pressure decreases. Several of these devices are described in the following sections.

Pneumatic and Electronic Alarm Devices

Many older anesthesia machines have a pneumatic alarm device that sounds a warning when the oxygen supply pressure decreases to a predetermined threshold value such as 30 psig. The 2000 ASTM F1850-00 standard mandated that a medium priority alarm be activated within 5 seconds when the oxygen pressure decreases below a manufacturer-specific pressure threshold.[37] Electronic alarm devices are now used to meet this guideline.

Oxygen Failure Cut Off (Failsafe) Valves

7 An oxygen failure cutoff valve is present in the gas line supplying each of the flowmeters except oxygen. Controlled by oxygen supply pressure, the valve shuts off (or proportionally decreases) the supply pressure of all other gases (e.g., nitrous oxide, air, CO_2, helium, nitrogen) as the oxygen supply pressure decreases. Unfortunately, the misnomer "failsafe" has led to the misconception that the valve prevents administration of a hypoxic mixture. Machines that are either not equipped with a flow-proportioning system (see "Proportioning Systems") or ones whose system may be disabled by the user can deliver a hypoxic mixture under normal working conditions. On such a system, the oxygen flow control valve can be closed intentionally or accidentally. Normal oxygen pressure will keep other gas lines open so that a hypoxic mixture can result.[28,29]

Many Datex-Ohmeda machines are equipped with a failsafe valve known as the *pressure-sensor shutoff valve* (Fig. 26-8). This valve operates in a threshold manner and is either open or

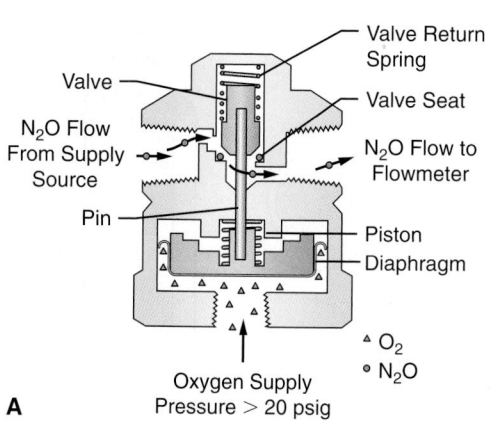

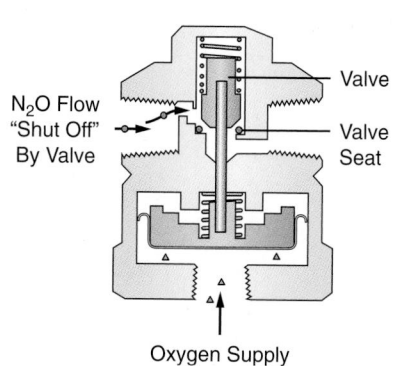

FIGURE 26-8. Pressure-sensor shutoff valve. The valve is open in **A** because the oxygen supply pressure is greater than the threshold value of 20 psig. The valve is closed in **B** because of inadequate oxygen pressure. (Redrawn from Bowie E, Huffman LM: The Anesthesia Machine: Essentials for Understanding. Madison, WI, Ohmeda, a Division of BOC Health Care, Inc, 1985, with permission.)

closed. Oxygen supply pressure opens the valve, and the valve return spring closes the valve. Figure 26-8 shows a nitrous oxide pressure-sensor shutoff valve with a threshold pressure of 20 psig. In Figure 26-8A, an oxygen supply pressure >20 psig is exerted on the mobile diaphragm. This pressure moves the piston and pin upward and the valve opens. Nitrous oxide flows freely to the nitrous oxide flow control valve. In Figure 26-8B, the oxygen supply pressure is <20 psig, and the force of the valve return spring completely closes the valve.[28] Nitrous oxide flow stops at the closed failsafe valve and it does not advance to the nitrous oxide flow control valve.

Dräger uses a different failsafe valve known as the *Oxygen Failure Protection Device* (OFPD) to interface the oxygen pressure with that of other gases, such as nitrous oxide or other inert gases. This is in contrast to Datex-Ohmeda's oxygen pressure-sensor shutoff valve because the OFPD is based on a proportioning principle rather than a threshold principle. The pressure of all gases controlled by the OFPD will decrease proportionally with the oxygen pressure. The OFPD consists of a seat-nozzle assembly connected to a spring-loaded piston (Fig. 26-9). The oxygen supply pressure in the left panel of Figure 26-9 is 50 psig. This pressure pushes the piston upward, forcing the nozzle away from the valve seat. Nitrous oxide and/or other gases advance toward the flow control valve at 50 psig. The oxygen pressure in the right panel is zero psig. The spring is expanded and forces the nozzle against the seat, preventing flow through the device. Finally, the center panel shows an intermediate oxygen pressure of 25 psig. The force of the spring partially closes the valve. The nitrous oxide pressure delivered to the flow control valve is 25 psig. There is a continuum of intermediate con-

figurations between the extremes (0 to 50 psig) of oxygen supply pressure. These intermediate valve configurations are responsible for the proportional nature of the OFPD. An important concept to be understood with these particular failsafe devices is that the Datex-Ohmeda Pressure Sensor Shutoff Valve is threshold in nature (all-or-nothing), whereas the Dräger OFPD is a variable, flow-type proportioning system.

Second-Stage Oxygen Pressure Regulator

Most contemporary Datex-Ohmeda workstations have a second-stage oxygen pressure regulator set at a specific value, ranging from 12 to 19 psig. Output from the oxygen flowmeter is constant when the oxygen supply pressure exceeds the threshold (minimal) value. The pressure-sensor shutoff valve of Datex-Ohmeda is set at a higher threshold value (20 to 30 psig) to ensure that oxygen is the last gas flowing if oxygen pressure failure occurs.

Flowmeter Assemblies

The flowmeter assembly (Fig. 26-10) precisely controls and measures gas flow to the common gas outlet. With traditional glass flowmeter assemblies, the flow control valve regulates the amount of flow that enters a tapered, transparent flow tube known as a *Thorpe tube*. A mobile indicator float inside the flow tube indicates the amount of flow passing through the associated flow control valve. The quantity of flow is indicated on a scale associated with the flow tube.[28,29] Some newer anesthesia

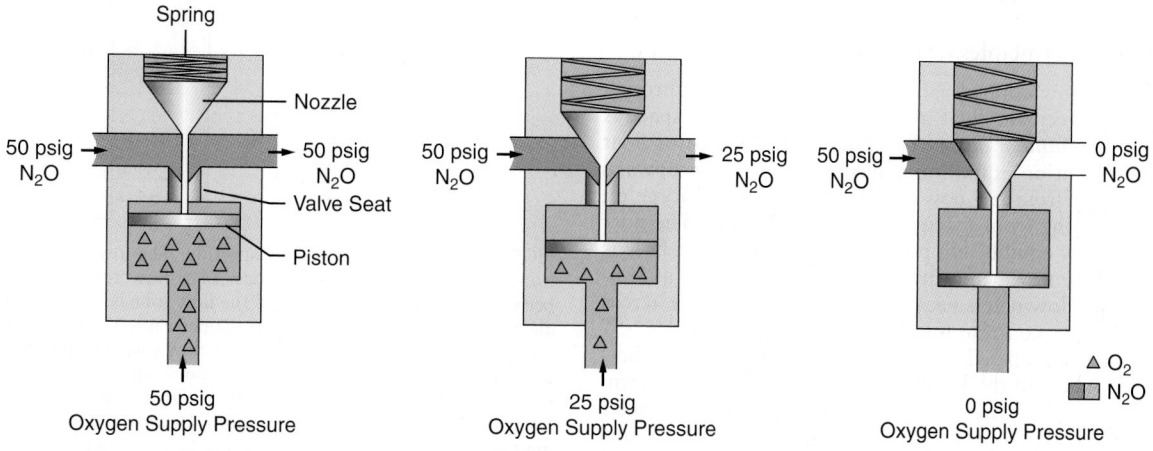

FIGURE 26-9. Oxygen failure protection device/sensitive oxygen ratio controller (OFPD/S-ORC), which responds proportionally to changes in oxygen supply pressure. (Redrawn from Narkomed 2A Anesthesia System: Technical Service Manual, 6th ed. Telford, PA, North American Dräger, June 1985, with permission.)

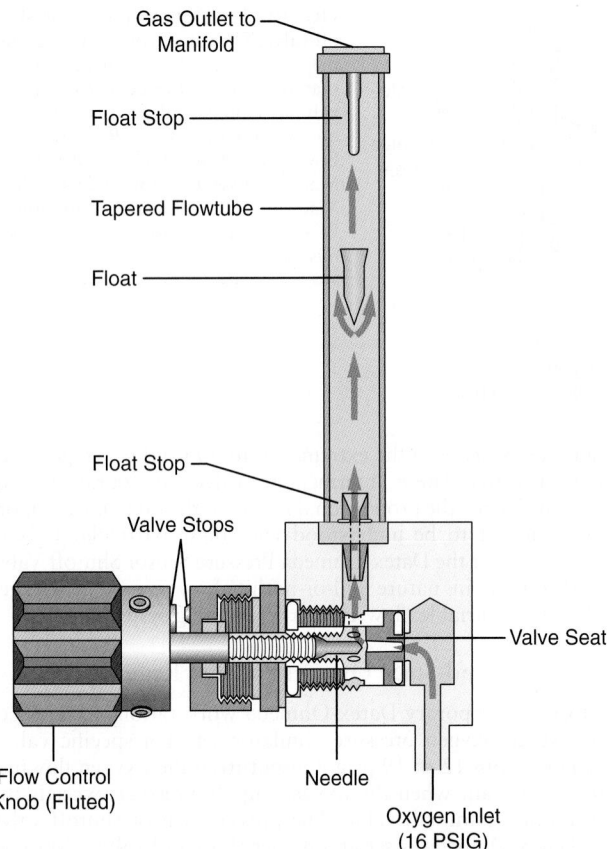

FIGURE 26-10.   Oxygen flowmeter assembly. The oxygen flowmeter assembly is composed of the flow control valve assembly plus the flowmeter subassembly. (Reproduced from Bowie E, Huffman LM: The Anesthesia Machine: Essentials for Understanding. Madison, WI, Ohmeda, a Division of BOC Health Care, Inc, 1985, with permission.)

workstations have now replaced the conventional glass flow tubes with electronic flow sensors that measure the flows of the individual gases. These flow rate data are then presented in either numerical format, graphical format, or a combination of the two. The integration of these "electronic flowmeters" is an essential step in the evolution of the anesthesia workstation if it is to become fully integrated with anesthesia data-capturing systems such as computerized anesthesia record keepers.

Operating Principles of Conventional Flowmeters

Opening the flow control valve allows gas to travel through the space between the float and the flow tube. This space is known as the *annular space* (Fig. 26-11). The indicator float hovers freely in an equilibrium position where the upward force resulting from gas flow equals the downward force on the float resulting from gravity at a given flow rate. The float moves to a new equilibrium position in the tube when flow is changed. These flowmeters are commonly referred to as *constant pressure* flowmeters because the pressure decrease across the float remains constant for all positions in the tube.[29,38,39]

Flow tubes are tapered, with the smallest diameter at the bottom of the tube and the largest diameter at the top. The term *variable orifice* designates this type of unit because the annular space between the float and the inner wall of the flow tube varies with the position of the float. Flow through the constriction created by the float can be laminar or turbulent, depending on the flow rate (Fig. 26-12). The characteristics of a gas that influence its flow rate through a given constriction are viscosity

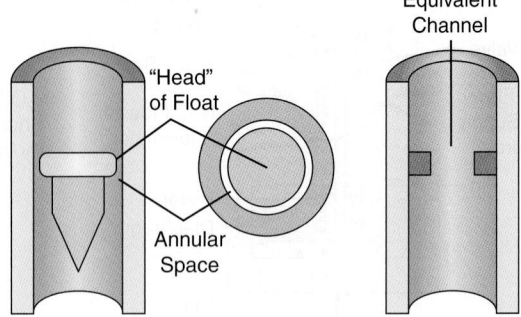

FIGURE 26-11.   The annular space. The clearance between the head of the float and the flow tube is known as the annular space. It can be considered an equivalent to a circular channel of the same cross-sectional area. (Redrawn from Macintosh R, Mushin WW, Epstein HG: Physics for the Anaesthetist, 3rd edition. Oxford, England, Blackwell Scientific Publications, 1963, with permission.)

(laminar flow) and density (turbulent flow). Because the annular space is tubular, at low flow rates laminar flow is present and *viscosity* determines the gas flow rate. The annular space simulates an orifice at high flow rates, and turbulent gas flow then depends predominantly on the *density* of the gas.[28,29]

Components of the Flowmeter Assembly

Flow Control Valve Assembly.   The flow control valve assembly is composed of a flow control knob, a needle valve, a valve seat, and a pair of valve stops (Fig. 26-10).[28] The assembly can receive its pneumatic input either directly from the pipeline source (50 psig) or from a second-stage pressure regulator. The location of the needle valve in the valve seat changes to establish different orifices when the flow control valve is adjusted.

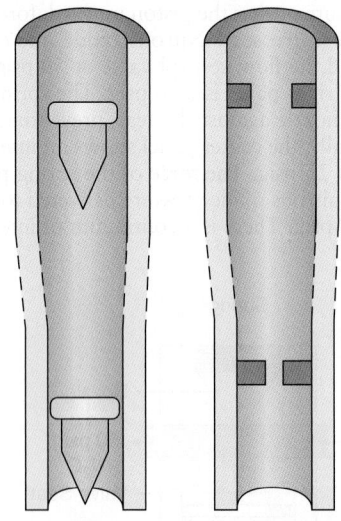

FIGURE 26-12.   Flow tube constriction. The lower pair of illustrations represents the lower portion of a flow tube. The clearance between the head of the float and the flow tube is narrow. The equivalent channel is tubular because its diameter is less than its length. Viscosity is dominant in determining gas flow rate through this tubular constriction. The upper pair of illustrations represents the upper portion of a flow tube. The equivalent channel is orificial (orificelike) because its length is less than its width. Density is dominant in determining gas flow rate through this orificial constriction. (Redrawn from Macintosh R, Mushin WW, Epstein HG: Physics for the Anaesthetist, 3rd edition. Oxford, England, Blackwell Scientific Publications, 1963, with permission.)

Gas flow increases when the flow control valve is turned counterclockwise, and it decreases when the valve is turned clockwise. Extreme clockwise rotation may result in damage to the needle valve and valve seat. Therefore, flow control valves are equipped with valve "stops" to prevent this occurrence.[29]

Safety Features.   Contemporary flow control valve assemblies have numerous safety features. The oxygen flow control knob is physically distinguishable from other gas knobs. It is distinctively fluted, projects beyond the control knobs of the other gases, and is larger in diameter than the flow control knobs of other gases. All knobs are color-coded for the appropriate gas, and the chemical formula or name of the gas is permanently marked on each. Flow control knobs are recessed or protected with a shield or barrier to minimize inadvertent change from a preset position. If a single gas has two flow tubes, the tubes are arranged in series and are controlled by a single flow control valve.[37]

In many of the new anesthesia workstations, the flowmeters have been replaced by electronic control panels that contain "soft keys." In order to adjust any gas flow, the operator must perform following steps: (1) select and press the soft key to identify the anesthetic agent selected, (2) turn the selector knob to adjust the desired flow level, and (3) press the selector knob again to confirm the selected flow level and anesthetic agent (see "Electronic Flowmeters").

Flowmeter Subassembly.   The flowmeter subassembly consists of the flow tube, the indicator float with float stops, and the indicator scale (Fig. 26-10).[29]

Flow Tubes.   Contemporary flow tubes are made of glass. Most have a single taper in which the inner diameter of the flow tube increases uniformly from bottom to top. Manufacturers provide double flow tubes for oxygen and nitrous oxide to provide better visual discrimination at low flow rates. A fine flow tube indicates flow from approximately 200 mL/min to 1 L/min, and a coarse flow tube indicates flow from approximately 1 L/min to 10 to 12 L/min. The two tubes are connected in series and supplied by a single flow control valve. The total gas flow is that shown on the higher flowmeter.

Indicator Floats and Float Stops.   Contemporary anesthesia machines use several different types of bobbins or floats, including plumb-bob floats, rotating skirted floats, and ball floats. Flow is read at the top of plumb-bob and skirted floats and at the center of the ball on the ball-type floats.[29] Flow tubes are equipped with float stops at the top and bottom of the tube. The upper stop prevents the float from ascending to the top of the tube and plugging the outlet. It also ensures that the float will be visible at maximum flows instead of being hidden in the manifold. The bottom float stop provides a central foundation for the indicator when the flow control valve is turned off.[28,29]

Scale.   The flowmeter scale can be marked directly on the flow tube or located to the right of the tube.[37] Gradations corresponding to equal increments in flow rate are closer together at the top of the scale because the annular space increases more rapidly than does the internal diameter from bottom to top of the tube. Rib guides are used in some flow tubes with ball-type indicators to minimize this compression effect. They are tapered glass ridges that run the length of the tube. There are usually three rib guides that are equally spaced around the inner circumference of the tube. In the presence of rib guides, the annular space from the bottom to the top of the tube increases almost proportionally with the internal diameter. This results in a nearly linear scale[29] Rib guides are employed on many Dräger Medical flow tubes.

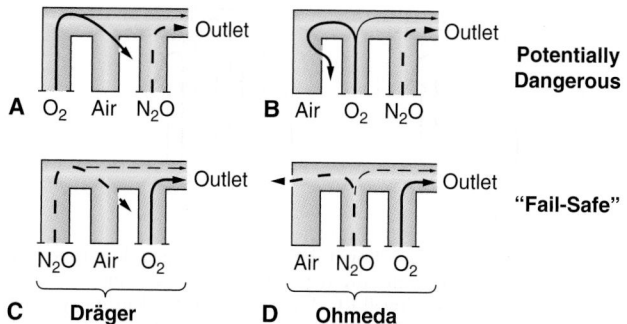

FIGURE 26-13.   Flowmeter sequence—a potential cause of hypoxia. In the event of a flowmeter leak, a potentially dangerous arrangement exists when nitrous oxide is located in the downstream position (*A* and *B*). The safest configuration exists when oxygen is located in the downstream position (*C* and *D*). See text for details. (Modified from Eger EI II, Hylton RR, Irwin RH, et al: Anesthetic flowmeter sequence—a cause for hypoxia. Anesthesiology 1963; 24: 396, with permission.)

Safety Features.   The flowmeter subassemblies for each gas on the Datex-Ohmeda Modulus I, Modulus II, Modulus II Plus, CD, and Aestiva are housed in independent, color-coded, pin-specific modules. The flow tubes are adjacent to a gas-specific, color-coded backing. The flow scale and the chemical formula (or name of the gas) are permanently etched on the backing to the right of the flow tube. Flowmeter scales are individually hand-calibrated using the specific float to provide a high degree of accuracy. The tube, float, and scale make an inseparable unit. The entire set must be replaced if any component is damaged.

Dräger Medical does not use a modular system for the flowmeter subassembly. The flow scale, the chemical symbol, and the gas-specific color codes are etched directly onto the flow tube. The scale in use is obvious when two flow tubes for the same gas are used.

Problems with Flowmeters

Leaks.   Flowmeter leaks are a substantial hazard because the flowmeters are located downstream from all machine safety devices except the oxygen analyzer.[40] Leaks can occur at the O-ring junctions between the glass flow tubes and the metal manifold or in cracked or broken glass flow tubes, the most fragile pneumatic component of the anesthesia machine. Even though gross damage to conventional glass flow tubes is usually apparent, subtle cracks and chips may be overlooked, resulting in errors of delivered flows.[41] The use of electronic flowmeters and the removal of conventional glass flow tubes from some newer anesthesia workstations (Datex-Ohmeda S/5 ADU and the Dräger Medical Fabius) may help to eliminate these potential sources of leaks (see "Electronic Flowmeters").

Eger et al.[42] in 1963 demonstrated that, in the presence of a flowmeter leak, a hypoxic mixture is less likely to occur if the oxygen flowmeter is located downstream from all other flowmeters. Figure 26-13 is a more contemporary version of the figure in the original publication of Eger et al. The unused air flow tube has a large leak. Nitrous oxide and oxygen flow rates are set at a ratio of 3:1. A potentially dangerous arrangement is shown in Figure 26-13A and 26-13B because the nitrous oxide flowmeter is located in the downstream position. A hypoxic mixture can result because a substantial portion of oxygen flow passes through the leak, and all nitrous oxide is directed to the common gas outlet. A safer configuration is shown in Figure 26-13C and 26-13D. The oxygen flowmeter is located in the downstream position. A portion of the nitrous oxide flow escapes through the leak, and the remainder goes toward the common gas outlet. A hypoxic mixture is less likely because all the

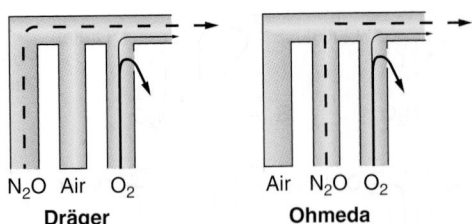

FIGURE 26-14. Oxygen flow tube leak. An oxygen flow tube leak can produce a hypoxic mixture regardless of flow tube arrangement. (Reproduced from Brockwell RC: Inhaled anesthetic delivery systems, Anesthesia, 6th edition. Edited by Miller RD. Philadelphia, Churchill Livingstone, 2004, p. 281, with permission.)

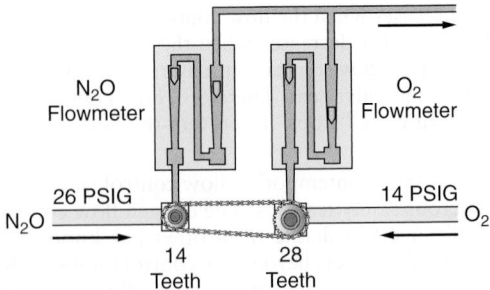

FIGURE 26-15. Ohmeda Link-25 proportion limiting control system. See text for details.

oxygen flow is advanced by the nitrous oxide.[42] North American Dräger flowmeters are arranged as in Figure 26-13C, and Datex-Ohmeda flowmeters are arranged as in Figure 26-13D.

A leak in the oxygen flow tube may result in creation of a hypoxic mixture even when oxygen is located in the downstream position (Fig. 26-14).[40,41] Oxygen escapes through the leak and nitrous oxide continues to flow toward the common outlet, particularly at high ratios of nitrous oxide to oxygen flow.

Inaccuracy. Flow measurement error can occur even when flowmeters are assembled properly with appropriate components. Dirt or static electricity can cause a float to stick, and the actual flow may be higher or lower than that indicated. Sticking of indicator float is more common in the low flow ranges because the annular space is smaller. A damaged float can cause inaccurate readings because the precise relationship between the float and the flow tube is altered. Back pressure from the breathing circuit can cause a float to drop so that it reads less than the actual flow. Finally, if flowmeters are not aligned properly in the vertical position (plumb), readings can be inaccurate because tilting distorts the annular space.[23,29,41]

Ambiguous Scale. Before the standardization of flowmeter scales and the widespread use of oxygen analyzers, at least two deaths resulted from confusion created by ambiguous scales.[23,41,43] The operator read the float position beside an adjacent but erroneous scale in both cases. Today this error is less likely to occur because contemporary flowmeter scales are marked either directly onto the flow tube or immediately to the right of it.[37] The possibility of confusion is minimized when the scale is etched directly onto the tube.

Electronic Flowmeters

As mentioned previously, some newer anesthesia workstations such as the Datex-Ohmeda S/5 ADU and the North American Dräger Fabius GS among others have conventional control knobs and flow control valves, but have electronic flow sensors and digital displays rather than glass flow tubes. The output from the flow control valve is represented graphically and/or numerically in liters per minute on the workstation's integrated user interface. These systems depend on electrical power to provide a precise display of gas flow. However, even when electrical power is totally interrupted, because the flow control valves themselves are not electronic, oxygen should continue to flow. Because these machines do not have individual flow tubes that physically quantify the flow of each gas, electronic flow sensors and often a small conventional pneumatic "fresh gas" or "total flow" indicators are provided that give the user an estimate of the total quantity of fresh gas flowing from all flow control valves. This miniature flow tube indicator serves to inform the user of the approximate quantity of gas that is leav-

ing the anesthesia workstation's common gas outlet, and is functional even in the event of a total power failure.

Proportioning Systems

Manufacturers equip anesthesia workstations with proportioning systems in an attempt to prevent creation and delivery of a hypoxic mixture. Nitrous oxide and oxygen are interfaced mechanically and/or pneumatically so that the minimum oxygen concentration at the common gas outlet is between 23 and 25% depending on manufacturer.

Datex-Ohmeda Link-25 Proportion Limiting Control System

Conventional Datex-Ohmeda machines use the Link-25 System. The heart of the system is the mechanical integration of the nitrous oxide and oxygen flow control valves. It allows independent adjustment of either valve, yet automatically intercedes to maintain a minimum 25% oxygen concentration with a maximum nitrous oxide–oxygen flow ratio of 3:1. The Link-25 automatically increases oxygen flow to prevent delivery of a hypoxic mixture.

Figure 26-15 illustrates the Datex-Ohmeda Link-25 System. The nitrous oxide and oxygen flow control valves are identical. A 14-tooth sprocket is attached to the nitrous oxide flow control valve and a 28-tooth sprocket is attached to the oxygen flow control valve. A chain physically links the sprockets. When the nitrous oxide flow control valve is turned through two revolutions, or 28 teeth, the oxygen flow control valve will revolve once because of the 2:1 gear ratio. The final 3:1 flow ratio results because the nitrous oxide flow control valve is supplied by approximately 26 psig, whereas the oxygen flow control valve is supplied by 14 psig. Thus, the combination of the mechanical and pneumatic aspects of the system yields the final oxygen concentration. The Datex-Ohmeda Link-25 proportioning system can be thought of as a system that *increases oxygen flow* when necessary to prevent delivery of a fresh gas mixture with oxygen concentration of less than 25%.

A few reports have described failures of the Datex-Ohmeda Link-25 system.[43–46] The authors of these reports describe failures that resulted in either inability to administer oxygen without nitrous oxide or that allowed creation of a hypoxic mixture.

North American Dräger Oxygen Ratio Monitor Controller/Sensitive Oxygen Ratio Controller System

North American Dräger's proportioning system, the Oxygen Ratio Monitor Controller (ORMC), is used on the North American Dräger Narkomed 2A, 2B, 3, and 4. An equivalent system is known as the Sensitive Oxygen Ratio Controller (S-ORC) on some newer Dräger anesthesia workstations such as the Dräger

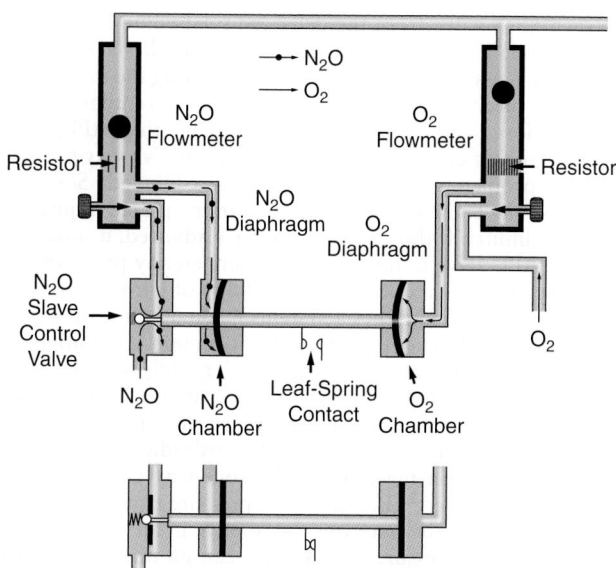

FIGURE 26-16. North American Dräger Oxygen Ratio Monitor Controller. See text for details. (Redrawn from Schreiber P: Safety Guidelines for Anesthesia Systems. Telford, PA, North American Dräger, 1984, with permission.)

Fabius GS and Narkomed 6000 series. The ORMC and the S-ORC are pneumatic oxygen–nitrous oxide interlock systems designed to maintain a fresh gas oxygen concentration of at least $25 \pm 3\%$. They control the fresh gas oxygen concentration to levels substantially higher than 25% at oxygen flow rates <1 L/min. The ORMC and S-ORC limit nitrous oxide flow to prevent delivery of a hypoxic mixture. This is unlike the Datex-Ohmeda Link-25, which actively increases oxygen flow.

A schematic of the ORMC is shown in Figure 26-16. It is composed of an oxygen chamber, a nitrous oxide chamber, and a nitrous oxide slave control valve. All are interconnected by a mobile horizontal shaft. The pneumatic input into the device is from the oxygen and the nitrous oxide flowmeters. These flowmeters are unique because they have specific resistors located downstream from the flow control valves. These resistors create back pressures directed to the oxygen and nitrous oxide chambers. The value of the oxygen flow tube resistor is 3 to 4 times that of the nitrous oxide flow tube resistor, and the relative value of these resistors determines the value of the controlled fresh gas oxygen concentration. The back pressure in the oxygen and nitrous oxide chambers pushes against rubber diaphragms attached to the mobile horizontal shaft. Movement of the shaft regulates the nitrous oxide slave control valve, which feeds the nitrous oxide flow control valve.

If the oxygen pressure is proportionally higher than the nitrous oxide pressure, the nitrous oxide slave control valve opens more widely, allowing more nitrous oxide to flow. As the nitrous oxide flow is increased manually, the nitrous oxide pressure forces the shaft toward the oxygen chamber. The valve opening becomes more restrictive and limits the nitrous oxide flow to the flowmeter.

Figure 26-16 illustrates the action of a single ORMC/S-ORC under different sets of circumstances. The back pressure exerted on the oxygen diaphragm, in the upper configuration, is greater than that exerted on the nitrous oxide diaphragm. This causes the horizontal shaft to move to the left, opening the nitrous oxide slave control valve. Nitrous oxide is then able to proceed to its flow control valve and out through the flowmeter. In the bottom configuration, the nitrous oxide slave control valve is closed because of inadequate oxygen back pressure.[30] To summarize, in contrast to the Datex-Ohmeda Link-25 system

that actively increases oxygen flow to maintain a fresh gas oxygen concentration >25%, the Dräger ORMC and S-ORC are systems that limit nitrous oxide flow to prevent delivery of a fresh gas mixture with an oxygen concentration of <25%.

Limitations

Proportioning systems are not foolproof. Workstations equipped with proportioning systems can still deliver a hypoxic mixture under certain conditions. Following is a description of some of the situations in which this may occur.

Wrong Supply Gas. Both the Datex-Ohmeda Link-25 and the Dräger ORMC/S-ORC will be fooled if a gas other than oxygen is present in the oxygen pipeline and will allow delivery of hypoxic gas mixtures. In the Link-25 System, the nitrous oxide and oxygen flow control valves will continue to be mechanically linked. Nevertheless, a hypoxic mixture can proceed to the common gas outlet. In the case of the Dräger ORMC or S-ORC, the rubber diaphragm for oxygen will reflect adequate supply pressure on the oxygen side even though the incorrect gas is present, and flow of both the wrong gas plus nitrous oxide will result. The oxygen analyzer is the only workstation monitor besides an integrated multigas analyzer that would detect this condition in either system.

Defective Pneumatics or Mechanics. Normal operation of the Datex-Ohmeda Link-25 and the North American Dräger ORMC/S-ORC is contingent on pneumatic and mechanical integrity.[47] Pneumatic integrity in the Datex-Ohmeda System requires properly functioning second-stage regulators. A nitrous oxide–oxygen ratio other than 3:1 will result if the regulators are not precise. The chain connecting the two sprockets must be intact; if the chain is cut or broken, a 97% nitrous oxide concentration can occur.[48] In the North American Dräger System, a functional OFPD is necessary to supply appropriate pressure to the ORMC. The mechanical aspects of the ORMC/S-ORC, such as the rubber diaphragms, the flow tube resistors, and the nitrous oxide slave control valve, must likewise be intact.

Downstream Leaks. The ORMC/S-ORC and the Link-25 function at the level of the flow control valves. A leak downstream from these devices, such as a broken oxygen flow tube (Fig. 26-14), can result in delivery of a hypoxic mixture to the common gas outlet. In this situation, oxygen escapes through the leak and the predominant gas delivered is nitrous oxide. The oxygen monitor and/or integrated multigas analyzer are the only machine safety devices that can detect this problem.[40] For the majority of its products, Dräger Medical recommends a preoperative positive pressure leak test to detect such a leak. However, in addition to this test, for many North American Dräger products, application of the negative-pressure leak test as well may provide a more sensitive way to detect such a leak. Datex-Ohmeda almost universally recommends a preoperative negative-pressure leak test for its workstations because of the frequently present check valve located at the common gas outlet (see "Checkout of the Anesthesia Workstation").

Inert Gas Administration. Administration of a third inert gas, such as helium, nitrogen, or CO_2, can cause a hypoxic mixture because contemporary proportioning systems link only nitrous oxide and oxygen.[49] Use of an oxygen analyzer is mandatory (or preferentially a multigas analyzer, when available) if the operator uses a third gas.

Dilution of Inspired Oxygen Concentration by Volatile Inhaled Anesthetics. Volatile inhaled anesthetics, like inert gases, are added to the mixed gases downstream from both the flowmeters and the proportioning system. Concentrations of less-potent inhaled anesthetics such as desflurane may account for a larger percentage of the total fresh gas composition than more potent agents. By examining the maximum vaporizer dial settings of the various volatile agents, one can assess the risk of this phenomenon (e.g., desflurane maximum dial setting 18% vs. isoflurane maximum dial setting of 5%). Because significant percentages of these inhaled anesthetics may be added downstream of the proportioning system, the resulting gas/vapor mixture may contain an inspired oxygen concentration that is <21% oxygen despite a functional proportioning system. The anesthesia provider must be aware of this possibility, particularly when high concentrations of less potent volatile inhaled anesthetics are used.

Oxygen Flush Valve

The oxygen flush valve allows direct communication between the oxygen high-pressure circuit and the low-pressure circuit (Fig. 26-3). Flow from the oxygen flush valve enters the low-pressure circuit downstream from the vaporizers and, most importantly, downstream from the Datex-Ohmeda machine outlet check valve. The spring-loaded oxygen flush valve stays closed until the operator opens it by depressing the oxygen flush button. Actuation of the valve delivers 100% oxygen at 35 to 75 L/min to the breathing circuit.[28]

The oxygen flush valve can provide a high-pressure oxygen source suitable for jet ventilation under the following circumstances: (1) the anesthesia machine is equipped with a one-way check valve positioned between the vaporizers and the oxygen flush valve, and (2) when a positive pressure relief valve exists downstream of the vaporizers, this pressure relief valve must be upstream of the outlet check valve. Because the Ohmeda Modulus II has such a one-way check valve and its positive pressure relief valve is upstream from the check valve, the entire oxygen flow of 35 to 75 L/min is delivered to the common gas outlet at a high pressure of 50 psig. On the other hand, the Ohmeda Modulus II Plus and some Ohmeda Excel machines are not capable of functioning as an appropriate oxygen source for jet ventilation. The Ohmeda Modulus II plus, which does not have the check valve, provides only 7 psig at the common gas outlet because some oxygen flow travels retrograde through an internal relief valve located upstream from the oxygen flush valve. The Ohmeda Excel 210, which does have a one-way check valve, also has a positive pressure relief valve downstream from the check valve and therefore is unsuitable for jet ventilation. Older North American Dräger machines such as the Narkomed 2A (which also does not have the outlet check valve) provide an intermediate pressure of 18 psig to the common gas outlet because some pressure is vented retrograde through a pressure relief valve located in the vaporizers.[50]

Several hazards have been reported with the oxygen flush valve. A defective or damaged valve can stick in the fully open position, resulting in barotrauma.[51] A valve sticking in a partially open position can result in patient awareness during general anesthesia because the oxygen flow from the incompetent valve dilutes the inhaled anesthetic.[26] Improper use of normally functioning oxygen flush valves also can result in problems. Overzealous intraoperative oxygen flushing can dilute inhaled anesthetics. Oxygen flushing during the inspiratory phase of positive pressure ventilation can produce barotrauma in patients if the anesthesia machine does not incorporate fresh gas decoupling or an appropriately adjusted inspiratory pressure limiter. Anesthesia systems (Dräger Narkomed 6000 series, Julian, Fabius GS and Datascope Anestar) with fresh gas decoupling are inherently safer from the standpoint of minimizing the chance of producing barotrauma from inappropriate oxygen flush valve use. These systems physically separate the fresh gas inflow from either the flowmeters or the

oxygen flush valve from the delivered tidal volume presented to the patient's lungs. With traditional anesthesia breathing circuits, excess volume cannot be vented during the inspiratory phase of mechanical ventilation because the ventilator relief valve is closed and the adjustable pressure limiting (APL) valve is either out-of-circuit or closed.[52] An alternative way to manage this problem can be seen on the Datex-Ohmeda S/5 ADU and Aestiva. These circle systems use an integrated adjustable pressure limiter. If this device is properly adjusted, it functions like the APL valve to limit the maximum airway pressure to a safe level, thereby reducing the possibility of barotrauma.

Some very old anesthesia systems made use of a freestanding vaporizer downstream from the common gas outlet; on these systems, oxygen flushing could rapidly deliver large quantities of inhaled anesthetic to the patient. Finally, inappropriate preoperative use of the oxygen flush to evaluate the low-pressure circuit for leaks can be misleading, particularly on Datex-Ohmeda machines with a one-way check valve at the common outlet.[25] Because back pressure from the breathing circuit closes the one-way check valve in an airtight manner, major low-pressure circuit leaks can go undetected with this leak test (see "Checkout of the Anesthesia Workstation").

WEB-BASED ANESTHESIA SOFTWARE SIMULATION, THE VIRTUAL ANESTHESIA MACHINE

The growth of Internet Web-based application technology as well as trends to incorporate simulation into anesthesia training and education has generated development of online simulation anesthesia simulation resources. The Virtual Anesthesia Machine (VAM) is a Web-based anesthesia simulation environment that provides information on the function of anesthesia machines along with tutorials and operational scenarios, including failure modes of new and traditional anesthesia workstations (Fig. 26-17).[53] It is available for use free of charge. The VAM allows the user to modify most of the controls found on a modern anesthesia workstation, such as gas flows and ventilator settings. The authors of the VAM, in collaboration with the Anesthesia Patient Safety Foundation (APSF), have created The Anesthesia Patient Safety Foundation Anesthesia Machine Workbook. The workbook provides additional information and tutorials covering six anesthesia machine subsystems: the high-pressure system, the low-pressure system, the breathing circuit, manual ventilation, mechanical ventilation, and the scavenging system.[54]

VAPORIZERS

As dramatically as the evolution of the anesthesia workstation has been in recent years, vaporizers have also changed from rudimentary ether inhalers and copper kettles to the present temperature-compensated, computer-controlled, and flow-sensing devices we use today. In 1993, with the introduction of desflurane to the clinical setting, an even more sophisticated vaporizer was introduced to handle the unique physical properties of this agent. Now, a new generation of anesthesia vaporizers blending both "old" copper kettlelike technology and "new" computerized control technology has emerged in the Datex-Ohmeda Aladin Cassette vaporizer system. Before the discussion of variable bypass vaporizers, the Datex-Ohmeda Tec 6 desflurane vaporizer, and the Datex-Ohmeda Aladin Cassette vaporizer, certain physical principles will be reviewed briefly to facilitate understanding of the operating principles, construction, and design of contemporary volatile anesthetic vaporizers.

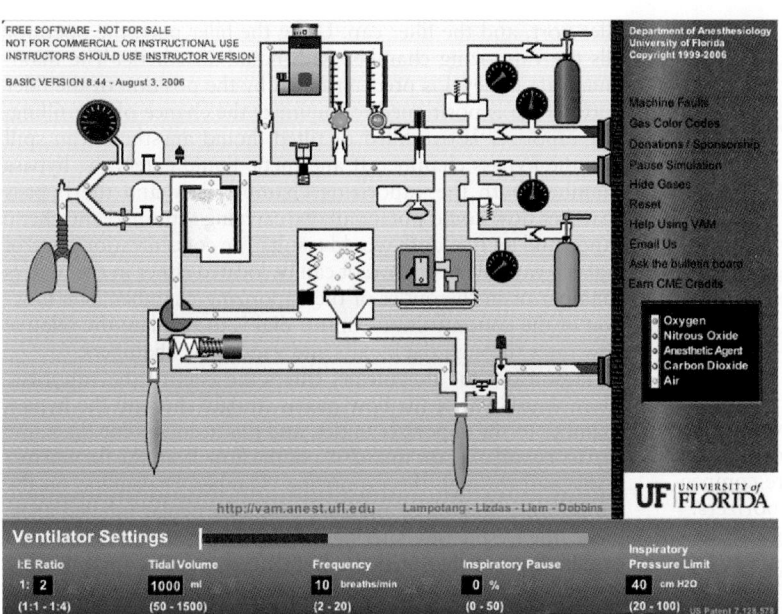

FIGURE 26-17. The Virtual Anesthesia Machine (VAM) simulator, an interactive model of an anesthesia machine. (Reproduced with permission from Lampotang S and Lizdas DE, Virtual Anesthesia Machine Website: http://vam.anest.ufl.edu/wip.html.)

PREANESTHETIC EVALUATION AND PREPARATION

Physics

Vapor Pressure

Contemporary inhaled volatile anesthetics exist in the liquid state at temperatures below 20°C. When a volatile liquid is in a closed container, molecules escape from the liquid phase to the vapor phase until the number of molecules in the vapor phase is constant. These molecules in the vapor phase bombard the wall of the container and create a pressure known as the *saturated vapor pressure*. As the temperature increases, more molecules enter the vapor phase, and the vapor pressure increases (Fig. 26-18). Vapor pressure is independent of atmospheric pressure and is contingent only on the temperature and physical characteristics of the liquid. The *boiling point* of a liquid is defined as that temperature at which the vapor pressure equals atmospheric pressure.[38,55,56] At 760 mm Hg, the boiling points for desflurane, isoflurane, halothane, enflurane, and sevoflurane are approximately 22.8, 48.5, 50.2, 56.5, and 58.5°C, respectively. Unlike other contemporary inhaled anesthetics, desflurane boils at temperatures that may be encountered in clinical settings such as pediatric and burn operating rooms. This unique physical characteristic alone mandates a special vaporizer design to control the delivery of desflurane. If agent-specific vaporizers are inadvertently misfilled with incorrect liquid anesthetic agents, the resulting mixtures of volatile agents may demonstrate unique properties from those of the individual component agents. The altered vapor pressure and other physical properties of the resulting azeotropic mixtures that result from the mixing of various agents may alter the output of the anesthetic vaporizer (see "Variable Bypass Vaporizers: Hazards and Misfilling").[57]

Latent Heat of Vaporization

When a molecule is converted from a liquid to the gaseous phase, energy is consumed because the molecules of a liquid tend to cohere. The amount of energy that is consumed for a given liquid as it is converted to a vapor is referred to as the *latent heat of vaporization*. It is more precisely defined as the number of calories required to change 1 g of liquid into vapor without a temperature change. The energy for vaporization must come either from the liquid itself or from an outside source. The temperature of the liquid itself will decrease during vaporization in the absence of an outside energy source. This energy loss can lead to significant decreases in temperature of the remaining liquid, and can greatly decrease subsequent vaporization.[38,55,58]

Specific Heat

The *specific heat* of a substance is the number of calories required to increase the temperature of 1 g of a substance by 1°C.[19,38,55] The substance can be a solid, liquid, or gas. The concept of specific heat is important to the design, operation, and construction of vaporizers because it is applicable in two ways. First, the specific heat value for an inhaled anesthetic is important because it indicates how much heat must be supplied to the liquid to maintain a constant temperature when heat is being lost during vaporization. Second, manufacturers select vaporizer component materials that have a high specific heat to minimize temperature changes associated with vaporization.

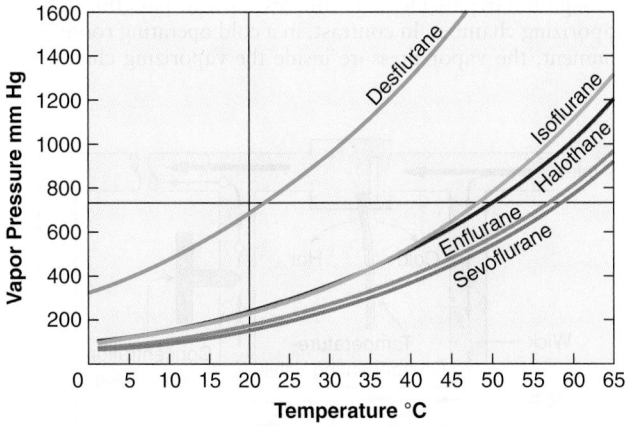

FIGURE 26-18. Vapor pressure versus temperature curves for desflurane, isoflurane, halothane, enflurane, and sevoflurane. The vapor pressure curve for desflurane is both steeper and shifted to higher vapor pressures when compared with the curves for other contemporary inhaled anesthetics. (From inhaled anesthetic package insert equations and from Susay SR, Smith MA, Lockwood GG: The saturated vapor pressure of desflurane at various temperatures. Anesth Analg 1996; 83: 864).

Thermal Conductivity

Thermal conductivity is a measure of the speed with which heat flows through a substance. The higher the thermal conductivity, the better the substance conducts heat.[55] Vaporizers are constructed of metals that have relatively high thermal conductivity, thus maintaining a uniform internal temperature.

Ambient Pressure Effects

See "Datex-Ohmeda Tec 6 Vaporizer for Desflurane: Factors that Influence Vaporizer Output: Varied Altitudes."

Variable Bypass Vaporizers

The Datex-Ohmeda Tec 4, Tec 5, and Tec 7, as well as the North American Dräger Vapor 19.n and 20.n vaporizers, are classified as variable bypass, flow-over, temperature-compensated, agent-specific, out-of-breathing circuit vaporizers.[55] *Variable bypass* refers to the method for regulating the anesthetic agent concentration output from the vaporizer. The concentration control dial setting determines the ratio of flow that goes through the bypass chamber and through the vaporizing chamber as fresh gas from the flowmeters enters the vaporizer inlet. The gas channeled through the vaporizing chamber flows over a wick system saturated with the liquid anesthetic and subsequently also becomes saturated with vapor. Thus, *flow-over* refers to the method of vaporization and is in contrast to a *bubble-through* system that may be seen in some copper kettle-type vaporizers of old. The Tec 4, Tec 5, and Tec 7, and the Dräger Vapor 19.n and 20.n are further classified as *temperature compensated*. Each of these is equipped with an automatic temperature-compensating device that helps maintain a constant vaporizer output over a wide range of operating temperatures. These vaporizers are *agent-specific* and *out-of-circuit* because each is designed to accommodate a single anesthetic agent and to be physically located outside the breathing circuit. Variable bypass vaporizers are used to deliver halothane, enflurane, isoflurane, and sevoflurane, but not desflurane.

Basic Operating Principles

A diagram of a generic, variable bypass vaporizer is shown in Figure 26-19. Vaporizer components include the concentration control dial, the bypass chamber, the vaporizing chamber, the

filler port, and the filler cap. Using the filler port, the operator fills the vaporizing chamber with liquid anesthetic. The maximum safe fill level is predetermined by the position of the filler port, which is positioned to minimize the chance of overfilling. If a vaporizer is overfilled or tilted, liquid anesthetic can spill into the bypass chamber. If anesthetic liquid enters the bypass chamber, both the vaporizing chamber flow and the bypass chamber flow could potentially be carrying saturated anesthetic vapor, and an overdose would result. The concentration control dial is a variable restrictor; it can be located either in the bypass chamber or in the outlet of the vaporizing chamber. The function of the concentration control dial is to regulate the relative flow rates through the bypass and vaporizing chambers.

Flow from the flowmeters enters the inlet of the vaporizer. More than 80% of the flow passes straight through the bypass chamber to the vaporizer outlet, and this accounts for the name *bypass chamber*. Less than 20% of the flow from the flowmeters is diverted through the vaporizing chamber. Depending on the temperature and vapor pressure of the particular inhaled anesthetic, the fresh gases entering the vaporizing chamber entrain a specific flow of the inhaled anesthetic agent. The mixture that exits the vaporizer is the combination of flow through the bypass chamber, flow through the vaporizing chamber, and flow of entrained anesthetic vapor. The final concentration of inhaled anesthetic is the ratio of the flow of the inhaled anesthetic to the total gas flow.[55,59] The amount of liquid volatile anesthetic (in milliliters) that a typical vaporizer uses is proportional to the flow rate and can be approximated from the following formula: $3 \times$ fresh gas flow (L/min) $\times$ volume % = mL liquid of volatile anesthetic per hour.[60]

The vapor pressure of an inhaled anesthetic depends on the ambient temperature (Fig. 26-18). For example, at 20°C the vapor pressure of isoflurane is 238 mm Hg, whereas at 35°C the vapor pressure almost doubles (450 mm Hg). Variable bypass vaporizers have an internal mechanism to compensate for variations in ambient temperature. The temperature-compensating valve of the Datex-Ohmeda Tec 4 is shown in Figure 26-20. At relatively high ambient temperatures, such as those commonly seen in operating rooms designated for the care of pediatric or burn patients, the vapor pressure inside the vaporizing chamber is high. To compensate for this increased vapor pressure, the bimetallic strip of the temperature-compensating valve leans to the right, decreasing the resistance to flow through the bypass chamber. This decreased resistance allows more flow to pass through the bypass chamber and less flow to pass through the vaporizing chamber. In contrast, in a cold operating room environment, the vapor pressure inside the vaporizing chamber is

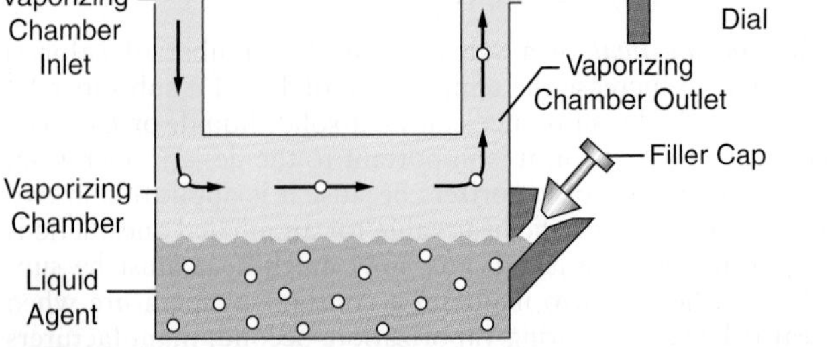

FIGURE 26-19. Generic variable bypass vaporizer. See text for details.

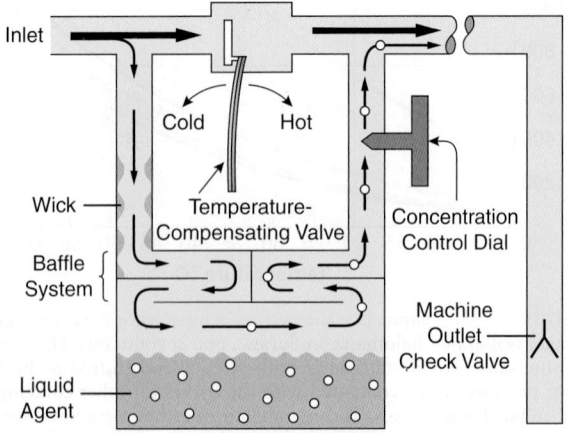

FIGURE 26-20. Simplified schematic of the Ohmeda Tec-Type Vaporizer. See text for details.

reduced. To compensate for this decrease in vapor pressure, the bimetallic strip leans to the left. This change increases the resistance to flow through the bypass chamber, causing more flow to pass through the vaporizing chamber and less to pass through the bypass chamber. The net effect in both situations is maintenance of relatively constant vaporizer output.

Factors That Influence Vaporizer Output

If an ideal vaporizer existed, with a fixed dial setting, its output would be constant regardless of varied flow rates, temperatures, back pressures, and carrier gases. Designing such a vaporizer is difficult because as ambient conditions change, the physical properties of gases and of vaporizers themselves can change.[59] Contemporary vaporizers approach ideal but still have some limitations. Even though some of the most sophisticated vaporizer systems now available use computer-controlled components and multiple sensors, they have yet to become significantly more accurate than conventional vaporizers. Several factors that affect vaporizer performance in general are described here.

Flow Rate. With a fixed dial setting, vaporizer output can vary with the rate of gas flowing through the vaporizer. This variation is particularly notable at extremes of flow rates. The output of all variable bypass vaporizers is less than the dial setting at low flow rates (<250 mL/min). This results from the relatively high density of volatile inhaled anesthetics. At low flow rates, insufficient turbulence is generated in the vaporizing chamber to advance the vapor molecules upwardly. At extremely high flow rates, such as 15 L/min, the output of most variable bypass vaporizers is less than the dial setting. This discrepancy is attributed to incomplete mixing and failure to saturate the carrier gas in the vaporizing chamber. Also, the resistance characteristics of the bypass chamber and the vaporizing chamber can vary as flow increases. These variations can result in decreased output concentration.[59]

Temperature. Because of improvements in design, the output of contemporary temperature-compensated vaporizers is almost linear over a wide range of temperatures. Automatic temperature-compensating mechanisms in the bypass chamber maintain a constant vaporizer output with varying temperatures.[28] As previously described, a bimetallic strip (of the temperature-compensating valve; Fig. 26-20) or an expansion element (Fig. 26-21) directs a greater proportion of gas flow through the bypass chamber as temperatures increase.[59] Additionally, the wick systems are placed in direct contact with the metal wall of the vaporizer to help replace energy (heat) consumed during vapor-

ization. The materials from which vaporizers are constructed are chosen because they have a relatively high specific heat and high thermal conductivity. These factors help minimize the effect of cooling of the liquid anesthetic during vaporization.

Intermittent Back Pressure. Intermittent back pressure that results from either positive pressure ventilation or use of the oxygen flush valve may result in higher than expected vaporizer output. This phenomenon, known as the *pumping effect*, is more pronounced at low flow rates, low dial settings, and low levels of liquid anesthetic in the vaporizing chamber.[55,59,61,62] Additionally, the pumping effect is increased by rapid respiratory rates, high peak inspired pressures, and rapid drops in pressure during exhalation.[38,52,55,56,63] Newer variable bypass vaporizers such as the Datex-Ohmeda Tec 4, Tec 5, and Tec 7, and North American Dräger Vapor 19.n and 20.n (Vapor 2000) are relatively immune from the pumping effect. One proposed mechanism for the pumping effect depends on retrograde pressure transmission from the patient circuit to the vaporizer during the inspiratory phase of positive pressure ventilation. Gas molecules are compressed in both the bypass and vaporizing chambers. When the back pressure is suddenly released during the expiratory phase of positive-pressure ventilation, vapor exits the vaporizing chamber via both the vaporizing chamber outlet and retrograde through the vaporizing chamber inlet. This occurs because the output resistance of the bypass chamber is lower than that of the vaporizing chamber, particularly at low dial settings. The enhanced output concentration results from the increment of vapor that travels in the retrograde direction to the bypass chamber.[59,61,62]

To decrease the pumping effect, the vaporizing chambers of newer systems are smaller than those of early variable bypass vaporizers such as the Fluotec Mark II (750 mL).[61] Therefore, no substantial volumes of vapor can be discharged from the vaporizing chamber into the bypass chamber during the expiratory phase. The North American Dräger Vapor 19.1 and 20.n (Fig. 26-21) have a long spiral tube that serves as the inlet to the vaporizing chamber.[61] When the pressure in the vaporizing chamber is released, some of the vapor enters this tube but does not enter the bypass chamber because of tube length.[56] The Tec 4 (Fig. 26-20) has an extensive baffle system in the vaporizing chamber, and a one-way check valve has been inserted at the common gas outlet to minimize the pumping effect. This check valve attenuates but does not eliminate the pressure increase because gas still flows from the flowmeters to the vaporizer during the inspiratory phase of positive pressure ventilation.[55,64]

Carrier Gas Composition. Vaporizer output is influenced by the composition of the carrier gas that flows through the vaporizer.[65–72] During experimental conditions, when the carrier gas is rapidly changed from 100% oxygen to 100% nitrous oxide, a sudden transient decrease in vaporizer output occurs, followed by a slow increase to a new steady-state value (Fig. 26-22B).[66,69] Because nitrous oxide is more soluble than oxygen in the halogenated liquid within the vaporizer sump, when this switch occurs the output from the vaporizing chamber is transiently reduced.[66] Once the anesthetic liquid is totally saturated with nitrous oxide, vaporizing chamber output increases somewhat, and a new steady state is established (Fig. 26-22C).

The explanation for the new steady-state output value is less well understood.[71] With contemporary vaporizers such as the North American Dräger Vapor 19.n and 20.n and the Ohmeda Tec–type conventional vaporizers, the steady-state output value is less when nitrous oxide rather than oxygen is the carrier gas (Fig. 26-22B). Conversely, the output of some older vaporizers is enhanced when nitrous oxide is the carrier gas instead of oxygen.[68,72] The steady-state plateau is achieved more rapidly with increased flow rates, regardless of the ultimate output value.[69] Factors that contribute to the characteristic steady-state response resulting when various carrier gases

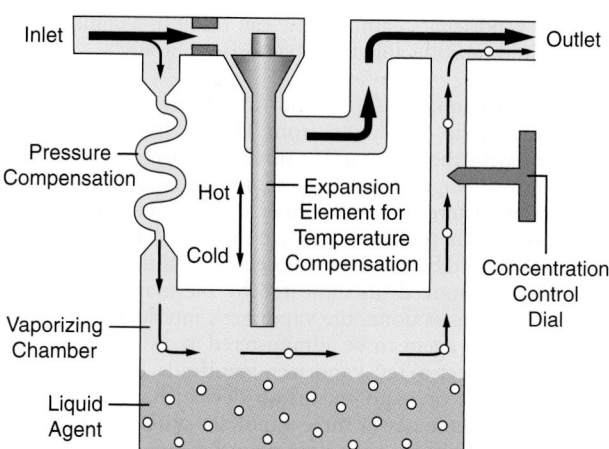

FIGURE 26-21.   Simplified schematic of the North American Dräger Vapor 19.1 vaporizer. See text for details.

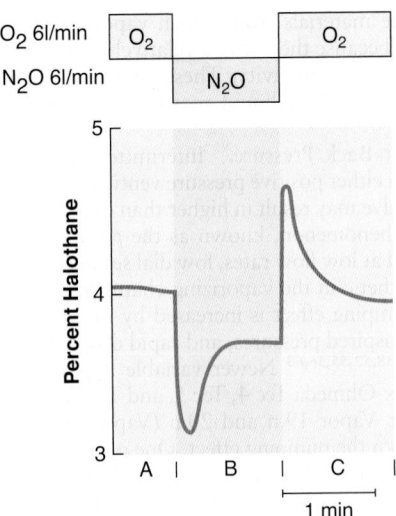

FIGURE 26-22.   Halothane output of a North American Dräger Vapor 19.1 vaporizer with different carrier gases. The initial output concentration is approximately 4% halothane when oxygen is the carrier gas at flows of 6 L/min (**A**). When the carrier gas is quickly switched to 100% nitrous oxide (**B**), the halothane concentration decreases to 3% within 8 to 10 seconds. Then, a new steady-state concentration of approximately 3.5% is attained within 1 minute. See text for details. (Modified from Gould DB, Lampert BA, MacKrell TN: Effect of nitrous oxide solubility on vaporizer aberrance. Anesth Analg 1982; 61: 939, with permission.)

are used include the viscosity and density of the carrier gas (depending on whether the flow is laminar or turbulent), the relative solubilities of the carrier gas in the anesthetic liquid, the flow-splitting characteristics of the specific vaporizer, and the concentration control dial setting.[66,68,69,71]

Safety Features

Newer generations of anesthesia vaporizers including the North American Dräger 19.n and 20.n, and the Datex-Ohmeda Tec 4, Tec 5, and Tec 7 now have built-in safety features that have minimized or eliminated many hazards once associated with variable bypass vaporizers. Agent-specific, keyed filling devices help prevent filling a vaporizer with the wrong agent. Overfilling of these vaporizers is minimized because the filler port is located at the maximum safe liquid level. Finally, today's vaporizers are firmly secured to a vaporizer manifold on the anesthesia workstation. Thus, problems associated with vaporizer tipping have become much less frequent. Contemporary interlock systems prevent administration of more than one inhaled anesthetic.

Hazards

Despite many safety features, some hazards are still associated with contemporary variable bypass vaporizers.

Misfilling.   Vaporizers not equipped with keyed fillers have been occasionally misfilled with the wrong anesthetic liquid.[73] A potential for misfilling exists even on contemporary vaporizers equipped with keyed fillers.[74–76] When a vaporizer misfilling occurs, patients inadvertently can be rendered inadequately, or excessively, anesthetized, depending on which drug is placed in the vaporizer. The use of a multigas analyzer may alert the user to such a problem.

Contamination.   Contamination of anesthetic vaporizer contents has occurred by filling an isoflurane vaporizer with a contaminated bottle of isoflurane. A potentially serious incident was avoided because the operator detected an abnormal acrid odor.[77]

Tipping.   Tipping of a vaporizer can occur when they are incorrectly "switched out" or moved. However, tipping is unlikely when a vaporizer is attached to the anesthesia workstation manifold short of the entire machine being turned over. Excessive tipping can cause the liquid agent to enter the bypass chamber and can cause output with extremely high agent concentration.[78] The Tec 4 is slightly more resistant to tipping than the North American Dräger Vapor 19.n because of its extensive baffle system. However, if either vaporizer is tipped, it should not be used until it has been flushed for 20 to 30 minutes at high fresh gas flow rates. During this procedure, having the vaporizer concentration control dial set at a low concentration maximizes bypass chamber flow and will aid in removal of any residual liquid anesthetic in that area.[55] After following this procedure, the use of a multigas analyzer is strongly recommended. The Dräger Vapor 20.n series vaporizers now have a transport ("T") dial setting that helps prevent tipping-related problems. When the dial is placed in this position, the vaporizer sump is isolated from the bypass chamber, thereby reducing the likelihood of tipping and a resulting accidental overdose. Therefore, any time one of these vaporizers is moved separate from the anesthesia workstation, the control dial should be placed in the T position.

The design of the Tec-6 and the Aladin Cassette vaporizer systems, both from Datex-Ohmeda, has practically eliminated the possibility of tipping from these products. Because the Aladin Cassette vaporizer's bypass chamber is physically separated from the "cassette," and permanently resides in the anesthesia workstation, the possibility of tipping is virtually eliminated. Tipping of the Aladin Cassettes themselves when they are not installed in the vaporizer is not problematic. Similarly, Dräger's D-Vapor vaporizer is hermetically tight and can be transported in any position without prior draining.

Overfilling.   Improper filling procedures combined with failure of the vaporizer sight glass can cause overfilling and patient overdose. Liquid anesthetic enters the bypass chamber and up to 10 times the intended vapor concentration can be delivered to the common gas outlet.[79] Most modern vaporizers are now relatively immune to overfilling because of side-fill rather than top-fill designs. Side-fill systems largely prevent overfilling.

Underfilling.   Just as with overfilling, underfilling of anesthetic vaporizers may also be problematic. When a Tec 5 sevoflurane vaporizer is in a low-fill state and used under conditions of high fresh gas flow rates (>7.5 L/min) and high dial setting (such as seen during inhalational inductions), the vaporizer output may abruptly decrease to <2%. The causes of this problem are most likely multifactorial. However, the combination of low vaporizer fill state (<25% full) in combination with the high vaporizing chamber flow can result in a clinically significant and reproducible fall in vaporizer output.[80]

Simultaneous Inhaled Anesthetic Administration.   On some older anesthesia machines from Datex-Ohmeda that are equipped with the Select-a-Tec three-vaporizer manifold that does not use a vapor-interlock system, two inhaled anesthetics can be administered simultaneously when the center vaporizer is removed. On such machines, either the left or the right vaporizer should be moved to the central position if the central vaporizer is removed (as indicated by the manifold warning label). Once this is done, the vaporizer's interlock system will allow only one agent to be administered at a time. More contemporary Select-a-Tec vaporizer manifolds have a built-in vapor-interlock or vapor-exclusion device that prevents this problem. On these newer three-vaporizer systems, a U-shaped plastic device links the vaporizer extension rods even when the vaporizers are not adjacent to one another on the manifold. On such a system, the manifold plus the vaporizers themselves comprise the vapor-interlock or vapor-exclusion system.

Leaks. Vaporizer leaks occur frequently, and can potentially result in patient awareness during anesthesia.[18,22,62,81] or in pollution of the operating room environment. A loose filler cap is the most common source of vaporizer leaks. With some key-filled Penlon and Dräger vaporizers, a loose filler screw clamp allows escape of saturated anesthetic vapor.[18] Leaks can occur at the O-ring junctions between the vaporizer and its manifold. To detect a leak within a vaporizer, the concentration control dial must be in the on position. Even though vaporizer leaks in Dräger systems potentially can be detected with a conventional positive-pressure leak test (because of the absence of an outlet check valve), a negative-pressure leak test is more sensitive and allows the user to detect even small leaks. Datex-Ohmeda recommends a negative-pressure leak testing device (suction bulb) to detect vaporizer leaks in the Modulus I, Modulus II, Excel, and the Aestiva workstations because of the check valve located just upstream of each machine's fresh gas outlet (see "Checkout of the Anesthesia Workstation").

Many newer anesthesia workstations are capable of performing self-testing procedures that, in some cases, may eliminate the need for the conventional negative-pressure leak testing. However, it is of vital importance that anesthesia providers understand that these self-tests may not detect internal vaporizer leaks on systems with add-on vaporizers. For the self-tests to determine if an internal vaporizer leak is present, the leak test must be repeated for each vaporizer sequentially, while its concentration control dial is turned to the on position. Recall that when a vaporizer's concentration control dial is set in the off position, it may not be possible to detect even major internal leaks such as an absent or loose filler cap.

Anesthesia Vaporizers and Environmental Considerations. Today more than ever, anesthetics are being administered to patients outside the operating room. One such location that has proved sometimes difficult to work in is the magnetic resonance imaging (MRI) suite. The presence of a powerful magnet field, the significant noise pollution, and limited access to the patient during the procedure all complicate care in this setting. It is imperative that only nonferrous (MRI-compatible) equipment be used in these settings. Some anesthesia vaporizers, although they may appear nonferrous by testing with a horseshoe magnet, may indeed contain substantial internal ferrous components. Inappropriate use of such a device in an MRI suite may potentially turn them into a dangerous missile if left unsecured.[82]

❽ ## The Datex-Ohmeda Tec 6 Vaporizer for Desflurane

Because of its unique physical characteristics, the controlled vaporization of desflurane required a novel approach to vaporizer design. Datex-Ohmeda developed the Tec 6 vaporizer, the first such system, and released it into clinical use in the early 1990s. The Tec 6 vaporizer is an electrically heated, pressurized device specifically designed to deliver desflurane.[83,84] The vapor pressure of desflurane is 3 to 4 times that of other contemporary inhaled anesthetics, and it boils at 22.8°C,[85] which is near room temperature (Fig. 26-18). Desflurane has a minimum alveolar anesthetic concentration (MAC) value of 6 to 7%.[85] Desflurane is valuable because it has a low blood gas solubility coefficient of 0.45 at 37°C, and recovery from anesthesia is more rapid than with many other potent inhaled anesthetics.[85] In 2004, Dräger Medical received FDA approval for its own version of the Tec 6 desflurane vaporizer, the D-Vapor. The operating principles described in the following discussion are applicable to either system, even though we refer to the Tec 6 specifically.

Unsuitability of Contemporary Variable Bypass Vaporizers for Controlled Vaporization of Desflurane

Desflurane's high volatility and moderate potency preclude its use with contemporary variable bypass vaporizers such as Datex-Ohmeda Tec 4, Tec 5, and Tec 7, or the North American Dräger Vapor 19.n or 20.n for two primary reasons[83]:

❾ 1. At 20°C the vapor pressure of desflurane is near 1 atmosphere (atm).

The vapor pressures of enflurane, isoflurane, halothane, and desflurane at 20°C are 172, 240, 244, and 669 mm Hg, respectively (Fig. 26-18).[85] Equal amounts of flow through a traditional vaporizer would vaporize many more volumes of desflurane than any other of the other agents. For example, at 1 atm and 20°C, 100 mL/min passing through the vaporizing chamber would entrain 735 mL/min desflurane versus 29, 46, and 47 mL/min of enflurane, isoflurane, and halothane, respectively.[83] Under these same conditions, to produce 1% desflurane output the amount of bypass flow necessary to achieve sufficient dilution of the large volume of desflurane saturated anesthetic vapor would be approximately 73 L/min, compared with ≤5 L/min for the other three anesthetics. Additionally, above 22.8°C at 1 atm, desflurane will boil. The amount of vapor produced would be limited only by the heat energy available from the vaporizer owing to its specific heat.[83]

2. Contemporary vaporizers lack an external heat source.

The latent heat of vaporization for desflurane is approximately equal to that of enflurane, isoflurane, and halothane; however, its MAC is 4 to 9 times higher than those of the other three inhaled anesthetics. Thus, the absolute amount of desflurane vaporized over a given time period is considerably greater than the other anesthetic drugs. Supplying desflurane via a conventional vaporizer in higher (equivalent MAC) concentrations would lead to excessive cooling of the vaporizer and would significantly reduce its output. In the absence of an external heat source, temperature compensation using traditional mechanical devices would be almost impossible. Because of the broad range of temperatures seen in the clinical setting, and because of desflurane's steep vapor pressure versus temperature curve (Fig. 26-18), the delivery of desflurane in a conventional anesthetic vaporizer at best would be unpredictable.[83]

Operating Principles of the Tec 6 and Tec 6 Plus

To achieve controlled vaporization of desflurane, Datex-Ohmeda introduced the Tec 6 vaporizer to widespread clinical practice in 1993. This was the first clinically available vaporizer to be electrically heated and pressurized. The physical appearance and operation of the Tec 6 are similar to contemporary vaporizers, but some aspects of the internal design and operating principles are radically different. The Tec 6 Plus represents a later version of the original Tec 6. The Tec 6 Plus has the same basic Tec 6 design, but also incorporates an enhanced audible alarm system not previously available on the Tec 6.

Functionally, the operation of the Tec 6 is more accurately described as a dual-gas blender than as a vaporizer. A simplified schematic of the Tec 6 is shown in Figure 26-23. The vaporizer has two independent gas circuits arranged in parallel. The fresh gas circuit is shown in gray, and the vapor circuit is shown in white. The fresh gas from the flowmeters enters at the fresh gas inlet, passes through a fixed restrictor (R1), and exits at the vaporizer gas outlet. The vapor circuit originates at the desflurane sump, which is electrically heated and thermostatically controlled to 39°C, a temperature well above the boiling point of desflurane. The heated sump assembly serves as a reservoir of desflurane vapor. At 39°C, the vapor pressure in the sump is approximately 1,300 mm Hg absolute,[86] or

FIGURE 26-23. Simplified schematic of the Tec 6 desflurane vaporizer. R1, fixed restrictor; R2, variable restrictor. See text for details. (From Andrews JJ: Operating Principles of the Ohmeda Tec 6 Desflurane Vaporizer: A Collection of Twelve Color Illustrations. Washington, DC, Library of Congress, 1996, with permission.)

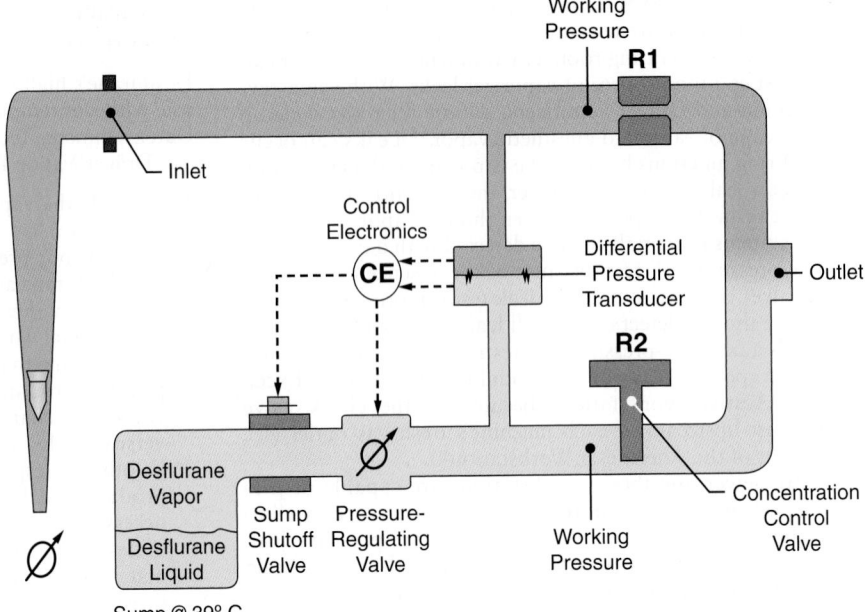

approximately 2 atm absolute (Fig. 26-18). Just downstream from the sump is the shutoff valve. After the vaporizer warms up, the shutoff valve fully opens when the concentration control valve is turned to the on position. A pressure-regulating valve located downstream from the shutoff valve regulates the pressure downward to approximately 1.1 atm absolute (74 mm Hg gauge) at a fresh gas flow rate of 10 L/min. The operator controls desflurane output by adjusting the concentration control valve (R2), which is a variable restrictor.[83]

The vapor flow through R2 joins the fresh gas flow through R1 at a point downstream from the restrictors. Until this point, the two circuits are physically divorced. They are interfaced pneumatically and electronically, however, through differential pressure transducers, a control electronics system, and a pressure-regulating valve. When a constant fresh gas flow rate encounters the fixed restrictor, R1, a specific back pressure, proportional to the fresh gas flow rate, pushes against the diaphragm of the control differential pressure transducer. The differential pressure transducer conveys the pressure difference between the fresh gas circuit and the vapor circuit to the control electronics system. The control electronics system regulates the pressure-regulating valve so that the pressure in the vapor circuit equals the pressure in the fresh gas circuit. This equalized pressure supplying R1 and R2 is the working pressure, and the working pressure is constant at a fixed fresh gas flow rate. If the operator increases the fresh gas flow rate, more back pressure is

exerted on the diaphragm of the control pressure transducer, and the working pressure of the vaporizer increases.[83]

Table 26-2 shows the approximate correlation between fresh gas flow rate and working pressure for a typical vaporizer. At a fresh gas flow rate of 1 L/min, the working pressure is 10 millibars, or 7.4 mm Hg gauge. At a fresh gas flow rate of 10 L/min, the working pressure is 100 millibars, or 74 mm Hg gauge. Therefore, there is a linear relationship between fresh gas flow rate and working pressure. When the fresh gas flow rate is increased tenfold, the working pressure increases tenfold.[83]

Listed in the following section are two specific examples to demonstrate the operating principles of the Tec 6.[83]

Example A: Constant fresh gas flow rate of 1 L/min, with an increase in the dial setting.

With a fresh gas flow rate of 1 L/min, the working pressure of the vaporizer is 7.4 mm Hg. That is, the pressure supplying R1 and R2 is 7.4 mm Hg. As the operator increases the dial setting, the opening at R2 becomes larger, allowing more vapor to pass through R2. Specific vapor flow rates at different dial settings are shown in Table 26-3.

Example B: Constant dial setting with an increase in fresh gas flow from 1 to 10 L/min.

At a fresh gas flow rate of 1 L/min, the working pressure is 7.4 mm Hg, and at a dial setting of 6% the vapor flow rate

TABLE 26-2

FRESH GAS FLOW RATE VERSUS WORKING PRESSURE

FRESH GAS FLOW RATE (L/min)	WORKING PRESSURE AT R1 AND R2 GAS INLET PRESSURE, PSIG		
	mbar	cm water	mm Hg
1	10	10.2	7.4
5	50	51.0	37.0
10	100	102.0	74.0

R1, fixed restrictor; R2, variable restrictor.
Reprinted from Andrews JJ, Johnston RV Jr: The new Tec 6 desflurane vaporizer. Anesth Analg 1993; 76: 1338, with permission.

TABLE 26-3

DIAL SETTING VERSUS FLOW THROUGH RESTRICTOR R2

■ DIAL SETTING (VOL%)[a]	■ FRESH GAS FLOW RATE (L/min)	■ APPROXIMATE VAPOR FLOW RATE THROUGH R2 (mL/min)
1	1	10
6	1	64
12	1	136
18	1	220

[a]Volume percent = [(vapor flow rate)/(fresh gas flow rate) + (vapor flow rate)] × 100%.
Reprinted from Andrews JJ, Johnston RV Jr: The new Tec 6 desflurane vaporizer. Anesth Analg 1993; 76: 1338, with permission.

through R2 is 64 mL/min (Tables 26-2 and 26-3). With a tenfold increase in the fresh gas flow rate, there is a concomitant tenfold increase in the working pressure to 74 mm Hg. The ratio of resistances of R2 to R1 is constant at a fixed dial setting of 6%. Because R2 is supplied by 10 times more pressure, the vapor flow rate through R2 increases tenfold to 640 mL/min. Vaporizer output is constant because both the fresh gas flow and the vapor flow increase proportionally.

Factors that Influence Vaporizer Output

Varied altitude and carrier gas composition influence Tec 6 output. Each is discussed in the following sections.

Varied Altitudes. Although ambient pressure changes affect conventional vaporizer output significantly in terms of volumes percent (%v/v; i.e., concentration), their effect on anesthetic potency (i.e., partial pressure) is minimal. This effect is illustrated using the example of isoflurane shown in Table 26-4. With a constant dial setting of 0.89%, at 1 atm (760 mm Hg), if perfectly calibrated, the volumes percent delivered would be

0.89% and the partial pressure of isoflurane would be 6.8 mm Hg. Maintaining the same dial setting and lowering ambient pressure to 0.66 atm or 502 mm Hg (roughly equivalent to 10,000 ft elevation) would result in an increase in the concentration output to 1.75% (almost double), but the partial pressure only increases to 8.77 mm Hg (only a 29% increase) because of the proportionate decline in ambient pressure (Fig. 26-24).

It is generally considered that the partial pressure of the anesthetic agent in the central nervous system, not its concentration, is responsible for the anesthetic effect. To obtain a consistent depth of anesthesia when gross changes in barometric pressure occur, the volumes percent must be changed in inverse proportion to the barometric pressure. For the most part, traditional variable bypass vaporizers automatically compensate for this change, and for practical purposes the effect of barometric pressure can generally be ignored.

This compensation should be considered in stark contrast to the response of the Tec 6 desflurane vaporizer at varied altitudes (Fig. 26-24 and Table 26-4). One must remember this device is more accurately described as a dual gas "blender" than a vaporizer. Regardless of the ambient pressure, the Tec 6

TABLE 26-4

PERFORMANCE OF TEC TYPE VAPORIZERS VERSUS THE TEC 6 DESFLURANE VAPORIZER AT VARYING AMBIENT PRESSURES[a]

		■ ISOFLURANE VAPORIZER WITH A DIAL SETTING OF 0.89%			■ TEC 6 DESFLURANE VAPORIZER WITH A DIAL SETTING OF 6%
■ ATMOSPHERES	■ AMBIENT PRESSURE (mm Hg)	■ MILLILITERS OF ISOFLURANE VAPOR ENTRAINED BY 100 mL O₂	■ OUTPUT CONCENTRATION (%)	■ PARTIAL PRESSURE OUTPUT (mm Hg)	■ PARTIAL PRESSURE OUTPUT OF DESFLURANE (mm Hg)
0.66 (2/3)	500 (10,000 feet)	91	1.753	8.77	30
0.74	560	74	1.429	8.0	33.6
0.80	608 (6,564 feet)	64.32	1.25	7.6	36.5
1.0	760	46	0.89	6.8	45.6
1.5	1,140	26.4	0.515	5.87	68.4
2	1,520	19	0.36	5.5	91.2
3	2,280	11.65	0.228	5.198	136

[a]The following were assumed: 5,000 mL bypass chamber flow, 100 mL vaporizing chamber flow, equivalent to an isoflurane dial setting of 0.89%.

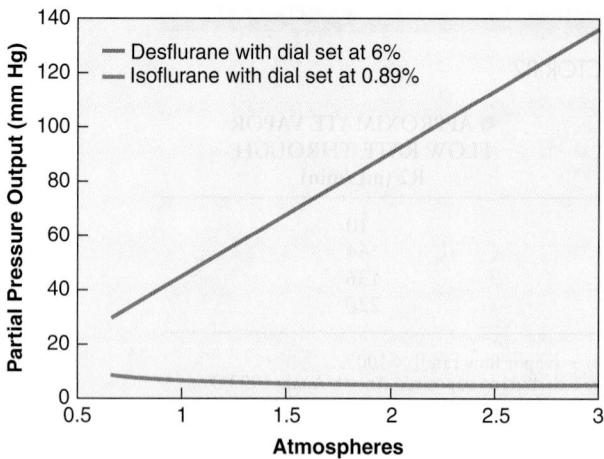

FIGURE 26-24.   Performance of TEC type vaporizer versus the Tec 6 desflurane vaporizer at varying ambient atmospheres (1 atmosphere = 760 mm Hg).

will maintain a constant concentration of vapor output (volumes percent), not a constant partial pressure. This means that at high altitudes, the partial pressure of desflurane for any given dial setting will be decreased in proportion to the atmospheric pressure divided by the calibration pressure (normally 760 mm Hg) per the following formula:

$$\begin{array}{c} \text{Required} \\ \text{dial} \\ \text{setting} \end{array} = \frac{\text{Normal dial setting (\%v/v)} \times 760 \text{ mm Hg}}{\text{Ambient pressure (mm Hg)}}$$

For example, at an altitude of 2000 m (6564 ft) where the ambient pressure is 608 mm Hg, the Tec 6 dial setting must be advanced from 10%v/v to 12.5%v/v to avoid underdosing that could potentially result in patient awareness. Conversely, the Tec 6's maintenance of a constant volumes percent in hyperbaric conditions could produce significant increases in partial pressure output, and if not accounted for, the potential for anesthetic overdose. Therefore, in hyperbaric settings the Tec 6 dial setting would need to be reduced to maintain the desired partial pressure output of desflurane.

Carrier Gas Composition.   Vaporizer output approximates the dial setting when oxygen is the carrier gas because the Tec 6 vaporizer is calibrated using 100% oxygen. At low flow rates when a carrier gas other than 100% oxygen is used, however, a clear trend toward reduction in vaporizer output emerges. This reduction parallels the proportional decrease in viscosity of the carrier gas. Nitrous oxide has a lower viscosity than oxygen, so the back pressure generated by resistor R1 (Fig. 26-23) is less when nitrous oxide is the carrier gas, and the working pressure is reduced. At low flow rates using nitrous oxide as the carrier gas, vaporizer output is approximately 20% less than the dial setting. This suggests that, at clinically useful fresh gas flow rates, the gas flow across resistor R1 is laminar, and the working pressure is proportional to both the fresh gas flow rate and the viscosity of the carrier gas.[87]

Safety Features

Because the vapor pressure of desflurane is near 1 atm, misfilling contemporary vaporizers with desflurane could theoretically result in both desflurane overdose and creation of a hypoxic gas mixture.[88] Datex-Ohmeda has introduced a unique, anesthetic-specific filling system to minimize occurrence of this potential hazard. The agent-specific filler of the desflurane bottle known as the *Saf-T-Fill* adapter is intended to

prevent its use with traditional vaporizers. The filling system also minimizes spillage of liquid or vapor anesthetic by maintaining a "closed system" during the filling process. Each desflurane bottle has a spring-loaded filler cap with an O-ring on the tip. The spring seals the bottle until it is engaged in the filler port of the vaporizer. Thus, this anesthetic-specific filling system interlocks the vaporizer and the dispensing bottle, preventing loss of anesthetic to the atmosphere. Despite these safety features designed to minimize filling errors, a case report described the misfilling of a Tec 6 desflurane vaporizer with sevoflurane. This error was possible because of similarities between a new type of keyed filler for sevoflurane and the desflurane Saf-T-Fill adapter. In this case, however, the desflurane vaporizer detected this error and automatically shut itself off.[74]

Major vaporizer faults cause the shutoff valve located just downstream from the desflurane sump (Fig. 26-23) to close, producing a no-output situation. The valve is closed and a "no-output" alarm is activated immediately if any of the following conditions occur: (1) the anesthetic level decreases to below 20 mL, (2) the vaporizer is tilted, (3) a power failure occurs, or (4) there is a disparity between the pressure in the vapor circuit versus the pressure in the fresh gas circuit exceeding a specified tolerance.

Summary

The Tec 6 vaporizer is an electrically heated, thermostatically controlled, constant-temperature, pressurized, electromechanically coupled dual circuit, gas-vapor blender. The pressure in the vapor circuit is electronically regulated to equal the pressure in the fresh gas circuit. At a constant fresh gas flow rate, the operator regulates vapor flow using a conventional concentration control dial. When the fresh gas flow rate increases, the working pressure increases proportionally. For a given concentration setting even when varying the fresh gas flow rate, the vaporizer output is constant because the amount of flow through each circuit remains proportional.[83]

The Datex-Ohmeda Aladin Cassette Vaporizer

The vaporizer system used in the Datex-Ohmeda S5/Anesthesia Delivery Unit (ADU) is unique in that the single electronically controlled vaporizer is designed to deliver five different inhaled anesthetics including halothane, isoflurane, enflurane, sevoflurane, and desflurane. The vaporizer consists of a permanent internal control unit housed within the ADU and an interchangeable Aladin agent cassette that contains anesthetic liquid. The Aladin agent cassettes are color-coded for each anesthetic agent, and they are also magnetically coded so that the Datex-Ohmeda ADU can identify which anesthetic cassette has been inserted. The cassettes are filled using agent-specific fillers.[55]

Although very different in external appearance, the functional anatomy of the S/5 ADU cassette vaporizer (Aladin, Fig. 26-25) is very similar to that of the Dräger vapor 19.1 and 20.n and the Datex-Ohmeda Tec 4, Tec 5, and Tec 7 vaporizers. The Aladin system is functionally similar to these conventional vaporizers because it is also made up of a bypass chamber and vaporizing chamber. A fixed restrictor is located in the bypass chamber, and flow measurement sensors are located both in the bypass chamber and in the outlet of the vaporizing chamber. The heart of the S/5 ADU cassette vaporizer is the electronically regulated flow control valve located in the vaporizing chamber outlet. This valve is controlled by a central processing unit (CPU). The CPU receives input from multiple sources including the concentration control dial, a pressure sensor located inside the vaporizing chamber, a temperature sensor located inside the vaporizing chamber, a flow

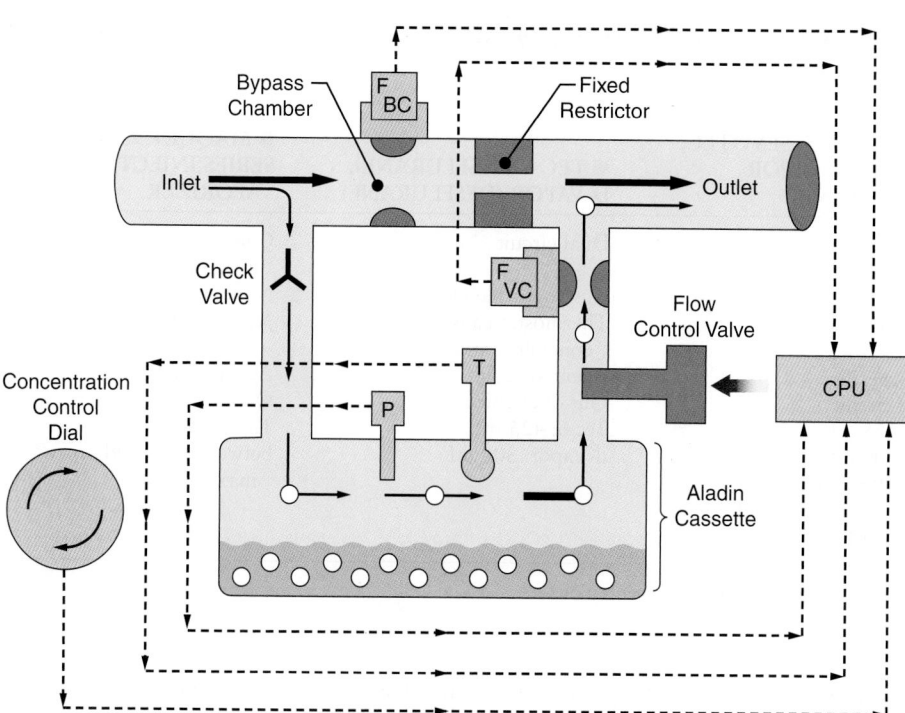

FIGURE 26-25. Simplified schematic of Datex-Ohmeda Aladin Cassette Vaporizer. The *black arrows* represent flow from the flowmeters, and the *white circles* represent anesthetic vapor. The heart of the vaporizer is the electronically controlled flow control valve located in the outlet of the vaporizing chamber. CPU, central processing unit; F_{BC}, flow measurement unit, which measures flow through the bypass chamber; F_{VC}, flow measurement unit, which measures flow through the vaporizing chamber; P, pressure sensor; T, temperature sensor. (Modified from Andrews, JJ: Operating Principles of the Datex-Ohmeda Aladin Cassette Vaporizer: A Collection of Color Illustrations. Washington, DC, Library of Congress, 2000.)

measurement unit located in the bypass chamber, and a flow measurement unit located in the outlet of the vaporizing chamber. The CPU also receives input from the flowmeters regarding the composition of the carrier gas. Using data from these multiple sources, the CPU is able to precisely regulate the flow control valve to attain the desired vapor concentration output. Appropriate electronic control of the flow control valve is essential to the proper function of this vaporizer.[55,89]

A fixed restrictor is located in the bypass chamber, and it causes flow from the vaporizer inlet to split into two flow streams (Fig. 26-25). One stream passes through the bypass chamber, and the other portion enters the inlet of the vaporizing chamber and passes through a one-way check valve. The presence of this check valve is unique to the Aladin system. This one-way valve prevents retrograde flow of the anesthetic vapor back into the bypass chamber, and its presence is crucial when delivering desflurane if the room temperature is greater than the boiling point for desflurane (22.8°C).[55] A precise amount of vapor-saturated carrier gas passes through the flow control valve, which is regulated by the CPU. This flow then joins the bypass flow and is directed to the outlet of the vaporizer.[55]

As mentioned in the discussion of the Tec 6, the controlled vaporization of desflurane presents a unique challenge, particularly when the room temperature is greater than the boiling point of desflurane (22.8°C). At higher temperatures, the pressure inside the vaporizer sump increases, and the sump becomes pressurized. When the sump pressure exceeds the pressure in the bypass chamber, the one-way check valve located in the vaporizing chamber inlet closes, preventing carrier gas from entering the vaporizing chamber. At this point, the carrier gas passes straight through the bypass chamber and its flow sensor. Under these conditions, the electronically regulated flow control valve simply meters in the appropriate flow of pure desflurane vapor needed to achieve the desired final concentration selected by the user. At least one case report has described a failure of the vaporizing chamber inlet check valve to function as designed. In this case, an anesthetic overdose occurred as a result of spillover of desflurane from the vaporiz-

ing chamber in a retrograde fashion into the bypass chamber. This report reminds ADU users to be cautious of this potential problem when desflurane is used.[89]

During operating conditions in which high fresh gas flow rates and/or high dial settings are used, large quantities of anesthetic liquid are rapidly vaporized. As a result, the temperature of the remaining liquid anesthetic and the vaporizer itself decrease as a result of energy consumption of the latent heat of vaporization. To offset this cooling effect, the S/5 ADU is equipped with a fan that forces warmed air from an "agent heating resistor" across the cassette (vaporizer sump) to raise its temperature when necessary. The fan is activated during two common clinical scenarios: (1) desflurane induction and maintenance, and (2) sevoflurane induction. A summary of the characteristics of various vaporizer models currently in use is found in Table 26-5.

The MAQUET 950 Series Injection Vaporizer

MAQUET, Inc. (Bridgwater, NJ) manufactures injection-type vaporizers for use with halothane, enflurane, and isoflurane. These vaporizers should be used with the MAQUET Servo Ventilator.[90] The injection vaporizer is similar in appearance to traditional variable bypass vaporizers and has a graduated concentration knob, keyed fill port with plug and locking screw, and a fill-level inspection window. In addition, there is an on/off switch with a safety lock.

Figure 26-26 describes the operation of the injection vaporizer. Mixed gas (1) flows into the vaporizer through a regulator valve (2) that prevents flow into the gas circuit when the ventilator bellows if full. When the bellows is empty, gas is allowed to flow into the vaporizer if the on/off switch (3) is set to on. In the vaporizer, an adjustable throttle valve (4) restricts gas flow, thus controlling pressure by directing excess gas into the liquid reservoir (5). Gas pressure within the reservoir forces anesthetic agent through a vaporization nozzle (6) and back into the gas stream. The pressure difference between the gas stream and the reservoir is proportional to the degree of throttling, which is controlled by the dial on the vaporizer.

TABLE 26-5

VAPORIZER MODELS AND CHARACTERISTICS

■ TYPE OF VAPORIZER	■ TEC 4, TEC 5, SEVOTEC, VAPOR 19.N, VAPOR 2000, ALADIN	■ TEC 6 (DESFLURANE), D-VAPOR (DESFLURANE)	■ MAQUET 950 SERIES INJECTION VAPORIZER
Carrier gas flow	Variable bypass	Dual circuit	Concentration-calibrated injector
Vaporization method	Flow-over	Gas/vapor blender	None; injected
Temperature compensation	Automatic	Thermostatically controlled at 39°C	None needed[a]
Calibration	Agent-specific	Agent-specific	Agent-specific
Position	Out of circuit	Out of circuit	Out of circuit
Fill capacity	Tec 4: 125 mL	Tec 6: 425 mL	125 mL (105 mL between min. and max. fill levels)
	Tec 5: 300 mL	d-Vapor: 300 mL	
	Vapor 19.n: 200 mL		
	Vapor 2000: 360 mL (dry wick)		
	Aladin: 250 mL		

[a]A 10°C increase in temperature will result in a 10% increase in output concentration.

The delivered concentration is mostly independent of the ventilator settings. There is normally no need for temperature compensation, as there is no vaporization of agent per se. The accuracy of the delivered agent is ±10% or 0.1 volume % (whichever is higher), and the concentration of the delivered anesthetic agent will deviate slightly depending on the mixture of the carrier gas.[90] The vaporizer should not be turned upside down or tilted sideways if there is liquid in the reservoir. Accumulation of the stabilization agent in halothane may interfere with normal operation, and vaporizers containing halothane should be emptied once every month. The vaporizer should be checked for leakage annually, according to MAQUET, Inc., and so should the concentration of the delivered anesthetic agent.[90]

FIGURE 26-26. Theory of operation of the MAQUET 950 series injection vaporizer. See text for details.

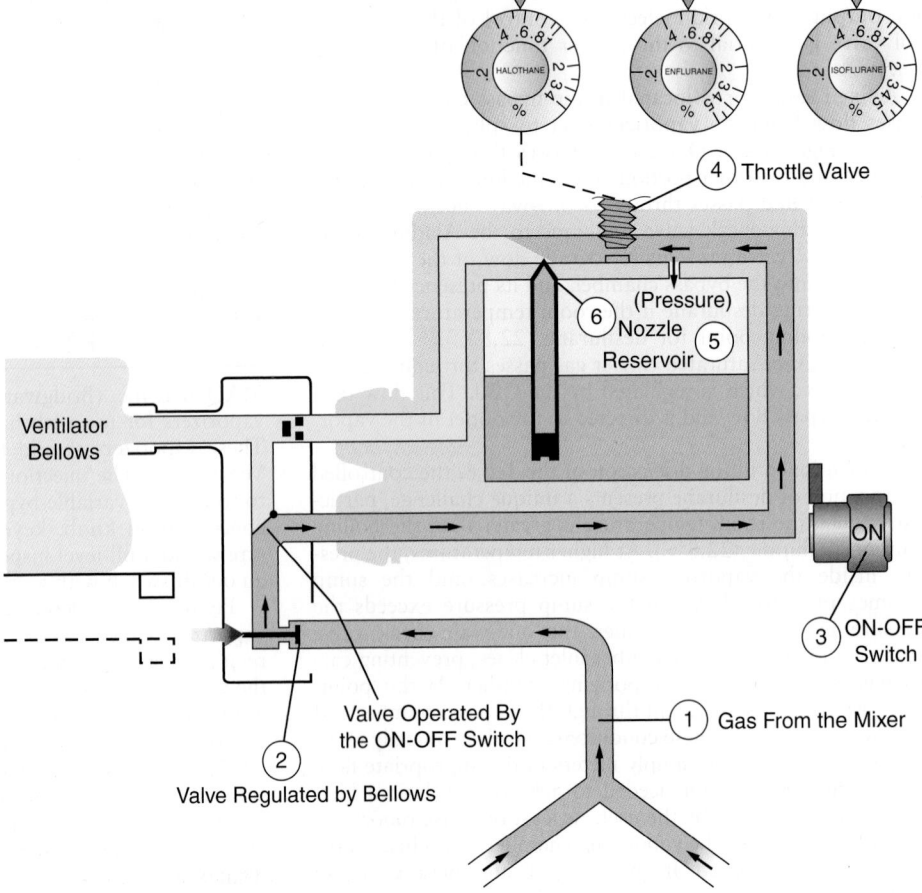

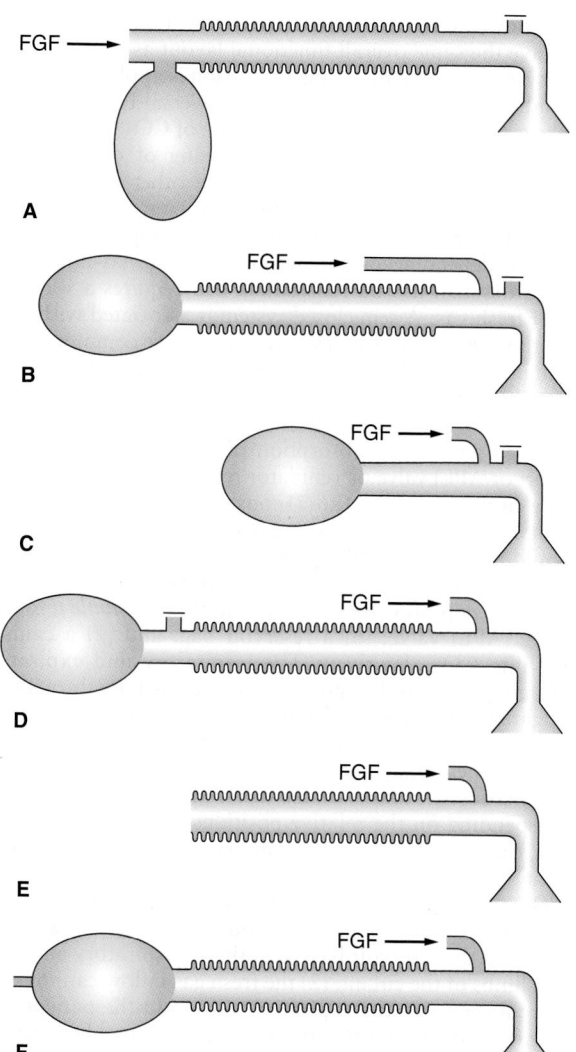

FIGURE 26-27. Mapleson breathing systems A-F. FGF, fresh gas flow. (Redrawn from Willis BA, Pender JW, Mapleson WW: Rebreathing in a T-piece: Volunteer and Theoretical Studies of the Jackson-Rees Modification of Ayre's T-piece during spontaneous respiration. Br J Anaesth 1975; 47: 1239, with permission.)

ANESTHETIC BREATHING CIRCUITS

As the prescribed mixture of gases from the flowmeters and vaporizer exits the anesthesia workstation at the common gas outlet, it then enters an anesthetic breathing circuit. The function of the anesthesia breathing circuit is not only to deliver oxygen and anesthetic gases to the patient, but also to eliminate CO_2. CO_2 can be removed either by washout with adequate fresh gas inflow or by the use of CO_2 absorbent media (e.g., soda lime absorption). The following discussion focuses on the semiclosed rebreathing circuits and the circle system.

Mapleson Systems

In 1954 Mapleson[91] described and analyzed five different semiclosed anesthetic systems; these are now classically referred to as the *Mapleson systems* and are designated with letters A through E (Fig. 26-27). Subsequently in 1975, Willis et al.[92] described the F system that was added to the original

five. The Mapleson systems consist of several common components. Theses components commonly include a face mask, a spring-loaded pop-off valve, reservoir tubing, fresh gas inflow tubing, and a reservoir bag. Within the Mapleson systems, three distinct functional groups can be seen: these include the A, the B/C, and D/E/F groups. The Mapleson A, also known as the *Magill Circuit*, has a spring-loaded pop-off valve located near the face mask, and the fresh gas flow enters the opposite end of the circuit near the reservoir bag. In the B and C systems, the spring-loaded pop-off valve is located near the face mask, but the fresh gas inlet tubing is located near the patient. The reservoir tubing and breathing bag serve as a blind limb where fresh gas, dead space gas, and alveolar gas can collect. Finally, in the Mapleson D/E/F group or "T-piece" group, the fresh gas enters near the patient, and excess gas is popped off at the opposite end of the circuit.

Even though the components and component arrangement are simple, functional analysis of the Mapleson systems can be complex.[93,94] The amount of CO_2 rebreathing associated with each system is multifactorial, and variables that dictate the ultimate CO_2 concentration include: (1) the fresh gas inflow rate, (2) the minute ventilation, (3) the mode of ventilation (spontaneous or controlled), (4) the tidal volume, (5) the respiratory rate, (6) the inspiratory to expiratory time ratio, (7) the duration of the expiratory pause, (8) the peak inspiratory flow rate, (9) the volume of the reservoir tube, (10) the volume of the breathing bag, (11) ventilation by mask, (12) ventilation through an endotracheal tube, and (13) the CO_2 sampling site.

The performance of the Mapleson systems is best understood by studying the expiratory phase of the respiratory cycle.[95] Illustrations of the various Mapleson system component arrangements may be found in Figure 26-27. During spontaneous ventilation, the Mapleson A has the best efficiency of the six systems, requiring a fresh gas inflow rate of only one times the minute ventilation to prevent rebreathing of CO_2. But it has the worst efficiency during controlled ventilation, requiring a minute ventilation as high as 20 L/min to prevent rebreathing. Systems DEF are slightly more efficient than systems BC. To prevent rebreathing CO_2, the DEF systems require a fresh gas inflow rate of approximately 2.5 times the minute ventilation, whereas the fresh gas inflow rates required for BC systems are somewhat higher.[93]

The following summarizes the relative efficiency of different Mapleson systems with respect to prevention of rebreathing, during spontaneous ventilation: A > D/F/E > C/B. During controlled ventilation, D/F/E > B/C > A.[91,93] The Mapleson A, B, and C systems are rarely used today, but the D, E, F systems are commonly employed. In the United States, the most popular representative from the D, E, and F group is the Bain circuit, and it will be discussed in the next section.

Bain Circuit

The Bain circuit is a coaxial circuit and a modification of the Mapleson D system. The fresh gas flows through a narrow inner tube within the outer corrugated tubing.[96] The central fresh gas tubing enters the outer corrugated hose near the reservoir bag, but the fresh gas actually empties into the circuit at the patient end (Fig. 26-28). Exhaled gases enter the corrugated tubing and are vented through the expiratory valve near the reservoir bag. The Bain circuit may be used for both spontaneous and controlled ventilation. The fresh gas inflow rate necessary to prevent rebreathing is 2.5 times the minute ventilation.

The Bain circuit has many advantages over other systems. It is lightweight, convenient, easily sterilized, and may be reusable. Scavenging of the gases from the expiratory valve is facilitated because the valve is located away from the patient. Exhaled gases in the outer reservoir tubing add warmth by countercurrent heat exchange to inspired fresh gases. The

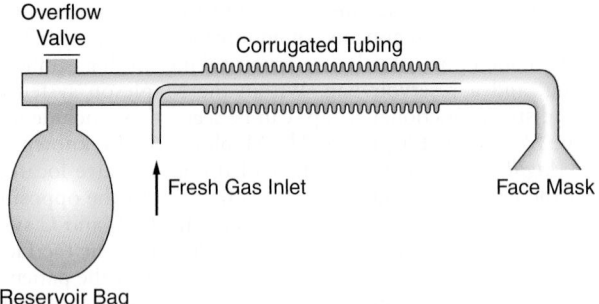

FIGURE 26-28.   The Bain circuit. (Redrawn from Bain JA, Spoerel WE: A streamlined anaesthetic system. Can Anaesth Soc J 1972; 19: 426, with permission.)

main hazards related to the use of the Bain circuit are either an unrecognized disconnection or kinking of the inner fresh gas hose. These problems can cause hypercarbia from inadequate gas flow or increased respiratory resistance. As with other circuits, an obstructed antimicrobial filter positioned between the Bain circuit and the endotracheal tube can result in increased resistance in the circuit, which in turn may produce hypoventilation and hypoxemia, and may even mimic the signs and symptoms of severe bronchospasm.[97]

The outer corrugated tube should be transparent to allow ongoing inspection of the inner tube. The integrity of the inner tube can be assessed as described by Pethick.[98] With his technique, high-flow oxygen is fed into the circuit while the patient end is occluded until the reservoir bag is filled. The patient end is opened, and oxygen is flushed into the circuit. If the inner tube is intact, the venturi effect occurs at the patient end. The venturi-induced decrease in pressure within the circuit results in the reservoir bag deflating. Conversely, a leak in the inner tube allows the fresh gas to escape into the expiratory limb, and the reservoir bag will remain inflated. This test is recommended as a part of the preanesthesia check if a Bain circuit is used.

Circle Breathing Systems

For many years, the overall design of the circle breathing system has changed very little from one anesthesia workstation manufacturer to the next. Both the individual components and the order in which they appeared in the circle system were consistent across major platforms. More recently, however, with the increasing technological complexity of the anesthesia workstation, the circle system has gone through some major changes as well. These changes have resulted in part from an effort to improve patient safety (as in the integration of fresh gas decoupling and inspiratory pressure limiters), but have also allowed the deployment of new technological advances. Examples of major new technologies include: (1) a return to the application of single-circuit piston-type ventilators, and (2) use of new spirometry devices that are located at the Y-connector instead of at the traditional location on the expiratory circuit limb. The following discussion focuses first on the traditional circle breathing system, and then follows a brief discussion of some variations in the designs of newer circle systems.

The Traditional Circle Breathing System

The circle system remains the most popular breathing system in the United States. It is so named because its components are arranged in a circular manner (Fig. 26-7). One version of the traditional circle system, referred to as either a *Universal F* or *single-limb circuit*, has increased in popularity over recent years. Although these systems appear very different externally, they have the same overall functional layout as the traditional circle system and the following discussion is applicable to both the traditional circle system and the Universal F system.

The circle system prevents rebreathing of CO_2 by use of CO_2 absorbents but allows partial rebreathing of other exhaled gases. The extent of rebreathing of the other exhaled gases depends on breathing circuit component arrangement and the fresh gas flow rate. A circle system can be semiopen, semiclosed, or closed, depending on the amount of fresh gas inflow.[99] A semiopen system has no rebreathing and requires a very high flow of fresh gas. A semiclosed system is associated with some rebreathing of exhaled gases and is the most commonly used system in the United States. A closed system is one in which the inflow gas exactly matches that being taken up, or consumed, by the patient. In a closed system, there is complete rebreathing of exhaled gases after absorption of CO_2, and the overflow (pop-off or APL) valve or ventilator relief valve remains closed.

The circle system (Fig. 26-7) consists of seven primary components, including: (1) a fresh gas inflow source; (2) inspiratory and expiratory unidirectional valves; (3) inspiratory and expiratory corrugated tubes; (4) a Y-piece connector; (5) an overflow or pop-off valve, referred to as the *adjustable pressure-limiting* (APL) valve; (6) a reservoir bag; and (7) a canister containing CO_2 absorbent. The inspiratory and expiratory valves are placed in the system to ensure gas flow through the corrugated hoses remains unidirectional. The fresh gas inflow enters the circle by a connection from the common gas outlet of the anesthesia machine.

Numerous variations of the circle arrangement are possible, depending on the relative positions of the unidirectional valves, the pop-off valve, the reservoir bag, the CO_2 absorber, and the site of fresh gas entry. However, to prevent rebreathing of CO_2 *in a traditional circle system*, three rules must be followed: (1) a unidirectional valve must be located between the patient and the reservoir bag on both the inspiratory and expiratory limbs of the circuit, (2) the fresh gas inflow cannot enter the circuit between the expiratory valve and the patient, and (3) the overflow (pop-off) valve cannot be located between the patient and the inspiratory valve. If these rules are followed, any arrangement of the other components will prevent rebreathing of CO_2.[100] Some newer anesthesia workstations now employ less traditional circle breathing systems. Two of these systems (the Datex-Ohmeda S/5 ADU breathing system and the Dräger Narkomed 6000 series and Fabius GS workstations breathing system) are discussed later in greater detail (see "Anesthesia Workstation Variations").

The most efficient circle system arrangement with the highest conservation of fresh gases is one in which the unidirectional valves are near the patient and the pop-off valve is located just downstream from the expiratory valve. This arrangement minimizes dead space gas and preferentially eliminates exhaled alveolar gases. A more practical arrangement, the one used on most conventional anesthesia machines (Fig. 26-7), is somewhat less efficient because it allows alveolar and dead space gases to mix before they are vented.[101,102]

The main advantages of the circle system over other breathing systems include its (1) maintenance of relatively stable inspired gas concentrations, (2) conservation of respiratory moisture and heat, and (3) prevention of operating room pollution. Additionally, the circle system can be used as a semiclosed system or as a closed system with very low fresh gas flows. The major disadvantage of the circle system stems from its complex design. Commonly, the circle system may have ten or more different connections. These multiple connection sites set the stage for misconnections, disconnections, obstructions, and leaks. In an ASA "Closed Claims" analysis of adverse anesthetic outcomes arising from gas delivery equipment, over one third (25/72) of malpractice claims resulted from breathing circuit misconnections or disconnections.[10] Malfunction of the circle system's unidirectional valves can result in life-threatening problems. Rebreathing can occur if the valves stick in the open position, and total occlusion of the circuit can occur if they are stuck shut. If the expiratory valve is stuck in the closed position, breath stacking and barotrauma or volutrauma can result. Obstructed filters located in the expiratory limb of the circle breathing system have caused increased airway pressures, hemodynamic collapse, and bilateral tension pneumothorax. Causes of circle system obstruction and failure include manufacturing defects, debris, patient secretions, and particulate obstruction from other odd sources such as albuterol nebulization.[103–106] Some systems, such as the Datex-Ohmeda 7900 SmartVent, use flow transducers located on both the inspiratory and expiratory limbs of the circle system. In one report, cracks in the flow transducer tubing used by this system produced a leak in the circle system that was difficult to detect.[107]

CO₂ ABSORBENTS

In the early 2000s, there were several reports of adverse chemical reactions between CO_2 absorbent materials and anesthetic agents. Some of these undesirable interactions are quite dramatic, such as sevoflurane interacting with desiccated Baralyme, resulting in fires within the breathing system and severe patient injury.[108,109] Although other sources of ignition and fire in the breathing system continue to be described,[110] the Baralyme-sevoflurane problem is somewhat unique in that nothing "unusual" is added to or removed from the breathing system for this to occur. Other reactions between agents such as desflurane or sevoflurane and desiccated strong base absorbents can produce more insidious patient morbidity and even death from the release of byproducts such as carbon monoxide or compound A.[111] Although absorbent materials may be problematic, they still represent an important component of the circle breathing system. Different anesthesia breathing systems eliminate CO_2 with varying degrees of efficiency. The closed and semiclosed circle system both *require* that CO_2 be absorbed from the exhaled gases to avoid hypercapnia. If one could design an ideal CO_2 absorbent, its characteristics would include lack of reactivity with common anesthetics, lack of toxicity, low resistance to air flow, low cost, ease of handling, and efficient in CO_2 absorption.

The Absorber Canister

On modern anesthesia machines, the absorber canister is composed of two clear plastic canisters arranged in series (Fig. 26-7). The canisters can be filled with either loose bulk absorbent or with absorbent supplied by the factory in prefilled plastic disposable cartridges called *prepacks*. Free granules from bulk absorbent can create a clinically significant leak if they lodge between the clear plastic canister and the O-ring gasket of the absorber. Leaks have also been caused by defective prepacks, which were larger than factory specifications.[112] Prepacks can also cause total obstruction of the circle system if the clear plastic shipping wrapper is not removed prior to use.[113] The newest workstations from GE Healthcare/Datex-Ohmeda incorporate proprietary CO_2 absorbent canisters that allow exchange of the canisters while maintaining the breathing circuit integrity.

Chemistry of Absorbents

Three formulations of CO_2 absorbents are commonly available today: soda lime, Baralyme (a mixture of calcium hydroxide and barium hydroxide), and calcium hydroxide lime (Amsorb). Of these agents, the most commonly used is soda lime. All serve to eliminate CO_2 from the breathing circuit with varying degrees of efficiency.

By weight, the approximate composition of "high moisture" soda lime is 80% calcium hydroxide, 15% water, 4% sodium hydroxide, and 1% potassium hydroxide (an activator). Small amounts of silica are added to produce calcium and sodium silicate. This addition produces a harder and more stable pellet and thereby reduces dust formation. The efficiency of the soda lime absorption varies inversely with the hardness; therefore, little silicate is used in contemporary soda lime. Sodium hydroxide is the catalyst for the CO_2 absorptive properties of soda lime.[114,115] Baralyme is a mixture of approximately 20% barium hydroxide and 80% calcium hydroxide. It may also contain some potassium hydroxide. Baralyme is the primary CO_2 absorbent implicated as an agent that may produce fires in the breathing system when used with sevoflurane. Calcium hydroxide lime is one of the newest clinically available CO_2 absorbents. It consists primarily of calcium hydroxide and calcium chloride and contains two setting agents: calcium sulfate and polyvinylpyrrolidone. The latter two agents serve to enhance the hardness and porosity of the agent.[116] The most significant advantage of calcium hydroxide lime over other agents is its lack of the strong bases, sodium and potassium hydroxide. The absence of these chemicals eliminates the undesirable production of carbon monoxide, the nephrotoxic substance known as *compound A*, and may reduce or eliminate the possibility of a fire in the breathing circuit.[117] The most significant disadvantages of calcium hydroxide lime are (1) less absorptive capacity—about 50% less than strong-base–containing absorbents, and (2) generally higher cost per unit than other absorbents.[118,119]

The size of the actual absorptive granules has been determined over time by trial and error. The current size particles represent a compromise between resistance to air flow and absorptive efficiency.[120] The smaller the granule size, the greater the surface area that is available for absorption. However, as particle size decreases, air flow resistance increases. The granular size of soda lime and Baralyme used in clinical practice is between 4 and 8 mesh, a size at which absorptive surface area and resistance to flow are optimized. Mesh size refers to the number of openings per linear inch in a sieve through which the granular particles can pass. A 4-mesh screen means that there are four quarter-inch openings per linear inch. Likewise, an 8-mesh screen has eight per linear inch.[114]

The absorption of CO_2 by absorbents such as soda lime occurs by a series of chemical reactions; it is not a physical process like soaking water into a sponge. CO_2 combines with water to form carbonic acid. Carbonic acid reacts with the hydroxides to form sodium (or potassium) carbonate and water. Calcium hydroxide accepts the carbonate to form calcium carbonate and sodium (or potassium) hydroxide. The equations are as follows:

1. $CO_2 + H_2O \Leftrightarrow H_2CO_3$
2. $H_2CO_3 + 2NaOH (KOH) \Leftrightarrow Na_2CO_3 (K_2CO_3) + 2H_2O$ + Heat
3. $Na_2CO_3 (K_2CO_3) + Ca(OH)_2 \Leftrightarrow CaCO_3 + 2NaOH$ (KOH)

Some CO_2 may react directly with $Ca(OH)_2$, but this reaction is much slower.

The reaction with Baralyme differs from that of soda lime because more water is liberated by a direct reaction of barium hydroxide and CO_2.

1. $Ba(OH)_2 + 8H_2O + CO_2 \Leftrightarrow BaCO_3 + 9H_2O$ + Heat
2. $9H_2O + 9CO_2 \Leftrightarrow 9H_2CO_3$
   Then by direct reactions and by KOH and NaOH,
3. $9H_2CO_3 + 9Ca(OH)_2 \Leftrightarrow CaCO_3 + 18H_2O$ + Heat

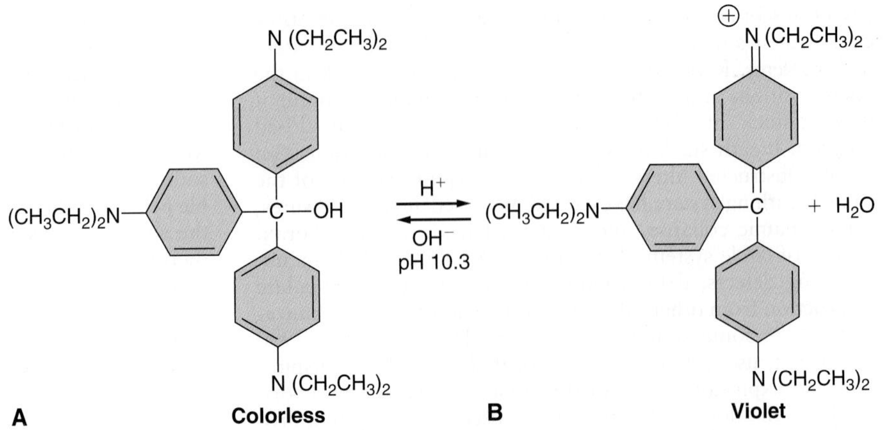

FIGURE 26-29.   A and B. Ethyl violet. See text for details. (Reprinted from Andrews JJ, Johnston RV Jr, Bee DE et al: Photodeactivation of ethyl violet: A potential hazard of Sodasorb. Anesthesiology 1990; 72: 59, with permission.)

A   Colorless   B   Violet

Absorptive Capacity

The maximum amount of CO_2 that can be absorbed by soda lime is 26 L of CO_2 per 100 g of absorbent. The absorptive capacity of calcium hydroxide lime is significantly less, and has been reported at 10.2 L per 100 g of absorbent.[116,118] However, as previously mentioned, absorptive capacity is the product of both available chemical reactivity and physical (granule) availability. As the absorbent granules stack up in the absorber canisters, small passageways inevitably form. These small passages channel gases preferentially through low-resistance areas. Because of this phenomenon, functional absorptive capacity of either soda lime or calcium hydroxide lime may be substantially decreased. In practice, because of channeling, the efficiency of soda lime may be reduced to allow only 10 to 20 L or less of CO_2 to actually be absorbed per 100 g of absorbent.[121]

Indicators

Ethyl violet is the pH indicator added to both soda lime and Baralyme to help assess the functional integrity of the absorbent. This compound is a substituted triphenylmethane dye with a critical pH of 10.3.[115] Ethyl violet changes from colorless to violet in color when the pH of the absorbent decreases as a result of CO_2 absorption. When the absorbent is fresh, the pH exceeds the critical pH of the indicator dye, and it exists in its colorless form (Fig. 26-29A). However, as absorbent becomes exhausted, the pH decreases below 10.3, and ethyl violet changes to its violet form (Fig. 26-29B) because of alcohol dehydration. This change in color indicates the absorptive capacity of the material has been consumed. Unfortunately, in some circumstances ethyl violet may not always be a reliable indicator of the functional status of absorbent. For example, prolonged exposure of ethyl violet to fluorescent lights can produce photodeactivation of this dye. When this occurs, the absorbent appears white even though it may have a reduced pH and its absorptive capacity has been exhausted.[122] Even in the absence of color changes, clinical signs that the CO_2 absorbent is exhausted include:

1. Increased spontaneous respiratory rate (only reliable when no muscle relaxant is used)
2. Initial increase in hemodynamics (blood pressure and heart rate), followed later by a decrease in both
3. Increased sympathetic drive: skin flushing, sweating, tachyarrhythmia, hypermetabolic state (increased CO_2 production; must rule out malignant hyperthermia)
4. Respiratory acidosis on arterial blood gas analysis
5. Increased surgical bleeding due to both hypertension and coagulopathy.

Interactions of Inhaled Anesthetics With Absorbents

10 It is important and desirable to have CO_2 absorbents that neither release toxic particles or fumes nor produce toxic compounds when exposed to common anesthetics. Soda lime and Baralyme generally fit this description, but inhaled anesthetics do interact with absorbents to some extent. Historically speaking, an uncommon anesthetic, trichloroethylene, reacts with soda lime to produce toxic compounds. In the presence of alkali and heat, trichloroethylene degrades into the cerebral neurotoxin dichloroacetylene, which can cause cranial nerve lesions and encephalitis. Phosgene, a potent pulmonary irritant, is also produced and phosgene can cause adult respiratory distress syndrome.[123]

Sevoflurane has been shown to produce degradation products on interaction with CO_2 absorbents.[111,124,125] The major degradation product produced is an olefin compound known as fluoromethyl-2,2-difluoro-1-(trifluoromethyl) vinyl ether, or compound A. During sevoflurane anesthesia, factors apparently leading to an increase in the concentration of compound A include (1) low flow or closed circuit anesthetic techniques, (2) the use of Baralyme rather than soda lime, (3) higher concentrations of sevoflurane in the anesthetic circuit, (4) higher absorbent temperatures, and (5) fresh absorbent.[124–127] Interestingly, the dehydration of Baralyme increases the concentration of compound A, but the dehydration of soda lime decreases the concentration of compound A.[128,129] Apparently, the degradation products released during clinical conditions do not commonly result in adverse effects in humans even during low-flow anesthesia,[127] but further studies are needed to verify this.[130–132]

11 Desiccated strong-base absorbents can also degrade contemporary inhaled anesthetics to clinically significant concentrations of carbon monoxide (CO) as well as trifluoromethane, which can interfere with anesthetic gas monitoring.[111] Under certain conditions, this process can produce very high carboxyhemoglobin concentrations, reaching 35% or more.[133] Higher levels of carbon monoxide are more likely after prolonged contact between absorbent and anesthetics, and after disuse of an absorber for at least 2 days, especially over a weekend. Thus, case reports describing carbon monoxide poisoning have been most common in patients anesthetized on Monday morning, presumably because continuous flow from the anesthesia machine dehydrated the absorbents over the weekend.[134,135] Fresh gas flow rates of ≥5 L/min through the breathing system and absorbent (without a patient connected) are sufficient to cause critical drying of the absorbent material. Dessication is even worse when the breathing bag is left off the breathing circuit. Absence of the reservoir bag facilitates retrograde flow through the circle system (Fig. 26-30).[133] Because the inspiratory

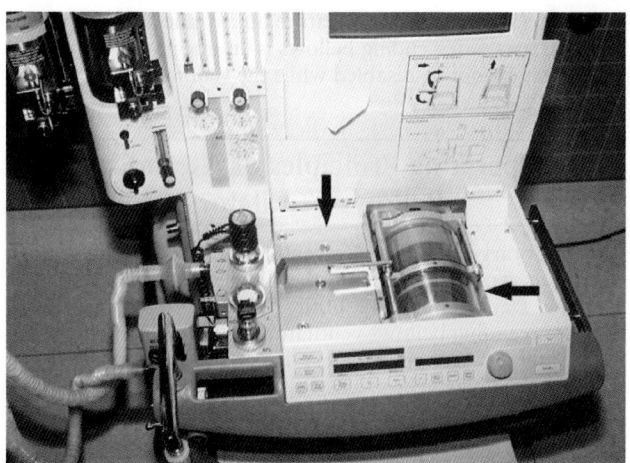

FIGURE 26-30. The Dräger Medical Narkomed 6000 with its single-circuit ventilator. The *horizontal arrow* indicates the piston cylinder unit of the Divan Ventilator. The *vertical arrow* indicates the rectangular valve manifold for fresh gas decoupling.

valve leaflet produces some resistance to flow, the fresh gas flow takes the retrograde path of least resistance through the absorbent and out the 22 mm breathing bag mount.

Several factors appear to increase the production of carbon monoxide and resulting elevated carboxyhemoglobin levels. Those factors include (1) the inhaled anesthetic used (for a given MAC multiple, the magnitude of CO production from greatest to least is desflurane ≥ enflurane > isoflurane >> halothane = sevoflurane); (2) the absorbent dryness (completely dry absorbent produces more CO than hydrated absorbent); (3) the type of absorbent (at a given water content, Baralyme produces more CO than does soda lime); (4) the temperature (increased temperature increases CO production); (5) the anesthetic concentration (more CO is produced from higher anesthetic concentrations)[136]; (6) low fresh gas flow rates; and (7) reduced experimental animal (patient) size[111,137] per 100 g of absorbent.

Several interventions have been suggested to reduce the incidence of carbon monoxide exposure in humans undergoing general anesthesia.[135] These interventions include (1) educating anesthesia personnel regarding the etiology of CO production, (2) turning off the anesthesia machine at the conclusion of the last case of the day to eliminate fresh gas flow that dries the absorbent, (3) changing CO_2 absorbent if fresh gas was found flowing during the morning machine check, (4) rehydrating desiccated absorbent by adding water to the absorbent,[118] (5) changing the chemical composition of soda lime to reduce or eliminate potassium hydroxide (such products now available include Dragersorb 800 plus, Sofnolime, and Spherasorb), and (6) using absorbent materials such as calcium hydroxide lime that are free of both sodium and potassium hydroxides. The elimination of sodium and potassium hydroxides from desiccated soda lime diminishes or eliminates degradation of desflurane to carbon monoxide and sevoflurane to compound A, but does not compromise CO_2 absorption.[117,138] Because of the increasing evidence that exposure of volatile anesthetics to desiccated CO_2 absorbents, the APSF convened in 2005 a conference entitled, "Carbon Dioxide Absorbent Desiccation: APSF Conference on Safety Considerations." The consensus statement following this conference included two broad recommendations: 1) the use of CO_2 absorbents that, when exposed to volatile anesthetics, do not result in significant degradation; and (2) that institutions have in place policies that address prevention of CO_2 desiccation if conventional CO_2 absorbents are used. In circumstances where absorbents that degrade volatile anesthetics are used (such as the strong-base absorbents), the APSF conference

experts agreed with the following recommendations: 1) turn off all gas flow when the machine is not in use, 2) change absorbents regularly (on Monday mornings, as the absorbent may have become desiccated over the weekend), 3) change absorbent whenever the color change indicates exhaustion, 4) change BOTH canisters in a two-canister system, 5) change absorbent whenever the fresh gas flow has been left on for an extensive or indeterminate period of time, and 6) if compact canisters are used, consider changing them more frequently.[139]

One extremely rare, but potentially life-threatening, complication related to CO_2 absorbent use is the development of fires within the breathing system. Specifically, this can occur as the result of interactions between the strong-base absorbents (particularly Baralyme) and the inhaled anesthetic, sevoflurane. In August 2003, Abbott Laboratories changed the package insert for sevoflurane to describe this rare phenomenon and the conditions under which it could occur. Almost 1 year later, in the fall of 2004, several case reports describing patient injuries related to this problem were published (all involving Baralyme). It seems that when desiccated strong-base absorbents are exposed to sevoflurane, absorber temperatures of several hundred degrees may result from their interaction.[109] The buildup of very high temperatures, the formation of combustible degradation byproducts (formaldehyde, methanol, and formic acid), plus the oxygen- or nitrous oxide–enriched environment provide all the substrates necessary for a fire to occur.[111] Avoidance of the use of the combination of sevoflurane with strong-base absorbents, particularly Baralyme, especially if it has become desiccated, is the best way to prevent this unusual and potentially life-threatening complication.

ANESTHESIA VENTILATORS

The ventilator on the modern anesthesia workstation serves as a mechanized substitute for the manual squeezing of the reservoir bag of the circle system, the Bain circuit, or another breathing system. As recently as the late 1980s, anesthesia ventilators were mere adjuncts to the anesthesia machine. Today, in newer anesthesia workstations, they have attained a prominent central role. In addition to the near ubiquitous role of the anesthesia ventilator in today's anesthesia workstation, many advanced intensive care unit–style ventilation features have also been integrated into anesthesia ventilators (Fig. 26-30). Although many similarities exist between today's anesthesia ventilator and intensive care unit ventilator, some fundamental differences in ventilation parameters and control systems still remain. This discussion focuses on the classification, operating principles, and hazards associated with contemporary anesthesia ventilators.

Classification

Ventilators can be classified according to their power source, drive mechanism, cycling mechanism, and bellows type.[140,141]

Power Source

The power source required to operate a mechanical ventilator is provided by compressed gas, electricity, or both. Older pneumatic ventilators required only a pneumatic power source to function properly. Contemporary electronic ventilators from Dräger Medical, Datex-Ohmeda, and other companies require either an electrical-only or both an electrical and a pneumatic power source.

Drive Mechanism and Circuit Designation

Double-circuit ventilators (in which one circuit contains patient gas and the other circuit contains drive gas) are used most commonly on modern anesthesia workstations. Generally, these conventional ventilators are pneumatically driven. In a double-circuit ventilator, a driving force such as pressurized gas compresses a component analogous to the reservoir bag known as the *ventilator bellows*. The bellows then in turn deliver ventilation to the patient. The driving gas in the Datex-Ohmeda 7000, 7810, 7100, and 7900 is 100% oxygen. In the North American Dräger AV-E and AV-2+, a venturi device mixes oxygen and air. Some newer pneumatic anesthesia workstations have the ability for the user to select whether compressed air or oxygen is used as the driving gas.

In recent years, with the introduction of circle breathing systems that integrate fresh gas decoupling, resurgence has been seen in the utilization of mechanically driven anesthesia ventilators. These "piston"-type ventilators use a computer-controlled stepper motor instead of compressed drive gas to actuate gas movement in the breathing system. In these systems, rather than having dual circuits, a single patient gas circuit is present. Thus, they are classified as piston-driven, single-circuit ventilators. The piston operates much like the plunger of a syringe to deliver the desired tidal volume or airway pressure to the patient. Sophisticated computerized controls are able to provide advanced types of ventilatory support such as synchronized intermittent mandatory ventilation, pressure-controlled ventilation, and pressure support–assisted ventilation, in addition to the conventional control mode ventilation. Because the patient's mechanical breath is delivered without the use of compressed gas to actuate a bellows, these systems consume dramatically less compressed gas during ventilator operation than traditional pneumatic ventilators. This improvement in efficiency may have clinical significance when the anesthesia workstation is used in a setting where no pipeline gas supply is available (e.g., remote locations or office-based anesthesia practices).

Cycling Mechanism

Most anesthesia machine ventilators are time-cycled and provide ventilator support in the control mode. Inspiratory phase is initiated by a timing device. Older pneumatic ventilators use a fluidic timing device. Contemporary electronic ventilators use a solid-state electronic timing device and are thus classified as time-cycled and electronically controlled. More advanced ventilation modes such as synchronized intermittent mandatory ventilation, pressure-controlled ventilation, and modes that use a pressure-support option may have an adjustable threshold pressure trigger as well. In these modes, pressure sensors provide feedback to the ventilator control system to allow it to determine when to initiate and/or terminate the respiratory cycle.

Bellows Classification

⑫ The direction of bellows movement during the expiratory phase determines the bellows classification. *Ascending (standing) bellows* ascend during the expiratory phase (Fig. 26-31B), whereas *descending (hanging) bellows* descend during the expiratory phase. Older pneumatic ventilators and some new anesthesia workstations use weighted descending bellows, while most contemporary electronic ventilators have an ascending bellows design. Of the two configurations, the ascending bellows is generally thought to be safer. An ascending bellows will not fill if a total disconnection occurs. However, the bellows of a descending bellows ventilator will continue its upward and downward movement despite a patient disconnection. The driving gas pushes the bellows upward during the inspiratory phase. During the expiratory phase, room air is entrained into the breathing system at the site of the disconnection because gravity acts on the weighted bellows. The disconnection pressure monitor and the volume monitor may be fooled even if a disconnection is complete.[40] Some contemporary anesthesia workstation designs have returned to the descending bellows to integrate fresh gas decoupling (Dräger Medical Julian and Datascope

Anestar). An essential safety feature on any anesthesia workstation that uses a descending bellows is an integrated CO_2 apnea alarm that cannot be disabled while the ventilator is in use.

Operating Principles of Ascending Bellows Ventilators

Contemporary examples of ascending bellows, double-circuit, electronic ventilators include the Dräger Medical AV-E, AV-2+, the Datex-Ohmeda 7000, 7800, and 7900 series. A generic ascending bellows ventilator is illustrated in Figure 26-31. It may be viewed as a breathing bag (bellows) located within a clear plastic box. The bellows physically separates the driving gas circuit from the patient gas circuit. The driving gas circuit is located outside the bellows, and the patient gas circuit is inside the bellows. During the inspiratory phase (Fig. 26-31A, *left*) the driving gas enters the bellows chamber, causing the pressure within it to increase. This increase in pressure is responsible for two events. First, the ventilator relief valve closes, preventing anesthetic gas from escaping into the scavenging system. Second, the bellows is compressed, and the anesthetic gas within the bellows is delivered to the patient's lungs. This compression action is analogous to the hand of the anesthesiologist squeezing the breathing bag.[52]

During the expiratory phase (Fig. 26-31B), the driving gas exits the bellows housing. This produces a drop to atmospheric pressure within both the bellows housing and the pilot line to the ventilator relief valve. The decrease in pressure to the ventilator relief valve causes the "mushroom valve" portion of the assembly to open. Exhaled patient gases refill the bellows before any scavenging can begin. The bellows refill first because a weighted ball (like those used in ball-type positive end-expiratory pressure [PEEP] valves) or similar device is incorporated into the base of the ventilator relief valve. This ball produces 2 to 3 cm water of back pressure; therefore, scavenging occurs only after the bellows fills completely and the pressure inside the bellows exceeds the pressure threshold of the "ball valve." This design causes all ascending bellows ventilators to produce 2 to 3 cm water pressure of PEEP within the breathing circuit when the ventilator is in use. Scavenging occurs only during the expiratory phase, as the ventilator relief valve is open only during expiration.[52]

It is important to understand that on most anesthesia workstations, gas flow from the anesthesia machine into the breathing circuit is continuous and independent of ventilator activity. During the inspiratory phase of mechanical ventilation, the ventilator relief valve is closed (Fig. 26-31A), and the breathing system's APL or pop-off valve is most commonly out of circuit. Therefore, the patient's lungs receive the volume from the bellows plus that from the flowmeters during the inspiratory phase. Factors that influence the correlation between set tidal volume and exhaled tidal volume include the flowmeter settings, the inspiratory time, the compliance of the breathing circuit, external leakage, and the location of the tidal volume sensor. Usually, the volume gained from the flowmeters during inspiration is counteracted by the volume lost to compliance of the breathing circuit, and set tidal volume generally approximates the exhaled tidal volume. However, certain conditions such as inappropriate activation of the oxygen flush valve during the inspiratory phase can result in barotrauma and/or volutrauma because excess pressure and volume may not be able to be vented from the circle system.[52]

Problems and Hazards

Numerous hazards are associated with anesthesia ventilators. These include problems with the breathing circuit, the bellows assembly, and the control assembly.

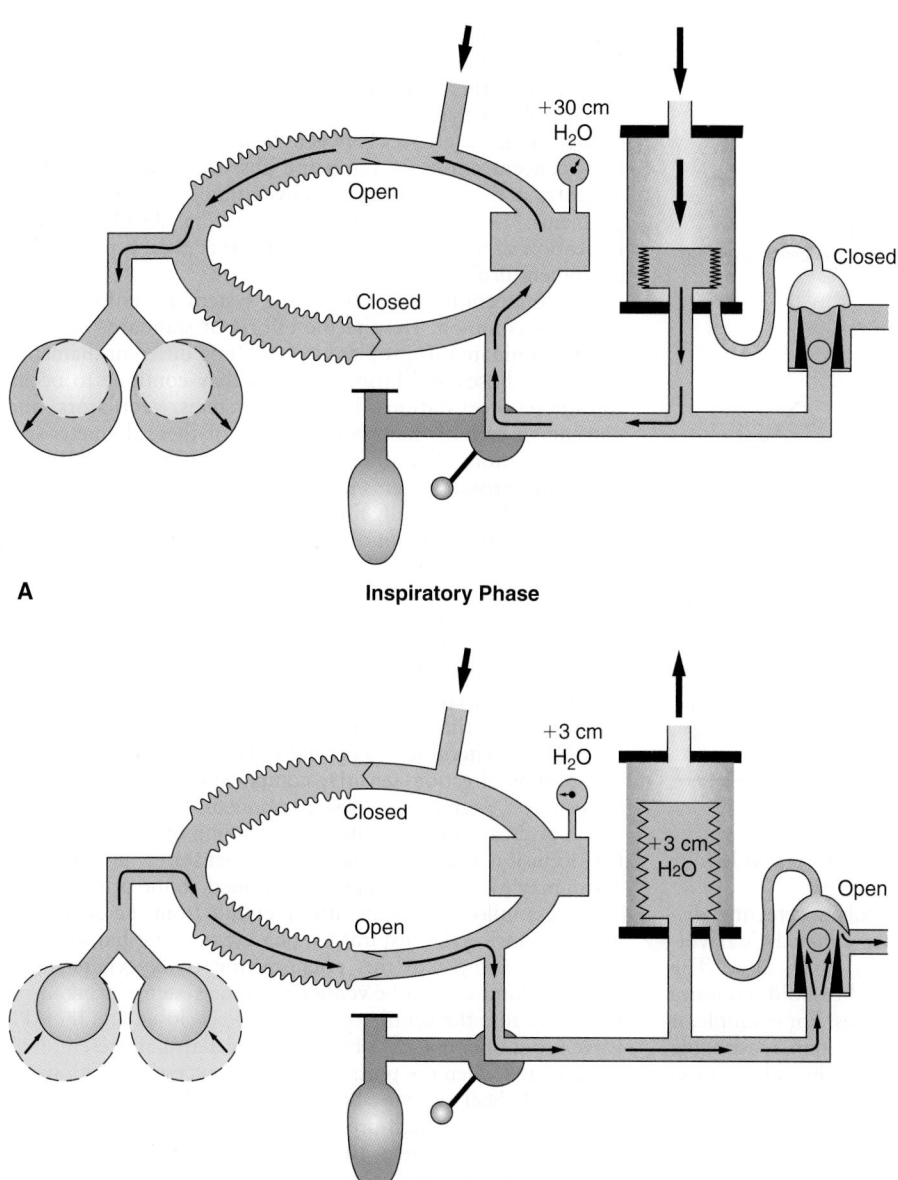

+30 cm H₂O

Open

Closed

Closed

A   **Inspiratory Phase**

+3 cm H₂O

Closed

+3 cm H₂O

Open

Open

B   **Expiratory Phase Late**

FIGURE 26-31. Inspiratory (**A**) and expiratory (**B**) phases of gas flow in a traditional circle system with an ascending bellows ventilator. The bellows physically separates the driving-gas circuit from the patient gas circuit. The driving-gas circuit is located outside the bellows and the patient gas circuit is inside the bellows. During inspiratory phase (**A**), the driving gas enters the bellows chamber, causing the pressure within it to increase. This causes the ventilator relief valve to close, preventing anesthetic gas from escaping into the scavenging system and the bellows to compress, delivering anesthetic gas within the bellows to the patient's lungs. During expiratory phase (**B**), pressure within the bellows chamber and the pilot line decreases to zero, causing the mushroom portion of the ventilator relief valve to open. Gas exhaled by the patient refills the bellows before any scavenging occurs because a weighted ball is incorporated into the base of the ventilator relief valve. Scavenging occurs only during the expiratory phase because the ventilator relief valve is open only during expiration. (Reprinted from Andrews JJ: The Circle System. A Collection of 30 Color Illustrations. Washington, DC, Library of Congress, 1998, with permission.)

Traditional Circle System Problems

Breathing circuit misconnections and disconnection are a leading cause of critical incidents in anesthesia.[10,142] The most common disconnection site is at the Y-piece. Disconnections can be complete or partial (leaks). In the past, a common source of leaks with older absorbers was failure to close the APL or pop-off valve on initiation of mechanical ventilation. On today's anesthesia workstations, the bag/ventilator selector switch has virtually eliminated this problem, as the APL valve is usually out of circuit when the ventilator mode is selected. Pre-existing undetected leaks can exist in compressed, corrugated, disposable anesthetic circuits. To detect such a leak preoperatively, the circuit must be fully expanded before the circuit is checked for leaks.[143] As previously mentioned, disconnections and leaks manifest more readily with the ascending bellows ventilator systems because they result in a situation in which the bellows will not refill.[40]

Several disconnection monitors exist, although none should replace vigilance. Monitoring of breath sounds and observation of chest wall excursion should continue despite use of both mechanical (spirometers and pressure sensors) and physiologic monitors.

Pneumatic and electronic pressure monitors are helpful in diagnosing disconnections. Factors that influence monitor effectiveness include the disconnection site, the pressure sensor location, the threshold pressure alarm limit, the inspiratory flow rate, and the resistance of the disconnected breathing circuit.[144,145] Various anesthesia workstations and ventilators have different locations for the airway pressure sensor and different values for the threshold pressure alarm limit. The threshold pressure alarm limit may be preset at the factory or adjustable. An audible or visual alarm is actuated if the peak inspiratory pressure of the breathing circuit does not exceed the threshold pressure alarm limit. When an adjustable threshold pressure alarm limit is available, such as on many workstations from Dräger Medical, the operator should set the pressure alarm limit to within 5 cm water of the peak inspiratory pressure. On systems that have an "autoset" feature, when activated, the threshold limit is automatically set at 3 to 5 cm water pressure below the current peak inspiratory pressure. On such systems, failure to reset the threshold pressure alarm limit may result in either an "Apnea Pressure" or "Threshold Low" alert. Figure 26-32 illustrates how a partial disconnection (leak) may be unrecognized by the low-pressure

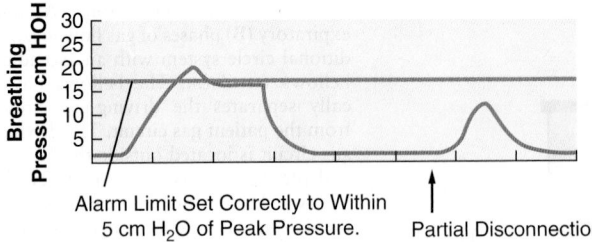

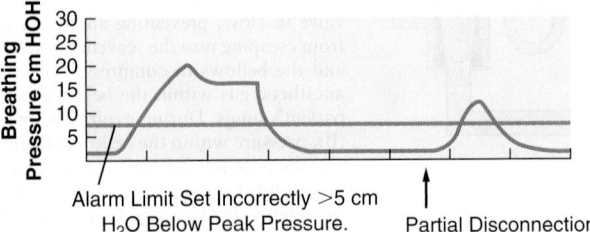

FIGURE 26-32. Threshold pressure alarm limit. *Top.* The threshold pressure alarm limit (*dotted line*) has been set appropriately. An alarm is actuated when a partial disconnection occurs (*arrow*) because the threshold pressure alarm limit is not exceeded by the breathing circuit pressure. *Bottom.* A partial disconnection is unrecognized by the pressure monitor because the threshold pressure alarm limit has been set too low. (Redrawn from Baromed Breathing Pressure Monitor: Operator's Instruction Manual. Telford, PA, North American Dräger, August 1986, with permission.)

monitor if the threshold pressure alarm limit is set too low or if the factory preset value is relatively low.

Respiratory volume monitors are useful in detecting disconnections. Volume monitors may sense exhaled tidal volume, inhaled tidal volume, minute volume, or all three. The user should bracket the high and low threshold volumes slightly above and below the exhaled volumes. For example, if the exhaled minute volume of a patient is 10 L/min, reasonable alarm limits would be 8 to 12 L/min. Many of the older Datex-Ohmeda ventilators are equipped with volume monitor sensors that use infrared light/turbine technology. These volume sensors are usually located in the expiratory limb of the breathing circuit and thus measure exhaled tidal volume. In the case of the Datex-Ohmeda S/5 ADU, a special attachment known as the D-lite spirometry connector is placed in the breathing circuit. This device is actually placed at or near the level of the patient connection and permits measurement of both inhaled and exhaled volumes and pressures (see "Anesthesia Workstation Variations"). With the older infrared type sensors, exposure to a direct beam of light from the overhead surgical lighting could cause erroneous volume readings as the surgical beam interfered with the infrared sensor.[146] Other types of expiratory volume sensors can be seen in systems such as the Datex-Ohmeda Aestiva, Aespire, and other workstations that incorporate the 7100 ventilator or 7900 SmartVent. These systems generally use differential pressure transduction technology to determine inhaled and exhaled volumes and to measure airway pressures. The Dräger Medical Narkomed 6000 series, 2B, and Fabius GS workstations commonly use an ultrasonic flow sensor located on the expiratory limb. Still other systems from Dräger measure exhaled volume using "hot wire" sensor technology. With this type of sensor, a tiny array of two platinum wires is electrically heated to a high temperature. As gas flows past the heated wires, they tend to be cooled. The amount of energy required to maintain the temperature of the wire is proportional to the volume of gas flowing past it. This system, however, has been associated in at least one report of accidental fire in the breathing circuit.[110]

CO_2 monitors are probably the best devices for revealing patient disconnections. CO_2 concentration is measured near the Y-piece either directly (mainstream) or by aspiration of a gas sample to the instrument (side-stream). Either a sudden change in the differences between the inspiratory and end-tidal CO_2 concentrations or the acute absence of measured CO_2 indicates a disconnection, a nonventilated patient, or other problems.[40] Importantly, an absence of exhaled CO_2 can be an indication of absent cardiac output rather than a mechanical equipment problem.

Misconnections of the breathing system are unfortunately relatively common. Despite the efforts of standards committees to eliminate this problem by assigning different diameters to various hoses and hose terminals, they continue to occur. Anesthesia workstations, breathing systems, ventilators, and scavenging systems incorporate many of these diameter-specific connections. The ability of anesthesia providers to outwit these "foolproof" systems has led to various hoses being cleverly adapted or forcefully fitted to inappropriate terminals and even to various other solid cylindrically shaped protrusions of the anesthesia machine.[40]

Occlusion (obstruction) of the breathing circuit may occur. Tracheal tubes can become kinked. Hoses throughout the breathing circuit are subject to occlusion by internal obstruction or external mechanical forces, which can impinge on flow and have severe consequences. For example, blockage of a bacterial filter in the expiratory limb of the circle system has resulted in bilateral tension pneumothorax.[104] Incorrect insertion of flow direction–sensitive components can result in a no-flow state.[40] Examples of these components include some PEEP valves and cascade humidifiers. Depending on the location of the occlusion relative to the pressure sensor, a high-pressure alarm may (or may not) alert practitioners to the problem.

Excess inflow to the breathing circuit from the anesthesia machine during the inspiratory phase can cause barotrauma. The best example of this phenomenon is oxygen flushing. Excess volume cannot be vented from the system during inspiration because the ventilator relief valve is closed and the APL valve is out of circuit.[52] A high-pressure alarm, if present, may be activated when the pressure becomes excessive. With many Dräger Medical systems, both audible and visual alarms are actuated when the high-pressure threshold is exceeded. In the Modulus II Plus System, the Datex-Ohmeda 7810 ventilator automatically switches from the inspiratory to the expiratory phase when the adjustable peak pressure threshold is exceeded.

On workstations equipped with adjustable inspiratory pressure limiters such as the Datex-Ohmeda S/5 ADU, Aestiva, and Aisys, and Dräger Medical's Narkomed 6000 series, 2B, 2C, GS, Fabius GS, and Apollo, maximal inspiratory pressure may be set by the user to a desired peak airway pressure. An adjustable pressure relief valve will open when the predetermined user-selected pressure is reached. This theoretically prevents generation of excessive airway pressure. Unfortunately, this feature depends on the user having preset the appropriate pop-off pressure. If the setting is too low, insufficient pressure for ventilation may be generated, resulting in inadequate minute ventilation; if set too high, the excessive airway pressure may still occur, resulting in barotrauma. The piston-driven Fabius GS, as well as others, may also include a factory-preset inspiratory pressure safety valve that opens at a preset airway pressure such as 75 cm of water pressure to minimize the risk of barotrauma. These strategies may reduce the risk of barotrauma and volutrauma; however, they are no substitute for vigilance.

Bellows Assembly Problems

Leaks can occur in the bellows assembly. Improper seating of the plastic bellows housing can result in inadequate ventilation because a portion of the driving gas is vented to the atmosphere. A hole in the bellows can lead to alveolar hyperinflation and possibly barotrauma in some ventilators because high-pressure driving gas can enter the patient circuit. The oxygen concentration of the patient gas may increase when the driving gas is 100% oxygen, or it may decrease if the driving gas is composed of an air–oxygen mixture.[147]

The ventilator relief valve can cause problems. Hypoventilation occurs if the valve is incompetent because the anesthetic gases are delivered to the scavenging system during the inspiratory phase instead of to the patient. Gas molecules preferentially exit into the scavenging system because it represents the path of least resistance, and the pressure within the scavenging system can be subatmospheric. Ventilator relief valve incompetency can result from a disconnected pilot line, a ruptured valve, or from a damaged flapper valve.[148,149] A ventilator relief valve stuck in the closed or partially closed position can produce either barotrauma or undesired PEEP.[150] Excessive suction from the scavenging system can draw the ventilator relief valve to its seat and close the valve during both the inspiratory and expiratory phases.[40] In this case, breathing circuit pressure escalates because excess anesthetic gas cannot be vented. It is worthwhile to note that during expiratory phase, some newer machines from Datex-Ohmeda (S/5 ADU, 7100 and 7900 SmartVent) scavenge both excess patient gases and the exhausted ventilator drive gas. That is, when the ventilator relief valve opens, and waste anesthetic gases are vented from the breathing circuit, the drive gas from the bellows housing joins with it to enter the scavenging system. Under certain conditions, the large volume of exhausted gases could overwhelm the scavenging system, resulting in pollution of the operating room with waste anesthetic gases (see "Scavenging Systems"). Other mechanical problems that can occur include leaks within the system, faulty pressure regulators, and faulty valves. Unlikely problems such as an occluded muffler on the Dräger AV-E ventilator can result in barotrauma. In this case, obstruction of driving gas outflow closes the ventilator relief valve, and excess patient gas cannot be vented.[151]

Control Assembly and Power Supply Problems

The control assembly can be the source of both electrical and mechanical problems. Electrical failure can be total or partial; the former is the more obvious. As anesthesia workstations are becoming more dependent on integrated computer-controlled systems, power interruptions become more significant. Battery backup systems are designed to continue operation of essential electronics during brief (up to several hours) outages. However, even with these systems, in the event of a failure, some time may be required to reboot after an electrical outage has occurred. During this time the availability of certain workstation features such as manual or mechanical ventilation can be variable. One cluster of electrical failures that could have potentially resulted in operating room fires was reported early on after the release of the Dräger Medical Narkomed 6000. Problems with the workstation's power supply printed circuit boards prompted a corrective recall action in November 2002.[152]

ANESTHESIA WORKSTATION VARIATIONS

The need for adaptation of current technology to successfully allow its integration into existing systems often comes with the introduction of new technology. Otherwise, a more comprehensive redesign of an entire anesthesia system "from the ground up" could be necessary. One such example of adaptation in the anesthesia workstation can be seen with two new design variations of the circle breathing system. The first of these is found on the Datex-Ohmeda S/5 ADU, and the second is incorporated into the Dräger Narkomed 6000 series and Fabius GS workstations. Because use of the circle system is fundamental to the day-to-day practice for most anesthesiologists, a comprehensive understanding of these new systems is crucial for their safe use.

The Datex-Ohmeda S/5 Anesthesia Delivery Unit and Aisys

The Datex-Ohmeda S/5 ADU debuted as the AS/3 ADU in 1998. Along with its more comprehensive safety features and integrated design that eliminated glass flow tubes and conventional anesthesia vaporizers in exchange for a computer screen with digital fresh gas flow scales and the built-in Aladin Cassette vaporizer system, the machine had a radically different appearance in general. It is not until closer inspection that the other unique properties of the ADU begin to stand out. The principal difference in the circle system of the ADU lies in the incorporation of the specialized D-lite flow and pressure transducer fitting into the circle at the level of the Y-connector. The D-lite spirometry module was redesigned to accommodate low-flow anesthesia and is currently a design feature of the GE Healthcare/Datex-Ohmeda Aisys workstation. On most traditional circle systems, exhaled tidal volume is measured by a spirometry sensor located in proximity to the expiratory valve. The placement of the D-lite fitting at the Y-connector provides a better location to perform exhaled volume measurement, allows airway gas composition and pressure monitoring to be done with a single adapter instead of with multiple fittings added to the breathing circuit, and it provides the ability to assess both inspiratory and expiratory gas flow and therefore generation of complete flow-volume spirometry. The relocation of the spirometer sensor to the Y-connector also makes it possible to move the location of the fresh gas inlet to the "patient" side of the inspiratory valve without adversely affecting accuracy of exhaled tidal volume measurement. On the other hand, placement of the D-lite sensor near the patient adds bulk and weight to the breathing circuit and may interfere with mask ventilation.

This atypical circle system arrangement with the fresh gas entering on the patient side of the inspiratory valve is advantageous for several reasons. It is likely to be more efficient in delivering fresh gas to the patient, while preferentially eliminating exhaled gases. Importantly, it is also less likely to cause desiccation of the CO_2 absorbent (see "Interactions of Inhaled Anesthetics with Absorbents"). Other notable changes on the S/5 ADU circle system include a compact proprietary CO_2 absorbent canister design that can be changed during ventilation without loss of circle system integrity and the relocation of the inspiratory and expiratory unidirectional valves from a horizontal position to a vertical position on the "compact block" assembly just below the absorbent canister. The reorientation of the unidirectional valves reduces the breathing circuit resistance encountered by a spontaneously ventilated patient. The vertically oriented unidirectional valves only have to be tipped away from the vertical position to be opened, unlike conventional horizontal valve discs, which have to be physically lifted off the valve seat against gravity to be opened. In the latest workstation, the Aisys, the inspiratory and expiratory check valves are positioned horizontally, but the circle system arrangement in which fresh gas enters the circuit downstream from the inspiratory valve is retained.

The Dräger Medical Narkomed 6000 Series, Fabius GS and Apollo Workstations

Several important differences exist between the traditional circle breathing systems of the newest Dräger products. At first

FIGURE 26-33. Inspiratory (A) and expiratory (B) phase of gas flows of a Dräger Narkomed 6000–type circle system with piston ventilator and fresh gas decoupling. NPR valve, negative-pressure relief valve. See text for details. (Reprinted from Brockwell RC: New Circle System Designs. A collection of figures privately published in Birmingham, AL, 2003, with permission.)

Inspiratory Phase–Mechanical Ventilation

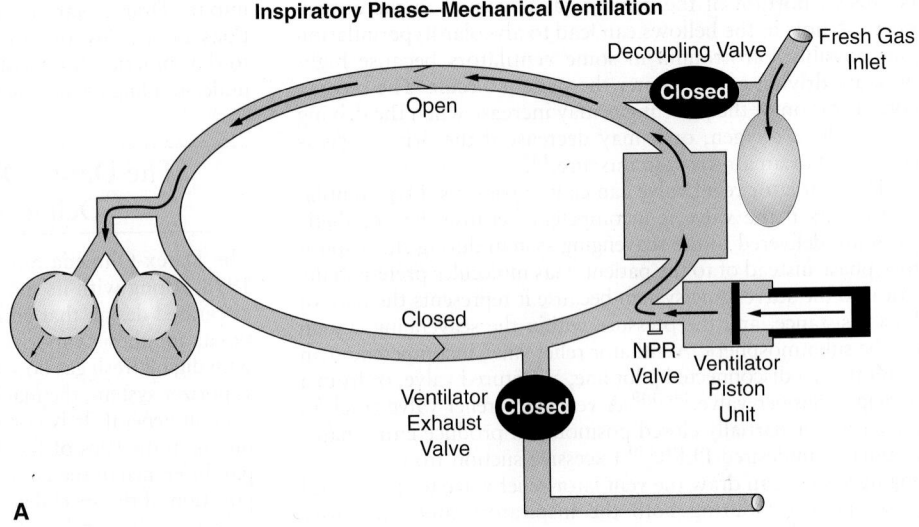

A

Expiratory Phase–Mechanical Ventilation

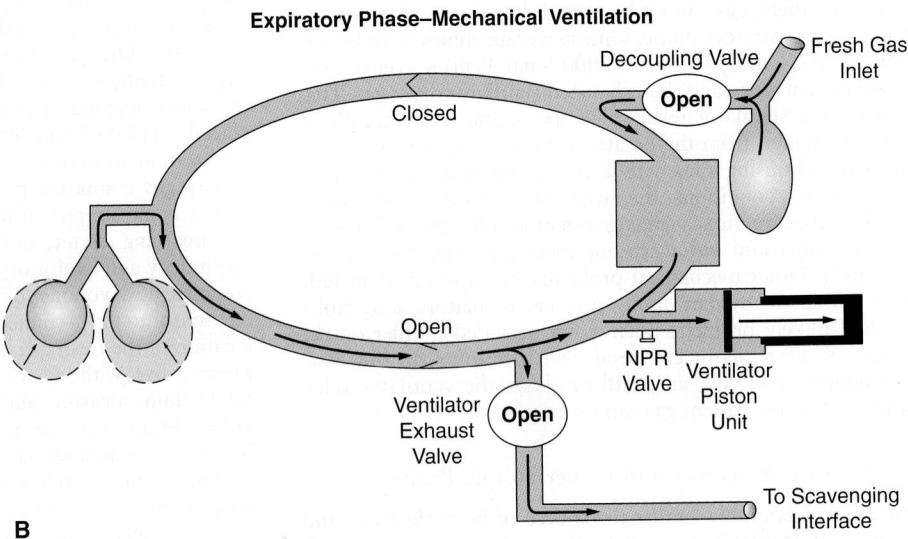

B

glance, the most notable difference lies in the appearance and design of the ventilators used with these systems. From the inconspicuous horizontally mounted Divan piston ventilator of the Narkomed 6000 to the vertically mounted and visible piston ventilator of the Fabius GS with its absent flow tubes and glowing electronic fresh gas flow indicators, these systems appear drastically different from traditional anesthesia systems. The piston ventilators of the Dräger Narkomed 6000 (Divan ventilator) and Fabius Series (E-Vent ventilator) anesthesia systems are classified as "electrically powered, piston driven, single circuit, electronically controlled with fresh gas decoupling." The ventilator found on the Apollo workstation, the E-Vent plus, is an electrically driven and electronically controlled, fresh gas decoupled, high-speed piston ventilator that requires no drive gas (unlike the traditional bellows ventilators). The E-Vent plus ventilator offers modes of ventilation previously found only in intensive care units: synchronized volume mode with adjustable flow trigger and pressure support.

The circle breathing systems used by these Dräger workstations incorporate a feature known as *fresh gas decoupling* (FGD). The incorporation of this patient safety-enhancing technology has required a significant redesign of the traditional circle system. A functional schematic of a circle system similar to the one used by the Dräger Narkomed 6000 series during both inspiratory and expiratory phase of mechanical ventilation can be seen in Figure 26-33, A and B. To understand the operating principles of FGD, it is important to have a good understanding

of gas flows in a traditional circle system both during inspiratory and expiratory phases of mechanical ventilation. A complete discussion of this was presented earlier in the section "Operating Principles of Ascending Bellows Ventilators."

The key concept of the fresh gas decoupled breathing system can be illustrated during the inspiratory phase of mechanical ventilation. With the traditional circle system, several events are occurring (Fig. 26-33A): (1) continuous fresh gas flow from the flowmeters and/or the oxygen flush valve is entering the circle system at the fresh gas inlet, (2) the ventilator is delivering the prescribed tidal volume to the patient's lungs, and (3) the ventilator relief valve (ventilator exhaust valve) is closed, so no gas is escaping the circle system except into the patient's lungs.[153] In a traditional circle system, when these events coincide and fresh gas inflow is coupled directly into the circle system, the total volume delivered to the patient's lungs is the sum of the volume delivered by the ventilator, plus the volume of gas that enters the circle via the fresh gas inlet. In contrast, when FGD is used, during the inspiratory phase (Fig. 26-33A) the fresh gas coming from the anesthesia workstation via the fresh gas inlet is diverted into the reservoir bag by a decoupling valve that is located between the fresh gas source and the ventilator circuit. The reservoir (breathing) bag serves as an accumulator for fresh gas until the expiratory phase begins. During expiratory phase (Fig. 26-33B), the decoupling valve opens, allowing the accumulated fresh gas in the reservoir bag to be drawn into the circle system to refill the piston ventilator chamber or descending bellows. Because the ventilator exhaust valve also opens during expiratory phase, excess fresh gas and exhaled patient gases are allowed to escape to the scavenging system.

Current fresh gas decoupled systems are designed with either piston-type or descending bellows–type ventilators. Because the bellows in either of these type of systems refills under slight negative pressure, it allows the accumulated fresh gas from the reservoir bag to be drawn into the ventilator for delivery to the patient during the next ventilator cycle. Because of this design requirement, it is unlikely that fresh gas decoupling, as described here, can be used with conventional ascending bellows ventilators, which refill under slight positive pressure.

13 The most significant advantage of circle systems using FGD is decreased risk of barotrauma and volutrauma. With a traditional circle system, increases in fresh gas flow from the flowmeters or from inappropriate use of the oxygen flush valve may contribute directly to tidal volume, which if excessive, may result in pneumothorax or other injury. Because systems with FGD isolate fresh gas coming into the system from the patient while the ventilator exhaust valve is closed, the risk of barotrauma is greatly reduced.

14 Modern ventilators compensate for the fresh gas flow as tidal volume is delivered. Thus, delivered tidal volume does not change as a function of fresh gas flow. This compensation is achieved either by fresh gas decoupling (in the Dräger 6000 series, Apollo and Fabius machines) or by fresh gas compensation in the GE Healthcare/Datex-Omeda machines.

Possibly the greatest disadvantage to the new anesthesia circle systems that use FGD is the possibility of entraining room air into the patient gas circuit. As previously discussed, in a fresh gas decoupled system the bellows or piston refills under slight negative pressure. If the volume of gas contained in the reservoir bag volume plus the returning volume of gas exhaled from the patient's lungs is inadequate to refill the bellows or piston, negative patient airway pressures could develop. To prevent this, a negative pressure relief valve is placed in the breathing system (Fig. 26-33, A and B). If breathing system pressure falls below a preset value such as -2 cm H_2O pressure, then the relief valve opens and ambient air is entrained into the patient gas circuit. If this goes undetected, the entrained atmospheric gases could lead to dilution of either or both the inhaled anesthetic agents or the enriched oxygen mixture (resulting in a lowering of the enriched oxygen concentration toward 21%). If unnoticed, this dilution of patient gases could lead to either intraoperative awareness or hypoxia.

High-priority alarms with both audible and visual alerts should notify the user that fresh gas flow is inadequate and room air is being entrained.

Another potential problem with an FGD system such as seen on the Narkomed 6000 series lies in its reliance on the reservoir bag to accumulate the incoming fresh gas. If the reservoir bag is removed during mechanical ventilation, or if it has a significant leak from poor fit on the bag mount or a perforation, room air may enter the breathing circuit as the ventilator piston unit refills during expiratory phase. This may also result in dilution of either or both the inhaled anesthetic agents or an enriched oxygen mixture, potentially resulting in awareness during anesthesia or hypoxia. Furthermore, this type of a disruption could lead to significant pollution of the operating room with anesthetic gases as fresh gases would be allowed to escape into the atmosphere. Other FGD designs, such as those seen in the Dräger Medical Fabius GS and the recently released Apollo anesthesia systems do not use the breathing bag as the fresh gas reservoir, but instead have an alternate location for fresh gas accumulation during the inspiratory phase.

SCAVENGING SYSTEMS

Scavenging is the collection and the subsequent removal of waste anesthetic gases from the operating room.[154] In most cases, the amount of gas used to anesthetize a patient for a given anesthetic far exceeds the minimal amount needed. Therefore, scavenging minimizes operating room pollution by removing this excess of gases. In 1977, the National Institute for Occupational Safety and Health (NIOSH) prepared a document entitled "Criteria for a Recommended Standard: Occupational Exposure to Waste Anesthetic Gases and Vapors."[155] Although it was maintained that a minimal safe level of exposure could not be defined, the NIOSH proceeded to issue the recommendations shown in Table 26-6.[155] It should be remembered that the 2 parts-per-million ceiling for volatile anesthetics was established in 1977, before desflurane and sevoflurane were introduced into clinical practice. However, this limit is likely to be applicable for the newer volatile anesthetics.[156] In 1991 the ASTM released the ASTM F1343-91 standard entitled "Standard Specification for Anesthetic Equipment—Scavenging Systems for Anesthetic Gases."[157] The document provided guidelines for devices that safely and effectively scavenge waste anesthetic gases to reduce

TABLE 26-6

NIOSH RECOMMENDATIONS FOR TRACE GAS LEVEL[a]

ANESTHETIC GAS	MAXIMUM TWA[b] CONCENTRATION (ppm)
Halogenated agent alone	2
Nitrous oxide	25
Combination of halogenated agent plus nitrous oxide:	
Halogenated agent	0.5
Nitrous oxide	25
Dental facilities (nitrous oxide alone)	50

NIOSH, National Institute for Occupational Safety and Health.
[a]Note: Despite being in clinical use for over 15 years, isoflurane, desflurane, and sevoflurane have not been tested for maximum recommended trace gas levels (see text).
[b]TWA, time-weighted average. Time-weighted average sampling, also known as time-integrated sampling, is a sampling method that evaluates the average concentration of anesthetic gas over a prolonged period of time, such as 1 to 8 hours.
Reprinted from U.S. Department of Health, Education, and Welfare: Criteria for a recommended standard: Occupational exposure to waste anesthetic gases and vapors. Washington DC, US Department of Health Education & Welfare, March 1977, with permission.

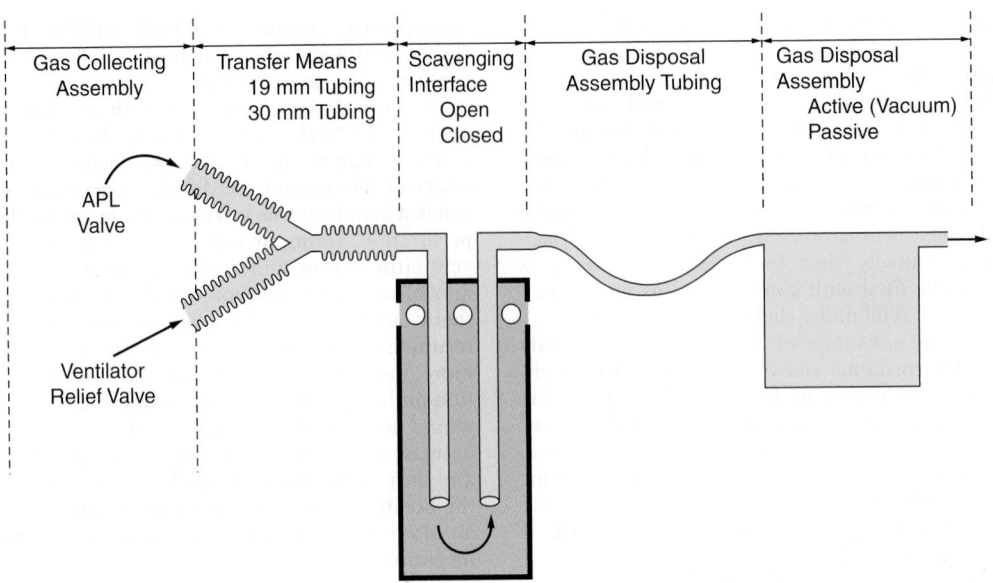

FIGURE 26-34.   Components of a scavenging system. APL, adjustable pressure limiting valve.

contamination in anesthetizing areas.[157] Because of lack of safety data on exposure to the new halogenated anesthetic agents (isoflurane, desflurane and sevoflurane), NIOSH has requested comments and information relevant to the evaluation of health risks associated with occupational exposure to these agents, in order to establish recommended exposure levels.[158] In 1999, the ASA Task Force on Trace Anesthetic Gases developed a booklet entitled *Waste Anesthetic Gases: Information for Management in Anesthetizing Areas and the Postanesthesia Care Unit*. This publication addresses analysis of the literature, the role of regulatory agencies, scavenging and monitoring equipment, and recommendations.[159]

The two major causes of waste gas contamination in the operating room are the anesthetic technique employed and equipment issues.[159,160] Regarding the anesthetic technique, the following factors cause operating room contamination: (1) failure to turn off gas flow control valves at the end of an anesthetic; (2) poorly fitting masks, flushing the circuit; (3) filling anesthetic vaporizers; (4) use of uncuffed endotracheal tubes; and (5) use of breathing circuits such as the Jackson-Rees, which are difficult to scavenge. Equipment failure or lack of understanding of proper equipment use can also contribute to operating room contamination. Leaks can occur in the high-pressure hoses, the nitrous oxide tank mounting, the high-pressure circuit and low-pressure circuit of the anesthesia machine, or in the circle system, particularly at the CO_2 absorber assembly. The anesthesia provider must be certain that the scavenging system is operational and adjusted properly to ensure adequate scavenging. If side stream CO_2 or multigas analyzers are used, the analyzed gas (withdrawn from the circuit at a rate of 50 to 250 mL/min) must be directed to the scavenging system or returned to the breathing system to prevent pollution of the operating room.[159,160]

Components

Scavenging systems generally have five components (Fig. 26-34): (1) the gas-collecting assembly, (2) the transfer means, (3) the scavenging interface, (4) the gas-disposal assembly tubing, and (5) an active or passive gas-disposal assembly.[155] An "active system" uses a central evacuation system to eliminate waste gases. The "weight" or pressure of the waste gas itself produces flow through a "passive system."

Gas-Collecting Assembly

The gas-collecting assembly captures excess anesthetic gas and delivers it to the transfer tubing.[140] Waste anesthetic gases are vented from the anesthesia system either through the APL valve or through the ventilator relief valve. All excess patient gas is either vented into the room (e.g., from a poor face mask fit or endotracheal tube leak) or exits the breathing system through one of these valves. Gas passing through these valves accumulates in the gas-collecting assembly and is directed to the transfer means. In some newer Datex-Ohmeda systems such as the S5/ADU and others that incorporate either the 7100 or 7900 ventilators, the ventilator drive gas is also exhausted into the scavenging system. Thus, it is important to recognize that under conditions of high fresh gas flows and high minute ventilation, the gases flowing into the scavenging interface may overwhelm the evacuation system. If this occurs, waste anesthetic gases may overflow the system via the positive-pressure relief valve (closed systems) or through the atmospheric vents (open systems), polluting the operating room. In contrast, most other pneumatic ventilators from both Datex-Ohmeda and Dräger exhaust their drive gas (100% oxygen or oxygen/air mixture) into the operating room through a small vent on the back of the ventilator control housing.

Transfer Means

The transfer means carries excess gas from the gas-collecting assembly to the scavenging interface. The tubing must be either 19 or 30 mm, as specified by the ASTM F1343-91 standard.[157] The tubing should be sufficiently rigid to prevent kinking, and as short as possible to minimize the chance of occlusion. Some manufacturers color code the transfer tubing with yellow bands to distinguish it from 22-mm breathing system tubing. Many machines have separate transfer tubes for the APL valve and for the ventilator relief valve. The two tubes frequently merge into a single hose before they enter the scavenging interface. Occlusion of the transfer means can be particularly problematic because it is upstream from the pressure-buffering features of the scavenging interface. If the transfer means is occluded, baseline breathing circuit pressure will increase, and barotrauma can occur.

Scavenging Interface

The scavenging interface is the most important component of the system because it protects the breathing circuit or ventilator from excessive positive or negative pressure.[154] The interface should limit the pressures immediately downstream from the gas-collecting assembly to between −0.5 and +10 cm water with normal working conditions.[157] Positive pressure relief is mandatory, irrespective of the type of disposal system used, to vent excess gas in case of occlusion downstream from the interface. If the disposal system is an "active system," negative pressure relief is necessary to protect the breathing circuit or ventilator from excessive subatmospheric pressure. A reservoir is highly desirable with active systems as it stores waste gases until the evacuation system can remove them. Interfaces can be open or closed, depending on the method used to provide positive and negative pressure relief.[154]

Open Interfaces. An open interface contains no valves and is open to the atmosphere, allowing both positive and negative pressure relief. Open interfaces should be used only with active disposal systems that use a central evacuation system. Open interfaces require a reservoir because waste gases are intermittently discharged in surges, whereas flow from the evacuation system is continuous.[154]

Many contemporary anesthesia machines are equipped with open interfaces like those shown in Figure 26-35, A and B.[161] An open canister provides reservoir capacity. The canister volume should be large enough to accommodate a variety of waste gas flow rates. Gas enters the system at the top of the canister and travels through a narrow inner tube to the canister base. Gases are stored in the reservoir between breaths. Positive and negative pressure relief is provided by holes in the top of the canister. The open interface shown in Figure 26-35A differs somewhat from the one shown in Figure 26-35B. The operator can regulate the vacuum by adjusting the vacuum control valve shown in Figure 26-35B.[161]

The efficiency of an open interface depends on several factors. The vacuum flow rate per minute must equal or exceed the minute volume of excess gases to prevent spillage. The volume of the reservoir and the flow characteristics within the interface are important. Spillage will occur if the volume of a single exhaled breath exceeds the capacity of the reservoir. The flow characteristics of the system are important because gas leakage can occur long before the volume of waste gas equals the reservoir volume if significant turbulence occurs within the interface.[162]

Closed Interfaces. A closed interface communicates with the atmosphere through valves. All closed interfaces must have a positive-pressure relief valve to vent excess system pressure if obstruction occurs downstream from the interface. A negative-pressure relief valve is mandatory to protect the breathing system from subatmospheric pressure if an active disposal system is used.[154] Two types of closed interfaces are commercially available. One has positive pressure relief only; the other has both positive and negative pressure relief. Each type is discussed in the following sections.

Positive Pressure Relief Only. This interface has a single positive-pressure relief valve and is designed to be used only with passive disposal systems (Fig. 26-36, *left*). Waste gas enters the interface at the waste gas inlets. Transfer of the waste gas from the interface to the disposal system relies on the "weight" or pressure of the waste gas itself as a negative pressure evacuation system is not used. The positive-pressure relief valve opens at a preset value such as 5 cm of water if an obstruction between the interface and the disposal system occurs.[163] On this type of system, a reservoir bag is not required.

Positive and Negative Pressure Relief. This interface has a positive-pressure relief valve, and at least one negative-pressure relief valve, in addition to a reservoir bag. It is used with active disposal systems. Figure 26-36 (*right*) is a schematic of the Dräger Medical closed interface for suction systems. A variable volume of waste gas intermittently enters the interface through the waste gas inlets. The reservoir intermittently accumulates excess gas until the evacuation system eliminates it. The operator should adjust the vacuum control valve so that the reservoir bag is properly inflated (A in Fig. 26-36), not over distended (B in Fig. 26-36), or completely deflated (C in Fig. 26-36). Gas is vented to the atmosphere through the positive-pressure relief valve if the system pressure exceeds +5 cm of water. Room air is entrained through the negative-pressure relief valve if the system pressure is more negative than −0.5 cm H_2O. On some systems, a backup negative-pressure relief valve opens at −1.8 cm H_2O if the primary negative-pressure relief valve becomes occluded.

The effectiveness of a closed system in preventing spillage depends on the rate of waste gas inflow, the evacuation flow rate, and the size of the reservoir. Leakage of waste gases into the atmosphere occurs only when the reservoir bag becomes fully inflated and the pressure increases sufficiently to open the positive pressure relief valve. In contrast, the effectiveness of an open system to prevent spillage depends not only on the volume of the reservoir but also on the flow characteristics within the interface.[162]

Gas-Disposal Assembly Conduit

The gas-disposal assembly conduit (Fig. 26-34) conducts waste gas from the scavenging interface to the gas-disposal assembly. It should be collapse-proof and should run overhead, if possible, to minimize the chances of accidental occlusion.[157]

Gas-Disposal Assembly

The gas-disposal assembly ultimately eliminates excess waste gas (Fig. 26-35). There are two types of disposal systems: active and passive.

The most common method of gas disposal is the active assembly, which uses a central evacuation system. A vacuum pump serves as the mechanical flow-inducing device that removes the waste gases usually to the outside of the building.

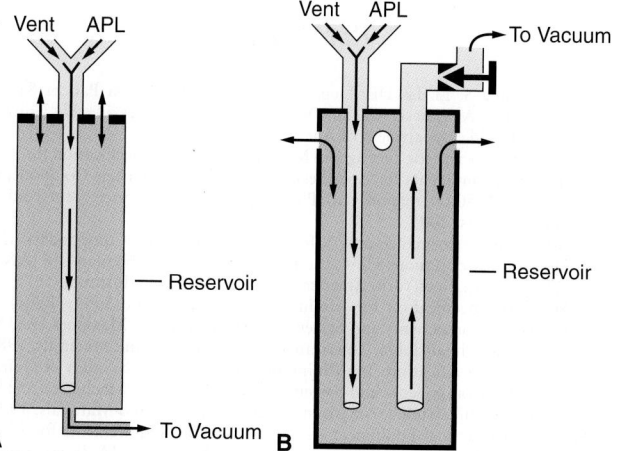

FIGURE 26-35. A and **B.** Two open scavenging interfaces. Each requires an active disposal system. APL, adjustable pressure limiting valve. See text for details. (Modified from Dorsch JA, Dorsch SE: Controlling trace gas levels, Understanding Anesthesia Equipment, 4th edition. Edited by Dorsch JA, Dorsch SE. Baltimore, Williams & Wilkins, 1999, p. 355, with permission.)

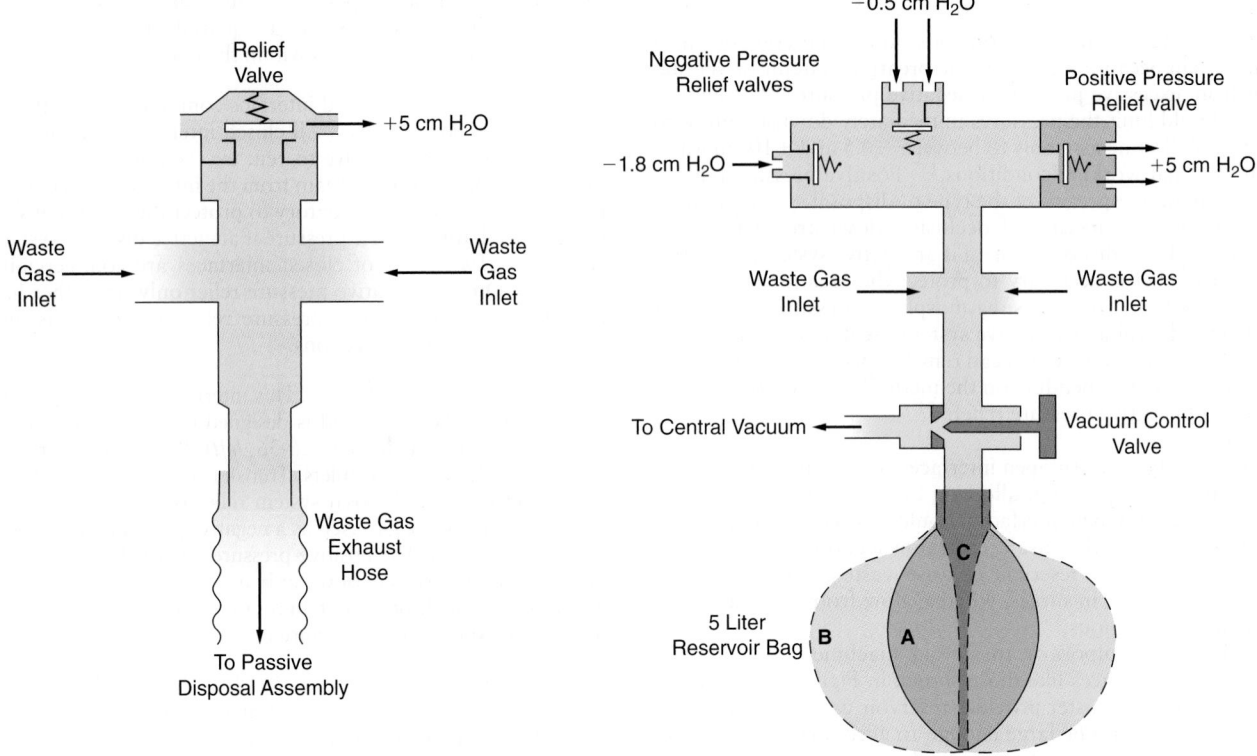

FIGURE 26-36.   Closed scavenging interfaces. *Left.* Interface used with a passive disposal system. *Right.* Interface used with an active system. See text for details. (Modified with permission (*left*) from Scavenger Interface for Air Conditioning: Instruction Manual. Telford, PA, North American Dräger, October 1984; (*right*) from Narkomed 2A Anesthesia System: Technical Service Manual. Telford, PA. North American Dräger, 1985.)

An interface with a negative-pressure relief valve is mandatory because the pressure within the system is negative. A reservoir is very desirable, and the larger the reservoir, the lower the suction flow rate needed.[154,162]

A passive disposal system does not use a mechanical flow-inducing device. Instead, the weight or pressure from the heavier-than-air anesthetic gases produces flow through the system. Positive-pressure relief is mandatory, but negative-pressure relief and a reservoir are unnecessary. Excess waste gases can be eliminated from the surgical suite in a number of ways. Some include venting through the wall, ceiling, floor, or to the room exhaust grill of a nonrecirculating air conditioning system.[154,162]

Hazards

Scavenging systems minimize operating room pollution, yet they add complexity to the anesthesia system. A scavenging system functionally extends the anesthesia circuit all the way from the anesthesia machine to the ultimate disposal site. This extension increases the potential for problems. Obstruction of scavenging pathways can cause excessive positive pressure in the breathing circuit, and barotrauma can occur. Excessive vacuum applied to a scavenging system can result in undesirable negative pressures within the breathing system. Finally, in 2004, another unusual problem that resulted from waste gas scavenging was reported by Allen and Lees.[164] They reported cases of fires in engineering equipment rooms that house the vacuum pumps used for waste anesthetic gas evacuation. It seems that in some hospitals, waste gases are not directly vented outside, but may be vented into machine rooms that have vents that open to the outside. Because some new anesthesia machines such as the Datex-Ohmeda S5/ADU and Aestiva, among others, now also scavenge ventila-

tor drive gas (which is 100% oxygen in most cases) in addition to gas from the breathing system, the environments in these machine rooms may become highly enriched with oxygen gas. The result of this has been the production of fires in these spaces outside the operating room. These sites may contain equipment or materials such as petroleum distillates (pumps/oil/grease) that in the presence of an oxygen-enriched atmosphere could be excessively combustible and a severe fire hazard.

References

1. Lampotang S, Lizdas DE, Liem EB et al: The Anesthesia Patient Safety Foundation Anesthesia Machine Workbook v1.1a. Gainesville, FL, University of Florida Department of Anesthesiology, 2007
2. American Society for Testing and Materials: Standard Specification for Particular Requirements for Anesthesia Workstations and Their Components (ASTM F1850-00, reapproved). Philadelphia, American Society for Testing and Materials, 2005
3. Minimum Performance and Safety Requirements for Components and Systems of Continuous Flow Anesthesia Machines for Human Use (ANSI Z79.8-1979). New York, American National Standards Institute, 1979
4. Standard Specification for Minimum Performance and Safety Requirements for Components and Systems of Anesthesia Gas Machines (ASTM F1161-88). Philadelphia, American Society for Testing and Materials, 1988
5. Standard Specification for Minimum Performance and Safety Requirements for Components and Systems of Anesthesia Gas Machines (ASTM 1161-94). Philadelphia, American Society for Testing and Materials, 1994
6. Medical Electrical Equipment — Part 1: General Requirements for Basic Safety and Essential Performance (60601-1). Worcester, MA, International Electrotechnical Commission, 2005
7. American Society of Anesthesiologists: Manual for Anesthesia Department Organization and Management. American Society of Anesthesiologists, Park Ridge, IL, 2007
8. James RH: 1000 anaesthetic incidents: Experience to date. Anaesthesia 2003; 58: 856
9. Kibelbek MJ: Cable trapped under Drager Fabius automatic pressure limiting valve causes inability to ventilate. Anesthesiology 2007; 106: 639

10. Caplan RA, Vistica MF, Posner KL et al: Adverse anesthetic outcomes arising from gas delivery equipment. Anesthesiology 1997; 87: 741
11. Olympio MA: Modern Anesthesia Machines Offer New Safety Features. APSF Newsletter 2003; 18: 17
12. Cooper JB: Toward prevention of anesthetic mishaps. Int Anesthesiol Clin 1984; 22: 167
13. Emergency Care Research Institute: Avoiding anesthetic mishaps through pre-use checks. Health Devices 1982; 11: 201
14. FDA Anesthesia Apparatus Checkout Recommendations 8th ed. Rockville, MD, Food and Drug Administration, 1986
15. Anesthesia Apparatus Checkout Recommendations. Rockville, MD, Food and Drug Administration, 1993
16. Spooner RB, Kirby RR: Equipment related anesthetic incidents. Int Anesthesiol Clin 1984; 22: 133
17. American Society of Anesthesiologists: Guideline for Designing Pre-Anesthesia Checkout Procedures. Park Ridge, IL, 2007, pp 1–16
18. Lewis SE, Andrews JJ, Long GW: An unexpected Penlon sigma elite vaporizer leak. Anesthesiology 1999; 90: 1221
19. Myers JA, Good ML, Andrews JJ: Comparison of tests for detecting leaks in the low-pressure system of anesthesia gas machines. Anesth Analg 1997; 84: 179
20. Dorsch JA, Dorsch SE: Hazards of anesthesia machines and breathing systems, Understanding Anesthesia Equipment, 5th ed. Edited by Dorsch JA, Dorsch SE. Baltimore, Lippincott Williams & Wilkins, 2007, p 404
21. Comm G, Rendell-Baker L: Back pressure check valves a hazard. Anesthesiology 1982; 56: 327
22. Peters KR, Wingard DW: Anesthesia machine leakage due to misaligned vaporizers. Anesth Rev 1987; 14: 36
23. Rendell-Baker L: Problems with anesthetic and respiratory therapy equipment. Int Anesthesiol Clin 1982; 20: 1
24. Yasukawa M, Yasukawa K: Hypoventilation due to disconnection of the vaporizer and negative-pressure leak test to find disconnection. Masui-Jpn J Anesthesiol 1992; 41(8): 1345
25. Dodgson BG: Inappropriate use of the oxygen flush to check an anaesthetic machine. Can J Anaesth 1988; 35: 436
26. Mann D, Ananian J, Alston T: Oxygen flush valve booby trap. Anesthesiology 2004; 101: 558
27. Dorsch JA, Dorsch SE: Equipment checking and maintenance, Understanding Anesthesia Equipment, 5th ed. Edited by Dorsch JA, Dorsch SE. Baltimore, Lippincott Williams & Wilkins, 2007, pp 931
28. Bowie E, Huffman LM: The Anesthesia Machine: Essentials for Understanding. Madison, Ohmeda The BOC Group Inc., 1985
29. Dorsch JA, Dorsch SE: The anesthesia machine, Understanding Anesthesia Equipment, 5th ed. Edited by Dorsch JA, Dorsch SE. Baltimore, Lippincott Williams & Wilkins, 2007, pp 83
30. Cicman JH, Jacoby MI, Skibo VF, Yoder JM: Anesthesia systems. Part 1: Operating principles of fundamental components. J Clin Monit 1992; 8: 295
31. Schumacher SD, Brockwell RC, Andrews JJ, et al.: Bulk liquid oxygen supply failure. Anesthesiology 2004; 100: 186
32. Feeley TW, Hedley-Whyte J: Bulk oxygen and nitrous oxide delivery systems: Design and safety. Anesthesiology 1976; 44: 301
33. Pelton DA: Non-flammable medical gas pipeline systems, Mechanical Misadventures in Anesthesia, 1st ed. Edited by Wyant GM. Toronto, University of Toronto Press, 1978, pp 8
34. Stassou A: Two die in Hospital Mix-up. WTHN News, New Haven, CT, 2002
35. Adriani J: Clinical application of physical principles concerning gases and vapor to anesthesiology, The Chemistry and Physics of Anesthesia, 2nd ed. Edited by Adriani J. Springfield, Illinois, Charles C Thomas, 1962, pp 58
36. Atlas G: A method to quickly estimate remaining time for an oxygen E-cylinder. Anesth Analg 2004; 98: 1190
37. American Society for Testing and Materials: Standard specification for particular requirements for anesthesia workstations and their components (ASTM F1850-00). Philadelphia, American Society for Testing and Materials West Conshohoken, 2000
38. Adriani J: Principles of physics and chemistry of solids and fluids applicable to anesthesiology, The Chemistry and Physics of Anesthesia, 2nd ed. Edited by Adriani J. Springfield, Illinois, Charles C Thomas, 1962, pp 7
39. Macintosh R, Mushin WW, Epstein HG, eds: Physics for the Anaesthetist, 3rd ed. Oxford, Blackwell Scientific Publications, 1963, pp 196
40. Schreiber P: Safety guidelines for anesthesia systems. Telford, Pennsylvania, North American Dräger, 1984
41. Eger EI, II, Epstein RM: Hazards of anesthetic equipment. Anesthesiology 1964; 24: 490
42. Eger EI, II, Hylton RR, Irwin RH, et al.: Anesthetic flowmeter sequence—a cause for hypoxia. Anesthesiology 1963; 24: 396
43. Mazze RI: Therapeutic misadventures with oxygen delivery systems: the need for continuous in-line oxygen monitors. Anesth Analg 1972; 51: 787
44. Cheng CJ, Garewal DS: A failure of the chain link mechanism of the Ohmeda Excel 210 anesthetic Machine. Anesth Analg 2001; 92: 913
45. Kidd AG, Hall I: Fault with an Ohmeda Excel 210 Anesthetic Machine (Letter and response). Anaesthesia 1994; 49: 83
46. Lohman G: Fault with an Ohmeda Excel 410 Machine (Letter and Response). Anaesthesia 1991; 46: 695
47. Richards C: Failure of a nitrous oxide-oxygen proportioning device. Anesthesiology 1989; 71: 997
48. Abraham ZA, Basagoitia B: A potentially lethal anesthesia machine failure. Anesthesiology 1987; 66: 589
49. Neubarth J: Another hazardous gas supply misconnection (Letter). Anesth Analg 1995; 80: 206
50. Gaughan SD, Benumof JL, Ozaki GT: Can an anesthesia machine flush valve provide for effective jet ventilation. Anesth Analg 1993; 76: 800
51. Anderson CE, Rendell-Baker L: Exposed O_2 flush hazard. Anesthesiology 1982; 56: 328
52. Andrews JJ: Understanding your anesthesia machine and ventilator, International Anesthesia Research Society 63rd Congress Lake Buena Vista, Florida, International Anesthesia Research Society, 1989, pp 59
53. Lampotang S, Lizdas DE, Liem EB: The Virtual Anesthesia Machine Website, University of Florida Department of Anesthesiology, Center for Simulation, Advanced Learning and Technology, Gainsville, FL, 2007. http://vam.anest.ufl.edu/
54. Lampotang S, Lizdas D, Liem E, Gravenstein J: The Anesthesia Patient Safety Foundation Anesthesia Machine Workbook v1.1a, University of Florida Department of Anesthesiology, 2007. http://vam.anest.ufl.edu/members/workbook/apsf-workbook-english.html
55. Dorsch JA, Dorsch SE: Vaporizers (anesthetic agent delivery devices), Understanding Anesthesia Equipment, 5th ed. Edited by Dorsch JA, Dorsch SE. Baltimore, Lippincott Williams & Wilkins, 2007, pp 121
56. Macintosh R, Mushin WW, Epstein HG: Physics for the Anaesthetist, 3rd ed. Oxford, Blackwell Scientific Publications, 1963, pp 68
57. Korman B, Richie IM: Chemistry of halothane-enflurane mixtures applied to anesthesia. Anesthesiology 1985; 63: 152
58. Macintosh R, Mushin WW, Epstein HG: Physics for the Anaesthetist, 3rd ed. Oxford, Blackwell Scientific Publications, 1963, p 26
59. Schreiber P: Anaesthetic equipment: Performance, classification, and safety. New York, Springer-Verlag, 1972
60. Dräger Medical: Dräger Vapor 2000 Anesthetic Vaporizer Operating Instructions. Telford, PA, 2001, pp 62
61. Hill DW: The design and calibration of vaporizers for volatile anaesthetic agents. Br J Anaesth 1968; 40: 648
62. Hill DW, Lowe HJ: Comparison of concentration of halothane in closed and semi-closed circuits during controlled ventilation. Anesthesiology 1962; 23: 291
63. Anonymous: Internal leakage from anesthesia unit flush valves. Health Devices 1981; 10: 172
64. Morris LE: Problems in the performance of anesthesia vaporizers. Int Anesthesiol Clin 1974; 12: 199
65. Diaz PD: The influence of carrier gas on the output of automatic vaporizers. Br J Anaesth 1976; 48: 387
66. Gould DB, Lampert BA, MacKrell TN: Effect of nitrous oxide solubility on vaporizer aberrance. Anesth Analg 1982; 61: 938
67. Lin CY: Assessment of vaporizer performance in low-flow and closed-circuit anesthesia. Anesth Analg 1980; 59: 359
68. Nawaf K, Stoelting RK: Nitrous oxide increases enflurane concentrations delivered by ethane vaporizers. Anesth Analg 1979; 58: 30
69. Palayiwa E, Sanderson MH, Hahn CEW: Effects of carrier gas composition on the output of six anaesthetic vaporizers. Br J Anaesth 1983; 55: 1025
70. Prins L, Strupat J, Clement J, Knill RL: An evaluation of gas density dependence of anaesthetic vaporizers. Can Anaesth Soc J 1980; 27: 106
71. Scheller MS, Drummond JC: Solubility of N2O in volatile anesthetics contributes to vaporizer aberrancy when changing carrier gases. Anesth Analg 1986; 65: 88
72. Stoelting RK: The effects of nitrous oxide on halothane output from Fluotec Mark 2 vaporizers. Anesthesiology 1971; 35: 215
73. Karis JH, Menzel DB: Inadvertent change of volatile anesthetics in anesthesia machines. Anesth Analg 1982; 61: 53
74. Broka SM, Gourdange PA, Joucken KL: Sevoflurane and desflurane confusion. Anesth Analg 1999; 88: 1194
75. George TM: Failure of keyed agent-specific filling devices. Anesthesiology 1984; 61: 228
76. Riegle EV, Desertspring D: Failure of the agent-specific filling device (Letter). Anesthesiology 1990; 73: 353
77. Lippmann M, Foran W, Ginsburg R, Lewis J: Contamination of anesthetic vaporizer contents. Anesthesiology 1993; 78: 1175
78. Munson WM: Cardiac arrest: A hazard of tipping a vaporizer. Anesthesiology 1965; 26: 235
79. Sinclair A: Vaporizer overfilling. Can J Anaesth 1993; 40: 77
80. Seropian MA, Robins B: Smaller than expected sevoflurane concentrations using the SevoTec 5 vaporizer at low fill states and high fresh gas glows. Anesth Analg 2000; 91: 834
81. Meister GC, Becker KE, Jr.: Potential fresh gas flow leak through Dräger vapor 19.1 vaporizer with key-index fill port. Anesthesiology 1993; 78: 211
82. Zimmer C, Janssen M, Treschan T, Peters J: Near-miss accident during magnetic resonance imaging. Anesthesiology 2004; 100: 1329
83. Andrews JJ, Johnston RV, Jr.: The new Tec 6 desflurane vaporizer. Anesth Analg 1993; 76: 1338
84. Weiskopf RB, Sampson D, Moore MA: The desflurane (Tec 6) vaporizer: Design, design considerations and performance evaluation. Br J Anaesth 1994; 72: 474
85. Eger EI: New inhaled anesthetics. Anesthesiology 1994; 80: 906
86. Susay SR, Smith MA, Lockwood GG: The saturated vapor pressure of desflurane at various temperatures. Anesth Analg 1996; 83: 864

87. Johnston RV, Jr., Andrews JJ: The effects of carrier gas composition on the performance of the Tec 6 desflurane vaporizer. Anesth Analg 1994; 79: 548

88. Andrews JJ, Johnston RV, Jr., Kramer GC: Consequences of misfilling contemporary vaporizers with desflurane. Can J Anaesth 1993; 40: 71

89. Hendrickx JF, Carette RM, Deloof T, De Wolf AM: Severe ADU desflurane vaporizing unit malfunction. Anesthesiology 2003; 99: 1459

90. Maquet Critical Care AB: Halothane 950, Enflurane 951, Isoflurane 952 Operating Manual. Solna, Sweden, Getinge, 2004

91. Mapleson WW: The elimination of rebreathing in various semiclosed anaesthetic systems. Br J Anaesth 1954; 26: 323

92. Willis BA, Pender JW, Mapleson WW: Rebreathing in a T-piece: Volunteer and theoretical studies of the Jackson-Rees modification of Ayre's T-piece during spontaneous respiration. Br J Anaesth 1975; 47: 1239

93. Froese AB, Rose DK: A detailed analysis of T-piece systems. Some Aspects of Paediatric Anaesthesia. Edited by Steward. Elsevier North-Holland Biomedical Press, 1982, pp 101

94. Rose DK, Froese AB: The regulation of PaCO2 during controlled ventilation of children with a T-piece. Canad Anaesth Soc J 1979; 26(2): 104

95. Sykes MK: Rebreathing circuits: A review. Br J Anaesth 1968; 40: 666

96. Bain JA, Spoerel WE: A streamlined anaesthetic system. Can Anaesth Soc J 1972; 19: 426

97. Aarhus D, Søredie E, Holst-Larsen H: Mechanical obstruction in the anaesthesia delivery-system mimicking severe bronchospasm. Anaesthesia 1997; 52: 992

98. Pethick SL: Letter to the Editor. Can Anaesth Soc J 1975; 22: 115

99. Moyers J: A nomenclature for methods of inhalation anesthesia. Anesthesiology 1953; 14: 609

100. Dorsch JA, Dorsch SE: The mapleson breathing systems, Understanding Anesthesia Equipment, 5th ed. Edited by Dorsch JA, Dorsch SE. Baltimore, Lippincott Williams & Wilkins, 2007, pp 207

101. Eger EI, II: Anesthetic systems: construction and function, Anesthetic Uptake and Action. Edited by Eger EI, II. Baltimore, Williams & Wilkins, 1974, pp 206

102. Eger EI, II, Ethans CT: The effects of inflow, overflow and valve placement on economy of the circle. Anesthesiology 1968; 29: 93

103. Chacon AC, Kuczkowski KM, Sanchez RA: Unusual case of breathing circuit obstruction: Plastic packaging revisited (Letter to the Editor). Anesthesiology 2004; 100: 753

104. McEwan AI, Dowell L, Karis JH: Bilateral tension pneumothorax caused by a blocked bacterial filter in an anesthesia breathing circuit. Anesth Analg 1993; 76: 440

105. Smith CR, Otworth JR, Kaluszyk GSW: Bilateral tension pneumothorax due to a defective anesthesia breathing circuit filter. J Clin Anesth 1991; 3: 229

106. Walton JS, Fears R, Burt N, Dorman BH: Intraoperative breathing circuit obstruction caused by albuterol nebulization. Anesth Analg 1999; 89: 650

107. Dhar P, George I, Sloan P: Flow transducer gas leak detected after induction. Anesth Analg 1999; 89: 1587

108. Kanno T, Aso C, Saito S, Yoshikawa D et al: A combustive destruction of expiration valve in an anesthetic circuit. Anesthesiology 2003; 98: 577

109. Laster M, Roth P, Eger E, II: Fires from the interaction of anesthetics with desiccated absorbent. Anesth Analg 2004; 99: 769

110. Fatheree RS, Leighton BL: Acute respiratory distress syndrome after an exothermic baralyme-sevoflurane reaction. Anesthesiology 2004; 101: 531

111. Holak E, Mei D, Dunning M, III, Gundamari R et al: Carbon monoxide production from sevoflurane breakdown. Anesth Analg 2003; 96: 757

112. Kshatri AM, Kingsley CP: Defective carbon dioxide absorber as a cause for a leak in a breathing circuit. Anes 1996; 84: 475

113. Norman PH, Daley MD, Walker JR, Fusetti S: Obstruction due to retained carbon dioxide absorber canister wrapping. Anesth Analg 1996; 83: 425

114. Adriani J: Carbon dioxide absorption, The Chemistry and Physics of Anesthesia, 2nd ed. Edited by Adriani J. Springfield, Illinois, Charles C. Thomas, 1962, pp 151

115. Dewey Almy Chemical Division: The Sodasorb Manual of CO2 Absorption. New York, W.R. Grace and Company, 1962

116. Murray JM, Renfrew CW, Bedi A, McCrystal CB et al: A new carbon dioxide absorbent for use in anesthetic breathing systems. Anesthesiology 1999; 91: 1342

117. Versichelen LF, Bouche MP, Rolly G et al: Only carbon dioxide absorbents free of both NaOH and KOH do not generate compound-A during in vitro closed system sevoflurane. Anesthesiology 2001; 95: 750

118. Higuchi H, Adachi Y, Arimura S, Satoh T: The carbon dioxide absorption capacity of Amsorb is half that of soda lime. Anesth Analg 2001; 93: 221

119. Sosis M: Why not use Amsorb alone as the CO2 absorbent and avoid any risk of CO production? (Letter to the Editor) Anesthesiology 2003; 98: 1299

120. Hunt HE: Resistance in respiratory valves and canisters. Anesthesiology 1955; 16: 190

121. Brown ES: Performance of absorbents: Continuous flow. Anesthesiology 1959; 20: 41

122. Andrews JJ, Johnston RV, Jr., Bee DE, Arens JF: Photodeactivation of ethyl violet: A potential hazard of Sodasorb. Anesthesiology 1990; 72: 59

123. Anonymous: Case History: Accidental use of trichloroethylene (Trilene, Trimar) in a closed system. Anesth Analg 1964; 43: 740

124. Kharasch ED, Powers KM, et al: Comparison of Amsorb, Sodalime, Baralyme® degradation of volatile anesthetics and formation of carbon monoxide and compound A in swine in vivo. Anesthesiology 2002; 96: 173

125. Morio M, Fujii K, Satoh N, Imai M et al: Reaction of sevoflurane and its degradation products with soda lime. Anesthesiology 1992; 77: 1155

126. Fang ZX, Kandel L, Laster MJ, Eger EI: Factors affecting production of compound-A from the interaction of sevoflurane with Baralyme® and soda lime. Anesth Analg 1996; 82: 775

127. Frink EJ, Jr., Malan TP, Morgan SE, Brown EA et al: Quantification of the degradation products of sevoflurane in two CO2 absorbents during low-flow anesthesia in surgical patients. Anesthesiology 1992; 77: 1064

128. Eger EI, II, Ionescu P, Laster MJ, Weiskopf RB: Baralyme dehydration increases and soda lime dehydration decreases the concentration of compound A resulting from sevoflurane degradation in a standard anesthetic circuit. Anesth Analg 1997; 85: 892

129. Steffey EP, Laster MJ, Ionescu P et al: Dehydration of baralyme® increases compound A resulting from sevoflurane degradation in a standard anesthetic circuit used to anesthetize swine. Anesth Analg 1997; 85: 1382

130. Bito H, Ikeuchi Y, Ikeda K: Effects of low-flow sevoflurane anesthesia on renal function: Comparison with high-flow sevoflurane anesthesia and low-flow isoflurane anesthesia. Anesthesiology 1997; 86: 1231

131. Eger EL, II, Koblin DD, Bowland T, Ionescu P et al: Nephrotoxicity of sevoflurane versus desflurane anesthesia in volunteers. Anesth Analg 1997; 84: 160

132. Kharasch ED, Frink EJ, Jr., Zager R, Bowdle TA et al: Assessment of low-flow sevoflurane and isoflurane effects on renal function using sensitive markers of tubular toxicity. Anesthesiology 1997; 86: 1238

133. Berry PD, Sessler DI, Larson MD: Severe carbon monoxide poisoning during desflurane anesthesia. Anesthesiology 1999; 90: 613

134. Baxter PJ, Kharasch ED: Rehydration of desiccated baralyme prevents carbon monoxide formation from desflurane in an anesthesia machine. Anesthesiology 1997; 86: 1061

135. Woehlck HJ, Dunning M 3rd, Connolly LA: Reduction in the incidence of carbon monoxide exposures in humans undergoing general anesthesia. Anesthesiology 1997; 87: 228

136. Fang ZX, Eger EI, Laster MJ, Chortkoff BS et al: Carbon monoxide production from degradation of desflurane, enflurane, isoflurane, halothane, and sevoflurane by soda lime and baralyme®. Anesth Analg 1995; 80: 1187

137. Bonome C, Belda J, Alavarez-Refojo F, Soro M et al: Low-flow anesthesia and reduced animal size increase carboxyhemoglobin levels in swine during desflurane and isoflurane breakdown in dried soda lime. Anesth Analg 1999; 89: 909

138. Neumann MA, Laster MJ, Weiskopf RB, Gong DH et al: The elimination of sodium and potassium hydroxides from desiccated soda lime diminishes degradation of desflurane to carbon monoxide and sevoflurane to compound A but does not compromise carbon dioxide absorption. Anesth Analg 1999; 89: 768

139. Olympio MA: Carbon Dioxide Absorbent Desiccation Safety Conference Convened by APSF. APSF Newsletter 2005; 20: 25

140. McPherson SP, Spearman CB: Respiratory Therapy Equipment, 3rd ed. St. Louis, C.V. Mosby, 1985, pp 230

141. Spearman CB, Sanders HG: Mechanical Ventilation. New York, Churchill Livingstone, 1985, pp 59

142. Cooper JB, Newbower RS, Kitz RJ: An analysis of major errors and equipment failures in anesthesia management: considerations for prevention and detection. Anesthesiology 1984; 60: 34

143. Reinhart DJ, Friz R: Undetected leak in corrugated circuit tubing in compressed configuration. Anesthesiology 1993; 78: 218

144. Raphael DT, Weller RS, Doran DJ: A response algorithm for the low-pressure alarm condition. Anesth Analg 1988; 67: 876

145. Slee TA, Pavlin EG: Failure of low pressure alarm associated with use of a humidifier. Anesthesiology 1988; 69: 791

146. Sattari R, Reichard PS, Riddle RT: Temporary malfunction of the Ohmeda modulus CD series volume monitor caused by the overhead surgical lighting. Anesthesiology 1999; 91: 894

147. Feeley TW, Bancroft ML: Problems with mechanical ventilators. Int Anesthesiol Clin 1980; 20: 83

148. Khalil SN, Gholston TK, Binderman J, Antosh S: Flapper valve malfunction in an Ohio closed scavenging system. Anaesth Analg 1987; 66: 1334

149. Sommer RM, Bhalla GS, Jackson JM: Hypoventilation caused by ventilator valve rupture. Anesth Analg 1988; 67: 999

150. Bourke D, Tolentino D: Inadvertent positive end-expiratory caused by a malfunctioning ventilator relief valve. Anesth Analg 2003; 97: 492

151. Roth S, Tweedie E, Sommer RM: Excessive airway pressure due to a malfunctioning anesthesia ventilator. Anesthesiology 1986; 65: 532

152. Usher A, Cave D, Finegan B: Critical incident with Narkomed 6000 anesthesia system (Letter to the Editor). Anesthesiology 2003; 99: 762

153. Dorsch JA, Dorsch SE: Anesthesia ventilators, Understanding Anesthesia Equipment, 5th ed. Edited by Dorsch JA, Dorsch SE. Baltimore, Lippincott Williams & Wilkins, 2007, pp 310.

154. Dorsch JA, Dorsch SE: Controlling Trace Gas Levels. In Dorsch JA, Dorsch SE (eds): Understanding Anesthesia Equipment, 5th ed, p 373. Baltimore, Lippincott Williams & Wilkins, 2007

155. US Department of Health, Education, and Welfare: Criteria for a Recommended Standard: Occupational Exposure to Waste Anesthetic Gases and Vapors. March ed. Washington, DC, US Department of Health, Education, and Welfare, 1977

156. Sessler DI, Badgwell JM: Exposure of postoperative nurses to exhaled anesthetic gases. Anaesth Analg 1998; 87: 1083

157. American Society for Testing and Materials: Standard Specification for Anesthetic Equipment-Scavenging Systems for Anesthetic Gases (ASTM F1343-91). Philadelphia, American Society for Testing and Materials, 1991
158. Hall A: Request for Information on Waste Halogenated Anesthetic Agents: Isoflurane, Desflurane, and Sevoflurane. Federal Register 2006; 71: 8859
159. ASA Task Force on Trace Anesthetic Gases: Waste Anesthetic Gases: Information for Management in Anesthetizing Areas and the Postanesthesia Care Unit (PACU), 1999. Edited by McGregor D. Park Ridge, Illinois, American Society of Anesthesiologists, pp 3

160. Kanmura Y, Sakai J, Yoshinaka H, Shirao K: Causes of nitrous oxide contamination in operating rooms. Anesthesiology 1999; 90: 693
161. Open Reservoir Scavenger: Operator's Instruction Manual. Telford, Pennsylvania, North American Dräger, 1986
162. Gray WM: Symposium on anaesthetic equipment. Scavenging equipment. Br J Anaesth 1985; 57: 685
163. Brockwell RC, Andrews JJ: Understanding your anesthesia machine, ASA Refresher Courses. Edited by Schwartz AJ. Lippincott Williams & Wilkins, Philadelphia, PA, 2002
164. Allen M, Lees DE: Fires in Medical Vacuum Pumps: Do you need to be concerned? ASA Newsletter 2004; 68(10): 22

APPENDIX A

1993 FDA Anesthesia Apparatus Checkout Recommendations

This checkout, or a reasonable equivalent, should be conducted before administration of anesthesia. These recommendations are valid only for an anesthesia system that conforms to current and relevant standards and includes an ascending bellows ventilator and at least the following monitors: capnograph, pulse oximeter, oxygen analyzer, respiratory volume monitor (spirometer), and breathing system pressure monitor with high- and low-pressure alarms. This is a guideline that users are encouraged to modify to accommodate differences in equipment design and variations in local clinical practice. Such local modifications should have appropriate peer review. Users should refer to the operator's manual for the manufacturer's specific procedures and precautions, especially the manufacturer's low-pressure leak test (step 5).

Emergency Ventilation Equipment

*1. **Verify Backup Ventilation Equipment is Available and Functioning**

High-Pressure System

*2. **Check Oxygen Cylinder Supply**
   a. Open O_2 cylinder and verify at least half full (about 1,000 psi).
   b. Close cylinder.
*3. **Check Central Pipeline Supplies**
   a. Check that hoses are connected and pipeline gauges read about 50 psi.

Low-Pressure System

*4. **Check Initial Status of Low-Pressure System**
   a. Close flow control valves and turn vaporizers off.
   b. Check fill level and tighten vaporizers' filler caps.
*5. **Perform Leak Check of Machine Low-Pressure System**
   a. Verify that the machine master switch and flow control valves are OFF.
   b. Attach "suction bulb" to common (fresh) gas outlet.
   c. Squeeze bulb repeatedly until fully collapsed.
   d. Verify that bulb stays fully collapsed for at least 10 seconds.
   e. Open one vaporizer at a time and repeat "c" and "d" as above.
   f. Remove suction bulb, and reconnect fresh gas hose.
*6. **Turn on Machine Master Switch and all other necessary electrical equipment.**
*7. **Test Flowmeters**
   a. Adjust flow of all gases through their full range, checking for smooth operation of floats and undamaged flow tubes.
   b. Attempt to create a hypoxic O_2/N_2O mixture and verify correct changes in flow and/or alarm.

Scavenging System

*8. **Adjust and Check Scavenging System**
   a. Ensure proper connections between the scavenging system and both adjustable pressure limiting (APL; pop-off) valve and ventilator relief valve.
   b. Adjust waste gas vacuum (if possible).
   c. Fully open APL valve and occlude Y-piece.
   d. With minimum O_2 flow, allow scavenger reservoir bag to collapse completely and verify that absorber pressure gauge reads about zero.
   e. With the O_2 flush activated, allow the scavenger reservoir bag to distend fully, and then verify that absorber pressure gauge reads <10 cm of H_2O.

Breathing System

*9. **Calibrate O_2 Monitor**
   a. Ensure monitor reads 21% in room air.
   b. Verify low O_2 alarm is enabled and functioning.

    c. Reinstall sensor in circuit and flush breathing system with O_2.

    d. Verify that monitor now reads >90%.

10. **Check Initial Status of Breathing System**

    a. Set selector switch to "Bag" mode.

    b. Check that breathing circuit is complete, undamaged, and unobstructed.

    c. Verify that CO_2 absorbent is adequate.

    d. Install breathing circuit accessory equipment (e.g., humidifier, positive end-expiratory pressure valve) to be used during the case.

11. **Perform Leak Check of the Breathing System**

    a. Set all gas flows to zero (or minimum).

    b. Close APL (pop-off) valve and occlude Y-piece.

    c. Pressurize breathing system to about 30 cm of H_2O with O_2 flush.

    d. Ensure that pressure remains fixed for at least 10 seconds.

    e. Open APL (pop-off) valve and ensure that pressure decreases.

Manual and Automatic Ventilation Systems

12. **Test Ventilation Systems and Unidirectional Valves**

    a. Place a second breathing bag on Y-piece.

    b. Set appropriate ventilator parameters for next patient.

    c. Switch to automatic ventilation (Ventilator) mode.

    d. Turn ventilator ON and fill bellows and breathing bag with O_2 flush.

    e. Set O_2 flow to minimum, other gas flows to zero.

    f. Verify that during inspiration bellows delivers appropriate tidal volume and that during expiration bellows fills completely.

    g. Set fresh gas flow to about 5 L/min.

    h. Verify that the ventilator bellows and simulated lungs fill and empty appropriately without sustained pressure at end expiration.

    i. Check for proper action of unidirectional valves.

    j. Exercise breathing circuit accessories to ensure proper function.

    k. Turn ventilator OFF and switch to manual ventilation (bag/APL) mode.

    l. Ventilate manually and assure inflation and deflation of artificial lungs and appropriate feel of system resistance and compliance.

    m. Remove second breathing bag from Y-piece.

Monitors

13. **Check, Calibrate, and/or Set Alarm Limits of all Monitors**

    a. Capnometer

    b. Oxygen analyzer

    c. Pressure monitor with high- and low-airway pressure alarms

    d. Pulse oximeter

    e. Respiratory volume monitor (spirometer)

Final Position

14. **Check Final Status of Machine**

    a. Vaporizers off.

    b. APL valve open.

    c. Selector switch to "Bag."

    d. All flowmeters to zero (or minimum).

    e. Patient suction level adequate.

    f. Breathing system ready to use.

*If an anesthesia provider uses the same machine in successive cases, these steps need not be repeated or may be abbreviated after the initial checkout.

APPENDIX B

Recommendations for Preanesthesia Checkout Procedures (2008)

Sub-Committee of ASA Committee on Equipment and Facilities

Task Force Members*
Russell C. Brockwell, MD
Jerry Dorsch, MD
Susan Dorsch, MD
James Eisenkraft, MD
Jeffrey Feldman, MD (Task Force Chair)
Julian Goldman, MD

Carolyn G. Holland, CRNA, MSN (AANA)
Tom C. Krejcie, MD
Samsun Lampotang, PhD
Donald Martin, MD (Chair, ASA Committee on Equipment & Facilities)
Julie Mills (GE Healthcare)
Michael A. Olympio, MD
Gerardo Trejo (American Society of Anesthesia Technicians and Technologists, ASATT)

Contributors (Individuals who have contributed in some fashion in the process of developing the new checkout guidelines)

Abe Abramovitch (Datascope)
Charles Biddle, CRNA, PhD
Robert Clark (Dräger Medical)
Ann Culp, CRNA, MSN
Chad Driscoll, CRNA, MHS
Ann Graham (FDA)
Marc Jans (Dräger Medical)
Michael Wilkening (Dräger Medical)
William Norfleet, MD (FDA)

*Task Force Members are ASA members unless otherwise indicated.

Guidelines for Preanesthesia Checkout Procedures

Background

Improperly checking anesthesia equipment prior to use can lead to patient injury and has also been associated with an increased risk of severe postoperative morbidity and mortality.[1,2] In 1993 a preanesthesia checkout (PAC) was developed and widely accepted as an important step in the process of preparing to deliver anesthesia care.[3] Despite the accepted importance of the PAC, available evidence suggests that the current version is neither well understood nor reliably used by anesthesia providers.[4–6] Furthermore, anesthesia delivery systems have evolved to the point that one checkout procedure is not applicable to all anesthesia delivery systems currently on the market. For these reasons, a new approach to the PAC has been developed. The goal was to provide guidelines applicable to all anesthesia delivery systems so that individual departments can develop a PAC that can be performed consistently and expeditiously.

General Considerations

The following document is intended to serve not as a PAC itself, but rather as a template for developing checkout procedures that are appropriate for each individual anesthesia machine design. When using this template to develop a checkout procedure for systems that incorporate automated checkout features, items that are not evaluated by the automated checkout need to be identified, and supplemental manual checkout procedures included as needed.

Simply because an automated checkout procedure exists does not mean it can completely replace a manual checkout procedure or that it can be performed safely without adequate training and a thorough understanding of what the automated checkout accomplishes. An automated checkout procedure can be incomplete and/or misleading. For example, the leak test performed by some current automated checkouts does not test for leaks at the vaporizers. As a result, a loose vaporizer filler cap, or a leak at the vaporizer mount, could easily be missed.

An ideally automated checkout procedure should clearly reveal to the user the functions that are being checked, any deficient function that is found, and recommendations to correct the problem. Documentation of the automated checkout process preferably should be in a manner that can be recorded on the anesthesia record.

Operator's manuals, which accompany anesthesia delivery systems, include extensive recommendations for equipment checkout. Although these recommendations are quite extensive and typically not used by anesthesia providers, they are nevertheless important references for developing machine-specific and institution-specific checkout procedures.

Personnel Performing the PreAnesthesia Checkout

The previously accepted Anesthesia Apparatus Checkout Recommendation placed all of the responsibility for pre-use checkout on the anesthesia provider. Sole reliance on one individual to complete the checkout process may increase the likelihood that one or more steps will be omitted or performed improperly. This guideline identifies those aspects of the PAC that could be completed by a qualified anesthesia and/or biomedical technician. Using technicians to perform some aspects of the PAC may improve compliance with the PAC. Steps completed by a technician may be part of the morning pre-use check or part of a procedure performed at the end of each day. Critical checkout steps (e.g., availability of backup ventilation equipment) will benefit from intentional redundancy (i.e., having more than one individual responsible for checking the equipment). ***Regardless of the level of training and support by technicians, the anesthesia care provider is ultimately responsible for proper function of all equipment used to provide anesthesia care.***

Adaptation of the PAC to local needs, assignment of responsibility for the checkout procedures, and training are the responsibilities of the individual anesthesia department. Training procedures should be documented. Proper documentation should include records of completed coursework (e.g.. a manufacturer course) or for in-house training, a listing of the competency items taught, and records of successful completion by trainees.

Objectives for a new PAC

- Outline the essential items that need to be available and functioning properly prior to delivering every anesthetic.
- Identify the frequency with which each of the items needs to be checked.
- Suggest which items may be checked by a qualified anesthesia technician, biomedical technician or a manufacturer-certified service technician.

Basic Principles

- The anesthesia care provider is ultimately responsible for ensuring that the anesthesia equipment is safe and ready for use. This responsibility includes adequate familiarity with the equipment, following relevant local policies for performing and documenting the PAC and being knowledgeable about those procedures.
- Depending on the staffing resources in a particular institution, anesthesia technicians and/or biomedical technicians can participate in the PAC. Biomedical technicians are often trained and certified by manufacturers to perform on-site maintenance of anesthesia delivery systems and therefore can be a useful resource for completing regular checkout procedures. Anesthesia technicians are not commonly trained to perform checkout procedures. Involving the anesthesia technicians is intended to enhance compliance with the PAC. Each department should decide whether or not the available technicians can or should be trained to assist with checkout procedures. Formal certification by the American Society of Anesthesia Technicians and Technologists is encouraged but does not necessarily guarantee familiarity with checkout procedures.
- Critical items will benefit from redundant checks to avoid errors and omissions.
- When more than one person is responsible for checking an item, all parties should perform the check if intentional redundancy is deemed important, or either party may be acceptable, depending on the available resources.
- Whoever conducts the PAC should provide documentation of successful performance. The anesthesia provider should include this documentation on the patient chart.
- Whenever an anesthesia machine is moved to a new location, a complete beginningof-the-day checkout should be performed.
- Automated checks should clearly distinguish the components of the delivery system that are checked automatically from those that require manual checkout.
- Ideally, the date, time, and outcome of the most recent check(s) should be recorded and the information made accessible to the user.
- Specific procedures for pre-use checkout cannot be prescribed in this document as they vary with the delivery systems. Clinicians must learn how to effectively perform the necessary pre-use check for each piece of equipment they use.
- Each department or health care facility should work with the manufacturer(s) of their equipment to develop pre-use checkout procedures that satisfy both the following guidelines and the needs of the local department.
- Default settings for ventilators, monitors, and alarms should be checked to determine if they are appropriate.
- These checkout recommendations are intended to replace the pre-existing FDA-approved Anesthesia Apparatus Checkout Recommendations. They are not intended to be a replacement for required preventive maintenance.
- The PAC is essential to safe care but should not delay initiating care if the patient needs are so urgent that time taken to complete the PAC could worsen the patient's outcome.

Guidelines for Developing Institution-Specific Checkout Procedures Prior to Anesthesia Delivery

These guidelines describe a basic approach to checkout procedures and rationale that will ensure that these priorities are satisfied. They should be used to develop institution-specific checkout procedures designed for the equipment and resources available. (Examples of institution-specific procedures for current anesthesia delivery systems are published on the same Web site as this document.)

Requirements for Safe Delivery of Anesthesia Care

- Reliable delivery of oxygen at any appropriate concentration up to 100%.
- Reliable means of positive pressure ventilation.
- Backup ventilation equipment available and functioning.
- Controlled release of positive pressure from the breathing circuit.
- Anesthesia vapor delivery (if intended as part of the anesthetic plan).
- Adequate suction.
- Means to conform to standards for patient monitoring.[7,8]

Specific Items

The following items need to be checked as part of a complete PAC. The intent is to identify what to check, the recommended frequency of checking, and the individual(s) who could be responsible for the item. For these guidelines, the responsible party would fall into one of four categories: provider, technician, technician or provider, or technician and provider. The designation "technician and provider" means that the provider must perform the check whether or not it has been completed by a technician. It is not intended to make the use of technician checks mandatory. The intent is not to specify how an item needs to be checked, as the specific checkout procedure will depend on the equipment being used.

Item 1: Verify that auxiliary oxygen cylinder and self-inflating manual ventilation device are available and functioning.
   Frequency: Daily.
   Responsible Parties: Provider and technician.

Rationale: Failure to be able to ventilate is a major cause of morbidity and mortality related to anesthesia care. Because equipment failure with resulting inability to ventilate the patient can occur at any time, a self-inflating manual ventilation device (e.g., Ambu bag) should be present at every anesthetizing location for every case and should be checked for proper function. In addition, a source of oxygen separate from the anesthesia machine and pipeline supply, specifically an oxygen cylinder with regulator and a means to open the cylinder valve, should be immediately available and checked. After checking the cylinder pressure, it is recommended that the main cylinder valve be closed to avoid inadvertent emptying of the cylinder through a leaky or open regulator.

Item 2: Verify patient suction is adequate to clear the airway.

Frequency: Prior to each use.

Responsible Parties: Provider and technician.

Rationale: Safe anesthetic care requires the immediate availability of suction to clear the airway if needed.

Item 3: Turn on anesthesia delivery system and confirm that AC power is available.

Frequency: Daily

Responsible Parties: Provider or technician

Rationale: Anesthesia delivery systems typically function with backup battery power if AC power fails. Unless the presence of AC power is confirmed, the first obvious sign of power failure can be a complete system shutdown when the batteries can no longer power the system. Many anesthesia delivery systems have visual indicators of the power source showing the presence of both AC and battery power. These indicators should be checked and connection of the power cord to a functional AC power source should be confirmed. Desflurane vaporizers require electrical power, and recommendations for checking power to these vaporizers should also be followed.

Item 4: Verify availability of required monitors and check alarms.

Frequency: Prior to each use.

Responsible Parties: Provider or technician.

Rationale: Standards for patient monitoring during anesthesia are clearly defined.[7,8] The ability to conform to these standards should be confirmed for every anesthetic. The first step is to visually verify that the appropriate monitoring supplies (e.g., blood pressure cuffs, oximetry probes) are available. All monitors should be turned on and proper completion of power-up self-tests confirmed. Given the importance of pulse oximetry and capnography to patient safety, verifying proper function of these devices before anesthetizing the patient is essential. Capnometer function can be verified by exhaling through the breathing circuit or gas sensor to generate a capnogram, or verifying that the patient's breathing efforts generate a capnogram before the patient is anesthetized. Visual and audible alarm signals should be generated when this is discontinued. Pulse oximeter function, including an audible alarm, can be verified by placing the sensor on a finger and observing for a proper recording. The pulse oximeter alarm can be tested by introducing motion artifact or removing the sensor.

Audible alarms have also been reconfirmed as essential to patient safety by American Society of Anesthesiologists, American Association of Nurse Anesthetists, Anesthesia Patient Safety Foundation, and Joint Commission on the Accreditation of Healthcare Organizations (currently named The Joint Commission).

Proper monitor functioning includes visual and audible alarm signals that function as designed.

Item 5: Verify that pressure is adequate on the spare oxygen cylinder mounted on the anesthesia machine.

Frequency: Daily

Responsible Parties: Provider and technician

Rationale: Anesthesia delivery systems rely on a supply of oxygen for various machine functions. At a minimum, the oxygen supply is used to provide oxygen to the patient. Pneumatically powered ventilators also rely on a gas supply. Oxygen cylinder(s) should be mounted on the anesthesia delivery system and determined to have an acceptable minimum pressure. The acceptable pressure depends on the intended use, the design of the anesthesia delivery system, and the availability of piped oxygen.

- Typically, an oxygen cylinder will be used if the central oxygen supply fails.
- If the cylinder is intended to be the primary source of oxygen (e.g., remote-site anesthesia), then a cylinder supply sufficient to last for the entire anesthetic is required. If a pneumatically powered ventilator that uses oxygen as its driving gas will be used, a full E oxygen cylinder may provide only 30 minutes of oxygen. In that case, the maximum duration of oxygen supply can be obtained from an oxygen cylinder if it is used only to provide fresh gas to the patient in conjunction with manual or spontaneous ventilation. Mechanical ventilators will consume the oxygen supply if pneumatically powered ventilators that require oxygen to power the ventilator are used. Electrically powered ventilators do not consume oxygen, so the duration of a cylinder supply will depend only on total fresh gas flow.
- The oxygen cylinder valve should be closed after it has been verified that adequate pressure is present, unless the cylinder is to be the primary source of oxygen (i.e., if piped oxygen is not available). If the valve remains open and the pipeline supply should fail, the oxygen cylinder can become depleted while the anesthesia provider is unaware of the oxygen supply problem. Other gas supply cylinders (e.g., Heliox, CO_2, air, N_2O) need to be checked only if that gas is required to provide anesthetic care.

Item 6: Verify that piped gas pressures are ≥50 psig.

Frequency: Daily

Responsible Parties: Provider and technician

Rationale: A minimum gas supply pressure is required for proper function of the anesthesia delivery system. Gas supplied from a central source can fail for a variety of reasons. Therefore, the pressure in the piped gas supply should be checked at least once daily.

Item 7: Verify that vaporizers are adequately filled and, if applicable, that the filler ports are tightly closed.

Frequency: Prior to each use.

Responsible Parties: Provider. Technician if redundancy desired.

Rationale: If anesthetic vapor delivery is planned, an adequate supply is essential to reduce the risk of light anesthesia or recall. This is especially true if an anesthetic agent monitor with a low agent alarm is not being used. Partially open filler ports are a common cause of leaks that may not be detected if the vaporizer control dial is not open when a leak test is performed. This leak source can be minimized by tightly closing filler ports. Newer vaporizer designs have filling systems that automatically close the filler port when filling is completed.

High and low anesthetic agent alarms are useful to help prevent over- or underdosage of anesthetic vapor. Use of these alarms is encouraged and they should be set to the appropriate limits and enabled.

Item 8: Verify that there are no leaks in the gas supply lines between the flowmeters and the common gas outlet.

Frequency: Daily and whenever a vaporizer is changed.

Responsible Parties: Provider or technician.

Rationale: The gas supply in this part of the anesthesia delivery system passes through the anesthetic vaporizer(s) on most anesthesia delivery systems. In order to perform a thorough leak test, each vaporizer must be turned on individually to check for leaks at the vaporizer mount(s) or inside the vaporizer. Furthermore, some machines have a check valve between the flowmeters and the common gas outlet, requiring a negative pressure test to adequately check for leaks. Automated checkout procedures typically include a leak test but may not evaluate leaks at the vaporizer, especially if the vaporizer is not turned on during the leak test. When relying on automated testing to evaluate the system for leaks, the automated leak test would need to be repeated for each vaporizer in place. This test should also be completed whenever a vaporizer is changed. The risk of a leak at the vaporizer depends on the vaporizer design. Vaporizer designs in which the filler port closes automatically after filling can reduce the risk of leaks.

Technicians can provide useful assistance with this aspect of the machine checkout as it can be time-consuming.

Item 9: Test scavenging system function.

Frequency: Daily

Responsible Parties: Provider or technician

Rationale: A properly functioning scavenging system prevents room contamination by anesthetic gases. Proper function depends on correct connections between the scavenging system and the anesthesia delivery system. These connections should be checked daily by a provider or technician. Depending on the scavenging system design, proper function may also require that the vacuum level is adequate, which should also be confirmed daily. Some scavenging systems have mechanical positive- and negative-pressure relief valves. Positive and negative pressure relief is important to protect the patient circuit from pressure fluctuations related to the scavenging system. Proper checkout of the scavenging system should ensure that positive- and negative-pressure relief is functioning properly. Because of the complexity of checking for effective positive and negative pressure relief, and the variations in scavenging system design, a properly trained technician can facilitate this aspect of the checkout process.

Item 10: Calibrate, or verify calibration of, the oxygen monitor and check the low oxygen alarm.

Frequency: Daily

Responsible Parties: Provider or technician.

Rationale: Continuous monitoring of the inspired oxygen concentration is the last line of defense against delivering hypoxic gas concentrations to the patient. The oxygen monitor is essential for detecting adulteration of the oxygen supply. Most oxygen monitors require calibration once daily, although some are self-calibrating. Self-calibrating oxygen monitors should be verified to read 21% when sampling room air. This is a step that is easily completed by a trained technician. When more than one oxygen monitor is present, the primary sensor that will be relied on for oxygen monitoring should be checked.

The low oxygen concentration alarm should also be checked at this time by setting the alarm above the measured oxygen concentration and confirming that an audible alarm signal is generated.

Item 11: Verify that carbon dioxide absorbent is not exhausted.

Frequency: Prior to each use

Responsible Parties: Provider or technician

Rationale: Proper function of a circle anesthesia system relies on the absorbent to remove carbon dioxide from rebreathed gas. Exhausted absorbent as indicated by the characteristic color change should be replaced. It is possible for absorbent material to lose the ability to absorb CO_2 yet the characteristic color change may be absent or difficult to see. Some newer absorbents do change color when desiccated. Capnography should be used for every anesthetic and, when using a circle anesthesia system, rebreathing carbon dioxide as indicated by an inspired CO_2 concentration >0 can also indicate exhausted absorbent. (See Note 2 to Appendix B.)

Item 12: Breathing system pressure and leak testing.

Frequency: Prior to each use.

Responsible Parties: Provider and technician.

Rationale: The breathing system pressure and leak test should be performed with the circuit configuration to be used during anesthetic delivery. If any components of the circuit are changed after this test is completed, the test should be performed again. Although the anesthesia provider should perform this test before each use, anesthesia technicians who replace and assemble circuits can also perform this check and add redundancy to this important checkout procedure. Proper testing will demonstrate that pressure can be developed in the breathing system during both manual and mechanical ventilation and that pressure can be relieved during manual ventilation by opening the adjustable pressure limiting valve.

Automated testing is often implemented in the newer anesthesia delivery systems to evaluate the system for leaks and also to determine the compliance of the breathing system. The compliance value determined during this testing will be used to automatically adjust the volume delivered by the ventilator to maintain a constant volume delivery to the patient. It is important that the circuit configuration that is to be used is in place during the test.

Item 13: Verify that gas flows properly through the breathing circuit during both inspiration and exhalation.

    Frequency: Prior to each use.

    Responsible Parties: Provider and technician.

    Rationale: Pressure and leak testing does not identify all obstructions in the breathing circuit or confirm proper function of the inspiratory and expiratory unidirectional valves. A test lung or second reservoir bag can be used to confirm that flow through the circuit is unimpeded. Complete testing includes both manual and mechanical ventilation. The presence of the unidirectional valves can be assessed visually during the PAC. Proper function of these valves cannot be visually assessed because subtle valve incompetence may not be detected. Checkout procedures to identify valve incompetence that may not be visually obvious can be implemented but are typically too complex for daily testing. A trained technician can perform regular valve competence tests. (See Note 4 to Appendix B) Capnography should be used during every anesthetic and the presence of carbon dioxide in the inspired gases can help to detect an incompetent valve.

Item 14: Document completion of checkout procedures.

    Frequency: Prior to each use.

    Responsible Parties: Provider and technician.

    Rationale: Each individual responsible for checkout procedures should document completion of these procedures. Documentation gives credit for completing the job and can be helpful if an adverse event should occur. Some automated checkout systems maintain an audit trail of completed checkout procedures that are dated and timed.

Item 15: Confirm ventilator settings and evaluate readiness to deliver anesthesia care. (ANESTHESIA TIME OUT)

    Frequency: Immediately prior to initiating the anesthetic.

    Responsible Parties: Provider

    Rationale: This step is intended to avoid errors due to production pressure or other sources of haste. The goal is to confirm that appropriate checks have been completed and that essential equipment is indeed available. The concept is analogous to the "time out" used to confirm patient identity and surgical site prior to incision. Improper ventilator settings can be harmful, especially if a small patient is following a much larger patient or vice versa. Pressure limit settings (when available) should be used to prevent excessive volume delivery from improper ventilator settings.

    Items to check:

- Monitors functional?
- Capnogram present?
- Oxygen saturation by pulse oximetry measured?
- Flowmeter and ventilator settings proper?
- Manual/ventilator switch set to manual?
- Vaporizer(s) adequately filled?

SUMMARY OF CHECKOUT RECOMMENDATIONS BY FREQUENCY AND RESPONSIBLE PARTY

ITEM TO BE COMPLETED	RESPONSIBLE PARTY
TO BE COMPLETED DAILY	
1: Verify that auxiliary oxygen cylinder and self-inflating manual ventilation device are available and functioning	Provider and technician
2: Verify patient suction is adequate to clear the airway	Provider and technician
3: Turn on anesthesia delivery system and confirm that AC power is available	Provider or technician
4: Verify availability of required monitors, including alarms	Provider or technician
5: Verify that pressure is adequate on the spare oxygen cylinder mounted on the anesthesia machine	Provider and technician
6: Verify that the piped gas pressures are ≥50 psig	Provider and technician
7: Verify that vaporizers are adequately filled and, if applicable, that the filler ports are tightly closed	Provider or technician
8: Verify that there are no leaks in the gas supply lines between the flowmeters and the common gas outlet	Provider or technician
9: Test scavenging system function	Provider or technician
10: Calibrate, or verify calibration of, the oxygen monitor and check the low oxygen alarm	Provider or technician
11: Verify carbon dioxide absorbent is not exhausted	Provider or technician
12: Breathing system pressure and leak testing	Provider and technician
13: Verify that gas flows properly through the breathing circuit during both inspiration and exhalation	Provider and technician
14: Document completion of checkout procedures	Provider and technician
15: Confirm ventilator settings and evaluate readiness to deliver anesthesia care (ANESTHESIA TIME OUT)	Provider
TO BE COMPLETED PRIOR TO EACH PROCEDURE	
2: Verify patient suction is adequate to clear the airway	Provider and technician
4: Verify availability of required monitors, including alarms	Provider or technician
7: Verify that vaporizers are adequately filled and, if applicable, that the filler ports are tightly closed	Provider

(continued)

11: Verify that carbon dioxide absorbent is not exhausted	Provider or technician
12: Breathing system pressure and leak testing	Provider and technician
13: Verify that gas flows properly through the breathing circuit during both inspiration and exhalation	Provider and technician
14: Document completion of checkout procedures	Provider and technician
15: **Confirm ventilator settings and evaluate readiness to deliver anesthesia care (ANESTHESIA TIME OUT)**	Provider

Appendix B References

1. Cooper JB, Newbower RS, Kitz RJ: An analysis of major errors and equipment failures in anesthesia management: Considerations for prevention and detection. Anesthesiology 1984; 60: 34
2. Arbous MS, Meursing AE, van Kleef JW et al: Impact of anesthesia management characteristics on severe morbidity and mortality. Anesthesiology 2005; 102: 257
3. Anesthesia Apparatus Checkout Recommendations, 1993. http://www.fda.gov/cdrh/humfac/anesckot.html
4. March MG, Crowley JJ: An evaluation of anesthesiologists' present checkout methods and the validity of the FDA checklist. Anesthesiology 1991; 75: 724
5. Lampotang S, Moon S, Lizdas DE et al: Anesthesia machine pre-use check survey: Preliminary results [abstract]. Anesthesiology 2005; A1195
6. Larson ER, Nuttall GA, Ogren BD et al: A prospective study on anesthesia machine fault identification. Anesth Analg 2007; 104: 154
7. American Society of Anesthesiologists: Standards for Basic Anesthetic Monitoring. October 25, 2005. http://www.asahq.org/publicationsAndServices/standards/02.pdf
8. Scope and Standards for Nurse Anesthesia Practice, in the Professional Practice Manual for the Certified Registered Nurse Anesthetist. Park Ridge, IL: American Association of Nurse Anesthetists, 2006.

APPENDIX (TO APPENDIX B)
ADDITIONAL NOTES ON PREANESTHESIA CHECKOUT

Notes

1. *Testing the flowmeters:* This step is present in the 1993 Checkout Recommendation and is intended to prompt checking of the oxygen/nitrous oxide proportioning system. It has been eliminated from the Preanesthesia Checkout in these guidelines because proper function is verified during the preventive maintenance and failures of this system in a properly maintained delivery system are rare.

2. *Desiccated carbon dioxide absorbent:* It has been well established that carbon dioxide absorbents that contain sodium, potassium, or barium hydroxide may become dangerous when desiccated, producing carbon monoxide and/or excessive heat leading to fires. Unfortunately, it is not possible to reliably identify when the absorbent material has been desiccated. Some departments elect to change all absorbent material on Monday morning to eliminate the possibility of using absorbent exposed to continuous fresh gas flow throughout the weekend. Other departments elect to use absorbent materials that do not pose a risk when desiccated. It is important to have a strategy to prevent the hazards related to using absorbents containing the problematic hydroxides that have desiccated. There are no steps that could be included in the checkout recommendation that can reliably identify desiccated absorbent. If a department uses absorbent that may be hazardous when desiccated, it may be prudent to change the absorbent material whenever the duration of time exposure to high fresh gas flow cannot be determined and is likely to have been prolonged.

    A protocol for preventing absorbent hazards should be part of every department's risk management strategy.

3. *Anesthesia information systems and automated record keepers:* These systems are being adopted by an increasing number of anesthesia departments and are the mainstay of the record keeping process in those departments. Reliably functioning systems are therefore important to the conduct of an anesthetic, although not essential to patient safety in the same fashion as the anesthesia delivery system and patient monitors. For departments that rely on these systems, it would be prudent to have a protocol for checking connections and the proper functioning of the associated computers, displays, and network function.

4. *Testing circle system valve competence:* As part of the test item 13 (Verify that gas flows properly through the breathing circuit during both inspiration and exhalation), the inspiratory and expiratory valves are visually observed for proper cycling (opening and closing fully). Visual inspection will also detect a missing valve leaflet. Ascertaining full closure of the valve is subjective. Incompetence of the valve may also be detected during item 13 through spirometry at the expiratory limb. For expiratory valve malfunction, a spirometer with reverse flow detection will alarm when gas flows retrograde in the expiratory limb. For inspiratory valve malfunction, the measured exhaled tidal volume will be less than the expected value. Capnography may also help to detect incompetence of the unidirectional valves. Intraoperatively, an inspiratory valve malfunction may not be indicated by an elevation of the inspired CO_2 baseline. If the delivered tidal volume exceeds the volume of gas in the inspiratory limb containing CO_2, rebreathing will appear on the capnogram as a gradual, instead of sharp, downstroke. An expiratory valve malfunction is indicated by an elevated CO_2 baseline as there is typically a large volume of exhaled gas containing CO_2 that can return to the patient.

ACKNOWLEDGMENT

Portions of this chapter have appeared with permission in Andrews JJ, Brockwell RC: Inhaled anesthesia delivery systems, Anesthesia, 6th edition. Edited by Miller RD. Philadelphia, Churchill Livingstone, 2004, p 273.

SECTION VI ■ ANESTHETIC MANAGEMENT

SECTION IV: ANATOMY

CHAPTER 27 ■ STANDARD MONITORING TECHNIQUES

STEVEN B. GREENBERG, GLENN S. MURPHY, AND JEFFERY S. VENDER

INSPIRATORY AND EXPIRED GAS MONITORING: OXYGEN
   Paramagnetic Oxygen Analysis
   Galvanic Cell Analyzers
   Polarographic Oxygen Analyzers
MONITORING OF EXPIRED GASES
   Carbon Dioxide
   Infrared Absorption Spectrophotometry
   Multiple Expired Gas Analysis
ARTERIAL OXYGENATION MONITORING
   Pulse Oximetry
BLOOD PRESSURE MONITORING
   Indirect Measurement of Arterial Blood Pressure

   Invasive Measurement of Vascular (Arterial Blood) Pressure
   Central Venous and Pulmonary Artery Monitoring
NONINVASIVE TECHNIQUES FOR CARDIAC OUTPUT/FLUID RESPONSIVENESS
   Indirect Fick Method
   Impedance Plethysmography
   Doppler Ultrasonography
   Arterial Pulse Contour Analysis/Transpulmonary
   Thermodilution/Lithium Dilution Technique
   Arterial Pulse Pressure/Systolic Pressure Variation
TEMPERATURE MONITORING
FUTURE TRENDS IN MONITORING

KEY POINTS

❶ Although the authors believe that electronic monitors augment clinical judgments when used properly, there is little high-grade evidence that electronic monitors, by themselves, reduce mortality or morbidity.

❷ Alterations in ventilation, cardiac output, distribution of pulmonary blood flow, and metabolic activity can all influence the capnograph display during carbon dioxide gas analysis.

❸ During direct invasive arterial pressure monitoring, systemic fidelity is optimized when the catheter and tubing are stiff, the mass of the fluid is small, and the length of the connecting tubing is not excessive. On the basis of available evidence, it is difficult to draw meaningful conclusions regarding the effectiveness of pulmonary artery catheter (PAC) monitoring in reducing morbidity and mortality in critically ill patients. Expert opinion suggests that perioperative complications may be reduced if PACs are used in the appropriate patients and settings, and if clinicians interpret and apply the data provided by the PAC correctly.

❹ New, noninvasive devices have been developed to generate similar parameters as the PAC as well as potentially to be able to predict fluid responsiveness.

Monitoring represents the process by which anesthesiologists recognize and evaluate potential physiologic problems in a timely manner. The term is derived from *monere,* which in Latin means to warn, remind, or admonish. In perioperative care, monitoring includes the following four essential features: observation and vigilance, instrumentation, interpretation of data, and initiation of corrective therapy when indicated.

Monitoring is an essential aspect of anesthesia care. It would seem that effective monitoring reduces the potential for poor outcomes that may follow anesthesia by identifying derangements before they result in serious or irreversible injury. Electronic monitors improve a physician's ability to respond because he or she is able to make repetitive measurements at higher frequencies than humans and do not fatigue or become distracted. Monitoring devices potentially increase the specificity and precision of clinical judgments. Our understanding of the physiologic effects of anesthesia and its inherent risks can be enhanced by the appropriate use of intraoperative physiologic monitoring.

This chapter discusses the methods by which anesthesiologists monitor organ function during anesthesia care. The descriptions of the technologic and scientific principles used in monitoring devices have been simplified for clarity.

Cost containment has been raised as a reason to discourage the use of expensive, technologically advanced monitoring systems. The value of a given monitor depends on the clinical expertise of the anesthesiologist, the clinical setting, the anesthetic technique, and the performance characteristics of the specific equipment in question. Monitoring devices should not be denied solely on the basis of expense.[1] Although it is appropriate for society to demand cost containment, anesthesiologists have a responsibility to assess how monitoring should be appropriately employed. Professional societies, regulatory agencies, and the legal profession have played important roles in establishing current monitoring practices.

Standards for basic anesthetic monitoring have been established by the American Society of Anesthesiologists (ASA). Since 1986, these standards have emphasized the evolution of technology and practice. Today's standards (last affirmed on October 25, 2005) emphasize the importance of regular and frequent measurements, integration of clinical judgment and experience, and the potential for extenuating circumstances that can influence the applicability or accuracy of monitoring systems.[2]

Standard I requires qualified personnel to be present in the operating room during general anesthesia, regional anesthesia, and monitored anesthesia care to monitor the patient continuously and modify anesthesia care based on clinical observations and the responses of the patient to dynamic changes resulting from surgery or drug therapy. Standard II focuses attention on continually evaluating the patient's oxygenation, ventilation, circulation, and temperature. Standard II specifically mandates the following:

1. Using an oxygen analyzer with a low concentration-limit alarm during general anesthesia.
2. Quantitatively assessing blood oxygenation during any anesthesia care.
3. Continuously ensuring the adequacy of ventilation by physical diagnostic techniques during all anesthesia care. Identification of expired carbon dioxide is performed unless nullified by the type of patient, procedure, or equipment. Quantitative monitoring of tidal volume and capnography is strongly encouraged in patients undergoing general anesthesia.
4. When administering regional anesthesia or monitored anesthesia care, sufficient ventilation should be assessed by qualitative clinical signs and/or monitoring of exhaled carbon dioxide.
5. Ensuring correct placement of an endotracheal intubation or laryngeal mask airway requires clinical assessment and qualitative identification of carbon dioxide in the expired gas. During general anesthesia, capnography and end-tidal carbon dioxide analysis is performed.
6. When using a mechanical ventilator, there should be a device that is able to detect a disconnection of any part of the breathing system.
7. The adequacy of circulation should be monitored by the continuous display of the electrocardiogram, and by determining the arterial blood pressure and heart rate at least at 5-minute intervals. During general anesthesia, circulatory function is to be continually evaluated by the quality of the pulse, either electronically or by palpation or auscultation.
8. During all anesthetics, the means for continuously measuring the patient's temperature must be available. When changes in body temperature are intended or anticipated, temperature should be continuously measured and recorded on the anesthesia record.

The ASA standards emphasize the melding of physical signs with instrumentation. Electronic monitoring, no matter how sophisticated or comprehensive, does not necessarily reduce the need for clinical skills such as inspection, palpation, and auscultation.

Although the authors believe that electronic monitors augment clinical judgments when used properly, there is little high-grade evidence that electronic monitors, by themselves, reduce mortality or morbidity. Moreover, there is considerable controversy regarding the need to apply specific monitors in unique clinical situations, particularly those that may add significant cost. Monitoring can be classified as invasive, minimally invasive, or noninvasive. Invasive monitors place patients at risk for complications related to their application and use. Anesthesiologists must balance the potential risk of instituting invasive monitoring with the presumed benefits derived from its application.

The variety of devices available for patient monitoring is expansive and changing as advances in biomedical engineering find their way into the marketplace. The Association for the Advancement of Medical Instrumentation has been effective in promoting design guidelines to ensure patient and operator safety and reduce stress and distractions often associated with medical monitoring.[3]

The proliferation of alarm tones during anesthesia care can be disturbing and may paradoxically impair clinical vigilance. Monitoring systems may lack adequate sensitivity and specificity to appropriately reject errors. During routine anesthesia care, a minimum of five alarms (inspired oxygen, airway pressure, pulse oximetry, blood pressure, and heart rate) should be operational. Unfortunately, spurious warnings occur with high frequency during routine anesthesia monitoring. The integration of alarm

signals is an important area in need of continuing evaluation and development. Loeb[4] reported that anesthesia providers have difficulty in accurately recognizing the source of an alarm tone. Alarm annunciators using unique sound and visual prompts are incorporated into newer anesthesia equipment. Warning signals for ventilation, oxygenation, drug administration, temperature, and cardiovascular parameters need to be designed so that problem identification is fast, simple, and relevant.

INSPIRATORY AND EXPIRED GAS MONITORING: OXYGEN

The concentration of oxygen in the anesthetic circuit must be measured. Measuring inspired oxygen does not guarantee the adequacy of arterial oxygenation.[5] Gas machine manufacturers place oxygen sensors on the inspired limb of the anesthesia circuit to ensure that hypoxic gas mixtures are never delivered to patients. Oxygen monitors require a fast response time (2 to 10 seconds), accuracy ($\pm 2\%$ of the actual level), and stability when exposed to humidity and inhalation agents.

Paramagnetic Oxygen Analysis

Oxygen is a highly paramagnetic gas. Paramagnetic gases are attracted to magnetic energy because of unpaired electrons in their outer shell orbits. Differential paramagnetic oximetry has been incorporated into a variety of operating room monitors. These instruments detect the change in sample line pressure resulting from the attraction of oxygen by switched magnetic fields. Signal changes during electromagnetic switching correlate with the oxygen concentration in the sample line.

Galvanic Cell Analyzers

Galvanic cell analyzers meet the performance criteria necessary for operative monitoring. These analyzers measure the current produced when oxygen diffuses across a membrane and is reduced to molecular oxygen at the anode of an electrical circuit. The electron flow (current) is proportional to the partial pressure of oxygen in the fuel cell. Galvanic cell analyzers require regular replacement of the galvanic sensor capsule. In the sensor, the electric potential for the reduction of oxygen results from a chemical reaction. Over time, the reactants require replenishment.[6]

Polarographic Oxygen Analyzers

Polarographic oxygen analyzers are commonly used in anesthesia monitoring. In this electrochemical system, oxygen diffuses through an oxygen-permeable polymeric membrane and participates in the following reaction: $O_2 + 2H_2O + 4e^- \rightarrow 4OH^-$. The current change is proportional to the number of oxygen molecules surrounding the electrode. Polarographic oxygen sensors are versatile and are important components of gas machine oxygen analyzers, blood gas analyzers, and transcutaneous oxygen analyzers.

MONITORING OF EXPIRED GASES

Carbon Dioxide

Monitoring the partial pressure of expiratory CO_2 has evolved as an important physiologic and safety monitor. CO_2 is usually

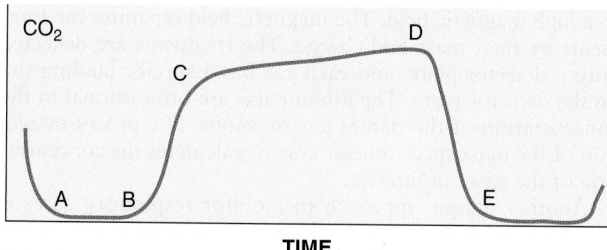

FIGURE 27-1. The normal capnogram. *Point D* delineates the end-tidal CO_2 (ETCO$_2$). ETCO$_2$ is the best reflection of the alveolar CO_2 partial measure.

❷ sampled near the endotracheal–gas delivery interface. Alterations in ventilation, cardiac output (CO), distribution of pulmonary blood flow, and metabolic activity influence end-tidal CO_2 concentration and the capnograph display obtained during quantitative expired gas analysis.

Capnometry is the measurement and numeric representation of the CO_2 concentration during inspiration and expiration. A *capnogram* is a continuous concentration–time display of the CO_2 concentration sampled at a patient's airway during ventilation.

Capnography is the continuous monitoring of a patient's capnogram. The capnogram is divided into four distinct phases (Fig. 27-1). The first phase (A–B in Fig. 27-1) represents the initial stage of expiration. Gas sampled during this phase occupies the anatomic dead space and is normally devoid of CO_2. At point B, CO_2-containing gas presents itself at the sampling site, and a sharp upstroke (B–C) is seen in the capnogram. The slope of this upstroke is determined by the evenness of expiratory ventilation and alveolar emptying. Phase C–D represents the alveolar or expiratory plateau. At this phase of the capnogram, alveolar gas is being sampled. Normally, this part of the waveform is almost horizontal. However, when ventilation and perfusion are mismatched, Phase C–D may take an upwards slope. Point D is the highest CO_2 value and is called the *end-tidal* CO_2 (ETCO$_2$). ETCO$_2$ is the best reflection of the alveolar CO_2 (PaCO$_2$). As the patient begins to inspire, fresh gas is entrained and there is a steep downstroke (D–E) back to baseline. Unless rebreathing of CO_2 occurs, the baseline approaches zero.

The utility of capnography depends on an understanding of the relationship between arterial CO_2 (PaCO$_2$), alveolar CO_2 (PACO$_2$), and ETCO$_2$. This concept assumes that ventilation and perfusion are appropriately matched, that CO_2 is easily diffusible across the capillary–alveolar membrane, and that no sampling errors occur during measurement. If these conditions are met, changes in ETCO$_2$ reflect changes in PaCO$_2$ even if it is assumed that all alveoli do not empty at the same time. In an upright, spontaneously breathing healthy person, one may assume the following idealized mathematical model of ventilation–perfusion, ETCO$_2 \approx$ PACO$_2 \approx$ PaCO$_2$. If the PACO$_2$–PaCO$_2$ gradient is constant and small, capnography provides a noninvasive, continuous, real-time reflection of ventilation. During general anesthesia, the ETCO$_2$–PaCO$_2$ gradient typically is 5 to 10 mm Hg. Dead space ventilation, a maldistribution of ventilation and perfusion ($\dot{V}/\dot{Q}$) where ventilation is disproportionally high relative to perfusion or problems in gas sampling may result in a widening of the ETCO$_2$–PaCO$_2$ gradient. Dead space $\dot{V}/\dot{Q}$ maldistribution is a common cause of an increased PACO$_2$–PaCO$_2$ gradient. Other patient factors that may influence the accuracy of ETCO$_2$ monitoring by widening the PaCO$_2$–ETCO$_2$ gradient include shallow tidal breaths, prolongation of the expiratory phase of ventilation, or uneven alveolar emptying.

Dead space (wasted) ventilation is the extreme example $\dot{V}/\dot{Q}$ of mismatch, where a complete absence of perfusion in the presence of adequate alveolar ventilation occurs. Because only perfused alveoli can participate in gas exchange, the non-perfused alveoli have a PaCO$_2$ of zero. The ventilation-weighted average of the perfused and nonperfused alveoli determines the ETCO$_2$. Therefore, conditions resulting in an increase of dead space ventilation lower the ETCO$_2$ measurement and increase the PaCO$_2$–ETCO$_2$ gradient. The common clinical causes associated with a widened PaCO$_2$–ETCO$_2$ gradient include embolic phenomena (thrombus, fat, air, amniotic fluid), hypoperfusion states with reduced pulmonary blood flow, and chronic obstructive pulmonary disease. In contrast, conditions that increase pulmonary shunt (perfusion in the absence of ventilation) result in minimal changes in the PaCO$_2$–ETCO$_2$ gradient.

Capnography is an essential element in determining the appropriate placement of endotracheal tubes. The presence of a stable ETCO$_2$ for three successive breaths indicates that the tube is not in the esophagus. A continuous, stable CO_2 waveform ensures the presence of alveolar ventilation but does not necessarily indicate that the endotracheal tube is properly positioned in the trachea. For example, the tip of the tube could be located in a main stem bronchus. In addition, a continuous CO_2 tracing can be evident when an endotracheal tube is proximally placed to the vocal cords. Capnography is also a monitor of potential changes in perfusion or dead space, is a very sensitive indicator of anesthetic circuit disconnection and gas circuit leaks, and is a method to detect the quality of CO_2 absorption. Increases in ETCO$_2$ can be expected when CO_2 production exceeds ventilation, such as in hyperthermia or when an exogenous source of CO_2 is present. Table 27-1 summarizes the common elements that may be reflected by changes in ETCO$_2$ during anesthesia care.

A sudden drop in ETCO$_2$ to near zero followed by the absence of a CO_2 waveform heralds a potentially life-threatening problem that could indicate malposition of an endotracheal tube into the pharynx or esophagus, sudden severe hypotension, massive pulmonary embolism, a cardiac arrest, or a disconnection or disruption of sampling lines. When a sudden drop of the ETCO$_2$ occurs, it is essential to quickly verify that there is pulmonary ventilation and to identify physiologic and mechanical factors that might account for then ETCO$_2$ of zero. During life-saving cardiopulmonary resuscitation, the generation of adequate circulation can be assessed by the restoration of the CO_2 waveform.

TABLE 27-1

FACTORS THAT MAY CHANGE END-TIDAL CO$_2$ (ETCO$_2$) DURING ANESTHESIA

▪ INCREASES IN ETCO$_2$	▪ DECREASES IN ETCO$_2$
▪ **ELEMENTS THAT CHANGE CO$_2$ PRODUCTION**	
Increases in metabolic rate	Decreases in metabolic rate
Hyperthermia	Hypothermia
Sepsis	Hypothyroidism
Malignant hyperthermia	
Shivering	
Hyperthyroidism	
▪ **ELEMENTS THAT CHANGE CO$_2$ ELIMINATION**	
Hypoventilation	Hyperventilation
Rebreathing	Hypoperfusion
	Pulmonary embolism

Whereas abrupt decreases in the $ETCO_2$ are often associated with an altered cardiopulmonary status (e.g., embolism or hypoperfusion), gradual reductions in $ETCO_2$ more often reflect decreases in $PaCO_2$ that occur when there exists an imbalance between minute ventilation and metabolic rate (i.e., CO_2 production), as commonly occurs during anesthesia at a fixed minute ventilation.

The size and shape of the capnogram waveform can be informative.[7] A slow rate of rise of the second phase (B–C in Fig. 27-1) is suggestive of either chronic obstructive pulmonary disease or acute airway obstruction as from bronchoconstriction (asthma) secondary to mismatching in ventilation to perfusion. A normally shaped capnogram with an increase in $ETCO_2$ suggests alveolar hypoventilation or an increase in CO_2 production. Transient increases in $ETCO_2$ are often observed during tourniquet release, aortic unclamping, or the administration of bicarbonate.

Several methods for the quantification of CO_2 have been applied to patient monitoring systems. One of the most commonly used methods is based on infrared absorption spectrophotometry.

Infrared Absorption Spectrophotometry

Asymmetric, polyatomic molecules like CO_2 absorb infrared light at specific wavelengths. Operating room infrared absorption spectrophotometry (IRAS) devices can detect CO_2, N_2O, and the potent inhaled anesthetic agents. Operating room instruments are designed to measure the unique energy absorbed by the gases and vapors of interest when a sample of the inspired and expired gas is placed into the optical path of an infrared beam.[8] The mixtures complicate the analysis because of interactions between the gases and vapors and the closeness of absorption spectra for the gases of interest. All anesthetic vapors absorb infrared light at 3.6 μm. Therefore, manufacturers using this signature cannot display with certainty the concentration of a specific anesthetic agent of interest. Optical filters and unique detection systems enhance the sensitivity of IRAS monitoring and permit estimation of CO_2, N_2O, and the specific potent inhalational agent present in the measurement chamber.

IRAS devices have five components: an infrared light source, a gas sampler, an optical path, a detection system, and a signal processor. The light source produces the infrared energy. The light is focused and filtered so that the quality of the photons with respect to the energy and frequency is stable over time. Narrow wavelengths are then presented to the gas stream. Once the sample has entered the measurement chamber, a detection system calibrated to determine the concentration of a specific gas or agent over time is activated. Changes in temperature, pressure, and acoustic characteristics in the detection chamber can be used to determine the concentration of the gas or agents of interest. Signal detectors create electrical currents analyzed by the signal processor, which transforms the current change to a measurement. The capnogram or agent waveform is an oscilloscopic representation of the electrical current changes over time. The signal-processing section of an IRAS instrument has a memory section that correlates the absorbed energy with a concentration as predicted by the Beer-Lambert law.

Multiple Expired Gas Analysis

Most operating room gas analyzers incorporate methods so that they can monitor concentrations of at least O_2, CO_2, and the inhaled anesthetic agents. *Mass spectrometry systems* bombard the gas mixture with electrons, creating ion fragments of a predictable mass and charge. These fragments are accelerated in a vacuum. A sample of this mixture enters a measurement chamber, where the fragment stream is subjected

to a high magnetic field. The magnetic field separates the fragments by their mass and charge. The fragments are deflected onto a detector plate, and each gas has a specific landing site on the detector plate. The ion impacts are proportional to the concentration of the parent gas or vapor. The processor section of the mass spectrometer system calculates the concentration of the gases of interest.

Another unique approach to monitor respiratory gases is based on *Raman scattering*. Raman scattering results when photons generated by a high-intensity argon laser collide with gas molecules. The scattered photons are measured as peaks in a spectrum that determine the concentration and composition of respiratory gases and inhaled vapors. O_2, N_2, N_2O, CO_2, H_2O vapors and inhaled anesthetic agents are all measurable using Raman scattering technology.[9]

Nitrogen monitoring provides quantification of washout during preoxygenation. A sudden rise in N_2 in the exhaled gas indicates either introduction of air from leaks in the anesthesia delivery system or venous air embolism. Critical events that can be detected by the analysis of respiratory gases and anesthetic vapors are listed in Table 27-2.

ARTERIAL OXYGENATION MONITORING

The assessment of arterial oxygenation is an integral part of anesthesia practice. Early detection and prompt intervention may limit serious sequelae of hypoxemia. The clinical signs associated with hypoxemia (e.g., tachycardia, altered mental status, cyanosis) are often masked or difficult to appreciate during anesthesia. The mechanisms responsible for hypoxemia are multifactorial. Oxygen analyzers assess oxygen delivery to the patient. Other noninvasive technologies detect the presence of arterial hypoxemia. Arterial oxygen monitors do not ensure adequacy of oxygen delivery to, or utilization by, the tissues, and should not be considered a replacement for arterial blood gas measurements when more definitive information regarding oxygenation is desired.

Pulse Oximetry

Pulse oximetry is one device suggested for monitoring oxygenation during anesthesia.[2] Pulse oximeters measure pulse rate and estimate oxygen saturation of hemoglobin (Hb; SpO_2) on a noninvasive, continuous basis. Figure 27-2 displays the oxyhemoglobin dissociation curve that defines the relationship of hemoglobin saturation and oxygen tension. On the steep part of the curve, a predictable correlation exists between SaO_2 and PaO_2. In this range, the SaO_2 is a good reflection of the extent of hypoxemia and the changing status of arterial oxygenation. Shifts in the oxyhemoglobin dissociation curve to the right or to the left define changes in the affinity of Hb for oxygen. Typically, at a PaO_2 of >75 mm Hg, the SaO_2 plateaus and loses its ability to reflect changes in PaO_2.

Pulse oximetry is based on several premises:

1. The color of blood is a function of oxygen saturation.

2. The change in color results from the optical properties of Hb and its interaction with oxygen.

3. The ratio of O_2Hb and reduced Hb can be determined by absorption spectrophotometry.

Pulse oximetry combines the technology of plethysmography and spectrophotometry. Plethysmography produces a pulse trace that is helpful in tracking circulation. Oxygen saturation is determined by spectrophotometry, which is based on the Beer-Lambert law. At a constant light intensity and Hb

TABLE 27-2

DETECTION OF CRITICAL EVENTS BY IMPLEMENTING GAS ANALYSIS

■ EVENT	■ GAS MEASURED BY ANALYZER
Error in gas delivery	O_2, N_2, CO_2, agent analysis
Anesthesia machine malfunction	O_2, N_2, CO_2, agent
Disconnection	CO_2, O_2, agent analysis
Vaporizer malfunction or contamination	Agent analysis
Anesthesia circuit leaks	N_2, CO_2 analysis
Endotracheal cuff leaks	N_2, CO_2
Poor mask or LMA fit	N_2, CO_2
Hypoventilation	CO_2 analysis
Malignant hyperthermia	CO_2
Airway obstruction	CO_2
Air embolism	CO_2, N_2
Circuit hypoxia	O_2 analysis
Vaporizer overdose	Agent analysis

LMA, laryngeal mask airway.
Modified from Knopes KD, Hecker BR: Monitoring anesthetic gases, Clinical Monitoring. Edited by Lake CL. Philadelphia, WB Saunders, 1990, p 24, with permission.

concentration, the intensity of light transmitted through a tissue is a logarithmic function of the oxygen saturation of Hb. Two wavelengths of light are required to distinguish O_2Hb from reduced Hb. Light-emitting diodes in the pulse sensor emit red (660 nm) and near infrared (940 nm) light. The percentage of O_2Hb and reduced Hb is determined by measuring the ratio of infrared and red light sensed by a photodetector. Pulse oximeters perform a plethysmographic analysis to differentiate the pulsatile "arterial" Hb saturation from the nonpulsatile signal resulting from "venous" absorption and other tissues such as skin, muscle, and bone. The absence of a pulsatile waveform during extreme hypothermia or hypoperfusion can limit the ability of a pulse oximeter to calculate the SpO_2.

The SpO_2 measured by pulse oximetry is not the same as the arterial saturation (SaO_2) measured by a laboratory co-oximeter. Pulse oximetry measures the "functional" saturation, which is defined by the following equation:

$$\text{Functional SaO}_2 = O_2Hb/(O_2Hb + \text{reduced Hb}) \times 100$$

Laboratory co-oximeters use multiple wavelengths to distinguish other types of Hb by their characteristic absorption. Co-oximeters measure the "fractional" saturation, which is defined by the following equation:

$$\text{Fractional SaO}_2 = O_2Hb/(O_2Hb + \text{reduced Hb} + COHb + MetHb) \times 100$$

In clinical circumstances where other Hb moieties are present, the SpO_2 measurement may not correlate with the actual SaO_2 reported by the blood gas laboratory. For example, methemoglobin absorbs red and infrared wavelengths of light in a 1:1 ratio corresponding to an SpO_2 of approximately 85%. Therefore, increases in MetHb produce an underestimation when $SpO_2 > 70\%$ and an overestimation when $SpO_2 < 70\%$. Similarly, carboxyhemoglobin also produces artificially high and misleading results. In fact, one study showed that at 70% COHb, the SpO_2 still measured 90%. In most patients, MetHb and COHb are present in low concentrations so that the functional saturation approximates the fractional value.[10]

Pulse oximetry has been used in all patient age groups to detect and prevent hypoxemia. The clinical benefits of pulse oximetry are enhanced by its simplicity. Modern pulse oximeters are noninvasive, continuous, and autocalibrating. They have quick response times and their battery backup provides monitoring during transport. The clinical accuracy is typically reported to be within ± 2 to 3% at 70 to 100% saturation and $\pm 3\%$ at 50 to 70% saturation. Published data from numerous investigations support accuracy and precision reported by instrument manufacturers.

The appropriate use of pulse oximetry necessitates an appreciation of both physiologic and technical limitations. Despite the numerous clinical benefits of pulse oximetry, other factors affect its accuracy and reliability. Factors that may be present during anesthesia care and that affect the accuracy and reliability of pulse oximetry include dyshemoglobins, dyes (methylene blue, indocyanine green, and indigo carmine), nail polish, ambient light, light-emitting diode variability, motion artifact, and background noise. Electrocautery can interfere with pulse oximetry if the radiofrequency emissions are sensed by the photodetector. Reports of burns or pressure necrosis exist but are infrequent. These complications can be reduced by inspecting the digits during monitoring.

Recent developments in pulse oximetry technology reportedly may permit more accurate measurements of SpO_2 during patient movement, low-perfusion conditions, and in the presence of dyshemoglobins. Some of these instruments use complex

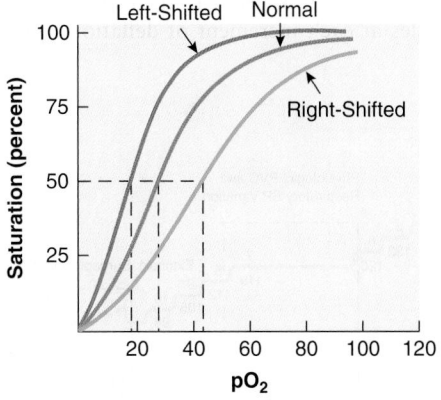

FIGURE 27-2. The oxyhemoglobin dissociation curve. The relationship between arterial saturation of hemoglobin and oxygen tension is represented by the sigmoid-shaped oxyhemoglobin dissociation curve. When the curve is left-shifted, the hemoglobin molecule binds oxygen more tightly. (Reproduced from Brown M, Vender JS: Non-invasive oxygen monitoring. Crit Care Clin 1988; 4: 493, with permission.)

signal processing of the two wavelengths of light to improve the signal-to-noise ratio and reject artifact. Studies in volunteers suggest that the performance of pulse oximeters incorporating this technology is superior to conventional oximetry during motion of the hand, hypoperfusion, and hypothermia.[11–13] Other pulse oximetry devices incorporate eight wavelengths of light to more accurately measure COHb and MetHb.[11–13]

Pulse oximetry has wide applicability in many hospital and nonhospital settings. However, there are no definitive data demonstrating a reduction in morbidity or mortality associated with the advent of pulse oximetry. An older large randomized trial did not detect a significant difference in postoperative complications when routine pulse oximetry was used.[14] However, the anesthesiologists using SpO₂ felt a greater level of comfort than those who did not use SpO₂. A reduction of anesthesia mortality, as well as fewer malpractice claims from respiratory events, coincident with the introduction of pulse oximeters suggests that the routine use of these devices may have been a contributing factor.

BLOOD PRESSURE MONITORING

Perioperative measurement of arterial blood pressure is an important indicator of the adequacy of circulation. Systemic blood pressure monitoring is commonly performed indirectly using extremity-encircling cuffs or directly by inserting a catheter into an artery and transducing the arterial pressure. Today, anesthesiologists have a variety of techniques available for measuring changes in systolic, diastolic, and mean arterial pressure (MAP).

Indirect Measurement of Arterial Blood Pressure

The simplest method of blood pressure determination estimates systolic blood pressure by palpating the return of the arterial pulse while an occluding cuff is deflated. Modifications of this technique include the observance of the return of Doppler sounds, the transduced arterial pressure trace, or a photoplethysmographic pulse wave as produced by a pulse oximeter.

Auscultation of the Korotkoff sounds permit estimation of both systolic (SP) and diastolic (DP) blood pressures. MAP can be calculated using an estimating equation (MAP = DP + 1/3 [SP–DP]). Korotkoff sounds result from turbulent flow within an artery created by the mechanical deformation from the blood pressure cuff. Systolic blood pressure is signaled by the appearance of the first Korotkoff sound. Disappearance of the sound or a muffled tone signals the diastolic blood pressure.

The detection of sound changes is subjective and prone to errors based on deficiencies in sound transmission or hearing. Cuff deflation rate also influences accuracy. Quick deflations underestimate blood pressure. Palpation and auscultatory techniques require pulsatile blood flow and are unreliable during conditions of low flow. These techniques are reasonably accurate when aneroid gauges are within calibration, the encircling cuff is appropriately sized and positioned, the inflation is above the true systolic pressure, and the Korotkoff sounds or pulse is properly identified.

The American Heart Association recommends that the bladder width for indirect blood pressure monitoring should approximate 40% of the circumference of the extremity. Bladder length should be sufficient to encircle at least 80% of the extremity. Falsely high estimates result when cuffs are too small, when cuffs are applied too loosely, or when the extremity is below heart level. Falsely low estimates result when cuffs are too large, when the extremity is above heart level, or after quick deflations.

Since 1976, microprocessor-controlled oscillotonometers have replaced auscultatory and palpatory techniques for routine perioperative blood pressure monitoring. Standard oscillometry measures mean blood pressure by sensing the point of maximal fluctuations in cuff pressure produced while deflating a blood pressure cuff. Most current instruments use oscillometric techniques to measure systolic, diastolic, and mean blood pressures by determining parameter identification points during cuff deflation.

In a generic noninvasive oscillometric monitor (*noninvasive blood pressure,* or NIBP), cuff pressure is sensed by a pressure transducer whose output is digitized for processing. After the cuff is inflated by an air pump, cuff pressure is held constant while oscillations are sampled. If no oscillations are sensed by the pressure transducer, the microprocessor switches open a deflation valve, and the next lower pressure level is sampled for the presence of oscillations. The microprocessor controlling the operation of the NIBP compares the amplitude of oscillation pairs and numerically displays the blood pressure estimate. Figure 27-3 depicts how a typical NIBP is obtained. In this example, the effect of respiratory variation, a premature ventricular complex, and cuff movement are demonstrated.

Automated oscillometry has been demonstrated to correlate well with direct intra-arterial measurement of MAP and diastolic blood pressure. Automated oscillometry may underestimate systolic blood pressure, with mean errors reported from −6.9 to −8.6 mm Hg compared with direct radial artery pressure measurements.

Oscillometry requires the careful evaluation of several cardiac cycles at each increment of deflation to smooth out

FIGURE 27-3. Diagram illustrating motion artifact, a premature ventricular contraction (PVC), and respiratory (RESP) artifact as sensed by a Dinamap noninvasive blood pressure (BP) monitor. (Reproduced from Ramsey M: Blood pressure monitoring: Automated oscillometric devices. J Clin Monit 1991; 7: 56, with permission.)

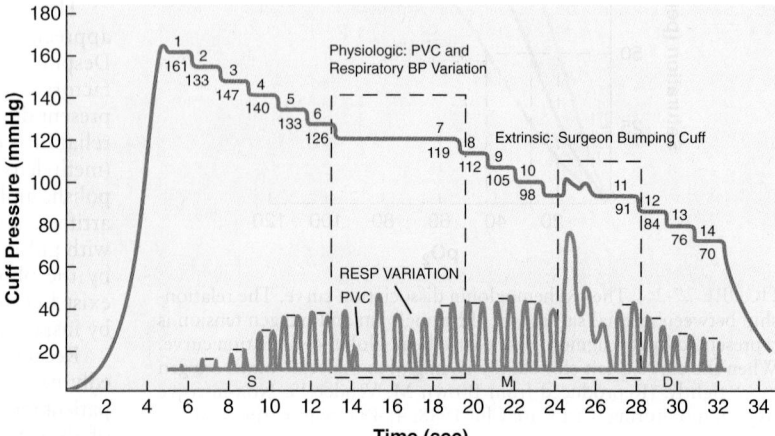

pronounced respiratory variations or motion artifacts. Cuff movement or erratic pulse transmission influences accuracy. In the anesthetized patient, automated oscillometry is usually accurate and versatile. A variety of cuff sizes makes it possible to use oscillometry in all age groups.

Problems With Noninvasive Blood Pressure Monitoring

Cuff-based pressure monitoring continues to be the standard method used in the perioperative period. Failure to deflate the cuff increases venous pressure. Hematomas have been described both beneath and distal to the cuff. Tremors or shivering can delay cuff deflation and prolong the deflation cycle. A compartment syndrome attributed to a prolonged inflation cycle has been described. Ulnar neuropathy has been reported after the use of automated cycled blood pressure cuffs. Compression of the ulnar nerve can be avoided by applying the encircling cuff proximal to the ulnar groove. Automated sequencing may alter the timing of intravenous drug administration when the access site is located in the same extremity. Hydrostatic errors result when blood pressure cuffs are placed on extremities that are above or below the level of the right atrium. The hydrostatic offset can be mathematically corrected by adding or subtracting 0.7 mm Hg for each centimeter that the cuff is off the horizontal plane of the heart.

Indirect Continuous Noninvasive Techniques

Several methods for monitoring blood pressure continuously and noninvasively have been designed and evaluated for intraoperative blood pressure surveillance. These techniques provide clinicians with a continuous blood pressure estimate and an accurate display of the arterial blood pressure trace. Indirect continuous noninvasive techniques continue to be evaluated to enable beat-to-beat blood pressure monitoring while reducing the inherent risks and costs of direct intra-arterial monitoring. Some clinical studies suggest that accuracy and precision of indirect continuous noninvasive techniques are satisfactory, even under conditions of rapidly changing hemodynamics.[15,16] However, one recent study using one of these devices illustrated variable agreement when compared with direct artery blood pressure monitoring during liver transplantation.[17] Therefore, randomized trials are needed to identify in which patient population and in which surgical environment the indirect continuous noninvasive techniques will be most efficacious.

Invasive Measurement of Vascular (Arterial Blood) Pressure

Indwelling arterial cannulation permits the opportunity to monitor arterial blood pressure continuously and to have vascular access for arterial blood sampling. Intra-arterial blood pressure monitoring uses fluid-filled tubing to transmit the force of the pressure pulse wave to a pressure transducer that converts the displacement of a silicon crystal into voltage changes. These electrical signals are amplified, filtered, and displayed as the arterial pressure trace. Intra-arterial pressure transducing systems are subject to many potential errors based on the physical properties of fluid motion and the performance of the catheter-transducer-amplification system used to sense, process, and display the pressure pulse wave.

The behavior of transducers, fluid couplings, signal amplification, and display systems can be described by a complex second-order differential equation. Solving the equation predicts the output and characterizes the fidelity of the system's ability to faithfully display and estimate the arterial pressure over time. The fidelity of fluid-coupled transducing systems is constrained by two properties: *damping* (ζ) and *natural frequency* (Fn). Zeta (ζ) describes the tendency for fluid in the measuring system to extinguish motion. Fn describes the tendency for the measuring system to resonate. The fidelity of the transduced pressure depends on optimizing ζ and Fn so that the system can respond appropriately to the range of frequencies contained in the pressure pulse wave. Analysis of high-fidelity recordings of arterial blood pressure indicates that the pressure trace contains frequencies from 1 to 30 Hz.

System fidelity is optimized when catheters and tubing are stiff, the mass of the fluid is small, the number of stopcocks is limited, and the connecting tubing is not excessive. Damping lowers the effective bandwidth of the transducer system, which promotes the potential for resonance. Figure 27-4 demonstrates the effect of damping on the character of the arterial pressure trace. In clinical practice, underdamped catheter–transducer systems tend to overestimate systolic pressure by 15 to 30 mm Hg and amplify artifact (catheter whip). Likewise, excessive increases in ζ reduce fidelity and underestimate systolic pressure. The presence of air bubbles in the coupling fluid reduces the natural frequency of the transducing system. For clinical use, it is sufficient to place the transducer at the level of the right atrium, open the stopcock to atmosphere, and balance the electronic amplifying system to display "zero." Periodic checks of the zero reference point ensure that transducer drift is eliminated.

The "fast flush" test is a method used at the bedside to determine the natural frequency and damping characteristics of the transducing system.[18] This test examines the characteristics of the resonant waves recorded after the release of a flush. Damping is estimated by the amplitude ratio of the first pair of resonant waves and the natural frequency is estimated by dividing the paper speed by the interval cycle.[18]

Arterial Cannulation

Multiple arteries can be used for direct measurement of blood pressure, including the radial, brachial, axillary, femoral, and dorsalis pedis arteries. The radial artery remains the most popular site for cannulation because of its accessibility and the presence of a collateral blood supply. In the past, assessment of the patency of the ulnar circulation by performance of an *Allen test* has been recommended before cannulation. An Allen test is performed by compressing both radial and ulnar arteries while the patient tightens his or her fist. Releasing pressure on each respective artery determines the dominant vessel supplying blood to the hand. The prognostic value of the Allen test in assessing the adequacy of the collateral circulation has not been confirmed.[19,20]

Radial artery cannulation and blood pressure monitoring have been associated with several problems. The radial artery pulse pressure wave is subject to inaccuracies inherent to its distal location. After separation from cardiopulmonary bypass, large pressure gradients between aortic and radial arteries have been described.[21]

Complications of Invasive Arterial Monitoring

Traumatic cannulation has been associated with hematoma formation, thrombosis, and damage to adjacent nerves. Abnormal radial artery blood flow after catheter removal occurs frequently. Studies suggest that blood flow normalizes in 3 to 70 days. Radial artery thrombosis can be minimized by using small catheters, avoiding polypropylene-tapered catheters, and reducing the duration of arterial cannulation. Flexible guidewires may reduce the potential trauma associated with catheters negotiating tortuous vessels. During cannula removal, the potential for thromboembolism may be diminished by compressing the proximal and distal arterial segment while aspirating the cannula during withdrawal.

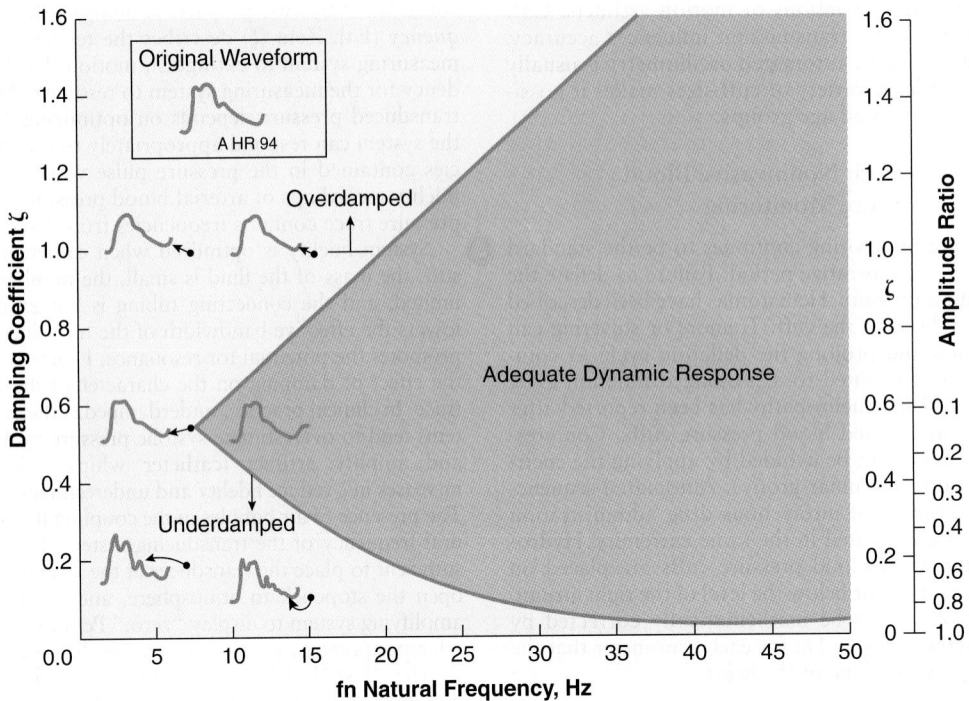

FIGURE 27-4. The relationship between the frequency of fluid-filled transducing systems and damping. The *shaded area* represents the appropriate range of damping for a given natural frequency (Fn). The size of the wedge also depends on the steepness of the arterial pressure trace and heart rate. (Reproduced from Gardner RM: Direct blood pressure measurement: Dynamic response requirements. Anesthesiology 1981; 54: 231, with permission.)

Many cannulation sites have been used for direct arterial blood pressure monitoring (Table 27-3). Three techniques for cannulation are common: direct arterial puncture, guidewire-assisted cannulation (Seldinger technique), and the transfixion–withdrawal method. A necessary condition for percutaneous placement is identification of the arterial pulse, which may be enhanced by a Doppler flow detection device in patients with poor peripheral pulses.

Arterial cannulation is regarded as an invasive procedure with documented morbidity. Ischemia after radial artery cannulation resulting from thrombosis, proximal emboli, or prolonged shock, albeit rare, has been described.[22] Contributing factors include severe atherosclerosis, diabetes, low CO, and intense peripheral vasoconstriction. Ischemia, hemorrhage, thrombosis, embolism, cerebral air embolism (retrograde flow associated with flushing), aneurysm formation, arteriovenous fistula formation, skin necrosis, and infection have reportedly occurred as the direct result of arterial cannulation, arterial blood sampling, or high-pressure flushing.

Continuous-flush devices are incorporated into disposable transducer kits and infuse at 3 to 6 mL/hr. In neonates, the infusion volume may contribute to fluid overload. Continuous-flush devices have little effect on the blood pressure measurement. However, pressurized flush systems may serve as a source of an air embolism. Removing air from the pressurized infusion bag, stopcocks, and tubing minimizes the potential for air embolism.

Direct arterial pressure monitoring requires constant vigilance. The data displayed must correlate with clinical conditions before therapeutic interventions are initiated. Sudden increases in the transduced blood pressure may represent a hydrostatic error because the position of the transducer was

TABLE 27-3

ARTERIAL CANNULATION AND DIRECT BLOOD PRESSURE MONITORING

ARTERIAL CANNULATION SITE	CLINICAL POINTS OF INTEREST
Radial artery	Preferred site for monitoring
	Nontapered catheters preferred
Ulnar artery	Complication similar to radial
	Primary source of hand blood flow
Brachial artery	Insertion site medial to biceps tendon
	Median nerve damage is potential hazard
	Can accommodate 18-gauge cannula
Axillary artery	Insertion site at junction of pectoralis and deltoid muscles
	Specialized kits available
Femoral artery	Easy access in low-flow states
	Potential for local and retroperitoneal hemorrhage
	Longer catheters preferred
Dorsalis pedis artery	Collateral circulation = posterior tibial artery
	Higher systolic pressure estimates

not adjusted after change in the operating room table's height. Sudden decreases often result from kinking of the catheter or tubing. Before initiating therapy, the transducer system should be "rezeroed" and the patency of the arterial cannula verified. This ensures the accuracy of the measurement and avoids the initiation of a potentially dangerous medication error.

Central Venous and Pulmonary Artery Monitoring

Central venous cannulas are important portals for intraoperative vascular access and for the assessment of changes in vascular volume. Central venous cannulas permit the rapid administration of fluids, insertion of pulmonary artery catheters (PACs) or central venous O_2 (ScvO$_2$) catheters, insertion of transvenous electrodes, monitoring of central venous pressure (CVP), and a site for observation and treatment of venous air embolism.

The right internal jugular vein is the most common site for cannulation by anesthesiologists because it is accessible from the head of the operating table, has a predictable anatomy, and has a high success rate in both adults and children.[23] The left-sided internal jugular vein is also available but is less desirable because of the potential for damaging the thoracic duct or difficulty in maneuvering catheters through the jugular–subclavian junction. Accidental carotid artery puncture is a potential problem with either location.

Three techniques (posterior, central, and anterior) have been described for internal jugular cannulation. Each insertion point is referenced to the triangle formed by the sternal and clavicular heads of the sternocleidomastoid muscle and the clavicle. Venipuncture using a 22-gauge "seeker" needle minimizes trauma to adjacent structures. When the location of the internal jugular vein is difficult to ascertain, ultrasonography can assist in identifying the proximity of internal jugular vein and the carotid artery. Some studies have suggested that ultrasound-guided placement of right internal jugular placed central venous catheters may reduce complications and improve first-attempt success rates.[24,25]

Alternatives to the internal jugular vein include the external jugular, subclavian, antecubital, and femoral veins. Although the Centers for Disease Control and Prevention suggests that the preferred site for central venous cannulation should be the subclavian site to potentially reduce bloodstream infections, this recommendation must be taken in context of the particular clinical situation.[26] The internal jugular approach may be superior in those patients with coagulopathies (where bleeding at the subclavian site may be more difficult to stop) or patients with severe acute lung injury (where the risk of pneumothorax may be heightened).[27] When comparing the subclavian approach with the femoral approach, the reported reduction in infection risk favors subclavian. However, there is a paucity of prospective randomized data when comparing subclavian to internal jugular.[28]

Central Venous Pressure Monitoring

The benefit of CVP monitoring has been the subject of considerable debate. Proponents of CVP monitoring believe that CVP pressures are essentially equivalent to right atrial pressures and serve as a reflection of right ventricular preload.[29] Conditions that affect right atrial pressure also influence the CVP pressure trace. The normal CVP waveform consists of three peaks (a, c, and v waves) and two descents (x, y), each resulting from the ebb and flow of blood in the right atrium (Fig. 27-5). Corresponding events occur in the left atrium and similar pressure contours are observed during monitoring of pulmonary artery pressure when the PAC is placed in the occluded position.

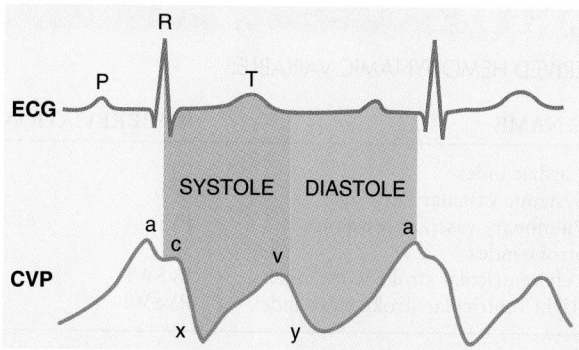

FIGURE 27-5. The normal central venous pressure (CVP) trace. ECG, electrocardiogram. (Redrawn from Mark JB: Central venous pressure monitoring: Clinical insights beyond the numbers. J Cardiothorac Anesth 1991; 5: 163, with permission.)

The character of the CVP trace depends on many factors, including heart rate, conduction disturbances, tricuspid valve function, normal or abnormal intrathoracic pressure changes, and changes in right ventricular compliance. In patients with atrial fibrillation, a waves are absent. When resistance to the emptying of the right atrium is present, large a waves are often observed. Examples include tricuspid stenosis, right ventricular hypertrophy as a result of pulmonic stenosis, or acute or chronic lung disease associated with pulmonary hypertension. Large a waves may also be observed when right ventricular compliance is impaired.

Tricuspid regurgitation typically produces giant v waves that begin immediately after the QRS complex. Large v waves are often observed when right ventricular ischemia or failure is present or when ventricular compliance is impaired by constrictive pericarditis or cardiac tamponade. A prominent v wave during CVP monitoring may suggest right ventricular papillary muscle ischemia and tricuspid regurgitation. When right ventricular compliance decreases, the CVP often increases with prominent a and v waves fusing to form an *m* or *w* configuration.

CVP monitoring is often unreliable for estimating left ventricular filling pressures, especially when cardiopulmonary disease processes alter the normal cardiovascular pressure–volume relationships. However, CVP monitoring is less invasive and less costly than pulmonary artery monitoring and offers unique understanding of right-sided hemodynamic events and the status of vascular volume.

Pulmonary Artery Monitoring

The development of the flow-directed, balloon flotation PAC was a major advance in hemodynamic monitoring, and it has been an important tool in the quantitative assessment of cardiopulmonary function. Numerous articles have reviewed the various applications and benefits of pulmonary artery monitoring.[30] Use should be guided by the information needed for enhanced diagnosis and therapy.[31] Today, PAC monitoring is commonly used in surgical patients to help evaluate and treat hemodynamic alterations, which contribute significantly to the morbidity and mortality inherent to the surgical care of high-risk patients.

In 1993, the ASA published practice guidelines that examined the evidence supporting the clinical effectiveness of PAC monitoring. These guidelines were updated in 2003.[32] Issues such as the timing of PAC monitoring, its effect on treatment decisions, patient selection and case mix, and evidence regarding PAC monitoring contribution to positive or negative outcomes were evaluated using stringent evidence-based methodology. This effort identified many flaws in the body of evidence,

TABLE 27-4

DERIVED HEMODYNAMIC VARIABLES

■ NAME	■ ABBREVIATION	■ CALCULATION	■ UNITS
Cardiac index	CI	CO/BSA	$1\ L/min/m^2$
Systemic vascular resistance	SVR	$(MAP - CVP/CO) \times 80$	dyne-cm/s
Pulmonary vascular resistance	PVR	$(MPAP - PCWP/CO) \times 80$	dyne-cm/s
Stroke index	SI	CI/heart rate	$mL/beat/m^2$
Left ventricular stroke work index	LVSWI	$SI \times (MAP - PCWP) \times 0.0136$	$g/beat/m^2$
Right ventricular stroke work index	RVSWI	$SI \times (MPAP - CVP) \times 0.0136$	$g/beat/m^2$

CO, cardiac output; BSA, body surface area; MAP, mean arterial pressure; CVP, central venous pressure; MPAP, mean pulmonary arterial pressure; PCWP, pulmonary capillary wedge pressure.

which made it difficult to draw meaningful conclusions regarding the effectiveness of PAC monitoring to reduce morbidity or mortality. The consensus opinion implies that PAC monitoring may reduce perioperative complications if critical hemodynamic data obtained during appropriate PAC monitoring are accurately interpreted and appropriate treatment is tailored to the conditions as they change over time.[32]

PACs permit the measurement of intracardiac pressures, thermodilution cardiac output (TCO), mixed venous oxygen saturation, intracavitary electrocardiograms, and lung water. This information can help define clinical problems, monitor the progression of hemodynamic dysfunctions, and guide the response of corrective therapy.

The measurement of intracardiac pressures can indirectly assess left ventricular preload, diagnose the existence of pulmonary hypertension, or differentiate cardiac and noncardiac causes of pulmonary edema. PACs allow for the rapid and reproducible measurements of TCO, calculation of oxygen delivery (CO × arterial O_2 content), and assessment of cardiac work. Hemodynamic measurements are often predicated on the manipulation of preload, afterload, and contractility. Several derived indices of hemodynamic function necessitate measurements commonly obtained from PAC monitoring (Table 27-4).

Access to mixed venous blood from the pulmonary artery port provides an indirect assessment of the balance between O_2 delivery and O_2 utilization. Mixed venous oxygen saturation (SvO_2) measurements are needed to calculate mixed venous oxygen content ($C\bar{v}O_2$). $C\bar{v}O_2$ is an important variable used for calculating intrapulmonary (first equation following) or intracardiac shunts (second equation following).

$$\frac{CcO_2 - CaO_2}{CcO_2 - C\bar{v}O_2} = \frac{\dot{Q}s}{\dot{Q}t}$$

$$\frac{SaO_2 - SraO_2}{SaO_2 - S\bar{v}O_2} = \frac{\dot{Q}p}{\dot{Q}s}$$

Where CcO_2 = end-capillary O_2 content, CaO_2 = arterial O_2 content, $C\bar{v}O_2$ = mixed venous O_2 content, $\dot{Q}s/\dot{Q}t$ = shunt fraction, SaO_2 = arterial O_2 saturation, $SraO_2$ = right atrial O_2 saturation, $S\bar{v}O_2$ = mixed venous O_2 saturation, and $\dot{Q}p/\dot{Q}s$ = pulmonary-to-systemic shunt.

The validity of PAC monitoring depends on a properly functioning pressure monitoring system, correctly identifying the "true" *pulmonary capillary occlusion pressure* (PCOP), and integration of the various factors that affect the relationship of PCOP, and the other cardiac pressures and volumes that are determinants of ventricular function. Figure 27-6 depicts the transduced pressure waves observed as a PAC is floated to the wedged position. Catheter placement is most commonly performed by observing the pressure waves as the catheter is floated from the CVP position through the right heart chambers into the pulmonary artery.

PAC monitoring necessitates an appreciation of the various physiologic determinants of CO and oxygen delivery. The PAC is used to continuously monitor the pulmonary artery pressure and intermittently monitor pulmonary wedge pressure. PCOP is used to assess left ventricular preload indirectly by reflecting changes in left ventricular end-diastolic pressure (LVEDP). Figure 27-7 depicts the relationship between the various pressures in the cardiopulmonary system.

It has been well demonstrated that right-sided pressures in the heart often are poor indicators of left ventricular filling, either as absolute numbers or in terms of the direction of change in response to therapy. The correlation of these pressures as estimates of LVEDP (or left ventricular end-diastolic volume [LVEDV]) is directly related to their proximity to the left ventricle and the status of ventricular compliance. Assuming an open conduit from the catheter tip to the left ventricle, when the PAC is occluded ("wedged"), the right-sided heart chambers and valves are bypassed. During end-diastole, there is cessation of forward blood flow, and a static fluid column is presumed to exist from the left ventricle to the PAC tip. Ideally, changes in LVEDP are reflected by all proximal pressures (left atrial, pulmonary venous, pulmonary artery end-diastolic

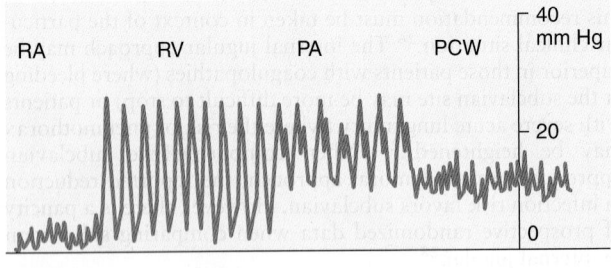
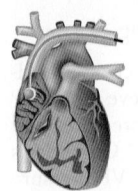
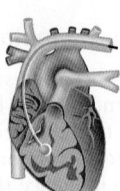
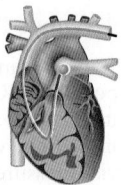
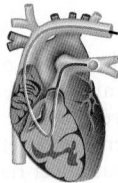

FIGURE 27-6. Pressure tracing observed during the flotation of a pulmonary artery catheter. RA, right atrium; RV, right ventricle; PA, pulmonary artery; PCW, pulmonary capillary wedge pressure. (Reproduced from Dizon CT, Barash PG: The value of monitoring pulmonary artery pressure in clinical practice. Conn Med 1979; 41: 622, with permission.)

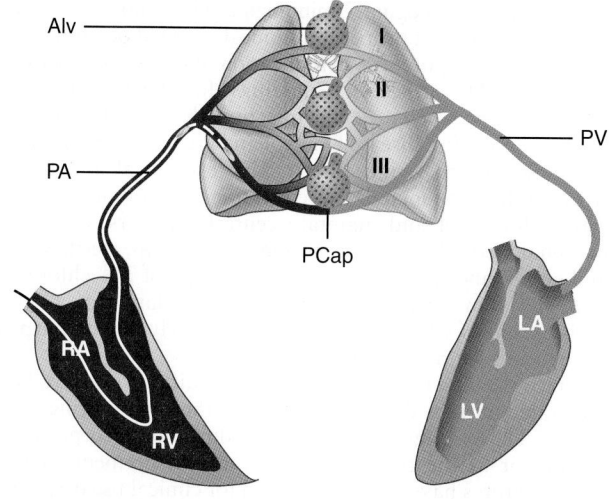

FIGURE 27-7. The anatomic position of a pulmonary artery catheter in the pulmonary artery. The *dashed line* positions the inflated balloon in the "wedged" position. RA, right atrium; RV, right ventricle; PA, pulmonary artery; Alv, alveolus; PCap, pulmonary capillary; PV, pulmonary vein; LA, left atrium; LV, left ventricle. I, II, and III characterize the relationship of $P_{aveolar}$, $P_{arterial}$, and P_{venous} as described by West et al.[33] The bottom of the figure shows a progressive correlation of vascular pressures. (Reproduced from Vender JS: Invasive cardiac monitoring. Crit Care Clin 1988; 4: 455, with permission.)

pressure, and PCOP). Alterations of internal or external forces applied to the open conduit during PCOP measurements may invalidate the PCOP-LVEDP-LVEDV relationship.

Factors Affecting the Accuracy of Pulmonary Artery Catheter Data

Pulmonary Vascular Resistance. Any disease process or condition that increases pulmonary vascular resistance has the potential to reduce pulmonary blood flow and alter the relationship between PCOP and pulmonary artery end-diastolic pressure (PAEDP). Pathologic conditions such as acute or chronic lung disease, pulmonary emboli, alveolar hypoxia, acidosis, and hypoxemia, and many vasoactive drugs increase pulmonary vascular resistance and have the potential to modify the PCOP–PAEDP relationship. Tachycardia shortens ventricular diastole and also increases pulmonary vascular resistance and the measure of pulmonary artery diastolic pressure.

Alveolar–Pulmonary Artery Pressure Relationships. West et al.[33] described a gravity-dependent difference between ventilation and perfusion in the lung. The variability in pulmonary blood flow is a result of differences in pulmonary artery (PA), alveolar (Palv), and venous pressures (PV) and is categorized into three distinct zones. Only Zone III (PA > PV> Palv) meets the criteria for uninterrupted blood flow and a continuous communication with distal intracardiac pressures. Increases in alveolar pressure, decreases in perfusion, or changes in the position of the patient can convert areas of zone III into either zone II or I. Flow-directed PACs usually advance to gravity-dependent areas of highest blood flow. The following characteristics suggest that the PAC tip is not in zone III: PCOP > PAEDP, nonphasic PCOP tracing, and inability to aspirate blood from the distal port when the catheter is wedged.

Respiratory Pattern and Airway Pressure. Changes in intrathoracic and intrapleural pressure affect transmural cardiac pressures. Transmural pressure is defined as the net distending pres-

sure of the left ventricle. Changes in intrathoracic pressure affect the PCOP–LVEDP relationship. Positive end–expiratory pressure (PEEP) therapy can induce changes in both intravascular and intrapleural pressures. PEEP increases alveolar pressure, potentially converting zone III areas to zone II. If PEEP is transmitted across the alveoli, intrapleural pressure increases. Pulmonary compliance determines the extent of this effect. PEEP alters ventricular distensibility and decreases venous return, which causes a disproportionate increase in PCOP (and LVEDP) compared with changes in LVEDV.

The effect of PEEP therapy on PCOP is minimal if the levels of PEEP are low ($\leq$10 cm H_2O) and the PAC is located in zone III. Higher levels of PEEP influence the PCOP–LVEDP relationship, depending on pulmonary compliance and transmission of alveolar pressures. During high PEEP therapy, esophageal pressure measurements can be measured to reflect intrapleural pressure. Alternatively, subtracting 1 to 2 mm Hg from the displayed "wedge" pressure for each 5 cm H_2O of PEEP therapy gives PCOP estimate when PEEP is above 10 cm H_2O.

Intracardiac Factors. Obstruction at the mitral valve from mitral stenosis, atrial myxoma, or clot can interfere with the ability of left atrial pressure to reflect LVEDP. Similarly, mitral regurgitation, a noncompliant left atrium, or left-to-right intracardiac shunting often is associated with large v waves[34] (see Chapter 62).

Decreases in left ventricular compliance, aortic regurgitation, or premature closure of the mitral valve may reverse the left atrial pressure–LVEDP pressure gradient. When this occurs, PCOP is not a valid reflection of LVEDV.

Figure 27-8 graphically depicts the relationship between LVEDP and LVEDV. The LVEDP–LVEDV relationship is not linear. A family of LVEDP–LVEDV compliance curves characterizes the effect of changing the stiffness of the left ventricle. Ventricular compliance is a dynamic factor influenced by many physiologic and pathologic variables. The LVEDP–LVEDV compliance curves suggest that at low preloads, larger increases in LVEDV produce smaller changes in LVEDP. Conversely, at higher preloads, a similar change in LVEDV produces a greater pressure change. For a given LVEDV, any decrease in ventricular compliance (e.g., ischemia) results in an increase in LVEDP. This explains the development of hydrostatic pulmonary edema at normal LVEDV. Factors that are associated with changes in ventricular compliance are listed in Table 27-5.

Complications of Pulmonary Catheter Monitoring

Adverse effects from PAC monitoring can be a result of accessing the central venous circulation, the catheterization procedure,

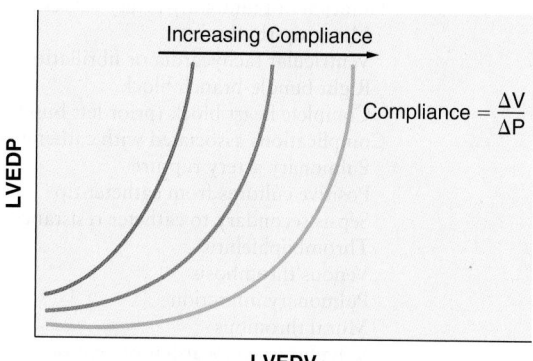

FIGURE 27-8. Typical ventricular compliance curve. LVEDP, left ventricular end-diastolic pressure; LVEDV, left ventricular end-diastolic volume. (Reproduced from Vender JS: Invasive cardiac monitoring. Crit Care Clin 1988; 4: 455, with permission.)

TABLE 27-5

DECREASED LEFT VENTRICULAR COMPLIANCE: COMMON ETIOLOGIES

Myocardial ischemia	Cardiac tamponade
Restrictive myopathies	Myocardial fibrosis
Right-to-left intraventricular shunts	Inotropic drugs
Aortic stenosis	Hypertension

or from use of the catheter after PAC placement. Central venous access represents an invasive process with inherent risks, some of which are rare but are potentially life-threatening.

Unintentional puncture of nearby arteries, bleeding, neuropathy, and pneumothorax may result from needle insertion into adjacent structures. Air embolism may occur if a cannula is open to the atmosphere and air is entrained during or after CVP placement. Dysrhythmias are common during the catheterization procedure, with a reported incidence of 4.7 to 68.9%.[32] Ventricular tachycardia or fibrillation may be induced during catheter advancement. Catheter advancement has been associated with right bundle-branch block and may precipitate complete heart block in patients with pre-existing left bundle-branch block. Table 27-6 summarizes the adverse effects as reported by the ASA Task Force on pulmonary artery catheterization.[32]

The rate of iatrogenic deaths associated with PAC monitoring is uncertain. The most dreaded complication associated with PAC monitoring is pulmonary artery rupture. Pulmonary hypertension, coagulopathy, and heparinization are often present in patients who have died of pulmonary artery rupture. Perforations and subsequent hemorrhage can be avoided by restricting "overwedging," minimizing the number of balloon inflations, and using proper technique during balloon inflations.

Infection is a potential complication of the continued use of CVP and PAC catheters. Guidelines for the prevention of intravascular catheter-related infections have been published by the Centers for Disease Control and Prevention.[26] Methods recommended to reduce the incidence of local and bloodstream infections include (1) education and training of clinicians who insert and maintain central catheters, (2) use of maximal sterile barrier precautions (mask, cap, sterile gloves and gown, and large sterile drape), (3) use of 2% chlorhexidine for skin preparation, and (4) avoidance of routine replacement of CVP and PAC catheters solely for the purpose of reducing the risk of infection.

Since the advent of PACs, several modifications have been integrated into the design that enhance their monitoring capabilities. The first significant design modification incorporated a thermistor at the tip, permitting the measurement of CO. Other features have been introduced for clinical use or evaluation. These include mixed venous oximetry, measurement of right ventricular ejection fraction, pacing options, and continuous CO monitoring.

Mixed Venous Oximetry

Continuous estimates of SvO_2 provide a reflection of total tissue oxygen balance. Oxygen delivery (DO_2) equals the arterial oxygen content multiplied by the CO (CO × [Hb 13.8 × SaO_2 + (PaO_2 × 0.0031)]), where 13.8 represents the volume of oxygen carried by Hb converted to grams per liter, SaO_2 represents the arterial oxygen saturation, PaO_2 represents the arterial pressure of oxygen, and 0.0031 represents the Bunsen solubility coefficient of dissolved oxygen per millimeters of mercury. Oxygen consumption (VO_2) is determined by the difference between arterial and venous oxygen delivery. The rela-

TABLE 27-6

ADVERSE EFFECTS ASSOCIATED WITH PULMONARY ARTERY MONITORING

▪ COMPLICATION	▪ REPORTED INCIDENCE (%)
Central venous access	
Arterial puncture	0.1–13
Postoperative neuropathy	0.3–1.1
Pneumothorax	0.3–4.5
Air embolism	0.5
Flotation of pulmonary artery catheter	
Minor dysrhythmias	4–68.9
Ventricular tachycardia or fibrillation	0.3–62.7
Right bundle-branch block	0.1–4.3
Complete heart block (prior left bundle-branch block)	0–8.5
Complications associated with catheter residence	
Pulmonary artery rupture	0.03–1.5
Positive cultures from catheter tip	1.4–34.8
Sepsis secondary to catheter resistance	0.7–11.4
Thrombophlebitis	6.5
Venous thrombosis	0.5–66.7
Pulmonary infarction	0.1–5.6
Mural thrombus	28–61
Valvular or endocardial vegetations	2.2–100
Deaths attributed to pulmonary artery catheter	0.02–1.5

From Practice Guidelines for Pulmonary Artery Catheterization: An updated report by The American Society of Anesthesiologists Task Force on Pulmonary Catheterization. Anesthesiology 2003; 99: 988, with permission.

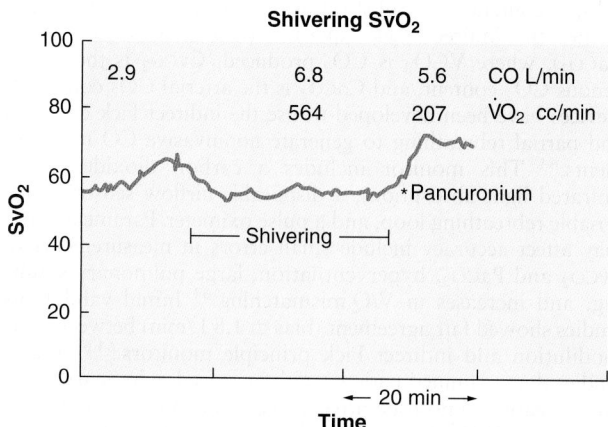

FIGURE 27-9. This $S\bar{v}O_2$ recording in a postcoronary artery bypass patient demonstrates the effects of shivering and its treatment, and the relationship between $S\bar{v}O_2$, cardiac output (CO), and metabolic rate ($S\dot{v}O_2$). *Pancuronium, a long acting muscle relaxant, used to eliminate shivering and improve $S\dot{v}O_2$. (Reproduced from Vender JS: Invasive cardiac monitoring. Crit Care Clin 1988; 4: 455, with permission.)

tionship between $S\bar{v}O_2$, $\dot{V}O_2$, and $\dot{D}O_2$ is demonstrated in the following equation derived from the Fick relationship:

$$S\bar{v}O = SaO_2 - \dot{V}O_2/Hb \times 13.8 \times CO$$

This equation indicates that changes in $S\bar{v}O_2$ vary directly with changes in CO, Hb, and SaO_2 and inversely with $\dot{V}O_2$. The normal is 75%, which denotes tissue oxygen extraction of 25%.

The oximetric PAC uses reflectance spectrophotometry in which several wavelengths are transmitted through optical fibers embedded in the PAC. The reflected intensity of light identifies the saturation of blood surrounding the tip of the PAC. Three-wavelength *in vivo* systems correlate well with simultaneous samples measured by co-oximetry.[35] An example of the utility of mixed venous oximetry is depicted in Figure 27-9.

Central Venous Oxygen Saturation and its Relation to Mixed Venous Oxygen Saturation

Although central venous O_2 saturation ($ScvO_2$) represents the amount of oxygen extraction from the upper part of the body and brain, some clinicians suggest the use of $ScvO_2$ as a surrogate measure of SvO_2.[36] $ScvO_2$ measurements are an appealing alternative because they can be taken from central venous catheters and do not require PAC insertion. Recent sepsis guidelines suggest using SvO_2 and $ScvO_2$ interchangeably for patients with septic shock.[37] However, others argue that $ScvO_2$ cannot be synonymously used in place of SvO_2 during septic shock.[36,38] The arguments against the use of $ScvO_2$ state that during septic shock, regional oxygen extraction in the gastrointestinal tract increases, but cerebral blood flow is maintained. This phenomenon may cause a less pronounced drop in $ScvO_2$ than SvO_2 during shock.[36,37] In addition, during cardiogenic or hypovolemic shock, mesenteric and renal flow decreases with an increase in oxygen extraction that may produce discrepancies between SvO_2 and $ScvO_2$.[36] Although studies in the septic shock patient population show mixed results, recent intraoperative data indicate that SvO_2 and $ScvO_2$ trends may correlate and this may aid in therapeutic decision making.[39] Therefore, further outcome data may be needed to address the affects of different patient populations and clinical situations on the utility of $ScvO_2$ when approximating SvO_2.

Indicator Dilution Applications

Indicator dilution determination of CO is based on a concept proposed by Stewart and tested by Hamilton and colleagues.[40,41]

Thermodilution cardiac output (TCO) determination is the most widely used adaptation of the indicator dilution principle, which was first described by Fegler[42] in 1954. Today, 0.9% saline or 5% dextrose mixtures can be used interchangeably as the indicator, producing similar CO measurements. A thermistor located at the PAC tip records the decrease in temperature as the bolus of cooled injectate passes through the pulmonary artery. Computers contend with the complexity of the TCO equation, which includes the following factors: specific heat of the blood and the indicator fluid, the volume of injectate, catheter size, specific gravity of the blood and indicator, and the area of the blood temperature curve. Comparison studies suggest that using either room-temperature or iced injectate provides acceptable estimates of CO. Iced injectate is often preferred because it produces a more exacting curve with a better signal-to-noise ratio.[43]

When properly performed, TCO measurements correlate well with direct Fick or dye dilution estimates of CO. In clinical practice, triplicate determinations are averaged to increase precision. TCO estimates can vary with the respiratory cycle. This variability can be reduced by performing measurements at peak inspiration or end expiration. Precision is enhanced by ensuring that the rate of injection and the volume are constant. Most CO computers delay the repeat measurement 30 to 90 seconds to stabilize the thermal environment of the PAC thermistor.

Adaptations for Continuous Cardiac Output Monitoring

Continuous CO monitoring offers the potential to identify acute changes in ventricular performance as they occur. A properly positioned PAC provides access to the right atrium, right ventricle, and pulmonary artery outflow tract. These locations provide many options for assessment of continuous CO monitoring. Several thermal techniques have been developed. Pulsed thermodilution uses a coiled right ventricular filament that applies a low-power heating signal to the right atrium and ventricle in a cyclical manner based on a proprietary sequence.[44] A thermistor at the tip of the PAC detects changes in blood temperature and sends the temperature information to a microcomputer that uses stochastic analysis to create a thermodilution curve. CO is computed continuously from a conservation of heat equation.[44]

Another technique applies heat to a thermistor located at the tip of a PAC. The right ventricular outflow subsequently cools the tip. The temperature changes registered are proportional to the decreased temperature produced by right ventricular blood flow. Both of these systems require calibration using standard thermodilution before initiating the continuous CO monitoring mode. Although a time lag can exist, continuous CO monitoring compares favorably with bolus CO measurements, even under conditions of varying patient temperature and CO.[45]

Right Ventricular Ejection Fraction

Calculation of right ventricular ejection fraction and end-diastolic volume may be performed with a special PAC that uses a rapid-response thermistor and a sophisticated computer system. This system analyzes the exponential decay of the pulmonary artery temperature over several cardiac cycles and calculates the ejection fraction by subtracting the mean residual fraction from the CO. Studies have demonstrated good correlation with *in vitro* techniques and clinical utility for detecting intraoperative right ventricular ischemia.[46–49] Other studies suggest acceptable agreement between right ventricular ejection fraction generated by this new PAC and transesophageal echocardiography only when heart rate is maintained below 100 beats per minute.[50] Right ventricular ejection fraction monitoring may be beneficial in conditions of right ventricular dysfunction. In addition, it may also be used for a more accurate assessment of right ventricular preload during orthotopic liver transplant.[51] Accuracy requires proper placement. Dysrhythmias and tricuspid regurgitation can affect the accuracy of the thermal decay methodology.

Clinical Benefits and Controversy of Pulmonary Artery Monitoring

The debate regarding the clinical benefit of PAC monitoring has persisted since the mid-1980s. Perioperative outcomes have been reported to be improved, worsened, or unchanged by PAC use. Several articles continue to illustrate insufficient evidence supporting an outcome benefit from utilization of the PAC.[52–55] However, proponents of the PAC site the many issues that surround the interpretation of PAC studies, including inadequate blinding, inadequate sample size for conclusions made, nonrandomization, selection bias, Hawthorne effect, crossover, violation of protocols without explanation, debatable end points of care, and statistical flaws.[56]

The proposed benefits of the PAC rely on providing additional data that may alter patient therapy to improve outcome. Still, the PAC is an instrument interpreted by health care staff, who oftentimes lack the knowledge to correctly translate the data into beneficial therapies for patients. Several studies have measured physician and nurse knowledge in the United States and Europe. These surveys revealed that knowledge of pulmonary artery catheterization is not uniformly good among intensive care unit physicians, with as many as half of respondents unable to interpret the PCWP correctly from a clearly marked tracing.[57,58] Changes in training and credentialing have been proposed to improve these deficiencies in knowledge.[59–61]

If the PAC is to be employed, it should be applied to the appropriate patient population, the correct clinical environment, and used in a timely fashion. Therefore, the patients should have significant comorbidities in jeopardy of sustaining further organ failure or death. Physiologic derangements must be present so that the PAC-derived variables can guide therapy to alter outcome. Finally, timely identification of disease progression should occur so that the health care professional interpreting the PAC data may have a chance to use it for patient clinical benefit before irreversible morbidity occurs. However, at present, the preponderance of studies for various reasons have had difficulty demonstrating outcome benefits.[56]

NONINVASIVE TECHNIQUES FOR CARDIAC OUTPUT/FLUID RESPONSIVENESS

❹ The consummate CO monitor would be noninvasive, reliable, and valid under a plethora of pathologic hemodynamic conditions. In addition, it should be easy to use, have continuous monitoring capabilities, and be inexpensive.

Indirect Fick Method

Almost two centuries ago, Adolf Fick reported that the uptake and release of material from an organ is the result of the blood flow to that organ and the arteriovenous concentration difference of the material.[62] This concept is represented as the Fick equation today:

$$CO = \dot{V}O_2/(CaO_2 - C\bar{v}O_2)$$

where CO equals cardiac output, $\dot{V}O_2$ is oxygen consumption, CaO_2 is arterial oxygen content, and $C\bar{v}O_2$ is mixed venous

oxygen content.[62,63] Substituting carbon dioxide for oxygen creates the indirect Fick equation ($CO = VCO_2/CvCO_2 - CaCO_2$), where VCO_2 is CO_2 produced, $CvCO_2$ is the mixed venous CO_2 content, and $CaCO_2$ is the arterial CO_2 content.[63] Devices have been developed to use the indirect Fick equation and partial rebreathing to generate noninvasive CO measurements.[64] This monitor includes a carbon dioxide sensor (infrared light absorption), a disposable airflow sensor, a disposable rebreathing loop, and a pulse oximeter. Parameters that may affect accuracy include small errors in measurements of $PvCO_2$ and $PaCO_2$, hyperventilation, large pulmonary shunting, and increases in $\dot{V}/\dot{Q}$ mismatching.[64] Initial validations studies showed fair agreement (bias ± 1.8 L/min) between thermodilution and indirect Fick principle monitors.[64,65] Other studies that examined patients with increased pulmonary shunt lung disease and postoperative atelectasis had dismal statistical agreement.[64,66,67] Therefore, this monitor may be best suited for critically ill patients with stable lung function.

Impedance Plethysmography

Impedance plethysmography is based on determining the pulsatile changes in resistance occurring during ventricular ejection. Classically, four electrodes are applied to the neck and thorax and a small electric current is applied. Impedance measurements (dZ/dT) are made using two thoracic electrode pairs. Changes in impedance correlate with stroke volume. CO is estimated by determining stroke volume and ventricular ejection time.[68] Electrode placement and appropriate contact with the skin are important sources of error. Other reported factors influencing bioimpedance measurements include intrathoracic fluid shifts, the presence of aortic regurgitation, extremes of heart rate, cardiac dysrhythmias, late liver cirrhosis, and changes in hematocrit.[69] More than 150 validation studies have been published, and both poor and good correlations between impedance plethysmography and a reference method have been reported.[70] Newer-generation impedance monitors attempt to overcome reported shortcomings of the device with upgraded computer technology and modified algorithms to calculate CO. Data are emerging from the critically ill and cardiac surgery literature suggesting that these newer devices have acceptable agreement (within 15%) with the thermodilution technique.[64,71]

Doppler Ultrasonography

Doppler ultrasonography can measure the velocity of blood in the ascending or descending aorta or outflow tract of the pulmonary artery. CO is calculated by multiplying the time-weighted average velocity of blood flow by an estimate of aortic or pulmonary artery cross-sectional area that can be directly measured or predicted from a nomogram.[72] Suprasternal, transtracheal, and transesophageal probes have been designed for clinical use.[64,73] Accuracy and precision depend on the estimate of the vessel diameter and the alignment of the Doppler probe. Velocity measurements are most accurate when the Doppler probe and the blood flow are parallel. If the alignment exceeds 25 degrees, velocity measurements lose precision. Other factors limiting the accuracy of this device include when CO is based on descending aortic blood flow only, when cross-sectional area of the aorta is dynamic (and not cylindrical as this device assumes for calculations), when turbulent flow occurs from tachycardia, when anemia exists, and when aortic valve disease is present.[64] It has been shown that changes in hemodynamics with the use of vasopressors and inotropes can reduce the accuracy of this device to measure stroke volume changes.[74] Still, the development of esophageal Doppler probes allows for continuous, minimally invasive estimation of CO,

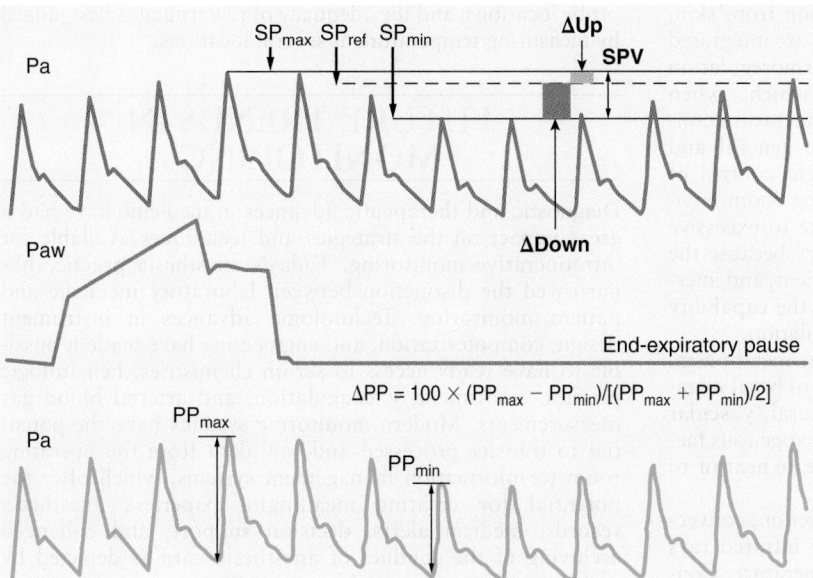

FIGURE 27-10. The figure represents both systolic pressure (SP) and pulse pressure (PP) variation throughout the respiratory cycle. The pulse pressure and systolic pressure are at the peak during inspiration and at minimum during expiration. By incorporating an expiratory pause during positive pressure mechanical ventilation, a reference systolic pressure and pulse pressure can be ascertained during expiration to differentiate between expiration and inspiration. SPV, systolic pressure variability; Pa, arterial pressure Paw, airway pressure (Reproduced from Michard F: Changes in arterial pressure during mechanical ventilation. Anesthesiology 2005; 103: 419, with permission.)

$$\Delta PP = 100 \times (PP_{max} - PP_{min})/[(PP_{max} + PP_{min})/2]$$

and may allow for optimization of intravascular volume status without the use of a CVP or PAC.[75–77]

Arterial Pulse Contour Analysis/ Transpulmonary Thermodilution/Lithium Dilution Technique

Pulse contour analysis of the arterial pressure waveform allows clinicians to determine beat-to-beat measurements of left ventricular output. Computer algorithms are used to calculate the area under the systolic portion of the arterial pulse waveform (from the end of diastole to the end of the ejection phase). Stroke volume is determined by dividing the resulting area by the aortic impedance. Therefore, pulse contour may not provide consistently reliable results in the setting of dysthymias or ill-defined arterial waveforms.[64]

Another limitation of arterial pulse contour analysis is that the technique requires calibration with another method of measuring CO. Reference CO determinations for calibration can be obtained using moderately invasive (TCO using a PAC or transpulmonary thermodilution using a central venous and arterial line) or minimally invasive (lithium dilution using a peripheral venous and arterial catheter) technology. Studies show reasonable agreement between the transpulmonary thermodilution and PAC thermodilution technique.[64,78] However, a femoral or axillary arterial line is often required for accurate measurements as the CO is generated from the change in temperature of iced saline in the aorta, when first injected into the central vein. Several other studies have compared lithium dilution (which measures CO in a similar fashion to the thermodilution technique) with pulmonary artery thermodilution and suggest appropriate agreement as well between the two.[79,80]

A number of clinical studies have demonstrated that the precision and accuracy of arterial pulse contour analysis is acceptable when compared with TCO measurements obtained by PACs and that it may also be able to predict fluid responsiveness.[81–84] New devices have been constructed to eliminate the need for calibration with thermodilution. This novel technology has shown to have variable levels of agreement with PAC measurements of CO under various clinical conditions.[85–87] Larger randomized controlled trials need to be performed to further validate the use of these technologies.

Arterial Pulse Pressure/Systolic Pressure Variation

Arterial pulse pressure/systolic pressure variation recently has been used as a relatively noninvasive way to predict fluid responsiveness (Fig. 27-10). Studies have examined the use of pulse pressure/systolic pressure respiratory variation in detecting patients who are hypovolemic.[88] Greater arterial pulse pressure/systolic pressure variation changes may occur in hypovolemic patients because of a drop in right ventricular preload, a greater increase in right ventricular afterload, and a decrease in left ventricular afterload.[88]

The clinical application of this concept has been examined. In 1978, Rick and Burke[89] discovered that a systolic pressure variation >10 mm Hg indicated hypovolemia. In addition, other studies have shown that systolic pressure variation has acceptable agreement with pulmonary artery occlusion pressures (as systolic pressure variation increases, PCOP decreases).[88,90] However, comparisons with echocardiography have produced mixed results. Although some investigators demonstrated an acceptable relationship between left ventricular end-diastolic area and the magnitude of systolic pressure variation during aortic surgery, others showed weak or no correlation between systolic pressure variation and left ventricular end-diastolic area in cardiovascular surgery.[88,91] Several factors may affect interpretation of pulse pressure/systolic pressure variation, including components of the arterial pressure monitoring device, arterial compliance, dysrhythmias, increased chest wall compliance, small tidal volumes, spontaneous breathing, and right/left ventricular failure. Nevertheless, arterial pulse pressure/systolic pressure variation may be used as a predictor of fluid responsiveness in patients undergoing most surgeries and critically ill patients who are deeply sedated undergoing conventional mechanical ventilation.[88]

TEMPERATURE MONITORING

The ability to monitor body temperature is a standard of anesthesia care. The continual observation of temperature changes in anesthetized patients allows for the detection of accidental heat loss or malignant hyperthermia. Humans maintain their core temperature by balancing heat production from metabolism and the many environmental factors that supply heat or cool the body. Regional temperature information from skin, muscle, the body cavities, spinal cord, and brain are integrated in the central nervous system. Conceptually, thermoregulation involves the integration of "set points," which, when exceeded, trigger temperature-dissipating, temperature-conserving, or heat-producing mechanisms. Both general and regional anesthesia inhibit afferent and efferent control of thermoregulation.[92,93] In addition, the operating room environment and surgical exposure often contribute to excessive heat losses. Heat loss is common during surgery because the surgical environment transfers heat from the patient, and anesthesia reduces heat production and diminishes the capability of patients to monitor and maintain thermoregulation.

Heat is produced as a consequence of cellular metabolism. In adults, thermoregulation involves the control of basal metabolic rate, muscular activity, sympathetic arousal, vascular tone, and hormone activation balanced against exogenous factors that determine the need for the body to create heat or to adjust the transfer of heat to the environment.

Heat losses may result from radiation, conduction, convection, and evaporation. Radiation refers to the infrared rays emanating from all objects above absolute temperature. Conduction refers to the transfer of heat from contact with objects. Convection refers to the transfer of heat from air passing by objects. Evaporation represents the heat loss that results when water vaporizes. For every gram of water evaporated, 0.58 kcal of heat is lost.

Perioperative hypothermia predisposes patients to increases in metabolic rate (shivering) and cardiac work, decreases in drug metabolism and cutaneous blood flow, and creates impairments of coagulation. Clinical studies have demonstrated that patients in whom intraoperative hypothermia develops are at a higher risk for development of postoperative myocardial ischemia and wound infection compared with patients who are normothermic in the perioperative period.[94,95] Anesthesiologists frequently monitor temperature and attempt to maintain central core temperature at near-normal values in all patients undergoing anesthesia.

Central core temperatures can be estimated using probes that can be placed into the bladder, distal esophagus, ear canal, trachea, nasopharynx, or rectum.[96] Pulmonary artery blood temperature is also a good estimate of central core temperature.

Temperature is usually measured using electrical probes containing calibrated thermistors or thermocouples that serve as temperature transducers. Thermistors respond to temperature changes by changing their electrical resistance. Thermocouples are constructed by passing current through a circuit where the electrodes are made of two dissimilar metals. The current measured is directly proportional to the temperature difference between the two metal junctions. Thermocouple temperature probes maintain one junction at a known temperature and place the second junction on the temperature probe tip. Skin temperature can also be monitored using liquid crystal thermometry. However, convenient, temperature strips do not correlate with core temperature measurements.[97]

Thermoregulatory responses are based on a physiologically weighted average reflecting changes in the mean body temperature. Mean body temperature is estimated by the following equation:

$$\text{Mean temperature} = 0.85\ T\ \text{core} + 0.15\ T\ \text{skin}$$

Skin temperature monitoring has been advocated to identify peripheral vasoconstriction but is not adequate to determine alterations in mean body temperature that may occur during surgery. Core temperature sites have been established as reliable indicators of changes in mean temperature. During routine noncardiac surgery, temperature differences between these sites are small. When anesthetized patients are being cooled, changes in rectal temperature often lag behind those of other probe locations, and the adequacy of rewarming is best judged by measuring temperature at several locations.

FUTURE TRENDS IN MONITORING

Diagnostic and therapeutic advances in medicine have had a great impact on the strategies and techniques available for intraoperative monitoring. Today's anesthesia practice has narrowed the distinction between laboratory medicine and patient monitoring. Technologic advances in instrument design, computerization, and engineering have made it possible to have ready access to serum chemistries, hematologic profiles, assessment of coagulation, and arterial blood gas measurements. Modern monitoring systems have the potential to transfer processed and raw data from the operating room to information management systems, which offer the potential for creating meaningful paperless anesthesia records, medical alerts, decision support, and enhanced archiving of the conduct of anesthesia care as depicted by real-time monitoring trends.

The U.S. Department of Health and Human Services proposed implementation of patient record systems in 1996.[98] Proprietary systems for automated anesthesia records are now in the marketplace. These offer file sharing so that information that is traditionally viewed as patient monitoring can also be used for billing, ordering supplies, and quality improvement. Although computerization of the hospital environment has direct and indirect costs, the benefits to physicians, patients, insurers, and hospital administrators indicate that, like in other business environments, information management is coming to operating room monitoring and anesthesiology.[99,100] The clinical and administrative data that can be obtained from anesthesia work stations integrated with hospital information systems could enhance the quality of care and improve the value of intraoperative monitoring of anesthetized patients.

References

1. Bodenheimer T: High and rising health care costs. Part 2: Technologic innovation. Ann Intern Med 2005; 142: 932
2. American Society of Anesthesiologists: Standards for Basic Anesthetic Monitoring. Park Ridge, IL American Society of Anesthesiologists, 2005
3. Association for the Advancement of Medical Instrumentation: Human Factors, Engineering Guidelines and Preferred Practices for the Design of Medical Devices. Arlington, VA Association for the Advancement of Medical Instrumentation, 1988
4. Loeb RG: A measure of intraoperative attention to monitor displays. Anesth Analg 1993; 76: 337
5. Barker L, Webb RK, Runciman EB et al: The Australian Incident Monitoring Study. The oxygen analyzer: Applications and limitations—an analysis of 200 incident reports. Anaesth Intensive Care 1993; 21: 570
6. Mayer RM: Oxygen analyzers: Failure rates and life-spans of galvanic cells. J Clin Monit 1990; 6: 196
7. Williamson JA, Webb RK, Cockings J et al: The Australian Incident Monitoring Study. The capnograph applications and limitations—an analysis of 2000 incident reports. Anaesth Intensive Care 1993; 21: 551
8. Walder B, Lauber R, Zbinden AM: Accuracy and cross-sensitivity of 10 different anesthetic gas monitors. J Clin Monit 1993; 9: 364
9. Westenskow DR, Smith KW, Coleman DL, et al: Clinical evaluation of a Raman scattering multiple gas analyzer for the operating room. Anesthesiology 1989; 70: 350
10. Haymond S, Cariappa R, Eby CS et al: Laboratory assessment of oxygenation in methemoglobinemia. Clin Chem 2005; 51: 434
11. Barker SJ, Curry J, Redford D et al: Measurement of carboxyhemoglobin and methemoglobin by pulse oximetry. Anesthesiology 2006; 105: 892
12. Barker SJ: "Motion resistant" pulse oximetry: A comparison of new and old models. Anesth Analg 2002; 95: 967
13. Nishiyama T: Pulse oximeters demonstrate different responses during hypothermia and changes in perfusion. Can J Anesth 2006; 53: 36
14. Moller JT, Pederson T, Rasmussen LS et al: Randomized evaluation of pulse oximetry in 20,802 patients: II. Perioperative events and postoperative complications. Anesthesiology 1993; 78: 445

ANESTHETIC MANAGEMENT

15. Janelle GM, Gravenstein M: An accuracy evaluation of the T-line Ten-symeter (continuous noninvasive blood pressure management device) versus conventional radial artery monitoring in surgical patients. Anesth Analg 2006; 102: 484

16. Hirschl MM, Binder M, Harken H, et al: Accuracy and reliability of noninvasive continuous finger blood pressure measurement in critically ill patients. Crit Care Med 1996; 24: 1684

17. Finlay JY, Gali B, Keegan MT, et al: Vasotrac® arterial blood pressure and direct arterial blood pressure monitoring during liver transplantation. Anesth Analg 2006; 102: 690

18. Kleinman B, Powell S, Kumar P, et al: The fast flush test measures the dynamic response for the entire pressure monitoring system. Anesthesiology 1992; 77: 1215

19. Slogoff S, Keats AS, Arlund C: On the safety of radial artery cannulation. Anesthesiology 1983; 59: 42

20. McGregor AD: The Allen test: An investigation of its accuracy by fluorescein angiography dye. J Hand Surg Br 1987; 12: 82

21. Kanazawa M, Fukuyama H, Kinefuchi Y, et al: Relationship between aortic-to-radial arterial pressure gradient after cardiopulmonary bypass and changes in arterial elasticity. Anesthesiology 2003; 99: 48

22. Vender JS, Watts RD: Differential diagnosis of hand ischemia in the presence of an arterial cannula. Anesth Analg 1982; 61: 465

23. Sanford TJ: Internal jugular vein cannulation versus subclavian vein cannulation. An anesthesiologist's view: The right internal jugular vein. J Clin Monit 1985; 1: 58

24. Karakitsos D, Labropoulos N, De Groot E, et al: Real-time ultrasound-guided catheterization of the internal jugular vein: a prospective comparison with the landmark technique in critical care patients. Crit Care 2006; 10: R162

25. Milling TJ, Rose J, Briggs WM, et al: Randomized, controlled trial of point-of-care, limited ultrasonography assistance of central venous cannulation: The third Sonography Outcomes Assessment Program (SOAP-3) Trial. Crit Care Med 2005; 33: 1764

26. O'Grady NP, Alexander M, Dellinger EP, et al: Guidelines for the prevention of intravascular catheter-related infections. MMWR Morb Mortal Wkly Rep 2002; 55: 1

27. Byrnes MC, Coopersmith CM: Prevention of catheter related bloodstream infection. Curr Opin Crit Care 2007; 13: 411

28. Hamilton HC, Foxcroft DR: Central venous access sites for the prevention of venous thrombosis, stenosis and infection in patients requiring long-term intravenous therapy. Cochrane Database of Systemic Reviews 2007; 3: CD004084

29. Mark JB: Central venous pressure monitoring: Clinical insights beyond the numbers. J Cardiothorac Anesth 1991; 5: 163

30. Vender JS: Pulmonary artery catheter monitoring. Anesthesiol Clin North Am 1988; 6: 743

31. Tuman KJ, Carroll GC, Ivankovich AD: Pitfalls of interpretation of pulmonary artery catheter data. J Cardiothorac Anesth 1989; 3: 625

32. Practice guidelines for pulmonary artery catheterization: An updated report by the American Society of Anesthesiologists Task Force on pulmonary artery catheterization. Anesthesiology 2003; 99: 988

33. West JB, Dollery CT, Naimark A: Distribution of blood flow in isolated lung: Relation to vascular and alveolar pressures. J Appl Physiol 1984; 19: 713

34. Davidson C: Cardiac catheterization, L Braunwald's Heart Disease, 8th ed. Edited by P.L. Saunders, Philadelphia, PA 2007, 449

35. Scuderi PE, MacGregor DA, Bowton DL, et al: A laboratory comparison of three pulmonary artery oximetry catheters. Anesthesiology 1994; 81: 245

36. Marx G, Reinhart K: Venous oximetry. Curr Opin Crit Care 2006; 12: 263

37. Dellinger RP, Carlet JM, Masur H, et al: Surviving sepsis campaign guidelines for management of severe sepsis and septic shock. Crit Care Med 2004; 32: 858

38. Varpula M, Karlsson S, Ruokonen E, et al: Mixed venous oxygen saturation cannot be estimated by central venous oxygen saturation in septic shock. Intensive Care Med 2006; 32: 1336

39. Dueck M, Klimek M, Appenrodt S, et al: Trends but not individual values of central venous oxygen saturation agree with mixed venous oxygen saturation during varying hemodynamic conditions. Anesthesiology 2005; 103: 249

40. Stewart GN: Researches on the circulation time and on the influences which affect it IV. The output of the heart. J Physiol 1897; 22:159

41. Hamilton WF, Moore JW, Kinsman JM, et al: Studies on the circulation IV. Further analysis of the injection method, and changes in hemodynamics under physiologic and pathological conditions. AM J Physiol 1932; 99: 534

42. Fegler G: Measurement of cardiac output in anesthetized animals by thermodilution method. Q J Exp Physiol 1954; 39: 153

43. Pearl RGB, Rosenthal MH, Mielson L, et al: Effect of injectate volume and temperature on thermodilution cardiac output determination. Anesthesiology 1986; 64: 798

44. Mihm FG, Gettinger A, Hansen WC, et al: A Multicenter evaluation of a new continuous cardiac output pulmonary artery catheter system. Crit Care Med 1998; 26: 1346

45. Mihm FG, Gettinger A, Hanson CW, et al: A multicenter evaluation of a new continuous cardiac output pulmonary artery catheter system. Crit Care Med 1998; 26: 1346

46. Hines R, Barash PG: Intraoperative right ventricular dysfunction detected with a right ventricular ejection fraction catheter. J Clin Monit 1986; 2: 206

47. Mukherjee R, Spinale FG, VonRecum AF, et al: In vitro validation of right ventricular thermodilution ejection fraction system. Ann Biomed Eng 1991; 19: 165

48. Dennis JW, Menawat S, Sobowale O, et al: Superiority of end-diastolic volume and ejection fraction measurements over wedge pressure in evaluating cardiac function during aortic reconstruction. J Vasc Surg 1992; 16: 372

49. Durand M, Chavanon O, Tessier Y, et al: Right ventricular function after coronary surgery with or without bypass. J Cardiac Surg 2006; 21: 11

50. Zink W, Noll J, Rauch H, et al: Continuous assessment of right ventricular ejection fraction: New pulmonary artery catheter versus transesophageal echocardiography. Anaesthesia 2004; 59: 1126

51. Siniscalchi A, Pavesi M, Piraccini E, et al: Right ventricular end diastolic volume index as a predictor of preload status in patients with low right ventricular ejection fraction during orthotopic liver transplantation. Tranplant Proc 2005; 37: 2541

52. Sandham JD, Hull RD, Brant RF, et al: A randomized, controlled trial of the use of pulmonary artery catheters in high-risk surgical patients. N Engl J Med 2003; 348: 5

53. Shah MR, Hasselblad V, Stevenson LW, et al: Impact of the pulmonary artery catheter in critically ill patients meta-analysis of randomized clinical trials. JAMA 2005; 294: 1664

54. Harvey S, Harrison DA, Singer M, et al: Assessment of clinical effectiveness of pulmonary artery catheters in the management of patients in intensive care (PAC-MAN): A randomized trial. Lancet 2005; 366: 472

55. Wheeler AP, Bernard GR, Thompson BT, et al: Pulmonary-artery versus central venous catheter to guide treatment of acute lung injury. New Engl J Med 2006; 354: 2213

56. Vender JS: Pulmonary artery catheter utilization: The use, misuse, or abuse. J Cardiothor Vasc Anesth 2006; 20: 295

57. Iberti TJ, Fischer EP, Leibowitz AB, et al: A multicenter study of physician's knowledge of the pulmonary artery catheter. JAMA 1990; 264: 2928

58. Gnaegi A, Feihl F, Perret C: Intensive care physicians insufficient knowledge of right-heart catheterization at the bedside: Time to act? Crit Care Med 1997; 25: 213

59. Papadakos PJ, Vender JS: Training requirement for pulmonary artery catheter utilization in adult patients. New Horiz 1997; 5: 287

60. Jacka M, Cohen MM, To T, et al: PAOP estimation—how confident are anesthesiologists? Crit Care Med 2002; 30: 1197

61. Ginosar Y, Thijs LG, Sprung CL: Raising the standard of hemodynamic monitoring: Targeting the practice or practitioner? Crit Care Med 1997; 25: 209

62. Chaney JC, Derdak S: Minimally invasive hemodynamic monitoring for the intensivist: Current and emerging technology. Crit Care Med 2002; 30: 2338

63. Laszlo G: Respiratory measurements of cardiac output: From elegant idea to useful test. J Appl Physiol 2004; 96: 428

64. Cholley BP, Payen D: Noninvasive techniques for measurements of cardiac output. Curr Opin Crit Care 2005; 11: 424

65. Kotake Y, Moriyama K, Innami Y, et al: Performance of noninvasive partial CO_2 rebreathing cardiac output and continuous thermodilution cardiac output in patients undergoing aortic reconstruction surgery. Anesthesiology 2003; 99: 283

66. Tachibana K, Imanaka H, Takeuchi M, et al: Noninvasive cardiac output measurement using partial carbon dioxide rebreathing is less acurate at settings of reduced minute ventilation and when spontaneous breathing is present. Anesthesiology 2003; 98: 830

67. Nilsson LB, Eldrup N, Berthelsen PG: Lack of agreement between thermodilution and carbon dioxide-rebreathing cardiac output. Acta Anaesthesiol Scand 2001; 45: 680

68. Young JD, McQuillan P: Comparison of thoracic electrical bioimpedance and thermodilution for the measurement of cardiac index in patients with severe sepsis. Br J Anaesth 1993; 70: 58

69. Suttner S, Schollhorn T, Boldt J, et al: Noninvasive assessment of cardiac output using thoracic electrical bioimpedance in hemodynamically stable and unstable patients after cardiac surgery: A comparison with pulmonary artery thermodilution. Intensive Care Med 2006; 32: 2053

70. Raaijmakers E, Faes TJ, Scholten RJ, et al: A meta-analysis of three decades of validating thoracic impedance cardiography. Crit Care Med 1999; 27: 1203

71. Schmidt C, Theilmeier H, Van Aken P, et al: Comparison of electrical velocimetry and transesophageal Doppler echocardiography for measuring stroke volume and cardiac output. Br J Anaesth 2005; 95: 603

72. Critchley LA, Peng ZY, Fok BS, et al: Testing the reliability of a new ultrasonic cardiac output monitor, the USCOM, by using aortic flowprobes in anesthetized dogs. Anesth Analg 2005; 100: 748

73. Perrino AC, O'Connor T, Luther M: Transtracheal Doppler cardiac output monitoring: Comparison to thermodilution during noncardiac surgery. Anesth Analg 1994; 78: 1060

74. Gunn S, Kook Kim H, Harrigan P, et al: Ability of pulse contour and esophageal Doppler to estimate rapid changes in stroke volume. Intensive Care Med 2006; 32: 1537

75. Chytra I, Pradl R, Bosman R, et al: Esophageal Doppler-guided fluid management decreases blood lactate levels in multiple-trauma patients: A randomized controlled trial. Critical Care 2007; 11: R24

76. Knobloch K, Lichtenberg A, Winterhalter M, et al: Non-invasive cardiac output determination by two-dimensional independent Doppler during and after cardiac surgery. Ann Thorac Surg 2005; 80: 1479

77. Monnet X, Rienzo M, Osman D, et al: Esophageal Doppler monitoring predicts fluid responsiveness in critically ill ventilated patients. Intensive Care Med 2005; 31: 1195

78. Halvorsen PS, Espinoza A, Lundblad R, et al: Agreement between PiCCO pulse contour analysis, pulmonary artery thermodilution and transthoracic thermodilution during off-pump coronary artery by-pass surgery. Acta Anaesthesiol Scand 2006; 50: 1050

79. Della Rocca G, Costa MG, Coccia C, et al: Cardiac output monitoring: aortic transpulmonary thermodilution and pulse contour analysis agree with standard thermodilution methods in patients undergoing lung transplantation. Can J Anaesth 2003; 50: 707

80. Chapman M, Gattas D, Suntharalingham G, et al: Health technology and credibility. Crit Care 2004; 8: 73

81. DeWall E, Kalkman CJ, Rex S, et al: Validation of new arterial pulse contour-based cardiac output device. Crit Care Med 2007; 35: 1904

82. Pittman J, Bar-Yosef S, SumPing J, et al: Continuous cardiac output monitoring with pulse contour analysis: A comparison with lithium indicator dilution cardiac output measurement. Crit Care Med 2005; 33: 2015

83. Rex S, Brose S, Metzelder S, et al: Prediction of fluid responsiveness in patients during cardiac surgery. Br J Anaesth 2004; 93: 782

84. Reuter DA, Goepfert MS, Goresch T, et al: Assessing fluid responsiveness during open chest conditions. Br J Anaesth 2005; 94: 318

85. Button D, Wiebel L, Reuthebuch O, et al: Clinical evaluation of the FloTrac/Vigileo™ system and two established continuous cardiac output monitoring devices in patients undergoing cardiac surgery. Br J Anaesth 2007; 99: 329

86. Mayer J, Boldt J, Schollhorn T, et al: Semi-invasive monitoring of cardiac output by a new device using arterial pressure waveform analysis: A comparison with intermittent pulmonary artery thermodilution in patients undergoing cardiac surgery. Br J Anaesth 2007; 98: 176

87. Sakka1 SG, Kozieras J, Thuemer O, et al: Measurement of cardiac output: a comparison between transpulmonary thermodilution and uncalibrated pulse contour analysis. Br J Anaesth 2007; 99: 337

88. Michard F: Changes in arterial pressure during mechanical ventilation. Anesthesiology 2005; 103: 419

89. Rick JJ, Burke SS: Respirator paradox. South Med J 1978; 71: 1376

90. Xu H, Zhou S, Ma W, et al: Prediction of pulmonary arterial wedge pressure from arterial pressure or pulse oximetry plethysmographic waveform. Chin Med J (Engl) 2002; 115: 1372

91. Dalibon N, Guenoun T, Journois D, et al: The clinical relevance of systolic pressure variation in anesthetized nonhypotensive patients. J Cardiothorac Vasc Anesth 2003; 17: 188

92. Sessler DI: Central thermoregulatory inhibition by general anesthesia. Anesthesiology 1991; 75: 557

93. Ozaki M, Kurz A, Sessler DI, et al: Thermoregulatory thresholds during epidural and spinal anesthesia. Anesthesiology 1994; 81: 282

94. Kurz A, Sessler DJ, Lenhardt R: Perioperative normothermia to reduce the incidence of surgical wound infection and shorten hospitalization. N Engl J Med 1996; 334: 1209

95. Frank SM, Fleisher LA, Breslow MJ, et al: Perioperative maintenance of normothermic reduces the incidence of morbid cardiac events: A randomized clinical trial. JAMA 1997; 277: 1127

96. Yamakage M, Kawanna S, Watanabe H, et al: The utility of tracheal temperature monitoring. Anesth Analg 1993; 76: 795

97. Vaughan MS, Cork RD, Vaughan RW: Inaccuracy of liquid crystal thermometry to identify core temperature trends in postoperative adults. Anesth Analg 1982; 61: 284

98. U.S. Department of Health and Human Services: Initiatives Toward the Electronic Health Care System of the Future. Washington, DC: U.S. Department of Health and Human Services, 1992

99. Smith NT: The M-15: A truly different workstation. J Clin Monit 1994; 10: 352

100. Gibby GL: Anesthesia information-management systems: Their role in risk-versus cost assessment and outcomes research. J Cardiothorac Vasc Anesth 1997; 11(2 Suppl 1): 2

CHAPTER 28 ■ ECHOCARDIOGRAPHY

ALBERT C. PERRINO, JR., WANDA M. POPESCU, AND NIKOLAOS J. SKUBAS

PRINCIPLES AND TECHNOLOGY OF
  ECHOCARDIOGRAPHY
TWO-DIMENSIONAL AND THREE-DIMENSIONAL
  TRANSESOPHAGEAL ECHOCARDIOGRAPHY
  EXAMINATION
DOPPLER ECHOCARDIOGRAPHY AND HEMODYNAMICS
ECHOCARDIOGRAPHIC EVALUATION OF SYSTOLIC
  FUNCTION

EVALUATION OF LEFT VENTRICULAR DIASTOLIC
  FUNCTION
EVALUATION OF VALVULAR HEART DISEASE
DISEASES OF THE AORTA
CARDIAC MASSES
CONGENITAL HEART DISEASE
ECHOCARDIOGRAPHY-ASSISTED PROCEDURES
EPICARDIAL AND EPIAORTIC ECHOCARDIOGRAPHY
ECHOCARDIOGRAPHY OUTSIDE THE OPERATING ROOM

KEY POINTS

1 Understanding the principles of ultrasound and echocardiographic instrumentation is essential in optimizing image quality.

2 Performing a comprehensive echocardiographic examination ensures that important pathologies are recognized.

3 Two-dimensional and Doppler techniques have complementary roles in the assessment of cardiovascular function.

4 Global left ventricular systolic function is influenced by load and contractility alterations; regional wall motion grading is based on systolic excursion and thickening.

5 Transmitral flow and pulmonary vein flow Doppler along with tissue Doppler imaging provide accurate diastolic function assessment.

6 Severity of aortic stenosis is based on the value of the aortic valve area calculated by continuity equation.

7 The ratio of the width of the regurgitant jet to the diameter of the left ventricular outflow tract is useful in assessing severity of aortic insufficiency. Diastolic flow reversal in the descending thoracic aorta is significant for severe aortic insufficiency.

8 Mitral regurgitation can be of structural or functional etiology. The jet's vena contracta and the effective regurgitant orifice area by proximal isovelocity surface area method help grade severity.

9 Aortic atheromas larger than 4 mm are harbingers of thromboembolic events.

10 The false lumen of aortic dissection does not have diastolic flow.

Echocardiography is the first imaging technique to enter the mainstream of intraoperative patient monitoring. A remarkably versatile tool, echocardiography provides a comprehensive evaluation of myocardial, valvular, and hemodynamic performance. These capabilities attracted the attention of anesthesiologists and surgeons challenged by the unique difficulties of perioperative cardiovascular management. Over the 30 years following the first report of intraoperative echocardiography to assess ventricular function by Barash and colleagues[1] in 1978, echocardiography has emerged as the technique of choice for a wide variety of intraoperative case challenges.

The benefit of intraoperative echocardiography in both cardiac and noncardiac surgical populations is supported by several case series.[2–8] Applications range from guiding the placement of intracardiac and intravascular catheters and devices, to the assessment of the severity of valve pathology and immediate evaluation of a surgical intervention, to the rapid diagnosis of acute hemodynamic instability and directing appropriate therapies.[9,10] Consequently, expertise in intraoperative echocardiography is highly desired among anesthesiology practitioners. The National Board of Echocardiography has established a certification pathway in perioperative trans-

esophageal echocardiography (TEE), http://www.echoboards. org/certification/certexpl.html. The American Society of Anesthesiologists is conjunction with the National Board of Echocardiography is establishing a second certification pathway in basic perioperative echocardiography, http://www.asahq.org/ publicationsAndServices/standards/TEE.pdf and, http://www. asahq.org/Newsletters/2008/01-08/savage01-08.html. These efforts are unique in intraoperative monitoring and attest to the critical role that accurate and thorough echocardiographic interpretation plays in current anesthetic practice.

PRINCIPLES AND TECHNOLOGY OF ECHOCARDIOGRAPHY

Echocardiography generates dynamic images of the heart from the reflections of sound waves. The echocardiography system transmits a brief pulse of high-frequency sound (i.e., ultrasound) that propagates through and is subsequently reflected from the cardiac structures encountered. The ultrasound transducer records the time delay and signal intensity for each returning reflection. Because the speed of sound in tissue is

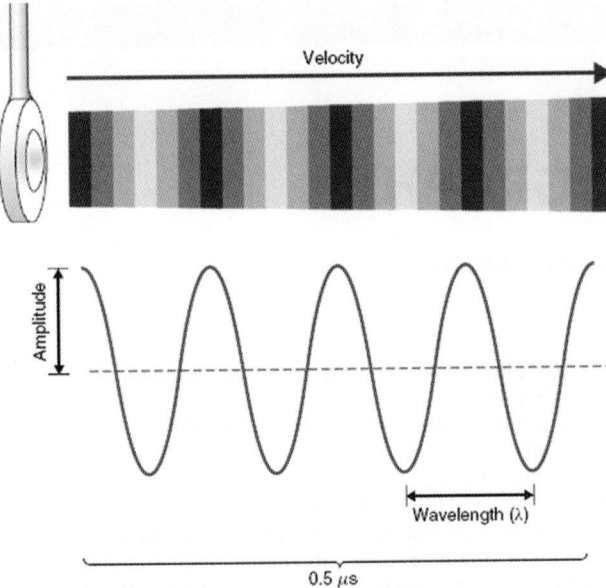

FIGURE 28-1. Sound wave. Vibrations of the ultrasound transducer create cycles of compression and rarefaction in adjacent tissue. The ultrasound energy is characterized by its amplitude, wavelength, frequency, and propagation velocity. In this example, four sound waves are shown in a period of 0.5 μs. The frequency can be calculated as four cycles divided by 0.5 μs and equals 8 MHz.

constant, the time delay allows the echo system to precisely calculate the location of cardiac structures and thereby create an image map of the heart.

Physics of Sound

Sound is vibration of a physical medium. In clinical echocardiography, a mechanical vibrator, known as the *transducer,* is placed in contact with the esophagus (transesophageal echocardiography), skin (transthoracic echocardiography), or the heart (epicardial echocardiography) to create tissue vibrations. The resulting tissue vibrations create a longitudinal wave with alternating areas of *compression* and *rarefaction* (Fig. 28-1).

The *amplitude* of a sound wave represents its peak pressure and is appreciated as loudness. The level of sound energy in an area of tissue is referred to as *intensity*. The intensity of the sound signal is proportional to the square of the amplitude and is an important factor regarding the potential for tissue damage with ultrasound. Because levels of sound pressure vary over a large range, it is convenient to use the logarithmic decibel (dB) scale:

$$\text{Decibel (dB)} = 10 \log_{10} I/Ir = 10 \log_{10} A^2/A_r^2$$

$$= 20 \log_{10} A/A_r$$

where A is the measured sound amplitude and A_r is a standard reference sound level; I is intensity and I_r is a standard reference intensity. The Food and Drug Administration limits the intensity output of cardiac ultrasound systems to be <720 W/cm^2 because of concerns of potential tissue injury.[11]

Sound waves are also characterized by their *frequency* (f), or pitch, expressed in cycles per second, or Hertz (Hz), and by their *wavelength* (λ). These attributes significantly impact the depth of penetration of a sound wave in tissue and the image resolution of the ultrasound system.

The propagation *velocity* of sound (v) is determined solely by the medium through which it passes. In soft tissue, the speed of sound is approximately 1,540 m/s. As the product of wavelength and frequency equals velocity: $V = \lambda \times f$ it becomes apparent that the wavelength and frequency are inversely related: $\lambda = v \times 1/f$ and that $\lambda = (1,540 \text{ m/s})f$. High-frequency, short-wavelength ultrasound is more easily focused and directed to a specific target location. Image resolution also increases with short wavelength sound waves; for these reasons, ultrasonic frequencies of 2 to 10 MHz are preferred in clinical echocardiography.

Properties of Sound Transmission in Tissue

The propagation of a sound wave through the body is markedly affected by its interactions with the various tissues encountered. These interactions result in reflection, refraction, scattering, and attenuation of the ultrasound signal and determine the resulting appearance of the two-dimensional image.

Echocardiographic imaging relies on the transmission and subsequent reflection of ultrasound energy back to the transducer. A sound wave propagates smoothly through uniform tissue until it encounters the interface between two tissues varying in acoustic impedance (a property largely related to the *density* [ρ] of the tissue and the speed that ultrasound travels). A large interface oriented perpendicular to the sound beam will produce a mirrorlike reflection of sound back toward the transducer with only a portion of the signal passing through the interface. Because cardiac structures are detected by their reflected echocardiography signal, echocardiographers adjust the position of the TEE transducer so that the direction of its beam is perpendicular to the cardiac structure of interest.

Refraction causes a change in direction of propagating sound and occurs when an interface lies oblique to the sound beam. Refraction is an important factor in the formation of artifacts as the transducer mistakenly interprets a reflection from the refracted beam as originating from a cardiac structure located within the *intended* scanning field.

Scattering reflections occur when an ultrasound beam encounters small or irregularly shaped surfaces, such as red blood cells. These reflectors scatter ultrasound energy in all directions, so that far less energy is reflected back to the transducer. This type of reflection is the basis of the Doppler analysis of blood flow (see following).

Even when traveling through uniform tissue, sound undergoes a steady loss (i.e., *attenuation*) in intensity as a consequence of dispersion and absorption. Attenuation results in less energy returning back to the transducer and low-quality images with poor signal-to-noise ratios. To combat attenuation echocardiographers select better penetrating low-frequency signals (e.g., 2.5 instead of 7.5 MHz) and choose an imaging window that is close to the structure of interest. Adjusting the gain controls to amplify the weak returning signals makes their appearance brighter on the display. Unfortunately, this increases the brightness of artifactual noise, which negatively impacts the image appearance.

Instrumentation

Transducers. Ultrasound transducers use piezoelectric crystals to create a brief pulse of ultrasound. Alternating electrical current stimulates polarized particles within the crystal's matrix to rapidly vibrate, generating ultrasound. Conversely, when a sound reflection strikes the crystal, the impact vibrates the polarized particles and generates an electric current. This property allows the piezoelectric crystal to function as both a transmitter and a receiver of ultrasound.

The shorter the length of the sound pulses, the better the axial resolution of the system. High-resolution imaging transducers emit sound pulses of just two to four cycles of short wavelength, high frequency sound.

Beam Shape. The ultrasound transducer emits a three-dimensional ultrasound beam similar to a movie projection (Fig. 28-2). The beam is narrow in the near field and then diverges into the far field zone. Focusing of the beam is used to improve spatial resolution by narrowing the ultrasound beam at the desired depth. The dense, narrow beam is preferred because it provides improved spatial resolution, produces high-intensity reflections, and reduces artifact. Echocardiographers adjust focal depth and focus to optimize the image resolution.

Resolution. Three parameters are evaluated when assessing the resolution of an ultrasound system: the resolution of objects lying along the axis of the ultrasound beam (*axial resolution*), the resolution of objects horizontal to the beam's orientation (*lateral resolution*), and the resolution of objects lying vertical to the beam's orientation (*elevational resolution*).

Short pulses of high-frequency ultrasound offer the greatest axial resolution but have a decreased tissue penetration. As resolution is highest along the axial plane, echocardiographic measurements are most precise when taken parallel to the beam's axis. Accordingly, echocardiographers select transmitted frequency based on the particular imaging need.

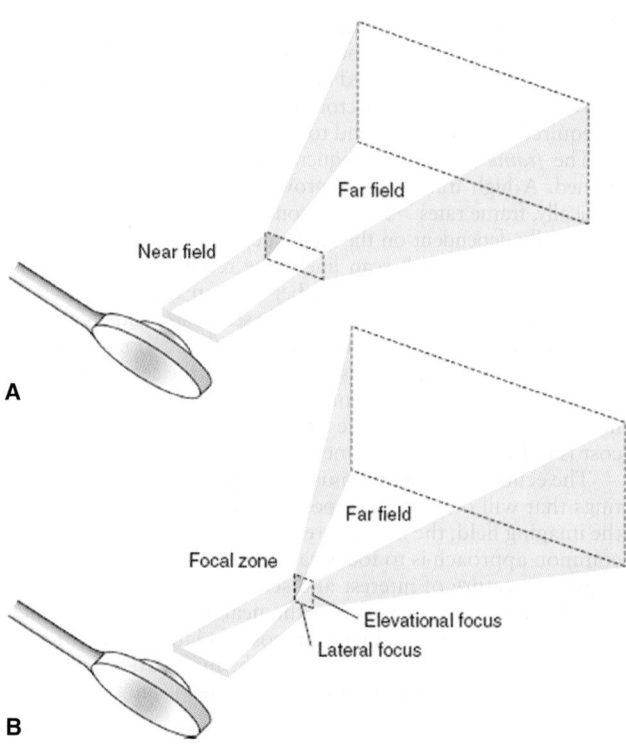

FIGURE 28-2. Three-dimensional beam. The ultrasound probe projects a three-dimensional beam. The dimensions of this projection have important effects on imaging resolution and artifact. Typically, a narrow profile is preferred. **A.** Unfocused beam. The beam is narrow in the near field and then diverges in the far field. **B.** Focused beam. Focusing has resulted in a narrower beam in both the lateral and elevational planes, so that the imaging resolution of structures in the focal zone is improved. Distal to the focal zone, the beam rapidly diverges, and the images of structures in this area will be of lower quality.

Beam size determines the lateral and elevational resolution. Broad beams produce a "smeared" image of two nearby objects, whereas narrow beams can identify each object individually. Beam size is reduced by selecting high-signal frequencies and minimizing imaging depth.

Signal Processing

To convert echoes into images, the returning ultrasound pulses are received, electronically processed, and displayed. The oscillator repeatedly cycles the transducer from a brief transmission to a relatively long receive mode. During the receive phase the reflected echocardiography signals are captured and converted to electrical signals by the piezoelectric crystal. The echocardiography system employs a series of controls including system gain, time gain compensation, compression, and postprocessing settings (not unlike those available with digital imaging software) to optimize the signal for display. Adjustments are used, for example, to emphasize edge detection versus tissue texture, or to improve the delineation of weaker reflectors. The choice of settings is dictated by the examination and the preferences of the echocardiographer.

Image Display

Ultrasonic imaging is based on the amplitude and time delay of the reflected signals. Because the velocity in tissue is a relatively constant 1,540 m/s, only the distance of the structure from the transducer alters the time required for the ultrasound wave to travel to and from the reflected structure. So by timing the interval between transmission and return of the reflections, the echocardiography system can precisely calculate the distance of a structure from the transducer.

Current imaging is based on brightness mode or *B-mode technology*. With B-mode the amplitude of the returning echoes from a single pulse determines the display brightness of the representative pixels. *M-mode* or motion mode adds temporal information to B-mode by displaying a series of sequentially collected B-mode images. M-mode echocardiography provides a one-dimensional, single-beam view through the heart but updates the B-mode images at a very high rate, providing dynamic real-time imaging. M-mode remains the best technique for examining the timing of cardiac events (Fig. 28-3).

Two-dimensional (2-D) echocardiography is a modification of B-mode echocardiography and the mainstay of the echocardiographic examination. Instead of repeatedly firing ultrasound pulses in a single direction, the transducer in 2-D echocardiography sequentially directs the ultrasound pulses across a sector of the cardiac anatomy. In this way, 2-D imaging displays a tomographic section of the cardiac anatomy, and unlike M-mode, reveals shape and lateral motion (Fig. 28-4).

Two-dimensional scanning is achieved using phased array technology, which sequentially activates each crystal in the array and thereby steers the beam without the transducer itself being moved. The two commonly used electronic scanning systems in medical ultrasound are the linear scanners and sector scanners.

The *linear scanner* uses a long linear array. Groups of crystals are activated sequentially from one end of the transducer to the other. The firing of each group of crystals creates an image of the structures directly in front of them. With sequential firing the anatomic features from one end of the transducer to the other are imaged (Fig. 28-5). The disadvantage of this approach is that the transducer face must be large to cover a broad anatomic area. The linear array is commonly used to guide vascular access and regional anesthetic procedures.

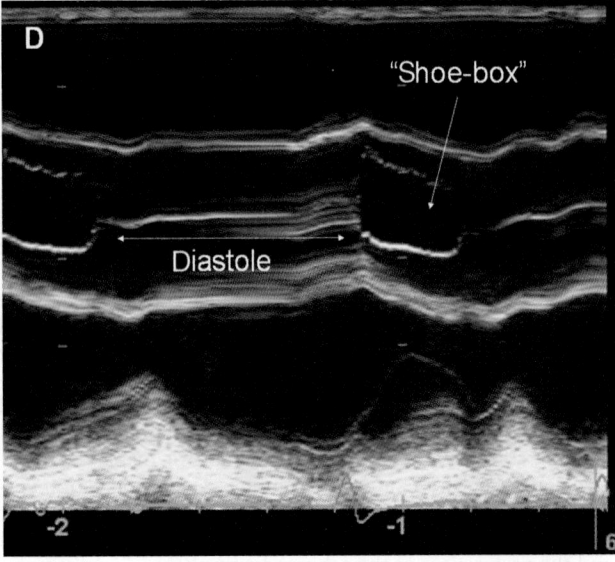

FIGURE 28-3.   Method-mode (M-mode) echocardiography of a normal aortic valve. The M-mode cursor is placed at the center of the aortic valve and the motion of the aortic cusps over time is shown. During diastolic coaptation the aortic valve cusps appear as a thick, bright white line (*long arrow*), while in systolic apposition they form a "shoebox" (*short arrow*).

The phased array *sector scanner* is the most commonly used in echocardiography. Here the ultrasound scan is sequentially directed in a fanlike arc. The resulting sector image known as a *frame* is similar in shape to that covered by a windshield wiper. The 2-D scanner then repeats the entire process to update the image and capture motion.

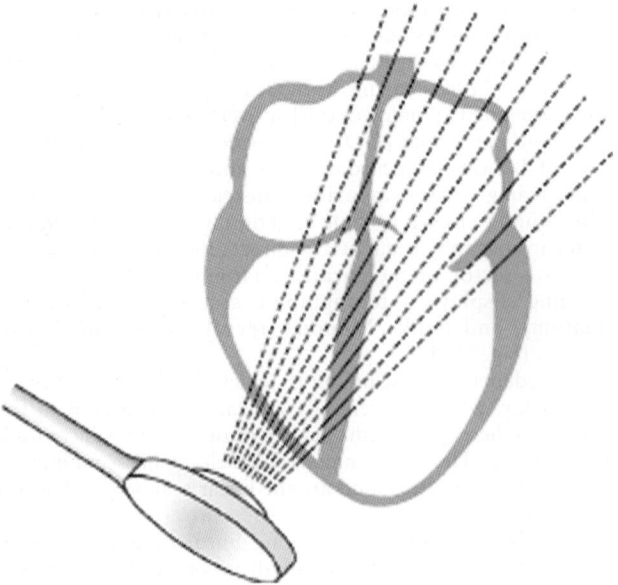

FIGURE 28-4.   Scan lines. Illustration of the arced sector from a phased array two-dimensional echocardiogram. Each dotted line represents an individual brightness mode scan line. Any structure that interacts with a scan line will create reflections (dark highlight); however, structures that lie between the scan lines are not interrogated, and the echocardiography system averages the neighboring signals to fill in this defect. Accordingly, the closer the scan lines, the better the image quality.

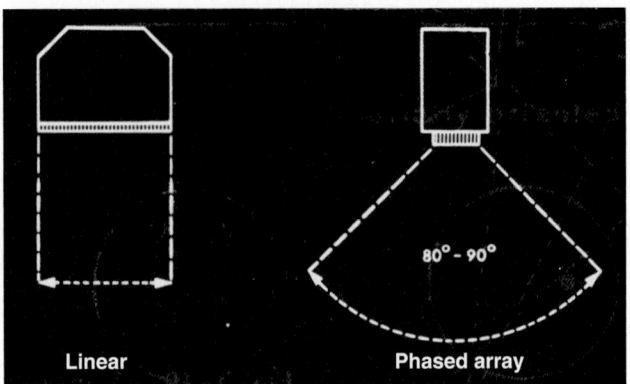

FIGURE 28-5.   Linear scanners image a rectangular section of anatomy compared with the arced sector imaged with phased array scanners.

Spatial versus Dynamic Image Quality

Expert echocardiographers select machine settings to optimize particular image qualities for the examination at hand. As discussed in the following sections, these selections will determine whether sector size, spatial resolution, or dynamic motion is best displayed.

The *pulse repetition frequency* is the rate at which sound pulses are triggered. The greater the pulse repetition frequency, the greater the number of scan lines that are emitted in a given period of time. This enhances motion display. Unfortunately, sector depth must be reduced because pulse repetition frequency is inversely related to the sector depth as a longer period of time is required for the ultrasound to travel the increased distances.

The *frame rate* is the frequency at which the sector is rescanned. A high frame rate improves the capture of movement. Typically, frame rates >30 per second are desired. The frame rate is critically dependent on the sector depth, which determines the time required for each scan line to be received, and the sector width, which increases the number of scan lines that must be transmitted. Consequently, increases in sector size and depth come at the cost of a decreased frame rate and poor motion imaging.

The number of scan lines per degree of the sector (*scan line density*) greatly affects the image resolution. Doubling the scan lines essentially doubles the lateral resolution. However, the cost is a decrease in the frame rate and motion imaging.

The echocardiographer must thoughtfully select among settings that will often have opposing effects between the size of the imaging field, the imaging resolution, and the frame rate. A common approach is to focus each part of the examination on a given structure of interest and select the imaging plane that best delineates the structure in the near field. Motion display can be then be enhanced without costs in lateral resolution by decreasing the sector angle and depth. In situations in which the maximal frame rate is desired, M-mode is chosen.

TWO-DIMENSIONAL AND THREE-DIMENSIONAL TRANSESOPHAGEAL ECHOCARDIOGRAPHY EXAMINATION

TEE is the favored approach to intraoperative echocardiography. Compared with transthoracic echocardiography (TTE), TEE offers additional "windows" to view the heart, often with improved image quality from the anatomic proximity of the esophagus and heart. In the operating room (OR), TEE is useful because the probe does not interfere with the operative field and can be left in situ, providing continuous, real-time hemodynamic information used to diagnose and manage critical cardiac events. TEE is also useful in situations in which the transthoracic examination is limited by various factors (obesity, emphysema, surgical dressings, and prosthetic valves) and for examining cardiac structures not well visualized with TTE (left atrial appendage). However, the diagnostic capability of TEE depends on image acquisition and interpretation.

This section is designed to introduce TEE image orientation and the diagnostic utility of each view. In addition, examination sequences useful for obtaining a comprehensive or targeted examination are provided. Readers are referred to *A Practical Approach to Transesophageal Echocardiography*[12] for a more detailed description of the TEE examinations described in this section.

Probe Insertion

The TEE probe is inserted in the anesthetized patient in a manner similar to insertion of an orogastric tube. For improved image quality, the stomach is emptied of gastric contents and air prior to probe insertion. The jaw is lifted with the left hand and the TEE probe, well lubricated, is inserted with the right hand by applying gentle but constant pressure. If significant resistance is encountered, additional force should be strictly avoided as oropharyngeal or esophageal injury may result. Rather, a decrease in neck extension and/or use of a laryngoscope to visualize the oropharyngeal structures often will allow easy passage of the probe. The TEE probe is advanced beyond the larynx and the cricopharyngeal muscle (around 25 to 30 cm from teeth) until a loss of resistance is appreciated. At this point, the TEE probe lies in the upper esophagus and the first cardiovascular images are seen. Extrinsic compression of the esophagus (e.g., osteophytes or an aortic aneurysm) may impede probe placement.[13]

Transesophageal Echocardiography Safety

TEE is a semi-invasive procedure. When performed by qualified operators TEE has a low incidence of complications. A retrospective study performed on 846 patients who underwent TEE described the following complications: three patients with pharyngeal abrasions, one patient with a chipped tooth, and few patients with transient vocal cord paresis.[14] Another retrospective study performed on a large case-series of 7,200 patients showed that the morbidity associated with TEE placement is 0.2% and the mortality is 0%.[15] The most common complaint (0.1%) was postoperative odynophagia. Various studies have suggested an association between swallowing dysfunction after cardiac surgery and the use of intraoperative TEE.[16,17] This fact is important as postoperative swallowing dysfunction is associated with pulmonary complications.[16]

Contraindication to Transesophageal Echocardiography Probe Placement

To maintain the safety profile of TEE, each patient should be evaluated before the procedure for signs, symptoms, or history of esophageal pathology. The most feared complication of TEE is esophageal or gastric perforation. For skilled practitioners this complication is extremely rare. Patients with extensive esophageal and gastric disease are at highest risk of perforation. Contraindications to TEE probe placement are represented by esophageal stricture, rings or webs,[18] esophageal masses (especially malignant tumors),[18] recent bleeding of esophageal varices,[18] Zencker diverticulum,[18] status post radiation to the neck,[13] and recent gastric bypass surgery. In the rare case in which TEE is essential and is the only alternative, placement of the TEE probe can be performed under direct visualization with a combined gastroscopic and echocardiographic examination.[13]

Probe Manipulation

Image acquisition depends on precise manipulation of the TEE probe. By advancing the shaft of the probe, the probe position can be moved from the upper esophagus to the midesophagus and into the stomach. The shaft can also be manually rotated to the left or to the right. By using the large knob on the probe handle, the head of the probe can be anteflexed (turning the knob clockwise) and retroflexed (turning the knob counter clockwise). The smaller knob, located on top of the large knob, is used to tilt the head of the probe to the right or to the left. Using the electronic switch on the probe handle, the operator can rotate the ultrasound beam from 0 degrees (transverse plane) to 180 degrees in 1-degree increments.

Orientation

The previously mentioned controls allow the experienced echocardiographers to perform comprehensive cardiac imaging. However, the diversity of imaging planes can confuse the less experienced echocardiographers, leaving them unable to recognize the various anatomic structures presented. Thus, an understanding of the basic rules of imaging orientation is essential to echocardiographic interpretation.

The ultrasound beam is always directed perpendicular to the probe face. The 2-D TEE image is displayed as a sector scan. The apex of the sector is in close proximity to the TEE probe and the structures seen in this area will be the posterior ones (e.g., left atrium). The arc of the sector will display the more distal and thereby more anterior structures. The angle of rotation of the imaging array determines the right and left orientation. An easy way to understand this orientation is to place your right hand in front of your chest with the palm facing down, the thumb oriented left and the fingers oriented anterior right. The scan lines that generate the TEE image start at your fingers and sweep toward the thumb. Consequently, the right anatomic structures will be displayed on the left side of the monitor (similar to chest x-ray orientation; Fig. 28-6).

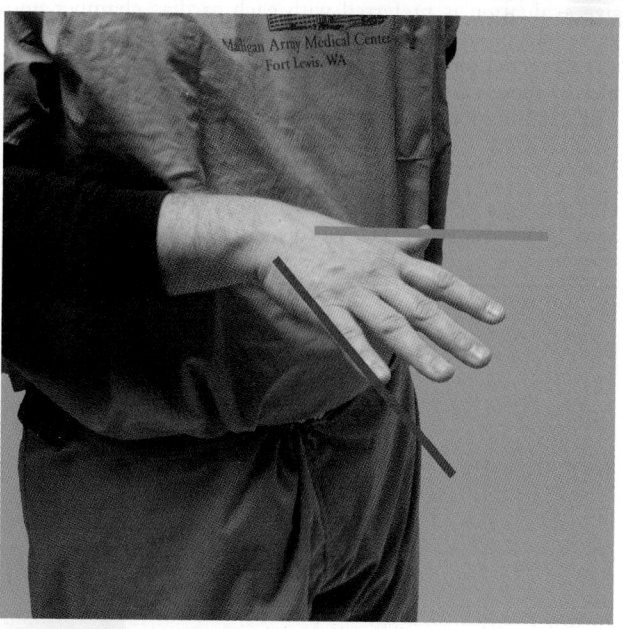

FIGURE 28-6. Orientation of hand, as described in the text, for an imaging plane of 0 degrees. The imaging plane is projected like a wedge anteriorly through the heart. The image is created by multiple scan lines traveling back and forth from the patient's left (green line) to the patient's right (red line). The resulting image is displayed on the monitor as a sector with the green edge (green line) on the right side of the monitor and the red edge (red line) on the left.

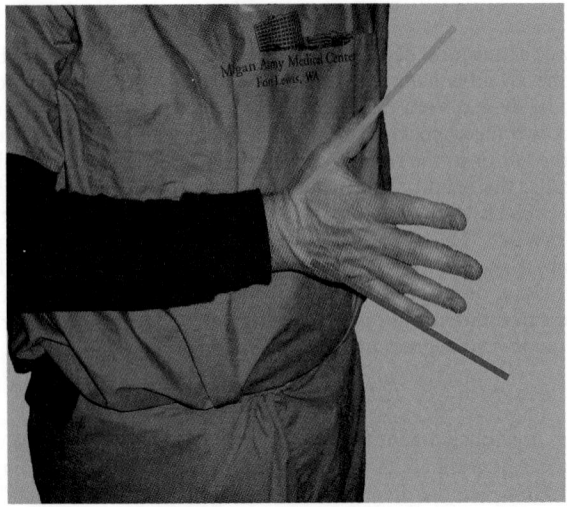

FIGURE 28-7.   Orientation of hand, as described in the text, for an imaging plane of 90 degrees. The imaging sector is rotated so that the green edge (green line) has moved clockwise and is now cephalad and the red edge is now caudad. As previously described, the green edge is displayed on the right side of the monitor and the red edge on the left.

Increasing the imaging plane angle produces clockwise rotation of the sector scan. This can be visualized by rotating your hand in a clockwise fashion. For example, at the 90-degree imaging plane the left side of the screen now displays posterior structures (note position of fingers) and the right side of the screen anterior structures (note position of thumb; Fig. 28-7).

Goals of the Two-Dimensional Examination

Each TEE examination is performed with the goal that no important diagnosis is missed. For this reason, a comprehensive evaluation is preferred with each cardiac chamber and valve imaged in at least two orthogonal planes. However, in an emergency situation, such examination may not be possible. In these cases, most echocardiographers will focus the TEE examination to those views most likely to provide a diag-

nosis: the transgastric short axis view of the left ventricle for diagnosing hypovolemia, coronary ischemia, or acute heart failure.

To achieve the goals of the intraoperative TEE examination, the Society of Cardiovascular Anesthesiologists together with the American Society of Echocardiography has published guidelines for performing a comprehensive intraoperative TEE examination.[19] These guidelines include 20 standardized 2-D echocardiographic views. Each TEE examination should be recorded (video tapes or digital media) along with a detailed report of the examination. Miller et al.[20] proposed a shortened version of the comprehensive examination that would meet the goals established by the these guidelines for basic intraoperative TEE proficiency and is particularly useful when time constraints preclude a more extensive examination. The sequence in which the views are acquired differs among echocardiographers. In the following section we detail the acquisition and anatomic features of the most commonly used intraoperative views.

1. The midesophageal ascending aorta short axis view.

   This view is obtained by advancing the probe slightly from the upper esophagus until the ascending aorta (AA) is seen and then rotating the multiplane angle from 0 to 45 degrees to obtain a true short axis. This "great vessel view" images the AA in short axis and the main pulmonary artery (PA) with its bifurcation and right PA in long axis (Fig. 28-8). If the multiplane angle is rotated to 90 degrees then the midesophageal AA long axis view is obtained, in which the AA is visualized in a longitudinal cut and the PA is visualized as a circular cross-sectional cut (Fig. 28-9). The main uses of the midesophageal ascending aorta short axis view view are to:
   a) Evaluate the AA for dimensions and presence of dissection flaps
   b) Evaluate the PA (position of catheter or rule out thrombus)
   c) Align the Doppler beam parallel to the blood flow in the main PA

2. The midesophageal aortic valve short axis view.

   This view is obtained from the previous view by advancing the probe until the aortic valve (AV) is visible, and then rotating the multiplane angle between 30 and 60 degrees. In the closed position, the three cusps of the AV

FIGURE 28-8.   Midesophageal ascending aortic short axis view. SVC, superior vena cava.

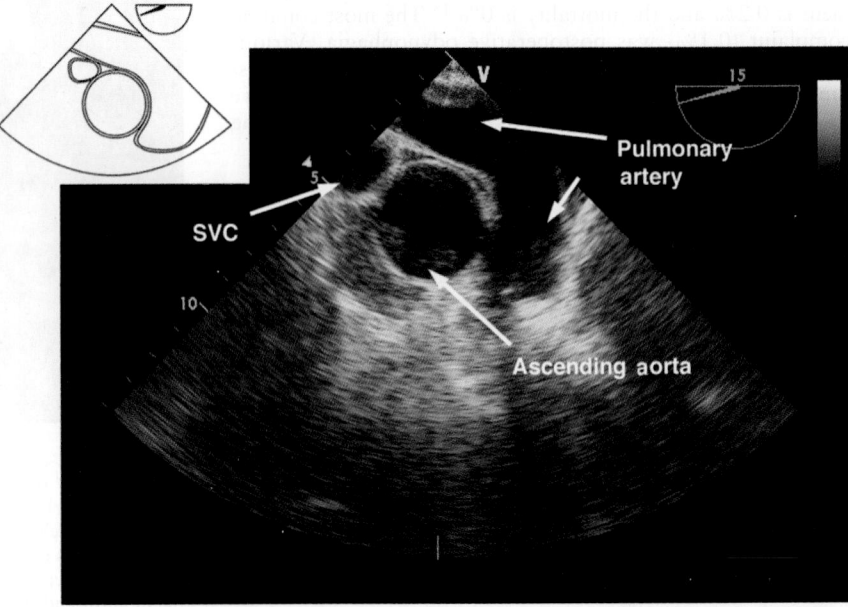

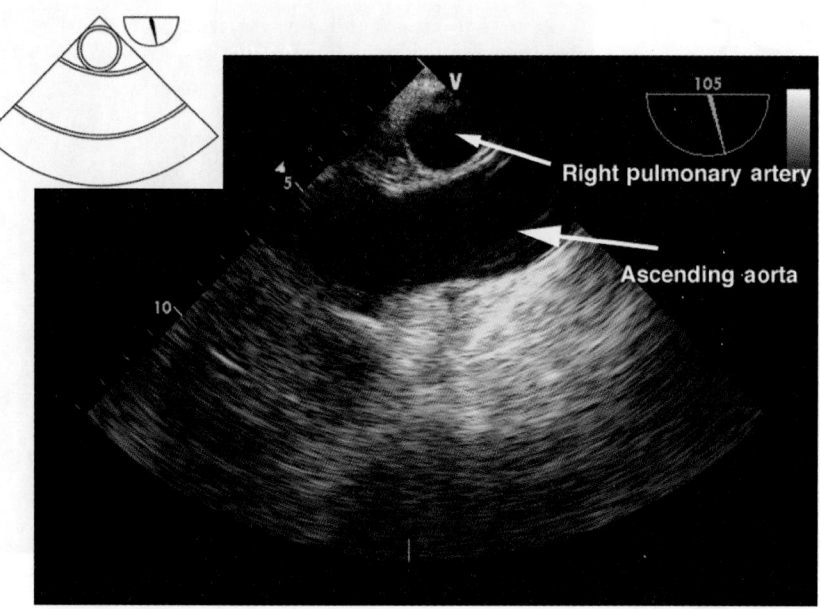

FIGURE 28-9.   Midesophageal ascending aortic long axis view.

form what is known as the "Mercedes Benz" sign (Fig. 28-10). This view is used to evaluate:

a) The AV cusps
b) Aortic stenosis and to measure the area of the AV orifice (planimetry)
c) Aortic insufficiency (AI) by applying color flow Doppler (CFD)
d) The interatrial septum for patent foramen ovale (PFO) or atrial septal defect (ASD)

3. The midesophageal aortic valve long axis view.
   This view is obtained from the previous position by rotating the multiplane angle to 120 to 160 degrees (Fig. 28-11). The view is used to assess:
   a) The AV annulus, sinus of Valsalva, sinotubular junction and AA dimensions
   b) AI by using CFD
   c) Vegetations or masses attached to the AV
   d) Left ventricular outflow tract (LVOT) pathology (e.g., hypertrophic septum with possible LVOT obstruction)

e) The presence of calcification or dissection flaps in the proximal AA

4. The midesophageal bicaval view.
   This view is obtained from the previous view by turning the probe shaft to the patient's right (Fig. 28-12). The view is used to:
   a) Assess the interatrial septum including CFD to detect a patent foramen ovale or ASD. The passage of air across the interatrial septum can be visualized.
   b) Guide placement of catheters and cannulas (PA catheter [PAC], pacemaker wires) or detect presence of thrombus or tumors.

5. The midesophageal right ventricular inflow-outflow view. This view is obtained from the previous view by decreasing the interrogation angle to approximately 60 to 90 degrees (Fig. 28-13). The main uses of the view are to evaluate the:
   a) Pulmonary valve (PV) by measuring the pulmonary annulus (required for Ross procedure) and to detect

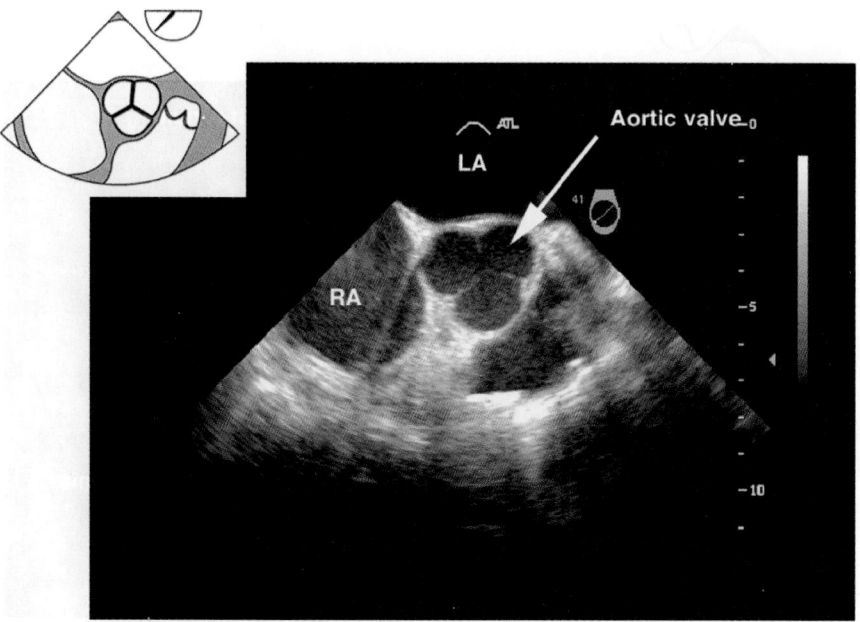

FIGURE 28-10. Midesophageal aortic valve short axis view. RA, right atrium; LA, left atrium.

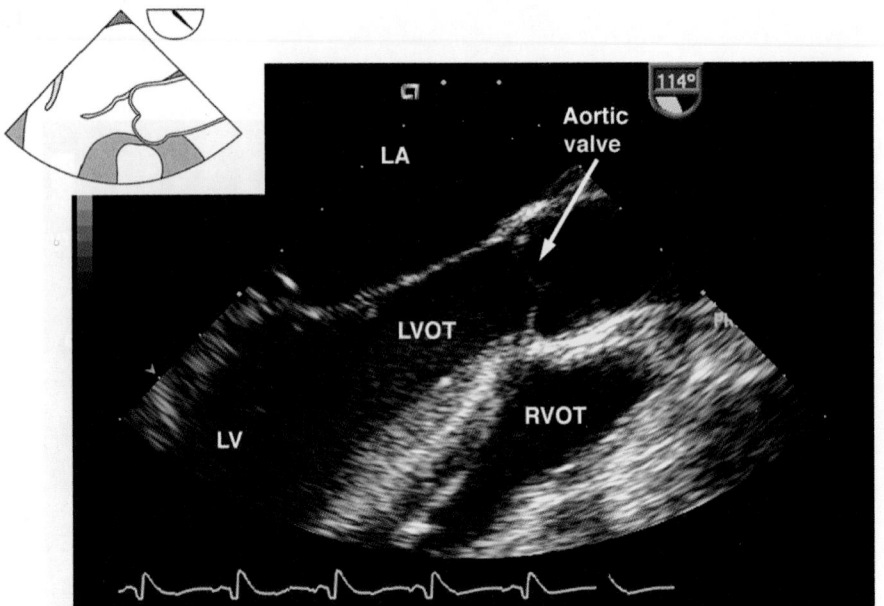

FIGURE 28-11. Midesophageal aortic valve long axis view. LA, left atrium; LV, left ventricle; LVOT, left ventricular outflow tract; RVOT, right ventricular outflow tract.

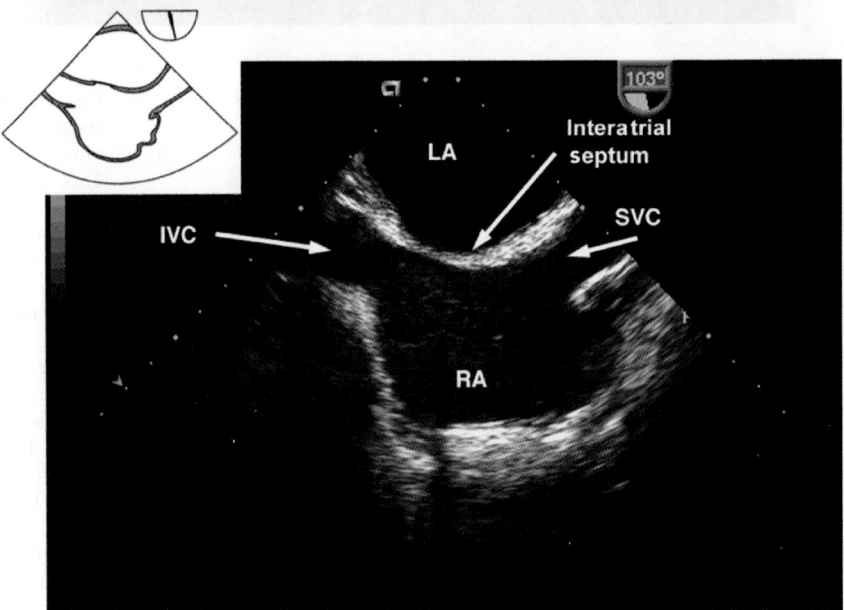

FIGURE 28-12. Midesophageal bicaval view. IVC, inferior vena cava; LA, left atrium, SVC, superior vena cava; RA, right atrium.

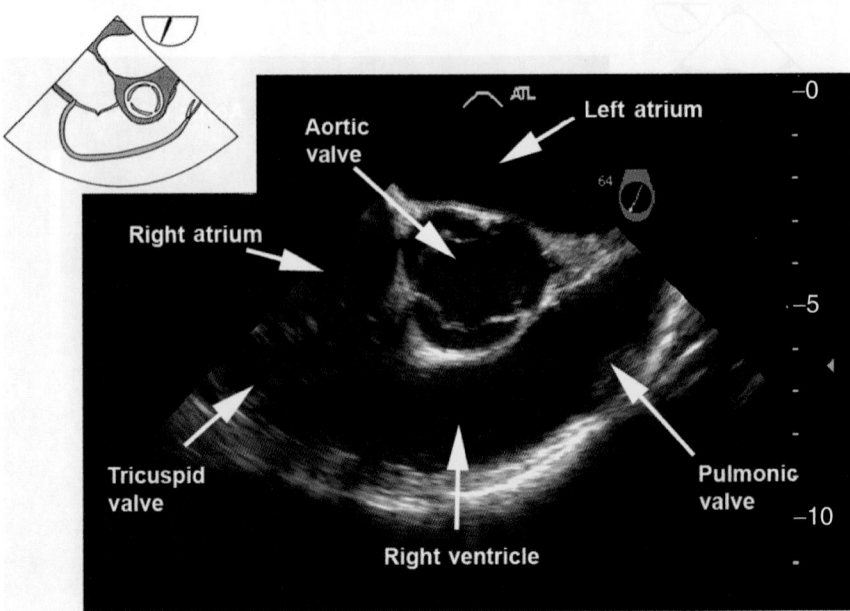

FIGURE 28-13. Midesophageal right ventricular inflow-outflow view.

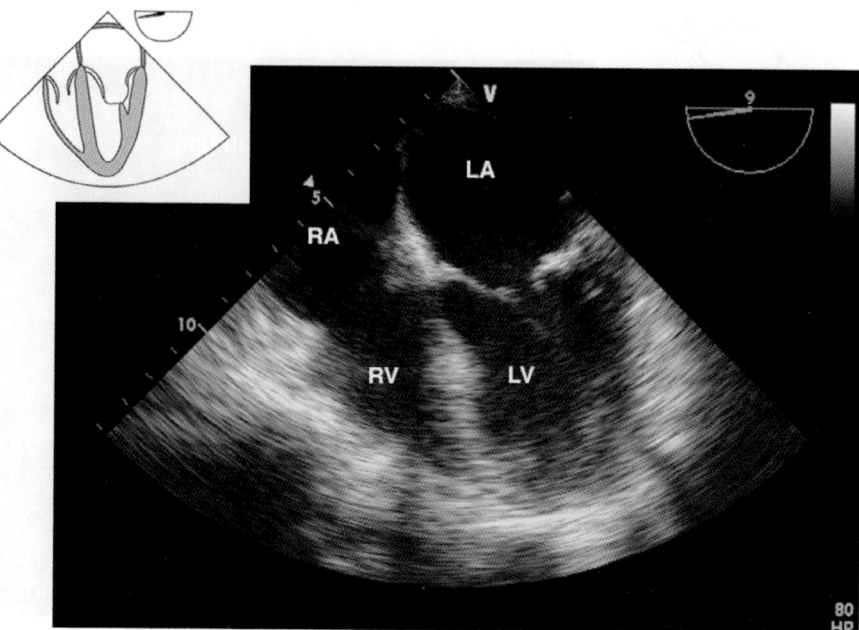

ANESTHETIC MANAGEMENT

FIGURE 28-14. Midesophageal four chamber view, RA, right atrium; RV, right ventricle; LA, left atrium; LV, left ventricle.

pulmonary insufficiency by applying CFD on top of 2-D view

b) RV and RVOT structure and function
c) Tricuspid valve (TV); this view offers the best Doppler beam alignment
d) PAC location

6. The midesophageal four-chamber view.

This view is obtained from the previous view by returning the imaging angle to 0 degree and slightly advancing the probe to the level of the mitral valve (MV). In this view the four cardiac chambers are visualized as well as the TV and MV (Fig. 28-14). Slight withdrawal or anteflexion of the probe will visualize the AV and represents the midesophageal five-chamber view. The midesophageal four-chamber view is one of the most recognizable and valuable diagnostic views. Its main uses are to evaluate the:

a) Left atrium, right atrium, RV, and the LV (inferoseptal and anterolateral walls) size and function

b) TV and MV structure and function; CFD will detect valvular pathology
c) Diastolic function

7. The midesophageal two-chamber view.

This view is obtained from the previous view by rotating the multiplane angle to 90 degrees. In this view the left atrial appendage is examined for presence of thrombus. Slight retroflexion is used to avoid a foreshortened view of the LV so as to visualize the LV apex (Fig. 28-15). If the multiplane angle is rotated to just 60 degrees then the midesophageal mitral commissural view is obtained (Fig. 28-16). The main uses of the midesophageal two-chamber view are to evaluate the:

a) LV anterior and inferior wall function b) LV apex as well as to diagnose apical thrombus

8. The midesophageal long axis view.

This view is obtained from the previous view by rotating the multiplane angle to 120 to 135 degrees (Fig. 28-17).

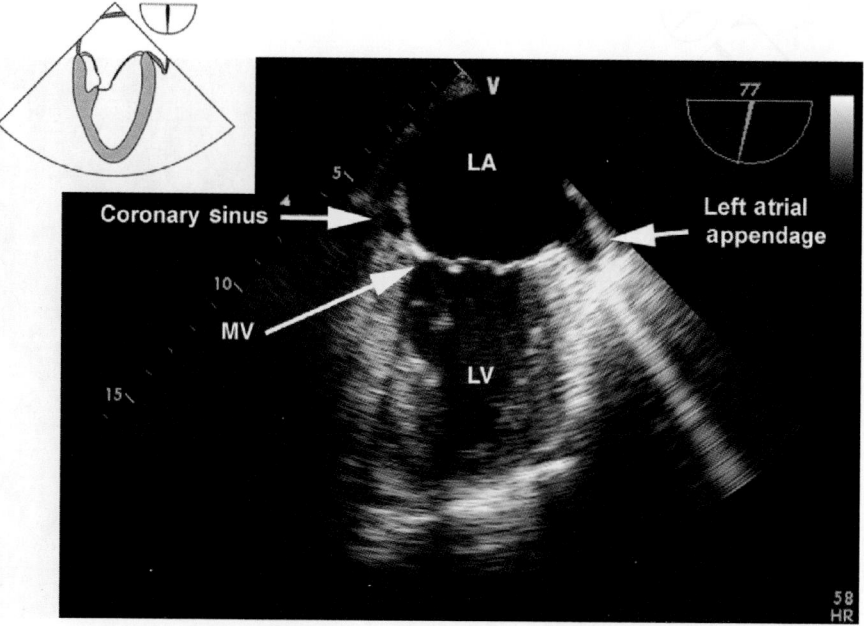

FIGURE 28-15. Midesophageal two chamber view. LA, left atrium; MV, mitral valve; LV, left ventricle.

FIGURE 28-16.   Midesophageal commissural view.

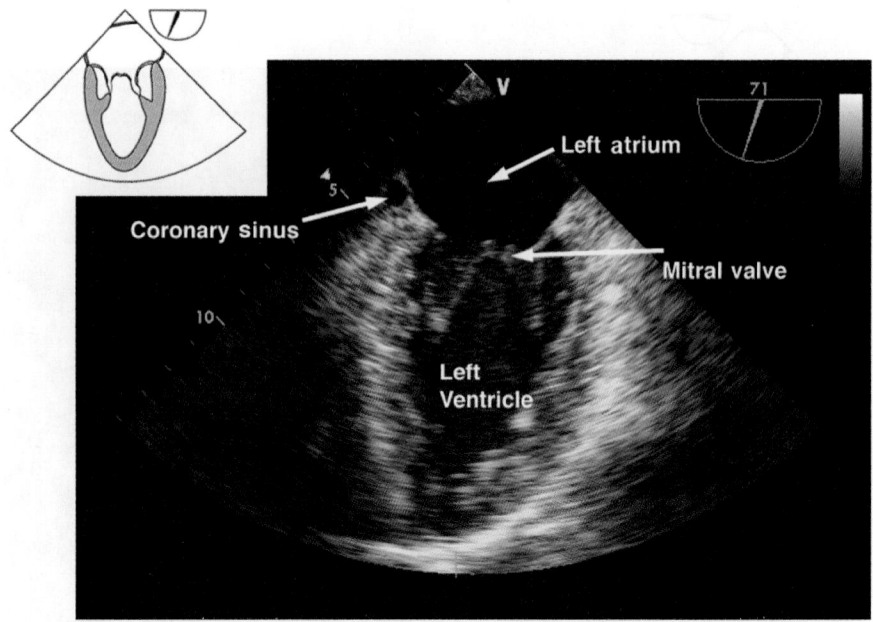

The main uses of the midesophageal long axis view are to evaluate the:
a) LV anteroseptal and posterior wall function
b) LV outflow tract pathology
c) MV pathology

9. The transgastric midpapillary short axis view.

The view is obtained by advancing the TEE probe from the midesophageal position into the stomach, anteflexing and then withdrawing until contact is made with the gastric wall. The LV is visualized as a doughnut shape in cross-section and both papillary muscles should be seen (Fig. 28-18). Additional anteflexion obtains the gastric basal short axis view (Fig. 28-19). Advancement of the probe allows visualization of the LV apex in cross-section. The transgastric midpapillary short axis view is unique in that it visualizes all the LV walls perfused by each of the three major coronary arteries. The view is considered to be the most useful one in situations of intraoperative

hemodynamic instability as it allows immediate diagnosis of hypovolemic state, pump failure, or coronary ischemia.

The primary uses of the transgastric midpapillary short axis view include assessment of the:
a) LV size (enlargement, hypertrophy) and cavity volume
b) Global ventricular systolic function and regional wall motion

10. The transgastric two-chamber view.

This view is obtained from the previous one by rotating the multiplane angle to 90 degrees. The LV is visualized in a longitudinal section with the apex at the left of the display and MV at the right (Fig. 28-20). The primary use of this view is to assess function of the LV anterior and, inferior walls.

11. The transgastric long axis view.

This view is obtained from the previous view by rotating the multiplane angle to 120 degrees (Fig. 28-21). The main uses of the view are to:

FIGURE 28-17.   Midesophageal long axis view. LA, left atrium; LV, left ventricle; RVOT, right ventricular outflow tract.

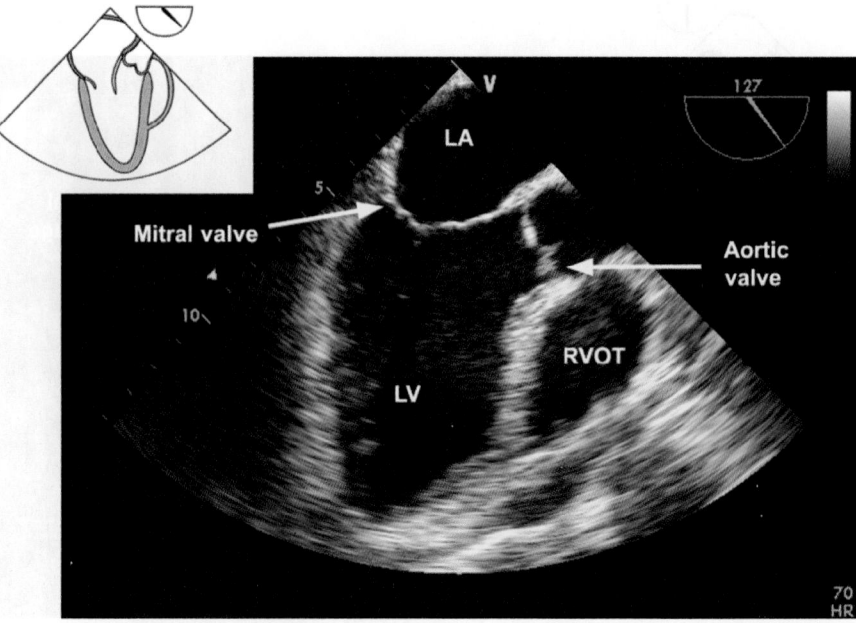

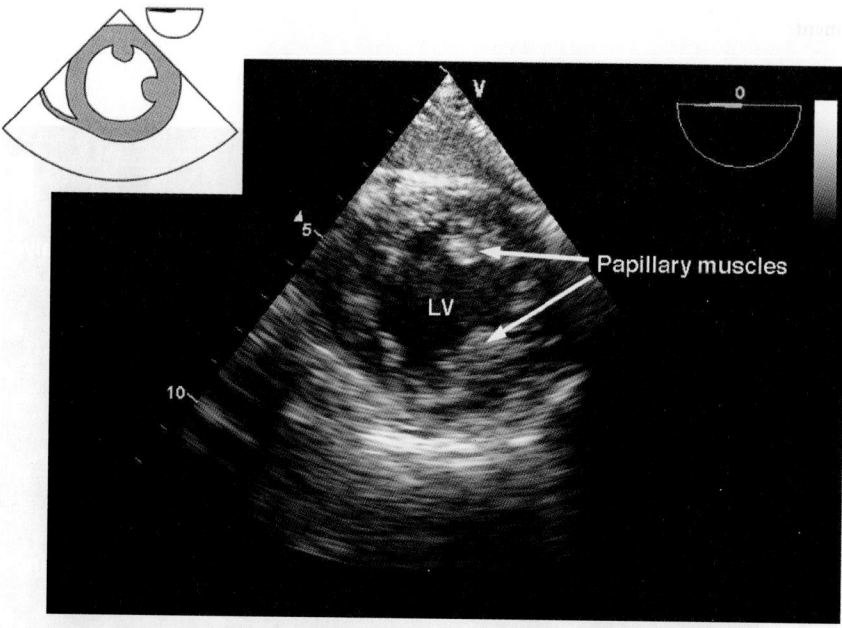

FIGURE 28-18. Transgastric short axis view. LV, left ventricle.

FIGURE 28-19. Transgastric basal short axis view. A1-3, anterior leaflet of mitral valve, scallops 1-3; P1-3, posterior leaflet of mitral valve, scallops 1-3.

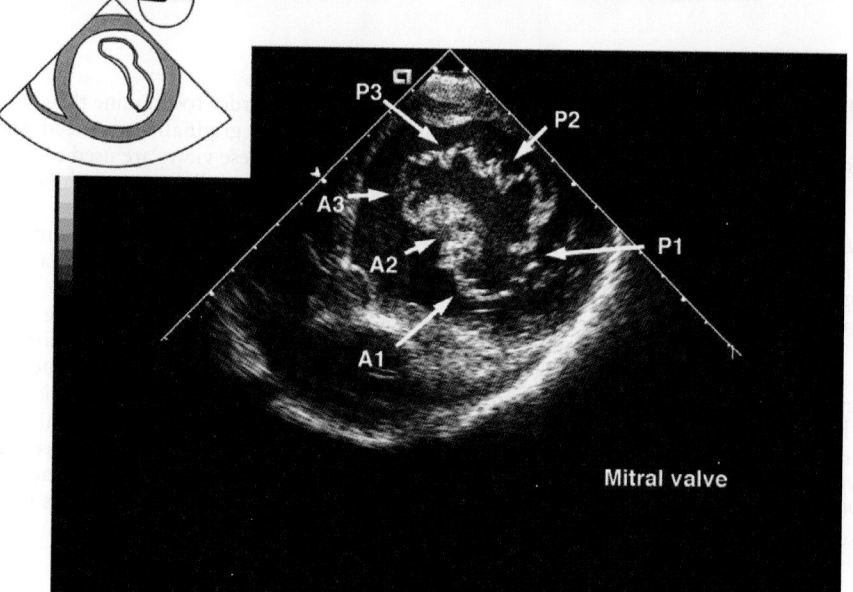

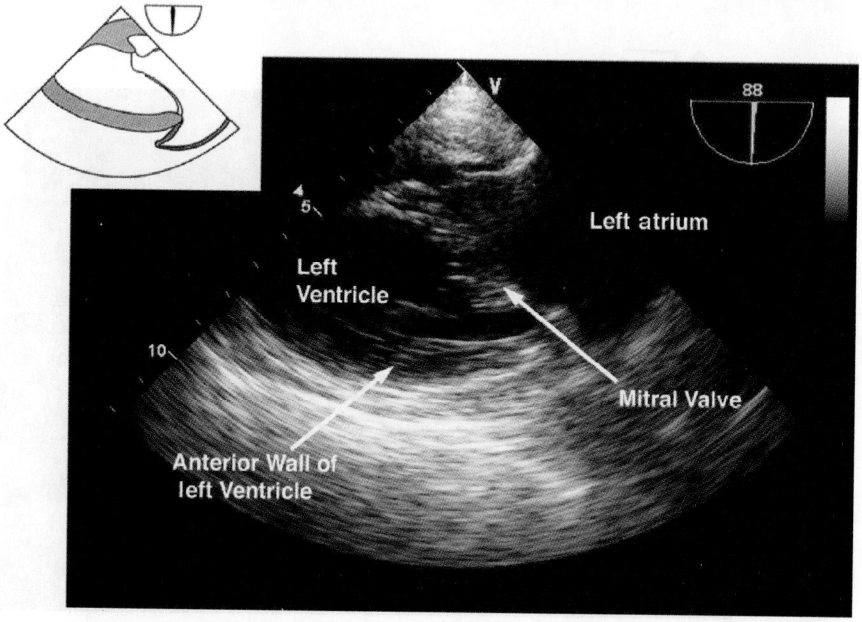

FIGURE 28-20. Transgastric two chamber view.

FIGURE 28-21.   Transgastric long axis view. LV, left ventricle; LVOT, left ventricular outflow tract.

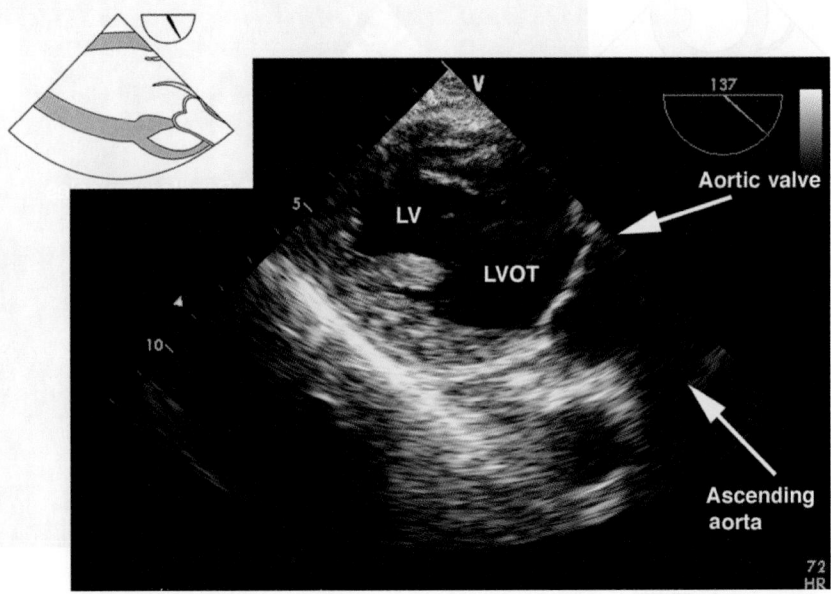

a) Position the Doppler beam parallel to blood flow across the LVOT and AV

b) Assess systolic function of the anteroseptal and posterior LV walls

12. The deep transgastric long axis view.

This view is obtained by advancing the probe deep in the stomach, toward the LV apex, and then anteflexing and slightly withdrawing the probe (Fig. 28-22). The main use of the view is Doppler assessment of LVOT and aortic blood velocities.

13. Descending short and long axis views.

The descending aortic short axis view is obtained from the midesophageal four-chamber view by turning the TEE probe to the left until a circular vascular structure is found, representing the descending aorta in cross-section (Fig. 28-23). Rotating the multiplane angle to 90 degrees visualizes the descending aorta in a longitudinal section (tubular vas-

cular structure; Fig. 28-24). In order to examine the entire descending aorta, the probe is gradually advanced and withdrawn in the esophagus. These views are used to:

a) Identify pathology of the descending aorta (atheroma, dissection flaps, aneurysm)

b) Assist with placement of guide wires and cannulas (intra-aortic balloon pump [IABP], aortic cannula)

14. Upper esophageal aortic arch short axis view.

The view is obtained from the descending aortic long axis view by withdrawing the probe in the upper esophagus and rotating it to the right until the tubular structure transforms into a circular one (Fig. 28-25). The view is used to assess the presence of pathology in the distal aortic arch and Doppler assessment of pulmonary arterial blood velocities. If the multiplane angle is rotated back to 0 degrees, the upper esophageal aortic arch long axis view is obtained (Fig. 28-26).

FIGURE 28-22.   Deep transgastric long axis view. LV, left ventricle; LVOT, left ventricular outflow tract.

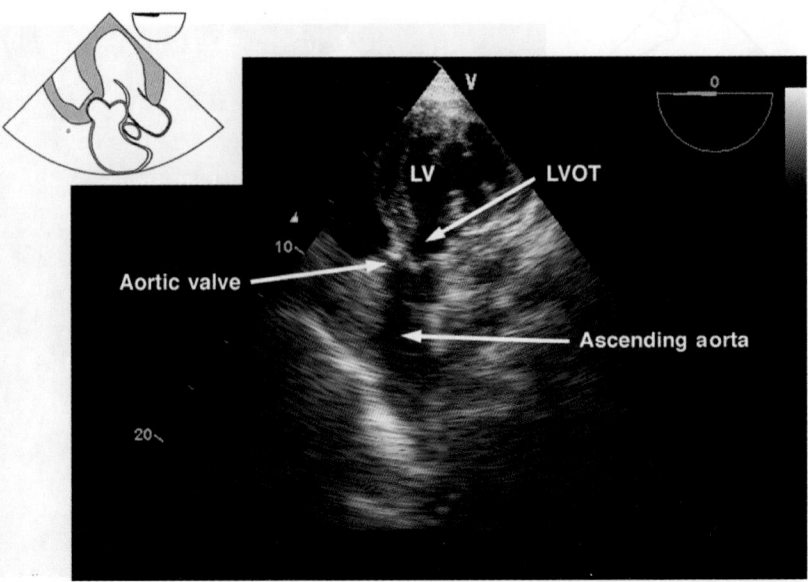

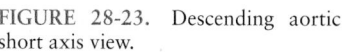

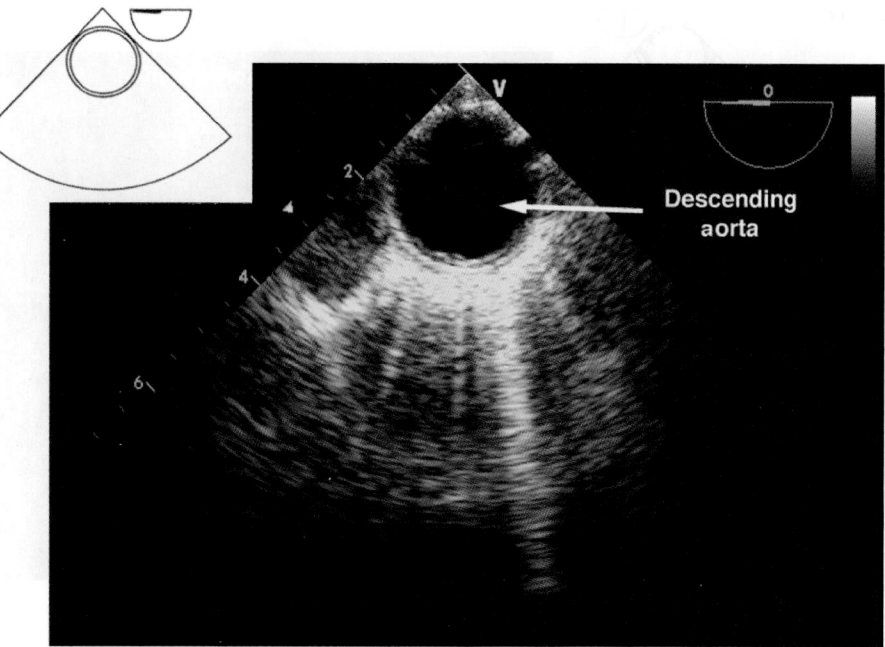

FIGURE 28-23. Descending aortic short axis view.

Three-Dimensional Echocardiography

In order to better conceptualize the morphology and pathology of the heart, three-dimensional (3-D) image presentation has been developed. The recent introduction of a real-time 3-D TEE probe makes this goal a reality for intraoperative echocardiographers. This technology is capable of acquiring full volumes of the left ventricle, of visualizing heart valves in three dimensions, and assessing the synchrony of LV contraction.

Uses of 3-D TEE are just emerging. The utility of 3-D imaging of the MV for a MV repair surgery is of particular interest.[21] The capacity of this probe to assess LV contraction synchrony in patients undergoing resynchronization therapy with biventricular pacing may offer a means to maximize their cardiac output. It is anticipated that additional intraoperative applications will emerge with this exciting advancement.

DOPPLER ECHOCARDIOGRAPHY AND HEMODYNAMICS

Use of 2-D echocardiography captures high-fidelity motion images of cardiac structures, but not blood flow. Blood flow indices such as blood velocities, stroke volume, and pressure gradients are the domain of Doppler echocardiography. Unlike 2-D imaging, which relies on the time delay and amplitude of reflected ultrasound, Doppler technologies are based on the change in frequency that occurs when ultrasound interacts with moving objects. Reflections from red blood cells are used to determine blood flow velocity and calculate hemodynamic parameters. The combination of 2-D images and quantitative Doppler measurements create a uniquely powerful diagnostic tool. Accordingly, Doppler assessments are an essential element of the echocardiographic examination.[22]

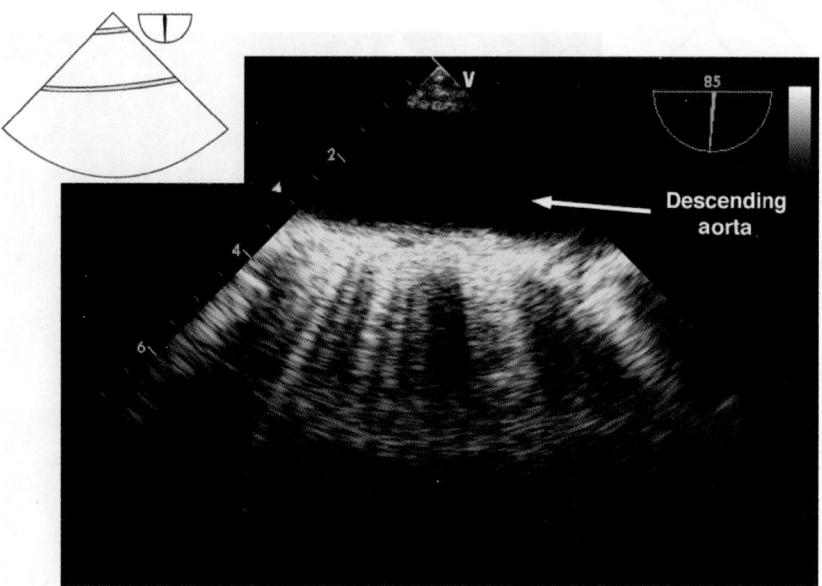

FIGURE 28-24. Descending aortic long axis view.

FIGURE 28-25. Upper esophageal aortic arch short axis view.

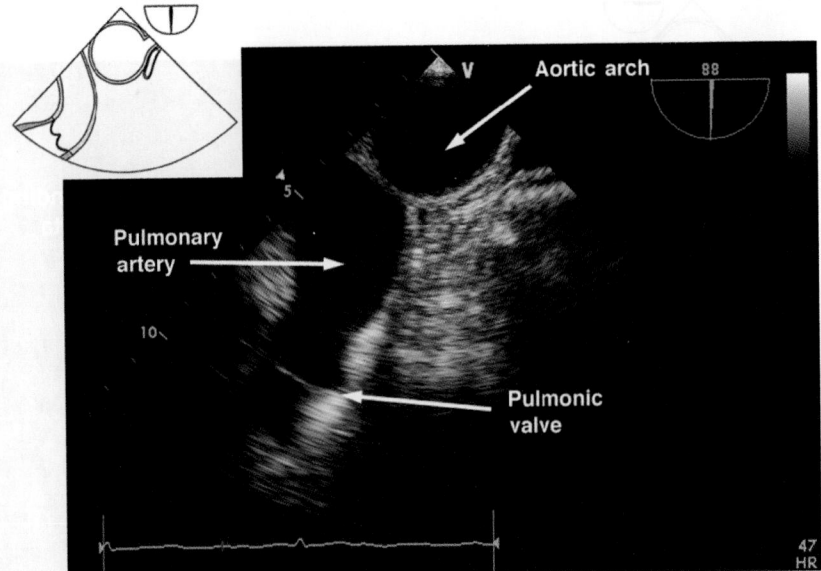

The motion of an object causes a sound wave to be compressed in the direction of the motion and expanded in the direction opposite to the motion. This alteration in frequency is known as the *Doppler effect*. By monitoring the frequency pattern of reflections of red blood cells, Doppler echocardiography can determine the speed, direction, and timing of blood flow. The *Doppler equation* describes the relationship between the alteration in ultrasound frequency and blood flow velocity (Fig. 28-27)

$$\Delta f = v \times \cos\theta \times 2f_t/c$$

where Δf is the difference between transmitted frequency (f_t) and received frequency, v is blood velocity, c is the speed of sound in blood (1,540 m/s), and θ is the angle of incidence between the ultrasound beam and blood flow. Conceptually, the equation is simplified by observing that the change in ultrasound frequency is related to just two variables: blood velocity and cos θ. For this reason the Doppler signal is shifted *only* by the component of the blood velocity that is in the direction of

the beam path (i.e., v cos θ). When the beam angle divergence is >30 degrees the value of cos θ decreases rapidly and the Doppler system will markedly underestimate blood velocity. The requirement of near-parallel orientation (cos 0 = 1) for Doppler examinations contrasts with the near-perpendicular orientation preferred for 2-D imaging. Consequently, the preferred imaging planes for Doppler will differ from those used for 2-D imaging.

Spectral Doppler

Two Doppler techniques, *pulsed wave* (PW) and *continuous wave* (CW), are commonly used to evaluate blood flow. A thorough understanding of the advantages and disadvantages of each technique is critical in selecting the one most appropriate for the clinical setting at hand.[23,24] In clinical practice, PW and CW Doppler are frequently used in conjunction with 2-D imaging. The 2-D image is used to identify the area of interest and guide the echocardiographer in precisely localizing the

FIGURE 28-26. Upper esophageal aortic arch long axis view.

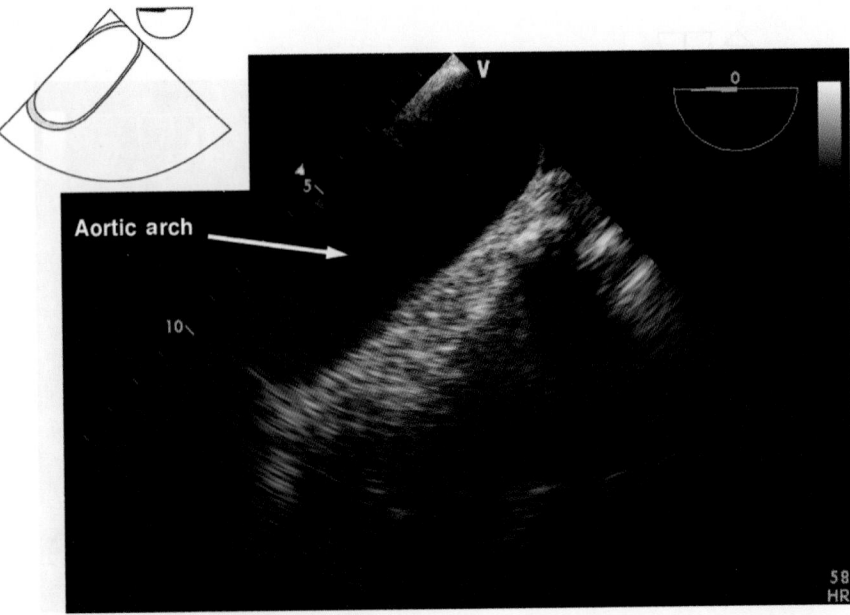

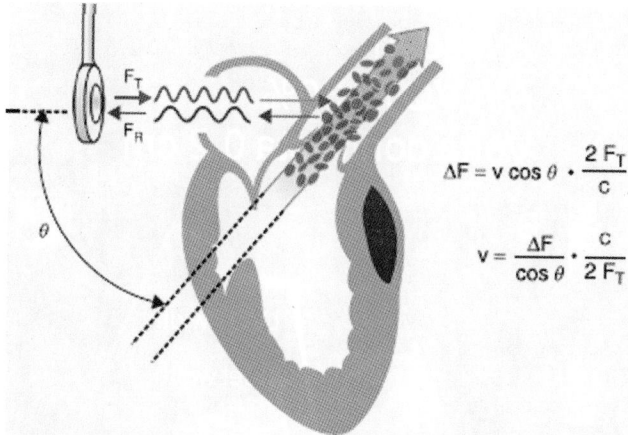

FIGURE 28-27.   Calculating blood flow velocity: the Doppler equation. The Doppler equation calculates blood flow velocity based on two variables: the Doppler frequency shift (ΔF) and the cosine (cos) of the angle of incidence between the ultrasound beam and the blood flow. The Doppler frequency shift is measured by the echocardiographic system, but cos θ is unknown, and manual entry by the echocardiographer is required for its estimation. v, flood blood flow velocity; F_T, transmitted signal frequency; F_R, reflected signal frequency; ΔF, difference between F_R, and F_T; c, speed of sound in tissue; θ, angle of incidence between the orientation of the ultrasound beam and that of the blood flow.

$$\Delta F = v \cos \theta \cdot \frac{2 F_T}{c}$$

$$v = \frac{\Delta F}{\cos \theta} \cdot \frac{c}{2 F_T}$$

sampling volume in a PW study or in directing the beam in a CW study.

Pulsed Wave Doppler.   PW Doppler offers the echocardiographer the ability to sample blood flow from a particular location. The PW transducer uses a single crystal as both the emitter and the receiver of ultrasound waves. Like the pulsed echocardiography system described for 2-D imaging, the PW Doppler system transmits a short burst of ultrasound toward the target and then switches to receive mode to interpret the returning echoes. Because the speed of sound (c) in tissue is constant, the time delay for a signal to reach its target and return to the transducer depends solely on the distance (d) to

the target. Consequently, reflected signals from locations more distant from the transducer return after a greater time interval. By *time gating*, the electronic circuitry of the PW transducer interprets returning echoes only after a predetermined time delay following the transmission of an ultrasound pulse. In this way, only those signals associated with a location, referred to as the *sample volume*, are selected for evaluation.

The pulsed Doppler system uses a repeating pattern of ultrasound transmission and reception. The rate at which the device repeatedly generates sound bursts is known as the *pulse repetition frequency*. Because the speed of sound through tissue is a constant, the pulse repetition frequency is directly related to the depth of the sample volume. The pulse repetition frequency is analogous to the frame rate of a movie camera. Like the multiple frames on a roll of movie film, each ultrasound pulse interacts with the blood flow for a brief period of time, and just as a series of movie frames display motion, a series of pulsed cycles are consecutively analyzed to determine the blood flow. The Doppler data is frequently presented as a velocity-time plot known as the *spectral display* (Fig. 28-28B).

Because the pulsed Doppler data are collected intermittently, the maximal frequency and blood flow velocity that can be accurately measured by PW Doppler are limited. The maximal frequency, which equals one-half the pulse repetition frequency, is known as the *Nyquist limit*. At blood velocities above the Nyquist limit, analysis of the returning signal becomes ambiguous, with the velocities appearing to be in the opposite direction. A similar effect is seen in movie animation, in which a rapidly spinning wheel appears to spin backward because of the slow frame rate. The ambiguous signal from frequencies above the Nyquist limit, known as *aliasing*, appears on the spectral display as a signal on the other side of the baseline, hence the term *wraparound*. This Nyquist limitation has led to an alternative approach for assessment of high-velocity blood flows, namely CW Doppler.

Continuous Wave Doppler.   The CW Doppler technique avoids the maximal velocity limitation of PW systems by using two crystals, one continuously transmitting and the other continuously receiving the reflected ultrasound signal. With continuous reception of the Doppler signal, the Nyquist limit is not applicable, and blood flows with very high velocities are recorded accurately. The CW mode receives reflected signals

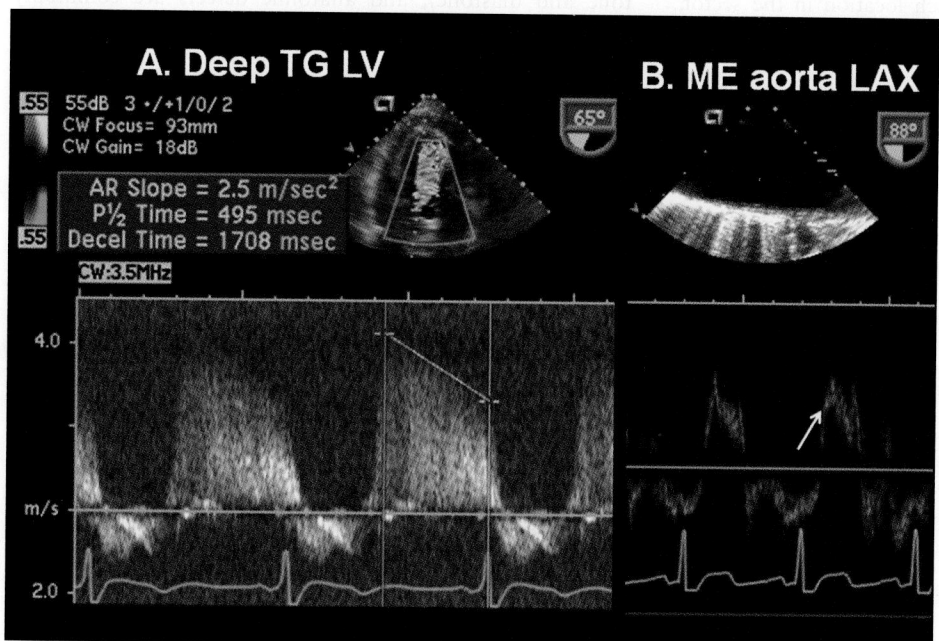

FIGURE 28-28.   Doppler echocardiography in aortic insufficiency. **A.** The deep transgastric (deep TG) view of the left ventricle (LV) is displayed. A color Doppler sector is placed over the aortic valve and LV outflow tract and the aortic insufficiency (AI) jet is imaged. The continuous wave (CW) Doppler cursor is positioned in the center of the AI flow and the spectral display of the AI jet is shown against time. The slope of the AI jet is used to calculate the pressure half time (P½ Time). A short P½ Time is associated with severe AI. **B.** The descending aorta is imaged in long axis (midesophageal [ME] aorta LAX). The sample volume of pulsed wave Doppler is placed upstream. There is a systolic wave above the baseline, as the blood moves toward the transesophageal echocardiography transducer, and a diastolic wave (*arrow*), indicating reversal of aortic flow because of severe AI. Decel, deceleration.

FIGURE 28-29. Evaluation of aortic insufficiency (AI). Color flow Doppler of the aortic valve (AV) in the midesophageal long axis view. AI is graded using (1) the relative ratio of the AI jet thickness to the diameter of left ventricular outflow tract (LVOT); both measurements are performed at the same site, usually within 0.5 to 1 cm proximal to the AV plane; and (2) the width of the AI jet as it crosses the AV cusps (vena contracta).

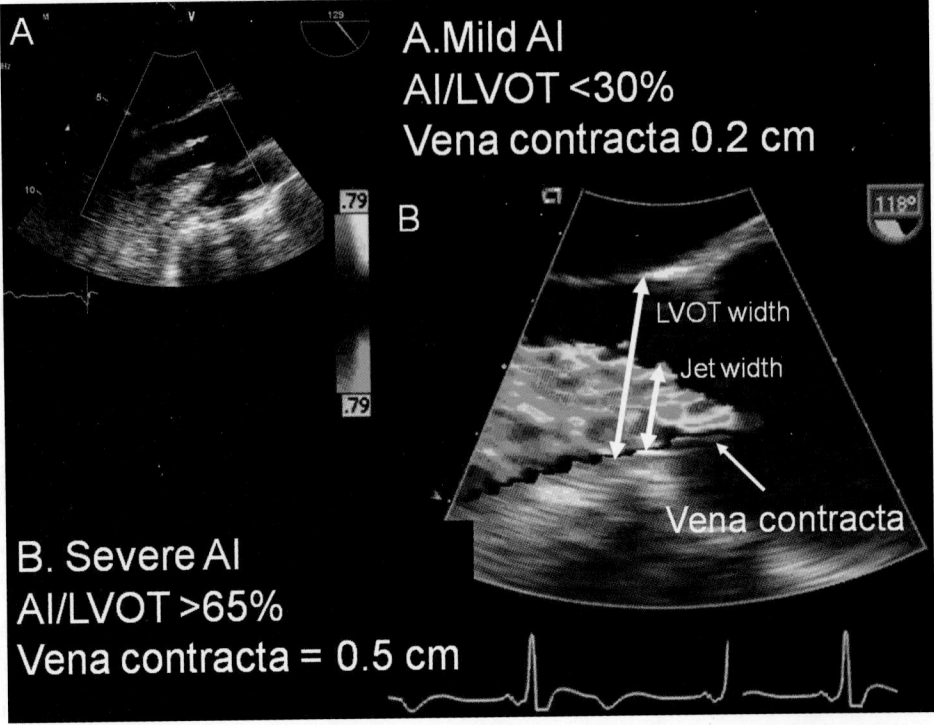

from blood flow throughout its beam path because it is not time-gated like the PW technique (Fig. 28-28A). The inability to select blood flow from a specific location favors the selection of CW Doppler primarily for detection of the highest velocities along the beam path, which is useful in applications such as determining the high velocity jet of aortic stenosis.

Color Flow Doppler

CFD provides a dramatic display of both blood flow and cardiac anatomy by combining 2-D echocardiography and PW Doppler methods (Fig. 28-29). The PW Doppler used for CFD differs from that previously discussed in two important ways. CFD performs *multiple* sample volume recordings along each scan line as the beam is swept through the sector. This approach provides flow data at each location in the sector, which can be overlaid on the structural data obtained by 2-D imaging. The Doppler velocity data from each sample volume are color-coded and superimposed on top of the gray scale 2-D image. In the most widely accepted color code, red hues indicate flow toward the transducer and blue hues indicates flow away from the transducer. The ability to provide a real-time, integrated display of flow and structural information makes CFD useful for assessing valvular function, aortic dissection, and congenital heart abnormalities. However, an important caveat to its use in the clinical setting must be noted. Because it relies on PW Doppler measurements, CFD is susceptible to alias artifacts. Aliasing in the color flow map is illustrated in Figure 28-30. This alias pattern can be useful to calculate blood flow in mitral valve disease using the proximal isovelocity surface area (PISA) method (Fig. 28-30).

Hemodynamic Assessments

Doppler echocardiography's ability to quantitatively measure blood velocity yields a wealth of information on the hemodynamic state. Stroke volume, chamber pressures, valvular disease, pulmonary vascular resistance, ventricular function (systolic and diastolic), and anatomic defects are commonly assessed with perioperative Doppler echocardiography.[25]

Volumetric Flow Assessments. Measurements such as stroke volume and cardiac output express the volume of blood ejected by the heart over time. Volumetric parameters are calculated using the principle that volumetric flow (Q) equals blood flow velocity (v) times the cross-sectional area (CSA) of the conduit,

FIGURE 28-30. Doppler evaluation of mitral regurgitation (MR) severity. MR severity is evaluated using color Doppler. **A.** MR jet is imaged with color flow Doppler (midesophageal two-chamber view). The Nyquist limit is moved upward to demonstrate flow acceleration inside the left ventricle and the neck (vena contracta) of the MR jet. **B.** Zoom of the proximal MR jet allows measurement of the proximal isovelocity surface area (PISA) radius and calculation of the incompetent mitral valve orifice.

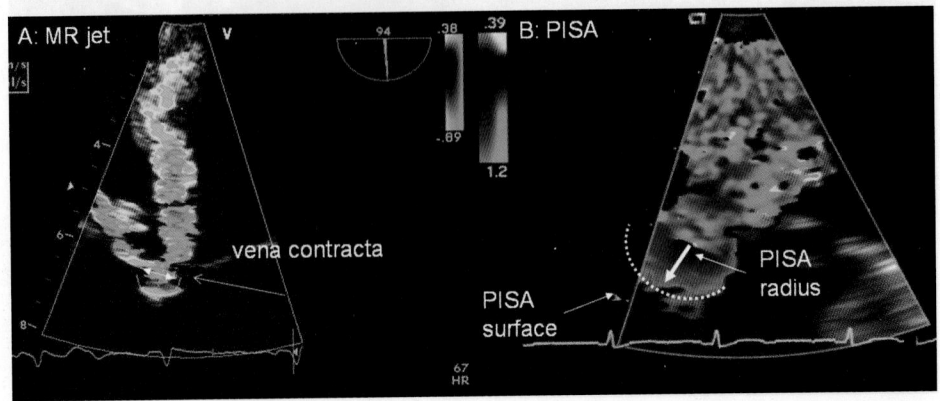

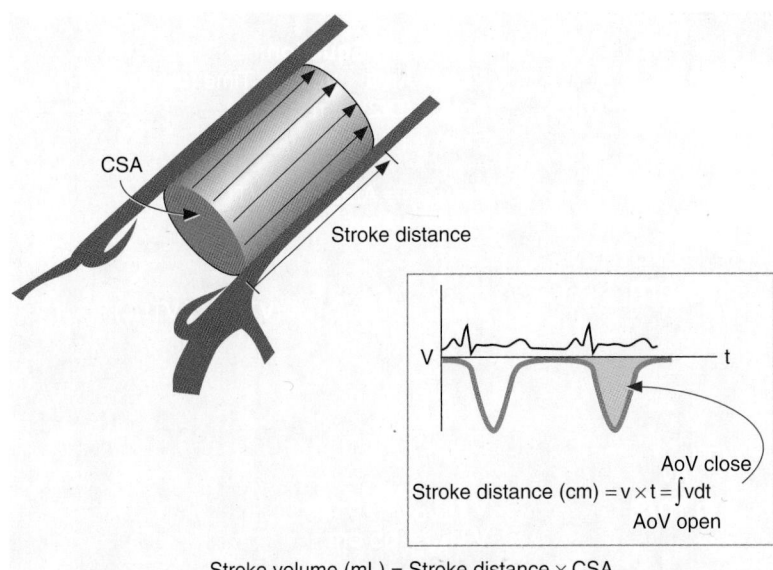

FIGURE 28-31. Determination of stroke volume. Volumetric flow can be determined from a combination of area and velocity measurements. In this example, flow through the ascending aorta is used to determine the stroke volume. Integrating the Doppler-derived flow velocities over time (known as the time-velocity integral) during a single cardiac cycle calculates the stroke distance. The cross-sectional area measurement is obtained by two-dimensional echocardiography. The product of these two measurements, conceptualized as a cylinder, is the stroke volume. CSA, cross-sectional area: AoV, aortic valve.

that is $Q = v \times CSA$. To determine volumetric flows with echocardiography, a Doppler measurement of the blood flow velocities and a 2-D measurement of the CSA are recorded.

Stroke Volume and Cardiac Output. To calculate stroke volume the instantaneous velocities during systole are traced from the spectral display and the echocardiographic system's internal software package calculates the time velocity integral (VTI, in centimeters). In effect the VTI represents the distance ($v \times t = d$) blood traveled during systole (i.e., stroke distance). By multiplying the VTI by the CSA (in square centimeters) of the conduit (e.g., aorta, MV, PA) through which the blood traveled, the stroke volume (in cubic centimeters) is obtained: $SV = VTI \times CSA$ (Fig. 28-31).[26-28] Cardiac output, which expresses volumetric flow in cubic centimeters per minute, is estimated from the product of SV and heart rate: $CO = VTI \times CSA \times$ HR. Figure 28-32 demonstrates calculation of cardiac output and stroke volume from the left ventricular outflow tract.

Valve Area. The Continuity Equation. The principle of conservation of mass is the basis of the *continuity equation*, which is commonly used to measure the aortic valve area.[29] The continuity equation simply states that the volume of blood passing through one site in the heart (e.g., the LVOT) is equal to the mass or volume of blood passing through another site (e.g., the aortic valve).

Volumetric Flow$_1$ = Volumetric Flow$_2$ therefore

$$CSA_1 \times VTI_1 = CSA_2 \times VTI_2 \text{ and}$$
$$CSA_1 = CSA_2 \times VTI_2 / VTI_1$$

Figure 28-33 demonstrates calculation of AV area using this approach.

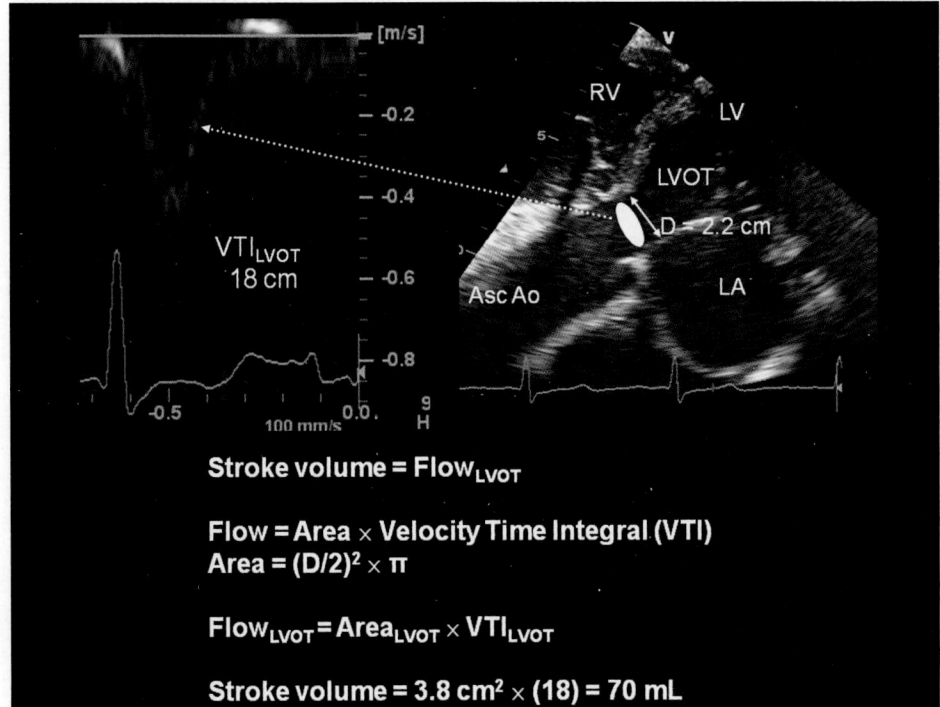

Stroke volume = Flow$_{LVOT}$

Flow = Area × Velocity Time Integral (VTI)
Area = $(D/2)^2 \times \pi$

Flow$_{LVOT}$ = Area$_{LVOT}$ × VTI$_{LVOT}$

Stroke volume = $3.8 \text{ cm}^2 \times (18) = 70 \text{ mL}$

FIGURE 28-32. Stroke volume calculation. Stroke volume is equal to the blood flow crossing the left ventricular outflow tract (LVOT). In the deep transgastric LV view, the LVOT orifice (*large oval*) can be calculated from the LVOT diameter (D). The blood flow velocity across the LVOT is measured with pulsed Doppler, and the velocity time integral (VTI) by tracing the velocity envelope. RV, right ventricle; LA, left atrium.

FIGURE 28-33. Evaluation of aortic stenosis. Calculation of aortic valve area using the "double envelope" technique. The cursor of continuous wave Doppler is placed in the middle of the blood flow traversing the stenosed aortic valve, and two envelopes are identified. The one with the slower velocity is from the left ventricular outflow tract (LVOT) and the one with the fastest is from the aortic valve (AV). The envelopes of the velocities are traced to derive the respective velocity time integrals (VTI). The aortic valve area is calculated using the continuity equation. D diameter.

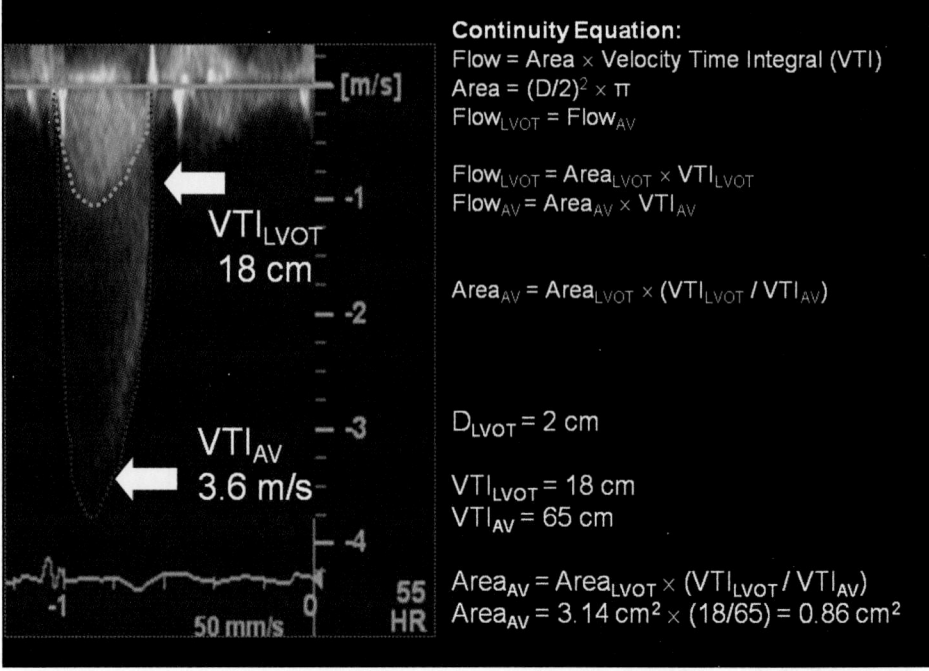

Pressure Assessment: The Bernoulli Equation. Pressure gradients are used to estimate intracavitary pressures and to assess conditions such as valvular disease (e.g., aortic stenosis), septal defects, outflow tract obstruction, and major vessel pathology (e.g., coarctation). As blood flows across a narrowed or stenotic orifice, blood flow velocity increases. The increase in velocities relates to the degree of narrowing. In the clinical situation, the *simplified Bernoulli equation* describes the relation between the increases in blood flow velocity and the pressure gradient across the narrowed orifice[11]: $\Delta P = 4V_{max}^2$ where ΔP in millimeters of mercury is the pressure gradient across the narrowed orifice and V_{max}^4 in meters per second is the maximum velocity across that orifice measured by Doppler.

Thus in clinical echocardiography, pressure gradient is obtained by the straightforward process of measuring the peak velocity of blood flow across the lesion of interest.[30,31] The measured peak velocity is then entered into the simplified Bernoulli equation to estimate the pressure gradient.

The Bernoulli equation is commonly employed to measure the pressure gradient across a stenotic valve. In addition, the rate of decline in the pressure gradient across the valve is related to the severity of disease.[32,33] This *pressure half-time* is the time required for the peak transvalvular pressure gradient to decrease by 50%. Typically, a larger orifice will have a shorter pressure half-time as pressure can equalize more quickly.

Measurement of Intracavitary Pressures. Intracavitary and pulmonary arterial pressures can be estimated by obtaining a Doppler-derived pressure gradient from a regurgitant jet of the valve separating two chambers.[34–36] The chamber pressure equals the pressure of the neighboring chamber plus the pressure gradient between them. Table 28-1 provides calculations for the heart chambers and PA.

❸   ECHOCARDIOGRAPHIC EVALUATION OF SYSTOLIC FUNCTION

Evaluation of LV systolic function is a primary component of every echocardiographic examination. Information about global as well regional LV performance is accomplished by

assessing the LV muscle contractile function and the size and shape of LV cavity. Both qualitative assessments (which are inherently subjective) and quantitative techniques (which produce hard numerical estimates) are useful. Modalities used are 2-D and motion mode (M-mode), which image the LV walls and cavity and Doppler echocardiography, which measures the velocity of blood flow and moving tissue.

Left Ventricular Walls

From the midesophageal position, the TEE imaging array is rotated electronically in a clockwise fashion to scan the entire circumference of the LV cavity and walls in a longitudinal orientation. Further advancement of the TEE probe to the transgastric position combined with anterior flexion (anteflexion) of the probe sequentially images the LV short axis from its base to apex. The LV cavity and walls at the basal, mid, and apical levels are evaluated in the midesophageal and transgastric views. The echocardiographic imaging of blood and myocardium is based on their different acoustic properties: muscle tissue is reflective and imaged in shades of gray, while ultrasound easily propagates through blood, resulting in the LV cavity appearing dark. Their interface is the endocardial

TABLE 28-1

CALCULATION OF CARDIOPULMONARY PRESSURES

■ PRESSURE	■ EQUATION
RVSP or PASP	$= 4(V_{TR}^2) + RAP$
PAMP	$= 4(V_{early\ PI})^2 + RAP$
PADP	$= 4(V_{late\ PI})^2 + RAP$
LAP	$= SBP-4(V_{MR})^2$
LVEDP	$= DBP-4(V_{AI\ end})^2$

RVSP, right ventricular systolic pressure; PASP, pulmonary artery systolic pressure; v, peak velocity; TR, tricuspid regurgitation; RAP, right atrial pressure; PAMP, pulmonary artery mean pressure; PI, pulmonic valve insufficiency; PADP, pulmonary artery diastolic pressure; LAP, left atrial pressure; SBP, systolic blood pressure; MR, mitral regurgitation; LVEDP, left ventricular end-diastolic pressure; DBP, diastolic blood pressure; AI, aortic insufficiency.

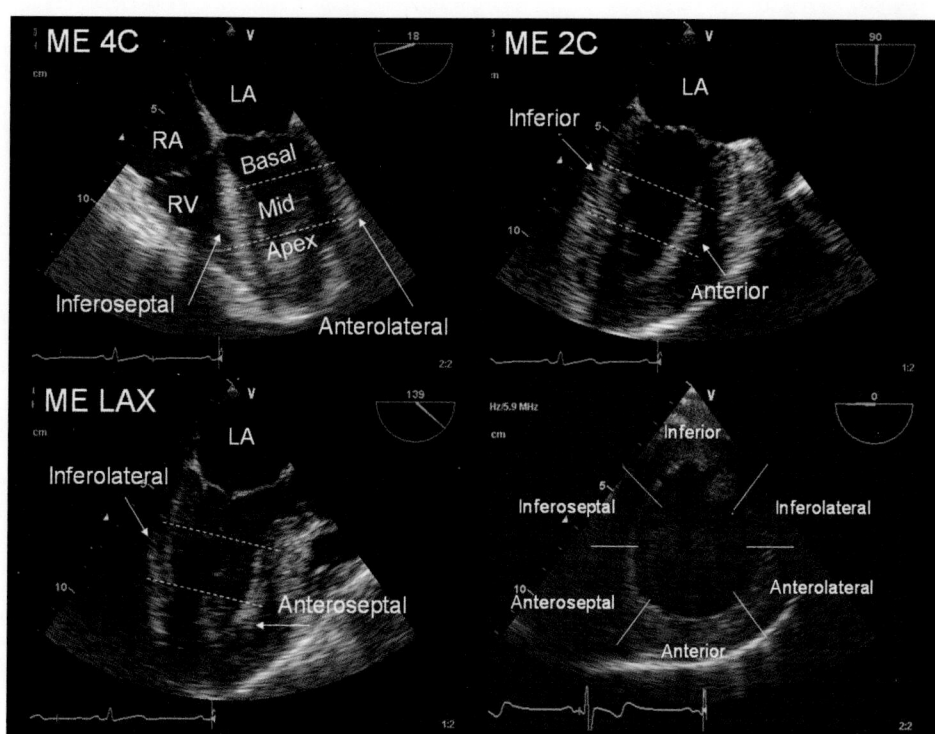

FIGURE 28-34. Left ventricular (LV) walls. In the esophagus, the transesophageal echocardiography (TEE) probe is rotated clockwise from 0 to 140 degrees to obtain the midesophageal (ME) views. Advancement of the TEE probe inside the stomach obtains the transgastric (TG) midpapillary short axis view. In the ME views, the LV is divided in basal, mid, and apical segments. 4C, four-chamber; 2C, two-chamber; LA, left atrium; RA, right atrium; RV, right ventricle. Note that the walls labeled "inferolateral" in this figure are referred to in the text as "posterior." These two terms are used interchangeably in many centers, but a recent consensus publication selected "posterior" as the official name.[43]

surface, which typically produces the brightest signal. The evaluation focuses on the shape, size, and motion of LV walls.

Shape.   The LV's longitudinal shape is evaluated in the midesophageal views (Fig. 28-34). It appears bullet-shaped with the mitral annulus and leaflets comprising its broad base, and the walls tapering toward its apex. In the midesophageal view at 0 degrees rotation (midesophageal four-chamber, midesophageal five-chamber) the lateral wall of the LV appears on the right of the TEE monitor screen and the septal wall on the left. Clockwise rotation of the TEE probe to about 90 degrees (midesophageal two-chamber) will image the long axis of the LV anterior and inferior walls presented on the right and left sides of the monitor, respectively. Further rotation to approximately 135 degrees will image the LV anteroseptal and posterior walls on the right and left sides of the screen.

The echocardiographer must be careful to image the LV along the true long axis in the midesophageal views. Often the imaging plane may cut obliquely in an anterior direction, which causes an increase in the wall thickness and foreshortens the LV cavity. This is avoided by confirming that the LV axis in each view approximates that of the longest LV axis obtained (as measured from the mitral annular plane to the apex, typically from the midesophageal two-chamber view). In many cases slight retroflection or imaging plane rotation from the 0 degree plane is helpful to achieve the best alignment. The LV walls are divided into three segments each—basal, mid, and apical—as defined by lines drawn perpendicular to the LV long axis at the tips and base of the papillary muscles.

From the transgastric position, the LV is seen along its short axis, and its shape resembles a doughnut. The basal segments are imaged in short axis with the TEE probe in the distal esophagus or very high up inside the stomach. At this depth, the mitral leaflets (base of heart) are seen "enface." Gradual advancement of the TEE probe into the stomach images the mid LV segments. Here, the anatomic landmark is the body of the papillary muscles at 2 o'clock (posteromedial) and 5 o'clock (anterolateral). Further advancement of the TEE probe will image the LV apex, much thicker and with smaller

cavity. In either midesophageal or transgastric imaging planes, the LV walls thicken in systole and thin in diastole. As seen in the midesophageal views, the LV base descends toward the LV apex and ascends at diastole.

Aneurysms.   Aneurysms appear as a dilated part of the LV perimeter with thinned wall(s) and decreased motion. Aneurysms are always pathologic and usually due to ischemia-related necrosis and weakening of the LV wall. Aneurysms are separated into true and false. If all myocardial layers (epi-, mid-, and endocardium) are present in the wall of the aneurysm, it is called a *true aneurysm*. The "neck" of a true aneurysm is usually wide, and the aneurysmal cavity shallow with a smooth transition from normal to aneurysmal walls. An aneurysm is called *false* or "pseudo" if the LV wall contains only some of the myocardial layers (usually the epicardium and part of the midwall). False aneurysms are caused by necrosis of the LV wall, usually from myocardial infarction. Sometimes, the wall of a false aneurysm consists only of the attached pericardium. False aneurysms have a narrower neck and the transition between healthy and diseased wall segments is abrupt. A false aneurysm is prone to rupture and is treated surgically. Blood flow is sluggish within aneurysms. Red blood cells clump together, which increases echogenicity and creates spontaneous echocardiography contrast, a smokelike appearance inside the LV cavity. Thrombus, appearing with brightness similar to that of myocardium but clearly separated from the LV wall, can also develop in aneurysms.

Texture.   The *texture* of the LV walls may offer additional information in patients with infiltrative cardiomyopathies, such as amyloid, where the thickened myocardium has a speckled appearance.

Wall Thickness.   LV hypertrophy is termed *concentric* if the cavity is not increased (usually resulting from increased pressure work) and *eccentric* when there is LV dilation (usually resulting from increased volume work). The diagnosis is made by summing the end-diastolic (ED) wall thickness of the

FIGURE 28-35. Two-dimensional evaluation of left ventricular (LV) global and regional function. Regional and global evaluation of the LV using the transgastric short axis view at the midpapillary level. Measurements are performed at end-diastole (ED) and end-systole (ES). **Top panels:** Measurement of diameters (D), areas (A), and wall thickness. Wall thickness is measured at ED in the anteroseptal and inferolateral wall segments. **Bottom panel:** Diameter and wall thickness measured using method mode with the cursor crossing the middle of inferior (top) and anterior (bottom) segments. The percent change of wall thickness of the midanterior wall segment can be used to grade its regional function. In this example, wall motion score (WMS) is 1 (normal) because the segment thickens >30%.

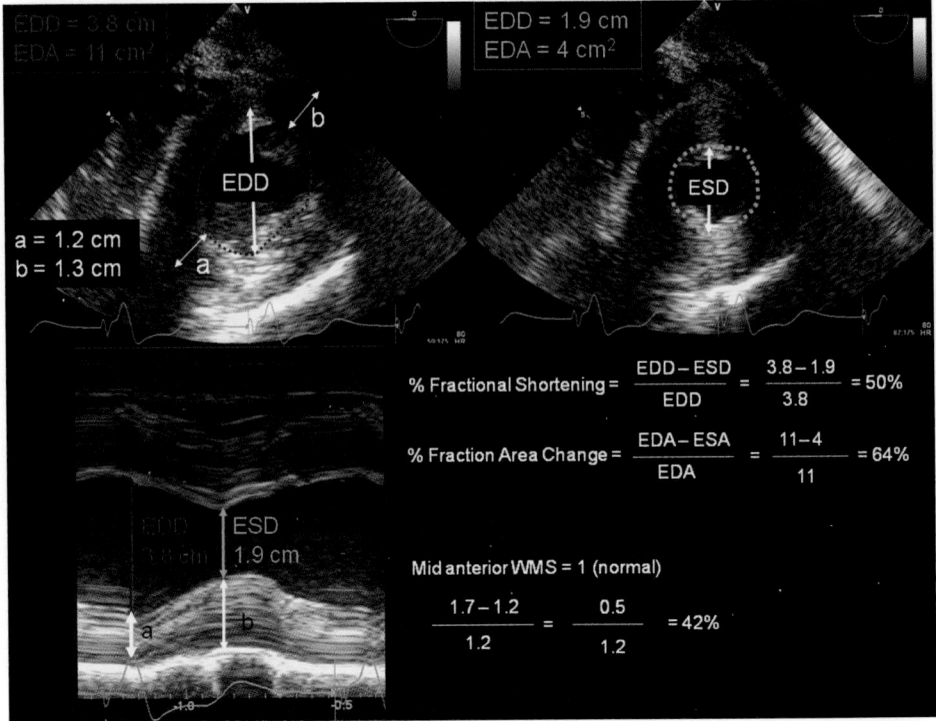

$$\% \text{ Fractional Shortening} = \frac{EDD - ESD}{EDD} = \frac{3.8 - 1.9}{3.8} = 50\%$$

$$\% \text{ Fraction Area Change} = \frac{EDA - ESA}{EDA} = \frac{11 - 4}{11} = 64\%$$

Mid anterior WMS = 1 (normal)

$$\frac{1.7 - 1.2}{1.2} = \frac{0.5}{1.2} = 42\%$$

anteroseptal and posterior LV segments in the basal transgastric short axis view, just at the tips of the papillary muscles (Fig. 28-35). Normal values are 18 ± 2 mm (men) and 15.5 ± 1.5 mm (women).

Segments and Regional Function. Abnormal myocardial wall thickening is a sensitive marker of myocardial ischemia that appears earlier than electrocardiographic and hemodynamic changes.[37–39] Regional LV systolic function reflects the regional myocardial blood flow.[40] The association of the regional LV wall motion with the underlying coronary artery distribution is used to diagnose local perfusion defects. The LV is divided in 17 regional segments[41] (Fig. 28-34). Along the longitudinal plane each wall is divided into basal, mid, and apical levels. The basal and mid levels are further divided into anterior, inferior, two septal (anteroseptal and inferoseptal), and two lateral (anterolateral and posterior) segments. The apical level is divided into four segments (anterior, inferior, septal, and lateral) and the apical cap is the seventeenth segment. To limit misdiagnosis, evaluation of each segment is done in at least two different views, ensuring that both endocardium and epicardium are visible. A midesophageal or transgastric view is digitally stored and played over time. The segmental (or regional) function is evaluated by noticing the presence or absence of endocardial excursion (toward the LV cavity) and degree of systolic wall thickening during one or two consecutive cardiac cycles (Fig. 28-35). The electrocardiogram is used to define systole and diastole. The function of each wall segment is scored as shown in Table 28-2.[42] The wall motion score index is the sum of all scores divided by the number of segments evaluated. The evaluation of segmental wall motion to detect ischemia is not error-free. In addition to being a subjective assessment, wall motion may be affected by tethering, regional loading conditions, and stunning.[43] Epicardial pacing of the free wall of the right ventricle (as in post-bypass period) produces a left bundle block and induces septal wall motion abnormalities. Interobserver reproducibility is better for normally contracting segments than for dysfunctional segments.[44] Because of these issues, wall thickening is a more reliable marker of regional function.

Left Ventricular Cavity

Diameters. The LV cavity is defined by its long and short axes. The LV major (or long) axis dimension is measured in the midesophageal views, from the base of the mitral annulus to the LV apex (Fig. 28-36) while the minor (or short) axis

TABLE 28-2

GRADING OF WALL FUNCTION

REGIONAL FUNCTION	GRADE	INWARD RADIAL MOTION (SYSTOLIC WALL THICKENING)
Normal	1	>30% (marked)
Hypokinetic	2	>10% to <30% (reduced)
Akinetic	3	<10% (negligible)
Dyskinetic	4	Paradoxical systolic motion (systolic thinning)
Aneurysmal	5	Diastolic deformation

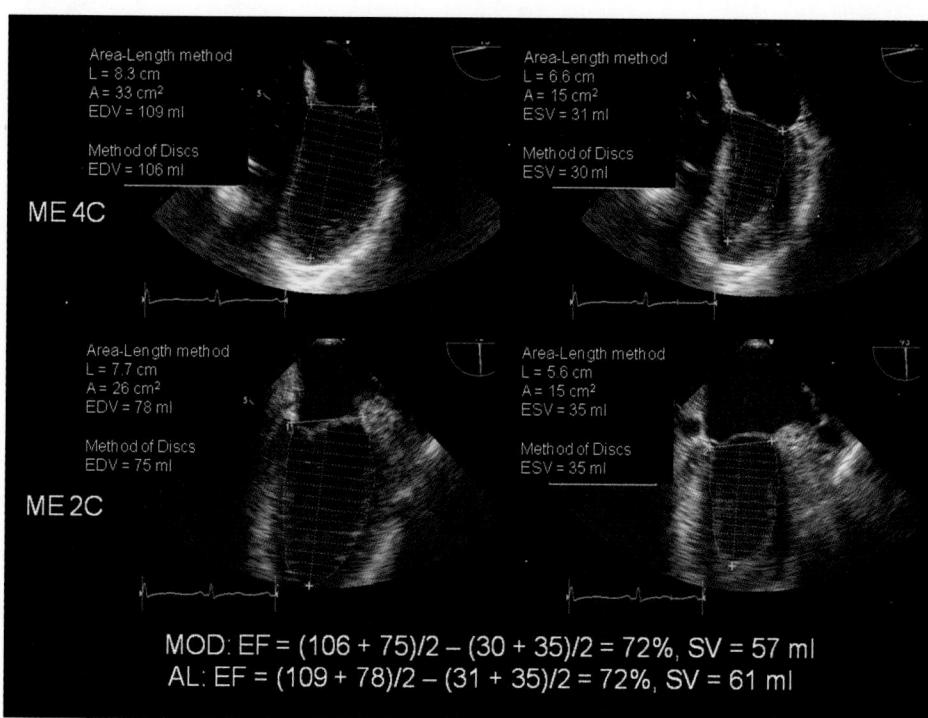

FIGURE 28-36. Quantitation of left ventricular (LV) systolic function. The midesophageal (ME) LV four-chamber (ME 4C) and two-chamber (ME 2C) views are obtained. The images are examined in end-diastole (ED) and end-systole (ES). The LV endocardium is traced. This automatically defines the LV area (A) and long axis (L). The system software will calculate LV volumes using either the method of discs (MOD) or the area-plane method (AL). EF, ejection fraction; EDV, end-diastolic volume, ESV, end-systolic volume SV, stroke volume.

dimension is measured in either the midesophageal or transgastric views, perpendicular to the long axis, at the height of the papillary muscle tips. The minor axis is equal to one half of the long axis measurement. Proper measurement of the LV minor axis is used to quantify the LV ED volume. Normal LV ED dimensions (EDDs) are 4.2 to 5.9 cm (men) and 3.9 to 5.3 cm (women). An increased LV EDD denotes LV dilation and volume overload, while a decreased LV EDD denotes hypovolemia and inadequate preload.

Global Systolic Function. This factor is responsible for delivering a sufficient amount of blood to the vessels at a high enough pressure to perfuse the tissues adequately. A variety of echocardiographic measurements are used to evaluate the components (preload, afterload, and contractility), which collectively define LV global systolic function. The techniques for LV evaluation are described in detail in references 45 and 46.

Percent Fractional Shortening (%FS). FS measures the relative change of the LV short axis diameter between ED and end-systole (ES; Fig. 28-35). FS is a one-dimensional, unitless measurement of systolic function. Measurements are done in the transgastric midpapillary short axis view, just above the papillary muscles. A larger number occurs when the LV has normal or increased systolic function. FS is not a substitute for ejection fraction (EF) and may overestimate systolic function if there is LV dilation or abnormal wall motion at another level. %FS = (LV EDD – LV ESD)/LV EDD and is normally 27 to 45%.

Volumes. LV volume measurements are used to calculate preload (ED volume [EDV]) as well as stroke volume (SV) and EF. The ED and ES LV volumes can be derived from manually tracing of the endocardial border in ED and ES, respectively.

LV volume is commonly measured using the modified Simpson or the area length method. The modified Simpson (or disc summation) method conceives a series of disks inside the LV cavity, which have equal thickness and are stacked like coins along the LV long axis dimension (Fig. 28-36). The diameter of each disk is defined by the short axis dimension from the LV endocardium tracing. Measurements are per-

formed in the midesophageal four- and two-chamber views. Alternatively, the area length method can be used to calculate LV volume: LV volume = 5/6 × [(area) × (length)]. This approach is performed in one of the previous views and calculates the LV volume using the endocardial-enclosed area and the LV major axis (Fig. 28-36). In most adults, an ED area <12 cm² indicates hypovolemia.[47] Reliable and correct visualization of the endocardial border is paramount for accurate measurement of LV volumes with either method. The methods underestimate LV volume when the LV cavity is "foreshortened."

Percent Fractional Area Change (FAC). FAC is the percent difference between ED and ES LV area (Fig. 28-35). The LV area is measured by manually tracing the endocardial border in the transgastric midpapillary short axis view in ED and in ES. The papillary muscles are not traced. Unlike LVEF measurements, FAC does not take into account the presence of wall motion abnormalities at a different level; for example, the function of the LV apex, which is frequently involved in coronary artery disease. Therefore, caution is advised when interpreting FAC. Normal values are 56 to 65%.[48]

Visual Estimation of FAC. The most frequently used technique to evaluate global LV function as well as preload is visual estimation of FAC, often referred to as the *eyeball* EF. Although highly subjective, it is practiced widely and is accurate in experienced echocardiographers, especially in normally contracting ventricles.[49] With LV dysfunction, visual evaluations of FAC become less reproducible among different observers.[50]

Ejection Fraction. EF is the most frequently used estimate of LV systolic function. The evaluation of EF provides prognostic information about mortality and morbidity.[51] EF and stroke volume are affected by factors such as preload, afterload, and heart rate, and thus are not always indicators of intrinsic systolic function. Typical clinical scenarios in which EF does not represent LV systolic function include the hypercontractile LV in mitral regurgitation (where more than half of ED volume may regurgitate inside the left atrium) or the hypocontractile LV in aortic stenosis (where LV systolic performance is poor despite preserved contractility).

Stroke Volume. Stroke volume is calculated as the difference between EDV and ESV, and percent EF is calculated as %EF = SV/EDV × 100 = (EDV − ESV)/EDV × 100. Normal values are EDV, 67 to 155 mL (men), 56 to 104 mL (women); ESV, 22 to 58 mL (men) and 19 to 49 mL (women); %EF, >55%.

Associated Findings. Sluggish flow will clump together red blood cells, producing spontaneous echocardiography contrast, which is imaged as "smoke." Thrombus is also found if there is blood stasis, such as inside an aneurysm or at the LV apex. These findings are often present when LV function is depressed.

Tissue Echocardiography—Myocardial Velocity. Tissue Doppler Imaging (TDI) measures the velocity of myocardial motion along the longitudinal axis and is a sensitive measurement of regional and global function and outcome.[52] The myocardial velocity is measured from the basal LV segments with the sample volume placed next to the mitral annulus. The velocities are comprised of a systolic (S') followed by, in the opposite direction, two diastolic waves, one early (E') and one following atrial contraction (A'). A reduced, or delayed S' velocity is associated with development of regional ischemia (Fig. 28-37).[53]

❹ EVALUATION OF LEFT VENTRICULAR DIASTOLIC FUNCTION

An increased recognition of the impact of LV diastolic function on cardiac function and outcome has driven efforts to both monitor and optimize diastolic performance in the perioperative period. Echocardiographic studies have suggested that patients with diastolic dysfunction presenting for cardiac surgery may be prone to intraoperative hemodynamic instability and worse outcomes.[54] The readmission and mortality rate in patients with diastolic heart failure are similar to those observed in systolic heart failure patients.[55] Doppler echocardiography is the preferred technique to assess diastolic performance and grade the severity of the disease process.

Diastolic dysfunction is defined as the inability of the LV to fill at normal left atrial (LA) pressures and is characterized by a decrease in relaxation and/or LV compliance. Diastolic dysfunction may be present in the absence of clinical symptoms of heart failure. When these symptoms occur in the presence of diastolic dysfunction, then the diagnosis of diastolic heart failure is made.

Diastolic Physiology

Traditionally, the cardiac cycle has been divided into two phases: systole, comprising isovolumic contraction and ejection, and diastole, comprising isovolumic relaxation, rapid filling, diastasis, and atrial contraction. Rather than a passive phase of the cardiac cycle when filling of the heart occurs, diastole is currently regarded as being intimately coupled and interdependent with systole. In this respect, Nishimura and Tajik[56] have proposed dividing the cardiac cycle into three phases: contraction, relaxation, and filling. Contraction encompasses the isovolumic contraction and the first half of ejection. The critical insight into the proposal of Nishimura and Tajik is that relaxation begins during the second part of *ejection*, and then continues during the isovolumic relaxation and rapid filling phases, illustrating the interdependency of systole and diastole. The filling phase consists of the early rapid filling phase, diastasis, and atrial contraction. The early filling phase coincides with and depends on the continuation of relaxation.

Ventricular filling is affected by load factors (preload and afterload) as well as mechanical factors such as ventricular relaxation and compliance, ventricular contraction, atrial contraction and MV dynamics, viscoelastic forces of the myocardium, and pericardial restraint.

The early manifestation of diastolic dysfunction is characterized by an impaired relaxation, implying that the rate and duration of decrease in LV pressure after systolic contraction is prolonged. This results in an inability of the LV to fill

FIGURE 28-37. Tissue Doppler imaging. Myocardial velocity of basal anterolateral segment of left ventricle is measured with pulsed wave tissue Doppler. ME, midesophageal; S', systolic velocity; E', early diastolic velocity; A', late diastolic velocity.

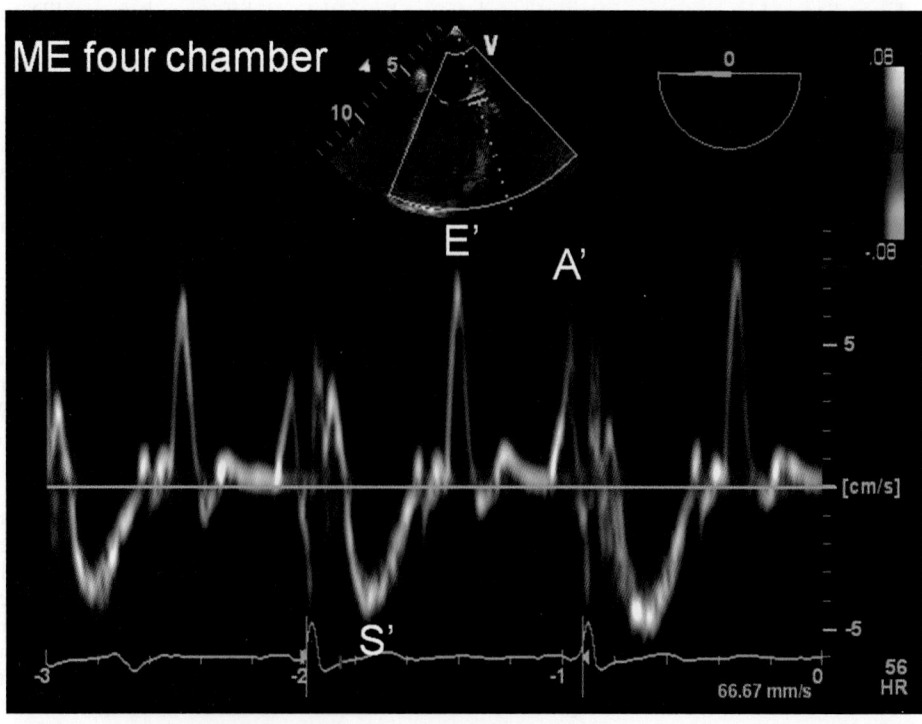

adequately during the rapid filling phase. A compensatory increase in filling occurs with atrial contraction. This stage of disease is known as *grade I diastolic dysfunction*. In more advanced stages of disease, grades II and III of diastolic dysfunction, a decrease in LV compliance ensues. Compliance is defined as a change of volume in respect to a change in pressure. Thus, a decrease in LV compliance will lead to a disproportionate increase in LV pressures and, ultimately, LA pressures.

Echocardiographic Assessment of Left Ventricular Diastolic Function

Echocardiography has become the diagnostic modality of choice for patients with diastolic dysfunction. Echocardiographic assessments have been validated by cardiac catheterization and correlate with clinical presentation.[57] A combination of different echocardiographic modalities is used to diagnosis diastolic dysfunction. These modalities are represented by 2-D echocardiography, pulsed-wave Doppler, M-mode color Doppler, and tissue Doppler. This section is limited to discussion of the two most commonly used methods: pulsed-wave Doppler of transmitral and pulmonary vein flows and TDI.

Imaging Views and Techniques.

The echocardiographic acquisition of the diastolic parameters is best done when integrated in a standard examination. The typical view used for both transmitral flow Doppler (TMF) as well as for the tissue Doppler imaging (TDI) is the midesophageal four-chamber view. Interrogation of the PV is usually performed in the midesophageal commissural or midesophageal two-chamber views. The interrogation volume sample should be placed at the tips of the MV for TMF assessment and 1 to 2 cm inside

the PV for the pulmonary vein flow (PVF) assessment. For TDI of myocardial velocity profiles, the sample volume is typically placed at the junction of the mitral annulus and the lateral wall.

Interpretation of Pulsed-Wave Doppler Flow Velocity Curves.

Relaxation, the active phase of diastole, commences with the dissociation of actin-myosin cross-bridges and a lowering of the intracellular calcium. LV pressure begins to fall and eventually becomes lower than ascending aortic pressure, resulting in closure of the AV. As the ventricle continues to relax, the LV pressure falls below LA pressure, reaching its nadir, and promotes opening of the MV. At this point, the pressure gradient between the LA and LV is maximal and early rapid filling phase of the LV occurs. This phase is responsible for 80 to 90% of LV filling. As the ventricle fills, the LV pressure gradually rises and equates the pressure in the LA; thus, minimal flow or diastasis occurs. With commencement of the atrial contraction phase, the pressure gradient between the LA and LV rises once again and blood flows from the LA to the LV. At the end of the LA systole, the pressure in the LV rises above the LA pressure and promotes closure of the MV (Fig. 28-38).

Doppler assessment of the TMF and PVF velocity reflects the instantaneous pressure gradient (see previous discussion of Bernoulli principle). Therefore, the displayed velocity waveforms parallel the changes in pressure gradient occurring in the left heart. The TMF profile consists of two waves, the "E" and "A" waves. The peak E wave represents the peak early filling velocity. The rate of decrease of velocity following the peak E velocity is known as the *deceleration time* (DT). The DT depends on how fast the pressure rises in LV during the rapid filling phase and represents a direct measure of ventricular compliance. Thus, if the ventricular compliance decreases, the

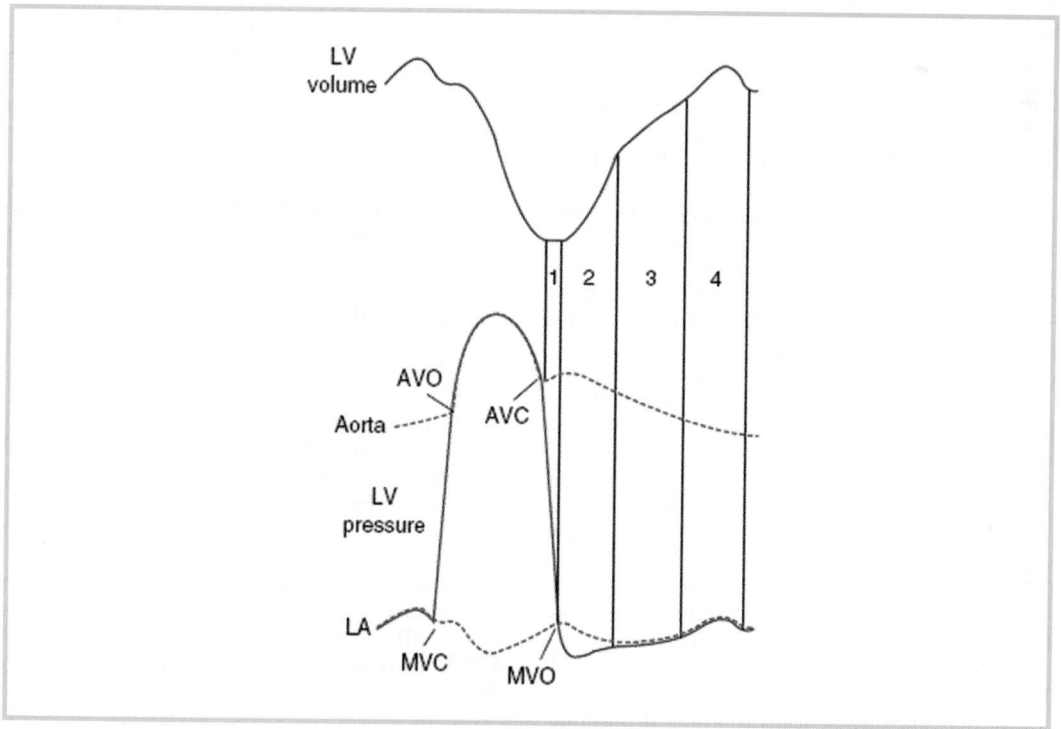

FIGURE 28-38. Diastolic phase of the cardiac cycle. During isovolumic relaxation (1) left ventricular (LV) pressure falls rapidly following aortic valve closure (AVC). When LV pressure decreases below left atrial (LA) pressure, the mitral valve opens (MVO), initiating early, rapid LV filling (2). Equilibration of LV and LA pressures results in diminished transmitral flow during diastasis (3) until atrial contraction (4). Diastole terminates with mitral valve closure (MVC). (Reproduced from Plotnick GD: Changes in diastolic function—difficult to measure, harder to interpret. Am Heart J 1989; 118: 637, with permission.)

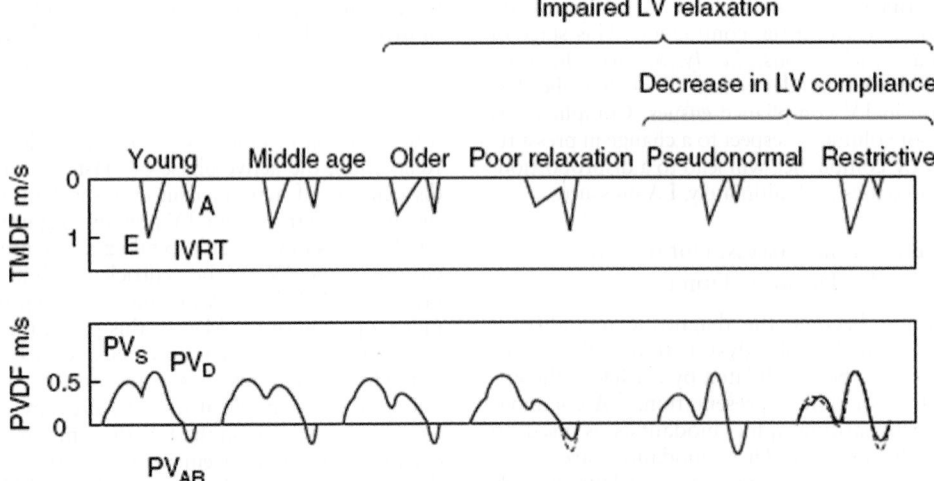

FIGURE 28-39. The impact of progressive left ventricular (LV) diastolic dysfunction on transmitral Doppler flow (TMDF) and pulmonary venous Doppler flow (PVDF). The transmitral pressure gradient is initially elevated in normal, young individuals because of vigorous LV relaxation and elastic recoil, before diminishing when relaxation becomes impaired and finally increasing again when left atrial pressure increases from an elevated LV end-diastolic pressure in the restrictive pattern of LV diastolic dysfunction. Respective changes are noted in pulmonary vein (PV) profile. E, E-wave; A, A-wave; IVRT, left ventricular isovolumic relaxation time; PV_{AR}, late diastolic retrograde velocity; PV_{S1}, first systolic component; PV_{S2}, second systolic component; PV_D, diastolic component.

DT shortens. The peak A wave represents the peak blood velocity during atrial contraction. In a normal individual the E wave is slightly larger than the A wave and the DT is 200 ± 40 msec (Fig. 28-39).

Similar events take place in the LA. Ventricular contraction lowers the MV annulus creating a suction effect and promoting blood flow from the PVs to the LA. Filling of the LA decreases the pressure gradient between the PVs and LA and blood flow plateaus. As the MV opens, an open conduit forms between the PVs, LA, and LV; thus, additional forward flow to the LA occurs. Subsequently, atrial contraction raises LA pressure above PV pressure and promotes backward blood flow into them. A normal PVF velocity curve consists of systolic forward flow representing the "S" wave, diastolic forward flow representing the "D" wave, and a reversal of velocity during atrial contraction representing the "a" wave (Fig. 28-36).

As diastolic dysfunction develops, the patterns of the flow velocity curves change in concordance with the pressure gradient changes in the PV-LA-LV system. In grade I diastolic dysfunction, as the LV is incompletely relaxed when early ventricular filling occurs, the pressure gradient, and thus E wave velocity, is less than normal. The delayed relaxation prolongs LV filling late into diastole, and therefore the DT is prolonged. A compensatory increase in TMF during atrial contraction, due to the higher residual atrial preload, generates a high A wave velocity. Thus, the TMF curve of an individual with abnormal relaxation is represented by a low E, high A, and prolonged DT. The increased residual atrial preload generates a smaller pressure gradient between the PVs and LA; thus, less flow to the LA occurs during the early filling phase. This is represented on the PVF curves as a higher S/D ratio as compared to normal (Fig. 28-39).

Progression of diastolic disease leads to grade II diastolic dysfunction, which is marked by decreases in LV compliance. LA pressure rises as a compensatory mechanism to normalize the pressure gradient across the MV. In this scenario, the TMF velocities resemble the normal curve; thus, this stage is known as *pseudonormal*. Because of the high LA pressure, less flow from the PVs occurs during ventricular systole, generating a lower S wave on the PVF curves, and thus a lower S/D ratio.

During atrial contraction a larger amount of blood is pushed back in the PVs, represented by a deeper a wave (Fig. 28-39).

Grade III diastolic dysfunction, known as the *restrictive phase*, is characterized by a significantly decreased LV compliance. The high LA-LV pressure gradient produces a fast acceleration of blood flow in the LV. This is represented by a high E velocity on the TMF curve. LV pressure increases rapidly during filling because of the increased LV stiffness resulting in a short DT. The forward filling velocity at atrial contraction is low (small A wave) because of the decreased compliance. The elevated LA pressures inhibit blood flow from the PVs to the LA during ventricular systole, and the PVF curves show a decreased S/D ratio (Fig. 28-39). One of the important caveats to assessing diastolic function using pulsed-wave Doppler is that the flow patterns depend on pressure gradients and therefore are affected by both preload and afterload. In settings in which the load conditions vary at a fast pace, such as the OR, changes in TMF or PVF velocities may be difficult to interpret. TDI, which directly measures myocardial velocities, provides a more load-independent method of diastolic function assessment.[58]

The normal mitral annular TDI profile has a biphasic diastolic component: the early diastolic wave E' related to the early filling and the late diastolic wave A' related to atrial contraction (Fig. 28-37). In a healthy patient, the TDI pattern mirrors the TMF pattern, except with lower velocities. E' reflects LV relaxation and values <8 cm/s are considered a sign of diastolic dysfunction.[59] Thus, in patients with pseudonormal or restrictive disease, in whom normal or elevated E wave TMF velocities occur despite advanced pathology, the TDI E' wave remains reduced, making it a useful approach to diagnosis.

Pericardial Disease: Constrictive Pericarditis and Pericardial Tamponade

Diastolic filling is also impacted by pericardial restraint. Pericardial pathologies, such as constrictive pericarditis or pericardial tamponade, impede diastolic flow.[60] On TMF Doppler profiles these diseases resemble the diastolic restrictive filling

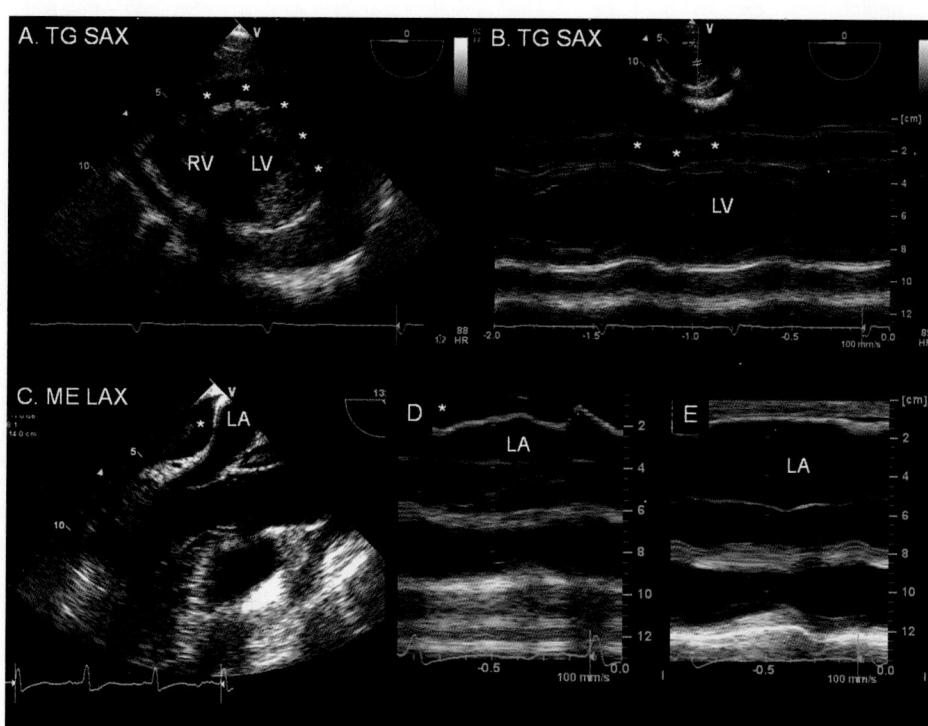

FIGURE 28-40. Echocardiographic findings in pericardial effusion. **A.** Global pericardial effusion (asterisks) surrounding both right ventricle (RV) and left ventricle (LV). Transgastric short axis (TG SAX) view. **B.** M-mode echocardiography demonstrates separation of the epicardium from the pericardium (asterisks) from pericardial effusion. **C.** Regional pericardial effusion (asterisks) compressing the left atrium (LA), seen in the midesophageal long axis (ME LAX) view. **D.** M-mode echocardiography reveals systolic compression (asterisk) of LA. **E.** After evacuation of the fluid collection, the LA size increases.

pattern. Two-dimensional echocardiography can be helpful in differentiating among these pathologies. In constrictive pericarditis the pericardium appears thick, fibrotic, calcified, and thus echogenic; the inferior vena cava is dilated and the ventricular septum has an abnormal motion.

Pericardial effusions can be global, surrounding the entire heart, or loculated, as seen mostly after cardiac surgery (Fig. 28-40). Because the intrapericardial volume is constant, cardiac chambers are compressed when at their lowest pressure (atria in systole, ventricles in diastole). Pericardial tamponade is characterized by the presence of a large pericardial effusion seen as an echo-free (black) space, a "swinging motion" of the heart, early diastolic RV collapse, and late diastolic right atrium (RA) collapse.

In summary, diastolic filling is an active process and a major component of effective cardiac performance. The presence of diastolic dysfunction, whether resulting from loss in fluid volume, LV disease, or pericardial restraint, is associated with potential deleterious surgical outcomes. Doppler echocardiography, in particular TDI, provides the anesthesiologist the means to rapidly diagnose and guide therapy of such patients in the perioperative period.

❺ EVALUATION OF VALVULAR HEART DISEASE

Two-dimensional echocardiography and Doppler are complementary methods in valve assessment. The 2-D echocardiography provides evaluation of valve anatomy and function and Doppler assesses the physiologic consequences and severity of the lesion.

Aortic Stenosis

Two-Dimensional and M-Mode Echocardiography. The normal aortic valve (AV) has three cusps, which open without restriction in systole, yielding an AV area 3 to 4 cm². The appearance of the valve and the systolic excursion of its cusps are imaged with 2-D and M-mode echocardiography. The AV is imaged enface in the midesophageal aortic valve short axis

view and its profile in the midesophageal aortic valve long axis view (Figs. 28-10, 28-11). With the TEE probe inside the stomach, the AV is imaged in the deep transgastric long axis and transgastric long axis views (Figs. 28-21, 28-22). Owing to the increased afterload, associated findings include concentric hypertrophy of the LV, decreased EF, as well as mitral regurgitation and left atrial dilatation.

Doppler Echocardiography. *Jet Velocity, Transvalvular Pressure Gradient.* The transvalvular pressure gradient can be calculated from the CWD measured velocity (V) using the modified Bernoulli equation: $\Delta P = 4 \times V^2$. The mean gradient, calculated from the VTI tracing is commonly reported as it correlates well with the angiographically determined pressure gradient.[61] However, for any given valve area, the flow velocity and pressure gradient vary with changes in stroke volume and cardiac output. An LV with normal function will generate a large pressure gradient across a critically stenosed AV, and a dysfunctional LV will not.[62]

Valve Area. Using the continuity equation, flow across the left ventricular outflow tract (LVOT) equals flow across the stenosed AV or $VTI_{LVOT} \times Area_{LVOT} = VTI_{AV} \times Area_{AV}$. By rearranging the equation, $Area_{AV} = (VTI_{LVOT} \times Area_{LVOT})/(VTI_{AV})$. The $area_{LVOT}$ is calculated using the LVOT diameter at the site of the Doppler measurement (Fig. 28-33). An error in the LVOT diameter measurement is geometrically increased as $Area_{LVOT} = \pi \times (D/2)^2$. The VTI_{LVOT}/VTI_{AV} ratio is often calculated to avoid this error as flow changes will be reflected proportionally across both the AV and LVOT (Doppler dimensionless index). An index value <0.25% indicates an AV area <0.75 cm². The echocardiographic cut-off values for grading aortic stenosis are shown in Table 28-3.[63]

❻ Mitral Stenosis

Two-Dimensional Echocardiography. The MV is imaged in the midesophageal views and in the basal transgastric short axis views. The leaflets can appear thickened and calcified (thus, strongly echogenic), while there may be fusion of the

TABLE 28-3

GRADING OF AORTIC STENOSIS

	■ Normal AV	■ Mild	■ Moderate	■ Severe
Peak AV velocity (m/s)	<1.7	<3.0	3.0–4.0	>4.0
Peak transvalvular gradient (mm Hg)		<36	36–64	>64
Mean transvalvular gradient (mm Hg)		<25	25–40	>40
AVA (cm²)	>2.5	1.5–2.5	1.0–1.5	<1.0

AV, aortic valve; AVA, AV area.

chordae and papillary muscles. The major and most striking finding in mitral stenosis (MS) is the inability of the two mitral leaflets to separate from each other in diastole. Instead, their tips remain opposed while the body of the leaflets bows toward the LV cavity because of the incoming blood (Fig. 28-41). The area of the MV orifice can be traced by planimetry in the transgastric basal short axis view.[64] Associated findings in MS are a dilated left atrium and left atrial appendage (because of increased pressure), and presence of thrombus or spontaneous echocardiographic contrast due to low flow in the LA. The LV cavity appears small, with a thickened and immobile interventricular septum. The right ventricle may be dilated and/or hypertrophied, with thickened walls, because of increased pressure work (Fig. 28-41 and Table 28-4).

Doppler Echocardiography. *Transvalvular Pressure Gradient.* The increased diastolic pressure gradient is measured with continuous Doppler in the midesophageal four-chamber or long axis view. The early diastolic velocity of the transmitral flow (E wave) is increased (usually >1.5 m/s). This is not specific to MS, as E velocity will also be elevated in the presence of increased blood flow, as in severe mitral regurgitation.[65] In severe MS, the mean pressure gradient is >10 mm Hg (Fig. 28-42).

Pressure Half-Time (PHT). The deceleration of E velocity is decreased, because in MS the equalization of transmitral valve pressures takes a longer time. PHT is the time required for the peak pressure to decrease to half value. The decaying velocity is traced on the CWD signal across the MV in diastole and the analysis package calculates the PHT. MV area (MVA) is calculated as 220/PHT. A prolonged PHT >220 ms is related to severe MS (calculated MVA <1 cm²) as smaller MV orifices will prolong the pressure decay across the valve.[66] When LV compliance is decreased or there is coexisting aortic regurgitation, the increased LV pressure results in a faster pressure equilibration across the stenosed MV. In such cases, PHT will be shortened, and the calculated MVA may be erroneously overestimated.[67]

Associated Findings. CFD will display a "rising sun" pattern of diastolic velocities inside the LA, indicating the high velocity (and increased pressure gradient) across the stenosed MV that exceeds the limits of the color scale (Fig. 28-42A). Associated

FIGURE 28-41. Two-dimensional echocardiographic findings in mitral stenosis. **A.** In the midesophageal four-chamber (ME 4C) view, echocardiographic signs of mitral stenosis include a dilated left atrium (LA) with a rightward displacement of the interatrial septum (indicating the elevated LA pressure), and a small left ventricle (LV). **B.** In the midesophageal bicaval view, red blood cell clumping creates spontaneous echocardiography contrast. Notice the rightward displacement of the interatrial septum toward the right atrium (RA). **C.** A zoom image of the mitral valve and neighboring structures in midesophageal four-chamber view. The anterior mitral leaflet exhibits diastolic doming while the posterior mitral leaflet is immobile. **D.** In the transgastric midpapillary short axis (TG mid SAX) view, the LV cavity is relatively small, as compared with the right ventricle (RV), and interventricular septum appears thickened.

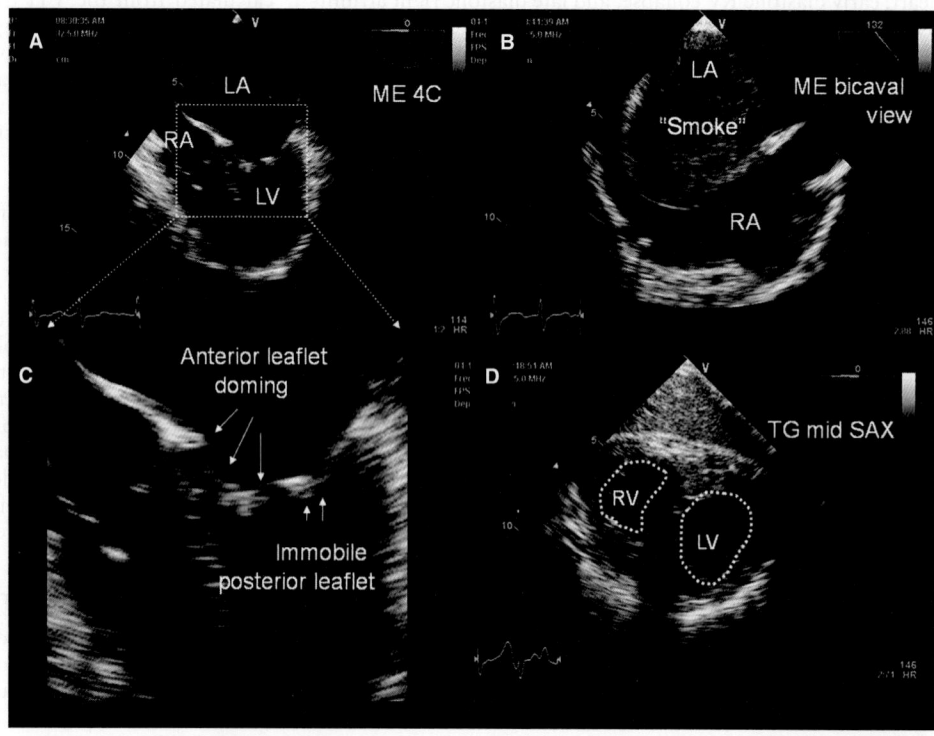

TABLE 28-4

GRADING OF MITRAL STENOSIS

	■ MILD	■ MODERATE	■ SEVERE
Mean pressure gradient (mm Hg)	≤6	6–10	>10
Pressure half time (ms)	≤100	100–220	>220
Mitral valve area (cm²)	1.6–2.0	1.0–1.5	<1.0

findings include pulmonary insufficiency due to pulmonary hypertension and tricuspid regurgitation.

Aortic Regurgitation

Two-Dimensional and M-Mode Echocardiography. The AV is imaged in the same views used for assessment of aortic stenosis. Associated findings may include dilated aortic root (Marfan's syndrome), endocarditis lesions, dilated ascending aorta, calcified AV, aortic dissection (may be associated with acute aortic insufficiency (AI)), fluttering of the anterior mitral leaflet and restricted diastolic opening of the MV from the AI jet, or a dilated LV in chronic AI (Table 28-5).

Doppler Echocardiography. *Color Flow.* In either of the midesophageal or the transgastric views of the AV, a CFD sector over the AV and the LVOT will demonstrate the presence or absence of the AI regurgitant jet. CFD reveals the characteristics of the AI jet as it enters the LVOT in diastole. The following techniques are used to grade the severity of AI:

Ratio of Jet Height to LVOT Diameter. The maximal height of the AI jet (within <1 cm from the AV plane) is compared with the LVOT diameter at the same point. The recommended view is the midesophageal aortic valve long axis view. A central jet usually is caused by aortic root dilation, whereas an eccentric jet implies an AV cusp lesion. The propagation of the jet into the LV does not correlate well with the angiographic degree of AI, and should not be used to grade AI (Fig. 28-29).[68]

Vena Contracta. Vena contracta is the narrowest "neck" of the AI jet as it traverses the AV plane, usually best appreciated in the midesophageal aortic valve long axis view. The largest diameter of the vena contracta in diastole is selected (Fig. 28-29). The size of vena contracta is relatively load-independent and provides a reliable way to quantitate AI intraoperatively, in the presence of fluctuating hemodynamics.[68]

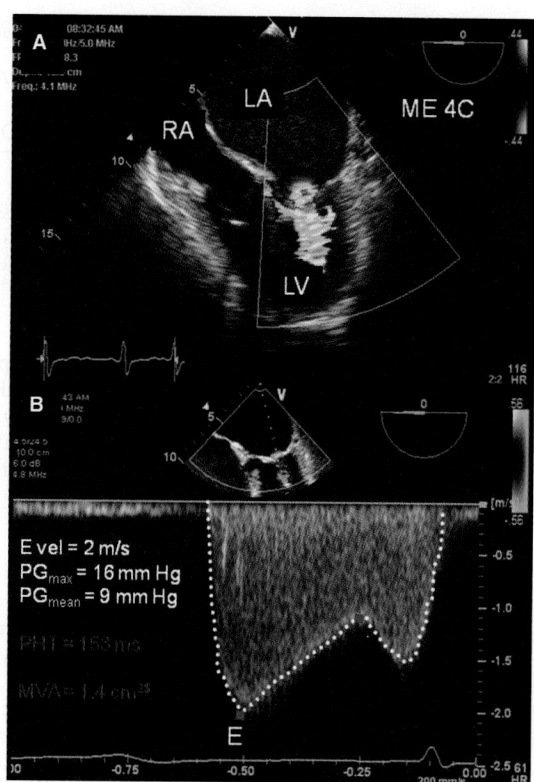

FIGURE 28-42. Doppler echocardiography findings in mitral stenosis. **A.** Diastolic blood acceleration upstream of the mitral valve is seen with color flow Doppler ("rising sun"). **B.** Spectral display of the diastolic velocity decay is imaged with a pulsed wave Doppler sample volume placed at the tips of mitral valve. Tracing of the velocity envelope (*white dots*) calculates the maximum and mean pressure gradient (PG). The pressure half-time (PHT) is calculated from the deceleration of the peak velocity (Evel) (*red dots*). The mitral valve area (MVA) is derived from the empiric formula: MVA = 220/PHT.

Pressure Half-Time. PHT of the AI jet is recorded in the transgastric long axis or deep transgastric long axis view. PHT expresses the pressure equilibration of the diastolic blood pressure ("driving" pressure) and the diastolic LV pressure ("resistance" pressure). A short PHT (<200 ms) is associated with severe AI. Factors associated with decreased LV compliance (e.g., LV failure with restrictive filling pattern) will cause the transaortic pressure gradient to dissipate faster and will overestimate the severity of AI (Fig. 28-28).

Aortic Diastolic Flow Reversal. Retrograde diastolic flow in the descending and abdominal aorta is sensitive and specific for severe AI. This is imaged with PWD in the midesophageal long axis view of the distal descending aorta (Fig. 28-28).[69]

TABLE 28-5

GRADING OF AORTIC INSUFFICIENCY (AI)

	■ TRACE	■ MILD	■ MODERATE	SEVERE
AI jet height/LVOT diameter (%)	<25	25–45	46–64	>65
Vena contracta (mm)	<3	—	—	>6
PHT (ms)	—	>500	200–500	<200
Aortic diastolic flow reversal	—	—	—	Holodiastolic

LVOT, left ventricular outflow tract; PHT, pressure half-time.

ANESTHETIC MANAGEMENT

TABLE 28-6

CARPENTIER CLASSIFICATION OF MITRAL REGURGITATION (MR)

■ CARPENTIER TYPE	■ MOTION LEAFLET	■ JET DIRECTION
1	Normal	Central
2	Excessive (prolapse, flail)	Away from lesion
3a	Restricted, structure is abnormal	Variable
3b	Restricted, structure is normal	

Other Findings. Severe AI rapidly elevates LV diastolic pressure and shortens the early transmitral flow velocity, resulting in a *restrictive LV filling pattern.* The *regurgitant volume* is calculated using the continuity equation and equals the difference between LVOT flow and the diastolic transmitral flow. Values >60 mL are consistent with severe AI.

Mitral Regurgitation

Two-Dimensional Echocardiography. The normal MV anatomy consists of two leaflets (anterior and posterior), their coaptation surface, the fibrous mitral annulus, the subvalvular apparatus with the two papillary muscles (anterolateral and posteromedial), and their chordae tendinae, which attach to the underside of the mitral leaflets. The competency of the MV depends on adequate coaptation between the D-shaped anterior leaflet and the crescent-shaped posterior leaflet. Common causes of mitral regurgitation (MR) are myxomatous valve degeneration, endocarditis, and ischemic, rheumatic and congenital heart disease.

The required TEE views for imaging of the MV include the midesophageal four-chamber, midesophageal commissural, midesophageal two-chamber, midesophageal aortic valve long axis view, and the basal transgastric short axis and two-chamber views (Figs. 28-14 through 28-20).[70] Echocardiographic findings may include any of the following: abnormal texture of leaflets (myxomatous degeneration), flail and/or prolapsing leaflet, ruptured chordae, papillary muscle dysfunction or rupture (secondary to ischemia), mitral annulus calcification, or endocarditis lesions. The leaflet motion is commonly reported using Carpentier's classification as described in Table 28-6.

Doppler Echocardiography. Color Flow Doppler. CFD is commonly used as a screening tool for the detection of MR. It provides an easy, qualitative technique but additional tests are advised to grade the severity of MR (Fig. 28-43). If the MR jet is >40% of the LA area, often times severe MR is present.[71] There are several limitations to this technique. It is difficult to visualize the entire LA with TEE. Secondly, eccentric jets that are in contact with the LA walls are underestimated (Coanda effect).[72] Third, machine settings such as frame rate and color Doppler scale influence the appearance of the MR jet. Fourth, despite its appearance, the color area associated with MR is not equivalent to regurgitant volume. CFD simply shows the area within the LA where blood has abnormal velocity and is dependent on the systolic pressure gradient between the LV (adequate LV systolic function) and the LA (chamber compliance). In acute MR, for example, the MR jet velocities are low because MR occurs in a noncompliant chamber.

Proximal Isovelocity Surface Area. During systole, blood inside the LV cavity accelerates as it converges toward the orifice of the incompetent MV (Fig. 28-30). This velocity pattern resembles concentric hemispheres, whose surfaces have the

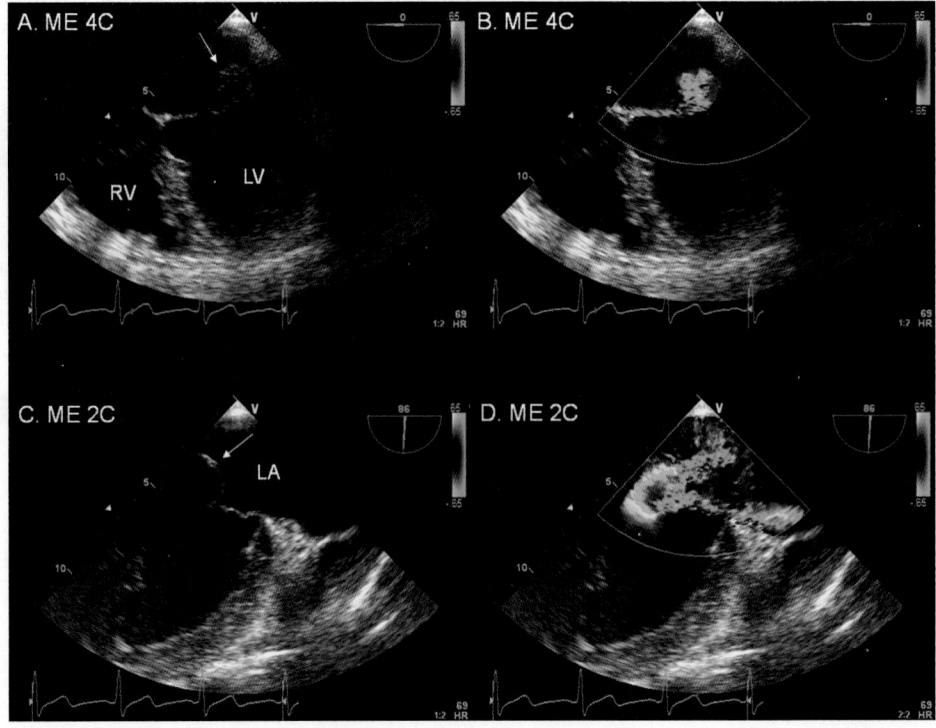

FIGURE 28-43. Mitral regurgitation. The anatomy of mitral valve (MV) is depicted with two-dimensional (**A** and **C**) echocardiographic imaging, and the presence of mitral regurgitation (MR) is imaged with color Doppler (**B** and **D**). The MV is incompetent because of posterior leaflet prolapse inside the left atrium (LA) during systole (arrows left in A and C). Left ventricular (LV) systolic contraction generates and anterior-directed MR jet, away from the MV lesion area. ME 4C, midesophageal four-chamber view; ME 2C, midesophageal two-chamber view.

ANESTHETIC MANAGEMENT

TABLE 28-7

GRADING OF MITRAL REGURGITATION

	■ MILD	■ MODERATE	■ SEVERE
Qualitative findings			
Jet area/LA area	<20%	—	>40%
Density of CW signal	—	—	Dense complete envelope
Pulmonary blood flow	—	S blunted (S/D < 1)	S reversed (S < 0)
Quantitative measurements			
Vena contracta (mm)	<3	3–7	≥7
EROA (cm^2)	<0.20	0.20–0.40	≥0.40
Regurgitant volume (ml)	<30	30–60	≥60
Regurgitant fraction (%)	<30	30–50	≥50

LA, left atrium; CW, continuous wave; S, S wave; S/D, Systolic wave of pulmonary vein flow to diastolic wave of pulmonary vein flow ratio; EROA effective regurgitant orrifice area

same velocity at a given distance (radius, R) from the MV orifice. Such an isovelocity surface is called *proximal isovelocity surface area* (PISA). Its velocity can be determined by the color Doppler system's aliasing velocity.[73] Based on the principle of conservation of mass (continuity equation), the flow through the MR orifice is the same as the flow of the PISA surface:

MR flow = PISA flow,

MR orifice × MR velocity = 2π(R^2) × Aliasing Velocity.

MR orifice = 6.28(R^2) × Aliasing Velocity/MR Velocity.

A simplified PISA equation—yields MR orifice = (PISA radius)^2/2 provided the Nyquist limit is set at 40 cm/s and that the MR jet has a velocity of 5 m/s.[74] Most significantly, a small error in measuring the PISA radius (R^2) will be squared in the equation.

Vena Contracta. Vena contracta is the narrowest part of the MR jet, and reflects the effective or physiologic area of the MR jet (Fig. 28-30). MR is severe if vena contracta is ≥7 mm.

Pulmonary Vein Inflow Pattern. The increased volume inside the LA will augment the transmitral diastolic pressure gradient and will produce a restrictive filling pattern in severe MR (E to A wave ratio >2). For the same reasons, the systolic filling of the LA via the pulmonary veins (S wave) will be decreased, in moderate and severe MR (Table 28-7).

Tricuspid Regurgitation

The tricuspid valve (TV) is evaluated concomitant with the right ventricle, using the midesophageal four-chamber, midesophageal right ventricular inflow-outflow, midesophageal bicaval, and transgastric RV long axis views. The TV plane is slightly higher than the MV plane. Tricuspid regurgitation (TR) is most commonly secondary to pulmonary hypertension from left-sided cardiac pathology, while endocarditis, carcinoid, Ebstein's anomaly, and rheumatic heart disease are less frequent causes of TR.

Two-Dimensional Echocardiography. The TV anatomy is examined for abnormal appearance (annular dilation, endocarditis vegetations, and thrombus) and motion (prolapsing or flailing leaflets). Structures proximal (inferior vena cava, right atrium, and interatrial septum) and distal (right ventricle and interventricular septum) to the TV are examined for signs of volume and pressure overload.

Doppler Echocardiography. CFD is applied to detect the presence, size, and direction of a TR jet, its vena contracta, and the PISA inside the RV. CWD is used to measure the TR jet velocity and calculate the RV and PA systolic pressure. PWD is used to record the hepatic vein flow pattern. Grading of severity of TR is shown in Table 28-8.

TABLE 28-8

GRADING OF TRICUSPID REGURGITATION

■ ECHOCARDIOGRAPHIC PARAMETER	■ MILD		■ SEVERE
TV morphology	Normal		Prolapse, mal-coaptation, endocarditis lesion, mass
IVC/RA/RV size	Normal		Dilated/increased
TR jet area (cm^2)	<5		>10
Vena contracta width (mm) (Nyquist limit 50–60 cm/s)	—	>7	
PISA radius (mm) (Nyquist limit ~28 cm/s)	<6	>9	
TR jet features	Soft, parabolic		Dense, triangular, early peak
Hepatic vein flow pattern	S > D		Systolic wave below baseline

TV, tricuspid valve; IVC, inferior vena cava; RA, right atrium; RV, right ventricle; PISA, proximal isovelocity surface area; TR, tricuspid regurgitation; S, Systolic wave of hepatic view flow; D, diastolic wave of hepatic vein flow.

TABLE 28-9

GRADING OF PULMONARY REGURGITATION

■ PARAMETER	■ MILD	■ SEVERE
PV morphology	Normal	Abnormal
RV size	Normal	Dilated
PR jet size	Length <1 cm, narrow origin	Large, wide origin
PR jet features	Soft, slow deceleration	Dense, rapid deceleration

PV, pulmonary vein; RV, right ventricle; PR, pulmonary regurgitation.

Pulmonic Valve Regurgitation

Pulmonic valve regurgitation (PR) is evaluated in the mid-esophageal right ventricular inflow-outflow, the upper esophageal aortic arch short axis, and in the modified deep transgastric RV views (approximately 60 to 70 degrees). PR is often an incidental finding. PR can develop because of right-sided endocarditis, or secondary to pulmonary hypertension. Grading of severity of PR is described in Table 28-9.

DISEASES OF THE AORTA

The evaluation of the aorta is an important part of perioperative TEE. In routine cases such as coronary artery bypass surgery, evaluation of the aorta may reveal previously unknown, significant atheromatous disease of the aorta and alter the surgical plan (off-pump bypass, alternative sites for cannulation). In emergencies, diagnosis of aortic pathology (dissection, aneurysm, transsection) may prove life-saving.

Two-Dimensional and Motion-Mode Echocardiography

The entire thoracic aorta can be imaged with TEE, apart from the distal ascending and proximal arch segments, where the interposition of the left main bronchus between the esophagus

and the left atrium prohibits the propagation of ultrasound. This blind spot can be imaged using epiaortic scanning.[75] The normal aorta has a smooth endothelial surface, and blood flow is laminar. Atherosclerotic plaques are irregularly shaped, often mobile protrusions inside the aortic lumen. The search for atheromas should be done by imaging the entire circumference of the aortic lumen (short axis views). Once a particular lesion is found, scanning in long axis view should be performed (Fig. 28-44). Plaques thicker than 4 mm are more likely to cause an embolic event.[76,77]

Aortic aneurysm is a dilatation of the aorta, usually >4 cm. Once the aneurysm is >5.5 cm, the probability of rupture increases (Fig. 28-45). Dissection is a separation between the intimal and medial layer of the aortic wall, creating a false lumen for blood flow[78] (Figs. 28-45 and 28-46). Both the true and false lumen fill with blood during systole, but only the true lumen has blood during diastole. Intramural hematoma is considered a precursor of dissection and should be treated similarly. Compared with an atheroma, an intramural hematoma has a smooth surface.

CARDIAC MASSES

Cardiac tumors can either originate from the heart or are metastases from other sites. They can embolize, cause arrhythmias, or

FIGURE 28-44. Aortic atheromas imaged in descending thoracic aorta short (**A** and **C**) and long (**B** and **D**) axis views.

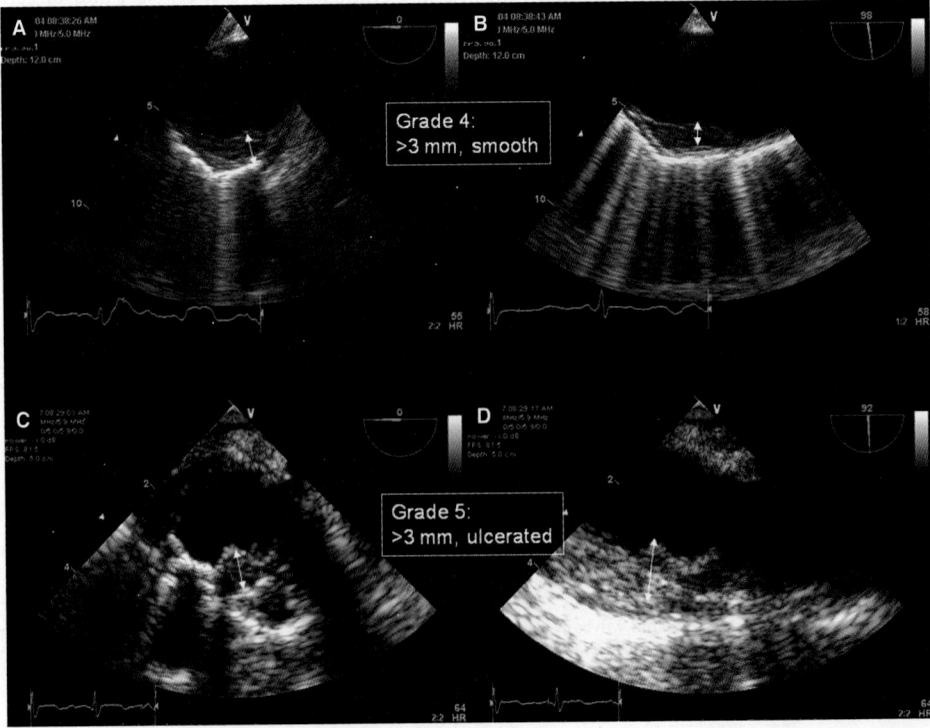

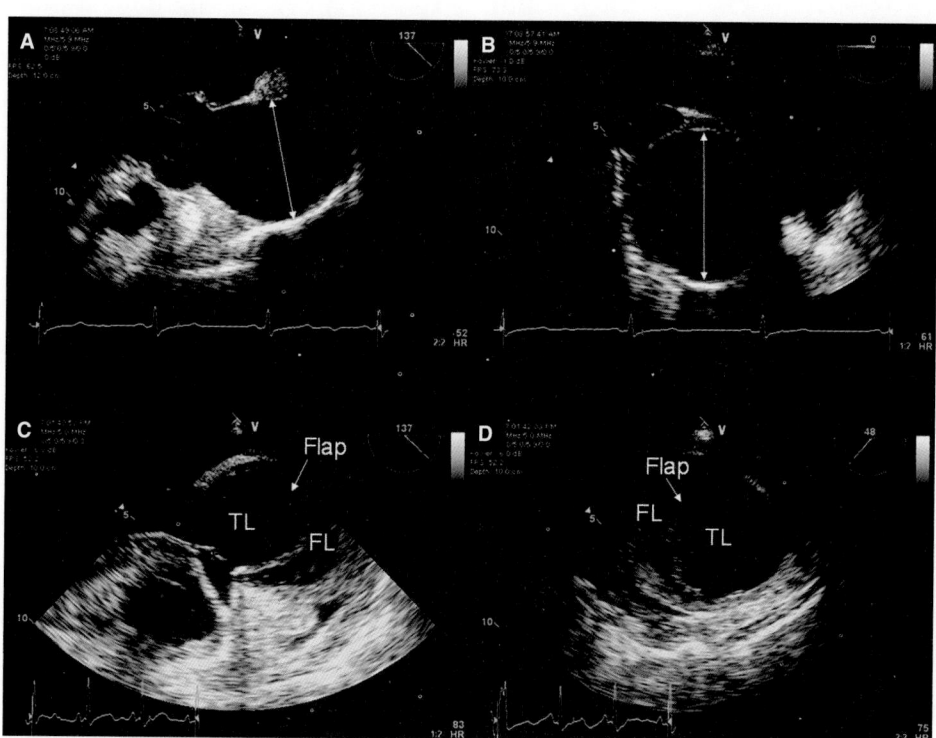

ANESTHETIC MANAGEMENT

FIGURE 28-45. Aortic disease. Ascending aorta aneurysm distal to the sinotubular junction (midesophageal ascending aorta long [A] and short [B] axis views). The diameter of the aorta is 5 cm. C. Ascending aorta dissection (Stanford type A) originating from the sinotubular junction. The true lumen (TL) expands in systole and the flap is convex toward the false lumen (FL). D. Descending aorta dissection (DeBakey type III).

cause heart failure. The most common primary tumor is myxoma, which is located most frequently at the interatrial septum. The potential of myxomas to obstruct the inflow or outflow region of a ventricle is demonstrated with Doppler echocardiography. The next most frequent tumor is fibroma of the ventricular wall. Fibromas are usually calcified, and can decrease the ventricular volume. Renal cell tumors often extend into the inferior vena cava and right atrium (Fig. 28-47). Pacemaker wires, thrombus, and normal anatomic structures that mimic the appearance of pathology (Eustachian valve, crista terminalis, Chiari network, or "Coumadin" ridge) should be differentiated from tumors.

CONGENITAL HEART DISEASE

The spectrum of congenital heart disease (CHD) seen in adult varies widely. Echocardiography is the primary imaging modality for diagnostic assessment of CHD. Advances in surgery have increased the survival rate of children with repaired CHD and, as a consequence, adults with repaired CHD are increasingly common in the OR. Common lesions evaluated with TEE include ASD, ventricular septal defect, patent ductus arteriosus, coarctation of the aorta, bicuspid AV, and repaired tetralogy of Fallot (Fig. 28-48).[79]

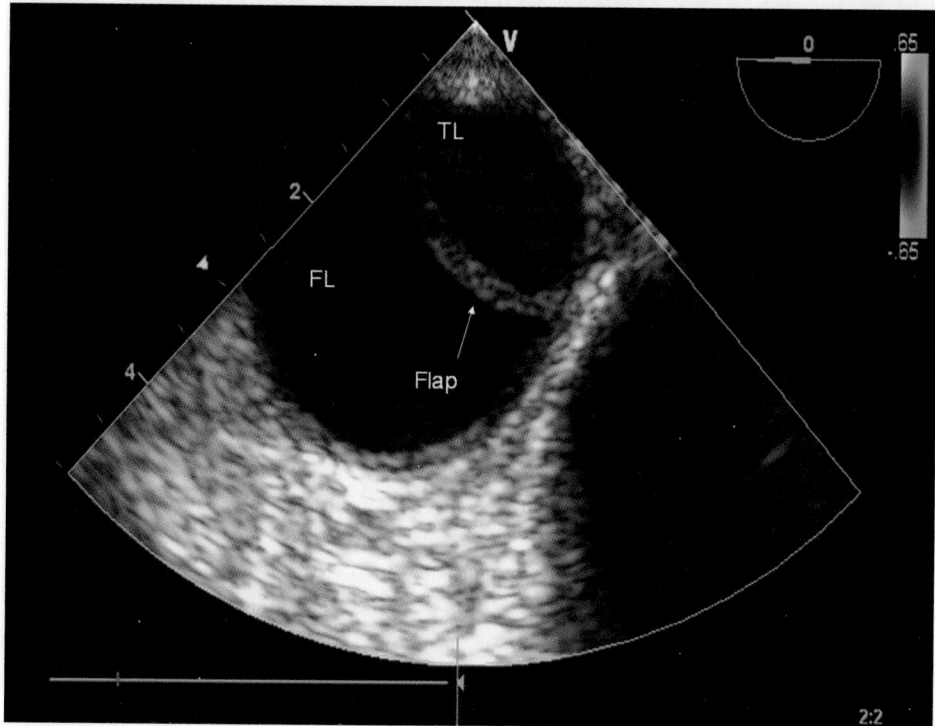

FIGURE 28-46. Aortic dissection. The descending aorta is seen in short axis. The aortic true lumen (TL) contains the aortic endothelium and has a smooth endoluminal surface. The intimal flap usually bows toward the false lumen (FL). Color flow Doppler demonstrates blood flow inside the true lumen (which expands in systole) and absence of flow inside the false lumen.

FIGURE 28-47. Cardiac masses. **A.** Left atrial (LA) myxoma seen in the midesophageal long axis view. **B.** Right atrial (RA) myxoma seen inside the right atrium (RA) in the midesophageal four-chamber view. **C.** Renal cell tumor occupying the inferior vena cava (IVC) and extending inside the RA. LVOT, left ventricular outflow tract; RV, right ventricle; SVC, superior vena cava.

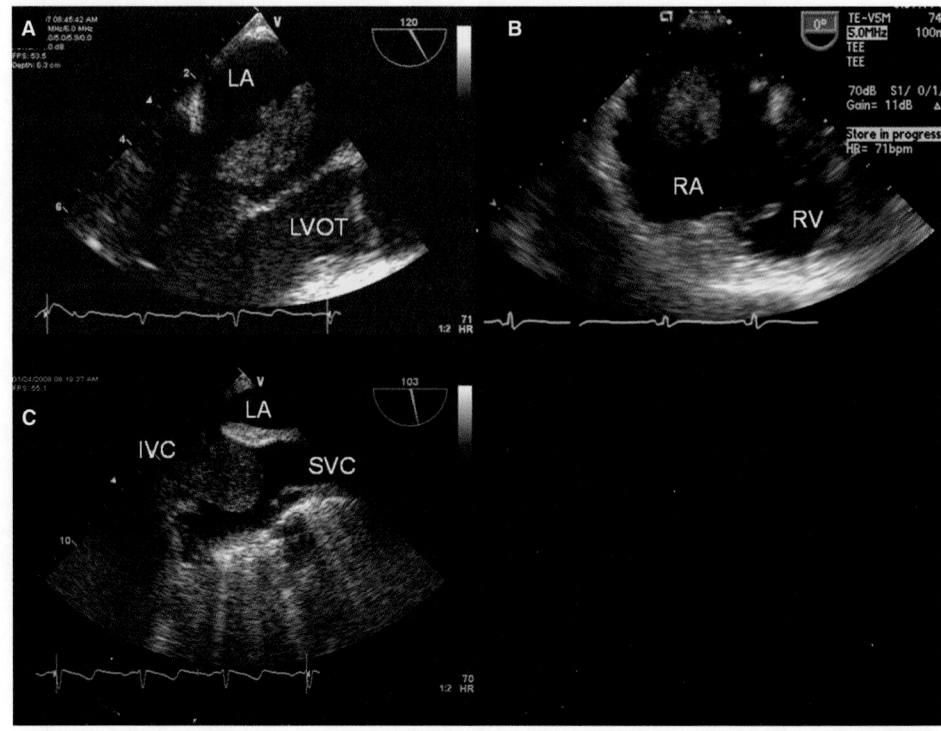

ECHOCARDIOGRAPHY-ASSISTED PROCEDURES

In addition to its role in diagnostics, echocardiography is also employed to assist various procedures such as placement of central venous catheter, intra-aortic balloon pump (IABP) catheter, coronary sinus cannula, and guidewires for other venous or arterial cannulas.

Ultrasound-Guided Central Vein Cannulation

The placement of central venous catheters is associated with complications including injury to vascular structures (carotid artery), pleura, nerve bundles, lymphatic system, and even the spinal canal. Historically, anatomic landmarks guided needle orientation during central venous access. However, multiple studies have demonstrated that the anatomic relationship between the internal jugular vein and carotid artery varies, and

FIGURE 28-48. Atrial septal defect (ASD). In the midesophageal four-chamber view, a color Doppler sector is positioned over the interatrial septum. An ASD with a left-to-right communication is shown in blue color, as the blood moves away from the transducer (top panel). Pulsed wave Doppler interrogation of the ASD measures a peak velocity gradient of 1 m/s.

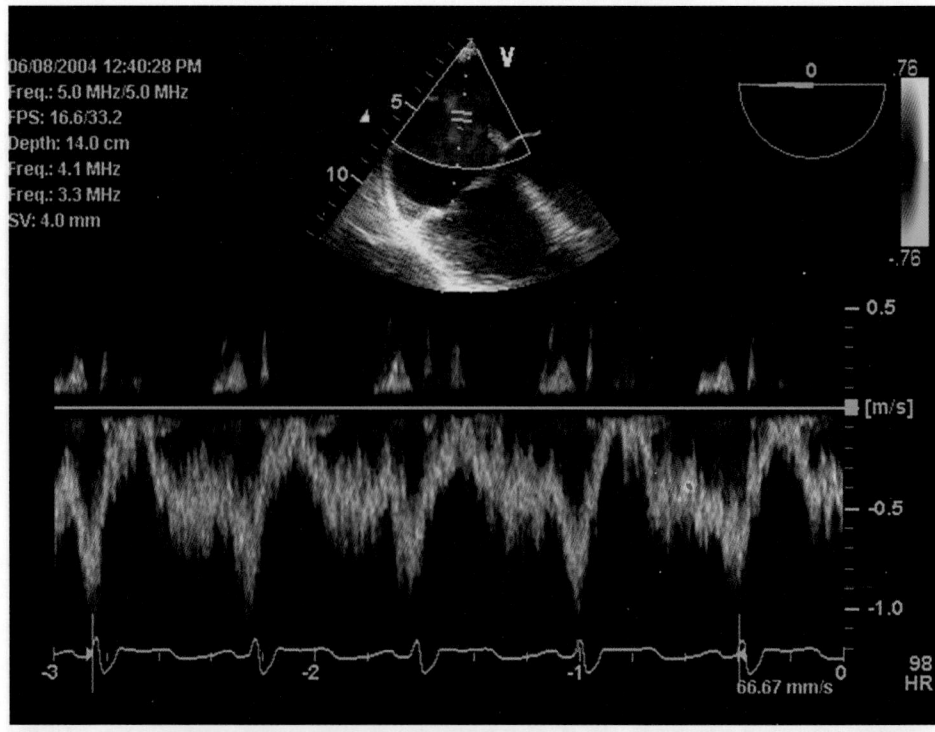

that even experienced physicians encounter complications.[80] Visual guidance by ultrasound provides real-time feedback, reducing the complication rate and the procedure time.[81] For patient safety reasons the National Institute for Clinical Excellence has recommended that central lines be placed under guidance of 2-D ultrasound imaging.[82]

A linear array hand-held transducer with high frequencies (7.5 to 12 MHz) is preferred for ultrasound-guided central line placement. The technique relies on placing the transducer over the traditional anatomic landmarks and identifying the internal jugular vein (IJ) and carotid artery (CA) in short axis and their anatomic relationship (Fig. 28-49). The 2-D criteria of differentiating the CA from the IJ vein are distensibility (the IJ increases in size with Valsalva maneuver and Trendelenburg position) and compressibility (the IJ will decrease in size with pressure applied over it by the transducer). Applying CFD with the transducer oriented slightly caudad displays the CA with red pulsating flow and the IJ with a continuous blue flow (Fig. 28-49). Note that if the transducer is oriented cephalad the colors are reversed. The needle insertion and venous puncture is performed under ultrasound guidance. The longitudinal view (Fig. 28-50) is then used to view the wire's placement in the vessel. TEE can confirm the guide wire's position in the superior vena cava (Fig. 28-50).

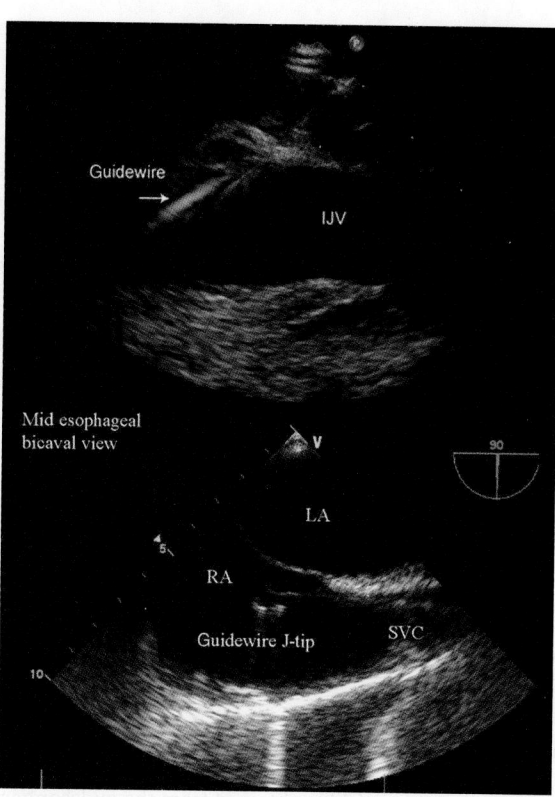

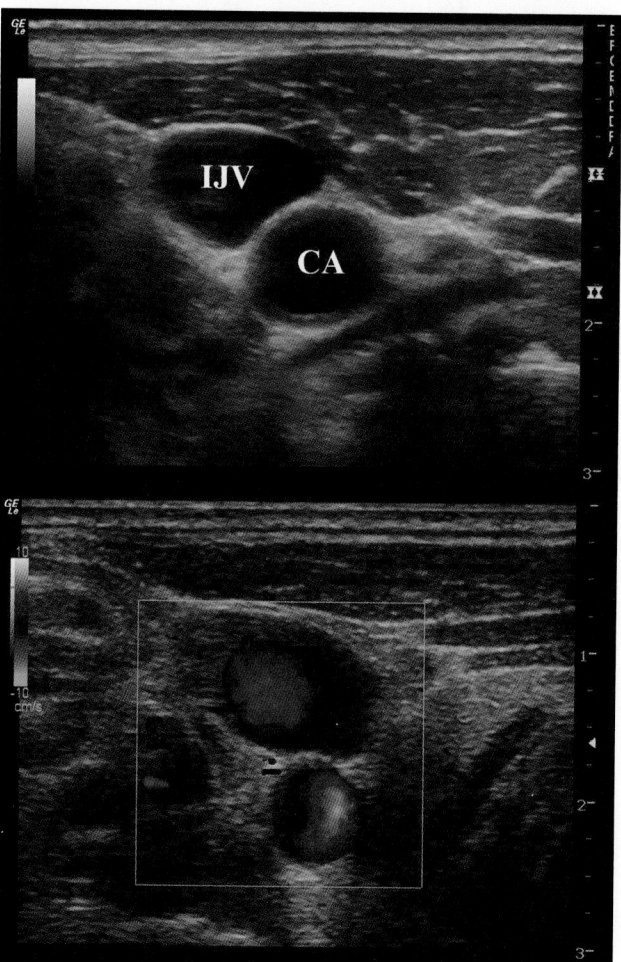

FIGURE 28-49. Internal jugular vein (IJV) and carotid artery (CA) and their anatomic relationship **Top panel.** Two-dimensional examination, using a linear scanner, showing the IJV lateral to the CA. **Bottom panel.** Color flow Doppler is applied showing continuous blue flow in the IJV and pulsating red flow in the CA (transducer oriented caudad).

FIGURE 28-50. **A.** Ultrasound confirmation of guidewire position. A sector scanner transducer is used to visualize the internal jugular vein (IJV) in long axis. The guidewire is seen as a thin echo-dense linear structure positioned in the lumen of the vein. **B.** Transesophageal echocardiographic confirmation of guidewire position. The midesophageal bicaval view is used. The guidewire is seen in the superior vena cava (SVC), with the tip in the right atrium (RA); LA, left atrium.

For PAC placement, TEE is useful in guiding the catheter through the right heart and confirming proper position in the PA. In the midesophageal right ventricular inflow-outflow view, the PAC can be followed from the RA, passing the TV into the RV, and then passing the PV into the PA. The midesophageal ascending aortic short axis view is used to position the PAC so that its tip lies in the right PA.

Although ultrasound can be a valuable tool in decreasing the number of complications, it does not eliminate the risk of the procedure. Experience and training are essential for enhancing patient safety with ultrasound.

Intra-Aortic Balloon Pump Placement

Use of TEE during IABP placement allows positioning of the catheter to the preferred location, distal to the left subclavian artery. Prior to its insertion, the echocardiographer should assess the descending thoracic aorta for presence of mobile atheroma or aortic dissections. These situations may represent contraindications to catheter placement. During cannulation, the presence of the guidewire in the descending aorta should be confirmed with TEE. Optimal function of the IABP requires that the tip lies 1 to10 cm distal to the left subclavian artery. The exact position of the IABP catheter tip is best visualized using the descending aortic long axis view.

Coronary Sinus Cannulation

TEE is helpful to guide the placement of the cannula and to check for proper position. Improper insertion of the cannula

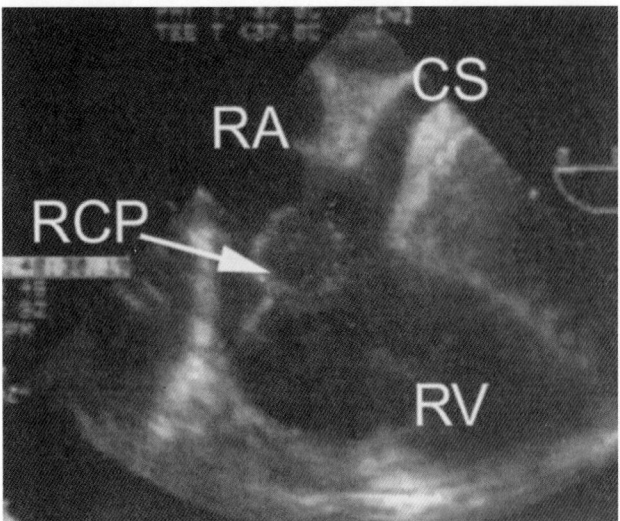

FIGURE 28-51. Probe retroflexion from the midesophageal four-chamber view is used to visualize the coronary sinus (CS). The *arrow* points to the balloon of the retrograde cannula (RCP), right atrium (RA), and right ventricle (RV).

can result in injury to the interatrial septum or to the crux of the heart, the fragile area joining the atria and ventricles. View of the coronary sinus (CS) is obtained from the midesophageal four-chamber view by retroflexing the probe (Fig. 28-51). After the cannula is positioned in the CS, the multiplane angle should be rotated to 90 degrees and the CS will be seen in cross section. The tip of the cannula will be displayed as a small echo-dense dot in the middle of the CS. This view will assure that the cannula is positioned at an appropriate depth.

Other Cannulation Techniques

TEE is useful in verifying the position of various other cannulas. For example, when femoral artery–femoral vein bypass is instituted, the venous cannula can be visualized as it advances in the inferior vena cava up to the level of the RA. Proper position of guidewires used to for aortic cannulation can be confirmed with TEE.

EPICARDIAL AND EPIAORTIC ECHOCARDIOGRAPHY

Epicardial Echocardiography

During surgeries performed via sternotomy or thoracotomy, epicardial echocardiography can be performed and is particularly valuable in those cases in which the TEE probe cannot be placed or is contraindicated. The epicardial views are similar to the ones obtained via TTE. The America Society of Echocardiography in collaboration with the Society of Cardiovascular Anesthesiologists has recently issued guidelines for the performance of epicardial echocardiography.[83] The epicardial probe uses high-frequency transducers (5 to 12 MHz) that may require a standoff device and/or saline in the mediastinum for best imaging. Epicardial imaging offers superior image quality as well as a better window to the anterior cardiac structures (aorta and AV, PA and PV).

Epiaortic Examination

Because of the interposition of the left bronchus, the distal AA and the proximal aortic arch cannot be visualized with TEE. The ascending aortic and proximal aortic arch are of particular interest during cardiac surgeries as they represent sites for aortic cannulation. Epiaortic scanning for atheroma is performed using a small footprint, linear array transducer. Guidelines for intraoperative epiaortic examination have been published.[75]

ECHOCARDIOGRAPHY OUTSIDE THE OPERATING ROOM

An understanding of echocardiography is also relevant to anesthesiologists in that many patients with a history of heart disease will have undergone an echocardiographic examination prior to surgery. The echocardiography report from a preoperative examination is useful for assessing surgical risk and developing the anesthetic plan. Echocardiography has also established itself as particularly valuable in assessment of postoperative hemodynamic instability. It offers rapid diagnosis by differentiating among the potential complications faced in postoperative care, such as hypovolemia, pericardial tamponade (Fig. 28-40), aortic dissection, myocardial infarction, endocarditis, and pulmonary embolism.

References

1. Barash PG, Glanz S, Katz JD, et al: Ventricular function in children during halothane anesthesia: an echocardiographic evaluation. Anesthesiology 1978; 49: 79
2. Click RL, Abel MD, Schaff HV: Intraoperative transesophageal echocardiography: 5-year prospective review of impact on surgical management. Mayo Clinic Proc 2000; 75: 241
3. Couture P, Denault AY, McKenty S, et al: Impact of routine use of intraoperative transesophageal echocardiography during cardiac surgery. Can J Anaesth 2000; 47: 20
4. Schmidlin D, Bettex D, Bernard E, et al: Transesophageal echocardiography in cardiac and vascular surgery: implications and observer variability: Br J Anaesth 2001; 86: 497
5. Perrino AC, Reeves ST: Echocardiographic assessment during non-cardiac surgery, Comprehensive Textbook of Intraoperative TEE. Edited by Savage RM, Aronson S. Philadelphia, Lippincott Williams & Wilkins, 2004
6. Suriani RJ, Neustein S, Shore-Lesserson L, et al: Intraoperative transesophageal echocardiography during noncardiac surgery. J Cardiothorac Vasc Anesth 1998; 12: 274
7. Kolev N, Brase R, Swanvelder M, et al: The influence of transesophageal echocardiography on intra-operative decision making. Anaesthesia 1998; 53: 767
8. Denault AY, Couture P, McKenty S, et al: Perioperative use of transesophageal echocardiography by anesthesiologists: impact in noncardiac surgery and in the intensive care unit. Can J Anesth 2002;49: 287
9. American Society of Anesthesiologists and the Society of Cardiovascular Anesthesiologists Task Force on Transesophageal echocardiography. Practice guidelines of perioperative transesophageal echocardiography. Anesthesiology 1996; 84: 986
10. Cheitlin MD, Armstrong WF, Aurigemma GP, et al: ACC. AHA. ASE. ACC/AHA/ASE 2003 Guideline Update for the Clinical Application of Echocardiography: summary article. A report of the American College of Cardiology/American Heart
11. Center for Devices and Radiological Health: Revised 510(k) Diagnostic Ultrasound Guidance for 1993. Rockville, MD, US Food and Drug Administration, 1993
12. Miller JP: Two-dimensional examination, A Practical Approach to Transesophageal Echocardiography, 2nd edition. Edited by Perrino AC, Reeves S. Philadelphia, Lippincott, Williams & Wilkins, 2007, p 24
13. Practice guidelines for perioperative transesophageal echocardiography: A report from the American Society of Anesthesiologists and the Society of Cardiovascular Anesthesiologists Task Force on Transesophageal Echocardiography. Anesthesiology 1996; 84: 986
14. Rafferty T, LaMantia KR, Davis E, et al: Quality assurance for intraoperative transesophageal echocardiography monitoring: A report of 846 procedures. Anesth Analg 1993; 76: 228
15. Kallameyer IJ, Collard CD, Fox JA, et al: The safety of intraoperative transesophageal echocardiography: A case series of 7200 cardiac surgical patients. Anesth Analg 2001; 92: 1126

16. Hogue CW, Lappas GD, Creswell LL, et al: Swallowing dysfunction after cardiac operations. J Thorac Cardiovasc Surg 1995; 110: 517

17. Rousou JA, Tighe DA, Garb JL, et al: Risk of dysphagia after trans-esophageal echocardiography during cardiac operations. Ann Thorac Surg 2000; 69: 486

18. Lighty GW, Kaplan DS, Hare CL: Training in transesophageal echocardiography: Esophageal disease considerations for the uninitiated echocardiographer. Video J Echocardiog 1991; 1: 9

19. Shanewise JS, Cheung AT, Aronson S, et al: ASE/SCA guidelines for performing a comprehensive intraoperative multiplane transesophageal echocardiographic examinations: Recommendations of the American Society of Echocardiography Council for Intraoperative Echocardiography and the Society of Cardiovascular Anesthesiologists Task Force for Certification in Perioperative Transesophageal Echocardiography. Anesth Analg 1999; 89: 870

20. Miller JP, Lambert AS, Shapiro WA, et al: The adequacy of basic intraoperative transesophageal echocardiography performed by experienced anesthesiologists. Anesth Analg 2001; 92: 1103

21. Ahmed S, Nanda NC, Miller AP, et al: Usefulness of transesophageal three-dimensional echocardiography in the identification of individual segment/scallop prolapse of the mitral valve. Echocardiography 2003; 20: 203

22. Perrino AC: Doppler technology and technique, A Practical Approach to Transesophageal Echocardiography, 2nd edition. Edited by Perrino AC, Reeves S. Philadelphia, Lippincott, Williams & Wilkins, 2007, p 109

23. Recommendations for Quantification of Doppler Echocardiography: A Report From the Doppler Quantification Task Force of the Nomenclature and Standards Committee of the American Society of Echocardiography: Miguel A. Quiñones, MD, Chair, Catherine M. Otto, MD, Marcus Stoddard, MD, Alan Waggoner, MHS, RDMS, and William A. Zoghbi, MD. J Am Soc Echocardiogr 2002; 15: 167

24. Nishimura RA, Miller FA, Callahan MJ, et al: Doppler echocardiography: theory, instrumentation, technique, and application: Mayo Clin Proc 1985; 60: 321

25. Maslow A, Perrino AC: Quantitative Doppler and hemodynamics, A Practical Approach to Transesophageal Echocardiography, 2nd edition. Edited by Perrino AC, Reeves S. Philadelphia, Lippincott, Williams & Wilkins, 2007, p 127

26. Perrino AC, Harris SN, Luther MA: Intraoperative determination of cardiac output using multiplane transesophageal echocardiography: A comparison to thermodilution. Anesthesiology 1998; 89: 350

27. Harris SN, Luther MA, Perrino AC: Multiplane transesophageal echocardiography acquisition of ascending aortic flow velocities: A comparison with established techniques. J Am Soc Echocardiogr 1999; 12: 754

28. Muhiudeen IA, Kuecherer HF, Lee E, et al: Intraoperative estimation of cardiac output by transesophageal pulsed Doppler echocardiography. Anesthesiology 1991; 74: 9

29. Otto CM, Pearlman AS, Comess KA, et al: Determination of the stenotic aortic valve area in adults using Doppler echocardiography. J Am Coll Cardiol 1986; 7: 509

30. Currie PJ, Seward JB, Reeder GS, et al: Continuous-wave Doppler echocardiographic assessment of severity of calcific aortic stenosis: a simultaneous Doppler-catheter correlative study in 100 adult patients. Circulation 1985; 71: 1162

31. Hatle L, Brubakk A, Tromsdal A, et al: Noninvasive assessment of pressure drop in mitral stenosis by Doppler ultrasound. Br Heart J 1978; 40: 131

32. Stamm RB, Martin RP: Quantification of pressure gradients across stenotic valves by Doppler ultrasound. J Am Coll Cardiol 1983; 2: 707

33. Teague SM, Heinsimer JA, Anderson JL, et al: Quantification of aortic regurgitation utilizing continuous wave Doppler ultrasound. J Am Coll Cardiol 1986; 8: 592

34. Lee RT, Lord CP, Plappert T, et al: Prospective Doppler echocardiographic evaluation of pulmonary artery diastolic pressure in the medical intensive care unit. Am J Cardiol 1989; 64: 1366

35. Gorcsan J III, Snow FR, Paulsen W, et al: Noninvasive estimation of left atrial pressure in patients with congestive heart failure and mitral regurgitation by Doppler echocardiography. Am Heart J 1991; 11: 858

36. Nishimura RA, Tajik AJ: Determination of left-sided pressure gradients by utilizing Doppler aortic and mitral regurgitation signals: validation by simultaneous dual catheter and Doppler studies. J Am Coll Cardiol 1988; 11: 317

37. Leung JM, O'Kelly BF, Mangano DT: Relationship of regional wall motion abnormalities to hemodynamic indices of myocardial oxygen supply and demand in patients undergoing CABG surgery. Anesthesiology 1990; 73: 802

38. Hauser AM, Gangadharan V, Ramos RG, et al: Sequence of mechanical, electrocardiographic and clinical effects of repeated coronary artery occlusion in human beings: Echocardiographic observations during coronary angioplasty. J Am Coll Cardiol 1985; 5: 193

39. Battler A, Froelicher VF, Gallagher KP, et al: Dissociation between regional myocardial dysfunction and ECG changes during ischemia in the conscious dog. Circulation 1980; 62: 735

40. Ross J Jr: Myocardial perfusion-contraction matching: implications for coronary artery disease and hibernation. Circulation 1991; 83: 1076

41. Cerqueira MD, Weissman NJ, Dilsizian V, et al: Standardized myocardial segmentation and nomenclature for tomographic imaging of the heart. A statement for healthcare professionals from the cardiac imaging committee of the Council on Clinical Cardiology of the American Heart Association. American Heart Association Writing Group on myocardial segmentation and registration for cardiac imaging. Circulation 2002; 105: 539

42. Lang RM, Bierig M, Devereux RB, et al: Recommendations for chamber quantification: A report from the American Society of Echocardiography's Guidelines and Standards Committee and the Chamber Quantification Writing group, developed in conjunction with the European Association of Echocardiography, a branch of the European Society of Cardiology. J Am Soc Echocardiogr 2005; 18: 1440

43. Lieberman AN, Weiss JL, Jugdutt BI, et al: Two-dimensional echocardiography and infarct size: relationship of regional wall motion and thickening to the extent of myocardial infarction in the dog. Circulation 1981; 63: 739

44. Bergquist BD, Leung, JM, Bellows WH: Transesophageal echocardiography in myocardial revascularization: I. Accuracy of intraoperative real-time interpretation. Anesth Analg 1996; 82: 1132

45. Odell DH, Cahallan MK: Assessment of left ventricular global and segmental systolic function with transesophageal echocardiography. Anesthesiology Clin 2006; 24: 755

46. London MJ: Assessment of left ventricular global systolic function by transesophageal echocardiography. Ann Card Anaesth 2006; 9: 157

47. Cheung AT, Savino JS, Weiss SJ, et al: Echocardiographic and hemodynamic index of left ventricular preload in patients with normal and abnormal ventricular function. Anesthesiology 1994; 81: 376

48. Skarvan K, Lambert A, Filipovic M: Reference values for left ventricular function in subjects under general anesthesia and controlled ventilation assessed by two-dimensional transoesophageal echocardiography. Eur J Anaesthesiol 2001; 18: 713

49. Swenson JD, Bull D, Stringham J: Subjective assessment of left ventricular preload using transesophageal echocardiography: corresponding pulmonary artery occlusion pressures. J Cardiothorac Vasc Anesth 2001; 15: 580

50. Bergquist BD, Leung JM, Bellows WH: Transesophageal echocardiography in myocardial revascularization: Accuracy of intraoperative real-time interpretation. Anesth Analg 1996; 82: 1132

51. Ditooe N, Stultz D, Schwartz BP, et al: Qualitative left ventricular systolic function: from chamber to myocardium. Crit Care Med 2007; 35: S330

52. Trambaiolo P, Tonti G, Salustri A, et al: New insights into regional systolic and diastolic left ventricular function with tissue Doppler echocardiography: from qualitative analysis to a quantitative approach. J Am Soc Echocardiogr 2001; 14: 85

53. Derumeaux G, Ovize M, Loufoua J, et al: Doppler tissue imaging quantitates regional wall motion during myocardial ischemia and reperfusion. Circulation 1998; 97: 1970

54. Bernard F, Denault A, Babin D, et al: Diastolic dysfunction is predictive of difficult weaning from cardiopulmonary bypass. Anesth Analg 2001; 92: 291

55. Bhatia RS, Tu JV, Lee DS, et al: Outcome of heart failure with preserved ejection fraction in a population-based study. N Engl J Med 2006; 355: 260

56. Nishimura RA, Tajik AJ: Evaluation of diastolic filling of left ventricle in health and disease: Doppler echocardiography is the clinician's Rosetta stone. J Am Coll Cardiol 1997; 30: 8

57. Gilman G, Nelson TA, Hansen WH: Diastolic function: a sonographer's approach to the essential echocardiographic measurements of left ventricular diastolic function. J Am Soc Echocardiogr 2007; 20: 199

58. Sutherland GR, Stewart MJ, Groundstroem KW, et al: Color Doppler myocardial imaging: a new technique for the assessment of myocardial function. J Am Soc Echocardiogr 1994; 7: 441

59. Pirracchio R, Cholley B, De Hert S, et al: Diastolic heart failure in anesthesia and critical care. Br J Anaesth 2007; 98: 707

60. Shernan SK: A Practical Approach to Transesophageal Echocardiography, 2nd edition. Edited by Perrino AC, Reeves S. Philadelphia, Lippincott, Williams & Wilkins, 2007, p 146

61. Baumgartner H, Stefenelli T, Niederberger J, et al: "Overestimation" of catheter gradients by Doppler ultrasound in patients with aortic stenosis: a predictable manifestation of pressure recovery. J Am Coll Cardiol 1999; 33: 1655

62. Burwash IG, Dickinson A, Teskey RJ: Aortic valve area discrepancy by Gorlin equation and Doppler echocardiography continuity equation: relationship to flow in patients with valvular aortic stenosis. Can J Cardiol 2000; 16: 985

63. Bonow RO, Carabello BA, Chatterjee KA, et al: ACC/AHA 2006 guidelines for the management of patients with valvular heart disease: A report of the American College of Cardiology/American Heart Association task force on practice guidelines. Circulation 2006; 114: e84

64. Henry WL, Griffith JM, Michaelis LL: Measurement of mitral orifice area in patients with mitral valve disease, by real-time, two-dimensional echocardiography. Circulation 1975; 51: 827

65. Bruce CJ, Nishimura RA: Clinical assessment and management of mitral stenosis, valvular heart disease. Cardiol Clin 1998; 16: 375

66. Libanoff AJ, Roadbard S: Atrioventricular pressure half-time: measure of mitral valve orifice area. Circulation 1968; 38: 144

67. Braverman AC, Thomas JD, Lee R: Doppler echocardiographic estimation of mitral valve area during changing hemodynamic conditions. Am J Cardiol 1991; 68: 1485

68. Perry GJ, Helmecke F, Nanda NC: Evaluation of aortic insufficiency by Doppler color flow mapping. J Am Coll Cardiol 1987; 9: 952

69. Takenaka K, Sakamoto T, Dabestani A: Pulsed Doppler echocardiographic detection of regurgitant blood flow in the ascending, descending and abdominal aorta of patients with aortic regurgitation. J Cardiol 1987; 17: 301

70. Lambert AS, Miller JP, Merrick SH: Improved evaluation of the location and mechanism of mitral valve regurgitation with a systemic transesophageal echocardiography examination. Anesth Analg 1999; 88: 1205

71. Helmcke F, Nanda NC, Hsiung MC: Color Doppler assessment of mitral regurgitation orthogonal planes. Circulation 1987; 75: 175

72. Schiller NB, Foster E, Redberg RF: Transesophageal echocardiography in the evaluation of mitral regurgitation. The twenty-four signs of severe mitral regurgitation. Cardiol Clin 1993; 11: 399

73. Simpson IA, Shiota T, Gharib M: Current status of flow convergence for clinical applications: is it a leaning tower of "PISA"? J Am Coll Cardiol 1996; 27: 504

74. Pu M, Prior DL, Fan X, et al: Calculation of mitral regurgitation orifice area with use of a simplified proximal convergence method: Initial clinical application. J Am Soc Echocardiogr 2001; 14: 180

75. Glas KE, Swaminathan M, Reeves ST, et al: Guidelines for the performance of a comprehensive intraoperative epiaortic ultrasonographic examination: recommendations of the American Society of Echocardiography and the Society of Cardiovascular Anesthesiologists; endorsed by the Society of Thoracic Surgeons. J Am Soc Echocardiogr 2007; 20: 1227

76. Massachusetts Medical Society: Atherosclerotic Disease of the Aortic Arch as a risk factor for recurrent ischemic stroke. The French study of aortic plaques in stroke groups. New Engl J Med 1996; 334: 1216

77. Weber A, Jones EF, Zavala JA, et al: Intraobserver and interobserver variability of transesophageal echocardiography in aortic arch atheroma measurement. J Am Soc Echocardiogr 2008; 21; 127

78. Vignon P, Spencer KT, Rambaud G, et al: Differential transesophageal echocardiographic diagnosis between linear artifacts and intraluminal flap of aortic dissection or disruption. Chest 2001; 119; 1778

79. Russell IA. Rouine-Rapp K, Stratmann G, et al: Congenital heart disease in the adult: a review with Internet-accessible transesophageal echocardiographic images. Anesth Analg 2006; 102: 694

80. Denys BG, Uretsky BF: Anatomical variations of internal jugular vein location: Impact on central venous access. Crit Care Med 1991; 19: 1516

81. Karakitsos D, Labropoulos N, De Groot E, et al: Real-time ultrasound-guided catheterization of the internal jugular vein: A prospective comparison with the landmark technique in critical care patients. Crit Care 2006; 10: R162

82. National Institute for Clinical Excellence (NICE). Guidance on the Use of Ultrasound Locating Devices for Placing Central Venous Catheters. London, UK, National Institute for Clinical Excellence 2002

83. Reeves ST, Glass KE, Eltzschig H, et al: Guidelines for performing a comprehensive intraoperative epicardial echocardiography examination: recommendations of the American Society of Echocardiography and the Society of Cardiovascular Anesthesiologists. J Am Soc Echocardiogr 2007; 20: 427

CHAPTER 29 ■ **AIRWAY MANAGEMENT**

WILLIAM H. ROSENBLATT AND WARIYA SUKHUPRAGARN

KEY POINTS

1 Management of the airway is paramount to safe perioperative care. Following a series of evaluation procedures affects outcomes in a favorable way.

2 The anatomically complex airway undergoes growth, and development and significant changes in its size, shape, and relation to the cervical spine between infancy and childhood.

3 A thorough airway-relevant history and physical examination must be obtained during the preoperative evaluation.

4 Preoxygenation (also commonly termed *denitrogenation*) should be practiced in all cases when time permits.

5 The advent of the laryngeal mask airway, as well as other supraglottic airways, has led some to question the relative safety of tracheal intubation.

6 The first attempt at laryngoscopy should be the "best attempt."

7 Successful laryngoscopy involves the distortion of the normal anatomic planes of the supraglottic airway to produce a line of direct visualization from the operator's eye to the larynx.

8 Analysis of laryngeal trauma cases has led some to question whether direct laryngoscopy is as benign and safe as we have always assumed.

9 The technique of rapid-sequence induction is performed to gain control of the airway in the shortest amount of time after the ablation of protective airway reflexes with the induction of anesthesia.

10 The period of extubation may be far more treacherous than that of induction and intubation.

11 The American Society of Anesthesiologists (ASA) algorithm for the approach to the difficult airway stands as a model for anesthesiologists and other health care specialties.

12 Awake intubation is usually successful if approached with care and patience.

13 Awake airway management remains a mainstay of the ASA's difficult airway algorithm.

14 Case studies applying the following technologies help clinicians to understand the modern airway armamentarium: video laryngoscopy, flexible and rigid fiberoptics, retrograde wire, and esophageal-tracheal Combitube.

15 An ever-increasing number of airway-management devices are commercially available.

16 When access to the airway from the mouth or nose fails, emergency access via the extrathoracic trachea is a feasible alternative.

PERSPECTIVES ON AIRWAY MANAGEMENT

In the 20 years since publication of the first edition of this text, the field of airway management has undergone a vigorous revolution. Although the airway manager of today may still employ many of the devices available in 1988, the array of devices, algorithms, and pharmaceuticals in the modern airway armamentarium can be daunting. Fortunately, expertise in a limited, albeit complementary, number of tools as well as careful thought given to planning, suffice in most cases. Although the final decade of the last century saw a resolute swing toward the application of supraglottic airways (SGA), a more recently introduced generation of devices reflect the application of video technology in the realm of tracheal intubation. The role of SGAs is firmly established in routine anesthetic care as well as airway rescue, but the advent of video laryngoscopy promises to remove many of the failings of a technique that has been in use for more than 100 years.

Techniques and practices in airway management have long been an important concern of the American Society of Anesthesiologists (ASA), as illustrated by the publication of original and revised difficult airway guidelines.[1] Analysis of the Society's closed claims database, in the periods before and after the 1993 publication of the ASA difficult airway guidelines, reveals both encouraging as well as disturbing trends.[2] A significant decrease in claims related to death/brain death at the induction of anesthesia is not matched with a decrease during emergence and the postoperative period. Although the closed claims data are useful, it has significant limitations, including its retrospective and nonrandom nature, and the lack of a denominator.[2]

Management of the airway is paramount to safe perioperative care, and the following steps become necessary to favorably affect outcome: (1) a thorough airway history and physical examination; (2) consideration of the ease of rapid tracheal intubation, by direct or indirect laryngoscopy; (3) formation of management plans for use of a supraglottic means of ventilation (e.g., face mask, SGA); (4) weighing the risk of aspiration of gastric contents; and (5) estimating the relative risk to the patient of failed airway maneuvers.[3] This chapter will reflect the need to consider these five factors when approaching any patient who requires or may require airway control.

Review of Airway Anatomy

The term *airway* refers to the upper airway—consisting of the nasal and oral cavities, pharynx, larynx, trachea, and principal bronchi. The airway in humans is primarily a conducting pathway. Because the oroesophageal and nasotracheal passages cross each other, anatomic and functional complexities have evolved for protection of the sublaryngeal airway against aspiration of food that passes through the pharynx. The anatomically complex airway undergoes growth and development and significant changes in its size, shape, and relation to the cervical spine between infancy and childhood.[4] As are other bodily systems, the airway is not immune from the influence of genetic, nutritional, and hormonal factors. Table 29-1 illustrates the anatomic differences in the larynx of infants and adult.

The laryngeal skeleton consists of nine cartilages (three paired and three unpaired); together, these house the vocal folds, which extend in an anterior–posterior plane from the thyroid cartilage to the arytenoid cartilages. The shield-shaped thyroid cartilage acts as the anterior "protective housing" of the vocal mechanism (Fig. 29-1). Movements of the laryngeal structures are controlled by two groups of muscles: the extrinsic muscles, which move the larynx as a whole, and the intrinsic muscles, which move the various cartilages in relation to one another. The larynx is innervated by two branches of each vagus nerve: the superior laryngeal and recurrent laryngeal nerves. Because the recurrent laryngeal nerves supply all of the intrinsic muscles of the larynx (with the exception of cricothyroid), trauma to these nerves can result in vocal cord dysfunction. As a result of unilateral nerve injury, airway function is usually unimpaired, although the protective role of larynx in preventing aspiration may be compromised.

The cricothyroid membrane provides coverage to the cricothyroid space. The membrane, which in the adult is typ-

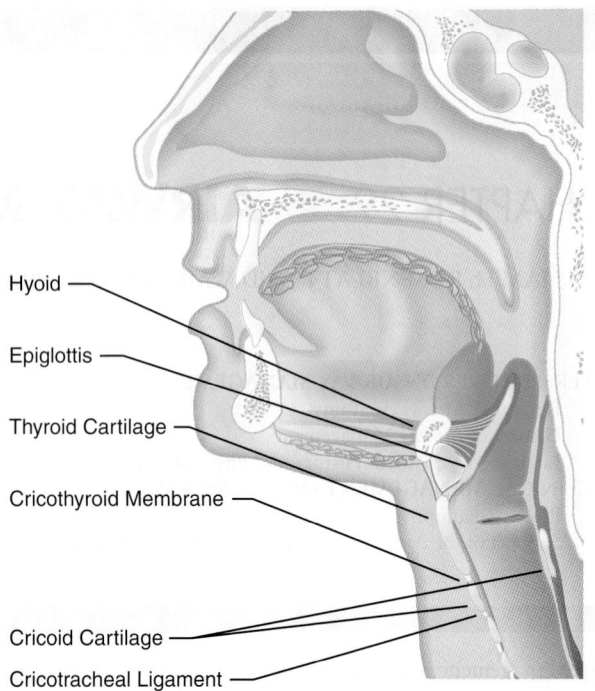

FIGURE 29-1. The major landmarks of the airway mechanism. Note that the cricoid cartilage is less than 1 cm in height in its anterior aspect, but may be 2 cm in height posteriorly (*small arrow*).

Labels:
- Hyoid
- Epiglottis
- Thyroid Cartilage
- Cricothyroid Membrane
- Cricoid Cartilage
- Cricotracheal Ligament

ically 9 mm in height and 3 cm in width, is composed of a yellow elastic tissue that lies directly beneath the skin and a thin facial layer. It is located in the anterior neck between the thyroid cartilage superiorly and the cricoid cartilage inferiorly. It can be identified 1 to 1.5 fingerbreadths below the laryngeal prominence (thyroid notch). It is often crossed horizontally in its upper third by the anastomosis of the left and right superior cricothyroid arteries. The membrane has a central portion known as the *conus elasticus* and two lateral, thinner portions. Directly beneath the membrane is the laryngeal mucosa. Because of anatomic variability in the course of veins and arteries and the membrane's proximity to the vocal folds (which may be 0.9 cm above the ligaments' upper border), it is suggested that any incisions or needle punctures to the cricothyroid membrane be made in its inferior third and be directed posteriorly (a posterior probing needles will strike the back side of the ring-shaped cricoid cartilage).

At the base of the larynx, suspended by the underside of the cricothyroid membrane, is the signet ring–shaped cricoid cartilage. This cartilage is approximately 1 cm in height anteriorly, but almost 2 cm in height in its posterior aspect as it extends in a cephalad direction creating the dorsal wall of the larynx at the level of the cricothyroid membrane and the thyroid cartilage (Fig. 29-1). The trachea is suspended from the cricoid cartilage by the cricotracheal ligament. The trachea measures approximately 15 cm in adults and is circumferentially supported by 17 to 18 C-shaped cartilages, with a membranous posterior aspect overlying the esophagus.

In the adult the first tracheal ring is anterior to the sixth cervical vertebrae. The tracheal cartilages are interconnected by fibroelastic tissue, which allows for expansion of the trachea both in length and diameter with inspiration/expiration and flexion/extension of the thoracocervical spine. The trachea ends at the carina (fifth thoracic vertebra), where it bifurcates into the principal bronchi. The right principal bronchus is

---

TABLE 29-1

ANATOMIC DIFFERENCES BETWEEN THE PEDIATRIC AND ADULT AIRWAYS

Proportionately smaller infant/child larynx

Narrowest portion: Cricoid cartilage in infant/child; vocal folds in adult

Relative vertical location: C3, C4, C5 in infant/child; C4, C5, C6 in adult

Epiglottis: Longer, narrower, and stiffer in infant/child

Aryepiglottic folds closer to midline in infant/child

Vocal folds: Anterior angle with respect to perpendicular axis of larynx in infant/child

Pliable laryngeal cartilage in infant/child

Mucosa more vulnerable to trauma in infant/child

larger in diameter than the left, and deviates from the plane of the trachea at a less acute angle. Aspirated materials, as well as a deeply inserted endotracheal tube (ETT), tend to gain entry into the right principal bronchus, although left-sided positioning should be excluded. Cartilaginous rings support the first seven generations of the bronchi.

History of Airway Management

Obstruction of the airway was a poorly understood phenomenon prior to 1874. Opening the mouth with a wooden screw and drawing the tongue forward with a forceps or a steel-gloved finger was the height of airway management.[5] Recognition that the base of the tongue falling against the posterior pharyngeal wall accounted for most airway obstruction did not occur until 1880. Credit for the first use of a true SGA is given to Joseph Thomas Clover (1825–1882), although it is possible that devices were used toward the end of the first millennium.[6] Clover used a nasopharyngeal tube for the delivery of chloroform anesthesia. The O'Dwyer tube was introduced in 1884. This device consisted of a curved metal conduit, with a conical end that could seal the laryngeal inlet when placed into the oropharynx. Although designed for the treatment of narcotic overdose, it was later modified to be used with volatile anesthetics. Over the next 50 years several modifications of the basic oropharyngeal airway were described. In the 1930s Ralph Waters introduced the now-familiar flattened tube oral airway. Gudel modified Waters' concept by fitting his airway within a stiff rubber envelope in an attempt to reduce mucosal trauma.

Tracheal intubation was first described in 1788 as a means of resuscitation of the "apparently dead,"[7] but was not used for the delivery of anesthesia until almost 100 years later. The forerunner of the modern ETT was designed by the German otolaryngologist, Dr. Franz Kuhn (1866–1929). Kuhn developed a flexo-metallic tube that resisted kinking and could be shaped to the patient's upper airway anatomy. It was inserted using a rigid stylet, and the hypopharynx was sealed with oiled gauze packing. Sir Ivan Magill and Stanley Rowbotham are credited with the initial development of modern tracheal intubation. Performing anesthesia for reconstructive facial surgery (during World Was I), they developed a two-tube nasal system. One narrow tube (gum elastic design) was passed through the nares and guided into the larynx using a surgical laryngoscope. The other tube was blindly passed into the pharynx to provide for the escape of gases. During use of this "Magill" tube, the exhaust lumen would occasional pass blindly into the larynx, leading Sir Ivan to describe "blind nasal intubation."[8]

Cuffed SGAs were initially described in the early part of the 20th century. Three factors led to the development of these devices: the introduction of cyclopropane (which was explosive and required an airtight circuit for appropriate gas containment), the fact that blind and laryngoscopic-guided tracheal intubation remained a difficult task, and a recognized need for protection of the lower airway from blood and surgical debris in the upper airway.[6] The Primrose cuffed oropharyngeal tube, the Shipway airway (a Gudel oropharyngeal airway fitted with a cuff, and a circuit connector designed by Sir Ivan MaGill) and the Lessinger airway were predecessors of the modern supraglottic devices. In 1937 Leech introduced a "pharyngeal bulb gasway" with a noninflatable cuff that fit snuggly into the hypopharynx.

The use of SGAs remained dominant until the introduction of curare in 1942, and the mass training of anesthesiologists in tracheal intubation in anticipation of casualties during World War II. The description by Mendelson[9] of gastric contents aspiration in obstetric cases (66 of 44,016 patients, with 2 deaths) further pushed the move toward tracheal intubation in most surgical procedures. Within a few years, proficiency in direct laryngoscopy and tracheal intubation became a mark of professionalism. The advent of succinylcholine (1951) furthered the dominance of tracheal intubation through providing rapid and profound muscle relaxation.

By 1981, two types of airway management prevailed: tracheal intubation or the anesthesia face-mask/Gudel airway. Although both were time-tested, each had its failings (apart from airway failure in a small number of patients). Tracheal intubation was associated with both dental and soft tissue injury and cardiovascular stimulation, and mask ventilation often required a hands-on-the-airway technique. These difficulties led to the reconsideration of SGAs.

Limitations of Patient History and Physical Examination

❸ A thorough airway-relevant history must be obtained during the preoperative evaluation. A search for documentation to confirm or dismiss manifest problems should be conducted. Signs and symptoms related to the airway should be sought. (Table 29-2). Many congenital and acquired syndromes are associated with difficult airway management (Table 29-3).

Over the last 2 decades, several physical evaluation measures have become popularized, although their reproducibility and predictability are disputed. The difficulty in developing the perfect airway evaluation tool lies in two interrelated areas: simplicity and interdependency. Simple bedside evaluation tools are useful, but adequate evaluation may require endoscopic, radiologic, or other currently uncommon examinations.[10,11] Interdependency refers to the predictive value of one airway examination measure based on the findings of another. This is discussed later in "Direct Laryngoscopy," under the topic of functional airway assessment (FAA). Details of the various examinations and their interdependency are discussed in that section.

Historically, airway assessment has been synonymous with evaluation for the ease of direct laryngoscopy (DL), the end point being the anticipated degree of visualization of the larynx. Unfortunately, these efforts have been only modestly successful. Shiga et al.[12] performed a meta-analysis of studies of the physical predictors of difficult DL. These authors concluded that, when used as individual test, currently used techniques of evaluation have only modest discriminative power (Tables 29-4 and 29-5).

Despite the disappointing usefulness of these individual indexes in identifying the difficult to intubate patient (by DL), other authors have recognized that combinations of tests can provide improved predictability. El-Ganzouri et al.[13] designed a statistical model for stratifying risk of difficult DL in a large population. This multivariate index assigned relative weights to each physical examination or historical finding based on the odds of a high-grade laryngeal view being achieved on DL with an increasing examination score. The authors noted that with increasing multivariate index scores, positive predictive value increased, but sensitivity decreased (i.e., higher multivariate index scores occur when there are more positive physical findings, but not all difficult laryngoscopy patients will manifest multiple findings). Compared with the Mallampati classification alone, the multivariate composite index had improved positive predictive and specificity values at equal sensitivity. Of course, some pathology will only present on the induction of anesthesia and/or attempts at laryngoscopy.[14,15] Other groups have used similar regimens to increase the predictability of multivariate indexes by incorporating imaging technologies.[16] In a small population of patients, Naguib

TABLE 29-2

SIGNS, SYMPTOMS AND DISORDERS WITH AIRWAY MANAGEMENT IMPLICATIONS

History related to airways problem
  Aspiration risk

- History of voice changes
- History of vocal cord polyps
- History of frequent pneumonias
- Coughing after eating/drinking
- Acute narcotic therapy
- Acute trauma
- Intensive care unit admission (current)
- Pregnancy (gestational age ≥12 weeks)
- Immediate postpartum (before second postpartum day)
- Systemic disease associated gastroparesis: diabetes mellitus, postvagotomy, collagen vascular disease, Parkinson disease, thyroid dysfunction, liver disease, CNS tumors, chronic renal insufficiency

Difficult laryngoscopy/S6A ventilation

- History of surgical manipulation in or around the airway
- History of radiation therapy of the head/neck
- Various congenital and acquired syndromes (Table 29-3)

Obstructive sleep apnea

- Body mass index >35 kg/m² (indicative)
- Loud snoring
- Pauses in breathing during normal sleep
- Sleep interruption (with choking)
- Daytime somnolence/napping
- Airway affecting craniofacial abnormalities

Lingual tonsil hyperplasia/supraglottic cyst or tumors

- Chronic sore throat
- Globus sensation
- Voice change
- Dysphagia
- Obstructive sleep apnea
- History of tonsillectomy (controversial)[10]

Thyroglossal duct cyst

- Asymptomatic anterior cervical mass that moves with deglutination
- Complications: cysts infection, fistula, spontaneous rupture, voice change, dysphagia, dyspnea, and snoring

Signs and symptoms related to the airway

- Snoring
- Changes in voice
- Dysphagia
- Stridor
- Bleeding
- Cervical spine pain or limited range of motion
- Upper extremity neuropathy
- Temporomandibular joint pain or dysfunction

Sequelae of previous intubation

- Chipped teeth
- Significant prolonged sore throat/mandible after a previous anesthetic

et al.[16] were able to achieve high predictive accuracy (90% or higher) when physical examination and imaging scores were weighted.

More recently some authors have argued against the efforts to devise methods to predict the ease or difficulty of DL, recognizing that the perfect test is elusive. Because all tests are likely to over- and/or underpredict the ease or difficulty of laryngoscopy in some patients, and because impossible intubation is relatively rare, the utility of these examinations is questioned. Similarly, because of the proliferation of new devices for supraglottic ventilation and tracheal intubation, the relevance of a predicted DL is questioned.[3]

Few studies have objectively determined those findings that identify the difficult-to-mask ventilate patient. This basic airway maneuver was examined in a control study by Langeron et al.[17] Of 1,502 patients (excluding planned rapid-sequence induction or emergency cases), 5% of patients were characterized as difficult to mask ventilate. Only one patient in the series was impossible to ventilate by face mask. Table 29-6 describes the criteria for defining difficult mask ventilation and the five independent clinical predictors found by Langeron et al.[17] The presence of two predictors indicted a high likelihood of difficult mask ventilation. Kheterpal et al.,[18] investigating 22,660 patients and using different criteria, found a difficult-to-mask ventilate incidence of 1.5%. In addition to the criteria used by Langeron et al., these authors found that a finding of a high Mallampati score and poor mandibular protrusion improved the prediction of difficult mask ventilation.

In general, tracheal intubation should be considered nonroutine under the following conditions: (1) the presence of equally important priorities to the management of the airway (such as "full stomach," "open globe"), (2) abnormal airway anatomy, (3) an emergency, or (4) direct injury to the upper airway and larynx and/or trachea. Although the finding of abnormal anatomy is not necessarily synonymous with the difficult airway, it should kindle a heightened level of suspicion. Several investigators have identified anatomic features as having unfavorable influences on the mechanics of DL; these are explainable on the basis of inability to create a line of site from the operator's eye to the aperture of the larynx.

Predicting difficulty in DL remains, in a large part, an enigma. As previously illustrated, the commonly used indexes may not only be less predictive than originally thought, but may be misleading. The advent of video laryngoscopy (discussed later) may make these deficits irrelevant; new criteria will need to be written.

CLINICAL MANAGEMENT OF THE AIRWAY

Preoxygenation

Preoxygenation (also commonly termed *denitrogenation*) should be practiced in all cases when time permits.[19] This procedure entails the replacement of the nitrogen volume of the lung (upward of 69% of the functional residual capacity) with oxygen in order to provide a reservoir for diffusion into the alveolar capillary blood after the onset of apnea. Preoxygenation with 100% O_2 via a tight-fitting face mask for 5 minutes in a spontaneously breathing patient can furnish up to 10 minutes of oxygen reserve following apnea (in a patient without significant cardiopulmonary disease and a normal oxygen consumption). In one study of healthy, nonobese patients who were allowed to breathe 100% O_2 preoperatively, subjects sustained an oxygen saturation of >90% for 6 ± 0.5 minutes, whereas obese patients experienced oxyhemoglobin desaturation to <90% in 2.7 ± 0.25 minutes.[20] Under ideal conditions, the patient breathing room air ($FIO_2 = 0.21$) will

ANESTHETIC MANAGEMENT

TABLE 29-3

SYNDROMES ASSOCIATED WITH DIFFICULT AIRWAY MANAGEMENT

■ PATHOLOGIC CONDITION	■ PRINCIPAL PATHOLOGIC CLINICAL FEATURES PERTAINING TO AIRWAY
CONGENITAL	
Pierre Robin syndrome	Micrognathia, macroglossia, glossoptosis, cleft soft palate
Treacher Collins syndrome	Auricular and ocular defects; malar and mandibular hypoplasia, microstomia, choanal atresia
Goldenhar syndrome	Auricular and ocular defects; malar and mandibular hypoplasia; occipitalization of atlas
Down syndrome	Poorly developed or absent bridge of the nose; macroglossia, microcephaly, cervical spine abnormalities
Klippel-Feil syndrome	Congenital fusion of a variable number of cervical vertebrae; restriction of neck movement
Alpert syndrome	Maxillary hypoplasia, prognathism, cleft soft palate, tracheobronchial cartilaginous anomalies
Beckwith syndrome	Macroglossia
Cherubism	Tumorous lesion of mandibles and maxillae with intraoral masses
Cretinism	Absent thyroid tissue or defective synthesis of thyroxine; macroglossia, goiter, compression of trachea, deviation of larynx/trachea
Cri du chat syndrome	Chromosome 5-P abnormal; microcephaly, micrognathia, laryngomalacia, stridor
Meckel syndrome	Microcephaly, micrognathia, cleft epiglottis
von Recklinghausen disease	Increased incidence of pheochromocytoma; tumors may occur in the larynx and right ventricle outflow tract
Hurler/Hunter syndrome	Stiff joints, upper airway obstruction due to infiltration of lymphoid tissue; abnormal tracheobronchial cartilages
Pompe disease	Muscle deposits, macroglossia
ACQUIRED	
Infections	
Supraglottitis	Laryngeal edema
Croup	Laryngeal edema
Abscess (intraoral, retropharyngeal)	Distortion and stenosis of the airway and trismus
Papillomatosis	Chronic viral infection forming obstructive papillomas
Ludwig angina	Distortion and stenosis of the airway and trismus
Arthritis	
Rheumatoid arthritis	Temporomandibular joint ankylosis, cricoarytenoid arthritis, deviation of larynx, restricted mobility of cervical spine
Ankylosing spondylitis	Ankylosis of cervical spine; less commonly ankylosis of temporomandibular joints; lack of mobility of cervical spine
Benign tumors	
Cystic hygroma, lipoma, adenoma, goiter	
Stenosis or distortion of the airway	
Malignant tumors	
Carcinoma of tongue/larynx/thyroid	Stenosis or distortion of the airway; fixation of larynx or adjacent tissues (e.g, infiltration or fibrosis from irradiation)
Trauma	
Head/facial/cervical spine	Cerebrospinal rhinorrhea, edema of the airway; hemorrhage; unstable fracture(s) of the maxillae and mandible; intralaryngeal damage
Miscellaneous conditions	
Morbid obesity	Short, thick neck and large tongue are likely to be present
Acromegaly	Macroglossia; prognathism
Acute burns	Edema of airway

TABLE 29-4

SUMMARY OF POOLED SENSITIVITY AND SPECIFICITY OF COMMONLY USED METHODS OF AIRWAY EVALUATION

■ EXAMINATION	■ SENSITIVITY (%)	■ SPECIFICITY (%)
Mallampiti classification	49	86
Thyromental distance	20	94
Sternomental distance	62	82
Mouth opening	46	89

Data derived from ref. 12.

TABLE 29-5

TECHNIQUES OF COMMON AIRWAY INDEXES MEASUREMENT

Thyromental distance: Measured along a straight line from tip of mentum to thyroid notch in neck-extended position

Mouth opening: Interincisor distance (or interalveolus distance when edentulous) with the mouth fully opened[13]

Mallampati score (see legend, Fig. 29-7)

Head and neck movement: The range of motion from full extension to full flexion[14]

Ability to prognath: Capacity to bring the lower incisors in front of the upper incisors[13]

experience oxyhemoglobin desaturation to a level of <90% after approximately 2 minutes of apnea. Patients in respiratory failure, or with conditions affecting metabolism or lung volumes, frequently evidence desaturation sooner, owing to increased O_2 extraction, decreased functional residual capacity, or right-to-left transpulmonary shunting. The most common reason for not achieving a maximum alveolar oxygen store during preoxygenation is a loose-fitting mask, allowing the entrainment of room air.[19]

Less time-consuming methods of preoxygenation have also been described. Using a series of four vital capacity breaths of 100% O_2 over a 30-second period, a high arterial PaO_2 (339 mm Hg) can be achieved, but the time to desaturation is consistently shorter as compared with traditional techniques.[19,21] A modified vital capacity technique, wherein the patient is asked to take eight deep breaths in a 60-second period, shows promise in terms of prolonging the time to desaturation.[19,21] The authors of the current chapter prefer the technique of applying a tight-fitting mask for 5 minutes or more of tidal volume breathing; the mask is placed immediately after the patient has been made comfortable on the operating room table, and remains in place during intravenous catheter insertion and the application of monitors. Pharyngeal insufflation of has been described to prolong the duration of oxyhemoglobin saturation (>90%) sustained during apnea. In this technique, oxygen is insufflated at a rate of 3 liters per minute via a catheter passed through the nares.[22] This technique relies on the phenomenon of apneic oxygenation, a process by which

TABLE 29-6

ASSESSMENT AND PREDICTABILITY OF DIFFICULT MASK VENTILATION[17]

Criteria for difficult mask ventilation

Inability for one anesthesiologist to maintain oxygen saturation >92%

Significant gas leak around face mask

Need for ≥4 Lites per minute gas flow (or use of fresh gas flow button more than twice)

No chest movement

Two-handed mask ventilation needed

Change of operator required

Independent risk factors for difficult mask ventilation	Odds ratio
Presence of a beard	3.18
Body mass index >26 ng/m²	2.75
Lack of teeth	2.28
Age >55 years	2.26
History of snoring	1.84

gases are entrained into the alveolar space during apnea, as long as there is a patent airway. In the obese patient, bilevel positive airway pressure as well as head-up position (approximately 25 degrees) has been advocated to both reach maximal preinduction arterial oxygenation and to delay oxyhemoglobin desaturation.[23,24] Surprisingly, the head-up position may not improve the efficacy of preoxygenation in the pregnant patient.[25]

Some circumstances can serve to decrease the effectiveness of preoxygenation. For example, the patient who experiences claustrophobia with the anesthesia face mask (which can almost always be overcome by patients holding the mask themselves) or the use of self-inflating breathing bags (which do not deliver an FIO_2 of 100% during spontaneous breathing) can decrease effectiveness of preoxygenation. Likewise, leaks between the face mask and patient's facial contours allow entrainment of air, thereby reducing the FIO_2. Leaks as small as 4 mm (cross-sectional) can cause significant reductions in the inspired oxygen content.[26]

Support of the Airway with the Induction of Anesthesia

With the induction of anesthesia and the onset of apnea, ventilation and oxygenation are supported by the anesthesiologist. Traditional methods include the anesthesia face mask, and the ETT. During the last 2 decades several SGA devices have been introduced into worldwide clinical practice. Of these, the laryngeal mask airway (LMA) has gained significant acceptance among anesthesiologists in the United States, with use rates as high as 35% of all general anesthesia cases in some settings.[27] These and more recently introduced SGAs, which have gained popularity in the United States, will also be discussed.

The Anesthesia Face Mask

The anesthesia face mask is the device most commonly used to deliver anesthetic gases and oxygen as well as to ventilate the patient who has been made apneic. The skillful use of a face mask may be challenging and, despite the many advances in airway management, remains a mainstay in the delivery of anesthesia and in resuscitation. When the induction of anesthesia is initiated, the patient's level of consciousness changes from the awake state, with a competent and protected airway, to the unconscious state, with an unprotected and potentially obstructed airway. This drug-induced central ventilatory drive and depression and relaxation of the musculature of the upper airway can rapidly lead to hypercapnia and hypoxia. Face mask ventilation is minimally invasive, virtually universal, and requires the least sophisticated equipment, thus making it critical to management of the airway.

The mask is gently held on the patient's face with the left hand, leaving the right hand free for other tasks (Fig. 29-2). Air leak around the edges of the mask is prevented by downward pressure. Most modern masks can be distorted by the operator's fingers in order to seal around the facial contours. Elastic "mask straps" may be used to help secure the mask in the awake or anesthetized patient who is breathing spontaneously and without obstruction, or to complement the left-hand grip. The mask straps can be particularly helpful for the clinician with short fingers. However, prolonged use of tight-fitting mask straps has been associated with motor and sensory neuropraxias. During a preoxygenation phase of anesthetic induction, gas leaks must be avoided; during inspiration, the patient may entrain air, limiting the efficacy of the preoxygenation maneuver.

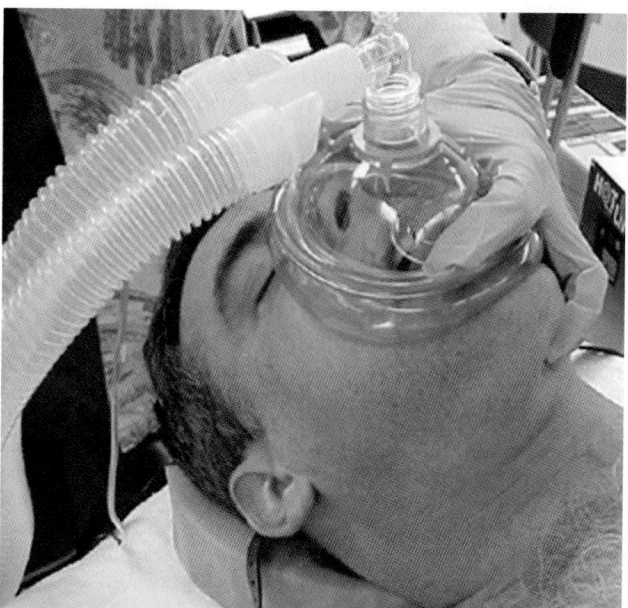

FIGURE 29-2. Holding the anesthesia mask on the face. The thumb and the first finger grip the mask in such a fashion that the anesthesia circuit (or Ambu bag) connection abuts the web between these digits. This allows the palm of the hand to apply pressure to the left side of the mask, while the tips of these three digits apply pressure over the right. The third finger helps to secure under the mentum, and the forth finger is under the angle of the mandible or along the lower mandibular ridge. Mask straps (on pillow) may be used to complement the hand grip by securing the right side of the mask.

In preparation for using the face mask for positive pressure ventilation (once apnea is induced), appropriate positioning of the patient is paramount. With the patient in the supine position, the head and neck are placed in the *sniffing* position, which is discussed extensively later. This position improves mask ventilation by anteriorizing the base of the tongue and the epiglottis. This has been demonstrated in endoscopic studies in anesthetized patients.[28]

After induction of anesthesia, a tight fit of the face mask is achieved by downward displacement of the mask between the thumb and first finger with concurrent upward displacement of the mandible with the remaining fingers. This latter maneuver, commonly known as a *jaw thrust*, raises the soft tissues of the anterior airway off the pharyngeal wall and allows for improved ventilation. In those patients who are obese, edentulous, or bearded, two hands or a mask strap may be required to ensure a tight-fitting mask seal. When two hands are required for holding the face mask, a second operator obviously will be required in order to ventilate the patient. If necessary, the second operator can lend a third hand to the mask fitting, providing for both jaw-thrust and chin lift.

One useful, albeit poorly characterized, maneuver that can aid in face mask ventilation is the *expiratory chin drop*. When positive pressure inspiration is successful, but is not followed by passive gas escape during expiration, allowing phasic head flexion and reducing chin/jaw lifting will often improve gas egress.

When a patient has presented with removable dentures, leaving the prosthetics in place can aid face mask ventilation.[29]

The patient with normal lung compliance should require no more than 20 to 25 cm H_2O pressure to inflate the lungs. If more pressure than this is required, the clinician should re-evaluate the adequacy of the airway, adjust the mask fit, seek the aid of a second operator in order to perform two- or three-handed mask holds, and/or consider other devices that aid in the creation of a open passage for air flow through the upper airway. Both rigid oral airways and soft nasal airways create an artificial passage to the hypopharynx. A variety of oral and nasal airways are available, but will not be discussed in detail. Nasal airways are less likely to stimulate cough, gag, or vomiting in the lightly anesthetized patient, but the risk of epistasis must always be weighted (especially in the anticoagulated patient). The nasal airway is inserted along the floor of the nose, in a directly anterior-posterior direction, and should always be lubricated. The turbinates of the lateral nasal cavity are avoided. Resistance to insertion should prompt repositioning of the airway bevel, reassessment of the direction of insertion forces, or change to the contralateral naris. The airway should be long enough to reach from the naris to the thyroid notch when placed alongside the face of the patient. Oral airways should likewise reach from the teeth (or alveolar ridge) to the mandibular angle. The typical rounded oral airway is placed with its longitudinal concavity rotated in a rostrad direction. Once the distal end of the airway has been inserted to the level of the oropharynx, the device is rotated 180 degrees as insertion continues, to reach its ultimate position. This maneuver avoids displacement of the tongue into the hypopharynx. A small oral aperture, an intrapharyngeal mass or foreign body, or light anesthesia may prevent its placement. As will be discussed later, some intubating oral airways are large and have a rectangular cross-section. These tend to be too large for intraoral rotation. They are inserted with the concavity facing caudad while the tongue is stabilized by a tongue depressor or held by the operator.

Obstruction to mask ventilation may be caused by laryngospasm, a reflex closure of the vocal folds. Laryngospasm occurs from local stimulation by a foreign body (e.g., oral or nasal airway), saliva, blood, or vomitus touching the glottis, or even a light plane of anesthesia. Hypoxia as well as noncardiogenic pulmonary edema can result if there is continued spontaneous ventilation against closed vocal cords (or other obstruction). Treatment of laryngospasm includes removal of an offending stimulus (if it can be identified), continuous positive airway pressure, deepening of the anesthetic state, and the use of a rapid-acting muscle relaxant.

If there are no contraindications (e.g., a full stomach or other aspiration risk), mask ventilation can be the technique employed for the duration of anesthesia maintenance. Otherwise, it is commonly used to administer anesthetic gases until the anesthetic state is adequate for use of another means of airway support (e.g., SGA, ETT). This decision is made after careful consideration of the patient's coexisting diseases and surgical requirements.

Supraglottic Airways

The LMA ushered in the first major use of SGAs in the United States. But by the time of its initial introduction in 1989 and approval by the U.S. Food and Drug Administration in 1991, it was being used in more than 500 hospitals in the United Kingdom. Although initially approved for use as a substitute for face mask ventilation, and when tracheal intubation was not achievable, it soon enjoyed wide use in surgical cases traditionally managed with tracheal intubation.[27]

Though other SGAs were available in the early 1990s (e.g., COPA, Mallinckrodt Medical, Athlone, Ireland), it was not until the patent of the original LMA design expired in 2002 that there was a proliferation of similar devices. A wealth of information exists on the LMA and its subsequent iterations (all by the original inventor, Dr. Archie Brain). Much of this knowledge may be applied to newer devices. This chapter will devote considerable text to the family of LMAs. This is not meant to infer preference, but rather the availability of information.

5 The advent of the LMA as well as other SGAs has led some to question the relative safety of tracheal intubation.[30] A recent study by Tanaka et al.[31] demonstrated vocal cord edema and increased airflow resistance in patients undergoing minor surgery with an ETT. These changes were not seen with LMA use. This, along with the ASA closed claims database information, lends support to the search for safe alternatives to tracheal intubation whenever possible.[32] Similarly, pharyngeal mucosal (traumatic) changes, as a result of SGA use appear to be markedly delayed when compared with the affects of the ETT in the trachea. In one animal study, mucosal injury from the LMA ProSeal (The Laryngeal Mask Company, Jersey, UK) did not occur until more than 9 hours of continuous use.[33]

The LMA Classic. The LMA is composed of a small "mask" designed to sit in the hypopharynx, with an anterior surface aperture overlying the laryngeal inlet (Fig. 29-3). The rim of the mask is composed of an inflatable silicone cuff that fills the hypopharyngeal space, creating a seal that allows positive pressure ventilation with up to 20 cm H_2O pressure. The adequacy of the seal depends on correct placement and appropriate size. It is less dependent on the cuff filling pressure or volume. Attached to the posterior surface of the mask is a barrel (airway tube) that extends from the mask's central aperture through the mouth and can be connected to a self-inflating resuscitation bag or anesthesia circuit.

LMA size selection is critical to its successful use, and to the avoidance of minor as well as more significant complications. Neonatal to large adult sizes are available. The manufacturer recommends that the clinician choose the largest size that will fit comfortably in the oral cavity, then inflate to the minimum pressure that allows ventilation to 20 cm H_2O without an air leak. The intracuff pressure should never exceed 60 cm H_2O (and should be periodically monitored if nitrous oxide is used

as part of the anesthetic). When an adequate seal cannot be obtained with 60 cm H_2O cuff pressure, the LMA may be malpositioned and/or sizing should be re-evaluated. Light anesthesia may also contribute to poor seal or partial or complete laryngospasm.

The insertion of the LMA as described by its inventor, Dr. Archie J. I. Brain, has been modified by a number of writers. Discussion of these various alternatives is beyond the scope of this text. In order to understand the insertion technique, we review the processes of deglutination, which the procedure mimics: lubrication with saliva; formation of a flat oval food bolus by the tongue; initiation of the swallowing reflex by stimulation of the palate; upward pressure by the tongue flattening the food bolus against the palate; directing of the food bolus toward the posterior pharyngeal wall and into the hypopharynx by the shape of the palate and pharyngeal wall; head extension and neck flexion, which enlarges the space behind the larynx to allow passage of the food bolus into the hypopharynx; and finally, opening of the upper esophageal sphincter to allow esophageal entry of the food bolus. These functions allow the food bolus to reach its mark blindly, while avoiding the anterior pharyngeal structures and avoiding reflex responses meant to protect the airway.

The currently recommended insertion technique is illustrated in Figure 29-4, and has 98% success rate. In this technique the mask is lubricated with a nonsilicone, non-local anesthetic–containing lubricant (simulating the saliva), and is fully deflated to form a thin, flat wedge shape (masticated food bolus). The operator's nondominant hand is placed under the occiput to flex the neck on the thorax and extend the head at the atlanto-occipital joint (creating a space behind the larynx; this action also tends to open the mouth).[34] The index finger of the dominant hand is placed in the cleft between the mask and barrel. The hard palate is visualized and the superior (nonaperture) surface of the mask is placed against it. Force is applied by the index finger in an upward direction toward the top of the patient's head. This will cause the mask to flatten out against the palate and follow the shape of the palate as it slides into the pharynx and hypopharynx. The index finger continues along this arc, continually applying an outward pressure until the resistance of the upper esophageal sphincter is met. The most common error made by clinicians is applying pressure with a posterior vector. This tends to catch the tip of the LMA on the posterior pharyngeal wall, causing folding with resultant misplacement and trauma.

Once insertion is complete, removal of the inserting hand is facilitated by gentle stabilization of the LMA barrel with the nondominant hand. Prior to attachment of the anesthesia circuit, the LMA is inflated with the minimum amount of gas to form an effective seal. Sixty centimeters of H_2O pressure is the maximum suggested pilot valve pressure. Accompanying the inflation, one should be able to observe a rising of the cricoid and thyroid cartilage and lifting of the barrel out of the mouth by approximately 1 cm as the mask is lifted off the upper esophageal sphincter. If a midline position is not possible owing to the nature of the patient position or surgical procedure, a flexible LMA (discussed later) should be considered. A bite block is recommend to prevent biting and occlusion of the LMA barrel.

Although the distal tip of the LMA mask sits in the esophageal inlet, it does not reliably seal it. The LMA was not designed to protect against the aspiration of gastric contents. Despite this, when used in patients at low risk for regurgitation, the rate of aspiration during LMA use is similar to that in all non-LMA general anesthetics (approximately 2 in 10,000 cases), although the incidence of gastroesophageal reflux may be increased when compared with use of the face mask.[35]

If regurgitated gastric contents are noted in the LMA barrel, maneuvers similar to those applied when using an ETT

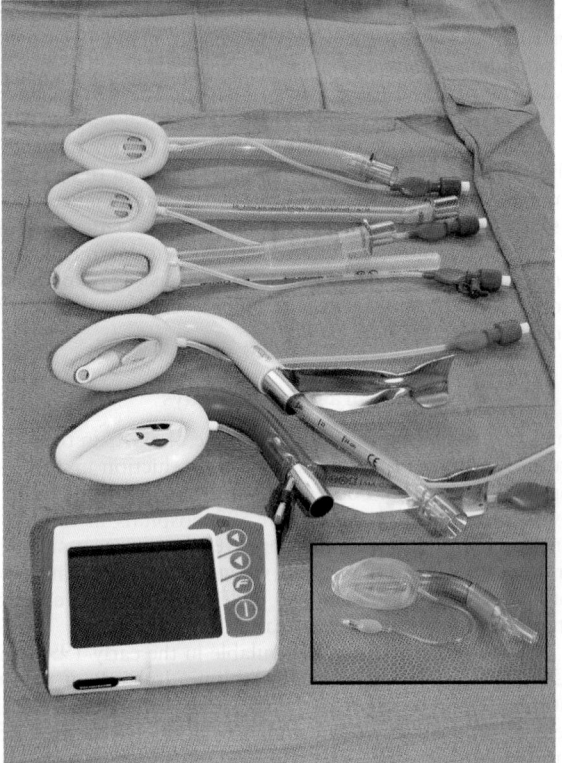

FIGURE 29-3. The family of laryngeal mask airways (from top): Classic, Flexible, ProSeal, Fastrach, CTrach with CTrach monitor, and Supreme (inset).

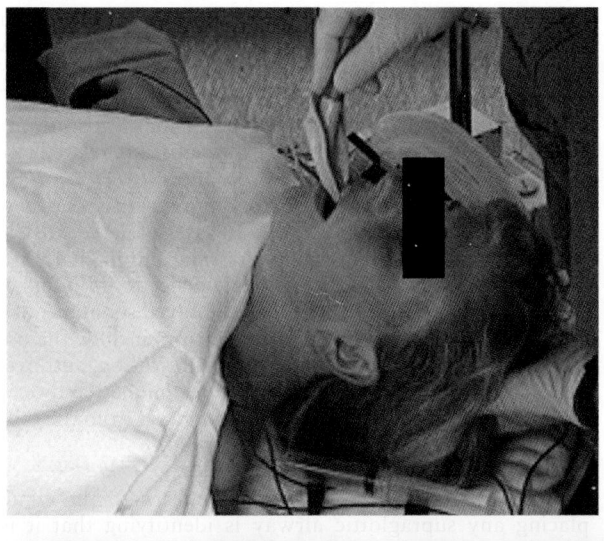
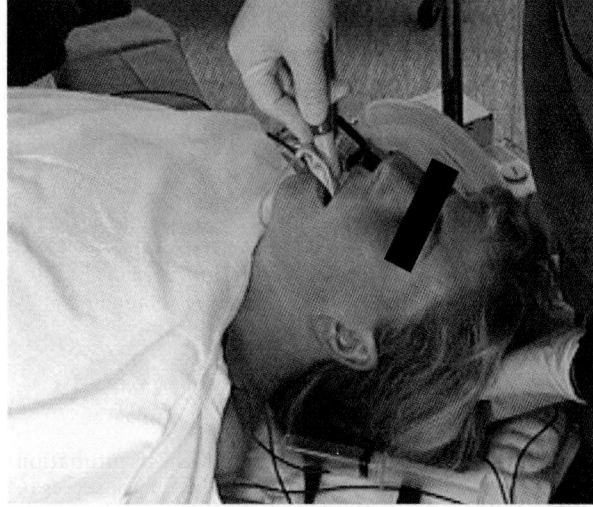
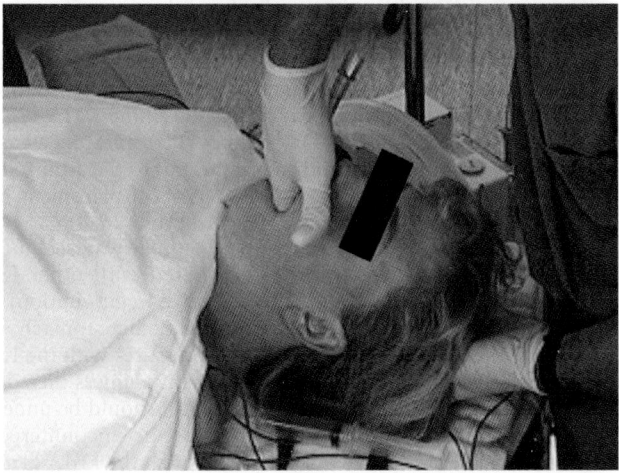
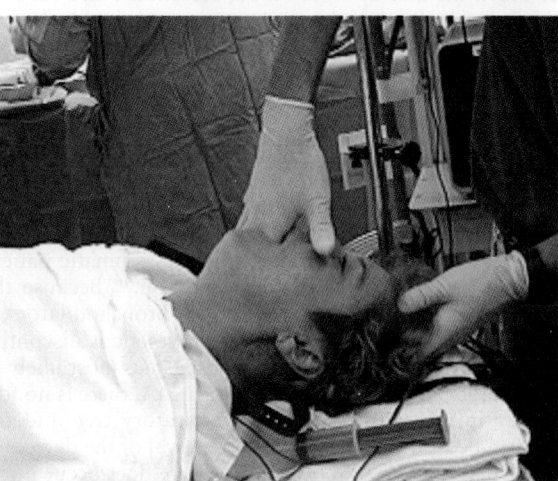

FIGURE 29-4. Insertion of the laryngeal mask airway (LMA). The LMA is inserted with the index finger of the dominant hand pressing with a force vector against the hard palate (**A** and **B**). The outward force vector is continued from the hard palate to the pharynx and hypopharynx (**C**) until the index finger meets resistance against the upper esophageal sphincter (**D**).

should be instituted: Trendelenburg position, administer 100% oxygen, leave the LMA in place and use a flexible suction device down the barrel, and if necessary, deepen the anesthetic.

When populations of patients considered to have a full stomach are studied (in controlled trials, prospective series, or anecdotally), there is a low incidence of aspiration noted with elective or emergency LMA use. Reports have included patients who are morbidly obese or experience frequent gastroesophageal reflux, those undergoing elective cesarean section or airway rescue during labor, and those presenting to emergency departments or paramedic crews.[36,37] During cardiopulmonary resuscitation, the incidence of gastroesophageal regurgitation is 4 times greater with a bag-valve mask than with the LMA.[38]

Although first introduced for use with spontaneous ventilation, the LMA has proved useful for cases in which positive-pressure ventilation is either desired or preferred.[39] Contrary to initial impression, positive-pressure ventilation can be safely accomplished with the LMA.[40,41] There is no difference found in gastric inflation with positive pressure (<17 cm H_2O) when comparing the LMA and the ETT.[42] When using the LMA, one should limit tidal volumes to 8 mL/kg and airway pressure to 20 cm H_2O. LMA use has been described with the supine,

prone, lateral, oblique, Trendelenburg, and lithotomy positions. Although the manufacturer recommends use for a maximum of 2 to 3 hours, reports of use lasting >24 hours can be found.[43]

The LMA Flexible. The introduction of the LMA Flexible (The Laryngeal Mask Company, Jersey, UK) (Fig. 29-3) has permitted extension of LMA use to a variety of cases in which the airway is shared with the surgical team (e.g., otolaryngologic surgery), or otherwise within the surgical field (e.g., ophthalmologic surgery.) The LMA Flexible differs from the original design by virtue of a thin-walled, small-diameter, wire-reinforced (kink-resistant) barrel, which can be positioned out of the midline without affecting the hypopharyngeal position of the mask. It was designed to be used with a tonsillar mouth gag employed in surgery on the mouth and pharynx.[44] The LMA Flexible has also proved useful when heavy drapes are placed over the head and airway (e.g., mastoidectomy, ophthalmic procedures), when there is movement of the head position during surgery (e.g., tympanostomy tubes), or when the LMA barrel cannot be secured in the midline (e.g., mid or lateral facial surgery). The use of this mask in surgery above the level of the hypopharynx, including tonsillectomy, affords a number of

Improved protection of the airway from blood and surgical debris
Reduced cardiovascular responses
Reduced coughing on emergence
Reduced laryngospasm after airway device removal
Improved oxygen saturation after airway device removal
Ability to administer oxygen until complete restoration of airway reflexes

clinically important advantages over tracheal intubation (Table 29-7). When correctly placed, the LMA mask serves to better block the airway from blood, secretions, and surgical debris above the level of the mask, as compared with the tracheal tube, which is known to not protect the trachea from liquids instilled into the pharynx.[45]

The LMA and Bronchospasm.   As an SGA, the LMA appears to be well suited to the patient with a history of bronchospasm. The LMA presents a unique opportunity for the clinician to conveniently and effectively control the airway without having to introduce a foreign body into the trachea. Thus, it may be an ideal airway tool in the asthmatic patient who is not at risk for reflux and aspiration.[46] Because the halogenated inhaled anesthetics are potent bronchodilators, it is at the time of emergence, when the anesthetic is discontinued, that the patient at risk for bronchospasm is most likely to wheeze. In the patient managed with the LMA, there is no foreign body in the sensitive bronchorespiratory tree and the patient can be fully emerged prior to removal of the device. In the event that uncontrollable bronchospasm does occur intraoperatively (e.g., from vagal stimuli such as traction on the peritoneum), intubation can be performed through the LMA or after its removal. When tracheal intubation is mandatory (for the surgical procedure) yet concerns regarding bronchospasm exist, the Bailey maneuver is employed.[47] In this maneuver, the deflated LMA is placed behind the in situ ETT. The ETT is removed and the LMA is inflated. The patient is then emerged on the LMA.

LMA Removal. Timing of the removal of the LMA at the end of surgery is critical.[47,48] The LMA should be removed either when the patient is deeply anesthetized or after protective reflexes have returned and the patient is able to open the mouth on command. Removal during excitation stages of emergence can be accompanied by coughing and/or laryngospasm. Many clinicians remove the LMA fully inflated; thus, it acts as a "scoop" for secretions above the mask, bringing them out of the airway.[49] This has been particularly useful in otolaryngologic surgery.

Contraindications to LMA Use. The primary contraindication to elective use of the LMA is a risk of gastric-contents aspiration (e.g., full stomach, hiatus hernia with significant gastroesophageal reflux, intestinal obstruction, delayed gastric emptying, poor history). Other contraindications include poor lung compliance or high airway resistance, glottic or subglottic airway obstruction, and limited mouth opening (<1.5 cm).[50]

LMA Use Complications. Apart from gastroesophageal reflux and aspiration, reported complications have included laryngospasm, coughing, gagging, retching, bronchospasm, and

other events characteristic of airway manipulation. The incidence of sore throat is approximately 10%, as compared with 30% with tracheal intubation, but has been reported with a range of 0 to 70%.[6] Also reported are hoarseness (4 to 47%) and dysphagia (4 to 24%). The LMA may cause transient changes in vocal cord function. This is possibly related to cuff overinflation during prolonged procedures.

There have been reports of nerve injury associated with LMA use. As of September 2007, 26 cases of nerve palsy have been reported: recurrent,[12] hypoglossal,[7] and lingual.[7,51] The injuries were first manifest from emergence to 48 hours after surgery. All but one of these injuries resolved spontaneously in 1 hour to 18 months. Predisposing factors include the use of small masks, nitrous oxide, lidocaine lubrication, cuff overinflation, difficult or alternate insertion techniques, and cervical bone or joint disease.[51] Pressure neuropraxia from the tube or cuff is the most common cause.

The LMA ProSeal.   A significant concern to the clinician placing any supraglottic airway is identifying that it is in proper position: the gold standards used to identify tracheal intubation by direct laryngoscopy (visualization of the vocal cords and end-tidal CO_2 detection) do not apply. Poor placement of the LMA has been blamed for gastric fluid aspiration, neuropraxias, and sore throat. In response, the LMA ProSeal was developed in 2001 by Dr. Brain by incorporating a gastric drain passing from the distal end of the cuff to the atmosphere. (Fig. 29-3). Several "tests" of LMA ProSeal placement have been described by Brain and others (Table 29-8).[52–55] The LMA ProSeal also increases the maximum airway seal during positive pressure ventilation as compared with other LMA devices (≥ 40 cm H_2O), and allows passive (regurgitation) and active (gastric tube insertion) emptying of the stomach.[53–55] Despite the ability to use high airway pressures with the LMA ProSeal, the clinician should remember that, unless there is an obvious cause (e.g., obesity) >20 cm H_2O should be unnecessary. When unexpectedly high pressure is encountered, a search for the cause is mandatory. Although the LMA ProSeal is typically inserted with the same method as a classic LMA, a metallic insertion device is available from the manufacturer. The advanced capabilities of the LMA have added to its use in airway resuscitation.[56,57]

Maltby et al.[58] have pioneered the use of the LMA ProSeal during laparoscopic cholecystectomy in obese patients. This surgical procedure has long been considered the prototypical case for contraindicated LMA use because of high intraperitoneal pressures, as well as intraoperative alimentary tract manipulation. Laparoscopic cholecystectomy was performed in 46 patients, 12 of whom had a body mass index of >30 kg/m². The median airway pressure at which a gas leak occurred was 34 cm H_2O (range, 18 to 45). Four obese patients crossed over to a control, tracheal tube group. Stomach size (e.g., distention) was equal between groups.

The Laryngeal Tube.   The Laryngeal Tube (VBM Medizintechnik, GmbH, Sulz, Germany) consists of a single lumen tube with an approximately 130-degree midshaft angle and two (distal and proximal) low-pressure cuffs (Fig. 29-5). An oval aperture between the cuffs serves as a ventilation orifice. The distal cuff encloses the distal end of the tube. When inserted correctly, the proximal cuff seals the oral and nasal pharynx whereas the distal cuff sits within the upper esophageal sphincter. Ventilation (spontaneous or positive pressure) occurs via an anterior surface orifice midway between the cuffs. The cuffs are inflated via a common pilot valve. The original laryngeal tube is available in single-use or reusable models, requires a mouth opening of at least 2.3 cm, and is inserted either blindly or with the aid of a laryngoscope. The Laryngeal Tube Suction is a modification of the Laryngeal Tube, with the addition of a

TABLE 29-8

FEATURES OF THE LARYNGEAL MASK AIRWAY PROSEAL

■ FEATURE	■ CLINICAL IMPACT
Gastric drain	Position confirmation
	Suprasternal notch test[a,52]
	No gas leak via gastric drain[53]
	Successfully passing gastric tube
	Active gastric emptying
	Passive gastric emptying
	Protection from gastric content aspiration
Posterior cuff	Increased seal pressure
Bite block	Prevents patient biting, obstruction
	Position confirmation
	50% or more of the bite block should be within the oral cavity[54]
Wire-reinforced airway barrel	Reduced overall size
	Decreased ability to tracheally intubate
Large barrel/bite block	First insertion less successful than LMA classic
	Confers rotational stability
	Size choice: size down from LMA classic

LMA, laryngeal mask airway.
[a]When a small amount of lubricant is used to occlude the gastric drain, gentle pressure on the suprasternal notch is reflected in movement of the lubricant meniscus.

second lumen for suction and gastric drainage (the orifice of which is at the distal aspect of the esophageal cuff). Six sizes (0 through 5) are suitable for neonates to large adults. Using Laryngeal Tube in children under 10 years old is less effective than the LMA during spontaneous or assisted ventilation and for fiberoptic evaluation of the airway.[59] The Laryngeal Tube is not recommended for children weighing <10 kg because of technical difficulties and inadequate ventilation.

Paramedics working in the operating room found insertion of the LT easy (success with ventilation at first attempt in 31 of 34 patients).[60] Insertion time of the Laryngeal Tube Suction is similar to that of the LMA ProSeal and significantly shorter than the Combitube (discussed later).[61] One study showed that the Laryngeal Tube Suction produced a greater and more sustained hemodynamic and catecholamine stress response than the LMA ProSeal.[62] Gaitini et al.[63] used the Laryngeal Tube in 175 patients presenting for elective surgery. Positive pressure ventilation was successful in 96.6% of cases. Successful ventilation in patients with unexpected difficult airways because of undiagnosed lingual tonsil hyperplasia and morbid obesity were reported.

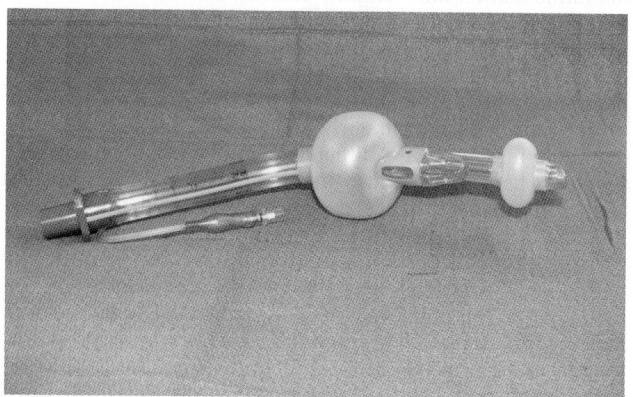

FIGURE 29-5.   The Laryngeal Tube.

The Laryngeal Tube can be used to facilitate fiberoptic tracheal intubation when combined with the Aintree intubation catheter (Cook Critical Care, Bloomington, Indiana). Rotation of Laryngeal Tube and jaw thrust maneuver can improve glottic visualization during this procedure. In one report the Laryngeal Tube was used for fiberoptic-aided intubation in a patient in whom laryngoscopy, conventional fiberoptic intubation, and insertion of an LMA had failed.[64]

A successful use of the Laryngeal Tube Suction was reported in an emergency airway situation in a pregnant woman with history of gastroesophageal reflux who underwent cesarean section but could not be intubated. The device improved oxygen saturation and drained gastric contents during the patient's emergence from rapid-sequence intubation.[65]

A study in 15 fresh cadavers showed that mucosal pressures in lateral pharynx, base of tongue, and posterior pharynx were similar between Laryngeal Tube and LMA ProSeal but pressure on posterior hypopharynx was always higher with the Laryngeal Tube. The investigators expressed concern that pressure from the Laryngeal Tube might impede pharyngeal perfusion more than LMA ProSeal.[66] A case of acute tongue and uvula ulceration after using Laryngeal Tube for hysteroscopy has been reported.[67]

The Cobra.   The Cobra perilaryngeal airway (CobraPLA, Engineered Medical Systems, Indianapolis, IN) is a disposable supralaryngeal airway device. It has a single lumen that terminates in a widened distal end. A pharyngeal cuff serves to occlude the upper airway from the oral cavity, and a series of slots in the widened end hold the epiglottis out of the barrel. A fiberscope and/or ETT may be passed through the barrel and the slots. This technique has been successfully used in patients presenting with difficult intubation/ventilation. Reports have demonstrated the use of the CobraPLA in airway rescue, as well as routine anesthetic care with spontaneous and positive pressure ventilation.[68] Some studies have shown the CobraPLA provides significantly higher airway sealing pressures than the LMA classic as well as a higher first-insertion success rate, although the incidence of blood on the device and sore throat were also higher.[69] Inspiratory tidal volume, expiratory tidal volume, end-tidal CO_2 concentration, and respiratory rate were not different between patients in the LMA and CobraPLA groups.[69]

Cookgas Air-Q Airway. Developed by Dr. Daniel Cook (Cookgas LLC, St Louis, MO), the Air-Q perilaryngeal airway functions as an elective SGA, or as a conduit for blind or fiberoptic-aided intubation of the trachea. The barrel of the airway is precurved and of wide diameter, and will accept a tracheal tube from 5.0 to 8.0 mm internal diameter (ID). The keyhole-shaped airway outlet is designed to steer the ETT toward the larynx. A cuff, grossly the shape of the LMA cuff, seals the perilaryngeal space. The device is inserted (cuff deflated) by a technique similar to that recommended for the LMA (see previous discussion). If, after insertion, the airway is obstructed, an up-down motion of the barrel will often realign the epiglottis. Blind tracheal intubation should be undertaken only if the airway is clear and the patient is muscle-relaxed and/or sufficiently anesthetized. The ETT cuff is completely deflated and lubricated. It is inserted 12 to 15 cm into the device barrel. Advancement past this point will be into the larynx. If resistance is met, the device can be repositioned. Once tracheal intubation is assured, the device can be removed with the help of a specialized stylet marketed by the manufacturer.

Tracheal Intubation

Routine Laryngoscopy. Preparing for Laryngoscopy and the "Best Attempt." Whether laryngoscopy is undertaken with the patient in an awake or unconscious state, repeated attempts at DL often result in trauma to the anterior upper airway structures (e.g., tongue, vallecula, epiglottis, laryngeal structures), potentially hindering subsequent attempts at visualization and causing increased airway obstruction. It is therefore important to assure that the first attempt at laryngoscopy is a "best attempt."

First, when faced with the critically ill patient, the most skilled laryngoscopist available should be positioned to perform the laryngoscopy. In less acute situations, it is not inappropriate for a trainee, clinician extender, or other skilled personnel to assume this role. Second, the availability of all the materials needed to perform laryngoscopy and intubation should be assured, as should the availability of devices needed to manage a failed intubation (Table 29-9).

Other devices that complete the equipment list, but may not be uniformly available, include: end-tidal CO_2 monitoring (e.g., capnography or colorimetric device such as Easy Cap II, Mallinckrodt), pulse oximetry, transtracheal jet ventilation catheter, and a high-pressure oxygen source.

The height of the supine patient's airway should be at the level of the laryngoscopists' xyphoid cartilage, with the bed or operating room table in a nonmovable mode (e.g., wheels locked). The clinician performing the intubation must have unobstructed access to the head.

Direct Laryngoscopy. Successful laryngoscopy involves the distortion of the normal anatomic planes of the upper airway to produce a line of direct visualization from the operator's eye to the larynx; this requires the creation of a new (nonanatomic) visual axis, through maximal alignment of the axes of the oral and pharyngeal cavities, and displacement of the tongue. Unanticipated failure of DL is primarily a problem of tongue displacement (inability to align the axes can be anticipated by physical examination).[11] Some investigators have focused the search for the cause of difficult DL on the relative position of the tongue. Chou and Wu[70] have found that a hypopharyngeal tongue (e.g., the greater mass of the tongue is within the hypopharynx) is accompanied by a cau-

---

TABLE 29-9

EQUIPMENT FOR LARYNGOSCOPY[a]

Oxygen source and self-inflating ventilation bag
(e.g., Ambu bag)
Face mask[b]
Oropharyngeal and nasopharyngeal airways[b]
Tracheal tubes[b]
Tracheal tube stylet
Syringe for tracheal tube cuff inflation
Suction apparatus
Laryngoscope handle (two), tested for working order
and battery freshness
Laryngoscope blades: Common blades include the curved
(Macintosh) and straight (Miller)[b]
Pillow, towel, blanket, or foam for head positioning
Stethoscope

---

[a]Equipment that should be immediately available in the ideal clinical setting.
[b]Presumed size as well as one larger and one smaller should be immediately available.

---

dad larynx, which is in turn determined by measurement of the mandibular hyoid distance (a measure of the cephalocaudad separation of the mandible and hyoid during fetal development). Benumof[71] eloquently explains this finding in terms of ontogeny and the descent of the larynx to create the phonics of the human pharyngeal space (ontogeny recapitulates phylogeny). A long descent of the larynx results in a large part of the tongue being in the hypopharynx. Poor descent of the larynx results in a small thyromental distance and can indicate a difficult DL.

Chou and Wu[72] also noted that the long mandibulohyoid distance can be partly due to a shortened mandibular ramus. A short ramus results in the floor of the mouth being more rostrad and less compliant, and therefore displacement of the tongue is more difficult. If a small thyromental distance as well as a large thyromental distance can both predict difficult laryngoscopy, then how can this measure be useful to the airway evaluator? As pointed out in the ASA Difficult Airway Practice Guidelines, no one measure may be adequate to determine difficulty of DL, and multiple measures must be integrated in order to make sensible airway management decisions.[1] Shiga et al.[12] published a meta-analysis of studies regarding airway physical examination scores, and cautioned on the poor sensitivity and only modest specificity of all routine tests.

Another mandibular dimension that has been examined is the mandibular depth index (the posterior depth of the mandible/mandibular length). Kikkawa et al.[73] have noted that a deep or short mandible (higher index) indicates a large hypopharyngeal tongue, and difficulty with displacement. Although the mandibular hyoid distance and the mandibular depth index are distinct measures, they approach the problem of difficulty with DL similarly: anatomic relationships of the mandible may predict a difficult to displace hypopharyngeal tongue. These authors also highlight that a single measure (e.g., thyromental distance) does not yield enough information to be predictive.

Even though congenital anatomic variation may occur, pathologic variations may mimic the same problem of hypopharyngeal tongue mass: Ovassapian et al.[11] have identified hyperplasia of the lymphoid tissue at the base of the tongue as the principle cause of unanticipated difficult laryngoscopy. Visualization of this tissue is currently the only method of diagnosis and may be done preoperatively. Often, lingual tonsil hyperplasia may be the cause of the difficult DL, but the diagnosis is not made because of the overlying position of the standard direct laryngoscope.

DL requires the creation of a line of site from the operator's eye to the aperture of the larynx. In 1944 Bannister and MacBeth proposed a three-axis model to explain the anatomic relationships involved in this operation. This explanation has been challenged by Adnet et al.,[74] who noted that, whereas extension at the atlanto-occipital joint maximally facilitated an oral cavity/pharyngeal alignment, no significant improvement was achieved with flexion of the cervical spine on the thorax. Chou and Wu[75] refined this approach by noting that laryngeal axis alignment is unnecessary. The end point of the effort to create an in-line space for tracheal intubation is the glottic aperture: alignment of the entire larynx is therefore unnecessary. These authors propose a two-axes/tongue-displacement model. This model does not depend on the alignment of all axes to create an in-line view of the larynx, but rather maximizes the spaces between the alveolar ridge and laryngeal aperture through oropharyngeal alignment and tongue displacement. This concept can be used to not only understand the problems that may hinder DL, but also why common indexes of airway assessment fail in their predictive power. This concept has been described previously and can be viewed as functional airway assessment (FAA).[76]

FAA is a method of examining the functional nature of each of the anatomic correlates of the commonly used assessment indices. FAA places an emphasis on the interdependence of these anatomic characteristics rather than on their individual size or functional integrity. As explained by Chou and Wu,[75] when the head and neck are in the neutral position, the oral and pharyngeal axes are perpendicular to each other. With maximal extension of a normal atlanto-occipital joint, 35 degrees or more of motion is attained (Fig. 29-6). This brings the angle between the oral and pharyngeal axis to 125 degrees. Although an improvement, it is certainly not the 180 degrees required for creation of a line of site to the glottis. A different space must be created. This space is created by displacement of the tongue with the laryngoscope. Although atlanto-occipital extension cannot by itself allow direct laryngeal vision, it does provide anterior displacement of the mass of the tongue and brings up the alveolar ridge into improved position relative to the tongue and larynx. The extension of the atlanto-occipital point also provides an advantage in mouth opening. Calder et al.[34] have shown that the maximal mouth opening is 26% greater in full

atlanto-occipital extension as compared with the neutral head position. Temporal-mandibular jaw function also contributes to the displacement of the tongue away from the required visual axis. Rotation and translation of the temporal-mandibular joint result in a relaxation of the tongue insertion, as well as creation of the aperture width needed for instrumentation.

Using the FAA approach to airway evaluation also helps to explain the value of the popular yet highly criticized Mallampati and thyromental distance indices.[77] These two measures have historically been considered important because they approximate the relative mass of the tongue (Mallampati) and the anterior-posterior borders of space in to which it will be displaced by the laryngoscope (Fig. 29-7). As noted elsewhere, these indices have shown to have poor and/or variable predictive power. Two groups have considered the interrelated nature of these measures in a way that reveals why they perform poorly when considered individually. Ayoub et al.[78] found a high Mallampati score to be predictive of a difficult DL when the thyromental distance was <4 cm. When the thyromental distance was >4 cm, relative tongue size (as determined by the Mallampati classification) was not predictive. Iohom et al.[79] found similar results using a thyromental distance cutoff of 6 cm. The finding that the predictive power of the Mallampati improves when the mandible is short is consistent with the concept of FAA: when the mandibular space is restricted, tongue size is important. When the space is large, a tongue of any nonpathologic size should be accommodated. An exception to this maybe hypopharyngeal tongue, as described by Chou and Wu[70]; although according to those authors, measurement of the mandibular hyoid distance should help in diagnosing this.

As noted above, a common cause of difficulty in DL is a pathologic increase in tongue size. Ovassapian et al.[11] have identified lingual tonsil hyperplasia as the most commonly undiagnosed cause of unanticipated difficult DL. They reviewed the cases of unanticipated difficult DL in their institution from 1999 to 2000. Thirty-three patients were identified. All patients were found to have lingual tonsil hyperplasia on fiberoptic examination (Fig. 29-8).

Devices that aid in placing the patient in a sniffing position have become available. These include the sniff position pillow (Popitz Pillow, Alimed, Dedham, MA), developed by Michael Popitz, and Pi's Pillow (American Eagle Medical, Holbrook, NY), which is comfortable for the awake patient but easily

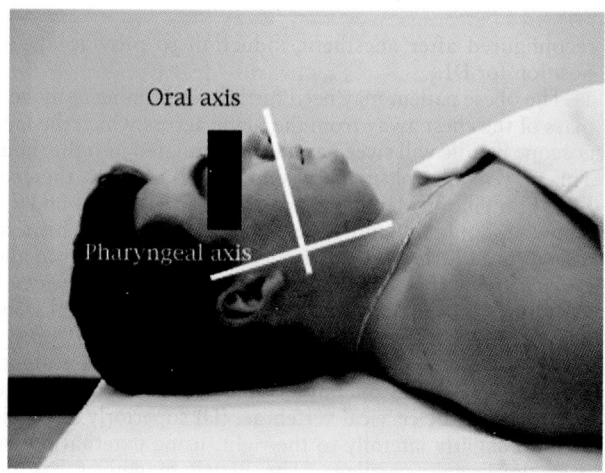
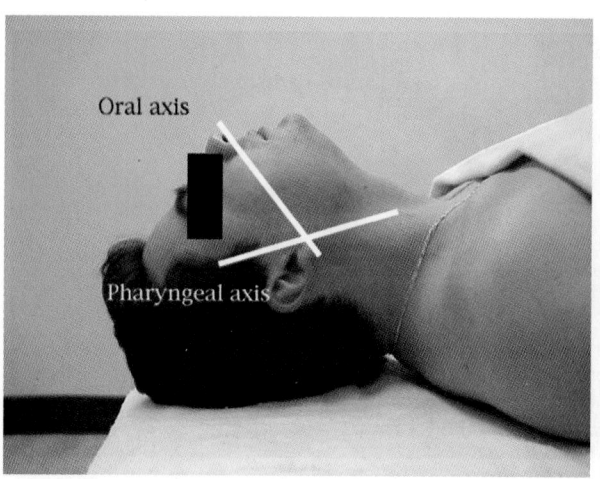

FIGURE 29-6.   A. With the patient supine, the oral and pharyngeal axes do not overlap. **B.** Extension at the atlanto-occipital joint maximally overlaps the oral and pharyngeal axes.

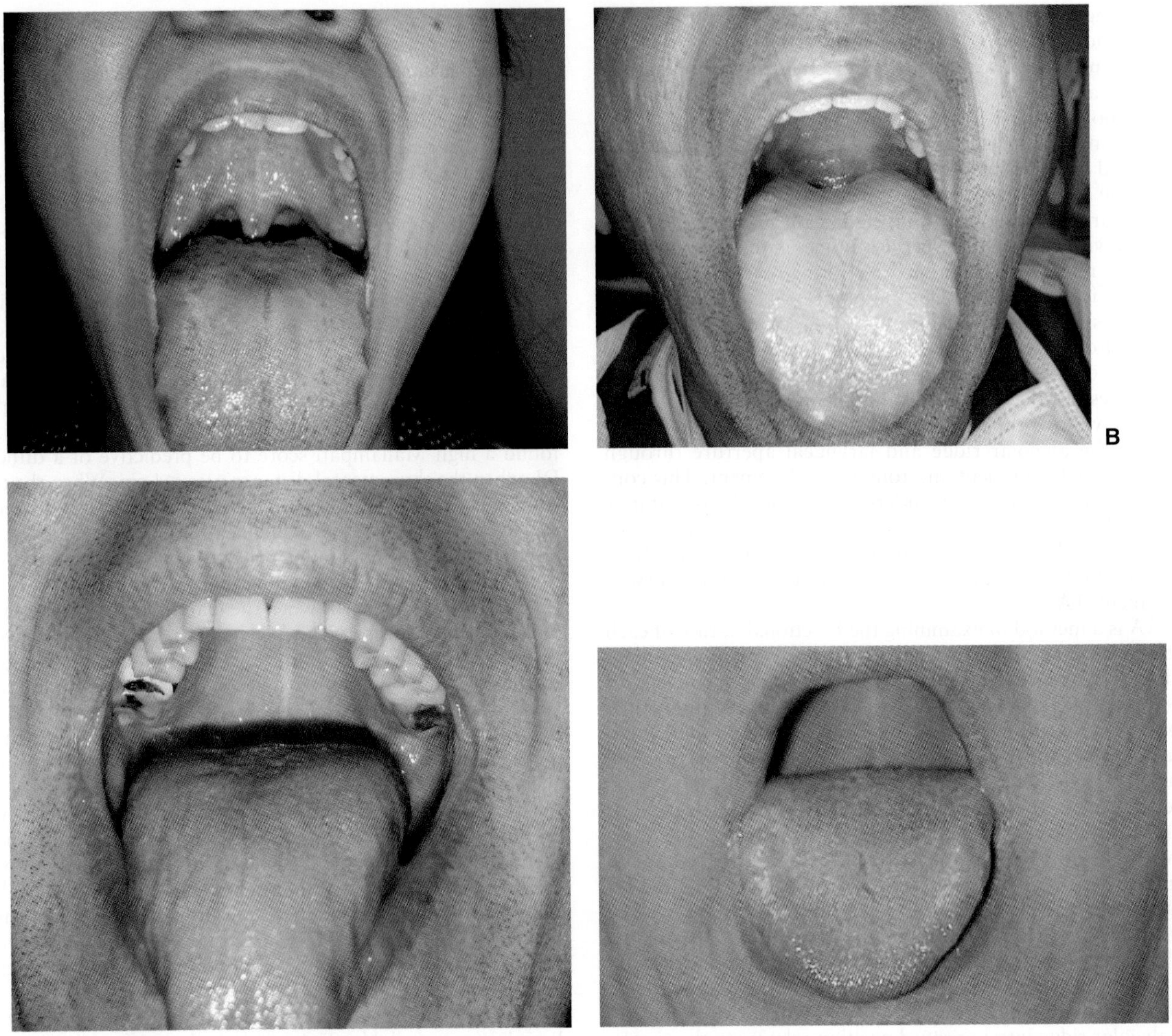

FIGURE 29-7. Mallampati/Samsoon–Young classification of the oropharyngeal view.[77] **A.** Class I: uvula, faucial pillars, soft palate visible. **B.** Class II: faucial pillars, soft palate visible. **C.** Class III: soft and hard palate visible. **D.** Class IV: hard palate visible only (added by Samsoon and Young).

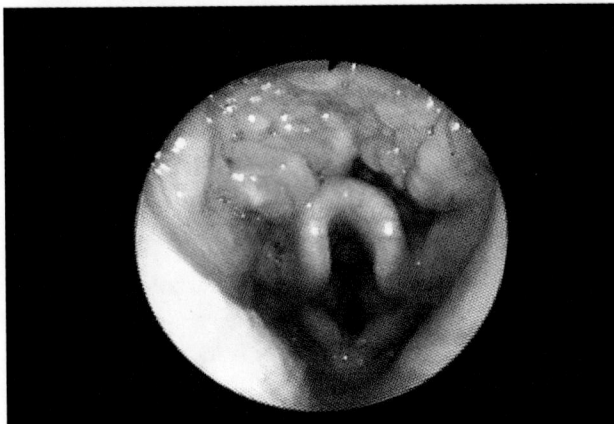

FIGURE 29-8. Lingual tonsil hyperplasia: the vallecula is filled with hyperplastic lymphoid tissue in a patient who had an unanticipated difficult direct laryngoscopy.

reconfigured after anesthetic induction to provide an ideal position for DL.

The obese patient may need further positioning to move the mass of the chest away from the plane across which the laryngoscope handle will sweep as it is manipulated into the mouth. This may require placing a wedge-shaped lift (e.g., the Troop Elevation Pillow, Mercury Medical, Clearwater, FL) under the scapula, shoulders, and nape of neck, raising the head and neck above the thorax and providing a grade in order to allow gravity to pull the pannus' weight away from the airway.

If during the laryngoscopy, a satisfactory laryngeal view is not achieved, the backward-upward-rightward pressure (BURP) maneuver may aid in improving the view. In this maneuver, a second operator displaces the larynx (B) backward against the cervical vertebrae, (U) superiorly as possible and (R) slightly laterally to the right, using external pressure over the cricoid cartilage. The BURP maneuver has been shown to improve the laryngeal view, decreasing the rate of difficult intubation in a study of 1,993 patients from 4.7 to 1.8%.[80] When a left-handed operator is using a left-handed laryngoscope blade, the lateral external pressure should displace the larynx to the left. Similarly, Benumof and Cooper[81] describe "optimal external laryngeal manipulation," which consists of pressing posteriorly and cephalad over the thyroid, hyoid, and cricoid, as improving laryngeal view by at least one Cormack and Lehane grade.[82]

Once alignment has been achieved, the mouth is opened by one of two techniques. The first method accomplishes hyperextension of the atlanto-occipital joint by the use of the dominant hand under the occiput. This maneuver leads to passive opening of the mouth, and can be accentuated by using the fifth finger of the nondominant hand (holding the laryngoscope) to apply pressure over the chin in a caudad direction. In the second technique, which tends to be more effective but requires contact of the (gloved) hand with the teeth and/or gum, caudad pressure is applied with the thumb of the dominant hand on the mandibular canine/bicuspids on the patient's same side while the first finger, crossed below the thumb, applies cephalad pressure to the ipsilateral maxillary canine/bicuspid. The ultimate goal of both techniques is rotation and translation of the temporomandibular joint in order to achieve the widest interincisor gap, and relaxation of the mandibular space. The patient, whether conscious or not, is now ready for laryngoscopy.

Although DL remains the most used method for tracheal intubation, it is far from successful in all cases and not always benign when successful. DL may be difficult or impossible in 8.5 and 1.8% of attempts, respectively.[83] The analysis of Domino et al.[32] of the ASA Closed Claims Database reveals that claims for laryngeal injury during DL arise more often in "easy" as opposed to difficult laryngoscopies. Among the 4,460 cases in the ASA Closed Claim Database, 87 instances of laryngeal trauma were recorded. Of these, 80% occurred during routine (nondifficult) tracheal intubation, in which no injury was suspected. This has led some to question whether routine tracheal intubation is as safe as assumed.[30]

Use of the Direct Laryngoscope Blade. Proper use of the laryngoscope blade is vital to the success of this basic airway management technique. Two blade types are commonly available and each is applied in a unique manner. Many other blades have been described but will not be discussed here; the reader is directed to some excellent reviews.[84]

The curved (Macintosh) blade is used to pull the epiglottis out of the line of sight by tensing the glossoepiglottic ligament, whereas the straight blade (Miller) compresses the epiglottis against the base of the tongue. Both blades include a flange along the left side of their length, which is used to sweep the tongue to the left side of the mouth. Blades with a right-sided flange are available for the left-handed practitioner, but they are not commonly found in practice.

Historically, choice of laryngoscopic blade has had a theoretical basis in airway innervation. The internal branch of the superior laryngeal nerve (a branch of the vagus) provides sensory innervation from the level of the vocal cords to the underside of the epiglottis. Stimulation of these structures (with the Miller blade) was believed to cause more vagally related reactions (laryngospasm, bradycardia, hypertension). The vallecula, stimulated by the curved, Macintosh blade is innervated by the glossopharyngeal nerve.

In most available systems the blade incorporates the light source, either a bulb placed near the distal blade aspect or a rigid fiberoptic cable that transmits light produced within the handle (see the history discussion, earlier in this chapter). In either case, these blades must be long enough to achieve their respective applications. Therefore, blade size needs to be chosen appropriately and, on occasion, exchanged after a failed attempt at DL. As a generalization, the Macintosh blade is regarded as advantageous whenever there is little room to pass

an ETT (e.g., small mouth), whereas the Miller blade is considered better in the patient who has a small mandibular space, large incisor teeth, or a large epiglottis.[85] The straight-against-the-tongue nature of the Miller blade affords maximal transfer of workforce from the operator's elbow and shoulder onto the surface of the tongue in order to displace it into a small mandibular space.

With the left hand holding the laryngoscope handle, the blade is inserted into the right side of the mouth, with care taken not to compress the upper lip against the teeth. As the blade is advanced toward the epiglottis, it is swept leftward, using the flange to displace the tongue to the left as the blade compresses it into the mandibular space. Once reaching the base of the tongue (the Macintosh blade tip in the vallecula, or the Miller blade compressing the epiglottis against the base of the tongue), the operator's arm and shoulder lift in an anterior and caudad direction (Fig. 29-9).

Importantly, the laryngoscopist must strive to avoid rotating the wrist and laryngoscope handle in a cephalad direction, bringing the blade against the upper incisor teeth. Extending either blade style too deeply can bring the tip of the blade to rest under the larynx itself, so that forward pressure lifts the entire airway from view.

Special considerations apply to the technique of laryngoscopy and intubation in the infant and child. Because of the

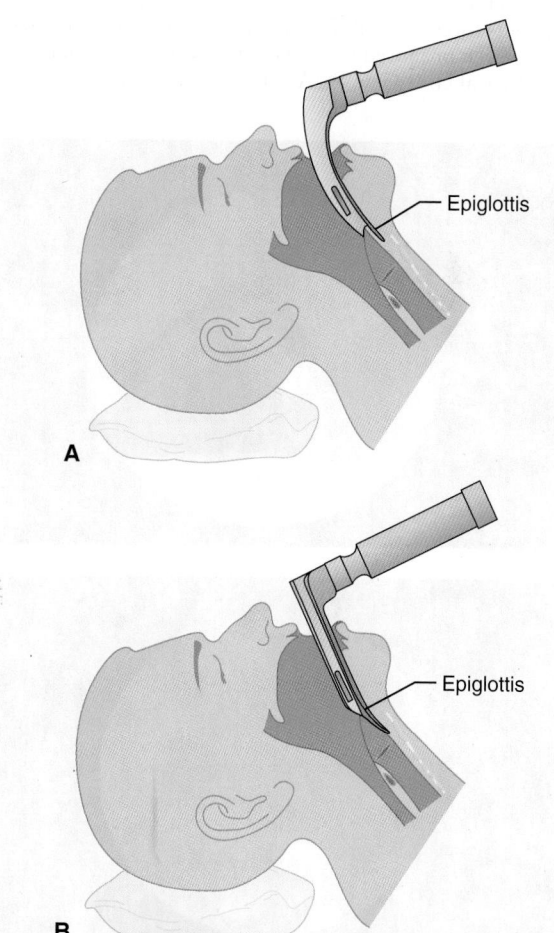

FIGURE 29-9. **A.** When a curved laryngoscope blade is used, the tip of the blade is placed in the vallecula, the space between the base of the tongue and the pharyngeal surface of the epiglottis. **B.** The tip of a straight blade is advanced beneath the epiglottis.

relatively larger size of the occiput in children, producing an anatomic sniffing position, elevation of the head (as done in the adult) is not required.[85] On occasion, one may need to elevate the thorax instead. The relatively short neck gives the impression of an anterior position of the larynx. Posterior cricoid pressure is often required to place the laryngeal inlet into view. A straight blade is more helpful in displacing the stiff, omega-shaped, and high epiglottis. Because the cricoid cartilage is the narrowest aspect of the airway until 6–8 years of age, the intubator must be sensitive to resistance to advancement of the ETT that has easily passed the vocal folds. Hyperextension at the atlanto-occipital joint, as done in adult, may cause airway obstruction from the relative pliability of the trachea. In the child, there is a higher risk of endobronchial intubation or accidental extubation with head movement owing to the short length of the trachea.

With laryngoscopy, the view of the larynx may be complete, partial, or impossible. A laryngeal view scoring system that has won general acceptance was developed by Cormack and Lehane,[82] who described four grades of laryngeal view. Grade 1 includes visualization of the entire glottic aperture; grade 2 includes visualization of only the posterior aspects of the glottic aperture; grade 3 is visualization of the tip of the epiglottis; and grade 4 is visualization of no more than the soft palate (Fig. 29-10). A Cormack-Lehane grade 3 or 4 is expected in 1.5 to 8.5% of adult laryngoscopies.[86]

This system has proved useful not only as a means of recording the laryngeal view on individual patients, but also as a clinical end point in the evaluation of preoperative airway assessments tools. A modification of the Cormack and Lehane score has been proposed by Koh et al.,[87] who noted that when a partial vocal cord view ("2A") is achieved, tracheal intuba-

tion was significantly easier than when only the arytenoids and epiglottis were visualized ("2B").

Once the larynx is visualized with a left-side–flanged blade, the tracheal tube is inserted from the right-hand side, care being taken not to obstruct the view of the vocal cords. Whenever possible, the action of the ETT passing through the vocal cords should be witnessed by the laryngoscopist. The tracheal tube should be inserted to a depth of at least 2 cm after the disappearance of the tracheal tube cuff into the larynx in order to approximate placement in the mid-trachea. This should present the 21- and 23-cm external markings at the teeth for the typical adult female and male, respectively.[88] Choice of adult tracheal tube size may be made by the generalization that for women, size 7 to 8 ID may be used, and for a male, size 8 to 9 ID. The larger tracheal tubes may be desirable if pulmonary toilet or diagnostic or therapeutic bronchoscopy is to be part of the clinical course. Pediatric laryngoscope blades and tracheal tube sizes are presented in detail in Table 29-10 (See also Chapter 45).

An alternative approach to DL has been described by Henderson.[88] In this approach to tongue displacement, a straight-bladed laryngoscope is introduced into the right side of the mouth. The blade is advanced between the tongue and palatine tonsil. The blade passes below the epiglottis, which is then elevated. This approach subjects the tongue to less compressive forces. It has been suggested that this technique may improve the view of the larynx in the presence of lingual tonsil hyperplasia.

Verification of successful tracheal tube placement is made by a variety of methods. The gold standard for confirmation of placement includes visualization of placement through the vocal folds and sustained detection of exhaled carbon dioxide as measured with capnography or a disposable chemical colorimetric

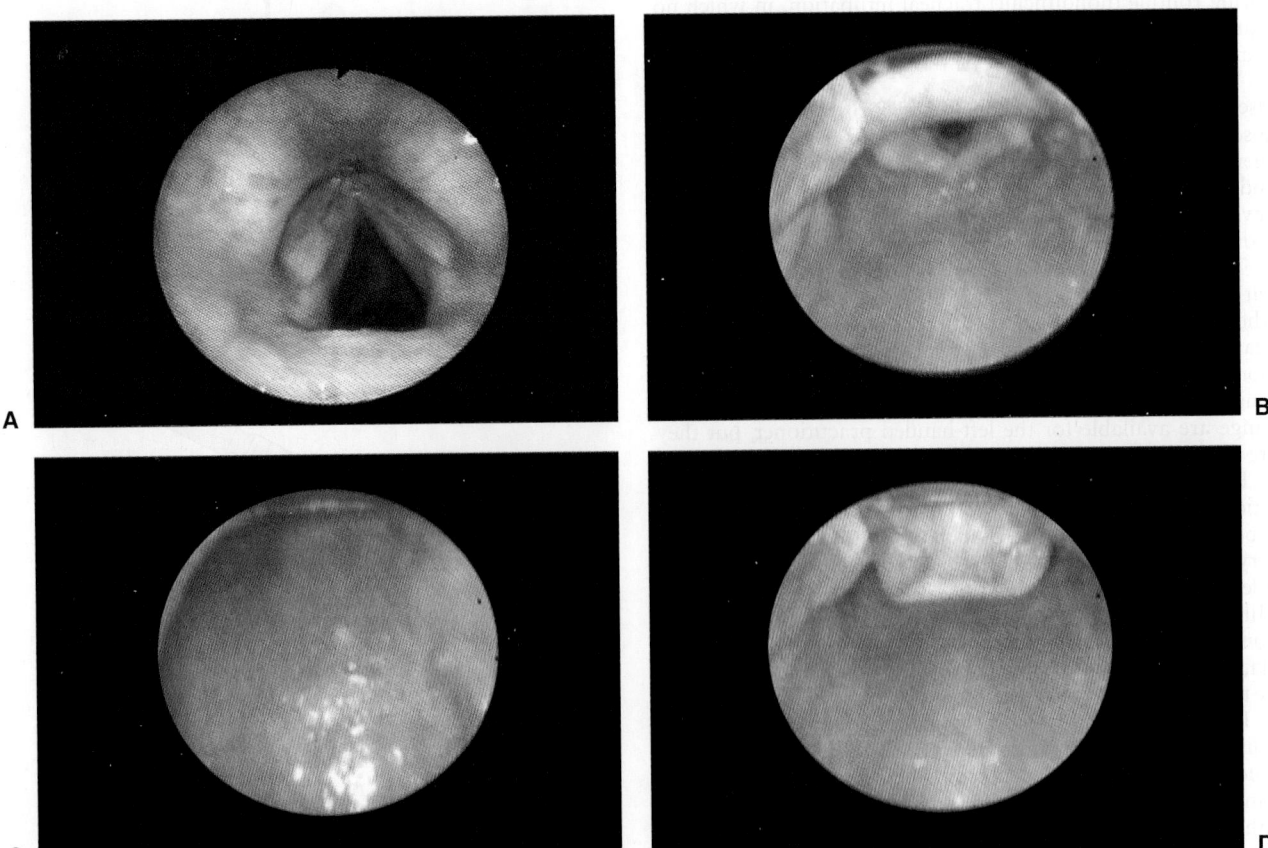

FIGURE 29-10.   The Cormack–Lehane laryngeal view scoring system: grade 1 (A), grade 2 (B), grade 3 (C), and grade 4 (D).

TABLE 29-10

SIZE AND LENGTH OF TRACHEAL TUBES RELATIVE TO AIRWAY ANATOMY

■ AGE	■ INTERNAL DIAMETER (mm)	■ DISTANCE FROM LIPS TO MIDTRACHEA[a] (cm)
Premature	2.5	8
Full term	3.0	10
1–6 mo	3.5	11
6–12 mo	4.0	12
2 yr	4.5	13
4 yr	5.0	14
6 yr	5.5	15
8 yr	6.5	16[b]
10 yr	7.0	17–18[c]
12 yr	7.5	18–20
14 yr	8.0–9.0	20–22

[a]Add 2 to 3 cm for nasal tubes.
[b]Females.
[c]Males.

ANESTHETIC MANAGEMENT

device such as the Easy Cap II. Other portable techniques include auscultation over the chest and abdomen, visualization of the chest excursion, observation of condensation in the ETT, use of a self-inflating bulb (TubeChek-B, Ambu, Linthicum, MD), lighted stylets (Trachlight, Laerdal Medical, Armonk, NY; Surch-Lite, Aaron Medical Industries, St. Petersburg, FL), and standard and dedicated fiberoptic devices used to identify the tracheal rings and carina (Foley Flexible Airway Stylet, Clarus Medical, Golden Valley, MN), ultrasound, or chest x-ray.[89]

NPO Status and the Rapid-Sequence Induction.   Induction of anesthesia in patients who have full stomachs or incompetent gastroesophageal sphincters can result in regurgitation and pulmonary aspiration. Individuals at risk include, pregnant women, diabetics, or others with gastroparesis or intestinal obstruction/ileus/distension, upper gastrointestinal tract hemorrhage, those who require emergency operations, patients presenting from the intensive care unit, patients receiving acute opioid therapy, patients with gastroesophageal reflux disease, and patients who have recently eaten or are experiencing nausea. Individuals experiencing emotional stress have increased gastric acid secretions and are also at an increased risk for aspiration.[90] A complete discussion of the pharmacologic therapy for aspiration prophylaxis is available elsewhere in this text. Obesity by itself, long taught as a risk factor for gastric contents aspiration, may not denote a risk in this regard. Though initial studies touted the increased volume of (more) acid secretions in the obese fasting patient, as compared with the lean control, others have refuted this claim.[91,92]

The technique of rapid-sequence induction is performed to gain control of the airway in the shortest amount of time after the ablation of protective airway reflexes with the induction of anesthesia. In the rapid-sequence technique, the administration of an intravenous anesthetic induction agent is immediately followed by a rapidly acting neuromuscular blocking drug. Laryngoscopy and intubation are performed as soon as muscle relaxation is confirmed. Cricoid pressure (Sellick maneuver) is applied by an assistant from the beginning of induction until confirmation of ETT placement. Cricoid pressure entails the downward displacement of the cricoid cartilage against the vertebral bodies. In this manner, the lumen of the esophagus is ablated, while the completely circular nature of the cricoid cartilage maintains the tracheal lumen. Early cadaveric studies showed that correctly applied cricoid pressure was effective in preventing gastric fluids under 100 cm H_2O pressure from leaking into the pharynx. Unfortunately, the esophagus is laterally displaced in a majority of normal patients.[93] Because cricoid pressure further lateralizes the esophagus, the adequacy of esophageal ablation has been questioned. Cricoid pressure is contraindicated with active vomiting (risk of esophageal rupture), cervical spine fracture, and laryngeal fracture. Historically face mask ventilation is not undertaken for the 40 to 90 seconds of time required to achieve adequate neuromuscular relaxation. This practice is based on minimal data and has recently been questioned.

If during rapid-sequence induction there are difficulties in securing the airway and oxyhemoglobin desaturation occurs, gentle positive pressure ventilation may be used while maintaining cricoid pressure. This positive pressure should require <25 cm H_2O pressure. Some authors argue that, because cricoid pressure is of dubious efficacy and may distort the laryngoscopist view, it be released if difficulties are encountered during the intubation attempt.[94]

The Intubating Laryngeal Mask Airway (LMA Fastrach).   Blind, fiberoptic-aided, stylet-guided, and laryngoscopy-directed tracheal intubation via the LMA has been widely reported in adults and children. Many limitations to this technique have been described. In an effort to overcome these limitations, Brain et al.[95] introduced a version of the LMA with a large-diameter (13 mm ID), short-length (14 cm), rigid stainless steel barrel curved to align the mask aperture to the glottic vestibule (Fig. 29-3).

The LMA Fastrach (Laryngeal Mask Company, Jersey, UK) mask incorporates a vertically oriented, semirigid bar fixed at the proximal end of the bowl aperture and positioned to sit beneath the epiglottis in the average adult. A handle at the proximal end of the barrel is used for insertion, repositioning, and removal. A secondary advantage of the handle is that the operator never needs to place fingers into the patient's mouth. The LMA Fastrach barrel can accommodate up to an 8.0-mm ID cuffed ETT, which can be inserted blindly or over a fiberscope or other stylet device. The LMA Fastrach is designed to be used with a straight tracheal tube manufactured in both single- and multiple-use models (Euromedics, Kedah, Malaysia), although standard or Parker Flex-Tip (Parker Medical, Englewood, CO) polyvinyl chloride tracheal tubes have been used.[96]

The LMA Fastrach is available in adult sizes with cuffs equivalent to the size 3, 4, and 5 LMAs. Experience has suggested that most adults between 40 and 70 kg are best managed with a size 4 LMA Fastrach; larger persons require the size 5.

The LMA Fastrach is indicated for routine, elective intubations and for anticipated and unanticipated difficult intubations. Because it was designed to facilitate blind tracheal intubation, the presence of airway secretions, blood, or edema (e.g., from previous intubation attempts or trauma) does not interfere with its use. Because the design of the barrel is based on the normal adult palate-to-glottis relationship, patients who are evaluated as being manageable with tracheal intubation by DL based on external examination, but subsequently are found to have a high Cormack–Lehane score (e.g., because of lingual tonsil hyperplasia or cervical spine immobility) should be successfully managed with the LMA Fastrach.[82] In a large trial of the LMA Fastrach, ventilation was satisfactory in 95% and unsatisfactory in 1% of 500 uses, and 96% of patients were intubated within three attempts (79.8% on first attempt, 12.4% on second, 4% on third).[97] Patients who are assessed as grossly abnormal on preoperative airway examination may often still be managed with the LMA Fastrach. The LMA Fastrach has been demonstrated to be useful as a ventilatory and intubating device after failed rapid sequence intubation.[98]

A large study has shown the utility of the LMA Fastrach in patients who were anticipated as well as unanticipated to be difficult to intubate. Ferson et al.[99] successfully intubated 234 patients over a 3-year period using the LMA Fastrach. Studied patients included those with normal-appearing airways on routine examination whose airways were unexpectedly difficult to manage, patients with a Cormack and Lehane laryngeal view grade 4 on laryngoscopic examination, patients with immobilized or traumatized cervical spines, and patients with airway tumors, prior airway surgery, or radiation. Successful blind intubation via the LMA Fastrach occurred in 97% of patients; the remaining patient intubations were facilitated with adjunct use of a fiberoptic intubation scope. A new design of the LMA Fastrach, the CTrach (Fig. 29-3), introduced in 2004, incorporates a fiberoptic cable and monitor into the LMA Fastrach design (discussed later).

Contraindications to the use of the LMA Fastrach are similar to those of the LMA. Because the end point of LMA Fastrach procedure is tracheal intubation, it may prove useful for the management of patients at moderate risk for gastroesophageal regurgitation and aspiration, or for high-risk patients on whom other techniques have failed.

The LMA Fastrach is inserted with the head in a neutral position. It can be used in the unconscious or awake patient (with the use of topical anesthetics). The mask of the LMA Fastrach is tested, deflated, and lubricated as described for the LMA. It is inserted into the mouth, with the handle held parallel to the chest, so the mask lies flat against the palate. Gentle pressure on the handle and barrel reproduces the palatal pressure described for insertion of the LMA. A smooth backward rotation of the handle toward the top of the head seats the tip of the mask in the hypopharynx, posterior to the cricoid cartilage. Once seated, the mask of the LMA Fastrach is inflated via the pilot cuff. An Ambu bag or anesthesia circuit is attached to the proximal end of the LMA Fastrach barrel and ventilation is attempted. By using the LMA Fastrach handle, the position of the device can be optimized by lateral and anterior-posterior manipulation. This action is termed the *Chandy maneuver* (after Dr. Chandy Verghese, Redding United Kingdom). A seemingly common cause of airway obstruction with the LMA Fastrach is the downfolding of the epiglottis. This can be relieved with a smooth rotational movement of the inflated LMA Fastrach out of the airway (6 cm

along the axis of the insertion) while the cuff remains inflated, and immediate replacement (the up-down maneuver).

After adequate ventilation is achieved, the ETT is advanced though the barrel. As the ETT exits the bowl aperture of the LMA Fastrach, the semirigid elevating bar is pushed anteriorly, carrying the epiglottis out of the way of the airway. If positioned correctly, the ETT can freely enter the glottis.

The second part of the Chandy maneuver may facilitate blind tracheal intubation. In this maneuver the handle is used to gently lift (without rotation) the LMA Fastrach anteriorly, sealing the bowl against the larynx.

When blind intubation fails (esophageal insertion or obstruction) several maneuvers are undertaken.[99] Early obstruction is typically caused by a downfolded epiglottis. An up-down maneuver, as described earlier, can be employed and tracheal intubation attempts repeated. Early resistance may also signify vallecular entrapment secondary to too large an LMA Fastrach size. The operator may remove the LMA Fastrach and place a smaller sized one. Later obstruction may signify entrapment or too small a device, and again, a change is indicated.

When intubation fails despite the Chandy or up-down maneuvers, or a change in the LMA Fastrach size, the clinician should recall that the LMA Fastrach is a ventilation device first! Typically, ventilation will be adequate despite failure to intubate. At this juncture the clinician can (1) continue with short surgical procedures using the LMA Fastrach as a simple SGA (procedures longer than 15 minutes may be ill advised because of the pressure exerted by the LMA Fastrach on tissues), (2) change to another LMA device, (3) diagnose the intubation impediment with the aid of another device (e.g., fiberoptic bronchoscope or Foley Flexible Airway Stylet), (4) remove the LMA Fastrach and employ DL or another technique of tracheal intubation, or (5) in the resuscitative situation, perform a surgical airway while continuing ventilation with the LMA Fastrach. This last procedure may be an underappreciated facility of all the SGAs. These devices may serve as a bridge while invasive airway procedures are performed.

Once intubation is achieved and confirmed (e.g., by auscultation or capnography), the ETT circuit adapter is removed and the LMA Fastrach is withdrawn over the ETT. During this removal procedure, the ETT is stabilized by one of two methods. A silicone stabilizing rod (supplied by the manufacturer) can be held against the ETT as the LMA Fastrach is retreated out of the mouth. In the second technique, described by Rosenblatt and Murphy,[98] a Magill forceps is used to hold the proximal tip of the ETT while the LMA Fastrach is removed. In the mid-removal position, a finger is placed in the mouth to identify and stabilize the ETT, while the Magill forceps is removed and the LMA Fastrach is fully retreated.

LMA CTrach. The LMA CTrach (The Laryngeal Mask Company, Bucks, UK) is functionally identical to the intubating LMA Fastrach, with the addition of integrated fiberoptic channels (image and light source) and a battery-powered monitor attached to the proximal airway tube via a magnetic latch connector, which provides a view of larynx to facilitate tracheal intubation (Fig. 29-3). A USB (universal serial bus) port on the monitor allows the video stream to be recorded on a personal computer. Both the CTrach and LMA Fastrach permit ventilation between intubation attempts.

There are reports of patients with known or unexpected difficult airways who were successfully intubated via CTrach under general anesthesia.[100–104] Even though successful ventilation with the CTrach is reliably achieved, initial glottic views are less certain.[105,106] Causes of poor CTrach view are a downfolding epiglottis (57%), obstruction by the arytenoids (7%), and secretions (5%).[107] Maneuvers to improve the view include the Chandy maneuvers, up-down maneuver, bimanual mandibular elevation, and medial-lateral-medial rotation. These maneuvers allow the operator to see the glottis in ≥80% of cases.[106,107] Over all intubation success rate is about 97%,[105–107] which is similar to that of the LMA Fastrach (96.5%).[99] The process of intubation with the CTrach is longer than DL (57 vs. 30 seconds), but it provides better oxygenation in morbidly obese patients compared with DL.[108] Awake intubation with the CTrach in three cases of unstable cervical spine[109] and three morbidly obese patients with obstructive sleep apnea[110] has been reported.

Extubation of the Trachea

Although a wealth of literature is focused on the field of tracheal intubation, few reviews have intensely contemplated the area of extubation after completion of surgery or prolonged ventilatory support. Indeed, the period of extubation may be far more treacherous than that of intubation (Table 29.11, section A).

Routine Extubation. Extubation of the trachea must not be considered a benign procedure. It is not simply the elimination or reversal of tracheal intubation. Extubation is fraught with its own set of potential complications (Table 29-11, section B). Appropriately trained personnel and equipment should be immediately available at the time of extubation. This may range from a postanesthetic care unit nurse or respiratory

TABLE 29-11

TRACHEAL EXTUBATION

A. Causes of Ventilatory Compromise During Tracheal Extubation
Residual anesthetic
Poor central respiratory effort
Decreased respiratory rate
Decreased respiratory drive in response to CO_2
Decreased respiratory drive in response to O_2
Reduced tone of upper airway musculature
Reduced gag and swallow reflex
Decreased threshold to laryngospasm
Surgical airway compromise
Surgical airway edema
Vocal cord paralysis
Arytenoid cartilage dislocation
Supraglottic edema with airway obstruction by the epiglottis
Retro arytenoid edema with limited vocal fold abduction
Subglottic edema
Tracheomalacia (from long-standing tracheal intubation)
Bronchospasm

B. Complications of Tracheal Extubation
Respiratory drive failure
Hypoxia (e.g., atelectasis)
Upper airway obstruction (e.g., edema, residual anesthetic)
Vocal fold–related obstruction (e.g., vocal cord paralysis)
Tracheal obstruction (e.g., subglottic edema)
Bronchospasm
Aspiration
Hypertension
Increased intracranial pressure
Increased pulmonary artery pressure
Increased bronchial stump pressure (e.g., after pulmonary resection)
Increased ocular pressure
Increased abdominal wall pressure (e.g., risk of wound dehiscence)

TABLE 29-12

CRITERIA FOR ROUTINE "AWAKE" EXTUBATION

Subjective Clinical Criteria
  Follows commands
  Clear oropharynx/hypopharynx (e.g., no active bleeding, secretions cleared)
  Intact gag reflex
  Sustained head lift for 5 seconds, sustained hand grasp
  Adequate pain control
  Minimal end expiratory concentration of inhaled anesthetics
Objective Criteria
  Vital capacity: ≥10 mL/kg
  Peak voluntary negative inspiratory pressure: >20 cm H_2O
  Tidal volume >6 cc/kg
  Sustained tetanic contraction (5 sec)
  T_1/T_4 ratio >0.7
  Alveolar-arterial PaO_2 gradient (on FIO_2 of 1.0): <350 mm Hg[a]
  Dead space to tidal volume ratio: ≤0.6[a]

[a]Used during weaning from mechanical ventilation in the intensive care setting.

therapist with a set of laryngoscopes to a surgeon prepared to perform an emergency tracheostomy.

Most adult patients are extubated after the return of consciousness and spontaneous respiration, the resolution of neuromuscular block, and the ability of the patient to follow simple commands (Table 29-12). The patient is asked to open the mouth, and a suction catheter is used to remove excessive secretions and/or blood. The airway pressure is allowed to rise to 5 to 15 cm of H_2O to facilitate a "passive cough," and the ETT is removed after the cuff (if present) is deflated.[85] If coughing or straining is contraindicated or hazardous (e.g., increased intracranial pressure), extubation may be performed while the patient is in a surgical plane of anesthesia. In patients at risk for gastric contents aspiration (e.g., full stomach) or upper airway obstruction, the clinician needs to assess the relative risk of each potential morbidity (e.g., coughing vs. obstruction). Murphy et al.[111] found that standard clinical criteria for adequacy of neuromuscular reversal such as 5-second head lift or hand grip, eye opening on command, negative inspiratory force more than –20 cm H_2O, or vital capacity breath of >15 cc/kg does not always represent acceptable neuromuscular recovery. Fifty-eight percent of patients in whom standard clinical criteria was achieved had a train-of-four ratio of <0.7 and 88% had a train-of-four ratio of <0.9. To reduce the risks of straining/coughing, a maneuver has been described in which an LMA is placed posterior to the ETT, which is then removed. This obviates the problem of upper airway obstruction, and may offer some protection against regurgitation and aspiration.[47,112] Because of the risks of atelectasis and diffusion hypoxia, the ability to administer oxygen should be available at the time of extubation.

Difficult Extubation. The patient who presented as having a difficult airway at the time of anesthetic induction must be considered as having a difficult airway at the time of extubation, even when corrective surgery was performed in the interim (e.g., uvulopalatoplasty in the obstructive sleep apnea patient).

Laryngospasm at extubation deserves special attention because of it prevalence in children and because it accounts for 23% of all critical postoperative respiratory events in adults.[85] Laryngospasm may be triggered by respiratory secretions, vomitus, blood, or a foreign body in the airway; pain in any part of the body; and pelvic or abdominal visceral stimulation. The cause of airway obstruction during laryngospasm is the contraction of the lateral cricoarytenoids, the thyroarytenoid, and the cricothyroid muscles. Management of laryngospasm consists of the immediate removal of the offending stimulus (if identifiable), administration of oxygen with continuous positive airway pressure, and if other maneuvers are unsuccessful, the use of a small dose of short-acting muscle relaxants.[85]

Negative-pressure pulmonary edema may result from any airway obstruction in a patient who continues to have a voluntary respiratory effort. Negative intrathoracic pressure is transmitted to the alveoli, which are unable to expand owing to the more proximal obstruction. Fluid is entrained from the pulmonary capillary bed. Negative-pressure pulmonary edema is treated as any other form of noncardiogenic edema.

Identification of Patients at Risk at Extubation. A number of well-known clinical situations may place patients at increased risk for complication at the time of extubation (Table 29-13). However, the clinician should evaluate every patient in terms of potential for problems, in the same manner that the anesthesiologist prepares for the unanticipated difficult intubation.

Approach to the Difficult Extubation. When there is a suspicion that a patient may have difficulty with oxygenation or ventilation after tracheal extubation, the clinician may choose from a number of management strategies. These may range from the preparation of standby reintubation equipment to the active establishment of a bridge or guide for reintubation and/or oxygenation. When the patient's intubation is without difficulty and there is no substantial reason to believe that an interim insult to the airway has occurred, extubation may be accomplished in a routine fashion, with a heightened state of readiness for reintubation. When there has been difficulty with intubation or there is a clinical suspicion that reintubation will be difficult, extubation over a guiding stylet may be a successful technique. Any number of devices can be used as a stylet (Table 29-14).

A popular test used to predict post extubation airway competency is the detection of a leak on deflation of the ETT cuff. A recent investigation has cast doubt on the reliability of this test as a predictor of airway incompetence: the absence of an airway leak on cuff deflation was not predictive of subsequent ventilatory failure after extubation.[113] Patients with a reduced cuff leak volume are at risk for postextubation stridor.[114]

A randomized control trial study in 2007 revealed that multiple-dose dexamethasone effectively reduced incidence of postextubation stridor in adult patients at high risk for postextubation laryngeal edema while single-dose injection of dexamethasone given 1 hour before extubation did not reduce the number of patients requiring reintubation.[115]

A fiberoptic bronchoscope may be used to view the tracheal structures during the removal of the ETT. If extubation is tolerated, the fiberoptic bronchoscope can be slowly withdrawn into the subglottic region. If secretions do not obstruct the objective lens, the vocal folds and other structures may be visualized and evaluated.

A number of obturators are available for use in trial extubation (where they may be left in place in the airway for extended periods) or ETT exchange (e.g., failure of the ETT cuff). Mort[116] found that the success of first-pass reintubation

---

TABLE 29-13

CLINICAL SITUATIONS PRESENTING INCREASED RISK FOR COMPLICATIONS AT EXTUBATION[a]

Paradoxical vocal cord motion (pre-existing)	Poorly understood mechanism
Thyroid surgery	4.3% recurrent laryngeal nerve injury
Local edema	
Tracheomalacia (from long-standing goiter)	
Laryngoscopy (diagnostic)	Edema, laryngospasm, especially with biopsy
Uvulopalatoplasty	Palatal and oropharyngeal edema
Obstructive sleep apnea syndrome (uncorrected)	
Carotid endarterectomy	Wound hematoma, glottic edema, nerve palsies
Maxillofacial trauma	Laryngeal fracture, reduced level of consciousness, requirements for mandibular/maxillary wires
Cervical vertebrae decompression	Supraglottic and hypopharyngeal edema
Parkinson disease	
Rheumatoid arthritis	
Generalized edema	Laryngotracheal narrowing
Angioneurotic edema	Laryngotracheal narrowing
Anaphylaxis	Laryngotracheal narrowing
Hypopharyngeal infections	Laryngotracheal narrowing
Hypoventilation syndromes[a]	
Hypoxemic syndromes[b]	
Inadequate airway protective reflexes	Aspiration risk

[a]Residual anesthetic or preoperative medications (including alcohol and illicit drugs), central sleep apnea, carotid endarterectomy, poliomyelitis, Guillain-Barré syndrome, myasthenia gravis, botulism, thoracic skeletal deformity, severe pain (with diaphragmatic splinting), morbid obesity, severe chronic obstructive pulmonary disease.
[b]Hypoventilation, ventilation-perfusion mismatch, intracardiac or intrapulmonary shunting, increased oxygen consumption, severe anemia, impaired alveolar oxygen diffusion.

ANESTHETIC MANAGEMENT

TABLE 29-14

DEVICES USED AS EXTUBATING STYLETS

■ DEVICE	■ ADVANTAGE	■ DISADVANTAGE
Fiberoptic bronchoscope	Visualize structures Oxygen can be insufflated	ETT cannot be exchanged
Eschmann catheter	Inexpensive, semirigid	Cannot visualize/oxygenate
Exchange catheter	Oxygen can be insufflated	Cannot visualize, may be to short

was significantly higher, and the incidence of hypoxia lower, in patients with a retained tracheal tube exchange catheter.

It is beyond the scope of this text to describe all the commercially available catheters. The Cook Airway Exchange Catheters (Cook Critical Care, Bloomington, IN) are manufactured with external diameters of 2.7, 3.7, 4.7, and 6.33 mm. The smallest diameter catheter (which can fit within a 3.0-mm ID ETT) is 45 cm long, whereas the others are 83 cm in length. They all have a central lumen and rounded, atraumatic ends. The catheters are graduated from the distal end. The proximal end is fitted with either a 15-mm or a Luer-lock Rapi-Fit adapter, which can be quickly removed and replaced for ETT removal or exchange. With these adapters an oxygen source can be used to provide insufflated or jet-ventilated oxygen if the patient fails extubation and/or if reintubation over the catheter fails.

The CardioMed endotracheal ventilation catheter (Gromley, Ontario, Canada) designed by Richard Cooper, MD, a Canadian anesthesiologist, is 85 cm in length and has inner and outer diameters of either 3 or 4 mm. An integral Luer-lock fitting adapter is found at the proximal end, whereas the blunted distal end incorporates eight helically arranged side holes in addition to the distal end hole. The arrangement of these holes is meant to center the catheter during oxygen insufflation and prevent traumatic "whipping" within the trachea. The use of this catheter for ETT exchange, tracheal reintubation, oxygen insufflation, jet oxygenation, and end-tidal

CO_2 detection after extubation has been documented by the inventor.[85]

Use of high-pressure oxygen insufflation via an exchange catheter causing bilateral pneumothorax has been reported.[117]

THE DIFFICULT AIRWAY

The Difficult Airway Algorithm

In 1993 the ASA Task Force on the Difficult Airway first published an algorithm that has become a staple of management for clinicians. This algorithm was reissued in 2003.[1] As will be discussed, the most dramatic change in the ASA Difficult Airway Algorithm (ASA-DAA) was the repositioning of the LMA from the emergency to the routine management pathway (Fig. 29-11). The ASA defines the difficult airway as the situation in which the "conventionally trained anesthesiologist experiences difficulty with intubation, mask ventilation or both." Based on available data, the incidence of difficult intubation by DL is 4.5 to 7.5%, whereas the incidence of failed intubation/inability to perform mask ventilation is 0.01 to 0.03%.[12]

The ASA algorithm stands as a model for the approach to the difficult airway for nurse anesthetists, emergency medicine physicians, and prehospital personnel, as well as for anesthesiologists. Although the algorithm largely speaks for itself, its salient features are discussed here. One statement in this document

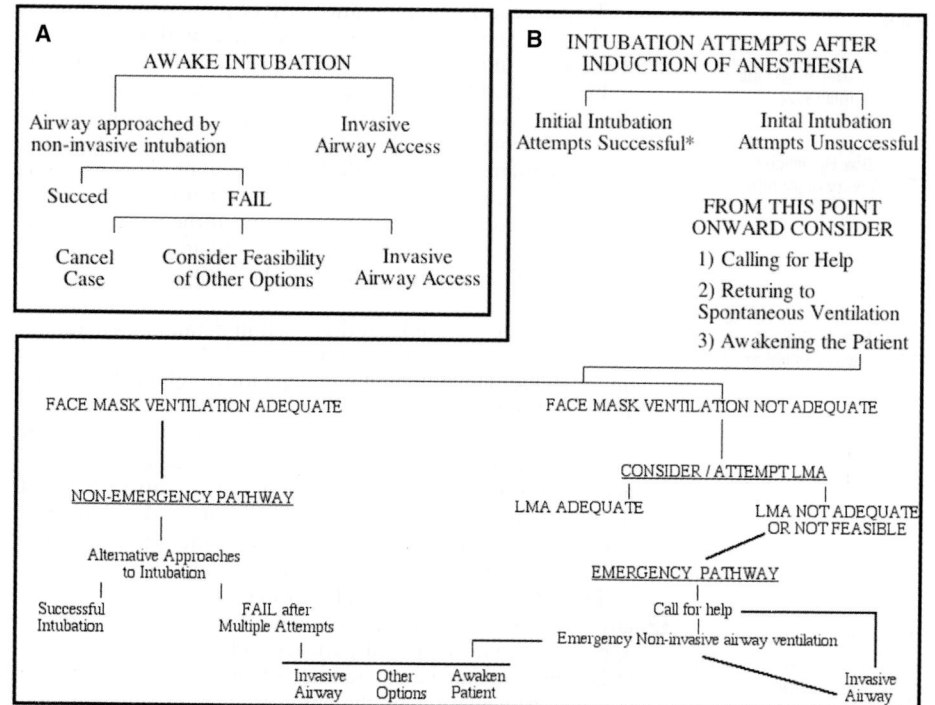

FIGURE 29-11. The American Society of Anesthesiologists Difficult Airway Algorithm. A. Awake intubation. B. Intubation attempts after induction of anesthesia.

summarizes the difficulty of writing and recommending practices in the difficult airway management: "The difficult airway represents a complex interaction between patient factors, the clinical setting and the skills of the practitioner."[1] It should be well recognized that though the ASA-DAA is a staple in the United States and much of the world, several groups worldwide have written their own airway algorithms emphasizing techniques and approaches native to their practice. Although the differences in these algorithms will not be discussed here, the reader is encouraged to explore these important alternative approaches.[86,118-122]

Entry into the algorithm begins with the evaluation of the airway. Although there is some debate as to the value of particular evaluation methods and indices, the clinician must use all available data and his or her own clinical experience to reach a general impression as to the difficulty of the patient's airway in terms of laryngoscopy and intubation, supraglottic ventilation techniques, aspiration risk, or apnea tolerance.

This evaluation should direct the clinician to enter the ASA-DAA at one of its two root points: awake intubation (Fig. 29-11A) or intubation attempts after the induction of general anesthesia (Fig. 29-11B). This highlights the misnomer of the algorithm: it is not only for difficult airways, but is relevant to all instances in which the airway is managed. Figure 29-11B describes the approach taken in the majority of tracheal intubations (and is applicable to face mask- and SGA-managed patients). The decision to enter the algorithm via either approach is a preoperative one. Box A (Fig. 29-11) is chosen when difficulty is anticipated that will place the patient at jeopardy, while box B is for the situation in which there may be anticipated difficulty with either ventilation or tracheal intubation, but an uncorrectable situation is not expected. This has been further delineated into a preoperative decision tree by Rosenblatt[3]: the airway approach algorithm (AAA). Figure 29-12 outlines the AAA, which is s simple one-pathway algorithm for entering in to the ASA-DAA. Branch choice, like the previously noted statement from the ASA practice guidelines, is highly dependent on the clinician's skill and experience. Details of the AAA can be found elsewhere and are summarized here.[3,123]

Airway Approach Algorithm

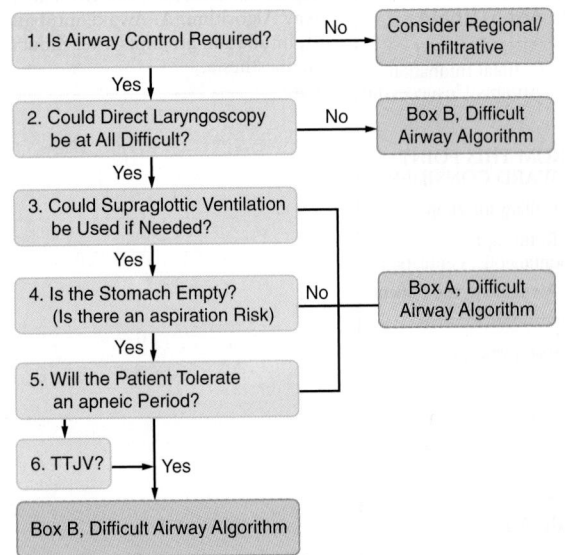

FIGURE 29-12.   The Airway Approach Algorithm: a decision tree approach to entry in to the American Society of Anesthesiologists Difficult Airway Algorithm. TTJV, transtracheal jet ventilation.

1. Is airway control necessary? No matter how routine sedation or general anesthesia become, whether or not to make a patient apneic should always be considered seriously and alternatives should be contemplated.

2. Could tracheal intubation be (at all) difficult? If there is no indication that rapid tracheal intubation by DL, in DL (e.g., video laryngoscopy or other means familiar to the operator) will be difficult, the clinician may proceed with any technique (induction, DL, LMA, and so forth) as clinically appropriate. This is the essence of box B of the ASA-DAA (prototypical case: rapid-sequence induction). If there is an indication, based on history or physical examination, that there may be difficulty with rapid tracheal intubation, the AAA is followed to the next question. By choosing to continue down the algorithm, the clinician is not assuming tracheal intubation difficulty, rather he or she is anticipating the viability of rescue maneuvers should difficultly occur.

3. Can SGA ventilation be used if needed? If the clinician thinks that there is a physical reason that SGA ventilation (by face mask, LMA, or other device) could be difficult, he or she is projecting the possibility that a juncture of "cannot intubate (question 2)—cannot ventilate (question 3)" could be reached. Because this is a preoperative algorithm, box A of the ASA-DAA may be the preferred root entry point.

4. Is there an aspiration risk? As discussed earlier, the patient at risk for aspiration is not a candidate for elective SGA use. Because the AAA is a preoperative algorithm, and therefore allows the luxury of discretionary paths, the juncture of "cannot intubate/should not ventilate" can be avoided by entering the ASA-DAA at box A.

5. Will the patient tolerate an apneic period? Question 3 is difficult to answer and is highly dependent on the skills and experience of the clinician. Should intubation fail, and SGA ventilation is inadequate, the patient's ability to sustain oxygen saturation will dictate the ability to tolerate an apneic period. Factors such as age, pregnancy, pulmonary status, abnormal oxygen consumption (e.g., fever), and choice of induction agents will influence this. If time to oxyhemoglobin desaturation is limited (limited time to correct hypoxemia), box A may be prophylactically chosen.

6. Can hypoxia be rapidly corrected through other means? Transtracheal jet oxygenation will be discussed later in this chapter. The question that arises here is with access to the patient's anterior trachea, the availability of equipment and knowledgeable personnel, and the experience of the operator. For example, if an error in judgment is made and the operator finds himself or herself in a cannot intubate/cannot ventilate scenario, will these conditions allow for using transtracheal jet ventilation (TTJV) to temporize the situation. All conditions may be right, but if the patient is morbidly obese or has had scarring or radiation over the larynx/trachea, this option may not be available.

These factors have been discussed in detail elsewhere.[3,123] To illustrate the clinical application of the AAA, the path through this algorithm will be traced for the clinical scenarios at the end of this chapter.

The exception to the AAA is the patient who is unable to cooperate owing to mental retardation, intoxication, anxiety, depressed level of consciousness, or age. This patient may still be approached by box A (Fig. 29-11), but awake intubation may need to be modified in favor of techniques that maintain spontaneous ventilation (e.g., inhalation induction).

Preparation of the patient for awake intubation is discussed later. In most instances, awake intubation is successful if approached with care and patience. When awake intubation fails, the clinician has a number of options. First, one can consider cancellation of the surgical case. In this situation,

TABLE 29-15

FACTORS TO CONSIDER IN PROCEEDING WITH REGIONAL ANESTHESIA (RA) AFTER THE PATIENT HAS BEEN JUDGED TO HAVE A DIFFICULT AIRWAY

■ MAY CONSIDER RA	■ SHOULD NOT CONSIDER RA
Superficial surgery	Cavity-invading surgery
Minimal sedation needed	Significant sedation needed
Local infiltration adequate	Extensive neuroaxial/local anesthetic required or risk of intravascular injection/absorption is high
Access to the airway	Poor access to the airway
Surgery can be halted at any time	Surgery cannot be stopped once started

specialized equipment or personnel can be assembled for a return to the operating room. Where cancellation is not an option, regional anesthetic techniques can be considered, or if demanded by the situation, a surgical airway (e.g., tracheostomy) may be called for.

The decision to proceed with regional anesthesia because the airway cannot be assessed or has been proven to be difficult to manage must be considered in terms of risks and benefits (Table 29-15). The ASA Closed Claims Database project has identified failure in regional anesthesia as a source of serious error when no airway strategy was prophylactically considered.[2]

The ASA-DAA truly becomes useful in the unanticipated difficult airway (box B in Fig. 29-11, unable to intubate by DL after the induction of anesthesia). When induction agents (with or without muscle relaxants) have been administered and the airway cannot be controlled, vital management decisions must be made rapidly. Typically, the clinician has attempted direct or video laryngoscopy and tracheal intubation after successful or failed anesthesia mask ventilation. Even if the patient's oxygen saturation remains adequate throughout these efforts, the number of laryngoscopy attempts should be limited to three. As discussed earlier, significant soft tissue trauma can result from multiple laryngoscopies, thereby worsening the situation. First, mask ventilation should be instituted. If face mask ventilation is adequate, the ASA-DAA nonemergency pathway is entered. The clinician may then turn to the most convenient and/or appropriate technique for establishing tracheal intubation, if needed. This might include, but is not limited to video laryngoscopy, intubation facilitated by a fiberoptic bronchoscope, LMA, LMA Fastrach, bougie, lighted stylet, or a retrograde wire. A surgical airway will sometimes be the most appropriate approach. (The most widely applied of these procedures, as well as new techniques, will be discussed within the clinical scenarios presented later.) When mask ventilation fails, the algorithm suggests supraglottic ventilation via any LMA. If successful, the nonemergency pathway of the ASA-DAA has again been entered and alternative techniques of tracheal intubation may be used, if needed (e.g., perhaps LMA ventilation is adequate for the remainder of the surgical procedure).

Should LMA ventilation fail to sustain the patient adequately, the emergency pathway is entered. The ASA-DAA suggests use of an esophageal-tracheal Combitube, rigid bronchoscopy, transtracheal oxygenation, or a surgical airway.

At any juncture, the decision to awaken the patient should be considered based on the adequacy of ventilation, the risk of aspiration, and the risk of proceeding with intubation attempts or the surgical procedure.

The repositioning of the LMA within the algorithm (in its 2003 revision) was based on more than 12 years of clinical use in the United States (and more than 20 years experience worldwide). Relatively few cases of LMA failure in the face of the cannot intubate/cannot ventilate situation have been reported.[15,124–130] Three broad categories account for these failures: acute oropharyngeal angle, obstruction at the level of the hypopharynx, and obstruction below the vocal folds. Conversely, many cases of LMA rescue of the failed airway have been reported. Although control studies are lacking, Parmet et al.[124] noted that all patients fitting the cannot intubate/cannot ventilate scenario (with the exception of an iatrogenic subglottic obstruction) occurring in a 2-year period in a single hospital were rescued with an LMA. As will be discussed later, there is evidence that many of the recently introduced SGAs will function with similar success.

Awake Airway Management

⓭ Awake airway management remains a mainstay of the ASA's difficult airway algorithm. Awake intubation provides many advantages over the anesthetic state, including maintenance of spontaneous ventilation in the event that the airway cannot be secured rapidly, increased size and patency of the pharynx, relative forward placement of the base of the tongue, posterior placement of the larynx, and patency of the retropalatal space.[131] The effect of sedatives and general anesthetics on airway patency may be secondary to direct effects on motoneurons and on the reticular activating system. The sleep apnea patient may be particularly prone to obstruction with minimal sedation. Additionally, the awake state confers some maintenance of upper and lower esophageal sphincter tone, thus reducing the risk of reflux. In the event that reflux occurs, the patient can close the glottis and/or expel aspirated foreign bodies by cough to the extent that these reflexes have not been obtunded by local anesthesia.[132] Lastly, patients at risk for neurologic sequelae (e.g., patients with unstable cervical spine pathology) may undergo active sensory-motor testing immediately after tracheal intubation. In an emergent situation, there may be cautions (e.g., cardiovascular stimulation in the presence of cardiac ischemia or ischemic risk, bronchospasm, increased intraocular pressure, increased intracranial pressure) but no absolute contraindications to awake intubation. Contraindications to elective awake intubation include patient refusal or inability to cooperate (e.g., child, profound mental retardation, dementia, intoxication) or allergy to local anesthetics.

Once the clinician has decided to proceed with awake airway management, the patient must be prepared both physically and psychologically. Most adult patients will appreciate an explanation of the need for an awake airway examination and will be more cooperative once they realize the importance of, and rationale for, any uncomfortable procedures. Patients understand safety and the discussion should emphasize the anesthesiologist's concerns. Once the airway has been prepared, patients will realize that they should experience no further discomfort during the intubation.

Apart from appropriate explanation, medication can also be used to allay anxiety. If sedatives are to be used, the clinician must keep in mind that producing obstruction or apnea in the difficult airway patient can be devastating and an overly sedated patient may not be able to protect the airway from regurgitated gastric contents, or cooperate with procedures. Although almost any sedative agent can be used, some rules should apply to all: judicious dosing in small amounts, avoid polypharmacy (try to use no more that two agents), and have reversal agents at hand. Small doses of benzodiazepines (diazepam, midazolam, lorazepam) are commonly used to alleviate anxiety without producing significant respiratory depression. These drugs may be given in intravenous or oral forms (when available) and may be reversed with specific antagonists (e.g., flumazenil). Opioid receptor agonists (e.g., fentanyl, alfentanil, remifentanil) can also be used in small, titrated doses for their sedative and antitussive effects, although caution must be exercised. A specific antagonist (e.g., naloxone) should always be immediately available. Ketamine, droperidol, and dexmedetomidine have also been popular among clinicians. Dexmedetomidine, a highly selective centrally acting α_2-adrenergic agonist, has been used for sedation and analgesia without respiratory depression in patients who underwent awake fiberoptic intubation because of difficult airways,[133] cervical spine problems,[133,134] and inability to cooperate with awake intubation. Combined with topical anesthesia dexmedetomidine sedation provided for a smooth intubation. A loading dose of dexmedetomidine is 1 μg/kg intravenously over 10 minutes, and maintenance infusion dose is 0.2 to 0.7 μg/kg/h.[85] Dexmedetomidine may cause hypotension, which can be corrected by phenylephrine or ephedrine. Deep sedation with dexmedetomidine should not be confused with awake intubation, during which the clinician strives to maintain airway protective reflexes and patient responsiveness to verbal commands and cooperation.

Administration of antisialagogues is important to the success of awake intubation techniques. As will be discussed later, clearing of airway secretions is essential to the use of indirect optical instruments (e.g., flexible or rigid fiberoptic laryngoscope, videolaryngoscope) because small amounts of any liquid can obscure the objective lens. The commonly used drugs atropine (0.5 to 1 mg intramuscularly or intravenously) and glycopyrrolate (0.2 to 0.4 mg intramuscularly or intravenously) have other significant effects: by reducing saliva production, these drugs increase the effectiveness of topically applied local anesthetics by removing a barrier to mucosal contact and reducing drug dilution. The clinician must wait until the patient subjectively reports the drying activity of the injected antisialagogue. Vasoconstriction of the nasal passages is required if there is to be instrumentation of this part of the airway. Oxymetazoline is a potent and long-lasting vasoconstrictor. In the authors' experience the nasal passages should always be included in the preparation for awake intubation: first, if during the course of the awake intubation, the plan is changed from the oral to nasal route, preparation is complete. Second, much of the preparation of the nose with local anesthesia (see later discussion), which can occur prior to the peak onset of the desiccant, will affect the pharyngeal airway. If the patient is at risk for gastric regurgitation and aspiration, prophylactic measures should be undertaken. It is also prudent to supply supplemental oxygen to the patient by nasal cannula (which can be placed over the nose or mouth).

Local anesthetics are a cornerstone of awake airway control techniques (see Chapter 21). The airway, from the base of the tongue to the bronchi, comprises an undeniably sensitive series of structures. Topical anesthesia and injected nerve block techniques have been developed to blunt the protective airway reflexes as well as to provide analgesia. As is well known to the anesthetic practitioner, local anesthetics are both effective and potentially dangerous drugs. The clinician should have a thorough understanding of the mechanism of action, metabolism, toxicities, and acceptable cumulative doses of the drugs that he or she chooses to employ in the airway. Because much of the agent used will be within the tracheal-bronchial tree and can travel to the alveoli, there is a potential for significant intravascular absorption with some techniques. In a human study on lidocaine toxicity, 400 or 800 mg was topically applied to the upper airway. Serial blood lidocaine levels were measured peaking 60 minutes later at 0.5 and 1.28 μg/mL, respectively. Toxic levels of lidocaine are considered to be 4.0 μg/mL.[135] In a recent study using the same dose of lidocaine administered by nebulizer, serum levels of 2.8 and 6.5 μg/mL were measured within 10 minutes of dose completion, respectively.[136]

Despite the myriad of local anesthetics available, only those most commonly used in airway preparation will be discussed here. In reality, the choice of local anesthetic employed has little to do with success of the technique of awake intubation; ignoring the other aspects of preparation outlined here lead to failure just as readily.[123]

Among otolaryngologists, cocaine is a popular topical agent. Not only is it a highly effective local anesthetic, but also it is the only local anesthetic that is a potent vasoconstrictor. It is commonly available in a 4% solution. The total dose applied to the mucosa should not exceed 200 mg in the adult. Cocaine should not be used in patients with a known cocaine hypersensitivity, hypertension, ischemic heart disease, pre-eclampsia, or those taking monoamine oxidase inhibitors. Because cocaine is metabolized by pseudocholinesterase, it is contraindicated in patients who are deficient in this enzyme.

Lidocaine, an amide local anesthetic, is available in a wide variety of preparations and doses (Table 29-16). Topically applied, peak onset is within 15 minutes.

Tetracaine is an amide local anesthetic with a longer duration of action than either cocaine or lidocaine. Solutions of 0.5%, 1%, and 2% are available. Absorption of this drug from the respiratory and gastrointestinal tracts is rapid, and toxicity after nebulized application has been reported with doses as low as 40 mg, although the acceptable safe dose in adults is 100 mg by other routes of application.[137]

Benzocaine is popular among some clinicians because of its very rapid onset (<1 minute) and short duration (approximately 10 minutes). It is available in 10%, 15%, and 20% solutions. It has been combined with tetracaine (Hurricaine) to prolong the duration of action. A 0.5-second aerosol administration of Hurricaine delivers 30 mg of benzocaine, the toxic dose being 100 mg. Another common preparation is Cetacaine spray, which combines benzocaine with tetracaine, butyl aminobenzoate, benzalkonium chloride, and cetyldimethylethyl ammonium bromide. Benzocaine may produce methemoglobinemia, which is treated by the administration of methylene blue (1 to 2 mg intravenously).

There are three anatomic areas to which the clinician directs local anesthetic therapy: the nasal cavity/nasopharynx,

TABLE 29-16

AVAILABLE LIDOCAINE PREPARATIONS

■ PREPARATION	■ DOSES (%)
Injectable/topical solution	1, 2, 4
Viscous solution	1, 2
Ointment	1, 5
Aerosol	10

the pharynx/base of tongue, and the hypopharynx/larynx/trachea. The nasal cavity is innervated by the greater and lesser palatine nerves (innervating the nasal turbinates and most of the nasal septum) and the anterior ethmoid nerve (innervating the nares and anterior third of the nasal septum). The two palatine nerves arise from the sphenopalatine ganglion, located posterior to the middle turbinate. Two techniques for nerve block have been described. The ganglion can be approached through a noninvasive nasal approach: cotton-tipped applicators soaked in local anesthetic are passed along the upper border of the middle turbinate until the posterior wall of the nasopharynx is reached. They are left in place for 5 to 10 minutes. In the oral approach, a needle is introduced into the greater palatine foramen, which can be palpated in the posterior lateral aspect of the hard palate, 1 cm medial to the second and third maxillary molars. Anesthetic solution (1 to 2 mL) is injected with a spinal needle inserted in a superior/posterior direction at a depth of 2 to 3 cm. Care must be taken not to inject into the sphenopalatine artery. The anterior ethmoid nerve can be blocked by cotton-tipped applicators soaked in local anesthetic placed along the dorsal surface of the nose until the anterior cribriform plate is reached. The applicator is left in place for 5 to 10 minutes.

The oropharynx is innervated by branches of the vagus, facial, and glossopharyngeal nerves. The glossopharyngeal nerve travels anteriorly along the lateral surface of the pharynx, its three branches supplying sensory innervation to the posterior third of the tongue, the vallecula, the anterior surface of the epiglottis (lingual branch), the walls of the pharynx (pharyngeal branch), and the tonsils (tonsillar branch). A wide variety of techniques may be used to anesthetize this part of the airway. The simplest techniques involve aerosolized local anesthetic solution, or a voluntary "swish and swallow." As long as the clinician has developed a plan to anesthetize all relevant structures, has allowed enough time for drying agents to work, and remains continually cognizant of the total dose of local anesthetics administered, most patients will be adequately anesthetized in this way.

Some patients may require a glossopharyngeal nerve block, especially when topical techniques do not adequately block the gag reflex. The branches of this nerve are most easily accessed as they transverse the palatoglossal folds. These folds are seen as soft tissue ridges that extend from the posterior aspect of the soft palate to the base of the tongue, bilaterally (Fig. 29-13).

A noninvasive technique employs anesthetic-soaked cotton-tipped applicators that are positioned against the inferior most aspect of the folds, and left in place for 5 to 10 minutes. When the noninvasive technique proves inadequate, local anesthetic can be injected. Standing on the side contralateral to the nerve to be blocked, the operator displaces the extended tongue to the contralateral side and a 25-gauge spinal needle is inserted into the membrane near the floor of the mouth. An aspiration test is performed. If air is aspirated, the needle has passed through-and-through the membrane. If blood is aspirated, the needle tip is redirected more medially. The lingual branch is most readily blocked in this manner, but retrograde tracking of the injectate has also been demonstrated.[132] Even though it provides a reliable block, this technique is reported to be painful and may result in a bothersome and persistent hematoma.[138] A posterior approach to the glossopharyngeal nerve has been described in the otolaryngologic literature (for tonsillectomy). It may be difficult to visualize the site of needle insertion as it is behind the palatopharyngeal arch where the nerve is in close proximity to the carotid artery. Because of the risk for arterial injection and bleeding, the technique will not be described here; however, the reader is referred to a more authoritative text.[85]

The internal branch of the superior laryngeal nerve, which is a branch of the vagus nerve, provides sensory innervation to

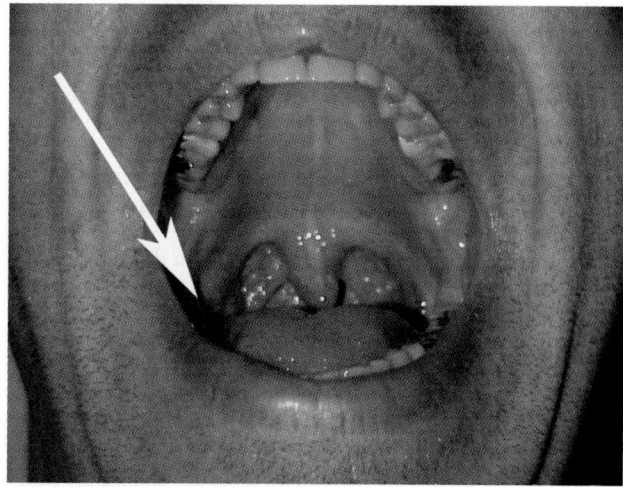

FIGURE 29-13. The palatoglossal arch (*arrow*) is a soft tissue fold that is a continuation of the posterior edge of the soft palate to the base of the tongue. A local anesthetic-soaked swab placed in the gutter along the base of the tongue is left in contact with the fold for 5 to 10 minutes.

the base of the tongue, epiglottis, aryepiglottic folds, and arytenoids. The branch originates from the superior laryngeal nerve lateral to the cornu of the hyoid bone. It then pierces the thyrohyoid membrane and travels under the mucosa in the pyriform recess. The remaining portion of the superior laryngeal nerve, the external branch, supplies motor innervation to the cricothyroid muscle. Several blocks of this nerve have been described. In many instances topical application of anesthetics in the oral cavity will provide adequate analgesia. An external block is performed with the patient supine with the head extended and the clinician standing on the side ipsilateral to the nerve to be blocked. The clinician identifies the superior cornu of the hyoid bone beneath the angle of the mandible. Using one hand, medially directed pressure is applied to the contralateral hyoid cornu, displacing the ipsilateral hyoid cornu toward the clinician. Caution must be taken to locate the carotid artery and displace it if necessary. The needle can be inserted directly over the hyoid cornu and then "walked" off the cartilage in an anterior-caudad direction until it can be passed through the ligament to a depth of 1 to 2 cm. Before the injection of local anesthetic, an aspiration test should be performed to ensure that one has not entered the pharynx or a vascular structure. Local anesthetic with epinephrine (1.5 to 2 mL) is injected in the space between the thyrohyoid membrane and the pharyngeal mucosa. The superior laryngeal nerve can also be blocked with a noninvasive internal technique. The patient is asked to open the mouth widely, and the tongue is grasped using a gauze pad or tongue blade. A right-angle forceps (e.g., Jackson-Krause forceps) with anesthetic-soaked cotton swabs is slid over the lateral tongue and into the pyriform sinuses bilaterally. The cotton swabs or sponge are held in place for 5 minutes.

Sensory innervation of the vocal folds and the trachea is provided by the recurrent laryngeal nerve. Transtracheal injection of local anesthetic can easily be performed to produce adequate analgesia, and the technique is described in detail later (see "Retrograde Intubation"). Lidocaine, 4 mL of 2% or 4% solution, is injected.

An effective and noninvasive technique of tracheal and vocal cord topical analgesia uses the working channel of the fiberoptic bronchoscope. A disadvantage of this technique is that solutions leaving the working channel can obscure the objective lens. This can be overcome by use of an epidural catheter, inserted through the working channel, as described by Ovassapian.[139] Not only does this prevent the obscuring of the view, but also allows specific "aiming" of the anesthetic stream. Multiorifice catheters should be trimmed in length so only the distal orifice exists.

Clinical Difficult Airway Scenarios

⓮ The clinician approaching the patient with a difficult airway has a vast armamentarium of techniques and instruments that can be applied to securing and maintaining oxygenation and ventilation.[140] Although this array can be confusing, textbook authors cannot dictate specific approaches in every situation; moreover, the variability of patient presentation makes specific recommendations difficult. Thus, in order to discuss management, the following section presents a number of brief clinical scenarios and the authors' own approach. The major alternative airway management techniques are discussed in this manner. All of the clinical cases described herein have been managed by the authors or a colleague. Other techniques that might be applied in each situation are also discussed, together with the authors' own "decision tree" regarding their applicability. In these cases, as in actual practice, the first technique applied may not have been the best one. The principle of flexibility (and a keen eye to the need to change course quickly) will be emphasized repeatedly. In view of the critical importance of the act of airway control, the clinician must be prepared to alter his or her approach as the situation demands. Table 29-17 shows the authors' route through the AAA (Fig. 29-12) with each case.

When DL and tracheal intubation fail, the clinician has a large armamentarium of tools to turn to. Because successful DL depends on sufficient tissue distortion (in order to create a line of site), techniques that do not require similar anatomic alignment may be successful after failed DL. Fiberoptic, video-coupled, supraglottic airway (SGA), stylet-assisted (e.g., lighted stylet), and retrograde techniques may provide a successful alternative. But these techniques also call upon alternative skill sets. In a difficult or critical situation it is unlikely that turning to an unpracticed technique will be helpful.[141]

Unfortunately, clinicians rarely employ alternative techniques until a difficult situation arises. Heidegger et al.[141] introduced a simple algorithm for incorporating flexible fiberoptic-aided tracheal intubation into daily practice as a routine alternative to DL. Their incidence of difficult intubation was 6 in 1,324 cases, or 0.049%, markedly lower than the 0.3% reported previously.[83]

Case 1: Video laryngoscopy

A 46-year-old obese woman (height, 153 cm; weight, 77 kg) is scheduled for craniotomy. On examination of her airway she is found to have a Mallampati grade of 2 and a thyromental distance of 4.0 cm. After induction of anesthesia and neuromuscular blockade, DL was performed and revealed a Cormack-Lehane score of 3. Repositioning of the patient's head and neck, and external laryngeal manipulation did not improve the view of the laryngeal anatomy. A GlideScope video laryngoscope was used and the arytenoids, but not glottic aperture, were displayed on the video screen. A second anesthesiologist applied external laryngeal pressure and the GlideScope display clearly showed that the arytenoids had been moved to the left. By watching the display, the second anesthesiologist was able to adjust the direction and force of external laryngeal pressure to bring the glottis into view. While observing the displayed image, the first anesthesiologist inserted a gum elastic bougie into the larynx over which a ETT was advanced. Both anesthesiologists were able to visually confirm ETT placement. Capnography and auscultation of the chest confirmed the correct ETT position.

GlideScope

The GlideScope (Verathon, Bothell, WA; Fig. 29-14A) provides an electronically projected image on a video monitor emanating from a video chip set at the distal end of a conventional-like laryngoscope blade, but with a more acute (60 degrees) distal angulation.[142] Illumination is likewise generated at the distal position. This configuration affords several advantages. (1) It may be handled with a skill set similar to that used with conventional DL. (2) The operator's point of sight (e.g., the video apparatus) is positioned close to the distal blade aspect. (3) The video apparatus is a charged coupled-like device (thereby eliminating fragile fiberoptic elements). The operator therefore "sees" at a position behind the tongue, and displacement as with conventional DL is not necessary in most cases. Similarly, lingual tonsil hyperplasia should not affect the visual axis as it does with conventional DL. (4) The video image of the airway is displayed on a lightweight portable screen, and allows for visualization by more than one individual (e.g., aid, mentor, student). (5) Less stress may be imposed on the airway by virtue of reduced compressive force directed to the tongue. (6) An external light source is not required.

When used by inexperienced operators the GlideScope provides better glottic exposure as compared with DL (Cormack-Lehane grade 1 view in 85.7% vs. 48.9%) and can obtain Cormack-Lehane grade 1 or 2 in 77% of patients in whom no glottic exposure was achieved by DL.[142] Although it can

TABLE 29-17

THE AIRWAY APPROACH ALGORITHM AS APPLIED TO CHAPTER CLINICAL CASES

■ CASE[a]	■ REQUIRE CONTROL?[b]	■ DL DIFFICULT?[b]	■ SGA POSSIBLE?[b]	■ STOMACH EMPTY?[b]	■ TOLERANCE APNEA[b]	■ BOX[b]
1	Yes	Yes	Yes	Yes	Yes	B
2	Yes	Yes	No[c]	—	—	A
3	Yes	Yes	Yes	Yes	No	A
4	Yes	No	—	—	—	B
5	Yes	No	—	—	—	B
6	Yes	Yes	Yes	No	—	B

DL, direct laryngoscopy; SGA, supraglottic airways.
[a]Refer to clinical cases.
[b]Refer to Figure 29-11.
[c]Once a "No" is reached a clinical decision (last column) is made.

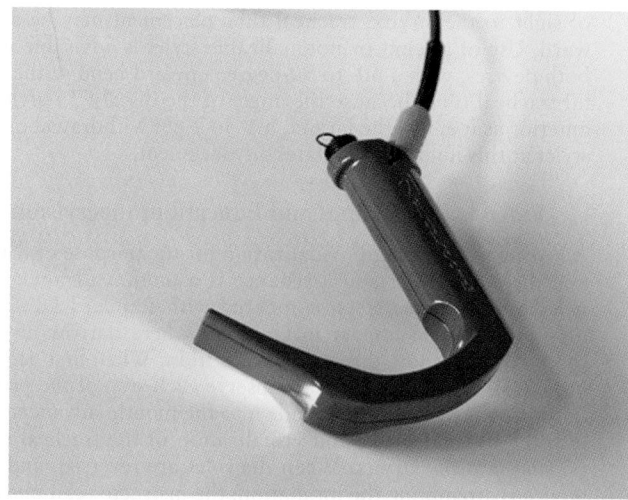

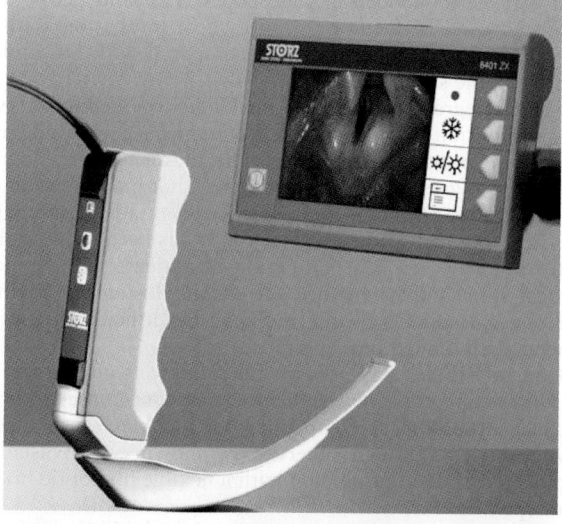

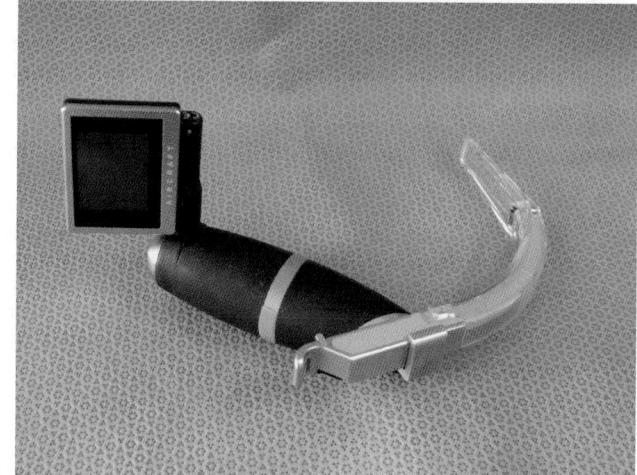

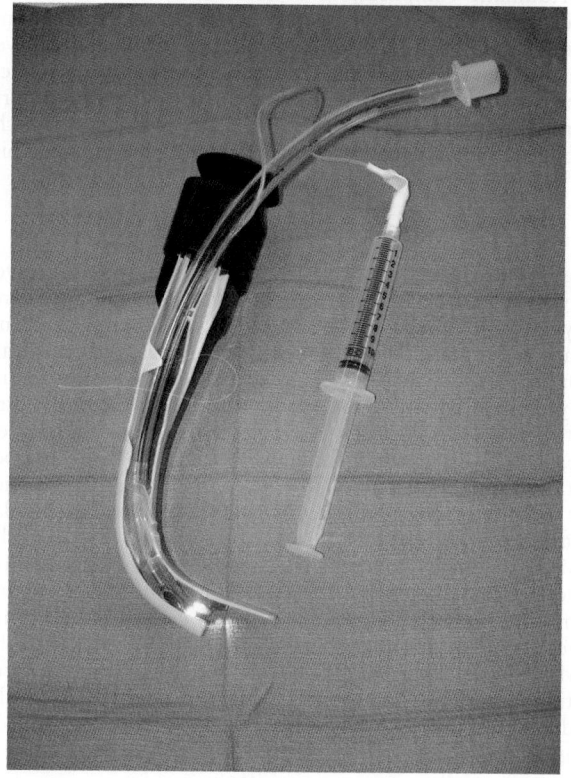

FIGURE 29-14. **A.** GlideScope. (Photograph courtesy of Dr. Richard Cooper.) **B.** C-Mac. (Photograph courtesy of Karl Storz Endoscopy, Culver City, CA). **C.** The McGrath Series 5 video laryngoscope (Courtesy of McGrath Medical, UK) **D.** Airtraq (Courtesy of King Systems).

improve the laryngeal view by one grade in many patients, this does not automatically imply more rapid tracheal intubation. In one study, placement of the ETT required an additional 16 seconds (average).[142,143]

The classic GlideScope insertion technique follows the midline approach. After the uvula is visualized, the blade is advanced midline into the vallecula or can be passed posterior to the epiglottis.[142] For patients with a limited mouth aperture, an alternative insertion has been described in which the blade is inserted like a Guedel airway; that is, the GlideScope blade concavity facing rostrad and rotated 180 degrees counterclockwise once the distal tip is in the oropharynx. This maneuver displaces the tongue to the left and minimizes neck movements.

Although achieving a good laryngeal view with the GlideScope appears relatively easy, ETT manipulation into the larynx may be more difficult because of the acute blade angulation. The use of a stylet is advised to deliver the ETT.[144,145] Different authors have suggested stylet shaping with a bend of 60-degree, 90-degree, a dynamic stylet, J, or "gear shift" shape. Reverse loading technique or use of a gum elastic bougie has also been described.[146] There is one study that evidenced that the angle of the ETT had greater impact on time to intubation than the Cormack and Lehane grade of the image.[147] Recently, a dedicated, nonmalleable stylet, the Glidescope reusable stylet (Verathon) has been introduced. This stylet has a 90-degree bend, and may be used with various video laryngoscopes. The GlideScope has also been used to facilitate nasotracheal intubation with a reduced time to intubation when compared with DL and a high first-time success rate.

The 60-degree angulation of the GlideScope reduces cervical spine motion by 50% at the C2-5 segments compared with Macintosh laryngoscopy. Theoretically, the airway axes do not need to be aligned to affect a good view, but manipulation of the GlideScope to the position to achieve an adequate image can cause cervical segment extension. It has been successfully used to achieve tracheal intubation in patients with limited cervical spine movement because of ankylosing spondylitis and cervical spine arthritis, but may be difficult to use in patients with limited oral aperture.[148,149]

Control studies have shown no significant advantage of the GlideScope in preventing hemodynamic responses to orotracheal intubation as compared with the Macintosh direct laryngoscope, although others have shown cardiovascular responses similar to intubation with a flexible fiberoptic bronchoscope.[150]

Traumatic complications associated with the use of the GlideScope video laryngoscope have been related to blind manipulation of the ETT as it enters the airway but is not yet visualized on the perilaryngeal image. Traumatic events, which appear to be more likely with the use of a rigid stylet, are primarily reported to involve the soft palate, palatoglossal arch, right palatopharyngeal arch, and right anterior tonsillar pillar.[151-155]

Video Macintosh

The Video Macintosh (VM; Karl Storz Endovision, Culver City, CA; Fig. 29-14B) consists of a conventional-appearing laryngoscope handle and blade fitted with illumination and image fiberoptics. The VM handle interfaces with the Karl Storz proprietary DCI camera system. The video image is displayed on a standard NTSC monitor. Although the image projected from the VM closely resembles that seen with the naked eye, (1) ETT placement is facilitated because the operator does not need to maintain an unobstructed line of sight (his or her eye using the video monitor), (2) external laryngeal manipulation can be observed by a second operator, and (3) use of the VM is identical standard DL, making the video facility uniquely valuable during supervised instruction. A comparison study of direct and video-assisted views of the larynx revealed significant improvement of the glottic view with the VM.[156] In controlled trials, the VM facilitated tracheal intubation in bariatric and thoracic surgery patients.[157] Recently, a digital version (CMOS) of the VA has been introduced (Fig. 29-14B).

McGrath

The McGrath Series 5 video laryngoscope (Aircraft Medical, Edinburgh, UK) was introduced to clinical practice in 2007 (Fig. 29-14C). At the time of this writing, no controlled clinical trials with this device have been published in the literature. The experience among users was extremely positive for use as a primary or rescue video laryngoscopy device. The unique features of the McGrath are (1) self-contained unit including laryngoscopic blade, handle, power source (1.5 v batteries), and 3.3 × 2.2 cm LCD (liquid crystal display) screen; (2) acute distal angle blade; (3) adjustable blade length; and (4) disposable patient contact blade. As with the GlideScope, the acute angle blade improves the Cormack and Lehane grade of the laryngeal view by affording the operator an oblique line of sight around the base of the tongue. In one uncontrolled series, tracheal intubation was successful in 98% of 150 elective surgery patients.[158] Because McGrath video laryngoscopy, as with the GlideScope, does not involve creation of a direct line

of sight to the larynx, tracheal tube placement may be awkward. Use of a semi- or nonmalleable stylet is advisable with both devices, with a 60- to 90-degree upward bend of the distal tracheal tube. Because the angle of the distal ETT-stylet is anterior as it enters the larynx, a 1- to 2-cm withdrawal of the stylet at this juncture facilitates advancement.

Video laryngoscopes and Education/Supervision

Allowing shared glottic visualization for the purpose of teaching, the supervising and assistance is a unique advantage of videolaryngoscopes when compared with standard DL. This may have special impact in children, where narrow airway spaces do not allow direct covisualization. When first acquiring DL skills, the student can observe each step of the procedure from insertion of the blade into the mouth, advancement into the hypopharynx, and visualization of the tracheal tube passing into the larynx. When the roles are reversed, and the novice is attempting the intubation, the instructor can observe the results of the efforts and can guide the novice through the entire process, as well as witness laryngeal passage of the ETT.[157] Video laryngoscopes may therefore provide important information to the instructor about the trainee's difficulties with DL and ETT insertion. Likewise, the progression of external laryngeal manipulation, its proper application, and effectiveness can be demonstrated and taught with these devices.[159,160]

The use of VM for teaching laryngoscopy in the patients with normal and anticipated difficult airways has been reported.[161] Recently, use of the GlideScope has been described in teaching fiberoptic bronchoscope-aided tracheal intubation.[162] The GlideScope image was used by the instructor to direct the novice operators' use of the fiberoptic bronchoscope.

Airtraq

The Airtraq optical laryngoscope (Prodol Meditec S.A., Vizcaya, Spain; Fig. 29-14D) is a single-use, anatomically shaped laryngoscope optical prism device, with a lateral guiding channel that holds and guides the ETT through the vocal cords. It has a built-in antifog system and a low temperature light.

Airtraq has been successfully used as a rescue device in seven patients after failed intubation with DL.[163] Reports of its use in awake patients, patients with cervical spine disease, and after failed DL have been published.[164] One study showed the need for fewer maneuvers to improve glottic exposure and fewer alterations in blood pressure and heart rate when compared with DL.[165]

Truview

The Truview EVO2 optical laryngoscope (Truphatek, Netanya, Israel), consists of a slim, straight laryngoscope blade with a distal upward curved tip (40 degrees). The proximal blade is fitted with a telescope that can be used with the naked eye or an endoscopic camera head. A lateral port may be connected to an oxygen source to provide defogging.[166] Two studies showed improved glottic view with Truview compared with Macintosh laryngoscope, but the time required for intubation was prolonged.[166] In two reports, patients who failed intubation with the Macintosh blade were successfully intubated with the Truview.[167]

Case 2: Flexible Fiberoptic-Aided Intubation

A 50-year-old man with symptomatic cervical vertebrae disk herniation presents for disk resection and spinal fixation. He has a history of tobacco use, alcohol consumption, and gastroesophageal reflux. In the preoperative holding area, 0.4 mg of intravenous glycopyrrolate is injected, and oxymetazoline is administered to the nasal cavity (commercial preparation: Afrin spray). Swabs of 5% lidocaine ointment (50 mg) are applied in to the nose. Fifteen minutes later, when the patient states that his oral secretions are minimized, topical anesthesia is administered to the remaining airway, as described. The patient receives 4 mg of intravenous midazolam. An intubating oral airway is placed without eliciting a gag reflex and a flexible fiberoptic bronchoscope is advanced into the airway. The vocal ligaments are visualized, and 4 mL of 4% lidocaine solution are injected through the accessory lumen of the fiberscope (using the Ovassapian catheter technique), being seen to bathe the laryngeal and sublaryngeal structures.[139] The distal end of the fiberscope is advanced into the larynx, and a 7.0-ID ETT, which had been threaded onto the insertion shaft of the fiberscope, is advanced into the trachea. The fiberscope is removed while the structures of the carina, trachea, and finally the tracheal tube are observed. The anesthesia circuit is attached to the tracheal tube and a steady output of carbon dioxide is detected by capnography. A brief sensory and motor neurologic examination is performed by the attending surgeon and general anesthesia is induced.

Use of the Fiberoptic Bronchoscope in Airway Management. The fiberoptic bronchoscope is a ubiquitous instrument in anesthesia, being available to 99% of surveyed active ASA members.[140] The technique of fiberoptic-aided intubation was first performed using a choledochoscope in a patient with Still's disease (idiopathic, adult-onset arthritis).[168] By the late 1980s it was recognized that the use of the flexible fiberoptic bronchoscope represented such a significant advancement in the management of the patient with a difficult airway that experts stated that no anesthesiologist could afford not to be facile with this technique.[169] It is now generally accepted that for a variety of clinical situations, the fiberoptic bronchoscope is a critical tool in the armamentarium of the anesthesiologist dealing with the awake or unconscious patient who is, or appears to be, difficult to intubate.[132] The fiberoptic bronchoscope has proven to be the most versatile tool available in this regard.[139]

There is no true or firm indication for fiberoptic bronchoscope-aided intubation, as there might be with DL (e.g., rapid-sequence induction for the full-stomach patient). There are, however, many clinical situations in which the fiberoptic bronchoscope can be of unparalleled aid in securing the airway, especially if the clinician has made an effort to master the necessary skills by using it in routine endotracheal intubations.[139,141] These include anticipated difficult intubation by history or physical examination findings, unanticipated difficult intubation (in which other techniques have failed), lower and upper airway obstruction, unstable or fixed cervical spine disease, mass effect in the upper or lower airways, dental risk or damage, and awake intubation.[139] Unlike the other devices used to intubate the trachea, the fiberoptic bronchoscope can also serve to visualize structures below the level of the vocal folds. For example, it can identify the placement of the tracheal tube or aid in placement of a double-lumen tracheal tube. It may be helpful in diagnosis within the trachea and bronchial tree or in pulmonary toilet (Fig. 29-15).

Contraindications to fiberoptic bronchoscope-aided intubation are relative, and revolve about the limitations of the device (Table 29-18).

Because the optical elements are small (the objective lens is typically 2 mm in diameter or smaller), minute amounts of airway secretions, blood, or traumatic debris can hinder visualization. Care must be taken to remove these obstacles from the airway beforehand; application of intramuscular or intravenous antisialagogues (e.g., glycopyrrolate, 0.2 to 0.4 mg; atropine, 0.5 to 1 mg) will produce a drying effect within 15 minutes, but caution should be taken in patients who may not

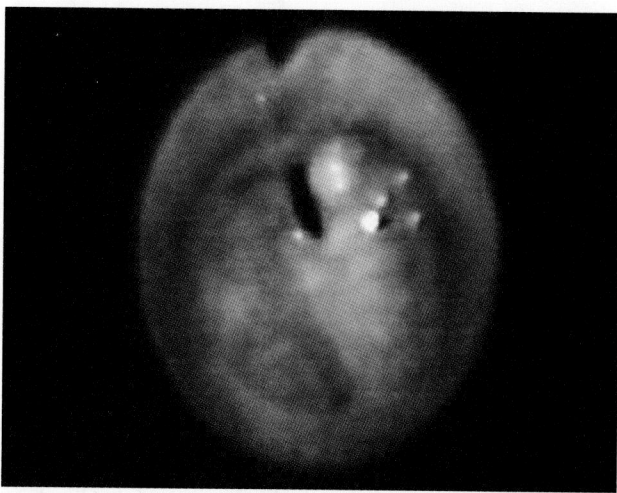

FIGURE 29-15. The fiberoptic bronchoscope may be useful for diagnosis and therapy below the level of the vocal ligaments, including bronchial segments examination and toilet. Laryngeal web is shown here.

be able to tolerate an increase in heart rate. Vasoconstriction of the nose using topical oxymetazoline, phenylephrine, or cocaine reduces the chances of bleeding if this route is chosen. If an awake intubation is planned using the fiberoptic bronchoscope, the patient must be able to cooperate—a "quiet" airway, with little motion of the head, neck, tongue, and larynx, is vital to success. Finally, because fiberoptic bronchoscope-aided intubation of the trachea can require significant time, especially if the clinician is not facile with the device, hypoxia or impending hypoxia is a contraindication, and a more rapid method of securing an airway (e.g., LMA or surgical airway) should be considered.

Elements of the Fiberoptic Bronchoscope. The fiberoptic bronchoscope is a fragile device with optical and nonoptical elements. The fundamental element consists of a glass-fiber bundle. Each fiber is 8 to 12 *microns* in diameter, and is coated with a secondary glass layer termed the *cladding*. The cladding aids in maintaining the image within each fiber as the light is reflected off the sidewall at a rate of 10,000 times per meter as it moves from the objective lens to the eyepiece lens in the operator's handle. The typical intubating fiberoptic bronchoscope has 10,000 to 30,000 such fibers encased in a 60-cm, water-impermeable insertion cord, with gradation marks every 10 cm. Although the fibers are allowed to rotate over each other throughout the length of the cord, they are fused together at the two ends in a coherent pattern; that is, the arrangement of the fibers at the eyepiece end is identical to the arrangement at the objective lens, where a diopter ring allows focusing. Therefore, one might envision that the image before the objective lens (i.e., the objective) is divided into 10,000

TABLE 29-18

CONTRAINDICATIONS TO FIBEROPTIC BRONCHOSCOPY

Hypoxia

Heavy airway secretions not relieved with suction or antisialagogues

Bleeding from the upper or lower airway not relieved with suction

Local anesthetic allergy (for awake attempts)

Inability to cooperate (for awake attempts)

individual and unique pictures, which independently travel down an unwieldy cord to be reassembled in front of the eyepiece lens. Broken fibers, which may occur because of bending of the insertion cord, entrapping the cord in other equipment, and dropping the fiberoptic bronchoscope, are readily apparent and are generally no more than a nuisance until the number of broken fibers interferes with the visual field.

The insertion cord also contains an *accessory lumen* ("working channel"): a lumen, up to 2 mm in diameter, which travels from the distal tip to the handle. It can be used for applying suction, or oxygen, and instilling lavaging fluids or drugs (e.g., local anesthetics). There is one report of gastric rupture attributed to the insufflation of oxygen through the working channel when the fiberoptic bronchoscope was within the esophagus.[170] In general, fiberoptic bronchoscopes that are <2 mm in external diameter (e.g., pediatric) do not have a working channel.

Two wires traveling from a lever in the handle down the length of the insertion cord control movement of the distal tip in the sagittal plane. The entire insertion cord is protected by a metal "wrap" until the level of the distal tip, which is hinged for movement. Coronal plane movement is accomplished by a combined use of the control lever and rotation of the entire fiberoptic bronchoscope from handle to distal end. Because the fibers are able to move over one another, except for where they are fused at the extreme ends of the optic cord, rotational control is maximized by reducing any curves in the fiberoptic bronchoscope shaft.

The final element of the fiberoptic bronchoscope is the light source. Illumination of the objective is provided by one or two noncoherent bundles of glass fibers that transmit light from the handle to the distal tip. The light is provided either by a "universal" cord that emerges from the handle and is inserted into a medical-grade endoscopic light source, or may be provided by a battery-operated light source on the handle.

Use of the Fiberoptic Bronchoscope. The fiberoptic bronchoscope is held in the nondominant hand, the thumb over the control lever and the index finger poised over the working channel valve. The dominant hand will be used to steady and hold the insertion cord as it is manipulated in the patient. Many operators are tempted to "switch" hands, but the thumb of the nondominant hand should be capable of controlling the gross movement of the control lever. Any experienced endoscopist will recognize that the fine control required to hold the shaft of the endoscope steady, advance the objective end into the airway, and make directional adjustments is where the art of endoscopy lies.

The insertion shaft is lubricated with a water-soluble lubricant and it is threaded through the lumen of an ETT, the objective end emerging from the main ETT orifice. A clinically appropriate ETT should be chosen, but the larger the ratio between the internal diameter of the ETT and the external diameter of the insertion shaft, the greater the risk of "hang-up" on airway structures, as occurs in 20 to 30% of attempts.[139]

Hang-up occurs when a cleft exists between these two devices because of the differential sizes. Hang-up may involve entrapment of the epiglottis, corniculate/arytenoid cartilages, the aryepiglottic folds, or the vocal folds, and can occur with any number of stylet-guided techniques (e.g., fiberoptic, retrograde wire, lighted stylet), although it is most thoroughly described with fiberoptic-aided intubation.[171,172] The orientation of the tracheal tube bevel is important in this regard. In orotracheal intubation, the bevel cleft is likely to entrap the right arytenoid cartilage when the ETT is in its typical concavity anterior position. Rotation of the ETT counterclockwise 90 degrees places the bevel facing posteriorly and improves passage. During nasotracheal intubation, the epiglottis may be

entrapped, and a bevel-up position (rotation of the ETT 90 degrees clockwise) may facilitate passage.

The type of tracheal tube may also affect passage. It has been suggested that the Parker Flex-Tip may pass the airway structures more easily than a standard ETT bevel.[173] The use of soft-tipped ETTs, asking the patient to inspire deeply during the ETT advancement, and the "double setup" ETT, which uses a small ETT (e.g., 5.0 ID) within a clinically adequate ETT (e.g., 7.5 ID) to overcome the clefts caused by size differentials have been described.[171]

The clinician chooses the route of intubation, either oral or nasal, based on clinical requirements, surgical needs, operator experience, and other intubation techniques available should fiberoptic bronchoscope-aided intubation fail. This last factor is important because should an attempt at nasal intubation fail, there may be significant bleeding, which may hinder other indirect visualization techniques. The nasal route is considered easier by many clinicians, although other cautions apply: vasoconstrictors should be applied to reduce bleeding; the turbinates (lateral walls) may obstruct ETT passage, bleed, or be painful when traumatized; small, lubricated, and softened (bathed in warm water) ETT should be employed.

A variety of intubating oral airways are commercially available. Their chief function is to provide a clear visual path from the oral aperture to the pharynx, keep the bronchoscope in the midline, prevent the patient from biting the insertion cord, and provide a clear airway for the spontaneously or mask-ventilated patient. The common characteristic of all intubating oral airways is a channel along the length of the airway large enough to allow the passage of the tracheal tube. The Ovassapian airway provides two sets of semicircular, incomplete flexible flanges that stabilize the ETT (up to size 9.0 ID) in the midline but allow its removal from the airway after intubation has been accomplished so that the intubating oral airway can be removed from the mouth. The flat lingual surface of the airway gives it good lateral and rotational stability. The Patil-Syracuse endoscopic airway and the Luomanen oral airway were also designed for fiberoptic-aided intubation. Each has a central groove, open at the lingual (Patil-Syracuse) or palatal (Luomanen) aspect, which allows easy removal of the ETT. The flat lingual surface provides good stability. Although this style of intubating oral airway provides superb access to the pharynx, it is larger than other airways and is often uncomfortable for the patient. The Williams airway and the Berman airway were both designed for blind oral intubation. It is often difficult to manipulate the tip of the fiberscope when it is within these narrow airways. Both are molded plastic with a complete circular internal lumen that guides the ETT toward the larynx. These airways have a small profile and are often better tolerated by the awake patient, but tend to be less stable on the tongue. Because the internal lumen is a complete circle, the Williams airway must be retreated off the ETT if it is going to be removed after intubation. This may pose difficulty if the ETT in use has a fused circuit adapter. The Berman airway solves this problem by being split along the length of one side. The plastic of the opposite side is thin and malleable. If the interincisor gap is adequate, the airway can be opened laterally to allow removal from the ETT.

After successful navigation through the oral airway, the endoscopist visualizes the vocal folds. If glottic closure, gag, or coughing occurs as the fiberoptic bronchoscope's distal tip stimulates the structures of the larynx, the operator can choose to apply local anesthetic through the working channel, administer more sedation, or withdraw the scope and reinforce preparatory procedures. The clinician might also decide to advance the fiberoptic bronchoscope into the larynx without further preparation. The actions taken must be dictated by the individual clinical situation; in the elective scenario, for example, there may be time for reinforced airway analgesia, whereas

TABLE 29-19

AIDS TO FIBEROPTIC-AIDED INTUBATION

■ TECHNIQUE	■ ADVANTAGE
Endoscopy mask	Controlled ventilation maintained during or between attempts at FOB-aided intubation
Laryngeal mask	Excellent view of the larynx and ability to ventilate during or between attempts at FOB-aided intubation
Fiberoptic-aided retrograde intubation	Guiding of the FOB with a wire known to be entering the trachea
Retrograde fiberoptic intubation	Changing a tracheostomy to an oral or nasal tracheal tube when antegrade intubation is difficult or impossible
FOB-aided intubation with the aid of a rigid laryngoscope	Helpful with an obstructing mass or large epiglottis

FOB, fiberoptic bronchoscope.

in the face of impending respiratory arrest, patient discomfort may need to be tolerated. Once the larynx is entered, the operator may choose a structure, such as the tracheal carina, to serve as an identifying landmark as the ETT is advanced. Simply because the fiberoptic bronchoscope has entered the trachea, there is no guarantee that the intubation will be successful. As previously noted, 20 to 30% of ETT advancements are accompanied by hang-up. Therefore, a patient with a critical airway should not be induced with a general anesthetic with the assumption that the ETT will be easy to pass.

The primary literature contains a number of variations and adjuncts to fiberoptic bronchoscope-aided intubation. Table 29-19, which is not meant to be exhaustive, lists several of these techniques.

Although fiberoptic bronchoscope-aided intubation is a versatile and vital technique, there are several pitfalls, most of which have been discussed. Table 29-20 lists the most common reasons for failure of fiberoptic bronchoscope-aided intubation.

Flexible fiberoptic aided intubation is a technology-intense technique. Apart from the delicate fiberoptic device, there are cameras, recorders, light sources, and a variety of disposable adjuncts that are typically required. Dedicated wheeled carts, designed to carry required and optional equipment in a functional arrangement, are available.

The Future Technology of the Flexible Fiberoptic Bronchoscope in Airway Management. The advent of the charge couple device technology was embraced in the manufacture of endoscopes used for diagnostic purposes. These devices required high-resolution images in order to detect small lesions or perform delicate procedures (e.g., venous dissection). This costly technology was slow to be incorporated into intubating flexible scopes, which work in a macro environment, not requiring the same micro resolution. Although some manufactures have produced these devices for the anesthesia market, CMOS technology, which may be produced at a far lower costs, promises to increase the number of available devices.

Rigid Fiberoptic Intubation Devices. Rigid fiberoptic devices allow indirect views of the larynx and act as an ETT guide for intubation. More than one third of all anesthesiologists have access to these devices.[140] The most commonly available of these devices include the Bullard (ACMI, Santa Barbara, CA) Upshur (Mercury Medical, Clearwater, FL) and WuScope (Pentax Precision Instruments, Orangeburg, NY) laryngoscopes. Although these laryngoscopes may be used in routine clinical situations, they are particularly useful when movement

of the patient's head and neck is impossible or contraindicated (e.g., atlanto-occipital joint disease and the spine-injured patient). They are also applicable when there is a limited oral aperture (0.64 cm in the case of the Bullard). These devices consist of a rigid, stainless steel laryngoscope-like blade that encases a fiberoptic cable with a proximal eyepiece and distal objective lens. The blades have an anatomic curve to match the neutral position of the human oral cavity-pharynx-hypopharynx relationship. Alignment of the oral, pharyngeal, and tracheal axes is not required. Illumination is provided by a second fiberoptic cable transmitting light from a battery-powered or freestanding light source.

The Bullard scope, which comes in adult and pediatric sizes, has been the best investigated. It features a fixed fiberoptic cable located on the posterior aspect of the blade. The eyepiece lens has an adjustable diopter. A working channel also runs the length of the blade. Once the larynx is visualized, the ETT is advanced using a detachable stylet, although other techniques have been described. The advantages of the Bullard scope over traditional laryngoscope blades in managing the spine-injured patient and the obese patient have been investigated.[174–176] Adequate exposure with the Bullard laryngoscope may be achieved after failed DL.

The Upsher scope (Mercury Medical, Clearwater, FL) is available in an adult size as of this writing. Instead of a stylet,

TABLE 29-20

COMMON REASONS FOR FAILURE DURING FIBEROPTIC-AIDED INTUBATION

Lack of experience: Not practicing on routine intubations
Failure to adequately dry the airway: Underdose or rushed technique
Failure to adequately anesthetize the airway of the awake patient: Secretions not dried; rushed technique
Nasal cavity bleeding: Inadequate vasoconstriction; rushed technique; forcible ETT insertion
Obstructing base of tongue or epiglottis: Poor choice of intubating airway; require chin lift/jaw thrust
Inadequate sedation of the awake patient
Hang-up: ETT too large
Fogging of the FOB: Suction or oxygen not attached to working channel; cold bronchoscope

ETT, endotracheal tube; FOB, fiberoptic bronchoscope.

the ETT is held and advanced through a C-shaped lumen in the blade. There is no working channel in this scope. The eyepiece is focusable.

The WuScope differs from the other devices in that a flexible fiberoptic endoscope is fitted into a passage within a three-part stainless steel handle and blade. A second, larger lumen accepts the ETT. A working channel is positioned alongside the endoscope lumen. Two adult sizes are manufactured. Once the larynx is visualized and the ETT is advanced into the trachea, the two stainless steel pieces of the laryngoscope blade are disassembled and removed from the mouth. Unlike the other two devices, the WuScope can also be used for nasal intubation by assembling only the anterior blade portion and the handle. An ETT, previously placed in the pharynx via the nares, can be fitted into the anterior portion of the blade.

A new generation of fiberoptic devices is focused on simplicity and portability by incorporating optical and light source elements into a single styletlike stainless steel sheath. The lack of a tongue-displacing blade and a suction/oxygen channel are potential disadvantages. The Bonfils Intubation Fiberscope (Karl Storz Endoscopy, Tuttingen, Germany; Fig. 29-16A) is a long, rigid tubular device with conventional optical and light-transmitting fiberoptic elements.[177] A proximal-end eyepiece (with adjustable diopter) can be used with the naked eye or fitted with a standard endoscopy camera. A cable (or battery-powered attachment) brings illumination from an external light source. The distal end has a 40-degree angulation. Suction may be applied through a working channel. The technique of use replicates the paraglossal approach of laryngoscopy discussed previously in this chapter. The Shikani Seeing Optical Stylet (SOS; Clarus Medical, Golden Valley, MN) has a similar configuration to the Bonfils, with the exception that the distal half of the stylet is malleable (Fig. 29-16B). The light source may be self-contained (a proprietary powered handle or a green line [Rusch Medical, Duluth, GA] laryngoscope handle), or cabled. Unlike the Bofils, a midline approach is recommended. A similar device, the Levitan FPS scope (Clarus Medical, Golden Valley, MN), a shorter (30-cm) version of the SOS, is designed to be used during DL when a high laryngeal view score is encountered (Fig. 29-16B). The shorter length allows more ergonomic positioning by the laryngoscopist.[178] Studies have investigated the use of the SOS as a substitute for the laryngoscope in routine anesthetic cases.[179] The hypothetical benefit of this practice is the reduction of unanticipated difficult intubations and the maintenance of alternative technique skills by incorporating this or similar devices in to daily practice.[141]

Case 3: Retrograde Wire Intubation

A 65-year-old woman with a 60-pack/year history of smoking and advanced rheumatoid arthritis presents to the emergency department in respiratory distress. Her oxygen saturation with a nonrebreather oxygen mask is 85%. She has a limited oral aperture (approximately 2.5 cm) and a thyromental distance of 6 cm. Although the cricothyroid membrane can be palpated, there is limited access to it and the tracheal rings owing to a significant cervical kyphosis. The sputum is noted to be blood-tinged and contains thickened bronchial secretions. Awake blind nasal intubation is attempted twice by the emergency medicine physicians, is unsuccessful, and results in epistaxis. Retrograde intubation of the airway is performed with the patient in a sitting position. After initial local anesthetic infiltration of the skin over the membrane, an 18-gauge angiocatheter is advanced over the mid-cricothyroid membrane at a angle of 45 degrees to the chest. After the free aspiration of air is noted, the Teflon sheath of the catheter is advanced into the trachea. A 0.035-inch radiologic guide wire 110 cm in length is advanced via the catheter until the proximal end emerges from the mouth. A 7.0 ETT is placed over the wire and is guided into the trachea. The wire is removed by pushing it into the percutaneous puncture site and retrieving it from the proximal end of the tracheal tube. Breath sounds are auscultated over the lung fields as ventilation is assisted with positive pressure. Once improved oxygen saturation is noted, the patient receives sedation with intravenous midazolam (in divided doses, titrating to the sedative effect).

Use of the Retrograde Wire Intubation in Airway Management. Retrograde wire intubation (RWI) involves the antegrade pulling or guiding of an ETT into the trachea using a wire that has been passed into the trachea via a percutaneous puncture through the cricothyroid membrane or the cricotracheal membrane, and blindly passed retrograde into the larynx, hypopharynx, pharynx, and out of the mouth or nose. In 1993 the technique was included in the ASA's Difficult Airway Algorithm. The basic equipment used in the retrograde intubation technique is listed in Table 29-21.

RWI has been described in a number of clinical situations as a primary intubation technique (elective or urgent) and after failed attempts at DL, fiberoptic-aided intubation, and LMA-guided intubation.[85] The most common indications are inability to visualize the vocal folds owing to blood, secretions, or anatomic variations, unstable cervical spine, upper airway malignancy, and mandibular fracture. Contraindications include lack of access to the cricothyroid membrane or

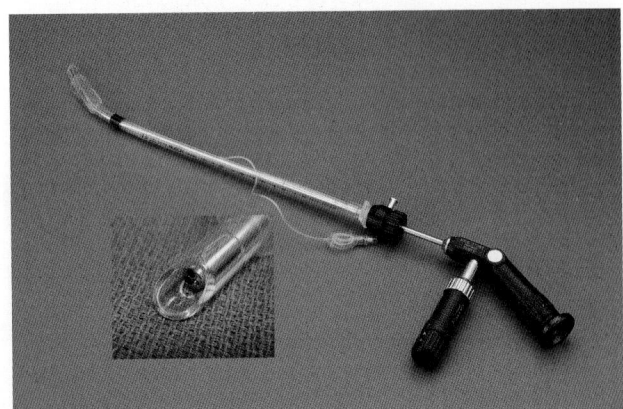
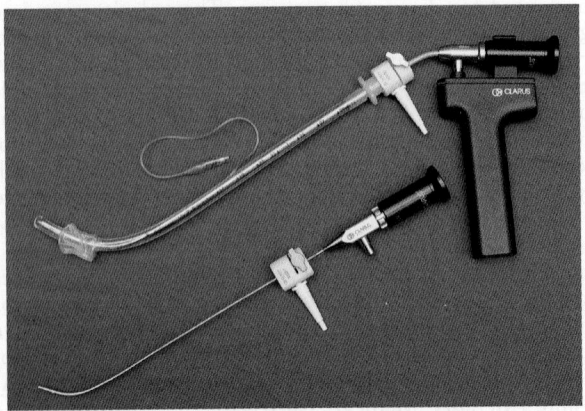

FIGURE 29-16.   **A.** The Bonfils (Karl Storz Endoscopy, Culver City, CA). Inset: Objective end within tracheal tube.
B. The Shikani Seeing Optical Stylet (Clarus Medical, Minneapolis, MN).

TABLE 29-21

EQUIPMENT FOR RETROGRADE WIRE INTUBATION

18 gauge or larger angiocatheter
Luer-lock syringe, 3 mL or larger
Guide wire:
 Preferably J-type end
 Length: at least 2.5 times the length of a standard ETT
  (typically 110–120 cm)
 Diameter: Capable of passing via angiocatheter being
  chosen
Other: Scalpel blade, nerve hook, Magill forceps, 30-inch silk
 suture, epidural catheter

ETT, endotracheal tube.

the cricotracheal ligament (because of severe neck deformity, obesity, mass), laryngotracheal disease (stenosis, malignancy, infection), coagulopathy, and skin infection.

The anatomic relationships to be considered in RWI have been described elsewhere in this chapter. Common complications reported with RWI include bleeding, subcutaneous emphysema, pneumomediastinum, pneumothorax, breath-holding, caudal traveling catheter, and trigeminal nerve trauma.

In the current patient (as in case 1), RWI was chosen in a setting in which the patient was not apneic and was therefore supporting her own ventilation and oxygenation, albeit poorly. The two cases differ in impending respiratory failure (case 2) versus fiberoptic bronchoscope-aided intubation undertaken in a stable situation (case 1). In many situations, where awake intubation is a preferred initial approach to securing the airway, there is little time for patient preparation (e.g., the administration of antisialagogues, topical anesthetics, and/or sedation). In this regard, RWI does not require a clear visual field or significant patient cooperation and can often be performed with little analgesia of the airway. The technique of RWI differs greatly from other methods of tracheal intubation familiar to the anesthesiologist. Preferably, RWI should be learned on a simulator/mannequin model before being attempted in a patient. In addition, unless RWI is practiced often, it may be time-consuming. For this reason, RWI may be a poor choice for rescue of an acutely compromised airway.

Performing Retrograde Wire Intubation. RWI is generally performed with the patient in a supine position, although the sitting position is often used for patients in respiratory distress (Fig. 29–17). Extension of the head or the neck displaces the

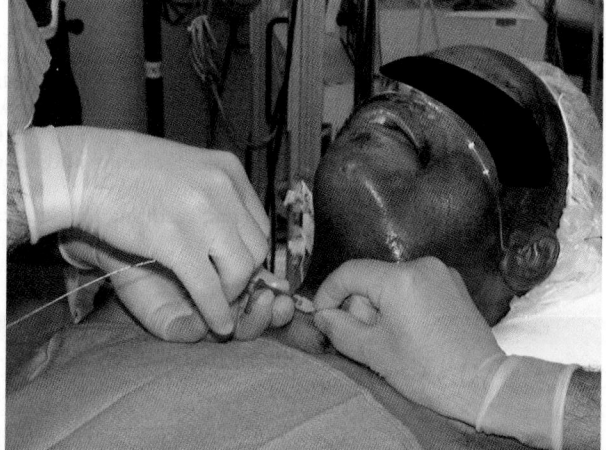
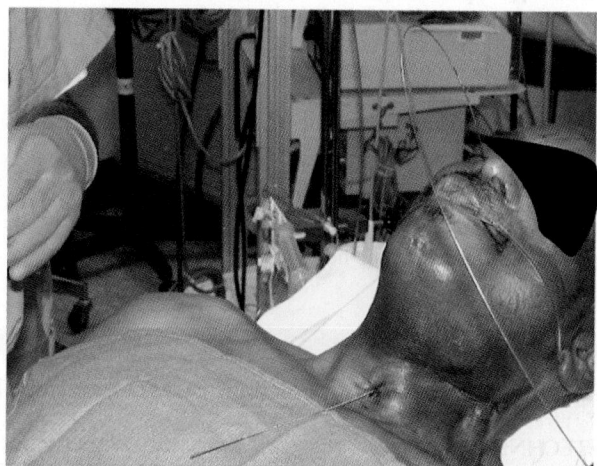
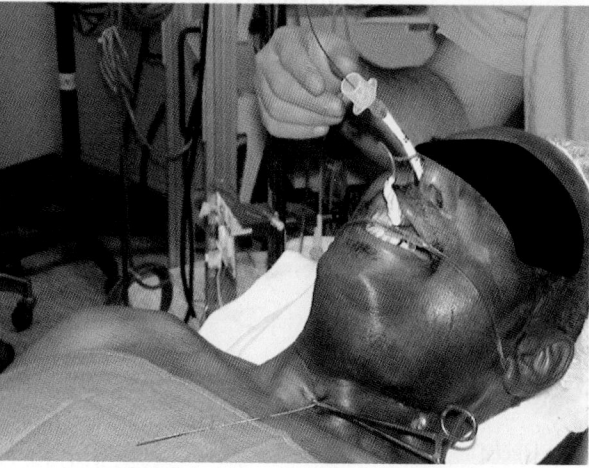
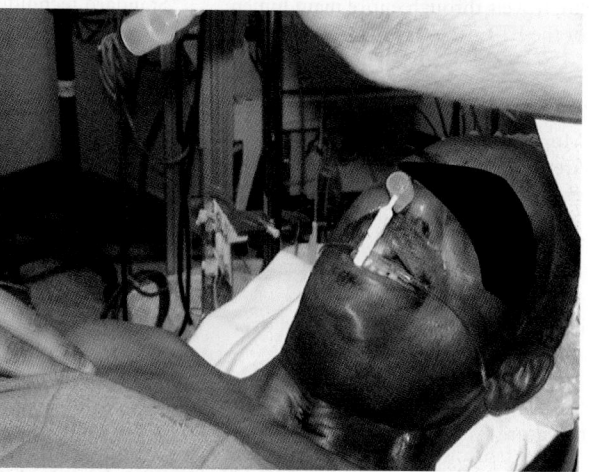

FIGURE 29-17. The sequence of retrograde wire intubation after the cricothyroid or cricotracheal ligament is identified and a percutaneous puncture is performed with air aspiration. **A.** The retrograde device (twisted wire) is advanced until (**B**) it emerges from the mouth or nose. **C.** The wire is clamped at the entrance site (*arrow*) and the endotracheal tube is advanced over the wire in an antegrade fashion. **D.** The wire is removed, leaving the tracheal tube in place.

cricoid and tracheal cartilages anteriorly and moves the sternocleidomastoid muscles laterally, although as in case 2, this may not always be possible. The skin should be prepared. If the patient is conscious, a local anesthetic skin wheel is made over the puncture site. Local anesthesia of the airway should be administered to prevent discomfort and to blunt airway reflexes as time permits. In general, topical anesthesia of the trachea, larynx, pharynx, and nasal passages is desirable. Translaryngeal anesthesia is a particularly convenient technique because a percutaneous entry of the trachea is required during the RWI. Structures above and below the vocal folds are anesthetized during the ensuing patient cough if a local anesthetic–filled syringe is used to facilitate the recognition of appropriate needle placement (with tracheal air bubbles) and then is injected to provide airway anesthesia.

As noted earlier, the cricothyroid membrane and cricotracheal ligament are both potential sites for translaryngeal puncture. Although the cricothyroid membrane has the advantage of being directly anterior to the large posterior surface of the cricoid cartilage, thereby protecting the esophagus from a puncturing needle, it places the needle in close proximity (0.9 to 1.5 cm) to the vocal folds, and hence allows for a somewhat smaller margin of error at the time of the intubation.

An atraumatic "J" guidewire is the preferred retrograde device. These guidewires are typically 0.032 to 0.038 inches in diameter, being able to pass though an 18-gauge intravenous catheter. The typical length is between 110 and 120 cm. The only requirement for length is that the wire be more than twice as long as the tracheal tube to be used. Kits are available that conveniently incorporate all the necessary equipment (Cook Critical Care).

The needle/catheter approaches the trachea at 90 degrees to the coronal and sagittal planes if possible (as it was not possible in case 2). In this orientation, the needle is likely to impact the posterior aspect of the cricoid cartilage if advanced too far, and not puncture the esophagus. Additionally, this angle will help to avoid trauma to the near-lying vocal folds.

After the percutaneous puncture is made and the trachea identified by free air aspiration, the catheter is angled cephalad and the wire is advanced (J-tip) into the trachea until it emerges from the mouth or nose. The wire may need to be retrieved from the mouth with a "sweeping" finger, Magill forceps, or nerve hook. Any obstruction to advancement of the wire should prompt re-evaluation of the angle of the catheter and the position of the head and neck (e.g., catheter directed posterior and/or caudad, neck flexed). Coughing typically heralds a caudad traveling of the wire. If the wire is retracted and found to be bent, it is prudent to procure a new one. When complaints of pain are encountered above the level of the larynx, it is typically because of the wire passing into an inadequately prepared nasal cavity. Options include retracting the wire modestly and asking the patient to open the mouth and maximally protrude the tongue during the readvancement, reaching into the oropharynx to retrieve the wire, or patiently repreparing the nasal passages. Once the wire is satisfactorily retrieved, placement of the tracheal tube may be performed using the wire in a number of fashions, depending on the operator's preference and previous experience. Table 29-22 lists common techniques, together with their advantages and disadvantages. Details of these techniques have been described elsewhere.[85]

In the case reported, other techniques may have been considered. Although indirect visual devices (flexible fiberoptic bronchoscope, rigid fiberoptic laryngoscope) also may have been helpful in this case, three elements worked against their use: (1) tissue trauma from repeated attempts at blind nasal intubation produced a bloody airway, frustrating the use of these devices; (2) the patient was unable to cooperate owing to her respiratory distress; and (3) because of the impending respiratory failure, there was little time for adequate airway analgesia. A coughing, gagging, conscious patient makes fiberoptic techniques nearly impossible. Straining and coughing during fiberoptic intubation attempts have resulted in Mallory-Weiss tears of the esophagus, resulting in significant hemorrhage.

TABLE 29-22

TECHNIQUES OF ENDOTRACHEAL TUBE (ETT) ADVANCEMENT OVER A RETROGRADE WIRE

■ TECHNIQUE	■ ADVANTAGE	■ DISADVANTAGE
Wire travels through entire main lumen of the ETT	Standard technique	• Margin of error[a] equals distance from vocal folds to puncture site • No stylet after removal of wire • "Railroading"[b] can occur
Wire placed into ETT lumen via Murphy eye	• Increased margin of error • Decreased railroading	• Cannot use stylet (below)
Wire enters distal end of ETT and exits via Murphy eye	• Decreased railroading	• Margin of error equals distance from vocal folds to puncture site • Cannot use stylet (below)
ETT "exchange" stylet is placed over wire, prior to placement of ETT	• Decreased railroading • Can use stylet to vastly increase margin of error once wire is removed	Cost
Fiberoptic bronchoscope is placed over wire prior to placement of ETT	• Decreased railroading • Can use stylet to vastly increase margin of error once wire is removed • Visualization	Cost
Silk suture	• No railroading • Margin of error issues reduced	May be difficult to place silk suture
Small ETT	Reduced railroading	May not be clinically adequate

[a]*Margin of error* refers to the distance below the vocal folds that the endotracheal tube extends at the time that the guidewire is removed. If this distance is not adequate, there is a risk of immediate extubation.
[b]*Railroading* refers to the differential size of the guidewire and the tracheal tube. A large discrepancy in size allows for a cleft, which may entrap the epiglottis, arytenoid cartilages, aryepiglottic folds, or vocal folds, hindering intubation attempts.

Blind nasal intubation was the first technique attempted in this patient. Until recently, blind nasal intubation has been a staple of airway control, especially in the emergency department, where it has been largely supplanted by rapid-sequence intubation. This technique requires significant analgesia of the nasal passages in the awake patient. Success is far more likely in the spontaneously breathing patient. With the head in the Magill position, the ETT is advanced into the nares, nasal passage (keeping the ETT bevel alongside the nasal septum), and into the pharynx. Breath sounds are auscultated from the ETT, and its position adjusted keep them maximized. The patient's head and larynx can be manipulated externally as necessary.

Case 4: Esophageal Tracheal Combitube

A 55-year-old man with a history of cirrhosis and esophageal varices requires airway control because of acute, recurrent upper gastrointestinal bleeding. Apart from fresh blood in the airway, physical examination of his external airway is consistent with a routine laryngoscopy. Furthermore, he had been intubated for similar events in the past. After a rapid-sequence induction, the larynx cannot be visualized on three laryngoscopies because of fresh blood emanating from the esophagus. On all three attempts, the ETT is advanced blindly, and the absence of breath sounds over the thorax together with the presence of copious blood in the ETT leads to the diagnosis of esophageal intubation. A large, adult-sized Esophageal Tracheal Combitube (Tyco Healthcare, Mansfield, NY) is requested, blindly inserted into the airway, and the pharyngeal and distal cuffs are inflated. Ventilation through the pharyngeal perforations lumen (blue) produces bilateral breath sounds to auscultation, and the oxygen saturation increases to >90%. Copious blood is suctioned from the esophageal lumen. The patient is transported to the angiography suite where his esophageal varices are embolized. The esophageal tracheal Combitube is removed and the patient is intubated with DL.

The Esophageal Tracheal Combitube (Combitube) was developed by Dr. Michael Frass, a critical care physician in Vienna, Austria, in 1986. Its design was meant to improve and replace the esophageal obturator airway, which was a rescue airway introduced in 1968. The Combitube is a double-lumen airway, the distal end of which is meant to be blindly placed into the esophagus. One lumen begins at this distal point with a large orifice, and travels to outside the patient where it opens to the atmosphere. This lumen serves as a gastric drain. The second lumen travels from outside the patient to a point in the hypopharynx. This lumen has a multiorifice opening that faces the larynx and acts as the airway. The Combitube has two cuffs, one within the esophagus and a second at the oropharynx/pharynx juncture. The Combitube is functional if introduced into the esophagus (ventilation being achieved through the esophageal lumen, via the hypopharyngeal perforations) or in the trachea (ventilation being achieved through the tracheal lumen, via the distal aperture). In either case, the proximal balloon seals both the oral and nasal passages, and the distal conventional tracheal tube cuff isolates the respiratory system from the gastrointestinal system. The device is available in two sizes: the 41-French size is used for larger adults (height >168 cm) and the 37-French size is used for adults 122–183 cm (Fig. 29-18).

Use of the Esophageal Tracheal Combitube. The Combitube is inserted "blindly." The operator lifts the lower jaw and tongue anteriorly with one hand, and the Combitube is inserted with a downward, caudad-curved motion until the proximal depth indicator (two black rings printed on the double-lumen tube) come to rest at the level of the teeth. The oropharyngeal balloon is inflated with 100 mL of air through a blue plastic pilot balloon (85 mL in the small adult size) while the distal cuff is

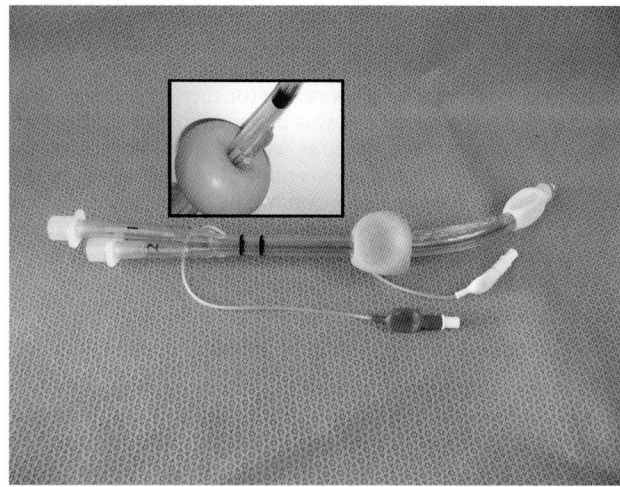

FIGURE 29-18.   The esophageal tracheal Combitube. Inset: The fiberoptic port of the Easy Tube.

inflated with 5 to 15 mL (via a white pilot balloon). An Ambu bag or anesthesia circuit is attached to the proximal end of the esophageal lumen (constructed of blue polyvinyl chloride), and ventilation is confirmed by auscultation or other means. Because 90% of Combitube placements result in an esophageal position, ventilation occurs via this lumen's hypopharyngeal perforations. If no breath sounds are auscultated and/or gastric inflation is noted, the Combitube has been positioned in the trachea. Without repositioning, ventilation is changed to the distal end of tracheal lumen (clear polyvinyl chloride). If no maneuver improves ventilation, the device is most likely in the esophagus but has been advanced too deeply, with the oropharyngeal cuff obstructing the airway. In this case, the cuffs should be deflated, the device withdrawn 2 cm, and the ventilation sequence repeated.

Advantages of the Combitube include rapid airway control, airway protection from regurgitation, ease of use by the inexperienced operator, no requirement to visualize the larynx, and the ability to maintain the neck in a neutral position, although cervical spine movement may be greater than that seen with the LMA, LMA Fastrach, and flexible fiberscope.[180] It has been shown to be useful in the patient with massive upper gastrointestinal bleeding or vomiting, and as a rescue device in failed rapid-sequence induction or unanticipated difficult intubation. It is also useful in the morbidly obese, in acute bronchospasm, during cardiopulmonary resuscitation, and for prolonged ventilation after airway rescue.[86,125–131,132,181–183] Several series have demonstrated the effectiveness Combitube in prehospital management of the airway.[184,185] Urtubia et al.[186] have used the esophageal tracheal Combitube for elective surgery with a high success and low complication rate.

Contraindications to use of the Combitube include esophageal obstruction or other abnormality, ingestion of caustic agents, upper airway foreign body or mass, lower airway obstruction, height <4 feet, and an intact gag reflex. Because the Combitube includes latex in its construction, it should not be used in patients with latex allergy.

Complications associated with the Combitube have included lacerations to the pyriform sinus and esophageal wall resulting in subcutaneous emphysema, pneumomediastinum, pneumoperitoneum, and esophageal rupture.[187–189]

A device similar to the Combitube has been available in many parts of the world since 2003.[190] The Easy Tube (Rusch International, Kernen, Germany) is distributed in two sizes, 41fr for patients above 130 cm in height and 28fr for patients

90 to 130 cm in height. Unlike the Combitube, the distal lumen of the Easy Tube is designed to resemble an ETT (including a Murphy eye). The pharyngeal aperture is designed to allow easy passage of a fiberscope (or suction catheter; Fig. 29-18, inset). The Easy Tube was designed for use during routine and emergency anesthetic as well as cannot intubate/cannot ventilate situations.[191] Contraindications to Easy Tube use are identical to those for the Combitube. Although it may be inserted blindly, it is designed to be used with a laryngoscope (much like a standard ETT). Unlike the Combitube, it is latex-free.

Case 5: Failed Rapid-Sequence Induction and the SGA

A 39-year-old man presents for elective uvulopharyngopalatoplasty. He has no previous surgical history. His maximal incisor gap is 5 cm, thyromental distance is 7 cm, and his oropharyngeal view is a Samsoon–Young class 2. There is no limitation in head and neck flexion and extension. During a sleep apnea study, he had 15 apneic events each hour. The patient has a significant history of gastroesophageal reflux, and rapid-sequence induction is planned. After the administration of pentothal, succinylcholine, and cricoid pressure (Sellick maneuver), DL with a Macintosh number 3 laryngoscope blade reveals a large epiglottis obscuring the view of the vocal folds (Cormack–Lehane grade 3).[82] Significant hyperplasia of the base of the tongue, which prevents its full displacement, is also noted. The BURP maneuver does not improve the view.[80] A Macintosh 4 and Miller 3 blades are used and do not improve the view. Oxygen saturation, which was 100% prior to induction, is now 92%, ansd face mask ventilation is initiated with the Sellick maneuver in place. Complete obstruction to ventilation is encountered, despite chin and/or jaw lift, two-person ventilation, and a reduction in the degree of cricoid pressure. The oxygen saturation falls to 85% and a size 5 LMA (which had been prepared prior to the induction of anesthesia) is inserted with the technique as described by the inventor. Immediately, a clear airway is established and the Sellick pressure remains in place. A second dose of Pentothal is administered, and the patient is intubated by the blind passage of a 7.0-ID ETT via the LMA. The LMA is then removed using a Cook airway exchange catheter as a stylet, and the surgical case proceeds.

The SGA in the Failed Airway. One clear advantage of SGA use is in the failed airway. There have been many reported (and unreported) cases of failed intubation and failure to ventilate by face mask in which the airway was rescued with an LMA, Laryngeal Tube, Cobra PLA or another SGA.[192–194]

Parmet et al.[124] estimate that 1 in 800,000 patients cannot be managed with an LMA, providing an 80-fold increase in margin of safety over the oft-noted 1 in 10,000 patients who cannot be ventilated by mask nor intubated by traditional means. Likewise, a wealth of literature describes the use of the various SGAs in elective difficult airway management in awake and unconscious patients, in anticipated and unanticipated situations, in cervical spine injury, and in pediatric dysmorphic syndromes.[56,57,116]

The characteristics of the SGAs that underlie their superiority as a tool in the difficult airway armamentarium are that they are well tolerated by the patient, simulating the natural distension of the hypopharyngeal tissues by food, and that its insertion follows an intrinsic pathway, requiring no tissue distortion (as with laryngoscopy), which may not be possible in all patients. Finally, it is a blind technique not hindered by blood, secretions, debris, and edema from previous attempts at laryngoscopy.[195] Because most of the ease of insertion of the SGA does not depend on anatomy that can be assessed on routine physical examination, typical airway assessment measures do not apply to its application.[196] The major disadvantage of the SGAs in resuscitation is the lack of mechanical protection from regurgitation and aspiration.[197,198]

Lower rates of regurgitation during cardiopulmonary resuscitation with a LMA (3.5%) than with the bag-valve mask ventilation (12.4%) have been shown.[199] Even in the face of regurgitation, pulmonary aspiration is a rare event.[200] Unfortunately, the use of the Sellick maneuver may prevent proper seating of the LMA in a minority of instances.[201] This may require the brief removal of the cricoid pressure until the LMA has been properly seated. Cricoid pressure is effective with an LMA in situ. Had it been available, the LMA Fastrack would also have been an ideal device in this case scenario.

Case 6: Deviation from the Difficult Airway Algorithm

Thirteen hours after admission to the intensive care unit, a 76-year-old woman who had sustained trauma to the face, head, and neck in a motor vehicle accident is noted to have progressive decline in her level of consciousness and respiratory effort. On examination, there appears to be an adequate interincisor gap and thyromental distance. The oropharyngeal view and range of motion of the head and neck cannot be evaluated. Because of the inability to fully evaluate the airway with respect to ease of intubation, an awake procedure is chosen. Fiberoptic devices are not considered usable because of the presence of fresh and clotted blood in the mouth as a result of continued epistaxis. Other airway techniques that require significant patient preparation are not considered because of the rapid progression of the patient's respiratory failure. Additionally, the presence of fresh blood in the oral and pharyngeal cavities will hinder adequate drying and analgesia. Blind nasal intubation is considered contraindicated based on the obvious facial trauma and the risk of cribriform plate disruption. Neither equipment for retrograde intubation nor the tracheal esophageal Combitube is readily available. A lighted stylet intubation guide is available, but no clinician present is experienced with this technique. Although the mental status change is believed to reflect an intracranial process (e.g., intracranial hypertension), the risk of complete loss of the airway is judged to be the primary clinical hazard. Awake DL is attempted with manual in-line stabilization of the neck. After clearing fresh blood from the pharynx with a Yankauer suction catheter, a Cormack–Lehane grade 3 laryngeal view is obtained, but because of patient resistance (biting on the laryngoscope and movement), tracheal intubation is not achieved. The decision is made to proceed with rapid-sequence induction and intubation, with preparations made for an emergency tracheostomy. After surgical preparation of the neck and preoxygenation, intravenous succinylcholine and etomidate are administered, DL is undertaken, the larynx is easily visualized, and the trachea is intubated.

Muscle Relaxants and Direct Laryngoscopy. In the case described, the use of muscle relaxants significantly improved the ability to visualize the larynx. In one study, the use of muscle relaxants during a DL increased the success rate of intubation and was associated with fewer incidents of airway trauma, intubation attempts, esophageal intubations, aspiration, and even death.[202] Intubating conditions with and without muscle relaxation have been investigated in few well-controlled trials because the superior intubating conditions achieved with muscle relaxants has discouraged inclusion of control groups.[203] The effects of muscle relaxation that improves laryngoscopic view include allowing complete temporomandibular joint relaxation and opening, anterior movement of the epiglottis, and widening of the laryngeal vestibule and laryngeal sinus.[204] In addition, the finding that laryngoscopic stimulation of the pharyngeal musculature causes the upper airway lumen to appear small is offset by the use of relaxants.

Leaving the Algorithm. The situation described in case 5 is unusual in that rapid-sequence induction was attempted because the clinical situation had deviated from the ASA-DA owing to the progressive nature of the airway compromise. The situation was more akin to the "crash" airway described by Walls.[205] In this case, the institution of muscle relaxation, which might be considered contraindicated in the apparently difficult-to-intubate patient, allowed for full visualization of the larynx. Knowing that failure to intubate in this case would result in probable loss of the airway, the clinician was prepared for cricothyroidotomy. Although the ASA-DAA is a valuable tool in the process of approaching the difficult airway, the clinician must always be prepared for the case that does not fit the mold. As stated earlier, adaptability in a rapidly changing clinical situation is critical to the success of airway management. Also of interest in this case was the availability of a lighted stylet for use in similar difficult airway scenarios. Although this device may have been useful in the current case, no clinician present was familiar with its operation. A critical situation is not an occasion for trying an unfamiliar technology.

Other Devices

⑮ An ever-increasing number of airway management devices are commercially available. Although encyclopedic coverage of these tools is beyond the scope of this chapter, a review of the more established equipment follows.

Lighted Stylets

These devices rely on transillumination of the airway. A light source introduced into the trachea will produce a well-circumscribed glow of the tissues over the larynx and trachea. The same light placed in the esophagus will produce no light or a diffuse light. A number of devices have become available, including disposable, partly disposable, and fully reusable systems. Although there are many reports of successful intubation using these devices, some common problems have been noted. In general, the operating theater lights must be dimmed to best appreciate the circumscribed glow; a stylet tip successfully placed in the trachea, but not pointing in an anterior direction, may give a false-negative impression; it is often difficult to remove the semirigid stylet from the ETT after intubation.

Airway Bougie

Airway bougies encompass a series of solid or hollow, semimalleable stylets that maybe be blindly manipulated in to the trachea. An ETT is then "threaded" over the bougie and into the trachea. These bougies are generally low in cost and highly portable. The Eschmann introducer (Eschmann Health Care, Kent, England) was introduced in 1949. It is 60 cm long, 15-French, and angled 40 degrees 3.5 cm from its distal end. It is constructed from a woven polyester base, which is malleable. It can be very helpful when the larynx cannot be visualized with laryngoscopy. The introducer (also known as the *gum elastic bougie*) can be manipulated under the epiglottis, its angled segment directed anteriorly toward the larynx.

Once it has entered the larynx and trachea, a distinctive "clicking" feel is elicited as the tip passes over the cartilaginous structures. A similar device, the Frova Intubating Introducer (Cook Critical Care) is disposable, has an optional "stiffening" stylet and a hollow bore. The internal lumen allows for the insufflation of oxygen, the detection of carbon dioxide, and the use of a self-inflating bulb to detect inadvertent esophageal placement.

Minimally Invasive Transtracheal Procedures

⑯ When access to the airway from the mouth or nose fails or is unavailable (e.g., maxillofacial, pharyngeal, or laryngeal trauma, pathology, or deformity), emergency access via the extrathoracic trachea is a feasible route to the airway. The clinician must be familiar with these alternative techniques of oxygenation and ventilation. The decision to proceed with an invasive procedure can be difficult, and most clinicians will hesitate, at potentially grave risk to the patient. One should consider becoming facile with at least one of these techniques in elective situations (such as transtracheal puncture for administering airway analgesia or elective retrograde intubation or, consider, for example, assisting a surgical colleague on a tracheostomy). Although tracheostomy and cricothyroidotomy are beyond the scope of this chapter, percutaneous techniques will be considered.

Cricothyroidotomy, cricothyrotomy, coniotomy, and minitracheostomy are synonyms for establishing an air passage through the cricothyroid membrane. The cricothyroid membrane is a fibroelastic membrane, lying over the tracheal mucosa. It is attached to the inferior border of the thyroid cartilage and superior edge of the cricoid cartilage. Although cricothyrotomy is the procedure of choice in an emergency situation, it may also apply to an elective situation when there is limited access to the trachea (e.g., severe cervical kyphoscoliosis). Cricothyrotomy is contraindicated in neonates and children younger than 6 years of age, and in patients with laryngeal fractures.

Percutaneous TTJV, as a form of cricothyroidotomy, is the most familiar to anesthesiologists. The ASA-DAA lists transtracheal jet ventilation as an option in the cannot mask ventilate/cannot intubate situation. TTJV is a simple and relatively safe means to sustain the patient's life in this critical situation.[85] It provides extra time for attempts to intubate the trachea either directly, optically or by a surgical airway, by maintaining arterial oxygenation.[206] A large bore catheter, attached to a 5-mL or larger empty or partially fluid-filled (saline or local anesthetic) syringe, should be used to enter the airway. The patient is positioned supine, with the head midline or extended on the neck and thorax (if not contraindicated by the clinical situation). After aseptic preparation, local anesthetic is injected over the cricothyroid membrane (if the patient is awake and time permits). The right-handed clinician stands on the right side of the patient, facing the head. The clinician can use his or her nondominant hand to stabilize the larynx. The catheter-needle is advanced at right angles to all planes in the caudad third of the membrane. From the moment of skin puncture there should be constant aspiration on the syringe plunger. Free aspiration of air confirms entrance into the trachea but does not indicate the direction that the catcher travels in the larynx; cephalad extension will not provide adequate oxygenation. Unless there is significant pulmonary fluid (e.g., blood, aspirated gastric contents, or water from drowning), the aspiration of tracheal air should be incontrovertible. The needle-catheter assembly should be advanced slightly, and subsequently the catheter advanced fully into the airway alone. Although this technique has been described with common angiocatheters (which may kink and obstruct), dedicated

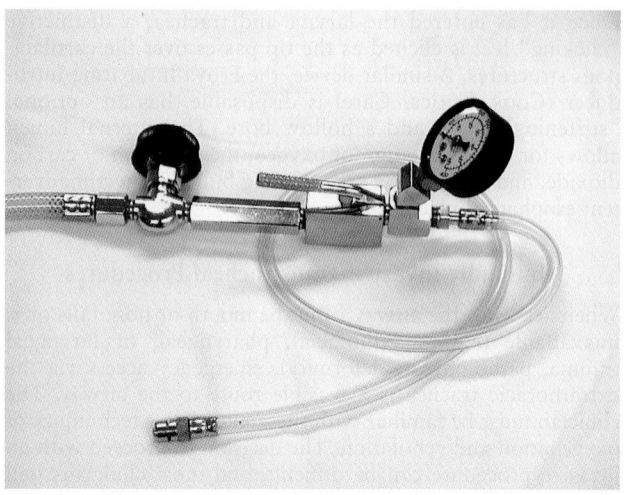

FIGURE 29-19.   System for regulation of a high-pressure oxygen source for transtracheal jet ventilation.

devices made of kink-resistant materials and with accessory ports are available such as the Cook Transtracheal jet ventilation catheter (Cook Critical Care, Bloomington, IN).

Once the catheter has been successfully placed in the airway, an oxygen source is attached. The clinician may have several options in this regard. If a high-pressure system is available—for example, a metered and adjustable oxygen source with a hand-controlled valve (Fig. 29-19) and a Luer-lock connector—15 to 30 psi of oxygen (central hospital supply or regulated cylinder) can be delivered directly through the catheter, with insufflations of 1 to 1.5 seconds at a rate of 12 insufflations per minute. If a 16-gauge catheter has been placed, this system will deliver a tidal volume of 400 to 700 mL. Low-pressure systems cannot provide enough flow to expand the chest adequately for oxygenation and ventilation (e.g., Ambu bag, 6 psi; common gas outlet, 20 psi). Hooker et al.[207] recommend connection to an unregulated oxygen source of at least 50 psi.

Low-pressure oxygen flow meters can be used for TTJV. These systems are capable of delivering a brief (0.5-second) 30-psi burst pressure, which quickly decays to 5 psi or less.[208] If this oxygen source is to be used, an inspiratory-to-expiratory ratio of 1:1 with a rate of 30 to 60 breaths per minute should be used to assure adequate burst pressures.

The Automatic Jet Ventilator (Mistral model, Acutronic, Hirzel, Switzerland) with a pause pressure alarm facility has been used safely for TTJV in two patients with upper airway obstruction.[209]

Specialized percutaneous cricothyroidotomy systems have been developed that improve the ease of this technique. These devices generally provide a large-bore access that is adequate for oxygenation and ventilation with low-pressure systems. The Melker emergency cricothyroidotomy catheter set (Cook Critical Care) uses a Seldinger—catheter-over-a-wire—technique familiar to most anesthesia practitioners. The set comes in a variety of cannula sizes (3.5-, 4-, and 6-mm ID, cuffed and uncuffed). Preparation and positioning of the patient are the same as with needle cricothyroidotomy. A 1- to 1.5-cm vertical incision of the skin only is made over the lower third of the cricothyroid membrane. Aiming 45 degrees caudad, a percutaneous puncture of the subcutaneous tissue and cricothyroid membrane is made with the provided 18-gauge needle-catheter assembly and syringe. After air is aspirated, the catheter is advanced into the trachea. The provided guidewire is inserted through the catheter and into the trachea. The catheter is removed and the tracheal cannula, fitted internally with a curved dilator, is threaded onto the wire. The dilator is advanced through the membrane using firm pressure. Significant resistance to its advancement may indicate that the skin incision needs to be extended. Once the cannula-dilator has been fully inserted, the dilator and wire are removed. The 15-mm circuit adapter end of the cannula is now attached to an Ambu bag or anesthesia circuit.

Other percutaneous systems include Nu-trake (Weiss Emergency Airway System; International Medical Devices) and the Quicktrach transtracheal catheter (VBM Medizintechnik). Nonneedle puncture techniques are beyond the current discussion.

Severe complications of TTJV are related to barotraumas such as cervicomediastinal emphysema, pneumothorax, or tension pneumothorax. Causes of penetration of air into paratracheal space include insufflation of gas through a misplaced cannula because of poor placement, multiple tracheal punctures, or migration due to coughing. Bilateral tension pneumothorax with high-frequency jet ventilation has been reported.[210]

The Hunsaker Mon-Jet tube (Xomed, Jacksonville, FL.) is a self-centering, nonflammable subglottic tube that allows continuous monitoring of end-expiratory and peak airway pressure and periodic sampling of ETCO2 during high-pressure, transglottic jet ventilation. The Hunsaker tube is used for elective laryngeal and supraglottic surgery. The distal end of the tube should be placed 7 to 8 cm below the glottis, ensuring that the CO_2/pressure monitor port is below vocal cords. The tube is self-centering in the trachea because of a basket-shaped distal extension that prevents malalignment and jet port contact with tracheal mucosa. An automatic jet ventilator that will automatically shut down if the end-expiratory or peak airway pressure rises above a preset level should be employed. The Hunsaker is composed of nonflammable fluoroplastic material making it safe to use in a 100% O_2 environment with CO_2, KTP (potassium-titanyl-phosphate), and Nd: Yag (neodymium: yttrium-aluminum-garnet) lasers. Orloff et al.[211] reviewed 84 patients in whom the Hunsaker Mon-Jet tube was used for microlaryngeal surgery. Anesthetic induction and recovery time were comparable with standard endotracheal intubation, but there was improved surgical exposure and reduced surgical time. Dr. J. Davis (personal communication, 2007) reviewed 552 patients cared for at Washington State University, in Seattle, Washington Three percent of patients required a change to a standard or laser ETT during the procedure because of hypoxia or hypercarbia. No barotrauma, submucosal injection of air, or tube ignition occurred in either study.

CONCLUSIONS

Apart from monitoring, the management of the "routine" patient airway is the most common task of the anesthesiologist—even during the administration of regional anesthesia, the airway must be monitored and possibly supported. Unfortunately, routine tasks often become neglected as the clinician becomes distracted. But the consequences of a lost airway are so devastating that the clinician can never afford a lackadaisical approach.

Although the ASA's Task Force on the Difficult Airway has given the medical community an immensely valuable tool in the approach to the patient with the difficult airway, the Task Force's algorithm must be viewed as a starting point only. Judgment, experience, the clinical situation, and available resources all affect the appropriateness of the chosen pathway through, or divergence from, the algorithm. The clinician does not need to be expert in all the equipment and techniques currently available. Rather, a broad range of approaches should be mastered so that the failure of one does not present a roadblock to success.

Whereas one may argue that the last decade of the 20th century was the decade of the SGA, the first decade of the 21st century is witnessing the proliferation of the video laryngoscope. A balance between supraglottic ventilation and video-assisted intubation is the challenge of the coming years.

The medical manufacturing community, and the far-sighted clinicians who supply it with concepts for airway management products, has supplied a vast array of devices. Many represent redundancy in concept, and each has its supporters and detractors. No one device can be considered superior to another when considered in isolation. It is the clinician and his or her resources (both equipment and personnel) and judgment that determine the effectiveness of any technique. In the management of the difficult airway, flexibility, and not rigidity, prevails.

References

1. Practice guidelines for the management of the difficult airway: An updated report by the American Society of Anesthesiologists Task Force on Management of the Difficult Airway. Anesthesiology 2003; 98: 1269
2. Peterson GN, Domino KB, Caplan RA et al: Management of the difficult airway: A closed claims analysis. Anesthesiology 2005; 103: 33
3. Rosenblatt W: The airway approach algorithm. J Clin Anesth 2004; 16: 312
4. Westhorpe RN: The position of the larynx in children and its relationship to the ease of intubation. Anaesth Intens Care 1987; 15: 384
5. Sykes WS: Essays on the first hundred years of anesthesia. London, Churchill Livingstone, 1982
6. Brimacombe JR (Ed): Laryngeal mask anesthesia: Principles and practice. Philadelphia, Saunders, 2005
7. Brandt L: The first reported oral intubation of the human trachea. Anesth Analg 1987; 66: 1198
8. Magill IW: Technique in endotracheal anaesthesia. Proc Roy Soc Med 1928; 22: 83
9. Mendelson CL: The aspiration of stomach contents into the lungs during obstetric anesthesia. Am J Obstet Gynecol 1946; 191
10. Breitmeier D, Wilke N, Schulz Y et al: The lingual tonsillar hyperplasia in relation to unanticipated difficult intubation: Is there any relationship between lingual tonsillar hyperplasia and tonsillectomy? Am J Forensic Med Pathol 2005; 26: 131
11. Ovassapian A, Glassenberg R, Randel GI et al: The unexpected difficult airway and lingual tonsil hyperplasia. A case series and a review of the literature. Anesthesiology 2002; 97: 124
12. Shiga T, Wajima Z, Inoue T et al: Predicting Difficult Intubation in Apparently Normal Patients: A Meta-analysis of Bedside Screening Test Performance. Anesthesiology 2005; 103: 429
13. El-Ganzouri AR, McCarthy RJ, Tuman KJ et al: Preoperative airway assessment: predictive value of a multivariate risk index. Anesth Analg 1996; 82: 1197
14. Wilson ME, Spiegelhalter D, Robertson J et al: Predicting difficult intubation. Br J Anaesth 1988; 61: 211
15. Patel SK, Whitten CW, Ivy R 3rd et al: Failure of the laryngeal mask airway: An undiagnosed laryngeal carcinoma. Anesth Analg 1998; 86: 438
16. Naguib M, Malabarey T, AlSatli RA et al: Predictive models for difficult laryngoscopy. A clinical, radiologic and three dimensional computer imaging study. Can J Anesth 1999; 46: 748
17. Langeron O, Masso E, Huraux C et al: Prediction of difficult mask ventilation. Anesthesiology 2000; 92: 1229
18. Kheterpal S, Han R, Tremper KK et al: Incidence and predictors of difficult and impossible mask ventilation. Anesthesiology 2006; 105: 885
19. Benumof JL: Preoxygenation: Best method for both efficacy and efficiency (editorial). Anesthesiology 1999; 91: 603
20. Jense HG, Dubin SA, Silverstein PI et al: Effect of obesity on safe duration of apnea in anesthetized humans. Anesth Analg 1991; 72: 89
21. Baraka AS, Taha SK, Aouad MT et al: Preoxygenation: Comparison of maximal breathing and tidal volume breathing techniques. Anesthesiology 1999; 91: 612
22. Taha SK, Siddik-Sayyid SM, El Khatib MF et al: Nasopharyngeal oxygen insufflation following pre-oxygenation using the four deep breath technique. Anaesthesia 2006; 61: 427
23. El-Khatib MF, Kanazi G, Baraka AS: Noninvasive bilevel positive airway pressure for preoxygenation of the critically ill morbidly obese patient. Can J Anaesth 2007; 54: 744
24. Dixon BJ, Dixon JB, Carden JR et al: Preoxygenation is more effective in the 25 degrees head-up position than in the supine position in severely obese patients: a randomized controlled study. Anesthesiology 2005; 102: 1110
25. Baraka AS, Hanna MT, Jabbour SI et al: Preoxygenation of pregnant and nonpregnant women in the head-up versus supine position. Anesth Analg 1992; 75: 757
26. Kwei P, Matzelle S, Wallman D et al: Inadequate preoxygenation during spontaneous ventilation with single patient use self-inflating resuscitation bags. Anaesth Intens Care 2006; 34: 685
27. Rosenblatt WH, Ovassapian A, Eige S: Use of the laryngeal mask airway in the United States: A randomized survey of ASA members. ASA Annual Meeting, Orlando, Florida, 1998
28. Isono S, Tanaka A, Ishikawa T et al: Sniffing position improves pharyngeal airway patency in anesthetized patients with obstructive sleep apnea. Anesthesiology 2005; 103: 489
29. Conlon NP, Sullivan RP, Herbison PG et al: The effect of leaving dentures in place on bag-mask ventilation at induction of general anesthesia. Anesth Analg 2007; 105: 370
30. Maktabi MA, Smith RB, Todd MM: Is routine endotracheal intubation as safe as we think or wish (Editorial). Anesthesiology 2003; 99: 247
31. Tanaka A, Isono S, Ishikawa T et al: Laryngeal resistance before and after minor surgery: Endotracheal tube versus laryngeal mask airway. Anesthesiology 2003; 99: 252
32. Domino KB, Posner KL, Caplan RA et al: Airway Injury during Anesthesia A Closed Claims Analysis. Anesthesiology 1999; 91: 1703
33. Goldmann K, Dieterich J, Roessler M: Laryngopharyngeal mucosal injury after prolonged use of the ProSealTM LMA in a porcine model: a pilot study. Can J Anaesth 2007; 54: 822
34. Calder I, Picard J, Chapman M et al: Mouth opening: a new angle. Anesthesiology 2003; 99: 799
35. Brimacombe JR, Berry A: The incidence of aspiration associated with the laryngeal mask airway: A meta-analysis of published literature. J Clin Anesth 1995; 7: 297
36. Yardy N, Hancox D, Strang TSO: A comparison of two airway aids for emergency use by unskilled personnel: The Combitube and laryngeal mask. Anaesthesia 1999; 54: 181
37. Han TH, Brimacombe JR, Lee EJ et al: The laryngeal mask airway is effective (and probably safe) in selected healthy parturients for elective Cesarean section: a prospective study of 1067 cases. Can J Anaesth 2001; 48: 1117
38. Stone BJ, Chantler PJ: The incidence of regurgitation during cardiopulmonary resuscitation: A comparison between the bag valve mask and laryngeal mask airway. Resuscitation 1998; 38: 3
39. Verghese C, Brimacombe J: Survey of laryngeal mask airway usage in 11,910 patients: Safety and efficacy for conventional and nonconventional usage. Anesth Analg 1996; 82: 129
40. Ho BY, Skinner HJ, Mahajan RP: Gastro-oesophageal reflux during day case gynaecological laparoscopy under positive pressure ventilation: Laryngeal mask vs. tracheal intubation. Anaesthesia 1999; 54: 93
41. Gursoy F, Algren JT, Skjonsby BS: Positive pressure ventilation with the laryngeal mask airway in children. Anesth Analg 1996; 82: 33
42. Brimacombe JR, Brain AI, Berry AM et al: Gastric insufflation and the laryngeal mask. Anesth Analg 1998; 86: 914
43. Brimacombe J, Shorney N: The laryngeal mask airway and prolonged balanced regional anaesthesia. Can J Anaesth 1993; 40: 360
44. Williams PJ, Bailey PM: Comparison of the reinforced laryngeal mask airway and tracheal intubation for adenotonsillectomy. Br J Anaesth 1993; 70: 30
45. Kaplan A, Crosby GJ, Bhattacharyya N: Airway protection and the laryngeal Mask Airway. The Laryngoscope 2004; 114: 652
46. Kim ES, Bishop MJ: Endotracheal intubation, but not laryngeal mask airway insertion, produces reversible bronchoconstriction. Anesthesiology 1999; 90: 391
47. Nair I, Bailey PM: Use of the laryngeal mask for airway maintenance following trachea extubation [letter]. Anaesthesia 1995; 50: 174
48. Erskine RJ, Rabey PG: The laryngeal mask airway in recovery. Anaesthesia 1992; 47: 354
49. Deakin CD, Diprose P, Majumdar R et al: An investigation into the quantity of secretions removed by inflated and deflated laryngeal mask airways. Anaesthesia 2000; 55: 478
50. Brimacombe JR: Advanced uses: clinical situations, The Laryngeal Mask Airway. A Review and Practical Guide. Edited by Brimacombe JR, Brain AIJ. London, WB Saunders, 2004, pp 138
51. Brimacombe J, Clarke G, Keller C: Lingual nerve injury associated with the ProSeal laryngeal mask airway: a case report and review of the literature. Br J Anaesth 2005; 95: 420
52. O'Connor CJ, Borromeo CJ, Stix MS: Assessing proseal laryngeal mask position: The suprasternal notch test. (Letter) Anesth Analg 2002; 94: 1374
53. Brain AIJ, Verghese C, Strube PJ: The LMA Proseal—a laryngeal mask with an oesophageal vent. Br J Anaesth 2000; 84: 650
54. Stix MS, O'Connor: Depth of insertion of the proseal laryngeal mask airway. Br J Anesth 2003; 90: 235
55. Brimacombe J, Keller C, Fullkrug B et al: A multicenter study comparing the proseal and classic laryngeal mask airway in anesthetized, non-paralyzed patients. Anesthesiology 2002; 96: 289
56. Rosenblatt WH: The use of the LMA-proseal in airway resuscitation. Anesth Analg 2004; 97: 1773
57. Awan R, Nolan JP, Cook TM: Use of the proseal laryngeal mask for airway maintenance during emergency cesarean section of the failed tracheal intubation. Br J of Anaesth 2004; 92: 144
58. Maltby JR, Beriault MT, Watson NC et al: The LMA-proseal is an effective alternative to tracheal intubation for laparoscopic cholecystectomy. Can J Anaesth 2002; 49: 857

59. Bortone L, Ingelmo PM, De Ninno G et al: Randomized controlled trial comparing the laryngeal tube and the laryngeal mask in pediatric patients. Paediatr Anaesth 2006; 16: 251

60. Asai T, Kawachi S: Use of the laryngeal tube by paramedic staff. Anaesthesia 2004; 59: 408

61. Bein B, Carstensen S, Gleim M et al: A comparison of the proseal laryngeal mask airway, the laryngeal tube S and the oesophageal-tracheal combitube during routine surgical procedures. Eur J Anaesthesiol 2005; 22: 341

62. Dahaba AA, Prax N, Gaube W et al: Haemodynamic and catecholamine stress responses to the laryngeal tube-suction airway and the proseal laryngeal mask airway. Anaesthesia 2006; 61: 330

63. Gaitini LA, Vaida SJ, Somri M et al: An evaluation of the laryngeal tube during general anesthesia using mechanical ventilation. Anesth Analg 2003; 96: 1750

64. Asai T: Use of the laryngeal tube for difficult fibreoptic tracheal intubation. Anaesthesia 2005; 60: 826

65. Zand F, Amini A: Use of the laryngeal tube-S for airway management and prevention of aspiration after a failed tracheal intubation in a parturient. Anesthesiology 2005; 102: 481

66. Keller C, Brimacombe J, Kleinsasser A et al: Pharyngeal mucosal pressures with the laryngeal tube airway versus ProSeal laryngeal mask airway. Anasthesiol Intensivmed Notfallmed Schmerzther 2003; 38: 393

67. Banchereau F, Delaunay F, Herve Y et al: Oropharyngeal ulcers following anaesthesia with the laryngeal tube S. Ann Fr Anesth Reanim 2006; 25: 884

68. Agro F, Carassitti M, Barzoi G et al: A first report on the diagnosis and treatment of acute postoperative airway obstruction with the cobra PLA. Can J Anesth 2004; 51: 640

69. Gaitini l, Yanovski B, Somri M et al: A comparison between the PLA Cobra and the Laryngeal Mask Airway Unique during spontaneous ventilation: a randomized prospective study. Anesth Analg 2006; 102: 631

70. Chou HC, Wu TL: Thyromental distance and anterior larynx: misconceptional and misname? Anesth Analg 2003; 96: 1526

71. Benumof JL: Both a large and small thyromental distance can predict difficult intubation, Anesth Analg 2003; 97: 1543

72. Chou HC, Wu TL: Mandibulohyoid distance in difficult laryngoscopy. Br J Anaesth 1993; 71: 335

73. Kikkawa YS, Koichi T, Nimi S: Prediction and surgical management of difficult laryngoscopy. The Laryngoscopy 2003; 114: 776

74. Adnet F, Borran SW, Lapostalle F et al: The Three axis alignment Theory and the sniffing position: Perpetuation of an anatomic myth? Anesthesiology 1999; 91: 1964

75. Chou HC, Wu TL: Rethinking the three axis alignment theory for direct laryngoscopy. Acta Anaesthesiol Scand 2001; 45: 261

76. Rosenblatt WH: Preoperative planning of airway management in critical care patients. Crit Care Med 2004; 32(4supp): 186

77. Mallampati SR, Gatt SP, Gugino LD et al: A clinical sign to predict difficult tracheal intubation: A prospective study. Can Anaesth Soc J 1985; 32: 429

78. Ayoub C, Baraka A, el-Khatib M, Muallem M, Kawkabani N, Soueide A: A new cut-off point of thyromental distance for prediction of difficult airway. Middle East J Anesthesiol 2000; 15: 619

79. Iohom G, Ronayne M, Cunningham AJ: Prediction of difficult tracheal intubation. Eur J Anaesthesiol 2003; 20: 31

80. Ulrich B, Listyo R, Gerig HJ et al: The difficult intubation: The value of BURP and 3 predictive tests of difficult intubation. Anaesthesist 1998; 47: 45

81. Benumof JL, Cooper SD: Quantitative improvement in laryngoscopic view by optimal external laryngeal manipulation. J Clin Anesth 1996; 8: 136

82. Cormack RS, Lehane J: Difficult tracheal intubation in obstetrics. Anaesthesia 1984; 39: 1105

83. Rose DK, Cohen MM: The airway: Problems and predictions in 18,500 patients. Can J Anaesth 1994; 41: 372

84. Levitan RM: Advanced Concepts in Laryngoscope Blade Design, The Airway Cam Guide to Intubation and Practical Emergency Airway Management. Edited by Levitan RM. Pennsylvania, Exton, 2004, pp 185

85. Hagberg CA (ed): Benumof's Airway management: Principles and Practice. Philadelphia, Mosby, 2007

86. Crosby ET, Cooper RM, Douglas MJ et al: The unanticipated difficult airway with recommendations for management. Can J Anaesth 1998; 45: 757

87. Koh LK, Kong CE, Ip-Yam PC: The modified Cormack-Lehane score for the grading of direct laryngoscopy: evaluation in the Asian population. Anaesth Intens Care 2002; 30: 48

88. Henderson JJ: The use of the paraglossal straight blade laryngoscopy in difficult tracheal intubation. Anaesthesia 1997; 52: 552

89. Cardoso MM, Banner MJ, Melker RJ et al: Portable devices used to detect endotracheal intubation during emergency situations: A review. Crit Care Med 1998; 26: 957

90. Bresnick WH, Rask-Madsen C, Hogan DL et al: The effect of acute emotional stress on gastric acid secretion in normal subjects and duodenal ulcer patients. J Clin Gastroenterol 1993; 17: 117

91. Juvin P, Fevre G, Merouche M et al: Gastric residue is not more copious in obese patients. Anesth Analg 2001; 93: 162

92. Harter RL, Kelly WB, Kramer MG et al: A comparison of the volume and pH of gastric contents of obese and lean surgical patients. Anesth Analg 1998; 86: 147

93. Smith KJ, Dombranowski J, Yip G et al: Cricoid pressure displaces the esophagus: an observational study using magnetic resonance imaging. Anesthesiology 2003; 99: 60

94. Alstrom HB, Belhage B: Cricoid pressure a.m. Sellick in rapid sequence intubation? Ugeskr Laeger 2007; 169: 2305

95. Brain AI, Verghese C, Addy EV et al: The intubating laryngeal mask. I: Development of a new device for intubation of the trachea. Br J Anaesth 1997; 79: 699

96. Kundra P, Sujata N, Ravishankar M: Conventional tracheal tubes for intubation through the intubating laryngeal mask airway. Anesth Analg 2005; 100: 284

97. Baskett PJ, Parr MJ, Nolan JP: The intubating laryngeal mask: Results of a multicentre trial with experience of 500 cases. Anaesthesia 1998; 53: 1174

98. Rosenblatt WH, Murphy M: The intubating laryngeal mask: Use of a new ventilating intubating device in the emergency department. Ann Emerg Med 1999; 33: 234

99. Ferson DZ, Rosenblatt WH, Johansen MJ, Osborne I, Ovassapian A: Use of the Intubating LMA-Fastrach in 254 Patients with Difficult-to-manage Airways. Anesthesiology 2001; 95: 1175

100. Goldman AJ, Rosenblatt WH: The LMA CTrach in airway resuscitation: Six case reports. Anaesthesia 2006; 61: 975

101. Goldman AJ, Rosenblatt WH: Use of the fibreoptic intubating LMA-CTrach in two patients with difficult airways. Anaesthesia 2006; 61: 601

102. Liu EH, Goy RW: The LMA-CTrach for unanticipated difficult intubation. Anaesthesia 2006; 61: 1015

103. Bjerkelund CE: Use of a new intubating laryngeal mask CTrach in patients with known difficult airways. Acta Anaesthesiol Scand 2006; 50: 388

104. Micaglio M, Ori C, Bergamasco C et al: Use of the LMA CTrach in unexpected difficult airway: A case report. Eur J Anaesthesiol 2006; 23: 445

105. Timmermann A, Russo S, Graf BM: Evaluation of the CTrach—an intubating LMA with integrated fibreoptic system. Br J Anaesth 2006; 96: 516

106. Goldman AJ, Wender R, Rosenblatt W, Theil D: The fiberoptic intubating LMA-CTrach: An initial device evaluation. Anesth Analg 2006; 103: 508

107. Liu EH, Goy RW, Chen FG: An evaluation of poor LMA-CTrach views with a fibreoptic laryngoscope and the effectiveness of corrective measures. Br J Anaesth 2006; 97: 878

108. Dhonneur G, Ndoko SK, Yavchitz A et al: Tracheal intubation of morbidly obese patients: LMA-CTrach vs direct laryngoscopy. Br J Anaesth 2006; 97: 742

109. Bilgin H, Yylmaz C: Awake intubation through the CTrach in the presence of an unstable cervical spine. Anaesthesia 2006; 61: 513

110. Wender R, Goldman AJ: Awake insertion of the fibreoptic intubating LMA CTrach in three morbidly obese patients with potentially difficult airways. Anaesthesia 2007; 62: 948

111. Murphy GS, Szokol JW, Marymont JH et al: Residual paralysis at the time of tracheal extubation. Anesth Analg 2005; 100: 1840

112. Asai T, Shingu K: Use of the laryngeal mask during emergence from anesthesia in a patient with an unstable neck. Anesth Analg 1999; 88: 469

113. Engoren M: Evaluation of the cuff-leak test in a cardiac surgery population. Chest 1999; 116: 1029

114. Jaber S, Chanques G, Matecki S et al: Post-extubation stridor in intensive care unit patients. risk factors evaluation and importance of the cuff-leak test. Intensive Care Med 2003; 29: 69

115. Lee CH, Peng MJ, Wu CL: Dexamethasone to prevent postextubation airway obstruction in adults: A prospective, randomized, double-blind, placebo-controlled study. Crit Care 2007; 11: R72

116. Mort TC: Continuous airway access for the difficult extubation: The efficacy of the airway exchange catheter. Anesth Analg 2007; 105: 1357

117. Nunn C, Uffman J, Bhananker SM: Bilateral tension pneumothoraces following jet ventilation via an airway exchange catheter. J Anesth 2007; 21: 76

118. Daucourt V, Michel P, Avargues P et al: Guidelines on difficult intubation in anesthesia: evaluation of 2 information diffusion methods. Rev Epidemiol Sante Publique 1999; 47: 353

119. Kroesen G: Guidelines for the advanced management of the airway and ventilation during resuscitation. A statement by the airway and ventilation management working group of the European Resuscitation Council, 1996 Resuscitation 1997; 35: 89

120. Petrini F, Accorsi A, Adrario E et al: Gruppo di Studio SIAARTI Vie Aeree Difficili; Recommendations for airway control and difficult airway management. Minerva Anestesiol 2005; 71: 617

121. Henderson J, Popat M, Latto P et al: Difficult Airway Society guidelines. Anaesthesia 2004; 59: 1242

122. Schalte G, Rex S, Henzler D: Airway management. Anaesthesist 2007; 56: 837

123. Rosenblatt WH. Awake intubation made easy! American Society for Anesthesiologists annual refresher courses, 2007, pp 218

124. Parmet JL, Colonna-Romano P, Horrow JC et al: The laryngeal mask airway reliably provides rescue ventilation in cases of unanticipated difficult tracheal intubation along with difficult mask ventilation. Anesth Analg 1998; 87: 661

125. Christian AS: Failed obstetric intubation (Case Reports). Anaesthesia 1990; 45: 995

126. Browning ST, Whittet HB, Williams A: Failure of insertion of a laryngeal mask airway caused by a variation in the anatomy of the thyroid cartilage. Anaesthesia 1999; 54: 884

127. Ishimura H, Minami K, Sata T et al: Impossible insertion of the laryngeal mask airway and oropharyngeal axes. Anesthesiology 1995; 83: 867

128. Gataure PS, Hughes JA: The laryngeal mask airway in obstetrical anaesthesia. Can J Anaesth 1995; 42: 130

129. Kokkinis K, Papageorgiou E: Failure of the laryngeal mask airway (LMA) to ventilate patients with severe tracheal stenosis. Resuscitation 1995; 30: 21

130. Busoni P, Fognani G: Failure of the laryngeal mask to secure the airway in a patient with Hunter's syndrome (mucopolysaccharidosis type II). Paediatr Anaesth 1999; 9: 153

131. Nandi PR, Charlesworth CH, Taylor SJ et al: Effect of general anaesthesia on the pharynx. Br J Anaesth 1991; 66: 157

132. Benumof JL: Management of the difficult adult airway: With special emphasis on awake tracheal intubation Anesthesiology 1991; 75: 1087

133. Bergese SD, Khabiri B, Roberts WD et al: Dexmedetomidine for conscious sedation in difficult awake fiberoptic intubation cases. J Clin Anesth 2007; 19: 141

134. Jooste EH, Ohkawa S, Sun LS: Fiberoptic intubation with dexmedetomidine in two children with spinal cord impingements. Anesth Analg 2005; 101: 1248

135. Nydahl PA, Axelsson K: Venous blood concentration of lidocaine after nasopharyngeal application of 2% lidocaine gel. Acta Anaesthesiol Scand 1988; 32: 135

136. Wieczorek PM, Schricker T, Vinet B et al: Airway topicalisation in morbidly obese patients using atomised lidocaine: 2% compared with 4%. Anaesthesia 2007; 62: 984

137. Weisel W, Tella RA: Reaction to tetracaine used as topical anesthetic in bronchoscopy: A study of 1000 cases. JAMA 1951; 147: 218

138. Sitzman BT, Rich GF, Rockwell JJ et al: Local anesthetic administration for awake direct laryngoscopy. Are glossopharyngeal nerve blocks superior? Anesthesiology 1997; 86: 34

139. Ovassapian A (ed): Fiberoptic Endoscopy and the Difficult Airway. Philadelphia, Lippincott-Raven, 1996, pp 47

140. Rosenblatt WH, Wagner PJ, Ovassapian A et al: Practice patterns in managing the difficult airway by anesthesiologists in the United States. Anesth Analg 1998; 87: 153

141. Heidegger T, Gerig HJ, Ulrich B et al: Validation of a simple algorithm for tracheal intubation: daily practice is the key to success in emergencies and analysis of 13,248 intubations. Anesth Anal 2001; 92: 517

142. Cooper RM, Pacey JA, Bishop MJ et al: Early clinical experience with a new videolaryngoscope (GlideScope) in 728 patients. Can J Anaesth 2005; 52: 191

143. Sun DA, Warriner CB, Parsons DG et al: The GlideScope video laryngoscope: Randomized clinical trial in 200 patients. Br J Anaesth 2005; 94: 381

144. Kramer DC, Osborn IP: More maneuvers to facilitate tracheal intubation with the GlideScope. Can J Anaesth 2006; 53: 737

145. Doyle DJ, Zura A, Ramachandran M: Video laryngoscopy in the management of the difficult airway. Can J Anaesth 2004; 51: 95

146. Dow WA, Parsons DG: 'Reverse loading' to facilitate glidescope intubation. Can J Anaesth 2007; 54: 161

147. Jones PM, Turkstra TP, Armstrong KP et al: Effect of stylet angulation and endotracheal tube camber on time to intubation with the GlideScope. Can J Anesth 2007; 54: 21

148. Turkstra TP, Craen RA, Pelz DM et al: Cervical spine motion: A fluoroscopic comparison during intubation with lighted stylet, GlideScope, and macintosh laryngoscope. Anesth Analg 2005; 101: 910

149. Gunaydin B, Gungor I, Yigit N et al: The glidescope for tracheal intubation in patients with ankylosing spondylitis. comment. Br J Anaesth 2007; 98: 408

150. Xue FS, Zhang GH, Li XY et al: Comparison of hemodynamic responses to orotracheal intubation with the GlideScope(R) video laryngoscope and the macintosh direct laryngoscope. J Clin Anesth 2007; 19: 245

151. Cross P, Cytryn J, Cheng KK: Perforation of the soft palate using the GlideScope(R) videolaryngoscope. Can J Anesth 2007; 54: 588

152. Hirabayashi Y: Pharyngeal injury related to GlideScope video laryngoscope. Otolaryngol Head Neck Surg 2007; 137: 175

153. Cooper RM: Complications associated with the use of the GlideScope video laryngoscope. Can J Anesth 2007; 54: 54

154. Choo MK, Yeo VS, See JJ: Another complication associated with video laryngoscopy. Can J Anesth 2007; 54: 322

155. Malik AM, Frogel JK: Anterior tonsillar pillar perforation during GlideScope video laryngoscopy. Anesth Analg 2007; 104: 1610

156. Kaplan MB, Hagberg CA, Ward DS et al: Comparison of direct and video-assisted views of the larynx during routine intubation. J Clin Anesth 2006; 18: 357

157. Kaplan MB, Ward D, Hagberg CA et al: Seeing is believing: The importance of video laryngoscopy in teaching and in managing the difficult airway. Surg Endosc 2006; 20 (Suppl 2): S479

158. Skippey B, Ray D, McKeown D: The McGrath Video laryngoscope — an initial clinical evaluation. Can J Anesth 2007; 54: 307

159. Weiss M, Schwarz U, Dillier CM et al: Teaching and supervising tracheal intubation in paediatric patients using video laryngoscopy. Paediatr Anaesth 2001; 11: 343

160. Asai T, Murao K, Shingu K: Training method of applying pressure on the neck for laryngoscopy: Use of a video laryngoscope. Anaesthesia 2003; 58: 602

161. Kaplan MB, Ward DS, Berci G: A new video laryngoscope—an aid to intubation and teaching. J Clin Anesth 2002; 14: 620

162. Doyle DJ: GlideScope-assisted fiberoptic intubation: A new airway teaching method. Anesthesiology 2004; 101: 1252

163. Maharaj CH, Costello JF, McDonnell JG et al: The airtraq as a rescue airway device following failed direct laryngoscopy: A case series. Anaesthesia 2007; 62: 598

164. Suzuki A, Toyama Y, Iwasaki H et al: Airtraq for awake tracheal intubation. Anaesthesia 2007; 62: 746

165. Maharaj CH, Buckley E, Harte BH et al: Endotracheal intubation in patients with cervical spine immobilization: A comparison of macintosh and airtraq laryngoscopes. Anesthesiology 2007; 107: 53

166. Barak M, Philipchuck P, Abecassis P et al: A comparison of the truview blade with the macintosh blade in adult patients. Anaesthesia 2007; 62: 827

167. Matsumoto S, Asai T, Shingu K: Truview video laryngoscope in patients with difficult airways. Anesth Analg 2007; 103: 492

168. Murphy P: A fibre-optic endoscope used for nasal intubation. Anaesthesia 1967; 22: 489

169. Ovassapian A, Yelich SJ, Dykes MH et al: Learning fibreoptic intubation: Use of simulators vs. traditional teaching. Br J Anaesth 1988; 61: 217

170. Hershey MD, Hannenberg AA: Gastric distention and rupture from oxygen insufflation during fiberoptic intubation. Anesthesiology 1996; 85: 1479

171. Rosenblatt WH: Overcoming obstruction during bronchoscope-guided intubation of the trachea with the double setup endotracheal tube. Anesth Analg 1996; 83: 175

172. Ovassapian A, Yellich J, Dykes MHM et al: Fiberoptic nasotracheal intubation: Incidence and causes of failure. Anesth Analg 1983; 62: 692

173. Kristensen MS: The Parker flex-tip tube versus a standard tube for fiberoptic orotracehal intubation: randomized double blind study. Anesthesiology 2003; 98: 334

174. Hastings RH, Vigil AC, Hanna R et al: Cervical spine movement during laryngoscopy with the Bullard, Macintosh, and Miller laryngoscopes. Anesthesiology 1995; 82: 859

175. Cohn AI, McGraw SR, King WH: Awake intubation of the adult trachea using the Bullard laryngoscope. Can J Anaesth 1995; 42: 246

176. Cohn AI, Hart RT, McGraw SR et al: The Bullard laryngoscope for emergency airway management in a morbidly obese parturient. Anesth Analg 1995; 81: 872

177. Halligan M, Charters P: A clinical evaluation of the Bonfils intubation fiberscope. Anaesthesia 2003; 58: 1087

178. Greenland KB, Liu G, Tan H et al: Comparison of the Levitan FPS Scope and the single-use bougie for simulated difficult intubation in anaesthetised patients. Anaesthesia 2007; 62: 509

179. Young CF, Rosenblatt WH: Comparison of the Shikani Optical Stylet to direct laryngoscopy for orotracheal intubation by a first year anesthesiology resident (abstract) Anesthesiology, 2008 (in press)

180. Brimacombe J, Keller C, Kunzel KH et al: Cervical spine motion during airway management: a cinefluoroscopic study of the posteriorly destabilized third cervical vertebrae in human cadavers. Anesth Analg 2000; 91: 1274

181. Kulozik U, Georgi R, Krier C: Intubation with the Combitube-TM in massive hemorrhage from the locus Kieselbachii. Anasthesiol Intensivmed Notfallmed Schmerzther 1996; 31: 191

182. Blostein PA, Koestner AJ, Hoak S: Failed rapid sequence intubation in trauma patients: Esophageal tracheal Combitube is a useful adjunct. J Trauma 1998; 44: 534

183. Frass M, Frenzer R, Mayer G et al: Mechanical ventilation with the esophageal tracheal combitube (ETC) in the intensive care unit. Arch Emerg Med 1987; 4: 219

184. Rumball CJ, MacDonald D: The PTL, Combitube, laryngeal mask, and oral airway: A randomized prehospital comparative study of ventilatory device effectiveness and cost-effectiveness in 470 cases of cardiorespiratory arrest. Prehosp Emerg Care 1997; 1: 1

185. Lefrancios DP, Dufour DG: Use of the esophageal tracheal Combitube by basic emergency medical technicians. Resuscitation 2002; 52: 77

186. Urtubia R, Medina J, Alzamora R et al: "Insertion of the Esophageal-Tracheal Combitube using Inhalational Induction of Anesthesia with Sevoflurane as single agent. Difficult Airway 2002; 3: 51

187. Richards CF: The pyriform sinus perforation during Esophageal Tracheal Combitube. J Emerg Med 1998; 16: 37

188. Vezina D, Lessard MR, Bussieres J et al: Complications associated with the use of the Esophageal-Tracheal Combitube. Can J Anaesth 1998; 45: 76

189. Klein H, Williamson M, Sue-Ling HM et al: Esophageal rupture associated with the use of the Combitube. Anesth Analg 1997; 85: 937

190. Thierbach AR: A new device for emergency airway management. The easy tube resuscitation 2004; 61: 347

191. Urtubia RM, Leyton P: Successful use of the Easy Tube for facial surgery in a patient with glottic and subglottic stenosis. J Clin Anesth 2007; 19: 77

192. Martin SE, Ochsner MG, Jarman RH et al: Laryngeal mask airway in air transport when intubation fails: Case report. J Trauma 1997; 42: 333

193. Brimacombe JR, De Maio B: Emergency use of the laryngeal mask airway during helicopter transfer of a neonate. J Clin Anesth 1995; 7: 689

194. Dimitriou V, Brimacombe J, Zogogiannis I et al: Success of the Cobra after failure of the Fastrach in the difficult airway. Can J Anaesth 2005; 52: 992

195. Asai T, Latto P: Role of the laryngeal mask in patients with difficult tracheal intubation and difficult ventilation, Difficulties in Tracheal Intubation. Edited by Latto IP, Vaughan RS. London, WB Saunders, 1997, pp 177

196. Brimacombe JR, Berry AM: Mallampati grade and laryngeal mask placement. Anesth Analg 1996; 82: 1112

197. Cook TM, Lee G, Nolan JP: The ProSeal laryngeal mask airway: a review of the literature. Can J Anaesth 2005; 52: 739

198. Agro F, Frass M, Benumof JL et al: Current status of the Combitube: a review of the literature. J Clin Anesth 2002; 14: 307

199. Verghese C, Prior Willeard PFS: Immediate management of the airway during cardiopulmonary resuscitation in a hospital without a resident anaesthesiologist. Eur J Emerg Med 1994; 1: 123

200. Keller C, Brimacombe J, Bittersohl J et al: Aspiration and Laryngeal mask airway: three cases and a review of the literature. Br J Anaesth 2004; 93: 579

201. Aoyama K, Takenaka I: Cricoid pressure impedes positioning and ventilation through the laryngeal mask. Can J Anaesth 1996; 43: 1035

202. Gnauck K, Lungo JB, Scalzo A et al: Emergency intubation of the pediatric medical patient: Use of anesthetic agents in the emergency department. Ann Emerg Med 1994; 23: 1242

203. Li J, Murphy-Lavoie H, Bugas C et al: Complications of emergency intubation with and without paralysis. Am J Emerg Med 1999; 17: 141

204. Sivarajan M, Joy JV: Effects of general anesthesia and paralysis on upper airway changes due to head position in humans. Anesthesiology 1996; 85: 787

205. Walls RM: Management of the difficult airway in the trauma patient. Emerg Med Clin North Am 1998; 16: 45

206. Mchugh R, Kumar M, Sprung J et al: Transtracheal jet ventilation in management of the difficult airway. Anaesth Intensive Care 2007; 35: 406

207. Hooker EA, Danzl DF, O'Brien D et al: Percutaneous transtracheal ventilation: Resuscitation bags do not provide adequate ventilation. Prehosp Disaster Med 2006; 21: 431

208. Gaughn SD, Gzaki GT, Benumof JL: Comparison in a lung model of low and high flow regulators for transtracheal jet ventilation. Anesthesiology 1992; 77: 189

209. McLeod AD, Turner MW, Torlot KJ et al: Safety of transtracheal jet ventilation in upper airway obstruction. Br J Anaesth 2005; 95: 560

210. Bellemain A, Ghimouz A, Goater P et al: Bilateral tension pneumothorax after retrieval of transtracheal jet ventilation catheter. Ann Fr Anesth Reanim 2006; 25: 401

211. Orloff LA, Parhizkar N, Ortiz E: The hunsaker mon-jet ventilation tube for microlaryngeal surgery: Optimal laryngeal exposure. Ear Nose Throat J 2002; 81: 390

CHAPTER 30 ■ PATIENT POSITIONING AND RELATED INJURIES

MARK A. WARNER

KEY POINTS

1 Sedated or anesthetized patients should be placed in positions that are comfortable while they are awake.

2 Padding provided by any number of different materials (e.g., gel or foam pads, blankets) should be used to widely disperse point pressure on body parts or tissues.

3 Elevated lower extremity positions (e.g., lithotomy) may reduce perfusion pressure in the elevated extremities and increase the opportunity for developing compartment syndromes, especially when the extremities are elevated for prolonged periods.

4 Brachial plexus neuropathy associated with sternotomy in anesthetized patients undergoing cardiac procedures may mimic as peripheral ulnar neuropathy.

5 The etiology of ulnar neuropathy is not always clear. Most commonly it develops postoperatively in men 40 to 70 years of age who undergo abdominal or pelvic procedures. There are anatomic and neurophysiologic reasons for men compared with women to develop this problem.

6 Excessive flexion or extension of the spine in anesthetized patients who are placed in unique surgical positions may contribute to spinal cord ischemia and catastrophic neurologic damage.

7 Perioperative vision loss occurs most frequently in anesthetized patients undergoing cardiac surgical procedures. Patients undergoing extensive spine procedures while positioned prone may develop vision loss, primarily from posterior ischemic optic neuropathy.

8 Neuropathies that result in motor function loss as well as sensory loss compared with those with isolated sensory loss generally are associated with more prolonged or permanent nerve dysfunction.

Positioning a patient for a surgical procedure is frequently a compromise between what the anesthetized patient can tolerate, both structurally and physiologically, and what the surgical team requires for access to their anatomic targets.[1] Establishment of the intended surgical posture may need to be modified to match the patient's tolerance. This chapter presents the significance of various positions in which a patient may be placed during an operation, briefly describes the techniques of establishing the positions, and discusses the potential complications of each posture.

It is very important for clinicians to understand the physiologic and potential pathologic consequences of patient positioning. In the past 2 decades, a number of studies of large surgical populations have provided new information on the frequency and natural history of rare perioperative events such as neuropathies and vision loss. However, these studies infrequently have provided sufficient data to allow speculation as to potential mechanisms of injury. Based on the findings of these studies, investigators are now seeking to confirm mechanisms of injury and the efficacy of novel interventions to decrease the frequency of, or to prevent, these perioperative events. Until these new investigations are complete, the mechanisms for many potential positioning-related complications remain unknown.

The lack of solid scientific information on basic mechanisms of positioning-related complications often leads to medicolegal entanglements. Notations on anesthesia and operating room records may be absent or uninformative.

Careful descriptive notations about positions used during anesthesia and surgery, as well as brief comments about special protective measures such as eye care and pressure-point padding, are useful to include on the anesthesia record. In potentially complicated or contentious circumstances, a separate brief description of care documented in the patient's record is advisable. Only in this manner can subsequent inquiries be properly answered on behalf of either the patient or the anesthesiologist. When credible, expanded knowledge that further delineates mechanisms of positioning-related complications is available, these issues and the care of patients will be improved.

DORSAL DECUBITUS POSITIONS

Variations of the Dorsal Decubitus Position

Supine

Horizontal. In the traditional horizontal supine position (dubbed "lying at attention"), the patient lies on his or her back with a small pillow beneath the head (Fig. 30-1A). The arms are either comfortably padded and restrained alongside the trunk or abducted on well-padded arm boards. Either arm (or both) may be extended ventrally and the flexed forearm

FIGURE 30-1. **A.** Supine adult with minimal gradients in the horizontal vascular axis. Pulmonary blood volume is greatest dorsally. Viscera displace the dorsal diaphragm cephalad. Cerebral circulation is slightly above heart level if the head is on a small pillow. **B.** Head-down tilt aids blood return from lower extremities but encourages reflex vasodilation, congests vessels in the poorly ventilated lung apices, and increases intracranial blood volume. **C.** Elevation of the head shifts abdominal viscera away from the diaphragm and improves ventilation of the lung bases. According to the gradient above the heart, pressure in arteries of the head and neck decreases; pressure in accompanying veins may become subatmospheric.

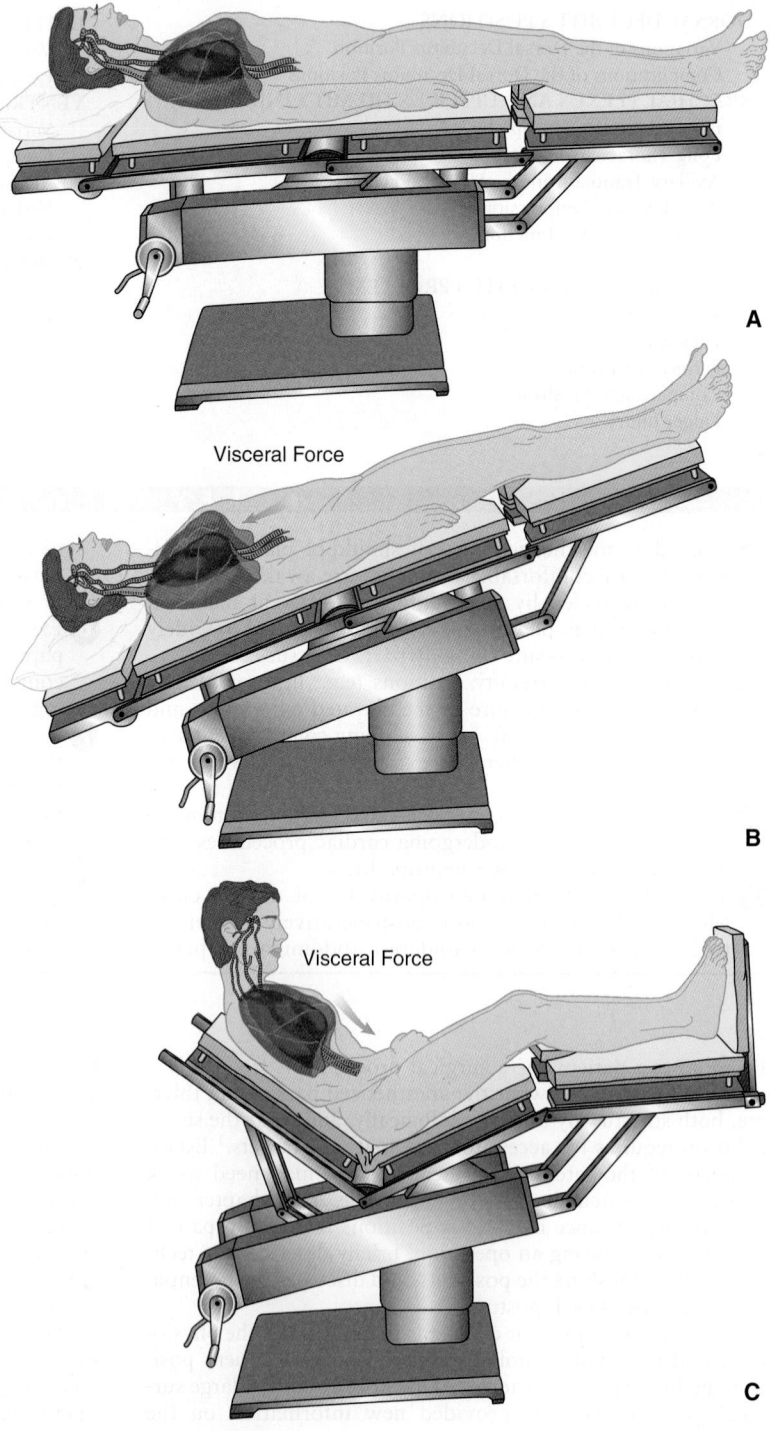

Visceral Force

Visceral Force

A

B

C

secured to an elevated frame in such a way that perfusion of the hand is not compromised, no skin-to-metal contact exists to cause electrical burns if a cautery is used, and the brachial neurovascular bundle is neither stretched nor compressed at the axilla. The lumbar spine may need padded support to prevent a postoperative backache (see "Complications of the Dorsal Decubitus Positions"). Bony contact points at the occiput, elbows, and heels should be padded. Fortunately, most modern surgical tables have mattress pads that are sufficiently buoyant and thick to allow dispersion of point pressure.

Although the horizontal supine posture has a long history of widespread use, it does not place hip and knee joints in neutral positions and is poorly tolerated for prolonged periods by an immobilized, awake patient.

Contoured. A contoured supine posture (Fig. 30-2C) has been termed the *lawn chair position*.[2] It is established by arranging the surface of the operating table so that the trunk–thigh hinge is angulated approximately 15 degrees and the thigh–knee hinge is angulated a similar amount in the opposite direction. Alternatively, a rolled towel, pillow, or blanket can be placed beneath the patient's knees to keep them flexed. The patient of average height then lies comfortably with hips and knees flexed gently. Quite often a person who

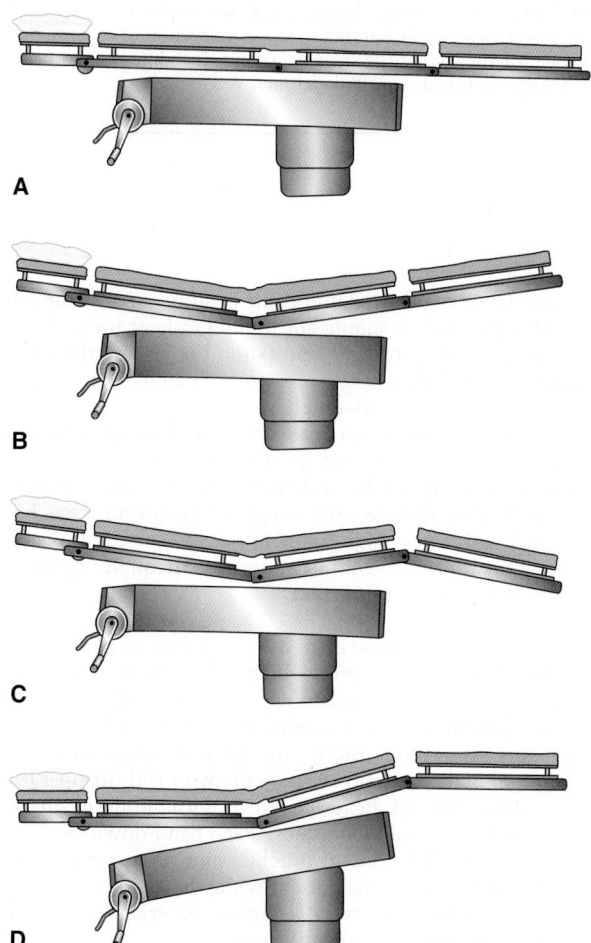

A

B

C

D

FIGURE 30-2. Establishment of the contoured supine ("lawn chair") position. **A.** Traditional flat supine tabletop. **B.** Thighs flexed on trunk. **C.** Knees gently flexed in final body position. **D.** Trunk section leveled to stabilize floor-supported arm board. (Reproduced from Martin JT, Warner MA [Eds]: Positioning in Anesthesia and Surgery, 3rd edition. Philadelphia, WB Saunders, 1997. p 42, with permission.)

has been required to lie motionless on a rigid horizontal table and then is changed to the contoured supine position offers an almost involuntary expression of relief and appreciation.

Lateral Uterine or Abdominal Mass Displacement. With a patient in the supine position, a mobile abdominal mass, such as a very large tumor or a pregnant uterus, can rest on the great vessels of the abdomen and compromise circulation. This is known as the *aortocaval syndrome* or the *supine hypotensive syndrome*. A significant degree of perfusion can be restored if the compressive mass is rolled toward the left hemiabdomen by leftward tilt of the tabletop or by a wedge under the right hip.[3]

Lithotomy

Standard. In the standard lithotomy position (Fig. 30-3), the patient lies supine with arms crossed on the trunk or with one or both arms extended laterally to <90 degrees on arm boards. Each lower extremity is flexed at the hip and knee, and both limbs are simultaneously elevated and separated so that the perineum becomes accessible to the surgeon. For many gynecologic and urologic procedures, the patient's thighs are flexed approximately 90 degrees on the trunk and the knees are bent sufficiently to maintain the lower legs nearly parallel to the floor. More acute flexion of the knees or hips can threaten to angulate and compress major vessels at either joint. In addition, hip flexion to >90 degrees on the trunk has been shown to increase stretch of the inguinal ligaments.[4] Branches of the lateral femoral cutaneous nerves often pass directly through these ligaments and can be impinged and become ischemic within the stretched ligament.

Numerous devices are available to hold legs that are elevated during obstetric delivery or perineal operations. Each device should be fitted to the stature of the individual patient. Care should be taken to ensure that angulations or edges of the padded holder do not compress the popliteal space or the upper dorsal thigh. Compartment syndromes of one or both lower extremities have resulted from prolonged use of the lithotomy position with some types of support devices.[5]

When the legs are to be lowered to the original supine position at the end of the procedure, they should first be brought together at the knees and ankles in the sagittal plane and then lowered slowly together to the tabletop. This minimizes torsion stress on the lumbar spine that would occur if each leg were lowered independently. It also permits gradual accommodation to the increase in circulatory capacitance, thereby avoiding sudden hypotension.

Low. For most urologic procedures and for many procedures that require simultaneous access to the abdomen and perineum, the degree of thigh elevation in the lithotomy position is only approximately 30 to 45 degrees (Fig. 30-4). This reduces perfusion gradients to and from the lower extremities and improves access to a perineal surgical site for members of the operating team who may need to stand at the lateral aspect of either leg.

High. Some surgeons prefer to improve access to the perineum by suspending the patient's feet from high poles. The effect is to have the patient's legs almost fully extended on the thighs (Fig. 30-5) and the thighs flexed 90 degrees or more on the trunk. The posture produces a significant uphill gradient for arterial perfusion into the feet, requiring careful avoidance of systemic hypotension. Less mobile patients may tolerate this posture poorly because of angulation and compression of the contents of the femoral canal by the inguinal ligament (Fig. 30-5A), or stretch of the sciatic nerve (Fig. 30-5B), or both.

ANESTHETIC MANAGEMENT

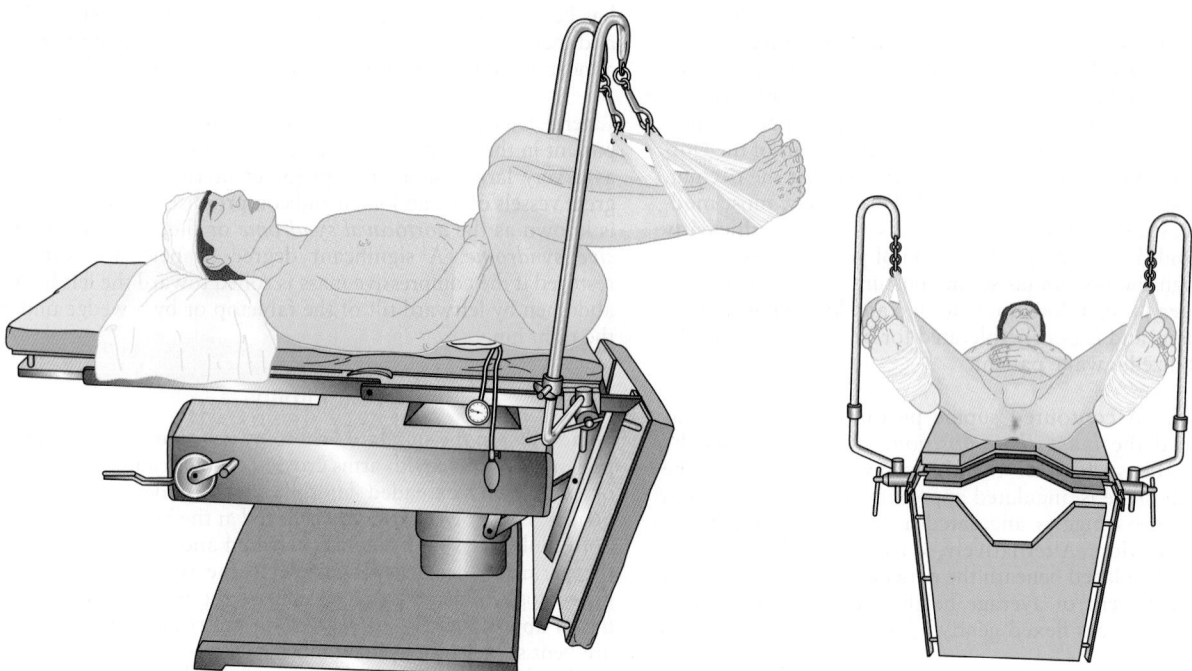

FIGURE 30-3. Standard lithotomy position with "candy cane" extremity support. Thighs are flexed approximately 90 degrees on abdomen; knees are flexed enough to bring lower legs grossly parallel to the torso section of the tabletop. Arms are retained on boards, crossed on the abdomen, or snugged at the sides of patient. (Modified from Martin JT, Warner MA [Eds]: Positioning in Anesthesia and Surgery, 3rd edition. Philadelphia, WB Saunders, 1997, pp 53, 66, with permission.)

Exaggerated. Transperineal access to the retropubic area requires that the patient's pelvis be flexed ventrally on the spine, the thighs almost forcibly flexed on the trunk, and the lower legs aimed skyward so they are out of the way (Fig. 30-6). The result places the long axis of the symphysis pubis almost parallel to

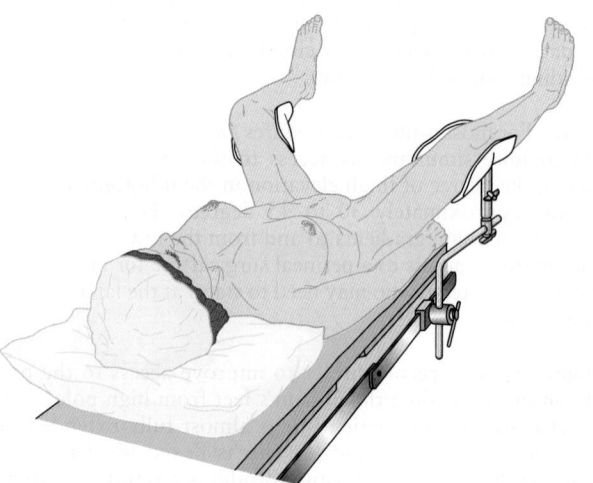

FIGURE 30-4. Low lithotomy position for perineal access, transurethral instrumentation, or combined abdominoperineal procedures. (Modified from Martin JT, Warner MA [Eds]: Positioning in Anesthesia and Surgery, 3rd edition. Philadelphia, WB Saunders, 1997, p 99, with permission.)

the floor. This exaggerated lithotomy position stresses the lumbar spine, produces a significant uphill gradient for perfusion of the feet, and may restrict ventilation because of abdominal compression by bulky thighs. It can be tolerated under anesthesia but rarely can be assumed by an awake patient. Control of ventilation is usually necessary. If pre-existing painful lumbar spine disease is present, an alternative surgical position may need to be chosen beforehand to avoid severely accentuating the lumbar distress after surgery. This position has been associated with a very high frequency of lower extremity compartment syndrome.[6] Maintenance of adequate perfusion pressure in the legs is important.

Tilted. Frequently, some degree of head-down tilt is added to one of the lithotomy positions. If the tilt is great enough, and particularly in the instance of the exaggerated lithotomy position, the patient may slide cephalad. Care must be taken to avoid this situation; there are several anecdotes from medicolegal actions involving patients who slid off operating tables with resulting head injuries. With modern surgical tables and procedural techniques, steep head-down tilt is not often warranted. The risk of brachial injuries associated with cephalad movement of the patient while the arms or shoulders are secured to the table with retention materials or shoulder braces is often present in this position.

Depending on the degree of head depression, the addition of tilt to the lithotomy position combines the worst features of both the lithotomy and the head-down postures. The weight of abdominal viscera on the diaphragm adds to whatever abdominal compression is produced by the flexed thighs of an obese patient or of one placed in an exaggerated lithotomy position. Ventilation should be assisted or controlled.

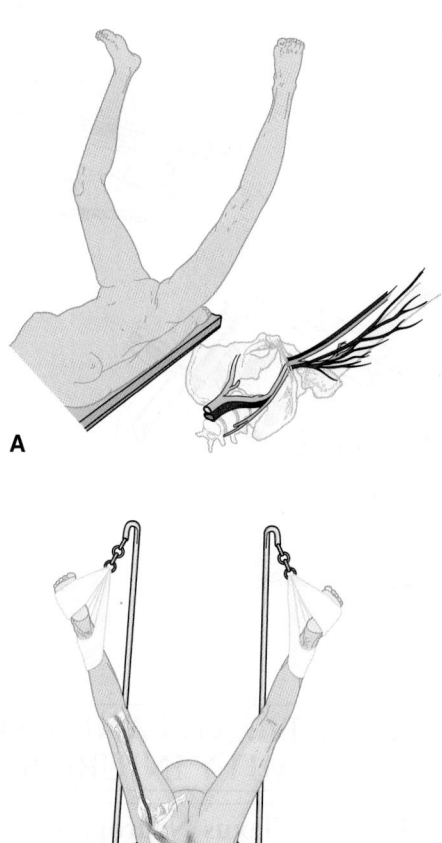

A

B

FIGURE 30-5. High lithotomy position. Note potential for angulation and compression/obstruction of contents of femoral canal (**A**, *inset*) or stretch of sciatic nerve (**B**). (**A** reproduced from McLeskey CH [Ed]: Geriatric Anesthesiology. Baltimore, Williams & Wilkins, 1997, p 146, with permission. **B** reproduced from Martin JT, Warner MA [Eds]: Positioning in Anesthesia and Surgery, 3rd edition. Philadelphia, WB Saunders, 1997, pp 61, 63, with permission.)

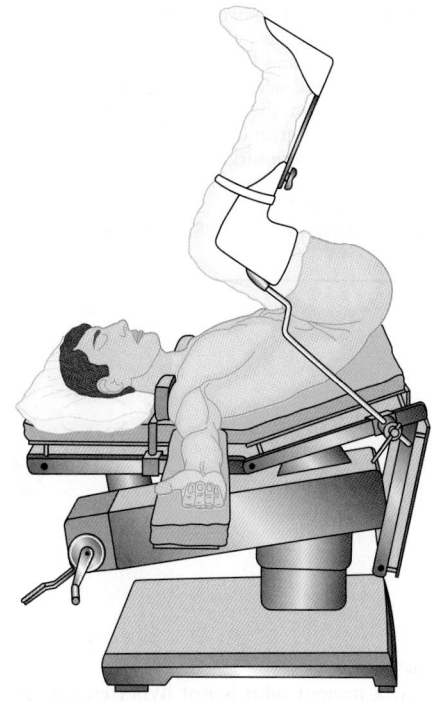

FIGURE 30-6. The exaggerated lithotomy position. Shoulder braces, usually needed to stabilize the torso, are placed over the acromioclavicular area to minimize compression of the brachial plexus and adjacent vessels. (Reprinted from Martin JT, Warner MA [Eds]: Positioning in Anesthesia and Surgery, 3rd edition. Philadelphia, WB Saunders, 1997, p 54, with permission.)

③ Because elevation of the lower extremities above the heart produces an uphill perfusion gradient, systemic hypotension and compressive leg wrapping may limit perfusion to the periphery, and both can be factors in the development of compartment syndromes in the legs of patients in the lithotomy position.[5] This perfusion gradient often is unpredictable and exaggerated, potentially increasing the risk of compartment syndrome.[7,8]

Cephalad displacement of the diaphragm and obstruction of its caudad inspiratory stroke accompany a head-down position because of gravity-shifted abdominal viscera. Consequently, the work of spontaneous ventilation is increased for an anesthetized patient in a posture that already worsens the ventilation–perfusion ratio by gravitational accumulation of blood in the poorly ventilated lung apices. During controlled ventilation, higher inspiratory pressures are needed to expand the lung.

Cranial vascular congestion and increased intracranial pressure can be expected to result from head-down tilt. For patients with known or suspected intracranial disease, the position should be used only in those rare instances in which a surgically useful alternate posture cannot be found. Maintenance of the position should then be as brief as possible.

Steep head-down tilt positions (e.g., 30 to 45 degrees of head-down tilt) may require some means of preventing the patient from sliding cephalad out of position. The use of bent knees is a satisfactory method of retaining the tilted patient in position (Fig. 30-7) if the flexed knee joints are placed sufficiently caudad of the leg–thigh hinge of the tabletop so that the adjacent firm edge of the depressed leg section of the table cannot indent either proximal calf or obstruct structures in the popliteal space. Compressive ischemia and phlebitis or a compartment syndrome may result if either occur.

Historically, shoulder braces also have been used to prevent cephalad sliding in steep head-down tilt positions. These braces are best tolerated if placed over the acromioclavicular joints, but care must be taken to see that the shoulder is not forced sufficiently caudad to trap and compress the subclavian neurovascular bundle between the clavicle and the first rib. If the braces are placed medially against the root of the neck, they may easily compress neurovascular structures that emerge from the area of the scalene musculature. For these and other reasons, the use of shoulder braces has waned in popularity and should not be used if possible.

For many of these reasons, steep head-down positions should be used only when a unique surgical issue requires it for optimal exposure and only for as long as needed for that exposure.

Complications of the Dorsal Decubitus Positions

Postural Hypotension

Postural hypotension may be seen when a head-elevated position is being established. If mean arterial pressure at the circle of Willis remains within the range of cerebral blood flow

FIGURE 30-7.   Head-down tilt. *Lower figure* shows traditional steep (30- to 45-degree) tilt described by Trendelenburg. Leg restraints and knee flexion stabilize the patient, avoiding the need for wristlets or shoulder braces that threaten the brachial plexus. *Upper figure* shows 10 to 15 degrees of head-down tilt, which is more common in modern surgical procedures. (Reprinted from Martin JT, Warner MA [Eds]: Positioning in Anesthesia and Surgery, 3rd edition. Philadelphia, WB Saunders, 1997, pp 98, 102, with permission.)

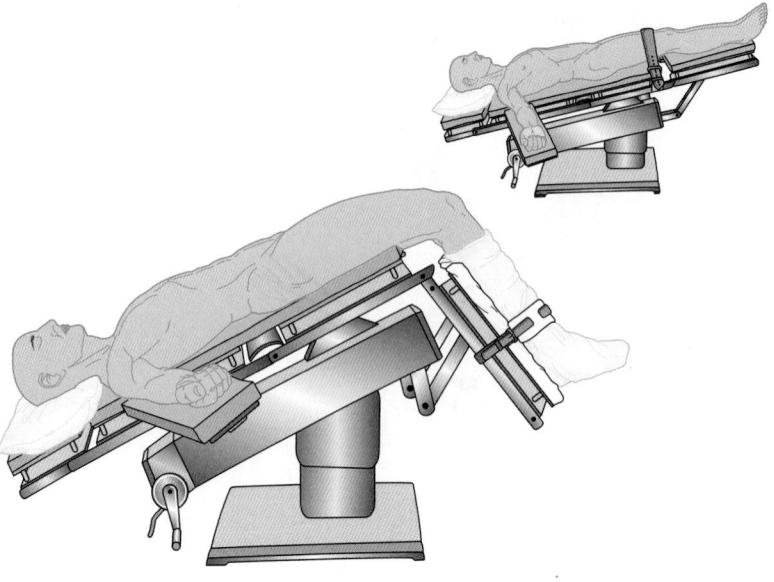

autoregulation in a patient who is not hypertensive, the postural hypotension may require little treatment other than to appropriately decrease the concentration of anesthetic drugs to preserve compensatory reflexes. If the degree of hypotension encountered is more severe, further head elevation should be delayed until the level of anesthetic is decreased; in addition, judicious use of fluids and vasopressors can re-establish effective perfusion.

Postural hypotension may also appear in the presence of inadequately replaced blood loss when the intravascular space has been functionally increased either by lowering the legs to horizontal at the termination of the lithotomy position or by returning a head-down tilt to horizontal. Volume repletion is the indicated therapy, although judiciously small doses of vasopressors may sometimes be needed initially.

Pressure Alopecia

Prolonged compression of hair follicles can produce hair loss. Abel and Lewis[9] described patients who had pain, swelling, and exudation where the occiput had been supporting the weight of the head for long periods in the Trendelenburg position. Alopecia occurred between the 3rd and 28th postoperative day; regrowth was complete within 3 months. Use of tight head straps to hold anesthetic face masks and prolonged hypotension and hypothermia have also been associated with compression alopecia.[10] Frequently turning the patient's head during long operations[11] and use of padded, soft head supports are recommended to reduce the risks of this complication.

Pressure-Point Reactions

Weight-bearing bony prominences can produce ischemic necrosis of overlying tissue unless proper padding is applied. Hypothermia and vasoconstrictive hypotension may enhance the process. The heels, the elbows, and the sacrum are particularly vulnerable. The use of a variety of pads (e.g., foam or gel) may disperse point pressure if used for protection. Although their use may protect against skin and soft tissue compression and ischemia, there are no studies that have proven their use to be beneficial in reducing peripheral neuropathies in the perioperative period.

BRACHIAL PLEXUS AND UPPER EXTREMITY INJURIES

Brachial Plexus Neuropathy

Root Injuries

Shoulder braces placed tight against the base of the neck can compress and injure the roots of the brachial plexus. Braces, if needed at all, are considered less harmful when placed more laterally over the acromioclavicular joint. In general, the use of shoulder braces should be discouraged.

The dorsal decubitus positions do not usually threaten structures in the patient's neck unless considerable lateral displacement of the head occurs. In that position, the roots of the brachial plexus on the side of the obtuse head–shoulder angle can be stretched and damaged. If the upper extremity is fixed at the wrist (e.g., by wrist wrap or a sheet or towel used to tuck the arm), the stretch injury of the plexus can be accentuated as the head moves laterally away from the anchoring point of the wrist. Similarly, exaggerated rotation of the head away from an extended arm can be associated with a brachial plexus injury.

Sternal Retraction

Frequently, the patient undergoing a median sternotomy has both arms padded and secured alongside the torso. An alternative is to have both arms abducted.[12] Vander Salm et al.[13,14] described first rib fractures and brachial plexus injuries associated with median sternotomies. They related the extent of the injury to the amount of retractor displacement of the rib, with the most severe injury being caused by displacement sufficient to produce a first rib fracture. Roy and associates,[15] in a study of 200 consecutive adults scheduled for cardiac surgery via a median sternotomy, positioned the left arm either abducted and padded on an arm board with the palm supinated or secured by a draw sheet alongside the trunk; the right arm was always placed alongside the trunk. They found a 10% incidence of upper extremity nerve injury that was not influenced by internal mammary artery harvest, internal jugular vein catheterization, or left arm position. Surgical manipulation was more contributory than extremity positioning in producing trauma to the brachial plexus. Jellish et al.[12] reported that there is less slowing of somatosensory evoked potentials (SSEPs) of the ulnar nerve during sternotomy when both arms are abducted instead of tucked at the sides. However, they found no differences in perioperative symptoms between patients in the arm-abducted versus arm-at-side groups.

Long Thoracic Nerve Dysfunction

A number of lawsuits have centered on postoperative serratus anterior muscle dysfunction and winging of the scapula (Fig. 30-8) alleged to be the result of position-related injuries to the long thoracic nerve of Bell, which arises from nerve roots C5, C6, and C7. Because C5 and C6 fibers of the nerve course through the middle scalene muscle and emerge from its lateral border to join the fibers from C7, it has been proposed that neuropathies of the long thoracic nerve are traumatic in origin.[16] Because the nerve is not routinely involved in a stretch injury of the brachial plexus and because the plexus is not routinely involved when long thoracic nerve dysfunction occurs, the relationship between postoperative long thoracic nerve palsy and patient positioning remains speculative. Based on evidence of Foo and Swann[17] plus data from litigations, Martin[18] concluded that in the absence of demonstrable trauma, postoperative dysfunctions of the long thoracic nerve were quite likely the result of coincidental neuropathies, possibly of viral origin.

Axillary Trauma from the Humeral Head

Abduction of the arm on an arm board to >90 degrees may thrust the head of the humerus into the axillary neurovascular bundle. The bundle is stretched at that point, and its neural structures may be damaged. In the same manner, vessels can be compressed or occluded and perfusion of the extremity can be jeopardized.

Radial Nerve Compression

The radial nerve, arising from roots C6-8 and T1, passes dorsolaterally around the middle and lower portions of the humerus in its musculospiral groove. At a point on the lateral aspect of the arm, approximately three fingerbreadths proximal to the lateral epicondyle of the humerus, the nerve can be compressed against the underlying bone and injured. Pressure from the vertical bar of an anesthesia screen or a similar device against the lateral aspect of the arm, excessive cycling of an automatic blood pressure cuff, and compression at the midhumerus level by restrictive sheets or towels used to tuck the arms have been implicated in causing damage to the radial nerve.

Median Nerve Dysfunction

Isolated perioperative injuries to the median nerve are uncommon and the mechanism is obscure.[19,20] A potential source of injury is iatrogenic trauma to the nerve during access to vessels in the antecubital fossa, as might occur during venipuncture. Anecdotally, this problem appears to occur primarily in men 20 to 40 years of age who cannot easily extend their elbows completely. Forced elbow extension after administration of muscle relaxants and while positioning the arms, with resultant stretch of the median nerve, has been suggested as one potential mechanism for this problem.

Ulnar Neuropathy

5 Improper anesthetic care and patient malpositioning have been implicated as causative factors in the development of ulnar neuropathies since reports by Büdinger[21] and Garriques[22] in the 1890s. These factors likely play an etiologic role for this problem in some surgical patients. Other factors, however, may contribute to the development of postoperative

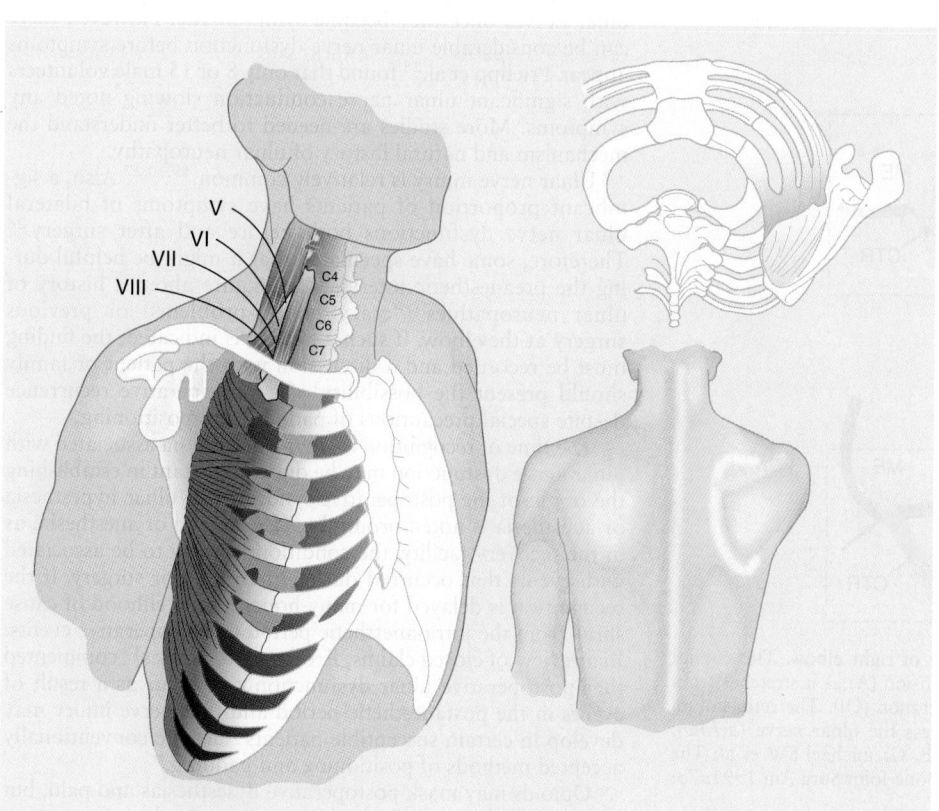

FIGURE 30-8. Scapular winging. The serratus anterior muscle (*upper right*) is supplied solely by the long thoracic nerve that branches immediately from C5, C6, C7, and sometimes C8 (*left figure*). Arising on the lateral ribs and inserting on the deep surface of the scapula, the muscle keeps the shoulder girdle approximated to the dorsal rib cage. Long thoracic nerve palsy allows dorsal protrusion of the scapula (*lower right*). See text for details. (Reproduced from Martin JT: Postoperative isolated dysfunction of the long thoracic nerve: A rare entity of uncertain etiology. Anesth Analg 1989; 69: 614, with permission.)

ulnar neuropathies. In a series of 12 inpatients with newly acquired ulnar neuropathy, Wadsworth and Williams[23] determined that external compression of an ulnar nerve during surgery was a factor in only two patients. Ulnar neuropathies develop in medical as well as surgical patients.[24] The mechanisms of ulnar neuropathy are unclear.

Typically, anesthesia-related ulnar nerve injury is thought to be associated with external nerve compression or stretch caused by malpositioning during the intraoperative period. Although this implication may be true for some patients, three findings suggest that other factors may contribute. First, patient characteristics (e.g., male sex, high body mass index [>38], and prolonged postoperative bed rest) are associated with these ulnar neuropathies.[25] Various reports suggest that 70 to 90% of patients who have this problem are men.[19,20,23–25] Second, many patients with perioperative ulnar neuropathies have a high frequency of contralateral ulnar nerve conduction dysfunction.[26] This finding suggests that many of these patients likely have asymptomatic but abnormal ulnar nerves before their anesthetics, and these abnormal nerves may become symptomatic during the perioperative period. Finally, many patients do not notice or complain of ulnar nerve symptoms until >48 hours after their surgical procedures.[25,26] A prospective study of ulnar neuropathy in 1,502 surgical patients found that none of the patients had symptoms of the neuropathy during the first 2 postoperative days.[27] It is not clear whether onset of symptoms indicates the time that an injury has occurred to the nerve. Prielipp et al.[28] found that 8 of 15 awake volunteers who had notable alterations in their ulnar nerve SSEP signals from direct ulnar nerve pressure did not perceive a paresthesia, even when the SSEP waveforms decreased as much as 72%.

Elbow flexion can cause ulnar nerve damage by several mechanisms. In some patients, the ulnar nerve is compressed by the aponeurosis of the flexor carpi ulnaris muscle and cubital tunnel retinaculum when the elbow is flexed by >110 degrees[29,30] (Fig. 30-9). In other patients, this fibrotendinous roof of the cubital tunnel is poorly formed and can lead to

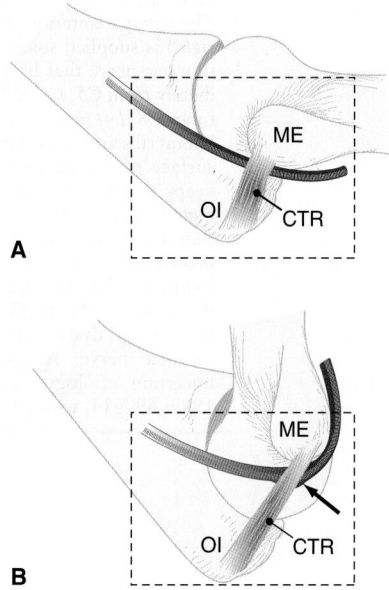

FIGURE 30-9. Medial-to-lateral view of right elbow. The cubital tunnel retinaculum (CTR) is lax in extension (**A**) as it stretches from the medial epicondyle (ME) to the olecranon (Ol). The retinaculum tightens in flexion (**B**) and can compress the ulnar nerve (*arrow*). (Reprinted from O'Driscoll SW, Horii E, Carmichael SW et al: The cubital tunnel and ulnar neuropathy. J Bone Joint Surg Am 1991; 73: 613, with permission.)

anterior subluxation or dislocation of the ulnar nerve over the medial epicondyle of the humerus during elbow flexion. This displacement has been observed in approximately 16% of cadavers in whom the flexor muscle aponeurosis and supporting tissues have not been dissected.[31,32] Ashenhurst[32] has speculated that the ulnar nerve may be chronically damaged by recurrent mechanical trauma as the nerve is in subluxation over the medial epicondyle.

External compression in the absence of elbow flexion also may damage the ulnar nerve.[33,34] Although compression within the medial epicondylar groove may be possible if the groove is shallower than normal, the bony groove usually is deep and the nerve is well protected from external compression.[35] External compression may occur distal to the medial epicondyle, where the nerve and its associated artery are relatively superficial. In an anatomic study, Contreras et al.[36] observed that the ulnar nerve and posterior recurrent ulnar artery pass posteromedially to the tubercle of the coronoid process, where they are covered only by skin, subcutaneous fat, and a thin distal band of the aponeurosis of the flexor carpi ulnaris.

Why are men more likely to have this complication? There are several anatomic differences between men and women that may increase the likelihood of perioperative ulnar neuropathy developing in men. First, two anatomic differences may increase the chance of ulnar nerve compression in the region of the elbow. The tubercle of the coronoid process is approximately 1.5 times larger in men than women.[36] In addition, there is less adipose tissue over the medial aspect of the elbow of men compared with women of similar body fat composition.[36–38] Second, men may be more likely to have a well-developed cubital tunnel retinaculum than women, and the retinaculum, if present, is thicker. A thicker cubital tunnel retinaculum may increase the risk of ulnar nerve compression in the cubital tunnel when the elbow is flexed.

Clinical manifestations of ulnar nerve dysfunction vary with the location and extent of the lesion.[39] Nearly all patients have numbness, tingling, or pain in the sensory distribution of the ulnar nerves once they become symptomatic. However, there can be considerable ulnar nerve dysfunction before symptoms appear. Prielipp et al.[28] found that only 8 of 15 male volunteers with significant ulnar nerve conduction slowing noted any symptoms. More studies are needed to better understand the mechanism and natural history of ulnar neuropathy.

Ulnar nerve injury is relatively common.[19,20,27] Also, a significant proportion of patients have symptoms of bilateral ulnar nerve dysfunctions both before and after surgery.[26] Therefore, some have speculated that it might be helpful during the preanesthetic interview to inquire about a history of ulnar neuropathies ("crazy bone" problems) or previous surgery at the elbow. If such a history is indicated, the finding must be recorded and a discussion with the patient or family should present the possibility of a postoperative recurrence despite special precautions of padding and positioning.

The time of recognition of digital anesthesia associated with ulnar nerve dysfunction may be quite important in establishing the origin of the postoperative syndrome. If ulnar hypesthesia or anesthesia is noted promptly after the end of anesthesia, as in the recovery facility, the condition is likely to be associated with events that occurred during anesthesia or surgery. If the recognition is delayed for many hours, the likelihood of cause shifts from the intra-anesthetic period to postoperative events. In a review of closed claims, Kroll and associates[19] commented that postoperative ulnar dysfunction can occur as a result of events in the postanesthetic period and that nerve injury may develop in certain susceptible patients "despite conventionally accepted methods of positioning and padding."

Opioids may mask postoperative dysesthesias and pain, but even strong analgesics do not appear to mask a loss of sensation as a result of nerve dysfunction. It may be helpful to assess ulnar nerve function and record these observations before discharging the patient from the recovery room.

OTHER DORSAL DECUBITUS PROBLEMS

Arm Complications

An arm that is hyperabducted can force the head of the humerus into the axillary neurovascular bundle and damage nerves and vessels to the arm. Abduction of the arm to >90 degrees from the trunk should be avoided. An arm board should be securely attached to the operating table to prevent its accidental release. An arm that is not properly secured can slip over the edge of the table or arm board, resulting in injury to the capsule of the shoulder joint by excessive dorsal extension of the humerus, fracture of the neck of an osteoporotic humerus, or injury to the ulnar nerve at the elbow. Conversely, in the unlikely event that the retaining strap is excessively tight across the supinated forearm (Fig. 30-10), the potential exists for pressure to compress the anterior interosseous nerve, a branch of the median nerve in the upper forearm that courses with its artery along the volar surface of the tough interosseous membrane. The result is an ischemic injury to the distribution of the nerve and artery that resembles a compartment syndrome in the lower extremity and may require prompt surgical decompression.[40–42]

Backache

Lumbar backache can be worsened by the ligamentous relaxation that occurs with general, spinal, or epidural anesthesia. Loss of normal lumbar curvature in the supine position is apparently the issue. Padding (Fig. 30-3) placed under the lumbar spine before the induction of anesthesia may help retain lordosis and make a patient with known lumbar distress more comfortable. Hyperlordosis should be avoided, however. Hyperextension of the lumbar spine, especially to an angulation of >10 degrees at the L2-3 apex of the lumbar spine, may result in ischemia of the spinal nerves.[43]

Elevation of the legs can worsen the pain of a herniated nucleus pulposus. When the lithotomy position is contemplated for a patient with a history of low back pain or a herniated lumbar disk, gentle passive attempts to have the patient

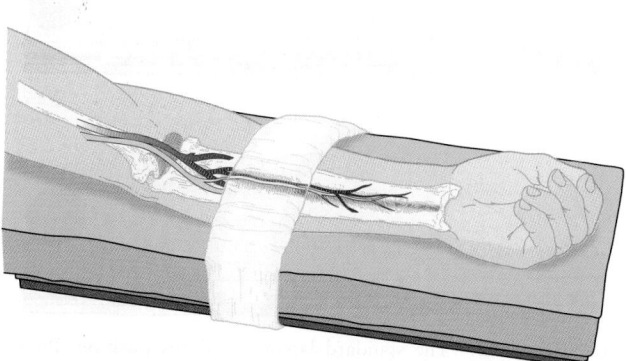

FIGURE 30-10. Arm restraint, if excessively tight, can compress the anterior interosseous nerve and vessel against the interosseous membrane in the volar forearm to produce an ischemic neuropathy. (Reproduced from McLeskey CH [Ed]: Geriatric Anesthesiology. Baltimore, Williams & Wilkins, 1997, p 155, with permission.)

assume the posture before anesthesia may be helpful in determining whether the position can be tolerated.

Perineal Crush Injury

The supine patient who is placed on a fracture table for repair of a fractured femur usually has the pelvis retained in place by a vertical pole at the perineum (Fig. 30-11), with the foot of the injured extremity fixed to a mobile rest. A worm gear on the rest lengthens the distance between the foot and the pelvis so that the bone fragments can be distracted and realigned. Unless the pole is well padded, severe pressure can be exerted on the pelvis, and damage can occur to the genitalia and the pudendal nerves. Complete loss of penile sensation has been reported after use of the fracture table.[44,45] The correct position for the pole is against the pelvis between the genitalia and the uninjured limb.[44]

Compartment Syndrome

If, for whatever reason, perfusion to an extremity is inadequate, a compartment syndrome may develop. Characterized by ischemia, hypoxic edema, elevated tissue pressure within fascial compartments of the leg, and extensive rhabdomyolysis, the syndrome produces extensive and potentially lasting damage to the muscles and nerves in the compartment.

Causes of a compartment syndrome that may be associated with positioning factors while a patient is in any of the dorsal decubitus positions include (1) systemic hypotension and loss of driving pressure to the extremity (augmented by elevation of the extremity); (2) vascular obstruction of major leg vessels by intrapelvic retractors, by excessive flexion of knees or hips, or by undue popliteal pressure from a knee crutch; and (3) external compression of the elevated extremity by straps or leg wrappings that are too tight, by the inadvertent pressure of the arm of a surgical assistant, or by the weight of the extremity against a poorly supportive leg holder. A tight strap on an arm as well as tight "draw sheets" for maintaining arms at the patient's sides may compress the anterior interosseous neurovascular bundle and may be associated with an anterior interosseous neuropathy or a forearm or a hand compartment syndrome.[41,42]

Several clinical characteristics seem to be associated with perioperative compartment syndrome. Prolonged lithotomy posture in excess of 5 hours has been a common factor in literature anecdotes of postlithotomy compartment syndromes. For lengthy procedures in the lithotomy position, well-padded holders that immobilize the limb by supporting the foot without compressing the calf or popliteal fossa seem to be the least threatening choice. There is considerable variability in the perfusion pressure of the lower extremity in elevated legs. Halliwill et al.[7] and Pfeffer et al.[8] found significant blood pressure variation at the ankle in volunteers placed in various lithotomy positions. Several volunteers had mean pressures of <20 mm Hg when positioned in the high lithotomy position. This pressure is less than intracompartment pressures commonly measured in many lithotomy positions.

Warner et al.[46] have shown that perioperative compartment syndromes occur in patients in positions other than lithotomy. The frequency of this problem appears to occur as often (approximately 1 in 9,000 patients) in anesthetized patients who are positioned laterally as in similar patients who are positioned in lithotomy. The difference between compartment syndromes in these two groups is that patients in a lateral decubitus position tend to have compartment syndromes of either arm, while those in a lithotomy position have compartment syndromes of the lower extremities.[46]

FIGURE 30-11. Traction table with perineal post stabilizing patient while leg is elongated to reposition bone ends. Elevated leg risks hypoperfusion; pelvic post threatens genitalia. (Reproduced from Martin JT, Warner MA [Eds]: Positioning in Anesthesia and Surgery, 3rd edition. Philadelphia, WB Saunders, 1997, p 54, with permission.)

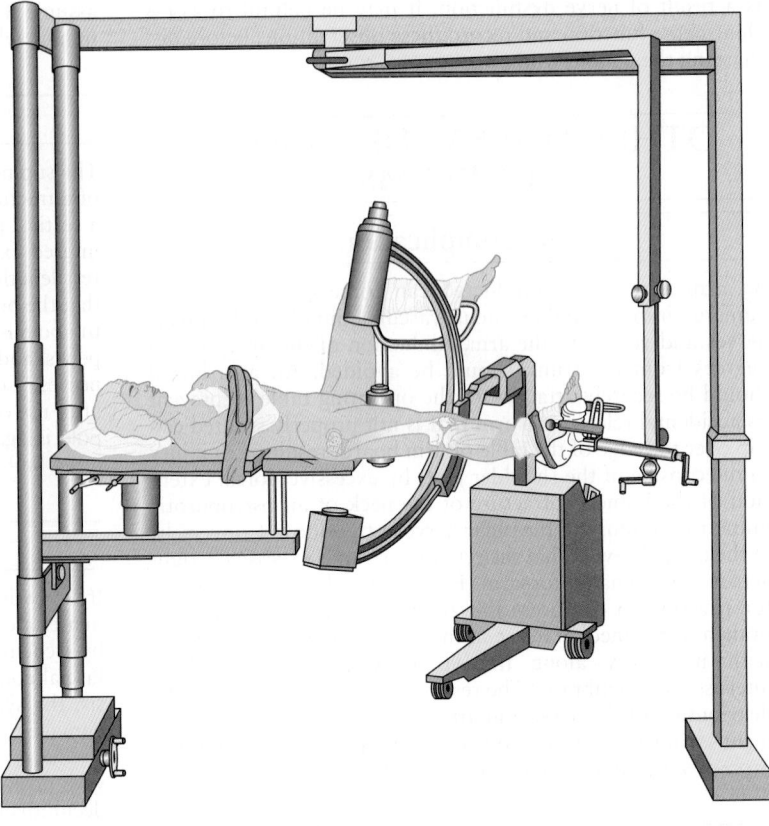

Finger Injury

Amputation of fingers has been reported when they were caught between the leg and thigh sections of the operating table as the leg section was returned to the horizontal position at the termination of an operation performed in the lithotomy position.[47] A towel used to create a boxing glove–like wrap on the hands of lithotomized patients or carefully removing the patient's hands from the risk position before raising the foot of the table may prevent such a tragic misadventure.

LATERAL DECUBITUS POSITIONS

There are several general positioning concepts to consider when placing a patient into a lateral decubitus position. Wrapping the legs and thighs in compressive bandages has been commonly used to combat venous pooling. Marked flexion of the lower extremities at knees and hips can partially or completely obstruct venous return to the inferior vena cava either by angulation of vessels at the popliteal space and inguinal ligament or by thigh compression against an obese abdomen. A small support placed just caudad of the down-side axilla can be used to lift the thorax enough to relieve pressure on the axillary neurovascular bundle and prevent disturbed blood flow to the arm and hand. However, this chest support (inappropriately called an *axillary roll* by some) has not been proven to reduce the frequency of ischemia, nerve damage, or compartment syndrome to the down-side upper extremity. It may, however, decrease shoulder discomfort postoperatively. Any padding should support only the chest wall and it should be periodically observed to ensure that it does not impinge on the neurovascular structures of the axilla.

Variations of the Lateral Decubitus Positions

Standard (Horizontal) Lateral Position

In the horizontal lateral decubitus position (Fig. 30-12), the patient is rolled onto one side on a flat table surface and stabilized in that posture by flexing the down-side thigh. The down-side knee is bent to retain the leg on the table and improve stabilization of the trunk. The common peroneal nerve of that

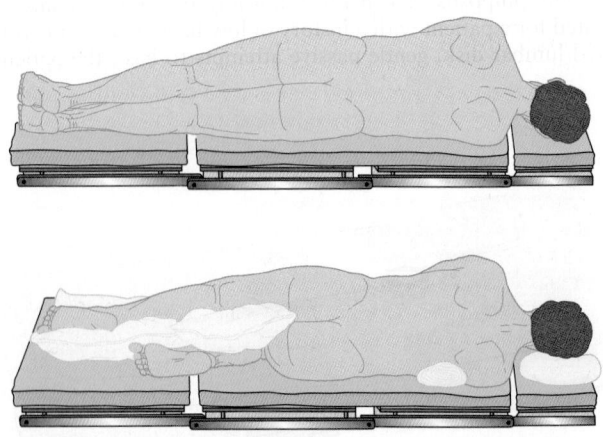

FIGURE 30-12. The standard lateral decubitus position. Proper head support, axillary roll, and leg pillow arrangement are shown on *lower figure*. Down-side leg is flexed at hip and knee to stabilize torso. Retaining straps and pad for down-side peroneal nerve are not shown. (Reproduced from Martin JT, Warner MA [Eds]: Positioning in Anesthesia and Surgery, 3rd edition. Philadelphia, WB Saunders, 1997, p 127, with permission.)

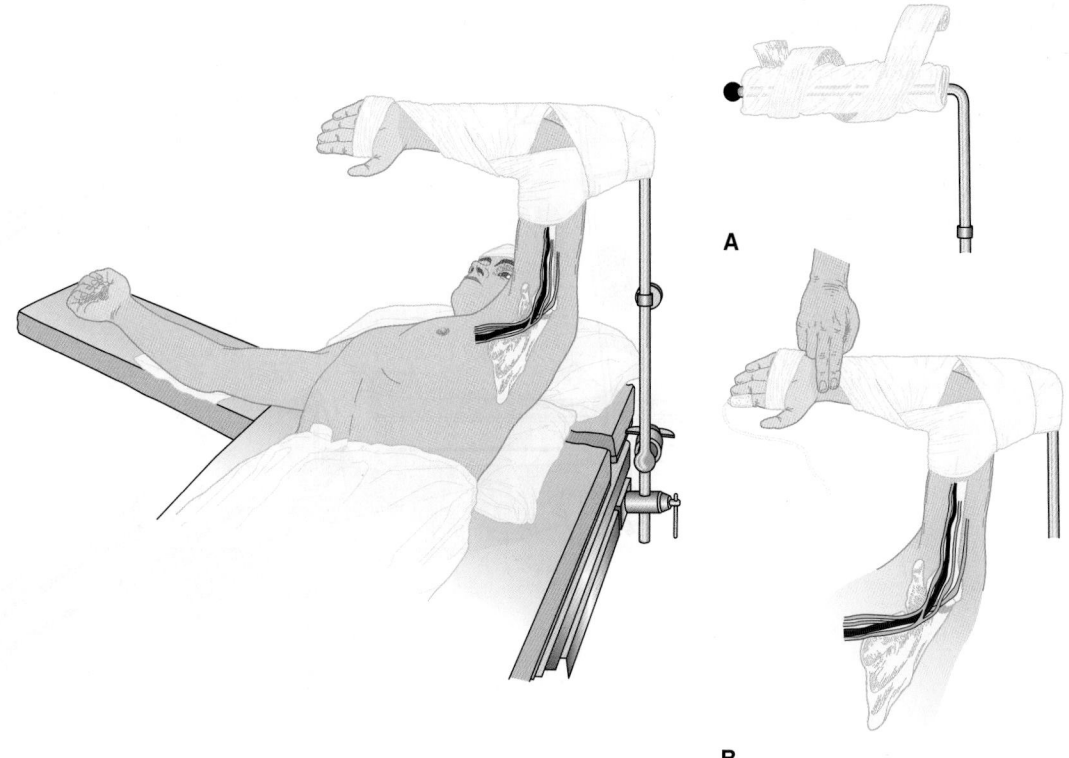

A

B

FIGURE 30-13.   The semisupine position with dorsal pads supporting the torso, the extended arm padded at the elbow, and the elevated arm restrained on a well-cushioned, adjustable overhead bar (**A**). Axillary contents (**B**) are not under tension and are not compressed by the head of the humerus, and a pulse oximeter ensures that the digital circulation is not compromised. The position is safe only if the arm does not become a hanging mechanism to support the torso. (Reproduced from Collins VJ [Ed]: Principles of Anesthesiology, 3rd edition. Philadelphia, Lea & Febiger, 1993, p 176, with permission.)

side is padded to minimize compression damage caused by the weight of the legs. The up-side thigh and leg are extended comfortably, and pillows are placed between the lower extremities. The head is supported by pillows or a headrest so that the cervical and thoracic spines are properly aligned. A small pad, thick enough to raise the chest wall and prevent excessive compression of the shoulder or entrapment/compression of the neurovascular structures of the axilla, is placed just caudad to the down-side axilla. This padding may support adequate perfusion of the down-side hand and minimize circumduction of the dependent shoulder, which might stretch its suprascapular nerve.

Arms may be extended ventrally and retained on a single arm board with suitable padding between them, or they may be individually retained on a padded two-level arm support that can also help to stabilize the thorax. An alternate method of arm arrangement is to flex each elbow and place the arms on suitable padding on the table in front of the patient's face.

The patient is stabilized in the lateral position by the use of one or more retaining tapes or straps stretched across the hip and fixed to the underside of the tabletop. Care must be taken to see that the hip tapes or straps lie safely between the iliac crest and the head of the femur rather than over the head of the femur. An additional restraining tape or strap may be used across the thorax or shoulders if needed.

Semisupine and Semiprone

The semilateral postures are designed to allow the surgeon to reach anterolateral (semisupine) and posterolateral (semiprone) structures of the trunk. In the semisupine position, the

up-side arm must be carefully supported so that it is not hyperextended and no traction or compression is applied to the brachial and axillary neurovascular bundles (Fig. 30-13). The supporting bar should be well wrapped to prevent electrical grounding contact (Fig. 30-13A). Sufficient noncompressible padding should be placed under the dorsal torso (Fig. 30-13, *large figure*) and hip to prevent the patient from rolling supine and stretching the anchored extremity. The pulse of the restrained wrist should be checked to ensure adequate circulation in the elevated arm and hand (Fig. 30-13B).

Flexed Lateral Positions

Lateral Jackknife.   The lateral jackknife position places the down-side iliac crest over the hinge between the back and thigh sections of the table (Fig. 30-14). The tabletop is angulated at that point to flex the thighs on the trunk laterally. After the patient has been suitably positioned and restrained, the chassis of the table is tipped so that the uppermost surface of the patient's flank and thorax becomes essentially horizontal. As a result, the feet are below the level of the atria, and significant amounts of blood may pool in distensible vessels in each leg.

The lateral jackknife position is usually intended to stretch the up-side flank and widen intercostal spaces as an asset to a thoracotomy incision. However, in terms of lumbar stress, restriction by the taut flank of up-side costal margin motion, and pooling of blood in depressed lower extremities, the position imposes a significant physiologic insult. Actually, its usefulness to the surgeon is brief, and its use should be limited. Once the rib-spreading retractor is placed in the incision, the position has reduced value for the rest of the operation.[48]

FIGURE 30-14. The lateral jackknife position, intended to open intercostal spaces. Note the properly placed restraining tapes (*large figure*) thrusting cephalad to retain the iliac crest at the flexion point of the table and prevent caudad slippage, which compresses the down-side flank (*inset*). (Reproduced from Martin JT, Warner MA [Eds]: Positioning in Anesthesia and Surgery, 3rd edition. Philadelphia, WB Saunders, 1997, 130, with permission.)

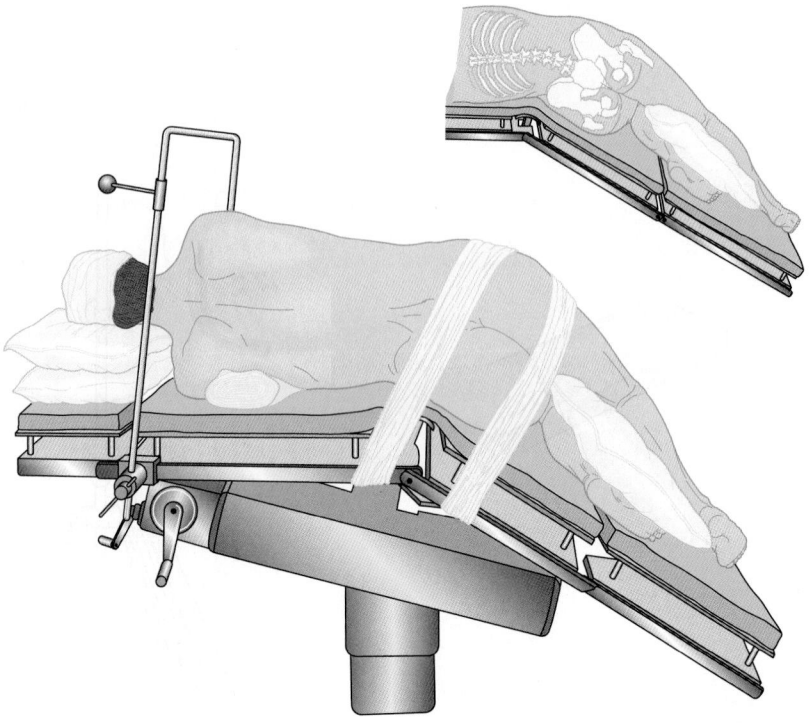

Kidney. The kidney position (Fig. 30-15) resembles the lateral jackknife position, but it adds the use of an elevated rest (the *kidney rest*) under the down-side iliac crest to increase the amount of lateral flexion and improve access to the up-side kidney under the overhanging costal margin. Unlike the lateral jackknife position, the kidney position does not have a useful alternative for a flank approach to the kidney. Thus, the physiologic insults associated with the posture need to be limited by vigilant anesthesia and rapid surgery. Strict stabilizing precautions should be taken to prevent the patient from subsequently shifting caudad on the table in such a manner that the elevated rest relocates into the down-side flank and becomes a severe impediment to ventilation of the dependent lung.

Complications of the Lateral Decubitus Positions

Eyes and Ears

Injuries to the dependent eye are unlikely if the head is properly supported during and after the turn from the supine to the lateral position. If the patient's face turns toward the mattress, however, and the lids are not closed or the eyes otherwise protected, abrasions of the ocular surface can occur. Direct pressure on the globe can displace the crystalline lens, increase intraocular pressure or, particularly if systemic hypotension is present, cause ischemia.

In the lateral position, the weight of the head can press the down-side ear against a rough or wrinkled supporting surface. Careful padding with a pillow or a foam sponge is usually sufficient protection against contusion of the ear. The external ear should also be palpated to ensure that it has not been folded over in the process of placing support beneath the head.

Neck

Lateral flexion of the neck is possible when the head of a patient in the lateral position is inadequately supported. If the cervical spine is arthritic, postoperative neck pain can be troublesome.

Pain from a symptomatic protrusion of a cervical disk can be intensified unless the head is carefully positioned so that lateral or ventral flexion, extension, or rotation is avoided.

Suprascapular Nerve

Ventral circumduction of the dependent shoulder can rotate the suprascapular notch away from the root of the neck (Fig. 30-16). Because the suprascapular nerve is fixed both paravertebrally and at the notch, circumduction can stretch the nerve and produce troublesome, diffuse, dull shoulder pain. The diagnosis is established by blocking the nerve at the notch and producing pain relief. Treatment may require resecting the ligament over the notch to decompress the nerve. A supporting pad placed under the thorax just caudad of the axilla and thick enough to raise the chest off the shoulder should prevent a circumduction stretch injury to the nerve.

Long Thoracic Nerve

Instances of postoperative winging of the scapula (Fig. 30-8) have followed use of the lateral decubitus position.[18] Although coincidental viral neuropathies of the long thoracic nerve may play a major etiologic role in postoperative appearances of scapular winging in patients for whom only a dorsal decubitus position was used, the possibility of trauma to the nerve while establishing the lateral position is difficult to refute. Lateral flexion of the neck may stretch the long thoracic nerve in the obtuse angle of the neck.

VENTRAL DECUBITUS (PRONE) POSITIONS

Variations of the Ventral Decubitus Position

Full (Horizontal) Prone

In the so-called *full* or *horizontal prone position* (Fig. 30-17), the requirement to elevate the trunk off the supporting surface

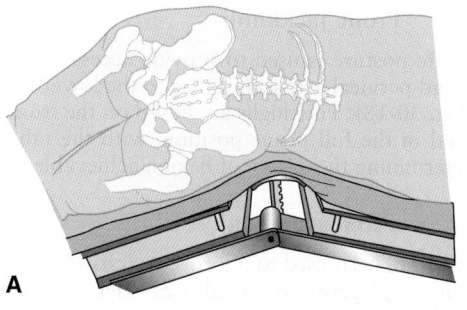

A

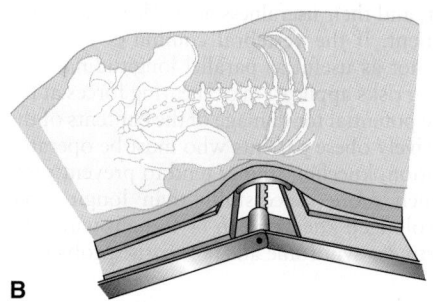

B

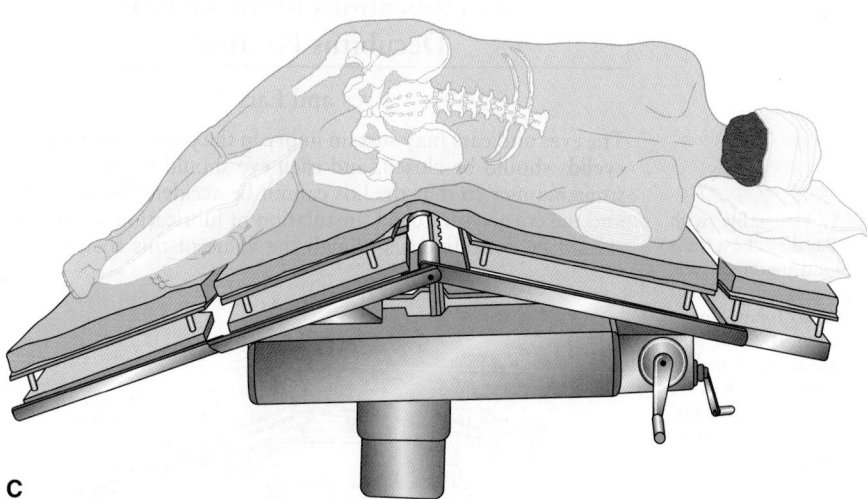

C

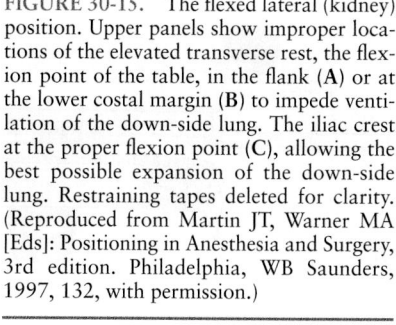

FIGURE 30-15.   The flexed lateral (kidney) position. Upper panels show improper locations of the elevated transverse rest, the flexion point of the table, in the flank (**A**) or at the lower costal margin (**B**) to impede ventilation of the down-side lung. The iliac crest at the proper flexion point (**C**), allowing the best possible expansion of the down-side lung. Restraining tapes deleted for clarity. (Reproduced from Martin JT, Warner MA [Eds]: Positioning in Anesthesia and Surgery, 3rd edition. Philadelphia, WB Saunders, 1997, 132, with permission.)

so that the ventral abdominal wall is freed of compression almost always results in the head and lower extremities being below the level of the spine. If the tabletop is angulated at the trunk–thigh hinge to remove the lumbar lordosis and separate the lumbar spinous processes, and if the chassis is then rotated head-up sufficiently to level the patient's back, a significant perfusion gradient may develop between the legs and the heart.[49] Wrapping the legs in compressive bandages, or the use of full-length elastic hosiery, minimizes pooling of blood in distensible vessels and supports venous return.

Various ventral supports, including parallel rolls of tightly packed sheets, padded and adjustable metal frames, and four-pillar frames, have been devised to free the abdomen from compression. Each has merit, and no specific unit has been shown to be better than the others for hemodynamic or respiratory maintenance. However, the use of frames may produce more opportunities for point pressure, and if they are used, careful padding of contact points should be considered. The choice of equipment is based on the physique of the patient, the requirements of the surgical procedure, and availability.

Pronated patients with limited mobility of the neck, a history of postural neck pain, or a history suggesting a symptomatic cervical disk should have their heads retained in the sagittal plane, either with a skull-pin head clamp or with a face rest.

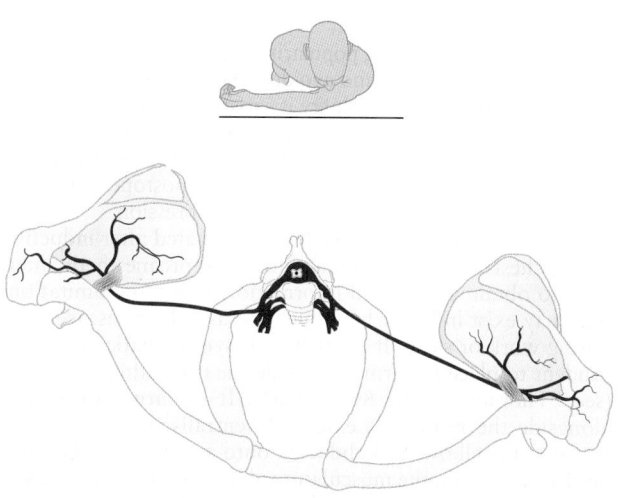

FIGURE 30-16.   Circumduction of the arm displacing the scapula and stretching the suprascapular nerve between its anchoring points at the cervical spine and the suprascapular notch. (Reproduced from Martin JT, Warner MA [Eds]: Positioning in Anesthesia and Surgery, 3rd edition. Philadelphia, WB Saunders, 1997, p 147, with permission.)

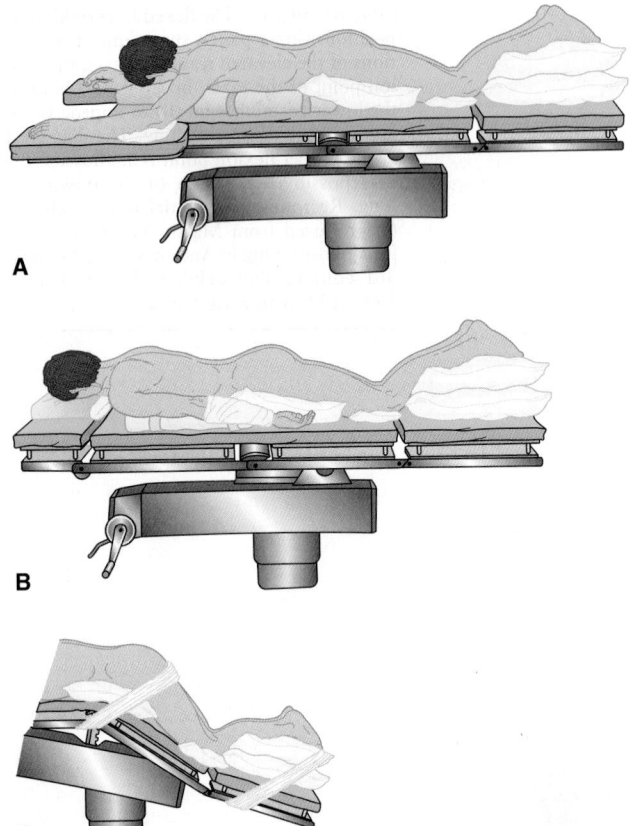

FIGURE 30-17. The classic prone position. **A.** Flat table with relaxed arms extended alongside patient's head. Parallel chest rolls extended from just caudad of clavicle to just beyond inguinal area, with pillow over pelvic end. Elbows and knees are padded, and legs are bent at the knees. Head is turned onto a C-shaped foam sponge that frees the down-side eye and ear from compression. **B.** Same posture with arms snugly retained alongside torso. **C.** Table flexed to reduce lumbar lordosis; subgluteal area straps placed after the legs are lowered to provide cephalad thrust and prevent caudad slippage. (Reproduced from Martin JT, Warner MA [Eds]: Positioning in Anesthesia and Surgery, 3rd edition. Philadelphia, WB Saunders, 1997, p 156, with permission.)

Face rests have fluctuating popularity. Excessive periocular pressure must be considered and avoided if a face rest is used. If the neck is pain-free and its mobility is satisfactory, the head can be turned laterally and supported to prevent pressure on the downside eye and ear. However, forced rotation of the pronated head should be carefully avoided lest it induce postoperative neck pain or cervical nerve root or vascular compression.

When a patient is scheduled to be pronated after induction of anesthesia, it is worthwhile during the preanesthetic interview to obtain and record information about any limitations that may exist in his or her ability to raise the arms overhead during work or sleep. If the patient is symptomatic, it may be prudent to place the arms alongside the torso after pronation (see "Thoracic Outlet Syndrome"). If the arms are placed alongside the head (i.e., extended ventrally at the shoulder, flexed at the elbow, and abducted onto arm boards; the "surrender" position), the musculature about the shoulders should be under no tension, neither humeral head should stretch or compress its axillary neurovascular bundle (i.e., shoulders should be abducted <90 degrees), ulnar nerves at the elbow should be padded, and the pulses at the wrists should remain full. Anterior (forward) flexion of the shoulders may reduce tension on the neurovascular structures of the axilla.

Prone Jackknife

The prone jackknife posture is used to provide access to the sacral, perianal, and perineal areas as well as to the lower alimentary canal (Fig. 30-18). The thighs are flexed on the trunk more than is usual in the full prone position, with the table surface hinges determining the degree of flexion achievable.

Prone Kneeling

Kneeling positions have been used to improve operative conditions in the lumbar and cervicooccipital areas (Fig. 30-19). Numerous frames have been constructed to support the weight of a kneeling patient, and their usefulness again depends on the physique of the patient. If the vertebral column is unstable, kneeling frames are not as useful as parallel longitudinal supports because kneeling risks application of shearing forces at the fracture site, with the potential for damage of the contents of the spinal canal. In massively obese patients who must be operated on in the prone position, kneeling frames tend to prevent pressure on the abdomen more successfully than longitudinal frames. However, prolonged kneeling can be fraught with hazards such as compartment syndrome and soft tissue problems.

Complications of the Ventral Decubitus Positions

Eyes and Ears

The eyes and ears may sustain injury in the prone position. The eyelids should be closed, and each eye should be protected in some manner so that the lids cannot be accidentally separated and the cornea scratched. Instillation of lubrication in the eyes should be considered, although the value of this treatment is

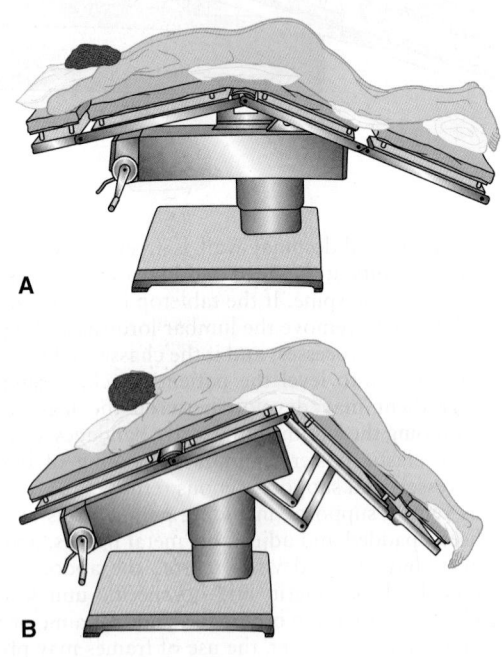

FIGURE 30-18. The prone jackknife positions. **A.** Low jackknife position with the trunk–thigh hinge of the table used as the flexion position and augmented by a pillow under the pelvis. **B.** Full jackknife position with the thigh–leg hinge of the table used as the flexion point to achieve more acute angulation of the hips on the torso. (Reproduced from Martin JT, Warner MA [Eds]: Positioning in Anesthesia and Surgery, 3rd edition. Philadelphia, WB Saunders, 1997, p 163, 164, with permission.)

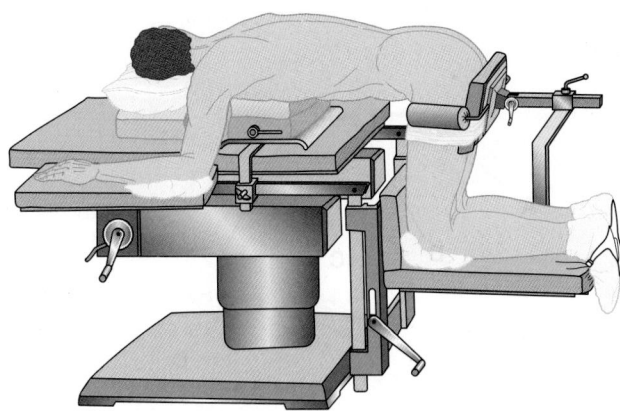

FIGURE 30-19.   The Andrews kneeling frame with Wiltse's thoracic jack in use. (Reproduced from Martin JT, Warner MA [Eds]: Positioning in Anesthesia and Surgery, 3rd edition. Philadelphia, WB Saunders, 1997, p 161, with permission.)

debated. The eyes should also be protected against the head turning after positioning and pressure being exerted on the globe. Monitoring wires and intravenous tubing should be checked after pronation to see that none has migrated beneath the head. If the head is retained in the sagittal plane, the eyes should be checked after positioning to ensure that they are safe from compression by any headrest.

Conjunctival edema usually occurs in the eyes of the pronated patient if the head is at or below the level of the heart. It is usually transient, inconsequential, and requires only re-establishment of the normal tissue perfusion gradients of the supine position, or of a slight amount of head-up tilt, to be redistributed. There does not appear to be any connection between this edema and the occurrence of posterior ischemic optic neuropathy.

❼ Blindness.   Permanent loss of vision can occur after nonocular surgical procedures, especially those performed in a ventral decubitus position.[50] The occurrence of this devastating complication is particularly associated with extensive surgical procedures done in the prone position, such as reconstructive spine surgery, where there is associated blood loss, anemia, and hypotension. Visual loss after neurovascular and cardiopulmonary bypass procedures is well recognized and may be related to embolic events produced by the surgical intervention itself, hypoperfusion, or other nonpositioning causes.[51–54] Visual loss after noncardiac, nonneurovascular procedures may initially be noticed by a loss of acuity, a loss of visual field, or both.

Speculated causes of significant permanent postoperative visual loss usually involve compromise of oxygen delivery to elements of the visual pathway and include ischemic optic neuropathy (anterior or posterior), retinal artery occlusion (central or branch), and cortical blindness.[55] No case series exist to provide information regarding the frequency of these events after nonocular, noncardiac surgery in a general surgical population. Brown et al.[56] identified three patients in whom postoperative ischemic optic neuropathy developed after noncardiac surgery over a 10-year period in one institution. Warner et al.[57] noted that none of nearly 11,000 prone-positioned patients developed perioperative vision loss. However, the institution of these authors subsequently has experienced several patients who have developed complete blindness after spinal surgery performed with patients positioned prone. Reflecting concern about the apparent increased incidence of perioperative blindness, the American Society of Anesthesiologists Committee on Professional Liability has created a formal registry to monitor and document the incidence of this complication.[50]

Positioning appears to be a risk factor for some of these events. A variety of studies noting a relative high frequency of postoperative visual loss in spinal surgery patients have implicated positioning as one causative factor. Use of the knee–chest position, the prone position, and the horseshoe headrest have been cited as potential causes of visual loss, perhaps by direct pressure on the globe increasing the intraocular pressure beyond the perfusion pressure of the retina. Other reports, including those of spinal surgery patients, describe visual loss after prolonged procedures, intraoperative hypotension, and massive blood loss, which may prevent adequate oxygen delivery to the visual apparatus. The American Society of Anesthesiologists Task Force on Perioperative Blindness reviewed studies current through 2005 and published an advisory (Table 30-1).[58]

ANESTHETIC MANAGEMENT

TABLE 30-1

SUMMARY OF PRACTICE ADVISORY FOR PERIOPERATIVE VISUAL LOSS ASSOCIATED WITH SPINE SURGERY

- There is a subset of patients who undergo spine procedures while they are positioned prone and receiving general anesthesia that has an increased risk for development of perioperative visual loss. This subset includes patients who are anticipated preoperatively to undergo procedures that are prolonged, have substantial blood loss, or both (high-risk patients).
- Consider informing high-risk patients that there is a small, unpredictable risk of perioperative visual loss.
- The use of deliberate hypotensive techniques during spine surgery has not been shown to be associated with the development of perioperative visual loss.
- Colloids should be used along with crystalloids to maintain intravascular volume in patients who have substantial blood loss.
- At this time, there is no apparent transfusion threshold that would eliminate the risk of perioperative visual loss related to anemia.
- High-risk patients should be positioned so that their heads are level with or higher than the heart when possible. In addition, their heads should be maintained in a neutral forward position (e.g., without significant neck flexion, extension, lateral flexion, or rotation) when possible.
- Consideration should be given to the use of staged spine procedures in high-risk patients.

Reproduced from American Society of Anesthesiologists Task Force on Perioperative Blindness. Anesthesiology 2006; 104: 1319, with permission.

FIGURE 30-20. Sources of potential injury to the brachial plexus and its peripheral components when the patient is in the prone position. **A.** Neck rotation, stretching roots of the plexus. **B.** Compression of the plexus and vessels between the clavicle and first rib. **C.** Injury to the axillary neurovascular bundle from the head of the humerus. **D.** Compression of the ulnar nerve before, beyond, and within the cubital tunnel. **E.** Area of vulnerability of the radial nerve to lateral compression proximal to the elbow. (Reproduced from Martin JT, Warner MA [Eds]: Positioning in Anesthesia and Surgery, 3rd edition. Philadelphia, WB Saunders, 1997, p 185, with permission.)

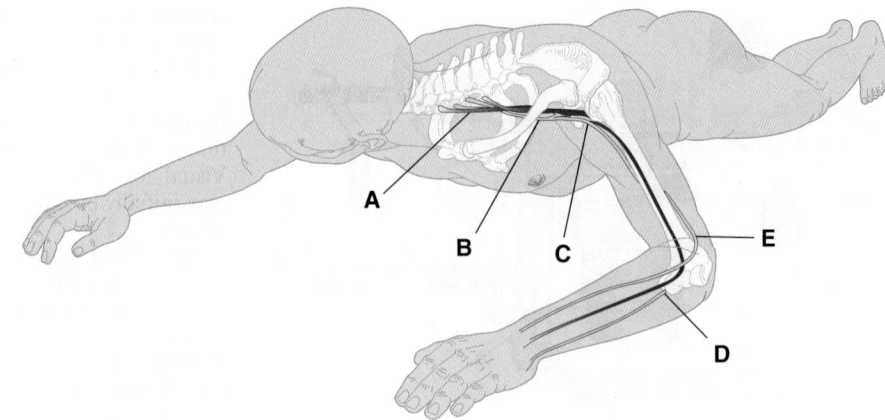

Neck Problems

Anesthesia impairs reflex muscle spasm that protects the skeleton against motion that would be painful if the patient were alert. Lateral rotation of the head and neck of an anesthetized, pronated patient, particularly one with an arthritic cervical spine, can stretch relaxed skeletal muscles and ligaments and injure articulations of cervical vertebrae. Postoperative neck pain and limitation of motion can result. The arthritic neck is usually best managed by keeping the head in the sagittal plane when the patient is prone.

Extremes of head and neck rotation can also interfere with flow in either the ipsilateral or contralateral vessels to and from the head. Excessive head rotation can reduce flow in both the carotid[59] and vertebral systems.[60] Impaired cerebral perfusion is the obvious consequence.

Brachial Plexus Injuries

Stretch injuries to the roots of the brachial plexus (Fig. 30-20A) on the side contralateral to the turned face are possible if the contralateral shoulder is held firmly caudad by a wrist restraint. If an arm is placed on an arm board alongside the head, care must be taken to ensure that the head of the humerus is not stretching and compressing the axillary neurovascular bundle (Fig. 30-20B,C).

When an arm is placed on an arm board alongside the head, the forearm naturally pronates. As a result, the ulnar nerve, lying in the cubital tunnel (the groove between the olecranon process and the medial epicondyle of the humerus), is vulnerable to being compressed by the weight of the elbow (Fig. 30-20D). Consequently, the medial aspect of the elbow must be well padded and its weight borne across a large area to avoid point pressure.

Asking patients about their ability to work or sleep with arms elevated overhead may identify patients with *thoracic outlet obstruction*. A useful preoperative test if the history is in question is to have the patient clasp hands behind the occiput during the interview (Fig. 30-21). If the patient describes dysesthesias, it may be prudent to keep the arms alongside the trunk in the prone position. Agonizing, debilitating, and unremitting postoperative pain has been known to follow overhead arm placement in pronated patients who have had prior discomfort in their arms in that position.

Breast Injuries

The breasts of a pronated woman, if forced laterally by ventral chest supports, can be stretched and injured along their sternal borders. Medial and cephalad displacement seems better tolerated. Direct pressure on breasts (particularly if breast prosthe-

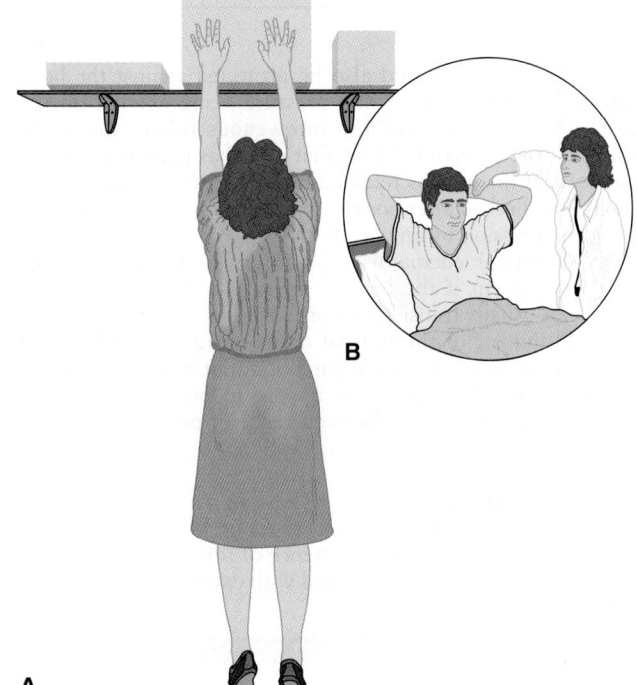

FIGURE 30-21. Assessment of a potential thoracic outlet syndrome. **A.** This patient has a history of distress when trying to work or sleep with arms over head. **B.** Interview carried out with this patient's hands clasped on occiput and radial pulses checked for damping. (Reproduced from McLeskey CH [Ed]: Geriatric Anesthesiology. Baltimore, Williams & Wilkins, 1997, p 186, with permission.)

ses are present) can cause ischemia to breast tissue and should be avoided.

Abdominal Compression

Compression of the abdomen by the weight of the prone patient's trunk can cause viscera to force the diaphragm cephalad enough to impair ventilation. If intra-abdominal pressure approaches or exceeds venous pressure, return of blood from the pelvis and lower extremities is reduced or obstructed. Because the vertebral venous plexuses communicate directly with the abdominal veins, increased intra-abdominal pressure is transmitted to the perivertebral and intraspinal surgical field in the form of venous distention and increased difficulty with

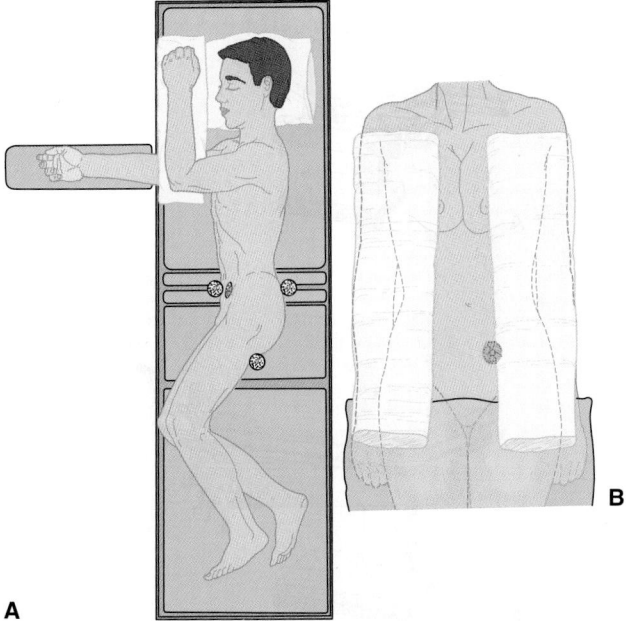

FIGURE 30-22. Postural supports compromising visceral stoma. Both the vertical abdominal support of a device designed to maintain a patient in the lateral position (**A**) and the longitudinal chest rolls supporting a pronated patient (**B**) can cause ischemic compression of a viscerocutaneous anastomosis and subsequent necrosis. Surgical repair of the stoma may be needed. (Modified from McLeskey CH [Ed]: Geriatric Anesthesiology. Baltimore, Williams & Wilkins, 1997, p 340, with permission.)

hemostasis. All of the various supportive pads and frames, when properly used, are designed to remove pressure from the abdomen and avoid these problems.

Viscerocutaneous Stomata

Stomata that drain visceral contents into containers affixed to the abdominal wall are at risk in the prone position if they lie against a part of the ventral supporting frame or pad (Fig. 30-22). Compressive ischemia of the stomal orifice can cause it to slough.

HEAD-ELEVATED POSITIONS

Variations of the Head-Elevated Positions

Sitting

The classic *sitting position* for surgery places the patient in a semireclining posture on an operating table, with the legs elevated to approximately the level of the heart and the head flexed ventrally on the neck (Fig. 30-23). Head flexion should not be sufficient to force the chin into the suprasternal notch (see "Midcervical Tetraplegia"). Elastic stockings or compressive wraps around the legs reduce pooling of blood in the lower extremities. The head often is held in place by some type of a face rest or by a three-pin skull fixation frame.

Supine—Tilted Head Up

A dorsal recumbent position with the head of the patient elevated is used for many operations involving the ventral and

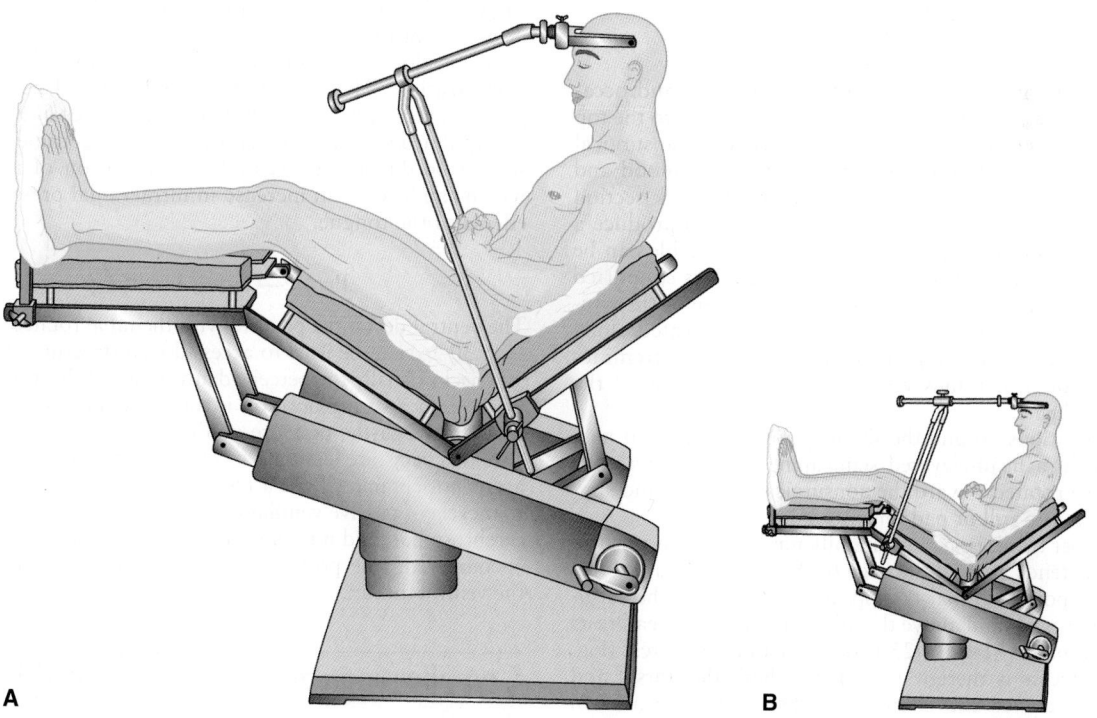

FIGURE 30-23. **A.** Conventional neurosurgical sitting position. The legs are at approximately the level of the heart and gently flexed on the thighs; the feet are supported at right angles to the legs; subgluteal padding protects the sciatic nerve. The frame of the head holder is *properly* clamped to the side rails of the back section in the event of hemodynamically significant air embolism. **B.** *Improper* attachment of the head frame to the table side rails at the thigh section. In this position, the patient's head could not be quickly lowered because it would require disengaging the skull clamp. (Reproduced from Martin JT, Warner MA [Eds]: Positioning in Anesthesia and Surgery, 3rd edition. Philadelphia, WB Saunders, 1997, p 72, with permission.)

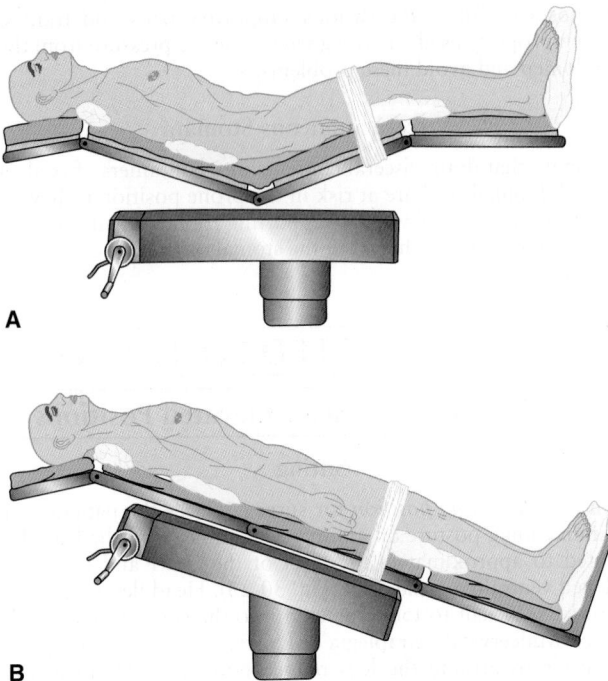

FIGURE 30-24. Head-elevated positions often used for operations about the ventral and ventrolateral aspects of the head, face, neck, and cervical spine. **A.** The legs are at approximately heart level and the gradient into the head is appreciable but slight. **B.** The flat table and foot rest are useful when a thyroidectomy is planned under regional anesthesia. (Reproduced from Martin JT, Warner MA [Eds]: Positioning in Anesthesia and Surgery, 3rd edition. Philadelphia, WB Saunders, 1997, p 89, with permission.)

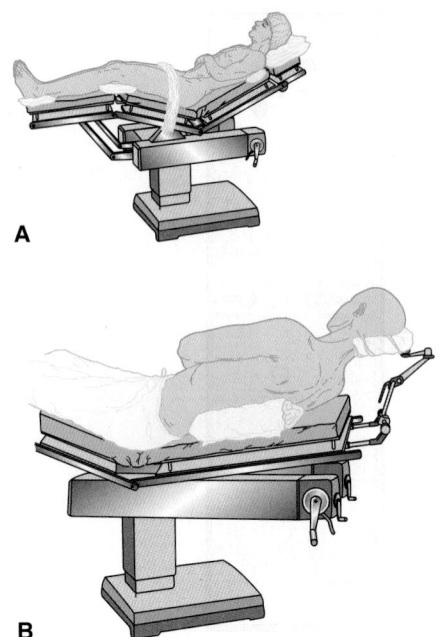

FIGURE 30-25. **A.** The barber chair position for surgery around the shoulder joint. **B.** The upper torso is rotated toward the nonsurgical shoulder and supported with a firm roll or pad.

lateral aspects of the head (Fig. 30-24) and neck, and occasionally with the neck flexed, for transcranial access to the top of the brain. Its purpose is to improve access to the surgical target for the operating team as well as to drain blood and irrigation solutions away from the wound. The back section of the surgical table can be elevated as needed to produce a low sitting position (Fig. 30-24A), or the entire table can be rotated head-high with the patient's extended legs supported by a foot rest (Fig. 30-24B). Although the degree of tilt typically is not great, small pressure gradients are created along the vascular axis that can pool blood in the lower extremities or entrain air in patulous vessels that are incised above the level of the heart.

For operations around the shoulder joint, the patient may be placed in a head-elevated semisupine position, with the upper torso rotated toward the nonsurgical shoulder and supported by a firm roll or pad (Fig. 30-25).

The upper trunk is moved laterally until the raised surgical shoulder extends beyond the edge of the operating table. The torso is supported so that the hips are on the table, the surgical shoulder is off and above the table edge, and the head rests on either a pillow (Fig. 30-25A) or a horseshoe headrest (Fig. 30-25B). Access is thereby provided to both the dorsal and ventral aspects of the shoulder girdle. The surgical arm remains on the ventral torso and is prepared and draped to be mobile in the surgical field.

Lateral—Tilted Head Up

The lateral decubitus position with the head somewhat elevated, a means of access to occipitocervical lesions, has also been referred to as the *park bench position*. All the stabilizing requirements needed for the usual lateral decubitus position

apply. The head may be held firmly in a three-pin skull fixation holder, which can be readjusted as needed during surgery, or supported by pillows or padding. Although the degree of head elevation used typically is <15 degrees, the position does not completely remove the threat of air embolization. The anesthesiologist has good access to the patient's face and ventral thorax for purposes of monitoring, manipulation, and resuscitation. Considerable attention should be directed to avoiding compression of neck veins, which can lead to an increase in intracranial pressure and to edema of the tongue.

Prone—Tilted Head Up

The ventral decubitus posture with the table rotated head high (Fig. 30-26) can be used to access dorsal structures of the head and neck. Usually the perceived advantage of this position compared with a sitting position is the avoidance of air embolization. Although the pressure gradients for air entrainment into patulous veins are less than in the full sitting position, the hazard is not eliminated. As a result of the positive-pressure inflation cycle of passive ventilation, a bothersome recurrent flux of cerebrospinal fluid into and out of the exposed wound may be encountered. The posture also restricts resuscitative access to the ventral thorax.

Complications of the Head-Elevated Positions

Postural Hypotension

In the anesthetized patient, establishing any of the head-elevated positions is frequently accompanied by some degree of reduction in systemic blood pressure. The normal protective reflexes are inhibited by drugs used during anesthesia. Measuring mean arterial pressures at the level of the circle of Willis is recommended to assess cerebral perfusion pressures more accurately.

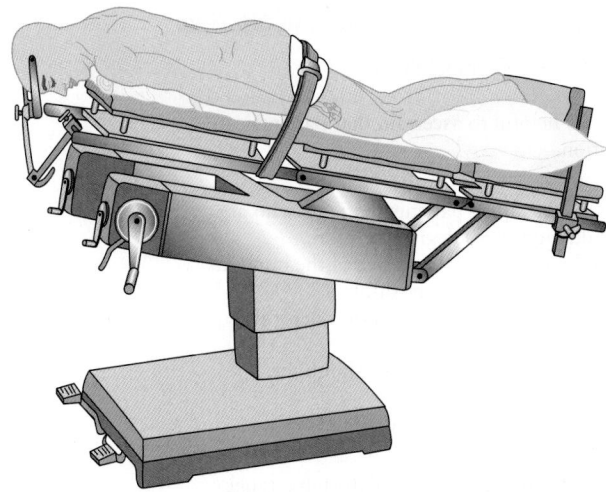

FIGURE 30-26.   The skull-pin headrest used to stabilize a patient in the head-elevated prone position. Note the chest rolls used to free the abdomen from compression and the gluteal strap to minimize caudad slippage after head-up tilt. (Reproduced from Martin JT, Warner MA [Eds]: Positioning in Anesthesia and Surgery, 3rd edition. Philadelphia, WB Saunders, 1997, p 88, with permission.)

Air Embolus

Air embolization is potentially lethal (see also Chapter 39). In the bloodstream, air migrates to the heart, where it creates a compressible foam that destroys the propulsive efficiency of ventricular contraction and irritates the conduction system. Air can also move into the pulmonary vasculature, where bubbles obstruct small vessels and compromise gas exchange, or it can cross through a patent foramen ovale to the left side of the heart and the systemic circulation.

The potential for venous air embolization increases with the degree of elevation of the operative site above the heart. Although the occurrence of air emboli is a relatively frequent phenomenon in head-elevated positions, most of the emboli are small in volume, clinically silent, and recognizable only by sophisticated Doppler detection techniques. Nevertheless, the potential for dangerous accumulations of entrained air requires immediate detection of the embolization, a careful search for its portal of entry, and prompt treatment of its clinical effects.

Pneumocephalus

In the usual craniotomy, most of the brain lies subjacent to the incision. After the dura is incised, cerebrospinal fluid is removed to improve working conditions, and the surgical field is open to the air. During closure of the craniotomy, most of the intracranial air escapes from the wound and any residual pneumocephalus is of little consequence. However, when an incision is made through the dura in the posterior fossa or cervical spine of a seated patient, the bulk of the brain lies above the incision. Cerebrospinal fluid drains downward out of the wound, and tissue retraction can allow air to bubble up over the surfaces of the brain to become trapped in the upper reaches of the cranium.[61] When brain mass is decreased by ventricular drainage, steroids, and diuresis, the space available to a pneumocephalus is enlarged. Diffusion of nitrous oxide into the accumulated air, or the warming of trapped gas, can produce a tension pneumocephalus with signs of increased intracranial pressure and delayed awakening from anesthesia.

Toung et al.[62] found postoperative pneumocephalus in all of a group of seated patients and in most of those who had been in the prone or the park bench position. Intraventricular air was present in most of the seated patients and was rare in those in the other positions. None of their group of 100 patients had neurologic changes attributable to the trapped intracranial air. Standefer et al.[63] reported a 3% incidence of symptomatic (tension) pneumocephalus in seated, anesthetized patients whose duras were opened.

Ocular Compression

Pressure from a padded headrest on the eyes of a patient who has been placed in a head-elevated position can dislocate a crystalline lens or render the globe ischemic. Modern skull-pin head clamps that grip firmly when properly applied have made ocular compression in the sitting position a rarity. In the head-elevated lateral decubitus or prone position, the threats to the eyes are those described in the preceding discussions of those nonelevated postures.

Edema of the Face, Tongue, and Neck

Severe postoperative macroglossia, apparently because of venous and lymphatic obstruction, can be caused by prolonged, marked neck flexion.[64] Postoperative need for a tracheostomy has been reported.[65] Try to avoid placing the patient's chin firmly against the chest and use an oral airway to protect the endotracheal tube. Extremes of neck flexion, with or without head rotation, have been widely used to gain access to structures in the posterior fossa and cervical spine, but their potential for damage should be understood and excessive flexion–rotation avoided if possible. Moore and associates[66] have suggested that the primary mechanism may be neurologically determined rather than being the result of either vascular obstruction or local trauma. This problem also has been described with the use of transesophageal echocardiography probes.

Midcervical Tetraplegia

This devastating injury occurs after hyperflexion of the neck, with or without rotation of the head, and is attributed to stretching of the spinal cord with resulting compromise of its vasculature in the midcervical area. An element of spondylosis or a spondylotic bar may be involved.[67,68] The result is paralysis below the general level of the fifth cervical vertebra. Although most reports in the literature have described the condition as occurring after the use of the sitting position, midcervical tetraplegia has also occurred after prolonged, nonforced head flexion for intracranial surgery in the supine position.

Sciatic Nerve

Stretch injuries of the sciatic nerve can occur in some seated patients if the hips are markedly flexed without bending the knees. Prolonged compression of the sciatic nerve as it emerges from the pelvis is possible in a thin, seated patient if the buttocks are not suitably padded. Foot drop may be the result of injuries to either the sciatic nerve or the common peroneal nerve and can be bilateral.

PERIOPERATIVE PERIPHERAL NEUROPATHIES

Prevention

The American Society of Anesthesiologists approved an advisory on peripheral neuropathies in 1999.[69] This advisory includes pertinent literature and a summary of the opinions of anesthesia providers on a variety of positioning and peripheral neuropathy issues. The paucity of literature related to these issues limited the advisory to recommendations based on opinions and current

TABLE 30-2

SUMMARY OF PERIOPERATIVE NEUROPATHY TASK FORCE CONSENSUS

Preoperative assessment: When judged appropriate, it is helpful to ascertain that patients can comfortably tolerate the anticipated operative position.

Upper Extremity Positioning
- Arm abduction should be limited to 90 degrees or less in supine patients. Patients who are positioned prone may comfortably tolerate arm abduction of 90 degrees or more.
- Arms should be positioned to decrease pressure on the postcondylar groove of the humerus (ulnar groove). When arms are tucked at the side, a neutral forearm position is recommended. When arms are abducted on arm boards, either supination or a neutral forearm position is acceptable.
- Prolonged pressure on the radial nerve in the spiral groove of the humerus should be avoided.
- Extension of the elbow beyond a comfortable range may stretch the median nerve.

Lower Extremity Positioning
- Lithotomy positions that stretch the hamstring muscle group beyond a comfortable range may stretch the sciatic nerve.
- Prolonged pressure on the peroneal nerve at the fibular head should be avoided.
- Neither extension nor flexion of the hip increases the risk of femoral neuropathy.

Protective Padding
- Padded arm boards may decrease the risk of upper extremity neuropathy.
- The use of chest rolls in laterally positioned patients may decrease the risk of upper extremity neuropathies.
- Padding at the elbow and at the fibular head may decrease the risk of upper and lower extremity neuropathies, respectively.

Equipment
- Properly functioning automated blood pressure cuffs on the upper arms do not affect the risk of upper extremity neuropathies.
- Shoulder braces in steep head-down positions may increase the risk of brachial plexus neuropathies.

Postoperative Assessment: A simple postoperative assessment of extremity nerve function may lead to early recognition of peripheral neuropathies.

Documentation: Charting specific positioning actions during the care of patients may result in improvements of care by (1) helping practitioners focus attention on relevant aspects of patient positioning and (2) providing information that continuous improvement processes can use to lead to refinements in patient care.

Reproduced from American Society of Anesthesiologists Task Force on Prevention of Perioperative Peripheral Neuropathies: Practice advisory for the prevention of perioperative peripheral neuropathies. Anesthesiology 2000; 92: 1168, with permission.

practices of a broadly representative group of anesthesia providers from around the United States. Additional input and opinions were obtained from consultants from around the world. A summary of the findings of the advisory is shown in Table 30-2.

Practical Considerations

Efforts to prevent perioperative neuropathies are frequently debated, and there often is confusion over how to manage a neuropathy once it has occurred. In general, there are no data to support recommendations on any of these issues. Therefore, the following opinions have been formulated by personal experience, guided by advice from neurologists who care primarily for patients with peripheral neuropathies, and seasoned or supported by speculation derived from anecdotal case reports.

Padding Exposed Peripheral Nerves

Many types of padding materials are advocated to protect exposed peripheral nerves. They often consist of cloth (e.g., blankets and towels), foam sponges (e.g., "eggcrate" foam), and gel pads. There are no data to suggest that any of these materials is more effective than any other, or that any is better than no padding at all. A good rule of thumb would be to position and pad exposed peripheral nerves to (1) prevent their stretch beyond normally tolerated limits while awake; (2) avoid their direct compression, if possible; and (3) distribute over as large an area as possible any compressive forces that must be placed on them.

Prolonged Duration in One Position

Prolonged duration in one position appears to increase the risk of neuropathy and other integumentary damage. For example, prolonged duration in lithotomy positions greatly increases the risk of lower extremity neuropathy.[70,71] When possible, it would appear prudent to limit as much as practical the time any patient spends in one position. However, intermittent movement of the limbs or head during the intraoperative period may increase the opportunity for a number of different problems, including but not limited to dislodging an endotracheal tube, abrading a cornea, or moving an extremity into a suboptimal position. Practitioners must judge the benefits versus risks of any intraoperative changes in a patient's position.

Course of Action for the Patient with a Neuropathy

8 Although each situation is unique and requires careful assessment, the following guidelines may suggest a basic course of action that will lead to appropriate care[72]:

- Is the neuropathy sensory or motor? Sensory lesions are more frequently transient than motor lesions. If the symptoms are numbness or tingling only, it may be appropriate to inform the patient that many of these neuropathies can be expected to resolve during the first 5 days.[27] The patient should be instructed to avoid postures that might compress or stretch the involved nerve. Arrangements should be made for frequent contact with the patient. A call to alert a neurologist is appropriate, and if the symptoms still persist on postoperative day 5, the neurologist should be consulted.

- If the neuropathy has a motor component, a neurologist should be consulted immediately. Electromyographic studies may be needed to assess the location of any acute lesion. This knowledge may direct an appropriate treatment plan. The studies may also demonstrate chronic abnormalities of the nerve or, if applicable, the contralateral nerve.

References

1. Martin JT, Warner MA (Eds): Positioning in Anesthesia and Surgery, 3rd edition. Philadelphia, WB Saunders, 1997
2. Warner MA: Supine positions, Positioning in Anesthesia and Surgery, 3rd edition. Edited by Martin JT, Warner MA. Philadelphia, WB Saunders, 1997, p 39
3. Smith BE: Obstetrics, Positioning in Anesthesia and Surgery, 3rd edition. Edited by Martin JT, Warner MA. Philadelphia, WB Saunders, 1997, p 267
4. Litwiller JP, Wells RE, Halliwill JR et al: Effect of lithotomy positions on strain of the obturator and lateral femoral cutaneous nerves. Clin Anat 2004; 17: 45
5. Martin JT: 1992—Compartment syndromes: Concepts and perspectives for the anesthesiologist. Anesth Analg 1992; 75: 275
6. Angermeier KW, Jordan GH: Complications of the exaggerated lithotomy position: A review of 177 cases. J Urol 1994; 151: 866
7. Halliwill JR, Hewitt SA, Joyner MJ et al: Effects of various lithotomy positions on lower extremity blood pressures. Anesthesiology 1999; 89: 1373
8. Pfeffer SD, Halliwill JR, Warner MA: Effects of lithotomy position and external compression on lower leg muscle compartment pressure. Anesthesiology 2001; 95: 632
9. Abel RR, Lewis GM: Postoperative alopecia. Arch Dermatol 1960; 81: 72
10. Gormley T, Sokoll MD: Permanent alopecia from pressure of a headstrap. JAMA 1967; 199: 157
11. Lawson NW, Mills NL, Ochsner JL: Occipital alopecia following cardiopulmonary bypass. J Thorac Cardiovasc Surg 1976; 71: 342
12. Jellish WS, Blakeman B, Warf P, Slogoff S: Hands-up positioning during asymmetric sternal retraction for internal mammary artery harvest: A possible method to reduce brachial plexus injury. Anesth Analg 1997; 84: 260
13. Vander Salm TJ, Cereda J-M, Cutler BS: Brachial plexus injury following median sternotomy. J Thorac Cardiovasc Surg 1980; 80: 447
14. Vander Salm TJ, Cutler BS, Okike ON: Brachial plexus injury following median sternotomy: Part II. J Thorac Cardiovasc Surg 1982; 83: 914
15. Roy RC, Stafford MA, Charlton JE: Nerve injury and musculoskeletal complaints after cardiac surgery: Influence of internal mammary artery dissection and left arm position. Anesth Analg 1988; 67: 277
16. Gregg JR, Labosky D, Harty M et al: Serratus anterior paralysis in the young athlete. J Bone Joint Surg Am 1979; 61: 825
17. Foo CL, Swann M: Isolated paralysis of the serratus anterior. J Bone Joint Surg Br 1983; 65: 552
18. Martin JT: Postoperative isolated dysfunction of the long thoracic nerve: A rare entity of uncertain etiology. Anesth Analg 1989; 69: 614
19. Kroll DA, Caplan RA, Posner K et al: Nerve injury associated with anesthesia. Anesthesiology 1990; 73: 202
20. Cheney FW, Domino KB, Caplan RA et al: Nerve injury associated with anesthesia. Anesthesiology 1999; 90: 1062
21. Büdinger K: Ueber Lähmungen nach Chloroform-Narkosen. Archiv für Klinische Chiruque 1894; 47: 121
22. Garriques HJ: Anaesthesia-paralysis. Am J Med Sci 1897; 133: 81
23. Wadsworth TG, Williams JR: Cubital tunnel external compression syndrome. BMJ 1973; 1: 662
24. Warner MA, Warner DO, Harper CM et al: Ulnar neuropathy in medical patients. Anesthesiology 2000; 92: 613
25. Warner MA, Warner ME, Martin JT: Ulnar neuropathy: Incidence, outcome, and risk factors in sedated or anesthetized patients. Anesthesiology 1994; 81: 1332
26. Alvine FG, Schurrer ME: Postoperative ulnar-nerve palsy: Are there predisposing factors? J Bone Joint Surg Am 1987; 69: 255
27. Warner MA, Warner DO, Matsumoto JY et al: Ulnar neuropathy in surgical patients. Anesthesiology 1999; 90: 54
28. Prielipp RC, Morell RC, Walker FO et al: Ulnar nerve pressure: Influence of arm position and relationship to somatosensory evoked potentials. Anesthesiology 1999; 91: 345
29. Campbell WW, Pridgeon RM, Riaz G et al: Variations in anatomy of the ulnar nerve at the cubital tunnel: Pitfalls in the diagnosis of ulnar neuropathy at the elbow. Muscle Nerve 1991; 14: 733
30. O'Driscoll SW, Horii E, Carmichael SW et al: The cubital tunnel and ulnar neuropathy. J Bone Joint Surg Am 1991; 73: 613
31. Childress HM: Recurrent ulnar nerve dislocation at the elbow. J Bone Joint Surg 1956; 38: 978
32. Ashenhurst EM: Anatomical factors in the etiology of ulnar neuropathy. CMAJ 1962; 87: 159
33. Macnicol MF: Extraneural pressures affecting the ulnar nerve at the elbow. Hand 1982; 14: 5
34. Morell RC, Prielipp RC, Harwood TN et al: Men are more susceptible than women to direct pressure on unmyelinated ulnar nerve fibers. Anesth Analg 2003; 97: 1183
35. Pechan J, Julis I: The pressure measurement in the ulnar nerve: A contribution to the pathophysiology of the cubital tunnel syndrome. J Biomech 1975; 8: 75
36. Contreras MG, Warner MA, Charboneau WJ et al: The anatomy of the ulnar nerve at the elbow: Potential relationship of acute ulnar neuropathy to gender differences. Clin Anat 1998; 11: 372
37. Shimokata H, Tobin JD, Muller DC et al: Studies in the distribution of body fat: I. Effects of age, sex, and obesity. J Gerontol 1989; 44: 66
38. Hattori K, Numata N, Ikoma M et al: Sex differences in the distribution of subcutaneous and internal fat. Hum Biol 1991; 63: 53
39. Chusid JG: Correlative Neuroanatomy and Functional Neurology. Los Altos, CA, Lange Medical Publications, 1985, p 149
40. Hill NA, Howard FM, Huffer BR: The incomplete anterior interosseous nerve syndrome. J Hand Surg [Am] 1985; 10: 4
41. Kies SJ, Danielson DR, Dennison DJ et al: Perioperative compartment syndrome of the hand. Anesthesiology 2004; 101:1232
42. Contreras MG, Warner MA, Carmichael SW et al: Perioperative anterior interosseous neuropathy. Anesthesiology 2002; 96: 243
43. Amoiridis G, Wöhrle JC, Langkafel M et al: Spinal cord infarction after surgery in a patient in the hyperlordotic position. Anesthesiology 1996; 84: 228
44. Hofmann A, Jones RE, Schoenvogel R: Pudendal nerve neuropraxia as a result of traction on the fracture table. J Bone Joint Surg Am 1982; 64: 136
45. Lindenbaum SD, Fleming LL, Smith DW: Pudendal nerve palsies associated with closed intramedullary femoral fixation. J Bone Joint Surg Am 1982; 64: 934
46. Warner ME, LaMaster LM, Thoeming AK et al: Compartment syndrome in surgical patients. Anesthesiology 2001; 94: 705
47. Courington FW, Little DM Jr: The role of posture in anesthesia. Clin Anesth 1968; 3: 24
48. Lawson NW, Meyer DJ Jr: The lateral decubitus position: Anesthesiologic considerations, Positioning in Anesthesia and Surgery, 3rd edition. Edited by Martin JT, Warner MA. Philadelphia, WB Saunders, 1997, p 127
49. Edgcombe H, Carter K, Yarrow S: Anaesthesia in the prone position. Br J Anaesth 2008; 100: 165
50. Lee LA, Roth S, Posner KL et al: The American Society of Anesthesiologists Postoperative Visual Loss Registry. Anesthesiology 2006; 105: 652
51. Sweeny PJ, Breuer AC, Selshorst JB et al: Ischemic optic neuropathy: A complication of cardiopulmonary bypass surgery. Neurology 1982; 32: 560
52. Shaw PJ, Bates D, Cartlidge NEF et al: Neurologic and neuropsychologic morbidity following major surgery: Comparison of coronary artery bypass and peripheral vascular surgery. Stroke 1987; 18: 700
53. Shapira OM, Kimmel WA, Lindsey PS et al: Anterior ischemic optic neuropathy after open heart operations. Ann Thorac Surg 1996; 61: 660
54. Nuttall GA, Garrity JA, Dearani JA et al: Risk factors for ischemic optic neuropathy after cardiopulmonary bypass: A matched case/control study. Anesth Analg 2001; 93: 1410
55. Roth S, Gillesberg I: Injuries to the visual system and other sense organs, Anesthesia and Perioperative Complications, 2nd edition. Edited by Benumof JL, Saidman LJ. St. Louis, Mosby, 1999
56. Brown RH, Schauble JF, Miller NR: Anemia and hypotension as contributors to perioperative vision loss. Anesthesiology 1994; 80: 222
57. Warner ME, Warner MA, Garrity JA et al: The frequency of perioperative vision loss. Anesth Analg 2001; 93: 1417

58. American Society of Anesthesiologists Task Force on Perioperative Blindness. Anesthesiology 2006; 104: 1319

59. Sherman DD, Hart RG, Easton JD: Abrupt change in head position and cerebral infarction. Stroke 1981; 12: 2

60. Toole JF: Effects of change of head, limb and body position on cephalic circulation. N Engl J Med 1968; 279: 307

61. Kitahata LM, Katz JD: Tension pneumocephalus after posterior fossa craniotomy, a complication of the sitting position. Anesthesiology 1976; 44: 448

62. Toung TKJ, McPherson RW, Ahn H: Pneumocephalus: Effects of patient position on incidence of aerocele after posterior fossa and upper cervical cord surgery. Anesth Analg 1986; 65: 65

63. Standefer M, Bay JW, Trusso R: The sitting position in neurosurgery: A retrospective analysis of 488 cases. Neurosurgery 1984; 14: 649

64. McAllister RG: Macroglossia: A positional complication. Anesthesiology 1974; 40: 199

65. Ellis SC, Bryan-Brown CW, Hyderally H: Massive swelling of the head and neck. Anesthesiology 1975; 42: 102

66. Moore JK, Chaudhri S, Moore AP, Easton J: Macroglossia and posterior fossa disease. Anaesthesia 1988; 43: 382

67. Hitselberger WE, House WF: A warning regarding the sitting position for acoustic tumor surgery. Arch Otolaryng 1980; 106: 69

68. Wilder BL: Hypothesis: The etiology of midcervical quadriplegia after operation with the patient in the sitting position. Neurosurgery 1982; 11: 530

69. American Society of Anesthesiologists Task Force on Prevention of Perioperative Peripheral Neuropathies: Practice advisory for the prevention of perioperative peripheral neuropathies. Anesthesiology 2000; 92: 1168

70. Warner MA, Martin JT, Schroeder DR et al: Lower extremity motor neuropathy associated with surgery performed on patients in a lithotomy position. Anesthesiology 1994; 81: 6

71. Warner MA, Warner DO, Harper CM et al: Lower extremity neuropathies associated with the lithotomy position. Anesthesiology 2000; 93: 938

72. Warner MA: Perioperative neuropathies. Mayo Clin Proc 1998; 73: 567

CHAPTER 31 ■ MONITORED ANESTHESIA CARE

SIMON C. HILLIER AND MICHAEL S. MAZUREK

KEY POINTS

1 The standards for preoperative evaluation, intraoperative monitoring, and the continuous presence of a member of the anesthesia care team, and so forth, are no different from those for general or regional anesthesia.[3]

2 If the level of sedation is deepened to the extent that verbal communication is lost, most of the advantages of monitored anesthesia care are lost and the risks of the technique approach those of general anesthesia with an unprotected and uncontrolled airway.

3 As a general principle, to avoid excessive levels of sedation, drugs should be titrated in small increments or by adjustable infusions rather than administered in larger doses according to predetermined notions of efficacy.

4 The context-sensitive half-time describes the time required for the plasma drug concentration to decline by 50% after terminating an infusion of a particular duration.

5 At the present time, no one inhaled or intravenous drug can provide all the components of monitored anesthesia care (i.e., analgesia, anxiolysis, and hypnosis) with an acceptable margin of safety or ease of titratability.

6 During monitored anesthesia care, the maximum benefit of opioid supplementation, in terms of potentiation of other administered sedatives, will accrue when the opioid is used in the analgesic dose range. Within this dose range there is great potential for adverse cardiorespiratory interaction.

7 The important mechanisms whereby respiratory function may be compromised during monitored anesthesia care include the effects of sedatives and opioids on respiratory drive, upper airway patency, and protective airway reflexes.

8 If anesthesiologists are not willing or able to provide these services, others, who are less well qualified, are prepared to assume that role.

During monitored anesthesia care the continuous attention of the anesthesiologist is directed at optimizing patient comfort and safety. Monitored anesthesia care usually involves the administration of drugs with anxiolytic, hypnotic, analgesic, and amnestic properties, either alone or as a supplement to a local or regional technique.

TERMINOLOGY

It is important to distinguish between "monitored anesthesia care" and "sedation/analgesia." In October 2004, the American Society of Anesthesiologists (ASA) House of Delegates approved a statement entitled "Distinguishing Monitored Anesthesia Care from Moderate Sedation/Analgesia."[1] *Sedation/ analgesia* is the term currently used by the ASA in their recently published *Practice Guidelines for Sedation and Analgesia by Non-Anesthesiologists.*[2] *Monitored anesthesia care* implies the potential for a deeper level of sedation than that provided by sedation/analgesia and is always administered by an anesthesiologist provider. **1** The standards for preoperative evaluation, intraoperative monitoring, and the continuous presence of a member of the anesthesia care team, and so forth, are no different from those for general or regional anesthesia.[3]

Conceptually, monitored anesthesia care is attractive because it should invoke less physiologic disturbance and allow a more rapid recovery than general anesthesia. It is instructive to review the ASA position statement that defines monitored anesthesia care as follows[3]:

> *Monitored anesthesia care is a specific anesthesia service for a diagnostic or therapeutic procedure. Indications for monitored anesthesia care include the nature of the procedure, the patient's clinical condition, and/or the potential need to convert to a general or regional anesthetic.*
>
> *Monitored anesthesia care includes all aspects of anesthesia care—a preprocedure visit, intraprocedure care, and postprocedure anesthesia management. During monitored anesthesia care, the anesthesiologist provides or medically directs a number of specific services, including but not limited to:*
>
> *Diagnosis and treatment of clinical problems that occur during the procedure*
> *Support of vital functions*
> *Administration of sedatives, analgesics, hypnotics, anesthetic agents, or other medications as necessary for patient safety*
> *Psychological support and physical comfort*
> *Provision of other medical services as needed to complete the procedure safely.*
>
> *Monitored anesthesia care may include varying levels of sedation, analgesia, and anxiolysis as necessary. The provider of monitored anesthesia care must be prepared and qualified to convert to general anesthesia when necessary. If the patient loses consciousness and the ability to respond purposefully, the anesthesia care is a general anesthetic, irrespective of whether airway instrumentation is required.*
>
> *Monitored anesthesia care is a physician service provided to an individual patient. It should be subject to the same level of payment as general or regional anesthesia. Accordingly, the ASA Relative Value Guide provides for the use of proper base procedural units, time units, and modifier units as the basis for determining reimbursement.*

The ASA also states that monitored anesthesia care should be requested by the attending physician and be made known to the patient, in accordance with accepted procedures of the institution. In addition, the ASA states that the service must include the following:

1. Performance of a preanesthetic examination and evaluation.
2. Prescription of anesthetic care.
3. Personal participation in, or medical direction of, the entire plan of care.
4. Continuous physical presence of the anesthesiologist or, in the case of medical direction, of the resident or nurse anesthetist being medically directed.
5. Proximate presence, or in the case of medical direction, availability of the anesthesiologist for diagnosis and treatment of emergencies.

Furthermore, the ASA states that all institutional regulations pertaining to anesthesia services shall be observed, and all the usual services performed by the anesthesiologist shall be furnished, including but not limited to:

1. Usual noninvasive cardiocirculatory and respiratory monitoring.
2. Oxygen administration, when indicated.
3. Administration of sedatives, tranquilizers, antiemetics, narcotics, other analgesics, beta-blockers, vasopressors, bronchodilators, antihypertensives, or other pharmacologic therapy as may be required in the judgment of the anesthesiologist.

PREOPERATIVE ASSESSMENT

The preoperative evaluation is an essential prerequisite to monitored anesthesia care and should be as comprehensive as that performed prior to any general or regional anesthetic (see Chapter 23). However, in addition to the usual evaluation for the patient who is planned to undergo general anesthesia, there are additional considerations unique to monitored anesthesia care that may ultimately determine the success or failure of the procedure. It is important to evaluate the patient's ability to remain motionless and, if necessary, actively cooperate throughout the procedure. Thus, it is important to evaluate the patient's psychological preparation for the planned procedure. It is also important to elicit the presence of coexisting sensorineural or cognitive deficits. These factors or the inability to communicate with the patient may occasionally make general anesthesia a more appropriate alternative. Verbal communication between physician and patient is very important for three reasons: (1) as a monitor of the level of sedation and cardiorespiratory function, (2) as a means of explanation and reassurance for the patient, and (3) as a mechanism of communication when the patient is required to actively cooperate. Although cardiorespiratory disease is often cited as an indication to perform a procedure using monitored anesthesia care rather than general anesthesia, there are occasions when cardiorespiratory disease may reduce the utility of monitored anesthesia care. For example, the presence of a persistent cough may make it very difficult for the patient to remain immobile, which can be particularly dangerous during ophthalmologic or awake neurosurgical procedures. Attempts to attenuate coughing with sedation techniques are likely to be unsuccessful and potentially harmful because a significant level of anesthesia is required to abolish the cough reflex. Similarly, some patients with significant cardiovascular disease may experience orthopnea and be unable to lie flat for an extended period.

TECHNIQUES OF MONITORED ANESTHESIA CARE

A variety of medications are commonly administered during monitored anesthesia care with the desired end points being providing patient comfort, maintaining cardiorespiratory stability, improving operating conditions, and preventing recall of unpleasant perioperative events. It is helpful to delineate and individualize the goals for each patient in order to formulate an appropriate regimen, which frequently involves the administration of either individual or combinations of analgesic, amnestic, and hypnotic drugs. There should be a minimal incidence of side effects, such as cardiorespiratory depression, nausea and vomiting, delayed emergence, and dysphoria, and there should be a rapid and complete recovery. Ideally, the patient should be able to communicate during the procedure. Clinical experience suggests that a level of sedation that allows verbal communication is optimal for the patient's comfort and safety. If the level of sedation is deepened to the extent that verbal communication is lost, most of the advantages of monitored anesthesia care are lost and the risks of the technique approach those of general anesthesia with an unprotected and uncontrolled airway. However, because monitored anesthesia care is provided by anesthesiologists, the range of sedation may be expanded to include significantly deeper sedation techniques than those provided by nonanesthesiologists during sedation/analgesia.

The preanesthetic evaluation and plan should strive to identify specific causes of and provide specific therapy for pain, anxiety, and agitation. Pain may be treated by local or regional analgesia, systemic analgesics, or removal of the painful stimulus. Anxiety may be reduced by the use of an anxiolytic such as a benzodiazepine and reassurance by the anesthesiologist. Patient agitation may be a result of pain or anxiety, but it is also vitally important to eliminate life-threatening factors such as hypoxia, hypercarbia, impending local anesthetic toxicity, and cerebral hypoperfusion. Other, less ominous, but often overlooked, causes of discomfort and agitation include a distended bladder, hypothermia, hyperthermia, pruritus, nausea, positional discomfort, uncomfortable oxygen masks and nasal cannulae, intravenous (IV) cannulation site infiltration, a member of the surgical team leaning on the patient, and prolonged pneumatic tourniquet inflation.

Pharmacologic Basis of Monitored Anesthesia Care Techniques—Optimizing Drug Administration

The ability to predict the effects of the drugs in our armamentarium demands an understanding of their pharmacokinetic and pharmacodynamic properties. This understanding is a fundamental prerequisite for the design of an effective sedation regimen and greatly increases the probability of producing the desired therapeutic effect. Context-sensitive half-time, effect–site equilibration time, and anesthetic/sedative drug interactions are fundamental concepts that are particularly useful in the context of monitored anesthesia care and will be discussed in some detail.

The ultimate objective of any dosing regimen is to deliver a therapeutic concentration of drug to its site of action, which is determined by the unique pharmacokinetic properties of that drug in that particular patient. The therapeutic response to a particular drug concentration is described by the pharmacodynamics of that particular patient-drug combination. There is a large degree of pharmacokinetic and pharmacodynamic variability, producing a significant variability in the dose-response relationship in clinical practice. Excessive sedation may result in cardiac or respiratory depression. Inadequate sedation may result in patient discomfort and potential morbidity from lack of cooperation. As a general principle, to avoid excessive levels of sedation, drugs should be titrated in small increments or by adjustable infusions rather than administered in larger doses according to predetermined notions of efficacy. In an ideal dosing regimen, an effective concentration of drug is achieved and then adjusted according to the magnitude of the noxious stimulus. If the noxious stimulus is increased or decreased, the concentration is increased or decreased accordingly. By the end of the procedure, the drug concentration should have decreased to a level compatible with rapid recovery. This approach requires the use of drugs that are easily titratable, such as propofol. When using drugs such as propofol, adjustable-rate continuous infusions are the most logical method of maintaining a desired therapeutic concentration. When the traditional method of intermittent bolus administration is used, significant fluctuations in drug concentration occur. Under these circumstances, the plasma concentrations are either above or below the desired therapeutic range for a significant proportion of the procedure (Fig. 31-1). Continuous infusions are superior to intermittent bolus dosing because they produce less fluctuation in drug concentration, thus reducing the number of episodes of inadequate or excessive sedation. Administration of drugs by continuous infusion rather than by intermittent dosing also reduces the total amount of drug administered and facilitates a more prompt recovery.[4]

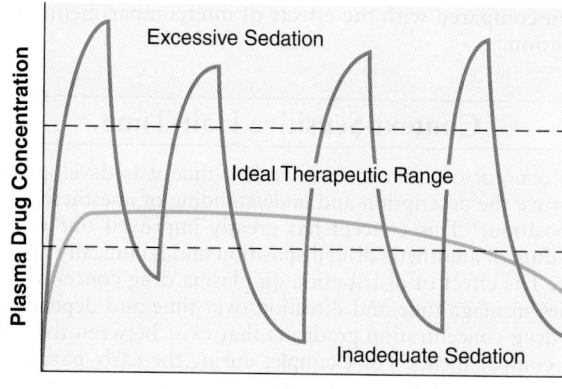

FIGURE 31-1. The changes in drug concentration during differing administration techniques. The *dark line* represents a continuous infusion of a drug. In this situation the drug is maintained within the therapeutic range for most of the procedure. The *lighter line* represents the drug concentration resulting from intermittent bolus administration. The drug concentration is significantly above or below the desired therapeutic level for most of the procedure.

Distribution, Elimination, Accumulation, and Duration of Action

Following the administration of IV anesthetic drugs, the immediate distribution phase causes a brisk decrease in plasma levels as the drug is transported to the rapidly equilibrating vessel-rich group of tissues. There is a simultaneously occurring distribution of drug to the less well-perfused tissues such as muscle and skin. Over time, the drug is also distributed to the poorly perfused tissues such as bone and fat. Although the latter compartments are poorly perfused, they may accumulate significant amounts of lipophilic drugs during prolonged administration. This peripheral depot may contribute to a delayed recovery when the drug is eventually released back into the central compartment after its administration is discontinued. Redistributive factors are important determinants of drug effect and influence the plasma concentration of a drug in a time-dependent fashion.

The Elimination Half-Life

Until recently, the elimination half-time was the predominant pharmacokinetic parameter used as the predictor of an anesthetic drug's duration of action. In everyday clinical practice, however, this parameter has not greatly enhanced our ability to predict anesthetic drug disposition. Only in single-compartment models does the elimination half-time actually represent the time required for a drug to reach half of its initial concentration after administration. In a single-compartment model, elimination is the only process that can alter drug concentration. Intercompartmental distribution cannot occur because there are no other compartments for the drug to be distributed to and from. Most drugs in the anesthesiologist's armamentarium are lipophilic and are therefore more suited to multicompartmental modeling than single-compartment modeling. Similarly, other pharmacokinetic parameters, such as distribution half-time, distribution volume, intercompartmental rate constants, and so forth, do not provide us with a practical means of predicting drug disposition. In multicompartmental models, the metabolism and excretion of some IV anesthetic drugs may have only a minor contribution to changes in plasma concentration when compared with the effects of intercompartmental distribution.

Context-Sensitive Half-Time

The concept of context-sensitive half-time was developed to improve the description and understanding of anesthetic drug disposition.[5] This concept has greatly improved our understanding of anesthetic drug disposition and is clinically applicable. The effect of distribution on plasma drug concentration varies in magnitude and direction over time and depends on the drug concentration gradients that exist between the various compartments. For example, during the early part of an infusion of a lipophilic drug, distributive factors will tend to decrease plasma concentrations as the drug is transported to the unsaturated peripheral tissues. Later, after the infusion is discontinued, drug will return from the peripheral tissues and re-enter the central circulation. The relative effect on plasma concentrations of distributive processes versus elimination varies over time and from drug to drug. The context-sensitive half-time describes the time required for the plasma drug concentration to decline by 50% after terminating an infusion of a particular duration. This parameter is calculated by using computer simulation of multicompartmental models of drug disposition (Fig. 31-2). The context-sensitive half-time reflects the combined effects of distribution and metabolism on drug disposition. There are several interesting aspects of these data. First, the data confirm the clinical impression that as the infusion duration increases, the context-sensitive half-time of all the drugs increases; this phenomenon is not described in any way by the elimination half-life. The increase in context-sensitive half-time is particularly marked with fentanyl and thiopental. In the case of fentanyl, drug that is irreversibly eliminated from the plasma by hepatic clearance is immediately replaced by drug returning from the peripheral compartments. Thus, although fentanyl has a shorter elimination half-life than that of sufentanil (462 vs. 577 minutes), its context-sensitive half-time is much greater than that of sufentanil after an infusion of longer than 2 hours. The storage and later release of fentanyl from peripheral binding sites delays the

decline in plasma concentration that would otherwise occur. The context-sensitive half-times of all the drugs bear no constant relationship to their elimination half-times. Compare also the context-sensitive half-times of propofol and thiopental (Fig. 31-2). Although the context-sensitive half-times of propofol and thiopental are comparable following a brief infusion, the context-sensitive half-time of thiopental increases rapidly following all but the shortest infusions. This finding confirms the clinical impression that thiopental is not an ideal drug for continuous infusion during ambulatory procedures. The context-sensitive half-time of propofol is prolonged to a minimal extent as the infusion duration increases. After an infusion of propofol, the drug that returns to the plasma from the peripheral compartments is rapidly cleared by metabolic processes and is therefore not available to retard the decay in plasma levels. This difference between thiopental and propofol is attributable to (1) the high metabolic clearance of propofol compared with thiopental, and (2) the relatively slow rate at which propofol returns to the plasma from peripheral compartments.

Alfentanil is the opioid that has, until recently, been most frequently studied, described, and promoted in the context of ambulatory techniques. Alfentanil has a very short elimination half-time, one-fifth that of sufentanil (111 vs. 577 minutes). However, despite the longer elimination half-time of sufentanil, its context-sensitive half-time is actually less than that of alfentanil for infusions up to 8 hours in duration. This phenomenon is explained in part by the huge distribution volume of sufentanil. After termination of a sufentanil infusion, the decay in plasma drug concentrations is accelerated not only by elimination but also by the continued redistribution of sufentanil into peripheral compartments. On the other hand, the small distribution volume of alfentanil equilibrates rapidly; therefore, peripheral distribution of drug away from the plasma is not a significant contributor to the decay in plasma concentration after an infusion. The data derived from computer simulation by Hughes et al.[5] show that the plasma decay of alfentanil is slower than that of sufentanil following infusions of similar duration to those used during conscious sedation. Thus, despite its short elimination half-time, alfentanil may not necessarily be superior to sufentanil for ambulatory sedation techniques.

How Does the Context-Sensitive Half-Time Relate to the Time to Recovery?

Although the context-sensitive half-time represents a significant advance in our ability to describe drug disposition, this parameter does not directly describe how long it will take the patient to recover from MAC. The context-sensitive half-time merely describes how long it will take for the plasma concentration of the drug to decrease by 50%. The time to recovery depends on other additional factors. The difference between the plasma concentration at the end of the infusion and the plasma concentration below which awakening can be expected is an obvious factor in determining time to recovery. For example, if the drug concentration is maintained at a level just above that required for awakening, the time to recovery will be more rapid than after an infusion during which the drug concentration is much greater than that required for awakening (Fig. 31-3). Furthermore, although context-sensitive half-time is a reflection of plasma drug decay, awakening from anesthesia is actually a function of effect–site (i.e., brain) concentration decay. Changes in effect–site concentration demonstrate a variable time lag behind changes in plasma drug concentration. Effect–site equilibration is a concept that is particularly relevant to IV sedation. When a drug is administered IV by bolus or infused rapidly, there is a delay before the onset of clinical effect. This delay occurs because the plasma is not

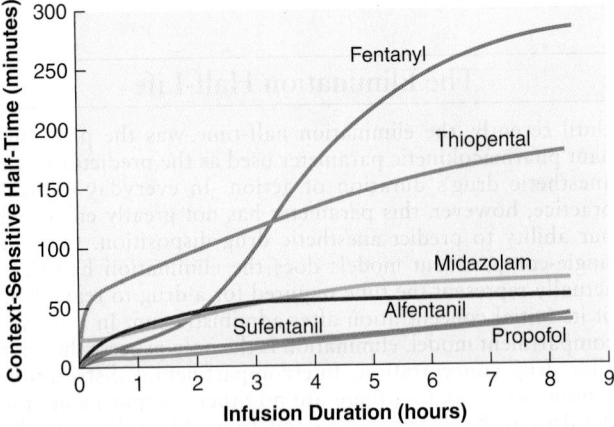

FIGURE 31-2. Context-sensitive half-times as a function of infusion duration. These data were generated from the computer model of Hughes et al.[5] It can be seen that the context-sensitive half-time of propofol demonstrates a minimal increase as the duration of the infusion increases. Also note that for infusions of short duration, sufentanil has a shorter half-time than alfentanil. (Reproduced from Hughes MA, Glass PSA, Jacobs JR: Context-sensitive half-time in multicompartment pharmacokinetic models for intravenous anesthetic drugs. Anesthesiology 1992; 76: 334, with permission.)

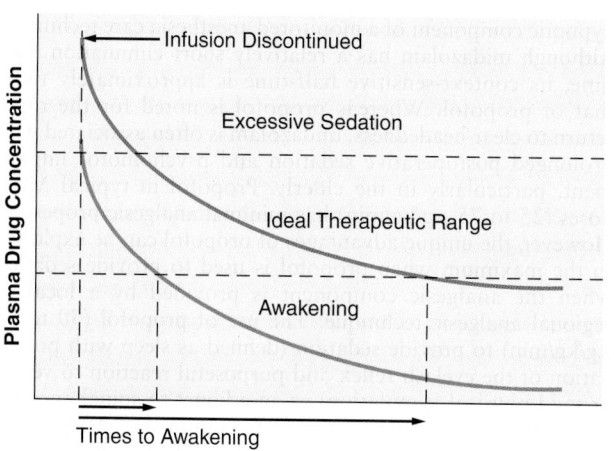

FIGURE 31-3. The context-sensitive half-time is not the sole determinant of the time it takes for the patient to awaken. This parameter merely reflects the time taken for the plasma concentration of a drug to decrease by 50%. The time to awakening is determined in addition by the difference in concentration at the end of the procedure and the concentration below which awakening will occur.

usually the site of action but is merely the route by which the drug reaches its effect site. If some parameter of drug effect can be measured (e.g., power spectrum electroencephalographic [EEG] analysis in the case of opioids), the half-time of equilibration between drug concentration in the blood and the drug effect can then be determined.[6] This parameter is abbreviated $t_{1/2}k_{e0}$. Drugs with a short $t_{1/2}k_{e0}$ will equilibrate rapidly with the brain and have a shorter delay in onset than drugs that have a longer $t_{1/2}k_{e0}$. Thiopental, propofol, and alfentanil have short $t_{1/2}k_{e0}$ values compared with midazolam, sufentanil, and fentanyl.

The $t_{1/2}k_{e0}$ allows predictions to be made of the time course of equilibration of the drug between the blood and the brain. A distinct time lag between the peak serum fentanyl concentration and the peak EEG slowing can be seen. In contrast, following alfentanil administration, the EEG changes closely parallel serum concentrations. The $t_{1/2}k_{e0}$ for fentanyl is 6.4 minutes compared with a $t_{1/2}k_{e0}$ of 1.1 minutes for alfentanil. If an opioid is required to blunt the response to a single brief stimulus, alfentanil might represent a logical choice over fentanyl. The $t_{1/2}k_{e0}$ is an important determinant of bolus spacing when titrating drugs to clinical effect. In the case of drugs like midazolam, which have a relatively long equilibration time (midazolam $t_{1/2}k_{e0}$ = 0.97 to 5.6 minutes), boluses of drug should be spaced far enough apart to allow the full peak effect to be clinically appreciated before further drug administration in order to avoid inadvertent overdosing.[7,8] For example, even if the shortest quoted equilibration half-time for midazolam (0.9 minute) is used, it will take 2.7 minutes for effect–site concentrations to be 87.5% equilibrated. Other factors are also important determinants of bolus size and spacing. For example, a low cardiac output will markedly delay drug arrival at the site of action. If sufficient time is not given for the drug to take effect before giving additional drug increments, significant cardiorespiratory compromise may occur. Furthermore, the effects of initial doses of most drugs in anesthetic practice are terminated by redistribution, which depends on blood flow to redistribution sites. If there is reduced blood flow to redistribution sites because of pre-existing and iatrogenic decreases in cardiac output, the dangerous adverse effects of these drugs are likely to be both delayed and markedly prolonged. An example of this scenario is the patient with a hemodynamic compromise caused by a tachydysrhythmia who requires sedation for cardioversion. Careful, well-spaced, small boluses of

drug should be given to induce the appropriate level of sedation, bearing in mind that it may take several minutes for the full effect of a small bolus dose to become apparent.

DRUG INTERACTIONS IN MONITORED ANESTHESIA CARE

5 At the present time, no one inhaled or IV drug can provide all the components of monitored anesthesia care (i.e., analgesia, anxiolysis, and hypnosis) with an acceptable margin of safety or ease of titratability. Therefore, patient comfort is usually maintained with a combination of drugs. By acting synergistically, combinations of drugs enable reductions in the dose requirements of individual drugs. For example, during general anesthesia, the combination of propofol and fentanyl by infusion has been shown to produce a more rapid recovery and better stress response abolition than the use of propofol alone.[9] However, synergistic interaction may also extend to the undesirable interactions of the drugs such as cardiorespiratory depression.

Drug interactions may have both a pharmacodynamic and a pharmacokinetic basis and may vary depending on the combination of drugs being coadministered, the dose range over which these drugs are administered, and the specific clinical effect that is measured. For example, because fentanyl is primarily an analgesic rather than a hypnotic, it reduces propofol requirements for suppression of response to skin incision to a much greater degree than it reduces propofol requirements for induction of anesthesia.[10] On the other hand, because midazolam has significant hypnotic properties, it displays significant synergism with propofol or thiopental when used to induce hypnosis.[11,12]

The plasma concentration of a drug at steady state that is required to abolish purposeful movement at skin incision in 50% of patients ($Cp_{ss}50$) is a measure of potency that is analogous to the familiar parameter of minimum alveolar concentration (MAC) of the volatile inhaled anesthetics. Intravenous anesthetic interactions may be evaluated by their effect on the $Cp_{ss}50$ in a manner analogous to the expression of the effects of opioids on volatile anesthetic requirements in terms of MAC reduction. For example, during general anesthesia, opioid requirements to suppress the responses to noxious stimuli are tenfold higher when used as the sole agent compared with when they are used in conjunction with a nitrous oxide/potent inhaled vapor technique. This interaction persists at the lighter levels of anesthesia encountered during MAC. Therefore, in an ambulatory conscious sedation setting, it is likely that a rapid recovery would be facilitated by using opioids in combination with other agents (e.g., propofol/midazolam) rather than as the sole drug.

Drug interactions are dose-dependent. For example, when fentanyl is combined with isoflurane, the greatest reduction in isoflurane MAC occurs within the analgesic concentration range of fentanyl (i.e., 1 to 2 ng/mL). At a fentanyl concentration of 1.7 ng/mL, the MAC of isoflurane is reduced by 50%.[13] Once the fentanyl concentration is increased beyond 3 ng/mL, there appears to be minimal further reduction with a maximum MAC reduction of 80%. Likewise, the MAC of desflurane is reduced by approximately 50% 25 minutes after a 3-μg/kg IV bolus of fentanyl.[14] However, when the fentanyl bolus is increased to 6 μg/kg, there is no significant further decrease in the MAC of desflurane. The interactions between propofol and opioids are important because these agents are frequently used during MAC. When analgesic concentrations of fentanyl (0.6 ng/mL) are used in combination with propofol for anesthesia, the $Cp_{ss}50$ of propofol is reduced by 50% compared with when propofol is used as the sole agent.[12] However, when the dose of fentanyl is increased, there is no significant further reduction of the $Cp_{ss}50$ for propofol beyond a fentanyl concentration of 3 ng/mL.

Although the data presented here pertain to patients under general anesthesia, these findings have important implications for monitored anesthesia care. These studies demonstrate that the potentiating effects of opioids on coadministered sedatives are pronounced within the dose range commonly used during MAC. Furthermore, the data suggest that the dose-response curve is likely to be steep within this dose range, thus supporting the clinical impression that significant increases in depth of sedation can occur with only modest increments in opioid or hypnotic/sedative dosage. The following clinical recommendations can be made: During MAC, the maximum benefit of opioid supplementation, in terms of potentiation of other administered sedatives, will accrue when the opioid is used in the analgesic dose range. Within this dose range there is great potential for adverse cardiorespiratory interaction.

Opioid and benzodiazepine combinations are frequently used to achieve the components of hypnosis, amnesia, and analgesia. This drug combination displays marked synergism in producing hypnosis. Approximately 25% of the median effective dose for each individual drug is required in combination to induce hypnosis in 50% of patients.[15] If the combination were simply additive, hypnosis would be induced in only approximately 25% of patients. Even subanalgesic doses of alfentanil (3 μg/kg) produce a profound reduction in midazolam requirements for hypnosis.[16] This synergism also extends to the unwanted effects of these drugs, producing the life-threatening complications of respiratory and cardiac depression.[17] Several fatalities have been reported after the use of midazolam, the majority of these being related to adverse respiratory events. In many of these cases, midazolam was used in combination with an opioid. The effects of midazolam and fentanyl on respiratory function in healthy volunteers have been examined by Bailey et al.[18] Whereas midazolam produced no significant respiratory effects alone, and fentanyl alone produced hypoxemia (oxyhemoglobin saturation 95%) in half of the subjects, the combination of midazolam 0.05 μg/kg and fentanyl 2.0 μg/kg resulted in hypoxemia in 11 of 12 subjects and apnea (no spontaneous respiratory effort for 15 seconds) in 6 of 12 subjects. The combination of midazolam and fentanyl places patients at high risk for developing hypoxemia and apnea. The respiratory depressant effects of this drug combination are likely to be even more significant in the patient with coexisting respiratory or central nervous system disease or at the extremes of age. In clinical practice, the clinical advantages of the synergy between opioids and benzodiazepines for the maintenance of patient comfort should be carefully weighed against the disadvantages of the potentially adverse effect of this drug combination on the cardiovascular and respiratory systems.

SPECIFIC DRUGS USED FOR MONITORED ANESTHESIA CARE

Propofol

Propofol has many of the ideal properties of a sedative–hypnotic for use in MAC. Its pharmacokinetic profile; that is, a context-sensitive half-time that remains short even after infusions of prolonged duration and a short effect–site equilibration time makes it an easily titratable drug with an excellent recovery profile. The quality of recovery and the low incidence of nausea and vomiting make propofol particularly well suited to ambulatory monitored anesthesia care procedures. A significant body of experience with the use of propofol for monitored anesthesia care has emerged. Propofol has significant advantages compared with benzodiazepines when used as the hypnotic component of a monitored anesthesia care technique. Although midazolam has a relatively short elimination half-time, its context-sensitive half-time is approximately twice that of propofol. Whereas propofol is noted for the rapid return to clear-headedness, midazolam is often associated with prolonged postoperative sedation and psychomotor impairment, particularly in the elderly. Propofol in typical MAC doses (25 to 75 μg/kg/min) has minimal analgesic properties. However, the unique advantages of propofol can be exploited to the maximum when propofol is used to provide sedation when the analgesic component is provided by a local or regional analgesic technique. The use of propofol (50 to 70 μg/kg/min) to provide sedation (defined as sleep with preservation of the eyelash reflex and purposeful reaction to verbal or mild physical stimulation) as an adjunct to spinal anesthesia for lower limb surgery has been examined.[19] After termination of infusions of approximately 100 minutes, patients regained consciousness in approximately 4 minutes. The authors also noted the ease with which general anesthesia could be induced if necessary by increasing the propofol infusion. The same group also compared propofol (60.5 μg/kg/min) with midazolam (4.3 μg/kg/min) as an adjunct to spinal anesthesia. The propofol group had faster immediate recovery than the midazolam group (2.3 vs. 9.2 minutes to spontaneous eye opening). Furthermore, psychomotor function was comparable with baseline values following propofol sedation but did not return to baseline until 2 hours after midazolam administration. Smith et al.[20] also compared propofol and midazolam sedation for local and regional anesthesia. These investigators examined several recovery parameters and demonstrated that propofol produced less postoperative sedation, drowsiness, confusion, and clumsiness than midazolam but that discharge times were similar.

The use of propofol for sedation has been examined in several diverse clinical settings, including propofol alone for upper gastrointestinal endoscopy[21] and magnetic resonance imaging in children,[22] with fentanyl for extracorporeal shock wave lithotripsy,[23] with alfentanil for transvaginal oocyte retrieval, and for sedation during the dental care to mentally and physically handicapped patients.[24,25]

There is a general clinical impression that patients recovering from propofol not only recover rapidly but often experience an increased sense of well-being. However, a study specifically addressing the issue of the subjective effects of low-dose propofol in volunteers could find no evidence for a euphoric effect of propofol.[26] The authors postulate that the sense of well-being arises from the feeling of relief that the procedure is over. This feeling of relief may be inhibited by the prolonged psychomotor impairment that often follows other anesthetic techniques.

General anesthesia with propofol is generally associated with less nausea and vomiting than most other anesthetic techniques. There is now evidence that even subhypnotic doses of propofol (a single 10-mg dose in an adult) also possess direct antiemetic properties.[27] Thus, it is likely that the beneficial effects of propofol upon nausea and vomiting will be a feature of monitored anesthesia care techniques using this drug. On the other hand, even during low-dose infusions used for sedation, pain during injection of propofol may be troublesome in 33 to 50% of patients.[28,29] Several strategies for reducing the pain of propofol administration are described in Table 31-1.[30]

Benzodiazepines

Benzodiazepines are commonly used during monitored anesthesia care for their anxiolytic, amnestic, and hypnotic properties. Midazolam has now displaced diazepam as the most commonly

TABLE 31-1

PUBLISHED STRATEGIES FOR REDUCING THE PAIN ON INTRAVENOUS INJECTION OF PROPOFOL

Using larger veins in antecubital fossa
Decreasing the speed of injection
Injection into a fast-running intravenous line
Diluting with 5% glucose or 10% intralipid
Adding lidocaine to propofol
Pretreating with lidocaine and venous occlusion
Pretreatment with opioid
Pretreatment with pentothal
Cooling propofol to 4°C prior to injection
Injecting cooled saline (4°C) prior to injection
Discontinuing intravenous fluid administration during injection

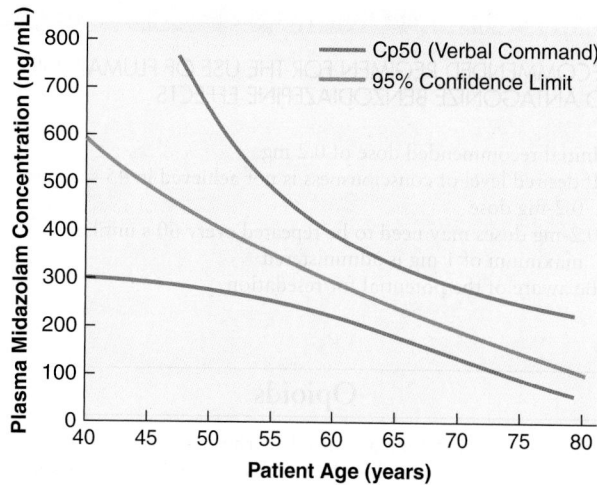

FIGURE 31-4. Midazolam Cp50 (the concentration at which 50% of subjects will fail to respond to a verbal command) as a function of age. There is a marked decrease in midazolam requirements as patient age increases. (Reproduced from Jacobs JR, Reves JG, Marty J et al: Aging increases pharmacodynamic sensitivity to the hypnotic effects of midazolam. Anesth Analg 1995; 80: 143, with permission.)

used benzodiazepine for conscious sedation. The important differences between midazolam and diazepam are listed in Table 31-2.[31] Although midazolam has a short elimination half-time, there is often significant and prolonged psychomotor impairment following sedation techniques using midazolam as a significant component. With the recent availability of propofol, midazolam may be better used in a modified role by using lower doses prior to the start of a propofol infusion to provide the specific amnestic and perhaps anxiolytic component of a "balanced" sedation technique rather than as the major hypnotic component.[32] This strategy allows the more evanescent and titratable propofol to provide the desired level of conscious sedation in an adjustable manner according to the specific stimulus. The analgesic component, if required, of a balanced monitored anesthesia care technique could be provided by regional/local techniques or opioids. Again, when using opioids with benzodiazepines, the potential for significant respiratory impairment should be considered.

Clinical experience suggests that the dose of a particular benzodiazepine required to reach a desired clinical end point is reduced in elderly compared with younger patients. This difference in dosing requirements in elderly patients is mainly related to pharmacodynamic factors, as demonstrated by the threefold decrease in plasma concentration of midazolam at which 50% of patients would be expected not to respond to verbal command (Cp50) in an 80-year-old patient compared with a 40-year-old patient (Fig. 31-4).[33]

Benzodiazepines are valuable components of monitored anesthesia care techniques because they enhance patient comfort, improve operating conditions, and provide amnesia.

However, recovery of psychomotor and cognitive function may be significantly prolonged following benzodiazepine sedation, especially when compared with sedative–hypnotic techniques using propofol as the major component.[34] The specific benzodiazepine antagonist flumazenil provides the potential to improve the recovery profile of benzodiazepines by permitting the active termination of their sedative and amnestic effects without invoking adverse side effects. However, the potential for resedation remains an obstacle to the routine use of benzodiazepine reversal, particularly in patients undergoing ambulatory procedures. The effects of midazolam may recur up to 90 minutes following the administration of flumazenil.[35] Thus it is possible that patients could be discharged prematurely to a less well-monitored area, or even out of the hospital in the case of ambulatory surgery, and later experience recurrence of benzodiazepine effects. An important additional issue is that of cost. The routine use of flumazenil-antagonized benzodiazepine sedation has a significant cost disadvantage. Ghouri et al.[35] demonstrated that flumazenil-antagonized midazolam sedation was more expensive than propofol sedation ($68.67 vs. $27.80). Typical dose requirements for use of flumazenil are listed in Table 31-3.

TABLE 31-2

COMPARISON OF THE IMPORTANT PROPERTIES OF MIDAZOLAM AND DIAZEPAM

■ MIDAZOLAM	■ DIAZEPAM
Water-soluble, does not require propylene glycol for solubilizing	Lipid-soluble, requires propylene glycol for solubilizing
Nonvenoirritant, usually painless	Venoirritant, pain on injection
Thrombophlebitis rare	Thrombophlebitis common
Short elimination half-time (1–4 h)	Long elimination half-time (>20 h)
Clearance unaffected by H₂ antagonists	Clearance reduced by H₂ antagonists
Inactive metabolites (1-hydroxy-midazolam)	Active metabolites (desmethyl-diazepam, oxazepam)
Resedation unlikely	Resedation more likely

RECOMMENDED REGIMEN FOR THE USE OF FLUMAZENIL TO ANTAGONIZE BENZODIAZEPINE EFFECTS

Initial recommended dose of 0.2 mg
If desired level of consciousness is not achieved in 45 s, repeat 0.2-mg dose
0.2-mg doses may need to be repeated every 60 s until a maximum of 1 mg is administered
Be aware of the potential for resedation

Opioids

Opioids are most logically used in the context of monitored anesthesia care to provide the specific analgesic component of a "balanced" technique rather than to provide the sedative component. Opioid analgesics are indicated when regional or local anesthetic techniques are inappropriate or ineffective. Opioids may also play an important role during the initial injection of local anesthetic solution or during other periods of intense patient discomfort. Pain relief may be required for factors other than the procedure itself, such as uncomfortable positioning, propofol injection, pneumatic tourniquet pain, or other pain not relieved by the local anesthetic technique.

A typical circumstance in which the patient must briefly cooperate and remain motionless is during the placement of a retrobulbar block prior to ophthalmic procedures. Patient movement during block placement may increase the incidence of complications such as brainstem anesthesia and cardiac arrest. Retrobulbar block placement affords an excellent opportunity to study the effects of drugs on the response to a standardized, ethically acceptable, brief painful stimulus. The ideal drug for block placement would provide a brief period of intense analgesia yet allow the patient to be awake and cooperative without causing cardiorespiratory depression or minimal nausea and vomiting, and not significantly prolong recovery.[36] Alfentanil (20 μg/kg) has a rapid onset and offset of intense analgesia and was compared with methohexital (0.5 mg/kg) for retrobulbar block placement.[36] Patients receiving methohexital were unresponsive to verbal command at the time of block placement and demonstrated more movement on injection than those receiving alfentanil, who were mostly (87%) awake and cooperative at the time of injection. The authors note that one elderly patient of the 15 who received alfentanil became apneic for 30 seconds, and suggested that the dose of opioids be reduced in elderly patients. They also noted that the personnel performing the block were accustomed to the patient being "asleep" during methohexital sedation, but took some time to become at ease with the awake yet comfortable and cooperative patient who had received alfentanil.

The well-described phenomenon of patient awareness and subsequent recall of intraoperative events following high-dose opioid anesthesia is taken as evidence that opioids lack significant amnestic properties. However, when the effects of low-dose fentanyl on memory were specifically examined in volunteers, it was found that although the subjects appeared to be awake during the fentanyl infusion, there was significant memory impairment.[37] However, the degree of stimulation was probably less than that experienced by a patient undergoing a painful surgical procedure. Recall for a painful stimulus may not be impaired to the same degree as recall for the less noxious stimuli experienced by the subjects of this study.

Alfentanil appears to have a pharmacokinetic advantage for the treatment of discrete stimuli because of its short effect–site equilibration time, which allows rapid access of the drug to the brain and facilitates titration. However, sufentanil may have a more favorable recovery profile when used over a longer period because of its shorter context-sensitive half-time. In clinical practice, however, there is a marked interpatient variability in opioid pharamacokinetics and dynamics. This interpatient variability may be more significant than the inter-drug differences, making it difficult to predict with any precision the effects of a given drug dose in an individual patient.

Remifentanil

In the context of monitored anesthesia care, the analgesic properties of opioids are extremely valuable. However, their adverse effects, including respiratory depression, muscle rigidity, and emesis, are undesirable in the spontaneously breathing patient with an unprotected airway and significantly limit the ability to consistently provide effective analgesic doses. A further complicating issue is that the ability to predict the effect of a given dose of opioid in a particular patient is limited by significant interpatient pharmacokinetic and pharmacodynamic variability. This problem is usually overcome in practice by the cautious incremental administration of small, carefully spaced boluses or by titrating infusions to the desired effect.

Remifentanil has pharmacodynamic properties similar to those of other potent μ-opioid receptor agonists such as fentanyl and alfentanil. However, remifentanil is predominantly metabolized by nonspecific esterases generating an extremely rapid clearance and offset of effect.[38] The context-sensitive half-time of remifentanil is consistently short, 3 to 5 minutes, increasing to a minimal degree with the duration of the infusion. Furthermore, remifentanil has a short effect–site equilibration time ($t_{1/2}k_{e0}$) of 1.0 to 1.5 minutes. This $t_{1/2}k_{e0}$ is slightly longer than that of alfentanil (0.6 to 1.2 minutes) but much shorter than that of fentanyl (4 to 5 minutes) and morphine (approximately 20 minutes), and makes the onset of effect after drug administration very rapid, thus facilitating titration of effect during monitored anesthesia care.

In clinical practice, remifentanil has been used successfully as the analgesic component of sedation techniques for regional and local anesthesia. Its unique pharmacokinetic profile makes it well suited for ambulatory monitored anesthesia care techniques. Published experience with the use of remifentanil suggests that it is possible to titrate remifentanil administration to provide effective analgesia with minimal respiratory depression. The published data can be used to generate some practical clinical guidelines,[39] which are discussed here.

1. As with other potent opioids used during sedation techniques, the most logical therapeutic end point for remifentanil administration is effective analgesia and patient comfort rather than sedation. When opioids are titrated to preconceived levels of sedation rather than patient comfort, an unacceptable degree of respiratory depression may occur. Drugs such as propofol or midazolam can be used in combination with remifentanil to provide the hypnotic-amnestic component of the sedation technique, remembering that the concomitant administration of midazolam decreases remifentanil dose requirements by up to 50%.[40]
2. Published data suggest that bolus administration of remifentanil is associated with an increased incidence of respiratory depression and chest wall rigidity. Because these side effects are likely to be related to high peak concentrations of drugs, it is recommended that remifentanil boluses be administered slowly (over 30 to 90 seconds) or avoided completely by using a pure infusion technique. Furthermore, the administration of remifentanil boluses during the concomitant administration of remifentanil infusions is also associated with an increased incidence of respiratory

depression, the most likely mechanism again being excessive peak drug concentrations. These episodes of respiratory depression are of significant concern, particularly in the spontaneously breathing patient with an unprotected airway. However, if promptly recognized and the remifentanil administration is reduced or discontinued, they should resolve within approximately 3 minutes. Thus, despite the pharmacokinetic advantages of remifentanil, the level of vigilance required for its administration should be no different from that for any other potent opioid. Although the offset time of remifentanil is rapid, it still requires the recognition of respiratory depression to trigger a downward adjustment in dosage. Similarly, the short $t_{1/2}k_{e0}$ of remifentanil suggests that sudden respiratory depression may occur in response to upward adjustments in dosage. Despite the potential for respiratory depression, the efficacy of remifentanil boluses during monitored anesthesia care has been investigated by several groups. The most logical scenario in which a bolus dose could be used is immediately prior to a brief but very painful stimulus, such as placement of a retrobulbar block.[41] A bolus of 1 μg/kg over 30 seconds was administered 90 seconds prior to block placement. More than three quarters of patients receiving remifentanil did not report any pain during subsequent block placement. However, 15% of the patients given a single bolus alone had significant respiratory depression (respiratory rates <8 breaths per minute), and 19% of those given a bolus followed by an infusion had significant respiratory depression.

3. The effects of coadministration of benzodiazepines and opioids are well documented. The addition of midazolam to provide the anxiolytic-sedative and amnestic components of a sedation technique has been shown to increase patient satisfaction and significantly reduce remifentanil dose requirements. The combination of remifentanil with midazolam significantly reduces patient anxiety when compared with the use of the opioid alone.[42] Even relatively low-dose midazolam (2 mg IV) produces significant reductions in remifentanil requirements and patient anxiety. During breast or lymph node biopsy, remifentanil infusion requirements were 0.065 μg/kg/min when preceded by midazolam compared with 0.123 μg/kg/min when used alone. The advantages of coadministration of small doses of midazolam include increased patient satisfaction, increased amnesia, decreased nausea and vomiting, and decreased anxiety. The disadvantages include a tendency toward increased respiratory depression, apnea, and excessive sedation.

4. Because most painful stimuli are of unpredictable duration and because the risk of adverse respiratory events is increased following bolus administration, the most logical method for the administration of remifentanil during monitored anesthesia care is by an adjustable infusion. This should ideally be preceded by a small bolus of midazolam. Most investigators have used infusion rates that start at 0.1 μg/kg/min approximately 5 minutes prior to the first painful stimulus. This initial "loading" infusion is then weaned to approximately 0.05 μg/kg/min to maintain patient comfort. The maintenance infusion is adjusted upward in response to pain or hemodynamic response or downward in response to excessive sedation, respiratory depression, or apnea. A typical incremental change in infusion rate is 0.025 μg/kg/min. The use of remifentanil infusions of 0.2 μg/kg/min is associated with an increased incidence of respiratory depression that is not necessarily associated with superior analgesia. As in the case of propofol administration, inadvertent interruption of remifentanil administration will result in abrupt offset of effect, which may result in patient discomfort, hemodynamic instability, and even morbidity due to patient movement. It is therefore very important to ensure that the drug delivery system is monitored carefully during the procedure. Remifentanil is supplied as a powder that must be reconstituted prior to use. It is particularly important when administering this drug to patients with an unsecured airway to ensure that there are no errors in drug dilution that would result in inadvertent dosing errors.

Typical adult dose recommendations for opioids and other drugs discussed in the text are listed in Table 31-4.

TABLE 31-4

TYPICAL DOSE RANGES OF SEDATIVE, HYPNOTIC, AND ANALGESIC DRUGS

■ DRUG	■ TYPICAL ADULT INTRAVENOUS DOSE RANGE (TITRATED TO EFFECT IN SMALL INCREMENTS)
Benzodiazepines	
Midazolam	1–2 mg prior to propofol or remifentanil infusion
Diazepam	2–8 mg as major component
	2.5–10 mg
Opioid analgesics	
Alfentanil	5–20-μg/kg bolus 2 min prior to stimulus
Fentanyl	0.5–2.0-μg/kg bolus 2–4 min prior to stimulus
Remifentanil	Infusion 0.1 μg/kg/min 5 min prior to stimulus
	Wean to 0.05 μg/kg/min as tolerated
	Adjust up or down in increments of 0.025 μg/kg/min
	Reduce dose accordingly when coadministered with midazolam or propofol
	Avoid boluses
Hypnotics	
Propofol	250–500-μg/kg boluses
	25–75 μg/kg/min infusion
Dexmedetomidine	Loading infusion: 0.5–1 μg/kg over 10–20 min
	Maintenance infusion: 0.2–0.7–1 μg/kg/h

Ketamine

Ketamine is a phencyclidine derivative and is an intense analgesic and is frequently used as a component of pediatric sedation techniques.[43,44] When used in small doses (0.25 to 0.5 mg/kg) its use is associated with minimal respiratory and cardiovascular depression. Ketamine produces a dissociative state in which the eyes remain open with a nystagmic gaze. However, as the dose of ketamine increases, or when used in combination with other sedatives, a state of deep sedation and/or general anesthesia may be inadvertently achieved. Increased oral secretions make laryngospasm more likely. The fear of laryngospasm is the underlying rationale for the frequent administration of atropine or glycopyrrolate. Ketamine is frequently combined with a benzodiazepine to reduce the incidence of hallucinations associated with its use. However, this practice is controversial.[45] Patient movement may make ketamine less than ideal for procedures requiring a completely motionless patient. Ketamine can elevate intracranial and intraocular pressure and is thus relatively contraindicated in patients with increased intracranial pressure and with glaucoma or open-globe injuries. Although it has been suggested that airway reflexes are relatively preserved with ketamine, there is no convincing evidence to support this notion.

Ketamine can be administered orally, intramuscularly, or intravenously. The oral dose of ketamine is 4 to 6 mg/kg. The onset of action typically occurs within 20 to 30 minutes and the duration of effect is between 60 and 90 minutes. The intramuscular dose is 2 to 4 mg/kg with an onset of action of 5 to 10 minutes and typically has a duration of effect of 30 to 120 minutes. When administered via the IV route, ketamine should be given in small (0.25 to 1.0 mg/kg) increments, titrating to effect with an onset of action of 1 to 2 minutes and an approximate duration of 20 to 60 minutes.

Dexmedetomidine

Dexmedetomidine is a selective α_2 receptor agonist. Stimulation of α_2 receptor depresses central sympathetic function and produces sedation and analgesia. The α_2 agonists potentiate opioid-induced analgesia, benzodiazepine-induced hypnosis, and have potent MAC-sparing effects when administered with volatile agents. Although currently approved in the United States for sedation of mechanically ventilated patients in an intensive care setting, dexmedetomidine has become an important addition to the anesthesiologist's armamentarium both as an adjunct to general anesthesia and as a component of procedural sedation techniques. However, the published experience with dexmedetomidine remains relatively limited and its role in monitored anesthesia care continues to evolve. There has also been recent interest in the use of dexmedetomidine for sedation provided by nonanesthesia professionals. To a degree, some of this interest was generated in response to the ASA statement on the safe use of propofol, the American Association of Nurse Anesthetists-ASA joint statement regarding propofol administration, the Astra-Zeneca Diprivan package insert, and prescriptive regulations in several states, all of which promote the position that the administration of propofol should be limited to those individuals trained in the administration of general anesthesia.[46]

Compared with other sedative and analgesic drugs, dexmedetomidine appears to have relatively minor effects on respiratory function when used in the typical dose range.[47] Of note, unlike during opioid-induced sedation, the hypercapnic arousal response, a feature of natural sleep, appears to be preserved during dexmedetomidine sedation. However, airway intervention to relieve obstruction and apnea may be required during dexmedetomidine administration, particularly when used in combination with other respiratory depressants.[48] Dexmedetomidine has been used for sedation during instrumentation of the difficult airway. Patients undergoing fiberoptic intubation sedated with dexmedetomidine are generally comfortable yet cooperative.[49] Administration of α_2 agonist is associated with a reduction of sympathetic outflow and an increase in cardiac vagal activity; therefore, it is not surprising that hypotension and bradycardia may occur during dexmedetomidine administration. Clinically significant episodes of bradycardia and sinus arrest have been associated with dexmedetomidine administration in young, healthy volunteers with high vagal tone, particularly during rapid IV or bolus administration.[50] The α_2 agonists do have peripheral vasoconstrictive effects that can occasionally precipitate hypertension. Despite this phenomenon, the incidence of hypertensive episodes requiring intervention is lower when compared with an equivalent propofol-based technique.[51]

Dexmedetomidine has been used successfully in both adult and pediatric patients for monitored anesthesia care during the awake portions of craniotomies requiring patient cooperation for cortical speech mapping.[52,53] Dexmedetomidine has been used as sedative supplementation to regional anesthesia during carotid endarterectomy. Under these circumstances, there were fewer fluctuations from the desired sedation level when compared with the combination of midazolam, fentanyl, and propofol.[54] Dexmedetomidine tends to decrease cerebral blood flow both directly via α_2-mediated constriction of cerebral blood vessels and indirectly via its effect on systemic pressure. However, there appears to be a concomitant decrease in cerebral metabolic rate.[55] To add further reassurance, the use of dexmedetomidine does not appear to be associated with an increase in the need for intracarotid shunting in patients undergoing awake carotid endarterectomy.[56]

The lack of pain on injection and its analgesic and minimal adverse respiratory properties would seem to make dexmedetomidine a useful alternative to propofol in certain circumstances. However, when compared with propofol, the target sedation level takes longer to achieve with dexmedetomidine (25 vs. 10 minutes).[57] Furthermore, if loading boluses of dexmedetomidine are used to accelerate the onset of sedation, bradycardia and hypotension may occur. Although the use of dexmedetomidine may result in greater sedation, lower blood pressure, and improved analgesia in the recovery room when compared with propofol, the time to postanesthesia care unit discharge is not significantly different.[57] Dexmedetomidine is most often delivered as an initial bolus followed by a continuous infusion. Initial bolus doses range from 0.5 to 1.0 μg/kg over 10 to 20 minutes, followed by a continuous infusion of 0.2 to 0.7 μ/kg/h.

Two large retrospective observational studies from a single children's hospital suggest that dexmedetomidine may be used for sedation for pediatric magnetic resonance imaging and computed tomography studies.[58,59] In these studies, the loading dose of dexmedetomidine was 2 to 3 μg/kg over 10 minutes, followed by an infusion of between 1 and 2 μg/kg/h. However, approximately 15% of patients required a second bolus in order to achieve satisfactory conditions to complete the scan. The analgesic properties of dexmedetomidine may make it a useful alternative to the use of propofol as a sole agent during painful procedures. However, the time taken to deliver the loading dose, the occasional need to rebolus, hypotension, bradycardia, and the relatively long recovery time may limit the utility of dexmedetomidine for very brief procedures such as computed tomography studies. On the other hand, the pain on injection of propofol and the legislative constraints on the administration of propofol by nonanesthesia-trained providers may make dexmedetomidine advantageous in certain circumstances.

Amnesia During Sedation with Dexmedetomidine or Propofol

Drugs with sedative-hypnotic properties reduce attention to stimuli during their administration as a direct consequence of depression of consciousness. Therefore, all sedative–hypnotics have the potential to impair memory formation because attention to stimuli is a crucial element of explicit memory formation.[60] However, like benzodiazepines, propofol has significant amnestic effects at subhypnotic doses, suggesting an additional amnestic mechanism that is separate from its sedative effect. In the case of propofol, drug-induced amnesia appears to be a consequence of lack of retention of information that was already successfully stored into long-term memory.[61] In contrast to propofol and benzodiazepines, it is unlikely that dexmedetomidine has amnestic properties at subhypnotic doses.[60] If amnesia is desired for a procedure performed during dexmedetomidine administration, loss of consciousness would be necessary if dexmedetomidine is used as the sole agent. Alternatively, amnestic doses of propofol or a benzodiazepine may be used to supplement dexmedetomidine. The properties of propofol and dexmedetomidine are compared in Table 31-5.

Patient-Controlled Sedation and Analgesia

Techniques that allow the direct patient control of the level of sedation may positively affect patient satisfaction.[62] The degree of sedation desired by the patient varies significantly and the individual response to drugs is variable. Patient-controlled sedation appears to be an attractive solution to this problem. One approach to patient-controlled sedation has been to use a conventional patient-controlled analgesia (PCA) delivery system set to deliver 0.7-mg/kg boluses of propofol with a 3-minute lockout period.[63] Other approaches include fixed-dose combinations of 0.5 mg midazolam and 25 μg fentanyl with a 5-minute lockout interval between doses.[64] This technique was as safe and effective as anesthesiologist-controlled drug delivery, but may be associated with greater postprocedure sedation.[65] The pharmacokinetic profile of alfentanil is ideal for the treatment of short, discrete episodes of pain. These properties have been exploited during vaginal ovum retrieval procedures, when ultrasonically guided needles are passed through the vaginal wall under monitored anesthesia care. Zelcer et al.[66] used a PCA delivery system to allow self-administration of alfentanil during this procedure. After midazolam premedication and a loading dose of alfentanil, patients received 5-μg/kg boluses of alfentanil via the PCA pump with a mandatory 3-minute lockout period. Patient acceptability, alfentanil dosage, respiratory variables, and pain scores were similar to those obtained with physician-controlled analgesia. From the limited data that are available, intraoperative PCA during monitored anesthesia care appears to be an effective alternative to physician-administered analgesia.

RESPIRATORY FUNCTION AND SEDATIVE–HYPNOTICS

During monitored anesthesia care there is significant potential for respiratory compromise mediated via several important mechanisms. These include adverse effects on respiratory drive, either directly as a result of sedative–hypnotic or opioid administration or indirectly as a consequence of brain stem hypoperfusion resulting from hypotension, such as that occurring during spinal or epidural anesthesia. There may also be a marked increase in the work of breathing because of increased upper airway resistance.[67] During sedation it is likely that protective airway reflexes will be attenuated. On the other hand, sedative doses of benzodiazepines appear to have variable effects on respiratory system mechanics, either decreasing, increasing, or having no effect on functional residual capacity.[68,69]

Sedation and Upper Airway Patency

The upper airway is located outside the thorax. During normal inspiration, the pressure within the upper airway is subatmospheric; thus, there is a tendency for the upper airway to collapse under the influence of the surrounding atmospheric pressure. However, in the normal subject this tendency for airway collapse is opposed by upper airway dilator muscle tone. These muscles probably both increase the diameter and reduce the compliance of the upper airway. An increase in upper airway dilator muscle tone occurs during inspiration, commencing just prior to diaphragmatic contraction.[70] Several studies have confirmed the importance of coordinated activation of the diaphragmatic and upper airway respiratory muscles in maintaining airway patency. Upper airway dilator muscle control appears to be extremely sensitive to sedative–hypnotic drug administration.[71] For example, sedative doses of midazolam have been reported to increase inspiratory subglottic airway resistance by three- to fourfold.[72] Sedative doses of diazepam selectively suppress genioglossal muscle activity to a greater degree than diaphragmatic activity; furthermore, this effect is exaggerated in elderly patients. In all these examples the increased upper airway resistance markedly increased the work of breathing. The response to this obstruction is a significant increase in intercostal and accessory muscle activity.

TABLE 31-5

A COMPARISON OF SOME IMPORTANT PROPERTIES OF PROPOFOL AND DEXMEDETOMIDINE

	PROPOFOL	DEXMEDETOMIDINE
Pain on injection	Yes	Minimal
Analgesic properties in subhypnotic doses	Minimal	Yes
Amnestic properties in subhypnotic doses	Significant	Insignificant
Time of onset with typical administration	Rapid	5–10 min
Restrictive regulations on use by nonanesthesia-trained providers	Yes	No
Potential for significant bradycardia	Minimal	Significant

However, this response is only partially effective because the increase in inspiratory force will further decrease intraluminal upper airway pressure, predisposing to further airway collapse. It is likely that these effects will be of greatest significance in patients with pre-existing respiratory compromise, such as elderly patients or those with chronic obstructive pulmonary disease. These patients often have limited respiratory reserve and are unable to increase their respiratory muscle activity in response to the increased work of breathing induced by sedation and may become hypercarbic, acidotic, and hypoxic.

Sedation and Protective Airway Reflexes

Competent laryngeal and upper airway reflexes are required to protect the lower airway from aspiration. Protective laryngeal and pharyngeal reflexes are depressed by anesthesia and sedation. Furthermore, it is also well documented that protective airway reflexes are compromised by advanced age and debilitation. Therefore, it is likely that significant depression of airway reflexes could occur during sedation in the elderly or debilitated patient. Aspiration of gastric contents could occur either in the operating room or during recovery, particularly if oral intake is allowed before the return of adequate upper airway protective reflexes. The time required for the return of protective reflexes varies considerably. Complete recovery of the swallowing reflex occurs approximately 15 minutes after the return of consciousness following propofol anesthesia.[73] However, the IV administration of 15 mg of diazepam has been shown to depress the swallowing reflex for up to 4 hours.[74] The swallowing reflex is significantly depressed for up to 2 hours following the administration of midazolam despite the return to a normal state of consciousness.[75] In otherwise healthy adult male volunteers the inhalation of 50% nitrous oxide was associated with marked depression of the swallowing reflex.[76]

It is apparent from the sources previously quoted that the protective airway reflexes alone cannot be relied on to protect the lower airway from aspiration during sedation. Thus, patients who are deemed to be at risk from aspiration of gastric contents should be maintained at the lightest level of sedation possible. Ideally, the patient should be awake enough to recognize the regurgitation of gastric contents and be able to protect his or her own airway. If the ability of the patient to protect his or her own airway cannot be reliably guaranteed and regurgitation/aspiration is thought to be a significant risk, placement of a cuffed endotracheal tube under general or local anesthesia should be seriously considered.

Sedation and Respiratory Control

Clinical experience would lead most anesthesiologists to predict that the administration of sedative–hypnotic drugs is associated with the depression of respiratory drive. However, the findings of scientific studies in this area are often conflicting and confusing, on occasion finding minimal, if any, effects of sedative drugs on ventilatory responsiveness. However, it is important to note that in many cases the methods used to measure respiratory drive may affect the outcome of the study by stimulating the subject, thus attenuating the negative effect of the drug on respiratory drive. In clinical practice it is likely that during regional anesthesia there is a degree of deafferentation that will potentiate the respiratory depressant effects of sedative–hypnotic drugs.[77] Most studies have demonstrated that opioids depress the ventilatory response to hypercapnia and hypoxia.[78] Reports of the effects of sedative doses of benzodiazepines on carbon dioxide responsiveness

have shown variable results, including no significant effect and clinically significant depression.[79,80] However, when opioids and benzodiazepines are used in combination, there appears to a consistent and marked negative effect on respiratory responsiveness.[17] Although the addition of sedative doses of propofol to opioids showed little potentiation of the respiratory effects of opioids, caution is still warranted when combinations of sedative–hypnotics are used.

SUPPLEMENTAL OXYGEN ADMINISTRATION

Hypoxia as a result of alveolar hypoventilation is a relatively common occurrence following the administration of sedatives, analgesics, and hypnotics. In the absence of significant lung disease, the administration of only modest concentrations of supplemental oxygen is frequently effective in restoring the patient's oxygen saturation to an acceptable level. This concept is well illustrated by reference to the familiar alveolar gas equation. An extreme example illustrates the point: an otherwise healthy adult male breathing room air receives a dose of an opioid that causes marked alveolar hypoventilation such that his alveolar PCO_2 is increased to 80 mm Hg. The alveolar gas equation predicts that his arterial PO_2 will fall to approximately 40 mm Hg as shown here:

$$PAO_2 = PIO_2 - PACO_2/R$$

$$PIO_2 = FIO_2 \times (P_B - PH_2O)$$

$$PIO_2 = 0.21 \times (760 - 47) = 150 \text{ mm Hg}$$

$$PAO_2 = 150 - 80/0.8$$

$$PAO_2 = 50 \text{ mm Hg}$$

Assuming a normal A–a gradient, his PaO_2 will be 40 mm Hg, corresponding to an arterial oxygen saturation of 75%. If while initiating definitive therapy for hypoventilation this patient were to receive only a modest increase in inspired oxygen, a marked improvement in arterial saturation would be achieved:

$$FIO_2 \text{ increased to } 28\%$$

$$PIO_2 = 0.28 \times (760 - 47) = 200 \text{ mm Hg}$$

$$PAO_2 = 200 - 80/0.8$$

$$PAO_2 = 100 \text{ mm Hg}$$

This theoretical example serves to highlight an important point. First, in isolated hypoventilation modest increases in inspired oxygen are remarkably effective at restoring oxygen saturation to acceptable levels. However, a patient who is receiving minimal supplemental oxygen and has an acceptable oxygen saturation may have significant undetected alveolar hypoventilation. Therefore, before making the decision to discharge patients to a less well-monitored environment without supplemental oxygen, it is useful to measure their oxygen saturation while breathing room air.

MONITORING DURING MONITORED ANESTHESIA CARE

American Society of Anesthesiologists Standards

The ASA standards for basic anesthetic monitoring are applicable to all levels of anesthesia care, including monitored anesthesia care. It is useful to review the components of the ASA standards that are pertinent to monitored anesthesia care as approved by the House of Delegates on October 21, 1986, and subsequently amended on October 25, 2005.[81] (See Chapter 2, Table 2-1, for the current ASA standards.)

Communication and Observation

A conscientious and well-trained anesthesia caregiver is the single most vital monitor in the operating room. However, his or her effectiveness will be markedly enhanced by the use of the basic quantitative and qualitative monitoring devices, which should be readily available in all operating rooms. It is important that the anesthesiologist continually evaluate the patient's response to verbal stimulation to effectively titrate the level of sedation and to allow the earlier detection of neurologic or cardiorespiratory dysfunction. Continuous visual, tactile, and auditory assessment of physiologic function should include observation of the rate, depth, and pattern of respiration; palpation of the arterial pulse; and assessment of peripheral perfusion by extremity temperature and capillary refill. In addition, the patient should be continually observed for diaphoresis, pallor, shivering, cyanosis, and acute changes in neurologic status.

Auscultation

Auscultation of heart and breath sounds has long been a vital component of monitoring during anesthesia. Placement of a precordial stethoscope near the sternal notch of a nonintubated patient provides important information concerning upper airway patency as well as a continuous monitor of heart sounds and ventilation. Continuous precordial auscultation is an inexpensive, effective, and essentially risk-free process that serves an additional important purpose by bringing the anesthesia care provider closer to the patient. If access to the patient is limited during the procedure, FM wireless or infrared remote transmission systems are now commercially available.

Pulse Oximetry

No monitor of oxygen transport has had a greater impact on the practice of anesthesiology than the pulse oximeter.[82] Pulse oximetry is noninvasive, safe, and comfortable to the awake patient; it is also technically simple to apply and interpret, and allows continuous real-time monitoring of arterial oxygenation. The use of a quantitative measure of oxygenation is specifically mandated by the ASA standards for intraoperative monitoring. The important mechanisms whereby respiratory function may be compromised during monitored anesthesia care include the effects of sedatives and opioids on respiratory drive, upper airway patency, and protective airway reflexes. Additional important risk factors for arterial desaturation include obesity, pre-existing upper airway obstruction and respiratory disease, the extremes of age, and the lithotomy position.[83] The fundamental importance of monitoring oxygenation during monitored anesthesia care can be appreciated from the closed-claim study of Caplan et al.,[77] who examined 14 cases of sudden cardiac arrest in otherwise healthy patients who received spinal anesthesia. These major anesthetic mishaps occurred before the routine adoption of pulse oximetry. One of the major findings of this study was that cyanosis frequently heralded the onset of cardiac arrest, suggesting that unappreciated respiratory insufficiency may have played an important role. Further support for the use of pulse oximetry comes from the ASA Committee on Professional Liability analysis of closed anesthesia claims, which reveals that respiratory events constitute the single largest source of adverse outcome. Furthermore, review of these cases suggests that pulse oximetry in combination with capnometry would have prevented the adverse outcome in most cases.

Capnography

Although capnography is most effective in the intubated patient, some useful information may be obtained from a spontaneously breathing, nonintubated patient. Sidestream capnographs have been adapted for use with face masks, nasal airways, and nasal cannulae and have been used successfully during monitored anesthesia care.[84–87] Nasal cannulae for oxygen delivery have been modified to provide an integral port for respiratory gas sampling and are available commercially. Alternatively, capnograph sampling lines can be attached to shortened IV catheters and inserted inside nasal oxygen probes.

Cardiovascular System

At a minimum, the electrocardiogram must be continually displayed and the blood pressure measured and recorded at least every 5 minutes during monitored anesthesia care. The pulse should be monitored by palpation, oximetry, or auscultation. The selection of additional hemodynamic monitoring is usually determined more by the cardiovascular status of the patient than the magnitude of the procedure. Most procedures performed under monitored anesthesia care do not involve major hemorrhage, fluid shifts, or major physiologic trespass. Decisions concerning choice of monitoring for myocardial ischemia and other adverse hemodynamic events will need to be individualized on a case-by-case basis.

Temperature Monitoring and Management During Monitored Anesthesia Care

The value of temperature monitoring is well established during general anesthesia, the perioperative period being frequently complicated by hypothermia and hyperthermia. Although sedation techniques used during monitored anesthesia care do not generally trigger malignant hyperthermia, there is potential for significant inadvertent hypothermia, particularly during neuraxial anesthesia. Even monitored anesthesia care techniques unaccompanied by regional anesthesia are associated with hypothermia at the extremes of age, both the old and very young having impaired thermoregulatory mechanisms. The elderly also have markedly reduced muscle mass and therefore basal heat production. Although the anesthesiologist may be able to exert some control over the ambient temperature in the operating room, he or she may be unable to influence the temperature at remote anesthetizing locations. Radiology suites are often maintained at lower temperatures to accommodate the computer systems that are used to reconstruct images. Radiant heating lamps, forced-air heaters, fluid warmers, or warming blankets, all common items in operating rooms, may be unavailable and unsuitable for use at remote locations. Forced-air heating has been shown to be an effective means of maintaining normothermia, and can be combined with IV fluid warming.[88] Even mild perioperative hypothermia (i.e., 1 to 2°C) accompanying general anesthesia is associated with adverse myocardial outcomes, increased bleeding tendency and transfusion requirements, wound infections, and delayed wound healing and hospital discharge.[89] There is no evidence suggesting that the morbidity associated with perioperative hypothermia is any less during monitored anesthesia care than during general anesthesia. The morbidity associated with perioperative hypothermia is well described in high-risk patients; this is a group of patients who are very likely to undergo procedures under monitored anesthesia care. When hypothermia is significant, shivering may interfere with the planned procedure and markedly increase oxygen requirements and predispose susceptible patients to myocardial ischemia or respiratory insufficiency. The major thermoregulatory defenses against hypothermia include vasoconstriction, shivering, and behavior. Vasoconstriction and shivering are impaired during major conduction anesthesia. Behavioral thermoregulation is impaired even in the conscious patient. Regional anesthesia has major effects on thermoregulation.[90] Lower extremity vasodilatation causes central cooling via a redistribution of heat from the core to the periphery. Afferent input to the hypothalamus from the warm peripheral compartment counteracts conflicting input from the cooling central compartment, thus delaying the initiation of compensatory thermoregulation. In the absence of reliable temperature monitoring it is possible that the first indication of hypothermia would be the onset of shivering, by which time considerable central cooling may have occurred.

Frank and coworkers[91] have examined the issue of temperature monitoring and management during neuraxial anesthesia and found that temperature monitoring is significantly underused, with only one third of patients being monitored. Furthermore, the method that was most frequently used to monitor temperature may not accurately reflect core temperature, the most important determinant of thermoregulatory response and perioperative morbidity. Forehead skin surface was the most commonly monitored site. The accuracy of these devices for perioperative temperature monitoring remains controversial; they do not reliably detect malignant hyperthermia and are not sufficiently accurate for fever screening purposes in children.[92] Sessler[90] recommends the use of a properly positioned axillary probe or intermittent oral temperature monitoring during neuraxial anesthetics.

Patients will frequently complain of feeling too warm when covered by heavy drapes. Although malignant hyperthermia is rare during monitored anesthesia care, hyperthermia is still possible as a result of thyroid storm or malignant neuroleptic syndrome. The subjective sensation of hyperthermia may also be the first indicator of important adverse events in evolution such as hypoxia, hypercarbia, cerebral ischemia, local anesthetic toxicity, and myocardial ischemia.

Bispectral Index Monitoring During Monitored Anesthesia Care

The bispectral index (BIS) is a processed EEG parameter that was developed specifically to evaluate patient response during drug-induced anesthesia and sedation. Sedation monitoring is attractive because of the potential to titrate drugs more accurately, avoiding the adverse effects of both over- and underdosing. BIS monitoring has some potential advantages over conventional intermittent techniques of patient assessment. Conventional assessment involves patient stimulation at frequent intervals to determine the level of consciousness, requires patient cooperation, and is subject to testing fatigue. An example of a conventional assessment tool is the Observer's Assessment of Alertness/Sedation Scale (Table 31-6).[93] The BIS has been shown to be a useful monitor of drug-induced sedation and recall in volunteers and has been shown to correlate with Observer's Assessment of Alertness/Sedation Scale scores during propofol-induced sedation in patients undergoing surgery with regional anesthesia.[94] An increasing depth of sedation was associated with a predictable decrease in the BIS. Absence of recall was associated with BIS values below 80. These findings correspond with those of Kearse et al.,[95] who found no intraoperative recall at BIS values below 79 during midazolam-, isoflurane-, and propofol-induced sedation. However, the inability to recall a nonnoxious stimulus such as a picture, as used in the previously mentioned studies, may not necessarily correspond to amnesia to noxious events such as surgical stimulation. Despite this caveat, Liu and coworkers[94] suggest that using a combination of propofol and midazolam to achieve a BIS value below 80 will minimize the possibility of intraoperative recall. Although the use of BIS to monitor sedation is appealing, conventional assessment of sedation is an important mechanism whereby continuous patient contact is maintained. Ideally, BIS monitoring will be employed in the future as an adjunct to clinical evaluation rather than as the primary monitor of consciousness.

Preparedness to Recognize and Treat Local Anesthetic Toxicity

Monitored anesthesia care is often provided in the context of regional or local anesthetic techniques. It is vitally important that the anesthesiologist responsible for the patient have a high index of suspicion and be fully prepared to recognize and

TABLE 31-6

OBSERVER'S ASSESSMENT OF ALERTNESS/SEDATION SCALE

■ RESPONSIVENESS	■ SPEECH	■ FACIAL EXPRESSION	■ EYES	■ COMPOSITE SCORE
Responds readily to name spoken in normal tone	Normal	Normal	Clear, no ptosis	5 (alert)
Lethargic response to name spoken in normal tone	Mild slowing or thickening	Mild relaxation	Glazed or mild ptosis (less than half the eye)	4
Responds only after name is called loudly or repeatedly	Slurring or prominent slowing	Marked relaxation (slack jaw)	Glazed and marked ptosis (half the eye or more)	3
Responds only after mild prodding or shaking	Few recognizable words			2
Does not respond to mild prodding or shaking				1 (asleep)

treat local anesthetic toxicity immediately (see Chapter 17). This point deserves special emphasis, particularly in view of the fact that monitored anesthesia care is often provided to the elderly or debilitated patient who has been deemed "unfit" for general anesthesia; these are the patients most likely to suffer adverse reactions to local anesthetic drugs. Even if the anesthesiologist does not perform the block personally, he or she is in a unique position to fulfill an important "preventive" role by advising the surgeon about the most appropriate volume, concentration, and type of local anesthetic drug or technique to be used.

Systemic local anesthetic toxicity occurs when plasma concentrations of drug are excessively high. Plasma concentrations will increase when the rate of entry of drug into the circulation exceeds the rate of drug clearance from the circulation. The clinically recognizable effects of local anesthetics on the central nervous system are concentration-dependent. At low concentrations, sedation and numbness of the tongue and circumoral tissues and a metallic taste are prominent features. As concentrations increase, restlessness, vertigo, tinnitus, and difficulty focusing may occur. Higher concentrations result in slurred speech and skeletal muscle twitching, which often herald the onset of tonic-clonic seizures.

The conduct of monitored anesthesia care may modify the individual's response to the potentially toxic effects of local anesthetic administration and adversely affect the margin of safety of a regional or local technique. For example, a patient with compromised cardiovascular function may experience a further decline in cardiac output during sedation. The resultant reduction in hepatic blood flow will reduce the clearance of local anesthetics that are metabolized by the liver and have a high hepatic extraction ratio, thereby increasing the likelihood of achieving toxic plasma concentrations. A patient receiving sedation may experience respiratory depression and a subsequent increase in arterial carbon dioxide concentration. Hypercarbia adversely affects the margin of safety in several ways. By increasing cerebral blood flow, hypercarbia will increase the amount of local anesthetic that is delivered to the brain, thereby increasing the potential for neurotoxicity. By reducing neuronal axoplasmic pH, hypercarbia increases the intracellular concentration of the charged, active form of local anesthetic, thus also increasing its toxicity. In addition, hypercarbia, acidosis, and hypoxia all markedly potentiate the cardiovascular toxicity of local anesthetics. Furthermore, the administration of sedative–hypnotic drugs may interfere with the patient's ability to communicate the symptoms of impending neurotoxicity. However, the anticonvulsant properties of

benzodiazepines and barbiturates may attenuate the seizures associated with neurotoxicity. In both of these circumstances, it is possible that the symptoms of cardiotoxicity will be the first evidence that an adverse reaction has occurred. Thus, appropriate treatment is delayed or inadvertent intravascular injection is continued because of the absence of any clinical evidence of neurotoxicity. Cardiovascular toxicity usually occurs at a higher plasma concentration than neurotoxicity, but when it does occur, it is usually much more difficult to manage than neurotoxicity. Although cardiotoxicity is usually preceded by neurotoxicity, it may occur de novo when bupivacaine is being used.

Sedation and Analgesia by Nonanesthesiologists

Although anesthesiologists have specific training and expertise to provide sedation and analgesia, in clinical practice these services are frequently provided by nonanesthesiologists. The specific reasons for nonanesthesiologist involvement differ from institution to institution and from case to case and include convenience, availability, and scheduling issues; perceived lack of anesthesiologist enthusiasm; perceived increased cost; and a perceived lack of benefit concerning patient satisfaction and safety when sedation and analgesia are provided by anesthesiologists. Despite our frequent noninvolvement in these cases, anesthesiologists are indirectly involved in the care of these patients by being required to participate in the development of institutional policies and procedures for sedation and analgesia. To assist anesthesiologists in this process, an ASA task force has developed practice guidelines for sedation and analgesia by nonanesthesiologists.[2]

Four levels of sedation are defined in the ASA practice guidelines and include minimal sedation, moderate sedation, deep sedation, and general anesthesia. The practice guidelines emphasize that sedation and analgesia represent a continuum of sedation wherein patients can easily pass into a level of sedation deeper than intended. The ASA House of Delegates issued a statement on this continuum of depth of sedation originally in October 1999, and most recently amended it in October 2004. This statement contains a chart representing the clinical progression along this continuum (Table 31-7).[96] When monitoring a sedated patient during a procedure, it is important to recognize when a patient becomes more deeply sedated than intended so that the care team can act appropriately to prevent cardiorespiratory compromise.

TABLE 31-7

CONTINUUM OF DEPTH OF SEDATION

	■ MINIMAL SEDATION	■ MODERATE SEDATION	■ DEEP SEDATION	■ GENERAL SEDATION
Responsiveness	Normal response to verbal stimulation	Purposeful response to verbal or tactile stimulation	Purposeful response following repeated or painful stimulation	Unarousable, even with a painful stimulus
Airway	Unaffected	No intervention required	Intervention may be required	Intervention often required
Spontaneous ventilation	Unaffected	Adequate	May be inadequate	Frequently inadequate
Cardiovascular function	Unaffected	Usually maintained	Usually maintained	May be impaired

Adapted from ASA House of Delegates: Continuum of Depth of Sedation, www.asahq.org, 2004.

The guidelines emphasize the importance of preprocedure patient evaluation, patient preparation, and appropriate fasting periods. The importance of continuous patient monitoring is discussed—in particular, the response of the patient to commands as a guide to the level of sedation. The appropriate monitoring of pulmonary ventilation, oxygenation, and hemodynamics is also discussed, and recommendations are made for the contemporaneous recording of these parameters. The task force strongly suggests that an individual other than the person performing the procedure be available to monitor the patient's comfort and physiologic status. Education and training of providers is recommended. Specific educational objectives include the potentiation of sedative- induced respiratory depression by concomitantly administered opioids, adequate time intervals between doses of sedative/analgesics to avoid cumulative overdosage, and familiarity with sedative/analgesic antagonists. The routine administration of supplemental oxygen is recommended. At least one person with advanced life support skills should be present during the procedure. This individual should have the ability to recognize airway obstruction, establish an airway, and maintain oxygenation and ventilation. The practice guidelines recommend that appropriate patient-size emergency equipment be readily available, specifically including equipment for establishing an airway and delivering positive pressure ventilation with supplemental oxygen, emergency resuscitation drugs, and a working defibrillator. The presence of reliable intravenous access until the patient is no longer at risk for cardiorespiratory depression will improve safety. Adequate postprocedure recovery care with appropriate monitoring must be provided until discharge. Certain high-risk patient groups (e.g., uncooperative patients, extremes of age, severe cardiac, pulmonary, hepatic, renal, or central nervous system disease, morbid obesity, sleep apnea, pregnancy, and patients who abuse drug or alcohol) will be encountered, and the guidelines recommend that preprocedure consultation with anesthesiologists, cardiologists, pulmonologists, and so forth be performed *before* administration of sedation and analgesia by nonanesthesiologists.

Controversy exists regarding the level of training required for nonanesthesiologists to be credentialed to provide moderate and deep sedation. The ASA released a statement in October 2005, amended in October 2006, suggesting a framework for granting privileges that will help ensure competence of individuals who administer or supervise the administration of moderate sedation.[97] This statement suggests that the practitioner should complete formal training in (1) the safe administration of sedative and analgesic drugs used to establish a level of moderate sedation, and (2) rescue of patients who exhibit adverse physiologic consequences of a deeper-than-intended level of sedation. Following is an excerpt from separate ASA statement concerning deep sedation released in October 2006.[98]

> *Because of the significant risk that patients who receive deep sedation may enter a state of general anesthesia, privileges to administer deep sedation should be granted only to practitioners who are qualified to administer general anesthesia or to appropriately supervised anesthesia professionals.*

Finally, it is instructive to review an excerpt from the joint statement released in 2004 by the American Association of Nurse Anesthetists and the ASA[46]:

> *Whenever propofol is used for sedation/anesthesia, it should be administered only by persons trained in the administration of general anesthesia, who are not simultaneously involved in these surgical or diagnostic procedures. This restriction is concordant with specific language in the propofol package insert, and failure to follow these recommendations could put patients at increased risk of significant injury or death.*

CONCLUSION

Through the use of monitored anesthesia care, an often terrifying and painful procedure can be made safe and comfortable for the patient. Monitored anesthesia care presents an opportunity for our patients to observe us at work. For the anesthesiologist, monitored anesthesia care presents an opportunity to provide a more prolonged and intimate level of care and reassurance to our patients that is in contrast to the more limited exposure that occurs during and after general anesthesia. Our airway management skills and our daily practice of applied pharmacology make us uniquely qualified to provide this service. Monitored anesthesia care presents us with an opportunity to display these skills and increase our recognition in areas outside the operating room. The availability of drugs with a more favorable pharmacologic profile allows us to tailor our techniques to provide the specific components of analgesia, sedation, anxiolysis, and amnesia with minimal morbidity and to facilitate a prompt recovery. As the population ages, increasing numbers of patients will become candidates for monitored anesthesia care. Significant advances in nonsurgical fields (e.g., interventional radiology) will increase the number of procedures that are ideally performed under monitored anesthesia care. It is our responsibility to clearly demonstrate to our nonanesthesia colleagues that anesthesiologist-provided monitored anesthesia care contributes to the best outcome for our patients. If anesthesiologists are not willing or able to provide these services, others, who are less well qualified, are prepared to assume that role.

References

1. American Society of Anesthesiologists: Distinguishing moderate anesthesia from moderate sedation/analgesia. www.asahq.org, 2004
2. American Society of Anesthesiologists Task Force: Practice guidelines for sedation and analgesia by non-anesthesiologists. Anesthesiology 2002; 96: 1004
3. American Society of Anesthesiologists: Position on monitored anesthesia care. www.asahq.org, 2005
4. Ausems ME, Vuyk J, Hug CC Jr et al: Comparison of a computer-assisted infusion versus intermittent bolus administration of alfentanil as a supplement to nitrous oxide for lower abdominal surgery. Anesthesiology 1988; 68: 851
5. Hughes MA, Glass PSA, Jacobs JR: Context-sensitive half-time in multicompartment pharmacokinetic models for intravenous anesthetic drugs. Anesthesiology 1992; 76: 334
6. Scott JC, Ponganis KV, Stanski DR: EEG quantitation of narcotic effect: The comparative pharmacodynamics of fentanyl and alfentanil. Anesthesiology 1985; 62: 234
7. Mandema JW, Tuk B, van Steveninck AL et al: Pharmacokinetic-pharmacodynamic modeling of the central nervous system effects of midazolam and its main metabolite α-hydroxy-midazolam in healthy volunteers. Clin Pharmacol Ther 1992; 521: 715
8. Buhrer M, Maitre PO, Crevoisier C et al: Electroencephalographic effects of benzodiazepines. II. Pharmacodynamic modeling of the effects of midazolam and diazepam. Clin Pharmacol Ther 1990; 48: 555
9. Glass P, Dyar O, Jhaveri R et al: TIVA-propofol and combinations of propofol with fentanyl [abstract]. Anesthesiology 1991; 75: A44
10. Smith C, McEwan AI, Jhaveri R et al: Reduction of propofol Cp50 by fentanyl [abstract]. Anesthesiology 1992; 77: A340
11. Short TG, Chui PT: Propofol and midazolam act synergistically in combination. Br J Anaesth 1991; 67: 539
12. Short TG, Plummer JL, Chui PT: Hypnotic and anesthetic interactions between midazolam, propofol and alfentanil. Br J Anaesth 1992; 69: 162
13. McEwan A, Smith C, Dyar O et al: MAC reduction of isoflurane by fentanyl [abstract]. Anesthesiology 1991; 75: A43
14. Sebel PS, Glass PSA, Fletcher JE et al: Reduction of the MAC of desflurane with fentanyl. Anesthesiology 1992; 76: 52
15. Vinik HR, Bradley EL, Kissin I: Midazolam–alfentanil synergism for anesthetic induction in patients. Anesth Analg 1989; 69: 213
16. Kissin I, Vinik HR, Castillo R et al: Alfentanil potentiates midazolam-induced unconsciousness in subanalgesic doses. Anesth Analg 1990; 71: 65
17. Federal Food and Drug Administration: Warning reemphasized in midazolam labeling. FDA Drug Bulletin 1987; 5
18. Bailey PL, Pace NL, Ashburn MA et al: Frequent hypoxemia and apnea after sedation with midazolam and fentanyl. Anesthesiology 1990; 73: 826

19. Mackenzie N, Grant IS: Propofol for intravenous sedation. Anaesthesia 1987; 42: 3
20. Smith I, Monk T, White PF et al: Propofol infusion during regional anesthesia: Sedative, hypnotic and amnestic properties. Anesth Analg 1994; 79: 313
21. Dubois A, Balatoni E, Peeters JP et al: Use of propofol for sedation during gastrointestinal endoscopies. Anaesthesia 1988; 43(Suppl): 75
22. Kain ZN, Gaal D, Jaeger DD et al: Sedation for MRI in children: Propofol vs. barbiturates [abstract]. Anesthesiology 1993; 79: A1158
23. Monk TG, Boure B, White PF et al: Comparison of intravenous sedative-hypnotic techniques for outpatient immersion lithotripsy. Anesth Analg 1991; 72: 616
24. Sherry E: Admixture of propofol and alfentanil: Use for intravenous sedation and analgesia during transvaginal oocyte retrieval. Anaesthesia 1992; 47: 477
25. Oei-Lim LB, Vermeulen-Cranch DME, Bouvry-Berends ECM: Conscious sedation with propofol in dentistry. Br Dent J 1991; 170: 340
26. Whitehead C, Sanders LD, Oldroyd G et al: The subjective effects of low dose propofol. Anaesthesia 1994; 49: 490
27. Borgeat A, Wilder-Smith OHG, Saiah M et al: Subhypnotic doses of propofol possess direct antiemetic properties. Anesth Analg 1992; 74: 539
28. White PF, Negus JB: Sedative infusions during local and regional anesthesia: A comparison of midazolam and propofol. J Clin Anesth 1991; 3: 32
29. Ghouri AF, Ramirez Ruiz MA, White PF: Effect of flumazenil on recovery after midazolam and propofol sedation. Anesthesiology 1994; 81: 333
30. Smith I, White PF, Nathanson M et al: Propofol: An update on its clinical use. Anesthesiology 1994; 81: 1005
31. Stoelting RK, Hillier SC: Benzodiazepines, Pharmacology and Physiology in Anesthetic Practice, 4th edition. Philadelphia, JB Lippincott, 2006
32. Taylor E, Ghouri AF, White PF: Midazolam in combination with propofol for sedation during local anesthesia. J Clin Anesth 1992; 4: 213
33. Jacobs JR, Reves JG, Marty J et al: Aging increases pharmacodynamic sensitivity to the hypnotic effects of midazolam. Anesth Analg 1995; 80: 143
34. Pratila MG, Fischer ME, Alagesan R et al: Propofol vs. midazolam for monitored sedation: A comparison of intraoperative and recovery parameters. J Clin Anesth 1993; 5: 268
35. Ghouri AF, Ramirez Ruiz MA, White PF: Effect of flumazenil on recovery after midazolam and propofol sedation. Anesthesiology 1994; 81: 333
36. Yee JB, Schafer PG, Crandall AS et al: Comparison of methohexital and alfentanil on movement during placement of retrobulbar nerve block. Anesth Analg 1994; 79: 320
37. Veselis RA, Reinsel RA, Feshchenko VA et al: Impaired memory and behavioural performance with fentanyl at low plasma concentrations. Anesth Analg 1994; 79: 952
38. Glass PSA, Gan TJ, Howell S: A review of the pharmacokinetics and pharmacodynamics of remifentanil. Anesth Analg 1999; 89(Suppl): S7
39. Servin F, Desmonts JM, Watkins WD: Remifentanil as an analgesic adjunct in local/regional anesthesia and monitored anesthesia care. Anesth Analg 1999; 89(Suppl): S28
40. Avramov MN, Smith I, White PF: Interactions between midazolam and remifentanil during monitored anesthesia care. Anesthesiology 1996; 85: 1283
41. Ahmad S, Leavell M, Fragen RJ et al: Remifentanil versus alfentanil as analgesic adjuncts during placement of ophthalmologic nerve blocks. Reg Analg Pain Med. 1999; 24: 331
42. Gold MI, Watkins WD, Sung YF et al: Remifentanil versus remifentanil/midazolam for ambulatory surgery during monitored anesthesia care. Anesthesiology 1997; 87: 51
43. Green SM, Klooster M, Harris T et al: Ketamine sedation for pediatric gastroenterology procedures. Pediatr Gastroenterol Nutr 2001; 32: 26
44. McCarty EC, Mencio GA, Walker LA et al: Ketamine sedation for the reduction of children's fractures in the emergency department. J Bone Surg 2000; 82: 912
45. Sherwin TS, Green SM, Khan A et al: Does adjunctive midazolam reduce recovery agitation after ketamine sedation for pediatric procedures? A randomized, double blind, placebo-controlled trial. Ann Emerg Med 2000; 35: 229
46. The American Society of Anesthesiologists: Position Statement on Safe use of Propofol. www.asahq.org 2004
47. Hsu YW. Cortinez LI. Robertson KM et al. Dexmedetomidine pharmacodynamics: part I: crossover comparison of the respiratory effects of dexmedetomidine and remifentanil in healthy volunteers. Anesthesiology. 2004; 101: 1066
48. Ho AM, Chen S, Karmakar MK: Central apnoea after balanced general anaesthesia that included dexmedetomidine. Br J Anaesth 2005; 95: 773
49. Maroof M, Khan RM, Jain D, et al: Dexmedetomidine is a useful adjunct for awake intubation. Can J Anaesth 2005; 52: 776-50
50. Videira RL, Ferreira RM: Dexmedetomidine and asystole. Anesthesiology 2004; 101: 1479
51. Talke P, Richardson CA, Scheinin M et al: Postoperative pharmacokinetics and sympatholytic effects of dexmedetomidine. Anesth Analg 1997; 85: 1136
52. Bekker AY, Kaufman B, Samir H et al: The use of dexmedetomidine infusion for awake craniotomy. Anesth Analg 2001; 92: 1251
53. Ard J, Doyle W, Bekker A: Awake craniotomy with dexmedetomidine in pediatric patients. J Neurosurg Anesthesiol 2003; 15: 263

54. Bekker AY, Basile J, Gold M et al: Dexmedetomidine for awake carotid endarterectomy: Efficacy, hemodynamic profile, and side effects. J Neurosurg Anesthesiol 2004; 16: 126
55. Drummond JC, Dao AV, Roth DM et al: Effect of dexmedetomidine on cerebral blood flow velocity, cerebral metabolic rate, and carbon dioxide response in normal humans. Anesthesiology 2008; 108: 225
56. Bekker A, Gold M, Ahmed R et al: Dexmedetomidine does not increase the incidence of intracarotid shunting in patients undergoing awake carotid endarterectomy. Anesth Analg 2006; 103: 955
57. Arain SR, Ebert TJ: The efficacy, side effects, and recovery characteristics of dexmedetomidine versus propofol when used for intraoperative sedation. Anesth Analg 2002; 95: 461
58. Mason KP, Zgleszewski SE: Hemodynamic effects of dexmedetomidine sedation for CT imaging studies. Paediatr Anaesth 2008; 18: 393
59. Mason KP, Zurakowski D, Zgleszewski SE et al: High dose dexmedetomidine as the sole sedative for pediatric MRI. Paediatr Anaesth 2008; 18: 403
60. Veselis RA, Reinsel RA, Feshchenko VA et al : Information loss over time defines the memory defect of propofol: A comparative response with thiopental and dexmedetomidine. Anesthesiology 2004; 101: 831
61. Veselis RA: Memory: A guide for anaesthetists. Best Pract Res Clin Anaesthes 2007; 21: 297
62. Perry F, Parker RK, White PF et al: Role of psychological factors in postoperative pain control and recovery with patient-controlled analgesia. Clin J Pain 1994; 10: 57
63. Rudkin GE, Osborne GA, Curtis NJ: Intraoperative patient controlled sedation. Anaesthesia 1991; 46: 90
64. Park WY, Watkins PA: Patient-controlled sedation during epidural anesthesia. Anesth Analg 1991; 72: 304
65. Cork R, Guillory E, Viswanathan S: Effect of patient-controlled sedation on recovery from ambulatory monitored anesthesia care [abstract]. Anesthesiology 1994; 81: A31
66. Zelcer J, White PF, Chester S et al: Intraoperative patient-controlled analgesia: An alternative to physician administration during outpatient monitored anesthesia care. Anesth Analg 1992; 75: 41
67. Montravers P, Duriel B, Molliex S et al: Effects of intravenous midazolam on the work of breathing. Anesth Analg 1994; 79: 558
68. Gelb A, Southorn P, Redher K et al: Sedation and respiratory mechanics in man. Br J Anaesth 1983; 57: 1104
67. Morel DR, Forster A, Bachmann M et al: Effect of intravenous midazolam on breathing pattern and chest wall mechanics in humans. J Appl Physiol 1983; 55: 419
68. Prato FS, Knill RL: Diazepam sedation reduces functional residual capacity and alters the distribution of ventilation in man. Anesth Analg 1982; 61: 209
69. Cohen MI: Phrenic and recurrent laryngeal discharge patterns and the Hering-Breuer reflex. Am J Physiol 1975; 228: 1489
70. Gottfried SR, Strohl KP, Van de Graaff W et al: Effects of phrenic stimulation on upper airway resistance in anesthetized dogs. J Appl Physiol 1983; 55: 419
71. Leiter JC, Knuth SL, Krol ZRC et al: The effects of diazepam on genioglossal muscle activity in normal subjects. Am Rev Respir Dis 1985; 132: 216
72. Montravers P, Dureuil B, Desmonts JM: Effects of i.v. midazolam on upper airway resistance. Br J Anaesth 1992; 68: 27
73. Rimaniol JM, D'Honneur G, Duvaldestin P: Recovery of the swallowing reflex after propofol anesthesia. Anesth Analg 1994; 79: 856
74. Groves ND, Rees JL: Effects of benzodiazepines on laryngeal reflexes. Anaesthesia 1987; 42: 808
75. Lambert Y, D'Honneur G, Abhay K et al: Depression of swallowing reflex two hours after midazolam [abstract]. Anesthesiology 1991; 75: A891
76. Nishino T, Takizawa K, Yokokawa N et al: Depression of the swallowing reflex during sedation and/or relative analgesia produced by inhalation of 50% nitrous oxide in oxygen. Anesthesiology 1987; 67: 995
77. Caplan RA, Ward RJ, Posner K et al: Unexpected cardiac arrest during spinal anesthesia: A closed claims analysis of predisposing factors. Anesthesiology 1988; 68: 5
78. Weil JV, McCullocugh RE, Kline JS et al: Diminished ventilatory response to hypoxia and hypercapnia after morphine in normal man. N Engl J Med 1975; 292: 1103
79. Power SJ, Morgan M, Chakrabarti MK: Carbon dioxide response curves following midazolam and diazepam. Br J Anaesth 1983; 55: 837
80. Jordan C, Lehane JR, Jones JG: Respiratory depression following diazepam: Reversal with high dose naloxone. Anesthesiology 1980; 53: 293
81. American Society of Anesthesiologists: Standards for Basic Intraoperative Monitoring. www.asahq.org, 2005
82. Barker SJ, Tremper KK: Pulse oximetry, Anesthetic Equipment: Principles and Applications. Edited by Ehrenworth J, Eisenkraft J. St Louis, CV Mosby, 1993, p 249
83. Raemer DB, Warren DL, Morris R et al: Hypoxemia during ambulatory gynecologic surgery as evaluated by the pulse oximeter. J Clin Monit 1987; 3: 244
84. Pressman MA: A simple method for measuring end-tidal CO_2 during MAC and major regional anesthesia. Anesth Analg 1988; 67: 900
85. Norman EA, Zeig NJ, Ahmad I: Better designs for mass spectrometer monitoring of the awake patient [letter]. Anesthesiology 1986; 64: 664
86. Bowe EA, Boysen PG, Brome JA et al: Accurate determination of end-tidal CO_2 through nasal cannulae. J Clin Monit 1989; 5: 105

ANESTHETIC MANAGEMENT

87. Goldmann JM: A simple and inexpensive method for monitoring end-tidal CO_2 through nasal cannulae [letter]. Anesthesiology 1987; 67: 606

88. Kurz A, Kurz M, Poeschl G et al: Forced-air warming maintains intra-operative normothermia better than circulating-water mattresses. Anesth Analg 1993; 77: 89

89. Frank SM, Fleisher LA, Breslow MJ et al: Perioperative maintenance of normothermia reduces the incidence of morbid cardiac events: a randomized trial. JAMA 1997; 277: 1127

90. Sessler DI: Temperature monitoring and management during neuraxial anesthesia. Anesth Analg 1999; 88: 243

91. Frank SM, Nguyen JM, Garcia CM et al: Temperature monitoring practices during regional anesthesia. Anesth Analg 1999; 88: 373

92. Scholefield JH, Gerber MA, Dwyer P: Liquid crystal forehead temperature strips. Am J Dis Child 1982; 136: 198

93. Chernik DA, Gillings D, Laine H et al: Validity and reliability of the observer's assessment of alertness/sedation scale: Study with intravenous midazolam. J Clin Psychopharmacol 1990; 10: 244

94. Liu J, Singh HS, White PF: Electroencephalographic bispectral index correlates with intraoperative recall and depth of propofol induced sedation. Anesth Analg 1997; 84: 185

95. Kearse LA, Manberg P, Chamoun N et al: Bispectral analysis of the electroencephalogram correlates with patient movement to skin incision during propofol/nitrous oxide anesthesia. Anesthesiology 1994; 81: 1365

96. American Society of Anesthesiologists: Continuum of depth of sedation, definition of general anesthesia and levels of sedation/analgesia. www.asahq.org, 2004

97. American Society of Anesthesiologists: Statement on granting privileges for administration of moderate sedation to practitioners who are not anesthesia professionals. www.asahq.org, 2006

98. American Society of Anesthesiologists: Statement on granting privileges to nonanesthesiologists practitioners for personally administering deep sedation or supervising deep sedation by individuals who are not anesthesia professionals. www.asahq.org, 2006

CHAPTER 32 ■ AMBULATORY ANESTHESIA

J. LANCE LICHTOR

PLACE, PROCEDURES, AND PATIENT SELECTION
PREOPERATIVE EVALUATION AND REDUCTION OF
    PATIENT ANXIETY
    Upper Respiratory Tract Infection
    Restriction of Food and Liquids Before
        Ambulatory Surgery
    Anxiety Reduction
MANAGING THE ANESTHETIC: PREMEDICATION
    Benzodiazepines
    Opioids and Nonsteroidal Analgesics

INTRAOPERATIVE MANAGEMENT: CHOICE OF
    ANESTHETIC METHOD
    Regional Techniques
    Sedation and Analgesia
    General Anesthesia
MANAGEMENT OF POSTANESTHESIA CARE
    Reversal of Drug Effects
    Nausea and Vomiting
    Pain
    Preparation for Discharging the Patient

KEY POINTS

1 Procedures appropriate for ambulatory surgery are those associated with postoperative care that is easily managed at home and with low rates of postoperative complications that require intensive physician or nursing management.

2 Whatever their age, ambulatory surgery is no longer restricted to patients of ASA physical status I or II. Patients of ASA physical status III or IV are appropriate candidates, providing their systemic diseases are medically stable.

3 In the 2006 ASA guidelines, the authors state that for patients with OSA, if a procedure is typically performed as an outpatient procedure and local or regional anesthesia is used, that the procedure can also be performed as an ambulatory procedure.

4 For adults, airflow obstruction has been shown to persist for up to 6 weeks after viral respiratory infections. For that reason, surgery should be delayed if an adult presents with a URI until 6 weeks have elapsed.

5 In 1999, the ASA published practice guidelines for preoperative fasting. The guidelines allow a patient to have a light meal up to 6 hours before an elective procedure and support a fasting period for clear liquids of 2 hours for all patients.

6 In a meta-analysis of peripheral nerve and centroneuraxial blocks compared to general anesthesia, time until discharge from the ambulatory surgery unit was no different for the three groups.

7 Postoperative pain control is best with regional techniques.

8 Nerve blocks using catheters can be placed before surgery that can be used to provide analgesia after the operation.

9 After induction doses of propofol or thiopental, impairment after thiopental can be apparent for up to 5 hours, but only for 1 hour after propofol.

10 Although many factors affect the choice of agents for maintenance of anesthesia, two primary concerns for ambulatory anesthesia are speed of wake-up and incidence of postoperative nausea and vomiting.

11 It is important to distinguish between wake-up time and discharge time. Patients may emerge from anesthesia with desflurane and nitrous oxide significantly faster than after propofol or sevoflurane and nitrous oxide, though the ability to sit up, stand, and tolerate fluids and the time to fitness for discharge may be no different.

12 Nausea, with or without vomiting, is probably the most important factor contributing to a delay in discharge of patients and an increase in unanticipated admissions of both children and adults after ambulatory surgery.

13 In addition to the PACU, many ambulatory surgery centers in the United States have another area, often known as a phase II recovery room, where patients may stay until they are able to tolerate liquids, walk, and/or void.

PLACE, PROCEDURES, AND PATIENT SELECTION

Ambulatory surgery occurs in a variety of settings. Some centers are within a hospital or in a freestanding satellite facility that is either part of or independent from a hospital. The independent facilities are often for-profit and not located in rural or inner-city areas. Some private companies acquire or build ambulatory facilities and then work usually with local surgeons who become the company's affiliated staff. Physicians' offices may also serve for procedures. Freestanding, independent facilities will continue to grow in number and popularity, although some consumers prefer care in units affiliated with hospitals.

A major concern of freestanding ambulatory surgery growth is that the surgery centers may force some hospitals out of business. This issue can be particularly problematic in areas in which population density or median income is low. Hospitals usually are nonprofit and care for patients who both can and cannot pay. Freestanding ambulatory facilities may also be nonprofit but usually do not provide charity care.

Some surgeons may work exclusively in a freestanding facility and not be on the staff of a hospital. A requirement for hospital staff privileges frequently is that a physician provides coverage for the hospital's emergency department. Some hospitals have lost emergency department coverage for an entire surgical specialty because that surgical specialty works exclusively in a freestanding facility.

The Centers for Medicare and Medicaid Services (CMS) is the U.S. federal agency that administers Medicare. CMS, in a set of regulations that were disclosed in July 2007, generally will pay ambulatory centers 65% of what hospital outpatient surgical facilities receive. For device-intensive procedures, though, ambulatory surgery centers will be paid the same as hospitals. For procedures that usually are performed in an office, ambulatory surgery centers will receive the lesser of 65% or Medicare's standard physician practice fee. This payment rate will be phased in from 2008 to 2011. The payment system may force some ambulatory facilities to decide whether they accept Medicare patients. At that time also, CMS added more than 700 procedures to the acceptable list of ambulatory procedures, making the total number of covered procedures about 3,300.

① Procedures appropriate for ambulatory surgery are those associated with postoperative care that are easily managed at home and with low rates of postoperative complications that require intensive physician or nursing management. Establishing a low rate of postoperative complication depends on the relative aggressiveness of the facility, surgeon, patient, and payer. For example, procedures that postoperatively result in intense pain may be treated with continuous regional techniques that are continued at home, whereas in other settings these procedures are limited to inpatients.

Scoring systems have been developed to help determine the likelihood of hospital admission after ambulatory surgery. One system is based on patients who were hospitalized after ambulatory surgery.[1] Patients receive one point if they are older than 65 years, have an operating time longer than 120 minutes, cardiac diagnoses, peripheral vascular disease, cerebrovascular disease, malignancy, positive human immunodeficiency virus status; and if regional anesthesia is used. Patients who receive general anesthesia get 2 points. Patients with a score of 3 have 21 times the odds of hospital admission of those with a score of 0 or 1, and patients with scores >3 have 32 times the odds.

Many facilities set a 4-hour limit as a criterion for performing a procedure. Patients undergoing longer procedures should have their operations earlier in the day, primarily because in most freestanding facilities, the anesthesiologist cannot leave until the last patient is discharged. The need for transfusion is also not a contraindication for ambulatory procedures. Some patients undergoing outpatient liposuction, for example, are given autologous blood. Because of blood banking issues, though, ambulatory procedures that require the use of a blood bank are more commonly performed in larger facilities. Freestanding dialysis facilities commonly receive blood shipped from a blood bank located elsewhere and the same can be set up with free standing ambulatory surgery facilities. The key is to have proper procedures established.

Some have wondered about the safety of performing liposuction in an office, following reports of death after the procedure in Florida. Thrombophlebitis was the cause of death in 9 of 11 patients who died in Florida from 2000 to 2006 after abdominoplasty and liposuction.[2] In a survey of 7,010 patients undergoing abdominal liposuction, the incidence of deep vein thrombosis was 0.04% and that of pulmonary embolus was 0.02%.[3] It is hoped that organizations will soon provide better guidelines for stratifying risk and strategies to prevent venous thromboembolism after liposuction surgery.

Infants whose postconceptual age is <46 weeks, or if their age is <60 weeks but they also have a history of chronic lung or neurologic disease, or who have anemia (hemoglobin <6 mmol/L) should be monitored for 12 hours after their procedure because they are at risk of developing apnea even without a history of apnea.[4] Infants older than 46 weeks and <60 weeks without disease should be monitored for 6 hours after their procedure. Some have found that spinal anesthesia without the use of other drugs intraoperatively or postoperatively is not associated with apnea;

although in one study of 62 premature and former-premature infants who underwent surgery using spinal anesthesia, postoperative apnea was seen in 5 of 55 premature infants.[5] Intravenous caffeine, 10 mg/kg, may help prevent apnea in infants (see also Chapter 44).

At the other extreme of life, advanced age alone is not a reason to disallow surgery in an ambulatory setting. Age, however, does affect the pharmacokinetics of drugs. Even short-acting drugs such as midazolam and propofol have decreased clearance in older individuals. In addition, as previously mentioned, increased age may be a factor that affects the likelihood of unanticipated admission.

Admission, by itself, is not necessarily bad if it results in a better quality of care or uncovers the need for more extensive surgery. With proper patient selection for ambulatory procedures, which are usually elective, the incidence of readmission should be very low. Most medical problems that older individuals may experience after ambulatory procedures are not related to patient age, but to specific organ dysfunction. For that reason, all individuals, whether young or old, deserve a careful preoperative history and physical examination.

② Whatever their age, ambulatory surgery is no longer restricted to patients of American Society of Anesthesiologists (ASA) physical status I or II. Patients of ASA physical status III or IV are appropriate candidates, providing their systemic diseases are medically stable. In a review of ASA III patients who were compared with ASA I or II patients undergoing outpatient surgery, no significant increase in unplanned admissions, unplanned contact with health professionals, and postoperative complications was found.[6] Certainly, not all life-threatening diseases have been studied as to how appropriate such patients with these diseases might be if they were to undergo ambulatory surgery. Yet, of those patients with such diseases who have been studied, the disease label itself does not seem to preclude an ambulatory surgical procedure.

Patients who are obese represent a special situation. They are not more likely to have adverse outcomes, although they have a higher incidence of obstructive sleep apnea (OSA). In a review of 258 morbidly obese patients who underwent outpatient surgery, compared with patients who were not morbidly obese, there was not a greater incidence of unplanned admissions, minor complications, or unplanned contact with health care professionals.[7] In another study, 3,900 patients received a risk factor questionnaire after ambulatory surgery; symptoms were not related to body mass index.[8] The ASA has published practice guidelines for the perioperative management of patients **③** with OSA.[9] In those guidelines, the authors state that for patients with OSA, if a procedure is typically performed as an outpatient procedure and local or regional anesthesia is used, the procedure can also be performed as an ambulatory procedure. Yet for patients who are at increased risk for perioperative complications, the procedure should not be performed in a freestanding ambulatory surgery facility. Table 32-1 presents a more complete list of recommended ambulatory procedures for patients with OSA, based on the ASA guidelines.

Patients who undergo ambulatory surgery should have someone to take them home and stay with them afterward to provide care. Before the procedure, the patient should receive information about the procedure itself, where it will be performed, laboratory studies that will be ordered, and dietary restrictions. The patient must understand that he or she will be going home on the day of surgery. The patient, or some responsible person, must ensure all instructions are followed. Once at home, the patient must be able to tolerate the pain from the procedure, assuming adequate pain therapy is provided. The majority of patients are satisfied with early discharge, although a few prefer a longer stay in the hospital. Patients for certain procedures such as laparoscopic cholecystectomy or transurethral resection of the prostate should live close to the ambulatory

TABLE 32-1

CONSULTANT OPINIONS REGARDING PROCEDURES THAT MAY BE PERFORMED SAFELY ON AN OUTPATIENT BASIS FOR PATIENTS AT INCREASED PERIOPERATIVE RISK FROM OBSTRUCTIVE SLEEP APNEA

■ TYPE OF SURGERY/ ANESTHESIA	■ CONSULTANT OPINION
Superficial surgery/local or regional anesthesia	Agree
Superficial surgery/general anesthesia	Equivocal
Airway surgery (adult, e.g., UPPP)	Disagree
Tonsillectomy in children <3 years old	Disagree
Tonsillectomy in children >3 years old	Equivocal
Minor orthopaedic surgery/local or regional anesthesia	Agree
Minor orthopaedic surgery/general anesthesia	Equivocal
Gynecologic laparoscopy	Equivocal
Laparoscopic surgery, upper abdomen	Disagree
Lithotripsy	Agree

UPPP, uvulopalatopharyngoplasty.
From Gross JB, Bachenberg KL, Benumof JL et al: Practice guidelines for the perioperative management of patients with obstructive sleep apnea: A report by the American Society of Anesthesiologists Task Force on Perioperative Management of patients with obstructive sleep apnea. Anesthesiology 2006; 104: 1081, with permission.

facility because postoperative complications may require their prompt return. "Reasonable" distance and time for the patient to get care if problems arise are not easily defined. This issue must be addressed by each facility and by each patient, and also depends on the type of surgery to be performed.

PREOPERATIVE EVALUATION AND REDUCTION OF PATIENT ANXIETY

Each outpatient facility should develop its own method of preoperative screening to be conducted before the day of surgery. The patient may visit the facility or staff members may telephone to obtain necessary information about the patient, including a complete medical history of the patient and family, the medications the patient is taking, and the problems the patient or the patient's family may have had with previous anesthetics. In a study of the usefulness of a preoperative screening telephone call, patients were less likely to cancel surgery if they had been screened beforehand.[10] The screening may uncover the need for transportation to the facility or the need for child care. The process also provides the staff with an opportunity to remind patients of arrival time, suitable attire, and dietary restrictions (e.g., nothing to eat or drink after midnight, no jewelry or makeup). Staff members can determine whether a responsible person is available to escort the patient to and from the facility and care for the patient at home after surgery. The screening is the ideal time for the anesthesiologist to talk with the patient, but if that is not possible, the anesthesiologist may review the screening record to determine whether additional evaluation by other consultants is necessary and whether laboratory tests must be obtained. Patients who do not show up for their clinic appointment may be more likely not to show up for their operation.[11]

Automated history-taking may also prove beneficial during the screening of a patient. Computerized questionnaires or checklists with plastic overlays automate the taking of patient histories, flag problem areas, and suggest laboratory tests to be ordered. Such devices can also be used in a surgeon's office, both to guide the surgeon in the selection of laboratory tests and to serve as a medical summary for the anesthesiologist. Such devices are particularly useful to control the cost of preoperative testing. They enable test ordering based on information obtained from a patient's responses to health questions, thus eliminating requests for tests that are not warranted by history or physical examination.

Upper Respiratory Tract Infection

For adults, airflow obstruction has been shown to persist for up to 6 weeks after viral respiratory infections. For that reason, surgery should be delayed if an adult presents with an upper respiratory infection (URI) until 6 weeks have elapsed. In the case of children, whether surgery should be delayed for that length of time is questionable. In one study of 1,078 children 1 month to 18 years of age, risk factors for adverse respiratory events in children with URIs were examined.[12] The authors could find no difference in laryngospasm or bronchospasm if the children had active URIs, a URI within 4 weeks, or no symptoms. But children with active or recent URIs had more episodes of breath holding, incidences of desaturation <90%, and more respiratory events compared with children without symptoms (Fig. 32-1). Although a case may be cancelled because a child is symptomatic, the child may develop another URI when the procedure is rescheduled. In children, URI has not been shown to be associated with an increased length of stay in the hospital after a procedure. Independent risk factors for adverse respiratory events in children with URIs include use of an endotracheal tube (versus use of a laryngeal mask airway [LMA] or face mask), history of prematurity, history of reactive airway disease, history of parental smoking, surgery involving the airway, presence of copious secretions, and nasal congestion. Generally, if a patient with a URI has a normal appetite, does not have a fever or an elevated respiratory rate, and does not appear toxic, it is probably safe to proceed with the planned procedure.

Restriction of Food and Liquids Before Ambulatory Surgery

To decrease the risk of aspiration of gastric contents, patients are routinely asked not to eat or drink anything (non per os

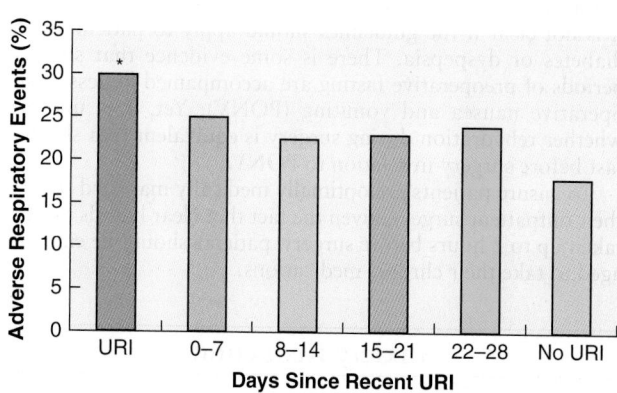

FIGURE 32-1. Adverse respiratory events are similar between children with an upper respiratory infection (URI) and a recent URI, and this similarity persists for at least 4 weeks after the URI.[12] *p <0.05 versus no URI. (Reprinted from Tait AR, Malviya S, Voepel-Lewis T et al: Risk factors for perioperative adverse respiratory events in children with upper respiratory tract infections. Anesthesiology 2001; 95: 299, with permission.)

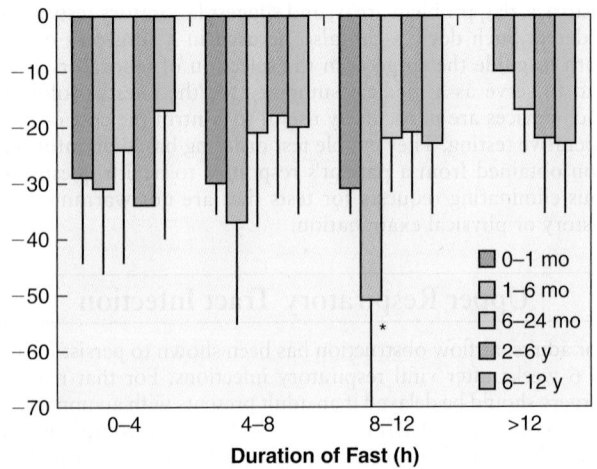

FIGURE 32-2.   Blood pressure is lower in children 1 to 6 months of age who fast more than 8 hours, compared with those who fast for less than 4 hours.[13] Illustrated are changes in systolic blood pressure from baseline to the time when 2 minimum alveolar concentration halothane was reached in 250 infants and children. *p <0.05 versus 0- to 4-hour fasting group. (Reprinted from Friesen RH, Wurl JL, Friesen RM: Duration of preoperative fast correlates with arterial blood pressure response to halothane in infants. Anesth Analg 2002; 95: 1572, with permission.)

[NPO] or "nothing by mouth") for at least 6 to 8 hours before surgery. However, prolonged fasting can be detrimental to a patient. Indeed, in one study infants who fasted longer had greater drops in intraoperative blood pressure (Fig. 32-2).[13] No trial has shown that a shortened fluid fast increases the risk of aspiration. Gastric volumes are actually less when patients are allowed to drink some fluids before surgery. Admittedly, though, the majority of studies have not been specifically performed in individuals who are at an increased risk for aspiration. An excellent review of this topic has been published.[14]

⑤   In 1999, the ASA published practice guidelines for preoperative fasting. The guidelines allow a patient to have a light meal up to 6 hours before an elective procedure and support a fasting period for clear liquids of 2 hours for all patients. Coffee and tea are considered clear liquids. Coffee and tea drinkers should follow fasting guidelines but should be encouraged to drink coffee prior to their procedure because physical signs of withdrawal (e.g., headache) can easily occur. It is not clear if the guidelines should apply to patients with diabetes or dyspepsia. There is some evidence that shorter periods of preoperative fasting are accompanied by less postoperative nausea and vomiting (PONV). Yet, it is unclear whether rehydration during surgery is equivalent to a shorter fast before surgery in relation to PONV.

To ensure patients are optimally medically managed before their outpatient surgery, given the fact that clear liquids can be taken up to 2 hours before surgery, patients should be encouraged to take their chronic medications.

Anxiety Reduction

Clearly, some patients scheduled to undergo surgery are anxious, and they are probably anxious long before they come to the outpatient area. Preoperative reassurance from nonanesthesia staff and providing booklets with information about the procedure also reduce preoperative anxiety. However, use of booklets is less effective than a preoperative visit by the anesthesiologist. Audiovisual instructions also reduce preoperative anxiety. However, not all outpatients are anxious. For

example, although insomnia and anxiety are related, in a study of sleep characteristics of outpatients before elective surgery, no differences in sleep quality were found between patients before surgery and a community control group,[15] Indeed, physicians often tend to overestimate the level of anxiety that patients are actually experiencing.[16] Some operations can certainly generate more anxiety than others. If in doubt about patient anxiety, ask the patient.

Like adults, children should have some idea of what to expect during a procedure. But much of a child's anxiety before surgery concerns separation from a parent or parents. A child is more likely to demonstrate problematic behavior from the time of separation from parents to induction of anesthesia if a procedure has not been explained preoperatively. Parents and children need to be involved in some preoperative discussions together so the anxiety of the parents is not transmitted to the child. The transmission of anxiety is at least as problematic as is the separation itself (e.g., experiences of children being left with babysitters). If the parents are calm and can effectively manage the physical transfer to a warm and playful anesthesiologist or nurse, premedication is not necessary. Semisedation may be awkward, and recovery after premedication may be prolonged.

If a child is accompanied by a parent during the induction of anesthesia, the child's anxiety can be reduced. Some parents can become upset when they see their anesthetized child, who appears to be dead, albeit breathing and with a beating heart. Separation anxiety on the part of the parents is probably no different if the child is awake or asleep. Those children who have preoperative instructions and coaching both for themselves and their families, and their parent/s present during induction have less anxiety preoperatively, less postoperative delirium, shortened discharge time after surgery, and reduced analgesic consumption after surgery.[17]

Family-centered care has become popular and is useful for decreasing preoperative anxiety in children. In one study, 408 children undergoing elective ambulatory surgery received either standard care, had a parent present during induction, received oral midazolam prior to surgery, or received family-centered care prior to surgery.[17] Family-centered therapy consisted of providing the families of children with a videotape, three pamphlets, and a mask practice kit during their preoperative visit. One pamphlet was designed to help parents understand what to expect on the day of surgery and some recommendations for them to decrease their anxiety and their child's anxiety. Another gave them instructions for distracting their child on the day of surgery. A third gave instructions to teach the child what to do when in the operating room (OR), such as getting on the OR bed, and using the mask for induction. Parents were also given an induction mask, and a hairnet. On the day of surgery, children in the family-centered therapy group were given toys, designed to be age-appropriate and distracting (e.g., puzzles, brainteasers), unlike the other children who were simply given toys. Patients in the family-centered group, compared with the other three groups, preoperatively were less anxious. Parents were also less anxious. In addition, the patients had less severe emergence delirium symptoms, needed less fentanyl postoperatively, and were discharged earlier.

MANAGING THE ANESTHETIC: PREMEDICATION

The outpatient is not that different from the inpatient undergoing surgery. In both, premedication is useful to control anxiety, postoperative pain, nausea and vomiting, and to reduce the risk of aspiration during induction of anesthesia. Because the outpatient is going home on the day of surgery, the drugs given before anesthesia should not hinder recovery afterward.

Most premedicants do not prolong recovery when given in appropriate doses for appropriate indications, although drug effects may be apparent even after discharge.

Benzodiazepines

Although historically many classes of drugs (e.g., barbiturates, antihistamines) have been used to reduce anxiety and induce sedation, benzodiazepines are currently the drugs most commonly used. Midazolam is the benzodiazepine most commonly used preoperatively. It can be used intravenously and orally. In adults, it can be used to control preoperative anxiety and, during a procedure alone or in combination with other drugs, for intravenous sedation. For children, oral midazolam in doses as small as 0.25 mg/kg produces effective sedation and reduces anxiety.[18] With this dose, most children can be effectively separated from their parents after 10 minutes and satisfactory sedation can be maintained for 45 minutes. Discharge may be delayed, though, when given before a short procedure. Oral diazepam is useful to control anxiety in adult patients, either the day before surgery or the day of surgery and before an intravenous line has been inserted.

Fatigue associated with the effects of anxiolytics may delay or prevent the discharge of patients on the day of surgery, although more frequently patients are not discharged because of the effects of the operation. With regard to anesthesia effects, patients normally stay in the hospital not because they are too sleepy but because they are nauseous. In adults, particularly when midazolam is combined with fentanyl, patients can remain sleepy for up to 8 hours (Fig. 32-3).[19] Although children may be sleepier after oral midazolam, discharge times are not affected.

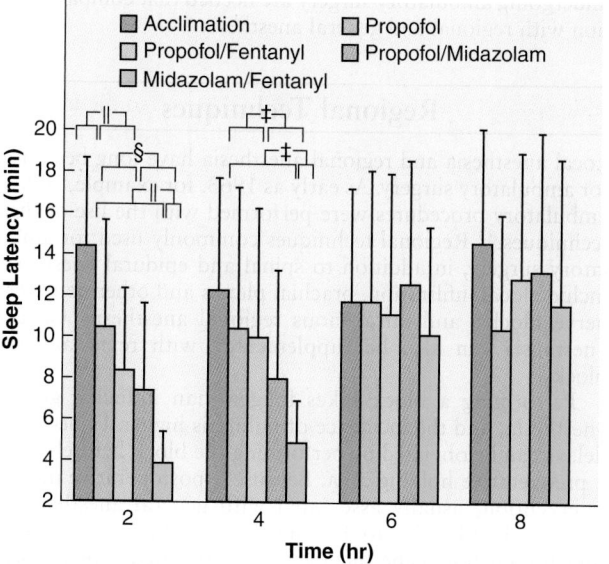

FIGURE 32-3. Patients can remain sleepy after receiving midazolam and fentanyl, even 8 hours after drug administration.[19] The abscissa represents time (hours) after sedation. The ordinate represents sleep latency (i.e., time to fall asleep). Data are the mean time to fall asleep. An individual is sleepier if less time is required to fall asleep. Subjects receiving the midazolam and fentanyl combination were much sleepier than the same subjects receiving other types of sedation. Although not seen in the figure, up to 8 hours after sedation, some subjects were still sleepier than before they received drug. (Reprinted from Lichtor JL, Alessi R, Lane BS: Sleep tendency as a measure of recovery after drugs used for ambulatory surgery. Anesthesiology 2002; 96: 878, with permission.)

At proper doses, neither midazolam nor diazepam place patients at any additional risk for cardiovascular and respiratory depression. Decreased oxygen saturation has been reported after injection of midazolam. Routine administration of supplemental oxygen with or without continuous monitoring of arterial oxygenation is recommended whenever benzodiazepines are given intravenously. This precaution is important not only when midazolam is given as a premedicant, but also when it is used alone or with other drugs for conscious sedation. The potential for amnesia after premedication is another concern, especially for patients undergoing ambulatory surgery. Anterograde amnesia certainly occurs. Although benzodiazepines facilitate retrograde memory, in one study there was no immediate retrograde amnesia after intravenous midazolam, 2 to 10 mg.[20] For benzodiazepines, the effects on memory are separate from the effects on sedation. In addition, amnesia is not simply an effect of drug administration but, among other factors, it is also a function of stimulus intensity.

Opioids and Nonsteroidal Analgesics

Opioids can be administered preoperatively to sedate patients, control hypertension during tracheal intubation, and decrease pain before surgery. Meperidine (but not morphine or fentanyl) is sometimes helpful in controlling shivering in the OR or the postanesthesia care unit (PACU), although treatment is usually instituted at the time of shivering and not in anticipation of the event. The effectiveness of opioids in relieving anxiety is controversial and probably nonexistent, particularly in adults.

Opioids are useful in controlling hypertension during tracheal intubation. Opioid premedication prevents increases in systolic pressure in a dose-dependent fashion. After tracheal intubation, systolic, diastolic, and mean arterial blood pressures sometimes decrease below baseline values.

Preoperative administration of opioids or nonsteroidal anti-inflammatory drugs (NSAIDs) may be useful for controlling pain in the early postoperative period. In one study, controlled-release oxycodone, 10 mg, when given before surgery, was effective in managing pain after laparoscopic tubal ligation surgery and was even associated with less PONV.[21] In a similar study of patients undergoing laparoscopic tubal ligation surgery, though, premedication with controlled-release oxycodone, 15 mg, did not improve the postoperative pain management.[22]

Celecoxib, up to 400 mg, is effective in reducing postoperative pain.[23] Ibuprofen or acetaminophen can be given rectally to children around the time of induction. If rectal acetaminophen is used in children, an initial loading dose of 40 mg/kg is appropriate; subsequent doses of 20 mg/kg every 6 hours can be used.[24] And, when preoperative rectal acetaminophen is combined with ketoprofen, particularly for more painful procedures, postoperative pain is less than when the drugs are given individually.[25]

Preoperative sedation is not needed for every patient. The following is our practice when patients require drugs to relieve anxiety. For the patient who has been seen at least 24 hours before a scheduled procedure and expresses a desire for medication to relieve anxiety or has anxiety that cannot be relieved with comforting, oral diazepam, 2 to 5 mg per 70 kg body weight, is prescribed for the night before and at 6:00 AM on the day of surgery (even if surgery is scheduled for 1:00 PM or later). For patients seen for the first time in the preoperative holding area who seem to need medication, midazolam, 0.01 mg/kg, is administered intravenously, or the patient is brought into the OR and propofol, 0.7 mg/kg, is injected intravenously. For children, when necessary, oral midazolam, 0.25 mg/kg, is administered in the preoperative holding area. When the child is asleep, acetaminophen, 40 mg/kg rectally, and ketorolac, 0.5 mg/kg intravenously, are administered prior to initiation of surgery.

INTRAOPERATIVE MANAGEMENT: CHOICE OF ANESTHETIC METHOD

There are several choices among anesthetic methods: general anesthesia, regional anesthesia, and local anesthesia. Regional and local anesthesia can be used with or without sedation. Except for obstetric cases, for which regional anesthesia may be safer than general anesthesia, all three types are otherwise equally safe. However, even for experienced anesthesiologists, there is a failure rate associated with regional anesthesia.

Certainly, some procedures are possible only with a general anesthetic. For others, the preference of patients, surgeons, or anesthesiologists may determine selection. The cost of sedation is usually less than the cost of a general or regional anesthetic. In a comparison of costs for patients undergoing inguinal hernia surgery in ten hospitals in Sweden, for example, intraoperative and postoperative costs were least in patients who received local anesthesia.[26] Those patients who received local anesthesia also spent less time in the OR, had less postoperative pain, and the least problems with urination. The three types of anesthesia, though, are not an option for all operations.

Time to recovery may also influence the choice of anesthetic method. In a study of patients undergoing prostate biopsy, discharge after general anesthesia was faster than after spinal anesthesia.[27] Conversely, in a study of patients undergoing shoulder surgery who received either general or regional anesthesia, patients who received regional anesthesia were more often able to bypass first-stage recovery, had less pain, were able to ambulate, and were eligible for discharge earlier than the general anesthesia group.[28] In a meta-analysis of peripheral nerve and centroneuraxial blocks compared with general anesthesia, time until discharge from the ambulatory surgery unit was no different for the three groups.[29] Interestingly also, postoperative nausea in the centroneuraxial block group was not different from the general anesthesia group. In a study of patients undergoing spinal or general anesthesia for knee surgery, recovery times were equivalent, but after spinal anesthesia, postoperative side effects were fewer.[30] When applying studies of regional anesthesia to everyday practice, remember that the studies come from centers where the authors are experienced in performing regional anesthesia and that might not be the case in other practices.

For some procedures such as arthroscopy, patients might prefer a regional anesthetic simply because they are curious and want to watch the surgery.[31] Postoperative pain is less after regional anesthesia, which is discussed in more detail later in this section. Also, with regional anesthesia or sedation, some of the side effects of general anesthesia can be avoided, although no form of medical care is without side effects. Whenever drugs are given that affect memory, patients might complain that they do not remember events that occur after the procedure. Although with regional anesthesia more time is required to place a block than it takes to induce a general anesthetic, a meta-analysis of several studies showed this increased time to be on average no more than 8 to 9 minutes.[29] In one survey of orthopaedic surgeons, the majority of surgeons who direct their patients' choice of anesthetic choose regional anesthesia, although the potential delay in establishing a block and perceived unpredictable success detracted from their enthusiasm with regional anesthesia (Fig. 32-4).[32]

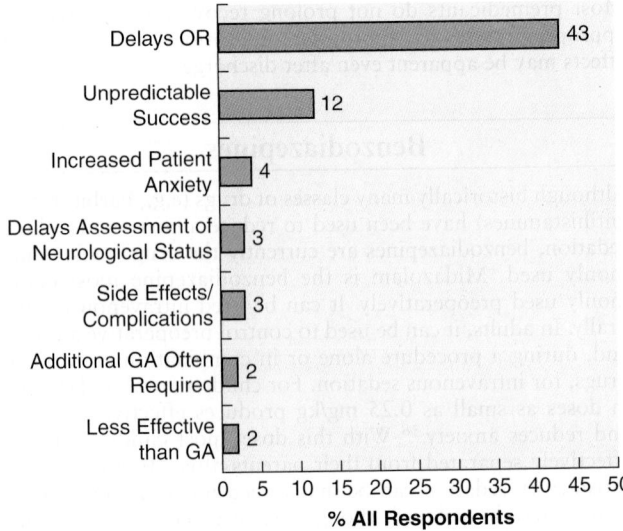

FIGURE 32-4.   Operating room (OR) delays are the major reasons orthopaedic surgeons do not favor regional anesthesia.[32] GA, general anesthesia. (Reprinted from Oldman M, McCartney CJ, Leung A et al: A survey of orthopedic surgeons' attitudes and knowledge regarding regional anesthesia. Anesth Analg 2004; 98: 1486, with permission.)

One adverse effect associated with spinal anesthesia is headache, but headaches are also experienced by patients after general anesthesia. The incidence of headache after either technique may be similar especially when smaller spinal needles are used. Patients may experience backache after spinal anesthesia, although sore throat and nausea are higher after general anesthesia than spinal type. Larger studies of patients undergoing ambulatory surgery are needed that compare sedation with regional and general anesthesia.

Regional Techniques

Local anesthesia and regional anesthesia have long been used for ambulatory surgery. As early as 1963, for example, 56% of ambulatory procedures were performed with the use of these techniques.[33] Regional techniques commonly used for ambulatory surgery, in addition to spinal and epidural anesthesia, include local infiltration, brachial plexus and other peripheral nerve blocks, and intravenous regional anesthesia. General anesthesia can also be supplemented with regional nerve blocks.

Performing a block takes longer than inducing general anesthesia, and the incidence of failure is higher. Unnecessary delays can be obviated by performing the block beforehand in a preoperative holding area. Because a postoperative nursing intervention, usually associated with general anesthesia, is associated with a 27- to 45-minute delay, the increased setup time for a regional anesthetic may be associated with a shorter time to discharge.[34] Postoperative pain control is best with regional techniques.

An occasional patient may experience syncope when the needle for the regional block is inserted. In the experience of oral and maxillofacial surgeons in Massachusetts in the late 1990s, 1 of 160 patients fainted when local anesthesia was injected.[35] When sedation accompanies local anesthesia injection, the incidence of syncope is reduced. Patients usually experience less postoperative pain when local or regional anesthesia has been used. Patients may still have a numb extremity (e.g., after a brachial plexus block) but otherwise meet all criteria for discharge. In such instances, the extremity must be well protected (e.g., with a sling for an upper extremity procedure) and patients must be cautioned to protect against injury because they are without normal sensations that would warn them of vulnerability. Reassurance that sensation will return should be provided.

Spinal Anesthesia

Children. Spinal anesthesia is used in some centers particularly for children undergoing inguinal hernia repair. One group described a series of >1,000 patients where spinal anesthesia was used for children aged 6 months to 14 years for procedures on the lower part of the body.[36] Muscle relaxation with the technique was excellent. In this series, all children left the OR awake and pain-free. The anesthesiology team used 0.5% hyperbaric bupivacaine at a dose of 0.2 mg/kg. Theoretically, PONV should be less after spinal anesthesia. That was the case in one study, although discharge times or patient satisfaction were no different when compared with patients who received general anesthesia.[37]

Adults. The use of spinal needles with pencil point, noncutting tips has prompted a resurgence of spinal anesthesia for ambulatory surgery in adults. Spinal anesthesia is suitable for pelvic, lower abdominal, and lower extremity surgery. One group described use of spinal anesthesia for ambulatory laparoscopic cholecystectomy with spinal needle insertion at L10, although even these authors recommended their technique not be used routinely because of the potential for direct contact of neural tissue by the spinal needle.[38]

Motor block of the legs may delay a patient's ability to walk. However, the use of a short-acting local anesthetic will minimize this problem. Nausea is much less frequent after epidural or spinal anesthesia than after general anesthesia.

Different drugs and drug concentrations have been used for spinal anesthesia. Lidocaine and mepivacaine are ideal for ambulatory surgery because of their short duration of action, although lidocaine use has been problematic because of transient neurologic symptoms. Transient neurologic symptoms can be seen after other local anesthetics, but the risk is 7 times more after intrathecal lidocaine than after bupivacaine, prilocaine, or procaine.[39]

Chloroprocaine spinal anesthesia has rapid onset and offset. In a study of nonpatient volunteers, after 40 mg of 2-chloroporcaine, the study participants could void after 110 minutes.[40] In that study, when 20 μg of fentanyl was included, regression time to L1 was lengthened and tourniquet tolerance was improved, although overall block length was minimally affected. Forty milligrams of preservative-free 2-chloroporcaine produces a similar onset time and block height when compared with 40 mg of lidocaine.[41] In one study, the authors showed that 40 and 50 mg of 2-chloroprocaine provided adequate spinal anesthesia for outpatient procedures lasting 45 to 60 minutes, whereas after 30 mg, the duration of block was inadequate.[42]

Both ropivacaine and bupivacaine have been used for ambulatory surgical procedures, but recovery time is relatively long. In a study comparing 7.5 mg bupivacaine and 15 mg ropivacaine for spinal anesthesia for knee arthroscopy, time to ambulation for both drugs was about 5 hours.[43]

Although headache is a common complication of lumbar puncture, smaller-gauge needles result in a lower incidence of postdural puncture headache. For those patients who do receive spinal anesthesia, it is incumbent on the anesthesiologist and the facility to have follow-up with telephone calls to ensure no disabling symptoms of headache have developed. If the headache does not respond to bed rest, analgesics, and oral hydration, the patient must return to the hospital for a course of intravenous caffeine therapy or an epidural blood patch.

Spinal anesthesia should not be avoided in ambulatory surgery patients simply because they may be more active postoperatively than inpatients. Bed rest does not reduce the frequency of headache. Indeed, early ambulation may decrease the incidence. Further study is needed to assess the relative risk–benefit ratio of spinal anesthesia as a technique for the ambulatory surgery patient.

Epidural and Caudal Anesthesia

Epidural anesthesia takes longer to perform than spinal anesthesia. Onset with spinal anesthesia is more rapid, although recovery may be the same with either technique. In one study of patients undergoing knee arthroscopy, spinal anesthesia with small-dose lidocaine and fentanyl was compared with 3% 2-chloroporcaine administered in the epidural space: intraoperative conditions, discharge characteristics and times, and recovery profiles were similar.[44] Also, failure rates for the two techniques, although low, were the same. Some studies suggest that bicarbonate can be added to solutions for faster onset of epidural anesthesia. An advantage of the epidural block is that it can be performed outside the OR, and after the surgical procedure is completed, the problem of postdural puncture headache is usually avoided.

Caudal anesthesia is a form of epidural anesthesia commonly used in children before surgery below the umbilicus as a supplement to general anesthesia and to control postoperative pain. Bupivacaine, 0.175 to 0.25%, or ropivacaine, 0.2%, in a volume of 0.5 to 1.0 mL/kg, may be used; a safe maximal dose is 2.5 mg/kg. Epinephrine, 1:200,000, when added to the anesthetic solution, may allow earlier detection of intravenous, rather than epidural, injection. Other useful albeit controversial additives for increasing duration of blockade include opioids, ketamine, clonidine, and neostigmine.[45] The block may be more difficult in children, particularly those who weigh >10 kg and are obese, if landmarks for the block are difficult to locate. The block is usually administered while the child is anesthetized. After injection, the depth of general anesthesia can be reduced. Because of better pain control after a caudal block, children can usually ambulate earlier and be discharged sooner than without a caudal block. Pain control and discharge times are no different whether the caudal block is placed before surgery or after it is completed.

Nerve Blocks

In a survey mailed to members of the Society for Ambulatory Anesthesia in 2001, there was shown to be widespread use of axillary and interscalene blocks for surgery in the upper extremity, and of ankle and femoral blocks for lower extremity surgery.[46] Nerve blocks improve postoperative patient satisfaction—PONV and postoperative pain are less. Costs are also less. One nonrandomized study of outpatients in a university setting showed that PACU admissions, hospital cost, and unexpected hospital admission were all reduced when nerve block was used for anterior cruciate ligament repair reconstruction.[47] For knee arthroscopy, psoas compartment block or spinal anesthesia is superior to general anesthesia in terms of postoperative pain management and patient satisfaction.[48] After more complex knee surgery, patients who received femoral-sciatic nerve block required fewer nursing interventions for pain; and, if patients received either that block or only a femoral nerve block, unplanned hospital admissions were less compared with patients who underwent the procedure without a block.[49] In a comparison of patients who underwent either infraclavicular brachial plexus block or general anesthesia for upper extremity surgery, after brachial plexus block more patients were able to bypass phase I PACU care, had less pain on PACU arrival, and were discharged much sooner (Fig. 32-5).[50]

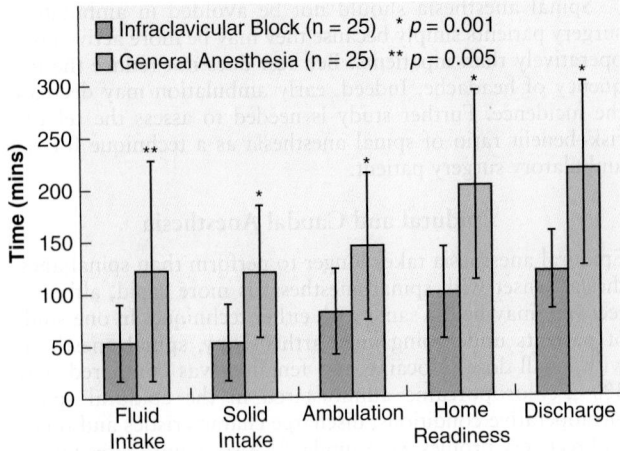

FIGURE 32-5. Recovery was faster when an infraclavicular brachial plexus block with a short-acting local anesthetic was used, compared with general anesthesia and wound infiltration for outpatients undergoing hand and wrist surgery.[50] Times are calculated from the end of anesthesia. (Reprinted from Hadzic A, Arliss J, Kerimoglu B et al: A comparison of infraclavicular nerve block versus general anesthesia for hand and wrist day-case surgeries. Anesthesiology 2004; 101: 127, with permission.)

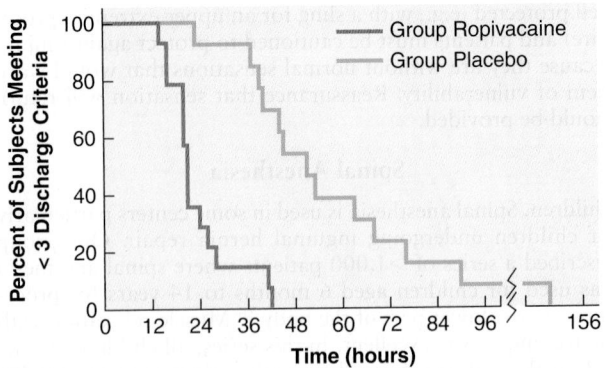

FIGURE 32-6. Patients who continued to receive an interscalene infusion of ropivacaine after surgery could be discharged home much earlier compared with patients who received postoperative narcotics.[55] Discharge criteria included adequate analgesia, independence from intravenous opioids, and the ability to tolerate at least 50% of passive shoulder motion targets during physical therapy. (Reprinted from Ilfeld, BM, Vandenborne, K, Duncan, PW, et al: Ambulatory continuous interscalene nerve blocks decrease the time to discharge readiness after total shoulder arthroplasty: A randomized, triple-masked, placebo-controlled study. Anesthesiology 2006; 105: 999, with permission.)

❽ Certain procedures can be quite painful, and hospitalization may be required to control pain. Nerve blocks using catheters that can be used to provide analgesia after the operation can be placed before surgery. Paravertebral somatic nerve block can be used for breast surgery, followed by a continuous perineural infusion of local anesthetic at home for 24 to 48 hours.[51] Perineural catheters in the sciatic nerve through the popliteal fossa can be used to control pain after foot surgery for both adults and children.[52,53] Femoral nerve catheters left in for about 2 days after anterior cruciate ligament reconstruction surgery after patients were discharged have been shown to decrease postoperative pain up to 4 days after surgery.[54] Interscalene perineural catheters, kept in for 4 days after surgery, have been used for patients undergoing moderately painful shoulder surgery.[55] Compared with patients who have regional anesthesia for surgery and then treatment afterward with narcotics, patients who go home with the interscalene perineural catheters attached to an infusion pump with ropivacaine can leave the hospital earlier the day after surgery, and once home have less pain and require less narcotics (Fig. 32-6). Continuous cervical paravertebral block may also be useful for analgesia after shoulder surgery.[56] Popliteal catheters have been used for lower extremity surgery such as hallux valgus surgery.[57]

Patients who go home with catheters inserted must be taught about pump function, understand signs of local anesthesia toxicity, and have someone else at home who can provide assistance. In addition, the patients must be able to communicate with someone by phone. The number of patients who have been sent home with catheters is increasing but is not large. More study is needed in order to demonstrate patient safety.

Sedation and Analgesia

Many patients who undergo surgery with local or regional anesthesia prefer to be sedated and to have no recollection of the procedure. Sedation is important, in part, because injection with local anesthetics can be painful and lying on a hard OR table can be uncomfortable. Levels of sedation vary from light,

during which a patient's consciousness is minimally depressed, to very deep, in which protective reflexes are partially blocked and response to physical stimulation or verbal command may not be appropriate. When patients are unsuitable for outpatient general anesthesia, surgery can often be performed if local or regional anesthesia is supplemented with conscious sedation. However, serious risk, such as death, is probably no different after sedation than after general anesthesia. Children who have surgery usually will not remain immobile unless they are deeply sedated or receive general anesthesia.

For adults, the proper dose might be selected by having the patient control the dosage. Yet, at least for ambulatory surgical procedures, patient-controlled sedation is not popular. This may be because a member of the anesthesia care team must be continuously present anyway.

General Anesthesia

The drugs selected for general anesthesia determine how long patients stay in the PACU after surgery, and for some patients, whether they can be discharged to go home.

Induction

The popularity of propofol as an induction agent for outpatient surgery in part relates to its half-life: the elimination half-life of propofol is 1 to 3 hours, shorter than that of methohexital (6 to 8 hours) or thiopental (10 to 12 hours). Although the effect of drugs given for induction seems to be transient, these drugs can depress psychomotor performance for several hours. **❾** After induction doses of propofol or thiopental, impairment after thiopental can be apparent for up to 5 hours, but only for 1 hour after propofol.

Pain on injection can be a problem with propofol. Pain is more likely on injection into dorsal hand veins and is minimized if forearm or larger antecubital veins are used. Some individuals, though, experience pain if the drug is injected into proximal larger veins. Nonetheless, thrombophlebitis does not appear to be a problem after intravenous administration of this agent, whereas it can be evident after thiopental.

Intravenous lidocaine, 0.2 mg/kg, can be used to decrease the incidence and severity of pain; other techniques have been tried, including ketamine, 0.1 mg/kg, immediately before propofol injection or lidocaine, 20 mg, plus metoclopramide, 10 mg.[58,59] Some have questioned the stability of mixing more than 20 mg lidocaine with 20 mL propofol.[60]

Most children and some adults prefer not to have an intravenous catheter inserted before the start of anesthesia. Sevoflurane has a relatively low blood-gas partition coefficient and the speed of induction is similar to, albeit somewhat slower than, that of propofol. Induction with sevoflurane can be hastened when the patient is told to breathe out to residual volume, take a vital capacity breath through a primed anesthesia circuit, and then hold the breath.

For short procedures, some patients may not require neuromuscular-blocking drugs; others may need brief paralysis (e.g., with succinylcholine) to facilitate tracheal intubation. Nondepolarizing drugs can be used to facilitate intubation and also during the procedure. Nondepolarizing drugs such as rocuronium have rapid onset times that are similar to those with succinylcholine. Of course, paralysis is not needed to insert an endotracheal tube; drug combinations such as propofol, alfentanil or remifentanil, and lidocaine obviate the need for paralysis.[61] Succinylcholine should be used with caution in children because of the possibility of cardiac arrest related to malignant hyperthermia or unsuspected muscular dystrophy, particularly Duchenne disease.

Maintenance

10 Although many factors affect the choice of agents for maintenance of anesthesia, two primary concerns for ambulatory anesthesia are speed of wake-up and incidence of PONV.

Anesthesia Maintenance and Wake-Up Times. Time to recovery may be measured by various criteria; however, for an ambulatory center, a patient may be considered awake when he or she is able to leave the center. Actual discharge from an ambulatory center, though, may depend on administrative issues such as a written order from a surgeon or anesthesiologist. The time necessary before a patient can be taken from the OR after completion of surgery, or a patient's ability to skip the PACU and go directly to a step-down unit, may be directly related to the anesthetic and may result in cost savings for an institution. Does choice of maintenance agent affect recovery after anesthesia? Propofol, desflurane, and sevoflurane have characteristics that make them ideal for maintenance of anesthesia for ambulatory surgery. Propofol has a short half-life and, when used as a maintenance agent, results in rapid recovery and few side effects. Desflurane and sevoflurane, halogenated ether anesthetics with low blood-gas partition coefficients, seem to be ideal for general anesthesia for ambulatory surgery. Sevoflurane, unlike desflurane, facilitates a smooth inhalation induction of anesthesia, the preferred technique to ensure rapid recovery of children in ambulatory surgery centers.

11 It is important to distinguish between wake-up time and discharge time. Patients may emerge from anesthesia with desflurane and nitrous oxide significantly faster than after propofol or sevoflurane and nitrous oxide, although the ability to sit up, stand, and tolerate fluids and the time to fitness for discharge may be no different. When the bispectral index (BIS) or other guide of anesthetic depth is used, the difference between drugs and wake-up times may not be as great.[62] Conversely, if fast wake-up times can translate to bypass of phase I, there may be cost savings.

Intraoperative Management of Postoperative Nausea and 12 *Vomiting.* Nausea, with or without vomiting, is probably the

most important factor contributing to a delay in discharge of patients and an increase in unanticipated admissions of both children and adults after ambulatory surgery. Patients hate vomiting. Studies have been performed in which patients are asked how much they would pay to avoid PONV or postoperative pain. Patients are willing to pay the most to prevent either of these outcomes, although the actual amount is a function, in part, on patient income.[63] Women, especially those who are pregnant, have a higher incidence of PONV. Other risk factors include a previous history of motion sickness or postanesthetic emesis, surgery within 1 to 7 days of the menstrual cycle, not smoking, and procedures such as laparoscopy, lithotripsy, major breast surgery, and ear, nose, or throat surgery. The greater the number of risk factors, the greater risk for nausea or vomiting after surgery. Inhalation agents are associated with an increased risk of PONV, particularly in the early stages of recovery; postoperative narcotic use is associated with PONV >2 hours after surgery.[64]

The vomiting pathway starts peripherally, where emerogenes through enterochromaffin cells in the gastrointestinal tract and/or other sensory neurons activate vagal afferents to the group of brainstem nuclei in the area postrema, the nucleus tractus solitarius, and the dorsal motor nucleus of the vagus. This area in the brain is otherwise known as the *vomiting center.* Although the pathways for vomiting are not completely understood, the area postrema is highly vascular, lacks a complete blood–brain barrier, and has receptors for neurotransmitters and hormones.[65] Receptor antagonists, specifically selective serotonin antagonists (ondansetron, dolasetron, and granisetron), have been shown to have similar efficacy to help alleviate nausea and vomiting. Dopamine antagonists, antihistamines, and anticholinergic drugs are useful and are generally less expensive, but are associated with extensive side effects. Neurokinin (NK1) receptor antagonists may also be useful to control PONV. Therapies useful in controlling PONV include acupuncture (Fig. 32-7).[66] supplemental fluid therapy,[67] clonidine (perhaps in part because it decreases anesthesia requirement),[68] and dexamethasone.[69,70] In one study, acupuncture therapy was effective in controlling both PONV and postoperative pain.[71] Acupressure is most effective when it is administered after surgery,[72] although if, intraoperatively, leads to

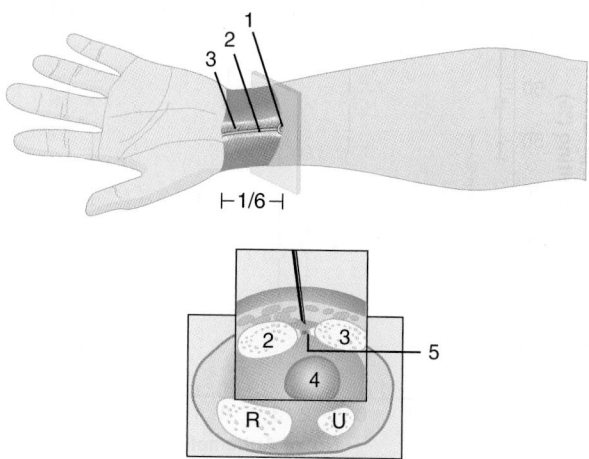

FIGURE 32-7. The P6 acupuncture point in relation to other hand structures is illustrated.[87] (1) P6 acupuncture point, (2) palmaris long tendon, (3) flexor carpi radialis tendon, (4) median nerve, and (5) palmar aponeurosis. (Reprinted from Wang SM, Kain ZN: P6 acupoint injections are as effective as droperidol in controlling early postoperative nausea and vomiting in children. Anesthesiology 2002; 97: 359, with permission.)

monitor patient paralysis are placed at the P6 acupuncture point, PONV is reduced.[73]

Combination therapy is probably the most effective way to control PONV. Therapy includes avoidance of nitrous oxide; avoidance of inhalation agents; avoidance of muscle relaxant reversal, if clinically indicated; avoidance of narcotics; fluid hydration; and administration of a 5-HT3 antagonist, an antiemetic from a different drug class, and dexamethasone. Risk, of course, is a function of other factors, as previously described. In one study in which combination therapy was used, nausea incidence was <10% and was even lower for certain procedures and types of patients.[74]

Because of its ability to decrease PONV, propofol is the best general anesthetic for ambulatory anesthesia. For example, in a study of 5,161 patients, propofol, compared with a volatile anesthetic, reduced nausea and vomiting by 19%; and nitrogen compared with nitrous oxide reduced the incidence by 12% (Fig. 32-8).[70] Propofol is now generic so the decision to use the drug should not be based on cost.

The use of nitrous oxide for ambulatory anesthesia is an issue because the incidence of emesis may be greater after nitrous oxide than after other inhalation agents. Although many studies have shown that nitrous oxide can be used successfully for ambulatory anesthesia, there is evidence that nitrous oxide should be avoided, except for inhalation induction of anesthesia. In one study of patients undergoing major, albeit not ambulatory, surgery, avoidance of nitrous oxide reduced postoperative complications, including postoperative fever, wound infection, pneumonia, pulmonary atelectasis, and severe nausea or vomiting.[75] Whether the changes found in that study would be as dramatic in ambulatory patients is not clear. Yet, many would argue that nitrous oxide is no longer needed except for inhalation induction of anesthesia.

Paralysis. Muscle paralysis for ambulatory anesthesia extends beyond the time of paralysis for intubation, particularly when nondepolarizing drugs are used. The duration of action of rocuronium, vecuronium, rapacuronium, and atracurium ranges from 25 to 40 minutes. Reversal agents must be used unless there is no doubt that muscle relaxation has been fully reversed.

Intraoperative Management of Postoperative Pain. Opioids, when given intraoperatively, are useful to supplement both intraoperative and postoperative analgesia. Fentanyl is probably the most popular drug, although all other available narcotics have been tried. All narcotics can cause nausea, sedation, and dizziness, which can delay a patient's discharge. Nonsteroidal analgesics are not effective as supplements during general anesthesia, although they are useful in controlling postoperative pain, particularly when given before skin incision. To control postoperative pain, combination therapy is most useful. (See also the previous discussion on opioids and nonsteroidal analgesics in "Opioids and Nonsteroidal Analgesics.")

Depth of Anesthesia. Use of BIS, and entropy, or auditory-evoked potential monitors can decrease anesthesia requirement without sacrificing amnesia during general anesthesia. Because less anesthesia is used, titration of anesthesia with these monitors results in earlier emergence from anesthesia. In a meta-analysis of BIS monitoring for ambulatory anesthesia, BIS monitoring was shown to reduce anesthetic use by 19%, with more modest decreases in PACU duration (4 minutes) and PONV (6%; Fig. 32-9).[76] Results are even more modest, albeit mixed, in terms of later recovery end points. Sympatholytic drugs, instead of anesthesia, can be used to control autonomic responses to anesthesia. In fact, recovery is faster and side effects are fewer in ambulatory patients whose blood pressure is controlled by sympatholytics instead of inhalation agents.[77] In a study of almost 5,000 patients who underwent general anesthesia and who were paralyzed and/or were intubated, awareness was significantly reduced in the group of patients who were monitored with a BIS compared with the group who were not monitored with the BIS.[78] Entropy, auditory-evoked potential, and cerebral state monitors are similar to BIS. Because these monitors result in less use of anesthesia, there is the possibility that intraoperative awareness and myocardial ischemia might be increased.

Airways. The use of an LMA, or similar type of airway, provides several advantages for allowing a patient to return to baseline

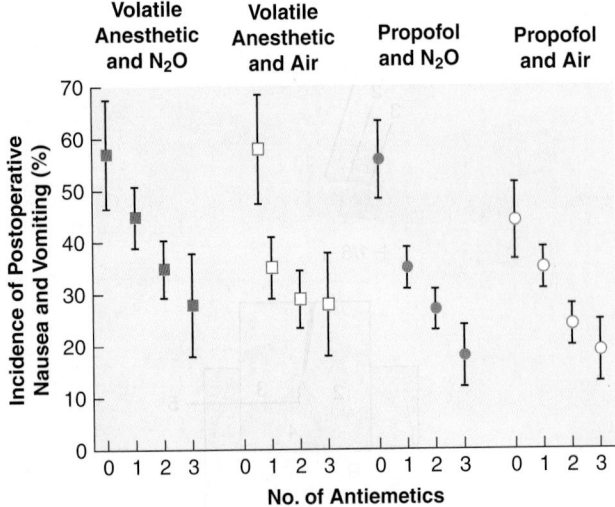

FIGURE 32-8. Postoperative nausea and vomiting (PONV) is least after a propofol anesthetic with air.[70] Illustrated is the incidence of PONV when different anesthetics and different numbers of prophylactic antiemetic treatments are administered. (Reprinted from Apfel CC, Korttila K, Abdalla M et al: A factorial trial of six interventions for the prevention of postoperative nausea and vomiting. N Engl J Med 2004; 350: 2441, with permission.)

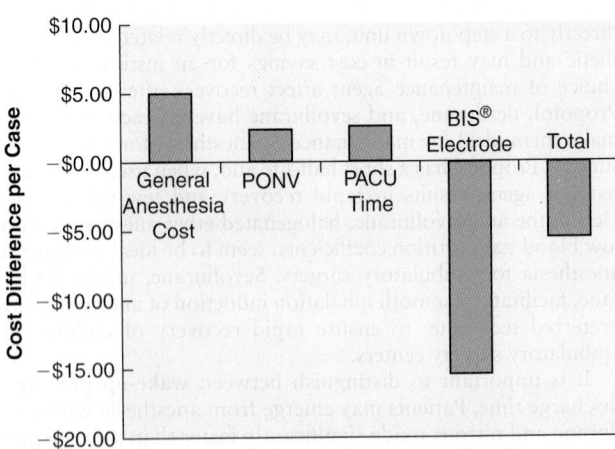

FIGURE 32-9. Bispectral index (BIS) (Aspect Medical Systems, Inc., Norwood, MA), monitoring reduces anesthetic consumption, cost to treat postoperative nausea and vomiting (PONV), and postanesthesia care unit (PACU) time; the cost of the electrode reverses cost savings.[76] The ordinate represents cost difference per case pooled from three studies (i.e., costs for the control group minus cost for the group that used BIS). The capital cost for the BIS monitor was not included. (Adapted from Liu SS: Effects of bispectral index monitoring on ambulatory anesthesia: A meta-analysis of randomized controlled trials and a cost analysis. Anesthesiology 2004; 101: 311, with permission.)

status quickly. Muscle relaxants required for intubation can be avoided. Coughing is less than with tracheal intubation. Anesthetic requirements are reduced. Hoarseness and sore throat are also reduced. Overall, cost savings result with the use of LMAs. Because of gastric insufflation, though, nausea and vomiting may be greater. The use of the LMA has been described for laparoscopic procedures, although the potential for aspiration exists because of an inflated abdomen during laparoscopy.

MANAGEMENT OF POSTANESTHESIA CARE

Many recovery issues are part of patient selection and perioperative management and must be considered before the patient enters the PACU. Managing common problems in the PACU quickly and effectively is as important as appropriate patient selection and choice of anesthetic technique if the patient is to return home on the day of surgery. The three most common reasons for delay in patient discharge from the PACU are drowsiness, nausea and vomiting, and pain. All three are a function of intraoperative management, but nausea, vomiting, and pain also can be treated in the PACU.

Reversal of Drug Effects

Reversal of muscle relaxants is not unique to the ambulatory surgery patient and is not discussed here. Reversal of opioids may sometimes be necessary. Flumazenil, a benzodiazepine receptor antagonist, has primarily been used to reverse the effects of sedation after endoscopy and spinal anesthesia. Reversal of psychomotor impairment with flumazenil is not complete, and the subjective experience of sedation is not necessarily attenuated. Reversal of amnesia with flumazenil is only partial, and the duration of the reversal effect may not be long enough to be clinically significant. Flumazenil should not be used routinely as a benzodiazepine antagonist, but may be used when sedation appears to be excessive. In addition, reversal of benzodiazepine-induced sedation by flumazenil should not replace appropriate ventilatory assistance and, if necessary, placement of an endotracheal tube.

Nausea and Vomiting

Nausea and vomiting are the most common reasons both children and adults have protracted stays in the PACU or unexpected hospital admission due to anesthesia. Nausea and vomiting are also the most common adverse effect in patients in the PACU. Much research has been undertaken to study prophylactic treatment of this problem before surgery, as well as techniques in the OR that can minimize nausea and vomiting in the PACU. The treatment of this problem, once it occurs in the PACU, has not received as much study. Yet, there are a variety of drugs that are effective in treating the problem. The 5-HT3 antagonists seem particularly effective. For example, in one study of children who underwent strabismus surgery and were then nauseous during the first 3 hours after recovery from anesthesia, emesis-free episodes were greater after granisetron, 40 μg/kg (88%), compared with droperidol, 50 μg/kg (63%), or metoclopramide, 0.25 mg/kg (58%).[79] In adults, granisetron, 40 μg/kg; metoclopramide, 0.2 mg/kg; or hydroxyzine, 25 mg, are also effective. Dexamethasone, 8 mg, given with other antiemetics can enhance treatment of established PONV in the PACU.[80]

Midazolam and propofol, although more commonly used for sedation, have antiemetic effects that are longer in duration than their effects on sedation. For example, when patients in the PACU were nauseous and then received either propofol, 15 mg, or midazolam, 1 or 2 mg, subsequent nausea was no different than with ondansetron, 4 mg.[81] Acupressure bands or acupressure stimulation in the region of the P6 acupuncture point can help reduce PONV. When a ReliefBand (Neurowave Medical Technologies,™ Chicago, IL) acustimulation device was compared with ondansetron for patients who were nauseous in the PACU after receiving metoclopramide or droperidol and undergoing laparoscopic surgery, nausea was most effectively treated with both the ReliefBand and ondansetron, although both therapies were equally effective individually in treating PONV.[82] If patients have already received ondansetron prophylaxis in the OR, and then are nauseous in the PACU, another repeat dose might not be effective. Based on a retrospective analysis of patients with nausea after receiving prophylactic ondansetron, established PONV was more effectively treated with promethazine than ondansetron; and promethazine, 6.25 mg intravenously, rather than higher doses was most effective.[83] More work is obviously needed to study effective therapies for treatment PONV in the PACU. Finally, because pain may be associated with nausea, treatment of pain frequently decreases nausea.

Pain

Postsurgical pain must be treated quickly and effectively. It is important for the practitioner to differentiate postsurgical pain from the discomfort of hypoxemia, hypercapnia, or a full bladder. Medications for pain control should be given in small intravenous doses (e.g., 1 to 3 mg/70 kg morphine or 10 to 25 μg/70 kg fentanyl). Intramuscular injection of opioid for pain control in the PACU is probably not necessary. Onset of action of drugs is faster after intravenous catheter administration than after oral administration. Control of postoperative pain may include administration of opioid analgesics or NSAIDs, which are not associated with respiratory depression, nausea, or vomiting. Fentanyl is the narcotic frequently used to control postoperative pain that ambulatory surgery patients experience, although the effects of morphine last longer. Patients who receive fentanyl for pain control may require additional injections and go home no sooner compared with patients who receive morphine. Nonsteroidal medications, such as ketorolac or ibuprofen, can also effectively control postoperative pain and, compared with narcotics, can give pain relief for a longer period and are associated with less nausea and vomiting. NSAIDs can increase bleeding, although there is no evidence at this time of such a danger for most ambulatory surgery procedures. When swelling and pain are problematic postoperatively, NSAIDs can be more effective than opioids in relieving both.

We manage pain in both adults and children initially either with a short-acting opioid analgesic such as fentanyl (25 μg/ 70 kg), or with an injection of ketorolac, 30 to 60 mg/70 kg intramuscularly or intravenously. Fentanyl is repeated at 5-minute intervals until pain is controlled. For children, we also use an elixir of acetaminophen containing codeine (120 mg acetaminophen and 12 mg codeine, in each 5 mL of solution). Five milliliters is administered to children between the ages of 3 and 6, and 10 mL to children between the ages of 7 and 12. Children are returned to parental care as soon as they are awake. We find frequently that infants younger than 6 months of age usually need to be reunited with their mothers for nursing or bottle feeding after a procedure not associated with severe pain. For older infants and young children in the PACU, acetaminophen, 60 mg per year of age (given orally or rectally), is commonly used to relieve mild pain. Intravenous fentanyl (up to a dose of 2 μg/kg) is preferred for more severe pain. Meperidine (0.5 mg/kg) and codeine (1 to 1.5 mg/kg) can be given intramuscularly if an intravenous route has not been established.

Preparation for Discharging the Patient

⓭ In addition to the PACU, many ambulatory surgery centers in the United States have another area, often known as a phase II recovery room, where patients may stay until they are able to tolerate liquids, walk, and/or void. With the anesthetics that are typically used in ambulatory surgery ORs, patients who are awakened in the OR and are evaluated as 9 or 10 according to the modified Aldrete scoring system may be transferred directly to phase II recovery from the OR. Patients who undergo procedures under monitored anesthesia care can usually go straight to the phase II area from the OR. After general anesthesia, LMA use and pain control using nonopioid analgesics facilitates fast-tracking. In one study, 35 to 53% of patients who underwent laparoscopic gynecologic surgery were able to bypass the PACU.[84] In that study, residual sedation was the most common reason the PACU was not bypassed. In another study of patients who underwent outpatient knee surgery bypassed the PACU and were in the phase II recovery area, 31% required nursing interventions and were 3 times more likely to need a nursing intervention, compared with 16% who required a nursing intervention who first went to the PACU. Yet, discharge times were faster and unplanned hospital admissions were fewer if patients were able to bypass the PACU.[85] In a similar study, those authors found that even though direct transfer to phase II recovery may decrease time spent in the hospital, nursing workload was no different than if patients first went to phase I recovery.[86]

Some criteria for discharge to home were created without scientific basis. One criterion is the ability to tolerate liquids before being discharged. Postoperative nausea may be greater if patients are required to drink liquids prior to discharge. Even though it is warranted after spinal or epidural anesthesia, the requirement that low-risk patients void before discharge may only lengthen stay in the hospital, particularly if patients are willing to return to a medical facility if they are unable to void. Practical criteria for patient discharge from the OR, from the PACU, and from the phase II recovery area are needed that in no way compromise patient safety. The value of psychomotor tests to measure different phases of recovery (except for research purposes) is questionable.

Although scoring systems may be used to guide transfer from the PACU to the phase II recovery room and from phase II recovery to home, they do little to test higher levels of function, such as the ability to use one's hands, to drive a car, or to remain alert long enough to drive. Patients may feel fine after they leave the hospital, but they should be advised against driving for at least 24 hours after a procedure. Patients and responsible parties should be reminded that the patient should not operate power tools or be involved in major business decisions for up to 24 hours. Once the patient leaves the medical facility, supervision may not be as good as it was in the hospital. Therefore, before a patient is discharged, dressings should be checked. It is wise to include the responsible person in all discharge instructions, which are best made available on printed forms.

Patients should also be informed that they may experience pain, headache, nausea, vomiting, or dizziness and, if succinylcholine was used, muscle aches and pains apart from the incision for at least 24 hours. A patient will be less stressed if the described symptoms are expected in the course of a normal recovery. Written instructions are important. The addition of written and oral education techniques at discharge has a significant impact on improving compliance.

For patients with a language barrier (e.g., in a population with a high percentage of immigrants), consent forms, procedural explanation, and discharge information may have to be written in languages other than English and the services of an interpreter may be necessary. Nursing staff should assess the adult who will take the patient home to determine whether he or she is a responsible person. A responsible person is someone who is physically and intellectually able to take care of the patient at home. Facilities should develop a method of follow-up after the patient has been discharged. At some facilities, staff members telephone the patient the next day to determine the progress of recovery; others use follow-up postcards.

Whenever we become innovative in the management of our outpatients, we must assess how a cost-effective, "no frills" approach to care affects patient safety. We must determine what we can do for the patient who lives alone, for the patient whose responsible person is unable to manage his or her needs, for the patient without means of transportation, and for the patient with limited insurance coverage. Hospital beds can be set aside for patients who require observation. Patients in these beds after an ambulatory surgical procedure are still considered outpatients. They are charged for the hours spent in the observation area. Some hospitals have joined with management firms to build a hospital hotel or medical motel close to the hospital itself. The hotel, usually a nonmedical facility, offers the outpatient a comfortable, inexpensive, and convenient place to recuperate while being cared for by family or nurses. Home health care nursing may be appropriate after surgical procedures such as reduction mammoplasty, abdominoplasty, vaginal hysterectomy, and major open ligament repairs of the knee. The various services for management and/or observation of outpatients after surgery stand today where techniques for management of outpatients during surgery stood in the health care delivery system 20 years ago. Prospective studies are needed to assess the quality of care and the effect that these innovative approaches have on patient safety.

Patient, procedure, availability and quality of aftercare, and anesthetic technique must be individually and collectively assessed to determine acceptability for ambulatory surgery. A delicate balance must be maintained between the physical status of the patient, the proposed surgical procedure, and the appropriate anesthetic technique, to which must be added the expertise level of the anesthesiologist caring for a patient.

Anesthesia for ambulatory surgery is a rapidly evolving specialty. Patients who were once believed to be unsuitable for ambulatory surgery are now considered to be appropriate candidates. Operations once believed unsuitable for outpatients are now routinely performed in the morning so patients can be discharged in the afternoon or evening. The appropriate anesthetic management before these patients come to the OR, during their operation, and then afterward is the key to success. The availability of both shorter-acting anesthetics and longer-acting analgesics and antiemetics enables us to care for patients in ambulatory centers effectively.

References

1. Fleisher LA, Pasternak LR, Lyles A: A novel index of elevated risk of inpatient hospital admission immediately following outpatient surgery. Arch Surg 2007; 142: 263
2. Clayman MA, Seagle BM: Office surgery safety: The myths and truths behind the Florida moratoria—six years of Florida data. Plast Reconstr Surg 2006; 118: 777
3. Matarasso A, Swift RW, Rankin M: Abdominoplasty and abdominal contour surgery: A national plastic surgery survey. Plast Reconstr Surg 2006; 117: 1797
4. Walther-Larsen S, Rasmussen LS: The former preterm infant and risk of post-operative apnoea: Recommendations for management. Acta Anaesthesiol Scand 2006; 50: 888

5. Shenkman Z, Hoppenstein D, Litmanowitz I et al: Spinal anesthesia in 62 premature, former-premature or young infants: Technical aspects and pitfalls. Can J Anaesth 2002; 49: 262

6. Ansell GL, Montgomery JE: Outcome of ASA III patients undergoing day case surgery. Br J Anaesth 2004; 92: 71

7. Davies KE, Houghton K, Montgomery JE: Obesity and day-case surgery. Anaesthesia 2001; 56: 1112

8. Mattila K, Toivonen J, Janhunen L et al: Postdischarge symptoms after ambulatory surgery: First-week incidence, intensity, and risk factors. Anesth Analg 2005; 101: 1643

9. Gross JB, Bachenberg KL, Benumof JL et al: Practice guidelines for the perioperative management of patients with obstructive sleep apnea: A report by the American Society of Anesthesiologists Task Force on Perioperative Management of patients with obstructive sleep apnea. Anesthesiology 2006; 104: 1081

10. Basu S, Babajee P, Selvachandran SN et al: Impact of questionnaires and telephone screening on attendance for ambulatory surgery. Ann R Coll Surg Engl 2001; 83: 329

11. Basson MD, Butler TW, Verma H: Predicting patient nonappearance for surgery as a scheduling strategy to optimize operating room utilization in a Veterans' Administration hospital. Anesthesiology 2006; 104: 826

12. Tait AR, Malviya S, Voepel-Lewis T et al: Risk factors for perioperative adverse respiratory events in children with upper respiratory tract infections. Anesthesiology 2001; 95: 299

13. Friesen RH, Wurl JL, Friesen RM: Duration of preoperative fast correlates with arterial blood pressure response to halothane in infants. Anesth Analg 2002; 95: 1572

14. Brady M, Kinn S, Stuart P: Preoperative fasting for adults to prevent perioperative complications. Cochrane Database Syst Rev 2003; 4: CD004423

15. Kain ZN, Caldwell-Andrews AA: Sleeping characteristics of adults undergoing outpatient elective surgery: a cohort study. J Clin Anesth 2003; 15: 505

16. Fekrat F, Sahin A, Yazici KM et al: Anaesthetists' and surgeons' estimation of preoperative anxiety by patients submitted for elective surgery in a university hospital. Eur J Anaesthesiol 2006; 23: 227

17. Kain ZN, Caldwell-Andrews AA, Mayes LC et al: Family-centered preparation for surgery improves perioperative outcomes in children: A randomized controlled trial. Anesthesiology 2007; 106: 65

18. Cote CJ, Cohen IT, Suresh S et al: A comparison of three doses of a commercially prepared oral midazolam syrup in children. Anesth Analg 2002; 94: 37

19. Lichtor JL, Alessi R, Lane BS: Sleep tendency as a measure of recovery after drugs used for ambulatory surgery. Anesthesiology 2002; 96: 878

20. Bulach R, Myles PS, Russnak M: Double-blind randomized controlled trial to determine extent of amnesia with midazolam given immediately before general anaesthesia. Br J Anaesth 2005; 94: 300

21. Reuben SS, Steinberg RB, Maciolek H et al: Preoperative administration of controlled-release oxycodone for the management of pain after ambulatory laparoscopic tubal ligation surgery. J Clin Anesth 2002; 14: 223

22. Jokela R, Ahonen J, Valjus M et al: Premedication with controlled-release oxycodone does not improve management of postoperative pain after day-case gynaecological laparoscopic surgery. Br J Anaesth 2007; 98: 255

23. Recart A, Issioui T, White PF et al: The efficacy of celecoxib premedication on postoperative pain and recovery times after ambulatory surgery: A dose-ranging study. Anesth Analg 2003; 96: 1631

24. Birmingham PK, Tobin MJ, Fisher DM et al: Initial and subsequent dosing of rectal acetaminophen in children: A 24-hour pharmacokinetic study of new dose recommendations. Anesthesiology 2001; 94: 385

25. Hiller A, Meretoja OA, Korpela R et al: The analgesic efficacy of acetaminophen, ketoprofen, or their combination for pediatric surgical patients having soft tissue or orthopedic procedures. Anesth Analg 2006; 102: 1365

26. Nordin P, Zetterstrom H, Carlsson P et al: Cost-effectiveness analysis of local, regional and general anaesthesia for inguinal hernia repair using data from a randomized clinical trial. Br J Surg 2007; 94: 500

27. Nishikawa K, Yoshida S, Shimodate Y et al: A comparison of spinal anesthesia with small-dose lidocaine and general anesthesia with fentanyl and propofol for ambulatory prostate biopsy procedures in elderly patients. J Clin Anesth 2007; 19: 25

28. Hadzic A, Williams BA, Karaca PE et al: For outpatient rotator cuff surgery, nerve block anesthesia provides superior same-day recovery over general anesthesia. Anesthesiology 2005; 102: 1001

29. Liu SS, Strodtbeck WM, Richman JM et al: A comparison of regional versus general anesthesia for ambulatory anesthesia: A meta-analysis of randomized controlled trials. Anesth Analg 2005; 101: 1634

30. Korhonen AM, Valanne JV, Jokela RM et al: A comparison of selective spinal anesthesia with hyperbaric bupivacaine and general anesthesia with desflurane for outpatient knee arthroscopy. Anesth Analg 2004; 99: 1668

31. Pelinka LE, Pelinka H, Leixnering M et al: Why patients choose regional anesthesia for orthopedic and trauma surgery. Arch Orthop Trauma Surg 2003; 123: 164

32. Oldman M, McCartney CJ, Leung A et al: A survey of orthopedic surgeons' attitudes and knowledge regarding regional anesthesia. Anesth Analg 2004; 98: 1486

33. Cohen DD, Dillon JB: Anesthesia for outpatient surgery. JAMA 1966; 196: 1114

34. Williams BA, Kentor ML: Making an ambulatory surgery centre suitable for regional anaesthesia. Best Pract Res Clin Anaesthesiol 2002; 16: 175

35. D'eramo EM, Bookless SJ, Howard JB: Adverse events with outpatient anesthesia in Massachusetts. J Oral Maxillofac Surg 2003; 61: 793

36. Puncuh F, Lampugnani E, Kokki H: Use of spinal anaesthesia in paediatric patients: A single centre experience with 1132 cases. Paediatr Anaesth 2004; 14: 564

37. Oddby E, Englund S, Lonnqvist PA: Postoperative nausea and vomiting in paediatric ambulatory surgery: Sevoflurane versus spinal anaesthesia with propofol sedation. Paediatr Anaesth 2001; 11: 337

38. van Zundert AA, Stultiens G, Jakimowicz JJ et al: Laparoscopic cholecystectomy under segmental thoracic spinal anaesthesia: a feasibility study. Br J Anaesth 2007; 98: 682

39. Zaric D, Christiansen C, Pace NL, Punjasawadwong Y: Transient neurologic symptoms after spinal anesthesia with lidocaine versus other local anesthetics: A systematic review of randomized, controlled trials. Anesth Analg 2005; 100: 1811

40. Vath JS, Kopacz DJ: Spinal 2-chloroprocaine: The effect of added fentanyl. Anesth Analg 2004; 98: 89

41. Kouri ME, Kopacz DJ: Spinal 2-chloroprocaine: a comparison with lidocaine in volunteers. Anesth Analg 2004; 98: 75

42. Casati A, Danelli G, Berti M et al: Intrathecal 2-chloroprocaine for lower limb outpatient surgery: A prospective, randomized, double-blind, clinical evaluation. Anesth Analg 2006; 103: 234

43. Boztug N, Bigat Z, Karsli B et al: Comparison of ropivacaine and bupivacaine for intrathecal anesthesia during outpatient arthroscopic surgery. J Clin Anesth 2006; 18: 521

44. Pollock JE, Mulroy MF, Bent E et al: A comparison of two regional anesthetic techniques for outpatient knee arthroscopy. Anesth Analg 2003; 97: 397

45. Lonnqvist PA: Adjuncts to caudal block in children—Quo vadis? Br J Anaesth 2005; 95: 431

46. Klein SM, Pietrobon R, Nielsen KC et al: Peripheral nerve blockade with long-acting local anesthetics: A survey of the Society for Ambulatory Anesthesia. Anesth Analg 2002; 94: 71

47. Williams BA, Kentor ML, Vogt MT et al: Economics of nerve block pain management after anterior cruciate ligament reconstruction: Potential hospital cost savings via associated postanesthesia care unit bypass and same-day discharge. Anesthesiology 2004; 100: 697

48. Jankowski CJ, Hebl JR, Stuart MJ et al: A comparison of psoas compartment block and spinal and general anesthesia for outpatient knee arthroscopy. Anesth Analg 2003; 97: 1003

49. Williams BA, Kentor ML, Vogt MT et al: Femoral-sciatic nerve blocks for complex outpatient knee surgery are associated with less postoperative pain before same-day discharge: A review of 1,200 consecutive cases from the period 1996-1999. Anesthesiology 2003; 98: 1206

50. Hadzic A, Arliss J, Kerimoglu B et al: A comparison of infraclavicular nerve block versus general anesthesia for hand and wrist day-case surgeries. Anesthesiology 2004; 101: 127

51. Buckenmaier CC 3rd, Klein SM, Nielsen KC et al: Continuous paravertebral catheter and outpatient infusion for breast surgery. Anesth Analg 2003; 97: 715

52. Zaric D, Boysen K, Christiansen J et al: Continuous popliteal sciatic nerve block for outpatient foot surgery—a randomized, controlled trial. Acta Anaesthesiol Scand 2004; 48: 337

53. Dadure C, Bringuier S, Nicolas F et al: Continuous epidural block versus continuous popliteal nerve block for postoperative pain relief after major podiatric surgery in children: A prospective, comparative randomized study. Anesth Analg 2006; 102: 744

54. Williams BA, Kentor ML, Vogt MT et al: Reduction of verbal pain scores after anterior cruciate ligament reconstruction with 2-day continuous femoral nerve block: A randomized clinical trial. Anesthesiology 2006; 104: 315

55. Ilfeld BM, Vandenborne K, Duncan PW et al: Ambulatory continuous interscalene nerve blocks decrease the time to discharge readiness after total shoulder arthroplasty: A randomized, triple-masked, placebo-controlled study. Anesthesiology 2006; 105: 999

56. Boezaart AP, De Beer JF, Nell ML: Early experience with continuous cervical paravertebral block using a stimulating catheter. Reg Anesth Pain Med 2003; 28: 406

57. Capdevila X, Dadure C, Bringuier S et al: Effect of patient-controlled perineural analgesia on rehabilitation and pain after ambulatory orthopedic surgery: A multicenter randomized trial. Anesthesiology 2006; 105: 566

58. Koo SW, Cho SJ, Kim YK et al: Small-dose ketamine reduces the pain of propofol injection. Anesth Analg 2006; 103: 1444

59. Fujii Y, Nakayama M: A lidocaine/metoclopramide combination decreases pain on injection of propofol. Can J Anaesth 2005; 52: 474

60. Masaki Y, Tanaka M, Nishikawa T: Physicochemical compatibility of propofol-lidocaine mixture. Anesth Analg 2003; 97: 1646

61. Jabbour-Khoury SI, Dabbous AS, Rizk LB et al: A combination of alfentanil-lidocaine-propofol provides better intubating conditions than fentanyl-lidocaine-propofol in the absence of muscle relaxants. Can J Anaesth 2003; 50: 116

62. Mayer J, Boldt J, Schellhaass A et al: Bispectral index-guided general anesthesia in combination with thoracic epidural analgesia reduces recovery time in fast-track colon surgery. Anesth Analg 2007; 104: 114563

63. Macario A, Fleisher LA: Is there value in obtaining a patient's willingness to pay for a particular anesthetic intervention? Anesthesiology 2006; 104: 906

ANESTHETIC MANAGEMENT

64. Apfel CC, Kranke P, Katz MH et al: Volatile anaesthetics may be the main cause of early but not delayed postoperative vomiting: A randomized controlled trial of factorial design. Br J Anaesth 2002; 88: 659

65. Saito R, Takano Y, Kamiya HO: Roles of substance P and NK(1) receptor in the brainstem in the development of emesis. J Pharmacol Sci 2003; 91: 87

66. Turgut S, Ozalp G, Dikmen S et al: Acupressure for postoperative nausea and vomiting in gynaecological patients receiving patient-controlled analgesia. Eur J Anaesthesiol 2007; 24: 87

67. Magner JJ, McCaul C, Carton E et al: Effect of intraoperative intravenous crystalloid infusion on postoperative nausea and vomiting after gynaecological laparoscopy: Comparison of 30 and 10 ml kg-1. Br J Anaesth 2004; 93: 381

68. Oddby-Muhrbeck E, Eksborg S, Bergendahl HT et al: Effects of clonidine on postoperative nausea and vomiting in breast cancer surgery. Anesthesiology 2002; 96: 1109

69. Henzi I, Walder B, Tramer MR: Dexamethasone for the prevention of postoperative nausea and vomiting: A quantitative systematic review. Anesth Analg 2000; 90: 186

70. Apfel CC, Korttila K, Abdalla M et al: A factorial trial of six interventions for the prevention of postoperative nausea and vomiting. N Engl J Med 2004; 350: 2441

71. Gan TJ, Jiao KR, Zenn M et al: A randomized controlled comparison of electro-acupoint stimulation or ondansetron versus placebo for the prevention of postoperative nausea and vomiting. Anesth Analg 2004; 99: 1070

72. White PF, Hamza MA, Recart A et al: Optimal timing of acustimulation for antiemetic prophylaxis as an adjunct to ondansetron in patients undergoing plastic surgery. Anesth Analg 2005; 100: 367

73. Arnberger M, Stadelmann K, Alischer P et al: Monitoring of neuromuscular blockade at the P6 acupuncture point reduces the incidence of postoperative nausea and vomiting. Anesthesiology 2007; 107: 903

74. Skledar SJ, Williams BA, Vallejo MC et al: Eliminating postoperative nausea and vomiting in outpatient surgery with multimodal strategies including low doses of nonsedating, off-patent antiemetics: Is "zero tolerance" achievable? Scientific World J 2007; 7: 959

75. Myles PS, Leslie K, Chan MT et al: Avoidance of nitrous oxide for patients undergoing major surgery: A randomized controlled trial. Anesthesiology 2007; 107: 221

76. Liu SS: Effects of Bispectral Index monitoring on ambulatory anesthesia: A meta-analysis of randomized controlled trials and a cost analysis. Anesthesiology 2004; 101: 311

77. White PF, Wang B, Tang J et al: The effect of intraoperative use of esmolol and nicardipine on recovery after ambulatory surgery. Anesth Analg 2003; 97: 1633

78. Ekman A, Lindholm ML, Lennmarken C et al: Reduction in the incidence of awareness using BIS monitoring. Acta Anaesthesiol Scand 2004; 48: 20

79. Fujii Y, Tanaka H, Ito M: Treatment of vomiting after paediatric strabismus surgery with granisetron, droperidol, and metoclopramide. Ophthalmologica 2002; 216: 359

80. Rusch D, Arndt C, Martin H et al: The addition of dexamethasone to dolasetron or haloperidol for treatment of established postoperative nausea and vomiting. Anaesthesia 2007; 62: 810

81. Unlugenc H, Guler T, Gunes Y et al: Comparative study of the antiemetic efficacy of ondansetron, propofol and midazolam in the early postoperative period. Eur J Anaesthesiol 2004; 21: 60

82. Coloma M, White PF, Ogunnaike BO et al: Comparison of acustimulation and ondansetron for the treatment of established postoperative nausea and vomiting. Anesthesiology 2002; 97: 1387

83. Habib AS, Reuveni J, Taguchi A et al: A comparison of ondansetron with promethazine for treating postoperative nausea and vomiting in patients who received prophylaxis with ondansetron: A retrospective database analysis. Anesth Analg 2007; 104: 548

84. Coloma M, Zhou T, White PF et al: Fast-tracking after outpatient laparoscopy: Reasons for failure after propofol, sevoflurane, and desflurane anesthesia. Anesth Analg 2001; 93: 112

85. Williams BA, Kentor ML, Williams JP et al: PACU bypass after outpatient knee surgery is associated with fewer unplanned hospital admissions but more phase II nursing interventions. Anesthesiology 2002; 97: 981

86. Song D, Chung F, Ronayne M et al: Fast-tracking (bypassing the PACU) does not reduce nursing workload after ambulatory surgery. Br J Anaesth 2004; 93: 768

87. Wang SM, Kain ZN: P6 acupoint injections are as effective as droperidol in controlling early postoperative nausea and vomiting in children. Anesthesiology 2002; 97: 359

CHAPTER 33 ■ OFFICE-BASED ANESTHESIA

LAURENCE M. HAUSMAN AND MEG A. ROSENBLATT

ADVANTAGES/DISADVANTAGES	**ANESTHETIC TECHNIQUES**
OFFICE SAFETY	Anesthetic Agents
PATIENT SELECTION	**POST ANESTHESIA CARE UNIT**
SURGEON SELECTION	**REGULATIONS**
OFFICE SELECTION	Business and Legal Aspects
Accreditation	**CONCLUSIONS**
PROCEDURE SELECTION	
Specific Procedures	

KEY POINTS

1. There is an increased risk of morbidity and mortality associated with an office-based anesthetic when compared with one performed in a freestanding ambulatory surgery center.

2. The Closed Claims Project database reveals that injuries during office-based procedures occur throughout the perioperative period and are multifactorial in etiology.

3. Patient selection remains a controversial topic among practicing office-based anesthesiologists because little morbidity and mortality data exist to support the inclusion or exclusion of specific populations.

4. Outpatient facilities have developed specific policies regarding acceptable patients for the outpatient setting, possibly excluding patients with obstructive sleep apnea syndrome.

5. The anesthesiologist should function as a zealous patient advocate in assuring that an anesthetic is performed only in a safe location.

6. Destinations for a patient in need of hospital admission must be identified.

7. The American Society of Plastic Surgeons has recommended that procedures be limited to 6 hours and be completed by 3 PM, thus allowing for a full patient recovery with maximum office staffing. In addition, when determining the suitability

of a procedure one must consider the possibility of hypothermia, blood loss, or significant fluid shifts.

8. Although no minimum age requirement for a child to undergo an office-based anesthetic has been established, patients >6 months of age and American Society of Anesthesiologists physical status 1 or 2 may be reasonable candidates.

9. The drugs should have a short half-life, be inexpensive, and not be associated with undesirable side effects such as nausea and vomiting.

10. There should be at least one Advanced Cardiac Life Support/Pediatric Advanced Life Support-certified member of the health care team present until the last patient has left the office.

11. Every anesthetic administered should be designed to maximize postoperative patient alertness and mobility and minimize the risks of the need for a prolonged postanesthesia care unit stay.

12. The anesthesiologist maintains the role of a zealous patient advocate and helps to educate the surgeon as to what constitutes a safe anesthetizing location.

13. Ignorance of the law offers no protection or excuse, and one should seek the advice of expert billing agencies even if one chooses not to outsource this responsibility.

The field of office-based anesthesia (OBA) has become an intrinsic and vital aspect within the field of anesthesiology. An office-based anesthetic is one that is performed in a location, usually an office or procedure room, that is not accredited by the state as an ambulatory surgery center (ASC) or as a hospital. In fact, in some parts of the country, the surgical office may have no accreditation at all. Additionally, the office must also house nonsurgical activities such as patient consultation and practice administration.

During the 1970s, <10% of all surgical/diagnostic procedures were performed on an ambulatory basis, and of these, virtually all were performed in hospitals. By 1987, approximately 25 million, or 40% of all procedures, were performed as ambulatory. In the United States between 1984 and 1990, the number of office-based procedures increased from 400,000 to 1.2 million, and by 1994, 8.5% of all procedures were performed in offices.[1] In the same year, a survey of the membership of the American Society of Plastic Surgeons (ASPS),

revealed that 55% of the respondents performed the majority or all of their procedures in an office.[2] By the year 2000, approximately 75% of all procedures were performed on an outpatient basis; 17% in freestanding ASCs, and 14 to 25% (approximately 8 to 10 million) in physicians' offices.[3–5] There are little exact data available; however it was estimated that in 2005 approximately 82% of all surgical procedures were outpatient and of these, 24% were office-based.[3,6]

Although an OBA practice may be an exciting alternative to the traditional hospital-based one, it requires the anesthesiologist to expand his or her role within the health care delivery system. Along with providing safe anesthetics across the spectrum of healthy-to-medically challenged patients undergoing increasingly complex procedures, the anesthesiologist must understand office safety and policy, as well as legal and financial issues such as billing and collection.[5,7] These are relatively new responsibilities for anesthesiologists, who historically have worked as members within a hospital department either in the private or academic setting. A further challenge to the office-based practitioner is that there is presently little to no training in OBA within the standard anesthesia residency program.[8]

ADVANTAGES/DISADVANTAGES

There are many advantages to an office-based procedure when compared with a traditional hospital-based one. The most obvious of these advantages is cost containment. Several components make up the actual cost of a given surgical procedure. In addition to surgical and anesthesia fees, which are usually negotiated prior to an elective procedure, there is a facility fee charged by the hospital or ASC. This fee generally covers the associated costs to the hospital/ASC, and includes overhead such as maintenance, equipment, and staff. It often constitutes a large component of the patient's overall charge. In an office, this amount can easily be predicted and is often minimal when compared with that of a hospital that, because of greater overhead costs, can be both enormous and unpredictable.[3,4,9,10] In 1994, Schultz[10] determined the cost of a laparoscopic inguinal hernia repair, when done in a hospital, to be $5,494. When the same procedure was performed in an office, the price was decreased to $1,533.84. Similarly, the average cost of an in-hospital open inguinal hernia repair was found to be $2,237, while the same procedure performed in a private office cost $894.79. Additionally, it has been reported that office-based ocular surgery performed under monitored anesthesia care (MAC) can cost 70% less than similar procedures performed in a hospital.[11] Realizing this cost savings, some insurance companies began offering incentives to surgeons who used an office location as their surgical venue. Other clear advantages of office-based procedures include ease of scheduling (often with less paperwork), patient and surgeon convenience, decreased patient exposure to nosocomial infections, and improved patient privacy and continuity of care (an office is usually staffed by a small, consistent group of personnel).[4,5,7,12,13]

There are potential disadvantages to office-based surgery, which usually relate to issues regarding patient safety and peer review. In some parts of the country, there are no regulations governing office-based surgery and OBA. Therefore, there may be little to no oversight regarding the certification/qualification of either the surgeon or anesthesiologist, the surgical office's policy regarding peer review, performance improvement, documentation, general policies and procedures, and the reporting of adverse outcomes. However, the number of states without such regulations is rapidly decreasing (Table 33-1).[14]

TABLE 33-1

STATES THAT HAVE REGULATIONS REGARDING OFFICE-BASED SURGERY AND ANESTHESIA AS OF DECEMBER 1, 2007

Alabama	Mississippi
Arizona[a]	New Jersey
California	New York
Colorado	North Carolina
Connecticut	Ohio
District of Columbia	Oklahoma
Florida	Oregon
Illinois	Pennsylvania
Indiana	Rhode Island
Kansas	South Carolina
Kentucky	Tennessee
Louisiana	Texas
Massachusetts	Washington

[a]In development.

Whether or not mandatory regulations exist, it is vital that the anesthesiologist consider all of these issues before selecting an office facility in which to deliver care.

OFFICE SAFETY

Media reports and newspaper articles raised the earliest questions regarding the safety of office-based procedures.[7,15,16] Data reveal that injuries and deaths occurring in offices are often multifactorial in causation. Reasons include overdosages of local anesthetics, prolonged surgery with occult blood loss, pulmonary embolism, accumulation of multiple anesthetics with oversedation, hypovolemia, hypoxemia, and the use of reversal drugs with short half-lives.[15,17,18] Both the Anesthesia Patient Safety Foundation and the American Society of Anesthesiologists (ASA) have emerged as leaders in the field of OBA safety and have advocated that the quality of care in an office-based practice be no less than that of a hospital or ASC.[19,20] Thus, it is imperative to ensure that all safety precautions one may take for granted in a hospital are present in the surgical office.[15]

In 1990 the mortality rate from anesthesia was approximately 1/100,000. By the year 2000, the rate had decreased to 1/250,000 in hospitals and 1/400,000 in freestanding ASCs.[5,15,21] Although the precision of these figures is open to debate, the decrease in mortality can be attributed, in part, to improvements in the training of the anesthesia providers, the safety profiles of the newer anesthetics, improved perioperative monitoring capabilities, and intrinsic safety mechanisms in place within the anesthetizing location. Because the majority of office-based patients are young and healthy, one would expect that an anesthetic performed in an office would be at least equally as safe as an anesthetic performed in a hospital, if not safer. However, reports of morbidity and mortality within office-based practices exist and vary dramatically. In 1997, Morello et al:[22] conducted a survey querying the office personnel of 418 accredited plastic surgeons. They had a 57% response rate and found that over a 5-year period, 400,675 office procedures were conducted; 63.2% were cosmetic and 36.8% were reconstructive. Several outcomes were reviewed including hemorrhage, hypertension, hypotension, wound infection, need for hospital admission, and reoperation. There was an overall complication rate of 0.24%, and seven deaths occurred. The causes of mortality were both surgery- and anesthesia-related. These deaths were from two cases of myocardial infarction, one following an augmentation mammaplasty and the other 4 hours after a rhinoplasty; one case of cerebral hypoxia during an abdominoplasty; one case of a tension pneumothorax during a breast augmentation; one case of a cardiac arrest during carpal tunnel surgery; one case of a stroke 3 days following a rhytidectomy and brow lift; and one unexplained death. This represents an overall mortality rate of 1 in 57,000. A report by Hoefflin et al,[23] however, found no complications after 23,000 plastic surgical procedures that occurred in an office under general anesthesia. Similarly, Sullivan and Tattini[24] retrospectively reviewed the results in an office performing >5,000 surgical procedures by five independent plastic surgeons. The anesthesia during this time consisted of deep sedation in conjunction with local anesthesia or regional block, and was performed by an anesthesiologist supervising a certified registered nurse anesthetist. No mortalities occurred during the 5-year period. Bitar et al:[25] retrospectively studied adverse outcomes in 3,615 consecutive patients undergoing 4,778 plastic surgery procedures in offices between 1995 and 2000, MAC with midazolam, propofol and an opioid, and no deaths were reported. Dyspnea occurred in 0.05% of patients, nausea and vomiting in 0.2%, and there was a 0.05% rate of hospital admissions. When analyzing these outcomes, it must be appreciated that because the mortality rate from anesthesia is so low, an extremely large cohort group would be necessary to provide real data regarding the relative risk of an office-based anesthetic. Recent data even suggests a 10-fold increased risk of morbidity and mortality associated with an office-based anesthetic when compared with one performed in a freestanding ASC. [17]

Other studies reveal a significant risk associated with an office-based procedure. Rao et al:[26] reported that according to closed malpractice claims in Florida, 830 deaths and 4,000 injuries were associated with OBA between 1990 and 1999. These claims accounted for 30% of all malpractice claims in that state. In a hospital operating room, the risks of an anesthetic are usually limited to the underlying medical condition of the patient, whereas in an office they may be increased because of factors such as inadequate standards and safeguards.[15] More recent Florida data have shown that office-based morbidity and mortality are usually the result of inadequate perioperative patient monitoring, oversedation, and thromboembolic events.[18,27,28] The challenge of acquiring accurate morbidity and mortality data for office-based anesthesia is complicated by the fact that many offices are not required to report adverse events. In addition, although an anesthesiologist may not even be administering the anesthetic in an office, many complications may still be reported as anesthetic-related.[29]

Traditional credentialing procedures, such as board certification and the granting or renewing of hospital privileges based on competency and proof of continuing medical education, may not be required in an office.[21] Within and among offices, health care providers of anesthesia may also have varying degrees of both education and expertise. The provider may be an anesthesiologist, a nurse anesthetist, a dental anesthetist, or a surgeon with little or no training in anesthesia.[30] Furthermore, safety within an anesthetizing location probably depends on the perioperative patient-monitoring capabilities. Although hospital patients receive defined standard of care for monitoring in the operating rooms and postanesthesia care units (PACUs), they may be lacking in an inadequately prepared surgical office.[25] There have been injuries to patients during office-based procedures resulting from the use of obsolete and/or malfunctioning anesthesia machines, as well as from alarms that have not been serviced and/or are not functioning properly.[4] The ASA created guidelines for defining obsolete anesthesia machines; the guidelines prohibit the use of any anesthesia machine that lacks essential safety features (e.g., oxygen ratio device, oxygen pressure failure alarm), has the presence of unacceptable features (e.g., copper kettles, or vaporizers with rotary concentration dials that increase vapor concentration when the dial is turned clockwise), or for which routine maintenance is no longer possible.[31]

A review of ASA Closed Claims Project data, which incorporates information from the 35 liability insurers that indemnify approximately 50% of the practicing anesthesiologists in the United States, reveals safety concerns in office-based practices are more than theoretical.[21] As of 2001 there were 753 (13.7%) claims for ambulatory procedures and 14 (0.26%) for office-based ones. This small number of claims most likely because of the 3- to 5-year time lag in reporting to the database.[21] ASA physical status 1 or 2 female patients who had undergone elective surgery under general anesthesia make up the majority of claims filed. This statistic parallels the profiles of trends seen in operating rooms and freestanding ASCs. The injuries that occur in offices tend to be of greater severity than those that occur in ASCs. Twenty-one percent of the reported injuries sustained in offices were temporary and nondisabling in nature and 64% were permanent or led to death, while 62% of the injuries sustained in ASCs were temporary and nondisabling and only 21% were permanent or led to death.[21] A

TABLE 33-2

CAUSES OF INJURY IN THE OFFICE-BASED PRACTICE

1. Inadequate resuscitation equipment
2. Inadequate monitoring
   a. Most commonly no pulse-oximetry
3. Inadequate preoperative or postoperative evaluation
4. Human error
   a. Slow recognition of an event
   b. Slow response to an event
   c. Lack of experience
   d. Drug overdosage

Data derived from Coté CJ, Karl HW, Notteman DA et al: Adverse sedation events in pediatrics: Analysis of medications used for sedation. Pediatrics 2000; 106: 663; and Coté CJ, Notteman DA, Karl HW et al: Adverse sedation events in pediatrics: A critical incident analysis of contributing factors. Pediatrics 2000; 105: 8

study by Coté et al:[32,33] revealed that the causes for injuries in an office ranged from human error to machine and equipment malfunction (Table 33-2).

The Closed Claims Project database reveals that injuries during office-based procedures occur throughout the perioperative period and are multifactorial in etiology. The majority, 64%, occurred intraoperatively, 14% occurred in the PACU, and 21% after discharge.[21] Half of these adverse events were respiratory in nature and included airway obstruction, bronchospasm, inadequate oxygenation and ventilation, and unrecognized esophageal intubation. The second most common group of events were drug-related, occurring 25% of the time. These included incorrect agent or dosage, allergy, and malignant hyperthermia. Cardiovascular injures and equipment-related injuries each occurred in 8% of incidents.[21]

An important point to consider when looking at adverse events is whether or not they were preventable. Again, according to the information in the Closed Claims Project database, 13% of the events that occurred in ASCs were considered preventable, whereas 46% of the office-based ones were deemed as preventable. Furthermore, all of the adverse respiratory events that occurred in the PACU of offices could have been prevented had pulse oximetry been used. Care was considered to be substandard in 50% of OBA claims and in 34% of ASC ones. In 2001, claims originating from an office-based procedure resulted in a monetary award 92% of the time, with a median payment of $200,000 (ranging between $10,000 and $2,000,000), whereas claims originating from ASC-based procedures were compensated only 59% of the time, with a median payout of $85,000 (ranging between $34 and $14,700,000).[21]

Ensuring office-based practice safety is critical. After several highly publicized office liposuction injuries and deaths in August 2000, the State of Florida attempted to address this problem by placing a 90-day moratorium on all office-based procedures that used anesthetic depths greater than conscious sedation. During that 90-day period a safety panel composed of surgeons, anesthesiologists, and other health care professionals was formed and charged with the task of developing recommendations to improve the safety record of office-based procedures. The panel's recommendations concerned factors including patient selection, preoperative evaluation and testing, procedures to be excluded, surgeon qualification, and facility standards.[13,34] Other major organizations that have played a leading role in developing standards for the office-based practitioner include the ASA, ASPS, the American Association of Nurse Anesthetists, and the American Medical Association.[13,19,24,34,36]

PATIENT SELECTION

Prior to presenting for an office-based procedure, the patient's medical condition should be optimally managed. He or she should have a preoperative history and physical examination recorded within 30 days, and all pertinent laboratory tests and any medically indicated specialist consultation(s) must be readily available. Consent for the procedure and the anesthetic must be in the chart. The anesthesiologist should have access to all of this information preoperatively and, when possible, should contact the patient prior to the scheduled procedure.

❸ Patient selection remains a controversial topic among practicing office-based anesthesiologists because little morbidity and mortality data exist to support the inclusion or exclusion of specific populations. A study by Meridy[37] in 1982 concluded that patients should not be excluded from undergoing ambulatory procedures based solely on their age, the type of procedure, or the duration of the planned procedure. Similar data are yet to exist regarding office-based practices; however, some recommendations have been made. The ASPS has acknowledged that the ideal patient for an office-based procedure has an ASA physical status of 1 or 2. They recommended that ASA physical status 3 patients undergo an office-based procedure only after an anesthesia consultation, and patients assigned an ASA physical status >3 should have an office-based procedure performed only under local anesthesia without sedation.[14] The ASA also has developed recommendations regarding patient selection.[38] It is important to realize that the office is often remote, and the anesthesiologist may be unable to get assistance should it be required. Thus, groups of patients in whom anticipated anesthetic problems may develop should be avoided (Table 33-3). Individual anesthesiologists should therefore consider excluding certain patients with significant comorbid conditions in order to avoid unanticipated problems.[15,39]

The morbidly obese and patients with obstructive sleep apnea syndrome (OSAS) present unique and increasingly frequent challenges to the office-based practitioner. Indeed, they are usually the same population, with estimates of 60 to 90% of all OSA patients being obese (body mass index ≥30 kg/m^2).[40,42] Confounding this problem is that the majority of the patients with OSAS have yet to be formally diagnosed.[43-45] These patients are likely to present major anesthetic problems throughout the perioperative period.[46] There may be failure to intubate or ventilate, they may have respira-

PATIENTS WHO MAY NOT BE GOOD CANDIDATES FOR AN OFFICE-BASED PROCEDURE

1. Poorly controlled diabetes
2. Expected significant blood loss or postoperative pain
3. History of substance abuse
4. Seizure disorder
5. Malignant hyperthermia susceptibility
6. Potential difficult airway
   a. Morbid obesity
   b. Obstructive sleep apnea syndrome
7. NPO <8 hours
8. No escort
9. Previous adverse outcome from anesthesia
10. Significant drug allergies
11. Aspiration risk

NPO, nothing by mouth.

TABLE 33-4

RISK FACTORS FOR THE DEVELOPMENT OF DEEP VEIN THROMBOSIS (DVT)

- Age >40
- Antithrombin III deficiency
- Central nervous system disease
- Family history of DVT
- Heart failure
- History of a DVT
- Hypercoagulable states
- Lupus anticoagulant
- Malignancy
- Obesity
- Oral contraceptive use
- Polycythemia
- Previous miscarriage
- Radiation therapy for pelvic neoplasms
- Severe infection
- Trauma
- Venous insufficiency

tory distress soon after extubation, or suffer from respiratory arrest with preoperative sedation or postoperative analgesia.[40] These patients tend to be exquisitely sensitive to the respiratory depressant effects of even small dosages of sedation or analgesics.[42,46,47] Furthermore, respiratory depression may not be reversible with pharmacologic antagonism.[48] One of the first steps in the ASA algorithm for management of the difficult airway is to call for help. In an office, this usually is not possible. It has been recommended that a postoperative observational unit with close monitoring of oxygen saturation or an intensive care unit setting be used for monitoring the OSAS

❹ patient postoperatively.[49] It has also been suggested that outpatient facilities develop specific policies regarding acceptable patients for the outpatient setting, possibly excluding patients with OSAS.[43] These recommendations would also clearly be relevant to the office-based practitioner.

Pulmonary embolism is a significant cause of perioperative morbidity and mortality from an office-based surgical procedure.[50,51] Reinisch et al:[52] found that 0.39% (37/9,493) of patients who underwent rhytidectomy developed a deep vein thrombosis. Of these, 40.5% (15/37) went on to form a pulmonary embolism. Although general anesthesia had accounted for only 43% of the anesthetic techniques used for the procedure, 83.7% of the embolic events were associated with the patient having undergone a general anesthetic (GA). Risk factors for the development of deep vein thrombosis appear in Table 33-4. [53] The ASPS recommends that patients be stratified according to risk and that the prophylactic treatment be directed by risk (Table 33-5).

As more persons in subspecialties begin to perform office-based procedures, they will treat older and sicker patients. The anesthesiologist must be the patient's advocate in the matter of safety. This advocacy can result only from a true understanding of how to adequately select appropriate patients for this unique surgical venue.

SURGEON SELECTION

The relationship between the surgeon and anesthesiologist must be one of mutual trust and understanding. Because the surgeon performing the procedure may also own the office, he or she must not put pressure on the anesthesiologist to perform an anesthetic if the anesthesiologist believes that the patient or procedure is not appropriate.

TABLE 33-5

RECOMMENDED TREATMENT FOR PREVENTION OF DEEP VEIN THROMBOSIS (DVT) IN PATIENTS, STRATIFIED BY RISK

■ COHORT	■ TREATMENT
Low Risk • No risk factors • Uncomplicated surgery • Short duration	• Comfortable position • Knees flexed at 5 degrees • Avoid constriction and external pressure
Moderate Risk • Age >40 with no other risks for the development of DVT • Procedure >30 min • Oral contraceptive use	• Proper positioning • Intermittent pneumatic compression of calf or ankle (prior to sedation and continued until patient is awake and moving) • Frequent alterations of the OR table
High Risk • Age >40 with other risk factors for the development of DVT • Procedure >30 min under general anesthesia • Oral contraceptive use	• Treatment as per patients with moderate risk • Preoperative hematology consultation with consideration of perioperative antithrombotic therapy

OR, operating room.

The surgeon must have a valid medical license, registration, and Drug Enforcement Administration (DEA) certificate. He or she should be either board-eligible or board-certified by a recognized member of the American Board of Medical Specialties,[34] and either have privileges to perform the proposed procedure in a local hospital, or have training and documented competency comparable to a practitioner who does have such privileges in a hospital. Although this requirement may sound intuitive, there have been cases reported of surgeons performing procedures for which they have little or no training.[4] In addition, the surgeon must have adequate liability insurance, at least equal to that carried by the anesthesiologist. If a lawsuit should arise and the surgeon is inadequately insured, the anesthesiologist may be held financially responsible and become the "deep pocket." Similarly, the facility itself should have adequate liability insurance.

In addition, there should be a system in place for monitoring continuing medical education as well as peer review and performance improvement, for both the surgeon and anesthesiologist. This is often not the case in an office-based practice.[4] If an anesthesia group provides care at more than one office, an overall peer review for the practice may be used; it need not be specific to each individual office site. Solo anesthesia practitioners should not be exempt from this process. He or she needs to align with the offices in which he or she provides services, and either participate in the office's process or help to organize an ongoing one. The peer review committee should include surgeons, anesthesiologists, and nursing staff. It should meet regularly and maintain a written record of minutes and recommendations. Similarly, continuing medical education should also be documented and, at a minimum, should be sufficient to meet relicensing requirements.

When formulating a quality assurance program, there should be key sentinel events that trigger a case review (Table 33-6). It is imperative that this review be an open forum to ensure continued quality improvement of care, and not be biased or hindered by fear of litigation. Legal counsel should be sought to determine whether information disclosed at these meetings is discoverable in a court of law, should a malpractice claim arise.

OFFICE SELECTION

❺ The anesthesiologist should function as a zealous patient advocate in assuring that an anesthetic is performed only in a safe location.[30] The office needs to be appropriately equipped, stocked, and maintained to perform a GA (Table 33-7). All supplies must be age- and size-appropriate for the patient population. If an anesthesia machine or ventilator is present, it must be regularly serviced and calibrated. If potent inhaled volatile agents or nitrous oxide (N_2O) are used, there must be a functioning waste gas scavenging system. This system may be exhausted via a window or roof vent. However, the exhaust must not be vented back into the office or into any other inhabited space and must be in accordance with Occupational

TABLE 33-6

ADVERSE OUTCOMES SIGNALING CASE REVIEW[a]

1. Dental injury
2. Corneal abrasion
3. Perioperative MI or stroke
4. Aspiration
5. Reintubation
6. Return to the operating room
7. Peripheral nerve injury
8. Adverse drug reaction
9. Uncontrolled pain or nausea/vomiting
10. Unexpected hospital admission
11. Cardiac arrest
12. Death
13. Incomplete charts
14. Controlled substance discrepancy
15. Patient complaints

MI, myocardial infarction.
[a]Sentinel events that should trigger a case review and be presented at a performance improvement/quality assurance meeting.

TABLE 33-7

EQUIPMENT REQUIRED FOR THE SAFE DELIVERY OF OFFICE-BASED ANESTHESIA

Monitors
  Noninvasive blood pressure with an assortment of cuff sizes
  Heart rate/ECG
  Pulse oximeter
  Temperature
  Capnography
Airway supplies
  Nasal cannulas
  Oral airways
  Face masks
  Self-inflating bag-mask ventilation device
  Laryngoscopes multiple sizes and styles (Macintosh and Miller)
  Handles
  Various sizes of tracheal tubes
  Stylettes
  Emergency airway equipment (LMAs, cricothyrotomy kit, transtracheal jet-ventilation equipment)
Suction catheters and suction equipment
Cardiac defibrillator
Emergency drugs
  ACLS drugs
  Dantrolene and malignant hyperthermia supplies
Anesthetic drugs
Vascular cannulation equipment

ECG, electrocardiogram; LMA, laryngeal mask airway; ACLS, Advanced Cardiac Life Support.

Safety and Health Administration standards. Air testing should also be done on a regular basis. In an office without an exhaust system, total intravenous anesthesia techniques should be employed. Similarly, all medical and hazardous waste must be disposed of in accordance with state and local laws.

All offices, especially those without ventilators or anesthesia machines, require a method to deliver positive pressure ventilation to the patient's lungs. This can be achieved using a self-inflating resuscitation device. An adequate supply of compressed oxygen must be present as well as a backup supply for use in an emergency. In offices that do not have a pipeline supply of oxygen, H-cylinders are usually used and several E-cylinders should be kept in reserve. A policy must be in place describing the transport, storage, and disposal of medical gases, consistent with state and local laws. All equipment described in the ASA algorithm for management of the difficult airway should be present.[54] A readily available means to create an emergency surgical airway and jet ventilation capability may be lifesaving.

Perioperative monitoring must adhere to the ASA standards for basic anesthetic monitoring.[55,56] These include continuous monitoring of heart rate and oxygen saturation, intermittent noninvasive blood pressure monitoring, end-tidal CO_2 monitoring and the capacity for both temperature monitoring and continuous electrocardiogram. Monitors must be routinely serviced, calibrated, and repaired as necessary. All monitors should have a backup battery supply and there should be an extra monitor available for an emergency.

All emergency drugs appearing on the American Heart Association Advanced Cardiac Life Support (ACLS) protocol should be available. The expiration dates for these agents should be checked on a regular basis and outdated drugs

replaced as necessary. A cardiac defibrillator with a battery backup must be immediately available and routinely checked, as should a source of suction including a pharyngeal suction catheter. The office-based anesthesiologist should be prepared to begin the initial treatment of malignant hyperthermia, which requires having at least 12 bottles of dantrolene. A complete listing of malignant hyperthermia supplies is available online at www.mhaus.org.

A protocol for the delivery and secure storage of controlled substances must be in place. A licensed anesthesiologist may supply these drugs in accordance with DEA regulations, as may any licensed physician with a current DEA registration certificate. Instead of transporting drugs, it is often more convenient to store them in the surgical office. In this situation, they must be stored in a double-locked storage cabinet, installed in a secure location, in accordance with state and local regulations. The office in which the controlled substances will be dispensed must also be properly registered with the DEA. Drug accounting must be performed in accordance with state and federal regulations. Individual states have different provisions and regulations regarding the dispensing of controlled substances, and it is the responsibility of the dispensing physician to assure that the office-based practice is in compliance.

A medical director, responsible for overall operations, should be identified for every office. There must also be a policy and procedures manual that outlines the responsibilities of each staff member, including nurses (circulating/scrub and postoperative), physician assistants, surgical technicians, office staff, and administrators. The manual should include a description of the infection control policy as well as anesthesia policies. All nurses should be licensed by the state and have training and education consistent with their responsibilities. Basic cardiac life support certification should be mandatory, and ACLS certification is preferable. In addition, either the anesthesiologist or the physician who supervises the anesthesia care provider must be certified in ACLS or Pediatric Advanced Life Support (PALS), depending on the patient population. There should always be at least one member of the health care team with ACLS/PALS certification present in the office until the last patient has been discharged.

Emergencies can, and do, occur in an office-based setting (Table 33-8). Each office must have a plan in place delineating the responsibilities of each staff member in the event of such an occurrence. The physical structure of the office is an important consideration. There should be a clear egress that would easily accommodate a stretcher carrying a mechanically ventilated

TABLE 33-8

EMERGENCIES THAT REQUIRE CONTINGENCY PLANS

1. Fire
2. Bomb/bomb threat
3. Power loss
4. Equipment malfunction
5. Loss of oxygen supply pressure
6. Cardiac or respiratory arrest in the waiting room, OR, or PACU
7. Earthquake
8. Hurricane
9. External disturbance such as a riot
10. Malignant hyperthermia
11. Massive blood loss
12. Emergency transfer of patient to a hospital

OR, operating room: PACU, postanesthesia unit.

patient. Adequate clearance and room for transport in an elevator must also be considered.

6 Destinations for a patient in need of hospital admission must be identified. Developing an office-hospital relationship is challenging, as hospitals may be reluctant to be involved in office mishaps. However, it is of utmost importance to have a formal written arrangement. Telephoning the emergency services number (911) is an acceptable plan for transportation, provided the response time is rapid. If 911 is unavailable in a specific city or has a slow response time, the office should have a contractual agreement with an ambulance company.

Ideally a 1-hour firewall should be in place. This wall would provide enough time to awaken and escort a patient to safety in the event of a fire. If a 1-hour firewall is not present, the office should, at a minimum, be in compliance with local fire codes. Additionally, the office must be in compliance with commercial construction codes and with maximum occupancy regulations.

There must be contingency plans in the event of a power supply interruption or electrical failure. Each office should have an emergency generator capable of running necessary equipment and monitors; monitors should have battery backup power that is routinely checked. Battery reserve power will usually last for 1 1/2 hours, but this needs to be verified for each piece of electrically powered equipment.

The office should keep patient records (including anesthesia records) in accordance with local laws, which is usually for a minimum of 5 years. Similarly, the anesthesiologist should maintain his or her own records, which include the preanesthesia history and physical, informed consent, intraoperative documentation, and postoperative care record, as well as discharge orders.

Accreditation

One way to objectively evaluate an office is to have it be accredited by a nationally recognized accrediting agency. The ASA has developed a classification of offices that stratifies them by the level of anesthetic depth that may be administered (Table 33-9).[38] Many states require offices to be accredited, and more states are following suit (Table 33-1). In states that do not require accreditation, there are benefits to voluntarily obtaining it. Oftentimes accreditation will allow the facility fee to be reimbursed by a third-party payer in medically necessary procedures.[57] In addition, the patient may feel more comfortable undergoing a procedure in an office that has been accredited. Finally, as more states require accreditation, if a surgeon's office proactively becomes accredited in a state that subsequently requires it, there would be no interruption of services.[7]

Currently there are three major accrediting bodies for office-based surgery offices, although several other agencies are also recognized. The Accreditation Association for Ambulatory Health Care (AAAHC) was the first major accrediting body, offering certification since 1998. The American Association for Accreditation of Ambulatory Surgical Facilities (AAAASF), originally the Accreditation Association for Ambulatory Plastic Surgical Facilities, was the second group, followed by the Joint Commission for Accreditation of Healthcare Organizations (JCAHO). To date, the most active organization is the AAAASF. Its requirements are simpler than those of AAAHC and JCAHO and accreditation is less expensive; however, changes are underway to allow AAAHC and JCAHO to be more competitive.[7] Each agency has different criteria for eligibility and different accreditation cycles pertaining to the time limit of a certificate.[58] The agencies deal with surgical conditions ranging from physical office design to patient issues (Table 33-10). In addition the AAAHC can accredit not only the surgical office, but also an anesthesia group that provides OBA.

TABLE 33-9

AMERICAN SOCIETY OF ANESTHESIOLOGISTS CLASSIFICATION OF SURGICAL PROCEDURES

Class A
  Minor surgical procedures
  Local, topical, or infiltration of local anesthetic
  No sedation preoperatively or intraoperatively
Class B
  Minor or major surgical procedures
  Sedation via oral, rectal, or intravenous sedation
  Analgesic or dissociative drugs
Class C
  Minor or major surgical procedures
  General anesthesia
  Major conduction block anesthesia

Data derived from American Society of Anesthesiologists Committee on Ambulatory Surgical Care and the American Society of Anesthesiologists Task Force on Office-Based Anesthesia: Office-based anesthesia: considerations for anesthesiologists in setting up and maintaining a safe office anesthesia environment. Park Ridge, IL, American Society of Anesthesiologists, 2000, with permission.

TABLE 33-10

FACTORS TO BE CONSIDERED IN ACCREDITING AN OFFICE FOR SURGICAL PROCEDURES[a]

1. Physical layout of the office
2. Environmental safety/infection control
3. Patient and personnel records
4. Surgeon qualification
   a. Training
   b. Local hospital privileges (surgical and admission)
5. Office administration
6. Anesthesiologist requirements
7. Staffing intraoperatively and postoperatively
8. Monitoring capabilities both intraoperatively and postoperatively
9. Ancillary care
10. Equipment
11. Drugs (emergency, controlled substances, routine medications)
12. BLS, ACLS/PALS certification
13. Temperature
14. Neuromuscular functioning
15. Patient positioning
16. Pre- and postanesthesia care/documentation
17. Quality assurance/peer review
18. Liability insurance
19. PACU evaluation
20. Discharge evaluation
21. Emergency procedure (e.g., fire/admission/transfer)

BLS, basic cardiac life support; ACLS, Advanced Cardiac Life Support; PALS, Pediatric Advanced Life Support; PACU, postanesthesia care unit.
[a]A complete listing of criteria can obtained from the individual agencies.

The accrediting agencies were developed, in part, to reduce some of the variability that exists among offices in regard to safety issues. Several professional societies are encouraging their members to perform procedures only in accredited facilities. The Society for Aesthetic Plastic Surgeons mandates that all of its members perform procedures only in offices that have either been accredited by one of the nationally recognized accrediting agencies, have been certified to participate in the Medicare program under Title XVIII, or are licensed by the state. The actual improvement in safety conferred by performing surgery in an accredited office has yet to be determined, and there are those who suggest that it provides no advantage.[22,59] As long as there is no mandatory reporting system in place, it will be impossible to determine true morbidity rates associated with an office-based practice. Clearly though, safety in an office depends on more than just accreditation; there must be constant vigilance by all members of the health care team.

PROCEDURE SELECTION

Early in the development of office-based surgery, procedures were generally noninvasive and of short duration. However, as newer surgical and anesthetic techniques have evolved, longer and more invasive procedures have been successfully performed.[30,60–65] Suitable office-based procedures range the gamut from incision and drainage of abscesses to microlaparoscopies.

Duration of procedure has long been correlated with the need for hospital admission, with procedures lasting >1 hour being associated with a higher incidence of unplanned admission.[67] Other data have shown that longer procedures are also often associated with an increased incidence of postoperative nausea and vomiting (PONV), postoperative pain, and bleeding,[68,69] which may warrant hospital admission. For these reasons the ASPS has recommended that procedures be limited to 6 hours and be completed by 3 PM, thus allowing for a full patient recovery with maximum office staffing.[34] In addition, when determining the suitability of a procedure, one must consider the possibility of hypothermia, blood loss, or significant fluid shifts.[34]

Specific Procedures

Liposuction

Liposuction is the second most commonly performed cosmetic procedure after breast augmentation, and is performed primarily by plastic surgeons and dermatologists.[70] It is accomplished by inserting hollow rods into small incisions in the skin and suctioning subcutaneous fat into an aspiration canister. Superwet and tumescent techniques, introduced in the mid 1980s, use large volumes (1 to 4 mL) of infiltrate solution (0.9% saline or Ringer lactate with epinephrine 1:1,000,000 and lidocaine 0.025 to 0.1%) for each 1 cm^3 of fat to be removed. Blood loss is generally 1% of the aspirate with these techniques.[71] The peak serum levels of lidocaine occur 12 to 14 hours after injection and decline over the subsequent 6 to 14 hours.[72,73] Although the maximum dose of lidocaine has been traditionally limited to 7 mg/kg, doses of 35 to 55 mg/kg have been used safely because the tumescent technique results in a single compartment clearance similar to that of a sustained-release medication.[73,74]

Liposuction is not a benign procedure. In 2000, a census survey of the 1,200 members of the American Society of Aesthetic Plastic Surgeons revealed an overall mortality rate of 19.1/100,000 liposuction procedures, with pulmonary embolism the diagnosis in 23.1% of deaths. Other causes of mortality included abdominal viscous perforation, anesthesia "causes," fat embolism, infection, and hemorrhage; 28.5% of all deaths in this study were reported as of unknown or confidential etiology.[75] Risk factors identified included the use of multiliter wetting solution infiltration, megavolume aspiration causing massive third spacing, multiple concurrent procedures, anesthetic sedative effects yielding hypoventilation, and permissive discharge policies. The management of the postoperative period, with attention to fluid and electrolyte balance and pain control, is critical to an optimal outcome after liposuction. The patient's fluid deficit, maintenance, intraoperative loss, and third spacing should guide fluid management throughout the perioperative period. Generally, an office liposuction should be limited to 5,000 mL of total aspirant, which includes supernatant fat and fluid.[34] It is also recommended that large-volume liposuction not be done in conjunction with other procedures.

Iverson et al:[13,34] developed the following considerations and recommendations regarding office-based liposuction:

1. Plastic surgeons should follow the current ASA Guidelines for Sedation and Analgesia.
2. GA can be used safely in the office setting.
3. GA has advantages for more complex liposuction procedures that include precise dosing, controlled patient movement, and airway management.
4. Epidural and spinal anesthesia in the office setting is discouraged because of the possibility of vasodilatation, hypotension, and fluid overload.
5. Moderate sedation/analgesia augments the patient's comfort and is an effective adjunct to the anesthetic infiltrate solutions.

Two hundred sixty-one respondents to a survey sent to the membership of The American Society for Dermatologic Surgery reported no mortalities among 66,570 liposuction procedures performed in hospitals, ASCs, and offices. The authors reported adverse events, which mirrored those in the American Society of Aesthetic Plastic Surgeons. They found that serious adverse events occurred more frequently with procedures performed in hospital and ASCs than those in offices. This may be partly because liposuction in hospitals is performed on sicker patients or that the procedures are associated with removal of a larger amount of fat. Interestingly, 71% of the offices surveyed were nonaccredited. Further, the authors reported that morbidity correlated better with the area of the body suctioned (abdomen and buttocks) than the facility in which the procedure took place.[76]

Aesthetics

Many facial aesthetic procedures such as blepharoplasty, rhinoplasty, and meloplasty are routinely performed in offices, usually under varying depths of MAC, but occasionally with GA. Facial plastic procedures that require use of a laser or even routine electrocautery pose a problem for the anesthesiologist. Supplemental nasal oxygen in patients receiving sedation is a fire hazard. Any supplemental oxygen must be turned off during periods of laser or electrocautery use about the face, and this requires vigilance by the anesthesiologist who must be in constant communication with the surgeon. Methods for delivering supplemental oxygen to a patient having a facial procedure include nasal cannula, an oxygen hood, or placement of oxygen tubing in an oral/nasal airway. The latter usually requires a deeper level of sedation. The avoidance of supplemental oxygen when medically appropriate is ideal.

Breast

Procedures such as breast biopsy or augmentation, implant exchanges, and completion of transverse rectus abdominal muscle flaps (e.g., nipple construction or revisions) are routinely performed in office settings. Breast augmentation entails separating the pectoralis muscles from the chest wall, which is painful and usually requires GA. This can be accomplished by using either a laryngeal mask airway or tracheal tube. The use of regional anesthesia with paravertebral nerve blocks has also been reported.[77] Breast surgery has a high incidence of PONV, thus it is likely that patients undergoing breast surgery will require antiemetic medication in addition to postoperative analgesics.[78]

Gastrointestinal Endoscopy

Procedures performed by gastroenterologists include esophageal, gastric, and duodenal endoscopies and colonoscopies. This patient population tends to be older, with significant comorbid conditions. Upper gastrointestinal procedures rarely require endotracheal intubation because, although many of these patients have gastroesophageal reflux, the stomach is emptied under direct visualization. The endoscopist requires patient participation to aid in insertion of the endoscope, which can usually be accomplished with sedation using small doses of propofol with or without midazolam.

Colonoscopy is painful secondary to the insertion and manipulation of the endoscope, and may be associated with cardiovascular effects, including dysrhythmia, bradycardia, hypotension, hypertension, myocardial infarction, and death. The mechanism of these cardiovascular effects is not known, but there is evidence that they may be mediated by the autonomic nervous system when stimulated by anxiety or discomfort.[79] Adding an opioid to midazolam during colonoscopy has been shown to improve patient tolerance of the procedure and decrease pain without increasing the frequency of respiratory events.[80] Interestingly, anesthetic techniques consisting of midazolam,[81] remifentanil/propofol, and fentanyl/propofol/midazolam[82] potentiate the low-frequency components of heart rate variability, which reflects sympathetic activation as seen on continuous electrocardiography, and may contribute to the number of cardiovascular events that occur during colonoscopy.

Recently, the gastroenterology community has sought to be able to provide moderate or even deep sedation with propofol without the assistance of a trained anesthesiologist.[83] However, because of safety concerns propofol may still only be given by an anesthesiologist as indicated in the product insert. Additionally, the Institute for Safe Medical Practices has indicated that propofol may be administered only by individuals who are "trained in the administration of drugs that cause deep sedation and GA" and who provide only the sedation (not also performing the procedure) and are proficient at tracheal intubation.[84] The AAAASF has likewise indicated that anesthesia professionals are best qualified to administer propofol sedation.

Dentistry and Oral and Maxillofacial Surgery

Nitrous oxide has been used for most of the world's office-based dental anesthetics since 1884, when Horace Wells, himself a dentist, had N_2O administered for a wisdom tooth extraction by a colleague. It was Harry Langa, another dentist, who pioneered the concept of using lower concentrations of N_2O in combination with local anesthetics. This idea of "relative analgesia" was the forbearer of "conscious sedation."[85]

The American Association of Oral and Maxillofacial Surgeons studied a prospective cohort study of patients who underwent oral and maxillofacial surgery between January and December 2001. Of the 34,191 patients included, 71.9% received deep sedation/GA, 15.5% conscious sedations, and 12.6% local anesthesia. The operating surgeon provided anesthesia services in 96% of cases; the anesthesia-specific hospitalization rate was 4/100,000, with no reported mortalities. The authors attributed this safety level to the use of pulse oximetry, blood pressure and ventilation monitoring, as well as administration of supplemental oxygen.[86] As anesthesiologists increase their presence in the dental/oral and maxillofacial surgery arena, one can expect an increased utilization of nontraditional agents for procedures.

Orthopaedics and Podiatry

The orthopaedic office provides an excellent location for the anesthesiologist who practices regional anesthesia. Although knee arthroscopies can be performed with intra-articular local anesthesia and MAC, a three-in-one block of the lumbar plexus with bupivacaine or ropivacaine, supplementing the intra-articular local anesthetic in an arthroscopically assisted anterior cruciate ligament repair will provide long-acting postoperative analgesia. Interscalene and axillary regional anesthetics avoid airway manipulations in patients undergoing upper extremity procedures, while ankle blocks or blocks of the sciatic nerve in the popliteal fossa provide anesthesia for operations on the lower extremity. All of these blocks can be supplemented with short-acting anxiolytic agents.

Spinal anesthetics in the office-based setting must be of short duration, secondary to limited PACU space. Lidocaine, which provides reliable short-acting analgesia, may be associated with an increased risk of transient neurologic symptoms in the ambulatory patient population,[87] whereas using procaine-fentanyl spinals are associated with nausea and vomiting as well as pruritus.[88] When the neuraxial anesthetic wears off, issues of postoperative pain management arise; therefore, the patient must be discharged with oral analgesics as well as contact information for both the surgeon and the anesthesiologist.

Gynecology and Genitourinary

Many procedures, such as dilation and curettage, vasectomy, and cystoscopy have been performed in offices for many years. Recently there has been an increase in more invasive procedures such as minilaparoscopies, ovum retrieval, prostate biopsies, and lithotripsy, necessitating an anesthesiologist's expertise. A variety of anesthetic options are available for these procedures and the anesthetic choice depends on the surgeon, patient, and anesthesiologist's preferences.

Ophthalmology and Otolaryngology

Ophthalmologic procedures suitable for the office include cataracts, lacrimal duct probing, and ocular plastics. Topical anesthesia and periorbital or retrobulbar blocks are frequently used to provide analgesia. Supplemental sedation may be required. Otolaryngology procedures include endoscopic sinus surgery, turbinate resection, septoplasty, and myringotomy. Again, combinations of topical and regional nerve blocks with supplemental sedation are commonly employed, but occasionally GA is used.

Pediatrics

Although no minimum age requirement for a child to undergo an office-based anesthetic has been established, patients >6 months of age and ASA physical status 1 or 2 may be reasonable candidates.[89] Appropriate OBA pediatric cases are usually dental, and chloral hydrate with N_2O has historically been the anesthetic choice of many dentists. However, the use of these agents is associated with significant morbidity. Ross and Eck[9] found that in children between the ages of 1 and 9 years, 70 mg/kg of chloral hydrate with 30% N_2O resulted in hypoventilation in 94% of patients, which increased to 97% of patients when the chloral hydrate was combined with 50% N_2O. This increase is significant in view of the findings of Coté et al.:[32,33] who reviewed 95 adverse sedation-related events in

ANESTHETIC MANAGEMENT

TABLE 33-11

GUIDELINES FOR THE PEDIATRIC PERIOPERATIVE ANESTHESIA ENVIRONMENT

Patient Care Facility and Medical Staff Policies
  Designation of operative procedures
  Categorization of pediatric patients undergoing anesthesia
  Annual minimal case volume to maintain clinical competence
Clinical Privileges of Anesthesiologists
  Regular privileges
  Special clinical privileges
  Pain management
Patient Care Units
  Preoperative evaluation and preparation units
  Operating room
  Anesthesiologists
  Other health care providers involved in perioperative care
  Clinical laboratory and radiologic services availability and
    capabilities
  Pediatric anesthesia equipment and drugs, including
    resuscitation cart
PACU
  Nursing staff
  Anesthesiologist/physician staff
  Pediatric anesthesia equipment and drugs
Postoperative Intensive Care

TABLE 33-12

DEFINITIONS OF LEVELS OF SEDATION/ANALGESIA BY THE AMERICAN SOCIETY OF ANESTHESIOLOGISTS

1. Minimal sedation (anxiolysis)
   a. Drug-induced sedation
   b. Patient responds normally to verbal commands
   c. Cognitive and motor function may be impaired
   d. Ventilatory and cardiovascular function maintained
      normally
2. Moderate sedation/analgesia (conscious sedation)
   a. Drug-induced sedation
   b. Patient responds purposefully to verbal commands
      either alone or with light tactile stimulation
   c. Patient maintains a patent airway and spontaneous
      ventilation
   d. Cardiovascular function maintained
3. Deep sedation/analgesia
   a. Drug-induced sedation
   b. Patient cannot be easily aroused but can respond
      purposefully to repeated or painful stimulation
   c. Ventilatory function may be impaired, requiring
      assistance in maintaining a patent airway, and
      spontaneous ventilation may be inadequate
   d. Cardiovascular function is usually maintained
4. General anesthesia
   a. Drug-induced loss of consciousness
   b. Patients cannot be aroused by painful stimulation
   c. Ventilatory function is often impaired; patient may
      require assistance in maintaining a patent airway.
   d. Spontaneous ventilation may be impaired as well as
      neuromuscular functioning
   e. Positive pressure ventilation is often required
   f. Cardiovascular function may be impaired.

Adapted from American Society of Anesthesiologists Task Force on Sedation and Analgesia by Non-Anesthesiologists. Practice guidelines for sedation and analgesia by non-anesthesiologists. Anesthesiology 2002; 96: 1004

pediatric patients. In the 93% of these cases that resulted in permanent neurologic injury or death, the anesthetic was delivered by either an oral surgeon, periodontist, or certified registered nurse anesthetist supervised by a dentist.

There are increasing numbers of ophthalmologic (examination under anesthesia, lacrimal duct probing), otolaryngology (myringotomy), cast/dressing changes, and minor plastics procedures being performed on children in offices. The American Academy of Pediatrics Section on Anesthesiology has developed guidelines for the pediatric perioperative environment that should be adhered to in the OBA setting (Table 33-11).[90]

ANESTHETIC TECHNIQUES

The ASA recommends that anesthetics be provided or supervised by a fully licensed anesthesiologist.[38] If an anesthesiologist is directing anesthesia care, he or she must be immediately available throughout the entire perioperative period. Regulations in several states have questioned the need for this level of anesthesia training in the delivery of OBA. Some states allow for an anesthetic to be performed by a nonphysician anesthesia provider supervised by a licensed physician. In this situation, the supervising physician must be qualified to perform a preanesthetic-focused history and physical examination as well as be immediately available throughout the perioperative period. He or she must know how to handle anesthetic-related emergencies and complications. The supervising physician must be ACLS-certified.

OBA may entail any type of anesthesia from MAC through regional and GA.[90] Anesthesia is, however, a continuum and it is often impossible to predict how a patient will react. The ASA has developed definitions regarding depths of anesthesia (Table 33-12). Patients will routinely drift between the anesthetic depths, thus it is imperative that the anesthesia provider or supervisor be able to rescue a patient from a deeper level of anesthetic than was anticipated.

When formulating an anesthetic plan, one must consider that all agents and techniques used should be short-acting,

and thus the patient should be ready for discharge home soon after the completion of the procedure.[5,91] Furthermore, any agents used should have a high safety profile as well as be cost-effective.[92] In choosing MAC over GA, one must not be under the false impression that MAC anesthesia is inherently safer than GA. In 1988, Cohen et al:[93] reviewed the data from 100,000 anesthetics. They found that the group with the greatest number of mortalities had undergone procedures with MAC, whereas MAC constituted only 2% of all cases. The complication rate related to MAC anesthetics is increasing as its use expands. The Closed Claims Project database reveals that in the 1970s MAC cases accounted for 1.6% of the claims, in the 1980s, 1.9%, and by the 1990s, 6% of the cases were MAC anesthetics.[94] In a recent review by Bhanaker, et al, it was found that injury during MAC ranges from temporary and non-disabling through death, with death accounting for 33% of all claims during MAC.[94a] The causes for injuries during MAC are varied (Table 33-13). The percentage of claims resulting from mortality was identical for both MAC and GA cases. In the 1990s, when injuries other than death occurred during MAC anesthetics, they were more likely to be permanent, whereas injuries occurring during GA were more frequently temporary.[94] MAC anesthetics also tend to lead to litigation. Suits were filed in 90% of the MAC claims; 65% were settled, 20% went to judgment, and 15% were discontinued. The range of payout was $2,000 to $6,300,000 with a median of $75,000.[94]

TABLE 33-13

CAUSES OF INJURIES DURING MONITORED ANESTHESIA CARE (n = 121)

Respiratory 29 (24%)
Equipment Failure/Malfunction 25 (21%)
Cardiovascular Event 17 (14%)
Inadequate Anesthesia/Patient Movement 13 (11%)
Medication Related 11 (9%)
Related to Regional Block 2 (2%)
Other Events 24 (20%)[a]

[a]Including surgical technique/patient condition, wrong operation/location, positioning, failure to diagnose.
Adapted from Bhananker SM, Posner KL, Cheney FW, et al. Injury and liability associated with monitored anesthesia care. A closed claims analysis. Anesthesiology 2006; 104: 228

Anesthetic Agents

Intravenous sedation (propofol, barbiturates, midazolam, fentanyl, meperidine) is the most-often used anesthetic technique in the OBA setting.[30] When selecting an anesthetic for an office-based procedure, one must consider factors such as duration of action, cost-effectiveness, and safety profile. The drugs should have a short half-life, be inexpensive, and not be associated with undesirable side effects such as nausea and vomiting.

Although fentanyl has been the mainstay for "short-acting" narcotics, recently the use of remifentanil has increased in popularity. This ultra–short-acting opioid, when combined with propofol for conscious sedation, has been shown to provide discharge readiness within 15 minutes after colonoscopy. This timeframe is a marked reduction from the 48 to 80 minutes reported after the traditional meperidine/midazolam technique.[95] Remifentanil is also an ideal drug for use during many office-based procedures, such as facial cosmetic procedures, which can be quite painful while the local anesthetic is being injected and after which it is relatively painless. An important caveat to the use of remifentanil is that it may cause nausea and vomiting as well as apnea. Additionally, it often requires the use of an infusion pump.

Ketamine, a phencyclidine derivative, has experienced a resurgence over the past several years in the OBA practice.[9] The use of ketamine-propofol sedation has been described as an excellent way to provide a relaxed surgical field in a quiet, immobile patient, often eliminating the need for supplemental oxygen.[96] Ketamine functions as both an anesthetic and an analgesic. It does not depress respiration and will increase laryngeal reflexes, thus decreasing the risk of aspiration. Furthermore, it is not associated with nausea and vomiting.[97] Ketamine can, however, cause an increase in secretions as well as cause hallucinations. The latter can be decreased or eliminated by adding propofol and midazolam.[97–100] Glycopyrrolate can be used as an antisialagogue. Another advantage of ketamine is that it is relatively inexpensive.

Clonidine has also been found to be useful in an office. Because it is an α_2-agonist, clonidine will help control blood pressure throughout the perioperative period, thus potentially minimizing blood loss.[101,102] In addition, it may decrease the total propofol usage.[100] However, its use may precipitate hypotension and oversedation during the perioperative period.

Any type of anesthesia from sedation through GA can be administered safely in an office setting. However, because anesthesia is a continuum, it is vital that the office be adequately equipped and staffed to rescue a patient from a deeper stage of anesthesia. Thus, if MAC is planned, GA must be anticipated.

Depth of anesthesia monitoring has been shown to decrease the time to extubation and discharge readiness.[103–105] A depth of anesthesia monitor has been described as useful in the office during MAC procedures, with a possible decrease in total propofol usage.[106] Whether this type of monitoring will prove to be cost-effective in the office-based situation remains to be seen.

POSTANESTHESIA CARE UNIT

Following an office-based procedure, the patient should be able to sit in a chair or ambulate to an examination room to dress, almost immediately postoperatively. A formal PACU may not be present, and the patient may be required to recover in the surgical suite. Regardless of where the patient recovers, it is important to adhere to all the ASA standards for monitoring and documentation throughout the postoperative period.[56] Staffing in the recovery area must be adequate, and the use of a pulse oximeter is imperative.[21,107] It is recommended that there be at least one ACLS/PALS-certified member of the health care team present until the last patient has left the office.

Because PACU space in an office is often limited and the anesthesiologist may have multiple locations to attend in a single day, problems of PONV and pain are of particular concern. The effect of these physiologic occurrences are not limited to the patient and anesthesiologist, but may also have a profound economic impact on an office surgical unit.[108] It is imperative that every anesthetic administered be designed to maximize postoperative patient alertness and mobility and minimize the risks of the need for a prolonged PACU stay.[109] Twersky has recommended that the postanesthesia discharge scoring system and clinical discharge criteria used in ambulatory surgery be also used in the office-based setting.[30] Interestingly, there is a trend to discharge patients, particularly after colonoscopy, without escorts. This has been sanctioned in some states. In New York, regulations require that all patients undergoing a procedure with anesthesia be "discharged in the company of a responsible adult, unless exempted by a physician."[110] Specific data confirming the safety of this practice do not exist.

Local anesthesia, conscious sedation supplemented by wound infiltration with local anesthetics, or peripheral nerve blocks often forms the basis for a multimodal strategy for postoperative pain management. These effective pain-relief techniques not only decrease the anesthetic and analgesic requirements during surgery but also reduce the need for opioid analgesics in the postoperative period, thus facilitating the recovery process.[111] Nonopioid analgesics (e.g., acetaminophen) and nonsteroidal anti-inflammatory drugs (e.g., ketorolac) are routinely used. Ketorolac decreases the incidence of PONV, and patients receiving it tolerate oral fluids and meet discharge criteria earlier than those receiving opioids.[112] In an effort to minimize the potential for postoperative bleeding and risk of gastrointestinal complications, more specific cyclooxygenase-2 inhibitors are being increasingly used as nonopioid adjuvants for minimizing postoperative pain.[113]

An optimal antiemetic regimen for OBA has yet to be established, but as the causes of PONV are multifactorial, combination therapies may be more beneficial in high-risk patients. Many of the traditional first-line therapies are associated with sedation, drowsiness, and extrapyramidal side effects, and have been supplanted by 5-hydroxytryptamine type 3 (5-HT$_3$) antagonists such as ondansetron, dolasetron,

ANESTHETIC MANAGEMENT

and granisetron.[114] Dexamethasone has been shown to improve the efficacy of both 5-HT$_3$ antagonists[115] as well as dopamine antagonists[116] Routine prophylaxis, though, has not been shown to offer any advantage over symptomatic treatment[117] and has direct costs associated with it. Ensuring adequate hydration (up to 20 mL/kg), to avoid orthostatic hypotension and thus prevent the release of emetogenic chemicals by decreased blood flow to the midbrain emetic centers is an intervention that may be useful in the prevention of PONV.[114]

REGULATIONS

Governmental oversight of office-based surgery varies among states; currently regulations exist in many states, and others are following in this direction. Whereas accreditation is often a voluntary certification of an office, regulations are governmental mandates imposed by the local or state government. It is imperative that any anesthesiologist embarking on an office-based practice familiarize himself or herself with any rules and regulations that govern practice in his or her particular state.

In 1994, California was the first state to adopt legislation regarding OBA, followed by New Jersey.[4] A closer look at these two states provides an example of the varied requirements being enforced by states throughout the country. California's regulations pertain to patients undergoing a GA and do not address procedures performed under local anesthetic, peripheral nerve block, or sedation/anxiolysis administered in doses that do not affect a patient's life-preserving reflexes.[118] The regulations deal with issues ranging from office policy and mandatory reporting of adverse outcomes, to surgeon and anesthesia provider qualifications.[119] California Health and Safety Code 1248-1248.85 mandates that surgical procedures occur only in offices that have been accredited or have been certified to participate in the Medicare Program under Title XVIII (42 U.S.C. Sec. 1395 et seq.), with very few exceptions.[120] In addition, the office must have a written plan in place that deals with issues regarding emergency admissions. The surgeon must have admitting privileges at a local licensed or accredited acute care hospital or have a written transfer agreement with a physician who does have such privileges. The office must have an agreement with the hospital for the admission, in accordance with the hospital's system of quality assurance and peer review. California law also requires that offices have adequate patient monitoring throughout the perioperative period, and have a system in place for the storage and maintenance of patient records. An office that fails to comply with the regulations in place risks sanctions ranging from reprimand with or without monetary penalties through criminal prosecution.

New Jersey's administrative Code 13: 35-4A.1-13: 35-4A.18 develops criteria for patient selection. Only ASA physical status 1 and 2 patients may undergo general or regional anesthesia. ASA physical status 3 patients can undergo only conscious sedation. The provider of GA must have credentials to do so by a hospital, and only a physician with appropriate credentials may supervise a certified registered nurse anesthetist. New Jersey law establishes guidelines regarding mandatory monitoring, emergency supplies that must be present, physician credentialing, and peer review. In contrast to California, New Jersey's regulations pertain to all patients undergoing a surgical procedure, regardless of the depth of anesthetic. However, similar to California, violations may result in fines ranging from reprimand to license revocation and criminal prosecution.[121]

Although most states have regulations in place regarding office-based surgical procedures, some still have none. Consequently, any physician who holds a valid medical license in an unregulated state may perform any procedure that he or she so chooses within an office. A surgeon may perform a procedure for which he or she may have had little to no training, and may sedate a patient without any training in anesthesia or airway management. In fact, there have been reported cases of patients undergoing a procedure without a preoperative evaluation, pertinent laboratory tests, informed consent, intraoperative or postoperative monitoring, or operative report, and without regard for sterile technique.[4] It is therefore imperative that the anesthesiologist continues to maintain the role of a zealous patient advocate and help to educate the surgeon as to what constitutes a safe anesthetizing location.

Business and Legal Aspects

It is in the anesthesia provider's best interest to seek legal counsel and create a valid business model before embarking on a career in OBA. This model must consider the overhead costs associated with staffing and running a safe surgical office as well as the potential and probable case load and patient insurance mix. An OBA division within a department may provide other benefits to an academic practice in addition to the monetary ones. There may be an intangible benefit to the community it serves, as well enhancing the anesthesia training program.[8] However, it would become necessary to involve the American Board of Anesthesiology as well as the American College of Graduate Education (ACGME) to ensure that any resident rotation outside the ACGME-approved hospital setting is acceptable.

Many OBA groups have formed either professional corporations or limited liability companies. Although not eliminating the need for liability insurance, both of these arrangements serve to protect the private assets of the anesthesiologist in the case of a malpractice claim.[7] Legal representation is thus an essential component formulating an OBA group. Legal counsel may also prove to be beneficial in creating a business plans that follows all state and federal laws regarding billing/collection and antitrust.[122]

It is imperative to have an aboveboard and legal relationship with every office in which a patient is sedated. Billing strategies must be legal and ethical. In this complex environment of third-party payers it is quite easy to make legal errors. Ignorance of the law offers no protection or excuse, and one should seek the advice of expert billing agencies even if one chooses not to outsource this responsibility. In calculating pricing one must include all overhead charges such as drugs, equipment, time, and business expenses including malpractice insurance. A pricing structure with the surgeon must exist before embarking on a business relationship. One must outline specifically what will be provided by the office (e.g., intravenous equipment, antibiotics, monitors) and what the anesthesiologist will supply. These decisions take on further legal implications when the office is charging a facility fee.

CONCLUSIONS

OBA continues to rapidly expand and pose unique challenges to anesthesiologists, who must not only provide medical care in new environments but also have a good business sense and an understanding of operating room management. It is imperative that, although regulations have not kept pace with the growth of OBA, anesthesia providers make it their responsibility to help ensure that every possible safety measure is afforded to their patients. Decisions about appropriate patient/procedure selection and equipping anesthetizing locations must be made in conjunction with the surgeon. All clinical decisions must take into consideration the need for rapid turnover and limited PACU availability. Any depth of anesthesia may be delivered as long as the proper safeguards are in place. The many advantages afforded by office-based surgery are fueling its evolution, and as more complex procedures are conducted on patients with increasing numbers of comorbidities the anesthesiologist's role as patient advocate is vital.

References

1. Lazarov SJ: Office-based surgery and anesthesia: Where are we now? World J Urol 1998; 16: 384
2. Courtiss EH, Goldwyn RM, Joffe JM et al: Anesthetic practices in ambulatory surgery. Plast Reconstr Surg 1994; 93: 792
3. Wetchler BV: Online shopping for ambulatory surgery: Let the buyer beware! Ambul Surg 2000; 8: 111
4. Quattrone MS: Is the physician office the wild, wild west of health care? J Ambul Care Manage 2000; 23: 64
5. Laurito CE: Report of educational meeting: The Society for Office-Based Anesthesia, Orlando, Florida, March 7, 1998. J Clin Anesth 1998; 10: 445
6. Johnston DL: Moratorium goes too far. USA Today. August 23, 2000, pp. 14A
7. Koch ME, Dayan S, Barinholtz D: Office-based anesthesia: An overview. Anesthesiol Clin North America 2003; 21: 417
8. Hausman LM, Levine AI, Rosenblatt MA: A survey evaluating the training of anesthesiology residents in office-based anesthesia. J Clin Anesth 2006; 18: 499
9. Ross AK, Eck JB: Office-based anesthesia for children. Anesthesiol Clin North America 2002; 20: 195
10. Schultz LS: Cost analysis of office surgery clinic with comparison to hospital outpatient facilities for laparoscopic procedures. Int Surg 1994; 79: 273
11. Bartamian, M, Meyer DR: Site of service, anesthesia, and postoperative practice patterns for oculoplastic and orbital surgeries. Ophthalmology 1996; 103: 1628
12. Anello S: Office-based anesthesia: advantages, disadvantages and the nurse's role. Plastic Surg Nurs 2002; 22: 107
13. Iverson RE, Lynch DJ, ASPS Task Force on Patient Safety in Office-Based Surgery Facilities: Patient safety in office-based surgery facilities: II. Patient selection. Plast Reconstr Surg 2002; 110: 1785
14. American Association for the Accreditation of Ambulatory Surgical Facilities. State laws and regulations for office-based surgery. http://www.aaaasf.org/pub/OBSstateregs.pdf
15. Arens J: Anesthesia for office-based surgery: are we paying too high a price for access and convenience? Mayo Clinic Proc 2000; 75: 225
16. Surgeons Leave OR and Go to the Office. New York Times. May 16, 1999: pp. 41
17. Vila H, Soto R, Cantor AB et al: Comparative Outcomes analysis of procedures performed in physician offices and ambulatory surgery centers. Arch Surg 2003; 138: 991
18. Clayman MA, Caffee HH. Office surgery safety and the Florida moratoria. Ann Plastic Surg 2006; 56: 78
19. American Society of Anesthesiologists, Directory of Members. Park Ridge, IL, ASA, 2000, pp. 480
20. Anesthesia Patient Safety Foundation. Office based anesthesia growth provokes safety fears. APSF 2000; 15: 1
21. Domino KB: Office-based anesthesia: lessons learned from the closed-claims project. ASA Newsletter 2001; 65: 9
22. Morello DC, Colon GA, Fredricks S, et al: Patient safety in accredited office surgical facilities. Plast Reconstr Surg 1997; 99: 1496
23. Hoefflin SM, Bornstein JB, Gordon M: General anesthesia in an office-based plastic surgical facility: a report on more than 23,000 consecutive office-based procedures under general anesthesia with no significant anesthetic complications. Plast Reconstr Surg 2001; 107: 243
24. Sullivan PK, Tattini CD: Office-based operatory experience: an overview of anesthetic technique, procedures and complications. Med Health RI 2001; 84: 392
25. Bitar G, Mullis W, Jacobs W, et al: Safety and efficacy of office-based surgery with monitored anesthesia care/sedation in 4778 consecutive plastic surgery procedures. Plast Reconstr Surg 2003; 111: 150
26. Rao RB, Ely SF, Hoffman RS: Deaths related to liposuction. N Engl J Med 1999; 340: 1471
27. Clayman MA, Caffee HH. Office surgery safety and the Florida moratoria. Ann Plastic Surg 2006; 56(1): 78
28. Clayman MA, Seagle BM. Office surgery safety: the myths and truths behind the Florida moratoria—six years of Florida data. Plast Reconstr Surg 2006; 118(3): 777
29. Twersky RS: Updates on office-based anesthesia: caveats on the professional finger-pointing. ASA Newsletter 2001; 65: 8
30. Twersky RS: Anaesthetic and management dilemmas in office-based surgery. Ambul Surg 1998; 6: 79
31. Dorsch JA. Anesthesia machine obsolescence guidelines published. ASA Newsletter 2004; 68; 14
32. Coté CJ, Karl HW, Notteman DA et al: Adverse sedation events in pediatrics: analysis of medications used for sedation. Pediatrics 2000; 106: 663
33. Coté CJ, Notteman DA, Karl HW, et al: Adverse sedation events in pediatrics: a critical incident analysis of contributing factors. Pediatrics 2000; 105: 805
34. Iverson R, ASPS Task Force on Patient Safety in Office-Based Surgery Facilities: Patient safety in office-based surgery facilities: I. Procedures in the office-based surgery setting. Plast Reconstr Surg 2002; 110: 1337
35. Tunajek SK: Office based procedure standards. AANA J 1999; 67: 115
36. American Medical Association House of Delegates at the I-01 Meeting: Office-based surgery core principles. American Society of Anesthesiologists Newsletter 2004; 68: 14
37. Meridy HW: Criteria for selection of ambulatory surgical patients and guidelines for anesthetic management: a retrospective of 1553 cases. Anesth Analg 1982; 61: 921
38. American Society of Anesthesiologists Committee on Ambulatory Surgical Care and the American Society of Anesthesiologists Task Force on Office-Based Anesthesia: Office-based anesthesia: considerations for anesthesiologists in setting up and maintaining a safe office anesthesia environment. Park Ridge, IL, American Society of Anesthesiologists, 2000
39. Twersky RS: Increase in office-based procedures begs caution among anesthesiologists. Anesthesiol News 1998; 24: 9
40. Benumof JL: Obstructive sleep apnea in the adult obese patient: implications for airway management. J Clin Anesth 2001; 13: 144
41. Bresnitz EA, Goldberg R, Kosinski RM: Epidemiology of obstructive sleep apnea. Epidemiol Rev 1994; 16: 210
42. Boushra NN: Anaesthetic management of patients with sleep apnea syndrome. Can J Anaesth 1996; 43: 599
43. Benumof JL: Policies & procedures needed for sleep apnea patients. APSF Newsletter, 2002–2003; Winter: 57
44. Young T, Evans L, Finn L et al: Estimation of the clinically diagnosed proportion of sleep apnea syndrome in middle-aged men and women. Sleep 1997; 20: 705
45. The American Society of Anesthesiologists Task Force on Peri-Operative Management of Patients with Obstructive Sleep Apnea: Practice guidelines for the perioperative management of patients with obstructive sleep apnea. A report by the American Society of Anesthesiologists Task Force on perioperative management with obstructive sleep apnea. Anesthesiology 2006; 104: 1081–1093
46. Lofsky A: Sleep apnea and narcotic postoperative pain medication: a morbidity and mortality risk. APSF Newsletter 2002; 17: 24
47. Esclamado RM, Glenn MG, McCulloch TM: Perioperative complications and risk factors in the surgical treatment of obstructive sleep apnea syndrome. Laryngoscope 1989; 99: 1125
48. Samuels SI, Rabinov W: Difficulty reversing drug-induced coma in a patient with sleep apnea. Anesth Analg 1986; 65: 1222
49. Benumof JL: Creation of observational unit may decrease sleep apnea risk. APSF Newsletter 2002; 17: 39
50. Coldiron B, Shreve E, Balkrishnan R: Patient injuries from surgical procedures performed in medical offices: Three years of Florida data. Dermatol Surg 2004; 30: 1435
51. Claymen MA, Seagle BM: Office surgery safety: The myths and truths behind the Florida moratoria-Six years of Florida data. Plast Reconstr Surg. 2006; 118: 777
52. Reinisch JF, Russo RF, Bresnick SD: Deep vein thrombosis and pulmonary embolism following face lift: A study of incidence and prophylaxis. Plastic Surg Forum 1998; 21: 159
53. Davison SP, Venturi ML, Attinger CE, et al: Prevention of venous thromboembolism in the plastic surgery patient. Plast Reconstr Surg 2004; 114; 43e
54. American Society of Anesthesiologists: Practice guidelines for the management of the difficult airway. An updated report by the American society of anesthesiologists task force on management of the difficult airway. Anesthesiology 2003; 98: 1269
55. American Society of Anesthesiologists: Standards for basic anesthetic monitoring. ASA Directory of Members, 2001. (Last amended October 21, 1998). Park Ridge, IL, American Society of Anesthesiologists, 2001, pp 493
56. American Society of Anesthesiologists: Standards for postanesthesia care. American Society of Anesthesiologists: Standards for basic anesthetic monitoring. ASA Directory of Members, 2001. (Last amended October 19 1994). Park Ridge, IL, American Society of Anesthesiologists, 2001, pp 494
57. Moss E: MD office regs stalled in New Jersey. APSF Newsletter 1997; Winter: 37
58. Yates JA, American Society of Plastic Surgeons: Office-based surgery accreditation crosswalk. Plastic Surg Nurs 2002; 22: 125
59. Coldiron B: Office surgical incidents: 19 months of Florida data. Dermatol Surg 2002; 28: 710
60. Bing J, McAuliffe MS, Lupton JR: Regional anesthesia with monitored anesthesia care for dermatologic laser surgery. Dermatol Clin 2002; 20: 123
61. Morris KT, Pommier RF, Vetto JT: Office-based wire-guided open breast biopsy under local anesthesia is accurate and cost effective. Am J Surg 2000; 179: 422
62. Jones JS, Streem SB: Office-based cystoureteroscopy for assessment of the upper urinary tract. J Endourol 2002; 16: 307
63. Friedman O, Deutsch ES, Reilly JS et al: The feasibility of office-based laser-assisted tympanic membrane fenestration with tympanostomy tube insertion: the du Pont Hospital experience. Int J Pediatr Otorhinolaryngol 2002; 62: 31

64. Goldblum TA, Summers CG, Egbert JE et al: Office probing for congenital nasolacrimal duct obstruction: a study of parental satisfaction. J Pediatr Ophthalmol Strabismus 1996; 33: 244

65. Jones JS, Oder M, Zippe CD: Saturation prostate biopsy with periprostatic block can be performed in the office. J Urol 2002; 168: 2108

66. Goldrath MH, Sherman AI: Office hysteroscopy and suction curettage: can we eliminate the hospital diagnostic dilitation and curettage? Am J Obstet Gynecol 1985; 152: 220

67. Mingus ML, Bodian CA, Bradford CN et al: Prolonged surgery increases the likelihood of admission of scheduled ambulatory surgery patients. J Clin Anesth 1997; 9: 446

68. Fortier J, Chung F, Su J: Unanticipated admission after ambulatory surgery-A prospective study. Can J Anaesth 1997; 45: 612

69. Gold BS, Kitz DS, Lecky JH et al: Unanticipated admission to the hospital following ambulatory surgery. JAMA 1989; 262: 3008

70. American Society of Plastic Surgeons. 2008 report of the 2007 statistics. American Society of Plastic Surgeons 2008. Arlington Heights, Illinois

71. Iverson RE, Lynch DJ, American Society of Plastic Surgeons Committee on Safety: Practice advisory on liposuction. Plast Reconstr Surg 2004; 113: 1478

72. Fodor PB, Watson JP: Wetting solutions in ultrasound assisted lipoplasty: a review. Clin Plast Surg 1999; 26: 289

73. Klein JA: Tumescent technique for regional anesthesia permits lidocaine doses of 35 mg/kg. J Dermatol Surg Oncol 1990; 16: 248

74. Ostad A, Kageyama N, Moy RL: Tumescent anesthesia with lidocaine dose of 55 mg/kg is safe for liposuction. Dermatol Surg 1996; 22: 921

75. Grazer FM, deJong RH: Fatal outcome from liposuction: census survey of cosmetic surgeons. Plast Reconstr Surg 2000; 105: 436

76. Housman TS, Lawrence N, Mellen BG et al: The safety of liposuction: results of a national survey. Dermatol Surg 2002; 28: 971

77. Conveney E, Weltz CR, Greengrass R et al: Use of paravertebral block anesthesia in the surgical management of breast cancer. Experience in 156 cases. Ann Surg 1998; 227: 496

78. Jaffe SM, Campbell P, Bellman M et al: Postoperative nausea and vomiting in women following breast surgery: an audit. Eur J Anaesth 2000; 17: 261

79. Vawter M, Vicaroi MD, Moorthy K et al: Electrocardiographic monitoring during colonoscopy. Am J Gastroenterol 1975; 63: 115

80. Radaelli F, Meucci G, Terruzzi V et al: Single bolus of midazolam versus bolus midazolam plus meperidine for colonoscopy: a prospective, randomized trial. Gastrointest Endosc 2003; 57: 329

81. Ristikankare M, Julkunen R, Laitinen T: Effect of conscious sedation on cardiac autonomic regulation during colonoscopy. Scand J Gastroenterol 2000; 9: 990

82. Petelenz M, Gonciarz M, Macfarlane P et al: Sympathovagal balance fluctuates during colonoscopy. Endoscopy 2004; 36: 508

83. Chutkan J, Cohen M, Abedi M, et al: Training guideline for use of propofol in gastrointestinal endoscopy. Gastrointest Endosc 2004; 60; 167

84. Institute for Medication Safety Practices. Propofol sedation. Who should administer? ISMP Medication Safety Alert! Acute Care Edition November 3, 2005. Institute for Safe Medication Practices. Horsham, PA

85. Finder RL: The art and science of office-based anesthesia in dentistry: a 150-year history. Int Anesthesiol Clin 2003; 41: 1

86. Perrott DH, Yuen JP, Andresen RV et al: Office-based ambulatory anesthesia: outcomes of clinical practices of oral and maxillofacial surgeons. J Oral Maxillofac Surg 2003; 61: 938

87. Freedman JM, Li DK, Drasner K, et al: Transient neurologic symptoms after spinal anesthesia: an epidemiologic study of 1,873 patients. Anesthesiology 1998; 89: 633

88. Mulroy MF, Larkin KL, Siddiqui A: Intrathecal fentanyl-induced pruritis is more severe in combination with procaine than with lidocaine or bupivicaine. Reg Anesth Pain Med 2001; 26: 252

89. Ross AK, Eck JB: Office-based anesthesia for children. Anesthesiol Clin North America 2002; 20: 195

90. Hackel A, Badgwell JM, Binding RR et al: Guidelines for the pediatric perioperative environment. American Academy of Pediatrics Section on Anesthesiology. Pediatrics 1999; 103: 572

91. Tang J, Chen L, White PF et al: Use of propofol for office-based anesthesia: effects of nitrous oxide on recovery. J Clin Anesth 1999; 11: 226

92. White PF: Ambulatory anesthesia advances into the new millennium. Anesth Analg 2000; 90: 1234

93. Cohen MM, Duncan PG, Tate RB: Does anesthesia contribute to operative mortality? JAMA 1988; 260: 2859

94. Domino KB: Trends in anesthesia litigation in the 1990's: monitored anesthesia care claims. ASA Newsletter 1997; 61: 17

94a. Bhananker SM, Posner KL, Cheney FW, et al. Injury and liability associated with monitored anesthesia care. A closed claims analysis. Anesthesiology 2006; 104: 228

95. Rudner R, Jalowiecki P, Kawecki P et al: Conscious analgesia/sedation with remifentanil and propofol versus total intravenous anesthesia with fentanyl, midazolam, and propofol for outpatient colonoscopy. Gastrointest Endosc 2003; 57: 657

96. Friedberg BL: Facial laser resurfacing with the propofol-ketamine technique: room air, spontaneous ventilation (RASV) anesthesia. Dermatol Surg 1999; 25: 569

97. Friedberg BL: Propofol-ketamine technique: Dissociative anesthesia for office surgery (a five year review of 1,264 cases). Aesthetic Plast Surg 1999; 23: 70

98. Friedberg BL: Propofol-ketamine technique. Aesthetic Plast Surg 1993; 17: 297

99. Friedberg BL: Hypnotic doses of propofol block ketamine-induced hallucinations. Plast Reconstr Surg 1993; 91: 196

100. Friedberg BL, Sigl JC: Clonidine premedication decreases propofol consumption during bispectral index (BIS) monitored propofol-ketamine technique for office-based surgery. Dermatol Surg 2000; 26: 848

101. Man D: Premedication with oral clonidine for facial rhytidectomy. Plast Reconstr Surg 1994; 94: 214

102. Baker TM, Stuzin JM, Baker TJ et al: What's new in aesthetic surgery? Clin Plast Surg 1996; 23: 16

103. Drover DR, Lemmens JH, Pierce ET et al: Patient state index: titration of delivery and recovery from propofol, alfentanil, and nitrous oxide anesthesia. Anesthesiology 2002; 97: 82

104. Gan TJ, Glass PS, Windsor A et al: Bispectral index monitoring allows faster emergence and improved recovery from propofol, alfentanil, and nitrous oxide anesthesia. Anesthesiology 1997; 87: 805

105. Song D, Joshi GP, White PF: Titration of volatile anesthetics using bispectral analysis index facilitates recovery after ambulatory anesthesia. Anesthesiology 1997; 87: 842

106. Friedberg B, Sigl JC: Bispectral index (BIS) monitoring decreases propofol usage during propofol-ketamine office based anesthesia. Anesth Analg 1999; 88 (S54): 54

107. Singer R, Thomas PE: Pulse oximeter in the ambulatory aesthetic surgical facility. Plast Reconstr Surg 1988; 82: 111

108. Tang J, Chen X, White PF et al: Antiemetic prophylaxis for office-based surgery—are the 5-HT3 receptor antagonists beneficial? Anesthesiology 2003; 98: 293

109. Chung FF, Chan VW, Ong D: A postanesthetic discharge scoring system for home readiness after ambulatory surgery. J Clin Anesth 1995; 7: 500

110. New York State Department of Health. Title X. Freestanding Ambulatory Surgical Services (Statutory Authority: Public Health Law, Section 2803) Section 755.6 Patient Admission and Discharge (f) 1985. Albany, NY

111. White PF: The role of non-opioid analgesic techniques in the management of pain after ambulatory surgery. Anesth Analg 2002; 94: 577

112. Ding Y, White PF: Comparative effects of ketorolac, dezocine and fentanyl as adjuvants during outpatient anesthesia. Anesth Analg 1992; 75: 566

113. Desjardins PJ, Shu VS, Recker DP et al: A single preoperative oral dose of valdecoxib, a new cyclooxygenase-2 specific inhibitor, relieves post-oral surgery or bunionectomy pain. Anesthesiology 2002; 97: 565

114. Kovac AL: Prevention and treatment of postoperative nausea and vomiting. Drugs 2000; 59: 213

115. Henzi I, Walder B, Tramer MR: Dexamethasone for prophylaxis of postoperative nausea and vomiting: a quantitative systematic review. Anesth Analg 2000; 90: 186

116. Eberhart LH, Morin AM, Georgieff M: Dexamethasone for prophylaxis of postoperative nausea and vomiting. A meta-analysis of randomized controlled studies. Anaesthetist 2000; 49: 713

117. Scuderi PE, James RL, Harris L et al: Antiemetic prophylaxis does not improve outcomes after outpatient surgery when compared to symptomatic treatment. Anesthesiology 1999; 90: 360

118. California Codes, Business & Professions Code, Division 2. Healing Arts, Chapter 5. Medicine Article 11.5. Surgery in certain outpatient settings, §2216. Restrictions on use of anesthesia. 2003

119. CAL Business & Professions Code, Div 2. Healing Arts, ch 5. Medicine: Art 11.5. Surgery in certain outpatient settings. §2215–40

120. CAL Health and Safety Code, Div 2. Licensing Provisions, ch 1.3. Outpatient settings: §1248.1

121. NJ Administrative Code: Title 13. Law and public safety: ch 35. Board of medical examiners: subch 4A. Surgery, special procedures, and anesthesia services performed in an office setting §18

122. Manchikanti L, McMahon EB: Physician refer thyself: Is stark II, Phase III the final voyage? Pain Physician 2007; 10: 725

CHAPTER 34 ■ ANESTHESIA PROVIDED AT ALTERNATE SITES

KAREN J. SOUTER

GENERAL PRINCIPLES
  The Environment
  Procedures
  Patients
ANESTHESIA CARE
RADIOLOGY AND RADIATION THERAPY
  Intravenous Contrast Agents
  Protection From Ionizing Radiation
SPECIFIC RADIOLOGIC PROCEDURES
  Interventional Neuroradiology
  Computed Tomography, Radiofrequency Ablation, and
    Magnetic Resonance Imaging
  Radiation Therapy
CARDIAC CATHETERIZATION

  Electrophysiological Procedures
  Automatic Implantable Cardioverter-
    Defibrillators
CARDIOVERSION
GASTROENTEROLOGY
  Upper Gastrointestinal Endoscopy
  Endoscopic Retrograde Cholangiopancreatography
  Transjugular Intrahepatic Portosystemic Shunt
ELECTROCONVULSIVE THERAPY
  Physiologic Response to Electroconvulsive Therapy
DENTAL SURGERY
TRANSPORT OF PATIENTS
SUMMARY

KEY POINTS

1 Alternate sites are locations remote from the operating room.

2 The number of requests for anesthetic services in alternate sites is increasing.

3 A three-step approach is useful in considering an anesthetic at an alternate site: the patient, the procedure, and the environment.

4 The American Society of Anesthesiologists (ASA) has defined guidelines to be applied to the administration of anesthesia at nonoperating room locations.

5 Environmental considerations include hazards such as radiation and the side effects of contrast media.

6 Procedural considerations are both general (e.g., duration, position, and level of discomfort) and specific to individual specialties.

7 Patient considerations include whether the patient will tolerate sedation or require general anesthesia, the ASA classification, significant comorbidities, and the level of monitoring.

8 Patients should receive the same standard of care at an alternate site as they do in the operating room.

9 The anesthetic and monitoring equipment must meet the same standards as equipment provided in the operating room.

10 Following anesthesia at an alternate site, the patient should be transported to an appropriate postanesthesia care unit, accompanied and monitored by anesthesia personnel.

---

1 This chapter discusses the challenges facing the anesthesiologist regarding the procedures, the patients, and the environment to better understand and develop a systematic approach to providing anesthesia at alternate sites. This chapter also describes the special considerations that apply to administering anesthesia at sites other than the operating room. These sites may be located within a large hospital, such as in a radiology department, endoscopy suite, or dental clinic, where the resources of the operating rooms are within the facility but are not close at hand. A discussion of the provision of anesthesia for surgical procedures performed in stand-alone ambulatory centers, or offices, appears in Chapters 32 and 33.

GENERAL PRINCIPLES

2 In recent years, the number of anesthetics being delivered to patients in areas other than the operating room has steadily

increased. This is mainly related to the development of large, complex equipment that cannot be transported to the operating room for both diagnostic and therapeutic procedures. Standards introduced by the Joint Commission on Accreditation of Healthcare Organizations require that the anesthesiology services of a hospital participate with other departments in setting up a uniform quality of care for patients undergoing sedation in all parts of the hospital.[1] To assist in this process The American Society of Anesthesiologists (ASA) has developed practice guidelines for sedation and analgesia by nonanesthesiologists.[2]

3 Anesthesiologists undertake most of their training in the operating room, surrounded by familiar equipment and staff experienced in the care of the anesthetized patient. Away from the operating room, the anesthesiologist may not have this support. A simple three-step paradigm can be used to **4** approach an anesthetic assignment in an alternate site (Fig. 34-1 and Table 34-1).

861

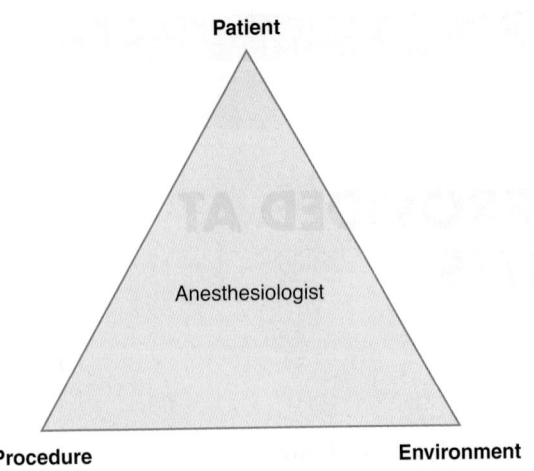

FIGURE 34-1.   A three-step paradigm for anesthesia at alternate sites.

The Environment

The ASA has developed standards to apply to anesthesia in remote locations[3] (Table 34-2). Before commencing an anesthetic in an alternate site, it is vital to confirm the presence and proper functioning of all equipment an anesthesiologist would expect to have in the operating room. This equipment includes a central oxygen supply, spare oxygen cylinders, wall suction, overhead lighting, gas scavenging systems, and electrical outlets. Replacement batteries should be available for any equipment that is battery-powered. The location of immediately

---

TABLE 34-1

A THREE-STEP APPROACH TO ANESTHESIA AT ALTERNATE SITES

1. Environment	Anesthetic equipment
	Anesthesia monitors
	Suction
	Resuscitation equipment
	Personnel
	Technical equipment
	Radiation hazard
	Magnetic fields
	Ambient temperature
	Warming blankets
2. Procedure	Diagnostic or therapeutic
	Duration
	Level of discomfort/pain
	Position of patient
	Special requirements (e.g., functional monitoring)
	Potential complications
	Surgical support
3. Patient	Ability to tolerate sedation versus general anesthesia
	ASA grade and comorbidity
	Airway assessment
	Allergies—IV contrast
	Monitoring requirements—simple versus advanced

ASA, American Society of Anesthesiologists; IV, intravenous.

---

available resuscitation equipment should be noted and protocols developed with the local staff for dealing with emergencies, including cardiopulmonary resuscitation and the management of anaphylaxis.

Anesthesia Equipment and Monitors

In some alternate sites, anesthesia machines and monitors are provided; in others, it may be necessary to bring anesthesia equipment to the location. Both situations can present problems. Anesthesia machines and monitors that remain in an outside location need to undergo routine maintenance, as does anesthesia equipment used in the main operating rooms. This equipment is not often used on a daily basis; therefore, before using the equipment, it is vital to conduct a thorough check. For example, attention should be paid to the freshness of the soda lime and whether any pieces of equipment or monitors have been removed or misplaced. Monitoring equipment found in alternate sites is often used by the staff to monitor patients who are not being anesthetized. These monitors may be different from monitors used in the operating room. Anesthesiologists should be aware of these differences. If more advanced monitors (e.g., an arterial line, central venous pressure or intracranial pressure [ICP] monitoring) are required, these devices should be readily available. Small, portable anesthesia machines and monitors are available. A pre-prepared cart containing essential equipment that is checked and restocked after each case is recommended to eliminate the need for anesthesia personnel to move between locations to collect equipment that has been forgotten or that is needed urgently.

Technical Equipment

The complex technical equipment used in alternate sites, particularly in radiology suites, is often bulky and fixed to the floor so the anesthesia team has to work around it (Fig. 34-2). Ionizing radiation related to both imaging and therapeutic procedures is a hazard to both staff and patients. Magnetic resonance imaging (MRI) creates its own environmental concerns related to magnetic fields. In all these areas, the equipment is kept at low temperatures, and patients may easily develop hypothermia. Patient-warming devices should be available. Radiation therapy rooms are heavily shielded, and staff are excluded from the room during treatment, requiring the anesthesiology team to monitor patients remotely, often with surveillance cameras.[4]

Procedures

Common procedures carried out in alternate sites for which the patient may require anesthesia or sedation are listed in Table 34-3. It is vital for the anesthesiologist to understand the nature of the procedure, the position of the patient, how painful the procedure will be, and how long the procedure will last. This will allow the development of an anesthesia plan to provide safe patient care and facilitate the procedure. Discussions with physicians, dentists, and others performing interventional procedures must include contingencies for adverse outcomes.

Patients

Patients may require anesthesia at alternate sites for a number of reasons (Table 34-4). The patient may have been unable to

TABLE 34-2

AMERICAN SOCIETY OF ANESTHESIOLOGISTS (ASA) GUIDELINES FOR NONOPERATING ROOM ANESTHETIZING LOCATIONS

1. Oxygen
   - Reliable source
   - Backup E-cylinder—full
2. Suction
   - Adequate and reliable
3. Scavenging system if inhalational agents are administered
4. Anesthetic equipment
   - Backup self-inflating bag to deliver positive-pressure ventilation
   - Adequate anesthetic drugs and supplies
   - Anesthesia machine with equivalent function to those in the operating rooms and maintained to the same standards
   - Adequate monitoring equipment to allow adherence to the ASA Standards for Basic Monitoring[9]
5. Electrical outlets
   - Sufficient for anesthesia machine and monitors
   - Isolated electrical power or ground fault circuit interrupters if "wet location"
6. Adequate illumination
   - Battery-operated backups
7. Sufficient space for
   - Personnel and equipment
   - Easy and expeditious access to patient, anesthesia machine, and monitoring
8. Resuscitation equipment immediately available
   - Defibrillator
   - Emergency drugs
   - Cardiopulmonary resuscitation equipment
9. Adequately trained staff to support anesthesia team
10. All building and safety codes and facility standards should be observed
11. Postanesthesia care facilities[7]
    - Adequately trained staff to provide postanesthesia care
    - Appropriate equipment to allow safe transport to main postanesthesia care unit

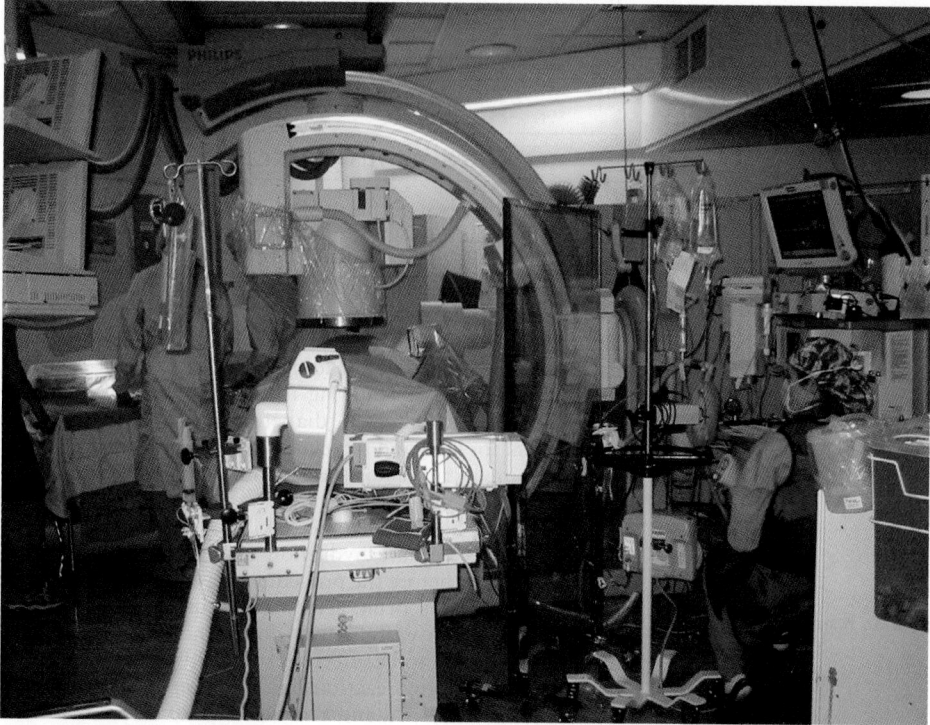

FIGURE 34-2. A radiology suite showing a maze of equipment and the necessity for the anesthesiologist to be remote from the patient's head.

COMMON PROCEDURES REQUIRING ANESTHESIA AT ALTERNATE SITES

Radiology
- Computed tomography
- Magnetic resonance imaging
- Interventional radiology (vascular and nonvascular)
- Interventional neuroradiology
- Functional brain imaging
- Positron emission tomography
- Radiofrequency ablation

Radiotherapy
- Radiation therapy
- Intraoperative radiotherapy
- Radiosurgery

Gastroenterology
- Upper gastroenterology endoscopy
- Endoscopic retrograde cholangiopancreatography
- Colonoscopy
- Liver biopsy
- Transjugular intrahepatic portosystemic shunt

Cardiology
- Cardiac catheterization
- Radiofrequency ablation
- Cardioversion
- Transesophageal echocardiography

Psychiatry
- Electroconvulsive therapy

tolerate the procedure without sedation or has failed with simple sedation administered by a nonanesthesiologist. Children represent a special group of patients who are more likely to require sedation or anesthesia for various diagnostic and therapeutic procedures. The term *pediatric procedural sedation* has been coined to describe this emerging field of practice.[5] Another group of challenging patients are those who are too ill to tolerate a major surgical procedure, but who may be able to undergo palliative, less-invasive procedures at alternate sites. These patients require a thorough preanesthetic assessment and often need invasive monitoring.

ANESTHESIA CARE

The terms *anesthesia, sedation, conscious sedation*, and *deep sedation* are commonly used. They span a continuum that

TABLE 34-4

PATIENT FACTORS REQUIRING SEDATION OR GENERAL ANESTHESIA AT ALTERNATE SITES

Anxiety and panic disorders
Claustrophobia
Developmental delay and learning difficulties
Cerebral palsy
Seizure disorders
Movement disorders
Severe pain
Acute trauma with unstable cardiovascular, respiratory, or neurologic function
Significant comorbidity
Child age

starts with a fully awake patient with a protected, patent airway and ends with general anesthesia and the need for interventions to maintain and protect the airway. The Joint Commission on Accreditation of Healthcare Organizations defines *anesthesia care* as the administration of intravenous, intramuscular, or inhalational agents that may result in the loss of the patient's protective reflexes. Patients who receive anesthesia or sedation at alternate sites should expect the same standard of care that they would receive in the operating room. The ASA has published guidelines and standards of care, including those for preanesthesia and postanesthesia care, as well as monitored anesthesia care,[6–8] and definitions of general anesthesia and levels of sedation[2] (Table 34-5). A patient's level of sedation frequently varies during the course of a procedure, and it is important that individuals administering a given level of sedation are able to rescue the patient whose level becomes deeper than initially intended. The ASA basic standards of monitoring should be adhered to in any location where anesthesia or sedation is being performed.[9] Standard I requires a qualified anesthesia provider to be present in the room throughout the conduct of anesthesia. Standard II calls for continual evaluation of the patient's oxygenation, ventilation, circulation, and temperature. The degree of invasive monitoring that should be used will depend on the patient's status and the procedure being undertaken.

At the conclusion of the procedure, patients should recover from anesthesia or sedation in a postanesthesia care unit (PACU) or similar setting.[7] Care should be supervised by personnel who are trained to take care of unconscious patients, with appropriate monitoring and resuscitation equipment immediately at hand.

RADIOLOGY AND RADIATION THERAPY

Developments in technology have meant that interventional radiologists now perform an increasing number of procedures that were once in the domain of surgeons. Anesthesiologists are increasingly required to take care of patients undergoing both diagnostic and therapeutic interventional procedures. Two important aspects of the radiologic environment are the side effects of contrast media, which are commonly used to enhance radiologic images, and the hazards of ionizing radiation.

Intravenous Contrast Agents

Intravenous contrast agents are iodinated compounds used for many radiologic procedures.[10] MRI contrast media are also now widely used; these agents are chelated metal complexes containing gadolinium, iron, and manganese.

Contrast media are eliminated via the kidneys, and contrast-induced nephropathy (CN) is a recognized complication of their use. CN is the third leading cause of hospital-acquired acute renal failure, accounting for 12% of cases.[11] Patients with chronic renal disease, diabetes, and hypovolemia are most at risk for CN, and patients taking metformin are at risk of developing lactic acidosis; adequate hydration, monitoring of urine output, and the use of low-osmolarity and nonionic contrast media help reduce the risk.[12] CN may be prevented by the use of adequate hydration and sodium bicarbonate infusions 1 hour before the procedure.[13] Antioxidants such as N-acetylcysteine, ascorbic acid may be useful in preventing CN. However, the vasodilators dopamine and fenoldopam have not be shown to be effective.[12] In 1990, the overall incidence of adverse drug reactions with nonionic contrast media was reported as 3.13% and the incidence of severe reactions

TABLE 34-5

DEFINITION OF GENERAL ANESTHESIA AND LEVELS OF SEDATION/ANALGESIA

	■ MINIMAL SEDATION "ANXIOLYSIS"	■ MODERATE SEDATION/ANALGESIA "CONSCIOUS SEDATION"	■ DEEP SEDATION/ ANALGESIA	■ GENERAL ANESTHESIA
Responsiveness	Normal response to verbal stimulation	Purposeful response to verbal or tactile stimulation	Purposeful response following repeated or painful stimulation	Unarousable even with painful stimulus
Airway	Unaffected	No intervention required	Intervention may be required	Intervention required
Spontaneous ventilation	Unaffected	Adequate	May be inadequate	Frequently inadequate
Cardiovascular function	Unaffected	Usually maintained	Usually maintained	May be impaired

is 0.04%.[14] These facts are shown in more detail in Table 34-6. Reactions are described as mild (e.g., urticaria, chills, fever, facial flushing, nausea, vomiting), moderate (e.g., edema, bronchospasm, hypotension seizures), and severe (e.g., dyspnea, prolonged hypotension, cardiac arrest, loss of consciousness, anaphylactic reactions). Patients with atopy or allergy to shellfish are more prone to contrast-related adverse reactions.[15] Pretreatment with oral methylprednisolone prior to intravenous administration of contrast medium[16] can reduce the incidence of adverse reactions. Treatment of severe reactions should include discontinuing the causative agent and supportive therapy, such as oxygen administration, securing the airway, and cardiovascular support with fluids, vasopressors, and inotropes. Bronchospasm should be treated with appropriate bronchodilators. Low-osmolarity, nonionic compounds with osmolarities ranging from 290 to 650 mOsm/kg have a lower incidence of adverse reactions compared with the older, high-osmolarity agents.[14,17] Adverse reactions to MRI contrast media are similar to those as other contrast media and have a similar incidence.[18] In some cases, there is cross-sensitivity between gadolinium-containing agents and iodinated ones.

Protection From Ionizing Radiation

Patients, physicians, and other health care workers are frequently exposed to ionizing radiation, usually in the form of x-rays. Exposure to gamma radiation, or rarely, alpha or beta radiation from radioactive isotopes, may also occur during implantation or removal procedures. Ionizing radiation exposure may occur directly from the source, as leakage from the ionizing device, or as scatter from the equipment. Direct exposure must be avoided. A *rad* (radiation-absorbed dose) is a measure of an absorbed dose of radiation. The total dose of x-rays is measured in roentgens, and a *rem* (roentgen-equivalent man) is the dose of ionizing radiation with the same biological tissue effect as 1 rad of x-rays.[19] The dose of radiation

TABLE 34-6

INCIDENCE OF CONTRAST-RELATED ADVERSE REACTIONS

	■ IODINATED CONTRAST MEDIA	
■ HIGH-OSMOLARITY CONTRAST MEDIA (%)	■ ADVERSE REACTIONS	■ LOW-OSMOLARITY CONTRAST MEDIA (%)
6.0	Nausea and vomiting	1.0
3.0	Urticaria	0.5
2.6	Hoarseness, sneezing, cough, dyspnea, facial edema	0.5
0.1	Hypotension	0.01

	■ MAGNETIC RESONANCE IMAGING CONTRAST MEDIA	
■ CONTRAST MEDIA	■ ADVERSE REACTIONS	■ INCIDENCE (%)
Gadolinium chelates	Mild (nausea and/or vomiting)	2.0
	Moderate	0.1
	Severe	0.01
Ferrous oxide	Aching muscles	8.0
	Others (including allergiclike reactions)	3.0
Manganese fodipir	Injection site discomfort	67.0
	Nausea and/or vomiting	14.0
	Headache	5.0
	Others	<1.0

Reprinted from King BF: Intravascular contrast media and premedication, Radiology Life Support. Edited by Bush WH, Krecke KN, King BF, et al. London, Arnold, 1999, p 13, with permission.

received during a chest radiograph is in the order of 8 mrem, a head computed tomography (CT) scan is 170 mrem, and an abdominal CT is 680 mrem.[20] Radiation exposure with fluoroscopy may be >75,000 mrem.[19] The effective dose received by the patient during intraoperative digital subtraction angiography was calculated as 76.7 mrem.[20] The exposure of health care workers to the radiation emitted from x-ray equipment is several orders of magnitude lower.[20] The National Council on Radiation Protection and Measurements has established guidelines governing medical radiation.[21] The recommended annual occupational exposure is 5,000 mrem. With the routine use of a lead apron, protective goggles, and thyroid shield, exposure to radiation can be kept to a low level. However, this protective clothing is cumbersome and can result in fatigue and discomfort, which can distract from patient care.

SPECIFIC RADIOLOGIC PROCEDURES

Cerebral and spinal angiography cause minimal discomfort and may be performed under local anesthesia with or without light sedation administered by nonanesthesiologists. Patients are required to remain completely motionless during these procedures, which may be lengthy, particularly spinal angiography. Neurologic disorders such as recent subarachnoid hemorrhage, stroke, and depressed level of consciousness or raised ICP may make it impossible for patients to tolerate these procedures unsedated. Deep sedation or general anesthesia with airway protection is often required. Angiography is usually performed via the femoral artery; the femoral vein may also be accessed when imaging arteriovenous malformations or dural venous abnormalities. Liberal use of local anesthetic at the puncture site precludes the need for intravenous analgesia. The injection of contrast media into the cerebral arteries may cause discomfort, burning, or pruritus around the face and eyes. Hypotension and bradycardia may also occur. Complications following angiography are described as neurologic and nonneurologic, and vary between 1 and 2.5%.[22]

During cerebral angiography, the patient is placed on a moving gantry and the radiologist positions the patient to track catheters as they pass from the groin into the cerebral vessels. It is vital to have extensions on all anesthesia breathing circuits, infusion lines, and monitors to prevent these from being accidentally dislodged as the radiologist swings the x-ray table rapidly back and forth. Care should be taken with positioning of radiopaque pieces of equipment. The electrocardiogram electrodes may interfere with imaging during spinal angiography, and little metallic coils in the cuffs of endotracheal tubes can cause interesting and annoying artifacts if they lie over the area being imaged.

Interventional Neuroradiology

A number of neurosurgical conditions may be treated by interventional neuroradiologic techniques.[23] The diseases amenable to endovascular treatment may be classified as emergent or elective, hemorrhagic or occlusive, and definitive, adjunctive, or palliative. Endovascular treatment of intracranial aneurysms with detachable platinum coils (Guglielmi detachable coils)[24] has become an acceptable alternative to surgery for reducing the risk of spontaneous recurrent hemorrhage following subarachnoid hemorrhage.[25] Endovascular treatment avoids the need for craniotomy and is often offered to patients with significant comorbidity or poor prognoses[26,27]; it may also reduce cognitive impairment and frontotemporal brain damage associated with craniotomy.[28]

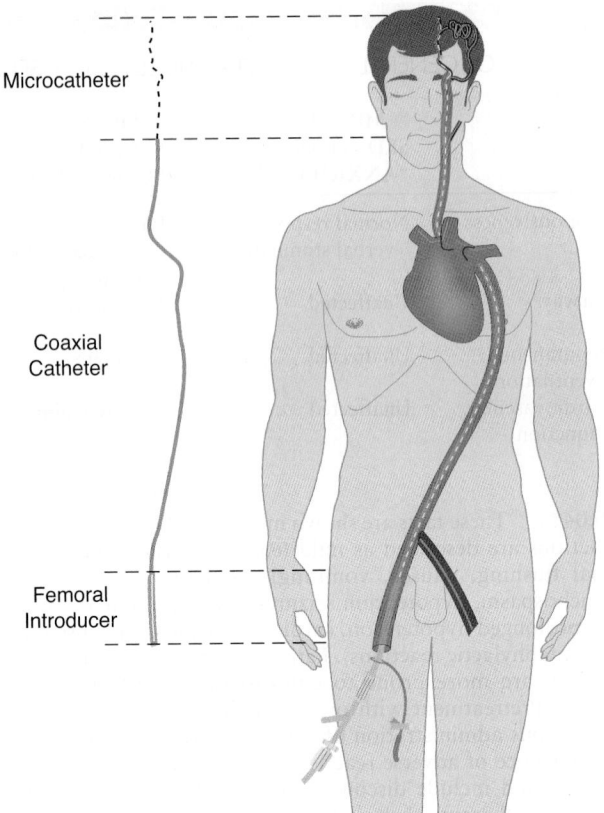

FIGURE 34-3. Representation of a superselective catheter. (Reprinted from Young WL, Pile-Spellman J: Anesthetic considerations for interventional neuroradiology. Anesthesiology 1994; 80: 427, with permission.)

Arteriovenous malformations (AVMs) are increasingly being treated endovascularly, either as the sole therapy or in conjunction with surgical resection or stereotactic radiosurgery.[29] Materials used for interventional neuroradiologic techniques include occlusive agents; detachable balloons, polyvinyl alcohol particles, coils (pushable, flow directed, and detachable), and liquid agents; and acrylic glues (N-butyl cyanoacrylates), nonadhesive polymerizing agents, and sclerosing agents.[29] For most interventional neuroradiologic procedures, arterial access is gained using a 6 or 7 French gauge sheath via the femoral or, rarely, the carotid or axillary artery[29,30] (Fig. 34-3). The umbilical vessels are an alternative route in neonates. A continuous infusion of heparinized saline is infused into the sheath via a side arm during the procedure. Continuous monitoring of blood pressure and sampling of arterial blood may be performed via the sheath, although most anesthesiologists prefer to insert a dedicated arterial catheter for monitoring the patient. The radiologic imaging techniques include high-speed fluoroscopy and digital subtraction angiography. Once the sheath is in place, a guide catheter is advanced through the sheath and a "road mapping" technique is employed, whereby a bolus of contrast medium is injected to outline the vascular anatomy. This image may be superimposed onto the live fluoroscopic imaging to guide the advancement of the microcatheters for placement of embolic materials into an aneurysm or the feeding vessels of an AVM.

Anticoagulation

Anticoagulation with heparin is required during and up to 24 hours after interventional radiologic procedures to prevent thromboembolism. The usual dose is between 3,000 and

5,000 U as an initial bolus, followed by an infusion. The activated clotting time is the preferred method of monitoring the effects of heparin and is generally maintained between 1.5 and 2.5 times the patient's baseline.[31]

Complications

Interventional neuroradiologic procedures are nonstimulating and generally well tolerated. Particular care should be exerted to prevent air embolism via the femoral sheath. Hematoma or hemorrhage may result from femoral artery puncture. There have also been reports of pulmonary embolic phenomena due to acrylic glues.[32] During angioplasty or stenting of carotid artery stenosis, the anesthesia team should be prepared to treat severe bradycardias or transient asystole. The two most catastrophic complications that can occur are intracranial hemorrhage or thromboembolic stroke. The incidence of these during coiling of cerebral aneurysms is 2.4 and 3.5%, respectively.[33] During embolization of AVMs, the incidence of catastrophic complications is between 1 and 8%.[34] The anesthesia team is vital in the expedient treatment of these life-threatening events (Table 34-7).

Anesthetic Technique

General anesthesia and conscious sedation are both suitable techniques for interventional neuroadiology depending on the complexity of the procedure, the need for blood pressure manipulation, and the need for intraprocedural assessment of neurologic function.[35]

General anesthesia is usually conducted with endotracheal intubation and intermittent positive-pressure ventilation, although the laryngeal mask airway (LMA) is a suitable alternative.[33] Conscious sedation techniques vary. Propofol infusions are widely used, as are combinations of a benzodiazepine (usually midazolam) and opioid (usually fentanyl). More

recently, dexmedetomidine has been evaluated as a sedative agent that does not cause significant respiratory depression in patients requiring neurologic testing.[35] Dexmedetomidine has many advantages as a sedative agent[36,37]; however, one study demonstrated impairment of cognitive testing in patients undergoing endovascular embolization of cerebral AVMs with dexmedetomidine as the sedative agent. Invasive monitoring is used less often in patients undergoing interventional neuroradiology compared with those having neurosurgical procedures. The anesthesia care team may facilitate the neuroradiologist in a number of ways by manipulating systemic blood pressure and controlling end-tidal carbon dioxide tension.[30,33] Controlled hypotension is often requested to facilitate embolization of AVMs. Esmolol, labetalol, metoprolol, and hydralazine are commonly used. Moderate hypertension may help reduce cerebral ischemia by maintaining cerebral perfusion; in this case, phenylephrine is the agent of choice.

Certain procedures require patients to be awake at least for part of the procedure. A superselective anesthesia functional examination, or SAFE,[30] may be performed prior to therapeutic embolization to determine whether the catheter has been placed in a vessel that supplies an eloquent area of the brain or spinal cord, such as speech or language areas. Following baseline neurologic examination, amobarbital 30 mg (for investigating the gray matter areas) or lidocaine 30 mg (to evaluate the integrity of the white matter tracts) mixed with contrast agent is injected via the catheter. The patient is then reassessed for neurologic deficits in the areas at risk; if the assessment is negative, embolization may proceed. A "sleep-awake-sleep" anesthetic technique using a propofol infusion allows the patient to be rapidly awakened for appropriate neurologic testing; once this is complete, the patient is again sedated or anesthetized while the definitive procedure is carried out.

Computed Tomography, Radiofrequency Ablation, and Magnetic Resonance Imaging

CT scanning and MRI are used for a wide array of diagnostic imaging and an increasingly large number of therapeutic procedures. The procedures are similar in that they are relatively painless and most adults can tolerate them without the need for sedation or anesthesia. However, there is an absolute requirement for the patient to remain motionless while the study is being performed. Children and adults with a variety of psychological or neurologic disorders may require sedation or anesthesia to enable them to tolerate the procedures (Table 34-4).

Patients with acute thoracic, abdominal, and cerebral trauma often require urgent imaging to facilitate diagnosis. It is not unheard of for these patients to develop hemorrhagic shock, raised ICP, depression of consciousness, and cardiac arrest in the CT scanner. Patients must be adequately resuscitated and stabilized before transportation to the radiology department.

Computed Tomography

Modern CT scanners obtain a cross-sectional image in just a few seconds, and spiral scanners can image a slice of the body in <1 second, minimizing the problems with motion artifacts. Contrast media may be required during CT imaging, and this is often administered orally. Anesthesiologists need to be aware that their patient may have just received a large volume of oral contrast media prior to the examination. Also, a nasogastric tube may be required to facilitate administration of the contrast medium in sedated or anesthetized patients. Occasionally, CT scanning may be employed to facilitate invasive procedures such as abscess localization and drainage, ablation

---

TABLE 34-7

ACUTE MANAGEMENT OF NEUROLOGIC CATASTROPHES

Initial resuscitation
Communicate with radiologists
Call for assistance
Secure the airway and hyperventilate with 100% O_2
Determine if problem is hemorrhagic or occlusive
  Hemorrhagic: immediate heparin reversal (1 mg of protamine for each 100 units of heparin given) and low normal pressure
  Occlusive: deliberate hypertension, titrated to neurologic examination, angiography, or physiologic imaging studies (e.g., TCD, CBF)
Further resuscitation
  Head up 15° in neutral position
  Titrate ventilation to a $Paco_2$ of 26–28 mm Hg
  0.5 g/kg mannitol, rapid intravenous infusion
  Anticonvulsants: Dilantin (give slowly, 50 mg/min) and phenobarbital
  Titrate thiopental infusion to electroencephalogram burst suppression
  Allow body temperature to fall as quickly as possible to 33–34°C
  Consider dexamethasone, 10 mg

TCD, transcranial Doppler; CBF, cerebral blood flow.
Reprinted from Young WL, Pile-Spellman J: Anesthetic considerations for interventional neuroradiology. Anesthesiology 1994; 80: 427

ANESTHETIC MANAGEMENT

of bony metastases, and radiofrequency ablation of lung or other malignancies.

Radiofrequency Ablation

Percutaneous radiofrequency ablation is carried out in the radiology suite for treatment of primary and metastatic hepatic tumors, as well as tumors in the lung, adrenal gland, kidney, breast, thyroid, prostate, kidney, and spleen. The majority of these procedures are tolerated without sedation. If an anesthesiologist does become involved in the care of these patients, they need careful evaluation. These patients may be in the later stages of their disease, have often failed surgical treatment, and may well have undergone extensive radiation therapy and/or chemotherapy. Percutaneous radiofrequency ablation of pulmonary lesions may be performed by radiologists as an outpatient procedure under conscious sedation or general anesthesia.[38] The incidence of complications is low; however, the "off-site" anesthesiologist should be aware of potential problems such as hemorrhage, pneumothorax, pleural effusion, infection, and bronchopleural fistula. During the procedure the surrounding tissues heat up, and the presence of a cardiac pacemaker is an absolute contraindication to the procedure.[39]

Magnetic Resonance Imaging

The physical principles of MRI are described in depth elsewhere.[40] Briefly, when atoms with an odd number of protons in their nuclei, notably hydrogen, are subjected to a powerful static magnetic field, they align themselves with the magnetic field. If they are then intermittently exposed to a radiofrequency wave, the nuclei change their alignment. As the radiofrequency pulses are discontinued, the protons return to their original alignment (i.e., they "relax") within the original magnetic field and, as they do, they release energy. The release of energy over time (the relaxation time) is specific for given tissues and is used to generate the MRI signal. The magnetic field strengths are measured in tesla (T; 1 T = 10,000 gauss). The earth's magnetic field is approximately 0.5 gauss. MRI scanners used for clinical purposes generate a field of 0.15 to 2.0 T,[41] and machines generating magnetic fields from 4 to 8 T are used in research. Despite extensive review,[42] no adverse effects have been described from human exposure to magnetic fields. Deaths and adverse outcomes in MRI scanners are entirely related to the presence of ferrometallic foreign bodies such as cerebral aneurysm clips or implanted devices such as pacemakers. Before entering the vicinity of the magnet, patients and staff need to complete a rigorous checklist to ensure they have no ferrometallic objects in their bodies. The magnetic field takes several days to establish and is constantly present. It decreases in strength with distance from the center of the magnet, quantified as a number of concentric rings termed *gauss lines*. This peripheral or fringe field around the magnet is responsible for malfunction of electrical equipment. The 5 gauss line, for example, is the point beyond which pacemakers will malfunction. Ferromagnetic anesthetic gas cylinders, if brought within the 50 gauss line, become potentially lethal projectiles; a number of near-miss incidents have been documented.[43] MRI-compatible anesthesia machines and monitors are available. The electrocardiogram is sensitive to the changing magnetic signals, and it is nearly impossible to eliminate all artifacts. The electrodes should be placed close together and toward the center of the magnetic field. The leads should be insulated from the patient's skin because they may heat up and cause thermal injury. All cables and wires should run a straight path and not be wound in loops to avoid induction heating effects. Noninvasive blood pressure monitors and transducers for invasive pressure monitoring are available. In the absence of MRI-compatible monitors, long sampling tubes can be connected to standard capnographs and anesthetic agent monitors. Most infusion pumps can be used outside the 30 gauss line,[44] and extra lengths of extension tubing should be available.

MRI takes upward of 30 minutes, and many patients find it difficult to stay still for long periods. It may become very warm within the coil of the magnet, often reaching 80°F, adding to patient discomfort. The MRI scanner emits a considerable amount of noise, up to 90 dB, and both the patient and the anesthesiologist should wear hearing protection. It is important to remember that once a scan sequence is initiated, no one may enter or leave the scan room. In the case of an emergency, the MRI technicians should be notified, the scan sequence stopped, and the patient rapidly removed. Resuscitation attempts should take place outside the scanner because equipment such as laryngoscopes, oxygen cylinders, and cardiac defibrillators cannot be taken close to the magnet.

Anesthetic Technique

Thirty percent of adult patients experience some degree of anxiety during MRI scanning,[45] and up to 10% experience severe panic and claustrophobia. Four percent of adult patients will terminate the procedure prematurely,[46] and 14% require some form of sedation to tolerate MRI scanning.[47] In most cases, this may be provided as either oral sedation with benzodiazepines or intravenous sedation administered under the supervision of the radiologist. Anesthesiologists are usually involved only with more complex patients, such as those with obesity, obstructive sleep apnea, raised ICP, movement disorders, developmental delay, and the potential for a difficult airway.

Most children younger than the age of 5 years and many as old as age 11[48] require sedation or general anesthesia to tolerate MRI and CT scanning. Twenty-two percent of children undergoing sedation for MRI or CT scans have been found to experience some sort of adverse event; oxygen desaturation occurred in 2.9%, and sedation was inadequate in 15%.[49] Adverse events are more common in children with a higher ASA classification who are undergoing sedation, and preselecting children who are unsuitable for oral sedation improves the efficiency of oral sedation programs. Oral sedation techniques, if appropriately administered, have a success rate of 93%.[48,49] Children who undergo general anesthesia for scans have a very low incidence of adverse reactions (<0.7%).[48,49] Oral chloral hydrate is a popular agent for sedation by nonanesthesiologists, and doses between 80 and 100 mg/kg have shown to be effective for children younger than 3 years of age who are undergoing CT scan.[50] Chloral hydrate can cause excessive sedation, agitation,[51] and respiratory depression; it may also have a prolonged effect in neonates.[52] Recently, a 20% failure rate with chloral hydrate as a sole agent for sedation of neurologically impaired children for MRI has been reported[53] although rescue sedation with sevoflurane, pentobarbital, midazolam, or ketamine was successful in most cases. Benzodiazepines such as midazolam administered either orally (0.25 to 0.75 mg/kg) or intravenously (0.05 to 0.15 mg/kg) are also commonly used for sedation. Deep sedation with propofol infusion, oxygen administration via nasal cannula, and end-tidal carbon dioxide monitoring is a successful technique.[48] Children are initially sedated with incremental propofol boluses up to 3 mg/kg with or without midazolam, 0.2 to 0.5 mg/kg, and then maintained with an infusion rate of propofol, 1 to 3 mg/kg/hr, with supplemental boluses of 1 mg/kg for movement.

Radiation Therapy

Two different types of radiation therapy commonly require anesthesia care: external beam radiation treatments, usually for children with malignancies, and intraoperative radiation

TABLE 34-8

COMMON RADIOSENSITIVE TUMORS IN CHILDREN

Primary CNS tumor—neuroblastoma, medulloblastoma
Acute leukemia—CNS leukemia
Radiosensitive ocular tumors—retinoblastoma
Intra-abdominal tumors—Wilms tumor
Rhabdomyosarcoma
Other tumors—Langerhans cell histiocytosis

CNS, central nervous system.

to tumor masses that cannot be completely resected. Radiosensitive malignancies occurring in children are shown in Table 34-8.

Tumors may involve a variety of vital areas, including the airway, thorax, mediastinum, and heart. Patients with central nervous system (CNS) tumors should be assessed for signs of raised ICP. Many children receive cytotoxic or immunosuppressive chemotherapy as well as radiotherapy. This may result in increased risk of sepsis, thrombocytopenia, and anemia. Patients are typically scheduled for a series of treatments over several weeks. Radiation doses are high, in the range of 180 to 250 cGy, and all medical personnel must leave the room during the treatment. Direct observation of the patient is not possible; an interfaced system of closed-circuit television and telemetric microphones is used with standard monitoring.[4] In the event of a problem, shutdown of the radiation beam and immediate access to the patient (within 20 to 30 seconds) are crucial.

The goals of anesthesia for pediatric radiotherapy have been defined as[54]:

1. Assurance of immobility
2. Rapid onset
3. Brief duration of action
4. Not painful to administer
5. Prompt recovery
6. Minimal interference with eating or drinking and playing
7. Avoidance of tolerance to the anesthetic agents
8. Maintenance of a patent airway in a variety of body positions

General anesthesia[54] or deep-sedation techniques with propofol[55] are preferable to prevent patient movement and to allow children to tolerate what can be fairly length procedures, some lasting at least 30 minutes. Most children will have indwelling intravenous access, avoiding the need for repeated intravenous puncture and inhalational induction.

Intraoperative radiation therapy treatments are provided after the masses are exposed to view. Patients with pancreatic, colon, and rectal cancers; radiation-sensitive sarcomas; and specific types of ovarian cancers receive this form of treatment. Doses of 5,000 to 6,000 cGy may be used during a single, intraoperative treatment. These patients typically suffer from advanced cancers and may have the attendant nutritional deficiency, dehydration, electrolyte imbalances, and coagulopathies that can complicate anesthetic management. Some hospitals are equipped with combination radiation therapy/operating room suites; however, most centers require that surgical exploration be performed in the traditional operating room. The anesthetized patient is subsequently transported to the radiology suite, which may be at a considerable distance. Portable monitors and methods for delivery of oxygen and agents to maintain general anesthesia during transport are required.[56] Requirements for patient monitoring for intraoperative radiation are comparable to those described for external beam radiation. Personnel must leave the room during the actual treatment. After treatment, patients must be

transported back to the operating room for surgical closure. Occasionally, closure can be performed in the radiology suite and the patient taken directly to the PACU.

CARDIAC CATHETERIZATION

Common interventions in the cardiac catheterization laboratory include[57]:

- Diagnostic cardiac catheterization
- Coronary angiography and stenting
- Electrophysiology studies and ablations
- Placement of pacing and defibrillator devices

In recent years the number and complexity of procedures performed have expanded rapidly.[58] New procedures have been developed, including, balloon dilation and stenting for valvular and subvalvular lesions, electrophysiological studies, and ablation of specific pathways (e.g., Wolff-Parkinson-White syndrome) or areas (e.g., atrial fibrillation), and biventricular pacing for heart failure. Many patients will tolerate these procedures with light or moderate sedation; however, general anesthesia is becoming more widely practiced, particularly as procedures become longer and more complex.

Cardiac catheterization is performed in children with congenital heart disease for both hemodynamic assessment and interventional procedures.[59] Careful cardiac assessment is essential, and the presence of a trained pediatric anesthesiologist is desirable. Patients often present with cyanosis, dyspnea, congestive heart failure, and intracardiac shunts. Hypoxia, hypercarbia, and sympathetic stimulation as a result of anxiety may exacerbate cardiopulmonary abnormalities. In patients with a patent ductus arteriosis, high oxygen tension can lead to premature closure and should be avoided. Prostaglandin infusions are often used to maintain duct patency. Meticulous attention must be paid to preventing air bubbles entering intravenous lines because they may cross to the arterial circulation via a right-to-left shunt. Diagnostic, noninterventional studies are often performed with sedation, and local anesthetic is injected at the site of femoral puncture. Oral sedation techniques include chloral hydrate, 75 to 100 mg/kg, or a mixture of meperidine, promethazine, and chlorpromazine.[59] Intravenous agents include midazolam, morphine, and ketamine. General anesthesia is necessary when children cannot tolerate sedation techniques and/or have significant cardiac or other morbidity, and when the procedure involves severe hemodynamic disturbances such as ventricular septal defect occlusion. Ketamine is useful in children with myocardial depression and can be used as an infusion together with propofol.[60] Fentanyl, midazolam, and etomidate are alternatives.

Electrophysiological Procedures

Electrophysiologic studies and ablation of abnormal conduction pathways are performed for treatment of dysrhythmias caused by aberrant conduction pathways. Cardiac catheters are inserted via the femoral and sometimes internal jugular routes, and multiple stimulations of the cardiac conducting system are carried out. Once identified, the abnormal conduction pathways are ablated using radiofrequency techniques. The volatile anesthetic agents and propofol have been shown not to interfere with cardiac conduction during these procedures.[61] Electrophysiologic studies are lengthy and can be painful; children usually require general anesthesia. Children undergoing radiofrequency ablation experience a high incidence of nausea and vomiting,[62] and this may be reduced using a propofol infusion technique rather than volatile anesthesia. The patient's antidysrhythmic therapy is stopped prior to the procedure, and cardiac dysrhythmias generated by the procedure are usually terminated using overdrive pacing via the catheters or, if unsuccessful, by external cardioversion. External defibrillation pads should be applied before the procedure.

Automatic Implantable Cardioverter-Defibrillators

In the late 1990s, a number of trials proved the benefit of automatic implantable cardioverter-defibrillators in reducing mortality of patients with ventricular tachyarrhythmias and left ventricular dysfunction following myocardial infarction or cardiac arrest.[63,64] Automatic implantable cardioverter-defibrillators are usually implanted in the electrophysiologic laboratory rather than in the operating room, under general anesthesia or sedation. The procedure itself is not particularly painful; however, ventricular fibrillation is induced to test the device during implantation, which is distressing for the patient.

CARDIOVERSION

Atrial fibrillation (AF) affects approximately 0.4% of the general population, its prevalence increasing with age.[65] AF is associated with a number of conditions, particularly hypertension, chronic heart failure, and valvular and ischemic heart disease, and is a frequent sequela of cardiothoracic surgery.[66] Transthoracic DC cardioversion is an accepted, often-used treatment for atrial dysrhythmias including AF and atrial flutter,[67] and in patients undergoing outpatient cardioversion; the success rate for conversion to sinus rhythm is 90%.[68] AF is associated with significant morbidity and mortality from thromboembolic stroke. Two strategies are employed to prevent thromboembolism following cardioversion in patients who have been in AF for longer than 48 hours. The conventional approach is to initiate anticoagulation 3 weeks before cardioversion, usually with Coumadin, and to continue for 4 weeks after cardioversion.[67,69] More recently, transesophageal echocardiography (TEE) has been recommended to determine whether patients are at low or high risk of thromboembolism.[70,71] In low-risk patients, the dose of anticoagulants can be reduced, whereas in patients considered to be high risk, cardioversion may be postponed to allow adequate anticoagulation.[72] Simple cardioversion takes a few seconds; however, it is distressing, and sedation is preferable except in life-threatening situations. The complication rate for cardioversion is reported as 2.6%.[68] Complications associated with cardioversion include thromboembolic phenomena, pulmonary edema, aspiration pneumonitis, and bradycardia.[68] Elective cardioversion is often performed in areas near the operating room, usually in the PACU. Alternatively, there may be a requirement for the anesthesiologist to provide sedation in the intensive care unit (ICU) for urgent cardioversion in an unstable patient.

A small bolus of intravenous induction agent is usually sufficient to sedate a patient for cardioversion. All currently available induction agents are effective. Etomidate produces less hypotension than propofol making it a better choice in patients with significant cardiac disease, although hypotension can be attenuated by using smaller doses of propofol (1 mg/kg).[73,74] Recently, propofol has been shown to provide more rapid recovery than midazolam following cardioversion in elderly patients,[74] and a propofol/remifentanil technique provided more hemodynamic stability and faster recovery than midazolam in patients undergoing cardioversion for AF following cardiac surgery.[75] When TEE is performed prior to cardioversion, the procedure takes 15 to 30 minutes and various sedation agents may be used to help the patient tolerate

the procedure. Airway control is important, and in most cases nasal cannulas are sufficient to provide supplemental oxygenation while the patient maintains his or her own airway.

A technique using deep propofol sedation together with a LMA to support the airway and allow ventilation has also been described.[76] In this study the LMA was inserted either at the beginning of the procedure or midway through if respiratory problems occurred. The presence of the LMA was not found to interfere with the TEE procedure. Thorough airway evaluation is important prior to TEE, and occasionally, endotracheal intubation may be the most prudent approach. Before TEE, local anesthetic, either 4% lidocaine or 20% benzocaine, is sprayed into the oropharynx to allow easy passage of the TEE probe. A bite block is inserted to prevent the patient from biting down on the probe, damaging both the teeth and the probe.

GASTROENTEROLOGY

The gastroenterology suite is another location where technology is expanding, and where an increasing number of diagnostic and therapeutic procedures are being performed. Procedures commonly performed in the gastrointestinal (GI) endoscopy suite are shown in Table 34-9.

A review in 2007 by the American Gastroenterological Association reports that 98% of endoscopists in the United States administer sedation for upper and lower endoscopies.[77] A wide variety of sedation techniques are used, and the complication rates for sedation are reported 0.54 to 0.1%.[78] The mortality rate is 0.03%.[79] Gastroenterologists are increasingly using propofol sedation techniques, and many have found it to be an effective and safe technique.[80] However, the American Gastroenterological Association recommendations call for appropriate training of endoscopists and the involvement of an anesthesiologist for patients in ASA categories IV and V or with histories of adverse or inadequate responses to sedation.[78]

Upper Gastrointestinal Endoscopy

Upper GI endoscopy is performed for diagnostic procedures, such as biopsy, and for therapeutic procedures, such as retrieval of foreign bodies, treatment of esophageal varices with sclerotherapy or band ligation, dilation of esophageal strictures, and placement of a percutaneous endoscopic gastrostomy. Patients may have a number of comorbidities, including disease of the esophagus and stomach, with a risk of reflux, biliary, and hepatic disease with esophageal varices, hepatic dysfunction, coagulopathy, and ascites. The procedure is tolerated without sedation in 66 to 81% of patients,[81] and conscious sedation is usually sufficient in the remainder. With general anesthesia, patients usually require endotracheal

---

TABLE 34-9

COMMON GASTROENTEROLOGIC PROCEDURES

Upper endoscopy
Sigmoidoscopy
Colonoscopy
Endoscopic retrograde cholangiopancreatography
Esophageal dilatation
Esophageal stenting
Percutaneous endoscopic gastrostomy tube placement
Transjugular intrahepatic portosystemic shunt

intubation to protect the airway and facilitate passage of the endoscope. The LMA has also been used successfully in adults[82] and children[83] as an alternative device for airway management. Local anesthetic is sprayed into the oropharynx to facilitate passage of the endoscope; this can abolish the gag reflex, increasing the risk of aspiration. A bite block is inserted to prevent the patient from biting down on the endoscope and damaging both the teeth and the endoscope. If the patient has received general anesthesia, care must be taken that the bite block and endoscope do not dislodge or obstruct the endotracheal tube. Procedures are performed in the prone or semiprone position with the patient's head rotated to the side. This position makes the airway less accessible. Care and attention should also be paid to pressure areas, particularly the eyes, lips, and teeth. Extreme rotation of the neck should be avoided. Most procedures are brief, lasting 10 to 30 minutes, and are generally painless.

Endoscopic Retrograde Cholangiopancreatography

Endoscopic retrograde cholangiopancreatography (ERCP) is important in the diagnosis and treatment of both biliary and pancreatic disease. During the procedure, the endoscope is advanced via the mouth into the stomach, and then into the duodenum where the ampulla of Vater is visualized. The biliary and pancreatic duct systems may then be instrumented, and therapeutic maneuvers such as the passage of stents or removal of stones carried out. Sphincter of Oddi manometry may also be performed. Patients usually experience discomfort during ERCP, particularly with instrumentation and stenting of the biliary and pancreatic ducts. Conscious or deep-sedation techniques are recommended for the procedure, which usually lasts between 20 and 80 minutes.[84] Only 5 to 8% of patients require general anesthesia.[82,85]

The airway and patient positioning considerations are similar to those for GI endoscopy. ERCP in the prone position can be particularly problematic if careful attention is not paid to maintenance of a patent airway. If sphincter of Oddi manometry is being performed, glycopyrrolate, atropine, and glucagon should be avoided[84] because they effect sphincter pressure. Opioids, particularly morphine[86] and fentanyl, cause spasm of the sphincter of Oddi, which may be relieved with naloxone.[87] Meperidine, in contrast, reduces the frequency of sphincter of Oddi contractions.[86]

Patients presenting for emergency ERCP may have significant comorbidity,[85] including acute cholangitis with septicemia, jaundice with liver dysfunction and coagulopathy, bleeding from esophageal varices resulting in hypovolemia, or biliary stricture following major hepatobiliary surgery, including liver transplantation. Transient bacteremia may occur during endoscopy, and antibiotic prophylaxis is recommended for patients with cardiac valvular abnormalities. Gastroenterologists frequently use antispasmodics to improve operating conditions during endoscopy.[88] Intravenous hyoscyamine given as a 0.5-mg bolus before the procedure has been shown to reduce the incidence of spasm, shorten the procedure, and improve patient comfort[88]; sinus tachycardia may occur.

Transjugular Intrahepatic Portosystemic Shunt

The transjugular intrahepatic portosystemic shunt (TIPS) is created via a catheter inserted in the internal jugular vein and directed into the liver. It connects the right or left portal vein through the liver parenchyma to one of the three hepatic

TABLE 34-10

PREOPERATIVE CONSIDERATIONS IN PATIENTS PRESENTING FOR THE TRANSJUGULAR INTRAHEPATIC PORTOSYSTEMIC SHUNT PROCEDURE

Airway—risk of aspiration	Recent gastrointestinal bleeding
	Raised intragastric pressure due to ascites
	Decreased level of consciousness due to hepatic encephalopathy
Respiratory system	Decreased functional residual capacity due to ascites
	Pleural effusion
	Intrapulmonary shunts
	Pneumonia
Cardiovascular system	Associated alcoholic cardiomyopathy
	Altered volume status
	Acute hemorrhage from esophageal varices
	Intraperitoneal hemorrhage
Hematologic system	Coagulopathy
	Thrombocytopenia
Neurologic system	Hepatic encephalopathy

veins.[89] The TIPS functions to decompress the portal circulation in patients with portal hypertension and is often performed in patients who have failed to respond to medical therapy. The TIPS has been found to be equally effective as other therapies in the secondary prophylaxis of bleeding varices and control of refractory cirrhotic ascites,[90] but with no improvement in mortality and an increased risk of development of encephalopathy. The TIPS has been used in children and found to be feasible and safe in providing temporary relief of portal hypertension while awaiting liver transplantation.[91] The TIPS procedure causes minimal stimulation, lasts between 2 and 3 hours, and may be performed under sedation or general anesthesia.[92]

Patients presenting for a TIPS procedure, in general, have significant hepatic dysfunction and require careful preoperative assessment. Considerations are outlined in Table 34-10 (see also Chapter 48). Chronic liver disease has a number of effects on the pharmacokinetics of anesthetic agents,[92] and the response to anesthetic agents may be unpredictable. Volume of distribution is increased, and protein binding, drug metabolism, and elimination are all decreased. CNS sensitivity is variably affected. Patients need careful monitoring; the use of an arterial catheter to monitor blood pressure and to allow frequent blood gas and chemistry analysis is recommended. Blood glucose should be monitored frequently as patients with hepatic disease are at risk for hypoglycemia because of depleted liver glycogen stores. Preoperative use of diuretics and intraoperative fluid shifts make these patients vulnerable to electrolyte abnormalities. Urine output should be closely monitored to prevent worsening of renal function and development of the hepatorenal syndrome.

ELECTROCONVULSIVE THERAPY

Electroconvulsive therapy (ECT) has had an important role in the management of psychiatric disorders since the 1930s. ECT is used to treat depression, mania, and affective disorders in schizophrenic patients, as well as a number of other psychiatric disorders. Typically, ECT is performed 3 times per week for 6 to 12 treatments, followed by weekly or monthly maintenance therapy to prevent relapses.[93]

Physiologic Response to Electroconvulsive Therapy

The physiologic response to an electrical current applied to the brain includes generalized motor seizures and an acute cardiovascular response. The grand mal seizure lasts several minutes and includes a short, 10- to 15-second tonic phase, followed by a more prolonged clonic phase, lasting 30 to 60 seconds. A minimum seizure duration of 25 seconds is recommended to ensure adequate antidepressant efficacy.[94] The cardiovascular response includes increased cerebral blood flow and ICP. Generalized autonomic nervous system stimulation results in an initial 10 to 15 seconds of bradycardia and occasional asystole, followed by a more prominent sympathetic response of hypertension and tachycardia. Occasionally, cardiac dysrhythmias, myocardial ischemia, infarction, or neurologic vascular events may be precipitated. Short-term memory loss is also common following ECT. Other sequelae include muscular aches, fracture/dislocations, headache, emergence agitation, status epilepticus, and sudden death.

Anesthetic Considerations

ECT is usually carried out in the PACU near the operating room; alternatively, psychiatric institutions may have an area set aside for treatments. Psychiatrists place scalp electrodes to monitor the electroencephalogram during the seizure, and a blood pressure cuff is applied to an extremity and inflated before the muscle relaxant is administered to monitor the seizure. Patients with depression presenting for ECT are often elderly, with a number of coexisting conditions; therefore, a thorough preoperative assessment and workup should be performed before the patient begins treatment.[95] First-line pharmacotherapeutic agents for the treatment of depression include tricyclic antidepressants, monoamine oxidase inhibitors, and selective serotonin-reuptake inhibitors. Patients may be taking a variety of drugs, which can have important interactions with the anesthetic agent. The monoamine oxidase inhibitors have the most significant interactions, although more modern drugs are superseding these. The anesthetic requirements for ECT include amnesia, airway management, prevention of bodily injury from the seizure, control of hemodynamic changes, and a smooth, rapid emergence.[93,95]

Most of the intravenous induction agents have been used to induce anesthesia for ECT. Methohexital (1 to 1.5 mg/kg) is considered the "gold standard,"[93] although it decreases seizure duration in a dose-dependant way. Etomidate (0.15 to 0.3 mg/kg) is generally associated with longer seizure duration, myoclonus, and delayed recovery, and is considered by some psychiatrists to be superior to propofol or methohexital.[96,97] Etomidate does not depress the cardiovascular system, so hypertensive and tachycardic responses may be accentuated.[93] Propofol is more effective at attenuating the acute hemodynamic responses to ECT[98] and recovery is rapid. Propofol, however, has anticonvulsant effects, although with a small dose (0.75 mg/kg) seizure duration is usually acceptable,[96] and studies have found that reduction in seizure duration by propofol does not adversely affect the outcome of ECT therapy.[99] Most other induction agents decrease seizure activity. Short-acting opioids, such as remifentanil, can be used to decrease the dose of induction agent and prolong seizure duration without reducing the depth of anesthesia.[100] Muscle relaxants are used to prevent musculoskeletal complications such as fractures or dislocations during the seizure. Succinylcholine, 0.75 to 1.5 mg/kg, is the most commonly used agent and is preferable to the longer-acting nondepolarizing agents.[93]

Anesthesia is induced and the patient is ventilated with 100% oxygen using an oral airway and a self-inflating bag and mask. Moderate hyperventilation is beneficial prior to the ECT to improve the quality and duration of seizures, and it has been suggested that the LMA may be useful to improve ventilation during ECT.[101] Before administering the seizure, a bite guard is placed to protect the teeth. In younger patients, 15 to 30 mg of intravenous ketorolac helps to reduce ECT-induced myalgia. Older patients, or those in whom ketorolac is contraindicated, may receive aspirin or acetaminophen orally before their treatment.[93] The parasympathetic effects of ECT, salivation, transient bradycardia, and asystole can be prevented by premedication with glycopyrrolate or atropine. A number of drugs have been used to attenuate the hypertensive and tachycardic responses that accompany ECT. Labetalol (0.3 mg/kg) and esmolol (1 mg/kg) both have been shown to ameliorate the hemodynamic responses, although esmolol has a lesser effect on seizure duration than labetalol.[102] The calcium channel antagonists nifedipine, diltiazem, and nicardipine all attenuate the hemodynamic responses to ECT, particularly in combination with labetalol. The α_2-adrenergic receptor agonists clonidine,[93] and more recently, dexmedetomidine[103] (1 μg/kg administered over 10 minutes just before induction of anesthesia) have been shown to be effective in controlling blood pressure without affecting seizure duration.

DENTAL SURGERY

Most dental procedures are performed in the office with no sedation and only local anesthesia. General anesthesia may be required during more complicated or prolonged cases and when patients are uncooperative, phobic, or mentally challenged. Patients may also present for dental clearance prior to undergoing cardiac surgery or heart transplantation with severe cardiomyopathy or valvular abnormalities. A number of genetic diseases result in mental deficiency, psychiatric diagnoses, and aberrant behavior. These patients commonly require sedation or general anesthesia to tolerate dental procedures. Genetic diseases are commonly associated with other medical problems, particularly those related to the cardiovascular system and the airway.[104] Down syndrome is commonly encountered, and the anesthesiologist should be aware of cardiac abnormalities, including conduction abnormalities and structural defects, the risk of atlanto-occipital dislocation, and a variety of potential airway problems, including macroglossia, hypoplastic maxilla, palatal abnormalities, or mandibular protrusion. If the patient is positioned head-up in the dental chair, vasodilation and myocardial depressant effects of anesthetics can be pronounced, especially in patients with cardiovascular diseases. Patients with neuromuscular diseases may have a history of aspiration and episodes of chronic recurrent pneumonitis that must be addressed before dental surgery.

The most challenging part of anesthesia for dental surgery is induction. Many patients, particularly children, are unable to cooperate because of learning disabilities or mental retardation. Ketamine is a useful induction agent. It may be given alone by a variety of routes (orally, intramuscularly, intravenously), or in combination with atropine and midazolam.[105] Doses are as follows: intravenously, 1 to 2 mg/kg; orally, 5 to 10 mg/kg; and intramuscularly, 2 to 4 mg/kg, with an onset time of 5 to 10 minutes. The rectal and intranasal routes have also been used. Ketamine is also advantageous in that it does not abolish upper airway reflexes. Oral midazolam is also popular. A dose of 0.5 mg/kg is dissolved in a small amount of liquid. In children and needle-phobic adults, the use of local anesthetic cream facilitates the placement of intravenous lines. Alternatively, an inhalation induction may be attempted.

During and after dental surgery blood, saliva, and dental debris are present in the upper airway. A throat pack is used to help protect the airway, and this must be removed at the end of surgery. Tracheal intubation, often via the nasal route, is required to protect the airway, although the LMA has been used successfully for both adults[106] and children[107] undergoing dental surgery. Anesthesia can be maintained with intravenous infusions or inhalation anesthesia. Patients need close observation during emergence and recovery. The immediate postoperative complications include bleeding, airway obstruction, and laryngeal spasm. Reanesthetizing the patient for treatment of dental hemorrhage can be very difficult because of the presence of blood in the airway and the risk of pulmonary aspiration. Later complications in ambulatory patients include drowsiness, nausea and vomiting, and pain.[108]

TRANSPORT OF PATIENTS

Patients who receive anesthesia or sedation at alternate sites may need to be transported to the PACU at the end of the procedure; this may be some distance away. During transport, patients should be accompanied by a member of the anesthesia team, who should continue to evaluate, monitor, and support the patient's medical condition.[9] Other patients transported within a hospital may require the care of an anesthesiologist for a variety of reasons. For example, surgery patients may be transferred to the ICU or the radiology department for imaging at the end of surgery, or critically ill patients may be transferred to the operating room from the ICU or the emergency department for urgent surgery. In these situations, the anesthesiologist should monitor the patients closely. These patients are often ventilated and receiving a number of drug infusions for both sedation and hemodynamic support. Portable ventilators are useful for transport; however, these are often oxygen-powered, and adequate supplies of oxygen must be available for the transfer, as well as a manual self-inflating bag to allow hand ventilation in the event of ventilator failure. Similarly, the infusion pumps and portable monitors should have adequate battery power to allow them to continue working in transit. The anesthesiologist should carry spare anesthetic and emergency drugs, equipment for intubation or reintubation, portable suction, and if the patient's condition requires, a portable defibrillator. It is useful to notify persons in the destination area that the patient is in transit so appropriate preparations to receive the patient can be made in advance. It is also useful to send personnel ahead to secure the elevators to prevent delays during transfer.

SUMMARY

The number and complexity of procedures that are performed at alternate sites is steadily increasing. This has led to an expansion of anesthesia services in areas remote from the operating room that may not be familiar to anesthesia providers. In preparing to administer anesthesia or sedation in an alternate site, a simple three-step approach can be followed. This involves giving careful consideration to the needs of the *patient*, the particular problems posed by the *procedure*, and the hazards and limitations of the *environment*. In all cases, the standards of anesthesia care and monitoring should be no different than those provided in the conventional operating room.

References

1. Joint Commission on Accreditation of Healthcare Organizations (JCAHO): Accreditation Manual for Hospitals. Oakbrook Terrace, IL, JCAHO, 1991, p 269
2. Practice Guidelines for Sedation and Analgesia by Non-Anesthesiologists An Updated Report by the American Society of Anesthesiologists Task Force on Sedation and Analgesia by Non-Anesthesiologists. Anesthesiology 2002; 96: 1004
3. American Society of Anesthesiologists (ASA): Guidelines for nonoperating room anesthetizing locations. Amended 2003. In ASA Guidelines, Standards, and Statements. American Society of Anesthesiologists, Park Ridge, Illinois
4. Bashein G, Russell AH, Momii ST: Anesthesia and remote monitoring for intraoperative radiation therapy. Anesthesiology 1986; 64: 804
5. Lawani K: Demographics and trends in nonoperating-room anesthesia. Curr Opin Anaesthesiol 2006; 19: 430
6. American Society of Anesthesiologists (ASA): Basic standards for preanesthesia care. (Approved by the House of Delegates on October 14, 1987, and amended October 25, 2005). In ASA Guidelines, Standards, and Statements. American Society of Anesthesiologists, Park Ridge, Illinois
7. American Society of Anesthesiologists (ASA): Standards for postanesthesia care. (Approved by House of Delegates on October 12, 1988 and last amended on October 27, 2004). In ASA Guidelines, Standards, and Statements. American Society of Anesthesiologists, Park Ridge, Illinois
8. American Society of Anesthesiologists (ASA): Position on monitored anesthesia care (Approved by the House of Delegates on October 21, 1986, and last amended on October 25, 2005). In ASA Guidelines, Standards, and Statements. American Society of Anesthesiologists, Park Ridge, Illinois
9. American Society of Anesthesiologists (ASA): Standards for basic anesthetic monitoring (Approved by the ASA House of Delegates on October 21, 1986, and last amended on October 25, 2005). In ASA Guidelines, Standards, and Statements. American Society of Anesthesiologists, Park Ridge, Illinois
10. King BF Jr: Intravascular contrast media and premedication, Radiology Life Support. Edited by Bush WH Jr, Krecke KN, King BH Jr, Bettmann MA. London, Arnold, 1999, p 1
11. Nash K, Hafeez A, Hou S: Hospital-acquired renal insufficiency. Am J Kidney Dis 2002; 39: 930
12. Pannu N, Wiebe N, Tonelli M: Prophylaxis strategies for contrast-induced nephropathy. JAMA 2006; 295: 2765
13. Merten GJ, Burgess WEP, Gray LV et al: Prevention of contrast-induced nephropathy with sodium bicarbonate: A randomized controlled trial. JAMA 2004; 291: 2328
14. Katayama H, Yamaguchi K, Kozuka T et al: Adverse reactions to ionic and nonionic contrast media. A report from the Japanese Committee on the Safety of Contrast Media. Radiology 1990; 175: 621
15. Goldberg M: Systemic reactions to intravascular contrast media. A guide for the anesthesiologist. Anesthesiology 1984; 60: 46
16. Lasser EC, Berry CC, Mishkin MM et al: Pretreatment with corticosteroids to prevent adverse reactions to nonionic contrast media. Am J Roentgenol 1994; 162: 523
17. Lasser EC, Lyon SG, Berry CC: Reports on contrast media reactions: Analysis of data from reports to the U.S. Food and Drug Administration. Radiology 1997; 203: 605
18. Murphy KJ, Brunberg JA, Cohan RH: Adverse reactions to gadolinium contrast media: A review of 36 cases. Am J Roentgenol 1996; 167: 847
19. Davies D: Subspeciality monitoring techniques—miscellaneous, Problems in Anesthesia Monitoring. Edited by Gravenstein N. Philadelphia, JB Lippincott, 1987, p 138
20. Derdeyn CP, Moran CJ, Eichling JO et al: Radiation dose to patients and personnel during intraoperative digital subtraction angiography. Am J Neuroradiol 1999; 20: 300
21. National Council on Radiation Protection and Measurements: Recommendations on limits for exposure to ionizing radiation. NCRP Report No. 116. Bethesda, MD, National Council on Radiation, 1993
22. Dion JE, Gates PC, Fox AJ et al: Clinical events following neuroangiography: A prospective study. Stroke 1987; 18: 997
23. Varma MK, Price K, Jayakrishnan V et al: Anaesthetic considerations for interventional radiology. Br J Anaesth 2007; 99: 775
24. Guglielmi G, Vinuela F, Dion J et al: Electrothrombosis of saccular aneurysms via endovascular approach. Part 2: Preliminary clinical experience. J Neurosurg 1991; 75: 8
25. McDougall CG, Halbach VV, Dowd CF et al: Endovascular treatment of basilar tip aneurysms using electrolytically detachable coils. J Neurosurg 1996; 84: 393
26. Kremer C, Groden C, Hansen HC et al: Outcome after endovascular treatment of Hunt and Hess grade IV or V aneurysms: Comparison of anterior versus posterior circulation. Stroke 1999; 30: 2617
27. Lai YC, Manninen PH: Anesthesia for cerebral aneurysms: A comparison between interventional neuroradiology and surgery. Can J Anaesth 2001; 48: 391
28. Hadjivassiliou M, Tooth CL, Romanowski CA et al: Aneurysmal SAH: Cognitive outcome and structural damage after clipping or coiling. Neurology 2001; 56: 1672
29. Deveikis JP: Endovascular therapy of intracranial arteriovenous malformations. Materials and techniques. Neuroimaging Clin N Am 1998; 8: 401
30. Young WL, Pile-Spellman J: Anesthetic considerations for interventional neuroradiology. Anesthesiology 1994; 80: 427
31. Kubalek R, Berlis A, Schwab M et al: Activated clotting time or activated partial thromboplastin time as the method of choice for patients undergoing neuroradiological intervention. Neuroradiology 2003; 45: 325
32. Pelz DM, Lownie SP, Fox AJ et al: Symptomatic pulmonary complications from liquid acrylate embolization of brain arteriovenous malformations. Am J Neuroradiol 1995; 16: 19
33. Osborn IP: Anesthetic considerations for interventional neuroradiology. Int Anesthesiol Clin 2003; 41: 69

ANESTHETIC MANAGEMENT

34. Martin NA, Khanna R, Doberstein C et al: Therapeutic embolization of arteriovenous malformations: The case for and against. Clin Neurosurg 2000; 46: 295

35. See JJ, Manninen PH: Anesthesia for neuroradiology. Curr Opin Anaesthesiol 2005; 18: 437

36. Hall JE, Uhrich TD, Barney JA et al: Sedative, amnesia and analgesic properties of small-dose dexmedetomidine infusions. Anesth Analg 2000; 90: 699

37. Bustillo MA, Lazar RM, Finck AD et al: Dexmedetomidine may impair cognitive testing during endovascular embolization of cerebral arteriovenous malformations: a retrospective case report series. J Neurosurg Anesthesiol 2002; 14: 209

38. Dupuy DE, Zagoria RJ, Akerley W et al: Percutaneous radiofrequency ablation of malignancies in the lung. Am J Roentgenol 2000; 174: 57

39. Vaughn C, Mychaskiw G 2nd, Sewell P: Massive hemorrhage during radiofrequency ablation of a pulmonary neoplasm. Anesth Analg 2002; 94: 1149

40. Menon DK, Peden CJ, Hall AS et al: Magnetic resonance for the anaesthetist. Part I: Physical principles, applications, safety aspects. Anaesthesia 1992; 47: 240

41. Patteson SK, Chesney JT: Anesthetic management for magnetic resonance imaging: Problems and solutions. Anesth Analg 1992; 74: 121

42. Schenck JF: Safety of strong, static magnetic fields. J Magn Reson Imaging 2000; 12: 2

43. Chaljub G, Kramer LA, Johnson RF III et al: Projectile cylinder accidents resulting from the presence of ferromagnetic nitrous oxide or oxygen tanks in the MR suite. Am J Roentgenol 2001; 177: 27

44. Peden CJ, Menon DK, Hall AS et al: Magnetic resonance for the anaesthetist. Part II: Anaesthesia and monitoring in MR units. Anaesthesia 1992; 47: 508

45. Melendez JC, McCrank E: Anxiety-related reactions associated with magnetic resonance imaging examinations. JAMA 1993; 270: 745

46. Flaherty JA, Hoskinson K: Emotional distress during magnetic resonance imaging. N Engl J Med 1989; 320: 467

47. Murphy KJ, Brunberg JA: Adult claustrophobia, anxiety and sedation in MRI. Magn Reson Imaging 1997; 15: 51

48. Keengwe IN, Hegde S, Dearlove O et al: Structured sedation programme for magnetic resonance imaging examination in children. Anaesthesia 1999; 54: 1069

49. Malviya S, Voepel-Lewis T, Eldevik OP et al: Sedation and general anaesthesia in children undergoing MRI and CT: Adverse events and outcomes. Br J Anaesth 2000; 84: 743

50. Greenberg SB, Faerber EN, Aspinall CL: High dose chloral hydrate sedation for children undergoing CT. J Comput Assist Tomogr 1991; 15: 467

51. Gooden CK, Dilos B: Anesthesia for magnetic resonance imaging. Int Anesthesiol Clin 2003; 41: 29

52. Merola C, Albarracin C, Lebowitz P et al: An audit of adverse events in children sedated with chloral hydrate or propofol during imaging studies. Paediatr Anaesth 1995; 5: 375

53. Cortellazzi P, Lamperti M, Minati L et al: Sedation of neurologically impaired children undergoing MRI: a sequential approach. Pediatr Anesth 2007; 17: 630

54. Fortney JT, Halperin EC, Hertz CM et al: Anesthesia for pediatric external beam radiation therapy. Int J Radiat Oncol Biol Phys 1999; 44: 587

55. Buehrer S, Immoos S, Frei M et al: Evaluation of propofol for repeated prolonged deep sedation in children undergoing proton radiation therapy. Br J Anaesth 2007; 99: 556

56. Mannaerts GH, Van Zundert AA, Meeusen VC et al: Anaesthesia for advanced rectal cancer patients treated with combined major resections and intraoperative radiotherapy. Eur J Anaesthesiol 2002; 19: 742

57. Shook DC, Gross W: Offsite anesthesiology in the cardiac catheterization lab. Curr Opin Anaesthesiol 2007; 20: 352

58. Reddy K, Jaggar S, Gillbe C: The anaesthetist and the cardiac catheterisation laboratory. Anaesthesia 2006; 61: 1175

59. Javorski JJ, Hansen DD, Laussen PC et al: Paediatric cardiac catheterization: Innovations. Can J Anaesth 1995; 42: 310

60. Kogan A, Efrat R, Katz J et al: Propofol-ketamine mixture for anesthesia in pediatric patients undergoing cardiac catheterization. J Cardiothorac Vasc Anesth 2003; 17: 691

61. Lavoie J, Walsh EP, Burrows FA et al: Effects of propofol or isoflurane anesthesia on cardiac conduction in children undergoing radiofrequency catheter ablation for tachydysrhythmias. Anesthesiology 1995; 82: 884

62. Erb TO, Hall JM, Ing RJ et al: Postoperative nausea and vomiting in children and adolescents undergoing radiofrequency catheter ablation: A randomized comparison of propofol- and isoflurane-based anesthetics. Anesth Analg 2002; 95: 1577

63. Bigger JT Jr, Whang W, Rottman JN et al: Mechanisms of death in the CABG patch trial: A randomized trial of implantable cardiac defibrillator prophylaxis in patients at high risk of death after coronary artery bypass graft surgery. Circulation 1999; 99: 1416

64. Higgins SL: Impact of the Multicenter Automatic Defibrillator Implantation Trial on implantable cardioverter defibrillator indication trends. Am J Cardiol 1999; 83: 79D

65. Kannel WB, Wolf PA, Benjamin EJ et al: Prevalence, incidence, prognosis, and predisposing conditions for atrial fibrillation: Population-based estimates. Am J Cardiol 1998; 82: 2N

66. Ommen SR, Odell JA, Stanton MS: Atrial arrhythmias after cardiothoracic surgery. N Engl J Med 1997; 336: 1429

67. Kerber RE: Transthoracic cardioversion of atrial fibrillation and flutter: Standard techniques and new advances. Am J Cardiol 1996; 78: 22

68. Botkin SB, Dhanekula LS, Olshansky B: Outpatient cardioversion of atrial arrythmias: Efficacy, safety, and costs. Am Heart J 2003; 145: 233

69. Albers GW, Dalen JE, Laupacis A et al: Antithrombotic therapy in atrial fibrillation. Chest 2001; 119: 194S

70. Klein AL, Grimm RA, Murray RD et al: Use of transesophageal echocardiography to guide cardioversion in patients with atrial fibrillation. N Engl J Med 2001; 344: 1411

71. Asher CR, Klein AL: Transesophageal echocardiography to guide cardioversion in patients with atrial fibrillation: ACUTE trial update. Card Electrophysiol Rev 2003; 7: 387

72. Troughton RW, Asher CR, Klein AL: The role of echocardiography in atrial fibrillation and cardioversion. Heart 2003; 89: 1447

73. Herregods LL, Bossuyt GP, De Baerdemaeker LE et al: Ambulatory electrical external cardioversion with propofol or etomidate. J Clin Anesth 2003; 15: 91

74. Parlak M, Parlak I, Erdur B et al: Age effect on efficacy and side effects of two sedation and analgesia protocols on patients goping through cardioversion: A randomized clinical trial. Acad Emerg Med 2006; 13: 493

75. Yildirim V, Doganci S, Bolcal C et al: Combined sedoanalgesia with remifentanil and propofol verus remifentanil and midazolam for elective cardioversion after coronary artery bypass grafting. Adv Ther 2007; 24: 662

76. Ferson D, Thakar D, Swafford J et al: Use of deep intravenous sedation with propofol and the laryngeal mask airway during transesophageal echocardiography. J Cardiothorac Vasc Anesth 2003; 17: 443

77. Cohen LB, Delegge MH, Aisenberg J et al: AGA Institute Review of Endoscopic Sedation. Gastroenterology 2007; 133: 675

78. Conigliaro R, Rossi A: Implementation of sedation guidelines in clinical practice in Italy: results of a prospective longitudinal multicenter study. Endoscopy 2006; 38: 1137

79. Arrowsmith JB, Gerstman BB, Fleischer DE et al: Results from the American Society for Gastrointestinal Endoscopy/U.S. Food and Drug Administration collaborative study on complication rates and drug use during gastrointestinal endoscopy. Gastrointest Endosc 1991; 37: 421

80. Byrne MF, Baillie J: Nurse-assisted propofol sedation: The jury is in! Am J Gastroenterol 2005;129: 1781

81. Zaman A, Hapke R, Sahagun G, Katon RM: Unsedated peroral endoscopy with a video ultrathin endoscope: Patient acceptance, tolerance, and diagnostic accuracy. Am J Gastroenterol 1998; 93: 1260

82. Osborn IP, Cohen J, Soper RJ et al: Laryngeal mask airway—A novel method of airway protection during ERCP: Comparison with endotracheal intubation. Gastrointest Endosc 2002; 56: 122

83. Gajraj NM: Use of the laryngeal mask airway during oesophago-gastro-duodenoscopy. Anaesthesia 1996; 51: 991

84. Wehrmann T, Kokabpick S, Lembcke B et al: Efficacy and safety of intravenous propofol sedation during routine ERCP: A prospective, controlled study. Gastrointest Endosc 1999; 49: 677

85. Martindale SJ: Anaesthetic considerations during endoscopic retrograde cholangiopancreatography. Anaesth Intens Care 2006; 35: 302

86. Thune A, Baker RA, Saccone GT et al: Differing effects of pethidine and morphine on human sphincter of Oddi motility. Br J Surg 1990; 77: 992

87. Butler KC, Selden B, Pollack CV Jr: Relief by naloxone of morphine-induced spasm of the sphincter of Oddi in a post-cholecystectomy patient. J Emerg Med 2001; 21: 129

88. Marshall JB, Patel M, Mahajan RJ et al: Benefit of intravenous antispasmodic (hyoscyamine sulfate) as premedication for colonoscopy. Gastrointest Endosc 1999; 49: 720

89. Ong JP, Sands M, Younossi ZM: Transjugular intrahepatic portosystemic shunts (TIPS): A decade later. J Clin Gastroenterol 2000; 30: 14

90. Boyer TD: Transjugular intrahepatic portosystemic shunt: Current status. Gastroenterology 2003; 124: 1700

91. Hackworth CA, Leef JA, Rosenblum JD et al: Transjugular intrahepatic portosystemic shunt creation in children: Initial clinical experience. Radiology 1998; 206: 109

92. Kelhoffer ER, Osborn IP: The gastroenterology suite and TIPS. Int Anesthesiol Clin 2003; 41: 51

93. Ding Z, White PF: Anesthesia for electroconvulsive therapy. Anesth Analg 2002; 94: 1351

94. American Psychiatric Association: The Practice of Electroconvulsive Therapy: Recommendations for Treatment, Training and Privileging. Washington, DC, American Psychiatric Press, 2000

95. Folk JW, Kellner CH, Beale MD et al: Anesthesia for electroconvulsive therapy: A review. J ECT 2000; 16: 157

96. Patel AS, Gorst-Unsworth C, Venn RM et al: Anesthesia and electroconvulsive therapy: a retrospective study comparing etomidate and propofol. J ECT 2006; 22: 179

97. Datto C, Rai AK, Ilivicky HJ et al: Augmentation of seizure induction in electroconvulsive therapy: A clinical reappraisal. J ECT 2002; 18: 118

98. Fredman B, d'Etienne J, Smith I et al: Anesthesia for electroconvulsive therapy: Effects of propofol and methohexital on seizure activity and recovery. Anesth Analg 1994; 79: 75

99. Fear CF, Littlejohns CS, Rouse E et al: Propofol anaesthesia in electroconvulsive therapy. Reduced seizure duration may not be relevant. Br J Psychiatry 1994; 165: 506

100. Smith DL, Angst MS, Brock-Utne JG et al: Seizure duration with remifentanil/methohexital vs. methohexital alone in middle-aged patients undergoing electroconvulsive therapy. Acta Anaesthesiol Scand 2003; 47: 1064

101. Nishihara F, Ohkawa M, Hiraoka H et al: Benefits of the laryngeal mask for airway management during electroconvulsive therapy. J ECT 2003; 19: 211

102. Weinger MB, Partridge BL, Hauger R et al: Prevention of the cardiovascular and neuroendocrine response to electroconvulsive therapy: I. Effectiveness of pretreatment regimens on hemodynamics. Anesth Analg 1991; 73: 556

103. Begec Z, Toprak HI, Demirbilek S et al: Dexmedetomidine blunts acute hyperdynamic responses to electroconvulsive therapy without altering seizure duration. Acta Anaesthesiol Scand 2008; 52: 302

104. Butler MG, Hayes BG, Hathaway MM et al: Specific genetic diseases at risk for sedation/anesthesia complications. Anesth Analg 2000; 91: 837

105. Bergman SA: Ketamine: Review of its pharmacology and its use in pediatric anesthesia. Anesth Prog 1999; 46: 10

106. Todd DW: A comparison of endotracheal intubation and use of the laryngeal mask airway for ambulatory oral surgery patients. J Oral Maxillofac Surg 2002; 60: 2

107. Dolling S, Anders NR, Rolfe SE: A comparison of deep vs. awake removal of the laryngeal mask airway in paediatric dental daycase surgery. A randomised controlled trial. Anaesthesia 2003; 58: 1224

108. Enever GR, Nunn JH, Sheehan JK: A comparison of post-operative morbidity following outpatient dental care under general anaesthesia in paediatric patients with and without disabilities. Int J Paediatr Dent 2000; 10: 120

ANESTHETIC MANAGEMENT

CHAPTER 35 ■ ANESTHESIA FOR THE OLDER PATIENT

G. ALEC ROOKE

KEY POINTS

1. The aging of America presents a medical and economic challenge to the entire health care system, including anesthesiologists, as older patients present for surgery in ever-increasing numbers.

2. The aging process affects connective tissue and cellular function, including the mitochondria, and inevitably leads to decreased function and, ultimately, frailty.

3. The rate at which diminished function and frailty develop is highly variable and lends credence to the concept of a measure of physiologic age.

4. Decreased organ reserve and increased sensitivity to anesthetic agents result from generalized body composition changes such as connective tissue stiffening and decreased muscle mass, plus central nervous system dysfunction including impaired swallowing, impaired autonomic reflexes, and increased sensitivity to drugs.

5. Preoperative preparation will more often involve evaluation of how best to enhance recovery of function after surgery, and discussions surrounding informed consents, living wills, and ethical treatment of the older patient.

6. Intraoperative management must take into account the increased sensitivity to drugs in the elderly patient, as well as an increased likelihood of hemodynamic, pulmonary, and thermoregulatory instability.

7. Analgesia is an important component of postoperative care, but is made more difficult by the increased likelihood of adverse consequences from the analgesic regimen.

8. Perioperative complications, most notably pulmonary, cardiac, and central nervous system complications such as delirium or cognitive decline, occur more commonly in the elderly patient because of an interaction between comorbid disease and the decreased physiological reserve of aging.

Age is not a particularly interesting subject. Anyone can get old. All you have to do is live long enough.

—*Don Marquis*

The above quote suggests that aging is dull. To many medical practitioners, it is far worse than "dull." It is overwhelming from the magnitude of care required by our ever-growing older population, frustrating from its complexity of care, and discouraging in its monetary reimbursement. Nevertheless, the impact of the aging population on the practice of medicine is far-reaching and profound, and therefore cannot be ignored. Just as children are not "little adults," the older patient is truly different from the younger adult counterpart. All caregivers, including anesthesiologists, should be knowledgeable of at least some aspects of aging in order to provide intelligent modification of their standard practice. More information is available than ever before, much of it electronically from the American Society of Anesthesiologists (www.asahq.org), the Society for the Advancement of Geriatric Anesthesia (www.sagahq.org), and the American Geriatrics Society (www.americangeriatrics.org). The politics, economics, and societal attitudes toward the elderly population must be reckoned with as well.

Lastly, caring for an older patient, although challenging, is usually fun and interesting. Anyone with a passing interest in physiology should enjoy the application of aging physiology to anesthetic management. Older patients are usually more relaxed about the prospect of surgery (often more so than their adult children!), and invariably have fascinating stories to tell about their lives. Yes, their care is often time-consuming and stressful, but more often than not it provides the anesthesia caregiver the opportunity to truly practice medicine and make a positive impact on a vulnerable patient's life.

DEMOGRAPHICS AND ECONOMICS OF AGING

1. When Social Security was initiated in 1935, only 6.1% of the U.S. population was older than 65 years.[a] By 2005 that percentage had more than doubled to 12.4%, and by 2035 it is

---

[a]www.census.gov, accessed Oct. 3, 2007

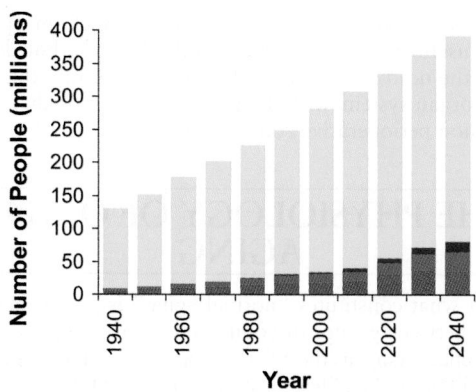

FIGURE 35-1.   The actual and estimated U.S. population from 1940 to 2040 is shown broken down by age range. Yellow bar = age <65; purple bar = age 65 to 74; green bar = age ≥75 for years 1940 to 1970, and age 75 to 84 from 1980 on; red bar = age ≥85. Data source: Statistical Abstract of the United States (www.census.gov).

ical direction is especially egregious for teaching institutions. Although Medicare will reimburse at 50% level for up to four concurrent medically directed procedures, academic programs are not permitted to staff more than two procedures simultaneously if any involve anesthesia residents. Fortunately, as of 2010, Medicare will reimburse academic institutions at 100% for two concurrent cases.

THE PROCESS OF AGING

You can't help getting older, but you don't have to get old.
—*George Burns*

❷ There are many theories of aging, and it is quite probable that each could play a role in the physiological changes with age and why death is inevitable. Some theories of programmed aging suggest that there are genetic codes that dictate how long a cell (and the organism as a whole) will live. This "killer gene" theory would have to confer an advantage to species survival for evolution to result in programmed death. Although this phenomenon does occur in nature (e.g., females of certain species of octopi), there is little evidence that such a mechanism applies to mammals. Another theory of limited cell viability is the attractive hypothesis of telomere shortening. Each time a cell divides, a telomere is cleaved off the DNA. When the DNA runs out of telomeres, the cell cannot divide and will eventually die.[4] Such limited cell division occurs in cultured mammalian cells, and although species life span correlates roughly with the number of allowable cell divisions, there is little evidence that telomere shortening affects human life span. Furthermore, aging involves more than just the death of the organism.

Mammalian aging clearly involves a gradual, cumulative process of damage and deterioration. The question could be posed: Why is such a process allowed in nature? Teleological reasoning would suggest that once offspring have been raised, there is no further need for continued survival of the individual. Protective mechanisms against aging are costly to the organism, so the "disposable soma" theory of aging states that antiaging mechanisms only need to be good enough to give the next generation the best opportunity to reproduce. In fact, most of the gains in average human life span have been as the result of reducing those factors that cause premature death: predation, accidents, and disease. The inability to thwart aging completely implies that the average human life span is limited, and that if everyone died only of "old age," the age at death would end up being a bell-shaped curve centered at a certain value, probably around age 85.[5] Nevertheless, it is possible that the bell-shaped curve could be shifting to a higher value, but how far it can be shifted is unclear.

A variety of deleterious processes continually attack DNA, proteins, and lipids (see Chapter 6). The primary culprits are free radicals and nonenzymatic glycosylation of sugars and amines. Free radicals are a by-product of oxidative metabolism, whereas glycosylation is enhanced by elevated glucose levels. Many of the changes associated with aging are the result of damage to protein. Collagen becomes stiffer from aromatic ring cleavage and by cross-linking to other collagen molecules. Elastin, once damaged and removed, is usually replaced by the stiffer collagen. In the cardiovascular system, arteries, veins, and the myocardium all stiffen with age. In contrast, lung parenchyma becomes less stiff because of loss of elastin without collagen substitution. DNA damage occurs as well and, curiously, mitochondrial DNA suffers more damage than nuclear DNA. In fact, one hypothesis of terminal aging and death is that we run out of energy as the mitochondria become less and less effective. Damage to lipids also appears to play a major role in senescence and life span.[6] Caloric restriction—well documented to increase life span in small mammals—probably does so by decreasing the rate of oxidative damage.

expected to be over 20% of the U.S. population. The percentage of people older than 85 is expected to double from 2005 (1.7%) to 2035 (estimated 3.3%). The growth of the older population is shown in Figure 35-1. The impact of these statistics is enormous with respect to medical care. The elderly account for over 44% of all inpatient days, an average per capita rate more than 5 times greater than people under age 65.[1] In 1996, there were an estimated 72 million surgical and nonsurgical procedures performed in the United States.[2] Of these, 47% were on patients older than 65 years. Although it is not clear if that percentage applies to the 47 million total surgical inpatient and outpatient procedures, of the 26.6 million inpatient surgical procedures in 2004, 33% were performed on elderly patients.[1] Even the lower percentage means that people over age 65 have surgery 3.5 times more often than people under age 65.

Federal spending for Medicare in 2005 was $286 billion.[b] This amount represents a 33% increase in total expenditure and a 29% increase per enrollee in comparison to the year 2000.[c] As impressive as that value may be, federal spending likely underestimates the total cost of all health care spending for people over age 65 to a considerable degree. It is estimated that people over age 65 account for nearly half of the nation's health care costs. For 2007, total U.S. health costs are estimated at $2.3 trillion, or approximately 16% of the gross national product.[d] In consequence, there is considerable pressure to contain health care costs in this country, including physician reimbursement, by both private insurance companies and the federal government. Unfortunately, federal reimbursement to anesthesiologists is especially poor. In 2002, Medicare reimbursed anesthesia care at approximately 39% of what commercial insurance companies paid. This percentage is in sharp contrast to all other specialties, for which Medicare reimbursement is approximately 83% of commercial rates.[3] By 2007, the conversion factor had fallen to $16.19, and now represented only 29% of private pay reimbursement.[e] Even the recent (late 2007) increase of 32%, as welcome as it is, does not restore Medicare payment to the 2002 relative level. The reduction in reimbursement for med-

[b]www.gpoaccess.gov/usbudget/fy05/pdf/budget/hhs.pdf, accessed Oct. 10, 2007

[c]www.gpoaccess.gov/usbudget/fy00/pdf/budget.pdf, accessed Oct. 10, 2007

[d]www.nchc.org/facts/cost.shtml, accessed Oct. 10, 2007

[e]www.asahq.org/news/ASACommentLetterFINAL1385P.pdf, accessed Oct. 10, 2007

ANESTHETIC MANAGEMENT

Functional Decline and the Concept of Frailty

Old age is no place for sissies.

—Bette Davis

Functional reserve represents the degree to which organ function can increase above the level necessary for basal activity. For healthy individuals, reserve peaks at approximately age 30, gradually declines over the next several decades, and then experiences more rapid decline beginning around the eighth decade. Assessment of reserve is something anesthesiologists perform all the time. For example, the ability to achieve the desired minimum of four metabolic equivalents presumably provides enough cardiovascular reserve to tolerate the stress of most surgical procedures.[7] Even without formal assessment, an intuitive sense of reserve is often obtained through simple observation. A person who looks and acts old presumably has suffered more from the aging process, regardless of chronologic age. The loss of subcutaneous tissue, unsteady or slowed gait, decreased cognition or memory, a stooped body habitus, and minimal muscle mass produce the impression of frailty. It turns out that some of these traits may well correlate with reserve. Sarcopenia is a serious problem for the very old patient, and when severe enough, can lead to an accelerated deterioration with further weight loss, mental and physical decline, and increased mortality.[8] Diminished mentation is a risk factor for postoperative delirium.[9] Oftentimes the anesthesiologist is the only caregiver prior to surgery to look at the patient as a whole. Whenever possible, we need to be aware of preoperative risk factors and probable perioperative adverse outcomes and assist the surgical team in handling identified issues.

Physiologic Age

If you didn't know how old you were, how old would you be?
—James Hubert 'Eubie' Blake

3 Although the effects of aging are inevitable and everyone will become "frail" if they live long enough, the rate at which a given individual ages is highly variable. Some age rapidly and suffer additional decrements from chronic diseases that interact with the effects of aging, whereas others remain remarkably active and vigorous late in life. Perhaps the greatest challenge facing the medical profession and society in general is not simply to keep people alive for a longer time, but to maintain function for as long as possible. Successful aging should be the goal, and it implies that physical and mental abilities remain at a level sufficient to maintain a lifestyle that is enjoyable and productive. It is the antithesis to the old adage that we have 20 years to learn, 40 years to earn, and the rest of the time to just sit around and wait. Unfortunately, how fast we age is to a great extent determined by our genetics and luck at avoiding illnesses, trauma, or environmental exposure that may contribute to functional loss. Nevertheless, successful aging can be promoted via good nutrition, regular exercise, and the avoidance of obesity.

Perhaps the most important point to be made about aging is that it is highly variable from one individual to the next. The older we get, the less likely our chronologic age reflects our physiological status and functional reserve. Ideally, an index of physiological age would be available. One interesting approach to this objective that is available to the lay public is to quantify many of the known modifiable and nonmodifiable factors that influence life expectancy.[f] By plugging one's individual data into the program, a measure of how old you are relative to your chronologic age is provided, plus tips on how you can improve

your health status and "lower" your age. Such an approach may be useful for promoting a healthy lifestyle, but does not address the need for an index that would quantify the reserve of each organ system, including the brain, and predict the risk of common perioperative complications.

THE PHYSIOLOGY OF ORGAN AGING

4 Defining what constitutes "normal aging" is problematic. Differences between groups of young and elderly subjects may not strictly reflect aging, as the elderly subjects may have experienced a much different diet, lifestyle, and environmental exposure than what the young group will experience by the time they become old. Following a group of healthy subjects over a long period is more likely to reveal the effects of aging, but not all available data come from such longitudinal studies. Studies that examine only the very old persons may actually underestimate the typical effects of aging because individuals generally do not achieve old age unless there is something intrinsically robust about them. Lastly, the reader is reminded that, as with the discussion of physiological age, the effects of aging described in this section will variably apply to any given patient, and that disease will interact with aging to further diminish functional organ reserve.

Changes in Body Composition, and Liver and Kidney Aging

Changes in body composition are primarily characterized by a gradual loss of skeletal muscle and an increase in body fat, although the latter is more prominent in women (Fig. 35-2).

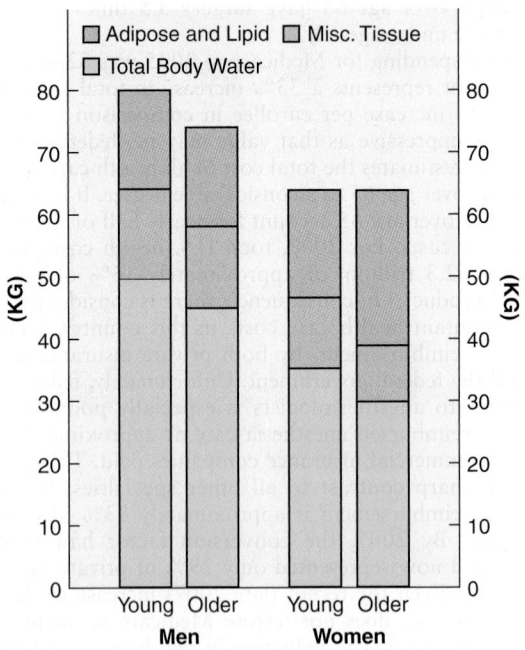

FIGURE 35-2.   Age-related changes in body composition are gender-specific. In women, total body mass remains constant because increases in body fat (*upper shaded segment*) offset bone loss (*middle segment*) and intracellular dehydration (*lower shaded segment*). In men, body mass declines despite maintenance of body lipid and skeletal tissue elements because accelerating loss of skeletal muscle and other components of lean tissue mass produces marked contraction of intracellular water (*lower shaded segment*).

---

[f]www.RealAge.com, accessed 12/15/07

Basal metabolism declines with age, with most of the decline accounted for by the change in body composition.[10] There is a reduction in total body water that reflects the reduction in cellular water that is associated with a loss of muscle and an increase in adipose tissue.[11] Aging causes a small decrease in plasma albumin levels; if anything, there is a small increase in α_1 acid glycoprotein.[12] The effect of these changes on drug protein binding and drug delivery, however, appear to be minimal.

Liver mass decreases with age, and accounts for most, but not all, of the 20 to 40% decrease in liver blood flow.[13] There is also a modest reduction in phase I drug metabolism and bile secretion with age. Even in the very old person, liver reserve should be more than adequate in the absence of disease, other than for the effect of aging on drug metabolism.

Renal cortical mass also decreases by 20 to 25% with age, but the most prominent effect of aging is the loss of up to half of the glomeruli by age 80.[14] The decrease in the glomerular filtration rate of approximately 1 mL/min/yr after age 40 typically reduces renal excretion of drugs to a level where drug dosage adjustment becomes a progressively important consideration beginning at approximately age 60. Nevertheless, the degree of decline in glomerular filtration rate is highly variable and is likely to be much less than predicted in many individuals, especially those who avoid excessive dietary protein.[15]

The aged kidney does not eliminate excess sodium or retain sodium when necessary as effectively as that of a young adult.[15] Part of the failure to conserve sodium when appropriate may be because of reduced aldosterone secretion. Similarly, the aged kidney does not retain or eliminate free water as rapidly as young kidneys when challenged by water deprivation or free water excess. Lastly, the sensation of thirst declines with age. In short, fluid and electrolyte homeostasis is more vulnerable in the older patient, particularly when an older patient suffers acute injury or disease and eating and drinking becomes more of a chore.

For the most part, functional endocrine decline does not interact with anesthetic management to any significant degree. However, aging is associated with decreased insulin secretion in response to a glucose load, and also increased insulin resistance, particularly in skeletal muscle.[16] Thus, even healthy elderly patients may require insulin therapy more often perioperatively than young adults. Aging also results in decreases in testosterone, estrogen, and growth hormone production.[17] The use of hormonal therapy to reduce sarcopenia, frailty in general, and cognitive decline and dementia is the subject of considerable current investigation, but has no current application to anesthetic management.

Central Nervous System Aging

Brain mass begins to decrease slowly beginning at approximately age 50 and declines more rapidly later, such that an 80-year-old brain has typically lost 10% of its weight.[18] Neurotransmitter functions suffer more significantly, including dopamine, serotonin, γ-aminobutyric acid, and especially the acetylcholine system.[19] The latter is especially important because of its connection to Alzheimer's disease. Response times increase, and learning is more difficult, but vocabulary, "wisdom," and past knowledge are better preserved.[18] Nevertheless, of those individuals age 85 and older, nearly half have significant cognitive impairment. In addition, some degree of atherosclerosis appears to be inevitable. Fortunately, and contrary to prior belief, the aged brain does make new neurons and is capable of forming new dendritic connections.[20]

Perhaps the best-known effect of brain aging as it applies to anesthesia is the approximately 6% decrease in MAC (minimum alveolar concentration) per decade after age 40.[21] This effect of aging is relatively simple to deal with in the clinical arena. Much more difficult is the potential interaction of anesthesia, the stress of surgery, and a brain with minimal reserve. Age is a major risk factor for postoperative delirium and/or cognitive decline (see "Perioperative Complications"). The other pertinent brain aging phenomenon is pharmacodynamic (see next section).

Drug Pharmacology and Aging

The effect of a drug in an older patient is often that of a more pronounced effect (see Chapter 7). The cause can be either pharmacodynamic, in which case the target organ (often the brain) is more sensitive to a given drug tissue level, or the cause can be pharmacokinetic, in which case a given dose of drug commonly produces higher blood levels in older patients.

Most intravenous anesthetic drugs follow a predictable pattern when administered as a bolus. If the drug was distributed only to the plasma on injection, then the initial drug concentration would be defined by the amount of drug given divided by the plasma volume. However, even as the drug is mixing into the plasma, some drug is leaving the plasma and entering tissue. The rate of transfer into a given piece of tissue depends on the rate of delivery (concentration times blood flow per gram of tissue), the concentration gradient of the drug between the blood and the tissue (obviously a high gradient initially), the ease with which the drug crosses the blood and tissue membranes, and the solubility of the drug in the tissue. Thus, the vessel-rich group (brain, heart, kidney, muscle) will acquire drug much more rapidly than the vessel-poor group (fat, bone). Protein binding may affect the rate of tissue transfer. Drugs that are highly protein-bound will have a lower free concentration and a slower rate of transfer.

Given this discussion, there are many ways for a bolus of drug to have a more pronounced initial effect on older patients. Typically, the initial blood concentration of bolus drugs is higher in older patients, partly because of a mildly contracted blood volume. Early redistribution of the drug from blood into tissue is often slower in older adults, perhaps partly because of the reduction in muscle mass. By diverting less drug into muscle and thereby keeping the drug blood concentration higher for a longer time, more drug will be driven into the other organs of the vessel-rich group such as the brain (often the target organ) or heart. A prime example of this phenomenon is sodium pentothal, and to a lesser degree, propofol.[22] If the drug is bound to albumin, the lower albumin level may increase the free drug concentration and further enhance target organ drug delivery.

Despite the typically enhanced effect of bolus drugs on older patients, there is a general impression that bolus drugs take longer to achieve that greater effect. It is not entirely clear why this is so. Slower circulation is sometimes hypothesized, but total blood flow to any organ does not appear to decrease beyond that expected from the decrease in organ mass. Another possibility is a slower rate of transfer into the target organ. The effect of a drug depends on its concentration in the target organ, not the blood level. It takes time, for example, for brain drug levels to equilibrate with blood levels. If a drug diffuses into the brain more slowly, or takes more time to alter the brain's function once in the tissue, then the peak drug effect would lag even further behind the time of peak blood concentration. The ease of transfer is often modeled as the variable k_{eo}. Blood-target organ equilibration half-life is therefore $0.693/k_{eo}$. Proof that k_{eo} decreases (and equilibration time increases) with age is limited, but has been documented for remifentanil.[23] Why k_{eo} should decrease with age is not understood.

Ultimately, though, the drug will distribute throughout the body based on tissue mass and solubility. Because most intravenous drugs used in anesthesia are highly lipid-soluble, most

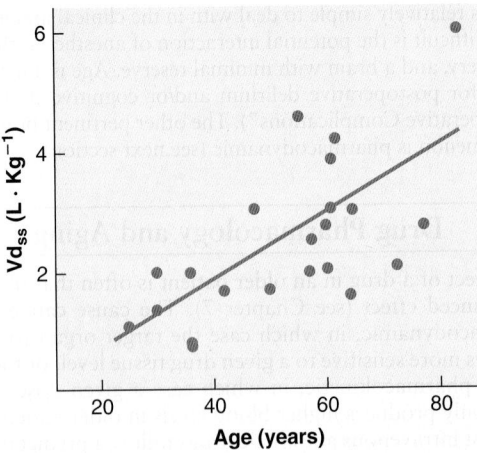

FIGURE 35-3. The effect of age on the volume of distribution at steady state (Vd$_{ss}$) for pentothal in women. (Reprinted from Jung D, Mayersohn M, Perrier D et al: Thiopental disposition as a function of age in female patients undergoing surgery. Anesthesiology 1982; 56: 263, with permission.)

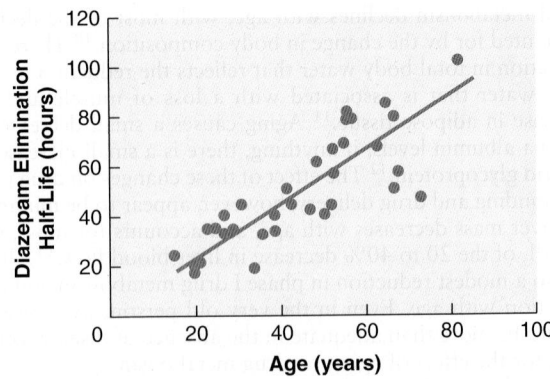

FIGURE 35-4. The effect of age on the elimination half-life of diazepam. The half-life in hours is equal to approximately the patient's age in years. (Reprinted from Klotz U, Avant GR, Hoyumpa A et al: The effects of age and liver disease on the disposition and elimination of diazepam in adult men. J Clin Invest 1975; 55: 347, with permission.)

of the drug will end up in fat. How completely the drug is dispersed out of the blood and into the tissue is reflected by Vd$_{ss}$, the drug's volume of distribution at steady state. This variable is expressed as the liters of plasma that would be necessary to dilute the amount of drug administered down to the concentration observed in the plasma. As such, drugs that are very fat-soluble can have a value for Vd$_{ss}$ that is several times greater than total body water. During the process of redistribution, drug will diffuse out of vessel-rich group tissue back into the blood, only to be soaked up by fat. In so doing, the target organ (e.g., brain) drug level will fall because the target organ is always in the vessel-rich group. Once a single therapeutic dose of a drug has fully distributed throughout the body, the blood and target organ drug levels are typically too low to have a meaningful clinical effect. However, very large doses, repeated doses, or infusions will eventually deliver enough drug to yield residual drug levels that produce therapeutic effects. At this point, the only way to decrease blood and target organ levels and eliminate the drug's effects is through metabolism. The elimination or metabolic half-life of a drug in the blood equals the volume of distribution at steady state (Vd$_{ss}$) divided by the clearance, where clearance represents the amount of blood from which drug is eliminated per minute.

Unfortunately, the most prominent pharmacokinetic effect of aging is a decrease in drug metabolism from both a decrease in clearance and an increase in Vd$_{ss}$ (Fig. 35-3). The increase in Vd$_{ss}$ with age is likely due to the increase in body fat. Clearance decreases with age for any drug metabolized by the liver or kidney. When drug metabolism is via the liver, decreased liver mass and blood flow will decrease clearance for both high and low extraction drugs. In addition, elderly patients are often on a host of chronic medications, a setup for drug interactions as well as for inhibition of drug metabolism. Drugs with primarily renal elimination will experience decreased metabolism because of reductions in glomerular filtration rate with aging. The net effect on drug metabolism is typically a doubling of the elimination half-life between old and young adults. However, with some drugs, the effect on half-life can be dramatic. In the case of diazepam, the half-life in hours is roughly equal to the patient's age (Fig. 35-4).[24] For a 72-year-old person, it would therefore require 3 days to metabolize half of a dose of diazepam. Such pharmacokinetics clearly illustrate why there is no place in modern medicine for the chronic use of diazepam and other drugs with similar half-lives

when the desired effect is supposed to be transient (e.g., as a sleeping aid).

When dealing with infusions—or for that matter a series of bolus injections—the time it takes to decrease the blood and target organ drug levels to below the therapeutic threshold will depend on many factors. This is where the concept of the context-sensitive half-time proves useful; that is, the time necessary for a 50% (or any desired percent) decrease in plasma concentration following termination of an infusion. At one extreme, if the residual level produced by the cumulative drug administration is still very low, and only a modest decrease in blood level is necessary to reverse the drug effect, then the to rapid redistribution of the most recently administered drug will lead to a rapid decrease in the blood level and termination of effect. At the other extreme, if there has been significant accumulation of drug in the body, and/or the maintenance blood level was high, then a long time may be required to decrease the drug levels enough to terminate the drug effect. As a general rule, the time to decrease the effect-site drug concentration is increased most dramatically by aging when a large percentage decrease in plasma level is necessary to dip below the therapeutic threshold.[25]

Review of the literature can yield a confusing picture when trying to sort out what pharmacologic variable is responsible for a given clinical effect. Fortunately, one does not need to know such details in order to use anesthetic drugs in an intelligent fashion with older patients. Table 35-1 summarizes some of this information for many of the common anesthetic drugs.[25–28] The effect of aging on sedative-hypnotic agents variably involves both pharmacodynamic and pharmacokinetic changes (Table 35-1). For the opioids, the older brain appears to be more sensitive than that of young adults, whereas the pharmacokinetics of opioids are largely unaffected by age.

Despite the loss of muscle and motor neurons with age, muscle relaxants do not appear to be more potent in the older patient when steady-state blood levels for a given level of paralysis are compared. Muscle relaxants often have a decreased initial volume of distribution, but this pharmacokinetic change does not seem to translate into smaller doses. For drugs eliminated by the liver or kidney, and where the effect of a bolus is eliminated primarily by redistribution, multiple doses will result in drug accumulation, and each subsequent dose will have a more prolonged effect. This phenomenon will be exaggerated in elderly patients because of decreased metabolic elimination, and will be most prominent with the long-acting

TABLE 35-1

EFFECT OF AGE ON DRUG DOSING

■ DRUG	■ BOLUS ADMINISTRATION	■ MULTIPLE BOLUSES OR INFUSION	■ COMMENTS[a]
Propofol	20–60% reduction, dose on lean body mass, 1 mg/kg in very old	50% reduction, infusions beyond 50 min progressively increase the time required to decrease the blood level by 50% (but effect-site levels may decrease faster in elderly)	↑ brain sensitivity (by some reports), decreased V_{cen}, slowed redistribution
Thiopental	20% reduction	20% reduction	= brain sensitivity, decreased V_{cen}, slowed redistribution
Etomidate	25–50% reduction	—	= brain sensitivity
Midazolam	Compared to age 20, modest reduction at age 60, 75% reduction at age 90	Similar to bolus (metabolic $t_{1/2}$ longer, but not meaningful unless very large doses are used)	↑↑ brain sensitivity
Morphine	Probably 50% reduction. Peak morphine effect is 90 min (though half of peak effect at 5 min)	Long effect-site equilibration time translates into very slow reduction in effect on termination of infusion (4 hr for 50% reduction)	Metabolite morphine-6-glucoronide build-up requires prolonged morphine use, but its renal excretion will make it very long-acting
Fentanyl	50% reduction	50% reduction	↑ brain sensitivity, minimal changes in pharmacokinetics; delayed absorption from fentanyl patch
Alfentanil, sufentanil	50% reduction	50% reduction	Probably ↑ brain sensitivity, minimal changes in pharmacokinetics
Remifentanil	50% reduction	50% reduction	Slower blood–brain equilibration, suggesting slower onset and offset, modest decreased V_{cen}
Hydromorphone	No studies on aging exist, but assume increased potency in elderly	Assume 50% reduction	Compared with morphine, no active metabolite, faster onset
Methadone	No studies on aging exist, but assume increased potency in elderly	Assume 50% reduction	
Meperidine	Use only for postoperative shivering	Do not use	Toxic metabolite normeperidine, whose renal excretion decreases with age
Vecuronium	Slower onset (≈33%)	Slower recovery times	Slightly greater liver metabolism than renal, age nearly doubles metabolic $t_{1/2}$
Mivacurium	Equally fast onset in young and old	Modest dose reduction for infusion, longer recovery time on repeated bolus	Elimination by plasma cholinesterase, modest prolongation of metabolic $t_{1/2}$ by age
Cisatracurium	Slower onset (≈33%)	No significant changes with age	Mostly Hoffmann elimination, modest prolongation of metabolic $t_{1/2}$ by age
Rocuronium	Minimally slower onset	—	Liver metabolism slightly greater than renal, modest increase in metabolic $t_{1/2}$ by age
Pancuronium	—	—	Primarily renal elimination, aging doubles metabolic $t_{1/2}$
Pipecuronium	Slower onset (≈50%), elderly may be less sensitive	—	Primarily renal elimination, no apparent change in metabolic $t_{1/2}$
Succinylcholine	Slower onset (≈40%)	—	
Edrophonium	Similar dosing and onset	—	↑ V_{cen}, primarily renal elimination, modest increase in metabolic $t_{1/2}$ by age
Neostigmine	Despite pharmacokinetic changes, some studies indicate need for increased dose with age	—	↑ V_{cen}, hepatic elimination, modest increase in metabolic $t_{1/2}$ by age

[a]V_{cen}, central volume of distribution or initial volume of distribution. Although V_{cen} does not have an anatomic correlate, a smaller V_{cen} will increase initial plasma levels and enhance transfer of the drug in the target organ (e.g., brain, muscle).

agents. Given the risk of residual neuromuscular blockade with long-acting drugs such as pancuronium, coupled with the muscle and nervous system changes of aging that increase the risk of ventilatory failure or aspiration postoperatively, it can be argued that long-acting neuromuscular blocking agents should be used very carefully in an older patient, if at all.

Cardiovascular Aging

A man is as old as his arteries.

—*Thomas Sydenham*

Virtually all components of the cardiovascular system are affected by the aging process. The major changes include (1) decreased response to β-receptor stimulation; (2) stiffening of the myocardium, arteries, and veins; (3) changes in the autonomic nervous system with increased sympathetic activity and decreased parasympathetic activity; (4) conduction system changes; and (5) defective ischemic preconditioning (see Chapter 10). Although atherosclerosis appears to affect everyone by virtue of the fact that the mechanisms of aging contribute to the development of atherosclerosis, it is not clear that it inevitably leads to functional impairment or disease.

Autonomic imbalance and dysfunction develops with age[29] (see Chapter 15). Sympathetic nervous system activity increases and vagal outflow decreases. The increased sympathetic activity is present at rest and there is often an exaggerated response to stimuli that increase sympathetic activity. Although there is some evidence of decreased responsiveness of α-receptors with age, it apparently is not enough to prevent excessive changes in vascular resistance from making a significant contribution to the lability in blood pressure observed during anesthesia or contribute to the decrease in blood pressure when anesthesia removes that sympathetic tone.[30] The decrease in vagal tone may limit the increase in heart rate after administration of atropine or glycopyrrolate.

Aging leads to a decrease in the response to β-receptor stimulation.[31] The mechanism does not appear to be a downregulation of β-receptors on the heart, but a defect in the intracellular coupling. Heart rate increases less in response to endogenous release or exogenous administration of catecholamines. The heart rate increase to exercise is therefore affected, as is maximal heart rate (often quoted as 220-age), and the decrement contributes to the decreased exertional capacity with age, even in trained individuals. Baroreflex control of heart rate is decreased and contributes to impaired regulation of blood pressure.[32] Chronic hypertension further decreases the baroreflex control of heart rate at any age.

Conductance artery (aorta to arterioles) stiffening typically leads to systolic hypertension via two mechanisms.[33] First, much of the stroke volume is stored in the thoracic aorta during ejection. Pressure must increase more to stretch out the stiffened aorta to accommodate that volume. Secondly, all arterial stiffening causes the pressure wave to transmit more rapidly in the arteries. In everyone, the wave reflects off the arterial walls and branch points, and the reflected waves travel back to the heart more quickly in an older person. In young people, the reflected waves do not reach the heart until after ejection is complete. These waves are responsible for the modest bump in pressure in the aortic root just after the dicrotic notch. But in older people, the reflected waves return to the heart in late ejection and increase the pressure against which the left ventricle must pump to complete the stroke volume. Normally at the end of ejection the ventricular contraction is weakening, so ideally the ventricle would like to push against an ever-decreasing pressure. When the ventricle must now pump against a higher pressure, this increased stress to the muscle stimulates hypertrophy.

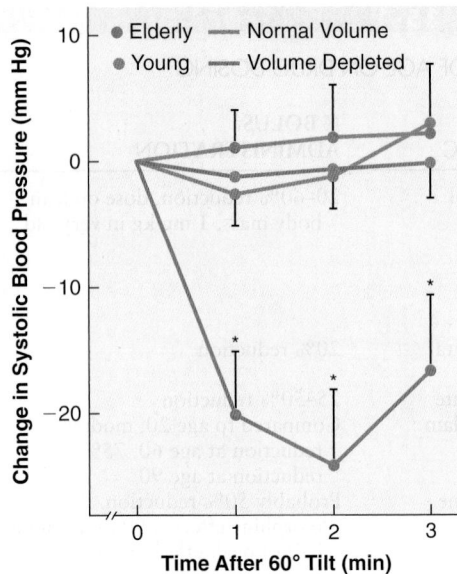

FIGURE 35-5. Young and elderly adults are subjected to a passive tilt test in their euvolemic state and after an approximate 2 kg of water and 100 mEq of sodium loss. With tilt, blood pools in the legs. Although young subjects tolerate tilt under both circumstances, the combination of hypovolemia and tilt exceeds the compensatory mechanisms of the older subjects. (Reprinted from Shannon RP, Wei JY, Rosa RM et al: The effect of age and sodium depletion on cardiovascular response to orthostasis. Hypertension 1986; 8: 438, with permission.)

Hypertrophy in and of itself stiffens the ventricle, but even worse, hypertrophy slows diastolic relaxation that, in turn, impairs ventricular filling in early diastole. The left ventricle is now more dependent on the atrial kick and left atrial pressure that control late diastolic filling. The increase in atrial pressure is present at rest, but can be quite dynamic with acute increases during stress such as tachycardia. This phenomenon, termed *diastolic dysfunction*, increases in severity with age. The majority of cases of congestive heart failure in very old persons are due to diastolic dysfunction and occur in the absence of clinically significant systolic dysfunction.[31,34]

Ventricular filling becomes more critical with age. The decreased response to β-receptor stimulation requires the ventricles to depend more on adequate end-diastolic volume to generate enough contractile strength via the length-tension (Frank-Starling) relationship. The diastolic dysfunction requires an increase in central blood volume and atrial pressure to maintain that end-diastolic volume. Therefore, maintenance of an adequate central blood volume to myocardial performance becomes more critical with age.

Unfortunately, the veins stiffen with age.[35] In everyone, the veins serve as a reservoir for blood and serve to buffer changes in blood volume in order to maintain central blood volume and ventricular filling at an appropriate level. Venous stiffening impairs this buffering capacity and creates a situation in which modest changes in venous blood volume may produce more dramatic changes in venous and cardiac filling. In short, the system has become inherently more unstable as illustrated by the development of postural hypotension in elderly persons but not in young adults with mild hypovolemia (Fig. 35-5).[36]

Rhythm disturbances may develop with age. Fibrosis of the conduction system may lead to conduction blocks, and loss of sinoatrial node cells may make the older patient more prone to sick sinus syndrome. The prevalence of atrial fibrillation exponentially climbs with age, perhaps partly because of atrial enlargement with age.

Lastly, aging appears to diminish or even eliminate any protective effect of ischemic preconditioning, a phenomenon whereby a brief period of myocardial ischemia will lessen the adverse effects of a subsequent, more prolonged ischemic event. "Warm-up angina" is the ability to achieve a higher level of exertion after first exercising to the point of angina. Starting around age 65 the increment in the level of exertion progressively diminishes with age. In younger adults, death or heart failure is a less frequent complication of a myocardial infarction if the patient had been experiencing angina within 2 weeks of the myocardial infarction. This protective effect of angina is not present in older adults.[31]

Pulmonary Aging

The most prominent effects of aging on the pulmonary system are stiffening of the chest wall and a decrease in elasticity of the lung parenchyma[37,38] (see Chapter 11). Chest wall stiffening increases the work of breathing and it also produces a more barrel-shaped thorax that leads to flattening of the diaphragm. Less diaphragmatic curvature provides a mechanical disadvantage for the generation of negative pressure in the intrapleural space. The stiffened chest wall, flattened diaphragm, and the loss of muscle mass from aging all combine to make the older patient more prone to fatigue when challenged by an increase in minute ventilation, and thus more likely to experience respiratory failure.

Although the decrease in lung tissue elasticity makes the lungs easier to inflate, there are several adverse effects of this increase in compliance. Small airways do not have enough inherent stiffness and depend on tethering by the surrounding tissue to remain open. The degree of outward pull by the tissue depends on the stiffness of the tissue and the degree of stretch of the tissue. As the tissue loses its springiness, greater lung inflation is needed to produce the same amount of outward pull on the airways. The need for greater lung inflation to prevent small airway collapse is reflected by the increase in closing capacity with age (Fig. 35-6). Closing capacity typically exceeds functional residual capacity in the mid-60s, and will eventually exceed the tidal volume at some later age. These changes, plus a modest reduction in alveolar surface area with age, contribute to a modest decline in resting PaO_2.[39]

Less-effective small airway tethering also leads to greater limitations during forced exhalation such as is present during exercise. At all ages, forced exhalation produces positive pressures in the intrapleural space that tend to compress intrathoracic airways. Only the airway connective tissue and lung tissue tethering oppose that compression. With less lung tissue tethering, airways compress at a larger lung volume in older subjects and produce a limitation in air flow during exhalation over a much larger percentage of the exhaled tidal volume (e.g., the last 45% in a 70-year-old person) than in a younger subject (e.g., 20% in a 30-year-old person).[40]

Changes within the nervous system further influence the respiratory system. Aging leads to an approximate 50% decrease in the ventilatory response to hypercapnia, and an even greater decrease in the response to hypoxia, especially at night.[41] Generalized loss of muscle tone with age applies to the hypopharyngeal and genioglossal muscles and predisposes elderly persons to upper airway obstruction. A high percentage, perhaps even 75%, of people over age 65 have sleep-disordered breathing, a phenomenon that may or may not be the same as sleep apnea, but certainly places the elderly people at increased risk of hypoxia postoperatively.[42] Aging also results in less-effective coughing and impaired swallowing. Aspiration is a significant cause of community-acquired pneumonia and may well play a role in the development of postoperative pneumonia.[43]

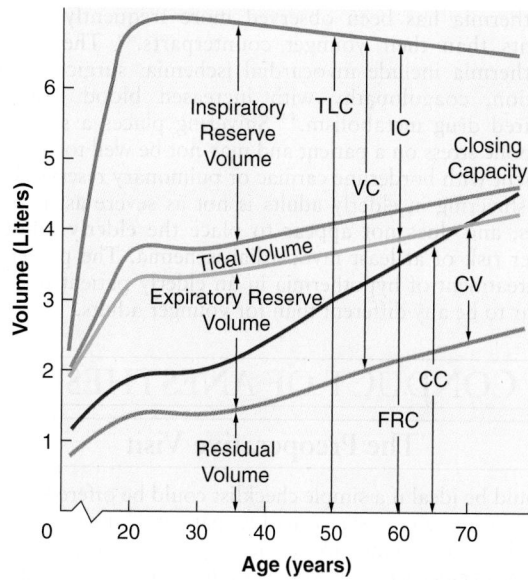

FIGURE 35-6. Effect of aging on lung volumes. With age, inspiratory capacity (IC) is compromised because of the combined effect of modest decreases in total lung capacity (TLC) and modest increase in functional residual capacity (FRC). Vital capacity (VC) decreases because of the decrease in IC and the increase in residual volume. However, the most dramatic change with aging is the increase in closing volume (CV) and closing capacity (CC) such that in very old persons, closing capacity exceeds functional residual capacity. (Reprinted from Smith TC: Respiratory system: Aging, adversity, and anesthesia, Geriatric Anesthesiology, 1st edition. Edited by McLeskey CH. Baltimore, Williams & Wilkins, 1997, p 85, with permission.)

Thermoregulation and Aging

In the past decade or so there has been heightened awareness of the adverse consequences of perioperative hypothermia as well as improved methods to prevent hypothermia. Even outside the operating room, elderly individuals are prone to hypothermia when stressed by modestly cold environments that would not affect younger individuals. The initial response to a cold environment is vasoconstriction, and if that response is insufficient and the subject becomes colder, then shivering is the second response. Both mechanisms are triggered by decreases in core and/or skin temperature. The two temperatures interact such that a decrease in skin temperature of 1 degree will initiate vasoconstriction or shivering at a core temperature approximately 0.2 degrees higher than would have otherwise occurred.[44] Aging has a variable effect on vasoconstriction and shivering, with some elderly individuals demonstrating responses identical to young individuals and other elderly individuals demonstrating a near-absent response. Overall, however, vasoconstriction and metabolic heat production are diminished in magnitude in the community dwelling elderly population.[45]

At all ages, both inhalational and some intravenous agents (e.g., propofol and alfentanil but not midazolam) alter the regulatory thresholds such that body temperature must fall by as much as 4°C (7°F) before initiation of vasoconstriction or shivering. Aging further impairs the thresholds, by approximately 1°C (2°F), not only during general anesthesia but during spinal anesthesia as well.[44]

The increased risk of intraoperative hypothermia in an elderly patient by less-effective vasoconstriction is compounded by the decreased basal metabolism (heat production) in elderly individuals. It is therefore not surprising that hypothermia has been observed more frequently in older patients than their younger counterparts.[46] The risks of hypothermia include myocardial ischemia, surgical wound infection, coagulopathy with increased blood loss, and impaired drug metabolism.[44] Shivering places a significant metabolic stress on a patient and may not be well tolerated by a patient with borderline cardiac or pulmonary reserve. However, shivering in elderly adults is not as severe as in young adults, and does not appear to place the elderly adults at greater risk of at least myocardial ischemia. The prevention and treatment of hypothermia in an elderly patient does not appear to be any different than for younger adults.

CONDUCT OF ANESTHESIA

The Preoperative Visit

It would be ideal if a simple checklist could be offered on how to administer anesthesia to an older patient. Unfortunately, the variability in response from one patient to another is more extreme in elderly than in young adults. Therefore, when managing the older patient, the art of anesthesia is an essential component of good care.

The preoperative visit can be extremely important in the care of the elderly patient. The visit should begin with a detailed understanding of the patient's medical history, current functional status of all vital organs, and medication list (see Chapter 23). Preoperative evaluation involves a search for factors that are associated with adverse outcomes, obtaining appropriate preoperative tests, and preparing the patient as much as possible in a fashion to reduce the likelihood of adverse outcomes. Studies that have examined only older patients have found preoperative risk factors that are similar to results from studies that examined the general population; for example, emergency surgery, American Society of Anesthesiologists classification of 3 or higher, low functional status, or clinical evidence of current congestive heart failure.[47] With respect to basic laboratory testing, there is growing evidence that for the general population such tests have little prognostic value and should be ordered based on the anticipated surgery or on medical issues identified at the preoperative visit. That basic laboratory testing is also not warranted for older persons has strong support from several studies, and it has been argued that the subsequent investigation of incidental abnormal test results may lead to more harm than good.[48]

5 There are some additional issues more prevalent among the elderly population that should be raised. For example, is the patient's living situation capable of providing the support necessary for a successful recovery? An aged spouse may not be physically capable of helping the patient if the surgery temporarily prevents the patient from self-management of some of the basic activities of daily living such as dressing and bathing. Furthermore, elderly patients may require a long time to return to their preoperative level of function. For example, after major abdominal surgery, most patients will need at least 3 months for activities of daily living (ADLs) and independent ADLs to return to baseline.[49] Persistent disability at 6 months will be present at an incidence that depends on the task, with only a 9% incidence of persistent ADL deficits, a 19% incidence of deficit in independent ADLs, and a 52% incidence of diminished grip strength.

Older patients often recognize that the end of their lives is no longer the theoretical consideration of youth, so they are more likely to have living wills, health care proxies, and health care directives in place at the time of surgery. The older patient's expectations from surgery may be much different than that of their younger counterparts, and the anesthesiologist must be careful not to judge a patient's decision making on the basis of more typical goals. This is particularly important

when questions of competence arise and the physician can be tempted to question competence when the patient's decision does not coincide with that of the physician.[50] A discussion of risks and benefits needs to include the probable degree of functional recovery and the speed with which that recovery is likely to occur. If health care directives prohibit various life-sustaining or resuscitative procedures, the patient/proxy and anesthesiologist must come to a mutual understanding of what will or will not be performed if an untoward event occurs.

Although beyond the scope of a single chapter on geriatric patients, there are several other issues that the practitioner should be alert to during the preoperative visit. Polypharmacy and drug interaction is a huge problem for older patients. In fact, one of the major goals of geriatric consult services to surgical patients is to pare down those medications whenever possible. The anesthesiologist can help by alerting the primary care team to this issue and suggest a consult. Dehydration, elder abuse, and malnutrition are all more common in the very old population than is generally appreciated. In the case of malnutrition, the deficit may be limited to isolated deficiencies such as vitamin D or B_{12}, or it may be more global and include inadequate caloric intake from poor oral hygiene or the "anorexia of aging," in which neuroendocrine changes lead to early satiety and diminished sense of taste.[51] Nutritional status is underappreciated as a risk factor for surgery. In fact, the Veterans Affairs National Surgical Quality Improvement Program found albumin to be as sensitive an index for mortality or morbidity as any other single indicator, including the American Society of Anesthesiologists status.[52]

Intraoperative Management

There are no magic bullets for the induction of general anesthesia in older patients. The effects of the initial dose on a single patient are highly variable, so admittedly there is a certain **6** amount of guesswork. Clearly, smaller doses are needed in comparison with young adults, and the efficacy of using less drug becomes more apparent if more time is allowed for the drug to get closer to its peak target organ (brain) effect. A given blood level of propofol causes a greater decrease in brain activity in an older patient, but the decrease in blood pressure is even more dramatic in comparison to the decrease observed in young adults.[53] Many strategies can be used to minimize the decrease in blood pressure, but most attempt to reduce the amount of propofol with the use of adjuncts such as opioids, or combining small doses of propofol with etomidate. Some advocate induction with a propofol infusion of 400 μg/kg/min to lessen the risk of overdose.[27] Etomidate has been observed to produce less hypotension than propofol in older patients.[54] Nevertheless, most any standard technique is safe if performed carefully. Hypo- or hypertension, or both, may occur during induction, intubation, and the postintubation, preincision period. Cycling the blood pressure cuff every minute should alert the practitioner to these changes sooner than would less frequent cycling. Although swings in blood pressure may not be desirable, there is no evidence that even major, but brief, changes in blood pressure lead to adverse outcomes.

Whether general or neuraxial anesthesia is used, induction and maintenance of anesthesia will commonly result in a significant decrease in systemic blood pressure, more so than typically occurs in younger patients.[55] Although decreases in both systemic vascular resistance and cardiac output likely occur, the decrease in vascular resistance is probably the largest contributor, although this observation has really been confirmed only during spinal anesthesia.[30] Figure 35-7 demonstrates this large decrease in vascular resistance and further shows that venous pooling is responsible for a decrease in preload that in turn decreases cardiac output. However, the afterload reduction from the decrease in blood pressure presumably allowed the

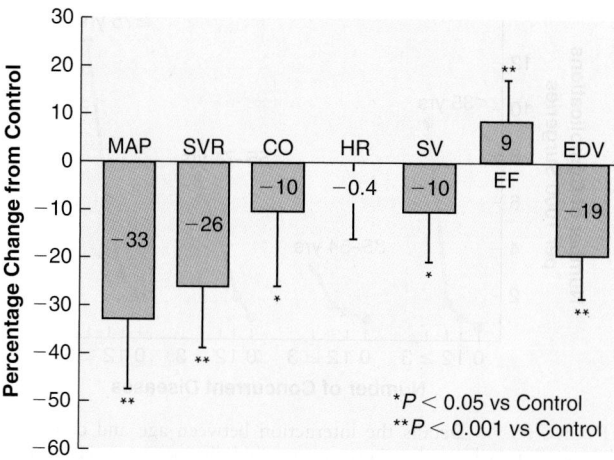

FIGURE 35-7. The response to total sympathectomy from spinal anesthesia is illustrated in older men with cardiac disease. Over 70% of the decrease in mean arterial blood pressure (MAP) was due to a decrease in systemic vascular resistance (SVR). Cardiac filling was markedly diminished, but its effect on stroke volume (SV) and cardiac output (CO) was ameliorated by an increase in ejection fraction (EF). Although heart rate (HR) increased in some subjects and decreased in others, the overall effect was no change. EDV, end-diastolic volume. (Reprinted from Rooke GA, Freund PR, Jacobson AF: Hemodynamic response and change in organ blood volume during spinal anesthesia in elderly men with cardiac disease. Anesth Analg 1997; 85: 99, with permission.)

ejection fraction to increase, thereby ameliorating the effect the decrease in end-diastolic volume had on stroke volume. Because vascular resistance contributes significantly to the decrease in blood pressure during anesthesia, it has been argued that the use of α-agonists is an appropriate therapy and may be more effective than volume alone.[31] α-Agonists also tend to promote venoconstriction, thereby shifting blood back to the central circulation and reducing the decrease in ventricular preload by venous pooling, and presumably reducing the need for at least some volume administration. Although no one would advocate vasoconstriction as a treatment for hypovolemia (except as a stopgap measure), the ventricle can only get so big; therefore, it is impossible for volume administration alone to raise cardiac output enough to compensate for a large decrease in vascular resistance. Furthermore, when sympathetic nervous system activity returns postoperatively, blood will shift from the periphery to the central circulation. Excess peripheral volume now becomes excess central volume and could push an elderly heart into diastolic heart failure. In short, volume administration to an older patient may be problematic, with a very fine line between too much and too little, and what was "just right" at one point may become "too much" later on.

The choice between an endotracheal tube versus a laryngeal mask airway involves many considerations, including body habitus, apparent frailty, surgical positioning, and duration of surgery (see Chapter 29). An endotracheal tube will likely have more adverse effects on mucociliary clearance and possibly on swallowing than a laryngeal mask, but an endotracheal tube will guarantee the ability to provide either a large tidal volume or positive end-expiratory pressure, the two maneuvers most likely to prevent intraoperative atelectasis.

Postoperative Care

The goals of emergence and the immediate postoperative period are no different for an elderly than for a young patient, they are just more difficult to achieve. Analgesia is a major goal, and it should be stated up front that there is no evidence that pain is any less severe or any less detrimental in an older patient than in young patients (see Chapter 57). Less drug may be required (or not), but given that the standard approach to analgesia is to titrate to the desired effect, the outcome should be good pain relief for patients of all ages. There are impediments to achieving adequate analgesia in an older patient, however.[56] Elderly patients sometimes underreport their pain level and may be more tolerant of their acute pain, perhaps partly because of the existence of chronic pain in their life. Older patients have more difficulty with visual analog scoring systems than verbal or numeric systems. If the patient is cognitively impaired, communication of pain is further impaired; indeed, demented patients often experience severe pain after hip surgery, but even mild cognitive impairment can lead to problems with pain assessment or with use of a patient-controlled analgesia machine.

Failure to achieve adequate levels of analgesia is associated with numerous adverse outcomes, including sleep deprivation, respiratory impairment, ileus, suboptimal mobilization, insulin resistance, tachycardia, and hypertension. The consequences include longer hospitalization and increased incidence of delirium.[56,57] The apparent paradox of adequate analgesia is that opioids are the mainstay of postoperative analgesia, and opioids are capable of producing many of those same adverse outcomes, including respiratory depression, sedation, ileus, and delirium, and those outcomes may be more frequent in the older patient. Therefore, as with all medical care of elderly patients, good judgment, caution, and frequent monitoring of analgesia and adverse effects are essential. A few studies have examined the choice of opioid in older patients, with the most prominent conclusion being to avoid the use of meperidine because of its association with delirium.[57,58] In fact, the only appropriate role of meperidine in elderly patients is the small dose used to treat postoperative shivering. Adjunctive medications such as nonsteroidal anti-inflammatory drugs have been shown to reduce opioid requirements and some of the opioid adverse effects, but often carry their own risks such as renal damage or gastrointestinal toxicity.[56] Epidural analgesia is well known to provide analgesia that is superior to intravenous therapy, a finding that has been specifically replicated in the elderly.[59,60] Although improved cardiopulmonary outcomes were equivocal, more rapid return of bowel function, earlier mobilization, and nutritional status were better with epidural analgesia.

Although most other aspects of postoperative care are generally more the purview of the surgeon or the internist, there are some things that the anesthesiologist could and probably should be watchful for when performing a postoperative visit on an older patient. If a patient had a surgery with major fluid requirements, it is important to look for signs of fluid overload, including rales, dyspnea, tachypnea, and orthopnea. A timely administration of a diuretic may prevent the patient from more florid pulmonary edema and the accompanying escalation of therapy and risk. Ask if the patient has experienced any chest pain. Vital signs can be reviewed with a particular eye to tachycardia. Feel the pulse: atrial fibrillation is often intermittent and the more often someone looks for it, the more likely it will be detected. Delirium often goes undetected in older patients, in part because the older patient is less likely to exhibit agitation than a young delirious patient. Take the time to chat with the patient for a few minutes. It should not be difficult to become suspicious if the patient demonstrates waxing and waning alertness, is inattentive or distractible, displays rambled or incoherent speech, is disoriented, or has perceptual disturbances. It has been demonstrated that overall recovery and avoidance of complications, including delirium, pneumonia, uncontrolled pain, infection, and length of stay, can be enhanced by comprehensive evaluation and management of each patient's risk factors.[61,62] Anesthesiologists should be prepared to support such programs as much as possible.

ANESTHETIC MANAGEMENT

PERIOPERATIVE COMPLICATIONS

My diseases are an asthma and a dropsy and, what is less curable, seventy-five.

—*Samuel Johnson*

8 The older patient is at increased risk for complications in the perioperative period. Part of that risk is certainly related to those comorbid diseases that are contributed to by the aging process. The other component of risk is typically thought of as the reduction in organ system reserve directly due to the aging process. Whether the aging process can be thought of as mere decreased reserve or subclinical disease is a matter of semantics. The result is the same: the elderly are at increased risk for almost every possible perioperative complication including cardiovascular, pulmonary, renal, central nervous system, wound infection, and death (Fig. 35-8).[63,64]

Because the mechanisms of aging contribute not only to normal aging but to the development and severity of disease, one might expect that age and disease would interact in their contribution to perioperative risk. Confirmation of such a hypothesis is provided by a prospective survey of nearly 200,000 anesthetics in France.[65] Both age and the number of chronic diseases were associated with an increased rate of complications, but what is particularly interesting is an apparent interaction of these two factors. Figure 35-9 demonstrates that, for any given age group, the number of complications increases with the number of comorbid diseases. Note that the ≤34-year-old group is somewhat of an outlier if that risk increases especially dramatically three or more comorbid diseases are present. It could be surmised that to be that sick at such a young age represents a special degree of risk. Connecting the dots of equal number of comorbid disease reveals a modest increase in risk with age for patients with zero comorbid disease, but examination of points of one, two, or three or more diseases reveals an effect of age that becomes increasingly larger. In other words, age appears to interact with comorbid disease to increase risk.

Complications of the cardiovascular and pulmonary systems are associated with the greatest perioperative mortality. The best database is provided by the Veterans Affairs National Surgical Quality Improvement Project, and much of the database involves examination of patients older than 80 (Table 35-2).[64] Although the perioperative complications of myocardial infarction or cardiac arrest carry higher associated mortality rates than pneumonia, prolonged intubation, or reintubation, the higher incidences of the pulmonary com-

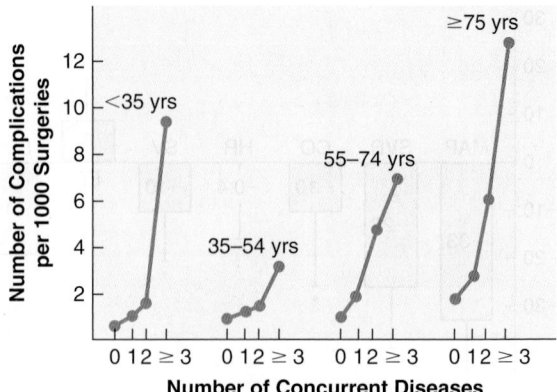

FIGURE 35-9. Details the interaction between age and comorbid disease. For each age bracket, as comorbid disease increases, so does the rate of complications. The effect of age on the complication rate is best visualized by examining points of equal comorbid disease. At zero disease, only a modest increase in complications is observed with increasing age. At ever-increasing degrees of comorbid disease, however, the increase in complications with age becomes more and more pronounced. (Reprinted from Tiret L, Desmonts JM, Hatton F et al: Complications associated with anaesthesia: A prospective survey in France. Can Anesth Soc J 1986; 33: 336, with permission.)

plications suggest that greater mortality results from pulmonary complications than cardiac complications. That pulmonary complications are so significant underscores the need for a better understanding of the mechanism of postoperative pneumonia, particularly the likely contribution of silent aspiration.[66]

Although anesthesiologists frequently focus on cardiovascular and pulmonary complications, central nervous system complications are also a major source of morbidity and mortality. The incidence of stroke in the general surgical population is approximately 0.5% (Table 35-2).[64,67,68] Age is a risk factor, as is atrial fibrillation, and a history of a prior stroke increases the risk of perioperative stroke by as much as 10-fold. Strokes typically occur well after surgery, on average 7 days later. In addition to coma or stroke, postoperative cognitive decline and postoperative delirium are receiving increased attention as significant sources of debilitating morbidity. Although these two entities may yet prove to be related to each other, at present they appear to be distinct clinical syndromes.

Postoperative delirium is an acute confusional state manifested by an acute onset (hours to days) and vacillating levels of attention and cognitive skill.[9,69] Disorientation, perceptual disturbances (from misinterpretation of the situation to hallucinations), disorganized thinking, and problems with memory may be manifested. Emergence delirium does not qualify as postoperative delirium. In fact, patients who go on to experience postoperative delirium have a defined period of normality after initial recovery from anesthesia. Several methods of diagnosis have been popularized, with the Confusion Assessment Method used most often, at least in research studies.[70] The risk of postoperative delirium after major surgery in older patients is somewhere on the order of 10%; however, the risk varies with the surgical procedure. Highest risk is hip surgery, with an approximate incidence of 35%. The cause of delirium is multifactorial. Patient risk factors include patient age, baseline low cognitive function (including dementia), depression, and possibly general debility including dehydration or visual/auditory impairment.[9,69] Virtually any drug with central nervous system effects has been implicated, including narcotics (especially meperidine), benzodiazepines (especially lorazepam), and drugs that possess anticholinergic properties (except

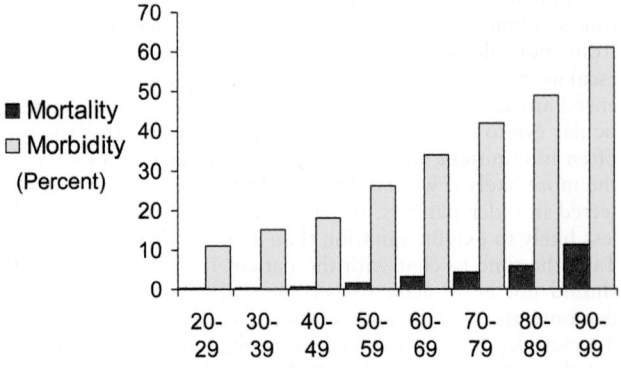

FIGURE 35-8. Shows the relationship between age and mortality and morbidity among a Veterans Affairs population. (Modified from Turrentine FE, Wang H, Simpson VB et al: Surgical risk factors, morbidity, and mortality in elderly patients. J Am Coll Surg 2006; 203: 865, with permission.)

TABLE 35-2

EFFECT OF AGE ON SELECTED PERIOPERATIVE COMPLICATIONS AND ASSOCIATED MORTALITY[a]

■ COMPLICATION	■ COMPLICATION RATE		■ MORTALITY RATE FROM THE COMPLICATION	
	Age <80	Age ≥80	Age <80	Age ≥80
Myocardial infarction	0.4	1.0	37.1	48.0
Cardiac arrest	0.9	2.1	80.0	88.2
Pneumonia	2.3	5.6	19.8	29.2
>48 hours on ventilator	2.1	3.5	30.1	38.5
Required reintubation	1.6	2.8	32.3	44.0
Cerebrovascular accident	0.3	0.7	26.1	39.3
Coma >24 hours	0.2	0.3	65.9	80.9
Prolonged ileus	1.2	1.7	9.2	16.0

[a]All differences between patients less than 80 versus 80 and older are significant at $p < 0.001$, except for coma mortality ($p = .004$).
Modified from Hamel MB, Henderson WG, Khuri SF et al: Surgical outcomes for patients aged 80 and older: morbidity and mortality from major noncardiac surgery. J Am Geriat Soc 2005; 53: 424, with permission.

glycopyrrolate). Other factors that likely contribute to delirium include sleep deprivation, being in an unfamiliar environment, postoperative pain, and perioperative blood loss. Choice of regional versus general anesthesia does not appear to be a factor, especially if sedation is used in conjunction with the regional technique. Once detected, management focuses on reversible risk factors such as current medications, pain management, and a better sleep environment. Haloperidol in doses no greater than 1.5 mg can be helpful, especially for agitated delirium, and when applied prophylactically, may reduce the severity and duration but not the incidence of delirium.[71] Special care programs designed to limit the reversible risk factors appear to reduce the incidence of delirium by 50%.[62] Prevention is not just an academic exercise. Delirium is associated with an increased duration of hospitalization and its attendant costs, poorer long-term functional recovery, and increased mortality.

Postoperative cognitive dysfunction is characterized by a long-term decrease in mental abilities after surgery. It is inherently more difficult to diagnose than delirium because it usually requires sophisticated neuropsychological testing, including baseline tests prior to surgery. Selection of tests, their timing, and what deficits are required to qualify for cognitive decline have proven problematic in the literature. Nevertheless, some basic observations can be made.[72] In comparison to nonsurgical control subjects, the cognitive decline lessens over time with perhaps a 10% incidence at 3 months in comparison with a 25% incidence at 1 week.[73] At 6 months and beyond there may be a prevalence of 1% of subjects with decline, but there is little evidence of decline in comparison with control subjects. Anesthetic management does not appear to affect cognitive decline when comparisons are made between general versus regional anesthesia, controlled hypotension versus normotension, or intravenous versus inhalation anesthesia.[72] Patient risk factors include age, lower levels of education, and prior history of stroke even without residual deficit.[74] Increased mortality at 1 year is associated with patients who demonstrate cognitive decline at both hospital discharge and at 3 months postoperatively. Interestingly, postoperative delirium was not found to be a risk factor for cognitive dysfunction at 3 months. Cognitive decline is a complication that is still in its infancy with respect to an understanding of the underlying mechanism(s) and the implications for patient quality of life.

THE FUTURE

I will never be an old man. To me, old age is always 15 years older than I am.

—*Francis Bacon*

Improvements in surgical and anesthetic techniques that reduce the overall stress to the patient are permitting more surgeries to be performed on older and sicker patients than ever before. Nevertheless, the older patient will continue to experience the majority of the adverse outcomes from surgery and anesthesia. Much remains to be accomplished in the quest to find ways to decrease the incidence and severity of those adverse outcomes.[66] The most pressing issues are arguably the prevention of postoperative delirium, cognitive decline, pneumonia, and respiratory failure. Improved pain-control techniques that also diminish side effects, especially to the brain and bowels, would be welcome. However, other realms of care are just in their infancy, most notably whether the functional status of frail patients can be improved prior to surgery. For example, can short courses of better nutrition, exercise regimens, or even medications reduce complications or speed recovery and improve functional recovery? When caring for the elderly, especially the frail elderly, the overriding goal should be to produce as little stress to the patient as possible during both surgery and the subsequent hospitalization and recovery. Complete care will often be multidisciplinary. No single specialty possesses the total perspective, and the anesthesiologist's expertise is an important component of that care.

References

1. National Center for Health Statistics: National hospital discharge survey: 2005 annual summary with detailed diagnosis and procedure data. Atlanta, GA, Centers for Disease Control and Prevention, 2006, Series 13, No. 162
2. National Center for Health Statistics: Ambulatory and inpatient procedures in the United States, 1996. Vital and Health Statistics. Atlanta, GA, Centers for Disease Control and Prevention, 1988, Series 13, No. 139
3. Bierstein K: Medicare is still the wrong benchmark. ASA Newslett 2002; 66: 25
4. Ahmed A, Tollefsbol T: Telomeres and telomerase: basic science implications for aging J Am Geriatr Soc 2001; 49: 1105
5. Fries JF: Aging, natural selection, and the compression of morbidity. N Engl J Med 1980; 303: 130

6. Hulbert AJ, Pamplona R, Buffenstein R et al: Life and death: metabolic rate, membrane composition, and life span of animals. Physiol Rev 2007; 87: 1175

7. Fleisher LA, Beckman JA, Brown KA et al: AHA/ACC 2007 guidelines on perioperative cardiovascular evaluation and care for noncardiac surgery. J Am Coll Cardiol 2007; 50: 1707

8. VanItallie TB: Frailty in the elderly: contributions of sarcopenia and visceral protein depletion. Metabolism 2003; 52(Suppl 2): 22

9. Dasgupta M, Dumbrell AC: Preoperative risk assessment for delirium after noncardiac surgery: A systematic review. J Am Geriatr Soc 2006; 54: 1578

10. Fukagawa NK, Bandini LG, Young JB: Effect of age on body composition and resting metabolic rate. Am J Physiol 1990; 259: E233

11. Doherty T: Invited review: aging and sarcopenia. J Appl Physiol 2003; 95: 1717

12. Grandison MK, Boudinot FD: Age-related changes in protein binding of drugs: implications for therapy. Clin Pharmacokinet 2000; 38: 271

13. Schmucker DL: Age-related changes in liver structure and function: implications for disease? Exper Gerontol 2005; 40: 650

14. Muhlberg W, Platt D: Age-dependent changes of the kidneys: pharmacologic implications. Gerontology 1999; 45: 243

15. Epstein M: Aging and the kidney. J Am Soc Nephrol 1996; 7: 1106

16. Scheen AJ: Diabetes mellitus in the elderly: insulin resistance and/or impaired insulin secretion? Diabetes Metab 2005; 31: 5S27

17. Paganelli R, Di Iorio A, Cherubini A et al: Frailty of older age: the role of the endocrine-immune interaction. Curr Pharm Des 2006; 12: 3147

18. Drachman DA: Aging of the brain, entropy, and Alzheimer disease. Neurology 2006; 67: 1340

19. Mrak RE, Griffin ST, Graham DI: Aging associated changes in human brain. J Neuropathol Exp Neurol 1997; 56: 1269

20. Shors TJ, Miesegaes G, Beylin A et al: Neurogenesis in the adult is involved in the formation of trace memories. Nature 2001; 410: 372

21. Mapleson WW: Effect of age on MAC in humans: A meta-analysis. Br J Anaesth 1996; 76: 179

22. Jung D, Mayersohn M, Perrier D et al: Thiopental disposition as a function of age in female patients undergoing surgery. Anesthesiology 1982; 56: 263

23. Minto CF, Schnider T, Egan T et al: Influence of age and gender on the pharmacokinetics and pharmacodynamics of remifentanil: I. Model development. Anesthesiology 1997; 86: 10

24. Klotz U, Avant GR, Hoyumpa A et al: The effects of age and liver disease on the disposition and elimination of diazepam in adult man. J Clin Invest 1975; 55: 347

25. Shafer SL: Pharmacokinetics and pharmacodynamics of the elderly, Geriatric Anesthesiology, 1st edition. Edited by McLeskey CH. Baltimore, Williams & Wilkins, 1997, p 123

26. Shafer SL, Flood P: The pharmacology of opioids, Geriatric Anesthesiology, 2nd edition. Edited by Silverstein JH, Rooke GA, Reves JG et al. New York, Springer, 2008, p 209

27. McEvoy MD, Reves JG: Intravenous hypnotic anesthetics, Geriatric Anesthesiology, 2nd edition. Edited by Silverstein JH, Rooke GA, Reves JG et al. New York, Springer, 2008, p 229

28. Lien CA, Suzuki T: Relaxants and their reversal agents, Geriatric Anesthesiology, 2nd edition. Edited by Silverstein JH, Rooke GA, Reves JG et al. New York, Springer, 2008, p 266

29. Folkow B, Svanborg A: Physiology of cardiovascular aging. Physiol Rev 1993; 73: 725

30. Rooke GA, Freund PR, Jacobson AF: Hemodynamic response and change in organ blood volume during spinal anesthesia in elderly men with cardiac disease. Anesth Analg 1997; 85: 99

31. Rooke GA: Cardiovascular aging and anesthetic implications. J Cardiothor Vasc Anesth 2003; 17: 512

32. Ebert TJ, Morgan BJ, Barney JA et al: Effects of aging on baroreflex regulation of sympathetic activity in humans. Am J Physiol 1992; 263: H798

33. Nichols WW, O'Rourke MF, Avolio AP et al: Effects of age on ventricular-vascular coupling. Am J Cardiol 1985; 55: 1179

34. Lakatta EG: Cardiovascular aging in health. Clin Geriatr Med 2000; 16: 419

35. Bouissou H, Julian M, Pieraggi M-Th et al: Structure of healthy and varicose veins, Return Circulation and Norepinephrine: An Update. Edited by Vanhoutte PM. Paris, John Libbey Eurotext, 1991, p 139

36. Shannon RP, Wei JY, Rosa RM et al: The effect of age and sodium depletion on cardiovascular response to orthostasis. Hypertension 1986; 8: 438

37. Crapo RO: The aging lung, Pulmonary Disease in the Elderly Patient. Edited by Mahler DA. New York, Marcel Dekker, 1993, p 1

38. Wahba WM: Influence of aging on lung function—clinical significance of changes from age twenty. Anesth Analg 1983; 62: 764

39. Zaugg M, Lucchinetti E: Respiratory function in the elderly. Anesthesiol Clin North Am 2000; 18: 47

40. DeLorey DS, Babb TG: Progressive mechanical ventilatory constraints with aging. Am J Respir Crit Care Med 1999; 160: 169

41. Kronenberg RS, Drage CW: Attenuation of the ventilatory and heart rate responses to hypoxia and hypercapnia with aging in normal men. J Clin Invest 1973; 52: 1812

42. Ancoli-Israel S, Coy T: Are breathing disturbances in elderly equivalent to sleep apnea syndrome? Sleep 1994; 17: 77

43. Marik PE, Kaplan D: Aspiration pneumonia and dysphagia in the elderly. Chest 2003; 124: 328

44. Sessler DI: Perioperative thermoregulation, Geriatric Anesthesiology, 2nd edition. Edited by Silverstein JH, Rooke GA, Reves JG et al. New York, Springer, 2008, p 107

45. Kenney, WL, Munce TA: Invited review: Aging and human temperature regulation. J Appl Physiol 2003; 95: 2598

46. Vaughan MS, Vaughan RW, Cork RC: Postoperative hypothermia in adults: relationship of age, anesthesia, and shivering to rewarming. Anesth Analg 1981; 60: 746

47. Leung JM, Dzankic S: Relative importance of preoperative health status versus intraoperative factors in predicting postoperative adverse outcomes in geriatric surgical patients. J Am Geriat Soc 2001; 49: 1080

48. Dzankic S, Pastor D, Gonzalez C et al: The prevalence and predictive value of abnormal preoperative laboratory tests in elderly surgical patients. Anesth Analg 2001; 93: 301

49. Lawrence VA, Hazuda HP, Cornell JP et al: Functional independence after major abdominal surgery in the elderly. J Am Coll Surg 2004; 199: 762

50. Rosenthal RA, Kavic SM: Assessment and management of the geriatric patient. Crit Care Med 2004; 32(Suppl): S92

51. Rosenthal RA: Nutritional concerns in the older surgical patient. J Am Coll Surg 2004; 199: 785

52. Gibbs J, Cull W, Henderson W et al: Preoperative serum albumin level as a predictor of operative mortality and morbidity. Arch Surg 1999; 134: 36

53. Kazama T, Ikeda K, Morita K et al: Comparison of the effect-site k_{eo}s of propofol for blood pressure and EEG bispectral index in elderly and younger patients. Anesthesiology 1999; 90: 1517

54. Reich DL, Hossain S, Krol M et al: Predictors of hypotension after induction of general anesthesia. Anesth Analg 2005; 101: 622

55. Forrest JB, Rehder K, Cahalan MK et al: Multicenter study of general anesthesia. III. Predictors of severe perioperative adverse outcomes. Anesthesiology 1992; 76: 3

56. Aubrun F: Management of postoperative analgesia in elderly patients. Reg Anesth Pain Med 2005; 30: 363

57. Morrison RS, Magaziner J, Gilbert M et al: Relationship between pain and opioid analgesics on the development of delirium following hip fracture. J Gerontol A Biol Sci Med Sci 2003; 58: 76

58. Fong HK, Sands LP, Leung JM: The role of postoperative analgesia in delirium and cognitive decline in elderly patients: a systematic review. Anesth Analg 2006; 102: 1255

59. Mann C, Pouzeratte Y, Bocarra G et al: Comparison of intravenous or epidural patient-controlled analgesia in the elderly after major abdominal surgery. Anesthesiology 2000; 92: 433

60. Carli F, Phil M, Mayo N et al: Epidural analgesia enhances functional exercise capacity and health related quality of life after colonic surgery. Results of a randomized trial. Anesthesiology 2002; 97: 540

61. Harari D, Hopper A, Dhesi J et al: Proactive care of older people undergoing surgery ('POPS'): designing, embedding, evaluating and funding a comprehensive geriatric assessment service for older elective surgical patients. Age Ageing 2007; 36: 190

62. Marcantonio ER, Flacker JM, Wright RJ et al: Reducing delirium after hip fracture: a randomized trial. J Am Geriatr Soc 2001; 49: 516

63. Turrentine FE, Wang H, Simpson VB et al: Surgical risk factors, morbidity, and mortality in elderly patients. J Am Coll Surg 2006; 203: 865

64. Hamel MB, Henderson WG, Khuri SF et al: Surgical outcomes for patients aged 80 and older: morbidity and mortality from major noncardiac surgery. J Am Geriat Soc 2005; 53: 424

65. Tiret L, Desmonts JM, Hatton F et al: Complications associated with anaesthesia—a prospective survey in France. Can Anesth Soc J 1986; 33: 336

66. Cook DJ, Rooke GA: Priorities in perioperative geriatrics. Anesth Analg 2003; 96: 1823

67. Kam PCA, Calcroft RM: Perioperative stroke in general surgical patients. Anaesthesia 1997; 52: 879

68. Selim M: Perioperative stroke. N Engl J Med 2007; 356: 706

69. Silverstein JH, Timberger BA, Reich DL et al: Central nervous system dysfunction after noncardiac surgery and anesthesia in the elderly. Anesthesiology 2007; 106: 622

70. Inouye SK, van Dyck CH, Alessi CA et al: Clarifying confusion: the confusion assessment method. Ann Intern Med 1990; 113: 941

71. Kalisvaart KJ, de Jonghe JF, Bogaards MJ et al: Haloperidol prophylaxis for elderly hip-surgery patients at risk for delirium: a randomized placebo-controlled study. J Am Geriatr Soc. 2005; 53: 1658

72. Newman S, Stygall J, Hirani S et al: Postoperative cognitive dysfunction after noncardiac surgery. Anesthesiology 2007; 106: 572

73. Moller JT, Cluitmans P, Rasmussen LS et al: Long-term postoperative cognitive dysfunction in the elderly: ISPOCD1 study. Lancet 1998; 351: 857

74. Monk TG, Weldon BC, Garvan CW et al: Predictors of cognitive dysfunction after major noncardiac surgery. Anesthesiology 2008; 108: 18

CHAPTER 36 ■ ANESTHESIA FOR TRAUMA AND BURN PATIENTS

LEVON M. CAPAN AND SANFORD M. MILLER

INITIAL EVALUATION AND RESUSCITATION
  Airway Evaluation and Intervention
  Management of Breathing Abnormalities
  Management of Shock
EARLY MANAGEMENT OF SPECIFIC INJURIES
  Head Injury
  Spine and Spinal Cord Injury
  Neck Injury
  Chest Injury
  Abdominal and Pelvic Injuries

Extremity Injuries
Burns
OPERATIVE MANAGEMENT
  Monitoring
  Anesthetic and Adjunct Drugs
  Management of Intraoperative Complications
EARLY POSTOPERATIVE CONSIDERATIONS
  Acute Renal Failure
  Abdominal Compartment Syndrome
  Thromboembolism

KEY POINTS

1 Initial evaluation of the trauma patient involves rapid overview, primary survey, and secondary survey.

2 Airway management is tailored to the type of injury, the nature and degree of airway compromise, and the patient's hemodynamic and oxygenation status.

3 Fast computed tomography technology with the capability of sagittal image reconstruction is replacing conventional multiple-view plain radiographic evaluation of cervical spine injury. Further, magnetic resonance imaging is replacing flexion/extension plain radiographic evaluation of the relatively infrequent ligamentous injuries of the cervical spine.

4 Morbidity and mortality of flail chest are primarily related to underlying pulmonary contusion that develops over a period of a few hours after injury. A too liberal indication for tracheal intubation of patients in this condition may be associated with increased morbidity and mortality.

5 "Lethal triad" or "bloody vicious circle" refers to the development of acidosis, hypothermia, and coagulopathy that, if untreated, may lead to death.

6 Approximately 10% of patients with hemorrhagic shock may have severe coagulopathy at the time of admission and the early operative phase, requiring hemostatic resuscitation with plasma, platelets, and coagulation factors.

7 Head injury and hemorrhagic shock are the most common causes of traumatic death.

8 The most important therapeutic maneuvers in head-injured patients are normalization of intracranial pressure, cerebral perfusion pressure, and oxygen delivery.

9 Brain ischemia is the most threatening consequence of head injury. By causing cerebral vasoconstriction, hyperventilation further aggravates ischemia.

10 Penetrating neck injuries usually present with obvious clinical manifestations, whereas blunt cervical trauma may be more subtle.

11 The term *blunt cardiac injury* has replaced *myocardial contusion* and encompasses varying degrees of myocardial damage, coronary artery injury, and rupture of the cardiac free wall, the septum, or a valve.

12 Extraperitoneal or preperitoneal pelvic packing may be helpful in diminishing the rate of severe pelvic fracture bleeding. Angiography and embolization may follow pelvic packing if there is arterial bleeding from a pelvic fracture.

13 Deep anesthesia and high airway pressures should be avoided before evacuation of the hemopericardium.

14 Hypermetabolism caused by major burn injuries can be reduced by early decompressive escharotomies and skin grafting. Other measures to decrease metabolism and catabolism include low-dose insulin infusion, beta-blockade, and anabolic oxandrolone.

15 Persistent hypotension following trauma is usually the result of one of four mechanisms: bleeding, tension pneumothorax, neurogenic shock, and cardiac injury.

16 Death is a much greater threat during emergency trauma surgery than it is in any other operative procedure.

According to data from the National Safety Council,[1] intentional and unintentional injuries killed 167,000 Americans in 2004. Intentional injuries (suicide, homicide, and assault) claimed 55,000 lives and unintentional mortality (e.g., motor vehicle, falls, drowning, and poisoning) accounted for 112,000 deaths, making trauma the third leading cause of death after heart disease and cancer. Unintentional injuries were the fifth, suicides the eleventh, and assault the fifteenth leading causes of death overall. For the age range between 15 and 31, accidents, suicide, and homicide were the three leading causes of death. Morbidity caused by injuries is far in excess of mortality; in 2005, a total of 27,156,734 emergency department visits were related to unintentional injuries. In 2006, the estimated cost of unintentional injuries alone was $652 billion, including the costs of fatal and nonfatal injuries, employer costs, vehicle damage, and fire losses. The additional cost of lost quality of life is estimated as $3,080 billion, bringing the total annual cost of trauma to $3,732 billion.[1]

Approximately 75% of the hospital mortality from trauma occurs within 48 hours after admission,[2] most commonly

FIGURE 36-1. Clinical sequence for initial management of the major trauma patient. CT, computed tomography; ER, emergency room; ICU, intensive care unit.

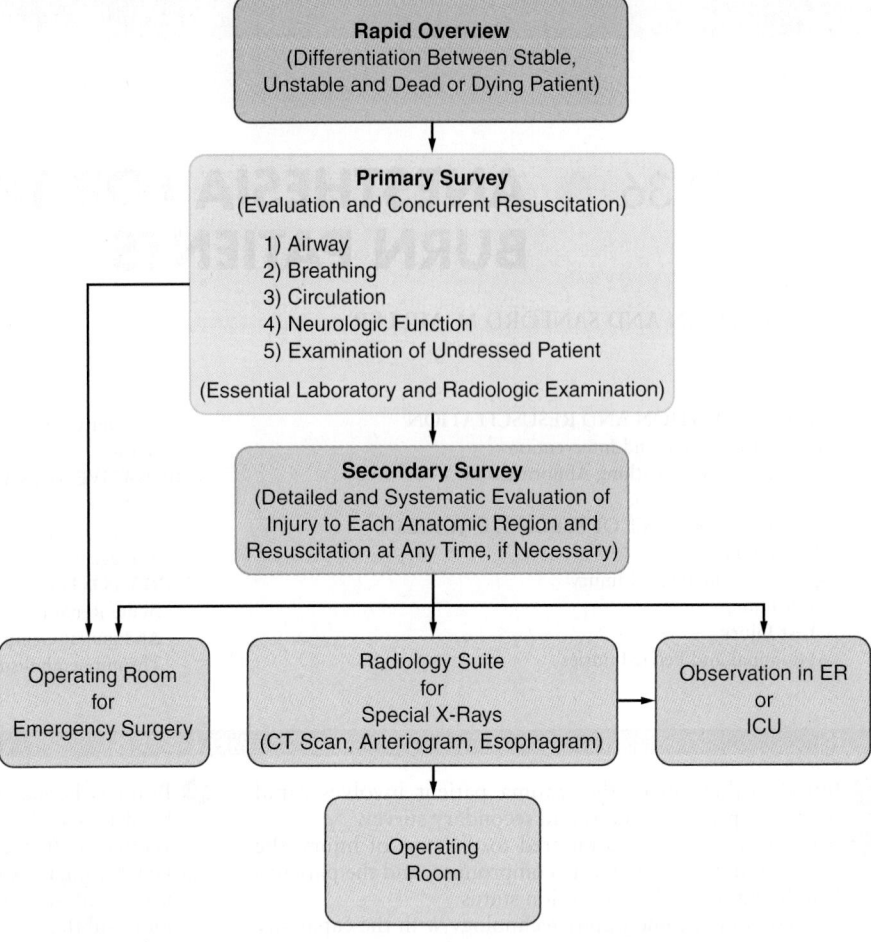

The *secondary survey* involves a more elaborate systematic examination of the entire body to identify additional injuries. Radiographic and other diagnostic procedures may also be performed if the stability of the patient permits. Within this general framework the anesthesiologist, aside from managing the airway, contributes as part of the team to evaluation and resuscitation, while gathering information needed for possible future anesthetic management.

Injuries may be missed during initial evaluation and even during emergency surgery, resulting in significant pain, complications, residual disability, delay of treatment, or death.[3] Reported missed diagnoses include cervical spine, thoracoabdominal, pelvic, nerve, and external soft-tissue injuries, and extremity fractures. Some of these injuries may present during anesthesia, such as spinal cord damage in a patient with unrecognized cervical spine injury, massive intraoperative bleeding from an unrecognized thoracoabdominal injury during extremity surgery, or sudden intraoperative hypoxemia in a patient with unrecognized pneumothorax. A *tertiary survey* within the first 24 hours after admission (which may include a period of anesthesia) can potentially diagnose the majority of clinically significant injuries missed during initial evaluation[3] by repeating the primary and secondary examinations and reviewing the results of radiologic and laboratory testing.

from central nervous system (CNS), thoracic, abdominal, retroperitoneal, or vascular injuries[2]; CNS injury and hemorrhage are the most common causes of early trauma mortality. Nearly one third of these trauma patients die within the first 4 hours after admission, representing the majority of operating room (OR) trauma deaths. Of the hospital deaths, 5 to 10% occur between the third and seventh day of admission, usually from CNS injuries,[2] and the remainder in subsequent weeks, most commonly as a result of multiorgan failure.[2] Pulmonary thromboembolism and infectious complications may also contribute to mortality during this phase.[2]

INITIAL EVALUATION AND RESUSCITATION

The strategy of initial management can be defined as a continuous, priority-driven process of patient assessment, resuscitation, and reassessment. The general approach to evaluation of the acute trauma patient has three sequential components: rapid overview, primary survey, and secondary survey (Fig. 36-1). Resuscitation is initiated, if needed, at any time during this continuum. *Rapid overview* takes only a few seconds and is used to determine whether the patient is stable, unstable, dying, or dead. The *primary survey* involves rapid evaluation of functions that are crucial to survival. The "ABCs" of airway patency, breathing, and circulation are assessed. Then a brief neurologic examination is performed and the patient is examined for any external injuries that might have been overlooked.

Airway Evaluation and Intervention

Airway evaluation involves the diagnosis of any trauma to the airway or surrounding tissues, recognition and anticipation of the respiratory consequences of these injuries, and prediction of the potential for exacerbation of these or other injuries by any contemplated airway management maneuvers (see Chapter 29). Although nontraumatic causes of airway difficulty, such as pre-existing factors, may be present, only the management of trauma-related problems is discussed in this section. Generally, the American Society of Anesthesiologists difficult airway algorithm can be applied with certain modifications to various trauma airway management scenarios. For instance, cancellation of airway management when difficulty arises may not be an option. Likewise, awake rather than asleep intubation or a surgical airway from the outset may be the preferred technique in some situations. The American Society of Anesthesiologists difficult airway algorithm as modified for various trauma conditions is available.[4]

Airway Obstruction

Airway obstruction is probably the most frequent cause of asphyxia and may result from posteriorly displaced or lacerated pharyngeal soft tissues, hematoma, bleeding, secretions, foreign bodies, or displaced bone or cartilage fragments. Bleeding into the cervical region may produce airway obstruction not only because of compression by the hematoma, but also from venous congestion and upper airway edema as a result of compression of neck veins. Signs of upper and lower airway obstruction include dyspnea, cyanosis, hoarseness, stridor, dysphonia, subcutaneous emphysema, and hemoptysis. Cervical deformity, edema, crepitation, tracheal tug and/or deviation, or jugular venous distention may be present before these symptoms appear and may help indicate that specialized techniques are required to secure the airway.

The initial steps in airway management are chin lift, jaw thrust, clearing of the oropharyngeal cavity, placement of an oropharyngeal or nasopharyngeal airway, and in inadequately breathing patients, ventilation with a self-inflating bag. Immobilization of the cervical spine and administration of oxygen should be applied simultaneously. Blind passage of a nasopharyngeal airway or a nasogastric or nasotracheal tube should be avoided if a basilar skull fracture is suspected; it may enter the anterior cranial fossa. A cuffed oropharyngeal airway or a laryngeal mask airway (LMA) may permit ventilation with a self-inflating bag, although neither provides protection against aspiration of gastric contents. They may be used as temporary measures, and if they do not provide adequate ventilation, the trachea must be intubated immediately using either direct laryngoscopy or a cricothyroidotomy, depending on the results of airway assessment.

Maxillofacial, neck, and chest injuries, as well as cervicofacial burns, are the most common trauma-related causes of difficult tracheal intubation. Airway assessment should include a rapid examination of the anterior neck for feasibility of access to the cricothyroid membrane. Tracheostomy is not desirable during initial management because it takes longer to perform than a cricothyroidotomy and requires neck extension, which may cause or exacerbate cord trauma in patients with cervical spine injuries. Conversion to a tracheostomy should be considered later to prevent laryngeal damage if a cricothyroidotomy will be in place for more than 2 to 3 days. Possible contraindications to cricothyroidotomy include age younger than 12 years and suspected laryngeal trauma; permanent laryngeal damage may result in the former, and uncorrectable airway obstruction may occur in the latter situation.

Full Stomach

A full stomach is a background condition in acute trauma; the urgency of securing the airway often does not permit adequate time for pharmacologic measures to reduce gastric volume and acidity. Thus, rather than relying on these agents, the emphasis should be placed on selection of a safe technique for securing the airway when necessary: rapid-sequence induction with cricoid pressure for those patients without serious airway problems, and awake intubation with sedation and topical anesthesia, if possible, for those with anticipated serious airway difficulties.

The probability of a full stomach precludes the use of an LMA or any other device that does not protect the trachea, as a definitive airway in trauma patients. However, these devices can serve as a bridge for a brief period to reestablish airway patency or to facilitate intubation aided by a flexible fiberoptic bronchoscope (FOB). In patients with maxillofacial injuries, aspiration of pharyngeal blood or secretions is more likely than aspiration of gastric contents. If it can be inserted in these circumstances, an LMA may protect the lungs. Although positive-pressure ventilation may be used with the LMA, patients with pulmonary contusion, edema, or aspiration may be difficult to ventilate with this device. An intubating laryngeal mask or similar laryngeal airways may permit rapid blind or FOB-guided tracheal intubation while allowing temporary ventilation. An important disadvantage of the intubating laryngeal mask is that its metal part may exert considerable pressure against the cervical vertebrae, potentially exacerbating an unstable injury in this region. In agitated and uncooperative patients, topical anesthesia of the airway may be impossible, whereas administration of sedative agents may result in apnea or airway obstruction, with an increased risk of aspiration of gastric contents and inadequate conditions for tracheal intubation. After locating the cricothyroid membrane and denitrogenating the lungs, a rapid-sequence induction may be used to permit securing the airway with direct laryngoscopy or, if necessary, with immediate cricothyroidotomy. Personnel and material necessary to perform translaryngeal ventilation or cricothyroidotomy must be in place before induction of general anesthesia.

Head, Open Eye, and Contained Major Vessel Injuries

The principles of tracheal intubation are similar for these injuries. Apart from the need to ensure adequate oxygenation and ventilation, patients with these injuries require deep anesthesia and profound muscle relaxation before airway manipulation. This helps prevent hypertension, coughing, and bucking, and thereby minimizes intracranial, intraocular, or intravascular pressure elevation, which can result in herniation of the brain, extrusion of eye contents, or dislodgment of a hemostatic clot from an injured vessel, respectively (see Chapter 51). The preferred anesthetic sequence to achieve this goal includes preoxygenation and opioid loading, followed by relatively large doses of an intravenous anesthetic and muscle relaxant. Hemodynamic responses to the opioid should be carefully monitored and promptly corrected. Systemic hypotension, intracranial pressure (ICP) elevation, and decreased cerebral perfusion pressure (CPP = mean arterial pressure – ICP) may occur whether cerebral autoregulation is present or absent in patients with head injuries, and if untreated can produce secondary ischemic insults.[5] Ketamine is usually contraindicated in patients with head and vascular injuries because it may increase both intracranial and systemic vascular pressures; however, no significant increase in intraocular pressure (IOP) has been documented. Any muscle relaxant, including succinylcholine, may be used as long as the fasciculation produced by this agent is inhibited by prior administration of an adequate dose of a nondepolarizing muscle relaxant. Alternatively, rocuronium can provide intubating conditions within 60 seconds with a dose of 1.6 to 2.0 mg/kg, although the neuromuscular blockade produced by this dose lasts approximately 2 hours.[6] Intravenous lidocaine has an attenuating effect on the pressor response to airway instrumentation, but it is mild and unpredictable. Of course, neither muscle relaxants nor intravenous anesthetics are indicated when initial assessment suggests a difficult airway. As in any other trauma patient, hypotension dictates either reduced or no intravenous anesthetic administration.

Cervical Spine Injury

Overall, 2 to 4% of blunt trauma patients have cervical spine injuries.[7] The most common causes include high-speed motor vehicle accidents, falls, diving accidents, and gunshot wounds. Head injuries, especially those with low Glasgow Coma Scores (GCS) and focal neurologic deficits, are likely to be associated with cervical spine injuries. Approximately 2 to 10% of head trauma patients have cervical spine injuries, while 25 to 50% of patients with cervical spine injuries have an associated head injury.[7] The incidence of assault-related injuries depends on the mechanism, being highest after gunshot wounds (1.35%), lowest after stab wounds (0.12%), and intermediate after blunt trauma (0.4%) to the cervicothoracic region. In conscious patients, neck pain, tenderness, and extremity paresthesias are strong indicators of spine injury. Accurate and timely evaluation is important because approximately 2 to 10% of blunt trauma-induced cervical spine injury patients develop new or worsening neurologic deficits after admission, attributable partly to delayed diagnosis and improper cervical spine protection and/or manipulation.[7] Often there is no time to evaluate the injury when emergency airway management is needed during the initial phase of management.

Immobilization of the neck in neutral position is indicated before airway management in all acute trauma patients suspected to have cervical spine injury based on mechanism and clinical presentation. Intubation may theoretically cause spinal cord damage during manipulation of the neck, although the available literature attests to the rare, possibly nonexistent, occurrence of this event.[7,8] Nevertheless, it is a priori necessary to protect the neck during airway maneuvers in any patient with a possibly unstable cervical spine.[7,8]

Initial Evaluation.   A patient who arrives in the hospital with a rigid collar and other neck-stabilizing devices that are routinely placed by the emergency medical service, but who is not in need of emergency airway management, should be evaluated for cervical spine injury. Clearance of the neck should be performed at the earliest possible time, not necessarily to facilitate airway management, but to minimize the risk of pressure ulceration by the collar.

The procedures for cervical spine clearance vary according to the patient's condition. In the conscious patient with a suspected injury, diagnosis is relatively easy. The American National Emergency X-Radiography Utilization Study (NEXUS) suggests that if, by careful clinical examination, the patient meets all of the following criteria, the injury may be ruled out: (1) no midline cervical tenderness, (2) no focal neurologic deficit, (3) normally alert, (4) not intoxicated, and (5) no distracting painful injury.[11] Of these criteria, distracting injury is the most difficult to evaluate. Spinal pain is not always localized to the level of injury, and not all distant painful injuries mask cervical pain. For example, upper torso injuries may be more painful and more likely to distract from reliable cervical spine examination than lower torso injuries.[9] The Canadian C-Spine Rule for Radiography after Trauma is another tool designed to determine low-risk patients.[10,11] Proper answers to the following three questions eliminate the possibility of injury and the need for radiographic studies: (1) Is there any high-risk factor mandating radiography? (2) Are there low-risk factors that permit safe evaluation of the range of motion of the neck? (3) Can the patient rotate the neck laterally for 45 degrees in each direction without pain? Comparison of these two sets of criteria showed that the Canadian

Rule is more reliable than NEXUS in diagnosing cervical spine injury in responsive patients.[11]

In awake patients with suggestive findings by the NEXUS or Canadian criteria, and those who are in coma or obtunded, the diagnosis of cervical spine injury necessitates the use of radiographic studies in addition to the clinical examination. The Eastern Association for the Surgery of Trauma (EAST) guidelines recommend a standard three-view (anteroposterior, lateral, and open mouth) series and examination of suspect or suboptimally visualized areas with limited, focused computed tomography (CT) scans.[12] With the development of fast, sophisticated CT scanners, it is clear that the diagnostic capability of the plain films recommended by the EAST guidelines is inferior to helical CT scans with sagittal and coronal reconstruction.[13–15] CT scans performed in this fashion provide reliable information about fractures and are able to differentiate fractures that can cause vertebral instability from those that are not likely to cause spinal cord damage. Stable fractures of the spine are spinous process fractures; isolated osteophyte, trabecular, transverse process, and avulsion fractures without ligament injury; and wedge compression fractures with loss of ≤25% of vertebral body height.[7] The advantages of CT examination include less reliance on plain films, which are frequently inadequate and difficult to obtain in uncooperative patients, almost 100% sensitivity in detecting an injury, the ability to scan other anatomic locations in the same session, and possibly reduced cost. Currently the EAST guidelines are still being updated; they will probably recommend CT scanning as a primary diagnostic measure. The ability of a CT scan to diagnose ligamentous injury is less than that to detect fractures.[16] The standard measure for diagnosing ligamentous injury is a flexion/extension series. This approach is cumbersome, not cost-effective, and perhaps hazardous. In addition, it is inadequate when, as in many acute trauma patients, the range of motion of the neck is limited. Magnetic resonance imaging (MRI) can be used instead for this purpose.[19–21] Although useful, MRI tends to overread the injury beyond the clinically significant range.[21] It is also impossible to perform in patients with multiple trauma patients who have metallic skeletal fixators. Fortunately, clinically significant ligamentous injuries are relatively rare, and thus the need for MRI is infrequent.

Two groups of trauma patients with normal CT results are difficult to evaluate: conscious patients with neck pain and obtunded or comatose patients. Obviously, the usual approach to diagnose ligamentous injury in these patients is evaluation by flexion/extension series or by MRI. It has been demonstrated that diagnosis may not require these additional studies, as long as conscious patients are neurologically intact, obtunded or comatose patients are able to move all of their extremities on admission, and the CT scan is performed with 3-mm cuts and sagittal reconstruction of the entire cervical spine.[22,23] Although this approach limits the need for MRI only to those who have neurologic deficits, it also emphasizes the importance of observing and documenting motor function before administration of anesthetic or muscle relaxant agents for airway management. Familiarity with these diagnostic strategies may help the anesthesiologist assess patients cleared for cervical spine injury before airway management.

Airway Management.   Almost all airway maneuvers including jaw thrust, chin lift, head tilt, and oral airway placement result in some degree of cervical spine movement[7] (see Chapter 29). Stabilization of the head, neck, and torso in neutral position for airway management in patients whose cervical spine is yet to be cleared is best accomplished by manual in-line immobilization. A hard cervical collar alone, which is routinely placed, does not provide absolute protection, especially for rotational movements of the neck. Manual in-line immobilization is best accomplished by having two operators in addition to the physician who is actually managing the airway. The first operator stabilizes and aligns the head in neutral position without applying cephalad traction, and the second operator stabilizes both shoulders by holding them against the table or stretcher. The anterior portion of the hard collar, which limits mouth opening, may be removed after immobilization.

An excellent review of airway management after cervical spine injury is provided by Crosby[7]; the reader is referred to it for more detailed information. Although controversy exists about the choice of technique in these patients, the selection should generally be based on the timing of airway management in relation to the injury and the familiarity of the operator with the specific technique. FOB-guided intubation produces the least distraction of the cervical spine, but in the acute phase of trauma factors such as full stomach, lack of patient cooperation, and time constraints may influence the operator to select conventional direct laryngoscopy, preferably after induction of anesthesia, in patients without anticipated airway difficulties. In-line stabilization, however, decreases the visibility of the larynx in a significant proportion of patients. The incidence of inadequate exposure of the larynx increases from <3% in the general population to approximately 10% with immobilization of the neck.[24] Furthermore, airway management may be difficult in some patients because of enlargement of the prevertebral space by a hematoma from vertebral fracture. Lateral neck films may help diagnose a retropharyngeal hematoma, which may cause tracheal deviation and complicate airway management. Using an alternate technique including cricothyroidotomy should be considered, if necessary, rather than causing excessive manipulation of the neck. Cricoid pressure should be applied with great care in the patient with a possible cervical spine injury as it may produce undue motion of the spine if excessive force is used.

Other devices and techniques, including the McCoy laryngoscope (Penlon America, Minnetonka, MN), rigid fiberoptic laryngoscopes (Bullard, ACMI Gyrus, Southborough, MA; GlideScope, Verethon, Bothell, WA; or WuScope, Achi Corporaton, San Jose, CA), flexible fiberoptic endoscope, light wand, translaryngeal (retrograde) intubation, and cricothyroidotomy, can be used to secure the airway in the acute phase in patients requiring cervical spine immobilization. The McCoy laryngoscope is able to lift the epiglottis and may improve the laryngeal view: the cuff of a Fogarty catheter attached to the tip of this device may further improve exposure. A gum elastic bougie passed through the endotracheal tube, or a satin-sheathed stylet placed through its Murphy aperture, may also be helpful; they can be inserted through the larynx more easily than the tube itself because their small diameter does not block the view of the glottis during direct laryngoscopy. The WuScope provides a consistently good laryngeal view with a high rate of successful intubation and minimal neck movement.[25] Flexible fiberoptic laryngoscopy and translaryngeal-guided intubation (see "Maxillofacial Injuries") cause almost no neck movement, but blood or secretions in the airway, a long preparation time, and difficulty in their use in comatose, uncooperative, or anesthetized patients reduce their utility during initial management.

Nasotracheal intubation carries the risks of epistaxis, failure of intubation, and the possibility of entry of the endotracheal tube into the cranial vault or the orbit if there is damage to the cranial base or the maxillofacial complex. Absence of the usual signs of cranial base fracture (Battle sign, raccoon eyes, or bleeding from the ear or the nose) cannot be relied on to exclude the possibility of its occurrence because these signs may not be immediately apparent with rapid prehospital transport.

In the subacute phase of cervical spine injury when time constraints, full stomach, and patient cooperation issues do not exist, the use of FOB in the awake, sedated patient with appropriate topical anesthesia is preferred. Advantages of this technique are minimal movement of the neck, positioning of the patient awake, maintenance of protective reflexes, and the ability to assess the neurologic status after intubation.

Direct Airway Injuries

Direct airway damage can occur anywhere between the nasopharynx and the bronchi; sometimes more than one site may be involved, resulting in persistent airway dysfunction after one of the problems is corrected.[26]

Maxillofacial Injuries.   In addition to soft-tissue edema of the pharynx and peripharyngeal hematoma, blood or debris in the oropharynx may be responsible for partial or complete airway obstruction in the acute stage of these injuries. Occasionally, teeth or foreign bodies in the pharynx may be aspirated into the airway, causing some degree of obstruction, which may occur or be recognized only during attempts at tracheal intubation. Another problem is the dynamic nature of soft-tissue injuries in this region. A hematoma or edema in the face, tongue, or neck may expand during the first several hours after injury and ultimately occlude the airway. Serious airway compromise may develop within a few hours in up to 50% of patients with major penetrating facial injuries or multiple trauma as a result of progressive inflammation or edema resulting from liberal administration of fluids. The face, head, and neck are vulnerable to missile and explosion injuries.[27] Although rare, massive hemorrhage, most frequently from the internal maxillary artery or its branches, may be life threatening, requiring angioembolization.[28] Prophylactic intubation of the trachea may avert airway compromise in these circumstances.

Fracture-induced encroachment on the airway or limitation of mandibular movement, pain, and trismus may limit mouth opening. Fentanyl in titrated doses of up to 2 to 4 μg/kg over a period of 10 to 20 minutes may produce an improvement in the patient's ability to open the mouth if mechanical limitation is not present.

The selection of an airway management technique in the presence of a maxillofacial fracture is based on the patient's presenting condition. Most patients with isolated facial injuries do not require emergency tracheal intubation. Surgery may be delayed for as long as a week with no adverse effect on the repair. Patients who present with airway compromise may be intubated using direct laryngoscopy; the decision about the use of anesthetics and muscle relaxants is based on the results of airway evaluation. When there is bleeding into the oropharynx, a flexible fiberoptic laryngoscope may be useless because of obstruction of the view. A retrograde technique, using a wire or epidural catheter passed through a 14-gauge catheter introduced into the trachea through the cricothyroid membrane, may be used if the patient can open his or her mouth. A surgical airway is indicated when there is airway compromise, when direct laryngoscopy has failed or is considered impossible, when the jaws will be wired, or when a tracheostomy will be performed anyway after definitive repair of the fracture. Nasogastric or nasotracheal intubation should be avoided when a basilar skull or maxillary fracture is suspected because of the possibility that the tube may enter the cranium or the orbital fossa. Hemorrhagic shock and life-threatening cranial, laryngotracheal, thoracic, and cervical spine injuries may accompany major facial fractures[9,29]; airway management must be tailored accordingly. The likelihood of cranial injury increases in midface fractures involving the frontal sinus, as well as the orbitozygomatic and orbitoethmoid complexes.

Cervical Airway Injuries.   Injury to the cervical air passages can result from blunt or penetrating trauma. The incidence of blunt and penetrating laryngotracheal injuries admitted to major trauma centers is 0.34% and 4%, respectively.[9] Similarly to maxillofacial injuries, wartime laryngotracheal injuries are more severe and occur more frequently (5 to 6%) than peacetime injuries (0.91%).[30] Although the pharynx and esophagus are close to the cervical air passages, their involvement in peacetime

ANESTHETIC MANAGEMENT

trauma is less likely than airway injuries (0.08% after blunt trauma and 0.9% after penetrating trauma).[9] Clinical signs such as escape of air, hemoptysis, and coughing are present in almost all patients with penetrating injuries, facilitating the diagnosis. In contrast, major blunt laryngotracheal damage may be missed, either because the patient is asymptomatic or unresponsive, or because suggestive signs and symptoms are missed in the initial evaluation.[26] The typical presentation includes hoarseness, muffled voice, dyspnea, stridor, dysphagia, odynophagia, cervical pain and tenderness, ecchymosis, subcutaneous emphysema, and flattening of the thyroid cartilage protuberance (Adam's apple). Whether the trauma is blunt or penetrating, attempts at blind tracheal intubation may produce further trauma to the larynx and complete airway obstruction if the endotracheal tube enters a false passage or disrupts the continuity of an already tenuous airway.[31] Thus, whenever possible, intubation of the trachea should be performed using an FOB, or the airway should be secured surgically. A CT scan of the neck provides valuable information and should be performed before any airway intervention in all stable patients with neck injury and without respiratory and hemodynamic compromise.

The strategy for tracheal intubation depends on the clinical presentation.[31] The tracheas of some patients with penetrating airway injuries, especially stab wounds, may be intubated through the airway defect without the need for anesthetics or optical equipment. The presence of cartilaginous fractures or mucosal abnormalities necessitates awake intubation with a FOB or awake tracheostomy. Laryngeal damage precludes cricothyroidotomy. Tracheostomy should be performed with extreme caution because up to 70% of patients with blunt laryngeal injuries may have an associated cervical spine injury.[31] Uncooperative or confused patients may not tolerate awake airway manipulation. It may be best to transport these patients to the OR, induce anesthesia with inhalational agents, and intubate the trachea without muscle relaxants.[31] Episodes of airway obstruction during spontaneous breathing under an inhalational anesthetic can be managed by positioning the patient upright in addition to the usual maneuvers. Complete transaction of the trachea is rare, but when it occurs it is life-threatening; the distal segment of the trachea retracts into the chest, causing airway obstruction either spontaneously or during airway manipulation. Surgery involves pulling up the distal end and performing an end-to-end anastomosis to the proximal segment or suturing it to the skin as a permanent tracheostomy. In extreme situations, such as complete or near-complete transection of the larynx and trachea, femoro-femoral bypass or percutaneous cardiopulmonary support may be considered if time permits.[32]

Thoracic Airway Injuries. Whereas penetrating trauma can cause damage to any segment of the intrathoracic airway, blunt injury usually involves the posterior membranous portion of the trachea and the mainstem bronchi, usually within approximately 3 cm of the carina. A significant number of these injuries result from iatrogenic causes such as tracheal intubation.[33] Pneumothorax, pneumomediastinum, pneumopericardium, subcutaneous emphysema, and a continuous air leak from the chest tube are the usual signs of this injury; they occur frequently but are not specific for thoracic airway damage. In patients intubated without the suspicion of a tracheal injury, difficulty in obtaining a seal around the endotracheal tube or the presence on a chest radiograph of a large radiolucent area in the trachea corresponding to the cuff suggests a perforated airway. Other radiographic findings include a radiolucent line along the prevertebral fascia due to air tracking up from the mediastinum, peribronchial air or sudden obstruction along an air-filled bronchus, and the "dropped lung" sign when complete intrapleural bronchial transection causes the apex of the collapsed lung to descend to the level of the hilum. Airway

management is similar to that of cervical airway injury. Anesthetics, and especially muscle relaxants, may produce irreversible obstruction, presumably because of relaxation of structures that maintain the airway patent in the awake patient; however, airway loss may also occur during attempts at awake intubation, often as a result of further distortion of the airway by the endotracheal tube, patient agitation, or rebleeding into the airway.[34] After intubation of the trachea, the adequacy of airway intervention is evaluated mainly by auscultation and capnography. Pulmonary contusion, atelectasis, diaphragmatic rupture with thoracic migration of the abdominal contents, and pneumothorax may complicate the interpretation of chest auscultation. Likewise, CO_2 elimination may be decreased or absent in shock and cardiac arrest.

The outcome after surgical repair of these injuries is often suboptimal and complicated by stump leak and empyema, suture line stenosis, or the need for tracheostomy or pneumonectomy. The recent trend is selective conservative management. Patients with lesions larger than 4 cm, cartilaginous rather than membranous injuries, concomitant esophageal trauma, progressive subcutaneous emphysema, severe dyspnea requiring intubation and ventilation, difficulty with mechanical ventilation, pneumothorax with an air leak through the chest drains, and/or mediastinitis are still managed surgically. Those without these problems may be treated nonoperatively with a reasonable outcome.[33]

Management of Breathing Abnormalities

Of the several causes that may alter respiration after trauma, tension pneumothorax, flail chest, and open pneumothorax are immediate threats to the patient's life and therefore require rapid diagnosis and treatment. Hemothorax, closed pneumothorax, pulmonary contusion, diaphragmatic rupture with herniation of abdominal contents into the thorax, and atelectasis from a mucous plug, aspiration, or chest wall splinting can also interfere with breathing and pulmonary gas exchange and deteriorate into life-threatening complications.

Although cyanosis, tachypnea, hypotension, neck vein distention, tracheal deviation, and diminished breath sounds on the affected side are the classic signs of tension pneumothorax, neck vein distention may be absent in hypovolemic patients and tracheal deviation may be difficult to appreciate. The definitive diagnosis is established by chest radiograph; however, in hypoxemic and hypotensive patients, immediate insertion of a 14-gauge angiocatheter through the fourth intercostal space in the midaxillary line or, at times, through the second intercostal space at the midclavicular line is essential. There is no time for radiologic confirmation in this setting.

A flail chest results from fractures of more than two sites of at least three adjacent ribs or rib fractures with associated costochondral separation or sternal fracture. An underlying pulmonary contusion with increased elastic recoil of the lung and work of breathing is the main cause of respiratory insufficiency or failure and resulting hypoxemia.[35] It often develops over a 3- to 6-hour period, causing gradual deterioration of the chest radiograph and arterial blood gases.[35] Coexisting hemopneumothorax, paradoxical chest wall movement, and/or pain-induced splinting may contribute to the gas exchange abnormalities. Repeated evaluation by physical examination, chest radiograph, and arterial blood gas determinations is essential for early recognition of these complications. The fraction of lung volume contused, as determined by chest radiograph or CT scan, may be predictive of the subsequent development of acute respiratory distress syndrome (ARDS); the likelihood increases abruptly once the contusion volume exceeds 20% of total lung volume[36] (see Chapter 56). Without significant gas exchange abnormalities, chest wall instability alone is not an indication for respiratory support. There is evidence that liberal use of tracheal intubation and mechanical ventilation in the presence of a flail chest or pulmonary contusion increases the rate of pulmonary complications and mortality, and prolongs the hospital stay.[35] Effective pain relief by itself can improve respiratory function and often avoid the need for mechanical ventilation. For this purpose, continuous epidural analgesia with local anesthetics and opioids, preferably directed to thoracic segments, provides better pain relief and ventilatory function than parenteral opioids, reducing morbidity and mortality in elderly patients with chest wall trauma[37] (see Chapter 57). Other therapeutic measures include supplemental oxygen, continuous positive airway pressure of 10 to 15 cm H_2O by face mask, airway humidification, chest physiotherapy, incentive spirometry, bronchodilators, airway suctioning (using fiberoptic bronchoscopy, if necessary), and nutritional support.[35] Overzealous infusion of fluids and transfusion of blood products may result in deterioration of oxygenation by worsening the underlying pulmonary injury.[35,38]

In patients with pulmonary contusion, respiratory insufficiency, or failure despite adequate analgesia, clinical evidence of severe shock, associated severe head injury, or injury requiring surgery, airway obstruction, and significant pre-existing chronic pulmonary disease are indications for tracheal intubation and mechanical ventilation. Positive end-expiratory pressure (PEEP) with low tidal volumes (6 to 8 mL/kg) and low inspiratory alveolar or plateau pressures should be used to decrease the likelihood of ARDS if ventilation is controlled. In intubated, spontaneously breathing patients, airway pressure release ventilation, in which spontaneous breathing is superimposed on mechanical ventilation by intermittent sudden, brief decrease of continuous positive airway pressure, provides improved $\dot{V}/\dot{Q}$ matching and systemic blood pressure, lower sedation requirements, greater O_2 delivery, and shorter periods of intubation.[35,39] Severe unilateral pulmonary contusion that is unresponsive to these measures may be treated by differential lung ventilation via a double-lumen endobronchial tube. In bilateral severe contusions with life-threatening hypoxemia, high-frequency jet ventilation may enhance oxygenation and cardiac function, which may be compromised by concomitant myocardial contusion or ischemia.[40]

Systemic air embolism occurs mainly after penetrating lung trauma and blast injuries, and less frequently after blunt thoracic trauma that produces lacerations of both distal air passages and pulmonary veins[41]; positive-pressure ventilation after tracheal intubation may then result in entrainment of air into the systemic circulation. Hemoptysis, circulatory, and CNS dysfunction immediately after starting artificial ventilation, as well as detection of air in blood from the radial artery, establishes the diagnosis. Air bubbles may also be seen in the coronary arteries during thoracotomy. Surgical management involves immediate thoracotomy and clamping of the hilum of the lacerated lung. Respiratory maneuvers that minimize or prevent air entry into the systemic circulation include isolating and collapsing the lacerated lung by means of a double-lumen tube, or ventilation with the lowest possible tidal volumes via a single-lumen tube.[41] Transesophageal echocardiography (TEE) of the left side of the heart may permit visualization of air bubbles and their disappearance with therapeutic maneuvers.

Management of Shock

Hemorrhage is the most common cause of traumatic hypotension and shock. Other causes are abnormal pump function (myocardial contusion, pericardial tamponade, pre-existing cardiac disease, or coronary artery or cardiac valve injury), pneumothorax or hemothorax, spinal cord injury, and, rarely, anaphylaxis or sepsis (Table 36-1).

Evaluation of the severity of hemorrhagic shock in the initial phase is based on a few relatively insensitive and nonspecific clinical signs. For example, tachycardia, which is traditionally used as an index of hypovolemia, may be absent in up to 30% of hypotensive trauma patients because of increased vagal tone, chronic cocaine use, or other reasons.[42] In contrast, by increasing catecholamine output, tissue injury and associated pain may maintain tachycardia and normal or elevated systemic blood pressure in the presence or absence of hypovolemia without necessarily increasing the cardiac index or tissue oxygen delivery. In fact, in this situation an increase in intestinal vascular resistance and a decrease in splanchnic blood flow may occur, and if prolonged, may allow entry of intestinal micro-organisms into the circulation and increase the likelihood of subsequent sepsis and organ failure.[43–45] Thus, equating a normal heart rate and systemic blood pressure with normovolemia during initial resuscitation may lead to loss of valuable time for treating underlying occult hypovolemia or hypoperfusion. Nevertheless, heart rate, systemic blood pressure, pulse pressure, respiratory rate, urine output, and mental status remain the available early clinical indicators of the severity of hemorrhagic shock[43,46] (Table 36-2).

Some of the proven markers of organ perfusion can be used during early management to set the goals of resuscitation. Of these, the base deficit and blood lactate level are the most useful and practical tools during all phases of shock, including the earliest. The base deficit reflects the severity of shock, the oxygen debt, changes in O_2 delivery, the adequacy of fluid resuscitation, and the likelihood of multiple-organ failure and survival with reasonable accuracy in *previously healthy* adult and pediatric trauma patients.[47,48] A base deficit between 2 and 5 mmol/L suggests mild shock, between 6 and 14 mmol/L indicates moderate shock, whereas >14 mmol/L is a sign of severe shock. An admission base deficit in excess of 5 to 8 mmol/L correlates with increased mortality.[47,48] Thus, normalization of the base deficit is one of the end points of resuscitation.[49,50]

Elevation of the blood lactate level is less specific than base deficit as a marker of tissue hypoxia because it can be generated in well-oxygenated tissues by increased epinephrine-induced skeletal muscle glycolysis, accelerated pyruvate oxidation, decreased hepatic clearance of lactate, and early mitochondrial dysfunction.[51] All these conditions may be present in the trauma patient. Nevertheless, in most trauma patients an elevated lactate level correlates with other signs of hypoperfusion, rendering it an important marker of dysoxia and an end point of resuscitation. The normal plasma lactate concentration is 0.5 to 1.5 mmol/L; levels above 5 mmol/L indicate significant lactic acidosis. The half-life of lactate is approximately 3 hours; thus, the level decreases rather gradually after correction of the cause. Failure to clear lactate within 24 hours after reversal of circulatory shock is a predictor of increased mortality.[52]

The response of the pulse and blood pressure to initial fluid therapy also aids in the assessment of hypovolemia.[43] In hypotensive and tachycardic patients, administration of lactated Ringer (LR) solution, 2,000 mL over 15 minutes in adults or 20 mL/kg in children, should normalize the vital signs if hemorrhage is mild (10 to 20%). A transient improvement after fluid infusion suggests a 20 to 40% decrease in circulating volume or continuing blood loss. More crystalloids and possibly blood transfusion are required in these patients. If the vital signs do not respond to initial fluid resuscitation, there has probably been severe (>40%) blood and/or volume loss, which must be replaced by rapid infusion of crystalloids, colloids, and blood. Traditionally, a systolic blood pressure ≤90 mm Hg is used to define shock during the early phase of trauma management, including the intraoperative period. Recent data from two trauma centers reviewing the relationship between initial systolic blood pressure and mortality, base deficit, length of stay, and infection rate suggest that a value of

TABLE 36-1

GUIDELINES FOR MANAGEMENT OF TRAUMATIC SHOCK

	■ ETIOLOGY					
	■ HEMORRHAGE OR EXTENSIVE TISSUE INJURY	■ CARDIAC TAMPONADE	■ MYOCARDIAL CONTUSION	■ PNEUMOTHORAX OR HEMOTHORAX	■ SPINAL CORD INJURY	■ SEPSIS
Primary mechanisms	Hypovolemia	Ventricular inflow restriction	Diminished ventricular performance and elevated pulmonary vascular resistance	Lung collapse Mediastinal shift, causing inflow and outflow obstruction of the heart	Vasodilatation and relative hypovolemia caused by loss of sympathetic tone	Intestinal perforation causing peritoneal contamination
Typical signs and symptoms	Tachycardia Narrow pulse pressure Cold, clammy skin from vasoconstriction	Tachycardia Hypotension Dilated and engorged neck veins Muffled heart sounds Diminished BP response to fluid challenge	Dysrhythmia Tachycardia Hypotension	Tachycardia Hypotension Dilated and engorged neck veins Absent breath sounds Hyperresonance to percussion Tracheal shift Dyspnea Subcutaneous emphysema	Hypotension without tachycardia, cutaneous vasoconstriction, or narrow pulse pressure	Develops mainly a few hours after colon injury In hypovolemic patients, signs and symptoms indistinguishable from hypovolemic shock In normovolemic patients, fever, modest tachycardia, warm, pink skin, near normal BP, wide pulse pressure Hypotension may develop
Treatment continuum, from least to most intense	Crystalloids initially Transfusion if 2,000 mL of crystalloid in 15 min does not restore BP	Pericardiocentesis Pericardial window Emergency department thoracotomy	Fluids Fluids and vasodilators Fluids and inotropes	Release of air with 14-gauge catheter Chest tube	Fluids Fluids and vasopressors Fluids, vasopressors, and inotropes, if myocardial damage is present	Fluids and antibiotics Fluids, antibiotics, and inotropes for hypotension

BP, blood pressure.

TABLE 36-2

ADVANCED TRAUMA LIFE SUPPORT CLASSIFICATION OF HEMORRHAGIC SHOCK[a]

	■ CLASS I	■ CLASS II	■ CLASS III	■ CLASS IV
Blood loss (mL)	≤750	750–1,500	1,500–2,000	≥2,000
Blood loss (% blood volume)	≤15	15–30	30–40	≥40
Pulse rate (per min)	<100	>100	>120	≥140
Blood pressure	Normal	Normal	Decreased	Decreased
Pulse pressure	Normal or increased	Decreased	Decreased	Decreased
Respiratory rate (breaths/min)	14–20	20–30	30–40	>35
Urine output (mL/hr)	≥30	20–30	5–15	Negligible
Mental status	Slightly anxious	Mildly anxious	Anxious and confused	Confused, lethargic
Fluid replacement (3:1 rule)[b]	Crystalloid	Crystalloid	Crystalloid + blood	Crystalloid + blood

[a]For a 70-kg male patient, based on initial presentation.
[b]The 3:1 rule is based on empiric observation that most patients require 300 mL balanced electrolyte solution for each 100 mL blood loss. Without other clinical and monitoring parameters, this guideline may result in excessive or inadequate fluid resuscitation.
Adapted from American College of Surgeons, Committee on Trauma: Shock, Advanced Trauma Life Support Course for Physicians. Chicago, American College of Surgeons, 1997, p 108. with permission.

≤110 mm Hg should be considered for this purpose[53,54] (Fig. 36-2).

Bickell et al.[55] showed that delaying fluid resuscitation until surgical control of bleeding in patients with penetrating trauma improved survival to hospital discharge and decreased the length of hospital stay. Vigorous fluid therapy increases arterial and venous pressures, dilutes clotting factors and platelets, and decreases blood viscosity, and thus may reinitiate bleeding already stopped by a soft thrombus. Although many experimental studies have confirmed these findings, it has also become clear that withholding fluids completely can result in as much harm as vigorous resuscitation.[56] In contrast, slow infusion of isotonic or hypertonic crystalloids, and preferably of packed red blood cells (PRBCs), titrated to lower than normal systemic pressure, had beneficial effects on animal survival without tissue injury or organ failure. A clinical study conducted subsequent to that of Bickell et al. failed to demonstrate any decrease in mortality.[57] Nevertheless, although this practice is contraindicated in traumatic brain and spinal cord injuries in which adequate perfusion is crucial, it emphasizes the useful fact that fluid administration in excess of that needed for achieving normovolemia prior to control of hemorrhage may be deleterious.

A reasonable transfusion threshold is a hematocrit <25% for young, healthy patients and <30% for older patients or those with coronary or cerebrovascular disease. Transfusion of PRBCs is shown to be an independent risk factor for mortality and intensive care unit (ICU) and hospital length of stay in

trauma patients; this finding was true independent of the severity of shock.[58] Nevertheless, this concern should not preclude timely and adequate administration of blood products. Normally, type-specific crossmatched blood can be available in most centers in about 30 minutes, including transport time. Type-specific uncrossmatched blood can be available in even less time for patients with severe hemorrhage. However, if the situation dictates immediate transfusion, type O Rh+ blood is satisfactory in most situations. Controversy exists about the use of uncrossmatched type O PRBCs because of concern about the development of alloantibodies and allergic reactions. Dutton et al.,[59] reviewing their experience in 161 patients receiving 581 units of universal donor blood, demonstrated that only one of the 10 Rh− male patients receiving O Rh+ blood developed alloantibodies. All four female patients in the series received type O Rh− blood without apparent problem.

One of the principal goals during early management of the hemorrhaging trauma patient is to avoid the development of the so called "vicious cycle" or "lethal triad," consisting of acidosis, hypothermia, and coagulopathy (Fig. 36-3). Both acidosis and hypothermia are major factors in the induction of coagulopathy. Resuscitation with fluids and PRBCs, which have no hemostatic activity, further adds to this effect by diluting platelets—already reduced in number and dysfunctional—and coagulation factors (see Chapter 16). Bleeding and intravascular coagulation further augment coagulopathy via loss or consumption of damaged or depleted platelets and coagulation

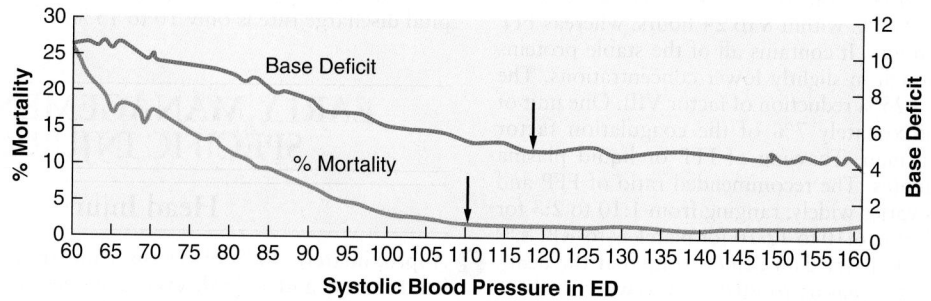

FIGURE 36-2. Relationship between emergency department (ED) systolic blood pressure, base deficit, and overall mortality rate of trauma patients; head injury patients are not included. Note that mortality and base deficit decrease as systolic blood pressure increases, stabilizing at 110 mm Hg rather than at the generally accepted 90 mm Hg. (Adapted from Eastridge BJ, Salinas J, McManus JG et al: Hypotension begins at 110 mm Hg: redefining "hypotension" with data. J Trauma 2007; 63: 291, with permission.)

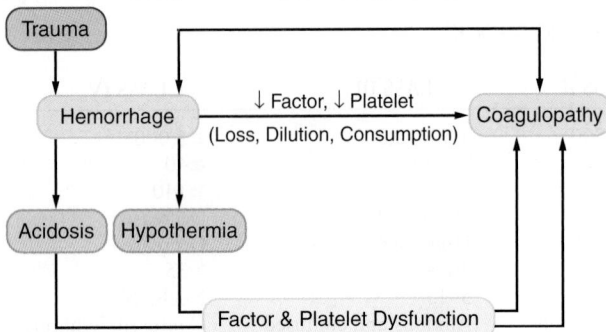

"Bloody Vicious Cycle" or "Lethal Triad"

FIGURE 36-3. Schematic representation of "bloody vicious cycle" or "lethal triad." Trauma-induced hemorrhage causes acidosis, hypothermia, and coagulopathy. Acidosis and hypothermia produce factor and platelet dysfunction enhancing coagulopathy, which in turn causes increased bleeding. The cycle continues until death ensues, unless effective treatment by timely control of bleeding and correction of acidosis, hypothermia, and coagulopathy is instituted.

factors. Augmented coagulopathy further increases the blood loss, necessitating additional fluid replacement and maintaining the vicious cycle.

The current practice of administering large volumes of crystalloids, colloids, and PRBCs with no hemostatic components for initial resuscitation is considered to be the major factor in the development of often lethal coagulopathy. Most trauma patients are hypercoagulable when admitted to the emergency department and do not develop coagulopathy when administration of hemostatic agents is delayed. However, in the estimated 10% of patients with severe trauma and shock who enter the hospital in a hypocoagulable state[60] or rapidly develop hypocoagulation, resuscitative fluids and PRBCs may further worsen the coagulopathy and facilitate the vicious cycle. A computer simulation study by Hirshberg et al.[61] clearly demonstrated that with current fluid resuscitation techniques, most major trauma patients are coagulopathic at the time they arrive to the OR. In their study, the prothrombin time (PT) would increase to below hemostatic levels after replacement of one blood volume, fibrinogen would decay at replacement of 1.25 blood volumes, and finally, platelets at a loss of 1.75 blood volumes. Experience gained from the Iraq and Afghanistan wars attests to the accuracy of the findings of Hirshberg et al.; Holcomb et al.[62] strongly recommend starting liquid plasma replacement along with fluids and PRBCs as soon as the patient arrives in the emergency department, and continuing it throughout surgery.

Liquid plasma differs from fresh-frozen plasma (FFP) in that it is frozen at −180°C within 8 to 24 hours, whereas FFP is frozen within 8 hours. It contains all of the stable proteins found in FFP, although in slightly lower concentrations. The major difference is a 25% reduction of factor VIII. One unit of FFP contains approximately 7% of the coagulation factor activity of a 70-kg man. Thawing of FFP or liquid plasma takes about 30 minutes. The recommended ratio of FFP and platelets to PRBCs varies widely, ranging from 1:10 to 2:3 for FFP-to-PRBCs and from 6:10 to 12:10 for platelets-to-RBCs.[63] Nevertheless, recent military data demonstrate that the death rate was 65% when the plasma-to-PRBCs ratio was 1:8, 34% when it was 1:2.5, and 19% when it was 1:1.4.[64]

Currently, many trauma centers use *hemostatic resuscitation protocols* during initial resuscitation of major traumatic hemorrhage in the emergency department and OR. These involve administering a relatively limited quantity of crystalloid solutions and volume replacement with liquid plasma and

PRBCs. In addition, platelets and cryoprecipitate are given regularly and, in special situations, recombinant factor VIIa (rFVIIa) is administered. Prothrombin complex concentrates are also likely to be added to this protocol in the near future.

One such protocol, used in Parkland Memorial Hospital in Dallas, Texas, involves regular shipment from the blood bank of packaged blood products, including 5 units of PRBCs, 2 units of thawed plasma, 5 units of platelets, and 10 units of cryoprecipitate in each package. Plasma and PRBCs are sent every 30 minutes, and platelets and cryoprecipitate every hour. Recombinant factor VIIa, if deemed necessary, is provided early during resuscitation. The number of units in each package can be doubled on request, if necessary.[65] Rapid establishment of venous access with large-bore cannulas placed in peripheral veins that drain both above and below the diaphragm is essential for adequate fluid resuscitation in the patient who is severely injured. When vascular collapse and extremity injury impair access to arm or leg vessels, percutaneous cannulation of the internal jugular, subclavian, or femoral veins can be performed. Ultrasound guidance may facilitate cannulation of the internal jugular vein and prevent needle entry and infusion of fluids into the pleural space in patients with a large hemothorax.[66] Ultrasound may also be used for infraclavicular access to the axillary vein,[67] or to the cephalic or basilic veins at the midarm level.[68] If necessary, a cutdown to a saphenous or arm vein can be rapidly performed in older children and adults. In children younger than 5 years of age, intraosseous cannulation has a high success rate and a low incidence of complications. Infusion rates comparable with those obtained with intravenous lines are possible in small children, although a pressure infusion device may be necessary to achieve flow.[69] A special screw-type needle or the needle of a 16- or 18-gauge angiocatheter is introduced into the bone marrow of the distal femur or proximal tibia at the level of its tuberosity. Care should be taken not to injure the epiphyseal plate during puncture. Proper placement is indicated by loss of resistance to fluid injection or aspiration of marrow.

Patients who arrive in the emergency department in cardiac arrest require advanced cardiac life support (see Chapter 59). However, the success rate of external cardiac massage in hypovolemic trauma patients is likely to be low.[70] Emergency department thoracotomy not only permits performance of open cardiac massage, but also aids resuscitation efforts by allowing drainage of pericardial blood, control of cardiac and great vessel bleeding, application of a cross-clamp to the aorta, and rapid administration of fluids through a small Foley catheter introduced into the right atrium, or in desperate situations, through a large-bore catheter or introducer in the descending aorta. This procedure is not indicated in blunt torso trauma; the mortality rate is similar regardless of whether it is attempted.[71] In penetrating injuries, depending on the presenting condition of the patient, the initial success rate may be as high as 70%, but the neurologically intact hospital discharge rate is only 10 to 15%.[71,72]

EARLY MANAGEMENT OF SPECIFIC INJURIES

Head Injury

Approximately 40% of deaths from trauma are caused by head injury, and indeed, even a moderate brain injury may increase the mortality rate of patients with other injuries. In nonsurvivors, progression of the damaged area beyond the directly injured region (secondary brain injury) can be demonstrated at autopsy.[73] The major factor in secondary injury is tissue hypoxia, which results in lactic acidosis, free radical generation, prostaglandin synthesis and release of excitatory

ANESTHETIC MANAGEMENT

TABLE 36-3

EFFECTS ON OUTCOME OF SECONDARY INSULTS OCCURRING FROM TIME OF INJURY THROUGH RESUSCITATION[a]

■ SECONDARY INSULTS	■ NO. OF PATIENTS	■ % OF TOTAL PATIENTS	■ 6-MONTH OUTCOME (%)		
			■ GOOD/ MODERATE	■ SEVERE/ VEGETATIVE	■ DEAD
Total cases	717	100	43.0	20.2	36.8
Neither	308	43.0	63.9	10.2	26.9
Hypoxia	161	22.4	50.3	21.7	28.0
Hypotension	62	11.4	32.9	17.1	50.0
Both	166	23.2	20.5	22.3	57.2

[a]Data from hospital emergency departments enrolled in Traumatic Coma Data Bank.
Reprinted from Prough DS, Lang J: Therapy of patients with head injuries: Key parameters for management. J Trauma 1997; 42(Suppl): 10S, with permission.

amino acids (primarily glutamate), lipid peroxidation and breakdown of cell membranes, entry of large quantities of sodium, calcium, and water into the cells, and leakage of fluid from the blood vessels into the extracellular space.[74,75] This process results in brain edema and both regional and global disturbances of the cerebral circulation. Thus, of all the possible secondary insults to the injured brain, decreased oxygen delivery as a result of hypotension and hypoxia has the greatest detrimental impact[76,77] (Table 36-3).

Brain injury by itself does not cause hypotension in adults except as a preterminal event. However, more than half of patients with severe head trauma have other injuries that render approximately 15% of them hypotensive; approximately 30% are hypoxic on admission as a result of central respiratory depression or associated chest injuries. Furthermore, exposure to these insults is likely to occur during any phase of the continuum of hospital care: in the radiology unit, the OR, the recovery room, the ICU, or elsewhere. The most common early complications of head trauma are intracranial hypertension, brain herniation, seizures, neurogenic pulmonary edema, cardiac dysrhythmias, bradycardia, systemic hypertension, and coagulopathy.

Diagnosis

Mental impairment after trauma may have any of several etiologies. However, the possibility of hypoxia and shock must always be considered first. If consciousness remains depressed despite ventilation and fluid replacement, a head injury is assumed to be present and the patient is managed accordingly. As noted, hypotension is the most important cause of death in the head-injured patient. Chesnut[77] demonstrated that a single episode of systolic blood pressure <90 mm Hg is associated with a 50% increase in mortality, and subsequent episodes or lower pressures[78] increase mortality even further. Therefore, every effort should be made to support the blood pressure with fluids and vasopressors (preferably phenylephrine, which does not constrict cerebral vessels), and ensure adequate oxygenation *before* the unconscious patient is evaluated. A baseline neurologic examination should be performed after initial resuscitation, but before any sedative or muscle relaxant agents are administered, and should be repeated at frequent intervals because the patient's condition may change rapidly. Anesthetic and adjunct drugs may render an adequate neurologic examination impossible; thus, long-acting muscle relaxants, opioids, sedatives, or hypnotics should be given selectively.[76,79]

Consciousness can be initially assessed within a few seconds using the AVPU system (*a*lert; responds to *v*erbal stimuli;

responds to *p*ain; *u*nresponsive; Table 36-4). More precise information is provided by the GCS score (Table 36-4), which provides a standard means of evaluating the patient's neurologic status. In this test, the sum of the scores obtained for eye opening, verbal response, and motor activity correlates with the state of consciousness, the severity of the head injury, and the prognosis.[79] Assessment of motor function should be performed on the extremity that responds best. The limb affected by neurologic injury is examined, but the result is not considered in the GCS score.

Dilatation and sluggish response of the pupil is a sign of compression of the oculomotor nerve by the medial portion of

TABLE 36-4

TWO-LEVEL INITIAL EVALUATION OF CONSCIOUSNESS

■ LEVEL 1. AVPU SYSTEM

A = Alert
V = Responds to verbal stimuli
P = Responds to painful stimuli
U = Unresponsive

■ LEVEL 2. GLASGOW COMA SCALE (GCS)[a]

Eye opening (E)	
Spontaneous, already open and blinking	4
To speech	3
To pain	2
None	1
Verbal response (V)	
Oriented	5
Answers but confused	4
Inappropriate but recognizable words	3
Incomprehensible sounds	2
None	1
Best motor response (M)	
Obeys verbal commands	6
Localizes painful stimulus	5
Withdraws from painful stimulus	4
Decorticate posturing (upper extremity flexion)	3
Decerebrate posturing (upper extremity extension)	2
No movement	1

[a]GCS ≤8 = deep coma, severe head trauma, poor outcome.
GCS 9–12 = conscious patient with moderate injury.
GCS >12 = mild injury.

the temporal lobe (uncus). A maximally dilated and unresponsive "blown" pupil suggests uncal herniation under the falx cerebri. The presence of similar findings in ocular injuries makes interpretation of pupillary findings difficult when eye and head injuries coexist. However, the pupillary reaction to light is usually more sluggish in the head-injured patient.

CT scanning is used for the diagnosis of most acute head injuries. Positive CT findings after acute head injury include midline shift, distortion of the ventricles and cisterns, effacement of the sulci in the uninjured hemisphere, and the presence of a hematoma at any location in the cranial vault. Subdural hematomas usually have a concave border, whereas epidural hematomas present with a convex outline classically termed a *lenticular* configuration. Patients in severe coma (GCS score <8) have a 40% likelihood of an intracranial hematoma. Those with higher GCS scores are less likely to have had intracranial bleeding, although it is evident that the significant incidence of this complication even in these patients necessitates a CT study, preferably with contrast enhancement. Other benefits of CT scanning include detection of intracranial air and depressed skull fractures.

Management

The primary objective of the early management of brain trauma is to prevent or alleviate the secondary injury process that may follow any complication that decreases the oxygen supply to the brain, including systemic hypotension, hypoxemia, anemia, raised ICP, acidosis, and possibly hyperglycemia (serum glucose >200 mg/dL; see Chapter 49). These insults cause exacerbation of trauma-induced cerebral ischemia and metabolic derangements, worsening the outcome.[80,81] *The most important therapeutic maneuvers in these patients are aimed at normalizing ICP, CPP, and oxygen delivery.* The Brain Trauma Foundation and the American Association of Neurological Surgeons have published evidence-based guidelines for the treatment of head-injured patients.[76] Primary therapy includes normalization of the systemic blood pressure (mean blood pressure >80) and maintaining the PaO_2 >95, the ICP <20 to 25 mm Hg, and the CPP 50 to 70 mm Hg. Maintaining the CPP at levels above 70 mm Hg, the former standard, is no longer advised as it may be associated with an increased incidence of ARDS.[76] The patient is kept at 30 degrees head elevation, sedation and neuromuscular blockers are given as necessary, and cerebrospinal fluid is drained through a ventriculostomy catheter, if available. Rapid and adequate restoration of the intravascular volume with isotonic crystalloid and, if necessary, with colloid solutions should be aimed at maintaining the CPP between 50 and 70 mm Hg while attempting to minimize further brain swelling. LR solution, which is slightly hypotonic (Na^+ = 130 mEq/L, osmolality approximately 255 mOsm/L), may promote swelling in uninjured areas of the brain if it is given in large quantities; edema tends to occur in injured brain regions regardless of the type of solution administered because of increased permeability of the blood–brain barrier. To minimize edema formation, it is wise to monitor serum osmolality and to replace LR solution with isotonic normal saline. If serum osmolality cannot be measured, this change can be made empirically after 3 liters of LR solution.

Effective reduction in ICP can be provided, or at least aided, by administration of mannitol, an important part of the management of severe head injury. It is administered in boluses of 0.25 to 0.5 g/kg, repeated every 4 to 6 hours as needed to control the ICP.[76] In addition to its osmotic diuretic effect, this agent may improve cerebral blood flow (CBF) and O_2 delivery by reducing the hematocrit and thus the blood viscosity, improving CBF and oxygen delivery.[76] There is a risk of hypovolemia and resultant hypotension when therapeutic doses of mannitol are used. If the ICP elevation persists, addi-

tional doses of mannitol should be given cautiously. Acute mannitol toxicity, manifested by hyponatremia, high serum osmolality, and a gap between calculated and measured serum osmolality >10 mOsm/L, may result when the drug is given in large doses (2 to 3 g/kg) or to patients with renal failure. Mannitol should be used with great care in the presence of hypotension, sepsis, nephrotoxic drugs, or pre-existing renal disease as these may also precipitate renal failure.[76] Further, the effects of mannitol result from its activity in regions of the brain where the blood–brain barrier is intact. It may exacerbate edema in injured areas in which it may easily enter the tissues.

Hyponatremia in these patients results from intravascular volume expansion rather than sodium loss; thus, treatment with saline solutions is not appropriate. Because of a synergistic action between mannitol and loop diuretics in improving the ICP, addition of furosemide may be a safer and more effective treatment than increasing the dose of mannitol when intracranial hypertension persists. Until about 1995, hyperventilation to a $PaCO_2$ of 25 to 30 mm Hg was a mainstay of the therapy of head injury. However, brain ischemia, which is probably the most threatening consequence of head injury, is likely to occur during the first 6 hours after trauma even when the CPP is maintained above the generally recommended 50 to 70 mm Hg.[82] This hypoperfusion seems to be caused largely by increased cerebral vascular resistance, which may be enhanced by hyperventilation. However, some degree of hyperventilation may be necessary for short periods of time in patients who have severe injuries and elevated ICP that does not respond to normal ventilation and diuretics, although this should not be used during the first 24 hours following injury.[76] Its use after the initial phase should be based on monitoring of the ICP and, if available, the jugular bulb O_2 saturation ($SjvO_2$) and arteriovenous O_2 difference ($AVDO_2$). It should be noted that hyperventilation in the severely brain-injured patient may also be associated with acute lung injury.[83]

Measurement of the $SjvO_2$ is used in some centers as a guide to therapy of the head-injured patient.[84] A catheter is passed retrograde into the jugular bulb under fluoroscopic control. The O_2 saturation may be measured with a co-oximeter or continuously by means of a fiberoptic sensor.[84] An $SjvO^2$ of <50% is considered critical desaturation. The $AVDO_2$ is a standard measure of the brain's oxygen supply/demand ratio. It is equal to $1.34 \cdot Hgb \cdot (SaO_2 - SjvO_2)$, with the saturations expressed as decimal values, and normally is approximately 6. An increase in this value is a sign of insufficient blood flow, whereas a subnormal level indicates hyperemia. A reduction in ICP with elevation of CPP during treatment is reflected by a rise in $SjvO_2$ and a narrowing of the $AVDO_2$, presumably reflecting an improvement in the circulation to the brain. Unfortunately, several shortcomings of the technique have hindered its universal acceptance. Because all of the cerebral veins drain into the cavernous sinus and from there into the jugular bulbs, $AVDO_2$ measures only global O_2 consumption, which may well be very different from the situation in the injured region. Indeed, Coles[82] has demonstrated by positron emission tomography scanning that a significant increase in the region of critical hypoperfusion resulting from hyperventilation was not necessarily associated with a correspondingly abnormal $SjvO_2$ or $AVDO_2$ (Fig. 36-4). Patient or catheter movement may also alter the measured $PjvO_2$. Thus, there may be a high proportion of inaccurate values—as high as nearly two-thirds—although recent advances in the technique have probably reduced these errors. Cruz[85] has suggested that jugular venous monitoring should be used only in sedated, paralyzed patients.

If the ICP remains elevated despite all of these measures, pentobarbital (3 to 10 mg/kg given over 0.5 to 2.5 hours, followed by a maintenance infusion of 0.5 to 3.0 mg/kg/hr, aimed at a serum concentration between 2.5 and 4.0 mg/dL) may be required. High-dose barbiturates are of no value in the routine

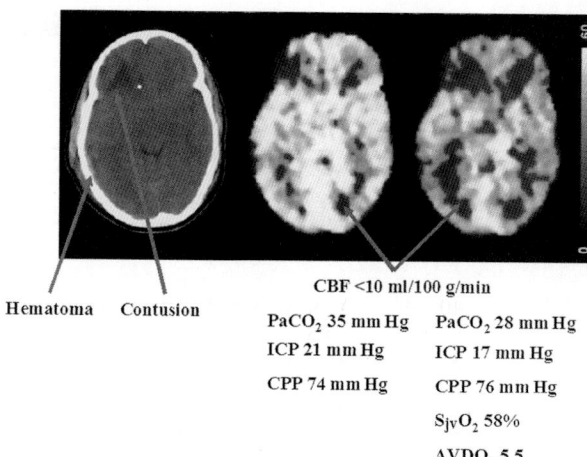

CBF <10 ml/100 g/min

PaCO$_2$ 35 mm Hg   PaCO$_2$ 28 mm Hg
ICP 21 mm Hg   ICP 17 mm Hg
CPP 74 mm Hg   CPP 76 mm Hg
                      SjvO$_2$ 58%
                      AVDO$_2$ 5.5

FIGURE 36-4. Effects of hyperventilation on cerebral blood flow (CBF). The left image is a computed tomography scan of the patient whose positron emission tomography scans are shown in the other two images. Note that there is a significant decrease in the CBF and an increase in the areas of hypoperfusion despite improvement in the intracranial pressure (ICP), and normal SjvO$_2$ and AVDO$_2$. CPP, cerebral perfusion pressure. (Adapted from Coles JP: Regional ischemia after head injury. Curr Opin Crit Care 2004; 10: 120, with permission.)

therapy of head injury, and should be used only for refractory ICP elevation. Whether active normalization of elevated serum glucose (a common occurrence in the head-injured patient) has any salutary effect on outcome is not known. Of course, immediate surgical decompression, especially of epidural hematomas, is an important factor in reducing morbidity and mortality.

If the patient is hemodynamically stable, a CT scan is performed; the strictest attention should be paid to ensuring adequate oxygenation, ventilation, blood pressure, and ICP control during the procedure. If the patient is hemodynamically unstable or requires emergency surgery for associated injuries, and has a history suggesting a head injury even though a significant intracranial hematoma is unlikely on clinical grounds, intraoperative ICP monitoring is indicated to permit rapid detection of ICP elevation. Both intracranial hematomas and hemorrhage in other regions have a high surgical priority. In the patient with multiple traumas, prioritization between the two is based on the severity of each injury. Because there is no time to obtain a CT scan of the head in patients with both profuse hemorrhage and brain herniation, the patient is brought directly to the OR for simultaneous control of the bleeding site and evacuation of the intracranial hematoma. The site of the craniotomy can be determined by a ventriculogram or an ultrasound examination with a pencil-tip probe; both tests may be performed under local anesthesia through a frontal burr hole.

The addition of relatively small volumes of hypertonic saline in concentrations between 3% (6 to 8 mL/kg) and 7.5% (4 mL/kg) followed by infusion of LR may be beneficial in multiple trauma patients with head injury.[86] Like mannitol, hypertonic saline draws fluid from the intracellular space and, thus, in addition to restoring the blood volume, it reduces brain edema and prevents elevation of the ICP.[87] On the other hand, hypertonic saline may, also like mannitol, increase edema in the injured region of the brain.[88] The intravascular volume expansion produced by hypertonic saline is transient; it can be prolonged by the addition of 6% dextran-70 or hetastarch to the solution. However, administration of hypertonic saline cannot be maintained for long periods. It may cause hypernatremia, hyperosmolality, or hyperchloremic acidosis, probably from renal bicarbonate loss secondary to increased

levels of Cl$^-$. Serum concentrations of Na$^+$ and Cl$^-$ and the patient's acid–base status should be followed, and the administration of hypertonic saline should be discontinued if plasma Na$^+$ reaches 160 mEq/L. Because of these considerations, and the fact that there has been no standardization of the concentration, the dose, or the duration of treatment, the use of hypertonic saline should still be considered experimental therapy.[76,89] Resuscitation with colloid solutions (hetastarch, pentastarch, pentafraction, human albumin 5% and 25%, or dextran) provides a sustained improvement in vital signs, but the increase in colloid osmotic pressure produced by these solutions may not have an important role in reducing brain edema.

It may be possible to improve the outlook for brain injured patients:

1. Cruz[90] and the Lund group[91] used widely different approaches, but the common factor in their treatments was not only maintenance of the CPP, but also avoidance, or at least limitation, of brain swelling. Cruz accomplished this by standard therapy augmented by monitoring the cerebral O$_2$ extraction (CeO$_2$ = SaO$_2$ − SjvO$_2$). Hyperventilation was used when this value decreased below the normal range of 24 to 42%, in order to constrict the circulation and thus decrease the ICP, while mannitol was used for increased CeO$_2$ to decrease ICP and improve the CBF. The Lund treatment involved a rather complex pharmacologic approach, both to control blood pressure and ICP, and to limit edema formation. The reported outcomes were very promising (Table 36-5). Unfortunately, because both of these approaches were reported in 1998, they have neither been confirmed by other groups nor followed up by the original authors.
2. The earlier definitive treatment is initiated, the better the outcome is likely to be. Rudehill et al.[92] have demonstrated improvement in outcomes in a large series of patients when care was initiated by anesthesiologists at the accident scene.
3. Meanwhile, the wide variety of types and severities of injury, and of responses to treatment—both among different patients and in the same patient at different times—imply that therapeutic interventions must be individualized.[93,94] These aims may be met, at least partly, by carefully structured intensive care.[95,96] Therapeutic goals should be set explicitly and reviewed, and altered if necessary, at every change of shift.

Indeed, early intervention and controlled management may explain much of the improvement in outcomes that has been obtained over the past 10 years, including the results obtained by Cruz[90] and the Lund group,[91] by Palmer et al.[95] using the Brain Trauma Foundation 1995 guidelines, and by Watts et al.[96] using the 2000 guidelines (Table 36-5).

Spine and Spinal Cord Injury

Initial Evaluation

The objective in the evaluation of spinal trauma is to diagnose instability of the spine and the extent of neurologic involvement (see Chapter 39). Not stabilizing the spine in the first hours after a major accident until a definitive diagnosis is established carries the risk of converting a neurologically intact patient into a paraplegic or quadriplegic. During transport to the hospital, the patient should be immobilized with a hard collar, a spine board, and tape. After admission, patients should not be left on a rigid spine board for longer than 1 hour, especially when they are paralyzed, because of the risk of decubitus ulcers.

In the conscious patient, the diagnosis is relatively easy: a history of a motor vehicle, industrial, or athletic accident, an act of violence, or a fall; penetrating trauma resulting in a neurologic deficit below a specific spinal level; or pain and tenderness

TABLE 36-5

SIX-MONTH OUTCOMES FOR PATIENTS WITH BRAIN INJURY IN VARIOUS STUDIES[a]

| | | | 6-MONTH OUTCOME (%) | | | |
NAME OF STUDY	N	YEAR PUBLISHED	GOOD/ MODERATE	SEVERE/ VEGETATIVE	DEAD	COMMENTS
Three-country (Jennett et al.[b])	700	1977	38	11	51	Various treatments, some untreated
Miller et al.[c]	158	1981	47	12	40	Vent, surgery, ICP monitoring, and Rx
Traumatic Coma Data Bank (TCDB)[86]	717	1997	43	20	37	Total patients, standard therapy
TCDB[86]	308	1997	54	19	27	Pts without hypotension or hypoxia
Rudehill et al.[92]	1,508	2002	69	11	20	Standard protocol
Cruz[90]	178	1998	74	17	9	CeO$_2$ group
Eker et al.[91]	53	1998	79	13	8	Lund treatment

[a]Results of various treatment protocols for brain injuries. The three-country study surveyed patients who had received a wide variety of treatment; some were untreated. Miller et al. relied on hyperventilation and, when necessary, barbiturates. The TCBD patients were treated similarly; note the difference in outcome of the patients who did not experience hypotension or hypoxia (see Table 36-3). The final three studies are described in the text.
[b]Jennett B, Teasdale G, Galbraith S: Severe head injuries in three countries. J Neurol Neurosurg Psychiatry 1977; 40: 291.
[c]Miller JD, Butterworth JF, Gudeman SK et al: Further experience in the management of severe head injury. J Neurosurg 1981; 54: 289.

over the involved vertebrae strongly suggest a spine injury. It should be noted, however, that spinal pain is not always localized to the level of injury.[97] Obviously, these symptoms are difficult to elicit in the comatose patient. In these circumstances, flaccid areflexia, loss of rectal sphincter tone, paradoxical respiration, and bradycardia in a hypovolemic patient suggest the diagnosis. In cervical spine trauma, an ability to flex but not to extend the elbow and response to painful stimuli above but not below the clavicle also indicate neurologic injury. Current guidelines consider absence of neck pain or paresthesia and a negative findings on physical examination—lack of tenderness with palpation and during voluntary flexion and extension of the neck—in a neurologically intact, conscious patient as adequate indications for ruling out a cervical spine injury without further radiologic studies. Alcohol intoxication and distracting associated injuries do not seem to alter these criteria as long as the patient is alert, conscious, and able to concentrate.

Depending on the degree of deficit, spinal cord injuries are categorized as *complete* or *incomplete*. Intact sensory perception over the sacral distribution and voluntary contraction of the anus (sacral sparing) are present in incomplete, but not in complete, injuries. There is practically no possibility of significant neurologic recovery in complete injury, whereas functional restoration may occur in up to 50% of patients after incomplete injuries. In some patients the development of *spinal shock*, which is manifested by absolute flaccidity and loss of reflexes, precludes distinguishing between complete and incomplete injuries during the initial phase of treatment. Therefore, even in the absence of sacral sparing, the possibility of neurologic recovery dictates that all possible efforts be made at this time to prevent further damage and to preserve cord function. A similar principle applies to the evaluation of the level of injury. After the first few days, spinal cord edema subsides and the final level is commonly a few segments lower than on initial presentation. Thus, early therapeutic efforts should not be abandoned even in the patient with a high-level injury, which carries a grim functional prognosis.

Spinal shock is probably caused by direct trauma to the spinal cord, and usually subsides within days to weeks. The term is frequently used as a misnomer for *neurogenic shock*, which is defined as hypotension and bradycardia caused by the loss of vasomotor tone and sympathetic innervation of the heart as a result of functional depression of the descending sympathetic pathways of the spinal cord. It is usually present after high thoracic and cervical spine injuries and improves within 3 to 5 days.

Initial Management

The spinal cord, a microcosm of the brain, is also vulnerable to a secondary injury process that may be a product of hypotension, hypoxia, and probably other physiologic complications.[98] Prompt recognition and aggressive treatment of these insults, which may also result from associated trauma, may minimize exacerbation of spinal cord lesions and improve the long-term outlook of these patients.[80,99]

Immobilization and Intubation.   Maintenance of immobilization of the injured spine is of paramount importance. If a cervical spine fracture is suspected, immobilization or manual inline stabilization of the neck is necessary before the patient is moved. If the patient has a thoracic or lumbar injury, a careful log-rolling maneuver should be used.[98,100]

About one third of paraplegic patients require airway management, mostly within the first 24 hours after injury. Signs of respiratory distress or fatigue, or a rising respiratory rate or PaCO$_2$, are major indications for ventilatory assistance. Severe bradycardia or dysrhythmias may result from unopposed vagal activity during tracheal intubation or suctioning: the patient must be preoxygenated and atropine (0.4 to 0.6 mg) should be given before any instrumentation. If bradycardia develops during airway management, treatment includes additional atropine, glycopyrrolate, isoproterenol, or, if necessary, cardiac pacing.

The techniques of intubation in spine-injured patients are discussed in the section "Airway Management."

Steroids.   For the past several years, high-dose methylprednisolone has been used in many centers in an attempt to improve the outcome from spinal cord injuries. The drug is given as a bolus of 30 mg/kg within 8 hours of injury, followed in 1 hour by an infusion of 5.4 mg/kg/hr for the next 23 to

47 hours. The National Acute Spinal Cord Injury Studies (NASCIS-2 and NASCIS-3)[101,102] indicated some improvement in motor function in treated patients who had partial sensory and motor loss. The results seemed to have been best in patients who received 24 hours of therapy starting within 3 hours of injury, and those receiving 48 hours of treatment starting within 3 to 8 hours of injury. There was virtually no improvement in sensory scores in any of the groups. There was little or no difference from untreated patients in groups with more severe injuries or in those who were treated after 8 hours, and the long-term improvement in the functional status of most of the patients was at best moderate. However, the findings of these studies have not been duplicated in any other prospective or retrospective trials,[103] and have been criticized because of multiple major deficiencies in the analysis of the data.

Furthermore, steroid therapy is associated with an increased rate of sepsis, pneumonia, and days of intensive care and positive-pressure ventilation,[104] and is also associated with increased mortality in the 36 to 74% of patients with spine injuries who also have head injuries.[105] Given these results, the *Guidelines for the Management of Acute Cervical Spine and Spinal Cord Injuries,*[106] states, "Treatment with methylprednisolone for either 24 or 48 hours is recommended as an option in the treatment of patients with acute spinal cord injuries that should be undertaken only with the knowledge that the evidence suggesting harmful side effects is more consistent than any suggestion of clinical benefit." Similarly, the National Association of Emergency Medical Physicians states that treatment with steroids should not be considered the standard of care, and that routine use of steroids in emergency medical services is not supported.[107]

Respiratory Complications

Respiratory complications are common in all phases of the care of spinal cord–injured patients and are the most frequent cause of death in the acute stage.[108,109] In the initial period these problems may be augmented by associated brain, neck, chest, or abdominal injury, alcohol intoxication, or the effects of self-administered or iatrogenic drugs. Injuries at C5 or lower are usually associated with normal tidal volumes because the function of the diaphragm is intact, whereas patients with levels at C4 or above may require permanent ventilatory assistance. Nevertheless, accessory respiratory muscle paresis may cause a significant loss of expiratory reserve even when the injury involves the lower spinal segments.[110] Pulmonary edema is another significant cause of respiratory dysfunction. A severe catecholamine surge follows acute trauma to the spinal cord.[111] Although the resultant severe hypertension lasts for only a few minutes, its effects persist; it may produce both pulmonary capillary damage, as a result of shifting of a large portion of the blood volume into the pulmonary circulation, and left ventricular dysfunction. Overzealous fluid therapy to treat the patient's initial hypotension may lead to acute pulmonary edema when the sympathetic activity returns approximately 3 to 5 days after the injury.

Paradoxical respiration in the quadriplegic patient results from partial chest wall collapse during inspiration; it may produce limitation of the tidal volume and an increased risk of hypoventilation.[110] The situation is aggravated when the patient is in an upright position. The diaphragm cannot maintain its normal domed shape, the only way it can contract efficiently, because the weight of the thoracic contents is not opposed by the normal tone of the abdominal muscles. Thus, in contrast to other diseases that produce respiratory insufficiency, the supine position improves respiration in persons with quadriplegia[110] (Fig. 36-5).

Other causes of inadequate respiration in the early phase of spinal cord injury are aspiration of gastric contents, atelectasis, pneumonia, and bronchoconstriction. Management includes

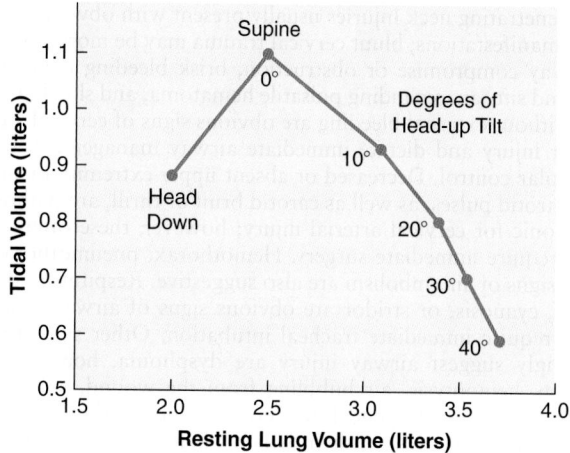

FIGURE 36-5. Effect of semi-Fowler position on ventilation in quadriplegic patients. (Reprinted from Winslow C, Bode RK, Felton D et al: Impact of respiratory complications on length of stay and hospital costs in acute cervical spine injury. Chest 2002; 121: 1548, with permission.)

careful observation of the patient's breathing and preparation to ventilate the lungs and intubate the trachea at the first sign of respiratory depression.[110]

Hemodynamic Management

Hemodynamic management of quadriplegic patients includes a complete assessment, with a pulmonary artery catheter if necessary, as early as possible after injury. In as many as 25% of patients with cervical spinal cord injuries, left ventricular dysfunction may contribute to the hypotension.[112] Decreased preload can be treated with fluid infusion using cardiac function curves as a guide. In general, volume may be safely replaced to a central venous or pulmonary capillary wedge pressure (PCWP) of 18 mm Hg.[112] This avoids, or at least limits, the severity of the pulmonary edema described previously. Hypotension despite adequate fluid infusion, acidosis, or low mixed venous P_{O_2} requires treatment with inotropes such as dopamine.

Anesthetic Considerations

Any anesthetic technique compatible with the patient's general condition is satisfactory for the spinal cord–injured patient. Hypotension is very common during anesthesia in quadriplegic patients. Placement of a central venous or pulmonary artery catheter may facilitate management of the patient's volume and blood pressure status.

Succinylcholine may produce a sudden, severe increase in serum K^+ in spine-injured patients (see Chapter 20). Levels as high as 14 mEq/L may be reached: the result may be irreversible ventricular dysrhythmias and cardiac arrest. Although succinylcholine is probably safe during the 4 to 7 days after injury, it is probably best to avoid it altogether in the paraplegic patient and to use rapid-onset nondepolarizing agents such as rocuronium when a rapid-sequence induction is required.

Neck Injury

Both penetrating and blunt trauma may injure the major structures in the neck: vessels, respiratory and digestive tracts, and nervous system. Hemorrhage, asphyxia, mediastinitis, paralysis, stroke, or death may result if these injuries are not promptly recognized and treated.

⑩ Penetrating neck injuries usually present with obvious clinical manifestations; blunt cervical trauma may be more subtle. Airway compromise or obstruction, brisk bleeding from the wound site, an expanding pulsatile hematoma, and shock with or without external bleeding are obvious signs of cervical vascular injury and dictate immediate airway management and vascular control. Decreased or absent upper-extremity or distal carotid pulses, as well as carotid bruit or thrill, are pathognomonic for cervical arterial injury; however, these often do not require immediate surgery. Hemothorax, pneumothorax, and signs of air embolism are also suggestive. Respiratory distress, cyanosis, or stridor are obvious signs of airway injury and require immediate tracheal intubation. Other signs that strongly suggest airway injury are dysphonia, hoarseness, cough, hemoptysis, air bubbling from the wound, subcutaneous crepitus, laryngeal tenderness, pneumothorax, and hemothorax. Because of their dynamic nature, cervical airway injuries may rapidly progress to obstruction; therefore, the patient should be observed carefully and the trachea intubated at the first sign of problems.

Esophageal injuries, whether in the neck or the chest, are insidious and difficult to diagnose. Dysphagia, odynophagia, hematemesis, subcutaneous crepitus, prevertebral air on a lateral cervical radiograph, and major concomitant injuries to other cervical structures suggest an esophageal injury and call for confirmation with an esophagram.

The neurologic manifestations of a penetrating neck injury vary depending on the injured structure. Partial spinal cord transection produces the Brown-Sequard syndrome with ipsilateral motor and contralateral sensory deficit below the injury. Complete spinal cord transection, depending on the level of injury, produces paraplegia or quadriplegia, usually with neurogenic shock. Occasionally, luminal occlusion of the carotid and vertebral arteries may lead to a hemispheric cerebrovascular accident; associated hypotension increases the likelihood of this event.

Patients with severe active bleeding, persistent hypotension, and air bubbling through the wound require immediate surgery without further diagnostic studies.[113] Controversy exists over the indications for surgical management of stable penetrating neck injuries. Mandatory exploration is associated with negative findings in approximately 70% of patients.[113] Thus, in many centers, patients are evaluated with noninvasive diagnostic tests and undergo surgery only when there are positive findings.[113]

Blunt cervical vascular injuries usually present with a hematoma that may compress the cervical veins, displace the airway, and produce pharyngeal and laryngeal congestion. Injury to an artery may produce an intimal tear, pseudoaneurysm, fistula, or thrombosis. If a carotid or vertebral artery is involved, cerebral ischemia may occur. Thrombosis often develops gradually over minutes to a few hours, thus the appearance of neurologic symptoms is delayed in approximately 40% of patients. Symptomatic patients may present with a cervical bruit, altered mental status, or lateralizing neurologic deficits including hemiparesis, transient ischemic attacks, amaurosis fugax, or Horner syndrome. The mortality rate associated with blunt carotid injury varies between 15 and 28%, and 15 to 50% of survivors have neurologic deficits.[114] Identification of a blunt carotid injury in an asymptomatic patient using CT, magnetic resonance angiography, or four-vessel arteriography not only allows early institution of antiplatelet therapy, systemic anticoagulation, endovascular intervention, or surgical repair,[114,115] but also occasionally prevents the neurologic deficits that may follow surgery for associated injuries in an unprotected patient.

Airway injuries after blunt trauma are rare, but carry an overall mortality rate of 2%.[115] Their severity varies from a simple mucosal tear or hematoma to a comminuted laryngeal cartilage fracture or complete cricotracheal separation. They frequently require primary laryngeal repair or tracheostomy. Anesthetic management is not only complicated by relatively complex airway management problems[31,32] (discussed in "Airway Evaluation and Intervention"), but also with associated skull base, intracranial, open neck, cervical spine, esophageal, or pharyngeal injuries.[115]

Chest Injury

Although a high percentage of thoracic injuries can be treated conservatively, patients who need surgery may have major intraoperative physiologic disturbances.

Chest Wall Injury

Rib, scapula, and sternal fractures, in addition to interfering with adequate respiration, may be associated with severe underlying thoracic, abdominal, and cranial injuries. The management principles for these injuries are similar to those previously described for flail chest, although the need for mechanical ventilation is less likely in single-rib fractures than in a flail chest. Effective pain relief, preferably with continuous thoracic epidural anesthetics or opioids, is central to management.[37]

Pleural Injury

Closed pneumothorax is easy to be missed in major trauma. The presence of subcutaneous emphysema, pulmonary contusion, and rib fractures should draw suspicion of coexisting pneumothorax.[116] Tension pneumothorax involving >50% of a hemithorax presents with dyspnea, tachycardia, cyanosis, agitation, diaphoresis, neck vein distention, tracheal deviation, and displacement of the maximal cardiac impulse to the contralateral side.

Although an upright plain chest radiograph provides the best opportunity for detection of pneumothorax, this position may be impossible or contraindicated in patients who are experiencing major hemorrhage or those with suspected spine injury. Air in the pleural space tends to accumulate anteriorly in supine or semirecumbent patients, often in the anteromedial sulcus. More recently, transthoracic ultrasound has been used for the diagnosis of pneumothorax. Normally, movement of the lung beneath the chest wall produces "comet tail" artifacts from echodense areas on the lung surface. In the presence of pneumothorax, neither lung motion nor comet tails can be seen. In one study of blunt and penetrating trauma patients, ultrasound was more sensitive than a supine chest film, but did not detect all pneumothoraces. Further, ultrasound detection of rib and sternal fractures also appeared to be more accurate than the chest radiograph. It was recommended that a chest film and the ultrasound can complement each other, but that chest CT be used as the definitive test.[117] Ultrasound examination may also be helpful in detecting residual pleural air after placement of thoracostomy tube. However, after 24 hours of tube placement, the accuracy of this technique decreases, probably because of adhesions between the lung and the pleura.[118]

Brasel et al. suggested that a small closed pneumothorax can be safely managed by observation alone, without a chest tube, even in those patients who require positive-pressure ventilation, as long as continuing vigilance is maintained.[118a] However, based on an earlier study[119] and our own experience, we strongly believe that once diagnosed, a traumatic pneumothorax, no matter how small, should be treated with thoracostomy drainage before tracheal intubation and positive-pressure ventilation.

Bleeding intercostal vessels are responsible for most hemothoraces. Severe airway deviation may be produced by a hemothorax, although it is not as common as it is after a pneumothorax. Treatment consists of drainage with a 30- to 40-French chest tube (26 to 32 French is used for pneumothorax). Initial drainage of 1,000 mL of blood, or collection of >200 mL/hr for several hours, is an indication for thoracotomy. Additional indications for thoracotomy are a "white lung" appearance on the anteroposterior chest radiograph, or a continuous major air leak from the chest tube, which may result from a direct airway injury or major lung laceration. Hemodynamically stable patients with persistent bleeding of <150 mL/hr are managed with video-assisted thoracoscopic surgery (VATS) to control bleeding. This procedure requires placement of a double-lumen tube to collapse the lung on the involved side; it can also be useful in diagnosis of suspected diaphragmatic, cardiac, or mediastinal injuries; evaluation of some bronchopleural fistulas; and evacuation of clotted blood or an empyema that does not drain with a chest tube. Use of VATS decreases the need for open thoracotomy and the number of negative explorations in stable trauma patients.[120]

Pulmonary Contusion

This entity often accompanies chest wall injury, but may also develop in isolation. Its management is discussed in the section on flail chest.

Penetrating Cardiac Injury

Pericardial tamponade, cardiac chamber perforation, and fistula formation between the cardiac chambers and the great vessels are the consequences of this type of trauma. Any penetrating wound of the chest, especially one within the "cardiac window" (midclavicular lines laterally, clavicles superiorly, and costal margins inferiorly), can cause this injury. Pneumopericardium visible on a plain chest radiograph after penetrating chest trauma should increase the suspicion, although it is not seen in all patients. Unstable patients require immediate sternotomy or left thoracotomy. Transthoracic echocardiography can be used for screening stable patients,[121] but it may be inconclusive in obese patients and in those with pneumothorax; TEE provides an accurate diagnosis in these patients, but it is impractical during the initial evaluation phase of trauma[122] (see Chapter 28). Of the alternative diagnostic measures, the central venous pressure (CVP) is not always accurate, and a subxiphoid pericardial window is invasive, must be performed in the OR under general anesthesia, takes longer, and cannot detect an intracardiac shunt.

Pericardial Tamponade

The classic findings of pericardial tamponade—tachycardia, hypotension, distant heart sounds, distended neck veins, pulsus paradoxus, or pulsus alternans—are difficult to appreciate or may be absent in a hypovolemic trauma patient. Transthoracic echocardiography or TEE can demonstrate blood in the pericardial sac and the presence of ventricular "diastolic collapse," which indicates at least a 20% reduction in cardiac output. Initial management consists of intravenous fluids and, if necessary, careful selection and titration of anesthetic agents, such as ketamine and etomidate, which produce relatively little myocardial depression. Evacuation of the pericardial blood by pericardiocentesis or surgery should be performed as soon as possible. If anesthesia is contemplated for surgery, its administration should be delayed until patient draping and preparation are completed.

Blunt Cardiac Injury

11 The term *blunt cardiac injury* has replaced *myocardial contusion* and encompasses varying degrees of myocardial damage, coronary artery injury, and rupture of the cardiac free wall, septum, or a valve following blunt trauma.[123] Myocardial injury consists of myofibrillar disintegration, edema, bleeding, or necrosis that, depending on its severity, presents as minor electrocardiogram (ECG) or enzyme abnormalities, complex dysrhythmias, or cardiac failure caused by direct mechanical impact or indirectly by coronary occlusion. Dysrhythmias last no more than a few days; ventricular wall motion abnormalities may persist for up to 1 year, but any increased risk of perioperative cardiac complications appears to last for no more than a month.

The prominent clinical findings are angina, sometimes responding to nitroglycerin, dyspnea, chest wall ecchymosis and/or fractures; dysrhythmias of any type; and right-sided or left-sided congestive heart failure. Orliaguet et al.[123] proposed an algorithm for the diagnosis and treatment of several clinical scenarios caused by this injury (Fig. 36-6). The diagnosis is based on the 12-lead ECG, troponin I level, and echocardiography. The ECG is very sensitive, although not specific. A normal trace cannot rule out the diagnosis, but it is the best screening test. Common ECG abnormalities include almost any type of dysrhythmia, ST or T-wave changes, and conduction

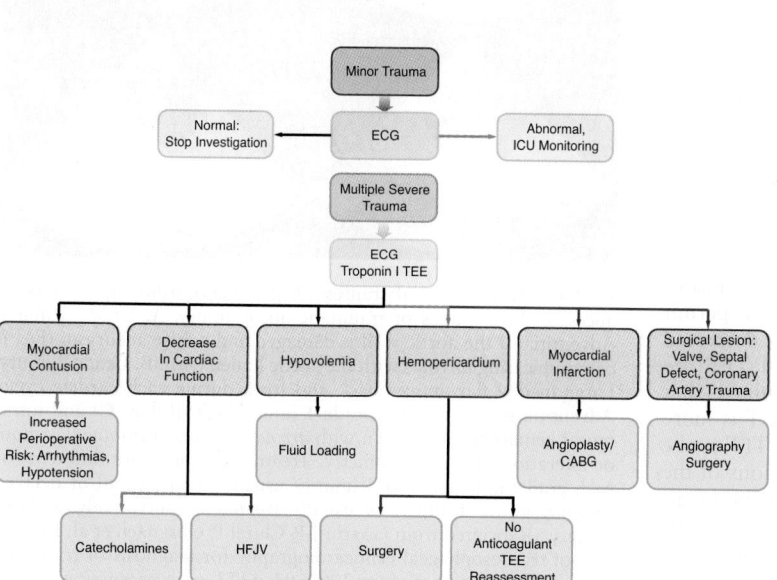

FIGURE 36-6. Algorithm for management of various clinical scenarios produced by severe blunt cardiac injury (BCI). Evaluation of severe multiple trauma-induced BCI uses electrocardiogram (ECG), troponin I, and transesophageal echocardiography (TEE). *Arrows* represent the frequency of occurrence of each scenario and the frequency of management measures. *Thick arrows* represent high frequency, *thin arrows* represent low frequency, and *dotted arrows* represent very rare occurrences. ICU, intensive care unit; CABG, coronary artery bypass graft; HFJV, high-frequency jet ventilation. (Adapted from Orliaguet G, Ferjani M, Riou B: The heart in blunt trauma. Anesthesiology 2001; 95: 544, with permission.)

ANESTHETIC MANAGEMENT

TABLE 36-6

COMMON CLINICAL, RADIOGRAPHIC, AND ULTRASOUND FEATURES OF THORACIC AORTIC INJURIES

■ CLINICAL	■ RADIOGRAPHIC	■ SPIRAL COMPUTED TOMOGRAPHY	■ ULTRASOUND
Increased arterial pressure and pulse amplitude in upper extremities	Widened mediastinum	Mediastinal hematoma	Intimal flap
Decreased arterial pressure and pulse amplitude in lower extremities	Blurring of the aortic contours	Aortic wall irregularity	Turbulent flow
Absent or weak left radial artery pulse	Widened paraspinal interfaces	Intimal flap	Dilated aortic isthmus
Osler's sign: discrepancy between left and right arm blood pressure	Left apical cap	False aneurysm	Acute false aneurysm
Retrosternal or interscapular pain	Opacified aortopulmonary window	Pseudocoarctation	Intraluminal medial flap
Hoarseness	Broadened paratracheal stripe	Intramural hematoma	Hemothorax
Systolic flow murmur over the precordium or medial to the left scapula	Displacement of the left main-stem bronchus	Intraluminal clot or medial flap	Hemomediastinum
Neurologic deficits in the lower extremities	Displaced SVC		
	Rightward deviation of the esophagus and trachea		
	Nasogastric tube shift		
	Left hemothorax		
	Sternal and/or upper rib fractures		
	Lung contusion		
	Pneumothorax		

SVC, superior vena cava.

delays. Patients with a normal ECG undergoing minor surgery do not require any further testing. Patients with severe injuries need measurement of troponin I and TEE to diagnose any abnormalities caused by the cardiac injury (Fig. 36-6). Troponin I has replaced serum creatine kinase and its myocardial band fraction because of its greater specificity for cardiac muscle damage. Echocardiography can demonstrate wall motion abnormalities, valve malfunction, hemopericardium, intracardiac thrombi, venous or systemic embolism, and end-diastolic and fractional ventricular wall area changes. Thus it aids not only in the diagnosis of blunt cardiac injury, but also in hemodynamic management. Treatment options depend on the diagnosis (Fig. 36-6). These options include antiarrhythmic agents, inotropes, fluid loading, high frequency jet ventilation to optimize cardiac function, and surgery for hemopericardium, valvular or septal lesions, or coronary artery injury or disease.

Thoracic Aortic Injury

This injury occurs at the isthmus—the junction between the free and fixed portions of the descending aorta—in 90% of cases, and carries an 80% mortality in the first hour following injury. There may be no clinical findings in the emergency department (Table 36-6). Only 20 to 30% of patients with mediastinal widening actually have thoracic aortic injury, although the negative predictive value of the finding is 98%. Measuring the left mediastinal width ($\geq$6 cm) and its fraction of the total mediastinal width ($\geq$0.6) may increase the specificity and positive predictive value of the plain film.[124] Contrast-enhanced spiral CT with volume-rendered image reconstruction techniques and ultrasound technologies permit reliable noninvasive diagnosis and have substantially decreased the need for biplanar aortography. Both CT and TEE are equally capable of diagnosing subadventitial aortic injuries that require surgical intervention[125] (see Chapter 28). CT is more likely to be used for diagnosis because introducing a TEE probe under these circumstances may be undesirable. Lesions of the intima and media that can be treated conservatively and concomitant blunt cardiac injuries are much more likely to be detectable by TEE and CT.[125] TEE is especially useful for the anesthesiologist when other injuries require immediate surgery without time for CT examination of the chest.

Based on TEE findings, traumatic aortic injury can be classified into three categories: grade 1 injury consists of an intramural hematoma, limited intimal flap and/or mural thrombus; grade 2 injury consists of subadventitial rupture, injury to the media, altered aortic geometry and/or small hemomediastinum; grade 3 injury consists of transsection with massive blood extravasation, intraluminal obstruction causing pseudocoarctation, and ischemia[126] (Fig. 36-7). Of these, grade 1 injuries can be treated nonoperatively with serial follow-ups using TEE. Grade 2 and 3

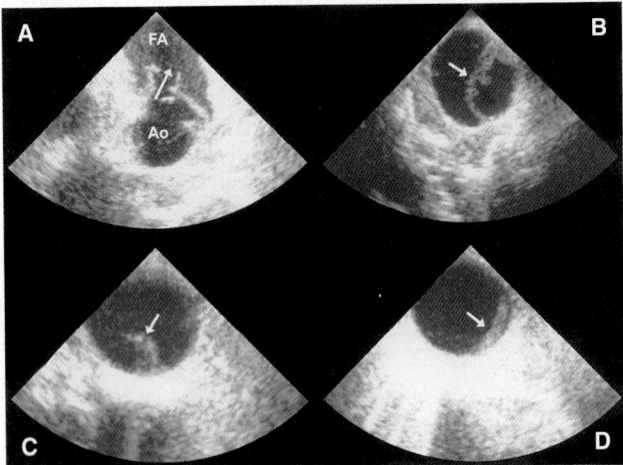

FIGURE 36-7. Typical transesophageal echocardiographic appearances of three grades of traumatic aortic injury. **A.** Grade 3 injury. Adventitia of the aortic wall is damaged and a false aneurysm (FA) is communicating (*arrow*) with the aortic lumen (Ao). **B.** Grade 2 injury. Large medial flap moves back and forth during each cardiac cycle. Adventitia is intact. **C,D.** Grade 1 injury. Intimal flap (C) and intramural hematoma (D, shown with *arrows*) without hemomediastinum or alteration of aortic geometry. Treatment choices are different for each grade: grades 2 and 3 injuries usually require rapid or delayed surgery; grade 1 injury is usually treated conservatively without surgery. (Reprinted from Goarin J-P, Cluzel P, Gosgnach et al: Evaluation of transesophageal echocardiography for diagnosis of traumatic aortic injury. Anesthesiology 2000; 93: 1373, with permission.)

injuries require immediate or delayed surgery based on clinical findings.[126,127] Severity grading may also be done by criteria involving measurement by TEE of maximum aortic diameter, the ratio between injured and normal aortic diameter, depth of pseudoaneurysm, esophagus-to-aortic isthmus distance, aortic isthmus-to-left visceral pleural distance, and the presence of hemothorax.[127]

Surgical prioritization when multiple injuries are present depends on the hemodynamic and neurologic status of the patient. Although the aorta should be repaired as early as possible, control of active hemorrhage from other sites and surgery for intracranial hematomas have a higher surgical priority, unless the aorta is leaking. In most instances, a blood clot between the aorta and the mediastinal pleura occludes the vessel. Any disturbance of the tamponaded region may reinitiate bleeding. A rapid flow of blood in a large artery tends to pull its endothelium with it and thus may rupture an injured vessel that is sealed with a clot or a hematoma. Such an increase in the aortic blood flow is usually caused by increased myocardial contractility; every effort should be made to prevent increased cardiac contractility and hypertension. Endovascular stent grafts have been used in many centers for repair of thoracic aortic injuries, with no risk of paraplegia, simpler anesthetic techniques, and many fewer of the complications associated with thoracotomy.[128]

Diaphragmatic Injury

Injury to the diaphragm may permit migration of abdominal contents into the chest where they may compress the lung, producing abnormalities of gas exchange, or the heart, resulting in dysrhythmias and/or hypotension. Because the defect produced by blunt injury is larger than that resulting from a penetrating injury, migration of abdominal contents, which requires a defect of at least 6 cm in diameter, is also more common after blunt trauma.[129] The liver protects the right side of the diaphragm, thus traumatic herniation is more common on the left side.[129]

The best method of diagnosing a diaphragmatic hernia is laparoscopy, or in selected cases, VATS. Nevertheless, noting that the end of a nasogastric tube is above the diaphragm on the chest radiograph is a certain sign that the stomach is displaced into the chest. A chest radiograph that shows intestinal markings and lung compression, or a contrast-enhanced abdominal CT scan that includes the lower third of the thorax, also can provide important information. Failure to retrieve the instilled fluid during diagnostic peritoneal lavage (DPL) or drainage of DPL fluid from a thoracostomy tube also indicates this injury.

Abdominal and Pelvic Injuries

Table 36-7 summarizes the strengths and weaknesses of the currently available diagnostic tools used for abdominal injuries.[130] Because of the unpredictable course of bullets in the body, exploratory laparotomy or, in selected cases, laparoscopy is required in most patients after a gunshot wound of the abdomen. Occasionally in hemodynamically stable patients, abdominal and flank gunshot wounds may be evaluated with an initial CT scan. Stab wounds may be managed with tractotomy to determine whether the peritoneum is involved. Laparoscopy, laparotomy, or DPL may be indicated after a positive tractotomy.

Patients with blunt abdominal trauma are evaluated by CT scan unless they are hemodynamically unstable and there are overt abdominal signs such as tenderness, guarding, and gross distention. Absence of abdominal distention, however, does not rule out intra-abdominal bleeding. At least 1 liter of blood can accumulate before the smallest change in girth is apparent, and the diaphragm can also move cephalad, allowing further significant blood loss without any change in abdominal circumference.

The diagnostic ability of focused assessment with sonography for trauma (FAST), popularized during the past decade, is inferior to CT scan evaluation, which has recently realized significant technologic improvements. FAST is operator-dependent, has good specificity but moderate sensitivity, can diagnose injuries associated with intraperitoneal fluid but not those without it, and cannot determine the severity of organ injury. Currently, many low-grade intra-abdominal solid-organ injuries that

---

TABLE 36-7

DIAGNOSTIC TOOLS IN ABDOMINAL TRAUMA: STRENGTHS AND WEAKNESSES

■ DIAGNOSTIC TOOL	■ STRENGTH	■ WEAKNESS
Physical examination	Expeditious, safe, and inexpensive; potential for serial examination	Diagnosis of specific injury (e.g., diaphragm)
Diagnostic peritoneal lavage	Expeditious, safe, and inexpensive	Diagnosis of diaphragmatic injury, hollow viscus injury, retroperitoneal injury; can be oversensitive and nonspecific
Computed tomography	Evaluation of peritoneum and retroperitoneum	Diagnosis of diaphragmatic injury, hollow viscus injury
	Staging of solid-organ injury	Expensive; controversial need for contrast
Ultrasonography	Expeditious, safe, and inexpensive; accurate for free peritoneal fluid	Diagnosis of diaphragmatic injury, hollow viscus injury, penetrating injury, good specificity, but moderate sensitivity
	Potential for serial examinations	Less accurate in the presence of large retroperitoneal hematomas
Laparoscopy	Diagnosis of peritoneal penetration, diaphragmatic injury	Diagnosis of hollow viscus injury, retroperitoneal injury
	Evaluation of bleeding or solid-organ injury Potential for therapy	Expensive
Video-assisted thoracic surgery	Evaluation of lung, diaphragm, mediastinum, chest wall, and pericardium; potential for treatment	Requires operating room; expensive Diagnosis of abdominal injuries

Reprinted from Villavicencio RT, Aucar JA: Analysis of laparoscopy in trauma. J Am Coll Surg 1999; 189: 11, with permission.

can be evaluated by CT but not FAST are treated conservatively without surgery. A recent Cochrane review reported that current data are insufficient to develop ultrasound-based clinical pathways to diagnose blunt abdominal injury. On the other hand FAST requires one third of the time and is less expensive to perform than CT, and is without the hazard of radiation.

Screening with abdominal ultrasonography is performed by placing a 3.0- to 5.0-MHz probe on four distinct areas of the abdomen: subxiphoid, to detect pericardial blood; right upper quadrant, for blood in the hepatorenal pouch; left upper quadrant, to detect perisplenic blood; and just above the pubic symphysis, for blood in the rectovesical pouch.

Laparoscopy is an excellent screening tool in abdominal trauma patients. An analysis showed that this method avoided laparotomy in 63% of patients and missed only 1% of the injuries.[130] It is also possible to repair diaphragmatic, bladder, and solid-organ injuries with this technique. The complication rate of laparoscopy in trauma is approximately 1%, including pneumothorax, small bowel injury, intra-abdominal vascular injury, and extraperitoneal CO_2 insufflation.[130]

Fractures of the Pelvis

Pelvic fractures occur in widely varied anatomic forms and physiologic severity. Major hemorrhage occurs in 25% and exsanguination in 1% of patients. They are usually associated with chest, brain, intra-abdominal, and long bone injuries, which increase the morbidity and mortality of pelvic fractures. A large database showed that the 3-month cumulative mortality of patients with pelvic fractures (14.2%) was almost 3 times higher than those without them (5.6%). In most of these fractures, bleeding results from venous disruption by fragments of bone. Retroperitoneal pelvic bleeding is self-limited in most patients with venous injuries because of tamponading, except those with open fractures. Approximately 18 to 20% of patients have arterial bleeding, which does not stop. The retroperitoneal space in these patients may serve as a distensible container, which expands superiorly and anteriorly and may totally obliterate the lower part of the abdominal cavity. Thus, DPL, as in pregnant trauma patients, should be performed above the umbilicus. Large retroperitoneal hematomas may also cause respiratory difficulty because of pressure on the diaphragm.

Following external pelvic fixation, which decreases the mobility of the bone fragments and thus helps control blood loss, angiography can indicate the type and location of bleeding. Arterial bleeding is treated with embolization; the angiography suite should be prepared in advance not only for anesthesia, but also for invasive monitoring and resuscitation. In hemodynamically unstable patients, deciding whether to transport the patient to the OR to control bleeding from associated injuries, or to proceed to interventional radiology for angiography and possible embolization is difficult. In most centers it takes at least 45 minutes to begin angiography, during which time a considerable amount of blood may be lost. Preliminary data from Europe suggest that external fixation and extraperitoneal packing of the pelvis in the OR followed by angiography and possible embolization is more beneficial than only external fixation and angiography.[131,132] In this manner, any intra-abdominal injuries may also be controlled. This concept contrasts with the traditional understanding that opening a retroperitoneal hematoma induced by a fractured pelvis must be avoided. Pelvic fractures may also injure the bladder and the urethra. Thus, a urethrogram should be performed before insertion of a urinary catheter.

Extremity Injuries

Surgical repair of extremity fractures, whether open or closed, should be performed as soon as possible (see Chapter 53).

Delayed fracture repair is associated with an increased risk of deep vein thrombosis (DVT), pneumonia, sepsis, and the pulmonary and cerebral complications of fat embolism. In open fractures, an additional important concern is infection. Wounds left unrepaired for more than 6 hours are likely to become septic.

Associated vascular trauma must be recognized early. Most vascular injuries exhibit at least some part of the classic syndrome of *pain, pulselessness, pallor, paresthesias,* and *paresis.* The definitive diagnosis is made with arteriography; in selected patients, a duplex ultrasound study may be used as a screening test. Patients with vascular trauma should be operated on expeditiously, often without preoperative angiography. These patients may bleed slowly but substantially both pre- and intraoperatively; thus, delayed surgery and prolonged skeletal repair may lead to unrecognized hemorrhagic shock, which may at times become irreversible. Damage control, that is, controlling bleeding and external fixation of the fractures, may be the management of choice.

Compartment syndrome, which is characterized by severe pain in the affected extremity, should be recognized early so that emergency fasciotomy can be effective in preventing irreversible muscle and nerve damage. In unconscious patients, swelling and tenseness of the extremity indicate the presence of this complication. The definitive diagnosis is made by measuring compartment pressures using a transducer attached to a fluid-filled extension tube and a needle inserted into the various compartments of the extremity. A pressure exceeding 40 cm H_2O is an indication for immediate surgery. Caution must be exercised when using epidural or nerve block analgesia for perioperative pain relief in the presence of extremity fractures. Absence of pain can delay the diagnosis of compartment syndrome.

Burns

Determination of the size and depth of a burn sets the guidelines for resuscitation, as well as the indications for surgical intervention.[133] A partial-thickness burn is red, blanches to touch, and is sensitive to painful stimuli and heat. Superficial partial-thickness (first-degree) burns involve the epidermis and upper dermis, and heal spontaneously. Deep partial-thickness (second-degree) burns involve the deep dermis and require excision and grafting to ensure rapid return of function. A full-thickness (third-degree) burn does not blanch even with deep pressure and is insensate. Complete destruction of the dermis requires wound excision and grafting to prevent wound infection that may lead to local sepsis and systemic inflammation. Fourth-degree burns involve muscle, fascia, and bone, necessitating complete excision and leaving the patient with limited function. Laser Doppler imaging can be used as an aid to judge burn wound depth.[134] The size of the burned area as a fraction of the total body surface area (TBSA) is estimated by the "rule of nines." In an adult, the head contributes to 9%; the upper extremities, 18%; the trunk, 36%; and the lower extremities, 36% of the TBSA. These proportions are somewhat different in children, depending on the age and size. To estimate the size of a burn, the palmar surface of a child (excluding the digits) represents about 0.5% of the TBSA over a wide range of ages.

Information about the mechanism of injury facilitates the diagnosis of associated clinical abnormalities. For example, thermal trauma caused by flames in a closed space is likely to be associated with airway damage. Burns resulting from motor vehicle, airplane, or industrial accidents may be complicated by other traumatic injuries. Finally, burns caused by electrocution may show little external evidence but may be associated with severe fractures, hematomas, visceral injury, and skeletal and cardiac muscle injury resulting in pain, myoglobinuria, and dysrhythmias or other ECG abnormalities.

Full-thickness burns involving >10% of the TBSA; partial-thickness burns covering >25% of TBSA in adults and over

20% at the extremes of age; burns involving the face, hands, feet, or perineum; inhalation, chemical, and electrical burns; and burns in patients with severe pre-existing medical disorders are considered to be major burns.[133] A severe burn is a systemic disease that stimulates the release of mediators such as interleukins, tumor necrosis factor, and neopterins, locally—producing wound edema—and into the circulation, resulting in immune suppression, hypermetabolism, protein catabolism, sepsis, and multisystem organ failure. Burns >40% TBSA consistently develop catabolism and weight loss that may last up to 1 year. Prevention of sepsis, maintenance of normal body temperature, and pain management may decrease the extent of catabolism. Pharmacologically, low-dose insulin infusion, beta-blockade, and the synthetic testosterone analogue oxandrolone can decrease catabolism or improve anabolism.[135]

Airway Complications

Respiratory distress in the initial phase of a burn is usually caused by airway injury involving the pharynx or the trachea. Singed facial hair, facial burns, dysphonia or hoarseness, cough, soot in the mouth or nose, and swallowing difficulties in patients without respiratory distress should increase the suspicion of upper (frequent) and lower (occasional) airway injury. In the upper airway, glottic and periglottic edema and copious, thick secretions may produce respiratory obstruction. This may be aggravated by fluid resuscitation even in the absence of significant inhalation injury.[136] In lower airway burns, decreased surfactant and mucociliary function, mucosal necrosis and ulceration, edema, tissue sloughing, and secretions produce bronchial obstruction, air trapping, and bronchopneumonia. The development of parenchymal lung injury takes approximately 1 to 5 days and presents with the clinical picture of adult respiratory distress syndrome. Pneumonia and pulmonary embolism (PE) are late complications that occur 5 or more days after burns. The presence of a lung injury markedly increases the mortality rate from thermal injuries.[137] Administration of the highest possible concentration of O_2 by face mask is the first priority in moderately to severely burned patients with a patent airway. In patients with massive burns, stridor, respiratory distress, hypoxemia, hypercarbia, loss of consciousness, or altered mentation, immediate tracheal intubation is indicated. The intubation technique selected depends on the operator's experience, the age of the patient, and the extent of airway compromise. In adults, awake fiberoptic intubation under adequate topical anesthesia is probably the safest approach, but other techniques (WuScope, Airtraq (King Systems, Nobelsville, IN), GlideScope, intubating LMA, retrograde intubation, or transtracheal jet ventilation) may be used. In most pediatric patients, awake intubation is not possible (see Chapter 29). An inhalation induction with O_2 and sevoflurane, followed by intubation using an FOB or conventional laryngoscope is appropriate.[133] A surgical airway entails a significant risk of pulmonary sepsis, late upper airway sequelae, and death in burned patients; it should be reserved for those whose airway management cannot be handled in any other way.[133,138] Immediately after securing the airway, ventilation with low levels of PEEP will prevent the pulmonary edema that may develop secondary to loss of laryngeal auto-PEEP in patients with significant airway obstruction before intubation. Airway humidification, bronchial toilet, and bronchodilators if needed for bronchospasm are also indicated.

The pediatric airway is particularly challenging because it may be occluded by minimal amounts of swelling because of its small diameter. Prophylactic intubation may therefore be required in children who are suspected of having an inhalation injury, even though they are not yet in respiratory distress. Prophylactic tracheal intubation may also be indicated in adults when the resources for careful follow-up are insufficient. Information obtained from radiologic, arterial blood gas, and endo-scopic examinations and pulmonary function testing may be useful to predict which patient will need tracheal intubation and possibly decrease the risks of airway manipulation.[139]

Fiberoptic laryngoscopy is easy to perform and can provide direct information about the glottic and periglottic structures. It may avoid tracheal intubation in patients who would otherwise be considered candidates for this procedure.[139] Fiberoptic bronchoscopy has the additional advantage of providing information about the lower airway, although it is more uncomfortable for the patient and requires topical anesthesia of the tracheobronchial tree. These studies should be performed every 3 to 4 hours for the first 12 hours after injury. In cooperative patients, pulmonary function testing may aid in the evaluation of airway obstruction. A saw-toothed or flattened inspiratory flow and an extrathoracic obstruction pattern on the flow/volume loop suggest upper airway obstruction. Decreased peak expiratory flow, forced vital capacity and pulmonary compliance, and increased airway resistance suggest lower airway injury.

The chest radiograph, arterial blood gases, and pulmonary function tests are usually normal in the immediate postburn period, even in patients with pulmonary complications.[17] However, these tests should be performed at this time for later comparison. As expected, the more extensive the pulmonary edema, the more severe are the functional abnormalities of the lungs. The treatment of smoke inhalation in burns involves ventilatory management, intensive care, and treatment of carbon monoxide (CO) and cyanide (CN^-) toxicity.

Ventilation and Intensive Care

Hypoxemia may persist despite tracheal intubation, ventilation with PEEP, bronchodilators, and suction of airway secretions (see Chapter 56). In the first 36 hours, this is caused by acute pulmonary edema. From the second to the fifth day, hypoxia may result from atelectasis, bronchopneumonia, and airway edema following mucosal necrosis and sloughing, viscous secretions, and distal airway obstruction. Later there may be nosocomial pneumonia, hypermetabolism-induced respiratory failure, and ARDS. Treatment of these complications is individualized, using ventilatory maneuvers such as low tidal volume (5 to 6 mL) with titrated PEEP, bronchoscopic lavage, antibiotics, chest physiotherapy, and other supportive measures. Prophylactic measures against DVT, gastric ulcers, and hypothermia should be used routinely. Lack of response to therapy because of severe ventilation–perfusion mismatching or shunt may be an indication for the use of nitric oxide, a potent, short-acting vasodilator, via the airway.[18] Patients with ARDS may benefit from high-frequency oscillatory ventilation both intraoperatively and in the ICU. Improvement in oxygenation has been reported in burn patients with this mode of ventilation; the beneficial effect on oxygenation was slower and less in patients with smoke inhalation than in those with burn injury only.[140]

Carbon Monoxide Toxicity

In burn victims, CO inhalation is almost always associated with smoke inhalation, which increases the morbidity and mortality compared with CO toxicity alone. CO produces tissue hypoxia primarily by its 200-fold greater affinity for hemoglobin than oxygen and by its ability to shift the hemoglobin dissociation curve to the left, impairing O_2 unloading to the tissues. It also interferes with mitochondrial function, uncoupling oxidative phosphorylation and reducing adenosine triphosphate production, thus causing metabolic acidosis. Probably because of this effect on the mitochondria, CO can be a direct myocardial toxin, preventing survival in patients who suffer cardiac arrest, even though they have been resuscitated and treated with hyperbaric oxygen.

A normal oxygen saturation on a pulse oximeter does not exclude the possibility of CO toxicity, although low arterial

SYMPTOMS OF CARBON MONOXIDE TOXICITY AS A FUNCTION OF THE BLOOD CARBOXYHEMOGLOBIN (COHb) LEVEL

■ BLOOD COHbc LEVEL (%)	■ SYMPTOMS
<15–20	Headache, dizziness, and occasional confusion
20–40	Nausea, vomiting, disorientation, and visual impairment
40–60	Agitation, combativeness, hallucinations, coma, and shock
>60	Death

O_2 saturation measured by a co-oximeter should raise the suspicion[141] (see Chapter 26). Recently introduced portable devices (Masimo Rad5, Masimo Corporation, Irvine, CA) are capable of measuring carboxyhemoglobin and methemoglobin levels noninvasively via a finger sensor along with pulse oximeter reading, alerting the clinician for high O_2 saturation values. The mixed venous oximeter catheters that are used for continuous in vivo measurement of SvO_2 overestimate oxyhemoglobin concentration in the presence of CO. If CO toxicity is not accompanied by a lung injury and thus by decreased PaO_2, tachypnea is absent; the carotid bodies are sensitive to the arterial O_2 tension and not to the O_2 content. The classic cherry-red color of the blood is also absent in most patients because it occurs only at carboxyhemoglobin (COHb) concentrations above 40%, and it may also be obscured by coexistent hypoxia and cyanosis.

The patient's inspired oxygen should be maintained at the highest possible concentration, even when there is no evidence of significant smoke-induced lung injury, until CO toxicity is ruled out by measurement of blood COHb. A high FIO_2 not only improves oxygenation, but also promotes elimination of CO; an FIO_2 of 1.0 decreases the blood half-life of COHb from the 4 hours seen in room air to 60 to 90 minutes, and to 20 to 30 minutes at 3 atm in a hyperbaric chamber.[133] The greater the blood concentrations of COHb, the more severe are the presenting symptoms (Table 36-8). Delayed neuropsychiatric disorders have been described in patients exposed to toxic levels of CO, and there is evidence to suggest that early hyperbaric O_2 treatment may prevent these symptoms.[133] The decision to institute this treatment should be based on comparing the risks of transport, decreased patient access, and delay in emergency treatment against the possible neurologic sequelae. Currently, hyperbaric O_2 is recommended for patients with COHb >30% at admission if the treatment of life-threatening problems—shock, neurologic injury, metabolic acidosis, myocardial ischemia, infarction, or arrhythmias—will not be compromised.

Cyanide Toxicity

Another cause of tissue hypoxia in burned patients is CN^- toxicity. Cyanide or hydrocyanic acid is produced by incomplete combustion of synthetic materials, and may be inhaled or absorbed through mucous membranes. As in CO toxicity, the usual clinical presentation is unexplained metabolic acidosis. Nonspecific neurologic symptoms such as agitation, confusion, or coma are also common findings. Elevated plasma lactate levels in severe burns may result from hypovolemia, CO toxicity, or CN^- toxicity. However, lactic acidosis after smoke inhalation in a patient without a major burn suggests CN^- toxicity.[142] The definitive diagnosis can be made only by determination of the blood cyanide level, which is toxic above 0.2 mg/L and lethal at levels beyond 1 mg/L. A spectrophotometric assay using methemoglobin as a colorimetric indicator provides a timely and reliable determination of blood CN^-.[143] The pulse oximetry reading will be accurate in the absence of CO toxicity and nitrate therapy-induced methemoglobinemia.

Increased CN^- in the blood can cause generalized cardiovascular depression and cardiac rhythm disturbances, especially in patients with lactic acidosis. Fortunately, the half-life of CN^- is short (approximately 1 hour),[142] and rapid improvement of hemodynamics should be expected after rescue of the victim from the toxic environment. Immediate administration of O_2, which is required for all burn victims, may be lifesaving for this complication. Although there are specific therapies for CN^- toxicity (e.g., amyl nitrate, sodium nitrite, thiosulfate), given the short half-life of the ion, it is not clear whether these measures offer significant help to the patient whose blood CN^- usually decreases to low levels during transport from the field to the hospital.[144] Of course, if circumstances permit, hyperbaric O_2 treatment can be used for all the complications of thermal injury: CO and CN^- poisoning, smoke-induced lung damage, and cutaneous burns.

Fluid Replacement

Immediately after a serious burn, microvascular permeability increases, causing the loss of a substantial amount of protein-rich fluid into the interstitial space. A major burn, a delay in initiation of resuscitation, or an inhalation injury increases the size of the leak.[133] Further, there seems to be a correlation between inhalation injury and cutaneous burns in the production of edema. Pulmonary edema increases cutaneous edema and vice versa.[145] If resuscitation is successful, edema formation stops within 18 to 24 hours.[145] This fluid flux is enhanced by increased intravascular hydrostatic and interstitial osmotic pressures and decreased interstitial hydrostatic pressure. In addition, cardiac contractility may decrease because of circulating mediators, a diminished response to catecholamines, decreased coronary blood flow, and increased systemic vascular resistance.[133] This may result in shock, whose origin is primarily hypovolemic and, to a much smaller extent, cardiogenic.[146] If the hypotension is treated appropriately with fluids, the hemodynamic picture is replaced within 24 to 48 hours by one resembling sepsis or septic shock, with increased cardiac output and diminished systemic vascular resistance caused by the release of inflammatory mediators.[146]

Fluid resuscitation is essential in the early care of the burned patient with an injury >15% of the TBSA. Smaller burns can be managed with replacement at 150% of the calculated maintenance rate and careful monitoring of fluid status. Intravascular volume should be restored with utmost care to prevent excessive edema formation in both damaged and intact tissues resulting from the generalized increase in capillary permeability caused by the injury. Edema from overaggressive resuscitation has many deleterious and potentially life-threatening effects. Mention has already been made of the facilitation of upper airway edema after rapid fluid infusion in large cutaneous burns with or without smoke inhalation.[136] Likewise, chest wall edema may develop after administration of large quantities of fluid, causing respiratory difficulties and necessitating excision of burned tissue from the anterior axillary line to improve breathing. Abdominal edema may also occur, and when resuscitation volume exceeds 300 mL/kg over 24 hours, increased intra-abdominal pressure may produce abdominal compartment syndrome with impedance of venous return.[147,148] Edema formation may also increase the tissue pressure in the burned area, resulting in reduction of blood flow to distal sites. This, together with decreased tissue oxygen tension, may produce necrosis of damaged but viable cells, increasing the extent of injury and the risk of infection.

Crystalloid solutions are preferred for resuscitation during the first day following a burn injury; leakage of colloids during this phase may increase edema. Nevertheless, crystalloid resuscitation, especially in children, may cause a rapid decline in plasma protein concentration and necessitate administration of 5% albumin in LR after the first day following a >30% burn and/or significant inhalation injury, when the capillary leak stops.[149] It is believed that this will moderate the tendency to edema formation associated with the administration of large amounts of isotonic (0.9% saline or LR) solutions, even though a 6% increase in the risk of mortality has been reported with the use of colloids in patients who are critically injured and burned. Some centers use plasma with crystalloid routinely and attribute the good outcome of their patients partly to this practice.[150] Administration of fluids in excess of the amount recommended by the Parkland formula appears to be relatively frequent in modern burn management and is termed "fluid creep." Avoidance of early overresuscitation, use of colloid routinely, adherence to protocols are recommended strategies to prevent fluid creep.[151] Alternatively, hypertonic saline solutions draw intracellular water into the bloodstream and thus decrease the fluid volume needed to maintain perfusion, maintain extracellular volume, and limit the severity of edema in patients with burns occupying >50% of the TBSA, circumferential extremity burns, or inhalational injury.[133] Unfortunately, hypertonic solutions cause hypernatremia and intracellular water depletion; patients and experimental animals receiving these fluids for burn therapy often did not show an overall fluid-sparing effect, and had an unacceptably high incidence of renal failure and death compared with those receiving LR.[152,153]

Of the many resuscitation formulas available, the Parkland (Baxter) and modified Brooke formulas are tailored to the clinical condition of the patient and are accepted in most centers[149] (Table 36-9). The addition of glucose is not necessary except in children, especially those weighing <20 kg. Albumin 5% may be administered after the first day following injury at a rate of 0.3, 0.4, or 0.5 mL/kg per percent burn per 24 hours for burns of 30 to 50%, 50 to 70%, or 70 to 100% of TBSA, respectively. These formulas are guidelines only, and none can be expected to provide adequate restoration of intravascular volume in all burn victims, especially small children and patients with inhalation injuries. Therefore, administration of fluids during the initial phase should be titrated to specific goals described in Table 36-9; and if a pulmonary artery catheter is placed, acceptable cardiac output, filling pressures, and a mixed venous oxygen tension (PvO_2) of 35 to 40 mm Hg. Careful monitoring of the hematocrit may also guide fluid management. An increase in hematocrit during the first day suggests inadequate fluid resuscitation because hemolysis and sequestration are actually expected to cause a decrease in this parameter. Acute anemia, as may occur during excision and grafting of burns, is usually well tolerated. Blood replacement is usually not initiated until the hematocrit is below 15 to 20% in healthy patients requiring limited operations, approximately 25% in those who are healthy but need extensive procedures, and 30% or more when there is a history of pre-existing cardiovascular disease.[154]

Although there is evidence that the standard clinical end points of resuscitation often provide inadequate information in major burns and that better information may be obtained from pulmonary artery catheter data,[155] there are also practical and methodologic problems associated with the latter, especially the risks of infectious complications and the requirement for additional vascular access.

When in rare instances fluid resuscitation fails despite administration of crystalloids in excess of 6 mL/kg/% TBSA, and invasive or semi-invasive monitoring suggests adequate intravascular volume, vasopressor and/or inotropic agents may be indicated. Dopamine in small doses (5 μg/kg/min) and/or β-adrenergic agents may improve urine output without further need for fluids.[149] Electrolyte abnormalities may occur after the first day for several reasons but are primarily a result of topical agents applied to control pain, decrease vapor loss, prevent desiccation, and slow bacterial growth.[149] Nonaqueous topicals (silver sulfadiazine), if administered without providing free water such as 5% dextrose, may result in hypernatremia and its CNS consequences, including intracranial bleeding. In contrast, aqueous topical agents such as 5% silver nitrate solution may cause hyponatremia and its consequences of cerebral edema and seizure secondary to electrolyte leaching. Central pontine demyelination may occur if the hyponatremia is corrected rapidly with salt solutions. Serum ionized calcium and magnesium should also be monitored.

OPERATIVE MANAGEMENT

Overall, nearly 25% of trauma patients present with pre-existing conditions such as cirrhosis; cardiovascular, pulmonary, and renal diseases; coagulation disorders; diabetes; and alcohol or drug abuse that may increase trauma-related morbidity and mortality and require additional care.[156] Premedication is rarely indicated, especially in those who are hypovolemic, head-injured, or intoxicated. If needed, small doses of opioid (morphine, 1 to 2 mg; fentanyl, 25 to 50 μg) or sedative (midazolam, 0.5 to 1.0 mg) may be administered with close monitoring of vital signs. Regional analgesia may be provided for stable patients with skeletal injuries awaiting surgery. Femoral nerve block, for example, provides excellent analgesia for femoral shaft fractures. Evaluation of the multiple trauma patient emergently transported to the OR involves reviewing pre-existing conditions, the vital signs, oxygenation, and preoperative fluid replacement, and confirmation of correct position and patency of a previously inserted endotracheal tube.

TABLE 36-9

GUIDELINES FOR INITIAL FLUID RESUSCITATION AFTER THERMAL INJURY

Adults and children >20 kg
Parkland formula[a]
  4.0 mL crystalloid per kg per % burn per first 24 hr
Modified Brooke formula[a]
  2.0 mL lactated Ringer per kg per % burn per first 24 hr
  Children <20 kg
  Crystalloid 2–3 mL/kg per % burn per 24 hr[a]
  Crystalloid with 5% dextrose at maintenance rate
  100 mL/kg for the first 10 kg and 50 mL/kg for the next
    10 kg for 24 hr
Clinical end points of burn resuscitation
  Urine output: 0.5–1 mL
  Pulse: 80–140 per min (age-dependent)
  Systolic BP: 60 mm Hg (infants); children 70–90 plus 2 × age
    in years mm Hg; adults MAP >60 mm Hg
  Base deficit: <2

BP, blood pressure; MAP, mean arterial pressure.
[a]50% of calculated volume is given during the first 8 hours, 25% is given during the second 8 hours, and the remaining 25% is given during the third 8 hours.

Monitoring

Table 36-10 lists monitoring techniques currently used in the OR and indicates their relative importance in the intraopera-

TABLE 36-10

TECHNIQUES TO MONITOR PHYSIOLOGIC PARAMETERS AND THEIR IMPORTANCE IN INTRAOPERATIVE MANAGEMENT OF THE TRAUMA PATIENT

■ PHYSIOLOGIC PARAMETER	■ DEGREE OF IMPORTANCE	■ MONITORING EQUIPMENT	■ SPECIFIC INTRAOPERATIVE USES IN THE TRAUMA PATIENT
Cardiac rate, rhythm, and myocardial ischemia	Essential	Five-lead electrocardiogram system with oscilloscope, digital display, recorder, and printer (three-lead system can be used)	Routine
Arterial blood pressure	Essential	Indirect Blood pressure cuff Doppler system Programmable oscillometric system Direct Pressure transducer with calibrated oscilloscope and recorder	Routine
Central venous pressure	Useful	Pressure transducer with calibrated oscilloscope and recorder	Hypovolemia Pericardial tamponade, myocardial contusion Air embolism Pulmonary contusion
Pulmonary artery pressures	Essential in multiple trauma	Pressure transducer with calibrated oscilloscope and recorder	Blunt chest injury (pericardial tamponade, myocardial contusion) Adult respiratory distress syndrome Differentiation of low-pressure and high-pressure pulmonary edema; traumatic (cardiac contusion) or preexisting heart failure
Cardiac output	Useful in some patients	Thermodilution cardiac output computer with recorder and printer	Same as pulmonary artery pressure measurement
Cardiac wall motion abnormalities, myocardial ischemia, flow through valves or septal defects	Useful in some patients	Transesophageal echocardiograph	Cardiac contusion Coronary artery injuries? Septal injuries Air embolism Thoracic aortic rupture Shock
Ventilation	Essential	End-tidal CO_2 monitor with waveform display and recording	Routine Head injury Air embolism
Arterial oxygenation	Essential	Airway pressure Pulse oximeter Arterial blood gases (intermittent or continuous)	Routine
Tissue oxygenation	Useful	Pulmonary artery catheter ($P\dot{v}O_2$) Arterial/venous lactate analyzer Base deficit	Low perfusion states
Renal function	Essential	Foley catheter and graduated container	In all major trauma patients
Temperature	Essential	Esophageal or rectal probe	Routine
Neuromuscular function	Essential	Peripheral nerve stimulator electromyograph	Head injury Open globe Sealed major vessel injury
Neurologic function	Useful	Intracranial pressure measurement with bolt, catheter, or fiberoptic sensor Jugular bulb O_2 saturation	Head injury
Depth of anesthesia		Bispectral index monitor	Intraoperative awareness
Blood coagulation	Useful	Prothrombin time/partial thromboplastin time/platelet count/fibrinogen, tube test, thrombelastograph	Shock Massive transfusion Pre-existing coagulation abnormalities

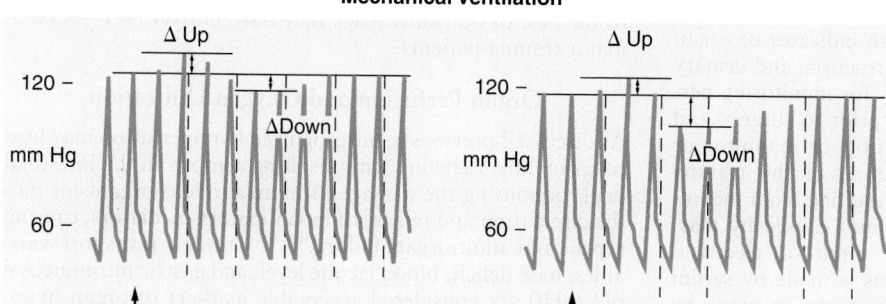

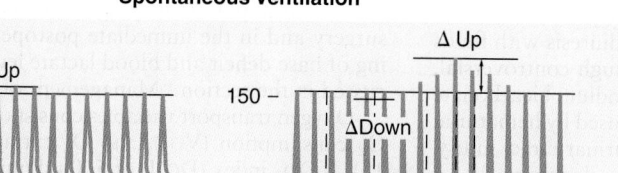

Baseline |← 5 Sec →| **1000 ml Blood Loss**

FIGURE 36-8. Arterial pressure records of a mechanically ventilated patient before (*left*) and after (*right*) 1,000 mL blood loss. Note the increase in systolic pressure variation and Δ down component following hemorrhage. Decrease in blood pressure occurs during exhalation with mechanical ventilation and inspiration in spontaneously breathing subjects (*upgoing arrow* defines inhalation). Δ Up is the difference between the end-expiratory systolic pressure and the maximum systolic pressure over a respiratory cycle. See text for definition of systolic pressure variation and Δ down component. (Reprinted from Rooke GA, Schwid HA, Shapira Y: The effect of graded hemorrhage and intravascular volume replacement on systolic pressure variation in humans during mechanical and spontaneous ventilation. Anesth Analg 1995; 80: 925, with permission.)

tive care of the trauma patient. Clearly, valuable time can be lost if the placement of invasive monitors takes precedence over resuscitation.

Hemodynamic Monitoring

Direct intra-arterial pressure monitoring, which permits beat-to-beat data acquisition and sampling for measurement of blood gases, should be in place before surgery (see Chapter 27). An ultrasound-guided technique or a surgical cutdown may be necessary to facilitate access. The radial artery is the vessel of choice in abdominal or chest trauma in which the aorta may be cross-clamped, making a femoral or dorsalis pedis cannula nonfunctional. The right radial artery is preferred in cases of chest trauma in which cross-clamping of the descending aorta might result in occlusion of the left subclavian artery. In mechanically ventilated patients, the magnitude of systolic pressure variation (the difference between the maximum and minimum systolic pressure over the respiratory cycle) and its Δ down component (the difference between systolic pressure at end expiration and the lowest value during the respiratory cycle) can provide reliable information about the intravascular volume status (Fig. 36-8). A systolic pressure variation >5 mm Hg and a Δ down >2 mm Hg suggest hypovolemia.[157]

Delaying emergent surgery to place a central venous line is rarely indicated unless a large-bore catheter is needed for volume resuscitation. However, if the patient is elderly, if there is a likelihood of myocardial damage, or if there is multiple-organ damage with requirement for prolonged surgery and massive fluid replacement, early placement of a CVP or pulmonary artery catheter is indicated before the development of coagulopathy renders it hazardous.

Several recently described dynamic measurement techniques may be useful in assessing hypovolemia and the response to fluid loading.[158] Of these, pulse contour analysis, using a mathematical algorithm, can determine the stroke volume, cardiac output, and systemic vascular resistance. The esophageal Doppler monitor can determine stroke volume and cardiac output; by using these parameters one can calculate aortic flow time, which correlates with preload, and peak velocity of blood flow, which correlates with myocardial contractility, enabling the clinician to assess intravascular volume, response to fluid loading, and myocardial performance. These techniques cannot be definitively recommended, however, as they have not been tested in trauma patients.

Volumetric assessment of preload appears to correlate better with cardiac index than the CVP or PCWP.[159] A pulmonary artery catheter equipped with a rapid-response thermistor and intracardiac electrodes is capable of measuring right ventricular (RV) cardiac output and ejection fraction, and calculating RV end-diastolic volume index. The latter appears to correlate with cardiac output better than CVP and PCWP in trauma patients. An RV end-diastolic volume index >130 mL/m² is considered optimal for organ perfusion.[159]

The mixed venous O_2 saturation can also convey important information about organ perfusion; it can be determined by analyzing blood from the pulmonary artery or continuously via a fiberoptic sensor at the junction of the superior vena cava and the right atrium. Of these parameters, systolic pressure variation and stroke volume appear to correlate best with intravascular volume status.

The TEE provides valuable diagnostic information in blunt cardiac injury, cardiac septal or valvular damage, coronary artery injury, pericardial tamponade, and aortic rupture.[160] It also permits assessment of cardiac function, including right and left ventricular volume, ejection fraction, wall motion abnormalities, pulmonary hypertension, and cardiac output, and detects acute ischemia more accurately than either ECG or pulmonary artery pressure monitoring. Monitoring left ventricular volume alone can provide information about the adequacy of the intravascular volume. This technique also allows visualization of fat and air entry into the right heart, or the left heart through a patent foramen ovale, during internal fixation of lower-extremity fractures.[161] In the trauma setting, it is possible that the TEE probe may be introduced into an unrecognized esophageal tear because the insidious nature of esophageal injury makes diagnosis difficult during the first 24 hours after trauma.

Urine Output

Urine output is routinely monitored as an indicator of organ perfusion, hemolysis, skeletal muscle destruction, and urinary tract integrity after trauma. Its reliability for monitoring perfusion is decreased by prolonged shock prior to surgery and osmotic diuresis caused by administration of mannitol or radiopaque dye. Dark, cola-colored urine in the trauma patient suggests either hemoglobinuria resulting from incompatible blood transfusion, or myoglobinuria caused by massive skeletal muscle destruction after blunt or electrical trauma. Although the definitive diagnosis is made by serum electrophoresis, rapid differential diagnosis can be made by centrifugation of a blood specimen. Pink-stained serum suggests hemoglobinuria, whereas unstained serum indicates myoglobinuria. Both of these conditions may result in acute renal failure. Prevention involves inducing diuresis with fluids and mannitol and, in myoglobinuria, although controversial, additional alkalinization of the urine with sodium bicarbonate to pH >5.6. Red-colored urine usually is caused by hematuria, which in the traumatized patient, suggests urinary tract injury. It should be investigated with intravenous pyelography.

Oxygenation

Frequently, most currently used older-generation pulse oximeters fail to provide accurate measurements in patients with O_2 saturation <90%, hypothermia, hypotension, decreased peripheral perfusion, or when excessive ambient light interferes with sensor function.[162] Trauma patients frequently develop these conditions, decreasing the usefulness of noninvasive O_2 saturation (SpO_2) monitoring. New-generation pulse oximeters are designed to be more accurate in these circumstances, although they are not absolutely exact. Two categories of these devices are available: forehead oximeters with reflectance mode sensors, produced primarily by Nellcor Pulse Oximetry, Nellcor Tyco Healthcare, Boulder, CO; and finger or earlobe pulse oximeters with transmission mode sensors, principally manufactured by Masimo. With the transmission mode sensor, the optical emitter and detector are positioned opposite to each other as on the finger, whereas in reflectance mode, the emitter and detector are positioned side by side. The forehead pulse oximeter is less affected by decreased perfusion because it senses the pulsation of the supraorbital artery, a branch of the carotid artery, which is presumably less affected by shock or hypothermia. However SpO_2 results with this monitor may be affected by venous pulsation, especially in patients receiving positive-pressure ventilation or in any situation that distends the tributaries of the superior vena cava.[163] It has been suggested that using these sensors with a head band that exerts 10- to 20-mm Hg pressure may minimize the inaccuracy.[163] The new-generation Masimo transmission mode pulse oximeters come in several types. Of these, the Masimo Blue Sensor attached to a Masimo Set Radical pulse oximeter appears to provide the most accurate results, comparable to those obtained with the forehead oximeter.[164,165]

With recent advances in technology, multiwavelength pulse co-oximeters are also capable of providing other physiologic data including pulse rate, SpO_2, perfusion index, carboxyhemoglobin, and methemoglobin. These monitors can also measure noninvasive continuous hemoglobin concentration ($SpHb$) with reasonable accuracy.[166] The ability of these new monitors (Masimo Rad 7 and Rad 57 Pulse CO-oximeter) to measure methemoglobin and carboxyhemoglobin concentration noninvasively renders them highly useful in acute burn injury management. A built-in algorithm also allows these monitors automatically to estimate the respiratory variations of the pulse oximetry curve, providing information about intravascular volume.[167] Although these monitors provide more accurate information than conventional pulse oximeters, to the best of our knowledge they have not yet been tested in major trauma patients.

Organ Perfusion and Oxygen Utilization

As discussed previously, unrecognized hypoperfusion may lead to splanchnic ischemia with resulting acidosis in the intestinal wall, permitting the passage of luminal micro-organisms into the circulation and release of inflammatory mediators, causing sepsis and multiorgan failure.[43–45] Oxygen transport variables, base deficit, blood lactate level, and gastric intramucosal pH (pHi) are considered acceptable markers of organ hypoperfusion in the *apparently* resuscitated patient and may be used to set the optimal end points of resuscitation.[45] Gastric intramucosal pH monitoring is too cumbersome to use during surgery and in the immediate postoperative period. Monitoring of base deficit and blood lactate level has already been discussed in the section "Management of Shock."

Oxygen transport variables consist of oxygen delivery (DO_2), O_2 consumption (VO_2), and O_2 extraction ratio (see Chapter 11). A DO_2 index (DO_2I) of 500 mL/min/m² has been shown to be an acceptable goal for optimal shock resuscitation,[168] performing as effectively as the previously recommended DO_2I of ≥600 mL/min/m². Selection of these specific numbers is based on the results of studies in which critically ill patients who could increase DO_2I above this level survived. At DO_2I ≥500 mL/min/m², patients received approximately 30% less crystalloids and blood transfusions than were required to attain the higher level. A computerized ICU bedside decision protocol developed to standardize shock resuscitation in some centers uses DO_2I >500 mL/min/m² as a goal.[168] This is a particularly useful end point because it integrates three important variables: hemoglobin concentration, arterial oxygen saturation, and cardiac output. The oxygen consumption index (VO_2I) is also an important variable. Subsequent organ failure may occur if it decreases below a value of 170 mL/min/m², indicating a flow-dependent phase of O_2 utilization.[45] Increasing DO_2I until VO_2I attains flow independence may prevent organ failure; however, this approach is not practical clinically, mainly because there are also DO_2I-independent regulators of VO_2.[168] Finally a global O_2 extraction ratio <0.25 to 0.3 suggests absence of dysoxia. However, it is possible that dysoxia may be present in an individual organ in the presence of a normal overall O_2 extraction ratio. Monitoring of O_2 transport variables, the most useful of which is DO_2I, is usually done in the ICU when invasive monitoring permits measurement of cardiac output and mixed venous O_2. These values can also be monitored in the OR whenever arterial and pulmonary artery lines are present.

A parameter that has been more recently used intraoperatively as a guide to resuscitation during emergency surgery for trauma patients is the end tidal–arterial CO_2 difference (Pa-ET) CO_2. Values >10 mm Hg after resuscitation predict mortality.[169] It may also be useful in the decision about when to perform damage control surgery and, intraoperatively, in guiding resuscitation with fluids, inotropes, and vasopressors.

Coagulation

Conventional blood coagulation monitoring includes a baseline and subsequent serial measurements of PT, activated partial thromboplastin time (aPTT), platelet count, blood fibrinogen level, and fibrin degradation products (FDP; see Chapter 16). Although trauma center laboratories cannot provide results of the standard coagulation tests within an hour, a blood sample should be sent to the laboratory to determine, at least retrospectively, the etiology of any coagulation abnormality. The "tube test," which involves obtaining a tube of blood with no anticoagulant and observing coagulation, clot retraction, and clot lysis, is a practical intraoperative method

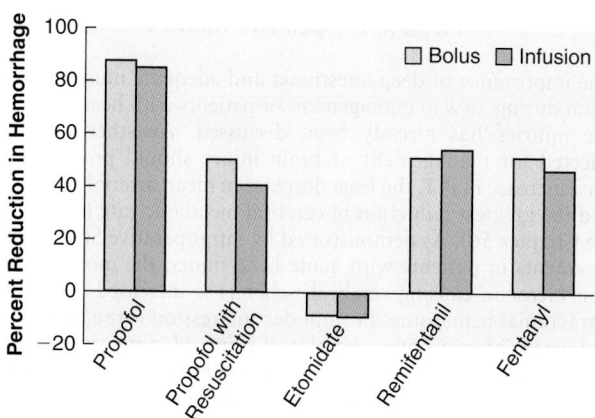

FIGURE 36-9. Calculated dose reduction of various anesthetics administered as a bolus or infusion in moderate hemorrhagic shock. Calculation is based on pharmacokinetic and pharmacodynamic studies performed in experimental hemorrhagic shock. (Reprinted from Shafer SL: Shock values. Anesthesiology 2004; 101: 567, with permission.)

of coagulation monitoring. If a good-quality clot does not form, or does so only after 10 to 20 minutes, clotting factor deficiency is the most likely cause. Failure of clot retraction within 1 hour after blood sampling suggests platelet depletion or dysfunction. Clot lysis earlier than 6 hours indicates fibrinolysis, which is infrequent in trauma patients. Disseminated intravascular coagulation (DIC) occurs frequently after trauma and is associated with absence of spontaneous clotting in the tube test. In addition to causing bleeding, it may prevent typing and cross-matching of blood.

Thrombelastography (TEG) is similar in principle to the tube test but provides a quantitative, graphic evaluation of clotting function.[170] TEG determines the time necessary for initial fibrin formation, the rapidity of fibrin deposition, clot consistency, the rate of clot formation, and the times required for clot retraction and lysis.[170] Basically, the R- and K-values are indices of formation, buildup, and cross-linking of fibrin, and depend on the function of coagulation factors. The maximum amplitude is the widest portion of the curve and indicates the absolute strength of the fibrin clot. It represents platelet function. The a-angle is the slope of the external divergence of the tracing from the R-value point, indicating the speed of clot formation and fibrin cross-linking. The value of this parameter is determined by both coagulation factors and platelets. Hypothermia can cause coagulopathy by interfering with both platelets and coagulation factors.[171] When the blood of a cold and coagulopathic patient is placed in the TEG cuvette, which is normally heated to 37°C, a near-normal trace may be obtained. Newer TEG devices are temperature-adjustable. Thus, the temperature in the cuvette can be adjusted to that of the patient.

Anesthetic and Adjunct Drugs

Apart from regional anesthesia techniques, which are used in patients with minor extremity injuries and stable hemodynamics, anesthetic and adjunct drugs for general anesthesia need to be tailored to five major clinical conditions. The varying contribution of these conditions to the clinical picture of a given patient necessitates priority-oriented planning.

Airway Compromise

Anesthetics and muscle relaxants should be avoided before the airway is secured if there is significant airway obstruction or if

there is doubt as to whether the patient's trachea can be intubated because of anatomic limitations. If time permits, lateral neck radiographs, CT scanning, and endoscopy can be used to better define the problem. Topical anesthesia with mild sedation can be used to secure the airway with a conventional blade or flexible FOB. If a rapid-sequence induction is contemplated, ketamine and etomidate may confer advantages over thiopental and propofol. In equipotent doses in normovolemic patients, they produce less cardiovascular depression. Although succinylcholine, with its short onset time and duration, is still the muscle relaxant of choice for rapid-sequence induction, rocuronium (0.9 to 1.2 mg/kg) has almost the same onset time and does not have the undesirable side effects associated with succinylcholine (e.g., increased intragastric pressure, intraocular pressure, and ICP; potassium release in patients with burns and neurologic diseases), its longer duration of action may be disadvantageous and may lead to hypoxia if both ventilation and intubation prove to be impossible (see Chapter 29). Under these circumstances, a Bullard blade, GlideScope, WuScope, Airtraq or other aids can be employed to overcome the problem; surgical standby for cricothyroidotomy maybe considered if other techniques fail.[172] Bradycardia, dysrhythmias, and cardiac arrest have been described after succinylcholine in the presence of hypoxia and hypercarbia; some of these complications may also follow an apparently uneventful intubation performed without succinylcholine.

Hypovolemia

Anesthetic agents not only have direct cardiovascular depressant effects, but also inhibit compensatory hemodynamic mechanisms such as central catecholamine output and baroreflex (neuroregulatory) mechanisms, which maintain systemic pressure in hypovolemia. Hemorrhage and hypovolemia lead to a higher than normal blood concentration following a given dose of intravenous agents, increased sensitivity of the brain to anesthetics, preferential distribution of the cardiac output to the brain and the heart, cerebral hypoxia, dilutional hypoproteinemia, and acidosis, all of which increase the effects of drugs on the brain and the heart.

The pharmacokinetic and pharmacodynamic responses of intravenous agent to experimental hemorrhagic shock vary (see Chapter 18). Because of the decrease in size of the central compartment and in systemic clearance, plasma concentrations of fentanyl and remifentanil are increased.[173] A decreased volume of distribution also increases the blood level of etomidate by 20% in shock,[174] and for propofol this effect is substantial. There is also variation in the extent of brain sensitivity to these agents. Although etomidate pharmacodynamics are unchanged,[175] a significant increase in the sensitivity of the brain and heart to propofol is noted in animals,[174] even after fluid resuscitation.[174] Based on these experimental findings, Shafer[176] calculated that in patients with shock, the dose of propofol should be only 10 to 20% of that given to a healthy patient. Although he calculated that etomidate dose should not require adjustment for shock, we decrease the dose by at least 25 to 50% when we suspect treated or untreated hypovolemia. Of the opioids, the calculated dose for fentanyl and remifentanil is approximately one half of that given to healthy patients[176] (Fig. 36-9). Of the remaining intravenous agents, thiopental and midazolam are also known to have significant cardiovascular depressant activity, whereas ketamine has stimulatory effects when the autonomic nervous system is intact.

There are also differences among anesthetics in the direction and extent of their effects on compensatory mechanisms. For example, the baroreceptor depression produced by intravenous agents is usually milder than that of inhalational agents (see Chapter 18). Opioid agents have little direct cardiovascular or baroreflex depressant effect; however, these agents can cause hypotension by inhibiting central sympathetic activity, especially in the hypovolemic trauma patient whose apparent hemodynamic stability is maintained by hyperactive sympathetic tone.

Two important principles in the use of anesthetic agents are accurate estimation of the degree of hypovolemia and reduction of doses accordingly. The presence of hypotension suggests uncompensated hypovolemia, in which case anesthetics almost invariably produce further deterioration of systemic blood pressure and sometimes cardiac standstill. Intravascular volume, to the extent possible, must be restored before their use. When time constraints or continuing hemorrhage prevent restoration of blood volume, the airway must be secured without the benefit of anesthesia (perhaps using only rapidly acting muscle relaxants and small doses of opioids, etomidate, or ketamine), even though this approach may result in recall of induction and intraoperative events in up to 40% of patients.[177] Hypothermia, alcohol intoxication, drug use before anesthesia, and metabolic disturbances in the acute trauma patient cannot reliably prevent recall. However, scopolamine, 0.6 mg, given before airway management may decrease the likelihood of this complication. Intraoperative use of the bispectral index monitor and, whenever possible, titrating anesthetics to bispectral index levels <60 may prevent recall in trauma patients.[178]

In normotensive but hypovolemic patients, restoration of volume and selection of an agent with the least cardiovascular depressant effect appears logical. Ketamine and etomidate are the preferred induction agents,[175] although at low doses other intravenous anesthetics are also unlikely to produce hypotension (see Chapter 18). Therefore, the use of any of these drugs in reduced doses is probably more important than the particular agent chosen. These principles may become especially important for the anesthesiologist if the concept of delayed fluid resuscitation, with hypovolemia prolonged until hemorrhage is controlled surgically, becomes widely accepted.[55]

Maintenance of anesthesia in the hypovolemic trauma patient raises concerns similar to those pertaining to induction. Recent experimental data has shown that depending on its severity hemorrhagic shock decreases minimum alveolar concentration (MAC) by approximately 25% (see Chapter 17). Restoration of intravascular volume did not, but administration of naloxone did, normalize MAC in the animals, suggesting that shock-induced release of endorphins is primarily responsible for reduction of isoflurane MAC.[179] Although the myocardial depressant effect of nitrous oxide (N_2O) is normally somewhat counterbalanced by its ability to increase sympathetic outflow, in acute hemorrhage there is already a dramatic increase in sympathetic activity and stimulation of baroreceptors. Under these circumstances, patients are unlikely to respond to the sympathetic effect of N_2O, and the cardiovascular depressant properties of the gas are unmasked; these may be similar to those of other inhalation agents. In addition, by reducing FIO_2, use of N_2O incurs a risk of hypoxemia in patients with reduced cardiac output or pulmonary compromise. Despite causing little impairment of reflex tachycardia and having a vasodilatory action that preserves organ blood flow in normovolemic patients, isoflurane can impair cardiac output and organ blood flow in hypovolemia—that is, it can cause cardiovascular depression. Desflurane and sevoflurane are not significantly better than isoflurane in this regard. However, because of their low solubility in blood, severe hemodynamic depression produced by these agents can be rapidly reversed, preventing suboptimal perfusion for a significant period of time. In summary, in the hypovolemic patient all inhalational agents may reduce both global and regional blood flows, and therefore, should be used only in small concentrations (<1 MAC). Opioid supplementation is usually well tolerated and often indicated.

Head and Open Eye Injuries

The importance of deep anesthesia and adequate muscle relaxation during airway management of patients with head or open eye injuries has already been discussed. Anesthetic agents selected for management of brain injury should produce the least increase in ICP, the least decrease in mean arterial pressure, and the greatest reduction in cerebral metabolic rate ($CMRO_2$; see Chapter 56). As demonstrated by intraoperative $SjvO_2$ measurements in patients with acute head injury, the most important factor in causing cerebral ischemia is increased ICP from intracranial hematoma. Prompt decompression is the most crucial means of ensuring cerebral well-being. Hypotension caused by anesthetics or other factors contributes to the development or progression of cerebral ischemia. Utmost attention should be paid during anesthesia to avoidance of hypotension (mean arterial pressure <60 mm Hg) and, more important, if reliable $SjvO_2$ monitoring is in place, to avoid values <55 to 60%. With the possible exception of ketamine, all intravenous anesthetics cause comparable degrees of cerebrovascular constriction.[180] Thiopental, midazolam, propofol, and etomidate therefore also produce a dose-dependent reduction in cerebrospinal fluid formation. Again, with the exception of ketamine, $CMRO_2$ is also reduced by all the available intravenous anesthetics.[180] An important drawback to these agents is that their cardiovascular depressant effects may reduce CPP.[180] This problem can be ameliorated by administering pretreatment doses of opioids (fentanyl, 2 to 3 $\mu g/kg$), which permit reduction of the anesthetic dose. This may also prevent the myoclonic movements associated with etomidate and occasionally with propofol, and thus reduce the risks of ICP and IOP increase. Nevertheless, myoclonus is best prevented by careful timing of the dose of muscle relaxants.[181] Another measure to preserve CPP during anesthesia is to administer vasopressors, being aware that hypovolemia may be masked by their use.

Ordinarily, administration of succinylcholine should follow pretreatment doses of nondepolarizing agents to prevent fasciculation-induced elevation of ICP and IOP[182] (see Chapter 20). Avoiding succinylcholine usually does not alleviate the problem because laryngoscopy and tracheal intubation produce a greater and longer-lasting increase in IOP and ICP.[183] Rocuronium, 0.9 to 1.2 mg/kg, has an onset time comparable with that of succinylcholine.[184] Mivacurium has a longer onset time than rocuronium and, unlike rocuronium, can cause vasodilatation and hypotension. None of the nondepolarizing muscle relaxants causes elevation of ICP or IOP in the absence of associated tracheal intubation.

All inhalation anesthetics may increase CBF, cerebral blood volume, and thus the ICP. Cerebral autoregulation, CO_2 responsiveness, and $CMRO_2$ are reduced. Unlike thiopental, which decreases both CBF and $CMRO_2$ in parallel, inhalational anesthetics decrease $CMRO_2$ while increasing the CBF. The extent of this uncoupling varies with the agent and the dose. Isoflurane has the least vasodilatory effect and thus is the most widely used inhalation anesthetic, although desflurane and sevoflurane have comparable effects on the cerebral circulation. In hyperventilated patients with cerebral tumors or mild edema, isoflurane does not raise the ICP if it is administered at an inspired concentration of <1 MAC. In the presence of severe head injury, when cerebral autoregulation and CO_2 responsiveness are impaired, isoflurane has the potential to increase CBF and ICP even at levels <1 MAC and with hyperventilation. Therefore, it may be prudent not to use this agent at high concentrations in the presence of elevated ICP, at least until the skull is opened and the ICP is controlled. In these patients, anesthesia can be maintained initially with opioids plus thiopental, propofol, midazolam, or etomidate.

Nitrous oxide may increase CBF, cerebral blood volume, and ICP when administered with inhalation anesthetics if the

PaCO$_2$ is normal or increased. This effect may be eliminated when this agent is administered with adequate doses of barbiturates or hyperventilation. The effect on CMRO$_2$ is variable: both an increase and a decrease have been observed. Thus, N$_2$O probably is not deleterious in patients with head injury with minimal ICP elevation, if it is used after a bolus dose or during infusion of intravenous anesthetics.

In a spontaneously breathing patient, opioids may produce hypoventilation with an associated increase in CBF and ICP; therefore, they should be used in head trauma only in mechanically ventilated patients (see Chapter 39). Some reports suggest that opioids and, to a smaller extent, opiates may interfere with CPP by increasing ICP, decreasing mean arterial pressure, or both.[5,185] Fentanyl and sufentanil are most implicated, and it appears that this phenomenon occurs when the head injury is severe.[186] Although the clinical significance of these findings is not yet clear, it is prudent to administer fentanyl or its analogs slowly, when the arterial pressure is normal or slightly elevated, ensuring preservation of systemic blood pressure with vasoactive agents, if necessary.

Cardiac Injury

If there is pericardial tamponade, preload and myocardial contractility should be maintained (see Chapter 41) as any decrease in these parameters may exacerbate an already existing RV inflow occlusion. A decrease in heart rate should also be treated promptly to maintain adequate cardiac output. Because all the available anesthetics can depress myocardial contractility and cause vasodilation, it is preferable to administer these agents after evacuation of pericardial blood under local anesthesia. If general anesthesia is required to relieve the tamponade, induction should be delayed until the patient is prepared and draped. Both anesthetics and controlled ventilation, particularly with PEEP, impair cardiac output. Deep anesthesia and high airway pressures should be avoided before evacuation of the hemopericardium. In chronic pericardial effusion, ketamine supports the cardiac index better than diazepam. In acute pericardial tamponade, even minor insults can bring cardiac activity to a halt. Ketamine thus remains the agent of choice. It should be given in small doses after adequate fluid infusion. Similar principles apply to the use of maintenance agents, which should be given in the smallest possible doses until the heart is decompressed. TEE monitoring may aid management between induction and pericardiotomy.

In blunt myocardial injury, the objective is not only to maintain cardiac contractility, but also to lower the elevated pulmonary vascular resistance that may result from concomitant pulmonary contusion, atelectasis or aspiration. Preferably, all anesthetics should be administered after restoration of intravascular volume and titrated to maintain adequate systemic blood pressure and cardiac output. If necessary, inotropes, preferably amrinone or milrinone, which produce some pulmonary vasodilation, may be used. Anesthetic maintenance by infusion of intravenous anesthetics and opioids to avoid the myocardial depression produced by inhalational agents should also be considered.

Burns

A hypermetabolic state characterized by tachycardia, tachypnea, catecholamine surge, increased O$_2$ consumption, and augmented catabolism follows the initial few hours of a burn and continues into the convalescent phase, necessitating increased oxygen, ventilation, and nutrition.[133] Early extensive and repeated escharotomies with coverage of skin grafts attenuate postburn hypermetabolic response, decrease fluid loss, and improve survival. It is usually performed between the second day and the second week, often necessitating massive transfusion, temperature control, and management of fluid,

electrolyte, and coagulation abnormalities. Usually either an autograft harvested from the patient, allograft from a cadaver, or both, is used. Recently, artificial skin, Integra (Integra Life Sciences, Plainsboro, NJ) consisting of dermal inner layer made of bovine collagen and chondroitin-6-sulfate and neoepidermal outer layer made of polysiloxane polymer is also used with more favorable reduction of resting energy expenditure and elevation of serum proteins as compared with cadaveric skin.[187]

Anesthetic management of escharotomies presents several difficulties. Burned tissue may prevent access for ECG, pulse oximeter, neuromuscular function, and noninvasive blood pressure monitoring; needle electrodes or surgical staples, a reflectance pulse oximeter, and an arterial catheter may be necessary. Large-bore intravenous catheters are essential. Hyperthermia occurs, but hypothermia is more likely in the OR and is to be avoided. Exposure and evaporative fluid loss necessitate maintenance of the OR temperature between 28 and 32°C, use of countercurrent fluid and blood-warming devices, surface heating with forced dry, warm air, and humidified inspired gases. Blood loss can be controlled by restricting the escharotomy to 15 to 20% of TBSA, use of extremity tourniquets, administering topical thrombin and fibrin sealants on the excised area,[188] applying dilute epinephrine solution topically (1:10,000) or by injection (0.5 mg per 1,000 mL), and using compression bandages. Epinephrine doses of up to 6.7 mg topically or 0.8 mg by injection to the surgical area are well tolerated; the affinity of β-adrenergic receptors to ligands is decreased after burns. The administration of a large amount of blood and blood products subjects the patient to complications of transfusion such as coagulopathy. Although citrate-induced hypocalcemia is a relatively rare complication of transfusion,[189] monitoring of Ca^{2+} and administration of calcium chloride (2.5 to 5.0 mg/kg) or gluconate (7.5 to 10.0 mg/kg) should be considered when blood products are administered rapidly.

Shock, hyperdynamic circulation, decreased serum albumin concentration, increased α_1-acid glycoprotein concentration, and altered receptor sensitivity alter the response to various drugs during the resuscitative and convalescent phases.[133] The doses of intravenous anesthetics should be reduced during the resuscitation phase to prevent excessive hemodynamic depression. Burn patients have excruciating pain and exceedingly high opioid requirements. A proven anesthetic regimen for excision and grafting of burns is isoflurane plus large doses of opioid. The response to depolarizing and nondepolarizing muscle relaxants remains unaltered during the first 24 hours after burn injury. However, after the first day, succinylcholine should be avoided for at least 1 year because it can result in a potentially lethal increase of serum K$^+$ when the burn size exceeds 10% of TBSA. The mechanism of this response is related to up-regulation (increase) of acetylcholine receptors, which ultimately occupy the entire muscle membrane, the additional expression of two new isoforms of acetylcholine receptor, and the recently described nicotinic (neural) α-7 acetylcholine receptors. The latter can be depolarized not only by acetylcholine and succinylcholine, but also by choline, which thus plays an important role in the development of hyperkalemia.[190] Resistance develops to all nondepolarizing muscle relaxants, except mivacurium in patients with burns of >30% TBSA starting approximately 1 week and peaking 5 to 6 weeks after injury, probably from pharmacodynamic causes.[133,134] Increasing the dose can partly overcome this resistance. For instance, rocuronium, which is important for rapid-sequence induction and treatment of laryngospasm when succinylcholine is contraindicated, has an onset time delayed by about 50 seconds (30% longer than patients without burn) when a 0.9 mg/kg dose is used. Increasing the dose to 1.2 mg/kg decreases the delay by 30 seconds but the onset time remains about 25 to 30 seconds longer than that observed in patients without burn.

Intubating conditions also improve by increasing the dose. Recovery time from block is shorter in burn patients than in normal individuals.[191]

For serial wound debridement, ketamine in intermittent doses, neuraxial or peripheral nerve blocks via an indwelling catheter, or sedation with opioids and intravenous agents may be employed.

Management of Intraoperative Complications

Persistent Hypotension

15 Persistent hypotension following trauma is usually the result of one of four mechanisms: bleeding, tension pneumothorax, neurogenic shock, and cardiac injury. Although many other causes, such as citrate intoxication (hypocalcemia), hypothermia, coronary artery disease, allergic reactions, or incompatible transfusion may be responsible for this complication, they occur infrequently.

Hypotension is most likely due to bleeding. The source may be obvious, such as external bleeding from the skull or an open vessel in the extremities, or hidden. The thoracic and abdominal cavities and the pelvic retroperitoneal space are the most common sites of occult hemorrhage that results in hypotension. Management includes early diagnosis and control of the bleeding site plus effective fluid resuscitation. The latter can best be accomplished using an infusion system with large-diameter tubing (5 mm) and a countercurrent heat exchanger. Up to 1,000 mL/min of crystalloid solution or 600 mL/min of packed cells can be given if a box-type pressure pump and a large-bore intravenous cannula are used. The system should be connected to 14-gauge or larger cannulas, preferably inserted into veins both above and below the diaphragm. The rapid infusor system (Belmont Instrument Corp., Bellerica, MA), which consists of a reservoir, countercurrent heating system, and roller pump, is capable of delivering up to 1,600 mL/min of warm fluids once the rate of infusion is programmed.

Of the isotonic crystalloid solutions, LR is preferred over normal saline. Experimental evidence shows that resuscitation with normal saline during uncontrolled hemorrhage is associated with greater urine output and thus greater fluid requirement compared with LR, resulting in hyperchloremic acidosis and dilutional coagulopathy.[192] Acidosis does not occur with LR, but tissue edema may result from its slight hypotonicity (273 mOsm/L), and neutralization of the citrate anticoagulant in PRBCs may occur because of its Ca^{2+} content.

Human serum albumin (5 and 25%) and hydroxyethyl starch are the most commonly used colloids. Hetastarch, a high-molecular-weight (670 kDa) polymeric glucose compound, is currently the most commonly used hydroxyethyl starch in the United States. Because of its molecular weight, it remains within the blood vessels and can restore the blood volume. However, it also has an adverse effect on coagulation, especially on platelets, factor VIII, and von Willebrand factor. Thus, the recommended dose should not exceed 20 mL/kg, although a review suggests that there is little support for this recommendation.[193] Its intravascular retention and adverse effects on coagulation are not only related to its molecular weight but also to molar substitution, which is defined as the number of hydroxyethyl groups per glucose subunit; the higher the molar substitution, the higher the intravascular retention and thus the more severe the coagulopathy. Efforts to reduce molecular weight and molar substitution in order to maintain intravascular retention and yet minimize coagulopathy recently resulted in the development of a new compound, hydroxyethyl starch 130/0.4 (Voluven; Fresnius Kabi, Bad Homburg, Germany), in Europe with a molecular weight of 130 kDa and molar substitution of 0.4. Although its use in major

trauma patients remains to be investigated, it appears to provide adequate vascular volume expansion with less coagulation abnormality in patients undergoing major orthopaedic surgery.

Although highly experimental, a new concept in hemorrhagic shock management is the combined use of fluid and vasopressor treatment. Theoretically, this strategy may rapidly restore blood pressure to normal levels while limiting the fluid volume infused. A moderate dose of norepinephrine with fluids has been shown to improve short-term survival in experimental animals.[194] Neurogenic shock from spinal cord injury may be missed during initial evaluation, especially in unconscious patients. However, differentiation of neurogenic shock from hemorrhagic shock is important[195]: patients with spinal cord injury are often bradycardic and readily respond to catecholamine administration. Mistaking neurogenic shock for hemorrhagic shock may lead to excessive fluid infusion and pulmonary edema. The reverse error may also occur: depriving patients with hemorrhagic shock of fluids because of misdiagnosis of neurogenic shock. Invasive central hemodynamic monitoring may be indicated in such patients.[112] In some patients, of course, hemorrhagic shock and neurogenic shock may coexist.

Cardiac causes of persistent hypotension include blunt cardiac injury and pericardial tamponade. Intraoperative TEE can be useful in the differential diagnosis. The RV is most commonly involved in blunt cardiac injury. If there is a concomitant increase in pulmonary vascular resistance (e.g., from an associated pulmonary contusion), the RV pressure increases while its output decreases, resulting in an increased CVP. The raised RV pressure causes the interventricular septum to shift toward the left, decreasing left ventricular compliance, increasing its diastolic pressure, and decreasing cardiac output (ventricular interdependence). These alterations in cardiac anatomy and ventricular dynamics can be displayed by TEE, information that can be useful during interpretation of elevated cardiac-filling pressures.

In the absence of TEE, a pulmonary artery catheter may be helpful. Equalization of pressures across the cardiac chambers during diastole suggests pericardial tamponade. A similar picture may also be seen in severe blunt cardiac injury, causing difficulty in differential diagnosis. This effect, however, is rare and is usually associated with critical hemodynamic instability. Differential diagnosis in these instances can be established by pericardiocentesis. Septal encroachment into the left ventricle from RV contusion results in an increase in pulmonary artery wedge pressure. Decreasing the rate of fluid infusion in these patients results in a further decrease in cardiac output. Treatment includes fluid infusion, pulmonary vasodilators if the systemic blood pressure is normal, and inotropic support if the systemic blood pressure is low. Absence of response to this treatment is an indication for placement of an intra-aortic balloon pump. Pulmonary artery catheterization may also help detect an oxygen step-up from septal injury. During thoracotomy, a distended RV should also raise the suspicion of a septal defect.

Hypothermia

Shock, alcohol intoxication, exposure to cold, fluid resuscitation, and abnormalities in thermoregulatory mechanisms render the major trauma patient hypothermic during the initial phase of injury. Admission hypothermia, which is present in approximately 50% of patients, is an independent risk factor after major trauma,[196] and the mortality rate increases with decreasing temperature. Severe hypothermia, which in the trauma patient is defined as core temperature below 32°C,[197] was associated with a 100% mortality rate in one study.[198] The intraoperative risk of hypothermia is also higher for the trauma patient than for electively operated patients.[199] Heat loss increases especially in patients with spinal cord, extensive soft-tissue, and burn injuries, and in those who consumed ethanol before surgery or patients undergoing body cavity surgery.

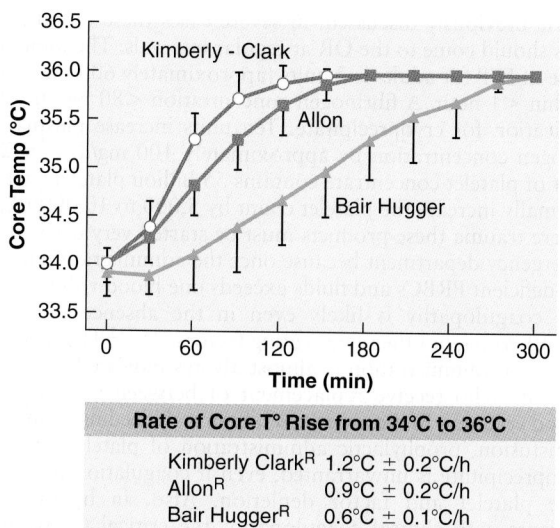

Rate of Core T° Rise from 34°C to 36°C	
Kimberly Clark[R]	1.2°C ± 0.2°C/h
Allon[R]	0.9°C ± 0.2°C/h
Bair Hugger[R]	0.6°C ± 0.1°C/h

FIGURE 36-10. The rate of rise in core temperature with circulating water and forced air devices used in healthy anesthetized volunteers. Circulating water devices warm the body faster than forced air devices. (Reproduced from Wadhwa A, Komatsu R, Orhan-Sungur M et al: New circulating water devices warm more quickly than forced-air in volunteers. Anesth Analg 2007; 105: 1681, with permission.)

Hypothermia causes cardiac depression, myocardial ischemia, dysrhythmias, peripheral vasoconstriction, impaired tissue oxygen delivery, elevated oxygen consumption during rewarming, blunted response to catecholamines, increased blood viscosity, metabolic acidosis, altered platelet and clotting function, abnormalities of K^+ and Ca^{2+} hemostasis, reduced drug clearance, and increased risk of infection.[196–199] Rewarming after hypothermia, especially at a rapid rate, may release accumulated metabolic products into the central circulation causing further myocardial depression, hypotension, and increased acidosis. Because of these adverse effects, deliberate hypothermia, although it is believed to be protective of organ function, has no indication during resuscitation from hemorrhagic shock and the management of head injury.

Prevention of hypothermia and correction of body temperature to normal appear to decrease mortality rate, blood loss, fluid requirement, organ failure, and length of ICU stay.[200] Convective warming with forced dry air at 43°C can prevent a temperature drop in most trauma patients but cannot effectively treat severe hypothermia; because the low specific heat of air has little heat content to give to the cold trauma patient, and often because of the nature of the surgical procedure, only a limited body surface area is exposed to warming.[200] Newly developed circulating-water warmers that occupy a relatively smaller body surface area than forced air warmers may produce faster rewarming[201] (Fig. 36-10). Airway warming can reduce the heat loss caused by the latent heat of vaporization, but this technique also transfers very little heat.[200] Administration of warm intravenous fluids is the most effective way to prevent and treat hypothermia in the trauma patient, provided that they are administered at a relatively rapid rate. For each liter of fluid given at 40°C to a patient with a body temperature of 33°C, 29.33 kJ of heat energy is gained; the specific heat of water is 4.19 kJ/L/°C. Countercurrent heat exchanging systems are more effective than dry heat or still-water bath warmers. They warm the fluid to 40°C, and the delivered fluid temperature is not affected by the rate of administration. The most effective method that may be used when rapid warming is intended, however, is continuous arteriovenous rewarming, which can be achieved using a modified level 1 countercurrent

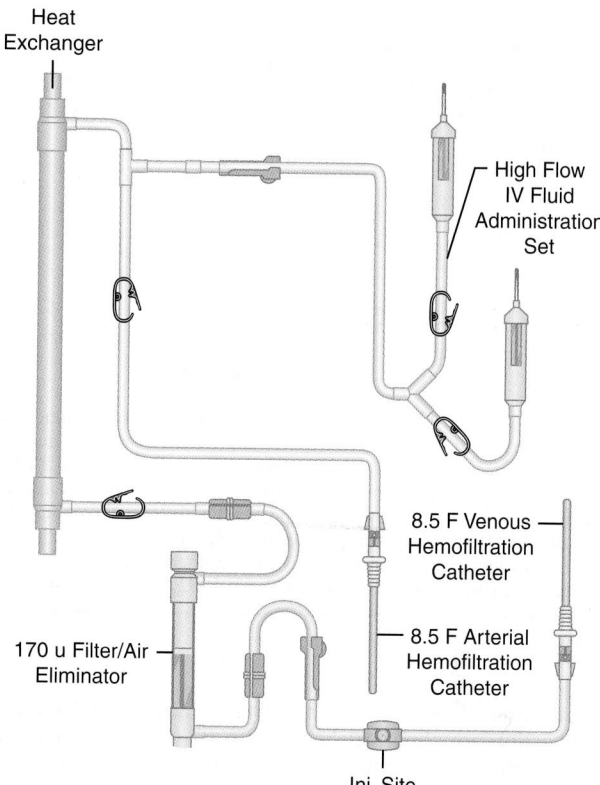

FIGURE 36-11. Schematic drawing of the system used for continuous arteriovenous rewarming. IV, intravenous; F, French; Injection (Reprinted from Gentilello LM, Cobean R, Offner PJ et al: Continuous arteriovenous rewarming: Rapid reversal of hypothermia in critically ill patients. J Trauma 1992; 32: 316, with permission.)

system (Fig. 36-11). The blood exits the body from a percutaneously placed femoral arterial catheter at the patient's pressure, and then is warmed in the infusion system and returned to the body through a venous cannula. Because the circuit tubing is heparin bonded, there is no need for heparinization. This technique can be used in the ICU and can rewarm a hypothermic patient (T <35°C) in approximately 40 minutes.[200,202]

Coagulation Abnormalities

In trauma, multiple factors may be responsible for coagulopathy: dilution of coagulation factors and platelets, disturbance of fibrinogen/fibrin polymerization by hydroxyethyl starch infusion,[203] tissue hypoperfusion, and hypoxia, hypothermia, acidosis, and DIC (see Chapter 16). DIC results from acute release of thromboplastin from injured brain, fat, amniotic fluid, or other sources, or subacutely from endothelial inflammation or failure interfering with clearance of activated coagulation factors, causing microthrombi and consumption coagulopathy.[204] It is also suggested that early coagulopathy, before fluid administration, is caused by tissue hypoperfusion, which increases thrombomodulin and diverts thrombin from fibrin generation to activation of protein C.[205] Hypothermia affects platelet morphology, function, and sequestration and retards enzyme activity, slowing the initiation and propagation of platelet plugs and fibrin clot, as well as enhancing fibrinolytic activity.[60,63] The mechanism of hypothermia-induced coagulopathy is complex and depends on the extent of temperature decrease. Down to 33°C there is little alteration in coagulation enzyme activity, explaining the practically unchanged values reported for aPTT.[206] Within this temperature range, coagulopathy results from altered platelet

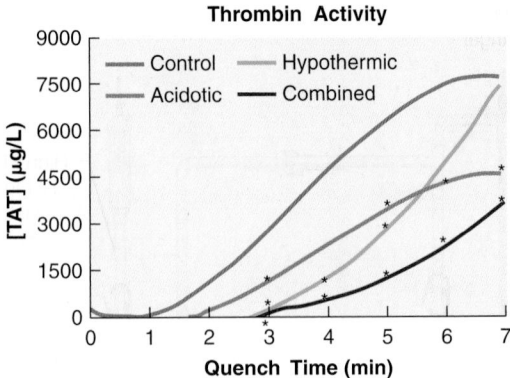

FIGURE 36-12. Thrombin generation rate in normal, acidotic, hypothermic, and acidotic and hypothermic swine. Thrombin generation was determined by measuring thrombin-antithrombin III (TAT) concentration in blood samples obtained at 1-minute intervals in each condition. Note that acidosis and hypothermia decrease thrombin generation rate. (Reproduced from Martini WZ, Pusateri AE, Uscilowicz JM et al: Independent contributions of hypothermia and acidosis to coagulopathy in swine. J Trauma 2005; 58: 1002, with permission.)

aggregation/adhesion.[206] Both enzymatic activity and platelet aggregation are abnormal below 33°C.[206] Thus, the aPTT at temperatures from 33 to 37°C does not provide any meaningful information about coagulation status, even when the test is performed at the hypothermic patient's temperature, because it does not measure platelet adhesion. In contrast, thrombelastography at the patient's temperature may be reflective of the degree of coagulopathy.[203]

Metabolic acidosis is probably a stronger coagulation enzyme inhibitor than hypothermia: it interferes with generation of thrombin, a factor essential in activating cofactors, platelets, and enzymes, in addition to converting fibrinogen to fibrin. This effect of acidosis is potentiated by hypothermia. Figure 36-12 shows the (indirectly determined) thrombin generation rate by measurement of thrombin-antithrombin III (TAT) complex concentrations in swine.[207] Perioperative diagnosis of coagulopathy is often made by observing bleeding from wounds or puncture sites, rather than by interpretation of laboratory tests. However, the differential diagnosis between consumptive and dilutional coagulopathy requires laboratory testing, although the results of these tests are usually delayed. In general, the inability to determine the type of coagulopathy does not present a problem because the initial treatment is similar for both conditions. Nevertheless, the diagnosis of DIC has prognostic significance because its treatment involves elimination of its cause(s). The presence of elevated circulating fibrin degradation products (FDP/fdp), especially when >40 mg/mL, is suggestive of DIC, but the result of this study will reach the clinician long after the completion of initial resuscitation. A fibrinogen level <100 mg/dL is also suggestive of DIC, but reduction to this value often takes a long time, decreasing the diagnostic value of the test, although serial measurements may be useful. A combination of platelet count, PT and partial thromboplastin time, fibrinogen, a few clotting factors and inhibitors and FDP/fdp measurement may be more useful than individual tests. A diagnostic scoring system consisting of platelet count, PT, fibrinogen level, and FDP/fdp measurements has been suggested to rule DIC in or out.[208] It has been shown that transfusion of PRBCs in elective surgery results in earlier depletion of coagulation factors than of platelets.[209,210] Thus it is not unreasonable to administer FFP, liquid plasma, or cryoprecipitate before or simultaneously with platelets during emergency trauma surgery.

As previously discussed, in severe cases these blood products should come to the OR at regular intervals. The minimum dose of FFP for adults is 2 units (approximately 600 mL) given within <1 hour. A fibrinogen concentration <80 mg/dL is an indication for cryoprecipitate. Ten units increase plasma fibrinogen concentration by approximately 100 mg/dL.[211] Each unit of platelet concentrate contains 55 billion platelets, which normally increase the platelet count by 5,000 to 10,000/μL. In severe trauma these products must be started very early in the emergency department because once the administration of factor-deficient PRBCs and fluids exceeds one blood volume, clinical coagulopathy is likely even in the absence of shock, hypothermia, or other aggravating factors.[211,212] Thus, platelet or factor administration is almost always indicated in trauma patients who receive replacement of between one and two blood volumes. In the absence of abnormal bleeding or massive transfusion, prophylactic administration of platelets, FFP, or cryoprecipitate is unwarranted, even if coagulation tests indicate platelet and factor depletion. Also, in hypothermic patients with clinical coagulopathy, the critical treatment is rewarming rather than platelet and coagulation factor administration, although some circumstances may require both.

Recombinant factor VIIa may be indicated for off-label use in selected patients with hemorrhage-induced coagulopathy. By activating factor X this agent produces a thrombin burst, which in turn converts fibrinogen to fibrin. The thrombin burst is augmented by platelet activation by factor X. Severe acidosis, hypothermia, and hemodilution block the effect of factor VIIa. Thus, to obtain benefit, it should be administered after correction of pH and hypothermia at least to 7.2 and 33°C, respectively.[213] Although numerous retrospective series and case reports suggest the usefulness of this agent in trauma-induced coagulopathy, so far there is only one phase II, multicenter, randomized controlled trial of rFVIIa in major trauma, using much higher (200 μg/kg) than usual doses (90 μg/kg for patients in shock and 1.2 mg in those not in shock).[214] The drug was able to reduce PRBC transfusion by 2.6 units in surviving victims of blunt trauma, but failed to produce any effect in penetrating trauma patients. Neither 48-hour nor 30-day survival was affected by rFVIIa and, when all surviving and nonsurviving patients were considered, the reduction in PRBC replacement was insignificant.

Because of its high cost, rFVIIa is used under strict protocol in many centers, in patients with survivable injury and/or medical disease, who are not in terminal shock as evidenced by pH <7.0 and K+ >6.0 mEq/L, nor in cardiac arrest or requiring vasoactive agents.[215] Based on these guidelines, patients must receive a large quantity of blood products before rFVIIa is considered.[215] This concept, however, recently has been challenged in a preliminary study conducted in Iraq and Afghanistan war victims, comparing early (after <8 U of PRBCs) and late (after >8 U of PRBCs), administration of the agent. Early administration reduced the overall requirement for PRBCs by 20% compared with late use of rFVIIa. Survival up to 30 days was not different between the groups, nor was the use of FFP, cryoprecipitate, platelets, and crystalloids.[216] Thromboembolic complications occur in about 3 to 5% of patients receiving the drug, usually not immediately, but within a few hours or days after administration. Both arterial and venous systems are vulnerable, and in fact, thrombosis can occur in central line or bypass circuit tubing.[215]

Recombinant factor VIIa also may be beneficial in patients receiving warfarin therapy with traumatic brain injuries and intracranial hematomas. In these patients the agent may successfully control potentially devastating bleeding and lower the international normalized ratio into a range permitting surgery, and in some cases, may obviate the need for surgery.[217] A multicenter study is underway to clarify further the indications for rFVIIa in trauma.

Electrolyte and Acid-Base Disturbances

Intraoperative hyperkalemia may develop as a result of three mechanisms. First, in patients with irreversible shock, cell membrane permeability is altered, thus massive K^+ efflux results in severe hyperkalemia; in this situation, survival is unlikely (see Chapter 14). Second, after repair of a major vessel, subsequent reperfusion of the ischemic tissues results in a sudden release of K^+ into the general circulation. Third, transfusion at a rate faster than 1 U every 4 minutes to an acidotic and hypovolemic patient may cause an increase in plasma K^+ levels. Frequent monitoring of serum K^+, gradual and intermittent unclamping of vascular shunts, and avoiding transfusion at higher rates than needed help reduce the rate of K^+ increase. If a rise in K^+ is detected, treatment with regular insulin, 10 U intravenously, with 50% dextrose, 50 mL, and sodium bicarbonate, 8.4%, 50 mL, is indicated. If there is a dysrhythmia, $CaCl_2$, 500 mg, should also be administered. Insulin and dextrose can be repeated 2 or 3 times at 30- to 45-minute intervals, if necessary. Hemodialysis may be indicated in desperate situations.

Metabolic acidosis is caused by shock in most trauma patients. Other rare causes of metabolic acidosis in this population are alcoholic lactic acidosis, alcoholic ketoacidosis, diabetic ketoacidosis, and CO or CN^- poisoning after inhalation injuries. The differential diagnosis between hypovolemic, diabetic, and alcoholic acidosis, all of which have anion gaps, requires measurement of blood lactate, urinary ketone bodies, blood sugar, and invasive monitoring to assess intravascular volume. Alcoholic ketoacidosis is treated with intravenous dextrose, whereas diabetic ketoacidosis is managed with insulin. No specific treatment except intravenous normal saline exists for alcoholic lactic acidosis.

Treatment of metabolic acidosis involves correction of the underlying cause: management of hypoxemia, restoration of intravascular volume, optimization of cardiac function, or treatment of CO or CN^- toxicity. Symptomatic treatment with sodium bicarbonate has serious disadvantages, including leftward shift of the oxyhemoglobin dissociation curve causing decreased O_2 unloading, a hyperosmolar state secondary to the excessive sodium load, hypokalemia, further hemodynamic depression, overshoot alkalosis a few hours after giving the drug, and intracellular acidosis if adequate ventilation or pulmonary blood flow cannot be provided. Nevertheless, because of the possibility that severe acidosis can cause dysrhythmias, myocardial depression, hypotension, and resistance to exogenous catecholamines, some clinicians administer bicarbonate to "buy time" if the pH is <7.2.

Intraoperative Death

16 Death is a much greater threat during emergency trauma surgery than it is in any other operative procedure. Approximately 0.7% of patients admitted for acute trauma die in the OR, accounting for approximately 8% of postinjury deaths.[218] Uncontrollable bleeding is the cause of approximately 80% of intraoperative mortality; brain herniation and air embolism are the most common causes of death in the remaining patients.[218] A multicenter, retrospective study has defined certain features that increase the likelihood of OR death[218] (Table 36-11). Rapid transport to the OR, rapidly stabilizing life-threatening injuries while deferring definitive surgery ("damage control"), simultaneous thoracotomy and laparotomy for thoracoabdominal injuries, appropriate management of retroperitoneal hematoma, and early correction of hypothermia and shock may reduce intraoperative mortality rates.[218]

Of these measures, the damage control principle has reduced not only the intraoperative, but also the overall mor-

TABLE 36-11

CLINICAL FEATURES ASSOCIATED WITH INTRAOPERATIVE MORTALITY

■ CATEGORY	■ CLINICAL FEATURES
Mechanism of injury	Gunshot wound
	Pedestrian injuries
Injury severity	Mean injury severity score >41
	Mean revised trauma score >3.0
Preoperative physiologic profile	Mean BP in the field <50 mm Hg
	Mean BP on arrival to ED <60 mm Hg
	Best systolic BP in the ED <90 mm Hg
	Circulatory shock time >10 min
	Best mean pH <7.18
	Mean preoperative crystalloid resuscitation >3,850 mL; mean red cell transfusion >834 mL
Type of injury	Significant head, chest, abdominal, and pelvic injuries individually or in combination after blunt trauma
	Significant chest and abdominal injuries individually or in combination after penetrating trauma
Organ injury	Brain
	Liver
	Aorta or other major vascular injury
	Cardiac injury
Operating room resuscitation and physiologic status	Systolic BP <90 mm Hg during first hour
	Systolic BP <90 mm Hg for >30 min
	Deterioration of mean pH from 7.19 to 7.01
	Mean intraoperative blood loss 5,172 mL; mean blood replacement 4,541 mL
	Mean platelet transfusion 784 mL
	Mean fresh frozen plasma 1,418 mL
	Mean intraoperative temperature 32.2°C
	Intraoperative cardiac arrest

BP, blood pressure; ED, emergency department.
Data from Hoyt DB, Bulger EM, Knudson MM et al: Death in the operating room: An analysis of a multi-center experience. J Trauma 1994; 37: 426.

tality from trauma surgery, although morbidity from sepsis, abscess formation, and gastrointestinal fistulas may increase.[219] Originally described in three stages, the current suggestion is that it should be managed in four phases. In the first phase, attention is directed in the emergency department to recognition of the pattern of injury, as well as to the decision to initiate damage control by activating rewarming and blood component replacement. The second phase occurs in the OR where, in addition to efforts to maintain the patient's intravascular volume, near-normal temperature, acid-base status, and coagulation, surgeons rapidly control bleeding and leave the abdominal cavity temporarily covered by a Vac-Pac dressing, which allows an enlarged space for edematous organs and controlled egress of fluid. The third phase takes place in the ICU where intravascular volume, hypothermia, acidosis, and coagulation abnormalities are corrected. In the fourth phase, the stabilized patient is returned to the OR for definitive surgery and abdominal closure. The damage control principle, originally proposed for abdominal trauma, is now applied to injuries at other anatomic sites including the chest, pelvis, extremities, and in soft tissues.[220]

EARLY POSTOPERATIVE CONSIDERATIONS

The concerns in the early postoperative period are similar to those of the intraoperative phase. Re-evaluation and optimization of the circulation, oxygenation, temperature, CNS function, coagulation, electrolyte and acid-base status, and renal function are the hallmarks of postoperative management. Pain control in this group of patients may have more than a humanitarian purpose; it can improve pulmonary function, ventilation, and oxygenation in patients with chest injury or a long abdominal incision (see Chapter 57). For sedation in mechanically ventilated patients, both propofol (25 to 75 μg/kg/min) and midazolam (0.1 to 20 μg/kg/min) infusions alone or in combination are equally effective and safe, although wake-up time in patients receiving midazolam is longer (660 $\pm$ 400 minutes) than in those receiving propofol alone (110 $\pm$ 50 minutes) or in both agents combined (190 $\pm$ 200 minutes).[221] Morphine, 0.02 to 0.04 mg/kg/hr, or fentanyl, 1 to 3 μg/kg/hr, may be added for analgesia. Small boluses of midazolam (3 to 5 mg), propofol (50 mg), morphine (2 to 3 mg), or fentanyl (25 to 50 μg) may also be given as required[221] (see Chapter 57).

Acute Renal Failure

Acute renal failure is a possibility if prolonged shock or crush syndrome occur during early management. In a study aimed at finding the predictors of acute renal failure after emergency noncardiac surgery, which includes trauma, prolonged hypotension was one of the seven independent predictors of this complication.[222] Following an episode of shock in patients who have not received an osmotic load (radiopaque material, mannitol) or diuretic, determination of 2- or 6-hour creatinine and free water clearances may help predict the development of posttraumatic renal dysfunction.[223] Creatinine clearance <25 mL/min and free water clearance $\geq$ –15 mL/hr suggest the likelihood of acute renal failure. Decreased urine flow rate is not a good predictor, and the blood urea nitrogen does not rise until at least 24 hours after surgery or trauma.[223]

The cause of renal failure in crush syndrome is probably rhabdomyolysis-induced myoglobin release into the circulation. Serum creatine kinase levels increase in these patients; levels above 5,000 U/L are associated with renal failure.[224] The differentiation of myoglobinuria from hemoglobinuria is described in "Urine Output.". A clear supernatant of the centrifuged blood sample suggests myoglobin, whereas a rose color indicates hemoglobin. The traditional prophylaxis for renal failure after rhabdomyolysis includes fluids, mannitol, and bicarbonate. However, more recent data suggest that bicarbonate and mannitol are ineffective.[224]

Abdominal Compartment Syndrome

Abdominal compartment syndrome results from intra-abdominal hypertension with organ dysfunction after major abdominal trauma and surgery (primary syndrome); patients also may develop the syndrome without surgery; for example, during massive fluid resuscitation following major trauma or burns (secondary syndrome).[225–228] It frequently follows hemorrhage.[227] The syndrome results from massive edema of intra-abdominal organs produced by shock-induced inflammatory mediators, fluid resuscitation, and surgical manipulation. The significant cardiac, pulmonary, renal, gastrointestinal, hepatic, and CNS dysfunction caused by this syndrome results in a high mortality rate[226] (Fig. 36-13). A damage control procedure with towel-clip closure of the fascia after laparotomy may increase its incidence from the 17% seen with bogata bag closure to 80%.[228]

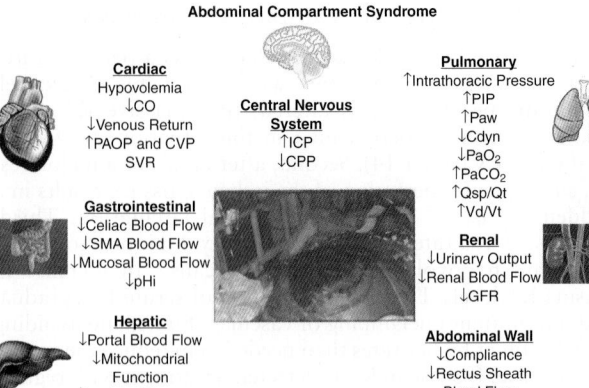

FIGURE 36-13. Physiologic effects of abdominal compartment syndrome. Image in the center is of a patient whose abdomen was left open but covered with nonadhesive dressing. CO, cardiac output; PAOP, pulmonary artery occlusion pressure; CVP, central venous pressure; SVR, systemic vascular resistance; ICP, intracranial pressure; CPP, cerebral perfusion pressure; PIP, peak inspiratory pressure; Paw, mean airway pressure; Cdyn, dynamic pulmonary compliance; Qsp/Qt, intrapulmonary shunt; Vd/Vt, dead space ventilation; SMA, superior mesenteric artery; pHi, intramucosal pH; GFR, glomerular filtration rate. (Adapted from Cheatham ML: Intra-abdominal hypertension and abdominal compartment syndrome. New Horiz 1999; 7: 96, with permission.)

Clinically, a tense, distended abdomen should direct the clinician to measure the intravesical pressure via a Foley catheter, which reflects the intra-abdominal pressure.[226] Values >20 to 25 mm Hg indicate inadequate organ perfusion and necessitate abdominal decompression, which, if delayed, results in progression to multiorgan failure and death.[225,228] Use of a volumetric pulmonary artery catheter for assessment of preload by left ventricular end-diastolic volume index determination may be more accurate than measuring CVP or PCWP in these patients.[226] Almost all these patients require mechanical ventilation. Attributing a relatively high PCWP to the ventilator and continuing high-volume fluid infusion may further increase intra-abdominal edema and increase mortality.[229] Interestingly, patients who will develop abdominal compartment syndrome often do not respond to fluid administration with elevated cardiac output despite an increasing PCWP.[229]

Thromboembolism

The overall incidence of DVT in the proximal femoral veins, the major source of PE, is approximately 18% in trauma patients.[230] However, DVT occurs in 24% of lower-extremity injuries, 27% of spine injuries, 20% of major head injuries, and 15% of serious injuries of the face, chest, or abdomen.[230] When injuries involve more than one of these high-risk regions, the likelihood of DVT is even higher.[230] Fortunately, only a relatively small fraction (approximately 0.3 to 2%) of severely injured patients have PE.[230–232] Almost half of all cases of PE occur within the first week, and in one study, 37% of the cases occurred within the first 4 days, suggesting that DVT develops shortly after trauma.[231,232] In most instances, DVT is asymptomatic, and in many of those in whom leg swelling develops, concurrent lower-extremity injuries may be implicated. The diagnosis of proximal DVT in symptomatic patients can be made by duplex ultrasonography, but this method has low sensitivity in the absence of symptoms.[233] Venography, which is the gold standard, can be performed in equivocal cases,

ANESTHETIC MANAGEMENT

although it is associated with complications and inherent logistical problems. Hypoxemia, even very early after injury, especially when sudden and associated with dyspnea and hemodynamic abnormalities, is highly suggestive of PE. The definitive diagnosis is established by spiral CT and pulmonary angiography. In hemodynamically unstable patients, resuscitation takes precedence over radiologic diagnosis. Management is symptomatic, and includes tracheal intubation, positive pressure ventilation with FIO_2 of 1.0, administration of fluids and inotropes (amrinone or milrinone), and continuous arterial and CVP or pulmonary artery monitoring. TEE is helpful because it may demonstrate RV performance, tricuspid regurgitation, or, in some cases, the thrombus within the pulmonary artery, the right heart chambers, or in transit through a patent foramen ovale to the left atrium.

In patients with relatively minor injuries, PE is treated with anticoagulants. Low-molecular-weight heparin may be used if bleeding is unlikely to exacerbate the injury. Consideration should be given to placement of a vena cava filter if the risk of bleeding is unacceptably high. Removable vena cava filters are now available[234] and are likely to be used prophylactically in high-risk patients more often than permanent filters, which are associated with long-term complications. In patients with severe hemodynamic depression or cardiac arrest that is unresponsive to resuscitative measures, thrombolytic agents may be considered despite the risk of hemorrhage. The current recommendation for prophylaxis in most trauma patients is low-molecular-weight heparin.[233] Low-dose unfractionated heparin appears to be ineffective in trauma patients.[235] Mechanical devices such as sequential compression boots should be applied as early as possible after injury. Late initiation of prophylaxis (>4 days after injury) because of massive transfusion, low anticipated risk because of absence of comorbidity, or because of fear of intracranial bleeding after severe head injury, has been shown to triple the risk of venous thromboembolism.[236]

References

1. National Safety Council: Injury Facts, 2008 edition. Chicago, National Safety Council, 2008
2. Acosta JA, Yang JC, Winchell RJ, et al: Lethal injuries and time of death in a level 1 trauma center. J Am Col Surgery 1998; 186: 528
3. Janjua KJ, Sugrue M, Deane SA: Prospective evaluation of early missed injuries and the role of tertiary trauma survey. J Trauma 1998; 44: 1000
4. Wilson WC: Trauma: Airway management. ASA difficult airway algorithm modified for trauma and five common intubation scenarios. ASA Newsletter 2005; 69: 9
5. de Nadal M, Munar F, Poca MA, et al: Cerebral hemodynamic effects of morphine and fentanyl in patients with severe head injury. Absence of correlation to cerebral autoregulation. Anesthesiology 2000; 92: 11
6. Heier T, Caldwell JE: Rapid tracheal intubation with large-dose rocuronium: a probability based approach. Anesth Analg 2000; 90: 175
7. Crosby ET: Airway management in adults after cervical spine trauma. Anesthesiology 2006; 104: 1293
8. McLeod AD, Calder I: Spinal cord injury and direct laryngoscopy—the legend lives on. Br J Anaesth 2000; 84: 705
9. Demetriades D, Velmahos GG, Asensio JA: Cervical pharyngoesophageal and laryngotracheal injuries. World J Surg 2001; 25: 1044
10. Heffernan DS, Schermer CR, Lu SW: What defines a distracting injury in cervical spine assessment? J Trauma 2005; 59: 1396
11. Stiell IG, Clement CM, McKnight RD, et al: The Canadian C-spine rule versus the NEXUS low-risk criteria in patients with trauma. N Engl J Med 2003; 349: 2510
12. Marion DW, Domeier R, Dunham CM, et al: Practice management guidelines for identifying cervical spine injuries following trauma, EAST Trauma Practice Guidelines http://www.east.org/tpg/chap3.pdf, 1998
13. Mathen R, Inaba K, Munera F, et al: Prospective evaluation of multislice computed tomography versus plain radiographic cervical spine clearance in trauma patients. J Trauma 2007; 62: 1427
14. Gale SC, Gracias VH, Reilly PM, et al: The inefficiency of plain radiography to evaluate the cervical spine after blunt trauma. J Trauma 2005; 59: 1121
15. Holmes JF, Akkinepalli R: Computed tomography versus plain radiography to screen for cervical spine injury: a meta-analysis. J Trauma 2005; 58: 902
16. Diaz JJ, Jr., Aulino JM, Collier B, et al: The early work-up for isolated ligamentous injury of the cervical spine: does computed tomography scan have a role? J Trauma 2005; 59: 897
17. Masanes MJ, Legendre C, Lioret N, et al: Fiberoptic bronchoscopy for the early diagnosis of subglottal inhalation injury: comparative value in the assessment of prognosis. J Trauma 1994; 36: 59
18. Sheridan RL, Hurford WE, Kacmarek RM, et al: Inhaled nitric oxide in burn patients with respiratory failure. J Trauma 1997; 42: 629
19. Ackland HM, Cooper DJ, Malham GM, et al: Magnetic resonance imaging for clearing the cervical spine in unconscious intensive care trauma patients. J Trauma 2006; 60: 668
20. Sundgren PC, Philipp M, Maly PV: Spinal trauma. Neuroimaging Clin North Am 2007; 17: 73
21. Stassen NA, Williams VA, Gestring ML, et al: Magnetic resonance imaging in combination with helical computed tomography provides a safe and efficient method of cervical spine clearance in the obtunded trauma patient. J Trauma 2006; 60: 171
22. Schuster R, Waxman K, Sanchez B, et al: Magnetic resonance imaging is not needed to clear cervical spines in blunt trauma patients with normal computed tomographic results and no motor deficits. Arch Surg 2005; 140: 762
23. Sanchez B, Waxman K, Jones T, et al: Cervical spine clearance in blunt trauma: evaluation of a computed tomography-based protocol. J Trauma 2005; 59: 179
24. Hastings RH, Vigil AC, Hanna R, et al: Cervical spine movement during laryngoscopy with the Bullard, Macintosh and Miller laryngoscopes. Anesthesiology 1995; 82: 859
25. Smith CE, Pinchak AB, Sidhu TS, et al: Evaluation of tracheal intubation difficulty in patients with cervical spine immobilization. Fiberoptic (Wu Scope) versus conventional laryngoscopy. Anesthesiology 1999; 91: 1253
26. Cicala RS, Kudsk KA, Butts A, et al: Initial evaluation and management of upper airway injuries in trauma patients. J Clin Anesth 1991; 3: 91
27. Wade AL, Dye JL, Mohrle CR, et al: Head, face, and neck injuries during Operation Iraqi Freedom II: results from the US Navy-Marine Corps Combat Trauma Registry. J Trauma 2007; 63: 836
28. Chen CC, Jeng SF, Tsai HH, et al: Life-threatening bleeding of bilateral maxillary arteries in maxillofacial trauma: report of two cases. J Trauma 2007; 63: 933
29. Kuttenberger JJ, Hardt N, Schlegel C: Diagnosis and initial management of laryngotracheal injuries associated with facial fractures. J Craniomaxillofac Surg 2004; 32: 80
30. Danic D, Prgomet D, Sekelj A, et al: External laryngotracheal trauma. Eur Arch Otorhinolaryngol 2006; 263: 228
31. O'Connor PJ, Russell JD, Moriarty DC: Anesthetic implications of laryngeal trauma. Anesth Analg 1998; 87: 1283
32. Yamazaki M, Sasaki R, Masuda A, et al: Anesthetic management of complete tracheal disruption using percutaneous cardiopulmonary support system. Anesth Analg 1998; 86: 998
33. Gomez-Caro A, Ausin P, Moradiellos FJ, et al: Role of conservative medical management of tracheobronchial injuries. J Trauma 2006; 61: 1426
34. Shearer VE, Giesecke AH: Airway management for patients with penetrating neck trauma: a retrospective study. Anesth Analg 1993; 77: 1135
35. Schweiger JW: The pathophysiology, diagnosis, and management strategies for flail chest injury and pulmonary contusion. Anesth and Analg 2001; 92 (Suppl., IARS Review Course Lectures): 86
36. Miller PR, Croce MA, Bee TK, et al: ARDS after pulmonary contusion: accurate measurement of contusion volume identifies high-risk patients. J Trauma 2001; 51: 223
37. Karmakar MK, Ho AM: Acute pain management of patients with multiple fractured ribs. J Trauma 2003; 54: 615
38. Plurad D, Green D, Demetriades D, et al: The increasing use of chest computed tomography for trauma: is it being overutilized? J Trauma 2007; 62: 631
39. McCunn M, Habashi NM: Airway pressure release ventilation in the acute respiratory distress syndrome following traumatic injury. Int Anesthesiol Clin 2002; 40: 89
40. Riou B, Zaier K, Kalfon P, et al: High-frequency jet ventilation in life-threatening bilateral pulmonary contusion. Anesthesiology 2001; 94: 927
41. Ho AM, Ling E: Systemic air embolism after lung trauma. Anesthesiology 1999; 90: 564
42. Demetriades D, Chan LS, Bhasin P, et al: Relative bradycardia in patients with traumatic hypotension. J Trauma 1998; 45: 534
43. American College of Surgeons Committee on Trauma: Shock, Advanced Trauma Life Support Instructor Manual. Edited by American College of Surgeons. Chicago, American College of Surgeons, 1997, p 97
44. Mackway-Jones K, Foex BA, Kirkman E, et al: Modification of the cardiovascular response to hemorrhage by somatic afferent nerve stimulation with special reference to gut and skeletal muscle blood flow. J Trauma 1999; 47: 481
45. Porter JM, Ivatury RR: In search of the optimal end points of resuscitation in trauma patients. A review. J Trauma 1998; 44: 908
46. Garrioch MA: The body's response to blood loss. Vox Sang 2004; 87 (Suppl 1): 74
47. Peterson DL, Schinco MA, Kerwin AJ, et al: Evaluation of initial base deficit as a prognosticator of outcome in the pediatric trauma population. Am Surg 2004; 70: 326

48. Randolph LC, Takacs M, Davis KA: Resuscitation in the pediatric trauma population: admission base deficit remains an important prognostic indicator. J Trauma 2002; 53: 838

49. Kincaid EH, Miller PR, Meredith JW, et al: Elevated arterial base deficit in trauma patients: a marker of impaired oxygen utilization. J Am Coll Surg 1998; 187: 384

50. Rutherford EJ, Morris JA, Reed GW, et al: Base deficit stratifies mortality and determines therapy. J Trauma 1992; 33: 417

51. James JH, Luchette FA, McCarter FD, et al: Lactate is an unreliable indicator of tissue hypoxia in injury or sepsis. Lancet 1999; 354: 505

52. McNelis J, Marini CP, Jurkiewicz A, et al: Prolonged lactate clearance is associated with increased mortality in the surgical intensive care unit. Am J Surg 2001; 182: 481

53. Eastridge BJ, Salinas J, McManus JG, et al: Hypotension begins at 110 mm Hg: redefining "hypotension" with data. J Trauma 2007; 63: 291

54. Edelman DA, White MT, Tyburski JG, et al: Post-traumatic hypotension: should systolic blood pressure of 90–109 mm Hg be included? Shock 2007; 27: 134

55. Bickell WH, Wall MJ, Pepe PE, et al: Immediate versus delayed fluid resuscitation for hypotensive patients with penetrating torso injuries. N Engl J Med 1994; 331: 1105

56. Stern SA: Low-volume fluid resuscitation for presumed hemorrhagic shock: helpful or harmful? Curr Opin Crit Care 2001; 7: 422

57. Dutton RP, Mackenzie CF, Scalea TM: Hypotensive resuscitation during active hemorrhage: impact on in-hospital mortality. J Trauma 2002; 52: 1141

58. Malone DL, Dunne J, Tracy JK, et al: Blood transfusion, independent of shock severity, is associated with worse outcome in trauma. J Trauma 2003; 54: 898

59. Dutton RP, Shih D, Edelman BB, et al: Safety of uncross matched type-O red cells for resuscitation from hemorrhagic shock. J Trauma 2005; 59: 1445

60. Tieu BH, Holcomb JB, Schreiber MA: Coagulopathy: its pathophysiology and treatment in the injured patient. World J Surg 2007; 31: 1055

61. Hirshberg A, Dugas M, Banez EI, et al: Minimizing dilutional coagulopathy in exsanguinating hemorrhage: a computer simulation. J Trauma 2003; 54: 454

62. Holcomb JB, Jenkins D, Rhee P, et al: Damage control resuscitation: directly addressing the early coagulopathy of trauma. J Trauma 2007; 62: 307

63. Spahn DR, Rossaint R: Coagulopathy and blood component transfusion in trauma. Br J Anaesth 2005; 95: 130

64. Borgman MA, Spinella PC, Perkins JG, et al: The ratio of blood products transfused affects mortality in patients receiving massive transfusions at a combat support hospital. J Trauma 2007; 63: 805

65. Forestner J: Massive transfusion: protocol for trauma. ASA Newsletter 2005; 69: 7

66. Wiklund CU, Romand JA, Suter PM, et al: Misplacement of central vein catheters in patients with hemothorax: a new approach to resolve the problem. J Trauma 2005; 59: 1029

67. Sharma A, Bodenham AR, Mallick A: Ultrasound-guided infraclavicular axillary vein cannulation for central venous access. Br J Anaesth 2004; 93: 188

68. Sandhu NP, Sidhu DS: Mid-arm approach to basilic and cephalic vein cannulation using ultrasound guidance. Br J Anaesth 2004; 93: 292

69. Neufeld JDG, Marx JA, Moore EE, et al: Comparison of intraosseous, central, and peripheral routes of crystalloid infusion for resuscitation of hemorrhagic shock in a swine model. J Trauma 1993; 34: 422

70. Luna GK, Pavlin EG, Kirkman T, et al: Hemodynamic effects of external cardiac massage in trauma shock. J Trauma 1989; 29: 1430

71. Durham LA, Richardson RJ, Wall MJ, et al: Emergency center thoracotomy: impact of prehospital resuscitation. J Trauma 1992; 32: 775

72. Millham FH, Gridlinger GA: Survival determinants in patients undergoing emergency room thoracotomy for penetrating chest injury. J Trauma 1993; 34: 332

73. Shackford SR, Mackersie RC, Davis JW, et al: Epidemiology and pathology of traumatic deaths occurring at a level I trauma center in a regionalized system; the importance of secondary brain injury. J Trauma 1989; 29: 1392

74. Verweij BH, Amelink GJ, Muizelaar JP: Current concepts of cerebral oxygen transport and energy metabolism after severe traumatic brain injury. Prog Brain Res 2007; 161: 111

75. Werner C, Engelhard K: Pathophysiology of traumatic brain injury. Br J Anaesth 2007; 99: 4

76. Brain Trauma Foundation, American Association of Neurologic Surgeons: Guidelines for the management of severe traumatic brain injury. J Neurotrauma 2007; 24(Suppl 1): S1

77. Chesnut RM: Avoidance of hypotension: Conditio sine qua non of successful head injury management. J Trauma 1997; 42(Suppl): 4S

78. McHugh GS, Engel DC, Butcher I, et al: Prognostic value of secondary insults in traumatic brain injury: results from the IMPACT study. J Neurotrauma 2007; 24: 287

79. American College of Surgeons Committee on Trauma: Head Trauma, Advanced Trauma Life Support Instructor Manual. Ed: American College of Surgeons. Chicago, 1999, 228

80. Chesnut RM: Management of brain and spine injuries. Crit Care Clin 2004; 20: 25

81. Duncan T, Krost WS, Mistovich JJ, et al: Beyond the basics: brain injuries. Emerg Med Serv 2007; 36: 65

82. Coles JP: Regional ischemia after head injury. Curr Opin Crit Care 2004; 10: 120

83. Mascia L, Zavala E, Bosma K, et al: High tidal volume is associated with the development of acute lung injury after severe brain injury: an international observational study. Crit Care Med 2007; 35: 1815

84. Chan KH, Dearden NM, Miller JD, et al: Multimodality monitoring as a guide to treatment of intracranial hypertension after severe brain injury. Neurosurgery 1993; 32: 547

85. Cruz J: Jugular venous oxygen saturation monitoring. J Neurosurg 1992; 77: 162

86. White H, Cook D, Venkatesh B: The use of hypertonic saline for treating intracranial hypertension after traumatic brain injury. Anesth Analg 2006; 102: 1836

87. Freshman SP, Battistella FD, Matteucci M, et al: Hypertonic saline (7.5%) versus mannitol: a comparison for treatment of acute head injuries. J Trauma 1993; 35: 344

88. Lescot T, Degos V, Zouaoui A, et al: Opposed effects of hypertonic saline on contusions and noncontused brain tissue in patients with severe traumatic brain injury. Crit Care Med 2006; 34: 3029

89. Doyle JA, Davis DP, Hoyt DB: The use of hypertonic saline in the treatment of traumatic brain injury. J Trauma 2001; 50: 367

90. Cruz J: The first decade of continuous monitoring of jugular bulb oxyhemoglobin saturation: Management strategies and clinical outcome. Crit Care Med 1998; 26: 344

91. Grände PO: The "Lund Concept" for the treatment of severe head trauma—physiological principles and clinical application. Intensive Care Med 2006; 32: 1475

92. Rudehill A, Bellander B, Weitzberg E, et al: Outcome of traumatic brain injuries in 1,508 patients: impact of prehospital care. J Neurotrauma 2002; 19: 855

93. Elf K, Nilsson P, Enblad P: Outcome after traumatic brain injury improved by an organized secondary insult program and standardized neurointensive care. Crit Care Med 2002; 30: 2129

94. Warner DS, Borel CO: Treatment of traumatic brain injury: one size does not fit all. Anesth Analg 2004; 99: 1208

95. Palmer S, Bader MK, Qureshi A, et al: The impact on outcomes in a community hospital setting of using the AANS traumatic brain injury guidelines. J Trauma 2001; 50: 657

96. Watts DD, Hanfling D, Waller MA, et al: An evaluation of the use of guidelines in prehospital management of brain injury. Prehosp Emerg Care 2004; 8: 254

97. Domeier RM, Evans RW, Swor RA, et al: Prehospital clinical findings associated with spinal injury. Prehosp Emerg Care 1997; 1: 11

98. Stevens RD, Bhardwaj A, Kirsch JR, et al: Critical care and perioperative management in traumatic spinal cord injury. J Neurosurg Anesthesiol 2003; 15: 215

99. Vale FL, Burns J, Jackson AB, et al: Combined medical and surgical treatment after acute spinal cord injury: results of a pilot study to assess the merits of aggressive medical resuscitation and blood pressure management. J Neurosurg 1997; 87: 239

100. Bernhard M, Gries A, Kremer P, et al: Spinal cord injury (SCI)—prehospital management. Resuscitation 2005; 66: 127

101. Bracken MB, Shepard MJ, Collins WF, Jr., et al: Methylprednisolone or naloxone treatment after acute spinal cord injury. Results of the Second National Acute Spinal Cord Injury Study. J Neurosurg 1992; 76: 23

102. Bracken MB, Shepard MJ, Holford TR, et al: Methylprednisolone or tirilazad mesylate after acute spinal cord injury: Results of the third National Acute Spinal Cord Injury randomized controlled trial. J Neurosurg 1998; 89: 699

103. Sayer FT, Kronvall E, Nilsson OG: Methylprednisolone treatment in acute spinal cord injury: the myth challenged through a structured analysis of published literature. Spine 2006; 6: 335

104. Gerndt SJ, Rodriguez JL, Pawlik JW, et al: Consequences of high-dose steroid therapy for acute spinal cord injury. J Trauma 1997; 42: 279

105. Tolonen A, Turkka J, Salonen O, et al: Traumatic brain injury is underdiagnosed in patients with spinal cord injury. J Rehabil Med 2007; 39: 622

106. Hadley MN, Walters BC, Grabb PA, et al: Guidelines for the management of acute cervical spine and spinal cord injuries. Clin Neurosurg 2002; 49: 407

107. Bledsoe BE, Wesley AK, Salomone JP: High-dose steroids for acute spinal cord injury in emergency medical services. Prehosp Emerg Care 2004; 8: 313

108. Berly M, Shem K: Respiratory management during the first five days after spinal cord injury. J Spinal Cord Med 2007; 30: 309

109. Brown R, DiMarco AF, Hoit JD, et al: Respiratory dysfunction and management in spinal cord injury. Respir Care 2006; 51: 853

110. Winslow C, Rozovsky J: Effect of spinal cord injury on the respiratory system. Am J Phys Med Rehabil 2003; 82: 803

111. Theodore J, Robin ED: Pathogenesis of neurogenic pulmonary edema. Lancet 1975; 2: 749

112. Mackenzie CF, Shin B, Krishnaprasad D, et al: Assessment of cardiac and respiratory function during surgery on patients with acute quadriplegia. J Neurosurg 1985; 62: 843

113. Demetriades D, Asensio JA, Velmahos G, et al: Complex problems in penetrating neck trauma. Surg Clin North Am 1996; 76: 661

114. Biffl WL, Moore EE, Ryu RK, et al: The unrecognized epidemic of blunt carotid arterial injuries. Early diagnosis improves neurologic outcome. Ann Surg 1998; 228: 462

115. Jewett BS, Shockley WW, Rutledge R: External laryngeal trauma: analysis of 392 patients. Arch Otolaryngol Head Neck Surg 1999; 125: 877

116. Ball CG, Kirkpatrick AW, Laupland KB, et al: Incidence, risk factors, and outcomes for occult pneumothoraces in victims of major trauma. J Trauma 2005; 59: 917

117. Kirkpatrick AW, Sirois M, Laupland KB, et al: Hand-held thoracic sonography for detecting post-traumatic pneumothoraces: The extended focused assessment with sonography for trauma (EFAST). J Trauma 2004; 57: 288

118. Dente CJ, Ustin J, Feliciano DV, et al: The accuracy of thoracic ultrasound for detection of pneumothorax is not sustained over time: a preliminary study. J Trauma 2007; 62: 1384

118a. Brasel KJ, Stafford RE, Weigelts JA, et al. Treatment of occult pneumothoraces from blunt trauma. J Trauma 1999; 46: 987

119. Enderson BL, Abdalla R, Frame SB, et al: Tube thoracostomy for occult pneumothorax: a prospective randomized study of its use. J Trauma 1993; 35: 726

120. Mineo TC, Ambrogi V, Cristino B, et al: Changing indications for thoracotomy in blunt chest trauma after the advent of videothoracoscopy. J Trauma 1999; 47: 1088

121. Rozycki GS, Feliciano DV, Ochsner G, et al: The role of ultrasound in patients with possible penetrating cardiac wounds: a prospective multicenter study. J Trauma 1999; 46: 543

122. Porembka DT, Johnson DJ, Hoyt BD, et al: Penetrating cardiac trauma: a perioperative role for transesophageal echocardiography. Anesth Analg 1993; 77: 1275

123. Orliaguet G, Ferjani M, Riou B: The heart in blunt trauma. Anesthesiology 2001; 95: 544

124. Wong YC, Ng CJ, Wang LJ, et al: Left mediastinal width and mediastinal width ratio are better radiographic criteria than general mediastinal width for predicting blunt aortic injury. J Trauma 2004; 57: 88

125. Vignon P, Boncoeur MP, Francois B, et al: Comparison of multiplane transesophageal echocardiography and contrast-enhanced helical CT in the diagnosis of blunt traumatic cardiovascular injuries. Anesthesiology 2001; 94: 615

126. Goarin JP, Cluzel P, Gosgnach M, et al: Evaluation of transesophageal echocardiography for diagnosis of traumatic aortic injury. Anesthesiology 2000; 93: 1373

127. Vignon P, Martaille JF, Francois B, et al: Transesophageal echocardiography and therapeutic management of patients sustaining blunt aortic injuries. J Trauma 2005; 58: 1150

128. Dunham MB, Zygun D, Petrasek P, et al: Endovascular stent grafts for acute blunt aortic injury. J Trauma 2004; 56: 1173

129. Symbas PN, Vlasis SE, Hatcher CR, Jr.: Blunt and penetrating diaphragmatic injuries with or without herniation of organs into the chest. Ann Thorac Surg 1986; 42: 158

130. Villavicencio RT, Aucar JA: Analysis of laparoscopy in trauma. J Am Coll Surg 1999; 189: 11

131. Cothren CC, Osborn PM, Moore EE, et al: Preperitoneal pelvic packing for hemodynamically unstable pelvic fractures: a paradigm shift. J Trauma 2007; 62: 834

132. Totterman A, Madsen JE, Skaga NO, et al: Extraperitoneal pelvic packing: a salvage procedure to control massive traumatic pelvic hemorrhage. J Trauma 2007; 62: 843

133. MacLennan N, Heimbach DM, Cullen BF: Anesthesia for major thermal injury. Anesthesiology 1998; 89: 749

134. Hemington-Gorse SJ: A comparison of laser Doppler imaging with other measurement techniques to assess burn depth. J Wound Care 2005; 14: 151

135. Pereira CT, Herndon DN: The pharmacologic modulation of the hypermetabolic response to burns. Adv Surg 2005; 39: 245

136. Haponik EF, Meyers DA, Munster AM, et al: Acute upper airway injury in burn patients: serial changes of flow-volume curves and nasopharyngoscopy. Am Rev Respir Dis 1987; 135: 360

137. Smith DL, Cairns BA, Ramadan F, et al: Effect of inhalation injury, burn size and age on mortality: A study of 1447 consecutive burn patients. J Trauma 1994; 37: 655

138. Jones WG, Madden M, Finkelstein J, et al: Tracheostomies in burn patients. Ann Surg 1989; 209: 471

139. Muehlberger T, Kunar D, Munster A, et al: Efficacy of fiberoptic laryngoscopy in the diagnosis of inhalation injuries. Arch Otolaryngol Head Neck Surg 1998; 124: 1003

140. Cartotto R, Ellis S, Smith T: Use of high-frequency oscillatory ventilation in burn patients. Crit Care Med 2005; 33: S175

141. Vegfors M, Lennmarken C: Carboxyhemoglobinaemia and pulse oximetry. Br J Anaesth 1991; 66: 625

142. Baud FJ, Barriot P, Toffis V, et al: Elevated blood cyanide concentrations in victims of smoke inhalation. N Engl J Med 1991; 325: 1761

143. Tung A, Lynch J, McDade WA: A new biological assay for measuring cyanide in blood. Anesth Analg 1997; 85: 1045

144. Breen PH, Isserles SA, Westley J, et al: Combined carbon monoxide and cyanide poisoning: A place for treatment? Anesth Analg 1995; 80: 671

145. Miller K, Chang A: Acute inhalation injury. Emerg Med Clin North Am 2003; 21: 533

146. Papp A, Uusaro A, Parviainen I, et al: Myocardial function and haemodynamics in extensive burn trauma: evaluation by clinical signs, invasive monitoring, echocardiography and cytokine concentrations. A prospective clinical study. Acta Anaesthesiol Scand 2003; 47: 1257

147. Namias N: Advances in burn care. Curr Opin Crit Care 2007; 13: 405

148. Ivy ME, Atweh NA, Palmer J, et al: Intra-abdominal hypertension and abdominal compartment syndrome in burn patients. J Trauma 2000; 49: 387

149. Sheridan RL: Burns. Crit Care Med 2002; 30: S500

150. Fodor L, Fodor A, Ramon Y, et al: Controversies in fluid resuscitation for burn management: literature review and our experience. Injury 2006; 37: 374

151. Saffle JI: The phenomenon of "fluid creep" in acute burn resuscitation. J Burn Care Res 2007; 28: 382

152. Huang PP, Stucky FS, Dimick AR, et al: Hypertonic sodium resuscitation is associated with renal failure and death. Ann Surg 1995; 221: 543

153. Elgjo GI, Poli de Figueiredo LF, Schenarts PJ, et al: Hypertonic saline dextran produces early (8–12 hrs) fluid sparing in burn resuscitation: a 24-hr prospective, double-blind study in sheep. Crit Care Med 2000; 28: 163

154. Mann R, Heimbach DM, Engrav LH, et al: Changes in transfusion practices in burn patients. J Trauma 1994; 37: 220

155. Dries DJ, Waxman K: Adequate resuscitation of burn patients may not be measured by urine output and vital signs. Crit Care Med 1991; 19: 327

156. Morris JR, MacKenzie EJ, Edelstein SL: The effect of preexisting conditions on mortality in trauma patients. JAMA 1990; 263: 1942

157. Rooke GA, Schwid HA, Shapira Y: The effect of graded hemorrhage and intravascular volume replacement on systolic pressure variation in humans during mechanical and spontaneous ventilation. Anesth Analg 1995; 80: 925

158. Welch G: Methods of hemodynamic monitoring. J Trauma 2007; 62: S109

159. Cheatham ML, Safcsak K, Block EF, et al: Preload assessment in patients with an open abdomen. J Trauma 1999; 46: 16

160. Porembka DT: Importance of transesophageal echocardiography in the critically ill and injured patient. Crit Care Med 2007; 35: S414

161. Capan LM, Miller SM, Patel KP: Fat embolism. Anesthesiol Clin North Am 1993; 11: 25

162. Reich DL, Timcenko A, Bodian CA, et al: Predictors of pulse oximetry data failure. Anesthesiology 1996; 84: 859

163. Agashe GS, Coakley J, Mannheimer PD: Forehead pulse oximetry: Headband use helps alleviate false low readings likely related to venous pulsation artifact. Anesthesiology 2006; 105: 1111

164. Tokuda K, Hayamizu K, Ogawa K, et al: A comparison of finger, ear, and forehead SpO2 on detecting oxygen saturation in healthy volunteers. Anesthesiology 2007; 107: A1544

165. Cox PN: New pulse oximetry sensors with low saturation accuracy claims—A clinical evaluation. Anesthesiology 2007; 107: A1540

166. Macknet MR, Kimball-Jones PL, Applegate RL, et al: Noninvasive measurement of continuous hemoglobin via pulse CO-oximetry. Anesthesiology 2007; 107: A1545

167. Cannasson M, Dellannoy B, Morand A, et al: New algorithm for automatic estimation of the respiratory variations in the pulse oximeter waveform. Anesthesiology 2007; 107: A451

168. McKinley BA, Kozar RA, Cocanour CS, et al: Normal versus supranormal oxygen delivery goals in shock resuscitation: the response is the same. J Trauma 2002; 53: 825

169. Tyburski JG, Carlin AM, Harvey EH, et al: End-tidal CO_2-arterial CO_2 differences: a useful intraoperative mortality marker in trauma surgery. J Trauma 2003; 55: 892

170. Mallett SV, Cox JA: Thromboelastography. Br J Anaesth 1992; 69: 307

171. Johnston TD, Chen Y, Reed RL: Functional equivalence of hypothermia to specific clotting factor deficiencies. J Trauma 1994; 37: 413

172. Capan LM: Airway management, Trauma Anesthesia and Intensive Care. Edited by Capan LM, Miller SM, Turndorf H. Philadelphia, Lippincott, 1991, p 43

173. Egar TD, Kuramkote S, Gong G, et al: Fentanyl pharmacokinetics in hemorrhagic shock. A porcine model. Anesthesiology 1999; 91: 156

174. Johnson KB, Egan TD, Kern SE, et al: The influence of hemorrhagic shock on propofol: a pharmacokinetic and pharmacodynamic analysis. Anesthesiology 2003; 99: 409

175. Johnson KB, Egan TD, Layman J, et al: The influence of hemorrhagic shock on etomidate: a pharmacokinetic and pharmacodynamic analysis. Anesth Analg 2003; 96: 1360

176. Shafer SL: Shock values. Anesthesiology 2004; 101: 567

177. Bogetz MS, Katz JA: Recall of surgery for major trauma. Anesthesiology 1984; 61: 6

178. Lubke GH, Kerssens C, Phaf H, et al: Dependence of explicit and implicit memory on hypnotic state in trauma patients. Anesthesiology 1999; 90: 670

179. Kurita T, Takata K, Uraoka M, et al: The influence of hemorrhagic shock on the minimum alveolar anesthetic concentration of isoflurane in a swine model. Anesth Analg 2007; 105: 1639

180. Smith I, White PF, Nathanson M, et al: Propofol. An update on its clinical use. Anesthesiology 1994; 81: 1005

181. Berry JM, Merin RG: Etomidate myoclonus and the open globe. Anesth Analg 1989; 69: 256

182. Libonati MM, Leahy MJ, Ellison N: The use of succinylcholine in open eye surgery. Anesthesiology 1985; 62: 637

183. Zimmerman AA, Funk K, Tidwell JL: Propofol and alfentanil prevent the increase in intraocular pressure caused by succinylcholine and endotracheal intubation during a rapid sequence induction of anesthesia. Anesth Analg 1996; 83: 814

184. Magorian T, Flannery KB, Miller RD: Comparison of rocuronium, succinylcholine, and vecuronium for rapid-sequence induction of anesthesia in adult patients. Anesthesiology 1993; 79: 913

185. Moss E: Alfentanil increases intracranial pressure when intracranial compliance is low. Anaesthesia 1992; 47: 134

186. Sperry RJ, Bailey PL, Reichman MV, et al: Fentanyl and sufentanil increase intracranial pressure in head trauma patients. Anesthesiology 1992; 77: 416

187. Branski LK, Herndon DN, Pereira C, et al: Longitudinal assessment of Integra in primary burn management: a randomized pediatric clinical trial. Crit Care Med 2007; 35: 2615

188. Foster K: The use of fibrin sealant in burn operations. Surgery 2007; 142: S50

189. Coté CJ, Drop LJ, Hoaglin DC, et al: Ionized hypocalcemia after fresh frozen plasma administration to thermally injured children: effects of infusion rate, duration, and treatment with calcium chloride. Anesth Analg 1988; 67: 152

190. Martyn JAJ, Fukushima Y, Chon Y, et al: Muscle relaxants in burns, trauma and critical illness. Int Anesthesiol Clin 2006; 44: 123

191. Han T, Kim H, Bae J, et al: Neuromuscular pharmacodynamics of rocuronium in patients with major burns. Anesth Analg 2004; 99: 386

192. Todd SR, Malinoski D, Muller PJ, et al: Lactated Ringer's is superior to normal saline in the resuscitation of uncontrolled hemorrhagic shock. J Trauma 2007; 62: 636

193. Warren BB, Durieux ME: Hydroxyethyl starch: safe or not? Anesth Analg 1997; 84: 206

194. Poloujadoff MP, Borron SW, Amathieu R, et al: Improved survival after resuscitation with norepinephrine in a murine model of uncontrolled hemorrhagic shock. Anesthesiology 2007; 107: 591

195. Zipnick RI, Scalea TM, Trooskin SZ, et al: Hemodynamic responses to penetrating spinal cord injuries. J Trauma 1993; 35: 578

196. Wang HE, Callaway CW, Peitzman AB, et al: Admission hypothermia and outcome after major trauma. Crit Care Med 2005; 33: 1296

197. Tsuei BJ, Kearney PA: Hypothermia in the trauma patient. Injury 2004; 35: 7

198. Jurkovich GJ, Greiser WB, Luterman A, et al: Hypothermia in trauma victims: An ominous predictor of survival. J Trauma 1987; 27: 1019

199. Smith C, Soreide, E: Hypothermia in trauma victims. ASA Newsletter 2005; 69: 17

200. Gentilello LM: Advances in the management of hypothermia. Surg Clin North Am 1995; 75: 243

201. Wadhwa A, Komatsu R, Orhan-Sungur M, et al: New circulating-water devices warm more quickly than forced-air in volunteers. Anesth Analg 2007; 105: 1681

202. Gentilello LM, Cobean R, Offner PJ, et al: Continuous arteriovenous rewarming: rapid reversal of hypothermia in critically ill patients. J Trauma 1992; 32: 316

203. Mittermayr M, Streif W, Haas T, et al: Hemostatic changes after crystalloid or colloid fluid administration during major orthopedic surgery: the role of fibrinogen administration. Anesth Analg 2007; 105: 905

204. Hess JR, Lawson JH: The coagulopathy of trauma versus disseminated intravascular coagulation. J Trauma 2006; 60: S12

205. Brohi K, Cohen MJ, Ganter MT, et al: Acute traumatic coagulopathy: initiated by hypoperfusion: modulated through the protein C pathway? Ann Surg 2007; 245: 812

206. Wolberg AS, Meng ZH, Monroe DM, 3rd, et al: A systematic evaluation of the effect of temperature on coagulation enzyme activity and platelet function. J Trauma 2004; 56: 1221

207. Martini WZ, Pusateri AE, Uscilowicz JM, et al: Independent contributions of hypothermia and acidosis to coagulopathy in swine. J Trauma 2005; 58: 1002

208. Levi M: Disseminated intravascular coagulation. Crit Care Med 2007; 35: 2191

209. Miller RD: Coagulation and packed red blood cell transfusions. Anesth Analg 1995; 80: 215

210. Murray DJ, Pennell BJ, Weinstein SL, et al: Packed red cells in acute blood loss: dilutional coagulopathy as a cause of surgical bleeding. Anesth Analg 1995; 80: 336

211. Murphy WG, Davies MJ, Eduardo A: The haemostatic response to surgery and trauma. Br J Anaesth 1993; 70: 205

212. Murray DJ, Olsen J, Strauss R, et al: Coagulation changes during packed red cell replacement of major blood loss. Anesthesiology 1988; 69: 839

213. Meng ZH, Wolberg AS, Monroe DM, 3rd, et al: The effect of temperature and pH on the activity of factor VIIa: implications for the efficacy of high-dose factor VIIa in hypothermic and acidotic patients. J Trauma 2003; 55: 886

214. Boffard KD, Riou B, Warren B, et al: Recombinant factor VIIa as adjunctive therapy for bleeding control in severely injured trauma patients: two parallel randomized, placebo-controlled, double-blind clinical trials. J Trauma 2005; 59: 8

215. Thomas GO, Dutton RP, Hemlock B, et al: Thromboembolic complications associated with factor VIIa administration. J Trauma 2007; 62: 564

216. Perkins JG, Schreiber MA, Wade CE, et al: Early versus late recombinant factor VIIa in combat trauma patients requiring massive transfusion. J Trauma 2007; 62: 1095

217. Bartal C, Freedman J, Bowman K, et al: Coagulopathic patients with traumatic intracranial bleeding: defining the role of recombinant factor VIIa. J Trauma 2007; 63: 725

218. Hoyt DB, Bulger EM, Knudson MM, et al: Death in the operating room: an analysis of a multi-center experience. J Trauma 1994; 37: 426

219. Nicholas JM, Rix EP, Easley KA, et al: Changing patterns in the management of penetrating abdominal trauma: the more things change, the more they stay the same. J Trauma 2003; 55: 1095

220. Leininger BE, Rasmussen TE, Smith DL, et al: Experience with wound VAC and delayed primary closure of contaminated soft tissue injuries in Iraq. J Trauma 2006; 61: 1207

221. Sanchez-Izquierdo-Riera JA, Caballero-Cubedo RE, Perez-Vela JL, et al: Propofol versus midazolam: Safety and efficacy for sedating the severe trauma patient. Anesth Analg 1998; 86: 1219

222. Kheterpal S, Tremper KK, Englesbe MJ, et al: Predictors of postoperative acute renal failure after noncardiac surgery in patients with previously normal renal function. Anesthesiology 2007; 107: 892

223. Shin B, Mackenzie CF, Helrich M: Creatinine clearance for early detection of posttraumatic renal dysfunction. Anesthesiology 1986; 64: 605

224. Brown CV, Rhee P, Chan L, et al: Preventing renal failure in patients with rhabdomyolysis: do bicarbonate and mannitol make a difference? J Trauma 2004; 56: 1191

225. Balogh Z, McKinley BA, Cocanour CS, et al: Secondary abdominal compartment syndrome is an elusive early complication of traumatic shock resuscitation. Am J Surg 2002; 184: 538

226. Cheatham ML: Intra-abdominal hypertension and abdominal compartment syndrome. New Horiz 1999; 7: 96

227. Maxwell RA, Fabian TC, Croce MA, et al: Secondary abdominal compartment syndrome: an underappreciated manifestation of severe hemorrhagic shock. J Trauma 1999; 47: 995

228. Balogh Z, McKinley BA, Holcomb JB, et al: Both primary and secondary abdominal compartment syndrome can be predicted early and are harbingers of multiple organ failure. J Trauma 2003; 54: 848

229. Balogh Z, McKinley BA, Cocanour CS, et al: Patients with impending abdominal compartment syndrome do not respond to early volume loading. Am J Surg 2003; 186: 602

230. Geerts WH, Code KI, Jay RM, et al: A prospective study of venous thromboembolism after major trauma. N Engl J Med 1994; 331: 1601

231. Menaker J, Stein DM, Scalea TM: Incidence of early pulmonary embolism after injury. J Trauma 2007; 63: 620

232. Owings JT, Kraut E, Battistella F, et al: Timing of the occurrence of pulmonary embolism in trauma patients. Arch Surg 1997; 132: 862

233. Jongbloets LM, Lensing AW, Koopman MM, et al: Limitations of compression ultrasound for the detection of symptomless postoperative deep vein thrombosis. Lancet 1994; 343: 1142

234. Morris CS, Rogers FB, Najarian KE, et al: Current trends in vena caval filtration with the introduction of a retrievable filter at a level I trauma center. J Trauma 2004; 57: 32

235. Geerts WH, Jay RM, Code KI, et al: A comparison of low-dose heparin with low-molecular-weight heparin as prophylaxis against venous thromboembolism after major trauma. N Engl J Med 1996; 335: 701

236. Nathens AB, McMurray MK, Cuschieri J, et al: The practice of venous thromboembolism prophylaxis in the major trauma patient. J Trauma 2007; 62: 557

CHAPTER 37 ■ EPIDURAL AND SPINAL ANESTHESIA

CHRISTOPHER M. BERNARDS

KEY POINTS

1. Clinicians must develop a three-dimensional mental picture of the spinal anatomy so that when they contact bony structures during attempted epidural or spinal needle placement they can redirect the needle in a reasoned and systematic manner and not subject the patient to random needle "pokes" in an effort to place the block.

2. The epidural fat and the epidural venous plexus do not form a continuous cylinder surrounding the spinal cord, as is often depicted. Rather, the epidural fat lies in discrete pockets in the posterior and lateral epidural space and the epidural veins travel primarily in the anterior and lateral epidural space and are normally absent in the posterior epidural space.

3. Serious systemic toxicity during attempted epidural block is almost always the result of inadvertent local anesthetic injection directly into the vasculature. Consequently, an appropriate test dose designed to identify intravascular injection is critical.

4. Physical characteristics (e.g., height, weight, cerebrospinal fluid volume) and age do have an effect on spinal and

epidural block characteristics. However, the magnitude of the effects are relatively small and of such low predictive power that these characteristics are not useful predictors of local anesthetic dose in any individual patient.

5. The risk of hemodynamic complications of epidural and spinal anesthesia increases with increasing block height.

6. Lidocaine appears to be worse than other local anesthetics in terms of the risk of neurologic toxicity (i.e., cauda equina syndrome and transient neurologic symptoms).

7. Human studies suggest that the preservative-free formulation of chloroprocaine may offer a viable alternative to lidocaine for short-duration spinal anesthesia.

8. Administration of drugs that impair coagulation can put patients at increased risk of spinal hematoma. Our understanding of the relative risk of different classes of drugs affecting the clotting system is constantly evolving. Clinicians are directed to the consensus statement from the American Society for Regional Anesthesia and Pain Medicine for the most recent recommendations.

There are no absolute indications for spinal or epidural anesthesia. However, there are clinical situations in which patient preference, patient physiology, or the surgical procedure makes central neuraxial block the technique of choice. There is also evidence that these techniques may improve outcome in selected situations. Spinal and epidural anesthesia have been shown to blunt the "stress response" to surgery,[1] to decrease intraoperative blood loss,[2,3] to lower the incidence of postoperative thromboembolic events,[2–5] and to decrease morbidity and mortality in high-risk surgical patients.[6,7] In addition, both spinal and epidural techniques can be used to extend analgesia into the postoperative period, where their use has been shown to provide better analgesia than can be achieved with parenteral opioids.[8] In addition, central neuraxial analgesia has become an indispensable technique to provide analgesia to nonsurgical patients. Thus, these techniques are an

FIGURE 37-1. Posterior (**A**) and lateral (**C**) views of the human spinal column. Note the inset (**B**), which depicts the variability in vertebral level at which the spinal cord terminates.

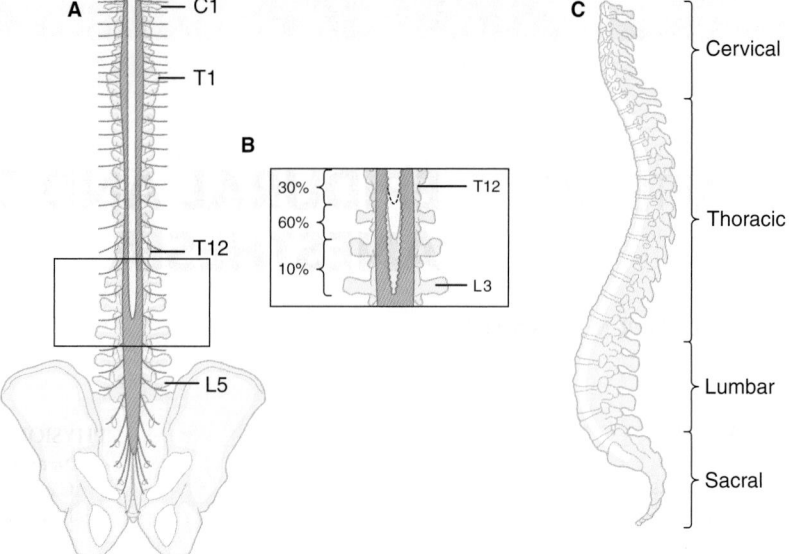

indispensable part of modern anesthetic practice, and every anesthesiologist should be adept at performing them.

ANATOMY

Proficiency in spinal and epidural anesthesia requires a thorough understanding of the anatomy of the spine and spinal cord. The anesthesiologist must be familiar with the surface anatomy of the spine but must also develop a mental picture of the three-dimensional anatomy of deeper structures. In addition, one must appreciate the relationship between the cutaneous dermatomes, the spinal nerves, the vertebrae, and the spinal segment from which each spinal nerve arises.

Vertebrae

The *spine* consists of 33 *vertebrae* (7 cervical, 12 thoracic, 5 lumbar, 5 fused sacral, and 4 fused coccygeal; Fig. 37-1). With the exception of C1, the cervical, thoracic, and lumbar vertebrae consist of a *body* anteriorly, two *pedicles* that project posteriorly from the body, and two *laminae* that connect the pedicles (Fig. 37-2). These structures form the *vertebral canal*, which contains the spinal cord, spinal nerves, and epidural space. The laminae give rise to the *transverse processes* that project laterally and the *spinous process* that projects posteriorly. These bony projections serve as sites for muscle and ligament attachments. The pedicles contain a superior and inferior *vertebral notch* through which the spinal nerves exit the vertebral canal. The superior and inferior *articular processes* arise at the junction of the lamina and pedicles and form joints with the adjoining vertebrae. The first cervical vertebra ("atlas") differs from this typical structure in that it does not have a body or a spinous process.

The five sacral vertebrae are fused together to form the wedge-shaped *sacrum*, which connects the spine with the iliac wings of the pelvis (Fig. 37-1). The fifth sacral vertebra is not fused posteriorly, giving rise to a variably shaped opening known as the *sacral hiatus*. Occasionally, other sacral vertebrae do not fuse posteriorly, giving rise to a much larger sacral hiatus. The *sacral cornu* are bony prominences on either side of the hiatus and aid in identifying it. The sacral hiatus provides an opening into the sacral canal, which is the caudal termination of the epidural space. The four rudimentary

coccygeal vertebrae are fused together to form the *coccyx,* a narrow triangular bone that abuts the sacral hiatus and can be helpful in identifying it. The tip of the coccyx can often be palpated in the proximal gluteal cleft, and by running one's finger cephalad along its smooth surface, the sacral cornu can be identified as the first bony prominence encountered.

Identifying individual vertebrae is important for correctly locating the desired interspace for epidural and spinal blockade. The spine of C7 is the first prominent spinous process encountered while running the hand down the back of the neck. The spine of T1 is the most prominent spinous process and immediately follows C7. The 12th thoracic vertebra can be identified by palpating the 12th rib and tracing it back to its attachment to T12. A line drawn between the iliac crests crosses the body of L5 or the 4-5 interspace.

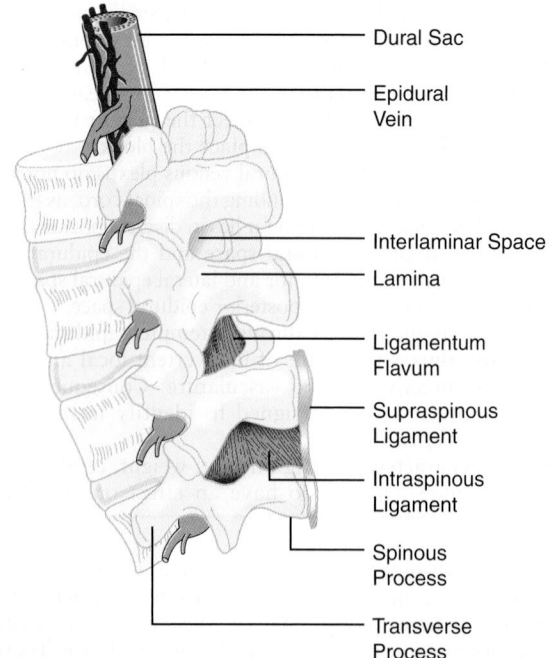

FIGURE 37-2. Detail of the lumbar spinal column and epidural space. Note that the epidural veins are largely restricted to the anterior and lateral epidural space.

Ligaments

The vertebral bodies are stabilized by five ligaments that increase in size between the cervical and lumbar vertebrae (Fig. 27-2). From the sacrum to T7, the *supraspinous ligament* runs between the tips of the spinous processes. Above T7 this ligament continues as the *ligamentum nuchae* and attaches to the occipital protuberance at the base of the skull. The *interspinous ligament* attaches between the spinous processes and blends posteriorly with the supraspinous ligament and anteriorly with the ligamentum flavum. The *ligamentum flavum* is a tough, wedge-shaped ligament composed of elastin. It consists of right and left portions that span adjacent vertebral laminae and fuse in the midline to varying degrees.[7,8] The ligamentum flavum is thickest in the midline, measuring 3 to 5 mm at the L2-3 interspace of adults. This ligament is also farthest from the spinal meninges in the midline, measuring 4 to 6 mm at the L2-3 interspace.[9] As a result, midline insertion of an epidural needle is least likely to result in unintended meningeal puncture. The anterior and posterior *longitudinal ligaments* run along the anterior and posterior surfaces of the vertebral bodies.

Epidural Space

The epidural space is the space that lies between the spinal meninges and the sides of the vertebral canal (Fig. 37-3). It is bounded cranially by the foramen magnum, caudally by the sacrococcygeal ligament covering the sacral hiatus, anteriorly by the posterior longitudinal ligament, laterally by the vertebral pedicles, and posteriorly by both the ligamentum flavum and vertebral lamina. The epidural space is not a closed space but communicates with the paravertebral space by way of the intervertebral foramina.[10] The epidural space is shallowest anteriorly where the dura may in some places fuse with the posterior longitudinal ligament. The space is deepest posteriorly, although the depth varies because the space is intermittently obliterated by contact between the dura mater and the ligamentum flavum or vertebral lamina. Contact between the dura mater and the pedicles also interrupts the epidural space laterally. Thus, the epidural space is composed of a series of discontinuous compartments that become continuous when the potential space separating the compartments is opened up by injection of air or liquid. A rich network of valveless veins (Batson plexus) courses

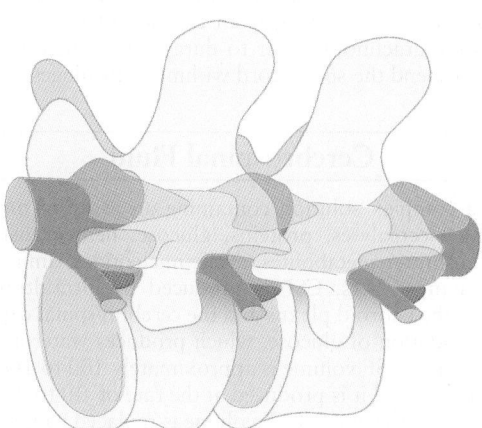

FIGURE 37-3. The compartments of the epidural space (*pink areas*) are discontinuous. Areas where no compartments are indicated represent a potential space where the dura mater normally abuts the sides of the vertebral canal. (Reprinted from Hogan Q: Lumbar epidural anatomy: A new look by cryomicrotome section. Anesthesiology 1991; 75: 767, with permission.)

through the anterior and lateral portions of the epidural space and only very rarely in the posterior epidural space (Fig. 37-2).[11] The epidural veins anastomose freely with extradural veins, including the pelvic veins, the azygous system, and the intracranial veins. The epidural space also contains lymphatics and segmental arteries running between the aorta and the spinal cord.

Epidural Fat

The most ubiquitous material in the epidural space is fat, which is principally located in the posterior and lateral epidural space (Fig. 37-3).[10] Interestingly, the epidural fat appears to have clinically important effects on the pharmacology of epidurally and intrathecally administered drugs. For example, using a pig model, Bernards et al.[12] showed that there is a linear relationship between an opioid's lipid solubility and its terminal elimination half-time in the epidural space, its mean residence time in the epidural space, and its concentration in epidural fat. In addition, net transfer of opioid from the epidural space to the intrathecal space was greatest for the least lipid-soluble opioid (morphine) and least for highly lipid-soluble opioids (fentanyl, sufentanil). In effect, increasing lipid solubility resulted in opioid "sequestration" in epidural fat, thereby reducing the bioavailability of drug in the underlying subarachnoid space and spinal tissue.

Epidural fat also appears to play a role in the pharmacokinetics of epidurally administered local anesthetics. Specifically, sequestration in epidural fat likely explains why a highly lipid-soluble local anesthetic like etidocaine is only approximately equipotent with lidocaine in the epidural space despite the fact that etidocaine is roughly 7 times more potent than lidocaine in vitro. Because of its much greater lipid solubility, etidocaine is more likely than lidocaine to be sequestered in epidural fat, thereby reducing the amount of drug available to produce block in the spinal nerve roots and spinal cord. Consistent with this hypothesis, Tucker and Mather[13] showed that after administering 80 mg of etidocaine and 50 mg of lidocaine into the epidural space of sheep, the amount of etidocaine still present in epidural fat 12 hours later was more than 100 times greater than the amount of lidocaine. Thus, sequestration in epidural fat appears to play an important role in the pharmacokinetics of local anesthetics just as it does for epidural opioids.

Meninges

The spinal meninges consist of three protective membranes (dura mater, arachnoid mater, and pia mater), which are continuous with the cranial meninges (Fig. 37-4).

Dura Mater

The dura mater is the outermost and thickest meningeal tissue. The spinal dura mater begins at the foramen magnum where it fuses with the periosteum of the skull, forming the cephalad border of the epidural space. Caudally, the dura mater ends at approximately S2, where it fuses with the filum terminale. The dura mater extends laterally along the spinal nerve roots and becomes continuous with the connective tissue of the epineurium at approximately the level of the intervertebral foramina. The dura mater is composed of randomly arranged collagen fibers and elastin fibers arranged longitudinally and circumferentially.[14] The dura mater is largely acellular except for a layer of cells that forms the border between the dura and arachnoid mater. Despite the lack of cellular elements, the inner edge of the dura mater is highly vascular,[15] which likely results in the dura mater being an important route of drug clearance from both the epidural space and the subarachnoid space.

There is controversy regarding the existence and clinical significance of a midline connective tissue band, the *plica medianis*

FIGURE 37-4. The spinal meninges of the dog, demonstrating the pia mater (PM) in apposition to the spinal cord, the subarachnoid space (SS), the arachnoid mater (AM), trabeculae (fibers stretching from arachnoid mater to pia mater), and the dura mater (DM). The separation between the arachnoid mater and the dura mater demonstrates the subdural space. The subdural space is only a potential space *in vivo* but is created here as an artifact of preparation. (Reprinted from Peters A, Palay SL, Webster H (Eds): The Fine Structure of the Nervous System: The Neurons and Supporting Cells. Philadelphia, WB Saunders, 1976, with permission.)

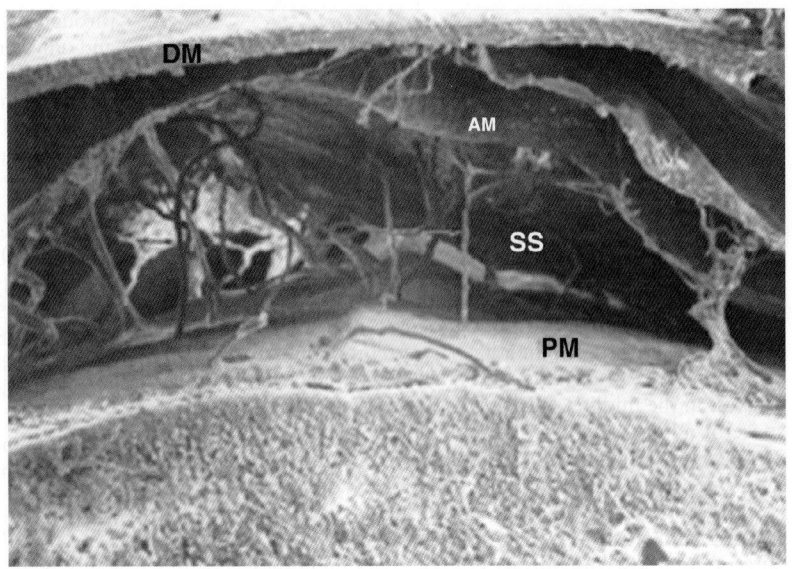

dorsalis, running from the dura mater to the ligamentum flavum. Anatomic studies using epiduroscopy[16] and epidurography[17] have demonstrated the presence of the plica medianis dorsalis and have led to speculation that this tissue band may on occasion be responsible for difficulty in inserting epidural catheters and for unilateral epidural block. However, using cryomicrotome sections to investigate the epidural space, Hogan[10] failed to find evidence of a substantial connection between the dura mater and the ligamentum flavum. He speculated that the injection of either air or contrast required for the earlier studies may have compressed epidural contents (e.g., fat) and produced an artifact mimicking a connective tissue band. In addition, Hogan[18] has shown in a clinical study that there is no significant impediment to spread of injectate across the midline. Thus, the plica medianis dorsalis does not appear to be clinically relevant with respect to clinical epidural anesthesia.

The inner surface of the dura mater abuts the arachnoid mater. There is a potential space between these two membranes called the *subdural space* (Fig. 37-4). Occasionally, a drug intended for either the epidural space or the subarachnoid space is injected into the subdural space.[19] Subdural injection has been estimated to occur in 0.82% of intended epidural injections.[20] The radiology literature suggests that the incidence of subdural injection during intended subarachnoid injection for myelography may be as high as 10%.[21]

Arachnoid Mater

The arachnoid mater is a delicate, avascular membrane composed of overlapping layers of flattened cells with connective tissue fibers running between the cellular layers. The arachnoid cells are interconnected by frequent tight junctions and occluding junctions. These specialized cellular connections likely account for the fact that the arachnoid mater is the principal anatomic barrier for drugs moving between the epidural space and the spinal cord.[22]

In the region where the spinal nerve roots traverse the dura and arachnoid membranes, the arachnoid mater herniates through the dura mater into the epidural space to form arachnoid granulations. As with the cranial arachnoid granulations, the spinal arachnoid granulations serve as a site for material in the subarachnoid space to exit the central nervous system (CNS). Although some have postulated that the arachnoid granulations are a preferred route for drugs to move from the

epidural space to the spinal cord, the available experimental data suggest that this is not the case.[23]

The *subarachnoid space* lies between the arachnoid mater and the pia mater and contains the cerebrospinal fluid (CSF). The spinal CSF is in continuity with the cranial CSF and provides an avenue for drugs in the spinal CSF to reach the brain. In addition, the spinal nerve roots and rootlets run in the subarachnoid space.

Pia Mater

The spinal pia mater is adherent to the spinal cord and is composed of a thin layer of connective tissue cells interspersed with collagen. Trabeculae connect the pia mater with the arachnoid mater and the cells of these two meninges blend together along the trabeculae. Unlike the arachnoid mater, the pia mater is fenestrated in places so that the spinal cord is in direct communication with the subarachnoid space. The pia mater extends to the tip of the spinal cord where it becomes the *filum terminale,* which anchors the spinal cord to the sacrum. The pia mater also gives rise to the dentate ligaments, which are thin connective tissue bands extending from the side of the spinal cord through the arachnoid mater to dura mater. These ligaments serve to suspend the spinal cord within the meninges.

Cerebrospinal Fluid

CSF is a complex solution containing an array of molecules including electrolytes, proteins, glucose, neurotransmitters, neurotransmitter metabolites, cyclic nucleotides, amino acids, among many others. CSF is produced by ultrafiltration of plasma in the choroid plexus and the cerebral/spinal capillaries and by oxidation of glucose, which produces water as a "byproduct." The CSF volume is approximately 100 to 160 mL in adult humans and it is produced at the rate of 20 to 25 mL/hr. Consequently, the entire CSF volume is replaced roughly every 6 hours. CSF is removed by arachnoid villi present in the superior sagittal sinus and along many spinal nerve roots.

Contrary to widely held view, CSF does not "flow" or "circulate" through the subarachnoid space. The development of cine-magnetic resonance imaging and cine-computed tomography techniques have shown that CSF oscillates in the cephalocaudal axis with a frequency equal to the heart rate.[24,25] CSF oscillates because cerebral expansion during systole displaces CSF caudally into the spinal canal and cerebral contraction during diastole causes the CSF displaced into the spinal canal to retreat back into the cranial vault. Net CSF movement is estimated at 0.04% per oscillation.

The clinical significance of this understanding of CSF motion is that CSF cannot be relied on to distribute drugs in the subarachnoid space. This is of little importance in single-shot spinal anesthesia because the kinetic energy of the injection and the baricity of the solution serve to distribute drug. However, the lack of significant net CSF motion explains why drug distribution during the very slow infusions used for chronic intrathecal analgesia results in very limited drug distribution.[26]

Spinal Cord

In the first-trimester fetus, the spinal cord extends from the foramen magnum to the end of the sacrum. Thereafter, the vertebral column lengthens more than the spinal cord so that at birth the spinal cord ends at about the level of the third lumbar vertebra. In the adult, the caudad tip of the spinal cord typically lies at the level of the first lumbar vertebra. However, in 30% of individuals the spinal cord may end at T12, while in 10% it may extend to L3 (Fig. 37-1).[27] A sacral spinal cord has been reported in an adult.[27] Flexion of the vertebral column causes the tip of the spinal cord to move slightly cephalad.

The spinal cord gives rise to 31 pairs of *spinal nerves*, each composed of an *anterior motor root* and a *posterior sensory root*. The nerve roots are in turn composed of multiple rootlets. The portion of the spinal cord that gives rise to all of the rootlets of a single spinal nerve is called a *cord segment*. The skin area innervated by a given spinal nerve and its corresponding cord segment is called a *dermatome* (Fig. 37-5). The

intermediolateral gray matter of the T1 through L2 spinal cord segments contains the cell bodies of the *preganglionic sympathetic neurons*. These sympathetic neurons run with the corresponding spinal nerve to a point just beyond the intervertebral foramen where they exit to join the sympathetic chain ganglia.

The spinal nerves and their corresponding cord segments are named for the intervertebral foramen through which they run. In the cervical region, the spinal nerves are named for the vertebra forming the caudad half of the intervertebral foramen; for example, C4 emerges through an intervertebral foramen formed by C3 and C4. In the thoracic and lumbar region, the nerve roots are named for the vertebrae forming the cephalad half of the intervertebral foramen; for example, L4 emerges through an intervertebral foramen formed by L4 and L5. Because the spinal cord usually ends between L1 and L2, the thoracic, lumbar, and sacral nerve roots run increasingly longer distances in the subarachnoid space to get from their spinal cord segment of origin to the intervertebral foramen through which they exit. Those nerves that extend beyond the end of the spinal cord to their exit site are collectively known as the *cauda equina* (Fig. 37-1).

TECHNIQUE

Spinal and epidural anesthesia should be performed only after appropriate monitors are applied and in a setting where equipment for airway management and resuscitation are immediately available. Before positioning the patient, all equipment for spinal block should be ready for use; for example, local anesthetics mixed and drawn up, needles uncapped, skin antiseptic solution available, and so on. Preparing all equipment ahead of time will minimize the time required to perform the block and thereby enhance patient comfort.

FIGURE 37-5. Human sensory dermatomes.

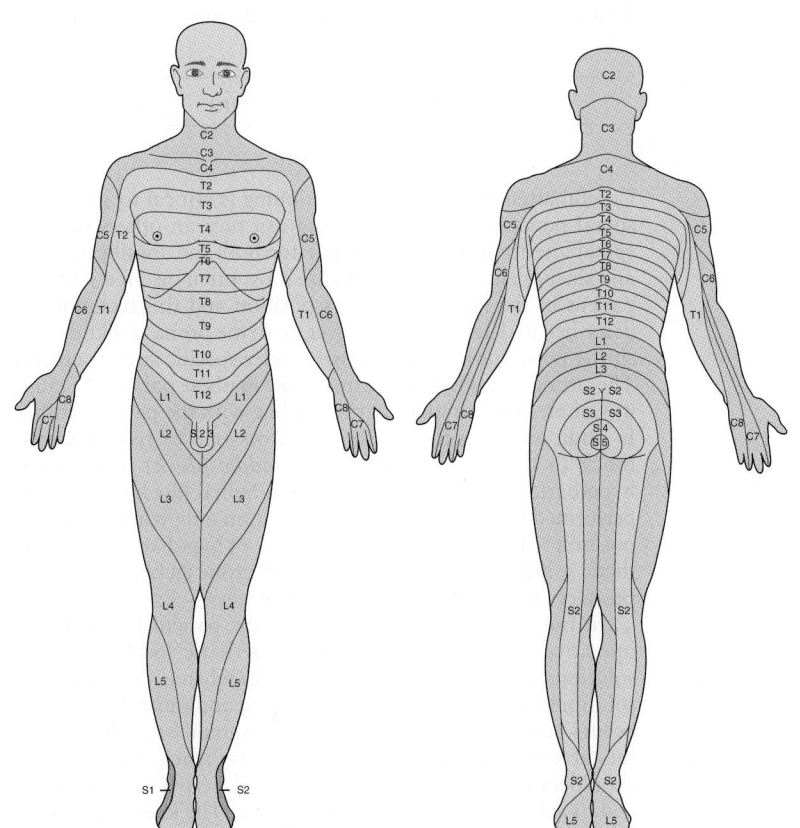

Needles

Spinal and epidural needles are classified by the design of their tips (Fig. 37-6). The Whitacre, Eldor, Marx, and Sprotte spinal needles have a "pencil-point" tip with one or two (Eldor) aperture(s) on the side of the shaft proximal to the tip. The Greene, Atraucan, and Quincke needles have beveled tips with cutting edges. The pencil-point needles require more force to insert than the bevel-tip needles but provide a better tactile "feel" of the various tissues encountered as the needle is inserted. In addition, the bevel has been shown to cause the needle to be deflected from the intended path as it passes through tissues while the pencil-point needles are not deflected.[28] Epidural needles have a larger diameter than spinal needles to facilitate the injection of fluid or air when using the "loss-of-resistance" technique to identify the epidural space. In addition, the larger diameter allows for easier insertion of catheters into the epidural space. The Tuohy epidural needle has a curved tip to help control the direction that the catheter moves in the epidural space. The Hustead needle tip is also curved, although somewhat less than the Tuohy needle. The Crawford needle tip is straight, making it less suitable for catheter insertion.

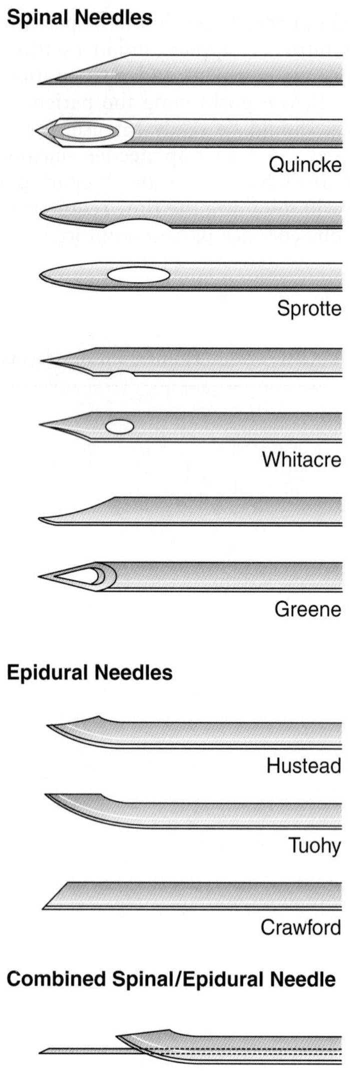

Spinal Needles

Quincke

Sprotte

Whitacre

Greene

Epidural Needles

Hustead

Tuohy

Crawford

Combined Spinal/Epidural Needle

FIGURE 37-6.   Some of the commercially available needles for spinal and epidural anesthesia. Needles are distinguished by the design of their tips.

The outside diameter of both epidural and spinal needles is used to determine their gauge. Larger gauge (i.e., smaller diameter) spinal needles are less likely to cause postdural puncture headaches (PDPH), but are more readily deflected than smaller gauge needles. Epidural needles are typically sized 16 to 19 gauge and spinal needles 22 to 29 gauge. Spinal needles smaller than 22 gauge are often easier to insert if an introducer needle is used. The introducer is inserted into the interspinous ligament in the intended direction of the spinal needle and the spinal needle is then inserted through the shaft of the introducer. The introducer prevents the spinal needle from being deflected or bent as it passes through the interspinous ligament.[28] Needles of the same outside diameter may have different inside diameters. This is important because inside diameter determines how large a catheter can be inserted through the needle and determines how rapidly CSF will appear at the needle hub during spinal needle insertion. All spinal and epidural needles come with a tight-fitting stylet. The stylet prevents the needle from being plugged with skin or fat and, importantly, prevents dragging skin into the epidural or subarachnoid spaces, where the skin may grow and form dermoid tumors.

Sedation

If the patient desires, light sedation is appropriate before placement of spinal or epidural block. Generally, the patient should not be heavily sedated because successful spinal and epidural anesthesia requires patient participation to maintain good position, evaluate block height, and to enable communication with the anesthesiologist should a paresthesia occur when the needle contacts neural elements. In addition, patient cooperation is required to properly evaluate an epidural test dose; sedation with as little as 1.5 mg of midazolam plus 75 μg of fentanyl has been shown to reduce the reliability of patient reports of subjective symptoms of intravenous (IV) local anesthetic injection.[29] Once the block is placed and adequate block height assured, the patient can be sedated as deemed appropriate.

Spinal Anesthesia

Position

Careful attention to patient positioning is critical to successful spinal puncture. Poor positioning can turn an otherwise easy spinal anesthetic into a challenge for both the anesthesiologist and the patient. Spinal needles are most often inserted with the patient in the lateral decubitus position and this technique is described in detail later. However, both the prone jackknife and sitting positions offer advantages under specific circumstances. The sitting position is sometimes used in obese patients because it is often easier to identify the midline with the patient sitting. In addition, the sitting position allows one to restrict spinal block to the sacral dermatomes (*saddle block*) when using hyperbaric local anesthetic solutions. Spinal block is generally performed in the prone jackknife position only when this is the position to be used for surgery. The use of hypobaric local anesthetic solutions with the patient in the prone jackknife position produces sacral block for perirectal surgery.

In the lateral decubitus position, the patient lies with the operative side down when using hyperbaric local anesthetic solutions and with the operative side up when using hypobaric solutions, thus assuring that the earliest and most dense block occurs on the operative side. The back should be at the edge of the table so that the patient is within easy reach. The patient's shoulders and hips are both positioned perpendicular to the bed to help prevent rotation of the spine. The knees are drawn to the chest, the neck is flexed, and the patient is instructed to actively curve the back outward. This will spread the spinous processes apart and maximize the size of the interlaminar foramen. It is useful to have an assistant who can help the patient maintain this position. Using the iliac crests as a landmark (a line drawn between the iliac crests crosses the body of L5 or the 4-5 interspace), the L2-3, L3-4, and L4-5 interspaces are identified and the desired interspace chosen for needle insertion. Interspaces above L2-3 are avoided to decrease the risk of hitting the spinal cord with the needle. Some find it helpful to mark the spinous processes flanking the desired interspace with a skin marker. This obviates the need to reidentify the intended interspace after the patient is prepared and draped.

The skin is prepared with an appropriate antiseptic solution and draped. All antiseptic solutions are neurotoxic, and care must be taken not to contaminate spinal needles or local anesthetics with the antiseptic solution. Chlorhexidine-alcohol antiseptic prevents colonization of percutaneous catheters better than does 10% povidone-iodine. Consequently, the American Society of Regional Anesthesia currently recommends chlorhexidine for skin antisepsis prior to regional anesthesia procedures.[a] How one drapes is a matter of personal preference, but clear plastic drapes offer the important advantage of permitting visualization of the entire back, which makes it easier to identify a rotated or inadequately flexed spine.

Midline Approach

For the midline approach to the subarachnoid space, the skin overlying the desired interspace is infiltrated with a small amount of local anesthetic to prevent pain when inserting the spinal needle. One should avoid raising too large a skin wheal because this can obscure palpation of the interspace, especially in obese patients. Additional local anesthetic (1 to 2 mL) is then deposited along the intended path of the spinal needle to a depth of 1 to 2 inches. This deeper infiltration provides additional anesthesia for spinal needle insertion and helps identify the correct path for the spinal needle. Infiltrating local anesthetic lateral to the midline is painful and generally unnecessary.

The spinal needle or introducer needle is inserted in the middle of the interspace with a slight cephalad angulation of 10 to 15 degrees (Fig. 37-7). The needle is then advanced, in order, through the subcutaneous tissue, supraspinous ligament, interspinous ligament, ligamentum flavum, epidural space, dura mater, and finally arachnoid mater. The ligaments produce a characteristic "feel" às the needle is advanced through them, and the anesthesiologist should develop the ability to distinguish a needle that is advancing through the high-resistance ligaments from one that is advancing through lower-resistance paraspinous muscle. This will allow early detection and correction of needles that are not advancing in the midline. Penetration of the dura mater often produces a subtle "pop" that is most easily detected with the pencil-point needles. Detection of dural penetration will prevent inserting the needle all the way through the subarachnoid space and contacting the vertebral body. In addition, learning to detect dural penetration will allow one to insert the spinal needle quickly without having to stop every few millimeters and remove the stylet to look for CSF at the needle hub.

Once the needle tip is believed to be in the subarachnoid space, the stylet is removed to see if CSF appears at the needle hub. With small-diameter needles (26 to 29 gauge) this generally requires 5 to 10 seconds, but may require ≥1 minute in some patients. Gentle aspiration may speed the appearance of CSF. If CSF does not appear, the needle orifice may be obstructed by a nerve root and rotating the needle 90 degrees may result in CSF flow. Alternatively, the needle orifice may not be completely in the subarachnoid space and advancing an

[a]See http://www.asra.com/consensus-statements/3.html.

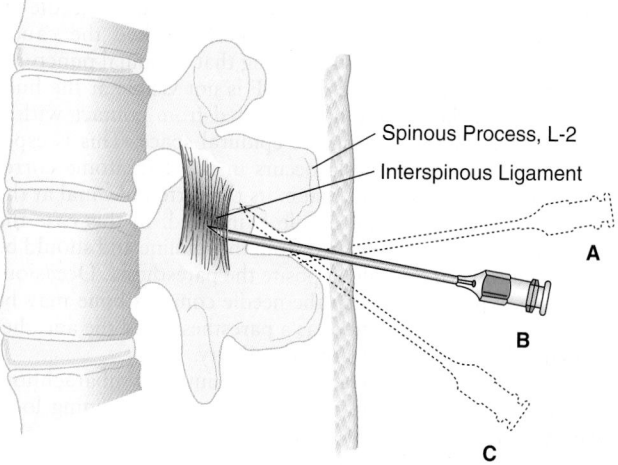

FIGURE 37-7. Midline approach to the subarachnoid space. The spinal needle is inserted with a slight cephalad angulation and should advance in the midline without contacting bone (**B**). If bone is contacted, it may be either the caudad (**A**) or the cephalad spinous process (**C**). The needle should be redirected slightly cephalad and reinserted. If bone is encountered at a shallower depth, the needle is likely walking up the cephalad spinous process. If bone is encountered at a deeper depth, the needle is likely walking down the inferior spinous process. If bone is repeatedly contacted at the same depth, the needle is likely off the midline and walking along the lamina. (Reprinted from Mulroy MF: Regional Anesthesia: An Illustrated Procedural Guide. Boston, Little Brown, 1989, with permission.)

additional 1 to 2 mm may result in brisk CSF flow. This is particularly true of pencil-point needles, which have their orifice on the side of the needle shaft proximal to the needle tip. Finally, failure to obtain CSF suggests that the needle orifice is not in the subarachnoid space and the needle should be reinserted.

If bone is encountered during needle insertion, the anesthesiologist must develop a reasoned, systematic approach to redirecting the needle. Simply withdrawing the needle and repeatedly reinserting it in different directions is not appropriate. When contacting bone, the depth should be immediately noted and the needle redirected slightly cephalad. If bone is again encountered at a greater depth, then the needle is most likely walking down the inferior spinous process and it should be redirected more cephalad until the subarachnoid space is reached. If bone is encountered again at a shallower depth, then the needle is most likely walking up the superior spinous process and it should be redirected more caudad. If bone is repeatedly encountered at the same depth, then the needle is likely off the midline and walking along the vertebral lamina (Fig. 37-7).

When redirecting a needle it is important to withdraw the tip into the subcutaneous tissue. If the tip remains embedded in one of the vertebral ligaments, attempts at redirecting the needle will simply bend the shaft and will not reliably change needle direction. When using an introducer needle, it also must be withdrawn into the subcutaneous tissue before being redirected. Changes in needle direction should be made in small increments because even small changes in needle angle at the skin may result in fairly large changes in position of the needle tip when it reaches the spinal meninges at a depth of 4 to 6 cm. Care should be exercised when gripping the needle to ensure that it does not bow. Insertion of a curved needle will cause it to veer off course.

If the patient experiences a paresthesia, it is important to determine whether the needle tip has encountered a nerve root in the epidural space or in the subarachnoid space. When the paresthesia occurs, immediately stop advancing the needle, remove the stylet, and look for CSF at the needle hub. The presence of CSF confirms that the needle encountered a cauda equina nerve root in the subarachnoid space and the needle tip is in good position. Given how tightly packed the cauda equina nerve roots are, it is surprising that all spinal punctures do not produce paresthesias. If CSF is not visible at the hub, then the paresthesia may have resulted from contact with a spinal nerve root traversing the epidural space. This is especially true if the paresthesia occurs in the dermatome corresponding to the nerve root that exits the vertebral canal at the same level that the spinal needle is inserted. In this case the needle has most likely deviated from the midline and should be redirected toward the side opposite the paresthesia. Occasionally, pain experienced when the needle contacts bone may be misinterpreted by the patient as a paresthesia and the anesthesiologist should be alert to this possibility.

Once the needle is correctly inserted into the subarachnoid space, it is fixed in position and the syringe containing local anesthetic is attached. CSF is gently aspirated to confirm that the needle is still in the subarachnoid space and the local anesthetic slowly injected (≤ 0.5 mL/sec). After completing the injection, a small volume of CSF is again aspirated to confirm that the needle tip remained in the subarachnoid space while the local anesthetic was deposited. This CSF is then reinjected and the needle, syringe, and any introducer removed together as a unit. If the surgical procedure is to be performed in the supine position, the patient is helped onto his or her back. To prevent excessive cephalad spread of hyperbaric local anesthetic, care should be taken to ensure that the patient's hips are not raised off the bed as they turn.

Once the block is placed, strict attention must be paid to the patient's hemodynamic status with blood pressure and/or heart rate supported as necessary. Block height should also be assessed early by pin prick or temperature sensation. Temperature sensation is tested by wiping the skin with alcohol, and may be preferable to pin prick because it is not painful. If, after a few minutes, the block is not rising high enough or is rising too high, the table may be tilted as appropriate to influence further spread of hypobaric or hyperbaric local anesthetics.

Paramedian Approach

The paramedian approach to the epidural and subarachnoid spaces is useful in situations where the patient's anatomy does not favor the midline approach, such as inability to flex the spine or heavily calcified interspinous ligaments. This approach can be used with the patient in any position and is probably the best approach for the patient in the prone jackknife position.

The spinous process forming the lower border of the desired interspace is identified. The needle is inserted approximately 1 cm lateral to this point and is directed toward the middle of the interspace by angling it approximately 45 degrees cephalad with just enough medial angulation (approximately 15 degrees) to compensate for the lateral insertion point. The first significant resistance encountered should be the ligamentum flavum. Bone encountered prior to the ligamentum flavum is usually the vertebral lamina of the cephalad vertebra and the needle should be redirected accordingly. An alternative method is to insert the needle perpendicular to the skin in all planes until the lamina is contacted. The needle is then walked off the superior edge of the lamina and into the subarachnoid space. The lamina provides a valuable landmark that facilitates correct needle placement; however, repeated needle contact with the periosteum can be painful.

Lumbosacral Approach

The lumbosacral (or Taylor) approach to the subarachnoid and epidural spaces is simply a paramedian approach directed at the L5-S1 interspace, which is the largest interlaminar space. This approach may be useful when anatomic constraints make other approaches unfeasible. The patient may be positioned laterally, prone, or sitting, and the needle inserted at a point 1 cm medial and 1 cm inferior to the posterior superior iliac spine. The needle is angled cephalad 45 to 55 degrees and just medial enough to reach the midline at the level of the L5 spinous process. As with the paramedian approach, the interspinous ligament is bypassed and the first significant resistance felt should be the ligamentum flavum.

Continuous Spinal Anesthesia

Inserting a catheter into the subarachnoid space increases the utility of spinal anesthesia by permitting repeated drug administration as often as necessary to extend the level or duration of spinal block. A common and reasonable recommendation for subsequent dosing or "topping up" of continuous spinal blocks is to administer half the original dose of local anesthetic when the block has reached two thirds of its expected duration.

The technique is similar to that described for "single-shot" spinal anesthesia except that a needle large enough to accommodate the desired catheter must be used. After inserting the needle and obtaining free-flowing CSF, the catheter is simply threaded into the subarachnoid space a distance of 2 to 3 cm. It is often easier to insert the catheter if it is directed cephalad or caudad instead of laterally. If the catheter does not easily pass beyond the needle tip, rotating the needle 180 degrees may be helpful or another interspace may be used. The catheter should not be withdrawn back into the needle shaft because of the risk of shearing the catheter off into the subarachnoid space.

A variety of catheters and needles are available for continuous spinal anesthesia. Commonly, 18-gauge epidural needles and 20-gauge catheters are used. However, needles and catheters this size carry a higher risk of PDPH, especially in young patients. Because of this risk, smaller needle and catheter combinations have been developed with catheters ranging in size from 24 to 32 gauge. Although smaller catheters decrease the risk of PDPH, they have also been associated with multiple reports of neurologic injury, specifically, cauda equina syndrome (see "Complications"). For this reason, the United States Food and Drug Administration has advised against using any catheter smaller than 24 gauge for continuous spinal anesthesia.

Epidural Anesthesia

For the novice, correct placement of an epidural needle can be technically more challenging than spinal needle placement because there is less room for error. However, with experience, epidural needle placement is often easier than spinal needle placement because the larger-gauge needles used for epidural anesthesia are less likely to be deflected from their intended path and they produce much better tactile feel of the interspinous and flaval ligaments. In addition, the loss of resistance technique provides a much clearer end point when entering the epidural space than does the subtle "pop" of a spinal needle piercing the dura mater.

Patient preparation, positioning, monitors, and needle approaches for epidural anesthesia are the same as for spinal anesthesia. Unlike spinal anesthesia, epidural anesthesia may be performed at any intervertebral space. However, at vertebral levels above the termination of the spinal cord, the epidural needle may accidentally puncture the spinal meninges and damage the underlying spinal cord. To prevent accidental meningeal puncture, the anesthesiologist must learn to identify the interspinous ligaments and the ligamentum flavum by their feel. In addition, epidural needles must be advanced slowly and, most importantly, under control.

After proper positioning, sterile skin preparation, and draping, the desired interspace is identified and a local anesthetic skin wheal is raised at the point of needle insertion. Because epidural needles are relatively blunt, it is sometimes helpful to pierce the skin with a ≥18-gauge hypodermic needle before inserting the epidural needle. For epidural anesthesia using the midline approach, the epidural needle is inserted through the subcutaneous tissue and into the interspinous ligament. The interspinous ligament has a characteristic "gritty" feel, much like inserting a needle into a bag of sand. This is especially true of younger patients. If the interspinous ligament is not clearly identified, then one should be suspicious that the needle is not in the midline. After engaging the interspinous ligament, the needle is advanced slowly through it until an increase in resistance is felt. This increased resistance represents the ligamentum flavum.

The epidural needle must now traverse the ligamentum flavum and stop within the epidural space before puncturing the spinal meninges. Numerous techniques for identifying the epidural space have been used successfully; however, the loss of resistance to fluid has the advantage of simplicity, reliability, and, most importantly, a higher success rate when compared to the use of air for loss of resistance.[30] In addition, use of fluid instead of air for loss of resistance decreases the risk of PDPH in the event of accidental meningeal puncture.[31]

A glass syringe or a specially designed low-resistance plastic syringe is filled with 2 to 3 mL of saline and a small (0.1 to 0.3 mL) air bubble. The syringe is attached to the epidural needle and the plunger is pressed until the air bubble is visibly compressed. If the needle tip is properly embedded within the ligamentum flavum, it should be possible to compress the air bubble without injecting fluid. In this way the air bubble serves as a gauge of the appropriate amount of pressure to exert on the syringe plunger. If the air bubble cannot be compressed without injecting fluid, then the needle tip is most likely not in the ligamentum flavum. In this case, the needle tip may still be in the interspinous ligament, or it may be off the midline in the paraspinous muscles. To differentiate between these possibilities, one can carefully advance the needle and syringe a few millimeters in an effort to engage the ligamentum flavum. If it is still not possible to compress the air bubble, withdraw the needle into the subcutaneous tissue and reinsert it.

Once the ligamentum flavum is identified, the needle is slowly advanced with the nondominant hand while the dominant hand maintains constant pressure on the syringe plunger (Fig. 37-8). Do not advance the needle with the hand compressing the plunger because this does not allow for adequate control of needle movement. As the needle tip enters the epidural space, there will be a sudden and dramatic loss of resistance as the saline is rapidly injected. Saline injection into the epidural space can be moderately painful and patients should be forewarned. If the needle is advancing obliquely through the ligamentum flavum, it is possible to enter into the paraspinous muscles instead of the epidural space. In this case the loss of resistance will be less dramatic. To help verify that the needle has entered the epidural space, 0.5 mL of air can be drawn into the syringe and injected. There will be virtually no resistance to air injection in the epidural space, while in the paraspinous muscles air injection will encounter demonstrable resistance.

After entering the epidural space, stop advancing the needle. Because the dura mater abuts the ligamentum flavum in many places, the dura may now be tented over the needle tip and advancing the needle any farther than necessary heightens the risk of accidental meningeal puncture, that is, "*wet tap*." When the syringe is disconnected from the needle, it is common to have a small amount of fluid flow from the needle hub. This is usually the saline flowing back out of the epidural space but it could be CSF if the needle accidentally entered the subarachnoid space. CSF can often be distinguished by the fact that CSF will usually flow out in a volume greatly exceeding that used for the loss of resistance, CSF will be warm compared with saline, and CSF will test positive for glucose.

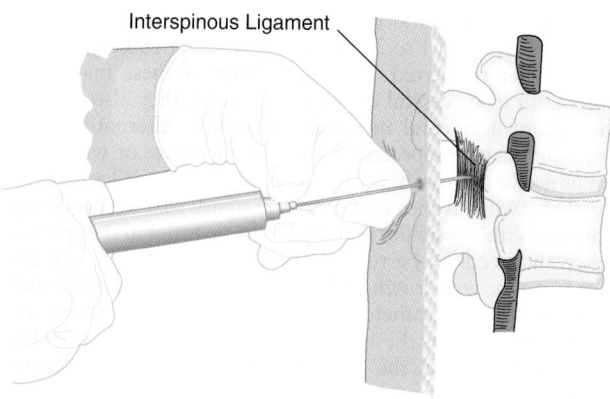

Interspinous Ligament

FIGURE 37-8.   Proper hand position when using the loss-of-resistance technique to locate the epidural space. After embedding the needle tip in the ligamentum flavum, a syringe with 2 to 3 mL of saline and an air bubble is attached. The left hand rests securely on the back and the fingers of the left hand grasp the needle firmly. The left hand advances the needle slowly and under control by rotating at the wrist. The fingers of the right hand maintain constant pressure on the syringe plunger but do not aid in advancing the needle. If the needle tip is properly engaged in the ligamentum flavum, it should be possible to compress the air bubble without injecting the saline. As the needle tip enters the epidural space, there will be a sudden loss of resistance and the saline will be suddenly injected. (Reprinted from Mulroy MF: Regional Anesthesia: An Illustrated Procedural Guide. Boston, Little Brown, 1989, with permission.)

If a single-shot technique is to be used, then a local anesthetic test dose should be administered to help rule out undetected subarachnoid or IV needle placement. After a negative test dose, the desired volume of local anesthetic should be administered in small increments (e.g., 5 mL) at a rate of 0.5 to 1 mL/sec. Slow, incremental injection decreases the risk of pain during injection and allows detection of adverse reactions to accidental IV or subarachnoid placement before the entire dose is administered.

Continuous Epidural Anesthesia

Use of a catheter for epidural anesthesia affords much greater flexibility than the single-shot technique because the catheter can be used to prolong a block that is too short, to extend a block that is too low, or to provide postoperative analgesia. On the downside, catheters may migrate into an epidural vein, into the subarachnoid space, or out an intervertebral foramen. Catheter use is also more likely to result in unilateral epidural block, a clinical fact shown to result from catheter tips that end up in the anterior epidural space or migrate out an intervertebral foramina.[18,32] An ever-changing selection of epidural catheters is commercially available. They differ in diameter, stiffness, location of injection holes, presence or absence of a stylet, construction material, and the like. Whichever catheter is chosen, it is important to verify that it passes easily through the epidural needle before the needle is placed in the epidural space. Epidural catheters are usually inserted through either Tuohy or Hustead needles because their curved tips help direct the catheter away from the dura mater. The needle bevel should be directed either cephalad or caudad, although the direction of the bevel does not guarantee that the catheter will travel in that direction. The catheter will typically encounter resistance as it reaches the curve at the tip of the needle, but steady pressure will usually result in passage into the epidural space. If the catheter will not pass beyond the needle tip, it is possible that the needle opening is not completely in the epidural space or that some structure in the epidural space is preventing catheter insertion (e.g., epidural fat). In this instance, the needle can be carefully advanced 1 to 2 mm more or rotated 180 degrees and the catheter reinserted. Although either of these maneuvers may result in successful catheter placement, they also increase the risk of accidental meningeal puncture. Alternatively, the procedure can be repeated at another interspace or with a different needle approach, for example, paramedian. Occasionally a catheter will advance only a short distance past the needle tip. This raises the possibility that the needle tip is not in the epidural space and needs to be repositioned. In this case, the catheter should not be withdrawn back into the epidural needle because of the risk that the catheter tip will be sheared off by the bevel's sharp edge. Rather, the needle and catheter should be pulled out in tandem and the procedure repeated. An alternative explanation for the inability to thread an epidural catheter is that the tip of the epidural needle was bent during bony contact and now partially occludes the needle lumen.

The catheter should be advanced only 3 to 5 cm into the epidural space. Placing a longer length of catheter in the epidural space increases the risk that it will form a knot,[33,34] enter an epidural vein, puncture the spinal meninges, exit an intervertebral foramen, wrap around a nerve root, or wind up in some other disadvantageous location. Once the catheter is appropriately positioned in the epidural space, the needle is slowly withdrawn with one hand as the catheter is stabilized with the other. After the needle is removed, the length of catheter in the epidural space is confirmed by subtracting the distance between the skin and the epidural space from the length of catheter below the skin. Documenting this distance is important when trying to determine if catheters used in the postoperative period have been dislodged.

An epidural test dose must be administered through the catheter to test for IV or subarachnoid placement before incrementally delivering the entire epidural drug dose. In addition, because of the risk of undetected IV or subarachnoid migration of the catheter over time, additional test doses must be administered before each top-up dose is given through the catheter. As with continuous spinal anesthesia, a reasonable guideline for top-up doses is to administer half the initial local anesthetic dose at an interval equal to two thirds the expected duration of the block.

Epidural Test Dose

The epidural test dose is designed to identify epidural needles or catheters that have entered an epidural vein or the subarachnoid space. Failure to perform the test may result in IV injection of toxic doses of local anesthetic or total spinal block. Aspirating the catheter or needle to check for blood or CSF is helpful if positive, but the incidence of false-negative aspirations is too high to rely on this technique alone.[35]

The most common test dose is 3 mL of local anesthetic containing 5 μg/mL of epinephrine (1:200,000). The dose of local anesthetic should be sufficient that subarachnoid injection will result in clear evidence of spinal anesthesia. Intravenous injection of this dose of epinephrine typically produces an average 30 beats per minute heart rate increase between 20 and 40 seconds after injection.[36,37] Heart rate increases may not be as evident in some patients taking beta-blocking drugs; reflex bradycardia usually occurs in these patients.[36,38] In beta-blocked patients, a systolic blood pressure increase of ≥20 mm Hg may be a more reliable indicator of IV injection.[36,38]

Importantly, the sensitivity of the standard 15 μg epinephrine test dose has been shown to be markedly diminished by preexisting high thoracic epidural anesthesia and/or concurrent general anesthesia.[39] Larger epinephrine doses may be effective at detecting IV injection in these settings, but that has not been shown experimentally.

Isoproterenol has also been used to detect intravascular injection.[40] In addition, air injection combined with a precordial Doppler to detect the characteristic murmur has been used successfully to test for IV placement of epidural catheters.[35] These techniques have been developed for use in laboring women in whom the sensitivity of epinephrine as a test dose is disturbingly low because maternal heart rate increases during contractions are often as large as those produced by epinephrine.[41] The clinical indications for these alternative tests of IV injection await additional larger studies.

Combined Spinal-Epidural Anesthesia

Combined spinal-epidural anesthesia (CSEA) is a useful technique by which a spinal block and an epidural catheter are placed simultaneously. This technique is popular because it combines the rapid onset, dense block of spinal anesthesia with the flexibility afforded by an epidural catheter. There are special epidural needles with a separate lumen to accommodate a spinal needle available for CSEA (Fig. 37-6). However, the technique is easily performed by first placing a standard epidural needle in the epidural space and then inserting an appropriately sized spinal needle through the shaft of the epidural needle and into the subarachnoid space. The desired local anesthetic is injected into the subarachnoid space, the spinal needle is removed, and a catheter placed in the epidural space via the epidural needle. The catheter can then be used to extend the height or duration of intraoperative block or can be used to provide postoperative epidural analgesia.

An interesting pharmacologic aspect of CSEA is the observation that after the peak spinal block height is established, both saline and local anesthetic injected into the epidural space are effective at pushing the block level higher.[42–44] This observation has been interpreted to indicate that the mechanism by which the epidural "top-up" increases block height is by a volume effect (i.e., compression of the spinal meninges forcing CSF cephalad) as well as a local anesthetic effect.

A potential risk of this technique is that the meningeal hole made by the spinal needle may allow dangerously high concentrations of subsequently administered epidural drugs to reach the subarachnoid space. Anecdotal case reports and in vitro animal studies suggest that this may be a legitimate concern.[41,45–47] Although CSEA is advantageous in some circumstances, additional prospective studies are necessary to identify the relative risks and limitations of the technique.

PHARMACOLOGY

Successful spinal or epidural anesthesia requires a block that is high enough to block sensation at the surgical site and last for the duration of the planned procedure. However, because variability between patients is considerable (Figs. 37-9 and 37-10), reliably predicting the height and duration of central neuraxial block that will result from a particular local anesthetic dose is difficult. Thus, recommendations regarding local anesthetic choice and dose must be viewed as approximate guidelines. The clinician must understand the factors governing spinal and epidural block height and duration to individualize local anesthetic choice and dose for each patient and procedure.

Spinal Anesthesia

Block Height

Table 37-1 lists some common surgical procedures that are readily performed under spinal anesthesia and the block height

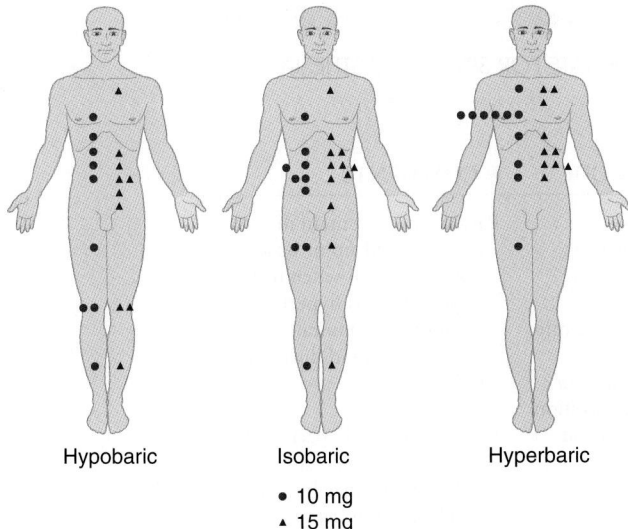

Hypobaric   Isobaric   Hyperbaric

• 10 mg
▲ 15 mg

FIGURE 37-9.   Peak spinal block height following 10- and 15-mg doses of hypobaric, isobaric, and hyperbaric tetracaine solutions injected at L3-4 with patients in the lateral horizontal position. Note that dose has no influence on block height and that there is considerable interindividual variability in peak block height, especially with the hypobaric solution. (Adapted from Brown DT, Wildsmith JA, Covino BG et al: Effect of baricity on spinal anaesthesia with amethocaine. Br J Anaesth 1980; 52: 589, with permission.)

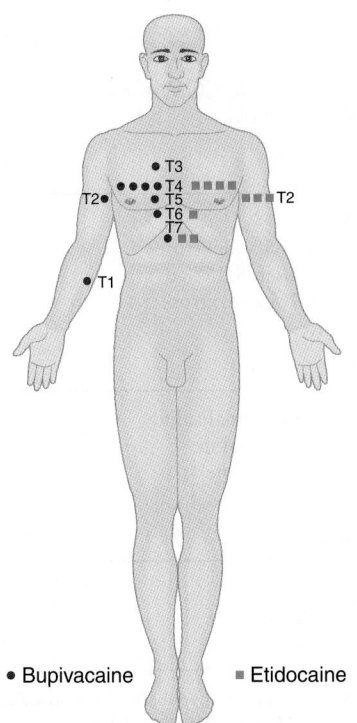

• Bupivacaine   ■ Etidocaine

FIGURE 37-10.   Peak epidural block height following 20 mL of 0.75% bupivacaine or 1.5% etidocaine injected via a catheter at the L1-2 interspace. Note that despite a well-controlled technique, the interindividual variability in block height is considerable and demonstrates the difficulty in accurately predicting block height in an individual patient. (Adapted from Sinclair CJ, Scott DB: Comparison of bupivacaine and etidocaine in extradural blockade. Br J Anaesth 1984; 56: 147, with permission.)

that is usually sufficient to ensure patient comfort. Also listed are techniques that are appropriate to achieve the desired block height. The rationale for these recommendations is explained in the following section.

Baricity and Patient Position.   The height of spinal block is thought to be determined by the cephalad spread of local anesthetic within the CSF. Table 37-2 lists some of the many variables that have been proposed to influence the spread of local anesthetics within the subarachnoid space. Many of these variables have been shown to be of negligible clinical importance. Of those factors that do exert significant influence on local anesthetic spread, the baricity of the local anesthetic solution relative to patient position is probably the most important. *Baricity* is defined as the ratio of the density (mass/volume) of the local anesthetic solution divided by the density of CSF, which averages 1.0003 ± 0.0003 g/mL at 37°C. Solutions that have the same density as CSF have a baricity of 1.0000 and are termed *isobaric*. Solutions that are more dense than CSF are termed *hyperbaric*, whereas solutions that are less dense than CSF are termed *hypobaric*.

Table 37-3 lists the baricity of local anesthetic solutions commonly used for spinal anesthesia. For practical purposes, solutions with a baricity <0.9990 can be expected to reliably behave hypobarically in all patients. Hypobaric solutions are typically prepared by mixing the local anesthetic solution with distilled water. Solutions with a baricity of ≥1.0015 can be expected to reliably behave hyperbarically. Hyperbaric solutions are typically prepared by mixing the local anesthetic in 5 to 8% dextrose. The baricity of the resultant solution depends on the amount of dextrose added; however, dextrose concentrations between 1.25 and 8% result in equivalent block heights.[48,49] Lower dextrose concentrations have been shown to have a concentration-dependent effect on block height, with 0.33% producing a block to T9.5 on average, 0.83% producing a block to T7.2, and 8% producing a block to T3.6.[50]

Baricity is important in determining local anesthetic spread and thus block height because gravity causes hyperbaric solutions to flow downward in CSF to the most dependent regions of the spinal column, whereas hypobaric solutions tend to rise in CSF. In contrast, gravity has no effect on the distribution of truly isobaric solutions. Thus, the anesthesiologist can exert considerable influence on block height by choice of anesthetic solution and proper patient positioning. Spinal block can be restricted to the sacral and low lumbar dermatomes ("*saddle block*") by administering a hyperbaric local anesthetic solution with the patient in the sitting position[51] or by administering a hypobaric solution with the patient in the prone jackknife position. Similarly, high thoracic to midcervical levels of anesthesia can be reached by administering hyperbaric solutions with the patient in the horizontal and Trendelenburg positions[52,53] or by administering hypobaric solutions with the patient in a semisitting position. However, this use of hypobaric solutions is not recommended because the high block achieved and the diminished venous return associated with the upright posture can lead to significant cardiovascular compromise.

The sitting, Trendelenberg, and jackknife positions have marked influences on the distribution of hypobaric and hyperbaric solutions because these positions accentuate the effect of gravity. However, most spinal anesthetics are administered as hyperbaric solutions injected while patients are in the horizontal lateral position, after which they are turned to the horizontal supine position. In this situation the influence of gravity is more subtle because the dependent areas of the spinal column do not deviate as much from the horizontal. While the patient is turned laterally, gravity has a small but measurable effect on local anesthetic distribution in that hyperbaric solutions will produce a denser, longer lasting block on the dependent side, while hypobaric solutions will have the opposite effect.[54] This

TABLE 37-1

REPRESENTATIVE SURGICAL PROCEDURES APPROPRIATE FOR SPINAL ANESTHESIA

SURGICAL PROCEDURE	SUGGESTED BLOCK HEIGHT	TECHNIQUE	COMMENTS
Perianal Perirectal	L1-2	Hyperbaric solution/sitting position Hypobaric solution/jackknife position Isobaric solution/horizontal position	Patients must remain in relative head-up or head-down position when using hypobaric and hyperbaric solutions to maintain restricted spread during the procedure
Lower extremity Hip Transurethral resection of the prostate Vaginal/cervical	T10	Isobaric solution	Hypobaric and hyperbaric solutions are also suitable but may produce higher blocks than necessary
Herniorrhaphy Pelvic procedures Appendectomy	T6-8	Hyperbaric solution/horizontal position	Isobaric solutions injected at L2-3 interspace may also be suitable
Abdominal Cesarean section	T4-6	Hyperbaric solution/horizontal position	Upper abdominal procedures usually require concomitant general anesthesia to prevent vagal reflexes and pain from traction on diaphragm, esophagus, and the like

TABLE 37-2

FACTORS THAT HAVE BEEN SUGGESTED AS POSSIBLE DETERMINANTS OF SPREAD OF LOCAL ANESTHETIC SOLUTIONS WITHIN THE SUBARACHNOID SPACE

CHARACTERISTICS OF THE LOCAL ANESTHETIC SOLUTION

Baricity
Local anesthetic dose
Local anesthetic concentration
Volume injected

PATIENT CHARACTERISTICS

Age
Weight
Height
Gender
Pregnancy
Patient position

TECHNIQUE

Site of injection
Speed of injection
Barbotage
Direction of needle bevel
Addition of vasoconstrictors

DIFFUSION

Adapted from Greene NM: Distribution of local anesthetic solutions within the subarachnoid space. Anesth Analg 1985; 64: 715, with permission.

TABLE 37-3

BARICITY OF SOLUTIONS COMMONLY USED FOR SPINAL ANESTHESIA

	BARICITY[a]
HYPERBARIC	
Tetracaine: 0.5% in 5% dextrose	1.0133
Bupivacaine: 0.75% in 8.25% dextrose	1.0227
Lidocaine: 5% in 7.5% dextrose	1.0265
Procaine: 10% in water	1.0104
ISOBARIC[b]	
Tetracaine: 0.5% in normal saline	0.9997
Bupivacaine: 0.75% in saline	0.9988
Bupivacaine: 0.5% in saline	0.9983
Lidocaine: 2% in saline	0.9986
HYPOBARIC	
Tetracaine: 0.2% in water	0.9922
Bupivacaine: 0.3% in water	0.9946
Lidocaine: 0.5% in water	0.9985

[a]Measured at 37°C, except for hypobaric 0.5% lidocaine measured at 25°C. At 37°C, this solution's baricity is less.
[b]These solutions are slightly hypobaric but are used clinically as if they were isobaric.
Data from Horlocker TT, Wedel DJ: Density, specific gravity, and baricity of spinal anesthetic solutions at body temperature. Anesth Analg 1993; 76: 1015; Lambert D, Covino B: Hyperbaric, hypobaric and isobaric spinal anesthesia. Resident Staff Physician 1987; 33: 79; Greene NM: Distribution of local anesthetic solutions within the subarachnoid space. Anesth Analg 1985; 64: 715; and Bodily N, Carpenter R, Owens B: Lidocaine 0.5% spinal anaesthesia: A hypobaric solution for short-stay perirectal surgery. Can J Anaesth 1992; 39: 770.

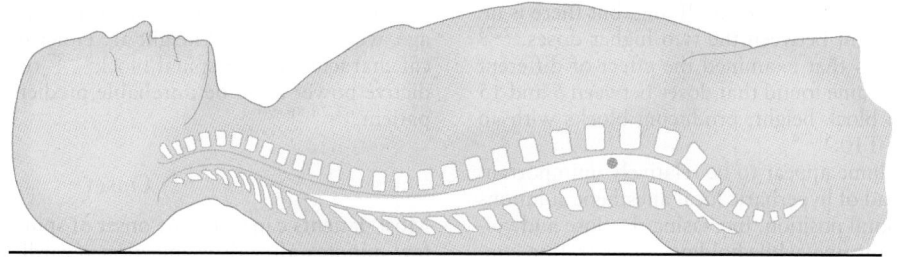

FIGURE 37-11. In the horizontal supine position, hyperbaric local anesthetic solutions injected at the height of the lumbar lordosis (*circle*) flow down the lumbar lordosis to pool in the sacrum and in the thoracic kyphosis. Pooling in the thoracic kyphosis is thought to explain the fact that hyperbaric solutions produce blocks with an average height of T4-6.

makes hypobaric solutions ideal for unilateral procedures performed in the lateral position (e.g., hip surgery). Hyperbaric solutions can be used to advantage for unilateral procedures performed in the supine position if the operative side is dependent during drug injection and the patient is left in the lateral position for at least 6 minutes.[54] Despite differences in block density and duration, peak block height will be comparable between the dependent and nondependent sides.

When the patient is turned supine following hyperbaric drug injection in the lateral position, the normal spinal curvature will influence subsequent movement of the injected solution. Hyperbaric solutions injected at the height of the lumbar lordosis will tend to flow cephalad to pool in the thoracic kyphosis and caudad to pool in the sacrum (Fig. 37-11). Pooling of hyperbaric local anesthetic solutions in the thoracic kyphosis has been evoked to explain the clinical observation that hyperbaric solutions tend to produce blocks with an average height in the midthoracic region (Fig. 37-9). In addition, hyperbaric solutions have also been observed to produce blocks with a bimodal distribution; that is, one group of patients with blocks centered in the low thoracic region and a second group of patients with blocks centered in the high thoracic region.[55,56] The presumed explanation for this observation is that the lumbar lordosis produces "splitting" of the local anesthetic solution with some portion flowing caudad toward the sacrum and the remainder flowing cephalad into the thoracic kyphosis. The cephalad extent of the block then depends on what fraction of the injected drug flows cephalad. Consistent with this hypothesis is the fact that eliminating the lumbar lordosis by maintaining the hips flexed has been shown to significantly reduce[56] or eliminate[55] the bimodal distribution of blocks without affecting maximal block height.

Obviously, gravity influences the distribution of hyperbaric and hypobaric solutions only until they are sufficiently diluted in CSF so that they become isobaric. At this point, the local anesthetic solution no longer moves in response to changes in patient position and the block is said to be "fixed." Interestingly, the time required for a local anesthetic solution to become fixed may be considerable. Povey et al.[51,52] showed that hyperbaric bupivacaine injected in the sitting position produces a saddle block that is restricted to the lumbar segments for as long as the subjects remained sitting. However, even 60 minutes after bupivacaine injection the block spread to midthoracic levels after turning the patients supine. Similarly, Bodily et al.[57] found that hypobaric lidocaine administered in the jackknife position rose as many as six dermatomes when patients were allowed to sit upright in the recovery room as long as 60 minutes after lidocaine injection. Whether it is also possible to affect spread so long after injecting hyperbaric or hypobaric solutions in the horizontal position is unclear. Nonetheless, these findings demonstrate that in some situations it may be possible to exert influence on block height by

adjusting patient position for at least 60 minutes after local anesthetic injection.

In contrast to the situation with hyperbaric solutions, patient position has no effect on the distribution of isobaric solutions because these solutions are not influenced by gravity. Consequently, isobaric solutions tend not to spread as far from the site of injection and produce blocks with an average height in the low thoracic region (Fig. 37-9).[49,58] The obvious caveat is that the local anesthetic solution must be truly isobaric in the patient in whom it is used. Because of the variability in CSF density among patients, it is difficult to produce reliably isobaric local anesthetic solutions. Nonetheless, as indicated in Table 37-3, several local anesthetic solutions are used as if they were isobaric. It is noteworthy that while isobaric solutions produce an average block height that is lower than comparable hyperbaric solutions,[49,58–60] the "isobaric" solutions produce blocks with a much greater variability in height.[61–63] Logan et al.[61] have termed plain bupivacaine "an unpredictable spinal anesthetic agent." The greater variability in spread may stem in part from the fact that these solutions are actually slightly hypobaric and their spread has been shown to be affected by patient position.[64,65] Temperature-related changes in baricity may also play a role in the variability in distribution of these nearly isobaric solutions. For example, Steinstra and van Poorten[66] have shown that the distribution of plain bupivacaine is significantly altered by changes in temperature of the injected solution. In addition, McClure et al.[67] have shown that increasing the volume and decreasing the concentration of isobaric tetracaine also increases the variability in block height. These and other unknown factors may play a role in the unpredictability of these nearly isobaric solutions. Although unpredictability is cause for concern, it should be pointed out that the lower average block height achieved offers potential advantages for surgical procedures below the umbilicus because of the decreased incidence of cardiovascular side effects associated with lower blocks. The isobaric solution that has been shown to most reliably produce a low thoracic block is 10 mg of tetracaine crystals diluted in 1- or 2-mL room temperature saline and injected in the horizontal position.[67]

Dose, Volume, and Concentration. Studies aimed at determining the effect of these three interdependent variables on block height are difficult to conduct and interpret because it is not possible to change one variable without simultaneously changing another. Nonetheless, it is possible to draw some conclusions regarding the effect of these variables on block height. Several studies with isobaric tetracaine and bupivacaine solutions have found that neither injected volume nor drug concentration affects block height when dose is held constant.[67–71] Drug dose does appear to play a small role in determining block height with isobaric bupivacaine. Two studies have found that 10 mg of isobaric bupivacaine results in significantly lower blocks than does 15 or 20 mg, but there is no difference in block height between the two higher doses.[72,73] In contrast, two studies that examined the effect of different doses of isobaric tetracaine found that doses between 5 and 15 mg had no effect on block height, producing blocks with an average height of T9-T10.[58,74]

Drug dose and volume appear to be relatively unimportant in predicting the spread of hyperbaric local anesthetic solutions injected in the horizontal position. Increasing the dose and volume of hyperbaric tetracaine, while holding concentration constant, does not affect block height when doses between 7.5 and 15 mg are used.[58,74,75] Similarly, increasing the dose and volume of hyperbaric 0.5% bupivacaine does not increase block height when doses between 10 and 20 mg are used.[76,77] However, doses of hyperbaric 0.5% bupivacaine <10 mg have been shown to result in blocks that are approximately two and one-half dermatomes lower than those achieved with doses >10 mg.[76] The fact that bupivacaine dose affects block height only at the extreme low end of the usual dose range is consistent with the experience with isobaric bupivacaine reported earlier. The fact that drug dose is relatively unimportant in determining block height with hyperbaric solutions likely results from an overwhelming effect of baricity and patient position in determining spread of these solutions.

Injection Site.   The site of injection can have an important effect on block height in some situations. In particular, sensory block height resulting from isobaric 0.5% bupivacaine is reduced by two dermatomes per interspace when comparing different groups of patients who received injections at the L2-3, L3-4, or L4-5 interspaces.[78,79] In an even more convincing study, this group of investigators performed repeated blocks in the same patient and found that by moving from the L3-4 to the L4-5 interspace means block height could be reduced from T6 to T10 when using isobaric 0.5% bupivacaine.[80] In contrast, Sundnes et al.[76] found no relationship between injection site and block height when using a hyperbaric bupivacaine solution, presumably because of the overwhelming effect of gravity and patient position on distribution of hyperbaric local anesthetics. Whether isobaric and hyperbaric solutions of other local anesthetics will behave similarly is not clear.

Patient Characteristics.   In young adults, it was determined that the most important variable governing block height with hyperbaric local anesthetic solutions may be lumbosacral CSF volume.[81] However, it is unclear if these findings can be extrapolated to other local anesthetics or patient ages.

Higuchi and colleagues[82] performed a detailed examination of the effect of lumbar CSF volume, CSF density, lumbar CSF motion, patient age, patient weight, patient height, and patient body mass index (BMI) on spinal block with isobaric bupivacaine. Multiple linear regression demonstrated that neither patient age nor height correlated with any clinical characteristic of spinal block. However, CSF volume and weight were correlated with peak block height. CSF volume was the only variable to correlate with time to voiding. BMI was the only significant predictor of time to onset of complete sensory block.

Although these variables were statistically significant predictors of several important aspects of spinal block, the coefficients of determination (R^2) were generally small (average, 0.23; range, 0.08 to 0.46), indicating that these variables account for a relatively small amount of the variability in each of the block outcomes examined. Clearly, other factors contribute significantly to the clinical characteristics of spinal block with isobaric bupivacaine.

Although these studies are mechanistically important, their clinical application is necessarily limited by the difficulty in determining an individual patient's CSF volume, CSF density, and velocity of CSF movement.

Importantly, several investigators have found that patient age, weight, BMI, and height are either not predictive of clinical characteristics of spinal block[83–87] or are of such low predictive power as to be unreliable predictors in any individual patient.[63,78,88–90]

Onset

Most patients can sense the onset of spinal block within a very few minutes after drug injection regardless of the local anesthetic used. However, there is a significant difference among drugs in the time to reach peak block height. Lidocaine and mepivacaine tend to reach peak block height between 10 and 15 minutes, whereas tetracaine and bupivacaine may require >20 minutes before peak block height is reached.

Duration

Spinal blocks do not end abruptly after a fixed period of time. Rather, they recede gradually from the most cephalad dermatome to the most caudad. As a result, surgical anesthesia lasts significantly longer at sacral levels than at thoracic levels. Therefore, when discussing the duration of spinal block it is necessary to distinguish between duration at the surgical site and the time required for the block to completely resolve. The former is important for providing adequate surgical anesthesia, and the latter is important for assuring a timely recovery. A thorough understanding of the factors that govern block duration is necessary if the clinician is to choose techniques that result in an appropriate duration of spinal blockade.

Local Anesthetic.   The principal determinant of spinal block duration is the local anesthetic drug employed. Procaine is the shortest-acting local anesthetic for subarachnoid use, lidocaine and mepivacaine are agents of intermediate duration, and bupivacaine and tetracaine are the longest-acting drugs. Table 37-4 lists the range of times required for sensory block to regress two dermatomes and to completely resolve with the local anesthetics most commonly used for spinal anesthesia. Although drug choice is the principal determinant of block duration, other variables are responsible for the wide range of block duration found in Table 37-4.

Drug Dose.   Increasing local anesthetic dose clearly increases the duration of spinal block.[72,73,75,91,92] For example, Brown et al.[58] demonstrated that duration of sensory block at L1 following 15 mg of tetracaine was approximately 20% greater than following 10 mg. Sheskey et al.[73] demonstrated an approximate 40% increase in block duration at L2 when comparing 10 mg of bupivacaine with 15 mg. Similarly, Axelsson et al.[91] found that duration of sensory block at L2 was nearly doubled when comparing 10 mg of bupivacaine with 20 mg.

Block Height.   If drug dose is held constant, higher blocks tend to regress faster than lower blocks.[92] Consequently, isobaric local anesthetic solutions will generally produce longer blocks than hyperbaric solutions using the same dose. The conventional wisdom is that greater cephalad spread results in relatively lower drug concentration in the CSF and spinal nerve roots. As a result, it takes less time for local anesthetic concentration to decrease below the minimally effective concentration.

Adrenergic Agonists.   Adrenergic agonists, such as epinephrine, phenylephrine, and clonidine, are added to local anesthetics in an effort to prolong the duration of spinal anesthesia. Their effectiveness depends on the local anesthetic with which they are combined. In addition, they are more effective at prolonging block in the lumbar and sacral dermatomes than in thoracic dermatomes.

TABLE 37-4

DOSE AND DURATION OF LOCAL ANESTHETICS USED FOR SPINAL ANESTHESIA

		■ DURATION OF SENSORY BLOCK		
■ DRUG	■ DOSE (mg)[a]	■ TWO-DERMATOME REGRESSION (min)[b]	■ COMPLETE RESOLUTION (min)[b]	■ PROLONGATION BY ADRENERGIC AGONISTS (%)[c]
Procaine	50–200	30–50	90–120	30–50
Chloroprocaine	30–100	30–50	70–150	NR
Lidocaine	25–100	40–100	140–240	20–50
Bupivacaine	5–20	90–140	240–380	20–50
Tetracaine	5–20	90–140	240–380	50–100

NR: Not recommended; see text for explanation.
[a]The lowest doses are used primarily for very restricted blocks (e.g., saddle block), lest they become too dilute to be effective.
[b]Duration is influenced by dose and block height. The duration of surgical anesthesia will obviously depend on the surgical site.
[c]The effect of adrenergic agonists depends on the dose and choice of agonist. Prolongation is greatest at lumbar and sacral dermatomes and least at thoracic dermatomes.

Epinephrine is typically administered in doses of 0.2 to 0.3 mg and phenylephrine in doses of 2 to 5 mg. There is evidence to suggest a relationship between the dose of vasoconstrictor added and the duration of spinal anesthesia; however, the relationship is not strong.[93–96] At the maximal doses used clinically, phenylephrine (5 mg) prolongs spinal block to a greater degree than epinephrine (0.5 mg).[97,98] At lower doses, epinephrine (0.2 to 0.3 mg) and phenylephrine (2 to 3 mg) appear to be equally effective in prolonging spinal block.[96,99] Thus, both choice of adrenergic agonist and dose administered appear to play a role in determining block duration. Clonidine, most commonly in a dose of 75 to 150 mg, is at least as effective as moderate doses of phenylephrine and epinephrine at prolonging sensory block but has been associated with greater decreases in blood pressure in some[100] but not all studies.[101] Interestingly, clonidine also prolongs spinal block when administered orally.[102–104]

Tetracaine is the local anesthetic that is most dramatically prolonged by addition of adrenergic agonists. The duration of tetracaine spinal block may be increased 70 to 100% at lumbar and sacral dermatomes by addition of phenylephrine. Epinephrine may prolong tetracaine spinal anesthesia by 40 to 60%. Clonidine prolongs tetracaine spinal block by 50 to 70%, with the larger effect occurring at lumbar dermatomes.

Bupivacaine spinal block is also prolonged by adrenergic agonists, although the effect is somewhat less than that seen with tetracaine (Table 37-4). Epinephrine in doses of 0.2 mg prolongs bupivacaine spinal block by 20 to 30%, but only in lumbar dermatomes. Larger doses of epinephrine (0.3 to 0.5 mg) prolong sensory block in thoracic dermatomes as well by 30 to 50%. Clonidine prolongs bupivacaine spinal block by 30 to 50% as well.

The effect of adrenergic agonists on the duration of lidocaine spinal block is controversial. Some clinical studies have demonstrated that adrenergic agonists clearly prolong lidocaine spinal block,[94,105–107] whereas others have concluded that adrenergic agonists do not produce clinically useful prolongation.[108,109] This discrepancy may be explained, in part, by the fact that spinal block duration is so variable that studies using small numbers of patients may lack sufficient statistical power to detect real differences in mean block duration between groups. This problem was obviated in an interesting study by Chiu et al.,[110] who used a crossover study design to demonstrate that 0.2 mg of epinephrine significantly prolonged lidocaine sensory block in lumbar and sacral der-

matomes. Thus, the available data suggest that adding epinephrine to lidocaine will result in a somewhat longer block, at least in lumbar and sacral dermatomes, than would be achieved if epinephrine were not added.

The mechanism by which adrenergic agonists prolong spinal block is not clear. Originally, epinephrine and phenylephrine were added to local anesthetics with the intent of reducing local spinal cord blood flow and thereby slowing the rate of drug elimination from the spinal cord and CSF. There are animal studies that support this mechanism[111,112] and others that do not.[113,114] Animal studies with clonidine indicate that it does reduce regional spinal cord blood flow.[115] There are no human studies that have investigated the effect of intrathecal adrenergic agonists on spinal cord blood flow. However, there are human studies that demonstrate that epinephrine decreases the rate of local anesthetic clearance from the CSF[116,117] and also slows the rate at which subarachnoid local anesthetic appears in the plasma.[105] These findings have been interpreted as evidence of a vasoconstrictor-mediated decrease in drug clearance from the spinal cord; however, they are not proof that this is the only, or even the principal, mechanism by which adrenergic agonists prolong spinal anesthesia. Alternatively, Kozody et al.[118] have shown that intrathecal epinephrine decreases blood flow in the dura mater without altering spinal cord blood flow, a finding most consistent with decreased drug clearance via the dural vasculature.

Adrenergic agonists are potent analgesic agents in their own right when administered into the subarachnoid space.[119] Analgesia results from inhibition of nociceptive afferents, an effect that is mediated by stimulation of α-adrenergic receptors in the spinal cord dorsal horn. In addition, large intrathecal doses of α-adrenergic agonists have been shown to produce flaccidity in animal models by hyperpolarizing motor neurons.[120] Thus, prolongation of motor and sensory block by adrenergic agonists may be partly because of direct inhibitory effects of these drugs on sensory and motor neurons.

Epidural Anesthesia

Any procedure that can be performed under spinal anesthesia can also be performed under epidural block and requires the same block height (Table 37-1). As with spinal anesthesia, there is a great deal of variability among patients in spread

TABLE 37-5

LOCAL ANESTHETICS USED FOR SURGICAL EPIDURAL BLOCK

	DURATION OF SENSORY BLOCK		
▪ DRUG[a]	▪ TWO-DERMATOME REGRESSION (min)	▪ COMPLETE RESOLUTION (min)	▪ PROLONGATION BY EPINEPHRINE (%)
Chloroprocaine 3%	45–60	100–160	40–60
Lidocaine 2%	60–100	160–200	40–80
Mepivacaine 2%	60–100	160–200	40–80
Ropivacaine 0.5–1.0%	90–180	240–420	No
Etidocaine 1–1.5%	120–240	300–460	No
Bupivacaine 0.5–0.75%	120–240	300–460	No

[a]These concentrations are recommended for surgical anesthesia; more dilute concentrations are appropriate for epidural analgesia.

(Fig. 37-10) and duration of epidural block (Table 37-5). Therefore, to choose the most appropriate local anesthetic and dose for a particular clinical situation, the anesthesiologist must be familiar with the variables that affect spread and duration of epidural anesthesia.

Block Spread

Injection Site. Unlike spinal anesthesia, epidural anesthesia produces a segmental block that spreads both caudally and cranially from the site of injection (Fig. 37-12). Thus, injection site is arguably the most important determinant of the spread of epidural block. *Caudal* epidural blocks are largely restricted to sacral and low lumbar dermatomes. Low thoracic levels can be reached with caudal injections if large volumes are used (e.g., 30 mL). However, the block at thoracic dermatomes tends to be patchy and short-lived following caudal injection.[121] *Lumbar* local anesthetic injections with volumes of 10 mL often extend caudad to include all sacral dermatomes, although the onset of block in the L5 and S1 roots is often delayed and may be patchy.[122] Twenty-milliliter volumes pro-

duce better-quality sacral anesthesia following lumbar injection. The slow onset at L5 and S1 is thought to result from their larger diameter and consequent slower drug penetration. Lumbar injections can be extended to midthoracic levels (T4-6) when 20-mL volumes of local anesthetic are used. *Thoracic* injections produce a symmetric segmental band of anesthesia, the width of which depends on the dose of local anesthetic administered. When using a mid-to-upper thoracic injection site, it is prudent to reduce the local anesthetic doses by approximately 30 to 50% relative to lumbar doses to prevent excessive cephalad spread. It is generally not feasible to produce surgical anesthesia in low lumbar and sacral dermatomes with midthoracic or higher injection sites. Thoracic epidural block is ideally suited for anesthesia of the chest and abdomen.

Dose, Volume, and Concentration. Within the range typically used for surgical anesthesia, drug concentration is relatively unimportant in determining block spread. However, drug dose and volume are important variables determining both spread and quality of epidural block. If drug concentration is held constant, increasing the volume of local anesthetic

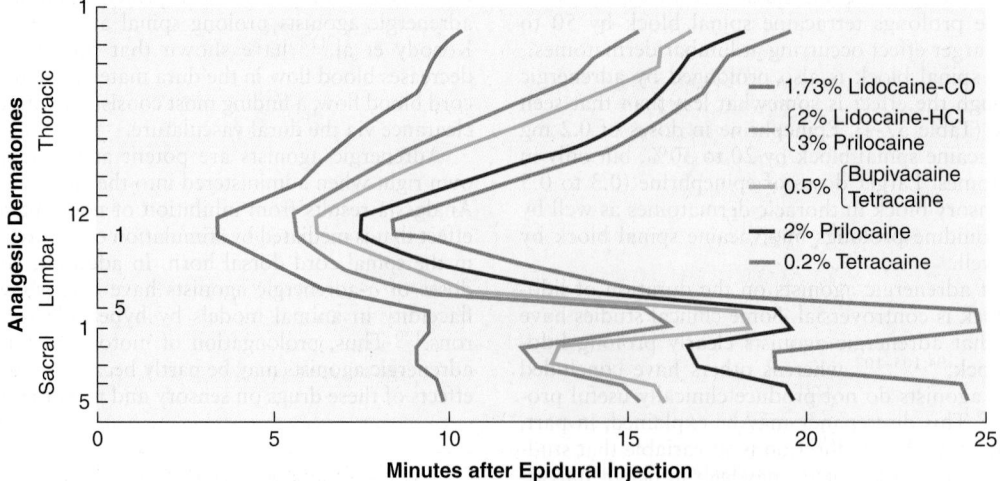

FIGURE 37-12. Spread of epidural sensory block over time following injection of various local anesthetic solutions at the L2-3 interspace. All solutions contained epinephrine 1:200,000. Sensory block spreads both cephalad and caudad from the site of injection with time. Note the delay in onset of block at the L5 and S1 dermatomes with all solutions tested. (Reprinted from Bromage PR: Epidural Analgesia. Philadelphia, WB Saunders, 1978, with permission.)

(and thereby the dose) will result in significantly greater average spread and greater block density. However, the relationship is nonlinear. For example, doubling the volume and dose of 1.5% lidocaine or 0.75% bupivacaine from 10 to 20 mL has been shown to increase spread by only three to four spinal segments.[122,123] Volume appears to be important in determining block spread independent of drug dose, but again the relationship is nonlinear. Erdemir et al.[124] showed that tripling the injected volume of lidocaine from 10 to 30 mL while holding the dose constant (300 mg) increased the cephalad extent of block by only 4.3 dermatomes. This tendency toward greater spread is thought to be explained by the observation that increasing the volume of solution injected into the epidural space increases cephalad distribution.[125]

Position.   When using a single-shot technique, maintaining patients in the lateral position during and after epidural injection of surgical doses of local anesthetics does not seem to have a clinically important effect on spread of the block from side to side.[126] Similarly, studies examining the effect of patient position on cephalad spread of epidural block have generally found that the effect of posture on spread is not clinically important.[127] Interestingly, Ponhold et al.[128] demonstrated that maintaining a 30-degree head-up position significantly increased the frequency of adequate block at the L5 and S1 nerve roots even though there was no effect on the cephalad extent of anesthesia.

Patient Characteristics

Age.   Most,[122,123,129–132] but not all,[133] studies that have examined the effect of age on epidural block have demonstrated greater spread in older patients. However, the effect of age is probably clinically significant only when comparing adults whose ages differ by ≥3 decades. Even so, the difference in block height is not likely to be more than three or four dermatomes. Greater spread in older patients is thought to be related to a less-compliant epidural space and diminished ability for epidural solutions to leak out of intervertebral foramina.[125,134] Both of these age-related changes would be expected to result in more extensive spread of solutions within the epidural space.

Height and Weight.   The correlation between patient height[122,123,132,133] or weight[132,133] and spread of epidural block is weak and of little clinical significance except perhaps in patients who are extremely tall, extremely short, or morbidly obese.

Pregnancy.   Studies examining the effect of pregnancy on spread of epidural block are conflicting. Some studies have demonstrated greater spread at term[135] and during early pregnancy,[129] suggesting that greater spread during pregnancy is not simply the result of anatomic changes associated with pregnancy. However, other studies have not found a significant difference in spread of epidural block between pregnant and nonpregnant women.[136–138]

Atherosclerosis.   Atherosclerosis was suggested as an important determinant of the spread of epidural block[135]; however, subsequent studies have failed to confirm this relationship.[123,129,139]

Given the myriad factors that have some effect on spread of epidural anesthesia, how should anesthesiologists choose an appropriate local anesthetic dose for a single-shot epidural block? A useful recommendation is to assume that a 20-mL volume of all local anesthetics intended for surgical anesthesia will produce a midthoracic block on average after lumbar injection. If there are multiple reasons to expect that the block may spread excessively in an individual patient (e.g., advanced

age, obesity, very short stature, high injection site) or if the procedure does not require a high block, then reduce the dose accordingly. If there are multiple reasons to expect that the spread may be reduced from the average, then increase the volume accordingly. Obviously, choice of the appropriate local anesthetic dose is obviated if an epidural catheter is used. In this situation, begin with a lower dose than one anticipates will be needed and administer additional local anesthetic as necessary to extend the block to the desired level.

Onset

The onset of epidural block with all local anesthetics can usually be detected within 5 minutes in the dermatomes immediately surrounding the injection site. The time to peak effect differs somewhat among local anesthetics. Shorter-acting drugs generally reach their maximum spread in 15 to 20 minutes, whereas longer-acting drugs require 20 to 25 minutes. Increasing the dose of local anesthetic speeds the onset of both motor and sensory block.

Duration

Local Anesthetic.   As with spinal anesthesia, choice of local anesthetic is the most important determinant of the duration of epidural block. Chloroprocaine is the shortest-duration drug used for epidural anesthesia; lidocaine and mepivacaine provide blocks of intermediate duration; and bupivacaine, ropivacaine, and etidocaine produce the longest-lasting epidural block. Table 37-5 lists local anesthetics commonly used for epidural block and approximate duration of surgical anesthesia. Of note, tetracaine and procaine are not generally used for epidural block because of the poor-quality block that these drugs produce.

Importantly, when used epidurally some local anesthetics exhibit considerable separation in both the intensity and duration of sensory and motor block. Etidocaine produces the most intense motor block and is unusual among local anesthetics in that motor block may considerably outlast sensory block.[140] The phenomenon of the postoperative patient who is in pain yet still unable to move his or her legs has led some anesthesiologists to abandon etidocaine for epidural use. This is unfortunate because etidocaine's superior muscle relaxation is sometimes beneficial intraoperatively. Bupivacaine has the opposite sensorimotor profile in that low concentrations of bupivacaine produce sensory block that is relatively more intense than motor block. This separation of sensory and motor block underlies the common practice of using dilute bupivacaine solutions for epidural analgesia.

Dose.   Increasing the dose of local anesthetic administered results in increased duration[122,141–143] and density[122,142,143] of epidural block.

Age.   Studies that have evaluated the effect of age on epidural block duration are inconclusive. Veering et al.[131] found that duration of epidural block with plain bupivacaine was not significantly affected by age. Nydahl et al.[130] found that epidural block using bupivacaine with epinephrine was actually shorter in older patients. In contrast, Park et al.[129] found that epidural block using lidocaine with epinephrine was slightly but significantly longer in older patients. Additional studies are necessary to clarify the effect of age on duration of epidural block.

Adrenergic Agonists.   Epinephrine, in a concentration of 5 μg/mL (1:200,000), is the most common adrenergic agonist added to epidural local anesthetics. It has been shown to prolong the duration of lidocaine and mepivacaine epidural block by as much as 80%.[144] Block is prolonged by decreased drug clearance from the epidural space,[145] probably as a result of reduced blood flow in the dura mater. As discussed earlier for spinal anesthesia, prolongation of motor and sensory block may be partly due to direct inhibitory effects of epinephrine on sensory and motor neurons.

Epinephrine does not significantly prolong the duration of anesthesia when added to concentrated solutions of bupivacaine,[146,147] etidocaine,[142,147] or ropivacaine[148] that are generally used for surgical anesthesia, probably because the inherent duration of these drugs exceeds the duration of epinephrine's effects. However, epinephrine does appear to prolong analgesia and improve the quality of block when added to more dilute solutions of these local anesthetics, such as those used for labor analgesia.[149–151]

Summary

The extent and duration of both spinal and epidural block are influenced by a number of variables, some of which are under the control of the anesthesiologist. Understanding the impact of these variables will allow the anesthesiologist to rationally select the most appropriate drug and dose for any clinical situation. However, even the most experienced anesthesiologist will still have blocks that are not adequate for the planned procedure. The frequency of failed blocks can be kept to a minimum if the clinician aims to produce blocks that are a little higher and a little longer than seems necessary. It is often easier to deal with a block that is too high or too long than to cover up for a block that is too low or too brief.

PHYSIOLOGY

Neurophysiology

The physiology of local anesthetic neural blockade is discussed in detail in Chapter 21. This section briefly presents aspects of the physiology of neural blockade that are unique to spinal and epidural anesthesia.

Site of Action

The site of action of spinal and epidural anesthesia is not precisely known. Following epidural administration, local anesthetic is found in the spinal nerves within the epidural space, in spinal nerve rootlets within the CSF, and in the spinal cord. Similarly, following intrathecal administration in animals, local anesthetic is found in all sites between the spinal nerve rootlets and the interior of the spinal cord.[152,153] Thus, neural blockade can potentially occur at any or all points along the neural pathways extending from the site of drug administration to the interior of the spinal cord.

In an interesting study in humans, Boswell et al.[154] demonstrated that patients are able to feel paresthesias during direct electrical stimulation of the spinal cord under spinal anesthesia. Cortical evoked potentials from direct spinal cord stimulation were also maintained under spinal anesthesia, although amplitudes were decreased. In contrast, paresthesias and cortical evoked potentials from tibial nerve stimulation were abolished by spinal anesthesia. These investigators concluded that neural pathways within the spinal cord were largely intact during spinal anesthesia and that the spinal nerve rootlets were the principal site of neural blockade.

The site of epidural block is less well localized. Monkey studies suggest that epidural block occurs largely at sites within the spinal meninges, including the cauda equina nerve roots, dorsal root entry zone, and the long tracts of spinal cord white matter.[155] However, these findings are not entirely consistent with the segmental onset of epidural anesthesia (Fig. 37-12) or with the limited segmental blocks that can be produced with small doses of lumbar epidural local anesthetics in humans. These clinical observations are most readily explained by block of the segmental spinal nerves as they traverse the epidural or paravertebral spaces. In reality, epidural block likely occurs at both extradural and subdural sites with extradural radicular block predominating early and subdural spinal block predominating later. This supposition is consistent with human studies by Urban,[156] who rigorously examined the anatomic pattern of analgesia that occurred during onset and regression of epidural block. He concluded that local anesthetics initially acted on radicular structures followed later by actions within the spinal cord.

Interestingly, human studies demonstrate that somatosensory evoked potentials are maintained during epidural anesthesia, although amplitudes are decreased and latencies are increased. This contrasts with spinal block in which evoked potentials are completely eliminated and supports the clinical impression that epidural block is generally less dense than that achieved with spinal anesthesia.

Differential Nerve Block

Differential block refers to a clinically important phenomenon in which nerve fibers subserving different functions display varying sensitivity to local anesthetic blockade. Sympathetic nerve fibers appear to be blocked by the lowest concentration of local anesthetic followed in order by fibers responsible for pain, touch, and motor function. This observation has led to the widely held belief that differences in sensitivity to local anesthetic blockade is explained solely by differences in fiber diameter, with smaller-diameter neurons exhibiting greater sensitivity than larger-diameter neurons. Although the mechanism for differential block in spinal and epidural anesthesia is not known, it is clear that fiber diameter is not the only, or perhaps not even the most important, factor contributing to differential block.[157,158]

Differential block occurs with both peripheral nerve blocks and central neuraxial blocks. In the peripheral nervous system, differential block is a temporal phenomenon with sympathetic block occurring first followed in time by sensory and motor block. In contrast, with spinal and epidural anesthesia differential block is manifest as a spatial separation in the modalities blocked. This is seen most clearly with spinal anesthesia in which sympathetic block may extend as many as two to six dermatomes higher than pin-prick sensation,[159] which in turn extends two to three dermatomes higher than motor block. This spatial separation is believed to result from a gradual decrease in local anesthetic concentration within the CSF as a function of distance from the site of injection. With epidural anesthesia, similar zones of differential sensory and sympathetic block are found.[160]

Perhaps the most troublesome consequence of differential block is the occasional patient who has intact touch and proprioception at the surgical site despite adequate blockade of pain sensation. Even the most stoic patients are likely to find this unpleasant and may lie in fear that the procedure will soon become painful. In no instance should the anesthesiologist downplay the distress this may cause patients. Reassurance and judicious sedation as necessary are usually sufficient to overcome this problem.

Another important neurophysiologic aspect of central neuroaxial block is that it produces sedation,[161] potentiates the effect of sedative hypnotic drugs,[162–164] and markedly decreases minimum alveolar concentration of volatile anesthetics.[165] The mechanism(s) underlying these effects is not known but "deafferentation," that is, the loss of ascending sensory input to the brain, is commonly invoked as causative.

Cardiovascular Physiology

5 Cardiovascular side effects, principally hypotension and bradycardia, are arguably the most important and most common physiologic changes during spinal and epidural anesthesia. Understanding the homeostatic mechanisms responsible for control of blood pressure and heart rate is essential for understanding and treating the cardiovascular changes associated with spinal and epidural anesthesia.

Spinal Anesthesia

Blockade of sympathetic efferents is the principal mechanism by which spinal anesthesia produces cardiovascular derangements. As would be expected, the incidence of significant hypotension or bradycardia is generally related to the extent of sympathetic blockade, which in turn parallels block height.[166,167] However, the severity of cardiovascular changes has been shown not to correlate with peak block height in one study[168] and to correlate poorly in another (Fig. 37-13).[166] Additional risk factors associated with hypotension include age >40 to 50 years, concurrent general anesthesia, obesity, hypovolemia, and addition of phenylephrine to the local anesthetic.[166,169]

Hypotension during spinal anesthesia is the result of both arterial and venodilation. Venodilation increases volume in capacitance vessels, thereby decreasing venous return and right-sided filling pressures.[168,170–172] This fall in preload is thought to be the principal cause of decreased cardiac output during high spinal anesthesia. Arterial dilation during spinal anesthesia results in significant decreases in total peripheral resistance (Fig. 37-14).[171,173] Thus, the hypotension that accompanies 30 to

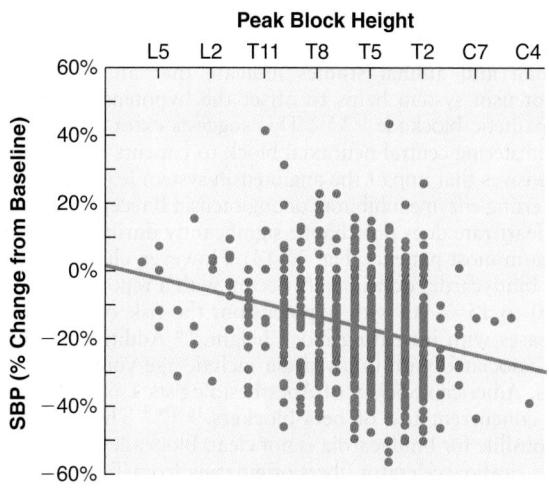

FIGURE 37-13. The relationship between peak block height and change in systolic blood pressure (SBP) during spinal anesthesia. Although there is a statistically significant correlation between block height and decrease in systolic blood pressure, the interindividual variability is so great that the relationship has little predictive value. This is reflected in the R^2 of 0.07 for the linear regression line. (From Carpenter RL, Caplan RA, Brown DL et al: Incidence and risk factors for side effects of spinal anesthesia. Anesthesiology 1992; 76: 906, with permission.)

ANESTHETIC MANAGEMENT

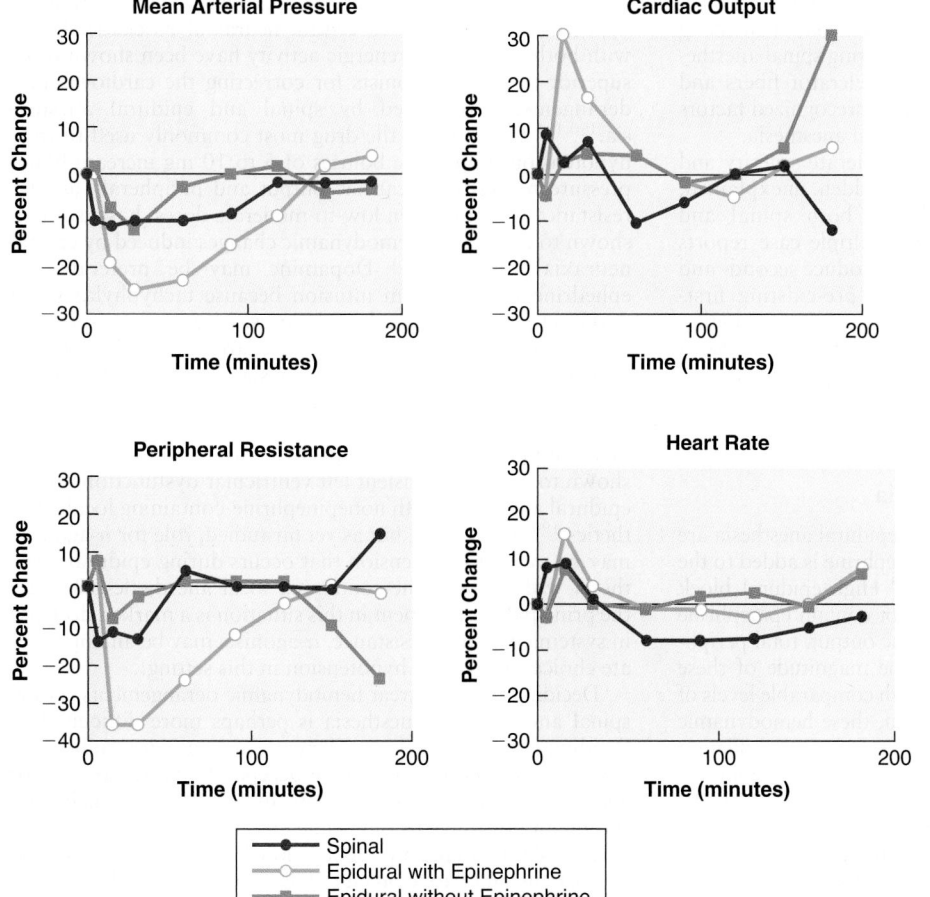

FIGURE 37-14. The cardiovascular effects of spinal and epidural anesthesia in volunteers with T5 blocks. The effects of spinal anesthesia and epidural anesthesia without epinephrine were generally comparable and are both qualitatively and quantitatively different from the effects of epidural anesthesia with epinephrine. (Modified from Bonica JJ, Kennedu WF Jr, Ward RJ et al: A comparison of the effects of high subarachnoid and epidural anesthesia. Acta Anaesthesiol Scand 1966; 23 (Suppl): 429.)

40% of spinal anesthetics may be the result of reductions in afterload, reductions in cardiac output, or both (Fig. 37-14). Human and animal studies indicate that an intact renin-angiotensin system helps to offset the hypotensive effects of sympathetic blockade.[174,175] This suggests extra caution when administering central neuraxial block to patients taking antihypertensives that impair the angiotensin system (e.g., angiotensin converting enzyme inhibitors or angiotensin II receptor blockers).

Heart rate does not change significantly during spinal anesthesia in most patients (Fig. 37-14). However, clinically significant bradycardia occasionally occurs with a reported incidence of 10 to 15%. As with hypotension, the risk of bradycardia increases with increasing block height.[166] Additional risk factors associated with bradycardia include age younger than 50 years, American Society of Anesthesiologists 1 physical status, and concurrent use of beta-blockers.[166,169] The mechanism responsible for bradycardia is not clear. Blockade of the sympathetic cardioaccelerator fibers originating from T1-4 spinal segments is often suggested as the cause. The fact that bradycardia is more common with high blocks supports this mechanism. However, significant bradycardia sometimes occurs with blocks that are seemingly too low to block cardioaccelerator fibers. Diminished venous return has also been proposed as a cause of bradycardia during spinal anesthesia. Intracardiac stretch receptors have been shown to reflexively decrease heart rate when filling pressures fall.[176] Consistent with this mechanism, Jacobsen et al.[177] demonstrated a significant reduction in left ventricular volumes and heart rate during hypotensive episodes in two patients during epidural anesthesia. They concluded that central volume depletion elicited a vagally mediated reflex slowing of heart rate. Similarly, Baron et al.[178] demonstrated that vagal activity is enhanced by decreased venous return during epidural anesthesia. However, this mechanism does not operate at all times in all patients. Anzai and Nishikawa[172] demonstrated significant heart rate increases in 40 patients who had their filling pressures suddenly decreased by body tilt during spinal anesthesia. In reality, both blockade of cardioaccelerator fibers and decreased filling pressures as well as other unrecognized factors likely contribute to bradycardia during spinal anesthesia.

Although bradycardia is usually of moderate severity and well tolerated, there have been reports of sudden, unexplained, severe bradycardia and asystole during both spinal and epidural anesthesia.[179,180] In addition, multiple case reports document that spinal anesthesia can also produce second- and third-degree heart block[181–183] and that pre-existing first-degree block may be a risk factor for progression to higher grade blocks during spinal anesthesia.[181] These reports document the need for continued vigilance with prompt and, if needed, aggressive treatment of the cardiovascular changes that accompany central neuraxial blockade.

Epidural Anesthesia

The hemodynamic changes produced by epidural anesthesia are largely dependent on whether or not epinephrine is added to the local anesthetic solution (Fig. 37-14).[184] High epidural block with local anesthetic solutions that do not contain epinephrine results in decreased stroke volume, cardiac output, total peripheral resistance, and arterial pressure. The magnitude of these changes is generally less than that seen with comparable levels of spinal block.[184] As with spinal anesthesia, these hemodynamic changes are believed to result from venous and arterial dilation induced by sympathetic blockade. In contrast, when epinephrine-containing solutions are used for epidural anesthesia, stroke volume and cardiac output increase significantly (Fig. 37-14).[184] However, peripheral resistance falls dramatically, resulting in a decrease in arterial pressure greater than that seen with non-epinephrine-containing solutions. β_2-adrenergic–mediated

vasodilatation produced by low doses of absorbed epinephrine accounts for the greater decrease in peripheral vascular resistance and blood pressure. Decreased peripheral resistance may also contribute to the marked increase in cardiac output. However, epinephrine-induced venoconstriction with a resultant increase in venous return may also play an important role in increasing cardiac output.[185]

Treating Hemodynamic Changes

Treatment of hypotension secondary to spinal and epidural block must be aimed at the root causes: decreased cardiac output and/or decreased peripheral resistance. Bolus crystalloid administration has often been advocated as a means of restoring venous return and thus cardiac output during central neuraxial blockade. However, the effectiveness of this therapy in normovolemic patients is controversial. Prehydrating patients with 500 to 1,500 mL of crystalloid does not reliably prevent hypotension, but it has been shown to decrease the incidence of hypotension during spinal anesthesia in some,[186,187] but not all, studies.[167,188] Thus, although judicious crystalloid preloading of patients before central neuraxial blocks may benefit some patients, this practice cannot be relied on to prevent clinically significant hypotension in all, or even most, patients. The reason for this is that increasing preload can only increase stroke volume, which has limited ability to restore blood pressure if heart rate or systemic vascular resistance remains low. In this regard colloid solutions offer an interesting alternative to crystalloids for preloading before central neuraxial blocks. Marhofer and colleagues[189] have shown that 500 mL of 6% hetastarch actually increases systemic vascular resistance index in elderly patients having spinal anesthesia, and 1,500 mL of crystalloid significantly decreases systemic vascular resistance index.

Vasopressors are a more reliable approach to treating hypotension secondary to central neuraxial blockade. Drugs with both α- and β-adrenergic activity have been shown to be superior to pure α-agonists for correcting the cardiovascular derangements produced by spinal and epidural anesthesia.[190,191] Ephedrine is the drug most commonly used to treat hypotension. Ephedrine boluses of 5 to 10 mg increase blood pressure by restoring cardiac output and peripheral vascular resistance. Dopamine, in low-to-moderate doses, has also been shown to correct the hemodynamic changes induced by central neuraxial block.[192,193] Dopamine may be preferable to ephedrine for long-term infusion because tachyphylaxis can develop to repeated ephedrine boluses. Pure α-adrenergic agonists, most commonly phenylephrine, are also used to correct hypotension during spinal anesthesia. However, α-agonists increase blood pressure largely by increasing systemic vascular resistance, sometimes at the expense of further decreasing cardiac output.[191] In addition, phenylephrine boluses have been shown to produce transient left ventricular dysfunction during epidural anesthesia with nonepinephrine-containing local anesthetics.[194] A potential, but as yet unstudied, role for α-agonists may be to treat hypotension that occurs during epidural anesthesia with epinephrine-containing local anesthetics. Because the principal derangement in this situation is a marked decrease in systemic vascular resistance, α-agonists may be an appropriate choice for treating hypotension in this setting.

Deciding *when* to treat hemodynamic derangements during spinal and epidural anesthesia is perhaps more difficult than deciding *how* to treat them. There are currently no studies that clearly define the lower limit of acceptable blood pressure or heart rate for any group of patients. In the absence of such data, several authors have recommended treating blood pressure if it decreases more than 25 to 30% below baseline or in normotensive patients, if systolic pressure falls below 90 mm Hg. Recommendations regarding bradycardia suggest initiating treatment if heart rate falls below 50 to 60 beats per minute. These recommendations are reasonable, although not universally applicable. Ultimately, anesthesiologists must decide what is an acceptable blood pressure and heart rate for an individual patient based on that patient's underlying medical condition.

Respiratory Physiology

Spinal and epidural blocks to midthoracic levels have little effect on pulmonary function in patients without pre-existing lung disease. Drugs used perioperatively for sedation during spinal or epidural block likely have a larger impact on pulmonary function than the block per se. In particular, lung volumes, resting minute ventilation, dead space, arterial blood gas tensions, and shunt fraction show little or no change during spinal or epidural anesthesia. Interestingly, the ventilatory response to hypercapnia is actually increased by spinal and epidural block.[195,196]

High blocks associated with abdominal and intercostal muscle paralysis can impair ventilatory functions requiring active exhalation. For example, expiratory reserve volume, peak expiratory flow, and maximum minute ventilation may be significantly reduced by high spinal and epidural blocks. The negative impact of high blocks on active exhalation suggests caution when using spinal or epidural anesthesia in patients with obstructive pulmonary disease, who need to cough to clear sputum, or who otherwise rely on their accessory muscles of respiration to maintain a clear airway and/or adequate ventilation.

Patients with high spinal or epidural blocks may complain of dyspnea despite normal or elevated minute ventilation. This likely results from the patient's inability to feel the chest wall move while breathing. This is understandably frightening to the patient, but reassurance is usually effective in alleviating the fear. The anesthesiologist must be alert to the possibility that the complaint of dyspnea stems from incipient respiratory failure secondary to respiratory muscle paralysis. A normal speaking voice, as opposed to a faint gasping voice, suggests ventilation is normal.

Gastrointestinal Physiology

The gastrointestinal effects of spinal and epidural anesthesia are largely the result of sympathetic blockade. The abdominal organs derive their sympathetic innervation from T6-L2. Blockade of these fibers results in unopposed parasympathetic activity by way of the vagus nerve. Consequently, secretions increase, sphincters relax, and the bowel becomes constricted. Some surgeons believe this improves surgical exposure. Nausea is a common complication of spinal and epidural anesthesia. The etiology is unknown but an increased incidence of nausea during spinal anesthesia is associated with blocks higher than T5, hypotension, opioid premedication, and a history of motion sickness.[166,169]

Endocrine-Metabolic Physiology

Surgery produces numerous endocrine and metabolic changes, including increased protein catabolism and oxygen consumption as well as increases in circulating concentrations of catecholamines, growth hormone, renin, angiotensin, thyroid-stimulating hormone, β-endorphin, glucose, and free fatty acids, among others.[1] These endocrine–metabolic changes have collectively been termed the *surgical stress response*.

The mechanisms responsible for the stress response are complex and incompletely understood. However, afferent sensory information from the surgical site plays an important role in initiating and maintaining these changes.[1] Not surprisingly, spinal and epidural anesthesia have been shown to inhibit many of the endocrine–metabolic changes associated with the stress response. The inhibitory effect is greatest with lower abdominal and lower extremity procedures and least with upper abdominal and thoracic procedures. The salutary effect of spinal and epidural anesthesia is believed to result from blockade of the afferent sensory information that helps initiate the stress response.

Although some aspects of the surgical stress response may be beneficial, it is generally viewed as maladaptive and possibly a contributor to postoperative morbidity and mortality.[1] Despite the ability of central neuraxial block to decrease the stress response, there is as yet no clear evidence that this results in decreased morbidity or mortality.

COMPLICATIONS

Backache

Although postoperative backache occurs following general anesthesia, it is more common following epidural and spinal anesthesia.[197] Compared with spinal anesthesia, back pain following epidural anesthesia is more common (11 vs. 30%) and of longer duration.[198] Importantly, back pain has been cited in one study as the most common reason for patients to refuse future epidural block.[198] The etiology of backache is not clear, although needle trauma, local anesthetic irritation, and ligamentous strain secondary to muscle relaxation have been offered as explanations.

Postdural Puncture Headache

PDPH is a common complication of spinal anesthesia with a reported incidence as high as 25% in some studies. The risk of PDPH is less with epidural anesthesia, but it occurs in up to 50% of young patients following accidental meningeal puncture with large-diameter epidural needles. The headache is characteristically mild or absent when the patient is supine, but head elevation rapidly leads to a severe fronto-occipital headache, which again improves on returning to the supine position. Occasionally, cranial nerve symptoms (e.g., diplopia, tinnitus) and nausea and vomiting are also present. The headache is believed to result from the loss of CSF through the meningeal needle hole, resulting in decreased buoyant support for the brain. In the upright position the brain sags in the cranial vault, putting traction on pain-sensitive structures. Traction on cranial nerves is believed to cause the cranial nerve palsies that are seen occasionally.

The incidence of PDPH decreases with increasing age (Fig. 37-15) and with the use of small-diameter spinal needles with noncutting tips.[199,200] Inserting cutting needles with the bevel aligned parallel to the long axis of the meninges has also been shown to decrease the incidence of PDPH.[200,201] Some authors have suggested that parallel insertion spreads dural fibers, whereas perpendicular insertion cuts the fibers, resulting in a larger meningeal hole. However, the collagen fibers of the dura mater are arranged randomly; therefore, as many fibers will be cut with parallel insertion as with perpendicular insertion. A more likely explanation arises from the fact that the dura mater is under longitudinal tension. Thus, a slitlike hole oriented perpendicular to this longitudinal tension will tend to be pulled open, and a hole oriented parallel to this tension will be pulled closed. Some studies have suggested that women are at greater risk of developing PDPH. However, if age differences are accounted for, there does not appear to be a gender difference in the incidence of PDPH.[200] Folklore aside, remaining supine following meningeal puncture does not decrease the

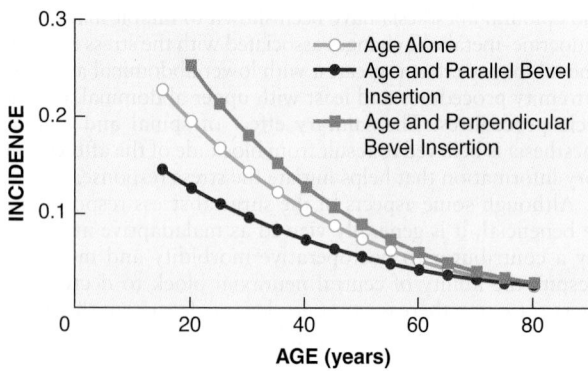

FIGURE 37-15. The incidence of postdural puncture headache decreases as patient age increases. When using beveled needles, the incidence is higher than average at any given age if the needle is inserted perpendicular to the spinal meninges and lower if inserted parallel to the spinal meninges. (Modified from Lybecker H, Møller JT, May O et al: Incidence and prediction of postdural puncture headache: A prospective study of 1021 spinal anesthesias. Anesth Analg 1990; 70: 389.)

incidence of PDPH. Finally, use of fluid, instead of air, for loss of resistance during attempted epidural anesthesia does not alter the risk of accidental meningeal puncture, but does markedly decrease the risk of subsequently developing PDPH.[31] PDPH usually resolves spontaneously in a few days to a week for most patients. However, there are reports of PDPH persisting for months following meningeal puncture. Initial treatment is appropriately conservative if this meets the patient's needs. Bed rest and analgesics as necessary are the mainstay of conservative treatment. Caffeine has also been shown to produce short-term symptomatic relief.[202]

Epidural Blood Patch

Patients who are unable or unwilling to await spontaneous resolution of PDPH should be offered epidural blood patch. Epidural blood patch is believed to form a clot over the meningeal hole, thereby preventing further CSF leak while the meningeal rent heals. Ten to 20 mL of autologous blood is aseptically injected into epidural space at or near the interspace at which the meningeal puncture occurred. This is effective in relieving symptoms within 1 to 24 hours in 85 to 95% of patients; approximately 90% of patients who fail an initial blood patch will respond to a second patch. The most common side effects of blood patch are backache and radicular pain, although transient bradycardia and cranial nerve palsies have also been reported.

The timing of epidural blood patch has been controversial. Early studies suggested that prophylactic blood patch in patients at high risk for PDPH was ineffective. This led several authors to suggest that blood patch should not be performed before patients develop symptoms of PDPH. Subsequent studies, which used larger volumes of blood in the epidural space (15 to 20 mL), have shown that prophylactic blood patch is effective in preventing PDPH in patients in whom the meninges were accidentally punctured during attempted epidural anesthesia.[203,204] Prophylactic blood patch is not appropriate for most patients but is worth considering in high-risk outpatients for whom a return trip to the hospital for epidural blood patch would be difficult.

Epidurally administered fibrin glue has been shown to be an effective alternative to blood administration for treatment of PDPH.[205] Whether it is superior to blood requires further study but it may be an attractive alternative for some patients.

Hearing Loss

Lamberg et al.[206] demonstrated that a transient (1 to 3 days) mild decrease in hearing acuity (>10 dB) is common after spinal anesthesia, with an incidence of roughly 40% and a 3:1 female-to-male predominance. Similarly, Gültekin et al.[207] demonstrated a 45% incidence of hearing impairment in subjects undergoing prilocaine spinal anesthesia but a much lower incidence (18%) in patients having bupivacaine spinal anesthesia. The mechanism of hearing loss in these studies is unclear, but the marked female predominance, the absence of PDPH, and the difference in incidence between prilocaine and bupivacaine suggest that CSF leak is not the cause.

Systemic Toxicity

Systemic toxicity of local anesthetics is discussed in detail in Chapter 21. Systemic toxicity does not occur with spinal anesthesia because the drug doses used are too low to cause toxic reactions even if injected intravenously. Both CNS and cardiovascular toxicity may occur during epidural anesthesia. CNS toxicity may result from local anesthetic absorption from the epidural space but more commonly occurs following accidental intravascular injection of local anesthetic. In contrast, cardiovascular toxicity from local anesthetics can probably only occur from unintended intravascular injection because the plasma concentrations of local anesthetics required to produce serious cardiovascular toxicity are very high. An adequate IV test dose and incremental injection of local anesthetics are the most important methods to prevent both CNS and cardiovascular toxicity during epidural anesthesia.

Total Spinal Anesthesia

Total spinal anesthesia occurs when local anesthetic spreads high enough to block the entire spinal cord and occasionally the brainstem during either spinal or epidural anesthesia. Profound hypotension and bradycardia are common secondary to complete sympathetic blockade. Respiratory arrest may occur as a result of respiratory muscle paralysis or dysfunction of brainstem respiratory control centers. Management includes vasopressors, atropine, and fluids as necessary to support the cardiovascular system, plus oxygen and controlled ventilation. If the cardiovascular and respiratory consequences are managed appropriately, total spinal block will resolve without sequelae.

Neurologic Injury

Serious neurologic injury is a rare but widely feared complication of epidural and spinal anesthesia. Multiple large series of spinal and epidural anesthesia report that neurologic injury occurs in approximately 0.03 to 0.1% of all central neuraxial blocks, although in most of these series the block was not clearly proven to be causative.[208] Persistent paresthesias and limited motor weakness are the most common injuries, although paraplegia and diffuse injury to cauda equina roots (*cauda equina syndrome*) do occur rarely. Injury may result from direct needle trauma to the spinal cord or spinal nerves, from spinal cord ischemia, from accidental injection of neurotoxic drugs or chemicals, from introduction of bacteria into the subarachnoid or epidural space, or very rarely from epidural hematoma.[208]

Importantly, local anesthetics intended for epidural and intrathecal use can themselves be neurotoxic in concentrations used clinically.[209] In particular, hyperbaric 5% lidocaine has been implicated as a cause of multiple cases of cauda equina syndrome following subarachnoid injection through small-bore ("microspinal") catheters during continuous spinal anesthesia.[210] Hyperbaric solutions injected through these high-resistance catheters have been shown to produce very little turbulence and thus poor mixing of the local anesthetic within CSF.[211] Nerve injury is believed to result from pooling of toxic concentrations of undiluted lidocaine around dependent cauda equina nerve roots. Consequently, the U.S. Food and Drug Administration has banned the use of these small-gauge catheters for continuous spinal anesthesia. Although the combination of microspinal catheters and high concentrations of lidocaine have clearly been implicated in causing cauda equina syndrome, this complication has also occurred when using larger (20-gauge) catheters,[210] 2% lidocaine,[212] and 0.5% tetracaine.[210] A common thread in all of these reports has been the apparent maldistribution of the local anesthetic within the CSF. Maldistribution should be suspected whenever spinal block is unexpectedly restricted, and maneuvers such as altering patient position or drug baricity should be employed to improve drug distribution before additional drug is injected through a continuous spinal catheter. If these maneuvers fail to improve drug distribution, an alternative anesthetic technique should be employed.

The mechanism by which local anesthetics produce cauda equina syndrome is not yet clear; however, in vitro evidence suggests that local anesthetics can produce excitotoxic damage by depolarizing neurons and increasing intracellular calcium concentrations.[213] Other studies demonstrate that local anesthetics can cause neuronal injury by damaging neuronal plasma membranes through detergentlike actions[214,215] or by activation of phospholipase-C.[216] It is also unclear as yet whether adjuncts added to local anesthetics (e.g., epinephrine) contribute to cauda equina syndrome. However, based on animal studies, it has been argued that epinephrine should not be added to intrathecal lidocaine.[217] Rather, if a prolonged duration of spinal anesthesia is necessary, then a longer-acting drug like bupivacaine should be used.

Transient Neurologic Symptoms

In addition to cauda equina syndrome, the occurrence of *transient neurologic symptoms* (TNS) or *transient radicular irritation* (TRI) has also emerged as a concern following central neuraxial blockade. TRI is defined as pain, dysesthesia, or both, in the legs or buttocks after spinal anesthesia and was first proposed as a recognizable entity by Schneider et al.[218] All local anesthetics have been shown to cause TRI, although the risk appears to be greater with lidocaine than other local anesthetics.[219–225]

In a large epidemiologic study of nearly 2,000 patients, Freedman et al.[226] characterized the clinical picture of TRI. They found that patients receiving lidocaine were significantly more likely to develop TRI than were patients receiving spinal tetracaine or bupivacaine, although TRI did occur with these latter two drugs as well. Other risk factors for TRI include addition of phenylephrine to 0.5% tetracaine,[227] surgery in the lithotomy position or with the leg flexed at the knee (as for meniscectomy), and outpatient status.[228] Evron et al.[229] reported the use of a double-orifice pencil-point needle was shown to significantly reduce the risk of TRI compared with a single orifice needle. Variables shown not to increase the risk of TRI included lidocaine dose, addition of epinephrine to lidocaine, presence of dextrose, paresthesia, hypotension, and blood-tinged CSF among others.

Pain from TRI **is** not trivial, with the majority of patients rating it as moderate (visual analogue scale = 4 to 7/10). The pain usually resolves spontaneously within 72 hours, but a few patients have required up to 6 months.[226]

The mechanism responsible for TRI is unknown; however, it is not simply a milder manifestation of cauda equina syndrome. Differences in clinical presentation and risk factors suggest that these are not simply two points along a continuum of the same process.

Chloroprocaine

Chloroprocaine was introduced into clinical practice in 1951 and was used for spinal anesthesia beginning that year. In the early 1980s, however, clinicians reported multiple cases of neurologic injury following intrathecal injection of chloroprocaine. Importantly, the chloroprocaine solution available at the time contained either methylparaben as an antimicrobial or bisulfite as an antioxidant. Subsequent animal studies aimed at determining the mechanism for spinal injury have been confusing, with some authors reporting that chloroprocaine itself does not cause neurologic injury but that bisulfite does, and others reporting that chloroprocaine can cause neurologic injury but that bisulfite is neuroprotective.[230–232] Nonetheless, concern about the potential for chloroprocaine-mediated neurotoxicity led to its nearly complete abandonment as a spinal anesthetic, in large part because lidocaine was perceived as a safer alternative.

However, we now recognize that lidocaine is not without risk of neurologic toxicity; in fact, it may be the most neurotoxic spinal anesthetic. This observation, coupled with the fact that a preservative-free chloroprocaine formulation is now available, has led to a re-evaluation of chloroprocaine as a short-acting spinal anesthetic. In 2004, Kouri and Kopacz[233] compared the block characteristics of 40 mg of plain 2% lidocaine with 40 mg of plain 2% preservative-free chloroprocaine in humans using a double-blind, randomized crossover study design. They found that both drugs produced identical average block heights (T8), but that chloroprocaine resulted in more rapid resolution of sensory block (103 ± 13 vs. 126 ± 16 minutes.) and faster attainment of discharge criteria (104 ± 12 vs. 134 ± 14 minutes). In addition, seven of eight volunteers experienced TNS following intrathecal lidocaine and none experienced TNS following 2% chloroprocaine. In other studies from the same research group, chloroprocaine spinal block height and duration were shown to be positively correlated with chloroprocaine dose[234] and addition of dextrose was shown not to alter spinal block characteristics, except that it increased postvoid bladder volume.[235] This group also performed studies to determine the effect of epinephrine and fentanyl as block-prolonging adjuvants to spinal chloroprocaine. Vath and Kopacz[236] found that the addition of 20 μg of fentanyl to 40 mg of chloroprocaine increased average peak block height (T5 vs. T9), prolonged the time for sensory block regression to L1 (78 ± 7 vs. 53 ± 19 minutes), and modestly increased the time to complete regression (104 ± 7 vs. 95 ± 9 minutes). Interestingly, Smith et al.[234] found that epinephrine (0.2 mg) increased chloroprocaine block duration but that its use was associated with a high incidence of myalgia, arthralgia, malaise, and anorexia that lasted up to 48 hours. The authors had no explanation for the epinephrine-associated side effects, but recommended against its use with intrathecal chloroprocaine. In a retrospective review of their experience with spinal chloroprocaine in 600 patients, Hejtmanek and Pollock[237] reported comparable clinical pharmacology, and no neurologic complications.

Thus, these studies, coupled with concerns about the potential for lidocaine-mediated neurotoxicity, raise the possibility that chloroprocaine will re-enter the mainstream as a spinal anesthetic, especially for ambulatory anesthesia.

Importantly, as of this writing, chloroprocaine is not specifically indicated for spinal anesthesia; therefore, its use is "off-label." But then, so is the use of multiple drugs that are routinely administered intrathecally, including plain bupiva-caine, plain lidocaine, hydromorphone, fentanyl, and sufen-tanil, among others.

Spinal Hematoma

Spinal hematoma is a rare but potentially devastating compli-cation of spinal and epidural anesthesia, with an incidence estimated to be <1 in 150,000. Patients most commonly pre-sent with numbness or lower extremity weakness, a fact that can make early detection difficult in patients receiving periop-erative spinal local anesthetics for pain control. Early detec-tion is critical because a delay of more than 8 hours in decom-pressing the spine reduces the odds of good recovery.[238]

Coagulation defects are the principal risk factor for epidural hematoma. This raises the legitimate question as to how to treat patients who are or who will be anticoagulated. This issue has been addressed in a Consensus Statement from the American Society for Regional Anesthesia and Pain Medi-cine[239] and the recommendations presented here are taken from this consensus statement. In brief, patients taking nons-teroidal anti-inflammatory drugs with antiplatelet effects (e.g., cyclooxygenase-1 inhibitors) or receiving subcutaneous unfractionated heparin for deep vein thrombosis prophylaxis are not viewed as being at increased risk of spinal hematoma.

In contrast, other classes of antiplatelet drugs, like thienopyridine derivatives (e.g., ticlopidine, clopidogrel) and glycoprotein IIb/IIIa antagonists (e.g., abciximab, eptifibatide, tirofiban) have a more potent effect on platelet aggregation, and neuraxial block should generally not be performed in patients taking these or similar medications. Further, the con-sensus statement recommends that ticlopidine be discontinued for 2 weeks and clopidogrel for 1 week before performing cen-tral neuraxial blocks. The glycoprotein IIb/IIIa antagonists have a shorter duration of action; thus, it is recommended that abciximab should be discontinued 24 to 48 hours before cen-tral neuraxial block, and eptifibatide and tirofiban should be discontinued 4 to 8 hours beforehand.

Patients receiving fractionated low-molecular weight heparin (e.g., enoxaparin, dalteparin, tinzaparin) are consid-ered to be at increased risk of spinal hematoma. Patients receiving these drugs preoperatively at thromboprophylactic doses should have the drug held for 10 to 12 hours before cen-tral neuraxial block. At higher doses, such as those used to treat established deep vein thrombosis, central neuraxial block should be delayed for 24 hours after the last dose. For patients in whom low-molecular-weight heparin is begun after surgery, single-shot central neuraxial blocks are not contraindicated provided that the first low-molecular-weight heparin dose is not administered until 24 hours postoperatively if using a twice-daily dosing regimen and 6 to 8 hours if using a once-daily dosing regimen. If an indwelling central neuraxial catheter is in place, it should not be removed until 10 to 12 hours after the last low-molecular-weight heparin dose, and the subsequent doses should not begin until at least 2 hours after catheter removal.

Patients who are "fully anticoagulated" (i.e., have elevated prothrombin time or partial thromboplastin time) or who are receiving thrombolytic or fibrinolytic therapy are considered to be at increased risk of spinal hematoma. These patients should not receive central neuraxial block except in very unusual circumstances when other options are not viable. Importantly for those patients who may have an epidural or intrathecal catheter placed, its removal is nearly as great a risk for spinal hematoma as its insertion, and the timing of removal and anticoagulation should be coordinated. Also, drugs/regimens not considered to put patients at increased risk of neuraxial bleeding when used alone (e.g., minidose unfrac-tionated heparin and nonsteroidal anti-inflammatory drugs) may in fact increase risk when combined.

CONTRAINDICATIONS

The only absolute contraindication to spinal or epidural anes-thesia is patient refusal. However, several pre-existing condi-tions increase the relative risk of these techniques and the anes-thesiologist must carefully weigh the expected benefits before proceeding. Some conditions that increase the apparent risk of central neuraxial block include the following:

1. Hypovolemia or shock increase the risk of hypotension.
2. Increased intracranial pressure increases the risk of brain her-niation when CSF is lost through the needle, or if a further increase in intracranial pressure follows injection of large vol-umes of solution into the epidural or subarachnoid spaces.
3. Coagulopathy or thrombocytopenia increase the risk of epidural hematoma.
4. Sepsis increases the risk of meningitis.
5. Infection at the puncture site increases the risk of meningitis.

Pre-existing neurologic disease, particularly diseases that wax and wane (e.g., multiple sclerosis), have been considered a contraindication to central-neuraxial block by some authors. Unfortunately, there are no well-controlled studies that answer the question as to whether spinal or epidural anesthesia alters the course of any pre-existing neurologic disease. However, Hebl et al.[240] conducted an uncontrolled retrospective chart review of 567 patients with pre-existing sensorimotor neu-ropathy or diabetic polyneuropathy who underwent spinal anesthesia. Two of these patients (0.4%; confidence interval: 0.1 to 1.3%) developed significant and persistent new neuro-logic symptoms: painful exacerbation of diabetic neuropathy and lumbar plexopathy superimposed on pre-existing sensori-motor neuropathy. In both cases, the role of spinal anesthesia in the patient's new symptoms was unknown; thus, it is diffi-cult to use these data to inform the decision whether or not to use central neuraxial block in patients with pre-existing peripheral neuropathy. Until more and better data are avail-able, it is prudent to inform patients that there may be a small risk that their neuropathy may worsen so that they can con-sider that when discussing their anesthetic choice.

SPINAL OR EPIDURAL ANESTHESIA?

Spinal and epidural anesthesia each have advantages and dis-advantages that may make one or the other technique better suited to a particular patient or procedure. Controlled studies comparing both techniques for surgical anesthesia have con-sistently found that spinal anesthesia takes less time to perform, produces more rapid onset of better-quality sensorimotor block, and is associated with less pain during surgery. Despite these important advantages of spinal anesthesia, epidural anesthesia offers advantages too. Chief among them are the lower risk of PDPH, less hypotension if epinephrine is not added to the local anesthetic, the ability to prolong or extend the block via an indwelling catheter, and the option of using an epidural catheter to provide postoperative analgesia.

References

1. Kehlet H: The stress response to surgery: Release mechanisms and the mod-ifying effect of pain relief. Acta Chir Scand Suppl 1988; 550: 22
2. Modig J, Borg T, Karlström G et al: Thromboembolism after total hip replacement: Role of epidural and general anesthesia. Anesth Analg 1983; 62: 174

3. Thornburn J, Louden J, Vallance R: Spinal and general anesthesia in total hip replacement: Frequency of deep vein thrombosis. Br J Anaesth 1980; 52: 1117

4. Christopherson R, Beattie C, Frank SM et al: Perioperative morbidity in patients randomized to epidural or general anesthesia for lower extremity vascular surgery. Anesthesiology 1993; 79: 422

5. Rosenfeld B, Beattie C, Christopherson R et al: The effects of different anesthetic regimens on fibrinolysis and the development of postoperative arterial thrombosis. Anesthesiology 1993; 79: 435

6. Yeager M, Glass D, Neff R, Brinck-Johnsen T: Epidural anesthesia and analgesia in high-risk surgical patients. Anesthesiology 1987; 66: 729

7. Moraca RJ, Sheldon DG, Thirlby RC: The role of epidural anesthesia and analgesia in surgical practice. Ann Surg 2003; 238: 663

8. Block BM, Liu SS, Rowlingson AJ et al: Efficacy of postoperative epidural analgesia: A meta-analysis. J Am Med Assoc 2003; 290: 2455

9. Zarzur E: Anatomic studies of the human lumbar ligamentum flavum. Anesth Analg 1984; 63: 499

10. Hogan Q: Lumbar epidural anatomy. A new look by cryomicrotome section. Anesthesiology 1991; 75: 767

11. Meijenhorst GC: Computed tomography of the lumbar epidural veins. Radiology 1982; 145: 687

12. Bernards CM, Shen DD, Sterling ES et al: Epidural, cerebrospinal fluid, and plasma pharmacokinetics of epidural opioids (part 1): Differences among opioids. Anesthesiology 2003; 99: 455

13. Tucker G, Mather L: Properties, absorption, and disposition of local anesthetic agents, Neural Blockade in Clinical Anesthesia and Management of Pain, 2nd edition. Edited by Cousins M, Bridenbaugh P. Philadelphia, JB Lippincott, 1988, p 47

14. Fink BR, Walker S: Orientation of fibers in human dorsal lumbar dura mater in relation to lumbar puncture. Anesth Analg 1989; 69: 768

15. Kerber CW, Newton TH: The macro and microvasculature of the dura mater. Neuroradiology 1973; 6: 175

16. Blomberg R: The dorsomedian connective tissue band in the lumbar epidural space of humans: An anatomical study using epiduroscopy in autopsy cases. Anesth Analg 1986; 65: 747

17. Savolaine ER, Pandya JB, Greenblatt SH et al: Anatomy of the human lumbar epidural space: New insights using CT-epidurography. Anesthesiology 1988; 68: 217

18. Hogan Q: Epidural catheter tip position and distribution of injectate evaluated by computed tomography. Anesthesiology 1999; 90: 964

19. Manchada V, Murad S, Shilyansky G et al: Unusual clinical course of accidental subdural local anesthetic injection. Anesth Analg 1983; 62: 1124

20. Lubenow T, Keh-Wong E, Kristof K et al: Inadvertant subdural injection: A complication of epidural block. Anesth Analg 1988; 67: 175

21. Jones M, Newton T: Inadvertent extra-arachnoid injections in myelography. Radiology 1983; 80: 818

22. Bernards C, Hill H: Morphine and alfentanil permeability through the spinal dura, arachnoid and pia mater of dogs and monkeys. Anesthesiology 1990; 73: 1214

23. Bernards C, Hill H: The spinal nerve root sleeve is not a preferred route for redistribution of drugs from the epidural space to the spinal cord. Anesthesiology 1991; 75: 827

24. Henry-Feugeas MC, Idy-Peretti I, Baledent O et al: Origin of subarachnoid cerebrospinal fluid pulsations: a phase-contrast MR analysis. Magn Reson Imaging 2000; 18: 387

25. Loth F, Yardimci MA, Alperin N: Hydrodynamic modeling of cerebrospinal fluid motion within the spinal cavity. J Biomech Eng 2001; 123: 71

26. Bernards CM: Cerebrospinal fluid and spinal cord distribution of baclofen and bupivacaine during slow intrathecal infusion in pigs. Anesthesiology 2006; 105: 169

27. Reiman R, Anson B: Vertebral level of termination of the spinal cord with report of a case of sacral cord. Anat Rec 1944; 88: 127

28. Drummond G, Scott D: Deflection of spinal needles by the bevel. Anaesthesia 1980; 35: 854

29. Moore JM, Liu SS, Neal JM: Premedication with fentanyl and midazolam decreases the reliability of intravenous lidocaine test dose. Anesth Analg 1998; 86: 1015

30. Evron S, Sessler D, Sadan O et al: Identification of the epidural space: Loss of resistance with air, lidocaine, or the combination of air and lidocaine. Anesth Analg 1999; 99: 245

31. Aida S, Taga K, Yamakura T et al: Headache after attempted epidural block: The role of intrathecal air. Anesthesiology 1998; 88: 76

32. Asato F, Goto F: Radiographic findings of unilateral epidural block. Anesth Analg 1996; 83: 519

33. Brichant JF, Bonhomme V, Hans P: On knots in epidural catheters: a case report and a review of the literature. Int J Obstet Anesth 2006; 15: 159

34. Gabopoulou Z, Mavrommati P, Chatzieleftheriou A et al: Epidural catheter entrapment caused by a double knot after combined spinal-epidural anesthesia. Reg Anesth Pain Med 2005; 30: 588

35. Leighton BL, Norris MC, DeSinome CA et al: The air test as a clinically useful indicator of intravenously placed epidural catheters. Anesthesiology 1990; 73: 610

36. Mackie K, Lam A: Epinephrine-containing test dose during beta-blockade. J Clin Monit 1991; 7: 213

37. Moore D, Batra M: The components of an effective test dose prior to epidural block. Anesthesiology 1981; 55: 693

38. Guinard J, Mulroy M, Carpenter R et al: Test doses: Optimal epinephrine content with and without acute beta-adrenergic blockade. Anesthesiology 1990; 73: 386

39. Liu SS: Hemodynamic responses to an epinephrine test dose in adults during epidural or combined epidural-general anesthesia. Anesth Analg 1996; 83: 97

40. Leighton B, DeSimone C, Norris M et al: Isoproterenol is an effective marker of intravenous injection in laboring women. Anesthesiology 1989; 71: 206

41. Leighton BL, Norris MC, Sosis M et al: Limitations of epinephrine as a marker of intravascular injection in laboring women. Anesthesiology 1987; 66: 688

42. Takiguchi T, Okano T, Egawa H et al: The effect of epidural saline injection on analgesic level during combined spinal and epidural anesthesia assessed clinically and myelographically [see comments]. Anesth Analg 1997; 85: 1097

43. Stienstra R, Dahan A, Alhadi BZ et al: Mechanism of action of an epidural top-up in combined spinal epidural anesthesia. Anesth Analg 1996; 83: 382

44. Stienstra R, Dilrosun-Alhadi BZ, Dahan A et al: The epidural "top-up" in combined spinal-epidural anesthesia: The effect of volume versus dose. Anesth Analg 1999; 88: 810

45. Myint Y, Bailey P, Milne B: Cardiorespiratory arrest following combined spinal epidural anaesthesia. Anaesthesia 1993; 48: 684

46. Bernards C, Kopacz D, Michel M: Effect of needle puncture on morphine and lidocaine flux through the spinal meninges of the monkey. Anesthesiology 1994; 80: 853

47. Hodgkinson R, Husain FJ: Obesity, gravity, and spread of epidural anesthesia. Anesth Analg 1981; 60: 421

48. Lee A, Ray D, Littlewood D, Wildsmith J: Effect of dextrose concentration on the intrathecal spread of amethocaine. Br J Anaesth 1988; 61: 135

49. Chambers WA, Edstrom HH, Scott DB: Effect of baricity on spinal anaesthesia with bupivacaine. Br J Anaesth 1981; 53: 279

50. Bannister J, McClure JH, Wildsmith JA: Effect of glucose concentration on the intrathecal spread of 0.5% bupivacaine. Br J Anaesth 1990; 64: 232

51. Povey HM, Jacobsen J, Westergaard-Nielsen J: Subarachnoid analgesia with hyperbaric 0.5% bupivacaine: Effect of a 60-min period of sitting. Acta Anaesthesiol Scand 1989; 33: 295

52. Povey HM, Olsen PA, Pihl H: Spinal analgesia with hyperbaric 0.5% bupivacaine: Effects of different patient positions. Acta Anaesthesiol Scand 1987; 31: 616

53. Sinclair CJ, Scott DB, Edström H: Effect of the Trendelenberg position on spinal anaesthesia with hyperbaric bupivacaine. Br J Anaesth 1982; 54: 497

54. Martin-Salvaj G, Van Gessel E, Forster A et al: Influence of duration of lateral decubitus on the spread of hyperbaric tetracaine during spinal anesthesia: A prospective time-response study. Anesth Analg 1994; 79: 1107

55. Smith T: The lumbar spine and subarachnoid block. Anesthesiology 1968; 29: 60

56. Logan MR, Drummond GB: Spinal anesthesia and lumbar lordosis. Anesth Analg 1988; 67: 338

57. Bodily M, Carpenter R, Owens B: Lidocaine 0.5% spinal anaesthesia: A hypobaric solution for short-stay perirectal surgery. Can J Anaesth 1992; 39: 770

58. Brown DT, Wildsmith JA, Covino BG et al: Effect of baricity on spinal anesthesia with amethocaine. Br J Anaesth 1980; 52: 589

59. Cummings GC, Bamber DB, Edstrom HH et al: Subarachnoid blockade with bupivacaine. A comparison with cinchocaine. Br J Anaesth 1984; 56: 573

60. Møller IW, Fernandes A, Edström HH: Subarachnoid anaesthesia with 0.5% bupivacaine: Effects of density. Br J Anaesth 1984; 56: 1191

61. Logan MR, McClure JH, Wildsmith JA: Plain bupivacaine: An unpredictable spinal anaesthetic agent. Br J Anaesth 1986; 58: 292

62. McKeown DW, Stewart K, Littlewood DG et al: Spinal anesthesia with plain solutions of lidocaine (2%) and bupivacaine (0.5%). Regional Anesth 1986; 11: 68

63. Cameron AE, Arnold RW, Ghorisa MW et al: Spinal analgesia using bupivacaine 0.5% plain. Variation in the extent of the block with patient age. Anaesthesia 1981; 36: 318

64. Kalso E, Tuominen M, Rosenberg PH: Effect of posture and some c.s.f. characteristics on spinal anaesthesia with isobaric 0.5% bupivacaine. Br J Anaesth 1982; 54: 1179

65. Tuominen M, Kalso E, Rosenberg P: Effects of posture on the spread of spinal anaesthesia with isobaric 0.75% or 0.5% bupivacaine. Br J Anaesth 1982; 54: 313

66. Stienstra R, van Poorten JF: The temperature of bupivacaine 0.5% affects the sensory level of spinal anesthesia. Anesth Analg 1988; 67: 272

67. McClure JH, Brown DT, Wildsmith JA: Effect of injected volume and speed of injection on the spread of spinal anaesthesia with isobaric amethocaine. Br J Anaesth 1982; 54: 917

68. Van Zundert AA, De Wolf AM: Extent of anesthesia and hemodynamic effects after subarachnoid administration of bupivacaine with epinephrine. Anesth Analg 1988; 67: 784

69. Nielsen TH, Kristoffersen E, Olsen KH et al: Plain bupivacaine: 0.5% or 0.25% for spinal analgesia? Br J Anaesth 1989; 62: 164

70. Bengtsson M, Malmqvist LA, Edström HH: Spinal analgesia with glucose-free bupivacaine—Effects of volume and concentration. Acta Anaesthesiol Scand 1984; 28: 583

71. Blomqvist H, Nilsson A, Arweström E: Spinal anaesthesia with 15 mg bupivacaine 0.25% and 0.5%. Regional Anesth 1988; 13: 165

ANESTHETIC MANAGEMENT

72. Mukkada TA, Bridenbaugh PO, Singh P et al: Effects of dose, volume, and concentration of glucose-free bupivacaine in spinal anesthesia. Regional Anesth 1986; 11: 98

73. Sheskey MC, Rocco AG, Bizzarri-Schmid M et al: A dose-response study of bupivacaine for spinal anesthesia. Anesth Analg 1983; 62: 931

74. Wildsmith J, McClure J, Brown D et al: Effects of posture on the spread of isobaric and hyperbaric amethocaine. Br J Anaesth 1981; 53: 273

75. Pflug AE, Aasheim GM, Beck HA: Spinal anesthesia: Bupivacaine versus tetracaine. Anesth Analg 1976; 55: 489

76. Sundnes KO, Vaagenes P, Skretting P et al: Spinal analgesia with hyperbaric bupivacaine: Effects of volume of solution. Br J Anaesth 1982; 54: 69

77. Chambers WA, Littlewood DG, Scott DB: Spinal anesthesia with hyperbaric bupivacaine: Effect of added vasoconstrictors. Anesth Analg 1982; 61: 49

78. Taivainen T, Tuominen M, Rosenberg PH: Influence of obesity on the spread of spinal analgesia after injection of plain 0.5% bupivacaine at the L3-4 of L4-5 interspace. Br J Anaesth 1990; 64: 542

79. Tuominen M, Kuulasmaa K, Taivainen T et al: Individual predictability of repeated spinal anaesthesia with isobaric bupivacaine. Acta Anaesthesiol Scand 1989; 33: 13

80. Tuominen M, Taivainen T, Rosenberg PH: Spread of spinal anaesthesia with plain 0.5% bupivacaine: Influence of the vertebral interspace used for injection. Br J Anaesth 1989; 62: 358

81. Carpenter RL, Hogan QH, Liu SS et al: Lumbosacral cerebrospinal fluid volume is the primary determinant of sensory block extent and duration during spinal anesthesia [see comments]. Anesthesiology 1998; 89: 24

82. Higuchi H, Hirata J, Adachi Y et al: Influence of lumbosacral cerebrospinal fluid density, velocity, and volume on extent and duration of plain bupivacaine spinal anesthesia. Anesthesiology 2004; 100: 106

83. Pargger H, Hampl KF, Aeschbach A et al: Combined effect of patient variables on sensory level after spinal 0.5% plain bupivacaine. Acta Anaesthesiol Scand 1998; 42: 430

84. Veering BT, Burm AG, van Kleef JW et al: Spinal anesthesia with glucose-free bupivacaine: effects of age on neural blockade and pharmacokinetics. Anesth Analg 1987; 66: 965

85. Pitkänen M, Haapaniemi L, Tuominen M et al: Influence of age on spinal anaesthesia with isobaric 0.5% bupivacaine. Br J Anaesth 1984; 56: 279

86. Norris M: Height, weight, and the spread of subarachnoid hyperbaric bupivacaine in the term parturient. Anesth Analg 1988; 67: 555

87. Norris MC: Patient variables and the subarachnoid spread of hyperbaric bupivacaine in the term parturient. Anesthesiology 1990; 72: 478

88. Wildsmith JA, Rocco AG: Current concepts in spinal anesthesia. Regional Anesth 1985; 10: 119

89. McCulloch WJ, Littlewood DG: Influence of obesity on spinal analgesia with isobaric 0.5% bupivacaine. Br J Anaesth 1986; 58: 610

90. Pitkänen MT: Body mass and spread of spinal anesthesia with bupivacaine. Anesth Analg 1987; 66: 127

91. Axelsson KH, Edström HH, Sundberg AE et al: Spinal anaesthesia with hyperbaric 0.5% bupivacaine: Effects of volume. Acta Anaesthesiol Scand 1982; 26: 439

92. Bengtsson M, Edström HH, Löfström JB: Spinal analgesia with bupivacaine, mepivacaine and tetracaine. Acta Anaesthesiol Scand 1983; 27: 278

93. Racle J, Benkhadra A, Poy J et al: Effect of increasing amounts of epinephrine during isobaric bupivacaine spinal anesthesia in elderly patients. Anesth Analg 1987; 66: 882

94. Vaida GT, Moss P, Capan LM et al: Prolongation of lidocaine spinal anesthesia with phenylephrine. Anesth Analg 1986; 65: 781

95. Egbert LD, Deas TC: Effect of epinephrine upon the duration of spinal anesthesia. Anesthesiology 1960; 21: 345

96. Concepcion M, Maddi R, Francis D et al: Vasoconstrictors in spinal anesthesia with tetracaine—A comparison of epinephrine and phenylephrine. Anesth Analg 1984; 63: 134

97. Meagher RP, Moore DC, DeVries JC: Phenylephrine: The most effective potentiator of tetracaine spinal anesthesia. Anesth Analg 1966; 45: 134

98. Caldwell C, Nielsen C, Baltz T et al: Comparison of high-dose epinephrine and phenylephrine in spinal anesthesia with tetracaine. Anesthesiology 1985; 62: 804

99. Park WY, Balingit PE, Macnamara TE: Effects of patient age, pH of cerebrospinal fluid, and vasopressors on onset and duration of spinal anesthesia. Anesth Analg 1975; 54: 455

100. Fukuda T, Dohi S, Naito H: Comparisons of tetracaine spinal anesthesia with clonidine or phenylephrine in normotensive and hypertensive humans. Anesth Analg 1994; 78: 106

101. Bonnet F, Brun-Buisson V, Saada M et al: Dose-related prolongation of hyperbaric tetracaine spinal anesthesia by clonidine in humans. Anesth Analg 1989; 68: 619

102. Dobrydnjov I, Samarutel J: Enhancement of intrathecal lidocaine by addition of local and systemic clonidine. Acta Anaesthesiol Scand 1999; 43: 556

103. Ota K, Namiki A, Ujike Y et al: Prolongation of tetracaine spinal anesthesia by oral clonidine. Anesth Analg 1992; 75: 262

104. Ota K, Namiki A, Iwasaki H et al: Dosing interval for prolongation of tetracaine spinal anesthesia by oral clonidine in humans. Anesth Analg 1994; 79: 1117

105. Axelsson K, Widman B: Blood concentration of lidocaine after spinal anaesthesia using lidocaine and lidocaine with adrenaline. Acta Anaesthesiol Scand 1981; 25: 240

106. Leicht CH, Carlson SA: Prolongation of lidocaine spinal anesthesia with epinephrine and phenylephrine. Anesth Analg 1986; 65: 365

107. Moore DC, Chadwick HS, Ready LB: Epinephrine prolongs libocaine spinal: Pain in the operative site is the most accurate method of determining local anesthetic duration. Anesthesiology 1987; 67: 416

108. Chambers WA, Littlewood DG, Logan MR et al: Effect of added epinephrine on spinal anesthesia with lidocaine. Anesth Analg 1981; 60: 417

109. Spivey DL: Epinephrine does not prolong lidocaine spinal anesthesia in term parturients. Anesth Analg 1985; 64: 468

110. Chiu AA, Liu S, Carpenter RL et al: The effects of epinephrine on lidocaine spinal anesthesia: a cross-over study. Anesth Analg 1995; 80: 735

111. Kozody R, Swartz J, Palahniuk RJ et al: Spinal cord blood flow following subarachnoid lidocaine. Can Anaesth Soc J 1985; 32: 472

112. Kozody R, Palahniuk RJ, Cumming MO: Spinal cord blood flow following subarachnoid tetracaine. Can Anaesth Soc J 1985; 32: 23

113. Kozody R, Ong B, Palahniuk RJ et al: Subarachnoid bupivacaine decreases spinal cord blood flow in dogs. Can Anaesth Soc J 1985; 32: 216

114. Denson DD, Bridenbaugh PO, Turner PA et al: Neural blockade and pharmacokinetics following subarachnoid lidocaine in the rhesus monkey. I. Effects of epinephrine. Anesth Analg 1982; 61: 746

115. Crosby G, Russo M, Szabo M et al: Subarachnoid clonidine reduces spinal cord blood flow and glucose utilization in conscious rats. Anesthesiology 1990; 73: 1179

116. Converse JG, Landmesser CM, Harmel MH: The concentration of pontocaine hydrochloride in the cerebrospinal fluid during spinal anesthesia, and the influence of epinephrine in prolonging the sensory anesthetic effect. Anesthesiology 1954; 15: 1

117. Mörch ET, Rosenberg MK, Truant AT: Lidocaine for spinal anesthesia. A study of the concentration in the spinal fluid. Acta Anaesthesiol Scand 1957; 1: 105

118. Kozody R, Palahniuk RJ, Wade JG et al: The effect of subarachnoid epinephrine and phenylephrine on spinal cord blood flow. Can Anaesth Soc J 1984; 31: 503

119. Reddy SV, Maderdrut JL, Yaksh TL: Spinal cord pharmacology of adrenergic agonist-mediated antinociception. J Pharmacol Exp Ther 1980; 213: 525

120. Phillis J, Tebecis A, York D: Depression of spinal motoneurons by noradrenalin, 5-hydroxytryptamine and histamine. Eur J Pharmacol 1968; 4: 471

121. Park W, Massengale M, Macnamara T: Age, height, and speed of injection as factors determining caudal anesthetic level and occurrence of severe hypertension. Anesthesiology 1979; 51: 81

122. Park WY, Hagins FM, Rivat EL et al: Age and epidural dose response in adult men. Anesthesiology 1982; 56: 318

123. Grundy EM, Ramamurthy S, Patel KP et al: Extradural analgesia revisited. Br J Anaesth 1978; 50: 805

124. Erdemir HA, Soper LE, Sweet RB: Studies of factors affecting peridural anesthesia. Anesth Analg 1965; 44: 400

125. Burn JM, Guyer PB, Langdon L: The spread of solutions injected into the epidural space. Br J Anaesth 1973; 45: 338

126. Apostolou GA, Zarmakoupis PK, Mastrokostopoulos GT: Spread of epidural anesthesia and the lateral position. Anesth Analg 1981; 60: 584

127. Park WY, Hagins FM, Massengale MD et al: The sitting position and anesthetic spread in the epidural space. Anesth Analg 1984; 63: 863

128. Ponhold H, Kulier A, Rehak P: 30 degree trunk elevation of the patient and quality of lumbar epidural anesthesia. Effects of elevation in operations on the lower extremities. Anaesthetist 1993; 42: 788

129. Park WY, Massengale M, Kim SI et al: Age and the spread of local anesthetic solutions in the epidural space. Anesth Analg 1980; 59: 768

130. Nydahl PA, Philipson L, Axelsson K et al: Epidural anesthesia with 0.5% bupivacaine: Influence of age on sensory and motor blockade. Anesth Analg 1991; 73: 780

131. Veering BT, Burm AG, van Kleef JW et al: Epidural anesthesia with bupivacaine: Effects of age on neural blockade and pharmacokinetics. Anesth Analg 1987; 66: 589

132. Hirabayashi Y, Saitoh K, Fukuda H et al: Effect of age on dose requirement for lumbar epidural anesthesia. Masui 1993; 42: 808

133. Duggan J, Bowler GM, McClure JH et al: Extradural block with bupivacaine: Influence of dose, volume, concentration and patient characteristics. Br J Anaesth 1988; 61: 324

134. Hirabayashi Y, Shimizu R, Matsuda I et al: Effect of extradural compliance and resistance on spread of extradural analgesia. Br J Anaesth 1990; 65: 508

135. Bromage P: Spread of analgesic solutions in the epidural space and their site of action: a statistical study. Br J Anaesth 1962; 34: 161

136. Fagraeus L, Urban BJ, Bromage PR: Spread of epidural analgesia in early pregnancy. Anesthesiology 1983; 58: 184

137. Grundy EM, Zamora AM, Winnie AP: Comparison of spread of epidural anesthesia in pregnant and nonpregnant women. Anesth Analg 1978; 57: 544

138. Kalas DB, Senfield RM, Hehre FW: Continuous lumbar peridural anesthesia in obstetrics. IV: Comparison of the number of segments blocked in pregnant and nonpregnant subjects. Anesth Analg 1966; 45: 848

139. Sharrock NE: Lack of exaggerated spread of epidural anesthesia in patients with arteriosclerosis. Anesthesiology 1977; 47: 307

140. Axelsson K, Nydahl PA, Philipson L et al: Motor and sensory blockade after epidural injection of mepivacaine, bupivacaine, and etidocaine—A double-blind study. Anesth Analg 1989; 69: 739

141. Kerkkamp HE, Gielen MJ, Wattwil M et al: An open study comparison of 0.5%, 0.75% and 1.0% ropivacaine, with epinephrine, in epidural anesthesia in patients undergoing urologic surgery. Regional Anesth 1990; 15: 53

142. Buckley FP, Littlewood DG, Covino BG et al: Effects of adrenaline and the concentration of solution on extradural block with etidocaine. Br J Anaesth 1978; 50: 171

143. Scott DB, McClure JH, Gaisi RM et al: Effects of concentration of local anaesthetic drugs in extradural block. Br J Anaesth 1980; 52: 1033

144. Bromage PR, Burfoot MF, Crowell DE et al: Quality of epidural blockade. I: Influence of physical factors. Br J Anaesth 1964; 36: 342

145. Bernards CM, Shen DD, Sterling ES et al: Epidural, cerebrospinal fluid, and plasma pharmacokinetics of epidural opioids (part 2): effect of epinephrine. Anesthesiology 2003; 99: 466

146. Kier L: Continuous epidural analgesia in prostatectomy: Comparison of bupivacaine with and without adrenaline. Acta Anaesthesiol Scand 1974; 18: 1

147. Sinclair CJ, Scott DB: Comparison of bupivacaine and etidocaine in extradural blockade. Br J Anaesth 1984; 56: 147

148. Cederholm I, Anskär S, Bengtsson M: Sensory, motor, and sympathetic block during epidural analgesia with 0.5% and 0.75% ropivacaine with and without epinephrine. Regional Anesth 1994; 19: 18

149. Abboud T, Sheik-ol-Eslam A, Yanagi T et al: Safety and efficacy of epinephrine added to bupivacaine for lumbar epidural analgesia in obstetrics. Anesth Analg 1985; 64: 585

150. Eisenach JC, Grice SC, Dewan DM: Epinephrine enhances analgesia produced by epidural bupivacaine during labor. Anesth Analg 1987; 66: 447

151. Finucane B, McCraney J, Bush D: Double-blind comparison of lidocaine and etidocaine during continuous epidural anesthesia for vaginal delivery. South Med J 1978; 71: 667

152. Cohen E: Distribution of local anesthetic agents in the neuroaxis of the dog. Anesthesiology 1968; 29: 1002

153. Post C, Freedman J, Ramsay C et al: Redistribution of lidocaine and bupivacaine after intrathecal injection in mice. Anesthesiology 1985; 63: 410

154. Boswell M, Iacono R, Guthkelch A: Sites of action of subarachnoid lidocaine and tetracaine: Observations with evoked potential monitoring during spinal cord stimulator implantation. Reg Anesth 1992; 17: 37

155. Cusick J, Myklebust J, Abram S: Differential neural effects of epidural anesthetics. Anesthesiology 1980; 53: 299

156. Urban B: Clinical observations suggesting a changing site of action during induction and recession of spinal and epidural anesthesia. Anesthesiology 1973; 39: 496

157. Fink BR: Mechanisms of differential axial blockade in epidural and subarachnoid anesthesia. Anesthesiology 1989; 70: 851

158. Fink BR, Cairns AM: Lack of size-related differential sensitivity to equilibrium conduction block among mammalian myelinated axons exposed to lidocaine. Anesth Analg 1987; 66: 948

159. Chamberlain D, Chamberlain B: Changes in skin temperature of the trunk and their relationship to sympathetic block during spinal anesthesia. Anesthesiology 1986; 65: 139

160. Brull SJ, Greene NM: Zones of differential sensory block during extradural anaesthesia. Br J Anaesth 1991; 66: 651

161. Gentili M, Huu PC, Enel D et al: Sedation depends on the level of sensory block induced by spinal anaesthesia. Br J Anaesth 1998; 81: 970

162. Ben-David B, Vaida S, Gaitini L: The influence of high spinal anesthesia on sensitivity to midazolam sedation [see comments]. Anesth Analg 1995; 81: 525

163. Tverskoy M, Shagal M, Finger J et al: Subarachnoid bupivacaine blockade decreases midazolam and thiopental hypnotic requirements. J Clin Anesth 1994; 6: 487

164. Tverskoy M, Shifrin V, Finger J, Fleyshman G, Kissin I: Effect of epidural bupivacaine block on midazolam hypnotic requirements. Reg Anesth 1996; 21: 209

165. Hodgson P, Liu S, Gras T: Does epidural anesthesia have general anesthetic effects? A prospective, randomized, double-blind, placebo-controlled trial. Anesthesiology 1999; 91: 1687

166. Carpenter RL, Caplan RA, Brown DL et al: Incidence and risk factors for side effects of spinal anesthesia. Anesthesiology 1992; 76: 906

167. Coe AJ, Revanäs B: Is crystalloid preloading useful in spinal anaesthesia in the elderly? Anaesthesia 1990; 45: 241

168. Phero JC, Bridenbaugh PO, Edström HH et al: Hypotension in spinal anesthesia: A comparison of isobaric tetracaine with epinephrine and isobaric bupivacaine without epinephrine. Anesth Analg 1987; 66: 549

169. Tarkkila P, Isola J: A regression model for identifying patients at high risk of hypotension, bradycardia and nausea during spinal anesthesia. Acta Anesthesiol Scand 1992; 36: 554

170. Shimosato S, Etsten BE: The role of the venous system in cardiocirculatory dynamics during spinal and epidural anesthesia in man. Anesthesiology 1969; 30: 619

171. Kennedy WF, Jr. , Bonica JJ, Akamatsu TJ et al: Cardiovascular and respiratory effects of subarachnoid block in the presence of acute blood loss. Anesthesiology 1968; 29: 29

172. Anzai Y, Nishikawa T: Heart rate responses to body tilt during spinal anesthesia. Anesth Analg 1991; 73: 385

173. Ward RJ, Bonica JJ, Freund FG et al: Epidural and subarachnoid anesthesia. Cardiovascular and respiratory effects. JAMA 1965; 191: 275

174. Carp H, Vadhera R, Jayaram A et al: Endogenous vasopressin and renin-angiotensin systems support blood pressure after epidural block in humans. Anesthesiology 1994; 80: 1000-7; discussion 27A

175. Peters J, Schlaghecke R, Thouet H et al: Endogenous vasopressin supports blood pressure and prevents severe hypotension during epidural anesthesia in conscious dogs. Anesthesiology 1990; 73: 694

176. Pathak CL: Autoregulation of chronotropic response of the heart through pacemaker stretch. Cardiology 1973; 58: 45

177. Jacobsen J, Søfelt S, Brocks V et al: Reduced left ventricular diameters at onset of bradycardia during epidural anaesthesia. Acta Anaesthesiol Scand 1992; 36: 831

178. Baron JF, Decaux-Jacolot A, Edouard A et al: Influence of venous return on baroreflex control of heart rate during lumbar epidural anesthesia in humans. Anesthesiology 1986; 64: 188

179. Caplan RA, Ward RJ, Posner K et al: Unexpected cardiac arrest during spinal anesthesia: A closed claims analysis of predisposing factors. Anesthesiology 1988; 68: 5

180. Mackey DC, Carpenter RL, Thompson GE et al: Bradycardia and asystole during spinal anesthesia: A report of three cases without morbidity. Anesthesiology 1989; 70: 866

181. Bernards CM, Hymas NJ: Progression of first degree heart block to high-grade second degree block during spinal anaesthesia. Can J Anaesth 1992; 39: 173

182. Jordi EM, Marsch SC, Strebel S: Third degree heart block and asystole associated with spinal anaesthesia. Anesthesiology 1998; 89: 257

183. Shen CL, Hung YC, Chen PJ et al: Mobitz type II AV block during spinal anesthesia. Anesthesiology 1990; 90: 1477

184. Bonica JJ, Kennedy WF, Jr., Ward RJ et al: A comparison of the effects of high subarachnoid and epidural anesthesia. Acta Anaesthesiol Scand 1966; 23: 429

185. Kerkkamp HE, Gielen MJ: Hemodynamic monitoring in epidural blockade: Cardiovascular effects of 20 ml 0.5% bupivacaine with and without epinephrine. Regional Anesth 1990; 15: 137

186. Graves CL, Underwood PS, Klein RL et al: Intravenous fluid administration as therapy for hypotension secondary to spinal anesthesia. Anesth Analg 1968; 47: 548

187. Venn PJ, Simpson DA, Rubin AP et al: Effect of fluid preloading on cardiovascular variables after spinal anaesthesia with glucose-free 0.75% bupivacaine. Br J Anaesth 1989; 63: 682

188. Rout CC, Rocke DA, Levin J et al: A reevaluation of the role of crystalloid preload in the prevention of hypotension associated with spinal anesthesia for elective cesarean section. Anesthesiology 1993; 79: 262

189. Marhofer P, Faryniak B, Oismuller C et al: Cardiovascular effects of 6% hetastarch and lactated Ringer's solution during spinal anesthesia. Reg Anesth Pain Med 1999; 24: 399

190. Butterworth J, Piccione W, Berrizbeitia L et al: Augmentation of venous return by adrenergic agonists during spinal anesthesia. Anesth Analg 1986; 65: 612

191. Ward RJ, Kennedy WF, Bonica JJ et al: Experimental evaluation of atropine and vasopressors for the treatment of hypotension of high subarachnoid anesthesia. Anesth Analg 1966; 45: 621

192. Lundberg J, Norgren L, Thomson D et al: Hemodynamic effects of dopamine during thoracic epidural analgesia in man. Anesthesiology 1987; 66: 641

193. Butterworth JF, 4th, Austin JC, Johnson MD et al: Effect of total spinal anesthesia on arterial and venous responses to dopamine and dobutamine. Anesth Analg 1987; 66: 209

194. Goertz AW, Seeling W, Heinrich H et al: Effect of phenylephrine bolus administration of left ventricular function during high thoracic and lumbar epidural anesthesia combined with general anesthesia. Anesth Analg 1993; 76: 541

195. Sakura S, Saito Y, Kosaka Y: Effect of lumbar epidural anesthesia on ventilatory response to hypercapnia in young and elderly patients. J Clin Anesth 1993; 5: 109

196. Steinbrook R, Concepcion M, Topulos G: Ventilatory responses to hypercapnia during bupivacaine spinal anesthesia. Anesth Analg 1988; 67: 247

197. Dahl JB, Schultz P, Anker-Møller E et al: Spinal anaesthesia in young patients using a 29-gauge needle: Technical considerations and an evaluation of postoperative complaints compared with general anaesthesia. Br J Anaesth 1990; 64: 178

198. Seeberger MD, Lang ML, Drewe J et al: Comparison of spinal and epidural anesthesia for patients younger than 50 years of age. Anesth Analg 1994; 78: 667

199. Halpern S, Preston R: Postdural puncture headache and spinal needle design. Anesthesiology 1994; 81: 1376

200. Lybecker H, Møller JT, May O et al: Incidence and prediction of postdural puncture headache. A prospective study of 1021 spinal anesthesias. Anesth Analg 1990; 70: 389

201. Flaatten H, Thorsen T, Askeland B et al: Puncture technique and postural postdural puncture headache. A randomised, double-blind study comparing transverse and parallel puncture. Acta Anaesthesiol Scand 1998; 42: 1209

202. Camann WR, Murray RS, Mushlin PS et al: Effects of oral caffeine on postdural puncture headache. A double-blind, placebo-controlled trial. Anesth Analg 1990; 70: 181

203. Cheek TG, Banner R, Sauter J et al: Prophylactic extradural blood patch is effective. Br J Anaesth 1988; 61: 340

204. Colonna-Romano P, Shapiro BE: Unintentional dural puncture and prophylactic epidural blood patch in obstetrics. Anesth Analg 1989; 69: 522

205. Crul BJ, Gerritse BM, van Dongen RT et al: Epidural fibrin glue injection stops persistent postdural puncture headache. Anesthesiology 1999; 91: 576

206. Lamberg T, Pitkanen MT, Marttila T et al: Hearing loss after continuous or single-shot spinal anesthesia. Reg Anesth 1997; 22: 539

207. Gültekin S, Yilmaz N, Ceyhan A et al: The effect of different anesthetic agents in hearing loss following spinal anaesthesia. Eur J Anaesthesiol 1998; 15: 61

208. Kane R: Neurologic deficits following epidural or spinal anesthesia. Anesth Analg 1981; 60: 150

209. Lambert LA, Lambert DH, Strichartz GR: Irreversible conduction block in isolated nerve by high concentrations of local anesthetics. Anesthesiology 1994; 80: 1082

210. Rigler M, Drasner K, Krejcie T et al: Cauda equina syndrome after continuous spinal anesthesia. Anesth Analg 1991; 72: 275

211. Ross B, Coda B, Heath C: Local anesthetic distribution in a spinal model: A possible mechanism of neurologic injury after continuous spinal anesthesia. Reg Anesth 1992; 17: 69

212. Drasner K, Rigler M, Sessler D et al: Cauda equina syndrome following intended epidural anesthesia. Anesthesiology 1992; 77: 582

213. Gold MS, Reichling DB, Hampl KF et al: Lidocaine toxicity in primary afferent neurons from the rat. J Pharmacol Exp Ther 1998; 285: 413

214. Johnson ME, Saenz JA, DaSilva AD et al: Effect of local anesthetic on neuronal cytoplasmic calcium and plasma membrane lysis (necrosis) in a cell culture model. Anesthesiology 2002; 97: 1466

215. Kitagawa N, Oda M, Totoki T: Possible mechanism of irreversible nerve injury caused by local anesthetics: detergent properties of local anesthetics and membrane disruption. Anesthesiology 2004; 100: 962

216. Raucher D, Sheetz MP: Phospholipase C activation by anesthetics decreases membrane-cytoskeleton adhesion. J Cell Sci 2001; 114: 3759

217. Drasner K: Lidocaine spinal anesthesia: A vanishing therapeutic index? [editorial; comment]. Anesthesiology 1997; 87: 469

218. Schneider M, Ettlin T, Kaufmann M et al: Transient neurologic toxicity after hyperbaric subarachnoid anesthesia with 5% lidocaine [see comments]. Anesth Analg 1993; 76: 1154

219. Hiller A, Rosenberg PH: Transient neurological symptoms after spinal anaesthesia with 4% mepivacaine and 0.5% bupivacaine. Br J Anaesth 1997; 79: 301

220. Liguori GA, Zayas VM, Chisholm MF: Transient neurologic symptoms after spinal anesthesia with mepivacaine and lidocaine [see comments]. Anesthesiology 1998; 88: 619

221. Martinez-Bourio R, Arzuaga M, Quintana JM et al: Incidence of transient neurologic symptoms after hyperbaric subarachnoid anesthesia with 5% lidocaine and 5% prilocaine [see comments]. Anesthesiology 1998; 88: 624

222. Hampl KF, Heinzmann-Wiedmer S, Luginbuehl I et al: Transient neurologic symptoms after spinal anesthesia: A lower incidence with prilocaine and bupivacaine than with lidocaine [see comments]. Anesthesiology 1998; 88: 629

223. Salmela L, Aromaa U: Transient radicular irritation after spinal anesthesia induced with hyperbaric solutions of cerebrospinal fluid-diluted lidocaine 50 mg/ml or mepivacaine 40 mg/ml or bupivacaine 5 mg/ml. Acta Anaesthesiol Scand 1998; 42: 765

224. Axelrod EH, Alexander GD, Brown M et al: Procaine spinal anesthesia: A pilot study of the incidence of transient neurologic symptoms. J Clin Anesth 1998; 10: 404

225. Bergeron L, Girard M, Drolet P et al: Spinal procaine with and without epinephrine and its relation to transient radicular irritation. Can J Anaesth 1999; 46: 846

226. Freedman JM, Li DK, Drasner K et al: Transient neurologic symptoms after spinal anesthesia: An epidemiologic study of 1,863 patients [published erratum appears in Anesthesiology 89(6) 1614, 1998]. Anesthesiology 1998; 89: 633

227. Sakura S, Sumi M, Sakaguchi Y et al: The addition of phenylephrine contributes to the development of transient neurologic symptoms after spinal anesthesia with 0.5% tetracaine [see comments]. Anesthesiology 1997; 87: 771

228. Pollock JE, Neal JM, Stephenson CA et al: Prospective study of the incidence of transient radicular irritation in patients undergoing spinal anesthesia [see comments]. Anesthesiology 1996; 84: 1361

229. Evron S, Gurstieva V, Ezri T et al: Transient neurological symptoms after isobaric subarachnoid anesthesia with 2% lidocaine: the impact of needle type. Anesth Analg 2007; 105: 1494

230. Gissen A, Datta S, Lambert D: The chloroprocaine controversy: II. Is chloroprocaine neurotoxic? Regional Anesthesia 1984; 9: 135

231. Ravindran RS, Turner MS, Muller J: Neurologic effects of subarachnoid administration of 2-chloroprocaine-CE, bupivacaine, and low pH normal saline in dogs. Anesth Analg 1982; 61: 279

232. Taniguchi M, Bollen AW, Drasner K: Sodium bisulfite: scapegoat for chloroprocaine neurotoxicity? Anesthesiology 2004; 100: 85

233. Kouri ME, Kopacz DJ: Spinal 2-chloroprocaine: A comparison with lidocaine in volunteers. Anesth Analg 2004; 98: 75

234. Smith KN, Kopacz DJ, McDonald SB: Spinal 2-chloroprocaine: a dose-ranging study and the effect of added epinephrine. Anesth Analg 2004; 98: 81

235. Warren DT, Kopacz DJ: Spinal 2-chloroprocaine: The effect of added dextrose. Anesth Analg 2004; 98: 95

236. Vath JS, Kopacz DJ: Spinal 2-chloroprocaine: The effect of added fentanyl. Anesth Analg 2004; 98: 89

237. Hejtmanek M, Pollock J: Chloroprocaine for Outpatient Surgery-Experience with 600 cases. Anesthesiology 2008 (in Press)

238. Vandermeulen EP, Van Aken H, Vermylen J: Anticoagulants and spinal-epidural anesthesia. Anesth Analg 1994; 79: 1165

239. Horlocker TT, Wedel DJ, Benzon H: Regional anesthesia in the anticoagulated patient: Defining the risks (the second ASRA Consensus Conference on Neuraxial Anesthesia and Anticoagulation). Reg Anesth Pain Med 2003; 28: 172

240. Hebl JR, Kopp SL, Schroeder DR et al: Neurologic complications after neuraxial anesthesia or analgesia in patients with preexisting peripheral sensorimotor neuropathy or diabetic polyneuropathy. Anesth Analg 2006; 103: 1294

CHAPTER 38 ■ PERIPHERAL NERVE BLOCKADE

BAN C.H. TSUI AND RICHARD W. ROSENQUIST

GENERAL PRINCIPLES AND EQUIPMENT
Setup and Monitoring
Common Techniques: Nerve Stimulation and Ultrasound
Imaging
Other Related Equipment
Avoiding Complications
Premedication and Sedation

SPECIFIC TECHNIQUES
Head and Neck Blocks
Upper Extremity Blocks
Trunk Blocks
Penile Blocks
Lower Extremity Blocks
ACKNOWLEDGMENTS

KEY POINTS

1 Peripheral nerve blocks provide effective anesthesia and analgesia in a site-specific manner with the potential for effects of long duration.

2 Accurate identification of target nerves and precise and adequate local anesthetic placement are paramount for performing safe and successful peripheral nerve blocks.

3 Ultrasound imaging has renewed interest in peripheral nerve blockade because it allows the needle to be directed toward the nerve structure(s) with real-time visualization, potentially avoiding critical structures in the path of the needle and reducing complications. Although highly desirable as an aid to the performance of regional anesthesia, this technology requires considerable training in addition to thorough knowledge of the equipment and regional nerve block anatomy.

4 Peripheral nerve stimulators are useful tools to facilitate nerve blockade, but they do not eliminate the risk of nerve injury. In

the adult patient, maintenance of responsiveness may allow reporting of nerve contact or pain during injection.

5 Nerve blocks associated with bony or vascular landmarks are more reliable and easy to perform than those that depend on surface landmarks alone.

6 Larger volumes of local anesthetic may increase the potential success of peripheral nerve blocks, but the total milligram dosage must be limited to avoid systemic toxicity. Higher concentrations of local anesthetics increase the degree of motor block, but larger volumes of more dilute solutions can be used with less risk of toxicity. Ultrasound imaging, through more accurate nerve localization and visualization of local anesthetic spread, may enable successful blocks to be performed with reduced volumes of local anesthetics, but this has yet to be proven.

1 Regional anesthesia enables site-specific, long-lasting, and effective anesthesia and analgesia. It is suitable for many surgical patients and can improve analgesia,[1] reduce morbidity, mortality, and the need for reoperation after major surgical procedures.[2] Peripheral nerve blocks (PNB) can be used as the only "surgical" anesthetic, as a supplement to provide analgesia and muscle relaxation along with general anesthesia, or as the initial step in the provision of prolonged postoperative analgesia such as with intercostal blocks or continuous peripheral nerve catheters. Compared with parenteral analgesics, single-shot or continuous PNB can provide superior analgesia and a lower incidence of side effects.[3–5] Optimal pain relief and minimal side effects (e.g., nausea and vomiting) after surgery can have a major impact on patient outcome, including patient satisfaction and earlier mobilization, as well as fulfilling the current need for streamlined surgical services with lower costs.[6] However, the safety and success of PNB techniques are highly dependent on

2 accurate delivery of the correct dose of local anesthetic. Unfortunately, there is an inherent failure rate associated with regional anesthesia even when applied in experienced hands,[7] with the (albeit rare) potential for systemic toxicity, infection, bleeding, permanent nerve injury, or other physical injury. In addition to the benefits of PNB, advances in knowledge (e.g., physiologic characteristics of solutions during electrical nerve

stimulation) and technology (e.g., the introduction of anatomically based ultrasound imaging) are attracting many anesthesiologists and surgeons to use PNB on a more frequent basis.

Medicine and the techniques associated with it are forever changing. Each new advance provides opportunities for improvement but we need to study these new advances and compare them to previously accepted techniques. In contrast to the rapid changes in medicine—and specifically anesthesiology—anatomic structures are static, and having a basic understanding of anatomic knowledge cannot be replaced by excellent technical skills and knowledge of the technique when performing regional anesthesia. Thus, this chapter provides an in-depth discussion of regional anatomy, while providing an overview of today's two most up-to-date techniques for nerve localization and block performance: nerve stimulation (NS) and ultrasound (US) imaging. Specific techniques that are practically useful for the anesthesiologist are described in sections grouped by anatomic location.

GENERAL PRINCIPLES AND EQUIPMENT

Regional anesthesia has long been regarded as an "art," and outstanding success with these techniques was confined to a small number of gifted individuals. The introduction of NS some 30 years ago was the first step toward transforming regional anesthesia into a "science." This technique relies on physiological responses of neural structures to electrical impulses. There is considerable interindividual variation in physiological responses to NS. Furthermore, a number of other factors influence responses to NS, including injectates, physiologic solutions (e.g., blood), and disease. Despite these limitations NS was one of the first objective methods available in regional anesthesia to place, with some reliability, a needle in close proximity to a target nerve. One of the most exciting advances in technology in relation to regional anesthesia in recent years has been the introduction of anatomically based US imaging. For the first time in nearly 100 years of regional anesthesia practice, we can actually visualize the target nerve. This quantum leap in technology may encourage many anesthesiologists who had previously abandoned these techniques to resume or increase their use of regional anesthesia.

However, despite initial excitement over this advancement, US visualization is still indirect and images are subject to individual interpretation depending on experience, training, and where that experience and training was obtained. Some individuals are gifted in their ability to interpret US images; however, this is not the case with the majority. There is a substantial learning curve associated with US-guided regional anesthesia. Consequently, in many situations, it is prudent to combine the two technologies of NS and US imaging in order to achieve the goal of 100% success with regional blocks. US may allow good visualization of the needle and nerve as well as a reasonable estimate of the spread of the full dose of the local anesthetic, yet the correct identity of the nerve may be unknown.[8] By stimulating that nerve we can objectively determine its identity by observing the motor response to NS.

Patient monitoring and other factors related to optimizing patient care and prevention of complications are similar to those for general anesthesia, with some important differences. Safe and successful performance of PNB requires careful selection of patients, administering an appropriate type and dose of local anesthetic in the correct location, and monitoring the patient during the procedure, prior to discharge, and in the case of ambulatory patients with homegoing catheters, observing them remotely until the catheter has been removed and the block has completely regressed.

Setup and Monitoring

Setup

Although regional blocks can be performed in the operating room setting just like general anesthesia, it is preferable and desirable to perform these techniques in a designated room or area outside the immediate operating room environment (Fig. 38-1). Because of the variable time required for regional anesthesia to work, a separate room allows variable "soak time," which is the time it takes for local anesthetics to cross the cell membrane and block action potentials without delaying the operating room. This designated area must contain the necessary equipment for safe monitoring and resuscitation, but must also contain all of the supplies and equipment to perform common and sophisticated regional block techniques. Some important considerations for this "block room" are described here.

- All supplies located in this area must be readily identifiable and accessible to the anesthesiologist.
- The area should be of ample size to allow block performance and monitoring and resuscitation of patients.
- There should be equipment for oxygen delivery, emergency airway management, and suction, and the area should have sufficient lighting.

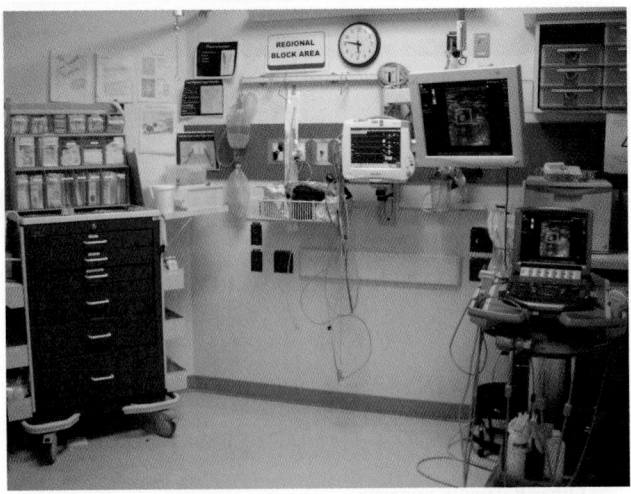

FIGURE 38-1.   Designated regional block room with labeled storage cart.

- A practically organized equipment storage cart (Fig. 38-1) is desirable and should contain all of the necessary equipment (including that required for emergency procedures), supplies, local anesthetics, needles, nerve stimulators, block trays, dressings, and resuscitation drugs.
- It is ideal to have a prepared specialty tray including items for sterile skin preparation and draping, a marking pen and ruler for landmark identification, needles and syringes for skin infiltration, and specific block needles and catheters.
- A selection of sedatives, hypnotics, and intravenous anesthetics should be immediately available to prepare patients for regional anesthesia. These drugs should be titrated to maximize benefits and minimize adverse effects (high therapeutic index); short-acting drugs with a high safety margin are desirable.
- Emergency drugs should include atropine, epinephrine, phenylephrine, ephedrine, propofol, thiopentone and succinylcholine, and amrinone and intralipid.

Monitoring

During the performance of regional anesthesia, it is vital to have skilled personnel monitor the patient at all times. At a minimum, standard monitoring should include electrocardiogram, noninvasive blood pressure, and pulse oximetry. In addition, the level of consciousness of the patient should be gauged frequently using verbal contact because vasovagal episodes are common with many regional procedures. At present there are no practical or effective devices that can detect rising blood levels of local anesthetic, although we can indirectly monitor local anesthetic blood levels by adding pharmacologic markers such as epinephrine to the local anesthetics. Close observation for systematic toxicity secondary to rapid intravenous injection (within 2 minutes) as well as delayed (approximately 20 minutes) absorption is essential. The patient should be monitored for at least 30 minutes postprocedurally.

- Standard electrocardiogram and pulse oximetry are essential monitors while performing regional anesthesia.
- Careful monitoring of the patient's heart rate (along with electrocardiogram measurement) is important to detect the tachycardia seen with epinephrine when it is included in a test dose. It is also useful as an indicator of systemic toxicity with bupivacaine and other potent local anesthetics.
- Before performing blocks with significant sympathetic effects, a baseline blood pressure reading should be obtained. Once the regional anesthesia procedure is

complete, the monitors should remain attached. In conscious patients, end-tidal carbon dioxide monitoring is not required; however, there are special nasal prongs available for monitoring patients when supplemental O_2 is indicated.

- At a minimum, stable vital signs must be present following regional anesthesia to fulfill discharge criteria from the recovery area. If the block has not begun to regress, appropriate protection for the anesthetized limb and complete instructions should be provided to the patient and his or her family if the patient is being discharged home. For inpatients, appropriate orders should be written to assure limb protection.
- Patients receiving perineural local anesthetic infusions should be visited regularly postoperatively by a qualified physician (i.e., acute pain service).

Common Techniques: Nerve Stimulation and Ultrasound Imaging

Nerve Stimulation

Basics of Technique and Equipment.   Electrical stimulation of nerve structures was introduced to regional anesthesia in the middle of the 20th century.[9,10] A low-current electrical impulse applied to a peripheral nerve produces stimulation of motor fibers and theoretically identifies proximity to the nerve without actual needle contact or related patient discomfort. When NS techniques are used it is not necessary to make actual contact with the nerve (in contrast to the paresthesia method). This notion theoretically infers that the risk of nerve injury should be less when using NS methods. However, this theory has not been proved. Stimulating catheters have recently been introduced and have increased our ability to accurately advance catheters along nerve structures for greater distances.[11,12]

4 Using motor responses to NS as a primary nerve-localization technique has drawbacks. The main limitations with NS are related to the inconsistent results of this technique[13,14] and the variance in electrical properties of different nerve stimulators.[15] Many variables affect the ability to stimulate nerves, including conductive area of the electrode (needle or stimulating catheter tip), electrical impedance of the tissues, electrode-to-nerve distance, current flow, and pulse duration.[16] Ultimately, the technique relies on the physiologic responses of neural structures to the stimulating current, which is subject to considerable interindividual variation.

Today's nerve stimulators have features to improve ease of use and success, such as maintaining a constant current with adjustable frequency, pulse width, and current intensity (in milliamperes [mA]). This consistency enables a stable current output (an important safety feature) in the presence of varied resistances from the needle, tissues, and connectors. A clear digital display indicating the actual current delivery is important, as is regular calibration and testing. Some nerve stimulators are equipped with low (up to 6 mA) and high (up to 80 mA) current output ranges. The lower range is primarily for localizing peripheral nerves, and the higher range is mainly used for monitoring neuromuscular blockade. Recently, higher ranges have been used for transcutaneous NS techniques[17] (2 to 5 mA) including percutaneous electrode guidance[18] and surface nerve mapping,[11,19] and the epidural stimulation test (1 to 10 mA).[20,21] Most nerve stimulators deliver an electrical pulse width of 100 μs or 200 μs for stimulating motor nerves. Similar to current amplitude, the length of time over which the current is delivered (pulse width) is usually considered important because currents of shorter duration can selectively stimulate motor components of mixed nerves while sparing the discomfort caused by sensory components. Some sophisticated devices

allow variable pulse widths from 50 μs to 1 ms in an attempt to provide such selective stimulation. The general rule is to use short-duration current of ≤100 μs for peripheral NS, although there is some evidence that duration does not impact patient discomfort[22] and that intensity (number of milliamperes) of the stimulation is perhaps the most important variable.[23]

Practical Guidelines.   During initial advancement of the needle, the nerve stimulator should be set to deliver a current of 1 to 2 mA in order to gauge the approximate distance to the nerve. Depolarization of the nerve can also be improved by using the positive (anode; red) pole of the stimulator as the ground (reference or surface electrode) electrode and the negative (cathode; black) lead as the connection to the needle itself (known as *cathodal preference*). The actual location of the ground is of little importance with the use of constant-current nerve stimulators.[23] Generally, the needle is in close proximity to the nerve when the threshold for motor response is between 0.3 and 0.5 mA; placing the needle to the point where a motor response only requires 0.1 to 0.2 mA may increase the chance of nerve puncture and should be avoided.[24] Once a low threshold response is obtained, 2 to 3 mL of local anesthetic is injected and the operator watches for disappearance of the motor twitch, which is a signal to inject the remainder of the proposed dose in divided aliquots. This "Raj test"[25] was originally thought to result from the physical displacement of the targeted nerve by the injection solution, but this response has recently also been attributed to a change in the electrical field at the needle-tissue interface. Electrically conducting solutions (e.g., local anesthetic or saline) reduces the current density at the needle tip, thereby increasing the current threshold for motor response, while nonconducting solutions (e.g., dextrose 5% in water [D5W]) increase the current density and maintain or augment the twitch response (Fig. 38-2).[26]

After nerve localization using a stimulating needle, introduction of a stimulating catheter with continuous stimulation of the nerve is suitable for provision of continuous analgesia. Similar current thresholds are applicable with the use of stimulating catheters. If an attempt to dilate the perineural space is undertaken, injection of D5W is preferable in order to maintain the motor response to stimulation.[27] The reader is

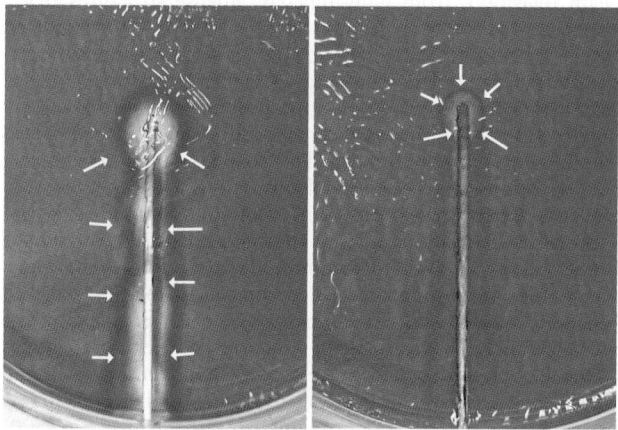

Insulated needle after saline injection   **Insulated needle after D5W injection**

FIGURE 38-2.   The current density is localized to the needle tip when using nonconducting solutions (e.g., dextrose 5% in water [D5W]), thereby maintaining the motor response to the threshold current level during nerve stimulation.

referred to the section "Other Related Equipment" for optimal features of stimulating catheters.

Ultrasound Imaging

Basics of Technique and Equipment. US imaging is rapidly emerging as a very promising regional anesthesia tool as the size, depth, and precise location of many nerves in their surrounding environment can be determined with correct interpretation of the visual image. Visualization of the moving needle, once inserted at an appropriate angle and within the plane of the US probe, as well as the spread of local anesthetic, provides valuable assistance to the anesthesiologist performing regional anesthesia. With US-guided PNB techniques, the operator can adjust the needle or catheter placement under in-direct vision (i.e., US imaging), which may lead to fewer needle attempts and ultimately improved motor and sensory block. Furthermore, visibility of vital structures (e.g., vessels and pleura) is advantageous in the quest to avoid complications. Today, technological advances have led to the development of US systems that can deliver high-frequency (10 MHz or higher) sound waves offering the high axial resolution required for visualization of nerves, which distinguishes them from the surrounding anatomic structures (e.g., tendons, muscles). The proposed benefits of US guidance, as compared with NS, for upper extremity blocks include improved block success[28] and completeness,[29] reduced block performance and onset times,[28–31] prolonged duration of blocks,[30] and reduction in complications.[32] Although the cumulative evidence may appear convincing, many of the studies show conflicting results for certain parameters, and the large variability in trial methods and application of different outcome measures account for many of the discrepancies. Indeed, the various end points used during research in regional anesthesia may bias outcomes when comparing multiple regional techniques.

US is defined as any sound with a frequency >20 kHz, although medical imaging generally requires between 3 and 15 MHz. Within the body, US scanners emit sound waves that produce an echo when they encounter a tissue interface. Therefore, US images reflect contours, including those of anatomic structures, based on differing acoustic impedances of tissue or fluids. Significant reflection of sound waves occurs at interfaces between substances of different acoustic impedance, resulting in good contour definition between different tissues. High US beam reflection, from high-impedance/dense structures (e.g., bone, connective tissue), results in a bright (hyperechoic) image, often with dorsal shadowing underneath; low-impedance structures reflect beams to a smaller extent and appear grey (hypoechoic); minimal impedance structures/spaces (e.g., fluid in vessels) appear black (anechoic).

Higher frequencies offer the best spatial resolution at superficial locations (e.g., brachial plexus at supraclavicular fossa), and lower frequencies are often required for structure delineation at deep locations (e.g., sciatic nerve at subgluteal region). Block location and depth of target nerve structures determine which transducer offers the best imaging and resolution. Several functions of the US system will be important to become familiar with, including field and gain functions as well as Doppler effect. Doppler effect can be very useful for identifying blood vessels during nerve localization using US guidance as many nerves are situated in close proximity to vascular structures.

Practical Guidelines. Both the probe and the skin of the patient should be prepared for maximum sterility and optimal imaging. Probe sterility is paramount if performing real-time, or dynamic, US guidance during block performance. Sterility can be maintained by standard sleeve covers but these can be expensive and cumbersome. For single-shot blocks, it is practical to use a sterile transparent dressing (e.g., Tegaderm; 3M Health Care, St. Paul, MN) without the full cover of a sterile sleeve (Fig. 38-3A).[33] An issue when using standard long covers is the potential for air to track between the probe and skin, which reduces image quality. The target area should be surveyed (scanned) using a generous amount of US gel (water-soluble conductivity gel is optimal) prior to sterile preparation. One of the most common reasons for poor visualization is lack of sufficient gel for skin-probe contact.

For nerve localization during US-guided PNB, it is effective to first identify one or more reliable anatomic landmarks (bone or vessel) with a known relationship to the nerve structure. The operator can then localize the nerve at a location near the landmark, and proceed to follow along or "trace" the nerve to the optimal block location (Table 38-1).[34,35] Generally, nerve structures are most visible when the angle of incidence is approximately 90 degrees to the US beam. Obtaining a transverse axis view of the nerve usually allows the best appreciation of the anatomic relationship of nerve with its surrounding structure. To obtain the best possible view of the shaft and tip of the needle, it is imperative to align the needle shaft to the longitudinal axis ("in-plane" [IP]) of the US transducer (probe) (Fig. 38-3B). The nerve structure is often placed at the edge of the US screen to ensure adequate viewing distance for the needle shaft. An alternative approach uses a transverse or tangential ("out-of-plane" [OOP]) alignment, which only allows appreciation of the needle in cross-section and usually only during movement (Fig. 38-3B). The nerve structure is often placed in the center of the screen to guarantee that aligning the needle puncture with the center of the probe will ensure close needle tip–nerve alignment. This approach can be beneficial in certain block locations (compact areas) and for inserting catheters (e.g., at the subgluteal area), but should never be used in areas where needle tip visibility in relation to vital structures is critical (e.g., supraclavicular fossa near the pleura).

After one observes that the needle is close to the nerve(s), a 1- to 2-mL test dose of local anesthetic or D5W can be injected to visualize the spread and perform a Raj test if a stimulating needle is being used. The solution will be seen as a hypoechoic expansion and will often illuminate the surrounding area, enabling better visibility of the nerves and block needle. If NS is being used to confirm nerve identity, it is useful to administer D5W in order to maintain accurate motor responses.[27] This response will be especially important during catheter introduction and advancement. If the test shows undesired application near or within vessels or cavities, subsequent injection of local anesthetic should be postponed until better needle localization is achieved. If suboptimal spread of injectate is observed, the needle can be repositioned to allow another injection.

There can be a lengthy learning curve for US-guided nerve blocks, and techniques to improve needle and catheter visibility during advancement are important in order to improve training for this technology. Two such approaches have been described experimentally:

- The first method is the "walk-down" approach to facilitate needle tip identification during OOP needling.[34,36] This technique involves calculating the required depth of puncture (with measurement to the desired neural structure recorded using US prior to the block) and using trigonometry with the shaft angle and length to calculate a "reasonable" location to place the initial needle puncture site. The initial shallow puncture will be easily seen as a bright dot on the screen, and the needle tip can be followed as it is "walked down" to the final calculated depth. For example, if the final depth of penetration for the block is 2 cm, the needle will ultimately obtain a 45-degree angle if the initial puncture site is 2 cm from the probe and the needle is incrementally angled to this level.
- A method of needle-probe alignment using a laser attachment for the probe has been reported; the laser line

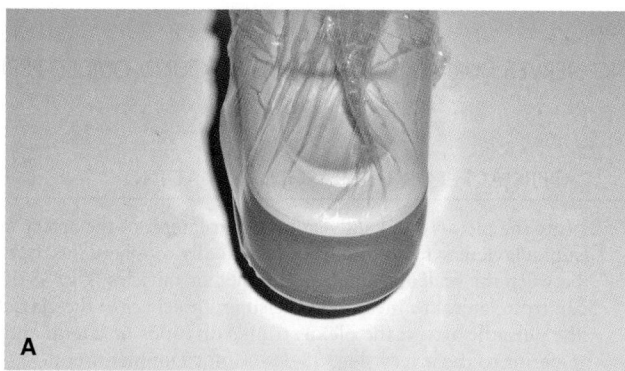

A

FIGURE 38-3. **A.** Probe sterility using a sterile transparent dressing (e.g., Tegaderm; 3M Health Care, St. Paul, MN) without the full cover of a sterile sleeve. Other dressings may create multiple small wells over the probe surface because of adhesive pockets and lead to poor image quality.[34] **B.** In-plane and out-of-plane needle alignment and the subsequent visibility of the needle.

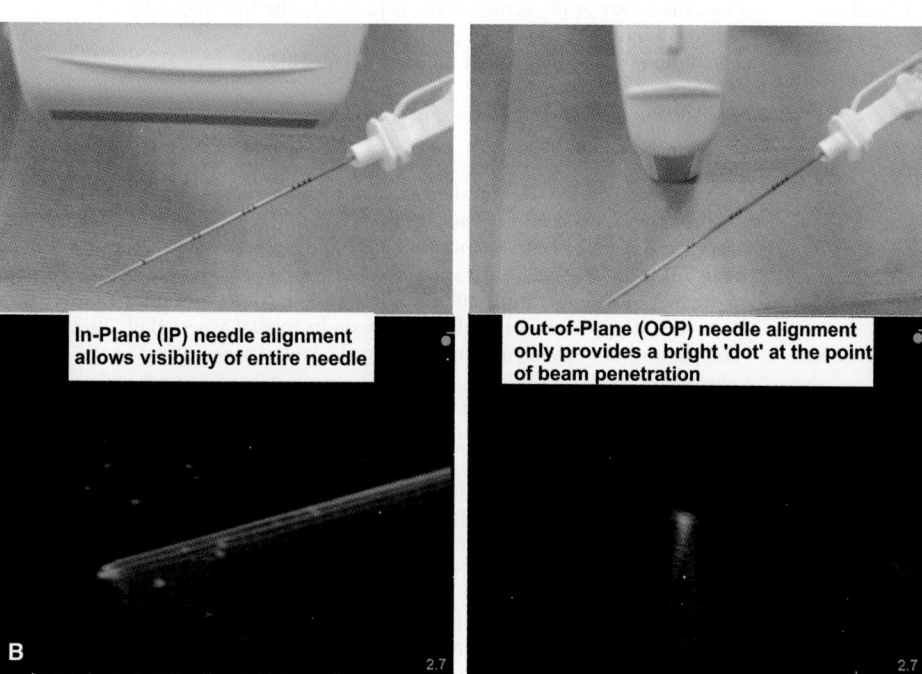

In-Plane (IP) needle alignment allows visibility of entire needle

Out-of-Plane (OOP) needle alignment only provides a bright 'dot' at the point of beam penetration

B

will project onto both the needle shaft and the midline of the probe, indicating an IP position.[34,37] Aligning the visible optical laser line with the longitudinal axis of the US probe will mimic the "invisible" beam from the US probe and allow improvements with IP needle alignment. With the laser-unit attachment, any misalignment of the needle to the US beam can be easily detected and adjusted in real time.

Other Related Equipment

Needles

Needles used for regional techniques are often modified from standard injection needles. Although reports may speculate that needle design is a determinant of nerve or other tissue injury, there is insufficient evidence to substantiate this claim. For peripheral nerve blocks, the "short bevel" (i.e., 30 to 45 degrees) or "B bevel" is often used to reduce the potential for injury to nerves.[38] Other modifications, such as the "pencil-point" needle, have been introduced in attempts to reduce nerve injury. Single-shot PNB techniques generally require using 22- to 24-gauge insulated needles with short bevels. If superficial and field blocks are performed, smaller gauge (e.g., 25- to 26-gauge) sharp needles can be used. Continuous blocks require larger-bore needles to facilitate catheter introduction (e.g., 18-gauge needles for 20-

gauge catheters). Blunt-tipped Tuohy-designed needles are commonly used for continuous PNB with success.[39] Short-bevel and Tuohy needles offer more resistance and give a better "feel" when traversing different tissues. Desired needle length will depend on each specific block and individual patient characteristics. Clear markings throughout the entire length of the needle are important for measuring depth of penetration, particularly for correspondence to US measurements.

Practical Tips. Techniques and devices have been proposed to limit injection pressure, as there is considerable variation among anesthesiologists in the amount of pressure they apply during injections[40] and high-pressure injections into the nerve (especially intrafascicular) have been associated with damage in animals.[41,42] Disposable, in-line injection pressure monitors are available, although their ability to prevent long-term injury is not well documented. Alternatively, a compressed air injection technique has been described to limit the generation of excessive pressure during injection. With this method, air is drawn into the syringe and compressed by 50% during the entire injection to maintain pressures of approximately 760 mm Hg (Boyle's law: pressure $\times$ volume = constant).[43]

Catheters

Continuous-infusion catheter kits suitable for PNB are available that include a standard polyamide catheter, such as those

TABLE 38-1

ANATOMICAL LANDMARKS USEFUL FOR LOCALIZING NERVES DURING COMMON ULTRASOUND-GUIDED PERIPHERAL NERVE BLOCKS

■ PERIPHERAL NERVE BLOCK LOCATION	■ ANATOMIC LANDMARK(S)	■ APPROACH FOR ULTRASOUND IMAGING
Interscalene	Subclavian artery and scalene muscles	Locate the plexus trunks/divisions superolateral to the artery at the supraclavicular fossa and trace proximally to where the roots/trunks lie between the scalenus anterior and medius muscles (Fig. 38-15).
Supraclavicular	Subclavian artery	Scan from lateral to medial on the superior aspect of the clavicle to locate the pulsatile artery; the plexus trunks/divisions lie lateral and often superior to the artery (Fig. 38-16). Color Doppler useful.
Infraclavicular	Subclavian/axillary artery and vein	Place the artery at the center of the field and locate the brachial plexus cords surrounding the artery (Fig. 38-17).
Axillary	Axillary artery	The terminal nerves surround the artery (Fig. 38-18).
Peripheral nerves:		
Median nerve at antecubital fossa	Brachial artery	The large anechoic artery lies immediately lateral to the nerve (Fig. 38-21).
Radial nerve at anterior elbow	Humerus at spiral groove and deep brachial artery	To confirm the nerve's identity at the elbow, trace the nerve proximally and posteriorly toward the spiral groove of the humerus, just inferior to the deltoid muscle insertion. The nerve is located here adjacent to the deep brachial artery and can be followed back to the anterior elbow (Fig. 38-19).
Ulnar at medial forearm	Ulnar artery	Scan at the anteromedial surface of the forearm approximately at the junction of its distal third and proximal two-thirds to capture the ulnar nerve as it approaches the ulnar artery on its medial aspect (Fig. 38-22).
Lumbar plexus	Transverse processes	The plexus lies between and just deep to the lateral aspect (tips) of the processes (Fig. 38-30).
Femoral	Femoral artery	The nerve lies lateral to the artery (vein most medial) (Fig. 38-31). Insert the needle above the branching of the deep femoral artery.
Sciatic		
Classic/Labat	Ischial bone and inferior gluteal or pudendal vessels	The nerve lies lateral to the thinnest aspect of the ischial bone. The inferior gluteal artery generally lies medial to and at the same depth as the nerve (Fig. 38-34).
Subgluteal	Greater trochanter and ischial tuberosity	The nerve lies between the two bone structures.
Popliteal	Popliteal artery	Trace the tibial and common peroneal nerves from the popliteal crease to where they form the sciatic nerve. At the crease, the tibial nerve lies adjacent to the popliteal artery. Scanning proximally to the sciatic bifurcation, the artery becomes deeper and at a greater distance from the nerve (Fig. 38-37).
Ankle		
Tibial (posterior tibial)	Posterior tibial artery	Nerve lies posterior to the artery (Fig. 38-38).
Deep peroneal	Anterior tibial artery	Nerve lies lateral to the artery (Fig. 38-39).

previously used for epidural analgesia, combined with an insulated Tuohy needle with NS capability. Recently, catheters have been advanced to the point of making them amenable to stimulation (an electrode is placed into the catheter tip). A stimulating catheter tip may enable more accurate advancement of catheters for substantial distances to provide continuous analgesia. Some studies have suggested that it may be helpful to inject a solution to dilate the perineural compartment to facilitate the advancement of catheter. The reader is referred to the discussion of practical guidelines of NS in the section "Common Techniques: Nerve Stimulation and Ultrasound Imaging" for discussion of injection solutions for perineural dilation. There are a number of continuous-infusion devices now available for both inpatient and outpatient use that allow delivery of dilute local anesthetic concentrations for as long as 72 hours after surgery. Standard precautions are required to maintain sterility of the catheter and insertion site, but complications have been rare with these techniques and new devices.

Avoiding Complications

Despite the excellent safety record of regional anesthesia in general with complication rates as low as 8 per 10,000 for seizures,[2] <0.1 to 1% for nerve injury[7,44] and rare case reports of severe chronic pain syndromes.[45] The incidence of some complications is often higher in PNB than other regional anesthesia/analgesia techniques, and results can be devastating. Choosing a suitable patient and applying the right dose of local anesthetic in the correct location are the primary considerations. Follow-up prior to and after discharge is equally important, although often overlooked.

Patient Selection

Patient selection is a critical element for the performance of safe and effective PNB. Not all patients are suitable candidates for PNB. In general, patients scheduled for extremity, thoracic, abdominal, or perineal surgery should be considered potential candidates for peripheral regional anesthetic techniques. Adamant refusal of regional anesthesia by a patient is a contraindication to the procedure.

Other contraindications include local infection, systemic anticoagulation, and severe systemic coagulopathy. In most cases, schizophrenic patients should receive regional techniques only if general anesthesia is also performed. The presence of pre-existing neurologic disease is a controversial topic. A limited amount of data is available in the case of spinal anesthesia, but the safety of PNB is unclear. One must be cognizant of the potential to compound existing neurologic deficit. Therefore, clear documentation of the deficits prior to the procedure and a careful discussion of the potential risks and benefits are critical. For every clinical situation, the use of regional anesthesia must be carefully evaluated as a matter of risk versus benefit. It is imperative to follow applicable national and international guidelines, such as those for monitoring by the American Society of Anesthesiologists, and for anticoagulated patients by the American Society for Regional Anesthesia and Pain Medicine.

Local Anesthetic Drug Selection, Toxicity, and Doses

This section will provide an overview of drug selection and toxicity during PNB. For a more detailed discussion of the pharmacology and toxicity of local anesthetics, the reader is referred to Chapter 21.

Rates of systemic and local toxicity in addition to nerve injury with PNB are generally low. However, use of available methods to reduce inadvertent intravascular and intraneural injections is clearly warranted. It is important to note that lower concentrations of local anesthetic (e.g., 1 to 1.5% lidocaine, 0.125 to 0.5% bupivacaine) than those used for epidural anesthesia are appropriate for peripheral nerves. Neural toxicity of these anesthetics appears to be concentration-dependent.[46] The use of highly concentrated solutions may be useful to increase motor block, but this increases the total milligram dose of local anesthetic. Lower concentrations are usually indicated when larger volumes are required to anesthetize poorly localized peripheral nerves or to block a series of nerves. Nevertheless, there is no clinical evidence that prolonged exposure (as with continuous PNB) of nerves to local anesthetic solutions of appropriate concentration predisposes to neurotoxic injury.[47]

Systemic toxicity is most often related to accidental intravascular injection and rarely to the administration of an excessive quantity of local anesthetic to an appropriate site. The risk of systemic toxic reactions is often related to the drug used. Ropivacaine (generally at 0.5%) is a recent example of a drug introduced into clinical practice in order to reduce central nervous system and cardiovascular toxicity through its physiochemical and stereoselective properties[48,49]; despite this, there are examples of ropivacaine toxicity during PNB.[50–53] One strategy to potentially reduce the volume and concentration of local anesthetic solution required to produce a successful block is using US imaging to more accurately position the needle in close proximity to the nerve and to visualize the spread of solution to ensure adequate exposure.[54,55] Of greatest importance is the ability to avoid intravascular injection. This risk may be reduced when using US, especially if combined with color Doppler for vessel localization.

The degree of systemic drug absorption and the duration of anesthesia can also vary depending on the site of injection (i.e., level of vascularization) and addition of vasoconstrictors. The highest blood levels of local anesthetic occur after intercostal blocks, followed by caudal, epidural, brachial plexus, intravenous regional, and lower extremity blockade. Equivalent doses of local anesthetic may produce only 3 to 4 hours of anesthesia when placed in the epidural space, but 12 to 14 hours in the arm and 24 to 36 hours when injected along the sciatic nerve. Many believe that the addition of epinephrine, 1:200,000 to 1:400,000, is advantageous in prolonging the duration of block and in reducing systemic blood levels of local anesthetic. Its use is not appropriate in the vicinity of "terminal" blood vessels, such as in the digits, penis, or ear, or when using an intravenous regional technique. PNB using significant quantities of local anesthetic should not be performed unless oxygen, suction, and appropriate resuscitation equipment is immediately available. When performing PNB, a test dose of an epinephrine-containing solution and small incremental injections are recommended to reduce the risk of unrecognized intravascular injection. Toxicity can also occur from peripheral absorption of excessive doses of local anesthetic. Patients should be observed carefully for at least 30 minutes following injection because peak blood levels may occur at this time.

Animal studies[56] and recent case reports[57,58] have shown successful resuscitation from local anesthetic toxicity by intravenous administration of Intralipid (20% lipid; not 10% lipid of propofol), using one or more boluses (each of 1 to 2 mL/kg or 100 mL) followed by a 30-minute infusion (0.5 mL/kg/min). It is important to use this strategy as an acute resuscitation agent, after standard measures have proven ineffective.

Nerve Damage and Other Complications

Peripheral nerve injury in humans may result from intraneural injection[59,60] or direct needle trauma,[61] although there are other causes including those related to the surgical procedures (e.g., patient positioning, proximity of nerve to surgical site, and tourniquet application).[62] Needle-related trauma without injection may result in injury of a lesser magnitude than that from injection injury.[63] In animal studies, nerve injury appears to occur when high injection pressures are applied intrafascicularly and particularly when highly concentrated local anesthetic solutions or their preservatives are used.[41,42,64] One major sequel from intrafascicular injection is endoneural ischemia.[65] Although in some cases these syndromes resolve uneventfully, full recovery of some peripheral injuries may never occur or may require several months as a result of slow regeneration of injured peripheral nerves.[66]

Other minor complications are reported following PNB, such as pain at the site of injection and local hematoma formation, but these are self-limited side effects and are best dealt with by communication with the patient and reassurance by the anesthesiologist. Hematoma around a peripheral nerve is not of the same significance as that occurring in the epidural or subarachnoid space. It is important to address concerns expressed by patients and to make every effort to relieve any pain or discomfort resulting from various interventions.

Discharge Criteria

Stable vital signs must be present in order to fulfill criteria for discharge from the recovery area. In some cases, acceptable evidence of regressing sensory and motor blockade should be present; however, if a long-lasting local anesthetic was used to perform the block or a continuous catheter with an infusion of local anesthetic is present, the block may not show evidence of regression at the time of discharge. Postoperative follow-up is important in confirming that neurologic function has returned to normal. If a deficit is suspected, early neurologic assessment is critical to determine the appropriate course of management.

Patients should have well-controlled pain on discharge; incorporating a standard level of pain relief (e.g., on a verbal rating scale) prior to discharge home or to the ward is prudent. Specific common risks for certain blocks should be discussed with the patient prior to discharge. When discharging patients from postanesthesia care units while an extremity is still anesthetized (e.g., the block was performed to provide extended analgesia), it will be necessary to provide in-depth instruction related to the risks and their prevention (e.g., risk of burns to anesthetized areas will require avoidance of certain forms of cooking, potential for developing pressure neuropathies). A clear understanding of the information provided is important for both the patient and the caregivers. Written instructions including expected course, common side effects, and 24-hour contact information should be provided.

Premedication and Sedation

The best preparation for a regional technique is careful patient selection as well as ensuring that the patient is adequately educated and informed about the anesthetic and surgical procedures. Supplemental medication is often helpful. Appropriate sedation and analgesia are an essential part of successful regional anesthesia in order to produce maximum benefit with minimal side effects. Effective sedation can be achieved with a variety of medications including but not limited to propofol, midazolam, fentanyl, ketamine, remifentanil, alfentanil, or a combination of these drugs. The dosages should be titrated to reach an appropriate level of sedation for the individual patient, specific nerve block procedure, and length of surgery. Some examples of adult dosages are listed here in bolus amounts:

- Midazolam, 1 to 2 mg (titrated up to 0.07 mg/kg)
- Fentanyl, 0.5 to 1 μg/kg
- Alfentanil, 7 to 10 μg/kg
- Ketamine, 0.1 to 0.5 mg/kg

In addition to the general comments about premedication discussed in earlier chapters, regional anesthesia techniques have special requirements. Sedation must be adjusted to the required level of patient cooperation. In the case of elicitation of a paresthesia (as during several blocks in the head and neck region) or electrical stimulation techniques, medication must be just sufficient enough to allow the patient to identify and report nerve contact. Although a low dose of opioid (50 to 100 μg of fentanyl or equivalent) will help ease the discomfort of nerve localization, patient responsiveness must be maintained. This goal for sedation does not preclude the use of an amnestic agent. Small doses of propofol or midazolam may provide excellent amnesia at levels of consciousness that still allow cooperation.

SPECIFIC TECHNIQUES

The remainder of this chapter is devoted to the anatomic and procedural details of the performance of specific blocks, arranged by anatomic regions of the body. In the sections discussing upper extremity, trunk, and lower extremity, details for using NS and US imaging during the blocks are included. The nerve stimulator is set to deliver variable currents with a frequency of 2 Hz and pulse width of 0.1 ms unless stated otherwise. The volumes of local anesthetic included are those suggested for blocks during which NS was used for nerve localization; US guidance may reduce the required volume in some instances. The figures in these sections will focus predominantly on using a combined US and NS stimulation-guided technique, although procedures for blind techniques using NS are also described. It is important to note that the figures illustrating technique in humans are representative of the clinical scenario, but without all of the sterile preparation required so as to facilitate observation of proper probe and needle handling. With each technique, there are comments, which include practical tips and evidence-based recommendations. In addition, most suggestions related to volume of local anesthetic

were based on conventional technique. Although it is not yet well established, many experts speculate that the use of US guidance may reduce the volume of local anesthetic required to achieve adequate block.

Head and Neck Blocks

Regional anesthesia for the head and neck is diverse, with many head and neck surgical procedures being amenable to some form of regional anesthesia. A regional technique may be the sole mode of anesthesia or may be incorporated into a balanced general anesthetic offering optimal postsurgical analgesia. Blocks can be used for ophthalmic, neurologic, ear/nose/throat, plastic, and endocrine surgery. Regional anesthesia techniques, such as trigeminal or occipital nerve block, may also be used for diagnostic and therapeutic purposes in acute and chronic pain syndromes. Block techniques range from local infiltration to field block to specific nerve blocks. The absence of definitive airway control is a frequent source of concern with regional techniques, as intraoperative airway control can be challenging.

Regional anesthesia of the head and neck primarily depends on local infiltration and/or specific nerve blocks placed with reliable anatomic landmarks. Elicitation of a paresthesia is the mainstay of nerve localization, while NS or US imaging has not yet been performed or reported to any extent for these blocks. Therefore, the description of techniques in this section will deviate from other areas where there is greater reliance on nerve localization modalities using NS and US imaging.

Clinical Anatomy

Trigeminal Nerve
- Sensory and motor innervation of the face is provided by the branches of the fifth cranial (trigeminal) nerve (Figs. 38-4 and 38-5).
- The roots of this nerve arise from the base of the pons and send sensory branches to the large semilunar (trigeminal or gasserian) ganglion, which lies on the dorsal surface of the petrous bone. Its anterior margin gives rise to three main branches: the ophthalmic, maxillary, and mandibular nerves.
- A smaller motor fiber nucleus lies behind the main trigeminal ganglion and sends motor branches to one terminal nerve, the mandibular nerve.
- The three major branches of the trigeminal nerve each have a separate exit from the skull.
- The uppermost *ophthalmic* branch passes through the sphenoidal fissure into the orbit. The main terminal fibers of this sensory nerve, the *frontal nerve*, run behind the center of the orbital cavity and bifurcate into the supratrochlear and supraorbital nerves. The *supratrochlear* branch traverses the orbit along the superior border and exits on the front of the face in the easily palpated supraorbital notch; the *supraorbital nerve* runs in a medial direction toward the trochlea.
- The *maxillary* nerve contains only sensory fibers. It exits the skull through the round foramen (foramen rotundum), passes beneath the skull anteriorly, and enters the sphenopalatine fossa. At this point, it lies medial to the lateral pterygoid plate on each side. At the anterior end of this channel, it again moves superiorly to re-enter the skull in the infraorbital canal in the floor of the orbit. It branches to form the zygomatic nerve to the orbit and the short sphenopalatine (pterygopalatine) nerves, and to give off the posterior dental branches. The anterior dental nerves arise from the main trunk as it passes through the infraorbital canal. The terminal infraorbital nerve penetrates through the inferior orbital fissure to

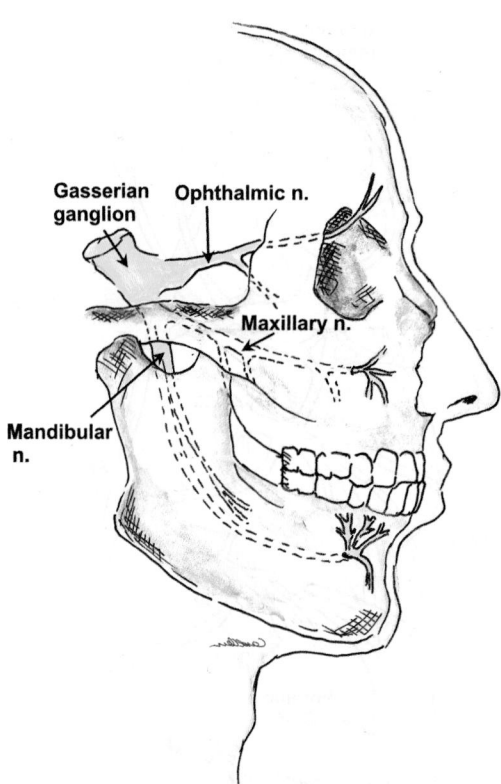

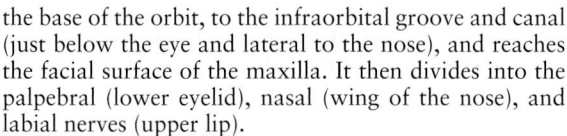

FIGURE 38-4. Major branches of the trigeminal nerve. The roots of this nerve arise from the pons and form the large gasserian (or semilunar) ganglion. The three major branches have separate exits from the skull. The main terminal fibers of the ophthalmic nerve, the frontal nerve, terminate as the supraorbital and supratrochlear nerves and exit their respective foramen. The maxillary and mandibular branches emerge from the skull medial to the lateral pterygoid plate; the maxillary terminating as the infraorbital nerve (through the infraorbital foramen) and the mandibular providing the inferior alveolar nerve (as well as motor branches), which exits at the mental foramen as the mental nerve.

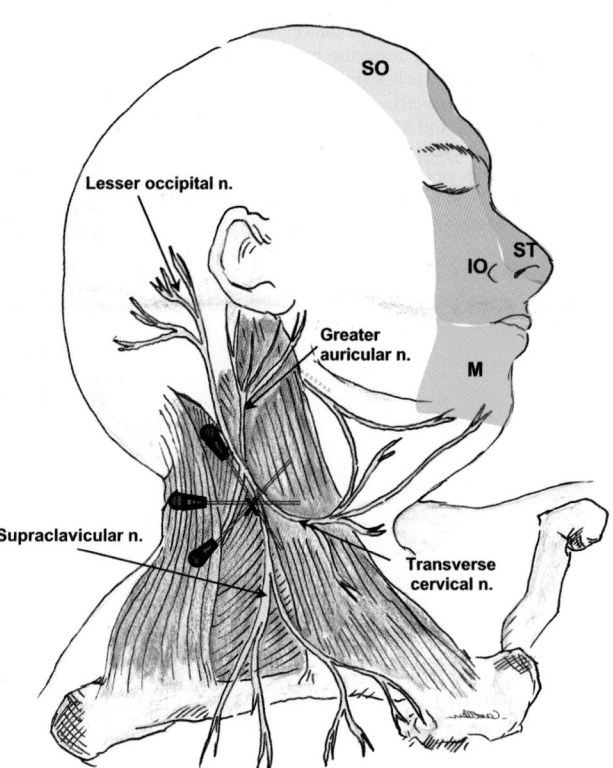

FIGURE 38-5. Lateral view of the surface of head, showing the cutaneous innervation of the superficial/distal trigeminal nerve branches to the face and the anatomy and block needle insertion angle of the superficial cervical block. The needle is initially inserted perpendicular to the skin at the midpoint of the lateral border of the sternocleidomastoid muscle (where it is crossed by the external jugular vein). Subsequently, the needle can be inserted in superior and inferior angulations to reach the entire plexus. SO, supraoribtal nerve; ST, supratrochlear nerve; IO, infraorbital nerve; M, mental nerve.

the base of the orbit, to the infraorbital groove and canal (just below the eye and lateral to the nose), and reaches the facial surface of the maxilla. It then divides into the palpebral (lower eyelid), nasal (wing of the nose), and labial nerves (upper lip).

■ The *mandibular* nerve is the third and largest branch of the trigeminal, and the only one to receive motor fibers. It exits the skull posterior to the maxillary nerve through the oval foramen (foramen ovale), forms a short thick trunk, and then divides into an anterior trunk, mainly motor, and a posterior trunk, which is mostly sensory. The main branch (posterior trunk) continues as the inferior alveolar nerve medial to the ramus of the mandible and innervates the molar and premolar teeth. This nerve curves anteriorly to follow the mandible and exits as a terminal branch (mental nerve) through the mental foramen. The *mental* nerve provides sensation to the lower lip and chin. Other terminal nerves include the lingual nerve (floor of mouth and anterior two thirds of tongue) and the auriculotemporal nerve (ear and temple).

Cervical Plexus

■ Sensory and motor fibers of the neck and posterior scalp arise from the anterior rami (branches) of the first four cervical (C1-4) spinal nerves. The reader is referred to the "Clinical Anatomy" of the upper extremity section for a description of the spinal nerve anatomy. The cervi-

cal plexus is unique in that it divides early into cutaneous branches (penetrating the cervical fascia) (Figs. 38-5 and 38-6) and muscular branches (deeper branches that innervate the muscles and joints), which can be blocked separately (Fig. 38-7). The dermatomes of the cervical nerves C2-4 are illustrated in Figure 38-8.

■ Classic cervical plexus anesthesia along the tubercles of the vertebral body produces both motor and sensory blockade. The transverse processes of the cervical vertebrae form peculiar elongated troughs for the emergence of their nerve roots. These troughs lie immediately lateral to a medial opening for the cephalad passage of the vertebral artery (Fig. 38-7). The trough at the terminal end of the transverse process divides into an anterior and a posterior tubercle, which often can be easily palpated.

■ These tubercles also serve as the attachments for the anterior and middle scalene muscles, which form a compartment for the cervical plexus as well as the brachial plexus immediately below. The compartment at this level is less developed than the one formed around the brachial plexus.

■ The deep muscular branches curl anteriorly around the lateral border of the anterior scalene and proceed caudally and medially. Many branches serve the deep anterior neck muscles, but other branches include the inferior descending cervical nerve, the trapezius branch of the plexus, and the phrenic nerve. They give anterior branches to the sternocleidomastoid muscle as they pass behind it.

FIGURE 38-6.   Schematic of the cervical plexus, which arises from the anterior primary rami of C2-4. The motor branches (including the phrenic nerve) curl anteriorly around the anterior scalene and travel caudad and medially to supply the deep muscles of the neck. The sensory branches exit at the lateral border of the sternocleidomastoid muscle to supply the skin of the neck and shoulder.

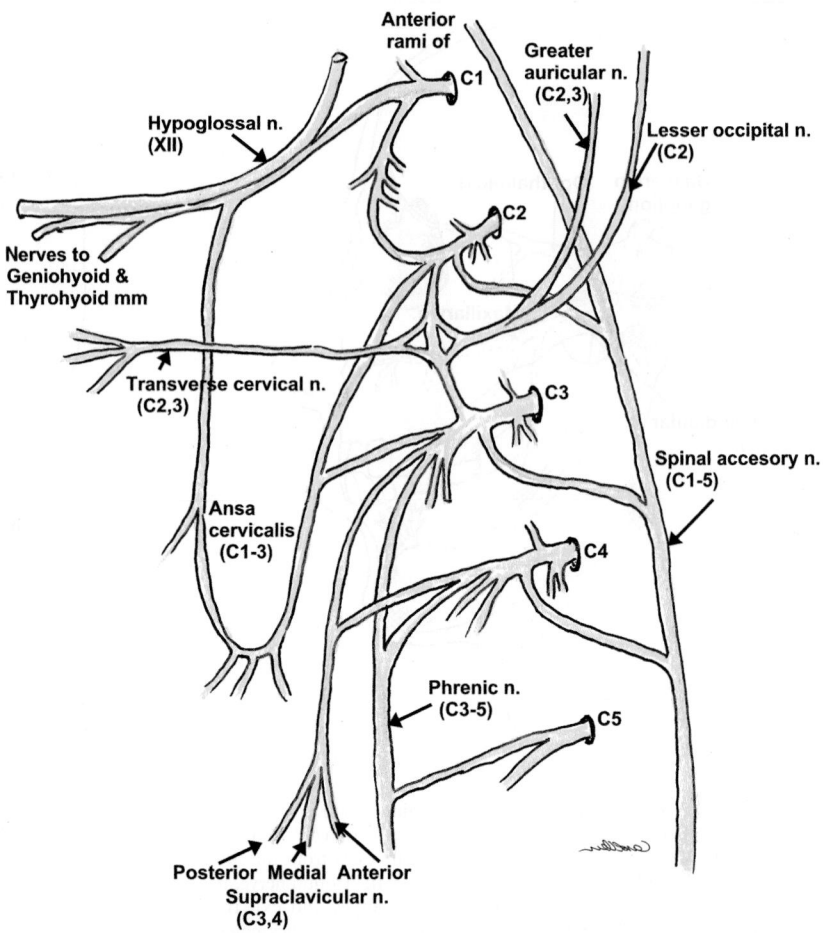

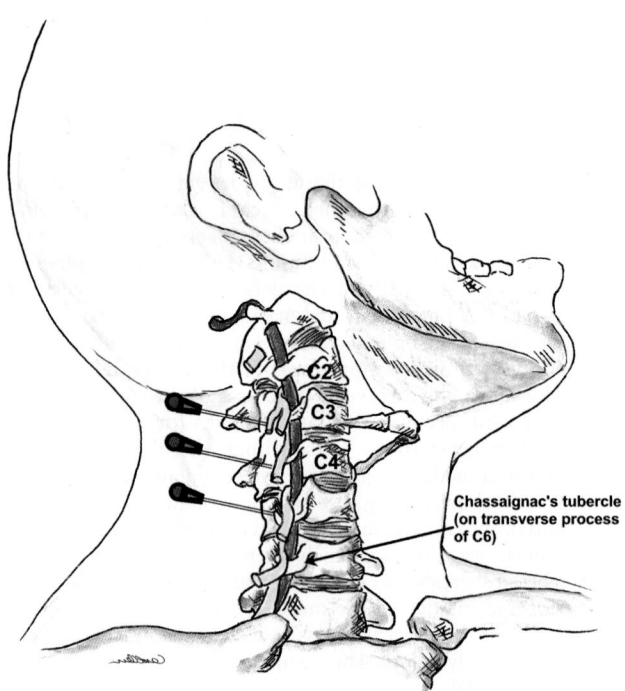

FIGURE 38-7.   Needle insertion points and angles for the deep cervical plexus blockade. The nerve roots exit the vertebral column via the troughs formed by the transverse processes. The needle is inserted at each of nerve roots of C2 through C4 using a caudad and posterior direction.

- The sensory fibers emerge behind the anterior scalene muscle but separate from the motor branches and continue laterally to emerge superficially under the posterior border of the sternocleidomastoid muscle. The branches, including the lesser occipital nerve, great auricular nerve, transverse cervical nerve, and the supraclavicular nerves (anterior, medial, posterior branches), innervate the anterior and posterior skin of the neck and shoulder.

Occipital Nerve
- The ophthalmic branch of the trigeminal nerve provides sensory innervation to the forehead and anterior scalp. The remainder of the scalp is innervated by fibers of the greater and lesser occipital nerves (Fig. 38-9).
- The *lesser occipital nerve* arises from the superficial (cutaneous) cervical plexus (Fig. 38-5) and traverses cephalad from the posterior edge of the sternocleidomastoid muscle toward the top of the head, dividing into several branches. The *greater occipital nerve* arises from the posterior ramus of the second cervical spinal nerve (the cervical plexus arises from the anterior rami) and travels in a cranial direction to reach the skin in the area of the superior nuchal line while giving branches to supply the head and laterally toward the ear.
- These nerves can be blocked by superficial injection at the point on the posterior skull where they emerge from below the muscles of the neck.

Techniques

For every procedure, prepare the needle insertion site and other applicable skin areas with an antiseptic solution and use sterile equipment.

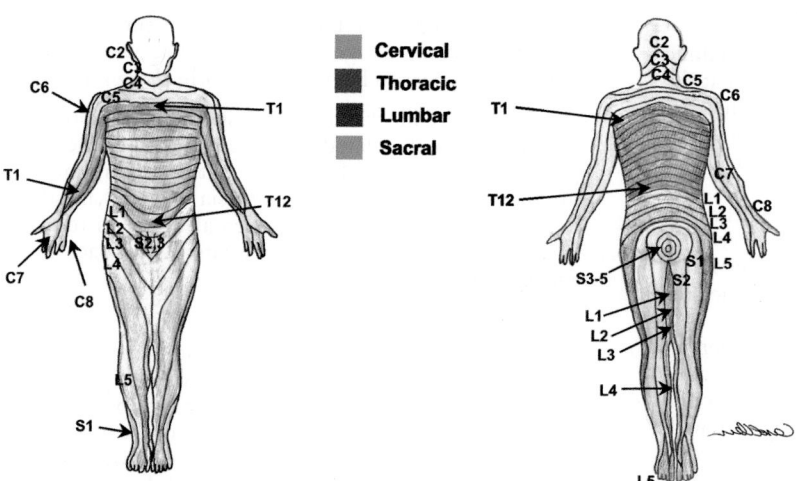

ANESTHETIC MANAGEMENT

Trigeminal Nerve Blocks.   All of the blocks described in this section use the extraoral route, although alternative intraoral routes may be suitable in many cases.

1. Semilunar (gasserian) ganglion block. The most comprehensive blockade of the trigeminal nerve targets the central ganglion (Fig. 38-4). This block is usually performed by neurosurgeons under fluoroscopic guidance for treatment of disabling trigeminal neuralgia. Few anesthesiologists perform this technically difficult block and it will not be described in detail here.
2. Superficial trigeminal nerve branch block. Trigeminal block can be easily performed by injection of the three individual terminal superficial branches (supraorbital, infraorbital, mental nerves). Each nerve is closely associated with its respective foramina, and all foramina lie in the same sagittal plane on each side of the face (approximately 2.5 cm lateral

to the midfacial line passing through the pupil) (Fig. 38-10). These foramina are readily palpable, and these nerves can be blocked with superficial injections of small quantities of local anesthetic. The bony landmarks are usually sufficient themselves for routine anesthetic purposes. However, paresthesias are desirable when performing neurolytic blocks with alcohol. An additional block of the supratrochlear nerve is required if the field of anesthesia is to cross the midline (Fig. 38-5). Generally, fine, short needles (e.g., 24 to 26 gauge, 2 to 3 cm) and small syringes (1 to 5 mL) will be suitable for these blocks. The block is usually performed with the patient in the supine position.

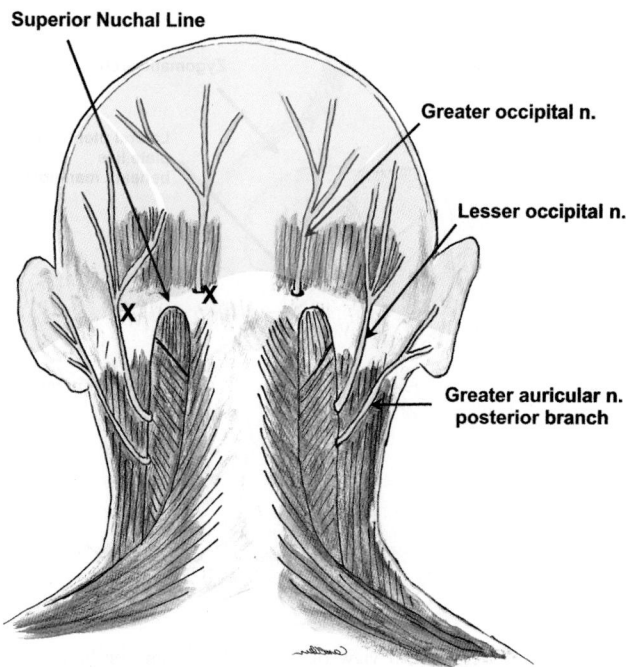

FIGURE 38-9.   Greater and lesser occipital nerve distribution, supply, and block needle insertion sites (X).

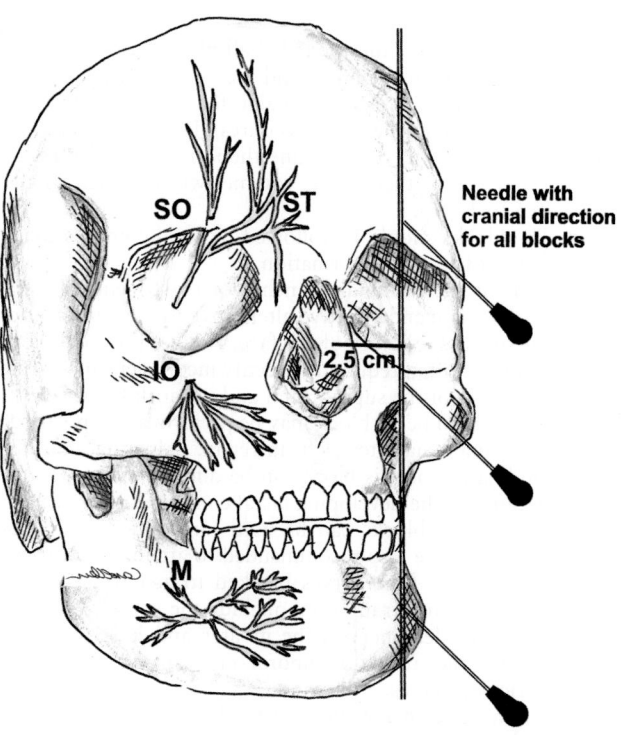

FIGURE 38-10.   Locations of foramen for the superficial/distal trigeminal nerve blocks. The supraorbital, infraorbital, and mental foramen all lay approximately 2.5 cm lateral to the midline of the face, in line with the middle of the pupil. SO, supraoribtal nerve; ST, supratrochlear nerve; IO, infraorbital nerve; M, mental nerve.

Procedure

- Supraorbital nerve (terminal nerve of ophthalmic branch). The supraorbital notch is easily palpated at the medial upper angle of the orbit. The needle is inserted and local anesthetic (see "Comments") is slowly injected after aspiration, slightly outside the notch and produces anesthesia of the ipsilateral forehead.
- Supratrochlear nerve (terminal nerve of ophthalmic branch). Anesthesia of the supratrochlear nerve is obtained with superficial infiltration of the upper internal angle of the orbital rim. This is needed if the field of anesthesia is to cross the midline.
- Infraorbital nerve (terminal branch of maxillary nerve). The infraorbital foramen lies about 1 cm below the middle of the lower orbital margin. If the foramen cannot be palpated directly, it can be sought by gently probing with a small-gauge needle. The needle should be introduced in a cranial direction through a skin wheal approximately 0.5 cm below the expected opening. After making contact with the bone and withdrawing slightly, injection of a small quantity of local anesthetic is performed. This block produces anesthesia of the middle third of the ipsilateral face.
- Mental nerve (sensory terminal branch of mandibular nerve). The mental nerve emerges from its foramen, which lies inferior to the outer lip at the level of the second premolar, midway between the upper and lower borders of the mandible. The mental canal angles medially and inferiorly so that, in this case, needle insertion should start approximately 0.5 cm above and 0.5 cm lateral to the anticipated location of the orifice if it cannot be palpated directly. Slow injection after aspiration at the opening of the canal produces anesthesia of the mandibular area. Injection directly into the canal should be avoided to reduce the risk of neural injury.

Comments

- Choice of local anesthetic for all blocks will depend on the purpose of the block and the duration of anesthesia required (e.g., 1% mepivacaine for shorter and 0.75% ropivacaine for longer procedures). For surgical anesthesia, 2 to 5 mL of local anesthetic may be used, while diagnostic or therapeutic volumes will be much smaller (0.5 to 1 mL).
- The blocks should be followed by local compression to prevent hematoma formation.
- PNB of the terminal branches of the trigeminal nerve offers a safe and effective alternative to local infiltration for soft-tissue injury of the face. Despite this, local infiltration is often required to rectify incomplete anesthesia, especially of the supraorbital and infraorbital nerves.[67]
- Infraorbital nerve block may be performed for postoperative analgesia after cleft lip repair. Palpating anatomic landmarks for this block can be difficult in the neonate because of the developing facial configuration.
- Skull nerve blocks can be used for craniotomy procedures and are also recommended to attenuate postoperative pain.[68] The nerves blocked to achieve successful anesthesia for craniotomy include the supraorbital and supratrochlear nerves, the greater and lesser occipital nerves, the auriculotemporal nerves, and the greater auricular nerves.
- Supraorbital nerve blocks have been associated with a high requirement for supplementation, perhaps because of the anatomic variation of the nerve. The nerve may exit the skull undivided or its medial and lateral branches may exit separately. For frame pin placement during stereotactic neurosurgery, failure to block the lateral branch may account for inadequate coverage.[69]

- During mental nerve block in older patients, resorption of the superior margin of the mandible will make the foramen appear to lie more superiorly along the ramus.

3. Maxillary nerve block. This block should be performed by practitioners with related and adequate experience. It is required when the superficial block of the infraorbital nerve does not produce adequate anesthesia or when anesthesia of the more proximal superior dental nerves is required. This block can be performed by a lateral approach to the sphenopalatine fossa.

Procedure

- The patient either sits with the mouth slightly open or lies supine with a small towel under the occiput and the head turned slightly away from the side to be blocked.
- Above the zygomatic arch. The center of the upper zygomatic arch is marked. A 6-cm needle is introduced at 45 degrees, caudally and medially, toward the contralateral molar teeth. After a paresthesia is elicited at the nostril, upper lip, and cheek, slow incremental injection of local anesthetic is performed after slight needle withdrawal and with frequent aspiration.
- Below the zygomatic arch (Fig. 38-11). The zygomatic arch is marked along its course, and the patient is asked to open and close the mouth slowly so that the curved upper border of the mandible can be identified. The mandibular fossa is palpated between the condylar and coronoid processes. The lowest point of the mandibular notch is palpated, and an X is marked at this spot, which is usually at the midpoint of the zygoma. A local anesthetic skin wheal is raised at the X after appropriate skin preparation.
- With the patient's jaw in the open position, a 6- to 9-cm needle is introduced through the X at a 45-degree angle toward the dorsal part of the eyeball (cephalad and slightly anterior).

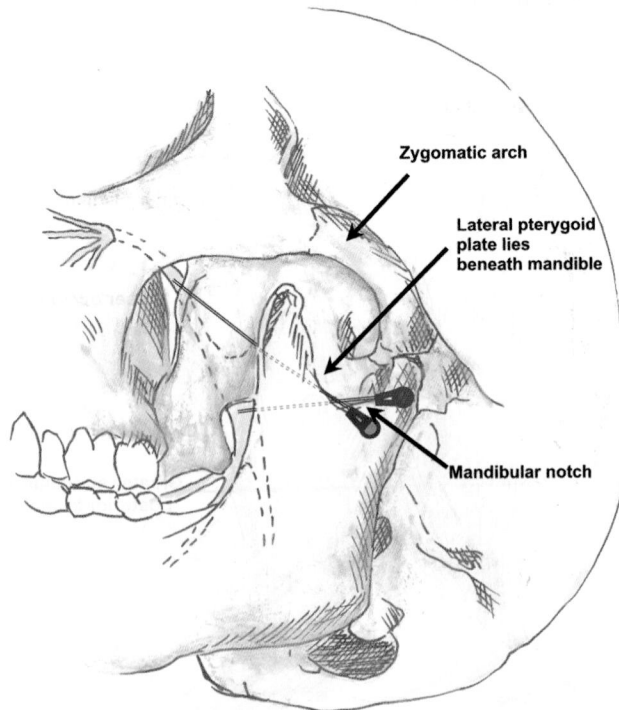

Zygomatic arch

Lateral pterygoid plate lies beneath mandible

Mandibular notch

FIGURE 38-11. Lateral view of the skull showing the bony landmarks and final needle insertion angles for the maxillary (*red needle*) and mandibular (*blue needle*) nerves. Each block procedure involves first reaching the lateral pterygoid plate (see text for details).

■ The needle should contact the lateral portion of the pterygoid process (pterygoid plate) at a depth of 4 to 5 cm. It is then withdrawn and redirected slightly cephalad and anteriorly until it passes beyond the pterygoid plate and enters the pterygopalatine fossa at an additional depth of no more than 1 cm. A paresthesia in the nose or the upper teeth confirms nerve localization. The pterygopalatine fossa is highly vascular, so care must be exercised to avoid intravascular injection.

■ Anesthesia can be achieved by injecting 5 ml into the pterygopalatine fossa, either on obtaining the paresthesia or blindly by advancing 1 cm beyond the plate.

Comments

■ One concern during this block is spread of local anesthetic to adjacent structures, especially to the nerves in the orbit. If pain occurs in the region of the orbit during the procedure, the injection should be stopped and the needle should be withdrawn.

■ Although the mainstay of treatment for trigeminal neuralgia continues to be pharmacologic or neuroablative, maxillary nerve block with extraoral mandibular nerve block has been reported to provide relief in some settings.[70]

4. Mandibular nerve block (Fig. 38-11). This nerve can be blocked for dental and maxillary surgery or for inferior dental pain, trigeminal neuralgia in the third branch, or temporomandibular joint dysfunction. It is the only branch of the trigeminal nerve where anesthesia carries the risk of loss of motor (mastication) function.

Procedure

■ The patient lies supine with the face in profile. Landmarks for location of the mandibular fossa are the same as those described for maxillary nerve blockade.

■ A 6- to 9-cm needle is introduced through the skin wheal and directed perpendicularly to the skin, without the cephalad angulation required for maxillary nerve anesthesia.

■ The depth should be noted when the pterygoid plate is contacted. The needle is then redirected posteriorly until it passes beyond the pterygoid plate. It should contact the nerve 0.5 to 1 cm deep to the point where the pterygoid plate is contacted.

■ Paresthesia of the lower jaw, lower lip, and lower incisors at a depth of approximately 4 to 4.5 cm confirms proximity to the nerve. Gentle exploration in a cephalad and caudad direction, from the initial point where the needle passes posterior to the plate, may be required. After slight needle withdrawal, 5 to 10 mL of solution is injected incrementally with repeated aspiration to avoid intravascular injection. As with maxillary blockade, paresthesias can be painful to the patient.

Comments

■ Anesthesia of the auriculotemporal nerve is often delayed.

■ Facial nerve anesthesia occasionally can be seen when large volumes are injected to block the mandibular nerve. This is of little consequence unless neurolytic agents are used.

■ A more serious complication is the possibility of intravascular injection in this highly vascularized area. Injection should be performed incrementally with small quantities and there should be constant observation for signs of toxicity.

Cervical Plexus Blocks. Anesthesia of either the deep or superficial cervical plexus, or both, can be used for procedures of the lateral or anterior neck such as parathyroidec-

tomy and carotid endarterectomy. In carotid surgery, local infiltration of the carotid bifurcation may be necessary to block reflex hemodynamic changes associated with glossopharyngeal stimulation.

1. Deep cervical plexus block

   Procedure
   ■ The patient is placed supine with a small towel under the head, which is turned 45 degrees to the opposite side with slight neck extension.

   ■ Landmarks include the posterior edge of the sternocleidomastoid muscle, the caudal portion of the mastoid process, the angle of the jaw, and the transverse processes of cervical vertebrae C2 through C5 (about 1.5 cm apart). If all transverse processes cannot be palpated, the most prominent tubercle of C6 (Chassaignac) is marked. A line is drawn from the mastoid process along the sternocleidomastoid muscle to reach the transverse process of C6. Each transverse process of C2 through C5 is marked approximately 0.5 to 1 cm behind the line; that of C2 lies about 1.5 cm inferior to the mastoid process.

   ■ Skin infiltration is carried out at the X marks of C2 through C4, and three needles (22-gauge, 3.5 to 5 cm) are introduced perpendicular to the skin and advanced about 30 degrees caudally with a slight posterior orientation (Fig. 38-7).

   ■ After confirming contact with the transverse process, the needle is withdrawn slightly and a syringe is connected to the needle. Two to 3 mL of local anesthetic solution is injected per segment for therapeutic or diagnostic purposes; 5 to 10 mL per segment may be sufficient for surgical block (limiting the total to approximately 20 mL if superficial blocks are also performed).

   Comments
   ■ The deep block may be performed by single injection at C3 or C4 as originally described by Winnie et al.[71] or by a standard three-injection technique.

   ■ Paresthesia occurring during these blocks has been associated with more effective anesthesia.[72]

   ■ Anesthesia for carotid endarterectomy may involve performing combined superficial and deep cervical plexus blocks, yet the benefit of combined over superficial block alone has been questioned.[73,74] There appears to be no difference between these two approaches in the amount of supplemental local anesthesia required.

   ■ There are several life-threatening complications that may arise from deep cervical plexus block. Injection may occur into the vertebral artery. Subarachnoid or epidural injections are possible if the needle is advanced too far medially into the vertebral foramen. This is more likely in the cervical region because of the longer dural sleeves that accompany these nerve branches. Careful monitoring of the patient should continue for 60 minutes after the block has been performed.

   ■ Phrenic nerve palsy leading to hemidiaphragmatic paresis is a common occurrence with this block.[75,76] This block is not indicated in any patient who depends on the diaphragm for tidal ventilation, nor is bilateral blockade ever recommended.

   ■ Other well-described side effects include Horner syndrome (if the superior cervical or cervicothoracic ganglion is blocked),[77] stellate ganglion block,[78] and hoarseness because of recurrent laryngeal nerve block.

2. Superficial cervical plexus block is performed in a similar position as deep cervical plexus block and results in anesthesia only of the sensory fibers of the plexus.

Procedure
- An X is made at the midpoint of the posterior border of the sternocleidomastoid muscle (Fig. 38-5).
- Local skin infiltration is performed with a fanlike injection using 10 to 20 mL of local anesthetic along the posterior border of the sternocleidomastoid muscle 4 cm above and below the level of the midpoint.

Comments
- The most common approach for minimally invasive parathyroidectomy (involving a small unilateral incision rather than bilateral neck exploration) includes a combination of C2 through C4 superficial cervical plexus block, infiltration along the incision line, and infiltration of the upper thyroid pedicle.[79] This approach can result in shorter anesthetic and operative times, leading to earlier hospital discharge as well as significantly better postoperative pain relief.[79,80]
- Thyroid surgery has been performed, using a modified surgical approach, under superficial cervical plexus block in combination with anterior field block.[81]
- Minimally invasive surgery may require conversion to general anesthesia when there is difficulty ensuring adequate protection of the recurrent laryngeal nerve or when intraoperative diagnosis of parathyroid carcinoma or multiglandular parathyroid hyperplasia occurs.
- Phrenic nerve paralysis leading to diaphragmatic dysfunction,[72] vagus nerve block with resultant recurrent nerve paralysis[82] and inadvertent intravascular injection have all been reported.[83]

Occipital Nerve Blocks. The greater and lesser occipital nerves can be blocked by superficial injection at the points on the posterior skull where they emerge from below the muscles of the neck. This block is rarely used for surgical procedures; it is more often applied as a diagnostic step in evaluating head and neck pain complaints.

Procedure (Fig. 38-9)
- The patient sits with the head tilted forward slightly to expose the prominent nuchal ridge of bone at the posterior base of the skull.
- The superior nuchal line is palpated at one third of the distance between the external occipital protuberance and the foramen magnum. A mark is placed on the nuchal line at the lateral border of the insertion of the erector muscles of the neck, usually 2.5 cm from the midline. The branches of the greater occipital nerve usually pass laterally from behind the muscle to cross the nuchal line at this point. The nerve is located directly lateral to the easily palpated occipital artery. During its ascent on the posterior skull, the lesser occipital nerve can be located at an additional 2.5 cm distance from the greater occipital nerve along the superior nuchal line; a mark should be placed here as well.
- A short, fine needle (e.g., 2.5 cm, 25 gauge) is introduced with a slight cranial angulation at each mark to the depth of the skull itself. After slight withdrawal, local anesthetic is injected (e.g., 0.5 to 1 mL of 1% lidocaine for diagnostic procedures or 1 to 3 mL of 0.75% ropivacaine for therapeutic procedures). Paresthesias are occasionally encountered but are not essential for obtaining simple skin anesthesia.
- If more anterior anesthesia of the scalp is required, the lesser occipital nerve branches are also blocked by advancing the needle subcutaneously from this point in an anterior direction toward the mastoid process. A band of anesthetic solution is deposited along the line between skin entry and the mastoid process using 2 to 3 mL of local anesthetic.

Comments
- Blocking the lesser occipital and the great auricular nerve (both blocked by subcutaneous injection from the angle of the mandible to the mastoid process) has been successful in providing postoperative analgesia after otoplasty.[84] Reducing the requirement for opioid analgesia (with its associated nausea and vomiting) is essential because of the high incidence of pain and vomiting on the first postoperative day related to the surgical procedure alone.
- The greater occipital nerve block is commonly used for primary headache syndromes; for chronic syndromes, the anterior region involving the trigeminal nerve is also blocked.[85] It has been reported for use with cervicogenic headache, occipital neuralgia, migraine, and cluster headache.[86]
- Complications with this technique are rare. Care must be taken not to advance the needle anteriorly under the skull as the foramen magnum might be entered unintentionally with a long needle. Local hematoma may be produced with superficial injection, but this is only a temporary problem.

Upper Extremity Blocks

Although many approaches to the brachial plexus have been described, there are traditionally four anatomic locations where local anesthetics are placed: (1) the interscalene groove near the cervical transverse processes, (2) the subclavian sheath at the first rib, (3) near the coracoid process in the infraclavicular fossa, and (4) surrounding the axillary artery in the axilla. The introduction of US imaging has greatly increased use of blocks at the supraclavicular fossa. Visualization of the subclavian artery and lung make these critical structures easier to avoid. It is important to stress that clear visibility of the needle is essential for this block (and generally for all blocks of the brachial plexus). The appropriate choice of approach depends not only on the patient's anatomy but on the site of surgery and the localization method.

The terminal branches can also be anesthetized by local anesthetic injection along their peripheral course where they lie in close proximity to easily identifiable structures (Table 38-1), or by the injection of a dilute local anesthetic solution intravenously below a pneumatic tourniquet on the upper arm ("intravenous regional" or Bier block). The use of US may increase the number of locations where the terminal nerves can be successfully blocked. For example, the ulnar nerve can be blocked effectively at the medial surface of the midforearm, which may reduce the risk of ulnar nerve palsy compared with block at the elbow near the cubital tunnel. As stated in the introduction to "Specific Techniques," the use of a combined US- and NS-guided technique is stressed in the figures, and the use of all necessary sterile precaution was not included for simplicity of viewing.

Clinical Anatomy

Spinal Nerves
- The spinal nerves are part of the peripheral nervous system, along with the cranial and autonomic nerves and their ganglia.
- There are 31 pairs of spinal nerves: 8 cervical (C1 through C8), 12 thoracic (T1 through T12), 5 lumbar (L1 through L5), 5 sacral (S1 through S5), and 1 coccygeal. These spinal nerves are formed by the union of the ventral (anterior) and dorsal (posterior) spinal roots.
- The spinal nerves are mixed nerves consisting of both motor and sensory fibers. In addition, all spinal nerves contain sympathetic fibers for supplying blood vessels, smooth muscle, and glands in the skin. The nerves give off

sympathetic branches immediately after leaving the intervertebral foramen. Gray and white rami communicantes connect the spinal nerves to the sympathetic chain ganglia to allow preganglionic sympathetic fibers leaving the spinal cord (T1 through L2/3) to enter the chain and leave it again to be distributed with spinal nerves at all levels.

■ Soon after exiting the intervertebral (spinal) foramina, each spinal nerve in turn divides into a larger ventral and a smaller dorsal ramus (branches). The ventral rami course laterally and anteriorly to supply the muscles, subcutaneous tissues (superficial fascia), and skin of the neck, trunk, and the upper and lower extremities (the dermatomes of the body are shown in Fig. 38-8). The dorsal rami course posteriorly and supply the paravertebral muscles, subcutaneous tissues, and skin of the back close to the midline.

■ It is important to realize that the first cervical (C1) nerve leaves the spinal cord and courses above the atlas (C1 vertebra); hence, the cervical nerves are numbered corresponding to the vertebrae inferior to them; for example, the C8 nerve exiting below C7 and above T1. From this point on, all the spinal nerves are named corresponding to the vertebral level above. For example, T3 and L4 spinal nerves exit below the T3 and L4 vertebrae, respectively.

Brachial Plexus

■ The brachial plexus (Fig. 38-12) classically arises from the anterior primary rami of C5-8 and T1 spinal nerves.

■ The plexus consists of five *roots*, three *trunks*, six *divisions* (two per trunk), three *cords*, and five major terminal nerves.

■ The C5-T1 nerve roots emerge from their corresponding intervertebral foramina and then travel along the grooves between the anterior and posterior tubercles of the corresponding transverse process. They finally emerge between the scalenus anterior and medius muscles, above the second part of subclavian artery and posterior to vertebral artery.

■ C5 and 6 nerve roots unite to form the *upper (superior) trunk*, C7 continues as the *middle trunk*, and C8 and T1 converge into the *lower (inferior) trunk*.

■ Fibrous sheaths (as part of the prevertebral fascia) surround the anterior and posterior parts of the plexus and continue to envelope the plexus between the scalene muscles more distally (called the *interscalene fascial sheath* proximally and the *axillary sheath* distally).

■ The three trunks travel inferolaterally and cross the base of the posterior triangle of the neck (superficial) and the first rib (upper and middle trunks above subclavian artery and lower trunk behind or below the artery). At the lateral border of first rib, each trunk bifurcates into *anterior* and *posterior divisions*.

■ Approximately at the level where the nerves course under the pectoralis minor muscle, the divisions converge to form three *cords*: *lateral cord*—anterior divisions of upper and middle trunks (C5-7); *medial cord*—anterior division of lower trunk (C8,T1); and *posterior cord*—posterior divisions of all three trunks (C5-T1).

■ The cords are grouped around the second part of the axillary artery (within 2.5 cm from its center).[87] There are three parts of the axillary artery named for their positions above (medial to), behind, and below (lateral to) the pectoralis minor muscle. Typically, with an US probe placed to view the transverse axis of the cords, the medial cord lies inferior, the lateral cord superior, and the posterior cord posterior to the first part of the axillary artery.

■ Immediately beyond the pectoralis minor muscle, the three cords diverge into the terminal branches; these include the median, ulnar, radial, axillary, and musculocutaneous nerves.

■ The phrenic nerve normally descends anterior to the scalenus anterior muscle; it crosses the muscle from lateral to medial as it descends and passes under the clavicle and through the superior thoracic aperture into the superior mediastinum just medial to the external jugular vein. However, there is anatomic variation of the course of the phrenic nerve and it is not always anterior to the scalenus anterior muscle.

Terminal Nerves.   The anatomy of the peripheral nerves is outlined here, although the clinically related innervation patterns are included in the discussion of each block's technique. Figure 38-13

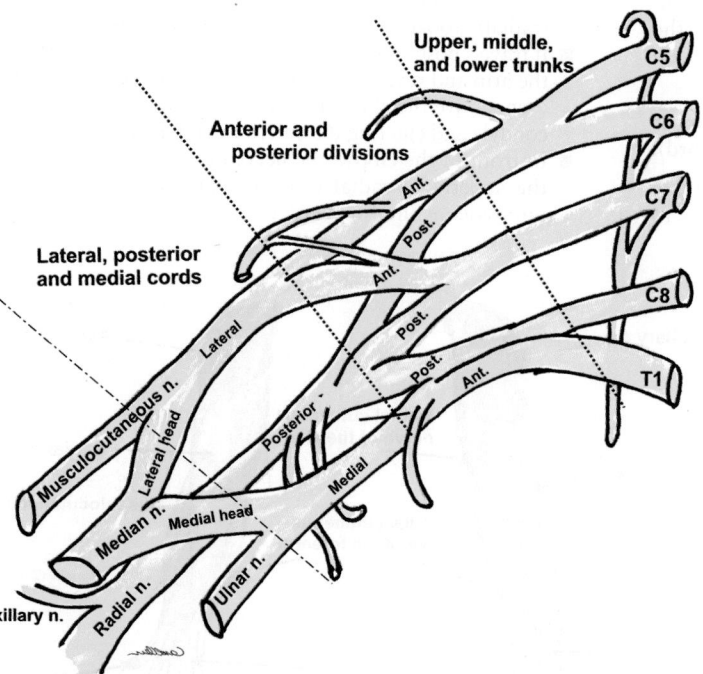

FIGURE 38-12. Schematic of the brachial plexus. Many branches, including the medial cutaneous nerves of the forearm and arm, which arise from the medial cord are not shown.

Upper, middle, and lower trunks

Anterior and posterior divisions

Lateral, posterior and medial cords

C5
C6
C7
C8
T1

Ant.
Post.
Ant.
Post.
Post.
Ant.

Musculocutaneous n.
Lateral
Lateral head
Median n.
Medial head
Posterior
Medial
Radial n.
Ulnar n.
Axillary n.

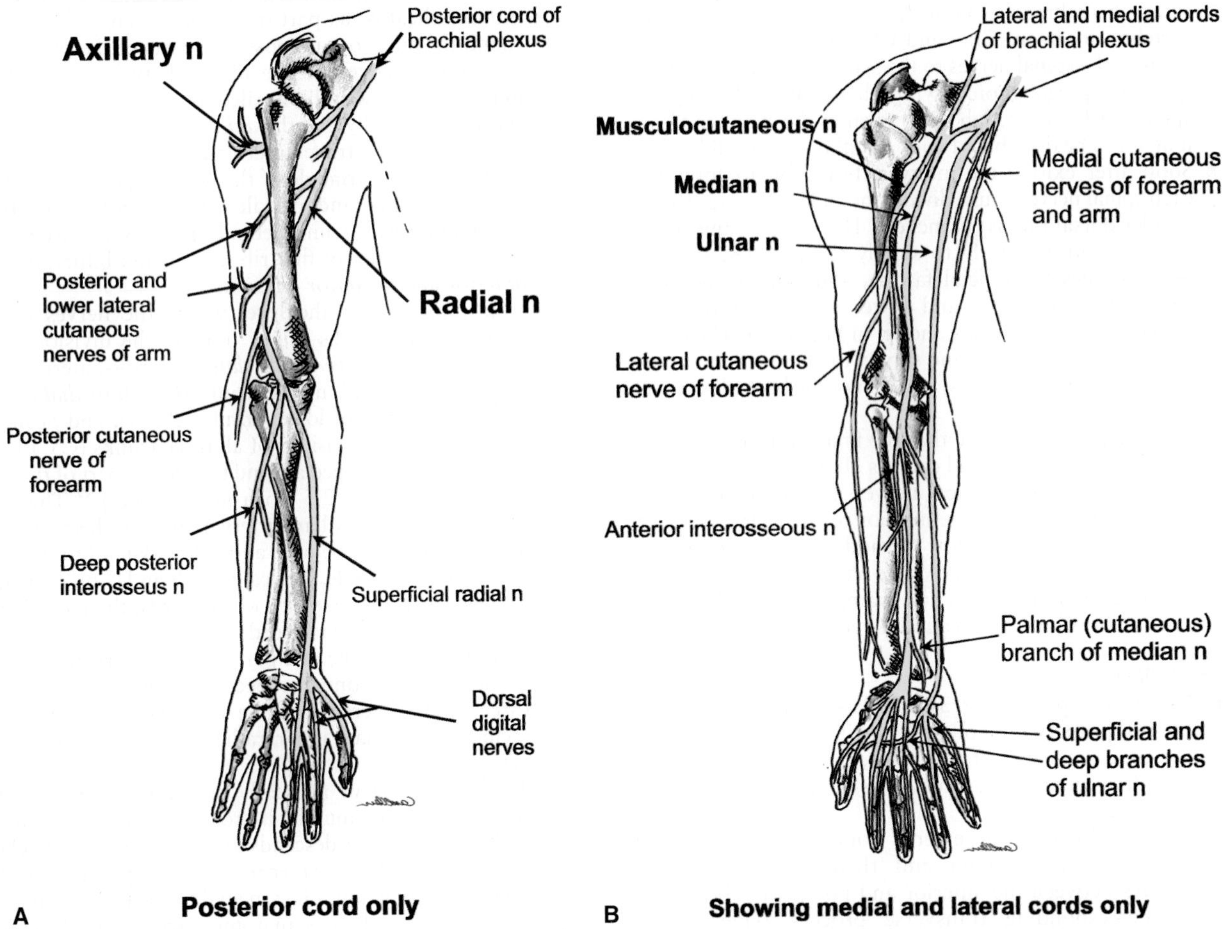

FIGURE 38-13. Courses of the terminal nerves of the upper extremity. The posterior view (**A**) illustrates the branches from the posterior cord (axillary and radial nerves), and the anterior view (**B**) illustrates the branches from the lateral (musculocutaneous and median nerves) and medial (median and ulnar nerves) cords.

illustrates the courses of these nerves within the upper extremity. Figure 38-14 illustrates the cutaneous innervation of the terminal nerves of the upper extremity. The axillary nerve is an additional terminal nerve of the upper extremity, but the anatomy and blocking of this nerve will not be discussed here.

1. Radial nerve (originates from C5-8 and T1 roots, upper and middle trunks, posterior divisions, and posterior cord).

   ■ It originates deep (often posteromedial)[88] to the axillary artery, descends within the axilla (giving off branches to

long head of the triceps brachii), passes between the medial and lateral heads of the triceps, and then descends obliquely across the posterior aspect of the humerus along the spiral (radial) groove at the level of the deltoid insertion.

■ It travels posterior and medial to the deep brachial artery of the arm and reaches the lateral margin of the humerus 5 to 7 cm above the elbow before crossing over the lateral epicondyle and entering the anterior compartment of the arm.

■ In front of the elbow, the nerve divides and continues as the superficial radial (sensory) and the deep posterior interosseous (motor) nerves.

FIGURE 38-14. Cutaneous innervation of the upper extremity nerves.

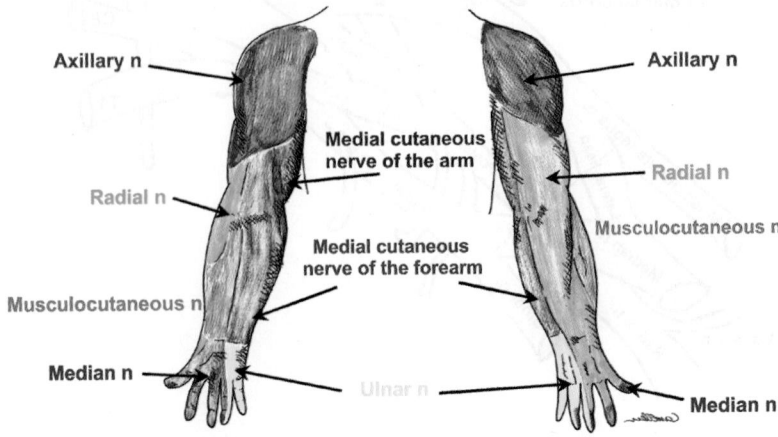

2. Median nerve (originates from C5-8, T1, all trunks, and lateral and medial cords).

- In the axilla, the nerve often lies anterolateral to the axillary artery.[88,89] The nerve descends along the medial aspect of the arm lateral to the brachial artery and crosses the artery, usually anteriorly, at the midpoint of the arm at the insertion of the coracobrachialis muscle.
- The nerve crosses the elbow lying medially on the brachialis muscle and just medial to the brachial artery and vein (all of these medial to the biceps brachii tendon).
- Distal to the antecubital fossa, the nerve gives off the anterior interosseous nerve and cutaneous sensory branches.

3. Musculocutaneous nerve (originates from C5-7 roots, upper and middle trunks, anterior divisions, lateral cord).

- This nerve leaves the fascial sheath of the plexus approximately at the level of the coracoid process, thus the infraclavicular location for brachial plexus block is generally the most distal block site for this nerve.
- Just distal (2 to 3 cm) to the pectoralis major muscle attachment, the nerve usually pierces the coracobrachialis muscle, after which it exits this muscle and comes to lie between the coracobrachialis muscle and the short and long heads of the biceps brachii muscle.
- Although it is difficult to observe using US, the nerve continues as the lateral cutaneous nerve of the forearm at the antecubital fossa and courses along the lateral aspect of the forearm providing subsequent anterior and posterior branches.

4. Ulnar nerve (originates from C7-8, T1 roots, lower trunk, anterior division, medial cord).

- Initially the nerve often courses between the axillary artery and vein (it may lie anteromedial to the artery and vein) and then along the medial aspect of the brachial artery to the midpoint of the humerus before passing posteriorly and following the anterior surface of the medial head of the triceps.
- It then passes behind the medial epicondyle of the humerus (in the condylar groove), divides between the humeral and ulnar heads of the flexor carpi ulnaris, and lies on the medial aspect of the elbow joint.
- During its descent through the forearm, the nerve courses anteriorly, to approach the ulnar artery directly anterior to the ulna at the junction of the lower third and upper two thirds of the forearm.
- At the wrist it crosses superficial to the flexor retinaculum and divides into superficial and deep branches; the ulnar artery lies anterolateral to the nerve at the wrist.

Anatomic Variation. There are many variations in formation of the brachial plexus,[90] as well as in the course of the terminal nerves and the vascular elements. Some of these variations may contribute to difficulty when performing PNB as there may be erroneous NS responses (e.g., if two nerves are conjoined) or poor localization by NS or by US imaging (e.g., if the nerve follows a substantially different path). Some examples are described here.

- The plexus may include anterior rami from C4 to C8 ("prefixed") or, less common, from C5 to T2 ("postfixed".)
- The existence and/or characteristics of the connective tissue sheath that invests the plexus at various regions are controversial. A continuous, tubular sheath has been shown unlikely, especially in the axillary region. A more convoluted and septated structure may be the cause of nonuniform distribution of local anesthetic in many cases, which supports the findings that multiple injection techniques may be superior.[91] US guidance can be very

valuable in this location to ensure circumferential spread of local anesthetic around the nerves.

- The interscalene groove may have variation in the relationship between the plexus roots and trunks and the muscles. For example, the C5 and/or C6 nerve roots may traverse either through or anterior to the anterior scalene muscle.[92]
- In many cadaveric specimens, no inferior trunk exists.[93] A single cord or a pair of cords may develop. It has been observed that no discrete posterior cord forms in some cases, with the posterior divisions diverging to form terminal nerves.[90]
- The terminal nerves may lie in various relations to the axillary vessels. The use of a combined NS- and US-guided technique to both confirm the nerve localization (NS) and obtain circumferential spread of local anesthetic around each of the nerves (US) may improve block success.[8] The musculocutaneous nerve may fuse to or have communications with the median nerve, which can result in its absence from within the coracobrachialis muscle.[94,95] Communication between the median and ulnar nerves in the forearm are common, with the median nerve replacing the innervation to various muscles normally supplied by the ulnar nerve.[96]
- There may also be large variations with respect to the vessels within the arm, with aberrant formations including double axillary veins, high origin of the radial artery, and double brachial arteries.[97–99]

Techniques

Brachial Plexus Blockade

1. Interscalene block as described by Winnie[100] in 1970, is indicated mostly for surgical anesthesia to the shoulder, upper arm, and forearm, but is often insufficient for the hand. It frequently spares the lowest branches of the plexus, the C8 and T1 fibers, which innervate the caudad (ulnar) border of the forearm. The patient is positioned supine, with the head faced slightly to the contralateral side. The main surface landmark (sternocleidomastoid muscle) used for this block can be accentuated by asking the patient to reach for the ipsilateral knee and by rotating the head approximately 45 degrees to the nonoperative side. The head should also be slightly elevated, and the patient should be instructed to take a deep breath because contraction of the scalenus muscles accentuates the interscalene groove. This groove lies immediately behind the lateral border of the clavicular head of the sternocleidomastoid muscle at the level of the cricoid cartilage (C6). As for all procedures of the upper extremity, prepare the needle insertion site and other applicable skin areas with an antiseptic solution and, if using US imaging, obtain sterility of the US probe with a standard sleeve cover or transparent dressing.

Procedure Using Nerve Stimulation Technique
- Landmarks: Using the maneuvers described, the interscalene groove is palpated by rolling the fingers posteriorly off the lateral border of the sternocleidomastoid muscle; mark the groove as high as possible. After the patient relaxes, the prominent transverse process of C6 can often be felt directly in the groove and should be marked.
- Needling: A skin wheal is raised in the interscalene groove at the level of the cricoid. A 22-gauge, 2.5-cm (or less) insulated needle is introduced through the wheal. The needle is directed medially, caudally, and slightly posteriorly in the direction of the C6 transverse process. The caudad tilt of the needle is important to avoid either entering the neural foramen or injection into the dural nerve root sheath, and thus high-spinal anesthesia or spinal cord injury.[101] Avoiding medial placement, by

FIGURE 38-15. Ultrasound-guided interscalene block using an in-plane needle alignment to a linear high-frequency probe. The needle is directed from lateral to medial with a slight caudal angle to avoid the intervertebral foramen. The roots/trunks of the plexus are usually seen as three or more round or oval-shaped hypoechoic structures sandwiched between scalenus anterior and medius muscles in the interscalene groove.

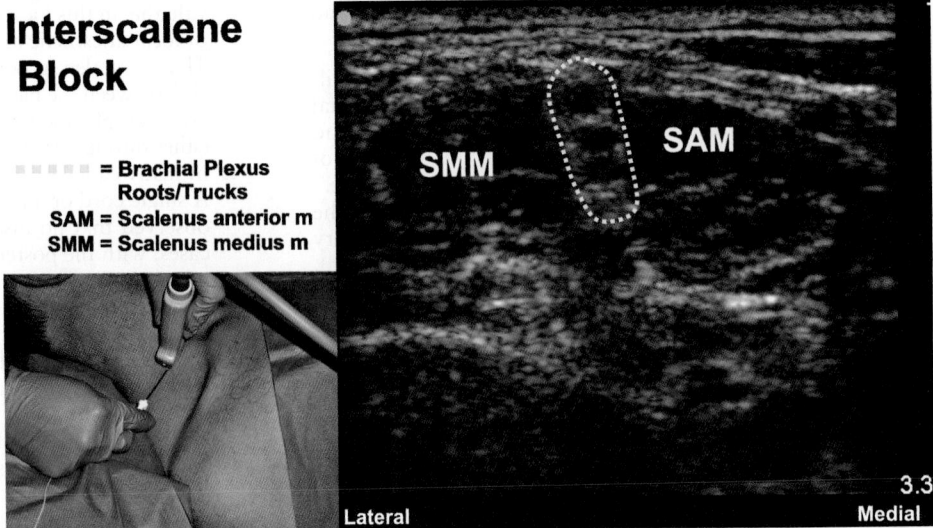

Interscalene Block

----- = Brachial Plexus Roots/Trucks
SAM = Scalenus anterior m
SMM = Scalenus medius m

using a mostly caudad and posterior direction, may reduce the risks even more. The superficial structures of the plexus have been shown to be located at an average, shallow depth of 5.5 mm.[102]

- Nerve localization: Applying an initial current of 0.8 mA is sufficient for stimulation of the plexus (usually at a depth of 1 to 3 cm), and the current is reduced to aim for a threshold current of 0.4 mA before injection after obtaining an appropriate motor response. Diaphragmatic or trapezius twitches should be avoided, as they are associated with cervical plexus stimulation; a diaphragmatic response indicates that the phrenic nerve is being stimulated and that the needle is too anterior.
- Injection: After careful aspiration, 25 to 30 mL of local anesthetic is injected in small increments to detect intraneural or intravascular placement of the needle.

Procedure Using Ultrasound Guidance
- Scanning: Two scanning techniques are recommended for viewing the brachial plexus at the interscalene level: (1) beginning anteriorly at the cricoid cartilage level (C6) with movement from anterior and medial to posterior and lateral towards the interscalene groove, and (2)

scanning proximally from the supraclavicular fossa to the interscalene location (Fig. 38-15).
- Appearance: At the supraclavicular fossa, the brachial plexus (trunks/divisions) can be seen in short axis as a tightly enclosed cluster (i.e., a honeycomb) superior and lateral to the subclavian artery (Fig. 38-16). After tracing the nerves in a proximal fashion toward the interscalene groove, the nerve structures (roots/trunks) in a sagittal oblique section are visualized as three (usually) or up to five round or oval-shaped hypoechoic (see "Common Techniques: Nerve Stimulation and Ultrasound Imaging") structures, sometimes with few internal punctate echoes, lying between the scalenus anterior and medius muscles. C8 and T1 roots may be difficult to identify because of their depth.[103,104]
- Needling: A skin wheal is raised in the groove at the level of the cricoid cartilage. A 22-gauge, 5-cm (or less) needle (insulated is recommended) is introduced either OOP (see "Common Techniques") or IP to the probe (Fig. 38-15) and advanced to a maximum of 3 cm for most patients. For OOP needle insertion technique, the clinician stands beside or cephalad to the probe and places the initial needle puncture site cranial to the probe. The

FIGURE 38-16. Ultrasound-guided supraclavicular block using an in-plane needle alignment to a small footprint curved probe, and directing the needle from lateral to medial in a slightly sagittal plane. Color Doppler can also be very valuable in locating the subclavian artery quickly, in order to locate the plexus trunks/divisions immediately superolateral to the vessel.

Supraclavicular Block

----- = Brachial Plexus trunks/divisions
----- = Subclavian artery

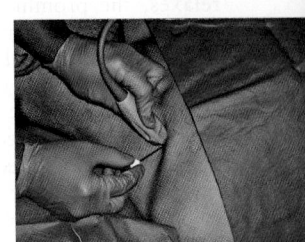

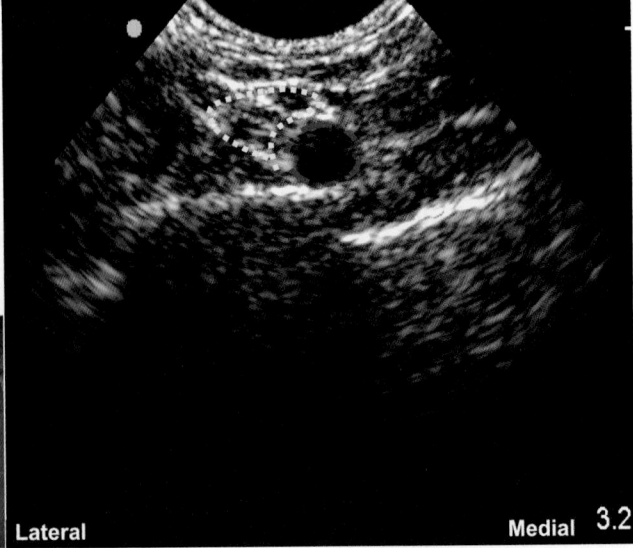

needle is typically angled somewhat caudally toward the US beam plane. For IP needle insertion technique, the needle is moved from lateral to medial (still slightly caudad) and will first penetrate the scalenus medius muscle before entering the interscalene groove. It is recommended to use NS to provide further nerve localization.

- Local anesthetic spread: A test injection of D5W is recommended and will help confirm nerve localization and estimate the pattern of local anesthetic spread. Local anesthetic should be deposited in the midst of the neural structures so that it spreads to surround the nerves circumferentially. Local anesthetic distention in this compartment can be seen by US as a hypoechoic (fluid) expansion.

Comments

- The use of long-acting local anesthetics may provide analgesia for 12 to 14 hours. For longer analgesia, insertion of a continuous catheter is effective for procedures such as total shoulder replacement, although securing the catheters in the mobile neck tissues is a challenge.
- Equal success has been achieved when any of the appropriate muscle responses is elicited as a positive stimulating test. Palpation of the muscle may confirm the response.
- Despite the fact that subarachnoid injection can occur even when the threshold current is >0.4 mA, it is advisable to avoid injecting when the current responses are present at <0.4 mA.
- The most commonly observed mistake is placement of the needle too anterior to the optimal skin insertion site. However, not infrequently the needle may be placed too posteriorly as well.
- Inadequate anesthesia is most likely to occur in the ulnar distribution. This may be reduced by using higher volumes (35 to 40 mL) of local anesthetic.
- If a continuous block is indicated, the needle entry point may be moved a centimeter cephalad and the corresponding angle of insertion is a little steeper and more tangential to the course of the plexus. The opening of the tip of the introducing needle should be directed laterally. When using a stimulating catheter, the perineural space may be dilated if necessary to facilitate catheter placement with D5W to monitor its advancement to a location where motor response is maintained at <0.5 mA.
- Securing catheters in the freely mobile neck is a challenge. Some prefer to secure the catheter by tunneling 3 to 4 cm below the skin by passing it back through an intravenous catheter that has been introduced subcutaneously near the entry site.
- During OOP US-guided technique, angling the needle more than 45 degrees should be avoided as the needle may be inserted too deep and directed toward the spinal cord.
- Complications from this approach are related to the structures located in the vicinity of the tubercle. The cupola of the lung is close, particularly on the right side, and can be contacted if the needle is directed too far caudally. Pneumothorax should be considered if cough or chest pain is produced while exploring for the nerve. If the needle is allowed to pass directly medially, it may enter the intervertebral foramen, and injection of local anesthetic may produce spinal or epidural anesthesia. The vertebral artery passes posteriorly at the level of the sixth vertebra to lie in its canal in the transverse process; direct injection into this vessel can rapidly produce central nervous system toxicity and convulsions. Careful aspiration and incremental injections are important to help avoid both of these potential problems.
- Even with appropriate injection, local anesthetic solution can spread to contiguous nerves. It may produce cervical plexus block, including motor fibers to the diaphragm, which may be a problem in patients with respiratory insufficiency. Horner syndrome is common because of spread to the sympathetic chain on the anterior vertebral body.
- Neuropathy of the C6 root is a potential problem because the needle may unintentionally pin the nerve root against the tubercle and predispose to intraneural injection. The needle should be withdrawn slightly if the first injection produces the characteristic "crampy" pain sensation.
- An alternative technique for blocking the roots of the brachial plexus is to perform a cervical paravertebral block,[105] which can use the bony landmarks of the vertebral column. This is a high-quality block, which is readily performed using US guidance. A lateral US view of the brachial plexus at the level of C6 allows visualization of the needle as it passes lateral to the C6 transverse process and into the interscalene space. This view avoids the challenges of attempting to view the brachial plexus from a posterior approach in which the bony structures may obscure the view of the needle and plexus.

2. Supraclavicular block targets the trunks and/or divisions of the brachial plexus depending on the location of the injection site and the patient's anatomy. Similar to the interscalene block, the patient is positioned supine with the head turned approximately 45 degrees to the contralateral side. Prepare the needle insertion site and other applicable skin areas with an antiseptic solution and obtain sterility of the US probe with a standard sleeve cover or transparent dressing.

Procedure Using Nerve Stimulation Technique

- Landmarks: The outline of the clavicle is drawn on the skin and the midpoint of the clavicle is marked. An X is placed posterior to this midpoint in the interscalene groove, usually 1 cm behind the clavicle. The subclavian artery pulse serves as a reliable landmark in thinner individuals as the plexus lies immediately cephaloposterior to the subclavian artery.
- Needling: Local infiltration is performed at the site of the nerve and a 2.5- to 5-cm, 22-gauge needle is introduced in the parasagittal plane at the superior border of the clavicle at the lateral edge of the sternocleidomastoid muscle insertion. An initial insertion angle of 45 degrees cephalad is recommended, with subsequent reductions in angle as necessary.[106] Less than 20 degrees may lead to the needle contacting the pleura and/or subclavian vein prior to the plexus. The rib may be contacted, with subsequent anteroposterior needle adjustment to contact the plexus, but avoiding rib contact may be most prudent. Careful lateral or medial exploration may be needed, but the greatest danger of contacting the pleura occurs when probing too medially.
- Nerve localization: The responses to NS can be very useful for confirmation of needle proximity to the separate trunks. Twitches of pectoralis, deltoid, biceps (upper trunk), triceps (upper/middle trunk), forearm (upper/middle trunk), and hand (lower trunk) muscles with current intensity of 0.4 mA (0.1 to 0.3 ms) are acceptable. Distal responses (hand or wrist flexion or extension) are best to confirm placement within the fascia. Multiple nerve responses are not required.
- Injection: If a nerve response is produced during the course of exploration, the anesthetic solution is injected while the needle is fixed in position. Twenty-five to 40 mL of local anesthetic will produce adequate analgesia.

Procedure Using Ultrasound Imaging

- Scanning: The probe is first placed in a coronal oblique plane at the lateral end of and just above the upper border of the clavicle (Fig. 38-16). It is then moved medially until an image of the subclavian artery appears on the screen. Some dorsal and ventral rotation of the probe may be necessary. With the subclavian artery in the middle of the screen, the plexus is located superolateral to the artery and the neurovascular structures are lying above the first rib.

- Appearance: The subclavian artery is anechoic, hypodense, pulsatile, and round; its identity can be further confirmed by color Doppler. Trunks/divisions of the brachial plexus appear as a cluster of hypoechoic "grapelike" structures consisting of usually three (more as one moves distally) hypoechoic nodules, all surrounded by a hyperechoic lining (presumably the connective tissues). With the probe in a coronal oblique plane, the plexus depth has been shown with magnetic resonance imaging to equal 1.65 cm in male patients and 1.45 cm in female patients.[106,107] Medial and deep to the artery, the rib may be seen as a hyperechoic line with dorsal shadowing. The anechoic subclavian vein may be seen inferomedial to the artery.
- Needling: The selected needle insertion site is often more lateral with the US-guided technique than when using NS techniques. The skin is infiltrated with local anesthetic and a 22-gauge, 5-cm (or less) needle (insulated is recommended) is introduced with IP needle alignment to a small footprint curved (Fig. 38-16) or linear probe. The needle is inserted immediately above the clavicle in a lateral-to-medial direction with a slight cephalad angle. It is recommended to follow NS procedure for additional confirmation of nerve localization.
- Local anesthetic spread: It is best to deposit local anesthetic next to the nerve structures immediately lateral to the subclavian artery on top of the first rib. Injection in this location will often lift the nerve structures superiorly away from the first rib and subclavian artery. The hypoechoic spread of local anesthetic surrounding the nerves may be seen on the US screen.

Comments

- It is recommended to use US imaging in addition to NS technique during this block to help avoid puncturing the pleura. It is critical to measure the skin-pleura distance with US prior to needle insertion. The responses to NS can be useful for confirmation of needle proximity to the separate trunks.
- The major challenge with US imaging in this region is the presence of a bony prominence (clavicle) and curved soft-tissue contour that can interfere with imaging of the brachial plexus in short axis. Despite disadvantages with current low-to-moderate frequency commercially available curved array probes (e.g., C11, Titan or MicroMaxx, Sonosite Inc., Bothell, WA); a curved array probe with a small footprint is extremely useful in this compact area.
- The lateral-to-medial IP needle approach will ensure the needle approaches the nerve structures prior to reaching the subclavian artery (i.e., less chance of inadvertent vascular puncture). Despite this, using a slightly sagittal plane (Fig. 38-16) may reduce the risk of pleural puncture. The needle should be viewed at all times when using a lateral-to-medial direction.
- The greatest fear when using this technique is the risk of pneumothorax as the cupola of the lung lies just medial to the first rib, not far from the plexus. The risk of pneumothorax is greater on the right side as the cupola of the lung is higher on that side. The risk is also greater in tall, thin patients.
- Other complications of PNB of the brachial plexus do not occur with any greater frequency with this block than with other methods of brachial plexus block.

3. Infraclavicular block targets the cords of the brachial plexus, and the nerves can be blocked next to the second part of the axillary artery at the level of the coracoid process. Brachial plexus block in the infraclavicular area offers excellent analgesia of the entire arm and allows introduction of continuous catheters to provide prolonged postoperative pain relief. The infraclavicular approach blocks the musculocutaneous and axillary nerves more consistently because these two nerves often branch off high in the axilla and are often missed with the axillary block approach. However, multiple injections may be required for successful infraclavicular and axillary blocks.

Infraclavicular blocks are indicated for forearm, elbow, and hand surgery. The patient is supine with the head turned approximately 45 degrees to the nonoperative side; the arm may either be at the side with hand on the abdomen or abducted with the palm placed behind the head. When preparing for this block, it is common to perform the block with the patient's elbow flexed and the hand resting on the abdomen to facilitate observation of motor responses generated with NS. Alternatively, externally rotating the arm and placing the hand behind the head stretches the cords and brings the nerves closer around the axillary artery, which may facilitate local anesthetic spread around the nerves. As always, prepare the needle insertion site and other applicable skin areas with an antiseptic solution and obtain sterility of the US probe with a standard sleeve cover or transparent dressing.

Procedure Using Nerve Stimulation Technique. Several approaches have been described for infraclavicular block, all with various needle puncture sites and angles of insertion.[108-113] Here we describe a lateral approach,[109] which may improve plexus cord localization and reduce risk of puncture to both the pleura and axillary artery.[114,115]

- Landmarks: With the patient's arm adducted and the hand resting on the abdomen, the medial aspect of the coracoid process is palpated as one slips the finger off the clavicle.
- Needling: After skin preparation and skin wheal, a 5- to 9-cm, 18- to 22-gauge needle is inserted where the clavicle meets the medial aspect of the coracoid process, directed generally at 0 to 15 degrees posterior to the horizontal plane (Fig. 38-17 illustrates this needle insertion when using US guidance). The 15-degree trajectory will likely increase the chances of contacting the more posteriorly located posterior or medial cords, which may improve analgesia. A greater angle may be required to achieve adequate responses to NS because local anesthetic injection at more than one cord may be beneficial. The cords should be reached at approximately 4 to 6 cm depth (more than 7.5 cm may risk pleural puncture).[109] The needle puncture site may be adjusted slightly caudad to this location, as with the technique of Kapral et al.[108] If the needle is placed at 2.5 cm caudad to the coracoid process, a laterally projected needle directed toward the axillary artery may be effective.[109]
- Nerve localization: The first response (elbow flexion) obtained is usually the musculocutaneous nerve arising from the lateral cord. For complete anesthesia of the hand, a separate distal response needs to be obtained from the medial (distal flexors) and posterior (distal and proximal extensors) cords.[116] A simplified approach to determining the specific cord distal responses during infraclavicular block has been described.[117] A close examination of the movements of the fifth digit can be useful to differentiate the cords, with lateral movement (i.e., pronation) representing the lateral cord, medial movement (i.e., flexion) representing the medial cord,

Infraclavicular Block

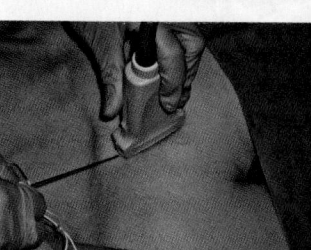

Axillary vein
Axillary artery
Lateral cord
Posterior cord
Medial cord

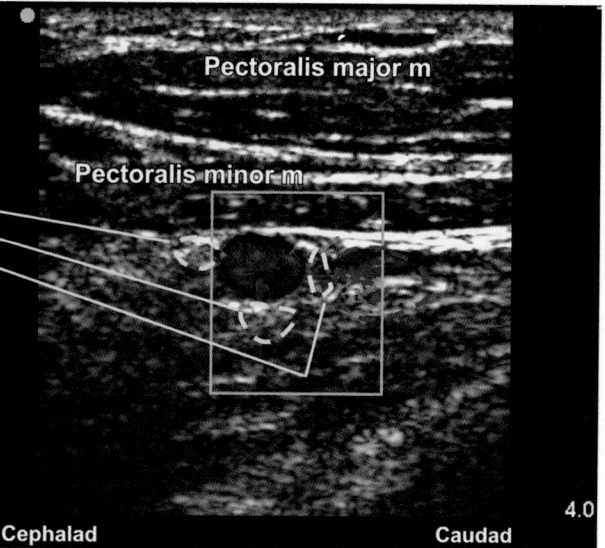

Pectoralis major m

Pectoralis minor m

Cephalad   Caudad
4.0

FIGURE 38-17. Ultrasound-guided infraclavicular block using an in-plane needle alignment to a linear probe, and directing the needle 15 degrees posteriorly in a cephalad-to-caudad direction. In contrast to the more proximal blocks, the nerves (cords) appear hyperechoic now because of their higher fascial content and because the surrounding tissue (muscle) is largely hypoechoic.

and dorsal movement (i.e., extension) representing the posterior cord.[117] Some also advocate that eliciting a forearm response (pronation via the lateral cord) is essential for a complete block.[118] The artery may be punctured easily at this point, and careful aspiration is required to prevent intravascular injection.

■ Injection: If a musculocutaneous nerve response is first obtained, the nerve or lateral cord can be blocked by an injection of 5 to 10 mL of local anesthetic. Once responses in the hand are obtained, a further 25 mL of local anesthetic can be injected along the posterior and medial cords.

Procedure Using Ultrasound Imaging
■ Scanning: Immediately medial and inferior to the coracoid process, position a linear or curved lower frequency transducer (4 to 7 MHz) in a parasagittal plane and capture the best possible short axis view of the brachial plexus cords and axillary vessels (Fig. 38-17). If the patient is quite thin or if using a more medial location (not described here) where the nerves are more superficial, a higher frequency probe may be used.
■ Appearance: The pectoralis major and minor muscles are separated by a hyperechoic lining (perimysium); the pectoralis major lies superficial and lateral to the pectoralis minor muscle. Deeper at a depth of approximately 4 to 5 cm lies the axillary neurovascular bundle; the large axillary vein lies medially and caudally to the artery. The lateral cord of the plexus is often readily visualized as a hyperechoic oval structure; the medial and posterior cords may not be readily identified because the medial cord lies between the axillary artery and vein, and the posterior cord can be hidden deep to an axillary artery acoustic shadow. In addition, the medial cord can be posterior or even slightly cephalad to the axillary artery. It is important to realize that there is a great deal of individual anatomic variation in the cord location around the artery. The nerve structures now appear hyperechoic, rather than hypoechoic as seen more proximally, presumably because of an increase in the number of fascicles and amount of (hyperechoic-appearing) connective tissue.[90]
■ Needling: The skin is infiltrated with local anesthetic. A 5- to 9-cm, 18- to 22-gauge insulated needle, if using NS, is used for single-shot technique; a 9-cm, 17- to 20-gauge needle is suitable for catheter placement. Using an IP

needle alignment will be most suitable in most cases; the block needle is inserted cephalad to the probe. It is then advanced caudally and posteriorly at approximately 30 degrees to the skin. The cords should be reached at a depth of 4 to 6 cm, similar to blind technique.[119] It is recommended to combine US with NS for accurate nerve localization (e.g., musculocutaneous nerve or specific cord) because of the high variability of cord location.
■ Local anesthetic spread: Aim to place the needle and local anesthetic posterior to the axillary artery next to the posterior cord (spread from this location is most optimal for complete block success). Performing a test dose with D5W is recommended prior to local anesthetic application to visualize spread and confirm nerve localization. Inject 20 to 25 mL of local anesthetic around the posterior cord. If local anesthetic spread is deemed inadequate to surround all cords, reposition the needle prior to injecting any additional local anesthetic.

Comments
■ In the past, numerous techniques were developed with modifications to localize nerves and avoid vessel and pleural punctures. Real-time guidance with US will address some of these issues, although US-guided blocks are going through a rapid development process to determine the safest and most successful approaches.
■ Techniques that incorporate multiple injections may be easier and potentially safer under combined US and NS guidance, which provides direct visualization of the anatomic structures.
■ If a catheter is to be threaded, the aim should be to elicit motor responses in the hand itself. The tip of the Tuohy needle (9 cm, 17 to 20 gauge) should be directed laterally to allow the catheter to run in the direction of the nerves.
■ As compared with blocks at more proximal locations, the infraclavicular block has the advantage of lower risk of blocking the phrenic nerve or stellate ganglion. However, in some cases, continuous catheters may lie along one cord and fail to provide complete anesthesia and analgesia of the entire brachial plexus with small-volume infusions. This may often be overcome to some degree by intermittent boluses of larger volumes of local anesthetic.
■ Vessel puncture is a potential complication; therefore, frequent aspiration should be performed. The lateral needle insertion will help avoid the risk of pneumothorax.

FIGURE 38-18. Ultrasound-guided axillary block using an in-plane needle alignment to a linear high-frequency probe. Typically, the block needle is advanced in sequence to reach each of the median, ulnar, and radial nerves.

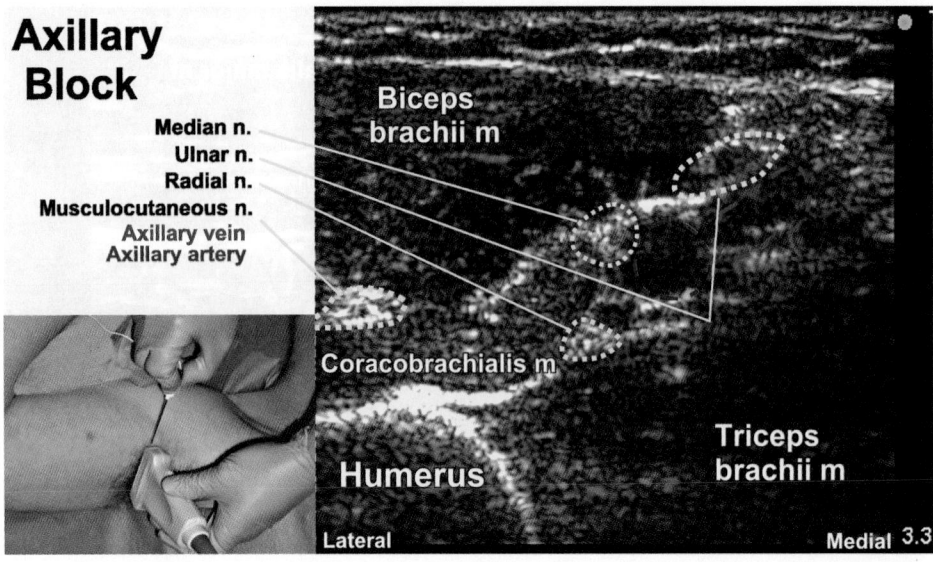

4. Axillary Block, The nerves targeted for the axillary block course distally with the axillary artery and vein along the humerus from the apex of the axilla (Fig. 38-13). This block is useful for surgery of the elbow, forearm, and hand. The ulnar, median, and radial nerves are the primary targets; the musculocutaneous nerve often leaves the plexus (via the lateral cord) proximal to this point and may be blocked separately during the axillary block (in the coracobrachialis muscle) or separately at midhumeral locations (along its diagonal course through or beyond the coracobrachialis muscle). Relative to the third part of the axillary artery, this is the usual course of the terminal nerves: the median nerve lies anterior and medial, the ulnar nerve lies posterior and medial, the musculocutaneous nerve lies anterior and lateral, and the radial nerve lies posterior and lateral. Because of the observation that the single sheath may be broken up into separate compartments by fascial septa surrounding individual nerves in the axilla, some advocate that local anesthetic should be injected at multiple sites in the axilla in contrast to the single injections possible with proximal approaches. The patient is positioned supine with the arm abducted at 70 to 80 degrees and externally rotated, the elbow flexed at 90 degrees, and the dorsum of the hand facing the table.

Procedure Using Nerve Stimulation Technique

- Landmarks: The axillary artery is marked as high in its course in the axilla as is practical. It is usually felt in the intramuscular groove between the coracobrachialis and the triceps muscles. It also passes between the insertions of the pectoralis major and the latissimus dorsi muscles on the humerus.
- Needling: A 3.5- to 5-cm, 22-gauge insulated needle is suitable for this block. After aseptic preparation, a skin wheal is raised over the proximal portion of the artery. The index and middle fingers of the nondominant hand straddle the artery just below this point, both localizing the pulsation and compressing the neurovascular bundle below the intended site of injection. The needle is inserted in a slight cephalad direction, in a two-step, four-injection process with puncture at locations just superior and inferior to the artery.
- Nerve localization: With NS technique, ideally, the nerves serving the area of proposed surgery are sought first. The median and the musculocutaneous nerves lie on the supe-

rior aspect of the artery (as viewed by the operator), whereas the ulnar and radial nerves lie below and behind the vessel. Obtaining a direct musculocutaneous nerve response (elbow flexion) indicates localization of this particular nerve, but not necessarily all nerves.
- Injection: Experience has shown that a multiple-injection technique around each individual nerve is the most reliable approach (10 to 15 mL at each nerve location); it may require less volume but the minimum required dose/volume per nerve is not known at this time.

Procedure Using Ultrasound Imaging

- Scanning: High-frequency, linear probes are generally recommended (10 to 15 MHz) for imaging because the nerves are superficial (1 to 2 cm) below the skin (Fig. 38-18). The most proximal location at the apex of the axilla may be the best for viewing all of the terminal branches of the brachial plexus. The probe is positioned perpendicular to the anterior axillary fold and in cross-section to the humerus at the bicipital sulcus (and at the level of the axillary pulse) to capture the transverse, or short-axis, view of the neurovascular bundle.
- Appearance: In cross-section:
  - The biceps brachii and coracobrachialis muscles are seen laterally; the triceps brachii muscle is medially, deeper than the biceps brachii muscle
  - The anechoic and circular axillary artery lies centrally, adjacent to both the biceps brachii and coracobrachialis muscles; it is surrounded by the nerves
  - The nerves appear round-to-oval in short axis; generally they appear as hyperechoic masses because of the large amount of connective tissue (epi- and perineurium) interspersed within the hypoechoic nerve fascicles
  - The *median* nerve is often located superficial and between the artery and biceps brachii muscle; the *ulnar* nerve is usually located medial and superficial to the artery; the *radial* nerve lies deep to the artery at the midline (clockwise: median, ulnar, radial, but there are many variations)
  - The *musculocutaneous* nerve is commonly located in the hyperechoic plane between the biceps brachii and coracobrachialis muscles
- Needling: A 5-cm, 22-gauge insulated (combined US and NS technique is recommended) needle is suitable. Both IP and OOP needle approaches can be used for axillary

block. An OOP approach, with the needle distal to the probe and in transverse axis to the nerve, is similar to the traditional blind procedure, except that the needle will be aligned at an angle to optimize needle visibility rather than more perpendicular to the skin. Using an angle of 30 to 45 degrees from the skin, with the needle placed approximately 1 to 2 cm caudally to the probe may allow optimal needle visibility (see the description of the walk-down technique in "Common Techniques: Nerve Stimulation and Ultrasound Imaging").[34,36] The IP approach involves inserting the needle at an acute angle (20 to 30 degrees) to the skin in a lateral-to-medial direction (Fig. 38-18). Typically, the block needle is advanced to contact the median nerve. It is then crossed over the axillary artery to contact the ulnar nerve superficially and then finally behind the artery to the deeper radial nerve. Follow the NS procedure if using this technique.

- Local anesthetic spread: Performing a test dose with D5W is recommended prior to local anesthetic application to visualize spread and confirm nerve localization. A proper injection is indicated by fluid spread completely around the nerve structure, with nerve movement away from the needle tip. Improper injection, such as injection outside the sheath, is indicated by a partial asymmetrical fluid expansion not immediately adjacent to the nerve structure.

Comments

- Although the multiple-injection NS technique has been used extensively for this and other blocks, it is important to consider that some spread of the local anesthetic solution will occur and hypesthesia can occur in an unpredictable fashion, limiting the identification of subsequent nerves.
- If forearm anesthesia is required and the musculocutaneous nerve was not localized previously, supplementary anesthesia of the musculocutaneous nerve should be attained using some reliable means of nerve localization (i.e., NS and/or US guidance) rather than blind injection into the coracobrachialis muscle. US imaging 1 to 2 cm distal to the axillary block location can clearly identify the muscle and usually the nerve.
- Intercostobrachial and medial antebrachial cutaneous nerve blocks can be achieved by subcutaneous injections (5 mL) on the medial surface of the upper arm all the way from the biceps to triceps muscles.
- Perivascular infiltration and transarterial approaches are also described for axillary block.
- For continuous nerve blocks, a catheter can be threaded centrally after nerve localization. A 17- to 18-gauge needle is required to facilitate catheter placement. Securing the catheter in the axilla may be challenging and may require a short tunnel to stabilize the catheter.
- Axillary approaches to the brachial plexus are associated with minimal complications compared with more proximal brachial plexus blocks. Neuropathy from needle puncture or intraneural injection of local anesthetic is the foremost consideration, although this may be reduced with US imaging and careful attention to injection pressures during the block. Hematoma can occur if the axillary artery is punctured, but this is self-limiting complication.

Terminal Upper Extremity Nerve Blocks. PNBs in the upper extremity are of particular value as rescue blocks to supplement incomplete surgical anesthesia and to provide long-lasting selective analgesia in the postoperative period. The peripheral nerves may be individually blocked at midhumeral, elbow, or wrist locations, depending on the specific nerve. If using US guidance, the elbow and forearm regions appear to be the

most suitable block regions and blocks at these sites may improve the accuracy of nerve localization and local anesthetic spread. The wrist is highly populated with tendons and fascial tissues (e.g., flexor and extensor retinaculae), which can be difficult to distinguish from, and may obscure the images of, the nerves. With the help of color Doppler, US can be used to clearly identify the nerves at many desirable locations as they are often situated near blood vessels (Table 38-1). This section will focus on those blocks where NS and US imaging are most amenable, but will comment on nerve blocks at the wrist for completion. Block of the musculocutaneous nerve at the midhumeral level is discussed in the section on axillary block. Figures 38-13 and 38-14 illustrate the courses and cutaneous innervation of the terminal nerves of the upper extremity.

1. Radial nerve can be blocked at the anterosuperior aspect of the lateral epicondyle of the humerus. The radial nerve supplies the posterior compartments of the arm and forearm including skin and subcutaneous tissues. It also supplies skin on the posterior aspect of the hand laterally near the base of the thumb and the dorsal aspect of the index and the lateral half of the ring finger up to the distal interphalangeal crease. The patient is positioned supine with the arm slightly abducted and laterally rotated and with the elbow extended.

Procedure Using Nerve Stimulation Technique

- Landmarks: A line is drawn on the anterior elbow between the medial and lateral epicondyles of the humerus. The radial nerve is located beneath this intracondylar line, approximately 1 to 2 cm lateral to the biceps tendon. This position should be marked with an X.
- Needling: A 3.5- to 5-cm, 22- to 24-gauge insulated needle is used and a skin wheal is raised at the X. The needle is then inserted perpendicular to the plane passing through the humeral epicondyles.
- Nerve localization: The correct response to radial NS at this location is extension (dorsiflexion) of the wrist and digits on the operative side. Elbow extension should not be elicited as the branch to the long head of the triceps has branched off proximally.
- Injection: Approximately 5 mL of local anesthetic is injected under low pressure.

Procedure Using Ultrasound Imaging

- Scanning: A linear probe in the frequency range of 5 to 10 MHz is suitable for scanning in most cases (Fig. 38-19). The radial nerve can first be located proximally at the level of the spiral (radial) groove of the humerus where it lies immediately adjacent the humerus and posteromedial to the deep brachial (profunda brachii) artery of the arm. The patient's arm should be internally rotated and placed with the hand over the abdomen on the opposite side of the body. The spiral groove lies immediately distal and posterior to the deltoid tubercle. Subsequent tracing of the nerve from this humeral location to the anterolateral elbow may facilitate its precise localization. The probe can be rotated slowly to scan the nerve both in the longitudinal and transverse planes at the elbow for confirmation of its location.
- Appearance: At the spiral groove of the humerus, the humerus is quite superficial and appears deep to the hypoechoic triceps brachii muscle as a clearly demarcated hyperechoic oval shape with dark shadowing in its interior (not shown in Fig. 38-19). The nerve appears oval and predominantly hyperechoic; it is located in the posterior aspect of the humerus and immediately adjacent to the small, pulsatile deep brachial (profunda brachii) artery (as verified with Doppler). At a point just proximal to the anterior compartment of the elbow, the

FIGURE 38-19. Ultrasound-guided radial nerve block using an out-of-plane needle alignment to a linear probe at the anterolateral elbow. The ideal placement will be a few centimeters above the elbow, where the nerve has not yet divided into superficial and deep branches.

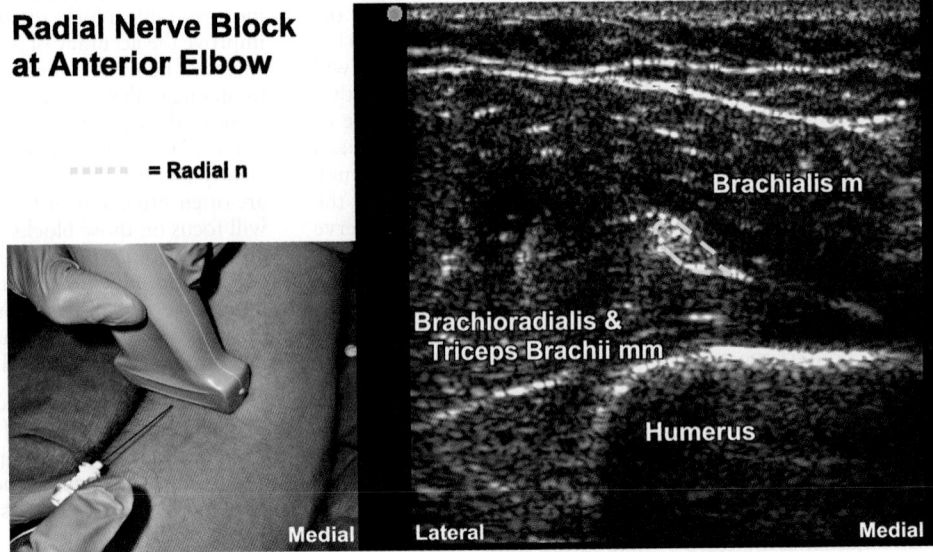

Radial Nerve Block at Anterior Elbow

----- = Radial n

humerus has changed in shape and appears smaller and almost rectangular in cross-section. The hyperechoic radial nerve now lies at some distance from the humerus and is sandwiched between the brachialis and brachioradialis muscles; it remains oval in shape.

- Needling: A 3.5- to 5-cm, 22-gauge insulated needle is suitable if using NS. The needle can be aligned both IP and OOP (Fig. 38-19) to the probe to block the nerve at the anterosuperior aspect of the lateral epicondyle of the humerus. The nerve should be blocked slightly above the elbow because it divides into deep and superficial branches approximately 2 cm above that site. The block needle is advanced to approach the target nerve on its side, preferably avoiding direct needle contact with the nerve.
- Local anesthetic spread: Performing a test dose with D5W is recommended prior to local anesthetic application to visualize spread and confirm nerve localization. The aim is to inject approximately 5 mL of local anesthetic and see spread around the nerve circumferentially.

Comments
- Needle contact with the humerus indicates that the needle is too deep, while deep needle penetration without bone contact indicates that the needle is lateral to the humerus (beyond the bone).
- The radial nerve can be blocked at the wrist or even lateral distal forearm adjacent to the radial artery. At the wrist, 3 mL of solution is injected into the anatomic "snuffbox" formed by the tendons of the extensor pollicis longus and extensor pollicis brevis tendons. A subcutaneous wheal is then raised from this point, extending over the dorsum of the wrist 3 to 4 cm onto the back of the hand. This approach is suboptimal for most procedures because the nerve divides immediately beyond the elbow and continues as the superficial radial (sensory) and the deep posterior interosseous (motor) nerves.

2. Median nerve can be blocked at the midline of the anterior elbow or at the mid-to-distal aspect of the anterior forearm (Fig. 38-20). The nerve is located adjacent (medial) to the brachial artery at the elbow, facilitating its localization here. In the forearm, the nerve can be located at its position lateral to the ulnar nerve. The nerve supplies the skin, anteriorly, on the medial surface of the thumb, palm, and digits two through four and posteriorly on the distal third

of the second through forth digits. It causes flexion at the metacarpophalangeal joints and extension at the interphalangeal joints of digits two and three. The nerve innervates muscles, which produce flexion and opposition of the thumb, middle and index fingers, and pronation and flexion of the wrist. For blocks at the anterior wrist or anterior distal forearm, the patient's arm should be positioned next to the torso, with the elbow flexed slightly and the hand free to allow a wrist or thumb flexion response elicited by NS.

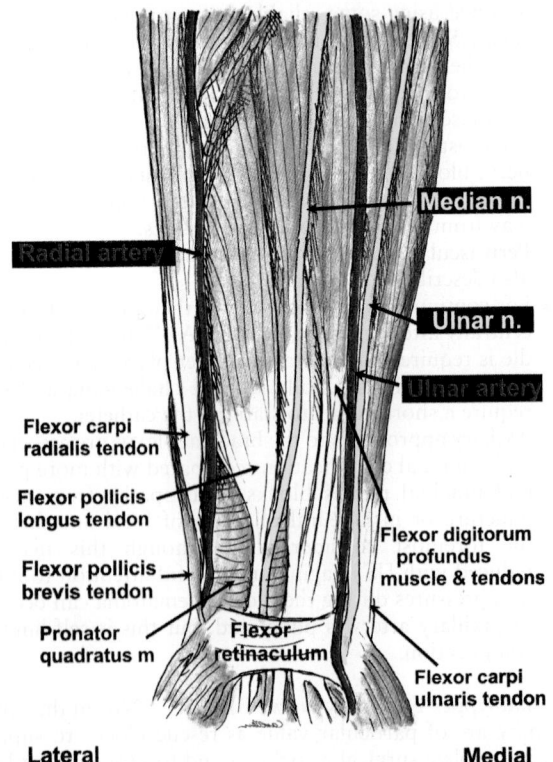

FIGURE 38-20. An illustration of the anterior forearm showing the courses of the median and ulnar nerves. The ulnar artery is a reliable landmark to localize the ulnar nerve when using ultrasound imaging.

Procedure Using Nerve Stimulation Technique at the Elbow
- Landmarks: The same intracondylar line is drawn as with the radial nerve block, and the nerve is located where this line crosses the pulsation of the brachial artery, usually 1 cm to the ulnar side of the biceps brachii tendon.
- Needling: Using a 3- to 5-cm insulated needle, a skin wheal is raised at the point designated with landmarking (above) and the needle is introduced perpendicularly at this point.
- Nerve localization: Nerve responses to electrical stimulation are sought immediately adjacent to the artery. The optimal NS response for median nerve block at the elbow location is any one of the following or a combination thereof: flexion and opposition of the thumb, middle and index fingers, flexion of the wrist, and pronation of the forearm.
- Injection: Injection of 5 mL of local anesthetic should suffice for blocking this nerve. Care should be taken to avoid intravascular and intraneural injection.

Procedure Using Nerve Stimulation Technique in the Forearm. It may be difficult to blindly locate this nerve in the forearm using NS, although the technique of transcutaneous electrical stimulation,[17] or similarly percutaneous electrode guidance,[18,120] can be used to locate the nerve using a probe placed on or indenting the skin's surface. Once the nerve has been localized, an insulated needle is inserted perpendicular to the plane of the forearm and NS responses are sought. A similar volume of local anesthetic should suffice.

Procedure Using Ultrasound Imaging (Elbow and Forearm)
- Scanning: A high-frequency (10 to 15 MHz) linear probe can be used to capture a transverse view of the nerve and localize the brachial artery (1) at the elbow where the nerve lies medial to both the artery and then the tendon of the biceps brachii muscle (Fig. 38-21), and (2) in the anterolateral forearm where it lies lateral to the ulnar nerve and artery (localizing the ulnar nerve first will help identify the median nerve) (Fig. 38-22). Color Doppler may be used to confirm the location of these arteries.
- Appearance: At the elbow, the median nerve can be identified at approximately 1 to 2 cm depth as a hyperechoic, yet distinctly honeycomb structure, lying medial to the anechoic pulsatile brachial artery. Deep to the neurovascular structures lies the musculature of the superior aspect of the elbow (pronator teres and brachialis muscles) as a hypoechoic homogeneous mass. At the fore-

arm, the nerve appears oval-shaped and lateral to the ulnar nerve and artery.
- Needling: Both OOP and IP techniques can be used for either block location. For OOP needling at the elbow (Fig. 38-21), after adjusting the US image to have the nerve located in the middle of the screen, insert a 3.5- to 5-cm insulated needle perpendicular to the transversely placed probe at a 45- to 60-degree angle. The NS procedure should be followed if using a combined technique. The IP technique, with the needle in a medial-to-lateral direction, may be advantageous at the elbow to allow easy tracking of the needle to ensure it avoids puncturing the brachial artery.
- Local anesthetic spread: After performing a test dose with D5W, the aim is to spread approximately 5 mL of local anesthetic around the nerve in a circular fashion to avoid nerve contact and obtain complete block.

Comments
- The median nerve lies deep to the flexor retinaculum at the wrist, and there is always the potential risk of causing carpal tunnel syndrome from elevated pressure within the tunnel from the injection solution. For this reason, the elbow or forearm locations for blocking the median nerve are the more logical choices.
- At the wrist, the median nerve lies between the tendons of the palmaris longus and the flexor carpi radialis muscles. If only the palmaris longus muscle can be felt, the nerve lies just to the radial side of this tendon. A skin wheal is raised, and a needle is inserted until it pierces the deep fascia. An injection of 3 mL of local anesthetic is sufficient to produce anesthesia.
- Blood aspirated into the tubing during elbow block indicates brachial artery puncture and the needle should be reinserted after applying pressure to the puncture site; contact with the humerus indicates that the needle is too deep; localized contraction of the arm muscles (e.g., elbow flexion and/or forearm pronation) indicates stimulation of the local muscles and that the needle is also likely too deep.

3. Ulnar nerve. In the periphery, the ulnar nerve can be blocked at the elbow, forearm, or wrist. Ulnar nerve block may be used for rescue analgesia or block of the fifth digit for surgery. At the junction of the distal third and proximal two thirds of the medial forearm, the nerve is commonly located just medial to the pulsatile ulnar artery (Fig. 38-20).

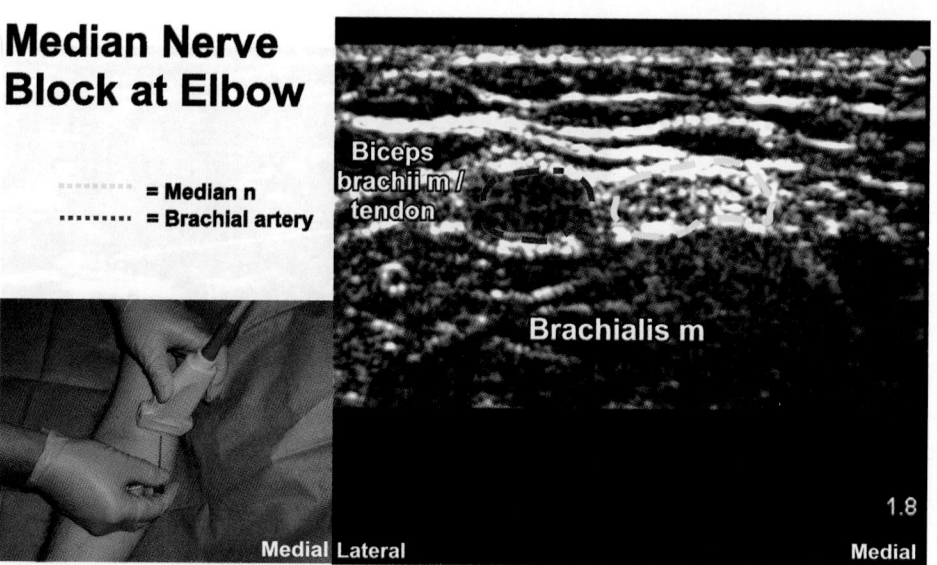

Median Nerve Block at Elbow

········· = Median n
········· = Brachial artery

Biceps brachii m / tendon

Brachialis m

1.8

Medial Lateral   Medial

FIGURE 38-21. Ultrasound-guided median nerve block using an out-of-plane needle alignment at the medial aspect of the anterior elbow. The nerve lies medial to the large anechoic brachial artery.

ANESTHETIC MANAGEMENT

US-guided technique is advised when using this block location in order to avoid the artery and localize the nerve more accurately. The ulnar nerve innervates muscles that produce flexion of the ring (fourth) and little (fifth) fingers and ulnar deviation of wrist. It supplies the skin over the medial surface (anterior and posterior) of the hand and digits four and five. The patient's arm is flexed at the elbow by 30 degrees, with the shoulder externally rotated and the forearm supinated. The forearm can rest on an armboard with an additional pillow under the wrist. Prepare the needle insertion site and skin surface with an antiseptic solution. Prepare the US probe surface by applying a sterile sheath or adhesive dressing to it prior to needling.

Procedure Using Nerve Stimulation Technique at the Elbow

■ Blocking the ulnar nerve at the elbow may be uncomfortable for patient. NS is not routinely used for localizing the ulnar nerve at the elbow as the nerve is easily located (and palpated) in the cubital tunnel (ulnar groove) between the medial epicondyle of the humerus and the olecranon process of the ulna. A small volume (1 to 4 mL) of local anesthetic should be injected if performing the block at this location.

Procedure Using Nerve Stimulation Technique in the Forearm

■ Similar to the median nerve, it may be difficult to blindly locate this nerve in the forearm using NS. Transcutaneous electrical stimulation[17] or percutaneous electrode guidance[18,19] can be used to locate the nerve. Once the nerve has been localized, an insulated needle attached to a nerve stimulator is inserted perpendicular to the plane of the forearm and appropriate motor responses are sought. The correct responses for ulnar nerve block at this location are flexion of the ring (fourth) and little (fifth) fingers and ulnar deviation of the wrist. Injection of 5 mL of local anesthetic is sufficient to block the nerve at the forearm. Combined US- and NS-guided technique provides good localization and accuracy with local anesthetic spread.

Procedure Using Ultrasound Imaging (Forearm)

■ Scanning: A high-frequency (10 to 15 MHz) linear probe is often used for this block. The probe is placed transversely just above the midforearm level to view the ulnar nerve in short axis as it approaches the ulnar artery (Fig. 38-22). It is positioned above the ulna and the belly of the flexor carpi ulnaris, on the anterior surface of the arm, rather than medially to contact the bone. The operator

scans downward slowly until the pulsatile artery and nerve are viewed adjacent to each other (Doppler may be very valuable here), and retracts the scan head slightly so the artery and nerve are separated somewhat (Fig. 38-22).

■ Appearance: The nerve in short axis is seen as a honeycomb, oval-shaped structure, including hypoechoic fascicular structures surrounded significantly by hyperechoic tissue. The adjacent ulnar artery appears anechoic and is roughly similar in size to the nerve and lateral to it. The median nerve may be seen at the lateral edge of the image and appears similar to the ulnar nerve in size and shape.

■ Needling: During IP needling, the image should be adjusted to move the image of the nerve to the most lateral edge of the screen for good visibility of the needle shaft (not shown in Fig. 38-22). A short (2- to 3-cm) needle can be used in a medial-to-lateral direction to reduce the risk of vascular puncture.

■ Local anesthetic spread: The aim is to spread approximately 5 mL of local anesthetic around the nerve in a circular fashion in order to avoid nerve contact but obtain a complete block. The local anesthetic injection will appear as an expansion of hypoechogenicity surrounding the nerve, which may separate the nerve from the artery.

Comments

■ During the elbow block, direct injection after eliciting a paresthesia or directly into the groove under pressure is not advised because of the risk of damage to the nerve. Small volumes (3 to 5 mL) of local anesthetic should be used.

■ During nerve block in the forearm, blood withdrawal into the tubing suggests ulnar artery puncture and the needle should be reinserted after holding pressure. Contact with the ulna indicates that the needle is too deep.

■ US imaging facilitates the unique approach of blocking the ulnar nerve in the forearm. This technique may reduce complications such as ulnar nerve neuritis or neurapraxia when compared with blocks at the cubital tunnel behind the medial epicondyle.

■ A linear or curved array US probe with a small footprint (26 mm; for example a "hockey stick" probe) may be used. This size probe is helpful for easy manipulation on the forearm and for good alignment of the needle using IP technique.

■ At the wrist, the ulnar nerve lies between the ulnar artery and the tendon of the flexor carpi ulnaris muscle. A skin wheal is raised at the level of the styloid process on the palmar side of the forearm between these two landmarks.

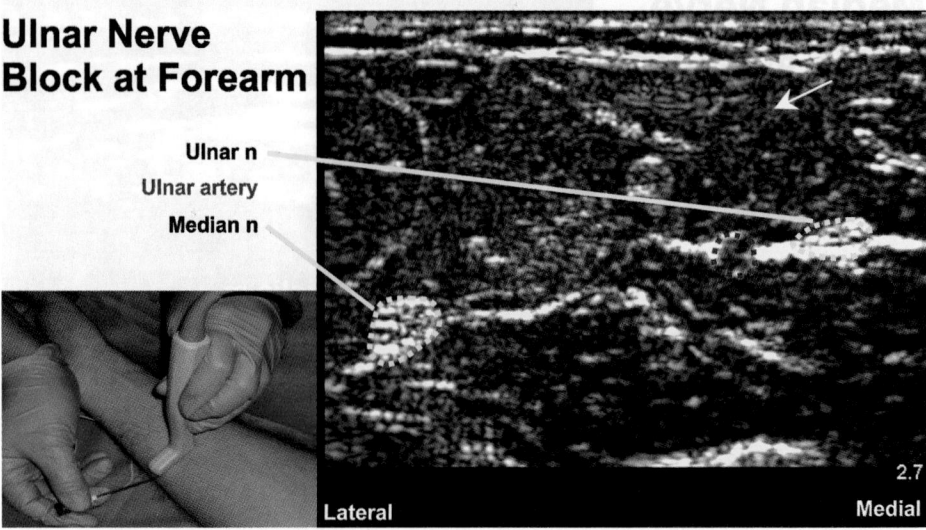

FIGURE 38-22. Ultrasound-guided ulnar nerve block in the middistal forearm using an in-plane needle alignment to a small footprint linear ("hockey stick") probe. The ideal block location, thereby avoiding arterial puncture, is where the nerve has yet to fully approach the ulnar artery.

Ulnar Nerve Block at Forearm

Ulnar n
Ulnar artery
Median n

2.7

Lateral   Medial

A small-gauge needle is inserted, and 3 mL of solution is injected into the area, with or without paresthesias.

Intravenous Regional Anesthesia (Bier Block).

Without using NS or US, arm anesthesia can be provided by the injection of local anesthetic into the venous system below an occluding tourniquet.

Procedure

- A small-gauge (20 or 22) intravenous catheter is inserted and taped on the dorsum of the hand in the arm to be blocked. A heparin lock or small syringe is attached and saline is injected to maintain patency. A pneumatic tourniquet is applied over the upper arm. The tourniquet pressure should be set to 2.5 times the systolic blood pressure. The tourniquet should be inflated to confirm that the pressure is sufficient to occlude distal arterial blood flow and deflated prior to starting the block.
- The arm is elevated to promote venous drainage. An Esmarch bandage is then wrapped tightly around the limb from distal to proximal to produce further exsanguination. After exsanguination, the tourniquet is inflated to 300 mm Hg or 2.5 times the patient's systolic blood pressure and is again tested for adequate occlusion of the distal radial pulse.
- The arm is returned to the horizontal position, a 50-mL syringe with 0.5% lidocaine is attached to the previously inserted cannula, and the contents are injected slowly. The forearm discolors, and the patient perceives a transient "pins and needles" sensation and warmth as anesthesia ensues over the following 5 minutes. Epinephrine should not be added to the local anesthetic solution.
- For short procedures, the cannula can be removed at this point. If surgery may extend beyond 1 hour, the cannula can be left in place and reinjected after 90 minutes.
- Beyond 45 minutes of surgery, many patients experience discomfort at the level of the tourniquet. Special "double-cuff" tourniquets are available for this block to alleviate this problem. The distal cuff is inflated first, followed by the proximal cuff. The distal cuff is then deflated, allowing anesthesia to be induced in the area under the distal cuff. If discomfort ensues, the distal cuff is inflated over the anesthetized area of skin, and the uncomfortable proximal cuff is released. This step is critical because the major risk of this procedure is premature release of the local anesthetic solution into the circulation. If a double cuff is used, both cuffs should be tested before starting and the proper sequence for inflation and deflation meticulously followed. The potential for leakage of anesthetic into the circulation is greater with the narrower cuffs used in the double setup. Because the shifting process also increases the potential for unintentional release of anesthetic, the use of a single, wider cuff may be better for short procedures.
- If surgery is completed in <20 minutes, the tourniquet is left inflated for at least that total period of time. If 40 minutes has elapsed, the tourniquet can be deflated as a single maneuver. Between 20 and 40 minutes, the cuff can be deflated, reinflated immediately, and finally deflated after 1 minute to delay the sudden absorption of anesthetic into the systemic circulation, although this may not truly lower the eventual peak plasma local anesthetic levels achieved.
- Duration of anesthesia is minimal beyond the time of tourniquet release. Although bupivacaine may produce a slight prolongation of analgesia, the cardiotoxicity of systemic levels of bupivacaine makes this drug contraindicated for a Bier block.

Comments

- The simplicity of this technique is offset by the potentially significant risk of systemic local anesthetic toxicity if the tourniquet fails or is released prematurely. Careful testing of the tourniquet and slow injection of solution into a peripheral (not antecubital) vein will reduce the chance of leakage under the tourniquet. Systemic blood levels are time-dependent, and careful attention should be paid to the sequence of tourniquet release and to patient monitoring during this period. A separate intravenous site for injection of resuscitation drugs is needed as well as ready availability of all appropriate resuscitative equipment. With careful attention to these details, this technique is one of the most effective and reliable available to the anesthesiologist.

Trunk Blocks

Anesthesia of the abdomen and chest is often most simply obtained with spinal and epidural injections of local anesthetics, but peripheral block of the spinal nerves in the paravertebral space or of the intercostal or inguinal nerves is quite suitable for many uses. Peripheral nerve blocks are particularly relevant when either a narrower band of anesthesia (intercostal or paravertebral) or when reduced motor block is preferable. Additionally, epidural injection may be hazardous because of the presence of infection or coagulopathy. Epidural anesthesia also carries concerns of systemic hypotension and epidural hematoma, which can limit its use for some patients.[121] In many clinical situations, it may be desirable to use intercostal blocks to separate anesthesia of the somatic and sympathetic fibers that occurs in combination when neuraxial blocks are performed. The sympathetic nerves separate from their somatic counterparts early in their course, which makes independent somatic and sympathetic blockade a practical consideration. Likewise, although paravertebral blocks may result in both somatic and sympathetic block, hemodynamic responses are often less than from epidural block. Sympathetic blocks are commonly performed at the major ganglia, particularly the stellate, celiac, and lumbar plexus. These blocks often require multiple injections and are technically more difficult than axial anesthesia, but they offer advantages in certain clinical situations. These blocks are not considered here, and the reader is referred to Chapter 56.

Ilioinguinal and iliohypogastric nerve blocks are used for procedures in the inguinal area, including hernia repair and orchidopexy. A separate block from that of the lumbar plexus is required because these nerves exit the plexus more cranially (L1 to L2) than those nerves targeted by the lumbar plexus block (L3 to L5). Transversus abdominis plane block[122,123] and rectus sheath block[124,125] can also be performed for abdominal, umbilical, or other midline surgical procedures and are often performed bilaterally. The approaches to the rectus sheath aim to block the terminal branches of the 9th, 10th, and 11th intercostal nerves within the rectus sheath. Ideally, the injection is between the posterior rectus sheath and the rectus abdominus muscle. The transversus abdominis plane block aims to block the innervation of the abdominal wall up to the level of T8 by injecting local anesthetic between the transversus abdominis and internal oblique muscles. Because the peritoneum is immediately beyond the posterior rectus sheath and transversus abdominis muscle, these two blocks have not been widely used. However, US imaging has been explored with success for these blocks.[126] Although promising, these blocks are not well established and are not described further here.

Traditionally, these blocks are performed blindly, with either sole use of landmarks, including a loss of resistance to needle penetration of the costotransverse ligament for paravertebral block, or a combined landmark and NS stimulation technique. US imaging may be beneficial for these blocks, particularly paravertebral block, in order to facilitate landmark localization. For example, preprocedural scanning can identify the tips of the transverse processes in order to identify correct needle insertion site. US may be particularly useful for performing blocks in obese patients (where the depth of needle insertion will be modified) or those with anatomic variation (e.g., scoliosis). This section provides a detailed description of the technique using NS guidance, also provides illustrations in the sections on paravertebral and inguinal blocks of US imaging prior to block performance.

Clinical Anatomy

An overview of the anatomy of the spinal nerves is described in "Upper Extremity, Clinical Anatomy." The dermatomal innervation of the thoracic and lumbar nerves is illustrated in Figure 38-7.

Orientation of the Vertebral Body Processes.   There are variations to the anatomy of the vertebral column that should be considered when determining the desired location for needle insertion for blocks of the trunk.

- The spinous processes lie in the midline, with T7 at the distal tips of the scapulae and L4 at the level of the iliac crests.
- The transverse processes approximately 2.5 cm lateral to the spinous processes: at T1, the transverse process is directly lateral to its corresponding spinous process but subsequent transverse processes are extended to increasingly cephalad locations (i.e., T7 transverse process is lateral to T6 spinous process).
- In the lumbar region, the spinous processes are straight, and the transverse processes lie opposite their own respective spinous process.

Paravertebral Space.   The paravertebral space is a bilateral wedge-shaped space between the individual vertebrae, on either side of and extending the entire length of the vertebral column. The spinal nerves pass through this space, giving off their sympathetic branch and also a small dorsal sensory branch after exiting from the intervertebral foramina. In the thoracic region, its boundaries are as follows:

- Medially it consists of the vertebral body, intervertebral disc and foramen, and spinous processes (angulation decreases from T1 to L4-5);
- Anterolaterally it is the parietal pleura; and
- Posteriorly lies the costotransverse process, approximately 2.5 cm from the tip of the spinous process, often in a slightly caudal orientation.

The intervertebral foramina at each level lie between the transverse processes and approximately 1 to 2 cm anterior to the plane formed by the transverse processes in their associated fasciae. At this point, the sympathetic ganglia lie close to the somatic nerves, and coincidental sympathetic blockade is usually attained.

Intercostal Nerves and Articulations
1. Intercostal Nerves.

- At the thoracic level, the anterior primary rami enter a neurovascular bundle with its respective artery and vein and travel along the intercostal groove along the ventral caudad surface of each rib.
- The fasciae of the internal and external intercostal muscles provide interior and external borders of this intercostal groove.
- As the intercostal nerves travel beyond the midaxillary line, they give off a lateral sensory branch while the main

trunk continues on to the anterior abdominal wall to provide sensory and motor innervation for the trunk and abdomen down to the level of the pubis.
- The intercostal groove becomes much less well defined anterior to the midaxillary line, and the nerve begins to move away from its protected position. The lowermost intercostal nerve (subcostal, the 12th) is much less closely applied to its accompanying rib and is not as easy to identify and anesthetize using a classic intercostal blockade technique.

2. Costovertebral Articulations. The ribs articulate through two synovial joints with the vertebral column, each enclosed in fibrous capsules that are reinforced by ligaments:

- *Costovertebral joint* is a synovial articulation of the head of the rib with the demifacets on the adjacent thoracic vertebral bodies and the corresponding intervertebral disc of the upper vertebral joint (except for 1st, 10th–12th ribs, which articulate with a single vertebral facet).
- *Costotransverse joint* is a synovial joint between the articular facets on the tubercles of the ribs and the transverse processes of the thoracic vertebrae (the 11th and 12th ribs lack this articulation because they do not possess tubercles). Penetration of the costotransverse ligament may occur during paravertebral block.

Lumbar Spinal Nerves and Plexus.   The spinal nerves at the lumbar level follow the same course as those of the thoracic level when leaving the intervertebral foramen, yet the anterior (ventral) rami form the lumbar plexus instead of continuing as intercostal nerves. The lumbar plexus (Fig. 38-23) is formed by the union of the anterior primary rami of L1-3 and part of L4.

- The upper nerve roots emerge from their foramina into a compartment lined by the fasciae of muscles anterior and posterior to it. In this case, the quadratus lumborum is posterior, while the posterior fascia of the psoas muscle provides the anterior border of the compartment before the nerves move into the body of the muscle.
- The lumbar plexus supplies the skin and muscles of the lower part of the anterior abdominal wall (including the external genitalia) and the skin and muscles of the anterior and medial compartments of the thigh. L1 bifurcates into an *upper* part (iliohypogastric and ilioinguinal nerves) and *lower* part, which joins with a branch from L2 to form the genitofemoral nerve. L3, with portions of L2 and L4, divides into *anterior* and *posterior divisions*: the anterior division forms the obturator (L2-4) and accessory obturator (L3-4, when present) nerves and the posterior division forms the lateral (femoral) cutaneous nerve of the thigh (L2-3) and the femoral nerve (L2-4).
- In anatomic relation to the psoas major muscle, the obturator (L2-4) and accessory obturator nerves emerge from its medial border; the genitofemoral (L1-2) pierces the muscle to lie on its anterior surface; all others emerge from its lateral border.

Inguinal Nerves.   The iliohypogastric nerve penetrates the transverse abdominis muscle just above the iliac crest, supplies it, and divides into anterior and lateral cutaneous branches: (1) the anterior branch pierces and supplies the internal oblique muscle just 2 cm medial to the anterior superior iliac spine; it then courses deep to the external oblique muscle and superior to the inguinal canal and pierces the external oblique aponeurosis about 2 to 3 cm above the superficial inguinal ring, terminating subcutaneously in the skin of the suprapubic region; and (2) the lateral cutaneous branch supplies the anterolateral portion of the gluteal skin after piercing both the oblique muscles. The ilioinguinal nerve pierces and supplies the internal oblique muscle and then enters the inguinal canal, in which it

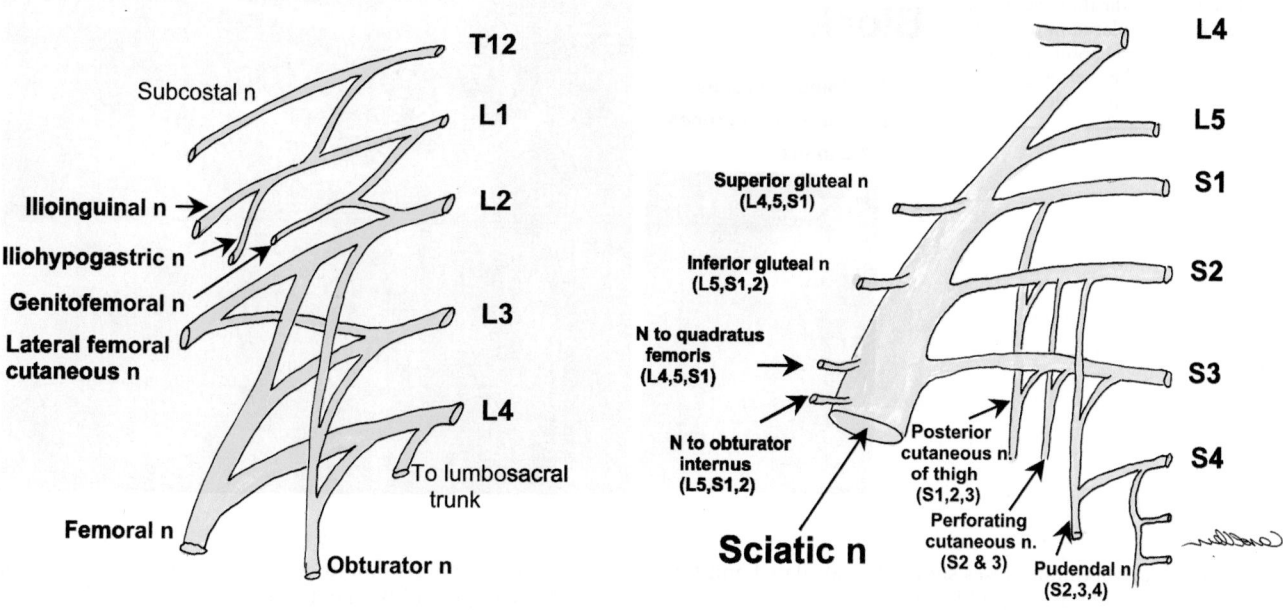

FIGURE 38-23. Lumbar (L1 through L4) and sacral (L4 through S4) plexuses.

traverses outside the spermatic cord, to emerge through the superficial (external) inguinal ring (the external oblique aponeurosis) where it provides cutaneous innervation to the skin of the scrotum (or labium majus) and adjacent thigh.

Techniques

Intercostal Nerve Blockade. Anesthesia of the intercostal nerves provides both motor and sensory anesthesia of the abdominal wall from the xiphoid to the pubis. Intercostal nerve blockade is used for various conditions of acute and chronic pain effecting the thorax and upper abdomen (e.g., postoperative analgesia after thoracotomies, various cardiac surgeries, and both open and laparoscopic cholecystectomies). It can be performed through several means, including continuous infusions into the subpleural space, through interpleural catheters, and by direct intercostal nerve block. The surgical site (i.e., intraoperative anatomic access) determines the available options.

These nerve blocks involve injections along the easily palpated sharp posterior angulation of the ribs, which occurs between 5 and 7 cm from the midline in the back. The blocks may be performed more laterally (8 to 10 cm from the midline)[127] or more medially (immediately beyond the transverse processes). The levels of T1 through T5 may be most amenable to paravertebral block because of the overlying scapula and bulky paraspinal musculature at this region. Establishing block of five or six levels of intercostal nerves is a useful anesthetic procedure for providing analgesia and motor relaxation for upper abdominal procedures such as cholecystectomy and gastric surgery. Unilateral blockade of these nerves is a useful treatment for the pain of rib fracture and also serves to reduce postoperative analgesia requirements in patients with subcostal incisions. Several segments must be blocked in each of these applications because of the overlap in supply of the intercostal nerves. This technique is also useful in reducing the pain associated with the insertion of chest tubes or percutaneous biliary drainage procedures.

For intercostal blocks, the patient may be in the lateral, sitting, or prone position. For operative anesthesia, the prone position is most practical. A pillow is placed under the abdomen to provide slight flexion of the thoracic spine. The arms are draped over the edge of the stretcher or operating table so that the scapula falls away laterally from the midline. The anesthesiologist stands at the patient's side. Most anesthesiologists prefer to stand on the side that allows their dominant hand to hold the syringe at the caudad end of the patient.

Procedure Using Landmark-Based Technique
- Landmarks: The reader is referred to the previous "Clinical Anatomy" section for descriptions of the locations of the relevant landmarks. The spinous processes in the midline from T6 through T12 are marked. The ribs are then identified along the line of their most extreme posterior angulation. The 6th and 12th ribs are marked first at their inferior borders and a line is drawn between these two points. The rest of the ribs between them are identified, and a mark is placed on the inferior border of each rib along the angled parasagittal plane identified by the first line between the 6th and 12th ribs.
- Needling: After aseptic preparation, light sedation is provided for the patient, and a skin wheal is raised at each mark on the inferior border of each respective rib. Starting with the lowest rib, the index finger of the cephalad hand retracts the skin above the identifying mark in a cephalad direction. The anesthesiologist's other hand inserts a needle (22 gauge, 3.75 cm) directly onto the rib, maintaining a constant 10-degree cephalad angulation. After contact is made with the rib, the cephalad traction is slowly released, the cephalad hand takes over the needle and syringe, and the needle is allowed to "walk" down to below the rib at the same angle. The needle is then advanced approximately 4 mm under the rib.
- Injection: Once in the groove, aspiration is performed and 3 to 5 mL of a local anesthetic solution is injected. The needling and injection procedure is repeated for each segmental level and for both sides if applicable. Because the intercostal space is highly vascularized, local anesthetics are absorbed rapidly and toxic levels of local anesthetic may be encountered when using large volumes and can quickly lead to neurologic or cardiovascular

FIGURE 38-24. Probe placement and ultrasound image during paravertebral block in the thoracic spine. The probe is first placed in the midline of the spine to capture a transverse view of the vertebral and costal (if thoracic spine) elements.

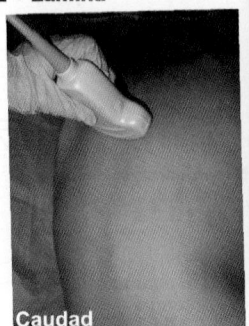

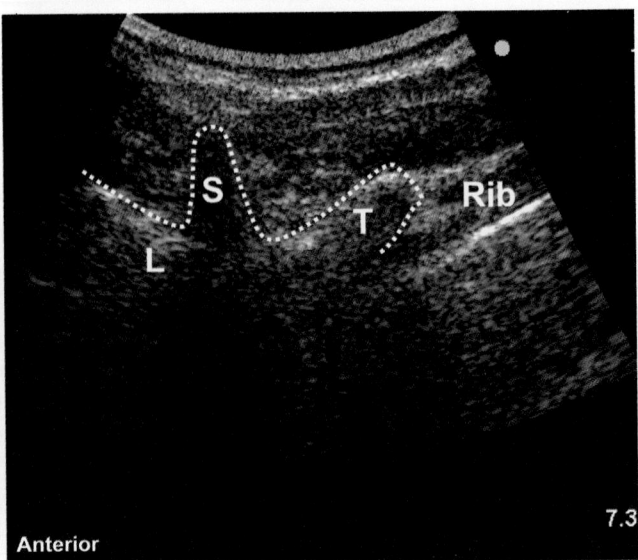

FIGURE 38-24. Probe placement and ultrasound image during paravertebral block in the thoracic spine. The probe is first placed in the midline of the spine to capture a transverse view of the vertebral and costal (if thoracic spine) elements.

Paravertebral Block

S = Spinous process
T = Transverse process
L = Lamina

sequelae. Maximum doses should be calculated and followed carefully for these blocks.

Procedure Using Ultrasound Imaging. Generally, the intercostal nerves are well localized with the blind landmark-based technique. Alternatively, the rib can be easily visualized with the use of US (Figs. 38-24 and 38-25). The remainder of the procedure will be similar to that of blind technique. If a more medial (proximal) intercostal nerve block is desired, such as to relieve the pain of herpes zoster or of proximal rib fractures, US imaging of the costotransverse joint and ribs may be helpful. The later section on paravertebral block describes and illustrates this imaging.

Comments
- Intercostal nerve blocks can be supplemented by a number of somatic paravertebral nerve blocks or sympathetic block of the celiac plexus. Care should be taken to adjust the total dose of drug in these combined techniques so that the maximal recommended amounts are not exceeded.
- The advantages with intercostal block over sole intravenous opioid use include superior analgesia, opioid sparing, improved pulmonary mechanics (including earlier extubation), reduced central nervous system depression, and avoidance of urinary retention.[127] Intercostal blocks are often used in addition to systemic analgesia (e.g., intravenous patient-controlled analgesia).
- Despite frequent concern about the incidence of pneumothorax with intercostal blocks, this complication is rare in experienced hands. This depends primarily on maintaining strict safety features of the described technique. Emphasis should be placed on absolute control of the syringe and needle at all times, particularly during injection.
- A common complication is related to the sedation required to perform this block in the prone position. Overdose can lead to airway obstruction and respiratory depression in the prone position. Attention must be paid to the patient's mental status because this block produces the highest blood levels of local anesthetics when compared with any other regional anesthetic technique. When the block is performed for postoperative pain relief, the dose should be reduced to 0.25% bupivacaine or ropivacaine to minimize the chance for toxicity.
- It is possible to produce partial spinal or epidural anesthesia if the injection is made close to the midline and the anesthetic tracks along a dural sleeve to the epidural or subarachnoid space. Respiratory insufficiency can also be seen if the intercostal muscles are blocked in a patient who depends on them for ventilation. Patients with chronic obstructive disease with ineffective diaphragm motion are not good candidates for this technique.

Paravertebral Block. This block technique is useful for segmental anesthesia, particularly of the upper thoracic segments. It is also useful if a more proximal (central) blockade than that of the intercostal nerves is needed, such as to relieve the pain of herpes zoster or of a proximal rib fracture. The thoracic paravertebral block is used for breast surgery and perioperatively for thoracic surgery. Thoracolumbar paravertebral anesthesia is commonly used for inguinal herniorrhaphy and postoperative analgesia following hip surgery. Lumbar paravertebral

FIGURE 38-25. Ultrasound images from scanning in a medial-to-lateral direction with a curved ultrasound probe placed in the longitudinal axis.

Longitudinal Scanning at Thoracic Spine

L = Lamina   A = Articular Process   T = Transverse Process   R = Rib
PS = Paravertebral Space   P = Pleural Space

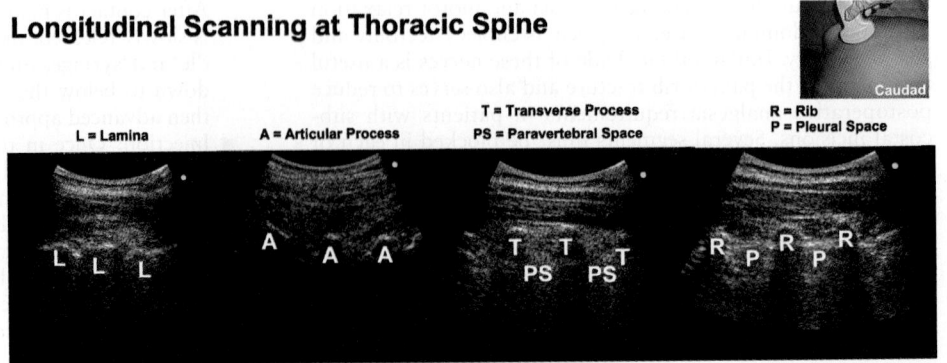

blockade has been used successfully for outpatient hernia operations, providing significant postoperative analgesia.

Single-injection paravertebral block used for surgical anesthesia has been shown to surpass general anesthesia with respect to postoperative pain relief, incidence of vomiting and pain during mobility.[128] Paravertebral blocks are considered "unilateral epidurals" because they selectively block spinal nerves on the side of anesthetic application, although they also have the potential for epidural spread (i.e., they can be bilateral if desired). The anesthesia includes both somatic and sympathetic effects, with a reduced hemodynamic response (e.g., hypotension) as compared with epidural anesthesia. This nerve block requires excellent knowledge of paravertebral anatomy, but can be easily performed with experience.

The upper five ribs are more difficult to palpate laterally, and blocks of their associated intercostal nerves is best performed with a paravertebral injection. This approach is technically more difficult and has slightly greater potential for complications because of the proximity of the lung and of the intervertebral foramina. The paravertebral block can be used at any level. At the lumbar spine, some prefer to perform lumbar plexus block to reduce the number of injections and avoid sympathetic block. The paravertebral block injection is made into the triangular paravertebral space where the spinal nerve has just left the intervertebral foramen. The nerve may be difficult to localize using bony landmarks in a blind fashion, and larger volumes of local anesthetic are often required. NS has been used to localize the nerve. US can be performed prior to the block to improve bony landmark identification, particularly for patients who have an obese habitus or a spinal deformity. However, real-time US guidance can be challenging and may offer limited additional value from preprocedural landmark identification, as the overriding bone tissue reflects the US beam and provides dorsal shadowing, which obscures imaging (especially of the needle) to the depth of the paravertebral space.

This block is performed with the patient in the lateral, sitting, or prone position, the latter using a pillow placed under the patient's abdomen to produce flexion of the thoracic and lumbar spine.

Procedure Using Nerve Stimulation or Loss-of-Resistance Technique

- Landmarks (Fig. 38-26): The paravertebral approach varies somewhat, depending on the spinal level and the respective orientation of the vertebral spinous and transverse processes (see "Clinical Anatomy"). Thus, paravertebral blocks in the upper thoracic region are performed at each level by identifying the spinous process of the vertebra above the level to be blocked; in the lumbar region, the spinous process of the level to be blocked is used to locate the transverse process. The appropriate spinous processes in the region to be blocked are marked and transverse lines are drawn across the cephalad border of the spinous processes and extended laterally to overlie the transverse process (approximately 2.5 cm). Finally, the transverse processes are marked individually or by drawing a vertical line parallel to the spine joining the ends of the transverse lines. For a diagnostic block, a single nerve may need to be anesthetized. For pain control, several levels must be identified. The injection of at least three segments (as in intercostal blockade) is required to produce reliable segmental block because of sensory overlap from multiple nerves.
- Needling: After aseptic skin preparation and patient sedation, skin wheals are raised at the marked transverse processes. A 22-gauge, 7.5-cm insulated needle is introduced through the skin wheal in the sagittal plane and directed slightly cephalad to contact the transverse process (usually at a depth of 2 to 4 cm in the thoracic region and 5 to 8 cm in the lumbar region), or oftentimes, likely the

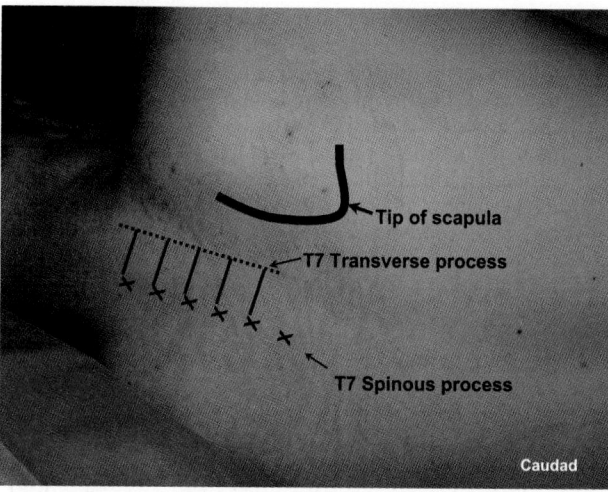

FIGURE 38-26. Landmarks for the paravertebral block at the thoracic spine. The spinous process of the level (e.g., T6) below the block (e.g., T7) is identified and a line is drawn horizontally from the cranial aspect of the spinous process to mark the transverse process. The needle is inserted at appropriate spinal levels at the lateral line marking the transverse processes.

costotransverse ligament. Gentle cephalad or caudad exploration may be required to identify the bone. The depth of the transverse process should be carefully noted on the needle shaft. The needle is now withdrawn from the transverse process to the skin level and reinserted 10 degrees superiorly (to target the spinal nerve corresponding to the spinous process) or inferiorly (corresponding to the vertebral level below the spinous process) and 1 cm deeper than the point of bone contact. The needle should be angled slightly medially to avoid causing pneumothorax. There will be a subtle "give" at the midpoint between these landmarks (spinous and transverse processes) indicating entrance into the paravertebral space.

- Nerve localization: For NS, an initial current of 2.5 to 5 mA is used and the needle is advanced until contractions of the appropriate muscles (e.g., abdominal muscles with lumbar paravertebral block) are observed, and the current intensity is then reduced to localize the nerves at 0.5 to 0.6 mA. A test dose of local anesthetic will confirm nerve localization with abolishment of the nerve response, resulting from the current dissipation at the needle tip from the conducting solution.[26] For loss of resistance, a 22-gauge Tuohy needle is used. After walking off the transverse processes, a "pop" or loss of resistance may be felt when entering the paravertebral space.
- Injection: When the needle has entered the paravertebral space, 3 to 7 mL of local anesthetic is injected after careful aspiration at each site, depending on number of sites and patient size. Attention must be paid to the total milligram dose injected. The volume required to block each level limits the concentration that can be used and the total number of levels that can be blocked. If lumbar paravertebral injections are combined with intercostal blocks, the concentration and total volume for both blocks may have to be reduced.

Procedure Using Ultrasound Imaging. Imaging for these blocks is often used before block performance (i.e., "preprocedural," "supported," or "off-line" imaging) rather than during (i.e., "real-time" or "on-line" imaging) to identify the deep bony landmarks, including the articular and transverse processes.

- Scanning: Placing the probe transversely at the midline will provide an overview of the vertebral lamina and processes, as well as costal structures if viewing the thoracic spine (Fig. 38-24). A medial-to-lateral scan using a longitudinally placed probe can then be used to locate and mark important bony landmarks (Fig. 38-25). For this, a 5 to 7 MHz curved-array US probe (lower frequency for obese patients and higher frequency linear probes for thin adult or pediatric patients) is positioned in the sagittal plane on top of the spinous processes of the target thoracic or lumbar region. Subsequent lateral scanning will allow consecutive identification of the lamina, articular and transverse processes and (in the thoracic spine) the ribs.

- Appearance: The initial transverse scan will show a hyperechoic outline of the vertebral spinous and transverse processes, the lamina, and (in the thoracic spine) associated rib. During the lateral scan with the probe placed longitudinally to the spine, the laminae will appear first, as largely overlapping linear structures. The articular processes in long axis appear as "multiple lumps" just lateral to the spinous processes and are short rectangular structures with hyperechoic lines with underlying hypoechoic bony shadowing. Moving laterally, the transverse processes appear and look similar to the articular processes; they will disappear from the view when the probe is moved beyond their tips, which can help distinguish them from the articular processes and mark the lateral block location. Beyond the transverse processes, the rib heads appear as long shadows within hyperechoic borders, deep to the linear hyperechoic muscle fibers of the paravertebral muscles. The paravertebral space lies deep to the transverse processes and the pleura can often be identified between and deep to the transverse process as well as deep to the ribs.
- Needling: Because multiple injections are generally needed to completely cover all the dermatomes of the surgical area in clinical practice, US imaging is more suitable for a preblock assessment ("supported" US) to visualize and measure the depth of needle penetration required for the needle to contact the transverse processes. Needling will be identical to that for blind technique, with the exception that the depth to the transverse process will be more accurately known. It is possible to perform real-time US guidance using either IP or OOP needle alignment. The reader is referred to the "Comments" section for advice related to important precautions when using US guidance.
- Local anesthetic spread: Local anesthetic spread will be difficult to view if using real-time guidance during this block. The overlying bones largely reflect the US beam and obstruct visibility beyond into the paravertebral space.

Comments
- Because the paravertebral space is well vascularized, inadvertent vascular puncture will often occur, which highlights the need for frequent aspiration and injection in small aliquots.[129]
- The complication of pneumothorax is more likely with a paravertebral technique than with intercostal block. The needle should be directed medially as it passes below the transverse process and never more than 2 cm beyond the transverse process. If cough or chest pain occurs, a chest radiograph should be performed to rule out pneumothorax.
- Subarachnoid injection is also more likely in the thoracic area because of the extension of the dural sleeves to the level of the intervertebral foramina. Careful aspiration is important but may not prevent the unintentional injection of local anesthetic into the subdural space. Total

spinal anesthesia can result with a 5- to 10-mL injection. Systemic toxicity is also a possibility because of the need for relatively large volumes of local anesthetic.
- If attempting real-time US guidance of paravertebral block, angulation of the needle is important to carefully observe and using an IP needle alignment to a longitudinal probe may be most prudent. The needle should not be inserted with a significant medial direction as there is a risk of spinal cord injury from intraforaminal insertion and injection. Likewise, a lateral direction bears the risk of pneumothorax. If choosing to use real time US-guidance during block procedure, please note: (1) with the probe placed in the sagittal/longitudinal plane, OOP needling may be more risky as it often requires the medial or lateral angulations previously described; and (2) an IP needling approach can be more risky when the probe is placed in the coronal/transverse plane.

Inguinal Nerve Block. This block is performed easily with blind technique, although US imaging may be performed to help improve the success rate of nerve localization and potentially reduce local anesthetic requirements and the risk of toxicity and other adverse effects.[55,130] The patient lies supine with the ipsilateral hand placed under the head.

Procedure Using Blind Technique (Single-Shot Fascial Click)
- Landmarks: The injection site is located at about 1 to 2 cm medial and 1 to 2 cm inferior to the anterior superior iliac spine.
- Needling and injection: A 25-gauge 3.75- to 5-cm needle is appropriate; a 22-gauge, 5-cm insulated needle is used if using NS. The needle is inserted from the anterior abdomen (vertically) until a fascial click is detected, presumably at the junction of the internal oblique and transverse abdominus muscles. An injection of about 10 to 15 mL local anesthetic (0.3 to 0.5 mL/kg) is performed.

Procedure Using Ultrasound Imaging.
This procedure has only been reported from studies in children.

- Scanning: Two different approaches have been used for US scanning of the ilioinguinal and iliohypogastric nerves.[55,131] In their clinical study, Willschke et al.[55] used a small footprint (hockey stick), 5 to 10 MHz probe, placed in transverse axis, just medial and superior to the anterior superior iliac spine. The cross-sectional view of the ilioinguinal nerve can be captured lying between the internal oblique and transverse abdominus muscles. In their cadaveric study, Eichenberger et al.[131] found a probe with 7.5 MHz to be superior to one having 10 MHz frequency. They used a position about 5 cm cranial and slightly posterior to the anterior superior iliac spine, where both nerves have been shown to be present between the previously mentioned muscles with a 90% probability. These authors visualized both nerves as distinct entities.
- Appearance: The nerves appear hypoechoic with many hyperechoic dots and a distinct hyperechoic rim. They have an oval, somewhat boomerang shape, and appear embedded between the fascicular hypoechoic-appearing muscles. In the more cranial position, the iliac bone may be captured, with its hyperechoic border and dorsal shadowing, on the medial aspect of the screen. The thin external oblique muscle lies superficial at the cranial position, but its even thinner component may not be visible more inferiorly.
- Needling: Both groups of authors used an OOP needling alignment, with the needle placed caudad to the probe in its center. This approach will only provide a view of the

needle tip, making good needle tracking within the tissue critical. Presumably, an IP alignment could be used as an alternative.

- Local anesthetic spread: Either one or two injections can be made, depending on the number of distinct nerves localized. The dose of local anesthetic may be lower (0.075 mL/kg has been shown effective for a single injection technique)[130] when using US imaging, as the nerves are well localized. A hypoechoic area of solution should be visualized adjacent to the nerve(s).

Comments

- The ilioinguinal and iliohypogastric nerves may exist as a common trunk at the level of the anterior superior iliac spine, which further supports the use of US guidance for localizing the single nerve.[131]
- Because there is high variability in the skin innervation from these nerves, it is impossible to confirm with clinical tests which nerve is blocked. Injecting lateral to the most laterally positioned ilioinguinal nerve, or medial to the iliohypogastric nerve, has been reported in an attempt to distinctly block these nerves.[131]
- Complications of this block are generally volume-related and include systemic toxicity and transient femoral nerve palsy.

Penile Blocks

A penile block is used in children and adults for surgical procedures of the glans and shaft of the penis. The dorsal nerves (terminal branches of pudendal nerve; S2 through S4) lie bilaterally on the outer aspect of the dorsal arteries of the penis. From the base of the penis, they divide several times and encircle the shaft of the penis before reaching the glans. This block is often performed as a circumferential infiltration of the root of the penis (ring block). Two skin wheals are raised at the dorsal base of the penis, one on each side just below and medial to the pubic spine. A 25-gauge, 3.75-cm needle is introduced on each side, and 5 mL of anesthetic (0.5 to 1 mL for infants) is deposited superficially and deep along the lower border of the pubic ramus to anesthetize the dorsal nerve. For a complete ring of infiltration, an additional 5 mL (adults) is infiltrated in the subcutaneous tissue around the underside of the shaft. A larger needle or a second injection site may be needed to complete the ring. Twenty to 25 mL of 0.75% lidocaine or 0.25% bupivacaine usually suffices in adults. Epinephrine-containing solutions should not be used to avoid compromising penile circulation.

Lower Extremity Blocks

Combined blocks of the lumbar and sciatic plexuses provide effective surgical anesthesia to the entire lower extremity. Prior to the 1990s an "anterior lumbar block" approach (aka, femoral three-in-one approach), first described by Winnie and colleagues in 1973,[132] was commonly performed, based on the assumption that a large-volume local anesthetic injection into the femoral nerve sheath would produce spread of the solution proximally to anesthetize the obturator and lateral femoral cutaneous nerves as well. Later reports of failures to obtain obturator nerve block with this approach,[133,134] however, have led to the femoral block being considered as an individual nerve block, and have advocated the posterior lumbar block approach for accessing the whole lumbar plexus.

PNB is indicated when spinal, caudal, or epidural techniques are contraindicated or when selective anesthesia of one leg or foot is needed. Because the anatomic landmarks identi-

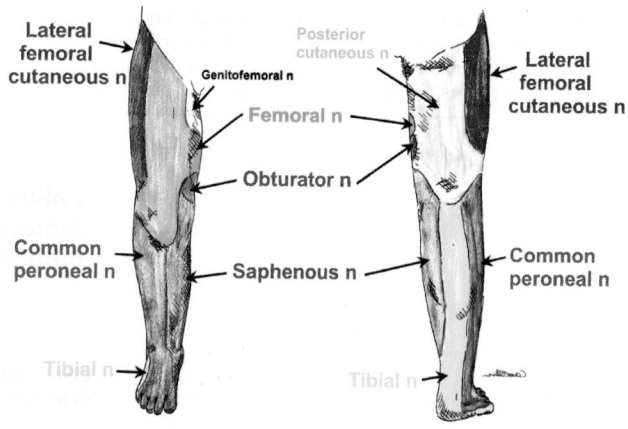

FIGURE 38-27. Cutaneous innervation from the terminal nerves of the lower extremity.

fying the fascial sheaths or compartments of the plexuses are not as clearly defined as those in the upper extremity, lower extremity blocks are often performed more distally, where the nerves have already separated into terminal branches. Thus, in addition to the fascial compartment approach (psoas block), there are peripheral approaches described at the anterior and posterior hip, knee, and ankle.

Clinical Anatomy

Together, the lumbar and sacral plexuses (Fig. 38-23) supply the lower limb. The formation of the lumbar plexus is discussed in "Trunk Block." Important landmarks that contain the plexus during its course include the psoas compartment, bordered posteriorly by the quadratus lumborum muscle and anteriorly by the posterior fascia of the psoas muscle, and more distally, the substance of the psoas major muscle. The anatomy of the terminal nerves is examined in the following section, as are the formation and branches of the sacral plexus. The cutaneous innervation in the lower extremity is shown in Figure 38-27. The lower extremity dermatomes are shown in Figure 38-8.

Terminal Nerves of the Lumbar Plexus

1. Genitofemoral nerve (L1,2). This nerve leaves the lumbar plexus at the lower border of the L3 vertebrae. It pierces and then lies anterior to the psoas major muscle, before descending subperitoneally and behind the ureter where it divides into two branches (genital and femoral), at a variable distance above the inguinal ligament. The genital branch crosses the external iliac artery and transverses the inguinal canal. It supplies the cremaster muscle and skin over the scrotum and adjacent thigh (males) or the skin over anterior part of labium majus and mons pubis (females). The femoral branch descends lateral to the external iliac artery, passes under the inguinal ligament, enters the femoral sheath lateral to the femoral artery, and pierces the anterior layer of the femoral sheath and fascia lata. It innervates the skin immediately below the crease of groin anterior to the upper part of the femoral triangle.

2. Lateral cutaneous nerve of thigh (aka, lateral femoral cutaneous nerve; L2,3). This nerve passes obliquely from the lateral border of the psoas major muscle over the iliacus to enter the thigh below or through the inguinal ligament, variably medial to the anterior superior iliac spine (Fig. 38-28). On the right side of the body, the nerve passes posterolateral to the cecum and on the left it traverses behind the lower part of the descending colon. The nerve lies on top of the sartorius muscle before dividing into anterior (supplies skin over the

FIGURE 38-28.   Illustration of the anterior thigh showing neuromuscular anatomy and block needle insertion sites (X) along the inguinal crease for the major branches of the lumbar plexus. ASIS, anterior superior iliac spine.

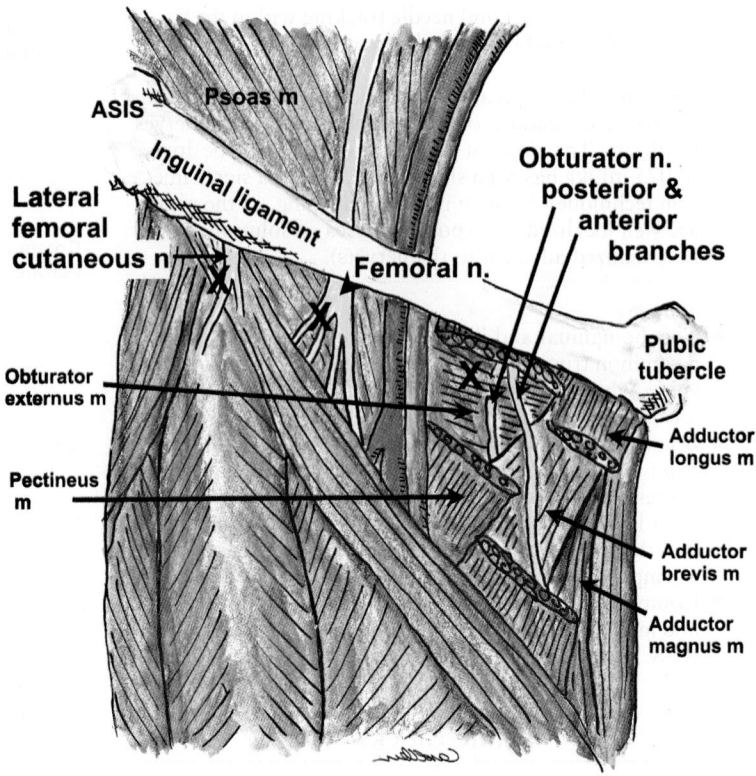

anterolateral aspect of the thigh) and posterior (supplies skin on the lateral aspect of thigh from the greater trochanter to the midthigh) branches. Occasionally, this nerve is a branch of the femoral nerve rather than its own nerve.

3. Femoral nerve (L2-4). The femoral nerve is the largest nerve of this plexus, supplying muscles and skin on the anterior aspect of the thigh. It descends through the psoas major muscle and emerges low at its lateral border, coursing inferiorly between the iliacus and psoas major muscles to enter the thigh under the inguinal ligament (Fig. 38-28). At the inguinal ligament (running between anterior superior iliac spine and the medial pubic tubercle) and just distal to it (in the femoral triangle), the nerve lies slightly deeper (0.5 to 1 cm) and lateral (approximately 1.5 cm) to the femoral artery; the vein is medial to the artery (VAN is the mnemonic for the anatomical relationship, starting medially). At the femoral (inguinal) crease (a few centimeters caudad to the inguinal ligament) the nerve lies underneath the fascia iliaca (iliopectineal fascia), deep to the fascia lata. Beyond the femoral triangle, it branches into anterior (quite proximally) and posterior divisions. The anterior division gives muscular branches to the pectineus and sartorius muscles and cutaneous branches (intermediate and medial cutaneous nerves of thigh) to the skin on the anterior aspect of the thigh. The posterior division sends muscular branches to the quadriceps femoris muscle and gives rise to the *saphenous nerve,* its largest cutaneous branch. The saphenous nerve follows the femoral artery, lying lateral to it within the adductor (Hunter, subsartorial) canal and then crossing it anteriorly to lie medial to the artery. Distal to the canal it leaves the artery to lie superficial at the medial aspect of the knee; the nerve then continues inferiorly (subcutaneously) with the long (great) saphenous vein along the medial aspect of the leg down to the tibial aspect of the ankle. The saphenous branch supplies the skin on the medial aspect of the leg below the knee and the skin on the medial aspect of the foot; it provides articular branches to the hip, knee and ankle joints.

4. Obturator nerve (L2-4). The obturator nerve emerges from the medial border of the psoas major muscle at the pelvic brim to pass behind the common iliac vessels and lateral to the internal iliac vessels. It then courses inferiorly and anteriorly along the lateral wall of the pelvic cavity on the obturator internus muscle toward the obturator canal, through which it enters the upper part of the medial aspect of the thigh above and anterior to the obturator vessels. It divides into its anterior and posterior branches near the obturator foramen (Fig. 38-28). The anterior branch passes into the thigh anterior to the obturator externus, descends in front of the adductor brevis, behind the pectineus and adductor longus muscle, with its terminal cutaneous branches emerging as it courses alongside the femoral artery. It supplies the adductor longus, gracilis, adductor brevis (usually), and pectineus (often) muscles. Its cutaneous branches supply the skin on the medial aspect of the thigh and perhaps to the medial knee. The nerve's posterior branch pierces the obturator externus muscle anteriorly and supplies it, then passes behind the adductor brevis muscle (sometimes supplies it) to descend on the anterior aspect of the adductor magnus muscle (medial to the anterior branch), which it supplies. There is no apparent cutaneous supply from this nerve. It then traverses the adductor canal with the femoral artery and vein to enter the popliteal fossa, where it terminates as an articular branch to the back of the knee joint capsule (oblique popliteal ligament).

5. Accessory obturator nerve (L3,4). This nerve is present in about 30% of individuals; it descends along the medial border of the psoas major muscle, crosses the superior pubic ramus behind the pectineus muscle, supplies it and gives articular branches to the hip joint.

Sacral Plexus: Formation and Branches.   At the medial border of the psoas major muscle, the lumbosacral trunk is formed by the union of a branch of L4 and the anterior ramus of L5. After exiting through the anterior sacral foramina, the anterior primary rami of S1-4 join the lumbosacral trunk to form the sacral plexus (Fig. 38-23). The nerves of the plexus converge toward the greater sciatic foramen anterior to the piriformis muscle on the posterior pelvic wall. The main terminal nerves are the sciatic nerve (continuation of the plexus) and the pudendal nerves (terminal branches); several other small branches are given off, including muscular branches (e.g., inferior and superior gluteal nerves and nerves to quadratus femoris, piriformis, obturator internus, and external sphincter muscles), cutaneous branches (e.g., posterior cutaneous nerve of the thigh), and visceral branches (pelvis splanchnic nerves). The gluteal vessels (superior and inferior) generally follow the course of the sacral nerves in the anterior plane and can be used to help identify the sciatic nerve at its proximal course. Additional vascular structures that may be identified under US imaging are the pudendal vessels, which pass from the greater to lesser sciatic foramen between the sciatic and pudendal nerves.

Sciatic, Tibial, and Common Peroneal Nerves. The sciatic nerve is the largest nerve of the body and is usually the conjunction of two trunks initially enveloped in a common sheath: a lateral trunk (L4 through S2), which eventually emerges as the common peroneal nerve and a medial trunk (L4 through S3), which later becomes the tibial nerve. These combined nerves exit through the sciatic notch and pass anteriorly to the piriformis muscle to then lie between the ischial tuberosity and the greater trochanter of the femur. They curve caudally and descend in the posterior thigh adjacent to the femur. At a variable distance within the posterior thigh (often high in the popliteal fossa), the sciatic nerve bifurcates into common peroneal and tibial nerves. The common peroneal nerve descends along the medial border of biceps femoris muscle and then on the lateral border of the gastrocnemius muscle. At the fossa it gives off the lateral sural nerve, which forms the lateral sural cutaneous nerve by joining the medial sural nerve supplied by the tibial nerve. It winds around the neck of the fibula and terminates as the deep and superficial peroneal nerves. In the posterior thigh, the tibial nerve is covered medially by the semitendinosus and semimembranosus muscles and laterally by the biceps femoris muscle. Beyond the knee joint, it is covered by both heads of the gastrocnemius muscle and then deep to the soleus muscle, before coming to an end on the tibialis posterior muscle and finally on the posterior surface of the tibial shaft medial to the medial malleolus. Within the fossa, it gives off muscular branches (gastrocnemius, soleus, popliteus, and plantaris muscles) as well as the medial sural nerve (to join its lateral counterpart from the common peroneal nerve). In the lower leg and foot, it gives off muscular, articular (ankle), and cutaneous branches, and terminates as medial and lateral plantar nerves. The nerve is often called the *posterior tibial nerve* in the lower leg.

Nerves at the Ankle. By the time the femoral, tibial, and common peroneal nerves reach the ankle, there are five branches that cross this joint to provide innervation for the skin and muscles of the foot.

1. Deep peroneal nerve (L5,S1). This nerve lies anterior to the tibia and interosseus membrane and lateral to the anterior tibial artery and vein at the ankle. It travels deep to and between the tendons of the extensor hallucis longus and extensor digitorum longus muscles. Beyond the extensor retinaculum it branches into medial and lateral terminal branches: the medial branch passes over the dorsum of the foot and supplies the first web space through two terminal digital branches and the lateral branch traverses laterally and terminates as the second, third, and fourth dorsal interosseus nerves.

2. Tibial nerve (aka, posterior tibial nerve; S1-3). On the posterior aspect of the knee joint, the tibial nerve joins the posterior tibial artery and then runs deep through to the lower third of the leg, where it emerges at the medial border of the calcaneal tendon (Achilles tendon). Behind the medial malleolus it lies beneath several layers of fascia and is separated from the Achilles tendon only by the tendon of the flexor hallucis longus muscle. The nerve is posteromedial to the posterior tibial artery and vein, which are in turn posteromedial to the tendons of the flexor digitorum longus and tibialis posterior muscles. Just below the medial malleolus, the nerve divides into the lateral and medial plantar nerves. The nerve innervates the ankle joint through its articular branches and the skin over the medial malleolus, the inner aspect of the heel (including Achilles tendon), and the dorsum of the foot (through the medial and lateral plantar nerves) with its cutaneous branches.

3. Superficial peroneal nerve. The superficial peroneal lies lateral to the deep peroneal nerve in the upper leg. In the anterolateral aspect of lower leg, it becomes superficial about 7 to 8 cm above the lateral malleolus and divides into medial and lateral dorsal cutaneous nerves to supply the dorsum of the foot.

4. Sural nerve. This nerve arises from tibial (medial sural nerve) and common peroneal (lateral sural nerve) nerves. It emerges to the superficial compartment at a similar but posterior level to the superficial peroneal nerve, 7 to 8 cm above the lateral malleolus and curves around the malleolus at some distance (1 to 1.5 cm) to enter and innervate the lateral aspect of the dorsal surface of the foot.

5. Saphenous nerve. The saphenous nerve is the superficial terminus of the femoral nerve, which supplies the skin over the lower medial leg (Fig. 38-27). It leaves the femoral nerve proximally in the femoral triangle (Scarpa triangle), descends within the adductor canal, and courses beneath the sartorius muscle with the femoral artery (beginning lateral of the vessel at first and then crossing to the medial side superior to the artery just proximal of the lower end of the adductor magnus muscle). Further distally, the femoral artery departs away from the sartorius muscle, traveling deep to continue as the popliteal artery at the adductor hiatus. At this location, the saphenous nerve continues its course under the sartorius muscle, traveling adjacent to the saphenous branch of the descending genicular artery. It runs superficial at the medial surface of the lower leg and in front of the heel.

Techniques

Psoas Compartment Block. Several techniques for blocking the lumbar plexus using a posterior approach have been described, although the approach at the psoas compartment, described first by Chayen et al.[135] in 1976, remains popular. This block is performed, often with a single injection, at a point some distance lateral to the spinous process of L4, as the nerves of the lumbar plexus are in close proximity between the transverse processes of L4 and L5. Continuous psoas compartment blocks have also been shown to be effective for anesthesia (with sciatic nerve block) and perioperative analgesia in patients with hip fractures[136] and after hip arthroplasty.[137] A more cephalad approach, near L3, as described by Parkinson et al.[134] may be used, although there have been reports of renal subcapsular hematomas with blocks performed at this level.[138] This block has the advantage of blocking the entire lumbar plexus and therefore provides anesthesia/analgesia of the anterolateral and medial thigh, the knee, and the cutaneous distribution of the saphenous nerve below the knee. Although the sacral nerve roots may be anesthetized, this block will likely not be complete and sciatic nerve block will usually need to be performed as well. The patient is placed in the lateral position, with the operative side up. Adequate sedation should be provided because the plexus lies deep and the needle will penetrate several muscles. Prepare the needle insertion

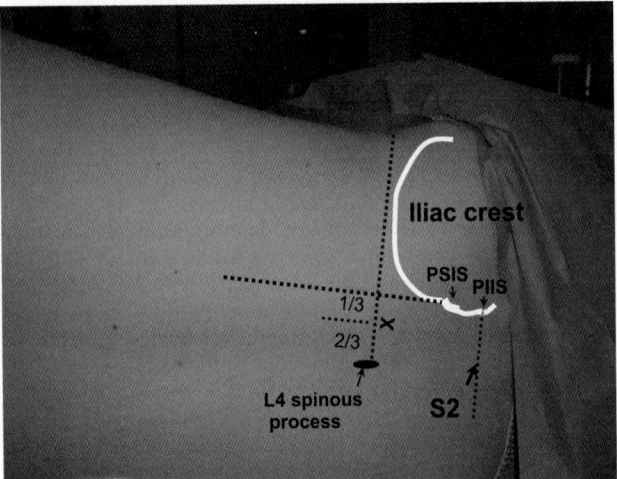

FIGURE 38-29. Surface landmarking for the psoas compartment block. The needle insertion site is one-third the distance along a horizontal line extending from the L4 transverse process to where it crosses a vertical line dissecting the posterior superior iliac spine (PSIS). PIIS, posterior inferior iliac spine.

site and skin surface with an antiseptic solution. Prepare the US probe surface by applying a sterile sleeve or adhesive dressing to it prior to needling.

Procedure Using Nerve Stimulation Technique

■ Landmarks: The landmarks developed by Capdevila et al.[137] using computed tomography are illustrated here (Fig. 38-29). As compared with the depth of the lumbar plexus or transverse processes, the distance between the L4 spinous process and the lumbar plexus was not affected by body mass index. The spinous process of L4 is estimated to lie approximately 1 cm cephalad to a line between the tops of the iliac crests (intercristal line); a horizontal line is drawn laterally from the L4 spinous processes to the far side of the body. A vertical line, running parallel to the spine, is then drawn at the point of the posterior superior iliac spine, to intersect the horizontal line. The lumbar plexus is then located with an X below a point on the horizontal line, at the junction between the lateral third and medial two-thirds between the spine and PSIS. The mean skin-to-lumbar plexus depth at the level of L4 is 8.4 cm in adult men and 7.1 cm in adult women, based on computed tomography assessment. The distance between the posterior edges of the transverse processes of the lumbar vertebrae and the lumbar plexus is about 1.8 cm.
■ Needling: A skin wheal is raised at the marked block site. An insulated needle (17 to 20 gauge, 9 to 10 cm long) is

inserted perpendicular to all planes at the X until contact with the L4 transverse process is obtained (approximately 5 to 6 cm deep). After contact, the needle is withdrawn and redirected caudad below the process to a maximum depth of 2 cm deep to the transverse process.
■ Nerve localization: With the nerve stimulator set to deliver an output current of 1 to 1.5 mA, a contraction of the quadratus femoris muscle (patellar twitch) is sought. The plexus is localized when the motor response is maintained at 0.3 to 0.5 mA. If a motor response is not obtained at first, cautiously moving the needle in a slight medial direction, without aiming toward the spinal cord, or in a 15-degree caudad or cephalad direction may help.
■ Injection: After the plexus is localized, 30 to 40 mL of local anesthetic is injected, using careful aspiration and administration of a test dose to rule out intravascular, epidural, or subarachnoid placement. Fifteen to 20 minutes may be required for spread of the anesthetic to all the roots of the lumbar plexus. It will take longer to produce anesthesia of the caudad branches (the lower sacral fibers that form the tibial nerve) and they may not be anesthetized at all.

Procedure Using Ultrasound Imaging. The lumbar plexus is difficult to view adequately as the target structures are located deep. Similar to paravertebral block, US imaging may be best for identifying the exact location and depth of the transverse processes prior to the block procedure. If there is desire to perform the block at L3–L4, viewing the kidneys prior to and/or during the block may help prevent renal injury and hematoma.

■ Scanning: A curved array probe (5 to 8 MHz) is placed in the midline at the level of the L4 spinous process to provide an overview of the L4 vertebra (Fig. 38-30). The probe should be rotated to the longitudinal axis, parallel to the spine, which will allow a lateral scan to be performed to identify the tips of the transverse processes. Without the continuation of ribs, the tips of the transverse processes are fairly easily delineated.
■ Appearance: The deep location of this block precludes clear visibility of the lumbar plexus. Indeed, the transverse processes (which are the primary landmarks) are still often very vaguely delineated. Therefore, it is important to switch between transverse and longitudinal scanning between the spinous processes and the tip of the transverse processes to survey the area. In the transverse scan, the spinous processes appear hypoechoic (likely from the dorsal shadowing effect) and extend superficially, while the transverse processes are hyperechoic masses/lines at the lateral edge of the vertebra. The fascicular-appearing musculature is evident surrounding the vertebra, yet poorly delineated by most compact US machines. In the longitudinal scan, the lateral tips of the transverse processes will be identified at the most lateral point where a hyperechoic nodule is viewed.

FIGURE 38-30. Ultrasound-assisted psoas compartment blockade. The curved array probe can be placed transversely to capture an overview of the spinal column (**left image**), while the longitudinal scan (**right image and clinical picture**) will help mark the block location: the tips of the transverse processes. If attempting real-time needle insertion, the safest needle alignment will be in-plane to a longitudinally placed probe over the L3-5 transverse processes.

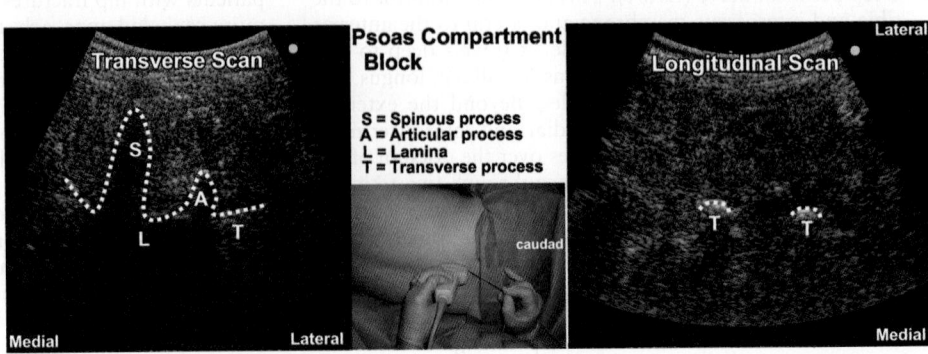

- Needling: Needling will be identical to that for blind technique, with the exception that the depth to the transverse process will be more accurately known. If choosing to perform a more cephalad approach above L4, real-time imaging may be helpful to view the kidneys (especially during inspiration when they fall toward L3-L4). An IP needle alignment to a longitudinal probe may be most suitable to avoid excessive medial or lateral needle angulation (see "Paravertebral Blockade" comments).
- Local anesthetic spread: It will be difficult to view local anesthetic spread when using US guidance. If seen, a hypoechoic mass will spread within the muscle mass lateral and deep to the transverse process.

Comments

- The psoas compartment block can be beneficial for placing a catheter to provide long-lasting analgesia; the catheter is securely fixed by the psoas muscles and kept away from any active joint region. After obtaining good localization with the stimulating needle (bevel facing caudad and lateral), a stimulating catheter is advanced 3 to 5 cm. In some cases, injecting a nonconducting solution such as D5W to expand the perineural space, while maintaining the electrical characteristics, is helpful.[27] The quadriceps muscle contraction should be maintained during catheter advancement with a stimulating catheter.
- Complications of this technique include hematoma in the muscle sheath, retroperitoneal space, or kidney, infection, and catheter placement within the peritoneum. Neuropathy of the nerves is possible. Unintended spread to the epidural or even subarachnoid space has also been reported. Inadequate anesthesia of some of the branches may occur more frequently than these rare complications.

Separate Blocks of the Terminal Nerves of the Lumbar Plexus. Anesthesia can be performed for four terminal nerves (lateral femoral cutaneous, femoral, obturator, and saphenous), although a lumbar plexus block is preferable if anesthesia of all these nerves is required. Anesthesia of the lateral femoral cutaneous nerve is occasionally used to provide sensory anesthesia for obtaining a skin graft from the lateral thigh. It can also be blocked as a diagnostic tool to identify cases of meralgia paresthetica. Obturator nerve block can be effective to prevent obturator reflex during transurethral bladder tumor resections, for treatment of pain in the hip area, for adductor spasm (as seen in multiple sclerosis patients), or as a diagnostic tool when studying hip mobility.[139] Saphenous nerve block often complements sciatic nerve block when anesthesia of the medial aspect of the ankle and foot are required. Procedures on the knee require anesthesia of the femoral and the obturator nerves, although postoperative analgesia of the knee can usually be provided by femoral nerve block alone. Single-shot femoral nerve block provides suitable postoperative analgesia after total knee arthroplasty, while sparing the side effects when compared with intrathecal morphine[140]; the use of a continuous technique can also reduce side effects as compared with continuous epidurals[141] and facilitate rehabilitation.[142] A US-guided infrapatellar nerve block has been described for use for postoperative analgesia after outpatient arthroscopic surgery,[143] but will not be included here. Because separate femoral nerve block is used extensively for analgesia and US guidance has been described for this block, this chapter will provide comprehensive description of this block. US guidance for obturator nerve block has been described and will be examined here. The other two nerve blocks will only be briefly discussed. The block sites for the femoral, lateral femoral cutaneous, and obturator nerves are illustrated in Figure 38-28.

1. Femoral Nerve/Fascia Iliacus Block: Procedure Using Nerve Stimulation.

- Landmarks: The patient is placed in the supine position, with slight external rotation of the femur. A pillow can be placed under the patient's hip to facilitate palpation of the femoral pulse and accentuate other pertinent landmarks for ease of palpation. Vloka et al.[144] studied cadavers using four common needle insertion sites for femoral nerve block and found that the point where the nerve lies beneath the inguinal crease, immediately lateral to the femoral artery, best localized the nerve. The artery descends at the midinguinal point, at the junction between the medial third and lateral two thirds of the inguinal ligament, although it is most superficial at the femoral crease. It lies approximately 1 to 1.5 cm medial to the nerve. The inguinal crease is the skin fold located caudally, approximately 2.5 cm, and parallel to the inguinal ligament (see "Clinical Anatomy" of lower extremity).
- Needling: A skin wheal is raised above the femoral nerve and a 5-cm, 22-gauge insulated needle is inserted perpendicular to the skin or using a cephalad angle of approximately 30 degrees. Aspiration is performed frequently because the femoral artery is situated close to the nerve.
- Nerve localization: For the femoral nerve using NS, a quadriceps femoris muscle response (patellar twitch preferably) is sought, with an end point of 0.5 mA used for accurate localization. Branches to the sartorius muscle arise just inferior to the inguinal ligament and leave the femoral nerve proximal to the main block location site. A response to stimulation of this muscle often indicates that the needle is too superficial and medial to the main femoral nerve. For a fasica iliacus block, loss-of-resistance technique is used instead of NS. The needle is placed vertically 5 cm lateral to the artery at the inguinal crease. Two pops are felt when the needle traverses the fascia lata and iliacus and enters the iliopsoas muscle.
- Injection: Injection of 20 mL (or less) of local anesthetic should suffice for sole femoral nerve anesthesia. Intermittent injection with interval aspiration should be performed.

Femoral Nerve/Fascia Iliacus Block: Procedure Using Ultrasound Imaging

- Scanning: A 10 MHz or higher transducer can be used for both blocks if the neurovascular structures are not located too deep (i.e., thin individuals) as this will show good distinction between the nerve and the surrounding structures (vessels and muscles). A midrange 5 to 8 MHz linear transducer is recommended if the nerve and artery are deep (>4 cm). Position the probe transverse to the nerve axis at the level of the inguinal crease (Fig. 38-31). The nerve should appear approximately 1 cm deep and 1.5 cm lateral to the femoral artery (color Doppler may be used to identify the femoral artery and vein).
- Appearance: The nerve lies about 1 cm lateral and deep to the large, circular, and anechoic femoral artery. It often appears triangular in shape and of variable size, because of its irregular course; early branching above the inguinal ligament can increase the transverse diameter of the nerve. The fascia lata (most superficial) and iliaca (immediately adjacent to the nerve and in fact separating the nerve from the artery) may be seen superficial to the femoral nerve and often appear bright and longitudinally angled.
- Needling: Place the nerve at the medial edge of the screen, with the probe capturing a transverse view of the neurovascular structures. A 5-cm, 22-gauge needle (for single-shot) can be inserted using either IP or OOP (Fig. 38-31) needle alignment, although OOP alignment will be beneficial if inserting a catheter. The needle should be inserted using an acute (30- to 45-degree) angle to maximize viewing. For iliacus block, the needle is generally placed more laterally than with the femoral nerve block.

FIGURE 38-31. Ultrasound-guided femoral nerve block. The probe is placed in a slightly oblique plane (at the level of and parallel to the inguinal crease) to capture the nerve in short-axis lateral to the femoral artery. The needle can be seen (not shown) as it transects the fascia lata and iliaca. In-plane needling should occur in a lateral-to-medial direction.

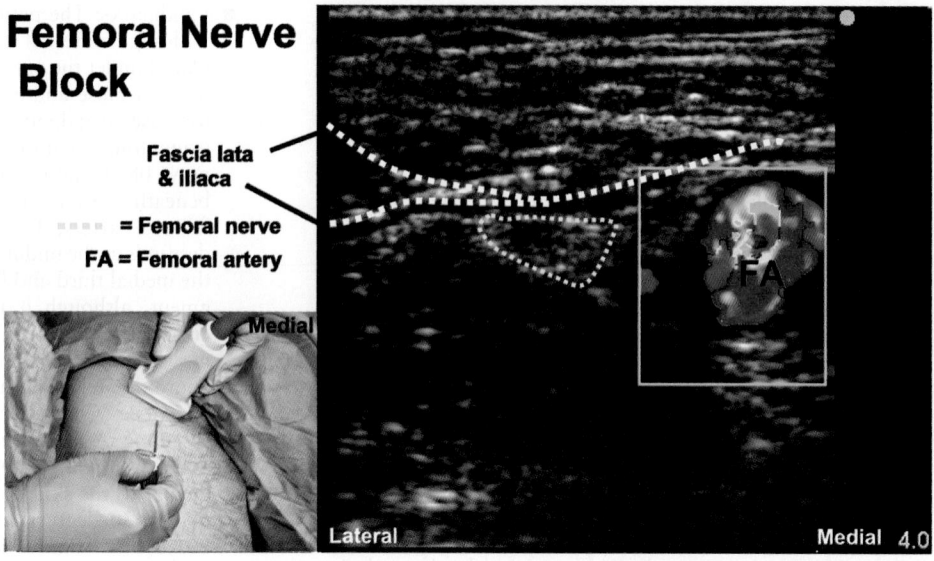

Femoral Nerve Block

Fascia lata & iliaca

---- = Femoral nerve

FA = Femoral artery

- Local anesthetic spread: Performing a test dose with D5W is recommended prior to local anesthetic application to visualize the spread and confirm nerve localization. Local anesthetic spread should occur within the fascial space surrounding the nerve. The solution may displace the nerve medially toward or laterally away from the artery.

Comments
- When inserting a catheter, it is debatable whether a stimulating catheter improves placement,[145,146] but using a solution to expand the perineural space has shown beneficial in some cases.[147] If using stimulating catheters, using D5W for tissue expansion will maintain motor responses to NS.[26,27]
- The lateral-to-medial needle insertion when using the IP needle alignment will ensure that the nerve is reached prior to reaching the femoral vessels.
- It is important to ensure that the US beam is perpendicular to the nerve's transverse axis to minimize anisotropic affects changing the echogenic properties of the structure. It has been shown that an approximate 10 degrees cephalad or caudad tilt of the transducer can make the nerve isoechoic (similar-appearing) to the underlying iliopsoas muscle.[148]

2. Lateral Femoral Cutaneous Nerve. Using NS technique, Shannon et al.[149] found that the lateral femoral cutaneous nerve can be localized at the inguinal crease, approximately 0 to 1 cm medial to the anterior superior iliac spine (Fig. 38-28), although this mark may be highly variant (some use 2.5 cm inferior and 2.5 cm medial to the spine) and should be confirmed with NS. An insulated needle (5 cm, 22 gauge is suitable) is inserted, using a perpendicular approach if the puncture is close to the anterior superior iliac spine but a lateral direction if it is at a distance. A "pop" may be felt as the needle penetrates the fascia lata. The primary end point for NS with this nerve is paresthesia over the lateral thigh (Fig. 38-27) with a current of approximately 0.5 to 0.6 mA. The sensory distribution may not extend proximal to the greater trochanter. Five to 10 mL of a local anesthetic is usually sufficient to obtain a block.

3. Obturator Nerve. Because the obturator nerve branches early after its descent from the obturator foramen, blocking this nerve before it branches, within the foramen near the superior pubic ramus, is often described for blind tech-

niques. The patient is placed supine with the hip slightly externally rotated; the hip may also be slightly flexed and abducted. If using US imaging a straight leg has been shown to be the best position. The public tubercle is located and a mark is placed 1.5 cm both inferior and lateral to it (this mark should resemble that shown in Fig. 38-28).

Procedure Using Nerve Stimulation Technique
- An insulated needle (18 to 22 gauge, 9 to 10 cm) is inserted perpendicularly until contact to the inferior pubic ramus is obtained. The needle is then redirected laterally and caudally to enter the obturator foramen and advanced 2 to 3 cm. NS using 0.5 mA for a current end point, with adductor muscle contraction, has been shown to greatly improve nerve localization.[139]

Procedure Using Ultrasound Imaging. The use of US to block the obturator nerve was recently introduced, although experience with this technique is limited. Soong et al.[150] used the Acuson Sequoia C256 machine from Siemens Medical Solutions (Mountain View, CA) and found that the anterior and posterior branches may be most easily visualized with the probe placed 2 cm laterally and distally to the pubic tubercle. The branches may be localized on either side of the adductor brevis muscle, if the fascial planes of the muscles are highly visible (hyperechoic). The depths of the anterior and posterior branches as measured during US guidance were 15.5 mm and 29.3 mm, respectively; tissue compression by the probe may influence this depth. The main (common) obturator nerve may be hard to view with US imaging. IP needling technique will be important to use, as will color Doppler, in order to avoid adjacent vessels.

Comment
- Aspiration is essential when injecting near the unbranched obturator nerve as the obturator artery lies adjacent to the nerve, and hemorrhage involving this artery can be life-threatening.[151]

4. Saphenous Nerve. Many approaches to blocking the saphenous nerve have been described, with needle placement at various locations including the midthigh, surrounding the knee or at the ankle (as discussed in "Ankle Block"). Using blind technique, a transarterial block described first by van der Wal et al.[152] has shown to be more effective as compared with block at the medial femoral condyle (paracondylar

Saphenous Nerve Block

S = Sartorius m
A = Femoral artery
▷ = Local anesthetic
AM = Adductor magnus m

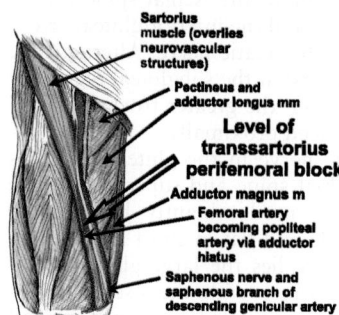

Sartorius muscle (overlies neurovascular structures)

Pectineus and adductor longus mm

Level of transsartorius perifemoral block

Adductor magnus m

Femoral artery becoming popliteal artery via adductor hiatus

Saphenous nerve and saphenous branch of descending genicular artery

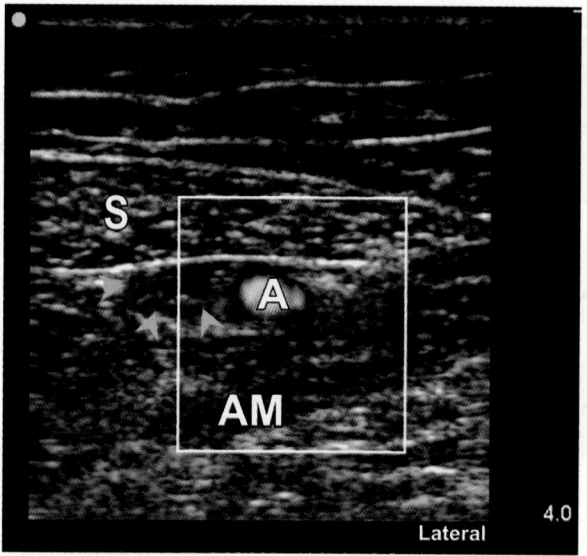

S

A

AM

Lateral   4.0

FIGURE 38-32. Ultrasound-guided saphenous nerve block using a transsartorius perifemoral approach. The probe is placed in the coronal plane at the location where the femoral nerve has yet to become the popliteal artery, approximately 10 to 12 cm proximal and 3 to 4 cm medial to the midpoint of the patella. Using the large femoral artery as a landmark may be beneficial to more distal approaches where the nerve lies adjacent to the smaller saphenous branch of the descending genicular artery.[148]

block) or tibial tuberosity (below-the-knee field block) for producing anesthesia to the medial aspect of the foot[153] and will be described here. US guidance has been used successfully with either a transsartorius perifemoral approach[154] or a perivenous (saphenous vein) approach[155,156]; the prior will be introduced here. Using the more proximally located larger femoral artery (rather than the more distal saphenous branch of the descending genicular artery) as a highly visible landmark seems to help identify the sartorius muscle and nerve.

Procedure Using Nerve Stimulation Technique (Transsartorial)

- Landmarks: The sartorius muscle is palpated at the medial aspect of the knee joint by asking the patient to raise the extended leg 5 to 10 cm off the table. The block location is marked by the end of a 4-cm vertical line drawn from this point in a proximal direction. (Benzon et al.[153] use a slightly more cephalad point 3 to 4 cm superior and 6 to 8 cm posterior to the superomedial border of the patella.)
- Needling: An insulated 22-gauge needle is inserted using an angle of 45 degrees with a slight posterior angle advanced from the medial aspect of the knee, in a slight posterior and caudad angle, to penetrate the sartorius muscle at a depth of approximately 2 to 3 cm.
- Nerve localization: Paresthesia referred to the medial malleolus should be elicited with the nerve stimulator at 0.6 mA or less at a depth of 3 to 5 cm.
- Injection: Following careful aspiration, 10 mL of local anesthetic (e.g., 1.5 to 2% lidocaine) is injected.

Procedure Using Ultrasound Imaging.
Using US,[154] the sartorius muscle can easily be identified as being a superficial roof to the relatively large landmark of the femoral artery before the artery travels deep and becomes the popliteal artery via the adductor hiatus. The nerve is located between the sartorius muscle and the artery in the thigh.

- Scanning: A high-frequency linear US transducer (e.g., L38, MicroMaxx, Sonosite, Bothell, WA) is placed transversely to the longitudinal axis of the extremity at the midthigh, approximately 10 to 12 cm proximal and 3 to 4 cm medial to the midpoint of the patella (Fig. 38-32). The femoral artery can be identified here with certainty by power Doppler; which in turn confirms the identity of the overlying sartorius muscle. The probe is then used to

scan distally until it captures the point just prior to where the femoral artery becomes the popliteal artery.
- Appearance: Using color Doppler is important to visualize the femoral artery, as a large hypoechoic (beneath the color) structure at a depth of approximately 2 to 3 cm in average-sized individuals. The sartorius muscle can then be identified as a highly delineated muscle immediately superficial to the artery, with hyperechoic borders. The nerve can be blocked as it lies sandwiched between the artery and muscle at this level. Alternatively, the nerve can be blocked more distally at the knee.
- Needling: A 22-gauge needle is inserted in either an IP or OOP fashion to penetrate the sartorius muscle to deposit local anesthetic immediately beneath the muscle and medial to the artery. Five to 10 mL of local anesthetic injected by the nerve should suffice.
- Local anesthetic spread: A small hypoechoic mass on the medial surface of the femoral artery should appear during injection.

Sciatic Nerve Blockade Using Posterior, Anterior and Posterior Popliteal Approaches. A sciatic nerve block can be used with lumbar plexus block for anesthesia of the lower extremity. Together with saphenous nerve block, the block produces adequate anesthesia to the sole of the foot and the lower leg. The large sciatic nerve is deep within the gluteal region and may be difficult to locate blindly or with US. Of benefit during US-guided blockade of the sciatic nerve and its terminal branches (tibial and common peroneal nerves) are the numerous bony and vascular landmarks that can be used for ease of identification. Knowledge of anatomy is paramount with these blocks, and the block location and approach will ultimately depend on the surgical requirement. For all blocks, prepare the needle insertion site and other applicable skin areas with an antiseptic solution and obtain sterility of the US probe with a standard sleeve cover or transparent dressing.

1. Posterior Sciatic Nerve Block: Classic Gluteal Approach. Position the patient semiprone (Sim position) with the hip and knee flexed and the operative side uppermost.

Procedure Using Nerve Stimulation
- Landmarks (Fig. 38-33): An oblique line is drawn joining the posterior superior iliac spine to the midpoint of the greater trochanter (on its medial aspect). Next, a horizontal line is drawn joining the greater trochanter

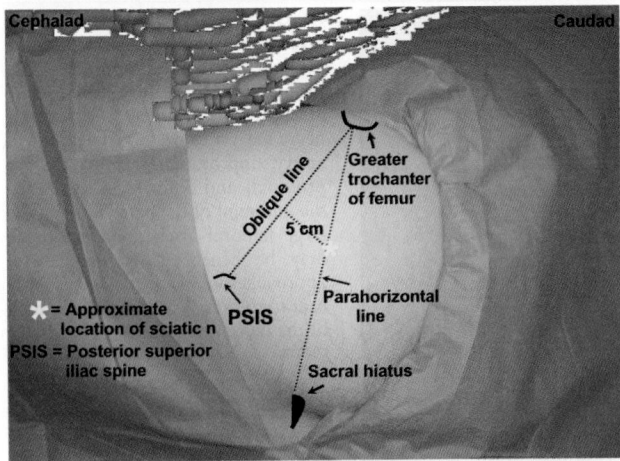

FIGURE 38-33. Landmarks for the sciatic nerve block using a posterior gluteal approach when using nerve stimulation-procedure. This location will serve as a reference point when applying ultrasound imaging. PSIS, posterior superior iliac spine.

(at above location) to the sacral hiatus. A perpendicular line drawn at the midpoint of the oblique line and reaching the parahorizontal line is the traditional puncture site (this intersection should be approximately 5 cm caudad along the perpendicular line).

- Needling: Raise a local anesthetic skin wheal after aseptic preparation. A 9- to 10-cm, 22-gauge needle, insulated if NS is desired, is inserted perpendicular to all planes.
- Nerve localization: Nerve responses of the lower leg and foot are sought. If they are not obtained at the full depth of the needle, the needle is withdrawn to the skin and reintroduced at a location perpendicular to the course of the nerve. Bone contact typically requires lateral needle adjustment.
- Injection: Injection of 20 to 30 mL of local anesthetic (e.g., 0.75% ropivacaine, 1% mepivacaine, 0.5% bupivacaine) is performed. If several blocks are required (i.e., lumbar plexus and/or saphenous nerve), a reduced concentration of local anesthetic may be necessary.

Procedure Using Ultrasound Imaging
- Scanning: A curved, lower frequency 2 to 5 MHz probe is generally used for scanning the gluteal region (Fig. 38-34).

Moving the probe cephalad and caudad in the gluteal region will help examine the ischial bone (a hyperechoic line with bony shadowing underneath), and the widest portion of this bone with the ischial spine medially should be located. The bulky gluteus maximus muscle will be seen superficial and posterior to the sciatic nerve. Vascular structures that may be useful to identify using color Doppler are the internal pudendal vessels (artery and vein) that are adjacent to the ischial spine that is medial to the sciatic nerve and the inferior gluteal artery immediately adjacent to the sciatic nerve. Alternatively, the nerve can be located first at the subgluteal region, at about the midpoint between the greater trochanter and ischial tuberosity, and traced proximally.

- Appearance: The sciatic nerve in the gluteal region is found lateral to the ischial spine and superficial to the ischial bone. It appears predominantly hyperechoic (bright) and is often wide and flat in short axis on US. Overlying the sciatic nerve lies the large gluteus maximus, which is quite distinct with the usual "starry night" appearance; the inner muscle layers (superior and inferior gemellus muscles, obturator internus muscle, and quadratus femoris muscle) are often indistinct.
- Needling: Both the IP and OOP approaches are appropriate for US-guided sciatic nerve block in the gluteal region. For OOP needling, the needle is inserted inferior to the probe in a cephaloanterior direction. A fairly steep angle of insertion will be required, but placing the needle slightly inferior to the probe will reduce the angle somewhat for better visibility of the needle. With the IP approach, the needle may be moved in a lateral-to-medial direction to penetrate the gluteus maximus muscle prior to reaching the sciatic nerve above the ischial bone (Fig. 38-34).
- Local anesthetic spread: Performing a test dose with D5W is recommended prior to local anesthetic application to visualize the spread and confirm nerve localization. It is generally recommended to deposit the local anesthetic solution so that it spreads completely around the sciatic nerve.

Comments
- For both IP and OOP needling approaches, scanning prior to needling will determine the angle, distance, and depth of needle penetration.
- The OOP approach is often used for catheter insertion and it is important to line up the site of needle insertion at the skin with the target nerve.

FIGURE 38-34. Ultrasound-guided sciatic nerve block using a posterior gluteal approach and an in-plane needle alignment to a curved low-frequency probe. The lateral-to-medial needle direction may help avoid puncture of the inferior gluteal or internal pudendal vessels.

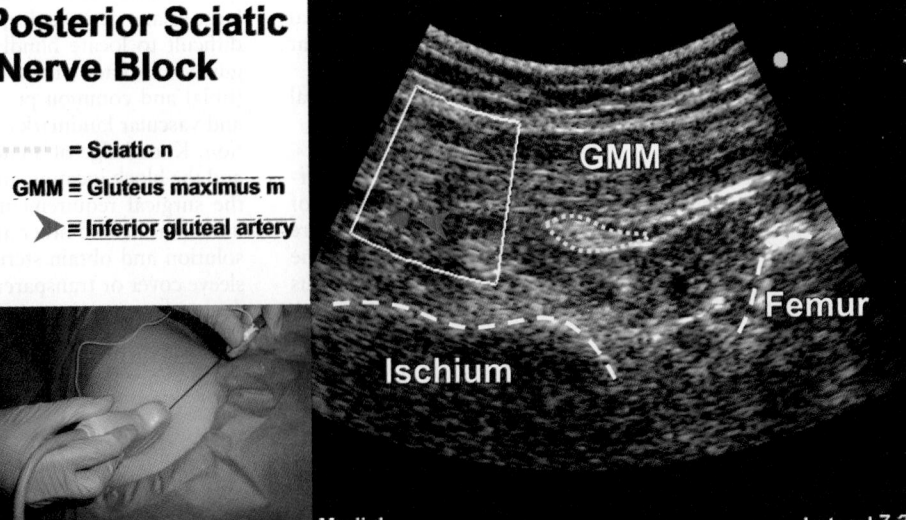

2. Posterior Sciatic Nerve Block: Subgluteal Approach. The patient is positioned semiprone (Sim position) with the hip and knee flexed and the foot resting on the dependent knee. In some patients, the supine position with the hip flexed and knee bent is either most comfortable or necessitated because of fracture or pain at the hip. This latter position requires an assistant to support the bent leg.

Procedure Using Nerve Stimulation Technique
- Landmarks: A horizontal line is drawn joining the medial aspect of the greater trochanter to the ischial tuberosity. The traditional puncture site is located on this line just medial to its midpoint.
- Needling: A 5- to 10-cm insulated needle is used, depending on patient size. The needle is inserted perpendicular to all skin planes.
- Nerve localization: Confirming sciatic nerve localization with NS is important prior to local anesthetic application. Similar responses as that for the classic gluteal approach are sought, with ankle responses preferable. It is important to distinguish the tibial (inversion or plantarflexion) and common peroneal (eversion or dorsiflexion) components of the nerve, and either obtain both or most importantly the tibial response.
- Injection: Injection of 20 to 30 mL of local anesthetic is sufficient. If additional blocks of the lower extremity are also performed, a solution with lower concentration should be considered.

Procedure Using Ultrasound Imaging
- Scanning: A curved, lower frequency 2 to 5 MHz probe or a linear 4 to 7 MHz probe is suitable for scanning the subgluteal region (Fig. 38-35). The center of the probe should be aligned with the midpoint of a line between the ischial tuberosity and the greater trochanter. If the sciatic nerve is difficult to localize at the subgluteal region, it can be traced proximally from the bifurcation point at or near the apex of the popliteal fossa.
- Appearance: On the lateral side of the screen, the medial aspect of the greater trochanter appears almost pear-shaped and hypoechoic when using a curved array probe. The sciatic nerve in the subgluteal region appears predominantly hyperechoic (bright) and is often elliptical in a short-axis view using US.
- Needling: Similar to the classic gluteal approach, both IP and OOP plane needling can be performed, with the needle directed from lateral to medial for the IP technique. Using an angle of insertion of approximately 45 degrees to the skin will provide the best view of the needle and reach the nerve, although 60 to 70 degrees may be required in certain obese individuals.
- Local anesthetic spread: The goal is to deposit local anesthetic (20 to 30 mL) next to, but not directly within, the sciatic nerve structure in the subgluteal region. A hypoechoic local anesthetic fluid collection is often seen around the hyperechoic nerve within the sheath compartment during injection.

Comments
- With the necessity of using a curved array probe in many cases, the needle tip as viewed by OOP needling will be even more difficult to identify than when using higher-resolution linear probes. Despite this, this approach is used often because indwelling catheters are commonly placed in the subgluteal area. It will be important to use NS in addition to US-guided technique to confirm the needle and local anesthetic placement.

3. Anterior Sciatic Nerve Block. This block is most suitable for those patients who cannot be positioned laterally. The block is indicated for surgery below the knee, with the only sensory deficiency being the medial strip of skin supplied by the saphenous nerve. The anterior block is performed on a short portion of the sciatic nerve close to the lesser trochanter of the femur. The patient is positioned supine, with the leg to be blocked externally rotated slightly.

Procedure Using Nerve Stimulation Technique
- Landmarks: A line is drawn connecting the anterior superior iliac spine with the pubic tubercle (inguinal ligament). A second line, parallel to the first, is drawn across the thigh from the greater trochanter. The nerve is usually located at the intersection on the lower line, with a line drawn downward from a point at the medial third of the upper line. Alternatively, the nerve is located lateral to the femoral artery pulse at the level of the inguinal crease.
- Needling: A 22-gauge, 12- to 15-cm insulated needle will be required for this deep block. The needle is inserted perpendicular to the skin and advanced until contact with the femur occurs; the needle is then withdrawn slightly, angulated slightly medial and cephalad, and introduced 5 cm further.

Subgluteal Sciatic Nerve Block

····· = Sciatic n
GMM = Gluteus maximus m
GT = Greater trochanter

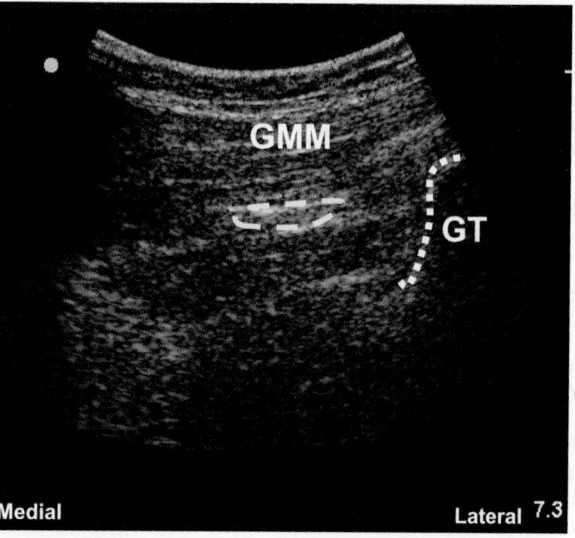

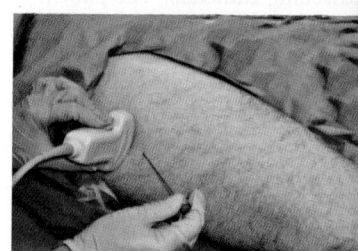

FIGURE 38-35. Ultrasound-guided sciatic nerve block from the subgluteal approach using out-of-plane needling to a curved probe. The medially positioned ischial tuberosity is not captured in this image, but will serve as a good bony landmark in most circumstances. Out-of-plane approaches often will be used as this block is often used for indwelling catheter placement.

FIGURE 38-36. Ultrasound-guided sciatic block from an anterior approach. The **clinical picture** and **upper image** show probe positioning and a short-axis view of the nerve that may be used. Using a longitudinally placed probe to capture the long axis of the nerve (**lower image**) may be beneficial if the transverse view is difficult to capture because of bony shadowing from the lesser trochanter.

Anterior Sciatic Nerve Block

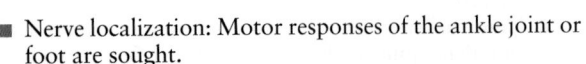 **&** = Sciatic n
FV = Femoral vessels
LT = Lesser trochanter of femur
AM = Adductor magnus m

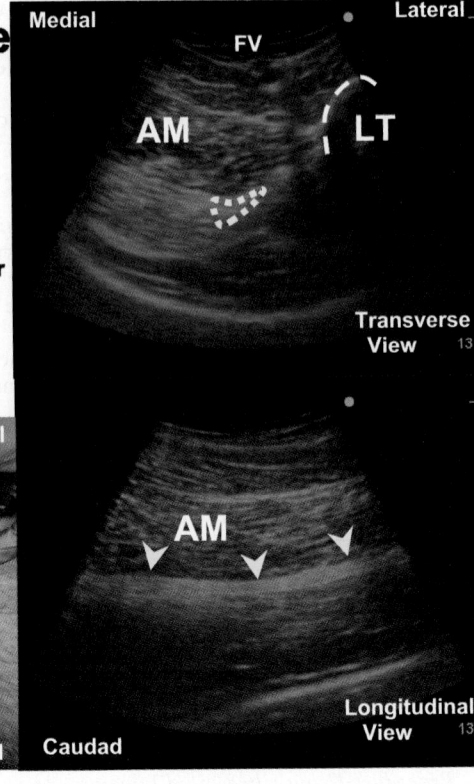

- Nerve localization: Motor responses of the ankle joint or foot are sought.
- Injection: Twenty to 30 mL of local anesthetic is injected after careful aspiration and administration of a test dose.

Procedure Using Ultrasound Imaging
- Scanning: It is most common to use a curved, lower frequency 2 to 5 MHz probe for scanning the sciatic nerve in the proximal thigh (Fig. 38-36). Place the probe over the proximal thigh approximately 8 cm distal to the femoral crease. A transversely placed probe is commonly used, although the nerve may be best visualized by placing the probe axis longitudinally along the course of the nerve, as capturing a longitudinal axis of the nerve may improve its identification. Moving in a medial-to-lateral direction may be helpful to capture an image of the nerve.
- Appearance: In transverse axis, the sciatic nerve often appears oval or round, predominantly hyperechoic, medial and posterior to the lesser trochanter, and deep to the adductor magus muscle. If using Doppler, the femoral neurovascular structures are seen superficially below the hyperechoic fascial tissue and lateral to the sciatic nerve in this projection when the leg is externally rotated. A longitudinal view captures a broad, linear, and hyperechoic cable of fibers and may allow easier identification of the nerve.[157]
- Needling: When using a probe positioned in transverse axis to the nerve, an IP approach includes advancing the needle in a medial-to-lateral and anterior-to-posterior direction, while an OOP approach involves inserting the needle along the midline of the probe at a location 2 to 3 cm inferior and perpendicular to the probe. If the probe is placed longitudinally, the needle direction for OOP alignment will be similar to that for the IP as previously described. With IP alignment, the needle should be placed a few centimeters caudad to the probe to improve needle visibility by reducing the angle of insertion. It is

highly recommended to use combined US and NS guidance for this procedure.
- Local anesthetic spread: After careful aspiration and injection of a small amount of D5W to visualize the probable anesthetic spread, inject the local anesthetic while ensuring that it spreads circumferentially around the nerve.

Comments
- Although depositing the local anesthetic around the nerve is desirable, it is technically challenging to reposition the needle on both sides of the nerve because of its depth within the muscle layers.
- Similar to other sciatic nerve blocks, if other blocks are being combined with this block, the local anesthetic may need to be diluted to reduce the risk of toxicity.
- Complications are rare, but include intravascular injection (e.g., femoral artery), infection in the injection area, hematoma formation, nerve injury. and potential CNS toxicity.

4. Posterior Popliteal Sciatic Block. The sciatic nerve can be blocked below the hip at the lateral midfemoral or lateral popliteal locations in addition to the posterior popliteal location,[158,159] but when using US guidance the posterior approach allows the needle to be placed closely to the probe and thus may improve needle tracking and visibility. Furthermore, the posterior popliteal approach is most amenable to inserting indwelling catheters. The patient is positioned laterally or prone with the operative leg slightly flexed. Ideally, the ankles should be positioned beyond the end of the table so that motor responses to NS can be readily observed. The landmarks become more visible when the knee is flexed against resistance.

Procedure Using Nerve Stimulation Technique
- Landmarks: The puncture site is often located at the tip of a triangle formed by the popliteal crease at the base, the biceps femoris tendon laterally, and the semimembranosus

Posterior Popliteal Block

Scanning proximally from the popliteal crease captures the sciatic nerve at its bifurcation point

SN = Sciatic n
    = Common peroneal n
    = Tibial n
➤ = Biceps femoris m
      Popliteal vein
      Popliteal artery

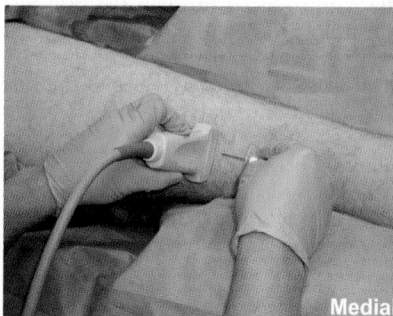

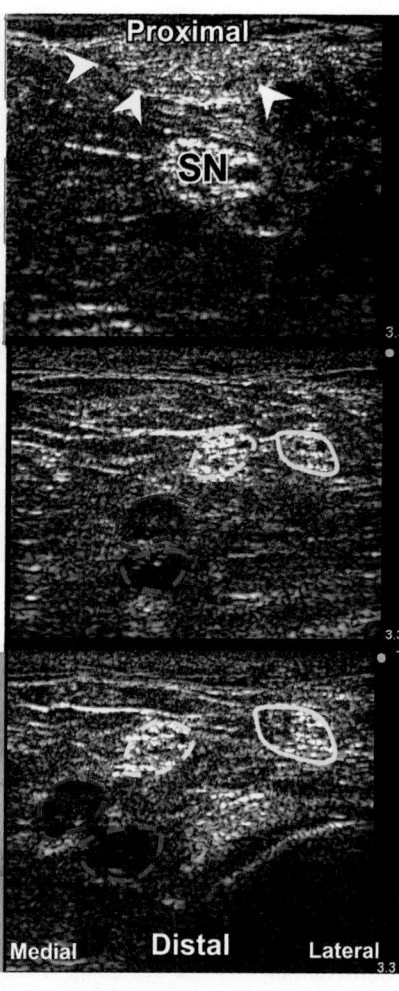

FIGURE 38-37. Ultrasound-guided popliteal nerve block. The probe is initially placed at the popliteal crease (**lower image**) and subsequently is used to scan proximally to capture the sciatic nerve just proximal to its bifurcation (i.e., the ideal block site) approximately 6 to 10 cm above the crease (**upper image**).

tendon medially (this tendon generally lies medial to the tendon of the semitendinosus at this location). Alternatively, drawing lines 8 cm long in the cephalad direction, from the insertion site of the medial and lateral tendons (above), the puncture point is at the midpoint of a line attaching the two (almost parallel) lines. It may be best to insert the needle at approximately 10 cm above the popliteal fossa in order to ensure the sciatic nerve is blocked before its bifurcation.

- Needling: Depending on the patient, a 5- to 10-cm insulated 22-gauge needle can be inserted using an angle 45 degrees cephalad to the skin. A fan-wise search is conducted perpendicular to this line until the nerve is contacted. If the femur is contacted by the needle, the depth is noted. The nerve should lie midway between the skin and the femur.
- Nerve localization: NS is used to localize the nerve by eliciting motor responses at the ankle or foot. The aim should be to localize the sciatic nerve before its bifurcation into tibial and common peroneal nerve components. If only ankle inversion and/or plantarflexion (tibial nerve) or eversion and/or dorsiflexion (common peroneal) is seen, it would be appropriate to adjust the needle insertion site a few centimeters cephalad to obtain complete ankle and foot movements. Otherwise, injecting after obtaining a sole tibial nerve response has been shown to provide similar success to that after both tibial and common peroneal responses (with two injections).[160] Maintaining a motor response with currents <0.5 mA will help ensure the nerve-needle distance is appropriate for successful block.[161]

- Injection: Twenty to 30 mL of local anesthetic should be deposited at the final needle location.

Procedure Using Ultrasound Guidance

- Scanning: A linear, higher frequency 10 to 15 MHz probe is commonly used for scanning the sciatic nerve transversely in the popliteal fossa (Fig. 38-37). A technique that uses a distal-to-proximal scan can effectively locate the sciatic nerve in the posterior popliteal fossa at a location where it has yet to bifurcate (Fig. 38-37). At the popliteal crease, the transverse probe captures the tibial and common peroneal nerves, with the prior being adjacent and lateral to the popliteal vessels (Doppler is very valuable here). During a proximal scan, the tibial and common peroneal nerves approach each other and finally join to form the sciatic nerve.
- Appearance: At the level of the popliteal crease, the tibial and common peroneal nerves lie superficial and lateral to the popliteal vessels (common peroneal nerve is the most lateral); both nerves appear round-to-oval and hyperechoic compared with the surrounding musculature. The hyperechoic border of the femur (condyles) may be apparent. During the proximal scan, the tibial nerve moves away from the vessels and approaches the common peroneal nerve. More cephalad in the posterior thigh, the biceps femoris muscle lies superficial to the joining nerves and appears as a larger, oval-shaped structure with less internal punctuate areas (hypoechoic spots) than the nerves. The sciatic nerve appears as a large, round to flat-oval hyperechoic structure.

FIGURE 38-38. Ultrasound-guided posterior tibial nerve block at the ankle using a small footprint linear probe. The nerve is captured adjacent to the posterior tibial artery, prior to its division into the medial and lateral plantar nerves.

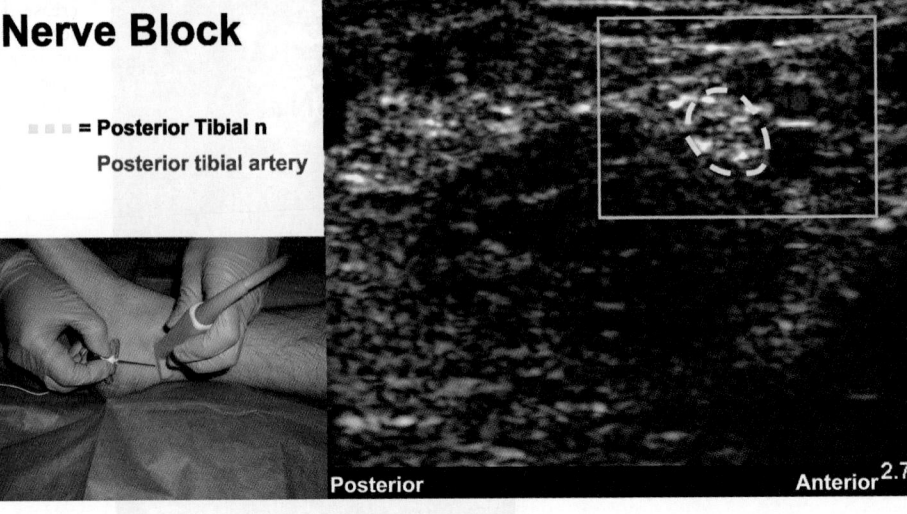

Posterior Tibial Nerve Block

▪ ▪ ▪ = Posterior Tibial n

Posterior tibial artery

Posterior   Anterior 2.7

▪ Needling: An OOP approach will be commonly performed, especially if placing indwelling catheters. The probe is positioned directly above the sciatic nerve at or slightly cephalad to its bifurcation point and so that the nerve is placed in the center of the image. The needle should be inserted at the caudal surface of probe, with the needle tip contacting the skin approximately 3 to 4 cm caudal to the probe surface.

▪ Local anesthetic spread: The correct response to proper injection is an expansion of hypoechoic fluid completely around the hyperechoic nerve structure, producing a "donut" sign; two separate injections (medial and lateral) may be required for complete circumferential spread.

Comments
▪ The US probe may be rotated 90 degrees to show the sciatic nerve in long axis. This is helpful to differentiate the sciatic nerve from other nonneural structures.

▪ During needle insertion using an OOP approach, it may be helpful to use incremental needle angulations: the needle may be best tracked within the tissue if an initial shallow angle is used to clearly identify the needle tip as a hyperechoic dot, which can be followed with subsequent steeper needle angulations (see the description of the "walk-down" technique under "Practical Approaches for Ultrasound Guidance").[34]

Ankle Block.   All five nerves of the foot can be blocked at the level of the ankle. The superficial nerves (sural, superficial peroneal, and saphenous nerves) can be blocked by simple infiltration techniques. US guidance can be useful for blocking the posterior tibial and deep peroneal (fibular) nerves as their locations can be easily identified next to reliable landmarks (i.e., bones and vessels) that are clearly visible.

1. Posterior Tibial Nerve

Procedure Using Landmark Technique
▪ Landmarks: The posterior tibial nerve is the major nerve to the sole of the foot. It can be approached with the patient either in the prone position or lying supine with the hip and knee flexed so that the foot rests on the bed. The medial malleolus is identified, along with the pulsation of the posterior tibial artery behind it. The nerve is located posterior to the artery.

▪ Needling: A needle is introduced through the skin just behind the posterior tibial artery and directed 45 degrees anteriorly, seeking a paresthesia in the sole of the foot. Although not typical, if NS is used, twitches of the first (medial plantar branch) and fifth (lateral plantar branch) toes will be sought.

▪ Injection: Five milliliters of a local anesthetic produces anesthesia if a paresthesia is identified. If not, a fan-shaped injection of 10 mL can be performed in the triangle formed by the artery, the Achilles tendon, and the tibia itself.

Procedure Using Ultrasound Imaging
▪ Scanning: A linear (hockey stick) 10 MHz probe with a small footprint is positioned in transverse (short) axis to the nerve just posterior and inferior to the medial malleolus (Fig. 38-38). Alternatively, the nerve can be identified 3 to 5 cm above the malleolus. Color Doppler is helpful to localize the nerve at these locations as the nerve lies posterior and deep to the posterior tibial artery at both locations. The nerve should be localized before it branches into the medial and lateral plantar nerves.

▪ Appearance: Immediately anterior to the artery lies the hypoechoic circular posterior tibial vein; this may be compressed and not apparent on the screen. Posterior to the artery, the nerve appears slightly more hyperechoic than the surrounding tissues and looks like a condensed honeycomb-appearing structure.

▪ Needling: A 3.5- to 5-cm needle is inserted using either an OOP approach with the needle caudal or an IP approach with the needle anterior to the transversely positioned probe.

2. Sural nerve. The patient is placed either in the prone position or supine with the hip and knee flexed so that the foot rests on the bed. The posteriorly located sural nerve can be blocked by injection on the lateral side. The subcutaneous injection of a ridge of anesthesia behind the lateral malleolus, filling the groove between it and the calcaneus, produces anesthesia of the sural nerve. This will require another 5 mL of local anesthetic.

3. Deep Peroneal Nerve.

Procedure Using Landmark Technique
▪ Landmarks: This is the major nerve to the dorsum of the foot and lies in the deep plane of the anterior tibial artery. The patient is positioned supine, generally with the leg

Deep Peroneal Nerve Block

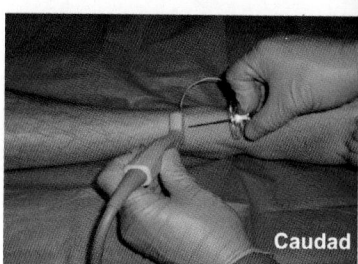

```
----- = Deep peroneal n
        Anterior tibial artery
```

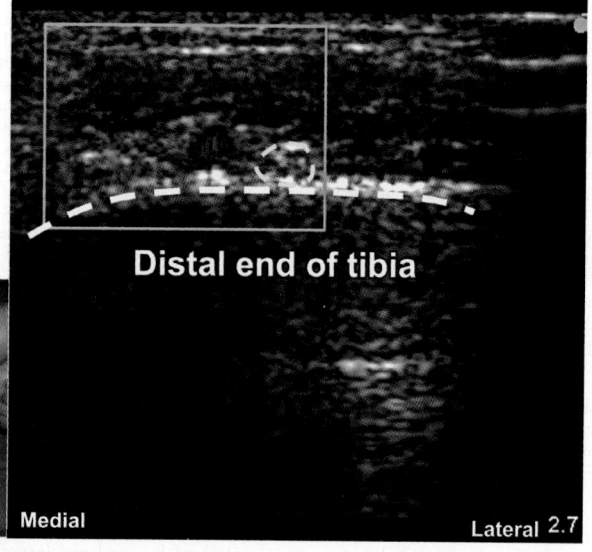

Distal end of tibia

Caudad   Medial   Lateral 2.7

FIGURE 38-39. Ultrasound-guided deep peroneal nerve block at the anterior ankle. It is helpful to use color Doppler to localize the anterior tibial artery lying immediately medial and adjacent to the nerve.

ANESTHETIC MANAGEMENT

extended. Pulsation of the artery is sought at the level of the skin crease on the anterior midline surface of the ankle. If the artery is not palpable, the tendon of the extensor hallucis longus can be identified (the nerve lies immediately lateral to this) by asking the patient to extend the big toe.

■ Needling and injection: If the artery pulse can be felt, 5 mL of local anesthetic is injected just lateral to this. If the artery is not palpable, the tendon of the extensor hallucis longus can be identified by asking the patient to extend the big toe. If using NS, toe extension is sought for this nerve. Injection can be made into the deep planes below the fascia using either one of these landmarks.

Procedure Using Ultrasound Imaging

■ Scanning: A small footprint linear (hockey stick) 10 MHz probe is placed in transverse (short) axis to the nerve at the anterior surface of the ankle joint (Fig. 38-39). Alternatively, the nerve can also be found 3 to 5 cm above the ankle joint. However, the nerve itself can be difficult to see and only the artery can be consistently located. Color Doppler can be used at both locations to illuminate the anterior tibial artery lying medial to the nerve.

■ Appearance: If seen, the nerve appears as a small cluster of hyperechoic fascicular-appearing fibers immediately lateral to the artery, with both adjacent to the well-demarcated distal end of the tibia.

■ Needling: An OOP approach will be most suitable here as the tendons lie on either side of the nerve. A 3.5- to 5-cm needle is inserted OOP and caudal to the transversely positioned small footprint probe.

■ Local anesthetic spread: Injection of 4 to 5 mL of local anesthetic solution lateral to the nerve will help avoid the anterior tibial artery. Aspiration is important to perform prior to injection.

4. Saphenous nerve. The patient is placed supine with the leg extended. The saphenous nerve is anesthetized by infiltrating 5 mL of local anesthetic around the saphenous vein at the level where this vein passes anterior to the medial malleolus. A wall of anesthesia between the skin and the bone itself suffices to block the nerve. See "Separate Blocks of the Terminal Nerves of the Lumbar Plexus" for blockade of this nerve more proximally in the thigh.

5. Superficial peroneal branches. Finally, a subcutaneous ridge of anesthetic solution is laid along the skin crease between the anterior tibial artery and the lateral malleolus. This sub-

cutaneous ridge overlies the previous subfascial injection for the deep peroneal nerve. Another 5 to 10 mL of local anesthetic may be required to cover this area.

6. Comments.

■ Anesthesia of the foot usually ensues within 15 minutes after performance of these five injections.

■ Complications of this block are rare, although neuropathy can be produced. Care should be taken not to pin any of the deep nerves against the bone at the time of injection, and intraneural injection should be avoided. Epinephrine should not be added to local anesthetics used for this block in order to avoid compromising the distal circulation.

■ US imaging for the deep nerves may help avoid bone contact and avoid the multiple injections of the infiltration technique.

ACKNOWLEDGMENTS

The authors thank Dr. Michael F. Mulroy, author of the Peripheral Nerve Block chapter in the fifth edition of this textbook, for providing an invaluable template from which this chapter was fashioned. Many of the simplified anatomic drawings for this chapter were produced by and used with permission from Ms. Carol Chan. Most figures were adapted from one of the author's (B.T.) textbooks, entitled "Atlas of Ultrasound and Nerve Stimulation-Guided Regional Anesthesia."[34]

References

1. Tziavrangos E, Schug SA: Regional anaesthesia and perioperative outcome. Curr Opin Anaesthesiol 2006; 19: 521

2. Brown DL, Ransom DM, Hall JA et al: Regional anesthesia and local anesthetic-induced systemic toxicity: Seizure frequency and accompanying cardiovascular changes. Anesth Analg 1995; 81: 321

3. Borgeat A, Schappi B, Biasca N et al: Patient-controlled analgesia after major shoulder surgery: Patient-controlled interscalene analgesia versus patient-controlled analgesia. Anesthesiology 1997; 87: 1343

4. Greengrass RA: Regional anesthesia for ambulatory surgery. Anesthesiol Clin North Am 2000; 18: 341

5. Singelyn FJ, Gouverneur JM: Postoperative analgesia after total hip arthroplasty: i.v. PCA with morphine, patient-controlled epidural analgesia, or continuous "3-in-1" block?: a prospective evaluation by our acute pain service in more than 1,300 patients. J Clin Anesth 1999; 11: 550

6. Nielsen KC, Steele SM: Outcome after regional anaesthesia in the ambulatory setting—is it really worth it? Best Pract Res Clin Anaesthesiol 2002; 16: 145

7. Auroy Y, Narchi P, Messiah A et al: Serious complications related to regional anesthesia: results of a prospective survey in France. Anesthesiology 1997; 87: 479

8. Tsui B: Ultrasound-guidance and NS: implications for the future practice of regional anesthesia. Can J Anaesth 2007; 54: 165

9. Greenblatt GM, Denson JS: Needle nerve stimulatorlocator: nerve blocks with a new instrument for locating nerves. Anesth Analg 1962; 41: 599

10. Sarnoff S: Functional localization of interspinal catheters. Anesthesiology 1950; 11: 360

11. Boezaart AP, De Beer JF, du Toit C et al: A new technique of continuous interscalene nerve block. Can J Anaesth 1999; 46: 275

12. Copeland SJ, Laxton MA: A new stimulating catheter for continuous peripheral nerve blocks. Reg Anesth Pain Med 2001; 26: 589

13. Perlas A, Niazi A, McCartney C et al: The sensitivity of motor response to nerve stimulation and paresthesia for nerve localization as evaluated by ultrasound. Reg Anesth Pain Med 2006; 31: 445

14. Urmey WF, Stanton J: Inability to consistently elicit a motor response following sensory paresthesia during interscalene block administration. Anesthesiology 2002; 96: 552

15. Hadzic A, Vloka J, Hadzic N et al: Nerve stimulators used for peripheral nerve blocks vary in their electrical characteristics. Anesthesiology 2003; 98: 969

16. Urmey WF: Using the nerve stimulator for peripheral or plexus nerve blocks. Minerva Anestesiologica 2006; 72: 467

17. Ganta R, Cajee RA, Henthorn RW: Use of transcutaneous nerve stimulation to assist interscalene block. Anesth Analg 1993; 76: 914

18. Urmey WF, Grossi P: Percutaneous electrode guidance: a noninvasive technique for prelocation of peripheral nerves to facilitate peripheral plexus or nerve block. Reg Anesth Pain Med 2002; 27: 261

19. Bosenberg AT, Raw R, Boezaart AP: Surface mapping of peripheral nerves in children with a nerve stimulator. Paediatr Anaesth 2002; 12: 398

20. Tsui BC, Gupta S, Finucane B: Confirmation of epidural catheter placement using nerve stimulation. Can J Anaesth 1998; 45: 640

21. Tsui BC, Finucane B: Epidural stimulator catheter. Tech Reg Anesth Pain Man 2002; 6: 150

22. Koscielniak-Nielsen ZJ, Rassmussen H et al: Effect of impulse duration on patients' perception of electrical stimulation and block effectiveness during axillary block in unsedated ambulatory patients. Reg Anesth Pain Med 2001; 26: 428

23. Hadzic A, Vloka JD, Claudio RE et al: Electrical nerve localization: effects of cutaneous electrode placement and duration of the stimulus on motor response. Anesthesiology 2004; 100: 1526

24. Borgeat A: Regional anesthesia, intraneural injection, and nerve injury: beyond the epineurium. Anesthesiology 2006; 105: 647

25. Raj PP, Rosenblatt R, Montgomery SJ: Use of the nerve stimulator for peripheral blocks. Reg Anaesth 1980; 5: 14

26. Tsui BC, Wagner A, Finucane B: Electrophysiologic effect of injectates on peripheral nerve stimulation. Reg Anesth Pain Med 2004; 29: 189

27. Tsui BC, Kropelin B, Ganapathy S et al: Dextrose 5% in water: fluid medium for maintaining electrical stimulation of peripheral nerves during stimulating catheter placement. Acta Anaesthesiol Scand 2005; 49: 1562

28. Sites BD, Beach ML, Spence BC et al: Ultrasound guidance improves the success rate of a perivascular axillary plexus block. Acta Anaesthesiol Scand 2006; 50: 678

29. Williams SR, Chouinard P, Arcand G et al: Ultrasound guidance speeds execution and improves the quality of supraclavicular block. Anesth Analg 2003; 97: 1518

30. Marhofer P, Sitzwohl C, Greher M et al: Ultrasound guidance for infraclavicular brachial plexus anesthesia in children. Anaesthesia 2004; 59: 642

31. Soeding PE, Sha S, Royse CE et al: A randomized trial of ultrasound-guided brachial plexus anaesthesia in upper limb surgery. Anaesth Intensive Care 2005; 33: 719

32. Liu FC, Liou JT, Tsai YF et al: Efficacy of ultrasound-guided axillary brachial plexus block: a comparative study with nerve stimulator-guided method. Chang Gung. Med J 2005; 28: 396

33. Tsui BC, Twomey C, Finucane BT: Visualization of the brachial plexus in the supraclavicular region using a curved ultrasound probe with a sterile transparent dressing. Reg Anesth Pain Med 2006; 31: 182

34. Tsui BC: Atlas of Nerve Stimulation and Ultrasound Guided Regional Anesthesia. New York, Springer, 2007

35. Tsui BC, Finucane BT: The importance of ultrasound landmarks: a "trace-back" approach using the popliteal blood vessels for identification of the sciatic nerve. Reg Anesth Pain Med 2006; 31: 481

36. Tsui BC, Dillane D: Needle puncture site and a "walkdown" approach for short-axis alignment during ultrasound-guided blocks. Reg Anesth Pain Med 2006; 31: 586

37. Tsui BC: Facilitating needle alignment in-plane to an ultrasound beam using a portable laser unit. Reg Anesth Pain Med 2007; 32: 84

38. Selander D, Dhuner KG, Lundborg G: Peripheral nerve injury due to injection needles used for regional anesthesia. An experimental study of the acute effects of needle point trauma. Acta Anaesthesiol Scand 1977; 21: 182

39. Steele SM, Klein SM, D'Ercole FJ et al: A new continuous catheter delivery system. Anesth Analg 1998; 87: 228

40. Claudio R, Hadzic A, Shih H et al: Injection pressures by anesthesiologists during simulated peripheral nerve block. Reg Anesth Pain Med 2004; 29: 201

41. Hadzic A, Dilberovic F, Shah S et al: Combination of intraneural injection and high injection pressure leads to fascicular injury and neurologic deficits in dogs. Reg Anesth Pain Med 2004; 29: 417

42. Selander D, Sjostrand J: Longitudinal spread of intraneurally injected local anesthetics. An experimental study of the initial neural distribution following intraneural injections. Acta Anaesthesiol Scand 1978; 22: 622

43. Tsui BC, Li LX, Pillay JJ: Compressed air injection technique to standardize block injection pressures. Can J Anaesth 2006; 53: 1098

44. Borgeat A, Blumenthal S: Nerve injury and regional anaesthesia. Curr Opin Anaesthesiol 2004; 17: 417

45. Kaufman BR, Nystrom E, Nath S et al: Debilitating chronic pain syndromes after presumed intraneural injections. Pain 2000; 85: 283

46. Selander D: Neurotoxicity of local anesthetics: animal data. Reg Anesth 1993; 18: 461

47. Ben-David B: Complications of peripheral blockade. Anesthesiol Clin North Am 2002; 20: 695

48. Graf BM, Abraham I, Eberbach N et al: Differences in cardiotoxicity of bupivacaine and ropivacaine are the result of physicochemical and stereoselective properties. Anesthesiology 2002; 96: 1427

49. Knudsen K, Beckman SM, Blomberg S et al: Central nervous and cardiovascular effects of i.v. infusions of ropivacaine, bupivacaine and placebo in volunteers. Br J Anaesth 1997; 78: 507

50. Muller M, Litz RJ, Huler M et al: Grand mal convulsion and plasma concentrations after intravascular injection of ropivacaine for axillary brachial plexus blockade. Br J Anaesth 2001; 87: 784

51. Petitjeans F, Mion G, Puidupin M et al: Tachycardia and convulsions induced by accidental intravascular ropivacaine injection during sciatic block. Acta Anaesthesiol Scand 2002; 46: 616

52. Reinikainen M, Hedman A, Pelkonen O et al: Cardiac arrest after interscalene brachial plexus block with ropivacaine and lidocaine. Acta Anaesthesiol Scand 2003; 47: 904

53. Ruetsch YA, Fattinger KE, Borgeat A: Ropivacaine-induced convulsions and severe cardiac dysrhythmia after sciatic block. Anesthesiology 1999; 90: 1784

54. Marhofer P, Schrogendorfer K, Wallner T et al: Ultrasonographic guidance reduces the amount of local anesthetic for 3-in-1 blocks. Reg Anesth Pain Med 1998; 23: 584

55. Willschke H, Marhofer P, Bosenberg A et al: Ultrasonography for ilioinguinal/iliohypogastric nerve blocks in children. Br J Anaesth 2005; 95: 226

56. Weinberg GL, VadeBoncouer T, Ramaraju GA et al: Pretreatment or resuscitation with a lipid infusion shifts the dose-response to bupivacaine-induced asystole in rats. Anesthesiology 1998; 88: 1071

57. Litz RJ, Popp M, Stehr SN et al: Successful resuscitation of a patient with ropivacaine-induced asystole after axillary plexus block using lipid infusion. Anaesthesia 2006; 61: 800

58. Rosenblatt MA, Abel M, Fischer GW et al: Successful use of a 20% lipid emulsion to resuscitate a patient after a presumed bupivacaine-related cardiac arrest. Anesthesiology 2006; 105: 217

59. Fremling MA, Mackinnon SE: Injection injury to the median nerve. Ann Plast. Surg 1996; 37: 561

60. Shah S, Hadzic A, Vloka JD et al: Neurologic complication after anterior sciatic nerve block. Anesth Analg 2005; 100: 1515

61. Selander D, Edshage S, Wolff T: Paresthesiae or no paresthesiae? Nerve lesions after axillary blocks. Acta Anaesthesiol Scand 1979; 23: 27

62. Winchell SW, Wolfe R: The incidence of neuropathy following upper extremity nerve blocks. Reg Anesth 1985; 10: 12

63. Enneking FK, Chan V, Greger J et al: Lower-extremity peripheral nerve blockade: essentials of our current understanding. Reg Anesth Pain Med 2005; 30: 4

64. Gentili F, Hudson AR, Hunter D et al: Nerve injection injury with local anesthetic agents: a light and electron microscopic, fluorescent microscopic, and horseradish peroxidase study. Neurosurgery 1980; 6: 263

65. Selander D: Peripheral nerve injury after regional anesthesia, Complications of Regional Anesthesia. Edited by Finucane BT. Philadelphia, Churchhill Livingstone, 1999, p 105

66. Fremling MA, Mackinnon SE: Injection injury to the median nerve. Ann Plast.Surg 1996; 37: 561

67. Pascal J, Charier D, Perret D et al: Peripheral blocks of trigeminal nerve for facial soft-tissue surgery: learning from failures. Eur. J Anaesthesiol 2005; 22: 480

68. Nguyen A, Girard F, Boudreault D et al: Scalp nerve blocks decrease the severity of pain after craniotomy. Anesth. Analg 2001; 93: 1272

69. Knize DM: A study of the supraorbital nerve. Plast Reconstr Surg 1995; 96: 564

70. Naja MZ, Al-Tannir M, Naja H et al: Repeated nerve blocks with clonidine, fentanyl and bupivacaine for trigeminal neuralgia. Anaesthesia 2006; 61: 70

71. Winnie AP, Ramamurthy S, Durrani Z et al: Interscalene cervical plexus block: a single-injection technic. Anesth. Analg 1975; 54: 370

72. Stoneham MD, Doyle AR, Knighton JD et al: Prospective, randomized comparison of deep or superficial cervical plexus block for carotid endarterectomy surgery. Anesthesiology 1998; 89: 907

73. de Sousa AA, Filho MA, Faglione W, Jr. et al: Superficial vs combined cervical plexus block for carotid endarterectomy: a prospective, randomized study. Surg. Neurol 2005; 63 Suppl 1: S22

74. Pandit JJ, Bree S, Dillon P et al: A comparison of superficial versus combined (superficial and deep) cervical plexus block for carotid endarterectomy: a prospective, randomized study. Anesth Analg 2000; 91: 781

75. Castresana EJ, Shaker IJ, Castresana MR: Incidence of shunting during carotid endarterectomy: Regional versus general anesthesia. Reg Anesth 1997; 22: 23S

76. Castresana MR, Masters RD, Castresana EJ et al: Incidence and clinical significance of hemidiaphragmatic paresis in patients undergoing carotid endarterectomy during cervical plexus block anesthesia. J Neurosurg Anesthesiol 1994; 6: 21

77. Masters RD, Castresana EJ, Castresana MR: Superficial and deep cervical plexus block: technical considerations. AANA J 1995; 63: 235

78. Stoneham MD, Knighton JD: Regional anaesthesia for carotid endarterectomy. Br J Anaesth 1999; 82: 910

79. Chen H, Sokoll LJ, Udelsman R: Outpatient minimally invasive parathyroidectomy: a combination of sestamibi-SPECT localization, cervical block anesthesia, and intraoperative parathyroid hormone assay. Surgery 1999; 126: 1016

80. Miccoli P, Barellini L, Monchik JM et al: Randomized clinical trial comparing regional and general anaesthesia in minimally invasive video-assisted parathyroidectomy. Br J Surg 2005; 92: 814

81. Spanknebel K, Chabot JA, DiGiorgi M et al: Thyroidectomy using local anesthesia: a report of 1,025 cases over 16 years. J Am Coll Surg 2005; 201: 375

82. Specht MC, Romero M, Barden CB et al: Characterisitcs of patients having thyroid surgery under regional anesthesia. J Am Coll Surg 2001; 193: 367

83. Tobias JD: Cervical plexus block in adolescents. J Clin Anesth 1999; 11: 606.

84. Burtles R: Analgesia for 'bat ear' surgery. Ann R Coll Surg Engl 1989; 71: 332

85. Afridi SK, Shields KG, Bhola R et al: Greater occipital nerve injection in primary headache syndromes—prolonged effects from a single injection. Pain 2006; 122: 126

86. Anthony M: Cervicogenic headache: prevalence and response to local steroid therapy. Clin Exp Rheumatol 2000; 18: S59

87. Sauter AR, Smith HJ, Stubhaug A et al: Use of magnetic resonance imaging to define the anatomical location closest to all three cords of the infraclavicular brachial plexus. Anesth Analg 2006; 103: 1574

88. Retzl G, Kapral S, Greher M et al: Ultrasonographic findings of the axillary part of the brachial plexus. Anesth Analg 2001; 92: 1271

89. Chan VWS, Perlas A, McCartney CJL et al: Ultrasound guidance improves success rate of axillary brachial plexus block. Can J Anesth 2007; 54: 176

90. Bonnel F: Microscopic anatomy of the adult human brachial plexus: an anatomical and histological basis for microsurgery. Microsurgery 1984; 5: 107

91. Klaastad O, Smedby O, Thompson GE et al: Distribution of local anesthetic in axillary brachial plexus block: a clinical and magnetic resonance imaging study. Anesthesiology 2002; 96: 1315

92. Kessler J, Gray AT: Sonography of scalene muscle anomalies for brachial plexus block. Reg Anesth Pain Med 2007; 32: 172

93. Uysal II, Seker M, Karabulut AK et al: Brachial plexus variations in human fetuses. Neurosurgery 2003; 53: 676

94. Orebaugh SL, Pennington S: Variant location of the musculocutaneous nerve during axillary nerve block. J Clin Anesth 2006; 18: 541

95. Venieratos D, Anagnostopoulou S: Classification of communications between the musculocutaneous and median nerves. Clin Anat 1998; 11: 327

96. Amoiridis G: Median—ulnar nerve communications and anomalous innervation of the intrinsic hand muscles: an electrophysiological study. Muscle Nerve 1992; 15: 576

97. Bigeleisen PE: The bifid axillary artery. J Clin Anesth 2004; 16: 224

98. Kutiyanawala MA, Stotter A, Windle R: Anatomical variants during axillary dissection. Br J Surg 1998; 85: 393

99. Uglietta JP, Kadir S: Arteriographic study of variant arterial anatomy of the upper extremities. Cardiovasc Intervent Radiol 1989; 12: 145

100. Winnie AP: Interscalene brachial plexus block. Anesth Analg 1970; 49: 466

101. Benumof JL: Permanent loss of cervical spinal cord function associated with interscalene block performed under general anesthesia. Anesthesiology 2000; 93: 1541

102. Yang WT, Chui PT, Metreweli C: Anatomy of the normal brachial plexus revealed by sonography and the role of sonographic guidance in anesthesia of the brachial plexus. AJR Am J Roentgenol 1998; 171: 1631

103. Demondion X, Herbinet P, Boutry N et al: Sonographic mapping of the normal brachial plexus. AJNR Am J Neuroradiol 2003; 24: 1303

104. Sheppard DG, Iyer RB, Fenstermacher MJ: Brachial plexus: demonstration at US. Radiology 1998; 208: 402

105. Boezaart AP, Koorn R, Rosenquist RW: Paravertebral approach to the brachial plexus: an anatomic improvement in technique. Reg Anesth Pain Med 2003; 28: 241

106. Klaastad O, VadeBoncouer TR, Tillung T et al: An evaluation of the supraclavicular plumb-bob technique for brachial plexus block by magnetic resonance imaging. Anesth Analg 2003; 96: 862

107. Apan A, Baydar S, Yilmaz S et al: Surface landmarks of brachial plexus: ultrasound and magnetic resonance imaging for supraclavicular approach with anatomical correlation. Eur J Ultrasound 2001; 13: 191

108. Kapral S, Jandrasits O, Schabernig C et al: Lateral infraclavicular plexus block vs. axillary block for hand and forearm surgery. Acta Anaesthesiol Scand 1999; 43: 1047

109. Klaastad O, Smith HJ, Smedby O et al: A novel infraclavicular brachial plexus block: the lateral and sagittal technique, developed by magnetic resonance imaging studies. Anesth Analg 2004; 98: 252

110. Raj PP, Montgomery SJ, Nettles D et al: Infraclavicular brachial plexus block—a new approach. Anesth Analg 1973; 52: 897

111. Rettig HC, Gielen MJ, Boersma E et al: A comparison of the vertical infraclavicular and axillary approaches for brachial plexus anaesthesia. Acta Anaesthesiol Scand 2005; 49: 1501

112. Whiffler K: Coracoid block—a safe and easy technique. Br J Anaesth 1981; 53: 845

113. Wilson JL, Brown DL, Wong GY et al: Infraclavicular brachial plexus block: parasagittal anatomy important to the coracoid technique. Anesth Analg 1998; 87: 870

114. Klaastad O, Lilleas FG, Rotnes JS et al: Magnetic resonance imaging demonstrates lack of precision in needle placement by the infraclavicular brachial plexus block described by Raj et al. Anesth Analg 1999; 88: 593

115. Koscielniak-Nielsen ZJ, Rasmussen H, Hesselbjerg L et al: Clinical evaluation of the lateral sagittal infraclavicular block developed by MRI studies. Reg Anesth Pain Med 2005; 30: 329

116. Groen GJ, Gielen MJ, Jack NT et al: At the cords, the pinkie towards: interpreting infraclavicular motor responses to neurostimulation. Reg Anesth Pain Med 2004; 29: 505

117. Borene SC, Edwards JN, Boezaart AP: At the cords, the pinkie towards: Interpreting infraclavicular motor responses to neurostimulation. Reg Anesth Pain Med 2004; 29: 125

118. Borene SC, Edwards JN, Boezaart A: Response to: At the cords, the Pinkie Towards: Interpreting Infraclavicular Motor Responses to Neurostimulation. Reg Anesth Pain Med 2004; 29: 505

119. Brull R, McCartney CJ, Chan VW: A novel approach to infraclavicular brachial plexus block: the ultrasound experience. Anesth Analg 2004; 99: 950

120. Urmey WF, Grossi P: Percutaneous electrode guidance and subcutaneous stimulating electrode guidance: modifications of the original technique. Reg Anesth Pain Med 2003; 28: 253

121. Horlocker TT: Peripheral nerve blocks-regional anesthesia for the new millennium. Reg Anesth Pain Med 1998; 23: 237

122. McDonnell JG, O'Donnell B, Curley G et al: The analgesic efficacy of transversus abdominis plane block after abdominal surgery: a prospective randomized controlled trial. Anesth Analg 2007; 104: 193

123. O'Donnell BD, McDonnell JG, McShane AJ: The transversus abdominis plane (TAP) block in open retropubic prostatectomy. Reg Anesth Pain Med 2006; 31: 91

124. Courreges P, Poddevin F, Lecoutre D: Para-umbilical block: a new concept for regional anaesthesia in children. Paediatr Anaesth 1997; 7: 211

125. Ferguson S, Thomas V, Lewis I: The rectus sheath block in paediatric anaesthesia: new indications for an old technique? Paediatr Anaesth 1996; 6: 463

126. Willschke H, Bosenberg A, Marhofer P et al: Ultrasonography-guided rectus sheath block in paediatric anaesthesia—a new approach to an old technique. Br J Anaesth 2006; 97: 244

127. Pourseidi B, Khorram-Manesh A: Effect of intercostals neural blockade with Marcaine (bupivacaine) on postoperative pain after laparoscopic cholecystectomy. Surgical Endoscopy 2007; 21: 1557

128. Pusch F, Freitag H, Weinstabl C et al: Single-injection paravertebral block compared to general anaesthesia in breast surgery. Acta Anaesthesiol Scand 1999; 43: 770

129. Naja Z, Lonnqvist PA: Somatic paravertebral nerve blockade. Incidence of failed block and complications. Anaesthesia 2001; 56: 1184

130. Willschke H, Bosenberg A, Marhofer P et al: Ultrasonographic-guided ilioinguinal/iliohypogastric nerve block in pediatric anaesthesia: what is the optimal volume? Anesth Analg 2006; 102: 1680

131. Eichenberger U, Greher M, Kirchmair L et al: Ultrasound-guided blocks of the ilioinguinal and iliohypogastric nerve: accuracy of a selective new technique confirmed by anatomical dissection. Br J Anaesth 2006; 97: 238

132. Winnie AP, Ramamurthy S, Durrani Z: The inguinal paravascular technic of lumbar plexus anesthesia: the "3-in-1 block". Anesth Analg 1973; 52: 989

133. Marhofer P, Nasel C, Sitzwohl C et al: Magnetic resonance imaging of the distribution of local anesthetic during the three-in-one block. Anesth Analg 2000; 90: 119

134. Parkinson SK, Mueller JB, Little WL et al: Extent of blockade with various approaches to the lumbar plexus. Anesth Analg 1989; 68: 243

135. Chayen D, Nathan H, Chayen M: The psoas compartment block. Anesthesiology 1976; 45: 95

136. Chudinov A, Berkenstadt H, Salai M et al: Continuous psoas compartment block for anesthesia and perioperative analgesia in patients with hip fractures. Reg Anesth Pain Med 1999; 24: 563

137. Capdevila X, Macaire P, Dadure C et al: Continuous psoas compartment block for postoperative analgesia after total hip arthroplasty: new landmarks, technical guidelines, and clinical evaluation. Anesth Analg 2002; 94: 1606

138. Aida S, Takahashi H, Shimoji K: Renal subcapsular hematoma after lumbar plexus block. Anesthesiology 1996; 84: 452

139. Magora F, Rozin R, Ben-Menachem Y et al: Obturator nerve block: an evaluation of technique. Br J Anaesth 1969; 41: 695

140. Sites BD, Beach M, Gallagher JD et al: A single injection ultrasound-assisted femoral nerve block provides side effect-sparing analgesia when compared with intrathecal morphine in patients undergoing total knee arthroplasty. Anesth Analg 2004; 99: 1539

ANESTHETIC MANAGEMENT

141. Barrington MJ, Olive D, Low K et al: Continuous femoral nerve blockade or epidural analgesia after total knee replacement: a prospective randomized controlled trial. Anesth Analg 2005; 101: 1824

142. Singelyn FJ, Deyaert M, Joris D et al: Effects of intravenous patient-controlled analgesia with morphine, continuous epidural analgesia, and continuous three-in-one block on postoperative pain and knee rehabilitation after unilateral total knee arthroplasty. Anesth Analg 1998; 87: 88

143. Lundblad M, Kapral S, Marhofer P et al: Ultrasound-guided infrapatellar nerve block in human volunteers: description of a novel technique. Br J Anaesth 2006; 97: 710

144. Vloka JD, Hadzic A, Drobnik L et al: Anatomical landmarks for femoral nerve block: a comparison of four needle insertion sites. Anesth Analg 1999; 89: 1467

145. Hayek SM, Ritchey RM, Sessler D et al: Continuous femoral nerve analgesia after unilateral total knee arthroplasty: stimulating versus nonstimulating catheters. Anesth Analg 2006; 103: 1565

146. Morin AM, Eberhart LH, Behnke HK et al: Does femoral nerve catheter placement with stimulating catheters improve effective placement? A randomized, controlled, and observer-blinded trial. Anesth Analg 2005; 100: 1503

147. Pham Dang C, Guilley J, Dernis L et al: Is there any need for expanding the perineural space before catheter placement in continuous femoral nerve blocks? Reg Anesth Pain Med 2006; 31: 393

148. Soong J, Schafhalter-Zoppoth I, Gray AT: The importance of transducer angle to ultrasound visibility of the femoral nerve. Reg Anesth Pain Med 2005; 30: 505

149. Shannon J, Lang SA, Yip RW et al: Lateral femoral cutaneous nerve block revisited. A nerve stimulator technique. Reg Anesth 1995; 20: 100

150. Soong J, Schafhalter-Zoppoth I, Gray AT: Sonographic imaging of the obturator nerve for regional block. Reg Anesth Pain Med 2007; 32: 146

151. Akata T, Murakami J, Yoshinaga A: Life-threatening haemorrhage following obturator artery injury during transurethral bladder surgery: a sequel of an unsuccessful obturator nerve block. Acta Anaesthesiol Scand 1999; 43: 784

152. van der Wal M, Lang SA, Yip RW: Transsartorial approach for saphenous nerve block. Can J Anaesth 1993; 40: 542

153. Benzon HT, Sharma S, Calimaran A: Comparison of the different approaches to saphenous nerve block. Anesthesiology 2005; 102: 633

154. Tsui B.C. Ultrasound-guided transsartorial perifemoral artery approach for a saphenous nerve block. Reg Anesth Pain Med 2007; *In Press*

155. de Mey JC, Deruyck LJ, Cammu G et al: A paravenous approach for the saphenous nerve block. Reg Anesth Pain Med 2001; 26: 504

156. Gray AT, Collins AB: Ultrasound-guided saphenous nerve block. Reg Anesth Pain Med 2003; 28: 148

157. Tsui BC, Ozelsel T. Ultrasound-guided anterior sciatic nerve block using a longitudinal approach: "expanding the view." Reg Anesth Pain Med 2008; 33: 275

158. Pham DC: Midfemoral block: a new lateral approach to the sciatic nerve. Anesth Analg 1999; 88: 1426

159. Zetlaoui PJ, Bouaziz H: Lateral approach to the sciatic nerve in the popliteal fossa. Anesth Analg 1998; 87: 79

160. March X, Pineda O, Garcia MM et al: The posterior approach to the sciatic nerve in the popliteal fossa: a comparison of single- versus double-injection technique. Anesth Analg 2006; 103: 1571

161. Vloka JD, Hadzic A: The intensity of the current at which sciatic nerve stimulation is achieved is a more important factor in determining the quality of nerve block than the type of motor response obtained. Anesthesiology 1998; 88: 1408

SECTION VII ■ ANESTHESIA FOR SURGICAL SUBSPECIALTIES

CHAPTER 39 ■ ANESTHESIA FOR NEUROSURGERY

M. SEAN KINCAID AND ARTHUR M. LAM

KEY POINTS

1. Anatomically, blood flow to the normal brain is supplied by the two carotid arteries and vertebral arteries. Collateral circulation is provided via the Circle of Willis.

2. Physiologically, blood flow to the brain is tightly regulated. The homeostatic mechanisms include flow-metabolism coupling, pressure autoregulation, and CO_2 reactivity.

3. These homeostatic mechanisms are affected by diseases as well as anesthetic drugs and techniques.

4. Multiple monitoring modalities are available to monitor brain function, perfusion, and oxygenation/metabolism. These include electroencephalogram, somatosensory evoked potentials, motor evoked potentials, electromyogram, intracranial pressure, transcranial Doppler ultrasonography, brain tissue oxygenation, and jugular venous oximetry. Although most are applicable for monitoring in the neurointensive care unit, many are useful in the operating room to increase patient safety and improve outcome.

5. Definitive cerebral protective therapy remains elusive, but many techniques have been investigated and some are frequently used in the operating room on theoretical grounds. These include the use of hypothermia, tight control of blood glucose, and maintenance of adequate perfusion. Anemia threshold for blood transfusion remains controversial.

6. Anesthetic management of the patient with neurologic disease mandates a thorough preoperative assessment as there are often multisystem manifestations.

7. Anesthetic techniques may influence brain relaxation conditions. In general intravenous agents cause more cerebral vasoconstriction than inhalation agents. There are no outcome studies demonstrating the superiority of any particular anesthetic agent. The use of intraoperative monitoring of evoked potentials makes an impact on the choice of anesthetic technique.

8. Movement of water into the brain is primarily determined by the osmotic gradient, which in turn is determined by serum osmolarity. Outcome studies do not provide guidance regarding the choice of crystalloids versus colloids. In patients with brain trauma the use of albumin for resuscitation is associated with increased mortality.

9. Common neurosurgical procedures requiring special understanding and expertise include tumor excision, transphenoidal or transcranial removal of pituitary lesions, extirpation of arteriovenous malformation, repair or clipping of aneurysms, carotid endarterectomy, craniotomy for traumatic brain lesions including epidural and subdural hematomas.

GOALS

The goal of this chapter is to provide the anesthesiologist with the requisite knowledge base with which to approach the anesthetic management of patients with disease of the central nervous system (CNS), including the brain and the spine. After an overview of neuroanatomy and neurophysiology, the focus of the chapter is on anesthesia for neurosurgical procedures and spine surgery, but the information should also be relevant to the patient with neurologic disease who is undergoing non-neurosurgical procedures.

NEUROANATOMY

A basic knowledge of neuroanatomy is essential for all anesthesiologists, particularly those caring for patients with disease of the CNS. Although the brain and spinal cord, which make up the CNS, are fragile organs, the bony structures that surround them provide protection. Yet by virtue of their protective nature, these structures are nondistensible. The intracranial volume is fixed, thereby providing little room for anything other than the brain, cerebrospinal fluid (CSF), and blood contained in the cerebral vasculature. Even the space in the spinal column, although not as restrictive as the cranium, is quickly exhausted by an expanding hematoma or abscess. It is in the context of the restrictive nature of the space in which the CNS is housed that all interventions must be considered.

❶   The blood supply to the brain is also unique. The carotid artery in the neck bifurcates into the external and internal carotid arteries, sending the internal branch through the base of the skull, perfusing the eye via the ophthalmic artery, and ultimately bifurcating into the anterior and middle cerebral arteries. These vessels define the anterior cerebral circulation. The posterior circulation results from the vertebral arteries, which ascend in the posterior aspect of the neck through foramina in the cervical vertebral bodies before exiting, coursing around the brainstem, and joining the contralateral vessel to form the basilar artery. The basilar artery ascends along the brainstem before dividing into the posterior cerebral arteries. The anterior and posterior circulations anastomose through the posterior communicating arteries to provide collateral flow; collateral circulation can also occur through the anterior communicating artery connecting the bilateral anterior cerebral arteries. This system of collateralization, named the *circle of Willis* (Fig. 39-1), was described by Thomas Willis (1621–1675) with the recognition of its purpose ". . . that there may be a manifold way, and that more certain, for the blood about to go into divers Regions of the Brain."

The spinal column is the bony structure made up of the 7 cervical, 12 thoracic, 5 lumbar vertebrae, as well as the sacrum. The spinal cord exits the skull through the foramen magnum and enters the canal formed by the vertebral bodies. In the adult, the cord typically ends at the lower aspect of the first lumbar vertebral body.

Blood supply to the entire cord is provided by several sources. The anterior spinal artery, which arises from the vertebral arteries, supplies the anterior two thirds of the spinal cord. This vessel runs the length of the cord, receiving contribution from radicular arteries via intercostal vessels. The artery of Adamkiewicz is the most important radicular vessel, typically joining the anterior spinal artery in the lower thoracic region and providing blood to the thoracolumbar cord. The posterior third of the cord is supplied by two posterior spinal arteries, which arise from the vertebral arteries and also receive contribution from radicular arteries (Fig. 39-2).

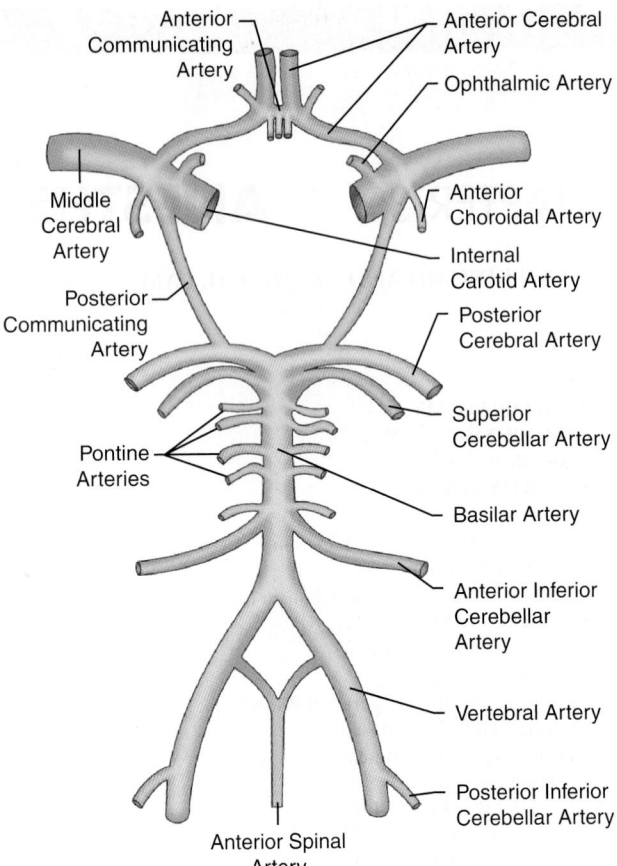

FIGURE 39-1.   Circle of Willis, and other blood supply to brain and spinal cord.

NEUROPHYSIOLOGY

Cerebral metabolic rate is directly related to the number and frequency of neuron depolarizations. Therefore, any activity or stimulation raises the metabolic rate. Cerebral blood flow (CBF) is tightly coupled to metabolism, on a regional as well on a global level. As an example, although visual stimulation may raise blood flow to the occipital cortex, mild hyperthermia, which raises global cerebral metabolic rate, increases flow to the entire brain.

The CSF occupies the subarachnoid space, providing a protective layer of fluid between the brain and the tissue that surrounds it. CSF is produced by the choroid plexus in the ventricles. CSF produced in the lateral ventricles travels into the third ventricle via the interventricular foramina. It subsequently transits through the cerebral aqueduct into the fourth ventricle, and then into the space around the brain via the foramina of Luschka and Magendie. It bathes both the spinal cord and the brain. Absorption into the dural venous sinuses occurs through the arachnoid granulations. Although CSF volume is approximately 150 mL, more than 3 times this amount is produced in a 24-hour period. This continuous flow of CSF from source to sink allows it to participate in many functions in addition to cushioning the brain. It maintains a milieu in which the brain can function by regulating pH and electrolytes, carrying away waste products, and delivering nutrients.[1,2]

Intracranial pressure (ICP) is low except in pathologic states. The Monroe-Kellie doctrine states that in the setting of a nondistensible cranial vault, the volume of blood, CSF, and brain tissue must be in equilibrium. An increase in one of these three elements,

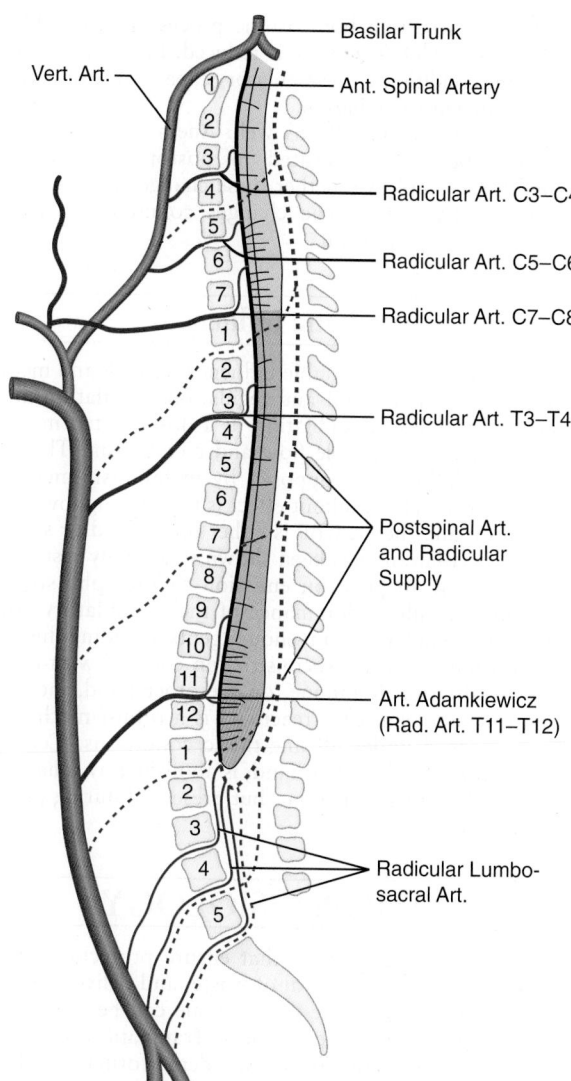

FIGURE 39-2.   Blood supply to the spinal cord. Both the single anterior spinal artery and the paired posterior spinal artery arise from the vertebral arteries. The radicular arteries and particularly the artery of Adamkiewicz are important contributors. The anterior spinal artery supplies the anterior two thirds of the spinal cord, with the posterior spinal artery supplying the rest. vert., vertebral; art., artery; ant., anterior.

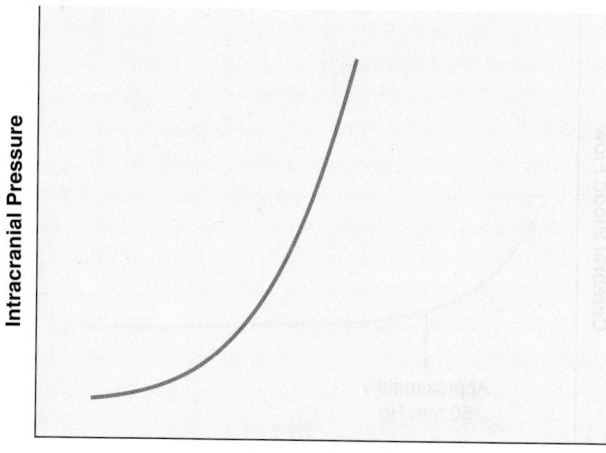

FIGURE 39-3.   Intracranial compliance (elastance) curve. The brain has minimal compensatory capacity, and any increase in mass from hematoma or brain swelling will result in an inordinate increase in intracranial pressure.

the brain or decrease ICP. This effect is thought to be short-lived, however. CSF pH normalizes over time, and vessel caliber returns to baseline. The exact duration of hypocapnic vasoconstriction is uncertain; a period of minutes to hours has been found in different patient populations.[3] Because the decrease in CBF occurs without a change in cerebral metabolic rate, the risk of ischemia is a theoretical concern. The significance of this concern is uncertain, however. We have no evidence of harm of moderate hyperventilation to the normal brain under general anesthesia. Early hyperventilation in traumatic brain injury (TBI) is associated with poor outcome, and the consequence of hyperventilation in TBI after the initial 24 hours is of uncertain consequence[4–6] (see Chapter 36).

In contrast to CO_2, O_2 has little effect on CBF except at abnormally low levels (Fig. 39-5). When PaO_2 falls below 50 mm Hg, CBF begins to increase sharply. A teleological explanation for this phenomenon is that CBF needs to increase only when O_2 content of the blood begins to decrease significantly.

CBF remains approximately constant despite modest swings in arterial blood pressure. The mechanism by which CBF is maintained, originally described by Lassen,[7] is called *autoregulation*

or the addition of a space-occupying lesion, can be accommodated initially through displacement of CSF into the thecal sac, but only to a small extent. Further increase, as with significant cerebral edema or accumulation of an extradural hematoma, will quickly lead to a marked increase in intracranial pressure due to the low intracranial compliance (Fig. 39-3).

As mentioned earlier, blood flow to the brain is tightly coupled to cerebral metabolism. As such, many factors affect CBF because of their effect on metabolism. Stimulation, arousal, nociception, and mild hyperthermia elevate metabolism and flow, while sedative-hypnotic agents and hypothermia decrease both metabolism and flow. A number of other factors govern CBF directly without changing metabolism. A potent determinant of CBF is arterial CO_2 tension ($PaCO_2$). Within physiologic range, CBF has an approximately linear relationship with $PaCO_2$. CBF changes by approximately 3% of baseline for each 1 mm Hg change in $PaCO_2$ (Fig. 39-4). As CBF changes, so does cerebral blood volume (CBV), which is why hyperventilation can be used for short periods of time to relax

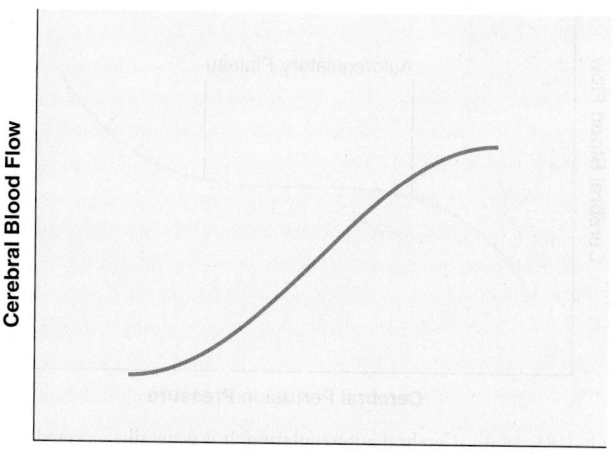

FIGURE 39-4.   Cerebrovascular response to change in $PaCO_2$ partial pressure. The change is linear between $PaCO_2$ of 25 and 65 mm Hg.

ANESTHESIA FOR SURGICAL SUBSPECIALTIES

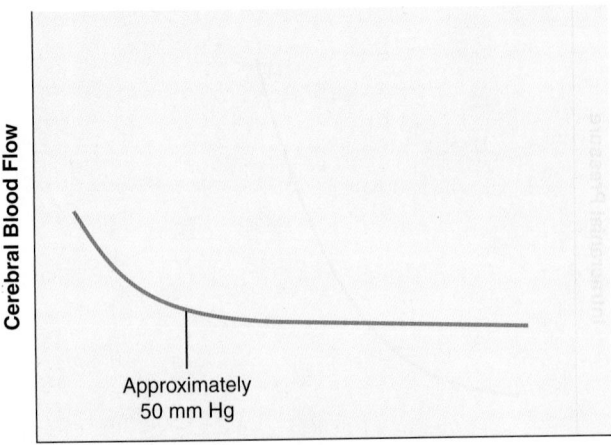

FIGURE 39-5. Cerebrovascular response to change in PaO_2 partial pressure. The response of cerebral blood flow to change in PaO_2 is flat until PaO_2 falls below 50 mm Hg.

of CBF, or at times, pressure autoregulation of CBF. As cerebral perfusion pressure (CPP), defined as the difference of mean arterial pressure (MAP) and ICP, changes, cerebrovascular resistance adjusts to maintain stable flow. The resistance is varied at the arteriolar level. The range of CPP over which autoregulation is maintained is termed the *autoregulatory plateau*. Although this range is frequently quoted as a MAP range of 60 to 150 mm Hg, there is significant variability between individuals, and these numbers are only approximate. At the low end of the plateau, cerebrovascular resistance is at a minimum, and any further decrease in CPP will compromise CBF. At the high end of the plateau, cerebrovascular resistance is at a maximum, and any further increase in CPP will result in hyperemia (Fig. 39-6). Various mechanisms have been proposed to account for autoregulation, including myogenic, neurogenic, and local metabolic mediators. However, the exact mechanism remains undefined.

There is interaction between CO_2 reactivity and pressure autoregulation, although the molecular mechanism is likely

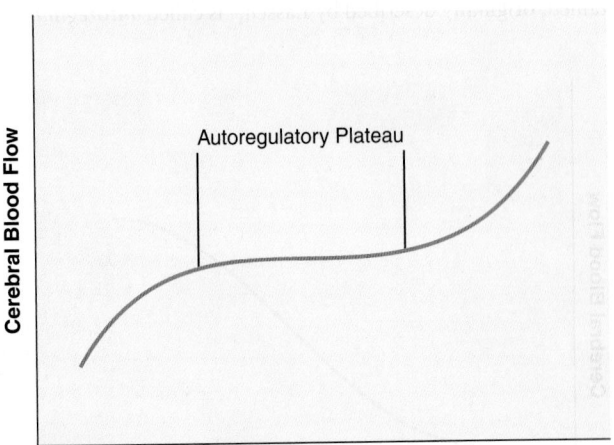

FIGURE 39-6. Cerebral autoregulation. It is generally accepted that cerebral blood flow is maintained constant between 60 and 160 mm Hg. However, these are average values, and there is considerable variation in both the lower and the upper limit of cerebral autoregulation among normal individuals.

different for these two homeostatic processes. When blood pressure is low, CO_2 reactivity is reduced. In contrast, under hypercapnic conditions, autoregulatory capacity is lost because of the concurrent vasodilation.

Other factors affect CBF as well. Anemia increases CBF, which has been demonstrated in postoperative cardiac patients, for example.[8] Whether these changes play a role in the perioperative neurologic changes common to cardiac surgery patients is uncertain.

Anesthetic Influences

Anesthetic agents have variable influence on CBF and metabolism, CO_2 reactivity, and autoregulation. Inhalation anesthetics tend to cause vasodilation in a dose-related manner, but do not per se uncouple flow and metabolism. Thus the vasodilatory influence is opposed by metabolism-mediated decrease in flow. The resultant effect is that during low doses of inhalation anesthesia, CBF is either unchanged or slightly increased. Sevoflurane has been shown to actually result in a decrease in CBF in positron emission tomography studies. Higher doses result in dominance of the vasodilatory effect and an increase in CBF. Intravenous agents including thiopental and propofol cause vasoconstriction coupled with reduction in metabolism. Ketamine, on the other hand, increases flow and metabolism. CO_2 reactivity is a robust mechanism and is preserved under all anesthetic conditions. Cerebral autoregulation, on the other hand, is abolished by inhalation agents in a dose-related manner but preserved during propofol anesthesia.

PATHOPHYSIOLOGY

The homeostatic mechanisms that ensure protection of the brain and spinal cord, removal of waste, and delivery of adequate oxygen and substrate to the tissue can be interrupted through a multitude of mechanisms. Traumatic insults may result in contusion with subsequent edema formation, direct injury from depressed skull fractures or spine fractures, diffuse injury to neurons from rapid deceleration, and disruption of the vasculature, resulting in ischemia or hemorrhage. All of these insults may ultimately compromise CNS perfusion.

Mass lesions, such as tumors, may compress adjacent structures, raise ICP, and obstruct normal flow of CSF. Hemorrhage may be spontaneous or traumatic. Depending on its location, they may cause mass effect, impair CSF circulation, or, in the case of subarachnoid blood, breakdown of the blood may lead to further ischemic injury by causing cerebral vasospasm.

Hydrocephalus is caused by an imbalance between CSF production and removal. It frequently results in elevation of ICP. Hydrocephalus is commonly divided into two categories: communicating hydrocephalus and obstructive hydrocephalus. The former is characterized by a failure to absorb CSF, typically because of dysfunctional arachnoid granulations. The latter may be caused by any direct obstruction or extrinsic compression of a passageway through which CSF must pass, such as the cerebral aqueduct. This obstruction, for example, may result from clot within the space or from tumor adjacent to it. Depending on the circumstances, hydrocephalus can have a subtle or dramatic presentation. For example, acute hydrocephalus following an intraventricular hemorrhage may result in rapidly progressive obtundation that improves dramatically with external ventricular drainage. In contrast, normal-pressure hydrocephalus may evolve over years, resulting in barely perceptible changes in cognition and gait.

MONITORING

❹ Anesthesia for neurosurgery and spine surgery requires the standard American Society of Anesthesiologists monitoring for physiologic parameters. The risk imposed to the CNS by these surgical procedures warrants more extensive monitoring, however. For many procedures, adequate oxygenation, ventilation, and systemic blood pressure do not ensure the well-being of the brain and spinal cord. Instead, the integrity of the CNS needs to be evaluated intraoperatively with monitors that specifically detect CNS function, perfusion, or metabolism. At times, the monitoring modalities can be combined to provide greater information regarding the well-being of the CNS.

Central Nervous System Function

Electroencephalogram

The electroencephalogram (EEG) is the quintessential cerebral function monitor. The depolarization of cortical neurons provides a pattern of electrical activity that can be measured on the scalp. Typically the activity is measured between two points on the scalp (bipolar), as there is no electrically neutral place from which to reference the signal. Other sources of electrical activity, such as that from the heart and muscles, must be filtered from the signal, otherwise they would overwhelm the small voltages generated by the cortical activity. Common-mode rejection, that is, rejection of signal common to both electrodes, allows interference from cardiac and muscle activity to be minimized.

Several standardized systems of electrode placement have been developed to facilitate reliable and consistent EEG monitoring, the most common of which is the International 10–20 System. In brief, artificial meridians are generated on the scalp running front to back and side to side, where the 10–20 refers to the percentage of the distance across the scalp, either from tragus to tragus or nasion to inion, that defines that meridian (Fig. 39-7). Electrodes can be placed at the intersection of each meridian. Each such intersection or point is given a name—either a combination of letters and a number, or two letters, where the final letter is Z. The letters are F for frontal, C for central, P for parietal, T for temporal, O for occipital, A for auricular, and Fp for frontal pole. A letter followed by an odd number is a point on the left hemisphere, while a letter followed by an even number is a point on the right hemisphere. Two letters, with the second letter a Z, indicate a point along midline.

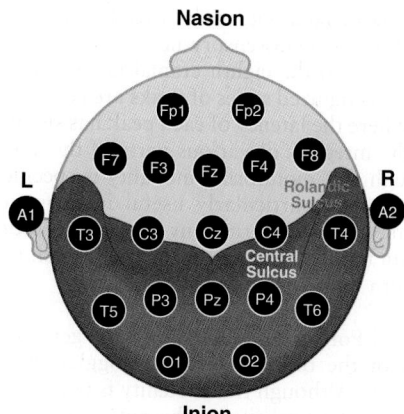

FIGURE 39-7. The international 10-20 system for electroencephalogram electrode montage. The odd numbers denote the left (L) hemisphere whereas the even numbers represent the right (R) hemisphere. See text for details.

TABLE 39-1

ELECTROENCEPHALOGRAM FREQUENCIES

WAVE	RANGE (Hz)	DESCRIPTION
Delta	0–3	Low frequency, high amplitude; present in deep coma, encephalopathy, and deep anesthesia
Theta	4–7	Not prominent in adults, although may be seen in encephalopathy
Alpha	8–12	Prominent in the posterior region during relaxation with eyes closed
Beta	>12	High frequency, low amplitude; the dominant frequency during arousal

Although sophisticated EEG monitoring for epilepsy evaluation may require recording of multiple channels, providing information on the activity between numerous points, the EEG monitoring performed during anesthesia frequently uses a broad montage with fewer channels (two or four) to evaluate hemispheric activity. Once the signal is recorded, it can be evaluated in several ways. Viewing raw EEG may be appropriate at times, but subtle changes are difficult to detect, particularly for the infrequent user. However, the EEG can be processed to yield readily interpretable information. A common method use is frequency domain analysis. Using Fourier analysis, the apparent random activity of raw EEG can be broken down into a series of wave frequencies, the summation of which gives the overall EEG pattern. The range of frequencies seen in EEG is described in Table 39-1. The power (amplitude squared) at each frequency can then be plotted as a spectral array, whereby the effect of various influences such as anesthetic agents or ischemic insult can be detected by how they modify the spectral analysis. A common parameter to include in analysis of EEG is the spectral edge frequency, which is the frequency below which 95% of the power resides.

A progressive reduction in CBF will produce a reliable pattern change in EEG, consisting of a loss of high-frequency activity, a loss of power, and the eventual progression to EEG silence. The monitor is therefore useful when surgical procedures jeopardize the perfusion of the brain, such as cross-clamp of the carotid artery during carotid endarterectomy (CEA). EEG is particularly useful in this setting because the spectral analysis on the at-risk side can be compared in real time with the unaffected side, thus facilitating detection of ischemia by the resultant asymmetry of the spectral edge frequency.

The changes in the EEG spectrum seen with ischemia can occur as a result of other influences, however. Intravenous anesthetic agents such as propofol and thiopental, as well as inhaled agents such as isoflurane, will cause a similar decrease in the spectral edge frequency, with eventual progression to a drug-induced isoelectric EEG in a dose-related manner. During certain surgical procedures, such as extracranial-to-intracranial bypass procedures, maximal suppression of cerebral metabolic rate is desirable to protect the brain during an ischemic insult. Under such circumstances, the anesthetic agent can be titrated against the EEG until the desired effect is achieved. Typically, instead of an isoelectric EEG, the goal is a state called *burst suppression*. In this state, periods of isoelectric EEG are punctuated by "bursts" of EEG activity. When burst suppression is the goal, a suppression ratio can be calculated as the percentage of an epoch in which the patient's EEG is isoelectric. The suppression ratio allows one to achieve near-complete suppression (>90%) of EEG activity, while remaining certain that regular EEG activity will return

TABLE 39-2

INDICATIONS FOR ELECTROENCEPHALOGRAM MONITORING

During anesthesia	1. Carotid endarterectomy
	2. Cardiopulmonary bypass procedures
	3. Cerebrovascular surgery
	   a. Aneurysm surgery involving temporary clipping
	   b. Vascular bypass procedures
	4. When burst suppression is desired for cerebral protection

In the intensive care unit	1. Barbiturate coma for patients with traumatic brain injury 2. When subclinical seizures are suspected

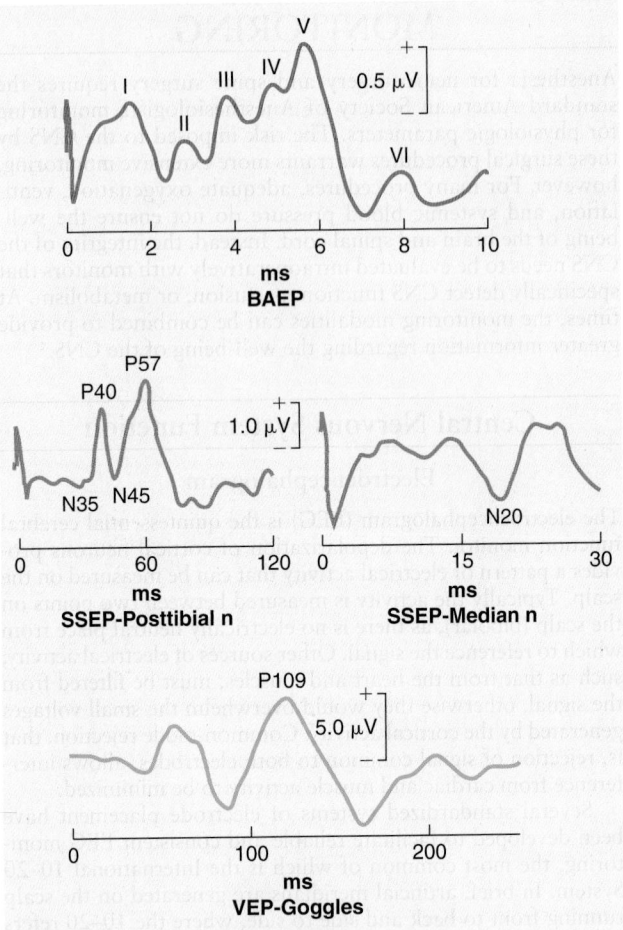

FIGURE 39-8. Representative tracings of multiple modalities of sensory evoked potential. BAEP, brainstem auditory evoked potential; n, nerve; SSEP, somatosensory evoked potential; VEP, visual evoked potential.

in a short while with cessation of administration of the drug. In contrast, when complete isoelectric EEG is achieved, time to arousal becomes unpredictable. Other settings in which EEG monitoring and burst suppression may be useful are listed in Table 39-2.

Evoked Potential Monitoring

Although EEG is a cerebral function monitor that detects spontaneous activity, evoked potential modalities detect signals that are the result of specific stimuli applied to the patient. These include somatosensory evoked potential (SSEP), brainstem auditory evoked potential (BAEP), visual evoked potential (VEP), and motor evoked potential (MEP).

Somatosensory Evoked Potential. SSEP is a signal that is detectable on EEG and that is generated in a time-locked fashion in response to a specific applied sensory input, typically a cutaneous electrical stimulation (i.e., of a peripheral sensory nerve, but also of a cranial nerve with a sensory pathway). As a result, an intact neural pathway from the periphery to the cerebral sensory cortex is essential for a signal to be generated. This monitoring modality has application in any surgical procedure that may jeopardize this pathway. Specifically, spine surgery in which the dorsal column of the spinal cord may be placed at risk is a particularly appropriate application, but it may also be used during other procedures such as craniotomy and carotid surgery where any part of the pathway may be subjected to ischemia or surgical retraction.

Because of the presence of spontaneous EEG activity, a single peripheral stimulus, which generates cortical activity of relatively low amplitude, would not be detectable amidst the background noise. Summation followed by signal averaging of repetitive stimuli is therefore necessary in order to extract meaningful signals.

Stimulation is typically done in the regions of the median nerve, ulnar nerve, and posterior tibial nerve to generate predictable and reliable signals. In theory, however, any sensory nerve could be used to generate SSEP. The SSEP is described by its polarity (the direction of the wave deflection) and its latency (the time required for a signal to be detected after the stimulus has been applied), and is quantified by both the amplitude of that signal and its latency. For example, N20 is the SSEP generated via stimulation of the median nerve that is expected to have a latency of approximately 20 ms and a negative displacement (Fig. 39-8).

Disruption of the neural pathway at any point will result in complete loss of SSEP. More commonly, ischemia, not mechanical disruption, is the intraoperative insult. As a result of ischemia, the amplitude of the signal decreases and the latency increases. A 50% decrease in signal amplitude is generally accepted as clinically significant, as is a 10% increase in latency.

Brainstem Auditory Evoked Potential. BAEP is a specialized type of sensory evoked potential. Instead of an electrical stimulus applied to a somatosensory nerve, a standardized sound (click) is applied to the eighth cranial nerve via the auditory apparatus. A recognized series of peaks are generated with this technique, where the latency of each peak has significance with respect to the integrity of various parts of the auditory pathway. Although this monitoring modality is specific to cranial nerve VIII, and is particularly useful in acoustic neuroma surgery, it may be used during any surgical procedure around the brainstem to infer its integrity, although such use is associated with both low sensitivity and specificity.

Visual Evoked Potential. VEP signals are generated via light stimulation of the retina. Typically, goggles that emit LED lights are worn. Although this modality is particularly appealing to monitor the integrity of the optic nerve in settings in which visual loss is a concern, such as in prone spine surgery, the signals are not robust. They are difficult to record in a consistent fashion during anesthesia. Research is ongoing with respect to its intraoperative use, particularly with regard to its interpretation.

Motor Evoked Potential.   MEP monitoring is different from the other evoked potential modalities described thus far. Whereas SSEP, BAEP, and VEP provide information about ascending sensory neural pathways (i.e., from the periphery to the cerebral cortex), MEP evaluates descending motor pathways (i.e., from the cerebral cortex, past the neuromuscular junction, to peripheral muscle groups). This difference allows MEP to complement SSEP, particularly in the setting of spine surgery, in which the two modalities provide information about the integrity of anatomically different areas of the spinal cord. With MEP, the stimulus is applied in a transcranial fashion over the motor cortex. The deflection, essentially an electromyographic signal, is then detected by electrodes embedded in the muscle belly. Although theoretically the stimulus can be delivered with either a magnetic or electrical source, transcranial magnetic stimulation is obliterated under anesthesia. The transcranial electrical signal is usually delivered as a rapid train of four or more stimuli, the voltage of which is adjusted to achieve adequate signals in both the upper and lower extremities. The MEP is typically detected at the thenar eminence and the abductor hallucis muscle. Transcranial electrical MEP is of substantially greater magnitude compared with SSEP, and signal averaging with repetitive stimuli is therefore not required. However, it is very sensitive to anesthetic agents, particularly the inhalation anesthetics. Its amplitude can be augmented by increasing the transcranial voltage, or the number of stimuli in the train. The stimulus can cause patient movement, so MEP signals are typically obtained intermittently at points during the surgery when slight patient movements are not problematic. A bite block is mandatory to prevent injury to the tongue during transcranial stimulation.

With MEP, latency of the signal is somewhat unreliable, and not typically used to make clinical decisions. Decision making is based on amplitude alone, where a 50% decrease is considered significant (Fig. 39-9). Although MEP can be used during any spine or intracranial surgical procedure, it is becoming increasingly used during cervical spine surgery.

MEP signals are much more sensitive to volatile anesthesia than SSEP. Although there is some evidence that MEP signals are adequate during desflurane anesthesia, more research on the efficacy of this technique is required, and total intravenous anesthesia is the preferred technique when MEP monitoring is required.[9] Some centers use partial neuromuscular blockade, but most centers avoid muscle relaxants altogether with MEP in order to avoid compromise of the signal.[10]

Spontaneous Electromyography

Spontaneous electromyography (EMG) is different from other evoked potentials in that a signal is not intentionally generated through stimulation at some point in a known neural pathway. Instead, it is a continuous recording of EMG activity in the muscle of regions innervated by nerve roots around which surgeons are working. Its purpose is to detect injury to those nerve roots by the surgical procedure. Impingement on a nerve root by an instrument will cause immediate motor activity that is easily detectable, which may allow the surgeon to modify his or her technique. Although spontaneous EMG is a robust signal that is tolerant of various anesthetic techniques, muscle relaxant must be avoided. Spontaneous EMG is frequently used during cervical and lumbar spine surgery where the brachial plexus and lumbosacral plexus are encountered.

Cranial Nerve Monitoring

Surgery in the posterior cranial fossa and adjacent to the brainstem places the surgeon in close proximity to cranial nerves. Although cranial nerve VIII can be monitored with BAEP as discussed earlier, several other cranial nerves can be monitored as well. Generally, only the integrity of nerves with motor components can be detected, either through spontaneous EMG or through EMG evoked by local electrical stimulation. These include cranial nerves V, VII, IX, XI, and XII.

Influence of Anesthetic Technique.   As mentioned previously, anesthetic agents can have profound influence on the amplitude and latency of evoked potentials. For instance, the quality of signals obtained with SSEP monitoring depends on the anesthetic agents used. Signals are obtainable under volatile anesthesia, but the anesthetic is typically kept at sub-MAC (minimum alveolar concentration) doses to avoid degradation in quality (increase in latency and decrease in amplitude), as amplitude of SSEP signals are depressed by volatile agents in a dose-related manner; they are recordable during low dose and obliterated with high doses. Potent volatile anesthetics should not be combined with nitrous oxide, as this technique will further compromise quality. The signals are unaffected by opioids, and opioid infusions are frequently used to facilitate low-dose volatile anesthesia. Signal quality is also excellent under intravenous anesthesia with propofol.

To summarize the influence of anesthetic agents on evoked potential monitoring, general statements can be made.

1. Inhalation agents including nitrous oxide generally have more depressant effects on evoked potential monitoring than intravenous agents.
2. Cortical evoked potentials with long latency involving multiple synapses are exquisitely sensitive to influence of anesthetic while short latency brainstem and spinal components are resistant to anesthetic influence. Thus, BAEP can be recorded under any anesthetic technique whereas VEP and SSEP are very sensitive.
3. Monitoring of MEP and cranial nerve EMG in general preclude the use of muscle relaxants, although use of a short-acting neuromuscular blocking agent for the purpose of tracheal intubation is not contraindicated as its effect usually wears off before monitoring and surgery begins.
4. MEP is exquisitely sensitive to the depressant effects of inhalation anesthetics including nitrous oxide. Although it can be recorded with low-dose agents, the signals are so severely attenuated that this practice is generally not advisable. Total intravenous anesthesia without nitrous oxide is the ideal anesthetic technique for monitoring of MEP.

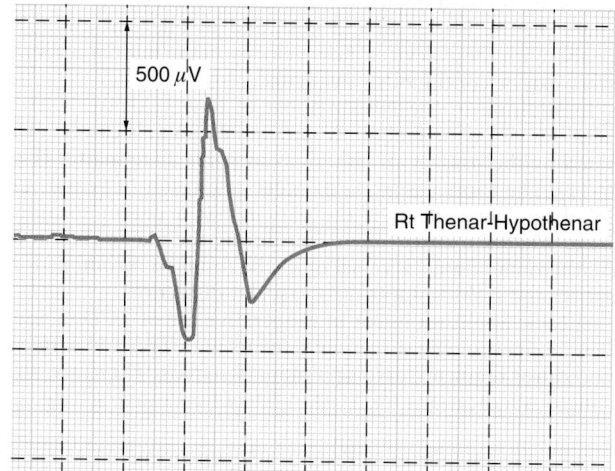

MEP from Stimulation of Left Cranium

500 μV

Rt Thenar Hypothenar

FIGURE 39-9.   Representative tracing of motor evoked potential (MEP) recorded from the thenar muscles in response to transcranial electrical stimulation.

FIGURE 39-10. Transcranial Doppler tracing with release of cross-clamp during carotid endarterectomy. The resultant hyperemia is accompanied with evidence of air emboli (vertical streaks on the tracing). MCA, middle cerebral artery; ICA, internal carotid artery.

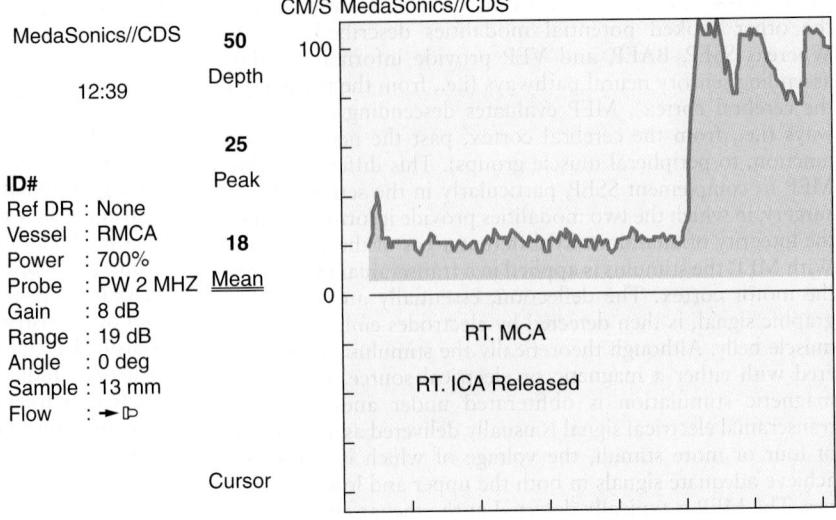

Cerebral Perfusion

Although adequate CBF does not guarantee the well-being of the CNS, it is one factor that is essential to its integrity. Measuring CBF is therefore an attractive method of monitoring the CNS. Currently available techniques for quantitative measurement of CBF are not practical as an intraoperative monitor, other methods for looking at relative changes in CBF do lend themselves to use in the operating room. Transcranial Doppler ultrasonography (TCD) and laser Doppler flowmetry are examples. Furthermore, as adequate CBF depends on an appropriate CPP, measuring intracranial pressure may be useful in certain patients to ensure conditions are adequate for sufficient CBF. Finally, numerous other modalities that evaluate CBF and that may not be practical in the operating room are used commonly in the perioperative setting.

Laser Doppler Flowmetry

Laser Doppler flowmetry is a technique that measures cortical blood flow in a small region of the brain adjacent to the placement of the device. Although it is useful for detecting relative changes in CBF, its utility is limited by several factors. First, it requires a burr hole for placement, which prevents its use in most patients. Second, it measures flow in only a small region of the brain; it could miss hypoperfusion in any area of the brain not directly monitored. Because of these limitations, laser Doppler flowmetry has found only limited applications.

5. Opioids and benzodiazepines have negligible effects on recording of evoked potentials.
6. Propofol and thiopental attenuate the amplitude of virtually all modalities of evoked potential but do not obliterate them. SSEP and MEP can be monitored even during burst suppression induced by these agents. BAEP can be recorded with any anesthetic technique.
7. During crucial events in which part of the central neural pathway is specifically placed at risk by surgical manipulation, as in placement of a temporary clip during aneurysm surgery, change in "anesthetic depth" should be minimized to avoid misinterpretation of the changes in evoked potential recorded.
8. Ketamine and etomidate have been reported to enhance the quality of signals in patients with weak baseline signals, although the clinical significance and interpretation of signals obtained under these circumstances remain unclear.

Transcranial Doppler Ultrasonography

TCD is a noninvasive monitor for evaluating relative changes in flow through the large basal arteries of the brain (i.e., the circle of Willis). TCD does not measure flow directly, and therefore cannot provide information regarding absolute CBF. TCD measures flow velocity (Fig. 39-10), which is directly proportional to flow if the diameters of these large vessels are constant. Except in well-known circumstances such as cerebral vasospasm following aneurysmal subarachnoid hemorrhage, these vessels are thought to be conductance vessels, where diameters of the basal arteries are stable.[11] Pressure autoregulation and CO_2 reactivity of CBF occur via changes in arteriolar diameter distal to these large vessels.

Although the vessels that can be evaluated with TCD include the middle cerebral artery, internal carotid artery, anterior cerebral artery, posterior cerebral artery, ophthalmic artery, vertebral artery, and basilar artery, not all of these vessels can be monitored continuously during surgical procedures. Many of these vessels can only be evaluated with a hand-held TCD probe, which is useful for providing a brief snapshot of flow velocity in that vessel. A commercially available device for fixation of the TCD probe is essential for continuous monitoring. These devices are available either as a headband or as a rack that remains attached via fixation points on the bridge of the nose and in bilateral auditory canals. With these devices, flow velocity in the middle cerebral artery can be continuously evaluated.

In addition to the measurement of flow velocity, TCD is useful for detecting emboli. Microembolic signals can be generated by the passage of either gas or particulate matter (Fig. 39-11). The former is likely to occur as a result of venous air embolism, particularly if the patient has a patent foramen ovale, while the latter may occur during the manipulation of an atheroma in a neck vessel or as the result of thrombus formation and dislodgement on a vascular dissection.

Specific applications for intraoperative use of TCD include CEA, nonneurologic surgery in patients with TBI, and surgical procedures requiring cardiopulmonary bypass. There are also numerous indications for TCD in the perioperative setting.

Intracranial Pressure Monitoring

Although monitoring ICP does not provide direct information about CBF, it allows one to calculate CPP, which must be in an appropriate range in order for CBF to be adequate. CPP is defined as the difference between MAP and ICP. In other words,

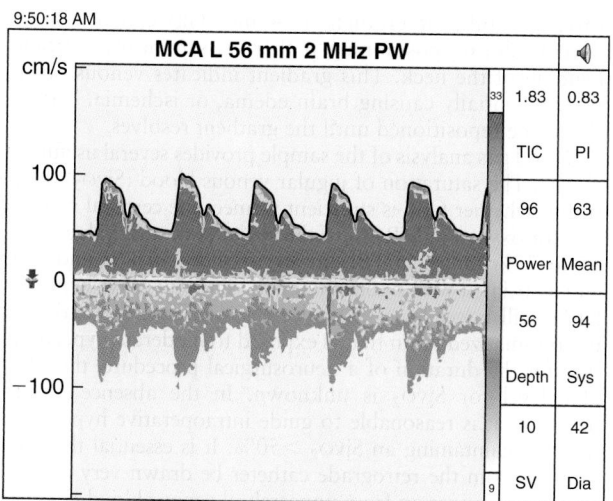
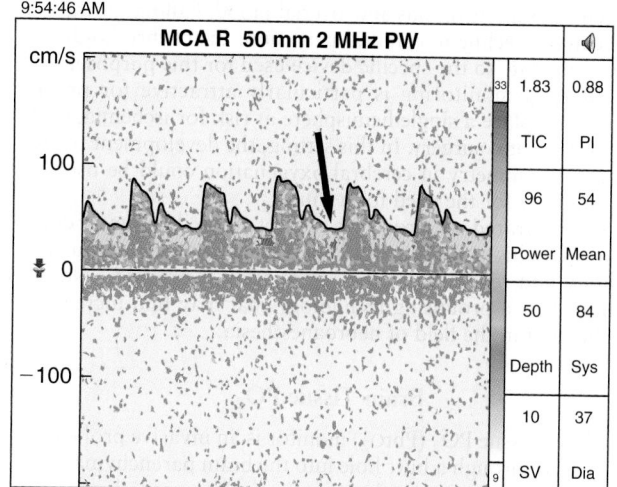
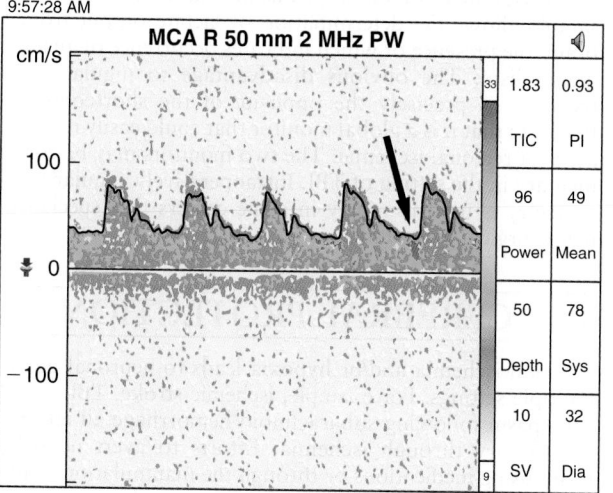
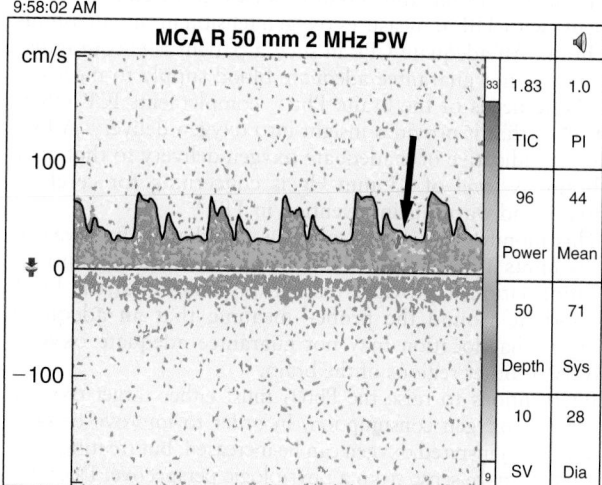

FIGURE 39-11.   Particulate emboli seen on transcranial Doppler in a patient with symptoms of transient ischemic attacks consistent with right carotid artery territory embolization. The emboli are denoted by the *arrows*. MCA, middle cerebral artery; PW, pulse wave.

it is the net pressure acting to move blood through the cerebral vasculature (assuming ICP is greater than right atrial pressure). CPP and CBF are not expected to be proportional, as there are other factors determining CBF (discussed elsewhere). In fact, within a physiologic range of CPP, CBF should remain approximately constant. A CPP that is too low will result in cerebral ischemia and CPP that is too high will cause hyperemia, however.

When ICP is high and CPP is low, interventions can target either ICP or MAP in order to restore a favorable balance of the two. Ideally, ICP should be maintained under 20 mm Hg. Interventions to lower ICP include suppression of cerebral metabolic activity, positional changes to decrease cerebral venous blood volume, drainage of CSF, removal of brain water with osmotic agents such as mannitol, and if absolutely essential, mild-to-moderate hyperventilation to further decrease CBV. MAP is raised via adequate intravascular resuscitation and with a vasopressor as needed. The goal CPP in TBI is >50 to 60 mm Hg.[12]

Other Modalities

Although seldom employed in the intraoperative setting, CT perfusion, single photon emission computed tomography, positron emission tomography, and cerebral angiography all have roles, experimental or clinical, in the evaluation of CBF.

These techniques are frequently used preoperatively and postoperatively in neurosurgical patients, however. On the other hand, intraoperative angiography is frequently used during neurovascular surgery to confirm placement of aneurysm clip or complete obliteration of arteriovenous malformation (AVM).

Cerebral Oxygenation/Metabolism Monitors

A number of invasive and noninvasive monitors provide insight into the metabolic state of the brain and the level of tissue oxygenation of the brain, both of which reveal the balance between blood supply and metabolic demands.

Near-Infrared Spectroscopy

Near-infrared spectroscopy is a noninvasive method of detecting the oxygenation of cerebral blood. Although it does not measure CBF specifically, it provides an indication of the balance between flow and metabolism. Typically, a sensor is applied to the forehead (over hairless skin). A light signal is transmitted through the skin, skull, and meninges into the cerebral cortex. A complex analysis of the reflected light allows calculation of the oxygenation of blood in the cortex, which is a mix of venous and arterial blood. Falling saturation indicates a decline in cerebral perfusion. Exact thresholds for concern relate to the specific device used for this purpose.

Bilateral monitoring is particularly attractive for procedures that place a single hemisphere at risk for ischemia, such as CEA carotid surgery. In this setting, the development of significant asymmetry in cerebral oxygenation could be used as an indicator for the need for a shunt.

Near-infrared spectroscopy has not entered common clinical use at this point, and there are some concerns about the validity and reliability of the information it provides. Nevertheless, it is a promising technology that may find increasing application in the field of neuroanesthesia.

Brain Tissue PO2

The brain tissue PO_2 ($PbtO_2$) monitor is an invasive probe that is inserted through a burr hole into the brain parenchyma, typically in conjunction with a fiberoptic intracranial pressure monitor. As a result, this monitor is used most commonly in patients with TBI. It measures oxygen tension in the surrounding brain. An adequate CPP in such a patient is encouraging, but it does not guarantee adequate blood supply to meet the metabolic needs of the brain. $PbtO_2$ complements ICP information in that it provides insight into oxygen delivery. A low $PbtO_2$ is indicative of inadequate oxygen delivery to that area of brain. A level of 15 mm Hg is concerning for cerebral hypoxia, and warrants intervention in TBI.[13]

This monitor has several obvious drawbacks. Its invasive nature limits its use to a small number of patients. In addition, the information it provides reflects oxygenation at the local level—right around the probe—meaning that an adequate $PbtO_2$ at that location may not guarantee adequate oxygen delivery to other regions of the brain.

Interventions to raise the $PbtO_2$ must either target oxygen delivery or oxygen consumption. In order to improve oxygen delivery, FIO_2 inspired oxygen can be increased, but treating anemia makes more sense from a physiologic perspective. Decreasing oxygen requirements can be accomplished by metabolic suppression with propofol or barbiturate, as well as by treating hyperthermia with external cooling, acetaminophen, and when appropriate, nonsteroidal anti-inflammatory medications.

Jugular Venous Oximetry

Although $PbtO_2$ gives a local view of the balance of oxygen supply and demand, jugular venous oximetry provides that same information for a larger portion, if not the complete, brain. For this monitor, a catheter is inserted into the jugular vein in a retrograde fashion so that its tip sits at the base of the skull in the jugular bulb. This allows continuous pressure monitoring as well as intermittent withdrawal of a jugular venous blood sample for gas analysis. Continuous monitoring can be achieved using an oximetric catheter inserted via a conduit sheath. Confirmation of location can be made with a lateral cervical spine film.

For best representation of the metabolic state of the brain, the catheter should be placed in the dominant jugular vein, most commonly the right side. In patients who have had a cerebral angiogram, the venous phase of the study will provide information on dominant venous drainage. Often the intra-arterial contrast will drain almost exclusively through one jugular vein, regardless of side of injection. Side dominance can also be predicted using ultrasound where the dominant vein may be larger. In the absence of this information, the right side is preferred.

Pressure transduction of the jugular bulb catheter allows comparison with the central venous pressure to rule out potential venous obstruction. In a supine patient with a neutral neck position, there should be no pressure gradient between the tip of the jugular bulb and the central venous catheter. Although rare, a significant gradient (>4 mm Hg) can occasionally develop during positioning if there is significant twisting or bending of the neck. This gradient indicates venous obstruction, potentially causing brain edema, or ischemia. The head should be repositioned until the gradient resolves.

Blood gas analysis of the sample provides several useful parameters. The saturation of jugular venous blood ($SjvO_2$) demonstrates whether CBF is sufficient to meet the cerebral metabolic rate for oxygen ($CMRO_2$) of the brain. A normal value is in the 65 to 75% range. In TBI, an $SjvO_2$ below 50% is undesirable and associated with poor outcome.[14] Intraoperative hyperventilation will lower $SjvO_2$ as it decreases CBF. In the setting of a nontraumatized brain that is exposed to moderate hyperventilation for the duration of a neurosurgical procedure, the acceptable level for $SjvO_2$ is unknown. In the absence of other demands, it is reasonable to guide intraoperative hyperventilation by maintaining an $SjvO_2$ >50%. It is essential that blood samples from the retrograde catheter be drawn very slowly to avoid contamination from noncerebral venous blood.[15]

Measurement of simultaneous arterial and jugular venous sample allows the determination of lactate output from the brain, the presence of which indicates occurrence of anaerobic metabolism. The obvious disadvantage to jugular venous oximetry is precisely the opposite of the shortcoming for $PbtO_2$, in that it is a global monitor that could easily miss small areas of regional ischemia. The two monitors may be complementary in the setting of TBI. Intraoperatively, jugular venous oximetry is used routinely in some centers that specialize in neurosurgical procedures.

CEREBRAL PROTECTION

5 Cerebral ischemia and/or hypoxia leads to neuronal death in multiple settings. For example, ischemic stroke, TBI, cerebral vasospasm following subarachnoid hemorrhage all effect cellular injury through ischemia. Efforts to avert neurologic insult using medications or through the manipulation of physiologic parameters have met with meager results. In the setting of ischemic stroke, for example, thrombolysis may restore perfusion and decrease infarct size, but it may also lead to expansion of the infarct, edema, and even hemorrhage as a result of ischemia-reperfusion injury. In general, a protective strategy that is effective in experimental cerebral ischemia has not been found to be useful in the clinical setting. Of recent advances that are intriguing and controversial, none matches that generated by the concept of cerebral protection by mild or moderate hypothermia.

Persons suffering out-of-hospital cardiac arrest have been shown to have improved neurologic outcome if they are made mildly hypothermic following resuscitation.[16,17] Therefore, it would seem that mild hypothermia is protective against global ischemia/hypoxia at least in the setting of cardiac arrest.

One problem with most settings in which cerebral ischemia is encountered is that the therapeutic intervention can be applied only after the insult has occurred, that is, during the reperfusion phase. Little opportunity exists to intervene before the ischemic event. The operating room is a unique environment in this respect, however. Many ischemic insults that patients suffer in the operating room are iatrogenic and anticipated. A temporary aneurysm clip on the middle cerebral artery is an example of a focal ischemic insult that could be predicted, and a brief period of circulatory arrest induced with adenosine to facilitate clipping of a basilar artery aneurysm is an example of a global insult. The value of anticipating such events is that it allows the anesthesiologist to intervene in advance.

Despite the luxury of planning the intervention for the ischemic insult, the options anesthesiologists have for cerebral protection are few and the evidence for benefit is modest;

much of this evidence has been extrapolated from animal research. Each technique will be examined in detail here.

Ischemia and Reperfusion

Ischemic insult to the brain results in energy failure. The brain depends on a continuous supply of glucose and oxygen to support aerobic metabolism, generation of adenosine triphosphate (ATP), and maintenance of cellular function. When this nutrient supply is interrupted, ATP is depleted. Cellular processes, such as those that maintain cellular membrane integrity, fail. It is reasonable then to attempt to minimize ischemic insult by lowering cerebral metabolic rate, thus decreasing the likelihood of exhausting ATP reserves during the period of ischemia. This has been the traditional paradigm for approaching the subject of intraoperative neuroprotection.

Unfortunately, further damage occurs as a result of processes that are initiated during the reperfusion stage. The reperfusion injury may be mediated via the generation of toxic oxygen species, release of excitotoxic amino acids such as glutamate, up-regulation of nitric oxide synthase, and initiation of cellular apoptosis. Further therapeutic interventions would need to target these pathways as well to provide protection. A shift in the focus of neuroprotection from metabolic suppression to targeting ischemic cascades has recently been advocated.[18]

Hypothermia

It is important to distinguish mild and profound hypothermia, as they have very different practical considerations and they likely modify cerebral function in different ways.

Profound hypothermia is well known for its neuroprotective effects. Anecdotes of successful resuscitation of hypothermic drowning and avalanche victims with good neurologic recovery have been reported.[19,20] Furthermore, extensive use of deep hypothermia with circulatory arrest has been used intraoperatively for repair of aneurysms of the thoracic aorta and for cerebral aneurysms.[21,22] When core body temperature is <20°C, circulatory arrest of <30 minutes appears to be well tolerated. This level of hypothermia not only decreases cerebral activity, but it also decreases the energy required for cellular housekeeping. The practical constraints against using deep hypothermia in settings in which cerebral ischemia is anticipated are numerous. Foremost is the need for cardiopulmonary bypass during the cooling and warming portion of the procedure. Hypothermia-induced coagulopathy is another concern during surgical procedures in the cold patient. Despite the drawbacks to this technique, it remains a reasonable anesthetic option to provide protection for the brain and other organs when the surgical procedure necessitates circulatory arrest.

Mild hypothermia (33 to 35°C) not only decreases cerebral metabolism, but likely modulates the immune and inflammatory response to ischemia, thus affecting the reperfusion portion of the injury as well. Animal studies have shown improved neurologic function following resuscitation from arrest.[23] This promising result in animals was later confirmed by two independent studies in humans, demonstrating that induction of hypothermia in cardiac arrest patients improved outcome.[16,17]

Although mild hypothermia is clearly beneficial in the setting of cardiac arrest, cerebral ischemia due to an arrest is an uncommon occurrence in patients under anesthesia. In contrast, the cerebral ischemia frequently encountered by the anesthesiologist is focal in nature because of the temporary occlusion of a cerebral vessel. Although there is considerable evidence in rats that mild hypothermia is beneficial here too,

there is a paucity of evidence in humans.[24] In fact, a large multicenter study (IHAST II—Intraoperative Hypothermia for Aneurysm Surgery Trial) evaluating patients undergoing cerebral aneurysm surgery found no benefit with mild intraoperative hypothermia.[25]

Nevertheless, hypothermia remains our most promising intervention for cerebral protection. There is a compelling physiologic rationale for its use, a clearly demonstrated effect in animals, and human data showing benefit in the setting of cardiac arrest. Unfortunately, inadequate evidence exists in humans outside cardiac arrest to recommend its routine use in the neurosurgical patient.

Despite the lack of evidence to support hypothermia in humans for cerebral protection, there is ample evidence that hyperthermia is associated with worse outcome in the setting of ischemic stroke, subarachnoid hemorrhage, cardiac arrest, and TBI.[26–29] A common extrapolation from these studies is the belief that concomitant hyperthermia and cerebral ischemia is deleterious. It is important to consider, however, that these studies demonstrate an association, not a causation, of poor outcome from fever. Nevertheless, it would seem reasonable to avoid hyperthermia and treat fever in any setting in which the brain is at risk.[30]

In the operating room, during neurosurgical procedures in which the brain is at risk for ischemic insult, a goal temperature of 35 to 36°C is reasonable. Mild hypothermia (33 to 35°C) may be appropriate in many patients, even recognizing that there may be no benefit to this therapy. Finally, deep hypothermia (<20°C) is appropriate in any situation in which a prolonged cardiac arrest is required.

Medical Therapy for Cerebral Protection

Volatile and intravenous anesthetic agents decrease cerebral metabolism, and thus seem like appropriate candidates for cerebral protection. However, evidence that the level of metabolic suppression does not correlate with the degree of protection has eroded the traditional belief in the mechanism of protection.[31] Nevertheless, numerous animal studies have found protective effects of volatile anesthetics, particularly isoflurane, in mitigating mild-to-moderate ischemic insult, although this effect may only be short-lived.[32–35] This effect may exist when applied during the insult, but also may be effective when administered prior to the insult as a preconditioning therapy.[36,37]

Barbiturates, such as thiopental, have been extensively researched in regard to cerebral protection. They have been shown to have at least short-term benefit on focal cerebral ischemia, while benefit in global ischemia remains controversial.[38–46] This effect may be mediated through reduction in glutamate activity and intracellular calcium, increase in γ-aminobutyric acid (GABA) activity, as well as N-methyl-D-aspartate (NMDA) antagonism.[47,48] Propofol likely has similar protective effects through its action on GABA receptors, as well as via free radical scavenging and limiting lipid peroxidation.[49,50] Again, the durability of this protection is unknown.

Current opinion is that anesthetic neuroprotection is primarily mediated through prevention of excitotoxic injury, not through termination of apoptotic pathways; it thus delays neuronal death and leaves a greater temporal window for intervention.[33] Without other therapeutic options to prevent eventual cell death, outcome is unlikely to be improved, save for perhaps the setting of mild ischemic insult in which apoptotic pathways are not initiated. Sufficient evidence in humans to guide clinical interventions, apart from mild hypothermia in cardiac arrest, is difficult to obtain.[18,51] Clinically, barbiturates and propofol are used intraoperatively to achieve burst suppression on EEG, although its neuroprotective action does not appear to be metabolically mediated.

Glucose and Cerebral Ischemia

Although hyperglycemia has long been recognized as a frequent occurrence in critically ill patients, it was commonly viewed as benign or even beneficial.[52] Hyperglycemia could facilitate cellular uptake of glucose through noninsulin-dependent mechanisms, and thus may benefit cellular metabolism. A subsequent recognition of its association with worse outcome in many settings, including acute coronary syndrome, stroke, TBI, and critical illness, forced the medical community to reconsider the burden of hyperglycemia.[53-58] Furthermore, animal studies suggested that hyperglycemia in the setting of both cerebral and myocardial ischemia increased infarct size.[59,60]

Although considerable evidence accumulated suggesting harm to hyperglycemia, evidence for benefit with normalization of serum glucose using insulin has been somewhat controversial. The most influential literature is from the intensive care unit (ICU) setting, not the operating room. A prospective study in surgical ICU patients (predominantly after cardiac surgery) showed that mortality and morbidity benefit with tight glycemic control (80 to 110 mg/dL).[61] This study spurred an unfettered enthusiasm for aggressive treatment of hyperglycemia, changing practice not only in the surgical ICU but the medical ICU, and in many cases, the operating room. A subsequent study evaluating this therapy in a much sicker medical ICU population showed no overall mortality benefit, however.[62] In fact, subgroup analysis revealed increased mortality in patients who stayed in the ICU <3 days, with an improvement only in those who had a longer ICU stay. In the heterogeneous patient population who present for neurological surgery, with operative times of several hours, not several days, it is inappropriate to extrapolate conclusions from a body of controversial ICU literature to the anesthetic environment, particularly when there is evidence for harm with short durations of therapy. Furthermore, a prospective study of intraoperative insulin therapy in cardiac surgery patients further eroded the basis for translating this ICU literature to the operating room; the insulin group had a higher incidence of death and stroke.[63]

Despite our reluctance to embrace intraoperative tight glycemic control given the current literature, it is worthwhile to consider the patient undergoing cerebrovascular surgery in particular. Given the preponderance of evidence that hyperglycemia and cerebral ischemia in combination are harmful, changing practice in these patients may be warranted. Hyperglycemia on the day of surgery for CEA is associated with worse outcome.[64] Patients who suffer from an ischemic stroke have an improved outcome if their glucose is treated aggressively.[65] Therefore, it may be appropriate to treat neurosurgical patients who will have a period of cerebral ischemia due to temporary vascular occlusion differently from other neurosurgical patients. Tight glycemic control is a reasonable goal in these patients; however, we cannot state at this time that this intervention is neuroprotective.

Promising Areas of Research

Continued research in the various excitotoxic and apoptotic pathways that lead to cell death with cerebral ischemia is essential to bring promising interventions to the clinical arena. It is likely that only a multimodality approach will create durable meaningful cerebral protection.[33] Mild hypothermia continues to hold promise, given its efficacy in certain circumstances. Several additional medical interventions show potential as well. Statins, which inhibit 3-hydroxy-3-methylglutaryl-coenzyme A (HMG-CoA) reductase, have nonlipid lowering effects such as improved endothelial function, as well as antithrombotic and anti-inflammatory activity, which may be neuroprotective.[66] Furthermore, the nonhematopoietic effects of erythropoietin include mitigation of lipid peroxidation and prevention of apoptosis.[67] Whether these medications will offer any benefit to neurosurgical patients remains to be determined.

A Practical Approach

In the absence of compelling evidence in humans regarding the benefit of one practice or another, it is difficult to present firm guidelines with respect to the prevention of intraoperative ischemic insult. For patients undergoing surgical procedures with an anticipated period of cerebral ischemia such as cerebral aneurysm surgery or cerebrovascular bypass procedures, either volatile anesthesia or an intravenous technique is appropriate. It is reasonable to administer additional propofol or thiopental prior to vessel occlusion. Even though this intervention can be guided by EEG monitoring with the goal of achieving burst suppression, this step may not be necessary or even beneficial. Euglycemia prior to vessel occlusion is desirable, but frequent glucose checks are essential throughout the anesthetic to avoid episodes of hypoglycemia if insulin is administered. Finally, hyperthermia should be avoided during this time, with the temperature kept at or below 36°C.

ANESTHETIC MANAGEMENT

Preoperative Evaluation

6 Evaluation of the patient who presents for neurologic or spine surgery requires the same thorough assessment appropriate to any person who will have an anesthetic. In addition, a number of considerations specific to this patient population are important.

It is prudent to consider the nature of the patient's disease that brings him or her to the operating room in the context of his or her medical and surgical history. A thorough history may be difficult to obtain from patients whose disease has resulted in a neurologic decline, such as those obtunded from TBI. Prior medical records and family members are both helpful in this context.

Preoperative risk stratification for cardiac complication is important to consider. The 2007 American College of Cardiology/American Heart Association guidelines has a simplified algorithm for considering whether a patient needs preoperative cardiac testing, such as stress echocardiography, or a nuclear medicine evaluation of myocardial perfusion.[68] Most spine and neurosurgical procedures fall into the intermediate-risk procedure category. The decision to perform a noninvasive cardiac test in patients with risk factors for coronary disease and poor functional status hinges on whether findings from that evaluation will affect management of the patient in the time before surgery. Changes in care of the patient include interventions such as coronary angiography and stenting, which may significantly delay surgery. Current guidelines include delaying surgery for at least 2 weeks following simple balloon angioplasty, 4 to 6 weeks for a bare metal stent, and a full year for a drug-eluting stent. Such a delay may be reasonable for some surgical procedures, but very few indicated spine and neurosurgical procedures can be delayed a year. Furthermore, the enthusiasm for perioperative beta-blockade has been tempered by further studies demonstrating no obvious benefit, as well as concerning preliminary adverse results on a large prospective trial evaluating perioperative metoprolol on all cause mortality (POISE trial described by Devereaux et al).[69,70] Beta-blockers are therefore appropriate primarily in two types of patients undergoing intermediate-risk surgical procedures: first, those already receiving a beta-blocker; second, those who are at high risk for perioperative myocardial infarction due to demonstrated reversible ischemia on a noninvasive study. Furthermore, patients previously receiving a statin should continue their statin in the perioperative period.

Further considerations in the preoperative visit should include issues that will affect choice of medications and anesthetic agents. Many patients presenting for spine surgery have weakness or paralysis that may present a contraindication to the use of succinylcholine. In addition, some neurosurgical patients may have suffered from a stroke resulting in a similar contraindication. Finally, many neurosurgical patients have been exposed to antiepileptic medications. Previous allergies or reactions to these medications, especially phenytoin, should be elucidated.

Induction and Airway Management

For most procedures, induction of anesthesia is an uncomplicated process with great flexibility of drug choice. With the exception of some minimally invasive spine surgery procedures and awake craniotomies, an endotracheal tube is essential for most surgical procedures of the brain and spinal cord.

During induction of anesthesia, there are three iatrogenic consequences that may be significant for the neurosurgical patient: hypotension, hypertension, and apnea. It is essential to understand how each of these will be tolerated by the patient. Brief mild hypotension is frequently encountered following induction of anesthesia. Although most patients tolerate this transient phenomenon well, it should be aggressively avoided in patients with brain injury in which any episode of hypotension is associated with unfavorable outcome.[71] Hypertension due to laryngoscopy, in contrast, would be poorly tolerated by patients following aneurysmal subarachnoid hemorrhage, as systolic hypertension is thought to be a cause of recurrent hemorrhage from the aneurysm.[72] Finally, apnea results in a predictable increase in $PaCO_2$, and corresponding cerebral vasodilation. Although most patients tolerate the increase in CBV, patients with intracranial hypertension may quickly decompensate from apnea, not to mention the decrease in cerebral perfusion.

TBI patients in particular are frequently intolerant of apnea. Unfortunately, many of these patients require a rapid-sequence induction. To further complicate matters, the presence of a cervical collar for known or suspected cervical spine injury may make intubation more difficult. Careful preparation for a difficult airway is essential. These patients are also particularly harmed by periods of hypotension, as noted earlier. Furthermore, these patients may have concomitant injuries with significant blood loss that may predispose to hypotension. Vigorous resuscitation with isotonic fluid and/or blood should be administered prior to induction and continued until the patient is euvolemic. A conservative dose of thiopental or etomidate may be appropriate for the induction agent, with succinylcholine a reasonable choice for the muscle relaxant in the setting of acute injury.

Because patients with subarachnoid hemorrhage are at risk for harm from hypertension, it is reasonable to place an arterial catheter for hemodynamic monitoring prior to induction. Unacceptable increases in blood pressure during laryngoscopy should result in discontinuing the attempt, returning to mask ventilation, and deepening the anesthesia. The latter can be accomplished either with a higher concentration of inspired volatile anesthetic, or a bolus of an intravenous agent such as propofol or remifentanil. In addition, esmolol (0.5 mg/kg) can be given prior to laryngoscopy to blunt the hypertensive response.

The choice of muscle relaxant used for induction deserves some consideration. Many neurosurgical and spine surgery patients have conditions in which succinylcholine is contraindicated. Muscle denervation from stroke, myelopathy, or spinal cord injury (SCI) results in up-regulation of acetylcholine receptor isoforms across the muscle belly. These receptors can be stimulated by acetylcholine, succinylcholine, and

choline.[73] The profound hyperkalemia that can result from the use of succinylcholine, described by Gronert and Theye[74] in 1975, is potentially lethal. Therefore, succinylcholine should be avoided in patients with significant denervation injuries. However, in the setting of acute stroke or SCI, it remains safe to use succinylcholine for approximately 48 hours from the time of injury. A nondepolarizing muscle relaxant is therefore appropriate in many neurosurgical patients to achieve acceptable intubating conditions. The criteria for deciding between the available options are similar to other circumstances, except duration of action is more significant if MEP, spontaneous EMG, or cranial nerve monitoring is planned.

Maintenance of Anesthesia

7 The primary considerations for maintenance of anesthesia include the type of monitoring planned for the procedure, brain relaxation, and the desired level of analgesia at the end of the surgical procedure.

Most neurosurgical and spine procedures can be performed using a balanced anesthetic with volatile agents. Opioids are frequently administered to reduce volatile anesthetic requirements. For both SSEP monitoring and brain relaxation, less than one MAC of volatile anesthetic is desired. For the opioid, an infusion of remifentanil, fentanyl, sufentanil, or alfentanil are all reasonable options. Remifentanil is most appropriate for neurosurgical procedures in which extubation is planned at the end of the surgery and minimal residual effect is desired to facilitate neurologic examination. Other opioids with longer duration of action are appropriate in spine surgery in which reasonable analgesia following the procedure is required.

Replacement of the volatile anesthetic with a continuous infusion of propofol is desirable in two settings. First, MEP monitoring virtually requires it to obtain excellent signal quality. Second, when brain relaxation is inadequate with a volatile anesthetic, propofol will provide better relaxation by further decreasing CBV.

The use of intraoperative muscle relaxant is of controversial utility for neurosurgical procedures. It should be avoided during MEP, spontaneous EMG, or cranial nerve monitoring. It may be used during isolated SSEP monitoring, however. Some are more comfortable managing a patient whose head is held in rigid fixation with muscle relaxant, but adequate anesthesia and avoidance of stimulating airway manipulations are far more important and should prevent unintended patient movement.

Ventilation Management

Hypocapnic cerebral vasoconstriction provides the anesthesiologist with a powerful tool for manipulating CBF and CBV. Hyperventilation is routinely employed to provide brain relaxation and optimize surgical conditions. Because hyperventilation decreases CBF, it has the theoretical potential for causing or exacerbating cerebral ischemia. Clinically it has been associated with harm only in the early period of TBI, but it is still recommended to be avoided in all patients with TBI except when necessary for a brief period to manage acute increases in intracranial pressure.[4,75,76] In the nontrauma population, it is not clear whether there is harm in mild-to-moderate hyperventilation, particularly for the duration of a typical anesthetic. As it appears to be well tolerated, it is reasonable during neurosurgical procedures to maintain a $PaCO_2$ between 30 and 35 mm Hg. Further brain relaxation should be accomplished with other modalities, such as mannitol, hypertonic saline, or intravenous anesthesia. Should hyperventilation to $PaCO_2$ below 30 mm Hg be required, it is appropriate to guide this therapy with jugular venous oximetry and the arterial-jugular lactate gradient.

The duration of effectiveness of hyperventilation is also controversial as normalization of CBF, and consequently CBV, has been reported to occur within minutes. Clinically, the effects of CBV appear to be sustained during most neurosurgical procedures of modest duration.

Fluid and Electrolytes

8 To maintain adequate cerebral perfusion, adequate intravascular volume should be maintained. With perhaps the exception of healthy patients with AVM, the aim should always be euvolemia or slight hypervolemia. Because of the presence of the blood–brain barrier, movement of water into the intracellular and interstitial compartments from the vascular compartment (unless the peripheral circulation) is primarily dependent on the osmotic pressure, and not on the oncotic pressure. Consequently, to minimize brain edema, it is important to maintain serum tonicity. The most important osmotic species in blood is sodium, so it is prudent to check serum sodium level on a regular basis in prolonged surgical procedures in which mannitol has been given. For the care of neurosurgical patient, hypotonic fluids including lactated Ringer solution should not be used, and colloid has no proven advantage over crystalloid. Moreover, hetastarch can result in coagulopathy, and although low doses in healthy individuals is well tolerated, this may not be the case with patients undergoing intracranial procedures as the brain is rich in thromboplastin, the release of which may initiate coagulation abnormalities.

Transfusion Therapy

There has been an increasing effort to conserve the limited resource of banked blood. This effort has been driven in part by concerns over the complications associated with transfusion, such as transfusion reaction, transfusion-related acute lung injury, and transmission of infections such a hepatitis and human immunodeficiency virus. The lower limit of acceptable hemoglobin or hematocrit has not been well defined. One study evaluated two different transfusion thresholds for hemoglobin in a heterogeneous ICU population—either 7 or 10 g/dL—and found that restrictive use of red cell transfusions was at least as good as or superior to a more liberal transfusion threshold.[77] Even though this study has been criticized for various reasons, including the poor representation of neurosurgical patients, it remains the best evidence to support avoidance of transfusion down to a hematocrit of approximately 21% except in the context of ongoing hemorrhage and possibly the early phase of resuscitation for septic patients.[78] Despite the lack of evidence to support the practice, many who care for neurosurgical patients have advocated for more liberal transfusion practices to maximize oxygen delivery to the CNS. But there is evidence to support a similar conservative transfusion threshold in both TBI and spine patients.[79,80]

Unfortunately, most of the evidence available on transfusion thresholds relates to critically ill but euvolemic patients. In the operating room with patients undergoing neurosurgical and spine procedures, ongoing hemorrhage may necessitate transfusion well before the hematocrit falls to 21%.

A practical approach is to consider the rate of surgical blood loss. If it is slow, then it may be appropriate simply to maintain a normal intravascular volume with isotonic crystalloid solution or with an appropriate colloid, recognizing that albumin should be avoided in patients with TBI.[81] Packed red blood cells can be administered when the hematocrit approaches 21%. As the rate of blood loss increases, blood transfusion should begin at a higher hematocrit to prevent

unintended profound anemia. In all circumstances, regardless of transfusion threshold, hypovolemia should be avoided.

Glucose Management

As discussed earlier, the combination of hyperglycemia and cerebral ischemia appears to be particularly deleterious. Although there is a paucity of evidence addressing the topic of intraoperative glucose management, logic would dictate that glucose should be normalized prior to periods of iatrogenic ischemia. Patients who present for cerebrovascular surgery should have a preoperative glucose check. Those who are hyperglycemic should be started on an insulin infusion. Unfortunately, the threshold for hyperglycemia that is associated with harm in the setting of cerebral ischemia is unknown because the definition of hyperglycemia varies dramatically between studies. Although the studies by van den Berghe et al.[61,62] on glycemic control in the ICU population used a goal range of 80 to 110 mg/dL, this level of control may be difficult to achieve in the operating room in the short period before, for example, a temporary clip is applied to the middle cerebral artery. For practical reasons, aiming for a glucose level of <140 g/dL is likely attainable in most patients, and 110 g/dL may be desirable. The presumed risk of tight glycemic control is inadvertent episodes of hypoglycemia. This risk is potentially greater in an anesthetized patient than an ICU patient, as the signs of hypoglycemia are masked by the anesthetic. Therefore, intraoperative glucose management with insulin requires frequent assessment of the serum glucose level.

In nonvascular neurosurgical procedures and spine procedures, the argument for tight glycemic control is less compelling. Many of these patients will be admitted to the ICU following their surgery. As the benefit from glycemic control appears to be realized only after several days of exposure to the therapy, it is reasonable to begin that therapy in the operating room. Furthermore, should the patient have come to the operating room from the ICU, it is also reasonable to continue aggressive glycemic control throughout the operation. However, given the possibility of harm with insulin therapy, the decision to initiate it should be carefully considered.

Even for patients in whom the benefits of tight control are unlikely to outweigh the risks (non-ICU patients and noncerebrovascular patients), glucose must be controlled sufficiently well to avoid glucosuria and the difficulty that arises from volume and electrolyte management with severe hyperglycemia. A target of under 180 mg/dL is adequate in most patients to achieve this goal.

Emergence

The decisions that need to be made with respect to emergence of neurosurgical and spine surgery patients hinge on whether the patient is an appropriate candidate for extubation. To determine this, one must evaluate what has changed over the duration of the procedure with respect to the patient's airway, oxygenation, and ventilation. In addition, one must consider whether this patient will tolerate the hemodynamic changes that occur with extubation. Finally, postoperative plans, such as cerebral angiography, should be taken into account.

For extensive prone spine surgeries, significant dependent edema frequently occurs. Although the predictive value of a cuff leak from the endotracheal tube is poor in general, the combination of pronounced facial edema and an absent cuff leak following prone surgery should make one suspicious for upper airway edema.[82–84] Delaying extubation of the trachea under these circumstances is appropriate. Other factors that may delay extubation in these patients include the development of pulmonary edema and hypoxemia from fluid administration, as well as persistent hemodynamic instability.

For neurosurgical cases, the desire usually is to allow the patient to emerge from anesthesia and extubate the trachea as soon after completion of the procedure as possible. This pathway provides an immediate neurologic examination and may obviate the need for postoperative CT scans. To facilitate emergence and extubation in the operating room, minimal use of opioids other than remifentanil is appropriate. Whether to give a longer-acting opioid, such as fentanyl or morphine, prior to emergence to treat postoperative pain is controversial. Opioids administration may delay emergence in a patient population that usually requires a relatively small amount of postoperative opioid for pain control.[85] The antitussive properties of opioids may be desirable during emergence.

Avoiding coughing and hemodynamic changes with emergence is important for all neurosurgical patients, and particularly those at high risk for postoperative hemorrhage, such as patients who have just had resection of an AVM. Coughing due to irritation of trachea can be minimized with intravenous lidocaine (1 to 1.5 mg/kg), and 4% lidocaine instilled in the cuff of the endotracheal tube for the duration of the procedure may achieve equivalent results.[86] Labetalol, hydralazine, and nicardipine are all reasonable options for controlling hypertension on emergence.

COMMON SURGICAL PROCEDURES

Surgery for Tumors

9 The fundamental anesthetic considerations in tumor surgery are proper positioning of the patient to facilitate the surgical approach, providing adequate relaxation of the brain to optimize surgical conditions, and avoiding well-known devastating complications, such as venous air embolism. In addition, patients with large tumors resulting in significant intracranial hypertension are at risk of cerebral ischemia as well as herniation. Preoperative review of level of consciousness and CT scan should always be performed and the results taken into consideration in the anesthetic plan.

Patient positioning can be very challenging for any neurosurgical procedure, particularly for surgery in the posterior fossa. Lateral, park bench, prone, and sitting positions are all used for surgical procedures in this region. When placing a patient in a complicated position for surgery, it is essential for the safety of the patient that all catheters and the endotracheal tube are secured particularly well. Ample help should be available at the time of positioning, particularly for large or obese patients. Padding adequately to avoid pressure necrosis is also essential. The head is typically secured in a Mayfield apparatus. Nothing should impinge on the nose, eyes, or chin.

As the sitting position confers the greatest risk for venous air embolism, plans should be made for treating it should it occur. A multiorifice catheter can be placed in the right atrium to evacuate air. Its location can be confirmed either electrocardiographically or with echocardiography. A patent foramen ovale increases the risk of paradoxical embolism; transpulmonary passage of air has been described, however, and its risk may be higher with volatile than intravenous anesthesia.[87–89] Patients to be placed in the sitting position should be evaluated for a patent foramen ovale, and an alternate position should be considered for those who have one.

The structures in the posterior fossa, most notably the brainstem and cranial nerves, are particularly vulnerable and intolerant of surgical invasion. BAEP and cranial nerve monitoring are appropriate when the surgical procedure places the cranial nerves or brainstem at risk. SSEP and MEP monitoring can be used for any tumor resection, whether supra or infratentorial; these modalities may be particularly useful in surgeries that place specific tracts at risk.[90,91]

The brainstem is intimately involved in systemic hemodynamics, and surgery in that region may effect rapid changes in blood pressure and heart rate. Hemodynamic lability should be anticipated and treated during surgery in this region. Bradycardia can be treated with atropine, but it should also prompt communication with the surgeon, as its development may affect surgical technique.

Adequate brain relaxation is typically achieved with a standard anesthetic including sub-MAC volatile anesthesia, an opioid infusion, mild-to-moderate hyperventilation, and mannitol. In addition, tumor edema may benefit from the administration of dexamethasone.[92] Further relaxation can be achieved with discontinuation of the volatile anesthetic and initiation of a propofol infusion. Hypertonic saline is a reasonable alternative to mannitol, particularly in the setting of anuric renal failure when mannitol is contraindicated. A recent randomized trial showed that 3% saline and mannitol have equivalent brain relaxation effects, but with the former having less electrolyte and vascular volume sequelae.[93] A brain that remains full may be the result of venous congestion. This problem can be mitigated with head-up tilt, but is best prevented during the positioning of the patient by minimizing excessive rotation or angulation of the neck. The central venous pressure and jugular venous pressure can be transduced to confirm the absence of a pressure gradient across the neck.

Vascular tumors such as meningioma may benefit from preoperative embolization, and large ones or ones that could not be embolized are still at risk of significant blood loss. Coagulopathy can also develop intraoperatively. It is important to perform frequent coagulation studies and administer clotting products and platelets promptly.

Pituitary Surgery

Masses in the region of the sella most commonly are of pituitary origin, although other benign (meningioma, craniopharyngioma) and malignant (germ cell tumor, lymphoma) tumors may occur in this region. These tumors are typically recognized as a result of the neurologic changes they effect as they compress adjacent structures, such as visual changes with impingement of the optic chiasm, or through the systemic effects they exert via a change in hormone secretion.

Although many patients with sellar tumors may undergo surgical resection with an uncomplicated general anesthetic, there are several preoperative considerations that will affect management of the patient. The patients should undergo a preoperative evaluation of their hormonal function to detect hypersecretion of pituitary hormones, common in pituitary adenomas, as well as panhypopituitarism. The hormones that may be secreted by pituitary tumors include prolactin, growth hormone, corticotropin, and thyroid-stimulating hormone. Patients with excess growth hormone eventually will develop acromegaly. The anesthesiologist should be prepared for a difficult airway, as well as postoperative respiratory complications in the acromegalic patient. Patients with a corticotropin-secreting adenoma will develop Cushing disease. These patients may have a typical "Cushingoid" habitus that may make airway management challenging. In addition, venous access may be difficult, and intraoperative hyperglycemia is likely. Patients with thyroid-stimulating hormone hypersecretion will exhibit signs of hyperthyroidism (e.g., tachycardia, weight loss). These patients should be managed in the preoperative period with antithyroid medications and beta-blockade. Close hemodynamic monitoring during surgery is essential.

Patients with panhypopituitarism will need hormone replacement, including cortisol, levothyroxine, and possibly DDAVP. These medications should be continued in the perioperative period.

Small pituitary tumors can be resected from a transsphenoidal approach, and larger tumors may require a craniotomy. Intraoperative monitoring of glucose and electrolytes is essential, particularly if the patient has pre-existing diabetes insipidus, or if the patient develops signs of diabetes insipidus during the surgery. Diabetes insipidus is a common complication of pituitary surgery due to loss of antidiuretic hormone production. It may be temporary or permanent, and may occur either in the intraoperative or postoperative period. It is initially suspected on the basis of copious urine output, as well as rising serum sodium. A urine specific gravity of <1.005 is confirmatory. Although infusions of intravenous fluids containing free water may mitigate the electrolyte changes, replacement of antidiuretic hormone with DDAVP (0.5 to 1 μg intravenously or subcutaneously) is an effective therapy for diabetes insipidus. Volume replacement therapy may be guided with the use of central venous pressure monitoring as well as the observation of systolic variation in blood pressure.

Arteriovenous Malformations

A cerebral AVM is an abnormal vascular connection between the arterial and venous circulation. The absence of an intervening capillary bed results in a low-resistance path for blood flow. Patients may present with hemorrhage, seizure, or focal neurologic deficit. Cerebral angiography remains the gold standard for AVM diagnosis. Although embolization of the AVM is commonly performed, either radiosurgery or an open surgical procedure is typically required subsequent to the embolization to cure the lesion. Although these lesions may be adjacent to vital structures, and an immediate postoperative neurologic examination may be desirable, emergence from anesthesia following resection of an AVM requires particular care. Because of local hemodynamic changes as a result of the AVM, the adjacent vessels must chronically vasodilate to preserve perfusion. When the low-resistance AVM has been occluded or resected, the adjacent vessels are exposed to higher pressures than they are accustomed to. These vessels may not be able to autoregulate appropriately within the normal blood pressure range, and "normal perfusion pressure breakthrough" may occur. This phenomenon is defined by regional hyperemia at a normal systemic blood pressure. Normal perfusion pressure breakthrough may result in vasogenic edema and hemorrhage. It can be minimized with careful blood pressure control; preoperative embolization likely decreases its incidence as well. Following resection of large AVMs or those in the posterior fossa, taking the patient to the ICU in a ventilated and sedated state may be appropriate. Should the decision be made between the surgeon and anesthesiologist to allow emergence and extubation of the trachea, aggressive management of blood pressure should be instituted, and coughing should be avoided. Intravenous labetalol and hydralazine may be adequate, but a nicardipine infusion may be appropriate for blood pressure control. Blood pressure control needs to be conducted using an anticipated and prophylactic approach rather than a reactive one, as the delay in treating hypertension may be detrimental. Intravenous lidocaine can be used to blunt coughing.

Cerebral Aneurysm Surgery and Endovascular Treatment

Cerebral aneurysms—abnormally shaped cerebral arteries—are relatively prevalent vascular abnormalities (approximately 5% incidence at autopsy) that arise from congenital weakness of the vessel wall as well as extrinsic influences such as hypertension and cigarette smoking. They are more prevalent in women than in men. Some aneurysms become clinically significant when they rupture, resulting in arterial bleeding into the subarachnoid space. This event typically causes severe headache, and may also cause focal neurologic deficit, lethargy, and coma. For patients who survive their hemorrhage, surgical or endovascular intervention to secure the aneurysm is essential to prevent further hemorrhage. In addition, many patients are incidentally found to have cerebral aneurysms, and they may need intervention to decrease the risk of an initial subarachnoid hemorrhage. Intervention for a cerebral aneurysm may include a craniotomy and surgical clipping, or endovascular coiling.

Anesthetic considerations for cerebral aneurysm surgery are somewhat different in those patients who have experienced a subarachnoid hemorrhage as compared with those who present for elective repair. Patients with aneurysmal subarachnoid hemorrhage are at risk for numerous complications that may affect the anesthetic plan. These include cardiac dysfunction, neurogenic or cardiogenic pulmonary edema, hydrocephalus, as well as further hemorrhage from the aneurysm. This last complication is perhaps the most devastating (see also Chapter 56).

Careful attention to hemodynamics, particularly during stimulating procedures, is essential to avoid recurrent hemorrhage. Laryngoscopy and placement of the head in the Mayfield device are two points at which the anesthesiologist must be particularly vigilant about maintaining adequate depth of anesthesia.

Following subarachnoid hemorrhage, cardiac dysfunction and pulmonary edema commonly resolve over time. The cardiac dysfunction may be severe, resulting in electrocardiogram changes, elevated troponin, and even cardiogenic shock. Echocardiography may reveal hypokinesis in a distribution not consistent with an anatomic vascular territory. Unfortunately, the need to secure the aneurysm in a timely fashion may require the anesthesiologist to provide anesthesia despite ongoing cardiac and pulmonary issues. Hemodynamic support with carefully titrated vasopressors may be necessary, recognizing the risk of elevating the blood pressure too much. Hypoxemia can often be managed with increased FiO_2 and positive end-expiratory pressure. With the exception of a hemodynamically unstable patient, surgical clipping of a ruptured aneurysm should rarely be postponed.

Once the aneurysm is secured with an aneurysm clip, the risk of recurrent hemorrhage from the aneurysm is removed. Although careful attention to hemodynamics as well as coughing during emergence is still important, the concern of devastating hemorrhage is diminished.

The patient presenting for an elective aneurysm procedure will typically have good brain conditions, with easily achievable relaxation using mannitol (0.5 to 1 g/kg), mild-to-moderate hyperventilation, and sub-MAC volatile anesthetic in combination with an opioid infusion. Following subarachnoid hemorrhage, brain relaxation may be more difficult to achieve; intravenous anesthesia may be required. Drainage of CSF via a lumbar drain or external ventricular drain can be used at the discretion of the surgeon.

In contrast to aneurysm surgery, endovascular treatment of aneurysms is a minimally invasive procedure performed in the interventional radiology suite. The interventional neuroradiologist or neurosurgeon accesses the aneurysm via an intra-arterial catheter and typically deploys coils into the aneurysm that cause it to thrombose. This technique requires a favorably shaped aneurysm that will retain the coils once they are deployed. Increasingly sophisticated techniques, such as placing a stent in the adjacent vessel and coiling through the stent, have increased the range of aneurysms that are amenable to endovascular therapy.

Despite the less invasive nature of this procedure, it can have equally severe complications as surgery, including further hemorrhage, stroke, and vessel dissection.

Although the procedure is not particularly stimulating, the general anesthetic needs to be performed with great care. Obviously, hypertension with laryngoscopy should be avoided. Furthermore, any patient movement during the procedure can incur devastating consequences because it may result in deployment of coils in a vessel rather than the aneurysm itself. Hyperventilation should be avoided, as it will decrease CBF and make access to the aneurysm more challenging. Heparin is commonly administered during this procedure. It is meant to decrease the risk of thromboembolic complications associated with the intra-arterial catheter. Protamine must be available should arterial rupture and extravasation occur. In addition, prompt transfer to an operating room for neurosurgical intervention should also be possible.

Carotid Surgery

Carotid stenosis is a common cause of transient ischemic attack and ischemic stroke. It is amenable to surgical intervention and endovascular stenting. In older studies, carotid endarterectomy (CEA) was found to be beneficial in reducing stroke rate in symptomatic patients (ipsilateral transient ischemic attack or nondisabling stroke) with ≥70% internal carotid artery stenosis and, to a lesser extent, in patients with 50 to 69% internal carotid artery stenosis.[94,95] In asymptomatic carotid stenosis, the benefit of surgical intervention over medical therapy appears to be somewhat smaller, and it depends on the incidence of perioperative stroke.[96,97] In addition, surgery is associated not only with a risk of stroke, but also myocardial infarction, wound infection, and so forth. At the time of the NASCET trial, medical therapy consisted primarily of daily aspirin. With advances in medical therapy, including more aggressive lipid-lowering drugs as well as other effective antiplatelet agents and better antihypertensive therapy, the margin of benefit of surgery may be even less.[98] Appropriate candidate selection for surgery has therefore become extremely important. Preoperative evaluation of the asymptomatic patient depends on assessment of the risk for progression to stroke and weighing that risk against the morbidity of the procedure.

Both general and regional anesthesia may be used for CEA. Regional anesthesia is accomplished with a superficial cervical plexus block, or a combination of superficial and deep block.[99,100] This technique allows continuous neurologic assessment during the surgery, which is particularly useful at the time of carotid cross-clamp. Some patients and surgeons may not be agreeable to this anesthetic technique, however. General anesthesia with an endotracheal tube is therefore a more common technique for CEA. These patients are at increased risk for perioperative complications, given their high prevalence of coronary artery disease, hypertension, chronic obstructive pulmonary disease, diabetes mellitus, and chronic kidney disease. Continuation of beta-blockers and statins is appropriate for patients who are receiving these medications preoperatively. Initiation of a beta-blocker prior to surgery, although theoretically indicated, must be considered within the context of the preliminary results from the POISE trial reporting higher mortality from stroke.[68] Blood pressure should be maintained as close to baseline as possible throughout the surgery. Without evidence to support it, some advocate raising the blood pressure during carotid cross-clamp to improve flow through collateral vessels. This practice presupposes that collateralization is marginal and will be helped by the elevation in pressure. Collateral flow may be marginal, but it may also be absent or entirely adequate. In the latter two situations, elevation in blood pressure through the use of phenylephrine will only increase myocardial oxygen demand.

However, evidence of hypoperfusion ipsilateral to the cross-clamp is reason to consider blood pressure elevation.

Several CNS monitors may be used during CEA under general anesthesia. EEG allows for easy detection of decline in spectral power on the hemisphere ipsilateral to the surgery, which would be concerning for ischemia. Near-infrared spectroscopy is also promising for its ability to demonstrate relative changes between the ipsilateral and contralateral hemispheres, but it has not come into common use as yet. TCD is particularly attractive, however, as it allows determination of changes in flow during carotid cross-clamp as well as detection of emboli. The former problem can be avoided with a shunt during the surgical procedure, but a shunt increases the risk of the latter problem. TCD is useful in providing real-time information on the nature of CBF during cross-clamp, and in guiding the decision on whether to shunt. A decrease in flow velocity of up to 60% is typically well tolerated in the anesthetized patient during this procedure. As the pulsatility of flow will decrease when it is supplied via collateral vessels, it is important to make decisions based on mean flow velocity, not systolic or diastolic velocity. Should a shunt be needed, the development of microembolic signals can provide feedback to the surgeon if there is a modifiable technique to the surgical procedure. At the end of the endarterectomy, during surgical closure, continued presence of a good flow velocity waveform on TCD provides confirmation of the stability of the graft and lack of an intimal flap, or thrombosis. Although each monitor has attractive features, ultimately user familiarity and comfort will determine its utility.[101] Sustained elevation of flow velocity exceeding 100% of baseline values is highly suggestive of the development of hyperperfusion syndrome, and should prompt lowering of systemic blood pressure.

Rapid emergence and tracheal extubation at the end of the procedure is desirable because it allows immediate neurologic assessment. Hemodynamic changes can occur in the postoperative period from denervation of the carotid baroreceptor. In addition, headache, obtundation, and/or focal neurologic deficit in the postoperative period should prompt one to consider hyperemia, hemorrhage, or ischemic stroke.

Carotid artery stenting may be used to treat carotid stenosis as well. It is an attractive procedure in that it is minimally invasive and can be performed under sedation. Noninferiority studies have not supported stenting as compared with CEA in symptomatic patients, however.[102,103] Yet the SAPPHIRE trial has indicated that stenting may be a reasonable option in asymptomatic patients with tight stenosis; currently, most centers reserve stenting for patients who are poor surgical candidates.[104,105] Anesthetic considerations for this procedure are important, even though it is typically performed under sedation. These patients tend to have significant medical comorbidities. Conversion to general anesthesia may incur significant risk. Furthermore, the procedure itself may induce significant hemodynamic changes, most notably bradycardia or asystole during balloon angioplasty of the internal carotid artery. Although pretreatment with atropine may prevent this complication, a brisk tachycardia is frequently not desirable in these patients.

Epilepsy Surgery and the Awake Craniotomy

Some intracranial neurosurgical procedures are performed on "awake" (that is, sedated and pain free, yet able to respond to verbal or visual command) patients in order to facilitate monitoring of the region of the brain on which the surgeon is operating. These procedures require particular attention on the part of the anesthesiologist to provide patient comfort and safety. Typically these surgeries are for tumors adjacent to eloquent cortex or for resection of an epileptic focus. Frequently the decision to perform the procedure awake has been made by the neurosurgeon prior to the patient meeting the anesthesiologist. It is the role of the anesthesiologist to determine whether the patient is an appropriate candidate for an awake procedure, to coordinate with the neurosurgeon the anesthetic plan, and to support and reassure the patient through the process.

Although the patient with a difficult airway, obstructive sleep apnea, or orthopnea may present a relative contraindication to an awake craniotomy, it is the patient with severe anxiety, claustrophobia, or other psychiatric disorder who may be particularly inappropriate for this type of procedure.

Preoperative evaluation should be complete and should include a thorough airway examination. Conversion to a general anesthetic remains a possibility at any point during the procedure. Extensive discussion with the patient regarding the plan is essential to prepare him or her for the experience in the operating room.

Although the patient may be kept awake for the entire surgery, to facilitate patient tolerance of the procedure, an asleep-awake-asleep pathway is often chosen. This anesthetic plan involves general anesthesia for the skin incision, initial craniotomy, and then for the closure in the end, while the patient is allowed to emerge from anesthesia for the middle portion of the surgery in which the surgeon is working around important structures. This general pathway can take on many forms, however. In particular, the asleep portions of the procedure may be performed without an airway, with a laryngeal mask airway (LMA), or with an endotracheal tube in place. For suitable candidates, spontaneous ventilation with propofol anesthesia is an attractive option, as it allows straightforward emergence with minimal coughing, gagging, or straining. In addition, propofol provides a nice anesthetic for these patients because of its low incidence of nausea and vomiting during the awake period. Benzodiazepines should be avoided as they may interfere with electrocorticography during epilepsy surgery. An LMA is a suitable alternative to no airway as it can frequently be removed with little movement of the patient as he or she emerges from anesthesia. Topical application of lidocaine to the airway prior to insertion of the LMA supplemented with lidocaine jelly on the LMA may improve patient tolerance during emergence.

An endotracheal tube provides the most secure airway, but it is also the most difficult to remove during the procedure, particularly with the patient's head secured in rigid fixation. If this pathway is chosen, several options exist to minimize coughing as the patient emerges. Prior to placement of the endotracheal tube, the larynx and trachea may be localized with lidocaine. In addition, the cuff of the endotracheal tube can be filled with 4% lidocaine rather than air. Finally, allowing the patient to emerge on an infusion of low-dose remifentanil or dexmedetomidine may facilitate extubation with little movement.

During the awake portion of the procedure, all sedatives are typically withheld. For particularly stimulating events (e.g., drilling) and in coordination with the surgeon, small boluses of propofol may be given. Antiemetics may be given for nausea and small doses of fentanyl for discomfort.

Following this critical portion of the surgery, the patient may be fully anesthetized for the surgical closure. Initiating a propofol infusion and continuing with spontaneous ventilation is again a good option. Otherwise, manipulation of the airway to place an LMA or endotracheal tube will be necessary while avoiding the sterile field.

For procedures in which the patient is kept awake throughout the process, planning in collaboration with the surgeon should include a discussion of sedation that allows continued participation of the patient in the neuromonitoring. Dexmedetomidine, a central α_2-agonist, is a useful medication that can be used as an infusion in these patients. It provides good sedation and blood pressure control without respiratory depression, and it allows the patient to respond to commands appropriately.

ANESTHESIA AND TRAUMATIC BRAIN INJURY

Overview of Traumatic Brain Injury

The presence of TBI is the primary determinant in quality of outcome for patients suffering from trauma.[12] Anesthesiologists are involved in the care of these patients in many different settings, including the initial resuscitation in the emergency department, anesthetic management in the operating room, and ongoing care in the ICU (see also Chapter 56).

Secondary injury includes insults resulting from inflammation, superoxide production, excitotoxic amino acid release, and apoptosis; these mechanisms are not preventable at this point.[12] The initial approach to patients with TBI should be similar to that of any trauma patient, as outlined in *Advanced Trauma Life Support* by the American College of Surgeons.

Airway and breathing are obviously of paramount importance in any critically ill patient but even more so in patients with head injuries, given the sensitivity of the brain to hypoxemia and hypercapnia. Prehospital intubation of the patient with TBI is controversial; outcome may be worsened by ultra-early hyperventilation.[106–108] If the patient arrives in the emergency department intubated, one must confirm proper placement of the endotracheal tube with a carbon dioxide detector. If the patient is not intubated, immediate attention should focus on assessing the airway and making preparations for intubation. Patients with TBI usually have several indications for intubation including: decreased level of consciousness, increased risk of aspiration, as well as concern for hypoxemia and hypercarbia. Sometimes these patients must be intubated and sedated simply to allow further diagnostic studies.

Patients with TBI have a 5 to 6% incidence of an unstable cervical spine injury.[109,110] Risk factors include a motor vehicle accident and Glasgow Coma Scale (GCS) score <8. Therefore, all attempts at intubation should include in-line neck stabilization to decrease the chance of worsening a neurologic injury.[111] This maneuver may worsen the view of the glottis, making intubation more difficult.[112] Therefore, one must always have a backup plan and device in mind when performing an emergency intubation including but not limited to laryngeal masks and fiberoptic or video technology. Patients with TBI should generally be intubated orally, as the potential presence of a basilar skull fracture could increase the risk associated with a nasal intubation. A surgical airway remains an appropriate procedure for patients with severe facial trauma and a difficult airway.

Minimizing the risk of aspiration during airway procedures is essential. The efficacy of cricoid pressure has not been demonstrated, and it may displace cervical fractures; nevertheless, it remains the standard of care during rapid-sequence intubation.[113,114]

Another important consideration is the choice of drugs to facilitate intubation. Hypotension is extremely detrimental to the injured brain, as discussed previously. Therefore, the choice of drugs must be tailored to each individual patient. Sodium thiopental in a dose of 3 to 6 mg/kg is a useful drug in euvolemic hemodynamically stable patients. Through its effect on $CMRO_2$, this drug decreases CBF, CBV, and ICP.[115,116] However, it also causes a large decrease in systemic vascular resistance, which may be deleterious to blood pressure in a hypovolemic patient.[117] Propofol has similar effects. Another choice to facilitate intubation is etomidate in doses of 0.2 to 0.3 mg/kg. This drug also decreases $CMRO_2$ and CBF but has less effect on blood pressure.[118,119] Care must be taken in the acutely unstable patient with the administration of any potent sedative hypnotic drug, as even etomidate can produce profound hypotension. Another drug that is useful to blunt the

TABLE 39-3

INTRAVENOUS FLUIDS

■ FLUID	■ OSMOLALITY (mOsm/kg)	■ ONCOTIC PRESSURE (mm Hg)	■ Na+ (mEq/L)	■ Cl− (mEq/L)	■ K+ (mEq/L)	■ Ca2+/Mg2+ (mEq/L)	■ GLUCOSE (g/L)
Plasma	289	21	141	103	4–5	5/2	—
Crystalloid							
0.9% NS	308	0	154	154	—	—	—
0.45% NS	154	0	77	77	—	—	—
3% NS	1,030	0	515	515	—	—	—
7.5% NS	2,400	0	1200	1200	—	—	—
LR	273	0	130	109	4	3/0	—
D5LR[a]	527	0	130	109	4	3/0	50
D5W[a]	252	0	—	—	—	—	50
D5 NS[a]	586	0	154	154	—	—	50
D50.45% NS[a]	406	0	77	77	—	—	50
Plasma-Lyte 148	294	0	140	98	5	0/3	—
Normosol-R	294	0	140	98	5	0/3	—
Mannitol (20%)	1,098	0	—	—	—	—	—
Colloid							
Hetastarch (6%)	310	31	154	154	—	—	—
Albumin (5%)	290	19	145	145	—	—	—

NS, normal saline; LR, lactated Ringer solution; D5W, 5% dextrose in water.
[a]In dextrose-containing solutions, it is important to distinguish between osmolality and tonicity.

ANESTHESIA FOR SURGICAL SUBSPECIALTIES

effects of laryngoscopy and intubation on ICP is lidocaine. In doses of 1.5 mg/kg this drug decreases ICP with minimal hemodynamic effects.[120] Finally, the choice of muscle relaxant is somewhat controversial. Administering muscle relaxants prevents coughing and the resultant spikes of ICP.[121] The main choice is between succinylcholine and rocuronium, the two agents with the fastest onset. The main drawback to rocuronium is the prolonged effect when a rapid-sequence dose is used (1.2 mg/kg), while the argument against succinylcholine is the potential increase in ICP.[122] However, Kovarik et al.[123] studied the effects of this drug in neurologically injured patients and found no increase on ICP. Once the trachea is intubated, the initial ventilation parameters should include 100% oxygen; arterial carbon dioxide should be maintained in the lower normal range (35 mm Hg), and should be guided by arterial blood gas analysis.

The goal of resuscitation in any trauma patient is to establish adequate circulation so that organ perfusion may be maintained. The long-standing belief that aggressive resuscitation in TBI patients should be avoided to minimize cerebral edema is no longer considered appropriate. The overwhelming evidence of harm from hypotension necessitates restoration of intravascular volume.[71] Isotonic fluids should be used to accomplish this goal; note that lactated Ringer solution is slightly hypotonic (Table 39-3). The goal is to maintain CPP in the range of 50 to 70 mm Hg, as recommended by the guidelines from the Brain Trauma Foundation in 2007.[124] Hypertonic fluids, such as 3% saline, may be useful in this setting, although there is insufficient evidence to justify routine use. Vasopressors and inotropes may be needed after fluid resuscitation to achieve the desired CPP, or to treat hypotension while volume restoration is ongoing. They should be used judiciously, as they are thought to increase the incidence of acute respiratory distress syndrome.[125] In the absence of ICP monitoring but with known TBI, an ICP of at least 20 should be assumed, and MAP should be kept above 60 mm Hg.

Patients with TBI are typically described by their localized Glasgow Coma Scale (GCS) score (Table 39-4).[126] This simple test facilitates communication between providers, and it provides prognostic information.[127] Mild head injury is represented by a score of 13 to 15, moderate head injury by a score of 9 to 12, and severe head injury by a score of ≤8. The score should be determined on postresuscitation information, as hypotension may depress mental status in any patient, even those without TBI. The pupil examination is also useful. The presence of a unilateral dilated pupil suggests brainstem compression and is a surgical emergency and the presence of dilated pupils bilaterally portends a dismal prognosis.[128]

Intracranial hypertension predisposes patients to poor outcomes, and elevated ICP refractory to therapy is associated with a worse prognosis.[129–131]

Some controversy exists regarding what constitutes the optimal ICP and CPP. Prior recommendations were to maintain the CPP at 70 mm Hg or above and to lower ICP when it exceeded 20 to 25 mm Hg.[132,133] Subsequently, CPP goals

TABLE 39-4

GLASGOW COMA SCALE

Eyes	1. No eye opening
	2. Opens to painful stimulus
	3. Opens to voice
	4. Spontaneous eye opening
Verbal	1. No sounds
	2. Incomprehensible sounds
	3. Inappropriate words
	4. Confused conversation
	5. Normal speech
Motor	1. No movement
	2. Extension to painful stimulus
	3. Abnormal flexion to painful stimulus
	4. Withdrawal from painful stimulus
	5. Localization of painful stimulus
	6. Follows commands

were redefined to the range between 60 and 70 mm Hg to avoid increased morbidity associated with acute respiratory distress syndrome.[125,134] The range was subsequently broadened to 50 to 70 mm Hg.[12,124]

Reduction of ICP in patients with head injuries can be accomplished effectively using osmotic diuretics. Mannitol is the most commonly used agent and is available for intravenous administration in either a 20 or 25% solution. Common dosages range from 0.25 to 1 g/kg of body weight. Mannitol may be used on a repeated schedule, but the serum osmolarity should not be allowed to exceed 320 mOsm. Furthermore, intravascular volume depletion should be avoided. The mechanism of ICP reduction by mannitol may be related to its osmotic effect in shifting fluid from the brain tissue compartment to the intravascular compartment as well as its ability to improve blood rheology by decreasing blood viscosity.[135,136] The latter effect has been postulated to cause reflex vasoconstriction, which keeps CBF constant while reducing CBV and ICP. In addition, mannitol, like other hypertonic fluids, decreases production of CSF. Some individuals may benefit from the use of furosemide in combination with mannitol, as the combination appears to increase the duration of their effect on ICP.[137]

Both hypertonic saline (HS) and HS-Dextran have been used to manage elevated ICP, primarily in the setting of intracranial hypertension refractory to mannitol therapy. As the blood–brain barrier reflection coefficient to sodium ions is approximately 1, HS establishes a gradient that facilitates the movement of water from the brain into the intravascular space. Recent evidence indicates that HS may be more effective in controlling ICP than mannitol.[138] In addition to efficacy, the proposed benefit of HS is lack of severe electrolyte disturbance, which is common with mannitol. The brisk diuresis seen with mannitol is absent from HS therapy. Although HS has been administered both as a bolus and as a continuous infusion, currently no firm guidelines have been established for its use. In addition, no standard concentration has been established for clinical use, although most clinical studies have used either 7.5 or 3% at an infusion at a rate of 20 to 40 mL/hr. Following prolonged infusion in the ICU, HS should be tapered off slowly to prevent subsequent hyponatremia and rebound edema. In addition, HS should be administered through a central line. In situations in which HS causes an unacceptable hyperchloremic acidosis, a mixture of sodium chloride and sodium acetate can be used.

Hyperventilation is an effective way to reduce ICP. It is useful in the setting of an acutely increased ICP that needs to be controlled until more definitive therapy can be initiated. Hyperventilation may be useful in the initial stages of resuscitation of head-injured patients or in a patient who suddenly demonstrates signs of herniation. Hyperventilation causes cerebral vasoconstriction, primarily in the small regulatory arteries in the brain; this vasoconstriction rapidly reduces the CBV and therefore the ICP. The reduction in CBV is achieved at the expense of CBF, however.

Hyperventilation in the setting of TBI remains controversial. The degree of hyperventilation that is acceptable is unknown, and the duration of hyperventilation that can be used safely and effectively is uncertain. The primary concern with hyperventilation is that it may exacerbate cerebral ischemia.[6] Current recommendations are that patients who are head-injured should be maintained at normocapnia except when hypocapnia is necessary to control acute increases in ICP.

Chronic hyperventilation should be avoided if possible. In situations in which prolonged hyperventilation is necessary because of failure of other agents to control ICP, monitoring $PbtO_2$, $SjvO_2$, and the arteriovenous lactate gradient is desirable.[139]

Moderate hypothermia has been considered as a therapeutic modality in head injury for many years. The theoretical benefits of hypothermia in preventing secondary brain injury may be related to its effects on attenuating the biochemical cascade that begins at the time of injury or on controlling intracranial hypertension. Despite these actions, a large multicenter clinical trial of head-injured patients demonstrated no benefit to induction of hypothermia.[140] A post hoc analysis of the data from this study did show that head-injured patients under 45 years of age who were mildly hypothermic ($<35°C$) on admission had a lower incidence of poor outcome if they were randomized to the hypothermia arm.[141] It was not clear, however, whether the benefit seen in this group of patients was from early hypothermia or from avoidance of the rewarming process. Given the rather limited situation in which hypothermia appears to be beneficial in head injury, it is not recommended for routine use.[142] In addition, hypothermia increases the risk of pneumonia and wound infection and may cause electrolyte and coagulation abnormalities.[143] Hypothermia does decrease ICP, however, primarily because it decreases cerebral metabolic rate and thus CBF. Despite the controversies surrounding the use of hypothermia in head injury, hypothermia remains a viable intervention for refractory intracranial hypertension.[144]

Barbiturates may be used as an adjunct to other therapy for controlling ICP. As discussed earlier, they lower ICP via their effect on $CMRO_2$. As long as the MAP is maintained, CPP will improve. Barbiturate therapy is appropriate only in patients who are hemodynamically stable and have been adequately resuscitated. It should not be employed if MAP and CPP cannot be maintained. Some patients with refractory elevations in ICP have sustained extensive neurologic injury, and their cerebral metabolic rate may already be low; failure to respond to barbiturates carries with it an ominous prognosis.[133] Propofol is a reasonable alternative to barbiturates for ICP management. Prolonged use of high-dose propofol is not recommended as it may cause propofol infusion syndrome, which imposes significant morbidity and mortality.[145]

Both barbiturates and propofol can be used in a dose-response manner to provide ICP control, ranging from mild sedation to induced coma. If maximal metabolic suppression is desired, the infusion rate can be guided by EEG burst suppression.

Decompressive craniectomy is another management option for refractory intracranial hypertension in TBI. Although this intervention decreases ICP and improves $PbtO_2$, outcome improvement has not been demonstrated for TBI in a prospective fashion.[146–150] RESCUE ICP is an ongoing prospective multicenter study that is meant to address this issue (see www.rescueicp.com) (Table 39-5).

TABLE 39-5

INTERVENTIONS FOR INADEQUATE CEREBRAL PERFUSION PRESSURE

Reduce brain water	1. Mannitol
	2. Hypertonic saline
	3. Furosemide
Remove cerebrospinal fluid	1. External ventricular drain
	2. Lumbar drain
	3. (Hypertonic fluid)
Decrease cerebral blood volume	1. Head-up tilt
	2. Neutral neck position
	3. Metabolic suppression (propofol or barbiturate)
	4. Mild to moderate hyperventilation
Elevate mean arterial pressure	1. Adequate intravascular volume resuscitation
	2. Support with vasopressor

Anesthetic Management

Patients with TBI requiring surgery can be subdivided into two major groups with different perioperative concerns. These groups include those who require emergent surgery and those who require nonemergent surgery. The emergent group can also be subdivided into neurosurgical procedures and nonneurosurgical procedures. The anesthetic management of these groups will be discussed here.

Emergent Surgery

Neurosurgical. These patients commonly arrive in the operating room with an endotracheal tube in place. If their airway has not yet been secured, then the same principles that were discussed in the airway section should be applied. Often there is little time allotted for the preoperative assessment; one's approach must be concise and focused to obtain the pertinent information in a brief amount of time. These patients may have other injuries that will affect their care. The neurologic condition of the patient can be determined rapidly by obtaining the GCS score, examining the pupils, and reviewing the CT scan. The hemodynamic status of the patient is also extremely important. Patients may demonstrate Cushing response of hypertension and bradycardia, which signifies brainstem compression from raised ICP. However, these classic findings may be masked by hypovolemia, and their absence does not rule out brainstem compression. An estimation of volume status is appropriate. Other important information includes oxygenation, which may be compromised because of pulmonary contusion; hematocrit, which may be low in the presence of additional injuries; and the extent of the evaluation obtained prior to the decision to proceed to the operating room. An incomplete evaluation, radiographic or otherwise, should leave one highly suspicious for missed injuries, such as pneumothorax or intra-abdominal hemorrhage.

Appropriate monitoring must be established rapidly so as not to delay surgical intervention. Standard monitors should be applied including electrocardiogram, pulse oximetry, capnography, and noninvasive blood pressure measurement. Two large-bore intravenous catheters are required at a minimum. Delay for placement of a central venous catheter should occur only if adequate peripheral access cannot be obtained. Consideration for a femoral venous catheter should be made, as it can be placed while preparation of the head for surgery is ongoing. An arterial catheter is desirable, but it is a secondary priority after venous access.

These patients usually do not have ICP monitors in place but one can assume the presence of intracranial hypertension in the setting of an acute space-occupying lesion. The presence of midline shift on CT scan and pupillary abnormalities on physical examination reinforce this diagnosis. Moderate hyperventilation should be used in these patients until the dura is opened, as the elevation in ICP is likely more detrimental than the short-term hyperventilation.

Blood pressure management in these patients is critical. They may arrive in the operating room in a hypertensive state. The hypertension is often a response to the stress of the injury as well as the elevated ICP. Unfortunately, this hypertension may mask an underlying volume deficit due to hemorrhage or high urine output from mannitol administered prior to arrival in the operating room. Profound hypotension may follow anesthesia induction, or more likely, after the craniectomy when the intrinsic stimulus for blood pressure elevation diminishes. Risk factors for postdecompressive hypotension include low GCS score, absence of basal cisterns on CT, and bilateral dilated pupils.[151] To avoid hypotension, intravenous volume loading in the early stages of the anesthetic is essential, particularly in patients with other injuries and significant blood loss.

The choice of anesthetic agents should be based on the clinical condition of the patient. Anesthetic requirement for the traumatized CNS is lower; adequate anesthesia should be administered without compromising hemodynamics. Volatile anesthesia is acceptable as it is easily titratable, whereas intravenous agents have the benefit of a greater reduction in CBV and ICP. Nitrous oxide should be avoided as it increases $CMRO_2$, CBF, and ICP in head-injured patients.[152–154] Narcotics can be used safely in these patients as long as blood pressure is not compromised and the patient is mechanically ventilated.

Nonneurosurgical. Trauma patients presenting for emergent surgical management of noncranial injuries who also have a concurrent TBI are complex to manage. The most immediately life-threatening condition must take priority but the presence of TBI should be considered, particularly in someone with depressed level of consciousness or an abnormal pupil examination. If the history and examination are consistent with TBI, and a complete evaluation was not possible prior to emergent management in the operating room, intraoperative neurosurgical consult for ICP monitoring is reasonable. The presence of dilated pupils bilaterally may suggest a devastating brain injury. TCD, if available, should be used to assess for nonviable CBF patterns.[155] A well-characterized progression of TCD waveform morphology has been described for increasing ICP with a corresponding decrease in CPP (Fig. 39-12).[156] Increasing pulsatility of the waveform is suggestive of high ICP. Appropriate intervention should be implemented when this morphology is seen (e.g., head-up and neutral neck position, elevation of MAP, administration of mannitol, conversion to intravenous anesthesia).

Nonemergent Surgery

Patients with TBI frequently have other injuries, especially fractures requiring operative fixation. The timing of surgery in these patients remains a controversial issue.[157] One must balance the need for operative fixation of these fractures to decrease the incidence of complications related to immobility such as atelectasis, pneumonia, and venous thromboembolism with the risks of performing surgery in patients with head injuries. These patients have altered physiologic mechanisms such as cerebral autoregulation; they are at risk for secondary injury, especially that from hypotension.[71,158,159] Although some studies favor early fixation and some favor delayed fixation, none provides sufficient evidence to guide management of these patients.

In the absence of definitive evidence to guide management, we offer several conservative recommendations. In the setting of refractory elevations in ICP or very labile ICP, only emergent surgery should be performed. Because patients with TBI cannot be examined clinically during anesthesia, there should be a low threshold for placing an ICP monitor in someone who will be going to the operating room, particularly for longer surgeries and those taking place in the first 48 hours after injury. When available, advanced neuromonitoring, including TCD, jugular bulb oximetry, and brain tissue oxygenation should be used for intraoperative management.

ANESTHESIA FOR SPINE TRAUMA AND COMPLEX SPINE SURGERY

Surgery on the spinal column has become increasingly complex and lengthy, with multilevel fusions, combined anterior and posterior approaches to the spine, as well as staged procedures. The anesthetic plan for these procedures is made more complicated by the increasing age of patients requiring spine surgery and the concomitant increase in comorbid disease, as well as the need for sophisticated monitoring of the spinal cord. In addition, SCI is a common traumatic injury often requiring surgical intervention.

FIGURE 39-12. Transcranial Doppler tracing illustrating the characteristic changes associated with increasing intracranial pressure. The occurrence of biphasic or oscillating flow signifies the onset of intracranial circulatory arrest. Transcranial Doppler is accepted as a confirmatory test for brain death. (Reprinted from Hassler W, Steinmetz H, Gawlowski J. Transcranial Doppler ultrasonography in raised intracranial pressure and in intracranial circulatory arrest. J Neurosurg 1988; 68: 745, with permission.)

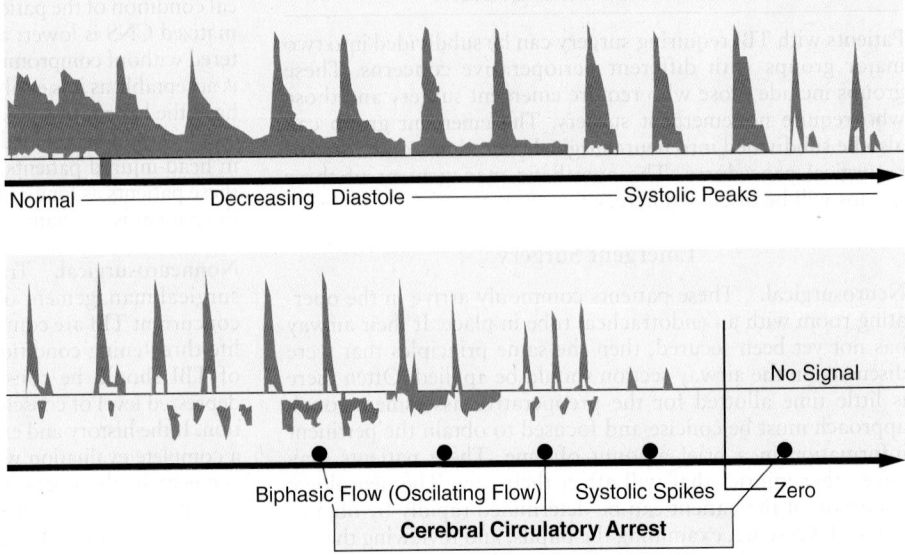

The anesthesiologist encounters many patients with disease of the spinal column, both in and out of the operating room. There are several aspects of their care, including airway management, resuscitation, and intraoperative management, that require a particular understanding of their disease. The focus of this section will be on anesthesia and SCI, but the anesthetic management will be relevant to all complex spine surgery.

Spinal Cord Injury

Primary Injury

SCI is analogous to TBI in that there is both a primary and secondary component. Initial injury typically involves damage to the bones and ligaments of the spinal column. Although SCI can occur without radiographic abnormality, which is referred to as *SCIWORA*, this phenomenon is more common in children than adults. Damage to the spinal column may occur without injury to the cord or it can cause SCI through various insults, including compression, hemorrhage, and vasospasm, all of which result in cord ischemia and infarction.

The nature of the bony injury is important as it will guide further management of the patient irrespective of the SCI. The purpose of the spinal column is to provide support to the individual while protecting the spinal cord and nerve roots. An unstable injury puts the neural elements at risk, and will necessitate some intervention to provide stability, which may be application of a brace or surgical intervention.

Secondary Injury

Secondary injury to the spinal cord is mediated through a cascade of deleterious events similar to that seen in TBI, including induction of nitric oxide synthase, release of excitotoxic amino acids, cellular influx of calcium, oxidative stress, and lipid peroxidation. Secondary injury may be exacerbated by hypotension due to hemorrhage or neurogenic shock.

Central, Anterior, Brown-Séquard, and Cauda Equina Injuries

Although a complete cord transection will result in disruption of afferent and efferent signals, many injuries damage only a portion of the spinal cord. The nature of this injury will determine its clinical manifestation. Several syndromes are well described for their classic cord lesion and corresponding signs.

Central cord syndrome is characterized by greater severity of paresis in the upper extremities than the lower, as well as bladder dysfunction and variable loss of sensory below the lesion. It is probably caused by a cervical spine lesion via hemorrhage into the cord following trauma.

Anterior cord syndrome is generally due to disruption of blood flow through the anterior spinal artery at the level of the injury. The anterior portion of the cord becomes ischemic, disrupting motor function below the level, with a variable effect on sensation. Pain and temperature tracts are typically interrupted as well, but proprioception remains intact. Brown-Séquard syndrome is characterized by interruption of a lateral half of the spinal cord, typically through penetrating trauma. Although a patient may not display all the classic findings of Brown-Séquard syndrome, these would include loss of motor and touch sensation ipsilateral to the lesion, with pain and temperature sensation lost contralateral to the lesion.

Cauda equina syndrome is the result of injury below the level of the conus, or caudal end of the cord, typically below L2. Compression of the cauda equina results in perineal anesthesia, urinary retention, fecal incontinence, and lower extremity weakness.

American Spinal Injury Association Classification

In an effort to categorize the nature of the injury, the American Spinal Injury Association (ASIA) classification was developed (Table 39-6). This system rates cord injuries with a letter from A through E. ASIA A is a complete cord lesion in which no motor or sensory is preserved in the sacral segments S4-S5. ASIA B is incomplete, with only sensory spared below the lesion, including S4-S5. ASIA C indicates an injury where more than half the important muscle groups below the injury have motor scores of <3. ASIA D is an injury where more than half the muscles groups have motor scores ≤3. ASIA E indicates a neurologically intact individual.

Comorbid Injuries

SCI frequently occurs in conjunction with other injuries. Cervical spine trauma is associated with blunt cerebrovascular injury, TBI, and facial fractures.[110,160,161] Thoracic trauma is

TABLE 39-6

AMERICAN SPINAL INJURY ASSOCIATION (ASIA) CLASSIFICATION FOR SPINAL CORD INJURY

■ CLASSIFICATION	■ DESCRIPTION
A	Complete cord injury. No motor or sensation in sacral nerve roots S4 and S5.
B	Incomplete cord injury. Sensory preserved below the level of the injury, including S4-S5.
C	Incomplete cord injury. Motor function preserved below the level of the injury, but with strength of less than 3 in half the major muscle groups.
D	Incomplete cord injury. Motor function preserved below the level of the injury, with strength of 3 or more in at least half the major muscle groups.
E	No cord injury. Motor and sensory intact.

also associated with vascular injury; in addition, one must consider the possibility of pneumothorax, myocardial contusion, pulmonary contusion, and so forth, with trauma to the thorax.[162] Lumbar spine fractures may be associated with bowel and solid viscus injury.[163]

Initial Management

Urgent Airway Management

Initial management of the patient with spine trauma follows the standard practices of care for trauma patients in general, with initial emphasis on airway, breathing, and circulation (as outlined in *Advanced Trauma Life Support* by the American College of Surgeons). Endotracheal intubation can be particularly difficult in the patient with SCI, especially if the lesion is in the cervical spine. In addition, intubation frequently needs to be accomplished before the presence or location of an injury can be confirmed. As a result, cervical spine injury should be presumed in trauma patients requiring intubation prior to complete physical and radiographic evaluation. Intubation should proceed with little movement of the cervical spine. A rapid-sequence induction with cricoid pressure and manual inline stabilization is appropriate, unless a difficult airway is anticipated.

Hemodynamic Stabilization

Restoration of intravascular volume is the first step in treatment of hypotension in the patient with SCI. Isotonic crystalloid resuscitation is appropriate. Concomitant injury with hemorrhage may necessitate blood product administration. Once euvolemia has been achieved, support of blood pressure with inotropic agents and/or vasopressors may be required.

The choice of pressor must be based on the clinical picture and individualized to the patient and his or her comorbidities. Patients with isolated injuries to the lower cord frequently do not require any such agents to maintain an adequate systemic blood pressure. Higher cord lesions result in greater sympathectomy, vasodilation, and thus vascular capacitance. Although volume is beneficial in this setting, a pure α-agonist

such as neosynephrine is a reasonable choice to restore vascular tone. Patients with higher lesions, in the upper thoracic or cervical spine, with concomitant hypotension and bradycardia should receive an agent such as dopamine or norepinephrine, which will restore both cardiac inotropy and chronotropy, as well as peripheral vascular tone.

Role for Steroids

Methylprednisolone has become a common therapy for patients with neurologic deficit resulting from SCI following the NASCIS II and III studies from the 1990s, which showed clinically important improvement in the motor function of patients with SCI.[164–166] The studies have been criticized, however, and some centers do not regard steroids as standard of care.[167] Furthermore, the difference in findings with respect to steroids in brain injury forces one to question why steroids would benefit one part of the CNS but harm another. A large multicenter study in patients with head injury found an increased risk of death in patients receiving methylprednisolone at both 2 weeks and 6 months.[168,169]

Timing of Surgical Intervention

The purpose of surgical intervention is to decompress the neural structures and stabilize the spinal column to prevent further injury to the cord. Management of the patient with SCI frequently requires intervention for comorbid life-threatening trauma, such as intra-abdominal or pelvic hemorrhage. Surgical decompression of the spinal cord with fixation of the spinal column must wait until the patient is clinically appropriate for the procedure. Persistent hemodynamic instability or severe acute respiratory distress syndrome may impose a significant delay on surgical intervention. Although early fixation of isolated SCI may decrease ICU length of stay, improved neurologic outcome has been demonstrated thus far primarily in animal models, not in humans; surgical fixation within 24 hours may be appropriate in patients with cervical SCI and tetraplegia, however.[170–173]

Intraoperative Management

Anesthetic Induction and Airway Management

If a patient with SCI did not require endotracheal intubation in the prehospital or emergency department setting, then he or she will need further airway management on presentation to the operating room. Given the less urgent nature of this setting, more options are available to the anesthesiologist.

If the patient's cervical spine has been radiographically and clinically cleared prior to arrival, then the technique for induction of anesthesia and endotracheal intubation should be determined by the patient's other injuries, comorbidities, and airway examination.

Patients with confirmed cervical spine injury require careful planning, however. These patients will undoubtedly be immobilized in either a cervical collar or Halo device. A rapid-sequence induction remains a viable option, particularly in someone who is unable to cooperate with an awake procedure. If the patient is fasted, a standard induction followed by intubation with inline stabilization may be a reasonable option as well.

The most conservative approach to airway management in this setting is the awake fiberoptic endotracheal intubation. This technique requires thorough application of topical anesthesia to the airway. The topical anesthetic of choice is plain lidocaine, as the complication of methemoglobinemia with benzocaine can obscure the clinical picture during airway management and harm the patient.[174]

Localization of an airway is time-consuming and difficult to accomplish in some patients who are particularly anxious or uncooperative. If such a patient is an appropriate candidate for mask ventilation, then fiberoptic intubation may be accomplished after induction of anesthesia.

The fiberoptic intubation can be accomplished either from the head of the bed or at the side of the patient. It is appropriate to develop proficiency with both techniques, as situations such as chin-on-chest deformity with ankylosing spondylitis may require fiberoptic intubation from the side.

Anesthetic Technique

Complex spine and trauma surgery imposes a significant risk of blood loss. An arterial catheter is essential for continuous hemodynamic monitoring and intermittent arterial blood gas and hematocrit analysis. In addition, the respiratory variation of the arterial line, or reversed pulsus paradoxus, is a useful indicator of a volume responsive state.[175,176] For many otherwise healthy patients presenting for spine surgery, the arterial line may be the only invasive monitor necessary.

Several medium- to large-bore peripheral intravenous catheters are appropriate for volume and blood product administration. In large thoracic or lumbar spine surgeries, particularly in the prone position, central venous access may be appropriate. In addition to providing more access for volume resuscitation, transducing a central venous pressure provides filling pressures of the right atrium. The value of the central venous pressure is controversial, however. It is neither a good indicator of end-diastolic volume nor a predictor of volume-responsiveness in hypotension.[177]

Although there is some literature suggesting a benefit to managing older patients with trauma with a pulmonary artery catheter (PAC), its use is not routinely recommended.[178] A recent large study has demonstrated that the complications associated with PAC use are similar to those of central line placement.[179] Therefore, although there may be few clear indications for their use, placement of a PAC can certainly be justified in sick patients with poor cardiac function, especially those in whom fluid management is difficult and vasopressor therapy is required. The recent development of arterial line-based cardiac output monitoring may further diminish the need for PAC use, however.[180]

Neuromonitoring

The goals of spine surgery, whether for trauma or other spine disease, are typically to decompress the cord and stabilize the spinal column. These goals must be accomplished without inflicting further injury to the cord. Monitoring cord function is appropriate for many surgical procedures. The details of this monitoring have been discussed already. Which modalities should be implemented is a decision made in conjunction with the spine surgeon and the electrophysiologist. The anesthetic plan must be tailored to accommodate these monitors.

Patient Positioning

The prone position provides unique challenges to the anesthesiologist with respect to achieving adequate protection of the patient from pressure points. Areas at particular risk include the eyes and face, the breasts, genitals, knees, and toes. Whether using the Mayfield device to hold the head in pins or a prone pillow, pressure on the eyes and nose must be avoided. Frequent confirmation that the eyes are free from contact is important, as the pillow may move over time. In addition, slight reverse Trendelenburg position may facilitate venous drainage from the head and reduce congestion and intraocular pressure.[181] Padding on the chest should not compress the neck, as this too may obstruct venous drainage. The breasts

and male genitals should be checked to ensure that they are free of undue pressure. Lower extremities must be padded adequately to prevent excess weight resting on the knees and toes.

Glucose Management

Apart from an animal study of SCI and hyperglycemia, there is little evidence to guide the management of glucose in patients with disease of the spine, particularly in the intraoperative setting.[182] In the absence of evidence, glucose management in spine surgery may be accomplished in a manner similar to that for neurosurgical procedures. It is reasonable to continue tight glycemic control in patients who arrive in the operating room from the ICU, and it is reasonable to start tight glycemic control on patients who will be admitted to the ICU following surgery. These recommendations assume that frequent glucose monitoring is an integral part of the anesthetic procedure. In SCI patients who are administered methylprednisolone, glucose control may be more difficult to achieve.

Complications of Anesthesia for Spine Surgery

Autonomic Hyperreflexia

Patients with chronic spinal cord lesion above the level of T7 may develop autonomic hyperreflexia when stimulated below the site of lesion. This is a condition characterized by intense vasoconstriction below the site of the lesion, accompanied by cutaneous vasodilation above the site, hypertension, and bradycardia. This is the result of reflex sympathetic stimulation below the lesion unmodulated by supraspinal influence from above. In severe cases, cerebral hemorrhage and myocardial ischemia can occur. To reduce the incidence of this complication, suppression of the afferent pathway by "deepening" anesthesia is necessary. To this end, a spinal anesthetic, if possible, may be the ideal anesthetic.

Postoperative Visual Loss

Although there are many potential complications of spine surgery, including massive hemorrhage, venous air embolism, myocardial infarction, pulmonary edema, and pressure necrosis, the complication of postoperative visual loss is of particular concern in prone spine surgery, although it can occur in other settings.[183] The visual loss is commonly bilateral and due to ischemic optic neuropathy, although retinal artery occlusion and cortical blindness may also occur.[184] These incidents of visual loss occur despite the absence of pressure on the eyes from positioning errors, which would result in central retinal artery thrombosis, and not anterior or posterior ischemic optic neuropathy. Ischemic optic neuropathy is associated with blood loss and hypotension, and most importantly, long duration, and most certainly has a multifactorial etiology, including anatomic variation in the vasculature of individual patients.[185] Given the increasing recognition of this problem, determining whether a patient has experienced any visual changes is an integral part of the postoperative evaluation. Visual complaints warrant an immediate retinal examination and ophthalmology consult. Currently there is no proven method to prevent it, nor is there a reliable method to monitor visual function during these procedures. A number of investigators have focused on monitoring of intraoperative intraocular pressure, which is unlikely to yield meaningful results. On the other hand, monitoring of VEP may provide more useful information. Staging of a complex spine procedure may be the most effective means of preventing this devastating complication, as limiting the duration of the procedure would also limit the risk of hypotension and blood loss.

References

1. Emerich DF, Vasconcellos AV, Ellitt RB et al: The choroid plexus: Function, pathology and therapeutic potential of its transplantation. Expert Opin Biol Ther 2004; 4: 1191

2. Praetorius J: Water and solute secretion by the choroid plexus. Pflugers Arch 2007; 454: 1

3. Steiner LA, Balestreri M, Johnston AJ et al: Sustained moderate reductions in arterial CO_2 after brain trauma time-course of cerebral blood flow velocity and intracranial pressure. Intensive Care Med 2004; 30: 2180

4. Warner KJ, Cushieri J, Copass MK et al: The impact of prehospital ventilation on outcome after severe traumatic brain injury. J Trauma 2007; 62: 1330

5. Diringer MN, Yundt K, Videen TO et al: No reduction in cerebral metabolism as a result of early moderate hyperventilation following severe traumatic brain injury. J Neurosurg 2000; 92: 76

6. Coles JP, Minhas PS, Fryer TD et al: Effect of hyperventilation on cerebral blood flow in traumatic head injury: clinical relevance and monitoring correlates. Crit Care Med 2002; 30: 1950

7. Lassen NA. Cerebral blood flow and oxygen consumption in man. Physiol Rev 1959; 39: 183

8. Floyd TF, McGarvey M, Ochroch EA et al: Perioperative changes in cerebral blood flow after cardiac surgery: influence of anemia and aging. Ann Thorac Surg 2003; 76: 2037

9. Lo YL, Chih HW, Yeh CY et al: Intraoperative monitoring study of ipsilateral motor evoked potentials in scoliosis surgery. Eur Spine J 2006; 15(Suppl 17): 656

10. Kakimoto M, Kawaguchi M, Yamamoto Y et al: Tetanic stimulation of the peripheral nerve before transcranial electrical stimulation can enlarge amplitudes of myogenic motor evoked potentials during general anesthesia with neuromuscular blockade. Anesthesiology 2005; 102: 733

11. Huber P, Handa J: Effect of contrast material, hypercapnia, hyperventilation, hypertonic glucose and papaverine on the diameter of the cerebral arteries. Angiographic determination in man. Invest Radiol 1967; 2: 17

12. Chesnut RM: Care of central nervous system injuries. Surg Clin North Am 2007; 87: 119

13. Valadka AB, Gopinath SP, Contant CF et al: Relationship of brain tissue PO2 to outcome after severe head injury. Crit Care Med 1998; 26: 1576

14. Robertson CS, Gopinath SP, Goodman JC et al: SjvO2 monitoring in head-injured patients. J Neurotrauma 1995; 12: 891

15. Matta BF, Lam AM: The rate of blood withdrawal affects the accuracy of jugular venous bulb. Oxygen saturation measurements. Anesthesiology 1997; 86: 806

16. Bernard SA, Gray TW, Buist MD et al: Treatment of comatose survivors of out-of-hospital cardiac arrest with induced hypothermia. N Engl J Med 2002; 346: 557

17. Hypothermic after Cardiac Arrest Study Group. Mild therapeutic hypothermia to improve the neurologic outcome after cardiac arrest. N Engl J Med 2002; 346: 549

18. Koerner IP, Brambrink AM: Brain protection by anesthetic agents. Curr Opin Anaesthesiol 2006; 19: 481

19. Fritz KW, Kasperczyk W, Galaske R: [Successful resuscitation in accidental hypothermia following drowning]. Anaesthesist 1988; 37: 331

20. Oberhammer R, Beikircher W, Hormann C et al: Full recovery of an avalanche victim with profound hypothermia and prolonged cardiac arrest treated by extracorporeal re-warming. Resuscitation 2008;76(3):474

21. Mack WJ, Ducruet AF, Angevine PD et al: Deep hypothermic circulatory arrest for complex cerebral aneurysms: lessons learned. Neurosurgery 2007; 60: 815

22. Kunihara T, Grun T, Aicher D et al: Hypothermic circulatory arrest is not a risk factor for neurologic morbidity in aortic surgery: a propensity score analysis. J Thorac Cardiovasc Surg 2005; 130: 712

23. Leonov Y, Sterz F, Safar P et al: Mild cerebral hypothermia during and after cardiac arrest improves neurologic outcome in dogs. J Cereb Blood Flow Metab 1990; 10: 57

24. Scholler K, Zausinger S, Baethmann A et al: Neuroprotection in ischemic stroke—combination drug therapy and mild hypothermia in a rat model of permanent focal cerebral ischemia. Brain Res 2004; 1023: 272

25. Todd MM, Hindman BJ, Clark WR et al: Intraoperative Hypothermia for Aneurysm Surgery Trial (IHAST) Investigators. Mild intraoperative hypothermia during surgery for intracranial aneurysm. N Engl J Med 2005; 352: 135

26. Reith J, Jorgensen HS, Pedersen PM et al: Body temperature in acute stroke: relation to stroke severity, infarct size, mortality, and outcome. Lancet 1996; 347: 422

27. Oliveira-Filho J, Ezzeddine MA, Segal AZ et al: Fever in subarachnoid hemorrhage: relationship to vasospasm and outcome. Neurology 2001; 56 1299

28. Zeiner A, Holzer M, Sterz F et al: Hyperthermia after cardiac arrest is associated with an unfavorable neurologic outcome. Arch Intern Med 2001; 161: 2007

29. Jiang JY, Macchiarelli G, Miyabayashi K et al: Early indicators of prognosis in 846 cases of severe traumatic brain injury. J Neurotrauma 2002; 19: 869

30. Aiyagari V, Diringer MN. Fever control and its impact on outcomes: what is the evidence? J Neurol Sci 2007; 261: 39

31. Warner DS, Takaoka S, Wu B et al: Electroencephalographic burst suppression is not required to elicit maximal neuroprotection from pentobarbital in a rat model of focal cerebral ischemia. Anesthesiology 1996; 84: 1475

32. Elsersy H, Sheng H, Lynch JR et al: Effects of isoflurane versus fentanyl-nitrous oxide anesthesia on long-term outcome from severe forebrain ischemia in the rat. Anesthesiology 2004; 100: 1160

33. Kawaguchi M, Furuya H, Patel PM. Neuroprotective effects of anesthetic agents. J Anesth 2005; 19: 150

34. Kawaguchi M, Kimbro JR, Drummond JC et al: Isoflurane delays but does not prevent cerebral infarction in rats subjected to focal ischemia. Anesthesiology 2000; 92: 1335

35. Soonthon-Brant V, Patel PM, Drummond JC et al: Fentanyl does not increase brain injury after focal cerebral ischemia in rats. Anesth Analg 1999; 88: 49

36. Blanck TJ, Haile M, Xu F et al: Isoflurane pretreatment ameliorates postischemic neurologic dysfunction and preserves hippocampal Ca2+/calmodulin-dependent protein kinase in a canine cardiac arrest model. Anesthesiology 2000; 93: 1285

37. Kapinya KJ, Lowl D, Futterer C et al: Tolerance against ischemic neuronal injury can be induced by volatile anesthetics and is inducible NO synthase dependent. Stroke 2002; 33: 1889

38. Drummond JC, Cole DJ, Patel PM et al: Focal cerebral ischemia during anesthesia with etomidate, isoflurane, or thiopental: a comparison of the extent of cerebral injury. Neurosurgery 1995; 37: 742

39. Michenfelder JD, Milde JH, Sundt TM Jr. Cerebral protection by barbiturate anesthesia. Use after middle cerebral artery occlusion in Java monkeys. Arch Neurol 1976; 33: 345

40. Selman WR, Spetzler RJ, Roski RA et al: Barbiturate coma in focal cerebral ischemia. Relationship of protection to timing of therapy. J Neurosurg 1982; 56: 685

41. Smith AL, Hoff JT, Nielsen SL et al: Barbiturate protection in acute focal cerebral ischemia. Stroke 1974; 5: 1

42. Bleyaert AL, Nemoto EM, Safar P et al: Thiopental amelioration of brain damage after global ischemia in monkeys. Anesthesiology 1978; 49: 390

43. Gisvold SE, Safar P, Hendrickx HH et al: Thiopental treatment after global brain ischemia in pigtailed monkeys. Anesthesiology 1984; 60: 88

44. Snyder BD, Ramirez-Lassepas M, Sukhum P et al: Failure of thiopental to modify global anoxic injury. Stroke 1979; 10: 135

45. Steen PA, Milde JH, Michenfelder JD: No barbiturate protection in a dog model of complete cerebral ischemia. Ann Neurol 1979; 5: 343

46. Todd MM, Chadwick HS, Shapiro HM et al: The neurologic effects of thiopental therapy following experimental cardiac arrest in cats. Anesthesiology 1982; 57: 76

47. Zhan RZ, Fujiwara N, Endoh H et al: Thiopental inhibits increases in [Ca2+]i induced by membrane depolarization, NMDA receptor activation, and ischemia in rat hippocampal and cortical slices. Anesthesiology 1998; 89: 456

48. Zhu H, Cottrell JE, Kass IS: The effect of thiopental and propofol on NMDA- and AMPA-mediated glutamate excitotoxicity. Anesthesiology 1997;87(4): 944

49. Rodriguez-Lopez JM, Sanchez-Conde P, Lozano FS et al: Laboratory investigation: effects of propofol on the systemic inflammatory response during aortic surgery. Can J Anaesth 2006; 53: 701

50. Young Y, Menon DK, Tisavipat N et al: Propofol neuroprotection in a rat model of ischaemia reperfusion injury. Eur J Anaesthesiol 1997; 14: 320

51. Fukuda S, Warner DS: Cerebral protection. Br J Anaesth 2007; 99: 10

52. Mizock BA: Alterations in carbohydrate metabolism during stress: a review of the literature. Am J Med 1995; 98: 75

53. Capes SE, Hunt D, Malmberg K et al: Stress hyperglycaemia and increased risk of death after myocardial infarction in patients with and without diabetes: a systematic overview. Lancet 2000; 355: 773

54. Capes SE, Hunt D, Malmberg K et al: Stress hyperglycemia and prognosis of stroke in nondiabetic and diabetic patients: a systematic overview. Stroke 2001; 32: 2426

55. Gore DC, Chinkes D, Heggers J et al: Association of hyperglycemia with increased mortality after severe burn injury. J Trauma 2001; 51: 540

56. Krinsley JS: Association between hyperglycemia and increased hospital mortality in a heterogeneous population of critically ill patients. Mayo Clin Proc 2003; 78: 1471

57. O'Neill PA, Davies I, Fullerton KJ et al: Stress hormone and blood glucose response following acute stroke in the elderly. Stroke 1991; 22: 842

58. Rovlias A, Kotsou S: The influence of hyperglycemia on neurological outcome in patients with severe head injury. Neurosurgery 2000; 46: 335

59. Chew W, Kucharczyk J, Moseley M et al: Hyperglycemia augments ischemic brain injury: in vivo MR imaging/spectroscopic study with nicardipine in cats with occluded middle cerebral arteries. AJNR Am J Neuroradiol 1991; 12: 603

60. Marfella R, D'Amico M, DiFilippo C et al: Myocardial infarction in diabetic rats: role of hyperglycaemia on infarct size and early expression of hypoxia-inducible factor 1. Diabetologia 2002; 45: 1172

61. van den Berghe G, Wouters P, Weekers F et al: Intensive insulin therapy in the critically ill patients. N Engl J Med 2001; 345: 1359

62. Van den Berghe G, Wilmer A, Hermans G et al: Intensive insulin therapy in the medical ICU. N Engl J Med 2006; 354: 449

63. Gandhi GY, Nuttell GA, Abel MD et al: Intensive intraoperative insulin therapy versus conventional glucose management during cardiac surgery: a randomized trial. Ann Intern Med 2007; 146: 233

64. McGirt MJ, Woodworth GF, Brooke BS et al: Hyperglycemia independently increases the risk of perioperative stroke, myocardial infarction, and death after carotid endarterectomy. Neurosurgery 2006; 58: 1066

65. Gentile NT et al: Decreased mortality by normalizing blood glucose after acute ischemic stroke. Acad Emerg Med 2006; 13: 174

66. Cimino M, Gelosa P, Gianelli A et al: Statins: multiple mechanisms of action in the ischemic brain. Neuroscientist 2007; 13: 208

67. Maiese K, Li F, Chong ZZ. New avenues of exploration for erythropoietin. JAMA 2005; 293: 90

68. Fleisher LA et al: ACC/AHA 2007 Guidelines on Perioperative Cardiovascular Evaluation and Care for Noncardiac Surgery: Executive Summary: A Report of the American College of Cardiology/American Heart Association Task Force on Practice Guidelines (Writing Committee to Revise the 2002 Guidelines on Perioperative Cardiovascular Evaluation for Noncardiac Surgery): Developed in Collaboration With the American Society of Echocardiography, American Society of Nuclear Cardiology, Heart Rhythm Society, Society of Cardiovascular Anesthesiologists, Society for Cardiovascular Angiography and Interventions, Society for Vascular Medicine and Biology, and Society for Vascular Surgery. Circulation 2007; 116: 1971

69. POISE trial investigators; Devereaux PJ, Yang H, Guyatt GH et al: Rationale, design, and organization of the PeriOperative ISchemic Evaluation (POISE) trial: a randomized controlled trial of metoprolol versus placebo in patients undergoing noncardiac surgery. Am Heart J 2006; 152: 223

70. Juul AB, Wetterslev J, Gluud C et al: Effect of perioperative beta blockade in patients with diabetes undergoing major non-cardiac surgery: randomised placebo controlled, blinded multicentre trial. BMJ 2006; 332: 1482

71. Chesnut RM, Marshall LE, Klauber MR et al: The role of secondary brain injury in determining outcome from severe head injury. J Trauma 1993; 34: 216

72. Fujii Y, Takeuchi S, Sasaki O et al: Ultra-early rebleeding in spontaneous subarachnoid hemorrhage. J Neurosurg 1996; 84: 35

73. Martyn JA, Richtsfeld M. Succinylcholine-induced hyperkalemia in acquired pathologic states: etiologic factors and molecular mechanisms. Anesthesiology 2006; 104: 158

74. Gronert GA, Theye RA: Pathophysiology of hyperkalemia induced by succinylcholine. Anesthesiology 1975; 43: 89

75. Davis DP, Dunford JV, Poste JC et al: The impact of hypoxia and hyperventilation on outcome after paramedic rapid sequence intubation of severely head-injured patients. J Trauma 2004; 57: 1

76. Guidelines for the management of severe traumatic brain injury. XIV. Hyperventilation. J Neurotrauma 2007; 24(Suppl 1): S87

77. Hebert PC, Wells G, Blajchman MA et al: A multicenter, randomized, controlled clinical trial of transfusion requirements in critical care. Transfusion Requirements in Critical Care Investigators, Canadian Critical Care Trials Group. N Engl J Med 1999; 340: 409

78. Rivers E, Nguyen B, Haustad S et al: Early goal-directed therapy in the treatment of severe sepsis and septic shock. N Engl J Med 2001; 345: 1368

79. Carlson AP, Schermer CR, Lu SW. Retrospective evaluation of anemia and transfusion in traumatic brain injury. J Trauma 2006; 61: 567

80. Wass CT, Long TR, Faust RJ et al: Changes in red blood cell transfusion practice during the past two decades: a retrospective analysis, with the Mayo database, of adult patients undergoing major spine surgery. Transfusion 2007; 47: 1022

81. SAFE Study Investigators; Australia and New Zealand Intensive Care Society Clinical Trials Group; Australian Red Cross Blood Service; George Institute for International Health; Myburgh J, et al: Saline or albumin for fluid resuscitation in patients with traumatic brain injury. N Engl J Med 2007; 357: 874

82. De Backer D: The cuff-leak test: what are we measuring? Crit Care 2005; 9: 31

83. Kriner EJ, Shafazand S, Colice GL: The endotracheal tube cuff-leak test as a predictor for postextubation stridor. Respir Care 2005; 50: 1632

84. Kwon B, Yoo JU, Furey CG et al: Risk factors for delayed extubation after single-stage, multi-level anterior cervical decompression and posterior fusion. J Spinal Disord Tech 2006; 19: 389

85. Dunbar PJ, Visco E, Lam AM: Craniotomy procedures are associated with less analgesic requirements than other surgical procedures. Anesth Analg 1999; 88: 335

86. Venkatesan T, Korula G: A comparative study between the effects of 4% endotracheal tube cuff lignocaine and 1.5 mg/kg intravenous lignocaine on coughing and hemodynamics during extubation in neurosurgical patients: a randomized controlled double-blind trial. J Neurosurg Anesthesiol 2006; 18: 230

87. Butler BD, Hills BA: Transpulmonary passage of venous air emboli. J Appl Physiol 1985; 59: 543

88. Vik A, Brubakk AO, Hennessey TR et al: Venous air embolism in swine: transport of gas bubbles through the pulmonary circulation. J Appl Physiol 1990; 69: 237

89. Yahagi N, Furuya H: The effects of halothane and pentobarbital on the threshold of transpulmonary passage of venous air emboli in dogs. Anesthesiology 1987; 67: 905

90. Glasker S, Pechstein U, Vongionkas VI et al: Monitoring motor function during resection of tumours in the lower brain stem and fourth ventricle. Childs Nerv Syst 2006; 22: 1288

91. Neuloh G, Pechstein U, Schramm J: Motor tract monitoring during insular glioma surgery. J Neurosurg 2007; 106: 582

92. Kaal EC, Vecht CJ: The management of brain edema in brain tumors. Curr Opin Oncol 2004; 16: 593

93. Rozet I et al: Effect of equiosmolar solutions of mannitol versus hypertonic saline on intraoperative brain relaxation and electrolyted balance. Anesthesiology, 2007; 107: 697

94. Beneficial effect of carotid endarterectomy in symptomatic patients with high-grade carotid stenosis. North American Symptomatic Carotid Endarterectomy Trial Collaborators. N Engl J Med 1991; 325: 445

95. Chaturvedi S, Bruno A, Feasby T et al: Carotid endarterectomy—an evidence-based review: report of the Therapeutics and Technology Assessment Subcommittee of the American Academy of Neurology. Neurology 2005; 65: 794

96. Endarterectomy for asymptomatic carotid artery stenosis. Executive Committee for the Asymptomatic Carotid Atherosclerosis Study. JAMA 1995; 273: 1421

97. Halliday A, Mansfield A, Marro J et al: MRC Asymptomatic Carotid Surgery Trial (ACST) Collaborative Group, et al. Prevention of disabling and fatal strokes by successful carotid endarterectomy in patients without recent neurological symptoms: randomised controlled trial. Lancet 2004; 363: 1491

98. Ederle J, Brown MM: The evidence for medicine versus surgery for carotid stenosis. Eur J Radiol 2006; 60: 3

99. de Sousa AA, Filho MA, Faglioni W Jr et al: Superficial vs combined cervical plexus block for carotid endarterectomy: a prospective, randomized study. Surg Neurol 2005; 63(Suppl 1): S22

100. Pandit JJ, Bree S, Dillon P et al: A comparison of superficial versus combined (superficial and deep) cervical plexus block for carotid endarterectomy: a prospective, randomized study. Anesth Analg 2000; 91: 781

101. Moritz S, Kasprzak P, Arlt M et al: Accuracy of cerebral monitoring in detecting cerebral ischemia during carotid endarterectomy: a comparison of transcranial Doppler sonography, near-infrared spectroscopy, stump pressure, and somatosensory evoked potentials. Anesthesiology 2007; 107: 563

102. SPACE Collaborative Group, Ringleb PA, Allenberg J, Bruckmann H et al: 30 day results from the SPACE trial of stent-protected angioplasty versus carotid endarterectomy in symptomatic patients: a randomised non-inferiority trial. Lancet 2006; 368: 1239

103. Mas JL, Chatellier G, Beyssen B et al: Endarterectomy versus stenting in patients with symptomatic severe carotid stenosis. N Engl J Med 2006; 355: 1660

104. Yadav JS, Wholey MH, Kuntz RT et al: Protected carotid-artery stenting versus endarterectomy in high-risk patients. N Engl J Med 2004; 351: 1493

105. McClelland S 3rd: Multimodality management of carotid artery stenosis: reviewing the class-I evidence. J Natl Med Assoc 2007; 99: 1235

106. Bulger EM, Copass MK, Sabath DR et al: The use of neuromuscular blocking agents to facilitate prehospital intubation does not impair outcome after traumatic brain injury. J Trauma 2005; 58: 718

107. Winchell RJ, Hoyt DB: Endotracheal intubation in the field improves survival in patients with severe head injury. Trauma Research and Education Foundation of San Diego. Arch Surg 1997; 132: 592

108. Davis DP, Hoyt DB, Ochs M et al: The effect of paramedic rapid sequence intubation on outcome in patients with severe traumatic brain injury. J Trauma 2003; 54: 444

109. Michael DB, Guyot DR, Darmody WR: Coincidence of head and cervical spine injury. J Neurotrauma 1989; 6: 177

110. Holly LT, Kelly DF, Counelis GJ et al: Cervical spine trauma associated with moderate and severe head injury: incidence, risk factors, and injury characteristics. J Neurosurg 2002; 96: 285

111. Lennarson PJ, Smith D, Todd MM et al: Segmental cervical spine motion during orotracheal intubation of the intact and injured spine with and without external stabilization. J Neurosurg 2000; 92: 201

112. Hastings RH, Wood PR: Head extension and laryngeal view during laryngoscopy with cervical spine stabilization maneuvers. Anesthesiology 1994; 80: 825

113. Donaldson WF 3rd, Towers JD, Doctor A et al: A methodology to evaluate motion of the unstable spine during intubation techniques. Spine 1993; 18: 2020

114. Butler J, Sen A: Best evidence topic report. Cricoid pressure in emergency rapid sequence induction. Emerg Med J 2005; 22: 815

115. Unni VK, Johnston RA, Young HS et al: Prevention of intracranial hypertension during laryngoscopy and endotracheal intubation. Use of a second dose of thiopentone. Br J Anaesth 1984; 56: 1219

116. Albrecht RF, Miletich DJ, Rosenberg R et al: Cerebral blood flow and metabolic changes from induction to onset of anesthesia with halothane or pentobarbital. Anesthesiology 1977; 47: 252

117. Eckstein JW, Hamilton WK, Mc CJ: The effect of thiopental on peripheral venous tone. Anesthesiology 1961; 22: 525

118. Renou AM, Vernhict J, Macrez P et al: Cerebral blood flow and metabolism during anaesthesia in man. Br J Anaesth 1978; 50: 1047

119. Gooding JM, Corssen G: Effect of etomidate on the cardiovascular system. Anesth Analg 1977; 56: 717

120. Bedford RF, Persing JA, Pobereskin L et al: Lidocaine or thiopental for rapid control of intracranial hypertension? Anesth Analg 1980; 59: 435

121. White PF, Schlobohm KM, Pitts LH et al: A randomized study of drugs for preventing increases in intracranial pressure during endotracheal suctioning. Anesthesiology 1982; 57: 242

122. Cottrell JE, Hartung J, Griffin JP et al: Intracranial and hemodynamic changes after succinylcholine administration in cats. Anesth Analg 1983; 62: 1006

123. Kovarik WD, Mayberg TS, Lam AM et al: Succinylcholine does not change intracranial pressure, cerebral blood flow velocity, or the electroencephalogram in patients with neurologic injury. Anesth Analg 1994; 78: 469

124. Guidelines for the management of severe traumatic brain injury. IX. Cerebral perfusion thresholds. J Neurotrauma 2007; 24(Suppl 1): S59

125. Contant CF, Valadka AB, Gopinath SP et al: Adult respiratory distress syndrome: a complication of induced hypertension after severe head injury. J Neurosurg 2001; 95: 560

126. Teasdale G, Jennett B: Assessment of coma and impaired consciousness. A practical scale. Lancet 1974; 2: 81

127. Klauber MR, Marshall LF, Barrett-Connor E et al: Prospective study of patients hospitalized with head injury in San Diego County, 1978. Neurosurgery 1981; 9: 236

128. Jennett B, Teasdale G, Braakman R et al: Prognosis of patients with severe head injury. Neurosurgery 1979; 4: 283

129. Juul N, Morris GF, Marshall SB et al: Intracranial hypertension and cerebral perfusion pressure: influence on neurological deterioration and outcome in severe head injury. The Executive Committee of the International Selfotel Trial. J Neurosurg 2000; 92: 1

130. Miller JD, Becker DP, Ward JD et al: Significance of intracranial hypertension in severe head injury. J Neurosurg 1977; 47: 503

131. Treggiari MM, Schutz N, Yanez ND et al: Role of intracranial pressure values and patterns in predicting outcome in traumatic brain injury: a systematic review. Neurocrit Care 2007; 6: 104

132. Rosner MJ, Rosner SD, Johnson AH: Cerebral perfusion pressure: management protocol and clinical results. J Neurosurg 1995; 83: 949

133. Eisenberg HM, Frankowski RF, Contant CF et al: High-dose barbiturate control of elevated intracranial pressure in patients with severe head injury. J Neurosurg 1988; 69: 15

134. Robertson CS, Valadka AB, Hannay HJ et al: Prevention of secondary ischemic insults after severe head injury. Crit Care Med 1999; 27: 2086

135. Muizelaar JP, Wei EP, Kontos HA et al: Mannitol causes compensatory cerebral vasoconstriction and vasodilation in response to blood viscosity changes. J Neurosurg 1983; 59: 822

136. Wise BL, Chater N: The value of hypertonic mannitol solution in decreasing brain mass and lowering cerebro-spinal-fluid pressure. J Neurosurg 1962; 19: 1038

137. Roberts PA, Pollay M, Engles C et al: Effect on intracranial pressure of furosemide combined with varying doses and administration rates of mannitol. J Neurosurg 1987; 66: 440

138. Battison C, Andrews PJ, Graham C et al: Randomized, controlled trial on the effect of a 20% mannitol solution and a 7.5% saline/6% dextran solution on increased intracranial pressure after brain injury. Crit Care Med 2005; 33: 196

139. Sheinberg M, Kanter MJ, Robertson CS et al: Continuous monitoring of jugular venous oxygen saturation in head-injured patients. J Neurosurg 1992; 76: 212

140. Clifton GL, Miller ER, Choi SC et al: Lack of effect of induction of hypothermia after acute brain injury. N Engl J Med 2001; 344: 556

141. Clifton GL, Miller ER, Choi SC et al: Hypothermia on admission in patients with severe brain injury. J Neurotrauma 2002; 19: 293

142. Clifton GL: Is keeping cool still hot? An update on hypothermia in brain injury. Curr Opin Crit Care 2004; 10: 116

143. Polderman KH: Application of therapeutic hypothermia in the intensive care unit. Opportunities and pitfalls of a promising treatment modality–Part 2: Practical aspects and side effects. Intensive Care Med 2004; 30: 757

144. Jiang J, Yu M, Zhu C: Effect of long-term mild hypothermia therapy in patients with severe traumatic brain injury: 1-year follow-up review of 87 cases. J Neurosurg 2000; 93: 546

145. Vasile B, Rasulo F, Candiani A et al: The pathophysiology of propofol infusion syndrome: a simple name for a complex syndrome. Intensive Care Med 2003; 29: 1417

146. Hutchinson PJ, Kirkpatrick PJ: Decompressive craniectomy in head injury. Curr Opin Crit Care 2004; 10: 101

147. Sahuquillo J, Arikan F: Decompressive craniectomy for the treatment of refractory high intracranial pressure in traumatic brain injury. Cochrane Database Syst Rev 2006: CD003983

148. Jaeger M, Soehle M, Meixensberger J: Effects of decompressive craniectomy on brain tissue oxygen in patients with intracranial hypertension. J Neurol Neurosurg Psychiatry 2003; 74: 513

149. Stiefel MF, Heuer GG, Smith MJ et al: Cerebral oxygenation following decompressive hemicraniectomy for the treatment of refractory intracranial hypertension. J Neurosurg 2004; 101: 241

150. Aarabi B, Hesdorffer DC, Ahn ES et al: Outcome following decompressive craniectomy for malignant swelling due to severe head injury. J Neurosurg 2006; 104: 469

151. Kawaguchi M, Sakamoto T, Ohnishi H et al: Preoperative predictors of reduction in arterial blood pressure following dural opening during surgical evacuation of acute subdural hematoma. J Neurosurg Anesthesiol 1996; 8: 117

152. Pelligrino DA, Miletich DJ, Hoffman WE et al: Nitrous oxide markedly increases cerebral cortical metabolic rate and blood flow in the goat. Anesthesiology 1984; 60: 405

153. Matta BF, Lam AM: Nitrous oxide increases cerebral blood flow velocity during pharmacologically induced EEG silence in humans. J Neurosurg Anesthesiol 1995; 7: 89

154. Moss E, McDowall DG: I.c.p. increases with 50% nitrous oxide in oxygen in severe head injuries during controlled ventilation. Br J Anaesth 1979; 51: 757

155. Wijdicks EF: The diagnosis of brain death. N Engl J Med 2001; 344: 1215

156. Hadani M, Bruk B, Ram Z et al: Application of transcranial doppler ultrasonography for the diagnosis of brain death. Intensive Care Med 1999; 25: 822

157. Grotz MR, Giannoudis PV, Pape HC et al: Traumatic brain injury and stabilisation of long bone fractures: an update. Injury 2004; 35: 1077

158. Hlatky R, Furuya Y, Valadka AB et al: Dynamic autoregulatory response after severe head injury. J Neurosurg 2002; 97: 1054

159. Pietropaoli JA, Rogers FB, Shackford SR et al: The deleterious effects of intraoperative hypotension on outcome in patients with severe head injuries. J Trauma 1992; 33: 403

160. Biffl WL, Egglin T, Benedetto B et al: Sixteen-slice computed tomographic angiography is a reliable noninvasive screening test for clinically significant blunt cerebrovascular injuries. J Trauma 2006; 60: 745

161. Hackl W, Hausberger K, Sailer R et al: Prevalence of cervical spine injuries in patients with facial trauma. Oral Surg Oral Med Oral Pathol Oral Radiol Endod 2001; 92: 370

162. McKevitt EC, Kirkpatrick AW, Vertesi L et al: Identifying patients at risk for intracranial and extracranial blunt carotid injuries. Am J Surg 2002; 183: 566

163. Rabinovici R, Ovadia P, Mathiak G et al: Abdominal injuries associated with lumbar spine fractures in blunt trauma. Injury 1999; 30: 471

164. Bracken MB, Holford TR. Neurological and functional status 1 year after acute spinal cord injury: estimates of functional recovery in National Acute Spinal Cord Injury Study II from results modeled in National Acute Spinal Cord Injury Study III. J Neurosurg 2002; 96(Suppl 3): 259

165. Bracken MB et al: A randomized, controlled trial of methylprednisolone or naloxone in the treatment of acute spinal-cord injury. Results of the Second National Acute Spinal Cord Injury Study. N Engl J Med 1990; 322: 1405

166. Bracken MB, Shephard MJ, Collins WF et al: Administration of methylprednisolone for 24 or 48 hours or tirilazad mesylate for 48 hours in the treatment of acute spinal cord injury. Results of the Third National Acute Spinal Cord Injury Randomized Controlled Trial. National Acute Spinal Cord Injury Study. JAMA 1997; 277: 1597

167. Sayer FT, Kronvall E, Nilsson OG: Methylprednisolone treatment in acute spinal cord injury: the myth challenged through a structured analysis of published literature. Spine J 2006; 6: 335

168. Edwards P, Arango M, Balica L et al: Final results of MRC CRASH, a randomised placebo-controlled trial of intravenous corticosteroid in adults with head injury-outcomes at 6 months. Lancet 2005; 365:1957

169. Roberts I, Yates D, Sandercock P et al: Effect of intravenous corticosteroids on death within 14 days in 10,008 adults with clinically significant head injury (MRC CRASH trial): randomised placebo-controlled trial. Lancet 2004; 364: 1321

170. Guest J, Eleraky MA, Apostolides PJ et al: Traumatic central cord syndrome: results of surgical management. J Neurosurg 2002; 97: 25

171. McKinley W, Meade MA, Kirshblum S et al: Outcomes of early surgical management versus late or no surgical intervention after acute spinal cord injury. Arch Phys Med Rehabil 2004; 85: 1818

172. Harris MB, Sethi RK: The initial assessment and management of the multiple-trauma patient with an associated spine injury. Spine 2006; 31(Suppl 11): S9

173. Fehlings MG, Perrin RG: The timing of surgical intervention in the treatment of spinal cord injury: a systematic review of recent clinical evidence. Spine 2006; 31: S28

174. Ash-Bernal R, Wise R, Wright SM: Acquired methemoglobinemia: a retrospective series of 138 cases at 2 teaching hospitals. Medicine (Baltimore) 2004; 83: 265

175. Massumi RA, Mason DT, Vera Z et al: Reversed pulsus paradoxus. N Engl J Med 1973; 289: 1272

176. Michard F: Changes in arterial pressure during mechanical ventilation. Anesthesiology 2005; 103: 419

177. Kumar A et al: Pulmonary artery occlusion pressure and central venous pressure fail to predict ventricular filling volume, cardiac performance, or the response to volume infusion in normal subjects. Crit Care Med 2004; 32: 691

178. Friese RS, Shafi S, Gentilello LM: Pulmonary artery catheter use is associated with reduced mortality in severely injured patients: a National Trauma Data Bank analysis of 53,312 patients. Crit Care Med 2006; 34: 1597

179. Harvey S, Harrison DA, Singer M et al: Assessment of the clinical effectiveness of pulmonary artery catheters in management of patients in intensive care (PAC-Man): a randomised controlled trial. Lancet 2005; 366: 472

180. Rubenfeld GD, McNamara-Aslin E, Rubinson L: The pulmonary artery catheter, 1967–2007: rest in peace? JAMA 2007; 298: 458

181. Ozcan MS, Praetel C, Bhatti MT et al: The effect of body inclination during prone positioning on intraocular pressure in awake volunteers: a comparison of two operating tables. Anesth Analg 2004; 99: 1152

182. Sala F, Menna G, Bricolo A et al: Role of glycemia in acute spinal cord injury. Data from a rat experimental model and clinical experience. Ann N Y Acad Sci 1999; 890: 133

183. Lee LA, Roth S, Posner KL et al: The American Society of Anesthesiologists Postoperative Visual Loss Registry: analysis of 93 spine surgery cases with postoperative visual loss. Anesthesiology 2006; 105: 652

184. Myers MA, Hamilton SK, Bogosian AJ et al: Visual loss as a complication of spine surgery. A review of 37 cases. Spine 1997; 22: 1325

185. Williams EL, Hart WM Jr, Tempelhoff R: Postoperative ischemic optic neuropathy. Anesth Analg 1995; 80: 1018.

CHAPTER 40 ■ ANESTHESIA FOR THORACIC SURGERY

STEVEN M. NEUSTEIN, JAMES B. EISENKRAFT, AND EDMOND COHEN

KEY POINTS

1 It is important to determine prior to the onset of anesthesia and surgery whether the patient will be able to tolerate the planned lung resection.

2 Preoperative assessment of vital capacity is critical because at least three times the tidal volume (VT) is necessary for an effective cough.

3 Smoking increases airway irritability, decreases mucociliary transport, and increases secretions. It also decreases forced vital capacity and forced expiratory flow 25 to 75%, thereby increasing the incidence of postoperative pulmonary complications.

4 The absolute indications for lung separation using a double-lumen tube have been for protection against spillage of blood, infectious material, or lavage fluid from one lung, or for ventilation in the case of bronchopleural fistula or bullae. A lobectomy or pneumonectomy is a relative indication.

5 The most important advance in checking the proper position of a double-lumen tube is the introduction of the pediatric flexible fiberoptic bronchoscope.

6 During one-lung ventilation (OLV), the dependent lung should be ventilated using a VT that results in a plateau airway pressure <25 cm H_2O at a rate adjusted to maintain $PaCO_2$ at 35 ± 3 mm Hg.

7 The choice of anesthetic technique for OLV must take into consideration the effects on oxygenation and therefore on hypoxic pulmonary vasoconstriction.

8 The need for OLV is much greater with video-assisted thoracoscopic surgery than with open thoracotomy because it is not possible to retract the lung during video-assisted thoracoscopic surgery as it is during an open thoracotomy.

9 The potential advantages offered by high-frequency positive-pressure ventilation during thoracic anesthesia are that lower VT and inspiratory pressures result in a quiet lung field for the surgeon, with minimal movements of airway, lung tissue, and mediastinum.

10 Myasthenia gravis, a disorder of the neuromuscular junction, is a chronic disorder characterized by weakness and fatigability of voluntary muscles with improvement following rest.

11 In addition to a more comfortable patient, important benefits of adequate pain relief are avoidance of postoperative atelectasis and limited inspiratory thoracic cage expansion.

Lung cancer has long been the most common cause of cancer mortality in the United States in men, and surpassed breast caner as the leading cause of cancer deaths in women in 1987.[1] The American Cancer Society has estimated that in 2007, cancer caused 289,550 deaths in men, and 270,100 deaths in women.[2] Lung cancer was the leading cause of death in men and women. The increased incidence of lung cancer has led to an increase in the amount of noncardiac thoracic surgery performed in the United States.

In this chapter, the physiologic, pharmacologic, and clinical considerations for the patient undergoing pulmonary surgery are reviewed, followed by sections on anesthesia for diagnostic and therapeutic procedures, high-frequency ventilation, and special situations, including bronchopleural fistula and tracheal reconstruction. A discussion of myasthenia gravis is included because of the relationship between the thymus gland and myasthenia, and because thymectomy is one of the most commonly performed surgical procedures in these patients. The chapter concludes with a review of the postoperative management of the patient who has undergone noncardiac thoracic surgery.

PREOPERATIVE EVALUATION

The preoperative evaluation of the patient for thoracic surgery should focus on the extent and severity of pulmonary disease and cardiovascular involvement (see Chapter 23). It is important to determine whether the patient will be able to tolerate the planned lung resection. To find out postoperatively that the patient cannot tolerate the resection would be catastrophic.

It is more difficult to predict postoperative pulmonary complications following elective cardiothoracic, compared with noncardiothoracic surgery.[3] Thoracic surgery is known to be associated with high risk, and patient factors that have been associated with increased risk include advanced age, poor general health status, and chronic obstructive pulmonary disease (COPD).[4]

History

Dyspnea

Dyspnea occurs when the requirement for ventilation is greater than the patient's ability to respond appropriately (see Chapter 11). Dyspnea is quantitated as to the degree of physical activity required to produce it, the level of activity possible (e.g., ability to walk on level ground or climb stairs), and management of daily activities. Severe exertional dyspnea usually implies a significantly diminished ventilatory reserve and a forced expiratory volume in 1 second (FEV$_1$) of <1,500 mL, with possible need for postoperative ventilatory support.

Cough

Recurrent productive cough for 3 months of the year for 2 consecutive years is necessary to make the diagnosis of chronic bronchitis. Cough indirectly increases airway irritability. If the cough is productive, the volume, consistency, and color of the sputum should be assessed. Sputum should be cultured to rule out infection and to establish whether there is a need for preoperative antibiotic therapy. Blood-stained sputum or episodes of gross hemoptysis should alert the anesthesiologist to the possibility of a tumor invading the respiratory tract (e.g., the main stem bronchus), which might interfere with endobronchial intubation.

Cigarette Smoking

Cigarette smoking increases the risk of chronic lung disease and malignancy, as well as the incidence of postoperative pulmonary complications. The number of pack-years (packs smoked per day multiplied by the number of years) is directly related to measurable changes in respiratory gas flow and closing capacity, making these patients prone to postoperative atelectasis and arterial hypoxemia.

Exercise Tolerance

Patients who can walk up three or more flights of stairs are at reduced risk, and those unable to climb two flights are generally at increased risk.[5] The best evaluation is actually the history of the patient's quality of life.[6] An otherwise healthy patient, with good exercise tolerance, generally does not require additional screening tests.

Risk Factors for Acute Lung Injury

In some cases, thoracic surgery may lead to acute lung injury postoperatively. Perioperative risk factors that have been identified include preoperative alcohol abuse and patients undergoing pneumonectomy. Intraoperative risk factors include high ventilatory pressures and excessive amounts of fluid administration.[7]

Physical Examination

The physical examination of the patient should address the following aspects.

Respiratory Pattern

The presence of cyanosis and clubbing, the breathing pattern, and the type of breath sounds should be noted.

Cyanosis.   The presence of peripheral cyanosis (in the fingers, toes, or ears) should be distinguished from causes of poor circulation (acrocyanosis). The presence of central cyanosis (in the buccal mucosa) is usually secondary to arterial hypoxemia. If cyanosis is present, the arterial hemoglobin saturation with oxygen is 80% or less (PaO$_2$ <50 to 52 mm Hg), which indicates a limited margin of respiratory reserve.

Clubbing.   Clubbing of fingers and toes is often seen in patients with chronic lung disease, malignancies, or congenital heart disease associated with right-to-left shunt.

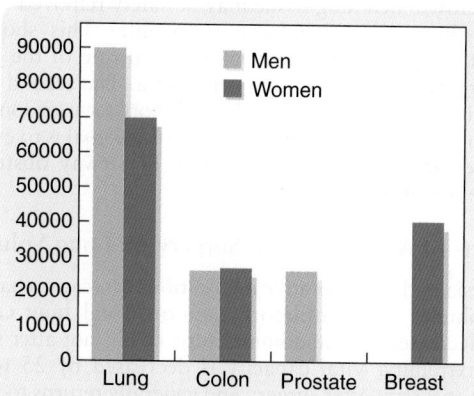

FIGURE 40-1. Lung cancer is the leading cause of cancer-related mortality. (Based on data from The American Cancer Society, Cancer statistics, 2007.)

Respiratory Rate and Pattern.   A patient's inability to complete a normal sentence without pausing for breath is an indication of severe dyspnea. Inspiratory paradox, the abdomen moving in while the chest moves out, suggests diaphragmatic fatigue and respiratory dysfunction. The patient should be assessed for paroxysmal retraction (Hoover sign), limited diaphragmatic movement because of hyperinflation, and asymmetry of chest movement secondary to phrenic nerve involvement, hemothorax, pleural effusion, and pneumothorax. The pattern and rate of breathing have important roles in distinguishing between obstructive and restrictive lung disease. For constant minute ventilation, the work done against airflow resistance decreases when breathing is slow and deep. Work done against elastic resistance decreases when breathing is rapid and shallow (e.g., as in pulmonary infarct or pulmonary fibrosis).

Breath Sounds.   Wet sounds (crackles) are usually caused by excessive fluid in the airways and indicate sputum retention or edema. Dry sounds (wheezes) are produced by high-velocity gas flow through bronchi and are a sign of airway obstruction. Distant sounds are an indication of emphysema and possibly bullae. The trachea should be in the midline. Displacement of the trachea may be secondary to a number of causes, including mediastinal mass, and should alert the anesthesiologist to a potentially difficult intubation of the trachea or airway obstruction on induction of anesthesia.

Evaluation of the Cardiovascular System

One of the most important factors in the evaluation of a patient scheduled for thoracic surgery is the presence of an increase in pulmonary vascular resistance secondary to a fixed reduction in the cross-sectional area of the pulmonary vascular bed. The pulmonary circulation is normally a low-pressure, high-compliance system capable of handling an increase in blood flow by recruitment of normally underperfused vessels. This acts as a compensatory mechanism that normally prevents an increase in pulmonary arterial pressure. In COPD, there is distention of the pulmonary capillary bed with decreased ability to tolerate an increase in blood flow (decreased compliance). Such patients demonstrate an increase in pulmonary vascular resistance when cardiac output increases because of a decreased ability to compensate for an increase in pulmonary blood flow. This results in pulmonary hypertension, signs of which include a narrowly split second heart sound, increased intensity of the pulmonary component of the second heart sound, and right ventricular and atrial hypertrophy. An increase in pulmonary vascular resistance is of significance in the management of the patient during anesthesia because several factors, such as acidosis, sepsis, hypoxia, and application of positive end-expiratory pressure (PEEP), all further increase the pulmonary vascular resistance and increase the likelihood of right ventricular failure.

In patients with ischemic or valvular heart disease, the function of the left side of the heart should also be carefully evaluated.

Electrocardiogram

A patient with COPD may present with electrocardiographic features of right atrial and ventricular hypertrophy and strain. These include a low-voltage QRS complex due to lung hyperinflation and poor R-wave progression across the precordial leads. An enlarged P wave ("P pulmonale") in standard lead II is diagnostic of right atrial hypertrophy. The electrocardiographic changes of right ventricular hypertrophy are an R/S ratio of greater than 1.0 in lead V_1 (i.e., R-wave voltage exceeds S-wave voltage).

Chest Radiography

Hyperinflation and increased vascular markings are usually present with COPD. Prominent lung markings often occur in bronchitis, whereas they are decreased in emphysema, particularly at the bases, where actual bullae may be present in severe cases. Hyperinflation, with an increased anteroposterior chest diameter, may be present, together with an enlarged retrosternal air space of >2 cm in diameter seen in a lateral chest radiograph.

The location of the lung lesion should be assessed by posteroanterior and lateral projections on chest radiography. In addition to tracheal or carinal shift, a mediastinal mass may indicate difficulty with ventilation, a difficult and bloody dissection, difficulty in placing a double-lumen tube (DLT; because of deviation of the main stem bronchus), or a collapsed lobe owing to bronchial obstruction with possible sepsis. Review of a computed tomography (CT) study is also useful, and often provides more information about tumor size and location than the chest radiograph.

Arterial Blood Gas Analysis

A common finding in arterial blood gas analysis of patients with COPD is hypoventilation and CO_2 retention. The "blue bloaters" (chronic bronchitics) are cyanotic, hypercarbic, hypoxemic, and usually overweight. They are in a state of chronic respiratory failure and have a decreased ventilatory response to CO_2. In these patients, the high $PaCO_2$ increases cerebrospinal fluid bicarbonate concentration, the medullary chemoreceptors become reset to a higher level of CO_2, and sensitivity to CO_2 is decreased. Such patients hypoventilate when given high oxygen concentrations to breathe because of a decreased hypoxic drive.

The "pink puffers" (patients with emphysema) are typically thin, dyspneic, and pink, with essentially normal arterial blood gas values. They present with an increase in minute ventilation to maintain their normal $PaCO_2$, which explains the increase in work of breathing and dyspnea. The preoperative PaO_2 correlates with the intraoperative PaO_2 during one-lung ventilation (OLV), but the intraoperative PaO_2 during two-lung ventilation correlates more closely.[8]

Pulmonary Function Testing and Evaluation for Lung Resectability

There are three goals in performing pulmonary function tests in a patient scheduled for lung resection. The first is to identify the patient at risk of increased postoperative morbidity and mortality. In thoracic surgery for lung cancer, the specific question is: How much lung tissue may be safely removed without making the patient a pulmonary cripple? This should be weighed against the 1-year mean survival rate of the patient with surgically untreated lung carcinoma. The second goal is to identify the patient who will need short-term or long-term postoperative ventilatory support. The third goal is to evaluate the beneficial effect and reversibility of airway obstruction with the use of bronchodilators.

Effects of Anesthesia and Surgery on Lung Volumes

Anesthesia and postoperative medications can cause changes in lung volumes and ventilatory pattern. Total lung capacity (TLC) decreases after abdominal surgery but not after surgery on an extremity. Vital capacity is decreased by 25 to 50% within 1 to 2 days after surgery and generally returns to normal after 1 to 2 weeks. Residual volume (RV) increases by 13%, whereas expiratory reserve volume decreases by 25% after lower abdominal surgery and 60% after upper abdominal and thoracic surgery. Tidal volume (V_T) decreases by 20% within

24 hours after surgery and gradually returns to normal after 2 weeks. Pulmonary compliance decreases by 33% with similar reductions in functional residual capacity (FRC) secondary to small airway closure. Most of the patients who undergo lung resection are smokers with a certain degree of COPD and are prone to postoperative complications in direct relation to the amount of lung to be resected (lobectomy or pneumonectomy) and to the severity of the preoperative lung disease.

Spirometry

2 Forced vital capacity (FVC), forced expired volume in 1 second (FEV$_1$), maximum voluntary ventilation (MVV), and RV/TLC correlate with outcome following thoracic surgery[9] (see Chapter 11). An abnormal preoperative vital capacity can be identified in 30 to 40% of postoperative deaths. A patient with an abnormal vital capacity has a 33% likelihood of complications and a 10% risk of postoperative mortality.

FEV$_1$ is a more direct indication of airway obstruction. In the past, an FEV$_1$ of <800 mL in a 70-kg man had been considered an absolute contraindication to lung resection. However, with the advent of thoracoscopic surgery and improved postoperative pain management, patients with smaller lung volumes are now successfully undergoing surgery. It is preferable to indicate the percentage of predicted value, rather than just using the actual results in liters. The percentage of predicted takes into account the age and size of the patient, and the same number may have a different implication in another patient. The ratio FEV$_1$/FVC is useful in differentiating between restrictive and obstructive pulmonary disease. It is normal in restrictive disease because both FEV$_1$ and FVC decrease, whereas in obstructive disease the ratio is usually low because the FEV$_1$ is markedly decreased. MVV is a nonspecific test and is an indicator of both restriction and obstruction. Although MVV has not been systematically evaluated as a predictor of morbidity, it is generally accepted that an MVV <50% of predicted value is an indication of high risk. A ratio of RV to TLC (RV/TLC) of >50% is generally indicative of a high-risk patient for pulmonary resection By multiplying the preoperative FEV$_1$ by the percentage of lung tissue expected to remain following resection, a predicted postoperative FEV$_1$ can be calculated. Patients with a predicted postoperative FEV$_1$ value >40% are at reduced risk, and those with predicted postoperative FEV$_1$ <30% are at increased risk.[10] Those patients who fall into the latter category are more likely to need postoperative ventilation.

Flow–Volume Loops

The flow–volume loop displays essentially the same information as a spirometer but is more convenient for measurement of specific flow rates (Fig. 40-2). The shape and peak airflow rates during expiration at high lung volumes are effort-dependent, but indicate the patency of the larger airways. Effort-independent expiration occurs at low lung volumes and usually reflects small airways resistance, best measured by forced expiratory flow (FEF) during the middle half of the FVC (FEF$_{25-75\%}$).

In general, patients with obstructive airways disease (Fig. 40-3), such as asthma, bronchitis, and emphysema, have grossly decreased FEV$_1$/FVC ratios because of increased airways resistance and a decrease in FEV$_1$. Peak expiratory flow rate and MVV are usually decreased, whereas total lung capacity increases secondary to increases in RV. In these patients, the effort-independent portion of the flow–volume curve is markedly depressed inward, with reduction of the flow rate at 25 to 75% of FVC.

In patients with restrictive disease (Fig. 40-3), such as pulmonary fibrosis and scoliosis, there is a decrease in FVC with a relatively normal FEV$_1$. Because the airways resistance is

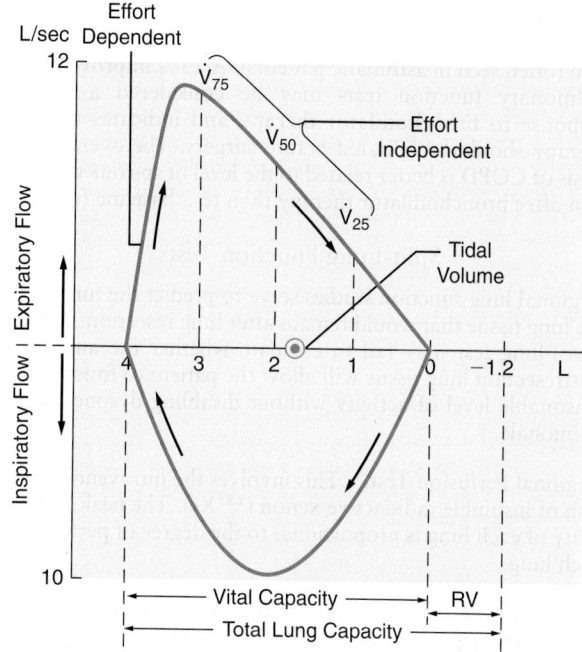

FIGURE 40-2. Flow–volume loop in a normal subject. $\dot{V}_{75}$, $\dot{V}_{50}$, and $\dot{V}_{25}$ represent flow at 75%, 50%, and 25% of vital capacity, respectively. RV, residual volume. (Reproduced from Goudsouzian N, Karamanian A: Physiology for the Anesthesiologist, 2nd edition. Norwalk, CT, Appleton-Century-Crofts, 1984, with permission.)

normal, FEV$_1$/FVC is also normal. TLC is markedly decreased, whereas MVV and FEF$_{25-75\%}$ are usually normal. The flow–volume curves of these patients are normal in shape, but the lung volumes and peak flow rates are decreased.

Significance of Bronchodilator Therapy. Pulmonary function tests are usually performed before and after bronchodilator therapy to assess the reversibility of the airways obstruction. This is useful in the assessment of the degree of airways obstruction and the patient's effort ability. After treatment

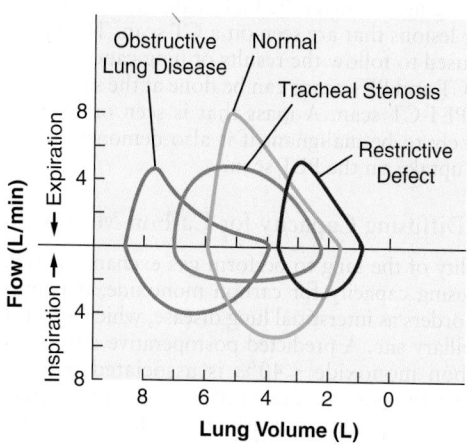

FIGURE 40-3. Flow–volume loops relative to lung volumes in a normal subject, in a patient with chronic obstructive pulmonary disease (COPD), in a patient with fixed obstruction (tracheal stenosis), and in a patient with pulmonary fibrosis (restrictive defect). Note the concave expiratory form in the patient with COPD and the flat inspiratory curve in the patient with a fixed obstruction. (Reprinted from Goudsouzian N, Karamanian A: Physiology for the Anesthesiologist, 2nd edition. Norwalk, CT, Appleton-Century-Crofts, 1984, with permission.)

with bronchodilators, increases in peak expiratory flow compared with a baseline indicate reversibility of airway obstruction (often seen in asthmatic patients). A 15% improvement in pulmonary function tests may be considered a positive response to bronchodilator therapy and indicates that this therapy should be initiated before surgery. The overall prognosis of COPD is better related to the level of spirometric function after bronchodilator therapy than to a baseline function.

Split-Lung Function Tests

Regional lung function studies serve to predict the function of the lung tissue that would remain after lung resection. A whole (two)-lung test may fail to estimate whether the amount of postresection lung tissue will allow the patient to function at a reasonable level of activity without disabling dyspnea or cor pulmonale.

Regional Perfusion Test. This involves the intravenous injection of insoluble radioactive xenon (^{133}Xe). The peak radioactivity of each lung is proportional to the degree of perfusion of each lung.

Regional Ventilation Test. Using an inhaled, insoluble radioactive gas, the peak radioactivity over each lung is proportional to the degree of ventilation. Combining radiospirometry with whole-lung testing (FEV$_1$, FVC, maximal breathing capacity) has resulted in a fair degree of correlation between predicted volumes and pulmonary function tests measured after pneumonectomy.

Computed Tomography and Positron Emission Tomography Scans. Patients normally undergo CT scanning. The CT scan provides anatomic sections through the chest and can delineate the size of the tumor. It can also reveal if there is airway or cardiovascular compression.

Positron emission tomography (PET) scans use a glucose analog that is labeled with a radionuclide positron emitter. This scan can detect tumor based on the metabolic activity. Because malignant tumors are growing at such a fast rate compared with healthy tissue, the tumor cells will use up more of the sugar that has the radionuclide attached to it. There is greater uptake by malignant mediastinal lymph nodes than benign nodes. PET may be more accurate than CT for mediastinal staging.[11] Currently, PET scans can be used to further evaluate lesions that are seen on a CT scan. The PET scan can also be used to follow the results of lung cancer treatments.[12]

The CT and PET scans can be done at the same time to produce a PET-CT scan. A mass that is seen on the CT scan is more likely to be malignant if it also demonstrates enhanced glucose uptake on the PET scan.

Diffusing Capacity for Carbon Monoxide

The ability of the lung to perform gas exchange is reflected by the diffusing capacity for carbon monoxide. It is impaired in such disorders as interstitial lung disease, which affects the alveolar-capillary site. A predicted postoperative diffusing capacity for carbon monoxide <40% is associated with increased risk. Predicted postoperative diffusing capacity percent is the strongest single predictor of risk of complications and mortality after lung resection. There is little interrelationship of predicted postoperative diffusing capacity percent and predicted postoperative FEV$_1$, indicating that these values should be assessed independently when estimating operative risk.[13]

Maximal Oxygen Consumption. The maximal oxygen consumption (VO$_2$ max) is a predictor of postoperative complications. Patients with a VO$_2$ max >15 to 20 mL/kg/min are at reduced risk.[14] A VO$_2$ max <10 mL/kg/min indicates very

high risk for lung resection.[15] A simpler test that can be performed is exercise oximetry—a decrease of 4% during exercise is associated with increased risk.[16] A 6-minute walk test <2,000 feet has been correlated both with a VO$_2$ max <15 mL/kg/min, and with a decrease in oximetry reading during exercise. It has been suggested that the percentage of predicted VO$_2$ max may be a better indicator for risk, and a threshold of 50 to 60% could be established without an increase in surgical mortality.[17] Brunelli and Fianchini[18] had patients climb the maximum number of stairs possible. Based on the results of this study, these authors recommended that patients who were able to climb >14 meters can safely undergo surgery, and those who were able to climb <12 meters, with predicted postoperative function FEV$_1$ <35% not be considered for major lung resection. The inability to do a maximal stair climbing has been correlated with an increased mortality following major lung resection.[19] The preoperative evaluation of the patient for lung resection is summarized in Figure 40-4.

PREOPERATIVE PREPARATION

The wide spectrum of physiologic changes that occur during thoracic surgery puts patients at great risk of developing postoperative complications. Morbidity and mortality increase when these changes are superimposed on an acutely or chronically compromised patient. Several conditions, including infection, dehydration, electrolyte imbalance, wheezing, obesity, cigarette smoking, cor pulmonale, and malnutrition, show particular correlations with postoperative complications. Proper, vigorous preoperative preparation can improve the patient's ability to face the surgery with a decreased risk of morbidity and mortality. It is important that conditions predisposing to postoperative complications be rigorously treated before surgery.

Smoking

There is a high prevalence of smoking among patients presenting for surgery, and there is extensive evidence that these patients are at increased risk for development of postoperative respiratory complications.[3] Approximately 33% of adult patients presenting for surgery are smokers, and there is extensive evidence that they are at increased risk for development of postoperative respiratory complications.[20] Smoking increases airway irritability, decreases mucociliary transport, decreases FVC and FEF$_{25-75\%}$, and increases secretions, thereby increasing the incidence of postoperative pulmonary complications. In contrast, cessation of smoking for a period of longer than 4 to 6 weeks before surgery is associated with a decreased incidence of postoperative complications.[20] Furthermore, cessation of smoking 48 hours before surgery has been shown to decrease the percentage of carboxyhemoglobin, to shift the oxyhemoglobin dissociation curve to the right, and to increase oxygen availability. It should be emphasized, however, that most of the beneficial effects of cessation of smoking, such as improvement in ciliary function, improvement in closing volume, increase in FEF$_{25-75\%}$, and reduction in sputum production, usually occur 2 to 3 months after smoking has ceased. In one study, there was no evidence of a paradoxical increase in postoperative complications in patients who stopped smoking within 2 months prior to undergoing thoracic resection for lung tumor.[21]

Infection

Acute or chronic infection should be vigorously treated before surgery. Broad-spectrum antibiotics are commonly used.

Whole-lung Function

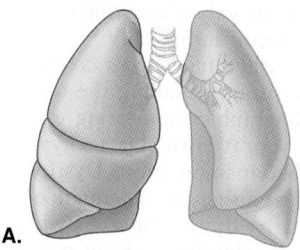

ABG (Fio$_2$ = 0.21)	Paco$_2$ >46 mm Hg
	Pao$_2$ <60 mm Hg
FVC	<50% or 1.5 mL/kg
FEV$_1$	<50%
VC	<2 L
MVV	<50% or <50 L/min
Lung Volume	RV/TLC >50%
DLco	<50%

A.

Split-lung Function

1. Split-lung Spirometry With DLT
2. Regional Lung Radiospirometry
   Regional Perfusion (^{133}Xe, ^{131}I-MAA)
   Regional Ventilation ^{133}Xe

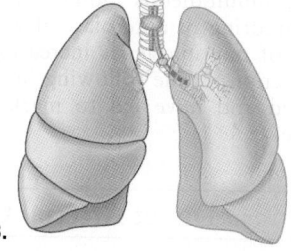

Predicted Postresection FEV$_1$ <800 mL

Blood Flow to the Resected Lung >70%

B.

FIGURE 40-4. The order of tests to determine the cardiopulmonary status of the patient and the extent of lung resection that would be tolerated. **A.** The whole-lung function test is a basic screening test. **B.** The split-lung function tests are regional tests to determine the involvement of the diseased lung to be removed. ABG, arterial blood gas; FVC, forced vital capacity; FEV$_1$, forced expiratory volume in 1 second; VC, vital capacity; MVV, maximum voluntary ventilation; RV/TLC, residual volume/total lung capacity; DLT, double-lumen tube. DL$_{CO}$, carbon monoxide diffusing capacity; (Adapted from Neustein SM, Cohen E: Preoperative evaluation of thoracic surgical patients, The Practice of Thoracic Anesthesia. Edited by Cohen E. Philadelphia, JB Lippincott, 1995, p 187, with permission.)

Treatment of the acutely ill patient depends on the results of the Gram stain of the sputum and blood cultures. Unless there are other modifying circumstances such as allergy history, or patients are already receiving antibiotics, cefazolin is routinely administered perioperatively. To be most effective, it needs to be given prior to skin incision.[22] In one prospective study, the incidence of mortality was lower in the group treated with prophylactic antibiotics compared with the untreated group (9% vs. 17%), and a lower incidence of postoperative pulmonary infection was also found.[23] Although not all surgeons routinely administer antibiotics prophylactically to their patients, any infection present before surgery should be vigorously treated.

Hydration and Removal of Bronchial Secretions

Correction of hypovolemia and electrolyte imbalance should be accomplished before surgery because adequate hydration decreases the viscosity of bronchial secretions and facilitates their removal from the bronchial tree. Humidification of inspired gas is extremely useful. The use of mucolytic drugs, such as acetylcysteine (Mucomyst), or oral expectorants (potassium iodide) can be beneficial to patients with viscous secretions. Commonly used methods for removing secretions from the bronchial tree include postural drainage, vigorous coughing, chest percussion, deep breathing, and the use of an incentive

spirometer. These modalities often require patient cooperation and frequent verbal encouragement to maximize the benefit.

Wheezing and Bronchodilation

The presence of acute wheezing represents a medical emergency, and elective surgery should be postponed until effective treatment has been instituted. Chronic wheezing is often seen in patients with COPD and is attributable to the presence of gas flow obstruction secondary to smooth muscle contraction, accumulation of secretions, and mucosal edema. Smooth muscle contraction may occur in small airways only (detectable by changes in FEF$_{25-75\%}$) or may be widespread, with a large reduction of FEV$_1$ and FVC. The efficacy of bronchodilators in reversing the bronchospastic component is extremely important. A trial of bronchodilators and measurement of their effects on pulmonary function should be performed in any patient who shows evidence of air flow obstruction. Several classes of bronchodilators are available.

Sympathomimetic Drugs

Sympathomimetic drugs increase the formation of 3'5'-cyclic adenosine monophosphate (cAMP). The balance between cAMP, which produces bronchodilation, and cyclic guanosine monophosphate, which produces bronchoconstriction, determines the state of contraction of the bronchial smooth muscle. Increasing cAMP production therefore causes relaxation of the bronchial tree. Sympathomimetic drugs, such as epinephrine, isoproterenol, isoetharine, and ephedrine, all have mixed β_1 and β_2 sympathetic agonist effects. The β_1 (cardiac effects) of these drugs are often undesirable in patients with COPD. Selective β_2 sympathomimetic drugs, such as albuterol, terbutaline, and metaproterenol, given as inhaled aerosols, are the preferred drugs for the treatment of bronchospasm, particularly in patients with cardiac disease.

Phosphodiesterase Inhibitors

Phosphodiesterase inhibitors inhibit the breakdown of cAMP by cytoplasmic phosphodiesterase. The methylxanthines, such as aminophylline, increase the level of cAMP, resulting in bronchodilation. In addition, aminophylline improves diaphragmatic contractility and increases the patient's resistance to fatigue. Therapeutic blood levels of aminophylline are 5 to 20 μg/mL and can be achieved by infusing a loading dose of 5 to 7 mg/kg over 20 minutes, followed by a continuous intravenous infusion of 0.5 to 0.7 mg/kg/hr. Aminophylline may cause ventricular dysrhythmias, and this side effect should be borne in mind when treating patients who have myocardial ischemia. Because newer medications have fewer side effects, aminophylline is now rarely used.

Steroids

Although not true bronchodilators, steroids are traditionally considered to decrease mucosal edema and may prevent the release of bronchoconstricting substances. They are of questionable benefit in acute bronchospasm. Steroids may be administered orally, parenterally, or in aerosol form, such as beclomethasone by inhaler.

Cromolyn Sodium

Cromolyn sodium stabilizes mast cells and inhibits degranulation and histamine release. It is useful in the prevention of bronchospastic attacks but is of little value in the treatment of the acute situation (see Chapter 12).

Parasympatholytic Drugs

Parasympatholytics include atropine and ipratropium (see Chapter 15). In the past, atropine has been avoided in patients with COPD and bronchitis because of concern regarding increases in the viscosity of mucus produced by this agent. However, atropine blocks the formation of cyclic guanosine monophosphate and therefore has a bronchodilator effect.

Pulmonary Rehabilitation

Sekine et al.[23] reported that pulmonary rehabilitation led to reduced hospital stay and improved postoperative FEV_1, compared with a historical control group. The pulmonary rehabilitation included education in a variety of areas such as breathing, exercise, and nutrition.

INTRAOPERATIVE MONITORING

All patients undergoing anesthesia for thoracic surgical procedures require use of standard American Society of Anesthesiologists or ASA monitors (see monitoring). These include an electrocardiogram (lead II and, if possible, V_5), chest or esophageal stethoscopes for heart and breath sound auscultation, and a temperature probe. A chest stethoscope may be placed over the dependent hemithorax to assess dependent lung ventilation. Pulse oximetry, which is a standard of care, is especially valuable during thoracic surgery because hypoxemia may occur during OLV.

Dysrhythmias occur commonly both during and after thoracic surgery, making the usual need for continuous electrocardiographic monitoring even more important. Intraoperative supraventricular tachyarrhythmias may be caused by cardiac manipulation. Dysrhythmias that occur during OLV may be a sign of inadequate oxygenation or ventilation. Postoperative dysrhythmias may be related to sympathetic nervous system stimulation from pain or to a decreased pulmonary vascular bed following lung resection. Patients who present for lung resection often have COPD due to cigarette smoking, have right-sided heart strain and are prone to multifocal atrial tachyarrhythmias.

The axis' of electrocardiogram lead II parallels that of the P wave, making this lead useful for dysrhythmia detection. The simultaneous monitoring of lead V_5 also allows for monitoring of anterolateral wall myocardial ischemia. The use of multiple leads increases the sensitivity for ischemia detection.[24] The following invasive monitors are also indicated and have led to marked improvements in patient care.

Direct Arterial Catheterization

Peripheral arterial catheterization has become an essential tool for the anesthesiologist in the management of patients undergoing major thoracic surgical procedures (see Chapter 27). It allows for continuous beat-to-beat measurement of blood pressure and frequent sampling for the determination of arterial blood gases. Continuous blood pressure readings are critical during thoracic surgery because surgical manipulations may result in cardiac compression and there may be sudden bleeding. Immediate recognition of these changes allows time for proper identification of the etiology and the institution of appropriate treatment.

Serial arterial blood gas determinations are performed as needed in the management of patients undergoing one-lung anesthesia or during cases in which a part of the lung may be "packed away" for a period. Arterial hypoxemia may occur because of shunting through the collapsed lung and inadequate hypoxic pulmonary vasoconstriction (HPV). Significant changes in acid-base status and hyperventilation or hypoventilation can also be identified.

A radial artery catheter (see monitoring Chapter 11) can be placed in either extremity during thoracic surgery. For a mediastinoscopic examination, one approach is to place the catheter in the right arm and to use it to monitor for possible compression of the innominate artery by the mediastinoscope. This can help avoid central nervous system complications that might result from inadequate cerebral blood flow via the right carotid artery (see "Mediastinoscopy"). The other approach would be to place the arterial catheter in the left radial artery, allowing for continuous blood pressure measurements, uninterrupted by innominate artery compression. If this is done, a pulse oximeter probe should be placed on the right upper extremity to monitor for innominate artery compression. During thoracotomy, placement of the arterial catheter in the dependent arm can be used to monitor for possible axillary artery compression, which may occur if the patient is not properly positioned.

Central Venous Pressure Monitoring

The central venous pressure (CVP) may reflect the patient's blood volume, venous tone, and right ventricular performance;

however, it is also affected by central venous obstructions and alterations of intrathoracic pressure such as PEEP (see Chapter 27). The CVP reflects right-sided heart function, not left ventricular performance. Catheters for measuring CVP may be placed for thoracotomies, and in particular, patients undergoing pneumonectomy. Uses of CVP catheters or large-bore introducers include (1) insertion of a transvenous pacemaker where necessary, (2) infusion of vasoactive drugs, and (3) insertion of a pulmonary artery (PA) catheter, which may subsequently be required during surgery or in the postoperative period. A recent study in healthy subjects indicated that, contrary to common belief, the CVP did not reflect intravascular volume status.[25]

The CVP catheter can be placed centrally from either the external or the internal jugular vein, from the subclavian veins, or from one of the arm veins. The success rate is highest using the right internal jugular vein, and a pacemaker or PA catheter can be inserted most easily from this vein. The major disadvantage of using the external jugular vein during thoracotomy is that the catheter often kinks when the patient is turned to the lateral decubitus position. The subclavian technique leads to a higher incidence of pneumothorax, which can be disastrous if it occurs in the dependent lung during OLV. If necessary, a subclavian catheter should be placed ipsilateral to the surgery, if possible.

Pulmonary Artery Catheterization

The PA catheter is most reliably inserted through the right internal jugular vein using a modified Seldinger technique (see Chapter 27). Insertion of the PA catheter through either the external jugular vein or the subclavian vein often leads to obstruction of the catheter when the patient is placed in the lateral decubitus position. Misinterpretation of data from a PA catheter is a real risk in a patient with cardiac and pulmonary disease undergoing thoracic surgery with OLV. These errors can be produced by altered ventilatory modes, the location of the PA catheter tip, ventricular compliance changes, or ventricular interdependence.[26] A major limitation of the PA catheter is the assumption that the pulmonary capillary wedge pressure (PCWP) provides a good approximation of left ventricular end-diastolic volume. The use of PCWP directly to assess preload assumes a linear relationship between ventricular end-diastolic volume and ventricular end-diastolic pressure. However, alterations in ventricular compliance affect this pressure–volume relationship during surgery. Decreases in ventricular compliance can occur with myocardial ischemia, shock, right ventricular overload, or pericardial effusion. Numerous investigators have demonstrated a poor correlation between PCWP and left ventricular end-diastolic volume in acutely ill patients.[27] This correlation is further worsened by the application of PEEP. Additionally, ventricular interdependence can cause misdiagnosis when the interventricular septum encroaches on the left ventricular cavity, leading to increased values of PCWP. A PCWP associated with a decreased cardiac output can be interpreted as left ventricular failure, when in fact, left ventricular end-diastolic volume may not be increased but decreased because of compression of the left ventricle by a distended right ventricle. This situation can occur with acute respiratory failure and high levels of PEEP. Techniques such as echocardiography, which directly measure ventricular dimensions, may facilitate resolution of this complex situation.

Because most of the pulmonary blood flow is to the right lower lobe, the tip of a flow-directed PA catheter is usually located in the right lower lobe. During a left thoracotomy with OLV, the catheter tip would then be in the dependent lung and should provide accurate hemodynamic measurements. However, during a right thoracotomy with OLV, the catheter tip would most likely be in the nondependent lung, and may not be accurate. The use of intraoperative mean pulmonary artery pressure has been reported to be an indicator of safety for lung resection under thoracotomy.[28] The authors concluded that following occlusion of the main PA, upper safety limits of 33 mm Hg for right, and 35 mm Hg for left thoracotomy could be used. The authors noted that the difference between sides was minimal, and less than expected. The monitoring of $S\bar{v}O_2$ has been evaluated in patients undergoing one-lung anesthesia.[29] Changes in $S\bar{v}O_2$ were mainly dependent on changes in SaO_2.

Transesophageal Echocardiography

Transesophageal echocardiography (TEE) is a useful intraoperative monitor for ventricular function, valvular function, and wall motion changes that might reflect ischemia (see Chapter 28). Its use in thoracic surgical patients has been limited, but it is widely used in patients undergoing lung transplant. In one study, central lung tumors were seen with TEE in nine of nine patients, peripheral lung tumors in one of three patients, and an anterior mediastinal mass in one of one patients.[30] In this study, TEE revealed PA compression in five patients and PA infiltration in two patients. In another study investigating echocardiographic recognition of mediastinal tumors, TEE revealed that the tumors were often adjacent to the heart and identified those patients in whom there was compression of the innominate vein or PA, or infiltration of the heart.[31]

Intraoperative TEE has also revealed tumor invasion of the heart, indicating that a resection by thoracotomy without cardiopulmonary bypass was not feasible.[32] In one case report, TEE monitoring during an attempted resection of a tumor invading the left atrium showed embolization of the tumor.[33] Fragments of the tumor were seen to pass through the aortic valve. This patient subsequently died of disseminated metastases. In an exploratory thoracotomy for hemothorax, intraoperative TEE revealed the presence of a subacute aortic dissection, which was believed to be the cause of the hemothorax.[34] TEE was used intraoperatively to evaluate a large anterior mediastinal mass, providing data on right ventricular outflow compression, and ventricular contractility and filling status.[35] In another recent report, a mediastinal mass was diagnosed intraoperatively using TEE; in that case, the mass had been misdiagnosed preoperatively with transthoracic echocardiography as a pericardial effusion.[36]

Monitoring of Oxygenation and Ventilation

Oxygenation

During the administration of all thoracic surgical anesthetics, the concentration of inspired oxygen in the breathing system must be measured using an oxygen analyzer with a low oxygen concentration limit alarm (see Chapter 26). Such analyzers vary in sophistication from fuel cells, polarographic and paramagnetic analyzers, to the Raman spectrometer that can monitor all the gases used during anesthesia. Adequacy of blood oxygenation must also be ensured, and adequate illumination and exposure of the patient are helpful to assess the color of shed blood or the presence of cyanosis of the lips, nail beds, or mucous membranes. Most patients undergoing thoracic surgical or diagnostic procedures have an arterial catheter in place for continuous monitoring of blood pressure and sampling of arterial blood for blood gas determinations.

Pulse oximetry is currently the standard of care for noninvasive assessment of blood oxygenation. The use of pulse oximetry is especially important during OLV, when rapid assessment of oxygenation is critical., A low SpO_2 reading provides the clinician with an indication for blood gas sampling and laboratory analysis of arterial blood. The traditional two-wavelength pulse oximeter may display spurious readings of SpO_2 in the presence of the dyshemoglobins methemoglobin and carboxyhemoglobin. Recently a multiwavelength (eight wavelength) pulse oximeter has become available that is capable of measuring carboxyhemoglobin, methemoglobin, and deoxygenated hemoglobin in addition to hemoglobin saturation with oxygen (HbO_2%).[37]

Ventilation

All patients must be continually monitored to ensure adequacy of ventilation. Monitoring includes qualitative signs such as chest excursion (visual observation of the lungs when the chest is open) and auscultation of breath sounds. In addition, during OLV, a stethoscope can be placed on the chest wall under the ventilated dependent lung. During controlled ventilation, circuit low-pressure and high-pressure alarms with an audible signal must be used. The respiratory rate, V_T, minute volume, and inflation pressures should be observed.

Adequacy of ventilation should be confirmed by monitoring arterial blood gases and $PaCO_2$, in particular. This may be estimated continuously and noninvasively by using a capnograph (see Chapter 27). The end-tidal CO_2 concentration represents alveolar CO_2 ($PACO_2$), which approximates $PaCO_2$. There is normally a small arterial-to-alveolar CO_2 difference (4 to 6 mm Hg), depending on alveolar dead space. The capnogram waveform is also helpful in diagnosing airway obstruction, incomplete relaxation, and even malposition of the DLT. In the latter application, a capnograph is coupled with each port of the DLT (one or two capnographs may be used), and the correct position of the DLT is identified by simultaneous and synchronous CO_2 readings on each of the two analyzers. The waveforms from each lung are examined for shape, height, and rhythm, depending on the correct position of the tube and on the ventilation/perfusion ($\dot{V}/\dot{Q}$) ratio for each lung.[38] During two-lung ventilation, a decrease in end-tidal CO_2 in the gas from one lumen of the DLT suggests that the tube may be malpositioned. During OLV, systemic hypoxemia is usually a greater problem than hypercarbia.[39] This is because CO_2 is approximately 20 times more diffusible than oxygen and $PaCO_2$ is more dependent on ventilation, compared with PaO_2, which is more dependent on perfusion.

Physiology of One-Lung Ventilation

Physiology of the Lateral Decubitus Position. Ventilation and blood flow in the upright position are discussed in Chapter 11. These variables will now be considered as they pertain to the lateral decubitus position under six circumstances that are encountered during thoracic surgery.

Lateral position, awake, breathing spontaneously, chest closed. In the lateral decubitus position, the distribution of blood flow and ventilation is similar to that in the upright position, but turned by 90 degrees (Fig. 40-5). Blood flow and ventilation to the dependent lung are significantly greater than to the nondependent lung. Good V/Q matching at the level of the dependent lung results in adequate oxygenation in the awake patient who is breathing spontaneously. There are two important concepts in this situation. First, because perfusion is gravity-dependent, the vertical hydrostatic pressure gradient is smaller in the lateral than in the upright position; therefore, zone 1 is usually less extended. Second, in regard to ventilation, the dependent hemidiaphragm is pushed higher into the chest by the abdominal contents compared with the nondependent lung hemidiaphragm. During spontaneous ventilation, the conserved ability of the dependent diaphragm to contract results in an adequate distribution of V_T to the dependent

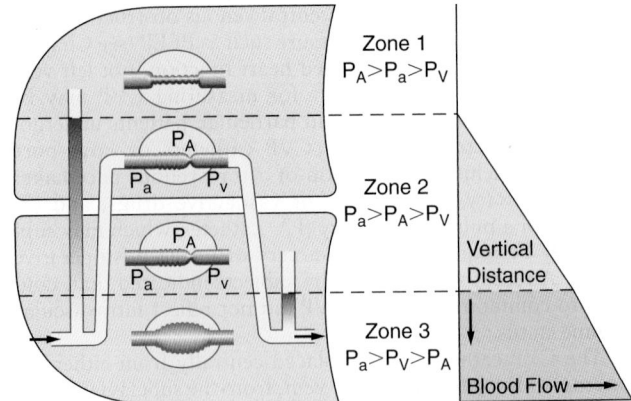

FIGURE 40-5. Schematic representation of the effects of gravity on the distribution of pulmonary blood flow in the lateral decubitus position. Vertical gradients in the lateral decubitus position are similar to those in the upright position and cause the creation of West zones 1, 2, and 3. Consequently, pulmonary blood flow increases with lung dependency, and is largest in the dependent lung and least in the nondependent lung. P_a, pulmonary artery pressure; P_A, alveolar pressure; P_v, pulmonary venous pressure. (From Benumof JL: Physiology of the open-chest and one lung ventilation, Thoracic Anesthesia, New York, Churchill Livingstone, 1983, p 288, with permission.)

lung. Because most of the perfusion is to the dependent lung, the V/Q matching in this position is maintained similar to that in the upright position.

Lateral position, awake, breathing spontaneously, chest open. Controlled positive-pressure ventilation is the most common way to provide adequate ventilation and ensure gas exchange in an open chest situation. Frequently, thoracoscopy is performed using intercostal blocks with the patient breathing spontaneously to allow proper lung examination. The thoracoscope provides an adequate seal of the open chest to prevent a "free" open-chest situation. Two complications can arise from the patient breathing spontaneously with an open chest. The first is mediastinal shift, usually occurring during inspiration (Fig. 40-6). The negative pressure in the intact hemithorax, compared with the less negative pressure of the open hemithorax, can cause the mediastinum to move vertically downward and push into the dependent hemithorax. The mediastinal shift can create circulatory and reflex changes that may result in a clinical picture similar to that of shock and respiratory distress. Sometimes, depending on the severity of the distress, the patient needs to be tracheally intubated immediately, with initiation of positive-pressure ventilation, and the anesthesiologist must be prepared to intubate in this position without disturbing the surgical field.

The second phenomenon is paradoxical breathing (Fig. 40-7). During inspiration, the relatively negative pressure in the intact hemithorax compared with atmospheric pressure in the open hemithorax can cause movement of air from the nondependent lung into the dependent lung. The opposite occurs during expiration. This gas movement reversal from one lung to the other represents wasted ventilation and can compromise the adequacy of gas exchange. Paradoxical breathing is increased by a large thoracotomy or by an increase in airways resistance in the dependent lung. Positive-pressure ventilation or adequate sealing of the open chest eliminates paradoxical breathing.

Lateral position, anesthetized, breathing spontaneously, chest closed. The induction of general anesthesia does not cause significant change in the distribution of blood flow, but it has an important impact on the distribution of ventilation. Most of the

Expiration

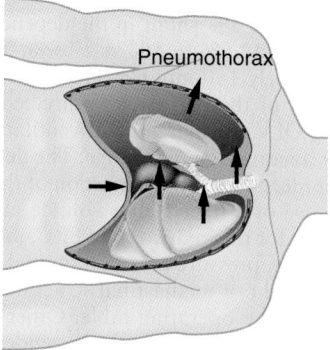

Inspiration

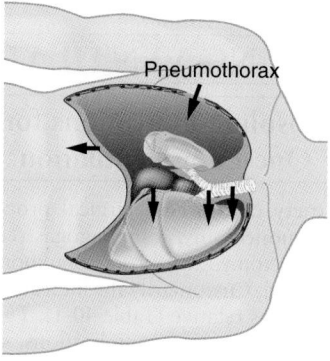

FIGURE 40-6. Schematic representation of mediastinal shift in the spontaneously breathing, open-chested patient in the lateral decubitus position. During inspiration, negative pressure in the intact hemithorax causes the mediastinum to move downward. During expiration, relative positive pressure in the intact hemithorax causes the mediastinum to move upward. (From Tarhan S, Moffitt EA: Principles of thoracic anesthesia. Surg Clin North Am 1973; 53: 813, with permission.)

Expiration

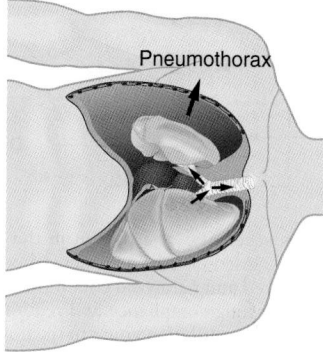

Inspiration

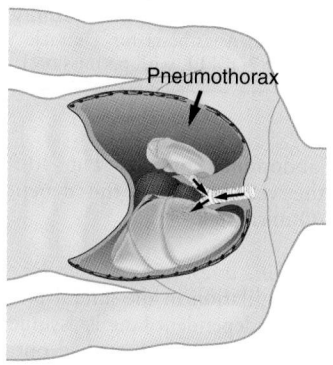

FIGURE 40-7. Schematic representation of paradoxical respiration in the spontaneously breathing, open-chested patient in the lateral decubitus position. During inspiration, movement of gas from the exposed lung into the intact lung and movement of air from the environment into the open hemithorax cause collapse of the exposed lung. During expiration, the reverse occurs, and the exposed lung expands. (From Tarhan S, Moffitt EA: Principles of thoracic anesthesia. Surg Clin North Am 1973; 53: 813, with permission.)

VT enters the nondependent lung, and this results in a significant V/Q mismatch. Induction of general anesthesia causes a reduction in the volumes of both lungs secondary to a reduction in FRC. Any reduction in volume in the dependent lung is of a greater magnitude than that in the nondependent lung for several reasons. First, the cephalad displacement of the dependent diaphragm by the abdominal contents is more pronounced and is increased by paralysis. Second, the mediastinal structures pressing on the dependent lung or poor positioning of the dependent side on the operating table prevents the lung from expanding properly. The aforementioned factors will move lungs to a lower volume on the S-shaped volume-pressure curve (Fig. 40-8). The nondependent lung moves to a steeper position on the compliance curve and receives most of the VT, whereas the dependent lung is on the flat (noncompliant) part of the curve.

Lateral position, anesthetized, breathing spontaneously, chest open.   Opening the chest has little impact on the distribution of perfusion. However, the upper lung is now no longer restricted by the chest wall and is free to expand, resulting in a further increase in V/Q mismatch as the nondependent lung is preferentially ventilated, owing to a now increased compliance.

Lateral position, anesthetized, paralyzed, chest open.   During paralysis and positive-pressure ventilation, diaphragmatic displacement is maximal over the nondependent lung, where there is the least amount of resistance to diaphragmatic movement

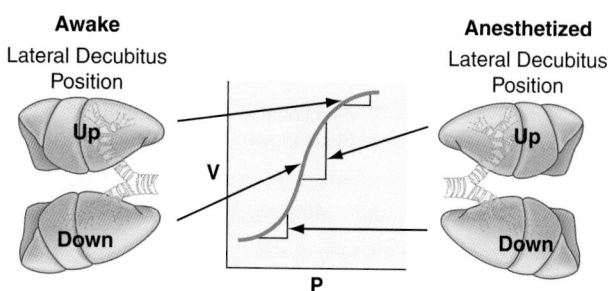

FIGURE 40-8. The **left** side of the schematic shows the distribution of ventilation in the awake patient (closed chest) in the lateral decubitus position, and the **right** side shows the distribution of ventilation in the anesthetized patient (closed chest) in the lateral decubitus position. The induction of anesthesia has caused a loss in lung volume in both lungs, with the nondependent (up) lung moving from a flat, noncompliant portion to a steep, compliant portion of the pressure–volume curve, and the dependent (down) lung moving from a steep, compliant part to a flat, noncompliant part of the pressure–volume curve. Thus, the anesthetized patient in the lateral decubitus position has most tidal ventilation in the nondependent lung (where there is the least perfusion) and less tidal ventilation in the dependent lung (where there is the most perfusion). V, volume; P, pressure. (From Benumof JL: Anesthesia for Thoracic Surgery, Philadelphia, WB Saunders, 1987, p 112, with permission.)

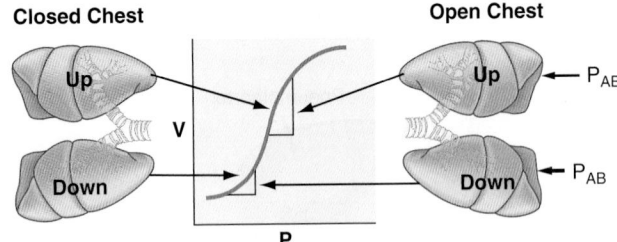

FIGURE 40-9. This schematic of a patient in the lateral decubitus position compares the closed-chested anesthetized condition with the open-chested anesthetized and paralyzed condition. Opening the chest increases nondependent lung compliance and reinforces or maintains the larger part of the tidal ventilation going to the nondependent lung. Paralysis also reinforces or maintains the larger part of tidal ventilation going to the nondependent lung because the pressure of the abdominal contents (P_{AB}) pressing against the upper diaphragm is minimal, and it is therefore easier for positive-pressure ventilation to displace this less resisting dome of the diaphragm. V, volume; P, pressure. (From Benumof JL: Anesthesia for Thoracic Surgery, Philadelphia, WB Saunders, 1987, p 112, with permission.)

caused by the abdominal contents (Fig. 40-9). This further compromises the ventilation to the dependent lung and increases the V/Q mismatch.

One-lung ventilation, anesthetized, paralyzed, chest open. During two-lung ventilation in the lateral position, the mean blood flow to the nondependent lung is assumed to be 40% of cardiac output, whereas 60% of cardiac output goes to the dependent lung (Fig. 40-10). Normally, venous admixture (shunt) in the lateral position is 10% of cardiac output and is equally divided as 5% in each lung. Therefore, the average percentage of cardiac output participating in gas exchange is 35% in the nondependent lung and 55% in the dependent lung.

OLV creates an obligatory right-to-left transpulmonary shunt through the nonventilated, nondependent lung because the V/Q ratio of that lung is zero. In theory, an additional 35% should be added to the total shunt during OLV. However, assuming active HPV, blood flow to the nondependent hypoxic lung will be decreased by 50% and therefore is (35/2) = 17.5%. To this, 5% must be added, which is the

obligatory shunt through the nondependent lung. The shunt through the nondependent lung is therefore 22.5% (Fig. 40-10). Together with the 5% shunt in the dependent lung, total shunt during OLV is 22.5% + 5% = 27.5%. This results in a PaO_2 of approximately 150 mm Hg (FiO_2 = 1.0).[40]

Because 72.5% of the perfusion is directed to the dependent lung during OLV, the matching of ventilation in this lung is important for adequate gas exchange. The dependent lung is no longer on the steep (compliant) portion of the volume-pressure curve because of reduced lung volume and FRC. There are several reasons for this reduction in FRC, including general anesthesia, paralysis, pressure from abdominal contents, compression by the weight of mediastinal structures, and suboptimal positioning on the operating table. Other considerations that impair optimal ventilation to the dependent lung include absorption atelectasis, accumulation of secretions, and the formation of a fluid transudate in the dependent lung. All these create a low V/Q ratio and a large $P(A\text{-}a)O_2$ gradient.

ONE-LUNG VENTILATION

Absolute Indications for One-Lung Ventilation

Currently, a variety of thoracic surgical procedures such as lobectomy, pneumonectomy, esophagogastrectomy, pleural decortication, bullectomy, and bronchopulmonary lavage are ❹ commonly performed. Customarily the indications are classified either as absolute or as relative (Table 40-1). *The absolute indications* include life-threatening complications, such as massive bleeding, sepsis, and pus, in which the nondiseased contralateral lung must be protected from contamination. Bronchopleural and bronchocutaneous fistulae are absolute indications because they offer a low-resistance pathway for the delivered tidal volume during positive-pressure ventilation. A giant unilateral bullae may rupture under positive pressure, and ventilatory exclusion is mandatory. Finally, during bronchopulmonary lavage for alveolar proteinosis or cystic fibrosis, prevention of drowning the contralateral lung is necessary.

During the last several years video-assisted thoracoscopy (VAT) was introduced to clinical practice. Unlike conventional thoracoscopy, VAT allows for an extensive variety of diagnostic

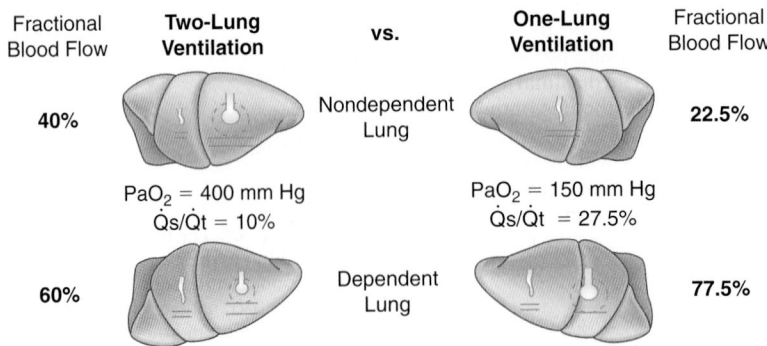

FIGURE 40-10. Schematic representation of two-lung ventilation versus one-lung ventilation (OLV). Typical values for fractional blood flow to the nondependent and dependent lungs, as well as PaO_2 and $\dot{Q}s/\dot{Q}t$ for the two conditions, are shown. The $\dot{Q}s/\dot{Q}t$ during two-lung ventilation is assumed to be distributed equally between the two lungs (5% to each lung). The essential difference between two-lung ventilation and OLV is that, during OLV, the nonventilated lung has some blood flow and therefore an obligatory shunt, which is not present during two-lung ventilation. The 35% of total flow perfusing the nondependent lung, which was not shunt flow, was assumed to be able to reduce its blood flow by 50% by hypoxic pulmonary vasoconstriction. The increase in $\dot{Q}s/\dot{Q}t$ from two-lung to OLV is assumed to be due solely to the increase in blood flow through the nonventilated, nondependent lung during OLV. (From Benumof JL: Anesthesia for Thoracic Surgery, Philadelphia, WB Saunders, 1987, p 112, with permission.)

ANESTHESIA FOR SURGICAL SUBSPECIALTIES

TABLE 40-1

INDICATIONS FOR ONE-LUNG VENTILATION

■ ABSOLUTE

1. Isolation of each lung to prevent contamination of a healthy lung
   a. Infection (abscess, infected cyst)
   b. Massive hemorrhage
2. Control of distribution of ventilation to only one lung
   a. Bronchopleural fistula
   b. Bronchopleural cutaneous fistula
   c. Unilateral cyst or bullae
   d. Major bronchial disruption or trauma
3. Unilateral lung lavage
4. Video-assisted thoracoscopic surgery

■ RELATIVE

1. Surgical exposure—high priority
   a. Thoracic aortic aneurysm
   b. Pneumonectomy
   c. Lung volume reduction
   d. Minimally invasive cardiac surgery
   e. Upper lobectomy
2. Surgical exposure—low priority
   a. Esophageal surgery
   b. Middle and lower lobectomy
   c. Mediastinal mass resection, thymectomy
   d. Bilateral sympathectomies

Modified from Benumof JL: Physiology of the open-chest and one lung ventilation, Thoracic Anesthesia. Edited by Kaplan JA. New York, Churchill Livingstone, 1983, p 299.

and therapeutic procedures. Improvements in video-endoscopic surgical equipment and a growing enthusiasm for minimally invasive surgical approaches have contributed to its use. In most cases general anesthesia with OLV is required. The lung should be well collapsed to provide the surgeon with an optimal view of the surgical field, and to facilitate palpation of the lesion in the lung parenchyma. In addition, it is difficult to place the stapler on a lung that is not completely collapsed, and there is an increase in incidence of postoperative air leak in these circumstances. The increased use of VAT has significantly increased the number of procedures that require lung separation. In some institutions, 80 to 90% of the procedures are performed using the thoracoscopic approach. In modern anesthesia practice, VAT is an absolute indication for lung separation.

Relative Indications for One-Lung Ventilation

In clinical practice, a DLT is commonly used for a lobectomy or pneumonectomy; these represent relative indications for lung separation when performed through an open thoracotomy. Upper lobectomy, pneumonectomy, and thoracic aortic aneurysm repair are high-priority indications. These procedures are technically difficult, and optimal surgical exposure and a quiet operative field are highly desirable. Lower or middle lobectomy and esophageal resection are of lower priority. There are a number of additional procedures that have not been traditionally included as indications for OLV. Nevertheless, many surgeons are accustomed to operating with the lung collapsed for these cases. OLV minimizes lung trauma from retractors and manipulation, improves visualization of lung anatomy, and facilitates identification and separation of

anatomic structures and lung fissures. These procedures include minimally invasive cardiac surgery, lung volume reduction, thoracic aneurysm repair, thoracic spinal procedures, mediastinal mass resection, thymectomies, and mediastinal lymph nodes dissection.

Methods of Lung Separation

Double-Lumen Endobronchial Tubes

Double-lumen endobronchial tubes are currently the most widely used means of achieving lung separation and OLV. There are several different types of DLT, but all are essentially similar in design in that two endotracheal tubes are "bonded" together. One lumen is long enough to reach a main stem bronchus, and the second lumen ends with an opening in the distal trachea. Lung separation is achieved by inflation of two cuffs: a proximal tracheal cuff and a distal bronchial cuff located in the main stem bronchus (see "Positioning Double-Lumen Tubes"). The endobronchial cuff of a right-sided tube is slotted or otherwise designed to allow ventilation of the right upper lobe because the right main stem bronchus is too short to accommodate both the right lumen tip and a right bronchial cuff.

Robertshaw Tube. The Carlens tube (which had a carinal hook) was the first clinically available DLT and was used by pulmonologists for split function spirometry testing (Fig. 40-11A). Subsequently, the Robertshaw design DLT (which lacked a carinal hook) was developed to facilitate thoracic surgery (Fig. 40-11B). This DLT is available in left-sided and right-sided forms. The absence of a carinal hook facilitates insertion. This tube design has the advantages of having D-shaped, large-diameter lumens that allow easy passage of a suction catheter, offer low resistance to gas flow, and have a fixed curvature to facilitate proper positioning and reduce the possibility of kinking. The original red rubber Robertshaw tubes were available in three sizes: small, medium, and large. Red rubber tubes are rarely used now and have been replaced by clear, polyvinyl chloride (PVC) disposable Robertshaw-design DLTs. These are available in both right-sided and left-sided versions and in 35 French (Fr), 37 Fr, 39 Fr, and 41 Fr. A 32-Fr left-sided DLT is available for small adults and a 28 Fr for use in pediatric cases. The advantages of the disposable tubes include relative ease of insertion and proper positioning, easy recognition of the blue color of the endobronchial cuff when fiberoptic bronchoscopy is used, confirmation of position on a chest radiograph using the radiopaque lines in the wall of the tube, and continuous observation of tidal gas exchange and respiratory moisture through the clear plastic. The right-sided endobronchial tube is designed to minimize occlusion of the opening of the right upper lobe bronchus. The right endobronchial cuff is doughnut-shaped and allows the right upper lobe ventilation slot to ride over the opening of the right upper lobe bronchus. The tube is also suitable for use in long-term ventilation in the intensive care unit because it has a high-volume, low-pressure cuff. These disposable PVC tubes are generally considered the tubes of choice for achieving lung separation and OLV.[41]

Recently, a new rubber-silicone left-sided DLT, Silbonco (Silbronco DLT, Fuji Systems, Tokyo, Japan), was introduced to clinical practice. It has a D-shaped wire reinforced lumen to maintain the tip at a 45-degree angle. The reinforced wall tends to prevent obstruction or kinking of the bronchial lumen, yet at the same time maintains flexibility. It is especially useful if the left main stem bronchus is angled at 90 degrees from the trachea, making it almost impossible to position a PVC DLT. This clinical scenario can be seen in patients who have previously undergone a left upper lobectomy and the

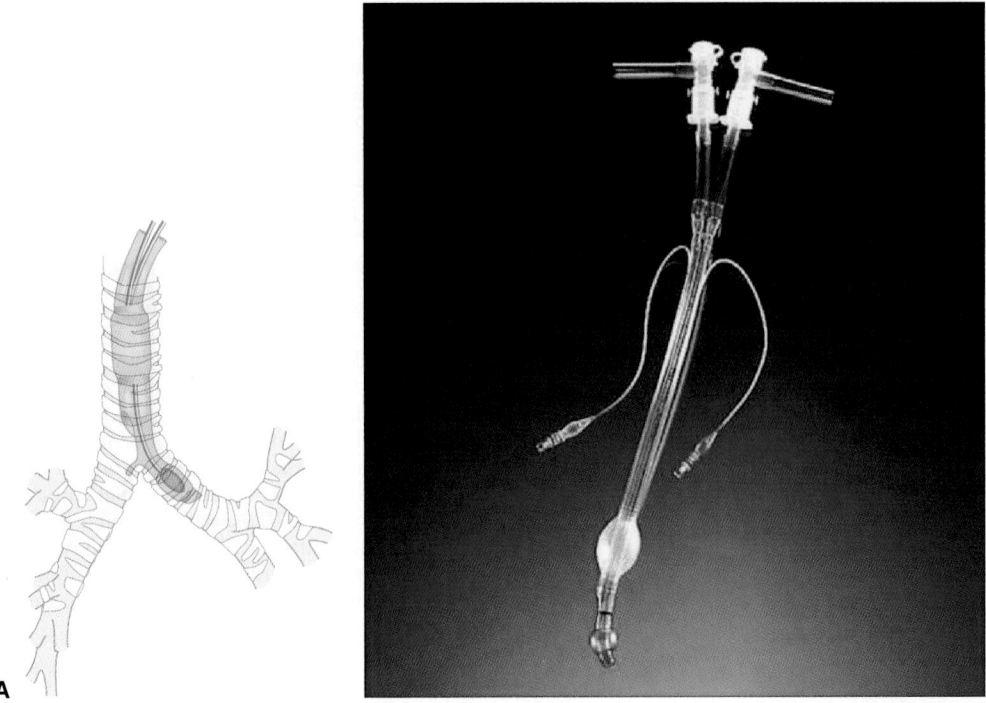

FIGURE 40-11. **A.** Left main stem endobronchial intubation using a Carlens tube. Note carinal "hook" used for correct positioning. **B.** A left-sided Robertshaw type double-lumen tube constructed from polyvinyl chloride. (**A,** From Hillard EK, Thompson PW: Instruments used in thoracic anaesthesia, Thoracic Anaesthesia. Edited by Mushin WW. Oxford, Blackwell Scientific, 1963, p 315. **B,** Courtesy of Nellcor Puritan Bennett, Inc., Pleasanton, California.)

expansion of the left lower lobe displaces the left main bronchus upward.[42]

As the left main bronchus is considerably longer than the right bronchus, there is a narrow margin of safety on the right main bronchus, with potentially a greater risk of upper lobe obstruction whenever a right-sided DLT is used. A left-sided DLT is preferred for both right- and left-sided procedures. A left-sided DLT was selected for 1,166 of the 1,170 patients in one report, and was used successfully in over 98% of those patients.[43] The authors recommended selecting the largest DLT that will safely fit the bronchus. This will provide less resistance to ventilation and is less likely to dislocate.

Some authors have suggested using the patient height as a basis for selecting a DLT. However, the correlation between airway size and height is extremely poor.[43] Tracheal and bronchial dimensions can be also directly measured from the chest radiograph or chest CT scan. It is possible to measure the diameter of the left bronchus from the chest radiograph in almost 75% of patients.[43] In patients in whom the left main bronchus cannot be directly measured, the left bronchial diameter can be accurately estimated by measuring tracheal width. The width of the left bronchus is directly proportional to tracheal width. The left bronchial width is estimated by multiplying the tracheal width by 0.68.[44]

Typically, most women will need a 37-Fr DLT and most men will be adequately managed with a 39-Fr DLT. In the past it was a more common practice to use the largest size DLT possible to avoid distal migration of the tube, and so that the pressure in the bronchial cuff could be minimized by needing less air for a seal. The common practice of fiberoptic bronchoscopy has lessened the risk of undetected distal placement or migration of the bronchial tip. A recent study demonstrated that the routine use of a 35-Fr DLT in adults regardless of height was not associated with an increase in hypoxemia or any other adverse clinical outcomes.[45]

The depth required for insertion of the DLT correlates with the height of the patient. For any adult 170 to 180 cm tall, the average depth for a left-sided DLT is 29 cm. For every 10 cm increase or decrease in height, the DLT is advanced or withdrawn 1.0 cm.[46]

Placement of Double-Lumen Tubes. This section concentrates on the insertion of disposable Robertshaw-design DLTs because they are the most widely used. Before insertion, the DLT should be prepared and checked. The tracheal cuff (high-volume, low-pressure) can accommodate up to 20 mL of air, and the bronchial cuff can be checked using a 3-mL syringe. The tube should be coated liberally with water-soluble lubricant and the stylet should be withdrawn, lubricated, and gently placed back into the bronchial lumen without disturbing the tube's preformed curvature. A Macintosh blade is preferred for intubation of the trachea because it provides the largest area through which to pass the tube. The insertion of the tube is performed with the distal concave curvature facing anteriorly. After the tip of the tube is past the vocal cords, the stylet is removed and the tube is rotated through 90 degrees. A left-sided tube is rotated 90 degrees to the left, and a right-sided tube is rotated to the right. Advancement of the tube ceases when moderate resistance to further passage is encountered, indicating that the tube tip has been firmly seated in the main stem bronchus. It is important to remove the stylet before rotating and advancing the tube to avoid tracheal or bronchial laceration. Rotation and advancement of the tube should be performed gently and under continuous direct laryngoscopy to prevent hypopharyngeal structures from interfering with proper positioning. Once the tube is believed to be in the proper position, a sequence of steps should be performed to check its location.

First the tracheal cuff should be inflated, and equal ventilation of both lungs established. If breath sounds are not equal,

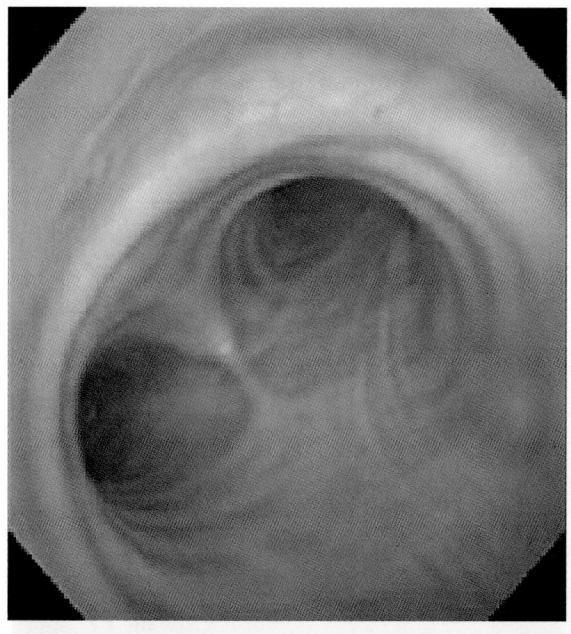

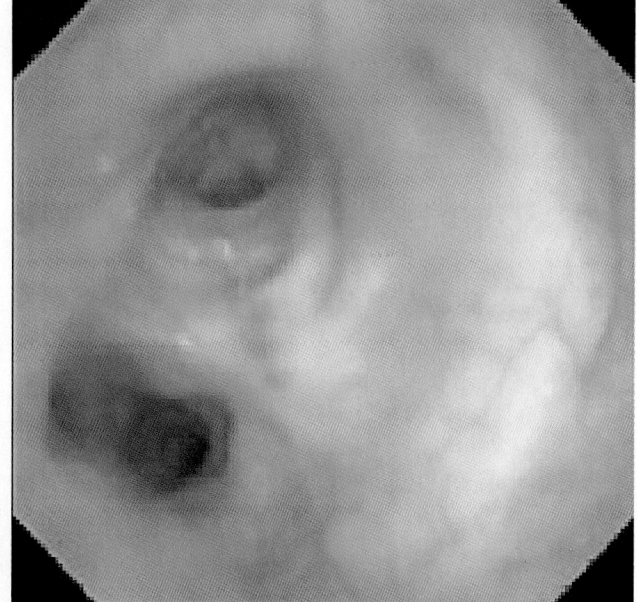

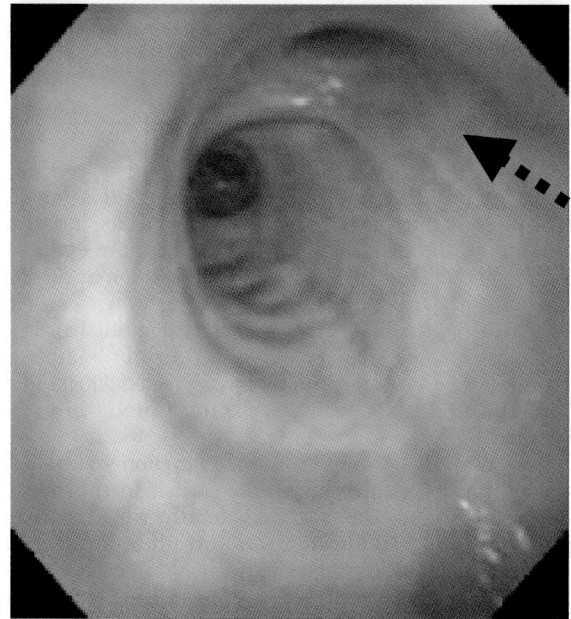

FIGURE 40-12.   Fiberoptic bronchoscopic view of the main carina (**A**), the "left bronchial carina" (**B**), and the right bronchus (**C**). Note right upper lobe orifice (*arrow*).

the tube is probably too far down, and the tracheal lumen opening is in a main stem bronchus or is lying at the carina. Withdrawal of the tube by 2 to 3 cm usually restores equal breath sounds. The second step is to clamp the right side (in the case of the left-sided tube) and remove the right cap from the connector. Then the bronchial cuff is slowly inflated to prevent an air leak from the bronchial lumen around the bronchial cuff into the tracheal lumen. This ensures excessive pressure is not applied to the bronchus and helps avoid laceration. Inflation of the bronchial cuff rarely requires >2 mL of air. The third step is to remove the clamp and check that both lungs are ventilated with both cuffs inflated. This ensures the bronchial cuff is not obstructing the contralateral hemithorax, either totally or partially. The final step is to clamp each side selectively and watch for absence of movement and breath sounds on the ipsilateral (clamped) side; the ventilated side should have clear breath sounds, chest movement that feels compliant, respiratory gas moisture with each tidal ventilation, and no gas leak. If peak

airway pressure during two-lung ventilation is 20 cm H_2O, it should not exceed 40 cm H_2O for the same VT during OLV.

Other methods that have been used for ensuring the correct placement of a DLT include fluoroscopy, chest radiography, selective capnography, and use of an underwater seal. Determination of the presence of gas leaks when positive pressure is applied to one lumen of a DLT is easily done in the operating room. If the bronchial cuff is not inflated and positive pressure is applied to the bronchial lumen of the DLT, gas leaks past the bronchial cuff and returns through the tracheal lumen. If the tracheal lumen is connected to an underwater seal system, gas will be seen to bubble up through the water. The bronchial cuff can then be gradually inflated until no gas bubbles are seen and the desired cuff seal pressure can be attained. This test is of extreme importance when absolute lung separation is needed, such as during bronchopulmonary lavage.

The most important advance in checking for proper position of a DLT is the introduction of the pediatric flexible

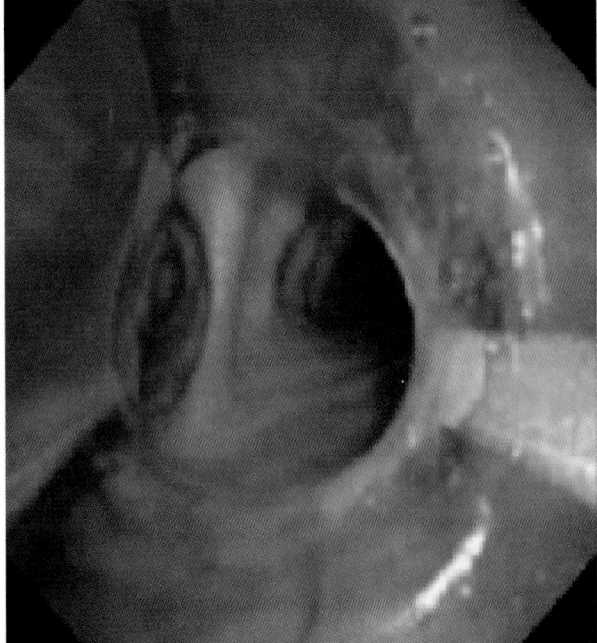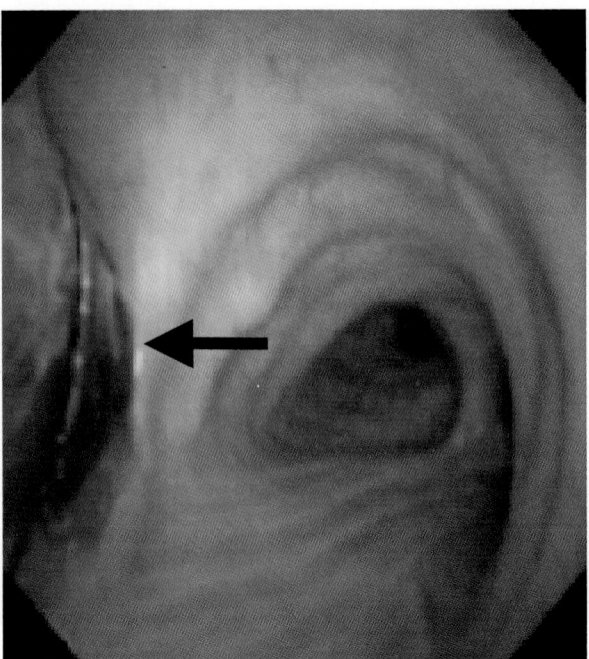

FIGURE 40-13. Malposition of the left bronchial limb of the double-lumen tube (DLT). **A.** The limb is too far into the left bronchus because the cuff is not evident. **B.** DLT withdrawn and balloon is now in view, indicating appropriate position of the DLT (*arrow*).

fiberoptic bronchoscope (Fig. 40-12). Smith et al.[47] showed that when the disposable DLT was believed to be in correct position by auscultation and physical examination, subsequent fiberoptic bronchoscopy showed that 48% of tubes were, in fact, malpositioned. Such malpositions, however, are usually of no clinical significance.[48] When using a left-sided DLT, the bronchoscope is usually first introduced through the tracheal lumen. The carina is visualized, but no bronchial cuff herniation should be seen. The upper surface of the blue endobronchial cuff should be just below the tracheal carina. The bronchial cuff of the disposable DLT is easily visualized because of its blue color. The bronchoscope should then be passed through the bronchial lumen, and the left upper lobe bronchial orifice should be identified. When a right-sided DLT is used, the carina should be visualized through the tracheal lumen but, more important, the orifice of the right upper lobe bronchus should be identified when the bronchoscope is passed through the right upper lobe ventilating slot of the DLT. Pediatric fiberoptic bronchoscopes are available in several sizes: 5.6, 4.9, and 3.6 mm in external diameter. The 4.9-mm diameter bronchoscope can be passed through DLTs of 37 Fr and larger. The 3.6-mm diameter bronchoscope is easily passed through all sizes of DLT. In general, it is recommended that the largest size that can pass through the lumen of a DLT be used because it provides better visualization and facilitates identification of the bronchial anatomy. Excellent fiberoptic images of the tracheobronchial tree can be seen by accessing the Web site thoracicanesthesia.com.

Problems of Malposition of the Double-Lumen Tube. The use of a DLT is associated with a number of potential problems, the most important of which is malposition. There are several possibilities for tube malposition. The DLT may be accidentally directed to the side opposite the desired main stem bronchus. In this case, the lung opposite the side of the connector clamp will collapse. Inadequate separation, increased airway pressures, and instability of the DLT usually occur. In addition, because of the morphology of the DLT curvatures,

tracheal or bronchial lacerations may result. If a left-sided DLT is inserted into the right main stem bronchus, it obstructs ventilation to the right upper lobe. It is therefore essential to recognize and correct such a malposition as soon as possible.

Second, the DLT may be passed too far down into either the right or the left main stem bronchus (Fig. 40-13). In this case, breath sounds are very diminished or not audible over the contralateral side. This situation is corrected when the tube is withdrawn and the opening of the tracheal lumen is above the carina.

Third, the DLT may not be inserted far enough, leaving the bronchial lumen opening above the carina. In this position, good breath sounds are heard bilaterally when ventilating through the bronchial lumen, but no breath sounds are audible when ventilating through the tracheal lumen because the inflated bronchial cuff obstructs gas flow arising from the tracheal lumen. The cuff should be deflated and the DLT rotated and advanced into the desired main stem bronchus.

Fourth, a right-sided DLT may occlude the right upper lobe orifice. The mean distance from the carina to the right upper lobe orifice is 2.3 ± 0.7 cm in men and 2.1 ± 0.7 cm in women.[49] With right-sided DLTs, the ventilatory slot in the side of the bronchial catheter must overlie the right upper lobe orifice to permit ventilation of this lobe. However, the margin of safety is extremely small, and varies from 1 to 8 mm.[49] It is therefore difficult to ensure proper ventilation to the right upper lobe and avoid dislocation of the DLT during surgical manipulation. When right endobronchial intubation is required, a disposable right-sided DLT is perhaps the best choice because of the slanted doughnut shape of the bronchial cuff, which allows the ventilation slot to ride off the right upper lobe ventilation orifice and increases the margin of safety.

Fifth, the left upper lobe orifice may be obstructed by a left-sided DLT. Traditionally, it was believed the take-off of the left upper lobe bronchus was at a safe distance from the carina and that it would not be obstructed by a left-sided DLT. However, the mean distance between the left upper lobe orifice and the carina is 5.4 ± 0.7 cm in men and 5.0 ± 0.7 cm in women.[50]

The average distance between the openings of the right and left lumens on the left-sided disposable tubes is 6.9 cm.[49] Therefore, an obstruction of the left upper lobe bronchus is possible while the tracheal lumen is still above the carina. There is also a 20% variation in the location of the blue endobronchial cuff on the disposable tubes because this cuff is attached to the tube at the end of the manufacturing process.

Bronchial cuff herniation may occur and obstruct the bronchial lumen if excessive volumes are used to inflate the cuff. The bronchial cuff has also been known to herniate over the tracheal carina, and in the case of a left-sided DLT, to obstruct ventilation to the right main stem bronchus.

Another rare complication with DLTs is tracheal rupture. Overinflation of the bronchial cuff, inappropriate positioning, and trauma owing to intraoperative dislocation that resulted in bronchial rupture have been described in association with the Robertshaw tube and the disposable DLT.[51] Therefore, the pressure in the bronchial cuff should be assessed and decreased if the cuff is found to be overinflated. If absolute separation of the lungs is not needed, the bronchial cuff should be deflated and then reinflated slowly to avoid excessive pressure on the bronchial walls. The bronchial cuff should also be deflated during any repositioning of the patient unless lung separation is absolutely required during this time.

In a recent prospective trial, 60 patients were randomly assigned to two groups. OLV was achieved with either an endobronchial blocker (blocker group) or a DLT (double-lumen group). Postoperative hoarseness and sore throat were assessed at 24, 48, and 72 hours after surgery. Bronchial injuries and vocal cord lesions were examined by bronchoscopy immediately after surgery. Postoperative hoarseness occurred significantly more frequently in the double-lumen group compared with the blocker group: (44% vs. 17%, respectively). Similar findings were observed for vocal cord lesions (44% vs. 17%). The incidence of bronchial injuries was comparable between groups.[52]

Lung Separation in the Patient with a Tracheostomy

Occasionally, a patient with a permanent tracheotomy is scheduled for surgery on the lung that requires isolation. Examples of such patients include those who have undergone resection of a tumor in the floor of the mouth or on the base of the tongue, followed by extensive reconstructive surgery with creation of a permanent tracheal stoma. Routine follow-up may reveal a lung lesion that requires a diagnostic procedure. Conventional double-lumen endobronchial tubes are designed to be inserted through the mouth, not through a tracheal stoma. The standard DLTs are usually too stiff to negotiate the curve required for insertion through a tracheal stoma and are difficult to position.[53] A separately inserted bronchial blocker may permit adequate lung separation.[54]

Saito et al.[55] described a spiral, wire-reinforced, double-lumen endobronchial tube made of silicone (Koken Medical, Tokyo, Japan) that is designed for placement through a tracheostomy. The middle section of the tube consists of two thin-walled silicone catheters with an internal diameter of 5 mm, glued together and reinforced with a stainless steel spiral wire and covered with a silicone coating with two pilot balloons. The distal section, which contains the bronchial lumen and the bronchial cuff, is made of wire-reinforced silicone to avoid excessive flexibility. The dimensions are based on the Mallinckrodt DLT (Hazelwood, MD). The bronchial cuff is located 1.2 cm from the tip, and the distance between the tip orifice and the tracheal orifice is 4.9 cm. In a clinical trial in patients with permanent tracheal stomas, the tubes functioned well in achieving lung separation, with no sign of kinking or movement, and permitted easy passage of a suction catheter.

Lung Separation in the Patient with a Difficult Airway

An airway may be recognized initially as difficult when conventional laryngoscopy reveals a grade III or IV view (see Chapter 29). When separation of the lungs is required and the patient has a clearly recognized difficult airway, then awake intubation using a flexible fiberoptic bronchoscope can be planned to place a double-lumen, Univent, or single-lumen tube. The single-lumen tube may then be exchanged for a double-lumen or Univent tube using a tube exchanger. Furthermore, depending on the expected extent and the duration of the surgical procedure and the degree of fluid shift, an airway not initially classified as difficult may become difficult secondary to facial edema, secretions, and laryngeal trauma from the initial intubation.[56,57]

A logical approach to lung separation is shown in Figure 40-14. When lung separation is mandated and the patient has a recognized difficult airway, awake intubation using flexible fiberoptic bronchoscopy can be attempted using a DLT, Univent, or single-lumen tube. The same approach may be used for the patient with an unrecognized difficult airway and a failure to intubate with conventional laryngoscopy. When using a DLT over a fiberoptic bronchoscope, the anesthesiologist should keep in mind that it is a bulky tube with a large external diameter, and because of the length of the DLT, only a limited part of the fiberoptic bronchoscope is available for manipulation. In addition, the mismatch between the flexibility of the fiberoptic bronchoscope and the rigidity of the DLT makes it more difficult to advance over the fiberoptic bronchoscope. The Univent tube has the same bulky external diameter and is also often difficult to pass between the vocal cords, particularly in a patient who is awake.

Single-Lumen Tube Can Be Successfully Placed

If a failure to provide lung separation could result in a life-threatening situation, there are two possibilities to provide OLV when a single-lumen tube is already in place. First, depending on the indication for lung isolation, a tube exchanger can be used to switch to a DLT or a Univent tube. The second possibility is to direct a bronchial blocker through the single-lumen tube into the selected main-stem bronchus. These two methods, however, offer limited protection or an inadequate seal in cases such a lung lavage, pulmonary abscess, or hemoptysis, where a DLT would be the tube of choice.

Use of a Tube Exchanger

Several tube exchangers are commercially available (Cook Critical Care, Bloomington, IN; Sheridan Catheter Corporation, Argyle, NY). On these tube exchangers, the depth is marked in centimeters; they are available in a wide range of external diameters and easily adapted for either oxygen insufflation or jet ventilation. The size of the tube exchanger and the size of the tube to be inserted should be tested before use in a patient. The 11-Fr tube changer will pass through a 35- to 41-Fr DLT, whereas the 14-Fr tube exchanger does not pass through a 35 Fr. To prevent lung laceration, the tube exchanger should never be inserted against resistance. Because the first generation of tube exchangers were very stiff, there was a risk for tracheal or bronchial laceration.[50] Recently a new tube exchanger with a soft flexible tip was released by Cook Critical Care that is safer to use and is less likely to cause airway laceration. Finally, when passing any tube over an airway guide, a laryngoscope should be used to facilitate passage of the tube over the airway guide past supraglottic tissues.

ANESTHESIA FOR SURGICAL SUBSPECIALTIES

FIGURE 40-14.   Lung separation in a patient with a difficult airway. LMA, laryngeal mask airway. (Adapted from Cohen E, Benumof JL. Lung separation in the patient with a difficult airway. Curr Opin in Anesthesiol 1999; 12: 29, with permission.)

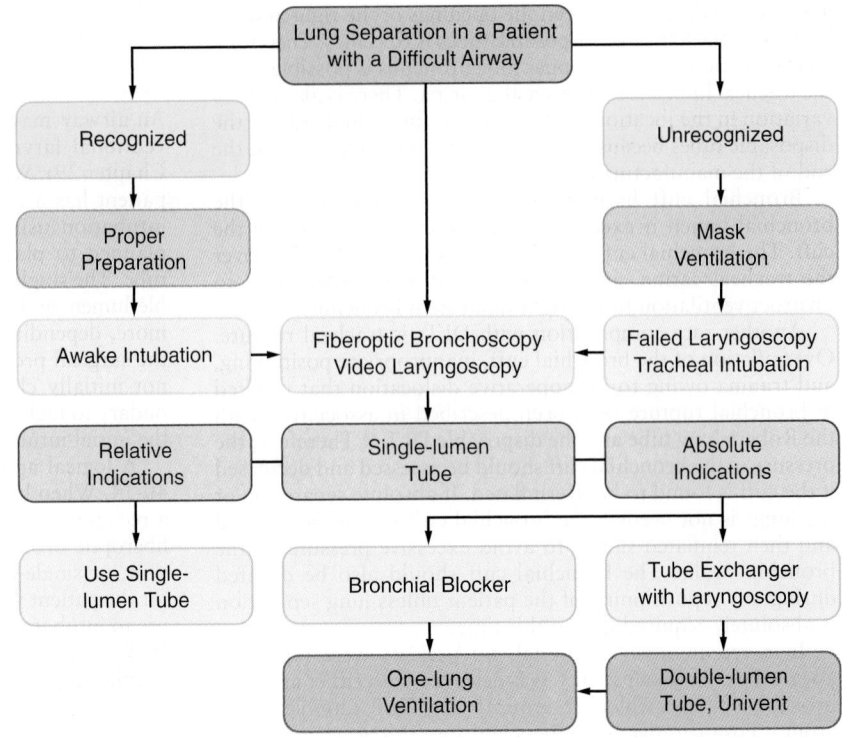

Use of Modern Bronchial Blockers

Bronchial Blocker (BB). Lung separation can be achieved with a reusable bronchial blocker. Sir Ivan Magill described an endobronchial blocker that is placed using a bronchoscope and directed to the nonventilated lung. Inflation of the cuff at the distal end of the blocker serves to block ventilation to that lung. The lumen of the blocker permits suctioning of the airway distal to the catheter tip. Depending on the clinical circumstance, oxygen can be insufflated through the catheter lumen. A conventional endotracheal tube is then placed in the trachea. This technique can be useful in achieving selective ventilation in children younger than 12 years of age. However, because the blocker balloon requires a high distending pressure, it easily slips out of the bronchus into the trachea, obstructing ventilation and losing the seal between the two lungs. This displacement can be secondary to changes in position or to surgical manipulation. The loss of lung separation can be a life-threatening situation if it was performed to prevent spillage of pus,

blood, or fluid from bronchopulmonary lavage. For this reason, bronchial blockers are rarely used in current practice.

The use of a bronchial blocker is discussed earlier in this chapter. An independently passed bronchial blocker may be used with a single-lumen tube to obtain lung isolation, thereby avoiding the use of a DLT in a patient with a difficult airway. The use of a bronchial blocker also eliminates the potential risk of needing to change a DLT to a single-lumen tube (SLI) at the conclusion of the procedure. The blockers are discussed later, in the chronological order in which they were developed, and came into practice. In the past, Fogarty vascular embolectomy catheters were used for lung separation, but there is no indication for their use in the current practice of thoracic anesthesia. The balloon of the Fogarty is high pressure, low volume, and there is no lumen to allow egress of gas from the lung to facilitate deflation.

Univent Tube.   The Univent (Fuji Systems Corp., Tokyo, Japan) is a single-lumen endotracheal tube with a movable endobronchial blocker (Fig. 40-15). In the Univent tube, the

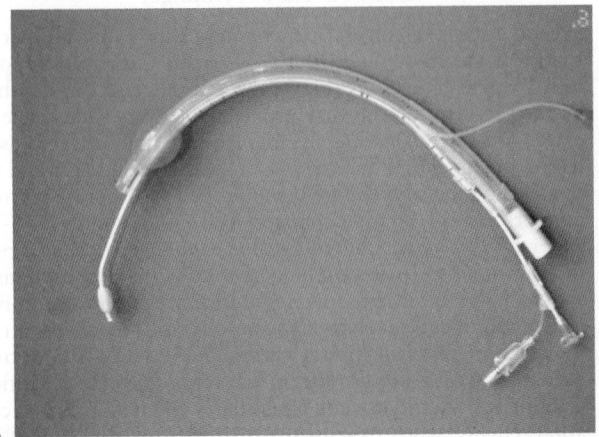
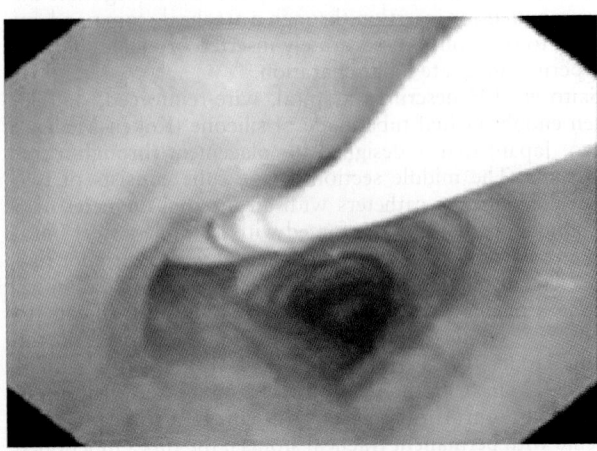

A   **B**

FIGURE 40-15.   **A.** The Univent tube also allows lung separation using a single-lumen endotracheal tube. **B.** The Univent bronchial blocker positioned in left main stem bronchus.

bronchial blocker is housed in a small channel bored in the wall of the tube. The blocker contains a high-volume, low-pressure balloon, and is angled to permit external direction into the desired bronchus under direct fiberoptic bronchoscopic (FB) vision. After intubation of the trachea, the movable blocker is manipulated into the desired main stem bronchus with the aid of a fiberoptic bronchoscope. The Univent tube may be ideal for cases in which a tube change (e.g., from single to double lumen) may be difficult (e.g., mediastinoscopy followed by thoracotomy), or in cases of bilateral lung transplantation. The Univent tube has the advantage common to all bronchial blockers: it is a single-lumen tube, and there is no need to change the tube at the end of the procedure if postoperative ventilatory support is required. This is particularly important in cases of difficult intubation, prolonged surgery with airway edema, such as thoracic aortic aneurysm surgery or extensive neurosurgical procedures on the spine with massive fluid replacement, and altered anatomy of the airway. It is also possible to suction through the blocker lumen or to apply continuous positive airway pressure (CPAP) to improve oxygenation in cases of hypoxemia.

The disadvantages of the Univent tubes are that correct positioning of the blocker may be difficult to achieve or maintain and that the external diameter is relatively large. Many anesthesiologists prefer to avoid postoperative ventilation with such a large-diameter tube, and in that case, change it to a standard tube at the conclusion of the surgery. The blocker can dislocate during surgical manipulation, and satisfactory bronchial seal and lung separation are sometimes difficult to achieve. The bronchial blocker is somewhat stiff and sometimes will not easily be directed into the main bronchus. This is particularly true for the left side. The bulky external diameter can also make it difficult to pass the tube between the vocal cords.

The first-generation Univent tube's bronchial blocker was difficult to direct into the selected main bronchus. The blocker would spin (torque) on its long axis, which made it difficult to control. The second generation, the Torque Control Blocker Univent, was introduced more recently. It consists of a silicon endotracheal tube that has a high friction coefficient. The Torque Control Blocker provides better control, which facilitates direction of the blocker into the target main stem bronchus.

The Arndt Endobronchial Blocker.   In an attempt to overcome the potential problems described previously, a snare-guided bronchial blocker has been introduced (Cook Critical Care) (Fig. 40-16). It is a wire-guided catheter with a loop snare. A fiberscope is passed through the loop of the bronchial blocker and then guided into the desired bronchus. The blocker is then slid distally over the fiberscope and into the selected bronchus. Bronchoscopic visualization confirms blocker placement and bronchial occlusion. This balloon-tipped catheter has a hollow lumen of 1.6 mm, which allows suction to facilitate the collapse of the lung and insufflation of oxygen to the nondependent lung. The balloon is available in spherical or elliptic shape. The set contains a multiport adapter, which allows uninterrupted ventilation during the positioning of the blocker. The wire may

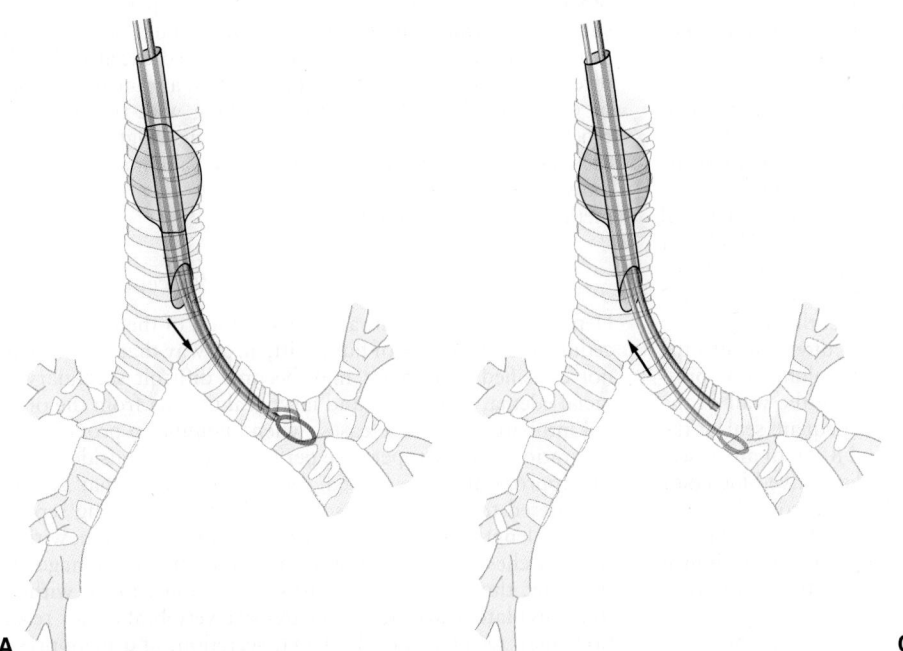

A

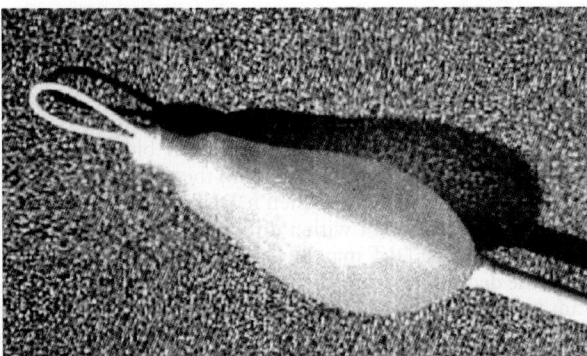

B

C

FIGURE 40-16. The Arndt endobronchial blocker is a wire-guided blocker that allows a direct placement with the use of a fiberoptic bronchoscope. The fiberoptic bronchoscope is inserted through the wire loop at the tip of the blocker, which is then slid over the bronchoscope into the selected bronchus. **A.** The fiberoptic bronchoscope is passed through the wire loop and guided into the left main bronchus. **B.** The wire loop at the tip of the blocker with the high-volume, low-pressure cuff. **C.** The bronchoscope is retracted leaving the blocker in place.

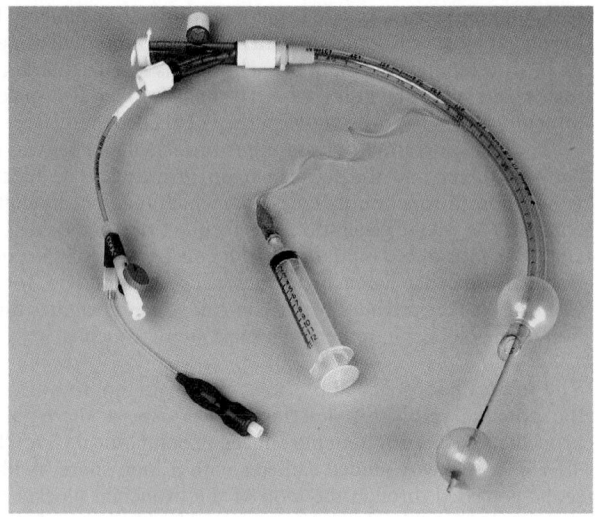
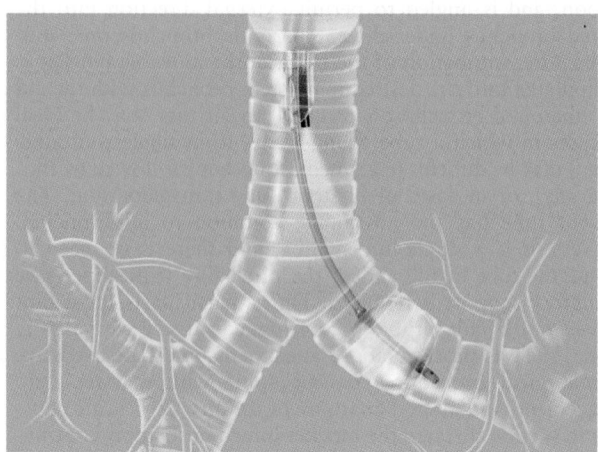

A   **B**

FIGURE 40-17.   Cohen Flexitip endobronchial blocker (**A**) allows flexion of the bronchial blocker tip and passage into the appropriate bronchial lumen (**B**). (Courtesy of Cook, Bloomington, Indiana.)

then be removed, and a 1.6-mm lumen may be used as a suction port or for oxygen insufflations. In the first generation of this device it was not possible to reinsert the string once it had been pulled out, losing the ability to redirect the bronchial blocker if necessary. External reinforcement of the wire now allows for its reintroduction through the lumen. Finally, the external diameter necessitates a large size single-lumen tube (at least 8.0 mm) to be able to accommodate the bronchial blocker. The Arndt blocker is available in 7 Fr and in a 5-Fr pediatric size.

One disadvantage of the Arndt Blocker is that it is advanced blindly over the FB into the desired main bronchus. In some occasions the tip of the blocker may get caught at the main carina or at the Murphy eye of the single-lumen tube.

The Cohen Flexitip endobronchial blocker (Cook Critical Care) is designed for use as an independent bronchial blocker. It is inserted through a single-lumen endotracheal tube with the aid of a small-diameter (4.0-mm) fiberoptic bronchoscope[58] (Fig. 40-17). The blocker has a rotating wheel that deflects the soft tip by more than 90 degrees and easily directs it into the desired bronchus. The blocker cuff is a high-volume, low-pressure balloon inflated via 0.4-mm lumen inside the wall of the blocker. It has a pear shape that provides adequate seal of the bronchus. Generally, it takes between 6 and 8 mL of air to seal the bronchus with the cuff. The cuff is a distinctive blue color that is easily recognizable by fiberoptic bronchoscopy. It is best to inflate the cuff under "direct vision" via the fiberoptic bronchoscope. The blocker size is 9 Fr It has a central main lumen (1.6 mm) that allows limited suctioning of secretions and insufflations of oxygen to the collapsed lung in case of hypoxemia. This blocker and the FB do not have to pass through the endotracheal tube at the same time for placement; the blocker can be passed ahead of the FB beyond the endotracheal tube tip. Therefore, it can be used with a 7.0-mm endotracheal tube.

Uniblocker.   Recently, the Fuji Systems introduced a new 9-Fr balloon-tipped, angled blocker with a multiple port adapter that is essentially the same design of the Univent tube blocker, but can be use as an independent blocker through a standard endotracheal tube with special connector.

One prospective randomized trial compared the effectiveness of lung isolation among three devices: the left-sided DLT Broncho-Cath, the torque control blocker Univent, and the wire-guided Arndt. There was no statistical difference in tube malpositions among the three groups: It took longer to position the Arndt blocker (3 minutes) compared with the left-sided DLT (2 minutes) and the Univent (2 minutes). Excluding the time for tube placement, the Arndt group also took longer for the lung to collapse (26 minutes), compared with the DLT group (17 minutes) or Univent group (19 minutes). Furthermore, unlike the other two groups, the majority of the Arndt patients required suction to achieve lung collapse. Once lung isolation was achieved, overall surgical exposure was rated excellent for the three groups. One minute longer to position a bronchial blocker or 6 minutes longer to collapse the lung with the bronchial blocker is insignificant when considering the length of the thoracic procedure. The risk benefit and the patient safety of each individual patient should be considered when choosing the methods for lung isolation.[59,60]

Conclusion of the Surgical Procedure

Depending on the extent and the duration of the surgical procedure and the degree of fluid shift, an airway that was initially not classified as difficult may become difficult secondary to facial edema, secretions, and laryngeal trauma from the original intubation. In these cases, when planning to provide lung separation, the postoperative period should be considered and the appropriate tube placed. Many procedures that are not considered to represent absolute indications for lung separation are lengthy and complex. Complex lung resection, with or without chest wall resection, thoracoabdominal esophagogastrectomy, thoracic aortic aneurysm resection with or without total circulatory arrest, or an extensive vertebral tumor resection, may result in facial edema, secretion, and hemoptysis, requiring postoperative ventilatory support. Other indications for postoperative ventilatory support are marginal respiratory reserve, unexpected blood loss or fluid shift, hypothermia, and inadequate reversal of residual neuromuscular blockade.

If a Univent tube was used to provide OLV, the blocker may be fully retracted and the Univent tube can be used as a single-lumen tube. If an independent bronchial blocker was used, then the blocker is removed, leaving the single-lumen tube in place. The problem arises when a DLT was inserted for lung separation. In a patient with a difficult airway and subsequent facial edema, the DLT may be left in place after surgery.

If the decision to leave the DLT in place is made, it is important to keep in mind that the intensive care unit staff is usually less experienced in managing such a tube, which may easily

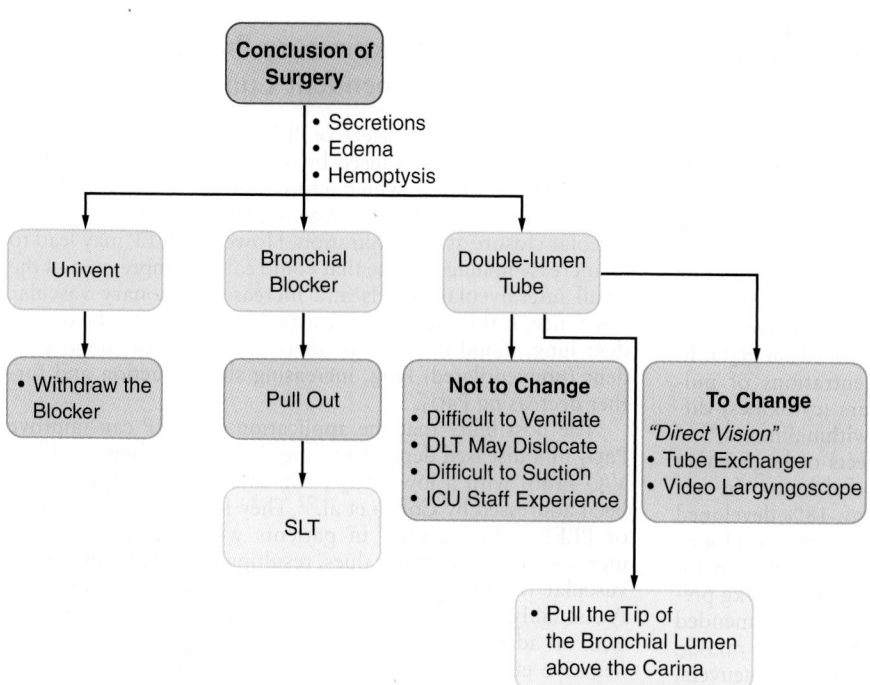

FIGURE 40-18. Conclusion of the surgical procedure. See text for discussion. SLT, single-lumen tube; DLT, double-lumen tube; ICU, intensive care unit.

become dislocated. In addition, it is more difficult to suction through the lumens, and a longer, narrower suction catheter is needed to reach the tip of the endobronchial lumen. Another possibility is to withdraw the DLT to place the 19- to 20-cm mark at the teeth so the endobronchial lumen is above the carina and both lungs can be ventilated via the bronchial lumen. Tracheal extubation from the DLT should be considered after diuresis and steroid therapy to allow reduction of the facial and airway edema.

If it is necessary to change the DLT to a single-lumen tube, a tube exchanger should be used to maintain access to the airway, as previously discussed. The tube exchanger can be passed through the bronchial limb of the DLT. Alternatively, the tube exchange may also be performed under direct vision using a Bullard or Wu laryngoscope (see Chapter 29). With these laryngoscopes, the tube exchanger can be placed under direct vision through the vocal cords alongside the existing tube to permit passage of a single-lumen tube (Fig. 40-18).

In summary, the clinician should be able to master different methods of lung separation and make himself or herself familiar with the devices available to provide OLV. In addition, one should always plan in advance for the postoperative period when choosing the method of lung separation. Finally, in these cases, a close dialog with the surgical team is of vital importance.

MANAGEMENT OF ONE-LUNG VENTILATION

This section discusses the management of OLV in a paralyzed patient in the lateral decubitus position with an open chest. Inspired oxygen fraction (FIO_2), VT and respiratory rate, dependent lung, PEEP, and nondependent lung CPAP are reviewed, and an approach to the management of OLV is presented.

Inspired Oxygen Fraction

An FIO_2 of 1.0 is usually used during OLV. This high-oxygen concentration serves to protect against hypoxemia during the procedure. Patients who have received bleomycin are at risk for oxygen toxicity, and the FIO_2 should be reduced as much as possible, without causing hypoxemia.

Tidal Volume and Respiratory Rate

It has been recommended that during OLV, the dependent lung be ventilated with a VT of 10 to 12 mL/kg. Tidal volumes ranging between 8 and 15 mL/kg produced no significant effect on transpulmonary shunt or PaO_2.[61] A VT <8 mL/kg can result in a decrease in FRC and enhanced formation of atelectasis in the dependent lung. A VT >15 mL/kg may recruit the atelectatic alveoli in the dependent lung. It will increase the pulmonary vascular resistance of the dependent lung (similar to the application of PEEP) and divert blood flow into the nondependent lung. It has been common practice during OLV to maintain the same tidal volume as during two-lung ventilation.

Recently, more attention has been directed toward protection of the ventilated lung (see Chapter 56). Data from studies conducted in the intensive care unit recommend the use of low tidal volume (VT) to avoid acute lung injury (ALI). That concept stimulated a debate over the optimal VT that should be used during OLV. A recent pro and con editorial argued that a (large) VT of 12 mL/kg during OLV may cause overdistension and stretching of the lung parenchyma and therefore would increase the risk of ALI.[62] However, a (small) VT of 6 mL/kg could lead to atelectasis in the dependent lung. Furthermore, a small VT with PEEP may cause dynamic hyperinflation secondary to the increase in respiratory rate necessary to maintain $PaCO_2$.[63]

Mechanical ventilation practice has changed over the past few decades, with tidal volumes decreasing significantly, especially in patients with ALI. The lungs of patients without ALI are still ventilated with large, and perhaps too large, tidal volumes. Studies of ventilator-associated lung injury in subjects without ALI demonstrate inconsistent results. Retrospective clinical studies, however, suggest that the use of large VT favors the development of lung injury in these patients.[64]

In a multicenter, prospective ARDS Network trial the results unambiguously confirmed that mechanical ventilation with smaller VT (6 mL/kg) rather than traditional VT (12 mL/kg) resulted in a significant increase in the number of ventilator-free days and reduction of in-hospital mortality.[65]

There is no evidence that these findings in patients with acute respiratory distress syndrome are applicable to patients undergoing a thoracic procedure requiring a relatively short period of controlled ventilation.

In one study, patients undergoing elective thoracotomy or laparotomy were randomly assigned to receive either mechanical ventilation with VT of 12 or 15 mL/kg, respectively, and without PEEP, or VT of 6 mL/kg with PEEP of 10 cm H_2O. In this study, neither time course nor concentrations of pulmonary or systemic inflammatory mediators (cytokines) differed between the two ventilatory settings within 3 hours.[66]

There are data indicating damaging effects of large VT in patients who were ventilated for only several hours. In one study of patients undergoing pneumonectomy, 18% developed postoperative respiratory failure. The patients who developed respiratory failure had been ventilated with larger intraoperative VT than those who did not (median, 8.3 vs. 6.7 mL/kg predicted body weight).[67] However, the authors recommended that protective lung ventilation with low VT 6 to 7 mL/kg, PEEP to the dependent lung, frequent recruitment maneuvers, and limited administration of fluid be used during OLV.

In patients undergoing general anesthesia, *lung recruitment maneuvers* proved to be easy to perform and effective in reversing alveolar collapse, hypoxemia, and decreased compliance. The beneficial effect of an alveolar recruitment strategy on arterial oxygenation and respiratory compliance in anesthetized patients undergoing nonthoracic surgery in the supine position has been demonstrated.[68]

In a study with a small number of patients undergoing lobectomy it was found that alveolar recruitment in the dependent lung augments PaO_2 values during OLV.[69]

Pressure-controlled ventilation (PCV) was also compared with volume-controlled ventilation (VCV) during OLV. The authors suggested that PCV may be preferred for management of OLV because the lower peak airway pressure was associated with greater perfusion of the dependent lung and smaller transpulmonary shunt.[70]

A recent study investigated whether PCV results in improved arterial oxygenation compared with VCV during OLV. Fifty-eight patients with good preoperative pulmonary function scheduled for thoracic surgery were prospectively randomized into two groups. Those in group A underwent OLV initially with VCV for 30 minutes followed by PCV for a similar period of time. Those in group B underwent OLV initially with PCV for 30 minutes followed by VCV for a similar duration. Airway pressures and arterial blood gases were obtained during OLV at the end of each ventilatory mode period. The authors found no differences in arterial oxygenation during OLV between VCV (PaO_2, 206.1 ± 62.4 mm Hg) and PCV (PaO_2, 202.1 ± 56.4 mm Hg; $p = 0.534$).[71]

The respiratory rate should be adjusted to maintain a $PaCO_2$ of 35 ± 3 mm Hg. Elimination of CO_2 is usually not a problem during OLV if the DLT is positioned correctly. The shunt during OLV has little influence on $PaCO_2$ values because the arteriovenous PCO_2 difference is normally only 6 mm Hg. Furthermore, CO_2 is 20 times more diffusible than O_2 and will be eliminated faster. It is also important not to hyperventilate the patient's lungs because hypocapnia increases vascular resistance in the dependent lung, inhibits nondependent lung HPV, increases shunt, and decreases PaO_2. Hypocarbia is believed to inhibit HPV secondary to a vasodilator effect. Because hypocarbia can only be achieved by hyperventilating the dependent lung, it raises the mean intra-alveolar pressure and therefore increases the vascular resistance in that lung.

Positive End-Expiratory Pressure to the Dependent Lung

The beneficial effect of selective PEEP 10 cm H_2O ($PEEP_{10}$) to the dependent lung is caused by an increased lung volume at end expiration (FRC), which improves the V/Q relationship in the dependent lung. The increase in FRC prevents airway and alveolar closure at end expiration. However, PEEP may lead to an increase in lung volume that could cause compression of the small interalveolar vessels and increase pulmonary vascular resistance. If this increase in resistance is limited to the dependent lung, blood flow can be diverted only to the nondependent (nonventilated) lung, increasing shunt fraction and further decreasing PaO_2.

The possibility that the application of PEEP can improve PaO_2 in a diseased dependent lung (low lung volume and low V/Q ratio) with a low PaO_2 (<80 mm Hg) during OLV has been addressed by Cohen et al.[72] They found that application of $PEEP_{10}$ during OLV in patients with a low PaO_2 may increase FRC to normal values, resulting in a lower pulmonary vascular resistance and in an improved V/Q ratio and PaO_2. Presumably, patients with a higher PaO_2 had a dependent lung with an adequate FRC, and the application of PEEP had the negative effect of redistributing blood flow away from the dependent ventilated lung (Fig. 40-19).

Continuous Positive Airway Pressure to the Nondependent Lung

The single most effective maneuver to increase PaO_2 during OLV is the application of CPAP to the nondependent lung.[73,74] A lower level of CPAP (5 to 10 cm H_2O) maintains the patency of the nondependent lung alveoli, allowing some oxygen uptake to occur in the distended alveoli. CPAP should be applied after delivering an inspiratory VT to the nondependent lung to keep it slightly expanded. CPAP, applied by insufflation

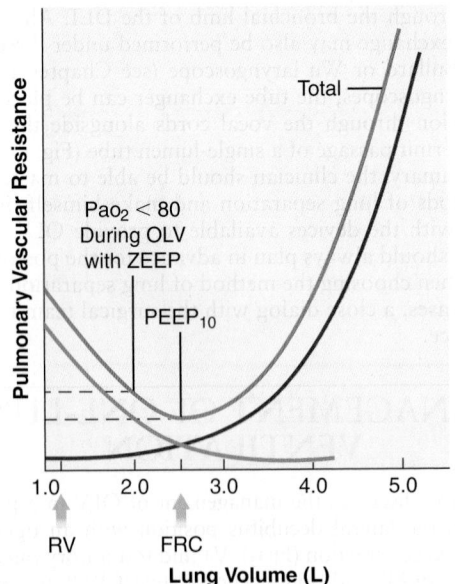

FIGURE 40-19. Effect of 10 cm H_2O positive end-expiratory pressure (PEEP) on functional residual capacity (FRC). It is postulated that, in patients having PaO_2 <80 mm Hg with zero end-expiratory pressure (ZEEP), FRC is low. $PEEP_{10}$ increases FRC and thereby increases PaO_2. OLV, one-lung ventilation; $PEEP_{10}$, positive end-expiratory pressure [10 cm H_2O]RV, residual volume.

of oxygen under positive pressure, keeps this lung "quiet" and prevents it from collapsing completely. Insufflation of oxygen without maintaining a positive pressure failed to improve PaO_2.[73.] Intermittent reinflation of the collapsed (nondependent) lung with oxygen also resulted in a significant improvement in PaO_2.[75]

Unfortunately most thoracic procedures are initiated thoracoscopically, and the application of CPAP to the nondependent lung is generally not acceptable to most surgeons. During VAT, the lung should be well collapsed to allow the surgeon an optimal view of the surgical field and to palpate the lesion in the lung parenchyma. In addition, it is difficult to place the stapler on a lung that is not completely collapsed, and there is an increase in incidence of postoperative air leak.

The beneficial effects of CPAP 10 cm H_2O ($CPAP_{10}$) are not attributable solely to the effect of positive pressure in diverting blood flow away from the collapsed lung because (in dogs) the hyperinflation of nitrogen into the nondependent lung under 10 cm H_2O failed to improve PaO_2.

The application of high-level CPAP (15 cm H_2O) is not beneficial. At this pressure, the lung becomes overdistended, which interferes with surgical exposure. Also, this level of CPAP might have hemodynamic consequences, whereas $CPAP_{10}$ has been shown to have no significant hemodynamic effects.[76]

CPAP can be applied to the nondependent lung using a number of simple systems, all of which have essentially the same features: an oxygen source, tubing to connect the oxygen source to the no ventilated lung, a pressure relief valve, and a pressure gauge. The catheter to the nondependent lung is usually insufflated with 5 L/min of oxygen using a modified Ayres T-piece (pediatric) circuit, and the valve on the expiratory limb is adjusted to the desired pressure as read on the attached gauge. Instead of a pressure gauge or manometer inserted into the circuit, a weighted pop-off valve, such as a ball or spring-loaded PEEP valve, can be used.

High-frequency ventilation with oxygen to the nondependent lung and conventional ventilation to the dependent lung has also been used to improve PaO_2 during OLV (see "High-Frequency Ventilation").

Clinical Approach to Management of One-Lung Ventilation

6 Once the patient is in the lateral position, the position of the DLT should be rechecked. Two-lung ventilation should be maintained for as long as possible, and when OLV needs to be instituted, it is generally recommended that an FIO_2 of 1.0 be used (Table 40-2). The lung should be ventilated using a V_T that results in a plateau airway pressure <25 cm H_2O at a rate adjusted to maintain $PaCO_2$ at 35 ± 3 mm Hg. This is usually monitored with the use of a capnometer or other multigas analyzer. It is recommended that protective lung ventilation with low V_T 6 to 7 mL/kg, PEEP to the dependent lung; frequent recruitment maneuvers and limited administration of fluid should be considered.[67]

After initiation of OLV, depending on the lung pathology and the intensity of hypoxic pulmonary vasoconstriction, PaO_2 can continue to decrease for up to 45 minutes. Frequent monitoring of arterial blood gases and use of a pulse oximeter continue throughout the operative period. It is also essential to work closely with the surgeon in case reinsufflation of the lung is necessary. If hypoxemia occurs during OLV, the position of the DLT should be rechecked using a fiberoptic bronchoscope. If the dependent lung is not severely diseased, a satisfactory PaO_2 on two-lung ventilation should not decrease to dangerously hypoxic

TABLE 40-2

CLINICAL APPROACH TO ONE-LUNG VENTILATION (OLV) MANAGEMENT

1. Use FIO_2 of 1.0
2. Ventilate with a TV of 6–8 mL/kg with PEEP 5 cm H_2O
3. Respiratory rate to maintain $PaCO_2$ between 35 and 40 mm Hg
4. Check the DLT/endobronchial blocker position subsequent to the lateral decubitus positioning
5. If peak airway pressure exceeds 40 mm Hg during OLV, DLT/endobronchial blocker malposition should be excluded
6. For hypoxemia, apply CPAP 10 cm H_2O to the nondependent lung (not during VAT)
7. If additional correction of hypoxemia is necessary add PEEP 5–10 cm H_2O to the ventilated lung
8. Frequent recruiting maneuvers
9. Avoid fluid overload
10. TIVA may be preferable to inhalation anesthetics
11. If necessary, intermittently inflate and deflate the operated lung

TV, tidal volume; PEEP, positive end-expiratory pressure; DLT, double-lumen tube; CPAP, continuous positive airway pressure; VAT, video-assisted thoracoscopy; TIVA, total intravenous anesthetic.

levels on OLV. If a left thoracotomy is being performed using a right-sided DLT, ventilation to the right upper lobe should be ensured. After the tube position has been confirmed as correct, $CPAP_{10}$ should be applied to the nondependent lung after a V_T that expands the lung. In most cases, the PaO_2 increases to a safe level. During thoracoscopy, application of CPAP is usually not possible because it impedes the surgeon. This is especially so during video-assisted thoracoscopic surgery (VATS) procedures. In this case, PEEP to the ventilated lung may be tried.

In the very rare case in which the PaO_2 remains low despite these maneuvers, intermittent two-lung ventilation can be reinstituted with the surgeon's cooperation. Also, depending on the stage of surgical dissection, if a pneumonectomy is being performed, ligation of the pulmonary artery eliminates the shunt.

During OLV, the peak airway pressure, the actual V_T delivered (measured by a spirometer), the shape of the capnogram, and, if available, the pressure–volume loop, should be checked continuously. A sudden increase in peak airway pressure may be secondary to tube dislocation because of surgical manipulation, resulting in impaired ventilation. In addition, the ability to auscultate by a stethoscope over the dependent lung is extremely important.

If any questions arise about the stability of the patient, or if the patient becomes hypotensive, dusky, or tachycardic, two-lung ventilation should be resumed until the problem has been resolved. Because of pericardial manipulation (during left thoracotomy in particular) and pulling on the great vessels, cardiac dysrhythmias and hypotension are not uncommon. Cardiotonic drugs should be prepared and kept available for use during any thoracic surgical procedure. Most thoracic surgical procedures represent only relative indications for OLV, and the benefits of OLV should always be weighed against the risks to the patient.

CHOICE OF ANESTHESIA FOR THORACIC SURGERY

7 The choice of anesthesia technique for a thoracic surgical procedure must take into account the patient's cardiovascular and respiratory status and the particular effects of anesthetic drugs on these and other organ systems. Thoracic surgical patients are more likely than others to have increased airway reactivity and a propensity to develop bronchoconstriction. This is because many of these patients are cigarette smokers and have chronic bronchitis or COPD. In addition, surgical manipulation of the airways and bronchial tree by instruments, a DLT, or the surgeon makes bronchoconstriction more likely to occur. The potent inhaled anesthetic agents have all been shown to decrease airway reactivity and bronchoconstriction provoked by hypocapnia or inhaled or irritant aerosols. Their mechanism of action is probably a direct one on the airway musculature itself, and potent inhaled anesthetic agents are therefore the drugs of choice in patients with reactive airways. For an inhalation induction, halothane or sevoflurane might be preferable because they are the least pungent of the three drugs, although once the patient is asleep, isoflurane may be the preferred drug because it raises the cardiac dysrhythmia threshold and provides greater cardiovascular stability than halothane (see Chapter 17). Fentanyl does not appear to influence bronchomotor tone, but morphine may increase tone by a central vagotonic effect and by releasing histamine.

In most patients, anesthesia is safely induced with thiopental or propofol (see Chapter 18). In patients with reactive airways, ketamine may be the drug of choice for induction because it has a bronchodilator effect and has been successfully used in the treatment of asthma. Thiopental has been associated with bronchospasm in asthmatic patients, although the reactivity in such cases may be related to inadequate levels of anesthesia before instrumentation of the airway. Shimizu et al.[77] compared the effects of isoflurane and sevoflurane on PaO_2 during OLV in 20 patients undergoing thoracotomy and found no significant difference between the groups in PaO_2, concluding that both agents can be used safely. In an in vitro study, Loer et al.[78] showed that desflurane inhibits HPV, with an ED_{50} of 1.6 minimum alveolar concentration (MAC). Propofol infused in doses of 6 to 12 mg/kg/hr does not abolish HPV during OLV in humans.[79] Propofol infusion in combination with remifentanil is probably the technique of choice for producing a stable OLV with no effect on HPV. Propofol is widely used during OLV and has been investigated in terms of its effect on oxygenation. Kellow et al.[80] compared the effects of propofol and isoflurane anesthesia on right ventricular function and shunt fraction during thoracic surgery and found that isoflurane, but not propofol, was associated with an increase in shunt fraction due to HPV inhibition. However, propofol was associated with a reduction in cardiac index and right ventricular ejection fraction.

The neuromuscular blocking drugs of choice for thoracic procedures are those that lack a histamine-releasing or vagotonic effect and that have some sympathomimetic effect (see Chapter 20). In this respect, pancuronium, vecuronium, rocuronium, and cisatracurium probably represent the drugs of choice. Succinylcholine is useful to provide rapid profound relaxation for intubation of the trachea and is not associated with an increase in airways reactivity.

Atropine or glycopyrrolate may be used to block the antimuscarinic effects of acetylcholine and thereby protect against cholinergically induced bronchoconstriction. It may be administered intravenously or in nebulized form (see "Bronchoscopy" and Chapter 15).

HYPOXIC PULMONARY VASOCONSTRICTION

Hypoxic pulmonary vasoconstriction was first described by Von Euler and Liljestrand[81] in 1946. They were studying changes in the pulmonary circulation of the cat in response to changes in inspired gas mixtures and found that 10.5% inspired O_2 (in N_2)

mixtures caused an increase in pulmonary artery pressure. Breathing 100% O_2 caused a decrease in pulmonary artery pressure. They concluded that the increased pressure during hypoxia was caused by a direct effect on the pulmonary vessels. Whereas they delivered hypoxic gas mixtures to both lungs, others have studied the effects of the size of the hypoxic segment and the size of the hypoxic stimulus on perfusion pressure and on flow diversion.[82] Pulmonary perfusion pressure (in dogs) increased with the size of the hypoxic segment from zero (smallest hypoxic segment) to approximately 2.2 times baseline for the hypoxic whole lung. Flow diversion, as a percentage of flow to the test segment under normoxic conditions, decreased with increasing size of the hypoxic test segment from a maximum of 75% for very small segments to zero when the whole lung was made hypoxic. Flow diversion increased linearly as PaO_2 was decreased over the range of 128 to 28 mm Hg. In both flow diversion and changes in perfusion pressure, the response to HPV was predictable, continuous, and maximal at a predicted PaO_2 of 30 mm Hg (4% oxygen). Thus, HPV causes an increase in both perfusion (pulmonary artery) pressure and flow diversion.[82]

The choice of anesthetic technique for OLV must take into consideration the effects on oxygenation and therefore on HPV. Normally, collapse of the nonventilated, nondependent lung results in activation of reflex HPV in this lung. This causes local increases in pulmonary vascular resistance and diversion of blood flow to other, better oxygenated parts of the pulmonary vascular bed (i.e., the dependent oxygenated and ventilated lung).

The relationship between PaO_2 and the size of the hypoxic segment (Fig. 40-20) shows that, when not much of the lung is hypoxic, HPV has little effect on PaO_2 because shunt is small in this situation. When most of the lung is hypoxic, there is no significant normoxic region to which the hypoxic region can divert flow, and then it does not matter, in terms of PaO_2, whether the hypoxic region has active HPV. When the amount of lung made hypoxic is 30 to 70%, such as occurs during OLV, there may be a large difference between the PaO_2 to be expected with normal HPV compared with that expected in its absence. HPV can raise PaO_2 from potentially dangerous levels to higher and safer ones. Conversely, inhibition of HPV may cause or contribute to hypoxemia during anesthesia.

The response is believed to be accounted for by each smooth muscle cell in the pulmonary arterial wall responding to the oxygen tension in its vicinity. The mechanism of HPV has been the subject of many studies and the current status (the Redox Theory) is summarized in some excellent reviews.[83-85]

Effects of Anesthetics on Hypoxic Pulmonary Vasoconstriction

The inhalation anesthetics and many of the intravenous drugs used in anesthesia have been studied for their effects on HPV. The results have not always been consistent. Benumof[86] classified the preparations used to study these effects as in vitro, in vivo nonintact, in vivo intact, and human studies. Based on the results of these three types of preparation, it is generally believed that inhaled agents inhibit HPV, whereas intravenous drugs do not have this effect.[87]

Rogers and Benumof[88] compared the effects of inhaled (isoflurane and halothane) with intravenous (methohexital and ketamine) anesthesia during OLV and concluded that the inhaled anesthetics at approximately 1 MAC do not significantly affect HPV in humans, as evidenced by a lack of significant differences in PaO_2 between use of the two techniques. The conclusions of this study have been questioned because the period of clinical exposure to the potent inhaled agents was very short. Thus, clinically relevant tissue concentrations of anesthetic may not have been achieved.

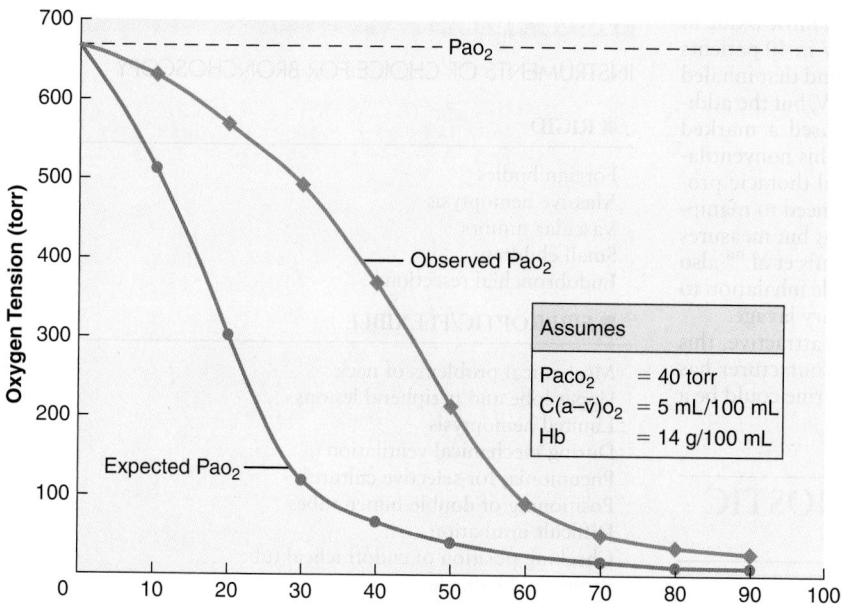

FIGURE 40-20. Role of hypoxic pulmonary vasoconstriction (HPV) in preserving Pao_2 (in dogs). Assumptions are shown in inset. Lung is ventilated with $Fio_2 = 1.0$, while increasing portions of lung are subjected to hypoxia or atelectasis. In the absence HPV, the expected Pao_2 would follow the *broken line*, whereas in the presence of an active HPV response, observed Pao_2 is maintained close to the *solid line*. Pao_2, alveolar Po_2; Pao_2, arterial Po_2. (Adapted from Marshall BE, Marshall C, Benumof JL et al: Hypoxic pulmonary vasoconstriction in dogs: Effects of lung segment size and alveolar oxygen tension. J Appl Physiol 1981; 51: 1543, with permission.)

In a subsequent study, Benumof et al.[89] investigated the changes in Pao_2 and shunt that occurred after conversion from 1 MAC halothane or isoflurane anesthesia to intravenous anesthesia (fentanyl, diazepam, and sodium thiopental) during OLV for thoracic surgery in 12 patients. In this study, they found that during one-lung atelectasis, 1 MAC halothane anesthesia slightly but significantly increased shunt and decreased Pao_2 (compared with intravenous anesthesia), whereas 1 MAC isoflurane anesthesia very slightly but non-significantly increased shunt and decreased Pao_2 (compared with intravenous anesthesia). Fundamental differences between the two studies[88,89] were in the duration of the periods of OLV with the potent inhaled agent and in the MAC multiples of the drugs used. In the earlier study,[88] end-tidal concentrations of halothane and isoflurane were kept constant for approximately 20 minutes at 1.45 and 1.15 MAC, respectively. In the later study,[89] patients were maintained on one-lung anesthesia with the potent inhaled agent (1 MAC) for 40 minutes before final measurements under these conditions were taken. The authors also concluded that halothane and isoflurane had only a small inhibitory effect on the one-lung HPV response.[89] A randomized crossover study during OLV with an Fio_2 of 1.0 found that 1 MAC isoflurane anesthesia was associated with greater Pao_2 values than was 1 MAC enflurane.[90] Shimizu et al.[77] compared the effects of isoflurane and sevoflurane on Pao_2 during OLV in 20 patients undergoing thoracotomy and found no significant difference between the groups in Pao_2, concluding that both agents can be used safely. In an in vitro study, Loer et al.[78] showed that desflurane inhibits HPV, with an ED_{50} of 1.6 MAC.

Beck et al.[91] studied 40 patients requiring OLV randomized to receive propofol (4 to 6 mg/kg/hr) or sevoflurane (1 MAC) for anesthesia maintenance. During OLV shunt fraction increased in both groups, but there was no significant difference between groups. It was concluded that inhibition of HPV by sevoflurane may only account for small increases in shunt fractions and that much of the overall shunt fraction during OLV has other causes.

Overall, the potent inhaled anesthetics are the drugs of choice during thoracic surgery. However, the technique chosen should always be dictated by the needs of the particular patient, so in the presence of cardiovascular instability or poor oxygenation when depression of HPV is a possibility, a balanced technique may be chosen.

Other Determinants of Hypoxic Pulmonary Vasoconstriction

Aside from potent inhaled agents, other drugs and maneuvers used during anesthesia may also have an inhibitory effect on regional or whole-lung HPV. Factors associated with an increase in pulmonary artery pressure antagonize the effect of increased resistance caused by HPV and result in increased flow to the hypoxic region. Such indirect inhibitors of HPV include mitral stenosis, volume overload, thromboembolism, hypothermia, vasoconstrictor drugs, and a large hypoxic lung segment. Direct inhibitors of HPV include infection, vasodilator drugs such as nitroglycerin and nitroprusside, hypocarbia, and metabolic alkalemia. All these potential inhibitors should be considered when evaluating a patient for hypoxemia during thoracic surgery.

Potentiators of Hypoxic Pulmonary Vasoconstriction

Whereas in the past most research effort has been directed to studying inhibition of HPV, more recent research has investigated substances that may potentiate it. Almitrine, a respiratory stimulant drug, has been found to improve Pao_2 in patients with COPD and to have this effect in the absence of ventilatory stimulation.

Nitric Oxide and One-Lung Ventilation

Nitric oxide is an endothelial-derived relaxing factor that is an important mediator for smooth muscle relaxation. HPV is inhibited by inhaled nitric oxide. Inhibition of nitric oxide synthase improved, but did not completely restore, HPV in dogs suffering from sepsis.[92] Frostell et al.[93] showed that inhalation of nitric oxide selectively induced vasodilation and reversed HPV in healthy humans without causing systemic vasodilatation. It was theorized that intravenous administration of almitrine (to increase HPV) causing vasoconstriction throughout the lung, together with inhalation of nitric oxide to inhibit HPV locally and cause increased flow in the ventilated regions, would improve V/Q matching and Pao_2 in patients with V/Q mismatching or during OLV.[94]

Moutafis et al.[95] studied the effects of inhaled nitric oxide in combination with almitrine infusion during OLV in 40 patients undergoing thoracoscopic procedures. They found that inhaled nitric oxide alone did not affect PaO_2 during OLV, but the additional infusion of almitrine 16 mg/kg/min caused a marked increase in PaO_2. These authors suggested that this nonventilatory technique should be of value during special thoracic procedures, such as thoracoscopy, where there is a need to manipulate the pulmonary circulation to improve PaO_2 but measures such as PEEP and CPAP cannot be used. Moutafis et al.[96] also reported the use of almitrine infusion/nitric oxide inhalation to improve PaO_2 during OLV for bronchopulmonary lavage.

Although the use of almitrine appears to be attractive, this drug is not without side effects.[97] Also, the manufacturer has not made it available outside France. Phenylephrine could be a possible alternative to almitrine.[98]

ANESTHESIA FOR DIAGNOSTIC PROCEDURES

Bronchoscopy

Early bronchoscopes were of the rigid type, but in 1966 the Machida and Olympus Companies introduced the first practical bronchofiberscopes. Since then, they have been improved dramatically and have simplified many otherwise complicated bronchoscopies. The indications for bronchoscopy are shown in Table 40-3 and the instruments of choice in Table 40-4. Operator preferences and experience may play a major role in the choice of instrument.

Before bronchoscopy is performed, the patient must be evaluated for chronic lung disease, respiratory obstruction, bronchospasm, coughing, hemoptysis, and infectivity of secretions. Medications should be reviewed, and the need for a more major procedure should always be anticipated. Thus, bronchoscopy may lead to thoracotomy or sternotomy. The planned technique for bronchoscopy should be discussed with the surgeon before the operation, and all equipment and con-

TABLE 40-3

INDICATIONS FOR BRONCHOSCOPY

■ DIAGNOSTIC	■ THERAPEUTIC
Cough	Foreign bodies
Hemoptysis	Accumulated secretions
Wheeze	Atelectasis
Atelectasis	Aspiration
Unresolved pneumonia	Lung abscess
Diffuse lung disease	Reposition endotracheal tubes
Preoperative evaluation	
Rule out metastases	Placement of endobronchial tubes
Abnormal chest radiograph	
Assess local disease recurrence	Laser surgery of the airway
Recurrent laryngeal nerve palsy	
Diaphragm paralysis	
Acute inhalation injury	
Exclude tracheoesophageal fistula	
During mechanical ventilation	
Selective bronchography	

Adapted from Landa JF: Indications for bronchoscopy. Chest 1978; 73(Suppl): 686, with permission.

TABLE 40-4

INSTRUMENTS OF CHOICE FOR BRONCHOSCOPY

■ RIGID
Foreign bodies
Massive hemoptysis
Vascular tumors
Small children
Endobronchial resections

■ FIBEROPTIC/FLEXIBLE
Mechanical problems of neck
Upper lobe and peripheral lesions
Limited hemoptysis
During mechanical ventilation
Pneumonia, for selective cultures
Positioning of double-lumen tubes
Difficult intubation
Checking position of endotracheal tube
Bronchial blockade

Adapted from Landa JF: Indication for bronchoscopy. Chest 1978; 73(Suppl): 686, with permission.

nectors should be checked for compatibility. Monitoring during bronchoscopy should include an electrocardiogram, a blood pressure cuff, a precordial stethoscope, and a pulse oximeter. If thoracotomy is planned, an arterial cannula should also be placed, as well as other monitors (e.g., PA or CVP catheters) that may be indicated by the patient's condition. Many anesthetic techniques are useful for bronchoscopy.

Local Anesthesia

The patient should first be pretreated with a drying agent. The local anesthetics most commonly used are lidocaine and tetracaine. In all cases, the total dose of anesthetic must be considered and the potential for toxicity recognized. A nebulizer can be used to spray the oropharynx and base of the tongue, or the patient may gargle with viscous (2%) lidocaine. The tongue is then held forward, and pledgets soaked in local anesthetic are held in each piriform fossa using Krause forceps to achieve block of the internal branch of the superior laryngeal nerve (see Chapter 29). Tracheal anesthesia is achieved by a transtracheal injection of local anesthetic, or by spraying the vocal cords and trachea under direct vision using a laryngoscope or through the suction channel of the bronchofiberscope. Alternatively, a superior laryngeal nerve block can be performed by an external approach, and a glossopharyngeal block can be used to depress the gag reflex. These blocks cause depression of airway reflexes, so patients must be kept on nothing by mouth status for several hours after the examination. If fiberoptic bronchoscopy is to be performed transnasally, the nasal mucosa should be pretreated topically with 4% cocaine, or viscous lidocaine may be administered through the nares. Local anesthesia for bronchoscopy has the advantages of a patient who is awake, cooperative, and breathing spontaneously. Sedatives may be added to make the patient more comfortable. Disadvantages of local anesthesia include poor tolerance of any bleeding by the patient and the occasional lack of patient cooperation.

General Anesthesia

General anesthesia for bronchoscopy is often combined with topical laryngeal anesthesia so less general anesthesia is needed. A balanced technique uses N_2O/O_2, incremental doses of an intravenous drug such as thiopental, an opioid, and a neuromuscular blocking drug. A potent inhaled anesthetic technique is also satisfactory. The use of N_2O and potent inhaled agents may create an operating room atmosphere contamination problem for the waste anesthesia gases, but limited scavenging may be possible by placing a suction catheter in the patient's oropharynx. Unless there is some contraindication, ventilation of the lungs is usually controlled. In any patient undergoing a thoracic diagnostic procedure for a suspected malignancy, the possibility of the myasthenic syndrome with sensitivity to nondepolarizing muscle relaxants must always be considered. The doses of neuromuscular blocking drugs should be titrated to effect using a neuromuscular monitoring system.

Rigid Bronchoscopy

A modern rigid ventilating bronchoscope is essentially a hollow tube with a blunted, beveled tip. Various sizes and designs are available; however, in all of them, a side arm is provided for connection to an anesthesia source. A number of techniques have been described for maintaining ventilation and oxygenation during rigid bronchoscopic examination.

Apneic Oxygenation.

After preoxygenation and induction of general anesthesia, skeletal muscle paralysis and cessation of intermittent positive-pressure breathing, the $PaCO_2$ increases. During the first minute the increase is approximately 6 mm Hg. Subsequently, the average rate of increase is 3 mm Hg/min. Oxygen is insufflated at 10 to 15 L/min through a small catheter placed above the carina. The apneic period should not be allowed to extend beyond 5 minutes, however, because the technique is limited by buildup of CO_2, respiratory acidosis, and cardiac dysrhythmias.

Apnea and Intermittent Ventilation.

Oxygen and anesthesia gases are delivered to the bronchoscope via the anesthesia circuit. Ventilation is possible only when the eyepiece is in place, which limits the period for instrumentation by the surgeon. Intermittent ventilation of the lungs is achieved by squeezing the reservoir bag. In this way, assuming a good bronchoscope fit in the airway, compliance is constantly monitored, the risk of barotrauma is reduced, and V_T may be estimated. The disadvantage of this technique is that there may be a leak around the bronchoscope, which could lead to hypoventilation and hypercarbia. Packing of the oropharynx can reduce the leak, and improve ventilation in the case of such a gas leak.

Sanders Injection System.

Oxygen from a high-pressure source (50 psig) is delivered, using a controllable pressure-reducing valve and toggle switch, to a 2.5- to 3.5-cm 18- or 16-gauge needle inside and parallel to the long axis of the bronchoscope. When the toggle switch is depressed, the jet of oxygen entering the bronchoscope entrains room air, and the air–oxygen mixture resulting at the distal tip of the bronchoscope emerges at a pressure to provide adequate ventilation and oxygenation. The intraluminal tracheal pressure depends on the driving pressure from the reducing valve, the size of the needle jet, and the length, internal diameter, and design of the bronchoscope. Increasing the size of the needle jet increases the total gas flow for any given driving pressure. For each combination of gas-driving pressure, jet orifice, and bronchoscope diameter, only one inflation pressure can be attained, regardless of the volume or compliance of the lung. As long as the proximal end of the bronchoscope is open, the system is strictly pressure limited, and the pressure does not increase because of obstruction at the distal end. Pressure varies inversely with the cross-sectional area of the bronchoscope, so insertion of a suction catheter or biopsy forceps into the lumen causes the intratracheal pressure to increase. Provided there is

not a tight fit between the bronchoscope and the airway, the risk of barotrauma is low. If the fit is tight, driving pressure should be decreased.

The advantages of the Sanders system are that because continuous ventilation is possible (because the presence of an eyepiece is not necessary for ventilation of the lungs), the duration of the bronchoscopy procedure is minimized, but the efficiency also permits extended bronchoscopy. A disadvantage is that entrainment of air by the oxygen jet results in a variable F_{IO_2} at the distal end of the bronchoscope, ventilation of the lungs may be inadequate if compliance is poor, and adequacy of ventilation may be difficult to assess.

Mechanical Ventilator.

Ventilation of the lungs may be achieved by connecting a mechanical ventilator to an anesthesia circuit that is connected to the bronchoscope side arm. One disadvantage of this ventilation technique is the presence of a leak of anesthesia gases, and consequentially, light anesthesia.

High-Frequency Positive-Pressure Ventilation.

HFPPV has been used in conjunction with rigid bronchoscopy and has been compared with the Sanders injector in patients with tracheobronchial stenosis. With HFPPV of up to 150 breaths/min, blood gases were identical with both techniques. At a frequency of 500 breaths/min, oxygenation deteriorated and CO_2 was not removed effectively. HFPPV has the advantage that the tracheobronchial wall remains immobilized during ventilation. A Food and Drug Administration–approved high-frequency jet ventilator is available from Acutronic Medical Systems AG (Hirzel, Switzerland).

Fiberoptic Bronchoscopy

The recent generations of fiberscopes, with their improved optics and smaller diameters, have revolutionized bronchoscopy. The flexibility has also been applied in preoperative assessment of the airway, management of difficult tracheal intubations, endotracheal tube positioning and change, bronchial toilet, correct positioning of DLTs, bronchial blockade, and evaluation of the larynx and trachea. Nasal fiberoptic bronchoscopy under topical anesthesia is well tolerated by most awake patients. The administration of an antisialogogue such as glycopyrrolate is useful in reducing secretions. Oral insertion is also possible in both awake and asleep patients and should be performed with a bite block in place to prevent damage to the bronchoscope.

Physiologic Changes Associated with Fiberoptic Bronchoscopy.

In all patients, insertion of the fiberoptic bronchoscope is associated with hypoxemia. The average decline in PaO_2 is 20 mm Hg and lasts for 1 to 4 hours after the procedure. By 24 hours, the blood gas tensions are usually back to normal. It is therefore recommended that if the initial PaO_2 is 70 mm Hg (F_{IO_2} = 0.21), bronchoscopy should be performed only with the administration of supplemental oxygen. This can be provided using mouth-held nasal prongs, a special face mask with a diaphragm through which the fiberscope can be passed, or an endotracheal tube with a T-piece diaphragm adapter.

During and after fiberoptic bronchoscopy, patients experience increased airway obstruction. Thus, in 35 patients, insertion of the bronchoscope was associated with an increase in FRC (17 to 30%) and decreases in PaO_2, vital capacity, FEV_1, and forced inspiratory flow.[99] All returned to baseline by 24 hours. These changes are believed to be secondary to direct mechanical activation of irritative reflexes in the airway and, possibly, to mucosal edema. They may be avoided if atropine, either intramuscular or aerosolized into the airway, is administered before the procedure.

The standard adult fiberoptic bronchoscope has an external diameter of 5.7 mm and a 2-mm diameter suction channel.

If suction at 1 atm is applied to the fiberscope, air is removed at a rate of 14 L/min. If the fiberscope is in the airway, this causes decreases in FIO_2, PaO_2, and FRC, leading to decreased PaO_2. Suctioning should therefore be kept brief. The adult fiberscope can be passed through endotracheal tubes of 7 mm or greater internal diameter. Clearly, passage through an endotracheal tube decreases the cross-sectional area available for ventilating the patient, so if fibroscopy is planned, an endotracheal tube of the largest possible diameter should be used.

Insertion of the bronchoscope also causes a significant PEEP effect that may result in barotrauma in ventilated patients. If PEEP is already being used, it should be discontinued before passage of the fiberscope. A postendoscopy chest radiograph is advisable to exclude the presence of mediastinal emphysema or pneumothorax. In patients whose tracheas are intubated with endotracheal tubes of <8 mm internal diameter, use of pediatric fiberscopes, which have smaller diameters, would be more appropriate.

The suction channel of the adult fiberoptic bronchoscope has been used to oxygenate and ventilate the lungs of patients. By attaching a jet ventilation system (similar to that used to drive the Sanders injector for rigid bronchoscopy) to the suction connection at the head of a fiberoptic bronchoscope, successful ventilation of the lungs of patients undergoing gynecologic procedures was achieved.[100] A driving pressure of 50 psig of oxygen was used with a ventilatory rate of 18 to 20 breaths/min. This technique permitted adequate ventilation of patients with normally compliant lungs and chest walls. Ventilation of the lungs should be performed only with the tip of the instrument in the trachea because a more peripheral location may produce barotrauma.

Neodymium-yttrium-aluminum garnet (Nd-YAG) lasers are used for the resection of obstructing and endobronchial lesions (see Chapter 50). This procedure is performed under general anesthesia. The lasers may be introduced into the bronchial tree through a fiberoptic bundle passed via the suction port of the fiberoptic bronchoscope. During laser resection, FIO_2 should be kept to a minimum and titrated against oxygen saturation (as continuously monitored by pulse oximeter) to make endotracheal fire less likely (see Chapter 8). Laser therapy of bronchial tumors is also possible using a rigid bronchoscope. HFPPV through a rigid bronchoscope provides satisfactory operating conditions for laser resection of tracheal tumors and has the advantage of producing airway immobility.

Complications of Bronchoscopy

Complications of rigid bronchoscopy include mechanical trauma to the teeth, hemorrhage, bronchospasm, loss of a sponge, bronchial or tracheal perforation, subglottic edema, and barotrauma. The incidence of complications is much lower with fiberoptic bronchoscopy. Nevertheless, complications may arise owing to overdose with topical anesthetic, insertion trauma, local trauma, hemorrhage, upper airway obstruction related to passage of the instrument through an area of tracheal stenosis, hypoxemia, and bronchospasm. In most cases, it is best to intubate the trachea with an endotracheal tube after bronchoscopy under general anesthesia. This permits avoidance or treatment of some of these problems, particularly the increased airway irritability. Intubation also facilitates effective suctioning of the trachea and bronchi, and allows the patient to recover more gradually from general anesthesia.

DIAGNOSTIC PROCEDURES FOR MEDIASTINAL MASS

Patients with an anterior mediastinal mass may present a special problem for the anesthesiologist. Although such masses

may cause obvious superior vena cava obstruction, they may also cause obstruction of major airways and cardiac compression, which are less obvious and may become apparent only on induction of anesthesia. Many cases of anesthetic-related airway compression from anterior mediastinal mass have been reported. In one case, total occlusion of the trachea starting 2 to 3 cm above the carina and extending to both main stem bronchi was observed, and a bronchoscope was passed through the obstruction.[101] In the second case of this report, extrinsic compression of the left main stem bronchus occurred on inspiration during recovery from anesthesia. In the third case, flow–volume studies were performed with the patient in the upright and supine positions, with marked reductions in FEV_1 and peak expiratory flow in the latter position. These findings suggested potential obstruction with onset of anesthesia; radiation therapy to the mediastinum was commenced, after which the flow–volume studies showed improved function. The planned surgical procedure was then performed under local anesthesia. In a more recent series of 105 patients with mediastinal masses, the incidence of intraoperative cardiorespiratory complications was 38%, and the incidence of postoperative respiratory complications was 11%.[102] No cases of airway collapse were reported during anesthesia. In this series, patients were at increased risk of complications if there were preoperative cardiorespiratory signs and symptoms, obstructive and restrictive dysfunction on pulmonary function tests, and >50% tracheal compression on CT scan.[103] In another series of patients with mediastinal mass, four patients had abnormal spirometry but underwent general anesthesia without sequealae.[104] In severe cases of airway compression, femoral vessels may be cannulated prior to induction to institute cardiopulmonary bypass.[105]

The mass may be sensitive to radiation therapy, which could shrink the tumor and make an induction of general anesthesia less hazardous. However, a serious potential disadvantage of preoperative radiation therapy is that it may affect tissue histologic appearance, thereby preventing an accurate diagnosis. Furthermore, if the patient is a child, it may be difficult to obtain tissue samples under local anesthesia. No fatalities occurred in a series of 44 patients aged 18 years of age or younger with anterior mediastinal masses who underwent general anesthesia before radiation or chemotherapy. However, seven patients did have airway compromise.[106] In another report in a series of children, it was found to be safe to induce general anesthesia if the CT scan revealed that the tracheal cross-sectional area and peak expiratory flow rates were at least 50% of predicted.[107]

Airway obstruction caused by an anterior mediastinal mass has been attributed to changes in lung and chest wall mechanics associated with changes in position or to onset of paralysis in muscles that previously maintained airway patency. Preoperative evaluation of a patient with an anterior mediastinal mass to avoid life-threatening total airway obstruction is shown in Figure 40-21.[101] It is important to determine in the history if the patient has dyspnea in the supine position and to examine the CT scan to determine the extent of the tumor and its effect on surrounding structures. If such obstruction occurs, it may be relieved by passage of a rigid bronchoscope or anode tube past the obstruction, by direct laryngoscopy,[108] or by changing the position of the patient.

In a situation in which the biopsy procedure cannot be performed under local anesthesia and there is concern that muscle paralysis may result in airway compression, fiberoptic intubation of the awake patient followed by general anesthesia with spontaneous ventilation has been described. Thus, during spontaneous inspiration, the normal transpulmonary pressure gradient distends the airways and helps maintain their patency, even in the presence of extrinsic compression.

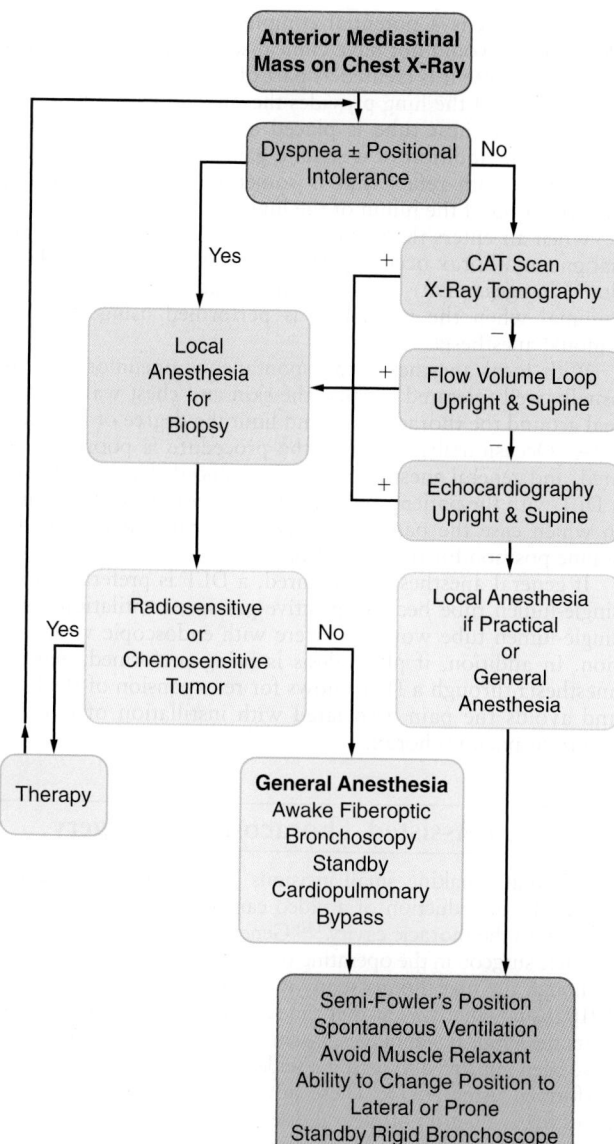

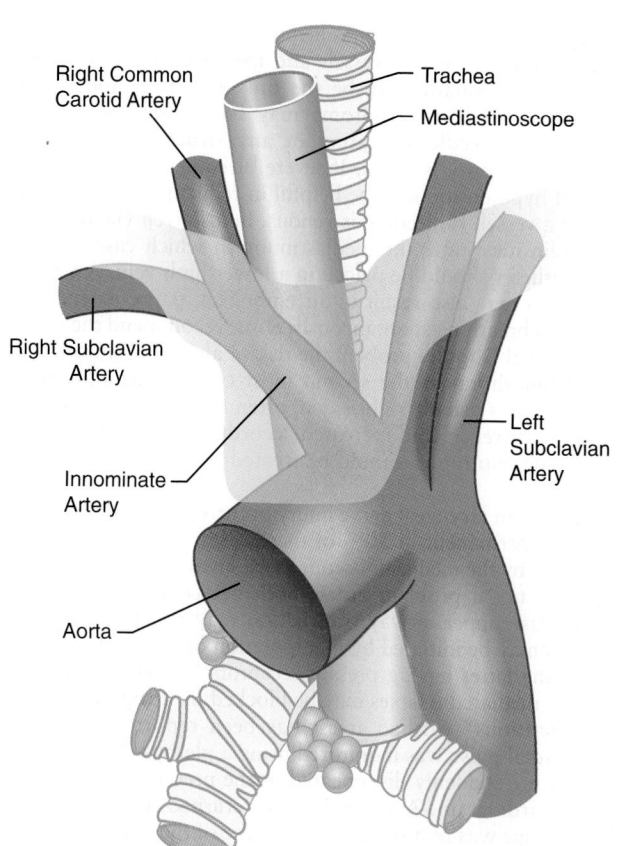

FIGURE 40-22.   Anatomic relationships during mediastinoscopy. Note the position of the mediastinoscope behind the right innominate artery and aortic arch and anterior to the trachea. (From Carlens E: Mediastinoscopy: A method for inspection and tissue biopsy in the superior mediastinum. Dis Chest 1959; 36: 343.)

FIGURE 40-21.   Flow chart describing the preoperative evaluation of the patient with an anterior mediastinal mass. +, indicates positive finding; –, indicates negative workup. (Reprinted from Neuman GG, Weingarten AE, Abramowitz RM et al: Anesthetic management of the patient with an anterior mediastinal mass. Anesthesiology 1984; 60: 144, with permission.)

Mediastinoscopy

Mediastinoscopy was introduced as a means of assessing spread of bronchial carcinoma. The lymphatics of the lung drain first to the subcarinal and paratracheal areas, and then to the sides of the trachea, the supraclavicular areas, and the thoracic duct. Examination of these nodes has provided a tissue diagnosis and greater selectivity of patients for thoracotomy. It is most useful in right-lung tumors because left-lung cancers tend to spread to subaortic nodes that are more accessible by an anterior mediastinoscopy in the second or third interspace (Chamberlain procedure). The transcervical approach to the thymus is an adaptation of mediastinoscopy.

The anesthetic considerations for mediastinoscopy follow naturally from an understanding of the anatomy of this procedure and its potential complications. For cervical medi-

astinoscopy, the patient is placed in a reverse Trendelenburg (i.e., head-up) position, and the mediastinoscope is inserted into the superior mediastinum through a transverse incision just above the suprasternal notch. The instrument is advanced along the anterior aspect of the trachea and passes behind the innominate vessels and the aortic arch (Fig. 40-22). The left recurrent nerve is vulnerable as it loops around the aortic arch, and any of these structures may be traumatized. Because of scarring, previous mediastinoscopy may be considered a contraindication to a repeat examination. Relative contraindications include superior vena cava obstruction, tracheal deviation, and aneurysm of the thoracic aorta.

Preoperative evaluation should include a search for airway obstruction or distortion. Review of a CT scan is very helpful in this regard. Evidence of impaired cerebral circulation, history of stroke, or signs of the Eaton-Lambert syndrome resulting from oat cell carcinoma should be sought. Blood must be available for the procedure because hemorrhage is a real risk and may be life-threatening.

Most surgeons and anesthesiologists prefer general anesthesia using an endotracheal tube and continuous ventilation because this offers a more controlled situation and greater flexibility in terms of surgical manipulation. The anesthetic technique should include a muscle relaxant to prevent the patient from coughing because this may produce venous engorgement in the chest or trauma by the mediastinoscope to surrounding structures.

The incidence of morbidity with mediastinoscopy has been reported as 1.5 to 3.0%, and that of mortality as 0.09%. The most common complication is hemorrhage (0.73%) because of the proximity of major vessels and the vascularity of certain tumors. Tamponade may be the only recourse, and thoracotomy or median sternotomy may be required to achieve hemostasis. Needle aspiration of any structure is essential before any biopsy is taken. If severe bleeding occurs, induced arterial hypotension may be helpful in reducing the size of the tear in a vessel. If bleeding is venous, fluids given via an upper limb vein may enter the mediastinum, in which case a large-bore catheter should be placed in a lower limb vein. A venous laceration may also result in air embolism, particularly if the patient is breathing spontaneously. Some recommend the use of a precordial Doppler probe if the risk of air embolism is likely.

Pneumothorax is the second most common complication (0.66%). It is usually right-sided, often recognized at the time of the occurrence, and is treated according to size. A symptomatic pneumothorax should be treated by chest tube decompression.

Recurrent laryngeal nerve injury occurred in 0.34% of cases and was permanent in 50% of these cases. The nerve may be damaged by the mediastinoscope or be involved in tumor. Such injury is not a problem unless both nerves are damaged, in which case upper airway obstruction may result. Autonomic reflexes may be initiated by manipulation of the trachea or the aorta, the latter having pressor receptors located in the arch. Vagally mediated reflexes may be blocked by atropine.

"Factitious" cardiac arrest has been reported when the right radial pulse was monitored using a plethysmograph, and the tracing suddenly disappeared in the presence of a normal electrocardiogram. A normal pulse returned after the mediastinoscope was removed, and the cause of the apparent arrest was pressure on the innominate artery by the instrument. Decreases in right arm as compared with left arm blood pressure have been reported in cases undergoing mediastinoscopy. Duration was 15 to 360 seconds. This is of particular significance if there is a history of impaired cerebral circulation or transient ischemic attacks, or if a carotid bruit is present, because transient left hemiparesis may occur after mediastinoscopy. It is therefore recommended that blood pressure be monitored in the left arm and that the right radial pulse be monitored continuously during mediastinoscopy. A decrease in the right radial pulse amplitude is an indication for repositioning the mediastinoscope, especially in a patient with a history of cerebrovascular disease.

Other reported complications include acute tracheal collapse, tension pneumomediastinum, mediastinitis, hemothorax, and chylothorax. A chest radiograph taken in the immediate postoperative period is a useful precaution in all patients after mediastinoscopy.

Thoracoscopy

Thoracoscopy (medical thoracoscopy) involves the insertion of an endoscope into the thoracic cavity and pleural space. It is used for the diagnosis of pleural disease, effusions, and infectious disease (especially in immunosuppressed patients and those with acquired immunodeficiency syndrome) and for staging procedures, chemical pleurodesis, and lung biopsy. It is usually performed by the pulmonary physician in the clinic, under local anesthesia. It is also used in therapeutic procedures such as CO_2 laser treatment of spontaneous pneumothorax or bullous emphysema[109] and Nd-YAG laser vaporization of malignant pleural tumors. A small incision is made in the lateral chest wall, and with the insertion of the instrument, fluid and biopsy specimens are easily obtained.

This procedure may be performed using local, regional, or general anesthesia, the choice depending on the expected duration of the procedure and the physical status of the patient.

Pneumothorax is a potential complication of an intercostal block, but it would not have clinical sequelae during a thoracoscopy because it is created as part of the surgical procedure. The collapse of the lung provides the surgeon with a working space, and a chest tube is placed at the conclusion of the surgery. The addition of a stellate ganglion block helps suppress the cough reflex that is sometimes provoked during manipulation of the hilum of the lung.

When air enters the pleural cavity under inspection, a partial pneumothorax occurs, permitting good surgical visualization. Changes in PaO_2, $PaCO_2$, and cardiac rhythm are usually minimal when the procedure is performed using local or regional anesthesia.

With local anesthesia, the spontaneous pneumothorax is usually well tolerated because the skin and chest wall form a seal around the thoracoscope and limit the degree of lung collapse. Occasionally, however, the procedure is poorly tolerated, and general anesthesia must be induced. The insertion of a DLT with the patient in the lateral position may be difficult, in which case the patient may be temporarily placed in the supine position for the intubation.

If general anesthesia is required, a DLT is preferable to a single-lumen tube because positive-pressure ventilation via a single-lumen tube would interfere with endoscopic visualization. In addition, if pleurodesis is being performed, general anesthesia through a DLT allows for re-expansion of the lung and avoids the pain associated with instillation of talc for recurrent pneumothorax.

Video-Assisted Thoracoscopic Surgery

VATS entails making small incisions in the chest wall, which allows the introduction of a video camera and surgical instruments into the thoracic cavity.[110] Generally, it is performed by a thoracic surgeon in the operating room under general anesthesia. Although the first thoracoscopy was performed by Jacobeus in 1910, using what was at that time a cystoscope, in more recent years the surgical techniques, instruments, and video technology have been improved to permit a wide variety of procedures to be performed using VATS. These now include diagnostic procedures for evaluation of pleural disease and effusions, staging of lung cancer, and the identification of parenchymal disease, including nodules, mediastinal tumors, and pericardial disease. They also include therapeutic procedures such as operations for pleural disease, including pleurodesis, decortication and drainage of empyema, resection of lung tissue or bullae, pericardial window or stripping, and esophageal surgery. Even lung lobectomies can now be performed by VATS.

Anesthesia Considerations

As with a traditional thoracotomy, the patient needs to be in the lateral decubitus position, and lung collapse is needed for adequate surgical exposure. This generally mandates the use of a lung-separation technique. VATS is most commonly performed under general anesthesia with OLV. The need for OLV is much greater with VATS than with open thoracotomy because it is not possible to retract the lung during VATS as it is during an open thoracotomy. The operated lung should be deflated as soon as possible after tracheal intubation and positioning because it may take over 30 minutes for complete lung collapse to occur. Also, the surgeon enters the thoracic cavity much sooner during VATS than with open thoracotomy. Suction applied to the airway can help facilitate a more rapid deflation of the lung. In some cases, carbon dioxide is insufflated into the pleural cavity to facilitate visualization. Insufflation pressures should be maintained as low as possible and the CO_2 inflow rate kept <2 L/min. Higher pressures can cause mediastinal shift, hemodynamic compromise, increases in airway pressure, and increases in end-tidal CO_2. Hemodynamic compromise presents a picture similar to that because of tension pneumothorax. Significant hemodynamic changes can be produced when pressures of as little as 5 mm Hg are used to insufflate CO_2 into the chest cavity.[111]

CPAP is commonly used for the treatment of hypoxemia during OLV for thoracotomy and is usually very effective. However, during VATS, CPAP interferes with the surgical exposure and is therefore best avoided. It would be preferable to use PEEP to the nonoperated (dependent lung). In addition, a lower PaO_2 may have to be tolerated during VATS compared with a thoracotomy.

Postoperative Concerns

There is less pain after VATS than open thoracotomy, and an epidural catheter is usually placed before surgery only if there is a likelihood that a thoracotomy may need to be performed. A lobectomy can be performed by VAT, but an open thoracotomy may be required. The patient's respiratory function is better preserved after VATS, and their recovery is faster. However, postoperative dysrhythmias, which commonly occur after thoracotomy, have also been reported after VATS.[112] Other complications that may occur include bleeding, pulmonary edema, and pneumonia.

ANESTHESIA FOR SPECIAL SITUATIONS

Management of patients with bronchopleural fistula (BPF), empyema, cysts, and bullae, as well as those requiring tracheal reconstruction, is considered here. Many of these patients are appropriately managed using high-frequency ventilatory techniques; therefore, these techniques are described first (see Chapter 29).

High-Frequency Ventilation

With conventional positive-pressure ventilation, V_T and rates usually exceed or approach those in the normal, spontaneously breathing patient. Gas transport to the alveoli occurs by convection in the larger airways, and then by convection and molecular diffusion in the more distal airways and alveoli. High-frequency ventilation differs from conventional positive-pressure ventilation in that smaller V_T and more rapid rates are used. Gas transport may depend more on molecular diffusion, high-velocity flow, and coaxial gas flow in the airways, with gas in the center moving distally and that in the periphery moving proximally.

There are three different types of high-frequency ventilation. HFPPV uses small V_T at rates of 60 to 120 breaths/min (1 to 2 Hz). The ventilator used has a negligible internal compliance so the V_T generated, which usually approximates the dead space volume, equals the volume set on the ventilator and represents all fresh gas. The high instantaneous gas flows generated facilitate gas exchange and movement in the conducting airways.

HFPPV may be delivered by an open or a closed system. An example of the former is the percutaneous placement of a transtracheal catheter or placement of a catheter through the nose or mouth with its distal end above the carina. Inflow is intraluminal and outflow is extraluminal. This technique has been used during bronchoscopy, tracheal resection, and reconstructive surgery. When open systems are used, the gas outflow pathway is not established mechanically and depends on natural airway patency. It is therefore subject to compromise. Also, aspiration is a potential complication with open systems.

The closed system is superior because it integrates both airway patency and outflow protection. A closed system is represented by a catheter placed in a short segment of an endotracheal tube for delivery of the HFPPV, whereas the remainder of the tube lumen represents the exit pathway for gas. A quadruple-lumen endotracheal tube (Hi-Lo Jet Tracheal Tube, Mallinckrodt, Inc.) has been designed specifically for delivery of HFPPV. One lumen is for the HFPPV delivery, one for gas outflow, one for cuff inflation, and one for measuring airway pressures at the distal end of the tube. The use of a closed system also permits application of PEEP, a situation not possible with an open arrangement.

High-frequency jet ventilation (HFJV) uses a pulse of a small jet of fresh gas introduced from a high-pressure source (50 psig) into the airway through a small catheter or additional lumen in an endotracheal tube. Rates used are usually 100 to 400 breaths/min. The fresh gas jet entrains gas from an injection cannula side-port reservoir. This system is somewhat analogous to the Sanders injector system described in the "Bronchoscopy" section, and FIO_2 is similarly variable. The jet and entrained gas flows cause forward motion of the mass of gas in the airways. HFJV can be used with an open system or with a closed arrangement, as described earlier. In the latter, PEEP may be added to enhance oxygenation. Also, with use of high fresh gas flows from an anesthesia circuit, inhaled anesthetics may be delivered as an entrained gas mixture.

High-frequency oscillation ventilation uses a mechanism that oscillates gas at rates of 400 to 2,400 breaths/min. It has not been described in association with thoracic surgical procedures. In this system, V_T is small (50 to 80 mL), and gas exchange occurs through enhanced molecular diffusion and coaxial airway flow.

The potential advantages offered by HFPPV during thoracic anesthesia are that lower V_T and inspiratory pressures result in a quiet lung field for the surgeon, with minimal movements of airway, lung tissue, and mediastinum. Thus, HFPPV has been used to ventilate both the nondependent and the dependent lung during thoracic surgical procedures, with adequate arterial blood gas measurements obtained throughout. At high frequencies (>6 Hz), however, CO_2 retention may become a problem.

HFJV has been used to ventilate the nondependent lung to improve PaO_2 during one-lung anesthesia, whereas the dependent lung was ventilated with conventional intermittent positive-pressure ventilation. PaO_2 increased compared with that obtained during simple collapse of the nondependent lung. A study comparing HFJV with CPAP to the nondependent lung during conventional intermittent positive-pressure ventilation to the dependent lung found that both improved PaO_2 significantly during closed and open stages of the surgery. When the chest was open, HFJV maintained satisfactory cardiac output, whereas CPAP usually decreased cardiac output; however, there were no significant differences in $PaCO_2$ between HFJV and CPAP. Because similar increases in PaO_2 may be obtained using selective CPAP to the nondependent lung and much simpler equipment than that necessary to deliver high-frequency ventilation, the use of CPAP would seem preferable to high-frequency ventilation to increase PaO_2 during most one-lung anesthesia situations.

The lower pressures and V_Ts associated with high-frequency ventilation result in a small leak through BPFs, and HFJV is now generally considered the conservative treatment of choice in this condition. Another advantage of high-frequency ventilation is that the rapid-rate small V_T can be delivered through small tubes or catheters so if an airway has to be divided, the passage of a small tube across the surgical field permits ventilation of the distal airway and lung tissue. This use has been applied during sleeve resection of the lung, tracheal reconstruction, and surgery for tracheal stenosis. In all three situations, the surgeon is able to work easily around the small catheter used to provide the high-frequency ventilation.

Bronchopleural Fistula and Empyema

A BPF is an abnormal communication between the bronchial tree and the pleural cavity. Occasionally, there is an additional communication to the surface of the chest, a cutaneous BPF. BPF occurs most commonly after pulmonary resection for carcinoma. Other causes include traumatic rupture of a bronchus or bulla (sometimes caused by barotrauma or PEEP), penetrating chest wound, or spontaneous drainage into the bronchial tree of an empyema cavity or lung cyst. The incidence of BPF is higher after pneumonectomy than following other types of lung resection. The problems associated with BPF and empyema are that positive-pressure ventilation may result in contamination of healthy lung, loss of air, decreased alveolar ventilation leading to CO_2 retention, and the development of a tension pneumothorax.

If an empyema is present, it should be drained under local anesthesia before any surgery to close the BPF. Drainage is performed with the patient sitting up and leaning toward the affected side. Empyemas are often loculated, and complete drainage is not always possible. A drain to an underwater seal system is left in the cavity before administration of anesthesia for surgery of the BPF, and after drainage of an empyema, a chest radiograph should be obtained to determine the efficacy of the procedure.

The priorities in the anesthetic management of BPF are the isolation of the affected side in terms of contamination and ventilation. The ideal approach is intubation of the trachea while the patient is awake using a DLT with the patient breathing spontaneously. Supplemental oxygen should be administered, and the patient should be constantly reassured. Neuroleptanalgesia is satisfactory in providing a suitably cooperative patient, and the airway is then pretreated with topical anesthesia. The endobronchial tube selected should be such that the bronchial lumen is on the side opposite the BPF. Selection of the largest possible tube provides a close fit in the trachea, which helps stabilize the tube. Once the tube is adequately positioned in the trachea, there may be a considerable outpouring of pus from the tracheal lumen if an empyema is present; therefore, this lumen should be immediately suctioned using a large-bore suction catheter. The healthy and possibly the affected lung may then be ventilated; adequacy of oxygenation and ventilation is assessed by pulse oximetry and arterial blood gas analysis.

An alternative technique is to insert the DLT under general anesthesia, with the patient breathing spontaneously to avoid a tension pneumothorax. With either technique, the chest drainage tube must be left unclamped to avoid any bouts of coughing and to prevent the buildup of a tension pneumothorax in the event that a predisposing valvular mechanism exists. In patients who do not have an empyema, use of a single-lumen tube has been described and may be satisfactory if the BPF and air leak are small. A rapid-sequence induction with ketamine or thiopental followed by a relaxant has also been described, but is associated with considerable risk of contamination and tension pneumothorax.

BPF may also be treated conservatively using various ventilatory techniques. Thus, the bronchus of the normal lung may be intubated and ventilated, allowing the BPF to rest and heal. This approach may result in an intolerable shunt, however, and PEEP may be necessary to maintain PaO_2. Differential lung ventilation using a DLT has also been described, the healthy lung being ventilated with normal Vt, while the affected lung is exposed to a smaller Vt or to CPAP with oxygen at pressures just below the critical opening pressure of the fistula. The critical opening pressure of the BPF can be assessed by determining the lowest level of CPAP that must be applied to the bronchus on the affected side to produce continuous bubbling through the underwater seal chest drain.

For a large BPF, HFJV may be the nonsurgical treatment of choice. The use of small Vts results in minimal gas loss through the fistula, which may heal more quickly. In addition, hemodynamic effects are usually minimal and spontaneous efforts at ventilation are usually abolished, thereby decreasing the work of breathing and eliminating the need for relaxants or excessive sedation.

Lung Cysts and Bullae

Air-filled cysts of the lung are usually bronchogenic, postinfective, infantile, or emphysematous. They may be associated with COPD or be an isolated finding. A *bulla* is a thin-walled space filled with air that results from the destruction of alveolar tissue. The walls are, therefore, composed of visceral pleura, connective tissue septa, or compressed lung tissue. In general, bullae represent an area of end-stage emphysematous destruction of the lung.

Patients may be considered for surgical bullectomy when dyspnea is incapacitating, when the bullae are expanding, when there are repeated pneumothoraces owing to rupture of bullae, or if the bullae compress a large area of normal lung. Most of these patients have severe COPD and CO_2 retention, and little functional respiratory reserve. The first consideration in management is maintenance of a high FIO_2. If the bulla or cyst communicates with the bronchial tree, positive-pressure ventilation may cause it to expand or even to rupture, if it is compliant, producing a situation analogous to tension pneumothorax. If the bulla is very compliant, most of the applied Vt may be wasted in this additional dead space. Nitrous oxide should be avoided because it causes expansion of any air spaces in the body, including bullae. Once the chest is open, even more of the Vt may enter the compliant bulla, which is no longer limited by chest wall integrity, and an increase in ventilation is needed until the bulla is controlled.

The anesthetic management of these patients is challenging, particularly if the disease is bilateral. Ideally, a DLT is inserted with the patient awake or under general anesthesia but breathing spontaneously. The avoidance of positive-pressure ventilation (when possible) helps decrease the likelihood of the potential problems described previously, although oxygenation may be precarious with spontaneous ventilation. Once the endotracheal tube is in place, each lung may be controlled separately, and adequate ventilation can be applied to the healthy lung if bilateral disease is not present. Gentle positive-pressure ventilation with rapid, small Vt and pressures not to exceed 10 cm H_2O may be used during the induction and maintenance of anesthesia, especially if the bullae have been shown to have no or only poor bronchial communication by preoperative ventilation scanning. While the surgery is being performed, as each bulla is resected, the operated lung can be separately ventilated to check for air leaks and the presence of additional bullae.

If positive-pressure ventilation is to be applied before the chest is opened, the possibility of a tension pneumothorax must be kept in mind, and treatment should be readily available. The diagnosis of pneumothorax may be made by a unilateral decrease in breath sounds (this may be difficult to distinguish in a patient with bullous disease), increase in ventilatory pressure, progressive tracheal deviation, wheezing, or cardiovascular changes. Treatment of a pneumothorax involves the rapid placement of a chest tube. An added risk of chest tube placement is the creation of a cutaneous BPF, which causes problems for ventilation. Alternatively, general anesthesia is induced only after the surgeon has prepared the operative field and draped the patient. In the event of sudden deterioration in the patient's condition during induction, the surgeon may perform an immediate median sternotomy. In any event, the time from induction of anesthesia to sternotomy must be kept to a minimum.

To avoid these problems in a patient with known bullae, HFJV has been used in a patient with a large bulla undergoing coronary artery bypass graft and in another patient undergoing bilateral bullectomy. If bilateral bullectomy is to be performed, a median sternotomy is usually used. Benumof[113] described the use of sequential OLV using a DLT in the management of a patient needing bilateral bullectomy. The side with the largest bulla and least lung function, as assessed before surgery by ventilation and perfusion scans, should be operated on first. In this way, the lung with the better function should support gas exchange first. If hypoxemia develops during this one-lung situation, application of CPAP to the nonventilated lung during the deflation phase of a tidal breath should increase PaO_2.

Unlike most cases of pulmonary resection, patients after bullectomy are left with a greater amount of functional lung tissue than was previously available to them, and the mechanics of respiration are improved. At the end of the procedure, the DLT is replaced by a single-lumen tube, and the patients generally require several days to be weaned from the ventilator. During this time, the positive airway pressure used should be minimized to avoid causing a pneumothorax owing to rupture of suture or staple lines or of residual bullae.

Anesthesia for Resection of the Trachea

Tracheal resection and reconstruction are technically difficult for the surgeon and challenging for the anesthesiologist. Indications for this type of procedure include congenital lesions (agenesis, stenosis), neoplasia (primary or secondary), injuries (direct or indirect), infections, and postintubation injuries (caused by an endotracheal tube or tracheotomy). For the surgical team, the major problems are maintenance of ventilation to the lungs while the airway is being operated on and postoperative integrity of the anastomoses. In this respect, the presence of lung disease sufficiently severe to require postoperative ventilatory support is a relative contraindication to tracheal resection or reconstruction.

Monitoring of these patients should include placement of an arterial cannula in the left radial artery to permit continuous measurement of blood pressure during periods of innominate artery compression. Steroids should be administered to help reduce any tracheal edema, and a high FIO_2 should be used throughout the procedure to ensure an adequate oxygen reserve at all times in the FRC so temporary interruptions of ventilation are less likely to produce hypoxemia.

Numerous methods have been reported to provide oxygenation and ventilation of the lungs during these procedures. A small-bore anode tube may be placed through and distal to an upper tracheal lesion so resection may occur around the tube. This technique is useful only in mild stenoses. Alternatively, an endotracheal tube may be passed through the glottis to above the stenosis, and a sterile endotracheal or bronchial tube may later be inserted into the trachea opened distal to the site of stenosis, with the sterile anesthesia tubing is being led across the surgical field. After resection of the lesion, the sterile and distally placed endotracheal tube is withdrawn, and the upper tube (originally passed through the glottis) is advanced across the anastomosis. With low tracheal or bronchial lesions, resection and reconstruction may be performed around an endobronchial or DLT. During these procedures, the patient is kept in a head-down position to minimize aspiration of blood and debris into the alveoli, and ventilation must be carefully monitored throughout the procedure.

Clearly, the presence of a large-bore tube in the airway may make these resections technically difficult, and the use of high-frequency ventilation techniques may improve surgical access. Thus, a small-diameter catheter or catheters may be placed across or through the stenotic lesion or transected airway(s) and ventilation to the distal airways and lungs maintained using HFPPV or HFJV. Potential disadvantages of these high-frequency ventilation techniques are that, by necessity, the system is "open" (see "High-Frequency Ventilation"), and egress of gas during exhalation may be compromised if the stenosis is tight. Also, the catheter may become occluded by blood and become displaced, and distal aspiration of debris or blood may occur. With complex resections, two anesthesia teams with two machines and anesthesia circuits or sets of ventilating equipment may be necessary to ensure adequate ventilation of the two distal airway segments, although during carinal resections, HFPPV to the left lung alone usually provides adequate oxygenation and ventilation.

After tracheal resection or reconstructive surgery, patients should be kept with the neck and head flexed to reduce tension on the anastomotic suture lines. In some cases, this is maintained by using sutures between the chin and the anterior chest wall. Extubation of the trachea is performed as early as possible to minimize tracheal trauma due to the endotracheal tube and cuff.

Bronchopulmonary Lavage

This procedure involves irrigation of the lung and bronchial tree, and is used as a treatment for alveolar proteinosis, radioactive dust inhalation, cystic fibrosis, bronchiectasis, and asthmatic bronchitis. Lung lavage is performed under general anesthesia using a DLT so one lung may be ventilated while the other is being treated with lavage fluid.[114]

The preoperative assessment of these patients should include ventilation–perfusion scans so lavage can be performed first on the more severely affected lung (i.e., the one with the least ventilation). If involvement is equal, the left lung is generally lavaged first because gas exchange should be better through the larger, right lung. Patients are premedicated and supplied with supplemental oxygen en route to the operating room.

Anesthesia is induced with an intravenous drug and maintained with an inhaled agent in oxygen to maintain the highest possible FIO_2. Muscle relaxation facilitates placement of the DLT, and the cuff seal should be checked to maintain perfect separation at a pressure of 50 cm H_2O to prevent leakage of lavage fluid around the cuff. A fiberoptic bronchoscope is useful to check the position of the bronchial cuff of the DLT. Monitoring should include an arterial catheter, and a stethoscope should be placed over the ventilated lung to check for rales, the presence of which may indicate leakage of lavage fluid into this lung.

The patient is maintained on an FIO_2 of 1.0 throughout the procedure. Before lavage, this serves to denitrogenate the lungs so only oxygen and carbon dioxide remain. Instillation of fluid then allows these gases to be absorbed, resulting in greater access by the fluid to the alveolar spaces than if the more insoluble nitrogen bubbles remained.

Once the trachea is intubated, the patient is turned so the side to be lavaged is lowermost, and the DLT position and seal are checked once again. With the patient in a head-up position, warmed heparinized isotonic saline is infused by gravity from a reservoir 30 cm above the midaxillary line into the catheter to the dependent lung, while the nondependent lung is ventilated. When fluid ceases to flow in (usually after 700 to 1,000 mL in an adult), the patient is placed in a head-down position and fluid is allowed to drain out. The lavage is continued until the effluent is clear (as opposed to the milky fluid that drains initially when lavage is being performed for alveolar proteinosis), at which point the lung is suctioned and ventilation is reestablished with large V_T (and pressures) because compliance is decreased owing to loss of surfactant. With each lavage, inflow and outflow volumes are monitored so the patient is not "drowned" in fluid, and there is no excessive absorption or leakage to the ventilated side. At least 90% of the saline volume should be recovered with each lavage. Two-lung ventilation is re-established and, as compliance improves, an air–oxygen mixture (addition of nitrogen) may be introduced to help maintain alveolar patency. After a further period of ventilation, in most patients, the trachea can be extubated in the operating room. In the posttreatment period, patients are encouraged to cough and engage in breathing exercises to fully re-expand the treated lung. From 3 days to 1 week after lavage of the first lung, the patient may return to the operating room for lavage of the other lung.

Problems sometimes encountered with this procedure include spillage of lavage fluid from the treated to the ventilated lung. This must be managed by stopping the lavage and ensuring functional separation of the lungs before continuing. DLT positioning is critical. Spillage may cause profound decreases in oxygenation, which may necessitate terminating the procedure and maintaining two-lung ventilation with oxygen and PEEP.

During periods when lavage fluid is being instilled into the dependent lung, oxygenation usually improves because the increased intra-alveolar pressure caused by the fluid produces diversion of the pulmonary blood flow to the nondependent, ventilated lung. Conversely, when the fluid is drained out of the dependent lung, hypoxemia may occur.[115] In some cases in which severe hypoxemia was anticipated during right lung lavage, the risk has been reduced by passing a balloon-tipped catheter into the right main pulmonary artery (checked by radiography) and inflating the balloon during periods of right lung drainage. In this way, blood flow to the dependent, right, nonventilated lung is minimized during periods of drainage. This technique is not without risk (e.g., pulmonary artery rupture) and is reserved for those patients considered to be at greatest risk for hypoxemia during lavage. If the patient has recently had a diagnostic open lung biopsy, a BPF may be present. If this is a possibility, a chest tube should be inserted on the side of the BPF, and this side should be lavaged first. The chest drain is removed several days later.

Limitations in the sizes of available DLTs preclude their use for lavage in patients weighing less than 40 kg. In such cases, cardiopulmonary bypass may be required to provide oxygenation during lavage.

Myasthenia Gravis

The thoracic anesthesiologist will most likely have to manage patients with myasthenia gravis (MG) for thymectomy, which is now considered the treatment of choice in most cases of MG. MG is a disorder of the neuromuscular junction, the function of which is altered routinely in the modern practice of anesthesia. The worldwide prevalence of the disease is 1 per 20,000 to 30,000 of the population; it is more common in women than men in a 6:4 ratio. People of any age may be affected, but peaks of incidence occur in the third decade for women and the fifth decade for men.[115] MG is a chronic disorder characterized by weakness and fatigability of voluntary muscles with improvement following rest.[116] Onset is usually slow and insidious, any skeletal muscle or group of muscles may be affected, and the condition is associated with relapses and remissions. The most common onset is ocular; if the disease remains localized to the eyes for 2 years, the likelihood of progression to generalized MG is low. In some cases, the disease is generalized and may

TABLE 40-5

CLINICAL CLASSIFICATION OF MYASTHENIA GRAVIS (MG)

■ CLASS	■ DESCRIPTION
I	Ocular myasthenia—Involvement of ocular muscles only. Mild with ptosis and diplopia. Electrophysiologic testing of other musculature is negative for MG.
IA	Ocular myasthenia with peripheral muscles showing no clinical symptoms but showing a positive electromyogram for MG.
II	Generalized myasthenia
IIA	Mild—Slow onset, usually ocular, spreading to skeletal and bulbar muscles. No respiratory involvement. Good response to drug therapy. Low mortality rate.
IIB	Moderate—As IIA but progressing to more severe involvement of skeletal and bulbar muscles. Dysarthria, dysphagia, difficulty chewing. No respiratory involvement. Patient's activities limited. Fair response to drug therapy.
III	Acute fulminating myasthenia—Rapid onset of severe bulbar and skeletal weakness with involvement of muscles of respiration. Progression usually within 6 months. Poor response to therapy. Patient's activities limited. Low mortality rate.
IV	Late severe myasthenia—Severe MG developing at least 2 years after onset of group I or group II symptoms. Progression of disease may be gradual or rapid. Poor response to therapy and poor prognosis.

Adapted from Osserman KE, Genkins G: Studies in myasthenia gravis—A review of a 20-year experience in over 1200 patients. Mt Sinai J Med 1971; 38: 497.

involve the bulbar musculature, causing problems with breathing and swallowing. Peripheral muscle involvement may cause weakness, clumsiness, and difficulty in holding up the head or in walking. The most commonly used clinical classification of MG is shown in Table 40-5.

In MG, there is a decrease in the number of postsynaptic acetylcholine receptors at the endplates of affected muscles. This causes a decrease in the margin of safety of neuromuscular transmission. MG is an autoimmune disorder, and most of the affected patients have circulating antibodies to the acetylcholine receptors. These antibodies may cause complement-mediated lysis of the postsynaptic membrane or direct blockade of the receptors, or may modulate the receptor turnover such that the degradation rate exceeds the resynthesis rate. Studies of the endplate area show loss of synaptic folds and a widening of the synaptic cleft.

The diagnosis of MG is suspected from the patient's history and confirmed by pharmacologic, electrophysiologic, or immunologic testing. Patients cannot sustain or repeat muscular contraction. The electrical counterpart of this is a decrement in the muscle action potentials evoked by repetitive stimulation of a motor nerve. Mechanical and electrical (electromyography) decrements improve with 2 to 10 mg of intravenous edrophonium (Tensilon test). MG patients characteristically are sensitive to nondepolarizer muscle relaxants. When the routine electromyographic results are equivocal, a regional nondepolarizer muscle relaxant test may be performed using a tourniquet to isolate the limb and limit the action of the drug. In the

TABLE 40-6

ANTICHOLINESTERASE DRUGS USED TO TREAT MYASTHENIA GRAVIS

■ DRUG	■ DOSE (mg)			■ EFFICACY
	■ ORAL	■ IV	■ IM	
Pyridostigmine (Mestinon)	60	2.0	2.0–4.0	1
Neostigmine (Prostigmin)	15	0.5	0.7–1.0	1

IV, intravenous; IM, intramuscular.

TABLE 40-7

DISORDERS ASSOCIATED WITH MYASTHENIA GRAVIS

Thymoma
Thyroid disease
  Hyperthyroidism
  Hypothyroidism
  Thyroiditis
Idiopathic thrombocytopenic purpura
Rheumatoid arthritis
Systemic lupus erythematosus
Anemias
  Pernicious
  Hemolytic
Multiple sclerosis
Ulcerative colitis
Leukemia
Lymphoma
Convulsive disorders
Extrathymic neoplasia
Sjögren syndrome
Scleroderma

regional nondepolarizer muscle relaxant test, electromyograms are performed before and after the administration of 0.2 mg of curare. In equivocal cases, a positive result of a test for anti-acetylcholine receptor antibodies is considered diagnostic.

Medical Therapy

Anticholinesterases are used to prolong the action of acetylcholine at the postsynaptic membrane and may also exert their own agonist effect at the acetylcholine receptors. They are the most commonly used therapy in MG (Table 40-6). Myasthenic patients learn to regulate their medication and titrate dose against optimum effect. Overdosage causes the muscarinic effects of acetylcholine and may cause a cholinergic crisis. Underdosage causes weakness or a myasthenic crisis. In a patient with weakness, distinction between the two types of crisis may be made by performing a Tensilon test or by examining pupillary size, which will be large (mydriatic) in a myasthenic crisis but small (miotic) in a cholinergic crisis. Muscarinic side effects are treatable with atropine (see Chapter 15).

The immunologic basis of MG has led to the use of immunosuppressive drugs such as steroids, azathioprine, cyclophosphamide, and, most recently, cyclosporine. Steroids often produce initial deterioration before an improvement. The usual regimen is prednisone 1 mg/kg on alternate days. The other drugs mentioned represent third and fourth lines of treatment.

Plasma exchange or plasmapheresis may produce dramatic but transient improvements in muscle strength with decreases in antiacetylcholine receptor antibody titers. Usually reserved for severe MG, plasma exchange has been shown to improve respiratory function in both operated and nonoperated patients with MG. Plasmapheresis causes a decrease in plasma cholinesterase levels that may prolong the effect of drugs such as succinylcholine that are normally broken down by this enzyme system.

Abnormalities are found in 75% of thymus glands removed from patients with MG (85% show hyperplasia, 15% show thymoma). After thymectomy, approximately 75% of patients either go into remission or show some improvement. Thymectomy is now considered the treatment of choice in most patients with MG, except for those in Osserman class I (Table 40-6).

Management of General Anesthesia

When possible, patients with MG should be admitted for elective surgery while in remission.[117] On admission, the patient's physical and emotional states should be optimized. Other diseases occasionally associated with MG should be excluded (Table 40-7). The patient's current drug therapy should be reviewed and possible drug interactions considered. Because patients are less active while in the hospital, their anticholinesterase dosage may need to be decreased. If the patient has a history of respiratory disease or bulbar involvement, preoperative evaluation should include respiratory function studies. Breathing exercises and instruction in the use of incentive spirometers may be indicated. Patients should be told of the possible need for postoperative intubation of the trachea and ventilation of the lungs. Ideally, patients with MG should be scheduled to be the first case of the day in the operating room. Patients receiving steroid therapy should receive perioperative coverage.

Because the trachea is to be intubated and the lungs ventilated for the planned procedure in the patient with MG, traditional practice is to withhold anticholinesterase therapy on the morning of surgery so that the patient is weak on arrival at the operating room.[118] This avoids interactions with other drugs used in the operating room. Anticholinesterase therapy may be continued if the patient is physically or psychologically dependent on it. Others recommend continuing pyridostigmine, including an oral dose just before induction.[119] Premedication is satisfactorily achieved with a benzodiazepine or barbiturate. Opioids are usually avoided because of the risk of producing respiratory depression.

Monitoring should be dictated by the patient's state and planned surgical procedure, but should include an assessment of neuromuscular transmission (by means of a mechanomyogram/twitch monitor, an integrated electromyographic monitor, or an accelograph monitor) if agents affecting neuromuscular transmission are to be used.

Induction of anesthesia is readily achieved with a short-acting barbiturate or propofol. In elective cases, intubation of the trachea, maintenance, and relaxation are readily achieved using potent inhaled anesthetics. Anesthesia may be deepened using a potent inhaled agent and the trachea intubated under its effect. Myasthenic patients are more sensitive than normal patients to the neuromuscular depressant effects of the potent inhaled agents. In patients with MG, isoflurane at 1.9 MAC end-tidal concentration induced a neuromuscular block of 30 to 50%, whereas halothane at 1.8 MAC induced a block of 10 to 20%. Both agents produced fade in the train-of-four ratio of 41% and 28%, respectively.[120] The less soluble inhaled agents, sevoflurane and desflurane, are even more easily administered and withdrawn; they are now the most commonly used anesthetic drugs for patients with MG. Nitahara et al.[121] studied the neuromuscular effects of sevoflurane in 16 myasthenic patients and 12 normal patients. As expected, they found a concentration-dependent decrease in T1 and T4/T1 values. The depressant effects of sevoflurane were more prominent in those myasthenic patients with baseline T4/T1 <0.90. Whichever agent is used, at the end of the procedure, the inhaled agent is discontinued and recovery of neuromuscular function begins.

Nondepolarizing Relaxants. In some cases, patients with MG cannot tolerate the cardiovascular depressant effects of the potent inhaled anesthetics, in which case neuromuscular blocking drugs may be used, titrating dose against monitored effect. Patients with MG are sensitive to the nondepolarizing relaxants. All nondepolarizing relaxants have been successfully and uneventfully used with careful monitoring in patients with MG (see Chapter 20). They should be titrated in 1/10 to 1/20 of the usual dose. Cis-atracurium may be preferred because of its short elimination half-life, small volume of distribution, lack of cumulative effect, and high clearance.[122] Sensitivity to nondepolarizing relaxants is increased during the coadministration of a potent inhaled anesthetic.[123]

Other intermediate-duration nondepolarizing agents such as vecuronium and rocuronium may be used; long-acting relaxants are best avoided in patients with MG. If necessary, the residual relaxation produced by nondepolarizers may be reversed by increments of anticholinesterase drugs, while neuromuscular transmission is carefully monitored to obtain maximum antagonism yet avoid a cholinergic crisis. All anticholinesterases have been safely used. Edrophonium may be the drug of choice because its onset of action is rapid and higher doses have a prolonged duration of action. The sensitivity of patients with MG to nondepolarizing relaxants is very variable, depending on the individual patient, the severity of MG, and the treatment. Mann et al.[124] showed that MG patients who have a T4/T1 ratio <0.9 in the preanesthetic period show increased sensitivity to atracurium. They suggest that neuromuscular monitoring using train-of-four stimulation should begin in the preinduction period following administration of adequate analgesia (fentanyl, 2 μg/kg). Itoh et al.[125] found that patients with ocular MG were less sensitive to vecuronium than were those with generalized MG. They also found that in patients with clinical MG, sensitivity to vecuronium was unrelated to presence or absence of antibodies to the acetylcholine receptor. Seronegative patients were as sensitive to vecuronium as seropositive patients.[126] There are conflicting reports as to the sensitivity of patients with MG in remission. All such patients should be considered sensitive to nondepolarizers until proven otherwise.[127]

Sugammadex is a novel cyclodextrin drug currently undergoing clinical trials worldwide, The molecule was designed to bind rocuronium with a great affinity. If approved for clinical use, this drug may simplify the management of relaxation in the myasthenic patient as it has been reported to provide very rapid, complete, and lasting recovery from deep levels of rocuronium-induced neuromuscular blockade.[128,129]

Succinylcholine. Myasthenic patients are resistant to the neuromuscular blocking effects of succinylcholine. The ED95 is 2.6 times normal in these patients.[130] Clinically, however, the use of succinylcholine has been without incident, with the usual clinical doses producing adequate relaxation for endotracheal intubation and a normal recovery time, despite the occasionally reported early onset of phase II block. Doses of 0.2 to 1.0 mg/kg have been used in a number of patients with MG, and most did not show fasciculation before becoming paralyzed. Fade in response to train-of-four stimulation was observed in some patients during recovery, but recovery was not delayed. Prior administration of an anticholinesterase may complicate the response to succinylcholine by delaying its metabolism.

When a rapid-sequence intubation of the trachea is required, rapid onset of muscle relaxation may be achieved with succinylcholine or with moderate doses of a nondepolarizer in the latter case, with an associated prolongation of effect. A succinylcholine (1.5 mg/kg)–vecuronium (0.01 mg/kg) sequence has been safely used in three patients with MG for thymectomy. The authors suggested that this technique may be particularly advantageous when rapid-sequence induction of anesthesia is indicated.[131]

Nonrelaxant Techniques. Because of concerns over the use of muscle relaxants in MG patients, there are many reports of successful use of nonrelaxant techniques. Della Rocca et al.[132] studied 68 consecutive MG patients undergoing transsternal thymectomy randomized to receive propofol/O2/N2O/fentanyl or sevoflurane/N2O/O2/fentanyl. All were tracheally extubated in the operating room, and none required intubation for postoperative respiratory depression. Madi-Jebara et al.[133] described the use of sevoflurane as the sole anesthetic combined with intrathecal sufentanil-morphine for analgesia in an adult patient who underwent transsternal thymectomy. Abe et al.[134] described propofol anesthesia combined with thoracic epidural anesthesia for thymectomy in 11 patients with MG. Chevalley et al.[135] reported use of propofol combined with epidural bupivacaine and sufentanil in 12 MG patients undergoing similar procedures. They commented that the shift away from use of muscle relaxants provided optimal operating condition and improved patient comfort. Lorimar and Hall[136] used a total intravenous anesthetic technique with propofol and remifentanil for transsternal thymectomy in an MG patient. Politis and Tobias[137] describe rapid-sequence intubation in a myasthenic patient with a full stomach using propofol, lidocaine, and remifentanil.

Baraka et al.[138] described a 19-year-old myasthenic patient with a thymoma who received remifentanil and sevoflurane anesthesia for a 2-hour thymectomy. Although the trachea was extubated 10 minutes after discontinuation of remifentanil, the patient was unresponsive to verbal stimuli and remained somnolent for 12 hours. Because the patient had been receiving pyridostigmine for the months prior to surgery, they suggest that the delayed arousal may have been the result of possible inhibition by pyridostigmine of the nonspecific esterases that normally hydrolyze remifentanil. Ingersoll-Weng et al.[139] reported use of a dexmedetomidine infusion/isoflurane technique for transsternal thymectomy in a 52-year-old woman. The patient was stable at the start of surgery but became asystolic on sternal retraction and received open cardiac massage. Resuscitation was successful, the dexmedetomidine infusion was discontinued, and surgery was completed uneventfully. Several factors may have contributed to the asystolic arrest, including a centrally mediated increase in parasympathetic activity resulting from dexmedetomidine in a patient who was also being treated with pyridostigmine, which also increases vagal tone. Thus, pyridostigmine may have interacted with dexmedetomidine in an additive or synergistic manner.

Other Drug Interactions. Medications with neuromuscular blocking properties should be used with caution in patients with MG, particularly if relaxants are being used concurrently. Such drugs include antiarrhythmics (quinidine, procainamide, calcium channel blockers), diuretics (by causing hypokalemia), nitrogen mustards, quinine, and aminoglycoside antibiotics. Dantrolene has been used safely in a patient with MG.

Recovery from Anesthesia. Recovery from anesthesia must be carefully monitored in these patients. Extubation of the trachea should be performed when the patients are responsive and able to generate negative inspiratory pressures of greater than –20 cm H2O. After extubation of the trachea, patients are carefully observed in the recovery area or the intensive care unit. As soon as possible, patients should resume their usual pyridostigmine regimen. Cases of mild respiratory depression may be treatable with parenteral anticholinesterase; more severe cases may require reintubation of the trachea and mechanical ventilation of the lungs. In the immediate postoperative period, postthymectomy patients often show a marked improvement in their condition and a decreased need for anticholinesterase therapy.

Postoperative Respiratory Failure

Myasthenic patients are at increased risk for development of postoperative respiratory failure. There have been several attempts to predict before surgery which patients with MG will require prolonged postoperative ventilation of the lungs.[140] For patients who underwent transsternal thymectomy, positive predictors were a duration of MG >6 years, history of chronic respiratory disease other than that directly caused by MG, pyridostigmine dosage >750 mg/day, and a preoperative vital capacity <2.9 L. This predictive system was not found useful when applied in patients with MG undergoing transsternal thymectomy at other centers, and of no value in patients with MG undergoing other types of surgical procedure.[140] In a study of 52 MG patients following thymectomy, Mori et al.[141] concluded that those patients who received >250 mg of pyridostigmine were at greater risk for respiratory failure requiring reintubation. Each patient should therefore be treated on his or her own merits.

A study of patients undergoing transsternal thymectomy suggested that the need for postoperative mechanical ventilation correlated best with preoperative maximum static expiratory pressure. It was concluded that expiratory weakness, by reducing cough efficacy and ability to clear secretions, was the main predictive determinant. Adequate clearance of secretions is essential in these patients and may occasionally necessitate bronchoscopy.

In general, the postoperative morbidity in terms of respiratory failure is lower after transcervical rather than transsternal thymectomy.[140] Techniques described that may be useful in reducing postoperative ventilatory failure include preoperative plasma exchange and high-dose perioperative steroid therapy. If the anticipated duration of the surgical procedure is 1 to 2 hours, preoperative oral anticholinesterase therapy may be of value because the peak effect of the drug coincides with the conclusion of the surgical procedure and attempts at tracheal extubation.

Postoperative Care

In the immediate postoperative period, pain relief for patients with MG is usually provided by opioid analgesics, such as meperidine, but in reduced doses. The analgesic effect of morphine and other opioid analgesics has been reported to be increased by anticholinesterases, which has led to the recommendation that the dose of opioid analgesics be reduced by one-third in patients receiving anticholinesterase therapy. Combined regional and general anesthesia techniques have also been used to provide good surgical conditions and improved postoperative analgesia in patients with MG undergoing thymectomy. Combined epidural–general anesthesia has been reported to provide excellent intraoperative and postoperative conditions for both surgeon and patient.[142,143]

Myasthenic Syndrome (Eaton-Lambert Syndrome)

The myasthenic syndrome is a very rare disorder of neuromuscular transmission with a prevalence of about 1 per 100,000.[144]

It is sometimes associated with small cell carcinoma of the lung. Complaints of weakness may be mistaken for MG, but in Eaton-Lambert syndrome, symptoms do not respond to administration of anticholinesterases or steroids, and activity improves strength. The defect in this condition is believed to be prejunctional, associated with diminished release of acetylcholine from nerve terminals, and improved by agents such as 4-aminopyridine, guanidine, and germine that increase repetitive firing. Affected patients are particularly sensitive to the effects of all muscle relaxants, which should be used with great caution or avoided entirely.[145]

The possibility of Eaton-Lambert syndrome should be considered in all patients with known malignant disease and those patients undergoing diagnostic procedures for suspected carcinoma of the lung. Anesthesia considerations in these patients are essentially the same as in those with MG.[146]

POSTOPERATIVE MANAGEMENT AND COMPLICATIONS

Postoperative Pain Control

After extubation of the trachea, respiratory therapy and pain management become critical components of postoperative care. Adequate postoperative pain control is necessary to ensure a good respiratory effort.[147] Administration of intravenous opioids has been the standard form of pain management for years. The administration of sufficient opioid to treat pain adequately may cause sedation and respiratory depression. Patient-controlled analgesia (PCA) has been reported to decrease the amount of postoperative pain, drug use, sedation, and pulmonary complications.[148] PCA also eliminates the delays associated with personnel-administered medications and in general is very well accepted by patients.

There are other intravenous medications that can be used for pain management in addition to opioids. Low-dose ketamine infusion at 0.05 mg/kg/hr was reported to be a useful adjunct to epidural analgesia for postthoracotomy pain management.[149] Small doses of ketamine added to morphine for PCA administration has been shown to reduce the amount of morphine administered, and improve respiratory parameters.[150] It reduced the incidence of oxygen desaturation below 90% during the first 3 postoperative nights. Gabapentin has also been successful in reducing pain following thoracic surgery, although side effects included dizziness and drowsiness.[151] Gabapentin may also reduce the incidence of postoperative delirium, and one approach could be to administer 900 mg 1 to 2 hours preoperatively.[152]

Intercostal nerve blocks can decrease pain and improve postoperative respiratory function. The intercostal blocks can be performed externally before or after surgery using a standard technique. However, the easiest method during thoracic surgery is to have the surgeon perform the blocks under direct vision from inside the thorax while the chest is open. Bupivacaine 0.5%, in doses of 2 to 3 mL, can be placed in the five intercostal spaces around the incision and in intercostal spaces where chest tubes will be placed. This provides 6 to 24 hours of moderate pain relief, but patients still complain of diaphragmatic and shoulder discomfort caused by the chest tubes. Larger volumes of local anesthetic (e.g., 5 to 10 mL) should not be used in the intercostal space because of the high absorption rate and attendant systemic toxicity that can be produced, as well as the possibility of pushing the drug centrally and producing a paravertebral sympathetic or epidural block with central sympatholysis and severe hypotension. The intraoperative placement of catheters in intercostal grooves allows for a continuous postoperative intercostal nerve block.

The technique reduces pain and improves pulmonary function. Placement of a catheter in the paravertebral space allows for blockade of multiple levels of intercostal nerves. This technique has been reported to provide good analgesia, and with fewer side effects than epidural analgesia.[153]

Another approach to postoperative pain control after thoracic surgery is the use of epidural or subarachnoid opioids (see Chapter 57). Epidural morphine produces profound analgesia lasting from 16 to 24 hours after thoracotomy and does not cause a sympathetic block or sensory or motor loss. These are significant advantages over opioids or local anesthetics. Epidural opioids are most effective at alleviating pain when administered at the thoracic level. Epidural morphine has been shown to decrease pain and improve respiratory function in postthoracotomy patients.[147]

Based on a meta-analysis of 100 studies in the National Library of Medicine's PubMed database from 1966 to 2002, Block et al.[154] concluded that epidural analgesia was superior to parenteral medication; this was true regardless of agent used in the epidural catheter or the level of catheter placement. There may be a reduction in both morbidity and mortality with epidural or spinal analgesia.[155] The technique most commonly employed in academic medical centers in the United States is an infusion of bupivacaine together with a narcotic such as fentanyl administered via a thoracic epidural catheter.[156] Data in the pediatric population are limited; in one study of adolescent patients, the use of thoracic epidural analgesia provided better postoperative pain relief following minimally invasive pectus excavatum repair.[157] Acetaminophen may be a useful adjunct to thoracic epidural for treatment of ipsilateral shoulder pain following thoracotomy.[158] Ketorolac may be given postoperatively, but carries a risk of bleeding if given intraoperatively.

Subarachnoid (intrathecal) morphine, in a dose of 10 to 12 μg/kg, has been successfully used after thoracic surgery.[159] With this technique, the drug acts directly on the spinal cord, and analgesia can be produced with a smaller dose than by the epidural or intravenous routes. When morphine is given intrathecally before the induction of anesthesia, a decrease in the dose of anesthetic drugs required may occur. All patients who have received subarachnoid or epidural opioids must be closely observed for potential side effects, including delayed respiratory depression, urine retention, pruritus, nausea, and vomiting. These effects appear to be dose-related and may be reversed with naloxone.

Noxious stimuli, including surgical incision, may lead to changes in the central nervous system that exacerbate postoperative pain. The administration of analgesic agents before surgery is termed *pre-emptive analgesia* and may prevent these neuroplastic changes, thereby decreasing postoperative pain. In an early study of pre-emptive analgesia, the administration of lumbar epidural fentanyl before thoracotomy incision reduced postoperative pain scores and use of PCA morphine by a small but significant amount, compared with administration of lumbar epidural fentanyl after skin incision.[160] Based on a meta-analysis of randomized controlled studies published between 1966 and 2004, Bong et al.[161] concluded that thoracic epidural pre-emptive analgesia did not provide a statistically significant reduction in postoperative pain, but was associated with a trend toward a reduction in the incidence of such pain.

Intrapleural analgesia is another technique for postoperative pain treatment. The injection of local anesthetic between the pleural layers can block multiple intercostal nerves and/or pain fibers traveling with the thoracic sympathetic chain. The surgeon can place the catheter under direct vision while the chest is open. The chest tubes should not be suctioned for approximately 15 minutes after injection of local anesthetic to avoid loss of the anesthetic into the drainage. There may be chronic pain following thoracotomy, and also following VAT, even though the incisions are smaller with this approach.[162,163] In one report, women were more likely than men to suffer from both perioperative postoperative pain and chronic pain.[164] If it occurs, it is important to treat this chronic postoperative pain early and aggressively.[165]

Complications Following Thoracic Surgery

Atelectasis

Patients who require thoracotomy often have pre-existing pulmonary disease that, when combined with the operative procedure, is likely to result in significant pulmonary dysfunction and possibly pneumonia. Atelectasis, the most significant cause of postoperative morbidity, has been reported to occur in up to 100% of patients undergoing thoracotomy for pulmonary resection. It occurs more commonly in the basal lobes than in the middle or upper lung regions. It may be secondary to reduction of normal respiratory effort due to splinting from pain, obesity, intrathoracic blood and fluid accumulation, and decreased compliance, all of which lead to rapid, shallow, constant V_T. Such a respiratory pattern produces small airway closure and obstruction with inspissated secretions, resulting ultimately in alveolar air resorption and terminal airway collapse. A poor cough and limited clearance of secretions add to the problem. Other sources of atelectasis include mucus plugging, which can obstruct a lobe or even an entire lung, and incomplete re-expansion of the remaining lung tissue after one-lung anesthesia.

The diagnosis of atelectasis can be made by clinical findings, chest radiography, or arterial blood gas analysis. This problem is best resolved by increasing resting lung volume or FRC. The latter can be increased by an increase in transpulmonary pressure (difference between airway pressure and interpleural pressure) or in lung compliance.

The tracheas of many patients can be extubated shortly after thoracic surgical procedures These patients should be observed in the operating room for at least 5 minutes following extubation, and many will require a high F_{IO_2} by face mask. Some patients with COPD undergoing extensive thoracic surgical procedures require postoperative ventilation to avoid atelectasis and other pulmonary complications. Mechanical ventilation increases airway pressure and, to a lesser extent, interpleural pressure; therefore, transpulmonary pressure increases.

The use of incentive spirometry and CPAP has been shown to reduce postoperative complications.[3] Additional modalities that may be helpful in preventing atelectasis include bronchodilator treatment, coughing and clearance of secretions, chest physiotherapy, mobilizing the patient, and providing adequate analgesia.[23] Atelectasis caused by collapse of lung tissue distal to a mucus plug can be treated by positioning the patient in the lateral decubitus position with the fully expanded lung in the dependent position. This improves V/Q matching and facilitates clearance of mucus from the nondependent obstructed lung. However, the patient should not be placed with the operative side in the dependent position after a pneumonectomy because of the risk of cardiac herniation.

The other major complications after thoracic surgery can be grouped into cardiovascular, pulmonary, and related problems.

Cardiovascular Complications

Cardiovascular complications are often the most difficult to manage in patients with associated respiratory insufficiency. The low cardiac output syndrome and postoperative cardiac dysrhythmias may be life-threatening. Invasive hemodynamic monitoring may be needed to assist in diagnosis and fluid management therapy. Other diagnostic modalities, such as echocardiography, may be required to rule out the presence of pericardial effusions or tamponade after opening the pericardium during certain types of thoracic surgical procedure. The low cardiac output syndrome must be differentiated from hypovolemia resulting from intrathoracic hemorrhage, tamponade, pulmonary emboli, or the effects of mechanical ventilation with PEEP. Postoperative fluid administration can lead to pulmonary edema resulting from the resection of lung tissue and the concomitant reduction of the pulmonary vascular bed. A postoperative pulmonary embolism can originate from the remaining pulmonary artery stump. Therapeutic interventions for postoperative myocardial dysfunction include inotropic drugs, vasodilators, and combinations of these drugs, as needed, to improve ventricular function. The goal is to shift the Starling function curve up and to the left by reducing preload of either the left or right side of the heart and increasing cardiac output. Vasodilators are very effective at decreasing right ventricular afterload and improving right ventricular function because this side of the heart is especially afterload-dependent. Combinations of inotropes and vasodilators, such as dopamine and nitroglycerin, or combined drugs, such as milrinone, can be especially useful in the treatment of right-sided heart failure.

Postoperative cardiac dysrhythmias are common after thoracic surgery. Patients following pulmonary resection have postoperative supraventricular tachycardias with a frequency and severity proportional to both their age and the magnitude of the surgical procedure. Many factors contribute to these dysrhythmias, including underlying cardiac disease, degree of surgical trauma, intraoperative cardiac manipulation, stimulation of the sympathetic nervous system by pain, a reduced pulmonary vascular bed, effects of anesthetics and cardioactive drugs, and metabolic abnormalities.

In a series of 300 thoracotomies for lung resection, atrial fibrillation occurred in 20% of patients with malignant disease but in only 3% with benign disease.[166] A similar incidence of dysrhythmias is observed after pneumonectomies. Multifocal atrial tachycardia often occurs in patients with COPD and concomitant right-sided cardiac dysfunction. The right side of the heart may be further strained by the reduction in the size of the pulmonary vasculature from the lung resection, especially after right pneumonectomy. The prophylactic use of digitalis in thoracic surgical patients is controversial, particularly in patients with signs of congestive heart failure. Arguments against its use include the potential toxic effects of the drug and the difficulty in assessing adequacy of digitalization in the absence of heart failure. A prospective, placebo-controlled, randomized study demonstrated no advantage to prophylactic digitalization of patients undergoing thoracic surgery.[167] Part of the argument for its use is the drug's efficacy in reducing the incidence of potentially fatal complications in older patients. In some studies, it has been reported to reduce the incidence of perioperative dysrhythmias. If digitalis therapy is to be instituted, normokalemia should be ensured to reduce the likelihood of digitalis toxicity.

Supraventricular tachycardias can also be treated with other agents such as beta-blockers or calcium channel-blocking drugs, after ruling out underlying reversible physiologic abnormalities, such as hypoxia. Verapamil has been the standard treatment for these problems until the introduction of the ultrashort-acting beta-blocker, esmolol. Esmolol has been shown to be equally effective in controlling the ventricular rate in patients with postoperative atrial fibrillation or flutter and in increasing the conversion rate to regular sinus rhythm from 8 to 34%. Owing to its short duration of action (β elimination half-life of 9 minutes) and β_1-cardioselectivity, it is the drug of choice in the postoperative period to control these dysrhythmias. Esmolol, in an intravenous loading dose of 500 μg/kg given over 1 minute followed by an infusion of 50 to 200 μg/kg/min, has been shown to be effective in the control of supraventricular tachycardias. Amio-

darone has been reported to be effective in restoring and maintaining sinus rhythm.[168]

Bleeding and Respiratory Complications

Hemorrhage and pneumothorax are always major concerns after intrathoracic surgery. Because of these problems, interpleural thoracostomy tubes with an underwater seal system are routinely used after thoracic surgery. Slippage of a suture on any major vessel or airway in the chest can lead to the slow or rapid development of hypovolemic shock or a tension pneumothorax. Drainage of more than 200 mL/hr of blood is an indication for surgical re-exploration for hemorrhage. Management of the pleural drainage system is fraught with confusion. The chest bottles must be kept below the level of the chest, and the tubes should not be clamped during patient transport. These tubes can be lifesaving, but errors in technique can lead to serious complications. The creation of a pneumothorax in the nonoperative chest by central venous catheter placement is very hazardous because this lung is essential both intraoperatively during one-lung anesthesia and postoperatively after contralateral lung resection. Dehiscence of the bronchial stump may lead to the formation of a BPF, which carries a mortality rate of 20%. Surgical treatment may be needed, in which case ventilation of the patient's lungs may be difficult because of loss of V_T through the fistula. A double-lumen endobronchial tube positioned in the contralateral main stem bronchus or the use of HFJV may be required for safe management. HFJV allows ventilation with lowered peak airway pressures. However, there have been reports in which ventilation by HFJV was difficult. If a double-lumen endobronchial tube is placed, the lung with the fistula can be ventilated independently with either CPAP or HFJV.

Neurologic Complications

Central and peripheral neurologic injuries can occur during intrathoracic procedures. Such injuries often result in serious and disabling loss of function. Peripheral nerves can also be injured, either in the chest or in other parts of the body, by pressure or stretching. The nerve injury may be apparent immediately after surgery or may not become obvious until several days later. These patients often complain of a variety of unpleasant sensations, including paresthesias, cold, pain, or anesthesia in the area supplied by the affected nerves. The brachial plexus is especially vulnerable to trauma during thoracic surgery, owing to its long superficial course in the axilla between two points of fixation, the vertebrae above, and the axillary fascia below. Stretching may be the primary cause of damage to the brachial plexus, with compression playing only a secondary role. Branches of the brachial plexus may also be injured lower in the arm by compression against objects such as an ether screen or other parts of the operating table. Intrathoracic nerves can be directly injured during a surgical procedure by being transected, crushed, stretched, or cauterized. The recurrent laryngeal nerve can become involved in lymph node tissue and injured at the time of a node biopsy, especially when the biopsy is performed through a mediastinoscope. This nerve can also be injured during tracheostomy or radical pulmonary dissections. The phrenic nerve may be injured during pericardiectomy, radical pulmonary hilar dissections, division of the diaphragm during esophageal surgery, or dissection of mediastinal tumors.

Prevention is the treatment of choice for these intraoperative nerve injuries. Analgesics may be necessary to control postoperative pain in the distribution of the nerve injury and to aid in maintaining joint mobility during the healing phase. Subsequent surgical procedures may be necessary to move a swollen ulnar nerve at the elbow or to stent a partially paralyzed vocal cord.

References

1. American Lung Association: Lung Cancer Fact Sheet. New York, American Lung Association, 2006
2. American Cancer Society: Cancer statistics 2007. A presentation from the American Cancer Society, 2007. www.cancer.org
3. Bapoje SR, Whitaker JF, Schulz T et al: Preoperative evaluation of the patient with pulmonary disease. Chest 2007; 132: 1637
4. Smetanta GW: Preoperative pulmonary evaluation: Identifying and reducing risks for pulmonary complications. Cleve Clin J Med 2006; 73(Suppl 1): S36
5. Slinger PD: Preoperative assessment for pulmonary resection. J Cardiothorac Vasc Anesth 2000; 4: 202
6. Reilly JJ: Evidence-based preoperative evaluation of candidates for thoracotomy. Chest 1999; 116: 474s
7. Licker M, Perrot M, Spiliopoulos A: Risk factors for acute lung injury after thoracic surgery for lung cancer. Anesth Analg 2003; 97: 1558
8. Slinger PD, Susssa S, Triolet W: Predicting arterial oxygenation during one-lung anaesthesia. Can J Anaesth 1992; 39: 1030
9. Slinger P Johnston M. Preoperative evaluation of the thoracic surgery patient. Semin Anesth 2002; 21: 168
10. Nakahara K, Ohno K, Hashimoto J et al: Prediction of postoperative respiratory failure in patients undergoing lung resection for cancer. Ann Thorac Surg 1988; 46: 549
11. Vansteenkiste J, Fischer BM, Dooms C et al: Positron-emission tomography in prognostic and therapeutic assessment of lung cancer: Systematic review. Lancet Oncol 2004; 5: 531
12. Gould MK, Kuschner WG, Rydzak CE et al: Test performance of positron emission tomography and computer tomography for mediastinal staging in patients with non-small-cell lung cancer: A meta-analysis. Ann Intern Med 2003; 139: 879
13. Ferguson MK, Reeder LB, Mick R: Optimizing selection of patients for major lung resection. J Thorac Cardiovasc Surg 1995; 109: 275
14. Walsh GL, Morice RC, Putnam JB: Resection of lung cancer is justified in high-risk patients selected by oxygen consumption. Ann Thorac Surg 1994; 58: 704
15. Bollinger CT, Wyser C, Roser H et al: Lung scanning and exercise testing for the prediction of postoperative performance in lung resection candidates at increased risk for complications. Chest 1995; 108: 341
16. Ninan M, Sommers KE, Landranau RJ et al: Standardized exercise oximetry predicts post pneumonectomy outcome. Ann Thorac Surg 1997; 64: 328
17. Win T, Jackson A, Sharples L et al: Cardiopulmonary exercise tests and lung cancer surgical outcome. *Chest* 2005; 127: 1159
18. Brunelli A, Fianchira A. Stair climbing test predicts cardiopulmonary complications after lung resection. Chest 2002; 121: 1106
19. Brunelli A, Sabbatini A, Xiume F et al: Inability to perform maximal stair climbing test before lung resection: a propensity score analysis on early outcome. Eur J Cardiothorac Surg 2005; 27: 367
20. Nakagawa M, Tanaka H, Tsukuma H. Relationship between the duration of the preoperative smoke-free period and the incidence of postoperative pulmonary complications after pulmonary surgery. Chest 2001; 120: 705
21. Barrera R, Shi W, Amar D. et al: Smoking and cessation: impact on pulmonary complications after thoracotomy. Chest 2005; 127: 1927
22. Mauermann WJ, Nemergut EC. The anesthesiologist's role in the prevention of surgical infections. Anesthesiology 2006; 105: 413
23. Sekine, Y, Chiyo, M, Iwata, T et al: Perioperative rehabilitation and physiotherapy for lung cancer patients with chronic obstructive pulmonary disease. Jpn J Thorac Cardiovasc Surg 2005; 53: 237
24. Landesberg G, Mosseri M, Wolf Y et al: The probability of detecting perioperative myocardial ischemia in vascular surgery by continuous 12-lead ECG. Anesthesiology 2002; 96: 264
25. Kumar A, Anel R, Bunnell E et al: Pulmonary artery occlusion pressure and central venous pressure fail to predict ventricular filling volume, cardiac performance, or the response to volume infusion in normal subjects. Crit Care Med 2004; 32: 691
26. Iberti TJ, Fischer EP, Leibowitz AB et al: A multicenter study of physician's knowledge of the pulmonary artery catheter. JAMA 1990; 264: 2928
27. Raper R, Sibbald WJ: Misled by the wedge. Chest 1986; 89: 427
28. Koji A: Mean pulmonary artery pressure under thoracotomy as an indicator of safety for lung resection. J Jpn Assoc Chest Surg 2001; 15: 561
29. Thys DM, Cohen E, Eisenkraft JB: Mixed venous oxygen saturation during thoracic anesthesia. Anesthesiology 1988; 69: 1005
30. Pothoft G, Curtius JM, Wassermann K et al: Transesophageal echography in staging of bronchial cancers. Pneumologie 1992; 446: 111
31. Manguso L, Pitrolo F, Bond F et al: Echocardiographic recognition of mediastinal masses. Chest 1988; 93: 144
32. Neustein SM, Cohen E, Reich DL et al: Transesophageal echocardiography and the intraoperative diagnosis of left atrial invasion by carcinoid tumor. Can J Anaesth 1993; 40: 664
33. Suriani RJ, Konstadt SN, Camunas J et al: Transesophageal echocardiographic detection of left atrial involvement in a lung tumor. J Cardiothorac Vasc Anesth 1993; 7: 73
34. Neustein SM, Narang J: Spontaneous hemothorax due to subacute aortic dissection. J Cardiothorac Vasc Anesth 1993; 7: 79
35. Redford D, Kim A, Barber B: Transesophageal echocardiography for the intraoperative evaluation of a large anterior mediastinal mass. Anesth Anlag 2006; 103: 578
36. Brooker RF, Zvara DA: Mediastinal mass diagnosed with intraoperative transeophageal echocardiography. J Cardiothorac Vasc Anesth 2007; 21: 257
37. Barker SJ, Curry J, Redford D et al: Measurement of carboxyhemoglobin and methemoglobin by pulse oximetry: a human volunteer study. Anesthesiology 2006; 105: 892
38. Shafieha MA, Sit J, Kartha R et al: End-tidal CO_2 analyzers in proper positioning of double-lumen tubes. Anesthesiology 1986; 64: 844
39. Yam PCI, Innes PA, Jackson M et al: Variation in the arterial to end-tidal PCO_2 difference during one-lung thoracic anaesthesia. Br J Anaesth 1994; 72: 21
40. Benumof JL: Isoflurane anesthesia and arterial oxygenation during one-lung ventilation. Anesthesiology 1986; 64: 419
41. Hurford WE, Alfille PH: A quality improvement study of the placement and complications of double-lumen endobronchial tubes. J Cardiothorac Vasc Anesth 1993; 7: 517
42. Lohser J, Brodsky J: Silibronco Double-Lumen Tube J Cardiothorac Vasc Anesth 2006; 20: 129
43. Brodsky JB, Lemmens HJM. Left double-lumen tubes: clinical experience with 1,170 patients. J Cardiothorac Vasc Anesth 2003; 17: 289
44. Brodsky JB, Lemmens HJM. Tracheal width and left double-lumen tube size: a formula to estimate left-bronchial width. J Clin Anesth 2005; 17: 267
45. Amar D, Desiderio D, Heerdt PM et al: Practice patterns in choice of left double-lumen tube size for thoracic surgery. Anesth Analg 2008; 106: 379
46. Chow MY, Go MH, Ti LK. Predicting the depth of insertion of left-sided double-lumen endobronchial tubes. J Cardiothorac Vasc Anesth 2002; 16: 456
47. Smith G, Hirsch N, Ehrenwerth J: Sight and sound: Can double-lumen endotracheal tubes be placed accurately without fiberoptic bronchoscopy? Br J Anaesth 1987; 54: 1317
48. Cohen E, Neustein SM, Goldofsky S et al: Incidence of malposition of PVC and red rubber left-sided double lumen tubes and clinical sequelae. J Cardiothorac Vasc Anesth 1995; 9: 122
49. Benumof JL, Partridge BL, Salvatierra C et al: Margin of safety in positioning modern double-lumen endotracheal tubes. Anesthesiology 1987; 67: 729
50. Thomas V, Neustein SN: Tracheal laceration after the use of an airway exchange catheter for double-lumen tube placement. J Cardiothorac Vasc Anesth 2007; 21: 718
51. Wagner DL, Gammage GW, Wong ML: Tracheal rupture following the insertion of a disposable double-lumen endotracheal tube. Anesthesiology 1985; 63: 698
52. Heike Knoll H, Stephan Ziegeler S, Jan-Uwe Schreiber JU et al: Airway Injuries after One-lung Ventilation: A Comparison between Double-lumen Tube and Endobronchial Blocker: A Randomized, Prospective, Controlled Trial: Anesthesiology 2006; 105: 471
53. Andros TG, Lennon PF: One-lung ventilation in a patient with a tracheostomy and severe tracheobronchial disease. Anesthesiology 1993; 79: 1127
54. Bellver J, Garcia-Aguado A, Andres JD et al: Selective bronchial intubation with the Univent system in patients with a tracheostomy. Anesthesiology 1993; 79: 1453
55. Saito T, Naruke T, Carney E et al: New double-lumen intrabronchial tube (Naruke tube) for tracheostomized patients. Anesthesiology 1998; 89: 1038
56. Cohen E, Benumof JL: Lung separation in the patient with a difficult airway. Curr Opin Anesthesiol 1999; 12: 29
57. Benumof JL: Difficult tubes and difficult airways. J Cardiothorac Vasc Anesth 1998; 12: 131
58. Cohen E. The Cohen Flextip Endobronchial Blocker: an alternative to a double lumen tube. Anesth Analg 2005; 101: 1877
59. Campos JH, Kernstine KH: A comparison of a left-sided Broncho-Cath with the torque control blocker Univent and the wire-guided blocker. Anesth Analg 2003; 96: 283
60. Campos JH: Progress in Lung Separation. Thorac Surg Clin 2005; 15: 71
61. Katz JA, Larlane RG, Fairly HB et al: Pulmonary oxygen exchange during endobronchial anesthesia: Effect of tidal volume and PEEP. Anesthesiology 1982; 56: 164
62. Slinger P, Low tidal volume is indicated during one-lung ventilation: Anesth Analg 2006; 103: 268
63. A. Gal T: Low tidal volume is not indicated during one lung ventilation: Anesth Analg 2006; 103: 271
64. Schultz, MJ, Jack J, Haitsma JJ et al: What Tidal Volumes Should Be Used in Patients without Acute Lung Injury? Anesthesiology 2007; 106: 1226
65. Wrigge H, Uhlig U, Zinserling J et al: The effects of different ventilatory settings on pulmonary and systemic inflammatory responses during major surgery. Anesth Analg 2004; 98: 775
66. Wrigge H, Zinserling J, Stuber F et al: Effects of mechanical ventilation on release of cytokines into systemic circulation in patients with normal pulmonary function. Anesthesiology 2000; 93: 1413
67. Fernandez-Perez ER, Keegan MT, Brown DR et al: Intraoperative tidal volume as a risk factor for respiratory failure after pneumonectomy. Anesthesiology 2006; 105: 14

68. Tusman G, Böhm SH, Vazquez da Anda G et al: "Alveolar recruitment strategy" improves arterial oxygenation during general Anaesthesia. Br J Anaesth 1999; 82: 8

69. Tusman J, Stephan H, Böhm SH et al: Alveolar Recruitment Strategy Increases Arterial Oxygenation During One-Lung Ventilation: Ann Thorac Surg 2002; 73: 1204

70. Tugrul M, Camici E, Karadeniz H et al: Comparison of volume control with pressure control ventilation during one-lung anaesthesia. Br J Anaesth 1997; 79: 306

71. Carmen MU, Casas J, Moral I et al: Pressure-Controlled Versus Volume-Controlled Ventilation During One-Lung Ventilation for Thoracic Surgery Anesth Analg 2007; 104: 1029

72. Cohen E, Thys DM, Eisenkraft JB et al: PEEP during one-lung anesthesia improves oxygenation in patients with low PaO_2. Anesth Analg 1985; 64: 200

73. Capan LM, Turndorf H, Patel K et al: Optimization of arterial oxygenation during one-lung anesthesia. Anesth Analg 1980; 59: 847

74. Hogue CW: Effectiveness of low levels of nonventilated lung continuous positive airway pressure in improving arterial oxygenation during one-lung ventilation. Anesth Analg 1994; 79: 364

75. Malmkvist G: Maintenance of oxygenation during one-lung ventilation. Effect of intermittent reinflation of the collapsed lung with oxygen. Anesth Analg 1989; 68: 763

76. Cohen E, Eisenkraft JB, Thys DM et al: Oxygenation and hemodynamic changes during one-lung ventilation. J Cardiovasc Vasc Anesth 1988; 2: 34

77. Shimizu T, Abe K, Kinovchik, Yoshiya I: Arterial oxygenation during one-lung ventilation. Can J Anaesth 1997; 44: 1162

78. Loer SA, Scheeren TWL, Tarnow J: Desflurane inhibits HPV in isolated rabbit lungs. Anesthesiology 1995; 83: 552

79. Van Keer L, Van Aken H, Vandermeersch E et al: Propofol does not inhibit HPV in humans. J Clin Anesth 1989; 1: 284

80. Kellow NH, Scott AD, White SA et al: Comparison of the effects of propofol and isoflurane anaesthesia on right ventricular function and shunt fraction during thoracic surgery. Br J Anesth 1995; 75: 578

81. Von Euler US, Liljestrand G: Observations on the pulmonary arterial blood pressure in the cat. Acta Physiol Scand 1946; 12: 301

82. Marshall BE, Marshall C, Benumof JL et al: Hypoxic pulmonary vasoconstriction in dogs: Effects of lung segment size and alveolar oxygen tensions. J Appl Physiol 1981; 51: 1543

83. Moudgil R, Michelakis ED, Archer SL. Hypoxic pulmonary vasoconstriction. J Appl Physiol 2005; 98: 390

84. Evans AM. Hypoxic pulmonary vasoconstriction. Essays in biochemistry 2007; 43: 61

85. Nagendran J, Stewart K, Hoskinson M et al: An anesthesiologist's guide to hypoxic pulmonary vasoconstriction: implications for managing single-lung anesthesia and atelectasis. Curr Opin Anesthesiol 2006; 19: 34

86. Benumof JL: One-lung ventilation and hypoxic pulmonary vasoconstriction: Implications for anesthetic management. Anesth Analg 1985; 64: 821

87. Eisenkraft JB: Effects of anesthetics on the pulmonary circulation. Br J Anaesth 1990; 65: 63

88. Rogers SM, Benumof JL: Halothane and isoflurane do not decrease PaO_2 during one-lung ventilation in intravenously anesthetized patients. Anesth Analg 1985; 64: 946

89. Benumof JL, Augustine SD, Gibbons JA: Halothane and isoflurane only slightly impair arterial oxygenation during one-lung ventilation in patients undergoing thoracotomy. Anesthesiology 1987; 67: 910

90. Slinger P, Scott WAC: Arterial oxygenation during one-lung ventilation: A comparison of enflurane and isoflurane. Anesthesiology 1995; 82: 940

91. Beck DH, Doepfmer UR, Sinemus C et al: Effects of sevoflurane and propofol on pulmonary shunt fraction during one-lung ventilation for thoracic surgery. Br J Anaesth 2001; 86: 38

92. Fischer SR, Deyo DJ, Bone HG et al: Nitric oxide synthase inhibition restores HPV in sepsis. Am J Respir Crit Care Med 1997; 156: 833

93. Frostell CG, Blomqvist H, Hedenstierna G et al: Inhaled nitric oxide selectively reverses human HPV without causing systemic vasodilation. Anesthesiology 1993; 78: 427

94. Troncy E, Francoeur M, Blaise G: Inhaled nitric oxide: Clinical applications, indications and toxicology. Can J Anaesth 1997; 44: 973

95. Moutafis M, Liu N, Dalibon N et al: The effects of inhaled nitric oxide and its combination with intravenous almitrine on PaO_2 during one-lung ventilation in patients undergoing thoracoscopic procedures. Anesth Analg 1997; 85: 1130

96. Moutafis M, Dalibon N, Colchen A et al: Improving oxygenation during bronchopulmonary lavage using nitric oxide inhalation and almitrine infusion. Anesth Analg 1999; 89: 32

97. B'chir A, Mebassa A, Losserm MR et al: Intravenous almitrine bimesylate reversibly inhibits lactic acidosis and hepatic dysfunction in patients with lung injury. Anesthesiology 1998; 89: 823

98. Doering EB, Hanson CW, Reily D et al: Improvement in oxygenation by phenylephrine and nitric oxide in patients with adult respiratory distress syndrome. Anesthesiology 1997; 87: 18

99. Matsushima Y, Jones RL, King EG et al: Alterations in pulmonary mechanics and gas exchange during routine fiberoptic bronchoscopy. Chest 1984; 86: 184

100. Satyanarayana T, Capan L, Ramanathan S et al: Bronchofiberscopic jet ventilation. Anesth Analg 1980; 59: 350

101. Neuman G, Weingarten AE, Abramowitz RM et al: The anesthetic management of the patient with an anterior mediastinal mass. Anesthesiology 1984; 60: 144

102. Bechard P, Letourneau L, Lacasse Y. Perioperative cardiorespiratory complications in adults with mediastinal mass: Incidence and risk factors. Anesthesiology 2004; 100: 826

103. Bechard P, Letourneau L, Lacasse Y. Perioperative cardiorespiratory complications in adults with mediastinal mass: Incidence and risk factors. Anesthesiology 2004; 100: 826

104. Oley LTC, Hnatiuk MC, Corcoran MC et al: Spirometry in surgery for anterior mediastinal masses. Chest 2001; 120: 1152

105. Tempe DK, Arya R, Dubey S et al: Mediastinal mass resection: Femoro-femoral cardiopulmonary bypass under induction of anesthesia in the management of airway obstruction. J Cardiothorac Vasc Anesth 2001; 15: 233

106. Ferrari LR, Bedford RF: General anesthesia prior to treatment of anterior mediastinal masses in pediatric cancer patients. Anesthesiology 1990; 72: 991

107. Shamberger RC: Preanesthetic evaluation of children with anterior mediastinal masses. Semin Pediatr Surg 1999; 8: 61

108. DeSoto H: Direct laryngoscopy as an aid to relieve airway obstruction in a patient with a mediastinal mass. Anesthesiology 1987; 67: 116

109. Barker SJ, Clarke C, Trivedi N et al: Anesthesia for thoracoscopic laser ablation of bullous emphysema. Anesthesiology 1993; 78: 44

110. Brodsky JB, Cohen E: Video-assisted thoracoscopic surgery. Curr Opin Anaesthesiol 2000; 13: 41

111. Plummer S, Hartley M, Vaughan RS: Anaesthesia for telescopic procedures in the thorax. Br J Anaesth 1998; 80: 223

112. Neustein SM, Kahn P, Krellenstein DJ et al: Incidence of arrhythmias and predisposing factors after thoracic surgery: Thoracotomy versus video-assisted thoracoscopy. J Cardiothorac Vasc Anesth 1998; 12: 659

113. Benumof JL: Sequential one-lung ventilation for bilateral bullectomy. Anesthesiology 1987; 67: 268

114. Cohen E, Eisenkraft JB: Bronchopulmonary lavage: Effects on oxygenation and hemodynamics. J Cardiothorac Anesth 1990; 4: 119

115. Hirsch NP. Neuromuscular junction in health and disease. Br J Anaesth 2007; 99: 132

116. Drachman DB: Myasthenia gravis: Review article. N Engl J Med 1994; 330: 1797

117. Eisenkraft JB, Neustein SM: Anesthesia for esophageal and mediastinal surgery, Thoracic Anesthesia, 3rd edition. Edited by Kaplan JA. New York, Churchill-Livingstone, 2003, p 269

118. Tripathi M, Kaushik S, Dubey P. The effect of use of pyridostigmine and requirement for vecuronium with myasthenia gravis. J Postgrad Med 2003; 49: 311

119. Dillon FX. Anesthesia issues in the perioperative management of myasthenia gravis. J Postgrad Med 2003; 49: 311

120. Nilsson E, Muller K: Neuromuscular effects of isoflurane in patients with myasthenia gravis. Acta Anaesthesiol Scand 1990; 34: 126

121. Nitahara K, Sugi Y, Higa K et al: Neuromuscular effects of sevoflurane in myasthenia gravis patients. Br J Anaesth 2007; 98: 337

122. Baraka A, Siddik S, Kawkabani N: Cisatracurium in a myasthenic patient undergoing thymectomy. Can J Anaesth 1999; 46: 779

123. Baraka AS, Taha SK, Kawkabani NI: Neuromuscular interaction of sevoflurane—cisatracurium in a myasthenic patient. Can J Anaesth 2000; 47: 562

124. Mann R, Blobner M, Jelen-Esselborn et al: Preanesthetic train-of-four fade predicts the atracurium requirement of myasthenia gravis patients. Anesthesiology 2000; 93: 346

125. Itoh H, Shibata K, Nitta S: Difference in sensitivity to vecuronium between patients with ocular and generalized myasthenia gravis. Br J Anaesth 2001; 87: 885

126. Itoh H, Shibata K, Nitta S: Sensitivity to vecuronium in seropositive and seronegative patients with myasthenia gravis. Anesth Analg 2003; 96: 1842

127. Basaranoglu G, Erden V, Delatioglu H. Anesthesia of a patient with cured myasthenia gravis. Anesth Analg 2003; 96: 1842

128. Naguib M. Sugammadex: Another milestone in clinical neuromuscular pharmacology. Anesth Analg 2007; 104: 575

129. Kopman AF. Sugammadex: A revolutionary approach to neuromuscular antagonism. Anesthesiology 2006; 104: 4

130. Eisenkraft JB, Book WJ, Papatestas AE et al: Resistance to succinylcholine in myasthenia gravis: A dose-response study. Anesthesiology 1988; 69: 760

131. Baraka A, Tabboush Z: Neuromuscular response to succinylcholine-vecuronium sequence in three myasthenic patients undergoing thymectomy. Anesth Analg 1991; 72: 827

132. Della Rocca G, Coccia C, Diana L et al: Propofol or sevoflurane anesthesia without muscle relaxants allow the early extubation of myasthenic patients. Can J Anesth 2003; 50: 547

133. Madi-Jebara S, Yazigi A, Hayek M et al: Sevoflurane anesthesia and intrathecal sufentanil-morphine for thymectomy in myasthenia gravis. J Clin Anesthesia 2002; 14: 558

134. Abe S, Takeuchi C, Kaneko T et al: Propofol anesthesia combined with thoracic epidural anesthesia for thymectomy for myasthenia gravis—a report of eleven cases. Masui 2001; 50: 1217

135. Chevalley C, Spiliopoulos A, dePerrot M et al: Perioperative medical management and outcome following thymectomy for myasthenia gravis. Can J Anesth 2001; 48: 446

136. Lorimer M, Hall R: Remifentanil and propofol total intravenous anaesthesia for thymectomy in myasthenia gravis. Anaesth Intens Care 1998; 26: 210

137. Politis GD, Tobias JD. Rapid sequence intubation without a neuromuscular blocking agent in a 14 year old female patient with myasthenia gravis. Pediatric Anesthesia 2007; 17: 285

138. Baraka AS, Haroun-Bizri ST, Georges FJ: Delayed postoperative arousal following remifentanil-based anesthesia in a myasthenic patient undergoing thymectomy. Anesthesiology 2004; 100: 460

139. Ingersoll-Weng E, Manecke GR, Thistlethwaite PA: Dexmedetomidine and cardiac arrest. Anesthesiology 2004; 100: 758

140. Eisenkraft JB, Papatestas AE, Kahn CH et al: Predicting the need for postoperative mechanical ventilation in myasthenia gravis. Anesthesiology 1986; 65: 79

141. Mori T, Yoshioka M, Watanabe K et al: Changes in respiratory condition after thymectomy for patients with myasthenia gravis. Ann Thorac Cardiovasc Surg 2003; 9: 93

142. Burgess FW, Wilcosky B: Thoracic epidural anesthesia for transsternal thymectomy in myasthenia gravis. Anesth Analg 1989; 69: 529

143. Gorback MS: Analgesic management after thymectomy. Anesthesiol Rep 1990; 2: 262

144. Petty R: Lambert Eaton myasthenic syndrome. Practical Neurology 2007; 7: 265

145. Itoh H, Shibata K, Nitta S: Neuromuscular monitoring in myasthenic syndrome. Anesthesia 2001; 56: 562

146. Telford RJ, Hollway TE: The myasthenic syndrome: Anesthesia in a patient treated with 3,4 diaminopyridine. Br J Anaesth 1990; 64: 363

147. Kavanagh BP, Katz J, Sandler AN: Pain control after thoracic surgery: A review of current techniques. Anesthesiology 1994; 81: 737

148. Whiting WG, Sandler AN, Lau LC et al: Analgesic and respiratory effects of epidural sufentanil in post-thoracotomy patients. Anesthesiology 1988; 69: 36

149. Suzuki M, Haraguti S, Sugimoto K et al: Low-dose intravenous ketamine potentiates epidural analgesia after thoracotomy. Anesthesiology 2006; 105: 111

150. Michelet P, Guervilly C, Helaine A: Adding ketamine to morphine for patient-contolled analgesia after thoracic surgery: influence on morphine consumption, respiratory function, and nocturnal desaturation. Br J Anaesth 2007; 99: 396

151. Sihoe AD, Lee TW, Wan IY et al: The use of gabapentin for post-operative and post-traumatic pain in thoracic surgery patients. Eur J Cardiothorac Surg 2006; 29: 795

152. Kong VKF, Irwin MG: Gabapentin: a multimodal perioperative drug? Br J Anaesth 2007; 99: 775

153. Davies RG, Myles PS, Graham JM: A comparison of the analgesic efficacy and side-effects of paravertebral vs epidural blockade for thoracotomy — a systematic review and meta-analysis of randomized controlled trials. Br J Anesth 2006; 96: 418

154. Block BM, Spencer SL, Rowlingson BA. et al: Efficacy of postoperative epidural analgesia. A meta-analysis. JAMA 2003; 290: 2455

155. Rodgers A, Walker N, Schug S et al: Reduction of postoperative mortality and morbidity with epidural or spinal anesthesia: results from an overview of randomized trials, Br Med J 2000; 321: 1

156. Minzler B, Grimm BJ, Johnson RF. et al: The practice of thoracic epidural analgesia: a survey of academic centers in the United States. Anesth Analg 2002; 95: 472

157. I. Weber T, Matzl J, Rokitansky A. et al: Superior postoperative pain relief with thoracic epidural analgesia versus intravenous patient-controlled analgesia after minimally invasive pectus excavatum repair. J of Thor and Cardiovasc Surg 2007; 132: 865

158. Mac TB, Girard F, Chouinard P et al: Acetaminophen decreases early post-thoracotomy ipsilateral shoulder pain in paients with thoracic epidural analgesia. J Cardiothorac Vasc Anesth 2005; 19: 475

159. Cohen E, Neustein SM: Intrathecal morphine during thoracotomy. J Thorac Cardiovasc Anesth 1993; 7: 154

160. Katz J, Kavanagh BP, Sandler AN et al: Preemptive analgesia. Anesthesiology 1992; 77: 439

161. Bong CL, Samuel M, Ng JM et al: Effects of preemptive epidural analgesia on post-thoracotomy pain. J Cardiothorac and Vasc Anesth 2005; 19: 786

162. Gotoda Y, Kambara N, Sakai T et al: The morbidity, time course and predictive factors for persistent post-thoracotomy pain. Eur J Pain 2001; 5: 89

163. Hutter J, Miller K, Moritz E. Chronic sequels after thoracoscopic procedures for benign diseases. Eur J Cardiothoracic Surg 2000; 17: 687

164. Ochroch EA, Gottschalk A, Troxel AB et al: Women suffer more short and long-term pain than men ater major thoracotomy. Clin J Pain 2006; 22: 491

165. Gottschalk A, Cohen S, Yang S et al: Preventing and treating pain after thoracic surgery. Anesthesiology 2006; 104: 594

166. Beck-Nielsen J, Sorensen HR, Alstrup P: Atrial fibrillation following thoracotomy for non-cardiac cases, in particular, cancer of the lung. Acta Med Scand 1973; 193: 425

167. Ritchie J, Bowe P, Gibbons JRP: Prophylactic digitalization for thoracotomy: A reassessment. Ann Thorac Surg 1990; 50: 86

168. Ciriaco P, Mazzone P, Canneto B et al: Supraventricular arrhythmia following lung resection for non-small-cell lung cancer and its treatment with amiodarone. Eur J Cardio-Thoracic Surg 2000; 18: 12

CHAPTER 41 ■ ANESTHESIA FOR CARDIAC SURGERY

NIKOLAOS J. SKUBAS, ADAM D. LICHTMAN, AARTI SHARMA, AND STEPHEN J. THOMAS

KEY POINTS

❶ When treating myocardial ischemia, decreasing O_2 demand is more important than modifying O_2 supply.

❷ Intraoperative ischemia is usually silent and is not usually accompanied by hemodynamic changes.

❸ Slow rate, small size, and adequate perfusion are the goals in patients with coronary artery disease.

❹ The pulmonary artery catheter does not always reliably detect ischemia.

❺ There is no "ideal" anesthetic in cardiac surgery.

❻ In aortic stenosis, a preload-dependent, hypertrophic ventricle requires adequate diastolic time and perfusion pressure.

❼ In chronic aortic insufficiency, a dilated ventricle requires increased preload and decreased afterload.

❽ In mitral stenosis, the left ventricle is "lazy" and "under-used," and requires a slow heart rate to fill.

❾ In mitral regurgitation, a preload-dependent and dilated left ventricle benefits from afterload reduction and fast heart rate.

❿ Maintenance of perfusion pressure should not take precedence over ventilation during cardiac anesthesia (never forget your ABCs).

⓫ Fast-track anesthetic techniques depend on higher concentration of inspired volatile agents, use of vasoactive medications (beta-blockers), and smaller doses of benzodiazepines and opioids.

⓬ The combination of systolic systemic and diastolic pulmonary pressures characterize the performance of the left ventricle, and the combination of systolic pulmonary and central venous pressures characterize the performance of the right ventricle.

Anesthetizing patients for open heart surgery is exciting, intellectually challenging, and emotionally rewarding. Competent and skillful clinical management requires a thorough understanding of normal and altered cardiac physiology; an intimate knowledge of the pharmacology of anesthetic, vasoactive, and cardioactive drugs; and a familiarity with the physiologic derangements associated with cardiopulmonary bypass (CPB) and the surgical procedures themselves. This chapter presents a brief overview of the subject to acquaint the reader with the critical physiologic and technical considerations when caring for cardiac surgical patients. The initial discussions concerning coronary artery and valvular heart disease lay the physiologic and some of the pharmacologic groundwork on which anesthetic planning and therapeutic decisions are based. First we describe the balance of myocardial oxygen supply and demand, with particular reference to the patient with coronary artery disease. Next we focus on those variables that regulate myocardial performance, specifically myocardial contractility, heart rate, and loading conditions (both preload and afterload). Then we discuss the mechanics of CPB. Following this, we describe anesthetic considerations relevant to all adults undergoing cardiac surgery either with or without CPB, including preoperative evaluation, choice of monitoring techniques, selection of anesthetic drugs, and the actual conduct of the anesthetic before, during, and after bypass. The chapter concludes with some special topics, as well as a brief introduction to the child with congenital heart disease. Some of the issues discussed are controversial because the field is continuously evolving. The authors have tried, whenever possible, to suggest what is the consensus about these topics, but, inevitably, the authors' own preferences will be apparent. For the sake of brevity, numerous tables are included that summarize data and provide readily accessible guidelines for the various phases of the operative procedure.

CORONARY ARTERY DISEASE

Prevention or treatment of ischemia during coronary artery bypass graft (CABG) surgery reduces the incidence of perioperative myocardial infarction. Hemodynamic management is tailored to avoid factors known to increase myocardial oxygen demand ($M\dot{V}O_2$), particularly during the vulnerable pre-CPB period. Optimizing oxygen delivery to the myocardium is equally important for the successful management of these patients because it is well recognized that most ischemic events occur with minimal or no change in $M\dot{V}O_2$.[1] The determinants of myocardial oxygen supply and demand are shown in Figure 41-1 and are also discussed in Chapter 10.

Myocardial Oxygen Demand

The principal determinants of $M\dot{V}O_2$ are wall tension and contractility.[2] Laplace law states that wall tension is directly proportional to intracavitary pressure and ventricular radius, and inversely proportional to wall thickness. Therefore, myocardial oxygen demand can be reduced by interventions that (1) prevent or promptly treat ventricular distention, and (2) decrease intraventricular pressure.

Myocardial Oxygen Supply

Increases in myocardial oxygen requirements can be met only by raising coronary blood flow. Blood oxygen content is important, as is oxygen extraction by the myocardium, but these are infrequent reasons for intraoperative ischemia because oxygenation and blood volume are usually well maintained during anesthesia. Blood in the coronary sinus is 50% saturated (PO_2 approximately 27 mm Hg), and although extraction can be increased somewhat under conditions of stress, it is inadequate to meet the continuously increasing demand. Therefore, the principal mechanism for matching oxygen supply to alterations in $M\dot{V}O_2$ is exquisite regulation and control of coronary blood flow.

Coronary Blood Flow

The critical factors that modify coronary blood flow are the perfusion pressure and vascular tone of the coronary circulation, the time available for perfusion (determined namely by heart rate), the severity of intraluminal obstructions, and the presence of (any) collateral circulation. The area most vulnerable to ischemia is the subendocardium of the left ventricle (LV), where metabolic requirements are increased because of greater systolic shortening.[3]

Perfusion of the LV subendocardium takes place almost entirely during diastole, whereas the right ventricular subendocardium is perfused mostly during systole, assuming pulmonary hypertension is not present. This temporal disparity is explained by the different intraventricular pressures developing during systole.

The LV coronary perfusion pressure is often defined as the difference between aortic diastolic pressure and left ventricular end-diastolic pressure. In the presence of intraluminal obstruction or increased vascular tone, this pressure gradient is reduced (Fig. 41-2). It is convenient and useful to consider the pulmonary artery occlusion pressure as the closest surrogate of left ventricular end-diastolic pressure. Therefore, a low left ventricular end-diastolic pressure is ideal both in terms of improving perfusion (higher pressure gradient) and of reducing $M\dot{V}O_2$ (decreased ventricular volume and wall tension). The consequences of systemic pressure are more difficult to predict; for example, increasing perfusion pressure may increase $M\dot{V}O_2$. However, it has been shown clinically that tachycardia is the most important trigger of intraoperative and perioperative ischemia.

Alterations in the tone of the small intramyocardial arterioles regulate diastolic vascular resistance, allowing the matching of oxygen supply with metabolic demand over a wide

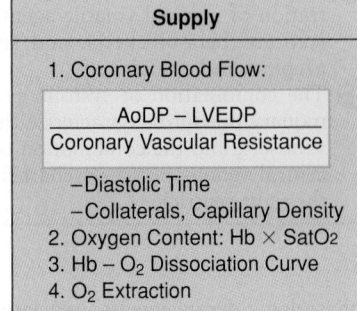

Demand	Supply

1. Wall Stress: $\frac{PR}{2h}$
  - Preload
  - Afterload
2. Heart Rate
3. Contractility
	1. Coronary Blood Flow:
	
	$$\frac{AoDP - LVEDP}{Coronary\ Vascular\ Resistance}$$
	
	  −Diastolic Time
	  −Collaterals, Capillary Density
	2. Oxygen Content: Hb × SatO₂
	3. Hb − O₂ Dissociation Curve
	4. O₂ Extraction

FIGURE 41-1. Determinants of myocardial oxygen balance. P, intracavitary pressure; R, ventricular radius; h, wall thickness; AoDP, diastolic arterial pressure; LVEDP, left ventricular end-diastolic pressure; Hb, hemoglobin; SatO₂ arterial oxygen saturation.

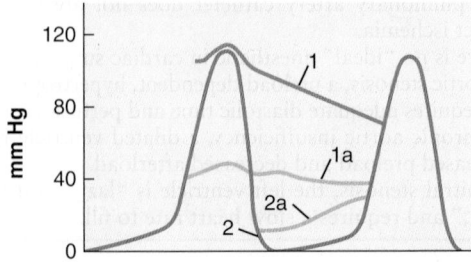

FIGURE 41-2. The pressure relationships between the aorta (1) and the left ventricle (2) determine coronary perfusion pressure. In coronary artery disease, myocardial perfusion may be compromised by decreased pressure distal to a significant stenosis (1a) (not quantifiable clinically) and/or by an increase in left ventricular end-diastolic pressure (2a). (Reprinted from Gorlin R: Coronary Artery Disease, Philadelphia, WB Saunders, 1976, p 75, with permission.)

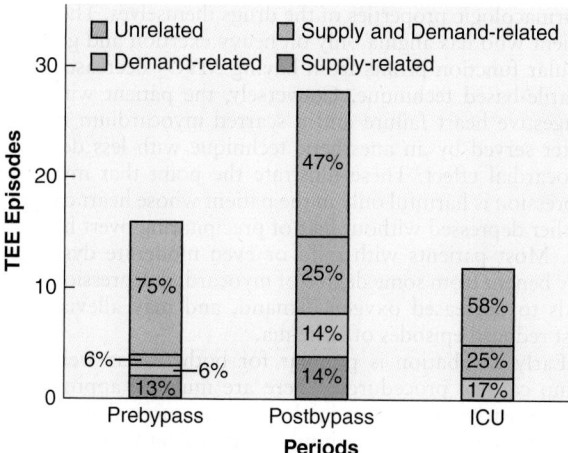

FIGURE 41-3. Association of transesophageal echocardiographic (TEE) wall motion changes with hemodynamic indices of supply and demand from continuous monitoring of 50 patients undergoing coronary artery bypass surgery. ICU, intensive care unit. (Reproduced from Leung JM, O'Kelly BV, Mangano DT et al: Relationship of regional wall motion abnormalities to hemodynamic indices of myocardial oxygen supply and demand in patients undergoing CABG surgery. Anesthesiology 1990; 73: 802, with permission.)

TABLE 41-1

CORONARY ARTERY DISEASE—HEMODYNAMIC GOALS

Preload	Keep the heart small: ↓ wall tension (diameter) and LVEDP; ↑ perfusion pressure gradient
Afterload	Maintain: hypertension better than hypotension
Contractility	Depression (if LV function is normal)
Rate	Slow
Rhythm	Sinus
MVO₂	Monitor for, and treat "supply"-related disturbances
CPB	Elevated filling pressures are usually not needed after CABG

↓, decrease; ↑, increase; LVEDP, left ventricular end-diastolic pressure; LV, left ventricular; MVO$_2$, myocardial oxygen consumption; CPB, postcardiopulmonary bypass; CABG, coronary artery bypass graft.

range of perfusion pressures.[4] The difference between autoregulated, baseline flow, and blood flow available under conditions of maximal vasodilation is termed *coronary vascular reserve*, and is normally 3 to 5 times higher than basal flow. As epicardial stenosis becomes more pronounced, progressive vasodilation of these resistance vessels allows preservation of basal flow, but at the cost of reduced reserve. Whenever demand increases above available reserve, signs, symptoms, and metabolic evidence of ischemia develop.

Prinzmetal et al.[5] first described angina and myocardial infarction in patients with angiographically normal coronary vessels. Subsequently, others have repeatedly emphasized the ❸ frequency with which reductions in oxygen supply cause ischemia, demonstrating that small adjustments in coronary vascular tone at the site of existing obstructions can cause substantial reductions in luminal cross-sectional area. Alterations in vessel diameter at the stenotic area are possible because at least two thirds of plaques or atheromas are not concentric. It is now apparent that anesthesia is not protective against "supply" ischemia, which occurs frequently during surgery (Fig. 41-3). The etiology of this is unclear, but may be caused by circulating catecholamines, local effects of blood components such as platelets at areas of unstable atherosclerotic plaques, or other as yet undetermined factors. It is not uncommon for an anesthetized patient to show signs of ischemia without any change in heart rate, blood pressure, or ventricular filling pressures. In fact, most ischemic episodes ❷ are not accompanied by hemodynamic changes. Drugs such as nitroglycerin or calcium entry blockers may be used to prevent and/or treat such episodes of coronary spasm, although prophylactic use of these agents is usually ineffective.

Hypotension, vasospasm, and acute thrombosis decrease coronary perfusion pressure, reduce coronary blood flow, and limit oxygen delivery to the myocardium. Unstable angina pectoris and/or acute coronary thrombosis are the results of plaque rupture with ensuing platelet activation and thrombus formation.[6] The presence of the potentially hyperreactive normal vessel wall adjacent to the thrombus may result in vasospasm and total occlusion of the vessel lumen in the presence of a previously nonocclusive eccentric plaque or thrombus. This type of acute thrombosis is believed to be the cause

of acute myocardial infarction and sudden death (mostly from ischemia-induced cardiac dysrhythmias).

Hemodynamic Goals

Although the precise relationship between intraoperative ischemia and postoperative myocardial infarction remains controversial, there is consensus that one of the primary goals of any successful anesthetic is prevention of myocardial ischemia. Failing that, prompt identification and treatment of new ischemic episodes is essential. As is evident from the previous discussion and from the summary in Table 41-1, anesthetic decisions are designed to reduce and control those factors that increase myocardial oxygen demand (heart rate, contractility, and wall tension). At the same time, every attempt is made to optimize coronary blood flow, notably, maintaining coronary ❸ perfusion pressure and increasing diastolic time. The goals for patients with coronary artery disease are "slow, small, and well perfused." Combinations of anesthetics, sedatives, muscle relaxants, and vasoactive drugs are selected to provide this hemodynamic milieu. Pharmacologic agents that may benefit coronary patients include statins and angiotensin-converting enzyme inhibitors (to stabilize the atherosclerotic plaque), and volatile anesthetics (anesthetic preconditioning).[7]

Monitoring for Ischemia

The ideal monitoring technique is not yet available. Analysis of the ST segment in multiple leads (most commonly leads II and V$_4$ or V$_5$) is currently the standard. Patients likely to develop right ventricular ischemia or those with disease of the right coronary artery might benefit from monitoring of leads V$_{4R}$ or V$_{5R}$. Computerized ST segment trending and interactive monitors that alarm when the ST segment deviates from the programmed algorithm aid in the detection of intraoperative events overlooked by even the most astute observer.

Multiple attempts have been made to determine ischemic thresholds using commonly measured hemodynamic variables. Among the earliest of these was the rate-pressure product (RPP = heart rate × peak systolic arterial pressure). The RPP was considered an easily determined index of MVO$_2$. Although RPP may correlate with oxygen demand, especially during exercise, it is not a sensitive or specific indicator of intraoperative ischemia; identical RPPs can be produced from multiple combinations of heart rate and blood pressure. Favorable conditions for oxygen balance are more likely those of lower heart rate and higher blood pressure than tachycardia and hypotension. Neither the pressure-rate *ratio* (P/RR: the ratio of pressure over heart rate), nor the mean arterial pressure (MAP)/heart rate ratio are any more predictive or reliable than the RPP.

Sudden elevations in pulmonary artery or capillary wedge pressure indicating systolic and/or diastolic left ventricular dysfunction, large *a* waves reflecting decreased ventricular compliance, and *v* waves indicative of increased left atrial pressure because of ischemia-induced papillary muscle dysfunction and/or mitral regurgitation are purported signs of ischemia that may be detected with a pulmonary artery catheter (PAC). PAC-based monitoring of filling pressures, saturation of mixed venous blood in oxygen, and thermodilution cardiac output is common practice in cardiac surgery centers. Several studies contradict this long-held dogma and demonstrate that the PAC is of little value as a monitor of myocardial ischemia. Leung et al.[8] found that only 10% of all regional wall motion abnormalities were associated with an acute rise in pulmonary capillary wedge pressure in 40 patients undergoing elective CABG surgery. Haggmark et al.[9] found that neither an increase in the pulmonary capillary wedge pressure nor the occurrence of an abnormal pulmonary capillary wedge pressure waveform was a sensitive indicator for myocardial ischemia in 53 patients with coronary artery disease undergoing vascular surgery. A prospective study of 1,094 patients by Tuman et al.[10] showed that even high-risk cardiac surgical patients may be safely managed without routine use of a PAC, and if the need for it developed intraoperatively, delayed placement of a PAC did not influence outcome. Fontes et al.[11] assessed the limitations of PAC in the management of critically ill patients in the intensive care unit (ICU). Compared with transesophageal echocardiography, PAC predicted normal left ventricular function well, but performed poorly in judging preload and ventricular dysfunction. A more recent study showed no benefit from PACs in high-risk surgical patients.[12] Nevertheless, the PAC is still frequently used in cardiac surgical patients to measure cardiac output and as a guide, albeit not ideal, to volume status. The most recent American Society of Anesthesiologists Practice Guidelines concluded that the evidence regarding the benefit that cardiac surgery patients receive from PAC is conflicting.[13]

Since its introduction in the 1980s, transesophageal echocardiography (TEE) has become an invaluable diagnostic and monitoring tool during cardiac surgery. TEE permits assessment of ventricular volume, global and regional function, estimation and quantitation of valvular pathology, measurement of valve gradients and calculation of filling pressures, visualization of the thoracic aorta, and detection of intracardiac air. Experienced cardiac anesthesiologists who are supported by continuous quality programs perform comprehensive TEE studies[14] and interpret TEE examinations at a level comparable with physicians whose primary practice is echocardiography.[15]

Multiple image planes are necessary to evaluate the three-dimensional structure of the heart. The American Society of Echocardiography/Society of Cardiovascular Anesthesiologists task force for intraoperative echocardiography has published guidelines for performing a comprehensive intraoperative echocardiographic examination.[16] These recommendations describe a series of 20 standard tomographic views of the heart and great vessels that should be included in a complete intraoperative echocardiographic examination. With experience, a thorough examination can be performed in <10 minutes.

Selection of Anesthetic

There is no one "ideal" anesthetic for patients with coronary artery disease. The choice of anesthetic should depend primarily on the extent of pre-existing myocardial dysfunction and the

pharmacologic properties of the drugs themselves. The healthy patient who has angina only on heavy exertion and good ventricular function profits from having $M\dot{V}O_2$ decreased with a volatile-based technique. Conversely, the patient with severe congestive heart failure and a scarred myocardium might be better served by an anesthetic technique with less depressant myocardial effect. These illustrate the point that myocardial depression is harmful only in the patient whose heart cannot be further depressed without fear of precipitating overt heart failure. Most patients with mild or even moderate dysfunction may benefit from some degree of myocardial depression, which leads to decreased oxygen demand, and may alleviate or at least reduced episodes of ischemia.

Early extubation is popular for both on- as well as off-pump cardiac procedures. There are multiple approaches to achieve early extubation in the cardiac surgical patient.[17,18] The choice of anesthetic should be based on known hemodynamic, pharmacologic, and pharmacokinetic effects of each drug as they apply to the particular patient, the experience of the anesthesiologist, and the relative cost-benefit of each agent. Volatile anesthetics with low-dose narcotics and total intravenous anesthesia with short-acting drugs (e.g., midazolam, alfentanil, remifentanil, propofol) have been used to effect early extubation. Another interesting approach is the combination of the opiates, sufentanil and morphine, instilled intrathecally before induction. Intraoperative clinical variables are important factors to be considered in the timing of postoperative extubation after fast-track cardiac surgery. Inotrope use and platelet transfusion were the most significant determinants of early (<10 hours postoperatively) tracheal extubation in a Veterans Administration population.[19]

Opioids

The primary advantages of opioids are lack of myocardial depression, maintenance of a stable hemodynamic state, and reduction of heart rate (except for meperidine). Notable side effects include (1) hypertension and tachycardia during surgical stimulation (sternotomy and aortic manipulation), especially in patients with good ventricular function; (2) predictable hypotension when combined with benzodiazepines; (3) lack of titratability when used in high doses; and (4) a low incidence of intraoperative recall if used as the sole anesthetic. An opioid-based technique may be of value in the patient with severe myocardial dysfunction, whereas in a patient with normal ventricle, it may be inadequate and need to be combined with other anesthetics or vasoactive drugs. The planned time of extubation is now one of the major factors determining the selection and dosage of opioid. Shorter-acting opioids (sufentanil and remifentanil) produce equally rapid extubation, similar ICU stay, and similar costs to fentanyl. Thus, any of these opioids can be used for fast-track cardiac surgery.[20]

Inhalation Anesthetics

The desirable features of volatile anesthetics include dose dependency, easy reversibility, titratable myocardial depression, amnesia, and suppression of sympathetic responses to surgical stress and cardiopulmonary bypass. Volatile anesthetics protect the myocardium from ischemia and reperfusion injury and reduce myocardial infarct size.[21] This beneficial effect has been shown when volatile anesthetics are administered before a period of prolonged ischemia ("anesthetic preconditioning') as well as during reperfusion ("anesthetic postconditioning").[22] Disadvantages include systemic hypotension (whether induced by decreased contractility or vasodilation) and lack of postoperative analgesia. Combinations of opioids and volatile anesthetics retain their advantages with minimal untoward effects. Any of the volatile agents can be used in a balanced technique.

Isoflurane is a coronary vasodilator, as are the other volatile anesthetics (although to a lesser degree). This dose-related effect is clinically insignificant in doses less than 1 MAC. Clinical studies using isoflurane to clinical rather than pharmacologic end points have not shown increased episodes of ischemia or a worsened outcome.[23]

Desflurane and sevoflurane have the fastest recovery of all volatile anesthetics. Desflurane has a rapid uptake and distribution, allowing it to be useful in cases in which hemodynamic swings are dramatic. It has a cardiac profile similar to that of isoflurane. Of concern is the fact that a sudden increase in inspired concentration can lead to a marked increase in heart rate, mean arterial pressure, and plasma epinephrine levels, making it riskier for use in patients with coronary artery disease. In patients undergoing noncardiac surgery, desflurane increases pulmonary artery pressure, wedge pressure, and pulmonary vascular resistance compared with isoflurane.[24] When studying sympathetic nervous system activity, Helman et al.[25] found an increase in sympathetic activity and myocardial ischemia in patients anesthetized with desflurane as the sole anesthetic agent for coronary artery bypass surgery compared with patients anesthetized with sufentanil. Compared with isoflurane, in a technique combining fentanyl with the inhalational anesthetic, sevoflurane had an acceptable cardiovascular profile prior to cardiopulmonary bypass and similar outcome data.[26]

Intravenous Sedative Hypnotics

An alternative adjuvant anesthetic to a low-dose opioid technique is a titratable intravenous infusion of a short-acting sedative, such as midazolam,[27] propofol, or dexmedetomidine.[28] These can be continued postoperatively in the ICU and afford a predictable and fairly rapid awakening after discontinuation.[29] When compared with volatile anesthetics, propofol was associated with less favorable cardiac function, higher need for inotropic support, and elevated plasma troponins after cardiac surgery in elderly patients.[30]

Treatment of Ischemia

The use of anesthetics or vasoactive drugs that enable the heart to return to the slower-rate, smaller-size, and well-perfused state is frequently essential during anesthesia. The principal vasoactive drugs are nitrates, beta-blockers, peripheral vasoconstrictors, and calcium-entry blockers. Clinical scenarios for their use are given in Table 41-2. These drugs are discussed briefly here. Volatile anesthetics can also be used to control blood pressure and reduce contractility.

Nitrates

Nitroglycerin (TNG) is the drug of choice for the acute treatment of coronary vasospasm. It is a systemic venodilator (reduces venous return and decreases wall tension and MVO_2) and a coronary arterial dilator (effective in both stenosed coronaries and in collateral beds).[31] The evidence for the prophylactic use of TNG is unconvincing for prevention of either intraoperative ischemic episodes or postoperative cardiac complications.[32] At higher doses, it dilates arterial beds and may cause systemic hypotension. Compensatory tachycardia increases heart rate and MVO_2. The recommended TNG dose is 0.5 to 3 μg/kg/min and is reduced in the presence of hepatic and/or renal disease. TNG may cause methemoglobinemia, especially in patients with methemoglobin reductase defi-

TABLE 41-2

TREATMENT OF INTRAOPERATIVE ISCHEMIA

■ CLINICAL MANIFESTATION

Increased demand	
↑ HR	Treat usual suspects, beta-blocker
↑ BP	↑ Anesthetic depth
↑ PCWP	Nitroglycerin
Decreased supply	
↓ HR	Atropine, pacing
↓ BP	↓ Anesthetic depth, vasoconstrictor
↑ PCWP	Nitroglycerin, inotrope
No changes	Nitroglycerin, calcium-channel blockers, ? heparin

↑, increase; ↓, decrease; HR, heart rate; BP, blood pressure; PCWP, pulmonary capillary wedge pressure.

ciency. TNG is administered via special intravenous tubing that does not adsorb the drug.

Sodium Nitroprusside

Sodium nitroprusside (SNP), which is comparable to other nitrovasodilators, decreases peripheral vascular resistance by metabolic or spontaneous reduction to nitric oxide. Similar to TNG, SNP improves ventricular compliance in the ischemic myocardium. The recommended SNP dose is 0.5 to 3 μg/kg per minute, and is reduced in the presence of hepatic and/or renal disease. Adverse effects include cyanide and thiocyanate toxicity, rebound hypertension, intracranial hypertension, blood coagulation abnormalities, increased pulmonary shunting, and hypothyroidism. In vitro findings suggest that cardiac surgical patients may be at increased risk of cyanide toxicity in response to the perioperative administration of SNP.[33] Cyanide is produced when SNP is metabolized; 1 mg of SNP contains 0.44 mg of cyanide. Toxic blood levels (>100 mg/dL) occur when >1 mg/kg SNP is administered within 2 hours or when >0.5 mg/kg/hr is administered within 24 hours. The presenting signs of cyanide toxicity include the triad of elevated mixed venous O_2 (PvO_2), requirements for increasing SNP dose (tachyphylaxis), and metabolic acidosis.[34] In addition, the patient may appear flushed. Greater risk of cyanide toxicity exists in patients who are nutritionally deficient in cobalamine (vitamin B_{12} compounds) or in dietary substances containing sulfur. Measurement of blood cyanide and pH will enable detection of abnormalities in high-risk patients for whom larger than recommended amounts of SNP have been used (8 to 10 μg/kg per minute). Treatment should consist of discontinuing infusion, administering 100% O_2, administering amyl nitrate (inhaler) or intravenous sodium nitrite and intravenous thiosulfate, except in those patients with abnormal renal function, for whom hydroxocobalamin is recommended. Circulating levels of thiocyanate increase when renal function is compromised, and central nervous system abnormalities result when thiocyanate levels reach 5 to 10 mg/dL. Lowering the SNP dose requirement can be achieved with captopril, trimethaphan, diltiazem, nicardipine, metoprolol, and esmolol, thereby reducing the consequent buildup of cyanide. SNP can also cause inhibition of platelet aggregation; however, this complication is reversible and transitory. Once dissolved, SNP deteriorates in the presence of light. The container, therefore, should be wrapped in aluminum foil. An unstable SNP ion in aqueous solution reacts with various substances within 3 to 4 hours, forming colored salts. Other drugs should not be infused in the same solution as SNP.

Vasoconstrictors

Vasoconstrictors are useful adjuncts in the prevention and treatment of ischemia because they increase systemic blood pressure. Administration of an α-adrenergic agent such as phenylephrine improves coronary perfusion pressure, albeit at the expense of increasing afterload and MVO_2. In addition, concomitant venoconstriction increases venous return and LV preload. TNG is sometimes added to counteract any increase in preload. In most situations, the increase in coronary perfusion pressure more than offsets any increase in wall tension. Peripheral vasoconstriction is indicated during episodes of systemic hypotension, especially those caused by reduced surgical stimulation or drug-induced vasodilation (e.g., when TNG results in unacceptably low arterial pressure). No one vasoconstrictor is superior to all others. Occasionally, a combination of vasoconstrictors (e.g., norepinephrine and vasopressin) may be needed to achieve the desired blood pressure.[35]

Beta Blockers

β-Adrenergic blockade improves myocardial oxygen balance by preventing or treating tachycardia and by decreasing contractility. Myocardial depression can result in increased ventricular end-systolic volume and wall tension. Clinically, this is not usually a problem. Indications for beta-blockers include treatment of sinus tachycardia not resulting from the usual causes (e.g., light anesthesia, hypovolemia), prophylaxis of, and slowing the ventricular response to, supraventricular dysrhythmias, decreasing heart rate and contractility in hyperdynamic states, and control of ventricular dysrhythmias.[36,37] The use of atenolol has been shown to improve long-term survival in patients with heart disease undergoing noncardiac surgery.[38,39] Intravenous preparations include propranolol, metoprolol, labetalol, and esmolol. Propranolol is a nonselective beta-blocker with an elimination half-life of 4 to 6 hours. Metoprolol is similar to propranolol but has the purported advantage of β_1 selectivity and is less likely to trigger bronchospasm in patients with reactive airway disease. Labetalol combines beta-blocking properties with those of α-blockade and is useful in treating hyperdynamic and hypertensive situations. Esmolol is a short-acting β_1-blocker that is cardioselective, with a half-life of only 9.5 minutes. It is particularly useful in treating transient increases in heart rate owing to episodic sympathetic stimulation.

Calcium Channel Blockers

Calcium channel blockers are useful in slowing the ventricular response in atrial fibrillation and flutter, as coronary vasodilators, and in the treatment of perioperative hypertension.[40,41] In vitro, all calcium entry blockers depress contractility, reduce coronary and systemic vascular tone, decrease sinoatrial node firing rate, and impede atrioventricular conduction. Unlike the beta-blockers, which are similar both in structure and pharmacodynamic effect, the calcium entry blockers vary remarkably in their predominant pharmacologic action. The negative inotropic effect is greatest with verapamil and less with nifedipine, diltiazem, and isradipine (in decreasing order). Verapamil is useful in the treatment of supraventricular tachycardia and slowing the ventricular response in atrial fibrillation and/or flutter; however, its myocardial depressant effects may limit its usefulness in some patients. In patients with reduced myocardial function, intravenous diltiazem is effective in the treatment of atrial fibrillation and flutter by slowing atrioventricular conduction with minimal myocardial depression. It is also useful in decreasing sinus rate. Nifedipine and diltiazem are coronary vasodilators used as antianginal agents and in the prevention of coronary vasospasm.

Nifedipine, isradipine, amlodipine, and nicardipine are prominent peripheral vasodilators. Owing to their systemic vasodilatory effects, intravenous isradipine and nicardipine have been shown to be effective in the treatment of postoperative hypertension in cardiac surgical patients, with minimal side effects.[42,43] Magnesium has use in the treatment of myocardial ischemia. It has coronary artery vasodilating properties, reduces the size of myocardial infarction in the setting of acute ischemia, and decreases mortality associated with infarction.[44] In addition, it is an antiarrhythmic and minimizes myocardial reperfusion injury.

VALVULAR HEART DISEASE

Alterations in loading conditions are the initial physiologic burdens imposed by valvular heart lesions, both stenotic and regurgitant. For example, the LV is pressure overloaded in aortic stenosis and volume overloaded in aortic insufficiency and mitral regurgitation. In mitral stenosis, however, the LV is both volume-underloaded and pressure-underloaded, whereas the right ventricle faces progressively increasing left atrial and pulmonary artery pressure. Compensatory mechanisms consist of chamber enlargement, myocardial hypertrophy, and variations in vascular tone and level of sympathetic activity. These mechanisms in turn induce secondary alterations, including altered ventricular compliance, development of myocardial ischemia, chronic cardiac dysrhythmias, and progressive myocardial dysfunction.

Myocardial contractility in patients with mitral insufficiency is often transiently depressed but may progress to irreversible impairment even in the absence of clinical symptoms. Conversely, the patient with aortic stenosis may complain of dyspnea, not because of impaired systolic function, but because of reduced ventricular compliance, increased left ventricular end-diastolic pressure, and increased pulmonary pressure.

The patient presenting for valve repair or replacement often has pulmonary hypertension, severe ventricular dysfunction, and chronic rhythm disorders. Anesthetic management is predicated on understanding the altered loading conditions, preserving the compensatory mechanisms, maintaining circulatory homeostasis, and anticipating problems that may arise during and after valve surgery. In this section, we briefly describe the pathophysiology, the desirable hemodynamic profile, and other pertinent anesthetic considerations for each valvular lesion.

TEE has become the standard of care in the perioperative management of patients undergoing valve surgery. TEE can further refine the preoperative diagnosis, identify valvular pathology and the mechanism of disease, and quantify the degree of stenosis and/or regurgitation. A detailed review of the perioperative role of TEE is presented in Chapter 28.

Aortic Stenosis

Aortic stenosis (AS) is the most common valvular disease in the United States. In a normal adult, the aortic valve (AV) is composed of three semilunar cusps attached to the wall of the aorta. The normal AV diameter is 1.9 to 2.3 cm with an aortic valve area of 2 to 4 cm^2. The outpouchings of the aortic wall immediately above the valve cusps are called the *sinuses of Valsalva*. These are symmetric with a diameter 0.2 to 0.3 cm greater than the AV annular diameter. The cusps and the corresponding sinuses are named according to their relation to the coronary ostia: left, right, and noncoronary (opposite the interatrial septum). On the ventricular side of the AV is the cylindrical LV outflow tract. Its borders are the inferior surface of the anterior leaflet of the mitral valve, the interventricular septum, and the LV free wall. The normal diameter of the LV outflow tract (LVOT) is 2.2 cm $\pm$ 0.2 cm.

Calcific AV disease has many similar features with coronary artery disease. What in the past was thought to be "degenerative" is a disease continuum, similar to atherosclerosis. Increased mechanical stress (higher on the aortic side of AV cusps, in the flexion area) causes endothelial disruption, which leads to lipoprotein deposition, chronic inflammation, and active cusp calcification.[45] These histologic changes result in macroscopic, progressive valve thickening. Increased calcification eventually leads to leaflet immobility and outflow obstruction. Clinical factors associated with aortic sclerosis include older age, male gender, smoking, hypertension, and hyperlipidemia. Patients with bicuspid AV (increased mechanical stress) or with altered mineral metabolism (Paget disease, renal failure) have a higher prevalence of calcific AS disease. Rheumatic disease (an autoimmune disease, rarely seen in developed countries, leading to calcification and fusion along the commissures) causes mixed AS and AV regurgitation, and usually coexists with mitral valve disease.

Pathophysiology

The classic symptoms of AS are angina (35%), syncope (15%), and dyspnea (50%) are harbingers of poor outcome (death) within 5, 3 and 2 years, respectively, unless the AV is replaced. The progressive narrowing of the AV orifice results in chronic obstruction to LV ejection. Intraventricular systolic pressure increases to preserve forward flow. "Concentric" ventricular hypertrophy, in which the wall gradually thickens but the chamber size remains unchanged, is the compensatory response normalizing the concomitant increase in wall tension. Contractility is preserved and ejection fraction is maintained at a normal range until late in the disease process (Fig. 41-4). Signs and symptoms of AS occur when the AV orifice is reduced to 0.8 cm^2.[46]

The costs of this concentric hypertrophy are decreased diastolic compliance and a precarious balance between myocardial oxygen supply and MVO_2. Hypertrophy-induced impairment of diastolic relaxation ("stiff" ventricle) impedes early left ventricular filling, and atrial contraction becomes critical for maintaining adequate ventricular filling and stroke volume.

The "atrial kick" may account for up to 30 to 40% of LV end-diastolic volume. The ventricular filling pressure, as reflected by pulmonary capillary wedge pressure, may vary widely with only small changes in ventricular volume (reduced compliance).

The enlarged muscle mass has increased basal MVO_2, while demand per beat rises because of the elevated intraventricular systolic pressure. Simultaneously, with a capillary density often inadequate for the hypertrophic muscle, reduction in perfusion pressure (as when the aortic diastolic pressure is decreased and/or the ventricular filling pressure is increased), may further compromise supply, and total vasodilator reserve. This situation is compounded in the presence of coronary obstruction. Patients with AS often present in heart failure.

There is an inverse relationship between wall stress (afterload) and LV ejection fraction. In patients with a substantial transvalvular pressure gradient (mean >40 mm Hg), AV replacement corrects the afterload excess and improves outcome. Decreased contractility results in decreased stroke volume, and a hemodynamically (and echocardiographically) decreased pressure gradient (<30 mm Hg: "pseudo-AS" or "low-gradient AS") despite the echocardiographic presence of AS. The response to pharmacologic intervention with dobutamine or nitroprusside will clarify the diagnosis: absence of change in calculated AV area indicates presence of true AS (therefore, AV replacement is indicated), stroke volume increase well out of proportion to the increase in valvular gradient indicates the presence of relative AS, while little or no response to stroke volume is diagnostic of severe and generally irreversible LV dysfunction and poor prognosis.[47]

Anesthetic Considerations

The ideal hemodynamic environment for the patient with AS is summarized in Table 41-3. Noncardiac surgery in patients with asymptomatic severe AS may not be associated with complications (one death in 23 patients with general anesthetic, no death in 25 patients with local anesthetic), provided that their hemodynamics are invasively monitored.[48] Subsequent larger studies

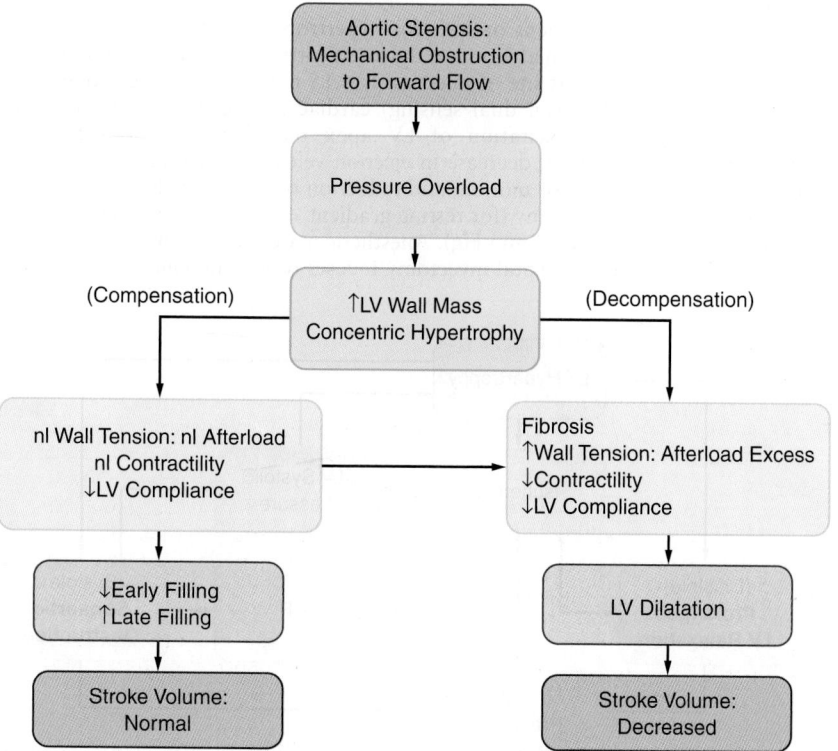

FIGURE 41-4. Pathophysiology of aortic stenosis. LV, left ventricle; nl, normal.

TABLE 41-3

AORTIC STENOSIS—HEMODYNAMIC GOALS

Preload	Full
Afterload	Maintain coronary perfusion gradient
Contractility	Usually not a problem, may require inotropic support if hypotension persists
Rate	Avoid bradycardia (↓ CO) and tachycardia (ischemia)
Rhythm	Sinus: may need cardioversion or beta-blockers
MV̇O₂	Avoid tachycardia and hypotension (ischemia is an ever-present risk)
CPB	Contractility augmentation may be required transiently secondary to myocardial stunning; blood pressure may need to be controlled later

↓, decrease; CO, cardiac output; CPB, cardiopulmonary bypass; MV̇O₂ myocardial oxygen consumption.

in this population present conflicting results. Some show a marked increase in perioperative death and infarction rates and others do not.[49,50] The reasons for these differences are not clear, but maintenance of adequate ventricular volume and sinus rhythm is crucial. Hypotension must be prevented and treated promptly if it develops. Anticipation of likely hemodynamic changes is essential (e.g., expected decreases in blood pressure following spinal or epidural anesthesia). Coronary perfusion pressure must be maintained to prevent the catastrophic cycle of hypotension-induced ischemia, subsequent ventricular dysfunction, and worsening hypotension. Bradycardia is a common clinical cause for hypotension in the patient with AS. Slowing the heart rate and increasing diastolic time will not increase stroke volume in the thick, concentrically hypertrophied LV. Therefore, bradycardia will induce a fall in total cardiac output and systemic arterial pressure. This is especially pertinent in the elderly patient, in whom sinus node disease and reduced sympathetic responses may predispose to significant bradycardia. Tachycardia must be avoided because it reduces the duration of diastolic coronary perfusion.

Ischemia may be difficult to detect because the characteristic electrocardiographic changes are often obscured by signs of LV hypertrophy and strain. Elevated LV filling pressures, although not necessarily reflecting increased volume, often require treatment to optimize coronary perfusion pressure.[47] TNG is useful in this regard, but it must be remembered that minimal reductions in ventricular volume are required; therefore, very low doses of TNG should be used and titrated to effect. In the presence of LV dysfunction, an arterial dilator,

such as SNP[51] (or perhaps nicardipine) carefully titrated will lower afterload without affecting ventricular volume. The utility of TEE in diagnosing and grading the severity of AS is described in Chapter 28.

Hypertrophic Cardiomyopathy

Hypertrophic cardiomyopathy (or idiopathic hypertrophic subaortic stenosis or asymmetric septal hypertrophy) is a genetically determined disease characterized by histologically abnormal myocytes and myocardial hypertrophy developing a priori, in the absence of a pressure or volume overload. The LV chamber is small and hyperdynamic.[52]

Pathophysiology

The physiologic consequences of hypertrophic cardiomyopathy (similar to those detailed for AS) are depicted in Figure 41-5. A subset of patients (20 to 30%) have some degree of subvalvular obstruction (hypertrophic obstructive cardiomyopathy). In patients with hypertrophic obstructive cardiomyopathy, systolic septal bulging into the LVOT, malposition of the anterior papillary muscle, drag forces, and hyperdynamic LV contraction (causing a Venturi effect) may contribute to creation of a LVOT gradient. This type of obstruction is dynamic and is accentuated by any intervention that reduces ventricular size. Therefore, increases in contractility and heart rate or decreases in either preload or afterload are harmful because they facilitate septal-leaflet contact. Blood is ejected rapidly through this area and the anterior mitral valve leaflet is pulled even closer to the septum (systolic anterior motion), resulting in a variable mitral regurgitation jet, which is directed posteriorly.[53]

In hypertrophic cardiomyopathy, myocardial oxygen balance is tenuous, and angina during exercise occurs even in the absence of epicardial coronary artery disease, when the coronary microcirculation is unable to supply the hypertrophied myocardium. In hypertrophic obstructive cardiomyopathy, angina results from the elevated LV systolic pressure.

Anesthetic Considerations

Treatment options for hypertrophic cardiomyopathy include alcohol ablation of the interventricular septum (if septal thickness at site of injection is <15 mm), DDD (dual mode, dual-chamber, dual sensing) cardiac pacing with short AV delay (pre-excitation of LV apex results in paradoxical septal motion, decrease in ejection velocity, amelioration of systolic anterior motion, and reduction of LVOT gradient), and septal myectomy (for resting gradient ≥30 mm Hg or exercise gradient ≥50 mm Hg). Anesthetic management for patients undergoing septal myectomy focuses on maintenance of ventricular

FIGURE 41-5. Pathophysiology of primary left ventricular (LV) hypertrophy in hypertrophic cardiomyopathy. BP, blood pressure.

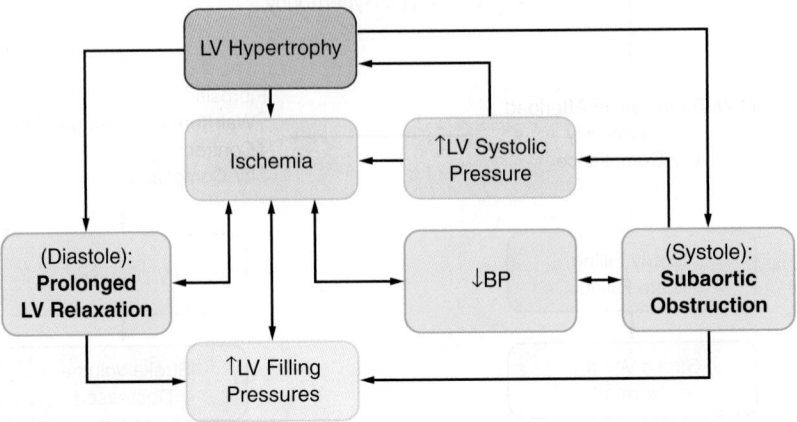

TABLE 41-4

HYPERTROPHIC CARDIOMYOPATHY—HEMODYNAMIC GOALS

Preload	Full: one of first treatments for hypotension
Afterload	Increased: treat hypotension aggressively with α-adrenergic agonists
Contractility	Prefer depression
Rate	Normal range; beta-blockers decrease LVOT gradient and increase LV end-diastolic pressure
Rhythm	Sinus rhythm is crucial: atrial pacing modalities (PAC, esophageal) may be helpful.
MV̇O₂	Not a problem
CPB	Start with volume and vasoconstrictors; avoid inotropes. Check carefully for residual gradient and SAM; rule out ventricular septal defect

LVOT, left ventricular outflow tract; LV, left ventricle; PAC, pulmonary artery catheter; MV̇O₂, myocardial oxygen consumption; CPB, cardiopulmonary bypass; SAM, systolic anterior motion.

filling and reduction in the factors predisposing to outflow tract obstruction or ischemia (Table 41-4). Myocardial depression is desirable, and volatile anesthetics are useful. Because of the dependence of preload on atrial contraction, these patients will benefit from atrial pacing if junctional rhythm occurs. Methods to achieve this include transesophageal pacing or use of a PAC with pacing capability. This permits the administration of volatile anesthetics without fear of compromising sinoatrial conduction. In addition, control of atrial rate and rhythm is beneficial during the prebypass period.

Although infrequent, hypertrophic cardiomyopathy occasionally coexists with valvular AS and may explain unanticipated difficulties in separating from bypass following seemingly uncomplicated AV replacement. If this is suspected, measurement of the gradient between the LV and the outflow tract will

resolve this dilemma. In addition, dynamic left ventricular outflow obstruction is occasionally observed following mitral valve repair. In this case, anterior septal motion of the mitral valve can be observed echocardiographically. Pharmacologic management of hypotension is with volume replacement and vasoconstrictors rather than inotropes and vasodilators.

Aortic Insufficiency

Aortic valve insufficiency (AI) is the result of annular dilatation or abnormal AV cusp motion. Annular dilatation can occur with aneurysms or dissections of the ascending aorta. Because the aortic cusp area is 40% greater than the cross-sectional area of a normal aortic root, small increases in the diameter of the aortic annulus can be accommodated before the valve becomes incompetent. Abnormal leaflet motion and coaptation is caused by calcific degeneration, rheumatic disease, bicuspid AV, endocarditis, trauma, or a jet lesion due to dynamic or fixed subvalvular stenosis. Moderate or severe AI is rare. Acute AI is caused by bacterial endocarditis, aortic dissection, or trauma.

Pathophysiology

The fundamental physiologic derangement in AI is diastolic blood flow from the aorta into the LV that leads to volume and pressure overload (Fig. 41-6). In chronic AI, LV chamber size increases gradually, sometimes to massive proportions increasing wall stress. The LV size increases to a greater magnitude than the ventricular wall thickness and the LV *hypertrophy* is termed *eccentric*. Despite the enormous increases in end-diastolic volume, end-diastolic pressures are usually within the normal range, evidence of a significant increase in chamber compliance. As a result, and in contrast to AS, considerable alterations in LV volume can occur with only minimal changes in LV filling pressure. Although the ventricle may pump more than twice the normal cardiac output, MV̇O₂ does not increase extraordinarily because the oxygen cost for muscle shortening (volume work) is low. The diastolic runoff and the

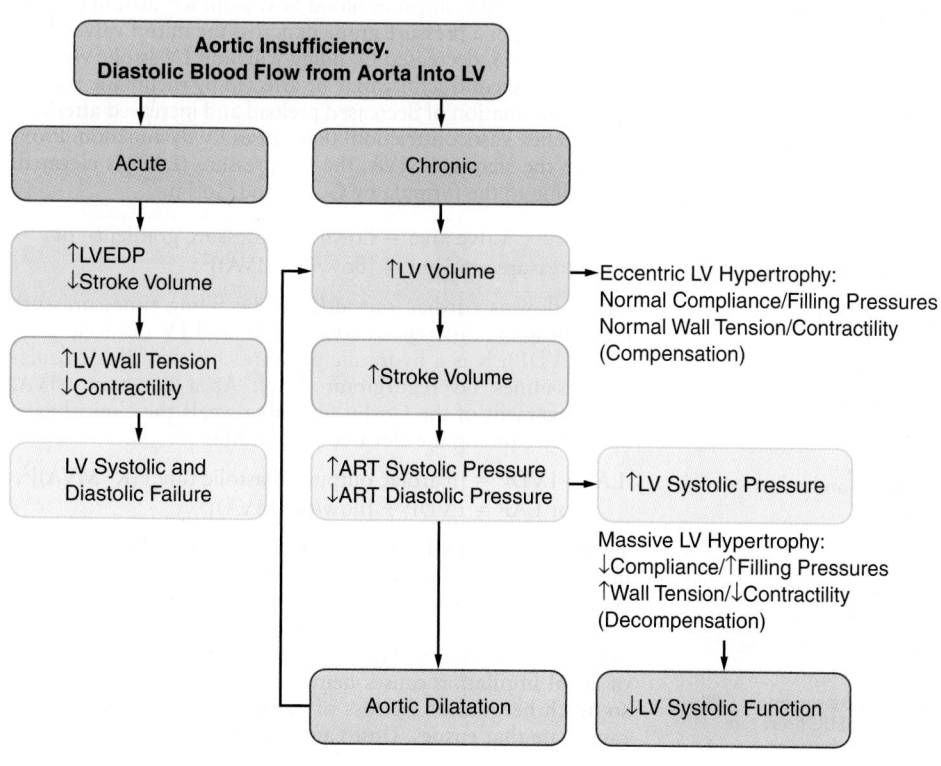

FIGURE 41-6. Pathophysiology of aortic insufficiency. LVEDP, left ventricular end-diastolic pressure; LV, left ventricle; ART, arterial.

moderate vasodilation reduce the ventricular afterload, and the arterial pulse pressure is increased. This will allow patients to be relatively symptom-free even when contractility is reduced so it is difficult to evaluate the myocardial contractile state from clinical signs and symptoms. This is important in terms of planning the anesthetic, but perhaps even more so with respect to the timing of AV replacement. Ideally, the valve should be replaced just prior to the onset of irreversible myocardial damage. The outcome is better in patients with LV ejection fraction >55% or an end-diastolic LV diameter <55 mm.[54] Therefore, continued follow-up of these patients emphasizes repeated noninvasive measurements of contractility, usually after some form of afterload stress, either pharmacologic-induced or exercise-induced.

In acute AI the previously normal-size and normally compliant LV is presented with a large regurgitant volume, and there is equilibration of aortic and LV pressures.[55] As a result LV end-diastolic pressure rises rapidly (along the steep portion of the diastolic pressure-volume relation). Severe congestive heart failure is the cardinal clinical sign. Myocardial contractility becomes impaired as LV end-diastolic pressure increases. Compensatory mechanisms include tachycardia and peripheral vasoconstriction, but occasionally hypotension and low cardiac output ensue. In acutely ill patients, emergency AV replacement is required, whereas in less severe circumstances, mild systemic vasodilation and inotropic support can return hemodynamics toward normal.

Anesthetic Considerations

The main goal is to avoid increased LV wall stress. Full, mildly vasodilated, and modestly tachycardic describe the optimal cardiovascular state for patients with AI (Table 41-5). Vasodilation (with an arterial dilator: nicardipine or SNP) promotes forward flow, although additional intravascular volume may be necessary to maintain preload. The ideal heart rate is somewhat controversial. It is likely that changes in heart rate alone will not alter forward or regurgitant flow; each will be proportionately reduced. Tachycardia reduces the diastolic runoff from the aorta to the LV and results in (1) reduction of the ventricular volume and wall tension, and (2) increase in the diastolic blood pressure and coronary perfusion gradient, thus offsetting any increase in $M\dot{V}O_2$ secondary to increased heart rate. Bradycardia should be avoided as it results in ventricular distention, elevations in left atrial pressure, and pulmonary congestion.

Ventricular distention may occur with the onset of CPB if the heart rate slows or if there is unexpected ventricular fibrillation. Monitoring of heart size, rate, rhythm, and ventricular filling pressure are especially important in these patients. If LV

distention occurs, insertion of an LV vent or immediate cross-clamping of the aorta should alleviate the problem. The presence of moderate-to-severe AI will affect the approach to CPB. After application of the aortic cross-clamp, cardioplegic solution is normally injected into the aortic root, delivering this solution to the coronary system, producing diastolic arrest of the heart. An incompetent AV prevents delivery of cardioplegia to the coronary system. Instead, cardioplegia will fill and distend the LV, increasing the ischemic insult incurred during CPB, and diastolic arrest of the heart becomes difficult. As a result, in the presence of AI the heart is arrested by injecting cardioplegia directly into the coronary ostia (after aortotomy) or into the coronary sinus ("retrograde").

Transesophageal Echocardiography in Aortic Insufficiency

Two-dimensional echocardiographic examination will demonstrate the structural findings associated with AI mentioned previously and the effects of volume overload on LV size and function. Doppler echocardiography will identify the AI jet, localize its site, and help grade its severity Accurate evaluation of AI is essential in determining the feasibility of performing an AV repair. Successful AV repairs are often performed during repair of aortic dissections and have been reported with aneurysms and bicuspid AVs.

Mitral Stenosis

Mitral valve stenosis (MS), usually caused by rheumatic fever, is rare in the United States. Chronic inflammation results to severe valve damage decades after the initial attack. MS develops from leaflet thickening, commissural fusion, and chordal shortening and fusion. Another cause of MS is atherosclerosis-associated mitral annular calcification.[56]

Pathophysiology

The spectrum of physiologic disruption in patients with MS is presented in Figure 41-7. Progressive decrease of the mitral valve area (MVA) impedes blood flow from left atrium (LA) to LV resulting in a pressure gradient across the mitral valve. With worsening MS, decreased LV filling will limit LV stroke volume. Although LV contractility may be affected by rheumatic fever, it is the combination of decreased preload and increased afterload (from reflex vasoconstriction) that causes LV dysfunction. Proximal to the stenosed MVA, the LA pressure (LAP) is elevated. According to the formula by Gorlin and Gorlin,[57]

$$\text{Valve area} = \text{flow}/(K \cdot \sqrt{\text{pressure gradient}}), \text{ or}$$
$$\text{Pressure gradient} = [\text{flow}/(K \cdot \text{MVA})]^2,$$

where flow is cardiac output/diastolic filling time; pressure gradient is the difference between LAP and LV diastolic pressure (LVDP); K is a hydraulic pressure constant (this calculation assumes no regurgitant flow). At a constant MVA, rearrangement of the Gorlin formula reveals the clinical variables determining the elevated LAP in MS:

$$\text{LAP} - \text{LVDP} = [(\text{cardiac output})/(\text{diastolic time})/(K \cdot \text{MVA})]^2,$$
$$\text{or LAP} = \text{LVDP} + [\text{flow}/(K \cdot \text{MVA})]^2$$

Therefore, increased cardiac output or decreased diastolic filling period result in increased LAP by the square of the original changes. This explains why tachycardia or increases in forward flow, seen classically with pregnancy, thyrotoxicosis, or infection, can precipitate pulmonary edema. Thus, the development of atrial fibrillation causes hemodynamic embarrassment, not so much because of the loss of atrial kick but because of the rapid rate that ensues. Upstream from the LA, the persistently

TABLE 41-5

AORTIC INSUFFICIENCY—HEMODYNAMIC GOALS

Preload	Normal to slightly ↑
Afterload	↓: with anesthetics or vasodilators (to decrease regurgitant fraction)
Contractility	Usually adequate
Rate	↑: reduces ventricular volume and raises diastolic aortic pressure
Rhythm	Usually sinus; not a problem
$M\dot{V}O_2$	Usually not a problem
CPB	Beware (and observe) for ventricular distention (pre- and post-AXC: regurgitant flow increases if ↓ HR or nonbeating heart)

↑, increase; ↓, decrease; $M\dot{V}O_2$, myocardial oxygen consumption; CPB, cardiopulmonary bypass; AXC, aortic cross-clamp; HR, heart rate.

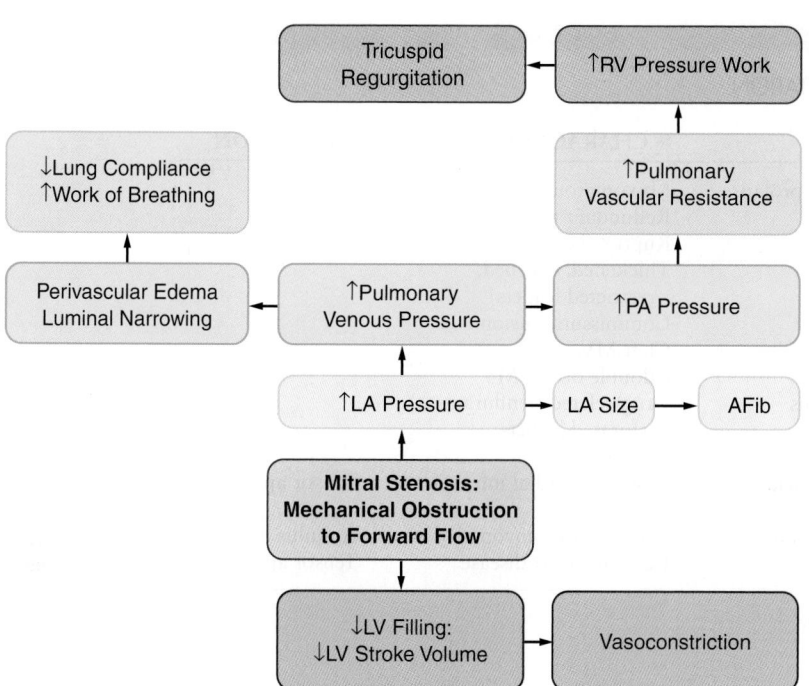

ANESTHESIA FOR SURGICAL SUBSPECIALTIES

elevated LAP (which leads to LA dilatation and atrial fibrillation, usually the first manifestation of MS) is reflected through the pulmonary circulation (pulmonary congestion and increased work of breathing), leading to right ventricular pressure overload with compensatory right ventricular hypertrophy and elevated strain. The progression and severity of pulmonary hypertension are variable and reflect further narrowing of the valve orifice and irreversible reactive changes in the pulmonary vasculature (rales on auscultation, hemoptysis). Once pulmonary hypertension has developed, operative risk is increased (12% vs. 3 to 8%).[58] Right ventricular dysfunction, tricuspid annular dilatation, and insufficiency (engorged neck veins) may develop as the right heart function worsens.

MS mimics left heart failure, with pulmonary congestion and decreased forward flow. The only definitive treatment is relief of obstruction with balloon valvuloplasty, open commissurotomy, or mitral valve replacement. Medical treatment is not inotropic or vasodilator therapy. Instead, the heart rate should be decreased (with beta- or calcium channel blockers) or the cause(s) responsible for the increased transmitral flow diagnosed and treated. The pulmonary capillary wedge pressure can be used as an index of LV filling, even during episodes of tachycardia or increased flow, keeping in mind that it is higher than the true LVDP at least by the amount of the pressure gradient.

Anesthetic Considerations

Pre-emption is the cornerstone of prebypass anesthetic management (Table 41-6). Avoiding tachycardia precludes episodes of left atrial and pulmonary hypertension with potential right ventricular dysfunction, as well as inadequate LV filling with concomitant systemic hypotension. Preoperative maintenance of rate-control and beta-blocking drugs, selection of anesthetics with no propensity to increase heart rate, and attainment of anesthetic levels deep enough to suppress autonomic responses are methods to achieve these goals. Episodes of pulmonary hypertension and potential right-sided heart failure stemming from pulmonary vasoconstriction must also be prevented. It is wise to avoid hypoxia, hypercarbia, and acidosis because they increase pulmonary vascular resistance.

Treatment of hypotension in patients with MS can present a challenging dilemma. Although these patients normally take diuretics, hypovolemia is not usually the cause; hence, the response to volume administration is often disappointing. Use of a vasoconstrictor to offset mild peripheral vasodilation is acceptable, bearing in mind the effect of pulmonary vasoconstriction on right ventricular function. It is often prudent to select a drug with some inotropic effect such as ephedrine or epinephrine instead of relying on a pure vasoconstrictor, such as phenylephrine. In separating from CPB, attention is on avoiding right ventricular failure (discussed subsequently); more commonly, however, there is LV dysfunction. This may be because of intraoperative injury or sudden increase in flow to and distention of the chronically underloaded LV. After bypass, prominent *v* waves may be present in the pulmonary

TABLE 41-6

MITRAL STENOSIS—HEMODYNAMIC GOALS

Preload	Maintain, avoid hypovolemia
Afterload	Prevent pulmonary vasoconstriction (hypoxia, hypercarbia)
	Inotropes may be required for systemic hypotension
Contractility	Usually intact. RV dysfunction may be a problem with long-standing pulmonary hypertension
Rate	Maintain at low end of normal. Avoid tachycardia
Rhythm	Keep ventricular response controlled in atrial fibrillation
$M\dot{V}O_2$	Not a problem
CPB	Post-MV replacement: LV preload and filling pressures may be elevated. Cardiac function does not improve immediately

RV, right ventricle; $M\dot{V}O_2$, myocardial oxygen consumption; CPB, cardiopulmonary bypass; MV, mitral valve; LV, left ventricle.

TABLE 41-7

CAUSES OF MITRAL REGURGITATION

	■ CAUSE	■ CHARACTERISTICS	■ LOCATION
Primary (structural)	Mitral valve prolapse	Myxomatous degeneration Redundant tissue Ruptured chordae	Leaflet
	Rheumatic	Thickened, calcified, restricted leaflets Commissural fusion	
	Congenital	Cleft MV, double orifice MV	
	Miscellaneous	Drug-related (fenfluramine)	
	Endocarditis	Perforated leaflets Vegetations	
	Papillary muscle rupture	Post–myocardial infarction	Tensor apparatus
Functional	Annular dilatation	Dilated cardiomyopathy	Annulus
	LV ischemia	Ischemic heart disease	Tensor apparatus

MV, mitral valve; LV, left ventricle.

capillary wedge pressure waveform. This almost always reflects increased LV filling rather than mitral regurgitation because cardiac output is increased after bypass when compared with preinduction values. The echocardiographic signs of MS are described in Chapter 28.

Mitral Regurgitation

Mitral regurgitation (MR) results from several mechanisms permitting systolic blood flow from the LV to the LA. Mechanical etiologies of MR include leaflet prolapse, restricted leaflet motion (rheumatic heart disease), and leaflet perforation (endocarditis), and changes in LV structure and function related to ischemia (ischemic MR). Acute MR occurs with papillary muscle dysfunction or chordal rupture following myocardial infarction and may require emergency surgical repair (Table 41-7).

Pathophysiology

Chronic volume overload similar to that described with AI is the cardinal feature of MR (Fig. 41-8). The LA acts as a low-pressure vent during LV ejection: there is no isovolumetric contraction period because blood is immediately ejected retrograde with the onset of ventricular systole. Total LV stroke volume consists of the forward flow (systemic) via the aorta and the retrograde flow into the LA. Atrial and ventricular chamber enlargement, ventricular wall hypertrophy, and increased blood volume are the compensatory responses. Ventricular compliance increases; thus, the large end-diastolic volume does not cause striking increases in LV end-diastolic pressure. The increase in oxygen cost (required for additional muscle shortening) is small because there is little pressure development. Thus, despite progressive myocardial dysfunction (decreased contractility), patients may have minimal symptoms. Ejection fraction, a parameter that is heavily afterload-dependent, can be misleading in

FIGURE 41-8. Pathophysiology of mitral regurgitation. LA, left atrial; LV, left ventricular.

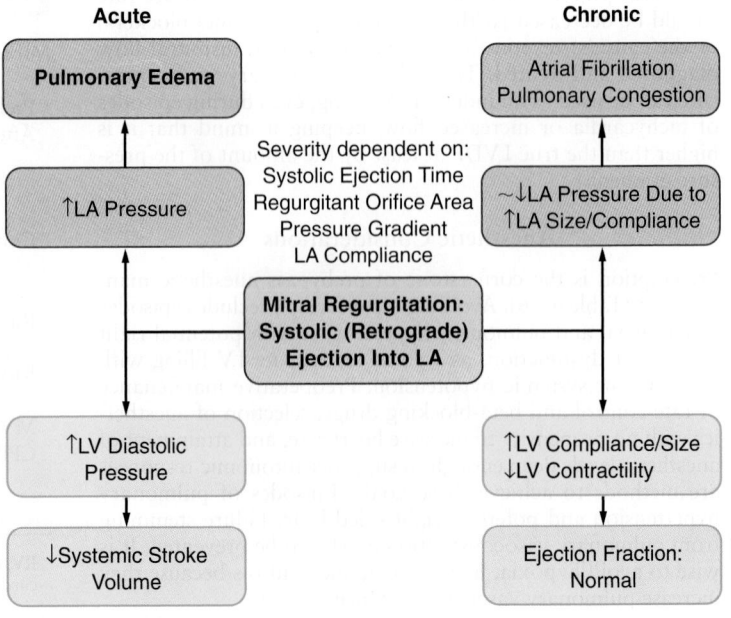

patients with MR: normal or minimally reduced ejection fraction can be present even with severe impairment of contractile function. The regurgitant blood volume is related to the size of the regurgitant orifice, the time available for retrograde flow, the pressure gradient across the valve and the compliance of the receiving chamber. Regurgitant orifice size, in turn, depends on ventricular size (LV enlargement causes mitral annulus dilatation and worsening MR). Therefore, both increases in heart rate and preload reduction decrease the amount of regurgitant flow by diminishing LV volume. Arterial dilators are effective by reducing the LV to LA systolic pressure gradient.

Repairing or replacing the valve increases LV afterload and often unmasks the dysfunction of the myocardium. Administration of inotropes and/or vasodilators, as well as judicious increase in preload, may be necessary to successfully separate from bypass.

Acute-onset MR has a different hemodynamic picture; acute left atrial and LV volume overload occurs in the absence of compensatory ventricular enlargement. Ventricular filling pressures increase dramatically, as do pulmonary pressures. Cardiac output decreases, and pulmonary edema develops. If this occurs in the setting of acute myocardial infarction, cardiac performance may be inadequate despite pharmacologic support. Intra-aortic balloon assistance and emergency surgery may be lifesaving.

Anesthetic Considerations

9 Selection of anesthetics that promote vasodilation and tachycardia is ideal in the patient with MR (Table 41-8). Active pharmacologic intervention is usually unnecessary because most patients with chronic MR are not teetering on the brink of myocardial failure. However, patients with acute MR require aggressive pharmacologic management. In the absence of acute deterioration, difficulties in management are usually limited to the postbypass period. Paradoxically, after the administration of vasodilators and inotropes, a patient occasionally deteriorates even further. This is seen after valve repair, not replacement. In these patients, the pathophysiological and clinical picture is that of hypertrophic cardiomyopathy, and systolic anterior motion of the anterior mitral leaflet is demonstrable by echocardiography. The risk of systolic anterior motion after repair is increased when the anteroposterior length of the anterior leaflet is longer than the transverse diameter, when there is excessive leaflet tissue, a nondilated LV cavity, and/or a narrow angle between the mitral and aortic annuli. If this scenario is suspected, a trial of volume expansion and vasoconstrictors is indicated. The approach to evaluation of MR severity is described in Chapter 28.

TABLE 41-8

MITRAL REGURGITATION—HEMODYNAMIC GOALS

Preload	Usually slightly increased; however: preload reduction may reduce regurgitant flow
Afterload	Decrease with anesthetics, vasodilators
Contractility	May be depressed, titrate myocardial depressants carefully
Rate	Slightly increased
Rhythm	If atrial fibrillation present: control ventricular response
$M\dot{V}O_2$	Compromised if MR coexists with ischemic heart disease
CPB	Newly competent valve increases afterload, often necessitating inotropic support

$M\dot{V}O_2$, myocardial oxygen consumption; MR, mitral regurgitation; CPB, cardiopulmonary bypass.

AORTIC DISEASES

Acquired (hypertension, inflammation, deceleration trauma, or iatrogenic factors) and genetic (Marfan syndrome, Ehlers-Danlos syndrome, bicuspid AV) conditions are the cause of aortic diseases: aortic dissection, intramural hematoma, and aortic aneurysm. All mechanisms weakening the media layers of the aorta (the term *cystic medial degeneration* denotes the disappearance of smooth muscle cells and the degeneration of elastic fibers) lead to higher wall stress, which can induce aortic dilatation and aneurysm formation, eventually resulting in intramural hemorrhage, aortic dissection, or rupture. Acute aortic dissection requires a tear in the aortic intima that commonly is preceded by medial wall degeneration or cystic medial necrosis.

Aortic Dissection

Acute aortic dissection affects men more than women in their fifth or sixth decade of life. Hypertension is the most common risk factor in older patients, while Marfan syndrome, bicuspid AV, or prior surgery are risk factors in younger patients (<40 years old). Acute aortic dissection is characterized by rapid development of an intimal flap separating the true and false lumens. The dissection can spread from the intimal tear in antegrade and retrograde fashion, often involving side branches and causing malperfusion syndromes, tamponade, or AI. Acute aortic dissection of the ascending aorta (type A) is highly lethal (mortality 1 to 2%/hr after symptom onset). Without surgery, (mortality exceeds 50% in 1 month). Uncomplicated descending aorta dissections (type B) have a 30-day mortality of 10% and may be managed medically or with stent placement. Intramural hematoma is considered a precursor to classic dissection and usually originates from ruptured vasa vasorum in the media.

Intramural hematoma has the same prognosis as aortic dissection and is treated similarly. Severe chest pain (chest pain usually in type A, back or abdominal pain in type B) is the single most common presenting complaint, although many patients have atypical symptoms mimicking stroke, myocardial infarction, vascular embolization, and abdominal pathology. Pulse and/or blood pressure variation is a significant finding related to impaired blood flow to an organ or limb induced by the original dissection or by propagation of the dissection. Syncope indicates development of dangerous complications (cardiac tamponade, cerebral hypoperfusion). A variety of diagnostic techniques (contrast-enhanced spiral computed tomography scanning, TEE, or magnetic resonance imaging) are extremely accurate in the diagnosis of acute aortic dissection, but selection should consider the information required, the access to, and the experience with the technique in the particular center.

Patients with a high clinical suspicion of acute aortic dissection may be sent directly to the operating room for TEE-based diagnostic workup and preparation for surgery, decreasing the time period before surgical intervention.[59] Two-dimensional TEE identifies the intimal tear in 61% of the patients.[60] Apart from direct visualization of intimal tear and flaps, the site of entry and re-entry, false lumen thrombosis, coronary involvement, intramural hematoma, pericardial effusion, and AI can be diagnosed with high sensitivity and specificity.[61] However, dissections in the distal ascending aorta and proximal arch are difficult to visualize because of interposition of the left main stem bronchus between the esophagus (TEE) and aorta. Surgery is the definitive treatment for patients with type A acute aortic dissection, with an aims to prevent aortic rupture and pericardial tamponade and to ameliorate concomitant AI. It involves implantation of a composite graft in the ascending aorta with or without reimplantation of the coronary arteries.

TABLE 41-9

ACUTE AORTIC DISSECTION—HEMODYNAMIC GOALS

Preload	May be increased if acute AI, increase if tamponade, combinations possible
Afterload	Decrease with anesthetics, analgesics, arterial dilators (nitroprusside, nicardipine): keep BP <120/60
Contractility	May be depressed; titrate myocardial depressants carefully
Rate	Decrease to <60 bpm: use beta-blocker (in COPD: use calcium-channel blocker); ensure contractility is adequate
Rhythm	If atrial fibrillation present: control ventricular response
$M\dot{V}O_2$	Compromised if aortic dissection involves coronary vessels
CPB	Alternate site of inflow (arterial) cannulation, deep hypothermic circulatory arrest possible if cerebral vessels are involved

AI, aortic insufficiency; BP, blood pressure; bpm, beats per minute; COPD, chronic obstructive pulmonary disease; $M\dot{V}O_2$, myocardial oxygen consumption; CPB, cardiopulmonary bypass.

Anesthetic Considerations

Acute aortic dissection is a surgical and anesthetic emergency. Adequate intravenous access and invasive hemodynamic monitoring, including TEE, are mandatory. The hemodynamic goals are shown in Table 41-9.

Aortic Aneurysm

Thoracic aneurysms (TAs) may involve one or more aortic segments (aortic root, ascending aorta, arch, descending aorta). Most patients are asymptomatic at the time of diagnosis. Aortic root TAs may cause AI (diastolic murmur or heart failure). When large, TAs may cause local mass effect such as compression of the trachea (cough), esophagus (dysphagia), and/or recurrent laryngeal nerve (hoarseness). Detection and sizing can be done with contrast-enhanced computed tomography scanning and magnetic resonance angiography. The risk for rupture increases abruptly as TAs reach a diameter of 6 cm.[62] Surgery is indicated for ascending aorta aneurysms >5.5 cm or descending TA >6 cm. Composite aortic repair (Bentall procedure) using a tube graft with a prosthetic AV sewn into one end is performed for aortic root TA associated with AI.[63] Alternatively, if AI is due to aortic root dilation, a valve-sparing procedure (preservation of the native AV cusps) is performed.[64]

The surgical replacement of aortic arch TA requires circulatory arrest during the creation of distal anastomosis and carries a risk of neurologic damage from global ischemic injury or embolization of atherosclerotic debris. Cerebral protection methods during replacement of the aortic arch include use of profound hypothermic circulatory arrest with or without arrest of cerebral circulation. Retrograde (via a superior vena cava cannula) or selective antegrade (direct cannulation of cerebral vessels) cerebral perfusion is employed to improve outcomes by providing nutrients and O_2 to the brain and flush out particulate matter from the cerebral and carotid arteries, with, so far, disputed results.[65]

Surgical replacement of the descending aorta is associated with postoperative paraplegia secondary to interruption of spinal cord blood supply (13 to 17%). A variety of methods

(cerebrospinal fluid drainage, reimplantation of critical spinal arteries, maintenance of distal aortic perfusion with the use of a LA-left femoral artery bypass circuit, intraoperative epidural cooling, or use of somatosensory evoked potentials) are being used to avoid this complication, although outcome is heavily influenced by hospital and surgeon volume.[66] Alternatively, a transluminally placed endovascular stent-graft can be inserted.[67] Chapter 42 reviews recent advances in vascular stenting.

Anesthetic Considerations

The anesthetic technique is centered around two major organ systems: (1) preservation of cardiac function (most crucial in surgery of descending TAs, where the "clamp-and-go" surgical technique imposes great fluctuations in systemic afterload and hemodynamic instability), and (2) neurologic integrity (in arch or descending TAs operations). Drainage of cerebrospinal fluid will augment the spinal cord perfusion pressure. Usually, increments of 10 mL are drained at a time and the cerebrospinal fluid pressure is monitored continuously, keeping a cerebrospinal fluid pressure <12 mm Hg at all times. Left heart bypass (LA to femoral artery) provides nonpulsatile retrograde aortic perfusion and supplements blood flow during aortic flow interruption, but does not perfuse the excluded aortic segment. Blood is actively removed via a cannula inserted inside the LA and advanced distal to the aortic interruption site. This technique ameliorates LV stress by reducing LV preload and afterload. The bypass flow depends on adequate preload (as assessed by the pulmonary arterial diastolic pressure or LV size via TEE) and low-normal afterload distal to the aortic cross-clamp. Too high flow of the bypass system will lead to hypotension, while increased pump flow will help decrease systemic hypertension proximal to the aortic interruption.

CARDIOPULMONARY BYPASS

Circuits

The cardiopulmonary bypass (CPB) circuit consists of (1) tubing (cannulae) to drain blood from and return blood and other fluids to the heart chambers; (2) reservoirs for collection of these solutions; (3) an oxygenator, where gas exchange takes place; and (4) pumps that allow the return of blood to the heart and patient's circulation (Fig. 41-9). Drainage of venous blood is accomplished by inserting a large-bore "dual-stage"

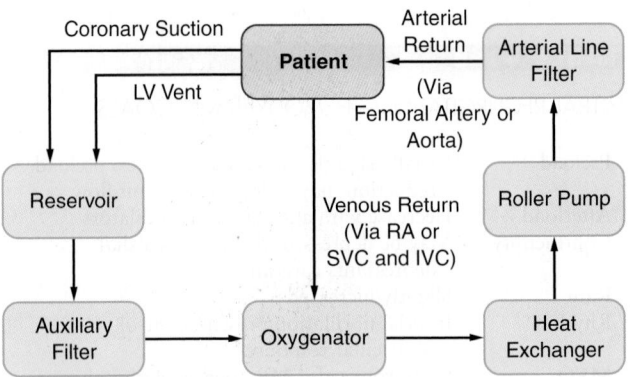

FIGURE 41-9.   The basic circuit for cardiopulmonary bypass. LV, left ventricle; RA, right atrium; SVC, superior vena cava; IVC, inferior vena cava. (Reprinted from Thomson IR: Technical aspects of cardiopulmonary bypass, Manual of Cardiac Anesthesia, 2nd edition. Edited by Thomas SJ. New York, Churchill Livingstone, 1993, p 480, with permission.)

cannula in the right atrium that drains blood from both right atrium and inferior vena cava. However, some blood is still left inside the heart. In open cardiac heart procedures, such as valve surgery, where total blood drainage is mandatory for a bloodless field, individual "single-stage" cannulae are placed into the superior and inferior vena cavae and then snared, thus preventing systemic venous blood from entering the heart. During CPB, the rate of venous drainage is passive and depends on several factors, such as proper placement of adequate diameter cannulae, intravascular volume status, and hydrostatic pressure gradient (how high is the right atrium above the venous reservoir). In the event of poor venous drainage, adjustment of cannulae, raising the height of the operating table, or application of suction will usually correct the problem.

From the venous reservoir, the blood enters the oxygenator/heat exchanger unit, where it is warmed/cooled, oxygenated, and carbon dioxide is removed. The now-oxygenated blood is returned to the arterial circulation via a large "arterial" cannulae. This blood cycle continues for the duration of CPB. Arterial cannulae may be placed in the ascending aorta, femoral, or axillary arteries. Surgeon preference, patient anatomy, and surgical procedure will dictate the location of the arterial cannula.

In addition to venous cannulae, additional sources of blood return to the CPB machine include suction cannulae, which scavenge blood from the surgical field, and vents used to decompress the LV and aspirate air from the heart during deairing procedures. Ventricular venting prevents ventricular distention that may lead to development of myocardial ischemia and is particularly important in patients with AI, large coronary sinus or bronchial blood flow, or when heart positioning restricts drainage. Common vent sites include the LV via a cannula placed in the left superior pulmonary vein (or, very rarely, the LV apex), or the aortic root via the antegrade cardioplegia cannula.

Modern CPB systems have additional components such as filters for removal of bubble and debris, in-line blood gas monitors, separate circuits to deliver cardioplegia, and volatile agent vaporizers. Monitors may be placed in key locations of the circuit to detect low blood levels in the venous reservoir/oxygenator (to prevent pumping of air to the arterial side of the circuit), and systemic line pressure (to detect possible arterial cannula obstruction/aortic dissection; both cause elevated line pressure).

Oxygenators

Oxygenators serve two main purposes: oxygenate venous blood and remove carbon dioxide. The two types of oxygenators are bubble and membrane. Bubble oxygenators are very efficient and work on the principle of direct gas-blood contact. Bubble oxygenators are divided into two sections. The first is a mixing chamber where fresh gas flows through a perforated plate or screen that forms the gas bubbles. Oxygen is relatively insoluble compared with carbon dioxide and requires a large surface area to ensure diffusion (or a high partial pressure). Diffusion takes place on the bubbles surface. By using many small gas bubbles, a large surface area develops and the driving force behind the diffusion of gases is simply the differential partial pressure between the gases in the bubble and dissolved gasses in the blood. After gas exchange occurs in the mixing chamber, the oxygenated blood is directed into the second section, which is a reservoir/heat exchanger. There it is allowed to settle and then is passed through a defoaming matrix. This causes the gas bubbles to destabilize and break down prior to the blood returning to the patient. Bubble oxygenators are not without problems. Prolonged CPB periods result in time-dependent destruction of blood elements. The gas-blood interface is responsible for hemolysis, platelet

destruction, and microemboli. This is seldom observed with CPB times that are <90 minutes.

Membrane oxygenators attempt to eliminate the destructive gas-blood interface by using microporous membranes that allow only a transient interaction between blood and gas. These micropores act as channels allowing the diffusion of both oxygen and carbon dioxide. Membrane oxygenators use bundles of hollow microporous polypropylene fibers contained in a plastic housing. Within this housing, blood flows around the fibers while fresh gas is passed though the microporous fibers. This allows fresh gas to diffuse though the micropores into the passing blood. With this arrangement oxygen tension is controlled by FIO_2 and carbon dioxide elimination by total gas flow.

Pumps

During extracorporeal circulation, a mechanical pump is required to circulate blood through the circuit tubing to the CPB machine and back to the patient. Roller and centrifugal pumps are the most common types used in clinical practice. Roller pumps are the simplest and earliest type of pump. A length of tubing (polyvinyl chloride, silicone rubber, latex rubber) is placed in the periphery of a 210-degree rigid curved housing. In the center of this housing are two metal arms set 180 degrees apart with rollers at each end. When the arm rotates, the tubing is alternately compressed and released against the housing so that one side of the arm is compressing, while the other is releasing the tubing. Alternately compressing and releasing the tubing generates forward flow without the possibility of retrograde flow. This permits constant flow over a range of arterial resistance. It is important to note that the roller head must be nonocclusive, because when the tubing is totally compressed destruction of blood elements will result.

The roller pump is simple and easy to use. Its disadvantages include destruction of blood elements, spallation (development of plastic microemboli due to tubing compression), and complications from inflow and outflow occlusion of the pump. If pump inflow is occluded, negative pressure will develop in the roller head causing cavitation or the development of microscopic bubbles. If pump outflow becomes occluded, excessive pressure may develop proximal to the occlusion, causing the tubing connections to separate or causing the tubing to burst. In modern cardiac surgery, roller pumps are most frequently used for delivering cardioplegia and providing vent/cardiotomy suction.

Centrifugal pumps have primarily replaced the roller pumps in daily practice. These pumps use a magnetically controlled impeller housed within a rigid plastic cone. This impeller is composed of stacked smooth plastic cones that rotate to provide flow. The impeller is magnetically coupled to an electric motor located in the CPB machine. By rotating rapidly, a pressure drop across the impeller is generated, which causes blood to be sucked into the housing and then ejected. One major difference between roller head and centrifugal pumps is that flow from centrifugal pumps will vary with changes in pump preload and afterload. It is for this reason that a flowmeter must be placed on the arterial side of the bypass circuit. Advantages of centrifugal pumps include less blood trauma, lower line pressures, less cavitation, lower risk of massive air emboli, and elimination of tubing wear and spallation.

Despite the reliability of both roller and centrifugal pumps to provide systemic pressure on CPB, neither is able to deliver physiologically significant pulsatile blood flow. Pulsatile flow is the native pattern of blood flow in the human body and its lack on CPB has been cited as a cause of renal dysfunction and production of ischemic metabolic byproducts. Studies show that in high-risk patients the use of pulsatile flow on CPB confers increased survival and may equate to a lower need for inotropes and mechanical support.[68] Until the controversy regarding the benefits of pulsatile flow is resolved, nonpulsatile flow will remain the most common type seen in cardiac surgery.

In the event of catastrophic CPB machine failure, a hand crank may be used to mechanically operate the head of a centrifugal pump to develop adequate pump flow and systemic blood pressure.

Heat Exchanger

A heat exchanger is a counter current device where, either heated or cooled, water is circulated around a conducting material with good thermal properties that is in contact with the patient's blood. The blood is subsequently warmed or cooled and maintained at a desired temperature. Separate heat exchangers are used in CPB circuits for the delivery of cardioplegia.

Prime

Prime is the fluid contained within the CPB tubing. Using crystalloid solutions, such as lactated Ringer, allows the CPB prime to achieve similar osmolarity and electrolyte composition as blood plasma. Other solutions such as albumin (to decrease postoperative edema), mannitol (to promote diuresis), additional electrolytes (calcium to prevent hypocalcemia due to citrate in transfused blood), corticosteroids (for anti-inflammatory effects), and heparin (to ensure a safe level of anticoagulation) may also be added to the priming solution. Many institutions use a standard volume prime for all adult patients, and others use a minimum volume based on body weight or body surface area. The average prime volume is 1,500 to 2,500 mL. To prevent excessive dilutional anemia and decrease in oxygen-carrying capacity, blood may be added to the pump prime prior to initiating CPB in children, small adults, and patients with preoperative anemia. The lowest safe hematocrit on CPB is debated, but hematocrits of 17% are well tolerated.[69] Despite limited data, the trend currently favors higher levels to avoid renal and neurologic consequences. Dilutional anemia on CPB is useful to the degree that it offsets changes in blood viscosity due to hypothermia. Thus, dilutional anemia may improve systemic flow.

Anticoagulation

To prevent any thrombosis of the CPB circuit (and the patient's death), systemic anticoagulation is required prior to insertion of cannulae and initiation of CPB. Contact between patient's blood and components of the CPB circuit initiate activation of the coagulation cascade. To avoid this, heparin is used as the anticoagulant of choice. Heparin is a polyionic mucopolysaccharide extracted from either bovine lung or porcine intestinal mucosa. Following intravenous injection, the peak onset of heparin is <5 minutes with a half-life of approximately 90 minutes in normothermic patients. In hypothermic patients, there is a progressive increase in the half-life proportional to the degree of hypothermia. The anticoagulant effect of heparin is derived from its ability to potentate the activity of antithrombin III (AT-III). The binding of heparin to AT-III alters its structural configuration and increases the AT-III-thrombin inhibitory potency greater than 1,000-fold. By inhibiting thrombin, AT-III prevents formation of fibrin clot via both the intrinsic and extrinsic pathways, in addition to inhibiting factors IX, Xa, XIa, XIIa, kallikrein, and plasmin. In patients receiving heparin preoperatively and those with congenital AT-III deficiencies, higher than expected doses of heparin are required to achieve adequate anticoagulation.

In the event of inadequate anticoagulation due to relative or absolute deficiency of AT-III, exogenous AT-III can be administered by transfusing fresh-frozen plasma or by a administering a commercial preparation of human AT-III concentrate (Thrombate III).[70] Patients exhibiting heparin resistance, defined by activated clotting time (ACT) <380 seconds after receiving 400 U/kg intravenous heparin, have benefited from the use of human recombinant AT-III. The increase in ACT is at least comparable to the increase achieved by the administration of fresh-frozen plasma and can be achieved without blood product administration and the possibility of viral transmission. Postoperative heparin rebound and subsequent bleeding are a concern following the administration of exogenous AT-III.

Partial thromboplastin time is not used in cardiac surgery to measure heparin level, as modern partial thromboplastin time assays are so sensitive, that heparin levels far lower than those used for safe initiation of CPB cause the sample blood to become almost unclottable within the time frame of the test. Currently, the two methods for determining adequate heparinization are measuring of ACTs or blood-heparin concentrations. The ACT consists of adding blood to tubes containing either diatomaceous earth (celite) or kaolin, warming and rotating the tube, and recording the time required for clot formation. Generally, ACTs >480 seconds are considered acceptable for the initiation of CPB. The exception to this is when the serine protease inhibitor aprotinin is used. If celite-containing tubes are used, ACTs >700 seconds are required because of the effect of aprotinin on the test (aprotinin delays activation of the intrinsic pathway via factor XIIa in addition to inhibiting kallikrein, and this prolongs the celite ACT artifactually). Adding kaolin activates the intrinsic pathway and binds to aprotinin, reducing its anticoagulant effect in vitro and producing a more accurate ACT.

Measuring heparin levels intraoperatively is an alternative method for determination of anticoagulation levels. In this method, known doses of protamine are added to a heparinized sample of blood sequentially, until the optimum dose of protamine that produces a clot in the shortest amount of time is determined. By knowing the neutralization ratio of heparin and protamine (usually 1 mg of protamine to 100 U of heparin), the heparin concentration in the sample can be determined. This method will correctly diagnose inadequate anticoagulation despite a therapeutic ACT (such as in hypothermia, hemodilution, and even surgical incision). However, heparin levels do not always correlate with anticoagulant effect. Thus, many centers prefer to use the ACT method, which also happens to be less expensive.

Allergies to heparin are rare; more commonly, patients may present with a history of heparin-induced thrombocytopenia. There are two subtypes of heparin-induced thrombocytopenia; the first is generally mild and there is a transient decrease in platelet count only. The second type is a more severe autoimmune-mediated decrease in the platelet count due to the formation of antigenic heparin compounds that activate platelets in the face of endothelial injury. This endothelial injury predisposes to platelet clumping and microvascular thrombosis. In patients with heparin-induced thrombocytopenia who require systemic anticoagulation, heparin alternatives should be used instead. These include defibrinogenating agents (ancrod obtained from pit viper venom), hirudin, bivalirudin, and factor inhibitors. Hirudin, which is isolated from the salivary gland of the medicinal leech (Hirudo medicinalis) and bivalirudin (Hirulog) are both direct inhibitors of thrombin. Their action is independent of AT-III. The use of these agents is uncommon and the reader is advised to consult one of the several reviews on this subject.[71]

Blood Conservation in Cardiac Surgery

Blood and blood components are finite resources that are increasingly difficult to replace because of declining donation and restrictions on those that may donate. In addition, patients are increasingly demanding "bloodless" surgeries to lessen the risks of blood transfusion (infection, incompatibility reactions, transfusion error). However, because of the nature of cardiac surgery, the risk of blood and blood product transfusion is high. Bleeding as the result of reoperation, use of anticoagulants/platelet function inhibitors, and ill-defined surgical bleeding contribute to this risk. Furthermore, the inherent risk of platelet dysfunction and coagulopathy due to CPB cannot be minimized. All of these have spurred the development of blood conservation techniques in cardiac surgery. In the past, these were the use of intraoperative autologous blood donation and the scavenging and reinfusion of shed blood. New techniques to reduce the need for homologous blood include the use of antifibrinolytics (ε-aminocaproic acid, tranexamic acid), aprotinin, ultrafiltration, blood fractionation, and the use of improved topical hemostatic agents.

Intraoperative autologous hemodilution is a well-described method of removing whole blood from a patient prior to systemic heparinization. Collecting whole blood, which is then retransfused following CPB, and returning red blood cells, active platelets, and coagulation factors that may mitigate surgical bleeding. Contraindications to intraoperative autologous blood donation include preoperative anemia, unstable angina/high-grade left main coronary artery disease, and AS. Blood salvage (cell washing) is an additional key method of intraoperative blood conservation in cardiac surgery. Cell washing is composed of four steps: harvesting of the patient's blood, processing of the shed blood and removal of the serum, storage of the red blood cells, and reinfusion of the high-hematocrit red blood cells. Final hematocrits of reinfused red cells may reach 70%. However, as platelets and coagulation factors are removed in the washing process, reinfusion of shed blood may worsen the CPB-associated coagulopathy by promoting a dilutional thrombocytopenia and reduction of clotting factors. Contraindications to the use of intraoperative cell salvage include infection, malignancy, and the use of topical hemostatic agents.

Antifibrinolytic use in cardiac surgery is the standard in most cardiac centers, with ε-aminocaproic acid being the primary agent used in the United States. The lysine analogues ε-aminocaproic and tranexamic acid bind to plasminogen and block its ability to bind at lysine residues of fibrinogen. Administration of these antifibrinolytics decreases bleeding after CPB and reduces the risk of blood transfusion.[72]

Until recently, aprotinin, a naturally occurring fibrinolytic possessing property that the synthetic lysine analogues do not have, was used in reoperation, aortic surgery, and whenever major bleeding was expected. These properties include the ability to inhibit kallikrein, preserve platelet glycoprotein receptors (GIb, GIIb/IIIa), inhibit the proinflammatory cytokine release associated with CPB, as well as the inhibition of plasmin and protein C. Because of its animal-derived protein structure, there is a small but significant risk of anaphylaxis with aprotinin use.

However, during the course of the marketing and use of aprotinin, disturbing questions have been raised in regard to its safety. Persistent questions have lingered about renal failure and increased patient mortality.[73] This culminated in November 2007 when, in response to initial patient data from the "Blood Conservation Using Antifibrinolytics: A Randomized Trial in a Cardiac Surgery Population" (BART) study, the Food and Drug Administration requested that Bayer, the manufacturer of aprotinin, suspend its marketing until a comprehensive review of its safety be performed. Early data demonstrated that there was a higher 30-day mortality associated with the use of aprotinin as opposed to ε-aminocaproic acid or tranexamic acid. As a result, aprotinin use has all but ceased except in extremely high-risk cases; whether it returns to clinical use is to be determined.

Hemodilution due to the CPB prime is one undesired byproduct of extracorporeal circulation. One method that has been used with success to avoid excess hemodilution and reduce the need for blood transfusion is retrograde autologous priming (RAP). In RAP, the crystalloid prime contained within the extracorporeal circuit is drained prior to the initiation of CPB and replaced by blood drained retrograde via the arterial cannula. RAP reduces hemodilution and diminishes the drop in systemic vascular resistance associated with the initiation of CPB. When using this technique, care must be taken to avoid acute hypovolemic hypotension. Reported benefits of RAP include reduced extravascular lung water and weight gain.[74]

Ultrafiltration is another technique used in conjunction with CPB to reduce postoperative bleeding and transfusion needs. During ultrafiltration (hemoconcentration), plasma water is separated from low-molecular-weight solutes, intravascular cell components, and plasma proteins using a semipermeable membrane, using a hydrostatic pressure differential created by external suction. The exact timing of the ultrafiltration process depends on the technique employed. Conventional ultrafiltration is initiated during rewarming and is based on the volume within the CPB circuit and exogenous fluid given. Modified ultrafiltration commonly used in pediatric cardiac surgery consists of ultrafiltration following separation from CPB when blood is pumped retrograde from the aortic cannula through the hemofilter/hemoconcentrator and returned to the right atrium. Advantages of hemoconcentration include a reduction in free water, preservation of hemostasis, and a decrease in levels of circulating inflammatory mediators. By employing hemoconcentration, levels of erythrocytes, platelets, and coagulation factors are augmented. This translates into an increase in hemoglobin and hematocrit concentrations and a decrease in postoperative bleeding and need for transfusion.[75]

Blood fractionation is similar to hemoconcentration: blood elements are removed and concentrated pre-bypass. These concentrates are then retuned to the patient following CPB, thereby avoiding dilutional coagulopathy and activation of these blood elements by CPB.

Because of the relative scarcity of blood and its products there is intensive research in the development of blood substitutes. These hemoglobin-based compounds are made from human or animal blood in which the hemoglobin is chemically extracted. The goal is to develop a shelf-stable product possessing the oxygen-carrying capacity of blood but devoid of the infectious complications of transfusion. Although they do not possess all the qualities of banked blood, these compound show great promise and are being actively studied.

Myocardial Protection

The most common method of myocardial protection used today is that of intermittent hyperkalemic cold cardioplegia and moderate systemic hypothermia. Systemic hypothermia is for myocardial and neurologic protection during cardiac surgery. The benefits of hypothermia are reduction in metabolic rate and oxygen consumption, preservation of high-energy phosphate substrates, and reduction in excitatory neurotransmitter release. For each degree Centigrade reduction in temperature, there is an 8% reduction in metabolic rate, so that at 28°C there is an approximate reduction in metabolic rate of 50%. Moderate systemic hypothermia can be achieved with either passive or active cooling. Using passive cooling, the patient's core temperature is allowed to equalize with ambient temperature. This may be a slow or rapid process depending on variables such as patient's body surface area exposed and ambient temperature. Most patients undergoing cardiac surgery are actively cooled and then rewarmed using a heat exchanger.

The fundamental concept of cold cardioplegia is that a cold solution (10 to 15°C) of either blood or crystalloid with a supranormal concentration of potassium is injected into the coronary arteries or veins to induce diastolic electrical arrest. Cardioplegia may be employed via an anterograde or retrograde route, or a combination of the two routes. Anterograde cardioplegia solution is injected via the aortic root following aortic cross-clamp and into the native coronaries. The cardioplegia follows the normal anatomic flow of blood. In patients with severe coronary disease or AI, anterograde cardioplegia may provide inadequate myocardial protection because the incompetent AV allows cardioplegia to flow inside the LV, bypassing the coronary ostia causing left ventricular distention and ischemia. In such cases, following aortic cross-clamping, an aortotomy is made and cardioplegia is delivered via hand-held cannulae placed in the individual coronary ostia under direct vision. During coronary artery bypass surgery, individual grafts may be used to deliver cardioplegia once distal anastomoses have been completed. Retrograde cardioplegia may also be employed for myocardial protection by the placement of a catheter inside the coronary sinus. Retrograde cardioplegia is then injected via the unobstructed cardiac venous system, bypassing obstructed coronaries and achieving greater myocardial protection. To maximize myocardial protection, both anterograde and retrograde are often used in combination. Depending on the time required for surgical repair, multiple injections of cardioplegia may be necessary to wash out metabolic by-products, add new high-energy and oxygen-carrying substrates, and maintain hypothermic diastolic arrest. Other techniques for myocardial protection include intermittent cross-clamp with periods of reperfusion, and hypothermic ventricular fibrillation.

For the anesthesiologist monitoring a patient on CPB, the sentinel events of cardioplegic electrical arrest and resumption of electrical activity must be observed closely. LV distention and lack of rapid electrical arrest may be evidence of poor myocardial protection and the possibility of difficulty in separation from CPB. Transesophageal echocardiography is particularly helpful in diagnosing ventricular distention and its relief by venting or manual decompression of the LV.

PREOPERATIVE AND INTRAOPERATIVE MANAGEMENT

The preoperative visit appropriately concentrates on the cardiovascular system but should also focus on the assessment of pulmonary, renal, hepatic, neurologic, endocrine, and hematologic functions. Equally invaluable is discussing with the patient the anticipated events on the day of surgery, including transport to the operating room, preoperative routines (O_2 mask, vascular cannulation, anesthetic induction), and finally, the awakening process in the recovery room or ICU. The importance of communicating to the anesthesiologist any symptoms such as chest pain, shortness of breath, or the need for nitroglycerin during transport or the preinduction period should be emphasized to the patient. The depth and detail of the explanation should be custom-tailored to each patient.

Data from history, physical examination, and laboratory investigations are used to define the cardiovascular anatomy and functional state. Pertinent findings suggestive of left and/or right ventricular dysfunction are described in Table 41-10. Increases in the severity or frequency of anginal attacks or the presence of ischemia-induced ventricular dysfunction suggest

TABLE 41-10

PREOPERATIVE FINDINGS SUGGESTIVE OF VENTRICULAR DYSFUNCTION

History
- CAD: Previous MI, chest pain/pressure
- CHF (intermittent or chronic): Fatigue, DOE, orthopnea, PND, ankle swelling

Physical examination
- Vital signs: hypotension, tachycardia (severe CHF)
- Engorged neck veins, apical impulse displaced laterally, S_3, S_4, rales, pitting edema, pulsatile liver, ascites

Electrocardiogram
- Ischemia/infarct, rhythm, conduction abnormalities

Chest X-ray
- Cardiomegaly, pulmonary vascular congestion/pulmonary edema, pleural effusion, Kerley B lines

Cardiovascular testing
- Catheterization data: LVEDP >18 mm Hg, EF <0.4, CI <2.0 L/min/m²

CAD, coronary artery disease; MI, myocardial infarction; CHF, congestive heart failure; DOE, dyspnea on exertion; PND, paroxysmal nocturnal dyspnea; LVEDP, left ventricular end-diastolic pressure; EF, ejection fraction; CI, cardiac index.

that large areas of myocardium are at risk. A history of dysrhythmias should be obtained, including the type, severity, associated symptoms, prior intervention, and successful treatment (including the presence/type/date of insertion of a rhythm device). Integration of this information leads to appropriate selection of monitoring devices and anesthetic techniques.

Conditions commonly associated with heart disease, such as hypertension, diabetes mellitus, and cigarette smoking, must also be evaluated. The latter is extremely important and may be useful in differentiating whether episodes of intraoperative pulmonary hypertension are caused primarily by pulmonary or cardiac factors. Higher systemic arterial pressures may be desirable throughout surgery in patients with a history or other evidence of carotid artery disease. Evidence for renal dysfunction must be sought because the most common cause of postoperative renal failure is pre-existing renal insufficiency. If renal reserve is reduced, intraoperative measures such as diuretics or dopamine may be used, although no data showing an improved outcome are available.

Current Drug Therapy

Almost without exception, cardiovascular drugs, including cardiac antiarrhythmics (e.g., amiodarone), beta-blockers or calcium channel blockers, and nitrates as well as aspirin, antilipidemics (statins), and ACE inhibitors are continued until the time of surgery.[76] Interactions between these drugs and anesthetics are more often beneficial than harmful in maintaining hemodynamic control during periods of surgical stress and reducing morbidity and mortality.

Concern about intraoperative hypotension and increased requirement for vasopressor support in patients receiving beta-blockers or calcium channel blockers or ACE inhibitors is unwarranted. Contrary to common belief, there is a potential long-term benefit of ACE inhibitors provided that dosing is adjusted so that hypotension is avoided.[77] Digoxin is prescribed, less frequently today, to suppress cardiac dysrhythmias, control the ventricular response to atrial fibrillation, and improve contractility in patients with congestive heart failure. Continuation until the time of surgery seems advisable for those patients in whom it is being used for rate or rhythm control. Signs or symptoms of digoxin excess, including ventricular ectopy, atrial tachydysrhythmias, and variable degrees of atrioventricular block should be sought. The latter is typically manifested by slowing and regularization of the ventricular response to atrial fibrillation. This represents digoxin-induced atrioventricular blockade with a regular junctional escape rhythm. Noncardiac symptoms include gastrointestinal distress or visual disturbances. Toxicity is more common in patients concomitantly receiving drugs that increase digoxin levels (e.g., nifedipine, verapamil, amiodarone) or reduce potassium levels (e.g., diuretics). Most cardiac antidysrhythmics should also be continued to the time of surgery.

Physical Examination

As mentioned previously, the physical examination seeks to elicit signs of cardiac decompensation such as an S_3 gallop, rales, jugular venous distention, or pulsatile liver. Routes for vascular access should be assessed, and the status of peripheral arteries should be evaluated. As always, the airway should be carefully evaluated with respect to ease of mask ventilation and intubation of the trachea. Other pertinent points are described in Table 41-11.

Premedication

Even the most thorough preoperative psychological preparation is often inadequate to assuage the anxieties and apprehensions of a patient facing cardiac surgery. Premedication will assist in providing a calm, anxiety-free but arousable and hemodynamically stable patient who is prepared for surgery. Selection of drug and dosage is predicated on the patient's age, cardiovascular state, level of anxiety, and location. If the patient is coming from home, often there is inadequate time for adequate premedication. Heavy premedication is ideal for the fit person scheduled for CABG (however, this patient is rarely in the hospital prior to surgery). Inadequate sedation may predispose to hypertension, tachycardia, or coronary vasospasm, all potential causes of myocardial ischemia. However, the frail, 50-kg, cachetic patient with severe valvular dysfunction fares better with light premedication to avoid possible respiratory depression or loss of endogenous catecholamine support. Additional sedation can always be given in the operating room under direct observation by the anesthesiologist.

Monitoring

We emphasize only those aspects of monitoring particularly relevant to cardiac surgery because the subject is discussed extensively in Chapters 27 and 38.

Pulse Oximeter

The need for multiple vascular cannulations and applications of numerous monitoring devices often prolongs the preinduction period. The pulse oximeter should be one of the first monitors placed prior to any other, invasive or not, intervention to detect clinically unsuspected episodes of hypoxemia, especially if additional intravenous sedation has been administered. Attention must be focused on the whole patient at all times.

Electrocardiogram

Regional ischemia may be localized by appropriate lead monitoring: lead II (and/or leads III, aVF: right coronary artery distribution) for the inferior, leads V_4, V_5 (left anterior descending [LAD] artery) for the anterior, and leads I and aVL (circumflex artery) for the lateral wall of the LV. If the standard leads prove inadequate for detection and analysis of cardiac dysrhythmia, esophageal or epicardial leads may be used. Occasionally, intraoperative myocardial injury causes substantial reductions in QRS voltage. Monitoring an electrocardiogram (ECG) via a surgically placed ventricular pacing wire provides adequate voltage to facilitate dysrhythmia analysis or to trigger an intra-aortic balloon pump, if necessary. A strip-chart recorder documents and facilitates detailed analysis of both ST segment alterations and complex dysrhythmias.

Temperature

Central temperature can be measured with nasopharyngeal, tympanic, and urinary bladder catheter probes or with a thermistor from a PAC.[78] Obviously, this last method is not reliable during the period of aortic cross-clamping when there is no flow through the heart. Rectal and toe probes record peripheral temperatures, which lag behind central measurements during both cooling and rewarming periods.

Arterial Blood Pressure

Systemic arterial pressure is always monitored invasively. The radial or femoral artery is usually cannulated, although the brachial and axillary arteries may also be used. The exact site is often a matter of personal or institutional preference. Criteria include convenience, selection of the fullest or most bounding pulse, and avoidance of the dominant hand. Occasionally, the site of surgery dictates appropriate placement; for example, the

TABLE 41-11

PREOPERATIVE PHYSICAL EXAMINATION

Vital Signs
- Current values and range

Height, weight
- For calculations of drug dosages, pump flow, cardiac index

Airway
- Evaluate, identify difficulties for ventilation, intubation

Neck
- Landmarks for jugular vein cannulation
- Vein engorgement (CHF)
- Bruits (carotid artery disease)

Heart
- Murmurs: characteristic of valve lesions, S_3 (elevated LVEDP), S_4 (decreased compliance), click (MVP prolapse)
- Lateral PMI displacement (cardiomegaly)
- Precordial heave, lift (hypertrophy, wall motion abnormality)

Lungs
- Rales (CHF)
- Rhonchi, wheezes (COPD, asthma)

Vasculature
- Peripheral pulses
- Sites for venous and arterial access

Abdomen
- Pulsatile liver (CHF, tricuspid regurgitation)

Extremities
- Peripheral edema (CHF)

Nervous System
- Motor or sensory deficits

CHF, congestive heart failure; LVEDP, left ventricular end-diastolic pressure; MVP: mitral valve prolapse; COPD, chronic obstructive pulmonary disease.

right radial artery should be used for procedures involving the descending thoracic aorta because the left subclavian artery may be included in the proximal aortic clamp. Following CPB, radial artery pressure is often misleading and may be as much as 30 mm Hg lower than central aortic pressure. The mechanism is believed to be peripheral vasodilation during rewarming. Whenever such a discrepancy is suspected, aortic pressure can be estimated by palpation by the surgeon, or if direct measurement is needed, a needle may be placed directly into the aorta. The gradient between aortic and radial pressure usually disappears within 45 minutes of separation from bypass.

Central Venous Pressure and Pulmonary Artery Catheter

Access to the central circulation is mandatory for infusion of cardioactive drugs. In addition, right atrial or central venous pressure accurately reflects right ventricular filling pressure and is of critical importance whenever right ventricular dysfunction is suspected. In patients with normal LV function, transduced right atrial pressure is often assumed to be a reliable guide of left-sided filling. This relationship is less predictable in the presence of severe LV dyssynergy, pulmonary hypertension, or reduced LV compliance. In these instances, insertion of a PAC for measurement of pulmonary capillary wedge pressure provides a somewhat better index of LV filling, although TEE data are far more valid because they provide volume information as well. In addition, determination of cardiac output and calculation of derived hemodynamic indices offer additional information to guide hemodynamic and anesthetic management.

Indications for pulmonary artery catheterization vary greatly among institutions. In some these catheters are used routinely, whereas in others they are limited to patients with specific disease states such as severe left ventricular dysfunction or pronounced pulmonary hypertension. Additional indications include combined procedures (valvular plus coronary) or those that require prolonged intraoperative time (cardiac reoperations or use of one or both internal mammary arteries). Insertion of a pacing PAC can be helpful whenever exact control of rate and rhythm is desirable; for example, in patients with hypertrophic cardiomyopathy or those with significant bradycardia secondary to beta-blockade.

When PACs are used, disagreement still exists as to whether they should be placed before or after the induction of anesthesia. In some patients, early insertion of the catheter and determination of baseline hemodynamic values can beneficially influence anesthetic selection and guide the induction sequence. However, the anxious and uncomfortable hypertensive patient is better served by a smooth anesthetic induction followed by catheter placement.

It must be remembered that the catheter often migrates toward the periphery of the lung with cardiac manipulation before and during CPB, as well as with acute preload changes. Therefore, it seems prudent to pull the catheter back a few centimeters prior to the initiation of bypass to prevent permanent wedging or possible pulmonary artery rupture.[79] Despite the controversy concerning the routine use of these catheters, there is no disagreement that the capability to measure both cardiac output and ventricular filling pressures must be available in any institution performing cardiac surgery. Whether this is done with a PAC or TEE is immaterial. The critically ill patient requires these measurements to determine the effectiveness of vasoactive drugs, adjust dosage, and evaluate the need for further pharmacologic or mechanical intervention.

Echocardiography

TEE is the newest, most complex, and most expensive diagnostic device. Detection of ischemia by online evaluation of new regional wall motion abnormalities and its utility in assessing valvular lesions (before and after repair) and the ascending aorta have been mentioned. Other applications specific to cardiac surgical patients are also useful. It is well known that, following CPB, ventricular filling pressure, irrespective of site of measurement (LV end-diastolic pressure, LA, pulmonary capillary wedge pressure), is a poor and often misleading indicator of ventricular volume status.[80] Direct estimation of left ventricular volume with two-dimensional TEE more appropriately directs fluid infusion and selection of vasoactive drugs in patients who are difficult to wean from bypass. In addition, residual valve lesions, intracardiac air, or new areas of ischemia are readily identified. Global dysfunction suggesting residual cross-clamp effect, inadequate cardioplegia, or reperfusion injury can be detected.

Central Nervous System Function and Complications

Monitoring of the brain during extracorporeal bypass is difficult, with a lack of standardized equipment or criteria. Neurologic complications after cardiac surgery can be devastating. The 1- and 5-year survival rates after stroke are about 65% and 45%, respectively, compared with >90% and 80 to 85% for patients not having stroke.[81] Thus, many investigators have more recently focused on methods to determine the etiology and improve the detection, prevention, and treatment of postoperative neurologic complications in patients undergoing cardiac surgery.

The incidence of stroke after CABG surgery ranges from <1% (for patients <64 years old) to >5 to 9% (for patients older >65 years).[82] There is a much higher incidence (60 to 70%) of subtle cognitive deficits that can be elicited by detailed neuropsychometric testing. It is known that the neuropsychiatric deficits do improve over the initial 2 to 6 months after cardiac surgery; however, a significant percentage of patients (13 to 39%) have residual impairment. The etiology of perioperative neurologic complications is believed to be predominantly secondary to emboli (air, atheroma, other particulate matter) than to hypoperfusion in susceptible patients (e.g., pre-existing cerebrovascular disease). Most overt strokes after cardiac surgery are focal and likely due to macroemboli, whereas the cognitive changes are subtle and probably result from microemboli. Risk factors for neurologic complications include advanced age (>70 years), pre-existing cerebrovascular disease (e.g., carotid artery stenosis >80%), history of prior stroke, peripheral vascular disease, ascending aortic atheroma, and diabetes. Operative factors include the duration of CPB, intracardiac procedure (e.g., valve replacement), excessive warming during and following CPB, and perhaps perfusion pressure on CPB.[83,84] Intraoperative hyperglycemia, which could theoretically result in worsened neurologic damage, has not been associated with poorer neurologic outcome.

The role of TEE in evaluating the ascending and descending aorta has been described previously. There are several management options undergoing investigation for patients with severely diseased aortas, especially those with mobile atheromas who are at increased risk of stroke. These include hypothermic fibrillatory arrest with left ventricular vent and no cross-clamp, single cross-clamp (i.e., distal and proximal grafts performed during same cross-clamp), relocation of proximal grafts to area of nondiseased aorta, no proximal grafts (internal mammary arteries only) either on CPB, or using off-pump coronary artery bypass, hypothermic ischemic arrest with resection, and graft replacement of diseased aorta. Cerebral protection is rather limited. Other than the use of 20–40 micron arterial line filters and membrane oxygenators, newer modifications of the basic CPB apparatus or the use of specialized equipment or procedures (including hypothermia and "tight" glucose control) have unproven benefit on neurologic outcomes.[85] Hypothermia is excellent in that it decreases cerebral metabolic rate and prolongs ischemic tolerance; however, profound hypothermia is not practical for routine cardiac surgery. Unfortunately, during routine CPB the patient is normothermic when the highest risk of embolization exists (unclamping, during rewarming, and with initial ventricular ejection). Sodium thiopental has been shown to be cerebroprotective in intracardiac procedures, but not in CABG surgery. This difference may be a result of the "reversible" neurologic impairment secondary to gas emboli, which is more likely during intracardiac procedures than CABG surgery.

Selection of Anesthetic Drugs

There are no data that document superiority of any anesthetic for either coronary or valvular surgery. The large outcome studies of Tuman et al.[86] and Slogoff et al.[87] indicate that the choice of anesthetic has no effect on outcome in CABG patients. As was previously emphasized, the most critical factor governing anesthetic selection is the degree of ventricular dysfunction. Anticipated difficulties during the tracheal intubation sequence, the expected length of surgery, and the anticipated time until extubation of the trachea also influence choice of anesthetic. It is desirable to be able to alter anesthetic depth to accommodate the varying intensity of surgical stress. During intubation of the trachea, incision, sternotomy, pericardiotomy, and manipulation of the aorta, there is intense stimulation and sympathetic response. The period of preparing and draping following intubation of the trachea requires minimal levels of anesthetic, as does the period of hypothermic bypass.

Volatile anesthetics are useful both as primary anesthetics and as adjuvants to treat or prevent "breakthrough" hypertension. The balance of myocardial oxygen supply and is usually altered favorably by reduction in contractility and afterload. Deleterious declines in perfusion must be prevented or treated, and the possibilities of increases in wall tension must be considered. Volatile agents have been used successfully in all types of valve surgery without untoward effects, although they are sometimes associated with more hemodynamic variability than is seen with opioids. The ability to rapidly increase and decrease concentrations permits easy adjustment to variable levels of surgical stimulation. Volatile anesthetics can be administered during bypass through a vaporizer mounted on the pump; they are also appropriate in the postbypass period, assuming cardiac function is adequate. Volatile anesthetics seem to be more important now, in combination with short-acting opiates or hypnotics, because the volume of off-bypass procedures is increasing and the urge to fast-track continues.

Opioids

The opioids lack negative inotropic effects in the doses used clinically and have thus found widespread use as the primary agents for cardiac surgery. This era began in 1969, when high doses of morphine were used to anesthetize patients for AV replacement.[88] However, hypotension, histamine release, increased fluid requirements and, often, inadequate anesthesia resulted in a decline in the use of morphine in favor of the more potent fentanyl derivatives. Aside from bradycardia, fentanyl and its analogs are relatively devoid of cardiovascular effects and have proved to be effective anesthetics. As a primary anesthetic agent, fentanyl (50 to 100 μg/kg) or sufentanil (10 to 20 μg/kg) and oxygen provide hemodynamic stability, although they do not consistently prevent a hypertensive response to periods of increased surgical stimulation. In patients with good ventricular function, although high doses of opioids produce unconsciousness and characteristic electrocardiographic slowing, recall of intraoperative events remains a potential problem.

Adjuvant agents are frequently used to supplement the opioids—benzodiazepines to provide amnesia and volatile anesthetics or vasodilators to control hypertension. Superiority of any one opioid has not been demonstrated for either coronary or valvular surgery. The use of high-dose opioids prolongs the time until emergence and extubation when compared with techniques primarily based on volatile anesthetics and is no longer in fashion. Alfentanil, with an elimination half-life shorter than that of fentanyl or sufentanil, is suitable for infusion techniques and may provide optimal conditions for early extubation of the trachea. Remifentanil, an ultrashort-acting opioid, is 30 times more potent than alfentanil and undergoes hydrolysis by nonspecific esterases in minutes. Its predictable and rapid elimination is unaffected by hepatic or renal disease, making it an optimal drug for infusion techniques.

Combinations of the fentanyl-type drugs and benzodiazepines, whether given concomitantly or as premedication, result in hypotension secondary to a fall in systemic vascular resistance. Any opioid in high doses can produce excessive bradycardia. Vecuronium or cis-atracurium may magnify this problem, whereas pancuronium is often useful in preventing it. Abdominal and chest wall rigidity commonly occur with rapid injection of high doses of opioids and can be severe enough to render ventilation impossible. A low dose (priming) of nondepolarizing muscle relaxant should be given prior to opioid administration.

Nitrous Oxide

In many centers, nitrous oxide is not used during cardiac surgery. Increases in pulmonary vascular resistance associated with nitrous oxide have been demonstrated, with the greatest response in patients with pre-existing pulmonary hypertension. Nitrous oxide is also a mild myocardial depressant and elicits a compensatory, sympathetically mediated increase in systemic vascular resistance. These minimal changes may not be well tolerated in patients with minimal cardiovascular reserve. It is well known that nitrous oxide increases the size of any air-filled cavity. The possibility of expansion of air introduced into the circulation either before or during bypass should preclude its use immediately before, during, or after bypass.

Induction Drugs

The benzodiazepines, barbiturates, propofol, and etomidate can be used as supplements to either inhalation or opioid anesthetics and, more important, are excellent as sole induction drugs in patients with cardiac disease. Obviously, dosage requirements must be altered to fit the clinical situation.

Neuromuscular Blocking Drugs

Muscle relaxants are part of an anesthetic plan for cardiac surgery. Although they are not essential to surgical exposure of the heart, muscle paralysis facilitates intubation of the trachea and attenuates skeletal muscle contraction during defibrillation. In addition, muscle relaxants are necessary to prevent or treat opioid-induced truncal rigidity. The chief criteria for selection are the hemodynamic and pharmacokinetic properties associated with each relaxant, the patient's myocardial function, the presence of coexisting disease, current pharmacologic regimen, and anesthetic technique.[89]

Intraoperative Management

In this section we describe the anesthetic management of a patient undergoing a cardiac surgical procedure from the time of arrival in the operating room until his or her care is transferred to ICU personnel. Because the physiologic and pharmacologic

TABLE 41-12

ANESTHETIC PREPARATION FOR CARDIAC SURGERY

Anesthesia machine
- Routine check

Airway
- Nasal cannula for O$_2$
- Ventilation/intubation equipment
- Suction
- Difficult airway anticipated?: special equipment
- Inspired gas humidifier

Circulatory access
- Catheters for peripheral and central intravenous and arterial access
- Intravenous fluids and infusion tubing and pumps
- Fluid warmer

Monitors
- Standard ASA: ECG leads, blood pressure cuff, pulse oximeter, neuromuscular blockade monitor
- Temperature: various probes (nasal, tympanic, bladder, rectal)
- Transducers (arterial, pulmonary and central venous pressure) calibrated and zeroed
- Cardiac output computer: proper constant inserted
- Anticoagulation (ACT)
- Recorder

Medications
- General anesthetic: hypnotic/induction, amnestic/benzodiazepine-volatile, opioid, muscle relaxant
- Heparin (predrawn)
- Cardioactive
  - In syringes: nitroglycerin, CaCl$_2$, phenylephrine/ephedrine, epinephrine
  - Infusions: nitroglycerin, inotrope
- Antibiotics

Miscellaneous
- Pacemaker with battery
- Compatible blood in operating room

ASA, American Society of Anesthesiologists; ECG, electrocardiogram; ACT, activated clotting time.

---

rationales for anesthetic selection are previously discussed, this is rather a sequential description of what occurs and what is required during surgery. Anticipation of needs specific to each stage of the procedure and immediate availability of necessary equipment and medications prevent untoward hemodynamic aberrations and last-minute rush-in decisions.

Preparation

The operating room must be readied prior to arrival of the patient. Heparin may be drawn up prior to induction of anesthesia in the unlikely event of the need to "crash" onto CPB. Typed and crossmatched blood should be available in the operating suite. Table 41-12 provides a checklist to aid in proper preoperative preparation of the operating room.

Preinduction Period

A conversation prior to entering the operating room serves to evaluate the patient's general status and level of anxiety, and to assess the effectiveness of premedication (if ordered). The patient is reminded to report if chest pain, shortness of breath, or other symptoms occur. Supplemental oxygen via nasal cannula should be administered once the patient has been transferred to the operating table; ECG leads, noninvasive blood pressure cuff, and peripheral oxygen saturation monitor are

placed, and a set of initial vital signs is recorded. Angina should be promptly treated with oxygen, sublingual or intravenous nitroglycerin, additional sedation, or if related to anxiety-induced hypertension or tachycardia, with beta-blocker and prompt induction of general anesthesia.

One or two large-bore intravenous cannulas are inserted after site infiltration with local anesthetic (additional routes for infusion are desirable in patients undergoing repeat cardiac surgery). In some centers, anesthesia is then induced, and following intubation of the trachea, arterial and central venous cannulas are inserted. In other centers, however, these cannulae are inserted prior to induction of anesthesia. Preinduction or postinduction insertion of central venous or pulmonary artery catheters has been discussed previously. Once they are inserted, however, initial values for all pressures and cardiac output should be recorded, and baseline determinations of arterial blood gases, hematocrit, blood glucose, and activated coagulation time should be obtained.

Throughout the preinduction period, while the intravenous and pressure monitoring catheters are inserted, the anesthesiologist must never divert his or her attention from the patient. Placing a functioning pulse oximeter with the volume loud enough to be easily heard should precede line placement. Continuous monitoring of the vital signs, careful observation of the patient, and periodic verbal contact facilitate detection of hemodynamic or ECG abnormalities, increased anxiety, or excessive response to intravenous sedation.

Induction and Intubation

The exact choice and sequence of drugs are a subtle—sometimes not so subtle—combination of art and science. The choice of specific agents (e.g., sedative, opioid, volatile drug, muscle relaxant), dose, and speed of administration depends primarily on the patient's cardiovascular reserve and desired cardiovascular profile. A smooth transition from consciousness to blissful sleep is desired without untoward airway difficulties (e.g., coughing, laryngospasm, truncal rigidity) or hemodynamic responses (e.g., hypotension from relative overdose, loss of sympathetic tone, or myocardial depression; hypertension caused by airway insertion; or jaw thrust). A "slow cardiac induction" sometimes causes, rather than alleviates, these potential problems. However, awake tracheal intubation, after proper sedation, may be appropriate in a bull-necked, obese patient if ventilation and intubation appear to be difficult. The necessity for individual approach to each patient cannot be overemphasized.

Deep planes of anesthesia, brief duration of laryngoscopy, and innumerable pharmacologic regimens have been proposed for eliminating the hypertension and tachycardia associated with intubation of the trachea. None is uniformly successful, and all drug interventions carry some degree of risk, even though they may be small. In addition, in some patients, especially those with a slow heart rate prior to induction of anesthesia, the reflex response to intubation of the trachea is primarily vagal, and severe bradycardia and rarely sinus arrest can occur. Furthermore, more recent evidence suggests that intubation of the trachea is a strong stimulus for coronary vasoconstriction irrespective of the anesthetic because LV blood flow is dramatically altered in the absence of hemodynamic changes. Therefore, the response to tracheal intubation may be variable, although usually short-lived. Nevertheless, identification of persistently abnormal hemodynamics or ischemia should be sought and treated.

Preincision Period

The period of time from tracheal intubation until skin incision is one of minimal stimulation as the surgical team attends to insertion of a bladder catheter, temperature probe, positioning, preparing, and draping. As a result, hypotension often develops, regardless of the anesthetic used. It may be necessary to reduce the anesthetic depth or alternatively support the systemic pressure with a vasoconstrictor. The potential risks of vasoconstriction in patients with poor left or right ventricular performance must be kept in mind. Deeper planes of anesthesia are obviously necessary immediately prior to incision and sternotomy.

Incision to Bypass

As previously emphasized, the prebypass period is characterized by periods of intense surgical stimulation that may cause hypertension and tachycardia, or induce ischemia. Anticipating these events and deepening the anesthetic may be effective, but a vasodilator or other adjuvant is often required. Hypotension can occur during the less stressful moments before bypass, but it is more commonly associated with cardiac manipulation in preparation for, and during, atrial cannulation. This may interfere with venous return or produce episodic ectopic beats or sustained supraventricular dysrhythmias. Atrial fibrillation is not uncommon. Depending on the blood pressure and heart rate response, appropriate treatment may range from nothing to vasoconstrictors, cardioversion, or rapid cannulation and institution of bypass. Maintaining adequate intravascular volume may attenuate the extent of blood pressure decrease. This is a critical period, and continual observation of the surgical field is essential.

Prebypass, ST segment analysis, and frequent TEE observation (if used) are important in identifying and localizing new ischemia. If it occurs, it should be treated appropriately and the surgeon notified. In rare cases in which a cardiac chamber is entered and bleeding is uncontrollable, heparin is administered, the femoral vessels are cannulated, and cardiopulmonary bypass is begun using coronary suction from the field as the major means of venous return. Communication between the anesthesiologist and the surgeon is necessary to keep both apprised of the situation and to ensure the heart gets a periodic "rest."

Cardiopulmonary Bypass

After heparin administration, the cannulae are inserted, and adequate levels of anticoagulation are checked to ensure the patient is ready for the institution of CPB (Table 41-13). Attention is focused on adequacy of venous drainage, unobstructed arterial return, sufficient gas exchange, and provision of necessary anesthetics and muscle relaxants. The anesthetic requirements are decreased if systemic hypothermia is used.

There is complete agreement that once full CPB is established, it is no longer necessary to ventilate the lungs. However, there is no such consensus about what exactly to do with the lungs during the period of bypass. Some anesthesiologists completely disconnect the patient from the anesthesia machine; others maintain the lungs slightly inflated with low levels of positive end-expiratory pressure using 100% oxygen or various mixtures of room air. No specific method is associated with superior postoperative pulmonary function.

During the initial minutes of bypass, systemic pressure initially drops to 30 to 40 mm Hg as pulsatile flow ceases and the hemodilution effect of the dilute prime becomes apparent. Once adequate mixing is obtained, blood pressure increases to levels determined primarily by flow rate, and secondarily by total vascular resistance (Table 41-14). There is no consensus as to what constitutes the ideal blood pressure or flow rate for adequate vital organ perfusion, especially of the brain, during bypass. Commonly, flow rates are maintained at approximately 50 to 60 mL/kg/min, with systemic blood pressures in the 50 to 60 mm Hg range. Some surgeons believe that a higher perfusion pressure affords better myocardial protection

---

TABLE 41-13

CHECKLIST BEFORE INITIATING CARDIOPULMONARY BYPASS

Laboratory values
- Heparinization adequate (ACT or other method)
- Hematocrit

Anesthetic
- Maintenance: amnestics, opioids, muscle relaxants are supplemented

Monitors
- Arterial pressure: initial hypotension and then return
- CVP: indicates adequate venous drainage
- PCWP:
  - Elevated?: LV distention (inadequate drainage, AI)
  - Pull back PAC 1–2 cm

Patient/field
- Cannulae in place:
  - No kinks or clamps or air locks
  - Arterial cannula is free of bubbles
- Face:
  - Suffusion?: inadequate SVC drainage
  - Unilateral blanching?: innominate artery cannulation
- Heart:
  - Signs of distention (AI, ischemia)

Support
- Usually not required

ACT, activated clotting time; CVP, central venous pressure; PCWP, pulmonary capillary wedge pressure; LV, left ventricle; AI, aortic insufficiency; PAC, pulmonary artery catheter; SVC, superior vena cava.

---

for the cold fibrillating heart, rather than cardioplegia. Others opt for a mean pressure equal to patient's age!

Monitoring and Management During Bypass

The common causes of blood pressure changes during CPB are listed in Table 41-14. Of primary importance is continuous observation of the surgical field and cannulae to ensure nothing mechanical is awry. Attention can then be directed to other causes of hypotension or hypertension and their appropriate treatment. Additional areas that require periodic monitoring and occasional intervention during bypass are also described in Table 41-14. Maintenance of adequate depths of anesthesia is obviously important during bypass, although clinical signs are few. Anesthetic requirements are decreased during the period of hypothermia but return toward normal when the patient is rewarmed.

Arterial pH and mixed venous oxygen saturation, often measured online, are used to assess the adequacy of perfusion. Urine output is also monitored, but so many variables (e.g., arterial and venous pressure, flow rate, temperature, diuretic history) influence this, that it is difficult to draw meaningful conclusions from this measurement.[90] In addition, postoperative renal failure develops from either aggravation of pre-existing renal dysfunction or persistent low cardiac output following bypass. Although many institutions administer diuretics routinely, they are just as assiduously avoided elsewhere.

Rewarming

When surgical repair is nearly complete, gradual rewarming of the patient begins. A gradient of approximately 10°C is maintained between the patient and the perfusate to prevent formation of gas bubbles, and blood temperature should be no greater than 37°C. Patient awareness becomes a possibility as the

TABLE 41-14

CHECKLIST DURING CARDIOPULMONARY BYPASS

Laboratory values
- Heparinization adequate (ACT or other method)
- ABGs (uncorrected): is there acidosis?
- Hematocrit, Na$^+$, K$^+$, ionized Ca^{++}, glucose

Anesthetic
- Discontinue ventilation

Monitors
- Arterial hypotension:
  - Inadequate venous return
    Venous cannula: malposition, clamp, kink, air lock
    Bleeding, hypovolemia, IVC obstruction, table too low
  - Pump: poor occlusion, low flow
  - Arterial cannula: misdirected, kinked, partially clamped, aortic dissection
  - Decreased vascular tone: anesthetics, hemodilution, idiopathic
  - Transducer/monitor malfunction: radial artery cannula malpositioned, dampened waveform
- Arterial hypertension:
  - Pump: high flow
  - Arterial cannula: misdirected
  - Vasoconstriction: light anesthetic plane, response to hypothermia
  - Transducer/monitor malfunction: radial artery cannula malpositioned/kinked
- Venous pressure:
  - Transducer higher than atrial level?
  - True obstruction to chamber drainage? (CVP: right, PCWP/LA: left heart)
- EEG
- Adequate body perfusion:
  - Flow and pressure?
  - Acidosis
  - Mixed venous blood oxygen saturation
- Temperature
- Urine output

Patient/field
- Conduct of the operation
- Heart: distention, fibrillation
- Cyanosis, venous engorgement, skin temperature
- Movement
- Signs of light anesthesia/hypercapnia: breathing/ diaphragmatic movement

Support
- Assist adequacy of pump flow:
  - Anesthetics/vasodilators for hypertension
  - Constrictors for hypotension

ACT, activated clotting time; ABGs, arterial blood gases; IVC, inferior vena cava; CVP, central venous pressure; PCWP, pulmonary capillary wedge pressure; LA, left atrium; EEG, electroencephalogram.

TABLE 41-15

CHECKLIST BEFORE SEPARATION FROM CARDIOPULMONARY BYPASS

Laboratory values
- Hematocrit, ABGs
- K$^+$: ? elevated (cardioplegia)
- Ionized Ca^{++}

Anesthetic/Machine
- Lung compliance: evaluate (hand ventilation)
- Lungs are ventilated (manual or mechanical)
- Vaporizers: off
- Alarms: on

Monitors
- Normothermia (37°C nasopharyngeal, 35.5°C bladder, 35°C rectal)
- ECG: rate, rhythm, ST
- Transducers recalibrated and zeroed
- Arterial and filling pressures
- Recorder (if available)

Patient/field
- LOOK AT THE HEART!
- De-aired: check lead II, TEE
- Eyeball contractility, size, rhythm
- LV vent clamped/removed, caval snares released
- Bleeding: no major sites (grafts, suture lines, LV vent site)
- Vascular resistance: CPB flow ∝ MAP ÷ Resistance

Support
- As needed

ABGs, arterial blood gases; ECG, electrocardiogram; TEE, transesophageal echocardiography; CPB, cardiopulmonary bypass; MAP, mean arterial pressure.

the de-airing process. The heart is defibrillated (if needed) and allowed to beat to replace some of the oxygen debt. The field is tidied up, and preparations are made to separate from CPB.

Discontinuation of Cardiopulmonary Bypass

Prior to discontinuing CPB, the patient should be normothermic, the surgical field must be dry, the appropriate laboratory values must be checked, the pulmonary compliance must be evaluated, and ventilation of the lungs begun (Table 41-15). If necessary, heart rate and rhythm are regulated either pharmacologically or electrically (appropriate pacing, defibrillation, cardioversion). The venous cannula(s) are then occluded incrementally and sufficient pump volume is transfused into the patient, while the bypass flow is slowly decreased (Fig. 41-10). During this time, the cardiac function is constantly evaluated from hemodynamic and TEE data and direct inspection of the heart, and the need for vasoactive or cardioactive drugs is assessed. The potential disparity, previously alluded to, between radial artery and aortic pressures must be kept in mind. Contractility, rhythm, and ventricular filling can all be estimated by careful observation of the beating heart, and assisted by TEE. For example, a low blood pressure and a vigorously contracting, relatively empty ventricle suggest that volume and perhaps a vasoconstrictor are all that is needed to wean the patient from bypass, whereas adequate blood pressure in the presence of a sluggish and overdistended heart may be treated with a vasodilator and/or a small dose of an inotrope. Figure 41-11 presents a general approach to termination of cardiopulmonary bypass.

Inadequate cardiac performance must prompt a search for possible causes (Table 41-16); structural defects require more than mere regulation of inotropes or vasodilators. If the clinical

potentiation of anesthetic effects due to hypothermia dissipates. If adequate doses of anesthetics have not been given, administration during rewarming should be considered to prevent recall of intraoperative events. Use of volatile anesthetics is helpful if a smooth postbypass course is anticipated and early weaning **11** from mechanical ventilation and extubation are planned. On completion of the surgical repair, various maneuvers are performed to remove any residual air in the ventricles. The anesthesiologist is called on to vigorously inflate the lungs to remove air from the pulmonary veins and aid in filling the cardiac chambers. TEE is particularly useful in assessing the effectiveness of

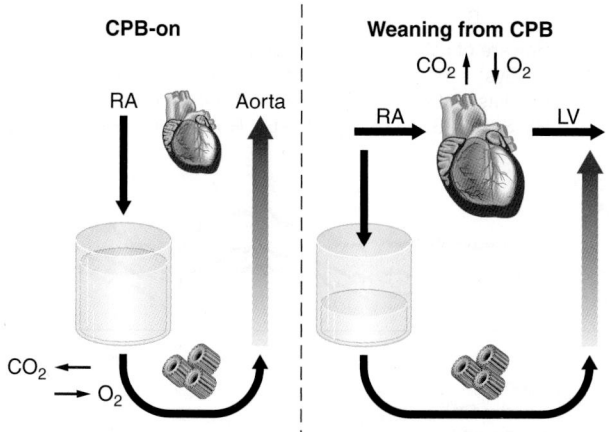

CPB-on | **Weaning from CPB**

FIGURE 41-10. Weaning from cardiopulmonary bypass. While on cardiopulmonary bypass (CPB), the venous return to the heart is diverted from the right atrium (RA) to the CPB reservoir. The drainage is passive (by gravity). From the venous reservoir, the blood is "ventilated," CO_2 is removed, and O_2 is added, and then returned to the patient, usually into the aorta but occasionally via the femoral or axillary arteries. During weaning from CPB, the venous return to the CPB is reduced by gradually occluding the venous cannula, directing more of its contents to the right heart and lungs. LV, left ventricle.

picture is suggestive of coronary air emboli with diffuse ST segment elevation and a hypocontractile heart, continuous support on CPB with a high perfusion pressure and an empty ventricle is indicated.

Our approach to patients with inadequate cardiac output is summarized in Table 41-17. The heart rate is adjusted. Following that, ventricular filling is optimized by transfusing blood from the CPB pump. It is important not to overdistend the heart by transfusing to an arbitrary level of filling pressure because this may result in further myocardial dysfunction. Looking at the heart (or better, imaging the cardiac chambers by TEE) to monitor the response to small incremental volume infusions is important. The ratio of systemic to pulmonary artery pressure is also helpful: both pressures should increase in the same direction (as in Fig. 41-12A). Change in opposite directions (e.g., pulmonary pressure increases and systemic pressure decreases; Fig. 41-12C) is suggestive of LV failure.

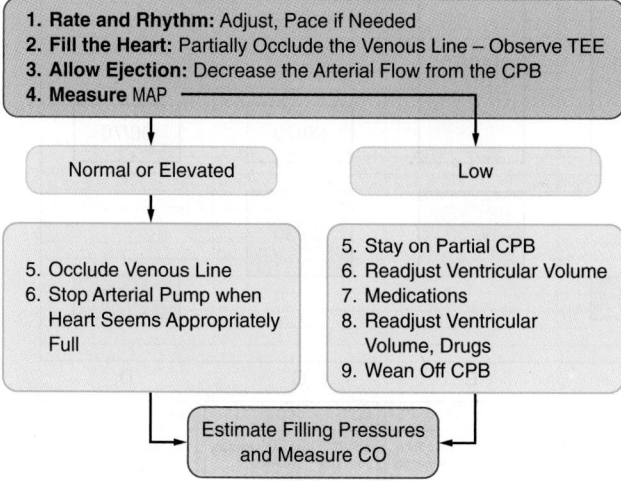

1. **Rate and Rhythm:** Adjust, Pace if Needed
2. **Fill the Heart:** Partially Occlude the Venous Line – Observe TEE
3. **Allow Ejection:** Decrease the Arterial Flow from the CPB
4. **Measure** MAP

Normal or Elevated | Low

5. Occlude Venous Line
6. Stop Arterial Pump when Heart Seems Appropriately Full

5. Stay on Partial CPB
6. Readjust Ventricular Volume
7. Medications
8. Readjust Ventricular Volume, Drugs
9. Wean Off CPB

Estimate Filling Pressures and Measure CO

FIGURE 41-11. General approach to termination of cardiopulmonary bypass (CPB). TEE, transesophageal echocardiographic; MAP, mean arterial pressure; CO, cardiac output.

TABLE 41-16

ETIOLOGY OF RIGHT OR LEFT VENTRICULAR DYSFUNCTION AFTER CARDIOPULMONARY BYPASS (CPB)

Ischemia
- Inadequate myocardial protection
- Intraoperative infarction
- Reperfusion injury
- Coronary spasm
- Coronary embolism (air, thrombus, calcium)
- Technical difficulties (kinked or clotted grafts)

Uncorrected structural defects
- Nongraftable vessels, diffuse coronary artery disease
- Residual or new valve pathology
- Hypertrophic cardiomyopathy
- Shunts
- Pre-existing cardiac dysfunction

CPB-related factors
- Excessive cardioplegia
- Unrecognized cardiac distention

If pharmacologic support is required, an integration of cardiac physiology (see Chapter 10) and pharmacology will lead to the rational selection of an appropriate drug or drugs. Numerous algorithms are available to guide decision making; one is presented in Figure 41-13. This algorithm uses systemic arterial and pulmonary artery pressures, and cardiac output. If TEE is available, myocardial contractility and valvular function can be more readily assessed. A search for new wall motion changes, paravalvular leaks, or new MR is appropriate. After integrating available data, a diagnosis is made and appropriate treatment is begun. Continual reassessment of the situation is necessary to document the efficacy of treatment or to suggest new diagnoses and therapeutic approaches. If cardiac output is low and systemic pressure is adequate (Fig. 41-13A), an arteriolar dilator may improve forward flow by decreasing afterload. If systemic pressure is too low (Fig. 41-13C,D), thus prohibiting the use of vasodilators, an inotrope should be selected instead. Each inotropic drug has a distinct profile with respect to its effects on rate, contractility, systemic and pulmonary vascular resistance, and cardiac dysrhythmogenic potential (Table 41-18). If these initial therapies are insufficient to promote adequate forward flow, various combinations of drugs may be tested. If systemic perfusion is still inadequate, mechanical circulatory support is required.

A therapeutic approach to right ventricular failure (Fig. 41-13D) is outlined in Table 41-19. When pulmonary arterial pressure is normal or decreased, the cause is usually severe

TABLE 41-17

STEPS FOR IMPROVING SYSTEMIC FLOW

1	Heart rate (A-, V-, A/V-pacing) and rhythm
2	Preload: optimize (beware of altered compliance postbypass)
3–4	Afterload reduction if blood pressure is high and/or contractility augmentation (inotrope if low CO)
5	Preload: recheck and adjust
6	Combine therapies
7	IABP
8	VAD

A, atrial; V, ventricular; CO, cardiac output; IABP, intra-aortic balloon pump; VAD, ventricular assist device.

FIGURE 41-12. Hemodynamic abnormalities at termination of cardiopulmonary bypass. LV, left ventricle; syst, systolic; diast, diastolic; RV, right ventricle; ART, arterial pressure; PA, pulmonary artery; CVP, central venous pressure.

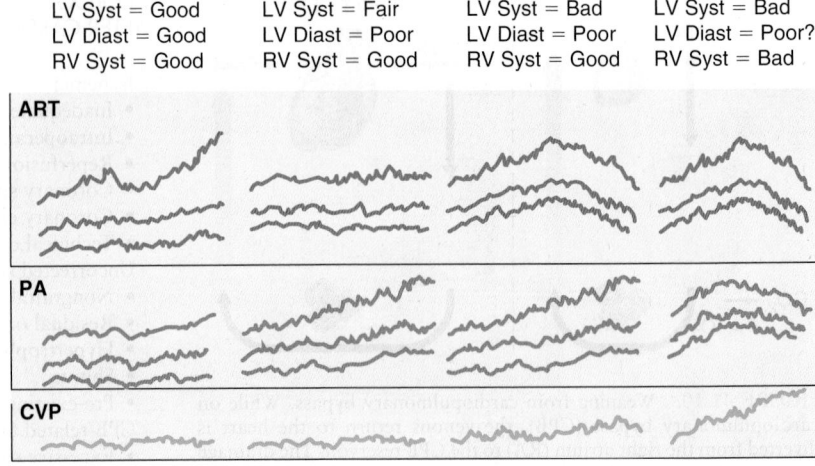

right ventricular ischemia secondary to intraoperative events or air. The initial response is to return to full bypass, improve perfusion, and await recovery and improvement of contractility. If this does not occur, inotropic and vasodilator therapy is established. In patients who have right ventricular failure secondary to high pulmonary vascular resistance, the mainstay of therapy is reduction of pulmonary vascular resistance with vasodilators, such as inhaled prostaglandin I_2 (PGE_1) or nitric oxide, and inotropic support. The phosphodiesterase III inhibitors, amrinone and milrinone, are particularly useful because they significantly decrease pulmonary vascular resistance and increase contractility. Overdistention of the ventricle must be assiduously avoided. Combination therapy with differential infusions refers to infusion of inotropes with vasoconstrictive properties into the left side of the circulation to maintain systemic perfusion, while avoiding an increase of the pulmonary circulation resistance. Persistent right ventricular failure precluding separation from CPB may require the insertion of a right ventricular assist device.

A retrospective study of 1,009 patients undergoing either CABG alone or in combination with valve surgery with CPB investigated the demographic, clinical, and echocardiographic factors associated with the use of inotropic support during separation from CPB. Wall motion score index, combined CABG and mitral valve surgery, LV ejection fraction <35%, reoperation, moderate-to-severe MR and aortic cross-clamp time were independent predictors for use of inotropes (39% of patients).[91]

Intra-Aortic Balloon Pump

The simplest and most readily available mechanical support device is the intra-aortic balloon pump.[92] It consists of a 25-cm long, sausage-shaped balloon composed of nonthrombogenic polyurethane mounted on a 90-cm vascular catheter. It is usually inserted into the femoral artery, either percutaneously or after surgical exposure, and advanced so the distal tip is below the left subclavian artery (to prevent emboli to the head vessels) and the proximal above the renal arteries. Occasionally, when peripheral

FIGURE 41-13. Algorithm for the diagnosis and treatment of hemodynamic abnormalities at termination of cardiopulmonary bypass. CO, cardiac output; SVR, systemic vascular resistance; vasc, vascular; IABP, intra-aortic balloon pump; LVAD, left ventricular assist device; CVP, central venous pressure; RV, right ventricle; NO, nitric oxide; PGI₂, prostacyclin.

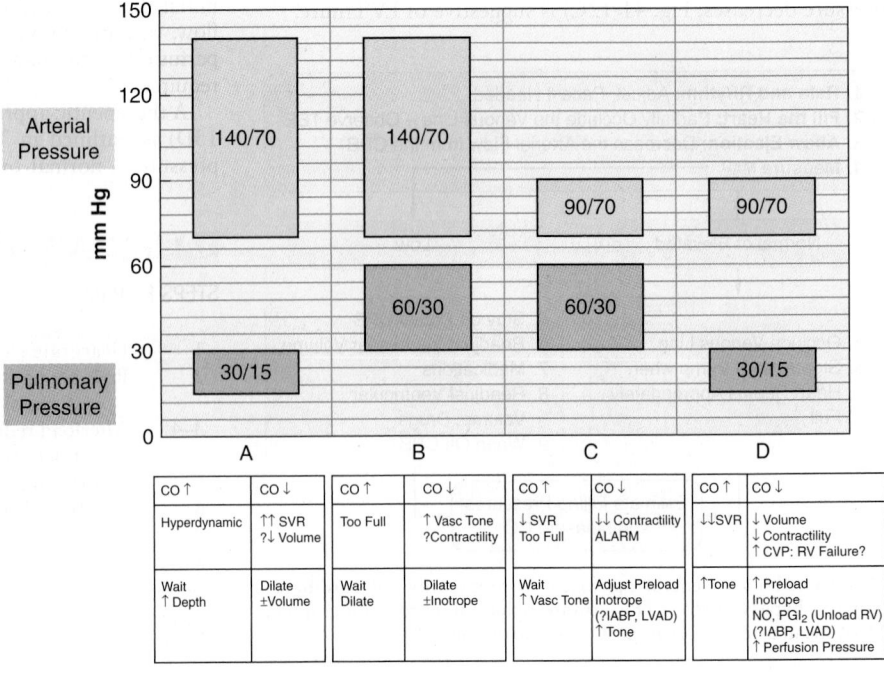

TABLE 41-18

MEDICATIONS GIVEN BY CONTINUOUS INFUSION

■ DRUGS	■ USUAL INITIAL DOSE (μg/kg/min)	■ USUAL DOSE RANGE (μg/kg/min)
Amrinone[a]	2–5	2–20
Dopamine	2–5	2–20
Dobutamine	2–5	2–20
Epinephrine	0.01	0.01–0.1
Isoproterenol[b]	0.05–1	0.1–1
Lidocaine	20	20–50
Milrinone	50 μg/kg (over 3 min)	0.3–0.7
Nitroglycerin	0.5	0.5–5
Nitroprusside	0.5	0.5–5
Norepinephrine	0.1	0.1–1
Phentolamine	0.1–1	0.5–5
Phenylephrine	1	1–3
Prostaglandin E$_1$	0.05–0.1	0.05–0.2
Trimethaphan	5	5–10
Vasopressin		0.0004

[a]Requires initial bolus of 750 μg/kg over 3 minutes before start of infusion.
[b]For chronotropic effect following cardiac transplantation, doses of 0.005 to 0.010 μg/kg/min are used.

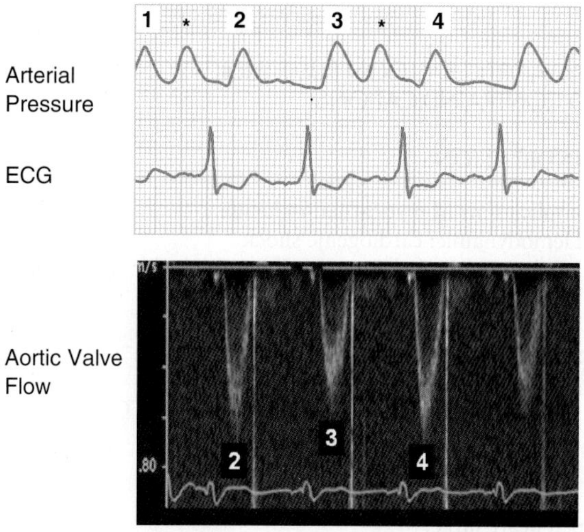

FIGURE 41-14.   The physiologic effects of intra-aortic balloon pump (IABP) counterpulsation. The IABP is inflated during diastole (*asterisk*), every other beat (rate 1:2). The arterial systolic pressure is decreased after IABP augmentation (compare beats 2 and 4 with beats 1 and 3). The diastolic arterial pressure is augmented during IABP inflation (*asterisk*). The flow through the aortic valve (approximate stroke volume) as demonstrated with pulsed wave Doppler echocardiography shows the increased forward flow after augmentation (beats 2 and 4). ECG, electrocardiogram.

vascular disease prohibits passage of the balloon via the femoral artery, it is inserted via the ascending aorta. The intra-aortic balloon pump is the only method that decreases myocardial oxygen demand and increases oxygen supply to the myocardium.

The intra-aortic balloon pump uses the principle of synchronized counterpulsation to assist a beating, ejecting heart: blood volume is moved in a direction "counter" to normal flow. The balloon is inflated during diastole and deflated during systole. The balloon inflation elevates aortic diastolic blood pressure (diastolic augmentation), thus increasing the coronary perfusion gradient proximally, and enhances forward flow distally. During the subsequent systole, the LV will eject facing a lower systemic diastolic pressure (systolic unloading, reduced MVO$_2$) (Fig. 41-14). Proper timing of balloon deflation is necessary to reduce end-diastolic pressure as much as possible to maximally offload the ventricle. The indications and contraindications for intra-aortic balloon pump placement are listed in Table 41-20. Myocardial function often improves with the use of the intra-

aortic balloon pump, and systemic perfusion and vital organ function are preserved.[93] It is crucial to control heart rate and suppress atrial and ventricular dysrhythmias to ensure proper balloon timing. As cardiac function returns, the assist ratio is gradually weaned from every beat to every other beat and so on and, assuming no further cardiac deterioration, it is removed.

Complications associated with the intra-aortic balloon pump are primarily related to ischemia distal to the site of balloon insertion. Direct trauma to the vessel, arterial obstruction, and thrombosis are most common, although aortic perforation and balloon rupture occur rarely. Platelet destruction and thrombocytopenia may also occur.

Ventricular Assist Device

Infrequently (1%), the heart is unable to meet systemic metabolic demands despite maximal pharmacologic therapy and insertion of the intra-aortic balloon pump. Under these circumstances,

TABLE 41-19

RIGHT VENTRICULAR FAILURE

	■ PULMONARY ARTERY PRESSURE			
	■ INCREASED		■ NORMAL OR DECREASED	
CVP	Increased	Decreased	Increased	Decreased
Diagnosis	RV and LV failure	LV failure		RV failure
Management	Inhaled NO or PGI$_2$, PDE-III		Support on CPB	
	Inotropes		High perfusion pressure	
	Differential infusions		Volume (if CVP low)	
	RVAD		? CABG	

CVP, central venous pressure; RV, right ventricle; LV, left ventricle; NO, nitric oxide; PGI$_1$, prostaglandin I$_2$; PDE-III, phosphodiesterase-III inhibitor; CPB, cardiopulmonary bypass; RVAD, right ventricular assist device; CABG, coronary artery bypass graft.

INTRA-AORTIC BALLOON PUMP INDICATIONS
AND CONTRAINDICATIONS

■ INDICATIONS

Complications of myocardial ischemia
• Hemodynamic: cardiogenic shock
• Mechanical: mitral regurgitation, ventricular septal defect
• Intractable dysrhythmias
• Extension of infarct: postinfarction angina
Acute cardiac instability
• Angina: unstable, preinfarction
• Catheterization laboratory mishap: failed PTCA
• Bridge to transplantation
• Cardiac contusion
• ? Septic shock
Open heart surgery
• Separation from cardiopulmonary bypass
• Ventricular failure: right or left
• Increasing inotropic requirement
• Progressive hemodynamic deterioration
• Refractory ischemia

■ CONTRAINDICATIONS

• Severe aortic insufficiency
• Inability to insert
• Irreversible cardiac disease (patient is not a transplant candidate)
• Irreversible brain damage

PTCA, percutaneous transluminal coronary angioplasty.

devices that actually pump blood and bypass either the LV or right ventricle are required. These devices are effective when the injury that produced myocardial dysfunction took place intraoperatively and, more important, if it is reversible. Markedly impaired cardiac function after bypass is not necessarily synonymous with cell death but, rather, may represent temporary "stunning" of the myocardium. Survival ranges from 20 to 30%, often with minimal or no decline in cardiac function.

A second group of patients who have shown benefit from assist devices are those with chronic heart failure. These devices allow for hemodynamic support as a temporizing measure prior to heart transplantation. In the failing heart, it is important to make decisions promptly and move swiftly to an assist device after the various therapeutic options are exhausted. Very often, mechanical support for one ventricle unmasks previously unrecognized failure in the other, necessitating additional pharmacologic or mechanical intervention.

Postcardiopulmonary Bypass

The procedure is not over when the patient is safely "off pump." Continued vigilance is mandatory during decannulation, protamine administration, "drying up," and chest closure. Anesthetics are administered as clinically indicated. Atrial or junctional dysrhythmias may be caused by removal of the atrial cannulae, but often disappear once they are out. Heparin is reversed with protamine following removal of the venous cannulae; the arterial return cannula remains in place for continued transfusion of pump contents. When this is completed and bleeding is controlled, the arterial cannula is removed, and after bleeding is considered to be under control, the chest is closed. During decannulation, the possibility exists for unexpected bleeding from the atrial or aortic suture lines, and this sometimes requires rapid transfusion. Continued vigilance for new ischemia (manifested by

ST segment changes, ectopy, atrial dysrhythmia, regional wall motion abnormalities by TEE) is important because it may indicate a correctable problem with the grafts. Valve patients should have the adequacy of the repair or replacement (i.e., perivalvular leak, residual stenosis) assessed by TEE.

Reversal of Anticoagulation

Protamine, a polycationic protein derived from salmon sperm, is used to neutralize heparin. The initial and total doses administered vary widely. Some use a fixed ratio of protamine to heparin, others use 2 to 4 mg/kg, and still others look to automated protamine titrations to suggest the initial dose. Regardless of the method selected, further requirements are assessed by repeated measures of the activated coagulation time or other clotting assay(s), as well as by the appearance of the surgical field.[94]

Protamine administration is associated with a broad spectrum of hemodynamic effects.[95] Idiosyncratic responses include type I anaphylactic reactions and both immediate and delayed anaphylactoid responses. True anaphylaxis, mercifully rare, is characterized by increased airway pressure, decreased systemic vascular resistance with systemic hypotension, and skin flushing. Increased incidence of reactions has been reported in patients sensitized to protamine from previous cardiac catheterization, hemodialysis, cardiac surgery, or exposure to neutral protamine Hagedorn insulin. Perhaps the most devastating complication associated with protamine is sudden and profound pulmonary hypertension accompanied by an elevated central venous pressure, a flaccid distended right ventricle, and systemic hypotension. This complication, which may occur in approximately 1% of patients, is mediated by release of thromboxane and C5a anaphylatoxin. The reaction is extremely short-lived, and although reinstitution of bypass is required on rare occasions, it is usually not necessary. Whether protamine is administered via the RA, LA, or aorta, or peripherally, probably makes no difference. However, slow administration into a peripheral venous site is advisable.

Postbypass Bleeding

Persistent oozing following heparin reversal is not uncommon. The usual causes include inadequate surgical hemostasis or reduced platelet count or function, and neither is identified by a prolonged activated coagulation time. Insufficient doses of protamine, dilution of coagulation factors, and, very rarely, "heparin rebound" belong in the differential diagnosis.

After adequate hemostasis is obtained, the chest is closed. This is occasionally associated with transient decreases in blood pressure, which usually respond to volume infusion. If hypotension persists, the chest should be reopened to rule out cardiac tamponade, a kinked graft, or other serious problems.

As the surgeon completes skin closure, the anesthesiologist prepares for an orderly, unhurried transfer of the patient from the operating room to the recovery room or ICU. Medicated infusions must be regulated, as clinically indicated, with portable infusion pumps. Additional syringes with emergency cardiac medications and necessary equipment for airway management should be carried, and blood pressure(s) and ECG are constantly monitored.

MINIMALLY INVASIVE CARDIAC SURGERY

Despite advantages in cardiac surgery and perfusion technology, the deleterious effects of CPB and aortic cross-clamping are well documented. The desire to avoid these complications as well as complications associated with sternotomy were factors leading to development of minimally invasive techniques not requiring CPB. As the population ages, older patients with multiple comorbid medical conditions requiring surgery are increasingly common. Avoidance of aortic manipulation and cross-clamping especially in elderly patients is associated with lower stroke rates.[96]

Newer procedures include MIDCAB (minimally invasive direct coronary artery bypass), OPCAB (off-pump coronary bypass), robotic surgery, and more recently, percutaneous valve repair/replacement performed in the catheterization laboratory. Initially, MIDACB was described as an alternative to angioplasty for single-vessel LAD coronary artery disease. To access the LAD and provide adequate exposure for graft anastomosis, MIDCAB was initially performed via a left thoracotomy using one-lung ventilation. MIDCAB success allowed the development of other forms of minimally invasive surgery. These include the use of parasternal and inframammary incisions, minithoracotomies, and partial sternotomy. Despite effectively decreasing complications seen from sternotomy (large scar, infection, brachial plexus palsy, and 4- to 8-week recovery period) these alternate incisions provide limited exposure and increase surgical difficulty. Another type of minimally invasive cardiac surgery uses port access technology. A small sternotomy is made and catheters are placed percutaneously in the femoral artery and internal jugular vein to facilitate CPB. These catheters include an endovascular aortic balloon that acts as cross-clamp, a PAC to act as vent, and a coronary sinus catheter placed for retrograde cardioplegia administration. This technique is used in only a few centers and is not commonly seen. Readers are directed to review articles on this subject.

Following success with minimally invasive surgery, the time was right for the development of OPCAB surgery, in which exposure is via a sternotomy but CPB is not used. The first experiences with off-pump surgery were "simple" left internal mammary artery (LIMA) to LAD grafts supplemented with angioplasty. OPCAB then developed into complete multivessel coronary revascularizations. During this period, the lack of specialized cardiac stabilization devices required the use of pharmacologic manipulation of heart rate and myocardial contractility. This facilitated surgery by allowing the surgeon to operate on a relatively slow and stable target(s) while not causing undue hypotension. With the development of improved retractors and stabilization devices, the need for bradycardia has for the most part disappeared. Other advances include the use of intracoronary shunts and sutureless anastomotic devices.

Changes in surgical technique have forced changes in anesthetic technique.[97] High-dose narcotics were abandoned in favor of shorter-acting agents that facilitate early extubation. In addition, the lull period seen on CPB was replaced by the need to constantly monitor hemodynamics and intervene rapidly in the face of changing hemodynamics. Use of an arterial line is mandatory as changes in hemodynamics occur rapidly and may be catastrophic during cardiac manipulation. Central access is also necessary for the infusion of drugs and volume. The use of a PAC is not mandatory but does provide information about filling pressures as well as cardiac output measurements. One major problem associated with OPCAB is that exposure of the diseased coronaries and subsequent graft placement often requires positioning of the heart that is associated with hypotension and ischemia. Unfortunately, standard monitors used in cardiac surgery may not be useful in detecting this ischemia. In OPCAB surgery, positioning and retraction of the heart often results in a low-amplitude ECG with axis deviation. These changes may cause ST-T wave changes to be obscured or falsely minimized. Because the heart is obscured by laporatomy pads in the pericardial well or being lifted out of the chest, transesophageal echocardiography may be unreliable in detecting regional wall motion changes signifying ischemia. Sudden changes in pulmonary artery pressure may be related to acute MR due to surgical positioning. In addition, displacement of the heart may cause falsely elevated central venous and pulmonary pressures despite the presence of hypovolemia. Direct observation of the heart and communication with the surgeon are critical in avoiding hemodynamic swings.

As a rule, the most critical lesion is bypassed last and the least critical performed first. The coronary artery to be anastomosed must be isolated proximally and distally. This is performed using either an occluder clip or a snare. Following occlusion, there is usually a period of myocardial ischemia distal to the occlusion. Pre-existing high-grade lesions might have caused formation of collateral circulation, which may ameliorate potential ischemia. Right coronary lesions will predispose to bradycardia, atrial dysrhythmias, and heart block. As a result, immediate access to cardiac pacing and cardioversion are essential. Left-sided coronary lesions may cause malignant ventricular dysrhythmias and hemodynamic collapse. Using inotropes, vasoconstrictors, and volume, sudden hemodynamic collapse may be rescued but may necessitate placement of an intra-aortic balloon pump or conversion to full CPB.

Several techniques are used to avoid rapid hemodynamic changes. These include optimizing preload prior to positioning, judicious use of inotropes and α-agonists, and placing the patient in Trendelenburg position, which allows redistribution of intravascular volume to support the heart in the vertical position.

Normothermia contributes to early extubation as well as prevention of coagulopathy. Aggressive pain control improves patient satisfaction and contributes to early extubation. Techniques for pain control in OPCAB and minimally invasive surgery include systemic opioids and nonsteroidal agents such as ketorolac (in patients without renal insufficiency), local infiltration of the surgical incision, and regional anesthesia. Regional techniques including thoracic epidurals and neuraxial narcotics are used with great success, although anticoagulation is a concern in patients with central regional anesthetics.[98] Anticoagulant protocols are controversial. Both heparin and protamine doses vary between centers. Some do not routinely reverse heparin or administer reduced doses of protamine because of the suspicion that OPCAB may cause hypercoagulability.[99]

Despite great interest in OPCAB as a way to decrease the complications associated with CPB, many remain skeptical as to the benefits. Several studies have shown the superiority of OPCAB in regard to improved neurologic outcome, while others have not.[100,101] Despite disappointing results in regard to neurocognitive and overall outcome, several short-term outcomes are improved following OPCABG. These include lower length of ICU stays, decreased utilization of hospital resources, and decreased incidence of atrial fibrillation.[102]

Many have argued that the advantages of traditional CABG on CPB include a still bloodless field allowing for a better anastomosis and long-term graft patency.[103] Other studies have refuted this to prove equal long-term graft patency rates. The proponents of OPCAB tend to be very familiar with the technique and perform off-pump surgery frequently. This frequency seems to make them technically facile in the peculiarities unique to OPCAB surgery. As such, this may account for varying results from center to center. Currently, there is no consensus as the superiority of standard CABG versus OPCAB.

Relatively new to the area of minimally invasive cardiac surgery is that of endoscopic and robotic cardiac surgery. In these techniques, trocars are placed in the chest in anatomic locations to allow the use of long-handled surgical instruments or manipulators. Supporters of its routine use cite decreased pain, faster healing, and greater patient satisfaction. Anesthetic considerations for endoscopic and robotic surgery are similar to those for standard minimally invasive off-pump surgery. These include one-lung ventilation, positioning issues, and normothermia.

POSTOPERATIVE CONSIDERATIONS

Bring Backs

Postoperative re-exploration is needed in 4 to 10% of cases. The indications are persistent bleeding, cardiac tamponade, and, infrequently, unexplained poor cardiac performance (rule out tamponade). Surgery is usually required within the first 24 hours but also later in cases of delayed tamponade. The possibility of cardiac tamponade must always be included in the differential diagnosis of the postoperative "dwindles" because the classic symptoms and signs are often absent.

Tamponade

In tamponade, the intracardiac pressures are deceptively elevated and do not reflect the actual volume state. Because the surrounding (intrapericardial) pressure is increased, the distending pressure (transmural pressure = intracavitary pressure – extracavitary pressure) is actually decreased. Cardiac chamber collapse is a critical feature of cardiac tamponade, and the chambers with the lowest intracardiac pressure (atria and right ventricle in diastole) are most likely to be compressed. The stroke volume is limited, and cardiac output depends on heart rate. Compensatory mechanisms include peripheral vasoconstriction to preserve venous return and systemic blood pressure, as well as tachycardia. Myocardial ischemia may occur because of the tachycardia and reduced coronary perfusion pressure.

Clinically, patients present with dyspnea, orthopnea, tachycardia, paradoxical pulse, and hypotension, but the intubated, sedated, mechanically ventilated patient in the postanesthesia care unit following cardiac surgery may have varied clinical and hemodynamic presentations. Owing to its often atypical presentation in the cardiac surgical patient, the diagnosis of tamponade should be considered whenever hemodynamic deterioration or signs of low-output failure occur in these patients. In postoperative cardiac patients, the pericardium is no longer intact, and loculated areas of clot may compress only one chamber, causing isolated increases in filling pressure (i.e., mimicking right and/or left ventricular dysfunction). Urine output is usually diminished. Serial chest films typically show progressive mediastinal widening. The diagnosis of tamponade may be confirmed by transthoracic echocardiography or TEE. Diastolic collapse of the RA and right ventricular and/or LV diastolic collapse are the most sensitive and specific signs of cardiac tamponade.[104] In addition, there is excessive respiratory variation of the Doppler flow velocities across the tricuspid and mitral valves. Because of the existing extracardiac compression, respiration increases the ventricular interdependence and affects the diastolic filling of the two ventricles differently. During mechanical inspiration, the increased intrathoracic pressure will impede the right ventricular and augment the LV filling, respectively. The pulsed-wave Doppler echocardiographic examination of the diastolic tricuspid flow will show marked decrease in the velocity of the early wave as the already compromised filling gradient between the extrathoracic veins and the intrathoracic right ventricle is further reduced. During the same time, the early diastolic mitral flow will increase as the increased intrathoracic pressure is transmitted to the intrathoracic pulmonary veins, increasing the filling gradient of the LV. The opposite effects take place during mechanical exhalation, when the effects of positive ventilation dissipate. The transthoracic echocardiography TTE approach may have important limitations: a retrosternal collection may be very difficult to be visualized in a postoperative patient, and subcostal views are rarely feasible early in the postoperative period because of the presence of chest tubes, pacemaker wires,

and/or local tenderness in the subxyphoid area. Therefore, TEE is a better diagnostic tool in the immediate postoperative period.

The cure for cardiac tamponade is surgical; anesthetics can only further depress cardiac function. Therefore, drugs are selected that will preserve the compensatory mechanisms sustaining forward flow. Drugs with vasodilator (either venous or arteriolar) or myocardial depressant properties should be avoided in patients with serious hemodynamic compromise; dosages of induction agents should be appropriately reduced. Ketamine, because of its sympathomimetic effects, may be helpful in preserving heart rate and blood pressure response. It is not, however, a panacea and can induce hypotension in patients under maximal sympathetic stress. If on reopening the chest there is minimal fluid or if the patient shows little improvement, a thorough search for other causes of inadequate cardiac performance, such as clotted or kinked grafts, myocardial ischemia, or valve malfunction, is indicated.

Pain Management

Early awakening and extubation have brought the problem of postoperative pain management in cardiac surgery into focus. The standard practice has been intravenous opioids given as needed followed by conversion to oral pain medications. However, the quest is on to find an ideal postoperative pain management technique to complement the goal of early extubation and maximize patient satisfaction.[105] Several studies have shown the benefits of intrathecal administration of opioids.[106] The addition of nonsteroidal anti-inflammatory agents may play an increasing role. In cardiac patients with severe pain associated with sternal fractures due to the sternal retraction device during internal mammary harvest, epidural analgesia has been shown to be safe and effective, and results in improved postoperative pulmonary function.

ANESTHESIA FOR CHILDREN WITH CONGENITAL HEART DISEASE

Because "anatomy dictates the physiology," the anesthetic management of children with congenital heart disease requires knowledge of anatomic defects, planned surgical procedures, and comprehensive understanding of the altered physiology. The overall incidence of congenital heart diseases varies between 4 and 12 per 1,000 live births. The best way to understand the impact of a congenital defect and how anesthetic agents will interact with this defect is to envision the path blood must follow to maintain flow to the pulmonary arteries and aorta. Congenital cardiac lesions can be cyanotic or not. Cyanotic lesions can be due a common mixing chamber, obstruction to pulmonary blood flow, or separation of the systemic and pulmonary circulation. Shunting of blood can cause volume overload on the ventricle and obstruction to the blood flow can cause pressure overload. Table 41-21 classifies various types of lesions by their physiologic impact; however it must be remembered that there is often more than one defect present.

Preoperative Evaluation

History

In infancy, heart failure usually becomes manifest through feeding difficulties, easy fatigability, vomiting, lethargy, and labored breathing. In the older child, heart failure causes easy

TABLE 41-21

PHYSIOLOGIC EFFECTS OF CONGENITAL CARDIAC LESIONS

Volume Overload of the Ventricle or Atrium Resulting in Increased Pulmonary Blood Flow
Atrial septal defect (high flow, low pressure)
Ventricular septal defect (high flow, high pressure)
Patent ductus arteriosus (high flow, high pressure)
Endocardial cushion defect (high flow, high pressure)

Cyanosis Resulting from Obstruction to Pulmonary Blood Flow
Tetralogy of Fallot
Tricuspid atresia
Pulmonary atresia

Pressure Overload to the Ventricle
Aortic stenosis
Coarctation of the aorta
Pulmonary stenosis

Cyanosis Due to a Common Mixing Chamber
Total anomalous venous return
Truncus arteriosus
Double outlet right ventricle
Single ventricle

Cyanosis Due to Separation of the Systemic and Pulmonary Circulation
Transposition of the great vessels

TABLE 41-22

CLASSIFICATION OF CARDIAC MURMURS

Systolic
• Stenotic semilunar valves
• Regurgitant atrioventricular valves
• Atrial septal defect
• Ventricular septal defect
• Coarctation of the aorta
• Still's murmur

Diastolic
• Regurgitant semilunar valves
• Stenotic atrioventricular valves
• Mitral flow rumble
• Tricuspid flow rumble

Continuous
• Patent ductus arteriosus
• Arteriovenous fistula
• Excessive bronchial collaterals
• Aortopulmonary window
• Venous hum
• Surgical shunt
• Severe peripheral pulmonic stenosis

fatigability, shortness of breath, and dyspnea on exertion. The presence of an upper respiratory tract infection in a child may be associated with an increased incidence of postoperative respiratory complications and an extended stay in the ICU. Each child should be carefully evaluated on a case-by-case basis, bearing in mind all the risk factors for adverse postoperative outcomes, including the child's age and weight, presence of an upper respiratory tract infection, baseline arterial saturation, and anticipated durations of surgery and CPB.[107]

In addition, a detailed medication and surgical history should be obtained. The previous surgical procedures may be key to understanding the patient's anatomy.

Physical Examination

The physical examination of a child should seek signs and symptoms of poorly compensated congenital cardiac lesions. These children most often present with failure to thrive, which could be due to pulmonary hypertension and/or poor peripheral oxygenation and organ perfusion. The physical examination should seek to discover other signs of congestive heart failure, such as irritability, diaphoresis, tachycardia, rales, jugular venous distention, and hepatomegaly. Clinical examination of extremities should include evaluation of cyanosis, clubbing, edema, pulse volume, and blood pressure. In children with Blalock-Taussig shunts, upper extremity pulses may be absent or reduced on the side of the shunt. It is important to measure blood pressure in the arms as well as in the legs in all patients in whom congenital heart disease is suspected; thus, coarctation of aorta will not be missed. Auscultation of the heart in these patients can reveal different types of murmurs depending on the lesions (Table 41-22).

All children undergoing cardiac surgery should have complete examination of the airway. Presence of macroglossia, hypoplastic mandible, narrow palate, enlarged tonsils, and laryngotracheal anomalies may compromise the anesthesiologist's ability to maintain a patent airway. This attention is particularly important in small children and in patients with already compromised hemodynamic status because their small functional residual capacity, in combination with higher oxygen consumption, provides a mechanism for rapid desatura-

tion and the potential for cardiovascular collapse. The possibility of associated congenital anomalies should be considered. The overall incidence of extracardiac anomalies among children with congenital heart disease may be as high as 20%.[108]

Laboratory Evaluations

The presence of anemia in these patients may require priming of the extracorporeal circuit with red blood cells. Children with cyanotic lesions manifest with polycythemia. Polycythemia results as a consequence of bone marrow stimulation (via release of erythropoietin from the kidneys) from arterial desaturation. Increased red cell mass can lead to hyperviscosity, peripheral sludging, and reduced oxygen delivery. The sludging is augmented by dehydration from preoperative fasting and by hypothermia from low ambient operating room temperatures. In patients with hematocrit >70%, consideration should be given to preoperative electrophoresis if symptomatic hyperviscosity is present. Cyanotic children with low hematocrit may exhibit hypoxic spells more readily than if the hematocrit were normal.

All children with congenital heart disease undergoing open heart surgical procedures are at risk for perioperative hemostatic derangements. Polycythemia can induce a low-grade disseminated intravascular coagulation with activation of fibrinolysis, degranulation of platelets, and consumption of coagulation factors. Newborns often have inadequate liver-dependent coagulation factors because of immaturity of hepatic function. Platelet count, prothrombin time, and partial thromboplastin time should be evaluated.

Children on diuretic therapy are at risk for hypokalemia, particularly if they are receiving digitalis. Infants, particularly those with congestive heart failure, are also at risk for both hypoglycemia and hypocalcemia. Children who have undergone major cardiac procedures earlier in their lives may have been exposed to blood or blood products and are at increased risk of having abnormal serum antibodies to various blood antigens. Hence, samples of a child's blood should be sent to the blood bank for possible cross-matching.

Cardiac Evaluations

Echocardiography delineates most of the cardiac anatomy and permits noninvasive measurement of ventricular size and function, cardiac output, and the severity of valve dysfunction. Cardiac catheterization is reserved for patients with poor echocardiographic windows and when there is intervening bone or air-filled lung (e.g., scoliosis or abnormalities of the peripheral pulmonary arteries). The chest radiograph of a child with congenital heart disease should be evaluated for cardiac position, size, shape, abnormal vessels, right aortic arch, scimitar syndrome (hypoplasia/aplasia of one or more lobes of right lung and hypoplasia of right pulmonary artery), aberrant pulmonary vessels, abnormal position of bronchi, vascular rings, or associated pulmonary abnormalities (e.g., pneumonia, atelectasis, or emphysema). The ECG should be reviewed for rate and rhythm abnormalities.

Premedication

The purpose of the premedication is to have a calm child without oversedation, loss of protective airway reflexes, or hemodynamic compromise. This will facilitate the separation of the child from the parents and ease the fear and anxiety associated with the perioperative period. Details on this topic are provided in Chapter 45.

Monitoring

In addition to standard monitors, additional monitors used during open heart procedures include peripheral and central temperature monitoring, invasive blood pressure monitoring, central venous pressure monitoring (which can include right atrial or left atrial pressure line placement by the surgeon intraoperatively), and transesophageal echocardiography.

Anesthetic and Intraoperative Management

Inhalational agents hold a prominent place as induction as well as maintenance agents in pediatric cardiac anesthesia. However, patients with poor ventricular function and those with critical dependence on systemic vascular resistance and/or pulmonary vascular resistance will need intravenous access preinduction, and avoidance or limitation of anesthetic agents that can further compromise hemodynamic function. The choice of anesthetic agents following induction is governed by ventricular function (presence or absence of congestive failure), the anticipated use of CPB, and the possibility of mechanical ventilation or tracheal extubation at the end of the case. Opioids are used routinely to limit the stress response in the prebypass phase of pediatric cardiac surgery. Neonates and infants undergoing cardiac surgery and deep hypothermic cardiopulmonary bypass can generate a significant hormonal stress response. No specific relationship between opioid dose and stress response has been established. Opioids that cause severe bradycardia should be used with caution in neonates with complex congenital cardiac lesions. Muscle relaxation is provided with standard agents. Details of dose and side effects are provided in Chapters 44 and 45. Of special note is the marked reduction in neuromuscular blocking requirements during hypothermic bypass.

The many advances in the CPB and surgical and anesthetic techniques have significantly improved the survival of children with congenital heart disease.[109] However, CPB produces marked hemostatic derangements including:

1. Dilution of blood clotting factors
2. Activation of the clotting cascade and consumption of clotting factors and platelets
3. Reduction in coagulation enzymatic activity
4. Activation of the fibrinolytic pathway

Aprotinin has been used to attenuate coagulopathy during pediatric cardiac surgery associated with cardiopulmonary bypass, but aprotinin has been withdrawn from the market after studies in adults demonstrated renal dysfunction and higher than expected mortality associated with its use.

Hemodilution is a prominent problem in CPB in pediatric and neonatal populations. Modified ultrafiltration during pediatric CPB reduces total body water and serum levels of inflammatory mediators. In neonates, modified ultrafiltration results in an elevated hematocrit, improved pulmonary compliance in the immediate postbypass period, and probably improved cerebral metabolic recovery after deep hypothermic circulatory arrest, although the long-term benefit on outcome is unclear.[110] Patients exposed to circulatory arrest during CPB may not recover normal cerebral metabolic activity. On the other hand, low-flow bypass may be associated with greater endothelial injury, as manifested by positive fluid balance after cardiopulmonary bypass compared with circulatory arrest. This accumulation of additional fluid may have an impact on cardiac and pulmonary performance postoperatively.

Separation from cardiopulmonary bypass will require pharmacologic and or pacing support in some patients. In lesions in which the presence of increased pulmonary vascular resistance is known or suspected, addition of nitric oxide may be of benefit. Inhaled nitric oxide works via cGMP, causing pulmonary vasodilatation. It is truly selective for the pulmonary vascular bed and, in addition, should improve the ventilation/perfusion matching in the lungs.

Drugs that are useful in the postbypass period are given in Table 41-18.

Tracheal Extubation and Postoperative Ventilation

Children with simple lesions who have undergone CPB for procedures that do not involve ventricular incisions (atrial septal defect, ventricular septal defect without failure repaired across the tricuspid valve) can often have the endotracheal tubes removed at the conclusion of surgery or shortly thereafter in the ICU.[111,112]

Children most at risk for ventilatory failure following cardiac surgery include:

- Patients with complex surgeries requiring long bypass time and circulatory arrest time
- Patients significantly younger in age and lighter in weight
- Patients with Down syndrome
- Patients with pulmonary hypertension requiring preoperative ventilatory support
- Patients with postoperative cardiovascular and pulmonary complications[113,114]

A thoracotomy incision in a young infant for ligation of a patent ductus arteriosus or placement of a Blalock shunt has been shown to decrease functional residual capacity, and postoperative respiratory support is indicated. In some cases, nasal continuous positive airway pressure can be employed instead of mechanical ventilation. In patients with Fontan physiology (passive pulmonary circulatory), decreasing pulmonary vascular resistance is paramount, and is very much dependent on adequate ventilation, usually through mechanical means. The potentially detrimental effects of endotracheal intubation and positive pressure ventilation offset this advantage. Positive pressure ventilation is known to have a deleterious effect on pulmonary blood flow in patients with Fontan physiology. Resumption of pain-free spontaneous respiration does enhance hemodynamic performance in these patients.[115]

Regional anesthetic techniques can be used to supplement intraoperative anesthesia and provide postoperative analgesia. For example, caudal (epidural) opioids can be used in repair of coarctation of the aorta in the older child or ligation of a patent ductus arteriosus. Some physicians have used caudal or intrathecal morphine for cases involving CPB (and concomitant heparin administration), although this is not a common practice. The recommendation has been made that one allow 60 minutes to elapse between placement of a neuraxial block and administration of heparin, although there is no evidence to support this time interval.[116] Reported benefits of regional techniques include decreased stress response, improved pulmonary and gastrointestinal function, and resultant potential for cost reduction.[117] However, it is difficult to establish the superiority of a regional technique compared with intravenous analgesia.[118]

Hybrid Procedures in Pediatric Cardiac Surgery

Hybrid pediatric cardiac surgery is an emerging field that reaches across interdisciplinary lines and combines skills and techniques traditionally used by pediatric cardiac surgeons and interventional pediatric cardiologists. Advantages of hybrid procedure are real-time feedback obtained by continuous transesophageal echocardiographic monitoring, avoidance of CPB, ventricular incisions, or muscle transections.[119]

References

1. Landesberg G: The pathophysiology of perioperative myocardial infarction: Facts and perspectives. J Cardiothorac Vasc Anesth 2003; 17: 90
2. Weber KT, Janicki JS: The metabolic demand and oxygen supply of the heart: Physiologic and clinical considerations. Am J Cardiol 1979; 44: 22
3. Hoffman J: Transmural myocardial perfusion. Prog Cardiovasc Dis 1987; 29: 429
4. Cheung AT: Exploring an optimum intra/postoperative management strategy for acute hypertension in the cardiac surgery patient. J Card Surg 2006; 21(Suppl 1): S8
5. Prinzmetal M, Kennamer R, Merliss R: Angina pectoris: A variant form of angina pectoris. Am J Med 1959; 27: 375
6. Hansson GK: Mechanisms of disease. Inflammation, atherosclerosis, and coronary artery disease. N Engl J Med 2005; 352: 1685
7. Nissen SE, Tuzcu EM, Schoenhagen P et al: Statin therapy, LDL cholesterol, C-reactive protein, and coronary artery disease. N Engl J Med 2005; 352: 29
8. Leung JM, O'Kelly B, Browner WS et al: Prognostic importance of postbypass regional wall-motion abnormalities in patients undergoing coronary artery bypass graft surgery. Anesthesiology 1989; 71: 16
9. Haggmark S, Hohner P, Ostman M et al: Comparison of hemodynamic, electrocardiographic, mechanical, and metabolic indicators of intraoperative myocardial ischemia in vascular surgical patients with coronary artery disease. Anesthesiology 1989; 70: 19
10. Tuman KJ, McCarthy RJ, Spiess BD et al: Effect of pulmonary artery catheterization on outcome in patients undergoing coronary artery surgery. Anesthesiology 1989; 70: 199
11. Fontes ML, Bellows W, Ngo L et al: Assessment of ventricular function in critically ill patients: Limitations of pulmonary artery catheterization. J Cardiothorac Vasc Anesth 1999; 13: 521
12. Sandham JD, Hull RD, Brant RF et al: A randomized, controlled trial of the use of pulmonary-artery catheters in high-risk surgical patients. N Engl J Med 2003; 348: 5
13. Practice guidelines for pulmonary artery catheterization. An updated report by the American Society of Anesthesiologists task force on pulmonary artery catheterization. Anesthesiology 2003; 99: 988
14. Miller JP, Lambert AS, Shapiro WA et al: The adequacy of basic intraoperative transesophageal echocardiography performed by experienced anesthesiologists. Anesth Analg 2001; 92: 1103
15. Mathew JP, Fontes ML, Garwood S et al: Transesophageal echocardiography interpretation: A comparative analysis between cardiac anesthesiologists and primary echocardiographers. Anesth Analg 2002; 94: 302
16. Shanewise JS, Cheung AT, Aronson S et al: ASE/SCA guidelines for performing a comprehensive intraoperative multiplane transesophageal echocardiographic examination: Recommendations of the American Society of Echocardiography council for intraoperative echocardiography and the Soci-
17. ety of Cardiovascular Anesthesiologists task force for certification in perioperative transesophageal echocardiography. Anesth Analg 1999; 89: 870
18. Cheng DC: Fast track cardiac surgery pathways: early extubation, process of care, and cost containment. Anesthesiology 1998; 88: 1429
19. Myles PS, Daly DJ, Djaiani G et al: A systematic review of the safety and effectiveness of fast-track cardiac anesthesia. Anesthesiology 2003; 99: 982
20. London MJ, Shroyer AL, Coll JR et al: Early extubation following cardiac surgery in a veterans population. Anesthesiology 1998; 88: 1429
21. Engoren M, Luther G, Fenn-Buderer N: A comparison of fentanyl, sufentanil, and remifentanil for fast-track cardiac anesthesia. Anesth Analg 2001; 93: 859
22. Jenkins DP, Pugsley WB, Alkhulaifi AM et al: Ischaemic preconditioning reduces troponin T release in patients undergoing coronary artery bypass surgery. Heart 1997; 77: 314
23. Tanaka K, Ludwig L, Kersten J et al: Mechanisms of cardioprotection by volatile anesthetics. Anesthesiology 2004; 100: 707
24. Belhomme D, Peynet J, Louzy M et al: Evidence for preconditioning by isoflurane in coronary artery bypass graft surgery. Circulation 1999; 100(19 Suppl): II340
25. Pagel S, Fu JL, Damask MC et al: Desflurane and isoflurane produce similar alterations in systemic and pulmonary hemodynamics and arterial oygenation in patients undergoing one-lung ventilation during thoracotomy. Anesth Analg 1998; 87: 800
26. Helman JD, Leung JM, Bellows WH et al: The risk of myocardial ischemia in patients receiving desflurane versus sufentanil anesthesia for coronary artery bypass graft surgery. Anesthesiology 1992; 77: 47
27. Searle N, Martineau RJ, Conzen P et al: Comparison of sevoflurane/fentanyl and isoflurane/fentanyl during elective coronary artery bypass surgery. Can J Anaeth 1996; 43: 890
28. Smith FJ, Bartel PR, Hugo JM et al: Anesthetic technique (sufentanil versus ketamine plus midazolam) and quantitative electroencephalographic changes after cardiac surgery. J Cardiothorac Vasc Anesth 2006; 20: 520
29. Dasta JF, Jacobi J, Sesti AM et al: Addition of dexmedetomidine to standard sedation regimens after cardiac surgery: An outcomes analysis. Pharmacotherapy 2006; 26: 798
30. Muellejans B, Matthey T, Scholpp J et al: Sedation in the intensive care unit with remifentanil/propofol versus midazolam/fentanyl: A randomised, open-label, pharmacoeconomic trial. Crit Care 2006; 10: R91
31. De Hert SG, Cromheecke S, ten Broecke PW et al: Effects of propofol, desflurane and sevoflurane on recovery of myocardial function after coronary surgery in elderly high-risk patients. Anesthesiology 2003; 99: 314
32. Smulyan H: Nitrates, arterial function, wave reflections and coronary heart disease. Adv Cardiol 2007; 44: 302
33. Ali I, Buth K, Maitland A: Impact of preoperative intravenous nitroglycerin on in-hospital outcomes after coronary artery bypass grafting for unstable angina. Am Heart J 2004; 148: 727
34. Cheung AT, Cruz-Shiavone GE, Meng QC et al: Cardiopulmonary bypass, hemolysis, and nitroprusside-induced cyanide production. Anesth Analg 2007; 105: 29
35. Zerbe NF, Wagner BKJ: Use of vitamin B_{12} in the treatment and prevention of nitroprusside-induced cyanide toxicity. Crit Care Med 1993; 21: 465
36. Egi M, Bellomo R, Langenberg C et al: Selecting a vasopressor drug for vasoplegic shock after adult cardiac surgery: A systematic literature review. Ann Thorac Surg 2007; 83: 715
37. Halonen J, Hakala T, Auvinen T et al: Intravenous administration of metoprolol is more effective than oral administration in the prevention of atrial fibrillation after cardiac surgery. Circulation 2006; 114(1 Suppl): I1
38. Booth JV, Ward EE, Colgan KC et al: Duke Heart Center Perioperative Desensitization Group. Metoprolol and coronary artery bypass grafting surgery: Does intraoperative metoprolol attenuate acute beta-adrenergic receptor desensitization during cardiac surgery? Anesth Analg 2004; 98: 1224
39. Mangano DT, Layug EL, Wallace A et al: Effect of atenolol on mortality and cardiovascular morbidity after noncardiac surgery. N Engl J Med 1996; 335: 1713
40. Warltier DC: β-Adrenergic-blocking drugs: Incredibly useful, incredibly underutilized [editorial comment]. Anesthesiology 1998; 88: 2
41. Opie L: Anti-ischemic properties of calcium-channel blockers: lessons from cardiac surgery. J Am Coll Cardiol 2003; 41: 1506
42. Wijeysundera DN, Beattie WS, Rao V et al: Calcium antagonists reduce cardiovascular complications after cardiac surgery: A meta-analysis. J Am Coll Cardiol 2003; 41: 1496
43. Brister NW, Barnette RE, Schartel SA et al: Isradipine for treatment of acute hypertension after myocardial revascularization. Crit Care Med 1991; 19: 334
44. Kaplan J: Clinical considerations for the use of intravenous nicardipine in the treatment of postoperative hypertension. Am Heart J 1990; 119: 443
45. Garcia LA, Dejong SC, Martin SM et al: Magnesium reduces free radicals in an in vivo coronary occlusion-reperfusion model. J Am Coll Cardiol 1998; 32: 536
46. Freeman RV, Otto CM: Spectrum of calcific aortic valve disease: Pathogenesis, disease progression, and treatment strategies. Circulation 2005; 111: 3316
47. Carabello BA: Clinical practice. Aortic stenosis. N Engl J Med 2002; 346: 677
48. Zile MR, Gaasch WH: Heart failure in aortic stenosis—improving diagnosis and treatment. N Engl J Med 2003; 348: 1735

48. O'Keefe JH Jr, Shub C, Rettke SR: Risk of noncardiac surgical procedures in patients with aortic stenosis. Mayo Clin Proc 1989; 64: 400

49. Kertai MD, Bountioukos M, Boersma E et al: Aortic stenosis: an underestimated risk factor for perioperative complications in patients undergoing noncardiac surgery. Am J Med 2004; 116: 8

50. Zahid M, Sonel AF, Saba S et al: Perioperative risk of noncardiac surgery associated with aortic stenosis. Am J Cardiol 2005; 96: 436

51. Khot UN, Novato GM, Popovic ZB et al: Nitroprusside in critically ill patients with left ventricular dysfunction and aortic stenosis. N Engl J Med 2003; 348: 1756

52. Ommen SR, Nishimura RA: Hypertrophic cardiomyopathy. Curr Probl Cardiol 2004; 29(5): 239

53. Fifer MA, Vlahakes GJ: Management of symptoms in hypertrophic cardiomyopathy. Circulation 2008; 117: 429

54. Borer JS, Bonow RO: Contemporary approach to aortic and mitral regurgitation. Circulation 2003; 108: 2432

55. Bekeredjian R, Grayburn PA: Valvular heart disease. Aortic regurgitation. Circulation 2005; 112: 125

56. Carabello BA: Modern management of mitral stenosis. Circulation 2005; 112: 432

57. Gorlin R, Gorlin SG: Hydraulic formula for calculation of area of the stenotic mitral valve, other cardiac valves, and central circulatory shunts. Am Heart J 1951; 41: 1

58. Cardoso LF, Grinberg M, Rati MA et al: Comparison between percutaneous balloon valvuloplasty and open commissurotomy for mitral stenosis: A prospective and randomized study. Cardiology 2002; 98: 186

59. Eltzschig HK, Rosenberger P, Lekowski RW Jr et al: Role of transesophageal echocardiography in patients with suspected aortic dissection. J Am Soc Echocardiogr 2005; 18: 1221

60. Mohr-Kahaly S, Erbel R, Rennollet H et al: Ambulatory follow-up of aortic dissection by transesophageal two-dimensional and color-coded Doppler echocardiography. Circulation 1989; 80: 24

61. Penco M, Paparoni S, Dagianti A et al : Usefulness of transesophageal echcocardiography in the assessment of aortic dissection. Am J Cardiol 2000; 86: 53G

62. Davies RR, Goldstein LJ, Coady MA et al:. Yearly rupture or dissection rates for thoracic aortic aneurysms: Simple prediction based on size. Ann Thorac Surg 2002; 73: 17

63. Isselbacher EM: Thoracic and abdominal aortic aneurysms. Circulation 2005; 111: 816

64. David TE, Ivanov J, Armstrong S et al: Aortic valve-sparing operations in patients with aneurysms of the aortic root or ascending aorta. Ann Thorac Surg 2002; 74: S1758

65. Hagl C, Ergin MA, Galla JD et al: Neurologic outcome after ascending aorta-aortic arch operations: Effect of brain protection technique in high-risk patients. J Thorac Cardiovasc Surg 2001; 121: 1107

66. Cowan JA Jr, Dimick JB, Henke PK et al: Surgical treatment of intact thoracoabdominal aortic aneurysms in the United States: Hospital and surgeon volume-related outcomes. J Vasc Surg 2003; 37: 1169

67. Conrad MF, Cambria RP: Contemporary management of descending thoracic and thoracoabdominal aortic aneurysms: endovascular versus open. Circulation 2008; 117: 841

68. Driessen JJ, Dhaese H, Fransen G et al: Pulsatile compared with nonpulsatile perfusion using a centrifugal pump for cardiopulmonary bypass during coronary artery bypass grafting. Effects on systemic haemodynamics, oxygenation, and inflammatory response parameters. Perfusion 1995; 10: 3

69. Fang WC, Helm RE, Krieger KH et al: Impact of minimum hematocrit during cardiopulmonary bypass on mortality in patients undergoing coronary artery surgery. Circulation 1997; 96(9 Suppl): II

70. Avidan MS, Lefy JH, Scholz J et al: A phase III, double-blind, placebo-controlled, multicenter study on the efficacy of recombinant human antithrombin in heparin-resistant patients scheduled to undergo cardiac surgery necessitating cardiopulmonary bypass. Anesthesiology 2005; 102: 276

71. Levy JH, Tanaka KA, Hursting MJ: Reducing thrombotic complications in the perioperative setting: an update on heparin-induced thrombocytopenia. Anesth Analg 2007; 105: 570

72. Hardy JF, Belisle S, Dupont C et al: Prophylactic tranexamic acid and epsilon-aminocaproic acid for primary myocardial revascularization. Circulation 2008; 108(Suppl 1): II15

73. Mangano DT, Miao Y, Vuylsteke A: Mortality associated with aprotinin during 5 years following coronary artery bypass graft surgery. JAMA 2007; 297: 471

74. Eising GP, Pfauder M, Niemeyer M et al: Retrograde autologous priming: Is it useful in elective on-pump coronary artery bypass surgery? Ann Thorac Surg 2003; 75: 23

75. Luciani GB, Menon T, Vecchi B et al: Modified ultrafiltration reduces morbidity after adult cardiac operations: a prospective, randomized clinical trial. Circulation 2001; 104(12 Suppl 1): I253

76. Filion KB, Pilote L, Rahme E et al: Perioperative use of cardiac medical therapy among patients undergoing coronary artery bypass graft surgery: A systematic review. Am Heart J 2007;154: 407

77. Lazar HL: All coronary artery bypass graft surgery patients will benefit from angiotensin-converting enzyme inhibitors. Circulation 2008; 117: 6

78. Grocott HP: Perioperative temperature and cardiac surgery. J Extra Corpor Technol 2006; 38: 77

79. Bussières JS: Iatrogenic pulmonary artery rupture. Curr Opin Anaesthesiol 2007; 20: 48

80. Hansen RM, Viquerat CE, Matthy MA et al: Poor correlation between pulmonary arterial wedge pressure and left ventricular end-diastolic volume after coronary artery bypass graft surgery. Anesthesiology 1986; 64: 764

81. Puskas JD, Winston D, Wright CE et al: Stroke after coronary artery operation. Incidence, correlates, outcome, and cost. Ann Thorac Surg 2000; 69: 1053

82. Ahonen J, Salmenperä M: Brain injury after adult cardiac surgery. Acta Anaesthesiol Scand 2004; 48: 4

83. Newman MF, Kirchner JL, Phillips-Bute B et al: The Neurological Outcome Research Group and the Cardiothoracic Anesthesiology Research Endeavors Investigators. Longitudinal assessment of neurocognitive fuction after coronary artery bypass surgery. N Engl J Med 2001; 344: 395

84. Grocott HP, Mackensen GB, Grigore AM et al: Postoperative hyperthermia is associated with cognitive dysfunction after coronary artery bypass graft surgery. Stroke 2002; 33: 537

85. Hogue CW Jr, Palin CA, Arrowsmith JE: Cardiopulmonary bypass management and neurologic outcomes: an evidence-based appraisal of current practices. Anesth Analg 2006; 103: 21

86. Tuman KJ, McCarthy RJ, Spiess BD et al: Does choice of anesthetic agent significantly affect outcome after coronary artery surgery? Anesthesiology 1989; 70(2): 189

87. Slogoff S, Keats AS, Dear WS et al: Steal-prone coronary anatomy and myocardial ischemia associated with four primary anesthetic agents in humans. Anesth Analg 1991; 72(1): 22

88. Lowenstein E, Hallowell P, Levine FH et al: Cardiovascular response to large doses of intravenous morphine in man. N Engl J Med 1969; 281: 1389

89. Murphy GS, Szokol JW, Marymont JH et al: Recovery of neuromuscular function after cardiac surgery: Pancuronium versus rocuronium. Anesth Analg 2003; 96: 1301

90. Garwood S: Renal insufficiency after cardiac surgery. Semin Cardiothorac Vasc Anesth 2004; 8: 227

91. McKinlay KH, Schinderle DB, Swaminathan M et al: Predictors of inotrope use during separation from cardiopulmonary bypass. J Cardiothorac Vasc Anesth 2004; 18: 404

92. Santa-Cruz RA, Cohen MG, Ohman EM: Aortic counterpulsation: a review of the hemodynamic effects and indications for use. Catheter Cardiovasc Interv 2006; 67: 68

93. Field ML, Rengarajan A, Khan O et al: Preoperative intra aortic balloon pumps in patients undergoing coronary artery bypass grafting. Cochrane Database Syst Rev 2007; 24: CD004472

94. Schulman S, Bijsterveld NR: Anticoagulants and their reversal. Transfus Med Rev 2007; 21: 37

95. Levy JH, Adkinson NF Jr: Anaphylaxis during cardiac surgery: Implications for clinicians. Anesth Analg 2008; 106: 392

96. Trehan N, Mishra M, Sharma OP: Further reduction in stroke after off-pump coronary artery bypass grafting: A 10-year experience. Ann Thorac Surg 2001; 72: S1026

97. Chassot PG, van der Linden P, Zaugg M et al: Off-pump coronary artery bypass surgery: Physiology and anaesthetic management. Br J Anaesth 2004; 92: 400

98. Fillinger MP, Yeager MP, Dodds TM et al: Epidural anesthesia and analgesia: Effects on recovery from cardiac surgery. J Cardiothorac Vasc Anesth 2002; 16: 15

99. Kurlansky PA: Is there a hypercoagulable state after off-pump coronary artery bypass surgery? What do we know and what can we do? J Thorac Cardiovasc Surg 2003; 126: 7

100. Lev-Ran O, Ben-Gal Y, Matsa M et al: 'No touch' techniques for porcelain ascending aorta: comparison between cardiopulmonary bypass with femoral artery cannulation and off-pump myocardial revascularization. J Card Surg 2002; 17: 370

101. Sharony R, Bizekis CS, Kanchuger M et al: Off-pump coronary artery bypass grafting reduces mortality and stroke in patients with atheromatous aortas: A case control study. Circulation 2003; 108(Suppl 1): II15

102. Cheng DC, Bainbridge D, Martin JE et al: Does off-pump coronary artery bypass reduce mortality, morbidity, and resource utilization when compared with conventional coronary artery bypass? A meta-analysis of randomized trials. Anesthesiology 2005; 102: 188

103. Kim KB, Lim C, Lee C, et al: Off-pump coronary artery bypass may decrease the patency of saphenous vein grafts. Ann Thorac Surg 2001; 72: S1033

104. Little WC, Freeman GL: Pericardial disease. Circulation 2006; 113: 1622

105. Roediger L, Larbuisson R, Lamy M: New approaches and old controversies to postoperative pain control following cardiac surgery. Eur J Anaesthesiol 2006; 23: 539

106. Chaney MA: Intrathecal and epidural anesthesia and analgesia for cardiac surgery. Anesth Analg 2006; 102: 45

107. Malviya S, Voepel-Lewis T, Siewert M et al: Risk factors for adverse postoperative outcomes in children presenting for cardiac surgery with upper respiratory tract infections. Anesthesiology 2003; 98(3): 628

108. Greenwood RD, Rosenthal LA, Parisi L et al: Extracardiac abnormalities in infants with congenital heart disease. Pediatrics 1975; 55: 485

109. Cho Ng, Goldman A: Management of the pediatric cardiac surgical patient, The Johns Hopkins Manual of Cardiothoracic Surgery. New York, McGraw Hill Medical, 2007, p 1019

110. Ungerleider RM: Effects of cardiopulmonary bypass and use of modified ultrafiltration. Ann Thorac Surg 1998; 65: S35

111. Davis S, Worley S, Mee R et al: Factors associated with early extubation after cardiac surgery in young children. Pediatr Crit Care Med 2004; 5(1): 63

112. Kloth RL, Baum VC: Very early extubation in children after cardiac surgery. Crit Care Med 2002; 30(4): 787

113. Ip P, Chiu CS, Cheung YF: Risk factors prolonging ventilation in young children after cardiac surgery: Impact of noninfectious pulmonary complications. Pediatr Crit Care Med 2002; 3: 269

114. Brown KL, Ridout DA, Goldman AP et al: Risk factors for long intensive care unit stay after cardiopulmonary bypass in children. Crit Care Med 2003; 31: 28

115. Lofland GK: The enhancement of hemodynamic performance in Fontan circulation using pain free spontaneous ventilation. E J Cardiothor Surg 2001; 20; 114

116. Peterson KL, DeCampli WM, Pike NA et al: A report of two hundred twenty cases of regional anesthesia in pediatric cardiac surgery. Anesth Analg 2000; 90: 1014

117. Hammer GB, Ngo K, Maracio A: A retrospective examination of regional plus general anesthesia in children undergoing open-heart surgery. Anesth Analg 2000; 90: 1020

118. Steven JM, McGowan Jr FX: Neuroaxial blockade for pediatric cardiac surgery: Lessons yet to be learned. Anesth Analg 2000; 90: 1011

119. Bacha BAM, Hijazi ZM: Hybrid procedures in pediatric cardiac surgery. Pediatr Cardiac Surg Ann 2005; 78

CHAPTER 42 ■ ANESTHESIA FOR VASCULAR SURGERY

SRINIVAS MANTHA, E. ANDREW OCHROCH, MICHAEL F. ROIZEN, JONATHAN C. KATZ, DAVID A. LUBARSKY, AND JOHN E. ELLIS

KEY POINTS

1 Excellent medical therapy with beta-blockers, angiotensin-converting enzyme inhibitors, statin drugs, aspirin, and control of hyperglycemia may reduce perioperative morbidity and mortality in vascular surgery patients.

2 Myocardial dysfunction remains the single most important cause of morbidity following vascular surgery.

3 The multicenter Coronary Artery Revascularization Prophylaxis Trial demonstrated no benefit of coronary revascularization over state-of-the-art medical therapy in elective vascular surgery patients.

4 Of the various risk-reducing strategies, evidence suggests that perioperative intensive cardiac troponin surveillance and aggressive beta-blockade therapy provides benefit in preventing cardiac morbidity and mortality.

5 Hypotension and hypoperfusion may not be the precipitating or sole cause of stroke after carotid endarterectomy; embolic events may be just as, or even more, important, and often occur postoperatively.

6 Phenylephrine doubles the incidence of wall motion abnormalities observed by echocardiography compared with the incidence in patients whose blood pressure is maintained simply by light anesthesia and endogenous vasoconstrictors.

7 The definitive preventive measures for spinal cord ischemia are short cross-clamping time, fast surgery, maintenance of normal cardiac function, and higher perfusion pressures. Other methods such as cerebrospinal fluid drainage, distal perfusion, and hypothermia may be beneficial in high aortic clamping.

8 As opposed to elective aortic reconstruction, in which preserving myocardial function is the primary goal, in emergency resection of the aorta the crucial factor for patient survival is first, rapid control of blood loss and reversal of hypotension, and then preservation of myocardial function.

9 Regional anesthesia may offer advantages, including avoidance of hyperdynamic responses to tracheal intubation and extubation, reduced postoperative respiratory and infectious complications, and reduced postoperative graft thrombosis.

10 Endovascular repair may reduce morbidity and mortality in the aortic and femoral circulations, but concerns persists about its durability. In the carotid circulation, concerns about distal embolization and stroke with carotid angioplasty and stenting suggest that traditional carotid endarterectomy may still be superior.

The increasing age of the population in Western societies will likely increase the number of vascular procedures performed. The morbidity from these procedures has decreased rapidly, from a 6-day mortality of >25% for major aortic reconstruction in the mid-1960s to as low as 3% mortality today. The anesthesiologist may have a greater influence in reducing the morbidity and costs of vascular surgery than in any other surgical procedure.

This chapter begins with a discussion of the pathophysiology of atherosclerotic vascular disease and the general medical problems common in patients with peripheral vascular disease, particularly coronary artery disease (CAD). Outcome after vascular surgery is determined essentially by patient factors, surgical factors, and institution-specific factors. The National Veterans Affairs Surgical Risk Study found that low serum albumin

TABLE 42-1

THE TEN MOST IMPORTANT PREOPERATIVE PREDICTORS OF POSTOPERATIVE 30-DAY MORTALITY AFTER VASCULAR SURGERY IN VETERAN'S AFFAIRS MEDICAL CENTERS[a]

■ PREDICTOR	■ ODDS RATIO
Ventilator dependent	2.71
ASA class	1.89
Emergency operation	2.40
DNR status	2.96
BUN >40 mg/dL	1.47
Albumin	0.61
Age	1.03
Creatinine >1.2 mg/dL	1.48
Esophageal varices	4.30
Operative complexity score	1.32

BUN, blood urea nitrogen; DNR, do not resuscitate.
[a]All variables are statistically significant ($p < 0.05$) and were selected after stepwise multivariable analysis.
Modified from Khuri SF, Daley J, Henderson W et al: Risk adjustment of the postoperative mortality rate for the comparative assessment of the quality of surgical care: Results of the National Veterans Affairs surgical risk study. J Am Coll Surg 1997; 185: 315

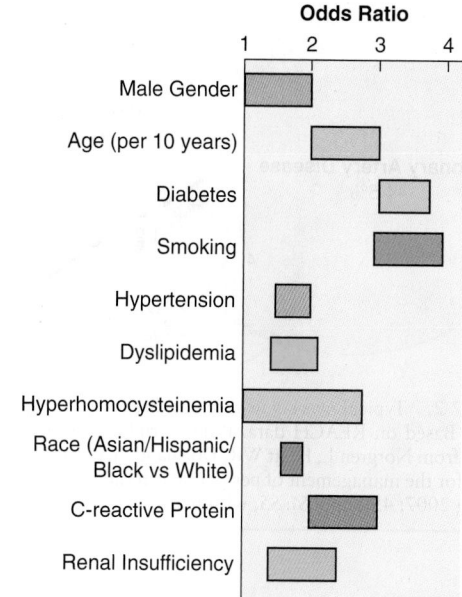

FIGURE 42-1.   Approximate range of odds ratios for risk factors for symptomatic peripheral arterial disease. Some of the factors are amenable for treatment and can help in secondary prevention of complications of vascular disease. (Reprinted from Norgren L, Hiatt WR, Dormandy JA et al: Inter-society consensus for the management of peripheral arterial disease (TASC II). J Vasc Surg 2007; 45(Suppl S): S5, with permission.)

values and high American Society of Anesthesiologists physical classification were among the best predictors of morbidity and mortality after vascular surgery (Table 42-1).[1] The specific surgical goals, anatomy, and complications for cerebrovascular, thoracic aortic, visceral, abdominal aortic, and lower extremity revascularization are placed in the context of optimal anesthetic management. New surgical techniques such as angioplasty and endovascular repair with the placement of stent grafts have revolutionized vascular surgery and promise to further reduce morbidity and mortality.[2]

VASCULAR DISEASE: EPIDEMIOLOGIC, MEDICAL, AND SURGICAL ASPECTS

Pathophysiology of Atherosclerosis

Atherosclerosis is a generalized inflammatory of the disorder arterial tree with associated endothelial dysfunction.[3] Putative causes are endothelial damage caused by hemodynamic shear stress, inflammation from chronic infections, hypercoagulability resulting in thrombosis, and the destructive effects of oxidized low-density lipoproteins (LDLs). Disruption of the fibrous cap over a lipid deposit can lead to plaque rupture and ulceration. Vasoactive influences can result in spasm and acute thrombosis. Platelets play a pivotal role in atherothrombosis after plaque rupture. Platelets internalize oxidized phospholipids and promote foam cell formation.[4] In fact, platelet polymorphisms are now found to be independent risk predictors for myocardial ischemia following vascular surgery.[5]

The development of atherosclerosis occurs in two stages: injury and response to injury. The primary injurious agents include LDL and other apolipoprotein B-containing lipoproteins. These lipoproteins filter into arterial intima through the endothelium. The entrapped lipoproteins get modified in such a way that they become proinflammatory. In the subendothelial space enriched with atherogenic lipoproteins, most

macrophages transform into foam cells. Foam cells aggregate to form the atheromatous core and as this process progresses, the atheromatous centers of plaques become necrotic, consisting of lipids, cholesterol crystals, and cell debris. Monocyte-derived macrophages act as scavenging and antigen-presenting cells and also produce several types of chemical mediators (e.g., cytokines, chemokines, growth regulating molecules) that are involved in inflammation. Adhesion molecules expressed by inflamed endothelium recruit leukocytes, including monocytes which then penetrate into the intima, predisposing the vessel wall to lipid accretion and vasculitis.

Predisposing risk factors for atherosclerosis include abdominal obesity, atherogenic dyslipidemia, raised blood pressure, insulin resistance, proinflammatory state, and prothrombotic state.[6] Major risk factors also include cigarette smoking, elevated LDL cholesterol (LDL-C), low high-density lipoprotein, family history of premature coronary heart disease, and aging; emerging risk factors include elevated triglycerides and small LDL particles. The relative contribution of these risk factors varies (Fig. 42-1).[7]

Natural History of Patients with Peripheral Vascular Disease

Atherosclerotic vascular disease (AVD) is one of the most important and common causes of death and disability in the United States and throughout the world. More than 25 million persons in the United States have at least one clinical manifestation of atherosclerosis. Throughout the past 50 years, coronary artery atherosclerosis has been a major focus for basic and clinical investigation. Yet, atherosclerosis is a systemic disease with important sequelae in many other regional circulations[8] (Fig. 42-2).

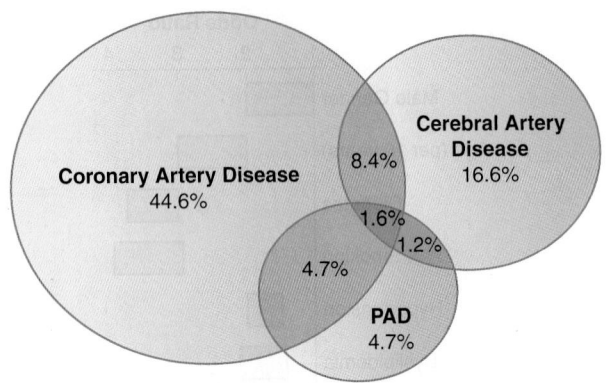

FIGURE 42-2.   Typical overlap in vascular disease affecting different territories. Based on REACH data. PAD, peripheral arterial disease. (Reprinted from Norgren L, Hiatt WR, Dormandy JA et al: Inter-society consensus for the management of peripheral arterial disease (TASC II). J Vasc Surg 2007; 45(Suppl S): S5, with permission.)

The prevalence of >25% carotid stenosis in patients older than 65 years of age was 43% in men and 34% in women in one of the Framingham studies. Stroke is the third leading cause of death and the principal cause of long-term disability in the United States today, with 600,000 new or recurrent strokes occurring annually. The risk of stroke is relatively uncommon (0.4% to 0.6% of patients) after noncarotid peripheral vascular surgery, but when it does occur it is associated with longer length of stay and higher mortality.[9] The principal clinical syndromes associated with aortic atherosclerosis are abdominal aortic aneurysms (AAAs), aortic dissection, peripheral atheroembolism, penetrating aortic ulcer, and intramural hematoma. Patients with atherosclerosis affecting the limb (i.e., peripheral arterial disease [PAD]) can develop disabling symptoms of claudication or critical limb ischemia. The prevalence of claudication is 2% among older adults, but 10 times as many elderly patients have asymptomatic lower extremity atherosclerosis, which can be detected by the ankle-brachial index. The ankle-brachial index is now regarded as the single best initial screening test to perform in a patient suspected of having PAD. The ankle-brachial index is the ratio of the highest systolic arm blood pressure to the highest systolic ankle blood pressure, obtained with a hand-held continuous-wave Doppler and blood pressure cuff. A ratio <0.9 is considered abnormal, and below 0.4 is often associated with limb-threatening ischemia.

Carotid intima-media thickness is increasingly used as a surrogate marker for atherosclerosis. A recent meta-analysis found carotid intima-media thickness to be a strong predictor of future vascular events.[10] Catheter-based angiography is the standard method for diagnosing the PAD, against which all other imaging modalities are compared for accuracy. However, recent advances in noninvasive angiography (magnetic resonance angiography and computed tomographic angiography) enable excellent noninvasive definition of the vascular anatomy.

AAAs occur in up to 5% of men older than 65 years of age; most of these aneurysms are small and require only infrequent follow-up. Data suggest that the risk of rupture is very low for AAAs ≤4.0 cm in diameter but rises exponentially for AAAs >5 cm. AAAs between 4 and 5 cm in diameter should be followed every 6 to 12 months to determine whether they are increasing in size. It is interesting to note that baseline hemoglobin concentration is independently associated with AAA size and reduced long-term survival following intervention for treatment. Thus, the presence or absence of anemia offers a potential refinement of existing risk stratification methods.[11]

Medical Therapy for Atherosclerosis

❶ Excellent medical therapy, including use of antihypertensives such as beta-blockers and angiotensin-converting enzyme (ACE) inhibitors, statin drugs, aspirin, and control of hyperglycemia with hypoglycemics and/or insulin, may reduce perioperative morbidity and mortality in vascular surgery. Prevention, including meticulous foot care in diabetic patients, is important to avoid infections and tissue loss. Lifestyle changes such as weight loss and exercise can forestall claudication. The use of statin drugs may reduce progression or even cause regression of atherosclerotic plaques, improve endothelial function, and reduce cardiovascular events in high-risk patients. Patients with high cardiac risk undergoing vascular surgery who received preoperative statin therapy were less likely to die.[12] Statin use is also associated with improved graft patency, limb salvage, and decreased amputation rate in patients undergoing infrainguinal bypass for AVD. Discontinuation of statin therapy after major vascular surgery is associated with an increased postoperative cardiac risk.[13] Furthermore, extended-release fluvastatin was associated with fewer perioperative cardiac events compared with other formulations of statins.[14] ACE inhibitors have numerous beneficial effects in patients with AVD, including plaque stabilization. Cessation of smoking may be the most effective "medical" therapy. The authors' recommendations for management of concomitant medical therapy in the perioperative period are listed in Table 42-2.

❷ Chronic therapy with aspirin or other anti-inflammatory drugs may retard the progression of atherosclerosis and prevent morbid cardiovascular events. A recent meta-analysis found the time interval between discontinuation of aspirin and occurrence of vascular events to be 14.3 ± 11.3 days for acute cerebral events, 8.5 ± 3.6 days for acute coronary events, and 25.8 ± 18.1 days for acute peripheral arterial syndromes.[15] The use in cyclooxygenase 2 (COX-2) inhibitors of patients with AVD is unclear at present, with studies suggesting increased cardiovascular events with long-term use.[16] In general, patients should continue to take aspirin until the day of surgery for carotid and lower extremity surgery, and individualize the choice for larger operations. In urgent situations when patients develop acute ischemia, systemic anticoagulation may be instituted.

Chronic Medical Problems and Management in Vascular Surgery Patients

Coronary Artery Disease in Patients with Peripheral Vascular Disease

Hertzer et al.[17] performed coronary angiography in 1,000 consecutive patients presenting for vascular surgery and identified severe correctable CAD in 25% of the entire series. The incidence of significant CAD (stenosis >70%) detected by angiography was 78% in those with clinical indications of CAD and 37% in patients without any clinical indications. However, subsequent analysis demonstrated that clinical risk factors still predicted the severity of CAD (Fig. 42-3). The absence of severe coronary stenoses can be predicted with a positive predictive value of 96% for patients without diabetes, prior angina, previous myocardial infarction (MI), or congestive heart failure (CHF).

Short-term postoperative cardiac morbidity and mortality after vascular surgery is higher than after other types of noncardiac surgery. Complications after carotid endarterectomy (CEA) are generally less frequent than after other types of vascular surgery, but still produce 50 to 100% of the mortality encountered. The presence of uncorrected CAD appears to

TABLE 42-2

CONCOMITANT MEDICAL THERAPY, SIDE EFFECTS OF POTENTIAL CONCERN PERIOPERATIVELY, AND THE AUTHORS' CURRENT RECOMMENDATIONS

■ MEDICATION OR DRUG CLASS	■ SIDE EFFECT OF POTENTIAL CONCERN IN THE PERIOPERATIVE PERIOD	■ RECOMMENDATION FOR PERIOPERATIVE USE
Aspirin	Platelet inhibition may increase bleeding; decreased GFR	Continue until day of surgery, especially for carotid and peripheral cases; monitor fluid and urine status
Clopidogrel	Platelet inhibition may increase bleeding Very rare thrombotic thrombocytopenic purpura	Hold for 7 d before surgery except for CEA and severe CAD and or DES. Consider cross-match of blood. Avoid neuraxial anesthesia if not held at least 7 d.
HMG CoA reductase inhibitors (statins)	Liver function test abnormalities Rhabdomyolysis	Assess liver function tests and continue through morning of surgery Check CPK if myalgias. *Resume therapy as soon as possible after surgery.* *Consider using extended-release fluvastatin formulation.*
Beta-blockers	Bronchospasm Hypotension Bradycardia, heart block	Continue through perioperative period
ACE inhibitors	Induction hypotension, cough	Continue through perioperative period; consider one-half dose on day of surgery
Diuretics	Hypovolemia, electrolyte abnormalities	Continue through morning of surgery; monitor fluid and urine status
Calcium channel blockers	Perioperative hypotension, especially with amlodipine	Continue through perioperative period; consider withholding amlodipine on the morning of surgery
Oral hypoglycemics	Hypoglycemia preoperatively and intraoperatively Lactic acidosis with metformin; *potential risk of water retention and congestive heart failure* with thiazolidinedione therapy (pioglitazone and rosiglitazone)	When feasible, switch to insulin preoperatively. Monitor glucose status perioperatively

GFR, glomerular filtration rate; CEA, carotid endarterectomy; CAD, coronary artery disease; DES, drug eluting stent; HMG, 3-hydroxy-3-methylglutaryl–coenzyme A reductase; CPK, creatine phosphokinase; ACE, angiotensin-converting enzyme.

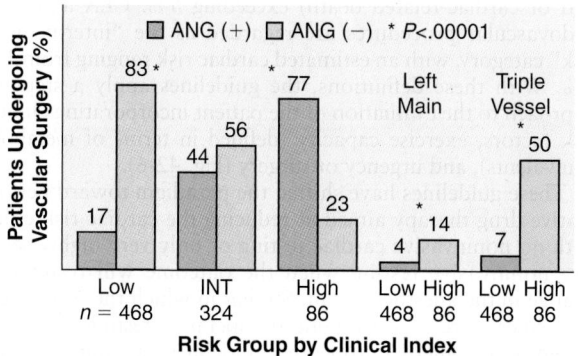

FIGURE 42-3. Clinical risk factors predict severe (left main or triple vessel) coronary artery disease. A preoperative clinical index (diabetes mellitus, prior myocardial infarction, angina, age older than 70 years, congestive heart failure) was used to stratify patients. ANG (+), angiogram positive for coronary artery disease; ANG (−), angiogram negative for coronary artery disease; INT, intermediate. (Based on data from Paul SD, Eagle KA, Kuntz KM et al: Concordance of preoperative clinical risk with angiographic severity of coronary artery disease in patients undergoing vascular surgery. Circulation 1996; 94: 1561; secondary analysis of data from Hertzer NR, Beven EG, Young JR et al: Coronary artery disease in peripheral vascular patients: A classification of 1000 coronary angiograms and results of surgical management. Ann Surg 1984; 199: 223.)

double 5-year mortality after vascular surgery. Previous percutaneous transluminal coronary angioplasty (PTCA) and stenting may or may not protect against perioperative cardiac events after vascular surgery. However, in the first 6 weeks after coronary stent placement, noncardiac surgery carries considerable risks. There are two basic types of stents: bare metal stents and drug-eluting stents. The latter have become increasingly popular as standard therapy as they reduce early stent restenosis. However, drug-eluting stents are slow to endothelialize, and the exposed stent material remains thrombogenic far longer than bare metal stents (Fig. 42-4).[18] Therefore, the duration of dual antiplatelet therapy (aspirin 325 mg/day and clopidogrel 75 mg/day) differs: 1 month for bare-metal stents, 12 months or more (perhaps forever) for drug-eluting stents. Aspirin is recommended for an indefinite period. Under the circumstances that prevent the use of clopidogrel for 1 year, the recommendations for duration of therapy are as follows: 3 months for sirolimus-eluting stents and 6 months for paclitaxel-eluting stents.[19] Nonfatal MI and cardiac-related death may result from discontinuation of antiplatelet therapy.[20] Whenever possible, noncardiac surgery should be delayed until 6 weeks after coronary bare metal stent placement, by which time stents are generally endothelialized[21] (Fig. 42-5). Longer delay is recommended for drug-eluting stents: initially, recommendations were for, at minimum, 3 months for sirolimus stents and 6 months for paclitaxel stents to allow effective dual antiplatelet therapy, although longer than a year may be ideal according to the most recent recommendations.[22]

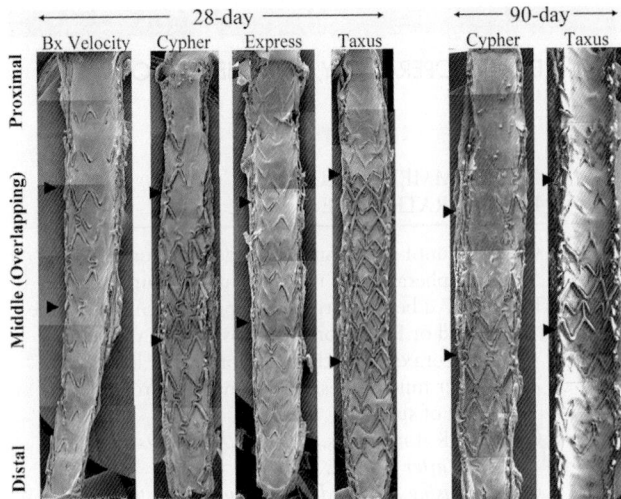

FIGURE 42-4. Scanning electron micrographs from overlapping bare metal stents (Bx) and drug-eluting stent DES) implanted in the rabbit iliac artery model for 28 and 90 days. Note significantly less endothelialization in Cypher and Taxus DES as compared with Bx Velocity and Express, especially at overlapping sites at 28 days. At 90 days the luminal surface in overlapping DES is still not fully endothelialized. *Arrows* indicate the overlapping regions. (Reprinted from Finn AV, Nakazawa G, Joner M et al: Vascular responses to drug eluting stents: Importance of delayed healing. Arterioscler Thromb Vasc Biol 2007; 27: 1500, with permission.)

Recently, two distinct types of perioperative myocardial infarction (PMI): "early" and "delayed" occurring after vascular surgery have been identified. Early PMI resembles that of acute nonsurgical MI and is probably due to acute coronary occlusion resulting from plaque rupture and thrombosis. The "delayed PMI" is associated with sustained elevation of heart rate, absence of chest pain, and prolonged premonitory episodes of ST segment depression before overt MI. The delayed PMI resembles that resulting from increase in oxygen demand in the setting of fixed coronary stenosis.[23] Myocardial

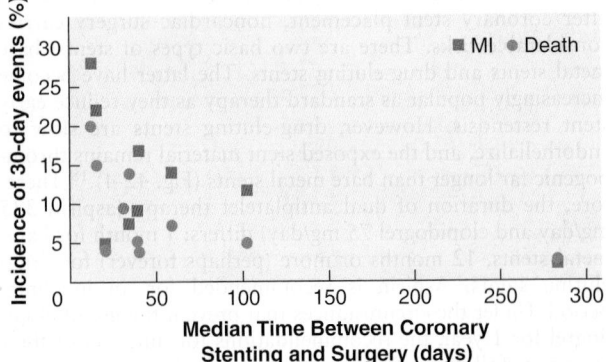

FIGURE 42-5. Incidence of perioperative cardiac complications in studies with different median times between percutaneous transluminal coronary angioplasty plus stenting and noncardiac surgery. Whenever possible, noncardiac surgery should be delayed until 6 weeks after coronary stent placement. These complications have recently been reported even with drug-eluting stents, and discontinuation of antiplatelet therapy happens to be the primary pathogenetic factor. MI, myocardial infarction. (Reprinted from Schouten O, Bax JJ, Damen J et al: Coronary artery stent placement immediately before noncardiac surgery: A potential risk? Anesthesiology 2007; 106: 1067, with permission.)

oxygen supply may be diminished by anemia or hypotension, whereas oxygen demand may be increased by tachycardia and hypertension resulting from postoperative pain, withdrawal of anesthesia, or shifts in intravascular volume. Even small changes in cardiac troponin-I (cTnI) or cardiac troponin-T (cTnT) after surgery are associated with a worse perioperative and 6-month outcome, with a dose-response relationship.[24] As a result, the new definition of MI requires the rise and fall of biochemical marker of myocardial necrosis together with one of the following clinical and electrocardiogram (ECG) criteria: ischemic symptoms, development of pathologic Q waves, ischemic ECG changes, or a coronary intervention.[25] Troponin screening is now recognized as an effective means of surveillance for perioperative myocardial ischemic damage.[26] In practical terms, the type of troponin that is used for surveillance, cTnI or cTnT is of little concern as both have similar diagnostic and risk stratification capabilities.

Controversy persists as to whether preoperative identification of patients most likely to have perioperative cardiovascular events related to myocardial ischemia benefits patients. However, in 2007, the American Heart Association and American College of Cardiology (AHA/ACC) published revised guidelines for perioperative cardiovascular evaluation before noncardiac surgery.[27] The guidelines classify the clinical predictors of increased perioperative cardiovascular risk (MI, CHF, and death) as "major," "intermediate," and "minor." The major predictors also defined in the guidelines as "active cardiac conditions" are acute MI (<7 days), recent MI (7 to 30 days), unstable angina, decompensated CHF, severe valvular disease and significant dysrhythmias. Active cardiac conditions, when present, mandate intensive management, which may result in delay or cancellation of surgery unless it is emergent. "Intermediate predictors" also defined in the guidelines as "clinical risk factors" are history of ischemic heart disease (e.g., current or prior angina pectoris or prior MI), past or compensated CHF, diabetes mellitus, renal insufficiency, or cerebrovascular disease. Minor predictors (recognized markers for cardiovascular disease that have not proven to increase perioperative risk independently) are age >70 years, abnormal ECG, rhythm other than sinus, and uncontrolled systemic hypertension. The guidelines place aortic and peripheral vascular surgery in the "high-risk" surgery category with an estimated cardiac risk (MI or cardiac-related death) exceeding 5%. CEA and most endovascular procedures are regarded as the "intermediate-risk" category, with an estimated cardiac risk ranging from 1 to 5%. With these definitions, the guidelines apply a stepwise approach to the evaluation of the patient incorporating clinical risk factors, exercise capacity (defined in terms of metabolic equivalents), and urgency of surgery (Fig. 42-6).

These guidelines have shifted the paradigm toward perioperative drug therapy aimed at reducing the cardiac risk either with no noninvasive cardiac testing or only very highly selective noninvasive testing when the outcome will result in a change in the anesthetic plan. Studies in which the AHA/ACC guidelines were used to guide preoperative testing have conflicted as to whether using the guidelines can improve outcome. Figure 42-7 summarizes the authors' recommendations for vascular surgery patients. Details regarding individual cardiac tests are covered in Chapter 23.

Preoperative Coronary Revascularization

Myocardial revascularization may have long-term benefits in patients with triple-vessel coronary disease or poor left ventricular function. However, mortality rates associated with these techniques are consistently higher in patients with peripheral vascular disease compared with those without. Whether preoperative coronary revascularization actually protects against perioperative cardiac events is controversial. The multicenter

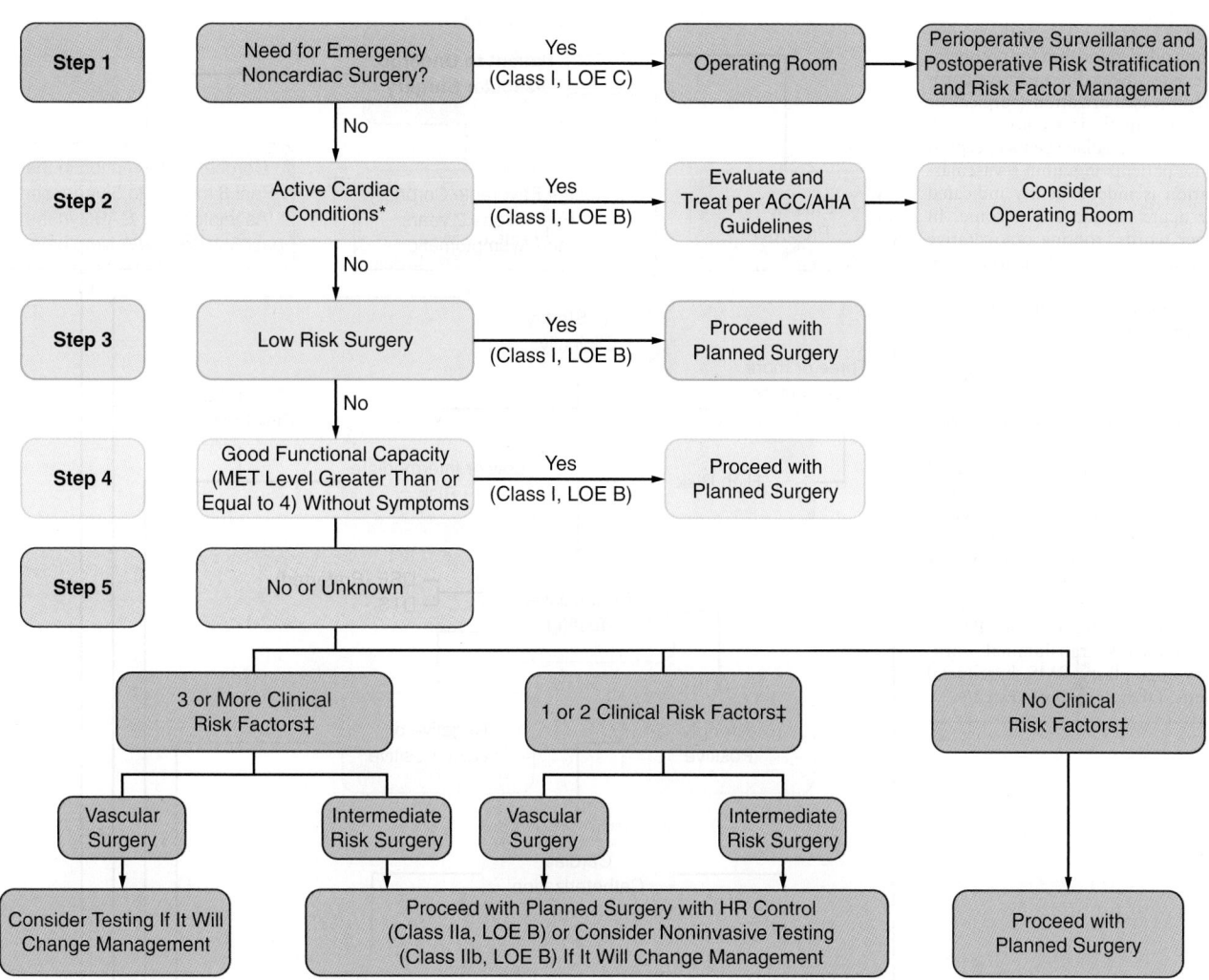

FIGURE 42-6. Cardiac evaluation and care algorithm for noncardiac surgery based on active clinical conditions, known cardiovascular disease, or cardiac risk factors for patients 50 years of age or greater. *See text for active clinical conditions. Clinical risk factors include ischemic heart disease, compensated or prior heart failure, diabetes mellitus, renal insufficiency, and cerebrovascular disease. Consider perioperative beta-blockade for populations in which this has been shown to reduce cardiac morbidity/mortality. ACC/AHA, American College of Cardiology/ American Heart Association; HR, heart rate; MET, metabolic equivalent. ACC/AHA 2007 Guidelines on Perioperative Cardiovascular Evaluation and Care for Noncardiac Surgery. Circulation 2007;116:e418–e500.

❸ Coronary Artery Revascularization Prophylaxis (CARP) Trial randomized patients with coronary disease (except left main disease or ejection fraction <20%) before elective vascular surgery to either coronary revascularization or medical therapy. With state-of-the-art aggressive medical therapy (>80% of patients on beta-blockers, >70% on aspirin, and >50% on statins in both groups), they could find no benefit to coronary revascularization.[28] A subsequent subgroup analysis of CARP trial examined the value of coronary artery bypass graft (CABG) versus PTCA in those requiring coronary revascularization. Patients having a CABG had fewer MIs and tended to spend less time in the hospital after vascular surgery than patients having PTCA.[29] The authors believed that complete revascularization in patients having CABG accounted for the intergroup differences. Interestingly, another recent study found that for multivessel CAD, CABG was associated with lower rates of revascularization, MI, and mortality when compared with drug-eluting stent coronary intervention.[30] Thus, preoperative coronary revascularization (surgical or interventional) may be of no value in preventing cardiac events except in those patients in whom revascularization is independently indicated for acute coronary syndrome. High-risk patients should have surveillance for myocardial ischemia (typically troponin I or T) and risk-reducing strategies (typically heart rate control). Should coronary revascularization be required prior to vascular surgery, then surgical revascularization is a suitable option compared with percutaneous coronary intervention. The safe time intervals between surgical revascularization and vascular surgery is 4 to 6 weeks for surgical coronary revascularization and 2 weeks for coronary angioplasty. The safe interval for stents is much longer (see previous discussion).

Management of Perioperative Myocardial Ischemia and Infarction in Vascular Patients

❹ The authors recently addressed cost-effectiveness of early aggressive treatment in a target population with a median age of 65 years with at least two clinical risk factors undergoing open abdominal aortic surgery.[31] In the model, patients would have cTnI surveillance on days 0, 1, 2, and 3. Those manifesting a value higher than 1.5 ng/mL, independent of other criteria for definite MI, would have aggressive beta-blockade therapy with close heart rate monitoring and routine coronary care in intensive

FIGURE 42-7. The authors' recommended algorithm for preoperative assessment. Preoperative coronary revascularization (surgical or interventional) is of no value in preventing cardiac events except in those patients in whom revascularization is independently indicated for acute coronary syndrome. In other words, routine preoperative coronary revascularization in patients with stable class III angina will not alter perioperative risk provided surveillance for myocardial ischemia (typically troponin I or T) and risk-reducing strategies (typically heart rate control) are employed. Should coronary revascularization be required prior to vascular surgery, then surgical revascularization is a suitable option compared with percutaneous coronary intervention. CABG, coronary artery bypass graft; DSE, dobutamine stress echocardiography; DTS, dipyridamole thallium scan; PTCA, percutaneous transluminal coronary angioplasty. BMS, bare-metal stents; DES, drug-eluting stents.

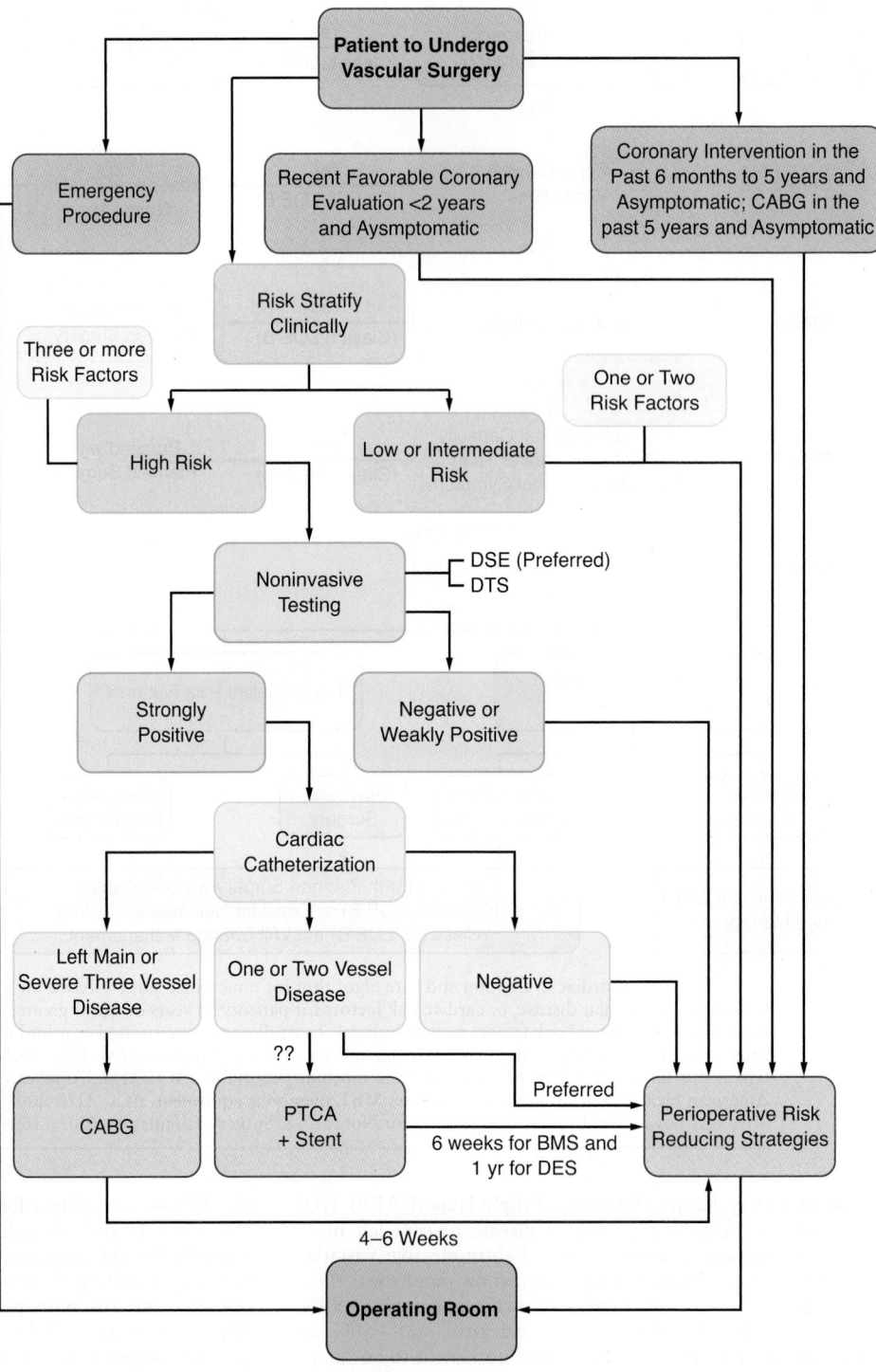

care unit (ICU) for an average period of 5 days. The base-case alternative strategy of standard care without cTnI surveillance was used for comparison. Not only the perioperative cardiac events but also the future events along with requirement for future coronary revascularization were modeled through the lifetime of the target population. The strategy was cost-effective and identified probability of MI and efficacy of aggressive beta-blocker therapy as key variables. Multivariate probabilistic sensitivity analysis revealed that the cTnI surveillance strategy was favored in 90.75% of simulations at a standard threshold of $50,000 per quality adjusted life year gained (Fig. 42-8). In addition, the authors recommend referral of patients with elevated troponins or documented severe postoperative myocardial ischemia (lasting longer than 2 hours; 2-mm ST segment depression) to a cardiologist because most adverse cardiac outcomes in a 2-year follow-up program were preceded by in-hospital postoperative ischemia.

Of the various pharmacologic risk-reducing strategies (Table 42-3), meta-analysis from randomized controlled trials suggests that perioperative beta-blockade therapy in noncardiac surgery is useful to reduce the rates of perioperative dysrhythmias and myocardial ischemia, but may not provide benefit with regard to MI, length of hospitalization, and mortality.[32] However Feringa et al.[33] found reduced myocardial ischemia and troponin release and improved long-term survival in an observational cohort study in 272 patients

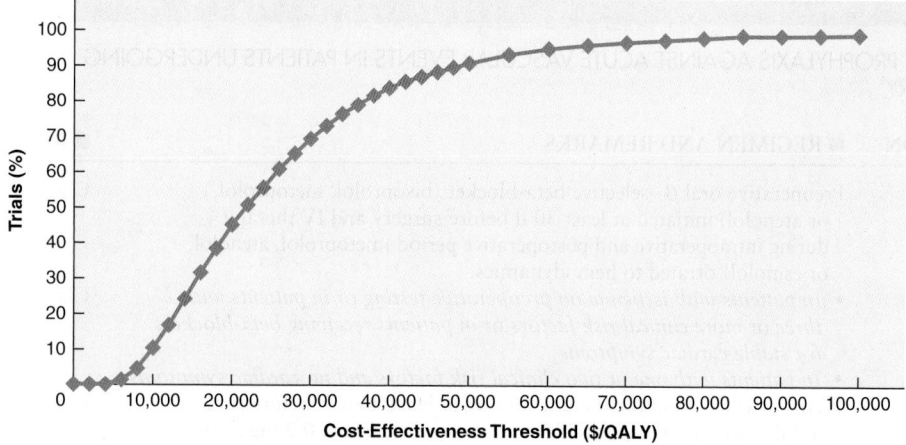

FIGURE 42-8. Cost-effectiveness acceptability curve based on the output of 10,000-simulation Monte Carlo analysis comparing cardiac troponin I (cTnI) surveillance with standard care in cost-effectiveness decision analysis model. In cTnI surveillance strategy, high-risk patients (cTnI >1.5 ng/mL) were modeled to receive aggressive beta-blocker therapy with close heart rate monitoring and routine coronary care in the intensive care unit. The graph depicts that the cTnI surveillance strategy was favored in 90.75% of simulations at a standard threshold of $50,000 per quality adjusted life year (QALY) gained. The y-axis depicts the proportion of trials for which cTnI surveillance resulted in net monetary benefit than standard care. See text for details. (Reprinted from Mantha S, Foss J, Ellis JE et al: Intense cardiac troponin surveillance for long-term benefits is cost effective in patients undergoing open abdominal aortic surgery: A decision analysis model. Anesth Analg 2007; 105: 1346, with permission.)

presenting for vascular surgery. Benefits of the therapy are best observed when oral preoperative therapy is extended to intraoperative and postoperative periods by intravenous therapy to titrate the heart rate ≤65 beats per minute. Typically, oral therapy has been initiated 7 to 30 days before surgery with either 50 to 100 mg atenolol daily or 5 to 10 mg of bisoprolol, whereas intraoperative and postoperative periods are best managed by intravenous administration of 5 to 10 mg atenolol or metoprolol twice daily. Alternatively, esmolol 100 to 500 μg/kg may be given intravenously over 1 minute followed by infusion of 50 to 300 μg/kg/min to achieve the target heart rate. In patients already taking beta-blockers, they are continued to the day of surgery followed by intravenous therapy to achieve the target heart rate as described previously.

Although older literature warns against use with any degree of reactive airway disease, insulin-dependent diabetes, and even peripheral vascular disease, newer data suggest that careful titration of β_1-selective agents is well tolerated in many of these patients. However, severe asthma or a strong reversible component with chronic obstructive airway disease remains a major contraindication, as do cardiac conduction disease in the absence of a pacemaker and previous documented drug sensitivities. It must be noted that hypovolemia can be poorly tolerated in the presence of beta-blockade and also that racial difference in response to beta-blockade can exist (blacks may respond less favorably).[34] Most recently, newer data suggest that patients with few or no risk factors may not benefit from beta-blockade and there may even be an increase in the risk of death, stroke, and clinically significant hypotension.[35]

α_2-Adrenergic agonists (clonidine or mivazerol) have been in use aimed at controlling the perioperative cardiac morbidity and mortality for more than a decade. The authors tested a regimen of a transdermal clonidine system (0.2 mg/day) the night prior to surgery, which was left in place for 72 hours, and 0.3 mg oral clonidine administered 60 to 90 minutes before surgery. Clonidine not only reduced intraoperative myocardial ischemia, but also reduced catecholamine (adrenaline and noradrenaline) levels as measured on the first postop-

erative day.[36] More recently, a meta-analysis demonstrated beneficial effects of perioperative α_2-agonists with regard to cardiac morbidity and death in patients undergoing vascular surgery (evidence level B).[37] In addition, a randomized trial suggested that perioperative clonidine administration during high-risk noncardiac surgery reduces mortality[38] in a fashion similar to atenolol.

Interest has focused on the use of statins aimed at controlling adverse cardiac events perioperatively and on those occurring during long-term follow-up for vascular surgery patients. A randomized trial demonstrated beneficial effects of statin use (atorvastatin 20 mg daily started 30 days before surgery and continued for roughly 2 weeks after surgery) with regard to primary end points (cardiac-related death, nonfatal MI, unstable angina, stroke) at 6-month follow-up.[39] Pleiotropic (non–lipid lowering) effects are thought to explain the perioperative beneficial effects of statins.[40] A meta-analysis found that preoperative statin therapy was associated with 59% reduction in relative risk of mortality after vascular surgery while no definitive conclusions could be drawn on cardiovascular morbidity.[12] A recent study found that discontinuation of statin therapy (>4 days) after major vascular surgery is associated with an increased postoperative cardiac risk, suggesting that statin therapy should be resumed early after major vascular surgery.[13] Another similar study confirming those findings identified that extended-release fluvastatin was associated with fewer perioperative cardiac events compared with atorvastatin, simvastatin, and pravastatin. Because statins are available only for enteral administration, administration of extended-release fluvastatin preoperatively appears ideal when prolonged postoperative ileus is expected, typically in AAA repair or aortobifemoral graft procedures.

ACE inhibitors also have several beneficial actions with regard to acute vascular events independent of their antihypertensive action in patients with atherosclerotic vascular disease. Currently there are no studies to provide evidence for their independent ability to reduce perioperative cardiac problems for their therapy aimed at risk reduction. However, if a patient is already taking ACE inhibitors, then they should be continued, realizing the potential for hypotension associated with general

TABLE 42-3

PHARMACOLOGIC PROPHYLAXIS AGAINST ACUTE VASCULAR EVENTS IN PATIENTS UNDERGOING VASCULAR SURGERY

■ INTERVENTION	■ REGIMEN AND REMARKS	■ RECOMMENDATION[a]
Perioperative beta-blockade	Preoperative oral β_1-selective beta-blocker (bisoprolol, metoprolol, or atenolol) initiated at least 30 d before surgery and IV therapy during intraoperative and postoperative period (metoprolol, atenolol, or esmolol) titrated to hemodynamics.	Class I
	• *In patients with ischemia on preoperative testing or in patients with three or more clinical risk factors or in patients receiving beta-blockers for stable cardiac symptoms*	Class IIa
	• *In patients with one or two clinical risk factors and no cardiac symptoms*	
α_2-Agonists	Pretreatment with oral clonidine 300 μg at least 90 min before surgery and therapy continued for 72 hr (oral or transdermal, 0.2 mg/d). IV clonidine 300 μg daily can also be administered for 72 hr.	Class IIa
Statin therapy	Typical dose of atorvastatin is 20 mg once daily initiated at least 45 d prior to surgery. Withdrawal of statin therapy for >4 d after vascular surgery is associated with increased risk of cardiac complications. Administration of extended-release fluvastatin preoperatively appears ideal when prolonged postoperative ileus is expected. Statin use is also associated with improved graft patency, limb salvage, and decreased amputation rate in patients undergoing infrainguinal bypass for atherosclerotic vascular disease.	Class IIa
ACE inhibitors	Potential benefits include decreased stroke rate (e.g., ramipril), limitation of ventricular remodeling that follows acute ST elevation MI, decreased long-term mortality following infrainguinal bypass surgery, and so forth. Ability to stabilize the atherosclerotic plaque by up-regulating type III collagen of the fibrous cap of the unstable plaque may explain some of these benefits.	Class IIb
Calcium channel blockers	Reduced perioperative adverse cardiac events; including supraventricular tachycardia in patients undergoing various types of noncardiac surgery (primarily diltiazem). Evidence limited in patients undergoing vascular surgery.	Class IIb
Nitroglycerin	Not indicated for myocardial ischemia prophylaxis or initial treatment. May be used to treat arterial hypertension or elevated cardiac filling pressures or suspected coronary vasospasm.	Class III

IV, intravenous; ACE, angiotensin-converting enzyme; MI, myocardial infarction.

[a]Class I recommendation refers to conditions for which there is evidence or general agreement that a given procedure or treatment is useful or effective; class III refers to conditions for which there is evidence and/or general agreement that the procedure/treatment is not useful/effective or in some cases may be harmful. Class II recommendations fall in between and indicate conditions for which there is conflicting evidence or a divergence of opinion about the usefulness/efficacy of a procedure/treatment. Class IIa indicates that the weight of evidence/opinion is in favor of usefulness/efficacy. Class IIb indicates that the usefulness/efficacy is less well established by evidence/opinion. In simple terms, class I recommendations are the "dos," class III recommendations are "don'ts," and class II recommendations are the "maybes." Refer to Figure 42-7 for the algorithm. Calcium channel blockers and ACE inhibitors, although not recommended as independent agents for the purpose, should be continued if a patient is receiving them. Refer to Table 42-2 for suggestions for precautions on their perioperative use.

anesthesia.[41] A systematic review and meta-analysis found that the relative risk of angio-edema from ACE inhibitors in black compared to nonblack patients was 3 (95% confidence interval 2.5 to 3.7).[42]

A meta-analysis suggested beneficial effects of calcium channel blockers in reducing perioperative adverse cardiac events (cardiac-related death, MI, ischemia, or supraventricular tachycardia) in patients undergoing different types of noncardiac surgery. The majority of these effects were attributable to diltiazem. Limited evidence was available from this meta-analysis for patients undergoing vascular surgery.[27] Large randomized trials are required to establish their benefits in vascular surgery patients. Currently, the authors do not recommend their use as independent drug therapeutic modality for the perioperative cardiac risk reduction. Similarly, prophylactic intravenous nitroglycerin 0.9 μg/kg/min failed to reduce the incidence of PMI in patients with known or suspected CAD undergoing noncardiac surgery.[43] In this study, the preponderance of myocardial ischemia occurred during emergence from

anesthesia, which is associated with acute increases in heart rate.

High-dose narcotic anesthetics reduce the stress response and may improve overall outcome after major surgery. Postoperative infusion of sufentanil 1 μg/kg/hr can reduce the severity of myocardial ischemia (ST segment changes) following CABG, although clinical outcome was not improved. High-dose narcotics may mandate overnight ventilation, which may not be cost-effective. In contrast, volatile anesthetics promote preconditioning, reduce troponin release, hasten extubation and hospital discharge in cardiac surgery, as well as reducing death and MI compared with intravenous anesthetics.[44,45] Whether these findings are transferable to vascular surgery is unclear.[46,47] Another approach using intensive analgesia involves the use of epidural analgesia. A meta-analysis suggests that thoracic epidurals may reduce PMI.[48] Epidural local anesthetics may reduce perioperative myocardial ischemia because preload and afterload are reduced, the postoperative adrenergic and coagulation responses are reduced, and with thoracic administration, the coronary arteries are dilated. Despite these effects on intermediate variables, improvement in cardiac outcomes have generally not been demonstrated in well-designed trials, suggesting that anesthetic technique does not affect cardiac outcome after abdominal aortic surgery, especially if heart rate is well controlled in the ICU.[49]

Anemia (hematocrit <28%) may increase the incidence of postoperative myocardial ischemia and cardiac events in high-risk patients undergoing noncardiac surgery.[50] Therefore, the authors are more likely to transfuse high-risk patients, those who demonstrate myocardial ischemia, and those with evidence of compromised end-organ perfusion with packed red blood cells, to augment the hematocrit to 30%. However, some work in ICU patients (with a relatively low percentage of patients with CAD) suggests that lower transfusion thresholds may be beneficial.[51] Hypothermia is also associated with increased adrenergic tone and postoperative myocardial ischemia and events in vascular surgery patients.[52] In addition, maintaining perioperative normothermia reduces blood loss and transfusion requirement by clinically important amounts.[53] Therefore, the authors recommend aggressively warming patients and conserving heat during and after such surgery, and attempting extubation in the operating room with the same attention to the control of hemodynamics as during induction. If patients require postoperative ventilation, adequate sedation, analgesia, and occasionally even paralysis (which can prevent shivering and its attendant increases in oxygen consumption) should be provided. Tachycardia should be treated aggressively, most often with β-adrenergic blocking agents after correction of other potential causes such as fever, pain, anemia, and hypovolemia.

Occasionally, in patients with evolving MI, an intra-aortic balloon pump may improve coronary blood flow while decreasing workload. Definitive studies of its effectiveness are lacking, and intra-aortic balloon pump placement can be difficult and risky in patients with peripheral vascular disease and abdominal or thoracic aortic pathology. Other patients may need emergent cardiac catheterization, selective thrombolysis, and percutaneous coronary intervention for unstable angina or evolving postoperative MI, understanding the challenges inherent in cardiologists' otherwise routine use of antiplatelet therapy in fresh postoperative patients.

Other Medical Problems in Vascular Surgery Patients

If hypertension is poorly controlled and time permits, consultation with the patient's internist or cardiologist may result in an improved antihypertensive regimen. Most often, this is accomplished with oral doses of atenolol or metoprolol, 25 to 200 mg daily. Additional therapy may include ACE inhibitors and statin drugs. Lowering blood pressure gradually before surgery (over days to weeks) allows for restoration of normal intravascular volume, cerebral autoregulation to return to a more normal range, and results in a more stable perioperative course. In the past few decades, many clinicians have chosen to postpone surgery in patients with elevated blood pressure before surgery, regardless of whether they receive chronic treatment for hypertension. A more recent meta-analysis of 30 observational trials of cardiovascular outcomes after surgery in hypertensive patients suggests a statistically but "not clinically significant" increase in events.[54]

Undiagnosed diabetes and abnormal glucose tolerance are common in vascular patients, and predicts perioperative myocardial ischemia.[55] Diabetic patients generally have higher risks of MI and wound infection compared with nondiabetics undergoing AAA. Glucose management during carotid and thoracic aortic procedures may be especially important, in situations in which hyperglycemia may exacerbate neurologic

injury. In addition, more recent randomized trials and large observational trials have suggested mortality reduction in surgical ICU patients and improved outcomes in cardiovascular surgery when insulin infusions are used to provide "tight" glucose control. The American College of Endocrinology recommends that preprandial glucose concentration should be <110 mg/dL, with maximal glucose not to exceed 180 mg/dL, in hospitalized patients, and that blood glucose concentration should be controlled to <110 mg/dL in the ICU. The use of intravenous insulin therapy and frequent glucose monitoring were recommended to maintain glycemic control in the perioperative period.[56]

Hypercoagulable states are more common in younger patients presenting for vascular surgery and in those with vascular thrombosis in unusual locations. Hypercoagulable responses to surgery may also predispose patients to vascular graft occlusion after surgery. Postoperative abnormalities include elevated fibrinogen levels, antithrombin III deficiency, impaired fibrinolysis, protein C deficiency, and protein S deficiency. Heparin-induced thrombocytopenia and thrombosis can occur (immunoglobulin G-mediated) after several days of exposure to heparin.[57] Treatment includes cessation of all heparin, full anticoagulation with a direct thrombin inhibitor, and 3 weeks of Coumadin to prevent arterial thrombosis. Coumadin alone is not recommended as it diminishes protein C and S activity and may initially promote thrombosis.

Patients with pre-existing renal insufficiency have an increased risk of postoperative renal failure, as well as cardiac complications and death. If patients receive chronic dialysis treatments, they should receive dialysis on the day before or the same day as surgery. Some patients will actually be hypovolemic as a result, which can contribute to hypotension with induction of general or regional anesthesia.

CAROTID ENDARTERECTOMY

In a recent review of anesthesia for CEA, Howell[58] notes that it "can yield significant benefit, but those with the most to gain from the operation also present the greatest challenge to the anesthetist." In addition to traditional CEA, carotid angioplasty and stenting (CAS) is increasingly used. Large randomized trials have more recently been reported, with varying results for stenting compared with traditional CEA. The disease is primarily a problem of embolization and rarely occlusion or insufficiency. Carotid disease may manifest itself only as an asymptomatic bruit, or as amaurosis fugax (transient attacks of monocular blindness) when the ophthalmic artery is embolized. Other patients may experience episodes of paresthesias, clumsiness of the extremities, or speech problems, which resolve spontaneously after a short period. These are the classic transient ischemic attacks (TIAs). An isolated, cervical bruit in asymptomatic patients also seems to be associated with a higher risk of stroke, but the correlation between the location of the bruits and the type of subsequent stroke is poor. Therefore, a bruit should prompt further testing.

The most common noninvasive test is the duplex scan, which combines B-mode anatomic imaging and pulse Doppler spectral analysis of blood flow velocity. The accuracy of duplex scanning reaches 95% in experienced hands when compared with angiography. Also, many surgeons use magnetic resonance angiography as the sole modality to detect disease.

Combined administration of aspirin and dipyridamole, when compared with placebo, reduces the incidence of TIAs more so than either drug alone.[59] More potent platelet inhibitors such a clopidogrel may offer further protection. Therefore, it is essential that patients presenting for CEA continue to receive aspirin and/or clopidogrel in the perioperative period. CEA, in conjunction with aspirin therapy, has proven superior to medical therapy alone in a large trial of symptomatic patients with a stenosis >70% in the North American trial (NASCET).[60] For asymptomatic patients with a stenosis of >60%, the Asymptomatic Carotid Atherosclerosis (ACAS) study also detected a substantial outcome benefit: ipsilateral stroke and any perioperative stroke or death was estimated to be 11.0% for patients treated medically and 5.1% for surgical patients after 5 years.[61] CEA is justifiable only if the operative morbidity and mortality are lower than the natural risk for ischemic events in the untreated patient. The number of asymptomatic patients who need to undergo CEA to prevent one stroke is approximately 20 to 40, leading some investigators to question its cost-effectiveness in this setting. The guidelines published for CEA by the AHA were last revised in 1998.[62]

A contemporary series showed good outcomes in 442 consecutive CEA procedures performed under general anesthesia (with routine shunting, patching, and completion duplex ultrasound imaging). At the 30-day follow-up, there were only two strokes, no deaths, and one MI.[63] A high-quality, prospectively collected database (primarily U.S. male veterans) identified predictors of outcome in 13,622 CEA operations. The composite stroke, death, or cardiac event rate was 4.0%; the stroke/death rate was 3.4%. Multivariate correlates of the composite outcome were age, diabetes, smoking, TIAs, history of stroke, creatinine >1.5 mg/dL, hypoalbuminemia, and long operative time; cardiopulmonary comorbid features did not affect the composite outcome. Regional anesthesia was used in 18% of cases, with a resultant relative risk reduction for stroke (17%), death (24%), cardiac event (33%), and the composite outcome (31%), compared with general anesthesia.[64] However, because retrospective studies do not address all confounding issues, these results are not conclusive but should guide future studies, wherein high-risk patients as identified here might be randomized to general versus regional anesthesia.

Preoperative Evaluation and Preparation

The authors do not delay urgent surgery that might prevent a stroke for extensive cardiac evaluation even in patients with known cardiac disease. However, the long-term risks of adverse cardiac events after CEA are related to progression of CAD. The approach to patients with both severe CAD and carotid occlusive disease is controversial. Because combined or staged operations are relatively rare (especially for symptomatic carotid disease), many case series suffer from the limitation of having been performed over many years, making generalizability to current practice difficult.

Monitoring and Preserving Neurologic Integrity

The two main goals of intraoperative management are to protect the brain and to protect the heart, yet these two goals often conflict. For example, increasing arterial blood pressure to augment cerebral blood flow can increase afterload or myocardial contractility, thereby increasing the oxygen demand of the heart. The rationale behind maintaining a stable, high-normal blood pressure throughout the procedure is based on the assumption that blood vessels in ischemic or hypoperfused areas of brain have lost normal autoregulation. Nonetheless, hypotension and hypoperfusion may not be the precipitating or sole cause of stroke after CEA; embolic events may be just as or even more important, and often occur postoperatively (Fig. 42-9).[33] However, the judicious use of phenylephrine to raise blood pressure only in specific instances of electroencephalogram (EEG)-detected reversible cerebral ischemia seems to be without detriment to the heart. Whatever the

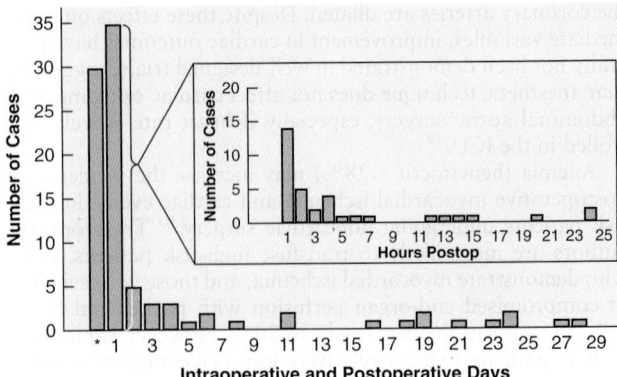

*Events Occurred Intraoperatively

FIGURE 42-9. Data from the North American Symptomatic Carotid Trial (NASCET). Of the perioperative strokes, 35% (30/85) occurred intraoperatively, whereas 65% (55/85) occurred after the patient left the operating room (delayed events). The figure illustrates the time of onset of the 92 surgical outcome events.

choice of vasopressor, EEG or other neurophysiologic monitoring may allow the anesthesiologist to use less vasopressor and to maintain a lower blood pressure during the period of temporary carotid occlusion than would be otherwise feasible.

Hypercapnia during CEA may be detrimental if it dilates vessels in normal areas of the brain while vessels in ischemic brain areas that are already maximally dilated cannot respond. The net effect, then, is a "steal" phenomenon (i.e., a diversion of blood flow from hypoperfused brain regions to normally perfused brain regions). Most authorities recommend the maintenance of normocarbia or moderate hypocarbia. Moderate hyperglycemia may worsen ischemic brain injury, and hyperglycemia has a documented association with worse outcome after CEA.[65] As a result, the authors recommend aggressive glucose control. Isovolemic hemodilution with dextran or hetastarch is of theoretical interest in cerebral ischemia because blood viscosity is reduced and attendant microcirculatory disturbances ameliorated.

Almost all commonly used anesthetic agents reduce cerebral metabolism, thereby decreasing the brain's requirements for oxygen. However, the notion that reduced cerebral metabolism is associated with cerebral protection has been challenged. Isoflurane, desflurane, and sevoflurane reduce cerebral oxygen requirements comparably, but the later two agents allow for faster emergence and recovery.[66] In addition, volatile anesthetics may provide preconditioning and neuronal protection by inducing nitric oxide synthase.[67]

Barbiturates may offer a degree of brain protection during periods of regional ischemia. Thiopental decreases cerebral metabolic oxygen requirements to about 50% of baseline. These maximally achievable reductions in oxygen requirements correspond to a silent (i.e., isoelectric) EEG. Beyond this point, additional doses of barbiturates are neither necessary nor helpful. In cases of massive global ischemia in which basal cellular metabolism has already deteriorated, even high doses of barbiturates will not improve neurologic outcome. Therefore, some clinicians use thiopental not only for induction of anesthesia, but also for continuous infusion and/or as a 4- to 6-mg/kg bolus just before carotid occlusion. The cardiac depressant effects of the barbiturates may require inotropic support. Unfortunately, no rigorous proof is available that the use of barbiturates in the described manner can improve neurologic outcome after CEA. Excellent results have been obtained for CEA using high doses of barbiturates during carotid occlusion, without neurophysiologic monitoring or shunt placement; on average, tracheal extubation was delayed until 2 hours after surgery was completed.

Both etomidate and propofol decrease brain electrical activity and thus decrease cellular oxygen requirements. Etomidate preserves cardiovascular stability and may be beneficial in a patient population whose cardiac reserves are often limited. Propofol also allows rapid awakening of the patient and neurologic assessment at the end of surgery. Propofol may be associated with a lower incidence of myocardial ischemia than a volatile-based anesthetic, but does not appear to affect overall clinical outcome.[68] Although the available evidence for the protective effects of etomidate or propofol during CEA is inconclusive, a small series in patients undergoing temporary ischemia for intracranial aneurysm clipping suggests that etomidate, propofol, or barbiturate use prolongs tolerable ischemia and reduces brain infarction.[69] Some animal studies have supported, and others refuted, the utility of α_2-agonists in reducing cerebral infarction in animal models.

Hypothermia can depress neuronal activity sufficiently to decrease cellular oxygen requirements below the minimum levels normally required for continued cell viability. In theory, hypothermia represents the most effective method of cerebral protection. Even a mild decrease in temperature of about 2 to 3°C at the time of arterial hypoxemia may reduce ischemic damage to the brain. The first reported CEA was performed with the patient's head covered by ice packs. Unfortunately, this method is cumbersome, unpredictable, and rarely used. The authors allow patients to cool passively in the operating room and avoid warming the operating suite, intravenous fluids, or inspired gases until the carotid repair has been completed. Afterward, forced-air warming may counteract the adrenergic response and increased incidence of myocardial ischemia associated with hypothermia in vascular surgery patients. The literature provides no definitive evidence to support the hypothesis that hypothermia protects the brain sufficiently to justify the myocardial risks imposed by hypothermia and shivering. In the setting of cerebral aneurysm surgery, intraoperative hypothermia did not improve the neurologic outcome after craniotomy among good-grade patients with aneurysmal subarachnoid hemorrhage.[70]

Temporary occlusion ("cross-clamping") of the carotid artery acutely disrupts blood flow, even if flow to the ipsilateral hemisphere of the brain was already markedly diminished by severe stenosis. Continued blood supply to the brain will depend entirely on adequate collateral blood flow through the circle of Willis if no shunt is used. If carotid stenosis has worsened gradually before CEA is performed, collaterals from the circle of Willis may have had time to develop, and the cerebral circulation may not be compromised by carotid occlusion during surgery. However, if collateral flow is compromised because of occlusive disease of the contralateral carotid artery and/or the vertebral arteries, the chances are greater that marked hypoperfusion of the brain will occur during carotid clamping. Indeed, patients with bilateral carotid disease have a higher risk of perioperative stroke after CEA than patients with unilateral disease only.

There are practice variations among surgeons in the use of shunts in carotid surgery. Surgeons who never use shunts usually rely on expedient surgery to avoid neurologic problems and do not report worse overall outcome statistics than those who do. Placement of a shunt is associated with an embolism-related stroke rate of at least 0.7% from the dislodgment and embolization of atheroma. The technical problems of shunting include air embolism, kinking of the shunt, shunt occlusion against the side of the vessel wall, and injury or disruption of the distal internal carotid artery. Patients with shunts may still develop EEG abnormalities; in these situations, shunt adjustments may be necessary. The shunt may impair surgical access to the artery, thereby increasing cross-clamp time. Most important, the use of

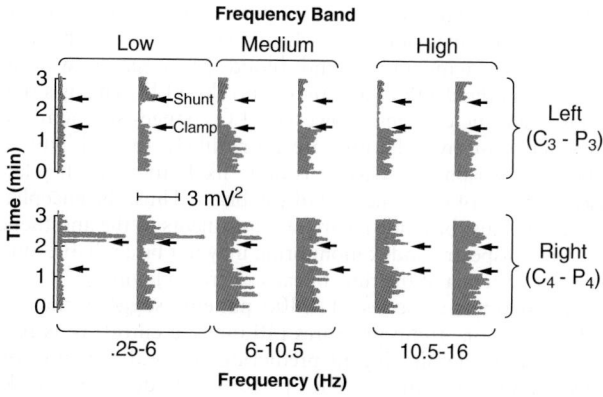

FIGURE 42-10. Acute cerebral ischemia following left carotid artery occlusion detected with processed electroencephalogram. The placement of a shunt in this case promptly reversed the ischemic changes. (Courtesy of Dr. Bruce L. Gewertz.)

a shunt is beneficial only if the cause of neurologic dysfunction is inadequate blood flow. However, the majority of studies suggest that as many as 65 to 95% of all neurologic deficits during CEA may be caused by thromboembolic events (Fig. 42-9). In the NASCET trial, shunting (used in 41% of patients) was not associated with a change in risk of stroke.

Surgeons who use shunts selectively need a monitoring device of cerebral perfusion to help them decide when to place the shunt. Monitoring approaches include assessment of the awake patient, transcranial Doppler, somatosensory evoked potential (SSEP), EEG, cerebral oximetry, and direct xenon cerebral blood flow measurement. In each case, the goal is to avoid unnecessary shunting. EEG monitoring is often used. EEG deterioration begins usually below a cerebral blood flow rate of about 15 mL/min/100 g brain tissue, but cellular metabolic failure does not seem to occur until blood flow falls below 10 to 12 mL/min/100 g brain tissue.[71] The most common manifestations of EEG ischemia during CEA are ipsilateral attenuation, ipsilateral slowing with attenuation, and ipsilateral slowing without attenuation. Figure 42-10 shows a processed EEG reflecting acute cerebral ischemia following left carotid artery occlusion; the placement of a shunt in this case promptly reversed the ischemic changes. However, as in all the cerebral monitoring techniques, the sensitivity in detecting perioperative stroke is limited by the fact that most strokes occur following surgery and are likely related to thromboembolic phenomena.[72] Rapid changes in anesthetic depth may also complicate interpretation.[73] This is particularly relevant in centers in which barbiturates or propofol infusions are used to induce EEG suppression. In the North American trial, 93% of patients underwent CEA with general anesthesia; 51% of patients had intraoperative cerebral monitoring (31% EEG, 14% stump pressure, 7% evoked potentials, and 3% transcranial Doppler). However, the use of monitoring was not associated with reduced risk of stroke.[74] The real value of cerebral monitoring may lie in the avoidance of the placement of shunts (which can cause stroke) and blood pressure augmentation (with its detrimental effects on the heart).

EEG monitoring has several limitations. One limitation is that deep brain structures are not monitored by EEG. Also, in patients with pre-existing or fluctuating neurologic deficits the EEG may be false-negative; that is, these patients can develop perioperative strokes despite the absence of major intraoperative EEG changes. In these patients, there may be cell populations that are electrically silent or immediately adjacent to regions of infarction, and therefore not monitored by the EEG. The still-viable regions may progress to irreversible deterioration in the course of the operative procedure. Furthermore, the EEG may not be an ischemia-specific monitor because decreases in temperature and blood pressure, as well as increases in the depth of anesthesia, produce EEG changes that mimic ischemic changes. However, EEG changes secondary to anesthetics or hypothermia are more likely to be bilateral, whereas hemispheric ischemia is more likely to affect the electrical activity of only one side of the brain. Thus, the encephalographer must be made aware of adjustments to the anesthetic regimen. Bispectral index monitoring may not be a reliable indicator of ischemia at the time of carotid cross-clamp.[75,76]

A retrospective series of >400 patients suggests that an "old" monitor, stump pressures (40 mm Hg cutoff) is as reliable as EEG monitoring in predicting cerebral ischemia on cross-clamp application in CEA performed under nerve block, with significant cost savings; whether these results are transferrable to general anesthesia is unclear.[77] In another study, when stump pressure and EEG were measured during CEA under regional anesthesia, both modalities had poor sensitivity as a guide to shunt placement (neurologic changes being the gold standard). Only 1.4% of patients with stump pressure >50 mm Hg required a shunt, while EEG identified cerebral ischemia in only 59.4% of patients needing shunt placement, with a false-positive rate of 1.0% and a false-negative rate of 40.6%. Again, whether these results are transferable to patients under general anesthesia is unclear.[78]

Recent work reports a comparison of four neuromonitoring modalities (transcranial Doppler [TCD] sonography, near-infrared spectroscopy, stump pressure, and SSEPs) in 48 patients under regional anesthesia; 12 patients developed ischemic changes. All parameters provided the ability to distinguish between ischemic and nonischemic patients. However, TCD monitoring was not possible in 21% and SSEP was not possible in 4% of patients.[79] Jugular bulb venous monitoring can also detect cerebral ischemia.[80]

TCD measures middle cerebral artery blood flow velocities. TCD can also detect and quantify embolic signals, which almost always arise during dissection and/or angioplasty. A large series of 1,058 patients found the following TCD predictors of stroke after CEA: emboli during wound closure, >90% decrease of middle cerebral artery peak systolic velocity at cross-clamping, and >100% increase of the pulsatility index of the Doppler signal at clamp release.[81] In a small case series, TCD predicted neurologic events despite a normal EEG.[82] However, compared with the awake patient as a gold standard, TCD may have a low positive predictive value for neurologic deficit accompanying carotid occlusion.[83] Other workers suggested that TCD is particularly useful in postoperative surveillance because most strokes occur after and not during CEA. TCD may also predict patients at risk of cerebral hyperperfusion syndrome following CEA or CAS.[84]

SSEP monitoring may be particularly useful in patients with cerebral ischemia in whom EEG interpretation is more difficult.[85] SSEP monitoring is based on the detection of cortical potentials after electrical stimuli are presented to a peripheral nerve. In contrast to the EEG, which interrogates only cortical function, SSEP monitoring also evaluates deep brain structures. Any damage to these neural structures results in characteristic changes in the SSEP, usually in a decrease in amplitude and/or an increase in latency. If neural damage is severe, the cortical evoked potential is completely abolished. Severe damage occurs at about one third of normal cerebral blood flow (i.e., at 15 mL/min/100 g brain tissue). Whereas some studies have been optimistic about the value of SSEP monitoring in the detection of cerebral ischemia, other investigators have concluded that SSEP is neither sensitive nor specific for the detection of ischemic injury during CEA. Virtually all commonly used anesthetics lead to SSEP changes that mimic changes produced by cerebral hypoxia. Therefore, a constant light plane of

anesthesia needs to be maintained if increased latencies and decreased amplitudes of evoked potentials are to be ascribed to inadequate cerebral perfusion. False-negative results may also occur. Based on the available data, the authors conclude that this monitoring system cannot yet be considered essential in CEA. Similarly, cerebral oximetry has had mixed results. It may not allow the definition of a threshold value indicating need for shunt placement[86] and if used alone might increase the number of unnecessary shunts because of its low specificity.[87]

Anesthetic and Monitoring Choices for Elective Surgery

In addition to routine monitors, the authors recommend an intra-arterial catheter for blood pressure monitoring and blood pressures measurement noninvasively in both arms because peripheral vascular disease can produce striking differences between the upper extremities. ECG monitoring should include continuous leads II and V_5 for ST-T segment assessment. In very high-risk patients, TEE may be used as an additional monitor, especially in those with acute stroke in whom source of embolus may be an issue or in those with left bundle branch block making ST-T segment evaluation impossible . Rarely is it necessary to use a central venous or pulmonary artery catheter, even if TEE is not available. The authors recommend restricting the use of central venous access to the rare patient with uncompensated CHF undergoing urgent CEA, and then insertion should be from the contralateral brachial or subclavian vein. One well-secured and well-running, medium-bore, intravenous catheter is sufficient because major blood loss or fluid shifts during CEA are rare.

If sedatives are deemed indispensable, the smallest effective dose of midazolam is chosen for premedication to facilitate early perioperative neurologic assessment. Blood pressure and heart rate determinations from the preoperative clinic, other hospital or clinic visits, and at the time of admission are assessed to determine the range of a patient's acceptable values. The authors seek to maintain hemodynamics within this range intraoperatively. Chronic antianginal, antihypertensive, and antiplatelet medications are generally continued on the day of surgery.

Often on the day of surgery, patients present hypertensive despite having taken their morning antihypertensive and antianginal medications. These patients appear to be the most prone to hypotension after the induction of general anesthesia. Propofol, thiopental, or etomidate may be used for induction. If thiopental is used, esmolol is particularly valuable to blunt hypertensive and tachycardic responses to intubation. Regardless of the induction agent, the clinician should be prepared to use pharmacologic blood pressure augmentation if blood pressure decreases excessively. Total fluid administration is limited in most patients to no more than 10 mL/kg of in a typical 2-hour operation because fluid overload may contribute to postoperative hypertension. Diastolic filling abnormalities are common in elderly surgical patients,[88] and limiting fluid administration may also lessen symptoms of congestion following surgery.

Because the respiratory depression and sedation caused by opioids may confound the results of early neurologic assessment, long-lasting opioids are restricted whenever possible (e.g., fentanyl ≤3 mcg/kg) or remifentanil is employed. The combined use of a cervical plexus block and/or surgeon-administered local anesthetic helps considerably in almost eliminating opiate requirements.

General anesthesia is maintained at a "light" level that permits EEG monitoring and results in blood pressures in the high range of normal. The trachea may be sprayed with 100 mg lidocaine to minimize stimulation by the endotracheal tube during surgery. Others have described the use of the laryngeal mask airway during CEA, which may reduce hypertensive and tachycardic episodes. The authors use 50% nitrous oxide in oxygen and light levels of desflurane or sevoflurane because of their salutary effects on the incidence of cerebral ischemia[66] rapid-awakening characteristics. Vasopressors are used as needed to treat hypotension or EEG changes. Because sudden onset of bradycardia and hypotension may be caused by baroreceptor reflexes with surgical irritation of the carotid sinus, some surgeons may infiltrate the carotid bifurcation with 1% lidocaine to attenuate this response. However, this practice may result in more postoperative hypertension. Relaxation is provided based on the clinical need and anesthesiologist's preference. Patients are almost always extubated at the end of the surgical procedure before or after neurologic integrity is confirmed. In patients who were easy to intubate, a deep extubation may limit the explosive hypertension that can accompany extubation. Neurologic integrity is always verified before the patient leaves the operating room. New neurologic deficits may lead to noninvasive imaging, contrast angiography, and/or surgical re-exploration. Using the approach presented here, the authors report their overall mortality as 1%, and stroke and MI, both 0.76%. Others achieved similar results using a nitrous oxide/opioid technique or a continuous infusion of thiopental. Intravenous techniques (propofol/remifentanil) may offer more hemodynamic stability[89] than volatile anesthetic techniques. When general anesthesia is used, remifentanil (0.5 μg/kg/min) may result in fewer episodes of intraoperative hypertension and less need for nitroglycerin compared with fentanyl (2 μg/kg).[90] There is no proof that any one general anesthetic technique provides a superior outcome.

Regional anesthesia is used by many centers for CEA. The necessary sensory blockade of the C2 to C4 dermatomes can be achieved by superficial or deep cervical block or by subcutaneous infiltration of the surgical field. Superficial and deep plexus blocks appear to be equivalent in providing good surgical conditions and patient satisfaction; deep plexus blocks are more effective when a paresthesia is obtained.[91] Proponents of regional anesthetic techniques claim the following advantages: greater stability of blood pressure during surgery, inexpensive and easy cerebral monitoring, avoidance of tracheal intubation in patients with chronic obstructive lung disease, and avoidance of negative inotropic anesthetic agents in patients with limited cardiac reserves. The use of regional techniques appears to be associated with fewer episodes of EEG ischemia compared with general anesthesia.[92] In addition, overall hospital costs associated with the use of regional anesthesia may be lower. Deep cervical plexus block may result in spread of local anesthetic to the phrenic nerve, resulting in respiratory embarrassment, particularly in patients with contralateral phrenic nerve palsy from previous cardiac surgery.[93] Deep cervical plexus block (and/or surgical nerve damage) can result in laryngeal nerve paralysis, which can cause respiratory distress in patients with contralateral laryngeal nerve palsy following previous neck surgery.[94] However, cervical plexus block is to be recommended over cervical epidural due to a much higher rate of complications (including life-threatening, inadvertent injection into the subarachnoid space or vertebral artery) of the latter.[95] Superficial cervical plexus block may be combined with general anesthesia, and reduces postoperative opiate requirements, reduces $PaCO_2$, and increases patients satisfaction with analgesia.[96] A systematic review comparing deep and superficial blocks concluded that superficial/intermediate block is safer than any method that employs a deep injection.[97] An updated systematic review published in 2007 concluded that the number of patients included in randomized controlled trials or even in prospective studies is too low to allow any conclusions on the differences in outcome between regional and general anesthetic techniques for CEA.[98]

α_2-Agonists may be used for sedation during CEA. A series of >100 patients showed a low rate of need for shunting (4.3%) and no strokes when dexmedetomidine (DEX) was used for sedation during CEA under nerve block.[99] DEX appears to reduce hypertension/tachycardia, but increases hypotension, such that the number of hemodynamic interventions is no different from placebo; analgesia requirements in the postanesthesia care unit, however, are reduced with DEX.[100] Clonidine 1 μg/kg/hr suppresses the hyperadrenergic response to CEA without adverse effects on hemodynamics or clinical neurologic monitoring.[101] The combination of superficial cervical plexus block and clonidine used to supplement general anesthesia results in an increase in hemodynamic stability after CEA and significant reductions in need for rescue medication postoperatively.[102]

Disadvantages of regional anesthesia are that potential pharmacologic brain protection with anesthetics cannot be provided and that in the case of panic, sudden loss of consciousness, or onset of seizures, control of the airway may be difficult. Although emergent intubation is uncommon, it may be difficult under these circumstances and complicate surgical management. Regional anesthesia requires that the patient remains highly cooperative throughout the operation, and sedation can be provided only to a limited extent during carotid occlusion. Based on the currently available evidence, the choice of anesthetic technique should take into account the preference of the surgeon and the experience and expertise of the anesthesiologist.

Carotid Angioplasty and Stenting

CAS may be performed by vascular surgeons, cardiologists, or radiologists. In some cases, this will involve sedation and monitoring provided by anesthesiologists; in other cases, no anesthesiologist will be involved. The subject needs to be arousable and responsive so that serial neurologic examinations can be conducted. Adequate heparinization is crucial, with most protocols seeking to maintain activated clotting time >300 seconds. Both CEA and CAS may cause blood pressure to fall immediately after reperfusion and into the postoperative period, because of alterations in baroreceptor function.[103] Throughout the development of CAS, concern had always been about risk and ramifications of cerebral emboli as a result of the angioplasty itself.[104] Consequently, two main areas have been pursued to decrease the risk of embolic stroke: proximal flow blockage and distal filters. Additionally, periprocedural antiplatelet and statin therapy have been considered but not tested adequately. Between 2001 and 2008, the results of four prospective randomized trials were published comparing CEA and CAS. Together they prove no clear outcome advantage of CAS over CEA.[105–109] Success rates for CEA and CAS of individual practitioners and institutions should dictate which procedure is chosen for a patient until more randomized trials resolve this controversial area. Given the long history and success of CEA, it remains the standard by which CAS must be judged.

Postoperative Management

Common problems arising after CEA or CAS include the onset of new neurologic dysfunction and hemodynamic instability; CEA may also be complicated by respiratory insufficiency. Other perioperative complications include temporary cranial nerve injuries (vagus, hypoglossal), temporary marginal mandibular nerve deficits, temporary and permanent posterior auricular nerve deficits, and mild cervical numbness, indicating injury to small sensory cervical nerves. Hematomas requiring return to surgery occurs in approximately 1% of patients. Headache, wound infections, and hyperperfusion syndrome manifesting as hypertension and headache may also occur.[63] Hyperperfusion syndrome is believed to result from blood flow to the brain that is greatly in excess of its metabolic need.

It may not occur until several days after surgery, when patients present with severe ipsilateral headache and can progress to develop signs of increased cerebral excitability or frank seizures. TCD may have a role in predicting which patients will develop this syndrome. Steroids may be used in the treatment of hyperperfusion syndrome.

Blood pressure abnormalities are common after CEA; hypertension is more common than hypotension. Severe hypertension seems to occur more often in patients with poorly controlled preoperative hypertension. Both acute tachycardia and hypertension may precipitate acute myocardial ischemia and failure, and hypertension may lead to cerebral edema and/or hemorrhage. Post-CEA hypertension is significantly associated with adverse events (stroke or death, with a statistical trend toward reduced cardiac complications), whereas postoperative hypotension and bradycardia do not appear to correlate with primary or secondary outcomes. Therefore, the authors recommend treatment of hypertension to reduce the work of the heart and in hope of decreasing neck hematoma. After excluding and/or treating other causes of hypertension such as bladder distention, pain, hypoxemia, and hypercarbia, systolic pressures of >140 mm Hg and diastolic pressures of >90 mm Hg are lowered to within the range of the patient's perioperative values, most often with labetalol in 5-mg increments. Because labetalol is not β_1-selective, other drugs are used in patients with reactive airways disease. Perioperative myocardial ischemia may occur in 15% of CEA patients; angina and hypertension may be important risk factors.[110] Usually, the hypertensive episode has its peak 2 to 3 hours after surgery, but in individual cases it may persist for 24 hours. Because significant hypertension and hypotension can be caused by myocardial ischemia or infarction, a 12-lead ECG should be obtained in the recovery room in hemodynamically unstable patients.

Postoperative respiratory insufficiency may be caused by recurrent laryngeal nerve or hypoglossal nerve injury, a neck hematoma, or deficient carotid body function. Wound hematomas develop in up to 2% of patients after CEA. Whereas small hematomas caused by venous oozing usually can be treated by reversing residual heparin with protamine or by applying gentle digital compression for a few minutes, an expanding hematoma must be carefully and immediately evaluated because tracheal compression and loss of the airway may ensue rapidly. In some cases, evacuation of the hematoma may not relieve the airway obstruction if lymphatic obstruction has produced massive pharyngolaryngeal edema.[111,112] Indeed, four patients (0.3%) in the NASCET trial died directly because of neck hematomas. Risk factors for neck hematoma may also include failure to reverse heparin and the presence of an endotracheal tube beyond the end of surgery. Hematomas are more common and delayed if a patch angioplasty has been performed. Therefore, some clinicians routinely reverse heparin with protamine in patients who have had a patch angioplasty. Some studies have suggested protamine may contribute to postoperative stroke. However, in the NASCET trial, heparin reversal using protamine (used in 40% of patients) was not associated with a change in risk of stroke.[74]

Surgical manipulation may also damage the nerve supply to the carotid body. Although unilateral loss of carotid body function is unlikely to be significant, a bilateral loss may prevent the patient from increasing ventilation in response to a decrease in PaO_2. Therefore, supplemental oxygen should be routinely used in the recovery area. Similarly, drugs that depress respiratory drive should be avoided as much as possible in postoperative pain management. Acetaminophen constitutes effective pain relief in most patients when skin infiltration or plexus block with local anesthetic was performed in the operating room.

Routine postoperative intensive care is unusual and has been questioned. In one study, postoperative intensive care surveillance was necessary only for patients with four or more of the following risk factors: stroke, CHF, chronic kidney failure, hypertension, dysrhythmia, and MI. Equally important, all patients requiring interventions or with adverse outcomes could be identified by the eighth postoperative hour.[113] Therefore, intensive care surveillance can be limited to high-risk patients.

Management of Emergent Carotid Surgery

The patient who awakens with a major new neurologic deficit or who develops a suspected stroke in the immediate postoperative period represents a surgical emergency. Although postoperative neurologic deficits may be due to inadequate collateral flow, carotid thrombosis may cause postoperative stroke; prompt surgical re-exploration can produce significant neurologic improvement. If a new neurologic deficit occurs in the postanesthesia recovery unit, most surgeons believe immediate reexploration is indicated, and logic would dictate utilization of pharmacologic methods of "cerebral protection;" however, this "logic" is controversial. Alternatively, if the deficit is deemed only focal and minor, it is most commonly because of microembolization. Consequently, noninvasive assessment of internal carotid flow and anticoagulation after exclusion of a hemorrhagic brain lesion usually constitute indicated treatment.

A patient undergoing emergency CEA may have a full stomach and thus may require protection against aspiration of gastric contents. Otherwise, an anesthetic technique similar to one for elective situations is used. For patients undergoing neck exploration for a wound hematoma following CEA, a tracheostomy or cricothyroidotomy tray should be immediately available, as well as other devices for management of the difficult airway. Esmolol is particularly useful to control hyperdynamic cardiovascular responses during awake intubation. If any difficulty is expected, the wound is opened and drained externally, and tracheal intubation is performed before general anesthesia is induced.

AORTIC RECONSTRUCTION

Each possible surgical approach to aortic reconstruction has risks and benefits. Surgery may be undertaken to correct aneurysmal or occlusive disease; sometimes the two coexist. Increasingly, endovascular repair of aortic aneurysms is supplanting traditional open repair.

Aneurysmal Disease

Aneurysms pose an ever-present threat to life because of their unpredictable tendency to rupture or embolize. Mortality from rupture may be as high as 85%, and even patients who receive emergent surgery have mortality rates one-half that. Therefore, early recognition and aggressive surgical management are warranted, even in the absence of symptoms.

Epidemiology and Pathophysiology of Abdominal Aortic Aneurysm

There are approximately 200,000 new AAAs diagnosed annually, with approximately 45,000 undergoing surgical repair per year in the United States. A population-based study in Norway in 1994 to 1995 used ultrasound to measure renal and infrarenal aortic diameters; an aneurysm was present in 8.9% of men and 2.2% of women ($p < 0.001$). Risk factors for aneurysm included advanced age, smoking >40 years, hypertension, low serum high-density lipoprotein cholesterol, high level of plasma fibrinogen, and low blood platelet count. In 2005, the U.S. Preventive Services Task Force recommended that AAA screening be done in men 65 to 75 years of age who have ever smoked, citing an increased incidence in this population. They also stated that no recommendations for women can be made because there is no evidence in the literature to support this recommendation.[114] Thoracoabdominal aneurysms also occur in patients with hypertension or other risk factors for atherosclerotic disease.

AAA represents a dilatation of the abdominal aorta generally below the level of the renal arteries. The risk of rupture of the AAA is directly related to the luminal diameter of the aortic aneurysm. The aneurysm can develop an inner lining of mural thrombus, thereby decreasing the effective luminal diameter, but the size of the mural thrombus has not been shown to significantly decrease the risk of rupture. The risk of aortic rupture is only related to the absolute diameter of the aortic aneurysm sac. The risk of rupture increases once the aneurysm is >4.5 to 5 cm in diameter. The size of the aneurysm is the most important predictor of subsequent rupture and mortality. A prospective study followed 300 consecutive patients (mean age, 70 years; 70% men) who presented with AAA (average size, 4.1 cm) and were initially managed nonoperatively. The diameter of the aneurysm increased by a median of 0.3 cm per year. The 6-year cumulative incidence of rupture was 1% among patients with aneurysms <4.0 cm and 2% for aneurysms 4.0 to 4.9 cm in diameter. By comparison, the 6-year cumulative incidence of rupture was 20% among patients with aneurysms >5.0 cm in diameter.[59] Larger aneurysms expand even more rapidly, and aneurysms >5 cm should be considered for surgical or endovascular repair. With frequent monitoring, watchful waiting may be preferable to repair in patients with AAAs of 4.0 to 5.4 cm in diameter. Unfortunately, in most patients with AAA rupture (surgical mortality approaching 50%), the diagnosis of AAA was unknown beforehand. These data reinforce the importance of screening of the high-risk population to permit elective repair at the appropriate time.

Pathophysiology of Aortic Occlusion and Reperfusion

Cardiovascular Changes

The classic investigations of Gelman[115] define the pathophysiology of hemodynamic changes during aortic cross-clamping and unclamping. Aortic cross-clamping increases the mean arterial pressure and systemic vascular resistance up to 50%. This is attributed to a sudden increase in impedance to aortic flow (afterload), activation of renin, and release of catecholamines, prostaglandins, and other active vasoconstrictors. Cardiac output initially decreases in the face of high systemic vascular resistance, and that decrease may be reinforced by the decrease in oxygen consumption below the aortic cross-clamp (Figs. 42-11 to 42-13, Table 42-4). Some of the initial changes

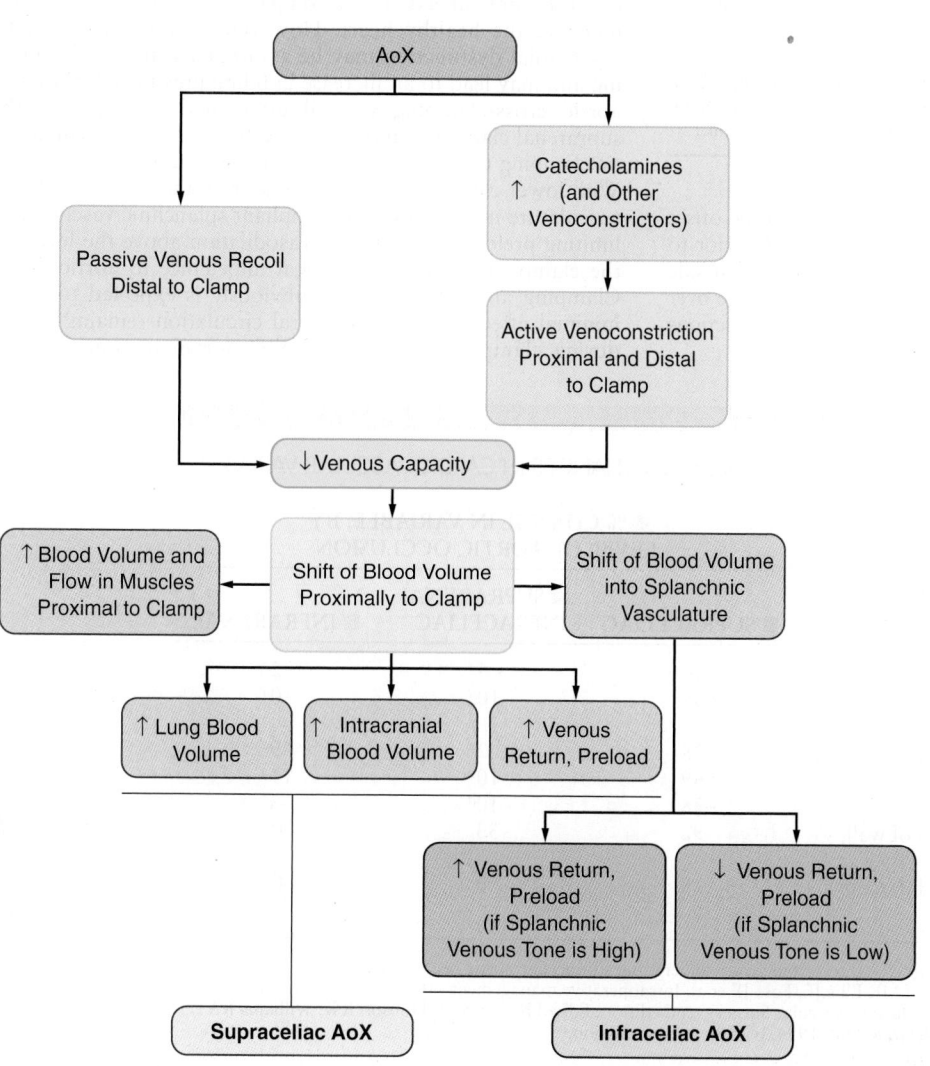

FIGURE 42-11. Blood volume redistribution during aortic cross-clamping (AoX). This schedule depicts the reason for the decrease in venous capacity, which results in blood volume redistribution from the vasculature distal-to-aortic occlusion to the vasculature proximal-to-aortic occlusion. If the aorta is occluded above the splanchnic system, the blood volume travels to the heart, increasing preload and blood volume in all organs and tissues proximal to the clamp. However, if the aorta is occluded below the splanchnic system, blood volume may shift into the splanchnic system or into the vasculature of other tissues proximal to the clamp. The distribution of this blood volume between the splanchnic and nonsplanchnic vasculature determines changes in preload. ↑ and ↓, increase and decrease, respectively. (Reprinted from Gelman S: The pathophysiology of aortic cross-clamping and unclamping. Anesthesiology 1995; 82: 1026, with permission.)

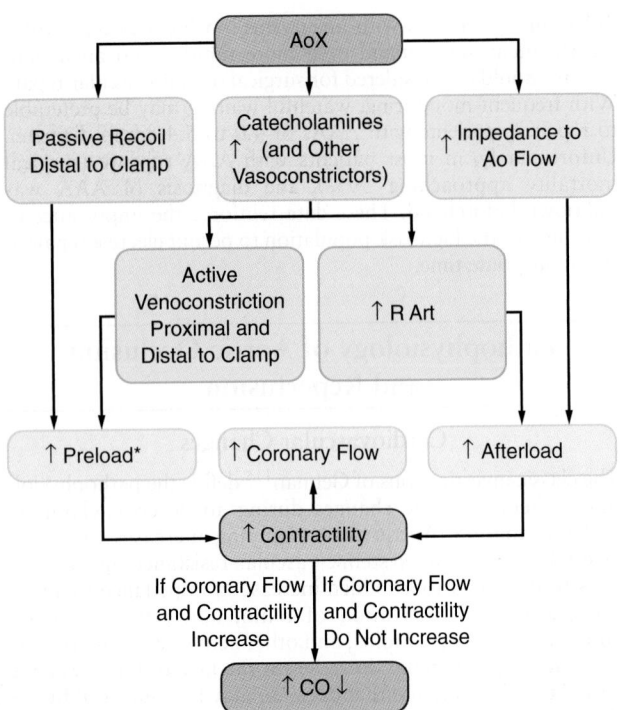

FIGURE 42-12. Systemic hemodynamic response to aortic cross-clamping (AoX). Preload does not necessarily increase. If during infrarenal aortic cross-clamping blood volume shifts into the splanchnic vasculature, preload does not increase (see Fig. 42-7). Ao, aortic; R art, arterial resistance; CO, cardiac output; ↑ and ↓, increase and decrease, respectively; *, different patterns are possible (see Fig. 42-7). (Reprinted from Gelman S: The pathophysiology of aortic cross-clamping and unclamping. Anesthesiology 1995; 82: 1026, with permission.)

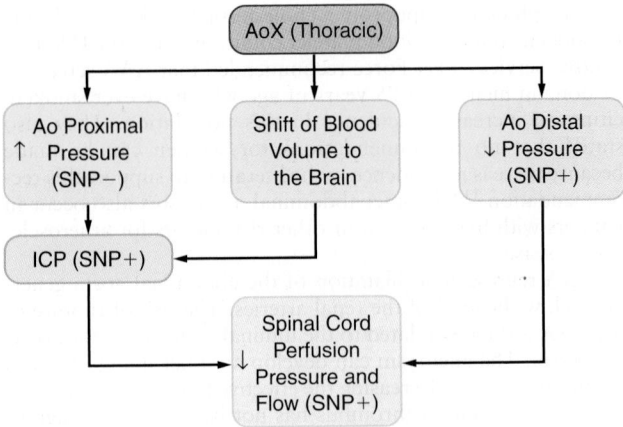

FIGURE 42-13. Spinal cord blood flow and perfusion pressure during thoracic aortic occlusion, with or without sodium nitroprusside (SNP) infusion. The changes (arrows) represent the response to aortic cross-clamping (AoX) per se. Ao, aortic; SNP−, SNP counteracts the effect of cross-clamping; SNP+, SNP aggravates the effect of cross-clamping; ICP, intercranial pressure; ↑ and ↓, increase and decrease, respectively. (Reprinted from Gelman S: The pathophysiology of aortic cross-clamping and unclamping. Anesthesiology 1995; 82: 1026, with permission.)

in hemodynamics associated with cross-clamping can be offset by boluses of a vasodilator administered immediately prior to placement of the clamp (e.g., 0.3 to 0.7 μg/kg of nitroprusside or 200 to 600 μg of nicardipine or 50 μg/kg of milrinone over 10 minutes). In this case, mechanical and pharmacologic actions cancel out each other while the body is allowed to adapt.

Preload changes are more variable than blood pressure changes. Higher central venous pressure and pulmonary artery occlusion pressures do not accompany the decrease in cardiac index in the healthy heart. However, in those with CAD, myocardial dysfunction may be associated with cross-clamping and may lead to an increase in filling pressures. Infrarenal aortic cross-clamping is well attenuated compared with suprarenal clamping, and during occlusive disease repair, aortic clamping usually has limited systemic hemodynamic effect. With lower clamping, blood volume from the infrasplanchnic vasculature may shift to the compliant splanchnic vasculature limiting preload changes, and vasodilation above the level of the clamp offsets the mechanical impedance to aortic flow. Clamping an occluded artery obviously is expected to have minimal effect. Existing collateral circulation remains intact during clamping and is responsible for maintaining lower

TABLE 42-4

EFFECT OF LEVEL OF AORTIC OCCLUSION ON CHANGES IN CARDIOVASCULAR VARIABLES

■ CARDIOVASCULAR VARIABLE	■ % CHANGE IN VARIABLE, BY LEVEL OF AORTIC OCCLUSION		
	■ SUPRACELIAC	■ SUPRARENAL INFRACELIAC	■ INFRARENAL
Mean arterial blood pressure	54	5[a]	2[a]
Pulmonary capillary wedge pressure	38	10[a]	0[a]
End-diastolic area	28	2[a]	9[a]
End-systolic area	69	10[a]	11[a]
Ejection fraction	−38	−10[a]	−3[a]
Abnormal motion of wall, % of patients	92	33	0
New myocardial infarctions, % of patients	8	0	0

[a]Statistically different (P <0.05) from group undergoing supraceliac aortic occlusion.
Adapted from Roizen MF, Ellis JE, Foss JF et al: Intraoperative management of the patient requiring supraceliac aortic occlusion, Vascular Surgery, 2nd edition. Edited by Veith FJ, Hobson RW, Williams RA et al. New York, McGraw-Hill, 1994, p 256, with permission.

body perfusion despite aortic cross-clamping. For higher clamps, nitrate therapy will not necessarily prevent wall motion abnormalities, and care should be exercised when using any vasodilator so perfusion pressure below the aortic cross-clamp remains at a level that will not potentiate visceral/spinal cord ischemia. Furthermore, utilization of a thoracic epidural at the start of the case may provide enough of a sympathectomy to mollify the increase in blood pressure seen with higher clamp levels. It may be acceptable to allow a systolic blood pressure as high as 180 to 200 mmHg as long as the surgeon has acceptable operating conditions. Even relative hypotension (<20% below resting pressure) probably should be avoided unless other means (shunts) are used to perfuse the lower part of the body and promote visceral/spinal cord blood flow.

Unclamping of the aorta can result in severe arterial hypotension unless aggressive therapy is undertaken prior to unclamping (Fig. 42-14). Various therapies are employed by anesthesiologists and surgeons, with no evidence one is superior to another. Most anesthesiologists employ some degree of fluid loading with or without vasoconstrictors such as neosynephrine (often 100 to 200 μg), norepinephrine (8 μg), or drugs such as calcium chloride (300 to 500 mg) that can offset the negative inotropic/dromotropic effects of an acute potassium and acid load (and possibly other mediators) on the heart immediately

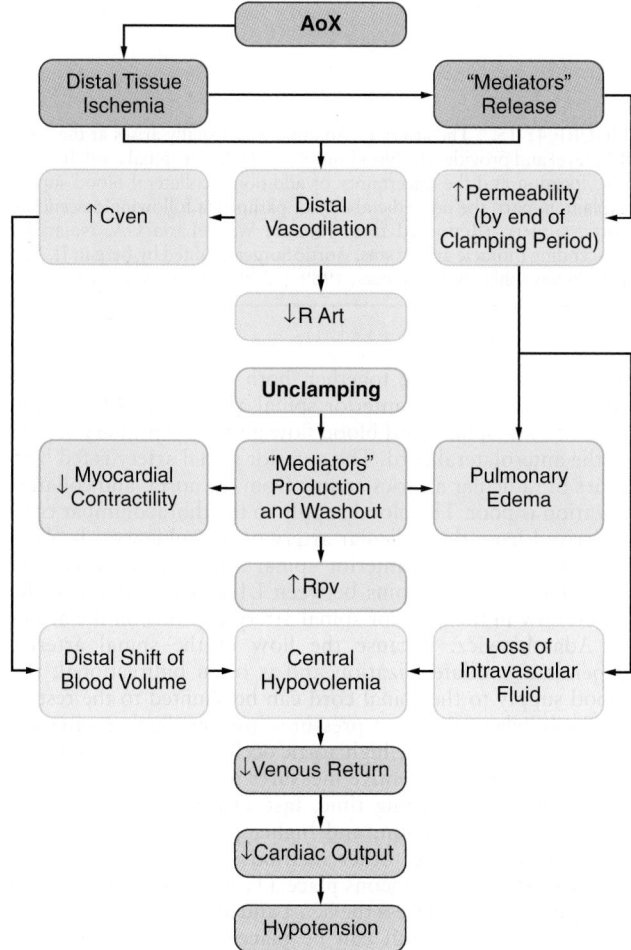

FIGURE 42-14. Systemic hemodynamic response to aortic unclamping. Preload does not necessarily increase. AoX, aortic cross-clamping; Cven, venous capacitance; R art, arterial resistance; Rpv, pulmonary vascular resistance; ↑ and ↓, increase and decrease, respectively. (Reprinted from Gelman S: The pathophysiology of aortic cross-clamping and unclamping. Anesthesiology 1995; 82: 1026, with permission.)

following reperfusion. Much preferable to pharmacologic manipulation is gradual unclamping, unclamping with gradual sequential release of bilateral femoral pressure, or restoring flow to one leg at a time in aortobifemoral grafts.

Renal Hemodynamics and Renal Protection

There is no renal protective strategy proven to yield superior outcome. The level of aortic clamping and the avoidance of prolonged hypotension are probably the most important of all the factors, as they markedly impact renal blood flow. The incidence of acute renal failure is approximately <5% postinfrarenal clamping but approaches 13% postsuprarenal clamping. Preoperative renal insufficiency and renal failure necessitating dialysis are probably the strongest predictors of mortality.[116] Postoperative mortality is four- to fivefold higher in those who develop acute renal failure when compared with those who do not. With suprarenal occlusion, renal blood flow decreases by 80%. Blood flow is not only reduced with aortic cross-clamping, but also redistributed, favoring the cortical and juxtamedullary layers over the hypoxia-prone renal medulla.[117] Even with an infrarenal aortic clamping, renal blood flow is 45% lower during cross-clamping. Renal vascular resistance increases by almost 70%. Interestingly, these renal hemodynamic changes do not immediately revert after the release of cross-clamping and persist for at least 30 minutes beyond the systemic cardiovascular return to baseline.

Many different methods of renal protection have been advocated, most of them centering on improving renal blood flow or glomerular flow. Mannitol increases diuresis (although physiologically unimportant, it often satisfies the surgeon's need to hear that there is some urine output) and functions as a hydroxyl free radical scavenger. Outcomes have not been shown to improve with its use and intraoperative urinary output is not predictive of postoperative renal function.[118] Rather, preoperative renal dysfunction is the most powerful predictor of postoperative renal dysfunction. Dopamine has been shown to lack specific renal hemodynamic effects and does not appear to improve postoperative renal dysfunction. Fenoldopam, despite its specific DA-1 activity, has not been shown to be of human clinical benefit.[119] One of the most important factors for preventing postoperative renal failure remains good hydration (as the most important factor for maintaining renal blood flow) during clamping and post-clamp release. If prolonged renal ischemia is anticipated, selective profound hypothermia with direct intra-arterial infusion of 4°C Ringer lactate into the kidneys may decrease the incidence of postoperative renal impairment.[120] Ali et al.[121] investigated the role of ischemic preconditioning on renal and myocardial injury in humans. Their findings suggest that intermittent cross-clamping of the internal iliacs prior to the insult may provide a stimulus for both renal and myocardial preconditioning. Using this technique, the incidence of renal insufficiency decreased by 23%.

Humoral and Coagulation Profiles

Although the most evident factor contributing to hypotension is volume redistribution to the lower body after aortic cross-clamp release, many humoral mediators are released from the underperfused areas and contribute to the hemodynamic changes. Among the many factors described are renin, angiotensin, epinephrine, norepinephrine, prostacyclin, endothelin, prostaglandin F1 (PGF-1), thromboxane A_2 and B_2, lactate, potassium, oxygen-free radicals, platelets activator, cytokines, activated complement (C3 and C4), and neutrophil sequestration. Administration of bicarbonate does not prevent immediate postunclamping hypotension and, in the authors' experience, can exacerbate it, probably because of the initial increase in intracellular myocardial acidity. Mannitol administration before and after unclamping may be beneficial because of its function as a hydroxyl free radical scavenger. Nonsteroidal anti-inflammatory drugs may counteract the effect of prostaglandins; however, their use remains controversial because of their potential detrimental antiplatelet and renal perfusion effects. The use of COX-2 inhibitors augments postoperative pain control and avoids any platelet effect, but still may have some renal perfusion effects that have not been studied in this context. Furthermore, although long-term COX-2 use can increase MI rate slightly,[122] there is no evidence that short-term COX-2 drugs are contraindicated in noncardiac surgery with cardiovascular disease. Taking this all into account, the authors often employ preoperative COX-2 inhibitors as part of a multimodal approach to postoperative pain control if a thoracic epidural is not employed.

A high incidence (5 to 14%) of pulmonary complications is a fact in thoracoabdominal aneurysm repair. Sequestration of microaggregates and neutrophils contributes to postoperative pulmonary dysfunction. Aortic reperfusion may result in pulmonary vasoconstriction from liberation of thromboxane A_2 and other vasoactive substances. Increased permeability and pulmonary edema are not uncommon. As noted previously, mannitol may attenuate these responses because of free radical scavenging, but no technique to date has been shown to be superior to another in this respect.

Thirty minutes after aortic cross-clamping, tissue plasminogen activator and tissue-type plasminogen activator antigen levels in the peripheral vascular bed are increased. This reflects the increase in adrenergic state. Thromboelastography studies have documented an increase in clotting factor activity during cross-clamping and decreased speed of solid clot formation after unclamping. These changes, along with a low fibrinogen level, are consistent with clotting factor consumption rather than fibrinolysis.

Visceral and Mesenteric Ischemia

Bowel ischemia is associated with a high postoperative mortality rate, approaching 25%. Factors contributing to the pathogenesis of visceral ischemia include pre-existing medical conditions, renal dysfunction, stage of aortic disease and level of aortic cross-clamping, the duration of cross-clamping, and perioperative hypotension. Hypoxic insult to the intestines during aortic occlusion leads to gut permeability and bacterial translocation as evidenced by activation of polymorphonuclear leukocytes. Peak plasma level of tumor necrosis factor and interleukin-6 are significantly higher in hypotensive patients and in those who die. With endovascular repair, intestinal ischemic events seem less profound. High doses of methylprednisolone at induction of anesthesia may be beneficial in reducing the inflammatory response, including C-reactive protein and T-cell activation levels, but have been shown to negatively impact postoperative renal function.[123] Anesthetic techniques appear to minimally influence inflammatory cytokine stress responses, which correlate most with increasing operative times. Further research is needed to determine if anti-inflammatory therapy can reduce morbidity and mortality **7** after aortic reconstructive surgery.

Central Nervous System and Spinal Cord Ischemia and Protection

Middle cerebral artery blood velocity decreases during aortic occlusion. Unclamping is followed by a transient dilation of cerebral pial arterioles, followed by a sustained vasoconstriction. These changes are due to the hemodynamic changes, CO_2 accumulation and washout, decreased pH, and release of thromboxane A_2, which is a powerful vasoconstrictor on cerebral vessels.

Spinal cord ischemia occurs in 1 to 11% of operations involving a distal aortic repair. The spinal cord is supplied by

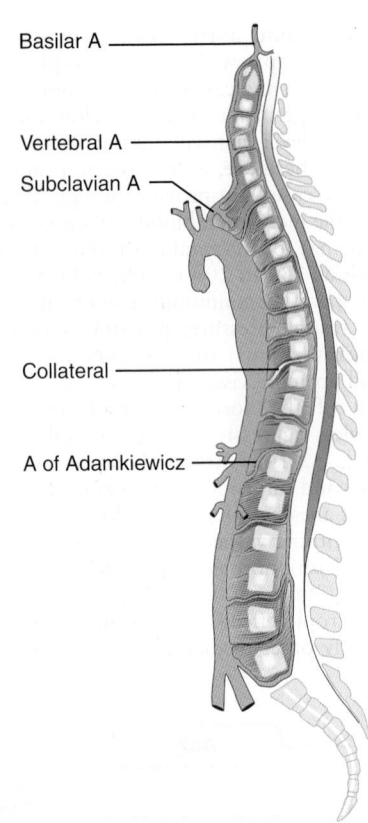

FIGURE 42-15. The artery of Adamkiewicz usually arises at the T11-T12 level and provides the blood supply to the lower spinal cord. Its variable location and the uncertainty of additional collateral blood supply explain, in part, the unpredictability of paraplegia following descending aortic surgery. (Reprinted from Piccone W, DeLaria GA, Najafi H: Descending thoracic aneurysms, Aortic Surgery. Edited by Bergan JJ, Yao JST. Philadelphia, WB Saunders, 1989, p 249, with permission.)

two posterior arteries; together, both supply 25% of spinal cord blood flow. The anterior spinal artery (Fig. 42-15) supplies 75% of spinal cord blood flow and is the primary supply to the anterolateral cord. The anterior spinal artery is fed by a series of radicular arteries arising from the aorta, and collateralization is poor. The blood supply to the thoracolumbar cord is derived from the radicular artery of Adamkiewicz. In 75% of cases, it joins the anterior spinal artery between T8 and T12, and in 10% it joins between L1 and L2. Much of the blood flow in the anterior spinal artery depends on the artery of Adamkiewicz. Because the flow in the spinal arteries depends on collateralization and is often bidirectional, the blood supply to the spinal cord can be shunted to the rest of the body when perfusion pressures are low. Such a situation may arise when a single high aortic occlusion clamp is applied.

The definitive preventive measures to spinal cord ischemia are short cross-clamping time, fast surgery, maintenance of normal cardiac function, and higher perfusion pressures. In high aortic clamping, other methods should be considered (Table 42-5). Some surgeons place a Gott shunt, a heparinized tube that can decompress the heart and also provide distal perfusion. The Gott shunt can be placed proximally into the ascending aorta (the most common site), aortic arch, descending aorta, or left ventricle, and inserted distally into the descending aorta (most commonly), femoral artery, or abdominal aorta. Even with a Gott shunt or partial bypass, there is an obligatory time of visceral ischemia when the visceral blood supply arises from a point between the proximal and distal clamps. Placement of a shunt may result in atheroembolism,

TABLE 42-5

METHODS OF SPINAL CORD PROTECTION DURING DESCENDING THORACIC AORTIC SURGERY

Limitation of cross-clamp duration
Distal circulatory support
Reattachment of critical intercostal arteries
CSF drainage
Hypothermia
  Moderate systemic (32–34°C)
  Epidural cooling
  Circulatory arrest
Maintenance of proximal blood pressure
  Pharmacotherapy
    Systemic
      Corticosteroids, barbiturates, naloxone, calcium channel antagonists, O_2 free radical scavengers, NMDA antagonists, mannitol, magnesium, vasodilators (adenosine papaverine, prostacyclin), perfluorocarbons, colchicine
    Intrathecal
      Papaverine, magnesium, tetracaine, perfluorocarbons
Avoidance of postoperative hypotension
Sequential aortic clamping
Enhanced monitoring for spinal cord ischemia
  Somatosensory evoked potentials
  Motor evoked potentials
  Hydrogen-saturated saline
  Avoidance of hyperglycemia

CSF, cerebrospinal fluid; NMDA, N-methyl-D-aspartate.
From Mas J-L, Chatellier G, Beyssen B et al: Endarterectomy versus stenting in patients with symptomatic severe carotid stenosis. N Engl J Med 2006; 355: 1660.

which can produce rather than prevent ischemic injury and death. Other surgeons may place a temporary ex vivo right axillofemoral bypass graft before positioning for thoracotomy. After the thoracic aortic surgery is completed, the axillofemoral graft is removed. The placement of a shunt or distal perfusion attenuates the hemodynamic response to aortic unclamping, reduces acidosis, and could conceivably ameliorate the hormonal and metabolic changes that accompany aortic occlusion.

Other groups have chosen to use partial bypass, either from the left atrium or ascending aorta to the iliac or femoral artery to provide distal perfusion and decompress the heart. A heat exchanger may be used to induce hypothermia, which may be neuroprotective. Segmental sequential surgical repair may minimize the duration of ischemia to any given vascular bed. Intercostal artery reattachment in hopes of preserving blood flow to the anterior spinal cord may also be beneficial. After reperfusion, the heat exchanger can be used to warm the patient. Other potential advantages of left atrial–left femoral artery shunt with centrifugal pump support are better operative field exposure, afterload reduction, maintenance of stable distal aortic perfusion, and reduced (but not eliminated) head and neck edema.

A markedly reduced incidence of neurologic deficits has been reported when distal aortic perfusion is combined with drainage of cerebrospinal fluid (CSF).[124] CSF drainage is used in the hope of improving the pressure gradient, allowing spinal cord blood flow as aortic occlusion lowers distal arterial pressures and increases the central venous pressure. The new endovascular techniques represent an alternative therapy when anatomy permits; lower paraplegia rates have been reported compared with open surgery.[125]

Traditional "Open" Surgical Procedures for Aortic Reconstruction

Perioperative (i.e., 30-day) mortality in elective aortic surgeries ranges between 0 and 12%, with a much higher probability of death in emergent surgery, especially in those situations in which preoperative hypotension (systolic blood pressure <90 mm Hg) exists. Hypotension increases the risk by threefold, whereas pre-existing heart disease, including CAD and CHF, increase the risk of mortality by 2.5-fold to fivefold. As stated previously, other identifiable risks for increased mortality are gender, with slight increase in women, age >80 years, and patients with serum creatinine above 2 mg/dL. The size alone of an aneurysm does not appear to influence operative mortality. Expeditious surgery with better graft materials, minimal clamp time, and blood conservation, along with better understanding of the pathophysiology of the disease, have made aortic surgery safer.

Arterial reconstruction surgery was developed based on normal anatomy. Although this is usually the easiest and best option, situations do occur that require circuitous revascularization procedures, such as axillofemoral or femoral-femoral bypass. These situations include graft infection, repeat surgery, and a hostile abdomen, such as one encounters with postradiation states, adhesions, sepsis, and malignancy. It should be emphasized that overall these procedures have lower long-term patency rates than anatomically correct procedures.

Approach

Abdominal aortic reconstruction can be performed through a transperitoneal or retroperitoneal exposure. In the first case, a thoracoabdominal midline incision is performed and the aorta is accessed through the peritoneum. This generous exposure is usually favored for complex aortic reconstruction or replacement. In the retroperitoneal approach, incision is made over the lateral border of the left rectus muscle, 2 cm below the umbilicus to the 12th rib. This will allow access to the aorta from the crux of the diaphragm to its bifurcation. The retroperitoneal technique allows a surgical exposure as good as the transperitoneal approach and is associated with less fluid shift, faster return of bowel function, lower pulmonary complications, shorter ICU stay, and lower overall hospital cost, with an average savings of $4,000 to $5,000.[126] The retroperitoneal approach is considered by many to be more appropriate in cases of truncal obesity, chronic obstructive pulmonary disease (COPD), hostile abdomen (e.g., previous surgeries), and juxtarenal aneurysm. However, the flank approach is not a panacea, as frequent chronic wound pain, incisional hernias, and abdominal bulges have been reported. Intraoperative blood loss during open AAA repair can be significant and depends on the size and complexity of the AAA. The postoperative course usually requires admission to the ICU for several days. The postoperative recovery period after the open repair can be several months.

Clamp Level

Infrarenal aortic clamping carries the lowest risk for patients; supraceliac clamping carries the highest. Anesthesiologists should be aware that 10 to 20% of "infrarenal" aortic disease will actually involve the suprarenal portion of the aorta, necessitating suprarenal clamping. Ruptured aneurysms often must be controlled initially by supraceliac clamping because of anatomic considerations.

Thoracic Aneurysm Repair

These operations are among the most challenging for anesthesiologists. Coincident CAD and COPD are common.

Lung isolation is required to facilitate surgical access to the aneurysm and to avoid an iatrogenic pulmonary contusion in the left lung. Lung isolation may be provided with either double-lumen tubes, bronchial blockers, or endotracheal tubes with incorporated bronchial blockers. Bronchial blockers might be advantageous when postoperative ventilation may be needed as a single-lumen endotracheal tube is already in place and there is no need to exchange the tube as with a double-lumen tube. Because edema of the head and neck frequently occur after high cross-clamping (even with distal perfusion), reintubation may be difficult at the end of the procedure. Generous exposure of the thoracic and abdominal aorta and its major branches can be obtained with a left thoracoabdominal incision and retroperitoneal dissection. The thoracoabdominal approach is favored for complex thoracoabdominal aortic replacement in the presence of stenotic or aneurysmal disease. The visceral branches are often excised from the parent aorta with a button of aortic wall. Identification of large intercostal vessels may warrant reanastomosis to the grafted section as well to optimize spinal cord perfusion after repair. If the patient also has mesenteric occlusive disease, endarterectomy of these branch vessels is performed before they are attached as "buttons" to the graft at appropriate positions. If only mesenteric revascularization is to be performed and aortic replacement is not used, endarterectomy of any or all the major branches of the aorta may be performed with this exposure.

Aortomesenteric Revascularization

Chronic mesenteric ischemia occurs because of atherosclerosis or dissection. Surgical revascularization is indicated only in symptomatic disease. This will occur when two of the main mesenteric vessels become occluded. Elective surgery for asymptomatic occlusive disease is not justified because of the high risk of perioperative mortality, which can range from 7 to 18%. Cardiac events, hemorrhage, and bowel infarction are the most dreaded complications. In symptomatic cases, elective surgical reconstruction with or without concomitant aortic replacement remains the best choice because percutaneous transluminal angioplasty and stenting are associated with a significant incidence of recurrence and should be reserved to specific cases. Partial cross-clamping of the aorta is preferred, if possible, and may mitigate hemodynamic changes.

Acute mesenteric ischemia differs in its genesis. It is usually the result of an acute embolic event or trauma. The presence or absence of intestinal infarction plays a major role in the patient's overall prognosis in this setting. Endarterectomy of the mesenteric arteries may be performed through a transaortic access for isolated disease, or before the attachment of the vessels to the aortic graft at appropriate positions. If single-vessel endarterectomy is performed, it may be carried out for either the celiac axis or the superior mesenteric artery.

Aortorenal Revascularization

Renal artery revascularization can be performed by endarterectomy, reimplantation, bypass, and ex vivo renal artery reconstruction. Extra-anatomic renal artery bypass may be best suited for sick, debilitated patients who would not tolerate aortic clamping. Percutaneous approaches have largely replaced surgery for isolated renal artery revascularization.

Infrarenal Operations

Reconstruction of the infrarenal aorta is performed by exposing the relevant portion of the aorta and the iliac arteries. Heparin is commonly administered through a central line to reduce the risk of thromboembolic events before aortic clamping. Although it is generally recognized that distal ischemic complications are due to dislodgment of atheromatous material off the diseased aorta and that the systemic use of heparin in the absence of distal occlusive disease is unnecessary, many centers still employ heparin before aortic clamping. Aortic repair is carried out by interposition of a graft with an end-to-end anastomosis. Collagen-impregnated polyester fiber (Dacron) grafts make up the majority of implanted grafts. Dacron grafts appear to be associated with rare episodes of anaphylactic reactions, which may be related to the stabilizers used in their manufacture. Polytetrafluoroethylene (PTFE) grafts are less porous and are gaining more widespread use. Aortobiiliac, aortobifemoral, and aortoiliac/femoral grafts are used in most cases. Straight grafting constitutes approximately 30% of cases.

Thoracic Aortic Surgery and Endovascular Repair

Traditional surgery for thoracic aortic aneurysm continues to be associated with higher morbidity and mortality than infrarenal AAAs. The analysis of large databases suggests that population-based perioperative mortality is higher than that reported in series from selected institutions.[127] Mortality may approach 20%; risk factors include diabetes mellitus, cerebrovascular disease, and renal insufficiency. Median hospital charges ($64,000) are also high. Therefore, endovascular thoracoabdominal aortic aneurysm repair (endoTAAR) has been advocated as an alternative to open surgery. Complications may be lower with endovascular approaches, with blood loss averaging 500 mL and 1 day in the ICU for uncomplicated cases. Although paraplegia still may occur after endoTAAR, its incidence seems reduced compared with open thoracic aortic aneurysm repair (TAAR).[125] One approach to attempt to lessen paraplegia after endoTAAR has been to place a temporary stent under SSEP monitoring; if SSEP is unchanged, a permanent stent may be placed. However, motor evoked potential monitoring would seem more appropriate for monitoring function of the anterior spinal column.[128]

Another possibility that has been shown to confer protection in animal models is intermittent aortic cross-clamping. Repetitive cycles of cross-clamping serve as the stimulus for spinal cord preconditioning. The periods of ischemia were followed with SSEPs. There were no cases of paraplegia in the repetitive exposure group.[129] In addition, a spinal drain may be placed pre-emptively to maintain low (≤ 8 cm H_2O) intrathecal pressures during the operation and allow for drainage of CSF, intraoperatively or postoperatively. Successful treatment of paraplegia with induced hypertension and CSF drainage following endoTAAR has been reported by several authors. The use of a single continuous subarachnoid catheter, first for local anesthetic injection to facilitate femoral or iliac arterial access in the groins and later for prophylactic removal of CSF, has been described during endoTAAR.[130] Aspiration of CSF does not result in loss of the sensory or motor blockade if performed 15 to 20 minutes after local anesthetic instillation.

Endovascular Abdominal Aortic Repair

Endovascular abdominal aortic repair (EVAAR) pioneered by Parodi et al.[131] in the 1980s has made significant progress in all aspects. In the early stages of development, stent grafts were hand-made and were used only to repair AAAs in patients deemed to be too high risk for conventional open aortic repair (OAR). With the advent of new technology, the rapid spread of the skill sets needed to place these grafts, and the demonstration that these grafts are not only safe but also becoming durable, EVAAR is now being used more commonly in patients who would otherwise undergo an open repair.

Development of Graft Technology and Patient Selection

The endovascular stents used in the early 1990s were unibody ("straight tube graft") polymer mesh fabrics. These could be used only in the small minority of patients who had ample normal aorta to seat the graft both below the renal arteries and above the iliac bifurcation. Subsequently, modular grafting systems allow extension above the renal arteries by means of suprarenal fixation (open metal framework) and distal touch down at or below the common iliacs. Currently in the United States three grafts are approved by the Food and Drug Administration: AneuRx (Medtronic, Minneapolis, MN), Excluder (W. L. Gore and Associates, Flagstaff, AZ), and Zenith (Cook Medical, Bloomington, IN). Many other grafts are currently in various stages of development. Risk of rupture and aneurysm-related death among all devices was extremely low at <1%, although there was an overall 15% requirement for secondary operative procedures.[132]

Patient eligibility for EVAAR depends on (1) the shape of the aneurysm, including involvement of the renal and iliac arteries and the size and shape of the neck of the aneurysm; (2) the feasibility of delivering the device through the femoral or iliac arteries; and (3) the ability of the patient to compensate for vascular exclusion (aortic branches that will not be supplied once the stent graft is in place). Preoperative evaluation for EVAAR should be as thorough as for open repair. Special attention needs to be focused on renal function by comparing preoperative creatinine levels to previous ones to determine if intravascular dye used in preoperative testing has decreased creatinine clearance. If there has been a decrease in renal function, sufficient time, typically 2 weeks, should be allowed between the last dye load and the time of operation. It is estimated that up to 60% of patients may be able to undergo EVAAR with the new, smaller modular grafts that are under development.

Outcome and Complications

With increasing experience and improved technology, some outcomes from EVAAR have improved. Intraoperative conversion to OAR because of aneurysm rupture, vascular injury, or inability to deliver or seal the device (endoleak; see later discussion) is now typically <2%.[133] Perioperative mortality is <5%, as compared with 5.4 to 8.2% for open repair. Cardiac and pulmonary morbidity is also <5%, and renal insufficiency is <3%.[133] In one study, aortic interruption was <1 minute for EVAAR as compared with 51 minutes for open repair, and there was significantly less tissue trauma and bleeding.[134] The patients who underwent EVAAR had no significant change in their heart rate, blood pressure, pulmonary capillary wedge pressure, stroke volume, or their stroke work index. Thirty minutes after aortic reperfusion, 57% of patients undergoing OAR had myocardial ischemia detected by ECG or regional wall motion abnormality on transesophageal echocardiogram as compared with 33% in EVAAR ($p = 0.01$). These changes were transient, and there were no differences in perioperative MI or death in this 120-patient cohort.[134,135] In patients at low risk for cardiopulmonary morbidity, there is a significantly lower rate of perioperative mortality in EVAAR rather than OAR (0% vs 1.7%, $p = 0.04$).[133] Patients who were deemed too high risk for OAR and underwent EVAAR had a similar rate of mortality as those patients who underwent OAR (4% vs. 4.4%). Length of stay after the initial operation is significantly shorter in EVAAR (5 vs. 8 days, $p = 0.009$), and ICU stay was shorter (1 vs. 3 days, $p = 0.03$).[136] Unfortunately, these benefits of mortality and shorter hospital stay do not translate into cost savings, primarily because of the high cost of the stents and the increased number of imaging studies. Furthermore, after EVAAR up to 20% of patients require reoperation for treatment of endoleak or malposition, as compared with a 5.4% rate of reoperation after OAR. Consequently, after 1 year of follow-up, there is no significant difference in mortality, total length of stay, or cost.[136]

New-onset or worsening of pre-existing renal failure is a significant source of perioperative morbidity and mortality in EVAAR. Approximately 6% of all patients undergoing EVAAR who present for surgery with normal renal function suffer a significant decrease in creatinine clearance, with 2% of patients requiring dialysis. The rate of significant worsening of renal function is 4 times more likely in those patients who start out with renal insufficiency.[137] This is very similar to traditional open repair in which the incidence of new-onset renal dysfunction is 5.4%, and that increases two- to threefold in patients with pre-existing renal insufficiency. Much of the renal dysfunction in EVAAR is believed to stem from the use of intravenous contrast pre- and intraoperatively. Limiting the amount of dye and ensuring intravascular hydration has been shown to reduce the worsening of creatinine clearance. Allowing adequate time for renal recovery between preoperative studies and EVAAR may be of benefit. Recently, magnetic resonance angiography or gadolinium-based contrast studies have been proposed for patients at risk for contrast-mediated nephropathy. The use of CO_2 as contrast media and endovascular ultrasound to limit the use of radio-opaque dye should help reduce nephropathy.

The variable anatomy of the aorta and its branches combined with the limited geometry of even the newest modular stents often results in the exclusion (nonperfusion) of even major aortic branches during EVAAR. Nonperfusion of the hypogastric artery can lead to abdominal complaints. The inferior mesenteric artery is occasionally excluded, and bowel ischemia can result if flow through the superior mesenteric artery is compromised. The artery of Adamkiewicz is typically excluded, and this can increase the risk of distal spinal cord ischemia, particularly in patients who have undergone thoracic aortic replacement. Currently there are no good data on the rate or severity of complications resulting from vascular exclusion, but bowel and pelvic ischemia should be strongly considered in patients suffering from lactic acidosis or diffuse abdominal or pelvic pain after EVAAR.

Endoleaks are leaks around or through the graft and are categorized by type (Fig. 42-16).[138] Type I endoleaks involve an inadequate proximal or distal seal. Type II endoleaks result from backflow from collaterals, such as lumbar arterial branches or the inferior mesenteric artery. Type III endoleaks arise from defects in the fabric or seal failures in which modular components overlap. Finally, type IV endoleaks are secondary to the porosity of graft fabrics and typically resolve after reversal of the anticoagulation employed for the EVAAR procedure. Any type I or III endoleaks are corrected as soon as they are detected, usually by placement of additional graft material. Conversely, type II and IV leaks are observed over weeks or months before intervention. Type II endoleaks are often treated by embolization.

Endoleaks are important because if there is continued pressurization of the aneurysm it can still expand and cause symptoms, cause compression or kinking of the graft, or it can even rupture the native aneurysm. Endoleaks occur in up to 20% of EVAAR, and account for the majority of secondary surgical interventions.[136]

Anesthetic Techniques

Most initial reports from the mid-1990s indicated that general anesthesia was used. Recently, many groups have reported using regional and local anesthetic infiltration combined with monitored anesthesia care sedation protocols with great success. The surgeon will require an immobile patient as he or she strives to position modular graft components. The surgeon will typically gain access to the aorta via the femoral or iliac arteries. Rarely, retroperitoneal vascular access is necessary,

FIGURE 42-16. Categories of endoleaks. Type I: inadequate proximal or distal seal. Type II: backflow from collaterals, such as lumbar arterial branches or the inferior mesenteric artery. Type III: defects in the fabric or seal failures where modular components overlap. Type IV: porosity of graft fabrics; typically resolve after reversal of the anticoagulation employed for the endovascular abdominal aortic repair procedure. (Reprinted from White GH, May J, Waugh RC et al: Type III and type IV endoleak: Toward a complete definition of blood flow in the sac after endoluminal AAA repair. J Endovasc Surg 1998; 5: 305, with permission.)

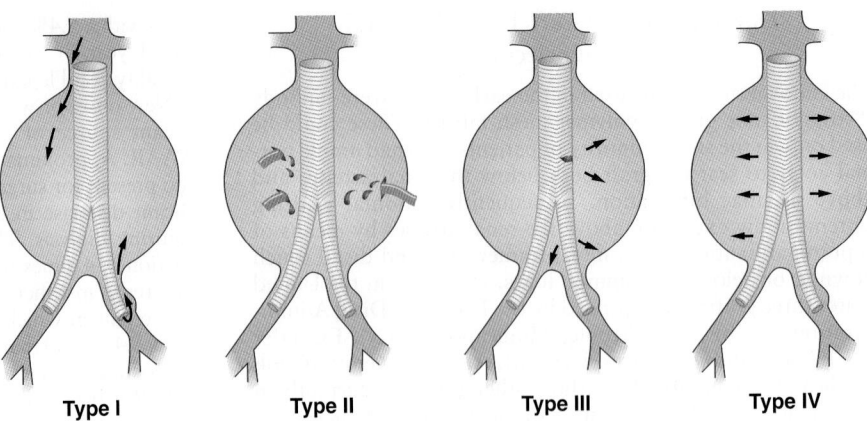

Type I   **Type II**   **Type III**   **Type IV**

which typically makes local anesthesia with monitored anesthesia care inadequate. A recent analysis by Ruppert et al.,[139] using the EUROSTAR database, found that patients who had local/regional anesthesia had lower morbidity and mortality than those having general anesthesia. Further, local/regional anesthesia was associated with shorter hospital stay and lower costs. However, anesthetic type was not randomly assigned and the "sicker" patients may have had general anesthesia. Consequently, anesthetic type remains a choice based on the preferences of the patient, anesthesiologist, and surgeon. Prior to device insertion, systemic anticoagulation will be started with a typical heparin dose of 5,000 units with a goal of activated coagulation time of ≥200 seconds. At the time of device deployment, awake patients will be asked to hold their breath, and mean arterial pressure is often lowered to decrease the risk of distal migration of the stent. After device deployment, anticoagulation is reversed and activated coagulation time rechecked. Typically, regardless of anesthetic choice, large-bore intravenous access, arterial line monitoring, and active warming are employed for all patients (Fig. 42-17).

Follow-Up and Costs

The DREAM trial[140] and the EVAR-1 trial[141] were two very high-quality studies that randomized 1,413 subjects between

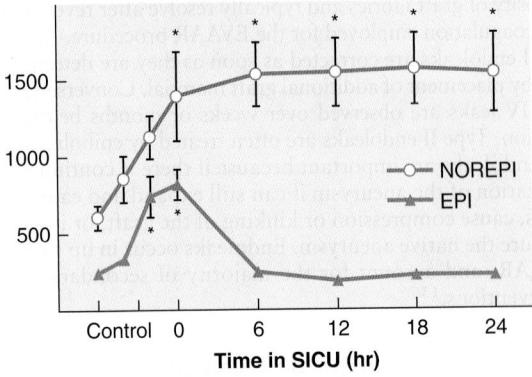

FIGURE 42-17. Aortic reconstructive surgery is associated with markedly elevated adrenergic tone. Epinephrine levels (in picograms per milliliter) rise with emergence from anesthesia but begin to fall by 6 hours after surgery. Norepinephrine levels (in picograms per milliliter) remain elevated for at least 1 day following surgery. NOREPI, norepinephrine; EPI, epinephrine; SICU, surgical ICU. (Reprinted from Breslow MJ: The role of stress hormones in perioperative myocardial ischemia. Int Anesthesiol Clin 1992; 30: 81, with permission.)

EVAAR and OAR of AAAs. Neither trial found a long-term all-cause mortality or quality of life advantage for EVAAR over OAR. EVAR-1 trial results indicated that graft rupture, infection, graft leak (including endoleak), thrombosis, and reoperation were 5 times more likely in the endovascular group (17.6 vs. 3.3 per 100 patient-years of follow-up). Reintervention through the 4-year follow-up was 3 times more common in endovascular group. The DREAM trial results indicated that rates of severe adverse events was similar between the two groups at 2 years (16.9% endovascular vs. 19.4% open). Schermerhorn et al.[142] studied 22,830 matched Medicare beneficiaries who underwent AAA repair between 2001 and 2004 with follow-up through 2005 and indicated that EVAAR and open OAR repair had similar outcomes. Perioperative mortality was lower after endovascular repair (1.2% vs. 4.8%, $p < 0.001$), with greater benefit for those who were 85 years of age or older, but survival became equivalent after 3 years.

Surprisingly, EVAAR has not reduced the cost of AAA repair. The cost of the initial hospitalization for surgery should be much less expensive for EVAAR than OAR because of the 3- to 5-day difference in the length of stay, but the cost of the device and the need for additional interventions, particularly radiologic follow-up of endovascular leaks, typically nullifies any cost savings.[143]

A cost analysis of the DREAM trial[144] indicates that at 1 year of follow-up, endovascular repair is associated with a euro 4293 (US $ 6500) greater direct cost ($p = 0.01$, 95% CI 2770–5830).

Conversion from EVAAR to OAR

Primary conversion, or the immediate alteration of the surgical plan from an endovascular approach to an open one, occurs in the setting of aneurysm rupture, stent migration or malposition, access site disruption with arterial wall dissection, and poor anatomic parameters for endovascular repair. For the anesthesiologist, the complexity of the operation will increase dramatically. Hemodynamic instability may ensue with either hemorrhage or aortic cross-clamping, or both. Secondary conversion may be performed where a stent has been placed and, on follow-up, either the aneurysm sac continues to enlarge or a persistent endoleak is noted. Another reason for secondary conversion is aneurysm rupture despite successful sac exclusion. Although the occurrence of some of these complications is low, the associated mortality is quite high. The incidence of late conversion is between 0.6 and 2%. Secondary conversion was found to have a perioperative mortality of 27% up to 50% if aneurysm rupture has occurred. Primary conversion may have a lower mortality, but is still considerable.

Monitoring and Anesthetic Choices for Aortic Reconstruction

Arterial catheters are placed in patients undergoing aortic reconstruction. In patients undergoing thoracic aortic clamping with distal perfusion, distal arterial pressure and CSF pressure may be measured. Pulmonary artery catheters are placed at the discretion of the anesthesiologist in patients undergoing suprarenal aortic cross-clamp, but rarely in patients when the clamp will be infrarenal. However, recent large randomized trials and observational studies have not been able to demonstrate any improvements in outcome with pulmonary artery catheters.[145]

For patients undergoing thoracic or thoracoabdominal aortic resection, a large double-lumen introducer in an internal jugular or subclavian vein provides two very large-bore routes for volume resuscitation and allows passage of a pulmonary artery catheter if desired. For a patient undergoing an infrarenal procedure, a simple 9-Fr introducer in the right internal jugular vein (with a triple-lumen central venous catheter or a pulmonary artery catheter) and a large-bore peripheral intravenous catheter are sufficient.

If CSF drainage is elected, a specialized silastic lumbar drainage catheters is placed into the intrathecal space at L3-L4 or L4-L5. These catheters have a one-way pressure valve that allows drainage only when the CSF pressure exceeds 5 to 10 mm Hg. Some clinicians have placed them the night before surgery in case a "bloody tap" results so clotting may be assured. Removal is planned after the likelihood of paraplegia has declined and after coagulopathy (which is common after thoracoabdominal repair) has resolved, usually on the second or third postoperative day. Communication with the ICU team regarding the CSF drain is critical as excessive drainage of CSF can be detrimental.

Virtually all anesthetic techniques and drugs have been used for aortic reconstructive surgery. The ability to maintain hemodynamic equilibrium and attend to detail is more crucial to outcome than is the choice of drugs. Volatile anesthetics provide a means of controlling afterload and preload but can lead to an increased need for intravascular volume. Perhaps the most important reason to routinely include volatile agents in general anesthetics is the increasing awareness that volatile anesthetics improve preconditioning mechanisms and reduce the size of MI, should it occur.[146] These effects have been documented in animal models and in CABG surgery in humans, but not in vascular surgery patients. In the authors' practice, a volatile anesthetic is combined with low doses of sufentanil (2 to 5 μg/kg) if an epidural is not used.

Combined general epidural and general spinal anesthetics have been used successfully for aortic reconstruction. For patients requiring thoracotomy, the analgesia provided by thoracic epidural infusion of narcotics and/or local anesthetics may be particularly helpful. Some clinicians are reluctant to use epidural anesthesia for supraceliac aortic reconstruction because of concerns about concurrent heparinization and the associated incidence of paraplegia. In such patients, the use of peridural narcotics without local anesthetics can preserve sensory and motor function and can allow early assessment of neurologic integrity. Intrathecal narcotics are a potential alternative after supraceliac aortic occlusion. Another disadvantage of epidural local anesthetics is that patients may require increased amounts of intravenous fluids.

Management of Elective Aortic Surgery

Prehydration may limit variations in blood pressure on induction of anesthesia. The anesthetic management is planned to keep the patient's vital signs within 20% of his or her normal range, as long as the heart rate does not exceed 80 to 90 beats per minute and signs of organ ischemia are absent. During the pre–cross-clamping phase, it is crucial to maintain temperature homeostasis (unless hypothermia is desired for its potential spinal cord protection), left ventricular end-diastolic volume as assessed by echocardiography, and stable hemodynamics. Increases in blood pressure or heart rate may be treated with 10 to 50 μg of sufentanil.

For the half-hour immediately before cross-clamping and aortic occlusion, the patient is kept slightly hypovolemic by examining the ventricular volume by means of echocardiography or by keeping pulmonary capillary wedge pressure at 5 to 15 mm Hg. At the time of occlusion, a vasodilating drug is available for immediate use if needed. Alternatively, the concentration of volatile anesthetic may be increased or local anesthetics injected into the epidural catheter. Both of these latter approaches require careful attention to avoid hypotension. A novel approach to reduce blood pressure in the face of aortic occlusion has been described using placement of 15-cm positive end-expiratory pressure immediately before cross-clamp, with removal just before unclamping.[147] This approach facilitates volume loading and reduces hypotension after unclamping. The authors' approach is different when there is concern about spinal cord perfusion. In these instances, some proximal hypertension while the aorta is occluded may provide higher distal perfusion pressures and prevent distal ischemia. This choice may come at the expense of myocardial well-being. In fact, 92% of the patients studied had ischemia, as evidenced by abnormal motion and thickening of the left ventricle (Table 42-4). Administration of exogenous vasoconstrictors is avoided, if possible. Adequate volume at the time of cross-clamp removal is best achieved by replacing blood that is lost during occlusion with crystalloid or colloid, warmed cell-saver blood, or banked blood to keep the hematocrit slightly above 30% because it will decrease to 30% in the postocclusion period.

The authors recommend the use of autotransfusion devices; they may not reduce transfusion of allogenic blood but only delay it. After the sixth unit of blood has been given and if more blood loss is anticipated, or after eight units of blood have been administered, ten units of platelets are requested for the patient (and occasionally two units of fresh-frozen plasma). Because a large part of the vascular tree is excluded from circulation during temporary aortic occlusion, blood loss can be considerable during supraceliac cross-clamping without the onset of hypotension or tachycardia. Evisceration of bowel, often necessary for optimal exposure of the thoracoabdominal aorta, further depletes intravascular volume. Blood loss into the pleural or retroperitoneal cavity may not be readily detected.

Immediately before removal of the cross-clamp, vasodilators are discontinued. The surgeon then opens the aorta gradually to ensure that severe hypotension or bleeding does not develop. Crystalloid, colloid, or blood is administered just before reperfusion guided by filling pressures or echocardiographic estimates of volume. Pulmonary artery pressures or central venous pressure may increase because reperfusion of ischemic tissues is associated with the release of lactic acid and other unknown mediators that can cause pulmonary vasoconstriction. Mannitol prophylaxis may prevent part of this response.

During emergence from anesthesia, infusions of nitroglycerin and esmolol or another β-adrenergic blocking agent are used if necessary to prevent hemodynamic variations outside the patient's normal range. If appropriate, the trachea is extubated at the conclusion of surgery. Prophylactic beta-blockade is continued into the postoperative period, as tolerated. In unstable patients, esmolol may be infused; in more stable patients, metoprolol 5 to 10 mg intravenously every 6 hours, as long as heart rate is >55 beats per minute and blood pressure is >110 mm Hg.

Anesthesia for Emergency Aortic Surgery

The most common cause of emergency aortic reconstruction is a leaking or ruptured aortic aneurysm. Ruptured aneurysms carry associated mortality roughly 10 times greater than elective repair. Symptoms of ruptured AAAs include pain, faintness or frank collapse, and vomiting. Pain in the back, abdomen, or both is almost always present. Therefore, many surgeons believe pain in combination with a known AAA or pulsatile abdominal mass indicates dissection or rupture and the immediate need for surgical exploration until proved otherwise. Ruptures most commonly occur into the retroperitoneum. This site permits tamponade of the hemorrhage; however, retroperitoneal hemorrhage and subsequent hematoma can displace the left renal vein, inferior vena cava, and intestine, possibly leading to damage to these structures during the surgical approach. Venous hemorrhage is often much more difficult to control than arterial hemorrhage. Approximately 25% of aneurysms rupture into the peritoneal cavity, a site associated with a great degree of exsanguination. Other sites of rupture include adjacent structures after formation of fistulae with the inferior vena cava, iliac veins, renal veins, or bowel.

Shock frequently accompanies rupture. However, the absence of hypotension does not rule out the possibility of rupture, and shock may occur suddenly. Rapid diagnosis with immediate laparotomy and control of the proximal aorta are of the highest priority. More recently, reports suggest significantly better results with a novel, multifaceted approach, which includes endovascular repair with a proprietary device, balloon inflation above the site of rupture to mimic "cross-clamping," hypotensive hemostasis, limited fluid resuscitation, and monitored anesthesia care. The endovascular approach to patients with ruptured AAAs may be limited because of the need for time-consuming measurement (angiography) and the expense of keeping multiple-size grafts in inventory. Future studies will define the role of endovascular therapy in emergent and rupture situations.

Because of hypothermia from massive fluid resuscitation and the aortic occlusion above the hepatic artery, replacement blood may not pass through the liver in amounts adequate to allow for metabolism of citrate. Therefore, if hypotension related to poor myocardial contractility or coagulopathy develops, administration of calcium may be therapeutic. In addition, vasopressin may be particularly effective in restoring blood pressure when hemorrhagic shock is resistant to catecholamines. As opposed to elective aortic reconstruction, in which preserving myocardial function is the primary goal, in emergency resection the crucial factor for patient survival is first, rapid control of blood loss and reversal of hypotension, and then preservation of myocardial function.

LOWER EXTREMITY REVASCULARIZATION

The number of patients undergoing lower extremity revascularization has increased as surgeons and proceduralists attempt to improve functional status in elderly patients. In a fashion similar to aortic surgery, lower-limb revascularization has been revolutionized by the diffusion of endovascular techniques.[148] Allaqaband et al.[149] have summarized the current landscape in epidemiology and treatment of PAD. They report that that 10 million people in the United States have symptomatic PAD; 20 to 30 million have asymptomatic PAD. The prevalence of intermittent claudication increases with age, affecting >5% of patients over age 70. The incidence of claudication doubles or triples in patients with diabetes. Today,

advances in minimally invasive percutaneous interventions have made endovascular procedures the primary modality for revascularization in most patients. Compared with open surgical procedures, endovascular interventions offer comparable or superior long-term rates of success with very low rates for morbidity and mortality.

In some cases, traditional and endovascular repair are used in tandem. One technique may be used for primary repair, while another for rescue. Alternatively, a percutaneous approach to superficial femoral artery occlusion may be combined with traditional surgery below the knee. The development of hybrid operating rooms, with a full array of imaging equipment, allows for real-time decision making and completion of the surgery in one sitting. Regional anesthesia may be appropriate for some patients undergoing these procedures, but the same clinical challenges remain: managing multiple comorbidities, preservation of renal function, and radiation safety. Drug-eluting stents in the femoral artery may limit restenosis, just as in the coronary circulation. For such patient presenting for subsequent surgery, it is unclear whether stopping antiplatelet therapy perioperatively produces adverse events; fortunately, femoral artery thrombosis is less common and less lethal than coronary thrombosis in stented vessels. Endovascular repair has also expanded to occlusive disease in the iliac arteries.

There are three clinical indications for elective surgery for chronic peripheral occlusive disease: (1) claudication, (2) ischemic rest pain or ulceration, and (3) gangrene. Patients with rest pain, ulceration, or gangrene are at variable risk for imminent limb loss and may have severe progressive ischemia. Thus, reconstruction for such patients is urgent. When a patient presents with a gangrenous (black) or pregangrenous (blue) toe, several causes other than progression of chronic arteriosclerotic occlusive disease must be considered. Emboli may originate from the heart, a proximal aneurysm, or any proximal atherosclerotic lesion. Intra-arterially administered lytic agents, particularly urokinase, may have been administered, precluding regional anesthesia. Local infection is particularly common in diabetic patients.

During surgery, tunneling of the graft may be more stimulating than other parts of the procedure and may cause hypertension or movement under general anesthesia. The patient is usually given heparin during the procedure. In most cases, the heparin effect is not antagonized because bleeding problems are rare and graft reocclusion is a concern. Graft patency is evaluated carefully in the recovery room. Most surgeons believe the patient's feet should be kept warm and that the patient should be well hydrated so peripheral vasoconstriction, which may limit outflow from the new graft, is prevented. If graft thrombosis develops early in the postoperative period, the patient is promptly returned to the operating room for graft thrombectomy, as well as for evaluation and correction of the cause of the thrombosis. It can be anticipated that, during graft thrombectomy, significant blood loss will occur with flushing of the graft. In a study of patients undergoing traditional surgery for lower-limb revascularization, early graft failure occurred in 4.9% of patients in the U.S. Veterans Administration NSQIP (National Surgical Quality Improvement Program) database. On multivariate analysis, risks for early graft failure included younger patients (age <70 years), black race, and diabetes mellitus. Femoral-to-popliteal bypass with vein or prosthetic graft was associated with better early graft patency than any of the tibial vessel bypass procedures except for popliteal-to-tibial bypass with autogenous vein.[150] Clinicians might especially consider catheter-based regional anesthetic techniques in patients at high risk for graft failure to facilitate anesthetic management should a return trip to the operating room be necessary.

Anesthetic Management of Elective Lower Extremity Revascularization

The morbidity and mortality following traditional distal operations approach those following infra-aortic reconstruction and are mainly of cardiac origin. Thus, although regional anesthesia is often used, the same management strategies and concerns previously described apply, with special attention to the postoperative period. It is during the postoperative period that most cardiac problems arise and pain relief and correction of hemodynamic and fluid disequilibria are most likely to be needed.

The choice of anesthetic for surgical lower extremity revascularization is individualized for each patient. Regional anesthesia may be poorly tolerated by patients who are orthopneic, uncomfortable lying still for many hours, or demented and uncooperative. Indeed, failed regional anesthesia (11% of spinal and 16% of epidural anesthesias) is associated with 9% mortality, compared with 2% for successful regional or general anesthesia for femoral bypass.[151] Regional anesthesia may offer several advantages, however, including avoidance of hyperdynamic responses to tracheal intubation and extubation, reduced incidences of postoperative respiratory and infectious complications, and reduced postoperative hypercoagulability and graft thrombosis.[152] Other studies refute any effects of regional anesthesia on thrombotic outcomes and suggest only higher costs for postoperative surveillance. In some cases, the combination of regional and general anesthesia may provide patients with the benefits of each technique.

New data on the effect of choice of anesthetic technique on outcome after lower extremity surgery comes from the NSQIP database: 14,788 patients (general anesthesia, 9,757 patients; subarachnoid block, 2,848 patients; epidural, 2,183 patients) underwent a lower extremity infrainguinal arterial bypass during the study period. Compared with subarachnoid block, the odds of graft failure were higher with general anesthesia. When compared with subarachnoid block and epidural, general anesthesia was associated with more cases of postoperative pneumonia. Compared with subarachnoid block, general anesthesia was associated with an increased odds of returning to the operating room. However, there was no significant difference in 30-day mortality among the three conditions.[153] Coagulopathy represents a relative contraindication to regional anesthesia. The degree of coagulopathy at which it becomes unsafe to perform regional anesthesia is unknown, is highly controversial, and must be part of the risk–benefit calculation in each patient. Please see Chapter 37 for further information on this issue.

General anesthesia for lower extremity revascularization has the advantage of obviating patient discomfort and lack of cooperation. Its use is virtually mandated in patients who are to have vein harvested from an arm. Peripheral nerve blocks ("three-in-one," femoral sciatic block) may also be useful during and after lower extremity revascularization. Compared with general anesthesia, combined sciatic and femoral nerve blocks reduced the frequency of intraoperative myocardial ischemia in a small series of patients undergoing lower extremity vascular surgery.[154]

Anesthesia for Emergency Surgery for Peripheral Vascular Insufficiency

Emergency surgery for peripheral vascular insufficiency is required when acute arterial occlusion results in severe ischemia and threatens the viability of a limb. With acute arterial occlusion, the involved extremity suddenly becomes cold and pulseless. Patients usually complain of coldness, pain, numbness, and paresthesias, and they may lose motion and sensation. Abnormal sensation in the toes, feet, and legs in response to light touch and pinprick, as well as abnormal proprioception and loss of motor function in the feet and toes, are hallmarks of acute ischemia and nonviability.

The cause of the vascular insufficiency is important in planning operative treatment and anesthetic management. If the cause is an arterial embolus, Fogarty embolectomy through a groin incision under local anesthesia may suffice. However, if the cause is thrombosis of severely diseased atherosclerotic arteries, bypass reconstruction may be required. Thus, the anesthesiologist must be prepared for a simple procedure or a complex, extended procedure. In addition, serum potassium levels can change quickly because cell death and release of intracellular potassium into the circulation. Myoglobin may also be released into the circulation, and the development of a compartment syndrome is a possibility. Free radical scavengers such as mannitol and N-acetyl cysteine may be requested to mitigate reperfusion responses; sodium bicarbonate may or may not be given at the time of reperfusion. Anticoagulants are commonly administered to patients suspected of having peripheral vascular occlusion. If a patient has received anticoagulants, the appropriateness of using regional anesthesia is controversial. However, the authors recommend that regional anesthesia should not be used when patients have received recent thrombolytic therapy.

CONCLUSION

Individuals undergoing vascular reconstruction are generally elderly patients with CAD and other major medical problems including diabetes, COPD, and renal insufficiency. The skills of the anesthesiologist can therefore greatly influence outcome. The considerations for preoperative patient evaluation are the same as for patients with cardiac disease undergoing other noncardiac procedures. The major morbidity relates to myocardial well-being; therefore, the heart should be the major focus of the anesthesiologist's attention. Attempts to segregate patients who have significant CAD by use of preoperative testing are controversial. The benefits of coronary revascularization are likely to persist long after vascular surgery in patients with triple-vessel CAD. In cerebrovascular surgery, the goals for anesthesia management (i.e., ensuring adequate myocardial and brain perfusion and a rapidly arousable patient) may be facilitated with the use of neurophysiologic monitoring. In aortic reconstruction, ensuring intact myocardial function is probably the best way of making certain that spinal cord, visceral, and renal perfusion will be adequate. In the case of peripheral occlusive disease, regional anesthesia plays a greater role, but the same attention to anesthetic and cardiovascular management is required.

References

1. Khuri SF, Daley J, Henderson W et al: Risk adjustment of the postoperative mortality rate for the comparative assessment of the quality of surgical care: results of the National Veterans Affairs Surgical Risk Study. J Am Coll Surg 1997; 185: 315
2. White CJ, Gray WA: Endovascular therapies for peripheral arterial disease: An evidence-based review. Circulation 2007; 116: 2203
3. Hansson GK: Inflammation, atherosclerosis, and coronary artery disease. N Engl J Med 2005; 352: 1685
4. Lindemann S, Kramer B, Seizer P et al: Platelets, inflammation and atherosclerosis. J Thromb Haemost 2007; 5(Suppl 1): 203
5. Faraday N, Martinez EA, Scharpf RB et al: Platelet gene polymorphisms and cardiac risk assessment in vascular surgical patients. Anesthesiology 2004; 101: 1291
6. Grundy SM, Cleeman JI, Daniels SR et al: Diagnosis and management of the metabolic syndrome: an American Heart Association/National Heart, Lung, and Blood Institute Scientific Statement. Circulation 2005; 112: 2735

7. Norgren L, Hiatt WR, Dormandy JA et al: Inter-Society Consensus for the Management of Peripheral Arterial Disease (TASC II). J Vasc Surg 2007; 45(Suppl S): S5

8. Bhatt DL, Steg PG, Ohman EM et al: International prevalence, recognition, and treatment of cardiovascular risk factors in outpatients with atherothrombosis. JAMA 2006; 295: 180

9. Axelrod DA, Stanley JC, Upchurch GR, Jr. et al: Risk for stroke after elective noncarotid vascular surgery. J Vasc Surg 2004; 39: 67

10. Lorenz MW, Markus HS, Bots ML et al: Prediction of clinical cardiovascular events with carotid intima-media thickness: a systematic review and meta-analysis. Circulation 2007; 115: 459

11. Diehm N, Benenati JF, Becker GJ et al: Anemia is associated with abdominal aortic aneurysm (AAA) size and decreased long-term survival after endovascular AAA repair. J Vasc Surg 2007; 46: 676

12. Hindler K, Shaw AD, Samuels J et al: Improved postoperative outcomes associated with preoperative statin therapy. Anesthesiology 2006; 105: 1260

13. Le Manach Y, Godet G, Coriat P et al: The impact of postoperative discontinuation or continuation of chronic statin therapy on cardiac outcome after major vascular surgery. Anesth Analg 2007; 104: 1326

14. Schouten O, Hoeks SE, Welten GM et al: Effect of statin withdrawal on frequency of cardiac events after vascular surgery. Am J Cardiol 2007; 100: 316

15. Burger W, Chemnitius JM, Kneissl GD et al: Low-dose aspirin for secondary cardiovascular prevention—cardiovascular risks after its perioperative withdrawal versus bleeding risks with its continuation—review and meta-analysis. J Intern Med 2005; 257: 399

16. Antman EM, DeMets D, Loscalzo J: Cyclooxygenase inhibition and cardiovascular risk. Circulation 2005; 112: 759

17. Hertzer NR, Beven EG, Young JR et al: Coronary artery disease in peripheral vascular patients. A classification of 1000 coronary angiograms and results of surgical management. Ann Surg 1984; 199: 223

18. Finn AV, Nakazawa G, Joner M et al: Vascular responses to drug eluting stents: importance of delayed healing. Arterioscler Thromb Vasc Biol 2007; 27: 1500

19. King SB, 3rd, Smith SC, Jr., Hirshfeld JW, Jr. et al: 2007 Focused Update of the ACC/AHA/SCAI 2005 Guideline Update for Percutaneous Coronary Intervention: a report of the American College of Cardiology/American Heart Association Task Force on Practice Guidelines: 2007 Writing Group to Review New Evidence and Update the ACC/AHA/SCAI 2005 Guideline Update for Percutaneous Coronary Intervention, Writing on Behalf of the 2005 Writing Committee. Circulation 2008; 117: 261

20. Schouten O, van Domburg RT, Bax JJ et al: Noncardiac surgery after coronary stenting: early surgery and interruption of antiplatelet therapy are associated with an increase in major adverse cardiac events. J Am Coll Cardiol 2007; 49: 122

21. Schouten O, Bax JJ, Damen J et al: Coronary artery stent placement immediately before noncardiac surgery: a potential risk? Anesthesiology 2007; 106: 1067

22. Brilakis ES, Banerjee S, Berger PB: Perioperative management of patients with coronary stents. J Am Coll Cardiol 2007; 49: 2145

23. Le Manach Y, Perel A, Coriat P et al: Early and delayed myocardial infarction after abdominal aortic surgery. Anesthesiology 2005; 102: 885

24. Kim LJ, Martinez EA, Faraday N et al: Cardiac troponin I predicts short-term mortality in vascular surgery patients. Circulation 2002; 106: 2366

25. Panteghini M: The new definition of myocardial infarction and the impact of troponin determination on clinical practice. Int J Cardiol 2006; 106: 298

26. Mohler ER, 3rd, Mantha S, Miller AB et al: Should troponin and creatinine kinase be routinely measured after vascular surgery? Vasc Med 2007; 12: 175

27. Fleisher LA, Beckman JA, Brown KA et al: ACC/AHA 2007 Guidelines on Perioperative Cardiovascular Evaluation and Care for Noncardiac Surgery. A Report of the American College of Cardiology/American Heart Association Task Force on Practice Guidelines. Circulation 2007; 116: 1971

28. McFalls EO, Ward HB, Moritz TE et al: Coronary-artery revascularization before elective major vascular surgery. N Engl J Med 2004; 351: 2795

29. Ward HB, Kelly RF, Thottapurathu L et al: Coronary artery bypass grafting is superior to percutaneous coronary intervention in prevention of perioperative myocardial infarctions during subsequent vascular surgery. Ann Thorac Surg 2006; 82: 795

30. Hannan EL, Wu C, Walford G et al: Drug-eluting stents vs. coronary-artery bypass grafting in multivessel coronary disease. N Engl J Med 2008; 358: 331

31. Mantha S, Foss J, Ellis JE et al: Intense cardiac troponin surveillance for long-term benefits is cost-effective in patients undergoing open abdominal aortic surgery: a decision analysis model. Anesth Analg 2007; 105: 1346

32. Wiesbauer F, Schlager O, Domanovits H et al: Perioperative (beta)-Blockers for Preventing Surgery-Related Mortality and Morbidity: A Systematic Review and Meta-Analysis. Anesth Analg 2007; 104: 27

33. Feringa HH, Bax JJ, Boersma E et al: High-dose beta-blockers and tight heart rate control reduce myocardial ischemia and troponin T release in vascular surgery patients. Circulation 2006; 114: I344

34. London MJ, Zaugg M, Schaub MC et al: Perioperative beta-adrenergic receptor blockade: physiologic foundations and clinical controversies. Anesthesiology 2004; 100: 170

35. Devereaux PJ, Yang H, Yusuf S et al: Effects of extended-release metoprotol succinate in patients undergoing non-cordiac surgery (POISE trial): a randomised controlled trial trial. Lancet 2008; 371: 1839

36. Ellis JE, Drijvers G, Pedlow S et al: Premedication with oral and transdermal clonidine provides safe and efficacious postoperative sympatholysis. Anesth Analg 1994; 79: 1133

37. Wijeysundera DN, Naik JS, Beattie WS: Alpha-2 adrenergic agonists to prevent perioperative cardiovascular complications: a meta-analysis. Am J Med 2003; 114: 742

38. Wallace AW, Galindez D, Salahieh A et al: Effect of clonidine on cardiovascular morbidity and mortality after noncardiac surgery. Anesthesiology 2004; 101: 284

39. Durazzo AE, Machado FS, Ikeoka DT et al: Reduction in cardiovascular events after vascular surgery with atorvastatin: a randomized trial. J Vasc Surg 2004; 39: 967

40. Leurs LJ, Visser P, Laheij RJ et al: Statin use is associated with reduced all-cause mortality after endovascular abdominal aortic aneurysm repair. Vascular 2006; 14: 1

41. Boccara G, Ouattara A, Godet G et al: Terlipressin versus norepinephrine to correct refractory arterial hypotension after general anesthesia in patients chronically treated with renin-angiotensin system inhibitors. Anesthesiology 2003; 98: 1338

42. McDowell SE, Coleman JJ, Ferner RE: Systematic review and meta-analysis of ethnic differences in risks of adverse reactions to drugs used in cardiovascular medicine. BMJ 2006; 332: 1177

43. Dodds TM, Stone JG, Coromilas J et al: Prophylactic nitroglycerin infusion during noncardiac surgery does not reduce perioperative ischemia. Anesth Analg 1993; 76: 705

44. Symons JA, Myles PS: Myocardial protection with volatile anaesthetic agents during coronary artery bypass surgery: a meta-analysis. Br J Anaesth 2006; 97: 127

45. Landoni G, Biondi-Zoccai GG, Zangrillo A et al: Desflurane and sevoflurane in cardiac surgery: a meta-analysis of randomized clinical trials. J Cardiothorac Vasc Anesth 2007; 21: 502

46. Landoni G, Fochi O, Zangrillo A: Cardioprotection by volatile anesthetics in noncardiac surgery? No, not yet at least. J Am Coll Cardiol 2008; 51: 1321

47. Kersten JR, Fleisher LA: Reply. J Am Coll Cardiol 2008; 51: 1321

48. Beattie WS, Badner NH, Choi P: Epidural analgesia reduces postoperative myocardial infarction: a meta-analysis. Anesth Analg 2001; 93: 853

49. Norris EJ, Beattie C, Perler BA et al: Double-masked randomized trial comparing alternate combinations of intraoperative anesthesia and postoperative analgesia in abdominal aortic surgery. Anesthesiology 2001; 95: 1054

50. Nelson AH, Fleisher LA, Rosenbaum SH: Relationship between postoperative anemia and cardiac morbidity in high-risk vascular patients in the intensive care unit. Crit Care Med 1993; 21: 860

51. Hebert PC, Wells G, Blajchman MA et al: A multicenter, randomized, controlled clinical trial of transfusion requirements in critical care. Transfusion Requirements in Critical Care Investigators, Canadian Critical Care Trials Group. N Engl J Med 1999; 340: 409

52. Frank SM, Fleisher LA, Breslow MJ et al: Perioperative maintenance of normothermia reduces the incidence of morbid cardiac events. A randomized clinical trial. JAMA 1997; 277: 1127

53. Rajagopalan S, Mascha E, Na J et al: The effects of mild perioperative hypothermia on blood loss and transfusion requirement. Anesthesiology 2008; 108: 71

54. Howell SJ, Sear JW, Foex P: Hypertension, hypertensive heart disease and perioperative cardiac risk. Br J Anaesth 2004; 92: 570

55. Dunkelgrun M, Schreiner F, Schockman DB et al: Usefulness of preoperative oral glucose tolerance testing for perioperative risk stratification in patients scheduled for elective vascular surgery. Am J Cardiol 2008; 101: 526

56. Garber AJ, Moghissi ES, Bransome ED, Jr. et al: American College of Endocrinology position statement on inpatient diabetes and metabolic control. Endocr Pract 2004; 10: 77

57. Levy JH, Tanaka KA, Hursting MJ: Reducing thrombotic complications in the perioperative setting: an update on heparin-induced thrombocytopenia. Anesth Analg 2007; 105: 570

58. Howell SJ: Carotid endarterectomy. Br J Anaesth 2007; 99: 119

59. Diener HC, Cunha L, Forbes C et al: European Stroke Prevention Study. 2. Dipyridamole and acetylsalicylic acid in the secondary prevention of stroke. J Neurol Sci 1996; 143: 1

60. Collaborators NASCET: Beneficial effect of carotid endarterectomy in symptomatic patients with high-grade carotid stenosis. North American Symptomatic Carotid Endarterectomy Trial Collaborators. N Engl J Med 1991; 325: 445

61. Atherosclerosis ECftAC: Endarterectomy for asymptomatic carotid artery stenosis. Executive Committee for the Asymptomatic Carotid Atherosclerosis Study. JAMA 1995; 273: 1421

62. Biller J, Feinberg WM, Castaldo JE et al: Guidelines for carotid endarterectomy: a statement for healthcare professionals from a Special Writing Group of the Stroke Council, American Heart Association. Circulation 1998; 97: 501

63. Flanigan DP, Flanigan ME, Dorne AL et al: Long-term results of 442 consecutive, standardized carotid endarterectomy procedures in standard-risk and high-risk patients. J Vasc Surg 2007; 46: 876

64. Stoner MC, Abbott WM, Wong DR et al: Defining the high-risk patient for carotid endarterectomy: an analysis of the prospective National Surgical Quality Improvement Program database. J Vasc Surg 2006; 43: 285

65. McGirt MJ, Woodworth GF, Brooke BS et al: Hyperglycemia independently increases the risk of perioperative stroke, myocardial infarction, and death after carotid endarterectomy. Neurosurgery 2006; 58: 1066

66. Umbrain V, Keeris J, D'Haese J et al: Isoflurane, desflurane and sevoflurane for carotid endarterectomy. Anaesthesia 2000; 55: 1052

67. Kapinya KJ, Lowl D, Futterer C et al: Tolerance against ischemic neuronal injury can be induced by volatile anesthetics and is inducible NO synthase dependent. Stroke 2002; 33: 1889

68. Jellish WS, Sheikh T, Baker WH et al: Hemodynamic stability, myocardial ischemia, and perioperative outcome after carotid surgery with remifentanil/propofol or isoflurane/fentanyl anesthesia. J Neurosurg Anesthesiol 2003; 15: 176

69. Lavine SD, Masri LS, Levy ML et al: Temporary occlusion of the middle cerebral artery in intracranial aneurysm surgery: time limitation and advantage of brain protection. J Neurosurg 1997; 87: 817

70. Todd MM, Hindman BJ, Clarke WR et al: Mild intraoperative hypothermia during surgery for intracranial aneurysm. N Engl J Med 2005; 352: 135

71. Sundt TM, Jr., Sharbrough FW, Piepgras DG et al: Correlation of cerebral blood flow and electroencephalographic changes during carotid endarterectomy: with results of surgery and hemodynamics of cerebral ischemia. Mayo Clin Proc 1981; 56: 533

72. de Borst GJ, Moll FL, van de Pavoordt HD et al: Stroke from carotid endarterectomy: when and how to reduce perioperative stroke rate? Eur J Vasc Endovasc Surg 2001; 21: 484

73. Heyer EJ, Adams DC, Moses C et al: Erroneous conclusion from processed electroencephalogram with changing anesthetic depth. Anesthesiology 2000; 92: 603

74. Ferguson GG, Eliasziw M, Barr HW et al: The North American Symptomatic Carotid Endarterectomy Trial: surgical results in 1415 patients. Stroke 1999; 30: 1751

75. Bonhomme V, Desiron Q, Lemineur T et al: Bispectral index profile during carotid cross clamping. J Neurosurg Anesthesiol 2007; 19: 49

76. Deogaonkar A, Vivar R, Bullock RE et al: Bispectral index monitoring may not reliably indicate cerebral ischaemia during awake carotid endarterectomy. Br J Anaesth 2005; 94: 800

77. Calligaro KD, Dougherty MJ: Correlation of carotid artery stump pressure and neurologic changes during 474 carotid endarterectomies performed in awake patients. J Vasc Surg 2005; 42: 684

78. Hans SS, Jareunpoon O: Prospective evaluation of electroencephalography, carotid artery stump pressure, and neurologic changes during 314 consecutive carotid endarterectomies performed in awake patients. J Vasc Surg 2007; 45: 511

79. Moritz S, Kasprzak P, Arlt M et al: Accuracy of cerebral monitoring in detecting cerebral ischemia during carotid endarterectomy: a comparison of transcranial Doppler sonography, near-infrared spectroscopy, stump pressure, and somatosensory evoked potentials. Anesthesiology 2007; 107: 563

80. Moritz S, Kasprzak P, Woertgen C et al: The accuracy of jugular bulb venous monitoring in detecting cerebral ischemia in awake patients undergoing carotid endarterectomy. J Neurosurg Anesthesiol 2008; 20: 8

81. Ackerstaff RG, Moons KG, van de Vlasakker CJ et al: Association of intraoperative transcranial doppler monitoring variables with stroke from carotid endarterectomy. Stroke 2000; 31: 1817

82. Costin M, Rampersad A, Solomon RA et al: Cerebral injury predicted by transcranial Doppler ultrasonography but not electroencephalography during carotid endarterectomy. J Neurosurg Anesthesiol 2002; 14: 287

83. McCarthy RJ, McCabe AE, Walker R et al: The value of transcranial Doppler in predicting cerebral ischaemia during carotid endarterectomy. Eur J Vasc Endovasc Surg 2001; 21: 408

84. Dalman JE, Beenakkers IC, Moll FL et al: Transcranial Doppler monitoring during carotid endarterectomy helps to identify patients at risk of postoperative hyperperfusion. Eur J Vasc Endovasc Surg 1999; 18: 222

85. Manninen PH, Tan TK, Sarjeant RM: Somatosensory evoked potential monitoring during carotid endarterectomy in patients with a stroke. Anesth Analg 2001; 93: 39

86. Beese U, Langer H, Lang W et al: Comparison of near-infrared spectroscopy and somatosensory evoked potentials for the detection of cerebral ischemia during carotid endarterectomy. Stroke 1998; 29: 2032

87. Grubhofer G, Plochl W, Skolka M et al: Comparing Doppler ultrasonography and cerebral oximetry as indicators for shunting in carotid endarterectomy. Anesth Analg 2000; 91: 1339

88. Phillip B, Pastor D, Bellows W et al: The prevalence of preoperative diastolic filling abnormalities in geriatric surgical patients. Anesth Analg 2003; 97: 1214

89. De Castro V, Godet G, Mencia G et al: Target-controlled infusion for remifentanil in vascular patients improves hemodynamics and decreases remifentanil requirement. Anesth Analg 2003; 96: 33

90. Kostopanagiotou G, Markantonis SL, Polydorou M et al: Recovery and cognitive function after fentanyl or remifentanil administration for carotid endarterectomy. J Clin Anesth 2005; 17: 16

91. Stoneham MD, Doyle AR, Knighton JD et al: Prospective, randomized comparison of deep or superficial cervical plexus block for carotid endarterectomy surgery. Anesthesiology 1998; 89: 907

92. Illig KA, Sternbach Y, Zhang R et al: EEG changes during awake carotid endarterectomy. Ann Vasc Surg 2002; 16: 6

93. D'Honneur G, Motamed C, Tual L et al: Respiratory distress after a deep cervical plexus block. Anesthesiology 2005; 102: 1070

94. Itobi E, Sutherland AD, Whinney D et al: Acute airway obstruction complicating unilateral carotid endarterectomy. Eur J Vasc Endovasc Surg 2005; 30: 152

95. Hakl M, Michalek P, Sevcik P et al: Regional anaesthesia for carotid endarterectomy: an audit over 10 years. Br J Anaesth 2007; 99: 415

96. Messner M, Albrecht S, Lang W et al: The superficial cervical plexus block for postoperative pain therapy in carotid artery surgery. A prospective randomised controlled trial. Eur J Vasc Endovasc Surg 2007; 33: 50

97. Pandit JJ, Satya-Krishna R, Gration P: Superficial or deep cervical plexus block for carotid endarterectomy: a systematic review of complications. Br J Anaesth 2007; 99: 159

98. Guay J: Regional or general anesthesia for carotid endarterectomy? Evidence from published prospective and retrospective studies. J Cardiothorac Vasc Anesth 2007; 21: 127

99. Bekker A, Gold M, Ahmed R et al: Dexmedetomidine does not increase the incidence of intracarotid shunting in patients undergoing awake carotid endarterectomy. Anesth Analg 2006; 103: 955

100. McCutcheon CA, Orme RM, Scott DA et al: A comparison of dexmedetomidine versus conventional therapy for sedation and hemodynamic control during carotid endarterectomy performed under regional anesthesia. Anesth Analg 2006; 102: 668

101. Schneemilch CE, Bachmann H, Ulrich A et al: Clonidine decreases stress response in patients undergoing carotid endarterectomy under regional anesthesia: a prospective, randomized, double-blinded, placebo-controlled study. Anesth Analg 2006; 103: 297

102. Wallenborn J, Thieme V, Hertel-Gilch G et al: Effects of clonidine and superficial cervical plexus block on hemodynamic stability after carotid endarterectomy. J Cardiothorac Vasc Anesth 2008; 22: 84

103. McKevitt FM, Sivaguru A, Venables GS et al: Effect of treatment of carotid artery stenosis on blood pressure: a comparison of hemodynamic disturbances after carotid endarterectomy and endovascular treatment. Stroke 2003; 34: 2576

104. Manninen HI, Rasanen HT, Vanninen RL et al: Stent placement versus percutaneous transluminal angioplasty of human carotid arteries in cadavers in situ: distal embolization and findings at intravascular US, MR imaging and histopathologic analysis. Radiology 1999; 212: 483

105. Endovascular versus surgical treatment in patients with carotid stenosis in the Carotid and Vertebral Artery Transluminal Angioplasty Study (CAVATAS): a randomised trial. Lancet 2001; 357: 1729

106. Yadav JS, Wholey MH, Kuntz RE et al: Protected carotid-artery stenting versus endarterectomy in high-risk patients. N Engl J Med 2004; 351: 1493

107. Gurm HS, Yadav JS, Fayad P et al: Long-term results of carotid stenting versus endarterectomy in high-risk patients. N Engl J Med 2008; 358: 1572

108. Mas J-L, Chatellier G, Beyssen B et al: Endarterectomy versus stenting in patients with symptomatic severe carotid stenosis. N Engl J Med 2006; 355: 1660

109. Group SC, Ringleb PA, Allenberg J et al: 30 day results from the SPACE trial of stent-protected angioplasty versus carotid endarterectomy in symptomatic patients: a randomised non-inferiority trial [erratum appears in Lancet. 2006 Oct 7; 368(9543): 1238]. Lancet 2006; 368: 1239

110. Kawahito S, Kitahata H, Tanaka K et al: Risk factors for perioperative myocardial ischemia in carotid artery endarterectomy. J Cardiothorac Vasc Anesth 2004; 18: 288

111. Munro FJ, Makin AP, Reid J: Airway problems after carotid endarterectomy. Br J Anaesth 1996; 76: 156

112. Carmichael FJ, McGuire GP, Wong DT et al: Computed tomographic analysis of airway dimensions after carotid endarterectomy. Anesth Analg 1996; 83: 12

113. Lipsett PA, Tierney S, Gordon TA et al: Carotid endarterectomy–is intensive care unit care necessary? J Vasc Surg 1994; 20: 403

114. Fleming C, Whitlock EP, Beil TL et al: Screening for abdominal aortic aneurysm: a best-evidence systematic review for the U.S. Preventive Services Task Force. Ann Intern Med 2005; 142: 203

115. Gelman S: The pathophysiology of aortic cross-clamping and unclamping. Anesthesiology 1995; 82: 1026

116. Lo A, Adams D: Ruptured abdominal aortic aneurysms: risk factors for mortality after emergency repair. N Z Med J 2004; 117: U1100

117. Wahlberg E, Dimuzio PJ, Stoney RJ: Aortic clamping during elective operations for infrarenal disease: The influence of clamping time on renal function. J Vasc Surg 2002; 36: 13

118. Alpert RA, Roizen MF, Hamilton WK et al: Intraoperative urinary output does not predict postoperative renal function in patients undergoing abdominal aortic revascularization. Surgery 1984; 95: 707

119. Oliver WC, Jr., Nuttall GA, Cherry KJ et al: A comparison of fenoldopam with dopamine and sodium nitroprusside in patients undergoing cross-clamping of the abdominal aorta. Anesth Analg 2006; 103: 833

120. Koksoy C, LeMaire SA, Curling PE et al: Renal perfusion during thoracoabdominal aortic operations: cold crystalloid is superior to normothermic blood. Ann Thorac Surg 2002; 73: 730

121. Ali ZA, Callaghan CJ, Lim E et al: Remote ischemic preconditioning reduces myocardial and renal injury after elective abdominal aortic aneurysm repair: a randomized controlled trial. Circulation 2007; 116: I98

122. FitzGerald GA, Patrono C: The coxibs, selective inhibitors of cyclooxygenase-2. N Engl J Med 2001; 345: 433

123. Turner S, Derham C, Orsi NM et al: Randomized clinical trial of the effects of methylprednisolone on renal function after major vascular surgery. Br J Surg 2008; 95: 50

124. Cheung AT, Pochettino A, Guvakov DV et al: Safety of lumbar drains in thoracic aortic operations performed with extracorporeal circulation. Ann Thorac Surg 2003; 76: 1190

125. Glade GJ, Vahl AC, Wisselink W et al: Mid-term survival and costs of treatment of patients with descending thoracic aortic aneurysms; endovascular vs. open repair: a case-control study. Eur J Vasc Endovasc Surg 2005; 29: 28

126. Ballard JL, Yonemoto H, Killeen JD: Cost-effective aortic exposure: a retroperitoneal experience. Ann Vasc Surg 2000; 14: 1

127. Derrow AE, Seeger JM, Dame DA et al: The outcome in the United States after thoracoabdominal aortic aneurysm repair, renal artery bypass, and mesenteric revascularization. J Vasc Surg 2001; 34: 54

128. Meylaerts SA, Jacobs MJ, van Iterson V et al: Comparison of transcranial motor evoked potentials and somatosensory evoked potentials during thoracoabdominal aortic aneurysm repair. Ann Surg 1999; 230: 742

129. Contreras IS, Moreira LF, Ballester G et al: Immediate ischemic preconditioning based on somatosensory evoked potentials seems to prevent spinal cord injury following descending thoracic aorta cross-clamping. Eur J Cardiothorac Surg 2005; 28: 274

130. Kim SS, Leibowitz AB: Endovascular thoracic aortic aneurysm repair using a single catheter for spinal anesthesia and cerebrospinal fluid drainage. J Cardiothorac Vasc Anesth 2001; 15: 88

131. Parodi JC, Palmaz JC, Barone HD: Transfemoral intraluminal graft implantation for abdominal aortic aneurysms. Ann Vasc Surg 1991; 5: 491

132. Sampram ES, Karafa MT, Mascha EJ et al: Nature, frequency, and predictors of secondary procedures after endovascular repair of abdominal aortic aneurysm. J Vasc Surg 2003; 37: 930

133. Lippmann M, Lingam K, Rubin S et al: Anesthesia for endovascular repair of abdominal and thoracic aortic aneurysms: a review article. J Cardiovasc Surg 2003; 44: 443

134. Cuypers PW, Gardien M, Buth J et al: Randomized study comparing cardiac response in endovascular and open abdominal aortic aneurysm repair. Br J Surg 2001; 88: 1059

135. Cuypers PW, Gardien M, Buth J et al: Cardiac response and complications during endovascular repair of abdominal aortic aneurysms: a concurrent comparison with open surgery. J Vasc Surg 2001; 33: 353

136. Carpenter JP, Baum RA, Barker CF et al: Durability of benefits of endovascular versus conventional abdominal aortic aneurysm repair. J Vasc Surg 2002; 35: 222

137. Walker SR, Yusuf SW, Wenham PW et al: Renal complications following endovascular repair of abdominal aortic aneurysms. J Endovasc Surg 1998; 5: 318

138. White GH, May J, Waugh RC et al: Type III and type IV endoleak: toward a complete definition of blood flow in the sac after endoluminal AAA repair. J Endovasc Surg 1998; 5: 305

139. Ruppert V, Leurs LJ, Rieger J et al: Risk-adapted outcome after endovascular aortic aneurysm repair: analysis of anesthesia types based on EUROSTAR data. J Endovasc Surg 2007; 14: 12

140. Prinssen M, Verhoeven EL, Buth J et al: A randomized trial comparing conventional and endovascular repair of abdominal aortic aneurysms. N Engl J Med 2004; 351: 1607

141. Participants ET: Endovascular aneurysm repair versus open repair in patients with abdominal aortic aneurysm (EVAR trial 1): randomised controlled trial. Lancet 2005; 365: 2179

142. Schermerhorn M, O'Malley A, Jhaveri A et al: Endovascular vs. Open Repair of Abdominal Aortic Aneurysms in the Medicare Population. N Engl J Med 2008; 358: 464

143. Jonk YC, Kane RL, Lederle FA et al: Cost-effectiveness of abdominal aortic aneurysm repair: a systematic review. Int J Technol Assess Health Care 2007; 23: 205

144. Prinssen M, Buskens E, de Jong SE et al: Cost-effectiveness of conventional and endovascular repair of abdominal aortic aneurysms: results of a randomized trial. J Vasc Surg 2007; 46: 883

145. Sandham JD, Hull RD, Brant RF et al: A randomized, controlled trial of the use of pulmonary-artery catheters in high-risk surgical patients. N Engl J Med 2003; 348: 5

146. Tanaka K, Ludwig LM, Kersten JR et al: Mechanisms of cardioprotection by volatile anesthetics. Anesthesiology 2004; 100: 707

147. Johnston WE, Conroy BP, Miller GS et al: Hemodynamic benefit of positive end-expiratory pressure during acute descending aortic occlusion. Anesthesiology 2002; 97: 875

148. Perera GB, Lyden SP: Current trends in lower extremity revascularization. Surg Clin North Am 2007; 87: 1135

149. Allaqaband S, Solis J, Kazemi S et al: Endovascular treatment of peripheral vascular disease. Curr Probl Cardiol 2006; 31: 711

150. Singh N, Sidawy AN, DeZee KJ et al: Factors associated with early failure of infrainguinal lower extremity arterial bypass. J Vasc Surg 2008; 47: 556

151. Bode RH, Jr., Lewis KP, Zarich SW et al: Cardiac outcome after peripheral vascular surgery. Comparison of general and regional anesthesia. Anesthesiology 1996; 84: 3

152. Breslow MJ: The role of stress hormones in perioperative myocardial ischemia. Int Anesthesiol Clin 1992; 30: 81

153. Singh N, Sidawy AN, Dezee K et al: The effects of the type of anesthesia on outcomes of lower extremity infrainguinal bypass. J Vasc Surg 2006; 44: 964

154. Yazigi A, Madi-Gebara S, Haddad F et al: Intraoperative myocardial ischemia in peripheral vascular surgery: general anesthesia vs. combined sciatic and femoral nerve blocks. J Clin Anesth 2005; 17: 499

CHAPTER 43 ■ OBSTETRICAL ANESTHESIA

FERNE R. BRAVEMAN, BARBARA M. SCAVONE, CYNTHIA A. WONG, AND ALAN C. SANTOS

KEY POINTS

1. As oxygen consumption increases during pregnancy, the maternal cardiovascular system adapts to meet the metabolic demands of a growing fetus.

2. Airway edema may be particularly severe in women with preeclampsia, in patients placed in the Trendelenburg position for prolonged periods, in those who have pushed during the second stage of labor, or with concurrent use of tocolytic agents.

3. A rapid-sequence induction of anesthesia, application of cricoid pressure, and intubation with a cuffed endotracheal tube are required for all pregnant women receiving general anesthesia after the first trimester.

4. The driving force for placental drug transfer is the concentration gradient of free drug between the maternal and fetal blood.

5. For cesarean delivery, the choice of anesthesia depends on the urgency of the procedure and the condition of the mother and fetus.

6. The case fatality rate (maternal mortality) with general anesthesia is almost 17 times greater than that with neuraxial anesthesia.

7. By virtue of age and gender, as well as reduced epidural pressure after delivery, pregnant women are at a higher risk for developing postdural puncture headache.

8. Pregnancy and parturition are considered "high risk" when accompanied by conditions unfavorable to the well-being of the mother, fetus, or both.

9. Preeclampsia is classified as severe if it is associated with severe hypertension, proteinuria, or end-organ damage.

10. Antepartum hemorrhage occurs most commonly in association with placenta previa and placental abruption.

11. Heart disease during pregnancy is a leading nonobstetric cause of maternal mortality.

12. Substance abuse with cocaine has implications for anesthetic management because it causes a heightened state of sympathetic tone.

13. Fetal asphyxia develops as a result of interference with maternal or fetal perfusion of the placenta.

14. There is an increased incidence of adverse obstetric outcome, particularly after nonobstetric operations during the first trimester.

PHYSIOLOGIC CHANGES OF PREGNANCY

During pregnancy, there are major alterations in nearly every maternal organ system. These changes are initiated by hormones secreted by the corpus luteum and placenta. The mechanical effects of the enlarging uterus and compression of surrounding structures play an increasing role in the second and third trimesters. This altered physiologic state has relevant implications for the anesthesiologist caring for the pregnant patient. The most relevant changes, involving hematologic, cardiovascular, ventilatory, metabolic, and gastrointestinal functions, are considered in Table 43-1.

Hematologic Alterations

Increased mineralocorticoid activity during pregnancy produces sodium retention and increased body water content. Thus, plasma volume and total blood volume begin to increase in early gestation, resulting in a final increase of 40 to 50% and 25 to 40%, respectively, at term. The relatively smaller increase in red blood cell volume (20%) accounts for a reduction in hemoglobin (to 11 to 12 g/dL) and hematocrit (to 35%).[1] The leukocyte count ranges from 8,000 to 10,000/mm³ throughout pregnancy. The platelet count is decreased in pregnant women, and 12% of pregnant women at term have a platelet count less than 150×10^9/L, compared with only 1% of age-matched nonpregnant controls.[2] Several procoagulant factor levels increase during pregnancy, most notably fibrinogen, which doubles in mass. Anticoagulant activity decreases, as evidenced by decreased protein S concentrations and activated protein C resistance, and fibrinolysis is impaired. Increases in D-dimer and thrombin-antithrombin complexes indicate increased clotting and probable secondary fibrinolysis. Indeed, pregnancy has been referred to as a state of *chronic compensated disseminated intravascular coagulation*.[3,4]

Serum cholinesterase activity declines to a level of 20% below normal by term and reaches a nadir in the puerperium. However, it is doubtful that moderate succinylcholine doses lead to prolonged apnea in otherwise normal circumstances.[5]

TABLE 43-1

SUMMARY OF PHYSIOLOGIC CHANGES OF PREGNANCY AT TERM

■ VARIABLE	■ CHANGE	■ AMOUNT
Total blood volume	↑	25–40%
Plasma volume	↑	40–50%
Fibrinogen	↑	100%
Serum cholinesterase activity	↓	20–30%
Cardiac output	↑	30–50%
Minute ventilation	↑	50%
Alveolar ventilation	↑	70%
Functional residual capacity	↓	20%
Oxygen consumption	↑	20%
Arterial carbon dioxide tension	↓	10 mm Hg
Arterial oxygen tension	↑	10 mm Hg
Minimum alveolar concentration	↓	32–40%

↑, increase; ↓, decrease.

Although the total amount of protein in the circulation increases, plasma protein concentration declines to <6 g/dL at term because of dilution from increased plasma volume.[6] The albumin–globulin ratio declines because of the relatively greater reduction in albumin concentration. A decrease in serum protein concentration may be clinically significant because the free fractions of protein-bound drugs can be expected to increase.

Cardiovascular Changes

As oxygen consumption increases during pregnancy, the maternal cardiovascular system adapts to meet the metabolic demands of a growing fetus. Decreased vascular resistance due to estrogens, progesterone, and prostacyclin may be the initiating factor.[7] Lowered resistance is found in the uterine, renal, and other vascular beds; at term, there is an increase in heart rate (15 to 25%) and cardiac output (up to 50%) above that of the nonpregnant state. Arterial blood pressure decreases slightly because the decrease in peripheral resistance exceeds the increase in cardiac output. Additional increases in cardiac output occur during labor (when cardiac output may reach 12 to 14 L/min) and also in the immediate postpartum period because of added blood volume from the contracted uterus. These changes are exaggerated in multiple gestation pregnancies.[8]

Supine hypotensive syndrome, which occurs in 10% of pregnant women, occurs because the supine position leads to vena cava occlusion and thus decreased preload to the heart, resulting in maternal tachycardia, arterial hypotension, faintness, and pallor. From the second trimester, aortocaval compression by the enlarged uterus becomes progressively more important, reaching its maximum at 36 to 38 weeks' gestation, after which it may decrease as the fetal head descends into the pelvis.[9] Studies of cardiac output, measured with the patient in the supine position during the last weeks of pregnancy, have indicated a decrease to nonpregnant levels; however, this decrease was not observed when patients were in the lateral decubitus position.[9] Compression of the lower aorta in this position may further decrease uteroplacental perfusion and result in fetal asphyxia. Therefore, uterine displacement or 15 degrees left lateral pelvic tilt should be applied routinely during the second and third trimesters of pregnancy; a minority of women may remain susceptible to vena cava compression even at this degree of tilt.[10]

Changes in the electrocardiogram may also occur. In addition to heart rate increases, left axis deviation is observed in the third trimester, possibly due to upward displacement of the heart by the gravid uterus. There is also a tendency toward premature atrial contractions, paroxysmal supraventricular tachycardia, and ventricular dysrhythmias.[11,12]

Ventilatory Changes

Increased extracellular fluid and vascular engorgement may lead to edema of the upper airway.[13] Many pregnant women complain of difficulty with nasal breathing, and the friable nature of the mucous membranes during pregnancy can cause severe bleeding, especially on insertion of nasopharyngeal airways or nasogastric and endotracheal tubes. Airway edema may be particularly severe in women with preeclampsia, in patients placed in the Trendelenburg position for prolonged periods, or with concurrent use of tocolytic agents. It may also be difficult to perform laryngoscopy in obese, short-necked parturients with enlarged breasts. Use of a short-handled laryngoscope may prove helpful.

The diaphragm is displaced cephalad as the uterus increases in size. This is accompanied by an increase in the anteroposterior and transverse diameters of the thoracic cage, so that total lung capacity decreases only slightly. From the fifth month, the

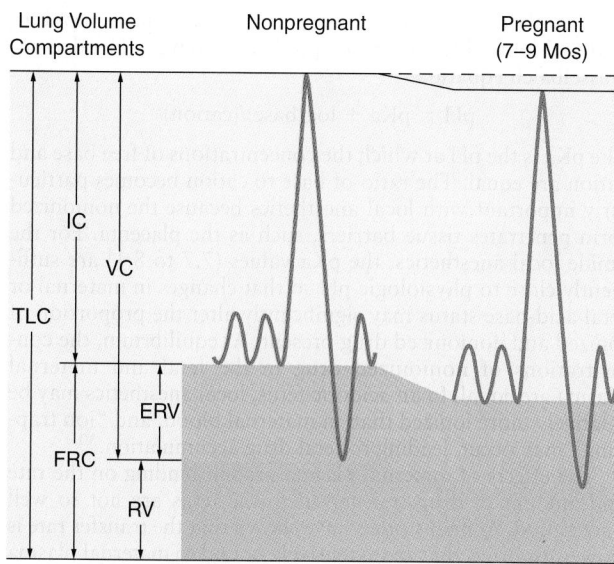

| | Nonpregnant | Pregnant (7–9 Mos) |

Lung Volume Compartments

TLC = Total Lung Capacity   IC = Inspiratory Capacity
FRC = Functional Residual Capacity   VC = Vital Capacity
ERV = Expiratory Reserve Volume   RV = Residual Volume

FIGURE 43-1. Lung volume and capacity changes during pregnancy. (Reprinted from Elkus R. Popovich J Jr: Respiratory physiology in pregnancy. Clin Chest Med 1992; 13: 555, with permission.)

expiratory reserve volume, residual volume, and functional residual capacity (FRC) decrease, the latter by 20% compared with the nonpregnant state. Concomitantly, there is an increase in inspiratory reserve volume[13] (Fig. 43-1). In most pregnant women, a decreased FRC does not cause problems, but those with pre-existing alterations in closing volume as a result of smoking, obesity, or scoliosis may experience early airway closure with advancing pregnancy, leading to hypoxemia. The Trendelenburg and supine positions also exacerbate the abnormal relationship between closing volume and FRC. The residual volume and FRC return to normal shortly after delivery.

Pregnancy is associated with physiologic changes that may influence maternal pharmacokinetics and the action of anesthetic drugs. These changes may be progressive during the course of gestation and are often difficult to predict. Alterations in ventilation and lung volumes have a significant effect on the rate of uptake and excretion of inhalation agents. Of most concern to the anesthesiologist is a 20% reduction in FRC that results in a shortened equilibration time between the alveolar and inspired concentrations of inhalation agents.[14]

Progesterone-induced relaxation of bronchiolar smooth muscle decreases airway resistance, whereas lung compliance remains unchanged. Minute ventilation increases from the beginning of pregnancy to a maximum of 50% above normal at term.[14] This is accomplished by a 40% increase in tidal volume and a 15% increase in respiratory rate. Dead space does not change significantly, and thus alveolar ventilation is increased by 70% at term. After delivery, as blood progesterone levels decline, ventilation returns to normal within 1 to 3 weeks.[15]

Metabolism

Basal oxygen consumption increases during early pregnancy, with an overall increase of 20% by term.[14] However, increased alveolar ventilation leads to a reduction in the partial pressure of carbon dioxide in arterial blood ($PaCO_2$) to 32 mm Hg and an increase in the partial pressure of oxygen in arterial blood (PaO_2) to 106 mm Hg. The plasma buffer base decreases from

47 to 42 mEq/L and, therefore, the pH remains practically unchanged. The maternal uptake and elimination of inhalational anesthetics is enhanced because of the increased alveolar ventilation and decreased FRC.[15] However, the decreased FRC and increased metabolic rate predispose the mother to development of hypoxemia during periods of apnea/hypoventilation, such as may occur during airway obstruction or prolonged attempts at tracheal intubation.[16]

Human placental lactogen and cortisol increase the tendency toward hyperglycemia and ketosis, which may exacerbate pre-existing diabetes mellitus. The patient's ability to handle a glucose load is decreased, and the transplacental passage of glucose may stimulate fetal secretion of insulin, leading in turn to neonatal hypoglycemia in the immediate postpartum period.[17]

Gastrointestinal Changes

Controversy exists as to when a pregnant woman becomes at risk for aspiration. Gastric secretions are more acidic and lower esophageal sphincter (LES) tone is decreased. Gastric emptying time is not prolonged during pregnancy, but overall gastrointestinal time is prolonged.[18] In two recent studies of obese and nonobese, nonlaboring parturients at term, gastric emptying did not differ after ingestion of a moderate amount (300 mL) of water versus after an overnight fast.[19,20] Recent obstetric anesthesia practice guidelines allow for oral intake of modest amounts of clear liquids in uncomplicated laboring patients, and for similar intake in patients scheduled for uncomplicated cesarean delivery up to 2 hours prior to induction of anesthesia.[21] However, the guidelines state that patients with additional risk factors for aspiration (e.g., morbid obesity, diabetes, difficult airway) or patients at increased risk for operative delivery (e.g., nonreassuring fetal heart rate pattern) may have further restrictions of oral intake.

The risk of regurgitation on induction of general anesthesia depends, in part, on the gradient between the LES and intragastric pressures. In most patients, the gradient increases after succinylcholine administration because the increase in LES pressure exceeds the increase in intragastric pressure. However, in parturients with "heartburn," the LES tone is greatly reduced.[22] The efficacy of prophylactic nonparticulate antacids may be diminished by inadequate mixing with gastric contents, improper timing of administration, and the tendency for antacids to increase gastric volume. Administration of histamine (H_2) receptor antagonists, such as ranitidine, requires careful timing. A good case can be made for the administration of intravenous metoclopramide before elective cesarean delivery. This dopamine antagonist hastens gastric emptying and increases resting LES tone in both nonpregnant and pregnant women.[23] However, conflicting reports have appeared on its efficacy and on the frequency of side effects such as extrapyramidal reactions and transient neurologic dysfunction.[24] These practice guidelines advise practitioners to consider the administration of nonparticulate antacids, H_2 receptor antagonists, and/or metoclopramide for aspiration prophylaxis before surgical procedures and to use neuraxial anesthesia whenever possible.[21] A rapid-sequence induction of anesthesia, application of cricoid pressure, and intubation with a cuffed endotracheal tube are recommended for pregnant women receiving general anesthesia from the 12th week of gestation.[25] These recommendations also pertain to women in the immediate postpartum period because there is uncertainty as to when gastric volume returns to normal.

Altered Drug Responses

The minimum alveolar concentration (MAC) for inhalation agents is decreased by 8 to 12 weeks gestation and may be related to an increase in progesterone levels.[26] In addition, maximal cephalad block level after neuraxial administration of local anesthetics is higher in the second and third trimesters of pregnancy.[27] Epidural venous engorgement, which decreases intrathecal volume, may lead to increased local anesthetic spread. Pregnancy increases median nerve sensitivity to lidocaine block[28] and *in vitro* preparations from pregnant animals demonstrate increased susceptibility to local anesthetic blockade.[29] This increased sensitivity may be due to progesterone or other hormonal mediators.

PLACENTAL TRANSFER AND FETAL EXPOSURE TO ANESTHETIC DRUGS

Most drugs, including many anesthetic agents, readily cross the placenta. Several factors influence the placental transfer of drugs, including physicochemical characteristics of the drug itself, maternal drug concentrations in the plasma, properties of the placenta, and hemodynamic events within the fetomaternal unit.

Drugs cross biologic membranes by simple diffusion, the rate of which is determined by the Fick principle, which states that:

$$Q/t = KA(C_m - C_f)/D$$

where Q/t is rate of diffusion, K is diffusion constant, A is surface area available for exchange, C_m is concentration of free drug in maternal blood, C_f is concentration of free drug in fetal blood, and D is thickness of the diffusion barrier.

The diffusion constant (K) of the drug depends on physicochemical characteristics such as molecular size, lipid solubility, and degree of ionization. Compounds with a molecular weight of <500 Da are unimpeded in crossing the placenta, whereas those with molecular weights of 500 to 1,000 Da are more restricted. Most drugs commonly used by the anesthesiologist have molecular weights that permit easy transfer.

Drugs that are highly lipid-soluble cross biological membranes more readily. The degree of ionization is important because the nonionized moiety of a drug is more lipophilic than the ionized one. Local anesthetics and opioids are weak bases, with a relatively low degree of ionization and considerable lipid solubility. In contrast, muscle relaxants are more ionized and less lipophilic, and their rate of placental transfer is therefore more limited.

The relative concentrations of drug existing in the nonionized and ionized forms can be predicted from the Henderson-Hasselbalch equation:

$$pH = pKa + log(base)/(cation)$$

The pKa is the pH at which the concentrations of free base and cation are equal. The ratio of base to cation becomes particularly important with local anesthetics because the nonionized form penetrates tissue barriers, such as the placenta. For the amide local anesthetics, the pKa values (7.7 to 8.1) are sufficiently close to physiologic pH so that changes in maternal or fetal acid-base status may significantly alter the proportion of ionized and nonionized drug present. At equilibrium, the concentrations of nonionized drug in the fetal and maternal plasma are equal. In an acidotic fetus, local anesthetics may be relatively more ionized than in maternal blood, and "ion trapping" may occur, leading to fetal drug accumulation.[30]

The effects of maternal plasma protein binding on the rate and amount of drug transferred to the fetus are not so well understood. Animal studies have shown that the transfer rate is slower for drugs that are extensively bound to maternal plasma proteins, such as bupivacaine.[31] In sheep, the low fetomaternal ratio of bupivacaine plasma concentrations has been attributed to the difference between fetal and maternal plasma protein binding, rather than to extensive fetal tissue uptake.[32] However, if enough time is allowed for fetomaternal equilibrium to be approached, substantial accumulation of highly protein-bound drugs, such as bupivacaine, can occur in the fetus.[33]

As already stated, the driving force for placental drug transfer is the concentration gradient of free drug between the maternal and fetal blood. On the maternal side, the following factors interact: the dose administered, the mode and site of administration, and, in the case of local anesthetics, the use of vasoconstrictors. The rates of distribution, metabolism, and excretion of the drug, which may vary at different stages of pregnancy, are equally important. In general, higher doses result in higher maternal blood concentrations. The absorption rate varies with the site of drug injection. Compared with other forms of administration, an intravenous bolus results in the highest blood concentrations. Increased maternal blood concentrations after repeated administration of a drug greatly depend on the dose and frequency of reinjection, in addition to the kinetic characteristics of the drug. The elimination half-life of amide local anesthetic agents is relatively long, so repeated injection may lead to accumulation in the maternal plasma[34] (Fig. 43-2). In contrast, 2-chloroprocaine, an

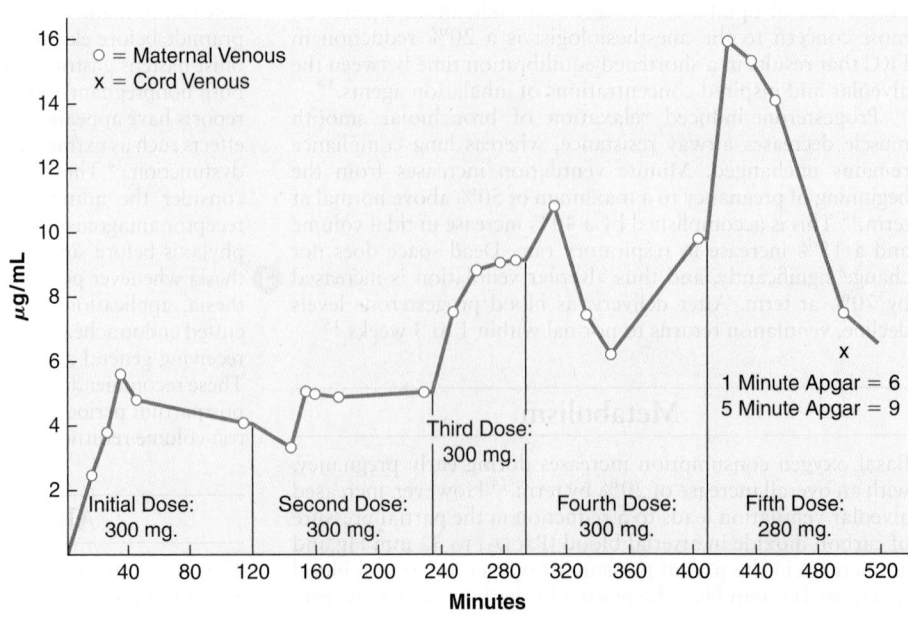

FIGURE 43-2. Increased levels of mepivacaine with each reinforcing dose in a patient receiving continuous caudal anesthesia during parturition. (Reprinted from Moore DC, Bridenbaugh LD, Bagdi PA et al: Accumulation of mepivacaine hydrochloride during caudal block. Anesthesiology 1968; 29: 585, with permission.)

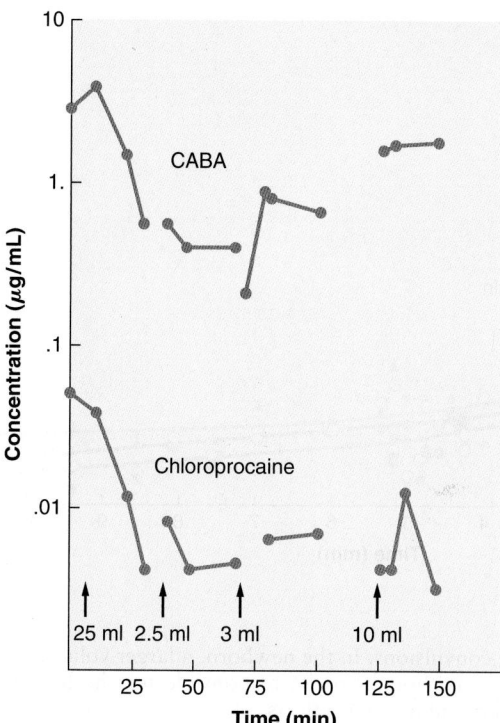

FIGURE 43-3. Plasma concentrations of chloroprocaine and chloroaminobenzoic acid (CABA) in a typical patient after epidural anesthesia (multiple injections) for vaginal delivery. (Reprinted from Kuhnert BR, Kuhnert PM, Prochaska AL et al: Plasma levels of 2-chloroprocaine in obstetric patients and their neonates after epidural anesthesia. Anesthesiology 1980; 53: 21, with permission.)

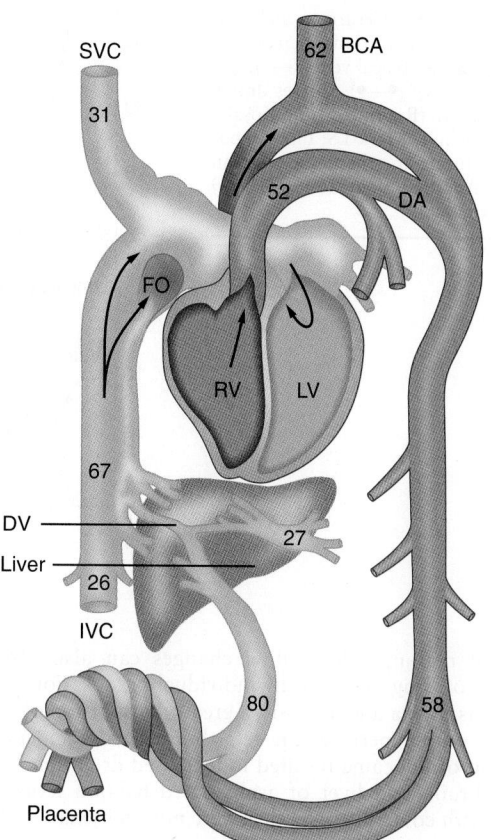

FIGURE 43-4. Diagram of the circulation in the mature fetal lamb. The numerals indicate the mean oxygen saturation (%) in the great vessels of six lambs: right ventricle (RV), left ventricle (LV), superior vena cava (SVC), inferior vena cava (IVC), brachiocephalic artery (BCA), foramen ovale (FO), ductus arteriosus (DA), ductus venosus (DV). (Reprinted from Born GVR, Dawes GS, Mott JC et al: Changes in the heart and lungs at birth. Cold Spring Harbor Symp Quant Biol 1954; 19: 103, with permission.)

ester local anesthetic, undergoes rapid enzymatic hydrolysis in the presence of pseudocholinesterase. After epidural injection, the mean half-life in the mother is approximately 3 minutes; after reinjection, 2-chloroprocaine can be detected in the maternal plasma for only 5 to 10 minutes, and no accumulation of this drug is evident[35] (Fig. 43-3).

Placenta

Maturation of the placenta can affect the rate of drug transfer to the fetus, as the thickness of the trophoblastic epithelium decreases from 25 to 2 mm at term. Uptake and biotransformation of anesthetic drugs by the placenta would decrease the amount transferred to the fetus. However, placental drug uptake is limited, and there is no evidence to suggest that this organ metabolizes any of the agents commonly used in obstetric anesthesia.

Hemodynamic Factors

Any factor decreasing placental blood flow, such as aortocaval compression, hypotension, or hemorrhage, can decrease drug delivery to the fetus. During labor, uterine contractions intermittently reduce perfusion of the placenta. If a uterine contraction coincides with a rapid decline in plasma drug concentration after an intravenous bolus injection, by the time perfusion has returned to normal, the concentration gradient across the placenta has been greatly reduced. When women were given an intravenous injection of diazepam, administered at the onset of contraction in one group and during uterine

diastole in the other, less drug was found in infants born to mothers in the former group.[36]

Several characteristics of the fetal circulation delay equilibration between the umbilical arterial and venous blood, and thus delay the depressant effects of anesthetic drugs (Fig. 43-4). The liver is the first fetal organ perfused by umbilical venous blood, which carries drug to the fetus. Substantial uptake by this organ has been demonstrated for a variety of drugs, including thiopental, lidocaine, and halothane. During its transit to the arterial side of the fetal circulation, the drug is progressively diluted as blood in the umbilical vein becomes admixed with fetal venous blood from the gastrointestinal tract, the lower extremities, the head and upper extremities, and, finally, the lungs. Because of this unique pattern of fetal circulation, continuous administration of anesthetic concentrations of nitrous oxide during elective cesarean sections caused newborn depression only if the induction-to-delivery interval exceeded 5 to 10 minutes. Rapid transfer of inhalation agents, including halothane, enflurane, and isoflurane, results in detectable umbilical arterial and venous concentrations after 1 minute.[37] Because of the rapid decline in maternal plasma drug concentrations, administration of thiopental or thiamylal as a single-bolus injection not exceeding 4 mg/kg was followed by fetal arterial concentrations of barbiturate below a level that would result in neonatal depression[38] (Fig. 43-5).

FIGURE 43-5. Cesarean delivery. Thiamylal concentrations in maternal vein (▲—▲), umbilical vein (○—○), and umbilical artery (●—●). Curves drawn by inspection. (Reprinted from Kosaka Y, Takahashi T, Mark LS: Intravenous thiobarbiturate anesthesia for cesarean section. Anesthesiology 1969; 31: 489 with permission.)

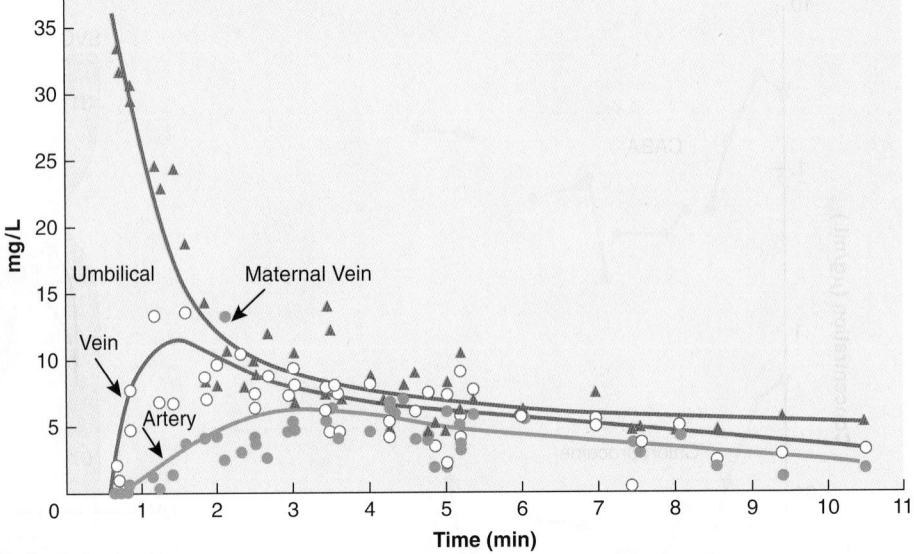

Fetal regional blood flow changes can also affect the amount of drug taken up by individual organs. For example, during asphyxia and acidosis, a greater proportion of the fetal cardiac output perfuses the fetal brain, heart, and placenta. Infusion of lidocaine resulted in increased drug uptake in the heart, brain, and liver of asphyxiated baboon fetuses compared with control fetuses that were not asphyxiated.[39]

Fetus and Newborn

Any drug that reaches the fetus undergoes metabolism and excretion. In this respect, the fetus has an advantage over the newborn in that it can excrete the drug back to the mother once the concentration gradient of the free drug across the placenta has been reversed. With the use of local anesthetics, this may occur even though the total plasma drug concentration in the mother may exceed that in the fetus because there is lower protein binding in fetal plasma.[32] There is only one drug, 2-chloroprocaine, that is metabolized in the fetal blood so rapidly that even in acidosis, substantial accumulation in the fetus is avoided.[35]

In both the term and the preterm newborn, the liver contains enzymes essential for the biotransformation of amide local anesthetics. A study comparing the pharmacokinetics of lidocaine among adult ewes and lambs (fetal and neonatal) showed that the metabolic clearance in the newborn was similar to, and renal clearance greater than, that in the adult.[39] Nonetheless, the elimination half-life was prolonged in the newborn. This was attributed to a greater volume of distribution of the drug. Similar results were reported in another study involving lidocaine administration to human infants in a neonatal intensive care unit.[40] Prolonged elimination half-lives in the newborn compared with the adult have been noted for other amide local anesthetics.

It is not completely understood whether the fetus and newborn are more sensitive than the adult to the depressant and toxic effects of local anesthetics. The relative central nervous and cardiorespiratory toxicity of lidocaine has been studied in adult ewes and lambs (fetal and neonatal).[41] The doses required to produce toxicity in the fetal and neonatal lamb were greater than those required in the adult, although serum concentrations at which toxicity occurred was not different. In the fetus, this was attributed to placental clearance of drug into the mother and better maintenance of blood gas tensions

during convulsions. In the newborn, a larger volume of distribution was thought to be responsible for the higher doses needed to induce toxic effects.

Bupivacaine has been implicated as a possible cause of neonatal jaundice because its high affinity for fetal erythrocyte membranes may lead to a decrease in filterability and deformability, rendering them more prone to hemolysis (see Chapter 44). However, a recent study failed to show increased bilirubin production in newborns whose mothers received bupivacaine for epidural anesthesia during labor and delivery.[42] Finally, observational neurobehavioral studies have revealed subtle changes in newborn neurologic and adaptive function. In the case of most anesthetic agents, these changes are minor and transient, lasting for only 24 to 48 hours.

ANESTHESIA FOR LABOR AND VAGINAL DELIVERY

Most women experience moderate-to-severe pain during parturition. In the first stage of labor, pain is caused by uterine contractions, associated with dilation of the cervix and stretching of the lower uterine segment. Pain impulses are carried in visceral afferent type C fibers accompanying the sympathetic nerves. In early labor, only the lower thoracic dermatomes (T11 to T12) are affected, but with progressing cervical dilation in the transition phase, adjacent dermatomes may be involved and pain referred from T10 to L1. In the second stage, additional pain impulses from distention of the vaginal vault and perineum are carried by the pudendal nerves, composed of lower sacral fibers (S2 to S4).

Well-conducted obstetric analgesia, in addition to relieving pain and anxiety, may benefit the mother. Pain may result in maternal hypertension and reduced uterine blood flow. During the first and second stages of labor, epidural analgesia blunts the increases in maternal cardiac output, heart rate, and blood pressure that occur with painful uterine contractions and "bearing-down" efforts.[43] In reducing maternal secretion of catecholamines, epidural analgesia may convert a previously dysfunctional labor pattern to normal. Maternal analgesia may also benefit the fetus by eliminating maternal hyperventilation, which often leads to reduced fetal arterial oxygen tension because of a leftward shift of the maternal oxygen-hemoglobin dissociation curve.

The most frequently chosen methods for relieving the pain of parturition are psychoprophylaxis, systemic medication, and regional analgesia. Inhalation analgesia, conventional spinal analgesia, and paracervical blockade are less commonly used. General anesthesia is rarely necessary, but may be indicated for uterine relaxation in some complicated deliveries. Labor varies in length and intensity, as do individual tolerance to pain and desire for pain relief. Women should be supported in their choice of labor analgesia, if any, and educated about the options. Neonatal outcome appears to be similar for healthy women who deliver without pharmacologic analgesia and for women who receive appropriate supplementary analgesia. Analgesia should not be withheld if requested.[44]

Nonpharmacologic Methods of Labor Analgesia

Nonpharmacologic methods to relieve the pain of childbirth include childbirth education, emotional support, massage, aroma therapy, audiotherapy, and therapeutic use of hot and cold. More specialized techniques that require specialized training or equipment include hydrotherapy, intradermal water injections, biofeedback, transcutaneous electrical nerve stimulation, acupuncture or acupressure, and hypnosis. Conclusions regarding the efficacy of most of these techniques are not possible, as the techniques have been inadequately studied because of methodologic flaws in many study designs.[45]

Prepared Childbirth and Psychoprophylaxis

The philosophy of prepared childbirth maintains that lack of knowledge, misinformation, fear, and anxiety can heighten a patient's response to pain and consequently increase the need for analgesics. The most popular method of prepared childbirth was introduced by Lamaze. It provides an educational program on the physiology of parturition and attempts to diminish cortical pain perception by encouraging responses such as specific patterns of breathing and focused attention on a fixed object.[46] Scientific data as to whether childbirth education and psychoprophylaxis are effective in reducing childbirth pain are inconsistent and lack scientific rigor. Education, intense motivation, and cultural influences can influence the affective and behavioral responses to pain, although they probably minimally affect actual pain sensation.[47]

Other Nonpharmacologic Methods

Continuous labor support refers to the presence during labor of nonmedical support by a trained person. Prospective, controlled trials and several systematic analyses have concluded that women who receive continuous labor support have shorter labors, fewer operative deliveries, fewer analgesic interventions, and overall satisfaction.[48] Systematic reviews of randomized controlled trials of hydrotherapy (water baths) have concluded that women experience less pain and use less analgesia, without change in the duration of labor, rate of operative delivery, or neonatal outcome.[49] Intradermal water injection consists of the injection of 0.05 to 0.1 mL of sterile water at four sites on the lower back to treat back pain during labor. Randomized controlled trials have found that the technique is effective in reducing severe back pain during labor, without any known side effects to the mother and fetus.[45] Hypnosis requires prenatal training of the mother by a trained hypnotherapist. A meta-analysis of five randomized controlled trials concluded that women randomized to hypnosis used pharmacologic analgesia methods at a lower rate compared with women in the control groups.[50] The results of studies using transcutaneous electrical nerve stimulation are inconsis-

tent, but in general, labor pain does not appear to be lessened, nor does it lower the use of other analgesic modalities.[45] In three randomized controlled trials of acupuncture conducted in Scandinavian countries, women who were randomized to acupuncture versus control (no or "false" acupuncture) had modestly lower pain scores, and lower use of epidural and systemic opioid analgesia.[51,52]

Systemic Medication

The advantages of systemic analgesics include ease of administration and patient acceptability. However, the drug, dose, time, and method of administration must be chosen carefully to avoid maternal or neonatal depression. Opioids are used most commonly, although tranquilizers and ketamine are used occasionally.

Opioids

Systemic opioids are commonly administered for labor analgesia, although existing data suggest that they provide little significant analgesia[53,54] (see Chapter 19). Meperidine is a commonly used systemic analgesic. It can be administered by intravenous injection (effective analgesia in 5 to 10 minutes) or intramuscularly (peak effect in 40 to 50 minutes). The major side effects are a high incidence of nausea and vomiting, maternal sedation, dose-related depression of ventilation, orthostatic hypotension, and the potential for neonatal depression. Meperidine may cause transient alterations of the fetal heart rate (FHR), such as decreased beat-to-beat variability and mild tachycardia. Among other factors, the risk of neonatal depression is related to the interval from the last drug injection to delivery. The placental transfer of an active metabolite, normeperidine, which has a long elimination half-life in the neonate (62 hours), has also been implicated in contributing to neonatal depression and subtle neonatal neurobehavioral dysfunction.

Synthetic opioids such as fentanyl, alfentanil, and remifentanil are more potent than meperidine; however, their use during labor is limited by their short duration of action. These drugs offer an advantage when analgesia of rapid onset but short duration is necessary (e.g., with forceps application). Alfentanil is not commonly used because of the finding of delayed elimination in newborn rhesus monkeys.[55] For more prolonged analgesia, fentanyl or remifentanil can be administered with patient-controlled delivery devices. Patient-controlled analgesia administration of opioid does carry with it the potential for drug accumulation and the risk of neonatal depression. Remifentanil has the theoretical advantage of rapid onset and offset compared with the other opioids. Bolus doses ranging from 0.2 to 1 μg/kg with lock-out intervals from 1 to 5 minutes[56,57] and background infusion rates from zero to 0.1 μg/kg/min[57] have been described. However, as with other systemic opioid techniques, it is unclear whether remifentanil patient-controlled analgesia can provide satisfactory analgesia without an unacceptably high incidence of maternal, fetal, and neonatal side effects.[56]

Opioid agonists–antagonists, such as butorphanol and nalbuphine, have also been used for obstetric analgesia. These drugs have the proposed benefits of a lower incidence of nausea, vomiting, and dysphoria, as well as a "ceiling effect" on depression of ventilation. Butorphanol, 1 to 2 mg, or nalbuphine, 10 mg by intravenous or intramuscular injection, are probably the most popular. Unlike meperidine, these are biotransformed into inactive metabolites and have a ceiling effect on depression of ventilation.

Naloxone, a pure opioid antagonist, should not be administered to the mother shortly before delivery to prevent neonatal ventilatory depression because it reverses maternal analgesia at a time when it is most needed and, in some instances, has caused maternal pulmonary edema and even cardiac arrest. If necessary, the drug should be given directly to the newborn intramuscularly (0.1 mg/kg).

Ketamine

Ketamine is a potent analgesic. However, it may also induce unacceptable amnesia that may interfere with the mother's recollection of the birth. Nonetheless, ketamine is a useful adjuvant to inadequate regional analgesia during vaginal delivery or for obstetric manipulations. In low doses (0.2 to 0.4 mg/kg), ketamine provides adequate analgesia without causing neonatal depression. Constant communication is required with the patient to ensure she is awake and able to protect her airway.

Regional Analgesia

Regional techniques provide excellent analgesia with minimal depressant effects on mother and fetus. The regional techniques most commonly used in obstetric anesthesia include central neuraxial blocks (spinal, epidural, and combined spinal/epidural [CSE]), paracervical and pudendal blocks, and, less frequently, lumbar sympathetic blocks. Hypotension resulting from sympathectomy is the most frequent complication of central neuraxial blockade. Therefore, maternal blood pressure should be monitored at regular intervals, typically every 2 to 5 minutes for approximately 15 to 20 minutes after the initiation of the block and at routine intervals thereafter. The use of regional analgesia may be contraindicated in the presence of coagulopathy, acute hypovolemia, or infection at the site of needle insertion. Chorioamnionitis without frank sepsis is not a contraindication to central neuraxial blockade in obstetrics, provided antibiotics have been administered.

Because of ethical considerations and methodologic difficulties, it is difficult to design clinical studies to examine the effects of neuraxial analgesia on the progress of labor and mode of delivery. Randomized controlled trials have found no difference in the rate of cesarean delivery in women who received neuraxial compared with systemic opioid labor analgesia.[58–60] The first stage of labor may be slightly prolonged by epidural analgesia; however, this is not of clinical consequence.[58,59] There has been concern that early initiation of epidural analgesia during the latent phase of labor (<4 cm cervical dilation) in nulliparous women may result in a higher incidence of dystocia and cesarean delivery.[60,61] However, several large, randomized studies found no difference in the rate of cesarean delivery in women randomized to early neuraxial compared with systemic opioid analgesia.[62–64] Neuraxial analgesia is, however, associated with prolongation of the second stage of labor in nulliparous women, possibly owing to a decrease in expulsive forces or malposition of the vertex.[58,59,65] Thus, in women with epidural analgesia, the American College of Obstetricians and Gynecologists have redefined an abnormally prolonged second stage of labor as >3 hours in nulliparous and 2 hours in multiparous women. Prolongation of the second stage may be minimized by the use of a dilute local anesthetic solutions in combination with opioid.[66]

Epidural Analgesia

Epidural analgesia may be used for pain relief during labor and vaginal delivery, and if necessary, converted to anesthesia for cesarean delivery. Effective analgesia during the first stage of labor may be achieved by blocking the T10 to L1 dermatomes with low concentrations of local anesthetic, usually combined with lipid-soluble opioids. Combining drugs allows the use of lower doses of both drugs, thus minimizing side effects and complications of each. For the second stage of

labor and delivery the nerve block should be extended to include the S2 to S4 segments in order to block pain for vaginal and perineal distension and trauma.

Long-acting amides such as bupivacaine or ropivacaine are most frequently used because they produce excellent sensory analgesia while sparing motor function, particularly at low concentrations (<0.1%). Analgesia for the first stage of labor may be achieved with 5 to 10 mL of bupivacaine or ropivacaine (0.125%) combined with fentanyl (50 to 100 μg) or sufentanil (5 to 10 μg). There is controversy regarding the need for a test dose when using dilute solutions of local anesthetic.[67] Because catheter aspiration is not always diagnostic, particularly when using single-orifice epidural catheters, some authors believe a test dose should be administered to improve detection of an intrathecally or intravascularly placed catheter.[68]

Analgesia may be maintained with a continuous infusion (8 to 12 mL/hr) of bupivacaine (0.0625 to 0.1%) or ropivacaine (0.08 to 0.15%). Addition of fentanyl, 1 to 2 μg/mL, or sufentanil, 0.3 to 0.5 μg/mL, is often required and will allow for more dilute local anesthetic solutions to be administered. Alternatively, analgesia may be maintained with patient-controlled epidural analgesia (PCEA) with similar solutions of local anesthetic and opioid. PCEA resulted in greater patient satisfaction,[69] a lower average hourly dose of bupivacaine (and therefore less motor block),[9,7] and less need for physician intervention[70,71] compared with a continuous epidural infusion. Protocols for PCEA vary widely. Data are conflicting as to whether a background infusion improves analgesia; however, a background infusion may be helpful in selected parturients (e.g., nulliparas with long labors).[72] Common PCEA parameters include a parturient administered bolus dose of 5 to 10 mL, a lock-out interval of 10 to 20 minutes, and a background infusion of 0 to 15 mL/hr. Thirty to 50% of the hourly dose is often administered as a background infusion.

Women with hemodynamic stability and preserved motor function who do not require continuous fetal monitoring may ambulate with the assistance of a partner during the first stage of labor. Before ambulation, women should be observed for 30 minutes after initiation of neuraxial blockade to assess maternal and fetal well-being.

During delivery, the sacral dermatomes may be blocked with 10 mL of bupivacaine (0.25 to 0.5%), lidocaine (1.0%), or 2-chloroprocaine (2 to 3%). Many parturients have adequate analgesia for delivery without an additional bolus dose, particularly if epidural analgesia has been maintained for a long interval (hours); however, instrumental vaginal delivery may require a more dense block than that obtained with dilute local anesthetic solutions.

Although some studies have found that ropivacaine is associated with less motor blockade than equipotent doses of bupivacaine,[73,74] there was no difference in the rate of instrumental vaginal delivery among women randomized to receive epidural levobupivacaine, bupivacaine, or ropivacaine for maintenance of labor analgesia.[75]

Spinal Analgesia

A single subarachnoid injection for labor analgesia has the advantage of fast and reliable onset of neural blockade, and it is technically easier to initiate compared with epidural analgesia. However, repeated intrathecal injections may be required for a long labor, thus increasing the risk of postdural puncture headache (PDPH). Spinal analgesia with fentanyl, 15 to 25 μg, or sufentanil, 2 to 5 μg, in combination with plain bupivacaine 1.25 to 2.5 mg, may be appropriate in the multiparous patient whose anticipated course of labor does not warrant a catheter technique (duration, 1.5 hours). A potential disadvantage of single-shot spinal analgesia is that the duration of labor, even in a rapidly progressing multiparous woman, may be longer than anticipated. Furthermore, if the woman requires an urgent cesarean delivery, a new anesthetic will need to be initiated. However, spinal anesthesia (a "saddle block") is a safe and effective alternative to general anesthesia or pudendal nerve block for instrumental delivery in parturients without pre-existing epidural analgesia.

Combined Spinal/Epidural Analgesia

CSE analgesia is an ideal analgesic technique for use during labor. CSE combines the rapid, reliable onset of profound analgesia resulting from spinal injection with the flexibility and longer duration associated with a continuous epidural technique. After identification of the epidural space using a conventional (or specialized) epidural needle, a longer (127-mm), pencil-point spinal needle is advanced into the subarachnoid space through the epidural needle. After intrathecal injection, the spinal needle is removed and an epidural catheter is inserted. Intrathecal injection of fentanyl, 10 to 25 μg, or sufentanil, 2.5 to 5 μg, alone or more commonly in combination with bupivacaine 1.25 to 2.5 mg, produces profound analgesia lasting for 90 to 120 minutes with minimal motor block. Opioid alone provides complete analgesia for the early latent phase of labor; however, the addition of bupivacaine is necessary for satisfactory analgesia during advanced labor. Continuous epidural analgesia or PCEA may be initiated within 10 to 20 minutes of the spinal injection. Alternatively, the epidural component may be activated when analgesia is again required.

The most common side effects of intrathecal opioids are pruritus, nausea, vomiting, and urinary retention. The incidence of pruritus is lower if opioid is coadministered with local anesthetic.[76] Rostral spread resulting in delayed respiratory depression is rare with fentanyl and sufentanil, and usually occurs within 30 minutes of injection. Transient nonreassuring FHR patterns may occur after initiation of both epidural and spinal analgesia, with and without opioids; however, the incidence may be higher after spinal opioid administration[77] and in multiparous women with rapidly progressing painful labors.[78] Presumably, uterine hypertonus and decreased uteroplacental perfusion occur as a result of a rapid decrease in circulating maternal epinephrine levels after initiation of analgesia, or as a result of hypotension after sympatholysis. The incidence of emergency cesarean delivery, however, is no greater after CSE than after conventional epidural analgesia.[79,80]

Mothers in early labor, or with preload dependent medical conditions (e.g., aortic stenosis), may particularly benefit from opioid-only CSE. Spinal opioid provides complete analgesia without the need for local anesthetic in early labor, thus avoiding an acute decrease in preload, and almost always allowing motivated women to ambulate because there is no motor block. Multiparous women with advanced cervical dilation also benefit from CSE analgesia in which both intrathecal opioid and local anesthetic are injected. The onset of sacral analgesia is accomplished significantly faster with much less drug than initiation of lumbar epidural analgesia. However, because the epidural component of a CSE is not initially tested, CSE analgesia should be used with caution in women who may require urgent cesarean delivery or are at increased risk from general anesthesia (e.g., morbidly obese or anticipated difficult airway).

Paracervical Block

Bilateral paracervical block interrupts transmission of nerve impulses from the uterus and cervix during the first stage of labor. Five to ten milliliters of dilute local anesthetic solution is injected submucosally via a needle guide in the vagina into the left and right lateral vaginal fornices. Although paracervical block effectively relieves pain during the first stage of labor, the technique has fallen out of favor during childbirth because it is

associated with a high incidence of fetal asphyxia and poor neonatal outcome, particularly with the use of bupivacaine. This may be related to uterine artery constriction or increased uterine tone, direct uptake of the drug into the uterine artery and hence the fetus, or direct fetal injection of local anesthetic. Performing the block with dilute local anesthetic solutions, allowing 5 to 10 minutes to elapse between injections on the left and right side, and limiting the block to women with <8 cm cervical dilation, may decrease the incidence of complications.

Paravertebral Lumbar Sympathetic Block

Paravertebral LSB is a reasonable alternative when contraindications exist to central neuraxial techniques. LSB interrupts the painful transmission of cervical and uterine impulses during the first stage of labor.[81] Although there is less risk of fetal bradycardia with LSB compared with paracervical blockade, unfamiliarity and technical difficulties associated with the performance of the block and risks of intravascular injection have decreased its use in standard practice.

Pudendal Nerve Block

The pudendal nerves, derived from the lower sacral nerve roots (S2 to S4), supply the vaginal vault, perineum, rectum, and parts of the bladder. The nerves are easily anesthetized transvaginally where they loop around the ischial spines. Ten milliliters of dilute local anesthetic solution deposited behind each sacrospinous ligament can provide adequate anesthesia for outlet forceps delivery and episiotomy repair.

Inhalation Analgesia and General Anesthesia

Inhalation labor analgesia is rare in the United States, although its use is more common in other parts of the world (see Inhaled Anesthetics, Chapter 17). Nitrous oxide, 50% by volume, is the most commonly used inhalation agent for analgesia during labor, and the mother is trained to intermittently self-administer the gas at the onset of a contraction. Studies are conflicting as to whether nitrous oxide provides benefit to the parturient[82,83]; however its use appears safe for the fetus and neonate. A major disadvantage of inhalation analgesia is the need for a waste gas scavenging system.

General anesthesia is rarely used for vaginal delivery, and precautions against gastric aspiration must always be observed (see "General Anesthesia" under "Anesthesia for Cesarean Delivery"). General anesthesia may be required when time constraints prevent induction of regional anesthesia. Potent inhalation drugs (1.5 to 2.0 MAC for short periods) can provide uterine relaxation for obstetric maneuvers such as second twin delivery, breech presentation, or postpartum manual removal of a retained placenta. However, in current practice, intravenous nitroglycerin (50 to 250 μg) has largely replaced the need for general anesthesia for uterine relaxation.

ANESTHESIA FOR CESAREAN DELIVERY

The most common indications for cesarean delivery include arrest of dilation, nonreassuring fetal status, cephalopelvic disproportion, malpresentation, prematurity, prior cesarean delivery, and prior uterine surgery involving the corpus.[84] The choice of anesthesia depends on the urgency of the procedure, the condition of the mother and fetus, and the mother's wishes.

A 2001 survey of obstetric anesthesia practices in the United States revealed that most patients undergoing cesarean delivery do so under spinal or epidural anesthesia.[85] Neuraxial techniques have several advantages: they avoid the necessity of airway manipulation, lessen the risk of gastric aspiration, avoid the use of depressant anesthetic drugs, allow the mother to remain awake during delivery, and may be associated with less operative blood loss. Compared with general anesthesia, there is less immediate neonatal depression after neuraxial compared with general anesthesia.

Neuraxial Anesthesia

Blockade to the T4 dermatome is necessary to perform cesarean delivery without maternal discomfort. The most common complication of neuraxial anesthesia is hypotension and the attendant risk of decreased uteroplacental perfusion (see "Hypotension" under "Anesthetic Complications"). Measures to decrease the incidence and severity of hypotension include left uterine displacement, intravenous fluid administration, and the liberal use of vasopressors to prevent and treat hypotension.

Most anesthesiologists administer a nonparticulate antacid before induction of anesthesia for pulmonary aspiration prophylaxis. Some practitioners also administer an H_2 receptor antagonist and metoclopramide. Sedative premedication is usually not necessary. Intraoperative monitoring mimics that for all anesthetics, although blood pressure should be measured frequently (every several minutes) for the first 20 minutes after initiation of anesthesia. Although supplemental oxygen is frequently administered, there is no evidence of benefit to the mother, fetus, or neonate.[86,87]

Multimodal analgesia, including systemic nonsteroidal anti-inflammatory drugs and neuraxial opioids and/or local anesthetics, is optimal for postoperative analgesia. Abdominal wall nerve block techniques have also been described after cesarean delivery.[88] Although postcesarean delivery analgesia should take the nursing infant into account, very small amounts of drugs administered to the mother actually cross into breast milk, and even smaller amounts are absorbed from the neonatal gut. Prolonged (12 to 24 hours) postoperative pain relief in the postpartum patient can be provided by intrathecal morphine (100 to 150 μg)[89] or epidural morphine (3.5 to 4.0 mg).[89] PCEA with a dilute solution of local anesthetic and lipid-soluble opioid is another option after epidural anesthesia. Side effects of neuraxial morphine include nausea, vomiting, and pruritus. Delayed respiratory depression is a rare but potentially devastating complication; therefore, the patient must be monitored carefully in the postoperative period. Morbidly obese women may be at higher risk for respiratory depression.[90]

Spinal Anesthesia

Subarachnoid block is probably the most commonly administered neuraxial anesthetic for cesarean delivery because of its simplicity, speed of onset, and reliability. It is an alternative to general anesthesia for almost all but the most emergent of cesarean deliveries. Hyperbaric 0.75% bupivacaine, 12.5 to 13.5 mg (1.6 to 1.8 mL), is the most commonly used local anesthetic in the United States. It reliably provides 90 to 120 minutes of surgical anesthesia.

Despite an adequate dermatomal level for surgery, women may experience varying degrees of visceral discomfort and nausea and vomiting, particularly during exteriorization of the uterus and traction on abdominal viscera. Improved perioperative anesthesia and analgesia can be provided with the addition of fentanyl, 10 to 20 μg, sufentanil, 2.5 to 5 μg, or morphine, 0.1 to 0.15 mg, to the local anesthetic solution. Fentanyl has a rapid onset, but is short-acting and provides little additional postoperative analgesia. In contrast, morphine has a longer latency than fentanyl, but will also provide anesthesia for 12 to 18 hours after delivery.

Lumbar Epidural Anesthesia

In contrast to spinal anesthesia, epidural anesthesia is associated with a slower onset of action and a larger drug requirement to establish adequate sensory block. The major advantages of epidural compared with spinal anesthesia are the ability to titrate the extent and duration of anesthesia. To avoid inadvertent intrathecal or intravascular injection, correct placement of the epidural needle and catheter is essential. This is especially true because epidural anesthesia for cesarean delivery necessitates the administration of large doses of local anesthetic.

Aspiration of the epidural catheter for blood or cerebrospinal fluid is not reliable for detection of catheter misplacement, particularly with single-orifice catheters. Thus, most anesthesiologists administer a test dose before the initiation of surgical anesthesia. A small dose of local anesthetic, for example, lidocaine, 45 mg, or bupivacaine, 5 mg, readily produces identifiable sensory and motor block if injected intrathecally. Addition of epinephrine (15 μg) with careful hemodynamic monitoring may signal intravascular injection if followed by a transient increase in heart rate and blood pressure. The use of an epinephrine test dose (15 μg) in obstetrics is controversial because false-positive results do occur (10% increase in heart rate) in the presence of uterine contractions. In addition, epinephrine may reduce uteroplacental perfusion. Rapid injection of 1 mL of air with simultaneous precordial Doppler monitoring appears to be a reliable indicator of intravascular catheter placement.[91] Fentanyl, 100 μg, has also been used to test epidural catheter placement (significant reduction in pain).[92] A negative test, although reassuring, does not eliminate the need for incremental administration of local anesthetic.

The most commonly used agents for obstetric epidural anesthesia are 3% 2-chloroprocaine and 2% lidocaine with epinephrine, 5 μg/mL (1:200,000). Adequate anesthesia is usually achieved with 15 to 25 mL of local anesthetic solution, administered in divided doses over 5 to 10 minutes. The 2-chloroprocaine provides rapid onset of a reliable block with minimal risk of systemic toxicity because of its extremely high rate of metabolism in maternal and fetal plasma, although 2% lidocaine with epinephrine and sodium bicarbonate (1 mEq/10 mL lidocaine) may also be used when the rapid conversion of pre-existing epidural labor analgesia to surgical anesthesia is required for urgent cesarean delivery. Lidocaine has an onset and duration intermediate to those of 2-chloroprocaine and bupivacaine. Lidocaine should be administered with epinephrine, as lidocaine without epinephrine does not consistently provide satisfactory surgical anesthesia. Bupivacaine is no longer commonly used for obstetric epidural *anesthesia* as it is associated with a greater risk of cardiac toxicity compared with other amide local anesthetics.[93] Unintentional intravascular injection of bupivacaine is associated with a high incidence of maternal mortality.[94] Ropivacaine 0.5% combined with fentanyl may be used for surgical anesthesia as the risk of toxicity is less than that of bupivacaine. The duration of motor block is shorter after ropivacaine compared with bupivacaine, but there are no differences in latency, quality of anesthesia, and duration of block.[95,96]

Combined Spinal-Epidural Anesthesia

Advantages of CSE anesthesia for cesarean delivery include the rapid onset of a dense block with a low anesthetic dose, and the ability to extend the duration of anesthesia, and perhaps to provide continuous postoperative analgesia. There is a lower incidence of breakthrough pain and intraoperative shivering, and maternal satisfaction was higher after CSE compared with epidural anesthesia for cesarean delivery.[97] Several variations of the CSE technique have been described. The standard technique uses the same spinal dose of local anesthetic as one would use for standard spinal anesthesia. In sequential CSE anesthesia a smaller spinal dose is expected to result in inadequate anesthesia for some patients. After 15 minutes, if anesthesia is inadequate, the block is extended by injecting supplemental local anesthetic via the epidural catheter.[98] Although the incidence of hypotension is lower with this technique compared with full-dose spinal anesthesia, the induction to incision time is prolonged. A third technique is also associated with a lower incidence of hypotension without prolonging onset time. A small dose of spinal local anesthetic is followed by the routine injection of additional anesthetic through the epidural catheter approximately 5 minutes after the intrathecal dose.[99] Bupivacaine doses from 6 to 12 mg have been described for CSE anesthesia.

General Anesthesia

General anesthesia may be necessary when contraindications or relative contraindications exist to neuraxial anesthesia (e.g., coagulopathy, or moderate or severe aortic stenosis), or when the need for emergency delivery precludes central neuraxial blockade. General anesthesia should be used cautiously in women with asthma, upper respiratory tract infection, obesity, or a history of difficult tracheal intubation. Preoperative airway evaluation is particularly important in pregnant women because inability to intubate the trachea and provide effective ventilation is the leading cause of maternal death related to anesthesia.[100] If airway difficulties are anticipated, a neuraxial anesthetic technique should be considered or an awake tracheal intubation performed. Pulmonary aspiration prophylaxis should be administered and the patient should be positioned with left lateral tilt to prevent aortocaval compression. Monitoring mimics that for all anesthetics.

To minimize the risk of hypoxemia during induction, denitrogenation for 3 to 5 minutes with a tight-fitting mask is essential. In an emergency, four deep breaths with 100% oxygen suffice. A "defasciculating" dose of a nondepolarizing muscle relaxant is not necessary. Rapid-sequence induction is performed with thiopental (4 mg/kg), propofol (2 mg/kg), ketamine (1 mg/kg), or etomidate (0.2 to 0.3 mg/kg), followed by succinylcholine (1 to 1.5 mg/kg) to facilitate tracheal intubation. Succinylcholine is the preferred muscle relaxant; however, when its use is contraindicated, rocuronium (0.6 mg/kg) is an acceptable alternative. Cricoid pressure is applied by a trained assistant until the airway is properly secured with a cuffed endotracheal tube. Once correct placement of the endotracheal tube is confirmed with capnography and auscultation, the obstetrician may proceed with incision.

If there is difficulty in securing the airway, cricoid pressure should be maintained throughout, and the mother ventilated with 100% oxygen before a subsequent attempt at tracheal intubation is made. The American Society of Anesthesiologists difficult airway algorithm[101] should be modified to include assessment of fetal status and the need for immediate delivery (Fig. 43-6). It is safer for the mother to allow her to awaken and to reassess the method of induction and intubation, rather than to persist with traumatic efforts at tracheal intubation. However, if the fetus is in extremis, airway management with a mask or laryngeal mask airway may be an acceptable alternative.[102,103]

In the interval between intubation and delivery, anesthesia is maintained with a 50:50 mixture of nitrous oxide in oxygen and a volatile anesthetic agent. In the past it was common to limit the volatile agent concentration to 0.5 MAC to limit fetal exposure before delivery, and limit uterine relaxation after delivery. However, the incidence of intraoperative awareness appears to be unacceptably high with this technique.[104] Indeed, a significant number of women had bispectral index values >60 during general anesthesia with sevoflurane 1% in nitrous oxide 50%.[105] Therefore, higher concentrations of volatile agent should be used before delivery. After delivery the nitrous

oxide concentration can be increased and/or an intravenous amnestic (e.g., midazolam) and opioids can be administered.

General anesthesia for cesarean delivery is associated with lower neonatal Apgar scores at 1 minute compared with neuraxial anesthesia[106,107]; however, the Apgar scores at 5 minutes are comparable. Therefore, an individual trained in neonatal resuscitation should be present at delivery of the infant. After delivery, intravenous oxytocin is administered to decrease the risk of uterine atony and anesthesia is deepened with an opioid and benzodiazepine, as necessary. At the end of the procedure, the mother's trachea is extubated once she is awake and extubation criteria have been met. The usual blood loss at a cesarean delivery is 750 to 1,000 mL, and transfusion is rarely necessary.

ANESTHETIC COMPLICATIONS

Maternal Mortality

6 A study of anesthesia-related deaths in the United States between 1979 and 1990 revealed that the case fatality rate with general anesthesia was 16.7 times greater than that with neuraxial anesthesia. Most anesthesia-related deaths were a result of cardiac arrest due to hypoxemia when difficulties securing the airway were encountered.[100] Pregnancy-induced anatomic and physiologic changes, such as reduced FRC, increased oxygen consumption, and oropharyngeal edema, may expose the patient to serious risks of desaturation during periods of apnea and hypoventilation (see "Physiologic Changes of Pregnancy").

Pulmonary Aspiration

The risk of inhalation of gastric contents may be increased in pregnant women, particularly if difficulty occurs with airway management. Women who have recently eaten, are laboring, received systemic opioids, or who have frequent heartburn are of greatest concern.[18,22] Comprehensive airway evaluation, prophylactic administration of nonparticulate antacids, and preferred use of regional anesthesia are essential. General anesthesia may be unavoidable occasionally; therefore, awake intubation may be indicated in women in whom airway difficulties are anticipated.

Hypotension

Neuraxial anesthesia is frequently associated with hypotension. Labor lowers the risk of hypotension in term pregnant women compared with nonlaboring women. Blood pressure should be monitored frequently (every 2 to 3 minutes) after the induction of neuraxial anesthesia. Techniques to reduce the incidence of hypotension during neuraxial anesthesia include intravenous fluid and vasopressor administration. Maintaining the maternal blood pressure close to baseline reduces the incidence of maternal nausea and vomiting and is associated with higher umbilical artery pH values.[108] The administration of an intravenous bolus of crystalloid solution (1,000 to 1,500 mL) at the time of induction of neuraxial analgesia (co-load) is more effective than administration of the same volume of solution prior to the initiation of anesthesia (preload).[109] Colloid (500 mL) is superior to crystalloid solution in preventing hypotension[110] and may be considered in woman at high risk for hypotension or its consequences.[111]

Recent evidence suggests that phenylephrine is equally efficacious to ephedrine for treating maternal hypotension, and results in less fetal acidosis.[112] Ephedrine may cross the placenta and increase fetal cerebral metabolic rate[113] although the clinical significance of this effect is not known.

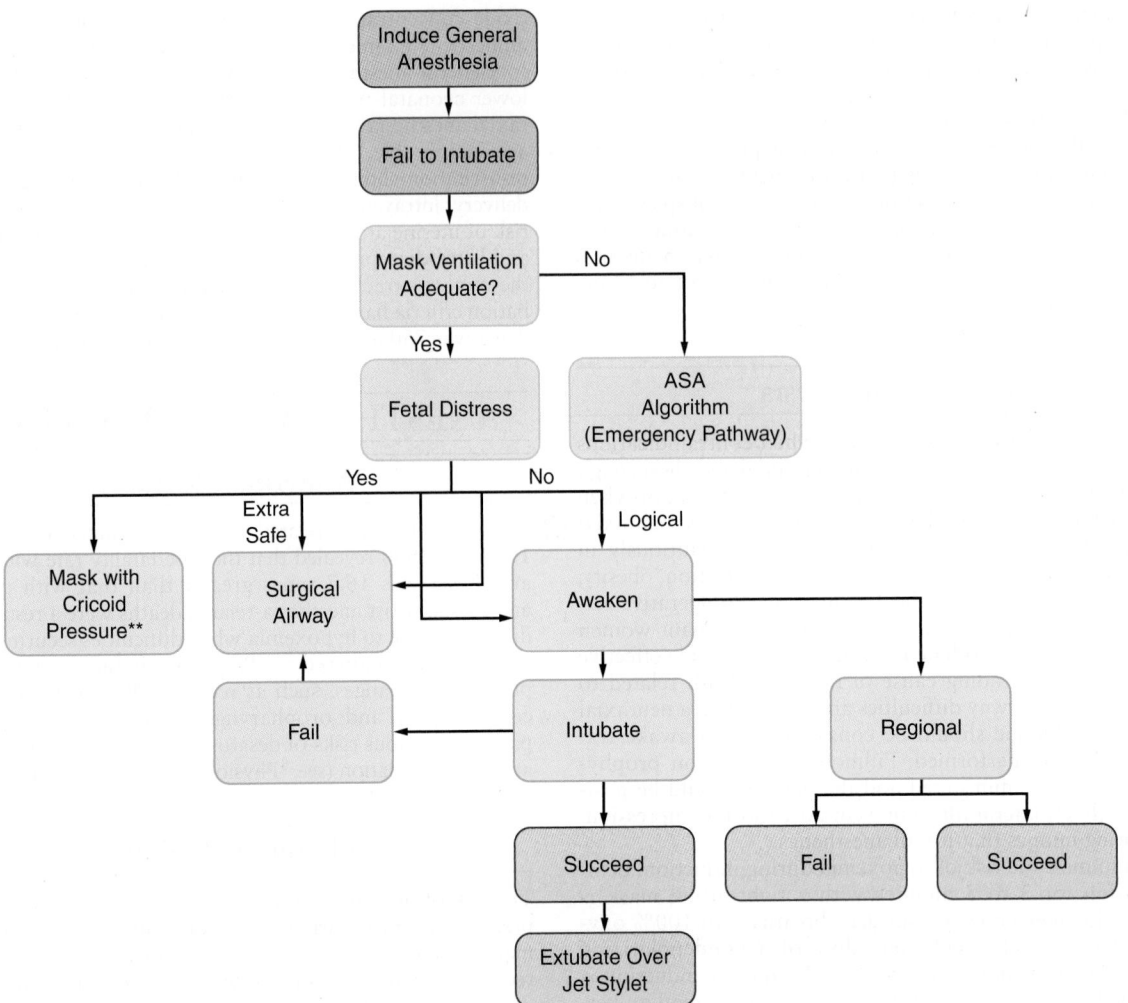

FIGURE 43-6.   Management of the difficult airway in pregnancy with special reference to the presence or absence of fetal distress. When mask ventilation is not possible, the clinician is referred to the American Society of Anesthesiologists (ASA) algorithm for the emergency airway management found in Chapter 22. (Reprinted from Kuczkowski KM, Reisner LS, Benumof JL: The difficult airway: Risk, prophylaxis, and management, Obstetric Anesthesia: Principles and Practice, 3rd edition. Edited by Chestnut DH. St. Louis, Elsevier-Mosby, 2004, p 550, with permission.)
**Conventional face mask or laryngeal mask airway.

Many anesthesiologists are currently using a combination of phenylephrine and ephedrine, depending on maternal heart rate. Ephedrine is commonly administered as an intravenous bolus (5 to 10 mg). Phenylephrine is shorter acting and may be administered as a bolus (50 to 100 μg) or continuous infusion (starting rate, 100 μg/min).

Total Spinal Anesthesia

High or total spinal anesthesia is a rare complication of intrathecal injection that occurs after excessive cephalad spread of local anesthetic in the subarachnoid or epidural space. Unintentional intrathecal administration of epidural medication as a result of dural puncture or catheter migration may also result in this complication. There is rapid ascent of sensory-motor blockade and patients may complain of dyspnea, inability to phonate, and difficulty swallowing. Profound hypotension may lead to brainstem and cerebral hypoperfusion and cause loss of consciousness. Immediate vasopressor administration, continued fluid administration, left uterine displacement, and leg elevation may be necessary to achieve hemodynamic stability. Reverse Trendelenburg position should not be used if hyper-

baric anesthetic solution was used for spinal blockade as there is a risk of cerebral hypoperfusion. Rapid control of the airway is essential, and endotracheal intubation may be necessary to ensure oxygenation without aspiration.

Local Anesthetic-Induced Seizures

Systemic toxicity may occur after unintended intravascular injection or drug accumulation (see Local Anesthetics). Resuscitation equipment (intravenous access, airway equipment, emergency drugs, and suction equipment) should always be available when using local anesthetics. To avoid systemic toxicity of local anesthetic agents, strict adherence to recommended dosages, methods to detect misplaced needles and catheters, and fractional administration of the induction dose are essential.

Despite these precautions, life-threatening convulsions and, more rarely, cardiovascular collapse may occur. Seizure activity should be treated with intravenous thiopental, 50 to 100 mg, or diazepam, 5 to 10 mg; larger doses may enhance local anesthetic-induced myocardial depression. Hemodynamics, ventilation, and oxygenation must be maintained. If cardiovascular collapse occurs, it should be treated according to advanced cardiac life support protocols. Amiodarone may be used to treat ventricular dysrhythmias, particularly those due to bupivacaine. A cesarean delivery may be required to relieve aortocaval compression and to ensure the efficacy of cardiac massage.[114] Recently, lipid emulsion therapy has been successfully used to treat cardiac arrest due to bupivacaine toxicity.[115] Protocols for lipid rescue may be found at www.lipidrescue.org.

Postdural Puncture Headache

7 By virtue of age and gender, pregnant women are at a higher risk for developing PDPH (see Spinal Epidural). In addition, after delivery, reduced epidural pressure may increase the risk of cerebrospinal fluid leakage through the dural opening, and estrogen withdrawal after delivery may exacerbate vascular headaches.

The incidence of PDPH is related to the diameter of the dural puncture, ranging from in excess of 70% after use of 16-gauge needles to <1% with the smaller 25- or 26-gauge spinal needles. The incidence of cephalalgia is reduced with the use of pencil-point needles (Whitacre or Sprotte), compared with cutting bevel (Quincke) needles. Conservative treatment is indicated in the presence of mild-to-moderate discomfort, and includes bed rest, hydration, and simple analgesics. Caffeine (500 mg intravenously or 300 mg orally) has also been used in treatment of PDPH, but the therapeutic effect is transient. Severe headache that does not respond to conservative measures for 24 hours is best treated with autologous blood patch. Using aseptic technique, 10 to 20 mL of the patient's blood is injected into the epidural space close to the site of dural puncture. This procedure may be repeated if necessary. A blood patch should not be performed for several hours after treatment with intravenous caffeine as this may precipitate a seizure. Prophylactic administration of autologous blood (after delivery, before removal of the epidural catheter) does not influence the incidence and severity of PDPH, although the duration of headache is less, compared with expectant management.[116]

Nerve Injury

Neurologic sequelae of central neuraxial blockade, although rare, have been reported. Pressure or trauma exerted by a needle or catheter on spinal nerve roots or the spinal cord produces immediate pain. Needle or catheter advancement should stop immediately on patient complaint of paresthesia or pain, and if the pain does not resolve within seconds the needle or catheter should be withdrawn and repositioned. Anesthetics should *not* be injected when there are paresthesias. Infections such as epidural abscess or meningitis are rare and may be a manifestation of systemic sepsis or local infection. Epidural hematoma can also occur, usually in association with coagulation defects. Nerve root irritation may have a protracted recovery, lasting weeks or months. Postpartum peripheral nerve injury as a result of instrumentation, lithotomy position, or compression by the fetal head is not uncommon and may occur even in the absence of neuraxial technique.[117]

MANAGEMENT OF HIGH-RISK PARTURIENTS

8 Pregnancy and parturition are considered "high risk" when accompanied by conditions unfavorable to the well-being of the mother, the fetus, or both. Maternal problems may be related to pregnancy, such as preeclampsia–eclampsia and other hypertensive disorders of pregnancy, or antepartum hemorrhage resulting from placenta previa or abruptio placen-

tae. Diabetes mellitus; cardiac, chronic renal, neurologic, or sickle cell disease; and asthma, obesity, and drug abuse are not related to pregnancy but are often affected by it. Advanced maternal age is associated with an increased risk of maternal and fetal complications. Prematurity (gestation of <37 weeks), postmaturity (≥42 weeks), intrauterine growth retardation, and multiple gestation are fetal conditions associated with risk. During labor and delivery, fetal malpresentation (breech, transverse lie), placental abruption, compression of the umbilical cord (prolapse, nuchal cord), precipitous labor, or intrauterine infection (prolonged rupture of membranes) may increase the risk to the mother or the fetus.

In general, the anesthetic management of the high-risk parturient is based on the same maternal and fetal considerations as the management of healthy mothers and fetuses. These include maintenance of maternal cardiovascular function and oxygenation, maintenance and possibly improvement of uteroplacental blood flow, and creation of optimal conditions for a painless, atraumatic delivery of an infant without significant drug effects. However, there is less physiologic reserve because many of these functions may be compromised before the induction of anesthesia. For example, significant acidosis is prone to develop in fetuses of diabetic mothers when delivered by cesarean with spinal anesthesia complicated by even brief maternal hypotension.[17] Because the high-risk parturient may have received a variety of drugs, anesthesiologists must be familiar with potential interactions between these drugs and the anesthetic drugs they plan to administer.

Preeclampsia–Eclampsia

Hypertensive disorders, which occur in approximately 7% of all late pregnancies, are a major cause of maternal mortality. Preeclampsia is diagnosed with the development of hypertension with proteinuria. Eclampsia is present if convulsions occur. Preeclampsia–eclampsia is a disease of unknown etiology but is unique to human pregnancy. Symptoms appear after the 20th week of gestation, earlier than that with a hydatidiform mole. The condition requires the presence of a trophoblast but not a fetus.

Many of the symptoms associated with preeclampsia, including placental ischemia, systemic vasoconstriction, and increased platelet aggregation, may result from an imbalance in placental production of prostacyclin and thromboxane (Figs. 43-7 and 43-8). During normal pregnancy the placenta produces equivalent quantities of these prostaglandins, whereas in preeclamptic pregnancy, there is 7 times more thromboxane than prostacyclin.[118] An alternative etiology may be related to an inhibition of the normal trophoblastic migration of placental arterioles during the second trimester, thus preventing a low-resistance, high-flow placental circulation from developing.[119] Endothelial injury is central to the development of preeclampsia and occurs as a result of reduced placental perfusion and a production and release of substances (possibly lipid peroxidases). Abnormal endothelial function contributes to an increase in peripheral resistance and other abnormalities noted in preeclampsia through a release of fibronectin, endothelin, and other substances.

Placental ischemia results in a release of uterine renin and an increase in angiotensin (Fig. 43-7). Widespread arteriolar vasoconstriction occurs, causing hypertension, tissue hypoxia, and endothelial damage. Adherence of platelets at sites of endothelial damage results in coagulopathy. Enhanced angiotensin-mediated aldosterone secretion may lead to an increased sodium reabsorption and edema. Proteinuria may also be attributed to placental ischemia, which would lead to local tissue degeneration and a release of thromboplastin with subsequent deposition of fibrin in constricted glomerular

FIGURE 43-7. Proposed scheme of pathophysiologic changes in toxemia of pregnancy. (Reprinted from Speroff L: Toxemia of pregnancy: Mechanism and therapeutic management. Am J Cardiol 1973; 32: 582, with permission.)

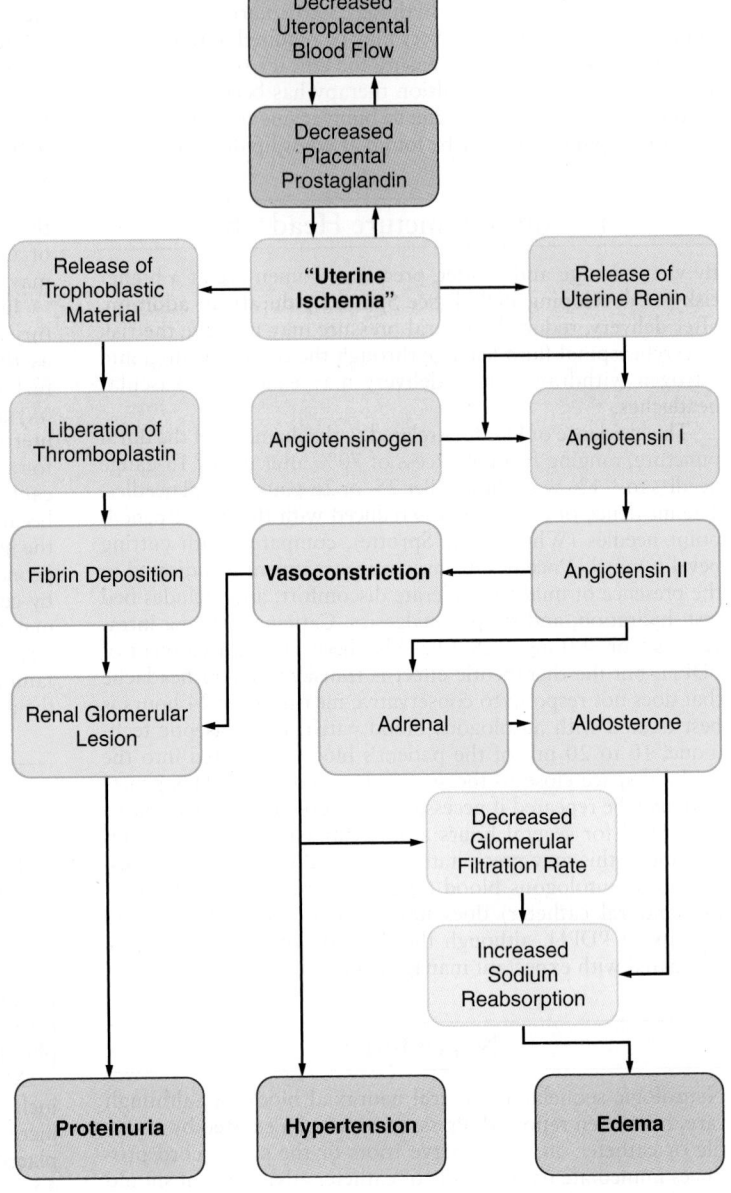

vessels, as well as increased permeability to albumin and other plasma proteins. Furthermore, there is believed to be a decreased production of prostaglandin E, a potent vasodilator secreted in the trophoblast, which normally would balance the hypertensive effects of the renin–angiotensin system. The HELLP syndrome is a particular form of severe preeclampsia characterized by *h*emolysis, *el*evated *l*iver enzymes, and *l*ow *p*latelet count (thrombocytopenia). In contrast to preeclampsia, elevations in blood pressure and proteinuria may be mild.

Preeclampsia is classified as severe if it is associated with any of the following:

1. Severe hypertension
   a. Systolic blood pressure of 160 mm Hg
   b. Diastolic blood pressure of 110 mm Hg
2. Severe proteinuria of 5 g/24 hr
3. Evidence of severe end-organ damage
   a. Refractory oliguria (400 mL/24 hr)
   b. Cerebral or visual disturbances
   c. Pulmonary edema or cyanosis
   d. Epigastric pain
   e. Intrauterine growth retardation

Severe preeclampsia–eclampsia is a multisystem disease. Global cerebral blood flow is not diminished, but focal hypoperfusion may occur. Postmortem examination has revealed hemorrhagic necrosis in the proximity of thrombosed precapillaries, suggesting intense vasoconstriction. Cerebral edema and small foci of degeneration have been attributed to hypoxia. Petechial hemorrhages are common after the onset of convulsions. Symptoms related to these changes include headache, vertigo, cortical blindness, hyperreflexia, and convulsions. Blood pressure elevation correlates poorly with the incidence of seizures. Cerebral hemorrhage and edema account for 50% of deaths with preeclampsia–eclampsia.

Intense ocular arteriolar constriction may cause blurred vision, even temporary blindness. Heart failure may result in severe cases as a result of peripheral vasoconstriction and increased blood viscosity secondary to hemoconcentration. Left ventricular hypertrophy, subendocardial hemorrhages, cloudy swelling, and fatty and hyaline degeneration may occur.

Decreased blood supply to the liver may lead to periportal necrosis. Subcapsular hemorrhages results in epigastric pain. Rarely, there is rupture of the overstretched liver capsule and massive hemorrhage into the abdominal cavity. There may be

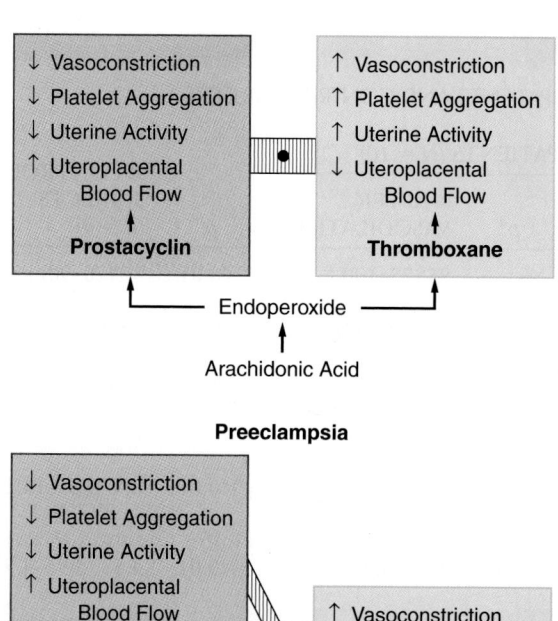

Preeclampsia

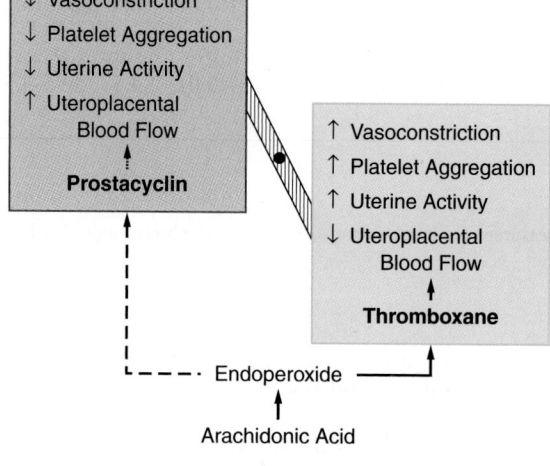

FIGURE 43-8. Comparison of the balance in the biological actions of prostacyclin and thromboxane in normal pregnancy with the imbalance of increased thromboxane and decreased prostacyclin in preeclamptic pregnancy. (Reprinted from Walsh SW: Preeclampsia: An imbalance in placental prostacyclin and thromboxane production. Am J Obstet Gynecol 1985; 152: 335, with permission.)

rate decrease, resulting in reduced uric acid clearance and, in severe cases, reduced clearance of urea and creatinine. Oliguria and proteinuria are characteristic symptoms of severe preeclampsia. The severity of renal involvement is reflected in the degree of proteinuria, which may reach nephrotic levels of 10 to 15 g/24 hr.

A mild pulmonary ventilation–perfusion imbalance has been reported in severe cases. It is not believed to be clinically important because the arterial oxygen tension was within normal limits. In contrast, airway edema, which may also occur in severe preeclampsia, is of great concern because it may lead to respiratory embarrassment and difficulty in tracheal intubation. Pulmonary edema occurs in approximately 2% of severe preeclamptic patients as a result of heart failure, circulatory overload, or aspiration of gastric contents during convulsions.

A reduction in intervillous blood flow may result from vasoconstriction or the development of occlusive lesions in decidual arteries, despite the elevated maternal blood pressure. Histologic examination of the placenta reveals nodular ischemia and varying stages of infarction. Necrosis of the supporting tissues may lead to a rupture of fetal cotyledonary vessels and hemorrhage. It may extend retroplacentally, resulting in placental abruption. Reduced placental blood flow leads to chronic fetal hypoxia and malnutrition. The risks of intrauterine growth retardation, premature birth, and perinatal death are substantially higher than in normal pregnancies and correlate with the severity of preeclampsia.

Although preeclampsia is accompanied by exaggerated retention of water and sodium, a shift of fluid and proteins from the intravascular into the extravascular compartment may result in hypovolemia, hypoproteinemia, and hemoconcentration. This phenomenon may be further affected by proteinuria. The risk of uteroplacental hypoperfusion and poor fetal outcome correlates with the degree of maternal plasma and protein depletion. The mean plasma volume in women with preeclampsia was found to be 9% less than normal, and in those with severe disease, 30 to 40% below normal.[120] The inverse relationship between the intravascular volume and the severity of hypertension was confirmed with measurements of central venous pressure (CVP) (Fig. 43-9). Patients with a diastolic pressure of 110 mm Hg may have a CVP as low as –4 cm H_2O and may require careful hydration to increase the CVP. A significant reduction in maternal plasma volume may precede the clinical appearance of preeclampsia in previously normotensive patients.

Hemodynamic changes in preeclampsia vary with the progression of the disease, whether patients are in labor or have

elevated aspartate aminotransferase, lactate dehydrogenase, and alkaline phosphatase, whereas bilirubin is unaltered.

In the kidneys, there is swelling of glomerular endothelial cells and deposition of fibrin, leading to a constriction of the capillary lumina. Renal blood flow and glomerular filtration

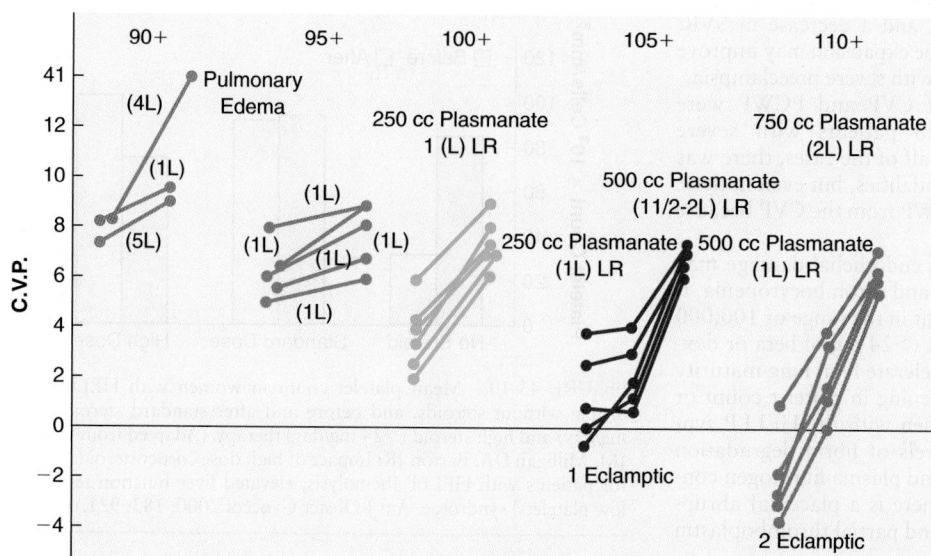

FIGURE 43-9. Initial central venous pressure measurements (three or more recordings of maternal diastolic pressure) and intravenous volume replacement required to attain the range of 6 to 8 cm H_2O in five groups of women with preeclampsia classified according to the severity of the disease (by diastolic blood pressure). LR, lactated Ringer solution. (Reprinted from Joyce TH III, Debnath KS, Baker EA: Preeclampsia: Relationship of CVP and epidural analgesia. Anesthesiology 1979; 51: S297, with permission.)

TABLE 43-2

HEMODYNAMIC VARIABLES (MEAN AND RANGE) IN PREECLAMPTIC PATIENTS AND CONTROL SUBJECTS

■ VARIABLE	■ INITIAL	PREECLAMPTIC PATIENTS (N = 10)					■ CONTROL SUBJECTS (n = 4)
		■ AFTER VOLUME EXPANSION	p^a	■ AFTER VASODILATION	p^b		
Diastolic blood pressure (mm Hg)	106 (100–120)	102 (90–120)	NS	85 (75–100)	<0.01		77 (70–90)
Mean arterial pressure (mm Hg)	121 (113–136)	116 (103–136)	<0.02	102 (97–116)	<0.01		95 (93–106)
Heart rate (beats/min)	100 (90–130)	81 (60–110)	<0.02	82 (70–100)	NS		84 (70–90)
Pulmonary capillary wedge pressure (mm Hg)	3.3 (1–5)	8 (7–10)	<0.01	8 (7–9)	NS		9 (6–12)
Systemic vascular resistance (dyne/sec/cm⁵)	1,943 (1,480–2,580)	1,284 (1,073–1,600)	<0.01	947 (782–1,028)	<0.01		886 (805–1,021)
Cardiac index (L/min/m²)	2.75 (1.97–3.33)	3.77 (3.26–4.05)	<0.01	4.40 (3.94–5.00)	<0.01		4.53 (3.96–4.97)

NS, not significant. Wilcoxon signed-rank test (two-tailed).
[a]As compared with initial values.
[b]As compared with values after volume expansion.
Reproduced from Groenendijk R, Trimbos MJ, Wallenberg HCS: Hemodynamic measurements in pre-eclampsia: Preliminary observations. Am J Obstet Gynecol 1984; 150: 232, with permission.

received therapy. Earlier studies, using pulmonary artery flow-directed catheters, suggested patients with severe preeclampsia were in a hyperdynamic state. However, these investigations were performed when patients were in labor or in the postpartum period, after treatment had been instituted. More recently, hemodynamic data were obtained in ten preeclamptic and four healthy pregnant women near term who were not in labor[121] (Table 43-2). In the preeclamptic women, measurements were made before treatment, after volume expansion, and after vasodilation was achieved with a continuous intravenous infusion of dihydralazine. Initial measurements revealed a low pulmonary capillary wedge pressure (PCWP), a low cardiac index, a high SVR, and an increased heart rate, indicating the existence of a low-output state in untreated preeclamptic women. Volume expansion resulted in an increase in PCWP and cardiac index, whereas the SVR and maternal heart rate decreased. The mean arterial pressure was significantly reduced, mainly because of a decrease in systolic pressure. Subsequent infusion of dihydralazine did not alter the capillary wedge pressure but led to an additional increase in cardiac index and a decrease in SVR. These data indicate that careful volume expansion may improve maternal tissue perfusion in patients with severe preeclampsia.

Simultaneous determinations of CVP and PCWP were obtained in another group of 18 patients with severe preeclampsia.[122] In approximately half of the cases, there was a linear relation between the two modalities, but even in these women it was difficult to predict PCWP from the CVP because of wide interindividual variations.

Adherence of platelets at sites of endothelial damage may result in consumption coagulopathy and thrombocytopenia. It is usually mild, with the platelet count in the range of 100,000 to 150,000/mm³. High-dose steroids (>24 mg of beta or dexamethasone in 24 hours) used to accelerate fetal lung maturity have been shown to prevent a worsening in platelet count or even increase platelet count in women with the HELLP syndrome[123] (Fig. 43-10). Elevated levels of fibrin degradation products are found less frequently, and plasma fibrinogen concentrations remain normal unless there is a placental abruption. Prolongation of prothrombin and partial thromboplastin times indicates consumption of procoagulant. Bleeding time is no longer considered a reliable test of clotting.

General Management

The definitive treatment of preeclampsia–eclampsia remains delivery of the fetus and placenta. Management is usually symptomatic until such time as the obstetrician determines that delivery is appropriate for the fetus. The goals are to prevent or control convulsions, improve organ perfusion, normalize blood pressure, and correct clotting abnormalities. Mild cases may be managed expectantly with bed rest, antihypertensive medication, and fetal surveillance until the pregnancy is closer to term. Delivery is indicated in refractory cases, if there is nonreassuring fetal status or if the pregnancy is already close to term. In severe cases, aggressive management should continue for at least 24 to 48 hours after delivery.

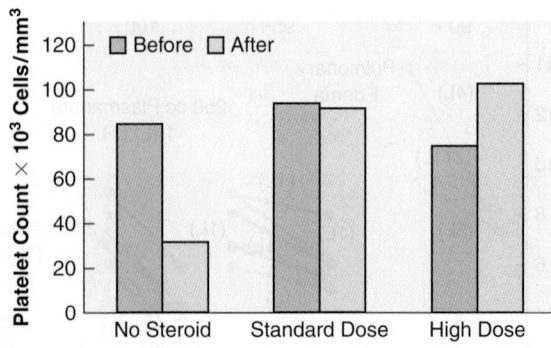

FIGURE 43-10. Mean platelet count in women with HELLP syndrome without steroids, and before and after standard steroid (<24 mg/day) and high steroid (>24 mg/day) therapy. (Adapted from O'Brien JM, Milligan DA, Barton JR: Impact of high dose corticosteroid therapy for patients with HELLP [hemolysis, elevated liver function tests, and low platelets] syndrome. Am J Obstet Gynecol 2000; 183: 921.)

The mainstay of anticonvulsant therapy is magnesium sulfate (see Chapter 14). The patient usually receives an intravenous loading dose of 4 g in a 20% solution over 5 minutes. Therapeutic blood levels are maintained by continuous infusion of 1 to 2 g/hr. Magnesium may cause mild peripheral arterial vasodilation. Magnesium ions cross the placenta readily, and may lead to fetal and neonatal hypermagnesemia. There is poor correlation between magnesium concentrations in the umbilical cord blood and the incidence of low Apgar scores and depression of ventilation at birth, which are more likely due to fetal asphyxia and prematurity.

Magnesium potentiates the duration and intensity of action of depolarizing and nondepolarizing muscle relaxants by decreasing the amount of acetylcholine liberated from the motor nerve terminals, diminishing the sensitivity of the end plate to acetylcholine, and depressing the excitability of the skeletal muscle membrane. Magnesium may also increase the severity of hypotension under regional anesthesia and make it more difficult to treat. Judicious hydration with a balanced salt solution may be required to replace intravascular volume. In all cases, careful monitoring of arterial pressure and urine output should be started as soon as possible. In severe cases, invasive central pressure monitoring may be required. A pulmonary artery catheter is preferred in patients with pulmonary edema, refractory hypertension, or oliguria.[122] Monitoring should be extended to the postpartum period.

Antihypertensive therapy in preeclampsia is used to lessen the risk of cerebral hemorrhage in the mother while maintaining, even improving, tissue perfusion. Plasma volume expansion combined with vasodilation fulfills these goals[121] (see Chapter 15). Hydralazine is the most commonly used vasodilator in preeclampsia because it increases uteroplacental and renal blood flows. Nitroprusside, a potent vasodilator of resistance and capacitance vessels, with an immediate but evanescent action, is useful in preventing dangerous elevations in systemic and pulmonary artery blood pressure during laryngoscopy and intubation, and is ideal for treatment of hypertensive emergencies. Infusion rates of nitroprusside 5 to 10 μg/kg/min, depending on the length of administration, can be maintained without undue risk of cyanide toxicity to the mother and fetus. Other agents used to control maternal blood pressure in preeclampsia include nitroglycerin and labetalol, a nonselective beta-blocker with some α_1-blocking effects.

Consumption coagulopathy may require infusion of fresh whole blood, platelet concentrates, fresh-frozen plasma, and cryoprecipitate (see Chapter 16). Neuraxial anesthesia is contraindicated in patients with severe coagulopathy because of the increased risk of an intraspinal hematoma.

Anesthetic Management

Epidural, spinal, or CSE analgesia or anesthesia for labor and delivery should no longer be considered contraindicated, provided there is no severe clotting abnormality or plasma volume deficit.[124] In volume-repleted patients positioned with left uterine displacement, neuraxial analgesia does not cause an unacceptable reduction in blood pressure and leads to a significant improvement in placental perfusion.[125] With the use of radioactive xenon, it was shown that the intervillous blood flow increased by approximately 75% after the induction of epidural analgesia (10 mL of bupivacaine 0.25%).[126] The total maternal body clearance of lidocaine may be prolonged in preeclampsia, and repeated administration can lead to higher blood concentrations than in normotensive patients.[127]

For cesarean delivery, the sensory level of anesthesia must extend to T3 to T4, making adequate fluid therapy and left uterine displacement even more critical. The use of spinal anesthesia in severely preeclamptic women has been discouraged in favor of the continuous epidural technique. The concern is related to the fact that severely preeclamptic women can have significant intravascular volume deficits related to widespread arteriolar vasoconstriction, which may result in catastrophic hypotension with the sudden onset of extensive sympathectomy associated with spinal anesthesia. In fact, women with severe preeclampsia appear to be at lower risk of hypotension than normotensive women having cesarean delivery.[128] Furthermore, studies to date have shown that the incidence and severity of hypotension is similar in women with severe preeclampsia having a cesarean delivery with spinal compared with epidural anesthesia.[129,130] Thus, spinal anesthesia is emerging as a suitable alternative to epidural anesthesia for cesarean delivery in severely preeclamptic women. It is important to note that severely preeclamptic women need to be adequately prepared prior to neuraxial anesthesia with judicious hydration and control of blood pressure.

General anesthesia in preeclamptic patients has its particular hazards. Rapid-sequence induction of anesthesia and intubation of the trachea are occasionally difficult because of a swollen tongue, epiglottis, or pharynx (see Chapter 29). In patients with impaired coagulation, laryngoscopy and intubation of the trachea may provoke profuse bleeding. Marked systemic and pulmonary hypertension occurring at intubation and extubation enhance the risk of cerebral hemorrhage and pulmonary edema (Fig. 43-11). However, these hemodynamic changes can be minimized with appropriate antihypertensive therapy, such as administration of labetalol or nitroprusside infusion. The use of ketamine and ergot alkaloids should be avoided. Magnesium may prolong the effects of all muscle relaxants through its actions on the myoneural junction. Therefore, relaxants should be administered with caution (using a nerve stimulator) to avoid overdosage. General anesthesia may be necessary in acute emergencies, such as abruptio placentae, and in patients who do not meet the criteria for neuraxial anesthesia.

Obstetric Hemorrhage

A working definition of *massive* hemorrhage is "difficult-to-control blood loss," which requires large-volume transfusions of fluid and blood products. Pregnancy-related hemorrhage, excluding early bleeding due to ectopic pregnancy or miscarriage, is one of the most common causes of maternal death. Although massive hemorrhage occurs in only approximately 1 in 1,000 deliveries, the event is life-threatening and demands that all labor and delivery units be prepared to handle it.

Antepartum hemorrhage occurs in association with placenta previa (abnormal implantation on the lower uterine segment and partial-to-total occlusion of the internal cervical os) and abruptio placentae. Placenta previa complicates between 0.3 and 0.5% of pregnancies, resulting in up to 0.9% incidence of maternal, and a 17 to 26% incidence of perinatal mortality. Risk factors for placenta previa include previous cesarean delivery, uterine surgery, or pregnancy termination. Other risk factors include smoking, advanced maternal age, multiparity, multiple gestation, and cocaine abuse. The risk for placenta previa increases in a "dose-dependent" manner with the number of previous cesarean deliveries and greater parity. The relative risk is 4.5 (95% confidence interval: 3.6–5.5) with one previous cesarean delivery and it increases to 44.9 (95% confidence interval: 13.5–139.5) with four prior cesarean deliveries.[131,132] It should be suspected whenever a patient presents with painless, bright red vaginal bleeding, usually after the seventh month of pregnancy. Placenta previa may also be associated with an unstable or abnormal lie. The diagnosis is confirmed by ultrasonography. If bleeding is not profuse and the fetus is immature, obstetric management is conservative to prolong pregnancy. Admission to a high-risk unit is advisable if contractions or acute bleeding are present.

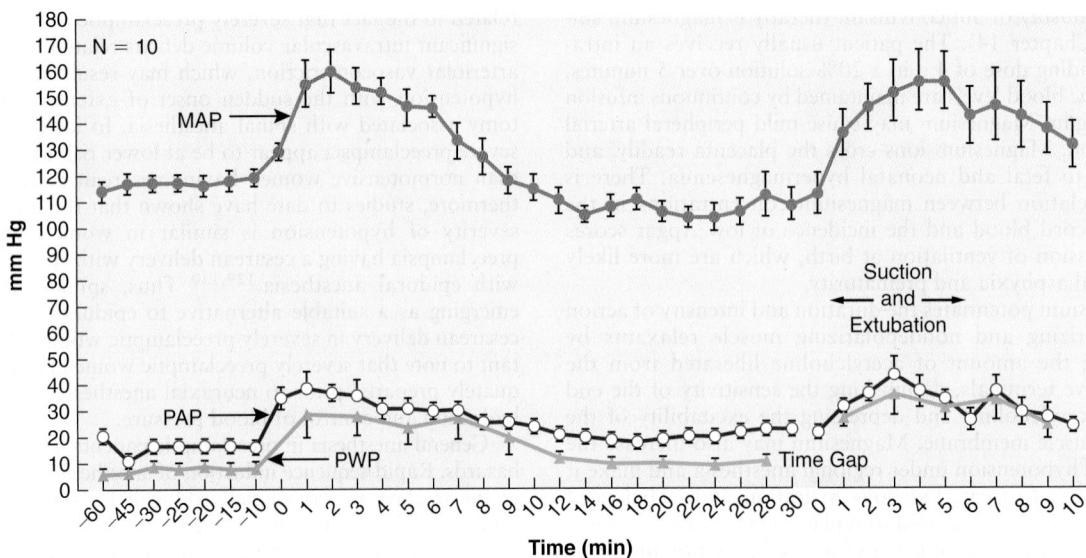

FIGURE 43-11. Mean and SE of mean arterial pressure (MAP), mean pulmonary artery pressure (PAP), and pulmonary wedge pressure (PWP) in patients with severe preeclampsia receiving thiopental and nitrous oxide (40%) with 0.5% halothane anesthesia for cesarean section. (Reprinted from Hodgkinson R, Husain FJ, Hayashi RH: Systemic and pulmonary blood pressure during cesarean section in parturients with gestational hypertension. Can Anaesth Soc J 1980; 27: 389, with permission.)

Intravenous access and typed and crossmatched blood should be available at all times. In severe cases, or if the fetus is mature at the onset of symptoms, prompt delivery is indicated, usually by cesarean.

Anesthesia for delivery of patients with placenta previa may be with neuraxial anesthesia, providing the mother is stable. Past recommendations for general anesthesia to provide "more control" are not supported by the literature, as there is no difference in complications between the two techniques, except that general anesthesia is associated with greater blood loss and greater need for transfusion. An emergency hysterectomy may be required if there is severe hemorrhage, even after delivery of the placenta, because of uterine atony. The risk of severe hemorrhage after attempted removal of the placenta is greatly increased in patients who have undergone prior uterine surgery, including cesarean delivery. This is related to a higher incidence of placenta accreta, which results from the penetration of myometrium by placental villi. After one previous cesarean delivery, placenta accreta was reported to occur in approximately 25% of patients with placenta previa, and after four or more prior cesarean deliveries, the incidence was >67%.[133] Indeed, placenta accreta is becoming the leading cause of cesarean hysterectomy.[134,135] The average blood loss during delivery of patients with placenta accreta is 3 to 5 L.

When placenta accreta is suspected or known, delivery is usually scheduled at 36 to 37 weeks' gestation. Under controlled, elective conditions, complications can be minimized. Some institutions now use occlusive balloon catheters placed in the internal iliac arteries prior to surgical delivery. In the face of bleeding with either placenta previa or accreta, when maintenance of fertility is desired, embolization, uterine compression sutures, and/or methotrexate therapy may be attempted to avoid hysterectomy.[136,137]

Abruptio placentae complicates approximately 1% of deliveries, usually in the final 10 weeks of gestation. Risk factors include smoking, trauma, cocaine abuse, multiple gestation, hypertension, preeclampsia, advanced maternal age, and preterm premature rupture of membranes. Complications include Couvelaire uterus (when extravasated blood dissects between the myometrial fibers), renal failure, disseminated intravascular coagulation, and anterior pituitary necrosis (Sheehan syndrome). The maternal mortality rate is high (1.8 to 11.0%), and the perinatal mortality rate is even higher, in excess of 50%. The diagnosis of abruptio placentae is based on the presence of uterine tenderness and hypertonus, as well as vaginal bleeding of dark, clotted blood. Bleeding may be concealed if the placental margins have remained attached to the uterine wall. If the blood loss is severe (>2 L), there may be changes in the maternal blood pressure and pulse rate, indicative of hypovolemia. Fetal movement may increase during acute hypoxia or decrease if hypoxia is gradual. Fetal bradycardia and death may ensue. When placental separation is >50%, stillbirth is the likeliest outcome. Management of abruption depends on presentation, gestational age, and the degree of compromise. Management of milder cases of abruption includes artificial rupture of amniotic membranes and oxytocin augmentation of labor, if required. Distant from term, expectant management with close observation is reasonable. In the presence of nonreassuring fetal status, an emergency cesarean delivery may be performed. If fetal death has occurred, usually with severe abruption, vaginal delivery is reasonable if the mother is stable.

The incidence of postpartum hemorrhage is estimated at 3 to 5% and is most commonly associated with retained products of conception, requiring evacuation of the uterus and/or uterine atony, requiring aggressive uterotonic therapy[138] (Table 43-3). Maternal resuscitation may require the administration of blood and blood products, especially if coagulopathy develops. If there is a need for dilation and curettage, the anesthesiologist may be asked to provide uterine relaxation. This can be accomplished with volatile agents if the patient is under general anesthesia or with intravenous nitroglycerine if regional anesthesia or general anesthesia is used.

In most cases of obstetric hemorrhage, the anesthesiologist is involved in both maternal resuscitation and provision of anesthesia. This may include placement of invasive monitoring (an arterial and a central venous catheter are usually adequate) and blood volume replacement, preferably through 14- or 16-gauge cannulae. If clotting abnormalities are present, fresh-frozen

TABLE 43-3

UTEROTONIC THERAPY

■ DRUG	■ DOSE	■ SIDE EFFECTS
Oxytocin	20–40 U in 1,000 mL LR by continuous intravenous infusion	Hypotension, tachycardia
Ergot alkaloids (Methergine)	0.2 mg IM q2–4 hr prn	Hypertension, vasoconstriction Coronary vasospasm Bronchospasm
Carboprost	0.25 mg IM q15–60 min prn	↑ Cardiac output ↑ Pulmonary vascular resistance Bronchospasm Nausea
Misoprostol	800–1,000 μg PR/PV/PO q2 hr	Fever Nausea
Dinoprostone	20 mg PO q2 hr	Hypotension Nausea

LR, Lactated Ringer solution; IM, intramuscularly; prn, as needed; PR, rectally; PV, vaginally; PO, orally.

plasma, cryoprecipitate, and platelet concentrates may be required. The anesthesiologist also performs the traditional role of providing appropriate anesthesia for a cesarean delivery, cesarean hysterectomy, or dilation and curettage. The choice of anesthetic technique depends on the anticipated duration of surgery, maternal condition and volume status, the potential for coagulopathy, and urgency of the procedure. General anesthesia is indicated in the presence of uncontrolled hemorrhage and/or severe coagulation abnormalities.[139] Neuraxial anesthesia, usually continuous epidural anesthesia, has been successfully used for hysterectomy in planned, controlled situations. A saddle block is an option for anesthesia when dilation and curettage for treatment of postpartum hemorrhage is indicated and the patient is hemodynamically stable.

Heart Disease

⑪ Heart disease during pregnancy occurs in about 1.6% of patients and is a leading nonobstetric cause of maternal morbidity and mortality, with a mortality rate ranging from 0.4% among patients in class I or II of the New York Heart Association's functional classification to 6.8% among those in classes III and IV. Medical and surgical advancements have changed the types of cardiac problems seen in pregnancy. For example, patients with congenital heart disease are reaching childbearing age and the number of patients with rheumatic heart disease has declined. The increase in the number of older parturients (advanced maternal age [AMA]) brings with it more patients with aortic stenosis and insufficiency associated with a bicuspid aortic valve. AMA and obesity are associated with coronary artery disease and myocardial ischemia, which occurred rarely during pregnancy 20 years ago. Peripartum cardiomyopathy continues to be associated with a high rate of maternal morbidity and mortality.[140]

Cardiac decompensation and death occur most commonly at the time of maximum hemodynamic stress, that is, in the third trimester of pregnancy, during labor and delivery, and during the immediate postpartum period. The increase in

maternal blood volume, which occurs at 20 to 24 weeks' gestation, may also precipitate cardiac decompensation. During labor, cardiac output increases progressively above antepartum levels. With each uterine contraction, approximately 200 mL of blood is squeezed out of the uterus into the central circulation. Consequently, stroke volume, cardiac output, and left ventricular work increase, and each contraction consistently increases cardiac output by 10 to 25% above that of uterine diastole. The greatest change occurs immediately after delivery of the placenta, when cardiac output increases to an average of 80% above prepartum values, and in some patients, it may increase by as much at 150%. These changes in cardiac output can be reduced by administration of neuraxial anesthesia. In patients managed with continuous caudal anesthesia, cardiac output increased only 24% above prepartum control values during the second stage and 59% immediately postpartum.[43]

Evaluation of pre-existing heart disease is crucial and a multidisciplinary approach is best when managing patients with complicated cardiac disease during pregnancy and parturition. For the anesthesiologist it is particularly important to understand how the hemodynamic consequences of different anesthetic techniques might adversely affect mothers with specific cardiac lesions. Invasive monitoring during labor and delivery is usually not necessary in the absence of cardiac symptoms. Exceptions are patients with pulmonary hypertension, right-to-left shunts, or coarctation of the aorta. Because hemodynamic changes observed during labor and delivery persist into the postpartum period, invasive monitoring should continue for 24 to 48 hours postpartum.

Congenital Heart Disease

Many patients with successful surgical repair of congenital heart defects are asymptomatic with minimal cardiac findings. Patients with uncorrected or partially corrected lesions may have serious cardiac decompensation with pregnancy. This includes patients with corrected tetralogy of Fallot who may have recurrence of a small ventricular septal defect or develop outflow obstruction. Neuraxial labor analgesia is recommended to prevent hemodynamic changes associated with pain. Maintenance of SVR and venous return is necessary to prevent an increase in right-to-left shunt. Phenylephrine should be used to prevent and/or treat reduction in SVR associated with sympathetic blockade.

Patients with corrected ventricular septal defects or atrial septal defects require no special care, similar to those with small asymptomatic atrial septal defects and ventricular septal defects. In symptomatic patients, neuraxial analgesia will prevent the increase in SVR associated with elevated catecholamines due to pain and may slightly decrease SVR, thus minimizing left-to-right shunting through the defect. Large ventricular septal defects or atrial septal defects are associated with pulmonary hypertension. Patients with these lesions require invasive monitoring and an analgesic technique that maintains SVR, heart rate, and pulmonary vascular resistance.

Eisenmenger syndrome occurs when uncorrected left-to-right shunt results in pulmonary hypertension, which, when severe, reverses flow to a right-to-left shunt. Pregnancy is not well tolerated and mortality is >30%, most commonly from embolic phenomena. Management of these patients is challenging. Invasive monitoring of arterial and cardiac filling pressures is indicated as the right ventricle is at greater risk of dysfunction than the left ventricle; thus measuring the right atrial pressure is useful in this setting. Implementing labor analgesia that does not lead to deleterious hemodynamic changes is a challenge; opioid-based neuraxial techniques (e.g., CSE, continuous spinal) combined with a dilute local anesthetic may be the best option.

TABLE 43-4

HEMODYNAMIC GOALS WITH VALVULAR LESIONS

■ LESION	■ GOAL
Aortic stenosis	Sinus rhythm
	Maintain HR
	Avoid ↓ SVR
	Maintain venous return
Aortic insufficiency	Mild ↑ HR
	Avoid ↑ SVR
Mitral stenosis	Sinus rhythm
	↓ HR
	Maintain SVR
	Maintain venous return
Mitral insufficiency	Sinus rhythm
	Mild ↑ HR
	Avoid ↑ SVR
	Avoid ↑ venous return

SVR, systemic vascular resistance; HR, heart rate.

General anesthesia is often elected for cesarean delivery in women with Eisenmenger syndrome. It should be recognized that arm-to-brain circulation times are rapid owing to right-to-left intracardiac shunts. Therefore, drugs given intravenously have a rapid onset of action. In contrast to parenteral drugs, the rate of rise of arterial concentrations of inhaled drugs is slow because of decreased pulmonary blood flow. Despite the slow onset, the myocardial depressant and vasodilating actions of volatile drugs may be hazardous in patients with Eisenmenger syndrome. Nitrous oxide may increase pulmonary vascular resistance and should be avoided. Positive-pressure ventilation of the lungs may also decrease pulmonary blood flow. Continuous spinal or epidural anesthesia for cesarean delivery may allow slow induction of anesthesia and thus maintenance of preload using phenylephrine and fluids, guided by CVP measurements. However, sympathetic blockade may lead to cardiovascular decompensation. Hemodynamic monitoring for 48 hours postpartum is essential.

Valvular Heart Disease

The decrease in incidence of rheumatic heart disease has resulted in fewer parturients with valvular heart disease compared with the past. Aortic stenosis is now likely associated with a bicuspid valve in the patient with AMA. Table 43-4 summarizes the goals of management of patients with valvular heart disease.

Coarctation of the Aorta

Coarctation of the aorta, similar to aortic stenosis, represents a fixed obstruction to the forward ejection of left ventricular stroke volume. Increases in cardiac output can be achieved primarily by increasing the heart rate. During periods of high demand the heart rate may not be able to increase to the extent necessary to maintain adequate cardiac output. This may result in acute left ventricular failure. Another hazard during labor and vaginal delivery is damage to the vascular wall of the aorta. Specifically, with the increased heart rate and myocardial contractility that accompany the pain of labor, the rate of ejection of blood from the left ventricle increases and may lead to dissection of the aorta.

Maintenance of heart rate, myocardial contractility, and SVR are important considerations in the management of anes-

thesia. As with aortic stenosis, analgesia for labor and vaginal delivery is often provided with systemic medications or inhalation analgesia and pudendal block. Likewise, general anesthesia is recommended for cesarean delivery. Invasive monitoring of arterial and cardiac filling pressures is helpful.

Primary Pulmonary Hypertension

Primary pulmonary hypertension is seen predominantly in young women. Pain during labor and vaginal delivery is especially detrimental because it may further increase pulmonary vascular resistance and decrease venous return. Neuraxial analgesia is useful for preventing pain-induced increases in pulmonary vascular resistance. Dilute local anesthetic solutions with the addition of opioids will minimize the decrease in SVR. General anesthesia has been recommended in the past for cesarean delivery, although epidural anesthesia is used successfully. Spinal anesthesia is not recommended for cesarean delivery because of the potential for sudden decreases in SVR. Potential risks of general anesthesia in these patients include increased pulmonary artery pressures during laryngoscopy and tracheal intubation, the adverse effects of positive-pressure ventilation on venous return, and the negative inotropic effects of volatile anesthetics. Nitrous oxide may further increase pulmonary vascular resistance. Predelivery assessment of the effects of vasodilators, inotropes, oxytocin, and fluid administration may be of value during subsequent anesthetic management. In addition to oxygen, the administration of isoproterenol, inhaled nitric oxide, calcium channel blockers, or sildenafil may be useful for decreasing pulmonary vascular resistance. Hemodynamic monitoring, including systemic and pulmonary arterial pressures, is indicated in these patients. Pulmonary artery rupture and thrombosis are risks of pulmonary artery catheters in the presence of pulmonary hypertension, but the benefits in these critically ill patients appear to offset these potential hazards. Maternal mortality is >50%, with most deaths due to congestive heart failure that occurs during labor and the early postpartum period.

Peripartum Cardiomyopathy

Peripartum cardiomyopathy occurs in approximately 1 in 3,000 births and is associated with a maternal mortality of 25 to 50%. It is a diagnosis of exclusion, and the etiology is thought to be related to myocarditis or an abnormal immune response. Risk factors include AMA, multiparity, multiple gestation, obesity, hypertension, and preeclampsia.[141,142] Good prognosis is expected if cardiac function returns to normal within 6 months of delivery. Intrapartum anesthetic management is directed at minimizing cardiac stress and thus decompensation.

Coronary Artery Disease and Myocardial Infarction

Acute myocardial infarction during pregnancy is rare, occurring in 1 in 10,000 to 30,000 women. It is associated with a maternal mortality as high as 37% as well as a high infant mortality rate. As more women with risk factors become pregnant, this complication will increase in frequency. The left anterior descending artery is most commonly affected, with 47% of infarcts associated with coronary spasm (i.e., normal angiogram) and another 16% associated with coronary artery dissection. Risk factors include smoking, obesity, AMA, diabetes, hypertension, and hyperlipidemia. Women over 35 years of age are at greatest risk. The ergot alkaloids should be avoided as they can lead to coronary vasospasm, as can cocaine use.[143]

Diagnosis may be difficult as symptoms of ischemia may mimic common nonspecific complaints during pregnancy. Thus, the greatest obstacle to diagnosis is a low index of suspicion. Cardiac troponin I levels are increased if cardiac muscle injury occurs; however, preeclampsia and gestational hypertension may also increase troponin levels. Therefore, electrocardiography (ECG) is an important diagnostic tool.

Delivery within 2 weeks of the infarct is associated with a high rate of reinfarction and death. Thus, delaying delivery, if possible, should be considered. Vaginal delivery is associated with lower morbidity and mortality than cesarean delivery. Intrapartum monitoring should mimic intraoperative monitoring of the nonobstetric patient with a recent myocardial infarction.

In the event of cardiac arrest in late pregnancy, left lateral displacement of the uterus should be achieved and if cardiopulmonary resuscitation is unsuccessful, the fetus should be delivered within 5 minutes to improve maternal and infant survival.[144]

Diabetes Mellitus

Gestational diabetes mellitus is diabetes or glucose intolerance that is first diagnosed during pregnancy (see Chapter 49). Three to eight percent of pregnant women develop gestational diabetes, and the incidence is increasing, in parallel with the increase in population obesity and type 2 diabetes.[145] Gestational diabetes mellitus is associated with increased adverse outcome, including macrosomia, neonatal hypoglycemia, hyperbilirubinemia, and intrauterine fetal demise, as well as an increased risk of obesity and diabetes in offspring later in life. Macrosomia is responsible for an increased risk of birth trauma, shoulder dystocia, and cesarean delivery. Women with gestational diabetes mellitus are at increased risk for development of type 2 diabetes later in life.

Pre-existing type 1 or 2 diabetes is also associated with adverse pregnancy outcomes, including congenital malformations. Vasculopathy, nephropathy, and retinopathy may be exacerbated by pregnancy. Tight glycemia control before and during pregnancy may decrease risk of adverse outcomes. Although diabetic ketoacidosis during pregnancy is rare, normal physiologic changes of pregnancy contribute to a propensity for diabetic women to develop diabetic ketoacidosis.[146] Maternal mortality from diabetic ketoacidosis is unusual, although fetal mortality remains high.

Guidelines for the management of pregnant diabetics vary somewhat, but generally insulin therapy is recommended if fasting blood sugar levels are >100 mg/dL.[147] Maternal insulin requirements increase progressively during the second and third trimesters. Fetal surveillance is more intense in diabetic women. Delivery at 38 weeks' gestation may be considered if estimated fetal weight exceeds 4,500 g or fetal surveillance indicates the need for delivery.

There is no compelling evidence that one analgesic or anesthetic technique is superior to another when caring for diabetic parturients. Neuraxial labor analgesia does not appear to alter peripartum insulin and glucose requirements. Intrapartum blood glucose levels should be monitored frequently and glucose administration and insulin therapy should be titrated to maintain maternal glucose concentration between 70 and 90 mg/dL. Insulin requirements decrease shortly after delivery.

Obesity

Obese women are more likely to have antenatal comorbidities, such as chronic hypertension, diabetes mellitus, and preeclampsia.[148] Obstetric outcome may also be affected by maternal obesity. For instance, there is a greater risk of congenital cardiac anomalies, macrosomia, and shoulder dystocia. There is also an increasing risk of cesarean delivery with increasing body mass index. Preanesthetic evaluation of the morbidly obese parturient

should be performed with anticipation of these complications and a multidisciplinary care plan should be generated. Careful airway evaluation is required and alternative airway equipment must be readily available. In addition, the extent of comorbidities such as hypertension and diabetes mellitus should be assessed. Despite technical challenges, continuous neuraxial analgesia has emerged as the preferred option for pain relief during labor because it provides excellent pain relief without sedation/obtundation, prevents additional demands on the cardiorespiratory system of the morbidly obese patient, and most importantly, a well-functioning neuraxial anesthetic for labor may also be used for anesthesia for instrumental vaginal or cesarean delivery, thus avoiding airway manipulation. For cesarean delivery, the choice of anesthetic depends on maternal and fetal condition. The panniculus must be positioned carefully to prevent cardiorespiratory embarrassment.[149] A continuous neuraxial anesthetic technique is preferred over a single-shot technique because there may be unpredictable spread of local anesthetic and because the procedure itself may outlast the effective anesthesia from the latter. In the postoperative period, there must be careful attention to adequate oxygenation, pain relief, and thromboprophylaxis.

Advanced Maternal Age

In 2002, almost 14% of all births in the United States occurred in women aged 35 years or older.[150] In 2003, the percentage of primiparas 35 years and older was 10%.[151] In Canada in 2002, live births to women 30 to 34 years old were 30.6% of all births; to women aged 35 to 39 years old, 14.1%; and 40 years of age or over, 2.6%.[152] Some studies have reported higher maternal morbidity as well as perinatal morbidity and mortality in older gravidas,[152–154] suggesting that pregnancy in older women may be a "medical problem."

Both patients and health care professionals hold the view that AMA results in poorer outcomes. Medically, this is rationalized by the higher prevalence of chronic medical conditions in older patients compared with younger ones. In one study, 47% of pregnant women over 45 years of age had pre-existing medical problems.[155] Cleary-Goldman et al.[154] found that 38% of 36,000 patients over 35 years of age took medication for pre-existing conditions. In addition, many older pregnant patients have been infertile or subfertile or had had a previous poor obstetric outcome. Seven percent had prior preterm delivery, and 26% had a previous miscarriage. As a result of these factors, patients with AMA are treated differently, even if healthy and regardless of whether there is scientific basis for this treatment.

AMA is independently associated with maternal morbidities including gestational diabetes, preeclampsia, placental abruption, and cesarean delivery. In addition, older gravidas are more likely to have a weight of >70 kg, hypertension, diabetes mellitus, and a bad obstetric history. These medical problems complicate the pregnancy and its management.

AMA is an independent risk factor for gestational diabetes mellitus and placental abruption. These have been discussed previously. Pregestational hypertension occurs more frequently in patients over 30 years of age.[156] Patients with chronic hypertension are more likely to develop superimposed preeclampsia (78%), deliver by cesarean (71%), and deliver before 37 weeks' gestation than the normotensive patient. Hypertensive parturients are at greater risk for placental abruption, congestive heart failure, pulmonary edema, and hypertensive encephalopathy.

Cesarean delivery is performed more frequently in those with AMA. In some patients the need for cesarean delivery is related to coexisting problems such as hypertension, preeclampsia, placental abruption, or fetal macrosomia. AMA is also independently associated with an increased likelihood for cesarean delivery. Lin et al.[157] reported that over a 5-year period "request cesarean delivery" rates rose steadily in all patients but rose disproportionately in patients with AMA. Women over age 34 years were twice as likely to request cesarean delivery compared with those age 25 years or younger. The cesarean delivery rate for mothers 30 to 34 years of age was 37% and for mothers >34 years it was 48%.[157] The complex sociodemographic explanation for the increased requests for cesarean delivery is yet to be fully ascertained and the long-term medical cost has yet to be defined. Cesarean delivery is associated with increased maternal risk compared with uncomplicated vaginal delivery. These include short-term risks of cesarean delivery such as hemorrhage, infection, ileus, and aspiration pneumonitis. Additionally, hysterectomy occurs 10 times more frequently following cesarean delivery compared with vaginal delivery. The risk of maternal death is 16 times greater. Long-term morbidity includes adhesions, bowel obstruction, bladder injury, and increased risk for placenta previa or ectopic pregnancy in subsequent pregnancies.[158]

Older women believe that their age makes their infant more vulnerable and, as such, believe a controlled cesarean delivery is safer than vaginal delivery. Other explanations for increased requests for cesarean delivery include concerns about physical stamina, protection of the pelvic floor from damage, refusal to undergo labor pain, and social convenience. Patient beliefs run counter to the many studies that show that cesarean delivery in the absence of clinical indications increases maternal mortality and perinatal morbidity.[158,159]

Perinatal complications are also significant in patients with AMA; multiple gestations,[160] both iatrogenic and naturally occurring, are more common in older gravidas. The incidence of miscarriage, congenital anomalies, preterm delivery, low birth weight, and intrauterine and neonatal death may also increase with age.

PRETERM DELIVERY

Preterm labor and delivery (before 37 completed weeks of gestation) present a significant challenge to the anesthesiologist because both mother and infant may be at risk. Although preterm deliveries occur in 8 to 10% of all births, they account for approximately 80% of early neonatal deaths. In general, the mortality and morbidity rates are higher among preterm infants than among small-for-gestational age infants of comparable weight. Severe problems that may develop in preterm infants are respiratory distress syndrome, intracranial hemorrhage, hypoglycemia, hypocalcemia, and hyperbilirubinemia. With improved neonatal intensive care, preterm infants who weigh >1,500 g often survive without severe long-term impairment. The very low birth weight infant (<1,500 g) is still at greater risk for significant long-term impairment.[161]

Obstetricians will try to stop preterm labor to enhance fetal lung maturity. Delaying delivery by even 24 to 48 hours may be beneficial if glucocorticoids are administered to the mother. Various agents have been used to suppress uterine activity (tocolysis), including ethanol, magnesium sulfate, prostaglandin inhibitors, β-sympathomimetics, and calcium channel blockers.

It is thought that the premature infant is more vulnerable than the term newborn to the effects of drugs used in obstetric analgesia and anesthesia. However, there have been few systematic studies to determine the maternal and fetal pharmacokinetics and dynamics of drugs throughout gestation. There are several postulated causes of enhanced drug sensitivity in the preterm newborn: less protein available for drug binding; higher levels of bilirubin, which may compete with the drug for protein binding; greater drug access to the central nervous system (CNS) because of a poorly developed blood–brain

barrier; greater total body water and lower fat content; and a decreased ability to metabolize and excrete drugs. However, these deficiencies of the preterm infant may not be as serious as we have been led to believe. Serum albumin and α_1-acid glycoprotein concentrations are lower in the preterm fetus; however, this would primarily affect drugs that are highly bound to these proteins. Most drugs used in anesthesia exhibit only low-to-moderate degrees of binding in the fetal serum: approximately 50% for etidocaine and bupivacaine, 25% for lidocaine, 52% for meperidine, and 75% for thiopental.

The placenta efficiently eliminates fetal bilirubin. Thus, the hyperbilirubinemia of prematurity normally occurs in the postpartum period. With the exception of diazepam, bilirubin does not compete with anesthetic drugs because most are bound to other serum proteins (e.g., meperidine and local anesthetics bind to α_1-acid glycoproteins). It seems likely that the human blood–brain barrier develops substantially in early gestation. Thus, factors such as tissue affinity changes may account for differences between immature and mature brain uptake of highly lipid-soluble drugs.

Greater total body water in the preterm fetus results in a greater volume of distribution for drugs (see Chapter 7). Thus, to achieve equal blood concentrations, the immature fetus must receive a greater amount of drug transplacentally than the mature fetus. A study of age-related toxicity of lidocaine in sheep showed that the greater the volume of distribution, the greater the dose required to achieve toxic blood concentrations of the drug.[41] Decreased ability to metabolize or excrete drugs that is associated with prematurity is certainly not a universal phenomenon. In a study comparing the pharmacokinetics of lidocaine in preterm newborns and adults, plasma clearance was similar in both groups.[40] Neonates excreted much more unchanged lidocaine than did adults. Similarly, although meperidine metabolism is more limited in the neonate than in the adult, urinary excretion of the unchanged drug is greater in the neonate.

Gestational changes in maternal serum albumin and α_1-acid glycoprotein concentrations, which tend to decrease, may also play a role in drug availability. Serial determinations of protein binding of diazepam, phenytoin, and valproic acid in maternal serum, performed in early (8 to 16 weeks), middle (17 to 32 weeks), and late pregnancy, showed a progressive increase in the unbound fraction of these drugs.[162] This increases drug availability for placental transfer. Placental permeability itself increases as pregnancy progresses because of the increased area and decreased thickness of tissue barriers.

It therefore appears that in selection of the anesthetic drugs and techniques for delivery of a preterm infant, concerns regarding drug effects on the newborn are far less important than prevention of asphyxia and trauma to the fetus. For labor and vaginal delivery, well-conducted neuraxial anesthesia is advantageous in providing good perineal relaxation. Preterm infants with breech presentation are usually delivered by cesarean as are very low birth weight infants (<1,500 g). If neuraxial anesthesia is used, nitroglycerin should be available for uterine relaxation. If vaginal delivery occurs with a breech infant and there is head entrapment, general anesthesia or nitroglycerine may be needed for uterine relaxation.

HUMAN IMMUNODEFICIENCY VIRUS AND ACQUIRED IMMUNODEFICIENCY SYNDROME

Women now represent nearly half of the people worldwide living with human immunodeficiency virus (HIV) (see Chapter 13). Thus, it is the rare labor and delivery unit that will not be caring for HIV-positive women. There is no evidence that pregnancy accelerates the progression of the disease. However, there is compelling interest to prevent vertical transmission of HIV from mother to fetus. The risk of intrauterine infection is 4.4%. Intrapartum transmission accounts for 60% of the risk of peripartum transmission and the remainder is through breastfeeding. However, when zidovudine prophylaxis is given to women with HIV perinatally, and to the newborn in the first weeks of life, vertical transmission is reduced to <2%.[163]

The choice of anesthetic technique for delivery should be based on maternal condition, obstetric considerations, and patient desires. HIV is a multiorgan disease, often with complex and changing medical management. Patients with high CD4 counts (>500 to 700/mm^3) often are not taking antiretroviral agents and have little or no end-organ damage. Patients with very low CD4 counts (<200/mm^3) are likely to be taking multiple antiretroviral and other medications. This group should have more extensive evaluation, with complete blood count, clotting studies, and liver and renal function tests. A history of cardiac or pulmonary dysfunction warrants obtaining ECG, echocardiogram, pulmonary function tests, and/or arterial blood gases in some patients.[164]

In the early years of the HIV/AIDS (acquired immunodeficiency syndrome) epidemic, concern was expressed regarding both general and neuraxial anesthesia, although there was no evidence of harm. Pulmonary disease was a concern for general anesthesia and there were early concerns of CNS HIV infection with neuraxial anesthesia. We now have extensive experience with neuraxial anesthesia in this patient population, without reports of unique complications.[165] There has been concern that an epidural blood patch, particularly if the viral load is high, may accelerate neurologic symptoms of the disease. In a more recent case series of six patients with HIV infection and PDPH requiring epidural blood patch, there was no evidence of acceleration of HIV symptoms.[166]

SUBSTANCE ABUSE

Nearly 90% of women with substance abuse are of childbearing age. The incidence of substance abuse during pregnancy has been steadily increasing over the past decade, mirroring the incidence in the general population. The most commonly abused substances in society as well as in pregnancy are alcohol, tobacco, cocaine, marijuana, opioids, caffeine, amphetamines, and to a lesser extent, hallucinogens and solvents. Substance abuse may significantly impact the intrapartum anesthetic management and may result in obstetric crises that require the intervention or assistance of an obstetric anesthesiologist. Diagnosis of the patient who is not under the effect of a substance at admission may be made when she, or her infant, develops withdrawal symptoms or the newborn is diagnosed with a syndrome related to in utero exposure.

Tobacco Abuse

Approximately 20% of pregnant women will continue to smoke during pregnancy. Smoking during pregnancy has been associated with miscarriages, intrauterine growth retardation, and increased risk premature rupture of membrane, placental previa, abruption placentae, preterm delivery, impaired respiratory function in newborns, and sudden infant death syndrome. The pregnant patient is at greater risk for bronchitis, pneumonia, and asthma. Nicotine causes vasoconstriction and thus may decrease placental blood flow and oxygen delivery to the fetus. The anesthetic management of a pregnant tobacco abuser is not unlike the management of a nonpregnant tobacco abuser.

Alcohol

In a pregnant female, heavy alcohol consumption may be associated with liver disease, coagulopathy, cardiomyopathy, and esophageal varices, and can alter drug metabolism. In the fetus, alcohol has been linked to fetal alcohol syndrome. The prevalence of fetal alcohol syndrome is up to 50% among the infants of moderate-to-heavy maternal drinkers (defined as the consumption of 1 to 2 ounces of absolute alcohol per day). The anesthetic management of the parturient who abuses alcohol should take into account that the individual is at further increased risk for aspiration compared with the average pregnant individual. She may have hepatic dysfunction, cardiac failure, or coagulopathy. Acute alcohol withdrawal may present within 6 to 48 hours of abstinence; thus, it may occur intrapartum or postpartum. The signs and symptoms of alcohol withdrawal include nausea and vomiting, hypertension, tachycardia, dysrhythmias, seizures, and cardiac failure. These are easily mistaken for other disease entities.

Opioids

Opioid abuse has multiple implications for both mother and fetus. The intravenous opioid abuser may have septic thrombophlebitis, HIV, endocarditis, or hepatitis. These patients are at an increased risk for developing preeclampsia and third-trimester bleeding. They will develop withdrawal symptoms should an agonist/antagonist be administered for pain relief in labor.

The anesthetic management of a chronic opioid user should include the continuation of opioids throughout labor and into the postpartum period to prevent acute opioid withdrawal. These patients are likely to have increased opioid requirements. Those patients with a history of opioid abuse who are on methadone maintenance should have a stable peripartum course. Neuraxial anesthesia is safe in these patients but one must continue a maintenance dose of parenteral opioid despite neuraxial labor analgesia. Neonates will have neonatal abstinence syndrome, which will require close observation and treatment.

Marijuana

Marijuana is frequently abused by women of childbearing age. Delta-9-tetrahydrocannabinol (THC) readily crosses the placenta and may directly affect the fetus. It has been associated with preterm labor and intrauterine growth retardation. The parturient who chronically uses marijuana has an increased incidence of respiratory problems including bronchitis and emphysema and thus may be at risk for respiratory complications related to general anesthesia. Acute marijuana use may be associated with cardiovascular stimulation at moderate doses and myocardial depression at higher doses. Thus, cardiovascular assessment is critical to the safe management of these patients.

Cocaine

Women abusing cocaine generally display euphoria, tachycardia, and hypertension. More serious manifestations may include seizure and coma, myocardial infarction, pulmonary edema, or subarachnoid hemorrhage. Sudden death may occur from a lethal ventricular dysrhythmia. Maternal cocaine use may also be harmful to the fetus. For instance, cocaine use in the first trimester may cause congenital anomalies. Later in pregnancy, cocaine use may be associated with premature labor, intrauterine growth retardation, and nonreassuring fetal status because of uteroplacental insufficiency or placental

TABLE 43-5

ANESTHETIC CONSIDERATIONS ASSOCIATED WITH COCAINE AND/OR AMPHETAMINE ABUSE

- Uncontrolled hypertension
- Cardiac dysrhythmias (ventricular tachycardia/fibrillation)
- Myocardial ischemia
- Ephedrine-resistant hypotension with neuraxial blockade (use direct-acting agent)
- Acute intake may increase MAC of volatile agents
- Chronic use may decrease dosage of anesthetic agents
- May have increased sensitivity to arrhythmogenic effects of volatile agents

MAC, minimum alveolar concentration.

abruption. Therapy is supportive, primarily aimed at controlling cardiovascular and CNS consequences of cocaine use. Pure β-antagonist drugs should be avoided because of the potential for worsening hypertension related to unopposed α-receptor stimulation by cocaine. The choice of anesthetic depends on maternal and fetal condition, the planned procedure (vaginal or cesarean delivery), and urgency. General anesthesia may be associated with uncontrolled hypertension/tachycardia and life-threatening dysrhythmias in women using cocaine. Neuraxial anesthesia is not without its hazards. Cocaine is a local anesthetic, and systemic toxicity may be additive when using amide local anesthetics for epidural anesthesia. Chronic cocaine use may also be associated with thrombocytopenia. The incidence and severity of hypotension related to neuraxial anesthesia may be greater in cocaine-using parturients compared with controls, and hypotension may be more difficult to treat.[167]

Amphetamines

Amphetamines are noncatecholamine sympathomimetic drugs. They are often abused in conjunction with other CNS stimulants such as cocaine. They can be taken orally or intravenously (methamphetamine) or smoked, as crystal methamphetamine. Ecstasy is an analog of methamphetamine that has become tremendously popular in young adults. Amphetamine use leads to an increased release of norepinephrine, leading to hypertension, tachycardia, dysrhythmias, dilated pupils, hyperpyrexia, proteinuria, agitation, confusion, and seizures. These signs and symptoms closely resemble those of cocaine abuse. Methamphetamine abuse has been associated with stroke in pregnant women as well as fetal and infant deaths. Amphetamines taken early in pregnancy can result in fetal anomalies. Later in pregnancy, placental abruption may lead to fetal death. The anesthetic management of patients who abuse amphetamines is similar to that of cocaine abusers (Table 43-5).

FETAL AND MATERNAL MONITORING

The development of biophysical monitoring of the fetus during labor and delivery has had a tremendous impact on obstetric practice since the early 1970s. Monitoring procedures are now performed routinely, and it is important that the anesthesiologist understand the basic principles of the technology, as well as the interpretation of results.

During the same period, there has been an explosion in monitoring technology in the fields of anesthesiology and

intensive care. The mother with serious medical problems requiring intensive care or the one whose infant is delivered in an operating room under an anesthesiologist's care is subject to the same standards of monitoring as any other surgical patient. It is generally agreed that the use of intensive peripartum monitoring is appropriate in a high-risk pregnancy. In contrast, patients with routine labor are frequently observed in the same way that patients were many generations ago (i.e., with intermittent blood pressure readings).

With the growing sophistication of electronic devices, and specifically the science of telemetry, we can look forward to better surveillance of both mother and fetus without the loss of maternal freedom and activity that monitoring currently entails.

Biophysical Monitoring

A fetal monitor is a two-channel recorder of FHR and uterine activity.[168] In the direct system, the fetal ECG is obtained from an electrode attached to the presenting part. Intrauterine pressure is measured continuously with a transducer connected to a saline-filled catheter that is inserted transcervically. Direct monitoring is quantitative but requires rupture of the membranes and a cervical dilation of at least 1.5 cm. In addition, the presenting part must be in the true pelvis. Indirect fetal monitoring uses data obtained from transducers secured to the mother's abdomen with adjustable straps. Ultrasound cardiography is the most commonly used indirect method of obtaining FHR signals. Uterine activity is monitored with a tocodynamometer triggered by the changing shape of the uterus during the contraction. Indirect monitoring is mostly qualitative. Its advantage is that it can be applied without rupture of membranes, even before the onset of labor.

The following variables are considered when fetal well-being is determined: baseline heart rate, beat-to-beat variability, periodic patterns, and uterine activity. The baseline FHR is measured between contractions and ranges between 120 and 160 beats per minute in the normal fetus. An acceleration of FHR in response to fetal stimulation during vaginal examination is a reassuring sign that the fetus is not acidotic. Persistently elevated rates may be associated with chronic fetal distress, maternal fever, or administration of drugs such as ephedrine and atropine. Abnormally low rates may be encountered in fetuses with congenital heart block or as a late occurrence during the course of fetal hypoxia and acidosis.

The baseline FHR variability, which is normally present, reflects the beat-to-beat adjustments of the parasympathetic and sympathetic nervous systems to a variety of internal and external stimuli and is mediated by the CNS, the peripheral nervous system, and the cardiac conduction system itself. Fetal CNS depression by asphyxia may decrease baseline variability. Therefore, a smooth FHR tracing may be an ominous finding. However, drugs that depress the CNS (tranquilizers, opioids, barbiturates, anesthetics) can also decrease FHR variability. Atropine may decrease variability by blocking the transmission of control impulses to the cardiac pacemaker. Ephedrine administration may increase beat-to-beat variability.

Periodic FHR patterns consist of decelerations or accelerations of relatively brief duration in association with uterine contractions (Fig. 43-12). There are three major forms of FHR deceleration: early, late, and variable. Early decelerations are U-shaped, with the heart rate usually not decreasing to <100 beats per minute. The fetal heart begins to slow with the onset of the contraction, the low point coincides with the peak of the contraction, and the rate usually returns to the baseline as the uterus relaxes. This type of deceleration has been attributed to fetal head compression, leading to increased vagal tone. It is not ameliorated by increasing fetal oxygenation but is blocked

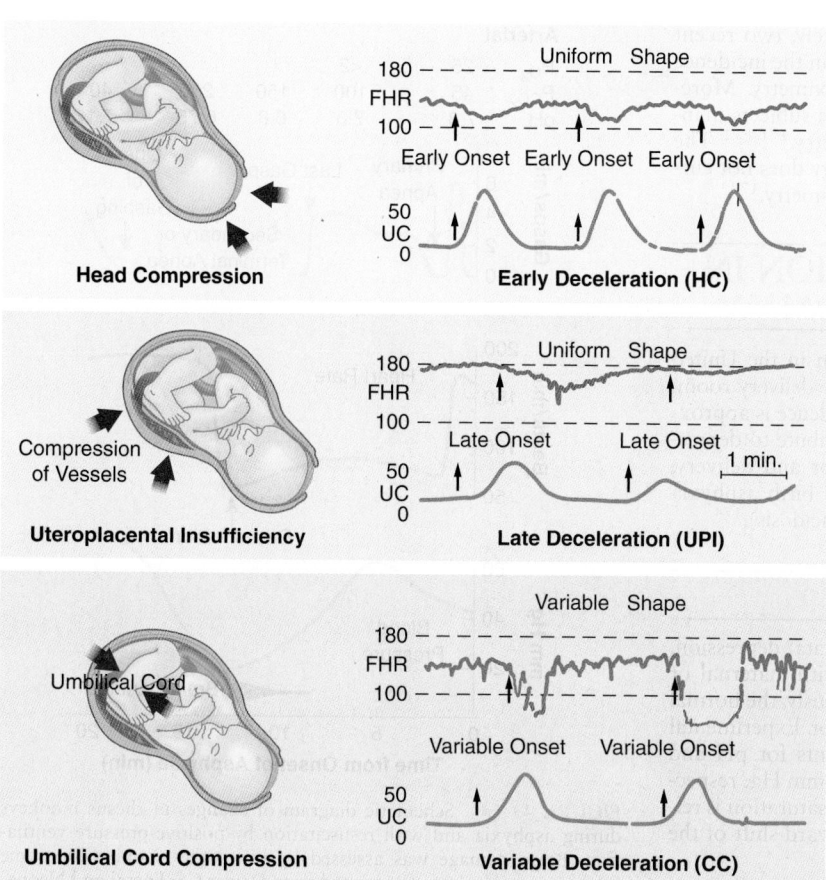

FIGURE 43-12. Classification and mechanism of fetal heart rate patterns. HC, head compression; UPI, uteroplacental insufficiency; CC, cord compression. (Reprinted from Hon EH: An Introduction to Fetal Heart Rate Monitoring. New Haven, CT, Harty Press, 1969, p 29, with permission.)

by atropine administration. Early decelerations are transient and well tolerated by the fetus because there is no systemic hypoxemia or acidosis.

Late decelerations are also U-shaped. However, they begin 20 to 30 seconds or more after the onset of uterine contraction and the low point of the deceleration occurs well after the peak of the contraction. Myocardial ischemia resulting from uteroplacental insufficiency and fetal hypoxemia is believed to cause late decelerations. Late decelerations can be corrected by improving fetal oxygenation, which may be accomplished with oxygen administration to the mother, correction of maternal hypotension or aortocaval compression, or by taking measures that reduce uterine activity. If late decelerations are repetitive, continuous, and progressive in severity, there is a significant correlation with fetal acidosis, and delivery may be required.

Variable decelerations are the most common periodic patterns observed in the intrapartum period. They are variable in shape and onset, with the rate usually decreasing to <100 beats per minute and >15 beats per minute below baseline, and they result from umbilical cord compression that results in activation of the carotid baroreceptor reflex. Although the initial FHR changes are of reflex origin, if the cord compressions are frequent or prolonged, fetal asphyxia may result in fetal hypoxemia and direct myocardial depression.

A prolonged deceleration is defined as an FHR decrease lasting >2 minutes but <10 minutes. All decelerations should be quantified based on deviation from baseline and duration.[169]

Cervical dilation and descent of the presenting part during the first stage of labor result primarily from uterine contractions. During the active phase, contractions should occur every 2 to 3 minutes, with peak intrauterine pressures of 50 to 80 mm Hg and resting pressures of 5 to 20 mm Hg.

Poor uterine contractility may result from overdistention (polyhydramnios, multiple gestation) or aortocaval compression. The addition of epinephrine to a local anesthetic solution may have a dose-related inhibitory effect on uterine activity. The effects of systemic opioid analgesia and neuraxial analgesia on the progress of labor are not well studied.

Currently, experts agree regarding the reassuring value of a normal FHR tracing with good beat-to-beat variability, without decelerations. There is also consensus regarding the potentially ominous nature of patterns that lack variability, and/or demonstrate persistent, severe, or prolonged decelerations. However, FHR patterns between these extremes present a clinical dilemma to the clinician.[170] A recent American College of Obstetrics and Gynecology Practice Bulletin recommends the use of continuous FHR analysis for high-risk conditions, although it allows for intermittent auscultation in an uncomplicated patient. Furthermore, it notes the high false-positive rate of nonreassuring FHR tracings for predicting adverse neonatal outcomes, and notes that the practice is associated with an increase in operative deliveries, without decreasing the incidence of cerebral palsy.[168]

Fetal Pulse Oximetry

Fetal pulse oximetry is a technique in which a sensor is placed through the cervix, in contact with fetal skin that evaluates intrapartum fetal oxygenation. Fetal O_2 saturation between 30 and 70% is considered normal, and saturation readings consistently <30% for a prolonged period of time may be associated with fetal acidemia. The technique was initially touted as an adjunct to FHR monitoring in the hope that it could reduce the incidence of unnecessary cesarean delivery associated with that methodology. Unfortunately, two recent large studies failed to demonstrate a reduction in the incidence of cesarean delivery with use of fetal pulse oximetry. Moreover, neonatal outcomes did not differ between subjects managed with versus without fetal pulse oximetry.[171,172] The American College of Obstetrics and Gynecology does not currently endorse the routine use of fetal pulse oximetry.[173]

NEWBORN RESUSCITATION IN THE DELIVERY ROOM

Of the approximately 3.5 million infants born in the United States each year, 6% require resuscitation in the delivery room. Among those weighing 1,500 g or less, the incidence is approximately 80%. The following factors may contribute to depression of the newborn: drugs used during labor and delivery, including anesthetic agents, birth trauma, and birth asphyxia (i.e., hypoxia and hypercapnia with metabolic acidosis).[174]

Fetal Asphyxia

Fetal asphyxia, the best-studied cause of neonatal depression, usually develops as a result of interference with maternal or fetal perfusion of the placenta. As stated previously, the normal fetus is neither hypoxic nor acidotic before labor. Experimental data have revealed that transplacental gradients for pH and PCO_2 are approximately 0.05 pH units and 5 mm Hg, respectively. Although oxygen tension is low, oxygen saturation is relatively high (80 to 85%) by virtue of the leftward shift of the fetal oxyhemoglobin dissociation curve.

During labor, uterine contractions decrease or even eliminate the blood flow through the intervillous space of the placenta. On the fetal side, cord compression occurs during the final stages of approximately one third of vaginal deliveries. Thus, mild degrees of hypoxia and acidosis occur even during normal labor and delivery, and play an important role in initiation of ventilation. On average, healthy, vigorous infants have an oxygen saturation of 21%, a pH of 7.24, and a PCO_2 of 56 mm Hg at birth.

Severe fetal asphyxia occasionally develops as a result of fetal and maternal complications, such as uterine hyperactivity, premature separation of the placenta, maternal hypotension, a tight nuchal cord, and a prolapsed cord. During asphyxia, changes in acid-base status are rapid. The decrease in pH results from accumulation of carbon dioxide (respiratory acidosis) and end products of anaerobic metabolism (metabolic acidosis). After oxygen stores are exhausted, the ability of fetal brain and myocardium to derive energy from anaerobic metabolism is essential for survival. However, anaerobic glycolysis is pH-dependent, and its rate is greatly diminished when the pH decreases below 7.0. Other untoward effects of severe hypoxia and acidosis include depression of the myocardium resulting from a decrease in its responsiveness to catecholamines, a shift to the right of the fetal oxyhemoglobin dissociation curve, resulting in reduced oxygen delivery, and an increase in pulmonary vascular resistance, which plays an important role during circulatory readjustment at birth.

Ventilatory and cardiovascular responses to controlled experimental asphyxia have been investigated extensively in newborn monkeys[175] (Fig. 43-13). During the initial phase of asphyxia, the unanesthetized animal exhibits respiratory efforts that increase in depth and frequency for up to 3 minutes. This period, called *primary hyperpnea*, is followed by primary apnea, which lasts for approximately 1 minute. Rhythmic gasping begins and is maintained at a fairly constant rate of approximately 6 gasps per minute for 4 to 5 minutes. Thereafter, the gasps become weaker and slower. Their cessation at approximately 8.5 minutes after the onset of asphyxia marks

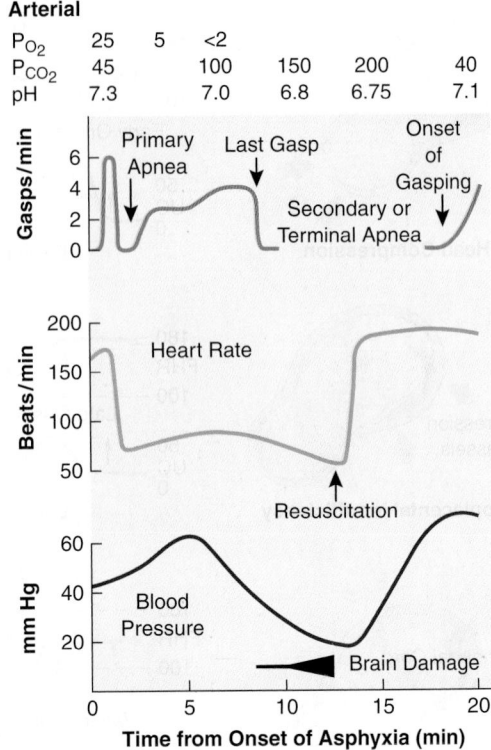

FIGURE 43-13. Schematic diagram of changes in rhesus monkeys during asphyxia and with resuscitation by positive-pressure ventilation. Brain damage was assessed by histologic examination some weeks or months later. (Reprinted from Dawes GS: Foetal and Neonatal Physiology: A Comparative Study of the Changes at Birth. Chicago, Year Book Medical, 1968, p 149, with permission.)

the beginning of secondary apnea. Administration of opioids and systemic anesthetic agents to the mother can abolish the period of primary hyperpnea and prolong primary apnea.

There is a linear relationship between the duration of asphyxia and the onset of gasping and rhythmic spontaneous breathing. In the newborn monkey, for each minute of asphyxia beyond the last gasp, 2 additional minutes of artificial ventilation is required before gasping begins again and 4 minutes before rhythmic breathing is established.[176] This indicates that the longer artificial ventilation of the lungs is delayed during secondary apnea, the longer it will take to resuscitate the infant. Furthermore, in the newborn monkey, prolongation of asphyxia for 4 minutes beyond the last gasp is accompanied by extensive damage to brainstem nuclei, whereas animals resuscitated before the last gasp show little or no brain damage.[176] Thus, a relatively short delay in resuscitation can have serious sequelae.

Neonatal Adaptations at Birth

During birth, and through the early hours and days of life, many morphologic and functional changes take place, with the cardiovascular and ventilatory systems undergoing the most dramatic alterations.[177] In the normal newborn, two events occur almost simultaneously and within seconds of delivery: the end of umbilical circulation through the placenta and expansion of the lungs. These events change the fetal circulation toward the adult type. Survival of the neonate depends primarily on prompt establishment of effective ventilation and expansion of the lungs.

The onset of ventilation and expansion of the lungs dilates the pulmonary vascular bed, resulting in decreased resistance and a significant increase in pulmonary blood flow. Pulmonary vascular resistance further decreases as oxygen tension increases and carbon dioxide levels decrease. As soon as pulmonary resistance decreases, the foramen ovale, which is a communication between the right and the left atrium, undergoes functional closure because of relative pressure changes across the valve of the foramen (Fig. 43-4). Cessation of the umbilical circulation reduces pressure in the inferior vena cava and right atrium, whereas the increase in pulmonary blood flow increases venous return and pressure in the left atrium. The ductus arteriosus does not constrict abruptly or completely after birth; functional closure may take hours, even days. Thus, shunting may still occur in the neonatal period, its direction depending on relative resistances in the pulmonary and systemic vascular beds. The smooth muscle of the ductus arteriosus constricts in response to increased oxygen tension in the newborn's blood. Catecholamines, which exist in increased concentrations in the newborn, particularly during the first 3 hours of life, also constrict the ductus arteriosus. In contrast, prostaglandins I_2 and E_2, produced by the wall of the ductus arteriosus, relax the ductal smooth muscle. Administration of prostaglandin synthesis inhibitors to fetal animals promotes closure of the ductus arteriosus.

Cardiac output and its distribution also increase; left ventricular output increases approximately 150 to 400 mL/kg/min, whereas right ventricular output increases less significantly. Cardiac output changes closely parallel the increase in oxygen consumption. The redistribution of cardiac output also leads to increases in myocardial, renal, and gastrointestinal blood flow, and decreases in cerebral, adrenal, and carotid flow.

During fetal life, respiratory gas exchange takes place through the placenta. Delivery of the infant's trunk relieves the thoracic compression that occurs as the infant passes through the birth canal, and the thorax and the lungs expand. Most infants initiate respiratory efforts a few seconds after birth. Negative pressures in excess of 40 cm H_2O bring about the initial entry of air into fluid-filled alveoli. In the mature, normal neonate, the lungs expand almost completely after the first few breaths, and the pressure–volume changes achieved with each respiration resemble those of the adult. After lung expansion, the FRC approximates 70 mL in the term newborn and changes little over the first 6 days of life. The tidal volume varies between 10 and 30 mL, the breathing frequency ranges from 30 to 60 breaths per minute, and minute ventilation exceeds 500 mL. After delivery and prompt lung expansion, reoxygenation is rapid, but it takes 2 to 3 hours to achieve a relatively normal acid-base balance, primarily by pulmonary excretion of carbon dioxide. By 24 hours, the healthy neonate has reached the same acid-base state as that of the mother before labor.

Resuscitation

The delivery room must be prepared for adequate and prompt treatment of severe neonatal depression at birth. Members of the delivery room team should be trained in resuscitation methods because both mother and infant may encounter difficulty simultaneously. Every piece of apparatus necessary for emergency resuscitation should be checked carefully before delivery (Table 43-6). An overview of resuscitation in the delivery room is provided in Figure 43-14.

Initial Treatment and Evaluation of All Infants

Immediately after delivery, the infant should be held head-down while the cord is clamped and cut. The infant should then be placed supine under a radiant heat source, with the

---

TABLE 43-6

RESUSCITATION EQUIPMENT IN THE DELIVERY ROOM

Radiant warmer
Suction with manometer and suction trap
Suction catheters
Wall oxygen with flow meter
Resuscitation bag ($\leq$750 mL)
Infant face masks
Infant oropharyngeal airways
Endotracheal tubes—2.5, 3.0, 3.5, and 4.0 mm
Endotracheal tube stylets
Laryngoscope(s) and blade(s)
Sterile umbilical artery catheterization tray
Needles, syringes, three-way stopcocks
Medications and solutions
    1:10,000 Epinephrine
    Naloxone hydrochloride
    Sodium bicarbonate
    Volume expanders

---

head kept low in the sniffing position, and the skin should be dried promptly. The scoring system introduced by Apgar is a useful method of clinically evaluating the infant, particularly at 1 and 5 minutes after delivery (Table 43-7). The initial appraisal of the newborn should start from the moment of birth, with particular attention paid to the first few breaths and the evenness and ease of respiration. Most infants are vigorous and cough or cry within seconds of delivery. Slapping the infant's soles lightly or rubbing its back frequently aids in initiating a deep breath or cry. An assistant should listen to the heart beat immediately, indicating the rate by finger movement, or the rate can be detected from pulsation of the umbilical cord. Normally, the newborn's heart rate is >100 beats per minute. At the same time, the resuscitator should aspirate the mouth, pharynx, and nose with a catheter. This suction should be brief, not exceeding 30 seconds.

The administration of free-flowing oxygen rapidly improves oxygenation and decreases pulmonary vascular resistance, and should be administered to newborns demonstrating central cyanosis (cyanosis of the extremities is a normal finding in newborns) or bradycardia. Mildly to moderately depressed infants constitute the largest group requiring some form of resuscitation at birth. These infants are pale or cyanotic, have not established sustained respiration even at 1 minute after delivery, and may be nearly flaccid. However, their heart rate is usually >100 beats per minute. The severely depressed

---

TABLE 43-7

APGAR SCORES

SIGN	0	1	2
Heart rate	Absent	<100 beats/min	>100 beats/min
Respiratory effort	Absent	Slow, irregular	Good, crying
Muscle tone	Limp	Some flexion of extremities	Active motion
Reflex irritability	No response	Grimace	Cough, sneeze, or cry
Color	Pale, blue	Body pink, extremities blue	Completely pink

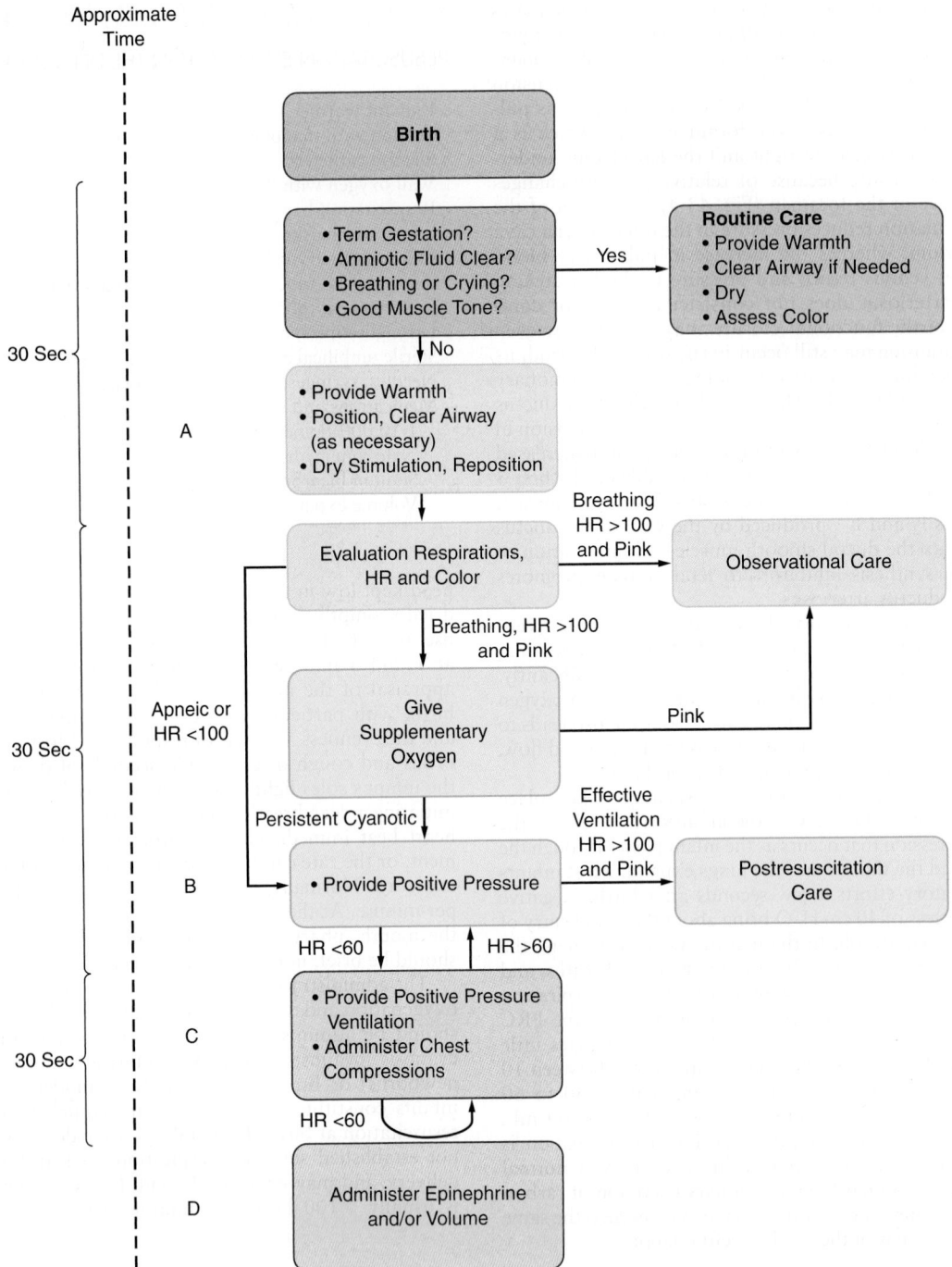

FIGURE 43-14. Algorithm for neonatal resuscitation. HR, heart rate. (Reprinted from 2005 American Heart Association [AHA] Guidelines for Cardiopulmonary Resuscitation [CPR] and Emergency Cardiovascular Care [ECC] of Pediatric and Neonatal Patients: Neonatal Resuscitation. Pediatrics 2006; 117: e1029, with permission.)

infant is flaccid, unresponsive, and pale, and may often have a heart rate <100 beats per minute.

Treatment of Moderately Depressed Infants

If initial resuscitative methods have produced no response, that is, the newborn does not demonstrate adequate respirations or heart rate remains <100 beats per minute, positive pressure ventilation by bag and mask with 100% oxygen should be instituted at a rate of 40 to 60 breaths per minute. The initial breath may require pressures of 30 to 40 cm H_2O. Subsequent inflation pressures should be reduced to 15 to 20 cm H_2O in an infant with normal lungs. A small plastic oropharyngeal airway may help maintain patency of the upper airway. If after 30 seconds of ventilation the heart rate is below 60 beats per minute, chest compressions should be initiated.[174]

Treatment of Severely Depressed Infants

Ventilation with 100% oxygen should be established without delay. If the amniotic fluid is meconium-stained, the glottis should be inspected immediately with the laryngoscope. If meconium is visible, the trachea should be suctioned through an endotracheal tube before the lungs are inflated. Severely depressed infants may require 3 to 8 minutes of artificial ventilation before spontaneous respiratory efforts are made. The endotracheal tube can be removed as soon as quiet and sustained respirations are established and heart rate is consistently >100 beats per minute.

Use of Cardiac Massage

If the blood pressure or heart rate is unduly low at the beginning of resuscitation, positive-pressure ventilation is unlikely to be successful unless cardiac massage is used. Chest compressions should be initiated if heart rate is <60 beats per minute despite adequate ventilation for 30 seconds. The recommended technique consists of a two-hand technique in which the fingers encircle the thorax and the two thumbs depress the sternum to a depth of one third the anterior-posterior diameter of the chest at a rate of 90 beats per minute. The ratio of chest compression to ventilation should be approximately 3:1 or 90 compressions and 30 breaths per minute. Cardiac massage and ventilation should be maintained until the heart rate exceeds 100 beats per minute.

Rapid Correction of Acidosis

Sodium bicarbonate use is not recommended during brief cardiopulmonary resuscitation. The hyperosmolarity and CO_2 generated may be detrimental to cerebral and myocardial function. In the case of persistent acidemia, administration should be guided by arterial blood gas measurements.

Other Drugs and Fluids

If it is believed that persistent depression has resulted from maternal opioid medication, naloxone should be given after adequate ventilation has been established (Table 43-8). The recommended dose of 0.1 mg/kg may be injected intravenously, intramuscularly, subcutaneously, or by endotracheal tube. The initial dose may be repeated as needed. Naloxone should be avoided in infants born to opioid-addicted mothers so as not to precipitate acute withdrawal. A severely asphyxiated newborn might require cardiotonic drugs during early resuscitation. Epinephrine should be used to treat asystole or persistent bradycardia (<60 beats per minute despite 30 seconds of effective ventilation and external cardiac massage). A dose of 0.1 to 0.3 mL/kg of a 1:10,000 solution should be injected intravenously or by endotracheal tube, and repeated every 5 minutes if necessary.

Hypovolemia frequently follows severe birth asphyxia because a greater-than-normal portion of fetal blood remains in the placenta. The infant may appear pale and have low arterial pressure, tachycardia, and tachypnea. Acute blood volume expansion may be accomplished with the intravenous administration of normal saline or lactated Ringer solution, 10 mL/kg over 5 to 10 minutes, or, when blood loss is suspected, a similar volume of O-negative blood. Albumin is no longer recommended.

Diagnostic Procedures

After the neonate is successfully resuscitated and stabilized, several diagnostic procedures are indicated. To rule out choanal atresia, each nostril should be obstructed. Because newborns must breathe through their noses, occlusion of the nostril on the patent side causes respiratory obstruction. To rule out esophageal atresia, a suction catheter is inserted into the stomach. Gastric contents are aspirated; volume in excess of 12 mL after vaginal delivery and 20 mL after cesarean delivery may result from an abnormality of the upper gastrointestinal tract.

EXIT Procedure

The EXIT procedure (ex utero intrapartum treatment), which maintains uteroplacental support for a period of time after partial delivery of the fetus, is employed for certain fetal conditions that pose an immediate threat to neonatal life on separation from the placental circulation. The most common indications are treatment of large fetal neck masses and reversal of tracheal occlusion from clips placed for congenital diaphragmatic hernia.[178] The usual procedure involves partial delivery of the fetus, surgical treatment of fetal pathology (e.g., attainment of a patent fetal airway), and, finally, delivery of the fetus and clamping of the umbilical cord.

Anesthetic considerations include maintenance of uterine relaxation during the phase of fetal manipulation, administration of fetal anesthesia, ensuring adequate fetal oxygenation, fetal monitoring, and rapid reversal of uterine relaxation after cord clamping to minimize maternal blood loss.[179] Most often the mother is anesthetized with deep inhalation general anesthesia following a standard rapid-sequence induction. Maintenance of anesthesia with high concentrations of volatile anesthetic agents provides for uterine relaxation during the procedure, although a recent report highlighted the use of intravenous nitroglycerin for this purpose.[180] The use of high inspired inhalational anesthesia may be associated with maternal hypotension; therefore, intravenous vasopressors may be required in order to ensure adequate uteroplacental blood flow. Use of volatile anesthetic concentrations <2 MAC is recommended to minimize untoward effects on uterine blood flow.[181] An FIO_2 of 1.0 helps maximize oxygen delivery to the placental unit.

ANESTHESIA FOR SURGICAL SUBSPECIALTIES

TABLE 43-8

THERAPEUTIC GUIDELINES FOR NEONATAL RESUSCITATION

■ DRUG OR VOLUME EXPANDER	■ CONCENTRATION	■ DOSAGE	■ ROUTE/RATE
Epinephrine	1:10,000	0.01–0.03 mg/kg	IV or IT Give rapidly
Volume expanders	PRBCs Normal saline Lactated Ringer	10 mL/kg	Give over 5–10 min
Naloxone hydrochloride	—	0.1 mg/kg	IV, IM, SC, or IT Give rapidly

IV, intravenously; IT, intratracheally; PRBCs, packed red blood cells; IM, intramuscularly; SC, subcutaneously.

Inhalational anesthetics rapidly cross the placenta and contribute to fetal anesthesia; intravenous opioids may be used to provide additional fetal anesthesia.[181] Intramuscular anesthetic agents, neuromuscular blocking agents, and atropine are administered to the fetus as needed after partial delivery. During the period of fetal manipulation, FHR and oxygenation can be monitored by sterile ultrasound and pulse oximetry sensors. A retrospective review of 31 EXIT procedures reported a mean FHR of 153 beats per minute and a mean fetal oxygen saturation of 71%.[178] After cord clamping, uterine relaxation must be reversed rapidly by decreasing the inspired concentration of inhalation agent and administering uterotonic agents such as oxytocin, so as to minimize maternal blood loss. The retrospective study previously referenced reported a mean maternal estimated blood loss of 848 mL and a mean duration of uteroplacental support of 30 minutes.[178]

Usually, two anesthetic teams are employed: one to tend to the mother and the other to tend to the fetus/newborn. Communication and coordination between surgical, pediatric, anesthesia, and nursing teams is mandatory for successful outcomes.

ANESTHESIA FOR NONOBSTETRIC SURGERY IN THE PREGNANT WOMAN

One to two percent of pregnant women in the United States undergo surgical procedures unrelated to pregnancy. The most frequent nonobstetric procedures are excision of ovarian cysts, appendectomy, breast biopsy, and surgery related to trauma. Treatment of an incompetent cervix (cervical cerclage) typically occurs early or mid pregnancy. Serious conditions such as intracranial aneurysms, cardiac valvular disease, and pheochromocytoma may rarely present and require surgery during pregnancy.

The objective for managing anesthesia in patients undergoing nonobstetric operative procedures is maternal safety, safe care of the fetus, and prevention of premature labor related to the surgical procedure or drugs administered during anesthesia. To achieve these goals, the effects of the patient's altered physiology must be recognized. Induction and emergence from anesthesia is more rapid than in the nonpregnant state because of increased minute ventilation, decreased FRC, and the decrease MAC of volatile agents, which may be seen as early as 8 to 10 weeks' gestation. Supine hypotensive syndrome can occur as early as the second trimester. The effects of altered physiology during pregnancy are not limited to general anesthesia. There is an increased effect of local anesthetics during pregnancy; thus, the amount of local anesthetic administered should be reduced by 25 to 30% during any stage of pregnancy.

Teratogenicity may be induced at any stage of gestation. However, most of the critical organogenesis occurs in the first trimester. Although many commonly used anesthetics are teratogenic at high doses in animals, few if any studies support teratogenic effects of anesthetic or sedative medications in the doses used for human anesthesia care. There is some evidence for a link between maternal high-dose diazepam injection in the first trimester and cleft palate[182]; however, medicinal doses of benzodiazepine are safe when needed to treat perioperative anxiety.

Nitrous oxide has also been suggested to be teratogenic in animals when administered for prolonged periods (1 to 2 days).[183] Its effect on DNA synthesis is of concern for its use in humans. Although teratogenesis has been seen only in animals under extreme conditions, not likely to be reproduced in clinical care, some believe nitrous oxide use is contraindicated in the first two trimesters.

Of all the information in the literature, two studies, although not new, still deserve mention. A review was taken of the entire population of the province of Manitoba, Canada, between the years 1971 and 1978.[184] State health insurance records were used to identify approximately 2,500 pregnant women who had undergone surgery during this period. Each patient was matched with a woman of similar age, living in the same area, with a pregnancy-related condition but no surgical intervention. As in earlier studies, there was no increase in the incidence of congenital anomalies in the offspring of mothers who had had surgery. However, there was an increased risk of spontaneous abortion in women who had received general anesthesia during the first or second trimesters, which was most evident after gynecologic operations. Few of the surgical group had had procedures to treat cervical incompetence, suggesting that factors other than the obstetric condition itself might be important. The results also might have been influenced by the fact that a small number of gynecologic procedures were performed with anesthesia other than general, so the effect of the surgical site alone could not be distinguished. The authors emphasized a multiplicity of factors other than choice of anesthetic agent (e.g., diagnostic radiologic procedures, antibiotics, analgesics, infection, decreased uterine perfusion, stress) that might have been responsible for the increased risk of abortion.

One of the largest studies regarding reproductive outcome after surgery during pregnancy is a Swedish registry review covering the years 1973 to 1981.[185] During this period, there were a total of 720,000 births, 5,405 of them after anesthesia and surgery during pregnancy. The results of this study are reassuring in that there was no increased incidence of congenital anomalies or stillbirths among infants exposed in utero to maternal surgery and anesthesia. However, in this group there was an increased frequency of very low and low birth weights, and of deaths within 168 hours after delivery. The reasons for this are unclear and are not related to any specific type of operation. The authors postulated that the maternal illness itself may have been a major contributor to adverse neonatal outcome.

Intrauterine fetal asphyxia is avoided by maintaining maternal PaO_2, $PaCO_2$, and uterine blood flow. $PaCO_2$ can affect uterine blood flow as maternal alkalosis may cause direct vasoconstriction. Alkalosis also shifts the oxyhemoglobin dissociation curve, resulting in the release of less oxygen to the fetus at the placenta. Maternal hypotension leads to a reduction in uterine blood flow and thus fetal hypoxia. Uterine hypertension, as occurs with increased uterine irritability, will also decrease uterine blood flow.

Anesthesia and surgery may also result in preterm labor during the intra- and postoperative periods. Abdominal and pelvic procedures are associated with the greatest incidence of preterm labor. Generally, elective surgery should be delayed until the patient is no longer pregnant and she has returned to her nonpregnant physiologic state (approximately 2 to 6 weeks postpartum). Procedures that can be scheduled with some flexibility but that cannot be delayed until postpartum are best scheduled in the midtrimester. This lessens the risk for teratogenicity (first trimester medication administration) or preterm labor (greater risk in the third trimester) (Fig. 43-15).

If emergency surgery is required, there is no proof that any well-conducted anesthetic is preferred over another, provided oxygenation and blood pressure are maintained and hyperventilation is avoided. Despite this statement, regional anesthesia should be considered as it minimizes fetal exposure to medications. Left uterine displacement should be used during the second and third trimesters, and aspiration prophylaxis should be administered to all pregnant patients. At a minimum, pre- and postoperative FHR and uterine activity should be assessed.[186]

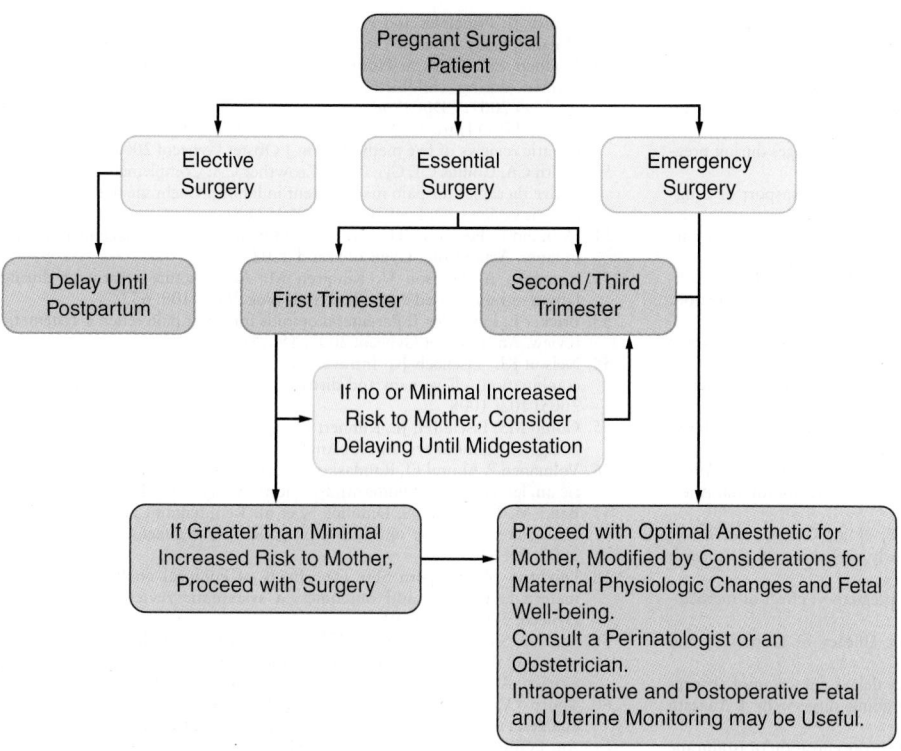

FIGURE 43-15. Recommendations for management of parturients and surgical procedures. (From Rosen MA: Management of anesthesia for the pregnant surgical patient. Anesthesiology 1999; 91: 1159. © 1999, Lippincott Williams & Wilkins, with permission.)

ANESTHESIA FOR SURGICAL SUBSPECIALTIES

Practical Suggestions

14 It is generally agreed that only surgical procedures that cannot be delayed for months, including emergency surgery, should be performed during pregnancy, particularly in the first trimester. The possibility of pregnancy should be considered in all female surgical patients of reproductive age. Based on the maternal and fetal hazards already described, the following approach to anesthesia is suggested (Fig. 43-15).

1. Anesthesiologists and surgeons should obtain consultation from an obstetrician before performing nonobstetric surgery in pregnancy.
2. The patient's apprehension should be allayed as much as possible by personal reassurance during the preanesthetic visit and by adequate sedation and premedication.
3. Pain should be relieved whenever present.
4. A nonparticulate antacid, 15 to 30 mL, should be administered within half an hour before induction of anesthesia. Ranitidine and metoclopramide may be useful.
5. Beginning in the second trimester, uterine displacement must be maintained at all times.
6. Hypotension related to spinal or epidural anesthesia should be prevented as much as possible by rapid intravenous infusion of crystalloid solution during induction of anesthesia. If the mother becomes hypotensive, ephedrine or phenylephrine should be promptly administered intravenously.
7. General anesthesia should be preceded by careful denitrogenation.
8. The risk of aspiration should be minimized by application of cricoid pressure and rapid tracheal intubation with a cuffed tube.
9. To reduce fetal hazard, particularly during the first trimester, it appears preferable to choose drugs with a long history of safety; these drugs include thiopental, morphine, meperidine, muscle relaxants, and low concentrations of nitrous oxide.
10. Avoid maternal hyperventilation and monitor end-expiratory $PaCO_2$ or arterial blood gases.
11. FHR may be monitored continuously or intermittently throughout surgery and anesthesia, provided that placement of the transducer does not encroach on the surgical field (this becomes technically feasible from the 16th week of pregnancy). The decision to monitor the fetus should be made in conjunction with the obstetrician based on the severity of maternal disease, the potential for fetal jeopardy, and whether the fetus is viable. Uterine tone may also be monitored with an external tocodynamometer if the uterus reaches the umbilicus or above.
12. Monitoring uterine activity should be continued after operation, and tocolytic agents may be required.

References

1. Taylor DJ, Lind T: Red cell mass during and after normal pregnancy. Br J Obstet Gynaecol 1979; 86: 364
2. Boehlen F, Hohlfeld P, Extermann P et al: Platelet count at term pregnancy: A reappraisal of the threshold. Obstet Gynecol 2000; 95: 29
3. Brenner B: Haemostatic changes in pregnancy. Thromb Res 2004; 114: 409
4. Cerneca F, Ricci G, Simeone R et al: Coagulation and fibrinolysis changes in normal pregnancy. Increased levels of procoagulants and reduced levels of inhibitors during pregnancy induce a hypercoagulable state, combined with a reactive fibrinolysis. Eur J Obstet Gynecol Reprod Biol 1997; 73: 31
5. Wildsmith JA: Serum cholinesterase, pregnancy and suxamethonium. Anaesthesia 1972; 27: 90
6. Coryell M, Beach E, Robinson A, et al: Metabolism of women during the reproductive cycle. XVII. Changes in electrophoretic patterns of plasma proteins throught the cycle and following delivery. J Clin Invest 1950; 29: 1559
7. Goodman RP, Killam AP, Brash AR, Branch RA: Prostacyclin production during pregnancy: comparison of production during normal pregnancy and pregnancy complicated by hypertension. Am J Obstet Gynecol 1982; 142: 817
8. Kametas NA, McAuliffe F, Krampl E, et al: Maternal cardiac function in twin pregnancy. Obstet Gynecol 2003; 102: 806
9. Kerr MG, Scott DB, Samuel E: Studies of the inferior vena cava in late pregnancy. Br Med J 1964; 1: 532
10. Kinsella SM: Lateral tilt for pregnant women: why 15 degrees? Anaesthesia 2003; 58: 835

11. Carruth JE, Mivis SB, Brogan DR, Wenger NK: The electrocardiogram in normal pregnancy. Am Heart J 1981; 102: 1075

12. Nakagawa M, Katou S, Ichinose M, et al: Characteristics of new-onset ventricular arrhythmias in pregnancy. J Electrocardiol 2004; 37: 47

13. Crapo RO: Normal cardiopulmonary physiology during pregnancy. Clin Obstet Gynecol 1996; 39: 3

14. Prowse CM, Gaensler EA: Respiratory and acid-base changes during pregnancy. Anesthesiology 1965; 26: 381

15. Moya F, Smith BE: Uptake, distribution and placental transport of drugs and anesthetics. Anesthesiology 1965; 26: 465

16. Archer GW Jr, Marx GF: Arterial oxygen tension during apnoea in parturient women. Br J Anaesth 1974; 46: 358

17. Datta S, Kitzmiller JL, Naulty JS, et al: Acid-base status of diabetic mothers and their infants following spinal anesthesia for cesarean section. Anesth Analg 1982; 61: 662

18. Chiloiro M, Darconza G, Piccioli E, et al: Gastric emptying and orocecal transit time in pregnancy. J Gastroenterol 2001; 36: 538

19. Wong CA, Loffredi M, Ganchiff JN, et al: Gastric emptying of water in term pregnancy. Anesthesiology 2002; 96: 1395

20. Wong CA, McCarthy RJ, Fitzgerald PC, et al: Gastric emptying of water in obese pregnant women at term. Anesth Analg 2007; 105: 751

21. Practice guidelines for obstetric anesthesia: an updated report by the American Society of Anesthesiologists Task Force on Obstetric Anesthesia. Anesthesiology 2007; 106: 843

22. Brock-Utne JG, Dow TG, Dimopoulos GE, et al: Gastric and lower oesophageal sphincter (LOS) pressures in early pregnancy. Br J Anaesth 1981; 53: 381

23. Wyner J, Cohen SE: Gastric volume in early pregnancy: effect of metoclopramide. Anesthesiology 1982; 57: 209

24. Cohen SE, Woods WA, Wyner J: Antiemetic efficacy of droperidol and metoclopramide. Anesthesiology 1984; 60: 67

25. Simpson KH, Stakes AF, Miller M: Pregnancy delays paracetamol absorption and gastric emptying in patients undergoing surgery. Br J Anaesth 1988; 60: 24

26. Gin T, Chan MT: Decreased minimum alveolar concentration of isoflurane in pregnant humans. Anesthesiology 1994; 81: 829

27. Hirabayashi Y, Shimizu R, Saitoh K, Fukuda H: Spread of subarachnoid hyperbaric amethocaine in pregnant women. Br J Anaesth 1995; 74: 384

28. Butterworth JF, IV, Walker FO, Lysak SZ: Pregnancy increases median nerve susceptibility to lidocaine. Anesthesiology 1990; 72: 962

29. Datta S, Lambert DH, Gregus J, et al: Differential sensitivities of mammalian nerve fibers during pregnancy. Anesth Analg 1983; 62: 1070

30. Brown WU Jr, Bell GC, Alper MH: Acidosis, local anesthetics, and the newborn. Obstet Gynecol 1976; 48: 27

31. Hamshaw-Thomas A, Rogerson N, Reynolds F: Transfer of bupivacaine, lignocaine and pethidine across the rabbit placenta: influence of maternal protein binding and fetal flow. Placenta 1984; 5: 61

32. Kennedy RL, Miller RP, Bell JU, et al: Uptake and distribution of bupivacaine in fetal lambs. Anesthesiology 1986; 65: 247

33. Kuhnert PM, Kuhnert BR, Stitts JM, Gross TL: The use of a selected ion monitoring technique to study the disposition of bupivacaine in mother, fetus, and neonate following epidural anesthesia for cesarean section. Anesthesiology 1981; 55: 611

34. Morishima HO, Daniel SS, Finster M, et al: Transmission of mepivacaine hydrochloride (carbocaine) across the human placenta. Anesthesiology 1966; 27: 147

35. Kuhnert BR, Kuhnert PM, Prochaska AL, Gross TL: Plasma levels of 2-chloroprocaine in obstetric patients and their neonates after epidural anesthesia. Anesthesiology 1980; 53: 21

36. Haram K, Bakke M, Johannessen KH, Lund T: Transplacental passage of diazepam during labor: influence of uterine contractions. Clin Pharmacol Ther 1978; 24: 590

37. Dwyer R, Fee JP, Moore J: Uptake of halothane and isoflurane by mother and baby during caesarean section. Br J Anaesth 1995; 74: 379

38. Kosaka Y, Takahashi T, Mark LC: Intravenous thiobarbiturate anesthesia for cesarean section. Anesthesiology 1969; 31: 489

39. Morishima HO, Finster M, Pedersen H, et al: Pharmacokinetics of lidocaine in fetal and neonatal lambs and adult sheep. Anesthesiology 1979; 50: 431

40. Mihaly GW, Moore RG, Thomas J, et al: The pharmacokinetics and metabolism of the anilide local anaesthetics in neonates. I. Lignocaine. Eur J Clin Pharmacol 1978; 13: 143

41. Morishima HO, Pedersen H, Finster M, et al: Toxicity of lidocaine in adult, newborn, and fetal sheep. Anesthesiology 1981; 55: 57

42. Gale R, Ferguson JE, 2nd, Stevenson DK: Effect of epidural analgesia with bupivacaine hydrochloride on neonatal bilirubin production. Obstet Gynecol 1987; 70: 692

43. Ueland K, Hansen JM: Maternal cardiovascular dynamics. III. Labor and delivery under local and caudal analgesia. Am J Obstet Gynecol 1969; 103: 8

44. Anonymous: ACOG Committe Opinion No. 339, June 2006. Analgesia and cesarean delivery rates. Obstet Gynecol 2006; 107: 1487

45. Simkin P, Bolding A: Update on nonpharmacologic approaches to relieve labor pain and prevent suffering. J Midwifery Womens Health 2004; 49: 489

46. Scott JR, Rose NB: Effect of psychoprophylaxis (Lamaze preparation) on labor and delivery in primiparas. N Engl J Med 1976; 294: 1205

47. Bonica JJ: Principles and Practice of Obstetric Analgesia and Anesthesia. Philadelphia, FA Davis, 1969

48. Hodnett ED, Gates S, Hofmeyr GJ, Sakala C: Continuous support for women during childbirth. Cochrane database of systematic reviews (Online) 2007: CD003766

49. Simkin PP, O'Hara M: Nonpharmacologic relief of pain during labor: systematic reviews of five methods. Am J Obstet Gynecol 2002; 186: S131

50. Smith CA, Collins CT, Cyna AM, Crowther CA: Complementary and alternative therapies for pain management in labour. Cochrane database of systematic reviews (Online) 2006: CD003521

51. Skilnand E, Fossen D, Heiberg E: Acupuncture in the management of pain in labor. Acta Obstet Gynecol Scand 2002; 81: 943

52. Ramnero A, Hanson U, Kihlgren M: Acupuncture treatment during labour–a randomised controlled trial. Bjog 2002; 109: 637

53. Bricker L, Lavender T: Parenteral opioids for labor pain relief: a systematic review. Am J Obstet Gynecol 2002; 186: S94

54. Nelson KE, Eisenach JC: Intravenous butorphanol, meperidine, and their combination relieve pain and distress in women in labor. Anesthesiology 2005; 102: 1008

55. Golub MS, Eisele JH, Jr., Kuhnert BR: Disposition of intrapartum narcotic analgesics in monkeys. Anesth Analg 1988; 67: 637

56. Volmanen P, Akural EI, Raudaskoski T, Alahuhta S: Remifentanil in obstetric analgesia: a dose-finding study. Anesth Analg 2002; 94: 913

57. Balki M, Kasodekar S, Dhumne S, et al: Remifentanil patient-controlled analgesia for labour: optimizing drug delivery regimens. Can J Anaesth 2007; 54: 626

58. Leighton BL, Halpern SH: The effects of epidural analgesia on labor, maternal, and neonatal outcomes: a systematic review. Am J Obstet Gynecol 2002; 186: S69

59. Sharma SK, McIntire DD, Wiley J, Leveno KJ: Labor analgesia and cesarean delivery: an individual patient meta-analysis of nulliparous women. Anesthesiology 2004; 100: 142; discussion 6A

60. Thorp JA, Hu DH, Albin RM, et al: The effect of intrapartum epidural analgesia on nulliparous labor: A randomized, controlled, prospective trial. Am J Obstet Gynecol 1993; 169: 851

61. Nageotte MP, Larson D, Rumney PJ, et al: Epidural analgesia compared with combined spinal-epidural analgesia during labor in nulliparous women. N Eng J Med 1997; 337: 1715

62. Wong CA, Scavone BM, Peaceman AM, et al: The risk of cesarean delivery with neuraxial analgesia given early versus late in labor. N Engl J Med 2005; 352: 655

63. Ohel G, Gonen R, Vaida S, et al: Early versus late initiation of epidural analgesia in labor: does it increase the risk of cesarean section? A randomized trial. Am J Obstet Gynecol 2006; 194: 600

64. Chestnut DH, McGrath JM, Vincent RD, et al: Does early administration of epidural analgesia affect obstetric outcome in nulliparous women who are in spontaneous labor? Anesthesiology 1994; 80: 1201

65. Halpern SH, Muir H, Breen TW, et al: A multicenter randomized controlled trial comparing patient-controlled epidural with intravenous analgesia for pain relief in labor. Anesth Analg 2004; 99: 1532

66. Chestnut DH, Laszewski LJ, Pollack KL, et al: Continuous epidural infusion of 0.0625% bupivacaine—0.0002% fentanyl during the second stage of labor. Anesthesiology 1990; 72: 613

67. Norris MC, Ferrenbach D, Dalman H, et al: Does epinephrine improve the diagnostic accuracy of aspiration during labor epidural analgesia? Anesth Analg 1999; 88: 1073

68. Birnbach DJ, Chestnut DH: The epidural test dose in obstetric patients: has it outlived its usefulness? [editorial]. Anesth Analg 1999; 88: 971

69. Curry PD, Pacsoo C, Heap DG: Patient-controlled epidural analgesia in obstetric anaesthetic practice. Pain 1994; 57: 125

70. van der Vyver M, Halpern S, Joseph G: Patient-controlled epidural analgesia versus continuous infusion for labour analgesia: a meta-analysis. Br J Anaesth 2002; 89: 459

71. Ledin Eriksson S, Gentele C, Olofsson CH: PCEA compared to continuous epidural infusion in an ultra-low-dose regimen for labor pain relief: a randomized study. Acta Anaesthesiol Scand 2003; 47: 1085

72. Halpern S: Recent advances in patient-controlled epidural analgesia for labour. Current opinion in anaesthesiology 2005; 18: 247

73. Zaric D, Nydahl P, Philipson L, et al: The effect of continuous lumbar epidural infusion of ropivacaine (0.1%, 0.2%, and 0.3%) and 0.25% bupivacaine on sensory and motor block in volunteers. Reg Anesth 1996; 21: 14

74. Lacassie HJ, Habib AS, Lacassie HP, Columb MO: Motor blocking minimum local anesthetic concentrations of bupivacaine, levobupivacaine, and ropivacaine in labor. Reg Anesth Pain Med 2007; 32: 323

75. Beilin Y, Guinn NR, Bernstein HH, et al: Local anesthetics and mode of delivery: bupivacaine versus ropivacaine versus levobupivacaine. Anesth Analg 2007; 105: 756

76. Asokumar B, Newman LM, McCarthy RJ, et al: Intrathecal bupivacaine reduces pruritus and prolongs duration of fentanyl analgesia during labor: a prospective, randomized controlled trial. Anesth Analg 1998; 87: 1309

77. Mardirosoff C, Dumont L, Boulvain M, Tramer MR: Fetal bradycardia due to intrathecal opioids for labour analgesia: a systematic review. Br J Obstet Gynaecol 2002; 109: 274

78. Cohen SE, Cherry CM, Holbrook RH, Jr, et al: Intrathecal sufentanil for labor analgesia–sensory changes, side effects, and fetal heart rate changes. Anesth Analg 1993; 77: 1155

79. Albright GA, Forster RM: Does combined spinal-epidural analgesia with subarachnoid sufentanil increase the incidence of emergency cesarean delivery? Reg Anesth 1997; 22: 400

80. Nielsen PE, Erickson JR, Abouleish EI, et al: Fetal heart rate changes after intrathecal sufentanil or epidural bupivacaine for labor analgesia: incidence and clinical significance. Anesth Analg 1996; 83: 742

81. Leighton BL, Halpern SH, Wilson DB: Lumbar sympathetic blocks speed early and second stage induced labor in nulliparous women. Anesthesiology 1999; 90: 1039

82. Yentis S: The use of Entonox® for labour pain should be abandoned. International Journal of Obstetric Anesthesia 2001; 10: 25

83. Carstoniu J, Levytam S, Norman P, et al: Nitrous oxide in early labor. Safety and analgesic efficacy assessed by a double-blind, placebo-controlled study. Anesthesiology 1994; 80: 30

84. Landon MB, Hauth JC, Leveno KJ, et al: Maternal and perinatal outcomes associated with a trial of labor after prior cesarean delivery. N Engl J Med 2004; 351: 2581

85. Bucklin BA, Hawkins JL, Anderson JR, Ullrich FA: Obstetric anesthesia workforce survey: twenty-year update. Anesthesiology 2005; 103: 645

86. Khaw KS, Ngan Kee WD, Lee A, et al: Supplementary oxygen for elective Caesarean section under spinal anaesthesia: useful in prolonged uterine incision-to-delivery interval? Br J Anaesth 2004; 92: 518

87. Backe SK, Kocarev M, Wilson RC, Lyons G: Effect of maternal facial oxygen on neonatal behavioural scores during elective Caesarean section with spinal anaesthesia. Eur J Anaesthesiol 2007; 24: 66

88. McDonnell JG, Curley G, Carney J, et al: The analgesic efficacy of transversus abdominis plane block after cesarean delivery: a randomized controlled trial. Anesth Analg 2008; 106: 186

89. Palmer CM, Nogami WM, Van Maren G, Alves DM: Postcesarean epidural morphine: A dose-response study. Anesth Analg 2000; 90: 887

90. Abouleish E, Rawal N, Rashad MN: The addition of 0.2 mg subarachnoid morphine to hyperbaric bupivacaine for cesarean delivery: a prospective study of 856 cases. Reg Anesth 1991; 16: 137

91. Leighton BL, Norris MC, DeSimone CA, et al: The air test as a clinically useful indicator of intravenously placed epidural catheters. Anesthesiology 1990; 73: 610

92. Morris GF, Gore-Hickman W, Lang SA, Yip RW: Can parturients distinguish between intravenous and epidural fentanyl? Can J Anaesth 1994; 41: 667

93. Tanz RD, Heskett T, Loehning RW, Fairfax CA: Comparative cardiotoxicity of bupivacaine and lidocaine in the isolated perfused mammalian heart. Anesth Analg 1984; 63: 549

94. Albright GA: Cardiac arrest following regional anesthesia with etidocaine or bupivacaine. Anesthesiology 1979; 51: 285

95. Crosby E, Sandler A, Finucane B, et al: Comparison of epidural anaesthesia with ropivacaine 0.5% and bupivacaine 0.5% for caesarean section. Can J Anaesth 1998; 45: 1066

96. Bjornestad E, Smedvig JP, Bjerkreim T, et al: Epidural ropivacaine 7.5 mg/ml for elective Caesarean section: a double-blind comparison of efficacy and tolerability with bupivacaine 5 mg/ml. Acta Anaesthesiol Scand 1999; 43: 603

97. Choi DH, Kim JA, Chung IS: Comparison of combined spinal epidural anesthesia and epidural anesthesia for cesarean section. Acta Anaesthesiol Scand 2000; 44: 214

98. Thoren T, Holmstrom B, Rawal N, et al: Sequential combined spinal epidural block versus spinal block for cesarean section: effects on maternal hypotension and neurobehavioral function of the newborn. Anesth Analg 1994; 78: 1087

99. Choi DH, Ahn HJ, Kim JA: Combined low-dose spinal-epidural anesthesia versus single-shot spinal anesthesia for elective cesarean delivery. Int J Obstet Anesth 2006; 15: 13

100. Hawkins JL, Koonin LM, Palmer SK, Gibbs CP: Anesthesia-related deaths during obstetric delivery in the United States, 1979–1990. Anesthesiology 1997; 86: 277

101. Practice guidelines for management of the difficult airway: an updated report by the American Society of Anesthesiologists Task Force on Management of the Difficult Airway. Anesthesiology 2003; 98: 1269

102. Awan R, Nolan JP, Cook TM: Use of a ProSeal laryngeal mask airway for airway maintenance during emergency Caesarean section after failed tracheal intubation. Br J Anaesth 2004; 92: 144

103. Crosby ET, Cooper RM, Douglas MJ, et al: The unanticipated difficult airway with recommendations for management. Can J Anaesth 1998; 45: 757

104. Lyons G, Macdonald R: Awareness during caesarean section. Anaesthesia 1991; 46: 62

105. Chin KJ, Yeo SW: Bispectral index values at sevoflurane concentrations of 1% and 1.5% in lower segment cesarean delivery. Anesth Analg 2004; 98: 1140

106. Ong BY, Cohen MM, Palahniuk RJ: Anesthesia for cesarean section–effects on neonates. Anesth Analg 1989; 68: 270

107. Marx GF, Luykx WM, Cohen S: Fetal-neonatal status following caesarean section for fetal distress. Br J Anaesth 1984; 56: 1009

108. Ngan Kee WD, Khaw KS, Ng FF: Comparison of phenylephrine infusion regimens for maintaining maternal blood pressure during spinal anaesthesia for Caesarean section. Br J Anaesth 2004; 92: 469

109. Dyer RA, Farina Z, Joubert IA, et al: Crystalloid preload versus rapid crystalloid administration after induction of spinal anaesthesia (coload) for elective Caesarean section. Anaesth Intensive Care 2004; 32: 351

110. Ko JS, Kim CS, Cho HS, Choi DH: A randomized trial of crystalloid versus colloid solution for prevention of hypotension during spinal or low-dose combined spinal-epidural anesthesia for elective cesarean delivery. Int J Obstet Anesth 2007; 16: 8

111. Dahlgren G, Granath F, Wessel H, Irestedt L: Prediction of hypotension during spinal anaesthesia for Cesarean section and its relation to the effect of crystalloid or colloid preload. Int J Obstet Anesth 2007; 16: 128

112. Lee A, Ngan Kee WD, Gin T: A quantitative, systematic review of randomized controlled trials of ephedrine versus phenylephrine for the management of hypotension during spinal anesthesia for cesarean delivery. Anesth Analg 2002; 94: 920

113. Riley ET: Editorial I: Spinal anaesthesia for Caesarean delivery: keep the pressure up and don't spare the vasoconstrictors. Br J Anaesth 2004; 92: 459

114. Kasten GW, Martin ST: Resuscitation from bupivacaine-induced cardiovascular toxicity during partial inferior vena cava occlusion. Anesth Analg 1986; 65: 341

115. Rosenblatt MA, Abel M, Fischer GW, et al: Successful use of a 20% lipid emulsion to resuscitate a patient after a presumed bupivacaine-related cardiac arrest. Anesthesiology 2006; 105: 217

116. Scavone BM, Wong CA, Sullivan JT, et al: Efficacy of a prophylactic epidural blood patch in preventing post dural puncture headache in parturients after inadvertent dural puncture. Anesthesiology 2004; 101: 1422

117. Wong CA, Scavone BM, Dugan S, et al: Incidence of postpartum lumbosacral spine and lower extremity nerve injuries. Obstet Gynecol 2003; 101: 279

118. Wang Y, Walsh SW, Kay HH: Placental lipid peroxides and thromboxane are increased and prostacyclin is decreased in women with preeclampsia. Am J Obstet Gynecol 1992; 167: 946

119. Meekins JW, Pijnenborg R, Hanssens M, et al: A study of placental bed spiral arteries and trophoblast invasion in normal and severe pre-eclamptic pregnancies. Br J Obstet Gynaecol 1994; 101: 669

120. Chesley LC: Plasma and red cell volumes during pregnancy. Am J Obstet Gynecol 1972; 112: 440

121. Bosio PM, McKenna PJ, Conroy R, O'Herlihy C: Maternal central hemodynamics in hypertensive disorders of pregnancy. Obstet Gynecol 1999; 94: 978

122. Cotton DB, Gonik B, Dorman K, Harrist R: Cardiovascular alterations in severe pregnancy-induced hypertension: relationship of central venous pressure to pulmonary capillary wedge pressure. Am J Obstet Gynecol 1985; 151: 762

123. O'Brien JM, Milligan DA, Barton JR: Impact of high-dose corticosteroid therapy for patients with HELLP (hemolysis, elevated liver enzymes, and low platelet count) syndrome. Am J Obstet Gynecol 2000; 183: 921

124. Hogg B, Hauth JC, Caritis SN, et al: Safety of labor epidural anesthesia for women with severe hypertensive disease. National Institute of Child Health and Human Development Maternal-Fetal Medicine Units Network. Am J Obstet Gynecol 1999; 181: 1096

125. Newsome LR, Bramwell RS, Curling PE: Severe preeclampsia: hemodynamic effects of lumbar epidural anesthesia. Anesth Analg 1986; 65: 31

126. Jouppila P, Jouppila R, Hollmen A, Koivula A: Lumbar epidural analgesia to improve intervillous blood flow during labor in severe preeclampsia. Obstet Gynecol 1982; 59: 158

127. Ramanathan J, Bottorff M, Jeter JN, et al: The pharmacokinetics and maternal and neonatal effects of epidural lidocaine in preeclampsia. Anesth Analg 1986; 65: 120

128. Aya AG, Mangin R, Vialles N, et al: Patients with severe preeclampsia experience less hypotension during spinal anaesthesia for elective Cesarean delivery than healthy parturients: a prospective cohort comparison. Anesth Analg 2003; 97: 867

129. Wallace DH, Leveno KJ, Cunningham FG, et al: Randomized comparison of general and regional anesthesia for cesarean delivery in pregnancies complicated by severe preeclampsia. Obstet Gynecol 1995; 86: 193

130. Hood DD, Curry R: Spinal versus epidural anesthesia for cesarean section in severely preeclamptic patients: a retrospective survey. Anesthesiology 1999; 90: 1276

131. Ananth CV, Smulian JC, Vintzileos AM: The association of placenta previa with history of cesarean delivery and abortion: a metaanalysis. Am J Obstet Gynecol 1997; 177: 1071

132. Miller DA, Chollet JA, Goodwin TM: Clinical risk factors for placenta previa-placenta accreta. Am J Obstet Gynecol 1997; 177: 210

133. Clark SL, Koonings PP, Phelan JP: Placenta previa/accreta and prior Cesarean section. Obstet Gynecol 1985; 66: 89

134. Crane JM, Van den Hof MC, Dodds L, et al: Maternal complications with placenta previa. Am J Perinatol 2000; 17: 101

135. Oyelese Y, Smulian JC: Placenta previa, placenta accreta, and vasa previa. Obstet Gynecol 2006; 107: 927

136. O'Brien JM, Barton JR, Donaldson ES: The management of placenta percreta: conservative and operative strategies. Am J Obstet Gynecol 1996; 175: 1632

137. ACOG Committee Opinion. Number 266, January 2002: Placenta accreta. Obstet Gynecol 2002; 99: 169

138. ACOG Practice Bulletin: Clinical Management Guidelines for Obstetrician-Gynecologists Number 76, October 2006: postpartum hemorrhage. Obstet Gynecol 2006; 108: 1039

139. Chestnut DH, Dewan DM, Redick LF, et al: Anesthetic management for obstetric hysterectomy: a multi-institutional study. Anesthesiology 1989; 70: 607

140. Arafeh JM, Baird SM: Cardiac disease in pregnancy. Crit Care Nurs Q 2006; 29: 32

141. Ro A, Frishman WH: Peripartum cardiomyopathy. Cardiol Rev 2006; 14: 35

142. Palmer DG: Peripartum cardiomyopathy. J Perinat Neonatal Nurs 2006; 20: 324

143. Baird SM, Kennedy B: Myocardial infarction in pregnancy. J Perinat Neonatal Nurs 2006; 20: 311; quiz 322

144. Mallampalli A, Guy E: Cardiac arrest in pregnancy and somatic support after brain death. Crit Care Med 2005; 33: S325

145. Hunt KJ, Schuller KL: The increasing prevalence of diabetes in pregnancy. Obstet Gynecol Clin North Am 2007; 34: 173, vii

146. Parker JA, Conway DL: Diabetic ketoacidosis in pregnancy. Obstet Gynecol Clin North Am 2007; 34: 533, xii

147. Mulholland C, Njoroge T, Mersereau P, Williams J: Comparison of guidelines available in the United States for diagnosis and management of diabetes before, during, and after pregnancy. Journal of women's health (2002) 2007; 16: 790

148. Perlow JH, Morgan MA, Montgomery D, et al: Perinatal outcome in pregnancy complicated by massive obesity. Am J Obstet Gynecol 1992; 167: 958

149. Tsueda K, Debrand M, Zeok SS, et al: Obesity supine death syndrome: reports of two morbidly obese patients. Anesth Analg 1979; 58: 345

150. Hamilton BE, Martin JA, Sutton PD: Births: preliminary data for 2002. Natl Vital Stat Rep 2003; 51: 1

151. Montan S: Increased risk in the elderly parturient. Curr Opin Obstet Gynecol 2007; 19: 110

152. Joseph KS, Allen AC, Dodds L, et al: The perinatal effects of delayed childbearing. Obstet Gynecol 2005; 105: 1410

153. Simchen MJ, Yinon Y, Moran O, et al: Pregnancy outcome after age 50. Obstet Gynecol 2006; 108: 1084

154. Cleary-Goldman J, Malone FD, Vidaver J, et al: Impact of maternal age on obstetric outcome. Obstet Gynecol 2005; 105: 983

155. Callaway LK, Lust K, McIntyre HD: Pregnancy outcomes in women of very advanced maternal age. Aust N Z J Obstet Gynaecol 2005; 45: 12

156. Vigil-De Gracia P, Montufar-Rueda C, Smith A: Pregnancy and severe chronic hypertension: maternal outcome. Hypertens Pregnancy 2004; 23: 285

157. Lin HC, Sheen TC, Tang CH, Kao S: Association between maternal age and the likelihood of a Cesarean section: a population-based multivariate logistic regression analysis. Acta Obstet Gynecol Scand 2004; 83: 1178

158. Amu O, Rajendran S, Bolaji, II: Should doctors perform an elective Caesarean section on request? Maternal choice alone should not determine method of delivery. BMJ 1998; 317: 463

159. Bell JS, Campbell DM, Graham WJ, et al: Do obstetric complications explain high Caesarean section rates among women over 30? A retrospective analysis. BMJ 2001; 322: 894

160. Oleszczuk JJ, Keith LG, Oleszczuk AK: The paradox of old maternal age in multiple pregnancies. Obstet Gynecol Clin North Am 2005; 32: 69, ix

161. Holcroft CJ, Blakemore KJ, Allen M, Graham EM: Association of prematurity and neonatal infection with neurologic morbidity in very low birth weight infants. Obstet Gynecol 2003; 101: 1249

162. Krauer B, Krauer F, Hytten F: Drug prescribing in pregnancy. Edinburgh, Churchill Livingstone, 1984

163. ACOG committee opinion number 304, November 2004. Prenatal and perinatal human immunodeficiency virus testing: expanded recommendations. Obstet Gynecol 2004; 104: 1119

164. Hughes SC: HIV and pregnancy: twenty-five years into the epidemic. Int Anesthesiol Clin 2007; 45: 29

165. Evron S, Glezerman M, Harow E, et al: Human immunodeficiency virus: anesthetic and obstetric considerations. Anesth Analg 2004; 98: 503

166. Tom DJ, Gulevich SJ, Shapiro HM, et al: Epidural blood patch in the HIV-positive patient. Review of clinical experience. San Diego HIV Neurobehavioral Research Center. Anesthesiology 1992; 76: 943

167. Birnbach DJ, Stein DJ: The substance-abusing parturient: implications for analgesia and anaesthesia management. Baillieres Clin Obstet Gynaecol 1998; 12: 443

168. ACOG Practice Bulletin. Clinical Management Guidelines for Obstetrician-Gynecologists. Number 62, May 2005. Intrapartum fetal heart rate monitoring. Obstet Gynecol 2005; 105: 1161

169. Parer JT: Efficacy and safety of intrapartum electronic fetal monitoring: an update. Obstet Gynecol 1996; 87: 476

170. Freeman RK: Problems with intrapartum fetal heart rate monitoring interpretation and patient management. Obstet Gynecol 2002; 100: 813

171. Bloom SL, Spong CY, Thom E, et al: Fetal pulse oximetry and Cesarean delivery. N Engl J Med 2006; 355: 2195

172. Garite TJ, Dildy GA, McNamara H, et al: A multicenter controlled trial of fetal pulse oximetry in the intrapartum management of nonreassuring fetal heart rate patterns. Am J Obstet Gynecol 2000; 183: 1049

173. ACOG Committee Opinion. Number 258, September 2001. Fetal pulse oximetry. Obstet Gynecol 2001; 98: 523

174. 2005 American Heart Association (AHA) guidelines for cardiopulmonary resuscitation (CPR) and emergency cardiovascular care (ECC) of pediatric and neonatal patients: neonatal resuscitation guidelines. Pediatrics 2006; 117: e1029

175. Dawes GS: Foetal and Neonatal Physiology: A Comparative Study of the Changes at Birth. Chicago, Year Book Medical, 1968

176. Adamsons K, Jr., Behrman R, Dawes GS, et al: Resuscitation by positive pressure ventilation and tris-hydroxymethylaminomethane of rhesus monkeys asphyxiated at birth. J Pediatr 1964; 65: 807

177. Carlton DP: Transitional changes in the newborn infant around the time of birth, Rudolph's Pediatrics. Edited by Bland RD. New York, McGraw-Hill, 2003

178. Bouchard S, Johnson MP, Flake AW, et al: The EXIT procedure: experience and outcome in 31 cases. J Pediatr Surg 2002; 37: 418

179. MacKenzie TC, Crombleholme TM, Flake AW: The ex-utero intrapartum treatment. Curr Opin Pediatr 2002; 14: 453

180. Rosen MA, Andreae MH, Cameron AG: Nitroglycerin for fetal surgery: fetoscopy and ex utero intrapartum treatment procedure with malignant hyperthermia precautions. Anesth Analg 2003; 96: 698

181. Gaiser RR, Cheek TG, Kurth CD: Anesthetic management of Cesarean delivery complicated by ex utero intrapartum treatment of the fetus. Anesth Analg 1997; 84: 1150

182. Safra MJ, Oakley GP, Jr.: Association between cleft lip with or without cleft palate and prenatal exposure to diazepam. Lancet 1975; 2: 478

183. Smith BE, Gaub ML, Moya F: Teratogenic effects of anesthetic agents: nitrous oxide. Anesth Analg 1965; 44: 726

184. Duncan PG, Pope WD, Cohen MM, Greer N: Fetal risk of anesthesia and surgery during pregnancy. Anesthesiology 1986; 64: 790

185. Mazze RI, Kallen B: Reproductive outcome after anesthesia and operation during pregnancy: a registry study of 5405 cases. American Journal of Obstetrics & Gynecology 1989; 161: 1178

186. ACOG Committee Opinion Number 284, August 2003: Nonobstetric surgery in pregnancy. Obstet Gynecol 2003; 102: 431

CHAPTER 44 ■ NEONATAL ANESTHESIA

STEVEN C. HALL AND SANTHANAM SURESH

KEY POINTS

1. Understanding the physiologic changes that occur during the transition from fetal to neonatal life is crucial to the anesthetic management of the neonate. The circulatory, pulmonary, hepatic, and renal systems are all affected in this process.

2. Important physiologic and anatomic factors account for the rapid rate of desaturation observed in neonates. These include an increase in oxygen consumption, a high closing volume, a high ratio of minute ventilation to functional residual capacity, and a pliable rib cage.

3. Persistent pulmonary hypertension of the newborn is a pathologic condition that can be primary but is often secondary to other conditions, including meconium aspiration, sepsis, congenital diaphragmatic hernia, or pneumonia. Understanding the pathophysiologic characteristics of this condition helps guide therapy.

4. Knowledge of the major anatomic differences between the infant and adult airway helps one understand why the infant's airway is often described as "anterior" and why airway management may be challenging. These differences include a relatively large tongue, a higher glottis with anterior slanting vocal folds, a larger occiput, and a narrowing at the cricoid ring.

5. Careful attention must be given to the choice of anesthetic agents and dosing of such agents in the neonatal popula-

tion. Ongoing maturational changes in the renal and hepatobiliary systems, which occur during the first 30 days of life, will affect the metabolism and elimination of many anesthetic agents.

6. Although a host of anesthetic techniques are available, including regional anesthesia, multiple factors are considered when choosing an anesthetic plan for the neonate. These include the surgical requirements, the need for postoperative ventilation, the cardiovascular stability of the neonate, and the anticipated method of postoperative pain control.

7. Special considerations must be addressed when planning an anesthetic for a neonate. Some of the controversial issues include the risk of postoperative apnea and the use of caffeine in treatment and prophylaxis, the role of oxygen concentration in the development of retinopathy of prematurity, and the neurodevelopmental effects of anesthetic agents on the fetal and neonatal brain.

8. True surgical emergencies are uncommon in the neonatal period. Knowledge of conditions with comorbidities, such as tracheoesophageal fistula, omphalocele, and congenital diaphragmatic hernia, and a thorough preoperative evaluation and stabilization of such neonates cannot be overemphasized.

PHYSIOLOGY OF THE INFANT AND THE TRANSITION PERIOD

An infant's first year of life is characterized by an almost miraculous growth in size and maturity. The body weight alone changes by a factor of three, and there is no other period in extrauterine life when changes occur so rapidly. Before birth, fetal growth and development depend on the genetic composition of the fetus, the mother's placental function, and potential exposure to chemicals or infectious agents that can affect mother, fetus, or both. After birth, the newborn must rapidly adjust to the extrauterine environment to survive. The dramatic changes in functions of several systems will determine the viability of the neonate, as well as its ability to grow and develop properly.

The newborn period has been defined as the first 24 hours of life, and the neonatal period as the first month. There is significant change in many physiologic systems during both of these periods. The first 72 hours are especially significant for the cardiovascular, pulmonary, and renal systems. The changes in these systems are interrelated; inadequate progression of change or a disease state altering one of these systems can quickly alter the maturation of one or more of the other systems. Understanding the differences in these systems from the older child, as well as the changes that occur in the neonatal period, is important in developing a comprehensive anesthetic approach.

The Cardiovascular System

Fetal Circulation

The fetal circulation is characterized by a parallel system in which both ventricles pump most of their output into the systemic circulation. Less than 10% of the combined cardiac output goes through the fetal pulmonary circulation via three main shunts through the placenta, foramen ovale, and ductus arteriosus (Fig. 44-1A). The placenta provides oxygenated blood into the ductus venosus, the inferior vena cava, and then into the right atrium. In the right atrium, the majority of the oxygenated blood primarily flows through the foramen ovale into the left atrium, bypassing the right ventricle and the pulmonary vascular bed. This preferential flow across the foramen occurs because of the relatively low pressure in the left atrium compared with that of the right atrium. Some blood from the right atrium does flow through the right ventricle and into the main pulmonary artery. The pulmonary vascular resistance is quite high in utero because of alveolar collapse and compression of blood vessels, inhibiting flow through the pulmonary circulation. The pulmonary vascular resistance is also high at this point because of the relatively low P_aO_2 and pH of the blood that does flow through the vessels. Some blood in the pulmonary artery does flow through the pulmonary circulation and then into the left atrium, but the majority of flow goes through the ductus arteriosus into the descending aorta.

Changes at Birth. After birth, all of these shunts are eliminated or start to close quickly.[1] The placental shunt is eliminated and the ductus venosus is closed. The newborn's left ventricle is now pumping blood into the higher pressure systemic circulation exclusively. Expansion of the lungs and initiation of

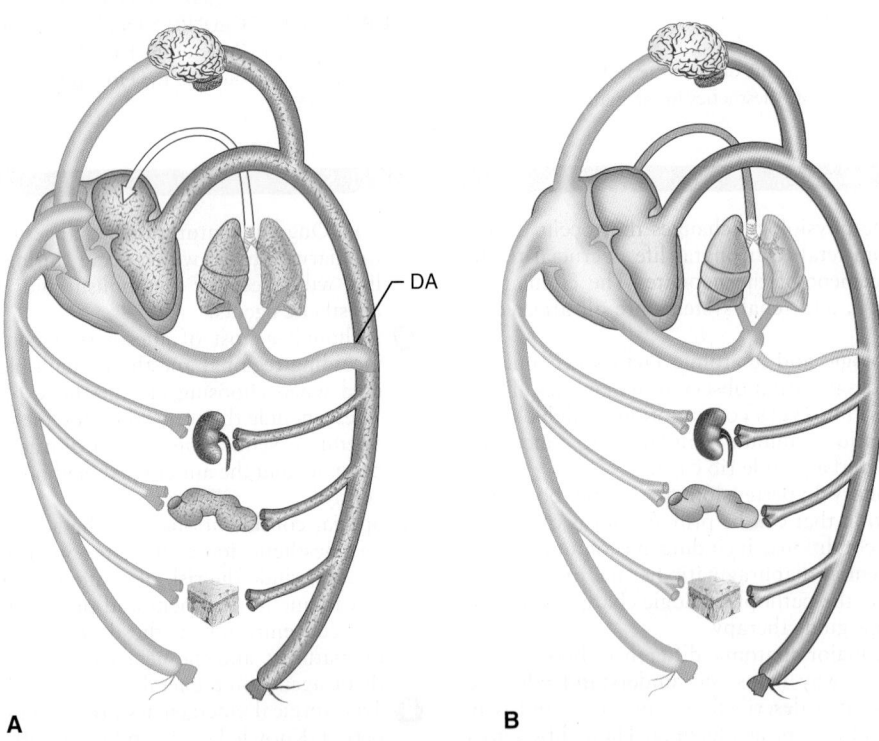

A   **B**

FIGURE 44-1.   **A.** Schematic representation of the fetal circulation. Oxygenated blood leaves the placenta in the umbilical vein (*vessel without stippling*). Umbilical vein blood joins blood from the viscera (represented here by the kidney, gut, and skin) in the inferior vena cava. Approximately half of the inferior vena cava flow passes through the foramen ovale to the left atrium, where it mixes with a small amount of pulmonary venous blood, and this relatively well-oxygenated blood (*light stippling*) supplies the heart and brain by way of the ascending aorta. The other half of the inferior vena cava stream mixes with superior vena cava blood and enters the right ventricle (blood in the right atrium and ventricle has little oxygen, which is denoted by *heavy stippling*). Because the pulmonary arterioles are constricted, most of the blood in the main pulmonary artery flows through the ductus arteriosus (DA) so the descending aorta's blood has less oxygen (*heavy stippling*) than does blood in the ascending aorta (*light stippling*). **B.** Schematic representation of the circulation in the normal newborn. After expansion of the lungs and ligation of the umbilical cord, pulmonary blood flow and left atrial and systemic arterial pressures increase. When left atrial pressure exceeds right atrial pressure, the foramen ovale closes so all inferior and superior vena cava blood leaves the right atrium, enters the right ventricle, and is pumped through the pulmonary artery toward the lung. With the increase in systemic arterial pressure and decrease in pulmonary artery pressure, flow through the ductus arteriosus becomes left to right, and the ductus constricts and closes. The course of circulation is the same as in the adult. (Reprinted from Phibbs R: Delivery room management of the newborn, Neonatology, Pathophysiology and Management of the Newborn. Edited by Avery GB. Philadelphia, JB Lippincott, 1981, p 184, with permission.)

breathing lead to dramatic changes in both the circulatory and pulmonary systems (Fig. 44-1B). As alveoli fill with air, the compression of the pulmonary alveolar capillaries is relieved, reducing pulmonary vascular resistance and promoting flow through the pulmonary circulation. This blood is now oxygenated, raising the arterial PO_2 and further reducing pulmonary vascular resistance. Although the change in the first minutes to hours is dramatic, it usually takes 3 to 4 days for the pulmonary vascular resistance to decrease to normal levels. The foramen ovale will usually functionally close in the first hour of life as the increase in left atrial pressure from increased pulmonary circulation after the initiation of breathing exceeds right atrial pressure. The foramen is closed by a flap of tissue that covers the foramen. This foramen can reopen if there is a relative increase in right atrial pressure, such as is seen with elevated pulmonary vascular resistance or fluid overload. Anatomic closure usually occurs in the first year of life, but may remain probe-patent into adulthood in 10 to 20% of patients. The ductus arteriosus starts to close in the first day of life and is usually functionally closed in the second day of life. In utero, patency of the ductus was determined by the combined relaxant effects of low oxygen tension and endogenously produced prostaglandins, especially prostaglandin E_2. In a full-term neonate, oxygen is the most important factor controlling ductal closure. When the P_aO_2 of blood in the ductus rises to about 50 mm Hg, the muscle in the vessel constricts. It should be noted that the ductus of a preterm infant is less responsive to increased oxygen, even though its musculature is developed.

Myocardial function is different in the neonate. The neonatal cardiac myocyte has less organized contractile elements than the child or adult.[2] Not only are there fewer myofibril elements, but they are not organized in parallel roles, as seen in the child and adult heart, making them less efficient. The neonate myocyte also has a less mature sarcoplasmic reticulum system. The underdeveloped sarcoplasmic reticulum is associated with a decrease in Ca^{2+}-adenosine triphosphatase activity, an important component of contractility. As the sarcoplasmic reticulum matures, the efficiency of calcium transport and subsequent contractility increases.[3] The neonatal myocardium cannot generate as much force as that of the older child and is relatively noncompliant. Consequently, there is limited functional reserve in the neonatal period, with afterload increases particularly poorly tolerated. After birth, there are dramatic changes in the myocardium. As the work of the ventricles increases secondary to high stroke volume and increased vascular resistance, these myocytes grow quickly in number and size. This growth is more dramatic in the left ventricle than the right ventricle because of the rise in systemic vascular resistance and fall in pulmonary vascular resistance, respectively.

Especially in the first 3 months of life, the parasympathetic nervous system influence on the heart is more mature than the sympathetic system and the myocardium does not respond to inotropic support as well as the older child or adult. There is animal evidence that there are maturational changes in β-adrenergic receptor function that explain the decreased responsiveness to inotropes in the neonate.[4] The neonatal myocardium does have increased glycogen stores and higher rates of anaerobic glycolysis, which may explain its relative resistance to hypoxia and better performance in the presence of an ischemic insult. Because the myocardium is relatively noncompliant in the newborn, preload changes can increase stroke volume and cardiac output, but not as effectively as in the older child.[5] In other words, the Frank-Starling relationship is present in the neonatal heart, but is not as effective as in the adult. The other clinical implication of a noncompliant ventricle is that, in the absence of significant increases in stroke volume, cardiac output is not well maintained in the presence of bradycardia. Lastly, neonates have immature baroreceptors.

The baroreceptor is responsible for the reflex tachycardia that occurs in response to hypotension. Therefore, the immaturity of this reflex would limit the neonate's ability to compensate for hypotension. In addition, the baroresponse of the neonate is more depressed than that of the adult at the same level of anesthesia.

In summary, the neonatal heart has some significant limitations. The resting cardiac output is much higher relative to body weight than in the adult because of the higher O_2 consumption per kilogram of body weight. Stimulation of the myocardium produces a limited increase in contractility and cardiac output. The sympathetic nervous system, which usually provides the important chronotropic and inotropic support to the mature circulation during stress, is severely limited in the neonate because of lack of development. Even in the absence of stress, the neonatal heart has limited ability to increase cardiac output compared with the mature heart (Fig. 44-2). The resting cardiac output of the immature heart is close to the maximal cardiac output, so there is a limited reserve. The mature heart can increase cardiac output by 300%, whereas the immature heart can only increase cardiac output by 30 to 40%.

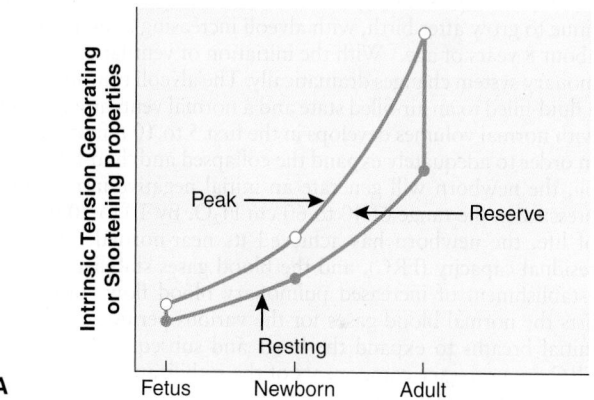

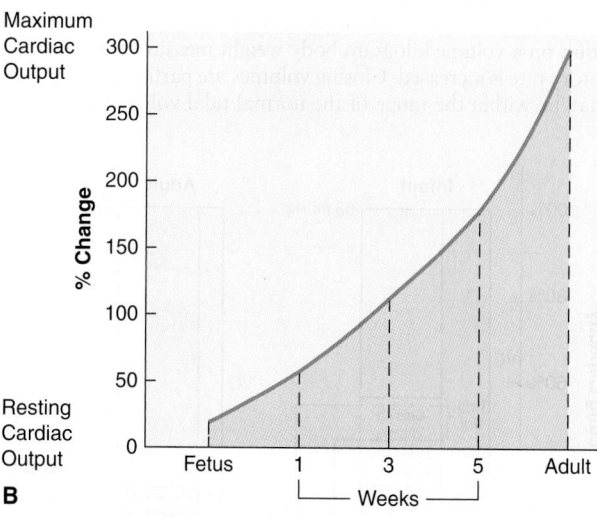

FIGURE 44-2.   Schema of reduced cardiac reserve in fetal and newborn animal hearts compared with adult hearts. A. In the newborn infant, resting cardiac muscle performance is close to a peak of ventricular function because of limitations in diastolic, systolic, and heart rate reserve. B. Similarly, pump reserve early in life is limited by these factors and by much higher resting cardiac output relative to body weight, compared with that in adults. (Reprinted from Friedman WF, George BL: Treatment of congestive heart failure by altering loading conditions of the heart. J Pediatr 1985; 106: 700, with permission.)

TABLE 44-1

NORMAL BLOOD GAS VALUES IN THE NEONATE

■ SUBJECT	■ AGE	■ PO_2 (mm Hg)	■ PCO_2 (mm Hg)	■ pH
Fetus (term)	Before labor	25	40	7.37
Fetus (term)	End of labor	10–20	55	7.25
Newborn (term)	10 min	50	48	7.20
Newborn (term)	1 hr	70	35	7.35
Newborn (term)	1 wk	75	35	7.40
Newborn (preterm, 1,500 g)	1 wk	60	38	7.37

The Pulmonary System

❷ The pulmonary system develops rapidly during the last trimester, with important changes in both the number of alveoli and the maturity of the pulmonary vascular system.[6] These systems have not matured enough to provide adequate gas exchange until about 24 to 26 weeks' gestation. The airways and alveoli continue to grow after birth, with alveoli increasing in number until about 8 years of age.[7] With the initiation of ventilation, the pulmonary system changes dramatically. The alveoli transition from a fluid-filled to an air-filled state and a normal ventilatory pattern with normal volumes develops in the first 5 to 10 minutes of life. In order to adequately expand the collapsed and fluid-filled alveoli, the newborn will generate an initial negative intrathoracic pressure in the range of 40 to 60 cm H_2O. By 10 to 20 minutes of life, the newborn has achieved its near-normal functional residual capacity (FRC), and the blood gases stabilize with the establishment of increased pulmonary blood flow. Table 44-1 lists the normal blood gases for the various periods of life. The initial breaths to expand the lungs and subsequently maintain FRC are necessary components of the stabilization of the ventilatory system, as well as the circulatory system. Failure to do so will quickly lead to deterioration of both systems.

Tidal volume is about the same in the neonate as the child or adult on a volume/kilogram body weight measure, but the respiratory rate is increased. Closing volumes are particularly high and may be within the range of the normal tidal volume (Fig. 44-3).

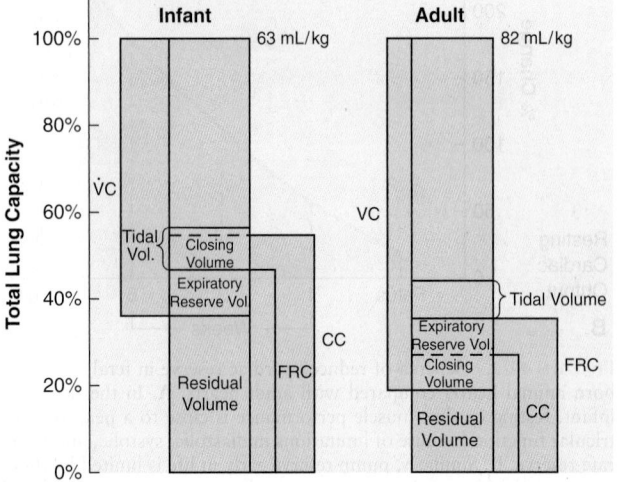

FIGURE 44-3. Static lung volumes of infants and adults. (Reprinted from Smith CA, Nelson NM: Physiology of the Newborn Infant, 4th edition. Springfield, IL, Charles C Thomas, 1976, p 207, with permission.)

TABLE 44-2

COMPARISON OF NORMAL RESPIRATORY VALUES IN INFANTS AND ADULTS

■ PARAMETER	■ INFANT	■ ADULT
Respiratory frequency (breaths/min)	30–50	12–16
Tidal volume (mL/kg)	7	7
Dead space (mL/kg)	2–2.5	2.2
Alveolar ventilation (mL/kg/min)	100–150	60
Functional residual capacity (mL/kg)	27–30	30
Oxygen consumption (mL/kg/min)	7–9	3

This increased minute ventilation mirrors the higher oxygen consumption in neonates, which is about double that seen in an adult. Because the FRC in the newborn is comparable to that of the older child or adult, but the minute ventilation is much higher, the ratio of minute ventilation to FRC is 2 to 3 times higher in the newborn. The clinical significance of this ratio is twofold. First, anesthetic induction with a volatile anesthetic agent should be faster, as should emergence. Second, the decrease in FRC relative to minute ventilation and oxygen consumption means that there is less "oxygen reserve" in the FRC compared to that of older children and adults. There will be a more rapid drop in arterial oxygen levels in the newborn in the presence of apnea or hypoventilation. Table 44-2 compares normal respiratory parameters in the normal newborn and adult.

Lung compliance is relatively low, but chest wall compliance is relatively high, compared to that of older children. The pliable rib cage gives less mechanical support than in the older child, leading to significant retractions with less efficient gas exchange and functional airway closure, thus increasing the work of breathing. The intercostal muscles are poorly developed at birth, with the diaphragm providing most of the gas exchange. The diaphragm in the neonate has two types of fibers, the type 1, slow twitch, high-oxidative fibers that give sustained contraction with very little fatigue, and the type 2, fast twitch, low-oxidative fibers that give quick contractions, but fatigue easily. The distribution of these fibers in the newborn shows only about 25% type 1 fibers, while 55% of the fibers are type 1 in the mature diaphragm at about 2 years of age. The preterm newborn has even fewer type 1 fibers at birth, in the 10% range. This relative lack of type 1 fibers means that the newborn, especially the preterm, is at risk for diaphragmatic fatigue in the presence of significant resistance to ventilation or periods of hyperventilation.

Lastly, the continued presence of surfactant is necessary to maintain both the distensibility of the alveoli and the maintenance of an FRC at exhalation. Decreased surfactant production, due to prematurity or other conditions such as maternal diabetes, can cause respiratory distress syndrome (RDS). The decreased surfactant can cause alveolar collapse, decrease in lung compliance, hypoxia, increased work of breathing, and respiratory failure.[8] Commercially available surfactant is extraordinarily useful to both treat and prevent RDS in susceptible patients. In addition, surfactant can improve gas exchange in preterms who may not have RDS, but are stressed by sepsis, heart failure, or other systemic problems.[9] Delivered through an endotracheal tube, it can be used prophylactically in the very preterm newborn to prevent RDS, as well as treat newborns who have developed RDS.

In addition to the mechanical aspects of the pulmonary system, control of breathing has unique aspects in the neonatal

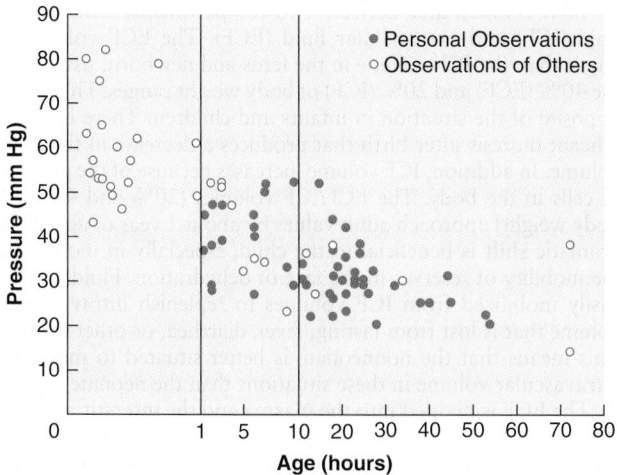

FIGURE 44-4. Correlation of mean pulmonary arterial pressure with age in 85 normal-term infants studied during the first 3 days of life. (Reprinted from Emmanouilides GC, Moss AJ, Duffie ER et al: Pulmonary arterial pressure changes in human newborn infants from birth to 3 days of age. J Pediatr 1964; 65: 327, with permission.)

period, especially in the preterm. Neonates respond less to hypercapnia than the older child. In addition, neonates respond to hypoxia with a brief period of hyperventilation, followed by hypoventilation. The initial hyperventilatory response can be prevented by hypothermia. Lastly, a periodic breathing pattern is common in neonates, especially in preterm newborns, that can persist up to a year of age.

Persistent Pulmonary Hypertension of the Newborn

3 The pulmonary circulation is known to be extremely sensitive to oxygen, pH, and nitric oxide, as well a variety of mediators such as adenosine and prostaglandins and mechanical factors such as lung inflation. Figure 44-4 illustrates the correlation of the mean pulmonary artery pressure with age during the first 3 days of life. Hypoxia and acidosis, along with inflammatory mediators, may cause pulmonary artery pressure either to persist at a high level or, after initially decreasing, to increase to pathologic levels. The result is termed *persistent pulmonary hypertension of the newborn*, sometimes referred to as *persistent fetal circulation*. Persistent pulmonary hypertension of the newborn occurs in term and preterm infants, usually caused by precipitating conditions such severe birth asphyxia, meconium aspiration, sepsis, congenital diaphragmatic hernia, and maternal use of nonsteroidal anti-inflammatory drugs with in utero constriction of the ductus arteriosus, although it is often idiopathic. Other risk factors include maternal diabetes or asthma, as well as cesarean delivery.[10] The elevated pulmonary vascular resistance causes both the ductus arteriosus and foramen ovale to remain open, with subsequent right-to-left (bypassing the pulmonary circulation) shunting. These changes result in profound hypoxia from right-to-left shunting and a normal or elevated P_aCO_2. The hypoxemia is often noted to be out of proportion to the other presenting signs of respiratory and cardiovascular compromise. Treatment starts with correcting any predisposing disease (hypoglycemia, polycythemia) and improving poor tissue oxygenation. The response to therapy is often unpredictable. However, the goals are to achieve a PaO_2 of 50 to 70 mm Hg and a P_aCO_2 of 50 to 55 mm Hg. In addition to standard mechanical ventilation, high-frequency ventilation, exogenous surfactant, inhaled nitric oxide, alkalinization, and extracorporeal membrane oxygenation have been used with varying degrees of success. Experimental therapy

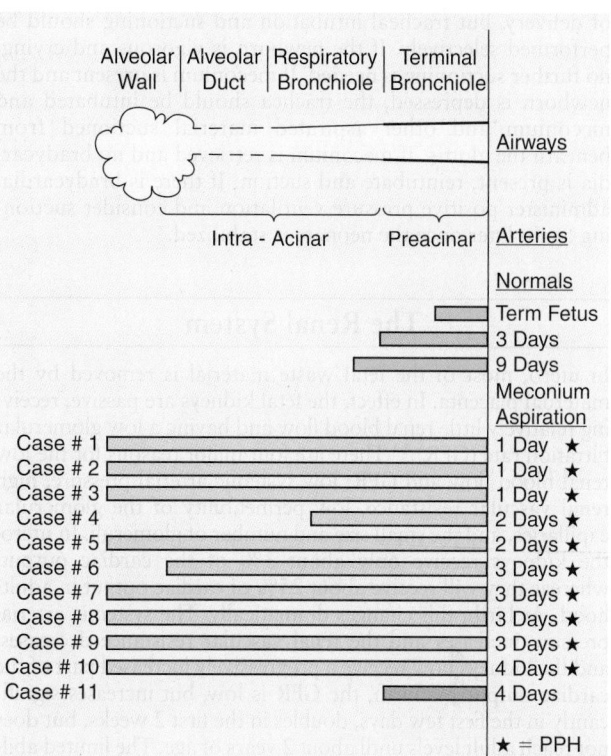

FIGURE 44-5. Diagram of muscle extension along pulmonary arterial branches (*shaded bars*). In the normal newborn, virtually no intra-acinar artery is muscular. In 9 of 10 infants with meconium aspiration and persistent pulmonary hypertension (PPH), muscle extended into the most peripheral arteries; the infant with meconium aspiration without PPH (case 11) had normal intra-acinar arteries. (Reprinted from Murphy JD, Vawter GF, Reid LM: Pulmonary vascular disease in fetal meconium aspiration. J Pediatr 1984; 104: 758, with permission.)

with other agents such as sildenafil continue to be evaluated.[11] Success in treatment and survival varies directly with the underlying cause. Significant prognostic factors are the ability of therapy to reduce pulmonary vascular resistance and associated complications, such as ischemic encephalopathy.

Meconium Aspiration

Another important pulmonary issue in the newborn period is *meconium aspiration*. Interference with the normal maternal placental circulation in the third trimester may cause fetal hypoxia. Fetal hypoxia can result in an increase in the amount of muscle in the blood vessels of the distal respiratory units. Figure 44-5 illustrates the muscle increase found in blood vessels of a series of 11 infants who died of persistent pulmonary hypertension.[12] Chronic fetal hypoxia leads to the passage of meconium in utero. The fetus breathes in utero so the meconium mixed with amniotic fluid enters the pulmonary system. Meconium aspiration can be a marker of chronic fetal hypoxia in the third trimester. This condition is different from the meconium aspiration that occurs during delivery. This meconium at birth is thick and tenacious, and mechanically obstructs the tracheobronchial system. Meconium aspiration syndrome leads to varying degrees of respiratory failure, which can be fatal in spite of all treatment modalities.

Current recommendations for intubation and suctioning for newborns at delivery with frank meconium aspiration or meconium staining (approximately 10% of newborns) emphasize a conservative approach.[13] Routine oropharyngeal suctioning of meconium is recommended immediately at the time of delivery, but tracheal intubation and suctioning should be performed selectively. If the newborn is vigorous and crying, no further suctioning is needed. If meconium is present and the newborn is depressed, the trachea should be intubated and meconium and other aspirated material suctioned from beneath the glottis. If meconium is retrieved and no bradycardia is present, reintubate and suction. If there is bradycardia, administer positive pressure ventilation and consider suctioning again later once the neonate is stabilized.

The Renal System

In utero, most of the fetal waste material is removed by the maternal placenta. In effect, the fetal kidneys are passive, receiving relatively little renal blood flow and having a low glomerular filtration rate (GFR).[14] There are four major reasons for the low renal blood flow and GFR: low systemic arterial pressure, high renal vascular resistance, low permeability of the glomerular capillaries, and the small size and number of glomeruli. In utero, the kidneys receive only about 3% of the cardiac output, whereas they will receive about 25% of cardiac output in adulthood. At birth, this changes dramatically. The systemic arterial pressure increases and the renal vascular resistance decreases, and the kidneys now receive a progressively increased part of the cardiac output. At birth, the GFR is low, but increases significantly in the first few days, doubles in the first 2 weeks, but does not reach adult levels until about 2 years of age. The limited ability of the newborn's kidney to concentrate or dilute urine results from this low GFR and decreased tubular function. However, during the first 3 to 4 days, the circulatory changes increase renal blood flow and GFR and improve the neonate's ability to concentrate and dilute the urine. Part of the improvement in renal function is the establishment of gradients in the medullary interstitium that promotes resorption of sodium. The maturation continues, and by the time the normal full-term infant is 1 month of age, the kidneys are approximately 60% mature. Urine output is low in the first 24 hours, but then increases to an expected level of at least 1 to 2 mL/kg/hr. Diuresis after the first day of life <1 mL/kg/hr should be considered indicative of either hypovolemia or decreased renal function for another reason.

Despite the rapid maturation of renal function and the increased capacity of the neonatal kidneys, they still have limitations.[15] From an anesthetic standpoint, the half-life of medications excreted by means of glomerular filtration will be prolonged.[16] The relative inability to conserve water means that neonates, especially in the first week of life, tolerate fluid restriction poorly. In addition, the inability to excrete large amounts of water means the newborn tolerates fluid overload poorly. The newborn kidney is better able to conserve sodium than excrete sodium, making hypernatremia a risk if excess sodium is administered. However, because of the lack of tonicity in the medullary interstitium shortly after birth, there will be some obligate sodium loss in the first days of life. This improves as the countercurrent multiplier is developed in the interstitium.

Fluid and Electrolyte Therapy in the Neonate

Total body water (TBW), which is usually described in terms of percent of body weight, varies by both age and gestational status. The highest TBW is found in the fetus, but decreases to about 75% of body weight for a term infant at birth. Preterm infants have a higher TBW than term infants, often in the 80 to 85% range. TBW decreases during the first 12 months of life to about 60 to 65% of body weight and stays at this level through childhood.

TBW is distributed between two compartments, intracellular fluid (ICF) and extracellular fluid (ECF). The ECF volume is larger than the ICF volume in the fetus and newborn, usually in the 40% (ECF) and 20% (ICF) of body weight ranges. This is the opposite of the situation in infants and children. There is a significant diuresis after birth that produces a decrease in the ECF volume. In addition, ICF volume increases because of the growth of cells in the body. The ECF/ICF volumes (20% and 40% of body weight) approach adult values by about 1 year of age. This dramatic shift is beneficial to the child, especially in increasing the mobility of reserves in the face of dehydration. Fluid can be easily mobilized from ICF volumes to replenish intravascular volume that is lost from fasting, fever, diarrhea, or other causes. This means that the nonneonate is better situated to maintain intravascular volume in these situations than the neonate.

The ECF is divided into the plasma and the interstitial fluid. The plasma water is usually about 5% of body weight and the related blood volume, assuming a hematocrit of 45%, is about 8% of body weight in infants and children. The water content is slightly higher in neonates and may approach 10% of body weight in preterms. The interstitial fluid, usually about 15% of body weight, can demonstrate large increases in disease states associated with liver failure, heart failure, renal failure, and other causes of conditions such as pleural effusions or ascites. The reason for this is the balance between oncotic and hydrostatic forces. Any condition that decreases oncotic pressure, such as loss of albumin in liver failure, promotes the loss of fluid into the interstitial fluid. On the other hand, raised hydrostatic pressures, such as seen in heart failure, can result in fluid leaving the plasma and accumulating in the interstitial space. Conditions that result in translocation of fluid from the plasma to the interstitial spaces, whether because of decreased oncotic pressure or increased oncotic pressure, are of significant consequence to the neonate. Loss of fluid from the plasma volume compromises the intravascular volume, potentially decreasing the perfusion of vital organs and systems.

The blood volume in the normal full-term newborn is approximately 85 mL/kg and approximately 90 to 100 mL/kg in the preterm, although estimates of these volumes can vary between studies. Approximately 50 mL/kg of this volume is the plasma volume. For all practical purposes, the electrolyte values in the neonatal period are the same as in the child and adult with the exception of potassium, which can be about 1 to 2 mmol/L higher than average for the first 2 days of life.[17]

Maintenance fluid requirements increase during the first days of life. They have been estimated to be 60, 80, 100, and 120 mL/kg/24 hr for the first 4 days of life, respectively. For the rest of the neonatal period, a maintenance rate of 150 mL/kg/24 hr is appropriate.

The appropriate type of maintenance fluid depends on several issues. Because of ongoing sodium loss secondary to the inability of the neonatal distal tubule to respond fully to aldosterone, intravenous fluids in the neonate must contain some sodium. Most operations on neonates involve loss of blood and extracellular fluid, which must be replaced with a fluid of similar electrolyte content (i.e., a balanced salt solution such as lactated Ringer or Plasma-Lyte). Hypotonic solutions should not be used to replace these losses because they can cause significant hyponatremia. Consequently, should a mixture of balanced salt solution and maintenance fluid be given during a surgical procedure? If the neonate is already stable on a maintenance solution, it is reasonable to continue this maintenance at a constant rate, adding balanced salt solution or colloid or blood products as needed.

The other issues for fluid choice in the neonate center on appropriate glucose administration. In most cases, maintenance fluids containing 10% glucose and 0.2 normal saline with 20 mmol/L of potassium are reasonable in the first 48 hours of life. Beyond that time period, full-term infants may do well with 5% glucose instead of 10%, although preterms will often require the higher glucose load longer. Newborns of diabetic mothers, those who are small for gestational age, and those who have had continuous glucose infusions stopped have particular problems with hypoglycemia. These infants need to have their blood glucose values monitored. Neonates who are scheduled for surgery and have been receiving hyperalimentation fluids or supplementary glucose must continue to receive that fluid during surgery or must have their glucose levels monitored because of concerns of hypoglycemia. There is little consensus on the issue of what constitutes hypoglycemia.[18]

The concern about hypoglycemia must be balanced against the potential augmentation of ischemic injury by the administration of glucose leading to hyperglycemia. Interestingly, there are observational reports examining neonates undergoing cardiac surgery in which high glucose concentrations during or after the surgery were not associated with worse neurodevelopmental outcomes.[19,20] These studies support the contention that avoiding hypoglycemia may be preferable to restricting glucose in newborns and risking hypoglycemia, at least in those having cardiac surgery.

Blood Component Therapy in the Neonate

Most of the basic principles of blood component therapy are the same in newborns and older children and adults. The first principle is to ensure adequate circulating intravascular volume and add components, as needed. However, there are a few important differences. These differences are related to the interconnection of maternal and fetal blood circulations and the flow of some, but not all elements, across the placenta, the incompletely developed immune system of the neonate, and the small blood volume of the neonate. The indications in the perioperative period for red blood cells are similar to those for adults, but the target values in available guidelines are higher.[21] Transfusion is indicated for a hemoglobin <10 g/dL for major surgery or in a newborn with moderate cardiopulmonary disease, while transfusion for a hemoglobin <13 g/dL is indicated in a newborn with severe cardiopulmonary disease. It is also recommended that platelets be kept above 50,000 for invasive procedures. These recommendations are based on expert consensus, not prospective studies.

The hemoglobin in transfused blood is hemoglobin A, as opposed to the hemoglobin F in the neonate at birth. An advantage of the transfused blood is better release of oxygen at the tissue level from hemoglobin A. Fresh blood cells have the advantage of lower potassium levels, especially during rapid transfusion, than older blood, although washed or frozen cells prevent this problem. Transfusion-associated graft-versus-host disease is a rare but potentially deadly complication of red blood cell transfusion. Transfused lymphocytes in the donor blood attack the recipient bone marrow and other tissues, causing fever, pancytopenia, diarrhea, and hepatitis. To prevent this, gamma irradiation of cellular blood components is used to destroy lymphocytes and prevent transfusion-associated graft-versus-host disease. For this reason, irradiated blood is routinely used for transfusion of preterm newborns and, in many centers, for all newborns under 6 months of age. Leukoreduction by filtration is also used to reduce cytomegalic virus transmission. Lastly, because there is very weak expression of the ABO antigens at birth, ABO typing, Rh typing, and an initial antibody screen are commonly done, although cross-matching is not.

The Hepatic System

The functional capacity of the liver is immature in the newborn, especially synthetic and metabolic functions. Although most enzyme systems for both normal function and drug metabolism are present at birth, the systems have not yet been induced.[22] In utero, the maternal circulation and metabolism were responsible for the majority of elimination of drugs. As the newborn develops, the different hepatic metabolic pathways mature at different rates. Conjugation by sulfation and acetylation are relatively well developed in the newborn, with conjugation with glutathione and glucuronidation less well-developed.[23] Some of these pathways do not achieve adult levels of activity until after 1 year of age.[24,25] Because of this immaturity, some drugs that undergo hepatic biotransformation, like morphine, have prolonged elimination half-lives in newborns.[26] Other drugs, such as lidocaine, do not undergo prolonged elimination in the newborn. In some drugs, such as caffeine, the lack of hepatic metabolism of the drug is balanced by excretion of an increased amount of unchanged drug through the kidney. Up to 85% of unmetabolized caffeine may be found in the urine in the newborn, compared with 1% in the adult.[27]

Lastly, decreased metabolism of a drug may actually increase its safety profile. Acetaminophen undergoes less biotransformation by the cytochrome P450 system in the newborn, producing less reactive metabolites that are toxic. Paradoxically, neonates can tolerate dosages of acetaminophen that would be hepatotoxic in adults.[28,29] Synthetic function of the liver is also altered in the neonatal period. Levels of albumin and other proteins necessary for binding of drugs are low in term newborns (and are even lower in preterm infants) and impacts the ability to bind drugs, producing greater levels of free drug. This phenomenon is especially true for the binding of alkaline drugs that bind to alpha$_1$—acid glycoprotein, such as synthetic opioids and local anesthetics. The ability to bind to existing albumin may also be altered by hyperbilirubinemia for some medications. The need for exogenous vitamin K in the newborn is another consequence of this decrease ability. Because of decreased synthetic function, neonatal hepatic glycogen stores are low, especially in the preterm, increasing the risk of hypoglycemia in response to stress.

Anatomy of the Neonatal Airway

The anatomic and maturational factors unique to the neonatal airway are important to understand in order to effectively manage the airway (Fig. 44-6). Although previous thinking

Complicating Anatomic Factors in Infants

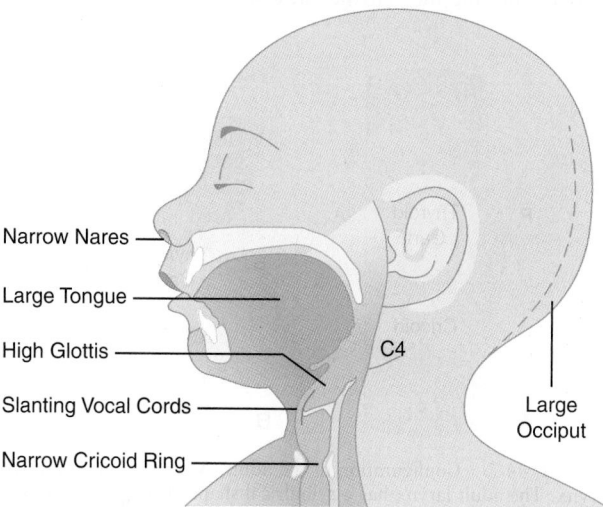

FIGURE 44-6. Complicating anatomic factors in infants. (Modified from Smith RM: Anesthesia for Infants and Children, 4th edition. St Louis, Mosby, 1980, p 16, with permission.)

suggested that all neonates, especially preterm babies, are *obligate* nasal breathers, the majority of neonates are actually *preferential* nose breathers.[30] Anything that obstructs the nares can compromise the neonate's ability to breathe.[31] For this reason, bilateral choanal atresia of the nasopharynx can be a life-threatening surgical problem for the neonate, and the airway needs to be secured or the atresia opened to ensure adequate ventilation. The large tongue occupies relatively more space in the infant's oropharynx, promoting both soft tissue obstruction of the upper airway and increasing the difficulty of laryngoscopic examination and intubation of the infant's trachea. In the normal adult, the glottis is at the level of C5-6. In the full-term infant, the glottis is at the level of C4, and in the premature infant, it is at the level of C3. The combination of a large tongue and a relatively high glottis means that on laryngoscopic examination it is more difficult to establish a line of vision between the mouth and larynx; there is relatively more tissue in less distance. Therefore, the infant's larynx appears to be "anterior", although the true description is cephalad. The epiglottis is omega- or tubular-shaped, with a stubby base and thick and bulky aryepiglottic folds, making it difficult to fix with laryngoscope blade. Because the tip of the epiglottis lies at C1, the close apposition with the soft palate allows the newborn to simultaneously suckle and breathe, and contributes to the preferential nasal breathing found in the neonate. The vocal cords are anterior-slanting, making visualization more difficult, but also occasionally providing some obstruction to the passage of the endotracheal tube. This phenomenon is especially true with either nasal or "blind" intubation attempts because the bevel of the blade may hang up in the anterior commissure of the angulated vocal cords instead of easily passing into the subglottic larynx.

The subglottic area is funnel-shaped, unlike the adult airway (Fig. 44-7). In adults, the narrowest aspect of the upper airway is at the vocal cords, but in the neonate there is further narrowing until the level of the cricoid ring, the first complete cartilaginous ring. Because this narrowing is susceptible to trauma from intubation or too large an endotracheal tube, uncuffed tubes have traditionally been used in the neonatal period, although cuffed tubes are increasingly popular beyond the first few months of life. A narrow cricoid ring is significant because it means that the narrowest portion of the neonate's airway is not the vocal cords but the cricoid ring.

Finally, the infant has a large occiput so the head flexes forward onto the chest when the infant is lying supine with its head in the midline. Further flexion of the neck can cause

obstruction. Extreme extension can also obstruct the airway, so a midposition of the head with slight extension is preferred for airway maintenance. Rarely, this may require placing a small roll at the base of the neck and shoulders.

Anesthetic Drugs in Neonates

The pharmacokinetics of drugs in neonates are different than in older children and adults. Factors affecting the metabolism of drugs in neonates include a larger volume of distribution, decreased protein binding, and decreased fat stores and immature renal and hepatic function. These physiological changes alter the amount of drugs used in neonates.

- Volume of distribution. Water is predominantly in greater proportion in premature and full-term infants,[32] which increases the need for larger doses of medications that are water-soluble.
- Protein binding. Neonates have decreased protein and hence have a decrease in protein binding of most drugs. This leads to increased free drug levels, which leads to increased toxicity of drugs that are predominantly protein-bound.[33]
- Fat content. Neonates have a decreased amount of fat and muscle mass, which leads to greater levels of drugs that are primarily redistributed to muscle and fat. Decreased renal and hepatic function predisposes neonates to increased blood levels from normal doses that are used for induction and maintenance of anesthesia.

Intravenous Agents

Anticholinergics. Anticholinergics like atropine and glycopyrrolate are used frequently in neonates. They may be helpful in decreasing secretions and decreasing the response to vagal stimulation on intubation. The dose of atropine is 10 μg/kg given intravenously and 20 μg/kg if given intramuscularly. It may be desirable intramuscularly in certain situations prior to induction of anesthesia, especially in emergency surgeries. Caution should be exercised if neonates have other associated congenital abnormalities, particularly narrow angle glaucoma in which case it could increase intraocular pressure. Glycopyrrolate, a synthetic quaternary ammonium compound, has a longer duration of action than atropine and may potentially have less central effects because of decreased penetration of the blood–brain barrier.

Midazolam. This is a water-soluble benzodiazepine that can be used for premedicating infants prior to surgery. Clearance of midazolam is lower in neonates and premature infants, and hence caution has to be exercised with the amount of midazolam used. If combined with opioids, intravenous midazolam can cause severe hypotension. A common modality for midazolam administration in neonatal intensive care units is by continuous infusion. If a patient is receiving midazolam infusion, care should be taken to avoid large doses of opioids. Our recommendation is to stop midazolam during surgery, although it is recommended to resume the infusion after surgery to avoid withdrawal symptoms.

Sedative/Hypnotics. The common sedative hypnotics used in neonates include propofol, thiopental, and ketamine.

Thiopental. Because of the large volume of distribution in neonates, it may be necessary to use large doses of thiopental for induction of anesthesia. However, because of their reduced clearance, the effect may last longer than anticipated. Thiopental can cause hypotension in neonates who are volume-depleted, especially in infants who are scheduled for

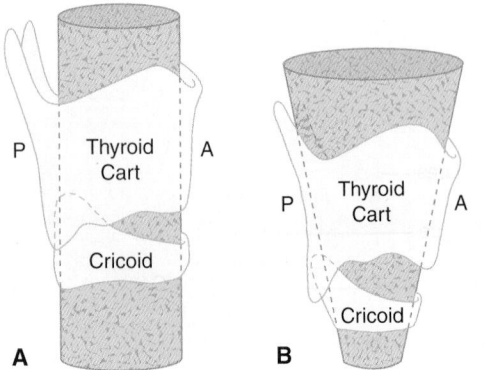

FIGURE 44-7. Configuration of the adult (**A**) versus the infant (**B**) larynx. The adult larynx has a cylindrical shape. The infant larynx is funnel-shaped because of the narrow, undeveloped cricoid cartilage. (Reprinted from the pediatric airway, A Practice of Anesthesia for Infants and Children, 2nd edition. Edited by Ryan JF, Coté CJ, Todres ID. Orlando, FL, Grune & Stratton, 1992, p 61, with permission.)

emergency surgery. It should be avoided in neonates with congenital heart disease because of its effect on myocardial function leading to hypotension. A dose of 2 to 4 mg/kg is usually well tolerated by most neonates for induction of anesthesia. When compared with intubation without any hypnotic, the use of intravenous thiopental demonstrated adequate maintenance of heart rate and blood pressure.[34]

Propofol.   Propofol, a phenyl sedative hypnotic, is a commonly used induction agent in infants and children. In a randomized trial comparing intravenous propofol with atropine, succinylcholine, and morphine, it was noted that propofol maintained adequate hemodynamics in neonates.[35] There is variability in elimination of propofol in neonates and preterm infants with longer elimination times.[36] Hence, while using propofol, it is important to reduce the dose to ensure early wake up and extubation.

Ketamine.   Ketamine, an N-methyl-D-aspartic acid (NMDA) antagonist, is used for induction of anesthesia in neonates who may have cardiovascular instability. An induction dose of 2 mg/kg intravenously with a higher dose of 4 to 5mg/kg is used intramuscularly. Although it produces hemodynamic stability, it can cause an increase in oral secretions. Recently, there have been significant alterations in excitotoxic cells in the animal model when exposed to NMDA receptor antagonists like ketamine with resultant concern about potential neurodegenerative changes with their exposure.[37,38] Ketamine is still used frequently in neonates with congenital heart disease for induction of anesthesia.[39]

Opioids

Opioids are used extensively in the management of anesthesia in neonates. The advantage of using opioids is their ability to maintain cardiovascular stability during major surgery. The common opioids used in neonates include fentanyl, morphine, and remifentanil. Infants who are on long-term doses of opioids may develop tolerance and may have to be placed on methadone, a longer-acting opioid.[40]

Fentanyl.   This synthetic opioid is commonly used for sedation in the neonate in the intensive care unit as well as in the operating room. A dose of 2 to 4 μg/kg/hr can maintain hemodynamic stability in these infants during surgery. The pharmacokinetics of fentanyl have been well studied in newborns.[41] The use of fentanyl in association with benzodiazepines may lead to hypotension and hemodynamic instability.[42] Caution must be exercised when the combination is administered during the perioperative period. Fentanyl may result in respiratory depression even with small doses. Continuous infusions may predispose to respiratory depression more frequently than bolus doses.[43] Chest wall rigidity and glottic rigidity has been described with fentanyl.[44] Small doses, as little as 1 to 2 μg/kg, can result in significant chest wall rigidity, leading to desaturation and need for mechanical ventilation. There is no significant maturational change on the brain associated with fentanyl compared with morphine. Hence, the sensitivity to fentanyl will not significantly change as the infant matures significantly. Fentanyl still continues to be the mainstay in newborns for sedation and analgesia.

Morphine.   The kinetics of morphine have been studied in newborns.[45] Premature babies have been shown to have decreased clearance. Morphine clearance (range, 0.8 to 6.5 mL/min/kg) correlated significantly with gestational age ($r = 0.60$; $p < 0.01$) and birth weight ($r = 0.55$; $p < 0.01$).[46] Because of decreased clearance, dosing in neonates, especially premature infants, should be adjusted to be provided every 6

hours to allow for clearance of the drug.[45] Morphine is used frequently in the intensive care unit for postoperative pain control. Morphine infusions in the perioperative period have resulted in minor prolongation of postoperative ventilation. However, the incidence of apnea or hypotension was not observed in neonates despite prolonged morphine infusions after successful extubation.[47] A large multicenter neonatal trial (NEOPAIN) demonstrated very little neurobehavioral changes associated with preemptive analgesia with morphine in neonates in the neonatal intensive care unit.[48]

Morphine is metabolized to morphine-3-glucuronide and morphine-6-glucuronide. Morphine-6-glucuronide predisposes to respiratory depression. The sensitivity to morphine-6-glucuronide increases with increase in age because of increased maturation of the neuronal receptors.[49] A minority of infants who are scheduled for surgery may have been on extracorporeal membrane oxygenation (ECMO). Kinetics of morphine have been carefully studied in neonates undergoing ECMO and do not show significant variability.[50]

Remifentanil.   Remifentanil is an ultra short-acting opioid that is metabolized by nonspecific esterases in plasma and tissues and has a half-life of <10 minutes. The pharmacokinetics of remifentanil in neonates are similar to that of older children.[51] Remifentanil is used for maintenance of anesthesia by avoiding volatile anesthetic agents. The use of remifentanil infusion facilitated tracheal extubation in infants in a randomized trial when compared with volatile agents.[52]

Methadone.   Methadone is a long-acting opioid that is used in neonates and infants in neonatal intensive care units, particularly when withdrawal from opioids is suspected. The pharmacokinetics of methadone has not been studied in neonates. However, it is used frequently in managing opioid tolerance.[40]

Neuromuscular Blocking Agents

Neuromuscular blocking agents (NMBAs) are frequently used during neonatal anesthesia to facilitate tracheal intubation, assist with controlled ventilation, relax abdominal musculature, and ensure immobility. Factors that influence the choice of agent include the time of onset, duration of action, cardiovascular effects, and mechanism of clearance/elimination.

Succinylcholine.   Succinylcholine, the only depolarizing muscle relaxant available, has the most rapid onset time of all the NMBAs. Neonates and infants have a larger extracellular fluid volume, leading to a larger volume of distribution and an increased dose requirement compared with children and adults. Thus, the recommended intravenous dose of succinylcholine for neonates and infants is 3 mg/kg, compared with 2 mg/kg in children, with an onset time of 30 to 45 seconds and duration of 5 to 10 minutes. The recommended intramuscular dose of succinylcholine is 4 mg/kg, with an onset time of 3 to 4 minutes and duration of approximately 20 minutes. Caution should be exercised when administering a second dose of succinylcholine because this can lead to vagally mediated bradycardia or sinus arrest. Pretreatment with atropine is recommended.[53]

The more recent succinylcholine controversy has called into question the use of succinylcholine in boys younger than 8 years of age.[54] The reports of hyperkalemia with cardiac arrest in such children with unrecognized muscular dystrophy have led some clinicians to take the position that succinylcholine should not be used routinely for this group of patients. The occurrence of this problem is somewhere in the range of 1 in 250,000 anesthetics, with a mortality rate of 50%. Although a concern in young children, it is not a problem in the neonatal period. Succinylcholine is still recommended in rapid-sequence situations, potential difficult airway, or if there are airway emergencies with progressive desaturation. When it is evident that a neonatal airway is obstructed by laryngospasm or other reason and no progress is made in ventilation, intramuscular or intravenous succinylcholine should be administered. Hyperkalemia can be recognized by peaked T waves. However, the clinician may not see this particular electrocardiographic change because it occurs 2 to 3 minutes after drug administration, when the anesthesiologist is attending to the airway. The hyperkalemia interferes with conduction, leading to a bradycardia and, if severe enough, cardiac arrest. The drug of first choice is intravenous calcium, 10 mg/kg. The use of sodium bicarbonate, 1 mEq/kg, to treat any metabolic acidosis that may occur with arrest is also believed to be useful because alkalosis decreases hyperkalemia. At the same time, the patient should be hyperventilated to reduce the CO_2, thereby encouraging a respiratory alkalosis. If there is refractory hypotension, an option is to administer epinephrine 5 to 10 μg/kg. One of the actions of epinephrine is to stimulate the sodium-potassium pump and cause the potassium to re-enter the cell, thereby reducing the serum level. If there is no response at this dose level, it should be increased incrementally until there is a response. Lastly, magnesium has been described as a treatment for hyperkalemia because it also antagonizes the effects of hyperkalemia, as does calcium.

Nondepolarizing Agents

⑤ The neonate's neuromuscular junction is more sensitive to nondepolarizing muscle relaxants, and the neonate has a larger volume of distribution because of a large extracellular fluid volume.[55] These two effects tend to balance each other so, roughly speaking, the dose of a nondepolarizing muscle relaxant for an infant is similar to that for a child on a milligram per kilogram basis. The ongoing organ maturation, which continues during the neonatal period, has a tremendous impact on the metabolism and clearance of the nondepolarizing agents. As a result, there is considerable variability and unpredictability in the duration of action of these agents in the neonatal period. Dosing should be titrated to effect and, when possible, guided by monitoring neuromuscular function with a nerve stimulator.

Intermediate Nondepolarizing Agents

Rocuronium.   Rocuronium appears to be the drug of choice among the intermediate-acting, nondepolarizing muscle relaxants for neonates. The intubating dose of rocuronium is 0.6 mg/kg. The length of action of rocuronium in the neonate is similar to that in the older infant or child following an equipotent dose. However, if a larger dose of rocuronium, 1.0 to 1.2 mg/kg, is administered to avoid using succinylcholine during a rapid-sequence induction, then rocuronium will be a relatively long-acting muscle relaxant. Rocuronium is metabolized by the liver; however, unlike vecuronium there are no active metabolites. Rocuronium has mild vagolytic properties and may slightly increase heart rate.

Vecuronium.   Although vecuronium is considered an intermediate-acting muscle relaxant in children and adults, in infants younger than 1 year of age it is considered a long-acting muscle relaxant. The duration of action of vecuronium is approximately twice that observed in children because of liver immaturity.[56] Vecuronium undergoes primarily hepatic metabolism with production of active metabolites that are dependent on renal excretion. The recommended dose of vecuronium is 0.1 to 0.15 mg/kg, with an onset time of 90 seconds and duration of action of 60 to 90 minutes in the neonate. Even with increased doses, vecuronium has no effect on the cardiovascular system.

Pancuronium.   Pancuronium is a long-acting NMBA with a pharmacokinetic profile similar to vecuronium. The recommended dose of 0.1 to 0.15 mg/kg has an onset time of 120 seconds and duration of 60 to 75 minutes. Unlike vecuronium, however, pancuronium primarily undergoes renal excretion.[57] Pancuronium has vagolytic and sympathomimetic actions that cause tachycardia and an increase in blood pressure.[58] In a relatively normal neonate with a normal blood pressure and normal blood volume, the use of pancuronium may result in hypertension, which has the potential to increase blood loss and increase the risk of hemorrhage in the extremely premature neonate. The risk for prolonged neuromuscular blockade in neonates, especially with altered renal function, makes pancuronium less desirable in neonates and infants undergoing minor outpatient surgical procedures.[59] The use of pancuronium for prolonged durations especially in the intensive care units can lead to muscle weakness. Prolonged use has also been associated with sensorineural hearing loss in infants.[60]

Reversal Agents.   The unpredictable nature of the NMBAs in the neonatal population, as well as the inability to accurately assess neuromuscular function in many situations, necessitates reversal of all nondepolarizing NMBA in neonates. The two commonly used reversal agents are edrophonium and neostigmine. Edrophonium in a dose of 1 mg/kg achieves a 90% reversal of a neuromuscular block in 2 minutes, whereas neostigmine in a dose of 0.07 mg/kg requires 10 minutes for a 90% reversal of neuromuscular block. This difference in time to peak effect allows the anesthesiologist to decide which agent is needed. Anticholinergic drugs like atropine or glycopyrrolate is coadministered to decrease the incidence of bradycardia. Neostigmine is the most common agent used for reversal of nondepolarizing muscle relaxants in neonates. The advantages of edrophonium over neostigmine are a more rapid reversal and fewer muscarinic side effects.

Volatile Agents

Volatile agents are used for maintenance of anesthesia in the neonatal period. Although halothane was the most commonly used volatile agent for many years and had a reasonable safety profile, the introduction of sevoflurane has clearly made a difference to the use of volatile agents in neonates. Desflurane, another potent volatile agent has limited application in children. Isoflurane is used for maintenance of anesthesia for longer surgical procedures. A brief synopsis of halothane followed by a more detail description of sevoflurane will be described in this chapter.

Halothane.   Halothane is still commonly used in many parts of the world as the primary inhaled anesthetic, although it is not currently used in the United States. Its long history for induction of anesthesia and its ease of use still make it a desirable agent in children. Halothane has a weak muscle relaxant property, facilitating induction and intubation without the use of a muscle relaxant. Halothane is a potent bronchodilator and may reduce the airway reflexes associated with intubation. The use of high doses of halothane for procedures including bronchoscopic evaluation of the airway may lead to significant myocardial depression and pump failure.[61] Infants <8 weeks old and with a history of RDS with longer period of preoperative fasting are prone to hypotension. Halothane also sensitizes the myocardium to cardiac dysrhythmias. Animal experiments demonstrate the increased sensitivity to epinephrine with halothane when compared with isoflurane or sevoflurane.[62] Hence, when concurrent exogenous catecholamines are administered (including epinephrine in local anesthetic solution), careful attention to the maximum dose should be carefully monitored. With the advent of sevoflurane, the use of halothane has decreased significantly in North America.

Isoflurane. Isoflurane has become a common maintenance volatile agent in neonates and infants. Its pungent odor does not allow its use for mask induction. Isoflurane increases the heart rate and hence may predispose to cardiac dysrhythmias. It has a greater effect in potentiation of muscle relaxation and hence plays an important role as a maintenance anesthetic. It is important to remember that the dose of muscle relaxants has to be reduced when isoflurane anesthesia is used. The dose of rocuronium bromide may have to be reduced to 0.45 mg/kg compared with a normal maintenance dose of 0.6 mg/kg.[63] Isoflurane has less myocardial depression when compared with halothane in neonates.[64]

Sevoflurane. This is the newer volatile agent that offers an advantage for rapid induction and rapid awakening. It has a less pungent smell than isoflurane. Its pharmacodynamics have been studied in neonates and children with a fairly reasonable safety profile.[65] In children with congenial cardiac disease, it has been shown to produce fewer hemodynamic changes when compared with isoflurane.[66] Although it produces less myocardial depression, it has a greater effect on respiratory depression compared with halothane. Minute ventilation and respiratory frequency were significantly lower during sevoflurane than halothane anesthesia (4.5 compared with 5.4 L/m^2/min, and 37.5 compared with 46.7 breaths per minute, respectively, $p < 0.05$). There was also significantly less thoracoabdominal asynchrony during sevoflurane anesthesia.[67]

Desflurane. Desflurane was touted to be the best volatile agent in children because of its partition coefficient being close to that of nitrous oxide, thereby allowing a rapid uptake. However, the pungent nature of the drug has made it difficult to use it for induction of anesthesia.[68] When compared with sevoflurane, infants who were preterm were noted to wake up sooner with desflurane, although there were no reductions in postoperative respiratory events.[69]

Local Anesthetic Solutions

Local anesthetic solutions are represented by two main classes, the amino-amides (amides) and the amino-esters (esters). The main difference between the two classes is that the amides undergo enzymatic degradation by the liver and the esters are hydrolyzed by plasma cholinesterases.[70]

Amides. These are commonly used local anesthetic solutions in neonates and infants. Local anesthetics used in common clinical practice belonging to this class include lidocaine, bupivacaine, ropivacaine and, more recently, levobupivacaine. The main characteristics differentiating these drugs are their speed of onset, duration of action, and potential for cardiac toxicity. The ability of neonatal liver enzymes to metabolize and their ability to oxidize and reduce these drugs are decreased when compared with adults.[32,71] At approximately 3 months of age, the conjugation of these drugs in the liver reaches adult levels. Older children can also achieve higher levels of local anesthetic solution than adults because of alteration in pharmacokinetics of the drugs. Local anesthetic solution levels have been shown to be higher in children undergoing intercostals nerve blocks compared with adults.[72] After caudal administration of local anesthetics, peak plasma level is obtained in children and adults in approximately 30 minutes.[73] The steady-state volume of distribution (Vd$_{SS}$) for amides is increased in children compared with adults, although clearance (CL) is similar.[73] Elimination half-life (t$_{1/2}$) is related to the volume of distribution and clearance as follows: t$_{1/2} = (0.693 \times Vd_{ss})/CL$. This results in a larger steady-state volume of distribution and prolongation of the elimination half-life, especially if a continuous infusion is used. The systemic absorption of local anesthetics is often based on the site of injection. On a decreasing scale, the incidence of complications with local anesthetic solution injections decrease, with the highest concentrations seen in the intercostal area followed by the caudal space, the epidural space, and peripheral nerve blocks. With newer technique in regional anesthesia, including ultrasound guidance, the volume and dose of local anesthetic solution can be significantly reduced.[74]

Toxicity of Local Anesthetic Solutions

Local anesthetic toxicity includes cardiac toxicity, central nervous system (CNS) toxicity, local reactions, and allergic reactions. Amide local anesthetic solutions may have a greater cardiac depressing effect than ester local anesthetic solution. Common local anesthetic compounds used in the neonatal and infant period include amide local anesthetics such as lidocaine, bupivacaine, ropivacaine, and levo-bupivacaine, and ester local anesthetics such as chloroprocaine. A brief description of each of these agents in children is provided here.

Bupivacaine. Bupivacaine is the most commonly used local anesthetic solution in infants and children in North America. The pharmacokinetics and the pharmacodynamics have been well studied in infants and children.[75] The concentration of the local anesthetic used depends on the site, the desired density of blockade (motor and sensory), postoperative "street readiness," and the potential for cardiovascular and neurotoxicity. The concomitant use of other local anesthetics including infiltration anesthesia has to be taken into consideration before a total volume of local anesthetic solution is taken into consideration. This is especially true in neonatal surgery in which large quantities of local anesthetic solution can sometimes be injected for skin infiltration. If upper safe limits are likely to be approached, it is reasonable to avoid local anesthetic solution for infiltration and use a dilute epinephrine solution instead. The preferred concentration for peripheral nerve blockade is 0.25% bupivacaine or 0.2% ropivacaine, and the preferred concentration for single dose bolus doses is 0.25% or 0.125% solution of bupivacaine or 0.2% ropivacaine. When a continuous infusion is desired, a 0.1% or 0.125% solution of bupivacaine is preferred. In premature infants and in infants weighing under 1 kg, we prefer using 0.0625% bupivacaine, or in some cases bolus doses given every 12 hours. Although clear guidelines do not exist for local anesthetic solutions, a rough rule of thumb is to use 0.2 mg/kg/hr for continuous infusions of bupivacaine and 2 mg/kg for bolus doses.[76]

Metabolism. Bupivacaine is bound to α_1-glycoprotein. This may be altered in the newborn period.[77] It is a racemic mixture of the levo and dextro enantiomers. Although the levo enantiomer is the active form that provides the clinical effect of the local anesthetic solution, the dextro enantiomer is responsible for the adverse effects related to local anesthesia, including cardiac toxicity and neurotoxicity.

Toxicity. The major adverse effect of bupivacaine is toxicity related to the cardiovascular and the CNS. Local anesthetics have the ability to cross the blood–brain barrier and can cause alterations in the CNS functions. Continuous infusions in neonates can predispose them to CNS toxicity sooner than older infants.[78] In pediatric patients, the incidence of cardiac toxicity occurs sooner than neurotoxicity,[78] which may be partly because children may be anesthetized and devastating neurotoxicity may not be noticed until significant cardiac toxicity is seen. Manifestation of bupivacaine toxicity may also be affected by the concomitant use of volatile agents for general anesthesia.

Dosage. Bupivacaine can be used for most peripheral nerve blocks as well as for epidural and caudal infusions in infants and children. The maximum dosage suggested for bolus injections in the caudal space or epidural space for older children is 4 mg/kg and for neonates and 2 mg/kg for infants.[76] Dosage recommendations for continuous infusions is 0.4 mg/kg/hr in older children and 0.2 mg/kg/hr in neonates and infants.[22] The concentration of the solution used for peripheral nerve blocks is usually 0.25 or 0.5%, bearing in mind the ceiling limit for maximum dosage. An example of a continuous infusion in a 4-kg neonate will be 0.2 mg/kg/hr; this will be equivalent to 0.8 mL/hr of a 0.1% solution of bupivacaine (1 mg/mL of bupivacaine).

Ropivacaine. Ropivacaine is a newer amide local anesthetic. It is a levo enantiomer with relatively less cardiovascular and CNS side effects compared with bupivacaine.[79] The pharmacokinetics of ropivacaine are such that caudal blocks with ropivacaine (2 mg/kg) in children (aged 1 to 8 years) result in plasma concentrations of ropivacaine well below toxic levels in adults.[79] This dose was also noted to produce less motor block, but provide adequate analgesia. Mean maximum plasma concentration of total ropivacaine at 2 mg/kg was 0.47 mg/L. A threshold of CNS toxicity was noted at a plasma concentration of 0.6 mg/L. Body weight-adjusted clearance was the same as in adults (5 mL/min/kg). Ropivacaine clearance depends on the unbound fraction of ropivacaine rather than the liver blood flow.

Toxicity. Although the safety of ropivacaine has been demonstrated in animal experiments, there have been reports of CNS toxicity and cardiac toxicity associated with the use of epidural ropivacaine. It is important to understand that an overdose of ropivacaine can cause toxicity, making close attention to dosage as important with ropivacaine as with other local anesthetics. Our recommended dose is bolus dose of 2 mg/kg and an infusion rate of 0.2 mg/kg/hr.

Levobupivacaine. Levobupivacaine is a newer levo enantiomer that has fewer adverse effects than bupivacaine.[80] There are fewer pediatric trials available in literature. Because of the common use of bupivacaine in children and its low incidence of complications, levobupivacaine is not used abundantly in general pediatric anesthesiology practice. It is currently not available for use in the United States, although it is widely used in other parts of the world.

Toxicity. Levobupivacaine, in the animal model, has been shown to have less cardiac toxicity with lower degree of myocardial depression than bupivacaine.[81]

Esters

Ester local anesthetics are metabolized by plasma cholinesterases.[82] As a result, in populations with lower pseudocholinesterases as in neonates, we see an increase in the duration of local anesthetic activity. This includes infants and neonates particularly. The duration of action of the drug is limited; hence, a continuous infusion of chloroprocaine is recommended.

Toxicity. Toxicity is based on the absence of pseudocholine esterase in the neonate.

Dosing. After a bolus dose of 1 mL/kg, a continuous infusion of chloroprocaine at 0.3 mL/kg of a 3% 2-chloroprocaine is recommended to achieve a level of T4 to T2.[83] This will be effective in producing complete surgical anesthesia for neonates undergoing hernia repair. Although the drug is not commonly used in pediatric practice, the advantage of its use is the capacity to provide complete motor block that is not prolonged.

Topical Anesthesia

Several local anesthetic preparations are now available for topical use. The most common local anesthetic preparations for topical use include lidocaine, tetracaine, benzocaine, and prilocaine. When these are applied to skin they produce effective but relatively short duration of analgesia. A topical anesthetic formulation EMLA (eutectic mixture of local anesthetic) is a mixture of lidocaine 2.5% and prilocaine 2.5%[84] and is used extensively for topical anesthesia in neonates, particularly for circumcision and venipunctures. The preparation has to applied under an occlusive bandage for 45 to 60 minutes to obtain effective cutaneous analgesia. Although the incidence of methemoglobinemia from prilocaine is not very common in neonates, caution should be exercised when applying large doses of EMLA and caution should be exercised while applying large doses for procedures.[85]

Newer topical anesthetic solutions are now available that may offer a faster rate of onset. LMX-4, a 4% liposomal lidocaine solution can be used as topical anesthesia. There is no need for an occlusive dressing when LMX-4 is used, and it has the same efficacy as EMLA.[86,87] Liposome-encapsulated lidocaine or tetracaine have been shown to remain in the epidermis after topical application, affording a fast and lasting anesthetic effect.

ANESTHETIC MANAGEMENT OF THE NEONATE

Effective evaluation, preparation, and anesthetic management of the neonate depends on appropriate knowledge, clinical skills, and vigilance by the anesthesiologist. For safe and effective care, the anesthesiologist must take extraordinary care to understand the current status of the patient, the nature of the planned surgery, and the potential need for stabilization and preparation before surgery. After ensuring that the patient has been adequately prepared, the anesthesiologist needs to develop a detailed plan that encompasses the issues of anesthetic equipment and monitoring, airway management, drug choice, fluid management, temperature control, anticipated surgical needs, pain management, and postoperative care.

Studies have shown that morbidity and mortality related to anesthesia is higher in infants, especially neonates, compared with infants, older children, and adults.[88–91] There are probably several causes for this higher complication rate, including the emergent nature of most surgical procedures that are performed at this age, the physiologic instability of the neonate, the relative lack of experience most clinicians have with patients in this age range, and the technical challenges of monitoring and treating a very small patient. Because of the specialized nature of neonatal surgery and care, it is important that each institution that provides care to these patients have the resources of equipment, critical care facilities, nursing, laboratory, blood bank, and social work necessary to meet the needs of these patients and their families, as well as systems in place to guarantee a robust quality-assurance emphasis on the provision of care. Both the American Academy of Pediatrics and the American Society of Anesthesiologists have provided guidance to many of the systems issues that should be addressed in institutions caring for these patients.[92] Physicians who agree to participate in this care need to have the preparation and ongoing experience needed to provide a consistent, high level of care.

In the distant past, concerns about physiologic instability and other challenges of caring for neonates led some practitioners to use minimal or no anesthesia for both minor and major procedures.[93–95] It is now widely recognized that neonates have stress responses similar to those of older patients, and the lack of adequate anesthetic care is as inhumane in the neonate as it is in the older child or adult.[96] Consequently, the same attention to adequate analgesia and anesthesia needs to be paid to the neonate as to other patients.

Preoperative Considerations

Preanesthetic Evaluation—History

The preanesthetic planning process starts with an evaluation of the course of intrauterine growth, followed by labor and delivery and the immediate postpartum course. The amount of history available to the anesthesiologist may vary widely. If the mother had received prepartum and postpartum care in the institution in which one is working, a significant amount of detail may be available. If the newborn is transferred from another institution, there may be limited information available. Best efforts should be made to get as much relevant information as possible, with an emphasis on maternal factors that may have affected fetal growth as well as the current status of the newborn. Additional history of the child's course since birth is important, with a particular focus on the signs that identified the surgical condition that is to be treated. Important factors include the history of feeding and hydration, need for oxygenation or ventilatory support, cardiovascular abnormalities and need for support, and any evidence of CNS problems such as seizures or intraventricular hemorrhage. Lastly, an estimation of the gestational status is made, with an emphasis on the issues of prematurity and intrauterine growth retardation with subsequent small-for-gestational age status.

The World Health Organization definition of prematurity as <37 weeks' gestation at birth. The determination of gestational age is based on the estimated date of full-term delivery, as well as physical examination of the newborn. Although these indicators are generally widely agreed on, they are subject to some degree of variation in interpretation. The greater the degree of prematurity, the more physiologic abnormalities will be expected. As one neonatologist explained, "Preterms obey no known law of physics" (Ogata E, personal communication 2008). The implications for anesthesiologists are that the more preterm a newborn, the greater the variability of responsiveness to anesthetic agents, fluids, cardioactive drugs, and the stress of the surgical procedure.

In addition to prematurity, there is a second, related classification system. Low birth weight, defined as a birth weight of ≤2,500 g, can be due to prematurity, poor intrauterine growth, or both. Prematurity and intrauterine growth retardation are associated with increased neonatal morbidity and mortality, and it is difficult to completely separate factors associated with prematurity from those associated with intrauterine growth retardation. For discussion purposes, preterm infants are often divided into subgroups. Newborns born at 35 to 37 weeks' gestation are considered near term. These newborns have a lower incidence of major physiologic abnormalities typical of the more preterm newborn. Although they usually do not have significant pulmonary abnormalities, they may have some feeding problems or hyperbilirubinemia. This degree of prematurity does not usually have a significant impact on anesthetic management. However, infants born between 30 and 34 weeks' gestation are much more likely to show some abnormalities related to prematurity that can complicate anesthetic management.[97]

Although RDS used to be a significant source of morbidity in this population, the widespread use of exogenous surfactant has decreased the incidence dramatically, as well as the later complications of chronic lung disease. This group does have more problems with inadequate feeding, persistent patency of the ductus arteriosus, apnea in response to stress, and temperature instability. However, infants born more premature than this begin to demonstrate significant physiologic abnormalities

TABLE 44-3

ABNORMALITIES ASSOCIATED WITH THE PRETERM—COMMON ANESTHETIC CONCERNS

Respiratory	Respiratory distress syndrome
	Apnea
	Pneumothorax, pneumomediastinum
	Pneumonia
	Pulmonary hemorrhage
	Bronchopulmonary dysplasia
Cardiovascular	Patent ductus arteriosus
	Hypotension
	Bradycardia
	Pulmonary hypertension
	Persistent transitional circulation
	Congenital heart disease
Central nervous system	Intraventricular hemorrhage
	Hypoxic-ischemic encephalopathy
	Seizures
	Kernicterus
	Drug withdrawal
Metabolic	Hypoglycemia
	Hyperglycemia
	Hypocalcemia
	Hypothermia
	Metabolic acidosis
Renal	Hyponatremia
	Hypernatremia
	Hyperkalemia
	Poor urine output
Gastrointestinal	Poor feeding
	Necrotizing enterocolitis
	Intestinal obstruction
Hematologic	Anemia
	Hyperbilirubinemia
	Vitamin K deficiency
Other	Retinopathy of prematurity
	Sepsis and infections

related to prematurity. For infants with very low birth weight, defined as <1,500 g, the presence of complicating problems and morbidity and mortality are inversely related to birth weight. RDS is found in approximately 80% of infants weighing 501 to 750 g, in 65% of those 751 to 1,000 g, in 45% between 1,001 and 1,250 g, and in 25% between 1,251 and 1,500 g. In addition, symptomatic intraventricular hemorrhage is found in about 25% of infants weighing 501 to 750 g, in 12% between 751 and 1,000 g, in 8% between 1,001 and 1,250 g, and in 3% between 1,251 and 1,500 g. Other complications, such as sepsis, necrotizing enterocolitis (NEC), and bronchopulmonary dysplasia, are very high in infants with very low birth weight. Table 44-3 lists some of the most common abnormalities found in the preterm population that have implications for anesthetic evaluation, preparation, and management.

Preanesthetic Evaluation—Physical Examination

Physical examination of the newborn is focused by the condition requiring surgical intervention. Hydration is often an important issue because of both fasting and losses related to the surgical lesion. Clinical signs of dehydration include a sunken fontanelle, poor skin turgor, dry mucus membranes, sunken eyes, poor skin perfusion, delayed capillary refill, hypothermia, and a history of tachycardia or absent urine output. If there are clinical signs of dehydration, efforts should be made to correct the deficits before surgery, except in extreme, life-threatening situations. Physical examination also focuses on the respiratory and cardiovascular systems. The presence of any cardiovascular abnormalities should be noted, including poor perfusion or pulses, abnormal rhythm or rate, a murmur or gallop, hepatomegaly, or other signs of either heart failure or poor perfusion. The presence of a murmur is of concern in the neonatal period and warrants further evaluation, which is best done by a pediatric cardiologist. An electrocardiogram and echocardiogram will help define whether there is significant cardiovascular disease present that can affect the anesthetic management. Although this evaluation may take some effort and time, it is worthwhile to ensure that the anesthesiologist can plan the child's care with full knowledge of the limitations cardiovascular disease can impose.

The respiratory system also must be examined in some detail. The presence of stridor or other evidence of airway obstruction, such as sternal or chest wall retractions, should be identified and investigated. Although upper airway obstruction is relatively rare in the newborn, laryngeal webs, cysts of the tongue or supraglottic region, vocal cord paralysis after a traumatic delivery, and hemangiomas of the airway can cause obstruction and need to be identified. In addition, newborns that have been previously intubated may have some degree of subglottic edema related to previous intubation. More likely are signs of lower airway disease, such as tachypnea, grunting, rhonchi, retractions, and cyanosis. This may be related to the early development of RDS, but may also represent meconium aspiration, pneumonia, pneumothorax, or heart failure. The cause of any respiratory distress needs to be evaluated expeditiously prior to anesthesia to identify treatable causes and begin therapy.

Preanesthetic Evaluation—Laboratory

Most laboratory investigations are related to the underlying surgical condition, such as radiologic investigations, computed tomography or magnetic resonance imaging studies, and echocardiography. However, most newborns will have, at a minimum, a blood count and glucose level drawn. The hemoglobin in a newborn is primarily fetal hemoglobin, which has a higher affinity for oxygen than adult hemoglobin. Because of this higher affinity, the hemoglobin dissociation curve is shifted to the left, releasing less oxygen to the tissues than adult hemoglobin. Newborns have a higher hemoglobin than the infant or child, often in the 15 to 18 g/dL range.[98] Rarely, a newborn will have significant polycythemia, with hemoglobin levels above 20 g/dL. If symptomatic, these patients may benefit from a lowering of the hemoglobin levels.

Glucose levels obtained close to the time of the proposed surgery are important. The stressed newborn, especially the stressed preterm or small-for-gestational age newborn, are at particular risk for hypoglycemia.[99] A glucose level between 60 and 80 mg/dL is expected in a full-term newborn, with a preterm often 10 mg/dL below that. Although there is some controversy about what actually constitutes hypoglycemia in these populations, most agree that levels <45 mg/dL warrant therapy with additional dextrose. Patients with diabetic mothers, those who have not been receiving either enteral or parenteral feeds, those who are very low birth weight, and those who have been septic are especially susceptible to hypoglycemia and require frequent monitoring and modification of parenteral fluids.

Other laboratory studies, such as electrolyte determinations and coagulation profiles, are indicated in specific patients. Hypocalcemia, in particular, can be troubling because signs of hypocalcemia are nonspecific. Unexplained hypotension, irritability, or even seizures can be presenting signs. Hypocalcemia is a problem with preterm newborns, but can also be seen in full-term newborns who have a delay in starting enteral feedings. Hyponatremia is not uncommon in newborns who have been receiving solutions with little or no salt in the first days of life, while hypernatremia may occur if there is inadequate resuscitation of the dehydrated patient when water loss is greater than salt loss. The longer a newborn has received parenteral fluids, the greater the chance of electrolyte abnormalities because of the difficulty in matching ongoing losses with replacement in the presence of an immature kidney.

Coagulation parameters are different in newborns compared with adults.[100] Although platelet counts in term newborns are usually similar to adult values, lower values are frequently seen in the preterm. Unexplained thrombocytopenia can be an early sign of sepsis, and a falling count should be an impetus to look for other signs of sepsis. Other coagulation tests are different in both the full-term and preterm newborn. The prothrombin time and partial thromboplastin time levels are about 10% longer in the newborn, but prothrombin time values approach adult levels in the first week of life and partial thromboplastin time levels within the first month of life.

Preanesthetic Plan

The anesthesiologist has a host of anesthetic techniques from which to choose and can tailor the anesthetic to the requirements of the surgery and the condition of the neonate. Major factors that should be considered in planning the anesthetic include (1) the need to have blood and blood products available before beginning the case, (2) the need for invasive monitoring, (3) the need for additional equipment for securing the airway or establishing vascular access, (4) the need to transport the child to and from the operating room, (5) the likelihood of postoperative ventilation, and (6) the plan for postoperative pain relief. Both the medical status of the patient and the planned surgical procedure will impact this planning. The anesthesiologist has the responsibility of clarifying any medical issues with the neonatologist before finalizing the plan, as well as clarifying any issues relates to the planned procedure with the surgeon. Occasionally, as planning progresses, it becomes obvious that the patient needs further medical resuscitation or evaluation before it is prudent to proceed with the procedure.

Once the anesthetic plan is clear, it should be discussed with the available parent or caregiver who has legal custody of the child. Informed consent is a process by which the anesthesiologist explains his/her understanding of the patient's status, the planned procedure, the plan for anesthetic management, alternatives to the plan, and some discussion of risks and benefits. Although there may be rare circumstances in which the legal guardian is not available to provide consent, efforts should be made in all except the most emergent of situations to have this discussion. It should be stressed that informed consent is a process, not a document. The goal of informed consent is to help the parent understand what care is being proposed, the risks and benefits involved, and reasonable alternatives. It is the discussion, in terms understandable to the parent, that is the basis of true informed consent.

Premedication

Premedication is not commonly used for neonatal anesthetics. Sedation is not usually appropriate, and analgesics are rarely indicated before taking the patient to the operating room. In the past, premedication with atropine was occasionally used, especially for older neonates, above a month of age, where an inhalation induction was considered. Because of the dominance of the parasympathetic nervous system, bradycardia on induction or in response to inhalation agents is of concern. There are some data that in the older neonate, the vagolytic activity of atropine does decrease the bradycardia and hypotension associated with volatile agents.[101,102] In older neonates, an inhalation agent may be the primary anesthetic for the case, making the additional of atropine useful. However, it is more common in neonates under a year of age to use opioids as the basis of the anesthetic, with lower doses of an inhalation agent titrated to effect. In this situation, atropine is less commonly indicated and can always be added intravenously as the anesthetic proceeds.

Intraoperative Considerations

Monitoring

Neonatal patients are at a disadvantage when it comes to perioperative monitoring because of their small size. Many of the monitoring modalities that are used in older children and adults are not available for the neonate. Examples of this include transesophageal echocardiography, pulmonary artery catheterization, and brain function monitoring. Other monitors that are used may occasionally not provide reliable information for technical reasons. Examples of this include neuromuscular blockade monitoring and automated blood pressure monitoring. Invasive monitoring such as arterial line and central venous line catheters may be technically difficult to insert, especially in the preterm. Consequently, the goal of monitoring should be to establish American Society of Anesthesiologists standard monitors of pulse oximetry, blood pressure, at the beginning of the case and add invasive monitoring, as appropriate.

Although physical observation of the patient is important in preanesthetic evaluation, it is difficult to use this monitor during a surgical procedure. Observation of the patient's color, capillary refill, warmth of skin, muscle tone, fullness of fontanelle, and chest expansion are useful monitors, but they are difficult to reliably observe once the patient is covered with surgical drapes. There is a large dependence on electronic monitors during the majority of the procedure. However, it should be remembered that heart and breath sounds heard through a precordial or esophageal stethoscope, the compliance determined during hand ventilation, the appearance of bleeding in the surgical field, and trends noted in the anesthetic record are all important observations that the anesthesiologist can use as part of the overall assessment of the patient.

Pulse oximetry is one of the most important monitors in neonatal anesthesia. Flexible probes designed for pediatric patients should be used. Placement is sometimes difficult because of the small fingers of the neonate. It may be necessary to place the probe across the web space between the thumb and first finger, around the lateral aspect of the hand, or on the foot. Many anesthesiologists will place and check two pulse oximeter probes at the beginning of the case because of the clinical experience of having one probe malfunctioning secondary to changes in perfusion during the case. Because there may be differences in preductal and postductal saturations, probes on the left hand or either leg may give lower values than a probe on the right hand.[103] Especially in the first 2 weeks of life, there is a preponderance of fetal hemoglobin. The pulse oximeter does not compensate for the left shift of the hemoglobin desaturation curve, and pulse oximeter values read about 2% higher than arterial blood saturations.[104]

The hallmark of the pediatric anesthesiologist has been the precordial stethoscope. It has the advantages of being simple and effective in allowing continuous monitoring of heart rate, heart rhythm, strength of heart sounds, and breath sounds. A softening of heart sounds often is indicative of a drop in blood pressure. The esophageal stethoscope is more secure and less susceptible to external noise as the precordial stethoscope, while also providing the ability to measure core temperature. Although there has been recent skepticism about the usefulness of the stethoscope,[105] the stethoscope continues to be a quick, continuously available monitor that can be used to detect changes in both the circulatory and ventilatory status of the newborn.

The electrocardiograph is useful primarily to assess heart rate and rhythm. It is sometimes difficult to get the leads to adhere properly, but wiping the skin with alcohol before placement is often helpful. These leads, once applied, can bind tightly to skin, and care must be taken when removing them to avoid removal of skin, especially in the preterm. ST-T wave abnormalities may be an indicator of significant electrolyte disturbances, but abnormalities related to myocardial ischemia are not common in the perioperative period.

Blood pressure measurements are important in the management of all newborns. Noninvasive automated machines are commonly used, but it is important that a proper-sized cuff—one half to two thirds of the length of the upper arm—be used, and that the arterial indicator, adjacent to the exit of the hoses, be place over the artery. The cuff should not be routinely cycled excessively, more than every 3 minutes, because of the danger of venous stasis, especially in preterms. In some cases, it is not possible to get reliable readings from an automated machine. An effective alternative is to use a manual cuff and place a Doppler probe over the brachial or radial artery. This system gives reliable systolic blood pressures over a very wide range; the Doppler probe can detect flow, even at very low blood pressures when the automated cuff may fail.

Direct arterial blood pressure monitoring offers the double advantage of accurate blood pressure readings and the ability to withdraw blood samples. A 22-gauge catheter is often used in full-term neonates and a 24-gauge catheter in preterms. A variety of sites can be used, including the radial, dorsal pedal, and posterior tibial arteries. Less commonly, the brachial or femoral arteries are used. Either percutaneous or cutdown can be used for access. Some patients may come to the operating room with an umbilical artery line in place. Although these can be used for monitoring, umbilical lines have both infectious and embolic risks, and may be in the way of the surgical field. All arterial lines should be flushed, either continuously or intermittently, with small amounts of heparinized saline, but caution should be used because even small amounts of flush can transmit significant pressure retrograde and cause embolic damage to the brain.

Central venous monitoring is occasionally used in neonatal surgery. Access to blood samples and central venous pressures can be especially useful in procedures, such as gastroschisis repair, in which there are anticipated large changes in both blood loss and third-space losses. Central catheters can also be used for the administration of blood, total parenteral nutrition, and cardioactive drug infusion. Insertion of these lines can be in a variety of sites, including the subclavian, internal jugular, femoral, or external jugular veins using special precautions to maintain sterile technique. The umbilical vein is not recommended as a site for central monitoring because of the risk of portal vein thrombosis. Percutaneous insertion may be assisted by ultrasound guidance. Central lines can be both challenging to insert, but also associated with significant complications related to infection, thrombosis, and emboli.[106] Meticulous technique with insertion and maintenance of the line will help minimize these complications.

Although there may be some differential between capnography and arterial PCO_2 readings, the trend data are accurate and the shape of the waveform can give significant information about changes in ventilation, obstruction, and rebreathing. Airway pressure measurements are particularly useful in assessing changes in resistance or compliance. Although it has been traditional that hand ventilation was important in determining changes in airway and chest compliance, there is controversy about the reliability of the "feel of the hand on the bag."[107,108] Airway pressure measurements are also useful in adopting adult anesthesia ventilators for use in neonatal and pediatric patients, using peak airway pressures as a guide for setting tidal volume.[109]

Anesthetic Systems

There is a long tradition in pediatric anesthesia of using semi-open, nonrebreathing systems for general anesthesia in newborns.[110,111] Circuits such as the Jackson-Rees adaptation of the Ayre's T-piece and the Bain circuit have been the most commonly used in the United States.[112] These and related circuits have the advantage of lightweight, easy-to-open valves or lack of valves, rapid changes in anesthetic concentration, minimal work of breathing, and high circuit compliance. On the other hand, they require relatively high gas flows and require some modification for mechanical ventilation. These circuits were especially popular when spontaneous ventilation was more commonly used than it is now in neonatal patients. As the use of these circuits has diminished, familiarity with their use and application has dropped in favor of the semiclosed, rebreathing circle systems used in adult patients. There will be slower change in anesthetic concentration, less circuit compliance, and larger compression volume with these circuits, but they give the advantage of using the same circuit on patients of all ages.

Because the loss of both heat and humidity through the endotracheal tube is of concern in the neonate, the anesthetic circuit should incorporate features to minimize water and heat loss. In the past, heated vaporizers were added to the circuit for this purpose. However, there is a danger of patient absorption of water and fluid overload with their use, as well as concerns about overheating the patient or an airway burn. It is now common to use a combination of low gas flows[113] and a disposable, neonatal humidity and heat exchanger to the circuit, with warming of the gases and retention of some of the exhaled humidity.[114,115]

Lastly, the anesthesia machine used for anesthetizing neonates should have the capacity to administer medical air. There are two reasons for this. First, if nitrous oxide is contraindicated, such as in the newborn with bowel obstruction, air is mixed with oxygen to prevent the administration of only 100% oxygen. This is also used to minimize the risk of retinopathy of prematurity by avoiding prolonged administration of 100% oxygen. Second, some patients, such as those with hypoplastic left heart syndrome, may benefit from the administration of air with additional oxygen. Without an air flowmeter in the system, this will not be possible.

Induction of Anesthesia.   There is no one method of induction and maintenance of anesthesia that is best for all patients. The current medical status of the patient, the surgical condition, the presence of ongoing fluid or blood losses, the gestational age of the patient, recent fasting, and the experience of the anesthesiologist are all important considerations. Most neonates who come to the operating room will have vascular access already established; if not, the first task before induction is to establish adequate vascular access after applying monitors. Although it may rarely be appropriate to use an inhalational induction if vascular access is difficult in the older newborn, near a month of age, it is mandatory to establish access first in the newborn who is preterm, medically unstable, has a full stomach, has a potentially difficult airway, or has ongoing fluid losses.

Airway Management.   Establishing the airway in the neonate requires an appreciation of the differences between the newborn and adult airway, as discussed earlier. It is rare to administer anesthesia in the newborn period without establishing an artificial airway. Although, with meticulous technique, a mask airway can successfully be used for short periods of time, the tolerances of mask fit, adequate airway pressure, and avoidance of gastric distention are small, making this a poor choice for any but the briefest of operations. In addition, controlled ventilation is used more commonly today than spontaneous ventilation for surgical procedures, making an artificial airway necessary.

Awake intubation has been used to secure the airway without the danger of loss of airway during the procedure, but it can be a traumatic experience for both the patient and the anesthesiologist, accompanied by pain, breath holding, desaturation, and tissue trauma.[116] The desaturation associated with this technique can be ameliorated by using an oxyscope, a Miller laryngoscope blade that has a side channel to allow insufflation of oxygen during the procedure.[117,118] However, this technique is usually reserved for patients with severe hemodynamic compromise, an extraordinarily distended and tense abdomen, or a presumed difficult airway, especially the newborn with micrognathia. In the latter situation, the addition of sedation with an opioid or topical application of local anesthetic can help decrease some of the trauma of the procedure. It has also been suggested that an awake intubation may be best for the anesthesiologist who is not very experienced in intubating newborns. It may be better to have a more experienced clinician, if available, attend to the airway in that situation.

Most newborns are intubated after a rapid-sequence induction. Preoxygenation is useful in adding additional safety to the procedure. Although there may be a minor concern about a period of hyperoxia in the preterm, there is no evidence that a short exposure such as preoxygenation will increase the risk of retinopathy of prematurity. Agents for induction and muscle relaxation are discussed later. If there is concern about the difficulty of intubation, it may be prudent to induce anesthesia, ensure adequacy of mask ventilation, and then give the muscle relaxant.

Positioning for intubation is based on the known differences in the neonatal airway. Because of the large occiput of the head, the newborn already has a flexed neck. No changes in position are usually needed, although additional extension of the head may be accomplished by a shoulder roll. A Miller no. 1 blade is commonly used for the full-term newborn and a Miller no. 0 in the preterm, although there are other available blades that individual practitioners may prefer. Sliding the blade down the right side of the mouth allows the blade to be seated with minimal overlap by the tongue (Fig. 44-8). The tip of the blade is advanced to lift the epiglottis directly instead of placing it in the vallecula, as is commonly done with older patients. Every patient's anatomy is different, but if the laryngoscope is advanced in the direction parallel to the handle, one will get the best visualization. If the glottis is not easily seen, cricoid pressure can be applied with the little finger of the hand holding the handle or by an assistant, often improving the view (Fig. 44-9).

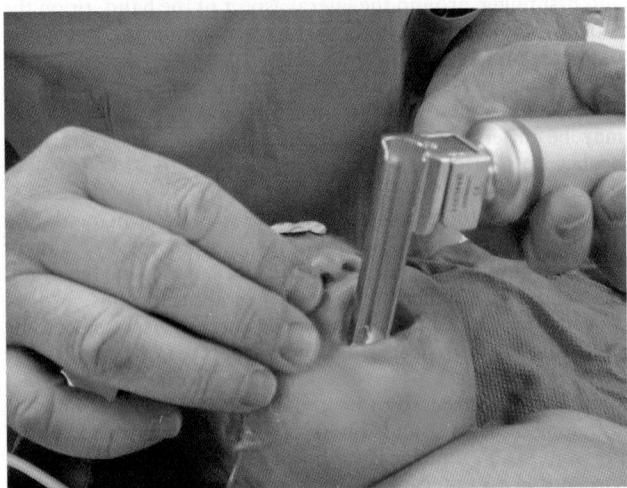

FIGURE 44-8.   Insertion of Miller blade down the right side of the tongue. The blade is then turned and pressure is applied in the direction of the handle.

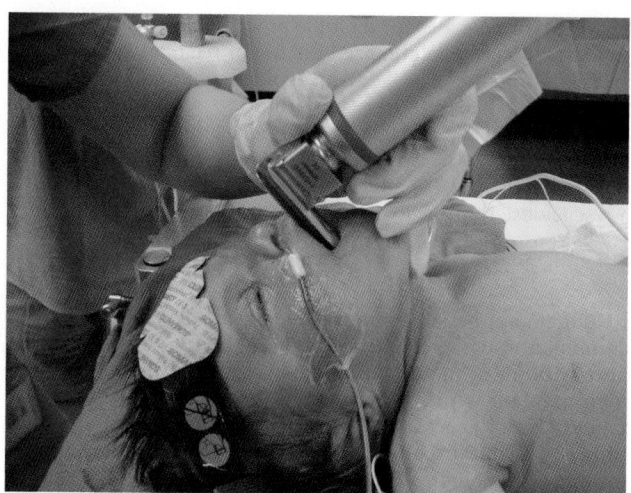

FIGURE 44-9. Cricoid pressure applied with little finger.

Uncuffed tubes have traditionally been used in newborns to minimize cuff pressure on the subglottic larynx, especially at the level of the cricoids. Although there has been interest in the use of cuffed tubes in newborns and infants,[119] most clinicians continue to use uncuffed tubes in newborns to maximize the internal diameter and gas flow characteristics for a given external diameter of tube. Although various formulas have been proposed for how far to advance an uncuffed tube, it is prudent to use the depth markers at the end of the tube to ensure under direct vision that the tip is advanced 2 or 3 cm past the vocal cords. A 3.0- or 3.5-mm internal diameter (ID) uncuffed tube is usually appropriate for a full-term newborn and a 2.5-mm ID tube is used in preterms, especially those under 1,500 g body weight. Once inserted, the presence of a positive capnograph tracing, bilateral expansion of the thorax, and bilateral breath sounds are used to ensure proper placement. Although some anesthesiologists prefer to advance the endotracheal tube past the carina and then withdraw until bilateral breath sounds are heard, there are two major disadvantages to the technique: trauma to the airway and lack of a guarantee that the tip of the tube is not sitting right at the carina, increasing the chance of migration into a bronchus with head movement. Lastly, listen for an air leak at an airway pressure of about 20 cm H_2O to ensure that the tube is not too large for the airway, increasing the chances of subglottic edema and damage.

If intubation proves difficult, there are a variety of options. A laryngeal mask airway (LMA) can be used to provide ventilation in newborns as small as 1 kg body weight as preparations are made to use other intubating techniques.[120] It is possible to use the LMA as a guide for blind intubations in newborns with the use of a styletted tube.[121] The light wand can also be used in newborns,[122] and can be particularly useful in the newborn with micrognathia or retrognathia because of the ability to mold the wand to a "hockey stick" configuration with a sharp angle. Fiberoptic laryngoscopy, the most flexible of intubating pools routinely used in older children and adults, can also be used in the newborn. Fiberscopes are currently available that accept endotracheal tubes as small as 2.5-mm ID, although these scopes do not currently have the ability to change direction and are useful more for confirmation of tube placement. Fiberscopes that can actively change direction accept a 3.5-mm ID tube at the smallest. Insertion of the fiberscope can be done directly or through an LMA. An LMA guide has been particularly useful in directly intubating newborns that could not be visualized by routine approaches.[123,124]

Lastly, an old technique that is used infrequently is digital intubation in which two fingers are advanced along the midline of the tongue and onto the epiglottis, with a styletted tube then advanced between the two fingers.[125] Once the airway is secured, ventilation is usually controlled during neonatal surgical procedures with hand ventilation or, more commonly, mechanical ventilation.[126] After establishing a baseline of acceptable ventilation, it is important to continuously monitor the peak airway pressures, chest expansion, return volume, pulse oximetry, and capnograph tracings for changes. Underlying pulmonary disease, a shift in the endotracheal tube, and surgical manipulation can be responsible for significant changes in compliance and ventilation. Initial tidal volumes of 10 mL/kg and rates of 20 to 25 breaths per minute are a reasonable starting point for most patients. With this rate and volume setting, it would be expected that peak airway pressures be approximately 20 cm H_2O. A level of positive end-expiratory pressure (PEEP) of 3 to 5 cm H_2O can be useful in preventing atelectasis. If the patient has significant pulmonary disease, he or she may require significantly higher volumes. The patient may have previously been ventilated in the neonatal intensive care unit with a ventilator modality not supported by the anesthesia ventilator. Consequently, parameters must be adjusted against physical examination and, if necessary, an arterial blood gas to ensure appropriate ventilation. If the patient has been dependent on special ventilator techniques such as high-frequency ventilation, oscillation, or nitric oxide inhalation, arrangements should be made to bring the needed equipment to the operating room and have a respiratory therapist or neonatologist who is familiar with the equipment assist in setup and, if necessary, troubleshooting.

Impact of Surgical Requirements on Anesthetic Technique

Every procedure has its own unique challenges. With any surgery, issues related to presurgical resuscitation, perioperative fluid and blood loss, heat loss from the surgical field, likely perioperative complications, and the likely need for postoperative intubation and ventilation should be anticipated, both on the basis of experience and communication about the unique needs of the upcoming procedure. There is a dramatic increase in the use of laparoscopic and thoracoscopic approaches to lesions, even in the smallest neonates. The considerations for these approaches are different from open procedures. There may be less blood, fluid, and heat loss, but there are additional issues related to positioning, insufflation pressures in the chest and abdomen, and prolonged surgical time. As new techniques evolve, close communication between the anesthesiologist and surgeon is necessary to ensure adequate preparation and resolution of problems or complications.

Uptake and Distribution of Anesthetics in Neonates

Various reasons for the faster uptake of anesthetics in infants have been proposed: (1) the ratio of alveolar ventilation to FRC is 5:1 in the infant and 1.5:1 in the adult; (2) in the neonate, more of the cardiac output goes to the vessel-rich group of organs, which includes the heart and brain; (3) the neonate has a greater cardiac output per kilogram of body mass; and (4) the infant has a lower blood gas partition coefficient for volatile anesthetics. One not well-recognized factor that may result in higher concentrations of volatile anesthetics being administered to infants has to do with the use of nonrebreathing systems such as the Bain or a Mapleson "D" circuit. When an adult circle system is used with infant tubes and bag, the clinician experienced with this equipment is used to reading the inspired, end-tidal, and dialed concentrations of the volatile anesthetic. In the circle system, the inspired concentration is a result of the combination of the end-tidal concentration that is rebreathed through the soda lime absorber and the dialed concentration. The inspired concentration is always lower than the dialed concentration, unless the flow rates are so high that a nonrebreathing system has been created. In the nonrebreathing system, the dialed concentration is the inspired concentration. Clinicians who use both systems are accustomed to these subtle differences. However, if the clinician switches back and forth between the circle system and a nonrebreathing circuit, but does so infrequently, there is a danger of not recognizing the possibility of excessive overpressure of volatile anesthetics with the nonrebreathing systems.

Anesthetic Dose Requirements of Neonates

Neonates and premature infants have lower anesthetic requirements than older infants and children.[32] The easiest way to remember the minimum alveolar concentration (MAC) values is that the MAC value in the mature state (i.e., late teenager or adult) is the same as for a full-term infant. By 6 months of age, the MAC value has increased by 50%. In the premature infant, the MAC value decreases by 20 to 30%.[33,34] The reasons for the lower MAC requirements are believed to be an immature nervous system, progesterone from the mother, and elevated blood levels of endorphins, coupled with an immature blood–brain barrier. The neonate has an immature CNS with attenuated responses to nociceptive cutaneous stimuli. These responses rapidly mature in the first several months of an infant's life, along with an increase in the MAC. Progesterone has been shown to reduce the MAC of the pregnant mother. The newborn infant has elevated progesterone levels, similar to those of the mother. Elevated levels of β-endorphin and β-lipotropin have been demonstrated in infants in the first few days of postnatal life. Endorphins do not cross the blood–brain barrier in adults; however, it is believed that the neonate's blood–brain barrier is more permeable and that endorphins might well pass into the CNS, thus elevating the pain threshold and reducing the MAC requirement.

Regional Anesthesia

There has been a tremendous increase in the use of regional anesthesia in infants and children. In general, regional techniques are combined with general anesthesia to permit early extubation and provide postoperative pain relief. Useful regional anesthesia techniques include spinal anesthesia, caudal anesthesia, epidural analgesia, penile block, and other peripheral nerve blocks (Table 44-4). Combined regional and general anesthesia is commonly

TABLE 44-4

REGIONAL ANESTHESIA TECHNIQUES USEFUL IN NEONATES

Central neuraxial
 Caudal
 Epidural (lumbar, thoracic, caudal)
 Spinal
Peripheral nerve blocks
 Infraorbital block
 Brachial plexus block (axillary, infraclavicular)
 Lateral femoral cutaneous block
 Penile block
 Ilioinguinal block
 Scalp blocks

provided for neonates for multiple procedures. The use of ultrasonography has revolutionized the use of regional anesthesia as vascular structures can be easily avoided while still providing a regional blockade.[127] It is important to remember that the dosage of local anesthetic solution used is limited and lipid solution is available to potentially treat any intravascular injections.[128] A dose of 1.5 mL/kg of intralipid has been suggested as a rescue dose for toxicity in children.

Spinal Anesthesia

Regional anesthesia can be provided as a sole anesthetic or in combination with general anesthesia. The use of sole regional anesthesia in neonates and infants is provided for the ex-premature infant with a potential for apnea. For patients receiving combined general and regional anesthesia, early extubation is possible because the addition of regional anesthetic techniques eliminates the need for intraoperative narcotics in neonates, reduces or eliminates the need for muscle relaxants, and reduces the concentration of volatile agents needed for relaxation.[129] Spinal anesthesia has been reported to be effective when used as the sole anesthetic technique in premature and high-risk infants, but this technique requires excellent cooperation between the anesthesiologist and an experienced surgeon.[130] Although this is technically feasible, because of increasing advancements in general anesthesia techniques, we may be able to provide safer anesthesia with fewer complications.[131,132] Even at a dose of 0.5 to 1 mg/kg, the effects of tetracaine last only approximately 90 minutes in the neonate.

In the authors' experiences, patients have additionally benefited by providing a caudal block in addition to the spinal anesthetic and seem to have a longer duration of surgical anesthesia. Total spinal anesthesia, produced either with a primary spinal technique or secondary to an attempted epidural puncture, will present as respiratory insufficiency rather than as hypotension because of the lack of sympathetic tone in infants. The exact mechanism for the lack of cardiovascular change with spinal anesthesia in infants and young children is not clear. Consequently, the first indication of a high spinal is falling oxygen saturation rather than a falling blood pressure. Sedation can be added to regional anesthesia but may cause problems of apnea in ex-premature infants.[133]

Caudal Block

Caudal epidural block is frequently used for abdominal surgery in neonates and is probably the most commonly used regional anesthetic technique in neonates and infants. There are several different techniques described for performing a caudal. The landmarks are the coccyx, the two sacral cornua, and the posterior superior iliac spines (Fig. 44-10). We prefer a styletted 22-gauge, short-bevel needle; the caudal space is identified both by the loss of resistance and the ease of administering the anesthetic. Once the sacrococcygeal membrane is penetrated and there is a loss of resistance, gentle aspiration is applied to the needle to determine if there is blood or cerebrospinal fluid. Injection of the anesthetic is then attempted. If there is difficulty in injecting the solution, the tip of the needle is not in the caudal space and it needs to be repositioned. If the anesthetic can be injected easily, this confirms placement in the epidural space. The needle is not advanced up the caudal canal after proper placement in the caudal epidural space has been accomplished. Other methods to identify the caudal space have been described, including stimulating technique[134] and ultrasound guidance.[135] Epinephrine is added to local anesthetic solutions for the purposes of determining if there is an intravascular injection of the anesthetic. Evidence of an intravascular injection includes (1) peaked T waves (which may be of relatively short duration, e.g., 30 seconds),[136] and (2) increase in heart

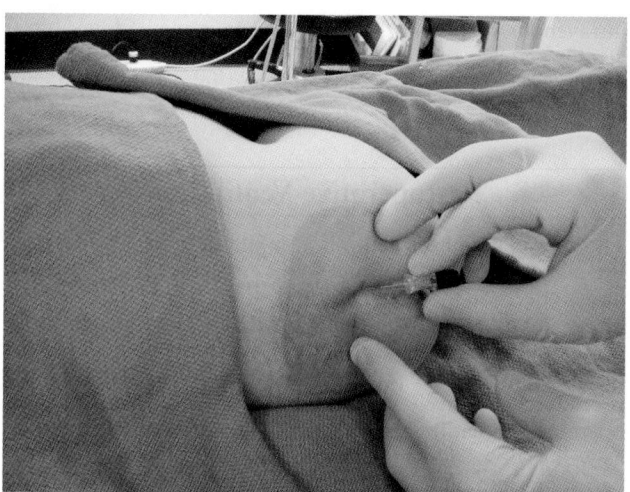

FIGURE 44-10. Caudal block. The sacral cornua are identified. A styletted needle is introduced into the caudal space through the sacral hiatus. A "pop" is felt as the sacrococcygeal ligament is accessed. After aspiration, 0.8 mL/kg of local anesthetic solution is injected. This provides analgesia for hernia repair, circumcisions, and lower abdominal surgeries.

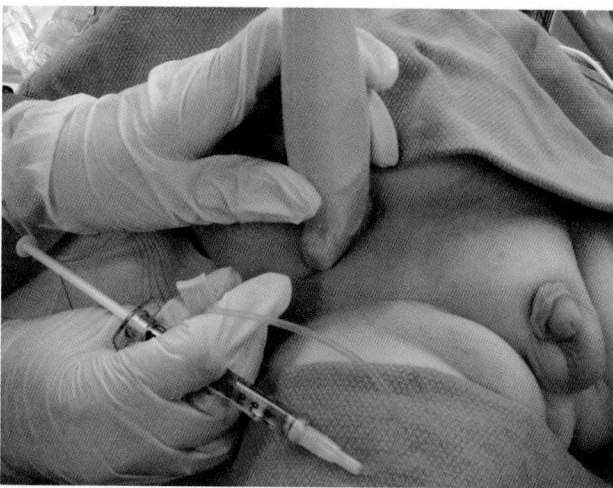

FIGURE 44-11. Ilioinguinal nerve block. Using a linear ultrasound probe, the anterior superior iliac spine is identified. The layers of the abdomen including the external oblique, transversus abdominis, and iliacus muscles are identified. The ilioinguinal and iliohypogastric nerves are located under the internal oblique muscle and in the plane between the internal oblique and the transversus abdominis muscle. A 27-gauge needle is inserted under ultrasound guidance in this plane. After aspiration, 0.1 mL/kg of local anesthetic solution is injected. This block can be used for pain relief following hernia surgery. (Reprinted from Langman J: Body cavities and serous membranes, Langman's Medical Embryology, 5th edition. Edited by Sadler TW. Baltimore, Williams & Wilkins, 1985, p 147, with permission.)

rate. The other technique to minimize the potential difficulties of an intravascular injection is to fractionate the dose by dividing the dose into three aliquots and waiting approximately 20 to 30 seconds between each aliquot before continuing the injection. Caudal anesthesia is particularly effective at reducing the concentrations of volatile anesthetics needed, as well as relaxants and opioids. In addition, a single-injection caudal anesthetic can provide analgesia for 6 to 8 hours. The two local anesthetics currently in use are 0.125% bupivacaine or 0.2% ropivacaine. Epinephrine, 1:200,000, is added to local anesthetics to assist in determining if there has been an intravenous injection. Ropivacaine has been reported to be less cardiodepressant than equipotent doses of bupivacaine. Occasionally, we place a caudal catheter for providing continuous analgesia in the postoperative period. If a caudal catheter is placed, an infusion of ropivacaine or bupivacaine can be administered and provide analgesia for several days. Current recommendations for infusions in neonates and young infants are for an initial loading dose of 0.2 to 0.25 mg/kg; after 1 to 2 hours, an infusion can be begun in a dose of 0.2 mg/kg/hr.[76] The addition of clonidine, 1.0 to 2.0 μg/kg, to local anesthetic for caudal block has been used, although this has not shown to greatly increase the duration of analgesia.[137] Opioids can occasionally be used for epidural infusions. However caution must be exercised in infants who may be prone to apnea with even moderate doses of opioids in the epidural space.

Epidural Analgesia

With the introduction of newer and smaller needles and epidural catheters we are now able to provide epidural analgesia in neonates and infants. Although most practitioners prefer using a caudal route to place catheters in the epidural space, we believe that with the introduction of ultrasound guidance, we are able to place lumbar catheters in neonates and infants easily.[138] It is imperative to limit the dose of local anesthetic solution in neonates and children to avoid toxicity.

Peripheral Nerve Blocks

Common peripheral nerve blocks in neonates include penile blocks, ilioinguinal nerve blocks, lateral femoral cutaneous blocks, brachial plexus blocks, and head and neck blocks for neurosurgical procedures.

Penile Block. This is a relatively simple block that can be performed easily. The dorsal nerves of the penis are located on either side of the shaft of the penis. A ring block using a non-epinephrine-containing solution can be used to provide analgesia following circumcision.[139]

Ilioinguinal Nerve Block. The ilioinguinal and iliohypogastric nerves supply sensory innervation to the inguinal area. These nerves can be easily visualized while operating. However, we find that blockade of these nerves can provide adequate postoperative analgesia (Fig. 44-11). The anterior superior iliac spine is identified. Immediately medial to the anterior superior iliac spine, a needle is inserted toward the umbilicus and local anesthesia is fanned into the area. The advantage with the use of ultrasonography is the ability to significantly reduce the dose of local anesthesia.[74] In our practice, we routinely use ultrasonography to localize the ilioinguinal nerve, which is then blocked with minimal quantity of local anesthesia solution. A new technique using ultrasonography can be used for these blocks.

Lateral Femoral Cutaneous Blocks. The lateral femoral cutaneous nerve is a sensory branch of the lumbar plexus that supplies the lateral aspect of the thigh. This block is particularly useful in neonates who undergo muscle biopsies of the muscle of the lateral thigh.[129]

Brachial Plexus Block. This is performed for major limb surgery including major hand and arm plastic surgical procedures. The axillary approach to the brachial plexus is our preferred approach in neonates and infants. Currently, we use ultrasonography to identify each one of the branches of the brachial

TABLE 44-5

POSTOPERATIVE PAIN CONTROL FOR NEONATES
AND INFANTS

Intravenous
  Opioids: morphine, fentanyl, methadone
  NSAIDs: ketorolac
Oral
  Acetaminophen
  Ibuprofen
  Hydrocodone
  Codeine
Rectal
  Acetaminophen
  Diclofenac
Regional and local anesthesia

NSAIDs, nonsteroidal anti-inflammatory drugs.

plexus to block them selectively,[140] thus allowing us to reduce the dose of local anesthesia needed for the block. For sustained pain relief, we prefer using an infraclavicular catheter.[141]

Neurosurgical Blocks.   Peripheral nerve blocks of the head and neck are useful for many surgical procedures. These may be useful in the sick neonate who requires a neurosurgical procedure. Peripheral nerve blocks of the trigeminal nerves, especially the frontal and occipital nerve branches, may be used to provide analgesia while avoiding general anesthesia.[142]

Postoperative Pain Management

The concepts of postoperative pain management are well known to most anesthesiologists. The use of intraoperative epidural anesthesia followed by postoperative epidural local anesthetics or opioids has been popular in older children and adults, and these techniques are being applied to neonates. In addition, most neonatologists are experienced with the intravenous administration of opioids for patient comfort. Each technique has its own risks and benefits.

Oral Routes.   Oral routes of medications have been used for decades in neonates and children for managing pain. The commonly used oral analgesics include nonsteroidal analgesics including acetaminophen (20 mg/kg) and ibuprofen (5 mg/kg), and opioids including codeine (0.5 mg/kg) and hydrocodone (0.1 mg/kg). There may be some pharmacogenetic changes associated with the use of codeine in infants.[143]

Rectal Routes.   Rectal suppositories are used frequently in neonates and infants for managing pyrexia. Rectal acetaminophen is commonly used for postoperative analgesia. A larger dose than is usually given orally is needed in infants to achieve good blood levels. A dose of 20 to 30 mg/kg is generally recommended for postoperative pain control.[144] Diclofenac, a commonly available rectal suppository in Europe, is frequently used in infants for postoperative pain control.[145]

Intravenous Analgesia.   Opioids are the mainstay of analgesia in neonates and infants in the postoperative period. Morphine and fentanyl are frequently used in the neonatal intensive care unit for analgesia. However, the potential for opioid tolerance after prolonged infusion of opioids is not uncommon. To decrease the likelihood of opioid tolerance,[40] one can rotate opioids or add other medications including continuous

intravenous naloxone[146] and intravenous methadone. Intravenous ketorolac, a nonsteroidal anti-inflammatory drug, has been used successfully in neonates and infants for pain control.[147]

Postoperative Ventilation

The choice of an anesthetic drug should be guided by the need for postoperative management of ventilation, as well as the drug's effects on the circulation and other organs. If the surgical procedure or the neonate's condition is such that postoperative ventilation is likely, the prolonged respiratory effects of opioids or any other drug are of little concern. However, if the surgical procedure is relatively short and by itself does not require postoperative ventilation, the clinician should carefully select drugs, as well as doses of anesthetic drugs and relaxants, that will not necessitate prolonged postoperative ventilation or intubation. Postoperative ventilation places the neonate at added risk because of the problems associated with mechanical ventilation, the trauma to the subglottic area, and the potential development of postoperative subglottic stenosis or edema. However, if there is any question about the neonate's ability to maintain protective airway reflexes or normal ventilation after anesthesia, the neonate should be returned to the recovery room or newborn intensive care unit with the trachea intubated, and either ventilated or treated with a small amount of PEEP (2 to 4 cm H_2O).

SPECIAL CONSIDERATIONS

Maternal Drug Use During Pregnancy

Many drugs taken during pregnancy can affect the fetus and neonate. One area of special concern is substance abuse. Maternal drug use during pregnancy of cocaine, marijuana, and others leads to a host of problems for the neonate. Cocaine use, for instance, results in a reduced catecholamine reuptake, which may result in the accumulation of catecholamines. This has circulatory effects on the uterus, the umbilical blood vessels, and the fetal cardiovascular system. Three major problems affecting the infant are premature birth, intrauterine growth retardation, and cardiovascular abnormalities, including low cardiac output.[148] The cardiac output and stroke volume are reduced on the first day of life but return to normal by the second day. The clinical implication of this finding is these neonates may be unstable enough in the first day of life that it may be advantageous to postpone surgery, if possible, until the second or third day of life. There is also an increase in structural cardiovascular malformations and electrocardiographic abnormalities. The most frequent lesions are peripheral pulmonic stenosis, right ventricular conduction delay, right ventricular hypertrophy, and ST segment and T-wave changes.[149] Preanesthetic history should elicit the use of drugs, including illicit use, if possible, to evaluate potential alteration of the anesthetic approach.

Temperature Control and Thermogenesis

The newborn is at risk for significant metabolic derangements caused by hypothermia. Newborns, and especially preterms, do not have the normal compensatory mechanisms that infants and children have when exposed to a cold environment. The newborn does not shiver, increase activity, or effectively vasoconstrict like older children or adults do in response to cold. In addition, the newborn has a larger body surface area-to-weight ratio that promotes heat loss, as well as low levels of subcutaneous fat for insulation. The primary mechanism the newborn has to respond to heat loss is nonshivering thermogenesis.[150] When there is a 2-degree Centigrade gradient between core and skin, there is a release of norepinephrine into the bloodstream. Norepinephrine stimulates increased metabolism in a specialized tissue, brown fat, that is high in mitochondria and has abundant vascular supply. Stimulated lipolysis results in heat production, with side effects of increased oxygen consumption and production of ketone bodies and water. Ketone production causes both a metabolic acidosis and osmotic dieresis. The aerobic activity results in diversion of cardiac output to the deposits of brown fat around the kidneys, under the sternum, and between the scapulae. Because the diuresis, diversion of cardiac output away from the core circulation, and metabolic acidosis are maladaptive, every effort should be made to prevent nonshivering thermogenesis in the newborn.

Efforts to minimize nonshivering thermogenesis in the newborn are based on minimizing heat loss, both during transport to and from the neonatal intensive care unit and in the operating room. Transport should be done with the newborn in an incubator, not an open bed with overhead heaters. This will prevent heat loss from conduction and radiation. In the operating room, the room temperature is raised to its maximal level to minimize loss by conduction. Placing the patient on a forced-air warming blanket can reduce conductive heat loss dramatically,[151] as well as using plastic wrap or commercially available covers and hats to minimize heat loss from the head and all other areas not in the surgical field. The goal of all these activities is to maintain a neutral thermal environment, minimizing the stress that hypothermia can induce in the perioperative period. A complicating factor is that anesthetic agents can reduce or eliminate thermogenesis, removing any ability to compensate for cold stress.[152,153]

Respiratory Distress Syndrome

Because of the enormous technical ability of the neonatologist and the resources of neonatal intensive care units, many small infants survive and some need surgery. One of the frequent problems of preterm infants is the occurrence of the RDS secondary to a deficiency of surfactant. As discussed earlier, the use of exogenous surfactant has been widely used in premature infants of low birth weight either to prevent or to treat RDS. As a result, fewer infants now die of this entity, and the incidence of complications related to RDS has dropped. One of the long-term consequences of RDS is bronchopulmonary dysplasia. *Bronchopulmonary dysplasia* refers to a continuum of chronic disease of the lung parenchyma and airways, as well as neurodevelopment that occurs in preterms, especially under 32 weeks gestation, who have survived RDS.[154] The theories of the cause of this condition include toxicity from oxygen administration, infection, inflammation, and barotrauma. Characteristics include airway smooth muscle hyperplasia, peribronchiolar fibrosis, enlarged alveoli, and disorganized pulmonary vasculature. Many patients improve as they age, but reactive airways, recurrent pulmonary infections, and a prolonged oxygen requirement are seen in some patients. Anesthetic concerns in these patients include evaluation of baseline oxygenation and potential presence of active bronchoconstriction. These patients often benefit from additional bronchodilator before induction. The baseline measure of oxygenation is important because these patients have less pulmonary oxygen reserve and may desaturate quickly with induction of anesthesia and hypoventilation. In patients with severe bronchopulmonary dysplasia, ventilatory management may be complicated by poor lung compliance and hyperinflation, as well as reactive airway disease. Although postanesthetic intubation is not usually required, a high index of suspicion should be used if there is significant clinical evidence of poor lung function preoperatively.

Postoperative Apnea

7 Apnea and bradycardia are well-recognized, major complications during and after surgery in neonates.[155] The infants at highest risk are those born prematurely, those with multiple congenital anomalies, those with a history of apnea and bradycardia, and those with chronic lung disease. The etiology of neonatal apnea is multifactorial. Decreased ventilatory control and hyporesponsiveness to hypoxia and hypercarbia may be potentiated by anesthetic agents. Respiratory muscle fatigue may also play a role because neonates have a smaller percentage of type I fibers in their diaphragm and intercostal muscles. In addition, hypothermia and anemia can also contribute to the development of postoperative apnea. The treatment of postoperative apnea or bradycardia may be as simple as tactile stimulation. However, some infants require mask ventilation or even prolonged intubation and ventilatory support. Infants with life-threatening apnea and bradycardia before surgery may be receiving CNS stimulants. Caffeine and theophylline (metabolized to caffeine) act by increasing central respiratory drive and lowering the threshold of response to hypercarbia, as well as stimulating contractility in the diaphragm. Caffeine is favored because of its wider therapeutic margin and decreased propensity for toxicity. Administering caffeine prophylactically to infants at risk of postoperative apnea to ensure adequate serum levels may prevent the need for prolonged periods of postoperative ventilatory support. The recommended loading dose is 10 mg/kg caffeine base.[156] Those infants at high risk for development of postoperative apnea may benefit from the use of a regional anesthetic as opposed to general anesthesia. Spinal anesthesia without supplemental sedation decreases the incidence of postoperative apnea and bradycardia in high-risk infants, but this advantage is lost if supplemental sedation is used.[157]

The question remains as to which infant should be admitted and monitored after outpatient surgery and for how long. The most conservative approach is to monitor all infants younger than 60 weeks postconceptual age overnight after surgery.[158] Although the incidence of significant apnea and bradycardia is highest in the first 4 to 6 hours after surgery, it can occur up to 12 hours after surgery. In addition, the incidence of apnea directly correlates to postconceptual age. The risk of apnea goes up the younger the gestational age. An insightful approach to interpreting the various small studies is to stratify the risk of apnea, as done by Cote et al.[159] Using a meta-analysis, the study determined that the risk of apnea could be correlated with a combination of gestational age and postconceptual age. Using 95% confidence limits, the authors found that the probability of apnea in nonanemic infants free of recovery room apnea was not <5% until postconceptual age was 48 weeks with gestational age of 35 weeks. This risk was not <1%, until a postconceptual age of 56 weeks with a gestational age of 32 weeks or a postconceptual age of 54 weeks and gestational age of 35 weeks. This type of analysis allows the clinician to determine which patients should be admitted not only on the criteria of gestational and postconceptual ages, but also the amount of risk they are willing to assume.

Retinopathy of Prematurity

As the survival rate of increasingly preterm infants has grown, there is increasing concern about the development of retinopathy of prematurity (ROP). The very preterm infant, especially those under 1,200 g of weight, are at highest risk, with an incidence of significant disease about 2%. Acute retinal changes are seen in about 45% of susceptible preterms, but there is spontaneous regression in most, permitting development of normal vision, but other infants will progress to a severe form of ROP and potential permanent blindness. Several complex factors may be responsible for the development of ROP. In the fetus, developing blood vessels grow gradually from the macula toward the edges of the developing retina. In full-term newborns, this process is complete at birth or in the first few weeks, but continues for a longer period in the preterm infant. These growing vessels are at risk for vasoconstriction and subsequent hemorrhage, followed by disorganized neovascularization or scarring. This scarring and lack of normal growth can eventually cause the retinal network to peel away, retinal detachment. The spectrum or stages of disease is classified as follows:

Stage I. Mildly abnormal blood vessel growth. Many children who develop stage I improve with no treatment and eventually develop normal vision.

Stage II. Moderately abnormal blood vessel growth. Many children who develop stage II improve with no treatment and eventually develop normal vision. The disease resolves on its own without further progression.

Stage III. Severely abnormal blood vessel growth. The abnormal blood vessels grow toward the center of the eye instead of following their normal growth pattern along the surface of the retina. Some infants who develop stage III disease improve with no treatment and eventually develop normal vision. However, when infants have a certain degree of stage III and "plus disease" develops, treatment is considered. Plus disease means that the blood vessels of the retina have become enlarged and twisted, indicating a worsening of the disease. Treatment at this point provides a good chance of preventing retinal detachment.

Stage IV. Partially detached retina

Stage V. Completely detached retina

The most common cited cause of ROP is hyperoxia from administered oxygen, but hypoxemia, hypotension, sepsis, intraventricular hemorrhage, and other stresses have been implicated. At one time, there was concern that exposure to bright ambient light could cause ROP, but this has been disproven.[160] Although there may be spontaneous regression in early stages, there may also be progression to advanced stages and retinal detachment. The most common therapies involve using cryotherapy or laser therapy to destroy peripheral areas of the retina, slowing or reversing the abnormal growth of blood vessels. This is done to preserve the central vision from continuing distortion of the abnormal vessels in the periphery, although there is some loss of peripheral vision with this therapy.[161] In advanced stages, partial retinal detachment can be treated with a scleral buckle or vitrectomy.

The cryotherapy and laser therapies, as well as advanced procedures, are usually performed under general anesthesia in the operating room, although it is occasionally done at bedside with sedation in ventilated patients. The surgical procedures do not involve blood loss or significant surgical stress, but they do depend on a still surgical field for periods ranging from 30 to 90 minutes. The primary anesthetic challenge in these patients is related to the extreme prematurity and small size of the patients. Adequate monitoring, vascular access, and thermal stability are common challenges to management.

The risks of the development of ROP from hyperoxia have been of concern to anesthesiologists who anesthetize preterm neonates for any type of surgery. Can supplemental oxygen during an anesthetic start the development of ROP in preterm patients? We do not have an absolute direct answer to this question, but some evidence from a large collaborative study may help provide some guidance. Premature infants with confirmed early stages of ROP and a median pulse oximetry <94% saturation were randomized to a conventional oxygen arm with pulse oximetry targeted at 89 to 94% saturation or a supplemental arm with pulse oximetry targeted at 96 to 99% saturation for at least 2 weeks.[162] The patients were then reexamined for progression of disease. Use of supplemental oxygen at pulse oximetry saturations of 96 to 99% did not cause additional progression of prethreshold ROP. This study demonstrates that the use of supplemental oxygen for a prolonged period of time, not just for the short duration of a general anesthetic, was not deleterious as long as the pulse oximetry readings were kept in the 96 to 99% range. Consequently, keeping pulse oximetry readings in this range during an anesthetic should not be responsible for causing a progression of ROP in susceptible patients.

Neurodevelopmental Effects of Anesthetic Agents

There has been recent concern about the potential deleterious impact of anesthetic drugs on the developing brain. A variety of studies have shown that prolonged exposure of animal models to anesthetic agents can lead to neurodegenerative changes in the developing brain of neonatal rats.[163] However, these exposures to volatile agents and ketamine were for prolonged periods, the equivalent of several weeks of continuous exposure in the human. Nonetheless, this is an area of great concern for anesthesiologists.[164] Animal experiments have demonstrated neurocognitive changes in animals exposed to NMDA receptor antagonists like ketamine, volatile agents like isoflurane, as well as other agents including midazolam. The collective data that are currently available in literature do not support the withdrawal of these drugs from the practice of pediatric anesthesia. The data seem to be reproducible in rodents but not in other species. Future prospective trials with prospective neurocognitive testing of infants exposed to anesthesia is needed to determine if this applies to the human neonate. At the time of writing this chapter, there was no conclusive evidence to demonstrate the deleterious effect of inhaled or intravenous anesthetics on neurocognitive function in neonates and infants.

SURGICAL PROCEDURES IN NEONATES

8 Surgical procedures in neonates are functionally divided into two periods: those performed in the first week and those performed in the first month. There has been a strong trend in recent years to put on emphasis of presurgical stabilization before taking the newborn to the operating room. This has reduced the emergent nature of newborn surgeries. Many procedures that used to be done an emergent basis, even in the middle of the night, such as repair of congenital diaphragmatic hernia or omphalocele, are now done days later after initial therapy has been instituted. Exceptions to this include gastroschisis, which is usually attended to within 12 to 24 hours, airway lesions such as webs that are causing significant airway obstruction, and acute subdural/epidural hematomas from traumatic delivery. In most cases, however, a period of 1 to 3 days can be allowed for stabilization of the newborn or transport to an appropriate pediatric center for treatment. There is more to neonatal emergency surgery than just the immediate anesthetic and surgical procedure. Many of these infants require the support services of specialized nursing units, pediatric radiologists, pediatric intensive care physicians, specialized laboratory facilities, and they must have their complete care be the main consideration of where their surgery should be done.

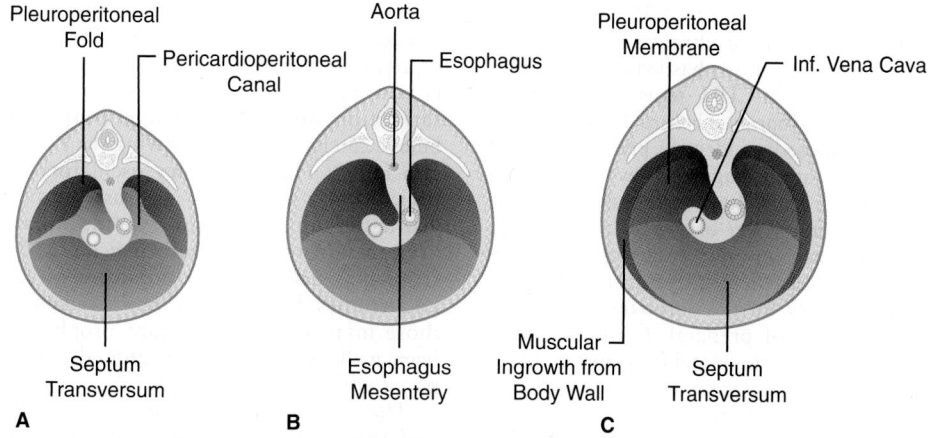

FIGURE 44-12.   Schematic drawings illustrating the development of the diaphragm. **A.** The pleuroperitoneal folds appear at the beginning of the sixth week. **B.** The pleuroperitoneal folds have fused with the septum transversum and the mesentery of the esophagus in the seventh week, thus separating the thoracic cavity from the abdominal cavity. **C.** In a transverse section at the fourth month of development, an additional rim derived from the body wall forms the most peripheral part of the diaphragm. (Reprinted from Langman J: Body cavities and serous membranes, Langman's Medical Embryology, 5th edition. Edited by Sadler TW. Baltimore, Williams & Wilkins, 1985, p 147, with permission.)

Surgical Procedures in the First Week of Life

The most frequent major surgical procedures performed in the first week of life are for congenital diaphragmatic hernia (CDH), omphalocele and gastroschisis, tracheoesophageal fistula (TEF), intestinal obstruction, and meningomyelocele. Some of these conditions, such as CDH, omphalocele and gastroschisis, and meningomyelocele, are obvious at birth. It may take hours or days for a TEF or intestinal obstruction to become manifest. Because of the lack of expertise many hospitals have in the care of these patients, the transfer of these neonates to hospitals with greater expertise is often prudent after initial stabilization of the patient. Most hospitals that have expertise in these patients have a transport team that is well qualified to help with stabilization and transport. Those that do not have transport teams often have extensive protocols and procedures to work with the other institution to help ensure the safe transfer of the patient.

Two confounding factors in neonatal surgery are prematurity and associated congenital anomalies. The presence of one congenital anomaly increases the likelihood of another one . In conditions such as TEF, the mortality rate from the associated congenital heart defect is higher than that from the surgical correction of the TEF. Prematurity, particularly when associated with RDS, may adversely affect surgical outcome. The use of surfactant in the treatment of the RDS has greatly increased the number of survivors and has decreased the complexity of the issues of the infant with a combination of TEF and RDS. A neonatologist should be consulted in the case of any neonate with a congenital defect who is considered for surgery. The most serious associated congenital lesion is that of the cardiovascular system. More than 10% of infants with an isolated CDH have a cardiac anomaly,[165] with a higher incidence in newborns with associated syndromes, and approximately 15 to 25% of infants with TEF have an associated congenital cardiac anomaly.[166]

Congenital Diaphragmatic Hernia

CDH occurs with an incidence of approximately 1 in 4,000 live births. Traditionally, the mortality rate from CDH was in the range of 40 to 50%. The new strategy of permissive hypercapnia and delayed surgical repair has resulted in survival rates of >75% in some centers.[167] However, the morbidity

remains high in survivors. A brief discussion of the embryologic characteristics of CDH will help the clinician understand the potentially enormous postoperative problems that may be encountered.

Embryology.   Early in fetal development, the pleuroperitoneal cavity is a single compartment. The gut is herniated or extruded to the extraembryonic coelom during the ninth to tenth weeks of fetal life. During this period, the diaphragm develops to separate the thoracic and abdominal cavities (Fig. 44-12). The development of the diaphragm is usually completed by the seventh fetal week. In the ninth to tenth weeks, the developing gut returns to the peritoneal cavity. If there is delay or incomplete closure of the diaphragm, or if the gut returns early and prevents normal closure of the diaphragm, a diaphragmatic hernia will develop, producing varying degrees of herniation of the intestinal contents into the chest. The left side of the diaphragm closes later than the right side, which results in the higher incidence of left-sided diaphragmatic hernias (foramen of Bochdalek). Approximately 90% of hernias detected in the first week of life are on the left side.

Clinical Presentation.   The clinical presentation and the outcome from a diaphragmatic hernia are varied. The bowel contents may compress the lung buds and prevent development, leading to bilateral hypoplastic lungs with very little chance for survival. In most instances, however, a moderately small diaphragmatic hernia may develop later in fetal life so the lung is normal but compressed by the abdominal viscera. At the mild end of the scale, the infant might have a relatively normal pulmonary vascular bed with varying degrees of persistent pulmonary hypertension that may rapidly revert to normal. In more severe defects, significant pulmonary hypoplasia and abnormal pulmonary vasculature lead to greater mortality.

After closure of the pleuroperitoneal membrane, muscular development of the diaphragm occurs. Incomplete muscularization of the diaphragm results in the development of a hernia sac because of intra-abdominal pressure. The condition is known as *eventration of the diaphragm*, and the diaphragm may extend well up into the thoracic cavity. The other possibility is that the innervation of the diaphragm is incomplete and the muscle is atonic. Eventration of the diaphragm is usually not symptomatic in the first week of life.

Antenatal Diagnosis. The diagnosis of CDH can be made prenatally by fetal ultrasonography or ultrafast fetal magnetic resonance imaging. Antenatal diagnosis has led to the identification of a "hidden mortality" in CDH, fetuses that did not survive gestation and neonates that died before diagnosis. Various factors have been proposed to identify predictability of survival, including early gestation diagnosis, severe mediastinal shift, polyhydramnios, a small lung-to-thorax transverse area ratio, and the herniation of liver or stomach. New techniques in fetal surgery, such as temporary endoscopic fetal tracheal occlusion, may prove beneficial to fetuses with CDH who are identified to be at risk for not surviving to term.[168] The other obvious advantage of prenatal diagnosis is that plans can be made for maternal or neonatal transport to a center with advanced neonatal critical care with availability of extracorporeal membrane oxygenation.

Clinical Presentation. The occurrence of symptoms depends on the degree of herniation and interference with pulmonary function. At times, the degree of interference is so great that the neonate's clinical condition begins to deteriorate immediately, whereas in other situations it may be several hours before the infant's condition is fully appreciated. In the severely involved newborn, the initial clinical findings are usually classic and readily discerned. The infant has a scaphoid abdomen secondary to the absence of intra-abdominal contents, which have herniated into the chest. Breath sounds on the affected side are reduced or absent. The diagnosis can be confirmed with a radiograph (Fig. 44-13). Immediate supportive care entails tracheal intubation and control of the airway, along with decompression of the stomach. Excessive airway pressure carries a high risk for pneumothorax and worsening of a bad situation.

Preoperative Care. CDH was traditionally treated as a surgical emergency. The infants were taken immediately to surgery for decompression and repair. The thought was that removing the abdominal viscera from the thorax would allow for re-expansion of the atelectatic lung and improved oxygenation. However, as the pathophysiology of CDH was more clearly defined—pulmonary hypoplasia associated with a hyperreactive pulmonary vasculature—a strategy of preoperative stabilization with delayed surgical repair was adopted.

The stabilization of an infant with CDH may require multiple treatment modalities. The use of aggressive ventilation strategies to induce hyperventilation alkalosis has been abandoned secondary to the high incidence of iatrogenic lung injury. Conventional ventilation with permissive hypercapnia is now favored. The goal is to maintain preductal arterial saturation above 85% using peak inspiratory pressures below 25 cm H_2O and allowing the PCO_2 to rise to 45 to 55 mm Hg.[167] High-frequency oscillatory ventilation, in addition to nitric oxide, has been used in place of conventional ventilation in an attempt to reduce barotraumas and has been demonstrated to be beneficial.[169] Neonates born with CDH may also have a component of surfactant deficiency, and studies have shown improvement in oxygenation in those infants given surfactant prophylactically. These have been well demonstrated in animal experiments when compared with tracheal ligation.[170]

The use of ECMO in infants with CDH was initiated in the mid-1980s. Despite extensive literature on the subject, there remains an ongoing debate as to whether ECMO improves survival in neonates with CDH. The Congenital Diaphragmatic Hernia Study Group analyzed data from the multicenter CDH Registry and determined that ECMO improves the survival rate in CDH neonates with a predicted high risk of mortality ($\geq$80%) based on birth weight and 5-minute Apgar score. A right-sided CDH may carry a higher mortality and morbidity compared with a left-sided defect, despite the use of ECMO.[171]

Perioperative Care. Because delayed surgical repair of CDH is now the norm, neonates with CDH frequently present to the operating room already intubated and on some form of ventilatory support. Despite a period of preoperative stabilization, some infants still have a component of reactive pulmonary hypertension. The goals of ventilatory management are to ensure adequate oxygenation and avoid barotrauma. Any sudden deterioration in oxygen saturation with or without associated hypotension should raise suspicion of pneumothorax. It is important to avoid hypothermia because this increases the oxygen requirement and could precipitate pulmonary hypertension. Blood loss and fluid shifts are usually not a problem, although maintenance of intravascular volume is essential to avoid acidosis, which could also precipitate pulmonary hypertension. More recently, these patients are being operated while on ECMO and mortality of these patients can be predicted based on fetal lung volumes.[172]

Anesthetic Technique. The anesthetic technique chosen depends on the size of the defect and the anticipated postoperative respiratory status. In those infants who will remain intubated after surgery, inhalation agents and narcotics may be used as tolerated. In those infants with a small defect who present to the operating room with little or no respiratory distress, it may be beneficial to avoid intraoperative narcotics and provide regional analgesia in anticipation of extubation. The use of nitrous oxide should be avoided, particularly in those situations in which abdominal closure could be difficult. Muscle relaxation is often needed to facilitate abdominal closure.

Postoperative Care. Most infants with CDH require intensive postoperative care. Recovery depends on the degree of pulmonary hypertension and pulmonary hypoplasia. It was previously believed that pulmonary hypoplasia was responsible for most deaths; however, it is now believed that potentially reversible pulmonary hypertension may be responsible for as much as 25% of reported deaths.

There is evidence to suggest that cardiac development is impaired in infants with CDH. Relative left ventricular hypoplasia with an attenuated muscle mass and cavity size have been described.

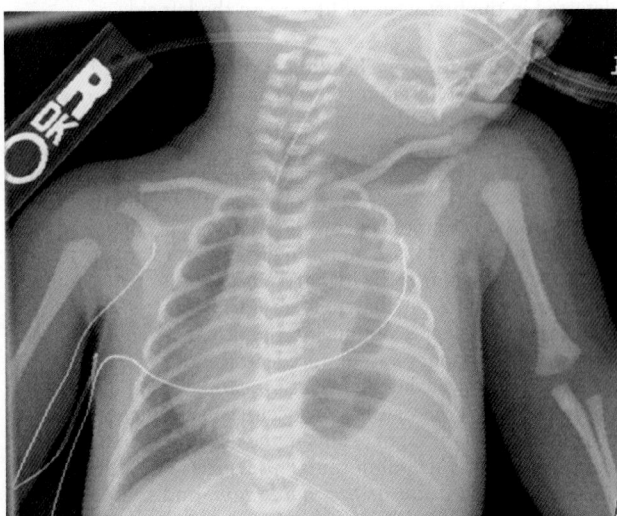

FIGURE 44-13. Infant with congenital diaphragmatic hernia. Note the loop of bowel gas in left hemithorax.

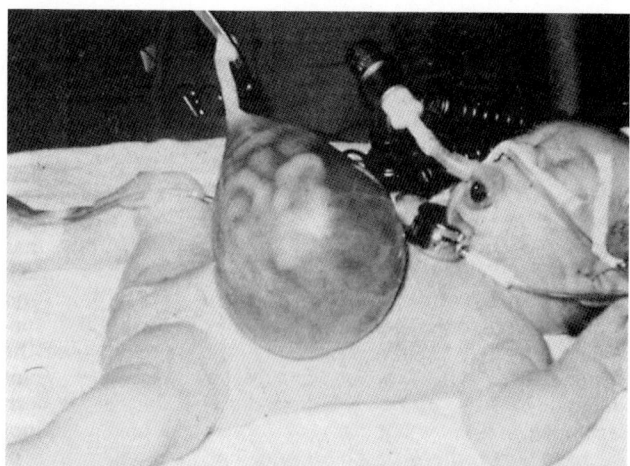

FIGURE 44-14.   Omphalocele. (Reprinted from Berry FA: Physiology and surgery of the infant, Anesthetic Management of Difficult and Routine Pediatric Patients. Edited by Berry FA. New York, Churchill Livingstone, 1990, p 152, with permission.)

Omphalocele and Gastroschisis

Although omphalocele and gastroschisis sometimes appear similar and may be confused, they have entirely different origins and associated congenital anomalies.[173] During the fifth to tenth weeks of fetal life, the abdominal contents are extruded into the extraembryonic coelom, and the gut returns to the abdominal cavity at approximately the tenth week. Failure of part of or all the intestinal contents to return to the abdominal cavity results in an omphalocele that is covered with a membrane called the *amnion* (Fig. 44-14). The amnion protects the abdominal contents from infection and the loss of extracellular fluid. The umbilical cord is found at approximately the apex of the sac. Gastroschisis, in contrast, develops later in fetal life, after the intestinal contents have returned to the abdominal cavity. It results from interruption of the omphalomesenteric artery, which results in ischemia and atrophy of the various layers of the abdominal wall at the base of the umbilical cord. The gut then herniates through this tissue defect. The degree of herniation may be slight, or major amounts of the abdominal viscera may be found outside the peritoneal cavity. The umbilical cord is found to one side of the intestinal contents (Fig. 44-15).

The intestines and viscera are not covered by any membrane and therefore are highly susceptible to infection and loss of extracellular fluid. There is a very high incidence of associated congenital anomalies with omphalocele, although much lower with gastroschisis.[174] The Beckwith-Wiedemann syndrome consists of mental retardation, hypoglycemia, congenital heart disease, a large tongue, and an omphalocele. Congenital heart lesions are found in approximately 20% of infants with omphalocele. Other associated congenital defects are found with gastroschisis and omphalocele; most involve the gastrointestinal tract and consist primarily of intestinal atresia or stenosis and malrotation. Because of the uncovered gut irritating the uterine lining, premature delivery is more common in gastroschisis patients.

Antenatal Diagnosis.   The overall incidence of these defects is about 1:5,00 live births. Screening for abdominal wall defects is accomplished through the use of maternal serum α-fetoprotein (AFP). AFP is a normal protein present in fetal tissues during fetal development. Closure of the abdominal wall and the neural tube (see "Meningomyelocele") prevents release of large quantities of this protein into the amniotic fluid. High levels of

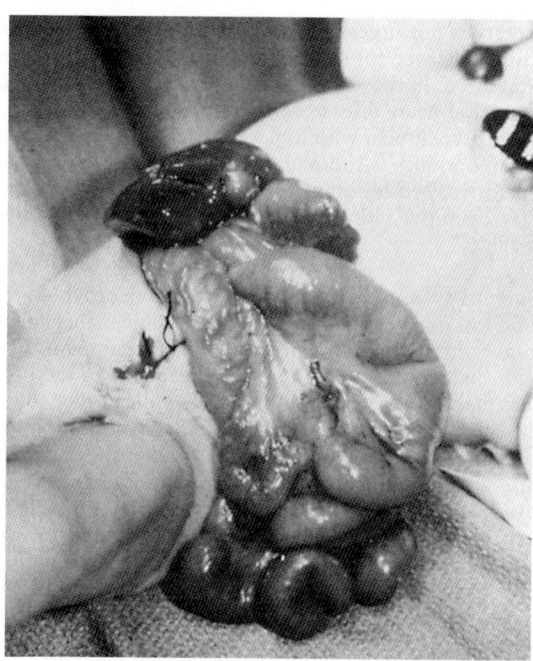

FIGURE 44-15.   Gastroschisis. (Reprinted from Berry FA: Physiology and surgery of the infant. Anesthetic Management of Difficult and Routine Pediatric Patients. Edited by Berry FA. New York, Churchill Livingstone, 1990, p 152, with permission.)

AFP in the amniotic fluid can cross the placenta and be detected in maternal blood. Thus, abnormal levels of maternal serum AFP in the mother raise concerns over the possibility of either an abdominal wall defect or a neural tube defect in the fetus, as do high levels of AFP in fluid obtained during amniocentesis. Levels tend to be higher when the defect is gastroschisis instead of omphalocele. The primary method of definitive fetal diagnosis of gastroschisis and omphalocele is ultrasonography. In a recent study, 88% of patients with gastroschisis and 69% with omphalocele were diagnosed prenatally with ultrasound.[175] An advantage of ultrasound is the ability to diagnosis other complicating abnormalities, such as cardiac defects.

Preoperative Care.   Most neonates with gastroschisis or omphalocele diagnosed prenatally are delivered by cesarean section. The advantages of this are the ability to prevent trauma to the exposed bowel and allow better coordination of the various medical specialties needed for immediate surgical management of the defect. Priorities in the delivery room care unique to an infant with gastroschisis are the need to protect the exposed bowel and minimize fluid and temperature loss. An effective way to achieve these goals involves placing the defect and lower body in a sterile, clear plastic bag to protect the defect and minimize heat and fluid loss. The bag can be filled with warm saline and a drawstring can be used to tighten the bag against the infant's body.

Preoperative stabilization of the neonate with an abdominal wall defect includes management of respiratory insufficiency, establishment of adequate intravenous access, and an assessment for associated congenital anomalies. It is expected that a significantly higher incidence in congenital anomalies will be found in omphalocele patients. Respiratory failure at birth in infants with omphalocele is a significant predictor of mortality.[176] Lung hypoplasia and abnormal thoracic development may be significant in infants with large omphaloceles. A difficult airway can be anticipated in the patient with Beckwith-Wiedemann syndrome because of the large tongue.

Surgery is not urgent in the neonate with an omphalocele and can be delayed for several days until the infant is assessed and stabilized. In those infants with severe respiratory distress or congenital heart disease who are too unstable for surgery, nonsurgical treatment with topical antiseptics and delayed closure is an option.[177] Although there has been some interest in nonoperative, bedside-staged closure of gastroschisis defects, primary operative closure continues to be the most common approach.[178]

Perioperative Care.   The two major perioperative concerns are fluid loss and ventilation. The fluid volume management of the infant often entails administration of large amounts of full-strength, balanced salt solution. The adequacy of the peripheral circulation and urine output is an indicator of the adequacy of the volume resuscitation. Both conditions may present an intraoperative challenge to the anesthesiologist because with an omphalocele, after the amniotic membrane is removed, large volumes of fluid may transude or exude from the exposed abdominal viscera. The fluid that is lost is extracellular fluid, which should be replaced with full-strength, balanced salt solution. An arterial line is often used for blood pressure monitoring and frequent blood gas monitoring to assess acid-base status.

If the defect in the abdominal wall is small, a primary repair of the deficit can be accomplished. However, with a large defect, it may be difficult to return the abdominal viscera to the peritoneal cavity because the muscle and peritoneum are underdeveloped. Because of concern for the increase in the volume of gas in the intestine, nitrous oxide should not be used. Muscle relaxation is necessary to allow closure of the abdomen. With moderate-size abdominal wall defects, it may not be possible to close the peritoneum, but there may be sufficient skin to close the defect. With large defects, the peritoneal cavity may be too small to contain the viscera, and attempted closure can impair circulation to the bowel, kidneys, and lower extremities, as well as compromise respiration. A pulse oximeter probe on the foot can be helpful in monitoring circulation to the lower extremities during abdominal wall closure.

Attempts have been made to find objective criteria by which to determine whether the infant will tolerate primary closure of the defect, and to avoid or minimize the circulatory and ventilatory problems. One method has been to measure intragastric pressure in infants who undergo primary closure. Intragastric pressure is measured by placing a nasogastric tube in the stomach and using a column of saline to measure the pressure.[179] Studies have used the criteria that if the intragastric pressure was ≤20 mm Hg, primary closure can proceed. Above 20 mm Hg pressures during closure, delayed closure and placement of a Dacron silo were used. With this approach, primary closure has been successful when used, with faster return to full feeds and shorter hospital length of stay compared with patients treated by delayed closure. Complications have been less with primary closure using this approach.

If primary closure is impossible, a silo is incorporated into the abdominal wall to contain and cover the abdominal viscera (Fig. 44-16). The repair is then staged from this point onward. Every 2 or 3 days, the size of the silo is reduced, in much the same fashion that a tube of toothpaste is squeezed. The infant may feel some degree of discomfort as the peritoneum and skin are stretched. Institutions vary in how they accomplish the delay closure, with some surgeons bringing the patient to the operating room for each stage and others doing this at bedside, often with the assistance of small doses of ketamine or other analgesics. Some of these patients remain on mechanical ventilation during this period, and others are extubated. In either case, both blood pressure and oxygen saturation should be closely monitored during and immediately after

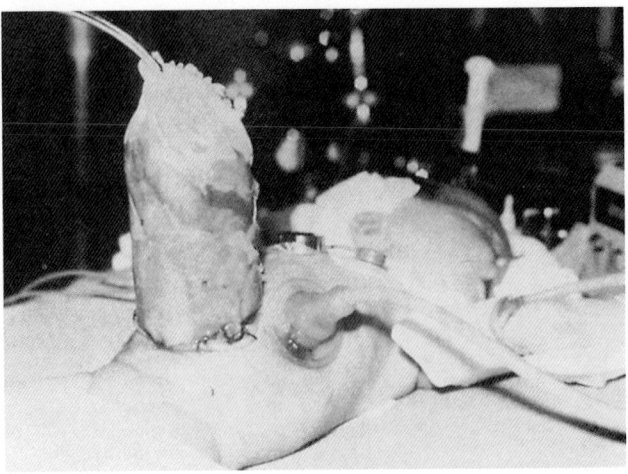

FIGURE 44-16.   Dacron silo for extruded viscera. (Reprinted from Berry FA: Physiology and surgery of the infant, Anesthetic Management of Difficult and Routine Pediatric Patients. Edited by Berry FA. New York, Churchill Livingstone, 1990, p 154, with permission.)

each stage of closure to ensure that the increase in abdominal and intrathoracic pressure does not significantly impede ventilation, oxygenation, and venous return. In some cases, further reduction must be delayed until there is more abdominal growth. This is a situation that requires clinical judgment. After several stages of silo reduction, the final operation is complete closure of the abdominal wall defect under full anesthesia with complete muscle relaxation.

Postoperative Care.   The postoperative care of infants with omphalocele or gastroschisis is critical. Some need tracheal intubation and assisted ventilation of the lungs for days to weeks. The ventilatory status of the patient is especially critical in omphalocele patients because up to half of these patients are born with pulmonary hypoplasia, making the balance of increased abdominal pressures and adequate ventilation and oxygenation especially challenging. Additional complications include postoperative hypertension and edema of the extremities. The increased abdominal pressure can reduce the circulation to the kidneys, which results in a release of renin. Renin activates the renin-angiotensin-aldosterone system, which is believed to cause the hypertension.

Tracheoesophageal Fistula

The treatment of esophageal atresia and TEF can be both challenging and satisfying for the anesthesiologist. Death in the perioperative period typically results from prematurity or from an associated congenital heart defect. TEF occurs in approximately 1 in 3,000 live births. Approximately 85% consist of a fistula from the distal trachea to the esophagus and a blind proximal esophageal pouch. In 10% of cases, there is a blind proximal esophageal pouch with no TEF (Fig. 44-17). The embryologic defect results from imperfect division of the foregut into the anteriorly positioned larynx and trachea and the posteriorly positioned esophagus; the division should occur between the fourth and fifth weeks of intrauterine life. Fifty percent of affected infants have associated congenital anomalies, of which approximately 15 to 25% involve the cardiovascular system.

Clinical Presentation.   Atresia of the esophagus leads to inability of the fetus to swallow amniotic fluid and the subsequent development of polyhydramnios. Ultrasound may well

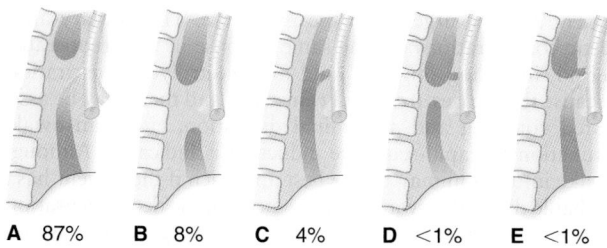

A 87%   **B** 8%   **C** 4%   **D** <1%   **E** <1%

FIGURE 44-17.   Diagrams of the five most commonly encountered forms of esophageal atresia and tracheoesophageal fistula, shown in order of frequency. (Reprinted from Herbst JJ: Gastrointestinal tract, Nelson Textbook of Pediatrics, 14th edition. Edited by Behrman RE, Kleigman RM, Nelson WE et al: Philadelphia, WB Saunders, 1992, p 942, with permission.)

raise the possibility of a congenital anomaly. For that reason, if polyhydramnios is present, attempts should be made to pass a nasogastric tube shortly after delivery. Passing a nasogastric tube is not routine in the delivery room; therefore, the diagnosis may not become apparent until the infant is fed. Cyanosis and choking with oral feedings should raise suspicion.

There are two major complications of esophageal atresia with a distal tracheal fistula: aspiration pneumonia and dehydration. The presence of a distal TEF increases the likelihood of reflux of gastric juice up the esophagus and into the pulmonary system. Dehydration results from the fact that the proximal esophagus does not communicate with the stomach. Therefore, preoperative preparation of these infants is aimed at evaluation and treatment of the pulmonary system, as well as at ensuring adequate hydration and electrolyte balance. Rarely, the degree of reflux and pneumonia is so great that a gastrostomy must be performed to protect the pulmonary system, and a period of several days is needed to improve the general condition of the infant. However, if the infant is in good condition, primary repair can be performed at 24 to 48 hours. This consists of ligation of the fistula and a primary repair with approximation of the two ends of the esophagus.

Anesthetic Considerations.   The repair of TEF can be done in the conventional method or by a thoracoscopic method. Both methods and the anesthetic implications for each technique will be described here. The presence of a gastrostomy reduces the potential for reflux of gastric juice during the surgical procedure. If a gastrostomy is present, the gastrostomy tube should be open to air and left at the head of the table under the anesthesiologist's observation to avoid kinking and obstruction.

Conventional Open TEF Closure.   There are three approaches to tracheal intubation after induction of anesthesia. One is to use an inhalation induction, followed by topical spray of lidocaine and intubation while the infant is breathing spontaneously. Another technique is to use an intravenous or inhalation induction and intubate the trachea after muscle paralysis. This technique may lead to distention of the fistula and stomach with excessive positive-pressure ventilation. When controlled ventilation of the lungs is used, attempts must be made to minimize the distention of the stomach and the potential for reflux. If a gastrostomy tube is in place, the point is moot. A third technique is to intubate the neonates awake with mild sedation. This can protect the airway while reducing the chances of aspiration. Alternatively, because the fistula is usually located just above the carina on the posterior wall of the membranous trachea, the endotracheal tube can be placed just distal to the TEF. To do this, the endotracheal tube is inserted until it enters one or the other main stem bronchi. This is judged by unilateral expansion of the chest and unilateral breath sounds. The endotracheal tube

is then slowly withdrawn until bilateral chest movement and breath sounds are confirmed.

The endotracheal tube might inadvertently enter the fistula when the infant is turned or during surgical manipulation. Intubation of the fistula should be suspected if there is increased difficulty in ventilation of the lungs, as well as decreased oxygen saturation and end-tidal CO_2. Because these findings may also be present when the lung is packed away to perform the surgery and because there are other explanations for these findings, intubation of the fistula should always be included in the differential diagnosis. Any time ventilation is difficult and desaturation is occurring, the surgeon must stop the procedure while the situation is clarified. The surgeon will be able to palpate the tip of the tube in the fistula if this is the problem.

The localization and isolation of H-type fistulas can be difficult. In this situation, direct laryngoscopy and bronchoscopy is performed by the surgeon, the fistula is identified, and a guidewire is fed through the fistula tract into the esophagus. The infant is then intubated, with care taken not to dislodge the guidewire. Once intubated esophagoscopy is performed, the guidewire is visualized and brought out through the mouth. In this way, the surgeon can use fluoroscopy to determine the level of the fistula and decide whether a cervical or thoracic approach is necessary. During surgery, the anesthesiologist can apply traction to the wire loop to facilitate the localization of the fistula by the surgeon.

Endoscopic TEF Repair.   The use of endoscopic methods for repair of TEF is being popularized in pediatric surgery.[180] The infant should be kept spontaneously breathing until the fistula is ligated. Maintenance of spontaneous ventilation can be challenging considering that these infants may not tolerate the use of potent inhalation agents while spontaneous ventilation is established. This approach may shorten the duration of surgical operating time while providing a minimally invasive method. The anesthetic management is still challenging.

Postoperative Care.   Although there have been great advances in the treatment of TEF and esophageal atresia, postoperative care can be complicated by associated congenital heart disease, RDS, and a need for continued postoperative ventilation. The compression of the lung for several hours, along with pre-existing aspiration pneumonia in some of these infants, suggest the need, in the more difficult cases, for a short period of postoperative ventilation, or at least intubation with PEEP, as the most conservative technique for postoperative airway management. Some infants are in excellent condition at the time of surgery with no complicating factors and, therefore, should be considered for extubation immediately at the end of surgery or shortly thereafter. If extubation of the trachea is planned for the end of surgery, the anesthetic technique must be tailored accordingly. Caudal anesthesia as part of the technique is useful in these situations, reducing the concentration of maintenance volatile anesthetics, the amount of muscle relaxants, and the need for intraoperative narcotics. We prefer placing caudal epidural catheters in these children for postoperative pain control. This offers good analgesia while at the same time avoiding the use of opioids, which may predispose these infants to apnea and respiratory depression.[181]

A high percentage of infants with esophageal atresia have residual difficulties of the tracheobronchial tree and esophagus for many years. These difficulties include tracheomalacia, gastroesophageal reflux, esophageal stricture, and recurrent fistulas.

Intestinal Obstruction

A useful way of classifying gastrointestinal obstruction is focus above and below the pylorus. Obstruction of the upper gastrointestinal tract is manifest by vomiting, especially after feeds, whereas obstruction of the lower gastrointestinal tract may present with abdominal distention, little or no stool passed, hematochezia, signs of pain, and vomiting.

Upper Gastrointestinal Tract Obstruction.   The most common cause of upper gastrointestinal obstruction in the newborn is pyloric stenosis, but pyloric stenosis does not usually present in the first week of life. Other rare causes of obstruction, such as congenital webs, may occur. If there has been persistent vomiting, this usually means that a deficit of fluids or electrolytes will develop in the infant. The stomach contains approximately 100 to 130 mEq/L of sodium and 5 to 10 mEq/L of potassium. Persistent vomiting results in the greatest deficit of sodium. Another major concern in the infant with upper gastrointestinal tract obstruction is aspiration of gastric contents.

The anesthetic management of these patients is directed toward ensuring adequate relaxation for abdominal exploration, repair of the congenital defect, and closure of the abdomen. Nitrous oxide can be used in high intestinal obstruction because there is essentially no gas in the upper gastrointestinal tract. The next concern is whether the infant's trachea should be extubated at the end of surgery. If the infant is robust, extubation of the trachea at the end of surgery can be anticipated. The preferred technique is for general anesthesia combined with caudal epidural anesthesia. This allows light levels of volatile agent and minimal muscle relaxant use, resulting in an early extubation. Opioids may be administered, although the impact on the ability to ventilate at the end of the procedure should be considered. If the infant is moderately debilitated or if the surgical incision is extensive, a period of postoperative ventilation may well be indicated, particularly if moderate doses of opioids have been used.

Lower Gastrointestinal Tract Obstruction.   Intestinal obstruction in the newborn can result from a variety of lesions. These include imperforate anus or anal atresia, duodenal atresia, jejunoileal atresia, intussusception, malrotation, volvulus, choledochal cyst, or meconium ileus. Although these are all different in etiology, their presentation is similar. The problems associated with lower gastrointestinal tract obstruction usually develop within 1 to 7 days after birth. It may take this long for the lesion to become evident because it is low in the gastrointestinal tract. An imperforate anus should be recognizable shortly after birth. However, once intestinal obstruction is diagnosed in the newborn, it becomes a surgical emergency. These patients may deteriorate rapidly. Some of these infants may have vomiting secondary to the obstruction, which poses a problem for fluid and electrolyte management. An enormous amount of fluid can be sequestered within the intestinal tract. This fluid is essentially extracellular fluid and has high sodium content. Therefore, these infants should be prepared expeditiously for surgery and have a serum sodium level of at least 130 mEq/L and a urine volume of 1 to 2 mL/kg/hr. In addition to fluid and electrolyte disturbances, delayed diagnosis or treatment of these patients can result in increased abdominal pressure, leading to respiratory embarrassment from pressure on the diaphragm and aspiration pneumonitis, as well as sepsis. Lastly, some of these conditions are associated with other congenital anomalies that complicate preanesthetic evaluation and anesthetic management.[182] Duodenal atresia, for instance, is often associated with Down syndrome, cystic fibrosis, imperforate anus, and renal abnormalities.

The preanesthetic evaluation and perioperative management is similar for all these lesions. Preanesthetic evaluation is focused on the stabilization of fluid and electrolyte status, ensuring adequate oxygenation and ventilation, hemodynamic support if the patient is septic, and identification of complicating issues such as other congenital abnormalities.

In the operating room, the need for invasive arterial and central venous monitoring is determined by the current status of the patient and the urgency of the procedure. The primary anesthetic considerations are the same as those in the preoperative period, including ongoing fluid and electrolyte resuscitation. Because these cases are usually emergent and there may be associated vomiting and abdominal distention, either an awake intubation or rapid-sequence induction is indicated. Although awake intubation may be the best approach if the patient has a probable difficult airway or has hemodynamic decompensation, a rapid-sequence induction after preoxygenation is the approach normally taken. Any induction agent can be used if judicious doses are chosen, but ketamine or etomidate are often chosen because of a concern about cardiovascular instability.

Anesthetic agents for maintenance during these cases is chosen on the basis of the patient's status and the likely surgical course. Nitrous oxide should not be used in any infant who has gaseous distention of the intestine, which is easily determined from the preoperative radiograph. Providing adequate muscle relaxation for surgery can be accomplished with various anesthetic techniques, such as volatile anesthesia, muscle relaxants, and caudal or epidural block.[183] There is increasing interest in the use of remifentanil in newborns and infants because of its titratability and short duration of action, potentially increasing the options for extubation at the end of the case for some patients.[184]

The criteria for tracheal extubation at the end of surgery are the same as those described for upper gastrointestinal tract obstruction. When in doubt, it is prudent to leave the tracheal tube in place and provide a period of postoperative ventilation during which the patient's status can be re-evaluated before deciding that extubation is safe.

Meningomyelocele

Clinical Presentation.   Myelomeningocele is the most common congenital primary neural tube defect. Despite the known ability of folic acid supplementation during pregnancy to largely prevent this defect, the lesion still occurs in approximately 0.5 to 1 of every 1,000 live births.[185] It results from failure of neural tube closure during the fourth week of gestation. Neural tube defects can be identified on prenatal ultrasound. Elevated maternal serum AFP detects 50 to 90% of open neural tube defects but has a false-positive rate of 5%. Amniotic fluid AFP is more reliable.

By definition, the lesion involves both the meninges and neural components, as compared with a meningocele, which does not contain neural elements. The infant is born with a cystic mass on the back comprising a neural placode, arachnoid, dura, nerve tissue and roots, and cerebrospinal fluid. The lesion most commonly occurs in the lumbosacral or sacral region, although it can extend to the thoracic region. The bony canal is also malformed, leading to multiple orthopaedic problems as the child matures. Urologic complications correlate with the level of the spinal lesion.

Newborns born with myelomeningocele have an associated anomaly of the brainstem known as the *Arnold-Chiari II (Chiari II) malformation*. The Chiari II malformation is characterized by caudal displacement of the cerebellar vermis through the foramen magnum, caudal displacement of the medulla oblongata and the cervical spine, kinking of the medulla, and obliteration of the cisterna magna.[186] The cause of Chiari II malformation rests in the small size of the skull housing the posterior fossa, forcing CNS contents out during development. Hydrocephalus requiring shunting develops in approximately 80 to 90% of infants with myelomeningocele. In contrast, only 20% of patients have symptoms of brainstem dysfunction as a result of the Chiari II malformation, but the mortality rate among those symptomatic patients is high. Complications of brainstem dysfunction include stridor, apnea and bradycardia, aspiration pneumonia, sleep-disordered breathing patterns, vocal cord paralysis, lack of coordination, and spasticity. If the symptoms are not improved by shunting, posterior fossa decompression is necessary.[187]

The infant with a myelomeningocele is usually operated on within the first 24 to 48 hours of life. This reduces the risk for development of ventriculitis or progressive neurologic deficits. Most centers close the defect and place a shunt at the same time. However, some centers may delay placement of a shunt until the infant shows symptoms of hydrocephalus. There is ongoing work to determine the benefits of intrauterine repair of myelomeningocele, hopefully with the benefits of decreased development of a Chiari II malformation, decreased hydrocephalus, and increased lower limb function. As these studies continue, the role of intrauterine repair will become clearer.[188]

Preoperative Care. The preoperative stabilization period focuses on the prevention of infection, maintenance of extracellular fluid volume, avoidance of hypothermia, and assessment for other congenital anomalies. The exposed neural placode is susceptible to trauma, leakage, and infection. The infant is usually placed in the prone position, and the placode is covered with warm saline-soaked gauze to prevent desiccation. Because of the high risk of infection, antibiotic therapy is initiated in the preoperative period. Rupture of the cyst on the back can lead to ongoing cerebrospinal fluid leakage. This fluid is replaced with full-strength, balanced salt solution. The infant is also assessed for any potentially life-threatening congenital anomalies.

Perioperative Care. The high prevalence of clinical latex allergy and latex sensitization in children with myelomeningocele has drawn much attention and led many individuals to believe that these patients have an impaired immune system that makes them more susceptible to latex allergy. The likely cause of the increased incidence of latex sensitization is repeated exposure to latex products through frequent hospitalizations and surgical procedures, as well as a program of daily bladder catheterization for those with neurogenic bladders.[189] Although it is reasonable to take special precautions to prevent latex exposure in these patients,[190] it is prudent to limit latex exposure to all patients, especially those who have repeated surgeries, bladder catheterizations, or other exposure to latex products.[191]

Positioning is critical in the infant with myelomeningocele. For induction of anesthesia, the infant may be placed supine with the defect resting in a "doughnut" to minimize trauma. Alternatively, the induction can be performed with the infant in the lateral position, although this makes intubation more challenging. The infant is turned prone for surgery. Rolls are positioned to ensure the abdomen and chest are free, avoiding pressure on the epidural venous plexus to minimize bleeding and allow adequate ventilation.

In most instances, the infant has an intravenous line placed before surgery and an intravenous induction is performed. Succinylcholine may be used to facilitate intubation without risking hyperkalemia.[192] Because increased intracranial pressure is rarely present before closure of the defect, inhalational induction is an alternative in the infant with difficult intravenous access. The anesthetic management of these newborns is rarely complicated unless there are other congenital anomalies that warrant special attention. There is no particular advantage of one technique over another because of the surgical lesion. Because these patients are usually extubated at the end of the case, a technique that allows this is usually chosen. Regional anesthesia has been reported as a safe adjunct or alternative to general anesthesia in the neonate with myelomeningocele. One small series has been published in which tetracaine spinals were used as the anesthetic for 14 infants undergoing repair of myelomeningocele.[193] In this series, there was no evidence of anesthetic-induced neurologic damage. Of note, 2 of the 14 infants had a postoperative res-

piratory event (1 transient apnea/bradycardia and 1 brief desaturation with bradycardia). Both of these infants had received intraoperative midazolam for sedation.

Postoperative Care. These infants must be monitored closely in the postoperative period. Respiratory complications, including stridor, apnea and bradycardia, cyanosis, and respiratory arrest, may develop after surgery in these infants with known brainstem abnormalities and potential disorders of central respiratory control. In addition, infants who were not shunted during repair may show signs of hydrocephalus, including lethargy, vomiting, seizures, apnea and bradycardia, or cardiovascular instability. These infants need to return to the operating room for insertion of a shunt. Although the majority of these patients will eventually require a shunt, a recent survey has shown that only about one third of the patients receive one during the initial hospitalization.[194]

Hydrocephalus

Hydrocephalus in the first month of life may have several causes. It may occur after closure of a meningomyelocele because of the Chiari II malformation; it may be congenital in origin; it may be related to intraventricular hemorrhage, especially in the very preterm newborn. The incidence of hydrocephalus has been stable in recent years, with a decrease related to Chiari II malformations, but an increase secondary to hemorrhage in the preterm.[195] The cranial sutures in the neonate are open, so intracranial pressure increases are blunted or minimized. However, infants with hydrocephalus eventually have an increase in head size and sometimes in intracranial pressure, resulting in lethargy, vomiting, and cardiorespiratory problems. The anesthetic approach and the technique for tracheal intubation depend on the infant's condition. The major concern is protection of the airway and control of intracranial pressure. Awake tracheal intubation, crying, struggling, and straining can increase intracranial pressure. A rapid-sequence induction of anesthesia to control the airway and intracranial pressure is preferred. Volatile drugs, nitrous oxide, and opioids are all reasonable choices for maintenance of anesthesia, with no evidence that one technique is superior. Noninvasive intracranial pressure measurements in neurologically normal preterm neonates have shown a decrease in intracranial pressure with all drugs, including ketamine, fentanyl, and isoflurane. The failure of volatile anesthetics and ketamine to increase intracranial pressure as in adults is attributed to the compliance of the neonate's open-sutured cranium. After surgery, the trachea of these infants may remain intubated if they were experiencing periods of apnea or bradycardia before surgery because of the intracranial abnormalities. If not, the trachea can be extubated as soon as the protective reflexes have recovered.

Surgical Procedures in the First Month of Life

Surgical procedures in the first month also are considered emergent, or at least urgent, surgery. The most frequent surgical procedures in the first month are exploratory laparotomy for NEC, inguinal hernia repair, correction of pyloric stenosis, patent ductus arteriosus (PDA) ligation, a shunt procedure for hydrocephalus, and placement of a central venous catheter.

Necrotizing Enterocolitis

Necrotizing enterocolitis is a disease that primarily affects premature infants who have survived the first days of life, although it can be seen in full-term newborns. One of the theories about NEC is that earlier, more rapid feeding places infants at greater risk for development of NEC. The incidence of NEC among very low birth weight infants varies between 5 and 15%.[196] The exact pathophysiology of NEC has been the source of much study and some controversy, although is likely multifactorial.[197] The condition is characterized by a cascade of pathologic events, beginning with an immature distal small and sometimes large intestine that has a decreased ability to absorb substrate, leading to stasis. The most common site is the ileocolic region, but can be seen in other areas and can be discontinuous, giving a patchy appearance. Stasis encourages bacterial proliferation, which leads to local infection. The picture is complicated by further pooling of fluid. The ischemia and infection may lead to necrosis of the intestinal mucosa, followed by perforation. The perforation leads to gangrene of the gut wall, fluid loss, peritonitis, septicemia, and disseminated intravascular coagulation. The first signs that NEC may be developing are abdominal distention, irritability, and the development of metabolic acidosis. This may be followed by radiologic evidence of pneumatosis intestinalis, portal venous air, or free abdominal air. NEC is primarily a medical disease and is treated by cessation of oral intake, administration of antibiotics, fluid and electrolyte therapy, insertion of an orogastric tube, hemodynamic support, and in some cases, the insertion of a peritoneal drain.[198] In nonresponsive cases, the infant becomes more septic with severe peritonitis, and the only solution is to perform an exploratory laparotomy to remove the gangrenous bowel and create an ileostomy.

The preoperative problems are an acute abdomen with severe peritonitis, necrosis, and gangrene of the intestine, septicemia, metabolic acidosis, and hypovolemia. These neonates may also have disseminated intravascular coagulation. Preparation of the patient is directed toward stabilization of these problems. By the time the newborn becomes a surgical candidate, the septicemia, coupled with the distended abdomen and the overall clinical deterioration of the infant, often has necessitated the use of intubation and ventilation in the neonatal intensive care unit. Appropriate laboratory investigations include an arterial blood gas, hemoglobin, glucose, electrolytes, and coagulation profile. The deteriorating status of the patient may compromise both resuscitation efforts and the desire to establish adequate vascular access and monitoring, but focused efforts should be made to provide multiple vascular access lines, an arterial line, and, if time allows, central venous line.

The anesthetic requirements are continuation of resuscitation, provision of abdominal relaxation for the surgery, and careful titration of anesthetic drugs. These infants are often so critically ill that they are very sensitive to the depressant effects of anesthesia. If the patient is not already intubated and ventilated, a rapid-sequence induction with ketamine and succinylcholine is often used. The only caution with this technique is that some patients with NEC have significant hyperkalemia secondary to dead bowel, making the use of succinylcholine problematic. High-dose rocuronium is a reasonable alternative in that situation. Maintenance of anesthesia is usually based on an opioid technique, supplemented with additional doses of ketamine or, if the patient's condition improves, low-dose inhalation agent. The use of nitrous oxide should be avoided because of the gas pockets in the abdomen.

These infants are among the most challenging cases in pediatric anesthesia. The fluid loss can be enormous, both because of surgical losses and third-space losses. Fluid management starts with full-strength, balanced salt solution for maintenance of blood pressure and urine output. Blood products are often needed during these cases. If the hematocrit is below 30 to 35%, red blood cells should be administered. Based on both preoperative and intraoperative laboratory work, fresh-frozen plasma, platelets, and cryoprecipitate may be needed. Inotropic support may be needed in addition to these measures. The surgical technique and length of surgery is variable, depending on the findings at laparotomy. A combination of bowel resection,

primary anastomoses, and enterostomies may be used. At the end of the procedure, these infants are returned intubated and ventilated to the intensive care unit, where resuscitation is continued.[199] Long-term survival is based on several factors, including the degree of prematurity, associated congenital abnormalities, the degree of surviving bowel, the total length of affected bowel, and subsequent complications. Mortality rates, especially in newborns weighing <1,500 g, are poor, with recent studies demonstrating 25 to 50% mortality before discharge.[199,200]

Inguinal Hernia Repair in the Neonate

The development of a hernia in the premature infant or neonate is a different clinical problem from the development of a hernia in an infant older than 1 year of age. In infants younger than 2 months of age who need inguinal hernia repair, there is a higher incidence of prematurity, history of RDS, history of incarceration, and congenital heart disease.[201] In preterms, the incidence of hernia may approach 20 to 30%. There is a concern about new or recurring incarceration in these patients, making hernia repair less an elective procedure than in older infants. Consequently, once identified, these patients usually are repaired within a relatively short time. If the patient is currently hospitalized, it is common to repair the hernia before discharge. Otherwise, the surgery should be scheduled within days to weeks of diagnosis.

Anesthetic Techniques for Hernia Repair. Surgical procedures below the umbilicus can be performed with either general or regional anesthesia. The choice of whether to use general or regional anesthesia depends on the preference of the surgeon and/or the anesthesiologist. However, the choice is influenced by the underlying status of the patient, previous complications, and the known risk of preterm patients to develop apnea and bradycardia during and after these procedures. As discussed earlier, there is a risk in any preterm for apnea and bradycardia after stressful procedures, but this has been most widely studied in association with inguinal hernia repair. Analysis of the many small studies have shown certain common elements.[159] Apneic events are inversely related to both gestational age and postconceptual age; the incidence is less in small-for-gestational age infants; anemia increases the incidence of apneic events; and apneic events at home are associated with a higher incidence in the perioperative period. There have been multiple studies that were recently analyzed to determine if the choice of regional or general anesthetic techniques decreased the incidence of apnea and bradycardia.[202] There is not a statistically significant difference in the studies in the incidence of apnea, bradycardia or oxygen desaturation in preterm infants, based on anesthetic technique. Consequently, the choice of anesthetic should not be based solely on the risk of preventing apneic spells. An adjunct that has some evidence in support of its use to minimize apneic spells is caffeine. The use of preservative-free caffeine in a single dose of 10 mg/kg has been suggested to decrease the incidence of apneic spells.[203]

Regional anesthesia can be used entirely for the surgery or as an adjunct to reduce general anesthetic requirements and provide postoperative analgesia. Other methods of providing intraoperative anesthesia and postoperative analgesia include the ilioinguinal-iliohypogastric nerve block or local infiltration. Ilioinguinal-iliohypogastric nerve block with 0.25% bupivacaine or 0.2% ropivacaine, with epinephrine, can be administered shortly after the induction of general anesthesia and affords excellent postoperative analgesia without the need for opioids.

Discharge after inguinal hernia repair to home is an area of some controversy. In particular, which patients can be discharged and which must be observed overnight for apnea and bradycardia? There is significant institutional variation on this issue, with the decision to admit overnight usually based on postconceptual age. There is a tendency to use 46 weeks' post-conceptual age as the limit for admission, but other centers will use up to 60 weeks' postconceptual age as the limit. In our own institution, we have used a different approach. In order to make the limit easily understandable and also understanding that the basis of determining gestational age is not precise, we have all preterms admitted until they are 6 months of age. This ensures 26 weeks added to gestational age and is a compromise between the 46-week and 60-week limits, but is easy to administer. No matter what limits are used, if the infant has apneic or bradycardic spells during the perioperative period, he or she should be monitored in-house until the infant has been symptom-free for at least 12 hours.

Pyloric Stenosis

Pyloric stenosis is a relatively frequent surgical disease of the neonate and infant. It can appear as early as the second week of life. The pathologic characteristics include hypertrophy of the pyloric smooth muscle with edema of the pyloric mucosa and submucosa. This process, which develops over a period of days to weeks, leads to progressive obstruction of the pyloric valve, causing persistent vomiting. The vomiting leads to varying losses of fluids and electrolytes. The diagnosis is usually made at an early stage in the development of symptoms, especially with the help of ultrasound, so it is rare to find an infant with severe fluid and electrolyte derangements. However, an infant is occasionally seen whose problem has developed slowly over a period of weeks, resulting in severe fluid and electrolyte derangements. The stomach contents contain sodium, potassium, chloride, hydrogen ions, and water. The classic electrolyte pattern in infants with severe vomiting is a hyponatremic, hypokalemic, and hypochloremic metabolic alkalosis with a compensatory respiratory acidosis. The anesthesiologist, pediatrician, and surgeon are all responsible for preparing these infants for surgery. Pyloric stenosis is a medical emergency, not a surgical emergency. The patient should not be operated on until there has been adequate fluid and electrolyte resuscitation. The infant should have normal skin turgor, and the correction of the electrolyte imbalance should produce a sodium level that is >130 mEq/L, a potassium level that is at least 3 mEq/L, a chloride level that is >85 mEq/L and increasing, and a urine output of at least 1 to 2 mL/kg/hr. These patients need a resuscitation fluid of full-strength, balanced salt solution and, after the infant begins to urinate, the addition of potassium.

Anesthetic Management.   It is prudent to pass a large orogastric tube and aspirate the stomach contents because of the significant volume that may be present.[204] This procedure greatly reduces the quantity of gastric fluid. A rapid-sequence induction is advisable because of the potential for additional volume in the stomach. Although awake intubation had been popular with some clinicians in the past, it is associated with a higher incidence of complications and is traumatic to the child.[116] These patients have been fully resuscitated before coming to surgery, so there is little reason for an awake intubation. Anesthesia can be maintained by almost any technique the clinician prefers. There has been a need for muscle relaxation only for a short period during open pyloromyotomy, especially during the delivery of the pylorus at the start of the procedure and during replacement of the pylorus back into the abdomen to begin closure. However, these cases are increasingly being performed laparoscopically. Controlled ventilation reduces or eliminates the need for muscle relaxants for this surgery. At the end of the case, the patient should be wide awake before extubation.

Ligation of a Patent Ductus Arteriosus

As the number of small premature infants who survive has increased, so also has the number of infants who have a PDA with heart failure and respiratory failure. Prostaglandins relax the smooth muscle of the ductus so it cannot constrict. Indomethacin, a prostaglandin synthetase inhibitor, is administered to encourage closure of the ductus. However, indomethacin is often unsuccessful in the small premature infant because of the lack of muscle within the ductus. Infants with a PDA and heart failure need maximal medical management with fluid restriction, diuretics, and inotropes. These infants are at special risk because of the reduced blood volume and precarious cardiopulmonary system. If the surgery is performed in the operating room, special attention is taken to maintain normothermia, ventilation, and oxygenation during transport. If the surgery is performed at bedside in the neonatal intensive care unit, the anesthesiologist must take time before the procedure to establish where he or she will be situated, where is all venous access, and that all drugs and fluids are already prepared. An opioid-based technique with muscle relaxant is a frequent choice for anesthesia. Probably the biggest challenge during these cases is the diagnosis and management of hypotension. There can be sudden, catastrophic blood loss if the ductus tears. Consequently, syringes of balanced salt solution and blood should be immediately available. The other common cause of hypotension is compression of the lungs, heart and great vessels by the surgeon as they are gaining exposure. This is a balance between stopping the procedure to allow the heart and blood pressure to recover versus the need to proceed with the operation. The answer comes in close communication between the anesthesiologist and surgeon. These patients usually remain intubated after procedure, without a need to reverse the muscle relaxant. Residual opioid will provide good analgesia for the immediate postoperative period.

There are two newer techniques for closing the PDA in infants that are increasing in popularity.[205] Video-assisted thoracoscopic surgery (VATS) uses small endoscopes inserted through a series of small thoracotomy incisions to guide instruments to ligate the ductus with a thoracotomy. VATS can be done either in the operating room or, rarely, at bedside. The other approach is used by cardiologists in the cardiac catheterization to occlude the ductus with a coil. In either case, the anesthetic challenge is not so much choice of drugs, but adapting to working in an unfamiliar environment, like the catheterization suite, or understanding how the positioning, lung deflation, and need to identify the recurrent laryngeal nerve requirements of the VATS will affect their anesthetic.

Placement of a Central Venous Catheter

The use of a central venous catheter for monitoring serum electrolytes, for hyperalimentation, and for administering medications is a well-established part of modern perioperative care. It can be placed either as part of the surgical procedure or at some other time as a separate procedure. The three major concerns in central venous catheter placement are airway management, pneumothorax, and bleeding. The airway should be secured by an endotracheal tube because of the difficulty in sharing the head, neck, and upper chest with the surgeon and as an adjunct for treating complications such as pneumothorax and bleeding. The anesthetic technique depends on the infant's condition. A pneumothorax may occur with attempts at subclavian vein puncture. The first indication of pneumothorax may be a decreasing oxygen saturation, hypotension, or difficulty with ventilation of the lungs. Because a fluoroscope is often used for central venous catheter placement, it can be used rapidly to diagnose a pneumothorax. If not, the chest should be rapidly aspirated for both diagnostic and therapeutic reasons. Bleeding is an unusual but serious complication of central venous catheter placement. It usually becomes manifest in the perioperative period as a hemothorax or as hypovolemia with a decreasing hematocrit or blood pressure. The establishment of intravenous access placed before proceeding with a central line is problematic for some patients. The reason for the central line may very well be the inability to obtain peripheral access, and the clinician is left with a trade-off between prolonged attempts at starting an intravenous catheter versus proceeding directly to obtain central venous line placement. This is a clinical judgment that depends not only on the time and effort that has been spent in obtaining peripheral access, but also the underlying status of the patient. If there is a question about how to proceed, the anesthesiologist and surgeon should discuss and agree on the approach. Strict attention to skin preparation, sterile glove and drape use, and minimizing access to the central line are components important to diminish catheter-related sepsis. Subclavian approach has a higher incidence of problems than an external or internal jugular approach.

SUMMARY

The anesthetic management of the newborn is among the most challenging in all of anesthesiology. A strong foundation in neonatal anatomy, physiology, and pharmacology is needed, as well as an appreciation of the disease states and surgical procedures that are unique to this population. A thorough preanesthetic evaluation and preparation, a concise plan, and meticulous technique are the basis of an effective approach. The patient's neonatologist or pediatrician and the surgeon are strong allies in providing the best care, and close communication with them is necessary. Lastly, the clinical status of a newborn can change remarkably quickly. Strict attention to detail and prospective management are the hallmarks of the anesthesiologist skilled in providing care in these difficult cases.

References

1. Friedman AH, Fahey JT: The transition from fetal to neonatal circulation: Normal responses and implications for infants with heart disease. Semin Perinatol 1993; 17: 106
2. Baum VC, Palmisano BW: The immature heart and anesthesia. Anesthesiology 1997; 87: 1529
3. Fu JD, Li J, Tweedie D et al: Crucial role of the sarcoplasmic reticulum in the developmental regulation of Ca^{2+} transients and contraction in cardiomyocytes derived from embryonic stem cells. Faseb J 2006; 20: 181
4. Auman JT, Seidler FJ, Tate CA et al: Are developing beta-adrenoceptors able to desensitize? Acute and chronic effects of beta-agonists in neonatal heart and liver. Am J Physiol Regul Integr Comp Physiol 2002; 283: R205
5. Kishkurno S, Takahashi Y, Harada K et al: Postnatal changes in left ventricular volume and contractility in healthy term infants. Pediatr Cardiol 1997; 18: 91
6. Hislop A: Developmental biology of the pulmonary circulation. Paediatr Respir Rev 2005; 6: 35
7. Mansell AL, Collins MH, Johnson E, Jr., Gil J: Postnatal growth of lung parenchyma in the piglet: morphometry correlated with mechanics. Anat Rec 1995; 241: 99
8. Merrill JD, Ballard RA: Pulmonary surfactant for neonatal respiratory disorders. Curr Opin Pediatr 2003; 15: 149
9. Engle WA: Surfactant-replacement therapy for respiratory distress in the preterm and term neonate. Pediatrics 2008; 121: 419
10. Hernandez-Diaz S, Van Marter LJ, Werler MM et al: Risk factors for persistent pulmonary hypertension of the newborn. Pediatrics 2007; 120: e272
11. Shah PS, Ohlsson A: Sildenafil for pulmonary hypertension in neonates. Cochrane Database Syst Rev 2007: CD005494
12. Murphy JD, Vawter GF, Reid LM: Pulmonary vascular disease in fatal meconium aspiration. J Pediatr 1984; 104: 758
13. Velaphi S, Vidyasagar D: Intrapartum and postdelivery management of infants born to mothers with meconium-stained amniotic fluid: evidence-based recommendations. Clin Perinatol 2006; 33: 29
14. Drukker A, Guignard JP: Renal aspects of the term and preterm infant: a selective update. Curr Opin Pediatr 2002; 14: 175
15. Bartelink IH, Rademaker CM, Schobben AF, van den Anker JN: Guidelines on paediatric dosing on the basis of developmental physiology and pharmacokinetic considerations. Clin Pharmacokinet 2006; 45: 1077
16. Alcorn J, McNamara PJ: Ontogeny of hepatic and renal systemic clearance pathways in infants: part I. Clin Pharmacokinet 2002; 41: 959
17. Nash PL: Potassum and sodium homeostasis in the neonate. Neonatal Netw 2007; 26: 125
18. Cornblath M, Ichord R: Hypoglycemia in the neonate. Semin Perinatol 2000; 24: 136
19. Ballweg JA, Wernovsky G, Ittenbach RF et al: Hyperglycemia after infant cardiac surgery does not adversely impact neurodevelopmental outcome. Ann Thorac Surg 2007; 84: 2052
20. de Ferranti S, Gauvreau K, Hickey PR et al: Intraoperative hyperglycemia during infant cardiac surgery is not associated with adverse neurodevelopmental outcomes at 1, 4, and 8 years. Anesthesiology 2004; 100: 1345
21. Wu Y, Stack G: Blood product replacement in the perinatal period. Semin Perinatol 2007; 31: 262
22. Alcorn J, McNamara PJ: Pharmacokinetics in the newborn. Adv Drug Deliv Rev 2003; 55: 667
23. Strassburg CP, Strassburg A, Kneip S et al: Developmental aspects of human hepatic drug glucuronidation in young children and adults. Gut 2002; 50: 259
24. de Wildt SN, Kearns GL, Leeder JS, van den Anker JN: Glucuronidation in humans. Pharmacogenetic and developmental aspects. Clin Pharmacokinet 1999; 36: 439
25. Leeder JS, Kearns GL: Pharmacogenetics in pediatrics. Implications for practice. Pediatr Clin North Am 1997; 44: 55
26. Lynn AM, Slattery JT: Morphine pharmacokinetics in early infancy. Anesthesiology 1987; 66: 136
27. Bory C, Baltassat P, Porthault M et al: Metabolism of theophylline to caffeine in premature newborn infants. J Pediatr 1979; 94: 988
28. Green MD, Fischer LJ: Hepatotoxicity of acetaminophen in neonatal and young rats. II. Metabolic aspects. Toxicol Appl Pharmacol 1984; 74: 125
29. Green MD, Shires TK, Fischer LJ: Hepatotoxicity of acetaminophen in neonatal and young rats. I. Age-related changes in susceptibility. Toxicol Appl Pharmacol 1984; 74: 116
30. deAlmeida VL, Alvaro RA, Haider Z et al: The effect of nasal occlusion on the initiation of oral breathing in preterm infants. Pediatr Pulmonol 1994; 18: 374
31. Miller MJ, Carlo WA, Strohl KP et al: Effect of maturation on oral breathing in sleeping premature infants. J Pediatr 1986; 109: 515
32. Mazoit JX: Pharmacokinetic/pharmacodynamic modeling of anesthetics in children: therapeutic implications. Paediatr Drugs 2006; 8: 139
33. McNamara PJ, Alcorn J: Protein binding predictions in infants. AAPS PharmSci 2002; 4: E4
34. Bhutada A, Sahni R, Rastogi S, Wung JT: Randomised controlled trial of thiopental for intubation in neonates. Arch Dis Child Fetal Neonatal Ed 2000; 82: F34
35. Ghanta S, Abdel-Latif ME, Lui K et al: Propofol compared with the morphine, atropine, and suxamethonium regimen as induction agents for neonatal endotracheal intubation: a randomized, controlled trial. Pediatrics 2007; 119: e1248
36. Allegaert K, Peeters MY, Verbesselt R et al: Inter-individual variability in propofol pharmacokinetics in preterm and term neonates. Br J Anaesth 2007; 99: 864
37. Bhutta AT: Ketamine: a controversial drug for neonates. Semin Perinatol 2007; 31: 303
38. Mellon RD, Simone AF, Rappaport BA: Use of anesthetic agents in neonates and young children. Anesth Analg 2007; 104: 509
39. Radnay PA, Hollinger I, Santi A, Nagashima H: Ketamine for pediatric cardiac anesthesia. Anaesthesist 1976; 25: 259
40. Suresh S, Anand KJ: Opioid tolerance in neonates: a state-of-the-art review. Paediatr Anaesth 2001; 11: 511
41. Santeiro ML, Christie J, Stromquist C et al: Pharmacokinetics of continuous infusion fentanyl in newborns. J Perinatol 1997; 17: 135
42. Burtin P, Daoud P, Jacqz-Aigrain E et al: Hypotension with midazolam and fentanyl in the newborn. Lancet 1991; 337: 1545
43. Vaughn PR, Townsend SF, Thilo EH et al: Comparison of continuous infusion of fentanyl to bolus dosing in neonates after surgery. J Pediatr Surg 1996; 31: 1616
44. Fahnenstich H, Steffan J, Kau N, Bartmann P: Fentanyl-induced chest wall rigidity and laryngospasm in preterm and term infants. Crit Care Med 2000; 28: 836
45. Bhat R, Chari G, Gulati A et al: Pharmacokinetics of a single dose of morphine in preterm infants during the first week of life. J Pediatr 1990; 117: 477
46. Saarenmaa E, Neuvonen PJ, Rosenberg P, Fellman V: Morphine clearance and effects in newborn infants in relation to gestational age. Clin Pharmacol Ther 2000; 68: 160
47. El Sayed MF, Taddio A, Fallah S et al: Safety profile of morphine following surgery in neonates. J Perinatol 2007; 27: 444
48. Rao R, Sampers JS, Kronsberg SS et al: Neurobehavior of preterm infants at 36 weeks postconception as a function of morphine analgesia. Am J Perinatol 2007; 24: 511
49. Murphey LJ, Olsen GD: Morphine-6-beta-D-glucuronide respiratory pharmacodynamics in the neonatal guinea pig. J Pharmacol Exp Ther 1994; 268: 110
50. Peters JW, Anderson BJ, Simons SH et al: Morphine metabolite pharmacokinetics during venoarterial extra corporeal membrane oxygenation in neonates. Clin Pharmacokinet 2006; 45: 705

51. Davis PJ, Cladis FP: The use of ultra-short-acting opioids in paediatric anaesthesia: the role of remifentanil. Clin Pharmacokinet 2005; 44: 787

52. Davis PJ, Galinkin J, McGowan FX et al: A randomized multicenter study of remifentanil compared with halothane in neonates and infants undergoing pyloromyotomy. I. Emergence and recovery profiles. Anesth Analg 2001; 93: 1380

53. Hannallah RS, Oh TH, McGill WA, Epstein BS: Changes in heart rate and rhythm after intramuscular succinylcholine with or without atropine in anesthetized children. Anesth Analg 1986; 65: 1329

54. Wang JM, Stanley TH: Duchenne muscular dystrophy and malignant hyperthermia–two case reports. Can Anaesth Soc J 1986; 33: 492

55. Meakin GH: Muscle relaxants in paediatric day case surgery. Eur J Anaesthesiol Suppl 2001; 23: 47

56. Meretoja OA, Wirtavuori K, Neuvonen PJ: Age-dependence of the dose-response curve of vecuronium in pediatric patients during balanced anesthesia. Anesth Analg 1988; 67: 21

57. Cook DR: Paediatric anaesthesia: pharmacological considerations. Drugs 1976; 12: 212

58. Gronert BJ, Brandom BW: Neuromuscular blocking drugs in infants and children. Pediatr Clin North Am 1994; 41: 73

59. Goudsouzian NG, Crone RK, Todres ID: Recovery from pancuronium blockade in the neonatal intensive care unit. Br J Anaesth 1981; 53: 1303

60. Cheung PY, Tyebkhan JM, Peliowski A et al: Prolonged use of pancuronium bromide and sensorineural hearing loss in childhood survivors of congenital diaphragmatic hernia. J Pediatr 1999; 135: 233

61. Diaz JH: Halothane anesthesia in infancy: identification and correlation of preoperative risk factors with intraoperative arterial hypotension and postoperative recovery. J Pediatr Surg 1985; 20: 502

62. Imamura S, Ikeda K: Comparison of the epinephrine-induced arrhythmogenic effect of sevoflurane with isoflurane and halothane. J Anesth 1987; 1: 62

63. Rapp HJ, Altenmueller CA, Waschke C: Neuromuscular recovery following rocuronium bromide single dose in infants. Paediatr Anaesth 2004; 14: 329

64. Murray DJ, Forbes RB, Mahoney LT: Comparative hemodynamic depression of halothane versus isoflurane in neonates and infants: an echocardiographic study. Anesth Analg 1992; 74: 329

65. Lerman J, Sikich N, Kleinman S, Yentis S: The pharmacology of sevoflurane in infants and children. Anesthesiology 1994; 80: 814

66. Russell IA, Miller Hance WC, Gregory G et al: The safety and efficacy of sevoflurane anesthesia in infants and children with congenital heart disease. Anesth Analg 2001; 92: 1152

67. Brown K, Aun C, Stocks J et al: A comparison of the respiratory effects of sevoflurane and halothane in infants and young children. Anesthesiology 1998; 89: 86

68. Taylor RH, Lerman J: Induction, maintenance and recovery characteristics of desflurane in infants and children. Can J Anaesth 1992; 39: 6

69. Sale SM, Read JA, Stoddart PA, Wolf AR: Prospective comparison of sevoflurane and desflurane in formerly premature infants undergoing inguinal herniotomy. Br J Anaesth 2006; 96: 774

70. Tucker GT: Pharmacokinetics of local anaesthetics. Br J Anaesth 1986; 58: 717

71. Anderson BJ, Palmer GM: Recent pharmacological advances in paediatric analgesics. Biomed Pharmacother 2006; 60: 303

72. Rothstein P, Arthur GR, Feldman HS et al: Bupivacaine for intercostal nerve blocks in children: blood concentrations and pharmacokinetics. Anesth Analg 1986; 65: 625

73. Ecoffey C, Desparmet J, Maury M et al: Bupivacaine in children: pharmacokinetics following caudal anaesthesia. Anesthesiology 1985; 63: 447

74. Willschke H, Bosenberg A, Marhofer P et al: Ultrasonographic-guided ilioinguinal/iliohypogastric nerve block in pediatric anesthesia: what is the optimal volume? Anesth Analg 2006; 102: 1680

75. Beauvoir C, Rochette A, Desch G, D'Athis F: Spinal anaesthesia in newborns: total and free bupivacaine plasma concentration. Paediatr Anaesth 1996; 6: 195

76. Berde CB: Convulsions associated with pediatric regional anesthesia. Anesth Analg 1992; 75: 164

77. Rapp HJ, Molnar V, Austin S et al: Ropivacaine in neonates and infants: a population pharmacokinetic evaluation following single caudal block. Paediatr Anaesth 2004; 14: 724

78. McCloskey JJ, Haun SE, Deshpande JK: Bupivacaine toxicity secondary to continuous caudal epidural infusion in children. Anesth Analg 1992; 75: 287

79. Hansen TG, Ilett KF, Reid C et al: Caudal ropivacaine in infants: population pharmacokinetics and plasma concentrations. Anesthesiology 2001; 94: 579

80. Chalkiadis GA, Eyres RL, Cranswick N et al: Pharmacokinetics of levobupivacaine 0.25% following caudal administration in children under 2 years of age. Br J Anaesth 2004; 92: 218

81. Simpson D, Curran MP, Oldfield V, Keating GM: Ropivacaine: a review of its use in regional anaesthesia and acute pain management. Drugs 2005; 65: 2675

82. Tucker GT, Mather LE: Clinical pharmacokinetics of local anaesthetics. Clin Pharmacokinet 1979; 4: 241

83. Tobias JD, O'Dell N: Chloroprocaine for epidural anesthesia in infants and children. Aana J 1995; 63: 131

84. Weise KL, Nahata MC: EMLA for painful procedures in infants. J Pediatr Health Care 2005; 19: 42; quiz 48

85. Couper RT: Methaemoglobinaemia secondary to topical lignocaine/prilocaine in a circumcised neonate. J Paediatr Child Health 2000; 36: 406

86. Lillieborg S, Otterbom I, Ahlen K: Topical anaesthesia in neonates, infants and children. Br J Anaesth 2004; 92: 450

87. Lehr VT, Taddio A: Topical anesthesia in neonates: clinical practices and practical considerations. Semin Perinatol 2007; 31: 323

88. Bhananker SM, Ramamoorthy C, Geiduschek JM et al: Anesthesia-related cardiac arrest in children: update from the Pediatric Perioperative Cardiac Arrest Registry. Anesth Analg 2007; 105: 344

89. Morray JP, Geiduschek JM, Caplan RA et al: A comparison of pediatric and adult anesthesia closed malpractice claims. Anesthesiology 1993; 78: 461

90. Braz LG, Modolo NS, do Nascimento P, Jr et al: Perioperative cardiac arrest: a study of 53,718 anaesthetics over 9 yr from a Brazilian teaching hospital. Br J Anaesth 2006; 96: 569

91. Murat I, Constant I, Maud'huy H: Perioperative anaesthetic morbidity in children: a database of 24,165 anaesthetics over a 30-month period. Paediatr Anaesth 2004; 14: 158

92. Hackel A, Badgwell JM, Binding RR et al: Guidelines for the pediatric perioperative anesthesia environment. American Academy of Pediatrics. Section on Anesthesiology. Pediatrics 1999; 103: 512

93. Howard CR, Howard FM, Garfunkel LC et al: Neonatal circumcision and pain relief: current training practices. Pediatrics 1998; 101: 423

94. Anand KJ, Sippell WG, Aynsley-Green A: Pain, anaesthesia, and babies. Lancet 1987; 2: 1210

95. Berry FA, Gregory GA: Do premature infants require anesthesia for surgery? Anesthesiology 1987; 67: 291

96. Anand KJ, Carr DB: The neuroanatomy, neurophysiology, and neurochemistry of pain, stress, and analgesia in newborns and children. Pediatr Clin North Am 1989; 36: 795

97. Tomashek KM, Shapiro-Mendoza CK, Davidoff MJ, Petrini JR: Differences in mortality between late-preterm and term singleton infants in the United States, 1995–2002. J Pediatr 2007; 151: 450

98. Ozyurek E, Cetintas S, Ceylan T et al: Complete blood count parameters for healthy, small-for-gestational-age, full-term newborns. Clin Lab Haematol 2006; 28: 97

99. Deshpande S, Ward Platt M: The investigation and management of neonatal hypoglycaemia. Semin Fetal Neonatal Med 2005; 10: 351

100. Lippi G, Salvagno GL, Rugolotto S et al: Routine coagulation tests in newborn and young infants. J Thromb Thrombolysis 2007; 24: 153

101. Friesen RH, Lichtor JL: Cardiovascular effects of inhalation induction with isoflurane in infants. Anesth Analg 1983; 62: 411

102. Murray DJ, Forbes RB, Dillman JB et al: Haemodynamic effects of atropine during halothane or isoflurane anaesthesia in infants and small children. Can J Anaesth 1989; 36: 295

103. Mariani G, Dik PB, Ezquer A et al: Pre-ductal and post-ductal O2 saturation in healthy term neonates after birth. J Pediatr 2007; 150: 418

104. Shiao SY: Effects of fetal hemoglobin on accurate measurements of oxygen saturation in neonates. J Perinat Neonatal Nurs 2005; 19: 348

105. Hubmayr RD: The times are a-changin': should we hang up the stethoscope? Anesthesiology 2004; 100: 1

106. Pandit PB, Pandit FA, Govan J, O'Brien K: Complications associated with surgically placed central venous catheters in low birth weight neonates. J Perinatol 1999; 19: 106

107. Schily M, Koumoukelis H, Lerman J, Creighton RE: Can pediatric anesthesiologists detect an occluded tracheal tube in neonates? Anesth Analg 2001; 93: 66

108. Spears RS, Jr., Yeh A, Fisher DM, Zwass MS: The "educated hand". Can anesthesiologists assess changes in neonatal pulmonary compliance manually? Anesthesiology 1991; 75: 693

109. Tobin MJ, Stevenson GW, Horn BJ et al: A comparison of three modes of ventilation with the use of an adult circle system in an infant lung model. Anesth Analg 1998; 87: 766

110. Nakae Y, Miyabe M, Sonoda H et al: Comparison of the Jackson-Rees circuit, the pediatric circle, and the MERA F breathing system for pediatric anesthesia. Anesth Analg 1996; 83: 488

111. Cote CJ: Pediatric breathing circuits and anesthesia machines. Int Anesthesiol Clin 1992; 30: 51

112. Spoerel WE, Bain JA: Anaesthetic breathing systems. Br J Anaesth 1986; 58: 819

113. Hunter T, Lerman J, Bissonnette B: The temperature and humidity of inspired gases in infants using a pediatric circle system: effects of high and low-flow anesthesia. Paediatr Anaesth 2005; 15: 750

114. Luchetti M, Pigna A, Gentili A, Marraro G: Evaluation of the efficiency of heat and moisture exchangers during paediatric anaesthesia. Paediatr Anaesth 1999; 9: 39

115. Monrigal JP, Granry JC: The benefit of using a heat and moisture exchanger during short operations in young children. Paediatr Anaesth 1997; 7: 295

116. Cook-Sather SD, Tulloch HV, Cnaan A et al: A comparison of awake versus paralyzed tracheal intubation for infants with pyloric stenosis. Anesth Analg 1998; 86: 945

117. Ledbetter JL, Rasch DK, Pollard TG et al: Reducing the risks of laryngoscopy in anaesthetised infants. Anaesthesia 1988; 43: 151

118. Todres ID, Crone RK: Experience with a modified laryngoscope in sick infants. Crit Care Med 1981; 9: 544

119. Salgo B, Schmitz A, Henze G et al: Evaluation of a new recommendation for improved cuffed tracheal tube size selection in infants and small children. Acta Anaesthesiol Scand 2006; 50: 557
120. Lonnqvist PA: Successful use of laryngeal mask airway in low-weight expremature infants with bronchopulmonary dysplasia undergoing cryotherapy for retinopathy of the premature. Anesthesiology 1995; 83: 422
121. Hansen TG, Joensen H, Henneberg SW, Hole P: Laryngeal mask airway guided tracheal intubation in a neonate with the Pierre Robin syndrome. Acta Anaesthesiol Scand 1995; 39: 129
122. Fisher QA, Tunkel DE: Lightwand intubation of infants and children. J Clin Anesth 1997; 9: 275
123. Cain JM, Mason LJ, Martin RD: Airway management in two of newborns with Pierre Robin Sequence: the use of disposable vs multiple use LMA for fiberoptic intubation. Paediatr Anaesth 2006; 16: 1274
124. Somri M, Barna Teszler C, Tome R et al: Flexible fiberoptic bronchoscopy through the laryngeal mask airway in a small, premature neonate. Am J Otolaryngol 2005; 26: 268
125. Moura JH, da Silva GA: Neonatal laryngoscope intubation and the digital method: a randomized controlled trial. J Pediatr 2006; 148: 840
126. Marraro G: Intraoperative ventilation. Paediatr Anaesth 1998; 8: 373
127. Marhofer P, Willschke H, Kettner S: Imaging techniques for regional nerve blockade and vascular cannulation in children. Curr Opin Anaesthesiol 2006; 19: 293
128. Weinberg GL, Ripper R, Murphy P et al: Lipid infusion accelerates removal of bupivacaine and recovery from bupivacaine toxicity in the isolated rat heart. Reg Anesth Pain Med 2006; 31: 296
129. Suresh S, Wheeler M: Practical pediatric regional anesthesia. Anesthesiol Clin North America 2002; 20: 83
130. Williams RK, Adams DC, Aladjem EV et al: The safety and efficacy of spinal anesthesia for surgery in infants: the Vermont Infant Spinal Registry. Anesth Analg 2006; 102: 67
131. Kim GS, Song JG, Gwak MS, Yang M: Postoperative outcome in formerly premature infants undergoing herniorrhaphy: comparison of spinal and general anesthesia. J Korean Med Sci 2003; 18: 691
132. Suresh S, Hall SC: Spinal anesthesia in infants: is the impractical practical? Anesth Analg 2006; 102: 65
133. Welborn LG, Rice LJ, Hannallah RS et al: Postoperative apnea in former preterm infants: prospective comparison of spinal and general anesthesia. Anesthesiology 1990; 72: 838
134. Tsui BC, Tarkkila P, Gupta S, Kearney R: Confirmation of caudal needle placement using nerve stimulation. Anesthesiology 1999; 91: 374
135. Marhofer P, Bosenberg A, Sitzwohl C et al: Pilot study of neuraxial imaging by ultrasound in infants and children. Paediatr Anaesth 2005; 15: 671
136. Freid EB, Bailey AG, Valley RD: Electrocardiographic and hemodynamic changes associated with unintentional intravascular injection of bupivacaine with epinephrine in infants. Anesthesiology 1993; 79: 394
137. Wheeler M, Patel A, Suresh S et al: The addition of clonidine 2 microg.kg-1 does not enhance the postoperative analgesia of a caudal block using 0.125% bupivacaine and epinephrine 1:200,000 in children: a prospective, double-blind, randomized study. Paediatr Anaesth 2005; 15: 476
138. Willschke H, Bosenberg A, Marhofer P et al: Epidural catheter placement in neonates: sonoanatomy and feasibility of ultrasonographic guidance in term and preterm neonates. Reg Anesth Pain Med 2007; 32: 34
139. Brady-Fryer B, Wiebe N, Lander JA: Pain relief for neonatal circumcision. Cochrane Database Syst Rev 2004: CD004217
140. Marhofer P, Greher M, Kapral S: Ultrasound guidance in regional anaesthesia. Br J Anaesth 2005; 94: 7
141. Marhofer P, Sitzwohl C, Greher M, Kapral S: Ultrasound guidance for infraclavicular brachial plexus anaesthesia in children. Anaesthesia 2004; 59: 642
142. Suresh S, Voronov P: Head and neck blocks in children: an anatomical and procedural review. Paediatr Anaesth 2006; 16: 910
143. Williams DG, Patel A, Howard RF: Pharmacogenetics of codeine metabolism in an urban population of children and its implications for analgesic reliability. Br J Anaesth 2002; 89: 839
144. Birmingham PK, Tobin MJ, Henthorn TK et al: Twenty-four-hour pharmacokinetics of rectal acetaminophen in children: an old drug with new recommendations. Anesthesiology 1997; 87: 244
145. Moores MA, Wandless JG, Fell D: Paediatric postoperative analgesia. A comparison of rectal diclofenac with caudal bupivacaine after inguinal herniotomy. Anaesthesia 1990; 45: 156
146. Cheung CL, van Dijk M, Green JW et al: Effects of low-dose naloxone on opioid therapy in pediatric patients: a retrospective case-control study. Intensive Care Med 2007; 33: 190
147. Papacci P, De Francisci G, Iacobucci T et al: Use of intravenous ketorolac in the neonate and premature babies. Paediatr Anaesth 2004; 14: 487
148. Rayburn WF: Maternal and fetal effects from substance use. Clin Perinatol 2007; 34: 559, vi
149. Lipshultz SE, Frassica JJ, Orav EJ: Cardiovascular abnormalities in infants prenatally exposed to cocaine. J Pediatr 1991; 118: 44
150. Hackman PS: Recognizing and understanding the cold-stressed term infant. Neonatal Netw 2001; 20: 35
151. Kongsayreepong S, Gunnaleka P, Suraseranivongse S et al: A reusable, custom-made warming blanket prevents core hypothermia during major neonatal surgery. Can J Anaesth 2002; 49: 605
152. Plattner O, Semsroth M, Sessler DI et al: Lack of nonshivering thermogenesis in infants anesthetized with fentanyl and propofol. Anesthesiology 1997; 86: 772

153. Bissonnette B, Sessler DI: The thermoregulatory threshold in infants and children anesthetized with isoflurane and caudal bupivacaine. Anesthesiology 1990; 73: 1114
154. Ehrenkranz RA, Walsh MC, Vohr BR, Jobe AH, Wright LL, Fanaroff AA, et al: Validation of the National Institutes of Health consensus definition of bronchopulmonary dysplasia. Pediatrics 2005; 116: 1353
155. Steward DJ: Preterm infants are more prone to complications following minor surgery than are term infants. Anesthesiology 1982; 56: 304
156. McNamara DG, Nixon GM, Anderson BJ: Methylxanthines for the treatment of apnea associated with bronchiolitis and anesthesia. Paediatr Anaesth 2004; 14: 541
157. Krane EJ, Haberkern CM, Jacobson LE: Postoperative apnea, bradycardia, and oxygen desaturation in formerly premature infants: prospective comparison of spinal and general anesthesia. Anesth Analg 1995; 80: 7
158. Kurth CD, Spitzer AR, Broennle AM, Downes JJ: Postoperative apnea in preterm infants. Anesthesiology 1987; 66: 483
159. Cote CJ, Zaslavsky A, Downes JJ et al: Postoperative apnea in former preterm infants after inguinal herniorrhaphy. A combined analysis. Anesthesiology 1995; 82: 809
160. Kennedy KA, Fielder AR, Hardy RJ et al: Reduced lighting does not improve medical outcomes in very low birth weight infants. J Pediatr 2001; 139: 527
161. Reynolds JD, Dobson V, Quinn GE et al: Evidence-based screening criteria for retinopathy of prematurity: natural history data from the CRYO-ROP and LIGHT-ROP studies. Arch Ophthalmol 2002; 120: 1470
162. Lloyd J, Askie L, Smith J, Tarnow-Mordi W: Supplemental oxygen for the treatment of prethreshold retinopathy of prematurity. Cochrane Database Syst Rev 2003: CD003482
163. Fredriksson A, Ponten E, Gordh T, Eriksson P: Neonatal exposure to a combination of N-methyl-D-aspartate and gamma-aminobutyric acid type A receptor anesthetic agents potentiates apoptotic neurodegeneration and persistent behavioral deficits. Anesthesiology 2007; 107: 427
164. Soriano SG, Anand KJ: Anesthetics and brain toxicity. Curr Opin Anaesthesiol 2005; 18: 293
165. Lin AE, Pober BR, Adatia I: Congenital diaphragmatic hernia and associated cardiovascular malformations: type, frequency, and impact on management. Am J Med Genet C Semin Med Genet 2007; 145: 201
166. Greenwood RD, Rosenthal A: Cardiovascular malformations associated with tracheoesophageal fistula and esophageal atresia. Pediatrics 1976; 57: 87
167. Harting MT, Lally KP: Surgical management of neonates with congenital diaphragmatic hernia. Semin Pediatr Surg 2007; 16: 109
168. Peralta CF, Jani JC, Van Schoubroeck D et al: Fetal lung volume after endoscopic tracheal occlusion in the prediction of postnatal outcome. Am J Obstet Gynecol 2008; 198: 60
169. Ng GY, Derry C, Marston L et al: Reduction in ventilator-induced lung injury improves outcome in congenital diaphragmatic hernia? Pediatr Surg Int 2008; 24: 145
170. Rodrigues CJ, Tannuri U, Tannuri AC et al: Prenatal tracheal ligation or intra-amniotic administration of surfactant or dexamethasone prevents some structural changes in the pulmonary arteries of surgically created diaphragmatic hernia in rabbits. Rev Hosp Clin Fac Med Sao Paulo 2002; 57: 1
171. Fisher JC, Jefferson RA, Arkovitz MS, Stolar CJ: Redefining outcomes in right congenital diaphragmatic hernia. J Pediatr Surg 2008; 43: 373
172. Neff KW, Kilian AK, Schaible T et al: Prediction of mortality and need for neonatal extracorporeal membrane oxygenation in fetuses with congenital diaphragmatic hernia: logistic regression analysis based on MRI fetal lung volume measurements. AJR Am J Roentgenol 2007; 189: 1307
173. Hwang PJ, Kousseff BG: Omphalocele and gastroschisis: an 18-year review study. Genet Med 2004; 6: 232
174. Ledbetter DJ: Gastroschisis and omphalocele. Surg Clin North Am 2006; 86: 249
175. Henrich K, Huemmer HP, Reingruber B, Weber PG: Gastroschisis and omphalocele: treatments and long-term outcomes. Pediatr Surg Int 2008; 24: 167
176. Tsakayannis DE, Zurakowski D, Lillehei CW: Respiratory insufficiency at birth: a predictor of mortality for infants with omphalocele. J Pediatr Surg 1996; 31: 1088
177. Lee SL, Beyer TD, Kim SS et al: Initial nonoperative management and delayed closure for treatment of giant omphaloceles. J Pediatr Surg 2006; 41: 1846
178. Owen A, Marven S, Jackson L et al: Experience of bedside preformed silo staged reduction and closure for gastroschisis. J Pediatr Surg 2006; 41: 1830
179. Olesevich M, Alexander F, Khan M, Cotman K: Gastroschisis revisited: role of intraoperative measurement of abdominal pressure. J Pediatr Surg 2005; 40: 789
180. Nguyen T, Zainabadi K, Bui T et al: Thoracoscopic repair of esophageal atresia and tracheoesophageal fistula: lessons learned. J Laparoendosc Adv Surg Tech A 2006; 16: 174
181. Hirabayashi Y, Yoshizawa Y, Inoue S, Shimizu R: Epidural analgesia for patients with tracheoesophageal fistula. Masui 1988; 37: 370
182. Dalla Vecchia LK, Grosfeld JL, West KW et al: Intestinal atresia and stenosis: a 25-year experience with 277 cases. Arch Surg 1998; 133: 490
183. Cucchiaro G, De Lagausie P, El-Ghoneimi A, Nivoche Y: Single-dose caudal anesthesia for major intraabdominal operations in high-risk infants. Anesth Analg 2001; 92: 1439
184. Welzing L, Roth B: Experience with remifentanil in neonates and infants. Drugs 2006; 66: 1339

185. Shaer CM, Chescheir N, Schulkin J: Myelomeningocele: a review of the epidemiology, genetics, risk factors for conception, prenatal diagnosis, and prognosis for affected individuals. Obstet Gynecol Surv 2007; 62: 471

186. McLone DG, Dias MS: The Chiari II malformation: cause and impact. Childs Nerv Syst 2003; 19: 540

187. McLone DG: Care of the neonate with a myelomeningocele. Neurosurg Clin N Am 1998; 9: 111

188. Sutton LN: Fetal surgery for neural tube defects. Best Pract Res Clin Obstet Gynaecol 2008; 22: 175

189. Shah S, Cawley M, Gleeson R et al: Latex allergy and latex sensitization in children and adolescents with meningomyelocele. J Allergy Clin Immunol 1998; 101: 741

190. Birmingham PK, Dsida RM, Grayhack JJ et al: Do latex precautions in children with myelodysplasia reduce intraoperative allergic reactions? J Pediatr Orthop 1996; 16: 799

191. Blum RH, Rockoff MA, Holzman RS et al: Overreaction to latex allergy? Anesth Analg 1997; 84: 467

192. Dierdorf SF, McNiece WL, Rao CC et al: Failure of succinylcholine to alter plasma potassium in children with myelomeningocoele. Anesthesiology 1986; 64: 272

193. Viscomi CM, Abajian JC, Wald SL et al: Spinal anesthesia for repair of meningomyelocele in neonates. Anesth Analg 1995; 81: 492

194. Sin AH, Rashidi M, Caldito G, Nanda A: Surgical treatment of myelomeningocele: year 2000 hospitalization, outcome, and cost analysis in the US. Childs Nerv Syst 2007; 23: 1125

195. Persson EK, Anderson S, Wiklund LM, Uvebrant P: Hydrocephalus in children born in 1999–2002: epidemiology, outcome and ophthalmological findings. Childs Nerv Syst 2007; 23: 1111

196. Lee JS, Polin RA: Treatment and prevention of necrotizing enterocolitis. Semin Neonatol 2003; 8: 449

197. Srinivasan PS, Brandler MD, D'Souza A: Necrotizing enterocolitis. Clin Perinatol 2008; 35: 251

198. Alfaleh K, Bassler D: Probiotics for prevention of necrotizing enterocolitis in preterm infants. Cochrane Database Syst Rev 2008: CD005496

199. Ehrlich PF, Sato TT, Short BL, Hartman GE: Outcome of perforated necrotizing enterocolitis in the very low-birth weight neonate may be independent of the type of surgical treatment. Am Surg 2001; 67: 752

200. Blakely ML, Lally KP, McDonald S et al: Postoperative outcomes of extremely low birth-weight infants with necrotizing enterocolitis or isolated intestinal perforation: a prospective cohort study by the NICHD Neonatal Research Network. Ann Surg 2005; 241: 984

201. Lau ST, Lee YH, Caty MG: Current management of hernias and hydroceles. Semin Pediatr Surg 2007; 16: 50

202. Craven PD, Badawi N, Henderson-Smart DJ, O'Brien M: Regional (spinal, epidural, caudal) versus general anaesthesia in preterm infants undergoing inguinal herniorrhaphy in early infancy. Cochrane Database Syst Rev 2003: CD003669

203. Walther-Larsen S, Rasmussen LS: The former preterm infant and risk of post-operative apnoea: recommendations for management. Acta Anaesthesiol Scand 2006; 50: 888

204. Cook-Sather SD, Tulloch HV, Liacouras CA, Schreiner MS: Gastric fluid volume in infants for pyloromyotomy. Can J Anaesth 1997; 44: 278

205. Jacobs JP, Giroud JM, Quintessenza JA et al: The modern approach to patent ductus arteriosus treatment: complementary roles of video-assisted thoracoscopic surgery and interventional cardiology coil occlusion. Ann Thorac Surg 2003; 76: 1421

ANESTHESIA FOR SURGICAL SUBSPECIALTIES

CHAPTER 45 ■ PEDIATRIC ANESTHESIA

JOSEPH P. CRAVERO AND ZEEV N. KAIN

KEY POINTS

1. A recent study found that most parents are very much interested in receiving all possible information about their child's surgery *and* that the parents were not overly anxious as a result of the detailed discussion regarding anesthetics plans and risks.

2. Multiple investigations have found that a child with a current upper respiratory infection (or recovering from such an infection) is at increased risk to develop laryngospasm, bronchospasm, oxygen desaturation, postextubation croup, and postoperative atelectasis.

3. Although most children who undergo tonsillectomy and adenoidectomy can be discharged home following 4 hours of postanesthesia care unit observation, children with severe obstructive sleep apnea require postoperative observation in the hospital.

4. Arrangements for overnight hospital monitoring following general anesthesia should be made for any infant considered to be at significant risk for postoperative apnea, particularly those with a history of severe respiratory illness or previous problems with apnea and bradycardia (regardless of postconceptual age).

5. Current standard of care dictates that healthy children undergoing elective minor surgery require *no* laboratory evaluation, and thus can be spared the anxiety and pain of blood drawing.

6. Solids are prohibited within 6 to 8 hours of surgery (generally after midnight), formula within 6 hours, breast milk within 4 hours of surgery, and clear liquids within 2 hours of surgery.

7. Over 85% of all preoperative sedation in the United States is performed using midazolam. It has rapid onset and predictable effect without causing cardiorespiratory depression.

8. Mask induction of general anesthesia remains the most common induction technique for pediatric anesthesia the United States. There is no question that inhalation induction of anesthesia is safe, but the incidence of bradycardia, hypotension, and cardiac arrest during this form of induction is higher in infants younger than age 1 year than in older children and adults.

9. Propofol is the most widely used intravenous agent for induction and maintenance of anesthesia or sedation in children. Although its safety is well established, its use in children is limited to the operating room environment and brief sedation outside the operating room. Prolonged infusion in the intensive care environment has been linked to acidosis, heart failure, and a number of fatalities.

10. Chest wall rigidity is not uncommon when administering bolus opioids, especially to drug-naive neonates and infants.

11. Postoperative nausea and vomiting is particularly prominent after certain surgeries such as orchidopexy, strabismus surgery, and tonsillectomy. There is no single therapy that is universally accepted as safe and effective.

12. Because the narrowest portion of the pediatric airway is at the level of the cricoid cartilage (and is therefore round), uncuffed tubes can be used and will create a functional seal when appropriately sized. Several formulas have been used for tube selection in children older than age 1 year, the most common being (16 + age)/4 or variations thereof.

13. The safety and efficacy of patient-controlled analgesia for children as young as 6 years have been shown. Although routinely used in children's hospitals, this technique is to be used *only* by highly trained medical personal who are knowledgeable in pediatric pain management.

14. The most commonly used form of regional anesthesia in children is the *caudal block*. This technique can provide postoperative analgesia following a wide variety of lower abdominal and genitourinary surgical procedures.

In order to deliver optimal anesthesia care to infants and children, one must appreciate the unique nature of this population and the impact that anesthesia can have on their developing physiology. There are numerous specific anatomic, physiologic, and psychological issues that should be understood prior to anesthetizing pediatric patients. These distinctive features form the basis for the techniques and pharmacology outlined in this chapter. A partial listing of the most important differences is presented in Table 45-1. Incorporating these facts into the anesthesia care of children is critical to achieving high quality. This chapter will focus on only the most salient issues relating to anesthesia delivery for pediatric patients. Important

TABLE 45-1

ANATOMIC AND PHYSIOLOGIC DISTINCTIONS BETWEEN ADULTS AND PEDIATRIC PATIENTS

■ PHYSICAL OR PHYSIOLOGIC VARIABLE	■ CONTRAST BETWEEN CHILD AND ADULT	■ ANESTHETIC IMPLICATION
Head size	Much larger head size relative to body	Consider roll under shoulders or neck for optimal intubation positioning
Tongue size	Larger size relative to mouth	Makes airway appear slightly anterior; oral airways particularly helpful during mask ventilation
Airway shape	Narrowest diameter is below the glottis at cricoid level in children	Uncuffed tubes can make seal when appropriately sized in children younger than 8 years of age
Respiratory physiology	Oxygen consumption is 2 to 3 times greater in infants than adults. FRC ranges from 8–13 mL/kg ≈ 1/3 as large as adults	Oxygen desaturation is extremely rapid following apnea
Cardiac physiology	Relatively fixed stroke volume in neonates and infants	Bradycardia must be treated aggressively in young age groups; consider atropine prior to airway management; heart rates less than 60 require circulatory support
Renal function	Limited GFR at birth; does not reach adult levels until infancy; total body water and % extracellular fluid are increased in the infant	Prolonged duration of action for hydrophilic drugs, particularly those that are renally excreted
Hepatic function	P450 system not fully developed in neonates and infants; liver blood flow decreased in newborns	Prolonged excretion for drugs, depending on hepatic metabolism
Body surface area	Larger surface-to-body ratio in newborns/infants/toddlers	Heat loss more prominent problem for these age groups
Psychological development	0–6 mo—stress on family 8 mo–4 yr—separation anxiety 4–6 yr—misconceptions of surgical mutilation 6–13 yr—fear of not "waking up" ≥13 yr—fear of loss of control, body image issues	Changes the manner in which each patient and family should be approached; must address issues with personal and systemic strategies

FRC, functional residual capacity; GFR, glomerular filtration rate.

topics such as neonatal anesthesia, pediatric pharmacology, and pediatric equipment are covered elsewhere in this textbook or in a number of textbooks that deal exclusively with pediatric anesthesiology.

THE PREOPERATIVE EVALUATION

The preoperative evaluation of the pediatric patient should consist of pertinent maternal history, birth and neonatal history, review of systems, physical examination, height, weight, and vital signs. Preoperative home use of medications such as bronchodilators, steroids, and chemotherapeutic agents has significant implications for the anesthetic management. The use of herbal medication and other alternative and complementary medicine modalities has to be assessed as well.[1] Many herbal remedies have anesthetic implications and the anesthesiologist should be fully informed about their effects. This topic is covered in further detail in Chapter 23. Special attention should be paid to the existence of malformations in the child and family. Issues such as anesthetic risks, anesthetic plans, recovery phenomena, postoperative analgesia, and discharge criteria have to be discussed in detail. A recent study found that most parents are very much interested in receiving all possible information about their child's surgery *and* that the parents were not overly anxious as a result of the detailed discussion regarding anesthetics plans and risks.[2]

It is important to appreciate that anesthesia and surgery cause an enormous amount of stress and hardship on both the child and parents. Anxiety in children undergoing surgery is characterized by subjective feelings of tension, apprehension, nervousness and worry, and may be expressed in many forms.[2] Some children verbalize their fears explicitly, while for others anxiety is expressed only behaviorally. Many children look scared, become agitated, breathe deeply, tremble, stop talking or playing, and may start to cry. These behaviors, which may prolong the induction of anesthesia, could give children some sense of control in the situation and thereby diminish a damaging sense of helplessness.[2] Coping with preoperative stress requires consistent communication between the child, the parents, and all health care providers involved in the perioperative period. Because parental anxiety increases child's anxiety, preoperative preparation should include the entire family.[2]

Both behavioral and pharmacologic interventions can be used to address the issue of preoperative anxiety in children and their parents. Behavioral interventions include tours of the operating room, written and audiovisual materials, coloring books, and patient care representatives skilled in the preoperative preparation of children.[2] To date, most studies suggest that preoperative preparation programs reduce anxiety and enhance coping in children.[2] Some hospitals allow parents to be present for the induction of anesthesia, but the efficacy of this intervention is uncertain and the availability of such programs is not universal.[2] Other nonpharmacologic interventions such as music, acupuncture, and hypnosis have been shown to reduce the anxiety in perioperative settings.[2,3] Pharmacologic interventions such as midazolam are very effective treatment for preoperative anxiety and will be discussed later in this chapter. Recent research has documented that a child's fear on the day of surgery might extend beyond the immediate operative period.[2] About 50% of all children undergoing routine outpatient surgery present at 2 weeks postoperatively with new-onset anxiety, nighttime crying, enuresis, separation anxiety, temper tantrums, and sleep or eating disturbances.[2] Most of these behaviors disappear within 3 to 4 weeks postoperatively. Primary health care providers should be aware of these behaviors and assure parents that these behavioral changes are self-limited. Children with postoperative behavioral changes that persist beyond 3 to 4 weeks after surgery should be referred to a trained mental health provider.

Coexisting Health Conditions

Upper Respiratory Infection

② Multiple investigations have found that a child with a current upper respiratory infection (URI; or recovering from a URI) is at increased risk to develop laryngospasm, bronchospasm, oxygen desaturation, postextubation croup, and postoperative atelectasis.[4,5] Although these complications usually do not cause significant morbidity in otherwise healthy children, they may be very significant in children with underlying conditions such as asthma and sickle cell disease. Children with asthma, infants/young children with bronchopulmonary dysphasia, children under 1 year of age, children with sickle cell disease, children who live in a household that includes smoking parents, and children who are to undergo bronchoscopy are at a higher risk of developing perioperative morbidity if suffering from a URI.[4] Patients in these categories should be carefully assessed and strong consideration should be given to postponing elective surgery. It is unclear how long surgery should be delayed following a URI, however, because bronchial hyperreactivity may exist for up to 7 weeks after such an infection.[6] The final decision must take into account the risk-to-benefit ratio of undergoing a surgical procedure in the patient's current state of health and the likelihood of acquiring another URI prior to rescheduled surgery. The technique used for anesthesia may impact the number of airway issues encountered. Mask anesthesia has been shown to be associated with a significantly lower rate of perioperative complications as compared with endotracheal tube. Conversely, the use of the laryngeal mask airway (LMA) has been associated with the same number of airway complications as the endotracheal tube in this population.[7]

Obstructive Sleep Apnea

Severe adenotonsillar hypertrophy with obstructive sleep apnea (OSA) is a frequent indication for tonsillectomy and adenoidectomy. OSA patients are at risk for airway obstruction with the use of preoperative sedative predication and during the induction process. Postoperatively, patients with severe OSA may exhibit worsening of their obstructive symptoms secondary to tissue edema, altered response to carbon dioxide, and residual effects of anesthetic agents.[8] Children under 3 years of age are at particularly high risk for respiratory complications.[9] **③** Although most children who undergo tonsillectomy and adenoidectomy can be discharged home following 4 hours of postanesthesia care unit (PACU) observation, children with severe OSA require postoperative observation in the hospital. Such issues have to be discussed a priori with the family and the surgeon.

OSA often accompanies obesity. All patients with markedly elevated body mass index should be questioned about sleep apnea symptoms. Obese children also have an increased incidence of difficult airway, upper airway obstruction in the PACU, extended PACU stays, and postoperative nausea and vomiting.[10,11]

Asthma

It is well established that children with asthma should be under optimal medical care prior to undergoing general anesthesia and surgery.[12] In fact, the more active the disease (as indicated by recent asthma symptoms, asthma medication usage, and recent treatment in an emergency department), the greater probability of perioperative complications.[13] All oral and inhaled medications, such as corticosteroids and β-agonists, should be continued up to and including the day of surgery. Recent data indicate that administration of inhaled short-acting β-agonists prior to induction of anesthesia eliminates the increase in airway pressure that is typically associated with intubation in asthmatic patients.[14]

The Former Preterm Infant

There are specific issues related to the perioperative period of infants with a history of preterm delivery. These concerns include (1) the impact that bronchopulmonary dysplasia might have on the patient's perioperative course and (2) the presence of anemia and the possibility of postoperative apnea. Perioperative complications from bronchopulmonary dysplasia generally involve reactivity of airways and the risk of severe hypoxia that can accompany bronchospastic episodes. Bronchodilators and inhaled corticosteroids should be continued up to and including the day of surgery. Parents should be questioned about the need for oxygen therapy at home and recent hematocrit data should be available. Data also indicate that former preterm infants are more likely to develop postoperative apnea following general anesthesia.[15,16] These reports indicate that risk of postoperative apnea is inversely related to postconceptional age and that infants with a history of apnea/bradycardia, respiratory distress, or mechanical ventilation may be at increased risk.[17] The question as to which of these infants needs to be admitted to the hospital (for observation) following general anesthesia is controversial. The age is generally agreed to be <52 to 60 weeks postconceptual age.[17] **④** Arrangements for overnight hospital monitoring following general anesthesia should be made for any infant considered to be at significant risk for postoperative apnea, particularly those with a history of severe respiratory illness or previous problems with apnea and bradycardia (regardless of postconceptual age).

Laboratory Evaluation

⑤ Current standard of care dictates that healthy children undergoing elective minor surgery require *no* laboratory evaluation, and thus can be spared the anxiety and pain of blood drawing.[18] Indeed, blood chemistry analyses are performed only for specific indications, such as measurement of ionized potassium in children on digoxin or diuretics. Hemoglobin measurement is not required for minor elective cases. For surgeries in which significant blood loss may be expected, an arbitrary value of 10 g/dL has been cited as acceptable for infants older than 3 months or age. When time allows, children whose hemoglobin values are less than this standard should have the cause of their anemia investigated and corrected. For younger infants and neonates, higher values may be desirable (depending on gestational age and general health status). Patients with sickle cell anemia or other hemoglobinopathies require special preoperative preparation including goal-directed transfusion. Routine chest radiographs and urinary analysis are unnecessary unless indicated by a specific symptom or known coexisting illness. Coagulation screening has been among the most debated of all laboratory tests. Although an undiagnosed coagulopathy could result in serious surgical morbidity, commonly used screening tests, such as bleeding time and prothrombin time, do *not* reliably predict abnormal perioperative bleeding.[19] Laboratory testing of coagulation should only be considered in selected situations including (1) children in whom either the history or medical condition suggests a possible hemostatic defect, (2) patients undergoing surgical procedures that might *induce* hemostatic disturbances (e.g., cardiopulmonary bypass), (3) cases in which an intact coagulation system is critical for adequate hemostasis, and (4) patients for whom even minimal postoperative bleeding could be life-threatening.

Although teratogenicity of anesthetic agents has not been firmly established, it is important to determine whether a postmenarchal female patient is possibly pregnant before the administration of anesthesia. This may be a difficult task as a reliable menstrual and sexual history may be difficult to obtain from an adolescent when a relationship of confidentiality with medical personnel has not been previously established. In addition, parents (or patients) may decline a request for a pregnancy test. At this point there are no clear national guidelines on the issue of pregnancy test screening of all female patients of childbearing age before the administration of anesthesia. Routine versus selective testing is a matter of policy at individual facilities. At the very least, patients should be warned of the possible danger that anesthesia poses to a fetus, and pregnancy testing should be offered if not required.

Preoperative Fasting Period

The risk of aspiration pneumonia in children is well recognized, and recent reports found an incidence of about 1 in 10,000 for this clinical phenomenon.[20] These reports also indicate that the outcome of children who developed aspiration pneumonia is excellent, unless these children had some major underlying problem such as abdominal or thoracic trauma.[20] In an effort to minimize aspiration injury, the American Society of Anesthesiologists has issued practice guidelines regarding preoperative fasting. Solids are prohibited within 6 to 8 hours of surgery (generally after midnight), formula within 6 hours, breast milk within 4 hours of surgery, and clear liquids within 2 hours of surgery.[21] Clear liquids such as apple or grape juice, flat cola, and sugar water may be encouraged up to 2 hours prior to the induction of anesthesia as their consumption has been shown to decrease the gastric residual volume. The issue of fasting time is of particular importance in pediatric anesthesiology as younger children have smaller glycogen stores and are more likely to develop hypoglycemia with prolonged intervals of fasting. Regardless of the length of fasting, there is a defined population of children who are at an increased risk for aspiration of stomach contents. This group includes those with delayed gastric-emptying times and abdominal pathology associated with outlet obstruction (pyloric stenosis), ileus, vomiting, or electrolyte disorders.

Preoperative Sedatives

Sedation before surgery is an effective method that is widely used for young children for decreasing anxiety.[2,22] The primary goals of premedication in children are to facilitate a smooth and anxiety-free separation from the parents and induction of anesthesia. Other effects that may be achieved by pharmacologic preparation of the patient include amnesia, anxiolysis, prevention of physiologic stress, and analgesia. In addition, children who are sedated before coming to the operating room may have fewer stress-related behavioral changes in the immediate postoperative time compared with groups of patients who receive no sedation (Fig. 45-1).

Oral

Midazolam is the most commonly used sedative premedicant used in the United States.[2] Over 85% of all preoperative sedation in the United States is performed using midazolam.[22] It has rapid onset and predictable effect without causing cardiorespiratory depression. In a dose of 0.5 to 0.75 mg/kg, midazolam effect peaks approximately 30 minutes after administration, and in surgery lasting an hour or more, oral midazolam in doses of 0.25 to 0.5 mg/kg does not appear to lengthen recovery room time.[5,22] Although it is very effective in most children, about 14% of children may not respond to a midazolam dose of 0.5 mg/kg.[23] This unresponsive group of children is reported to be younger (4.2 ± 2.3 vs. 5.9 ± 2.0 years) and to have high levels of preoperative emotionality. Higher doses of midazolam (0.75 mg/kg) may be more appropriate in these nonresponders. Although midazolam has a short duration that generally does not delay emergence from general anesthesia or discharge from PACU, some reports indicate that the use of this agent with children undergoing ultra-short procedures such myringotomies may delay hospital discharge.[24] Although serious side effects after oral midazolam are uncommon, strict adult supervision is necessary in children who receive this drug. Midazolam has been shown to be superior to parental presence in decreasing perioperative stress for patients and families, although the addition of parental presence will result in increased parental satisfaction from the overall perioperative experience.[2] Midazolam can be reversed with flumazenil, which antagonizes benzodiazepines competitively. The initial recommended dose in children is 0.05 mg/kg given intravenously titrated up to 1.0 mg total.[25]

Oral ketamine has also been used as a sedation medication in doses of 5 to 6 mg/kg for children 1 to 6 years of age.[22] Maximal sedation occurred within 20 minutes. The combination of ketamine and midazolam has also been used as an oral sedative premedication mixture. Funk et al.[26] reported that the combination of midazolam and ketamine administrated orally had a 90% success rate of satisfactory anxiolysis compared with <75% with either drug alone. Nausea and vomiting rates were slightly increased in children who received oral ketamine.

Oral transmucosal fentanyl was the first commercial attempt to deliver medication to children by the transmucosal oral route and was shown to sedate children prior to induction of anesthesia.[22] Side effects include facial pruritus, high incidence of postoperative nausea and vomiting, and arterial oxygen desaturation. Thus, this drug is not currently used routinely in the perioperative settings.

Clonidine is an α_2-agonist that, when given in combination with atropine, produces satisfactory preoperative sedation, easy separation from parents, and mask acceptance within 45 minutes.[27] Orally administered clonidine in a dose of 4 μg/kg has been demonstrated to reliably cause sedation, decrease anesthetic requirements, and decrease requirement for postoperative analgesics. It also attenuates the hemodynamic response to tracheal intubation. With the recommended dose, perioperative hypotension is not observed.[22] The major disadvantage of this sedative is slow onset as compared with midazolam.

Most recently, dexmedetomidine, a more selective α_2-agonist than clonidine, has gained some popularity as a preoperative

FIGURE 45-1. **A.** Frequency of sedative premedication practice in the United States as of 2002. **B.** Frequency of sedative premedication practice in the United States as of 1996. Data reported are medians (range, 0 to 100%). (From Kain ZN, Caldwell-Andrews AA, Krivuta DM et al: Trends in practice of parental presence during induction of anesthesia and the use of preoperative sedative premedication in the United States, 1995–2002: Results of a follow-up national survey. Anesth Analg 2004; 98: 1252, with permission.)

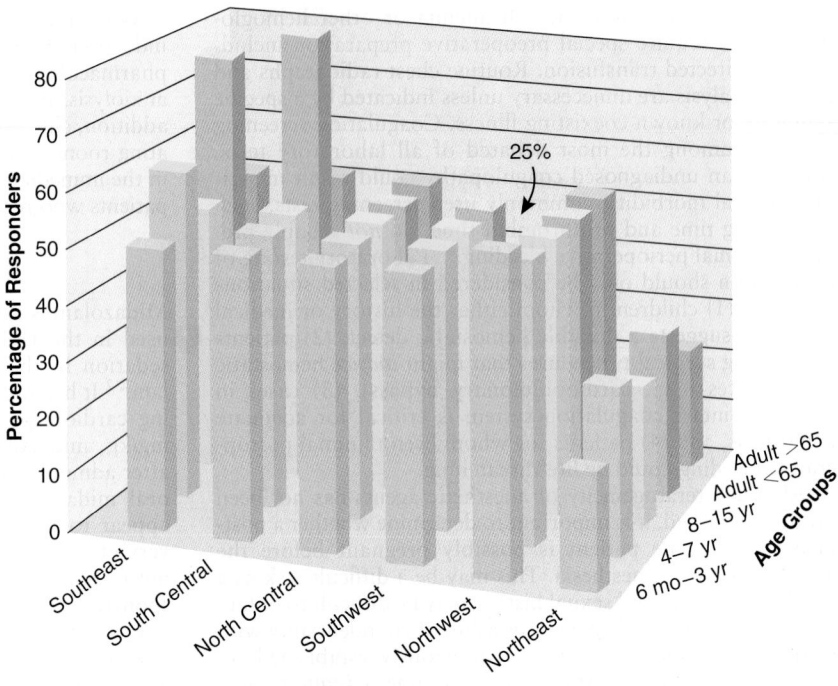

A   **Geographical Region**

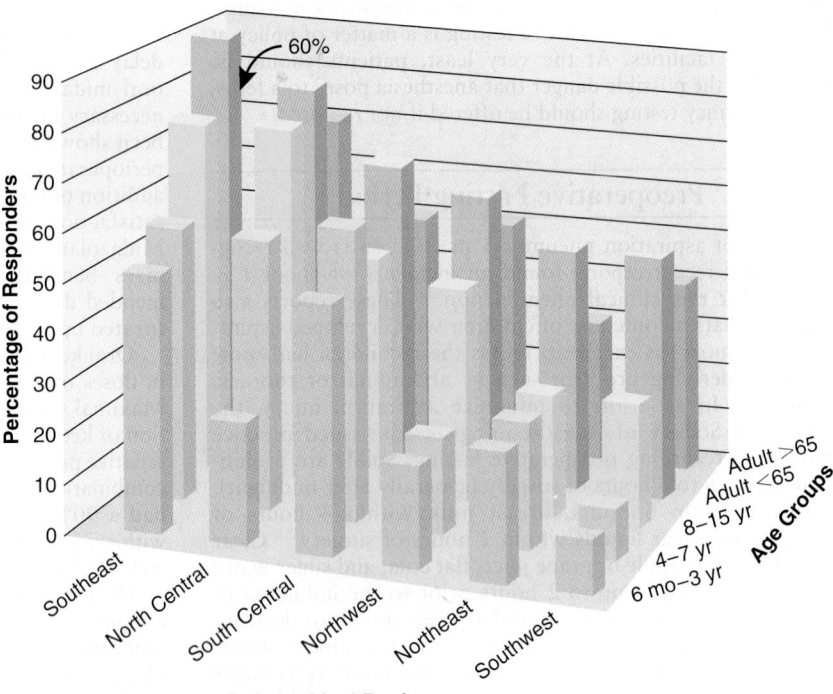

B   **Geographical Region**

sedative for children. When used at 1 μg/kg transmucosally or 3 to 4 μg/kg orally, this drug has a similar sedative and anxiolytic effect to clonidine or midazolam. Similar to clonidine, dexmedetomidine has the effect of lowering pain scores in the postanesthesia time frame.[1]

Nasal

A major disadvantage of intranasally administered sedative medications is that *most* children cry on administration because it transiently irritates the nasal passages. Rapid absorption as well as avoidance of first-pass hepatic metabo-

lism of medications are advantages of this route of administration. When required, midazolam can be administered intranasally in a dose of 0.2 mg/kg. The use of sufentanil and other sedatives intranasally has been abandoned because of untoward side effects including chest wall rigidity and hypoxia (Table 45-2).

Rectal

Rectal administration of midazolam in doses of 0.5 to 1.0 mg/kg effectively reduces the anxiety of children prior to induction.[22] Care must be taken, however, that the medication is not

TABLE 45-2

PREMEDICATION—DRUGS OPTIONS AND DOSES

■ MEDICATION	■ ROUTE	■ DOSE (mg/kg)	■ TIME TO ONSET (min)	■ ELIMINATION HALF-LIFE T½ (hr)
Midazolam	Oral	0.25–1.0	10	2
	Intranasal	0.2–0.3	<10	2–3
	Rectal	0.3–1.0	10	2–3
Ketamine	Oral	3.0–6.0	10	2–3
	Intranasal	3.0–5.0	<10	3
	Rectal	5.0–6.0	20–30	3
Clonidine	Oral	0.002–0.004	45	8–12

expelled immediately. Both methohexital and thiopental have also been used in rectal formulations in a dose of 25 mg/kg. Onset of sedation requires approximately 10 minutes. Respiratory depression and oxygen desaturation may occur because of variable absorption of the medication in the rectum.

Intramuscular

Parenteral administration of sedation may be the only alternative in a child who refuses to cooperate with other modalities. Intramuscular midazolam in a dose of 0.3 mg/kg provides anxiolysis in 5 to 10 minute. Ketamine in an intramuscular dose of 3 to 4 mg/kg provides a quiet, breathing, yet minimally responsive patient in approximately 5 minutes.

It is important to note that the oral route is by far the most commonly used and preferred route of sedative administration for children. Nasal, rectal, and intramuscular routes should be used only under special circumstances such as cognitively challenged children.

ANESTHETIC AGENTS

Potent Inhalation Agents

Mask Induction Pharmacology

8 Mask induction of general anesthesia remains the most common induction technique for pediatric anesthesia the United States. There is no question that inhalation induction of anesthesia is safe, but the incidence of bradycardia, hypotension, and cardiac arrest during this form of induction is higher in infants younger than age 1 year than in older children and adults.[28] This difference in outcome is due to the extremely rapid uptake of inhalation agents in infants compared with adults as a result of the much greater ratio of alveolar ventilation to funcional residual capacity and the altered distribution of cardiac output. High inspired concentrations (overpressure) are often used early in induction, yielding very high tissue concentrations of anesthetic that can lead to severe cardiac depression and junctional rhythms.[29] In light of these facts, mask induction of anesthesia in this age group should be accompanied by monitoring of blood pressure, electrocardiogram, oxygenation, and ventilation.

Minimal Alveolar Concentration. The minimum alveolar concentration (MAC) of anesthetic required in pediatric patients differs with age. There is actually a small increase in MAC between birth and 2 to 3 months of age, which represents the age of highest MAC requirement. After that time MAC slowly decreases with age. For sevoflurane the change in MAC is marked, with a value of approximately 2.5% for young infants compared with 2% for adolescents and adults.[30]

Intracardiac Shunts. Children with unrepaired or partially repaired congenital heart malformations may safely undergo inhaled induction of anesthesia. Although intracardiac shunts can, in theory, alter the uptake of anesthetic agents and affect the speed of induction, this is rarely clinically evident. A right-to-left shunt slows the inhaled induction of anesthesia because anesthetic concentration in the arterial blood increases more slowly. A left-to-right shunt should have the opposite effect; volatile agent induction is more rapid because the rate of anesthetic transfer from the lungs to the arterial blood is increased. In practice, decreased delivery of anesthetic to the target tissues largely negates the increased uptake with this type of shunt.

Inhaled Agents for Induction of Anesthesia. The only two potent anesthetic agents currently in use that are compatible with inhaled induction are sevoflurane and halothane.[31] Both of these agents have acceptable odor and can be used for smooth inhaled induction in children. In the United States sevoflurane is the only potent inhalation agent available for inhalation induction. Its advantages (including rapid onset and low frequency of dysrhythmias or hypotension) allowed it to completely dominate the U.S. market.[32,33] Some of these (clinically noted) differences may, in fact, be due to vaporizer design owing to the fact that it is possible to deliver a much higher MAC multiple of halothane versus sevoflurane.[33] Halothane has been shown to have a greater depressive effect on the myocardial contractility than sevoflurane during standard inhaled induction techniques.[34,35]

Sevoflurane undergoes ex vivo degradation reaction in the clinical setting through direct contact with CO_2 absorbents (i.e., soda lime or Baralyme) in the anesthesia circuit. This reaction produces pentafluoroisopropenyl fluoromethyl ether (PIFE), also known as Compound A, and trace amounts of pentafluoromethoxy isopropyl fluoromethyl ether (PMFE, Compound B). Mean maximum concentrations in pediatric patients with soda lime are about half those found in adults. Although the level of compound A at which toxicity occurs is not known, sevoflurane use with fresh gas flows of 1 L/min appears to be safe in children. Finally, while emergence from anesthesia is more rapid with sevoflurane than with more soluble agents such as halothane or isoflurane, there is a growing literature supporting the fact that agitation behaviors in children on emergence are more common with this agent. The exact reason for this disturbance is not known, but there is evidence that is may occur with or without pain as a factor.[36] A number of medications have been used to decrease the problem of emergence agitation after sevoflurane (including midazolam, ketorolac, fentanyl, propofol, and dexmedetomidine). Careful attention to pain control and supportive environments are indicated.

Halothane (where it is still available) has a long history of safety and efficacy as an inhaled agent for pediatric anesthesia.

Although there has been some concern regarding sensitization of the myocardium to catecholamines, there is little problem in the absence of hypercarbia or light anesthesia. Up to 10 μmg/kg of epinephrine may be used with minimal risk of cardiac dysrhythmia in normocarbic pediatric patients.

Isoflurane also has a long track record as a safe and efficacious agent for maintenance of anesthesia in infants and children. Like halothane, it decreases blood pressure in pediatric patients. Although myocardial depression in children is less than that caused by halothane, isoflurane reduces peripheral vascular resistance, whereas halothane does not. (In neonates, equal myocardial depression has been demonstrated with both drugs.[37]) The major disadvantage of isoflurane is its pungent odor and high incidence of laryngospasm when this agent is used for inhaled induction of anesthesia. For this reason it should not be used for inhaled induction of anesthesia.

Desflurane is also a safe and effective agent for maintenance of anesthesia in infants and children. Unfortunately, as with isoflurane, an unacceptable incidence of coughing, increased secretions, and laryngospasm preclude its use as a mask induction agent.[38] Although desflurane appears to be associated with faster initial awakening when used as a maintenance anesthetic agent in pediatric patients, studies have shown no difference between halothane and desflurane in time to discharge after ambulatory surgery. As is the case with sevoflurane, emergence agitation has been reported with desflurane use in children.[38]

Intravenous Agents

Sedative Hypnotics

Sedative hypnotic agents may be employed after inhaled induction of anesthesia (for instance, to deepen anesthesia for airway management) or they may be used as primary induction and maintenance agents in children who have an intravenous line in place. Intravenous line placement may be made easier for the awake patient through the use of topical anesthetics such as the eutectic mixture of local anesthetics, topical liposomal lidocaine cream, or other topical local anesthetic creams.[39,40] As with inhaled agents previously mentioned, the doses of intravenous agents used in infants and toddlers will often need to be increased by 25 to 40% in order to obtain the same level of sedation/anesthesia in children as compared with adults.

Propofol, thiopental, methohexital, etomidate, midazolam, and ketamine have all been used to produce effective intravenous induction of anesthesia or sedation in infants and children. Propofol is the most widely used agent for induction and maintenance of anesthesia or sedation in children. Although its safety is well established, its use in children is limited to the operating room environment and brief sedation outside the operating room. Prolonged infusion in the intensive care environment has been linked to acidosis, heart failure, and a number of fatalities.[41,42] Propofol induction doses range from 3 to 4 mg/kg for children younger than 2 years to approximately 2.5 to 3 mg/kg for older children. Maintenance of general anesthesia requires 200 to 300 μg/kg/min.[43] Onset is rapid but may be accompanied by some random movement and cough. Bag-mask ventilation is generally easily performed. Pain on injection of propofol is marked. This problem may be minimized by infusing the largest vein possible and running carrier fluid as rapidly as possible. Lidocaine preceding (or mixed with) the propofol bolus can be employed to decrease the pain with intravenous injection. Other techniques to decrease discomfort include fentanyl premedication, ketamine premedication, and nitrous oxide inhalation.[43] Propofol will cause mild-

to-moderate decreases in blood pressure when used at recommended doses.[45]

The emergence profile of propofol in children shows clear advantages over other intravenous agents and inhaled anesthetics. Emergence from deep sedation/anesthesia is clearly faster than that from most other sedative agents and most inhaled agents, especially after prolonged administration. In addition, even though time to awakening may not be faster than sevoflurane or desflurane, the emergence from propofol is associated with less nausea and vomiting[46] and it is accompanied by less emergence agitation,[47] so readiness for discharge is at least as rapid.[48]

Although it was first described 40 years ago, ketamine has been increasingly reported for use in anesthesia, procedural sedation, and sedation the intensive care environment for children. It is the only intravenous agent that offers both potent hypnosis *and* analgesia. Other unique aspects include the fact that ketamine preserves airway reflexes, maintains respiratory drive, increases endogenous catecholamine release, and results in a small amount of bronchodilation. Induction doses of 1 mg/kg intravenously yields effective analgesia and sedation with rapid onset. Intramuscular doses of 3 to 4 mg/kg result in a similar state with significant analgesia, appropriate for minor procedures such as intravenous starts or fracture manipulation.[49]

Simultaneous administration of an anticholinergic will minimize oral secretions. Emergence from ketamine sedation/anesthesia can be marked by diplopia, occasional disturbing dreams, and nausea/vomiting, although these are less common in children than adults.[50] The use of concomitant midazolam 0.025 to 0.50 mg/kg to decrease some of these side effects has a mixed record of success and should not be considered reliable. On the other hand, a recent investigation suggested that a single dose of ketamine may decrease emergence agitation after sevoflurane anesthesia,[51] and another indicated an induction with ketamine may decrease the incidence of oculocardiac reflex during ophthalmologic surgery.[52]

Note on Toxicity of Anesthetic Agents

The Food and Drug Administration (FDA) has completed a review of the data available from animal studies involving inhalation and intravenous anesthetic agents.[53] The conclusions of the study find that "neurodegeneration, with possible cognitive sequelae, is a potential long-term risk of anesthetics in neonatal and young pediatric patients." The review goes on to suggest that drugs that act at the NMDA (N-methyl-D-aspartic acid) receptor as well as at the γ-aminobutyric acid receptors have been identified as potentially neurotoxic in infant animal models. There is currently not enough information available to suggest that operative anesthesia is harmful in humans, and there is also not enough evidence to suggest that one type of anesthetic agent is safer than another. Observation human studies have been initiated but there is likely to be debate over the safety of anesthetic agents, especially in the context of long-term exposure in very young (neonatal) patients for some years to come.

Opioids

Opioids are important elements of balanced anesthesia and sedation in children. Their use for surgical anesthesia will decrease MAC of inhaled agents, smooth hemodynamics during airway management, or stimulating procedures, and provides postoperative analgesia. Usual recommended doses include fentanyl, 5 to 1 μg/kg; morphine, 0.10 mg/kg; sufentanil, 1 μg/kg; and alfentanil, 50 to 100 μg/kg. Remifentanil has also been shown to be an effective part of anesthesia and sedation protocols for a variety of procedures at 0.25 to 1.0

μg/kg/min.[54,55] Because of its very short half-life, remifentanil does not offer effective postoperative analgesia when used in this manner.

10 Chest wall rigidity is not uncommon when administering bolus opioids, especially to drug-naive neonates and infants. This effect can severely embarrass respiration, and providers must be prepared to provide muscle relaxation and general airway support when delivering these medications in this manner. Opioids are also well known to depress central respiratory effort. Newborns and infants younger than 6 months are particularly susceptible to this effect because of the immature blood–brain barrier and increased levels of free drug. These facts highlight the need to carefully monitor pediatric patients given opioids; however, they do not argue for withholding pain medications. In fact, after 6 months of age there is evidence that infants and children are no more susceptible to central depression from opioids than adults given equivalent doses.[56] It should be noted that opiate delivery via patient-controlled analgesia is well studied and effective in most developmentally normal patients 5 years of age or older.[57] Other modalities such as nurse-controlled analgesia and parent-controlled analgesia are also employed in some centers under carefully controlled conditions.[58]

Muscle Relaxants

Succinylcholine has been used as part of pediatric anesthesia and airway management for over 60 years. When given in a dose of 1.5 to 2.0 mg/kg it produces excellent intubating conditions (reliably) in 60 seconds. Recovery occurs in 6 to 7 minutes. Succinylcholine can also be given intramuscularly at 4 mg/kg in emergencies when intravenous access is not available. Its use is absolutely contraindicated in a variety of patients, particularly in those with muscular dystrophy, recent burn injury, spinal cord transaction, and/or immobilization, as well as any child with a family history of malignant hyperthermia because of the risk of rhabdomyolysis, hyperkalemia, masseter spasm, and malignant hyperthermia. In addition, the drug is currently listed as relatively contraindicated for use in

all children by the FDA. This is because of the infrequent, but well-reported cases in which succinylcholine has been administered to children with risk factors that are not clinically apparent or unappreciated. The requirement for succinylcholine has also been decreased by the availability of fast-onset, nondepolarizing agents such as rocuronium. For all these reasons, succinylcholine can be recommended only in situations in which ultrarapid onset and short duration of action is of paramount importance (laryngospasm) or when muscle relaxation required when intravenous access is not available and intramuscular administration is required.

All nondepolarizing muscle relaxants used in adults are effective for pediatric patients. Because they have a larger percentage of total body water and larger extracellular fluid volume, neonates and young infants have a larger volume of distribution for these hydrophilic drugs than older children and adults. On the other hand, these patients are slightly more sensitive to these drugs. The result is a pharmacokinetic and pharmacodynamic profile in which the recommended doses of these agents are identical for children and adults but the duration of action tends to be slightly longer (Table 45-3).

In selecting a muscle relaxant, one must consider the possible side effects of each medication, its route of metabolism, and the possible duration of action. For instance, pancuronium has a vagolytic effect that may be desirable in many neonates. On the other hand, it is dependent on renal excretion and therefore may have a markedly extended duration of action in neonates when glomerular filtration rate is relatively decreased. Rocuronium has the lowest potency and the fastest onset of action of the currently available nondepolarizing relaxants (60 seconds for a 1-mg/kg dose) and is therefore the logical choice for rapid-sequence intubation.[59,60] Atracurium and cis-atracurium are popular nondepolarizing muscle relaxants for children largely because they are eliminated by Hofmann elimination, a process only dependent on pH and temperature. The onset and offset of these drugs appear faster in neonates than in infants or children.[61] Cis-atracurium is a stereoisomer of atracurium, which has more specificity in

TABLE 45-3

ONSET, DURATION, CARDIOVASCULAR EFFECTS, COST, AND SPECIAL CONSIDERATIONS OF NONDEPOLARIZING NEUROMUSCULAR-BLOCKING AGENTS IN CHILDREN

	■ RECOMMENDED DOSE (μg/kg)	■ ONSET	■ DURATION	■ CARDIOVASCULAR EFFECTS	■ COST	■ SPECIAL CONSIDERATIONS
Atracurium	500	Intermediate	Intermediate	Rare hypotension	Intermediate	Mild erythema common
Cis-atracurium	80–200	Slow-intermediate	Intermediate–long	Absent	Inexpensive-intermediate	
Mivacurium	250–400	Intermediate	Short	Rare hypotension	Intermediate	Mild erythema common
Pancuronium	100	Intermediate	Intermediate–long	Tachycardia, occasional hypertension	Inexpensive	Effect prolonged in renal failure
Rocuronium	500–1,200	Rapid	Intermediate	Slight increase in heart rate	Intermediate	Deltoid injection facilitates tracheal intubation
Vecuronium	100–400	Intermediate (rapid with large doses)	Intermediate (long with doses >150 μg/kg)	Absent	Intermediate	

Doses are the authors' preference and, in some instances, exceed those recommended in the package insert. For onset and duration, specific values are omitted because of the difficulty in comparing studies and the influence of anesthetic technique.
From Fisher DM: Neuromuscular blocking agents in paediatric anaesthesia. Br J Anaesth 1999;83:58.

action and is associated fewer side effects related to histamine release.

The need for reversal of muscle blockade should be carefully considered in each patient. The risks associated with inadequate ventilation in small children are great, especially in cases in which the work of breathing may be increased, as is the case with intercurrent illness as well as chest/abdominal procedures. Muscle twitch should be monitored and reversal agents (i.e., neostigmine, 0.05 mg/kg, with 0.015 mg/kg of atropine or 0.01 mg/kg of glycopyrrolate) administered if residual weakness is detected. Clinical signs of adequate strength for ventilation in this age group include the ability to flex hips.

Antiemetics

In children, the postoperative nausea and vomiting (PONV) rate can be twice as high as in adults, which suggests a greater need for PONV prophylaxis in this population.[29] Unfortunately, this is a complex clinical problem to manage, with many factors influencing its frequency. PONV is particularly prominent after certain surgeries such as orchidopexy, strabismus surgery, and tonsillectomy. There is no single therapy that is universally accepted as safe and effective. In fact, all antiemetic therapies for children are shown to have efficacy only in high-risk groups and surgeries; their use in lower risk situations is suspect. The type of anesthetic employed for a particular surgery will also influence the incidence of PONV. For instance, when propofol is used in place of inhaled agents as the primary anesthetic, there is evidence that PONV less common, particularly for high-risk surgeries such as tonsillectomy.[62]

All of the antiemetics used in adults including phenothiazines, antihistamines, anticholinergics, benzamides, butyrophenones and 5-HT$_3$ antagonists have been used in children and (to one extent of the other) have been shown to have some effectiveness. The 5-HT$_3$ antagonists are general considered equivalent as a group; however, ondansetron has been most thoroughly studied in children and at 0.05 to 0.15 mg/kg has been found to be effective in tonsillectomy and strabismus models.[63] Its effectiveness as a "rescue" medication is not proven. Dexamethasone, 0.15 to 1.0 mg/kg, appears to be effective in limiting PONV after oral pharyngeal surgery (tonsillectomy) but there are much less data on its use in other types of procedures.[64]

The most effective prophylaxis strategy in children at moderate or high risk for PONV is to use combination therapy that includes a 5-HT$_3$ antagonist and a second drug such as low-dose dexamethasone. Antiemetic rescue therapy should be administered to children who vomit after surgery. The current Society for Ambulatory Anesthesia consensus statement on PONV recommends that if vomiting occurs within 6 hours postoperatively, patients should not receive a repeat dose of the same prophylactic antiemetic because of lack of evidence for effectiveness in this time frame.[65] The guidelines recommend using a drug that is of a different class than those used for prophylaxis, such as promethazine.[65] It should be noted, however, that much of this information is derived from studies

of adult patients, and repeat dosing of 5-HT$_3$ agents is likely not dangerous in this time frame.

Complete reviews of antiemetic use in children are available[65]; however, droperidol deserves special mention. Its use and effectiveness in children as antiemetic is well documented.[66] Its current use in children is limited because in 2003 the FDA issued a report warning of prolonged QT syndrome and possible torsades de pointes with its use, and suggesting prolonged monitoring (6 hours) for patients given this drug. A black box warning has been placed on this medication to this effect. The frequency of this problem in children is unknown but is thought to be extremely low; nevertheless, use of the drug has decreased significantly in light of this warning.

Unfortunately, the issue of antiemetic efficacy and cost-effectiveness remains largely unanswered in spite of the hundreds of studies that exist concerning their use in children. The use at least one of the drugs mentioned here with known antiemetic action is indicated for surgeries associated with a high incidence of nausea and vomiting, especially in high-risk age groups. In addition, the practice of *requiring* patients to eat and/or drink prior to discharge will only increase PONV rates and does not appear to improve outcomes. Likewise, the use of pain control modalities in lieu of opioids (acetaminophen or nonsteroidal anti-inflammatory drugs [NSAIDs], and regional anesthesia) will likely decrease the overall risk of PONV.

FLUID AND BLOOD PRODUCT MANAGEMENT

Perioperative fluid and blood product management for pediatric patients must take into account fluid deficits, translocation of fluids and blood loss during surgery, and maintenance fluid requirements. A patient's fluid deficit prior to starting a case can be simply calculated by multiplying his or her calculated maintenance requirement by the number of hours since the last fluid intake by mouth. The calculation for maintenance fluids depends directly on metabolic demand; each calorie of energy expended requires 1 mL of H$_2$O for metabolism. Relating this energy requirement to patient weight results in an hourly fluid requirement that may be estimated as in Table 45-4.

Immediate intravascular volume expansion may be accomplished with a 10 mL/kg bolus of isotonic fluid. The balance of the calculated fluid deficit can be provided over 1 or 2 hours and is often provided in the form isotonic fluid or a 5% dextrose solution in 0.9% normal saline. There are conflicting data concerning the need for glucose-containing solutions in this setting. In our current era with liberalized recommendations for intake of clear fluids (generally up to 2 hours prior to surgery), there is little evidence of hypoglycemia in children related to fasting prior to surgery. Indeed, most children who are given non–glucose-containing fluids during surgery actually experience a rise in blood glucose because of sympathetic activation. Hyperglycemia has been documented in children given 5% dextrose solutions to replace deficits or fluid losses

TABLE 45-4

MAINTENANCE FLUID REQUIREMENTS FOR PEDIATRIC PATIENTS

WEIGHT (kg)	HOURLY FLUID	24-hr FLUID
<10	4 mL/kg	100 mL/kg
11–20	40 mL+2 mL/kg > 10 kg	1,000 mL+50 mL/kg > 10 kg
>20	60 mL+1 mL/kg > 20 kg	1,500 mL+20 mL/kg > 20 kg

intraoperatively. This is particularly problematic for patients with intracranial injury in whom hyperglycemia may result in worsening outcomes. In addition, hyperosmolar diuresis caused by significant hyperglycemia may also confuse diuretic and fluid therapy. On the other hand, life-threatening *hypo*glycemia would be undetectable on clinical grounds under anesthesia.

To optimize fluid administration and glucose delivery, a balanced salt solution containing 2.5% glucose may be used (although not commercially available). Another approach would be to provide 5% dextrose in 0.45% normal saline (D_5 0.45 normal saline) for maintenance, piggybacked into a balanced salt solution for the deficit and third-space fluid. The exact composition of fluids used is less important than being aware of the issue of glucose control.[67] Intraoperative monitoring of blood glucose is appropriate for newborns, former premature infants, and any high risk pediatric patients.

Surgical manipulation is associated with the isotonic transfer of fluids from the extracellular fluid compartment to the nonfunctional interstitial compartment. Estimated third-space loss during intra-abdominal surgery varies from 6 to 15 mL/kg/hr, whereas in intrathoracic surgery it is less (4 to 7 mL/kg/hr) and during intracranial or cutaneous surgery it is negligible (1 to 2 mL/kg/hr). These third-space losses should be estimated and replaced on an hourly basis. As these losses are derived from extracellular fluid it is important to replace with a balanced salt solution to avoid hyponatremia that would result from using hypotonic replacement. Lactated Ringer solution is frequently used as normal saline contains an excessive chloride and acid load for infants.

Indications for blood or blood component therapy in pediatric patients are not always clear-cut. Decisions must be based on considerations of the patient's blood volume, preoperative hematocrit, general medical condition, ability to provide oxygen to tissues, the nature of the surgical procedure, and the risks versus benefits of transfusion. All blood loss should be measured as accurately as possible and accounted for with some form of volume replacement in order to maintain intravascular volume and perfusion. If an isotonic solution is chosen to replace some element of blood loss it should be given in a ratio of 3 mL of solution for each milliliter of blood lost.

Many major procedures in children will be accompanied by significant blood loss and require transfusion of red blood cells and other blood products. In these cases, calculation of acceptable blood loss is vital to any replacement plan. The concept of the maximum allowable blood loss (MABL) takes into account the patients total blood volume, starting hematocrit, and estimated "target" hematocrit, that which represents the lowest acceptable hematocrit for this patient considering age and comorbid conditions. In general, blood volume is estimated at 100 mL/kg for the preterm infant, 90 mL/kg for the term infant, 80 mL/kg for the child 3 to 12 months of age, and 70 mL/kg for the patient older than 1 year. These estimates of blood volume can be used in calculating the individual patient's blood volume by multiplying the child's weight by the estimated blood volume (EBV) per kilogram:

$$\text{MABL} = \frac{\text{EBV} \times (\text{starting hematocrit} - \text{target hematocrit})}{\text{Starting hematocrit}}$$

As the MABL is approached, the patient's hematocrit should be checked to confirm estimated blood losses and volumes.

Packed red blood cells have a hematocrit between 55 and 70%. On the average, 1 mL/kg of packed red blood cells increases the hematocrit by 1.5%. Units of blood can be subdivided into pediatric packs of 50 to 100 mL; thus, the remainder of a single unit is not wasted. Administration of other products such as cryoprecipitate or fresh-frozen plasma should be based on laboratory evidence of coagulopathy and

should be aimed at replacement of identifiable deficiencies of factors relating to hemostasis. Rapid administration of citrated blood products (particularly fresh-frozen plasma) can result in hypocalcemia as well as hypothermia. Although under most circumstances mobilization of calcium and hepatic metabolism of citrate are sufficiently rapid to prevent precipitous decreases in ionized calcium, infants have smaller stores of calcium.

As always, the end point of fluid and blood therapy is adequate blood pressure, tissue perfusion, and urine volume (0.5 to 1 mL/kg/hour). Careful attention to these goals through the examination of clinical (capillary refill time, urine output) and laboratory (e.g., blood gasses) examination are more important than adherence to any one particular clinical protocol.

AIRWAY MANAGEMENT

Appropriate airway management remains the single most important aspect of delivering safe pediatric anesthesia. At any age, operative cases can be performed with face mask, LMA, or endotracheal tube placement. The choice of airway will depend on the age of the child, patient position during surgery, the time since last intake by mouth, coexisting illness, and the procedure to be performed. Each case must be considered on its own merits, but trends and guidelines have been established:

1. As a general rule, endotracheal tubes are preferred for premature infants and most neonates in maintaining general anesthesia because of the slightly greater difficulty of providing effective face mask ventilation and the risk of filling the stomach with air while providing mask ventilation.

2. Cases in which recent oral intake or pathology (such as pyloric stenosis or intestinal obstruction) raise the probability that the stomach contains food or acid (and therefore risk aspiration injury) are best managed with a rapid-sequence induction and intubation regardless of age.

3. LMAs and other pharyngeal airways come in a range of sizes that can be employed in infants, toddlers, and older children for almost any procedure that does not involve opening the abdomen or thoracic cavity. Although their use is standard for lower extremity, inguinal, cutaneous, or eye procedures, the application this airway for oral procedures such as tonsillectomy/adenoidectomy varies from center to center. Use of the LMA in neonates and premature infants is less common and depends on provider experience and preference. Aspiration and laryngospasm with the airway in place are not common but are possible, and plans to quickly manage these events must always be in place.[4] The LMA has become a critical part of the difficult airway algorithm for pediatric patients. This device can be used to ventilate patients in whom conventional mask ventilation is difficult as well as providing a conduit for fiber optic assisted intubation.

4. Because the narrowest portion of the pediatric airway is at the level of the cricoid cartilage (and is therefore round), uncuffed tubes can be used and will create a functional seal when appropriately sized.[68] Several formulas have been used for tube selection in children older than age 1 year, the most common being (16 + age)/4 or variations thereof. One may also estimate the size by comparing the size of the fifth digit or the opening of a nare. Once the tube is in place, it should be checked to determine at what pressure air can escape around the tube. Air should leak out at no lower than approximately 10 cm H_2O (to allow adequate ventilation) and no higher than 25 to 30 cm H_2O (to minimize risk of postextubation croup). Cuffed tubes can also be safely used in infants and young children by selecting a

tube 0.5 mm smaller in internal diameter than the uncuffed choice (as previously mentioned).[68] Care should be taken to check the pressure in the cuff to assure it does not exceed 20 cm H_2O.

5. Intubation in children can be safely accomplished after inhaled induction with or without the use of muscle relaxant. Intubating conditions after 3 minutes of 8% sevoflurane or a dose of propofol and opiate[69,70] may produce acceptable views of the larynx. In fact, a survey of pediatric anesthesiologists revealed the majority do not use muscle relaxants for elective surgery.[71] The use of muscle relaxants should be based on the specific issues related to the child and the procedure to be performed.

PEDIATRIC BREATHING CIRCUITS

Much has been written about the advantages and disadvantages of various anesthesia circuits for use in pediatric patients. Pediatric circuit design has been directed to the physiology of the neonate and ways of reducing the work of breathing while preventing rebreathing. Nonrebreathing circuits minimize the work of breathing because they have no valves to be opened by the patient's respiratory effort. In addition, because the total volume of the circuit is less, the partial pressure of inhaled agent increases faster. Compression volumes are also decreased compared with a standard breathing circuit.

A number of combinations of the simple T-piece tubing, reservoir bag, and sites of fresh gas entry and overflow are possible. Mapleson classified the various combinations into five types. The Jackson-Reese modification is functionally identical to the Mapleson D, as are coaxial systems. Carbon dioxide is removed most effectively in the D configuration when controlled ventilation is used, whereas spontaneous ventilation is most effective in the A system.

Circle breathing systems can also be used very effectively in infants and children. Newer anesthesia machines use valves with much less resistance than older models. In addition, most neonates and small infants (for whom resistance would be the biggest problem) are ventilated mechanically during surgery, making work of breathing a nonissue. Dead space in these systems is no more than that of the Mapleson circuits.[72]

MONITORING

Monitoring decisions for pediatric patients are similar in many respects to those for adults. The pediatric patient should be monitored continuously with precordial or esophageal stethoscope. This simple device allows the anesthesiologist to detect changes in the rate, quality, and intensity of the heart sounds. Pulse oximetry, capnography, blood pressure (measured *appropriately* sized cuffs), temperature, and electrocardiogram should also be monitored routinely in children as in adults. More invasive or sophisticated monitoring should be used in appropriate circumstances. One should note that patient pathophysiology may contribute to an increased gradient between end-tidal and arterial CO_2 measurements usually by increasing shunt ($\dot{V}/\dot{Q}$ mismatch) and increasing dead space (V_D/V_T). That is, in children with cyanotic congenital heart disease, $ETCO_2$ underestimates $PaCO_2$ as venous blood passes directly into the arterial circulation *without* going through the lungs. Low tidal volumes, rapid respiratory rates, and changing intrapulmonary shunts make $ETCO_2$ inaccurate for infants and premature neonates with respiratory distress syndrome. It is important to note that transesophageal echocardiography has become an important tool for intraoperative assessment of cardiac function, flow defects, cardiac morphology, and adequacy of repair during and after surgical procedures for congenital

heart disease. Although placement of the probe in the anesthetized infant is usually the responsibility of the anesthesiologist, interpretation of the echocardiogram occurs in collaboration between surgeons, cardiologists, and anesthesiologists. Finally, the use of pulmonary artery catheters (Swan-Ganz) is quite limited in the pediatric population because of size issues as well as to the fact that left- and right-sided pressures are very similar.

Awareness and Level of Consciousness Monitoring

Historically, pediatric patients have not been considered high risk for awareness during anesthesia. Recent reports indicate that children may experience awareness as often as 0.3 to 1.7% of anesthetics.[72a] Although there (as yet) has not been shown to be significant psychological trauma associated with awareness in children, the issue has brought the question of consciousness monitoring in children to new light. Monitors of depth of anesthesia that have been validated in children include the Bispectral Index (BIS), Spectral Entropy, Narcotrend Index, A-line ARX Index, Cerebral State Index, and electroencephalogram. General concepts concerning the use of these monitors include the following: (1) They track level of sedation/anesthesia in children much as they do in adults. (2) Performance in infants is significantly different than that found in children and none of these monitors can be considered a reliable measure in infants and neonates. (3) There is no clear "best" monitor among those mentioned here. (4) No monitors have been evaluated in terms of their ability to decrease awareness in children. (5) BIS and A-line ARX have been demonstrated to reduce anesthetic dose and speed recovery, but no direct comparison studies exist and no difference in other outcomes have been demonstrated.[22]

PAIN MANAGEMENT AND REGIONAL ANESTHESIA

Neonates, infants, and children experience pain, just like adults, regardless of their age. Recent studies indicate that neonates have considerable maturation of pain transmission by 26 weeks of gestation and respond to injury with specific behaviors, autonomic, hormonal, and metabolic signs of stress and distress.[73] In fact, recent data indicate that extreme pain experienced during the neonatal period may have life long-lasting adverse effects.[31,73] Pain in children can be assessed by self-reporting, observational, and physiological assessment tools.[73,74] Self-reporting pain is considered the gold standard, but this assessment method cannot be used in infants, younger children, and in children who suffer from developmental delay. In these children, the clinicians often need to rely on parental report.[74] Children older than 4 to 6 years of age can usually self-report pain using a face scale. Younger children are usually assessed using a behavioral or physiologic-behavioral scale.[74]

Of the over 5 million children who undergo surgery in the United States, it is estimated that up to 65% will experience significant pain while in the hospital.[75] Postoperative pain continues to be prevalent when children return home, with one study indicating that 56% of children report immediate postoperative pain at home and up to 33% continue to experience pain 1 week following surgery.[76] Unfortunately, many studies indicate that pain in children is underestimated by health care professionals, and therefore children often receive subtherapeutic doses of analgesics. The issue of undermedication appears to be particularly problematic in the postoperative setting.[76] The undertreatment of pain in the postoperative setting is particularly significant as medical procedure distress in children has been linked years later to adults' reports of pain and anxiety regarding medical events.[77] In addition, early painful procedures have been associated with changes in sensitivity to later medical procedures.[78]

Several studies have indicated that younger children experience more distress and pain from procedures than older children.[79] Children's temperament has also been shown to be related to postoperative pain.[80] Schechter et al.[81] found a relation between "difficult" temperament and pain. Hsu et al.[82] suggested the existence of a "pain-sensitive temperament" that includes perceptual sensitivity and avoidance of sensations. Recent clinical and experimental research has demonstrated a relation between children's coping styles and their pain.[83] Specifically, children's preference for monitoring coping (e.g., watching procedure) has been found to be related to higher procedural distress.[84] Further, interventions matched to children's coping styles appear to be more effective than those not considering children's coping style.[85] Anticipatory anxiety has been reported by Palermo et al.[86] to be related to children's postoperative pain. Kain et al.[87] have completed a study that has confirmed these results. In this study of over 300 patients, children who reported more anxiety before surgery were found to be significantly more likely to experience higher pain after surgery both by self-report as well as parent and nursing report.[87]

Pharmacologic Treatment of Pain

The most common oral analgesic used in children continues to be acetaminophen. This medication has been shown to be safe and efficacious in neonates as well as older children. Doses of 10 to 15 mg/kg orally every 4 hours or 30 to 40 mg/kg rectally as a loading dose followed by 10 to 15 mg/kg every 6 hours, with a maximum dose of 90 mg/24 hr, produce therapeutic plasma levels with good analgesia.[88] The plasma concentrations effective for fever control and analgesia are 10 to 20 μg/mL.[89] Rectal administration is associated with delayed and erratic uptake; single doses of 35 to 45 mg/kg generally produce therapeutic plasma concentrations.[73] Subsequent rectal doses, however, should not exceed 20 mg/kg and the interval between doses should be extended to at least 6 to 8 hours. The rectal route of administration can be particularly effective for children with no intravenous access, such as pressure-equalizing ear tube placement (Table 45-5).

Ketorolac has been shown to be an effective and safe analgesic for pediatric patients.[73,90] It may be administered intramuscularly (0.75 mg/kg) or intravenously with a loading dose of 1 mg/kg followed by a maintenance dose of 0.5 mg/kg every 6 hours. Ketorolac has the disadvantage of prolonging bleeding time because of its effect on platelet aggregation. As with other NSAIDs, ketorolac should be avoided in patients with pre-existing nephropathy or bleeding diathesis. Ibuprofen is the most popular NSAID given orally to children. It comes in several palatable preparations. When given in the recommended oral dose of 10 mg/kg it has similar analgesic effects as acetaminophen or ketorolac. Gastrointestinal side effects are uncommon.

The safety and efficacy of patient-controlled analgesia for children as young as 6 years has been shown.[91] While routinely used in children's hospitals, this technique is to be used *only* by highly trained medical personal who are knowledgeable in pediatric pain management. For infants and children younger than 6 years, nurse-controlled analgesia is now widely used as a pain management modality. Finally, it should be noted that while parent-controlled analgesia is now accepted in palliative care, its use for postoperative pain is controversial because of the potential for overdosing.

Behavioral Treatment of Pain

Behavioral interventions such as imagery[92] and relaxation have received empirical attention and their efficacy has been supported in the postoperative settings. Although behavioral interventions are important in the optimal management of postoperative pain, it is important to note that these types of strategies also have some limitations. One significant issue is the lack of dissemination of evidence-based nonpharmacologic pain management strategies to providers and families.[94] Behavioral strategies such as imagery and distraction have been found to be effective in the management of postoperative pain, but are not widely used by parents following surgery. This is likely because of the lack of training in these strategies; children must understand the instructions on how to use relaxation or imagery and must actually engage in the intervention

TABLE 45-5

MANAGEMENT OF POSTOPERATIVE PAIN

| DRUG | DOSE | | | MAXIMAL DAILY DOSE | |
	PATIENTS <60 kg (mg/kg)	PATIENTS ≥60 kg (mg)	INTERVAL (hr)	PATIENTS <60 kg (mg/kg)	PATIENTS ≥60 kg (mg)
Acetaminophen	10–25	650–1,000	4	100[a]	4,000
Ibuprofen	6–10	400–600[b]	6	40[b,c]	2,400[b]
Naproxen	5–6[b]	250–375[b]	12	24[b,c]	1,000[b]
Aspirin[d]	10–15[b,d]	650–1000[b]	4	80[b–d]	3,600[b]

[a]The maximal daily doses of acetaminophen for infants and neonates are a subject of current controversy. Provisional recommendations are that daily dosing should not exceed 75 mg/kg per day for infants, 60 mg/kg per day for term neonates and preterm neonates of more than 32 weeks of postconceptional age, and 40 mg/kg per day for preterm neonates 28 to 32 weeks of postconceptional age. Fever, dehydration, hepatic disease, and lack of oral intake may all increase the risk of hepatotoxicity.
[b]Higher doses may be used in selected cases for treatment of rheumatologic conditions in children.
[c]Dosage guidelines for neonates and infants have not been established.
[d]Aspirin carries a risk of provoking Reye's syndrome in infants and children. If other analgesics are available, aspirin should be restricted to indications for which an antiplatelet or antiinflammatory effect is requird, rather than being used as a routine analgesic or antipyretic in neonates, infants, or children. Dosage guidelines for aspirin in neonates have not been established.
From Berde CB, Sethna NF: Analgesics for the treatment of pain in children. N Engl J Med 2002; 347: 1094.

in order for it to be effective.[95] Behavioral pain strategies work best when children have had the opportunity to practice and build mastery in their use. Given that most surgeries today are conducted on an outpatient basis and little preparation is offered,[96] children's opportunities to learn and practice these pain-reduction behavioral techniques are limited.

Regional Anesthesia

Chapters 37 and 38 discuss regional anesthesia and analgesia in detail. Most regional anesthetic techniques can be very useful for children undergoing anesthesia and surgery. Because of obvious developmental and cognitive issues, regional techniques are rarely used as a sole anesthetic and most often used as adjuncts to general anesthesia and providing postoperative analgesia. Regional anesthetic techniques (e.g., spinal and epidural) may also be used as the sole anesthetic in premature infants at risk for postoperative apnea undergoing abdominal or lower extremity procedures. Simple techniques such as ilioinguinal–iliohypogastric nerve block, ring block of the penis, or caudal block can be very useful for common pediatric surgical procedures. Direct local infiltration of surgical wounds can also be very helpful. The types of blocks that can be used safely in children are limited only by the skill of the anesthesiologist. The use of ultrasound as an aid in placement of local anesthesia for nerve blocks is rapidly gaining popularity over conventional landmark-based techniques with or without neurostimulation.[97,98] Ultrasound localization actually allows a lower dose/volume of local anesthetic to be used, which is particularly important in infants and children in whom total dose is limited by weight-based dosing.

Because of the unique anatomic and physiological considerations, strict attention must be paid to the dose of local anesthetic, dose of epinephrine, and technique of administration. More sophisticated techniques such as continuous caudal or epidural analgesia using combinations of opioids and local anesthetics are useful for inpatients after thoracic, abdominal, or lower extremity procedures. These regional techniques usually are used in combination with general anesthesia (catheters are placed after the child is induced) and the regional block is maintained for postoperative pain control. Ultrasound-based nerve blocks are routinely performed after the induction of anesthesia. Close postoperative monitoring of the child must take place when these continuous infusions are used.[99]

(14) The most commonly used form of regional anesthesia in children is the *caudal block*. This technique can provide postoperative analgesia following a wide variety of lower abdominal and genitourinary surgical procedures. For single-dose administration (outpatient surgeries) bupivacaine, 0.25 to 0.175%[100] solution, or ropivacaine, 0.2 to 0.175%,[101] at a dose of 1 mL/kg is commonly used. Postoperative analgesia typically lasts 4 to 6 hours and is not associated with a motor paralysis at these concentrations. This route can be used for either a single-dose injection or for catheter advancement for continuous infusion.[102]

Spinal anesthesia may be used for procedures involving surgical dermatomes below T_6.[103] It is important to note that the dural sac migrates cephalad during the first year of life and in a neonate it is at S_3 while over the age of 1 year it is at the S_1 level. The sitting position may be especially helpful in neonates to maintain midline needle position and free flow of spinal fluid. It may be easier for the novice assistant to hold the infant more securely in the lateral decubitus position. As previously mentioned, spinal anesthetic is a particular good option for premature infants who undergo surgery as the incidence of postoperative apnea has been shown to be reduced in these infants with the use of this technique.

POSTANESTHESIA CARE

Recovery of the young child in the PACU can be hindered by a variety of challenges. Hypothermia is a common perioperative problem, particularly in infants and young children. The inability to regulate body temperature under general anesthesia, cold large operating rooms, and continued heat loss are major reasons for hypothermia. Although minor hypothermia (34 to 36°C) has not been found to influence the recovery period, it is best to restore normothermia prior to discharge from the PACU. More significant hypothermia can result in increased oxygen consumption, cardiovascular manifestations of hypothermia,[104,105] prolonged metabolism, and excretion of anesthetic drugs and delayed wound healing.

Emergence agitation refers to the presence of thrashing, crying, screaming, and disorientation that can accompany emergence from anesthesia in any age group, but is particularly common in children. The frequency of this problem varies with age, anesthetics used, and the surgery performed. In general, younger children are more at risk, as are children who have had strabismus surgery or tonsillectomy or adenoidectomy. As mentioned in the section on anesthetic agents, many reports have linked a higher incidence of agitation with the use of pure sevoflurane anesthesia.[37] This phenomenon is not strictly related to pain. There are reports of effective treatment with a variety of medications including fentanyl, dexmedetomidine, midazolam, and ketamine.[106–108] The incidence is clearly lower after propofol-based anesthesia.[109] With few exceptions, the behaviors stop within 30 to 45 minutes after surgery.

Nausea and vomiting occur frequently after eye or ear surgery but can occur after any surgical procedure or anesthetic. Some studies quote an overall incidence of 20 to 30%, while others have found that the problem is even more widespread (39 to 73%).[65] The physiological mechanisms for postoperative nausea include central causes (opiates), gastrointestinal malfunction (ileus or gastric distention), the surgical procedure itself (eye and ear, most commonly), and postoperative pain.[110] Control of nausea and vomiting no longer remains purely within the domain of the PACU, but begins in the selection of agents/techniques used for anesthesia.[111] For example, induction and maintenance of anesthesia with propofol-air-oxygen is associated with only a 23% incidence of nausea and vomiting, as compared with a 50% incidence using halothane-N_2O-droperidol for strabismus surgery.[65]

Special attention should be paid to the treatment of pain in the PACU. Although pain self-report is considered the best assessment modality in older children, physiological responses such as tachycardia, hypertension, nausea, vomiting, and agitation may be important indicators of analgesic needs in the preverbal child. Intravenous opiates such as fentanyl or morphine are used most commonly to treat moderate to severe pain in the PACU. Carefully titrated intravenous narcotics present few untoward effects. Pretreatment with ondansetron, 0.15 mg/kg; droperidol, 0.075 mg/kg; or metoclopramide, 0.15 mg/kg, has been very successful in reducing nausea and vomiting for patients at higher risk, such as those undergoing tonsillectomy or strabismus repair. Ondansetron, a selective serotonin antagonist, is particularly effective in reducing postoperative nausea and vomiting when used prophylactically. Although more expensive than other antiemetics, its significant efficacy makes it cost-effective when used for procedures with a high incidence of nausea and vomiting.

Finally, many children are terrified in the recovery room. They awaken in a strange place with unfamiliar people and may be disoriented from residual effects of the anesthesia. Some children may experience nightmares, develop enuresis, or have behavioral problems after a surgical procedure.[2]

Measures taken to calm and comfort the child may reduce the incidence of these sequelae and aid in the overall recovery. Many institutions have found that allowing parents to soothe the child during recovery is beneficial.

References

1. Lin Y, Bioteau A, Ferrari L. The use of herbs and complementary and alternative medicine in pediatric preoperative patients. J Clin Anesth 2004; 16: 406

2. Kain ZN C-AA, Maranets I, McClain B et al: Preoperative anxiety and emergence delirium and postoperative maladaptive behaviors. Anesth Analg 2004; 99: 1648

3. Wang SM HM, Kain ZN: An alternative method to alleviate postoperative nausea and vomiting in children. J Clin Anesth 1999; 11: 231

4. Tait AR, Pandit UA, Voepel-Lewis T et al: Use of the laryngeal mask airway in children with upper respiratory tract infections: A comparison with endotracheal intubation. Anesth Analg 1998; 86: 706

5. Cote CJ CI, Suresh S, Rabb M et al: A comparison of three doses of a commercially prepared oral midazolam syrup in children. Anesth Analg 2002; 94: 37

6. Collier A, Pimmel R, Hasselblad V et al: Spirometric changes in normal children with upper respiratory infections. Am Rev Respir Dis 1978; 117: 47

7. von Ungern-Sternberg BS, Boda K, Schwab C et al: Laryngeal mask airway is associated with an increased incidence of adverse respiratory events in children with recent upper respiratory tract infections. Anesthesiology 2007; 107: 714

8. Helfar M, Wilson D: Obstructive sleep apnea, control of ventilation, and anesthesia in children. Pediatr Clin North Am 1994; 41: 131

9. Statham MM, Elluru RG, Buncher R et al: Adenotonsillectomy for obstructive sleep apnea syndrome in young children: prevalence of pulmonary complications. Arch Otolaryng Head Neck Surg 2006; 132: 476

10. Setzer N, Saade E: Childhood obesity and anesthetic morbidity. Paediatr Anaesth 2007; 17: 321

11. Nafiu OO, Reynolds PI, Bamgbade OA et al: Childhood body mass index and perioperative complications. Obesity (Silver Spring). 2008; [Epub ahead of print].

12. Szefler S: Current concepts in asthma treatment in children. Curr Opin Pediatr 2004; 16: 299

13. Warner D, Warner M, Barnes R et al. Perioperative respiratory complications in patients with asthma. Anesthesiology 1996; 85: 460

14. Scalfaro P, Sly P, Sims C et al: Salbutamol prevents the increase of respiratory resistance caused by tracheal intubation during sevoflurane anesthesia in asthmatic children. Anesth Analg 2001; 93: 898

15. Kurth C, Spitzer A, Broennle A et al. Postoperative apnea in preterm infants. Anesthesiology 1987; 66: 483

16. Welborn L, Ramirez N, Oh T et al: Postanesthetic apnea and periodic breathing in infants. Anesthesiology 1986; 65: 658

17. Walther-Larsen S, Rasmussen LS: The former preterm infant and risk of post-operative apnoea: recommendations for management. Acta Anaesthesiol Scand 2006; 50: 888

18. Maxwell L, Yaster M: Perioperative management issues in pediatric patients. Anesthesiol Clin North Am 2000; 18: 601

19. Gabriel P, Mazoit X, Ecoffey C: Relationship between clinical history, coagulation tests, and perioperative bleeding during tonsillectomies in pediatrics. J Clin Anesth 2000; 12: 288

20. Warner M, Warner M, Warner D et al: Perioperative pulmonary aspiration in infants and children. Anesthesiology 1999; 90: 66

21. Practice guidelines for preoperative fasting and the use of pharmacologic agents to reduce the risk of pulmonary aspiration: application to healthy patients undergoing elective procedures: A report by the American Society of Anesthesiologist Task Force on Preoperative Fasting. Anesthesiology 1999; 90: 896

22. McCann ME, Kain ZN: The management of preoperative anxiety in children: an update. Anesth Analg 2001; 93: 98

23. Kain ZN, MacLaren J, McClain BC et al: Effects of age and emotionality on the effectiveness of midazolam administered preoperatively to children. Anesthesiology 2007; 107: 545

24. Viitanen H, Annila P, Viitanen M et al: Premedication with midazolam delays recovery after ambulatory sevoflurane anesthesia in children. Anesth Analg 1999; 89: 75

25. Shannon M, Albers G, Burkhart K et al: Safety and efficacy of flumazenil in the reversal of benzodiazepine-induced conscious sedation. J Pediatr 1997; 131: 582

26. Funk W, Jakob W, Reidl T et al: Oral preanaesthetic medication for children: Double-blind randomized study of a combination of midazolam and ketamine vs midazolam or ketamine alone. Br J Anaesth 2000; 84: 335

27. Nishina K, Mikawa K, Shiga M et al: Clonidine in paediatric anaesthesia. Paediatr Anaesth 1999; 9: 187

28. Keenan RL SJ, Dawson K: Frequency of anesthetic cardiac arrests in infants: Effect of pediatric anesthesiologists. J Clin Anesth 1991; 3: 433

29. Lerman J: Pharmacology of inhalational anaesthetics in infants and children. Paediatr Anaesth 1992; 2: 191

30. Katoh T, Ikeda K: Minimum alveolar concentration of sevoflurane in children. Br J Anaesth 1992; 68: 139

31. Black A, Sury MR, Hemington L et al: A comparison of the induction characteristics of sevoflurane and halothane in children. Anaesthesia 1996; 51: 539

32. Goa KL, Noble S, Spencer CM: Sevoflurane in paediatric anaesthesia: A review. Paediatr Drugs 1999; 1: 127

33. Lerman J: Inhalational anaesthetics. Paediatr Anaesth 2004; 14: 380

34. Holzman RS, van der Velde ME, Kaus SJ et al: Sevoflurane depresses myocardial contractility less than halothane during induction of anesthesia in children. Anesthesiology 1996; 85: 1260

35. Wodey E, Pladys P, Copin C et al: Comparative hemodynamic depression of sevoflurane versus halothane in infants: An echocardiographic study. Anesthesiology 1997; 87: 795

36. Cravero J, Surgenor S, Whalen K. Emergence agitation in paediatric patients after sevoflurane anaesthesia and no surgery: a comparison with halothane. Paediatr Anaesth 2000; 10: 419

37. Friesen RH, Henry DB: Cardiovascular changes in preterm neonates receiving isoflurane, halothane, fentanyl, and ketamine. Anesthesiology 1986; 64: 238

38. Welborn LG HR, McGill WA et al: Induction and recovery characteristics of desflurane and halothane anaesthesia in paediatric outpatients. Paediatr Anaesth 1994; 4: 359

39. Eichenfield LF FA, Fallon-Friedlander S, Cunnigham BB: A clinical study to evaluate the efficacy of ELA-Max (4% liposomal lidocaine) as compared with eutectic mixture of local anesthetics cream for pain reduction of venipuncture in children. Pediatrics 2002; 109: 1093

40. Kleiber C SM, Whiteside K, Gronstal BA et al: Topical anesthetics for intravenous insertion in children: a randomized equivalency study. Pediatrics 2002; 110: 758

41. Wolf A, Weir P, Segar P et al: Impaired fatty acid oxidation in propofol infusion syndrome. Lancet 2001; 357: 606

42. Vasile B, Rasulo F, Candiani A et al: The pathophysiology of propofol infusion syndrome: A simple name for a complex syndrome. Intens Care Medicine 2003; 29:1417

43. McFarlan CS, Anderson BJ, Short TG: The use of propofol infusions in paediatric anaesthesia: a practical guide. Paediatr Anaesth 1999; 9: 209

44. Bryson GL, Chung F, Cox RG et al: Patient selection in ambulatory anesthesia—an evidence-based review: Part II. Can J Anaesth 2004; 51: 782

45. Guard BC, Sikich N, Lerman J et al: Maintenance and recovery characteristics after sevoflurane or propofol during ambulatory surgery in children with epidural blockade. Can J Anaesth 1998; 45: 1072

46. Erb TO, Hall JM, Ing RJ et al: Postoperative nausea and vomiting in children and adolescents undergoing radiofrequency catheter ablation: a randomized comparison of propofol- and isoflurane-based anesthetics. Anesth Analg 2002; 95: 1577

47. Nakayama S, Furukawa H, Yanai H: Propofol reduces the incidence of emergence agitation in preschool-aged children as well as in school-aged children: A comparison with sevoflurane. J Anesth 2007; 21: 19

48. Picard V, Dumont L, Pellegrini M: Quality of recovery in children: sevoflurane versus propofol. Acta Anaesthesiol Scand 2000; 44: 307

49. Bergman SA: Ketamine: review of its pharmacology and its use in pediatric anesthesia. Anesth Progr 1999; 46: 10

50. McGonagle M, Kennedy TL: Laryngospasm induced pulmonary edema. Laryngoscope 1984; 94: 1583

51. Abu-Shahwan I, Chowdary K: Ketamine is effective in decreasing the incidence of emergence agitation in children undergoing dental repair under sevoflurane general anesthesia. Paediatr Anaesth 2007 17: 846

52. Choi SH, Lee SJ, Kim SH et al: Single bolus of intravenous ketamine for anesthetic induction decreases oculocardiac reflex in children undergoing strabismus surgery. Acta Anaesthesiolog Scand 2007; 51: 759

53. Mellon RD, Simone AF, Rappaport BA: Use of anesthetic agents in neonates and young children. Anesth Analg 2007 104: 509

54. Roulleau P, Gall O, Desjeux L et al: Remifentanil infusion for cleft palate surgery in young infants. Paediatr Anaesth 2003; 13: 701

55. Ganidagli S, Cengiz M, Baysal Z: Remifentanil vs alfentanil in the total intravenous anaesthesia for paediatric abdominal surgery. Paediatr Anaesth 2003; 13: 695

56. Bhatt-Mehta V, Rosen DA: Management of acute pain in children. Clin Pharm 1991; 10: 667

57. Lehr VT, BeVier P: Patient-controlled analgesia for the pediatric patient. Orthopaed Nurs 2003; 22: 298

58. Monitto CL, Greenberg RS, Kost-Byerly S et al: The safety and efficacy of parent-/nurse-controlled analgesia in patients less than six years of age. Anesth Analg 2000; 91: 573

59. Fuchs-Buder T, Tassonyi E: Intubating conditions and time course of rocuronium-induced neuromuscular block in children. Br J Anaesth 1996; 77: 335

60. Woloszczuk-Gebicka B, Wyska E, Gabowski T: Pharmacokinetic-pharmacodynamic relationship of rocuronium uncer stable nitrous oxide-fentanyl or nitrous oxide-sevoflurane anaesthesia in children. Paediatr Anaesth 2006; 16: 761

61. Meakin G, Meretoja O, Perkins R: Comparison of atracurium-induced meruomuscular blockade in neonates, infants, and children. Br J Anaesth 1988; 60: 171

62. Ved SA, Walden TL, Montana J et al: Vomiting and recovery after outpatient tonsillectomy and adenoidectomy in children. Comparison of four anesthetic techniques using nitrous oxide with halothane or propofol. Anesthesiology 1996; 85:4

63. Culy CR, Bhana N, Plosker GL: Ondansetron: A review of its use as an antiemetic in children. Paediatr Drugs. 2001; 3: 441

64. Steward DL, Welge JA, Myer CM: Steroids for improving recovery following tonsillectomy in children. Cochrane Database Syst Rev 2003; (1): CD003997

65. Gan TJ YT, Apfel CC, Chung F et al. Consensus guidelines for managing postoperative nausea and vomiting. Anesthesia & Analgesia 2003; 97: 62

66. Henzi I, Sonderegger J, Tramer MR: Efficacy, dose-response, and adverse effects of droperidol for prevention of postoperative nausea and vomiting. Can J Anaesth 2000; 47: 537

67. Berleur M, Dahan A, Murat I et al: Perioperative infusions in paediatric patients: rationale for using Ringer-lactate solution with low dextrose concentration. J Clin Pharm Ther 2003; 28: 31

68. Khine HH, Corddry DH, Kettrick RG et al: Comparison of cuffed and uncuffed endotracheal tubes in young children during general anesthesia. Anesthesiology 1997; 86: 627

69. Blair JM, Hill DA, Bali IM et al: Tracheal intubating conditions after induction with sevoflurane 8% in children. A comparison with two intravenous techniques. Anaesthesia 2000; 55: 774

70. Simon L, Boucebci KJ, Orliaguet G et al: A survey of practice of tracheal intubation without muscle relaxant in paediatric patients. Paediatr Anaesth 2002; 12: 36

71. Politis GD, Tobin JR, Morell RC et al: Tracheal intubation of healthy pediatric patients without muscle relaxant: a survey of technique utilization and perceptions of safety. Anesth Analg 1999; 88: 737

72. Conterato JP, Lindahl SG, Meyer DM et al: Assessment of spontaneous ventilation in anesthetized children with use of a pediatric circle or a Jackson-Rees system. Anesth Analg 1989; 69: 484

72a. Davidson AJ. Awareness and paediatric anaesthesia. Paediatr Anaesth 2002; 12: 567

73. Berde C, Sethna N: Analgesics for the treatment of pain in children. N Engl J Med 2002; 347: 1094

74. Franck L, Greenberg C, Stevens B: Pain assessment in infants and children. Pediatr Clin North Am 2000; 47: 487

75. Cummings E, Reid G, Finley G et al: Prevalence and source of pain in pediatric inpatients. Pain 1996; 68: 25

76. Hamers J, Abu-Saad H, van den Hout M et al: Are children given insufficient pain-relieving medication postoperatively? J Adv Nurs 1998; 27: 37

77. Pate J, Blount R, Cohen L, Smith A. Childhood medical experience and temperament as predictors of adult functioning in medical situations. Child Health Care 1996; 25: 281

78. Taddio A, Goldbach M, Ipp M et al: Effect of neonatal circumcision on pain responses during vaccination in boys. Lancet 1995; 345: 291

79. Kotzer M: Factors predicting postoperative pain in children and adolescents following spine fusion. Issues Comp Pediatr Nurs 2000; 23: 83

80. Helgadottir HL, Wilson ME: Temperament and pain in 3 to 7-year-old children undergoing tonsillectomy. J Pediatr Nurs 2004; 19: 204

81. Schechter N, Bernstein B, Beck A et al: Individual differences in children's response to pain: role of temperament and parental characteristics. Pediatrics 1991; 87: e1184

82. Hsu YW, Pan MH, Huang CJ et al: Comparison of inhalation induction with 2%, 4%, 6%, and 8% sevoflurane in nitrous oxide for pediatric patients. Acta Anaesthesiol Sinica 2000; 38: 73

83. Piira T, Hayes B, Goodenough B et al: Effects of attentional direction, age, and coping style on cold-pressor pain in children. Behav Res Ther 2006; 44: 835

84. Russell IA, Miller Hance WC, Gregory G et al: The safety and efficacy of sevoflurane anesthesia in infants and children with congenital heart disease. Anesth Analg 92: 1152

85. Fanurik D, Zeltzer L, Roberts M et al: The relationship between children's coping styles and psychological interventions for cold pressor pain. Pain 1993; 53: 213

86. Palermo T, Drotar D, Lambert S: Psychosocial predictors of children's postoperative pain. Clin Nurs Res 1998; 7: 275

87. Kain Z, Mayes L, Caldwell-Andrews A et al: Preoperative anxiety and postoperative pain and behavioral recovery in young children undergoing surgery. Pediatrics 2006; 118: 651

88. Anderson B, Holford N, Woollard G et al: Perioperative pharmacodynamics of acetaminophen analgesia in children. Anesthesiology 1999; 90: 411

89. Schachtel B, Thoden W: A placebo-controlled model for assaying systemic analgesics in children. Clin Pharmacol Ther 1993; 53: 593

90. Rusy L, Houck C, Sullivan L et al: A double-blind evaluation of ketorolac tromethamine versus acetaminophen in pediatric tonsillectomy: analgesia and bleeding. Anesth Analg 1995; 80: 226

91. Berde C, Lehn B, Yee J et al: Patient-controlled analgesia in children and adolescents: a randomized, prospective comparison with intramuscular administration of morphine for postoperative analgesia. J Pediatr 1991; 118: 460

92. Huth MM, Broome ME, Good M: Imagery reduces children's post-operative pain. Pain 2004; 110: 439

93. Dubois MC, Piat V, Constant I et al: Comparison of three techniques for induction of anaesthesia with sevoflurane in children. Paediatr Anaesth 1999; 9: 19

94. Maclaren JE, Cohen LL: Teaching behavioral pain management to health-care professionals: a systematic review of research in training programs. J Pain 2005; 6: 481

95. MacLaren JE, Cohen LL: A comparison of distraction strategies for venipuncture distress in children. J Pediatr Psychol 2005; 30: 387

96. Kain ZN, Caldwell-Andrews AA: Preoperative psychological preparation of the child for surgery: an update. Anesthesiol Clin North Am 2005; 23: 597

97. Robers S: Ultrasonographic guidance in pediatric regional anesthesia. Part 2: techniques. Paediatr Anaesth 2006; 16: 1112

98. Marhofer PF: Ultrasonographic guidance in pediatric regional anesthesia. Part 1: theoretical background. Paediatr Anaesth 2006; 16: 1008

99. Giaufre E, Dalens B, Gombert A: Epidemiology and morbidity of regional anesthesia in children: A 1-year prospective survey of the French-Language Society of Pediatric Anesthesiologists. Anesth Analg 1996; 83: 904

100. Schrock CR, Jones MB: The dose of caudal epidural analgesia and duration of postoperative analgesia. Paediatr Anaesth 2003; 13: 403

101. Khalil S, Lingadevaru H, Bolos M et al: Caudal regional anesthesia, ropivacaine concentration, postoperative analgesia, and infants. Anesth Analg 2006; 102: 395

102. Gunter J, Watcha M, Forestner J et al: Caudal epidural anesthesia in conscious premature and high-risk infants. J Pediatr Surg 1991; 26: 9

103. Williams RK, Adams DC, Aladjem EV et al: The safety and efficacy of spinal anesthesia for surgery in infants: The Vermont Infant Spinal Registry. Anesth Analg 2006; 102: 67

104. Kurz A, Sessler DI, Lenhardt R: Perioperative normothermia to reduce the incidence of surgical-wound infection and shorten hospitalization. Study of Wound Infection and Temperature Group. N Engl J Med 1996; 334: 1209

105. Kurz A, Sessler DI, Narzt E, Bekar A et al. Postoperative hemodynamic and thermoregulatory consequences of intraoperative core hypothermia. J Clin Anesth 1995; 7: 359

106. Ibacache ME, Munoz HR, Brandes V et al: Single-dose dexmedetomidine reduces agitation after sevoflurane anesthesia in children. Anesth Analg 2004; 98: 60

107. Hollman GA: Oral midazolam and emergence delirium. Ann Emerg Med 1995; 25: 853

108. Cravero JP, Beach M, Thyr B et al: The effect of small dose fentanyl on the emergence characteristics of pediatric patients after sevoflurane anesthesia without surgery. Anesth Analg 2003; 97: 364

109. Picard V, Dumont L, Pellegrini M: Quality of recovery in children: Sevoflurane versus propofol. Acta Anaesthesiolog Scand 2000; 44: 307

110. Eberhart L, Morin A, Guber D et al: Applicability of risk scores for postoperative nausea and vomiting in adults to paediatric patients. Br J Anaesth 2004; 93: 386

111. Olutoye O, Watcha M: Management of postoperative vomiting in pediatric patients. Internat Anesthesiol Clin 2003; 41: 99

CHAPTER 46 ■ GASTROINTESTINAL DISORDERS

BABATUNDE O. OGUNNAIKE AND CHARLES W. WHITTEN

KEY POINTS

1. The difference between the lower esophageal sphincter (LES) pressure and gastric pressure is "barrier pressure," which is more important than the LES tone in the production of gastroesophageal reflux.

2. The American Society of Anesthesiologists recommends a fasting period of 4 hours for breast milk, 6 hours for both nonhuman milk and infant formula, and 6 hours for a light solid meal. Clear liquids may be consumed up to 2 hours prior to anesthesia.

3. Application of cricoid pressure reduces LES tone and may cause the esophagus to be displaced to the side rather than to be compressed. Compression in the backward and upward direction improves laryngoscopy.

4. Anastomotic site dehiscence may be caused by a variety of factors including a reduction of blood supply to the anastomotic site. There is no statistically significant evidence to indicate that epidural analgesia with local anesthetic, or the use of neostigmine, increases the incidence of anastomotic dehiscence in patients undergoing colorectal surgery.

5. Epidural analgesia that includes local anesthetics is effective in minimizing postoperative ileus. Other beneficial adjuncts include use of minimally invasive surgical techniques, early enteral nutrition, and early mobilization.

6. Carcinoid crises can be precipitated by physical or chemical factors that can potentially trigger mediator release. Examples include stress, tumor necrosis from hepatic artery ligation or embolization, chemotherapy, and succinylcholine-induced fasciculations. Octreotide effectively treats intraoperative carcinoid crises.

GASTROINTESTINAL DISORDERS

Esophagus

The adult esophagus extends from the cricopharyngeal sphincter at the level of the C6 vertebra to the gastroesophageal junction. An inner circular layer surrounded by an outer longitudinal layer makes up the musculature. The upper third of the inner circular muscle is striated and the lower two-thirds are smooth.

The cricopharyngeus muscle, one of the two inferior muscles of the pharynx, together with the circular fibers of the upper esophagus, acts as the functional *upper esophageal sphincter* (UES) at the pharyngoesophageal junction. The UES extends from one side of the cricoid arch to the other and is continuous with the circular muscular coat of the esophagus. This sphincter is in a state of tonic contraction with a resting pressure of 15 to 60 cm H_2O, preventing air from entering the esophagus under normal circumstances. The UES also helps prevent aspiration by sealing off the upper esophagus from the hypopharynx in conscious healthy patients. UES function is impaired during both normal sleep and anesthesia. Most anesthetic agents, except ketamine, will reduce UES tone and

increase the likelihood of regurgitation of material from the esophagus into the hypopharynx. Impaired swallowing and reduction in tone of the UES from partial neuromuscular blockade increase the risk of aspiration.[1] Video manometry studies have shown a significant delay in relaxation of the UES following contraction of the inferior constrictor muscle during partial neuromuscular blockade, suggesting that conscious patients in the recovery room may still be at risk of aspiration even with clinically adequate neuromuscular transmission.[2] Subhypnotic concentrations of intravenous (IV) and inhalational anesthetics increase the incidence of pharyngeal dysfunction.[3] Both intrinsic and extrinsic nerves supply the esophagus. The intrinsic nerve supply includes the myenteric plexus of Auerbach (which lies between the outer longitudinal and middle circular layers of muscle) and the submucosal plexus of Meissner (which lies between the circular layer and the mucosa). The extrinsic nerve supply is derived from parasympathetic fibers from the vagi with sympathetic fibers from the superior and inferior cervical and fourth and fifth thoracic sympathetic ganglia.

The border between the stomach and esophagus is formed by the *lower esophageal sphincter* (LES). It is a band of circular muscle fibers surrounding the lower end of the esophagus and has a resting tone of 10 to 15 cm H_2O with an approximate

TABLE 46-1

FACTORS AFFECTING LOWER ESOPHAGEAL SPHINCTER TONE

■ DECREASE TONE	■ INCREASE TONE	■ NO CHANGE IN TONE
• Inhaled anesthetics	• Anticholinesterases—	• H$_2$-receptor antagonists—
• Opioids	neostigmine,	cimetidine, ranitidine
• Anticholinergics—	edrophonium	• Nondepolarizing muscle relaxants—
atropine,	• Cholinergics	atracurium, vecuronium
glycopyrrolate	• Acetylcholine	• Propranolol
• Thiopental	• Succinylcholine	
• Propofol	• α-Adrenergic	
	stimulants	
• β-Agonists	• Antacids	
• Ganglion blockers	• Metoclopramide	
• Tricyclic	• Gastrin	
antidepressants		
• Secretin	• Serotonin	
• Glucagon	• Histamine	
• Cricoid pressure	• Pancreatic polypeptide	
• Obesity	• Metoprolol	
• Hiatal hernia		
• Pregnancy	—	—

length of 3 cm. The left margin of the lower esophagus makes an acute angle with the gastric fundus and contraction of the right crus of the diaphragm forms a sling around the abdominal esophagus. The LES, the major barrier to gastroesophageal reflux, is histologically similar to the rest of the esophagus but functionally different. The LES appears as an area of increased pressure on gastroesophageal manometry. During swallowing, the LES is relaxed, whereas there is peristalsis in the remainder of the esophagus. The major physiological derangement in gastroesophageal reflux is a reduction in LES pressure. The sphincteric pressure is affected by both the intrinsic nerve plexus and by gastrin released by the mucosa of the gastric antrum in response to the presence of acid. Gastrin increases the sphincter pressure, as well as α-adrenergic agents, acetylcholine, serotonin, histamine, and pancreatic polypeptide. Dopamine, secretin, glucagons, and β-adrenergic agents decrease the LES sphincter pressure among other factors (Table 46-1).

❶   The difference between the LES pressure (about 25 mm Hg) and gastric pressure (5 to 10 mm Hg) is *barrier pressure,* which is more important than the LES tone in the production of gastroesophageal reflux. Adequately high intragastric pressure can overcome the LES and lead to reflux. Regurgitation occurs if the barrier pressure becomes negative as may occur with obstruction to gastric emptying (e.g., pyloric stenosis). This is unlikely in healthy individuals whose LES pressure usually rises in response to increased intragastric pressure. Low-to-normal barrier pressures are characteristic of patients with gastroesophageal reflux with no distinct cutoff point. Vagal denervation does not seem to affect the active function or resting tone of the LES, but reduced tone can be clinically seen with obesity, hiatal hernia, and pregnancy. Anesthetic agents that may reduce the barrier pressure, thereby reducing LES pressure, include thiopental, propofol, opioids, anticholinergics, and inhaled anesthetics. In contrast, antiemetics, cholinergics, antacids, and succinylcholine increase LES pressure. Nondepolarizing muscle relaxants and H$_2$-receptor antagonists have no effect on LES pressure. Cricoid pressure in both conscious and unconscious patients decreases LES tone as a result of a significant reduction in esophageal barrier pressure while gastric pressure remains normal.[4] The evidence that succinylcholine increases LES tone, while cricoid pressure decreases LES tone, makes the necessity for application of

cricoid pressure during a rapid-sequence induction questionable.

Stomach

Digestion begins in the stomach by mixing of ingested food with gastric secretions. It is very distensible with the capacity to store large amounts of material (up to 1.5 L of fluid) without a significant increase in intragastric pressure. Electrical activity that originates at a "pacemaker" located near the midpoint of the greater curvature of the stomach initiates mechanical activity that spreads toward the pylorus. Pyloric relaxation, in response to the waves of gastric activity, expels gastric contents into the duodenum in small amounts.

Obesity, bedridden states, pregnancy, shock, trauma, and pain are examples of pathologic states associated with high gastric content volume. Bowel handling during laparotomy increases gastric emptying time for up to 24 hours. Gastric secretion is predominantly hydrochloric acid with a pH of between 1.0 and 3.5, high potassium content, and a rate of production of about 50 to 100 mL/hr. A gastric volume of 0.4 mL/kg and gastric pH of <2.5 increase the risk and severity of aspiration pneumonitis; however, the volume of fluid aspirated does not necessarily relate to the volume in the stomach. Adequately starved patients have been anesthetized with >0.5 mL/kg gastric volumes without evidence of aspiration. There is a dose-response relationship in the severity of aspiration pneumonitis for both gastric volume and acidity that directly reaches the lung. Human breast milk predisposes to an increased severity of aspiration pneumonitis when compared with other types of milk. Soy-based formula causes a less severe form of acute lung injury than human milk or dairy formula.[5]

Protective Airway Reflexes

The main protective airway reflexes include the following: (1) Apnea with laryngospasm causes closure of both the false and true vocal cords. Prolonged laryngospasm maintains the true cords in spasm while the false cords relax. (2) Coughing, which is a brief period of inspiration followed by a forceful expiratory effort. Expiration is accompanied by wider opening of the false cords than inspiration. (3) The expiration reflex, which induces a closure of the false cords preceded by sudden opening of the glottis. It is a forceful expiration without prior preceding inspiration. (4) Spasmodic panting, which is a reflex involving the glottis opening and closing rapidly and involves shallow breathing at approximately 60 breaths per minute for <10 seconds. These reflexes, except for laryngospasm, can be blunted by opioids, such as fentanyl. Premedicated and anesthetized patients, and elderly patients, have reduced airway reflexes, putting them at an increased risk for perioperative aspiration pneumonitis.[6]

REDUCING PERIOPERATIVE ASPIRATION RISK

This involves the control of gastric contents (volume and acidity) and prevention of pulmonary aspiration (e.g., cricoid pressure and cuffed endotracheal intubation). Controlling gastric volume and acidity helps minimize the effects of aspiration if it occurs (Table 46-2).

Control of Gastric Contents

Control of gastric contents involves (1) minimizing intake, (2) increasing gastric emptying with prokinetics, and (3) reducing gastric volume and acidity with a nasogastric tube, antacids, H_2-receptor antagonists, and proton pump inhibitors (PPIs). Clear liquids may be consumed up to 2 hours prior to anesthesia without increased risk for regurgitation and aspiration.[7] Gastric emptying is slower for milk than for clear liquids. Human breast milk is cleared more rapidly than other milk products.[8] Altered physiological states (e.g., pregnancy and diabetes mellitus) and gastrointestinal (GI) pathology (e.g., bowel obstruction and peritonitis) adversely affect the rate of gastric emptying, thereby increasing aspiration risk. The extent of delayed gastric emptying with diabetes mellitus correlates well with the presence of autonomic neuropathy, but not with age, duration of disease, preprandial HbA_{1C}, or peripheral neuropathy. The time difference in the delay between diabetic and healthy patients ranges from 30 minutes to 2 hours.[9] The American Society of Anesthesiologists recommends a fasting period of 4 hours for breast milk, 6 hours for

both nonhuman milk and infant formula, and also 6 hours for a light solid meal.[7]

Reduction of gastric acidity may be achieved with the aid of H_2-receptor antagonists and PPIs, which also reduce gastric volume. Famotidine effectively reduces gastric volume and increases gastric pH better than ranitidine given a few hours before surgery.[10] The PPIs rabeprazole, lansoprazole, and omeprazole are most effective when given in two successive doses, in the evening before and on the morning of anesthesia.[11,12] When given as a single dose, rabeprazole and lansoprazole should be administered on the morning of anesthesia as they are not sufficiently effective when given the previous night, but single-dose omeprazole can be given the previous night because it is not as effective when given on the morning of anesthesia.[11–13] Sodium citrate, best administered within 1 hour preoperatively in a dose of 15 to 30 mL, increases gastric pH to >2.5, and when combined with metoclopramide (10 mg IV), it reduces gastric contents to <25 mL. A nasogastric (NG) tube may be used to reduce gastric volume prior to induction of anesthesia, especially in an emergency situation, but also in elective patients with a high risk of regurgitation and aspiration. The insertion of an NG tube does not guarantee an "empty stomach" and may impair the function of the LES and UES, but it does not diminish the effectiveness of cricoid pressure.[14] The NG tube also provides a direct connection to the outside for passive drainage of gastric contents and is best left in place and open to freely drain during induction of anesthesia.

Prevention of Pulmonary Aspiration

Although the effectiveness of the technique is controversial, the application of cricoid pressure is recommended to occlude the upper end of the esophagus to prevent passive regurgitation of gastric contents and decrease the risk of pulmonary aspiration during rapid-sequence induction intubation technique. However, application of cricoid pressure reduces LES tone and may cause the esophagus to be displaced to the side rather than to be compressed.[15] Application of cricoid pressure was first described by Dr. Brian Sellick[16] in 1961, who stated that, "the maneuver consists in temporary occlusion of the upper end of the esophagus by backward pressure of the cricoid cartilage against the bodies of the cervical vertebrae." It was further clarified as compression generated with downward pressure exerted by the forefinger while the thumb and middle finger prevent lateral displacement of the cricoid ring (Fig. 46-1). Compression in the backward and upward direction has since been found to improve laryngoscopy. The force applied to the cricoid cartilage should be sufficient to prevent aspiration but not so great as to cause airway obstruction or allow the possibility of esophageal rupture if vomiting occurs. The recommended force is estimated to range between 20 and 44 newtons (N); however, cricoid deformation occurs at 44 N with associated cricoid occlusion, vocal cord closure, and difficult ventilation. A force of 1 N will give a mass of 1 kg an acceleration of 1 meter per second squared (i.e., 1 N = 1 kg/m/s/s). Cricoid occlusion may also occur at 20 and 30 N but to a lesser degree.[17] Cricoid deformation, vocal cord closure, and associated difficult ventilation may be caused by improperly applied cricoid pressure. Awake patients experience pain, coughing, and retching with pressures >20 N, so this amount of force should be applied only after loss of consciousness. A reasonable approach is to apply 10 N force to the cricoid in the awake state and increase to 30 N after loss of consciousness.[14] Cricoid pressure by itself, before laryngoscopy and intubation, increases the incidence of hypertension and tachycardia during induction of anesthesia.[18] The upward and backward direction of application of cricoid pressure, which improves laryngoscopy, is associated with a

---

TABLE 46-2

METHODS TO REDUCE THE RISK OF REGURGITATION AND PULMONARY ASPIRATION

1. Minimize intake
   Adequate preoperative fasting
   Clear liquids only if necessary
2. Increase gastric emptying
   Prokinetics (e.g., metoclopramide)
3. Reduce gastric volume and acidity
   Nasogastric tube
   Nonparticulate antacid (e.g., sodium citrate)
   H_2-receptor antagonists (e.g., famotidine)
   Proton pump inhibitors (e.g., lansoprazole)
4. Airway management and protection
   Cricoid pressure
   Cuffed endotracheal intubation
   Esophageal-tracheal combitube
   ProSeal laryngeal mask airway

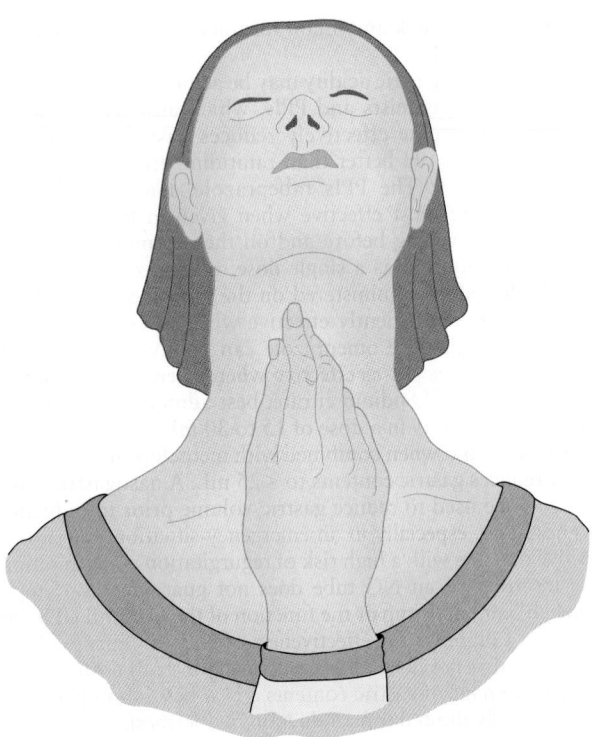

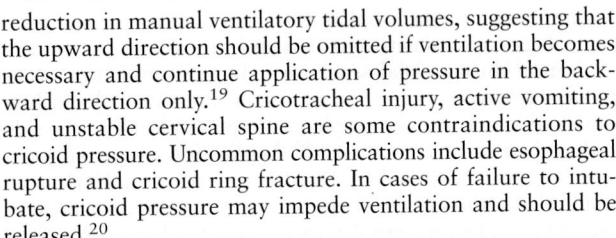

FIGURE 46-1. Cricoid pressure (Sellick's maneuver). Pressure is exerted by the forefinger while the thumb and middle finger prevent lateral displacement of the cricoid ring.

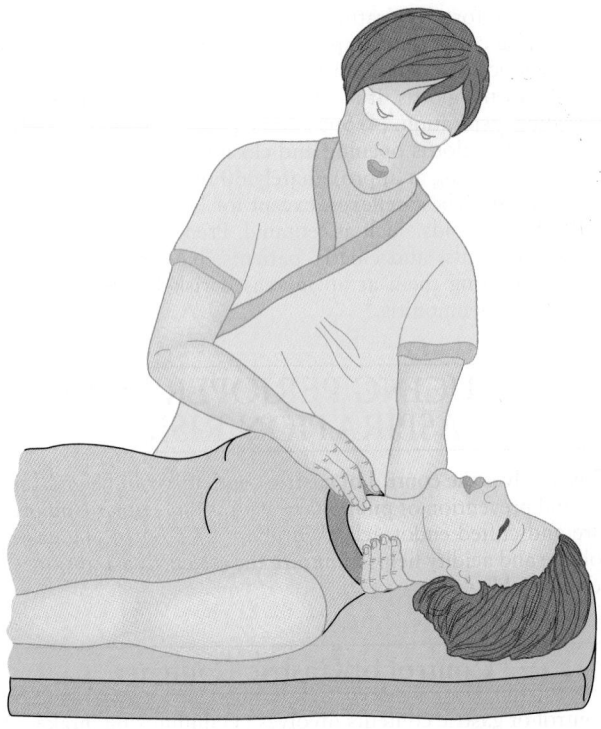

FIGURE 46-2. Bimanual cricoid pressure. Counterpressure is applied with a hand beneath the cervical vertebrae supporting the neck and minimizing distortions of the head position.

reduction in manual ventilatory tidal volumes, suggesting that the upward direction should be omitted if ventilation becomes necessary and continue application of pressure in the backward direction only.[19] Cricotracheal injury, active vomiting, and unstable cervical spine are some contraindications to cricoid pressure. Uncommon complications include esophageal rupture and cricoid ring fracture. In cases of failure to intubate, cricoid pressure may impede ventilation and should be released.[20]

Bimanual cricoid pressure (Fig. 46-2), described as counterpressure with a hand beneath the cervical vertebrae to support the neck, minimizes the distortions of the position of the head and the alignment of the trachea, which can complicate cricoid pressure performed with one hand. A hyperextended vertebral column forms an arch based on the scapulae fixed below and a mobile rotating occiput above. The cricoid forms the apex of this arch, which if disrupted, complicates the maintenance of an unobstructed airway and good glottic view at laryngoscopy. Significant cricoid pressure with the neck extended tends to collapse the arch by downward apical pressure, making the occipital base of the arch to rotate and flex the head on the neck, reducing the glottic view with the tongue blocking the pharynx. The use of two hands balances pressure, facilitates the "sniffing" position, and aids laryngoscopy and intubation. Caution should be exercised with this technique in patients with suspected cervical spine trauma or fracture, cervical spine arthritis, immobile neck, and laryngotracheal pathology. No difference in laryngoscopic view was found in some patients when bimanual cricoid pressure was compared with the single-handed technique.[21]

The likelihood of reflux may be reduced by tilting the upper part of the body 30 to 45 degrees, a position that may promote aspiration of gastric contents if regurgitated. However, this position may have no effect on intragastric-esophageal barrier pressure nor reduce the incidence of gastroesophageal reflux.[22] Minimal head-down tilt at induction may increase the risk of

passive regurgitation but should minimize aspiration, and has been recommended by some practitioners.[23]

Airway Protection

Cuffed endotracheal intubation is the mainstay of prevention of regurgitated material from reaching the trachea and lungs. The high-volume, low-pressure cuffs in current widespread use may not completely prevent regurgitated material from reaching the airway. Leakage from the subglottis via the longitudinal folds of the cuff into the trachea may be prevented by cuff lubrication.[24] Of the other airway devices used, the laryngeal mask airway (LMA™, LMA North America Inc. San Diego, CA) reduces barrier pressure at the LES with an increased incidence of reflux in comparison with the cuffed endotracheal tube.[25] The use of the LMA™ with unusual positions, such as the lithotomy position, increases the incidence of gastroesophageal reflux.[26] Some LMA™ devices have an esophageal vent for passage of a nasogastric tube and through which regurgitated material can pass to the outside. An incorporated dorsal cuff also allows for provision of a better seal around periglottic tissues. These improvements help to better isolate the airway from the GI tract.

THE INTESTINES

The small intestine is the site of most of the absorption of fluids and nutrients from the GI tract. Parasympathetic stimulation and antagonism increases and decreases the activity of the small intestine, respectively. Suppression of sympathetic activity increases small intestine activity and stimulation results in a decrease. Bowel denervation results in minimal change in intestinal activity, lending credence to the possibility that humoral secretions (e.g., somatostatin and pancreatic polypeptides) play a major role in intestinal activity. Hypokalemia, peritonitis, and laparotomy all suppress intestinal activity for up to 48 hours. In addition, laparotomy decreases small intestine absorptive ability.

Absorption is the predominant function of the colon. A pacemaker in the transverse colon controls colonic motility. The vagus nerve supplies neural control to the colon down to the splenic flexure, after which the sacral parasympathetic outflow takes over. Sympathetic supply is from T_{6-10}, which decreases colonic motility when stimulated in contrast to parasympathetic stimulation, which increases motility. Neostigmine increases colonic activity while morphine and other opioids decrease both activity and tone.

Splanchnic Blood Flow

Splanchnic blood flow is influenced predominantly by the autonomic nervous system. α-Adrenergic stimulation leads to vasoconstriction and β_2-adrenergic stimulation causes vasodilation. Stimulation of dopaminergic receptors produces vasoconstriction, which predominates over the mild vasodilation produced by β_2-adrenergic stimulation. Parasympathetic stimulation increases metabolism, which increases blood flow. Autoregulation normally maintains blood flow to the small intestine. With prolonged sympathetic stimulation, there is an initial decrease in blood flow, which is not sustained because of an "escape" phenomenon in the mesenteric circulation whereby the blood flow gradually increases toward normal after a few minutes. Severe stress induces the release of vasoconstrictors, including vasopressin, angiotensin II, and catecholamines, which all reduce visceral blood flow. Reduced blood flow results in sympathetic stimulation, which preferentially diverts blood to the muscularis while reducing mucosal perfusion.

It is difficult to maintain adequacy of blood flow after colonic resection, especially in the sigmoid region. This is not usually a problem with small intestinal or stomach surgery. Hypoxia, inadequate oxygen-carrying capacity from anemia, or impairment of blood supply, may lead to further reductions in oxygen supply, causing ischemia at the anastomotic suture line and consequent anastomotic damage. Splanchnic vascular resistance increases with severe hemorrhage, which helps divert blood flow to other vital organs. Hypocapnia significantly reduces splanchnic blood flow while hypercapnia does the opposite; therefore, hyperventilation to produce hypocapnia is better avoided during colonic surgery and in the perioperative period. Neostigmine reduces mesenteric blood flow because of induced exaggerated contraction. Atropine partially offsets the blood flow reduction. Morphine decreases splanchnic vascular resistance, thereby increasing splanchnic blood flow, an effect that can be reversed by naloxone. Thoracic epidural block reduces mean colonic serosal red cell flux and inferior mesenteric artery flow in proportion to a reduction in the mean arterial blood pressure, a situation that does not improve with fluid resuscitation but responds to vasopressor therapy.[27]

Postoperative Anastomotic Leakage

Anastomotic leakage after colon surgery may be related to patient factors (anemia, comorbidity), surgical factors (bowel preparation, operative expertise), and anesthesia and pain management-related factors (e.g., morphine, epidural analgesia, neostigmine).[28] Risk factors for leakage include the male gender, low anastomoses, smoking, excessive alcohol consumption, and preoperative chemotherapy and/or radiotherapy.[29] The theoretical mechanism by which anesthesia-related factors increase the incidence of anastomotic dehiscence is through increased intestinal motility and intraluminar pressure. In addition, epidural analgesia may reduce blood supply to the anastomotic site. However, there is no statistically significant evidence to indicate that epidural analgesia with local anesthetic increases the incidence of anastomotic dehiscence when compared with epidural or IV opioids in patients undergoing colorectal surgery.[30] On the contrary, thoracic epidural analgesia may decrease the incidence of anastomotic leakage after esophagectomy by improving microvascular perfusion of the gastric conduit in the anastomotic area.[31,32] Neostigmine is an anticholinesterase that increases parasympathetic activity, which increases bowel peristalsis. Vagotomy reduces this effect. Postoperative use of neostigmine after bowel anastomosis has generated controversy as a result of the unsubstantiated suggestion that it increases the incidence of anastomotic disruption because of its prokinetic effect. Neostigmine increases the frequency and magnitude of colonic pressure waves, an effect that can be magnified by bowel disease. Anticholinergics such as atropine and glycopyrrolate reduce these effects. Sugammadex, a modified γ-cyclodextrin compound that encapsulates rocuronium, (and other steroid-based neuromuscular blockers to a lesser extent), does not stimulate bowel peristalsis and may be substituted for neostigmine for reversal after bowel anastomotic surgery.[33] Prokinetics such as metoclopramide have been associated with colonic anastomotic dehiscence in rats during the early postoperative period[34]; however, clinical observations and animal studies have largely discounted the suggestions that neostigmine has a deleterious effect on bowel anastomosis.[35]

Postoperative Ileus

Multiple mechanisms contribute to ileus after intestinal surgery (Table 46-3). Abdominal pain activates a spinal reflex that inhibits GI motility, which is further inhibited by the stress of surgery that induces sympathetic hyperactivity. Other contributing factors include excessive handling of bowel, parenteral opioids, electrolyte imbalance, immobility, lack of enteral feeding, and intestinal wall swelling from excessive fluid administration.[36] Thoracic epidural analgesia that includes local anesthetics blocks sympathetic outflow to increase GI parasympathetic activity with subsequent increased motility and decreased duration of ileus. Epidural opioids may delay enteric transit time in a manner similar to parenteral opioids, and because it may also cause nausea, it may be incorrectly attributed to paralytic ileus. Low thoracic and lumbar epidural blockade are not as beneficial for minimizing postoperative ileus as is upper thoracic epidural blockade. The colon, beyond the splenic flexure, and the rectum receive their parasympathetic supply from sacral nerve roots and are therefore more susceptible to ileus when lumbar epidural blockade is initiated. Opioids depress GI motility through μ-opioid receptors within the bowels, an effect that can be reversed by naloxone (a tertiary opioid-receptor antagonist). Peripherally acting quaternary opioid-receptor antagonists, such as methylnaltrexone and alvimopan, are a class of drugs that show almost exclusive binding to μ-opioid receptors in the GI tract to reduce the duration of postoperative ileus.[37] They do not cross the blood–brain barrier and are therefore unable to reverse analgesic effects of opioids. Minimally invasive surgery (including laparoscopy) reduces inflammatory responses, thereby reducing ileus; as does early enteral nutrition and early mobilization.[38] "Sham feeding by chewing a stick of gum represents a form early enteral nutrition that is thought to accelerate bowel function by increasing vagal cholinergic stimulation of the gut, leading to release of GI hormones such as gastrin, neurotensin,

TABLE 46-3

MANAGEMENT OF POSTOPERATIVE ILEUS

■ ETIOLOGY	■ COMMENTS	■ MANAGEMENT
Abdominal pain	• Activation of spinal reflex that inhibits gastrointestinal motility • Sympathetic hyperactivity	• Thoracic epidural analgesia • Minimally invasive surgery • Use of NSAIDs in place of opioids
Surgical stress	• Induces sympathetic hyperactivity to inhibit GI motility	• Thoracic epidural analgesia; blocks sympathetic outflow to increase GI parasympathetic activity
Parenteral opioids	• Depression of GI motility through μ-opioid receptors within the bowels • Inhibition of GI nervous system and musculature	• Tertiary opioid receptor antagonists (e.g., naloxone; may reverse opioid analgesia) • Quaternary opioid receptor antagonists (e.g., methylnaltrexone, alvimopan) • Use of NSAIDs in place of opioids
Electrolyte imbalance (hypokalemia, hypomagnesemia, hyponatremia)	• Nonspecific inhibition of intrinsic GI nervous system and musculature	• Correct electrolyte abnormalities before invasive procedures
Excessive bowel handling	• Temporary abolition of contractions—change in gastric pacemaker • Bowel edema and inflammation	• Minimally invasive surgery (e.g., laparoscopy) to minimize bowel handling • Anticholinesterases (e.g. neostigmine, edrophonium) and cholinergic agonists (e.g., bethanechol, carbachol, methacholine); increase parasympathetic tone
Bowel edema	• Inflammation • Excessive hydration • Nonspecific inhibition of intrinsic GI nervous system and musculature	• Avoid excessive hydration • NSAIDs to reduce inflammation
Nothing by mouth	• Lack of diet-induced GI stimulation	• Early postoperative feeding • Chewing gum, a form of early "sham feeding"
Immobility	• Nonspecific inhibition of GI nervous system and musculature	• Early mobilization
Hypoxia	• Increased risk with prolonged postoperative hypoxemia • Inadequate reperfusion and hypoxia leads to injury	• Supplemental oxygen therapy • Hyperbaric oxygen therapy; improves microcirculation and oxygenation of hypoxic intestinal tissue

NSAIDs, nonsteroidal anti-inflammatory drugs; GI, gastrointestinal.

and pancreatic polypeptide.[39] Gum chewing also increases gastric pH but will also increase gastric fluid volume.[40] Hyperbaric oxygen therapy may have a prophylactic effect on postoperative paralytic ileus.[41] Oxygen under pressure enhances inert gas diffusion form the closed intestinal lumen into blood, leading relaxation of the distended intestinal loop and improvement of microcirculation and oxygenation of hypoxic intestinal tissue, which leads to preservation of intestinal viability and recovery of motility.

Mesenteric Traction Syndrome

The mesenteric traction syndrome consists of sudden tachycardia, hypotension, and cutaneous hyperemia during traction on the mesentery; hypoxia may also be present.[42] Clinical features suggest that the syndrome results from a release of vasoactive amines (mainly prostacyclin [PGI_2]) from the mesenteric vascular bed because the hemodynamic changes coincide with an increase in plasma concentrations of 6-keto-prostaglandin F_1 (a stable metabolite of prostacyclin) and thromboxane B_2 (a stable metabolite of thromboxane). In addition, traction on the small intestine can cause histamine release from the mesenteric mast cells. Nonsteroidal anti-inflammatory drugs and aspirin, which inhibit cyclo-oxygenase, significantly ameliorate these

clinical features, further suggesting a prostacyclin-mediated etiology. Intravenous ketorolac has been successfully used to treat persistent hypotension and flushing associated with mesenteric traction syndrome.[43] Prophylactic administration of H_1 and H_2 antihistamines also reduce the incidence of dysrhythmias due to mesenteric traction syndrome. In addition, they reduce the need for stabilizing interventions.[42] High-dose phenylephrine (up to 15 times the usual effective dose) has been successfully used to treat mesenteric traction syndrome.[44] Significant decreases in mean arterial pressure related to central and/or autonomic nervous reflexes occur during operations on upper abdominal viscera.[45] These hypotensive responses to visceral traction appear to be transmitted along afferent fibers contained within the splanchnic nerves. However, deafferentation of the splanchnic nerves, as occurs with epidural anesthesia, does not influence prostacyclin release, hypotension, or hypoxemia during mesenteric traction, lending further credence that prostacyclin is involved in the etiology of the syndrome.

Nitrous Oxide and the Bowel

Because nitrous oxide is 30 times more soluble than nitrogen in blood, nitrous oxide diffuses into gas-containing body cavities from the bloodstream faster than the nitrogen in those cavities can diffuse out into circulation. This may contribute to excessive distension of gas-containing bowels, possible bowel ischemia, and increased difficulty with surgical exposure.[46,47] Factors that determine the extent of distention include the amount of gas within the bowel, the duration of nitrous oxide administration, and the concentration of nitrous oxide used. There is a linear increase in bowel cavity size with time during administration of nitrous oxide such that after about 4 hours a 100 to 200% increase in gaseous bowel volume is observed with nitrous oxide anesthesia.[48]

Use of 80% nitrous oxide may potentially result in a fivefold increase in bowel gas, whereas use of a 50% concentration results in no more than a doubling of bowel gas. Nitrous oxide is best avoided in situations in which the bowels are already distended and during prolonged abdominal surgical procedures. On the other hand, use of low concentrations of nitrous oxide during short elective abdominal operations in which no significant amount of gas is present in the bowels is reasonable.[49,50]

CARCINOID TUMORS

Carcinoid tumors were so named for their resemblance to carcinoma. It is a slow-growing, benign, small intestinal tumor capable of metastasis, but with a good prognosis. The GI tract is the usual site of origin of carcinoid tumors, which are derived from enterochromaffin cells but may be found in any tissue derived from the endoderm. Intestinal carcinoid (appendix and ileum) is the usual source of metastasis.[51] Carcinoid tumors are usually asymptomatic, although nonspecific symptoms such as abdominal pain, diarrhea, intermittent intestinal obstruction, and GI bleeding are occasionally seen. Non-metastatic carcinoid tumors secrete hormones that are usually transported to the liver through the portal vein where they are subsequently inactivated. Although symptoms are sometimes caused by mechanical effects of the tumors, most symptoms are produced by the effects of hormones and substances secreted into the GI tract or into the systemic circulation. Carcinoid tumors, especially those arising in the midgut, secrete a variety of hormones, mediators, and biogenic amines including large quantities of serotonin that produce increased platelet serotonin levels and increased urinary levels of 5-hydroxy-indole-acetic-acid (5-HIAA), a metabolite of serotonin. Other secreted substances include histamine, substance P, catecholamines (including dopamine), bradykinin, tachykinin, motilin, corticotrophin, prostaglandins, kallikrein, and neurotensin. Bradykinin produces cutaneous flushing, bronchospasm and hypotension and serotonin causes hypertension or hypotension. Histamine also produces flushing.

Carcinoid Syndrome

Metastatic carcinoid tumor releases vasoactive peptides into the systemic circulation, which leads to signs and symptoms collectively known as the *carcinoid syndrome*. It generally indicates the presence of pulmonary or hepatic metastasis, although access to the systemic circulation can occur without hepatic metastasis. Carcinoid syndrome occurs when massive amounts of circulating hormones produced by the tumor reach the systemic circulation. It occurs in approximately 20% of patients with carcinoid tumors.[51] The overall clinical manifestations of carcinoid syndrome include cutaneous flushing of the head, neck, and upper thorax (most common); bronchoconstriction; hypotension; diarrhea; and carcinoid heart disease. Hypertension may also be seen. Serotonin increases the chronotropic and inotropic activity of the heart, and when coupled with vasocon-

striction, will lead to hypertension. The diagnosis of carcinoid syndrome may be confirmed by urinary excretion of 5-HIAA, and serial values of this metabolite can be used to monitor tumor progression. A 24-hour urine sample containing >30 mg of 5-HIAA suggests carcinoid syndrome (normal level is 3 to 15 mg per 24 hours). There is, however, no correlation between the blood level of serotonin and the severity of symptoms. Serotonin increases the tone and motility of the jejunum causing diarrhea, the major feature of increased serotonin level.

Carcinoid Heart Disease

Carcinoid heart disease is seen in up to 60% of patients with carcinoid syndrome. Cardiac involvement combines with flushing and diarrhea to make up the classic "carcinoid triad." Cardiac involvement is usually right-sided, affecting tricuspid and pulmonary valves. Left-sided cardiac involvement is rare. There are plaquelike deposits of fibrous tissue on the endocardium of right-sided valvular cusps and leaflets, as well as the right atrium and ventricle.[52] Two-dimensional echocardiography is the diagnostic tool of choice. Tricuspid regurgitation is the predominant finding, although tricuspid stenosis and pulmonary valve regurgitation or stenosis can also occur. Tricuspid and/or pulmonary valve fibrosis with retraction and fixation of the leaflets may lead to regurgitation.[53] Intramyocardial metastases may lead to cardiac dysrhythmias. Over 50% of carcinoid deaths are a result of cardiac failure. The predominance of right-sided cardiac lesions suggests that the substances secreted from liver metastasis into the hepatic vein never reach the left side of the heart because of pulmonary metabolism. Carcinoid plaques can damage cardiac valves. They are caused by the actions of serotonin and tachykinin on platelets and endothelium. The now-banned appetite-suppressant drugs fenfluramine and dexfenfluramine interfere with serotonin metabolism to produce cardiac valve lesions similar to carcinoid valvular lesions.[54] Patients with carcinoid heart disease have higher levels of serum serotonin and urinary 5-HIAA, but it is debatable whether serotonin is responsible for the cardiac lesions. Also, treatment that reduces 5-HIAA excretion does not lead to regression of cardiac lesions.

Perioperative Management of the Carcinoid Patient

Complete surgical excision is the most effective treatment for carcinoid tumors (Table 46-4). Chemotherapy results are marginal at best. Biotherapy with interferon and octreotide may reduce tumor bulk and attenuate the release of vasoactive amines. Management should focus on blocking histamine and serotonin receptors and avoidance of drugs that facilitate mediator release from tumor cells. Mediator release can be triggered by opioids and muscle relaxants that release histamine, including succinylcholine, mivacurium, atracurium, and d-tubocurarine. Epinephrine, norepinephrine, histamine, dopamine, and isoproterenol have all been known to also provoke carcinoid crises. Perioperative management should include acquisition of the knowledge and severity of the specific features of the syndrome in each specific patient. Therapy should be directed at preventing the release of mediator substances from the tumor or antagonizing their effects. There is a positive correlation between the presence of carcinoid heart disease or high urinary output of 5-HIAA and postoperative complications.[55] Patients with carcinoid may have diarrhea and high gastric output.[56] Therefore, fluid resuscitation may be required, and serum electrolytes and glucose should be measured at regular intervals.

TABLE 46-4

PATIENTS WITH CARCINOID TUMORS

Diagnosis of carcinoid syndrome
- Cutaneous flushing of head, neck, and upper thorax
- Bronchoconstriction
- Hypotension
- Diarrhea
- ± Hypertension
- ± Carcinoid heart disease

Confirmation: >30 mg of 5-HIAA per 24 hour urine sample
(normal = 3–15 mg/24 hr)

Diagnosis of carcinoid heart disease
- Plaquelike deposits of fibrous tissue on right heart valvular cusps, atrium, and ventricle
- Tricuspid and/or pulmonary regurgitation
- Cardiac dysrhythmias

Confirmation: Two-dimensional echocardiography

Management
1. Perioperative blockade of serotonin receptors
2. Pay attention to procedures, treatments, and drugs that may stimulate release of vasoactive substances from tumor cells. These include:
   - Tumor-debulking surgery to reduce tumor size
   - Hepatic artery embolization to reduce tumor size
   - Biotherapy (e.g., interferon for tumor shrinkage)
   - Chemotherapy for systemic spread
3. Treat effects of hormone release as necessary.
   - Long-acting somatostatin analogues (e.g., octreotide), the mainstay of perioperative therapy
   - Anxiolytics to prevent stress-triggered release of serotonin
   - H_1- and H_2-blockers to block the effects of histamine
   - Symptomatic therapy (e.g., bronchodilators for wheezing)
   - H_2-blockers, diphenhydramine, and steroids inhibit the action of bradykinin
   - Aprotinin (kallikrein inhibitor) to treat hypotension refractory to refractory to octreotide

5-HIAA, 5-hydroxy-indole-acetic-acid.

Many carcinoid tumor specimens contain somatostatin receptors. Somatostatin is a GI regulatory peptide that reduces the production and release of gastropancreatic hormones. It reduces the amount of serotonin released from carcinoid tumors, which subsequently reduces the levels of urinary 5-HIAA. Somatostatin has a very short half-life of about 3 minutes and must therefore be given as infusion. Octreotide is a synthetic somatostatin analogue with approximately 50 times the half-life of somatostatin and is useful in treatment of symptoms and perioperative management of carcinoid syndrome. It has a half-life of approximately 2.5 hours. Subcutaneous octreotide at a dose of 50 to 500 μg every 8 hours may be titrated to effect for relief of symptoms or prevention of hypotension. Alternatively, 10 to 100 μg IV can be administered slowly 1 hour preoperatively. Preoperative preparation should also include 100 μg octreotide subcutaneously 3 times daily in the preceding 2 weeks and, if necessary, should be weaned slowly over 1 week postoperatively. Preoperative anxiolytics should be administered to prevent stress-triggered release of serotonin, and patients receiving octreotide preoperatively should continue with their normal dose on the morning of surgery. A combination of H_1- and H_2-blocking drugs may be used to block the effects of histamine. Histamine release is most likely to occur with gastric carcinoids; therefore, antihistamines may not be needed for carcinoid tumors originating in other areas.[51] H_2-blockers, diphenhydramine, and steroids inhibit the action of bradykinin.

6 Carcinoid crises can be precipitated by physical or chemical factors that can potentially trigger mediator release. Examples include stress, tumor necrosis from hepatic artery ligation or embolization, chemotherapy, and succinylcholine-induced fasciculations. Octreotide effectively treats intraoperative carcinoid crises. An octreotide infusion at a rate of 50 to 100 μg/hr can be administered during surgery; if more is required, IV boluses of 25 to 100 μg can be administered to the desired effect. Bolus IV doses have been associated with severe bradycardia and heart block through an effect on the cardiac conduction system.[57] Aprotinin, a kallikrein inhibitor, may be employed for hypotension if there is a refractory response to octreotide.[58]

The availability of newer, titratable, and short-acting anesthetic agents precludes the use of older, long-acting, and potentially histamine-releasing anesthetic agents. Any of the currently available induction agents and muscle relaxants including propofol, etomidate, vecuronium, cis-atracurium, and rocuronium can be used successfully. Caution should be exercised with drugs such as thiopental and succinylcholine that can release histamine. The short-acting synthetic opioids sufentanil, alfentanil, fentanyl, and remifentanil are all acceptable for use.[59] All current inhalation agents may be successfully used; however, desflurane may be the better choice in patients with liver metastasis because of its low rate of metabolism. Increased levels of serotonin have been associated with delayed awakening from general anesthesia. Administration of octreotide prior to manipulation of the tumor will attenuate adverse hemodynamic responses. Epidural analgesia is safe in patients who have been adequately treated with octreotide, provided that local anesthetic is administered in a graded manner, with careful hemodynamic monitoring, and in a diluted concentration.[59] The sympathetic blockade produced by epidural or spinal anesthesia may worsen hypotension, which can be minimized by dosing the epidural catheter with opioids or dilute local anesthetic solutions. Intraoperative hypotension from sympathetic blockade should be treated with volume expansion and IV infusion of octreotide. Although sympathomimetics such as ephedrine, epinephrine, and norepinephrine have been implicated in triggering the release of vasoactive amines from carcinoid tumors, there is evidence to suggest that they can be safely used to treat hypotension in patients who have been adequately treated with somatostatin analogues.[60,61] Octreotide infusion can also be used for intraoperative hypertension in combination with increasing doses of volatile anesthetic. Ondansetron, a serotonin antagonist, is a useful and logical antiemetic choice.

Invasive arterial blood pressure monitoring may be necessary during the intraoperative management of patients with carcinoid syndrome because of rapid changes in hemodynamic variables. Other useful monitors may include central venous or pulmonary artery catheters and transesophageal echocardiography. Intense hemodynamic monitoring and octreotide administration should continue into the postoperative period as secretion of vasoactive substances can still occur from residual tumor or metastases. Emotional and physical stress that may trigger vasoactive substance release is minimized by effective postoperative analgesia.

References

1. Ng A, Smith G: Gastroesophageal reflux and aspiration of gastric contents in anesthetic practice. Anesth Analg 2001; 93: 494
2. Sundman E, Witt H, Olsson R et al: The incidence and mechanisms of pharyngeal and upper esophageal dysfunction in partially paralyzed humans: Pharyngeal videoradiography and simultaneous manometry after atracurium. Anesthesiology 2000; 92: 977
3. Sundman E, Witt H, Sandin R et al: Pharyngeal function and airway protection during sybhypnotic concentrations of propofol, isoflurane and

sevoflurane: volunteers examined by pharyngeal videoradiography and simultaneous manometry. Anesthesiology 2001; 95: 1125

4. Garrard A, Campbell AE, Turley A et al: The effect of mechanically induced cricoid force on lower esophageal sphincter pressure in anaesthetized patients. Anaesthesia 2004; 59: 435

5. Chin C, Lerman J, Endo J: Acute lung injury after tracheal instillation of acidified soy-based or Enfalac formula or human breast milk in rabbits. Can J Anaesth 1999; 46: 282

6. Caranza R, Nandwani N, Tring JP et al: Upper airway reflex sensitivity following general anesthesia for day-case surgery. Anaesthesia 2000; 55: 367

7. American Society of Anesthesiologists Task Force on Preoperative Fasting: Practice guidelines for preoperative fasting and the use of pharmacologic agents to reduce the risk of pulmonary aspiration: Application to healthy patients undergoing elective procedures. Anesthesiology 1999; 79: 482

8. Van Den Driessche M, Peeters K, Marien P et al: Gastric emptying in formula-fed and breast-fed infants measured with 13C-octanoic acid breath test. J Pediatr Gastroenterol Nutr 1999; 29: 46

9. Merio R, Festa A, Bergmann H et al: Slow gastric emptying in Type I diabetes: Relation to autonomic and peripheral neuropathy, blood glucose, and glycemic control. Diabetes Care 1997; 20: 419

10. Kulkarni PN, Batra VK, Wig J: Effects of different combinations of H2 receptor antagonist with gastrokinetic drugs on gastric fluid pH and volume in children—a comparative study. Int J Pharmacol Ther 1997; 35: 561

11. Nishina K, Mikawa K, Takao Y et al: A comparison of rabeprazole, lansoprazole and ranitidine for improving preoperative gastric fluid property in adults undergoing elective surgery. Anesth Analg 2000; 90: 717

12. Nishina K, Mikawa K, Maekawa N et al: A comparison of lansoprazole, omeprazole and ranitidine for reducing preoperative gastric secretion in adult patients undergoing elective surgery. Anesth Analg 1996; 82: 832

13. Escolano F, Castano J, Lopez R et al: Effects of omeprazole, ranitidine, Famotidine and placebo on gastric secretion in patients undergoing elective surgery. Br J Anaesth 1992; 69: 404

14. Vanner RG, Asai T: Safe use of cricoid pressure. Anaesthesia 1999; 54: 1

15. Smith KJ, Dobranowski J, Yip G et al: Cricoid pressure displaces the esophagus: An observational study using magnetic resonance imaging. Anesthesiology 2003; 99: 60

16. Sellick BA: Cricoid pressure to control regurgitation of stomach contents during induction of anaesthesia. Lancet 1961; 2: 404

17. MacG Palmer JH, Ball DR: The effect of cricoid pressure on the cricoid cartilage and vocal cords: An endoscope study in anaesthetized patients. Anaesthesia 2000; 55: 263

18. Saghaei M, Masoodifar M: The pressor response and airway effects of cricoid pressure during induction of general anesthesia. Anesth Analg 2001; 93: 787

19. Hartsilver EL, Vanner RG: Airway obstruction with cricoid pressure. Anaesthesia 2000; 55: 208

20. Harry RM, Nolan JP: The use of cricoid pressure with the intubating laryngeal mask. Anaesthesia 1999; 54: 656

21. Vanner RG, Clarke P, Moore WJ et al: The effect of cricoid pressure and neck support on the view at laryngoscopy. Anaesthesia 1997; 52: 896

22. Jeske HC, Borovicka J, von Goedecke A et al: The influence of postural changes on gastroesophageal reflux and barrier pressure in nonfasting individuals. Anesth Analg 2005; 101: 597

23. Apfel CC, Roewer N: Ways to prevent and treat pulmonary aspiration of gastric contents. Curr Opin Anaesthesiol 2005; 18: 157

24. Young PJ, Basson C, Hamilton D et al: Prevention of tracheal aspiration using the pressure-limited tracheal tube cuff. Anaesthesia 1999; 54: 559

25. Valentine J, Stakes AF, Bellamy MC: Reflux during positive pressure ventilation through the laryngeal mask. Br J Anaesth 1994; 73: 543

26. McCrory CR, McShane AJ: Gastroesophageal reflux during spontaneous respiration with the laryngeal mask airway. Can J Anaesth 1999; 46: 268

27. Gould TH, Grace K, Thorne G et al: Effect of thoracic epidural anaesthesia on colonic blood flow. Br J Anaesth 2002; 89: 446

28. Ng A, Smith G: Anesthesia and the gastrointestinal tract. J Anesth 2002; 16: 51

29. Alberts JC, Parvaiz A, Moran BJ: Predicting risk and diminishing the consequences of anastomotic dehiscence following rectal resection. Colorectal Dis 2003; 5: 478

30. Holte K, Kehlet H: Epidural analgesia and risk of anastomotic leakage. Reg Anesth Pain Med 2001; 26: 111

31. Michelet P, D'Journo X, Roch A et al: Perioperative risk factors for anastomotic leakage after esophagectomy: influence of thoracic epidural analgesia. Chest 2005; 128: 3461

32. Michelet P, Roch A, D'Journo XP et al: Effect of thoracic epidural analgesia on gastric blood flow after esophagectomy. Acta Anaesthesiol Scand 2007; 51: 587

33. Sacan O, White PF, Tufanogullari B et al: Sugammadex reversal of rocuronium-induced neuromuscular blockade: A comparison with neostigmine-glycopyrrolate and edrophonium-atropine. Anesth Analg 2007; 104: 569

34. Garcia-Olmo D, Paya J, Lucas FJ et al: Effects of the pharmacological manipulation of postoperative intestinal motility on colonic anastomosis. An experimental study in a rat model. Int J Colorectal Dis 1997; 12: 73

35. Garcia-Olmo DC, Garcia-Rivas M, Garcia-Olmo D: Does neostigmine have deleterious effect on the resistance of colonic anastomoses? Eur J Anaesthesiol 1998; 15: 38

36. Fotiadis RJ, Badvie S, Weston MD et al: Epidural analgesia in gastrointestinal surgery. Br J Surg 2004; 91: 828

37. Goodman AJ, Le Bourdonnec B, Dolle RE. Mu opioid receptor antagonists: Recent developments. Chem Med Chem 2007; 2: 1552

38. Baig MK, Wexner SD: Postoperative ileus: a review. Dis Colon Rectum 2004; 47: 516

39. Schuster R, Grewal N, Greaney GC et al: Gum chewing reduces ileus after elective open sigmoid colectomy. Arch Surg 2006; 141: 174

40. Schoenfelder RC, Ponnamma CM, Freyle D et al: Residual gastric volume and chewing gum before surgery. Anesth Analg 2006; 102: 415

41. Ambiru S, Furuyama N, Kimura F et al: Hyperbaric oxygen therapy as a prophylactic and treatment against ileus and recurrent intestinal obstruction soon after surgery to relieve adhesive intestinal obstruction. J Gastroenterol Hepatol 2008; 23(8 Pt 2): e379

42. Duda D, Lorenz W, Celik I: Histamine release in mesenteric traction syndrome during abdominal aortic aneurysm surgery: prophylaxis with H1 and H2 antihistamines. Inflamm Res 2002; 51: 495

43. Latson TW, Reinhart DJ, Allison PM et al: Ketorolac tromethamine may be efficacious in treating hypotension from mesenteric traction. J Cardiothorac Vasc Anesth 1992; 6: 456

44. Woehlck H, Antapli M, Mann A: Treatment of refractory mesenteric traction syndrome without cyclooxygenase inhibitors. J Clin Anesth 2004; 16: 542

45. Brinkmann A, Seeling W, Wolf CF et al: The effect of thoracic epidural anesthesia on the pathophysiology of the eventration syndrome. Anaesthesist 1994; 43: 235

46. El-Galley R, Hammontree L, Urban D et al: Anesthesia for laparoscopic donor nephrectomy: Is nitrous oxide contraindicated? J Urol 2007; 178: 225

47. Reinelt H, Marx T, Schirmer U et al: Diffusion of xenon and nitrous oxide into bowel during mechanical ileus. Anesthesiology 2002; 96: 512

48. Akca O, Lenhardt R, Fleischmann E et al: Nitrous oxide increases the incidence of bowel distension in patients undergoing elective colon resection. Acta Anaesthesiol Scand 2004; 48: 894

49. Orhan-Sungur M, Apfel C, Akca O: Effects of nitrous oxide on intraoperative bowel distension. Curr Opin Anaesthesiol 2005; 18: 620

50. Brodsky JB, Lemmens HJM, Collins JS et al: Nitrous oxide and laparoscopic bariatric surgery. Obes Surg 2005; 15: 494

51. Dierdorf SF: Carcinoid tumor and carcinoid syndrome. Curr Opin Anaesthesiol 2003; 16: 343

52. Bernheim AM, Connolly HM, Hobday TJ et al: Carcinoid heart disease. Prog Cardiovasc Dis 2007; 49: 439

53. Simula DV, Edwards WD, Tazolaar HD et al: Surgical pathology of carcinoid heart disease: a study of 139 values from 75 patients spanning 20 years. Mayo Clin Proc 2002; 77: 139

54. Khan MA, Herzog CA, St Peter JV et al: The prevalence of cardiac valvular insufficiency assessed by transthoracic echocardiography in obese patients treated with appetite suppressant drugs. N Engl J Med 1998; 339: 713

55. Kinney MA, Warner ME, Nagorney DM et al: Perianesthetic risks and outcomes of abdominal surgery for metastatic carcinoid tumors. Br J Anaesth 2001; 87: 447

56. Pandharipande PP, Reichard PS, Vallee MF: High gastric output as a perioperative sign of carcinoid syndrome. Anesthesiology 2002; 96: 755

57. Dilger JA, Rho EH, Que FG et al: Octreotide-induced bradycardia and heart block during surgical resection of a carcinoid tumor. Anesth Analg 2004; 98: 318

58. Cortinez FLI: Refractory hypotension during carcinoid resection surgery. Anaesthesia 2000; 55: 505

59. Farling PA, Durairaju AK: Remifentanil and anaesthesia for carcinoid syndrome. Br J Anaesth 2004; 92: 893

60. Neustein SM, Cohen E: Anesthesia for aortic and mitral valve replacement in a patient with carcinoid heart disease. Anesthesiology 1995; 82: 1067

61. Hamid SK, Harris DN: Hypotension following valve replacement surgery in carcinoid heart disease. Anaesthesia 1992; 47: 490

CHAPTER 47 ■ ANESTHESIA AND OBESITY

BABATUNDE O. OGUNNAIKE AND CHARLES W. WHITTEN

KEY POINTS

1. Expiratory reserve volume is the most sensitive indicator of the effect of obesity on pulmonary function.

2. Many morbidly obese patients have clinically significant obstructive sleep apnea, which in the long term may result in the obesity hypoventilation syndrome. Obstructive sleep apnea predisposes to airway difficulties during anesthesia.

3. Angina or exertional dyspnea may rarely present because morbidly obese patients often have limited mobility and may appear asymptomatic even when they have significant cardiovascular disease.

4. Adipose tissue releases a large number of bioactive mediators that can result in abnormal lipids, insulin resistance, inflammation, and coagulopathies. Obese patients have impaired fibrinolysis and elevated fibrinogen.

5. Nonalcoholic fatty liver disease and elevated liver function tests (mostly elevated alanine aminotransferase) are seen in a significant number of obese patients. Despite these histologic and enzymatic changes, no clear correlation exists between abnormalities of routine liver function tests and the capacity of the liver to metabolize drugs.

6. Rhabdomyolysis is sometimes seen in morbidly obese patients undergoing prolonged operative procedures. Unexplained elevations in serum creatinine and creatine phosphokinase levels or complaints of buttock, hip, or shoulder pain in the postoperative period may indicate that rhabdomyolysis has occurred.

7. Patients scheduled for repeat bariatric surgery may have long-term vitamin and nutrient deficiencies, which may lead to acute postgastric reduction surgery neuropathy, a polynutritional multisystem disorder characterized by protracted postoperative vomiting, hyporeflexia, and muscular weakness.

8. Morbid obesity is a major independent risk factor for deep venous thrombosis and sudden death from acute postoperative pulmonary embolism. Subcutaneous heparin reduces the risk of deep venous thrombosis; however, low-molecular-weight heparins are currently popular for thromboembolism prophylaxis because of their bioavailability when injected subcutaneously.

9. Neck circumference has been identified as the single best predictor of problematic intubation in morbidly obese patients. A larger neck circumference is associated with the male sex, a higher Mallampati score, grade 3 views at laryngoscopy, and obstructive sleep apnea.

10. Forearm blood pressure is a fairly good predictor of upper arm blood pressure in most patients, but in obese patients, forearm measurements with a standard cuff may overestimate both systolic and diastolic blood pressures.

11. The head-elevated laryngoscopy position elevates the obese patient's head, upper body, and shoulders above the chest and can improve laryngoscopy and intubation.

12. Positive end-expiratory pressure is the only ventilatory parameter that has consistently been shown to improve respiratory function in obese patients but it decreases venous return, cardiac output, and subsequent oxygen delivery.

OBESITY

Obesity is at epidemic proportions worldwide and it comes with adverse health implications, including increased risk for hypertension, coronary artery disease, hyperlipidemia, diabetes mellitus, coagulopathy, gallbladder disease, degenerative joint disease, obstructive sleep apnea (OSA), and psychological and socioeconomic impairment. *Obesity* is characterized by an abnormally high percentage of body weight as fat. *Overweight* is an increase in body weight above a standard related to height.

Varying pathophysiologic consequences are associated with the anatomic distribution of body fat. In *android* (central) obesity, adipose tissue is located predominantly in the upper body (truncal distribution) and is associated with increased oxygen consumption and increased incidence of cardiovascular disease. Visceral fat is particularly associated with cardiovascular disease and left ventricular dysfunction. In *gynecoid* (peripheral) obesity, adipose tissue is located predominantly in the hips, buttocks, and thighs. This fat is less metabolically active so it is less closely associated with cardiovascular disease.

Ideal body weight (IBW) is a concept derived by life insurance companies by referencing height-weight tables. It is the weight associated with the lowest mortality rate for a given height and gender and can be estimated using Broca's index:

$$IBW \text{ (kg)} = \text{height (cm)} - x$$

where x is 100 for adult males and 105 for adult females. Lean body weight (LBW) is the total body weight (TBW) minus the adipose tissue. It is a combination of body cell mass, extracellular water, and nonfat connective tissue. It approximates 80% and 75% of TBW for males and females, respectively. In morbidly obese patients, increasing the IBW by 20 to 30% gives an estimate of LBW. In the nonobese and not overtly muscular individuals, TBW approximates IBW.[1,2] When reversed, the BMI equation can be used to estimate IBW by relating the "normal" BMI average of 22 (normal = 18 to 24.9) to a known height, and rearranging the equation to read IBW = 22 × height².[2] This equation yields weights that fall midway within the range of values obtained with other IBW formulae.[3]

In clinical practice, *body mass (Quetelet's) index* (BMI) is used to estimate the degree of obesity:

$$BMI = \frac{body\ weight\ (kg)}{height^2\ (m)}$$

Obesity and *morbid obesity* are BMI ≥30 and ≥40 kg/m², respectively. Obesity is further classified into three levels according to systemic disease risk (Table 47-1). BMI differentiates obese from nonobese adults and it reliably measures body fat because it adjusts for height while strongly correlating with body weight; however, it cannot distinguish between overweight and overfat, as heavily muscled individuals can be easily classified as overweight using BMI. Therefore, other factors such as age and fat distribution should be taken into consideration, among other health risk predictors that use the concept of BMI. Weight loss reduces the risk associated with obesity, and men are at a higher risk than women for a given level of obesity. Immediate preoperative weight loss has not been shown to reduce overall perioperative morbidity and mortality.

Body circumference indices such as waist circumference, waist-to-height ratio, and waist-to-hip ratio can identify patterns of obesity (e.g., android obesity) and correlate strongly with mortality and the risk for developing obesity-related diseases. Waist circumference strongly correlates with abdominal fat and is an independent risk predictor of disease. A waist circumference exceeding 102 cm in men and 88 cm (35 inches) in women indicates increased risk in overweight and obese individuals (Table 47-2). A waist-to-hip ratio >0.9 in women and >1.0 in men is associated with a higher risk of morbidity and mortality than a more peripheral distribution of body fat (waist-to-hip ratio <0.75 in women and <0.85 in men). Alcohol encourages central (android) pattern of fat distribution.

Pathophysiology of Obesity

Table 47-3 provides a succinct listing of the bodily systems that are adversely affected by obesity. Each system will be discussed separately in this section.

Respiratory System

Fat accumulation on the thorax and abdomen decreases chest wall and lung compliance. Decreased lung compliance is partially explained by increased pulmonary blood volume because

TABLE 47-1

CLASSIFICATIONS OF OBESITY

BMI (kg/m²)	DESCRIPTION
<18.5	Underweight
18.5–24.9	Normal
25.0–29.9	Overweight
30.0–34.9	Obesity (class I)
35.0–39.9	Obesity (class II)
≥40	Morbid obesity (class III)

BMI, body mass index.

TABLE 47-2

SYSTEMIC DISEASE RISK ACCORDING TO WAIST CIRCUMFERENCE

BMI (kg/m²)	WAIST CIRCUMFERENCE/RISK	
	Male: <102 cm Female: <88 cm	Male: ≥102 cm Female: ≥88 cm
18.5–24.9	Average	Average
25.0–29.9	Increased	High
30.0–34.9	High	Very high
35.0–39.9	Very high	Very high
≥40	Extremely high	Extremely high

BMI, body mass index.

TABLE 47-3

MEDICAL CONSEQUENCES OF OBESITY

SYSTEM	PATHOLOGY
Respiratory	Obstructive sleep apnea, obesity-hypoventilation syndrome, asthma, pulmonary hypertension
Cardiovascular	Dysrhythmias, atherosclerosis, cardiac failure, coronary artery disease, peripheral vascular disease, sudden cardiac death, systemic hypertension, thromboembolism, varicose veins
Gastrointestinal	Colon cancer, gallbladder disease, gastroesophageal reflux disease, hernias, nonalcoholic fatty liver disease, nonalcoholic steatohepatitis
Endocrine/metabolic	Diabetes mellitus, dyslipidemia, hyperinsulinemia, hypothyroidism, insulin resistance, metabolic syndrome
Genitourinary	End-stage renal disease, macrosomia, menorrhagia, preeclampsia and eclampsia, prostate cancer, urinary incontinence
Neurologic	Carpal tunnel syndrome, pseudotumor cerebri, stroke
Hematology	Hypercoagulability, polycythemia
Musculoskeletal	Acanthosis nigricans, gout, osteoarthritis, rheumatoid arthritis
Psychology/psychiatry	Depression, reduced self-esteem, social stigma

of an overall increase in blood volume as more volume is required to perfuse the additional body fat. Polycythemia of chronic hypoxemia contributes to increased total blood volume. Increased elastic resistance and decreased compliance of the chest wall further reduces total respiratory compliance while supine, leading to shallow and rapid breathing, increased work of breathing, and limited maximum ventilatory capacity. Respiratory muscle efficiency is below normal in obese individuals. Decreased pulmonary compliance leads to decreased functional residual capacity (FRC), vital capacity, and total lung capacity. Reduction in FRC is primarily a result of reduced expiratory reserve volume (ERV), but the relationship between FRC and closing capacity, the volume at which small airways begin to close, is adversely affected (Fig. 47-1). Decreases in FRC and ERV are the most commonly reported abnormalities of pulmonary function in obese patients.[4] Residual volume and closing capacity are unchanged. Reduced FRC (due to decreased ERV) can result in lung volumes below closing capacity in the course of normal tidal ventilation, leading to small airway closure, ventilation-perfusion mismatch, right-to-left shunting, and arterial hypoxemia. Anesthesia worsens this situation such that up to a 50% reduction in FRC occurs in the obese anesthetized patient compared with 20% in the nonobese individual. Forced expiratory volume in 1 second and forced vital capacity are usually within normal limits. ERV is the most sensitive indicator of the effect of obesity on pulmonary function.

Obesity increases oxygen consumption and carbon dioxide production even at rest. This is because of the metabolic activity of excess fat and the increased workload on supportive tissues. The body attempts to meet these metabolic demands by increasing both cardiac output and alveolar ventilation. Basal metabolic activity is usually within normal limits in relation to body surface area and normocapnia is usually maintained by an increase in minute ventilation. This requires increased oxygen consumption because most obese patients retain their normal response to hypoxemia and hypercapnia. Arterial oxygen tension in morbidly obese patients' breathing room air is lower than that predicted for similarly aged nonobese subjects in both sitting and supine positions. Chronic hypoxemia may lead to pulmonary hypertension and cor pulmonale.

Obstructive Sleep Apnea (OSA).   Obese patients may suffer from an upper airway obstruction syndrome that is classified into three categories: OSA, obstructive sleep hypopnea, and increased upper airway resistance. Up to 5% of obese patients have clinically significant OSA. It is characterized by periodic, partial, or complete obstruction of the upper airway during sleep.[5] In addition, there are frequent episodes of apnea or hypopnea, snoring, and daytime symptoms, including sleepiness, impaired concentration, memory problems, and morning headaches. Apnea is defined as 10 seconds or more of total cessation of airflow, ≥5 times per hour of sleep, despite continuous respiratory effort against a closed glottis, in combination with a decrease in arterial oxygenation of >4% (Fig. 47-2). Hypopnea is a 50% reduction in airflow for >10 seconds, occurring ≥15 seconds per hour of sleep and sufficient enough to cause a 4% decrease in arterial oxygen saturation. The apnea-hypopnea index, which quantifies the severity of OSA, is the total number of apneas and hypopneas per hour.[6] An apnea-hypopnea index >30 signifies severe OSA and values of 5 to 15 and 16 to 30 define mild and moderate OSA, respectively. The total arousal index is the total number of arousals per hour. The sum of the apnea-hypopnea index and total arousal index is the respiratory disturbance index.

Physiologic abnormalities resulting from OSA include hypoxemia, hypercapnia, pulmonary and systemic vasoconstriction, and secondary polycythemia (from recurrent hypoxemia). These result in an increased risk of ischemic heart disease and cerebrovascular disease. Right ventricular failure can occur from hypoxic pulmonary vasoconstriction. Respiratory acidosis is usually limited only to periods of sleep.

Obesity Hypoventilation (Pickwickian) Syndrome.   This syndrome may result from long-term OSA and is seen in 5 to 10% of morbidly obese patients. Obesity hypoventilation syndrome (OHS) is a combination of obesity and chronic hypoventilation that ultimately results in pulmonary hypertension and cor

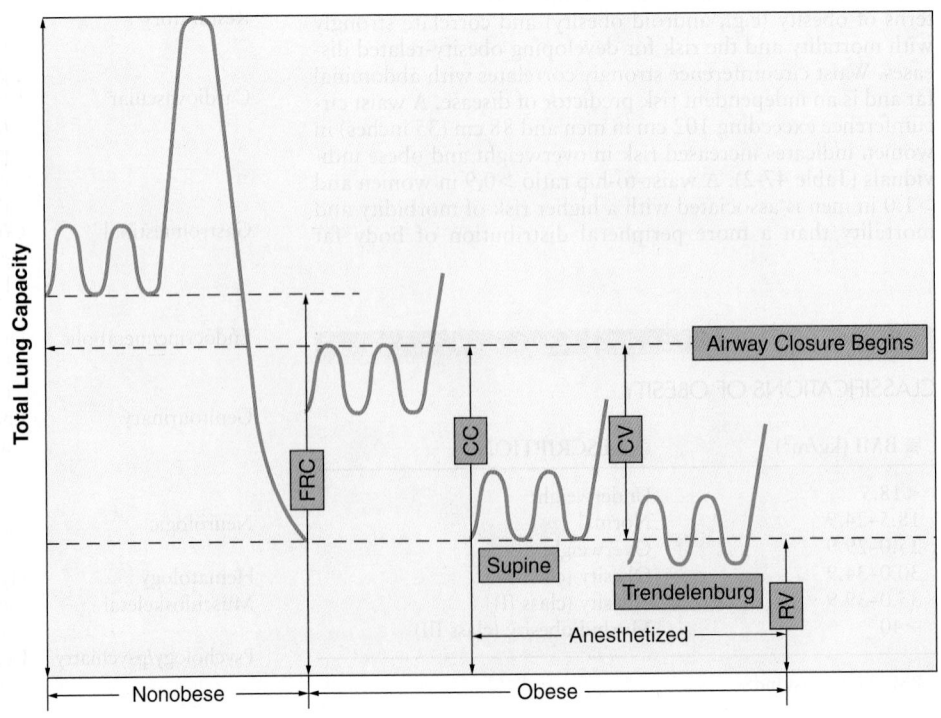

FIGURE 47-1.   Effects of obesity, positioning, and anesthesia on lung volumes. FRC, functional residual capacity; CC, closing capacity; CV, closing volume; RV, residual volume.

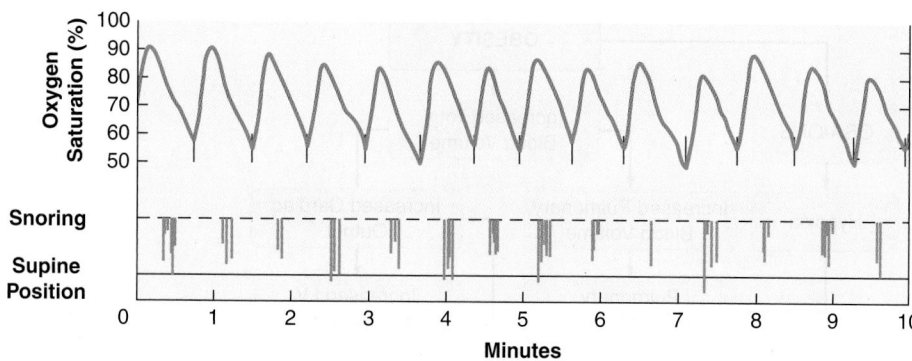

FIGURE 47-2. Pattern of oxygen saturation in a patient with severe sleep apnea. The vertical lines below the oxygen saturation values indicate respiratory disturbances. Episodes of snoring are shown. Patient is in supine position. (Reprinted from Flemons WW: Obstructive sleep apnea. N Engl J Med 2002; 347: 498, with permission.)

pulmonale.[7] The presence of both obesity (BMI >30 kg/m^2) and awake arterial hypercapnia (PaCO$_2$ >45 mm Hg) in the absence of known causes of hypoventilation supports the diagnosis (Table 47-4). Prolonged OSA also alters the control of breathing, leading to CNS-mediated apneic events. This increases reliance on hypoxic drive for ventilation. The main ventilatory impairment of OHS is alveolar hypoventilation independent of intrinsic lung disease in a patient with obesity, daytime hypersomnolence, hypercapnia, hypoxemia, and polycythemia. Right ventricular failure eventually ensues. These patients also have an increased sensitivity to the respiratory depressant effects of general anesthetics.

Cardiovascular and Hematologic Systems

Total blood volume is increased in the obese individual, but on a volume-to-weight basis, it is less than in nonobese individuals (50 mL/kg compared with 70 mL/kg). Most of this extra volume is distributed to the adipose tissue. Renal and splanchnic blood flows are increased. Cardiac output increases with increasing weight by as much as 20 to 30 mL/kg of excess body fat because of ventricular dilatation and increases in stroke volume. The resulting increased left ventricular wall stress leads to hypertrophy, reduced compliance, and impairment of left ventricular filling (diastolic dysfunction) with elevated left ventricular and diastolic pressure and pulmonary edema, but when left ventricular wall thickening fails to keep pace with dilatation, systolic dysfunction ("obesity cardiomyopathy") and eventual biventricular failure results (Fig. 47-3). Obesity accelerates atherosclerosis. Symptoms such as angina or exertional dyspnea occur only occasionally because morbidly obese patients often have very limited mobility and may appear asymptomatic even when they have significant cardiovascular disease.

Blood flow to fat is 2 to 3 mL/100 g of tissue. An excess of fat requires an increase in cardiac output, to parallel an increase in oxygen consumption, leading to a systemic arteriovenous oxygen difference that remains normal or slightly above normal. Intraoperative ventricular failure may occur from rapid intravenous fluid administration (indicating left ventricular diastolic dysfunction), the negative inotropy of anesthetic agents, or pulmonary hypertension precipitated by hypoxia or hypercapnia. Cardiac dysrhythmias may be precipitated by fatty infiltration of the conduction system, hypoxia,

TABLE 47-4

SIMPLIFIED COMPARISON OF OBSTRUCTIVE SLEEP APNEA (OSA) AND OBESITY HYPOVENTILATION SYNDROME (OHS) PARAMETERS

■ PARAMETER	■ OHS	■ OSA
Gender distribution	Males = females	Males > females
Obesity (BMI ≥30 kg/m^2)	Yes	Maybe (risk increases with obesity)
Ventilation pattern	Hypoventilation	Normal (except during apnea)
PaCO$_2$ (mm Hg)	Increased (>45 mm Hg)	Normal (increased during apnea)
PaO$_2$ (mm Hg)	Decreased; most severe during REM sleep	Normal (decreased during apnea)
SaO$_2$ (%)	Decreased	Normal (decreased during apnea)
Nocturnal upper airway obstruction	No (except with coexisting OSA)	Yes; choking or gasping during sleep
Recurrent awakenings from sleep	No	Yes
Pulmonary hypertension	More common and more severe	Less common
Nocturnal monitoring	Increased PaCO$_2$ during sleep to >10 mm Hg from awake supine values. O$_2$ desaturation during sleep not explained by apnea or hypopnea	≥5 obstructive breathing events per hour of sleep

BMI, body mass index; REM, rapid eye movement.

FIGURE 47-3. Interrelationship of cardiovascular and pulmonary sequelae of obesity. OSA, obstructive sleep apnea; OHS, obesity hypoventilation syndrome; LV, left ventricular; RV, right ventricular.

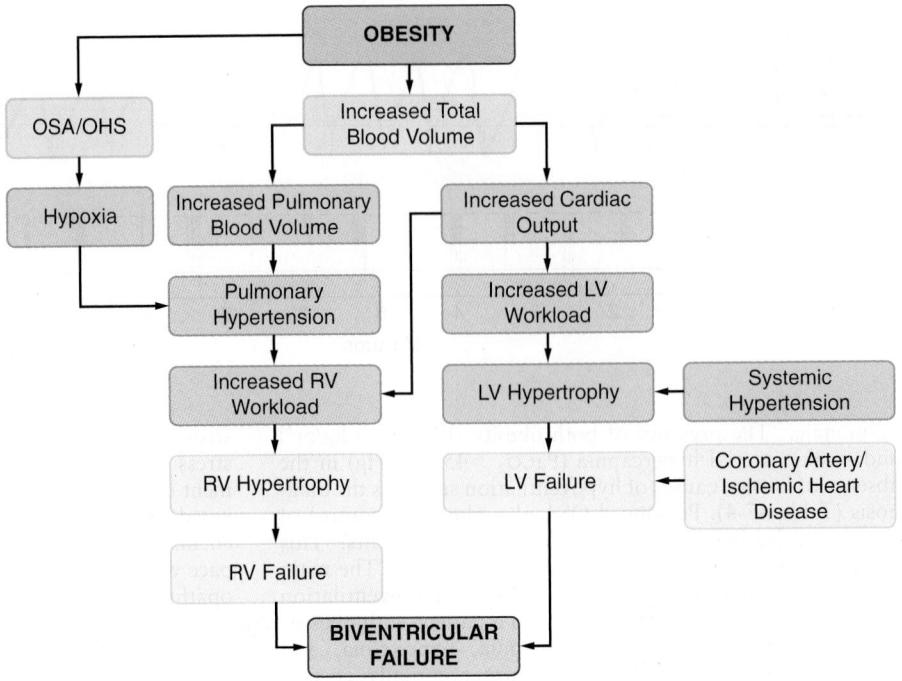

hypercapnia, electrolyte imbalance, coronary artery disease, increased circulating catecholamines, OSA, and myocardial hypertrophy. Frequent electrocardiogram (ECG) findings seen in morbidly obese patients include low QRS voltage, multiple criteria for left ventricular hypertrophy (LVH) and left atrial enlargement, and T-wave flattening in the inferior and lateral leads.[8] In addition, there is a leftward shift of the P-wave, QRS complex, and T-wave axes, lengthening of the corrected QT interval, and prolonged QT interval duration. Substantial weight reduction reverses many of these ECG abnormalities.[9]

Cardiac output rises faster in response to exercise in the morbidly obese and is often associated with a rise in left ventricular end-diastolic pressure and pulmonary capillary wedge pressure. Similar changes occur during the perioperative period, which should prompt a low threshold for performing detailed cardiac investigations. Many obese patients have mild-to-moderate hypertension, with a 3- to 4-mm Hg increase in systolic and a 2-mm Hg increase in diastolic arterial pressure for every 10 kg of weight gained. Normotensive obese patients have reduced systemic vascular resistance, which rises with the onset of hypertension. Their expanded blood volume causes an increased cardiac output with a lower calculated systemic vascular resistance for the same level of arterial blood pressure. The rennin-angiotensin system plays a major role in the hypertension of obesity by increased circulating levels of angiotensinogen, aldosterone, and angiotensin-converting enzyme. As little as 5% reduction in body weight leads to a significant reduction in activity of the rennin-angiotensin system in both plasma and adipose tissue, contributing to a reduction in blood pressure.[10]

Obese patients have normal-to-increased level of sympathetic nervous system activity, which predisposes to insulin resistance, dyslipidemia, and hypertension.[11] Obesity-induced insulin resistance enhances the pressor activity of norepinephrine and angiotensin II.[12] Hyperinsulinemia further activates the sympathetic nervous system, causing sodium retention and contributing to the hypertension of obesity.[13] Hypertension causes concentric hypertrophy of the ventricle in normal-weight individuals but causes eccentric dilatation in obese individuals.[14] It is associated with increased preload and stroke work. The combination of obesity and hypertension

causes left ventricular wall thickening and a larger heart volume; therefore, there is increased likelihood of cardiac failure (Fig. 47-4).

Obese individuals are also prone to cardiovascular disease because adipose tissue releases a large number of bioactive mediators. These can result in abnormal lipids, insulin resistance, inflammation, and coagulopathies.[15] Obese individuals have higher levels of fibrinogen (a marker for the inflammatory process of atherosclerosis), factor VII, factor VIII, von Willebrand factor, and plasminogen activator inhibitor-1 (PAI-1). Increased levels of fibrinogen, factor VII, factor VIII, and hypofibrinolysis are associated with hypercoagulability. Correction of impaired fibrinolysis requires substantial (>40%) weight loss.[16] High factor VIII levels are associated with increased cardiovascular mortality. High fasting triglyceride levels correlate with increased factor VII concentrations, and postprandial lipemia causes activation of factor VII. Endothelial dysfunction induced by insulin increases von Willebrand factor and factor VIII levels, predisposing to fibrin formation. PAI-1 is secreted by the endothelium, vascular smooth muscle cells, hepatocytes, and adipocytes. Increased secretion of PAI-1 inhibits the fibrinolytic system and is associated with visceral obesity.[17]

Gastrointestinal System

Gastric volume and acidity are increased, hepatic function is altered, and drug metabolism is adversely affected by obesity. Many fasted morbidly obese patients presenting for elective surgery have gastric volumes in excess of 25 mL and gastric fluid pH <2.5 (the generally accepted volume and pH indicative of high risk for pneumonitis should regurgitation and aspiration occur). Delayed gastric emptying occurs because of increased abdominal mass that causes antral distention, gastrin release, and a decrease in pH with parietal cell secretion. An increased incidence of hiatal hernia and gastroesophageal reflux also increase aspiration risk.

Gastric emptying is faster with high energy content intake such as fat emulsions, but because of larger gastric volume (up to 75% larger), the residual volume is increased. Both the faster gastric emptying and the larger gastric volume can be

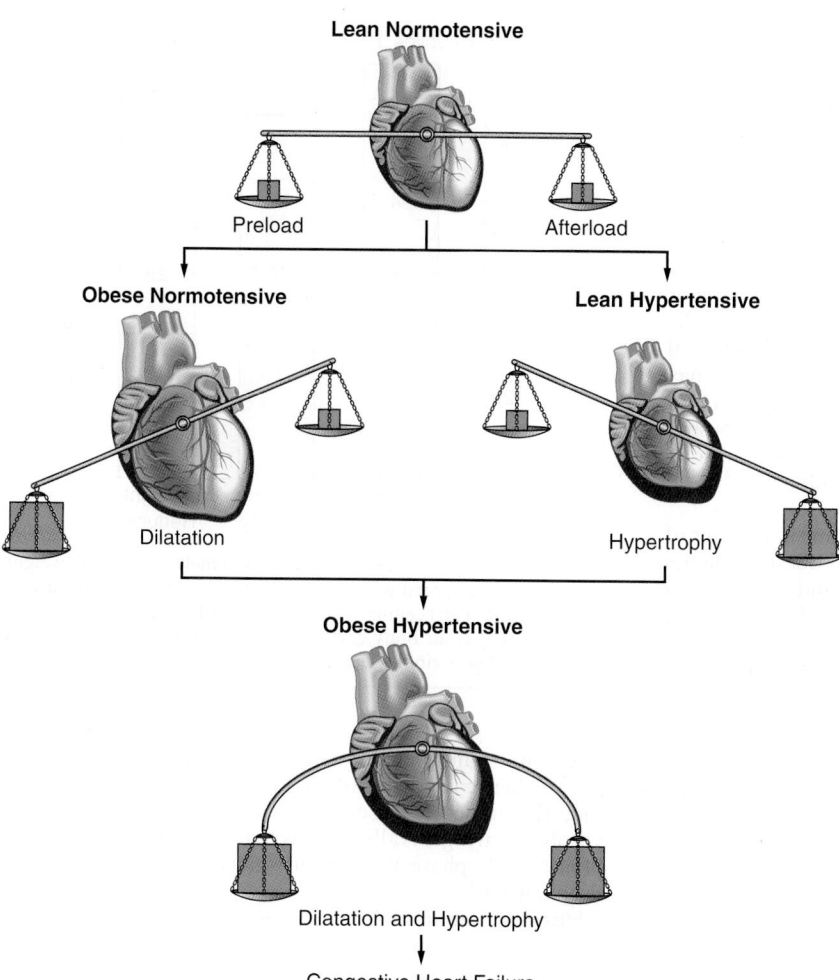

FIGURE 47-4.   Adaptation of the heart to obesity and hypertension. (Reprinted from Messerli FH: Cardiovascular effects of obesity and hypertension. Lancet 1982; 1: 1165, with permission.)

ANESTHESIA FOR SURGICAL SUBSPECIALTIES

partially reversed by weight loss.[18] Nonpremedicated, nondiabetic fasting obese surgical patients who are free from significant gastroesophageal pathology are unlikely to have high volume, low pH gastric contents after routine preoperative fasting.[19] They should follow the same fasting guidelines as nonobese patients and be allowed to drink clear liquids until up to 2 hours before elective surgery.[20] A positive correlation exists between obesity and frequent gastroesophageal reflux symptoms and esophageal erosions.[21] Abdominal obesity increases intragastric pressure, increasing the frequency of transient lower esophageal sphincter relaxation, and/or hiatal hernia formation. An increase >3.5 kg/m^2 in BMI is associated with a 2.7-fold increase in risk for developing new reflux symptoms.[22] Weight loss significantly improves gastroesophageal reflux symptoms.[23] The combination of hiatal hernia, gastroesophageal reflux, and delayed gastric emptying, coupled with increased intra-abdominal pressure and a high-volume/low pH gastric content, puts the obese at risk for increased incidence of severe pneumonitis should aspiration occur.

5 Peculiar morphologic and biochemical abnormalities of the liver that are associated with obesity include fatty infiltration (high prevalence of nonalcoholic fatty liver disease), inflammation, focal necrosis, and cirrhosis. Fatty infiltration reflects the duration rather than the degree of obesity. Histologic and liver function test abnormalities are relatively common, but clearance usually is not reduced. Abnormal liver function tests are seen in up to one third of obese patients who have no evidence of concomitant liver disease, of which increased alanine

aminotransferase is most frequently seen. Weight loss results in sustained improvement in liver enzymes in direct proportion to the extent of weight reduction.[24] Despite these histologic and enzymatic changes, no clear correlation exists between routine liver function tests and the capacity of the liver to metabolize drugs.[25] Morbidly obese patients who have undergone intestinal bypass surgery have a particularly high prevalence of hepatic dysfunction and cholelithiasis, which is also common in the general obese population and of which abnormal cholesterol metabolism is partially to blame.

The high prevalence of nonalcoholic fatty liver disease (NAFLD) and cirrhosis necessitates careful assessment for preexisting liver disease in patients scheduled for surgery.[26] Obesity is a major risk factor for NAFLD and nonalcoholic steatohepatitis. Features of NAFLD include hepatomegaly, elevated liver enzymes, and abnormal liver histology (steatosis, steatohepatitis, fibrosis, and cirrhosis).[27]

Renal and Endocrine Systems

Impaired glucose tolerance in the morbidly obese is reflected by a high prevalence of type II diabetes mellitus as a result of resistance of peripheral fatty tissues to insulin. More than 10% of obese patients have an abnormal glucose tolerance test, which predisposes them to wound infection and an increased risk of myocardial infarction during periods of myocardial ischemia.[28] Exogenous insulin may be required perioperatively even in obese patients with type II diabetes mellitus to oppose the catabolic response to surgery.

Subclinical hypothyroidism occurs in about 25% of all morbidly obese patients.[29] Thyroid-stimulating hormone levels are frequently elevated, suggesting the possibility that obesity leads to a state of thyroid hormone resistance in peripheral tissues.[30,31] Hypothyroidism may be associated with hypoglycemia, hyponatremia, and impaired hepatic drug metabolism. Reduction of thyroxine requirements is seen with a decrease in BMI.[32]

Obesity is associated with glomerular hyperfiltration as evidenced by increased renal plasma flow and increased glomerular filtration rate. Excessive weight gain increases renal tubular resorption and impairs natriuresis through activation of the sympathetic and renin-angiotensin system as well as physical compression of the kidney. With prolonged obesity, there may be a loss of nephron function, with further impairment of natriuresis and further increases in arterial pressure. Obesity-related glomerular hyperfiltration decreases after weight loss, which decreases the incidence of overt glomerulopathy.[33,34]

Metabolic Syndrome. The metabolic syndrome is a cluster of metabolic abnormalities including abdominal obesity, glucose intolerance, hypertension, and dyslipidemia, and is associated with an increased risk of vascular events. Individuals with this syndrome have up to a fivefold greater risk of developing type 2 diabetes mellitus (if not already present) and are also twice as likely to die from a heart attack or stroke compared with those without the syndrome. Diagnostic components of this syndrome include central obesity plus any two of the following four factors: raised serum triglycerides, reduced serum high density lipoprotein-cholesterol level, hypertension, or an elevated fasting plasma glucose.[35]

PHARMACOLOGY

General pharmacokinetic principles dictate, with certain exceptions, that drug dosing should take into consideration the *volume of distribution* (V_D) for administration of the loading dose, and on the *clearance* for the maintenance dose.[36] A drug that is mainly distributed to lean tissues should have the loading dose calculated based on LBW. If the drug is equally distributed between adipose and lean tissues, dosing should be calculated based on TBW. For maintenance, a drug with similar clearance values in both obese and nonobese individuals should have the maintenance dose calculated based on LBW, and a drug whose clearance increases with obesity should have the maintenance dose calculated according to TBW.

The volume of the central compartment in which drugs are first distributed remains unchanged in obese patients, but absolute body water content is decreased and lean body and adipose tissue mass are increased, affecting lipophilic and polar drug distribution (Fig. 47-5). The V_D in obese patients is affected by reduced total body water, increased total body fat, increased lean body mass, altered protein binding, increased blood volume, increased cardiac output, increased blood concentrations of free fatty acids, triglycerides, cholesterol, and α_1-acid glycoprotein, lipophilicity of the drug, and organomegaly.[37] Increased distribution of a drug prolongs its elimination half-life even when clearance is unchanged or increased. Hyperlipidemia and an increased concentration of α_1-acid glycoprotein may affect protein binding, leading to a reduction in free drug concentration. Plasma albumin and total plasma protein concentration and binding are not significantly changed by obesity, but when compared with normal-weight individuals, a relative increase in plasma protein binding may be evident. Splanchnic blood flow, blood volume, and cardiac output are all increased in obese patients. In contrast to the expected decrease in bioavailability of orally administered medication because of increased splanchnic blood flow,

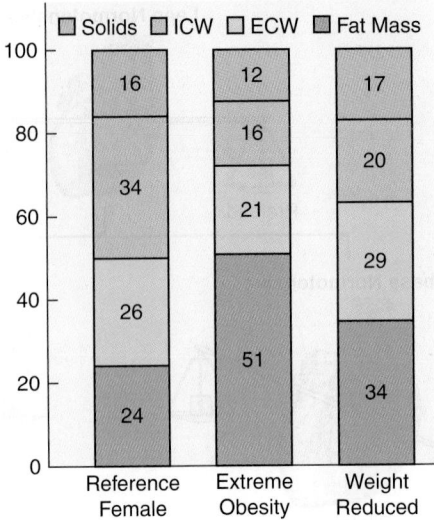

FIGURE 47-5. Body composition in extremely obese and weight-reduced states compared with reference female values. ICW, intracellular water; ECW, extracellular water. (Reprinted from Das SK, Roberts SB, Kehayias JJ et al: Body composition methods in extreme obesity. Am J Physiol Endocrinol Metab 2003; 284: E1080, with permission.)

there is no significant difference in absorption and bioavailability when comparing obese and normal-weight subjects. Drugs that undergo phase I metabolism (oxidation, reduction, hydrolysis) are generally unaffected by changes induced by obesity, while phase II reactions (glucuronidation, sulfation) are enhanced.[37]

Histologic abnormalities of the liver are common in the obese, with concomitant deranged liver function tests, but drug clearance is not usually affected. Renal clearance of drugs is increased in obesity because of increased renal blood flow and glomerular filtration rate.[33,34] As a result of both increased glomerular filtration rate and increased tubular secretion, drugs such as cimetidine and aminoglycoside antibiotics that depend on renal excretion may require increased dosing. Highly lipophilic substances such as barbiturates and benzodiazepines show significant increases in V_D for obese individuals.[37] These drugs have a more selective distribution to fat stores and therefore a longer elimination half-life but with comparable clearance values to normal individuals. Less lipophilic compounds have little or no change in V_D with obesity. Exceptions to this rule include the highly lipophilic drugs digoxin, procainamide, and remifentanil.[38–40] Drugs with weak or moderate lipophilicity may be dosed on the basis of LBW. Adding 20% to the estimated IBW dose of hydrophilic medications is sufficient to include the obese patient's extra lean mass. Nondepolarizing muscle relaxants can be dosed in this manner.

Specific Intravenous Agents

Table 47-5 presents dosing of intravenous agents used in obese patients. Further information is also provided in this section.

1. **Thiopental.** Prolonged somnolence with thiopental is expected because it is highly lipophilic and has a larger V_D in the obese patient. However, increased blood volume, cardiac output, and muscle mass necessitate an increase in the initial induction dose based on LBW.
2. **Propofol.** There is no difference in initial V_D between obese and nonobese patients with propofol. Increased V_D at steady state and increased clearance offsets any increase in

TABLE 47-5

INTRAVENOUS DRUG DOSING IN OBESITY

■ DRUG	■ DOSING	■ COMMENTS
Thiopental	Induction: LBW (somewhat increased)	Increased V_D, increased blood volume, cardiac output, and muscle mass. Increased absolute dose. Prolonged duration of action. Elimination half-life longer. Adjust loading/induction dose accordingly.
Propofol	Induction: LBW (somewhat increased) Maintenance infusion: TBW	Highly lipophilic. Total clearance and V_D at steady state correlate with TBW. Negative cardiovascular effects. High affinity for well perfused organs. Titrate to effect.
Succinylcholine	TBW	Larger extracellular fluid compartment in obese patients. Pseudocholinesterase activity increases with increasing weight.
Rocuronium	LBW	Faster onset and longer duration when dosed according to TBW. Pharmacokinetics and pharmacodynamics not altered in obese patients.
Vecuronium	LBW	Prolonged action when dosed according to TBW. Obesity does not alter distribution or elimination of the drug
Atracurium	LBW	V_D, absolute clearance, and elimination half-life unchanged by obesity. Unchanged dose per unit body weight without prolongation of recovery because of organ-independent elimination
Cis-atracurium	LBW	Pharmacokinetics similar to atracurium but prolonged duration of action when dosed according to TBW.
Fentanyl	LBW	Measured total body clearance has a nonlinear relationship to TBW. Fentanyl dosing based on a derived "pharmacokinetic mass" correlates better with clearance. Dosing based on TBW overestimates dose requirements in the obese patient.
Sufentanil	LBW	Increased V_D and prolonged elimination half-life, which correlates with degree of obesity. Clearance similar in obese and nonobese patients. Overestimation of plasma concentration occurs in the morbidly obese range (BMI >40 kg/m^2).
Remifentanil	LBW	Pharmacokinetics similar in obese and nonobese patients. Systemic clearance and V_D corrected per kilogram of TBW is significantly smaller in the obese patient. Consider age and lean body mass for dosing.
Dexmedetomidine	TBW	Lacks significant effect on respiration. Very good analgesic adjuvant in the morbidly obese patient. Sympatholytic properties.

LBW, lean body weight; V_D, volume of distribution; TBW, total body weight; BMI, body mass index.
Adapted from Ogunnaike BO, Jones SB, Jones DB et al: Anesthetic considerations for bariatric surgery. Anesth Analg 2002; 95: 1793.

elimination half-life without evidence of accumulation. Total clearance and V_D at steady state correlate to body weight during maintenance infusion. The dose should be increased based on LBW. Propofol has high affinity for excess fat and other well-perfused organs. High hepatic extraction and conjugation relates to TBW.[41]

3. **Benzodiazepines.** Benzodiazepines persist long after discontinuation because they are highly lipophilic drugs with a larger V_D in obese patients. Midazolam, although considered short acting, has the potential for prolonged sedation in obese patients because larger initial doses are required to achieve adequate serum concentrations.

4. **Neuromuscular Blocking and Reversal Agents.** Pseudocholinesterase activity increases linearly with increasing weight and larger extracellular fluid compartment; therefore, the dose of succinylcholine should be increased somewhat. Nondepolarizing muscle relaxants should be administered according to LBW to prevent delayed recovery because of increased V_D and impaired hepatic clearance. The pharmacokinetics and pharmacodynamics of rocuronium are not altered by obesity in female patients; however, in the general obese population, the onset time is shorter and duration slightly prolonged.[42–44] The V_D, absolute clearance, and elimination half-life of atracurium are unchanged and dosing may be based on actual body weight

without prolongation of recovery because of organ function-independent breakdown.[45] Cis-atracurium duration may be prolonged if administered on the basis of actual body weight.[46] Prompt early reversal but slow full recovery has been documented in overweight and obese patients during neostigmine-induced reversal of vecuronium dosed according to TBW.[44] Sugammadex, a modified γ-cyclodextrin compound that encapsulates rocuronium, (and other steroid-based neuromuscular blockers to a lesser extent), may prove invaluable for more rapid and complete neuromuscular blockade reversal in obese patients.[47]

5. **Opioids.** Application of nonweight-scaled pharmacokinetic models for fentanyl derived from normal-weight patients overestimates the plasma concentration of fentanyl as body weight increases from normal to morbid obesity. Fentanyl dosing should be based on LBW or a similar size metric such as a derived "pharmacokinetic mass" (derived pharmacokinetic body weight for dosing), which correlates better with total body clearance than with TBW-based dosing.[48,49] Sufentanil, a highly lipid soluble opioid, has an increased V_D and a prolonged elimination half-life that correlates positively with the degree of obesity. It distributes extensively in excess body fat as in lean tissues; therefore, dosing should account for total body mass. Pharmacokinetic parameters derived from nonobese subjects accurately

predict plasma sufentanil concentrations in obese (30 to 39.9 kg/m²) patients, but at the morbidly obese (≥40 kg/m²) range, overestimation of plasma sufentanil concentration rises with increasing BMI.[50] Remifentanil pharmacokinetics are more closely related to lean body mass than to TBW; therefore, dosing should be based on LBW.[38]

6. **Dexmedetomidine.** Dexmedetomidine is a highly selective α_2-adrenergic agonist with sedative-hypnotic, anesthetic-sparing, analgesic, and sympatholytic properties but with no significant effects on respiration. It may be ideally suitable as an analgesic adjuvant in morbidly obese patients in whom opioid-induced respiratory depression may be catastrophic.[51] When used as part of balanced anesthesia, infusion rates of 0.2 to 0.7 µg/kg/hr produces clinically effective sedation with decreased analgesic and anesthetic requirements.

Increased blood volume in the obese patient decreases the plasma concentrations of rapidly injected intravenous drugs. Fat, however, has poor blood flow, and doses calculated on actual body weight could lead to excessive plasma concentrations. Calculating initial doses based on LBW with subsequent doses determined by pharmacologic response to the initial dose is a reasonable approach. Repeated injections may accumulate in fat, leading to a prolonged response because of subsequent release from this large depot.

MEDICAL THERAPY FOR OBESITY

Medications used to treat obesity are formulated to reduce energy intake, increase energy utilization, or decrease absorption of nutrients. Indications for drug treatment include a BMI ≥30 kg/m² or a BMI between 27 and 29.9 kg/m² in conjunction with an obesity-related medical complication. The combination of phentermine and fenfluramine (Phen-Fen) was popular for the treatment of obesity until it became evident that it was associated with valvular heart disease and pulmonary hypertension.

Sibutramine and orlistat are newer antiobesity medications approved for long-term use. Sibutramine inhibits the reuptake of norepinephrine to increase satiety after the onset of eating rather than reduce appetite. It does not promote the release of serotonin, unlike fenfluramine and dexfenfluramine, which primarily increase the release of serotonin in brain synapses and also inhibit reuptake to cause anorexia. These differences in mechanisms of action may explain why thus far there have been no reports of sibutramine causing cardiac valvular lesions. Because sibutramine does not deplete neural synapses of catecholamines, dangerous hypotension unresponsive to indirectly acting vasopressors, as seen with fenfluramine and dexfenfluramine, does not generally occur.[52] The most frequent adverse effects of sibutramine include dry mouth, insomnia, anorexia, and constipation. Sibutramine may cause transient dose-related increases in systolic and diastolic blood pressure by an average of 2 to 4 mm Hg and a slight increase in heart rate of 3 to 5 beats per minute.[53]

Orlistat blocks the absorption and digestion of dietary fat by binding lipases in the gastrointestinal tract. Cardiovascular risk factors associated with obesity, including blood pressure, waist circumference, fasting blood glucose levels, and lipid profile, all improve with orlistat treatment.[54] Gastrointestinal complaints of oily spotting, liquid stools, fecal urgency, flatulence, and abdominal cramping are most common and are induced by fat malabsorption. Chronic dosing of orlistat results in an increase in warfarin's anticoagulant effect because of decreased absorption of vitamin K.[55] This leads to an abnormal prothrombin time with a normal partial thromboplastin time because of deficiency of clotting factors II, VII, IX, and X. The resulting coagulopathy should be corrected 6 to 24 hours before elective surgery with a vitamin K analogue such

as phytonadione and fresh-frozen plasma for emergency surgery or active bleeding.

Rimonabant, a selective cannabinoid-1 receptor antagonist, decreases appetite, leading to significant weight loss, reduced waist circumference, improvements in lipid profile and glucose control, and a reduced incidence of the metabolic syndrome.[56] Psychiatric disorders, including anxiety and depression, are significant side effects that should be considered during the perioperative period. Other notable side effects include nausea, dizziness, diarrhea, arthralgia, and back pain.

BARIATRIC SURGERY

Bariatric surgery is currently the most effective treatment for morbid (class III) obesity. It is classified into malabsorptive, restrictive, or combined. *Malabsorptive procedures* (jejunoileal bypass and biliopancreatic diversion) are rarely used today. *Restrictive procedures* include vertical-banded gastroplasty and adjustable gastric banding. Roux-en-Y gastric bypass (RYGB) combines gastric restriction with a minimal degree of malabsorption. Vertical-banded gastroplasty, adjustable gastric banding, and RYGB can all be performed laparoscopically, albeit with difficulty in patients weighing >180 kg, because of technical considerations.

Gastric restriction (gastroplasty) creates a small upper pouch (15 to 30 mL) in the stomach, which restricts food intake and communicates with the remainder of the stomach through a narrow channel, or stoma. RYGB is performed by anastomosing the proximal gastric pouch to a segment of the proximal jejunum, bypassing most of the stomach and the entire duodenum (Fig. 47-6). It is the most effective bariatric

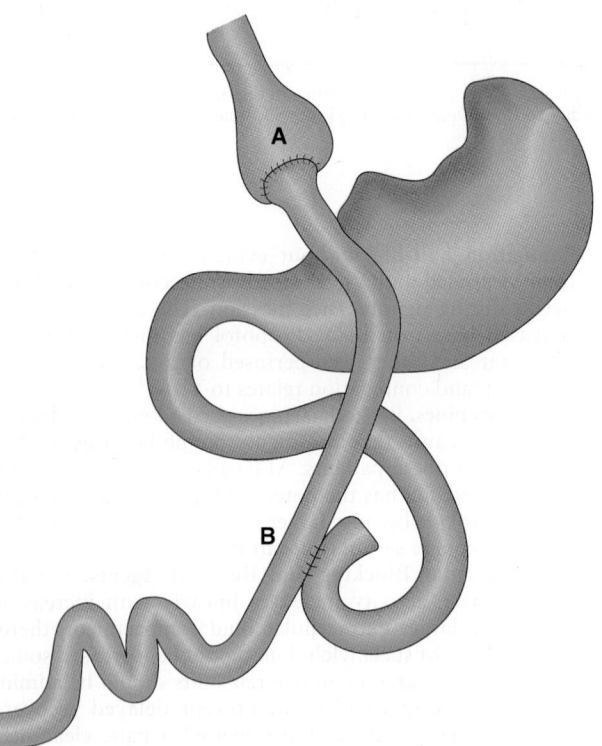

FIGURE 47-6. Roux-en-Y gastric bypass. **A.** A 15- to 30-mL gastric pouch with connected jejunal limb. **B.** Site of jejunojejunostomy. (Reprinted from Ogunnaike BO, Jones SB, Jones DB et al: Anesthetic considerations for bariatric surgery. Anesth Analg 2002; 95; 1794 with permission.)

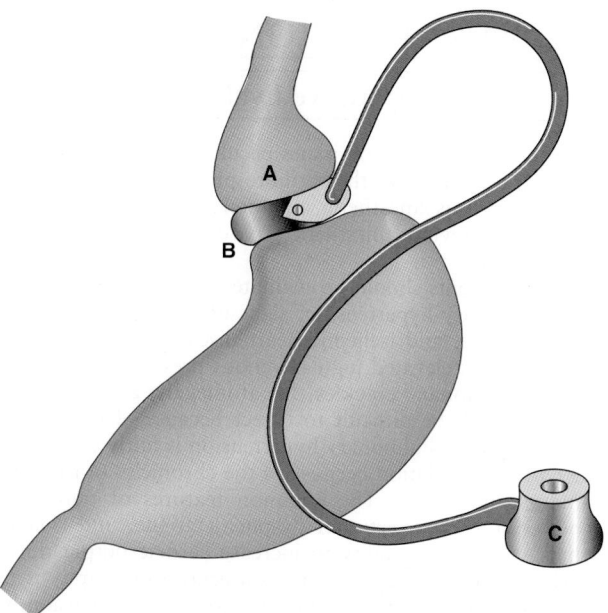

FIGURE 47-7. Adjustable gastric banding. **A.** Proximal pouch. **B.** Adjustable band. **C.** Needle access port through which saline is injected or removed to vary the size of the adjustable band. (Reprinted from Ogunnaike BO, Jones SB, Jones DB et al: Anesthetic considerations for bariatric surgery. Anesth Analg 2002; 95; 1795, with permission.)

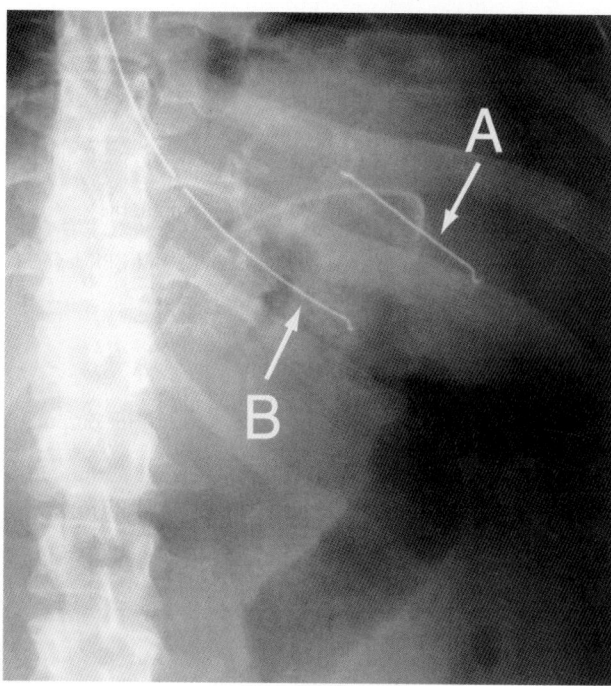

FIGURE 47-8. Radiograph of postoperative gastrografin swallow. **A.** Transected end of nasogastric (NG) tube left in the gastric remnant. **B.** New properly placed NG tube replacing the transected one. (Reprinted from Ogunnaike BO, Jones SB, Jones DB et al: Anesthetic considerations for bariatric surgery. Anesth Analg 2002; 95; 1801, with permission.)

ANESTHESIA FOR SURGICAL SUBSPECIALTIES

procedure to produce safe short- and long-term weight loss in severely obese patients. With RYGB, patients lose an average of 50 to 60% excess body weight and show a BMI decrease of approximately 10 kg/m² during the first 12 to 24 postoperative months. Type II diabetes resolves in the majority of patients.[57] Adjustable gastric banding is a restrictive gastric operation usually done by a laparoscopic approach. An adjustable inflatable band is placed around the proximal stomach to limit stomach capacity (Fig. 47-7). The band can be made tighter or less so by adding or removing saline with adjustments made to meet patients' individual weight loss needs.

Laparoscopic bariatric surgery is associated with less postoperative pain, lower morbidity, and faster recovery. It is performed through five or six small abdominal incisions with a pneumoperitoneum and gravity displacement of the abdominal viscera. Patients appreciate laparoscopic bariatric surgery because it reduces postoperative pain and the duration of convalescence.[58] Accumulation of "third-space" fluid, which correlates with the extent of surgical trauma, is significantly lower after laparoscopic RYGB than after open RYGB.[58]

Profound muscle relaxation is important during laparoscopic bariatric procedures to facilitate ventilation and to maintain an adequate working space for visualization and safe manipulation of laparoscopic instruments. It also facilitates extraction of excised tissues. Collapse of the pneumoperitoneum and tightening of the patient's musculature around port sites are early indications of inadequate muscle relaxation.[59]

Laparoscopic bariatric surgery requires maneuvering the operating table into various surgically favorable positions. These maneuvers could cause a very large patient to slip off the operating table, with disastrous consequences. The use of a malleable "bean-bag," in addition to belts and straps, may help to keep the patient secured. Anesthesia personnel may be asked to facilitate the proper placement of an intragastric balloon to help the surgeon size the gastric pouch and also facilitate performance of leak tests with saline or methylene blue through a nasogastric tube. Care should be taken to ensure a tight seal of the endotracheal tube cuff, otherwise aspiration of saline or methylene blue can occur. All endogastric tubes should be completely removed (not just merely pulled back into the esophagus) before gastric division to avoid unplanned stapling and transection of these devices (Fig. 47-8). After the gastric pouch is created, blind insertion of a nasogastric tube should be avoided by viewing the laparoscope monitor and carefully watching to avoid disruption of the anastomosis.[59] Cephalad displacement of the diaphragm and carina from a pneumoperitoneum during laparoscopy can cause a firmly secured endotracheal tube to displace into a main stem bronchus.[60]

Rhabdomyolysis is more common in morbidly obese patients undergoing laparoscopic procedures when compared with the open procedure. Long duration of surgery is one of the risk factors. Unexplained elevations in serum creatinine and creatine phosphokinase (CPK) levels or complaints of buttock, hip, or shoulder pain in the postoperative period is suggestive of rhabdomyolysis (Table 47-6). Serum CPK measured pre- and postoperatively aids in early diagnosis and treatment. The complication of myoglobinuric acute renal failure can be as high as 30% with serum CPK >5,000 IU/L.[61]

Gastric electrical stimulation by means of an implantable gastric stimulator (IGS) is another weight-loss procedure performed laparoscopically. Electrical impulses stimulate smooth muscles of the stomach to stop peristalsis so that the patient feels full.[62] A lead with two electrodes implanted in the lesser curvature of the stomach is connected to an electrical pulse generator implanted subcutaneously on the abdominal wall

TABLE 47-6

RHABDOMYOLYSIS

Diagnosis
- Presence of major risk factors—morbid obesity, prolonged operative time
- Complaints of buttock, hip, or shoulder pain in the postoperative period
- Unexplained elevations in serum creatinine and CPK levels

Prevention and treatment
- Proper positioning and padding of pressure areas
- Reduced total operative time
- Maintain a high index of suspicion
- Aggressive hydration (administration of volume)
- Stimulation of diuresis with mannitol (target urine output of 1.5 mL/kg/hr)
- Alkalinization of urine to prevent myoglobin deposition in renal tubules (alkalinization increases solubility of myoglobin in a pH-dependent manner)
- Hemofiltration may be necessary for rapid clearance of myoglobin

CPK, creatine phosphokinase.

(Fig. 47-9). Implications of this procedure for the anesthesiologist include possible lead dislodgement from violent stomach contractions during postoperative nausea and vomiting. The stimulating pulses emitted by the IGS can be picked up on the ECG, which may lead to false readings. The IGS can also be adversely affected by defibrillation, electrocautery, lithotripsy, magnetic resonance imaging, and therapeutic radiation.

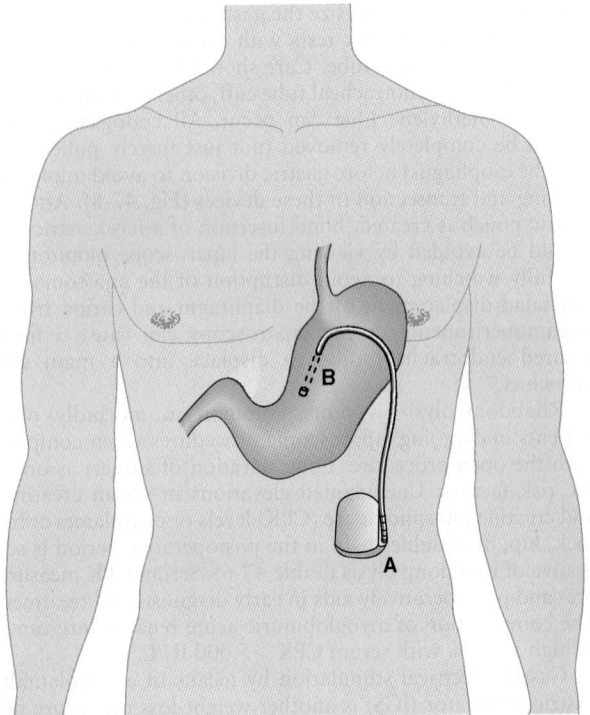

FIGURE 47-9. Illustration of the implantable gastric stimulator. A pulse generator **A.** implanted subcutaneously sends impulses to a lead with two electrodes **B.** implanted in the lesser curvature of the stomach.

PREOPERATIVE CONSIDERATIONS

Preoperative Evaluation

Attention should focus on issues peculiar to the obese patient including evaluation of the cardiorespiratory systems and the airway. Previous anesthetic experiences as detailed by the patient and previous anesthetic records are useful sources of information.

Obese patients should be evaluated for systemic hypertension, pulmonary hypertension, signs of right and/or left ventricular failure, and ischemic heart disease. Signs of cardiac failure such as elevated jugular venous pressure, added heart sounds, pulmonary crackles, hepatomegaly, and peripheral edema may all be difficult to detect because of masking by excess adiposity. Pulmonary hypertension is fairly common in this patient population because of the chronicity of their pulmonary impairment. The common features of pulmonary hypertension are exertional dyspnea, fatigue, and syncope (which reflect an inability to increase cardiac output during activity). Tricuspid regurgitation on echocardiography is the most useful confirmatory test of pulmonary hypertension but should be combined with clinical evaluation.[63] An ECG may demonstrate signs of right ventricular hypertrophy such as tall precordial R waves, right axis deviation, and right ventricular strain. The higher the pulmonary artery pressure the more sensitive the ECG. Chest radiographs may show evidence of underlying lung disease and prominent pulmonary arteries.

Patients scheduled for repeat bariatric surgery should be screened preoperatively for long-term metabolic and nutritional abnormalities. Common deficiencies include vitamin B_{12}, iron, calcium, and folate. Vitamin and nutritional deficiencies can lead to a collective form of postoperative polyneuropathy, known as *acute postgastric reduction surgery neuropathy,* a polynutritional multisystem disorder characterized by protracted postoperative vomiting, hyporeflexia, and muscular weakness.[64] Differential diagnoses of this disorder include thiamine deficiency (Wernicke encephalopathy, beriberi), vitamin B_{12} deficiency, and Guillain-Barré syndrome. Acute postgastric reduction surgery neuropathy should cause anesthesiologists to pay close attention to dosing and monitoring neuromuscular blocking agents. Electrolyte and coagulation indices should be checked before surgery, particularly in poorly compliant or acutely ill patients because chronic vitamin K deficiency may lead to coagulation abnormalities. Administration of vitamin K analog or fresh-frozen plasma may be required.

Evidence of OSA and OHS should be sought preoperatively because they are frequently associated with difficult laryngoscopy. A history of hypertension or a neck circumference >40 cm correlates with an increased probability of OSA. OSA is a legitimate reason to delay surgery for a proper workup.[65] The severity may be quantified by a formal sleep study. OSA patients should generally be treated as inpatients; however, outpatient surgery can be considered under certain circumstances, including mild OSA, use of local or regional anesthesia with minimal sedation, availability of a 23-hour observation postanesthesia care unit, and when patients can resume oral medication at the time of discharge. OSA patients on a continuous positive airway pressure (CPAP) device at home should be instructed to bring it with them to the hospital as it may be needed postoperatively. The possibility of invasive monitoring, prolonged intubation, and postoperative mechanical ventilation should be discussed with obese patients. Arterial blood gas measurements help evaluate ventilation, as well as the need for perioperative oxygen administration and postoperative ventilation. Routine pulmonary function tests and liver function tests are not cost-effective in asymptomatic obese patients. Blood glucose abnormalities should be corrected if present.

Concurrent, Preoperative, and Prophylactic Medications

Patients' usual medications should be continued until the time of surgery, with the possible exception of insulin and oral hypoglycemics. Antibiotic prophylaxis is usually indicated because of an increased incidence of wound infections in the obese.[66] Anxiolysis and prophylaxis against both aspiration pneumonitis and deep vein thrombosis (DVT) should be addressed at premedication. Oral benzodiazepines are reliable for anxiolysis and sedation. Intravenous midazolam can also be titrated in small doses for anxiolysis during the immediate preoperative period. Dexmedetomidine, because of its minimal respiratory depressant effects, should be considered. Pharmacologic intervention with H_2-receptor antagonists, nonparticulate antacids, or proton pump inhibitors will reduce gastric volume, acidity, or both, thereby reducing the risk and severity of aspiration pneumonitis.

Morbid obesity is a major independent risk factor for sudden death from acute postoperative pulmonary embolism. Subcutaneous heparin 5,000 IU administered before surgery and repeated every 8 to 12 hours until the patient is fully mobile reduces the risk of DVT. Four important risk factors, namely venous stasis disease, BMI $\geq$60, truncal obesity, and OHS and/or OSA, are significant in the development of postoperative DVT, and if present, preoperative prophylactic placement of an inferior vena cava filter should be considered.[67] Many bariatric surgeons prefer low-dose unfractionated heparin as their method of thromboprophylaxis. Use of a protocol for heparin dosing in gastric bypass patients, as opposed to a fixed dose, is preferred. Dosing based on height and weight initially, and then adjusted based on peak antifactor Xa activity, results in better thromboprophylaxis and few side effects.[68] Low-molecular-weight heparins have gained popularity for thromboembolism prophylaxis during bariatric surgery because of their bioavailability when injected subcutaneously. Enoxaparin, 40 mg, injected subcutaneously every 12 hours rather than the often recommended 30 mg every 12 hours decreases the incidence of postoperative DVT without an increase in bleeding complications.[69] It has also been suggested that enoxaparin dosing in obese patients be varied with age and lean body mass.[70] A combination of short duration of surgery, lower extremity pneumatic compression, and routine early ambulation, may preclude mandatory heparin anticoagulation, except in patients with a history of previous DVT, a known hypercoagulable state, or a significant family history of DVT.[71]

AIRWAY

Anatomic changes associated with obesity that contribute to a potentially difficult airway include limitation of movement of the atlantoaxial joint and cervical spine by upper thoracic and low cervical fat pads; excessive tissue folds in the mouth and pharynx; short, thick neck; suprasternal, presternal, and posterior cervical fat; and a very thick submental fat pad. The history obtained from the patient and examination of previous records may help predict airway difficulties. OSA predisposes to airway difficulties during anesthesia. Excess pharyngeal tissue deposited in the lateral pharyngeal walls may not be noticed during routine airway examination.[72] Overall, the magnitude of BMI does not seem to have much influence on the difficulty of laryngoscopy. Such difficulty correlates better with increased age, male sex, temporomandibular joint

pathology, Mallampati classes 3 and 4, history of OSA, and abnormal upper teeth.[73] The patient's neck circumference has been identified as the single biggest predictor of problematic intubation in morbidly obese patients.[74] The probability of a problematic intubation is approximately 5% with a 40-cm neck circumference compared with a 35% probability at 60-cm neck circumference. A larger neck circumference is associated with the male sex, a higher Mallampati score, grade 3 views at laryngoscopy, and OSA.

AMBULATORY ANESTHESIA

Previous guidelines issued by the Royal College of Surgeons of England deemed patients with BMI >30 kg/m^2 unsuitable for ambulatory surgery.[75] Subsequent evaluation of adherence to these guidelines discovered that >85% of ambulatory surgery units in England and a significant number in other countries continued to routinely anesthetize patients with BMI >30 kg/m^2.[76,77] A significant number of anesthesiologists believe that morbidly obese patients with comorbidities and no patient escort are unsuitable for ambulatory anesthesia because many are in suboptimal health. The presence of cardiovascular or respiratory comorbidity significantly reduces the willingness of anesthesiologists to provide ambulatory care to the obese patient.[78] There is no evidence to suggest increased morbidity in morbidly obese patients with stable concomitant diseases; therefore, they should not be excluded from day-case surgery based solely on absolute weight or BMI.[79] Individual evaluation and proper selection is important in determining which obese patients can undergo ambulatory anesthesia and surgery. Airway surgery, such as uvulopalatopharyngoplasty and tonsillectomy, should not be performed on an outpatient basis.[6] Use of regional blocks, where feasible, rapidly dissipating anesthetic agents, and appropriate-sized equipment and procedures for positioning and monitoring should be combined with the availability of prolonged observation and overnight admission facility for optimum safety.[80,81] Obese patients do not have a higher incidence of contact with health care professionals after discharge from the ambulatory surgery unit; neither do they have a higher postambulatory surgery, unplanned hospital admission rate than the general population.[82] Obesity is associated with a higher regional block failure and complication rates during ambulatory anesthesia. However, blocks are often successful, with high overall satisfaction; therefore, obese patients should not be arbitrarily excluded from use for ambulatory procedures.[83]

INTRAOPERATIVE CONSIDERATIONS

Positioning

Specially designed tables or two regular operating tables may be required for safe anesthesia and surgery in obese patients. Regular operating tables have a maximum weight limit of approximately 200 kg, but operating tables capable of holding up to 455 kg, with a little extra width to accommodate the extra girth, are available. Strapping obese patients to the operating table in combination with a malleable bean bag helps keep them from falling off the operating table. Particular care should be paid to protecting pressure areas because pressure sores, neural injuries, and rhabdomyolysis may occur. Brachial plexus and lower extremity nerve injuries are frequent. Carpal tunnel syndrome is the most common mononeuropathy after bariatric surgery.[84] Other reported neurologic complications include encephalopathy (Wernicke), optic neuropathy, and myelopathy associated with vitamin B_{12} and copper deficiencies.[85]

Supine positioning causes ventilatory impairment and inferior vena cava and aortic compression in obese patients. FRC and oxygenation are decreased further with supine positioning. Head-down positioning, often required during bariatric procedures, further worsens FRC and should be avoided if possible. Simply changing the obese patient from a sitting to supine position can cause a significant increase in oxygen consumption and cardiac output. The head-up position provides the longest safe apnea period during induction of anesthesia.[86] The extra time gained may help preclude hypoxemia if intubation is delayed. Both intraoperative positive end-expiratory pressure (PEEP) and the head-up position significantly decrease alveolar-arterial oxygen tension difference and increase total respiratory compliance to a similar degree in the obese patient, but the head-up position results in lower airway pressures. Both, however, decrease cardiac output significantly, which partially counteracts the beneficial effects on oxygenation.[87] Prone positioning, rarely required in the obese patient, should be correctly performed with freedom of abdominal movement to prevent detrimental effects on lung compliance, ventilation, and arterial oxygenation. Lateral decubitus positioning allows for better diaphragmatic excursion and should be favored over prone positioning whenever the surgical procedure permits.

Monitoring

Invasive arterial pressure monitoring may be indicated for the super morbidly obese patient, for those patients with cardiopulmonary disease, and for those patients on whom the noninvasive blood pressure cuff may not fit properly. Blood pressure measurements can be falsely elevated if a cuff is too small. Cuffs with bladders that encircle a minimum of 75% of the upper arm circumference or, preferably, the entire arm, should be used. Forearm measurements with a standard cuff overestimate both systolic and diastolic blood pressures in obese patients.[88] Central venous and pulmonary artery catheters can be used selectively in patients with significant cardiopulmonary disease or in patients undergoing extensive surgery. Central venous catheterization may also be required for intravenous access, which can be problematic in this patient population.[89]

Induction, Intubation, and Maintenance

Adequate preoxygenation is vital in obese patients because of rapid desaturation after loss of consciousness related to increased oxygen consumption and decreased FRC. Application of positive pressure ventilation during preoxygenation decreases atelectasis formation and improves oxygenation.[90] Four vital capacity breaths with 100% oxygen within 30 seconds have been suggested as superior to the usually recommended 3 minutes of 100% preoxygenation in obese patients.[91]

Larger doses of induction agents may be required by obese patients because blood volume, muscle mass, and cardiac output increase linearly with the degree of obesity. An increased dose of succinylcholine is necessary because of an increase in activity of pseudocholinesterase. Myalgia is not frequently seen following succinylcholine in morbidly obese patients; therefore, it is highly recommended for tracheal intubation.[92] Any of the commonly available intravenous induction agents may be employed after taking into consideration problems peculiar to individual patients.

If a difficult intubation is anticipated, awake intubation using topical or regional anesthesia is a prudent approach.

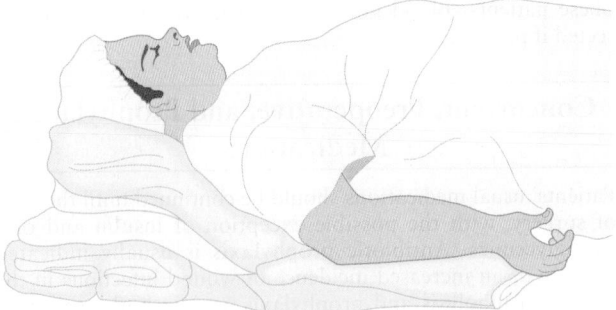

FIGURE 47-10. "Stacking" using towels and blankets.

During awake intubation, sedative-hypnotic medications should be reduced to a minimum. Sedation with dexmedetomidine during awake intubation provides adequate anxiolysis and analgesia without respiratory depression.[93] If endotracheal intubation under general anesthesia is selected, hypoxia and aspiration of gastric contents should be prevented at all costs. An experienced colleague who is immediately available or, better still, in the room during induction and airway management can help with mask ventilation or attempts at intubation. A surgeon capable of accessing the airway surgically should be readily available. Towels or folded blankets under the shoulders and head can compensate for the exaggerated flexed position of posterior cervical fat (Fig. 47-10). The object of this maneuver, known as "stacking," is to position the patient so that the tip of the chin is at a higher level than the chest to facilitate laryngoscopy and intubation. The *head-elevated laryngoscopy position* (HELP) is a step beyond stacking. It significantly elevates the obese patient's head, upper body, and shoulders above the chest to the extent that an imaginary horizontal line connects the sternal notch with the external auditory meatus to better improve laryngoscopy and intubation.[94] To facilitate proper HELP placement, the preformed Troop Elevation Pillow (C&R Enterprises, Frisco, TX) may be used in place of folded towels or blankets (Fig. 47-11, A–C). The advantage of this preformed pillow is that it can be prepositioned, inserted, and removed much faster with less effort than that required to build and dismantle a ramp made from blankets and towels.[95] An inflatable, multichambered pillow may more easily facilitate HELP placement without the need for additional lifting of the morbidly obese patient[96] (Fig. 47-12).

Continuous infusion of a short-acting intravenous agent, such as propofol, or any of the inhalation agents, or a combination, may be used to maintain anesthesia. Desflurane, sevoflurane, and isoflurane are minimally metabolized and are therefore useful agents in the obese patient, with desflurane possibly providing better hemodynamic stability and faster washout.[97,98] Metabolism of volatile anesthetics is greater in obese than in normal-weight patients, but even sevoflurane, which when undergoing biotransformation can result in significant elevations in plasma fluoride levels, is safe in obese patients.[99] Rapid elimination and analgesic properties make nitrous oxide (N_2O) an attractive choice for anesthesia in obese patients, but high oxygen demand in this patient population limits its use. N_2O does not cause noticeable bowel distention during short-duration laparoscopic bariatric procedures.[100]

Short-acting opioids, combined with a low-solubility inhalation anesthetic, facilitate a more rapid emergence without increasing opioid-related side effects.[101] Cis-atracurium possesses an organ-independent elimination profile and is a favorable nondepolarizing muscle relaxant for use during maintenance of anesthesia. Vecuronium and rocuronium are also useful choices. Dexmedetomidine, an α_2-agonist with

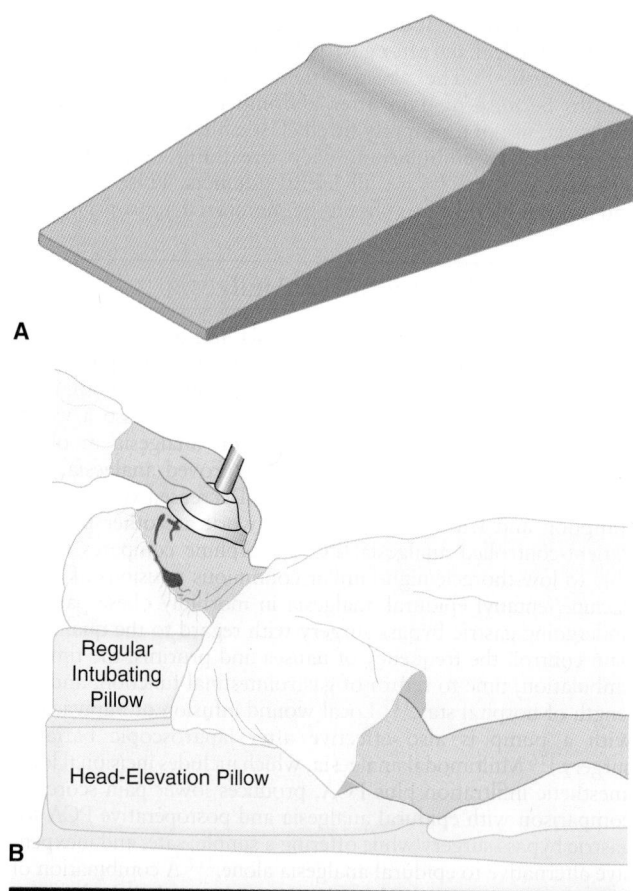

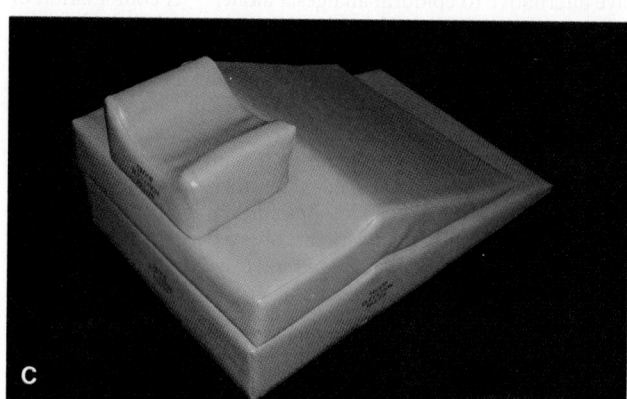

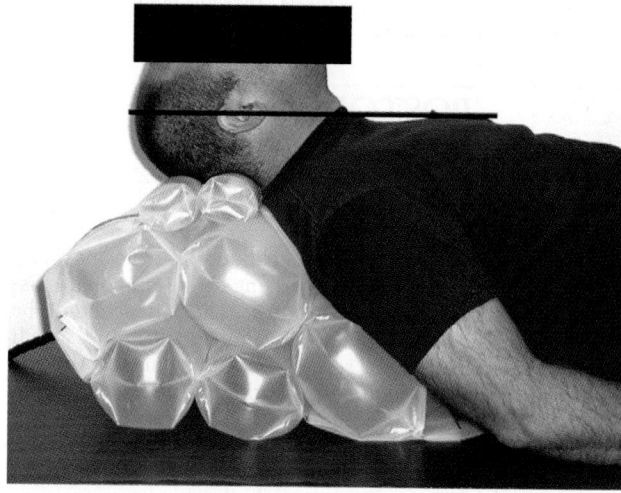

FIGURE 47-12. Prototype of the inflatable, multichambered pillow for proper head-elevated laryngoscopy position (HELP) placement of the obese patient. (Reprinted from Nissen MD, Gayes JM: An inflatable multichambered upper body support for the placement of the obese patient in the head-elevated laryngoscopy position. Anesth Analg 2007; 104: 1305, with permission.)

FIGURE 47-11. **A.** Illustration of the preformed Troop elevation pillow. **B.** Proper head-elevated laryngoscopy position (HELP) placement with the Troop elevation pillow combined with a standard intubating pillow as described in the text. **C.** Photograph of the Troop elevation pillow with additional layer (for extra-large patients) and preattached intubating pillow.

sedative and analgesic properties, has no clinically significant adverse effects on respiration and is an attractive anesthetic adjunct in obese patients.[102] Furthermore, it reduces postoperative opioid analgesic requirements.[102,103]

Ventilatory tidal volumes >13 mL/kg offer no added advantages during ventilation of anesthetized morbidly obese patients. Further increasing tidal volumes only increases the peak inspiratory airway pressure, end-expiratory (plateau) airway pressure, and lung compliance without significantly improving arterial oxygen tension.[104,105] PEEP is the only ventilatory parameter that consistently has been shown to improve respiratory function in obese subjects.[106] PEEP may, however, decrease venous return and cardiac output.

Excess adipose tissue may mask peripheral perfusion, making fluid balance difficult to assess. Blood loss is usually greater in the obese than in the nonobese patient for the same type of surgery, because technical difficulties of accessing the surgical site necessitate larger incisions and more extensive dissection. Early infusion of colloids and blood products may be necessary because obese patients are less able to compensate for small volumes lost, but rapid infusion of excessive amounts should be avoided because pre-existing congestive cardiac failure is common in the obese patient.

Regional Anesthesia

A regional anesthetic technique is a useful alternative to general anesthesia in the morbidly obese patient as it may help avoid potential intubation difficulties. It can, however, be technically difficult because of inability to identify usual bony landmarks. Central neuraxial block is easier in the lumbar region because the midline in this area has a thinner layer of fat than other areas of the spinal column. Longer needles and the sitting position are other useful tools that facilitate central neuraxial anesthesia. Ultrasound[107] and fluoroscopy[108] have been used to guide a needle or catheter into the epidural space. Epidural vascular engorgement and fatty infiltration reduce the volume of the space, making dose requirements of local anesthetics for epidural anesthesia 20 to 25% less in obese patients. Subarachnoid blocks are not technically as difficult as epidural blocks but the height of a subarachnoid block in obese patients can be unpredictable because of considerable upward spread within a short time, causing cardiovascular and respiratory compromise. A continuous catheter subarachnoid block therefore seems an attractive choice that allows careful titration of the local anesthetic to desired effect and level.[109] Spirometric parameters such as peak expiratory flow rate and maximum mid expiratory flow are reduced in obese patients receiving subarachnoid block.[110]

Combined epidural and general anesthesia allows for better titration of anesthetic drugs, use of larger oxygen concentration, and optimal muscle relaxation. It also allows for continuation of postoperative analgesia through the same catheter used to provide surgical anesthesia, thereby facilitating early postoperative mobilization.

POSTOPERATIVE CONSIDERATIONS

Emergence

Prompt extubation reduces the likelihood that the morbidly obese patient, who may have underlying cardiopulmonary disease, will become ventilator-dependent. The patient should be preferably extubated in the semirecumbent position, which has less adverse effect on respiration. Supplemental oxygen should be administrated after extubation. Lifting devices such as the HoverMatt (Patient Handling Technologies, Allentown, PA), the Patient Transfer Device (PTD; Alimed, Dedham, MA), and gantry-style mechanical lifting devices that use a sling are useful for transporting morbidly obese patients onto or off the operating table. The PTD can be combined with the Walter Henderson Maneuver (Fig. 47-13) to safely and gently transfer obese patients onto their postoperative beds.[111]

There is an increased incidence of atelectasis in morbidly obese patients after general anesthesia, which persists into the postoperative period.[112] Consequently, initiation of CPAP or bilevel positive airway pressure has been advocated. Postoperative CPAP may improve oxygenation but does not facilitate

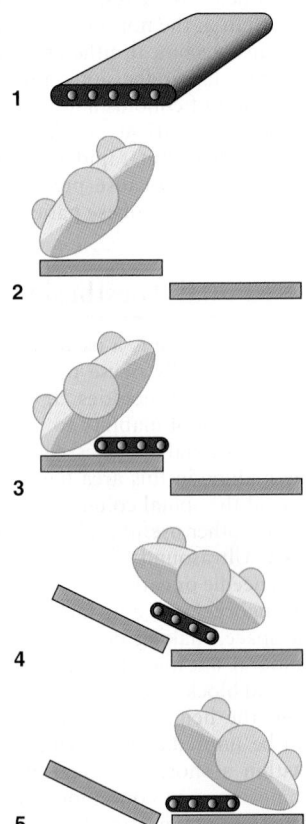

FIGURE 47-13. Illustration of the Walter Henderson maneuver. 1, Patient Transfer Device (PTD; a.k.a. patient roller); 2, patient tilted to slip roller underneath; 3, roller slipped under patient; 4, table tilted to roll patient "downhill" onto bed; 5, patient rolled onto bed. (Reprinted from Ogunnaike BO, Whitten CW: In response to Rosenblatt MA, Reich DL, Roth R et al: [letter]. Anesth Analg 2004; 98: 1809, with permission.)

CO_2 elimination.[113] It does not increase the incidence of major anastomotic leakage after gastric bypass surgery despite a theoretical risk.[114] The obese patient may avoid taking deep breaths because of pain after abdominal surgery. Adequate analgesia, use of a properly fitted elastic binder for abdominal support, early ambulation, deep breathing exercises, and incentive spirometry are all useful adjuncts. Pulse oximetry and arterial blood gases should be monitored appropriately.

Postoperative Analgesia

Perioperative use of regional anesthesia and analgesia reduces the incidence of postoperative respiratory complications. Epidural analgesia with local anesthetics, opioids, or both, is an effective form of analgesia. Intrathecal opioid is also a viable option. Potential advantages of epidural analgesia in obese patients include prevention of DVT, improved analgesia, and earlier recovery of intestinal motility. Decreased oxygen consumption and left ventricular stroke work are other benefits. Patient-controlled analgesia (PCA) morphine compares favorably to low-thoracic/high-lumbar continuous infusions of bupivacaine/fentanyl epidural analgesia in morbidly obese patients undergoing gastric bypass surgery with regard to the quality of pain control, the frequency of nausea and pruritus, the time to ambulation, time to return of gastrointestinal function, and the length of hospital stay.[115] Local wound infusion of bupivacaine with a pump is also effective after laparoscopic bariatric surgery.[116] Multimodal analgesia, which includes incisional local anesthetic infiltration plus PCA, produces lower pain scores in comparison with epidural analgesia and postoperative PCA for gastric bypass surgery while offering a simple, safe, and inexpensive alternative to epidural analgesia alone.[117] A combination of intraoperative nonopioid analgesics and anesthetic adjuvants (ketorolac, clonidine, ketamine, lidocaine, magnesium sulfate, and methylprednisolone) that produce analgesia by mechanisms different from opioids decreases sedation during recovery from anesthesia and reduces postoperative morphine requirements when compared with intraoperative fentanyl anesthesia in morbidly obese patients.[118] Delayed respiratory depression with centrally administered neuraxial opioids, when coupled with a potentially difficult airway in the obese patient, suggests that close monitoring in a step-down or intensive care unit is prudent.

RESUSCITATION

The possible need for cardiopulmonary resuscitation should be entertained when anesthetizing the morbidly obese patient. There are both equipment and technical concerns. Chest compressions may not be effective and mechanical compression devices may be required. The maximum 400 J of energy on regular defibrillators is sufficient for morbidly obese patients[119] because their chest wall is usually not much thicker, but the higher transthoracic impedance from the fat may obligate several attempts. Mask ventilation is more difficult because of poor mask fit, redundant oropharyngeal tissues, and reduced chest wall compliance. Regurgitation of gastric contents is also likely. Consideration should be given to employment of airway adjuncts, such as the gum-elastic bougie, the laryngeal mask airway™ (LMA North America, Inc. San Diego, CA) and the esophageal tracheal Combitube™, (Sheridan Catheter Corporation, Argyle, NY). The intubating laryngeal mask airway (Fastrach™ (LMA North America, Inc. San Diego, CA)) is better for both intubation and keeping the airway open for ventilation because of its rigidity and noncollapsible tubing. Tracheostomy, percutaneous cricothyrotomy, transtracheal jet ventilation, and retrograde wire intubation are all time-consuming and technically difficult procedures in such emergency situations and should be reserved as final options to be performed by experienced practitioners.[120]

References

1. Lemmens HJ, Brodsky JB: Anesthetic drugs and bariatric surgery. Expert Rev Neurotherapeutics 2006; 6: 1107
2. Pai MP, Paloucek FP: The origin of the "ideal" body weight equations. Ann Pharmacother 2000; 34: 1066
3. Lemmens HJ, Brodsky JB, Bernstein DP: Estimating ideal body weight—a new formula. Obes Surg 2005; 15: 1082
4. Jubber AS: Respiratory complications of obesity. Int J Clin Pract 2004; 58: 573
5. American Society of Anesthesiologists (ASA) Task Force on Perioperative Management of Patients with Obstructive Sleep Apnea (Report): Practice guidelines for the perioperative management of patients with obstructive sleep apnea. Anesthesiology 2006; 104: 1081
6. Flemons WW: Obstructive sleep apnea. N Engl J Med 2002; 347: 498
7. Olson AL, Zwillich C: The obesity hypoventilation syndrome. Am J Med 2005; 118: 948
8. Fraley MA, Bircham JA, Senkottaiyan N et al: Obesity and the electrocardiogram. Obes Rev 2005; 6: 275
9. Alpert MA, Terry BE, Hamm CR et al: Effect of weight loss on the ECG of normotensive morbidly obese patients. Chest 2001; 119: 507
10. Engeli S, Böhnke J, Gorzelniak K et al: Weight loss and the reninn-angiotensin-aldosterone system. Hypertension 2005; 45: 356
11. van Baak MA: The peripheral sympathetic nervous system in human obesity. Obes Rev 2001; 2: 3
12. Thomas F, Bean K, Pannier B et al: Cardiovascular mortality in overweight subjects. The key role of associated risk factors. Hypertension 2005; 46: 654
13. Wolf C, Tanner M: Obesity. West Med J 2002; 176: 23
14. Bray GA: Medical consequences of obesity. J Clin Endocrinol Metab 2004; 89: 2583
15. Van Gaal LF, Mertens IL, DeBlock CE: Mechanisms linking obesity with cardiovascular disease. Nature 2006; 444: 875
16. Primrose JN, Davies JA, Prentice CR et al: Reduction in factor VII fibrinogen and plasminogen activator inhibitor-1 activity after surgical treatment of morbid obesity. Thromb Haemost 2002; 68: 396
17. Birgel M, Gottschling-Zeller H, Röhrig K, et al: Role of cytokines in the regulation of plasminogen activator inhibitor-1 expression and secretion in newly differentiated subcutaneous human adipocytes. Arterioscler Thromb Vasc Biol 2000; 20: 1682
18. Tosetti C, Corinaldesi R, Stranghellini V et al: Gastric emptying of solids in morbid obesity. Int J Obes Relat Metab Disord 1996; 20: 200
19. Harter RL, Kelly WB, Kramer MG et al: A comparison of the volume and pH of gastric contents of obese and lean surgical patients. Anesth Analg 1998; 86: 147
20. Maltby JR, Pytka S, Watson NC et al: Drinking 300 ml of clear fluid two hours before surgery has no effect on gastric fluid volume and pH in fasting and non-fasting obese patients. Can J Anesth 2004; 51: 111
21. El-Serag HB, Graham DY, Satia JA, et al: Obesity is an independent risk factor for GERD symptoms and erosive esophagitis. Am J Gastroenterol 2005; 100: 1243
22. Nilsson M, Johnsen R, Ye W, et al: Obesity and estrogen as risk factors for gastroesophageal reflux symptoms. JAMA 2003; 290: 66
23. Frezza EE, Ikramuddin S, Gourash W, et al: Symptomatic improvement in gastroesophageal reflux disease (GERD) following laparoscopic Roux-en-Y gastric bypass. Surg Endosc 2002; 16: 1027
24. Hickman IJ, Jonsson JR, Prins JB et al: Modest weight loss and physical activity in overweight patients with chronic liver disease results in sustained improvements in alanine aminotransferase, fasting insulin, and quality of life. Gut 2004; 53: 413
25. Cheymol G: Effects of obesity on pharmacokinetics: implications for drug therapy. Clin Pharmacokinet 2000; 39: 215
26. Cotler SJ, Vitello JM, Guzman G, et al: Hepatic decompensation after gastric bypass surgery for morbid obesity. Dig Dis Sci 2004; 49: 1563
27. Matteoni C, Younossi ZM, McCullough A: Non alcoholic fatty liver disease: a spectrum of clinical pathological severity. Gastroenterology 1999; 116: 1413
28. Rosenberg DE, Jabbour SA, Goldstein BJ: Insulin resistance, diabetes and cardiovascular risk: approaches to treatment. Diabetes Obes Metab 2005; 7: 642
29. Moulin de Moraes CM, Mancini MC, de Melo ME, et al: Prevalence of subclinical hypothyroidism in a morbidly obese population and improvement after weight loss induced by Roux-en-Y gastric bypass. Obes Surg 2005; 15: 1287
30. Reinehr T, Andler W: Thyroid hormones before and after weight loss in obesity. Arch Dis Child 2002; 87: 320
31. Douyon L, Schteingart DE: Effect of obesity and starvation on thyroid hormone, growth hormone, and cortisol secretion. Endocrinol Metab Clin North Am 2002; 31: 173
32. Raftopoulos Y, Gagné DJ, Papasavas P, et al: Improvement in hypothyroidism after laparoscopic Roux-en-Y gastric bypass for morbid obesity. Obes Surg 2004; 14: 509
33. Chagnac A, Weinstein T, Herman M et al: The effects of weight loss on renal function in patients with severe obesity. J Am Soc Nephrol 2003; 14: 1480
34. Hall JE: The kidney, hypertension, and obesity. Hypertension 2003; 41: 625
35. Alberti KG, Zimmet P, Shaw J: The metabolic syndrome-a new worldwide definition. Lancet 2005; 366: 1059
36. Casati A, Putzu M: Anesthesia in the obese patient: pharmacokinetic considerations. J Clin Anesth 2005; 17: 134
37. Blouin RA, Warren GW: Pharmacokinetic considerations in obesity. J Pharm Sci 1999; 88: 1
38. Egan TD, Huizinga B, Gupta SK et al: Remifentanil pharmacokinetics in obese versus lean patients. Anesthesiology 1998; 89: 562
39. Abernethy DR, Greenblatt DJ, Smith TW: Digoxin disposition in obesity: Clinical pharmacokinetic investigation. Am Heart J 1981; 102: 740
40. Christoff PB, Conti DR, Naylor C et al: Procainamide disposition in obesity. Drug Intell Clin Pharm 1983; 17: 516
41. Servin F, Farinotti R, Haberer JP et al: Propofol infusion for maintenance of anesthesia in morbidly obese patients receiving nitrous oxide. A clinical pharmacokinetic study. Anesthesiology 1993; 78: 657
42. Leykin Y, Pellis T, Lucca M, et al: The pharmacodynamic effects of rocuronium when dosed according to real body weight or ideal body weight in morbidly obese patients. Anesth Analg 2004; 99: 1086
43. Puhringer FK, Keller C, Kleinsasser A et al: Pharmacokinetics of rocuronium bromide in obese female patients. Eur J Anaesthesiol 1999; 16: 507
44. Suzuki T, Masaki G, Ogawa S: Neostigmine-induced reversal of vecuronium in normal weight, overweight, and obese female patients. Br J Anaesth 2006; 97: 160
45. Varin F, Ducharme J, Theoret Y et al: Influence of extreme obesity on the body disposition and neuromuscular blocking effect of atracurium. Clin Pharmacol Ther 1990; 48: 18
46. Leykin Y, Pellis T, Lucca M, et al: The effects of cisatracurium on morbidly obese women. Anesth Analg 2004; 99: 1090
47. Sacan O, White PF, Tufanogullari B et al: Sugammadex reversal of rocuronium-induced neuromuscular blockade: a comparison with neostigmine-glycopyrrolate and edrophonium-atropine. Anesth Analg 2007; 104: 569
48. Shibutani K, Inchiosa MA, Sawada K et al: Accuracy of pharmacokinetic models for prediction plasma fentanyl concentrations in lean and obese surgical patients. Derivation of dosing weight ("pharmacokinetic mass"). Anesthesiology 2004; 101: 603
49. Han PY, Duffull SB, Kirkpatrick CM et al: Dosing in obesity: a simple solution to a big problem. Clin Pharmacol Ther 2007; 82: 505
50. Slepchenko G, Simon N, Goubaux B et al: Performance of target-controlled sufentanil infusion on obese patients. Anesthesiology 2003; 98: 65
51. Feld JM, Hoffman WE, Stechert MM et al: Fentanyl or dexmedetomidine combined with desflurane for bariatric surgery. J Clin Anesth 2006; 18: 24
52. Rich JM, Njo L, Roberts KW et al: Unusual hypotension and bradycardia in a patient receiving fenfluramine, phentermine, and fluoxetine. Anesthesiology 1997; 88: 529
53. Perrio MJ, Wilton LV, Shakir SA: The safety profiles of orlistat and sibutramine: results of prescription-event monitoring studies in England. Obesity (Silver Spring) 2007; 15: 2712
54. Bray GA, Ryan DH: Drug treatment of the overweight patient. Gastroenterology 2007; 132: 2239
55. MacWalter RS, Fraser HW, Armstrong KM: Orlistat enhances warfarin effect. Ann Pharmacother 2003; 37: 510
56. Patel PN, Pathak R: Rimonabant: A novel selective cannabinoid-1 receptor antagonist for treatment of obesity. Am J Health Syst Pharm 2007; 64: 481
57. Rubino F, Gagner M, Gentileschi P et al: The early effect of the Roux-en-Y gastric bypass on hormones involved in body weight regulation and glucose metabolism. Ann Surg 2004; 240: 236
58. Nguyen NT: Open vs. laparoscopic procedures in bariatric surgery. J Gastrointest Surg 2004; 8: 393
59. Ogunnaike BO, Jones SB, Jones DB et al: Anesthetic considerations for bariatric surgery. Anesth Analg 2002; 95: 1793
60. Ezri T, Hazin V, Warters D et al: The endotracheal tube moves more often in obese patients undergoing laparoscopy compared with open abdominal surgery. Anesth Analg 2003; 96: 278
61. Mognol P, Vignes S, Chosidow D et al: Rhabdomyolysis after laparoscopic bariatric surgery. Obes Surg 2004; 14: 19
62. Cigaina V: Gastric pacing as therapy for morbid obesity: preliminary results. Obes Surg 2002; 12: S12
63. Elliot C, Kiely DG: Pulmonary hypertension: Diagnosis and treatment. Clin Med 2004; 4: 211
64. Chang C, Adams-Huet B, Provost DA: Acute post-gastric reduction surgery (APGARS) neuropathy. Obes Surg 2004; 14: 182
65. Benumof JL: Obesity, sleep apnea, the airway, and anesthesia. Curr Opin Anaesth 2004; 17: 21
66. Kabon B, Nagele A, Reddy D et al: Obesity decreases perioperative tissue oxygenation. Anesthesiology 2004; 100: 274
67. Sapala JA, Wood MH, Schuhknecht MP et al: Fatal pulmonary embolism after bariatric operations for morbid obesity: A 24-year retrospective analysis. Obes Surg 2003; 13: 819
68. Shepherd MF, Rosborough TK, Schwartz ML: Heparin thromboprophylaxis in gastric bypass. Obes Surg 2003; 13: 249
69. Scholten DJ, Hoedema RM, Scholten SE: A comparison of two different prophylactic dose regimens of low molecular weight heparin in bariatric surgery. Obes Surg 2002; 12: 19

ANESTHESIA FOR SURGICAL SUBSPECIALTIES

70. Green B, Duffull SB: Development of a dosing strategy for enoxaparin in obese patients. Br J Clin Pharmacol 2003; 56: 96

71. Gonzalez QH, Tisher DS, Plata-Munoz JJ et al: Incidence of clinically evident deep venous thrombosis after laparoscopic Roux-en-Y gastric bypass. Surg Endosc 2004; 18: 1082

72. Kim JA, Lee JJ: Preoperative predictors of difficult intubation in patients with obstructive sleep apnea syndrome. Can J Anesth 2006; 53: 393

73. Ezri T, Medalion B, Weisenberg M et al: Increased body mass per se is not a predictor of difficult laryngoscopy. Can J Anesth 2003; 50: 179

74. Brodsky JB, Lemmons HJM, Brock-Utne JG et al: Morbid obesity and tracheal intubation. Anesth Analg 2002; 94: 732

75. Commission on the Provision of Surgical Services: Guidelines for Day Case Surgery. A report of the Royal College of Surgeons of England, revised edition. London, Royal College of Surgeons of England, 1992

76. Atkins M, White J, Ahmed K: Day surgery and body mass index: results of a national survey. Anaesthesia 2002; 57: 169

77. Bryson GL, Chung F, Cox RG, et al: Patient selection in ambulatory anesthesia—an evidence-based review: part II. Can J Anesth 2004; 51: 782

78. Friedman Z, Chung F, Wong DT: Ambulatory surgery adult patient selection criteria—a survey of Canadian anesthesiologists. Can J Anesth 2004; 51: 437

79. Montgomery KF, Watkins BM, Ahroni JH et al: Outpatient laparoscopic adjustable gastric banding in super-obese patients. Obes Surg 2007; 17: 711

80. Servin F: Ambulatory anesthesia for the obese patient. Curr Opin Anaesthesiol 2006; 19: 597

81. Qadir N, Smith I: Day surgery: how far can we go and are there still limits?: Curr Opin Anaesthesiol 2007; 20: 503

82. Davies KE, Houghton K, Montgomery JE: Obesity and day-case surgery. Anaesthesia 2001; 56: 1112

83. Nielsen KC, Guller U, Steele SM, et al: Influence of obesity on surgical regional anesthesia in the ambulatory setting: an analysis of 9038 blocks. Anesthesiology 2005; 102: 181

84. Thaisetthawatkul P, Collazo-Clavell ML, Sarr MG et al: A controlled study of peripheral neuropathy after bariatric surgery. Neurology 2004; 63: 1462

85. Juhasz-Pocsine K, Rudnicki SA, Archer RL et al: Neurologic complications of gastric bypass surgery for morbid obesity. Neurology 2007; 68: 1843

86. Boyce JR, Ness T, Castroman P: A preliminary study of the optimal positioning for the morbidly obese patient. Obes Surg 2003; 13: 4

87. Perilli V, Sollazzi L, Modesti C et al: Comparison of positive end-expiratory pressure with reverse Trendelenburg position in morbidly obese patients. Obes Surg 2003; 13: 605

88. Pierin AM, Alavarce DC, Gusmao JL et al: Blood pressure measurement in obese patients: Comparison between upper arm and forearm measurements. Blood Press Monit 2004; 9: 101

89. Juvin P, Blarel A, Bruno F et al: Is peripheral line placement more difficult in obese than in lean patients? Anesth Analg 2003; 96: 1218

90. Coussa M, Proietti S, Schnyder P et al: Prevention of atelectasis formation during the induction of general anesthesia in morbidly obese patients. Anesth Analg 2004; 98: 1491

91. Goldberg ME, Norris MC, Larijani GE et al: Preoxygenation in the morbidly obese: A comparison of two techniques. Anesth Analg 1989; 68: 520

92. Lemmens HJ, Brodsky JB: The dose of succinylcholine in morbid obesity. Anesth Analg 2006; 102: 438

93. Abdelmalak B, Makary L, Hoban J et al: Dexmedetomidine as sole sedative for awake intubation in management of the critical airway. J Clin Anesth 2007; 19: 370

94. Levitan RM, Mechem CC, Ochroch EA et al: Head-elevated laryngoscopy position: Improving laryngeal exposure during laryngoscopy by increasing head elevation. Ann Emerg Med 2003; 41: 322

95. Rich JM: Use of an elevation pillow to produce the head-elevated laryngoscopy position for airway management in morbidly obese and large-framed patients. Anesth Analg 2004; 98: 264

96. Nissen MD, Graves JM: An inflatable, multichambered upper body support for the placement of the obese patient in the head-elevated laryngoscopy position (letter). Anesth Analg 2007; 104: 1305

97. De Baerdemaeker LE, Struys MM, Jacobs S et al: Optimization of desflurane administration in morbidly obese patients: A comparison with sevoflurane. Br J Anaesth 2003; 91: 638

98. La Colla L, Albertin A, La Colla G et al: Faster wash-out and recovery for desflurane vs sevoflurane in morbidly obese patients when no premedication is used. Br J Anaesth 2007; 99: 353

99. Frink EJ, Malan TP, Brown EA et al: Plasma inorganic fluoride levels with sevoflurane anesthesia in morbidly obese and nonobese patients. Anesth Analg 1993; 76: 1333

100. Brodsky JB, Lemmens HJM, Collins JS et al: Nitrous oxide and laparoscopic bariatric surgery. Obes Surg 2005; 15: 494

101. Song D, Whitten CW, White PF: Remifentanil infusion facilitates early recovery for obese outpatients undergoing laparoscopic cholecystectomy. Anesth Analg 2000; 90: 1111

102. Feld JM, Hoffman WE, Stechert MM et al: Fentanyl or dexmedetomidine combined with desflurane for bariatric surgery. J Clin Anesth 2006; 18: 24

103. Hofer RE, Sprung J, Sarr MG et al: Anesthesia for a patient with morbid obesity using dexmedetomidine without narcotics. Can J Anesth 2005; 52: 176

104. Bardoczky GI, Yernault JC, Houben JJ et al: Large tidal volume ventilation does not improve oxygenation in morbidly obese patients during anesthesia. Anesth Analg 1995; 81: 385

105. Sprung J, Whalley DG, Falcone T et al: The effects of tidal volume and respiratory rate on oxygenation and respiratory mechanics during laparoscopy in morbidly obese patients. Anesth Analg 2003; 97: 268

106. Pelosi P, Ravagnan I, Giurati G et al: Positive end-expiratory pressure improves respiratory function in obese but not in normal subjects during anesthesia and paralysis. Anesthesiology 1999; 91: 1221

107. Grau T, Leipold RW, Fatehi S et al: Real time ultrasonic observation of combined spinal-epidural anaesthesia. Eur J Anaesthesiol 2004; 21: 25

108. Johnson TW, Morgan R, Smalley P: Radiographic guided epidural placement. Anaesthesia 2003; 58: 485

109. Michaloudis D, Fraidakis O, Petrou A et al: Continuous spinal anesthesia/analgesia for perioperative management of morbidly obese patients undergoing laparotomy for gastroplastic surgery. Obes Surg 2000; 10: 220

110. Regli A, von Ungern-Sternberg BS, Reber A et al: Impact of spinal anaesthesia on perioperative lung volumes in obese and morbidly obese female patients. Anaesthesia 2006; 61: 215

111. Ogunnaike BO, Whitten CW: Bariatric surgery and the prevention of postoperative respiratory complications (in reply). Anesth Analg 2004; 98: 1809

112. Eichenberger A, Proietti S, Wicky S et al: Morbid obesity and postoperative pulmonary atelectasis: An underestimated problem. Anesth Analg 2002; 95: 1788

113. Gaszynski T, Tokarz A, Piotrowski D et al: Boussignac CPAP in the postoperative period in morbidly obese patients. Obes Surg 2007; 17: 452

114. Huerta S, DeShields S, Shpiner R et al: Safety and efficacy of postoperative continuous positive airway pressure to prevent pulmonary complications after Roux-en-y gastric bypass. J Gastrointest Surg 2002; 6: 354

115. Charghi R, Backman S, Christou N et al: Patient controlled IV analgesia is an acceptable pain management strategy in morbidly obese patients undergoing gastric bypass surgery. A retrospective comparison with epidural analgesia. Can J Anesth 2003; 50: 672

116. Cottam DR, Fisher B, Atkinson J et al: A randomized trial of bupivacaine pain pumps to eliminate the need for patient controlled analgesia pumps in primary laparoscopic Roux-en-Y gastric bypass. Obes Surg 2007; 17: 595

117. Schumann R, Shikora S, Weiss JM et al: A comparison of multimodal perioperative analgesia to epidural pain management after gastric bypass surgery. Anesth Analg 2003; 96: 469

118. Feld JM, Laurito CE, Beckerman M et al: Non-opioid analgesia improves pain relief and decreases sedation after gastric bypass surgery. Can J Anesth 2003; 50: 336

119. DeSilva RA, Lown B: Energy requirement for defibrillation of a markedly overweight patient. Circulation 1978; 57: 827

120. Brunette DD: Resuscitation of the obese patient. Ann J Emerg Med 2004; 22: 40

CHAPTER 48 ■ HEPATIC ANATOMY, FUNCTION, AND PHYSIOLOGY

BRIAN S. KAUFMAN AND J. DAVID ROCCAFORTE

KEY POINTS

1 The hepatic buffer response, in which the hepatic artery blood flow changes reciprocally with changing portal venous flow, is the mechanism by which total oxygen delivery to the liver is maintained. This response is limited in its ability to compensate during conditions of hypoperfusion, inflammation, or shock.

2 Hepatitis associated with volatile anesthetics is rare overall and is most commonly associated with halothane. The disorder appears to be immune-mediated and is best avoided by eliminating halothane from clinical use.

3 Because of the liver's central role in the inflammatory response, the metabolic demands greatly increase whenever acute-phase proteins are being produced. These

demands occur when hepatic oxygen delivery is likely to be compromised, placing the liver in a highly vulnerable situation.

4 The risk of developing perioperative hepatic dysfunction varies with the pre-existing hepatic reserve status; presence of comorbid conditions; and the type, duration, and location of surgery. Commonly employed general and regional anesthetic techniques impart minimal additional stress to the liver.

5 Currently, there is no commonly available hepatic replacement therapy for acute liver failure. The most effective support for the liver is the maintenance of adequate perfusion and oxygenation and avoidance of toxic insults.

The liver provides a diverse spectrum of vital physiologic functions and plays an essential role in maintaining perioperative homeostasis.[1] Patients with advanced liver disease are at high risk for excessive morbidity and mortality following surgery because of failure of one or more of these essential functions. For example, the normal liver moderates the hypotensive response to acute blood loss and hypovolemia through its reservoir function, and helps minimize blood loss through synthesis of coagulation factors and degradation of fibrinolytic substances. Failure of these functions contributes to intraoperative and postoperative hypoperfusion, tissue ischemia, and activation of the systemic inflammatory response, setting the stage for the postoperative development of multisystem organ failure.

The liver is a remarkably resilient organ, with unparalleled regenerative capacity and substantial physiologic reserves. Normal function may be present in humans when as much as 80% of the organ has been resected. Insidious hepatic diseases such as chronic hepatitis C (HCV) can progress silently and destroy the majority of the liver before symptoms develop. Identifying patients with marked limitation of hepatic reserve, but without overt hepatic failure, is important but often difficult. A careful preoperative history and physical examination will help identify patients in whom laboratory evaluation of liver function is appropriate. These patients are often at increased risk for perioperative morbidity and mortality, including development of overt liver dysfunction postoperatively, particularly after major procedures. Thus, anesthesiologists must understand the interactions between liver disease, surgical procedures, and anesthetic interventions so an appropriate therapeutic plan can be developed and implemented to optimize patient outcome (Table 48-1).

HEPATIC HOMEOSTASIS

Vascular Supply

The liver receives about 25% of the cardiac output, and therefore has an average blood flow between 100 and 130 mL/min/100 g. There are two major sources of blood to the liver: the hepatic artery and the portal vein. The common hepatic artery arises from the celiac trunk and sends off the cystic artery before entering the liver (Fig. 48-1). The portal vein is formed by the confluence of the splenic and superior mesenteric veins, and receives blood from the entire digestive tract, spleen, pancreas, and gallbladder. The hepatic artery

---

TABLE 48-1

MAJOR PHYSIOLOGIC FUNCTIONS OF THE LIVER

■ FUNCTION	■ DETAILS	■ ANESTHETIC RELEVANCE
Blood reservoir	10–15% of total blood volume can be sequestered and quickly released after sympathetic stimulation	Many anesthetics suppress sympathetic tone and response.
Blood coagulation	Both pro- and anticlotting factors are synthesized in the liver. Vitamin K absorption depends on bile excretion. Liver-produced thrombopoietin modulates platelet production.	Coagulopathies may lead to increased perioperative bleeding requiring aggressive correction and resuscitation.
Endocrine control	Synthesizes and secretes: insulinlike growth factor-1, angiotensinogen, thrombopoietin, thyroid-binding globulin. Converts T_4 to T_3. Inactivates: corticosteroids, aldosterone, estrogen, androgens, insulin, and antidiuretic hormone.	Perioperative endocrine abnormalities may be more common in patients with liver disease.
Bilirubin excretion	Absorbs bilirubin from the bloodstream, conjugates, and excretes it into the biliary system. Synthesizes haptoglobin and scavenges hemoglobin.	Hyperbilirubinemia detected by preoperative screening tests may detect occult liver disease.
Carbohydrate metabolism	Stores and releases glycogen. Site of gluconeogenesis from amino acids, lactate, and glycerol.	Abnormal glycemic control is common in patients with liver disease and may manifest as perioperative hyper- or hypoglycemia.
Lipid metabolism	Major site of fatty acid synthesis, and cholesterol and lipoprotein metabolism.	Dysfunction leads to wide-reaching systemic abnormalities of cellular function, involving cell membranes, and hormones, possibly affecting pharmacokinetics and pharmacodynamics of anesthetic agents.
Amino acid metabolism	Major site of protein and amino acid metabolism, and urea production.	Dysfunction leads to elevated ammonia levels and associated encephalopathy.
Protein synthesis	Production of albumin, acute-phase proteins, coagulation factors, and globulins.	Alterations of pharmacokinetics and pharmacodynamics of many anesthetic agents.
Immunologic modulation	Largest reticuloendothelial organ. Filters out toxins, bacteria and debris from the GI tract. Hepatic macrophages, T cells, and Kupffer cells then trigger and amplify the systemic inflammatory response.	Immunocompromise associated with liver disease renders patients susceptible to perioperative infection and sepsis.

GI, gastrointestinal.

delivers about 25% of the total hepatic blood flow but nearly 50% of the hepatic oxygen delivery. The portal vein provides the remaining 75% of total hepatic blood flow and 50% of hepatic oxygen delivery. Because portal venous blood has already perfused the preportal organs (stomach, intestines, spleen, and pancreas; Fig. 48-1), it is partially deoxygenated and enriched with nutrients and other substances absorbed from the gastrointestinal tract.

The portal vein has numerous tributaries, which are usually of little importance. When patients develop portal hypertension, however, these normally rudimentary connections form large portosystemic shunts, permitting portal venous blood to return to the systemic circulation without traversing the liver. These shunts produce many of the pathologic findings and severe complications of portal hypertension (e.g., esophageal varices).

Hepatic arterial pressure is similar to aortic pressure, while the mean portal vein pressure is approximately 6 to 10 mm Hg. These two afferent vascular systems merge in the sinusoids where the pressure is normally 2 to 4 mm Hg above that of the inferior vena cava (IVC). The hepatic sinusoids connect the terminal portal vessels with the hepatic venules. The continuity of the sinusoidal wall is interrupted by fenestrations, which facilitate transfer of solutes to the space of Disse for uptake by hepatocytes. Flow through the sinusoids is influenced by several factors, the most important of which may be local control by shrinking or swelling of endothelial and Kupffer cells.

Blood drains from the hepatic sinusoids into the central vein and then flows through sublobular veins that join to form one of the three major hepatic veins (right, middle, and left). A short extrahepatic segment joins each major hepatic vein to the IVC. The caudate lobe drains directly into the IVC through small posterior caudate veins. If thrombosis of the major hepatic veins occurs (Budd-Chiari syndrome), the caudate veins become the key to drainage of hepatic blood into the IVC.

Periportal hepatocytes located close to the terminal vascular branches of the portal vein and hepatic artery are the first to be supplied with oxygen and nutrients (*zone 1*). The perivenular (centrilobular) area, which is most distant from these terminal vascular branches, has the least resistance to metabolic and anoxic damage (*zone 3*). The intermediate area is termed *zone 2*. The oxygen content and nutritive value of the blood progressively decreases as blood flows from zone 1 to zone 3.

The sequential perfusion of hepatocytes in the liver cell plate allows a progressive qualitative and quantitative modification of the composition of sinusoidal blood as it traverses the liver. There are ultrastructural differences between hepatocytes located in zones 1 and 3, and these hepatocytes attain different functional capabilities. Hepatocytes in zone 1 contain numerous large mitochondria and have the highest concentrations of Krebs cycle enzymes. These cells are adapted for high oxidative activities such as gluconeogenesis, β-oxidation of fatty acids, amino acid catabolism, ureagenesis, cholesterol synthesis, and bile acid secretion. Zone 3 hepatocytes are relatively anaerobic. Smooth endoplasmic reticulum is more abundant in these cells. Zone 3 is a primary site for glycolysis and lipogenesis. It is also the site for general detoxification and biotransformation of drugs, chemicals, and toxins. The anaerobic milieu of zone 3, however, is also its Achilles heel because these cells are exquisitely susceptible to injury from systemic hypoperfusion and hypoxemia. Sharply defined zone 3 necrosis is also characteristic of injury resulting from accumulation of toxic products of biotransformation as seen in toxicity from acetaminophen and halothane.

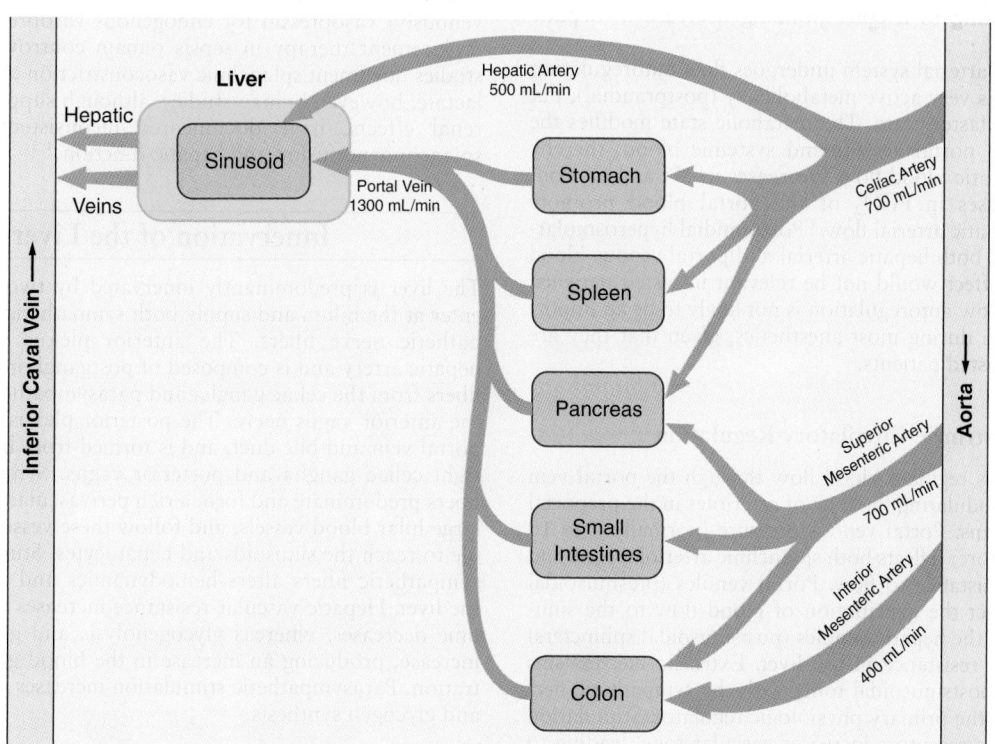

FIGURE 48-1.   Schematic representation of splanchnic circulation. (Reprinted from Gelman S: Effects of anesthetics on splanchnic circulation, Cardiovascular Action of Anesthetics and Drugs Used in Anesthesia. Edited by Altura BM, Halevy S. Basel, Karger, 1986, p 127, with permission.)

Hepatic Blood Flow

Blood flow and oxygen supply to the liver are regulated to fulfill two separate demands. The first is to supply the liver itself with necessary energy substrates and oxygen for its own maintenance needs. The second is to provide vital services to the rest of the body. Although the liver as a whole receives 25% of the cardiac output, regional blood flow within the organ is such that certain areas are highly prone to ischemia. The hepatic circulation is regulated by both intrinsic (regional microvascular) and extrinsic (neural and hormonal) mechanisms.[2]

Intrinsic Circulatory Regulation

The liver lacks the ability to directly regulate portal venous flow; therefore, regional microvascular regulatory mechanisms must operate almost exclusively by modulating hepatic arteriolar tone. The primary mechanism by which this occurs is called the *hepatic arterial buffer response,* whereby hepatic arterial flow varies reciprocally with changes in portal venous flow. This response is limited, however, to a 50% reduction of portal venous flow and a corresponding twofold increase in hepatic artery flow. Fortunately, because the hepatic artery carries higher oxygen content, this is usually an effective mechanism for protecting the liver from ischemic insults.

The hepatic buffer response appears to be mediated via adenosine. Presumably, this potent arteriolar dilator is synthesized at a constant rate and continuously secreted in the vicinity of the terminal hepatic arterioles and portal venules.[2] As flow through the portal vein decreases, less of the perivascular adenosine is "washed out," leading to its accumulation around hepatic arterioles. The result is increased arteriolar dilatation and an increase in hepatic arterial flow. Conversely, an increase in portal vein flow decreases the periarteriolar adenosine, leading to a corresponding decrease in hepatic artery flow.

The hepatic arterial system undergoes flow autoregulation when the liver is very active metabolically (postprandial), but not during the fasted state. The metabolic state modifies the composition of portal venous and systemic blood, thereby influencing hepatic blood flow. Decreases in pH and O_2 content, or increases in PCO_2 of the portal blood promote increases of hepatic arterial flow.[3] Postprandial hyperosmolarity can increase both hepatic arterial and portal venous blood flow, but this effect would not be relevant in fasted patients. Thus, hepatic flow autoregulation is not likely to be an important mechanism during most anesthetics, given that they are performed in fasted patients.

Extrinsic Circulatory Regulation

Extrinsic factors regulate blood flow through the portal vein indirectly by modulating the tone of arterioles in the preportal splanchnic organs. Portal venous pressure (normally 7 to 10 mm Hg), therefore, reflects both splanchnic arteriolar tone and intrahepatic resistance to flow. Portal venules (presinusoidal sphincters) affect the distribution of blood flow to the sinusoids; however, the hepatic venules (postsinusoidal sphincters) control venous resistance in the liver. Extrinsic mechanisms modulate this postsinusoidal tone, with the sympathetic nervous system as the primary physiologic regulator. Stimulation of α_1-adrenergic receptors increases vascular tone, leading to constriction and a reduction in both blood flow and blood volume in the sinusoids.

Hepatic arteriolar tone is the main determinant of resistance in the hepatic arterial tree. Blood flow through the liver decreases with stimulation of certain arteriolar receptors (α_1-adrenergic and type 1 dopaminergic) and increases with activation of others (β_2-adrenergic).

Humoral Regulators

Myriad humoral substances alter liver blood flow, including gastrin, glucagon, secretin, bile salts, angiotensin II, vasopressin, and catecholamines. In addition, during inflammatory or septic states, cytokines, interleukins, and other inflammatory mediators have been implicated in the alteration of normal splanchnic and hepatic blood flow. Of the systemic hormones, epinephrine is most likely to attain concentrations producing vasoactive effects. Both α-adrenergic and β-adrenergic receptors exist in the hepatic arterial bed, whereas the portal vasculature has only α receptors. An injection of epinephrine directly into the hepatic artery causes vasoconstriction (α_1-adrenergic effect), followed by vasodilation (β_2-adrenergic effect). When injected into the portal vein, epinephrine produces only vasoconstriction. During activation of the sympathetic nervous system, the hepatic circulatory effects of epinephrine and norepinephrine far exceed those of dopamine, which probably has little if any importance as a physiologic modulator of the hepatic circulation. Glucagon induces a graded, long-lasting dilation of hepatic arterioles; it also antagonizes arterial constrictor responses to a wide range of physiologic stimuli, including stress-induced sympathoadrenal outflow. Angiotensin II markedly constricts both hepatic arterial and portal beds, and significantly reduces mesenteric outflow; the result is a substantial decrease in total hepatic blood flow. Vasopressin also intensely constricts splanchnic vessels, markedly reducing flow into the portal vein. This action accounts for the efficacy of high-dose vasopressin (0.2 to 0.4 U/min intravenously) to alleviate portal hypertension and decrease bleeding from esophageal varices. The splanchnic and hepatic effects of low-dose (0.02 to 0.04 U/min intravenously) vasopressin for endogenous vasopressin deficiency replacement therapy in sepsis remain controversial. Animal studies document splanchnic vasoconstriction and increases in lactate; however, human studies, although supporting positive renal effects, have documented inconsistent benefits on splanchnic perfusion and hepatic function.[4,5]

Innervation of the Liver

The liver is predominantly innervated by two plexuses that enter at the hilum and supply both sympathetic and parasympathetic nerve fibers. The anterior plexus surrounds the hepatic artery and is composed of postganglionic sympathetic fibers from the celiac ganglia and parasympathetic fibers from the anterior vagus nerve. The posterior plexus surrounds the portal vein and bile duct, and is formed from branches of the right celiac ganglia and posterior vagus. Sympathetic nerve fibers predominate and form a rich perivascular plexus around large hilar blood vessels, and follow these vessels to each lobule to reach the sinusoids and hepatocytes. Stimulation of the sympathetic fibers alters hemodynamics and metabolism of the liver. Hepatic vascular resistance increases and blood volume decreases, whereas glycogenolysis and gluconeogenesis increase, producing an increase in the blood glucose concentration. Parasympathetic stimulation increases glucose uptake and glycogen synthesis.

Pharmacokinetics

Drug metabolism is primarily a hepatic event. The liver influences the plasma concentration and systemic availability of most orally and parenterally administered drugs. Through its synthesis of drug-binding proteins, the liver affects the partitioning of drugs into the various compartments of the body (apparent volume of distribution, V_d). Plasma proteins, especially albumin and α_1-acid glycoprotein, act as sinks to decrease free drug concentrations. Consequently, changes in the concentration of plasma proteins often modify dose-response relationships of drugs.

Hepatic clearance is the sum of all processes by which the liver eliminates a drug from the body. Hepatic biotransformation refers to the metabolism of drugs by hepatocytes with the goal of changing them into inactive water-soluble substances that can be excreted into the bile or urine for elimination from the body. A series of reactions that have been classified as phase 1 and phase 2 participate in these processes. Most drugs contain lipophilic functional groups to facilitate penetration of membrane barriers, thereby expediting gastrointestinal absorption. These same lipophilic groups inhibit excretion, owing to a high degree of protein binding and renal tubular reabsorption. By converting lipophilic substances to metabolites that can be excreted, hepatic enzymes detoxify drugs and terminate their pharmacologic activity. In general, phase 1 reactions (oxidation, reduction, N-dealkylation) modify structural features of drugs to render them more polar than the original compound. Most phase 1 reactions involve the participation of a group of cytochrome P450 isozymes, which are localized in the hepatic microsomes. In phase 2 reactions, catalyzed by transferase enzymes, the water solubility of the product is enhanced beyond that achieved by phase 1 reactions alone. The chemical groups generated by phase 1 reactions serve as receptors for conjugation with polar substances such as sulfate, glucuronic acid, and glutathione. The products of phase 2 reactions are usually less toxic and less biologically active than those of the parent compound. Phase 1 reactions are much more susceptible to inhibition by advanced age or hepatic diseases than are phase 2 reactions.

The ability of the liver to metabolize a drug is referred to as its *intrinsic metabolic clearance*.[6] Intrinsic clearance, which reflects the fraction of the delivered drug load that is metabolized or extracted during a single pass through the liver, provides the basis for classifying drugs as high-, intermediate-, or low-clearance compounds. High-clearance drugs (e.g., lidocaine, diphenhydramine, or metoprolol) are so efficiently metabolized that their hepatic clearance approaches the rates at which they traverse the liver (i.e., total hepatic blood flow) (Fig. 48-2). Therefore, hepatic blood flow determines the liver's ability to eliminate high-clearance drugs. Low-clearance drugs (e.g., diazepam), however, are metabolized at rates that are usually far below their flow rates through the liver; therefore, their hepatic clearances are relatively independent of hepatic blood flow (Fig. 48-2). Factors that increase the free fraction of drugs (e.g., hypoalbuminemia) are much more consequential for low-extraction than high-extraction drugs. The clearance of low-extraction drugs increases almost linearly as the free fraction increases (Fig. 48-3). Patients with significant liver disease may have marked alterations of pharmacokinetics and pharmacodynamics. Portosystemic shunts allow orally administered drugs to bypass the liver, thereby reducing first-pass clearance. This and the reduction in total hepatic blood flow seen in patients with liver disease prolong the terminal half-life and increases the systemic effects of high-extraction drugs. The dosage of these agents should be reduced by as much as 50%. Hypoalbuminemia causes an increase in the free plasma drug concentration, not only increasing drug effects, but also facilitating elimination of compounds with low hepatic extraction ratios. The volume of distribution of some drugs will be increased in patients with hypoalbuminemia and ascites.

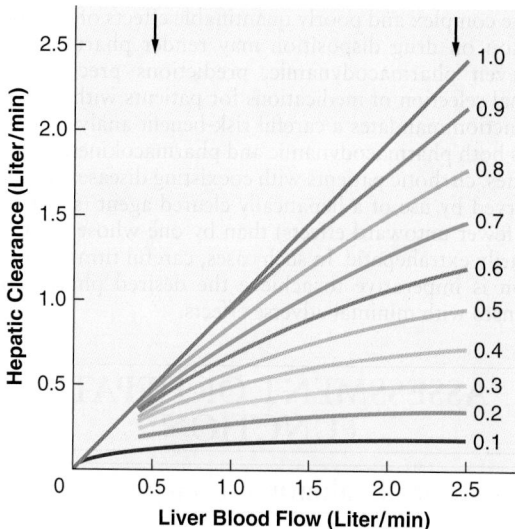

FIGURE 48-2. Relationship between hepatic clearance (*ordinate, on left*) and liver blood flow (*abscissa*) as determined by the extraction ratios of the drug (*ordinate, on right*). Hepatic clearances of compounds with low extraction ratios are nearly independent of liver blood flow, whereas the clearances of compounds with high extraction ratios vary almost directly with changes in hepatic blood flow. The *arrows* indicate the normal physiologic range of liver blood flow. (Reprinted from Wilkinson GR, Shand DG: A physiological approach to hepatic drug clearance. Clin Pharmacol Ther 1975; 18: 377, with permission.)

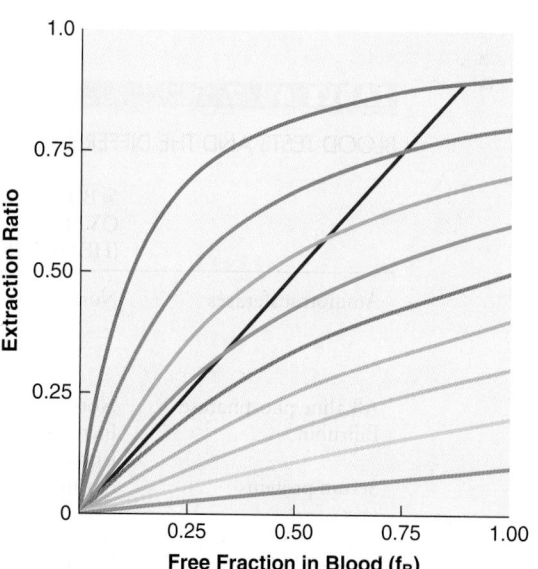

FIGURE 48-3. Relationship between hepatic extraction and fraction of unbound drug in blood: increasing free fraction (more unbound drug) usually produces increased extraction. This phenomenon is of greater importance for low-extraction drugs (with almost a direct linear change in extraction ratio with increasing free fraction) than for high-extraction drugs because the latter are almost completely cleared, regardless of extent of binding (nonrestrictive binding). The hepatic clearance (CL) reflects the changes in extraction ratio (E) if blood flow (Q) is constant (CL = Q · E). (Reprinted from Wilkinson GR, Shand DG: A physiological approach to hepatic drug clearance. Clin Pharmacol Ther 1975; 18: 377, with permission.)

The complex and poorly quantifiable effects of hepatic dysfunction on drug disposition may render pharmacokinetic, and even pharmacodynamic, predictions precarious. The rational selection of medications for patients with severe liver dysfunction mandates a careful risk-benefit analysis that integrates both pharmacodynamic and pharmacokinetic concerns. At times, cirrhotic patients with coexisting diseases will be better served by use of a hepatically cleared agent (superior efficacy, fewer untoward effects) than by one whose clearance is primarily extrahepatic. In such cases, careful titration of medication is imperative to achieve the desired pharmacologic responses with minimal adverse effects.

ASSESSMENT OF HEPATIC FUNCTION

Laboratory Evaluation of Hepatic Function

A broad array of biochemical tests is available to assess the multiple functions of the liver (Table 48-2) and to evaluate patients with suspected or established liver disease.[7] Although collectively called *liver function tests* (LFTs), many (e.g., aspartate aminotransferase [AST] and alanine aminotransferase [ALT]) do not assess a function of the liver but rather are indicative of liver cell injury or dysfunction. LFTs are used to screen for the presence of liver disease, suggest a general category of disease as the etiology, assess prognosis, and monitor the effectiveness of therapy. Many of the routine tests are not specific for liver disease; however, when combined in a battery of tests, the sensitivity and specificity for liver disease is high.

LFTs can be classified into several broad categories. These include tests that reflect (1) hepatocellular damage; (2) obstructed bile flow; (3) hepatic synthetic function; (4) hepatic uptake, conjugation, and excretion; and (5) other aspects of liver function.

Indices of Hepatocellular Damage

Increased serum activities of AST (formerly, serum glutamic oxalacetic transaminase or SGOT) and ALT (formerly, serum glutamic pyruvic transaminase or SGPT) are detected when there is hepatocellular injury and necrosis. Serum levels of AST and ALT are elevated in almost all types of hepatic disease. ALT is localized primarily to the liver, whereas AST is present in a wide variety of tissues, including liver, heart, skeletal muscle, kidney, and brain. An isolated elevation of the AST level is typically seen in cardiac or muscle disease. Mild elevations of ALT and AST (less than threefold) are seen in fatty liver, nonalcoholic steatohepatitis, drug toxicity, and chronic viral hepatitis. Larger increases (3- to 22-fold) are seen in patients with acute hepatitis or exacerbation of chronic hepatitis (alcoholic hepatitis). The highest concentrations are seen in drug-induced or toxin-induced hepatocellular necrosis (including anesthetics), severe viral hepatitis, and ischemic hepatitis complicating circulatory shock.

AST and ALT levels do not correlate with prognosis. A declining level may reflect either recovery from injury or a poor prognosis because of a paucity of surviving hepatocytes. The serum AST/ALT ratio may be helpful diagnostically. A ratio of >2 is characteristically found in alcoholic liver disease, while in viral hepatitis the ratio is typically <1.

Lactate dehydrogenase (LDH) is usually included in liver biochemistry panels. Markedly increased serum levels may be seen in hepatocellular necrosis, shock liver, or hemolysis associated with liver disease. However, LDH has poor diagnostic specificity for liver disease and even measurement of LDH isoenzymes has limited clinical usefulness.

TABLE 48-2

BLOOD TESTS AND THE DIFFERENTIAL DIAGNOSIS OF HEPATIC DYSFUNCTION

	■ BILIRUBIN OVERLOAD (HEMOLYSIS)	■ PARENCHYMAL DYSFUNCTION	■ CHOLESTASIS
Aminotransferases	Normal	Increased (may be normal or decreased in advanced stages)	Normal (may be increased in advanced stages)
Alkaline phosphatase	Normal	Normal	Increased
Bilirubin	Increased Unconjugated	Increased Conjugated	Increased Conjugated
Serum proteins	Normal	Decreased	Normal (may be decreased in advanced stages)
Prothrombin time	Normal	Decreased (may be normal in early stages)	Normal (may be prolonged in advanced stages)
Blood urea nitrogen	Normal	Normal (may be decreased in advanced stages)	Normal
Sulfobromophthalein/ indocyanine green	Normal	Retention	Normal or retention

From Gelman S: Anesthesia and the liver, Clinical Anesthesia, 3rd edition. Edited by Barash P, Cullen B, Stoelting, R. Philadelphia, Lippincott-Raven, 1997, p 1011.

Glutathione S-transferase (GST) is found in multiple organs, but plasma elevation of isoenzyme B is a sensitive indicator of liver damage. GST is rapidly released into the circulation following hepatic injury, and because of its short plasma half-life (90 minutes), monitoring of plasma GST concentrations permits rapid identification of continuing or resolving cellular damage. GST is most abundant in centrolobular (zone 3) hepatocytes, which are most susceptible to injuries from circulatory disturbances and toxic products of drug metabolism.[8] Following such injuries, GST elevations may be disproportionately greater than increases of serum transaminases, which are more highly localized to the periportal (zone 1) hepatocytes.

Indices of Obstructed Bile Flow

Alkaline phosphatase (AP) is a family of isoenzymes found in multiple organs, including the liver, bone, kidney, intestines, placenta, and leukocytes. In healthy individuals, most circulating AP originates from the liver or bone. In the liver, AP is concentrated in the microvilli of the bile canaliculi and the sinusoidal surface of hepatocytes. Elevations of serum AP disproportionate to changes of AST and ALT occur with intrahepatic or extrahepatic obstruction to bile flow. It is a highly sensitive test for assessing the integrity of the biliary system. Elevated serum levels of AP may also result from infiltrative liver diseases such as metastatic cancer. Mildly elevated levels of serum AP are nonspecific and may be seen in cirrhosis, hepatitis, or congestive heart failure. The liver is the source of an elevated AP in the majority of cases, but in up to one-third, no evidence of liver disease is found. During pregnancy, AP can nearly double from placental release of the enzyme.

5'-Nucleotidase (5'NT) is an alkaline phosphatase that degrades specific nucleotides. Although it is present in most human tissues, elevated serum levels are believed to be solely of hepatobiliary origin and may reflect the detergent action of bile salts on plasma membranes, which is needed for release of the enzyme into the circulation. 5'NT is markedly increased with intrahepatic or extrahepatic biliary obstruction, with more modest increases seen with other hepatocellular disorders. Serum levels correlate closely with AP levels, and because serum 5'NT is so specific for liver diseases, it is used to determine if an elevated serum AP level is of hepatic origin.

γ-Glutamyl transferase (GGT) is a membrane-bound enzyme widely distributed in a variety of tissues, including the liver. It is found in high concentrations in epithelial cells lining biliary ductules. Serum GGT is the most sensitive laboratory indicator of biliary tract disease. However, because it is ubiquitous, an elevated GGT has limited usefulness because of its poor specificity and has largely been replaced by 5'NT measurements to determine if an elevated AP is of hepatic origin.

Bilirubin is an endogenous organic anion derived primarily from the degradation of hemoglobin released from aging red blood cells. Measurement of serum bilirubin levels is central to the evaluation of hepatobiliary disorders. Serum levels of bilirubin are determined by the van den Bergh reaction, which separates bilirubin into two fractions: a water-soluble, direct-reacting form representing conjugated bilirubin and a lipid-soluble, indirect-reacting form representing unconjugated bilirubin.

Serum bilirubin levels are measured to confirm the severity of jaundice and to determine the extent of its conjugation. Hyperbilirubinemia has a wide variety of causes (Table 48-3) and is classified as either predominantly unconjugated or predominantly conjugated. Serum concentrations of unconju-

TABLE 48-3

CAUSES OF HYPERBILIRUBINEMIA

■ UNCONJUGATED (INDIRECT)

Excessive bilirubin production (hemolysis)
Immaturity of enzyme systems
    Physiologic jaundice of newborn
    Jaundice of prematurity
Inherited defects
    Gilbert syndrome
    Crigler-Najjar syndrome
Drug effects

■ CONJUGATED (DIRECT)

Hepatocellular disease (hepatitis, cirrhosis, drugs)
Intrahepatic cholestasis (drugs, pregnancy)
Benign postoperative jaundice, sepsis
Congenital conjugated hyperbilirubinemia
    Dubin-Johnson syndrome
    Rotor syndrome
Obstructive jaundice
    Extrahepatic (calculus, stricture, neoplasm)
    Intrahepatic (sclerosing cholangitis, neoplasm, primary biliary cirrhosis)

From Friedman L, Martin P, Munoz S: Liver function tests and the objective evaluation of the patient with liver disease, Hepatology: A Textbook of Liver Disease, 3rd edition. Edited by Zakim D, Boyer T. Philadelphia, WB Saunders, 1996, p 791, with permission.

gated bilirubin between 1 and 4 mg/dL usually indicate a disorder of bilirubin metabolism, such as excessive production (hemolysis), impaired transport into hepatocytes, or defective conjugation by hepatocytes. Even in cases of severe hemolysis, the total serum bilirubin is rarely above 5 mg/dL in the presence of normal liver function. Serum bilirubin levels above 5 mg/dL, or lower levels in association with other LFT abnormalities, usually signify the presence of liver disease. Conjugated hyperbilirubinemia results from impaired intrahepatic excretion of bilirubin or extrahepatic obstruction. With complete biliary tract obstruction, the maximal serum bilirubin level will rarely exceed 35 mg/dL because of renal excretion of conjugated bilirubin. Therefore, total bilirubin levels above 35 mg/dL usually signify severe parenchymal liver disease in association with hemolysis or renal failure.

Indices of Hepatic Synthetic Function

The liver synthesizes and releases a variety of proteins, including albumin and the coagulation factors. Measurement of serum albumin level and assays of coagulation function are the most widely used methods for assessing hepatic synthetic function. Proper interpretation of these tests requires an understanding of the patient's clinical status. Many factors influence the serum albumin level independent of hepatic synthesis. Protein-losing enteropathy, burns, nephrotic syndrome, increased vascular permeability, nutritional deficiency, increased catabolism, and fluid retention can all depress serum albumin levels. A decreasing serum albumin concentration indicates worsening hepatic function in patients with chronic liver disease if none of these other factors is present. Because the half-life in serum is as long as 20 days, the serum albumin level is not a reliable indicator of hepatic protein synthesis in acute liver disease.

In contrast, the prothrombin time (PT) and international normalized ratio (INR) are sensitive indicators of severe

ANESTHESIA FOR SURGICAL SUBSPECIALTIES

hepatic dysfunction (whether patients have acute or chronic liver disease) because of the short half-life of factor VII. However, because most of the coagulation factors are present in quantities that far exceed requirements for normal coagulation, mild-to-moderate hepatic disease may not be detected by measurement of the PT. In acute or chronic hepatocellular disease, the PT may be a useful prognostic indicator. A progressively increasing PT is usually ominous in patients with acute hepatocellular disease, suggesting an increased likelihood of acute hepatic failure. Prolongation of the PT also suggests a poor long-term prognosis in chronic liver disease.

PT depends on normal hepatic synthesis of clotting factors and sufficient uptake of vitamin K. Absorption of vitamin K from the gastrointestinal tract requires adequate biliary secretion of bile salts. In patients with obstructive jaundice, a prolonged PT may be a manifestation of vitamin K deficiency rather than of impaired hepatic synthetic function. Prolongation of the PT is not specific for liver disease. It may result from congenital coagulation factor deficiencies, disseminated intravascular coagulopathy, vitamin K deficiency, or the use of drugs that antagonize the prothrombin complex, such as warfarin.

Indices of Hepatic Blood Flow and Metabolic Capacity

Elimination of the dye indocyanine green (ICG) from the blood provides an estimate of hepatic perfusion and hepatocellular function because it is highly extracted (70 to 95% by the liver following an intravenous injection). Acute changes in hepatic circulation and function can be detected by this test and the ICG method has been a standard technique for comparing effects of various anesthetics on hepatic blood flow.

Hepatic function can also be assessed with substances that are metabolized selectively by the liver. Lidocaine is metabolized by oxidative N-demethylation to monoethylglycinexylidide (MEGX). Its concentration 15 to 30 minutes after intravenous injection of a single dose of lidocaine can be used as a quantitative measure of liver function. The MEGX test may have prognostic value in patients with end-stage liver disease; in one study of well-compensated cirrhotic patients, this test was able to identify patients at increased risk for developing postoperative complications following hepatic resection for carcinoma.[9]

Additional metabolic tests for assessing hepatic function include antipyrine clearance from plasma, aminopyrine breath test, caffeine breath test, galactose elimination capacity, and the maximum rate of urea synthesis. These tests have not gained wide acceptance in the United States, and their precise role in clinical practice remains uncertain.

Miscellaneous Tests

Several other laboratory tests are available for the diagnosis of liver disease but provide no specific information about hepatic function. These include specific serologic tests for hepatitis viruses, autoantibody measurements useful for the diagnosis of primary biliary cirrhosis and the classification of autoimmune hepatitis; specific protein measurements (ceruloplasmin, ferritin, α_1-antitrypsin, and α-fetoprotein) useful for the diagnosis of Wilson disease; hemochromatosis; α_1-antitrypsin deficiency and hepatocellular carcinoma, respectively; and serum ammonia often followed in patients with, or at risk for, developing hepatic encephalopathy.

Hepatobiliary Imaging

Selection of the most appropriate hepatobiliary imaging technique in a patient depends on the clinical presentation (history,

physical examination, and LFT results), an understanding of the uses and limitations of each technique, and whether the test is for diagnosis alone or for therapeutic intervention as well.

Plain radiography has a limited role in the evaluation of hepatobiliary disease. Abdominal radiographs can be useful for calcified or gas-containing lesions that may be overlooked or misinterpreted by ultrasonography. These lesions include calcified gallstones, chronic calcific pancreatitis, gas-containing liver abscesses, portal venous gas, and emphysematous cholecystitis.

Ultrasonography is the primary screening test for hepatic disease, gallstones, and biliary tract disease that may be suspected because of symptoms, abnormal LFT, hepatomegaly, jaundice, or suspicion of a mass lesion. It is the best method for detecting gallstones and confirming the presence of extrahepatic biliary obstruction. It also may be useful for determining the thickness of the gallbladder wall, detecting the presence of ascites, demonstrating portal or hepatic vein thrombosis, evaluating the patency of portosystemic shunts in patients with recurrent variceal bleeding after shunt surgery, and directing thin-needle biopsy of hepatic mass lesions. Its major limitations are its dependence on the operator's skill and its inability to penetrate bone or air (including bowel gas), which may prevent complete examination of the abdominal organs.

A variety of radioisotopes can be used to study the anatomy and function of the liver and biliary system. Radioisotope scanning of the liver seldom provides a precise diagnosis, and these tests have largely been supplanted by ultrasonography and computed tomography (CT) scanning. However, radioisotope scanning of the biliary tract remains an important investigative tool in patients with suspected acute cholecystitis. Radioisotopes that are cleared rapidly by hepatocytes and excreted into bile permit rapid visualization of the biliary tract. Visualization of the gallbladder rules out obstruction of the cystic duct, while visualization of the biliary tree and common bile duct without the gallbladder confirms obstruction of the cystic duct and presence of cholecystitis.

CT is a complementary examination to ultrasonography and provides information on liver texture, gallbladder disease, bile duct dilatation, and mass lesions of the liver and pancreas. It provides better and more complete anatomic definition than ultrasonography and is less operator-dependent. Lesions can be biopsied under CT guidance. The disadvantages of CT scanning are radiation exposure and cost.

The role of magnetic resonance imaging (MRI) for the evaluation of hepatobiliary disease is evolving. The algorithm for noninvasive biliary imaging has been markedly altered by the development of magnetic resonance cholangiopancreatography, which has dramatically reduced the need for direct cholangiography for visualization of the bile and pancreatic ducts, and for delineating the most proximal extent of biliary tract obstruction when planning for operative resection or drainage.

Percutaneous transhepatic cholangiography (THC) involves the direct percutaneous injection through a 22-gauge needle of contrast into bile ducts in the liver under fluoroscopic guidance. THC may be used to determine the level and cause of biliary obstruction, confirm the presence of cholestasis without obstruction, and evaluate whether a proximal cholangiocarcinoma is surgically resectable. THC can be used for balloon dilation of biliary strictures via a catheter inserted through the tract, for placement of an internal stent to relieve obstruction, or for placement of an external drain.

Endoscopic retrograde cholangiopancreatography (ERCP) uses endoscopy to visualize the ampulla of Vater and guide insertion of a guidewire and catheter through the ampulla to permit selective injection of contrast material into the pancreatic and common bile ducts, which are then imaged radiographically. ERCP has the advantage over THC of not requiring dilation of the biliary tree to achieve a very high procedural success rate. ERCP is the imaging technique of choice in patients with choledocholithiasis because a sphincterotomy and stone extraction can often be performed. Stones can also be removed with this technique in patients with acute cholangitis and severe gallstone pancreatitis. ERCP also permits biopsies, brushings, balloon dilation, and stent insertion to relieve biliary obstruction caused by tumors.

Liver Biopsy

Liver biopsy continues to have a central role in the evaluation of patients with suspected liver disease because it provides the only means of determining the precise nature of hepatic damage (necrosis, inflammation, steatosis, or fibrosis). Liver biopsy plays a key role in the evaluation of otherwise unexplained abnormalities of liver enzymes in patients with or without hepatomegaly. It is used in patients with chronic hepatitis to determine the nature and extent of hepatic injury and degree of inflammation, which for patients with chronic HCV will be used to determine if antiviral therapy should be initiated. Liver biopsy is also an important tool for determining the etiology of abnormal LFT in the postliver transplant patient (see Chapter 54). The presence of coagulopathy (e.g., PT that is 3 seconds greater than control, platelet count <60,000 cells/μL), however, contraindicates percutaneous liver biopsy, although transjugular liver biopsy can be performed safely in these patients.

HEPATIC AND HEPATOBILIARY DISEASES

Classification of Liver Diseases

For the purposes of the following discussion, liver diseases are divided into two large heterogeneous groups: parenchymal diseases (e.g., viral hepatitis, steatohepatitis, cirrhosis) and cholestatic diseases (e.g., intrahepatic and extrahepatic biliary obstruction). Some diseases are characterized by features of both parenchymal dysfunction and cholestasis.

Prevalence of Hepatobiliary Disease

More than 100 distinct hepatic diseases have been described. Currently, nearly 10% of the American population (25 million) has some form of hepatobiliary disease. Hepatitis B or C afflicts more than 5 million Americans. About 50% of those with HCV may develop cirrhosis, which currently accounts for between 13,000 and 15,000 deaths each year. Alcoholic liver disease remains a problem, becoming severe in 10 to 15% of those who consume large amounts of alcohol over a prolonged period.

PARENCHYMAL DISEASES

Viral Hepatitis

Acute hepatitis usually results from a viral infection, although it may also be caused by drugs and toxins. Viral hepatitides are important causes of perioperative hepatic dysfunction. The diagnosis of viral hepatitis depends on the appearance of clinical signs and symptoms, laboratory findings, serologic assays, and, on occasion, liver biopsy. During the incubation period,

patients are often asymptomatic and may undergo surgical procedures. When increased ALT and AST and/or jaundice develop postoperatively, it is essential that a comprehensive serologic evaluation be performed to document the viral origin for the liver damage.

Classic acute hepatitis is caused by one of five viruses: hepatitis A (HAV), hepatitis B (HBV), hepatitis C (HCV), hepatitis D (HDV, delta), and hepatitis E (HEV). In the United States, approximately 50% of reported cases of acute viral hepatitis are caused by HBV, 30% by HAV, and 20% by HCV. Chronic hepatitis can occur following HBV, HCV, and HDV infections. All five types of viral hepatitis have similar clinical and laboratory features. Patients may remain asymptomatic, develop influenzalike symptoms, became jaundiced, or develop acute hepatic failure.

HAV infection (infectious hepatitis) is a highly contagious enterovirus transmitted by the intake of fecal-contaminated food. It is not transmitted by blood transfusion. Viremia is present for several days prior to the onset of clinical symptoms. Virus is shed in stool for 14 to 21 days before the onset of jaundice. Patients are usually not infectious after 21 days. There are no chronic carriers, and chronic liver disease does not occur. Fulminant hepatic failure is rare (0.14 to 2%) in the absence of pre-existing liver disease. Patients with HBV who acquire a HAV infection typically have an uncomplicated clinical course. In contrast, 41% of patients with chronic HCV who acquire a HAV superinfection progress to fulminant hepatitis with a 35% fatality rate.[10]

HBV is primarily transmitted through percutaneous inoculation of infected serum or blood products. HBV is present in the serum and body secretions of most patients early in the course of acute HBV. The surface coat of the virus is composed of a polypeptide that acts as the major HBV surface antigen (HBsAg). Development of serum antibodies to HbsAg (anti-HbsAg) confirms immunity. Individuals who have detectable HbsAg for >6 months have a chronic HBV infection.

HCV (formerly, non-A, non-B hepatitis), which was discovered in 1989, was the major cause of transfusion-related hepatitis until the 1990s. It is also transmitted by percutaneous inoculation of infected serum or blood products, occupational exposure to blood or blood products, and intravenous drug abuse. HCV is the most common blood-borne infection in the United States; it accounts for 40% of chronic liver disease. Fortunately, serologic tests for HCV now exist.[11] Because of their use in screening donated blood, HCV has almost been eliminated as a cause of posttransfusion hepatitis. HDV is an RNA strand that coinfects with and requires the helper function of HBV for its replication and expression. HDV may be acquired simultaneously with HBV or may be a superinfection of a patient with prior HBV infection. HBV and HDV coinfection substantially increases the likelihood of fulminant hepatitis and death.

HEV is an enterically transmitted virus that has epidemiologic features resembling HAV. HEV infections occur primarily in Asia, Africa, and Central America.

Other important but infrequent causes of viral hepatitis include cytomegalovirus, Epstein-Barr virus, and herpes simplex. These viruses typically produce benign, anicteric disease and often escape detection preoperatively. However, in rare circumstances, particularly in immunocompromised patients, they can disseminate, causing acute hepatitis, fulminant hepatic failure, and death.

Acute viral hepatitis occurs after an incubation period that varies with the specific virus involved. The mean incubation period for HAV is 4 weeks, for HBV 12 weeks, and for HCV 7 weeks. Clinical disease is often heralded by the development of constitutional symptoms such as anorexia, nausea, vomiting, and low-grade fever. Dark urine and clay-colored stools usually precede the onset of jaundice. At this point, the liver may be enlarged and tender. Recovery usually takes weeks to months. Many patients with acute viral hepatitis never become clinically jaundiced. AST and ALT levels begin to rise during the prodromal phase and usually reach a peak between 400 and 4,000 IU when the patient is clinically jaundiced. Serologic tests are the mainstay for the diagnosis of viral hepatitis. The diagnosis of HAV is based on the detection of serum immunoglobulin M (IgM) antibody to the HAV capsid or HAV RNA in stool during acute illness; recovery is associated with immunoglobulin G anti-HAV antibody, which confers long-lasting immunity to recurrent HAV infection. The diagnosis of HBV infection is usually made by identifying HbsAg in serum. HbsAg may be present in serum as early as 7 days after HBV infection. Infrequently, levels of HbsAg are too low to be detected during acute HBV infection, and in such cases, the diagnosis can be established by the identification of IgM antibody to the HBV core antigen (IgM anti-Hbc). Hepatitis Be antigen (HbeAg) follows the pattern of HbsAg, and recovery is heralded by the disappearance of this antigen, while persistence of HbeAg identifies patients whose blood remains infective. Development of antibody to HbsAg (anti-Hbs) is seen in recovered patients.

The serologic diagnosis of HCV can be made by demonstrating the presence in serum of anti-HCV or the presence of HCV RNA. HBD infection can be identified by demonstrating the presence of anti-HDV antibody.

Nonviral Hepatitis

Toxin- and Drug-Induced Hepatitis

Acute hepatitis may follow the ingestion, inhalation, or parenteral administration of pharmacologic and chemical agents. Drugs and chemicals that are directly toxic to the liver (carbon tetrachloride, acetaminophen, α-amanitin from the toxic mushroom, *Amanita phalloides*) predictably produce dose-dependent liver injury. Each of these direct hepatotoxins produces a pattern of histologic injury that is reasonably characteristic and reproducible. Clinical manifestations of liver injury usually occur within 1 to 2 days of exposure. Acetaminophen not only causes fulminant hepatic failure following ingestion of extremely large doses (suicide attempts), but can also produce chronic liver injury with analgesic doses in susceptible individuals (malnutrition, chronic alcoholism).[12]

Other drugs (nonsteroidal anti-inflammatory agents, volatile anesthetics, antibiotics, antihypertensives, anticonvulsants) infrequently cause liver injury. These idiosyncratic drug reactions are unpredictable, and the response is not dose-dependent. Hepatitis may develop during or shortly after exposure to the drug, but more commonly, clinical signs of liver dysfunction occur 2 to 6 weeks after initiation. Treatment of toxin-induced and drug-induced hepatitis is largely supportive. Failure to discontinue the offending drug promptly may result in progressive hepatitis and death. Hemodialysis may be useful following ingestion of *A. phalloides*, whereas *N*-acetylcysteine is used to treat patients with potentially hepatotoxic ingestions of acetaminophen. Liver transplantation may be lifesaving in patients with fulminant hepatitis, resulting from toxin or drug ingestion.

Toxic Acute Hepatitis and Volatile Anesthetics

Halothane was introduced in the United States in 1958; concerns linking this agent to acute hepatitis were raised shortly thereafter. To determine the incidence of massive hepatic necrosis after halothane anesthesia, the Committee on Anesthesia of the National Academy of Sciences launched one of the largest epidemiologic studies ever completed: the National Halothane Study.[13] From 1959 to 1962, 856,000 anesthetics were retrospectively reviewed. The incidence of fulminant hepatic necrosis terminating in death associated with halothane was found to be 1 per 35,000 anesthetics. The incidence of nonfatal hepatitis, however, may be as high as 1 in 3,000.[14] The association prompted a dramatic decrease in the use of halothane, especially in adult patients. Other volatile anesthetic agents have been reported to cause hepatitis, but at a much lower rate.[15]

The classic presentation of volatile anesthetic-associated hepatitis includes fever, anorexia, nausea, chills, myalgias, and rash, followed by the appearance of jaundice 3 to 6 days later. The syndrome characteristically develops after minor uneventful procedures of brief duration (<30 minutes). Overt jaundice indicates severe disease and portends a mortality rate as high as 40%. Other predictors of poor prognosis include a short latency between the anesthetic and the onset of symptoms, certain demographic factors (age >40, obesity), and severe hepatic dysfunction.

The single most important risk factor for halothane hepatitis is prior exposure to halothane. Previous exposure has also been reported as a factor in isoflurane-associated hepatitis.[16] Of the patients who develop jaundice after halothane, 71 to 95% have had at least one prior exposure to this agent.[17] Severe reactions occur nearly 10 times more often in patients who have had multiple exposures to halothane than in those having their first halothane anesthetic.[18]

Demographic factors also provide important information about the risk of developing halothane hepatitis. Obese women appear to be more likely than their nonobese counterparts to contract halothane hepatitis. The disease may also have a genetic basis.[19] Some ethnic groups, such as Mexican Americans, seem to be at greater risk, and chromosomal differences have been noted between patients who recovered from halothane hepatitis and halothane-treated patients who never had the disease.[20,21] For reasons that are not yet clear, age is also a significant risk factor. Approximately 50% of the cases of halothane-associated fulminant hepatic failure occur in patients older than 50, whereas children are highly resistant to the development of halothane hepatitis.[18,22,23] The rare cases documented in children have involved multiple exposures to halothane.[24] Notably, neither pre-existing liver disease nor concomitant administration of medication has been identified as a risk factor for halothane hepatitis.

Although the incidence of hepatitis appears to correlate with the degree of metabolism of the various agents, the paucity of cases reported with anesthetics other than halothane has cast doubt that any of these anesthetics was actually involved in the hepatic complications.

Isoflurane metabolism yields highly reactive intermediates (TF-acetyl chloride; acyl ester) that bind covalently to hepatic proteins The likelihood that isoflurane causes hepatitis via production of these intermediates appears to be extremely low, however, as just 0.2% of the isoflurane taken up into the body is actually metabolized. Only trace amounts of isoflurane-derived adducts are bound to hepatic proteins following isoflurane anesthesia.

Desflurane, which is similarly biotransformed to trifluoroacetyl metabolites, appears even less likely than isoflurane to cause immune injury because only 0.02 to 0.2% of this agent is metabolized (1/1,000th that of halothane). Desflurane metabolites are usually undetectable in plasma, except after prolonged administration. Furthermore, although antibodies from patients with halothane hepatitis clearly react with proteins isolated from halothane-treated or enflurane-treated rats, they do not appear to react with hepatic proteins from desflurane-treated or isoflurane-treated rats.[25]

Sevoflurane is metabolized more extensively than is isoflurane or desflurane, slightly less than enflurane, and much less

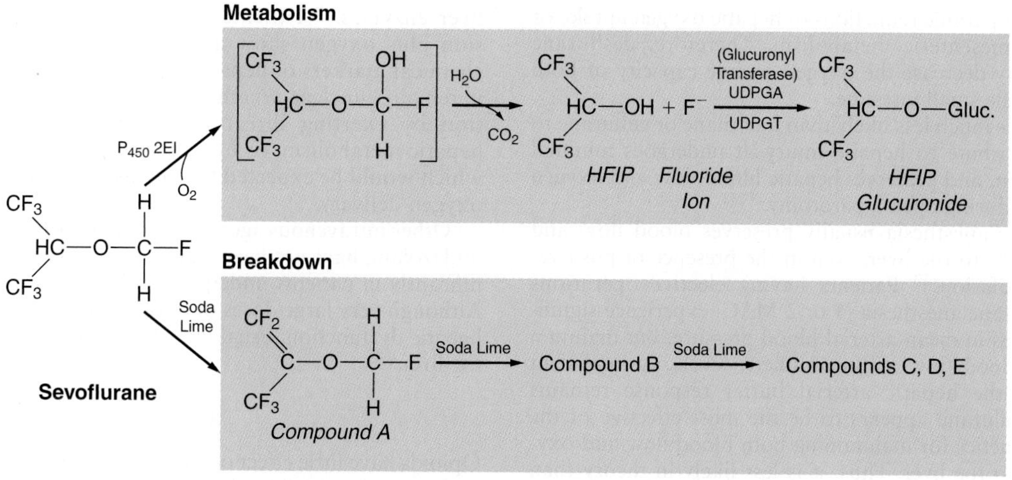

Metabolism

Breakdown

Sevoflurane

Compound A

FIGURE 48-4. Cytochrome P450 2E1-catalyzed biotransformation of sevoflurane produces inorganic fluoride and hexafluoroisopropanol (HFIP). The liver rapidly metabolizes HFIP to HFIP-glucuronide. Sevoflurane also undergoes breakdown in soda lime, yielding compound A, which is nephrotoxic but does not appear to be hepatotoxic. (Modified from Mushlin PS, Gelman S: Liver dysfunction after anesthesia, Anesthesia and Perioperative Complications, 2nd edition. Edited by Benumof JL, Saidman LJ. St. Louis, MO, Mosby, 1999, p 442, with permission; modified from Frink EJ Jr: The hepatic effects of sevoflurane. Anesth Analg 1995; 81[suppl 6]: S46.)

ANESTHESIA FOR SURGICAL SUBSPECIALTIES

than halothane.[26] The metabolism of sevoflurane (primarily via cytochrome P450 2E1) is rapid (1.5 to 2 times faster than enflurane) and produces detectable plasma concentrations of fluoride and hexafluoroisopropanol (HFIP) within minutes of initiating the anesthetic. The liver conjugates most of the HFIP with glucuronic acid, which is then excreted by the kidney (Fig. 48-4). An important distinction between sevoflurane and the other volatile agents is that sevoflurane produces neither highly reactive metabolites nor fluoroacetylated liver proteins. There is no evidence that any sevoflurane metabolites cause severe hepatic injury.

Volatile Agents and Hepatic Blood Flow and Oxygen Delivery

Because halogenated anesthetics depress cardiac output and most surgical procedures stimulate catecholamine-induced vasoconstriction, hepatic blood flow and oxygen delivery decrease during general anesthesia and surgery. The degree to which hepatic metabolic demands are also depressed with the various agents determines the relative impact on the hepatic supply-demand relationship, and consequently, the potential of each agent for causing hepatic ischemia.

Other perioperative conditions also contribute to hepatic blood flow, oxygen delivery, and metabolic requirements: hemoglobin concentration, oxygen saturation, systemic inflammation, volume status, and temperature. Additional insults such as direct hepatic trauma and hepatotoxic drug exposure, as well as occult pre-existing hepatic insufficiency, can obscure the independent effects of the volatile agent.

Both animal and human studies indicate that halothane is more likely than other inhaled anesthetics to produce liver injury, probably because it causes the most cardiovascular and respiratory depression, as well as the greatest reduction in hepatic arterial flow (Fig. 48-5). Consequently, halothane is the most likely of the clinically used vapors to produce, or exacerbate, hepatic hypoxia when blood flow to the liver is critically limited and the adequacy of the oxygen supply-to-demand balance is in question.

Excluding halothane, enflurane decreases hepatic blood flow and splanchnic perfusion more than any other halogenated vapor in clinical use. It induces dose-dependant

decreases in portal venous blood flow and either reduces or leaves unchanged hepatic arterial blood flow.[27,28] Splanchnic perfusion decreases in parallel with decreased mean arterial pressure and cardiac output. Enflurane also increases splanchnic oxygen extraction, and lowers both hepatic venous and mixed venous oxygen saturation.

Desflurane decreases hepatic blood flow in both experimental and clinical settings. Administration of 1 minimum alveolar concentration (MAC) desflurane to patients prior to skin incision reportedly decreases hepatic blood flow by 30% (measured by ICG), similar to the reduction associated with 1 MAC of halothane or isoflurane.[29] Desflurane can markedly reduce oxygen delivery to the liver and small intestine without

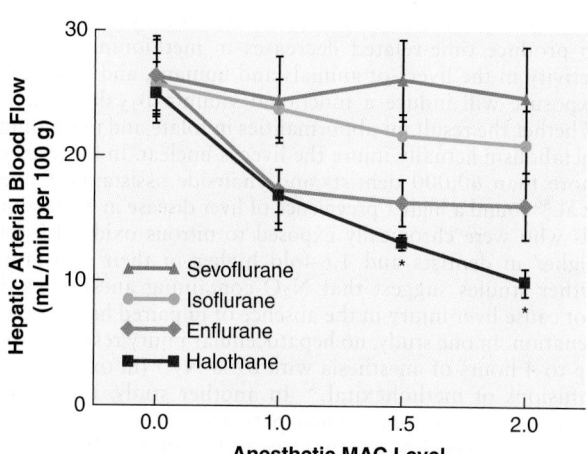

FIGURE 48-5. Dose-dependent effects of inhaled anesthetics on hepatic arterial flow in chronically instrumented dogs in the absence of a surgical stress. Sevoflurane and isoflurane preserve hepatic arterial flow even at the higher minimum alveolar concentration (MAC) levels. *Differs from sevoflurane and isoflurane at same MAC values ($p < 0.05$). †Differs from sevoflurane at same MAC value ($p < 0.05$). (Reprinted from Frink EJ Jr: The hepatic effects of sevoflurane. Anesth Analg 1995; 8[suppl 6]: S46, with permission.)

producing comparable reductions of hepatic oxygen uptake or hepatic and mesenteric metabolism. Therefore, desflurane anesthesia may decrease the oxygen reserve capacity of both the liver and the small intestine.

Isoflurane is much less likely than halothane or enflurane to cause or contribute to hepatic injury. It undergoes minimal biodegradation, and preserves hepatic blood flow and oxygen delivery even during open laparotomy.[30,31]

Sevoflurane anesthesia usually preserves blood flow and oxygen delivery to the liver, even in the presence of positive-pressure ventilation.[32] Patients having elective operations under sevoflurane anesthesia (1 or 2 MAC) experience significant reductions in mean arterial blood pressure, but maintain the hepatic blood flow at preanesthetic levels. Animal data suggest that the hepatic arterial buffer response remains intact.[33] Sevoflurane appears to be the most effective of the inhaled anesthetics for maintaining both blood flow and oxygen delivery to the liver. Thus, it is less likely in theory than either halothane or enflurane to induce liver injury and is no more toxic than desflurane or isoflurane. Its metabolic products are less reactive, and therefore probably less injurious, than those resulting from halothane, enflurane, isoflurane, or even desflurane.[34] Other than sevoflurane, desflurane is the least likely of the halogenated vapors to cause severe hepatic injury, based on the immune theory of anesthesia-induced hepatitis. Nonetheless, desflurane produces a greater reduction of hepatic blood flow and oxygen delivery than either isoflurane or sevoflurane. Hence, it may be more likely than the latter agents to cause liver injury in the setting of marginal hepatic oxygenation.

Anesthetics and Hepatic Functions

Nitrous Oxide

Nitrous oxide (N_2O) produces a mild increase in sympathetic nervous system tone. Consequently, one would expect mild vasoconstriction of the splanchnic vasculature, leading to a decrease in portal blood flow, and mild vasoconstriction of the hepatic arterial system. In addition, N_2O is a known inhibitor of the enzyme methionine synthase, which could potentially produce toxic hepatic effects. Even brief exposures to N_2O at concentrations used clinically are sufficient to produce time-related decreases in methionine synthase activity in the livers of animals and humans, and prolonged exposure will induce a functional vitamin B_{12} deficiency.[35] Whether the resultant abnormalities in folate and methionine metabolism actually injure the liver is unclear. In a survey of more than 60,000 dentists and chairside assistants, Cohen et al.[36] found a higher prevalence of liver disease in professionals who were chronically exposed to nitrous oxide: 1.7-fold higher in dentists and 1.6-fold higher in their assistants. Other studies suggest that N_2O-containing anesthetics do not cause liver injury in the absence of impaired hepatic oxygenation. In one study, no hepatocellular injury resulted from up to 4 hours of anesthesia with 67% N_2O (in oxygen) and infusions of methohexital.[37] In another study, no hepatic dysfunction developed when patients with mild alcoholic hepatitis received N_2O-opioid or N_2O-enflurane anesthetics for peripheral or superficial operations.[38] There is no convincing evidence that nitrous oxide per se causes hepatotoxicity in the absence of a precarious oxygen supply-demand ratio in the liver.[39]

Nonopioid Sedative-Hypnotic Agents

Because it is a sympathomimetic agent, ketamine may produce a moderate increase in serum concentrations of some liver enzymes.[40] Patients anesthetized with ketamine infusion plus oxygen show a dose-dependent increase in biochemical markers of hepatic injury.[41] Despite these findings, it remains unclear whether ketamine causes liver dysfunction by exerting direct hepatotoxic effects, by altering hepatic metabolism, or by increasing serum catecholamines, which would be expected to decrease hepatic blood flow and oxygen delivery.

Other intravenous agents, such as propofol, etomidate, and midazolam, have not been shown to alter hepatic function significantly in patients undergoing minor operative procedures. Although very large doses of thiopental (>750 mg) may cause hepatic dysfunction, usual induction doses have little effect on the liver.[42]

Opioids

Opioids have little effect on hepatic function, provided they do not impair hepatic blood flow and oxygen supply. All opioids increase tone of the common bile duct and the sphincter of Oddi, as well as the frequency of phasic contractions, leading to increases in biliary tract pressure and biliary spasm. The effect on the sphincter of Oddi does not favor one opioid over another and is not considered an absolute contraindication to narcotic analgesia, even in cases of pancreatitis.[43]

NONPHARMACOLOGIC CAUSES OF PERIOPERATIVE LIVER DYSFUNCTION

Inflammation and Sepsis

❸ The liver occupies a central position in the inflammatory response, especially when the inflammation is secondary to intra-abdominal sepsis. Because of its location downstream from the splanchnic circulation, bacteria, endotoxin, and proinflammatory cytokines (interleukin 1, interleukin 6, and tumor necrosis factor-α) are carried directly to the liver. These interact with sinusoidal Kupffer cells and stimulate hepatocytes to decrease production of certain proteins (mainly albumin), called *negative acute-phase reactants*, and increase production of others (mainly C-reactive protein and serum amyloid A), called *acute-phase reactants*. In addition, especially following blunt trauma and burns, complement and coagulation factor production also increase in the liver. Some, such as C-reactive protein and serum amyloid A, up to 30,000-fold, greatly increase the liver's metabolic demands (Fig. 48-6). With inflammation, the resulting changes in systemic vascular resistance; regional blood flow distribution; tissue oxygen extraction; coagulation status; glucose, fat, and protein metabolism; and catecholamine sensitivity can be far-reaching and profound.[44] In sepsis, hepatic arterial flow changes in a biphasic manner: an initial transient decrease followed by a marked and sustained increase in flow. The increase in hepatic artery flow occurs independent of changes in portal venous flow, suggesting a dysregulation of the physiologic hepatic arterial buffer response.[45] In sepsis, and inflammation in general, hypovolemia and splanchnic hypoperfusion are common, predictably decreasing oxygen delivery to the liver.

Hypoxia and Ischemia

The liver is exquisitely sensitive to hypoxia. In one study, patients with chronic lung disease whose blood oxygen content fell below 9 mL/dL all developed liver injury without

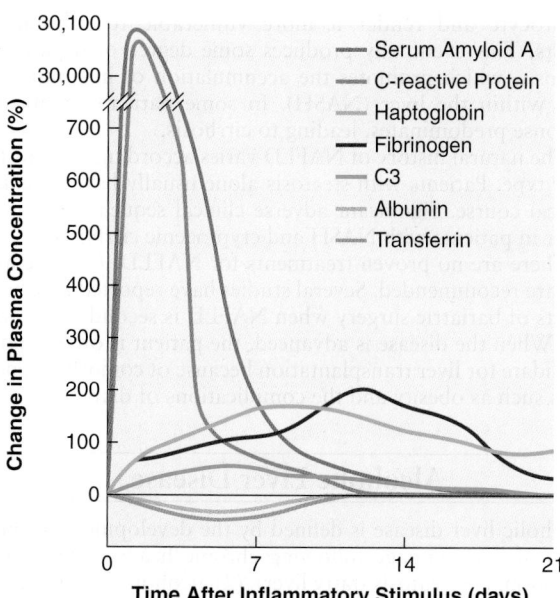

FIGURE 48-6. Characteristic patterns of change in plasma concentrations of some acute-phase proteins after a moderate inflammatory stimulus. (Reprinted from Giltin JD, Colten HR: Molecular biology of the acute phase plasma proteins, Lymphokines. Vol 14. Edited by Pick E, Landy M. San Diego, Academic Press, 1987, p 123, with permission.)

developing overt myocardial or cerebral damage.[46] The detrimental effects of oxygen deprivation on perioperative hepatic function can occur independent of anesthetic techniques.[47] In addition, if moderate hypotension occurs, a hepatitis-like illness (ischemic hepatitis) may follow. Patients develop jaundice, systemic symptoms, and large increases of serum transaminases, which may persist for 3 to 11 days. Liver biopsy shows centrilobular necrosis with little or no inflammatory response.[48]

Patients with ischemic hepatitis typically have a history of inadequate systemic perfusion, along with marked increases of serum aminotransferases. The increases are usually of greater magnitude than those associated with viral hepatitis. Prolonged shock or sepsis can cause extreme liver injury; a hepatic lobe or the entire liver may become infarcted, even in the absence of portal venous or hepatic arterial occlusion.[49] The mechanism of ischemic hepatitis is unknown, but it may involve free radical production because hepatocytes contain very high concentrations of xanthine oxidase. Ischemia and reperfusion increase xanthine oxidase activity; this enzyme catalyzes the oxidation of purines to uric acid and the associated reduction of O_2 to superoxide anion, which initiates toxic free radical reactions.

Cardiac Disease

Severe congestive heart failure may be associated with liver dysfunction.[50] The most common cause is ischemic hepatitis from decreased hepatic blood flow secondary to low cardiac output. Cardiac cirrhosis (fibrosis) may result from prolonged recurrent congestive heart failure. Acute liver failure is more likely to occur in patients with pre-existing cirrhosis, severe chronic heart failure, or sustained hepatic ischemia, although passive hepatic congestion and fulminant hepatocellular necrosis has been reported from acute, severe elevations of central venous pressures.[51]

Surgical Stress

The surgical stress response includes stimulation of the sympathetic nervous system, activation of the renin-angiotensin-aldosterone system, and the nonosmotic release of vasopressin; each of these responses may compromise the splanchnic circulation. These effects may persist for many hours or even days after surgery. Laboratory studies indicate that laparotomy, in particular, induces marked mesenteric vasoconstriction and decreases gastrointestinal and hepatic blood flow.[52] In addition to the surgical stress response, laparotomy independently decreases blood flow through the intestine and the liver, probably as a result of traction and manipulation of the viscera.[53]

Although reducing the surgical stress response and minimizing tissue injury and inflammation, laparoscopic procedures are not entirely benign with respect to the liver. The increased intra-abdominal pressures induced with insufflation appear to significantly decrease splanchnic perfusion and hepatic blood flow.[54]

Procedures performed under cardiopulmonary bypass, with low-flow states and nonpulsatile perfusion, can aggravate pre-existing hepatic dysfunction. Administration of catecholamines to improve cardiac performance, either before or after bypass, may decrease hepatic oxygen delivery. Hypothermia during cardiopulmonary bypass probably limits the hepatic injury caused by the abnormal hemodynamics. Hypotension and hemorrhage decrease portal blood flow, but the hepatic arterial buffer response and pressure-flow autoregulation tend to preserve hepatic arterial flow and oxygen delivery. Perfusion at 28°C increases portal flow and slightly decreases hepatic arterial flow. A pump flow rate of 2.4 L/min/m^2 maintains total blood flow to the liver better than does a rate of 1.2 L/min/m^2. Only at low rates does pulsatile flow appear to be more advantageous than nonpulsatile perfusion in terms of hepatic blood flow.[55]

CHRONIC HEPATITIS

Chronic hepatitis refers to a group of liver disorders of varying etiologies and severity in which hepatic inflammation and necrosis continue for at least 6 months. Chronic hepatitis was previously classified based on liver biopsy as chronic persistent or chronic active hepatitis. When this early classification was devised, chronic persistent hepatitis was considered to have a good prognosis, whereas chronic active hepatitis was considered a progressive disorder with a poor outcome. However, the prognostic value of these histologic distinctions has been found to be limited; thus, this classification has been supplanted by one based on cause, grade, and stage. Clinical and serologic features allow the establishment of an etiology for chronic hepatitis by HBV, HBV plus HDV, HCV, autoimmune hepatitis, drug-associated chronic hepatitis, and a category of cryptogenic chronic hepatitis. Histologic features on liver biopsy are necessary for grading and staging chronic hepatitis. The grade is determined by an assessment of the degree of necrosis and inflammation, and the stage reflects the level of progression of the disease, which is determined by an assessment of the degree of fibrosis.

Patients with chronic HBV infection who are asymptomatic and have normal serum transaminases are called *HbsAg carriers*. Those with chronic HBV infection who have clinical, laboratory, or pathologic evidence of chronic hepatic disease are diagnosed as having chronic HBV. An estimated 0.2 to 0.5% of the American population are chronic carriers of HbsAg. These HBV carriers are at risk for developing cirrhosis and hepatocellular carcinoma. The goal of treatment of chronic

HBV is to eradicate HBV infection, and thereby prevent the development of cirrhosis and hepatocellular carcinoma. Current therapy of chronic HBV has limited long-term efficacy and does not yet achieve these goals. However, available therapies can suppress HBV replication and lead to laboratory and histologic improvement.[56,57] The decision to initiate treatment depends on balancing the patient's age, severity of disease, likelihood of response, and potential adverse effects and complications. Treatment is not recommended for inactive HbsAg carriers. To date, six drugs have been approved for treatment of chronic HBV: interferon alfa-2b, lamivudine, adefovir, entecavir, pegylated interferon alfa-2a, and telbivudine.[58]

Chronic HCV infection follows acute HCV infection in 85% of patients; an estimated 1.8% of the United States population are carriers of HCV. Although the progression of chronic HCV infection to cirrhosis is characteristically slow, end-stage liver disease due to HCV-associated cirrhosis is the most common indication for liver transplantation. At least six distinct genotypes of HCV have been identified by nucleotide sequencing, and differences exist among these genotypes in responsiveness to antiviral therapy. Chronic HCV infection is usually treated with the combination of ribavirin and pegylated interferon alfa-2a.[59]

Autoimmune hepatitis is a chronic disease characterized by a wide spectrum of clinical symptoms, seroimmunologic manifestations, and continued hepatocellular necrosis and inflammation, which often progresses to cirrhosis. Extrahepatic features of autoimmunity, seroimmunologic abnormalities, and association with other autoimmune disorders all support an autoimmune pathogenesis. The clinical and laboratory features of autoimmune hepatitis are often similar to those described for chronic hepatitis. Patients with autoimmune hepatitis, however, usually have hypergammaglobulinemia, rheumatoid factor, and other circulating autoantibodies. Immunosuppressive therapy using corticosteroids with or without azathioprine is the mainstay of treatment and leads to symptomatic, clinical, biochemical, and histologic improvement, along with increased survival.

Fatty Liver Disease

Nonalcoholic fatty liver disease (NAFLD) is the most common cause of chronic liver disease in the United States.[60] NAFLD is defined as fat accumulation in the liver exceeding 5% by weight.[61] It has been estimated that up to 24% of American adults have NAFLD. It usually becomes manifest in the fifth and sixth decades of life and is more common in women.[62] The two major risk factors for NAFLD are type II diabetes and obesity. In a consecutive autopsy series, 70% of obese patients had fatty liver. Among type II diabetics, it is estimated that 75% have some form of fatty liver.

NAFLD includes a spectrum of hepatic pathology that ranges from fatty liver (steatosis) at its most clinically indolent extreme to the intermediate stage of nonalcoholic steatohepatitis (NASH), characterized by steatosis with lobular inflammation and perisinusoidal fibrosis, to its most severe form, cirrhosis. NAFLD is now believed to be responsible for most cases of what was once classified as cryptogenic cirrhosis, a form that accounts for half of the annual liver-related deaths.

Most patients with NAFLD are asymptomatic, and the presence of an abnormality is often detected by abnormal LFT or hepatomegaly on a routine physician's office visit. The most common LFT abnormality is a two- to fivefold elevation of the AST and ALT. The AST/ALT ratio is reported to be <1 in 65 to 90% of patients with NAFLD, which distinguishes it from alcohol-related liver injury.

The pathophysiology of NAFLD is unknown, but present data suggest multiple causes in which common initial insults promote hepatic steatosis (e.g., obesity, subclinical insulin resistance), and the increased hepatic fat appears to stress the

hepatocyte and render it more vulnerable to subsequent insults. This eventually produces some degree of hepatocyte necrosis, which promotes the accumulation of inflammatory cells within the liver (NASH). In some patients, a fibrotic response predominates, leading to cirrhosis.

The natural history of NAFLD varies according to its histologic type. Patients with steatosis alone usually have a benign clinical course. Significant adverse clinical sequelae, however, occur in patients with NASH and cryptogenic cirrhosis.

There are no proven treatments for NAFLD. Exercise and diet are recommended. Several studies have reported beneficial effects of bariatric surgery when NAFLD is secondary to obesity. When the disease is advanced, the patient is often a poor candidate for liver transplantation because of comorbid conditions such as obesity and the complications of diabetes.

Alcoholic Liver Disease

Alcoholic liver disease is defined by the development of three types of liver damage following chronic heavy alcohol consumption: (1) steatosis (fatty liver), (2) alcoholic hepatitis, and (3) cirrhosis.[63] The clinical features and laboratory values frequently do not distinguish among these because compensatory mechanisms can mask extensive liver disease. A liver biopsy is often necessary to arrive at a definitive diagnosis.

Alcoholic steatosis occurs commonly after ingestion of moderate-to-large amounts of alcohol for even a short period of time. When severe, patients may be symptomatic, with malaise, nausea, anorexia, weakness, abdominal discomfort, and tender hepatomegaly. Mild transaminase and AP elevations may be present. Alcoholic steatosis is usually a benign disorder, and the liver abnormalities will usually resolve with abstinence from alcohol. In contrast, alcoholic hepatitis is a precursor of cirrhosis. Although symptoms may overlap with those of alcoholic steatosis, patients with alcoholic hepatitis may be febrile and jaundiced. There may be up to a 10-fold elevation of the aminotransferases with the AST level characteristically higher than the ALT. Hypoalbuminemia, prolongation of the PT, and marked elevations of the AP may be present. Treatment of alcoholic hepatitis consists of abstinence from alcohol, bed rest, and intake of a normal or high-protein diet if hepatic encephalopathy is not present. Corticosteroids are often used to treat patients with severe alcoholic hepatitis, although their use for this indication remains controversial. It should be noted that alcohol abusers have a two- to threefold increase in perioperative morbidity (Fig. 48-7).[64]

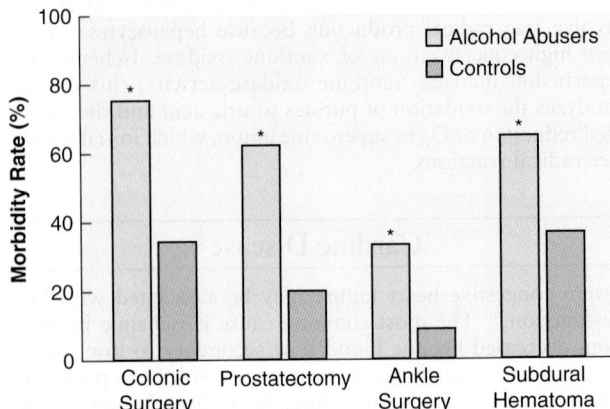

FIGURE 48-7. Prospective studies of postoperative morbidity in alcohol abusers and control subjects. *$p < 0.05$ versus control subjects. (Reprinted from Tonnesen H, Kehlet H: Preoperative alcoholism and postoperative morbidity. Br J Surg 1999; 86: 869, with permission.)

TABLE 48-4

UNCOMMON CAUSES OF CIRRHOSIS

Wilson disease[147]: Hereditary copper accumulation
Hereditary hemochromatosis[148,149]: Excessive iron absorption and deposition
Primary biliary cirrhosis[150]: Unknown etiology
α_1-Antitrypsin deficiency[151]: Often associated with emphysema
Budd-Chiari syndrome[152,153]: Vascular hepatic outflow obstruction

CIRRHOSIS: A PARADIGM FOR END-STAGE PARENCHYMAL LIVER DISEASE

This section discusses the pathophysiology of parenchymal liver disease, typified by hepatic cirrhosis, as it relates to anesthesia. Cirrhosis affects more than 3 million Americans and is the 12th leading cause of death. The most frequent causes of cirrhosis in the United States are chronic HCV infection and alcoholism, although many less common causes have been described (Table 48-4). The most common symptoms are anorexia, weakness, nausea, vomiting, and abdominal pain. Signs include hepatosplenomegaly, ascites, jaundice, spider nevi, and metabolic encephalopathy. Advanced parenchymal hepatic disease alters the function of nearly every organ and body system.

Cardiovascular Abnormalities

Characteristically, patients with cirrhosis and portal hypertension have a hyperdynamic circulation with a high cardiac output, low peripheral vascular resistance, low-to-normal arterial blood pressure, normal to increased stroke volume, normal filling pressures, and a mildly elevated heart rate (Table 48-5).[65] The total blood volume is usually increased, but with an altered distribution in which the central "effective" blood volume is decreased, while the splanchnic bed is hypervolemic. Extensive arteriovenous collateralization occurs in many

TABLE 48-5

CARDIOVASCULAR FUNCTION IN HEPATIC CIRRHOSIS

Decreased vascular resistance (peripheral vasodilation, increased arteriovenous shunting)
Increased cardiac output
Maintained arterial blood pressure, filling pressures, and heart rate (deterioration is late)
Blood volume maintained or increased, but redistributed (splanchnic hypervolemia, central hypovolemia)
Possible cardiomyopathy
Increased O_2 content in mixed venous blood; decreased difference in the O_2 contents of arterial and venous blood
Diminished responsiveness to catecholamines
Increased blood flow in splanchnic (extrahepatic), pulmonary, muscular, and cutaneous tissues
Decreased total hepatic blood flow
   Maintained hepatic arterial blood flow
   Decreased portal venous blood flow
Maintained or decreased renal blood flow

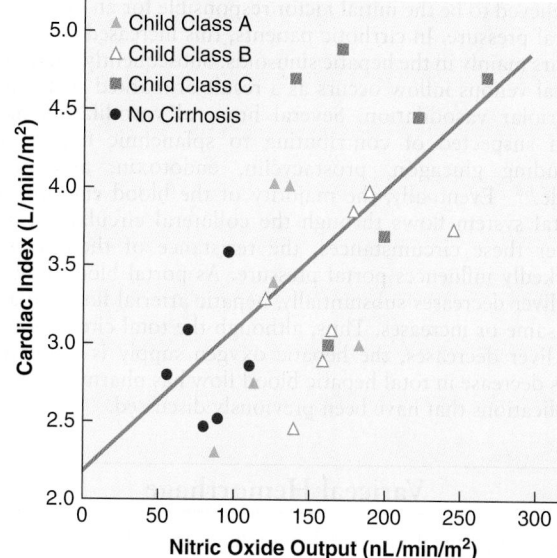

FIGURE 48-8. Relationship between nitric oxide in exhaled air and the cardiac index in 25 patients who had either normal hepatic function or cirrhosis with varying degrees of hepatic dysfunction. (Severity of liver dysfunction increases progressively from Child class A to class C.) A positive correlation exists between nitric oxide output (expressed in nanoliters per minute per square meter of body surface area) and cardiac index (expressed in liters per minute per square meter). $r = 0.62$ and $p < 0.001$. (Reprinted from Matsumoto A, Ogura K, Hirata Y et al: Increased nitric oxide production in the exhaled air of patients with decompensated cirrhosis. Ann Intern Med 1995; 123: 110, with permission.)

organs and tissues, leading to increased oxygen tension and saturation of the peripheral and mixed venous blood, and a decrease in the arteriovenous oxygen content difference. The mechanism by which these collaterals develop is complex and not completely understood, but may be related to increased plasma levels of glucagon and vasoactive intestinal polypeptide, which can induce peripheral vasodilation, decrease vascular resistance, and increase arteriovenous shunting. Glucagon also reduces the vascular responsiveness to infused catecholamines and other vasopressors in experimental animals.[66] Nitric oxide may also be an important mediator of the hyperdynamic changes that occur in cirrhosis and portal hypertension. Data from normal subjects and patients with cirrhosis reveal a positive correlation between exhaled concentrations of nitric oxide and cardiac index (Fig. 48-8).[67] Some causes of liver disease are also associated with cardiomyopathy (alcoholic liver disease, hemochromatosis); these patients may develop signs and symptoms of congestive heart failure, including decreased peripheral blood flow.

Hepatic Circulatory Dysfunction

Portal hypertension can complicate the course of many chronic liver diseases but is a hallmark of end-stage cirrhosis. Portal hypertension is a pathologic increase in portal venous pressure, resulting in the formation of portosystemic collaterals, which develop by dilatation and hypertrophy of pre-existing vascular channels. It plays an important role in the pathogenesis of ascites and hepatic encephalopathy, leads to the development of esophageal varices, and contributes to the enhanced susceptibility to bacterial infections and altered drug metabolism found in these patients.

In patients with cirrhosis, portal hypertension may result from increased vascular resistance to portal blood flow, which is believed to be the initial factor responsible for an increase in portal pressure. In cirrhotic patients, this increased resistance occurs mainly in the hepatic sinusoids. Subsequently, increased portal venous inflow occurs as a result of marked splanchnic arteriolar vasodilation. Several humeral vasodilators have been suspected of contributing to splanchnic hyperemia, including glucagon, prostacyclin, endotoxin, and nitric oxide.[68] Eventually, the majority of the blood entering the portal system flows through the collateral circulation, and under these circumstances, the resistance of these vessels markedly influences portal pressure. As portal blood flow to the liver decreases substantially, hepatic arterial flow remains the same or increases. Thus, although the total circulation of the liver decreases, the hepatic oxygen supply is preserved. This decrease in total hepatic blood flow has pharmacokinetic implications that have been previously discussed.

Variceal Hemorrhage

Gastroesophageal variceal hemorrhage is probably the most dreaded complication of portal hypertension. Varices are portosystemic collaterals formed after pre-existing vascular channels have been dilated by portal hypertension. They permit the passage of splanchnic venous blood from the high-pressure portal venous system to the low-pressure azygos and hemiazygous veins. Gastroesophageal varices are present in 40 to 60% of cirrhotic patients, and 25 to 35% of these will bleed. Up to 30% of initial bleeding episodes are fatal, and as many as 70% of survivors of an initial hemorrhage will have a recurrence.[69]

Variceal ruptures typically present as acute severe upper gastrointestinal hemorrhage. Prompt aggressive fluid resuscitation, blood transfusion, and correction of hemostatic abnormalities are essential, and are usually implemented in an intensive care unit. Endotracheal intubation for airway protection is frequently necessary. Empiric pharmacologic therapy (e.g., with octreotide) is indicated in situations in which variceal bleeding is likely. Subsequent esophagogastroduodenoscopy will define the site of bleeding and permit endoscopic therapy if appropriate.

Treatment of patients with gastroesophageal varices includes prevention of the initial bleeding episode (primary prophylaxis), control of active hemorrhage, and prevention of recurrent bleeding after a first episode (secondary prophylaxis).[70]

The goal of pharmacologic treatment is to reduce portal and intravariceal pressures. The nonselective beta-blockers, propranolol and nadolol, are effective agents for primary prophylaxis as they produce sustained decreases in portal venous pressure and decrease the risk of bleeding by 40 to 50%. Isosorbide mononitrate added to a beta-blocker may not only produce a further decrease in portal pressure, but also cause increased side effects. Endoscopic band ligation is an acceptable option for primary prophylaxis in patients at high risk for variceal bleeding who cannot tolerate medical therapy.

Patients with acute gastrointestinal bleeding of probable variceal origin are initially treated with intravenous somatostatin or its synthetic analogue octreotide. These drugs stop variceal hemorrhage in up to 80% of patients by reducing portal pressure. The variceal origin of the bleeding is then confirmed endoscopically, and the varices are subsequently treated either by band ligation or sclerotherapy. Current endoscopic therapies are capable of stopping bleeding in approximately 90% of patients.

If variceal bleeding persists or recurs despite endoscopic and pharmacologic therapy, balloon tamponade with a Sengstaken-Blakemore or Minnesota tube may be attempted. These modified nasogastric tubes are infrequently used, but when applied properly, achieve hemostasis in most cases.

Because rebleeding frequently occurs after balloon decompression, it should be used as a rescue technique and a bridge to more definitive treatment.

Transjugular intrahepatic portal systemic shunt (TIPS) was introduced in the 1990s, and its use has nearly eliminated the need for emergency shunt surgery. TIPS has become the preferred therapy for most bleeding patients who are not controlled by other nonoperative therapies. TIPS effectively decompresses the portal venous circulation with low short-term mortality, but late TIPS failure rates are high.[71]

A surgical portocaval shunt is considered in cases of continued hemorrhage or recurrent bleeding that cannot be controlled by endoscopic and pharmacologic means, and when TIPS is not available or technically feasible. When performed emergently, mortality approaches 40% but is substantially less when the procedure can be performed electively. Liver transplantation is often offered to patients with Childs B and C cirrhosis soon after or even before they bleed from varices. Secondary prophylaxis with nonselective beta-blockers, plus isosorbide mononitrate and band ligation of varices, reduces the incidence of rebleeding.

Pulmonary Dysfunction

A variety of disorders may produce hypoxemia in patients with advanced cirrhosis, including intrinsic cardiopulmonary disorders such as congestive heart failure, interstitial lung disease, obstructive airway disease, pleural effusions, and pulmonary vascular disease (Table 48-6). Fluid retention may cause interstitial edema, airway edema, and large-volume ascites, all of which may contribute to the development of hypoxemia through ventilation-perfusion mismatch and intrapulmonary shunting from compression of the basal regions of the lung.

In the absence of primary lung disease, the major causes of arterial hypoxemia in patients with advanced cirrhosis may be intrapulmonary vascular dilatations (IPVDs). The clinical triad of chronic liver disease, increased alveolar-arterial oxygen gradient, and evidence of IPVDs is defined as the *hepatopulmonary syndrome* (HPS). IPVD encompasses two types of vascular abnormalities: (1) vascular dilatation at the precapillary level close to the alveoli, and (2) vascular dilatation resulting in larger arteriovenous communications that may or may not be in proximity to gas exchange units.[72] Supplemental oxygen significantly increases the PaO_2 when precapillary IPVD is contributing to hypoxemia, but has minimal effects when larger arteriovenous communications are the primary cause of hypoxemia. The pathogenesis of IPVD in HPS is incompletely understood, but enhanced pulmonary production of nitric oxide likely plays a role.

IPVD is most commonly detected using contrast-enhanced echocardiography. In normal patients, injection of microbubbles results in transient echogenicity in the right heart with no

---

TABLE 48-6

HYPOXEMIA IN PATIENTS WITH CIRRHOSIS

Intrapulmonary shunting caused by intrapulmonary vascular dilatations (precapillary or arteriovenous)

Ventilation-perfusion mismatch caused by impaired hypoxic pulmonary vasoconstriction, pleural effusions, ascites, and diaphragm dysfunction

Decreases in pulmonary diffusion capacity secondary to increased extracellular fluid, interstitial pneumonitis, and/or pulmonary hypertension

contrast in the left heart. Patients with dilated precapillary pulmonary vessels show delayed opacification in the left atrium approximately three to six contractions after visualization of the right ventricle.[72]

As many as 40% of patients with cirrhosis have detectable IPVD, and up to 15% have hypoxemia and functional limitation.[72] Survival of patients with HPS is reduced compared with cirrhotic patients of similar Child-Pugh class without HPS. Severe hypoxemia from HPS increases intraoperative and postoperative risks in liver transplantation. IPVD often resolves completely after liver transplantation.

Hepatic hydrothorax occurs in 4 to 10% of cirrhotic patients. These patients characteristically have pleural effusions in the absence of cardiopulmonary disease, secondary to transfer of ascitic fluid from the peritoneal cavity into the pleural space through diaphragmatic defects.[73] The initial treatment of hepatic hydrothorax consists of sodium restriction, diuretics, and thoracentesis; TIPS may be required in refractory cases. Because most of these patients have end-stage liver disease, liver transplantation becomes the preferred treatment if the previous options fail.[73]

Portopulmonary hypertension refers to the development of pulmonary artery hypertension in patients with portal hypertension. It is usually defined as a mean pulmonary artery pressure >25 mm Hg with a normal pulmonary capillary wedge pressure and an elevated pulmonary vascular resistance (>120 dyne/sec/cm^{-5}). Portopulmonary hypertension affects between 4 and 6% of patients referred for liver transplantation. Patients with mean pulmonary artery pressures >35 mm Hg are considered to be high-risk transplant candidates.[74]

Ascites, Renal Dysfunction, and the Hepatorenal Syndrome

Ascites and Edema

Ascites is the most common of the major complications of cirrhosis. Nearly 50% of cirrhotic patients develop ascites within 10 years of being diagnosed.[75] Because 50% of cirrhotic patients with ascites die within 3 years, the development of ascites is a clear indication for evaluation for liver transplantation.

The pathogenesis of ascites in cirrhosis is complex and multifactorial. Portal hypertension and sodium and water retention play a key role.

The initial treatment for patients with ascites resulting from cirrhosis is reduction of sodium intake and diuretic therapy.[76] Fluid intake should be restricted if the patient has severe dilutional hyponatremia. The diuretics of choice are either spironolactone or amiloride. Furosemide should be used with caution because of the risk of excessive diuresis, which may lead to potentially serious complications including renal failure of prerenal origin, precipitation of hepatorenal syndrome, hyponatremia, hypokalemia, and encephalopathy.

Refractory ascites occurs in 5 to 10% of ascitic patients and is defined as a lack of response to high dose of diuretics (spironolactone, 400 mg/day plus furosemide 160 mg/day).[77] The main clinical features include marked abdominal distention, frequent recurrence of ascites after paracentesis, an increased risk of developing hepatorenal syndrome, and a poor prognosis. Repeated large-volume paracentesis with use of plasma volume expanders is the most widely accepted therapy for refractory ascites.[78] Removal of large amounts of ascitic fluid without the administration of plasma volume expanders is associated with paracentesis-induced circulatory dysfunction, characterized by reduction of effective arterial blood volume due to shift of intravascular fluid to the peritoneal cavity, with progressive reaccumulation of ascites and

marked activation of the renin-angiotensin-aldosterone system.[79]

The hemodynamic status of patients with tense ascites who undergo rapid total paracentesis without fluid resuscitation typically improves for the first 3 hours following the procedure, as a result of release of compression of the IVC and right atrium. Cardiac output increases, whereas pulmonary artery wedge pressure is unchanged and right atrial pressure decreases.[79] Other studies have demonstrated that along with the early increase in cardiac output, there is a decrease in plasma renin and aldosterone levels, a decrease in serum creatinine and blood urea nitrogen, and reduced portal pressures.[80] However, these beneficial effects are transient.

After 3 hours, the hemodynamic status is determined by the development of a relative hypovolemia caused by progressive reaccumulation of ascites. Twenty-four hours after total paracentesis, there is a significant decrease in cardiac output and cardiac filling pressures, accompanied by increased plasma renin and aldosterone concentrations. This effect is prevented by intravenous albumin infusion.[81] Although the use of albumin in this setting remains controversial because of its high cost and the lack of documented improvement in survival, albumin has a greater protective effect on the circulatory system than other expanders. More recent studies suggest that 50% of the plasma expander should be infused immediately after paracentesis, and the other half, 6 hours later.[82] The prevalence of paracentesis-induced circulatory dysfunction also depends on the amount of ascitic fluid removed because it is an uncommon complication following a low-volume paracentesis. It can be anticipated that similar hemodynamic changes may occur following emergent laparotomy in patients with tense ascites.

Placement of a peritoneal-venous shunt (Le Veen or Denver) was the first treatment specifically designed for patients with refractory ascites. Le Veen introduced the first prosthesis in 1974. It consists of a perforated intra-abdominal tube connected via a one-way valve to a second tube that traverses the subcutaneous tissue to the jugular vein. This creates a continuous passage of ascites into the systemic circulation. Poor long-term patency and excessive complications have led to the near abandonment of this procedure. A TIPS procedure is effective for preventing recurrence of ascites in patients with refractory ascites. TIPS decreases the activity of sodium-retaining mechanisms and improves the renal response to diuretics. This procedure is better than repeated large-volume paracentesis for the long-term control of ascites, but it has several disadvantages, including a high rate of shunt stenosis, which can lead to recurrence of ascites, a high incidence of severe hepatic encephalopathy, a high cost, and lack of availability in some centers. Survival is not improved by TIPS compared with repeated large-volume paracentesis. Thus, TIPS is not considered the first-line treatment for refractory ascites. Liver transplantation may also be a consideration in these patients.

Spontaneous Bacterial Peritonitis

Spontaneous bacterial peritonitis (SBP) is characterized by the spontaneous infection of ascitic fluid in the absence of an intra-abdominal source of infection. Its prevalence among patients with ascites ranges between 10 and 30%. SBP is diagnosed when there are ≥250 polymorphonuclear (PMN) cells/mm^3 of ascitic fluid. Bacterascites is diagnosed when there are positive ascitic fluid cultures and the neutrophil count is <250 cells/mm^3. SBP develops secondary to translocation of bacteria from the intestinal lumen to regional lymph nodes with subsequent bacteremia and infection of the ascitic fluid. Aerobic Gram-negative bacteria are most commonly isolated, but Gram-positive isolates are being recovered with increasing frequency. Ascitic fluid should be obtained by paracentesis and should be directly inoculated into blood culture bottles at the bedside rather than be cultured by conventional methods. Prospective clinical trials have demonstrated that cultures will be positive in approximately 80% of instances with the former approach versus 50% with the latter in patients with ≥250 PMN cells/mm³ of ascitic fluid.

Because ascitic fluid PMN count can be assessed much more rapidly than cultures and accurately determines who can benefit from empiric antibiotic coverage, patients with a PMN count ≥250 cells/mm³ in a clinical setting that is compatible with ascitic fluid infection should receive empiric antibiotic therapy. Delaying antibiotic therapy until positive ascitic fluid cultures are present likely increases the risk of the patient developing severe sepsis. Patients with ascitic PMN counts <250 cells mm³ with clinical signs or symptoms of infection should also be treated with empiric antibiotics until ascitic culture results are available. Cefotaxime, a third-generation cephalosporin, appears to be the antibiotic of choice for suspected SBP because it covers 95% of the responsible flora, including the three most common isolates, which are *Escherichia coli*, *Klebsiella pneumonia*, and the pneumococcus.

In a retrospective analysis of 252 episodes of SBP, renal insufficiency developed in 33%.[83] The renal dysfunction was transient in 25%, stable in 33%, and progressive in 42%. The overall mortality for an episode of SBP was 24%, but was 54% versus 9% in those with and without the development of renal insufficiency. The development of renal impairment is therefore an important clinical event in the course of SBP. Sepsis-induced decrease in the effective arterial blood volume with subsequent baroreceptor-mediated stimulation of the renin-angiotensin and sympathetic nervous systems, and vasopressin release contribute to the development of renal dysfunction. Direct stimulation of renal vasoconstrictors by endotoxin may also play a role. Sort et al.[84] demonstrated in a randomized, controlled clinical trial of 126 patients with SBP that interventions directed at maintaining effective arterial blood volume (1.5 g/kg albumin within 6 hours of diagnosis of SBP followed by 1 g/kg on day 3) were associated with a significant decrease in development of hepatorenal syndrome (HRS), and in both the in-hospital and 30-day mortality rates. Data do not exist regarding the efficacy of lower doses of albumin or other plasma volume expanders in preventing HRS.

Long-term antibiotic prophylaxis with a quinolone is recommended following resolution of SBP because there is an estimated 70% probability of recurrence within the first year, and antibiotic prophylaxis has a beneficial effect on patient survival. Short-term quinolone prophylaxis is also recommended for patients with low-protein ascites and gastrointestinal bleeding because bleeding increases bacterial translocation and SBP.

Pathogenesis of Renal Dysfunction

The three main renal functional abnormalities in cirrhosis are reduction in sodium excretion, reduction in free water excretion, and a decrease in renal perfusion and glomerular filtration.[76]

The arterial vasodilation characteristic of cirrhosis, with its associated decrease in effective plasma volume, leads to baroreceptor-mediated activation of the sympathetic nervous system. This causes the kidney to release renin, which results in an increased production of angiotensin II and aldosterone. Both aldosterone and increased sympathetic nervous system outflow enhance tubular sodium resorption. In addition, through their vasoconstrictive actions, norepinephrine and angiotensin II cause a redistribution of renal blood flow, which further decreases sodium elimination.

Water homeostasis is disturbed in up to 75% of patients with advanced cirrhosis and ascites (decompensated cirrhosis).

In these patients, water retention, increased total body water, and dilutional hyponatremia develop when fluid intake exceeds the impaired renal capacity to excrete free water. Reduced glomerular filtration secondary to impaired perfusion, elevated vasopressin levels caused by nonosmotic hypersecretion and decreased metabolic clearance, and impaired renal production of prostaglandin E2 also contribute to the impairment of free water excretion.

The major consequence of reduced sodium excretion is the development of edema and ascites. When free water clearance becomes significantly reduced, dilutional hyponatremia develops. The main consequence of decreased renal perfusion and glomerular filtration rate (GFR) is development of the HRS.

Hepatorenal Syndrome

HRS is a functional prerenal failure that occurs in up to 10% of patients with advanced cirrhosis and ascites, and less commonly in patients with acute liver failure. HRS is characterized by intense vasoconstriction of the renal circulation, low glomerular filtration, preserved renal tubular function, and normal renal histology. Progression to development of HRS in patients with cirrhosis may be a result of a sustained decrease in cardiac output (due to both decreased cardiac preload and impaired chronotropic function), in combination with severe splanchnic dilatation.[85]

HRS may be diagnosed after other causes of renal failure are ruled out. The International Ascites Club has suggested five major criteria to confirm the diagnosis of HRS: (1) chronic or acute liver disease with advanced hepatic failure and portal hypertension; (2) a low GFR as assessed by serum creatinine >1.5 mg/dL or creatinine clearance below 40 mL/min; (3) absence of shock, ongoing bacterial infection, fluid losses, or treatment with nephrotoxic drugs; (4) no sustained improvement in renal function after oral diuretic withdrawal and plasma volume expansion; and (5) <500 mg/day proteinuria with no ultrasonographic evidence of parenchymal renal disease or urinary obstruction.[86]

HRS has been classified clinically into two types based on its intensity and presentation. Type 1 HRS is characterized by progressive oliguria and a rapid rise in the serum creatinine concentration. Type 1 HRS develops in 5% of cirrhotic patients hospitalized for acute upper gastrointestinal bleeding, 30% of those admitted for SBP, 10% of patients with ascites treated with total paracentesis, and 25% of patients with severe acute alcoholic hepatitis.[87] SBP commonly precipitates the development of type 1 HRS. The prognosis of type 1 HRS is poor, with a median survival of <1 month without therapeutic intervention. Type 2 HRS is usually seen in patients with refractory ascites, and is characterized by a moderate and more stable impairment of renal function.

Pathophysiologically, intense renal vasoconstriction is the final consequence of extreme vasodilation of the splanchnic arterial circulation that reduces the effective arterial blood volume (that sensed by the central arterial circulation). The resulting abnormal distribution of arterial volume is associated with reduced flow to all extrasplanchnic areas, including the kidneys. Splanchnic arterial vasodilation is related to an increased level of both endothelial (prostacyclin and nitric oxide) and nonendothelial vasodilators (e.g., glucagon). Increased activity of the renin-angiotensin and sympathetic nervous systems mediate renal vasoconstriction, which is counterbalanced by increased intrarenal production of vasodilating prostaglandins and kallikreins.[88]

The development of type 1 HRS was once considered to be an irreversible clinical condition, which in the absence of an emergent liver transplant was associated with rapid progression to death. However, there are recent data demonstrating that the combination of albumin infusion and vasoconstrictors may improve renal function.[89,90] Because HRS develops as a consequence of splanchnic arterial vasodilation, drugs that produce splanchnic vasoconstriction are used to treat this syndrome. Several different vasoconstrictors (vasopressin analogs, catecholamines), usually combined with albumin infusion, have been evaluated in small nonrandomized clinical trials. Vasoconstrictor therapy results in an increased arterial blood pressure, near-normalization of the activity of the major endogenous vasoconstrictor systems, and marked increases in renal plasma flow, GFR, and urine volume in approximately two thirds of patients. These studies have demonstrated that a prolonged improvement in circulatory function, with 1 to 2 weeks of administration of intravenous albumin and vasoconstrictors, is required to reverse HRS, with a lag between the normalization of systemic circulation and the improvement in renal perfusion and GFR. Recurrence of HRS in responding patients after withdrawal of therapy is uncommon.[89,90]

Octreotide, an inhibitor of the release of gastrointestinal vasodilator peptides such as glucagon and vasoactive intestinal peptide, when combined with midodrine and intravenous albumin, has been shown to have beneficial effects on renal function in a clinical study of five patients with type 1 HRS.[90]

Patients showing an improvement in renal function after vasoconstrictor therapy survive significantly longer than patients who do not respond. Treatment with vasoconstrictors may thus increase the likelihood that patients with HRS will survive long enough to undergo liver transplantation. Transplant survival may be significantly reduced in cirrhotic patients with preoperative renal failure. Therefore, reversal of HRS with vasoconstrictor therapy is an important tool in patients waiting for a liver transplant.

Acute Renal Failure and Acute Tubular Necrosis

Cirrhotic patients are also at risk for developing acute renal failure from acute tubular necrosis (ATN), especially following infection or hypotensive episodes. ATN occurs more frequently after surgical procedures to relieve obstructive jaundice than it does following similar operations on nonjaundiced patients. The impaired vasoconstrictor response to hypovolemia seen in patients with hepatic parenchymal disease and obstructive jaundice limits the normal redistribution of splanchnic blood to the central circulation that occurs with hemorrhage. Therefore, even moderate hemorrhage may produce severe hypotension and cause ATN. In addition, conjugated bilirubin appears to be toxic to renal tubules and may contribute to the development of ATN in jaundiced patients.

The differential diagnosis of acute azotemia in patients with liver disease is outlined in Table 48-7. Of note is the remarkable similarity of the urinary characteristics of prerenal azotemia and HRS. Prompt detection and treatment of hypovolemia may rapidly improve renal function in prerenal azotemia, but this response does not if HRS is present.

Hematologic and Coagulation Disorders

The liver is the site of synthesis of all clotting factors with the exception of von Willebrand factor, an endothelial product. Anticoagulant (antithrombin III, proteins C and S), and fibrinolytic factors are also products of the liver. Acute or chronic liver disease results in a variable level of impairment of hemostasis from multiple causes: decreased production of coagulation and inhibitor factors, synthesis of dysfunctional clotting factors, quantitative and qualitative platelet defects, vitamin K deficiency, decreased clearance of activated factors, hyperfibrinolysis, and disseminated intravascular coagulation.

Vitamin K is an essential cofactor for the production in the liver of factors II, VII, IX, and X, and also proteins C and S. The precursors of vitamin K-dependent coagulation factors are also synthesized in the liver. Vitamin K is needed for conversion of these factors to active forms by gamma carboxylation of glutamic acid residues in the amino terminal region of the precursors. The carboxylated residues permit the binding of calcium ions that are essential for their functional activity.

Vitamin K is a fat-soluble vitamin requiring bile salts for absorption from the intestines. Thus, deficiency of the vitamin K-dependent factors results when there is impaired bile secretion from either intrahepatic or extrahepatic cholestasis.

Thrombocytopenia occurs in approximately 30 to 64% of patients with advanced chronic liver disease; however, the platelet count is rarely <30,000 cells/μL, and spontaneous bleeding is uncommon. The primary cause of thrombocytopenia in cirrhosis is portal hypertension-induced splenomegaly because up to 90% of circulating platelets may be sequestered in the enlarged spleen. Decreased hepatic synthesis and serum levels of the cytokine thrombopoietin are also believed to have a causative role in cirrhotic patients with thrombocytopenia. Increased destruction of platelets by immune mechanism; coexistent, low-grade, disseminated intravascular coagulation; sepsis; and direct suppression of bone marrow thrombopoiesis by ethanol, folate deficiency, and other drugs may all contribute to the development of thrombocytopenia in patients with chronic liver disease.

Dysfibrinogenemia is the most common qualitative abnormality of clotting factors in patients with liver disease. The abnormal functioning of fibrinogen is caused by an increased degree of sialylation of the molecule. This produces abnormal

TABLE 48-7

DIFFERENTIAL DIAGNOSIS OF ACUTE AZOTEMIA IN PATIENTS WITH LIVER DISEASE: IMPORTANT DIFFERENTIAL URINARY FINDINGS

	PRERENAL AZOTEMIA	HEPATORENAL SYNDROME	ACUTE RENAL FAILURE (ACUTE TUBULAR NECROSIS)
Urinary sodium concentration	<10 mEq/L	<10 mEq/L	>30 mEq/L
Urine-to-plasma creatinine ratio	>30:1	>30:1	<20:1
Urinary osmolality	Exceeds plasma osmolality by at least 100 mOsm	Exceeds plasma osmolality by at least 100 mOsm	Equal to plasma osmolality
Urinary sediment	Normal	Unremarkable	Casts, cellular debris

From Epstein M: Renal functional abnormalities in cirrhosis: Pathophysiology and management, Hepatology: A Textbook of Liver Disease. Edited by Zakim D, Boyer TD. Philadelphia, WB Saunders, 1982, p 460, with permission.

polymerization of fibrin monomers and leads to a disproportionate prolonged thrombin time, despite mild prolongation of the PT and partial thromboplastin (PTT) and normal amount of fibrinogen.

Hyperfibrinolysis is a common finding in patients with advanced liver disease and results from decreased hepatic clearance of plasminogen activator. This complication may be documented by the finding of decreased whole-blood euglobulin clot lysis time, with elevated levels of D-dimer, fibrin, and fibrinogen degradation products.

Diagnosing disseminated intravascular coagulation in cirrhotic patients is difficult. The diagnosis is suggested when there is a known triggering event associated with progressive worsening of coagulation test results and platelet counts, as well as a disproportionate reduction of factor V with a concomitant decreased level of a previously normal factor VIII.

Disorders of coagulation rapidly develop in patients with severe acute liver failure because of the brief half-life of some of the clotting factors. Factors II, V, VII, IX and X are all reduced in acute liver failure. As a consequence, the PT and INR become markedly elevated, serving as prognostic indicators and predictors of the need for transplantation. Reduced concentrations of the vitamin K-dependent factors are due predominantly to a combination of decreased hepatic synthesis and increased consumption of coagulation factors, rather than to vitamin K deficiency.

Quantitative and qualitative abnormalities of fibrinogen are also seen, and there is often evidence of excessive thrombin activity, increased fibrinogen turnover, and fibrinolysis, but the relative contributions of disseminated intravascular coagulopathy and impaired hepatic synthesis/clearance to the development of hemostatic abnormalities in acute liver failure remains unclear.

Spontaneous bleeding occurs infrequently in patients with advanced liver disease, and prophylactic treatment is not generally required. Bleeding, however, accounts for 60% of all deaths in cirrhotic patients having abdominal surgery; therefore, correction of coagulation abnormalities is appropriate prior to major surgical procedures and invasive diagnostic studies. A PT prolonged by >3 seconds or a platelet count of <50,000 cells/μL is considered contraindications to elective surgery.[91]

Perioperative management includes blood component therapy guided by laboratory studies. Fresh-frozen plasma contains all the clotting factors, and administration of 10 to 20 mL/kg will usually correct the PT to nearly normal levels but the effect lasts for no more than 12 to 24 hours. Vitamin K may improve the PT in patients with cholestatic disease. In these instances, 10 mg of subcutaneous vitamin K should be given for 3 consecutive days. Platelets should be infused prophylactically prior to elective surgery when the platelet count is <60,000 cells/μL.[92]

Endocrine Disorders

The presence of advanced cirrhosis invariably leads to abnormal regulation and function of multiple endocrine systems. The prevalence and severity of endocrine dysfunction are increased in diseases such as hemochromatosis, in which both the liver and endocrine organs are damaged by a common pathophysiologic process. Cirrhotic patients often have abnormal glucose utilization. The mechanism of this phenomenon is rather complex and includes increased fatty acid concentration in the plasma, which antagonizes the effects of insulin on glucose uptake by skeletal muscles. In addition, plasma levels of growth hormone and glucagon are often increased, and undoubtedly contribute to the glucose intolerance and other derangements of intermediary metabolism that occur in

patients with hepatic dysfunction. Patients with cirrhosis are also prone to hypoglycemia. This may reflect glycogen depletion secondary to malnutrition or alcohol-induced glycogenolysis and interference with gluconeogenesis. Severe cirrhosis may also impair hepatic conversion of lactate to glucose.

Abnormal metabolism of sex hormones causes gonadal dysfunction in both men and women. Men undergo feminization, often developing gynecomastia along with a decrease in the size of their testes and prostate gland. The frequency of impotence increases, and sperm counts typically decrease. Women with liver dysfunction commonly exhibit oligomenorrhea or amenorrhea.

Hepatic Encephalopathy

Hepatic encephalopathy (HE) is a complex reversible metabolic encephalopathy presenting as a wide spectrum of neuropsychiatric abnormalities in patients with hepatocellular failure and/or increased portal-systemic shunting. The clinical manifestations are highly variable and range from minimal changes in personality or altered sleep patterns without overt signs of HE (minimal HE), to confusion, lethargy, somnolence, and coma. Thirty to 60% of cirrhotic patients have at least minimal HE. Several well-recognized factors can precipitate HE in patients with cirrhosis who were previously stable (Table 48-8). A large dietary protein load, gastrointestinal hemorrhage, constipation, hypokalemia, diuretics, and azotemia produce an increased blood ammonia level. Surgery, associated with anesthesia and dehydration, can precipitate an episode of HE because of decreased hepatic perfusion. Sepsis can precipitate HE through increased ammonia production due to protein catabolism, impaired hepatic perfusion, and the effects of cytokines on the central nervous system. Psychoactive drugs can also precipitate HE. The diagnosis has to be

TABLE 48-8

FACTORS THAT MAY PRECIPITATE
HEPATIC ENCEPHALOPATHY

■ PRECIPITATING FACTOR	■ POSSIBLE MECHANISMS
Excessive dietary protein	Increased ammonia production
Constipation	—
Gastrointestinal bleeding	—
Infection	—
Azotemia	—
Diarrhea and vomiting Diuretic therapy Paracentesis	Dehydration with electrolyte and acid-base imbalance, increased ammonia generation, and decreased hepatic perfusion, increasing blood ammonia level
Hypoxia	Adverse effect on liver and brain function
Hypotension	—
Anemia	—
Hypoglycemia	—
Sedatives/hypnotics	Action at the GABA$_A$/benzodiazepine receptor complex
Creation of portal-systemic shunt	Reduced hepatic metabolism

made on the basis of clinical findings. Several other conditions that may present in a similar fashion must be excluded, including chronic subdural hematoma, Wernicke encephalopathy, and electrolyte disturbances.

It is commonly believed that HE is caused by substances that under normal circumstances are efficiently metabolized by the liver, rather than by insufficient synthesis of substrates essential for normal neurologic function. This notion is consistent with the development of HE in patients following portosystemic bypass who do not have significant intrinsic liver disease. More than 20 different compounds have increased blood concentrations when liver function is impaired. Of these, ammonia has been considered the most important factor in the genesis of HE. Ammonia is produced in the intestine by catabolism of proteins, amino acids, and biogenic amines. Forty percent is derived from intestinal bacterial metabolism of nitrogenous substances, and most of the remainder from digestion of dietary protein. The concentration of ammonia in portal venous blood is high, and a high degree of extraction occurs in the liver, where the ammonia is converted to urea and glutamine. This detoxification is impaired in cirrhotic patients as a result of impaired conversion by the liver and marked portal-systemic shunting. Increased ammonia levels in blood results in increased diffusion of ammonia into the brain. Variation in the transfer of ammonia across the blood–brain barrier may explain the poor relationship between the blood ammonia level and the degree of hepatic encephalopathy. Ammonia has many deleterious effects on brain function. Although this ion seems to play a central role, the clinical features of HE differ from those of pure ammonia intoxication, and therefore other mechanisms must be involved.

The clinical and neurophysiologic manifestations of HE seem to reflect a global depression of central nervous system function caused by an increase in inhibitory neurotransmission. The observation of an improvement in mental status after the administration of flumazenil, a benzodiazepine receptor antagonist, in some patients with advanced HE who have not taken benzodiazepines supports a role for an increased GABAergic tone. One possible mechanism is an increased availability of agonist ligands of the GABA receptor complex. These are called *natural benzodiazepines* and bind to the benzodiazepine site of the GABA receptor. Natural benzodiazepines accumulate in the brains of patients with HE, and it has been suggested that they may induce a decrease in consciousness.

Other putative mechanisms include the effects of a group of potentially neurotoxic compounds of colonic origin (mercaptans, short-chain fatty acids, manganese), impairment of cerebral energy metabolism, gliopathy secondary to astrocyte swelling, and disruption of the blood–brain barrier. Patients with liver failure have an increase in plasma levels of aromatic amino acids and a decrease in branched-chain amino acids. It has been proposed that this imbalance enhances the entry of aromatic amino acids into the brain and that these are channeled into the synthesis of abnormal biogenic amines, which are released along with, or instead of, normal neurotransmitters. These *false neurotransmitters* (octopamine, phenylethanolamine) are relatively inactive. However, this hypothesis has not been supported by in vivo or postmortem studies. Administration of intravenous branched-chain amino acids does not produce beneficial effects in acute HE.

The main principles of treatment of HE have not been evaluated by randomized clinical trials but rather have been accepted on the basis of clinical observation.[93,94] Most episodes of HE in patients with cirrhosis are initiated by an identifiable precipitating factor. Because effective methods exist to control most of these, a key component of the treatment of HE is to identify and treat the precipitating cause. Often, the elimination of these factors leads to an improve-

ment without need for any additional therapy. If no precipitating factor can be identified or if rapid improvement does not occur with treatment, therapy should be initiated to reduce the production and absorption of ammonia. Dietary protein intake should be restricted to an extent dependent on the severity of HE. However, severe restriction of dietary protein is no longer recommended because of the adverse effects of severe malnutrition on liver function and short-term prognosis.[95]

Lactulose (β-galactosidofructose) is a nonabsorbable disaccharide that is not broken down by intestinal enzymes following oral administration, but is metabolized by enteric bacteria in the cecum to lactate and acetate. This produces a reduction of ammonia absorption from the large intestine (because it is converted to ammonium) and net movement of NH_3 from the blood into the bowel. In addition, lactulose enhances the growth of non–urease-producing bacteria, thereby reducing the bacterial production of ammonia, and it also has cathartic activity.

Neomycin is an alternative to lactulose for patients who do not tolerate the disaccharide or have unsatisfactory results. It reduces the intestinal production of ammonia by reducing the population of urease-producing bacteria and may also have nonbacterial effects. Prolonged use should be avoided because of possible toxicity from the small amount of drug that is absorbed. Neomycin is as effective as lactulose.

Zinc deficiency is common in cirrhotic patients from increased urinary excretion and malnutrition. Two of the five enzymes responsible for the metabolism of ammonia to urea are zinc-dependent; thus, it has been suggested that zinc deficiency contributes to the development of HE. Whether zinc supplementation in this population is beneficial has not been established. Flumazenil, a selective antagonist of the central benzodiazepine receptor, produces a transient improvement in the mental status of some patients with HE, but has no sustained benefits. The dopamine agonists, bromocriptine and levodopa, were introduced to restore the decreased activity of central neurotransmitters caused by false neurotransmitters. Although the false neurotransmitter hypothesis is now questioned, these drugs may help chronic HE patients with extrapyramidal manifestations, which are believed to develop as a result of manganese accumulation in the basal ganglia.

It appears clear that encephalopathic changes are associated with clinically important alterations in pharmacodynamics and pharmacokinetics of various medications. For example, cerebral uptake of benzodiazepines increases substantially, which may reflect an increase in the density or affinity of benzodiazepine receptors or a leaky blood–brain barrier. Drugs administered to patients with advanced hepatic disease require careful titration against effect.

Orthotopic liver transplantation cures HE. Medical management for HE is mainly used for patients who do not yet meet the criteria for liver transplantation, who are waiting for a transplant, or who are not transplant candidates. Without transplantation, overt HE in the patient with chronic liver disease has a poor prognosis, with a survival rate of 42% at 1 year and 23% at 3 years.

HEPATOCELLULAR CARCINOMA

Primary hepatocellular carcinoma (HCC) is one of the most common tumors in the world and the third most frequent cause of death from cancer. It occurs in the United States with an incidence of 2.4 individuals per 100,000 population. HCC usually arises in a cirrhotic liver. Cirrhosis secondary to chronic viral hepatitis accounts for the large majority of HCC worldwide but only 30 to 40% of reported cases in America. Thus, there are many individuals in whom no obvious cause can be identified. Inherited metabolic diseases, including hemochromatosis, α1-antitrypsin deficiency, and Wilson disease, are well known to be risk factors for the development of HCC. Another implicated factor is alcohol. Alcoholic cirrhosis may clearly result in HCC, but it is uncertain whether alcohol is directly carcinogenic or whether associated hepatocellular injury and regeneration, iron accumulation, or coexistent HCV infection is responsible.

HCC may escape early clinical detection because it occurs in patients with underlying cirrhosis, and the clinical findings may suggest progression of the underlying disease. The most common presenting complaint is abdominal pain, and the most frequent finding on physical examination is an abdominal mass. Serum α-fetoprotein (AFP) values are >500 μg/L in about 70 to 80% of patients with HCC. Unfortunately, AFP has a low specificity and levels may be elevated in pregnancy, germ cell tumors, and acute or chronic hepatitis. Hepatic ultrasound has greater sensitivity and specificity than AFP levels when used for HCC screening. Three imaging procedures are in common use for diagnosing HCC: ultrasonography, helical CT, and MRI. The sensitivity and specificity of radiologic studies for detection of HCC is unknown.

Chemoembolization is widely used for treatment of HCC. No studies have shown a long-term survival advantage in treated versus untreated patients. Surgical resection offers a chance for cure; however, few patients have a resectable tumor at the time of presentation. Patients with two or fewer lesions, each smaller than 5 cm, which are encapsulated and have no evidence of macroscopic vascular invasion are the best candidates for hepatic resection. Operative mortality in carefully selected patients should be <3%. The absence of significant portal hypertension (hepatic vein pressure <10 mm Hg) and normal bilirubin concentration are the best predictors of excellent outcomes after surgery.[96] Liver transplantation may be considered as a therapeutic option for patients who have a single lesion ≤5 cm or three or fewer lesions ≤3 cm. Survival after transplantation in these groups is similar to that of patients transplanted for nonmalignant disease.

PREGNANCY-RELATED DISORDERS

Well-known disorders of pregnancy that can cause fulminant hepatic failure during the third trimester or in the immediate postpartum period include acute fatty liver of pregnancy (AFLP) and the HELLP syndrome (hemolysis, elevated liver enzymes, low platelets). In addition, parturients are unusually susceptible to morbidity and mortality from HEV infection and herpes simplex hepatitis.

Acute Fatty Liver of Pregnancy

AFLP occurs in the late stages of pregnancy. Although severe cases are rare (frequency of 1/6,659 deliveries in a 1999 report), it is now recognized to exist in a broad clinical spectrum ranging from mild to severe hepatic disease[97]. The pathogenesis is unclear, but an association between inherited defects in β-oxidation of fatty acids and AFLP is now well established. Some affected patients have an inherited long-chain 3-hydroxyacyl-CoA dehydrogenase deficiency, which causes a defect in intramitochondrial β-oxidation of fatty acids. Other patients with AFLP have a defect in β-oxidation caused by deficiency of carnitine palmitoyltransferase I.

Affected women usually present in the third trimester with symptoms related to hepatic failure. Initial symptoms are variable and include nausea, vomiting, abdominal pain, and

encephalopathy. Modest elevations of serum transaminases (<750 U/L) are usual. Jaundice is common as is laboratory evidence of renal dysfunction and leukocytosis. Prolongation of the PT and other laboratory findings of disseminated intravascular coagulation are often present and help distinguish AFLP from HELLP syndrome. Severely affected patients have complications typical of any form of fulminant hepatic failure, including hepatic coma and renal failure. Some patients are asymptomatic, with the diagnosis made during evaluation of abnormal LFTs. Imaging techniques have not been consistently useful for confirming the diagnosis of AFLP. Although a liver biopsy can be diagnostic, it is often contraindicated because of coagulopathy. Therefore, the diagnosis of AFLP is clinical. When a biopsy is available, the characteristic histologic finding is microvesicular fatty infiltration most prominent in the central zone, with sparing of the periportal hepatocytes.

When AFLP is diagnosed, delivery of the fetus is expedited, usually by induction of labor or, occasionally, cesarean section, because AFLP improves in response to termination of pregnancy. After delivery, maximal supportive care is required as the liver recovers. Most affected women recover completely, although in severe cases the patients may require prolonged intensive care. On rare occasions, liver transplantation has been necessary. Recurrence of AFLP with future pregnancy is uncommon, but genetic screening for defects in fatty acid oxidation of the offspring of women with AFLP is warranted.[98]

Preeclampsia and HELLP Syndrome

HELLP syndrome is a common and potentially ominous complication of preeclampsia, affecting 10% of women with this disorder and 20% of women with severe preeclampsia. The presence of HELLP syndrome is associated with an increased risk of maternal (1%) and perinatal (up to 20.4%) death.[99] The diagnosis of HELLP syndrome is made clinically by the presence of signs of preeclampsia and laboratory evidence of hemolysis (elevated serum LDH level, schistocytes, and burr cells on peripheral smear), elevated serum transaminases due to ischemic hepatocellular necrosis (up to several thousand international units), and thrombocytopenia (<100,000 cells/μL). Hyperbilirubinemia occurs in approximately 40% of cases of HELLP and may be caused by hemolysis and liver dysfunction. The presence of full-blown coagulopathy is rare and should raise concern for the presence of hepatic failure caused by AFLP. It should be noted that there is considerable disagreement in the medical literature about the diagnostic criteria for the HELLP syndrome.[99]

Liver biopsy is rarely warranted, but when performed, the specimens usually demonstrate periportal hemorrhage and fibrin deposition with periportal hepatic necrosis. Both macrovesicular and microvesicular fat are present, but steatosis is usually modest and is unlike the pericentral microvesicular fat seen in AFLP. The liver involvement in HELLP syndrome is most frequently misdiagnosed as viral hepatitis, although thrombocytopenia is an uncommon finding in the latter disease. AFLP also should be considered, but is usually associated with more severe liver failure and not necessarily with thrombocytopenia. All affected patients should be considered to have severe preeclampsia. Once the diagnosis is made, management is primarily supportive. There is a consensus of opinion that prompt delivery is indicated if the syndrome develops beyond 34 weeks' gestation, or earlier if life-threatening morbidity develops in the mother. When HELLP syndrome develops prior to 34 weeks' gestation, management is controversial with the choice of either providing supportive care with close monitoring of mother and fetus until the fetus is mature, or administration of corticosteroids to accelerate fetal lung maturity followed by delivery after 24 hours.[99]

In most affected patients, all abnormalities associated with preeclampsia and HELLP syndrome resolve after delivery, leaving no hepatic sequelae. Rarely, the condition worsens progressively after delivery with further diminution of the platelet count and development of sepsis with multisystem organ failure.

Hepatic Rupture, Hematoma, and Infarct

These conditions occur in preeclampsia and may be the extreme end of the spectrum of HELLP syndrome. Patients with spontaneous rupture of the liver present close to term with abdominal pain and distention, as well as cardiovascular collapse. The rupture results from extravasation of blood, presumably from one or several microscopic areas of periportal hemorrhage with subsequent separation of Glisson's capsule from the liver surface and eventual capsule rupture. The diagnosis depends on a high index of suspicion and identification of hemoperitoneum on abdominal ultrasonography, CT scan, or MRI. If the rupture goes undiagnosed, death results for both mother and fetus. Aggressive management is essential, with vigorous hemodynamic support, rapid delivery of the fetus, and surgical repair of the liver. Some patients may have a contained subcapsular hematoma without frank rupture into the peritoneum. These patients may be managed expectantly with serial hepatic CT scans.

Hepatic infarction typically occurs in the third trimester and presents with right upper quadrant pain, fever, leukocytosis, and marked elevations of serum transaminases. The infarcts can be seen on abdominal CT scan. Management is supportive.

CHOLESTATIC DISEASE

Cardiovascular Dysfunction

The presence of bile salts in circulating blood (cholemia) can impair myocardial contractility.[100] Cholemia also blunts the response to norepinephrine, angiotensin II, and isoproterenol, probably by interfering with their binding to membrane receptors.[101] Less severe hemodynamic perturbations occur in patients with biliary obstruction than in those with cirrhosis. However, the pattern of the pathophysiologic change is remarkably similar: increases in peripheral vasodilatation, cardiac output, and portal venous pressure, and a decrease in portal venous blood flow.

Coagulation Disorders

Cholestatic disease predisposes the patient toward development of coagulopathy primarily related to vitamin K deficiency. During even brief episodes of biliary obstruction, coagulopathy can result from a deficiency of coagulation factors whose activation depends on the presence of vitamin K. Absorption of vitamin K depends on the excretion of bile into the gastrointestinal tract. Long-lasting biliary obstruction can cause liver injury, with subsequent deterioration in the hepatic synthesis of proteins, including coagulation factors. Usually, the coagulation disorders are moderate, and parenteral vitamin K corrects the problem. If this treatment is not fully effective, one should suspect that the disease is not purely cholestatic and that hepatic parenchymal injury exists. If such patients need urgent surgery, the coagulopathy will require immediate treatment with fresh-frozen plasma. The failure of parenteral

vitamin K to correct a prolonged PT time typically indicates the presence of severe hepatic parenchymal dysfunction and portends a poor prognosis.

PREOPERATIVE AND PERIOPERATIVE MANAGEMENT

Hepatic Evaluation and Preparation

While obtaining the history, inquiry should be made about risk factors and the presence of symptoms attributable to chronic liver disease. The history should include questions about prior episodes of jaundice and their relationship to surgical procedures and the anesthetic techniques used, blood product transfusions, use of alcohol and other recreational drugs, current medications (including herbal preparations), family history of jaundice or liver disease, travel history, and an occupational history (exposure to hepatotoxins). In the review of systems, the patient should be asked about easy bruising, anorexia, weight loss or gain, fatigue, nausea, vomiting, pain with fatty meals, pruritus, abdominal distention, and episodes of gastrointestinal bleeding.

The capacity of pharmacologic agents to injure the liver is an important perioperative concern. Some 500 to 1,000 therapeutic agents have been implicated in causing a broad spectrum of liver diseases.[102] These diseases may be classified in accordance with whether the drug produces primarily direct cell toxicity (necrosis), cholestasis, or steatosis. Most forms of drug-induced liver disease are benign and of little consequence (e.g., estrogen-induced cholestasis), producing only transient alterations of LFT. Severe drug toxicities, which are typically dose-related (acetaminophen) or idiosyncratic (halothane), are responsible for 15 to 30% of cases of fulminant hepatic failure and 20 to 50% of cases of chronic nonviral hepatitis. Moreover, when drug reactions produce hepatocellular necrosis, the estimated case fatality approaches 50%.

Drugs known to produce hepatocellular injury and centrilobular necrosis include acetaminophen, isoniazid, and methyldopa. Other cytotoxic drugs include oxyphenisatin, rifampin, papaverine, phenytoin, indomethacin, monoamine oxidase inhibitors, and amitriptyline. The use of dantrolene for treatment of muscle spastic disorders has been associated with the development of hepatic failure in patients receiving the drug for >60 days. Cholestatic reactions often result from drugs such as chlorpromazine, phenylbutazone, and androgenic and anabolic steroids. In at least one case, erythromycin (ethylsuccinate form) has caused hepatic failure.[103]

A drug's potential to cause hepatotoxicity is influenced by various pharmacologic (other drugs) or pathophysiologic (hepatitis) factors. For example, the combination of trimethoprim and sulfamethoxazole is nearly 5 times more frequently associated with hepatotoxicity than sulfamethoxazole alone. By inducing hepatic microsomal drug-metabolizing systems, some drugs can markedly increase the injurious potential of others by altering their metabolism to favor the production of toxic metabolites. For example, phenobarbital increases the hepatotoxicity of various drugs, including chemotherapeutic agents (methotrexate) and antibiotics (tetracycline).[104]

Although elective surgery is not contraindicated in patients with alcoholic steatosis, the mortality from acute alcoholic hepatitis, even without surgery, is significant. Therefore, if alcoholic hepatitis is suspected, further examination of liver function is warranted before performing an elective operation.

The physical examination of the patient with chronic liver disease is particularly valuable because the patient may appear ill before there is laboratory evidence of hepatic dysfunction.

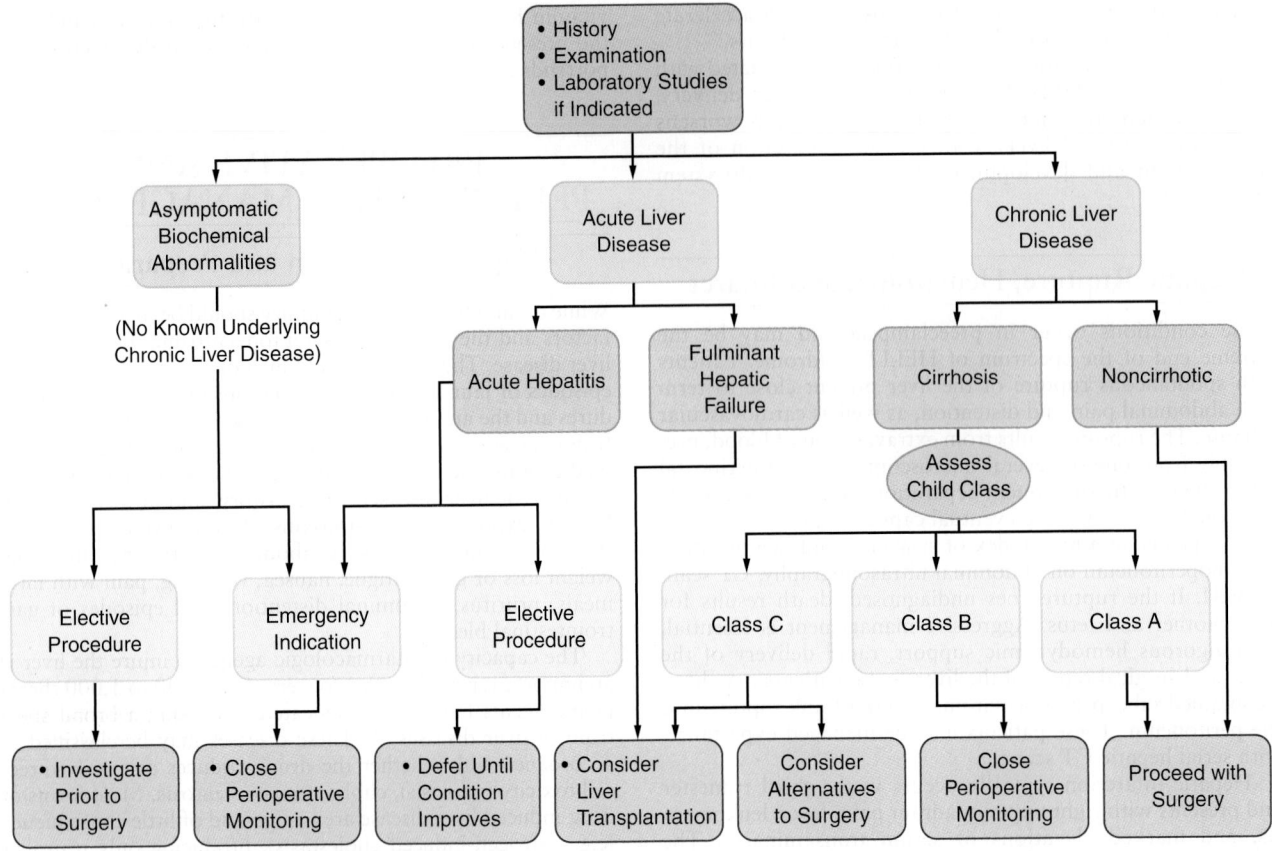

FIGURE 48-9. Preoperative approach to a patient with known or suspected liver disease. (Modified from Patel T: Surgery in the patient with liver disease. Mayo Clin Proc 1999; 74: 593, with permission.)

The examination should focus on signs such as scleral icterus, jaundice, ascites, splenomegaly, palmar erythema, gynecomastia, asterixis, testicular atrophy, spider angiomata, petechiae, and ecchymosis. The liver may be enlarged with a tender soft and smooth edge if the patient has hepatitis, or firm and nodular with presence of cirrhosis or malignancy. Patients with chronic hepatitis often have extrahepatic manifestations, including arthritis, skin rashes, and thyroiditis.

Acute liver failure has a distinct clinical presentation. Typically, nonspecific symptoms such as nausea and malaise are followed by the rapid onset of jaundice and subsequently altered mental status, which may progress to coma with clinical and radiologic evidence of cerebral edema.

If no suspicion of liver dysfunction arises from a thorough history and physical examination, then laboratory tests for liver function do not need to be routinely obtained because of the low prevalence of disease. Routine testing may yield false-positive results, engendering patient anxiety and prompting the performance of expensive, unnecessary, and potentially dangerous invasive tests. If, however, hepatic dysfunction is known or suspected, then the degree of dysfunction should be quantified by applying either the Child-Pugh or Model of End-stage Liver Disease (MELD) scoring system. A dilemma arises when a patient without any risk factors or stigmata of liver disease is found to have one or more abnormal LFT on a recent blood test (e.g., routine yearly employment health assessment). The prudent action may be to delay surgery and repeat the tests later. This conservative approach helps ensure a patient is not in the early stages of a disease process (e.g., hepatitis) that may abruptly worsen and may minimize the medical-legal risk for the anesthesiologist. Acute hepatitis (viral, alcoholic, ischemic, or drug-related) is associated with increased perioperative risk and

mortality. For nonemergent procedures, supportive care allowing an improvement in the overall condition will diminish the perioperative risk. Therefore, in the presence of acute hepatic disease, elective surgery should be postponed (Fig. 48-9).

Perioperative Risk Associated with Acute and Chronic Liver Disease

Because of our limited ability to support a failing liver, the perioperative risks associated with acute and chronic liver disease present significant challenges.[105] The increased surgical morbidity and mortality associated with varying degrees of liver insufficiency have been described in detail for over 4 decades.[106–111] What remains less clear, however, is whether perioperative outcomes can be improved with proactive interventions.

Regardless of the cause, an increased magnitude of liver dysfunction is associated with a higher probability of morbidity and mortality.[112] Thus, it is important to quantify and grade preoperative liver dysfunction. Most risk assessment studies about liver disease address expected lifespan in reference to the prioritization of candidates for liver transplant. In 1999, a new classification system called *MELD* was designed to predict the outcome of decompressive therapy for portal hypertension.[111] MELD integrates weighted values of three parameters: serum bilirubin, INR, and serum creatinine:

$$\text{MELD score} = 0.957 \times \log_e (\text{creatinine mg/dL}) + 0.378 \times \log_e (\text{bilirubin mg/dL}) + 1.120 \times \log_e (\text{INR}) + 0.643$$

The model was developed from prospective data. MELD has since been adopted by the United Network of Organ Sharing

TABLE 48-9

MODIFIED CHILD-PUGH SCORE

	POINTS[a]		
PRESENTATION	1	2	3
Albumin (g/dL)	>3.5	2.8–3.5	<2.8
Prothrombin time			
Seconds prolonged	<4	4-6	>6
International normalized ratio	<1.7	1.7–2.3	>2.3
Bilirubin (mg/dL)[b]	<2	2–3	>3
Ascites	Absent	Slight-moderate	Tense
Encephalopathy	None	Grade I–II	Grade III–IV

[a]Class A = 5–6 points; B = 7–9 points; C = 10–15 points.
[b]Cholestatic diseases (e.g., primary biliary cirrhosis) produce bilirubin elevations that are disproportionate to the hepatic dysfunction. Thus, the following adjustments should be made: assign 1 point for a bilirubin level of 4 mg/dL; 2 points for bilirubin concentrations between 4 and 10 mg/dL; and 3 points for bilirubin >10 mg/dL.
From Kamath PS: Clinical approach to the patient with abnormal liver test results. Mayo Clin Proc 1996; 71: 1089, with permission.

in the United States to prioritize patients for liver transplantation.

Child and Turcotte[106] first described their classification system in 1964. They selected five parameters—serum albumin, serum bilirubin, ascites, encephalopathy, and nutritional status—each graded at one of three levels of severity, and combined to generate an assignment to one of three classes (A to C). Mortality was assessed following portosystemic shunt operations. In 1972, Pugh et al.[114] modified the Child-Turcotte system, replacing the subjective assessment of nutritional status with the more objective system listed in Table 48-9.

It is important to note that surgical mortality from hepatic shunt and transplant procedures is less than that from other major surgery.[115,116] In 1997, Rice et al.[110] reported a retrospective analysis of 40 consecutive patients over a 5-year period undergoing general anesthesia for surgery, including 28 abdominal procedures, 2 coronary artery bypass grafts, 5 orthopedic procedures, and 5 miscellaneous procedures. By multiple logistic regression analysis, an INR >1.6 and encephalopathy were associated with a greater than 10- and 35-fold increased mortality risk, respectively. However, Child classification and Pugh score failed to predict 30-day mortality. Also in 1997, Mansour et al.[111] studied mortality of patients with liver disease undergoing abdominal surgery. Their retrospective analysis from a single institution reported operative 30-day mortality on 92 cirrhotic patients during a 12-year period. Types of surgery were divided into four categories: cholecystectomy, hernia repair, gastrointestinal, and miscellaneous procedures. Twenty-six percent of operations were performed as emergencies. Child class A was associated with 10% mortality, class B with 30%, and class C with 82%. Gastrointestinal procedures and emergent operations were associated with the highest mortality. For comparison, the 3-month mortality in patients hospitalized for liver complications but not undergoing surgery was 4% for Child class A, 14% for class B, and 51% for class C.

MELD score has shown comparable prediction of short-term, nonoperative mortality in advanced cirrhosis when compared with the Child classification. Except for liver transplantation and shunt procedures, MELD is not commonly used to predict perioperative morbidity and mortality.[117]

The scoring of liver disease is only one component of evaluating perioperative risks. Other considerations are the patient's age, coexisting diseases, and the type, location, and duration of the surgery. Accurate assessment and communication of perioperative risks is an essential condition of informed consent.

Scant data exist to support lengthy preoperative admissions for "optimization," especially for patients with mild hepatic dysfunction having minor operative procedures. Patients with severe or long-standing hepatic dysfunction, however, may benefit from aggressive inpatient correction of certain abnormalities. Liver-related conditions that may benefit from preoperative correction or optimization include ethanol dependency, coagulopathy, malnutrition, anemia, SBP, and hepatic encephalopathy.[118] Esophageal varices can be treated as previously discussed. Preoperative coagulopathy warrants particular attention. Ideally, coagulation abnormalities should be corrected preoperatively, and this should help minimize intraoperative blood loss and thereby decrease the risk of major complications, including development of postoperative HRS. Significant coagulation abnormalities must be corrected prior to performing a spinal or epidural anesthetic. Increased PT or INR in patients with either cholestasis or obstructive jaundice may respond to a few days of vitamin K therapy, but if unsuccessful or if the urgency of surgery does not allow adequate time for a response, administration of fresh-frozen plasma is indicated. Platelet transfusion should be considered for patients with evidence of platelet dysfunction or thrombocytopenia (<100,000 cells/μL).

Minor operations do not cause postoperative liver dysfunction in healthy patients. Even patients with marginal hepatic function usually tolerate peripheral procedures without hepatic complications, including those who receive halothane anesthesia.[119] A randomized study in patients with mild alcoholic hepatitis compared spinal with general anesthesia (enflurane plus N_2O plus opioid) and found no anesthesia-related differences in values of LFTs following peripheral or superficial surgery.[38]

Major operations (especially laparotomy) are often associated with hepatic dysfunction or injury. The magnitude of the abnormality depends more on the type of operation than on a particular anesthetic technique.[120] Nonetheless, hepatic dysfunction subsequent to major surgery is rarely of concern in healthy patients. In contrast, patients with advanced hepatic disease (marginal hepatic function) who undergo major operations, such as laparotomy, have extremely high postoperative morbidity and mortality.[105]

Medications needed to control the myriad complications of severe liver disease should be continued throughout the perioperative period. Preoperative sedatives, when indicated, should be used in lower doses because of the marked derangements in pharmacokinetics and pharmacodynamics associated with advanced liver disease. These patients may have a full stomach, even if they have not taken food or fluid for several hours, because of hiatal hernia, massive ascites, and decreased gastric and intestinal motility. Therefore, premedication may include an H_2-receptor blocker, metoclopramide, as well as sodium citrate.

Anticipated Pharmacokinetic and Pharmacodynamic Alterations

Drugs administered to patients with advanced hepatic disease require careful titration against effect. It appears clear that encephalopathic changes are associated with clinically important alterations in the pharmacodynamics and pharmacokinetics of various medications. For example, cerebral uptake of benzodiazepines increases substantially, which may reflect an increase in the density or affinity of benzodiazepine receptors or a leaky blood–brain barrier. Data concerning the pharmacokinetics of midazolam in patients with advanced liver disease are conflicting. One study demonstrated a significant decrease in clearance and elimination half-life, whereas another study demonstrated only slightly impaired disposition in cirrhotic patients.[121,122] The pharmacokinetics of single doses of sufentanil and propofol were found to be similar in cirrhotic patients and those with normal hepatic function, although some differences in elimination time were observed.[123,124] Such findings imply that administering infusions or multiple doses of certain intravenous drugs can result in prolonged pharmacologic effects because of impaired hepatic elimination in patients with advanced hepatic disease. The differences in the results of these studies are probably a consequence of certain differences in the binding proteins, as well as in the accumulation of endogenous binding inhibitors such as bilirubin. These findings might explain a smaller degree of midazolam protein binding in cirrhotic individuals, with a subsequent increase in the free fraction of the drug and enhancement of the pharmacologic effect in cirrhotic patients.

For thiopental, total plasma clearance and total apparent volume of distribution at the steady state are unchanged in cirrhotic patients. Therefore, the elimination half-life is not prolonged.[125] Thiopental has a low extraction ratio, so its clearance is independent of hepatic blood flow. Nonetheless, decreases in plasma protein binding, which are often unpredictable, may cause excessive pharmacologic responses to standard doses of the various agents used to induce anesthesia.

The plasma clearance of fentanyl is significantly lower in cirrhotic patients than in control subjects. The total apparent volume of distribution does not change, but the elimination half-life increases owing to decreased plasma clearance. With alfentanil, the free fraction also increases, and this agent exerts prolonged and pronounced effects in cirrhotic patients with advanced liver disease.[126] The data regarding morphine pharmacokinetics in cirrhotic patients are contradictory. For example, Patwardhan et al.[127] reported that the pharmacokinetics of morphine in cirrhotic patients and healthy people are similar. They suggested that the "reported intolerance to the central effects of morphine cannot be explained by impaired drug elimination and increased availability of morphine to cerebral receptors." Other investigators, however, reported that the clearances of free morphine and its metabolites are decreased and their half-lives prolonged in cirrhotic patients compared with healthy control subjects.[128]

Although hepatic disease often produces substantial pharmacokinetic changes, it can also lead to important pharmacodynamic alterations. Patients with cirrhosis, particularly those with hepatic encephalopathy, are much more sensitive to sedatives (e.g., opioids, benzodiazepines) than are healthy people. For example, at equal plasma concentrations of diazepam, more pronounced encephalographic alterations occur in those with severe hepatic disease than in healthy individuals.[129] By contrast, pharmacologic responses to some medications decrease in patients with cirrhosis and portal hypertension as a result of the pathophysiologic changes associated with the disease. Increases in plasma concentrations of certain vasodilatory substances antagonize responses to catecholamines and other vasoconstrictors. Patients, as well as animals with portal hypertension, have elevations of plasma glucagon, which substantially reduces the responses of a variety of blood vessels to catecholamines.[66,68] Thus, while patients with advanced liver disease often require reduced doses of central nervous system depressants, they require increased doses of catecholamine or addition of a nonadrenergic vasoconstrictor (vasopressin) when such therapy is needed to support blood pressure.

INTRAOPERATIVE MANAGEMENT

Monitoring and Vascular Access

In addition to using the routine array of monitors required by the American Society of Anesthesiologists (ASA), the need for invasive monitoring and degree of vascular access will be dictated by the severity of the liver disease and type of surgery. For severely ill patients or major operative procedures, cannulation of an artery is important for continuous blood pressure monitoring, as well as for periodic determinations of blood gases, electrolytes, hematocrit, and other laboratory data as needed during surgery. Because patients with advanced liver disease may present with multiple complex hemodynamic abnormalities, a central venous catheter or even a pulmonary artery catheter may be of utility for confirming diagnoses of hypovolemia, abdominal compartment syndrome, distributive shock, or congestive heart failure, as well as for following responses to therapeutic intervention and for monitoring trends as the case progresses. In addition, because coagulopathies can accompany even mild hepatic insufficiency, the surgical bleeding encountered may be far in excess of that anticipated based on normal circumstances. Large-bore vascular access is encouraged for all but the most minor of procedures. Intraoperative monitoring of coagulation status presents formidable challenges; baseline values may be abnormal despite lack of bleeding. Intraoperative PT, PTT, and platelet count usually take too long for results to be of much utility during a large blood-loss operation. Assessing the activated clotting time and thromboelastography may be helpful, although clinical assessment remains the standard for intraoperative diagnosis of coagulopathy.[130]

Selection of Anesthetic Technique

For most cases, the presence of liver disease will not alter the choice of anesthetic technique based on other common considerations. Regional anesthesia is generally the preferred technique in patients without coagulation abnormalities who are undergoing peripheral surgery. However, it would be difficult to justify using regional anesthesia or analgesia for patients with overt coagulopathies or for those having major or lengthy operations. Local anesthesia with sedation is usually the least invasive for relatively minor procedures, such as sclerotherapy. Adequate sedation is essential to minimize sympathetic stimulation and resultant decreases in hepatic blood flow and oxygen delivery. A short-acting benzodiazepine, such as midazolam combined with remifentanil, or a low dose of fentanyl, will usually provide sedation, anxiolysis, and analgesia. As mentioned, patients with advanced hepatic disease have extensive pharmacodynamic and pharmacokinetic abnormalities, so each medication should be titrated carefully to achieve the desired effect.

Induction of General Anesthesia

Rapid-sequence induction (or awake intubation of the trachea) is indicated in patients perceived to be at risk for aspiration pneumonitis (full stomach). All widely used intravenous induction agents have been administered to patients with advanced hepatic disease. For patients who do not require rapid-sequence induction, careful titration of the anesthetic will minimize hemodynamic lability while achieving the desired anesthetic effect. Succinylcholine is a reasonable choice to facilitate endotracheal intubation, after screening for the usual contraindications (e.g., prolonged immobility or critical illness, hyperkalemia). Although severe liver dysfunction can markedly decrease cholinesterase activity and may prolong the effect of succinylcholine somewhat, this rarely causes a clinical problem. When using nondepolarizing neuromuscular blocking agents to induce anesthesia, consider that the initial dose to achieve total relaxation may be higher than in healthy patients. This increased dose requirement results primarily from pharmacokinetic alterations and pertains to relaxants such as rocuronium, atracurium, and pancuronium, but not to vecuronium.

Maintenance of Anesthesia

Intraoperative liver injury can develop from oxygen deprivation, the stress response, drug toxicity, blood transfusion, and infection. An impairment of hepatic oxygen supply can occur at any step in the process of delivering oxygen to the liver. Hypoxic hypoxia may result from inadequate FIO_2, right-to-left-shunting, or $\dot{V}/\dot{Q}$ mismatch. Anemic hypoxia may develop when the oxygen-carrying capacity of the blood (hematocrit) is inadequate. Circulatory hypoxia may result from systemic (hypovolemia, arterial hypotension, reduction in cardiac output) or regional (decrease in hepatic blood flow and oxygen supply) hemodynamic disorders. Delivery of blood and oxygen to the liver may decrease owing to systemic circulatory disturbances, surgical manipulation of the liver or adjacent structures, or from endogenous vasoconstrictors (e.g., renin-angiotensin, catecholamines, antidiuretic hormone). Anesthetics, exogenous vasoconstrictors, and other medications that impair electron transport or cellular metabolism could also induce histotoxic hypoxia.

In addition to ensuring adequate blood flow and oxygen supply, one must always consider the oxygen supply-demand relations in the liver. Experimental data indicate that severe surgical stress during fentanyl (moderate-dose) anesthesia can produce a somewhat higher hepatic oxygen supply and uptake than an identical stress during isoflurane anesthesia; this results in similar values of hepatic oxygen supply-uptake ratio with the two anesthetics.[31] Taking this into consideration, the guiding principle is to maintain adequate pulmonary and cardiovascular function, including cardiac output, blood volume, and perfusion pressures. One should strive to prevent arterial hypotension by adequate blood and volume replacement, and by avoidance of relative overdoses of anesthetics or other blood pressure-lowering drugs. Vasodilation, a reduced perfusion pressure, and a decrease in blood velocity will inevitably

increase oxygen extraction in all tissues, including those in the preportal area. A decrease in blood velocity and increased oxygen extraction will cause a decrease in venous oxygen content—in this case, decreased oxygen content in the portal venous blood. A reduction in portal blood oxygen content or flow usually leads to a compensatory increase in hepatic arterial flow. Thus, hepatic injury after moderate systemic arterial hypotension is a relatively rare event. However, in the presence of severe liver dysfunction, the ability of autoregulatory mechanisms to increase hepatic arterial blood flow may be diminished or abolished. Therefore, with severe hepatic disease, the hepatic arterial blood flow may not increase appropriately when portal blood flow or oxygen content decreases. This might lead to hepatic oxygen deprivation. Thus, the lesson is clear: take all precautions to avoid arterial hypotension and low cardiac output states.

A particular challenge exists when the operative procedure is on the splanchnic tissues or on the liver itself. In these cases, one objective is to minimize potential for hemorrhage by decreasing the portal blood pressures. Judicious limitation of fluids during the operative resection to maintain a low central venous pressure (<5 mm Hg) has been associated with significantly decreased blood loss while maintaining renal function in a retrospective analysis of hepatic resection cases.[131]

When performing general anesthesia, it seems prudent to avoid halothane, and possibly enflurane, because they cause the most prominent decreases in hepatic blood and oxygen supply and are associated with the highest incidences of postoperative hepatic dysfunction. Isoflurane and probably sevoflurane appear to be the anesthetics of choice for inhalation anesthesia. Nitrous oxide does not appear to be associated with major hepatic complications in patients with advanced liver disease, despite its abilities to produce sympathomimetic effects and to limit the maximum oxygen content of arterial blood.

Opioids are reasonable to include in the anesthetics of patients with hepatic disease. Despite certain pharmacokinetic concerns (decreased clearance and prolonged half-life), fentanyl is probably the opioid of choice. Interestingly, fentanyl neither decreases the hepatic oxygen or blood supply nor prevents an increase in hepatic oxygen requirements when used in moderate doses. Therefore, the oxygen supply-demand relation in the liver is no better with a fentanyl-based anesthetic than during anesthesia with isoflurane.[31] It seems that anesthetic management using inhaled agents (especially isoflurane or sevoflurane) alone or in combination with nitrous oxide and small doses of fentanyl would be the method of choice, provided that adequate hemodynamic parameters are maintained. Many other agents also have favorable risk-benefit profiles for patients with advanced hepatic disease.

Because substantial alterations in pharmacokinetics occur in patients with advanced hepatic disease, dose requirements for a variety of medications can be unpredictable. For example, the half-life of lidocaine may be increased by >300% and benzodiazepines by >100%. Drugs that bind to proteins usually have a decreased volume of distribution, so a lower initial dose would be required. The volume of distribution of other agents, such as muscle relaxants, may increase substantially for various reasons, including an increase in γ-globulin concentration or the presence of edema. These factors appear to account for the so-called resistance to such agents and explain why the initial dose requirements of these medications are increased in cirrhotic patients. However, subsequent dose requirements may be decreased, and drug effects prolonged, owing to decreases in hepatic blood flow and impaired hepatic clearance and possible concurrent renal dysfunction. Advanced hepatic disease does not appear to significantly affect the pharmacokinetics of vecuronium, although some dose-dependent pharmacokinetic alterations may occur. These alterations may be the result of a limited hepatic uptake capacity, which is usually exceeded at doses >0.15 mg/kg. At lower doses, hepatic dysfunction does not affect the pharmacokinetics or duration of action of vecuronium.[132]

Severe hepatic dysfunction per se does not contraindicate the use of any specific muscle relaxant. Atracurium (and cis-atracurium) have a theoretical advantage because their elimination occurs mainly by Hofmann decomposition, making their clearance relatively independent of renal or hepatic function. Despite elimination and clearance profiles, which match those in healthy patients, the volumes of distribution of these agents are larger in cirrhosis and, accordingly, the distribution half-life is shorter in patients with hepatorenal dysfunction compared with normal individuals. The only situation that appears to prolong the elimination half-life of atracurium is marked metabolic acidosis, which may decrease the rate of Hofmann decomposition.[133]

The pharmacokinetics of many muscle relaxants in conditions of cholestasis and obstructive jaundice may be altered: prolonged duration of action has been demonstrated.[134] However, especially when postoperative ventilation is planned, any nondepolarizing agent can be used successfully. Titration of any relaxant must be made according to transcutaneous nerve-stimulation monitoring. Although pharmacokinetic studies in patients with hepatic cirrhosis provide interesting data that are helpful in understanding the pathogenic aspects of chronic liver disease, the results do not necessarily have significant value for predicting the safety of a drug. The degree of hepatic dysfunction affects the degree of pharmacokinetic disorder, and both are dynamic processes that may vary during the course of a procedure; therefore, the best way to avoid complications when administering medications is to titrate to effect.

Fluids and Blood Products

Standard indications for intravascular resuscitation and transfusion of blood products apply to the patient with hepatic insufficiency. No prospective data exist, demonstrating superiority of either a crystalloid-based or colloid-based resuscitation strategy. Because of this lack of conclusive data, the choice of fluid continues to engender spirited opinion and debate. Clearly, colloids represent a higher cost, and some may contribute to coagulopathy, especially at higher doses; however, despite these limitations and lack of documented benefit, they remain the resuscitation fluid of choice for some practitioners.[135] Normovolemic hemodilution has been described as a blood conservation technique for hepatic resections with some success, but is not routinely used for nonhepatic cases in patients with liver insufficiency.[136]

Monitoring of central filling pressures may assist in administering proper fluid therapy and maintaining renal perfusion. The contents of infused solutions should be initially selected and then adjusted based on periodic determinations of serum electrolyte concentrations.

Vasopressors

Patients with hepatic disease, either parenchymal or cholestatic, have peripheral vasodilatation, systemic shunting, and a reduced sensitivity to vasopressor drugs. The exact reason for the decreased pressor sensitivity is unclear. However, data from in vitro and in vivo experiments indicate that bile acids contribute to the vasodilatation and hypotension that often occur in patients with biliary obstruction.[100] Conceivably, a decreased responsiveness to vasoactive substances (including

catecholamines) is responsible for the interesting and clinically important observation that patients with biliary obstruction are often intolerant of even small blood losses. A moderate loss (10%) of blood volume in animals with experimentally induced biliary obstruction causes severe (approximately 50%) arterial hypotension. Intact animals respond to such blood loss with an approximately 15% decrease in blood volumes in both the pulmonary and splanchnic vascular beds. Animals with biliary obstruction have only a 7% decrease of their pulmonary blood volume and no change in splanchnic blood volume.[100] If we can extrapolate these results to humans, patients with biliary obstruction would have an impaired hemodynamic response to blood loss. An impairment of the ability to translocate blood from pulmonary and splanchnic blood reservoirs to the systemic circulation would render patients highly susceptible to arterial hypotension from bleeding. Furthermore, the results would indicate the urgency of expeditiously replacing perioperative volume losses in this patient population. The anesthesiologist should be aware that biliary decompression can be accompanied by severe cardiovascular collapse.[137]

POSTOPERATIVE MANAGEMENT

Liver Dysfunction and Management

Postoperative liver dysfunction is common but rarely severe (Table 48-10). Although it is usually asymptomatic, it may progress to overt liver failure on rare occasions. Mild, transient increases in serum concentrations of hepatic enzymes are often detectable within hours of surgery, but do not usually persist for >2 days. Such subclinical hepatocellular injury occurs in as many as 20% of patients who receive enflurane anesthesia, and in nearly 50% of those receiving halothane. Jaundice rarely occurs in healthy patients following minor operations, but appears in up to 20% of patients after major surgical procedures.[138] Jaundice is typically the earliest sign of serious hepatic or hepatobiliary dysfunction and therefore requires prompt medical attention. Marked increases of serum aminotransferase activities are an ominous finding, reflecting extensive hepatocellular necrosis.

Some cases of severe postoperative liver dysfunction are apparent hours after surgery (e.g., with hypoxic injury), whereas other cases are delayed in onset for days to weeks (e.g., with anesthesia-induced hepatitis). With severe postoperative liver

TABLE 48-10

CAUSES OF POSTOPERATIVE LIVER DYSFUNCTION

Hepatocellular	Drugs
	Anesthetics
	Ischemia
	Shock, hypotension, iatrogenic injury
	Viral hepatitis
Cholestasis	Benign postoperative cholestasis
	Sepsis
	Bile duct injury
	Drugs
	Antibiotics, antiemetics
	Choledocholithiasis or pancreatitis
	Cholecystitis
	Gilbert syndrome

dysfunction, residual liver function may fall below a critical threshold, leading to the development of hepatic encephalopathy. If encephalopathy occurs within 2 weeks of the onset of jaundice or within 8 weeks of the initial manifestation of hepatic disease, the disorder is defined as *fulminant hepatic failure*. Fulminant hepatic failure has a variety of causes.[139] The mortality rate from fulminant hepatic failure correlates with the severity of encephalopathy. The shorter the interval between the appearance of jaundice and presentation of encephalopathy, the worse the prognosis.

Successful treatment of patients with fulminant hepatic failure requires the clinician to make prompt and accurate predictions about the outcome of the disease. Proper recognition of reversible disease obviates unnecessary orthotopic liver transplantation. Irreversible cases of fulminant hepatic failure require immediate identification. Otherwise, the severe complications of fulminant hepatic failure that develop may render patients unacceptable candidates for orthotopic liver transplantation. Several bioartificial liver devices are in various stages of development to provide "liver replacement therapy."[140] Most use porcine or human hepatocytes as a bridge to transplantation or regeneration. Other artificial liver devices are based on albumin dialysis and are undoubtedly effective in removing protein-bound toxins, and uncontrolled evidence shows some survival benefit. Although initial animal studies demonstrated survival benefit of bioartificial liver devices, to date, no prospective randomized trial has shown improved survival using these devices.[141]

Hemolysis and Transfusion

Reabsorption of large surgical or traumatic hematomas and transfusions of red blood cells are major causes of postoperative jaundice in the absence of overt hepatocellular dysfunction. At least 10% of transfused erythrocytes hemolyze within the initial 24 hours following a blood transfusion (the bilirubin load is about 250 mg per unit transfused). A normal liver readily clears the bilirubin that results from mild hemolysis. With severe hemolysis, the excessive bilirubin leads to unconjugated hyperbilirubinemia, which persists until the liver conjugates and excretes the excess bilirubin. Excessive bilirubin loads can also result from severe hemolytic disorders, including hemoglobinopathies (e.g., sickle cell disease) or derangements of erythrocyte metabolism (e.g., glucose-6-phosphate dehydrogenase [G6PD] deficiency). These problems may be seen in the perioperative period as a result of hypovolemia, hypoxia, hypothermia or stress, exacerbations of sickle cell disease, or G6PD deficiency. Other causes of significant hemolysis include transfusion reactions and prosthetic cardiac valves.

CAUSES OF POSTOPERATIVE LIVER DYSFUNCTION UNRELATED TO PERIOPERATIVE FACTORS

Asymptomatic and Pre-Existing Hepatic Injury

Although postoperative liver dysfunction can clearly result from anesthetic or surgical interventions, it is often unrelated to perioperative factors. For example, it can arise from preexisting liver disease that has escaped preoperative detection. According to a study by Schemel,[142] the prevalence of acute, asymptomatic liver disease in a healthy-appearing surgical population may approach 0.25%.

During a 1-year period, Schemel and coworkers performed multiple laboratory screening tests in 7,620 patients (ASA physical status I) scheduled for elective surgical procedures. Eleven of these patients (approximately 1 per 700) were found to have abnormal increases of AST, ALT, and LDH, and the proposed surgeries were cancelled. All 11 proved to have overt hepatic disorders (infectious mononucleosis, viral hepatitis, cirrhosis, or alcoholic hepatitis), and 3 later became clinically jaundiced (overall incidence of jaundice of 1: 2,540). If any of these three patients actually received a halogenated anesthetic, with the subsequent development of overt hepatic disease between the 6th and 14th postoperative days, their diseases may well have been diagnosed erroneously as anesthesia-induced hepatitis. None of the 7,609 patients who underwent anesthesia and surgery exhibited laboratory evidence of pre-existing hepatic disease, and none developed unexplained postsurgical jaundice. Another clinical study[143] has documented a prevalence of unsuspected preoperative hepatic dysfunction similar to that reported by Schemel.[142] Thus, it appears that approximately 1 of every 2,500 healthy patients who undergo surgery and anesthesia may have clinically significant postoperative liver dysfunction that is totally unrelated to surgery or anesthesia, and that a pre-existing disease is more likely than an anesthetic agent to cause severe postoperative liver dysfunction.

Congenital Disorders

Gilbert's syndrome (familial unconjugated hyperbilirubinemia) is the most common cause of jaundice in the United States. It is a benign metabolic disorder characterized by a decrease in the activity of the hepatic enzyme bilirubin glucuronyltransferase, which is required for hepatocyte uptake of unconjugated bilirubin. Affected individuals may have modest increases in their unconjugated bilirubin level preoperatively, but become jaundiced postoperatively secondary to exacerbation of the condition by commonly occurring postoperative factors such as stress, fasting, fever, and infection. The diagnosis is suggested by the combination of clinical (jaundice without dark urine) and laboratory (unconjugated hyperbilirubinemia) abnormalities.

Crigler-Najjar syndrome (congenital nonhemolytic jaundice) is a much less common congenital disorder that exhibits either an absence (type 1) or marked decrease (type 2) of bilirubin glucuronyltransferase producing unconjugated hyperbilirubinemia. Surgical and anesthesia-related problems are apparently minimal in patients with either Gilbert or Crigler-Najjar syndrome.

Conjugated bilirubin is excreted into the bile by a rate-limited, energy-requiring mechanism. Dubin-Johnson and Rotor syndromes are congenital disorders that exhibit a defect in the biliary excretory mechanism, resulting in an increased conjugated bilirubin level. Surgery can exacerbate these abnormalities.

CONCLUSION: PREVENTION AND TREATMENT OF POSTOPERATIVE LIVER DYSFUNCTION

Identifying patients at high risk for developing liver dysfunction or for having an exacerbation of pre-existing liver disease is of utmost importance for minimizing the morbidity and mortality in such patients. Thus, a careful preoperative evaluation is required to detect pre-existing liver disease and to identify important risk factors for anesthesia-induced hepatic injury. Perioperative physicians who are armed with an understanding of the interactions among liver disease, surgical procedures, the physiologic stress response, and anesthetic interventions can formulate and orchestrate therapeutic plans to optimize patient outcome.

When liver abnormalities are recognized preoperatively, it is prudent to defer elective procedures until the course of the disease can be determined. For operations that cannot be deferred, clinically significant pathophysiologic changes associated with the liver disease (e.g., coagulopathy, fluid and electrolyte abnormalities) should be corrected as soon as practical.

Which anesthetic technique best preserves the function of the liver? The choice of anesthesia is usually an insignificant issue for peripheral or minor surgery (operations that do not affect splanchnic blood flow), even in patients with severe liver disease. Regional anesthetic techniques, when appropriate (e.g., absence of coagulopathy), are often preferred because they minimize the cardiovascular and pulmonary perturbations associated with anesthesia. In addition, at least for certain types of procedures such as laparoscopic cholecystectomy, the addition of epidural anesthesia to a general anesthetic technique may decrease the circulating levels of endogenous catecholamines by mitigating the surgical stress response.[144] This effect seems to persist into the postoperative period, when epidural pain management is maintained.[145] The selection of pharmacologic anesthetic agents may also have important implications, especially in patients undergoing major operations. A rational approach to general anesthesia would include the use of agents that preserve cardiac output and do not adversely affect the oxygen supply-demand relationships of the liver (e.g., isoflurane, sevoflurane, fentanyl, remifentanil). Throughout the perioperative period, medications must be carefully titrated to achieve the desired pharmacologic effects while minimizing untoward effects; this can be challenging because pharmacokinetics and pharmacodynamics of many drugs are often unpredictable in patients with hepatobiliary dysfunction.

A primary goal during the maintenance of anesthesia is to ensure the adequacy of splanchnic, hepatic, and renal perfusion, especially in patients with severe liver disease who undergo major abdominal operations. Although well tolerated in the absence of liver disease, hepatic hypoperfusion in patients recovering from infectious hepatitis or chronic alcoholics can have devastating consequences. These patients may be highly susceptible to hepatic ischemia because of critically compromised liver blood flow, impaired pressure-flow autoregulation, and a dysfunctional hepatic arterial buffer response. In such cases, invasive monitoring of the circulation may be indicated so acute hypoperfusion can be rapidly detected and expeditiously treated.

Although anesthesia-induced hepatitis rarely occurs, we must remain aware of the association between this disorder and the use of halogenated vapors. As halothane usage for inhalation inductions and general anesthesia maintenance is increasingly supplanted by other agents, the incidence of this complication decreases with each passing year.[146] In the final analysis, completely avoiding the use of halothane is perhaps the single most effective way to decrease the incidence of anesthesia-induced hepatitis.

When postoperative hepatic injury occurs, the mainstay of therapy is supportive. A thorough search is required to identify any reversible cause of the injury. The hepatotoxic potentials of all medications merit consideration. Discontinue any medication that is suspect. Investigate all potential sources of sepsis because the presence of sepsis mandates rapid, aggressive therapy. Consider extrahepatic biliary obstruction in the differential diagnosis because this may require prompt surgical intervention. In some cases, identifying the pathogen or documenting the type of hepatic injury requires a percutaneous liver biopsy. Judicious use of biochemical tests and imaging studies, which can help delineate hepatocellular from cholestatic dysfunction, usually shortens the list of diagnostic possibilities and provides useful prognostic information.

Unfortunately, fulminant hepatic failure is often survived only with orthotopic liver transplantation. Given that organ donors are far fewer than those needing organ transplants, many must endure our currently inadequate means of supporting this essential organ when it fails. Caring for patients whose liver is failing can be a frustrating endeavor. Perhaps the future holds promise for a supportive intervention as dialysis has provided for renal failure. In the meantime, our efforts at mitigating the tragedy of liver failure will continue to be best directed at prevention.

ACKNOWLEDGMENT

The authors are indebted to Dr. Simon Gelman for his permission to use text, figures, and tables from this chapter in previous editions of *Clinical Anesthesia*.

References

1. Jones AL: Anatomy of the normal liver, Hepatology: A Textbook of Liver Disease, 3rd edition. Edited by Zakim D, Boyer T. Philadelphia, WB Saunders, 1996, p 3
2. Lautt WW: The 1995 Ciba-Geigy award lecture: Intrinsic regulation of hepatic blood flow. Can J Physiol Pharmacol 1996; 74: 233
3. Gelman S, Ernst EA: Role of pH, PCO_2, and O_2 content of portal blood in hepatic circulatory autoregulation. Am J Physiol 1977; 233: E255
4. Martikainen TJ, Tenhunen JJ, Uusaro A et al: The effects of vasopressin on systemic and splanchnic hemodynamics and metabolism in endotoxin shock. Anesth Analg 2003; 97: 1756
5. Asfar P, De Backer D, Meier-Hellmann A et al: Clinical review: Influence of vasoactive and other therapies on intestinal and hepatic circulations in patients with septic shock. Crit Care 2004; 8: 170
6. Adedoyin A, Branch RA: Pharmacokinetics, Hepatology: A Textbook of Liver Disease, 3rd edition. Edited by Zakim D, Boyer T. Philadelphia, WB Saunders, 1996, p 307
7. Friedman LS, Martin P, Munoz SJ: Laboratory evaluation of the patient with liver disease, Hepatology: A Textbook of Liver Disease, 3rd edition. Edited by Zakim D, Boyer T. Philadelphia, WB Saunders, 1996, pp 791
8. Redick JA, Jakoby WB, Baron J: Immunohistochemical localization of glutathione S-transferases in livers of untreated rats. J Biol Chem 1982; 257: 15200
9. Ercolani G, Grazi GL, Calliva R et al: The lidocaine (MEGX) test as an index of hepatic function: Its usefulness in liver surgery. Surgery 2000; 127: 464
10. Vento S, Garofano T, Renzini C et al: Fulminant hepatitis associated with hepatitis A virus superinfection in patients with chronic hepatitis C. N Engl J Med 1998; 338: 286
11. Scott JD, Gretch DR: Molecular diagnostics of hepatitis C virus infection: a systematic review. JAMA 2007; 297: 724
12. Eriksson LS, Broome U, Kalin M, Lindholm M: Hepatotoxicity due to repeated intake of low doses of paracetamol. J Intern Med 1992; 231: 567
13. Anonymous: Summary of the National Halothane Study: Possible association between halothane anesthesia and postoperative hepatic necrosis. JAMA 1966; 197: 775
14. Kenna JG, Jones RM: The organ toxicity of inhaled anesthetics. Anesth Analg 1995; 81(Suppl 6): S51
15. Martin JL: [Volatile anesthetics and liver injury: a clinical update or what every anesthesiologist should know.]. Can J Anaesth 2005; 52: 125
16. Turner GB, O'Rourke D, Scott GO, Beringer TR: Fatal hepatotoxicity after re-exposure to isoflurane: A case report and review of the literature. Eur J Gastroenterol Hepatol 2000; 12: 955
17. Inman WH, Mushin WW: Jaundice after repeated exposure to halothane: An analysis of reports to the Committee on Safety of Medicines. BMJ 1974; 1: 5
18. Neuberger J, Williams R: Halothane anaesthesia and liver damage. BMJ 1984; 289: 1136
19. Hoft R, Bunker JP, Goodman HI, Gregory PB: Halothane hepatitis in three pairs of closely related women. N Engl J Med 1981; 304: 1023
20. Brown BJ, Gandolfi A: Adverse effects of volatile anaesthetics. Br J Anaesth 1987; 59: 14
21. Otsuka S, Yamamoto S, Kasuya H et al: HLA antigens in patients with unexplained hepatitis following halothane anesthesia. Acta Anaesthesiol Scand 1985; 29: 497
22. Warner LO, Beach TP, Garvin JP, Warner EJ: Halothane and children: The first quarter century. Anesth Analg 1984; 63: 838

23. Hassall E, Israel DM, Gunasekaran T, Steward D: Halothane hepatitis in children. J Pediatr Gastroenterol Nutr 1990; 11: 553

24. Kenna J, Neuberger J, Mieli-Vergeni G et al: Halothane hepatitis in children. BMJ 1987; 294: 1209

25. Njoku D, Laster MJ, Gong DH et al: Biotransformation of halothane, enflurane, isoflurane, and desflurane to trifluoroacetylated liver proteins: Association between protein acylation and hepatic injury. Anesth Analg 1997; 84: 173

26. Shiraishi Y, Ikeda K: Uptake and biotransformation of sevoflurane in humans: A comparative study of sevoflurane with halothane, enflurane, and isoflurane. J Clin Anesth 1990; 2: 381

27. Frink EJ Jr, Morgan SE, Coetzee A et al: The effects of sevoflurane, halothane, enflurane, and isoflurane on hepatic blood flow and oxygenation in chronically instrumented greyhound dogs. Anesthesiology 1992; 76: 85

28. Bernard JM, Doursout MF, Wouters P et al: Effects of enflurane and isoflurane on hepatic and renal circulation in chronically instrumented dogs. Anesthesiology 1991; 74: 298

29. Schindler E, Muller M, Zickmann B et al: Blood supply to the liver after 1 MAC desflurane in comparison with isoflurane and halothane (in German). Anasthesiol Intensivmed Notfallmed Schmerzther 1996; 31: 344

30. Kanaya N, Nakayama M, Fujita S, Namiki A: Comparison of the effects of sevoflurane, isoflurane and halothane on indocyanine green clearance. Br J Anaesth 1995; 74: 164

31. Gelman S, Dillard E, Bradley EL Jr: Hepatic circulation during surgical stress and anesthesia with halothane, isoflurane, or fentanyl. Anesth Analg 1987; 66: 936

32. Conzen PF, Vollmar B, Habazettl H et al: Systemic and regional hemodynamics of isoflurane and sevoflurane in rats. Anesth Analg 1992; 74: 79

33. Bernard JM, Doursout MF, Wouters P et al: Effects of sevoflurane and isoflurane on hepatic circulation in the chronically instrumented dog. Anesthesiology 1992; 77: 541

34. Frink EJ Jr: The hepatic effects of sevoflurane. Anesth Analg 1995; 81(Suppl 6): S46

35. Nunn JF: Clinical aspects of the interaction between nitrous oxide and vitamin B12. Br J Anaesth 1987; 59(1): 3

36. Cohen EN, Gift HC, Brown BW et al: Occupational disease in dentistry and chronic exposure to trace anesthetic gases. J Am Dent Assoc 1980; 101: 21

37. Prys-Roberts C, Sear JW, Low JM et al: Hemodynamic and hepatic effects of methohexital infusion during nitrous oxide anesthesia in humans. Anesth Analg 1983; 62: 317

38. Zinn SE, Fairley HB, Glenn JD: Liver function in patients with mild alcoholic hepatitis, after enflurane, nitrous oxide-narcotic, and spinal anesthesia. Anesth Analg 1985; 64: 487

39. Brodsky JB: Toxicity of nitrous oxide, Nitrous Oxide/N2O. Edited by Eger EI. New York, Elsevier, 1985, pp 265

40. Gelman S: General anesthesia and hepatic circulation. Can J Physiol Pharmacol 1987; 65: 1762

41. Dundee JW, Fee JP, Moore J et al: Changes in serum enzyme levels following ketamine infusions. Anaesthesia 1980; 35: 12

42. Clarke RS, Kirwin MJ, Dundee JW et al: Clinical studies of induction agents: XIII. Liver function after propanidad and thiopentone anaesthesia. Br J Anaesth 1965; 37: 415

43. Thompson DR: Narcotic analgesic effects on the sphincter of Oddi: A review of the data and therapeutic implications in treating pancreatitis. Am J Gastroenterol 2001; 96: 1266

44. Tenhunen JJ, Uusaro A, Karja V et al: Apparent heterogeneity of regional blood flow and metabolic changes within splanchnic tissues during experimental endotoxin shock. Anesth Analg 2003; 97: 555

45. Schiffer ER, Mentha G, Schwieger IM, Morel DR: Sequential changes in the splanchnic circulation during continuous endotoxin infusion in sedated sheep: Evidence for a selective increase of hepatic artery blood flow and loss of the hepatic arterial buffer response. Acta Physiol Scand 1993; 147: 251

46. Refsum H: Arterial hypoxaemia, serum activity of GO-T, GP-T and LDH, and central lobular liver cell necrosis in pulmonary insufficiency. Clin Sci 1963; 25: 369

47. Sims J, Morris L, Orth O et al: The influence of oxygen and carbon dioxide levels during anesthesia upon postsurgical hepatic damage. J Lab Clin Med 1951; 38: 388

48. Gibson PR, Dudley FJ: Ischemic hepatitis: Clinical features, diagnosis and prognosis. Aust N Z J Med 1984; 14: 822

49. Bynum TE, Boitnott JK, Maddrey WC: Ischemic hepatitis. Dig Dis Sci 1979; 24: 129

50. Giallourakis CC, Rosenberg PM, Friedman LS: The liver in heart failure. Clin Liver Dis 2002; 6: 947

51. Szawarski P, Sensky PR, Doshi M, Hudson I: Fulminant liver failure: An indicator of silent myocardial rupture. Postgrad Med J 2004; 80: 553

52. McNeill JR, Pang CC: Effect of pentobarbital anesthesia and surgery on the control of arterial pressure and mesenteric resistance in cats: Role of vasopressin and angiotensin. Can J Physiol Pharmacol 1982; 60: 363

53. Gelman SI: Disturbances in hepatic blood flow during anesthesia and surgery. Arch Surg 1976; 111: 881

54. Kotake Y, Takeda J, Matsumoto M et al: Subclinical hepatic dysfunction in laparoscopic cholecystectomy and laparoscopic colectomy. Br J Anaesth 2001; 87: 774

55. Mathie RT: Hepatic blood flow during cardiopulmonary bypass. Crit Care Med 1993; 21: S72

56. Liaw YF, Sung JJY, Chow WC et al: Lamivudine for patients with chronic hepatitis B and advanced liver disease. N Engl J Med 2004; 351: 1521

57. Lok ASF, McMahon BJ: AASLD practice guideline: Chronic hepatitis B: Update of recommendations. Hepatology 2004; 39: 857

58. Feld JJ, Ghany MG: Evolution of therapy for chronic hepatitis B: progressing from the simple to the complex. Ann Intern Med 2007; 147: 806

59. Dienstag JL, McHutchison JG: American Gastroenterological Association medical position statement on the management of hepatitis C. Gastroenterology 2006; 130: 225

60. Solga SF, Diehl AM: Non-alcoholic fatty liver disease: Lumen-liver interactions and possible role for probiotics. J Hepatol 2003; 38: 681

61. Neuschwander-Tetri BA, Caldwell SH: Nonalcoholic steatohepatitis: Summary of an AASLD single topic conference. Hepatology 2003; 37: 1202

62. Falck-Ytter Y, Younossi ZM, Marchesini G, McCullough AJ: Clinical features and natural history of nonalcoholic steatosis syndromes. Semin Liver Dis 2001; 21: 17

63. Stewart SF, Day CP: The management of alcoholic liver disease. J Hepatol 2003; 38: S2

64. Tonnesen H, Kehlet H: Preoperative alcoholism and postoperative morbidity. Br J Surg 1999; 86: 869

65. Murray JF, Dawson AM, Sherlock S: Circulatory changes in chronic liver disease. Am J Med 1958; 24: 358

66. Bomzon A, Blendis L: Vascular reactivity in experimental portal hypertension. Am J Physiol 1987; 252: G158

67. Matsumoto A, Ogura K, Hirata Y et al: Increased nitric oxide production in the exhaled air of patients with decompensated cirrhosis. Ann Intern Med 1995; 123: 110

68. Benoit JN, Granger DN: Splanchnic hemodynamics in chronic portal hypertension. Semin Liver Dis 1986; 6: 287

69. Sharara AI, Rockey DC: Gastroesophageal variceal hemorrhage. N Engl J Med 2001; 345: 669

70. Bosch J, Abraldes JG, Groszmann R: Current management of portal hypertension. J Hepatol 2003; 38: S54

71. Salerno F, Camma C, Enea M, Rossle M, Wong F: Transjugular intrahepatic portosystemic shunt for refractory ascites: a meta-analysis of individual patient data. Gastroenterology 2007; 133: 825

72. Palma DT, Fallon MB: The hepatopulmonary syndrome. J Hepatol 2006; 45: 617

73. Lazaridis KN, Frank JW, Krowka MJ, Kamath PS: Hepatic hydrothorax: Pathogenesis, diagnosis, and management. Am J Med 1999; 107: 262

74. Krowka M, Plevak D, Findlay J et al: Pulmonary hemodynamics and perioperative cardiopulmonary-related mortality in patients with portopulmonary hypertension undergoing liver transplantation. Liver Transpl 2000; 6: 443

75. Jalen R, Hayes PC: Hepatic encephalopathy and ascites. Lancet 1997; 350: 1309

76. Moore KP, Aithal GP: Guidelines on the management of ascites in cirrhosis. Gut 2006; 55(Suppl 6): vi1

77. Runyon BA: AASLD practice guidelines: Management of adult patients with ascites caused by cirrhosis. Hepatology 1998; 27: 264

78. Moore KP, Wong F, Gines P et al: The management of ascites in cirrhosis: Report on the consensus conference of the International Ascites Club. Hepatology 2003; 38: 258

79. Panos MZ, Moore K, Vlavianos P et al: Single total paracentesis for tense ascites: Sequential hemodynamic changes and right atrial size. Hepatology 1990; 11: 662

80. Luca A, Garcia-Pagan JC, Bosch J et al: Beneficial effects of intravenous albumin infusion on the hemodynamics and humoral changes after total paracentesis. Hepatology 1995; 22: 753

81. Sola-Vera J, Minana J, Ricart E et al: Randomized trial comparing albumin and saline in the prevention of paracentesis-induced circulatory dysfunction in cirrhotic patients with ascites. Hepatology 2003; 37: 1147

82. Gines A, Fernandez-Esparrach G, Monescillo A et al: Randomized trial comparing albumin, dextran 70, and polygeline in cirrhotic patients with ascites treated by paracentesis. Gastroenterology 1996; 111: 1002

83. Follo A, Llovet JM, Navasa M et al: Renal impairment after spontaneous bacterial peritonitis in cirrhosis: Incidence, clinical course, predictive factors and prognosis. Hepatology 1994; 20: 1495

84. Sort P, Navasa M, Arroyo V et al: Effect of intravenous albumin on renal impairment and mortality in patients with cirrhosis and spontaneous bacterial peritonitis. N Engl J Med 1999; 341: 403

85. Ruiz-del-Arbol L, Monescillo A, Arocena C et al: Circulatory function and hepatorenal syndrome in cirrhosis. Hepatology 2005; 42: 439

86. Arroyo V, Gines P, Gerbes AL et al: Definition and diagnostic criteria of refractory ascites and hepatorenal syndrome in cirrhosis. Hepatology 1996; 23: 164

87. Moreau R, Lebrec D: Acute renal failure in patients with cirrhosis: Perspectives in the age of MELD. Hepatology 2003; 37: 233

88. Wadei HM, Mai ML, Ahsan N, Gonwa TA: Hepatorenal syndrome: pathophysiology and management. Clin J Am Soc Nephrol 2006; 1: 1066

89. Duvoux C, Zanditenas D, Hezode C et al: Effects of noradrenalin and albumin in patients with type I hepatorenal syndrome: A pilot study. Hepatology 2002; 36: 374

90. Angeli P, Volpin R, Gerunda G et al: Reversal of type I hepatorenal syndrome with the administration of midodrine and octreotide. Hepatology 1999; 29: 1690

ANESTHESIA FOR SURGICAL SUBSPECIALTIES

91. Friedman LS: The risk of surgery in patients with liver disease. Hepatology 1999; 29: 1617

92. Amitrano L, Guardascione MA, Brancaccio V, Balzano A: Coagulation disorders in liver disease. Semin Liver Dis 2002; 22: 83

93. Wright G, Jalan R: Management of hepatic encephalopathy in patients with cirrhosis. Best Pract Res Clin Gastroenterol 2007; 21: 95

94. Riordan SM, Williams R: Treatment of hepatic encephalopathy. N Engl J Med 1997; 337: 473

95. Plauth M, Merli M, Weimann A et al: ESPEN guidelines for nutrition in liver disease and transplantation. Clin Nutr 1997; 16: 43

96. Bruix J, Sherman M: Management of hepatocellular carcinoma. Hepatology 2005; 42: 1208

97. Castro MA, Fassett MJ, Reynolds TB et al. Reversible peripartum liver failure: A new perspective on the diagnosis, treatment, and cause of acute fatty liver of pregnancy, based on 28 consecutive cases. Am J Obstet Gynecol 1999; 181: 389

98. Ibdah JA: Acute fatty liver of pregnancy: an update on pathogenesis and clinical implications. World J Gastroenterol 2006; 12: 7397

99. Sibai BM: Diagnosis, controversies, and management of the syndrome of hemolysis, elevated liver enzymes, and low platelet count. Obstet Gynecol 2004; 103: 981

100. Better OS: Renal and cardiovascular dysfunction in liver disease (clinical conference). Kidney Int 1986; 29: 598

101. Bomzon A, Monies-Chass I, Kamenetz L, Blendis L: Anesthesia and pressor responsiveness in chronic bile-duct-ligated dogs. Hepatology 1990; 11: 551

102. Bonkovsky HL, Jones DP, LaBrecque DR, Shedlofsky SI: Drug-induced liver disease, Hepatology: A Textbook of Liver Disease, 5th ed. Edited by Zakim D, Boyer T. Philadelphia, WB Saunders: 503

103. Sullivan D, Csuka ME, Blanchard B: Erythromycin ethylsuccinate hepatotoxicity. JAMA 1980; 243: 1074.

104. Charney DS, Mikic J, Harris RA: Hypnotics and Sedatives, The Pharmacological Basis of Therapeutics, 11th ed. Edited by Goodman, Gilman A. Philadelphia, McGraw Hill, 2006: 417

105. Ziser A, Plevak DJ, Wiesner RH et al: Morbidity and mortality in cirrhotic patients undergoing anesthesia and surgery. Anesthesiology 1999; 90: 42

106. Child CG, Turcotte JG: Surgery and portal hypertension, The Liver and Portal Hypertension: Volume I, Major Problems in Clinical Surgery. Edited by Child CG. Philadelphia, WB Saunders, 1964, pp 50

107. Aranha GV, Sontag SJ, Greenlee HB: Cholecystectomy in cirrhotic patients: A formidable operation. Am J Surg 1982; 143: 55

108. Doberneck RC, Sterling WA, Allison DC: Morbidity and mortality after operation in nonbleeding cirrhotic patients. Am J Surg 1983; 146: 306

109. Garrison RN, Cryer HM, Howard DA, Polk HC: Clarification of risk factors for abdominal operations in patients with hepatic cirrhosis. Ann Surg 1984; 199: 648

110. Rice HE, O'Keefe GE, Helton WS, Johanson K: Morbid prognostic features in patients with chronic liver failure undergoing nonhepatic surgery. Arch Surg 1997; 132: 880

111. Mansour A, Watson W, Shayani V, Pickleman J: Abdominal operations in patients with cirrhosis: Still a major surgical challenge. Surgery 1997; 122: 730

112. Knaus WA, Draper EA, Wagner DP, Zimmerman JE: APACHE II: A severity of disease classification system. Crit Care Med 1985; 13: 818

113. Freeman RB Jr, Wiesner RH, Harper A et al: UNOS/OPTN Liver Disease Severity Score, UNOS/OPTN Liver and Intestine, and UNOS/OPTN Pediatric Transplantation Committees. The new liver allocation system: Moving toward evidence-based transplantation policy. Liver Transpl 2002; 8: 851

114. Pugh RNH, Murray-Lyon IM, Dawson JL et al: Transection of the oesophagus for bleeding oesophageal varices. Br J Surg 1973; 60: 646

115. Iwatsuki S, Starzl TE, Todo S et al: Liver transplantation in the treatment of bleeding esophageal varices. Surgery 1988; 104: 697

116. Orloff MJ, Orloff MS, Rambotti M, Girard B: Is portal-systemic shunt worthwhile in Child's class C cirrhosis? Long-term results of emergency shunt in 94 patients with bleeding varices. Ann Surg 1992; 216: 256

117. Kamath PS, Wiesner RH, Malinchoc M et al: A model to predict survival in patients with end-stage liver disease. Hepatology 2001; 33: 464

118. Wiklund RA: Preoperative preparation of patients with advanced liver disease. Crit Care Med 2004; 32: S106

119. Clarke RS, Doggart JR, Lavery T: Changes in liver function after different types of surgery. Br J Anaesth 1976; 48: 119

120. Viegas O, Stoelting RK: LDH5 changes after cholecystectomy or hysterectomy in patients receiving halothane, enflurane, or fentanyl. Anesthesiology 1979; 51: 556

121. MacGilchrist AJ, Birnie GG, Cook A et al: Pharmacokinetics and pharmacodynamics of intravenous midazolam in patients with severe alcoholic cirrhosis. Gut 1986; 27: 190

122. Trouvin JH, Farinotti R, Haberer JP et al: Pharmacokinetics of midazolam in anesthetized cirrhotic patients. Br J Anaesth 1988; 60: 762

123. Chauvin M, Ferrier C, Haberer JP et al: Sufentanil pharmacokinetics in patients with cirrhosis. Anesth Analg 1989; 68: 1

124. Servin F, Desmonts JM, Haberer JP et al: Pharmacokinetics and protein binding of propofol in patients with cirrhosis. Anesthesiology 1988; 69: 887

125. Pandele G, Chaux F, Salvadori C et al: Thiopental pharmacokinetics in patients with cirrhosis. Anesthesiology 1983; 59: 123

126. Ferrier C, Marty J, Bouffard Y et al: Alfentanil pharmacokinetics in patients with cirrhosis. Anesthesiology 1985; 62: 480

127. Patwardhan RV, Johnson RF, Hoyumpa A Jr et al: Normal metabolism of morphine in cirrhotics. Gastroenterology 1981; 81: 1006

128. Mazoit JX, Sandouk P, Zetlaoui P, Scherrmann JHM: Pharmacokintics of unchanged morphine in normal and cirrhotic subjects. Anesth Analg 1987; 66: 293

129. Branch R, Morgan M, James J et al: Intravenous administration of diazepam in patients with chronic liver disease. Gut 1976; 17: 975

130. Clayton DG, Miro AM, Kramer DJ et al: Quantification of thromboelastographic changes after blood component transfusion in patients with liver disease in the intensive care unit. Anesth Analg 1995; 81: 272

131. Melendez JA, Arsian V, Fischer ME et al: Perioperative outcomes of major hepatic resection under low central venous pressure anesthesia: Blood loss, blood transfusion, and the risk of postoperative renal dysfunction. J Am Coll Surg 1998; 187: 620

132. Arden J, Cannon J, Lynam D et al: Vecuronium pharmacokinetics and pharmacodynamics in hepatocellular disease. Anesth Analg 1987; 66: S3

133. Ward S, Neill E: Pharmacokinetics of atracurium in acute hepatic failure (with acute renal failure). Br J Anaesth 1984; 28: 401

134. Westra P, Houwertjes C, DeLange A et al: Effect of experimental cholestasis on neuromuscular blocking drugs in cats. Br J Anaesth 1980; 52: 747

135. Redai I, Emond J, Brentjens T: Anesthetic considerations during liver surgery. Surg Clin North Am 2004; 84: 401

136. Matot I, Scheinin O, Jurim O, Eid A: Effectiveness of acute normovolemic hemodilution to minimize allogeneic blood transfusion during major liver resections. Anesthesiology 2002; 97: 794

137. Tamakuma S, Wada N, Ishiyama M et al: Relationship between hepatic hemodynamics and biliary pressure in dogs: Its significance in clinical shock following biliary decompression. Jap J Surg 1975; 5: 255

138. Evans C, Evans M, Pollack AV: The incidence and causes of postoperative jaundice: A prospective study. Br J Anaesth 1974; 46: 520

139. Lee WM: Acute liver failure in the United States. Semin Liver Dis 2003; 23: 217

140. Van de Kerkhove MP, Hoekstra R, Chamuleau RA, Van Gulik TM: Clinical application of bioartificial liver support systems. Ann Surg 2004; 240: 216

141. Sens S, Williams R: New liver support devices in acute liver failure: A critical evaluation. Semin Liver Dis 2003; 23: 283

142. Schemel WH: Unexpected hepatic dysfunction found by multiple laboratory screening. Anesth Analg 1976; 55: 810

143. Wataneeyawech M, Kelly K: Hepatic disease: Unsuspected before surgery. N Y State J Med 1975; 75: 1278

144. Aono H, Takeda A, Tarver SD, Goto H: Stress responses in three different anesthetic techniques for carbon dioxide laparoscopic cholecystectomy. J Clin Anesth 1998; 10: 546

145. Adams HA, Saatweber P, Schmitz CS, Hecker H: Postoperative pain management in orthopaedic patients: No differences in pain score, but improved stress control by epidural anaesthesia. Eur J Anaesthesiol 2002; 19: 658

146. Tarpey J, Lawler PG: Volatile agent use: Perception and practice. A survey of agent use over a 3-year period. Anaesthesia 1989; 44: 596

147. Roberts EA, Schilsky ML: A practice guideline on Wilson disease. Hepatology 2003; 37: 1475

148. Pietrangelo A: Hereditary hemochromatosis—A new look at an old disease. N Engl J Med 2004; 350: 2383

149. Rouault TA: Hereditary hemochromatosis. JAMA 1993; 269: 3152

150. Kaplan MM: Primary biliary cirrhosis. N Engl J Med 1996; 335: 1570

151. Mulgrew AT, Taggart CC, McElvaney NG. Alpha-1-antitrypsin deficiency: current concepts. Lung 2007; 185: 191

152. Menon KVN, Shah V, Kamath PS: The Budd-Chiari syndrome. N Engl J Med 2004; 350: 578

153. Mentha G, Giostra E, Majno PE et al: Liver transplantation for Budd-Chiari syndrome: A European study on 248 patients from 51 centres. J Hepatol 2006; 44: 520

CHAPTER 49 ■ **ENDOCRINE FUNCTION**

JEFFREY J. SCHWARTZ, SHAMSUDDIN AKHTAR, AND STANLEY H. ROSENBAUM

KEY POINTS

❶ The major risk of anesthesia in the poorly controlled thyrotoxic patient is thyroid storm, which must be aggressively treated with beta-blockers, iodide, and antithyroid drugs.

❷ Asymptomatic or mild hypothyroidism does not appear to significantly increase anesthetic risk and is not a contraindication to surgery. Moderate-to-severe hypothyroidism should be corrected before surgery to prevent multisystem complications.

❸ Patients who have received corticosteroids for >1 week in the past year may have adrenal suppression and should receive supplemental steroids in the perioperative period.

❹ Preoperative preparation of the pheochromocytoma patient with alpha-blockers decreases intraoperative hemodynamic instability.

❺ Pheochromocytoma manipulation is associated with severe hypertension that should be treated aggressively with nitroprusside, phentolamine, or other rapidly acting vasodilators.

❻ The major perioperative risks to the diabetic patient come from coexisting disease, especially coronary artery disease. Coexisting disease must be aggressively sought and optimized.

❼ Maintenance of blood glucose levels near euglycemia appears to reduce cardiac, wound, neurologic, and septic complications.

❽ Endotracheal intubation may be unpredictably difficult in patients with acromegaly.

THYROID GLAND

The thyroid gland secretes thyroid hormones, thyroxine (T_4), and $3,3',5$ triiodothyronine (T_3), which are the major regulators of cellular metabolic activity. Thyroid hormones exert a variety of actions by regulating the synthesis and activity of various proteins. They are necessary for proper cardiac, pulmonary, and neurologic function during both health and illness.

Thyroid Metabolism and Function

The production of thyroid hormone is initiated by the active uptake and concentration of iodide in the thyroid gland

(Fig. 49-1). Dietary iodine is reduced to iodide in the gastrointestinal (GI) tract. Circulating iodide is taken up by the thyroid gland, where it is then bound to tyrosine residues to form various iodotyrosines. After organification, monoiodotyrosine or diiodotyrosine is coupled enzymatically by thyroid peroxidase to form either T_3 or T_4. These hormones are attached to the thyroglobulin protein and stored as colloid in the gland. The release of T_3 and T_4 from the gland is accomplished through proteolysis from the thyroglobulin and diffusion into the circulation. Thyrotropin (thyroid-stimulating hormone or TSH) is produced in the anterior pituitary gland, and its secretion is regulated by thyrotropin-releasing hormone produced in the hypothalamus. TSH is responsible for maintaining the uptake of iodide and proteolytic release of thyroid hormone. Excess iodine inhibits the synthesis and secretion of thyroid hormone.

FIGURE 49-1. Thyroid hormone biosynthesis consists of four stages: (1) organification, (2) binding, (3) coupling, and (4) release. TSH, thyroid-stimulating hormone; T_3, triiodothyronine; T_4, thyroxine.

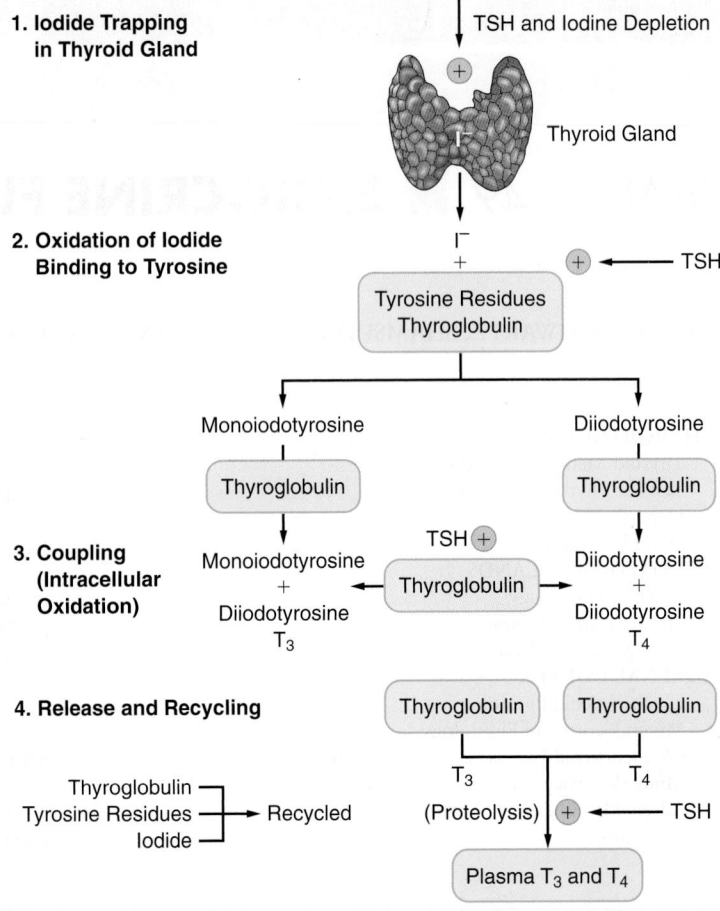

Circulating thyroid hormone inhibits thyroid-releasing hormone and TSH secretion in a negative feedback loop. The thyroid gland is solely responsible for the daily secretion of T_4 (80 to 100 μg/day). The half-life of T_4 in the circulation is 6 to 7 days.

Approximately 80% of T_3 is produced by the extrathyroidal deiodination of T_4 and 20% is produced by direct thyroid secretion. The half-life of T_3 is 24 to 30 hours. Most of the effects of thyroid hormones are mediated by the more potent and less protein-bound T_3. The degree to which these hormones are protein bound in the circulation is the major factor influencing their activity and degradation. T_4 is metabolized by monodeiodination to either T_3 or reverse T_3 (rT_3). T_3 is biologically active, whereas rT_3 is inactive. The major fraction of circulating hormone is bound to thyroxine-binding globulin (TBG), with a smaller fraction bound to albumin and thyroid-binding prealbumin. Less than 0.1% is present as free, unbound hormone. Changes in serum-binding protein concentrations have a major effect on total T_3 and T_4 serum concentrations. The plasma normally contains 5 to 12 μg/dL of T_4 and 80 to 220 ng/dL of T_3. Many drugs can affect thyroid function, including amiodarone and dopamine.[1]

Although the thyroid hormone is important to many aspects of growth and function, the anesthesiologist is most often concerned with the cardiovascular manifestations of thyroid disease. Thyroid hormones affect tissue responses to sympathetic stimuli and increase the intrinsic contractile state of cardiac muscle.

β-Adrenergic receptors are increased in number, and cardiac α-adrenergic receptors are decreased by thyroid hormone.[2]

Tests of Thyroid Function

Serum Thyroxine

The serum T_4 assay is a standard test for evaluation of thyroid gland function (Table 49-1). The total T_4 is elevated in approximately 90% of patients with hyperthyroidism, and it is low in 85% of those who are hypothyroid. The concentration of T_4 is measured by radioimmunoassay (RIA). The serum T_4 concentration is influenced by thyroid hormone protein-binding capacity. An increase or decrease in TBG levels or in protein binding may therefore alter the total T_4 but not the concentration of the free T_4. Because of the effect of TBG on circulating total T_4, the T_4 levels should never be used alone to evaluate thyroid disease. Elevations in the TBG concentration are the most common cause of hyperthyroxinemia in euthyroid patients. Increases in TBG due to acute liver disease, pregnancy, or drugs (oral contraceptives, exogenous estrogens, clofibrate, opioids) may be the causative factor. Because a total T_4 can be misleadingly high in euthyroidism or normal in hypothyroidism, some measure of free thyroid hormone activity (free T_4) must also be used.

Serum Triiodothyronine

The serum T_3 is also measured by RIA. Serum T_3 levels are often determined to detect disease in patients with clinical evidence of hyperthyroidism in the absence of elevations of T_4. T_3 may be the only thyroid hormone produced in excess. T_3 concentrations may be depressed by factors that impair the peripheral conversion of T_4 to T_3 (sick euthyroid syndrome).

TABLE 49-1

TESTS OF THYROID GLAND FUNCTION

	■ T₄	■ T₃	■ THBR	■ TSH
Hyperthyroidism	Elevated	Elevated	Elevated	Normal or low
Primary hypothyroidism	Low	Low or normal	Low	Elevated
Secondary hypothyroidism	Low	Low	Low	Low
Sick euthyroidism (decreased peripheral conversion of T₄ to T₃)	Normal	Low	Normal	Normal
Pregnancy	Elevated	Normal	Low	Normal

T_4, total serum thyroxine; T_3, serum triiodothyronine; THBR, thyroid hormone-binding rate; TSH, thyroid-stimulating hormone.

In 50% of hypothyroid patients, the serum T_3 concentration is low; in the remaining 50%, it is normal.

Tests for Assessing Thyroid Hormone Binding

It is necessary to find some measure of thyroid-binding proteins, mostly TBG, to interpret correctly total thyroxine levels. The "T_4 uptake" test measures the ability of the patient's serum to bind exogenously introduced T_4 and reflects the amount of TBG and the extent of T_4 saturation on TBG. The T_4 uptake is inversely related to the degree of unsaturation of TBG. The T_4 uptake can be used to calculate the T_4-binding capacity, which is directly related to the degree of unsaturation of TBG. The T_4 uptake or T_4-binding capacity can be used to calculate the thyroid hormone binding ratio, which can be used to calculate the free T_4 index, which reflects the free T_4 concentration in the blood independent of binding proteins.

Thyroid-Stimulating Hormone

The RIA for this hormone has improved in sensitivity and specificity enough to become the first test in evaluating suspected thyroid dysfunction. It is often higher than 20 μIU/mL in primary hypothyroidism (normal, 8 μIU/mL). Hyperthyroidism can be suspected from depressed TSH levels. A condition characterized by elevated TSH and normal T_4 may represent subclinical hypothyroidism. A low TSH level in a clinically hypothyroid patient indicates disease at the pituitary or hypothalamic level. The goal of thyroid replacement therapy is to normalize TSH levels.[3] Starvation, fever, stress, corticosteroids, and T_3 or T_4 can all depress TSH levels.

Radioactive Iodine Uptake

The thyroid gland has the ability to concentrate large amounts of inorganic iodide. The oral administration of radioactive iodine (^{131}I) can be used to indicate thyroid gland activity. Thyroid uptake is elevated in hyperthyroidism unless the hyperthyroidism is caused by thyroiditis, in which case the uptake is low or absent. Because of overlap in values, it is difficult to distinguish euthyroid from hypothyroid people. Radioactive iodide uptake may be increased by a variety of factors, including dietary iodine deficiency, renal failure, and congestive heart failure. Because uptake is under TSH control, elevated free T_4 levels and corticosteroids decrease radioactive iodide uptake. Functioning ("hot") thyroid tissue is rarely malignant. Nonfunctioning ("cold") tissue may be malignant or benign.

Hyperthyroidism

Hyperthyroidism results from the exposure of tissues to excessive amounts of thyroid hormone (Table 49-2). The most common cause is the multinodular diffuse goiter of Graves disease. This typically occurs between the ages of 20 and 40 years, and is predominant in women. Most patients with this condition demonstrate a syndrome characterized by diffuse glandular enlargement, ophthalmopathy, dermopathy, and clubbing of the fingers. A thyroid-stimulating autoantibody may be present. Thyroid adenoma is the second most common cause. Another cause of increased thyroid hormone synthesis is thyroiditis. Subacute thyroiditis frequently follows a respiratory illness and is characterized by a viral-like illness with a firm, painful gland. This type of thyroiditis is frequently treated with anti-inflammatory agents alone. Rarely, subacute thyroiditis may occur in a patient with a normal-size, painless

TABLE 49-2

CAUSES OF HYPERTHYROIDISM

■ **INTRINSIC THYROID DISEASE**

Hyperfunctioning thyroid adenoma
Toxic multinodular goiter

■ **ABNORMAL TSH STIMULATOR**

Graves disease
Trophoblastic tumor

■ **DISORDERS OF HORMONE STORAGE OR RELEASE**

Thyroiditis

■ **EXCESS PRODUCTION OF TSH**

Pituitary thyrotropin (rare)

■ **EXTRATHYROIDAL SOURCE OF HORMONE**

Struma ovarii
Functioning follicular carcinoma

■ **EXOGENOUS THYROID**

Iatrogenic
Iodine induced

TSH, thyroid-stimulating hormone.

gland. Hashimoto's thyroiditis is a chronic autoimmune disease that usually produces hypothyroidism but may occasionally produce hyperthyroidism. Hyperthyroidism may also be associated with pregnancy, ^{131}I therapy, thyroid carcinoma, trophoblastic tumors, or TSH-secreting pituitary adenomas. Iatrogenic hyperthyroidism may follow thyroid hormone replacement or may occur after iodide exposure (angiographic contrast media) in patients with chronically low iodide intake (Jod-Basedow phenomenon). The antiarrhythmic agent amiodarone is iodine-rich and is another cause of iodine-induced thyrotoxicosis.[4]

The major manifestations of hyperthyroidism are weight loss, diarrhea, skeletal muscle weakness and stiffness, warm and moist skin, heat intolerance, and nervousness. Cardiovascular manifestations include increased left ventricular contractility and ejection fraction, tachycardia, elevated systolic blood pressure, and decreased diastolic blood pressure. Hypercalcemia, thrombocytopenia, and a mild anemia may be present. Elderly patients may present with heart failure, atrial fibrillation, or other cardiac dysrhythmias. They may also present with apathetic hyperthyroidism characterized by depression and withdrawal, without the usual systemic signs or symptoms.

Treatment and Anesthetic Considerations

The most important goal in managing the hyperthyroid patient is to make the patient euthyroid before any surgery, if possible. The drugs propylthiouracil and methimazole are thiourea derivatives that inhibit organification of iodide and the synthesis of thyroid hormone.[5] Propylthiouracil also decreases the peripheral conversion of T_4 to T_3. Normal thyroid glands usually contain a store of hormone that is large enough to maintain a euthyroid state for several months, even if synthesis is abolished. Therefore, hyperthyroid patients are unlikely to be regulated to a euthyroid state with antithyroid drugs alone in <6 to 8 weeks. Toxic reactions from these drugs are uncommon but include skin rash, nausea, fever, agranulocytosis, hepatitis, and arthralgias.

Inorganic iodide inhibits iodide organification and thyroid hormone release—the Wolff-Chaikoff effect. Iodide is also effective in reducing the size of the hyperplastic gland and has a role in the preparation of the patient for emergency thyroid surgery. Antithyroid drugs should be started before iodide treatment because of the possibility of worsening the thyrotoxicosis.

β-Adrenergic antagonists are effective in attenuating the manifestations of excessive sympathetic activity and should be used in all hyperthyroid patients unless contraindicated. β-Adrenergic blockade alone does not inhibit hormone synthesis, but specifically propranolol does impair the peripheral conversion of T_4 to T_3 over 1 to 2 weeks. Propranolol given over 12 to 24 hours decreases tachycardia, heat intolerance, anxiety, and tremor. Any beta-blocker may be used, and long-acting agents may be more convenient. The combination of propranolol (in doses titrated to effect) plus potassium iodide (two to five drops every 8 hours) is frequently used before surgery to ameliorate cardiovascular symptoms and reduce circulating concentrations of T_4 and T_3. Preoperative preparation usually requires 7 to 14 days. Heart failure secondary to poorly controlled paroxysmal atrial fibrillation may improve with slowing of the ventricular rate, but abnormalities of left ventricular function secondary to hyperthyroidism may not be corrected with the use of β-antagonists. If a hyperthyroid patient with clinically apparent disease requires emergency surgery, β-adrenergic blockade should be administered to achieve a heart rate <90 beats per minute. Beta-blockers do not prevent thyroid storm. Glucocorticoids such as dexamethasone (8 to 12 mg/day) are used in the management of severe thyrotoxicosis because they reduce thyroid hormone secretion and the peripheral conversion of T_4 to T_3.

Iopanoic acid, a radiographic contrast agent that decreases peripheral conversion of T_4 and releases iodine that inhibits synthesis, is useful for emergency preparation.

Radioactive iodine therapy is an effective treatment for some patients with thyrotoxicosis.[6] However, it should not be administered to patients who are pregnant because it crosses the placenta and may destroy the fetal thyroid. A side effect of RIA therapy is hypothyroidism; 10 to 60% of cases occur in the first year of therapy, and an additional 2% occur per year thereafter.

A variety of anesthetic techniques and drugs have been used for hyperthyroid patients undergoing surgery. All antithyroid medications are continued through the morning of surgery. The goal of intraoperative management in the hyperthyroid patient is to achieve a depth of anesthesia that prevents an exaggerated sympathetic response to surgical stimulation while avoiding the administration of medication that stimulates the sympathetic nervous system. Pancuronium should be avoided. It is best to avoid using ketamine, even when a patient is clinically euthyroid. Hypotension that occurs during surgery is best treated with direct-acting vasopressors rather than a medication that provokes the release of catecholamines. The incidence of myasthenia gravis is increased in hyperthyroid patients; thus, the initial dose of muscle relaxant should be reduced and a twitch monitor should be used to titrate subsequent doses. Regional anesthesia is an excellent alternative when appropriate; however, epinephrine-containing solutions should be avoided.

① *Thyroid storm* is a life-threatening exacerbation of hyperthyroidism that most commonly develops in the undiagnosed or untreated hyperthyroid patient because of the stress of surgery or nonthyroid illness.[7] Operating on an acutely hyperthyroid gland may provoke thyroid storm, although this is probably not due to mechanical release of hormone.[8] Its manifestations include hyperthermia, tachycardia, dysrhythmias, myocardial ischemia, congestive heart failure, agitation, and confusion. It must be distinguished from, or considered with, pheochromocytoma, malignant hyperthermia, and light anesthesia. Although free T_4 levels are often markedly elevated, no laboratory test is diagnostic. Treatment involves large doses of propylthiouracil and supportive measures to control fever and restore intravascular volume. Hemodynamic monitoring (pulmonary artery catheter, arterial catheter) is especially useful in guiding the treatment of patients with significant left ventricular dysfunction (Table 49-3). Again, it is essential to remove or treat the precipitating event.

Anesthesia for Thyroid Surgery

Subtotal thyroidectomy as an alternative to prolonged medical therapy is used less frequently now than in the past. Indica-

---

TABLE 49-3

MANAGEMENT OF THYROID STORM

Administer IV fluids.
Administer sodium iodide, 250 mg PO or IV q6h.
Administer propylthiouracil, 200–400 mg PO or via NGT q6h.
Administer hydrocortisone, 50–100 mg IV q6h.
Administer propranolol, 10–40 mg PO q4–6h, or esmolol infusion to treat hyperadrenergic signs.
Cooling blankets and acetaminophen and meperidine (25–50 mg) IV q4–6h may be used to prevent shivering.
Use digoxin for heart failure especially in the presence of atrial fibrillation with rapid ventricular response.

IV, intravenous(ly); PO, oral(ly); NGT, nasogastric tube.

tions include failed medical therapy, underlying cancer, and symptomatic goiter. It is usually performed under general endotracheal anesthesia, although the use of the laryngeal mask airway is increasing.[9] Use of a laryngeal mask airway allows real-time visualization of vocal cord function because the patient is allowed to breathe spontaneously. Limited thyroidectomy may also be performed under bilateral superficial cervical plexus block. The anesthesiologist must be prepared to manage an unexpected difficult intubation because the incidence of difficult intubation during goiter surgery is 5 to 8%.[10] Thyroid cancer increases the risk, but the size of the goiter is not predictive. Airway obstruction is a potential problem in the patient with a large substernal goiter, although rarely a problem with goiters exclusively in the neck. Evidence of significant airway obstruction or tracheal deviation or narrowing may warrant inhalation induction or awake fiberoptic intubation. The complications after subtotal thyroidectomy include recurrent laryngeal nerve damage, tracheal compression secondary to hematoma or tracheomalacia, and hypoparathyroidism. Hypoparathyroidism secondary to the inadvertent surgical removal of parathyroid glands is most frequently seen after total thyroidectomy. The symptoms of hypocalcemia develop within the first 24 to 96 hours after surgery[11] (see Chapter 14). Laryngeal stridor progressing to laryngospasm may be one of the first indications of hypocalcemic tetany. The intravenous administration of calcium chloride or calcium gluconate is warranted in this situation. Magnesium levels should also be monitored and corrected if low. Bilateral recurrent laryngeal nerve injury is an extremely rare injury and necessitates reintubation. Unilateral nerve injury is more common and is often transient.[12] Unilateral damage to the recurrent laryngeal nerve is characterized by hoarseness and a paralyzed vocal cord, whereas bilateral injury causes aphonia (see Chapter 29). It is wise to evaluate vocal cord function before and after surgery by laryngoscopy or by asking the patient to phonate by saying the letter "e." Routine postoperative visualization of the vocal cords is not warranted. Postoperative extubation of the trachea should be performed under optimal conditions. Intraoperative laryngeal nerve injury or collapse of the tracheal rings from previous weakening may mandate emergency reintubation.

Hypothyroidism

Hypothyroidism is a relatively common disease (0.5 to 0.8% of the adult population) that results from inadequate circulating levels of T_4 or T_3, or both.[13] The development of hypothyroidism is often slow and progressive, making the clinical diagnosis difficult, especially in the more subtle cases. Hypofunctioning of the thyroid gland has many causes (Table 49-4). Primary failure of the thyroid gland refers to decreased production of thyroid hormone, despite adequate TSH production, and accounts for 95% of all cases of thyroid dysfunction. The remainder of the cases are caused by either hypothalamic or pituitary disease (secondary hypothyroidism) and are associated with other pituitary deficiencies.

A lack of thyroid hormone produces a variety of signs and symptoms. These early findings are often nonspecific and difficult to recognize. A history of RIA therapy, external neck irradiation, or the presence of a goiter is helpful in diagnosis. There is a generalized reduction in metabolic activity, resulting in lethargy, slow mental functioning, cold intolerance, and slow movements. The cardiovascular manifestations of hypothyroidism reflect the importance of thyroid hormone for myocardial contractility and catecholamine function. These patients exhibit bradycardia, decreased cardiac output, and increased peripheral resistance.[14] The accumulation of a cholesterol-rich pericardial fluid produces low voltage on the elec-

TABLE 49-4

CAUSES OF HYPOTHYROIDISM

■ PRIMARY HYPOTHYROIDISM

Autoimmune
Irradiation to the neck
Previous ^{131}I therapy
Surgical removal
Thyroiditis (Hashimoto disease)
Severe iodine depletion
Medications (iodines, propylthiouracil, methimazole)
Hereditary defects in biosynthesis
Congenital defects in gland development

■ SECONDARY OR TERTIARY HYPOTHYROIDISM

Pituitary
Hypothalamic

Reproduced from Petersdorf RG, ed: Harrison's Principles of Internal Medicine, 10th edition. New York, McGraw-Hill, 1983, with permission.

trocardiogram (ECG). Heart failure only rarely occurs in the absence of coexisting heart disease. Angina pectoris itself is unusual in hypothyroidism but can appear when thyroid hormone treatment is initiated. Ventilatory responsiveness to hypoxia and hypercapnia is depressed in hypothyroid patients. This depression is potentiated by sedatives, opioids, and general anesthesia. Postoperative ventilatory failure requiring prolonged ventilation is rarely seen in hypothyroid patients in the absence of coexisting lung disease, obesity, or myxedema coma. Other abnormalities found in hypothyroidism include anemia, coagulopathy, hypothermia, sleep apnea, and impaired renal free water clearance with hyponatremia. Decreased GI motility can compound the effect of postoperative ileus. In long-standing or severe disease, the stress response may be blunted and adrenal depression may occur.

Treatment and Anesthetic Considerations

Treatment of symptomatic hypothyroidism is with hormone replacement therapy.[15] Controversy remains regarding the preoperative anesthetic management of the hypothyroid patient. Although it seems logical, given the multisystem effects of thyroid hormone, to recommend that all hypothyroid surgical candidates be restored to a euthyroid state before surgery, such a recommendation is, in general, based on individual case reports. There have been few controlled studies to support the position that most hypothyroid patients are unusually sensitive to anesthetic drugs, have prolonged recovery times, or have a higher incidence of cardiovascular instability or collapse.

No increase in serious complications in patients with mild or moderate hypothyroidism undergoing general anesthesia has been noted.[16] One study[17] noted a higher incidence of intraoperative hypotension and postoperative GI and neuropsychiatric complications in mild and moderately hypothyroid patients undergoing noncardiac surgery, but still noted there were no compelling clinical reasons to postpone surgery in these patients. Surgery in severely hypothyroid patients should be postponed when possible until these patients are at least partially treated.

The management of hypothyroid patients with symptomatic coronary artery disease has been a subject of particular controversy.[18] The need for thyroid hormone replacement therapy

TABLE 49-5

MANAGEMENT OF MYXEDEMA

Tracheal intubation and controlled ventilation as needed
Levothyroxine, 200–300 μg IV over 5–10 min initially, and
    100 μg IV q24h
Hydrocortisone, 100 mg IV, then 25 mg IV q6h
Fluid and electrolyte therapy as indicated by serum
    electrolytes
Cover to conserve body heat; no warming blankets

IV, intravenous(ly).

must be weighed against the risk of precipitating myocardial ischemia. Several studies and a literature review found no differences in the frequency of intraoperative or postoperative complications when mild or moderately hypothyroid patients underwent cardiac surgery. In symptomatic patients or unstable patients with cardiac ischemia, thyroid replacement should probably be delayed until after coronary revascularization.

There appears to be little reason to postpone elective surgery in patients who have mild or moderate hypothyroidism. However, thyroid replacement therapy is indicated for patients with severe hypothyroidism or myxedema coma and for pregnant patients who are hypothyroid. Untreated hypothyroidism in pregnant patients is associated with an increased incidence of spontaneous abortion and mental and physical abnormalities in the offspring.

A number of anesthetic medications have been used without difficulty in hypothyroid patients. Although ketamine has been proposed as the ideal induction agent, thiopental has also been used in the hypothyroid patient. The maintenance of anesthesia may be safely achieved with either intravenous or inhaled anesthetics. There appears to be little if any decrease in the minimum alveolar concentration for volatile agents. Regional anesthesia is a good choice in the hypothyroid patient, provided the intravascular volume is well maintained. Monitoring is directed toward the early recognition of hypotension, congestive heart failure, and hypothermia. Scrupulous attention should be paid to maintaining normal body temperature.

Myxedema coma represents a severe form of hypothyroidism characterized by stupor or coma, hypoventilation, hypothermia, hypotension, and hyponatremia. This is a medical emergency with a high mortality rate (25 to 50%), and as such, requires aggressive therapy (Table 49-5). Only lifesaving surgery should proceed in the face of myxedema coma. Intravenous thyroid replacement is initiated as soon as the clinical diagnosis is made. An intravenous loading dose of T_4 (sodium levothyroxine, 200 to 300 μg) is given initially and followed by a maintenance dose of T_4, 50 to 200 μg/day intravenously.[19] Alternatively, T_3 may be used because it has a more rapid onset. Improvements in heart rate, blood pressure, and body temperature may occur within 24 hours. However, replacement therapy with either form of thyroid hormone may precipitate myocardial ischemia. There is also an increased likelihood of acute primary adrenal insufficiency in these patients, and they should receive stress doses of hydrocortisone. Steroid replacement continues until normal adrenal function can be confirmed.

PARATHYROID GLANDS

Calcium Physiology

The normal adult body contains approximately 1 to 2 kg of calcium (Ca^{2+}), of which 99% is in the skeleton.[20] Plasma calcium is present in three forms: (1) a protein-bound fraction (50%), (2) an ionized fraction (45%), and (3) a diffusible but nonionized fraction (5%) that is complexed with phosphate, bicarbonate, and citrate (see Chapter 14). This division is interesting because it is the ionized fraction that is physiologically active and homeostatically regulated. The normal total serum calcium concentration is 8.8 to 10.4 mg/dL. Albumin binds approximately 90% of the protein-bound fraction of calcium, and total serum Ca^{2+} consequently depends on albumin levels. In general, an increase or decrease in albumin of 1 g/dL is associated with a parallel change in total serum Ca^{2+} of 0.8 mg/dL. The serum ionized Ca^{2+} concentration is affected by temperature and blood pH through alterations in Ca^{2+} protein binding to albumin. Acidosis decreases protein binding (increases ionized Ca^{2+}), and alkalosis increases protein binding (decreases ionized Ca^{2+}). The concentration of free Ca^{2+} ion is of critical importance in regulating skeletal muscle contraction, coagulation, neurotransmitter release, endocrine secretion, and a variety of other cellular functions. As a consequence, the maintenance of serum Ca^{2+} concentration is subject to tight hormonal control by parathyroid hormone (PTH) and vitamin D (Fig. 49-2).

PTH acts to maintain the extracellular fluid Ca^{2+} concentration through direct effects on bone resorption and renal Ca^{2+} resorption at the distal tubule, and indirectly through its effects on the synthesis of 1,25-dihydroxyvitamin D. The renal effects of PTH include phosphaturia and bicarbonaturia, in addition to enhanced Ca^{2+} and magnesium resorption. Most evidence suggests that rapid changes in blood Ca^{2+} levels are primarily the result of hormonal effects on bone and, to a lesser extent, to renal Ca^{2+} clearance, whereas maintenance of Ca^{2+} balance depends more on the indirect effects of the hormone on intestinal calcium absorption.

PTH secretion is primarily regulated by the serum ionized Ca^{2+} concentration. This negative feedback mechanism is exquisitely sensitive in maintaining calcium levels in a normal range. Release of PTH is also influenced by phosphate, magnesium, and catecholamine levels. Acute hypomagnesemia directly stimulates PTH release, whereas chronic magnesium depletion appears to inhibit proper functioning of the parathyroid gland. The plasma phosphate concentration has an indirect influence on PTH secretion by causing reciprocal changes in the serum ionized Ca^{2+} concentration.

Vitamin D is absorbed from the GI tract and can be produced enzymatically by ultraviolet irradiation of the skin. Vitamin D (cholecalciferol) is made from cholesterol metabolites and is inactive. Calciferol is hydroxylated in the liver to 25-hydroxycholecalciferol (25-OHD) and in the kidney is further hydroxylated to 1,25-dihydroxycholecalciferol [1,25(OH)$_2$D] or 24,25-dihydroxycholecalciferol [24,25(OH)$_2$D]. 25-OHD is the major circulating form of vitamin D. The synthesis of this hormone is not regulated by a hormone or by Ca^{2+} or phosphate levels. 1,25(OH)$_2$D and 24,25(OH)$_2$D are the major active metabolites of vitamin D, and their production is reciprocally regulated at the kidney. Hypocalcemia and hypophosphatemia cause an increased production of 1,25(OH)$_2$D and a decreased production of 24,25(OH)$_2$D. 1,25(OH)$_2$D stimulates bone, kidney, and intestinal absorption of calcium and phosphate. Vitamin D deficiency can lead to decreased intestinal absorption of Ca^{2+} and secondary hyperparathyroidism.

Hyperparathyroidism

Primary hyperparathyroidism is most commonly due to a benign parathyroid adenoma (90% of cases) or hyperplasia (9%) and very rarely to a parathyroid carcinoma. Primary hyperparathyroidism may also exist as part of a multiple

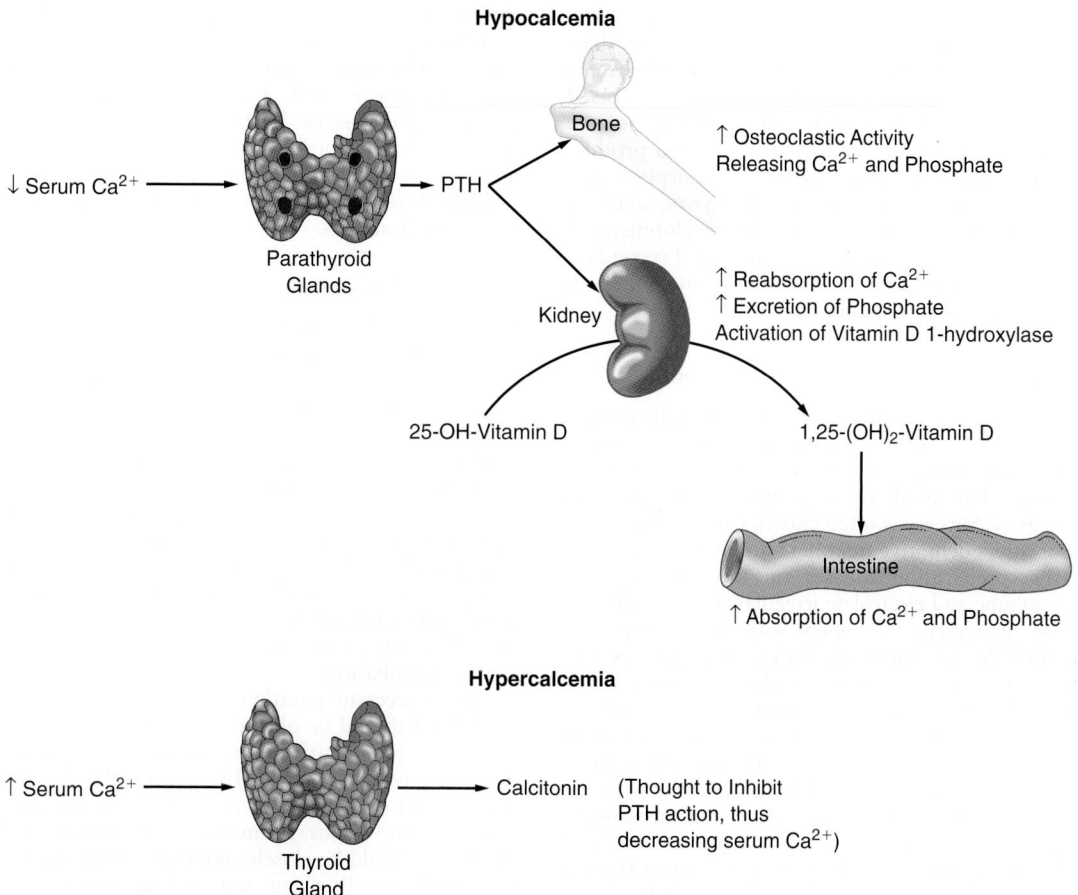

Hypocalcemia

↓ Serum Ca^{2+} → Parathyroid Glands → PTH → Bone

↑ Osteoclastic Activity Releasing Ca^{2+} and Phosphate

Kidney

↑ Reabsorption of Ca^{2+}
↑ Excretion of Phosphate
Activation of Vitamin D 1-hydroxylase

25-OH-Vitamin D   1,25-$(OH)_2$-Vitamin D

Intestine

↑ Absorption of Ca^{2+} and Phosphate

Hypercalcemia

↑ Serum Ca^{2+} → Thyroid Gland → Calcitonin   (Thought to Inhibit PTH action, thus decreasing serum Ca^{2+})

FIGURE 49-2.   Parathyroid hormone (PTH) and vitamin D metabolism and action. 25-OH, 25-hydroxycholecalciferol; 1,25-$(OH)_2$, 1,25-dihydroxycholecalciferol. (From McClatchey KD: Clinical Laboratory Medicine, 2nd edition. Philadelphia, Lippincott Williams & Wilkins, 2002.)

endocrine neoplastic (MEN) syndrome. Hyperplasia usually involves all four glands. Although most patients with primary hyperparathyroidism are hypercalcemic, most are asymptomatic at the time of diagnosis. When symptoms occur, they usually result from the hypercalcemia that accompanies the disease. Primary hyperparathyroidism occurring during pregnancy is associated with a high maternal and fetal morbidity rate (50%). The placenta allows the fetus to concentrate calcium, promoting fetal hypercalcemia and leading to hypoparathyroidism in the newborn. Pregnant women with primary hyperparathyroidism should generally be treated with surgery.

Hypercalcemia is responsible for a broad spectrum of signs and symptoms. Nephrolithiasis is the most common manifestation, occurring in 60 to 70% of patients. Polyuria and polydipsia are also common complaints. An increase in bone turnover may lead to generalized demineralization and subperiosteal bone resorption; however, only a small group of patients (10 to 15%) have clinically significant bone disease. Patients may experience generalized skeletal muscle weakness and fatigability, epigastric discomfort, peptic ulceration, and constipation. Psychiatric manifestations include depression, memory loss, confusion, or psychosis. Between 20 and 50% of patients are hypertensive, but this usually resolves with successful treatment of the disease. Cardiac function is enhanced in the early stages of hypercalcemia. Calcium flux into the cells is reflected in the plateau phase of the action potential (phase 2). As extracellular calcium increases, the inward flux is more rapid, and phase 2 is shortened (see Chapter 10). The corresponding ECG change is a shorter QT interval. Cardiac con-

tractility may increase until a level between 15 and 20 mg/dL is reached. At this point, there is a prolongation of the PR segment and QRS complex that can result in heart block or bundle-branch block. Bradycardia also occurs.

An elevated serum Ca^{2+} concentration is a valuable diagnostic indicator of primary hyperparathyroidism. The serum phosphate concentration is nonspecific, with many patients having normal or near-normal levels. The reported incidence of hyperchloremic acidosis varies widely in primary hyperparathyroidism, but most patients usually have a serum chloride concentration in excess of 102 mEq/L. Rarely does a patient with hypercalcemia secondary to ectopic PTH production (malignancy) present with hyperchloremic acidosis. The definitive diagnosis of primary hyperparathyroidism is made by RIA demonstration of an elevation in PTH levels in the presence of hypercalcemia. An elevated nephrogenous cyclic adenosine monophosphate is noted in >90% of patients with primary hyperparathyroidism.

Hypercalcemia may also result from the ectopic production of PTH or PTH-like substances from lung, genitourinary, breast, GI, and lymphoproliferative malignancies. Tumors may also produce hypercalcemia through direct bone resorption or the production of osteoclast-activating factor. In the absence of a clinically obvious neoplasm, there may be difficulty in differentiating between PTH-producing malignancies and primary hyperparathyroidism. PTH fragments from malignant tissue differ from native PTH, so precise clinical identification may aid in distinguishing between ectopic PTH production and primary hyperparathyroidism.

Secondary hyperparathyroidism represents an increase in parathyroid function as a result of conditions that produce hypocalcemia or hyperphosphatemia. Chronic renal disease is a common cause of hyperphosphatemia (due to decreased phosphate excretion) and decreased vitamin D metabolism. The hypocalcemia that results leads to an increased production of PTH. GI disorders accompanied by malabsorption may also lead to a secondary increase in parathyroid activity. Tertiary hyperparathyroidism refers to the development of hypercalcemia in a patient who has had prolonged secondary hyperparathyroidism that has caused adenomatous changes in the parathyroid gland and unregulated PTH.

Treatment and Anesthetic Considerations

Surgery is the treatment of choice for the patient with symptomatic disease. However, there is considerable controversy surrounding the choice of treatment in the asymptomatic patient. It is not clear that mild primary hyperparathyroidism decreases longevity. Surgery is often chosen over medical therapy because it offers definitive treatment and is generally safe.

Preoperative preparation focuses on the correction of intravascular volume and electrolyte irregularities. It is particularly important to evaluate the patient with chronic hypercalcemia for abnormalities of the renal, cardiac, or central nervous systems. Emergency treatment of hypercalcemia is undertaken before surgery when the serum Ca^{2+} concentration exceeds 15 mg/dL (7.5 mEq/L). Lowering of the serum Ca^{2+} concentration is initially accomplished by expanding the intravascular volume and establishing a sodium diuresis. This is achieved with the intravenous administration of normal saline and furosemide. Rehydration alone is capable of lowering the serum Ca^{2+} level by ≥ 2 mg/dL. Hydration dilutes the serum Ca^{2+}, and a sodium diuresis promotes Ca^{2+} excretion through an inhibition of sodium and Ca^{2+} resorption in the proximal tubule. Hypokalemia and hypomagnesemia may result.

Another element in the treatment of hypercalcemia is the correction of hypophosphatemia. Hypophosphatemia increases GI absorption of Ca^{2+}, stimulates the breakdown of bone, and impairs the uptake of Ca^{2+} by bone. Low serum phosphate levels impair cardiac contractility and may contribute to congestive heart failure. Hypophosphatemia also causes skeletal muscle weakness, hemolysis, and platelet dysfunction.

Other medications that have a role in lowering the serum Ca^{2+} include bisphosphonates, mithramycin, calcitonin, and glucocorticoids. Bisphosphonates are pyrophosphate analogs that inhibit osteoclast action. They are the drugs of choice for severe hypercalcemia. Toxic effects include fever and hypophosphatemia. Mithramycin, a cytotoxic agent, inhibits PTH-induced osteoclast activity and can lower the serum Ca^{2+} levels by ≥ 2 mg/dL in 24 to 48 hours. Toxic effects include azotemia, hepatotoxicity, and thrombocytopenia. Calcitonin is useful in transiently lowering the serum Ca^{2+} level 2 to 4 mg/dL through direct inhibition of osteoclastic bone resorption. The advantages of calcitonin are the mild side effects (urticaria, nausea) and the rapid onset of activity. Calcitonin resistance usually develops within 24 to 48 hours. Glucocorticoids are effective in lowering the serum Ca^{2+} concentration in several conditions (sarcoidosis, some malignancies, hyperthyroidism, vitamin D intoxication) through their actions on osteoclast bone resorption, GI absorption of calcium, and the urinary excretion of calcium. Glucocorticoids are usually of no benefit in the treatment of primary hypercalcemia. Finally, hemodialysis or peritoneal dialysis can be used to lower the serum Ca^{2+} level when alternative regimens are ineffective or contraindicated.

There is no evidence that a specific anesthetic drug or technique has advantages over another. A thorough knowledge of the clinical manifestations attributable to hypercalcemia is of

the greatest value in choosing an anesthetic technique. Special monitoring is usually not required. Because of the unpredictable response to neuromuscular blocking drugs in the hypercalcemic patient, a conservative approach to muscle paralysis makes sense. There is an increased requirement for vecuronium, and probably all nondepolarizing muscle relaxants, during onset of neuromuscular blockade.[21] Careful positioning of the osteopenic patient is necessary to avoid pathologic bone fractures.

Anesthesia for Parathyroid Surgery

General anesthesia is most commonly used for parathyroid surgery, but cervical plexus block and local anesthesia with hypnosis have been used successfully.[22] Some centers use an intraoperative rapid PTH assay to help determine when a hyperfunctioning gland has been removed. There is in vitro evidence that propofol can interfere with the assay, so many surgeons prefer that propofol not be used within 15 minutes of an assay. Postoperative complications include recurrent laryngeal nerve injury, bleeding, and transient or complete hypoparathyroidism. Unilateral recurrent laryngeal nerve injury is characterized by hoarseness and usually requires no intervention. Bilateral recurrent laryngeal nerve injury is a rare complication, producing aphonia and requiring immediate tracheal intubation.

After successful parathyroidectomy, a decrease in the serum Ca^{2+} level should be observed within 24 hours. Patients with significant preoperative bone disease may have hypocalcemia after removal of the PTH-secreting glands. This "hungry bone" syndrome comes as a result of the rapid remineralization of bone.[23] Thus, serum Ca^{2+}, magnesium, and phosphorus levels should be closely monitored until stable. The serum Ca^{2+} nadir usually occurs within 3 to 7 days.

Hypoparathyroidism

An underproduction of PTH or resistance of the end-organ tissues to PTH results in hypocalcemia (<8 mg/dL). The normal physiologic response to hypocalcemia is an increase in PTH secretion and $1,25(OH)_2D$ synthesis with an increase in Ca^{2+} mobilization from bone, GI absorption, and renal tubule reclamation. The most common cause of acquired PTH deficiency is inadvertent removal of the parathyroid glands during thyroid or parathyroid surgery. Other causes of acquired hypoparathyroidism include ^{131}I therapy for thyroid disease, neck trauma, granulomatous disease, or an infiltrating process (malignancy or amyloidosis). Severe hypomagnesemia (<0.8 mEq/L) from any cause can produce hypocalcemia by suppressing PTH secretion and interfering with PTH action. Renal insufficiency leads to phosphorus retention and impaired $1,25(OH)_2D$ synthesis, which results in hypocalcemia. These patients are commonly treated with vitamin D, which increases intestinal calcium absorption and suppresses secondary increases in PTH secretion. Hypocalcemia due to pancreatitis and burns results from the suppression of PTH and from the sequestration of calcium.

Clinical Features and Treatment

The clinical features of hypoparathyroidism are a manifestation of hypocalcemia. Neuronal irritability and skeletal muscle spasms, tetany, or seizures reflect a reduced threshold of excitation. Latent tetany may be demonstrated by eliciting Chvostek or Trousseau sign. Chvostek sign is a contracture of the facial muscle produced by tapping the facial nerve as it passes through the parotid gland. Trousseau sign is contraction of the fingers and wrist after application of a blood pressure cuff inflated above the systolic blood pressure for approximately 3 minutes. Other common complaints of hypocalcemia include fatigue, depression, paresthesias, and skeletal muscle cramps. The acute onset of hypocalcemia after thyroid or parathyroid surgery may manifest as stridor and apnea. Cardiovascular manifestations of hypocalcemia include congestive heart failure, hypotension, and a relative insensitivity to the effects of β-adrenergic agonists (see Chapter 10). Delayed ventricular repolarization results in a prolonged QT interval on the ECG. Although prolongation of the QT interval may be a reliable sign of hypocalcemia in an individual patient, the ECG is relatively insensitive for the detection of hypocalcemia.

The treatment of hypoparathyroidism consists of electrolyte replacement. The objective is to have the patient's clinical symptoms under control before anesthesia and surgery. Hypocalcemia caused by magnesium depletion is treated by correcting the magnesium deficit. Serum phosphate excess is corrected by the removal of phosphate from the diet and the oral administration of phosphate-binding resins (aluminum hydroxide). The urinary excretion of phosphate can be increased with a saline volume infusion. Ca^{2+} deficiencies are corrected with Ca^{2+} supplements or vitamin D analogs. Patients with severe symptomatic hypocalcemia are treated with intravenous calcium gluconate (10 to 20 mL of 10% solution) given over several minutes and followed by a continuous infusion (1 to 2 mg/kg/hr) of elemental Ca^{2+}. The correction of serum Ca^{2+} levels should be monitored by measuring serum Ca^{2+} concentrations and following clinical symptoms. When oral or intravenous calcium is inadequate to maintain a normal serum ionized calcium level, vitamin D is added to the regimen.

ADRENAL CORTEX

The adrenal cortex functions to synthesize and secrete three types of hormones. Endogenous and dietary cholesterol is used in the adrenal biosynthesis of glucocorticoids (cortisol), mineralocorticoids (aldosterone and 11-deoxycorticosterone), and androgens (dehydroepiandrosterone). Cortisol and aldosterone are the two essential hormones, whereas adrenal androgens are of relatively minor physiologic significance in adults. The major biologic effects of adrenal cortical hyperfunction or hypofunction occur as a result of cortisol or aldosterone excess or deficiency. Abnormal function of the adrenal cortex may render a patient unable to respond appropriately during a period of surgical stress or critical illness.

Glucocorticoid Physiology

Cortisol (hydrocortisone) is the most potent endogenous glucocorticoid and is produced by the inner portions of the adrenal cortex. Cortisone is a glucocorticoid produced in small amounts. Cortisol is produced under the control of adrenocorticotropic hormone (ACTH; corticotropin), a polypeptide synthesized and released by the anterior pituitary gland. Glucocorticoids exert their biological effects by diffusing into the cytoplasm of target cells and combining with specific high-affinity receptor proteins.

The daily production of endogenous cortisol is approximately 20 mg. The maximal output is 150 to 300 mg. Most of the circulating hormone is bound to the α-globulin transcortin (cortisol-binding globulin). It is the relatively small amount of free hormone that exerts the biological effects. Endogenous glucocorticoids are inactivated primarily by the liver and are excreted in the urine as 17-hydroxycorticosteroids. Cortisol is also filtered at the glomerulus and may be excreted unchanged

in the urine. Although the rate of cortisol secretion is decreased by approximately 30% in the elderly patient, plasma cortisol levels remain in a normal range because of a corresponding decrease in hepatic and renal clearance.

Cortisol secretion is directly controlled by ACTH, which in turn is regulated by the corticotropin-releasing factor from the hypothalamus. ACTH is synthesized in the pituitary gland from a precursor molecule that also produces β-lipotropin and β-endorphin. The secretion of ACTH and corticotropin-releasing factor is governed chiefly by glucocorticoids, the sleep–wake cycle, and stress. Cortisol is the most potent regulator of ACTH secretion, acting by a negative-feedback mechanism to maintain cortisol levels in a physiologic range. ACTH release follows a diurnal pattern, with maximal activity occurring soon after awakening. This diurnal pattern of activity occurs in normal subjects and in those with adrenal insufficiency. Psychological or physical stress (trauma, surgery, intense exercise) also promotes ACTH release, regardless of the level of circulating cortisol or the time of day.

Cortisol has multiple effects on intermediate carbohydrate, protein, and fatty acid metabolism, as well as maintenance and regulation of immune and circulatory function. Glucocorticoids enhance gluconeogenesis, elevate blood glucose, and promote hepatic glycogen synthesis. The catabolic effect of glucocorticoids is partially blocked by insulin. The net effect on protein metabolism is enhanced degradation of muscle tissue and negative nitrogen balance. In supraphysiologic amounts, glucocorticoids suppress growth hormone secretion and impair somatic growth. The anti-inflammatory actions of cortisol relate to its effect in stabilizing lysosomes and promoting capillary integrity. Cortisol also antagonizes leukocyte migration inhibition factor, thus reducing white cell adherence to vascular endothelium and diminishing leukocyte response to local inflammation. Phagocytic activity does not decrease, although the killing potential of macrophages and monocytes is diminished. Other diverse actions include the facilitation of free water clearance, maintenance of blood pressure, a weak mineralocorticoid effect, promotion of appetite, stimulation of hematopoiesis, and induction of liver enzymes.

Mineralocorticoid Physiology

Aldosterone is the most potent mineralocorticoid produced by the adrenal gland. This hormone binds to receptors in sweat glands, the alimentary tract, and the distal convoluted tubule of the kidney. Aldosterone is a major regulator of extracellular volume and potassium homeostasis through the resorption of sodium and the secretion of potassium by these tissues. The major regulators of aldosterone release are the renin–angiotensin system and serum potassium (Fig. 49-3). The juxtaglomerular apparatus that surrounds the renal afferent arterioles produces renin in response to decreased perfusion pressures and sympathetic stimulation. Renin splits the hepatic precursor angiotensinogen to form the decapeptide, angiotensin I, which is then altered enzymatically by converting enzyme (primarily in the lung) to form the octapeptide angiotensin II. Angiotensin II is the most potent vasopressor produced in the body. It directly stimulates the adrenal cortex to produce aldosterone. The renin–angiotensin system is the body's most important protector of volume status. Other stimuli that increase the production of aldosterone include hyperkalemia and, to a limited degree, hyponatremia, prostaglandin E, and ACTH.

Glucocorticoid Excess (Cushing Syndrome)

Cushing syndrome, caused by either the overproduction of cortisol by the adrenal cortex or exogenous glucocorticoid

FIGURE 49-3. The interrelationship of the volume and potassium feedback loops on aldosterone secretion. (Reprinted from Petersdorf RG, ed: Harrison's Principles of Internal Medicine, 10th edition. New York, McGraw-Hill, 1983, with permission.)

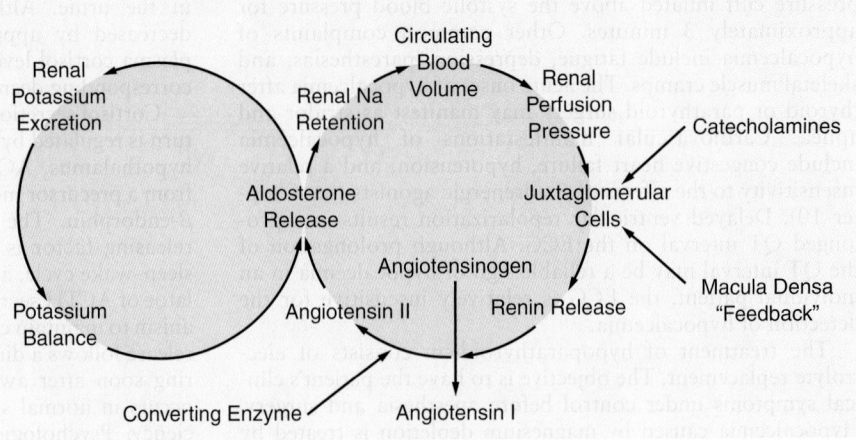

therapy, results in a syndrome characterized by truncal obesity, hypertension, hyperglycemia, increased intravascular fluid volume, hypokalemia, fatigability, abdominal striae, osteoporosis, and muscle weakness. Most cases of Cushing syndrome that occur spontaneously are due to bilateral adrenal hyperplasia secondary to ACTH produced by an anterior pituitary microadenoma or nonendocrine tumor (e.g., of the lung, kidney, or pancreas) (see Chapter 39). The primary overproduction of cortisol and other adrenal steroids is caused by an adrenal neoplasm in approximately 20 to 25% of patients with Cushing syndrome. These tumors are usually unilateral, and approximately half are malignant. When Cushing syndrome occurs in patients older than 60 years of age, the most likely cause is an adrenal carcinoma or ectopic ACTH produced from a nonendocrine tumor. Finally, an increasingly common cause of Cushing syndrome is the prolonged administration of exogenous glucocorticoids to treat a variety of illnesses.

The signs and symptoms of Cushing syndrome follow from the known actions of glucocorticoids. Truncal obesity and thin extremities reflect increased muscle wasting and a redistribution of fat in facial, cervical, and truncal areas. Impaired calcium absorption and a decrease in bone formation may result in osteopenia. Sixty percent of patients have hyperglycemia, but overt diabetes mellitus (DM) occurs in <20%. Hypertension and fluid retention are seen in most patients. Profound emotional changes ranging from emotional lability to frank psychosis may be present. An increased susceptibility to infection reflects the immunosuppressive effects of corticosteroids. Hypokalemic alkalosis without distinctive physical findings is common when adrenal hyperplasia is caused by ectopic ACTH production from a nonendocrine tumor.

The laboratory diagnosis of hyperadrenocorticism is based on a variable elevation in plasma and urinary cortisol levels, urinary 17-hydroxycorticosteroids, and plasma ACTH. Once the diagnosis is established, simultaneous measurement of plasma ACTH and cortisol levels can determine whether the Cushing syndrome is due to primary pituitary or adrenal disease.[24]

Alternatively, a dexamethasone suppression test can be used. Patients with pituitary adenomas frequently show depression in cortisol and 17-hydroxycorticosteroid levels when a high dose of dexamethasone is administered because the tumor retains some negative feedback control, while adrenal tumors do not.

Anesthetic Management

General considerations for the preoperative preparation of the patient include treating hypertension and diabetes and nor-

malizing intravascular fluid volume and electrolyte concentrations. Diuresis with the aldosterone antagonist spironolactone helps mobilize fluid and normalize the potassium concentration. Careful positioning of the osteopenic patient is important to avoid fractures. Intraoperative monitoring is planned after evaluation of the patient's cardiac reserve and consideration of the site and extent of the proposed surgery. When either unilateral or bilateral adrenalectomy is planned, glucocorticoid replacement therapy is initiated at a dose equal to full replacement of adrenal output during periods of extreme stress (see "Steroid Replacement During the Perioperative Period"). The total dosage is reduced by approximately 50% per day until a daily maintenance dose of steroids is achieved (20 to 30 mg/day). Hydrocortisone given in doses of this magnitude exerts significant mineralocorticoid activity, and additional exogenous mineralocorticoid is usually not necessary during the perioperative period. After bilateral adrenalectomy, most patients require 0.05 to 0.1 mg/day of fludrocortisone (9-α-fluorohydrocortisone) starting around day 5 to provide mineralocorticoid activity. Slightly higher doses may be needed if prednisone is used for glucocorticoid maintenance because it has little intrinsic mineralocorticoid activity. The fludrocortisone dose is reduced if congestive heart failure, hypokalemia, or hypertension develops. For the patient with a solitary adrenal adenoma, unilateral adrenalectomy may be followed by normalization of function in the contralateral gland over time. Treatment plans should therefore be individualized, and adjustments in dosage may be necessary. The production of glucocorticoids or ACTH by a neoplasm may not be eliminated if the tumor is unresectable. These patients often need continuous medical therapy with steroid inhibitors such as metyrapone to control their symptoms.

There are no specific recommendations regarding the use of a particular anesthetic technique or medication in patients with hyperadrenocorticism. When significant skeletal muscle weakness is present, a conservative approach to the use of muscle relaxants is warranted. Etomidate has been used for temporizing medical treatment of severe Cushing syndrome because of its inhibition of steroid synthesis.

Mineralocorticoid Excess

Hypersecretion of the major adrenal mineralocorticoid aldosterone increases the renal tubular exchange of sodium for potassium and hydrogen ions. This leads to hypertension, hypokalemic alkalosis, skeletal muscle weakness, and fatigue. Possibly as many as 1% of unselected hypertensive patients have primary hyperaldosteronism. The increase in renal sodium reabsorption and extracellular volume expansion is partly responsible for the high incidence of diastolic hypertension in these patients. Patients with primary hyperaldosteronism (Conn syndrome) characteristically do not have edema. Secondary aldosteronism results from an elevation in renin production. The diagnosis of primary or secondary hyperaldosteronism should be entertained in the nonedematous hypertensive patient with persistent hypokalemia who is not receiving potassium-wasting diuretics. Hyposecretion of renin that fails to increase appropriately during volume depletion or salt restriction is an important finding in primary aldosteronism. The measurement of plasma renin levels is useful in distinguishing primary from secondary hyperaldosteronism. It is of limited value in differentiating patients with primary aldosteronism from those with other causes of hypertension because renin activity is also suppressed in approximately 25% of patients with essential hypertension.

Anesthetic Considerations

Preoperative preparation for the patient with primary aldosteronism is directed toward restoring the intravascular volume and the electrolyte concentrations to normal. Hypertension and hypokalemia may be controlled by restricting sodium intake and administration of the aldosterone antagonist spironolactone. This diuretic works slowly to produce an increase in potassium levels, with dosages in the range of 25 to 100 mg every 8 hours. Total-body potassium deficits are difficult to estimate and may be in excess of 300 mEq. Whenever possible, potassium should be replaced slowly to allow equilibration between intracellular and extracellular potassium stores. The usual complications of chronic hypertension need to be assessed.

Adrenal Insufficiency (Addison Disease)

The undersecretion of adrenal steroid hormones may develop as the result of a primary inability of the adrenal gland to elaborate sufficient quantities of hormone or as the result of a deficiency in the production of ACTH.

Clinically, primary adrenal insufficiency is usually not apparent until at least 90% of the adrenal cortex has been destroyed. The predominant cause of primary adrenal insufficiency used to be tuberculosis; however, today, the most frequent cause of Addison disease is idiopathic adrenal insufficiency secondary to autoimmune destruction of the gland. Autoimmune destruction of the adrenal cortex causes both a glucocorticoid and a mineralocorticoid deficiency. A variety of other conditions presumed to have an autoimmune pathogenesis may also occur concomitantly with idiopathic Addison disease. Hashimoto's thyroiditis in association with autoimmune adrenal insufficiency is termed *Schmidt syndrome*. Other possible causes of adrenal gland destruction include certain bacterial, fungal, and advanced human immunodeficiency virus infections; metastatic cancer; sepsis; and hemorrhage. Secondary adrenal insufficiency occurs when the anterior pituitary fails to secrete sufficient quantities of ACTH. Pituitary failure may result from tumor, infection, surgical ablation, or radiation therapy. Pituitary surgery may cause transient adrenal insufficiency requiring supplemental glucocorticoids.[25]

Patients receiving chronic corticosteroid therapy will not generally have frank adrenal insufficiency, but may have hypothalamic-pituitary-adrenal (HPA) suppression and may develop acute adrenal insufficiency during the stress of the perioperative period. Relative adrenal insufficiency is a common finding in critically ill surgical patients with hypotension requiring vasopressors.[26]

Clinical Presentation

The cardinal symptoms of idiopathic Addison disease include chronic fatigue, muscle weakness, anorexia, weight loss, nausea, vomiting, and diarrhea. Hypotension is almost always encountered in the disease process. Female patients may exhibit decreased axillary and pubic hair growth because of the loss of adrenal androgen secretion. An acute crisis can present as abdominal pain, severe vomiting and diarrhea, hypotension, decreased consciousness, and shock. Diffuse hyperpigmentation occurs in most patients with primary adrenal insufficiency and is secondary to the compensatory increase in ACTH and β-lipotropin. These hormones stimulate an increase in melanocyte production. Mineralocorticoid deficiency is characteristically present in primary adrenal disease; as a result, there is a reduction in urine sodium conservation. Hyperkalemia may be a cause of life-threatening cardiac dysrhythmias. Adrenal insufficiency secondary to pituitary disease is not associated with cutaneous hyperpigmentation or mineralocorticoid deficiency. Salt and water balance is usually maintained unless severe fluid and electrolyte losses overwhelm the subnormal aldosterone secretory capacity. Organic lesions of pituitary origin require a diligent search for coexisting hormone deficiencies. Acute adrenal insufficiency from inadequate replacement of steroids on chronic steroid therapy is rare and can present as refractory, distributive shock. In critically ill patients, adrenal insufficiency may not present with classic symptoms. The clinical picture may resemble that of sepsis without a source of infection.[27] A high degree of suspicion must be maintained if the patient has cardiovascular instability without a defined cause.[28,29]

Diagnosis

The patient's pituitary-adrenal responsiveness should be determined when the diagnosis of primary or secondary adrenal insufficiency is first suspected. Biochemical evidence of impaired adrenal or pituitary secretory reserve unequivocally confirms the diagnosis. Patients who are clinically stable may undergo testing before treatment is initiated. Those believed to have acute adrenal insufficiency should receive immediate therapy.

Plasma cortisol levels are measured before and 30 and 60 minutes after the intravenous administration of 250 μg of synthetic ACTH. There are multiple determinants for adequate adrenal reserve; usually the plasma cortisol rises at least 9 mg/dL or to a total of at least 18 g/dL 60 minutes after the injection of the synthetic ACTH.[30] Patients with adrenal insufficiency usually demonstrate little or no adrenal response.

Treatment and Anesthetic Considerations

Normal adults secrete about 20 mg of cortisol (hydrocortisone) and 0.1 mg of aldosterone per day. Glucocorticoid therapy is usually given twice daily in sufficient dosage to meet physiologic requirements. A typical regimen in the unstressed patient may consist of prednisone, 5 mg in the morning and 2.5 mg in the evening, or hydrocortisone, 20 mg in the morning and 10 mg in the evening. The daily glucocorticoid dosage is typically 50% higher than basal adrenal output to cover the patient for mild stress. Replacement dosages are adjusted in response to the patient's clinical symptoms or the occurrence of intercurrent illnesses. Mineralocorticoid replacement is also administered on a daily basis; most patients require 0.05 to 0.1 mg/day of fludrocortisone. The mineralocorticoid dose may be reduced if severe hypokalemia, hypertension, or congestive heart failure develops, or it may be increased if postural hypotension is demonstrated.

TABLE 49-6

MANAGEMENT OF ACUTE ADRENAL INSUFFICIENCY

Hydrocortisone, 100 mg IV bolus, followed by
  hydrocortisone, 100 mg q6h for 24 hr
Fluid and electrolyte replacement as indicated by vital signs,
  serum electrolytes, and serum glucose

IV, intravenous(ly).

TABLE 49-7

MANAGEMENT OPTIONS FOR STEROID REPLACEMENT IN THE PERIOPERATIVE PERIOD

Hydrocortisone, 25 mg IV, at time of induction followed by
  hydrocortisone infusion, 100 mg over 24 hr
Hydrocortisone, 100 mg IV before, during, and after surgery

IV, intravenous(ly).

Secondary adrenal insufficiency often occurs in the presence of multiple hormone deficiencies. A decrease in ACTH production results in the decreased secretion of cortisol and adrenal androgens, but aldosterone control by more dominant mechanisms remains intact. A liberal salt diet is encouraged. Glucocorticoid substitution follows the same guidelines previously outlined for primary adrenal insufficiency.

Immediate therapy of acute adrenal insufficiency is mandatory, regardless of the etiology, and consists of electrolyte resuscitation and steroid replacement (Table 49-6). Initial therapy begins with the rapid intravenous administration of an isotonic crystalloid solution. One hundred milligrams of hydrocortisone is administered as an intravenous bolus over several minutes. Steroid replacement is continued during the first 24 hours with 100 mg of intravenous hydrocortisone given every 8 hours. If the patient is stable, the steroid dose is reduced starting on the second day. After adequate fluid resuscitation, if the patient continues to be hemodynamically unstable, inotropic support may be necessary. Invasive monitoring is extremely valuable as a guide to both diagnosis and therapy.

Steroid Replacement During the Perioperative Period

Perioperatively, patients with adrenal insufficiency and those with HPA suppression from chronic steroid use require additional corticosteroids to mimic the increased output of the normal adrenal gland during stress. The normal adrenal gland can secrete up to 100 mg/m² of cortisol per day or more during the perioperative period.[31] The pituitary-adrenal axis is usually considered to be intact if a plasma cortisol level of >19 µg/dL is measured during acute stress but there is no precise threshold. The degree of adrenal responsiveness has been correlated with the duration of surgery and the extent of surgical trauma. The mean maximal plasma cortisol level measured during major surgery (colectomy, hip osteotomy) was 47 µg/dL. Minor surgical procedures (herniorrhaphy) resulted in mean maximal plasma cortisol levels of 28 µg/dL. Adrenal activity may also be affected by the anesthetic technique used. Regional anesthesia is effective in postponing the elevation in cortisol levels during surgery of the lower abdomen and extremities.[32] Deep general anesthesia may also suppress the elevation of stress hormones such as ACTH and cortisol during the surgical procedure.

Although symptoms indicative of clinically significant adrenal insufficiency have been reported during the perioperative period, these clinical findings have rarely been documented in direct association with glucocorticoid deficiency.[33] There is evidence in adrenally suppressed primates that subphysiologic steroid replacement causes perioperative hemodynamic instability and increased mortality.

❸   Identifying which patients require steroid supplementation can be difficult. Provocative testing with ACTH stimulation is too costly to justify compared with the risk of brief steroid supplementation. HPA suppression can occur after five daily doses of prednisone ≥20 mg. Recovery of HPA function occurs gradually and can take up to 9 to 12 months. HPA

suppression can occur with topical, regional, and inhaled steroids. Alternate-day therapy decreases the risk of HPA suppression.[34]

The clinical problem is how much steroid to give. There is no proven optimal regimen for perioperative steroid replacement (Table 49-7). A "low-dose" cortisol replacement program using an intravenous infusion of 25 mg of cortisol before the induction of anesthesia, followed by a continuous infusion of cortisol (100 mg) in the next 24 hours has been advocated[35] (Fig. 49-4). This low-dose cortisol replacement program was used in patients with proven adrenal insufficiency and resulted

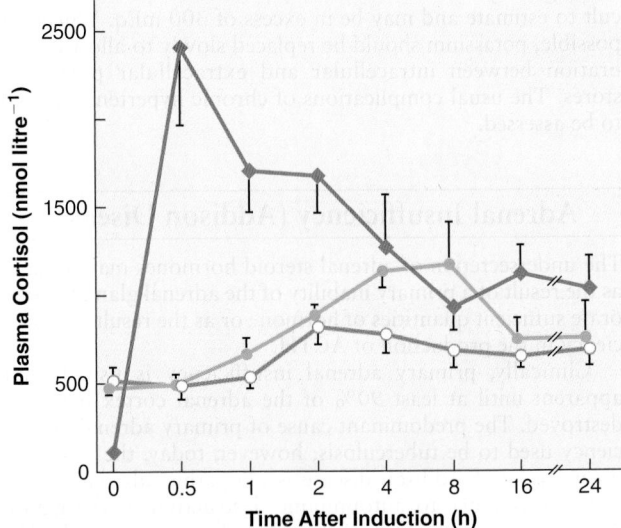

FIGURE 49-4.   Plasma cortisol concentrations (mean ± SEM) were measured in three groups of patients undergoing elective surgery. Group I control patients, n = 8 (closed circles), had never received corticosteroids. Group II patients, n = 8 (open circles), received preoperative corticosteroids with a normal response to preoperative adrenocorticotropic hormone (ACTH; corticotropin) stimulation testing. These patients and control patients received no corticosteroid substitution during the perioperative period. Group III, n = 6 (asterisks), consisted of patients receiving long-term corticosteroid therapy with an abnormal response to ACTH stimulation testing during the perioperative period. These patients (group III) received intravenous (IV) cortisol, 25 mg, after the induction of anesthesia plus a continuous IV infusion of cortisol, 100 mg, during the next 24 hours. Plasma cortisol levels in group III were significantly lower than in the other two groups before the induction of anesthesia. After IV administration of cortisol to group III patients, plasma concentrations were significantly higher than in groups I and II for the next 2 hours (p <0.01). Thereafter, the mean plasma concentrations were similar for all groups. There were no clinical signs of circulatory insufficiency in any group. (Reprinted from Symreng T, Karlberg BE, Kagedol B et al: Physiological cortisol substitution of long-term steroid-treated patients undergoing major surgery. Br J Anaesth 1981; 53: 949, with permission.)

in plasma cortisol levels as high as those seen in healthy control subjects subjected to a similar operative stress. One study with a limited number of patients found no problems with cardiovascular instability if patients received their usual dose of steroids.[36] An extensive review concluded that the best evidence was that patients should receive their usual daily dose but no supplementation.[37] Although the low-dose approach appears logical, many clinicians are unwilling to adopt this regimen until further trials have been undertaken in patients receiving physiologic steroid replacement. A popular regimen calls for the administration of 200 to 300 mg of hydrocortisone per 70 kg body weight in divided doses on the day of surgery. The lower dose is adjusted upward for longer and more extensive surgical procedures. Patients who are using steroids at the time of surgery receive their usual dose on the morning of surgery and are supplemented at a level that is at least equivalent to the usual daily replacement. Glucocorticoid coverage is rapidly tapered to the patient's normal maintenance dosage during the postoperative period. Although no conclusive evidence supports an increased incidence of infection or abnormal wound healing when supraphysiologic doses of supplemental steroids are used acutely, the goal of therapy is to use the minimal drug dosage necessary to adequately protect the patient.

Exogenous Glucocorticoid Therapy

The therapeutic use of supraphysiologic doses of glucocorticoids has expanded, and the anesthesiologist should be familiar with the various preparations (Table 49-8). Dexamethasone, methylprednisolone, and prednisone have less mineralocorticoid effect than cortisone or hydrocortisone. Prednisone and methylprednisolone are precursors that must be metabolized by the liver before anti-inflammatory activity can occur and should be used cautiously in the presence of liver disease.

Mineralocorticoid Insufficiency

Isolated mineralocorticoid insufficiency has been reported as a congenital biosynthetic defect, after unilateral adrenalectomy for removal of an aldosterone-secreting adenoma, during protracted heparin therapy, and in patients with a deficiency in renin production. This syndrome is commonly seen in patients with mild renal failure and long-standing DM. A feature common to all patients with hypoaldosteronism is a failure to increase aldosterone production in response to salt restriction or volume contraction.

Most patients present with hypotension, hyperkalemia that may be life-threatening, and a metabolic acidosis that is out of proportion to the degree of coexisting renal impairment. Patients with low renin secretion, hypoaldosteronism, and renal dysfunction respond to ACTH stimulation. Nonsteroidal anti-inflammatory drugs, which inhibit prostaglandin synthesis, may further inhibit renin release and exacerbate the condition. Patients with isolated hypoaldosteronism are given fludrocortisone orally in a dose of 0.05 to 0.1 mg/day. Patients with low renin secretion usually require higher doses to correct the electrolyte abnormalities. Caution should be observed in patients with hypertension or congestive heart failure. An alternative approach in these patients is the administration of furosemide alone or in combination with mineralocorticoid.

ADRENAL MEDULLA

The adrenal medulla is derived embryologically from neuroectodermal cells. As a specialized part of the sympathetic nervous system, the adrenal medulla synthesizes and secretes the catecholamines epinephrine (80%) and norepinephrine (20%). Preganglionic fibers of the sympathetic nervous system bypass the paravertebral ganglia and pass directly from the spinal cord to the adrenal medulla. The adrenal medulla is analogous to a postganglionic neuron, although the catecholamines secreted by the medulla function as hormones, not as neurotransmitters.

The synthesis of norepinephrine begins with hydroxylation of tyrosine to dopa (Fig. 49-5). This rate-limiting step in catecholamine biosynthesis is regulated so synthesis is coupled to release. In the adrenal medulla and in those rare central neurons using epinephrine as a neurotransmitter, most of the norepinephrine is converted to epinephrine by the enzyme phenylethanolamine-N-methyltransferase. It is likely that the capacity of the adrenal medulla to synthesize epinephrine is influenced by the flow of glucocorticoid-rich blood from the adrenal cortex through the intra-adrenal portal system

TABLE 49-8

GLUCOCORTICOID PREPARATIONS

GENERIC NAME	ANTI-INFLAMMATORY	MINERALOCORTICOID	APPROXIMATE EQUIVALENT DOSE (mg)
SHORT ACTING			
Hydrocortisone	1.0	1.0	20.0
Cortisone	0.8	0.8	25.0
Prednisone	4.0	0.25	5.0
Prednisolone	4.0	0.25	5.0
Methylprednisolone	5.0	—	4.0
INTERMEDIATE ACTING			
Triamcinolone	5.0	—	4.0
LONG ACTING			
Dexamethasone	30.0	—	0.75

Relative milligram comparisons with cortisol. The glucocorticoid and mineralocorticoid properties of cortisol are set as 1.0.

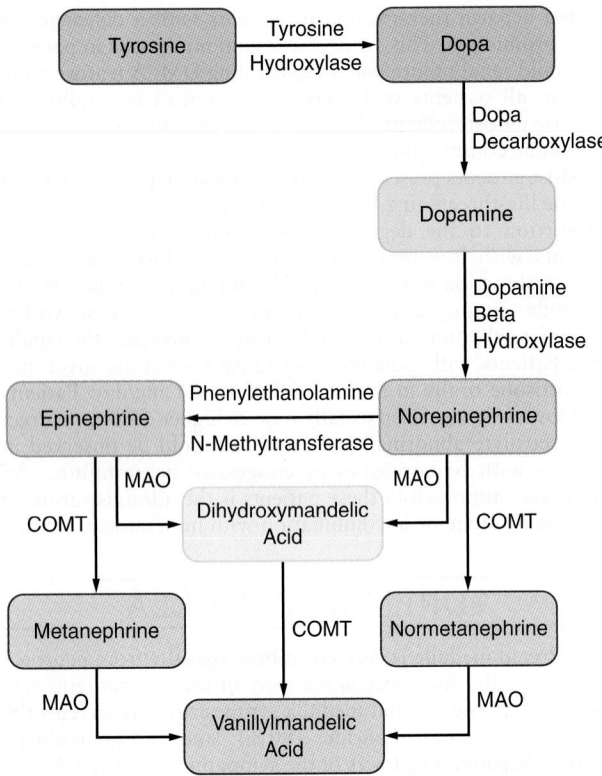

FIGURE 49-5. The synthesis and metabolism of endogenous catecholamines. COMT, catechol-O-methyltransferase; MAO, monoamine oxidase. (Reprinted from Stoelting RK, Dierdorf SF, eds: Anesthesia and Co-existing Disease. New York, Churchill-Livingstone, 1983, with permission.)

because it is known that high concentrations of glucocorticoid are able to induce the enzyme phenylethanolamine-N-methyltransferase.

In the adrenal medulla, catecholamines are stored in chromaffin granules complexed with adenosine triphosphate and Ca^{2+}. The normal adrenal releases epinephrine and norepinephrine by exocytosis in response to stimulation by preganglionic sympathetic neurons. The circulatory half-life (10 to 30 seconds) of these catechols is considerably longer than the brief receptor activity of norepinephrine released as a neurotransmitter from postganglionic sympathetic nerve endings. Biotransformation of circulating norepinephrine and epinephrine is accomplished chiefly by the enzyme catechol-O-methyltransferase, located in the liver and kidney. Monoamine oxidase is of less importance in the metabolism of circulating catechols. Metanephrine and vanillylmandelic acid are the major end products of catecholamine metabolism. These metabolites and a small amount of unchanged catecholamine (1%) appear in the urine.

The outflow of postganglionic sympathetic neurotransmitters and circulating catecholamine from the adrenal medulla is coordinated by higher cortical centers connected to the brainstem. The intrinsic activity of the brainstem sympathetic areas is modulated by higher cortical functions, emotional reactions (anger, fear), and various physiologic stimuli, including changes in the physical and chemical properties of the extracellular fluid (hypoglycemia, hypotension). The adrenal medulla and sympathetic nervous system are often stimulated together in a generalized fashion, although many physiologic conditions exist in which they act independently.

Pheochromocytoma

The only important disease process associated with the adrenal medulla is pheochromocytoma. These tumors produce, store, and secrete catecholamines. Most pheochromocytomas secrete both epinephrine and norepinephrine, with the percentage of secreted norepinephrine being greater than that secreted by the normal gland. Although pheochromocytomas occur in <0.2% of hypertensive patients, it is important to aggressively evaluate the patient with clinically suspect symptoms because surgical extirpation is curative in >90% of patients and complications are often lethal in undiagnosed cases.[38] Postmortem series have reported high perioperative mortality rates in undiagnosed patients undergoing relatively minor surgical procedures. Most deaths are from cardiovascular causes. Perioperative morbidity is related to tumor size and the degree of catecholamine secretion.[39]

Most (85 to 90%) pheochromocytomas are solitary tumors localized to a single adrenal gland, usually the right. Approximately 10% of adults and 25% of children have bilateral tumors. The tumor may originate in extra-adrenal sites (10%), anywhere along the paravertebral sympathetic chain; however, 95% are located in the abdomen, and a small percentage is located in the thorax, urinary bladder, or neck. Malignant spread of these highly vascular tumors occurs in approximately 10% of cases.

In approximately 5% of cases, this tumor is inherited as a familial autosomal dominant trait. It may be part of the polyglandular syndrome referred to as *MEN type IIA or IIB*. Type IIA includes medullary carcinoma of the thyroid, parathyroid hyperplasia, and pheochromocytoma; Type IIB consists of medullary carcinoma of the thyroid, pheochromocytoma, and neuromas of the oral mucosa. Pheochromocytomas may also arise in association with von Recklinghausen neurofibromatosis or von Hippel-Lindau disease (retinal and cerebellar angiomatosis). The pheochromocytoma of the familial syndromes is rarely extra-adrenal or malignant. Bilateral tumors occur in approximately 75% of cases. When these patients present with a single adrenal pheochromocytoma, the chances of subsequent development of a second adrenal pheochromocytoma are sufficiently high that bilateral adrenalectomy should be considered. Every member of a MEN family should be considered at risk for pheochromocytoma.

Clinical Presentation

Pheochromocytoma may occur at any age, but it is most common in young to mid-adult life. The clinical manifestations are mainly due to the pharmacologic effects of the catecholamines released from the tumor. These tumors are not innervated, and catecholamine release is independent of neurogenic control. Most patients have sustained hypertension, although occasionally it is paroxysmal.[40] When true paroxysms occur, the blood pressure may rise to alarmingly high levels, placing the patient at risk for cerebrovascular hemorrhage, heart failure, dysrhythmias, or myocardial infarction. Headache, palpitations, tremor, profuse sweating, and either pallor or flushing may accompany an attack. Pheochromocytoma can masquerade as malignant hyperthermia. Physical examination of the patient with pheochromocytoma may be unrevealing during the period between attacks unless the patient presents with symptoms and signs of sequelae related to long-standing hypertension. A catecholamine-induced cardiomyopathy may be accompanied by heart failure and cardiac dysrhythmias. Paroxysms are commonly not associated with clearly defined events but may be precipitated by displacement of the abdominal contents or, in the case of a bladder tumor, by micturition.

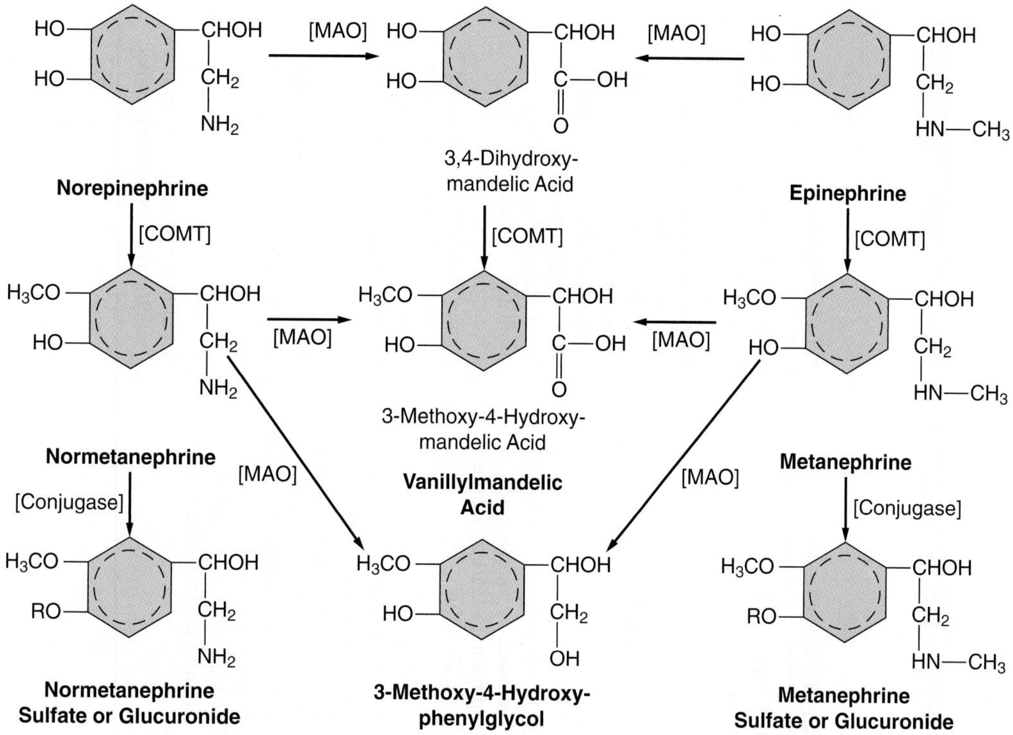

FIGURE 49-6.   Catabolism of norepinephrine and epinephrine.

Diagnosis

Biochemical determination of free catecholamine concentration and catecholamine metabolites in the urine is the most common screening test used to establish the diagnosis of pheochromocytoma.[41] Urinary vanillylmandelic acid and unconjugated norepinephrine and epinephrine levels are measured in a 24-hour urine collection and are expressed as a function of the creatinine clearance (Fig. 49-6). Excess production of catecholamines is diagnostic for pheochromocytoma. Free catecholamines represent <1% of the originally released hormone, and urinary levels are not always elevated to a significant degree. Hence, differentiation from normal subjects may be difficult. A change in the ratio of unconjugated epinephrine to norepinephrine may be the only biochemical finding. Certain drugs interfere with urinary assays, and some patients with paroxysmal hypertension have normal values between attacks.

Although routine laboratory data are unlikely to provide specific diagnostic insight, the ECG, chest radiograph, and complete blood cell count can provide valuable information to the clinician who entertains the diagnosis. Left ventricular hypertrophy and nonspecific T-wave changes are two of the more common ECG findings. Evidence of acute myocardial infarction or tachyarrhythmia has also been reported. The chest radiograph may reveal cardiomegaly, and the blood count often shows an elevated hematocrit consistent with a reduced intravascular volume and hemoconcentration. Standardized imaging methods such as computed tomography and magnetic resonance imaging are used in the noninvasive localization of these tumors.[42] Improvements in imaging may obviate the need for abdominal exploration or venous sampling to localize the tumor in selected patients.[43] Ultrasound and magnetic resonance imaging are especially useful in pregnant patients. ^{131}I-Metaiodobenzylguanidine scintigraphy is also effective in localizing recurrent or extra-adrenal masses.

Anesthetic Considerations

4 Preoperative Preparation. The reduction in perioperative mortality rates from a high of 45% to between 0% and 3%, with the excision of pheochromocytoma followed the introduction of α-antagonists for preoperative therapy. Perioperative blood pressure fluctuations, myocardial infarction, congestive heart failure, cardiac dysrhythmias, and cerebral hemorrhage all appear to be reduced in frequency when the patient has been treated before surgery with alpha-blockers and the intravascular fluid compartment has been reexpanded. Extended treatment with α-antagonists is also effective in treating the clinical manifestations of catecholamine myocarditis. However, alpha-blocker therapy has never been studied in a controlled way, and there are some groups that question its necessity in light of the availability of potent titratable vasodilators for intraoperative use.[44] A list of drugs frequently used in the management of pheochromocytoma is given in Table 49-9.

α-Adrenergic blockade is initiated once the diagnosis of pheochromocytoma is established (see Chapter 15). Phenoxybenzamine, a long-acting (24 to 48 hours), noncompetitive presynaptic (α_2) and postsynaptic (α_1) blocker, has traditionally been used at doses of 10 mg every 8 hours. Increments are added until the blood pressure is controlled and paroxysms disappear. Most patients need between 80 and 200 mg/day. The absorption after oral administration is variable, and side effects are common. Certain cardiovascular reflexes such as the baroreceptor reflex are blunted, and postural hypotension is common. Selective competitive α_1-blockers, such as doxazosin, terazosin, and prazosin, have also been used effectively. Because postural hypotension can be pronounced with the commencement of therapy, the initial 1-mg dose is given at bedtime. Postural changes are also seen with maintenance therapy. A comparison of patients with pheochromocytoma receiving phenoxybenzamine or prazosin has shown both

TABLE 49-9

DRUGS USED IN THE MANAGEMENT OF PHEOCHROMOCYTOMA

DRUG	ACTION	PREOPERATIVE BLOOD PRESSURE CONTROL	PRESSOR CRISIS	COMMENT
Phentolamine	Nonselective α-antagonist	—	1–5 mg IV; 0.5–1 mg/min IV	Short duration of action ~5 min
Phenoxybenzamine	Nonselective α-antagonist	20 mg/d PO up to 160 mg/d in divided doses	—	Long half-life; may accumulate
Doxazosin (terazosin dosing similar)	Selective α₁-antagonist	1 mg/d PO up to 8 mg/d PO	—	First-dose phenomena; may cause syncope
Propranolol	Nonselective β-antagonist	40 mg/d PO up to 480 mg/d in divided doses to control tachycardia	1–2 mg IV bolus	Should never be given without first creating α-blockade
Atenolol	Selective β₁-antagonist	50–100 mg/d PO	—	Long-acting drug eliminated; unchanged by kidney
Esmolol	Selective β₁-antagonist	—	250–500 μg/kg/min IV loading followed by maintenance infusion 25–250 μg/kg/min	Short acting; elimination half-life ~9 min
Labetalol	α-antagonist and β-antagonist	200 mg/d PO in divided doses up to 800 mg/d	10 mg IV bolus	A much weaker alpha-blocker than beta-blocker; may cause hypertensive response
Nitroprusside	Direct vasodilator	—	0.5–1.5 μg/kg/min initially, increased to maximum of 8 μg/kg/min; titrate to effect	Powerful vasodilator; short acting
Magnesium sulfate	Direct vasodilator and membrane stabilizer	—	2–4 g IV bolus followed by 1–2 g/hr and additional 1–2 g boluses as needed	May potentiate neuromuscular blockade
Nicardipine	Calcium channel antagonist	—	1–2 μg/kg/min increased to 7.5 μg/kg/min; titrate to effect	—
α-Methyltyrosine	Inhibitor of biosynthesis of catecholamine	1–4 g/d PO in divided doses	—	Suitable for patients not amenable to surgery; may be nephrotoxic

IV, intravenous(ly); PO, oral(ly).

drugs to be equally effective in controlling the blood pressure. Although the optimal period of preoperative treatment has not been established, most clinicians recommend beginning α-blockade therapy at least 10 to 14 days before the proposed surgery; however, periods as short as 3 to 5 days have been used.[45] During this time, the contracted intravascular volume and hematocrit return toward normal and the blood pressure is stabilized. Despite the real possibility of hypotension after vascular isolation of the tumor, most clinicians continue alpha-blockers up until the morning of surgery.

β-Adrenergic blockade is occasionally added after α-blockade has been established. This addition is considered in patients with persistent tachycardia or cardiac dysrhythmias that may be caused by nonselective α-blockade or epinephrine-secreting tumors. Beta-blockers should not be given until adequate α-blockade is ensured to avoid the possibility of unopposed α-mediated vasoconstriction. There is no clear preoperative advantage of one β antagonist over another, although the short half-life of esmolol may allow better control of heart rate and arrhythmias in the perioperative setting. Labetalol, a β-adrenergic antagonist with α-blocking activity, is effective as a second-line medication, but can increase blood pressure when this drug is used alone.

α-Methyl tyrosine is an agent that inhibits the enzyme tyrosine hydroxylase, the rate-limiting step in catecholamine biosynthesis. This medication is currently reserved for patients with metastatic disease, or for situations in which surgery is contraindicated and long-term medical therapy is required. When α-methyl tyrosine is used in combination with α-adrenergic-blocking agents, there is a significant reduction in catecholamine biosynthesis.

Unrecognized pheochromocytoma during pregnancy may be life-threatening to the mother and fetus. Although the safety of adrenergic-blocking agents during pregnancy has not been established, these agents probably improve fetal survival in pregnant patients with pheochromocytoma. The trend is to perform surgery during the first trimester or at the time of cesarean delivery. There is no reason to terminate an early pregnancy, but the patient should be aware of the risk of spontaneous abortion resulting from abdominal surgery to remove the tumor.[46]

Perioperative Anesthetic Management Symptomatic patients continue to receive medical therapy until tachycardia, cardiac dysrhythmias, and paroxysmal elevations in blood pressure are well controlled. If it is not possible to initiate α-blocking therapy before surgery, or if the patient has received <48 hours of intensive treatment, it may be necessary to infuse nitroprusside during the induction of anesthesia. A low-dose infusion is often initiated in anticipation of the marked blood pressure elevations that can occur with laryngoscopy and surgical stimulation.

Improvements in imaging now allow most patients with solitary tumors without evidence of metastases or local invasion to undergo a laparoscopic retroperitoneal approach. If the surgeon needs to assess for bilateral disease or the dissection is too difficult, then the procedure can be converted to an open one. During laparoscopic surgery, creation of the pneumoperitoneum may cause release of catecholamines and large changes in hemodynamics that can be controlled with a vasodilator.[47]

Although there is no clear advantage to one anesthetic technique over another, drugs that are known to liberate histamine are avoided. Because of the potential for ventricular irritability, halothane is not administered. A potent sedative-hypnotic, in combination with an opioid analgesic, is used for induction. It is extremely important to achieve an adequate depth of anesthesia before proceeding with laryngoscopy to minimize the sympathetic nervous system response to this maneuver. Maintenance is provided with an opioid analgesic and a potent ⑤ inhalation agent. Manipulation of the tumor may produce marked elevations in blood pressure. Acute hypertensive crises are treated with intravenous infusions of nitroprusside or phentolamine or any vasodilator mentioned later. Phentolamine is a short-acting α-adrenergic antagonist that may be given as an intravenous bolus (2 to 5 mg) or by continuous infusion. Tachydysrhythmia is controlled with intravenous boluses of propranolol (1-mg increments) or by a continuous infusion of the ultrashort-acting selective β1-adrenergic antagonist esmolol. The disadvantage of long-acting beta-blockers may be persistence of bradycardia and hypotension after the tumor is removed. Even esmolol may be problematic because there are cases of cardiac arrest after clamping of the venous drainage in patients receiving large doses of esmolol. Almost every vasodilator has been tried and recommended as an adjuvant to control hypertension. Magnesium sulfate given as an infusion with intermittent boluses has successfully controlled blood pressure.[48] Nicardipine, nitroglycerin, diltiazem, fenoldopam, and prostaglandin E_1 have all been used anecdotally. The reduction in blood pressure that may occur after ligation of the tumor's venous supply can be dangerously abrupt and should be anticipated through close communication with the surgical team. Restitution of any intravascular fluid deficit is the initial therapy in this situation. After replenishment of the intravascular volume, if the patient remains hypotensive, phenylephrine is administered. After surgery, catecholamine levels return to normal over several days. Approximately 75% of patients become normotensive within 10 days.

DIABETES MELLITUS

A fasting glucose level below 100 mg/dL is considered normal. Individuals with documented fasting glucose levels above 126 mg/dL are considered diabetics and those with levels between 100 and 125 mg/dL are considered prediabetics.[49] An estimated 20.8 million Americans (7% of the U.S. population) have DM and about 40 million Americans have prediabetes. DM is the most commonly occurring endocrine disease found in surgical patients.[50] Although the most serious complications of DM are related to its character as a chronic disease, it can cause difficulties in the short-term management of acute illness. Occasionally, DM remains clinically inapparent until exacerbated by the stress of trauma or surgery.

The principles of the treatment of DM will be easier to understand if we review the physiology of glucose metabolism and the stress response and then consider some of the specific pathologic entities that comprise the clinical picture of DM.

Classification

DM is primarily a disease of glucose metabolism; however, it has numerous manifestations and has a range of endocrinologic effects. Despite a variety of etiologic factors, its hallmark is a deficiency, either absolute or relative, in the amount of insulin effect to the tissues.

DM is often divided into two broad types. Type I (formerly called *insulin-dependent diabetes mellitus*) accounts for 5 to 10% of all DM cases and is distinguished from type II (formerly called *non–insulin-dependent diabetes mellitus*), which accounts for the remaining 90 to 95% of all DM cases. The patient with type I DM typically experiences the onset of disease early in life.[51] Consequently, this form is also referred to as *juvenile-onset diabetes*. In general, the patient with type I DM is not obese, had an abrupt onset of the disease, and has very low levels of circulating insulin. Disease in these patients cannot be controlled with diet or oral hypoglycemic agents;

rather, it mandates treatment with insulin as there is an absolute deficiency of insulin. It is difficult to maintain an optimal glucose level in patients with type I DM; they are more likely to become ketotic and are likely to sustain the end-organ complications of diabetes if they live long enough.

Patients with type II DM, also called *adult-onset diabetes*, typically experience a gradual onset of the disease later in life. However, because of the obesity epidemic, adolescents and teenagers are presenting more frequently with this disorder. Patients with type II DM are often obese, have resistance to the effects of insulin (commonly referred to as *insulin resistance*), and hence may have normal or even elevated levels of insulin. In milder forms, this version of diabetes can often be treated with diet, lifestyle modifications, and oral hypoglycemic agents. Because these patients are relatively resistant to ketosis, their disease may be clinically inapparent until exacerbated by the stress of surgery or intercurrent illness.

This classification of DM is only a generalization. The milder type II form can occur in young people, and many older adults can acquire a severe and brittle form of type I. Secondary DM can be a result of a disease that damages the pancreas and thus impairs insulin secretion. Pancreatic surgery, chronic pancreatitis, cystic fibrosis, and hemochromatosis can damage the pancreas and impair insulin secretion sufficiently to produce clinical DM. DM can also result from one of the endocrine diseases that produces a hormone that opposes the action of insulin. Hence, a patient with a glucagonoma, pheochromocytoma, or acromegaly may be diabetic. An increased effect of glucocorticoids, either from Cushing disease or steroid therapy, may also oppose the effect of insulin enough to elicit clinical diabetes and would certainly complicate the management of pre-existing diabetes. Gestational diabetes is a common medical problem of pregnancy and may presage future type II DM.

Physiology

Insulin has multiple and complex interactions with lipid, protein, and glucose metabolism. It also has many nonmetabolic functions.[52] For our purposes, it is easiest to regard the effects of insulin on glucose metabolism as primary and to view its effects on other metabolic functions only as they relate to glucose.

Insulin is a small protein produced by the β cells of the islets of Langerhans in the pancreas. The basal rate of insulin secretion is about 1 U/hr, which can increase by five- to tenfold after ingestion of food. Normal production in the adult human is approximately 40 to 50 U/day. Insulin acts through specific receptors on cells. The half-life of insulin in the circulation is roughly 5 minutes. However, it may clinically appear to have a longer duration of action, owing to delays in binding and release from the cellular receptors. These facts lead to the important principle that once a high level of insulin saturates all the binding sites, insulin will not have a more potent effect, just a more long-lasting effect.

Insulin is metabolized in the liver and kidney. In patients with hepatic dysfunction, the loss of gluconeogenesis and a prolongation of insulin effect increase the risk of hypoglycemia. Similarly, in patients with renal disease, the action of insulin is prolonged and they are more prone to hypoglycemia. Exogenous insulin should be administered judiciously in diabetic patients with renal disease.

Insulin release is related to a number of events. Glucose and amino acids directly stimulate insulin release. The mechanism involves interaction with hormones from the GI tract released during enteral feeding. The autonomic nervous system, through vagal stimulation, increases insulin release, as do β-adrenergic stimulation and α-adrenergic blockade. Nitric oxide stimu-

lates insulin secretion. Potassium depletion decreases insulin secretion.

The most fundamental action of insulin is to stimulate increased cellular uptake of glucose in skeletal muscle cells, adipose tissue, and cardiac cells. This is particularly important in skeletal muscle cells, in which muscle activity also increases glucose uptake and is an important variable in the management of the physically active diabetic patient. The brain, liver, and immune cells are exceptions, as insulin does not affect glucose transport. Hence, the diabetic patient has hyperglycemia because of inadequate cellular uptake of glucose. Along with glucose, potassium enters the cells under the influence of insulin, so the diabetic patient is also likely to have an imbalance of potassium concentrations across cell membranes.

Other important metabolic functions of insulin include the stimulation of glycogen formation, as well as the suppression of gluconeogenesis and lipolysis. The patient with insulin deficiency has low glycogen stores and active gluconeogenesis. This implies that in the diabetic patient with a deficiency of glycogen, protein must be broken down to make glucose. Insulin also increases the uptake of amino acids into muscle cells. Hence, insulin deficiency leads to catabolism and negative nitrogen balance.

Fat metabolism is also abnormal in the diabetic state, with acceleration of lipid catabolism and increased formation of ketone bodies. Insulin deficiency leads to increased fatty acid liberation from adipose tissue. These fatty acids have multiple metabolic effects, including interference with carbohydrate phosphorylation in muscle, which leads to further hyperglycemia. Low concentrations of insulin, which may be inadequate to prevent hyperglycemia, are often sufficient to block lipolysis. This effect explains the common clinical situation in which a patient is hyperglycemic without being ketotic.

Glucagon is a polypeptide released from the α cells of the pancreas, and acts to oppose some of the effects of insulin. It has both a direct and indirect ability to increase circulating glucose levels. In some patients, after total pancreatic resection, glucose balance is not as poor as might be expected because of the concomitant absence of glucagon. Glucagon release is stimulated by hypoglycemia, as well as by epinephrine and cortisol, and is suppressed by glucose ingestion.

The metabolic effects of stress are intricately involved with the same pathways as those involved in DM. During stress, elevations in the circulating levels of cortisol, glucagon, catecholamines, and growth hormone all act to cause hyperglycemia. In addition, glucagon and adrenergic stimulation exert a suppressive effect on insulin release. Furthermore, inflammatory mediators released during stress enhance the release of the counterregulatory hormones and directly affect the intracellular signaling pathways of insulin, culminating in significant insulin resistance.[53,54] Hence, mild hyperglycemia may occur in the stressed patient who does not have DM. In the diabetic patient, stress makes the hyperglycemia more difficult to control. In a patient with minimal or subclinical DM before the stressful episode, the hyperglycemia may become difficult to manage during the stress-related event.

Treatment

Patients with type I DM require insulin to survive. The risk of microvascular complications can be decreased if tight glycemic control is maintained near normal levels of blood glucose. Patients may be on a range of doses of short-, intermediate-, and long-acting insulin, with doses given one to six times per day, depending on the desire for tight control. In some clinical situations, an insulin pump may be used to administer constant levels of insulin.

Patients with type II DM initially may be treated with diet control and exercise. If this fails to control glucose levels or the diabetes worsens, therapy with an oral agent is indicated.[55] Sulfonylureas (glyburide, glipizide, glimepiride) and glinides (repaglinide, nateglinide) enhance β-cell insulin secretion. Metformin is a biguanide that decreases hepatic glucose output and enhances the sensitivity of both hepatic and peripheral tissues to insulin.[56] Rosiglitazone (Avandia) and pioglitazone (Actos) are thiazolidinediones that increase insulin sensitivity. α-Glucosidase inhibitors (acarbose, miglitol) decrease postprandial glucose absorption. Amylin analogs (pramlinide [Symlin]) suppress glucagon secretion and slow gastric emptying, while incretin mimetics (exenatide [Byetta]), as the name implies, emulate natural incretin hormones (glucagonlike peptide 1, glucose-dependent insulinotropic polypeptide) and increase insulin production, inhibit glucagon secretion, and decrease glucose absorption. Dipeptidyl-peptidase 4 inhibitors (sitagliptin [Januvia]) also slow degradation of incretin hormones and improve postprandial hyperglycemia. If oral agents cannot maintain acceptable glucose levels, insulin is required.

Anesthetic Management

6 Successful management of the diabetic patient depends as much, if not more, on the proper management of the chronic complications of the disease as on acute glycemic management.

Preoperative

A thorough preoperative search must be done for end-organ complications of DM. In addition to a thorough history and physical examination, a recent ECG, blood urea nitrogen, potassium, creatinine, glucose, and urinalysis are essential.

Atherosclerosis develops earlier and is more widespread in diabetic patients compared with nondiabetic patients. Manifestations include coronary artery disease, peripheral vascular disease, cerebrovascular disease, and renovascular disease. The incidence of postoperative myocardial infarction is increased in diabetic patients, and the complication rate is higher. Coronary artery disease can manifest at a young age or atypically in type I diabetics. Silent myocardial ischemia and infarction occur more commonly in diabetic patients, perhaps because of sensory neuropathy of the visceral afferents to the heart. DM may be associated with a cardiomyopathy in the face of angiographically normal coronary arteries, possibly with diffuse disease in arteries too small to be visualized (see Preoperative Evaluation). The American College of Cardiology/American Heart Association guidelines recognize DM as a moderate clinical risk factor when evaluating patients for noncardiac surgery.[57] Preoperative hyperglycemia, as documented by increased hemoglobin A1c, has been associated with poor perioperative outcomes in a variety of clinical situations.

Laryngoscopy can be difficult in up to 40% of juvenile patients with DM presenting for renal transplantation.[58] This may be because of diabetic stiff joint syndrome, a frequent complication of type I DM leading to decreased mobility of the atlanto-occipital joint. The "prayer sign," an inability to approximate the palmar surfaces of the interphalangeal joints, is associated with stiff joint syndrome and may predict difficult laryngoscopy.

Diabetic nephropathy eventually occurs in up to 40 to 50% of patients with DM. Albuminuria usually precedes a steady decline in renal function.

Diabetic patients with autonomic neuropathy are at increased risk for intraoperative hypotension and perioperative cardiorespiratory arrest.[59–61] There may be an exaggerated pressor response to tracheal intubation.[62] Autonomic function may be tested by measuring the beat-to-beat variation in heart rate during breathing, heart rate response to a Valsalva maneuver, and orthostatic changes in diastolic blood pressure and heart rate. Autonomic neuropathy predisposes to intraoperative hypothermia.[63]

Diabetic patients may have delayed gastric emptying as a result of diabetic autonomic neuropathy, and therefore an increased risk of pulmonary aspiration of gastric contents. Autonomic function tests can predict the presence of solid food particles in gastric contents but not increased gastric volume or acidity.[64] Metoclopramide may be useful in emptying the stomach of solid food.

It is axiomatic that the patient should attain the best possible preoperative metabolic control. If the patient's glucose level has been unstable, especially with episodes of hypoglycemia, adjustment of insulin therapy is required. Traditionally, oral hypoglycemics have been held before surgery because of fear of hypoglycemia in the fasted patient. With modern shorter-acting agents, this may be unnecessary because the risk is much reduced. It is desirable to discontinue metformin preoperatively because it has been associated with severe lactic acidosis during episodes of hypotension, poor perfusion, or hypoxia. However, a recent study did not show an increase in morbidity and mortality after cardiac surgery in patients who did not discontinue metformin preoperatively.[65] Unless the patient has a surgical emergency, patients with diabetic ketoacidosis or hyperosmolar coma should receive intensive medical management before coming to the operating room (see "Emergencies").

Intraoperative

The details of the anesthetic plan depend intimately on the end-organ complications. Invasive monitoring may be indicated for the patient with heart disease, awake intubation may be necessary if a difficult intubation is predicted, fluid management and drug choices may depend on renal function, and pulmonary aspiration must be considered if there is gastroparesis.

Blood glucose levels should be measured before and after surgery. The need for additional measurements is determined by the duration and magnitude of surgery, as well as the brittleness of the diabetes. Hourly measurements are reasonable in high-risk patients.

The standard glucose dosage for an adult patient is 5 to 10 g/hr (100 to 200 mL of 5% dextrose solution hourly). Intraoperative administration of glucose should be guided by patient's glucose level and with the goal of preventing hypoglycemia or hyperglycemia. Routine administration of glucose-containing intravenous fluids is not recommended. It is best to monitor and record the dextrose administered separately from the fluids given.

Monitoring of the patient who arrives in the operating room with significant metabolic impairment, such as diabetic ketoacidosis, is similar to management in the medical intensive care unit, including hourly determinations of blood glucose, arterial pH, electrolytes, and fluid balance. Frequent reassessments, with medical consultation as needed, guide the use of fluids, electrolytes, especially potassium, insulin, phosphate, and glucose.

Another area of patient monitoring that is extremely important in the diabetic patient is positioning on the operating table. Injuries to the limbs or nerves are more likely in the patient who arrives in the operating room already compromised by diabetic peripheral vascular disease or neuropathy. The peripheral nerves may already be partly ischemic and therefore particularly vulnerable to pressure or stretch injuries.[66]

Glycemic Goals

Insulin secretion can be decreased by the direct effects of anesthetics, while significant insulin resistance develops postoperatively. Insulin resistance implies that despite adequate, or even increased, levels of insulin, there is a submaximal effect, and glucose levels are not normalized. Perioperatively, inflammatory mediators and increased catabolic hormones contribute significantly to insulin resistance.[54] The degree of insulin resistance is directly related to surgical trauma. Intraoperative and postoperative hyperglycemia is predicable in patients who present for cardiac and high-risk noncardiac surgery and/or have poor glycemic control preoperatively (e.g., diabetics, or patients who have an ongoing metabolic insult secondary to trauma or sepsis). Hyperglycemia significantly impairs chemotaxis, phagocytosis, generation of reactive oxygen species, and intracellular killing of bacteria.[67] Vascular reactivity is also decreased by hyperglycemia and is proposed to be related to decreased nitric oxide production. Acute hyperglycemia has also been shown to lead to poor outcomes in the setting of myocardial infarction and stroke.

In view of the ubiquitous nature of the hyperglycemic response, until recently it was considered acceptable not to treat perioperative hyperglycemia unless blood glucose was >200 to 250 mg/dL, or even higher. However, this practice has been seriously challenged by recent studies. Hyperglycemia is associated with poor perioperative outcomes. The evidence for improvement in perioperative outcomes predominantly comes from the studies in critically ill patients or patients who have undergone cardiac surgery.

The study that revolutionized the practice of hyperglycemic control in critically ill patients was published by Van den Berghe et al.[68] In intensive care unit (ICU) patients, most of whom were postsurgery and mechanically ventilated, ICU mortality, renal dysfunction, need for dialysis, and neuropathic changes were decreased in patients undergoing intensive insulin therapy compared with those who had their glucose levels maintained at 180 to 210 mg/dL. These results were supported by other observational studies. A study of medical and surgical ICU patients demonstrated significant reductions in mortality, renal dysfunction, and red blood cell transfusion in patients with glucose levels <150 mg/dL.[69] Although other studies have not been able to replicate these findings, especially in the medical ICU settings, these initial studies provide significant evidence in support of tight glycemic control in critically ill patients.

The best evidence for the benefits of glycemic control comes from patients undergoing cardiac surgery[70–73] (see Chapter 41). In one large study, glycemic control was achieved by continuous insulin infusion in the treatment group versus subcutaneous insulin in the control group.[73] Morbidity and mortality increased significantly once glucose levels increased >175 mg/dL. For each 18-mg/dL increase in glucose, adverse events increased by 17%. Another study found that for each 20-mg/dL increase in glucose levels, risk of adverse events increased by 30%.[74] Poor cardiac and noncardiac outcomes have been associated with intraoperative hyperglycemia.[75] A mortality benefit has been demonstrated by maintaining glucose between 150 and 200 mg/dL in diabetic patients who underwent cardiac surgery.[76]

Although glycemic control has been associated with improved outcomes, the benefits of tight intraoperative glycemic control are much less clear. Achieving glycemic control during cardiopulmonary bypass can be difficult. A study of patients undergoing cardiopulmonary bypass found no difference in composite outcomes in patients who received continuous insulin to achieve euglycemia compared with conventional treatment to keep glucose <200 mg/dL.[77] Indeed, more

deaths and strokes were noted in the intensive treatment group. This study definitely puts to question the efficacy of tight *intraoperative* glycemic control in patients undergoing cardiac surgery (see Chapter 41). Some have cautioned against tight intraoperative glycemic control (<110 mg/dL) and consider it to be experimental and of limited value in the setting of tighter glycemic control postoperatively.[78]

Retrospective data in noncardiac surgery also suggest that perioperative hyperglycemia portends poor outcome. Increased levels of HbA1c and/or development of hyperglycemia have been associated with poorer perioperative outcomes after vascular, orthopaedic, trauma, and subarachnoid hemorrhage. Again, the data investigating the role of intraoperative glucose control in noncardiac surgery are limited. At the present time, tight intraoperative glucose control cannot be advocated.

One of the major drawbacks of tight glycemic control is hypoglycemia. In surgical ICU patients the incidence of severe hypoglycemia (<40 mg/dL) may be 7 times higher in an intensive insulin treatment group compared with those receiving conventional treatment. In medical ICU patients the absolute incidence of hypoglycemia was far greater (25.1% in the treatment group vs 3.9% in the control group).[79] The Efficacy of Volume Substitution and Insulin Therapy in Severe Sepsis (VISEP) study[80] and the Glucontrol studies were both stopped because of the concerns of significant hypoglycemia. An association between hypoglycemia and mortality in an ICU population has also been reported.[81] A meta-analysis of randomized controlled trials found that perioperative insulin infusion may reduce mortality but increases hypoglycemia.[82]

In summary, association between perioperative hyperglycemia and poor outcomes is strong. Poor glycemic control is probably a marker of significant metabolic perturbation, which is beyond the regulatory capacity of the body. Although hyperglycemia develops frequently in patients who undergo cardiac or high-risk noncardiac surgery, the value of controlling glucose levels tightly *intraoperatively* has not been proven conclusively. Many endocrinologic societies recommend maintaining glycemic levels to <110 mg/dL in the ICU patients and <150 mg/dL in diabetic patients undergoing cardiac surgery (Table 49-10). Similar recommendations have been adopted by ACC/AHA in their guidelines for perioperative management of patients undergoing noncardiac surgery. Until the results of current trials are available it seems prudent to maintain glucose levels <180 mg/dL, especially in the perioperative period.

Management of Perioperative Hyperglycemia

Many factors influence the glucose levels in the perioperative period. Endogenous insulin secretion, exogenous insulin administration, insulin resistance, endogenous glucose production, exogenous glucose administration, and overall glucose consumption are some of the key factors that determine glucose levels in a patient. Insulin resistance can be modified not only by the stress of surgery and the inflammatory state, but also by diet and physical activity. Postoperative ambulation and physical activity can alter glucose consumption acutely. In view of the complex nature of glycemic control in the perioperative period, maintaining glucose levels within a specific range can be demanding. The narrower the desired glycemic range, the more resource-intensive the protocol will be.

Insulin can be administered in many different ways. The simplest route is to administer it subcutaneously. Few studies have adopted this route and they have not been very successful in maintaining tight or timely control. In the perioperative set-

ANESTHESIA FOR SURGICAL SUBSPECIALTIES

TABLE 49-10

CURRENT RECOMMENDATIONS FOR GLYCEMIC CONTROL

■ LOCATION	■ AMERICAN COLLEGE OF ENDOCRINOLOGY (2004)	■ CANADIAN DIABETIC ASSOCIATION (2003)	■ AMERICAN DIABETIC ASSOCIATION (2007)	■ AHA/ACC (2007)
ICU	Close to 110 mg/dL; generally <180 mg/dL	<110 mg/dL	<110 mg/dL	110–180 mg/dL
Intraoperatively	<150 mg/dL	90–180 mg/dL	??	
Perioperatively	(Noncritically ill: 90–130 mg/dL)	90–180 mg/dL	??	?

AHA, American Heart Association; ACC, American College of Cardiology; ICU, intensive care unit.

ting, the state of peripheral perfusion is extremely variable and peripheral vasoconstriction is common. Hence, absorption of any drug administered subcutaneously can be erratic and unreliable. Similarly, sliding scale protocols have also been disappointing. Most study protocols that have demonstrated desirable glycemic control in the acute care setting have used continuous intravenous insulin infusion combined with intravenous bolus injections. Targeted glucose levels can be achieved effectively using these dynamic scale protocols combined with frequent blood glucose determinations.

Blood glucose can be determined by central laboratory, blood-gas analysis machines, or various point-of-care testing devices that use capillary blood (fingerstick). Point-of-care devices are most commonly used in many acute care areas for glucose monitoring and management. The practitioners should keep in mind that the accuracy varies with each handheld meter. Glucose meter analysis (arterial and capillary blood) may provide higher glucose values, whereas blood gas analysis of arterial blood may yield lower glucose values, compared with central laboratory values. The hemodynamic state of the patient may also affect the accuracy of the blood glucose measurement by the point-of-care devices.[83] Furthermore, whole-blood glucose values and plasma glucose values are different, and the same is true for arterial and venous blood. Therefore, a real possibility exists of overdosing or underdosing a patient with insulin. Hence, aberrant glucose values should be confirmed by central laboratory measurements, and practitioners should be aware of the performance of these point-of-care devices in their institutions.[84]

Although it is possible to institute protocols that can be followed by nurses without much physician input and to control glucose levels, the practice can be significantly resource-intensive. By some estimates, each point-of-care glucose measurement adds 3.5 to 9 minutes to patient care. Aggregate time spent by the caregivers to perform glucose monitoring and achieve target glucose levels safely may be substantial.

Type I Diabetes

Type I diabetics require insulin or they will rapidly develop ketoacidosis and its complications. This treatment can be given by administering one half to two thirds of the patient's usual intermediate-acting insulin subcutaneously on the morning of surgery. In addition to this basal insulin, a regular insulin sliding scale (RISS) can be added and titrated to blood glucose measurement.[85] Alternatively, an insulin infusion of 1 to 2 U/hr (100 U regular insulin in 100 mL normal saline at 1 to 2 mL/hr) can meet basal metabolic needs and be adjusted to maintain blood glucose at the desired level.[86] With either method, a slow glucose infusion (dextrose 5% in water at 75 to 100 mL/hr) will prevent hypoglycemia while the patient is fasting. Some authorities recommend a combination glucose-insulin or glucose-insulin-potassium infusions.

Type II Diabetes

The hospitalized type II diabetic patient may find glucose control improved because of stricter dietary control. Fasting patients will not have postprandial hyperglycemia. Sulfonylureas should be held while the patient is NPO (nothing per mouth) to decrease the risk of hypoglycemia and because they interfere with the cardioprotective effect of ischemic preconditioning. Metformin probably should also be held, especially if there is a risk of decreased renal function perioperatively because of a risk of lactic acidosis. Thiazolidinediones can be continued because they do not predispose to hypoglycemia. α-Glucosidase inhibitors should be held because they work only when taken with meals. For type II patients taking oral agents alone, RISS can be added to control blood glucose levels.

Patients receiving chronic insulin can be treated similarly to the type I patient by giving one-half the usual NPH (neutral protamine Hagedorn) dose the morning of surgery, supplemented by a RISS, or an insulin infusion titrated to blood glucose. The use of a RISS as the sole method of control is to be discouraged because it can predispose to wide glucose variations.[87]

Because of the multiple approaches and varied data, many institutions have instituted collaborative insulin infusion protocols designed to achieve strict glycemic control in medical ICU patients.[88] These protocols emphasize the need to consider the current blood glucose value as well as the rate of change of blood glucose level when adjusting the infusion.

Postoperatively, as the patient resumes oral intake, therapy can be transitioned to the patient's chronic regimen. Type II diabetics who have had gastric bypass can have rapid resolution of their glucose intolerance and will often need their oral agents and insulin reduced or even discontinued in the postoperative period. This effect appears to be due to changes in the incretin hormones such as glucose-dependent insulinotropic polypeptide and glucagonlike peptide 1, rather than weight loss.[89]

Emergencies

Patients may present with metabolic instability, or it may develop perioperatively. Stress, trauma, and infection may all lead to increased insulin requirements and insulin resistance.

Hyperosmolar Nonketotic Coma

An occasional elderly patient with minimal or mild DM may present with remarkably high blood glucose levels (>600 mg/dL) and profound dehydration. Such patients usually have enough endogenous insulin activity to prevent ketosis; even with blood sugar concentrations of 1,000 mg/dL, they are not in ketoacidosis. Presumably, it is the combination of an impaired thirst response and mild renal insufficiency that allows the hyperglycemia to develop. The marked hyperosmolarity may lead to coma and seizures, with the increased plasma viscosity producing a tendency to intravascular thrombosis. It is characteristic of this syndrome that the metabolic disturbance responds quickly to rehydration and small doses of insulin. One to 2 L of isotonic fluid should be infused over 1 to 2 hours if there are no cardiovascular contraindications. Insulin, by bolus or infusion, should be administered. With rapid correction of the hyperosmolarity, cerebral edema is a risk, and recovery of mental acuity may be delayed after the blood glucose level and circulating volume have been normalized.

Diabetic Ketoacidosis

If the diabetic patient has insufficient insulin effect to block the mobilization and metabolism of free fatty acids, the metabolic byproducts acetoacetate and β-hydroxybutyrate accumulate.[90] These ketone bodies are organic acids and cause a metabolic acidosis with an increased unmeasured anion gap. Clinically, the patient often presents because of intercurrent illness, trauma, or the untoward cessation of insulin therapy. Although hyperglycemia is almost always present, the degree of hyperglycemia does not correlate with the severity of the acidosis. Blood sugar levels are often in the 300 to 500 mg/dL range. The patient is always dehydrated because of the combination of the hyperglycemia-induced osmotic diuresis and the nausea and vomiting typical of this syndrome. Because leukocytosis, abdominal pain, GI ileus, and mildly elevated amylase levels are all common in ketoacidosis, an occasional patient is misdiagnosed as having an intra-abdominal surgical problem.

Treatment of diabetic ketoacidosis includes insulin administration and fluid and electrolyte replacement (Table 49-11). An intravenous bolus of 10 to 20 U of insulin achieves rapid maximal effect. Further insulin can be administered by intravenous infusion or intermittent bolus every 30 to 60 minutes. When blood glucose levels decrease below 250 mg/dL, glucose should be added to the intravenous fluid while insulin therapy continues. Fluid requirements can be marked; 1 to 2 L of isotonic fluid, should be given over 1 to 2 hours. Further deficits can be replaced more gradually. Potassium replacement is a key concern in patients with diabetic ketoacidosis. Because of the diuresis, the total-body potassium stores are reduced. However, acidosis by itself causes a shift of potassium ions out of the cell. Thus, the serum potassium concentration may be normal or even slightly elevated while the patient is acidotic.

As soon as the metabolic acidosis is corrected, the potassium ions shift back into the cells. Consequently, the serum potassium concentration can decline acutely. Therefore, early and vigorous potassium replacement is required in these patients, with the exception of those patients in renal failure. Hypophosphatemia also occurs with the correction of the acidosis and, if severe, may cause impairment of ventilation, resulting from skeletal muscle weakness in the vulnerable patient. Instead of diabetic ketoacidosis, the diabetic patient with a metabolic acidosis may have lactic acidosis, which results from poor tissue perfusion or sepsis. It is diagnosed by the presence of an increased serum lactate concentration without an elevated ketone concentration.

Diabetic ketoacidosis must also be distinguished from the syndrome of alcoholic ketoacidosis. This typically occurs in the poorly nourished alcoholic patient after acute intoxication. Except for the presence of chemical ketoacidosis, alcoholic ketoacidosis is not clinically related in any way to DM. The alcoholic patient may be hypoglycemic or mildly hyperglycemic. The predominant ketone in this syndrome is β-hydroxybutyrate, which tends to react less sensitively in the standard laboratory nitroprusside reaction measurement of ketones. Hence, the diagnosis may be obscured. Administration of dextrose and parenteral fluids is the specific treatment for alcoholic ketoacidosis; insulin is not indicated (except in the rare circumstance in which the patient also has clear-cut DM).

Hypoglycemia

Hypoglycemia is the clinical occurrence most feared in the management of diabetic patients. The precise level at which symptomatic hypoglycemia occurs is variable. The normal, fasted patient may have blood sugar levels lower than 50 mg/dL without symptoms. However, the diabetic patient who has a chronically elevated blood sugar level may be symptomatic at levels significantly above this glucose concentration. Hypoglycemia is almost impossible to diagnose clinically in the unconscious patient.

In the awake patient, hypoglycemia often produces central nervous system changes ranging from light-headedness to coma with seizures. Often, the patient recognizes the symptoms and can tell that the blood sugar is low before any overt clinical signs develop. With hypoglycemia, there is a reflex catecholamine release that produces overt sympathetic hyperactivity causing tachycardia, lacrimation, diaphoresis, and hypertension. In the anesthetized patient, these signs of sympathetic hyperactivity can be easily misinterpreted as inadequate or "light" anesthesia. In the anesthetized, sedated, or seriously ill patient, the mental changes of hypoglycemia are also unrecognizable. Furthermore, in patients being treated with β-adrenergic blocking agents or in patients with advanced diabetic autonomic neuropathy, the sympathetic hyperactivity of hypoglycemia may be obscured. Thus, the clinical diagnosis of hypoglycemia in the surgical patient may be difficult to make, and only a high degree of suspicion and frequent blood glucose checks can prevent this complication. Treatment is with 25 g of intravenous dextrose (1 amp of dextrose 50% in water) or 1 mg of intramuscular glucagon if the patient is not alert, and 8 oz of juice if the patient is alert.

Hypoglycemia is more likely to occur in the diabetic surgical patient if insulin or sulfonylureas are given without supplemental glucose. With renal insufficiency, the action of insulin and oral hypoglycemic agents is prolonged.

TABLE 49-11

MANAGEMENT OF DIABETIC KETOACIDOSIS

- Regular insulin, 10 U IV bolus, followed by an insulin infusion nominally at (blood glucose/150) U/hr
- Isotonic IV fluids as guided by vital signs and urine output; anticipate 4–10 L deficit
- When urine output is >0.5 mL/kg/hr, give potassium chloride, 10–40 mEq/hr (with continuous ECG monitoring when the rate is >10 mEq/hr)
- When serum glucose decreased to 250 mg/dL, add dextrose 5% at 100 mL/hr
- Consider sodium bicarbonate to correct pH <6.9

IV, intravenous(ly); ECG, electrocardiogram.

PITUITARY GLAND

The pituitary gland is located below the base of the brain in a bony structure called the *sella turcica*. The pituitary gland and the hypothalamus together form a central unit that regulates the release of various hormones. The pituitary gland is divided into two components. The *anterior pituitary* (adenohypophysis) secretes prolactin, growth hormone, gonadotropins (luteinizing hormone and follicle-stimulating hormone), TSH, and ACTH. The *posterior pituitary* (neurohypophysis) secretes the hormones vasopressin and oxytocin. Hormone release from the anterior and posterior pituitary is regulated by the hypothalamus. Regulatory peptides or preformed hormones from the hypothalamus are transported to the pituitary gland through vascular or tissue connections.

Anterior Pituitary

Hyposecretion of anterior pituitary hormones is usually due to compression of the gland by tumor. This may begin as an isolated deficiency, but it usually develops into multiglandular dysfunction. Male impotence or secondary amenorrhea in the woman is an early manifestation of panhypopituitarism. Panhypopituitarism after postpartum hemorrhagic shock (Sheehan syndrome) is due to necrosis of the anterior pituitary gland. Radiation therapy delivered to the sella turcica or nearby structures and surgical hypophysectomy are other causes of panhypopituitarism. Panhypopituitarism is treated with specific hormone replacement therapy, which should be continued in the perioperative period. Stress doses of corticosteroids are necessary for patients receiving steroid replacement because of inadequate ACTH.

The hypersecretion of various anterior pituitary hormones is usually caused by an adenoma. Excess prolactin secretion with galactorrhea is a common hormonal abnormality associated with pituitary adenoma. Cushing disease may occur secondary to excess ACTH production, and gigantism or acromegaly may occur as a consequence of excess growth hormone production in the child or adult, respectively. Excessive secretion of TSH is rare.

Acromegaly in the adult patient may pose several problems for the anesthesiologist.[91] Hypertrophy occurs in skeletal, connective, and soft tissues.[92] The tongue and epiglottis are enlarged, making the patient susceptible to upper airway obstruction. The incidence of difficult intubation is 20 to 30%, and may be clinically unpredictable.[93] Hoarseness may reflect thickening of the vocal cords or paralysis of a recurrent laryngeal nerve due to stretching. Dyspnea or stridor is associated with subglottic narrowing. Peripheral nerve or artery entrapment, hypertension, and DM are other common findings. The anesthetic management of these patients is complicated by distortion of the facial anatomy and upper airway. Induction of general anesthesia may put the patient at increased risk if mask fit or vocal cord visualization is impaired. When the preoperative history suggests upper airway or vocal cord involvement, it is prudent to consider intubation of the trachea while the patient is awake.

Posterior Pituitary

The posterior pituitary, or neurohypophysis, is composed of terminal nerve endings that extend from the ventral hypothalamus. Vasopressin (antidiuretic hormone or antidiuretic hormone [ADH]) and oxytocin are the two principal hormones secreted by the posterior pituitary. Both hormones are synthesized in the supraoptic and paraventricular nuclei of the hypothalamus. They are bound to inactive carrier proteins, neurophysins, and transported by axons to membrane-bound storage vesicles located in the posterior pituitary. ADH is a nonapeptide that circulates as a free peptide after its release. The primary functions of ADH are the maintenance of extracellular fluid volume and regulation of plasma osmolality. Oxytocin elicits contraction of the uterus and promotes milk secretion and ejection by the mammary glands.

Vasopressin

ADH promotes resorption of solute-free water by increasing cell membrane permeability to water alone. The target sites for ADH are the collecting tubules of the kidneys. A decrease in free water clearance causes a decrease in serum osmolality and a corresponding increase in circulating blood volume. Under normal conditions, the primary stimulus for the release of ADH is an increase in serum osmolality.

Osmoreceptors located in the hypothalamus are sensitive to changes in the normal serum osmolality of as little as 1% (normal osmolality is approximately 285 mOsm/L). Stretch receptors in the left atrium and perhaps pulmonary veins, which are sensitive to moderate reductions in the blood volume, are also capable of stimulating ADH secretion. The need to restore plasma volume may at times override osmotic inhibition of ADH release. Various physiologic and pharmacologic stimuli also influence the secretion of ADH. Positive-pressure ventilation of the lungs, stress, anxiety, hyperthermia, β-adrenergic stimulation, and any histamine-releasing stimulus can promote the release of ADH.

ADH also has other actions. It can increase blood pressure by constricting vascular smooth muscle (see Chapter 41). This activity is most significant in the splanchnic, renal, and coronary vascular beds, and provides the rationale for administering exogenous vasopressin in the management of hemorrhage due to esophageal varices. Caution must be taken when this drug is used in patients with coronary artery disease. ADH (even in small doses) can precipitate myocardial ischemia through vasoconstriction of the coronary arteries. It is unclear whether selective arterial infusion is safer than systemic administration with regard to cardiac and vascular side effects. ADH is also often used in vasodilatory shock as an adjuvant to other pressor agents.

ADH also promotes hemostasis through an increase in the level of circulating von Willebrand factor and factor VIII. Desmopressin (DDAVP), an analog of ADH, is commonly used to treat some types of von Willebrand disease (see Chapter 16). DDAVP is also frequently used to reverse the coagulopathy of renal failure.

Diabetes Insipidus

This disorder results from inadequate secretion of ADH or resistance on the part of the renal tubules to ADH (nephrogenic diabetes insipidus). Failure to secrete adequate amounts of ADH results in polydipsia, hypernatremia, and a high output of poorly concentrated urine. Hypovolemia and hypernatremia may become so severe as to be life-threatening. This disorder usually occurs after destruction of the pituitary gland by intracranial trauma, infiltrating lesions, or surgery (see Chapter 39). Patients in whom diabetes insipidus develops secondary to severe head trauma or subarachnoid hemorrhage often have impending brain death.[94] The treatment of diabetes insipidus depends on the extent of the hormonal deficiency. During surgery, the patient with complete diabetes insipidus receives an intravenous infusion of aqueous ADH (100 to 200 mU/hr), combined with administration of an isotonic crystalloid solution. The serum sodium and plasma osmolality are measured on a regular basis and therapeutic changes are made accordingly. ADH may also be given intramuscularly (as vasopressin tannate in oil). DDAVP administered intranasally has prolonged antidiuretic activity (12 to 24 hours) and is associated with a low incidence of pressor effects. As a consequence of the large outpouring of ADH in response to surgical stress, patients with a residually functioning gland usually do not need parenteral ADH during the perioperative period unless the plasma osmolality rises above 290 mOsm/L. Nonhormonal agents that have efficacy in the treatment of incomplete diabetes insipidus include the oral hypoglycemic chlorpropamide (200 to 500 mg/day). This drug stimulates the release of ADH and sensitizes the renal tubules to the hormone. Hypoglycemia is a serious side effect that limits the usefulness of the drug. Clofibrate, a hypolipidemic agent, is also capable of stimulating ADH release and has been used in the outpatient setting. None of these medications is effective in the patient with nephrogenic diabetes insipidus. Paradoxically, the thiazide diuretics exert an antidiuretic action in patients with this disorder.

Inappropriate Secretion of Antidiuretic Hormone

The inappropriate and excessive secretion of ADH may occur in association with a number of diverse pathologic processes, including head injuries, intracranial tumors, pulmonary infections, small cell carcinoma of the lung, and hypothyroidism (see Chapter 39). The clinical manifestations occur as a result of a dilutional hyponatremia, decreased serum osmolality, and a reduced urine output with a high osmolality. Weight gain, skeletal muscle weakness, and mental confusion or convulsions are presenting symptoms. Peripheral edema and hypertension are rare. The diagnosis of the syndrome of inappropriate ADH secretion is one of exclusion, and other causes of hyponatremia must be ruled out first. The prognosis is related to the underlying cause of the syndrome.

The treatment of patients with mild or moderate water intoxication is restriction of fluid intake to 800 mL/day. Patients with severe water intoxication associated with hyponatremia and mental confusion may require more aggressive therapy, with the intravenous administration of a hypertonic saline solution. This may be administered in conjunction with furosemide. Caution must be observed in patients with poor left ventricular function. Isotonic saline is substituted for hypertonic solutions once the serum sodium is brought into a safe range. Too-rapid correction of hyponatremia may induce central pontine myelinolysis and cause permanent brain damage. Serum sodium should not be raised by more than 12 mEq/L in 24 hours. Other drugs that may be used in the patient with syndrome of inappropriate ADH are demeclocycline and lithium. Demeclocycline interferes with the ability of the renal tubules to concentrate urine and is frequently used in outpatients. Lithium usually is not used because of the high incidence of toxicity.

ENDOCRINE RESPONSE TO SURGICAL STRESS

Anesthesia, surgery, and trauma elicit a generalized endocrine metabolic response characterized by an increase in the plasma levels of cortisol, ADH, renin, catecholamines, and endorphins, and by metabolic changes such as hyperglycemia and a negative nitrogen balance.[95,96] Various neural and humoral factors (e.g., pain, anxiety, acidosis, local tissue factors, hypoxia) play a role in activating this stress response. There is an acute response to critical illness that is characterized by normal pituitary function but target organ insensitivity. During the chronic phase of critical illness there is generalized endocrine hypofunction probably of a hypothalamic origin.[97]

The induction of anesthesia increases the levels of circulating catecholamines and is a form of metabolic stress. Regional anesthesia may block part of the metabolic stress response during surgery, probably by blockade of the neural communi-

cations from the surgical area. It is theorized that the persistently high levels of circulating catecholamines in trauma and critical illness lead to stress hyperglycemia through a direct inhibition of insulin release. Bypass of the gut hormonal actions in patients receiving intravenous glucose feedings, especially if given in large amounts, contributes to the impairment of insulin release during illness and can create a particularly difficult management problem for diabetic patients.

Endorphins are a group of endogenous peptides with opioid activity that have been isolated from the central nervous system. It is well documented that β-endorphin is released from the anterior pituitary, where it is contained as part of β-lipoprotein, a 91-chain amino acid, which is a cleavage product of the precursor peptide for ACTH. Large increases in the central nervous system and plasma concentrations of endorphins in response to emotional or surgical stimuli suggest that these substances play a role in the body's response to stress. These substances modulate painful stimuli by binding to opiate receptors located throughout the brain and spinal cord.

Numerous experiments have focused on the stress response and its relationship to the depth of anesthesia. Regional anesthesia and general anesthesia appear to blunt the release of various stress hormones during the period of surgical stimulation in a dose-dependent fashion. Historically, anesthesiologists have relied on the indirect measurement of hemodynamic variables such as blood pressure and heart rate to evaluate the level of autonomic activity in response to anesthesia and surgery. It is assumed that the physiologic manifestations of stress are potentially harmful, especially in patients with limited functional reserve. As such, anesthetic techniques and pain management strategies are designed to limit this neurohormonal response in the hope of providing the patient with some benefit. Further investigations are needed to assess the impact of these efforts on perioperative morbidity and mortality.

References

1. Surks MI, Sievert R: Drugs and thyroid function. N Engl J Med 1995; 333: 1688
2. Klein I, Danzi S: Thyroid disease and the heart. Circulation 2007; 116: 1725
3. Mandel SJ, Brent GA, Larsen PR: Levothyroxine therapy in patients with thyroid disease. Ann Intern Med 1993; 119: 492
4. Mulligan DC, McHenry CR, Kinney W et al: Amiodarone-induced thyrotoxicosis: Clinical presentation and expanded indications for thyroidectomy. Surgery 1993; 114: 1114
5. Langley RW, Burch HB: Perioperative management of the thyrotoxic patient. Endocrinol Metab Clin North Am 2003; 32: 519
6. Franklyn JA: The management of hyperthyroidism. N Engl J Med 1994; 330: 1731
7. Smallridge RC: Metabolic and anatomic thyroid emergencies: A review. Crit Care Med 1992; 20: 276
8. Hermann M, Richter B, Roka R et al: Thyroid surgery in untreated severe hyperthyroidism: Perioperative kinetics of free thyroid hormones in the glandular venous effluent and peripheral blood. Surgery 1994; 115: 240
9. Farling PA: Thyroid disease. Br J Anaesth 2000; 85: 15
10. Bouaggad A, Nejmi SE, Bouderka MA et al: Prediction of difficult tracheal intubation in thyroid surgery. Anesth Analg 2004; 99: 603
11. Szubin L, Kacker A, Kakani R et al: The management of post-thyroidectomy hypocalcemia. Ear Nose Throat J 1996; 75: 612
12. Wagner HE, Seiler C: Recurrent laryngeal nerve palsy after thyroid gland surgery. Br J Surg 1994; 81: 226
13. Lindsay RS, Toft AD: Hypothyroidism. Lancet 1997; 349: 413
14. Stathatos N, Wartofsky L: Perioperative management of patients with hypothyroidism. Endocrinol Metab Clin North Am 2003; 32: 503
15. Toft AD: Thyroxine therapy. N Engl J Med 1994; 331: 174
16. Bennett-Guerrero E, Kramer DC, Schwinn DA: Effect of chronic and acute thyroid hormone reduction on perioperative outcome. Anesth Analg 1997; 85: 30
17. Ladenson PW, Levin AA, Ridgway EC et al: Complications of surgery in hypothyroid patients. Am J Med 1984; 77: 261
18. Whitten CW, Latson TW, Klein KW et al: Anesthetic management of a hypothyroid cardiac surgical patient. J Cardiothorac Vasc Anesth 1991; 5: 156
19. Weinberg AD, Ehrenwerth J: Anesthetic considerations and perioperative management of patients with hypothyroidism. Adv Anesth 1987; 4: 185

20. Mihai R, Farndon JR: Parathyroid disease and calcium metabolism. Br J Anaesth 2000; 85: 29
21. Roland EJ, Wierda JM, Eurin BG et al: Pharmacodynamic behaviour of vecuronium in primary hyperparathyroidism. Can J Anaesth 1994; 41: 694
22. Meuriaaw M, Hamoir E, Defechereux T et al: Bilateral neck exploration under hypnosedation. Ann Surg 1999; 229: 401
23. Al-Zahrani A, Levine MA: Primary hyperparathyroidism. Lancet 1997; 349: 1233
24. Vaughan ED Jr: Diseases of the adrenal gland. Med Clin North Am 2004; 88: 443
25. Inder WJ, Hunt PJ: Glucocorticoid replacement in pituitary surgery: Guidelines for perioperative assessment and management. J Clin Endocrinol Metab 2002; 87: 2745
26. Rivers EP, Gaspari M, Abi Saad G et al: Adrenal insufficiency in high-risk surgical ICU patients. Chest 2001; 119: 889
27. Lamberts SWJ, Bruining HA, DeJong FH: Corticosteroid therapy in severe illness. N Engl J Med 1997; 337: 1285
28. Bennett N, Gabrielli A: Hypotension and adrenal insufficiency. J Clin Anesth 1999; 11: 425
29. Sutherland FWH, Naik SK: Acute adrenal insufficiency after coronary artery bypass grafting. Ann Thorac Surg 1996; 62: 1516
30. Oelkers W: Adrenal insufficiency. N Engl J Med 1996; 335: 1206
31. Coursin DB, Wood KE: Corticosteroid supplementation for adrenal insufficiency. JAMA 2002; 287: 236
32. Engquist A, Brandt MR, Fernandes A et al: The blocking effect of epidural analgesia on the adrenocortical and hyperglycemic responses to surgery. Acta Anaesthesiol Scand 1977; 21: 330
33. Salem M, Tainsh RE Jr, Bromberg J et al: Perioperative glucocorticoid coverage: A reassessment 41 years after emergence of a problem. Ann Surg 1994; 219: 416
34. Axelrod L: Perioperative management of patients treated with glucocorticoids. Endocrinol Metab Clin North Am 2003; 32: 367
35. Symreng T, Karlberg BE, Kagedal B et al: Physiological cortisol substitution of long-term steroid-treated patients undergoing major surgery. Br J Anaesth 1981; 53: 949
36. Glowniak JV, Loriaux DL: A double-blind study of perioperative steroid requirements in secondary adrenal insufficiency. Surgery 1997; 121: 123
37. Brown CJ, Buie WD: Perioperative stress dose steroids: Do they make a difference? J Am Coll Surg 2001; 193: 678
38. Prys-Roberts C: Phaeochromocytoma: Recent progress in its management. Br J Anaesth 2000; 85: 44
39. Kinney MAO, Warner ME, van Heerden JA et al: Perianesthetic risks and outcomes of pheochromocytoma and paraganglioma resection. Anesth Analg 2000; 91: 1118
40. Kinney MAO, Narr BJ, Warner MA: Perioperative management of pheochromocytoma. J Cardiothorac Vasc Anesth 2002; 16: 359
41. Giffird RW Jr, Manger WM, Bravo EL: Pheochromocytoma. Endocrinol Metab Clin North Am 1994; 23: 387
42. Witteles RM, Kaplan EL, Roizen MF: Sensitivity of diagnostic and localization tests for pheochromocytoma in clinical practice. Arch Intern Med 2000; 160: 2521
43. Geoghegan JG, Emberton M, Bloom R et al: Changing trends in the management of phaeochromocytoma. Br J Surg 1998; 85: 117
44. Ulchaker JC, Goldfarb DA, Bravo EL et al: Successful outcomes in pheochromocytoma surgery in the modern era. J Urol 1999; 161: 764
45. Pacak K: Preoperative management of the pheochromocytoma patient. J Clin Endocrinol Metab 2007; 92: 4069
46. Hamilton A, Sirrs S, Schmidt N et al: Anaesthesia for phaeochromocytoma in pregnancy. Can J Anaesth 1997; 44: 654
47. Joris JL, Hamoir EE, Hartstein GM et al: Hemodynamic changes and catecholamine release during laparoscopic adrenalectomy for pheochromocytoma. Anesth Analg 1999; 88: 16
48. James MF, Cronje L: Pheochromocytoma crisis: The use of magnesium sulfate. Anesth Analg 2004; 99: 680
49. American Association of Clinical Endocrinologists medical guidelines for clinical practice for the management of diabetes mellitus. Endocr Pract 2007; 13(Suppl 1): 1
50. Gusberg RJ, Moley J: Diabetes and abdominal surgery. Yale J Biol Med 1983; 56: 285
51. Atkinson MA, Maclaren NK: The pathogenesis of insulin-dependent diabetes mellitus. N Engl J Med 1994; 331: 1428
52. Kim JA, Montagnani M, Koh KK et al: Reciprocal relationships between insulin resistance and endothelial dysfunction: Molecular and pathophysiological mechanisms. Circulation 2006; 113: 1888
53. Biddinger SB, Kahn CR: From mice to men: insights into the insulin resistance syndromes. Annu Rev Physiol 2006; 68: 123
54. Bagry HS, Raghavendran S, Carli F: Metabolic syndrome and insulin resistance: perioperative considerations. Anesthesiology 2008; 108: 506
55. DeFronzo RA: Pharmacologic therapy for type 2 diabetes mellitus. Ann Intern Med 1999; 131: 281
56. Bailey CJ, Turner RC: Metformin. N Engl J Med 1996; 334: 574
57. Fleisher LA, Beckman JA, Brown KA et al: ACC/AHA 2007 Guidelines on Perioperative Cardiovascular Evaluation and Care for Noncardiac Surgery: A Report of the American College of Cardiology/American Heart Association Task Force on Practice Guidelines (Writing Committee to Revise the 2002 Guidelines on Perioperative Cardiovascular Evaluation for Noncardiac Surgery): Developed in Collaboration With the American Society of Echocardiography, American Society of Nuclear Cardiology, Heart Rhythm Society, Society of Cardiovascular Anesthesiologists, Society for Cardiovascular Angiography and Interventions, Society for Vascular Medicine and Biology, and Society for Vascular Surgery. Circulation 2007; 116: e418
58. Hogan K, Rusy D, Springman SR: Difficult laryngoscopy and diabetes mellitus. Anesth Analg 1988; 67: 1162
59. Charlson ME, MacKenzie CR, Gold JP: Preoperative autonomic function abnormalities in patients with diabetes mellitus and patients with hypertension. J Am Coll Surg 1994; 179: 1
60. Latson TW, Ashmore TH, Reinhart DJ et al: Autonomic reflex dysfunction in patients presenting for elective surgery is associated with hypotension after anesthesia induction. Anesthesiology 1994; 80: 326
61. Page MM, Watkins PJ: Cardiorespiratory arrest and diabetic autonomic neuropathy. Lancet 1978; 1: 14
62. Vohra A, Kumar S, Charlton AJ et al: Effect of diabetes mellitus on the cardiovascular responses to induction of anesthesia and tracheal intubation. Br J Anaesth 1993; 71: 258
63. Kitamura A, Hoshino T, Kon Tadashi T et al: Patients with diabetic neuropathy are at risk of a greater intraoperative reduction in core temperature. Anesthesiology 2000; 92: 1311
64. Ishihara H, Singh H, Giesecke AH: Relationship between diabetic autonomic neuropathy and gastric contents. Anesth Analg 1994; 78: 943
65. Duncan AI, Koch CG, Xu M et al: Recent metformin ingestion does not increase in-hospital morbidity or mortality after cardiac surgery. Anesth Analg 2007; 104: 42
66. Harati Y: Diabetic peripheral neuropathies. Ann Intern Med 1987; 107: 546
67. Inzucchi SE: Clinical practice. Management of hyperglycemia in the hospital setting. N Engl J Med 2006; 355: 1903
68. Van den Berghe G, Wouters P, Weekers F et al: Intensive insulin therapy in critically ill patients. N Engl J Med 2001; 345: 1359
69. Krinsley JS: Effect of an intensive glucose management protocol on the mortality of critically ill adult patients. Mayo Clin Proc 2004; 79: 992
70. Estrada CA, Young JA, Nifong LW et al: Outcomes and perioperative hyperglycemia in patients with or without diabetes mellitus undergoing coronary artery bypass grafting. Ann Thorac Surg 2003; 75: 1392
71. Guvener M, Pasaoglu I, Demircin M et al: Perioperative hyperglycemia is a strong correlate of postoperative infection in type II diabetic patients after coronary artery bypass grafting. Endocr J 2002; 49: 531
72. Quinn DW, Pagano D, Bonser RS et al: Improved myocardial protection during coronary artery surgery with glucose-insulin-potassium: a randomized controlled trial. J Thorac Cardiovasc Surg 2006; 131: 34
73. Furnary AP, Gao G, Grunkemeier GL et al: Continuous insulin infusion reduces mortality in patients with diabetes undergoing coronary artery bypass grafting. J Thorac Cardiovasc Surg 2003; 125: 1007
74. Gandhi GY, Nuttall GA, Abel MD et al: Intraoperative hyperglycemia and perioperative outcomes in cardiac surgery patients. Mayo Clin Proc 2005; 80: 862
75. Ouattara A, Lecomte P, Le Manach Y et al: Poor intraoperative blood glucose control is associated with a worsened hospital outcome after cardiac surgery in diabetic patients. Anesthesiology 2005; 103: 687
76. D'Alessandro C, Leprince P, Golmard JL et al: Strict glycemic control reduces EuroSCORE expected mortality in diabetic patients undergoing myocardial revascularization. J Thorac Cardiovasc Surg 2007; 134: 29
77. Gandhi GY, Nuttall GA, Abel MD et al: Intensive intraoperative insulin therapy versus conventional glucose management during cardiac surgery: A randomized trial. Ann Intern Med 2007; 146: 233
78. Van den Berghe G: Does tight blood glucose control during cardiac surgery improve patient outcome? Ann Intern Med 2007; 146: 307
79. Van den Berghe G, Wilmer A, Hermans G et al: Intensive insulin therapy in the medical ICU. N Engl J Med 2006; 354: 449
80. Brunkhorst FM, Engel C, Bloos F et al: Intensive insulin therapy and pentastarch resuscitation in severe sepsis. N Engl J Med 2008; 358: 125
81. Krinsley JS, Grover A: Severe hypoglycemia in critically ill patients: Risk factors and outcomes. Crit Care Med 2007; 35: 2262
82. Gandhi GY, Murad MH, Flynn DN et al: Effect of perioperative insulin infusion on surgical morbidity and mortality: Systematic review and meta-analysis of randomized trials. Mayo Clin Proc 2008; 83: 418
83. Desachy A, Vuagnat AC, Ghazali AD et al: Accuracy of bedside glucometry in critically ill patients: Influence of clinical characteristics and perfusion index. Mayo Clin Proc 2008; 83: 400
84. Kroll HR, Maher TR: Significant hypoglycemia secondary to icodextron peritoneal dialysate in a diabetic patient. Anesth Analg 2007; 104: 1473
85. Coursin DB, Connery LE, Ketzler JT: Perioperative diabetic and hyperglycemic management issues. Crit Care Med 2004; 32: S116
86. Inzucchi SE: Diabetes facts and guidelines 2007. http://info.med.yale.edu/intmed/endocrin/yale_diab_ctr.html
87. Metchick LN, Petit WA Jr, Inzucchi SE: Inpatient management of diabetes mellitus. Am J Med 2002; 113: 317
88. Goldberg PA, Siegel MD, Sherwin RS et al: Implementation of a safe and effective insulin infusion protocol in a medical intensive care unit. Diabetes Care 2004; 27: 461
89. Cummings DE, Overduin J, Foster-Schubert KE: Gastric bypass for obesity: Mechanisms of weight loss and diabetes resolution. J Clin Endocrinol Metabol 2004; 89: 2608

90. Foster DW, McGarry JD: The metabolic derangements and treatment of diabetic ketoacidosis. N Engl J Med 1983; 309: 159

91. Melmed S: Acromegaly. N Engl J Med 1990; 322: 966

92. Kitahata LM: Airway difficulties associated with anaesthesia in acromegaly. Br J Anaesth 1971; 43: 1187

93. Schmitt H, Buchfelder M, Radespiel-Troger M et al: Difficult intubation in acromegalic patients: Incidence and predictability. Anesthesiology 2000; 93: 110

94. Wong MF, Chin NM, Lew TW: Diabetes insipidus in neurosurgical patients. Ann Acad Med Singapore 1998; 27: 340

95. Weissman C: The metabolic response to stress: An overview and update. Anesthesiology 1990; 73: 308

96. Woolf PD: Hormonal responses to trauma. Crit Care Med 1992; 20: 216

97. Langouche L, Van Den Berghe G: The dynamic neuroendocrine response to critical illness. Endocrinol Metab Clin N Am 2006; 35: 777

CHAPTER 50 ■ ANESTHESIA FOR OTOLARYNGOLOGIC SURGERY

LYNNE R. FERRARI AND ALEXANDER W. GOTTA

KEY POINTS

1. The restricted spaces in the airway require an understanding and cooperative relationship between surgeon and anesthesiologist, and the use of specially adapted equipment suitable to these cramped areas.

2. Despite only mild-to-moderate tonsillar enlargement on physical examination, children with obstructive sleep apnea have upper airway obstruction while awake and apnea during sleep. The clinician should not underestimate the severity of the problem based on tonsillar size alone.

3. Posttonsillar hemorrhage may result in unappreciated large volumes of swallowed blood originating from the tonsillar fossa. These patients must be considered to have a full stomach, and anesthetic precautions addressing this situation must be taken.

4. The middle ear and sinuses are air-filled, nondistensible cavities. During procedures in which the eardrum is replaced or perforation is patched, nitrous oxide should be discontinued or, if this is not possible, limited to a maximum of 50% during the application of the tympanic membrane graft to avoid pressure-related displacement.

5. In a LeFort III fracture, the fracture line may pass through the cribriform plate of the ethmoid bone, creating a fistula between the nasopharynx and the subarachnoid space within the skull. Clinical and radiographic studies are mandated to determine the integrity of the cribriform plate.

6. Upper airway tumors may be friable and lead to significant hemorrhage during intubation. Prior radiation therapy may lead to fibrosis and ankylosis in the temporomandibular joint, rendering orotracheal intubation difficult.

7. Prior to extubation after temporomandibular arthroscopy, the oral cavity and neck must be examined carefully to rule out the presence of extracapsular extravasation of irrigation fluid. Extravasation can lead to airway closure.

8. After extensive facial trauma or resection of tumors of the upper airway, it is prudent to keep the patient intubated until edema has subsided. Extraoral facial edema should lead the physician to suspect intraoral edema and possible airway compromise.

EVALUATING THE AIRWAY

Air flows through the upper respiratory passages, into the trachea, bronchi, bronchioles, and into alveoli in the healthy human. Air flow occurs seemingly without either thought or effort, and the actual work of respiration in the unobstructed airway is minimal. However, airway obstruction due to malformation, tumor, infection, or trauma may significantly alter the clinical presentation and make gas exchange a laborious, energy-consuming process. The increased work of breathing can leave the patient exhausted, incapable of maintaining adequate gas exchange, and finally succumbing to ventilatory failure. Significant obstruction and anatomic distortion may be present in a patient with minimal evidence of disease because clinically evident upper airway obstruction is a late sign. It is a most unwelcome experience for the anesthesiologist to discover a large, unexpected, obstructed upper airway at the time of attempted tracheal intubation.

In the presence of tumor, other mass lesions, or infection in the airway, it may be useful to obtain radiologic evaluation of the airway with plain films of the tracheal and laryngeal air columns or computed tomography and magnetic resonance imaging studies of the airway. Significant anatomic distortion is usually evident and may help the anesthesiologist determine the most appropriate technique for securing the airway.

ANESTHESIA FOR PEDIATRIC EAR, NOSE, AND THROAT SURGERY

Particularly challenging to the anesthesiologist is the safe management of the pediatric patient undergoing surgery of the ear, nose, and throat. The restricted spaces in the airway of the child require an understanding and cooperative relationship between surgeon and anesthesiologist, and the use of specially adapted equipment suitable to these cramped areas.

Tonsillectomy and Adenoidectomy

Untreated adenoidal hyperplasia may lead to nasopharyngeal obstruction, causing failure to thrive, speech disorders, obligate mouth breathing, sleep disturbances, orofacial abnormalities with a narrowing of the upper airway, and dental abnormalities. Surgical removal of the adenoids is usually accompanied by tonsillectomy; however, purulent adenitis, despite adequate medical therapy, and recurrent otitis media with effusion secondary to adenoidal hyperplasia are improved with adenoidectomy alone.

Tonsillectomy is one of the more commonly performed pediatric surgical procedures.[1] Chronic or recurrent acute tonsillitis, peritonsillar abscess, tonsillar hyperplasia, and obstructive sleep apnea syndrome are the major indications for surgery.[2–4] In addition, patients with cardiac valvular disease are at risk for endocarditis from recurrent streptococcal bacteremia secondary to infected tonsils. Tonsillar hyperplasia may lead to chronic airway obstruction resulting in sleep apnea, carbon dioxide (CO_2) retention, cor pulmonale, failure to thrive, swallowing disorders, and speech abnormalities. These risks are eliminated with removal of the tonsils.

Obstruction of the oropharyngeal airway by hypertrophied tonsils leading to apnea during sleep is an important clinical constellation referred to as *obstructive sleep apnea syndrome*. Despite only mild-to-moderate tonsillar enlargement on physical examination, these patients have upper airway obstruction while awake and apnea during sleep. The goals of treatment are to relieve airway obstruction and increase the cross-sectional area of the pharynx, which is successful in two thirds of pediatric cases.[5] Some patients require the use of nasal continuous positive airway pressure during sleep, whereas others may require a tracheostomy to bypass the chronic upper airway obstruction that is present. The two most frequent levels of obstruction during sleep are at the soft palate and the base of the tongue.[6] Most children have tremendous improvement in their symptoms after tonsillectomy.

In children with long-standing hypoxemia and hypercarbia, increased airway resistance can lead to cor pulmonale (Fig. 50-1). Patients have electrocardiographic evidence of right ventricular hypertrophy, with one third of them having chest radiographs consistent with cardiomegaly. Each apneic episode causes progressively increasing pulmonary artery pressure with significant systemic and pulmonary artery hypertension, leading to ventricular dysfunction and cardiac dysrhythmias.[7] These patients often have dysfunction in the medulla or hypothalamic areas of the central nervous system causing persistently elevated CO_2, despite relief of airway obstruction. This group of patients has a hyperreactive pulmonary vascular bed, and the increased pulmonary vascular resistance and myocardial depression in response to hypoxia, hypercarbia, and acidosis are far greater than what is expected for that degree of physiologic alteration in the normal population. Cardiac enlargement is frequently reversible with digitalization and surgical removal of the tonsils and adenoids.

Preoperative Evaluation

A thorough history is the basis for the preoperative evaluation. Because patients requiring tonsillectomy and adenoidectomy have frequent infections, the parent should be questioned for current use of antibiotics, antihistamines, or other medicines. A history of sleep apnea should be sought. The physical examination should begin with observation of the patient. The presence of audible respirations, mouth breathing, nasal quality of the speech, and chest retractions should be noted. Mouth breathing may be the result of chronic nasopharyngeal obstruction. An elongated face, retrognathic mandible, and a high-arched palate may be present.[8] The oropharynx should be inspected for evaluation of tonsillar size to determine the ease of mask ventilation and tracheal intubation (Fig. 50-2). The presence of wheezing or rales on auscultation of the chest may be a lower respiratory manifestation of pharyngitis or tonsillitis. The presence of inspiratory stridor or prolonged expiration may indicate partial airway obstruction from hypertrophied tonsils or adenoids.

Measurement of hematocrit and coagulation parameters is suggested. Many nonprescription cold medications and antihistamines contain aspirin, which may affect platelet function, and this potential anticoagulation should be taken into consideration. Chest radiographs and electrocardiograms (ECGs) are not required unless specific abnormalities are elicited during the history, such as recent pneumonia, bronchitis, upper respiratory infection (URI), or history consistent with cor pulmonale, which is seen in children with obstructive sleep apnea syndrome. In those children with a history of cardiac abnormalities, an echocardiogram may be indicated.

Anesthetic Management

The goals of the anesthesia for tonsillectomy and adenoidectomy are to render the child unconscious in the most atraumatic manner possible, provide the surgeon with optimal operating conditions, establish intravenous access to provide a route for volume expansion and medications when necessary, and to provide rapid emergence so the patient is awake and able to protect the recently instrumented airway. Premedication may be used as determined by the anesthesiologist during the preanesthetic visit. Sedative premedication should be avoided in children with obstructive sleep apnea, intermittent obstruction, or very large tonsils. Use of antisialagogue will minimize secretions in the operative field.

Anesthesia is usually induced with a volatile anesthetic agent, oxygen, and nitrous oxide (N_2O) by mask. Parental presence in the operating room (OR) during mask induction is often helpful in the anxious unpremedicated child. Tracheal intubation is best accomplished under deep inhalation anesthesia or aided by a short-acting nondepolarizing muscle relaxant. Many clinicians may choose to eliminate the

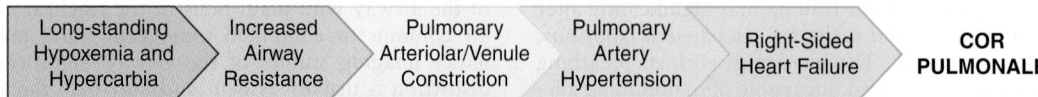

FIGURE 50-1.   Events leading to cor pulmonale.

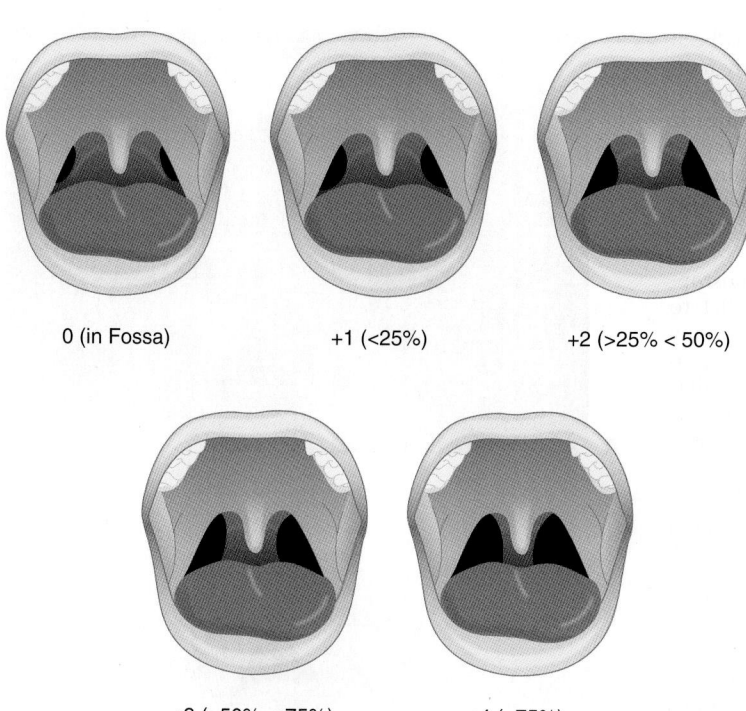

0 (in Fossa)   +1 (<25%)   +2 (>25% < 50%)

+3 (>50% < 75%)   +4 (>75%)

FIGURE 50-2. Classification of tonsil size, including percentage of oropharyngeal area occupied by hypertrophied tonsils.

ANESTHESIA FOR SURGICAL SUBSPECIALTIES

neuromuscular blocking agent in favor of enhancing the depth of anesthesia with the use of propofol. Blood in the pharynx may enter the trachea during the surgical procedure. For this reason, the supraglottic area may be packed with petroleum gauze, or a cuffed endotracheal tube may be used. If a cuffed endotracheal tube is selected, careful attention to the inflation pressure of the cuff is essential if postextubation croup is to be avoided. Monitoring consists of precordial stethoscope, ECG, automated blood pressure, pulse oximetry, and end-tidal capnography.

Emergence from anesthesia should be rapid, and the child should be alert before transfer to the recovery area. The child should be awake and able to clear blood or secretions from the oropharynx as efficiently as possible before removal of the endotracheal tube. Maintenance of airway and pharyngeal reflexes is essential in the prevention of aspiration, laryngospasm, and airway obstruction. There is no difference in the incidence of airway complications on emergence between patients who are extubated awake or deeply anesthetized.[9]

The use of the laryngeal mask airway (LMA) for adenotonsillectomy was described in 1990; however, it was not until the widespread availability of a streamlined flexible model that it was widely used for this purpose.[10,11] There is an emerging trend to use the flexible LMA for tonsillectomy, which protects the vocal cords from blood or secretions that may be present in the oropharynx.[12] The wide, rigid tube of the standard LMA model does not fit under the mouth gag and is easily compressed or dislodged during full mouth opening. The flexible model has a soft, reinforced shaft that easily fits under the mouth gag without becoming dislodged or compressed. Adequate surgical access can be achieved, and the lower airway is protected from exposure to blood during the procedure.[13,14]

Insertion is possible after either the intravenous administration of 3 mg/kg of propofol or when sufficient depth of anesthesia is achieved using a volatile agent administered by mask. The same depth of anesthesia should be obtained during insertion of the LMA as would be required for performing laryngoscopy and endotracheal intubation. Positive-pressure ventilation should be avoided when the LMA is used during

tonsillectomy, although gentle assisted ventilation is both safe and effective if peak inspiratory pressure is kept below 20 cm H_2O.

Tonsillar enlargement can make LMA insertion difficult, so care in placement is essential.[15] Maneuvers to overcome this difficulty include increased head extension, lateral insertion of the mask, anterior displacement of the tongue, pressure on the tip of the LMA using the index finger as it negotiates the pharyngeal curve, or use of the laryngoscope if all else fails. Dislodgment of the device does not occur during extreme head extension, assuming good position and ventilation were obtained before changes in head position.[16]

Advantages of the LMA over traditional endotracheal intubation are a decrease in the incidence of postoperative stridor and laryngospasm and an increase in immediate postoperative oxygen saturation. If the child is breathing spontaneously at a regular rate and depth, the LMA may be removed before emergence from anesthesia. The oropharynx should be gently suctioned with a soft, flexible catheter, the LMA deflated and removed, an oral airway inserted, and the respirations assisted with 100% oxygen delivered by mask. It is often distressing for young children to awaken with the LMA still in place. Although the device is an appropriate substitute for an oral airway in the adult population, this is not so in children. If the practitioner wants to remove the LMA when the child has emerged from anesthesia, it should be deflated and removed as soon as possible after the return to consciousness.

Complications

The incidence of emesis after tonsillectomy ranges from 30 to 65%.[17] Whether emesis is due to irritant blood in the stomach or stimulation of the gag reflex by inflammation and edema at the surgical site remains unclear. Central nervous system stimulation from the gastrointestinal tract, as may be seen with gastric distention from the introduction of swallowed or insufflated air, may trigger the emetic center. Decompressing the stomach with an orogastric tube may be helpful in preventing this response. Treatment with ondansetron, 0.10 to

0.15 mg/kg, either with or without dexamethasone, has been shown to be very effective in reducing posttonsillectomy nausea and vomiting.[18,19] Postoperative administration of meperidine increases the probability of emesis, and other analgesic agents should be administered. Dehydration secondary to poor oral intake as a result of nausea, vomiting, or pain can occur after tonsillectomy in 1% of cases. Vigorous intravenous hydration during surgery can offset the physiologic effects of lower postoperative fluid intake.

3 The most serious complication of tonsillectomy is postoperative hemorrhage, which occurs at a frequency of 0.1 to 8.1%. The recent innovation of coblation tonsillectomy may result in an incidence of posttonsillectomy hemorrhage up to 11.1%.[4,20,21] Approximately 75% of postoperative tonsillar hemorrhage occurs within 6 hours of surgery. Most of the remaining 25% occurs within the first 24 hours of surgery, although bleeding may be noted until the sixth postoperative day.[22,23] Sixty-seven percent of postoperative bleeding originates from the tonsillar fossa, 26% in the nasopharynx, and 7% in both. Initial attempts to control bleeding may be made using pharyngeal packs and cautery. If this fails, patients must return to the OR for exploration and surgical hemostasis.

Unappreciated large volumes of blood originating from the tonsillar bed may be swallowed. These patients must be considered to have a full stomach, and anesthetic precautions addressing this situation must be taken. A rapid-sequence induction accompanied by cricoid pressure and a styletted endotracheal tube is controversial but may be of benefit in some circumstances. Because the amount of blood swallowed can be considerable, blood pressure must be checked in both the erect and supine positions to look for orthostatic changes resulting from decreases in vascular volume. Intravenous access and hydration must be established before the induction of anesthesia. A variety of laryngoscope blades and endotracheal tubes, as well as functioning suction apparatus, should be prepared in duplicate because blood in the airway may impair visualization of the vocal cords and cause plugging of the endotracheal tube.

Pain after adenoidectomy is usually minimal, but pain after tonsillectomy is severe. This contributes to poor fluid intake and overall discomfort of patients. An increase in postoperative pain medication requirements has been noted in patients having laser or electrocautery as part of the operative tonsillectomy compared with those who have had sharp surgical dissection and ligation of blood vessels to achieve hemostasis.[7,24] Intraoperative administration of corticosteroids may decrease edema formation and subsequent patient discomfort. Although infiltration of the peritonsillar space with local anesthetic and epinephrine has been shown to be effective in reducing intraoperative blood loss, it does not decrease postoperative pain.

Peritonsillar abscess, or quinsy tonsil, is a condition that may require immediate surgical intervention to relieve potential or existing airway obstruction. An acutely infected tonsil may undergo abscess formation, producing a large mass in the lateral pharynx that can interfere with swallowing and breathing (Figs. 50-3 through 50-5). Fever, pain, and trismus are frequent symptoms. Treatment consists of surgical drainage of the abscess, either with or without tonsillectomy, and intravenous antibiotic therapy. Although the airway seems compromised, the peritonsillar abscess is usually in a fixed location in the lateral pharynx and does not interfere with ventilation of the patient by mask after induction of general anesthesia. Visualization of the vocal cords should not be impaired because the pathologic process is supraglottic and well above the laryngeal inlet. Laryngoscopy must be carefully performed, avoiding manipulation of the larynx and surrounding structures. Intubation should be gentle because the tonsillar area is

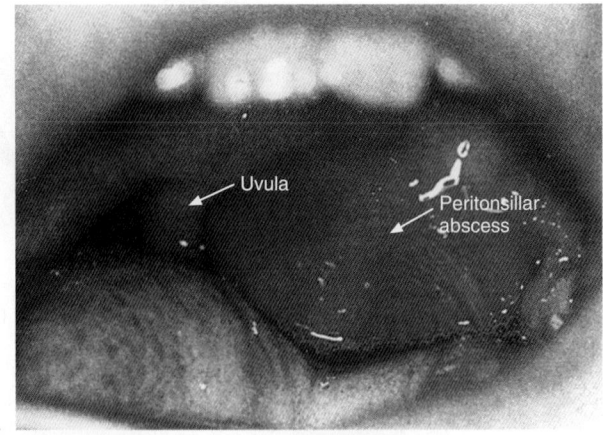

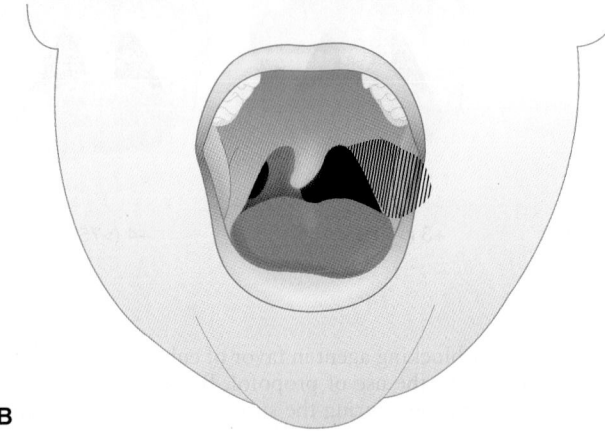

FIGURE 50-3. **A.** Patient with a peritonsillar abscess on the left side. **B.** Note the displacement of the uvula. (Courtesy of Michael Cunningham, MD, Boston, MA.)

tense and friable and inadvertent rupture of the abscess can occur, leading to spillage of purulent material into the trachea.

Acute postoperative pulmonary edema is an infrequent but potentially life-threatening complication encountered when airway obstruction is suddenly relieved. One proposed mechanism is that during inspiration before adenotonsillectomy, the negative intrapleural pressure that is generated causes an increase in venous return, enhancing pulmonary blood volume. In the healthy child without airway obstruction, pleural pressure ranges from –2.5 cm to –10.0 cm H_2O during inspiration. Intrapleural pressure generated in the child with airway obstruction can be as much as –30 cm H_2O, which causes disruption of the capillary walls of the pulmonary microvasculature when transmitted to the interstitial peribronchial and perivascular spaces. Concurrent with a negative transpulmonary gradient is an increase in venous return to the right side of the heart, thus increasing preload, which in the setting of "leaky capillaries" facilitates transudation of fluid into the alveolar space. To counterbalance this negative gradient, positive intrapleural and alveolar pressure is generated during exhalation, which decreases pulmonary venous return and blood volume. This phenomenon is similar to an expiratory "grunt" mechanism in which the transpleural pressures generated are similar to those present during a Valsalva maneuver.

The rapid relief of airway obstruction results in decreased airway pressure, an increase in venous return, an increase in pulmonary hydrostatic pressure, hyperemia, and finally pulmonary edema. The all-important counterbalance of the expiratory grunt in limiting pulmonary venous return is lost when

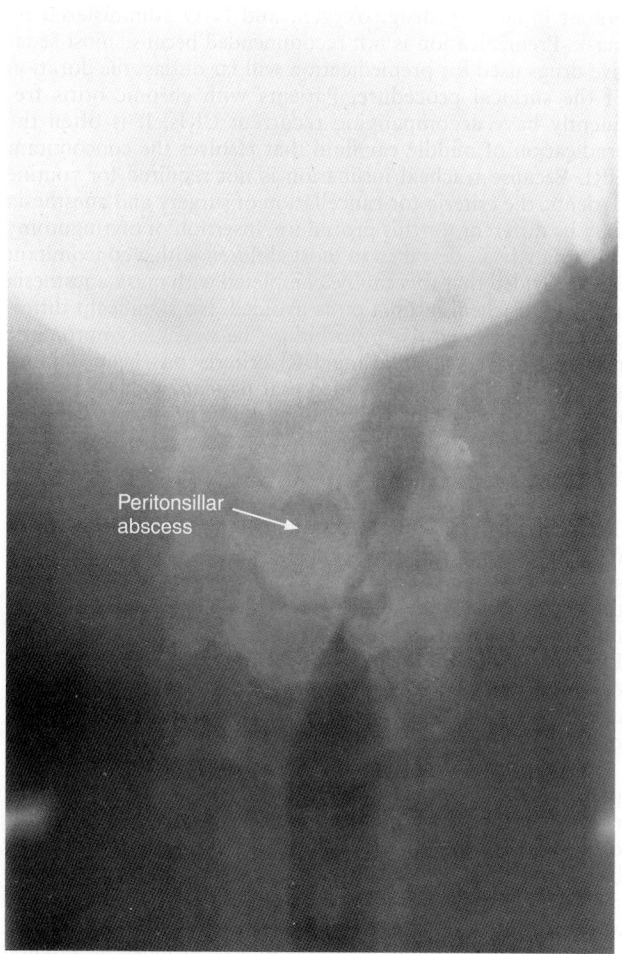

FIGURE 50-4. Neck radiograph of a patient with a peritonsillar abscess (*arrow*).

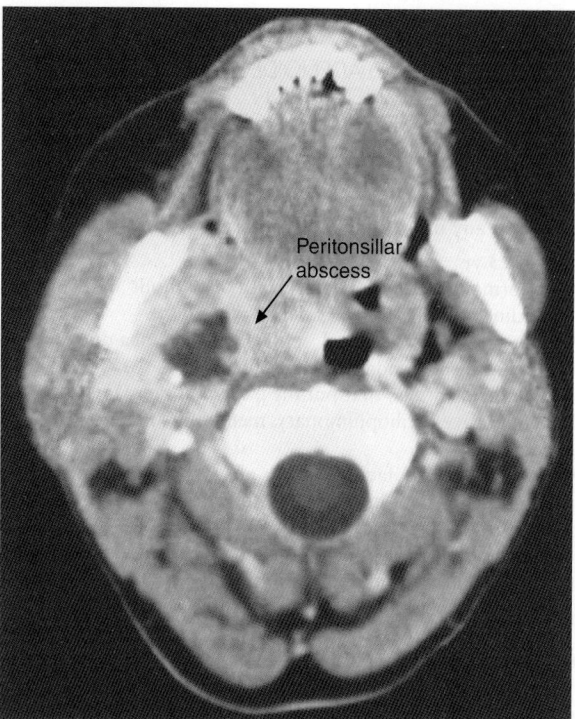

FIGURE 50-5. Computed tomography scan of a patient with a peritonsillar abscess (*arrow*).

the obstruction is relieved. Contributing factors are the increased volume load on both ventricles, as well as the inability of the pulmonary lymphatic system to remove acutely large amounts of fluid. The anesthesiologist may attempt to prevent this situation during induction of anesthesia by applying moderate amounts of continuous positive pressure to the airway, thus allowing time for circulatory adaptation to take place. This physiologic sequence is similar to that seen in patients with severe acute airway obstruction secondary to epiglottitis or laryngospasm.

Negative-pressure pulmonary edema is signaled by the appearance of frothy pink fluid in the endotracheal tube of an intubated patient or the presence of a decreased oxygen saturation, wheezing, dyspnea, and increased respiratory rate in the immediate postoperative period in a previously extubated patient. Mild cases may present with minimal symptoms. The differential diagnosis of negative-pressure pulmonary edema includes aspiration of gastric contents, adult respiratory distress syndrome, congestive heart failure, volume overload, and anaphylaxis. A chest radiograph illustrating diffuse, usually bilateral interstitial pulmonary infiltrates combined with an appropriate clinical history will confirm the diagnosis.[7,25,26]

Treatment is usually supportive, with maintenance of a patent airway, oxygen administration, and diuretic therapy in some cases. Endotracheal intubation and mechanical ventilation with positive end-expiratory pressure may be necessary in severe cases. Resolution is usually rapid and may occur within

hours of inception. Most cases resolve within 24 hours without treatment. There is currently no reliable method for predicting which children will experience this clinical syndrome after their airway obstruction has been resolved.

Adenoidectomy patients may be safely discharged on the same day after recovering from anesthesia. Although most tonsillectomy patients previously required postoperative admission to the hospital for observation, administration of analgesics, and hydration, many centers are discharging tonsillectomy patients on the day of surgery without adverse outcomes, and this trend will likely continue.[26,27] Patients should be observed for early hemorrhage for a minimum of 4 to 6 hours and be free from significant nausea, vomiting, and pain prior to discharge. The ability to take fluid by mouth is not a requirement for discharge home. However, intravenous hydration must be adequate to prevent dehydration. Excessive somnolence and severe vomiting are indications for hospital admission. There are patients for whom early discharge is not advised, and those patients should be admitted to the hospital after tonsillectomy. The characteristics of such patients are listed in Table 50-1.

Ear Surgery

The ear and its associated structures are target organs for many pathologic conditions. General anesthesia for surgery of the ear has its own set of unique considerations that must be addressed.

Myringotomy and Tube Insertion

Chronic serous otitis in children can lead to hearing loss, and drainage of accumulated fluid in the middle ear is effective treatment for this condition. Myringotomy, which creates an opening in the tympanic membrane for fluid drainage, may be

TABLE 50-1

TONSILLECTOMY AND ADENOIDECTOMY INPATIENT GUIDELINES: RECOMMENDATION OF THE AMERICAN ACADEMY OF OTOLARYNGOLOGY–HEAD AND NECK SURGERY PEDIATRIC OTOLARYNGOLOGY COMMITTEE

Admit patients to the hospital after adenotonsillectomy if they meet any of the following criteria:

- Age ≤3 yr
- Abnormal coagulation values with or without an identified bleeding disorder in the patient or family
- Evidence of obstructive sleep disorder or apnea due to tonsillar or adenoidal hypertrophy
- Systemic disorders that put the patient at increased preoperative cardiopulmonary, metabolic, or general medical risk
- Child with craniofacial or other airway abnormalities including, but not limited to, syndromic disorders such as Treacher Collins syndrome, Crouzon syndrome, Goldenhar syndrome, Pierre Robin anomalad, CHARGE syndrome, achondroplasia, and, most prominently, Down syndrome, as well as isolated airway abnormalities such as choanal atresia and laryngotracheal stenosis
- When the procedure is being done for acute peritonsillar abscess
- When extended travel time, weather conditions, and home social conditions are not consistent with close observation, cooperation, and ability to return to the hospital quickly at the discretion of the attending physician

CHARGE, coloboma of the eye, heart defects, atresia of the choanae, retardation of growth and/or development, genital and/or urinary abnormalities, and ear abnormalities.

performed alone. During healing, the drainage path may become occluded; therefore, ventilation tube placement is usually included. The insertion of a small plastic tube in the tympanic membrane serves as a vent for the ostium and allows for continued drainage of the middle ear until the tubes are naturally extruded in 6 months to 1 year, or surgically removed at an appropriate time (Fig. 50-6).

Myringotomy and tube insertion is a relatively short procedure, and anesthesia may be effectively accomplished with a potent inhalation drug, oxygen, and N₂O administered by mask. Premedication is not recommended because most sedative drugs used for premedication will far outlast the duration of the surgical procedure. Patients with chronic otitis frequently have accompanying recurrent URIs. It is often the eradication of middle ear fluid that resolves the concomitant URI. Because tracheal intubation is not required for routine patients, the criteria for cancellation of surgery and anesthesia may be different for this procedure. Insertion of myringotomy tubes may be undertaken in most children with a concomitant URI provided that this can be completed with mask anesthesia and endotracheal intubation is avoided. No significant difference in perioperative morbidity between asymptomatic patients and those fulfilling URI criteria has been demonstrated.[28,29] It is recommended that patients with URI symptoms receive supplemental postoperative oxygen.

Middle Ear and Mastoid

Tympanoplasty and mastoidectomy are two of the most common procedures performed on the middle ear and accessory structures. To gain access to the surgical site, the head is positioned on a headrest, which may be lower than the operative table, and extreme degrees of lateral rotation may be required. Extreme tension on the heads of the sternocleidomastoid muscles must be avoided. The laxity of the ligaments of the cervical spine and the immaturity of odontoid process in children make them especially prone to C1–C2 subluxation.

Ear surgery often involves surgical identification and preservation of the facial nerve, which requires isolation of the nerve by the surgeon and verification of its function by means of electrical stimulation (Fig. 50-7). This is accomplished by brainstem auditory-evoked potential and electrocochleogram monitoring, which requires that complete muscle relaxation be avoided.[30] If an opioid-relaxant technique is chosen, however, at least 30% of the muscle response, as determined by a twitch monitor, should be preserved. This fact suggests that it is not mandatory to avoid skeletal muscle relaxants in the anesthetic management of patients undergoing surgical procedures when monitoring of facial nerve function is necessary.

Bleeding must be kept to a minimum during surgery of the small structures of the middle ear. Relative hypotension, keeping the mean arterial pressure 25% below baseline, is effective.

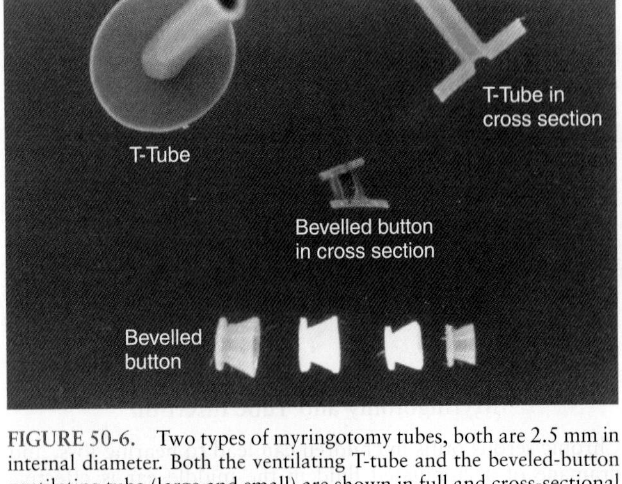

FIGURE 50-6. Two types of myringotomy tubes, both are 2.5 mm in internal diameter. Both the ventilating T-tube and the beveled-button ventilating tube (large and small) are shown in full and cross-sectional views. (Courtesy of Michael Cunningham, MD, Boston, MA.)

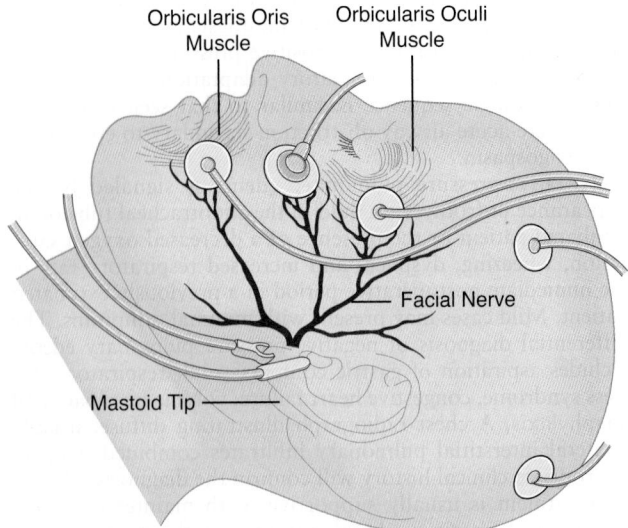

FIGURE 50-7. Illustration of facial nerve and monitoring electrodes. (Courtesy of Steve Ronner, PhD, Boston, MA.)

TABLE 50-2

CAUSES OF STRIDOR

■ SUPRAGLOTTIC AIRWAY	■ LARYNX	■ SUBGLOTTIC AIRWAY
Laryngomalacia	Laryngocele	Tracheomalacia
Vocal cord paralysis	Infection (tonsillitis, peritonsillar abscess)	Vascular ring
Subglottic stenosis	Foreign body	Foreign body
Hemangiomas	Choanal atresia	Infection (croup, epiglottitis)
Cysts	Cyst	
	Mass	
	Large tonsils	
	Large adenoids	
	Craniofacial abnormalities	

Concentrated epinephrine solution, often 1:1,000, can be injected in the area of the tympanic vessels to produce vasoconstriction. Close attention should be paid to the volume of injected epinephrine so that dysrhythmias and wide swings in blood pressure may be avoided.

4 The middle ear and sinuses are air-filled, nondistensible cavities. An increase in the volume of gas in these structures results in an increase in pressure. N_2O diffuses along a concentration gradient into the air-filled middle ear spaces more rapidly than nitrogen moves out. Passive venting occurs at 20 to 30 cm H_2O pressure, and it has been shown that use of N_2O results in pressures that exceed the ability of the eustachian tube to vent the middle ear within 5 minutes, leading to pressure buildup.[31] During procedures in which the eardrum is replaced or a perforation is patched, N_2O should be discontinued or, if this is not possible, limited to a maximum of 50% during the application of the tympanic membrane graft to avoid pressure-related displacement.

After N_2O is discontinued, it is quickly reabsorbed, creating a void in the middle ear with resulting negative pressure. This negative pressure may result in serous otitis, disarticulation of the ossicles in the middle ear (especially the stapes), and hearing impairment, which may last up to 6 weeks after surgery. The use of N_2O is related to a high incidence of postoperative nausea and vomiting, which is a direct result of negative middle ear pressure during recovery. The vestibular system is stimulated by traction placed on the round window by the negative pressure that is created. Although all patients have the potential for nausea and vomiting after surgery, children younger than 8 years of age seem to be most affected. If the use of N_2O cannot be avoided, vigorous use of antiemetics is warranted.

Airway Surgery

Stridor

Noisy breathing due to obstructed airflow is known as *stridor*. Inspiratory stridor results from upper airway obstruction; expiratory stridor results from lower airway obstruction; and biphasic stridor is present with midtracheal lesions. The evaluation of a patient with stridor begins with a thorough history. The age of onset suggests a cause: laryngotracheomalacia and vocal cord paralysis are usually present at or shortly after birth, whereas cysts or mass lesions develop later in life (Table 50-2). Information indicating positions that make the stridor better or worse should be obtained, and placing a patient in a position that allows gravity to aid in reducing obstruction can be of benefit during anesthetic induction.

Physical examination reveals the general condition of a patient and the degree of the airway compromise. Laboratory examination may include assessment of hemoglobin, a chest radiograph, and barium swallow, which can aid in identifying lesions that may be compressing the trachea. Other radiologic examinations such as magnetic resonance imaging and computed tomography scan may be indicated in isolated instances but are not routinely ordered. Specific note of the signs and symptoms listed in Table 50-3 should be made.

Laryngomalacia is the most common cause of stridor in infants. It is most often due to a long epiglottis that prolapses posteriorly and prominent arytenoid cartilages with redundant aryepiglottic folds that obstruct the glottic opening during inspiration.[32] The definitive diagnosis is obtained by direct laryngoscopy and rigid or flexible bronchoscopy. Preliminary examination is usually carried out in the surgeon's office. A small, flexible fiberoptic bronchoscope is inserted through the nares into the oropharynx, and the movement of the vocal cords is observed. Alternatively, it may be accomplished in the OR before anesthetic induction in an awake patient or in a lightly anesthetized patient during spontaneous respiration. Patients must be spontaneously breathing so the vocal cords move freely. After deepening anesthesia, a rigid bronchoscope is inserted through the vocal cords and the subglottic area is inspected; the lower trachea and bronchi are evaluated with a rigid or flexible fiberoptic bronchoscope.

Bronchoscopy

Small infants may be brought into the OR unpremedicated. Older children and adults may experience respiratory depression and worsening of airway obstruction if heavy premedication is administered, so only light sedation is suggested. The airway must be protected from aspiration of gastric contents during prolonged airway manipulation; therefore, premedication with the full regimen of acid aspiration prophylaxis may be indicated.

TABLE 50-3

CLINICAL COMPONENT OF THE EVALUATION OF PATIENTS WITH STRIDOR

Respiratory rate	Chest retractions
Heart rate	Nasal flaring
Wheezing	Level of consciousness
Cyanosis	

TABLE 50-4

COMPARISON OF EXTERNAL DIAMETER OF STANDARD ENDOTRACHEAL TUBES VERSUS RIGID BRONCHOSCOPE

■ ENDOTRACHEAL TUBE		■ RIGID BRONCHOSCOPE
■ INTERNAL DIAMETER (mm)	■ EXTERNAL DIAMETER (mm)	■ EXTERNAL DIAMETER (mm)
2.5	3.5	4.2
3.0	4.3	5.0
3.5	4.9	5.7
4.0	5.5	6.7
5.0	6.8	7.8
6.0	8.2	8.2

The goals of the anesthetic are analgesia, an unconscious patient, and a "quiet" surgical field.[33] Coughing, bucking, or straining during instrumentation with the rigid bronchoscope may cause difficulty for the surgeon and result in damage to the patient's airway. At the conclusion of the procedure, patients should be returned to consciousness quickly, with airway reflexes intact. For most patients, a pulse oximeter, blood pressure cuff, ECG, and precordial stethoscope are applied before induction of anesthesia. Inhalation induction by mask is accompanied by oxygen and a volatile agent administered in increasing concentrations in children and intravenous drugs in adults. Patients should be placed in the position that produces the least adverse effect on airway symptoms (often the sitting position). An intravenously administered antisialagogue may help decrease secretions that might compromise the view through the bronchoscope.

The size of a bronchoscope refers to the internal diameter. Because the external diameter may be significantly greater than in an endotracheal tube of similar size (Table 50-4), care must be taken to select a bronchoscope of proper external diameter to avoid damage to the laryngeal structures. A rigid bronchoscope can be used for ventilation of the lungs during examination of the airway. It is inserted through the vocal cords, and ventilation is accomplished through a side port, which can be attached to the anesthesia circuit. During ventilation with the viewing telescope in place, high resistance may be encountered as a result of partial occlusion of the lumen. High fresh gas flow rates, large tidal volumes, and high inspired volatile anesthetic concentrations are often necessary to compensate for leaks around the ventilating bronchoscope and the high resistance encountered when the viewing telescope is in place. Manual ventilation at higher-than-normal rates is most effective in achieving adequate ventilation. Adequate time for exhalation must be provided for passive recoil of the chest.[34]

An alternative method of ventilation is the jet ventilation technique, which involves intermittent bursts of oxygen delivered under pressure through a 16-gauge catheter attached to a rigid bronchoscope.[35] Intermittent flow is accomplished by depressing the lever of an on–off valve. The use of jet ventilation techniques is associated with the additional risks of pneumothorax or pneumomediastinum due to rupture of alveolar blebs or a bronchus.[36] Because ventilation may be intermittent and at times suboptimal, oxygen should be used as the carrier gas during bronchoscopic examination. Intravenous drugs that cause excessive respiratory depression should be avoided. It is wise to ask the surgeon if movement of the vocal cords will be required at the conclusion of the procedure or if tracheal or bronchial dynamics will be evaluated during the procedure so the anesthetic may be planned accordingly

(i.e., spontaneous respirations preserved during light levels of anesthesia versus no respiratory efforts and the use of short-acting muscle relaxants).

Maintenance of anesthesia is usually accomplished with a volatile anesthetic. Intravenous anesthetics combined with muscle relaxation best maintain a constant level of anesthesia because the delivery of volatile anesthetics through the bronchoscope may be interrupted, and anesthetic depth can vary. At the conclusion of rigid bronchoscopy, an endotracheal tube is usually placed in the trachea to control the airway during recovery of anesthesia. Securing the airway is particularly important if muscle relaxants have been used because passive regurgitation of gastric contents may be more likely to occur in paralyzed patients. An additional advantage of placing an endotracheal tube is that if the surgeon should want to examine the distal airways, a small, flexible fiberoptic bronchoscope can be passed through the endotracheal tube.

Pediatric Airway Emergencies

Upper airway emergencies may be life-threatening and demand immediate treatment. Rapid respiratory failure can occur in patients with croup, epiglottitis, or foreign body aspiration, and few clinical situations are more challenging to the anesthesiologist.

Epiglottitis

Acute epiglottitis is one of the most feared infectious diseases in children and adults, and is the result of *Haemophilus influenzae* type B. It can progress with extreme rapidity from sore throat to airway obstruction to respiratory failure and ultimately to death if proper diagnosis and intervention are not rapidly implemented. Patients are usually between 2 and 7 years of age, although epiglottitis has been reported in younger children and in adults. Vaccination against *H. influenzae* type B polysaccharide is now recommended before 2 years of age to provide immunity before the greatest period of vulnerability in pediatric patients.

Characteristic signs and symptoms of acute epiglottitis include sudden onset of fever, dysphagia, drooling, thick muffled voice, and preference for the sitting position with the head extended and leaning forward. Retractions, labored breathing, and cyanosis may be observed in cases in which respiratory obstruction is present. However, in the early stages, the patient may be pale and toxic without respiratory distress. *Supraglottitis* may be a more appropriate designation because it is the tissues of the supraglottic structures—from the vallecula to the arytenoids—that are involved in the infectious process. At no time, especially in the emergency department or radiography suite, should direct visualization of the epiglottis be attempted in the unanesthetized patient. The differential resulting from negative pressure inside and atmospheric pressure outside the extrathoracic airway results in slight narrowing during normal inspiration. The pressure differential on inspiration is exaggerated in the patient with airway obstruction. This dynamic collapse of the airway may become life-threatening in the struggling, agitated patient, and every attempt should be made to keep the patient calm. Blood drawing, intravenous catheter insertion, and excessive manipulation of the patient, as well as sedation, should be avoided before securing the airway to avoid the possibility of total obstruction.

If the clinical situation allows, oxygen should be administered by mask, and lateral radiographs of the soft tissues in the neck may be obtained. Thickening of the aryepiglottic folds and swelling of the epiglottis may be noted (the "thumbprint" sign). Radiologic examination should be carried out only if skilled personnel and adequate equipment accompany the patient at all times. The patient with severe airway compromise should proceed from the emergency department directly to the operating suite accompanied by both the anesthesiologist and surgeon. Parental presence in this situation may calm an anxious and frightened child.

In all cases of epiglottitis, an artificial airway is established by means of tracheal intubation. In some centers in which personnel experienced in the management of the compromised airway are not available, tracheostomy is a less-favored alternative. In the OR, the child is kept in the sitting position while monitors are placed. A pulse oximeter and precordial stethoscope are essential. If it is believed to be helpful, one parent may accompany the child and remain in the OR during the induction of general anesthesia. The OR must be prepared with equipment and personnel for laryngoscopy, rigid bronchoscopy, and tracheostomy. Anesthetic induction is accomplished by inhalation of oxygen and increasing concentrations of sevoflurane. After loss of consciousness occurs, intravenous access should be secured and the child lowered into the supine position. Laryngoscopy followed by oral tracheal intubation is then accomplished without the use of muscle relaxants. The endotracheal tube chosen should be at least one size (0.5 mm) smaller than would normally be chosen, and a stylette is often useful. Once the surgeon has examined the larynx, noting the appearance of the epiglottis, aryepiglottic folds, and surrounding tissues, the endotracheal tube may be changed to a nasotracheal tube and secured. Tissue and blood cultures are taken, and antibiotic therapy is initiated. The child is then transferred to the intensive care unit for continued observation and radiographic confirmation of tube placement. Sedation is appropriate at this time. Tracheal extubation is usually attempted 48 to 72 hours later in the OR, when a significant leak around the nasotracheal tube is present and visual inspection of the larynx by flexible fiberoptic bronchoscopy confirms reduction in swelling of the epiglottis and surrounding tissues.

Laryngotracheobronchitis

Laryngotracheobronchitis (LTB), or croup, occurs in children from 6 months to 6 years of age, but is primarily seen in children younger than 3 years of age. It is usually viral in etiology, and its onset is more insidious than that of epiglottitis. The child presents with low-grade fever, inspiratory stridor, and a "barking" cough. Radiologic examination confirms the diagnosis, and subglottic narrowing of the airway column secondary to circumferential soft-tissue edema produces the "steeple" sign characteristic of LTB. Approximately 6% of patients with LTB require admission to the hospital. Treatment includes cool, humidified mist and oxygen therapy, usually administered in a tent for mild-to-moderate cases. More severe cases of LTB are accompanied by tachypnea, tachycardia, and cyanosis. Racemic epinephrine administered by nebulizer is beneficial. The use of steroids has been surrounded by a great deal of controversy, but current opinion is that a short course of steroids may be beneficial. In rare circumstances, thick secretions are present in the airway, and the child requires intubation to allow pulmonary toilet and suctioning to be performed. Management in the intensive care unit and extubation are carried out in the same fashion as for epiglottitis.

Foreign Body Aspiration

A major cause of morbidity and mortality in children and adults is aspiration of a foreign body. Any history of coughing, choking, or cyanosis while eating should suggest the possibility of foreign body aspiration. Peanuts, popcorn, jelly beans, and hot dogs are some of the ingested items most commonly associated with pulmonary aspiration. Any patient who presents to the emergency department with refractory wheezing should be suspected of this diagnosis. Physical findings include decreased breath sounds, tachypnea, stridor, wheezing, and fever. These signs indicate an obstructive process with inflammation present in the airway. Some foreign bodies are identifiable on radiologic examination; however, 90% are radiolucent, and air trapping, infiltrate, and atelectasis are all that are noted.

The most common site of foreign body aspiration is the main stem bronchus, the right being more frequent than the left. Food particles comprise the majority of aspirated items; however, beads, pins, and small toys are not unusual. Each type of aspirated item has potential complications associated with it. Vegetable items expand with moisture encountered in the respiratory tract and can fragment into multiple pieces, thus creating a situation in which the original foreign body is in one bronchus and, with coughing, a fragment is dislodged and transported to the other bronchus. Oil-containing objects, such as peanuts, cause a chemical inflammation, and sharp objects cause bleeding in addition to the obstruction.

All aspirated foreign bodies in the airway should be removed in the OR and considered to be emergency situations. No sedation should be administered to patients before removal of the foreign body. If the patient has recently eaten, full-stomach precautions must be taken and anesthesia should be induced intravenously (topical anesthetic cream may be applied to the skin before intravenous catheter insertion in small children) by rapid sequence, and gentle cricoid pressure maintained during intubation of the trachea. If the child has not eaten recently, anesthesia may be induced by inhalation of sevoflurane in oxygen by mask. Inhalation induction can be prolonged secondary to obstruction of the airway, and N_2O should be avoided to reduce air trapping distal to the obstruction. After evacuation of the stomach by orogastric tube, the airway may be given over to the surgeon, who introduces a rigid bronchoscope and removes the aspirated object.

Spontaneous ventilation should be preserved until the location and nature of the foreign body have been determined. Ventilation via the bronchoscope requires careful attention. Hypoxia and hypercarbia may occur because of inadequate ventilation caused by an excessively large leak around the bronchoscope or, more commonly, inability to provide adequate gas exchange through a narrow-lumen bronchoscope fitted with an internal telescope. These conditions are remedied by frequent removal of the telescope and withdrawal of the bronchoscope to the midtrachea, allowing effective ventilation. Bronchospasm may occur during examination of the respiratory tract and should be treated with increasing depths of anesthesia, nebulized albuterol, or intravenous bronchodilators. Although rare, pneumothorax should be suspected if acute deterioration occurs during the procedure.

Once the foreign body has been removed, examination of the entire tracheobronchial tree is carried out to detect any additional objects or fragments. Often, vigorous irrigation and suctioning distal to the obstruction are required to remove secretions and prevent the possibility of postobstructive pneumonia. Steroids are administered if inflammation of the airway mucosa is observed. Close postoperative observation of the patient is required so that early intervention may be instituted in the event of respiratory compromise secondary to airway edema or infection.

ANESTHESIA FOR PEDIATRIC AND ADULT SURGERY

Certain surgical procedures are commonly performed in both adults and children, including nasal surgery and laser surgery of the airway. Surgery for maxillofacial trauma and upper airway tumors or infection, as well as temporomandibular joint (TMJ) arthroscopy, are conducted more commonly in adults.

Laser Surgery of the Airway

One of the greatest advances in airway surgery has been the use of the laser (*l*ight *a*mplification by *s*timulated *e*mission of *r*adiation). For use in the airway, the laser provides precision in targeting lesions, minimal bleeding and edema, preservation of surrounding structures, and rapid healing. The laser consists of a tube with reflective mirrors at either end and an amplifying medium between them to generate electron activity, resulting in the production of light.[37] The CO_2 laser is the most widely used in medical practice, having particular application in the treatment of laryngeal or vocal cord papillomas, laryngeal webs, resection of redundant subglottic tissue, and coagulation of hemangiomas. The laser is an especially useful modality for the surgeon because the invisible beam of light affords an unobstructed view of the lesion during resection. The energy emitted by a CO_2 laser is absorbed by water contained in blood and tissues. Human tissue is approximately 80% water, and laser energy absorbed by tissue water rapidly increases the temperature, denaturing protein and vaporizing the target tissue. The thermal energy of the laser beam cauterizes capillaries as it vaporizes tissues; thus, bleeding and postoperative edema are minimized.

The properties that give the laser a high degree of specificity also supply the route by which a misdirected laser beam may cause injury to a patient or to unprotected OR personnel.[38] The eyes are especially vulnerable, and all OR personnel should wear laser-specific eye goggles with side protectors to prevent injury. Because of the limited penetration (0.01 mm) of the CO_2 laser, it may cause injury only to the cornea. Other lasers such as the neodymium–yttrium-aluminum-garnet (Nd:YAG) have deeper penetration, and may cause retinal injury and scarring. The eyes of a patient undergoing laser treatment must be protected by taping them shut, followed by the application of wet gauze pads and a metal shield. Any stray laser beam is absorbed by the wet gauze, preventing penetration of the eyes. Laser radiation increases the temperature of absorbent material, and flammable objects such as surgical drapes must be kept away from the path of the laser beam. To avoid cutaneous burns from deflected beams, wet towels should be applied to exposed skin of the face and neck when the laser is being used in the airway. Laser smoke plumes may cause damage to the lungs; interstitial pneumonia has been reported with long-term exposure. In addition, it has been postulated that cancer cells and virus particles, including human immunodeficiency virus, are vaporized during laser application, and the resultant smoke plume, if inhaled, may be a vehicle for spread. The use of specially designed surgical masks for filtering laser smoke is recommended.

Most anesthetic techniques are suitable for laser surgery, provided that patients are immobile and the laser beam can be directed at a target that is entirely still and in full view. Both N_2O and oxygen support combustion; therefore, the primary gas for anesthetic maintenance should consist of blended air and oxygen or helium and oxygen. A pulse oximeter should be used at all times to ensure adequate oxygenation at the lowest possible inspired concentration of oxygen.

Anesthesia during laser surgery may be administered with or without an endotracheal tube. The choice of endotracheal tube used during laser surgery can affect the safety of the technique. All standard polyvinyl chloride (PVC) endotracheal tubes are flammable and can ignite and vaporize producing hydrochloric aced when in contact with the laser beam. Red rubber endotracheal tubes wrapped with reflective metallic tape do not vaporize but deflect the laser beam instead; however, the introduction of commercially available laser-specific endotracheal tubes has essentially replaced the use of these endotracheal tubes. Cuffed endotracheal tubes should be inflated with sterile saline to which methylene blue has been added so that a cuff rupture from a misdirected laser spark is readily detected by the blue dye and extinguished by the saline.[39] Endotracheal tubes have been manufactured specifically for use during laser surgery. Some have a double cuff to ensure protection of the airway in the event of a cuff rupture, and some have a special matte finish that effectively prevents reflected laser beam scattering; some have both. Nonreflective flexible metal endotracheal tubes are also specifically manufactured for use during laser surgery. The outer diameter of each size of metal laser tube is considerably greater than the PVC counterpart, especially in the small sizes used for pediatric anesthesia (Table 50-5).

TABLE 50-5

COMPARISON OF STANDARD PLASTIC VERSUS METAL ENDOTRACHEAL TUBES

■ INTERNAL DIAMETER (mm)	■ EXTERNAL DIAMETER (mm)	
	■ PLASTIC	■ METAL
3.0 (uncuffed)	4.3	5.2
3.5 (uncuffed)	4.9	5.7
4.0 (uncuffed)	5.5	6.1
4.5 (cuffed)	6.2	7.0
5.0 (cuffed)	6.8	7.5
5.5 (cuffed)	7.5	7.9
6.0 (cuffed)	8.2	8.5

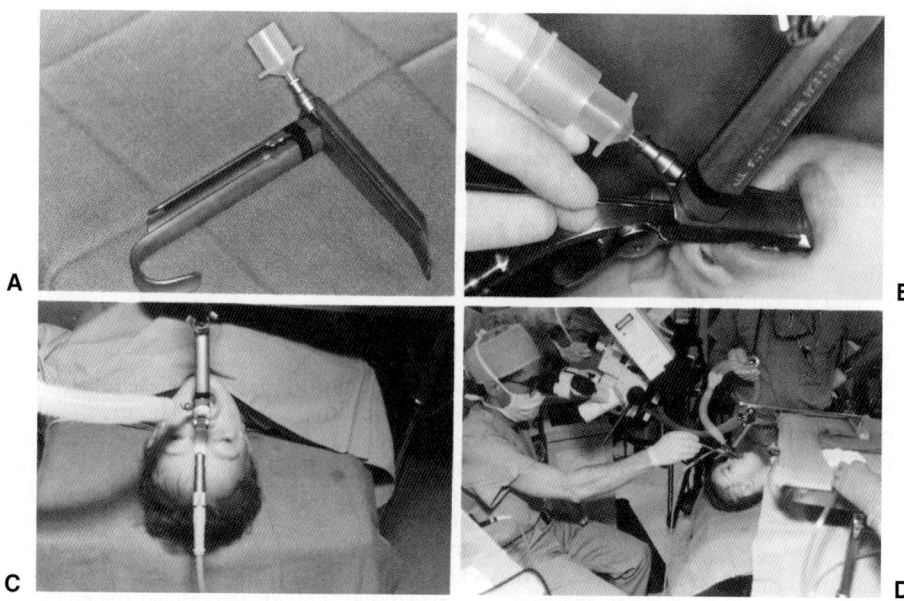

FIGURE 50-8.   **A.** The surgical laryngoscope fitted with an endotracheal tube connector. **B.** The surgical laryngoscope positioned in the patient's pharynx and connected to the anesthesia circuit. **C.** Surgical view of the anesthetized, spontaneously breathing patient. **D.** Laser-aided resection of vocal cord lesion.

An apneic technique is preferred by some surgeons, especially when working on the airway of small infants and children. The advantage of this technique is an unobstructed surgical field to the absence of an endotracheal tube, which may obscure the surgical field. In this circumstance, a child is anesthetized and rendered immobile by use of a muscle relaxant or deep inhalation of a volatile anesthetic. The patient's trachea is not intubated, and the airway is given over to the surgeon, who uses the laser for brief periods. Between laser applications, the patient's lungs are ventilated by mask. Because apnea is a component of this technique, it is prudent to ventilate the lungs with oxygen. Although this technique has been widely used with safety, there is a greater potential for debris and resected material to enter the trachea, as well as the potential for airway trauma as a result of repeated endotracheal intubation.

The use of a jet ventilator is a modification of the apneic technique that does not require tracheal intubation but does provide for oxygenation; ventilation during laser surgery uses a jet ventilator. The operating laryngoscope is fitted with a catheter through which oxygen is delivered under pressure through a variable reducing valve. Additional room air is entrained, and the patient's lungs are ventilated with this combination of gases. This technique produces a quiet surgical field because large chest excursions of the diaphragm are eliminated and ventilation is uninterrupted. In morbidly obese patients and those with severe small airway disease, effective ventilation is difficult to impossible with this technique, and an alternate technique should be used.

The final technique that may be used is spontaneous ventilation without the aid of an endotracheal tube (Figs. 50-8 and 50-9). In this technique, a surgical laryngoscope fitted with an oxygen insufflation port is inserted into the larynx. Anesthesia may be induced with a volatile agent by mask but is maintained with total intravenous agents without muscle relaxant in the spontaneously breathing patient. Propofol may be infused with or without a short-acting narcotic, and the vocal cords may be sprayed with 4% lidocaine to decrease reactivity. This technique is advantageous in that longer periods of uninterrupted laser application may be provided. Disadvantages include the absence of complete control of the airway, limited protection from laryngospasm, limited protection from debris entering the airway, vocal cords motion, and difficult scavenging.

Nasal Surgery

Nasal surgery may be successfully accomplished under either general anesthesia or conscious sedation. Whichever method is selected, profound intranasal vasoconstriction is required. Cocaine packs, local anesthetics, and epinephrine infiltration are often used simultaneously. All three of these agents can cause cardiac irritability, and both epinephrine and cocaine are known to produce varying degrees of hypertension. The simultaneous use of these medications causes cumulative and often dangerous side effects. Young, healthy patients may be able to tolerate these effects. The older patient, or one who has known cardiovascular compromise, may benefit from slow, sequential administration of these medications guided by heart rate, cardiac rhythm, and blood pressure. The potent inhalation anesthetics do have varying degrees of dysrhythmogenic potential and should be used with caution in the face of pharmacologically induced alterations in cardiac rhythm.

A moderate degree of controlled hypotension combined with head elevation decreases bleeding in the surgical site, but

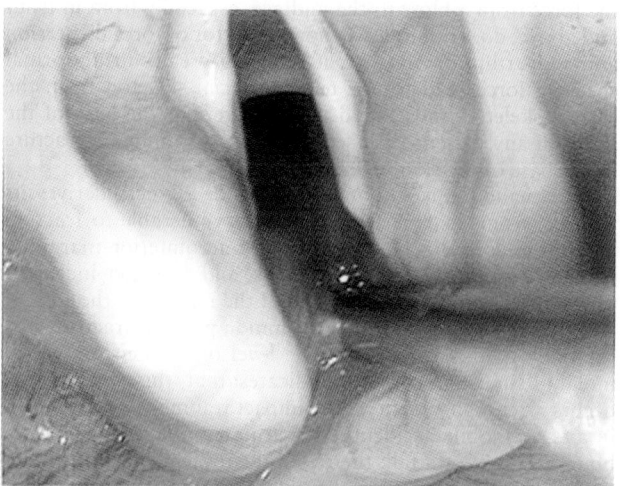

FIGURE 50-9.   Unrepaired posterior laryngeal cleft.

some blood may passively enter the stomach. The placement of an oropharyngeal pack at the beginning of the operation, or suctioning of the stomach at the conclusion, may attenuate postoperative retching and vomiting.

Maxillofacial Trauma

Traumatic disruption of the bony, cartilaginous, and soft-tissue components of the face and upper airway challenges the anesthesiologist to recognize the nature and extent of the injury and consequent anatomic alteration, create a plan for securing the airway safely, implement the plan without doing further damage, maintain the airway during the administration of an anesthetic, and determine when and how to extubate the patient's trachea. Also necessary is the creation of a comfortable environment for both surgeon and anesthesiologist in a limited work space.

Anatomy

It is conventional to divide the facial skeleton into thirds. The lower third consists of the mandible, with its subdivisions of midline symphysis, body, angle, ramus, condyle, and coronoid process. The middle third contains the zygomatic arch of the temporal bone, blending into the zygomaticomaxillary complex, the maxillae, nasal bones, and orbits. The superior third consists of the frontal bone. Great forces are generated within the facial skeleton during the normal physiologic process of mastication. To prevent injury of one skeleton against the other, there is a series of bony buttresses built into the articulation between the two skeletons. Horizontal posterior displacement of the facial skeleton is limited by the zygomatic process of the temporal bone, oblique posterior displacement by the pterygoid process of the sphenoid bone, and vertical posterior displacement by the greater wing of the sphenoid bone. Upward displacement is held in check by the zygomatic process of the frontal bone, the nasal part of the frontal bone, and the roof of the mandibular fossa. In addition there are two arches lending stability to the craniofacial skeleton. An arch extends from the mandibular condyle to the coronoid process, and another arch is created by the zygomatic arch of the temporal bone extending into the zygomaticomaxillary complex.

This combination of bony buttresses and arches creates a normal vector of force dispersion and distribution. Thus, a blow to the mandible may be of sufficient magnitude to fracture the mandible at the point of impact or elsewhere, but does not extend the fracture line into the base of the skull. However, the force from a blow to the midface, especially from in front and above, does not follow a normal vector of force dispersion and redistribution. Rather, it tends to create an abnormal shearing force, which may tear the facial skeleton from the cranial skeleton and extend the fracture into the base of the skull. In any patient with severe midfacial trauma, a fracture of the base of the skull must be considered.

The mandible is a tubular bone and, as such, derives its strength from the cortices and is least vulnerable to fracture where the cortex is thickest at the anteroinferior margin.[40] Moving posteriorly, the cortex thins, and a greater incidence of fractures is found at the angle of the mandible, the ramus, and the condyle.[41–43] Another common point of fracture is in the body of the mandible at the level of the first or second molar. Clinical experience indicates that this distribution occurs after high-velocity, high-impact trauma, such as occurs in an automobile accident. After trauma inflicted by a fist, a blunt weapon, or a fall, there is a greater tendency for a fracture of the symphysis, parasymphysis, and body to occur. This difference may result not only from lesser versus greater energy impact and redistribution, but also from the person's tendency to turn the head away from an impending blow and thus take the force of impact on the side of the face and the body of the mandible rather than on the symphysis.[44]

The mandible has a unique, horseshoe shape that causes forces to gather at points of vulnerability, often distant from the point of impact. If this phenomenon is unrecognized, it can create serious problems in diagnosis. It may be known, for example, that the patient was struck on the symphysis, but it must also be recognized that he or she may have a fracture of the condyle, perhaps with involvement of the TMJ and limitation of jaw mobility.

LeFort Classification of Fractures

In 1901, Rene LeFort[45] of Lille, France, published the results of a series of rather bizarre experiments. He attempted to determine if there is a reliable means of detecting facial fractures by examining facial soft-tissue injuries and by using the nature and extent of these injuries as indicators of bony disruption. He concluded that extensive soft-tissue injury does not necessarily indicate bony trauma, and conversely, serious fractures may exist with relatively little soft-tissue disruption. In the course of his studies, LeFort determined the common lines of midface fracture, which are thus eponymous and called LeFort I, LeFort II, and LeFort III fractures.

The LeFort I fracture is a horizontal fracture of the maxilla, passing above the floor of the nose but involving the lower third of the septum, mobilizing the palate, maxillary alveolar process, and the lower third of the pterygoid plates and parts of the palatine bones. The fracture segment may be displaced posteriorly or laterally or rotated about a vertical axis.

The LeFort II fracture is pyramidal, beginning at the junction of the thick upper part of the nasal bone, with the thinner portion forming the upper margin of the anterior nasal aperture. The fracture crosses the medial wall of the orbit, including the lacrimal bone beneath the zygomaticomaxillary suture; crosses the lateral wall of the antrum; and passes posteriorly through the pterygoid plates. The fracture segment may be displaced posteriorly or rotated about an axis.

In a LeFort III fracture, the line of fracture parallels the base of the skull, separating the midfacial skeleton from the base of the cranium. The line of fracture passes through the base of the nose and the ethmoid bone in its depth, and through the orbital plates. The cribriform plate of the ethmoid may or may not be fractured. The fracture line crosses the lesser wing of the sphenoid, then downward to the pterygomaxillary fissure and sphenopalatine fossa. From the base of the inferior orbital fissure, the fracture extends laterally and upward to the frontozygomatic suture and downward and backward to the root of the pterygoid plates. A LeFort III fracture results from massive force applied to the midface. The zygomata are displaced, applying rotational force to the zygomatic arches. The arches are usually fractured as a result.

With a LeFort III fracture, the midface is mobilized and often distracted posteriorly. The normal convexity of the face becomes concave, giving rise to the characteristic "dish face deformity" of a LeFort III fracture. Even if this facial concavity is not clinically evident, the presence of a LeFort III fracture should be suspected if the incisive edges of the maxillary and mandibular teeth are apposed, instead of the normal position in which the maxillary incisors shingle over the mandibular incisors. This apposition serves as a subtle clue to minimal posterior displacement of the midface.

Tumors

Neoplastic growths can occur anywhere within the upper airway and may achieve significant size with little evidence of airway obstruction. These tumors are often friable and bleed readily. Attempted tracheal intubation can induce significant hemorrhage and edema and cause severe compromise of the airway. Prior radiation therapy may cause extensive fibrosis, **6** increased intraoperative bleeding, and ankylosis of the TMJ, making tracheal intubation using rigid laryngoscopy difficult or impossible. Consultation with a surgeon as to the nature and extent of the tumor, and its potential to bleed, together with review of appropriate radiographs and prior therapy, are important in determining techniques for airway management. Tumors of the head and neck are usually associated with abuse of both cigarettes and alcohol, with consequent abnormalities of both pulmonary and hepatic function.

Upper Airway Infection

Infectious processes in the upper airway may be of sufficient size to mimic neoplasms and present the same problems of airway distortion, compression, and compromise. The same precautions must be taken in dealing with airway abscesses as with tumors. An added problem is the ability of an abscess to leak spontaneously, introducing purulent material into the lungs, contaminating and infecting them, and producing scattered areas of pneumonitis; or to rupture during tracheal intubation, flooding the lungs with purulent material.

Ludwig Angina

Ludwig angina is an overwhelming generalized septic cellulitis of the submandibular region.[46,47] It frequently occurs after dental extraction, especially of the second or third molars, whose roots lie below the mandibular attachment of the mylohyoid muscle. The infection is bilateral and involves three fascial spaces: submandibular, submental, and sublingual. Ludwig angina is characterized by brawny induration of the upper neck, usually without obvious fluctuation, and the patient has a typical open-mouthed appearance. Involvement of the sublingual space pushes the tongue upward and backward, and it usually protrudes from the open mouth. Soft-tissue swelling in the suprahyoid region, coupled with upward and posterior displacement of the tongue, as well as the frequent presence of laryngeal edema, can obstruct the airway and asphyxiate the patient.

Early signs and symptoms include chills, fever, drooling of saliva, inability to open the mouth, and difficulty in speaking. The cause is often hemolytic streptococci, but may be a mixture of aerobic and anaerobic organisms, including gas-forming bacteria. Although fluctuation is rarely appreciated, abscesses may be present but their presence hidden by the thick, indurated tissue of the neck. The infectious process may spread into the thorax, causing empyema, pericarditis, pericardial effusion, and pulmonary infiltrates.

Patients with Ludwig angina often require incision and drainage of whatever purulent material is present, coupled with airway decompression. Airway management may be extremely difficult. Although inhalation anesthesia and intubation have been advocated, preliminary tracheostomy using local anesthesia in the awake patient is the safest course. The patient with Ludwig angina is commonly septic, extremely ill, and often poorly hydrated.

Temporomandibular Joint Arthroscopy

Open surgery of the human TMJ was first described in 1887 in a discussion of operative repair of displaced interarticular cartilage of the joint.[48] Although open surgery of the joint is still sometimes considered necessary, the development of small-

gauge arthroscopes and lasers has made arthroscopic surgery of the TMJ an increasingly popular technique, frequently performed on an ambulatory basis. Common indications for arthroscopic correction of TMJ lesions include internal joint derangement with closed lock, internal joint derangement with painful clicking, osteoarthritis, hypermobility, fibrous ankylosis, chondromalacia, synovitis and arthralgia.

TMJ disease is usually caused by spasm of the muscles of mastication secondary to chronic tensing of these muscles as an involuntary mental tension–relieving mechanism. The patient population is unique in that 86% of patients with chronic TMJ dysfunction have significant psychopathology, with major depression in 74% and somatoform disorder in 50%.[49] A total of 40% of the patients are preoccupied with facial pain, yet have no physical findings accounting for the pain. Many of these patients habitually use mood-altering or tension-abating drugs such as benzodiazepines, phenothiazines, or lithium.

Nasotracheal intubation is usually preferred, allowing the surgeon the option of intraoral manipulation during surgery. Complications of TMJ arthroscopy are rare but include partial or total hearing loss, infection, hemorrhage requiring open arthrotomy, and temporary or permanent deficits of the fifth and eighth cranial nerves and temporary seventh nerve paresis.[49,50]

7 Of particular importance to the anesthesiologist is partial or even complete closure of the airway due to extracapsular extravasation of the fluid used to irrigate the joint during arthroscopy.[51] Significant amounts of fluid can leak into the soft tissues of the neck and compromise the airway. After TMJ arthroscopy, the patient's trachea should not be extubated until the oral cavity, especially on the affected side, and neck have been examined carefully and no evidence of unusual swelling that might indicate extravasated fluid is found.

Patient Evaluation

The patient who has sustained facial trauma or whose airway is clearly distorted by tumor or infection may present with an obvious pathologic process that can distract the physician from completing a total evaluation of the patient. In the patient with facial trauma, other injuries may not be as apparent but may represent a greater threat to the patient's well-being. One study revealed that in patients with maxillofacial injury due to low-velocity, low-impact blows, 4% had additional major life-threatening injuries and 10% had additional minor injuries. With high-velocity, high-impact accidents, 32% had major additional injuries and 31% had minor additional injuries.[52] Of great importance, cervical spine fractures occurred in 1.2% of high-velocity injuries. Another study has reported a 5.5% incidence of cervical spine injury in patients with facial skeletal trauma.[53] Any level of the cervical spine may be involved, but injuries at C2 (31%) and C6–C7 (50%) predominate. Cranial fractures and intracranial injury also are not uncommon.

INTUBATING THE TRACHEA

In most instances of anesthesia for head and neck surgery, tracheal intubation is effected without significant problems. Significant difficulties can arise in patients with tumor, infection, or other facial trauma. If the normal anatomy of the airway has been altered, awake tracheal intubation or preliminary tracheostomy should be considered. History, physical examination, appropriate radiographs, and surgical consultation are the foundation of airway evaluation and choice of intubating technique. The technique of an "awake look" before a decision to anesthetize and paralyze a patient is particularly hazardous and misleading. Muscle tone and labored respiration in the awake patient help identify the rima glottis or some seemingly familiar anatomic structure, but disappear once anesthesia and paralysis have been induced and it may be impossible to identify the entrance to the airway and intubate the trachea.

For the anesthesiologist to be able to intubate the trachea of a patient under direct vision, the patient must be able, at a minimum, to open the mouth and extend the tongue beyond the incisors. After maxillofacial trauma, there may be serious limitation in mobility owing to one or more factors, including pain, trismus, edema, and mechanical dysfunction of the TMJ. If the patient suffers from pain but has no injury that interferes with jaw mechanisms, using anesthesia and muscle relaxant will be satisfactory for tracheal intubation.

Trismus is spasm of the masseter muscles, binding the jaw closed, secondary to trauma or infection. Trismus, too, succumbs to an anesthetic and muscle relaxant, but with an important caveat. If the trismus has been present for 2 weeks or if the jaw has been closed for some other reason for 2 weeks, the masseter muscles acquire a degree of fibrosis that limits jaw opening and is not overcome by general anesthetic and muscle relaxant. A jaw closed for 2 weeks for any reason merits consideration for awake tracheal intubation. Edema varies in severity and consequences from mild to extreme, and may occasionally cause serious limitation in jaw mobility.

Mechanical dysfunction in the jaw arises from several causes. A fracture of the condyle in its articulation in the TMJ may create a situation in which the jaw is mechanically locked closed. General anesthesia and muscle relaxant will not overcome these mechanisms. A fracture of the zygomatic arch of the temporal bone will always causes some decrease in jaw mobility. This bone is well protected and is enveloped in the tough temporal fascia. Nonetheless, a severe blow to the side of the head may fracture the bone, pushing bony segments down onto the coronoid process of the mandible. There is a biphasic motion in the mandible, rotation about an axis passing through the condyles, and anterior-posterior motion (translation). This anterior motion is limited by the bony impingement on the coronoid process, and TMJ function is thus restricted by the limitation in translation. Although the decrease in TMJ function is not usually severe enough to make tracheal intubation impossible, it occasionally does prevent mouth opening. Thus, the decision to anesthetize and paralyze the patient or perform awake tracheal intubation may be difficult. If in doubt, the anesthesiologist is cautioned to act conservatively.

Patients with TMJ dysfunction undergoing arthroscopic surgery may present with either closed or open lock and be unsuitable for intubation of the trachea with rigid laryngoscopy after induction of anesthesia. Patients with large cervical abscesses may require awake intubation or tracheostomy. If the abscess has caused anatomic distortion or respiratory difficulty, awake intubation or tracheostomy is usually mandatory. Early tracheostomy in Ludwig angina is preferred, and no patient should ever be observed to the point of airway compromise.[54] In any instance in which awake intubation is elected in the infected patient, provision must be available for immediate tracheostomy.

Awake Intubation

Passing an endotracheal tube through the mouth or nose and into the larynx and trachea of an awake patient is a formidable procedure that the patient resists fiercely and that is compounded by the protestations of highly sensitive airway reflexes. To overcome these reflexes, the airway must be anesthetized using a combination of topical local anesthetic and superior laryngeal nerve block.

The *superior laryngeal nerve* is a branch of the vagus arising from the nodose ganglion and coursing with the main trunk of the vagus until it reaches the level of the larynx, where it springs forward and terminates in two branches, internal and external. The external branch of the superior laryngeal nerve penetrates and innervates the cricothyroid muscle, a tensor of the vocal cords. The internal branch penetrates the thyrohyoid membrane, ramifies, and provides sensory innervation from the base of the tongue to the vocal cords.[55] Once it has penetrated the thyrohyoid membrane, it lies in a closed space, bounded medially by the laryngeal mucosa, laterally by the thyrohyoid membrane, superiorly by the inferior border of the hyoid bone, and inferiorly by the superior surface of the thyroid cartilage. The anatomic landmarks for superior laryngeal nerve block are as follows:

1. The hyoid bone, a freely movable bone in the upper part of the neck, articulating with no other bone
2. The thyroid cartilage, the largest component of the larynx, usually easily identified
3. The thyrohyoid membrane, binding the two together

With the patient lying supine, a 22-gauge needle attached to a syringe containing 2 mL of 2% lidocaine is aimed directly at the hyoid, traveling parallel to the operating table. When the needle strikes the hyoid, the operator can appreciate the characteristic gritty feeling of a needle on bone, similar to striking the rib while doing an intercostal block. The needle is then walked caudad until it just slips off the bone, penetrating the thyrohyoid membrane. After negative aspiration, lidocaine may be injected and the block repeated on the other side.[56]

Contraindications to a superior laryngeal nerve block are relative, not absolute, and include the following:

1. A full stomach, because of the possibility of vomiting and aspiration into an airway whose protective reflexes have been partially obtunded
2. Tumor at the site of block
3. Infection at the site of block

Tumor and infection are considered to be relative contraindications because of the possibility of dissemination of either tumor or infection secondary to the manipulation associated with the block. Risks must be weighed against benefits. Protection against aspiration can be increased by the presence of knowledgeable help, an operating table that can swing quickly into the Trendelenburg position, and efficient suction apparatus.

Local anesthetic may be instilled into the nose for nasotracheal intubation and into the mouth and oropharynx for either nasal or oral intubation. A vasoconstrictor, such as 0.5% phenylephrine hydrochloride or 0.05% oxymetazoline, should also be instilled into the nose to shrink the nasal mucosa, decrease the risk of trauma, and create a larger passage for tracheal intubation. Topical anesthetic may be applied to the trachea below the level of the vocal cords by introducing a 22-gauge needle attached to a syringe containing 4 mL of 2% lidocaine and injecting the drug rapidly into the trachea at the end of the maximal expiration. The injection of the drug excites a vigorous cough reflex, spraying the local anesthetic along the tracheal side walls and inferior surface of the vocal cords. As a supplement to direct tracheal instillation of local anesthetic and bilateral superior laryngeal nerve block, local anesthetic (e.g., 2% lidocaine) may be nebulized in a handheld nebulizer and inhaled by the patient. Local anesthetic nebulization is a tedious process, demanding long, slow breaths and inhalation of the nebulized anesthetic over the course of at least 20 minutes. The endotracheal tube may then be passed into the anesthetized airway using a guided, fiberoptic technique or blindly. Complications of superior laryngeal nerve block include intravascular injection of local anesthetic. The carotid sheath lies just posterior to the site of block and, if the needle is angled posteriorly, the sheath may be entered and the anesthetic injected directly into the carotid artery or internal jugular vein.

The LMA may be useful in temporarily securing a compromised airway. However, in any situation in which the airway is jeopardized by blood or pus, or the anatomy is distorted by trauma, the airway must be secured with a cuffed endotracheal or tracheostomy tube. This frequently is accomplished by guiding an endotracheal tube over a bronchoscope introduced through the standard LMA. The intubating LMA may facilitate awake intubation.[57] The flexible LMA is unsafe in head and neck surgery in the presence of foreign material such as blood, bone fragments, or pus.[58]

A modification of the LMA is the LMA ProSeal (LMA North America), which has a double cuff and a double-lumen design that separates the airway and the alimentary tract, thus providing a safe escape channel for regurgitated fluids. Incorporated in its design is an independent drain tube that opens at the upper esophageal sphincter, permitting drainage of gastric fluids and allowing blind insertion of an orogastric tube. However, only a properly placed endotracheal tube offers complete airway protection.

The LMA Fastrach (LMA North America) is a modification of the intubating LMA, designed specifically for the anatomically difficult airway, especially the patient who cannot open his or her mouth fully. When used with the LMA Fastrach, endotracheal tube intubation can be effected without moving the patient. This tube is a straight, silicone, wire-reinforced, cuffed tube, not exceeding 8 mm internal diameter, and capable of being passed entirely through an LMA Fastrach. The use of this device may make possible an otherwise very difficult intubation.

LeFort III Fractures

A LeFort III fracture may involve the cribriform plate of the ethmoid bone, thus violating the separation of nasopharynx and base of the skull and allowing entrance into the intracranial subarachnoid space. Nasotracheal intubation risks the introduction of foreign material from the nasopharynx into the subarachnoid space and the consequent development of meningitis. More important, it risks the introduction of the endotracheal tube into the substance of the brain, with direct mechanical damage. Even positive-pressure bag and mask ventilation is contraindicated because the increase in volume and pressure within the nasopharynx can force foreign material or air into the skull.[59]

The problems of securing the airway in a patient with a LeFort III fracture are ordinarily obviated by doing a preliminary tracheostomy using local anesthetic in an awake patient. This method has the added advantage of separating surgeon and anesthesiologist and allowing each an adequate working space. Nasotracheal intubation can be performed in a patient with a LeFort III fracture provided that there is absence of clinical and radiologic evidence of basal skull fracture, and a compelling reason for doing so.

Anesthetic Management of the Traumatized Upper Airway

After tracheal intubation has been achieved or tracheostomy performed, general or intravenous anesthetics may be used. The use of ketamine as a sole anesthetic in an attempt to obviate the necessity of performing a difficult tracheal intubation is perilous and should be avoided. Ketamine is a potent respiratory depressant in bolus doses, increases intracranial pressure (ICP), and causes focal alterations in the cerebral metabolic rate.[60,61] Because there is a significant incidence of intracranial trauma associated with maxillofacial trauma, the brain must be protected and alterations in ICP avoided. Opioids have little effect on ICP and are useful in anesthetic management. However, the dose may be difficult to determine because of the high incidence of drug abuse associated with trauma. Inhalation anesthetics are safe and effective, and ICP can be moderated by altering the $PaCO_2$.

A recent development in the management of the traumatized airway when awake fiberoptic intubation is the preferred method of securing the airway is the use of dexmedetomidine. Dexmedetomidine is an α_2-agonist that results in a moderate level of conscious sedation without causing respiratory distress or hemodynamic instability during fiberoptic intubation.[62] Patients at risk for cervical spine cord compression had excellent cooperation for postintubation neurologic examination when treated with a loading dose of 1 µg/kg bolus over 10 minutes followed by an infusion of 0.2 to 0.7 µg/kg/hr.[63] Side effects of hypertension, hypotension, and bradycardia may occur.[64]

Extubation

When tracheostomy has been incorporated into the anesthetic-surgical plan, it is maintained at the termination of the procedure, and the only decision facing the anesthesiologist is whether to allow spontaneous respiration or to create suitable conditions for continued mechanical ventilation by maintaining the patient in an anesthetized and paralyzed state. This decision is contingent on such factors as the nature and duration of surgery, the patient's prior physical condition, and concurrent respiratory disease, a frequent concomitant of head and neck tumors.

After trauma, infection, or extensive oral resection for tumor, the endotracheal tube must not be removed until there is clearly subsidence of any edema that might compromise the unprotected airway. Particular attention must be given to the submandibular area, where extensive edema pushes the tongue upward and posteriorly and risks the airway. An edematous tongue protruding past the incisors is an ominous warning of dangerous edema. If substantial edema is present, a waiting period of 24 to 36 hours is usually indicated. Serious infection may require a longer period of time to resolve. An oral endotracheal tube may be removed over a tube changer. When removing a nasotracheal tube, a useful technique is to place a fiberoptic bronchoscope through the tube and into the airway and to remove the tube over the bronchoscope so it can be replaced immediately if necessary.

References

1. Brodsky L: Modern assessment of tonsils and adenoids. Pediatr Clin North Am 1989; 36: 1551
2. Berkowitz RG, Zaltzal GH: Tonsillectomy in children under 3 years of age. Arch Otolaryngol Head Neck Surg 1990; 116: 685
3. Ferrari L: Anesthesia for pediatric ENT procedures. Danamiller Memorial Education Foundation. Progr Anesthesiol 2001; 15: 15
4. Deutsch E: Tonsillectomy and adenoidectomy changing indications. Pediatr Clin North Am 1996; 43: 1319
5. Clinical Practice Guideline: Diagnosis and management of childhood obstructive sleep apnea syndrome. Pediatrics 2002; 109: 704
6. Chaban R, Cole P, Hoffstein V: Site of upper airway obstruction in patients with idiopathic obstructive sleep apnea. Laryngoscope 1988; 98: 641
7. Blum R, McGowan F: Chronic upper airway obstruction and cardiac dysfunction: Anatomy, pathophysiology and anesthetic implications. Pediatr Anesth 2004; 14: 75
8. Smith R, Gonzalez C: The relationship between nasal obstruction and craniofacial growth. Pediatr Clin North Am 1989; 36: 1423

9. Patel R, Hannallah R, Norden J: Emergence airway complications in children: A comparison of tracheal extubation in awake and deeply anesthetized patients. Anesth Analg 1991; 73: 266

10. Alexander C: A modified Intavent laryngeal mask for ENT and dental anaesthesia. Anaesthesia 1990; 45: 892

11. Haynes S, Morton N: The laryngeal mask airway: A review of its use in paediatric anaesthesia. Paediatr Anaesth 1993; 3: 65

12. Johr M: Anaesthesia for tonsillectomy. Curr Opin Anaesthesiol 2006; 19: 260

13. Nair I, Bailey P: Comparison of the reinforced laryngeal mask airway and tracheal intubation for adenotonsillectomy. Br J Anaesth 1993; 30: 1993

14. Nair I, Bailey P: Review of the uses of the laryngeal mask airway in ENT anaesthesia. Anaesthesia 1995; 50: 898

15. Mason D, Bingham R: The laryngeal mask airway in children. Anaesthesia 1990; 45: 760

16. Goudsouzian N, Cleveland R: Stability of the laryngeal mask airway during marked extension of the neck. Paediatr Anaesth 1993; 3: 117

17. Gunter JB, McAuliffe JJ, Beckman EC et al: A factorial study of ondansetron, metoclopramide, and dexamethasone for emesis prophylaxis after adenotonsillectomy in children. Paediatr Anaesth 2006; 16: 1153

18. Sukhani R, Pappas AL, Lurie J et al: Ondansetron and dolasetron provide equivalent postoperative vomiting control after ambulatory tonsillectomy in dexamethasone-pretreated children. Anesth Analg 2002; 95: 1230

19. Randall DA, Hoffer ME: Complications of tonsillectomy and adenoidectomy. Otolaryngol Head Neck Surg 1998; 118: 61

20. Windfuhr JP, Deck JC, Remmert S: Hemorrhage following coblation tonsillectomy. Ann Otol Rhinol Laryngol 2005; 114: 749

21. Windfuhr JP, Chen YS, Remmert S: Hemorrhage following tonsillectomy and adenoidectomy in 15,218 patients. Otolaryngol Head Neck Surg 2005; 132: 281

22. Crysdale W, Russel D: Complications of tonsillectomy and adenoidectomy in 9,409 children observed overnight. CMAJ 1986; 135: 1139

23. Linden BE, Gross CW, Long TE et al: Morbidity in pediatric tonsillectomy. Laryngoscope 1990; 100: 120

24. Broadman L, PAtel R, Feldman B: The effects of peritonsillar infiltration on the reduction of intraoperative blood loss and post-tonsillectomy pain in children. Laryngoscope 1989; 99: 578

25. Mehta VM, Har-El G, Goldstein NA: Postobstructive pulmonary edema after laryngospasm in the otolaryngology patient. Laryngoscope 2006; 116: 1693

26. Brigger MT, Brietzke SE: Outpatient tonsillectomy in children: A systematic review. Otolaryngol Head Neck Surg 2006; 135: 1

27. Pizzuto M, Volk M, Kingston L: Common topics in otolaryngology. Pediatr Clin North Am 1998; 45: 973

28. Tait A, Malviya S, Voepel-Lewis T et al: Risk factors for perioperative adverse respiratory events in children with upper respiratory tract infections. Anesthesiology 2001; 95: 299

29. Tait A, Malviya S: Anesthesia for the child with an upper respiratory tract infection: Still a dilemma? Anesth Analg 2005; 100: 59

30. Levine RA, Ronner SF, Ojemann RG: Auditory evoked potential and other neurophysiologic monitoring techniques during tumor surgery in the cerebellopontine angle, Intraoperative Monitoring Techniques in Neurosurgery. Edited by Levine RA, Ronner SF, Ojemann RG. New York, McGraw-Hill, 1994, p 175

31. Casey WF, Drake-Lee AB: Nitrous oxide and middle ear pressure. A study of induction methods in children. Anaesthesia 1982; 37: 896

32. Zalzal GH: Stridor and airway compromise. Pediatr Clin North Am 1989; 36: 1389

33. Ferrari L, Vasallo S: Anesthesia for otorhinolaryngology procedures, A Practice of Anesthesia for Infants and Children. Edited by Cootie C, Toddies I, Goudsouzian N et al. Philadelphia, WB Saunders, 1992, p 318

34. Soriano S, Kim C, Jones D: Surgical airway, rigid bronchoscopy and transtracheal jet ventilation in the pediatric patient. Anesth Clin North Am 2005; 16: 827

35. Sanders RD: Two ventilating attachments for bronchoscopes. Delaware Medical Journal 1967; July: 170

36. Steward DJ: Percutaneous transtracheal ventilation for laser endoscopic procedures in infants and small children. Can J Anaesth 1987; 34: 429

37. Hermens J, Bennett M, Hirshman C: Anesthesia for laser surgery. Anesth Analg 1983; 62: 218

38. McLesky C: Anesthestic management of patients undergoing laser surgery. San Diego, IARS Review Course Lectures, 1988, p 135

39. Sosis M, Dillon F: Saline-filled cuffs help prevent laser-induced polyvinylchloride endotracheal tube fires. Anesth Analg 1991; 72: 187

40. Haskell R: Applied surgical anatomy, Maxillo Facial Injuries. Edited by Haskell R. Edinburgh, Churchill Livingstone, 1985, p 3

41. Halazonetis JA: The 'weak' regions of the mandible. Br J Oral Surg 1968; 6: 37

42. Huelke DF, Patrick LM: Mechanics in the production of mandibular fractures: Strain-gauge measurements of impacts to the chin. J Dent Res 1964; 43: 437

43. Nahum AM: The biomechanics of facial bone fracture. Laryngoscope 1975; 85: 140

44. Olson RA, Fonseca RJ, Zeitler DL et al: Fractures of the mandible: A review of 580 cases. J Oral Maxillofac Surg 1982; 40: 23

45. LeFort R: Etude experimentale sur les fractures de la machoire superieure. Rev Chir 1901; 23: 208

46. Ballenger JJ: Diseases of the Nose, Throat, Ear, Head and Neck. Philadelphia, Lea & Febiger, 1991

47. Burke J: Angina Ludovici: A translation, together with a biography of Wilhelm Frederick von Ludwig. Bull Hist Med 1939; 7: 1115

48. Annandale T: On displacement of the inter-articular cartilage of the lower jaw, and its treatment by operation. Lancet 1887; 1: 411

49. Kinney RK, Gatchel RJ, Ellis E et al: Major psychological disorders in chronic TMJ patients: implications for successful management. J Am Dent Assoc 1992; 123: 49

50. Sanders B: Arthroscopic surgery of the temporomandibular joint: Treatment of internal derangement with persistent closed lock. Oral Surg Oral Med Oral Pathol 1986; 62: 361

51. Hendler BH, Levin LM: Postobstructive pulmonary edema as a sequela of temporomandibular joint arthroscopy: a case report. J Oral Maxillofac Surg 1993; 51: 315

52. Luce EA, Tubb TD, Moore AM: Review of 1,000 major facial fractures and associated injuries. Plast Reconstr Surg 1979; 63: 26

53. Davidson JS, Birdsell DC: Cervical spine injury in patients with facial skeletal trauma. J Trauma 1989; 29: 1276

54. Har-El G, Aroesty JH, Shaha A et al: Changing trends in deep neck abscess. A retrospective study of 110 patients. Oral Surg Oral Med Oral Pathol 1994; 77: 446

55. Durham CF, Harrison TS: The surgical anatomy of the superior laryngeal nerve. Surg Gynecol Obstet 1964; 118: 38

56. Gotta AW, Sullivan CA: Superior laryngeal nerve block: An aid to intubating the patient with fractured mandible. J Trauma 1984; 24: 83

57. Ferson DZ, Brimacombe J, Brain AI et al: The intubating laryngeal mask airway. Int Anesthesiol Clin 1998; 36: 183

58. Bailey P, Brimacombe JR, Keller C: The flexible LMA: Literature considerations and practical guide. Int Anesthesiol Clin 1998; 36: 111

59. Dacosta A, Billard JL, Gery P et al: Posttraumatic intracerebral pneumatocele after ventilation with a mask: Case report. J Trauma 1994; 36: 255

60. Ben Yehuda Y, Watemberg N: Ketamine increases opening cerebrospinal pressure in children undergoing lumbar puncture. J Child Neurol 2006; 21: 441

61. Sehdev RS, Symmons DA, Kindl K: Ketamine for rapid sequence induction in patients with head injury in the emergency department. Emerg Med Australas 2006; 18: 37

62. Bergese S, Khabiri B: Dexmedetomidine for conscious sedation in difficult awake fiberoptic intubation cases. J Clin Anesth 2007; 19: 141

63. Avistian R, Lin J: Dexmedetomidine and awake fiberoptic intubation for possible cervical spine myelopathy: A clinical series. J Neurosurg Anesthesiol 2005; 17: 97

64. Gerlach A, Dasta J: Dexmedetomidine: An updated review. Ann Pharmacother 2007; 41: 245

CHAPTER 51 ■ ANESTHESIA FOR OPHTHALMOLOGIC SURGERY

KATHRYN E. McGOLDRICK AND STEVEN I. GAYER

KEY POINTS

1 Although apprehension is predictable in potentially blind patients awaiting surgery, this problem is often exacerbated in the elderly, whose coping mechanisms may be diminished by depression or dementia.

2 Inhalation anesthetics cause dose-related reductions in intraocular pressure (IOP). The exact mechanisms are unknown, but postulated causes include depression of a control center in the diencephalon, reduction of aqueous humor production, enhancement of aqueous outflow, or relaxation of the extraocular muscles.

3 The oculocardiac reflex is triggered by pressure on the globe and by traction on the extraocular muscles, as well as on the conjunctiva or on the orbital structures. This reflex, the afferent limb of which is trigeminal and the efferent limb is vagal, may also be elicited by performance of a retrobulbar block, by ocular trauma, and by direct

pressure on tissue remaining in the orbital apex after enucleation.

4 Ophthalmic drugs may significantly alter the patient's reaction to anesthesia. Similarly, anesthetic drugs and maneuvers may dramatically influence intraocular dynamics.

5 Several anesthetic options are available for many types of ocular procedures, including general anesthesia, retrobulbar block, peribulbar anesthesia, sub-Tenon (episcleral) block, topical analgesia, and intracameral injection.

6 The complications of ophthalmic anesthesia can be both vision- and life-threatening.

7 With intraocular procedures, profound akinesia and meticulous control of IOP are requisite. However, with extraocular surgery, the significance of IOP fades, whereas concern about elicitation of the oculocardiac reflex assumes prominence.

Anesthesia for ophthalmic surgery presents many unique challenges (Table 51-1). In addition to possessing technical expertise, the anesthesiologist must have detailed knowledge of ocular anatomy, physiology, and pharmacology. It is essential to appreciate that ophthalmic drugs may significantly alter the

reaction to anesthesia and that, concomitantly, anesthetic drugs and maneuvers may dramatically influence intraocular dynamics. Patients undergoing ophthalmic surgery may represent extremes of age and coexisting medical diseases (e.g., diabetes mellitus, coronary artery disease, essential hypertension,

TABLE 51-1

REQUIREMENTS OF OPHTHALMIC SURGERY

Safety
Akinesia
Analgesia
Minimal bleeding
Avoidance or obtundation of oculocardiac reflex
Control of intraocular pressure
Awareness of drug interactions
Smooth emergence

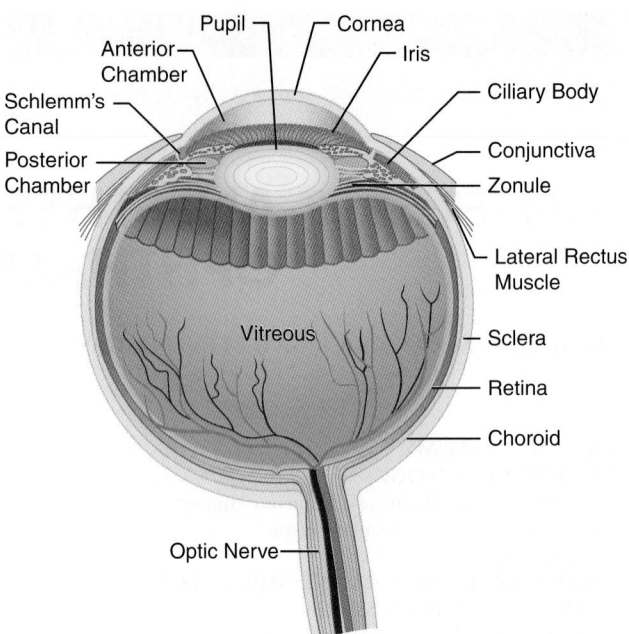

FIGURE 51-1.   Diagram of ocular anatomy.

chronic lung disease), but they are likely to be in the elderly age group. Indeed, the elderly constitute the most rapidly growing subset of the U.S. population, with the 2002 Census reporting 4.2 million Americans age 85 years or older, an increase of 30% since 1990. Moreover, the elderly are a uniquely vulnerable group with reduced functional reserve and a myriad of age-related diseases. The economic implication of these age-related diseases is staggering. For example, age-related macular degeneration is the leading cause of blindness in individuals older than 65 years of age in the United States, affecting more than 1.75 million people. Because of the rapid aging of our population, this number will increase to almost 3 million by 2020.[1] More recent prevalence studies suggest that the number of persons with Alzheimer disease in the United States is 4.5 million. Given that the percentage of individuals with Alzheimer disease increases by a factor of 2 with approximately every 5 years of age, 1% of persons who are 60 years old and about 30% of those who are 85 years old have the disease. Without advances in therapy, the number of symptomatic cases in the United States is predicted to increase to 13.2 million by 2050.[2] Current annual expenditures on care for patients with Alzheimer disease exceed $84 billion,[3] a statistic that underscores the urgency of seeking more effective therapeutic and prophylactic interventions. Moreover, although apprehension is predictable in blind or potentially blind patients awaiting surgery, this problem is often exacerbated in the elderly, whose coping mechanisms may be diminished by depression or dementia.

It is mandatory to be knowledgeable about the numerous surgical procedures that are unique to the specialty of ophthalmology. Although the list of ocular surgical interventions is lengthy, these procedures may, in general, be classified as *extraocular* or *intraocular*. This distinction is critical because anesthetic considerations are different for these two major surgical categories. For example, with intraocular procedures, profound akinesia (relaxation of recti muscles) and meticulous control of intraocular pressure (IOP) are requisite. However, with extraocular surgery, the significance of IOP fades, whereas concern about elicitation of the oculocardiac reflex assumes prominence.

OCULAR ANATOMY

The anesthesiologist should be knowledgeable about ocular anatomy to enhance his or her understanding of surgical procedures and to aid the surgeon in the performance of regional blocks when needed[4] (Fig. 51-1). Salient subdivisions of ocular anatomy include the orbit, the eye itself, the extraocular muscles, the eyelids, and the lacrimal system.

The orbit is a bony box, or pyramidal cavity, housing the eyeball and its associated structures in the skull. The walls of

the orbit are composed of the following bones: frontal, zygomatic, greater wing of the sphenoid, maxilla, palatine, lacrimal, and ethmoid. A familiarity with the surface relationships of the orbital rim is mandatory for the skilled performance of regional blocks.

The optic foramen, located at the orbital apex, transmits the optic nerve and the ophthalmic artery, as well as the sympathetic nerves from the carotid plexus. The superior orbital fissure transmits the superior and inferior branches of the oculomotor nerve; the lacrimal, frontal, and nasociliary branches of the trigeminal nerve; the trochlear and abducens nerves; and the superior and inferior ophthalmic veins. The inferior orbital or sphenomaxillary fissure contains the infraorbital and zygomatic nerves and communication between the inferior ophthalmic vein and the pterygoid plexus. The infraorbital foramen, located about 4 mm below the orbital rim in the maxilla, transmits the infraorbital nerve, artery, and vein. The lacrimal fossa contains the lacrimal gland in the superior temporal orbit. The supraorbital notch, located at the junction of the medial one third and temporal two thirds of the superior orbital rim, transmits the supraorbital nerve, artery, and vein. The supraorbital notch, the infraorbital foramen, and the lacrimal fossa are clinically palpable and function as major landmarks for administration of regional anesthesia.

The eye itself is actually one large sphere with part of a smaller sphere incorporated in the anterior surface, constituting a structure with two different radii of curvature. The coat of the eye is composed of three layers: sclera, uveal tract, and retina. The fibrous outer layer, or *sclera*, is protective, providing sufficient rigidity to maintain the shape of the eye. The anterior portion of the sclera, the cornea, is transparent, permitting light to pass into the internal ocular structures. The double-spherical shape of the eye exists because the corneal arc of curvature is steeper than the scleral arc of curvature. The focusing of rays of light to form a retinal image commences at the cornea.

The *uveal tract*, or middle layer of the globe, is vascular and in direct apposition to the sclera. A potential space, known as the *suprachoroidal space*, separates the sclera from the uveal tract. This potential space, however, may become filled with blood during an expulsive or suprachoroidal hemorrhage, often associated with surgical disaster. The iris, ciliary body, and choroid compose the uveal tract. The iris includes the pupil, which controls the amount of light entering the eye by contractions of three sets of muscles. The iris dilator is sympathetically innervated; the iris sphincter and the ciliary muscle have parasympathetic innervation. Posterior to the iris lays the ciliary body, which produces aqueous humor (see "Formation and Drainage of Aqueous Humor"). The ciliary muscles, situated in the ciliary body, adjust the shape of the lens to accommodate focusing at various distances. Large vessels and a network of small vessels and capillaries known as the *choriocapillaris* constitute the choroid, which supplies nutrition to the outer part of the retina.

The *retina* is a neurosensory membrane composed of ten layers that convert light impulses into neural impulses. These neural impulses are then carried through the optic nerve to the brain. Located in the center of the globe is the vitreous cavity, filled with a gelatinous substance known as *vitreous humor.* This material is adherent to the most anterior 3 mm of the retina, as well as to large blood vessels and the optic nerve. The vitreous humor may pull on the retina, causing retinal tears and retinal detachment.

The crystalline lens, located posterior to the pupil, refracts rays of light passing through the cornea and pupil to focus images on the retina. The ciliary muscle, whose contractile state causes tautness or relaxation of the lens zonules, regulates the thickness of the lens.

In addition, six extraocular muscles move the eye within the orbit to various positions. The bilobed lacrimal gland provides most of the tear film, which serves to maintain a moist anterior surface on the globe. The lacrimal drainage system—composed of the puncta, canaliculi, lacrimal sac, and lacrimal duct—drains into the nose below the inferior turbinate. Blockage of this system occurs frequently, necessitating procedures ranging from lacrimal duct probing to dacryocystorhinostomy, which involves anastomosis of the lacrimal sac to the nasal mucosa.

Covering the surface of the globe and lining the eyelids is a mucous membrane called the *conjunctiva.* Because drugs are absorbed across the membrane, it is a popular site for administration of ophthalmic drugs.

The eyelids consist of four layers: (1) the conjunctiva, (2) the cartilaginous tarsal plate, (3) a muscle layer composed mainly of the orbicularis and the levator palpebrae, and (4) the skin. The eyelids protect the eye from foreign objects; through blinking, the tear film produced by the lacrimal gland is spread across the surface of the eye, keeping the cornea moist.

Blood supply to the eye and orbit is by means of branches of both the internal and external carotid arteries. Venous drainage of the orbit is accomplished through the multiple anastomoses of the superior and inferior ophthalmic veins. Venous drainage of the eye is achieved mainly through the central retinal vein. All these veins empty directly into the cavernous sinus.

The sensory and motor innervations of the eye and its adnexa are very complex, with multiple cranial nerves supplying branches to various ocular structures. A branch of the oculomotor nerve supplies a motor root to the ciliary ganglion, which in turn supplies the sphincter of the pupil and the ciliary muscle. The trochlear nerve supplies the superior oblique muscle. The abducens nerve supplies the lateral rectus muscle. The trigeminal nerve constitutes the most complex ocular and adnexal innervation. In addition, the zygomatic branch of the facial nerve eventually divides into an upper branch, supplying the frontalis and the upper lid orbicularis, whereas the lower branch supplies the orbicularis of the lower lid.

OCULAR PHYSIOLOGY

Despite its relatively diminutive size, the eye is a complex organ, concerned with many intricate physiologic processes. The formation and drainage of aqueous humor and their influence on IOP in both normal and glaucomatous eyes are among the most important functions, especially from the anesthesiologist's perspective. An appreciation of the effects of various anesthetic manipulations on IOP requires an understanding of the fundamental principles of ocular physiology.

Formation and Drainage of Aqueous Humor

Two thirds of the aqueous humor is formed in the posterior chamber by the ciliary body in an active secretory process involving both the carbonic anhydrase and the cytochrome oxidase systems (Fig. 51-2). The remaining third is formed by passive filtration of aqueous humor from the vessels on the anterior surface of the iris.

At the ciliary epithelium, sodium is actively transported into the aqueous humor in the posterior chamber. Bicarbonate and chloride ions passively follow the sodium ions. This active mechanism results in the osmotic pressure of the aqueous humor being many times greater than that of plasma. It is this disparity in osmotic pressure that leads to an average rate of aqueous humor production of 2 μL/min.

Aqueous humor flows from the posterior chamber through the pupillary aperture and into the anterior chamber, where it mixes with the aqueous formed by the iris. During its journey into the anterior chamber, the aqueous humor bathes the avascular lens and, once in the anterior chamber, it also bathes the corneal endothelium. Then the aqueous humor flows into the peripheral segment of the anterior chamber and exits the eye through the trabecular network, Schlemm canal, and episcleral venous system. A network of connecting venous channels eventually leads to the superior vena cava and the right atrium. Thus, obstruction of venous return at any point from the eye to the right side of the heart impedes aqueous drainage, elevating IOP accordingly.

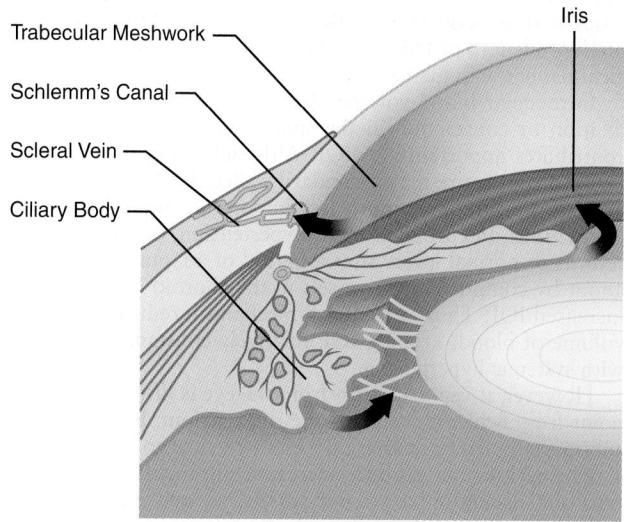

FIGURE 51-2. Ocular anatomy concerned with control of intraocular pressure.

Maintenance of Intraocular Pressure

IOP normally varies between 10 and 21.7 mm Hg and is considered abnormal above 22 mm Hg. This level varies 1 to 2 mm Hg with each cardiac contraction. Also, a diurnal variation of 2 to 5 mm Hg is observed, with a higher value noted on awakening. This higher awakening pressure has been ascribed to vascular congestion, pressure on the globe from closed lids, and mydriasis—all of which occur during sleep. If IOP is too high, it may produce opacities by interfering with normal corneal metabolism.

During anesthesia, a rise in IOP can produce permanent visual loss. If the IOP is already elevated, a further increase can trigger acute glaucoma. If penetration of the globe occurs when the IOP is excessively high, rupture of a blood vessel with subsequent hemorrhage may transpire. IOP becomes atmospheric once the eye cavity has been entered, and any sudden rise in pressure may lead to prolapse of the iris and lens, and loss of vitreous. Thus, proper control of IOP is critical.

Three main factors influence IOP: (1) external pressure on the eye by the contraction of the orbicularis oculi muscle and the tone of the extraocular muscles, venous congestion of orbital veins (as may occur with vomiting and coughing), and conditions such as orbital tumor; (2) scleral rigidity; and (3) changes in intraocular contents that are semisolid (lens, vitreous, or intraocular tumor) or fluid (blood and aqueous humor). Although these factors are significant in affecting IOP, the major control of intraocular tension is exerted by the fluid content, especially the aqueous humor.

Sclerosis of the sclera, not uncommonly seen in the elderly, may be associated with decreased scleral compliance and increased IOP. Other degenerative changes of the eye linked with aging can also influence IOP, the most significant being a hardening and enlargement of the crystalline lens. When these degenerative changes occur, they may lead to anterior displacement of the lens–iris diaphragm. A resultant shallowness of the anterior chamber angle may then occur, reducing access of the trabecular meshwork to aqueous. This process is usually gradual, but, if rapid lens engorgement occurs, angle-closure glaucoma may transpire.

Changes in the nature of the vitreous that affect the amount of unbound water also influence IOP. Myopia, trauma, and aging produce liquefaction of vitreous gel and a subsequent increase in unbound water, which may lower IOP by facilitating fluid removal. However, under different circumstances, the opposite may occur; that is, the hydration of more normal vitreous may be associated with elevation of IOP. Hence, it is often prudent to produce a slightly dehydrated state in the surgical patient with glaucoma.

Intraocular blood volume, determined primarily by vessel dilation or contraction in the spongy layers of the choroid, contributes importantly to IOP. Although changes in arterial or venous pressure may secondarily affect IOP, excursions in arterial pressure have much less importance than do venous fluctuations. In chronic arterial hypertension, ocular pressure returns to normal levels after a period of adaptation brought about by compression of vessels in the choroid as a result of increased IOP. Thus, a feedback mechanism reduces the total volume of blood, keeping IOP relatively constant in patients with systemic hypertension.

However, if venous return from the eye is disturbed at any point from Schlemm canal to the right atrium, IOP increases substantially. Trendelenburg position, cervical collar, and even a tight necktie can produce increased intraocular blood volume and distention of orbital vessels, as well as attenuated aqueous drainage.[5] Straining, vomiting, or coughing greatly increase venous pressure and raise IOP as much as 40 mm Hg or more. The deleterious implications of these activities cannot be overemphasized. Laryngoscopy and tracheal intubation may also elevate IOP, even without any visible reaction to intubation, but especially when the patient coughs. Topical anesthesia of the larynx may attenuate the systemic hypertensive response to laryngoscopy but does not reliably prevent associated increases in IOP.[6] Ordinarily, the pressure elevation from such increases in blood volume or venous pressure dissipates rapidly. However, if the coughing or straining occurs during ocular surgery when the eye is open, as in penetrating keratoplasty, the result may be a disastrous expulsive hemorrhage, at worst, or a disconcerting loss of vitreous, at best.

Despite the notable role of venous pressure, scleral rigidity, and vitreous composition, maintenance of IOP is determined primarily by the rate of aqueous formation and the rate of aqueous humor outflow. The most important influence on formation of aqueous humor is the difference in osmotic pressure between aqueous humor and plasma. This fact is illustrated by the equation:

$$IOP = K[(OPaq - OPpl) + CP] \qquad (51\text{-}1)$$

where K is coefficient of outflow, OPaq is osmotic pressure of aqueous humor, OPpl is osmotic pressure of plasma, and CP is capillary pressure. Hypertonic solutions such as mannitol are used to lower IOP because a small change in the solute concentration of plasma can markedly influence the formation of aqueous humor and hence IOP.

Fluctuations in aqueous humor outflow may also produce a dramatic alteration in IOP. The most significant factor controlling aqueous humor outflow is the diameter of Fontana spaces, as illustrated by the equation:

$$A = \frac{r^4(Piop - Pv)}{8\eta L} \qquad (51\text{-}2)$$

where A is volume of aqueous outflow per unit of time, r is radius of Fontana spaces, Piop is IOP, Pv is venous pressure, η is viscosity, and L is length of Fontana spaces. When the pupil dilates, Fontana spaces narrow, resistance to outflow is increased, and IOP rises. Because mydriasis is undesirable in both closed-angle and open-angle glaucoma, miotics such as pilocarpine are applied conjunctivally in patients with glaucoma.

Glaucoma

Glaucoma is a condition characterized by elevated IOP, resulting in impairment of capillary blood flow to the optic nerve with eventual loss of optic nerve tissue and function. Two different anatomic types of glaucoma exist: open-angle or chronic simple glaucoma, and closed-angle or acute glaucoma. (Other variations of these processes occur but are not especially germane to anesthetic management.)

With open-angle glaucoma, the elevated IOP exists with an anatomically open anterior chamber angle. It is believed that sclerosis of trabecular tissue results in impaired aqueous humor filtration and drainage. Treatment consists of medication to produce miosis and trabecular stretching. Commonly used eyedrops are epinephrine, timolol, dipivefrin, and betaxolol. Closed-angle glaucoma is characterized by the peripheral iris moving into direct contact with the posterior corneal surface, mechanically obstructing aqueous humor outflow. People who have a narrow angle between the iris and posterior cornea are predisposed to this condition. In these patients, mydriasis can produce such increased thickening of the peripheral iris that corneal touch occurs and the angle is closed. Another mechanism producing acute, closed-angle glaucoma is swelling of the crystalline lens. In this case, pupillary block occurs, with the edematous lens blocking the flow of aqueous humor from the posterior to the anterior chamber. This situation can also develop if the lens is traumatically dislocated anteriorly, thus physically blocking the anterior chamber.

It was previously believed by some clinicians that patients with glaucoma should not be given atropine. However, this claim is untenable. Atropine in the dose range used clinically has no effect on IOP in either open-angle or closed-angle glaucoma. When 0.4 mg of atropine is given parenterally to a 70-kg person, approximately 0.0001 mg is absorbed by the eye.[7] Garde et al.[8] reported, however, that scopolamine has a greater mydriatic effect than atropine and recommended not using scopolamine in patients with known or suspected closed-angle glaucoma.

Equation 51-2, describing the volume of aqueous outflow per unit of time, clearly demonstrates that outflow is exquisitely sensitive to fluctuations in venous pressure. Because a rise in venous pressure produces an increased volume of ocular blood and decreased aqueous outflow, it is obvious that considerable elevation of IOP occurs with any maneuver that increases venous pressure. Hence, in addition to preoperative instillation of miotics, other anesthetic goals for the patient with glaucoma include perioperative avoidance of venous congestion and overhydration. Furthermore, hypotensive episodes are to be avoided because these patients are allegedly vulnerable to retinal vascular thrombosis.

Primary congenital glaucoma is classified according to age of onset, with the infantile type presenting any time after birth until 3 years of age. The juvenile type presents between the ages of 37 months and 30 years. Moreover, childhood glaucoma may also occur in conjunction with various eye diseases or developmental anomalies such as aniridia, mesodermal dysgenesis syndrome, and retinopathy of prematurity.

Successful management of infantile glaucoma critically depends on early diagnosis. Presenting symptoms include epiphora, photophobia, blepharospasm, and irritability. Ocular enlargement, termed *buphthalmos,* or "ox eye," and corneal haziness secondary to edema are common. Buphthalmos is rare, however, if glaucoma develops after 3 years of age because by then the eye is much less elastic.

Because infantile glaucoma is frequently associated with obstructed aqueous humor outflow, management of it often requires surgical creation, by goniotomy or trabeculotomy, of a route for aqueous humor to flow into Schlemm canal. However, advanced disease may be unresponsive to even multiple goniotomies, and the more radical trabeculectomy or some other variety of filtering procedure may be necessary.

The juvenile form of glaucoma, in which the cornea and eye size are normal, is commonly associated with a family history of open-angle glaucoma and is treated similarly to primary open-angle glaucoma.

In cases of pediatric secondary glaucoma, goniotomy and filtering may be unsuccessful, whereas cyclocryotherapy may effect a reduction in IOP, pain, and corneal edema. The ciliary body is destroyed with a cryoprobe cooled to −70°C, thus dramatically decreasing aqueous formation.

It is essential to appreciate that the high IOP frequently encountered in infantile glaucoma can be reduced by >15 mm Hg when surgical anesthesia is achieved. However, one study demonstrated minimal effect of halothane on IOP when the concentration ranged narrowly between 0.5 and 1.0%.[9] Some clinicians maintain that ketamine is a useful drug to use for examination under anesthesia when infantile glaucoma is part of the differential diagnosis because ketamine does not appear to reduce IOP, giving a spuriously low reading. Moreover, even normal infants sporadically have pressures in the mid-20s. Hence, diagnosis is not based exclusively on the numerical pressure recorded under anesthesia. Other factors such as corneal edema and increased corneal diameter, tears in Descemet membrane, and cupping of the optic nerve are considered in making the diagnosis. If these aberrations are noted,

surgical intervention may be mandatory, even in the setting of a reputedly normal IOP.

EFFECTS OF ANESTHESIA AND ADJUVANT DRUGS ON INTRAOCULAR PRESSURE

Central Nervous System Depressants

Inhalation anesthetics purportedly cause dose-related decreases in IOP. The exact mechanisms are unknown, but postulated causes include depression of a central nervous system (CNS) control center in the diencephalon, reduction of aqueous humor production, enhancement of aqueous humor outflow, or relaxation of the extraocular muscles.[7] Moreover, virtually all CNS depressants—including barbiturates, neuroleptics, opioids, tranquilizers,[7] and hypnotics, such as etomidate and propofol—lower IOP in both normal and glaucomatous eyes. Etomidate, despite its proclivity to produce pain on intravenous injection and skeletal muscle movement, is associated with a significant reduction in IOP.[10] However, etomidate-induced myoclonus may be hazardous in the setting of a ruptured globe.

Controversy surrounds the issue of ketamine's effect on IOP. Administered intravenously or intramuscularly, ketamine initially was believed to increase IOP significantly, as measured by indentation tonometry.[11] Corssen and Hoy[12] also reported a slight but statistically significant increase in IOP that appeared unrelated to changes in blood pressure or depth of anesthesia. However, nystagmus made proper positioning of the tonometer difficult and may have resulted in less-than-accurate measurements.

Conflicting results arose from a study in which 2 mg/kg of ketamine given intravenously to adults failed to have a significant effect on IOP.[13] Furthermore, a pediatric study reported no increase in IOP after an intramuscular ketamine dose of 8 mg/kg. Indeed, values obtained were similar to those reported with halothane and isoflurane.[14,15]

Some of the confusion may arise from differences in premedication practices and from the use of different instruments to measure IOP. More recent studies have used applanation tonometry rather than indentation tonometry. However, even if future studies should confirm that ketamine has minimal or no effect on IOP, ketamine's proclivity to cause nystagmus and blepharospasm makes it a less-than-optimal agent for many types of ophthalmic surgery.

Ventilation and Temperature

Hyperventilation decreases IOP, whereas asphyxia, administration of carbon dioxide, and hypoventilation have been shown to elevate IOP.[16]

Hypothermia lowers IOP. On initial consideration, hypothermia might be expected to raise IOP because of the associated increase in viscosity of aqueous humor. However, hypothermia is linked with decreased formation of aqueous humor and with vasoconstriction; hence, the net result is a reduction in IOP.

Adjuvant Drugs

Ganglionic Blockers, Hypertonic Solutions, and Acetazolamide

Ganglionic blockers such as tetraethylammonium and pentamethonium cause a dramatic decrease in IOP. Trimethaphan also substantially lowers IOP in normal subjects, despite mydriasis.

Intravenous administration of hypertonic solutions such as dextran, urea, mannitol, and sorbitol elevates plasma osmotic pressure, thereby decreasing aqueous humor formation and reducing IOP. As effective as urea is in reducing IOP, intravenous mannitol has the advantage of fewer side effects. Mannitol's onset, peak (30 to 45 minutes), and duration of action (5 to 6 hours) are similar to those of urea. Moreover, both drugs may produce acute intravascular volume overload. Sudden expansion of plasma volume secondary to efflux of intracellular water into the vascular compartment places a heavy workload on the kidneys and heart, often resulting in hypertension and dilution of plasma sodium. Furthermore, mannitol-associated diuresis, if protracted, may trigger hypotension in volume-depleted patients.

Intravenous administration of acetazolamide inactivates carbonic anhydrase and interferes with the sodium pump. The resultant decrease in aqueous humor formation lowers IOP. However, the action of acetazolamide is not limited to the eye, and systemic effects include loss of sodium, potassium, and water secondary to the drug's renal tubular effects. Such electrolyte imbalances may then be linked to cardiac dysrhythmias during general anesthesia.

An advantage of acetazolamide is its relative ease of administration. Whereas large volumes of hypertonic solutions must be infused to reduce IOP, acetazolamide is easily given as a typical adult dose of 500 mg dissolved in 10 mL of sterile water. Acetazolamide may also be given orally, and topical carbonic anhydrase inhibitors are commercially available.

Neuromuscular Blocking Drugs

Neuromuscular blocking drugs have both direct and indirect actions on IOP. Hence, a paralyzing dose of d-tubocurarine directly lowers IOP by relaxing the extraocular muscles. The same is true of equipotent doses of the other nondepolarizing drugs, including pancuronium[17] (Fig. 51-3). However, if paralysis of the respiratory muscles is accompanied by alveolar hypoventilation, the latter secondary effect may supervene to increase IOP.

In contrast to nondepolarizing drugs, the depolarizing drug succinylcholine elevates IOP. Lincoff et al.[18] reported extrusion of vitreous after succinylcholine administration to a patient with a surgically open eye. An average peak IOP increase of about 8 mm Hg is produced within 1 to 4 minutes of an intravenous dose. Within 7 minutes, return to baseline usually transpires.[19] The ocular hypertensive effect of succinylcholine has been attributed to several mechanisms, including tonic contraction of extraocular muscles,[7] choroidal vascular dilation, and relaxation of orbital smooth muscle. One study speculates that the succinylcholine-induced increase in IOP is multifactorial

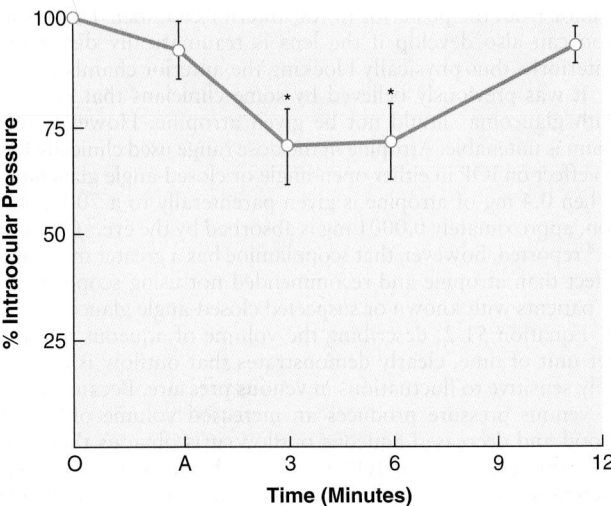

FIGURE 51-3.   Mean intraocular pressure after administration of thiopental, 3 to 4 mg/kg, and pancuronium, 0.08 mg/kg at 0. A, loss of lid reflex; *$p < 0.05$. (Reprinted from Litwiller RW, DiFazio CA, Rushia EF: Pancuronium and intraocular pressure. Anesthesiology 1975; 42: 750, with permission.)

but primarily the result of the cycloplegic action of succinylcholine, producing a deepening of the anterior chamber and increased outflow resistance.[20] Because they studied eyes with the extraocular muscles detached and still observed an elevation in IOP, these investigators proposed that changes in extraocular muscle tone do not contribute significantly to the increase in IOP observed after succinylcholine administration.

A variety of methods have been advocated to prevent succinylcholine-induced elevations in IOP. However, although some attenuation of the increase results, none of these techniques consistently and completely block the ocular hypertensive response. Prior administration of such drugs as acetazolamide, propranolol, and nondepolarizing neuromuscular blocking drugs has been suggested. The efficacy of pretreatment with nondepolarizing drugs is controversial.

In 1968, using indentation tonometry, Miller et al.[21] reported that pretreatment with small amounts of gallamine or d-tubocurarine prevented succinylcholine-associated increases in IOP. However, in 1978, using the more sensitive applanation tonometer, Meyers et al.[22] were unable to consistently circumvent the ocular hypertensive response after similar pretreatment therapy (Table 51-2). In addition, Verma[23] claimed that a "self-taming" dose of succinylcholine was protective,

TABLE 51-2

EFFECTS OF SUCCINYLCHOLINE ON INTRAOCULAR PRESSURE: DOUBLE-BLIND d-TUBOCURARINE OR GALLAMINE PRETREATMENT

		■ INTRAOCULAR PRESSURE (mm Hg, MEAN ± SE)		
■ PRETREATMENT[a]	■ MEAN AGE (yr)	BASELINE	■ 3 MIN AFTER PRETREATMENT	■ 1 MIN AFTER SUCCINYLCHOLINE[b]
d-Tubocurarine	13.4	13.0 ± 1.0	12.3 ± 1.2	24.0 ± 1.3
Gallamine	8.7	10.9 ± 1.1	10.6 ± 1.0	23.4 ± 2.3

[a]d-Tubocurarine, 0.09 mg/kg, or gallamine, 0.3 mg/kg.
[b]1 to 1.5 mg/kg intravenously.
Reprinted from Meyers EF, Krupin T, Johnson M et al: Failure of nondepolarizing neuromuscular blockers to inhibit succinylcholine-induced increased intraocular pressure: A controlled study. Anesthesiology 1978; 48: 149, with permission.

but in a controlled study using applanation tonometry, Meyers et al.[24] challenged this claim. Although intravenous pretreatment with lidocaine, 1 to 2 mg/kg, may blunt the hemodynamic response to laryngoscopy,[6,25] such therapy does not reliably prevent the ocular hypertensive response associated with succinylcholine and intubation.[26] However, Grover et al.[27] claimed that pretreatment with lidocaine, 1.5 mg/kg intravenously, 1 minute before induction with thiopental and succinylcholine offered protection from IOP increases because of succinylcholine and may therefore be of value in rapid-sequence induction for open eye injuries.

Certainly, no one would disagree that succinylcholine—if unaccompanied by pretreatment with a nondepolarizing neuromuscular blocking drug—is contraindicated in patients with penetrating ocular wounds and should not be given for the first time after the eye has been opened. Nonetheless, it is no longer valid to recommend that succinylcholine be used only with extreme reluctance in ocular surgery. Clearly, any succinylcholine-induced increment in IOP is usually dissipated before surgery is started. Of concern, however, is the warning of Jampolsky[28] that succinylcholine should be avoided in patients undergoing repeat strabismus surgery because the forced duction test (FDT) does not return to baseline for approximately 30 minutes after administration of the drug. More recent and quantitatively sophisticated studies by Dell and Williams[29] supported this caveat, although the latter investigators suggest waiting only 20 minutes after administration of succinylcholine before performing the FDT.

OCULOCARDIAC REFLEX

3 Bernard Aschner and Guiseppe Dagnini first described the oculocardiac reflex in 1908. This reflex is triggered by pressure on the globe and by traction on the extraocular muscles, as well as on the conjunctiva or the orbital structures. Moreover, the reflex may also be elicited by performance of a retrobulbar block,[30] by ocular trauma, and by direct pressure on tissue remaining in the orbital apex after enucleation. The afferent limb is trigeminal, and the efferent limb is vagal. Although the most common manifestation of the oculocardiac reflex is sinus bradycardia, a wide spectrum of cardiac dysrhythmias may occur, including junctional rhythm, ectopic atrial rhythm, atrioventricular blockade, ventricular bigeminy, multifocal premature ventricular contractions, wandering pacemaker, idioventricular rhythm, asystole, and ventricular tachycardia.[31] This reflex may appear during either local or general anesthesia; however, hypercarbia and hypoxemia are believed to augment the incidence and severity of the problem, as may inappropriate anesthetic depth.

Reports on the alleged incidence of the oculocardiac reflex are remarkable in their striking variability. Berler[30] reported an incidence of 50%, but other sources quote rates ranging from 16 to 82%. Commonly, those articles disclosing a higher incidence included children in the study population, and children tend to have more vagal tone.

A variety of maneuvers to abolish or obtund the oculocardiac reflex have been promulgated. None of these methods has been consistently effective, safe, and reliable. Inclusion of intramuscular anticholinergic drugs such as atropine or glycopyrrolate in the usual premedication regimen for oculocardiac reflex prophylaxis is ineffective.[32]

Atropine given intravenously within 30 minutes of surgery is believed to reduce incidence of the reflex. However, reports differ concerning dosage and timing. Moreover, some anesthesiologists claim that prior intravenous administration of atropine may yield more serious and refractory cardiac dysrhythmias than the reflex itself. Clearly, atropine may be considered a potential myocardial irritant. A variety of cardiac dysrhythmias[33] and several conduction abnormalities,[34] including ventricular fibrillation, ventricular tachycardia, and left bundle-branch block, have been attributed to intravenous atropine.

Although administration of retrobulbar anesthesia may provide some cardiac antidysrhythmic value by blocking the afferent limb of the reflex arc, such a regional technique is not devoid of potential complications, which include, but are not limited to, optic nerve damage, retrobulbar hemorrhage, and stimulation of the oculocardiac reflex arc by the retrobulbar block itself.

It is generally believed that the aforementioned prophylactic measures, fraught with inherent hazards, are usually not indicated in adults. If a cardiac dysrhythmia appears, initially the surgeon should be asked to cease operative manipulation. Next, the patient's anesthetic depth and ventilatory status are evaluated. Commonly, heart rate and rhythm return to baseline within 20 seconds after institution of these measures. Moreover, Moonie et al.[35] noted that, with repeated manipulation, bradycardia is less likely to recur, probably secondary to fatigue of the reflex arc at the level of the cardioinhibitory center. However, if the initial cardiac dysrhythmia is especially serious or if the reflex tenaciously recurs, atropine should be administered intravenously, but only after the surgeon stops ocular manipulation.

For pediatric strabismus surgery, however, some anesthesiologists administer intravenous atropine, 0.02 mg/kg, before commencing surgery.[36] Alternatively, glycopyrrolate, 0.01 mg/kg administered intravenously, may be associated with less tachycardia than atropine in this setting.

ANESTHETIC RAMIFICATIONS OF OPHTHALMIC DRUGS

4 There is considerable potential for drug interactions during administration of anesthesia for ocular surgery. Topical ophthalmic drugs may produce undesirable systemic effects or may have deleterious anesthetic implications. Systemic absorption of topical ophthalmic drugs may occur from either the conjunctiva or the nasal mucosa after drainage through the nasolacrimal duct. In addition, from spillover, some percutaneous absorption through the immature epidermis of the premature infant may transpire.[37] Occluding the nasolacrimal duct by pressing on the inner canthus of the eye for a few minutes after each instillation greatly decreases systemic absorption. Some of the potentially worrisome topical ocular drugs include acetylcholine, anticholinesterases, cocaine, cyclopentolate, epinephrine, phenylephrine, and timolol. In addition, intraocular sulfur hexafluoride and other intraocular gases have important anesthetic ramifications. Furthermore, certain ophthalmic drugs given systemically may produce untoward sequelae germane to anesthetic management. Drugs in this category include glycerol, mannitol, and acetazolamide.

Acetylcholine

Acetylcholine is sometimes used intraocularly after lens extraction to produce miosis. The local use of this drug occasionally may result in such systemic effects as bradycardia, increased salivation, and bronchial secretions, as well as bronchospasm. The side effects, including hypotension and bradycardia, that may develop in patients given acetylcholine after cataract extraction may be rapidly reversed with intravenous atropine. Furthermore, vagotonic anesthetic agents such as halothane can accentuate the effects of acetylcholine.

Anticholinesterase Agents

Echothiophate, also known as *phospholine iodide*, is a long-acting anticholinesterase miotic that lowers IOP by decreasing resistance to the outflow of aqueous humor. It is used to treat glaucoma that is refractory to other therapies and also to treat some children with accommodative esotropia. It is absorbed into the systemic circulation after instillation in the conjunctival sac. Any of the long-acting anticholinesterases may prolong the action of succinylcholine because, after ≥1 month of therapy, plasma pseudocholinesterase activity may be <5% of normal. It is said, moreover, that normal enzyme activity does not return until 4 to 6 weeks after discontinuation of the drug.[38] Hence, the anesthesiologist should anticipate prolonged apnea after a usual dose of succinylcholine. In addition, a delay in metabolism of ester local anesthetics should be expected.

Cocaine

Cocaine, introduced to ophthalmology in 1884 by Koller, has limited topical ocular use because it can cause corneal pits and erosion. However, as the only local anesthetic that inherently produces vasoconstriction and shrinkage of mucous membranes, cocaine is commonly used in nasal packs during dacryocystorhinostomy. The drug is so well absorbed from mucosal surfaces that plasma concentrations are achieved that are comparable to those after direct intravenous injection. Because cocaine interferes with catecholamine uptake, it has a sympathetic nervous system potentiating effect.

The usual maximal dose of cocaine used in clinical practice is 200 mg for a 70-kg adult, or 3 mg/kg. Although 1 g is considered to be the usual lethal dose for an adult, considerable variation occurs. Furthermore, systemic reactions may appear with as little as 20 mg.

Meyers[39] described two cases of cocaine toxicity during dacryocystorhinostomy, underscoring that cocaine is contraindicated in hypertensive patients or in patients receiving drugs such as tricyclic antidepressants or monoamine oxidase inhibitors. In addition, sympathomimetics, such as epinephrine or phenylephrine, should not be given with cocaine.

Obviously, before administering cocaine or another potent vasoconstrictor for dacryocystorhinostomy, the physician should carefully search out possible contraindications. To avoid toxic levels, doses of dilute solutions should be meticulously calculated and carefully administered. If serious cardiovascular effects occur, labetalol should be used to counteract them.[40] Propanolol should not be administered in this situation owing to the potential to exacerbate hypertension as a result of unopposed α-adrenergic stimulation. Labetalol offers the advantages of combined α-blockade and β-blockade. Additionally, labetalol is preferable to esmolol because of its longer duration of action. It is important to appreciate, however, that labetalol has not been shown to reverse coronary artery vasoconstriction in humans. In the setting of cocaine-associated chest pain and/or myocardial infarction, β-blockers should not be administered acutely. Rather, nitroglycerin should be given.

Cyclopentolate

Despite the popularity of cyclopentolate as a mydriatic, it is not without side effects, which include CNS toxicity. Manifestations include dysarthria, disorientation, and frank psychotic reactions. Purportedly, CNS dysfunction is more likely to follow use of the 2% solution as opposed to the 1% solution. Furthermore, cases of convulsions in children after ocular instillation of cyclopentolate have been reported. Hence, for pediatric use, 0.5 to 1.0% solutions are recommended. At higher concentrations, cyclopentolate also causes cycloplegia.

Epinephrine

Although topical epinephrine has proved useful in some patients with open-angle glaucoma, the 2% solution has been associated with such systemic effects as nervousness, hypertension, angina pectoris, tachycardia, and other dysrhythmias.[41]

Some anesthesiologists have maintained that it is unwise to use topical or intraocular epinephrine in patients being anesthetized with a halogenated hydrocarbon. However, the iris, with its rich supply of adrenergic receptors, is able to capture with extreme rapidity the epinephrine given into the eye. Apparently, there is not much systemic absorption from the globe.

Phenylephrine

Pupillary dilation and capillary decongestion are reliably produced by topical phenylephrine. Although systemic effects secondary to topical application of prudent doses are rare,[42] severe hypertension, headache, tachycardia, and tremulousness have been reported.

In patients with coronary artery disease, severe myocardial ischemia, cardiac dysrhythmias, and even myocardial infarction may develop after topical 10% eyedrops. Those with cerebral aneurysms may be susceptible to cerebral hemorrhage after phenylephrine in this concentration. In general, a safe systemic level follows absorption from either the conjunctiva or the nasal mucosa after drainage by the tear ducts. However, phenylephrine should not be given in the eye after surgery has begun and venous channels are patent.

Children are especially vulnerable to overdose and may respond in a dramatic and adverse fashion to phenylephrine drops. Hence, the use of only 2.5%, rather than 10%, phenylephrine is recommended in infants and the elderly, and the frequency of application should be strictly limited in these patient populations.

Timolol and Betaxolol

Timolol, a nonselective β-adrenergic blocking drug, historically has been a popular antiglaucoma drug. Because significant conjunctival absorption may occur, timolol should be administered with caution to patients with known obstructive airway disease, congestive heart failure, or greater than first-degree heart block. Life-threatening asthmatic crises have been reported after the administration of timolol drops to some patients with chronic, stable asthma.[43] The development of severe sinus bradycardia in a patient with cardiac conduction defects (left anterior hemiblock, first-degree atrioventricular block, and incomplete right bundle branch block) has been reported after timolol.[44] Moreover, timolol has been implicated in the exacerbation of myasthenia gravis[45] and in the production of postoperative apnea in neonates and young infants.[46]

In contrast to timolol, a newer antiglaucoma drug, betaxolol, a β$_1$-blocker, is said to be more oculospecific and have minimal systemic effects.[47] However, patients receiving an oral beta-blocker and betaxolol should be observed for potential additive effect on known systemic effects of β-blockade. Caution should be exercised in patients receiving catecholamine-depleting drugs. Although betaxolol has produced only minimal effects in patients with obstructive airway disease, caution should be exercised in the treatment of patients with excessive restriction of pulmonary function. Moreover, betaxolol is contraindicated in patients with sinus bradycardia, congestive heart failure, greater than first-degree heart block, cardiogenic shock, and overt myocardial failure.

TABLE 51-3

DIFFERENTIAL SOLUBILITIES OF GASES

	■ BLOOD: GAS PARTITION COEFFICIENTS
Sulfur hexafluoride	0.004
Nitrogen	0.015
Nitrous oxide	0.468

Intraocular Sulfur Hexafluoride

For a patient with a retinal detachment, intraocular sulfur hexafluoride or other gases, such as certain perfluorocarbons, may be injected into the vitreous to facilitate reattachment mechanically. These recommendations do not apply to open-eye procedures, during which volume and pressure changes are readily compensated for by fluid and gas leak.

Stinson and Donlon[48] suggested terminating nitrous oxide 15 minutes before gas injection to prevent significant changes in the size of the intravitreous gas bubble. The patient is then given virtually 100% oxygen, or a combination of oxygen and air (admixed with a small percentage of volatile agent), for the balance of the operation without adversely affecting intravitreous gas dynamics. Furthermore, if a patient requires reoperation and general anesthesia after intravitreous gas injection, nitrous oxide should be avoided for 5 days subsequent to air injection and for 10 days after sulfur hexafluoride injection[49] (Table 51-3).

Perfluoropropane and octafluorocyclobutane may also be used in vitreoretinal surgery to support the retina. Like sulfur hexafluoride, these gases are relatively insoluble and require discontinuance of nitrous oxide at least 15 minutes before injection. If the patient requires reoperation, it must be remembered that perfluoropropane lingers in the eye for longer than 30 days.[50] A Medic-Alert bracelet might be helpful in these circumstances.

Systemic Ophthalmic Drugs

In addition to topical and intraocular therapies, various ophthalmic drugs given systemically may result in complications of concern to the anesthesiologist. These systemic drugs include glycerol, mannitol, and acetazolamide. For example, oral glycerol may be associated with nausea, vomiting, and risk of aspiration. Hyperglycemia or glycosuria, disorientation, and seizure activity may also occur after oral glycerol.

The recommended intravenous dose of mannitol is 1.5 g/kg given over a 30- to 60-minute interval. However, serious systemic problems may result from rapid infusion of large doses of mannitol. These complications include renal failure, congestive heart failure, pulmonary congestion, electrolyte imbalance, hypotension or hypertension, myocardial ischemia, and, rarely, allergic reactions. Clearly, the patient's renal and cardiovascular status must be thoroughly evaluated before mannitol therapy.

Acetazolamide, a carbonic anhydrase inhibitor with renal tubular effects, should be considered contraindicated in patients with marked hepatic or renal dysfunction or in those with low sodium levels or abnormal potassium values. As is well known, severe electrolyte imbalances can trigger serious cardiac dysrhythmias during general anesthesia. Furthermore, people with chronic lung disease may be vulnerable to the development of severe acidosis with long-term aceta-

zolamide therapy. Topically active carbonic anhydrase inhibitors have been developed, are now commercially available, and appear to be relatively free of clinically important systemic effects.

PREOPERATIVE EVALUATION

Establishing Rapport and Assessing Medical Condition

Preoperative preparation and evaluation of the patient begin with the establishment of rapport and communication among the anesthesiologist, the surgeon, and the patient. Most patients realize that surgery and anesthesia entail inherent risks, and they appreciate a candid explanation of potential complications, balanced with information concerning probability or frequency of permanent adverse sequelae. Such an approach also fulfills the medicolegal responsibilities of the physician to obtain informed consent.

A thorough history of the patient and physical examination are the foundation of safe patient care. Questionnaires, in lieu of medical evaluation, lack sensitivity to detect pertinent medical issues.[51] A complete list of medications that the patient is currently taking, both systemic and topical, must be obtained so potential drug interactions can be anticipated and essential medication will be administered during the hospital stay. Naturally, a history of any allergies to medicines, foods, or tape should be documented. Clearly, knowledge of any personal or family history of adverse reactions to anesthesia is mandatory. The requisite laboratory data vary, depending on the medical history and physical status of the patient, as well as the nature of the surgical procedure. Indeed, the American Society of Anesthesiologists (ASA) task force on preoperative evaluation concluded that routine preoperative tests are commonly not useful in assessing and managing patients' perioperative experience. In a more recent multicenter study of cataract patients, for example, Schein et al.[52] demonstrated that "routine" testing does not improve patient safety or outcome. Some physicians and laypersons misinterpreted the results and conclusions of this investigation, believing that patients having cataract surgery need no preoperative evaluation. It is vital to note that all patients in this trial received regular medical care and were evaluated by a physician preoperatively. Patients whose medical status indicated a need for preoperative laboratory tests were excluded from the study. Clearly, testing should be based on the results of the history and physical examination. Because "routine" testing for the >1.5 million cataract operations in the United States is estimated to cost $150 million annually, the favorable economic impact of this "targeted" approach is obvious.

Many elderly adult candidates for ophthalmic surgery are on antiplatelet or anticoagulant therapy because of a history of coronary or vascular pathology. Such patients are at higher risk for perioperative hemorrhagic events, including retrobulbar hemorrhage, circumorbital hematoma, intravitreous bleeding, and hyphema. Traditionally, antiplatelet and anticoagulant medications were withheld for an appropriate length of time before eye surgery. However, this strategy may increase the risk of such adverse events as myocardial ischemia or infarction, cerebrovascular accident, and deep venous thrombosis. Several studies exploring this controversial issue suggest that cataract and other ophthalmic procedures can be safely performed under regional anesthesia without discontinuing anticoagulants,[53,54] especially if the prothrombin time is approximately 1.5 times control.[55] A more recent multicenter study of almost 20,000 cataract patients older than 50 years of age attempted to establish the risks and benefits of continuing aspirin or warfarin therapy.[56] Despite the large population studied, the rate of complications was so low that absolute differences in risk were minimal. Patients who continued therapy did not have more ocular hemorrhage; those who discontinued treatment did not have a greater incidence of medical events. Nonetheless, it is critical to appreciate that these investigations focused specifically on cataract operations. Oculoplastic or retinal surgery may be another matter.

Another area of potential concern involves patients whose coronary artery disease is being managed with drug-eluting stents. Although bare-metal stents are susceptible to in-stent restenosis, drug-eluting stents are more vulnerable to stent thrombosis, a complication with a high mortality rate. Thus, patients with drug-eluting stents are typically on dual antiplatelet therapy with aspirin and clopidogrel for extended periods of time. Although prospective trials are clearly needed, a conclusion that is emerging is that the risk of thrombotic complications in patients with drug-eluting stents appears to heavily outweigh the risk of bleeding complications.[57] Therefore, given current information, a convincing case can be made for continuing dual antiplatelet therapy in the perioperative period.[58]

Eye surgery patients are often at the extremes of age, ranging from premature babies with retinopathy of prematurity to nonagenarians. Hence, special age-related considerations such as altered pharmacokinetics and pharmacodynamics apply. In addition, elderly patients frequently have multiple comorbidities that include thyroid dysfunction, cardiopulmonary, and renal diseases. Hypertension is encountered in the majority of geriatric patients. Those with poorly controlled blood pressure should not receive dilating eye drops, such as phenylephrine, without consulting an anesthesiologist. Systemic absorption of high concentrations (e.g., >2.5% phenylephrine) or improperly instilled mydriatics can precipitate a hypertensive crisis with potentially devastating consequences.

As our society becomes increasingly geriatric, the number of ophthalmic surgery patients presenting with implanted cardiac defibrillators (ICDs) and pacemakers grows. The theoretical possibility of eye injury from patient movement in the event of ICD discharge during surgery exists. Although there is a broad spectrum of ophthalmic surgical procedures, the majority of cases use minimal bipolar cautery. For some, such as clear-corneal cataract surgery, no cautery is used. Thus, there is low risk of electromagnetic interference precipitating device discharge. Despite multitudinous procedures performed each year, there have not been any case reports of ICD activation during ophthalmic surgery and none of the device manufacturers have documented such an incident.[59,60] A retrospective survey of ophthalmic-anesthesia providers found that >80% did not use a magnet to reprogram or inactivate an ICD before surgery.[60]

Perioperative movement is a possible cause of patient eye injury and potential anesthesiologist liability. An analysis of ophthalmic monitored anesthesia care (MAC) closed claims cases that resulted in blindness or poor visual outcome found that >80% were associated with inadequate anesthesia and/or patient movement either during the block or intraoperatively.[61] Cough, orthopnea, and restlessness are the most common precipitators of excessive motion. Intraoperative movement during general anesthesia may also induce dire visual consequences. Because most ophthalmic surgical procedures are elective, should an enhanced risk of perioperative movement be noted during the preoperative assessment, the prudent course may be to postpone surgery until the patient is in optimal condition to remain relatively still,[62] or to perform the procedure under general anesthesia. Deliberate patient selection is requisite in order to prescribe the optimal anesthesia care plan.

The anesthesiologist must be aware of the anesthetic implications of congenital and metabolic diseases with ocular manifestations. Diabetic patients often present with ocular complications, and the anesthesiologist must be knowledgeable about the systemic disturbances of physiology that affect these patients. Indeed, the list of congenital and metabolic diseases associated with ocular pathologic effects that have important anesthetic implications is lengthy. A partial summary includes syndromes such as Crouzon, Apert, Goldenhar (oculoauriculovertebral dysplasia), Sturge-Weber, Marfan, Lowe (oculocerebrorenal syndrome), Down (trisomy 21), Wagner-Stickler, and Riley-Day (familial dysautonomia). Other diseases in this category are homocystinuria, malignant hyperthermia, myotonia dystrophica, and sickle cell disease.[63]

Anesthesia Options

The requirements of ophthalmic surgery include safety, akinesia, analgesia, minimal bleeding, avoidance or obtundation of the oculocardiac reflex, prevention of intraocular hypertension, awareness of drug interactions, and a smooth emergence devoid of vomiting, coughing, or retching (Table 51-1). Moreover, the exigencies of ophthalmic anesthesia mandate that the anesthesiologist be positioned remote from the patient's airway, sometimes creating certain logistic problems.

A number of anesthetic options exist, including general anesthesia, retrobulbar block, peribulbar anesthesia, sub-Tenon (episcleral) block, topical anesthesia, and intracameral injection. General anesthesia is administered for most children. Some adolescent and most adult patients can be cared for with regional or topical anesthesia and MAC, with or without sedation. The choice of anesthesia technique should be individualized based on the patient's needs and preferences, the nature and duration of the procedure, and the preferences and skills of the anesthesiologist and the surgeon.

Traditionally, the most commonly selected regional anesthetic technique for cataract surgery had been the retrobulbar block. Since the mid-1990s, peribulbar injection has surpassed retrobulbar block in popularity because of a relatively superior safety profile. Recently, however, topical analgesia has become more commonly used for cataract surgery in the United States (59% vs. 41% for block techniques),[64] and sub-Tenon blocks have surged in popularity in the United Kingdom and New Zealand.[65] Anesthesia for adult patients undergoing retina surgery is still accomplished primarily with peribulbar or retrobulbar block,[66] although some surgeons prefer general anesthesia for certain patients. More recently, anesthesiologists have had increasing interest in administering ocular anesthesia, and workshops in ophthalmic regional anesthesia are often conducted at major regional and national meetings. Many ophthalmologists and administrators encourage anesthesiologists to administer the blocks to facilitate operating room efficiency.

When a regional anesthetic of the orbit is administered, either by the anesthesiologist or the ophthalmologist, it is the responsibility of the anesthesiologist to monitor the patient's vital signs, electrocardiogram (ECG), and oxygen saturation. Sedation may be administered before performance of the block and/or initiation of surgery. The anesthesiologist must be vigilant for the oculocardiac reflex, signs of brainstem anesthesia, and the need for airway support or other interventions.

Side of Anesthesia and Surgery

In an attempt to ensure proper patient, side, site, and procedure selection, The Joint Commission (formerly known as the Joint Commission on Accreditation of Healthcare Organizations) held a "Wrong Site Summit" in May 2003 in which they developed a "Universal Protocol for Preventing Wrong Site,

Wrong Procedure, Wrong Person Surgery." The policy is tripartite, involving preoperative verification, marking of the intended site, and a "time-out" immediately before the start of surgery.[67] Patient involvement and effective communication are key components.

Ophthalmologic surgery and regional anesthesia confer greater risk than many other surgical procedures owing to the potential for laterality errors. Patients (and medical staff) may be confused as to the side, site, or actual procedure. Sedatives or anesthetic agents may enhance the likelihood of error. Some patients, such as children and infants, may lack the competence to intervene. Similarity of names can be conducive to mistakes. Procedural factors may be contributory; a wrong side may be draped or prepared, a patient's cap may obscure a clearly marked surgical site. Human factors play a key role in the problem. Failure to cross-check consent forms, patient charts, and patients, tragically, occasionally still occurs. Our distraction-rich environment, coupled with dysfunctional verbal/written communication, and lack of proper adherence to safety protocols also play a role.

Anesthesia Techniques

More than 40 years ago, it was common for ophthalmic procedures to involve large ocular incisions. General endotracheal anesthesia, with deep and sustained neuromuscular paralysis and placement of sandbags to surround the patient's head, were typical strategies to ensure perioperative immobility. In more recent years, general anesthesia typically has been reserved for children and adults who are unable to communicate, cooperate, or remain suitably stationary. Although endotracheal anesthesia is necessary for patients at risk of aspiration, the laryngeal mask airway (LMA) has been increasingly accepted as a means to secure the airway in patients with no risk factors for aspiration who are having eye surgery with general anesthesia.[68] The LMA is not only safe and effective in this setting, but it also offers the advantage of less increase in IOP on insertion and removal than is encountered with an endotracheal tube.[69] Similarly, less bucking and coughing on emergence and during the recovery phase have been noted.[70] Vigilance must be maintained, however, to detect initial misplacement or intraoperative displacement of the LMA. In addition, intraoperative laryngospasm in infants and neonates is not uncommon with an LMA.

Retrobulbar and Peribulbar Blocks

Needle-based ophthalmic regional anesthesia was first described by Knapp[71] in 1884. Then, in the early 20th century, Atkin-

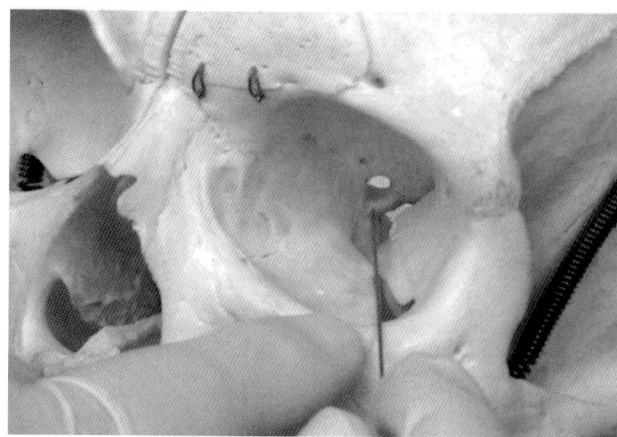

FIGURE 51-5. Needle placement for retrobulbar block.

son[72] introduced the retrobulbar block. Retrobulbar block is a practical means to achieve analgesia and profound akinesia of the globe. The peribulbar block is a more recently introduced needle-based technique that varies from the retrobulbar block in terms of the depth and angulation of needle placement within the orbit. Traditionally, the four rectus muscles, along with connective tissue septae, were believed to create a defined compartment known as the *orbital cone*. This so-called cone extends from the rectus muscle origins around the optic foramen at the apex of the orbit to the attachment of the muscles to the globe anteriorly. Retrobulbar blocks are accomplished by directing a needle toward the orbital apex with sufficient depth and angulation such that the cone is penetrated (Figs. 51-4 and 51-5).[73] Local anesthetic is then instilled in the cone, behind the eye. Cadaveric dissections, however, have shown the fallacy of the classic concept of the cone. There is no complete intermuscular septum encircling the rectus muscles, linking them together to form an impermeable compartment behind the globe akin to the brachial plexus sheath in the axilla.[74]

Ripart et al.[75] clearly demonstrated that extraconal injections of dye into cadaveric specimens diffused into the intraconal space, and solutions placed within the cone distributed to the extraconal space. Thus, the peribulbar block is executed by directing a needle to less depth and with minimal angulation, parallel to the globe, toward the greater wing of the sphenoid bone (Figs. 51-6 and 51-7). Local anesthetic instilled in this extraconal space will eventually penetrate toward the optic nerve and other structures, establishing conduction anesthesia.

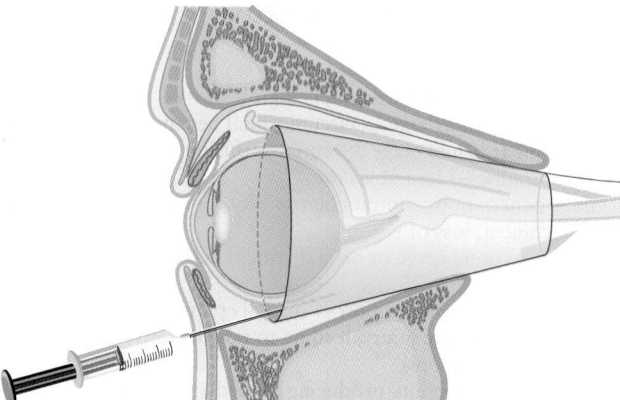

FIGURE 51-4. Retrobulbar (intraconal) block and schematic representation of the intraorbital muscle cone.

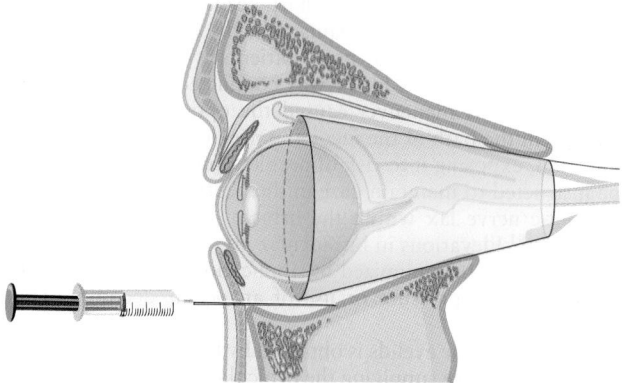

FIGURE 51-6. Peribulbar (extraconal) block and schematic representation of the intraorbital muscle cone.

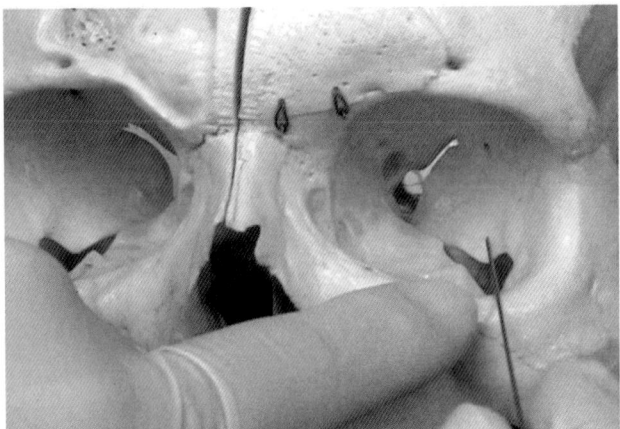

FIGURE 51-7.   Needle placement for peribulbar block.

The peribulbar block is theoretically safer because the needle tip is kept at a greater distance from vital intraorbital structures and brain.

A retrobulbar, or so-called intraconal block, positions local anesthetics deep within the orbit proximate to the nerves and muscle origins. Thus, it requires low volume, has rapid onset, and yields intense depth of anesthesia. The peribulbar, or extraconal block, placed further from the optic and other orbital nerves, requires larger volumes of local anesthetic and has longer latency of onset. The needle entry point for both blocks is at the same inferotemporal location. The junction of the lateral third and medial two thirds of the inferior orbital rim in line with the lateral limbal margin has been the conventional access point. However, locating the needle entry point more laterally may serve to decrease the likelihood of injecting local anesthetics into the delicate inferior rectus muscle. This is important because intramuscular injection of anesthetics has been postulated as a potential cause of postoperative strabismus.[76] Medial approaches at the caruncle have also been popularized more recently.[77] Supplementation of anesthesia with an injection above the globe may not be prudent because the preponderance of vessels lie in the superior orbit. In addition, the belly of the superior oblique muscle and the trochlear muscle can be encountered superonasally.

Katsev et al.[78] demonstrated that the tips of commonly used 1.5-inch (38-mm) needles can reach critical structures in the densely packed apex of the orbit in almost 20% of retrobulbar blocks. Consequently, 1.25-inch (31-mm) needles are appropriate. Controversy exists over the advantages of sharp versus dull needles. Dull needles may require more force to penetrate the globe. However, sharp needles are less painful to insert and may cause less damage in the face of inadvertent globe puncture.[79] In the past, patients were asked to gaze superonasally while a block was conducted. Unsold et al.[80] found that this maneuver caused the optic nerve to stretch directly in the path of the incoming needle during retrobulbar injection, exposing it to risk of needle trauma. Patients should be instructed to maintain gaze in the neutral position, leaving the optic nerve lax within the orbit in the course of needle insertion.[81] Elevations in intraocular pressure after a retrobulbar block can be minimized by application of gentle noncontinuous digital pressure or use of an ocular decompression device.[82]

Akinesia of the eyelids is obtained by blocking the branches of the facial nerve supplying the orbicularis muscle. Lid akinesia is often a direct consequence of the larger volume of local anesthetic used for peribulbar blocks. Retrobulbar blocks, in contrast, often leave the orbicularis oculi fully functional.

Thus, a facial nerve block is performed in conjunction with retrobulbar block to prevent squeezing of the eyelid that could result in extrusion of intraocular contents during corneal transplantation, for example. Since facial nerve block was first used for ophthalmic surgery by Van Lint in 1914, numerous methods of facial nerve blockade have been described. These techniques block the facial nerve after its exit point from the skull in the stylomastoid foramen. Moving distally to proximally to the foramen, the techniques include the Van Lint, Atkinson, O'Brien, and Nadbath-Rehman methods. Although each has advantages and disadvantages, the Nadbath-Rehman approach can potentially produce the most serious systemic consequences. With this approach, a 27-gauge, 12-mm needle is inserted between the mastoid process and the posterior border of the mandibular ramus. Because of the proximity of the jugular foramen (10 mm medial to the stylomastoid foramen) to the injection site, ipsilateral paralysis of cranial nerves IX, X, and XI can occur, producing hoarseness, dysphagia, pooling of secretions, agitation, respiratory distress, or laryngospasm. Moreover, because the Nadbath-Rehman block produces complete hemifacial akinesia that interferes with oral intake, this approach is not recommended for outpatients.

6 Complications associated with needle-based ophthalmic anesthetics may be local or systemic, and may result in blindness or even death (Table 51-4). Bleeding may be superficial or deep, arterial or venous. Superficial hemorrhage may produce an unsightly circumorbital hematoma. Retrobulbar hemorrhage, when arterially based, may produce precipitous bleeding and a palpable, dramatic increase in IOP, as well as globe proptosis and entrapment of the upper lid. With the globe's vascular supply in jeopardy, the patient's long-term ultimate visual acuity may be quickly compromised. Consultation with an ophthalmologist should be immediately sought, and fundoscopic examination, tonometric measurement of IOP, ultrasound to assess presence/location of blood, and even a lateral canthotomy may be warranted. Continuous ECG monitoring is indicated because the oculocardiac reflex may occur as blood extravasates from the muscle cone. The decision to proceed with surgery in the presence of a mild or moderate hemorrhage depends on numerous factors, including the degree of bleeding, the nature of the planned ophthalmologic surgery, and the patient's condition.

Penetration of the sclera is a distinct, although rare, possibility with needle-based anesthesia techniques. Mechanical trauma, with potential retinal detachment, and chemical

---

TABLE 51-4

COMPLICATIONS OF NEEDLE-BASED OPHTHALMIC ANESTHESIA

Stimulation of oculocardiac reflex arc
Superficial hemorrhage → circumorbital hematoma
Retrobulbar hemorrhage ± retinal perfusion compromise → loss of vision
Globe penetration ± intraocular injection → retinal detachment, loss of vision
Trauma to optic nerve or orbital cranial nerves → loss of vision
Optic nerve sheath injection → orbital epidural anesthesia
Extraocular muscle injury, leading to postoperative strabismus, diplopia
Intra-arterial injection, producing immediate convulsions
Central retinal artery occlusion
Inadvertent brainstem anesthesia → contralateral amaurosis, neurocardiopulmonary compromise

injury to delicate retina tissue caused by local anesthetics can occur. Blindness or very poor vision may be the result. Globe puncture is defined as a single entry into the eye, whereas perforation is caused by two full-thickness wounds—an entry and a subsequent exit. The globe's posterior pole is the most commonly penetrated area. Risk factors for posterior pole needle injury include presence of an elongated globe, recessed orb, and/or atypical-shaped eye. The anteroposterior distance of an eye may be long because of myopia or presence of globe-enveloping intraorbital hardware such as a scleral buckle. Some patients have an abnormal outpouching of the eye, termed *staphyloma*. Most staphyloma are located at the posterior of the globe, surrounding the juncture of the eye with the optic nerve. By definition, a retrobulbar anesthetic is conducted by purposefully angling the needle steeply and deeply within the orbit behind the globe. If the globe is longer than one assumes, it is at greater risk of penetration or puncture by the retrobulbar needle. In one study, ultrasound detection determined that the tip of the needle, placed in retrobulbar fashion, can be much closer to the posterior pole of the globe than presupposed by physicians.[83] Peribulbar anesthesia entails shallower placement of the needle without directing the needle inward toward the orbital apex; thus, it is associated with a lower incidence of globe-needle injury. Be aware, however, that it is still possible to engage the needle with sclera laterally.

The risk of penetrating the sclera with a needle is also inversely proportional to the anesthesiologist's education and experience. This notion is affirmed by several reports of globe injuries rendered by inadequately educated or trained personnel in the early 1990s.[84] In a survey of 284 directors of anesthesiology and ophthalmology programs, no formal training or education in ophthalmic regional anesthesia techniques was provided to anesthesia residents in most academic programs.[85] This survey concluded that anesthesiologists who perform needle-based ophthalmic blocks should have knowledge of orbital anatomy and the ocular risk factors that were noted previously. Thus, appropriate preanesthesia history-taking includes direct interrogation concerning myopia or previous scleral buckle surgery, as both imply increased globe length. Physical examination of surface anatomy should note the position of the globe within the orbit and whether enophthalmos is present. A recessed eye is at greater risk of needle-tip misadventure. The most important laboratory examination is the preoperative ultrasound. For patients undergoing cataract surgery, an ultrasound is *always* performed to calculate the appropriate intraocular lens to insert intraoperatively. Additionally, it reveals the length and shape of the eye. An axial length >26 mm confers greater risk of perforation. In the event that the ultrasound report is not found in the patient's chart, the anesthesiologist should inquire about the results before embarking on a needle-based block.

In the future, portable real-time ultrasonography may have a role in reducing the risk of penetrating injury (Fig. 51-8). The eye is easily accessible, its geometry and surrounding elements are relatively straightforward, and the tissue contents of the orbit lack gas-filled or osseous structures, making this an ideal area for ultrasonic imaging. Suitable transducers need to be developed and machines need to be more readily available.[86]

Brainstem anesthesia and inadvertent intravascular injection of local anesthetics are two additional potentially devastating consequences of needle-based ocular anesthesia. In the course of accidental intravascular arterial injection, local anesthetics flow from the needle via a branch of the ophthalmic artery in retrograde fashion to the internal carotid artery and then to the Circle of Willis. Rapid redistribution of local anesthetic to the brain results in immediate onset of convulsions, and cardiopulmonary instability may also occur. Although the incidence of brainstem anesthesia is rare, it is even less common with peribulbar versus retrobulbar blocks. Brainstem

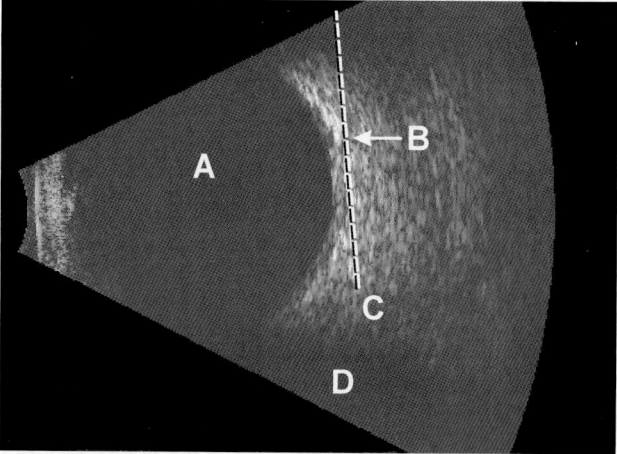

FIGURE 51-8. Ultrasound-guided block with overlay. **A.** Globe. **B.** Needle shaft. **C.** Needle tip. **D.** Optic nerve.

anesthesia is a consequence of the direct spread of local anesthetic agents to the brain along the meningeal sheath surrounding the optic nerve. In contradistinction to intra-arterial injection, symptoms are not always immediate. There is a continuum of sequelae dependent on the concentration and volume of drug that gains access centrally, as well as the specific areas into which the anesthetic spreads (Fig. 51-9). One case report described the insidious onset of unconsciousness and apnea over 7 minutes, without concomitant seizures or cardiovascular collapse.[87] Nicoll et al.[88] reported 16 cases of apparently central spread of anesthetics in a series of 6,000 retrobulbar blocks. Eight patients developed respiratory arrest. Other protean CNS signs may include violent shivering; contralateral amaurosis; eventual loss of consciousness; apnea; and hemiplegia, paraplegia, quadriplegia, or hyperreflexia.

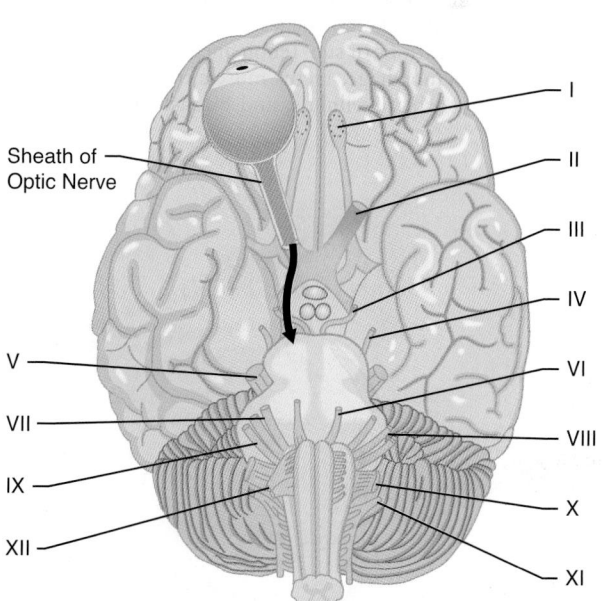

FIGURE 51-9. Base of the brain and the path that local anesthetic agents might follow if inadvertently injected into the subarachnoid space. This route includes the cranial nerves, pons, and midbrain. (Reprinted from Javitt JC, Addiego R, Friedberg HL et al: Brain stem anesthesia after retrobulbar block. Ophthalmology 1987; 94: 718, with permission).

Blockade of cranial nerves VIII to XII results in deafness, vertigo, vagolysis, dysphagia, aphasia, and loss of neck muscle power. It is axiomatic that personnel skilled in airway maintenance and ventilatory and circulatory support should be immediately available whenever retrobulbar or other needle-based anesthetic blocks are administered.

Cannula-Based Techniques

Cannula-based ophthalmic regional anesthesia was first described by Swan[89] in 1956. The sub-Tenon block was rediscovered and popularized in the 1990s as another practical means to achieve analgesia and akinesia of the globe, while offering potential advantages in certain circumstances over needle-based blocks.[90] Imaging studies have shown that local anesthetics instilled beneath Tenon capsule spread into the posterior orbit.[91] The block is accomplished by inserting a blunt cannula through a small incision in the conjunctiva and Tenon capsule, also known as the *episcleral membrane*, with subsequent infusion of local anesthetics (Fig. 51-10). Onset of analgesia is rapid. The ultimate extent of globe akinesia is proportional to the volume of local anesthetic injected. One large prospective study by Guise[92] of 6,000 such blocks found this technique to be highly effective. Advantages, particularly for very myopic patients who have elongated axial lengths, include decreased risk of posterior pole perforation because needles are not placed into the posterior orbit.

After application of topical anesthetic, the episcleral space can be accessed from all quadrants with blunt-tipped scissors; however, the incision is most commonly made in the inferonasal quadrant. The cannula is guided through the opening with the aid of a toothless forceps. It is common for local anesthetics to leak retrograde out of the incision site. Conjunctival bleeding, chemosis, and ballooning up of the conjunctiva are common. Fortunately, these are cosmetic issues that rarely affect outcome. Guise[92] estimated the incidence of minor hemorrhage to be <10% and had to abandon only one case because of a large subconjunctival hemorrhage that was not sight-threatening. Thus, the sub-Tenon block may be a prudent ocular anesthesia technique for the anticoagulated patient at risk for retrobulbar hemorrhage.

Major complications of sub-Tenon anesthesia include globe perforation,[93] hemorrhage, rectus muscle trauma, postoperative strabismus, orbital cellulitis, and brainstem anesthesia.[94]

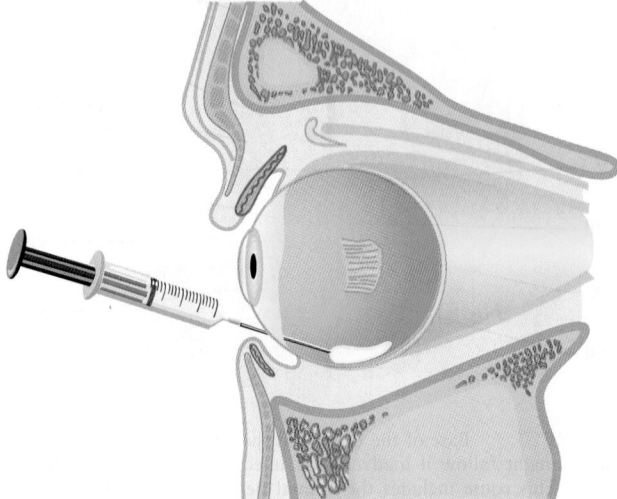

FIGURE 51-10. Sub-Tenon (episcleral) block with blunt cannula.

More complications are reported with longer (18 to 25 mm), rigid, metallic cannulae. Shorter (12 mm), more flexible, plastic cannulae may be preferable; however, they are associated with a higher incidence of conjunctival hemorrhage and chemosis. Variations of sub-Tenon blocks include ultrashort cannulae (6 mm) and needle-based episcleral block techniques.[95] There has been a report of a death associated with a sub-Tenon block, potentially secondary to central spread of local anesthetic.[96] However, the definitive pathogenesis remains an enigma.[97]

Topical Analgesia

Ophthalmologists have also been returning to a technique that was popularized during the early 1900s—the use of topical anesthetic agents, particularly when the surgical incision is being made through clear cornea. Indeed, surface analgesia was the technique of choice for cataract surgery until the evolution of effective needle-based methods of regional anesthesia and improved safety of general anesthesia in the 1930s. Multiple advances in cataract surgery that have enabled faster operations, with greater control and less trauma, have allowed ophthalmologists to re-examine the use of topical anesthesia for this procedure. Phacoemulsification, with its small incisions, is clearly the procedure of choice in using topical anesthesia; however, planned extracapsular procedures can also be performed under topical anesthesia, thereby circumventing potential complications of peribulbar or retrobulbar block.

Fully anticoagulated patients may be excellent candidates for topical analgesia, as are monocular patients who are spared the trauma of prolonged local anesthetic-induced postoperative amaurosis. Potential disadvantages of topical anesthesia include eye movement during surgery, patient anxiety or discomfort, and, rarely, allergic reactions. Patient selection is critical and should be restricted to individuals who are alert and able to follow instructions, and who can control their eye movements. Patients who are demented or photophobic, or who cannot communicate, are inappropriate candidates, as are those with an inflamed eye. Similarly, patients with dense cataracts or with small pupils who may require significant iris manipulation or those who need large scleral incisions may be contraindicated for topical anesthesia.

Topical analgesia can be achieved with local anesthetic drops or gels. Anesthetic gels produce greater levels of drug in the anterior chamber than equal doses of drops and may afford superior surface analgesia.[98] Intracameral injection of 0.1 to 0.2 mL of 1% preservative-free lidocaine into the anterior chamber supplements the analgesic effects but may be deleterious to corneal endothelium.[99] Concerns about increased potential for postoperative endophthalmitis with gel-based topical analgesia exist because gels might theoretically form a barrier to bactericidal agents. Therefore, if administered, gels should be applied after antiseptic solutions, taking care to apply anesthetic drops before the use of caustic bactericidal preps.

Choice of Local Anesthetics, Block Adjuvants, and Adjuncts

Anesthetics for ocular surgery are selected on the basis of onset and duration needed. Fast-onset, brief-duration local anesthetics are optimal for procedures such as cataract surgery or pterygium excision. Longer-acting agents are indicated for lengthier operations such as vitreoretinal surgery. A tradition of mixing different local anesthetics to produce a block with shorter latency of onset, yet longer duration of effect, has been a paradigm of ophthalmic anesthesia. Vasoconstrictors may improve the quality of the block by delaying washout of drug from the orbit. There is concern, however, that epinephrine, the most common vasoconstrictor additive, may compromise retinal perfusion[100]; it is best avoided in patients with glaucomatous optic nerve damage.

Sodium bicarbonate, morphine sulfate, clonidine, and even vecuronium have been used as local anesthetic adjuvants in ophthalmic surgery. Without question, however, hyaluronidase has been the most popular ancillary agent used to modify ocular local anesthetic actions since it was introduced by Atkinson in 1949. It acts by hydrolyzing hyaluronic acid, a natural substance that binds cells together, keeping them cohesive. Thus, hyaluronidase increases tissue permeability, serves to promote dispersion of local anesthetics through tissues within the orbit, reduces the increase in orbital pressure associated with the volume of injected anesthetics, and enhances the quality of orbital blockade. Furthermore, hyaluronidase may reduce the risk of local anesthetic-induced extraocular muscle injury because clustered increases of postoperative diplopia were reported after national shortages of the drug in 1998 and 2000.[101] Studies since that time have supported these findings.[102,103] However, it is possible that many who were administering orbital blocks may have modified their technique in response to the absence of hyaluronidase by placing needles deeper, using more injections, or depositing larger volumes of local anesthetics.

Intravenous osmotic agents, such as mannitol and glycerin, as well as carbonic anhydrase inhibitors can be given to reduce vitreous volume and decrease IOP after it is artificially increased by local anesthetics. Digital pressure to soften the globe was described almost 50 years ago.[104] Mechanical devices that apply pressure to the globe were developed shortly thereafter; and a number of these devices are commercially available. Essentially, they are all variations on a ball, balloon, or bag theme. The Super Pinky ball, the Honan IOP Reducer (The Lebanon Corporation, Lebanon, Indiana), and the Buys Mercury Reducer (soon to be eliminated because of pollutant concerns expressed by the U.S. Environmental Protection Agency) are examples.[82] Immediately after administration of regional orbital anesthesia, the compression device may be positioned on the eye for 5 to 20 minutes. Reduction of IOP to below baseline levels is not uncommon. However, excessive pressure on the globe by these devices may impede blood flow, causing ischemic optic neuropathy or central retinal artery occlusion, possibly leading to blindness.[105] The Honan device addresses this potentially catastrophic complication with a pneumatic bellows that maintains even compression of the globe coupled to a manometric gauge that indicates a numeric value of applied pressure. A safety valve limits the amount of inflation of the bellows. With the increasing popularity of smaller incisions, lower-profile prosthetic lenses, and topical analgesia for cataract surgery, there is less need for IOP-reducing devices.

General Principles of Monitored Anesthesia Care

Many advocate the intravenous administration of an appropriate agent immediately prior to ocular regional anesthesia to provide comfort and amnesia. Polypharmacy and deep sedation in the form of high doses of opioids, benzodiazepines, and hypnotics may be unwise because of the pharmacologic vagaries in the geriatric population and the attendant risks of respiratory depression, airway obstruction, hypotension, CNS aberrations, and prolonged recovery time. This undesirable technique has all the disadvantages of a general anesthetic in the absence of an endotracheal tube or LMA without the advantage of controllability that general anesthesia offers. After the block has been performed, the patient should be relaxed but sufficiently responsive to avoid head movement associated with snoring or sudden abrupt movement on awakening. Perioperative patient movement is a leading cause of patient eye injury and anesthesiologist liability.[61] Clearly, patients under conscious sedation must be capable of remaining relatively still, responding rationally to commands, and maintaining airway patency. Undersedation should likewise be avoided because tachycardia and hypertension may have deleterious effects, especially in patients with coronary artery disease. Moreover, patients with orthopaedic deformities or arthritis must be meticulously positioned and given comfortable padding on the operating table. Adequate ventilation about the face is essential to avoid carbon dioxide accumulation, particularly as supplemental oxygen can delay signs of desaturation.[106] Use of exogenous oxygen can also contribute to surgical fire, particularly during oculoplastic surgery performed with electrocautery. Tightly occluded drapes may also promote accumulation of oxygen. In fact, burn injuries during facial surgery with supplemental oxygen account for nearly 20% of MAC closed claims cases.[61] Patients must be comfortably warm as the hazards of shivering in patients having delicate eye surgery are well known. Further, shivering causes a risk for patients with coronary artery disease. Continuous ECG monitoring is vital, lest performance of the retrobulbar block, pressure on the orbit, or tugging on the extraocular muscles stimulates the oculocardiac reflex arc and produces dangerous cardiac dysrhythmias. Likewise, pulse oximetry is essential. Unequivocally, MAC should reflect "maximum anesthesia caution, not minimal anesthesiology care."[107]

Studies have confirmed that most cataract operations performed in the United States are conducted with the patient under some form of local anesthesia (either retrobulbar, peribulbar, sub-Tenon, or topical analgesia), with monitoring equipment used in 97% of cases and an anesthesiologist present in 78% of cases.[108] An international survey of ophthalmologists reported routine use of anesthesia-trained personnel in 96% and 97% of cases in the United States and Australia, respectively.[109] On the other side of the spectrum, ophthalmologists from Malaysia and Thailand had anesthesia monitoring 31% and 18% of the time, respectively. Indeed, many anesthesiologists fear that the Centers for Medicare and Medicaid Services will decide not to reimburse for MAC for "routine" cataract cases.

An important study by Rosenfeld et al.[110] assessed the need for MAC in cataract surgery. These investigators prospectively studied the incidence and nature of interventions required by anesthesia personnel in 1,006 consecutive cataract operations (both phacoemulsification and extracapsular techniques were included) performed under peribulbar block. They also analyzed germane information, including patient demographic data, medical history, and preoperative laboratory tests, for ability to predict those patients at greatest risk for intervention. They found that 37% of patients required some type of intervention and that, in general, the majority of those interventions could not have been predicted before surgery. Patients younger than 60 years required intervention in >60% of cases. The interventions ranged from minor forms, such as verbal reassurance and hand holding, to administering such intravenous medications as supplemental sedation or antihypertensive, pressor, or antiarrhythmic agents, or to providing respiratory assistance. Although hypertension, lung disease, renal disease, and a diagnosis of cancer were related to interventions, these four conditions combined accounted for only a small portion of the needed interventions. Moreover, although many of the interventions were relatively minor, several were more serious, and 30% of the interventions were considered (by the involved anesthesia personnel) to be critical to the success of the operation. The investigators concluded that MAC by qualified anesthesia personnel is reasonable and justified and contributes to the quality of patient care when cataract surgery is performed with local anesthesia. Fung et al.[111] examined satisfaction scores for community-based cataract surgery via topical anesthesia and discovered that patients' value and regard for the anesthesiologist's role actually increased from the preoperative to the postoperative interview. In view of the fact that topical anesthesia produces analgesia that is less profound and provides operating conditions that are less ideal than regional or general anesthesia, it seems likely that anesthesia care is equally appropriate to provide comfort, support, and indicated drugs for these patients as well. For both ethical and surgical reasons, the ophthalmologist's attention must not be distracted from the microsurgical field.

ANESTHETIC MANAGEMENT IN SPECIFIC SITUATIONS

General Concepts and Objectives

Most patients undergoing eye surgery are either younger than 10 years of age or older than 55 years of age. In children, operations on the ocular adnexa, including lid surgery, repair of lacrimal apparatus, and adjustment of extraocular muscles, are common. However, surgery on the anterior segment, such as cataract removal, glaucoma procedures, and trauma repair, is not limited to the adult population. Nor are posterior segment operations such as scleral buckling and vitrectomy the exclusive domain of geriatrics.

Most ocular procedures demand profound analgesia but minimal skeletal muscle relaxation. The airway must be protected from obstruction, and the anesthesiologist must work at a distance—along with anesthetic apparatus—from the surgical field. The anesthesiologist and surgeon should agree on the selection of local or general anesthesia. Additional preparation must include identification of underlying diseases, such as asthma, diabetes mellitus, or nephropathy. The patient should also be prepared emotionally for the recovery period, when he or she may awaken with one or both eyes closed by bandages. This preparation is important not only to spare the patient fear and anxiety but to prevent much of the thrashing about that fright might produce, to the detriment of the eye.

Preoperative sedation is chosen carefully and is usually administered intravenously immediately before surgery because most ophthalmic procedures are performed on an ambulatory basis. Except for strabismus correction, retinal detachment surgery, and cryosurgery, ophthalmic procedures are usually associated with little pain. Thus, the routine use of opioid premedication, replete with emetic potential, is ill-advised. Rather, premedication should be prescribed with a view toward amnesia, sedation, and antiemesis.

7 Analgesia and akinesia are then secured through either local or general anesthesia, with careful attention paid to proper control of IOP and to the possible appearance of the oculocardiac reflex. The anesthesiologist strives to provide a smooth intraoperative course and to prevent coughing, retching, and vomiting, lest harmful increases in IOP transpire that could hinder successful surgery. If general anesthesia is elected, extubation of the trachea should be accomplished before there is a tendency to cough. The administration of intravenous lidocaine, 1.5 to 2 mg/kg, before extubation of the trachea is helpful in attenuating coughing. If the patient is deemed to be at extremely high risk for postoperative nausea and vomiting, prophylactic multimodal antiemetic therapy may be selected in conjunction with total intravenous anesthesia with propofol.

"Open-Eye, Full-Stomach" Encounters

The anesthesiologist involved in caring for a patient with a penetrating eye injury and a full stomach confronts special challenges. He or she must weigh the risk of aspiration against the risk of blindness in the injured eye that could result from elevated IOP and extrusion of ocular contents.

As in all cases of trauma, attention should be given to the exclusion of other injuries, such as skull and orbital fractures, intracranial trauma associated with subdural hematoma formation, and the possibility of thoracic or abdominal bleeding.

Although regional anesthesia is often a valuable alternative for the management of trauma patients who have recently eaten, this option had traditionally been considered contraindicated in patients with penetrating eye injuries because of the potential to extrude intraocular contents via pressure generated by local anesthetics. Nonetheless, some anecdotal case reports of successful use of ophthalmic blocks in this setting have been published.[112] Recognizing that there are several distinct permutations of eye injuries, Scott et al.[113] developed techniques to safely block patients with *select* open-globe injuries. In a 4-year period, 220 disrupted eyes were repaired via regional anesthesia at Bascom Palmer Eye Institute. A significant number of injuries were caused by intraocular foreign bodies and dehiscence of cataract or corneal transplant incisions. Blocked eyes tended to have more anterior, smaller wounds than those repaired via general anesthesia. There was no outcome difference—that is, change of visual acuity from initial evaluation until final examination—between the eyes repaired via regional versus general anesthesia. Moreover, combined topical anesthesia and sedation for *selected* patients with open-globe injuries has also been reported.[114]

Nonetheless, it is not always possible to determine the extent of disruption preoperatively, and general anesthesia is typically considered prudent in this setting. Preoperative prophylaxis against aspiration may involve administering H_2 receptor antagonists to elevate gastric fluid pH and to reduce gastric acid production. Metoclopramide may be given to induce peristalsis and enhance gastric emptying.

Frequently, a barbiturate, nondepolarizing neuromuscular blocking drug technique is described as the method of choice for the emergency repair of an open eye injury; the nondepolarizing drug pancuronium in a dose of 0.15 mg/kg has been shown to lower IOP. However, this method has its disadvantages, including risk of aspiration and death during the relatively lengthy period—ranging from 75 to 150 seconds—during which the airway is unprotected. Performance of the Sellick maneuver during this interval affords some protection. Furthermore, a premature attempt at intubation of the trachea produces coughing, straining, and a dramatic rise in IOP, emphasizing the need to confirm the onset of drug effect with a peripheral nerve stimulator while appreciating, nonetheless, that muscle groups vary in their response to muscle relaxants. Moreover, the cardiovascular side effects of tachycardia and hypertension may prove worrisome in patients with coronary artery disease. Also, the long duration of action of intubating doses of pancuronium may mandate postoperative mechanical ventilation of the lungs. Intermediate-acting nondepolarizing drugs such as vecuronium have briefer durations of action, and less dramatic, if any, circulatory effects, but nevertheless have an onset of action similar to that of pancuronium.

Several studies have explored the use of extremely large doses of nondepolarizing muscle relaxants to accelerate the onset of adequate relaxation for endotracheal intubation. Using vecuronium doses of 0.2 and 0.4 mg/kg, Casson and Jones[115] found mean onset times of 95 and 87 seconds, respectively. Ginsberg et al.[116] found that by increasing the vecuronium dose from 100 to 400 μg/kg the corresponding times to endotracheal intubation decreased from 183 to 96 seconds.

Succinylcholine offers the distinct advantages of swift onset, superb intubating conditions, and brief duration of action. If administered after careful pretreatment with a nondepolarizing drug and an induction dose of thiopental (4 to 6 mg/kg), succinylcholine produces only small increases in IOP.[117] Although the advisability of this technique has been debated vociferously, there are no published reports of loss of intraocular contents from a pretreatment barbiturate–succinylcholine sequence when used in this setting.[118] Moreover, in 1993, McGoldrick[119] pointed out that the 1957 watershed article of Lincoff et al.[18] states: "Various communications have been received from ophthalmologists who have used succinylcholine in surgery. This includes several reports of cases in which succinylcholine was given to forestall impending vitreous prolapse only to have a prompt expulsion of vitreous occur." Under such desperate circumstances, it is extremely difficult to attribute the expulsion of vitreous directly to succinylcholine.[119]

Rocuronium, with its purportedly rapid onset, may prove to be a useful drug in these circumstances, provided adequate doses (1.2 mg/kg intravenously) are administered. Unfortunately, it has an intermediate duration of action that could be disadvantageous, compared with succinylcholine, in a patient with an unrecognized difficult airway. Sugammadex may provide a solution. It is an oligosaccharide chelating agent that rapidly reverses the effects of aminosteroid neuromuscular blocking agents, particularly rocuronium. Recovery of >90% train-of-four responses may be accomplished in <120 seconds.[120] Thus, in the future, a new paradigm for the "openglobe, full-stomach" scenario may entail rapid-sequence induction with high-dose rocuronium to achieve swift onset of superb intubating conditions, followed by quick termination of neuromuscular blocking effect by sugammadex if the situation is encountered in which one cannot intubate or cannot ventilate.[121]

It was hoped that rapacuronium, with its swift onset, would emerge as a viable alternative to succinylcholine. However, rapacuronium is no longer available in the United States because of its role in triggering intractable bronchospasm in some patients. New ultrashort-acting nondepolarizing alternatives to succinylcholine are currently undergoing clinical investigation in human volunteers. Perhaps the wisest approach to the management of open-eye, full-stomach situations is summarized by Baumgarten and Reynolds,[122] who wrote in 1985:

It may be possible to devise a combination of intravenous anesthetics and nondepolarizing relaxants that totally prevents coughing after rapid intubation. Until this combination is devised and confirmed in a large, controlled double-blind series, clinicians should not apply the priming principle to the open eye-full stomach patient. Use of a blockade monitor to predict intubating conditions may be unreliable, since muscle groups vary in their response to nondepolarizing relaxants. At this time, succinylcholine with precurarization probably remains the most tenable compromise in the open eye-full stomach challenge.

Patients with open-globe injuries requiring general anesthesia whose airway assessment is reassuring may occasionally have a contraindication to succinylcholine, such as malignant hyperthermia susceptibility, Duchenne muscular dystrophy, or certain types of myotonia. These patients may be managed using appropriately large doses of a nondepolarizing neuromuscular blocker to enable accelerated onset of paralysis and satisfactory intubating conditions. Maintenance could then be accomplished with a total intravenous anesthetic technique.

When confronted with a patient whose airway anatomy or anesthetic history suggests potential difficulties, the anesthesiologist should consult with the ophthalmologist concerning the probability of saving the injured eye. In selected instances, general anesthesia may be avoided by using topical or regional anesthesia. If this approach is not feasible, awake fiberoptic laryngoscopy and intubation may be the safest option, realizing that substantial increases in IOP may occur if the patient gags or coughs. These risks, which can be minimized by thorough topical anesthesia of the airway, assume relative unimportance when balanced against the risk of being unable to ventilate and oxygenate the patient.

Strabismus Surgery

Approximately 3% of the population has malalignment of the visual axes, which may be accompanied by diplopia, amblyopia, and loss of stereopsis (Table 51-5). Indeed, strabismus surgery is the most common pediatric ocular operation performed in the United States, and it entails a variety of techniques to weaken an extraocular muscle by moving its insertion on the globe (recession) or to strengthen an extraocular muscle by eliminating a short strip of the tendon or muscle (resection).

Infantile strabismus occurs within the first 6 months of life and is often observed in the neonatal period. Although most patients with strabismus are healthy, normal children, the incidence of strabismus is increased in those with CNS dysfunction such as cerebral palsy and meningomyelocele with hydrocephalus. Moreover, strabismus may be acquired secondary to oculomotor nerve trauma or sensory abnormalities such as cataracts or refractive aberrations.

In addition to the well-known propensity of strabismus surgery to trigger the oculocardiac reflex (previously discussed), there is also an increased incidence of malignant hyperthermia in patients with conditions such as strabismus or ptosis. This observation is consistent with the impression that people susceptible to malignant hyperthermia often have localized areas of skeletal muscle weakness or other musculoskeletal abnormalities. Other aspects of strabismus surgery of interest to anesthesiologists include succinylcholine-induced interference with the FDT and an increased incidence of postoperative nausea and vomiting.

In formulating a surgical treatment plan for incomitant strabismus, ophthalmologists often find the FDT to be exquisitely helpful in differentiating between a paretic muscle and a restrictive force preventing ocular motion. To perform the FDT, the surgeon grasps the sclera of the anesthetized eye with a forceps near the corneal limbus and moves the eye into each field of gaze, concomitantly assessing tissue and elastic properties. This simple test provides valuable clues to the presence and site of mechanical restrictions of the extraocular muscles and is most valuable in patients who have previously undergone strabismus surgery, in those who may have paralysis of one of the extraocular muscles, and in those who have sustained orbital trauma.

France et al.[123] quantitated the magnitude and duration of change of the FDT after succinylcholine administration. They

TABLE 51-5

CONCERNS WITH VARIOUS OCULAR PROCEDURES

■ PROCEDURE	■ CONCERNS
Strabismus repair	Forced duction testing
	Oculocardiac reflex
	Oculogastric reflex
	Malignant hyperthermia
Intraocular surgery	Proper control of IOP
	Akinesia
	Drug interactions
	Associated systemic disease
Retinal detachment surgery	Oculocardiac reflex
	Proper control of IOP
	Nitrous oxide interaction with air, sulfur hexafluoride, or perfluorocarbons

IOP, intraocular pressure.

demonstrated that quantification of the force necessary to rotate the globe remained notably increased over control for 15 minutes, even though the rise in IOP and the skeletal muscle paralysis lasted <5 minutes. Because succinylcholine interferes with FDT, its use is contraindicated <20 minutes before testing. Hence, France et al.[123] suggested performing the FDT on the anesthetized patient either while mask inhalation anesthesia is being administered, before intubation of the trachea; after intubation, facilitated by nondepolarizing neuromuscular blocking drugs; or after intubation under moderately deep inhalation anesthesia, unaided by succinylcholine.

Eye movement under general anesthesia is well documented, and in nonaligned eyes this tendency is augmented such that divergent squints diverge more and convergent squints converge less. Another recent report discloses that surgeons at a regional eye teaching hospital in the United Kingdom who specialize in strabismus surgery are increasingly requesting that, if the FDT is being used, nondepolarizing neuromuscular blockade be incorporated into the anesthetic management so muscle tone is minimal or absent during testing.[29]

Once intubation of the trachea has been accomplished, anesthesia is commonly maintained with halothane, desflurane, sevoflurane or isoflurane, nitrous oxide, and oxygen. The patient is carefully monitored with a precordial stethoscope, ECG, blood pressure device, pulse oximeter, end-tidal carbon dioxide measurement, and temperature probe. If bradycardia occurs, the surgeon is asked to discontinue ocular manipulation, and the patient's ventilatory status and anesthetic depth are quickly assessed. If additional intravenous atropine is indicated, it is not given while the oculocardiac reflex is active in case even more dangerous cardiac dysrhythmias are triggered.

The LMA is gaining popularity for strabismus surgery in the United States, provided the patient is not at risk for aspiration. The laryngeal mask can be inserted without the use of muscle relaxants, causes less hemodynamic perturbation, and is associated with less straining and coughing on removal.

Vomiting after eye muscle surgery is common, giving credibility to the existence of the oculogastric reflex. The administration of droperidol, 0.075 mg/kg at induction of anesthesia before manipulation of the eye, has been shown to reduce the incidence of vomiting after strabismus surgery to a clinically acceptable level of approximately 10% without prolonging recovery time.[124] Moreover, a lower dose of droperidol, 0.02 mg/kg intravenously, administered immediately after anesthetic induction in patients with strabismus may decrease both the incidence and severity of nausea and vomiting.[125] Many physicians have stopped using droperidol owing to the U.S. Food and Drug Administration (FDA) "black box" warning. However, the droperidol doses used for postoperative nausea and vomiting are extremely low and unlikely to be associated with notable cardiovascular events. Indeed, considerable concern has been expressed about the quality and quantity of evidence and the validity of the FDA conclusion.[126]

Prophylactic intravenous administration of a serotonin receptor antagonist such as ondansetron, dolasetron, or granisetron also appears to be efficacious. Combination therapy consisting of one or two antiemetics, each with a different mechanism of action, plus a glucocorticoid such as dexamethasone, has been shown to be efficacious and safe in patients at high risk for postoperative nausea and vomiting.[126] Moreover, a total intravenous technique with propofol has also been associated with a low incidence of emesis after strabismus surgery.[127] In addition, avoiding narcotics may be helpful. One study demonstrates that the nonopioid analgesic ketorolac, in a dose of 0.75 mg/kg intravenously, provides analgesia comparable with that of morphine in pediatric patients with strabismus, but with a much lower incidence of nausea and vomiting in the first 24 hours.[128]

Intraocular Surgery

Advances in both anesthesia and in technology now permit a level of controlled intraocular manipulation that was not possible one-quarter century ago (Table 51-5).

Proper control of IOP is crucial for such intraocular procedures as glaucoma drainage surgery, open sky vitrectomy, penetrating keratoplasty (corneal transplantation), and traditional intracapsular cataract extraction. Before scleral incision (when IOP becomes equal to atmospheric pressure), a low-normal IOP is essential because abrupt decompression of a hypertensive eye could result in iris or lens prolapse, vitreous loss, or expulsive choroidal hemorrhage. Available data have not demonstrated a major difference in the rate of complications such as vitreous loss and iris prolapse between local anesthesia and general anesthesia.

Many anesthetic techniques may be safely used for elective intraocular surgery. If general anesthesia is selected, virtually any of the inhalation drugs may be given after intravenous induction of anesthesia with a barbiturate or propofol, neuromuscular blocking drug, and topical laryngeal lidocaine. Because complete akinesia is essential for delicate intraocular surgery, nondepolarizing drugs are administered, followed by neuromuscular function monitoring to ensure a 90 to 95% twitch suppression level during surgery. Because proper control of IOP is critical, controlled ventilation of the lungs is used, along with end-tidal carbon dioxide monitoring to ensure avoidance of hypercarbia.

Maximal pupillary dilation is important for many types of intraocular surgery and can be induced by continuous infusion of epinephrine 1: 200,000 in a balanced salt solution, delivered through a small-gauge needle placed in the anterior chamber. Almost simultaneous with its administration, the drug is removed by aspirating it from the anterior chamber. The iris usually dilates immediately on contact with the epinephrine infusion, and drug uptake is presumably limited by the associated intense vasoconstriction of the iris and ciliary body. However, epinephrine may also be potentially absorbed by drainage through Schlemm canal into the venous system or by spillover of the infusion into the conjunctival vessels or drainage to the nasal mucosa.

At the completion of surgery, any residual neuromuscular blockade is reversed. On resumption of spontaneous ventilation, the patient's trachea is extubated (often in the lateral position) with the patient still deeply anesthetized and after intravenous administration of lidocaine to prevent coughing. Atropine and neostigmine may be safely used to reverse neuromuscular blockade, even in patients with glaucoma because this combination of drugs, in conventional doses, has minimal effects on pupil size and IOP.

Retinal Detachment Surgery

Surgery to repair retinal detachments involves procedures affecting intraocular volume, frequently using a synthetic silicone band or sponge to produce a localized or encircling scleral indentation (Table 51-5). Furthermore, internal tamponade of the retinal break may be accomplished by injecting an expandable gas such as sulfur hexafluoride into the vitreous. Because of blood gas partition coefficient differences, the administration of nitrous oxide may enhance the internal tamponade effect of sulfur hexafluoride intraoperatively, only to be followed by a dramatic drop in IOP and volume on discontinuation of nitrous oxide. The injected sulfur hexafluoride bubble, in the presence of concomitant administration of nitrous oxide, can cause a rapid and dramatic rise in IOP, reaching a peak within 20 minutes[48,49] (see "Intraocular

Sulfur Hexafluoride"). Because the resultant rise in IOP may compromise retinal circulation, Stinson and Donlon[48] recommended cessation of nitrous oxide administration 15 minutes before gas injection to prevent significant changes in the volume of the intravitreous gas bubble. Furthermore, Wolf et al.[49] stated that if a patient requires anesthesia after intravitreous gas injection, nitrous oxide should be omitted for 5 days after an air injection and for 10 days after sulfur hexafluoride injection. In cases in which perfluoropropane has been injected, the nitrous oxide proscription should be in effect for longer than 30 days. Alternatively, silicone oil, a vitreous substitute, may be injected to achieve internal tamponade of a retinal break.

It should be emphasized that resorption time is not always uniform or predictable. For example, reports have appeared where a 19-year-old woman with type 1 diabetes injected with sulfur hexafluoride 25 days before subsequent surgery and a 37-year-old man with insulin-dependent diabetes injected with perfluoropropane gas 41 days before subsequent surgery were given nitrous oxide and developed central retinal artery occlusion and permanent blindness in the affected eye.[129] Because the pressure in the retinal arterial vessels is lower in patients with diabetes, the elderly, and those with atherosclerosis, these patients are likely at higher risk for this devastating complication.[130–132] The international distributors of medical-grade gases, in cooperation with the American distributors and the FDA, has begun to provide hospital band-type warning bracelets for patients who receive intraocular gas injection to alert health professionals to the presence of the bubble and the need to avoid nitrous oxide administration.

Retinal detachment operations are basically extraocular but may briefly become intraocular if the surgeon elects to perforate and drain subretinal fluid. Furthermore, rotation of the globe with traction on the extraocular muscles may elicit the oculocardiac reflex, so the anesthesiologist must be vigilant about potential cardiac dysrhythmias. In addition, because it is desirable to have a soft eye while the sclera is being buckled, intravenous administration of acetazolamide or mannitol is common during retinal surgery to lower IOP.

These patients are usually managed in the same manner as those having intraocular surgery, except that maintenance of intraoperative skeletal muscle paralysis is not as critical as during intraocular surgery. Hence, inhalational anesthetics need not be accompanied during surgery by nondepolarizing neuromuscular blocking drugs.

Principles of Laser Therapy

In 1957, in a laboratory at Columbia University, the first design for the laser was born. The invention has revolutionized industry, refined scientific measurements, provided therapy for countless medical and surgical conditions, and inspired 13 Nobel Prizes. The principle is based on the consequences of a photon meeting an electron in an excited state. Sometimes the collision produces a second photon that has the same color and direction as the original. When repeated on a large scale, this process creates an orderly beam of light. The term *laser* was coined to describe this photon-cloning effect, and the acronym signifies *light amplified by stimulated emission of radiation*.

Laser radiation has many notable properties. Because it is monochromatic, all the photons have the same wavelength, energy, and frequency. It is coherent, with all the photons in phase. Moreover, laser radiation is collimated, so its beam is nondivergent. These properties allow the precision that is associated with laser surgery. The amount of radiant energy (joules) absorbed by tissues is the product of power (watts) multiplied by duration (seconds). Surgical lasers typically are used in either a continuous or a pulsed mode.

The effect that a particular laser beam exerts on tissue depends predominantly on its wavelength and power density. A specific laser's wavelength depends on its lasing medium, which also gives the laser its name. In general, the longer the wavelength, the more strongly absorbed the light. The converse is true; the shorter the wavelength, the more scattered the light. The power of the laser beam is converted to heat at a shallow depth. Coherent light of high-power density excels in cutting or vaporizing tissue. Lower-power densities are used to photocoagulate tissue and promote hemostasis. Of course, another variable that can be manipulated to produce a given effect is the duration of contact between laser beam and tissue. Additional uses of lasers of low-power density include the photoactivation of systemically administered dyes to precisely treat localized disease sites, such as with age-related macular degeneration.

Lasers are used to treat a wide spectrum of eye conditions, including three of the most common causes of visual loss in the United States: diabetic retinopathy, glaucoma, and age-related macular degeneration. Recently, the use of lasers expanded to include the rapidly growing field of refractive surgery. Argon, krypton, diode, dye-tuned, neodymium: yttrium-aluminum-garnet (Nd: YAG), and excimer lasers are among those commonly used for ophthalmic surgery. Owing to concern that indirect exposure to laser energy could cause ocular damage to operating room personnel, staff working with or near the laser wear protective goggles designed to block the particular wavelength of light emitted by the laser in use.

The argon laser emits blue-green light with a wavelength of approximately 488 to 515 nm (approximately 0.5 μm). This laser has low maximum power and is easily transmitted by fiberoptic bundles. Light from the argon laser is strongly absorbed by hemoglobin, melanin, and other pigments, rendering it useful in retinal detachment surgery to photocoagulate or cauterize pigment epithelium and the adjacent neurosensory retina, thus creating an adhesion between the retina and the "wall of the eye" to keep the retina attached. This photocoagulative property of the argon and similar lasers achieves its therapeutic effect in the treatment of diabetic retinopathy by focal and controlled necrosis of a limited amount of ischemic retina. The argon laser is also used with some efficacy to treat the late complications that can develop in the natural history of retinal vein occlusion. Because emissions of the argon laser can penetrate the cornea and lens, causing severe retinal damage, personnel in the vicinity of the argon laser should wear orange protective goggles.

The Nd: YAG, commonly called the *YAG laser*, emits light in the infrared range (wavelength, 1,064 nm [1.06 μm]) and is useful in posterior lens-capsule surgery. The Nd: YAG laser has high-power density and is efficacious in creating an opening in opacified posterior capsule membranes that develop in approximately one third of cases after phacoemulsification or other extracapsular cataract surgery. Personnel working in the vicinity of this laser should wear green goggles and realize that their ability to detect cyanosis will be impaired.

An excimer laser (sometimes, and more correctly, called an *exciplex laser*) is a form of high-power, ultraviolet chemical laser frequently used in delicate refractive surgery (LASIK), commonly referred to as *laser corrective surgery*. The term *excimer* is short for "excited dimer," and *exciplex* is short for "excited complex." An excimer laser generally uses a combination of inert gas (argon, krypton, or xenon) and a reactive gas (fluorine or chlorine). Under appropriate conditions of electrical stimulation, a pseudomolecule called a *dimer* is generated, which can exist only in an energized state and gives rise to laser light in the ultraviolet range, typically with wavelengths of 125 to 200 nm. The ultraviolet light from an excimer laser is well absorbed by biological matter and organic compounds. Instead of burning or cutting material, the excimer laser supplies enough energy to disrupt the molecular bonds of surface tissue through ablation. This property allows removal of exceptionally fine layers of surface material with almost no heating or change to neighboring tissue. These lasers are usually operated with a pulse rate of around 100 Hz and a pulse duration of 10 ns, although some may operate as high as 8 kHz and 30 ns.

Age-related macular degeneration is the most common cause of blindness in the elderly and has become alarmingly prevalent. The treatment of the generally more severe wet form of age-related macular degeneration has interestingly progressed over the years from the initial photocoagulation of the neovascular membrane that develops in the central retina or macula. Cauterization obliterates this membrane, but can also damage the adjacent healthy macular tissue. The next modality used to treat age-related macular degeneration was the cold laser to photoactivate an intravenously injected drug, verteporfin, which chemically changed on light exposure of 693 nm in the presence of oxygen. By precisely applying the cold laser light to the area of the neovascular membrane, the photoactivated verteporfin produced highly reactive oxygen radicals and "selectively" necrosed the diseased tissue. Because of ill effects on nearby healthy tissue, this approach has been superseded by a more effective, nonlaser treatment with intravitreous injection of monoclonal antibody drugs such as ranibizumab (FDA-approved) or bevacizumab (off-label).

POSTOPERATIVE OCULAR COMPLICATIONS

The incidence of eye injuries associated with nonocular surgery is low. In a study by Roth et al.[133] of 60,965 patients undergoing nonocular surgery from 1988 to 1992, the incidence of eye injury was 0.056% (34 patients). Twenty-one of these 34 patients sustained corneal abrasion, although other injuries included conjunctivitis, blurry vision, red eye, chemical injury, direct ocular trauma, and blindness. Independent risk factors for greater relative risk of ocular injury were protracted surgical procedures, lateral intraoperative positioning, head or neck surgery, general anesthesia, and (for some unknown reason) surgery on a Monday. A specific mechanism of injury could be identified in only 21% of cases. In the ASA Closed Claims Study published in 1992 (which analyzed only cases involving litigation), eye injuries represented merely 3% of all claims, but the serious nature of some of the injuries was reflected in large financial awards.[134] Similar to the findings of Roth et al., in the Closed Claims Study the specific mechanism of injury could be ascertained in only a minority of cases. Another Closed Claims Study published in 2004 and examining injuries associated with regional anesthesia reported that the proportion of regional anesthesia claims linked to eye blocks increased from 2% in the 1980s to 7% in the 1990s.[135] These injuries were typically permanent and related to the block technique. More than half of the claims resulted in blindness. Almost all these claims involved retrobulbar or peribulbar block performed by anesthesiologists. Topical anesthesia for cataract removal is becoming more common and may result in a reduced prevalence of these complications.

Although infrequent and often transient, eye injuries occasionally can result in blindness or more limited, but nonetheless permanent, visual impairment. Postoperative complications after nonocular surgery include corneal abrasion and minor visual disturbances, chemical injuries, thermal or photic injury, and serious visual disturbances, including blindness. Serious injury may result from such diverse conditions as acute corneal epithelial edema, glycine toxicity and other visual disturbances associated with transurethral resection of the prostate, retinal ischemia, ischemic optic neuropathy, cortical blindness, and acute glaucoma. It appears that certain types of surgery, including complex spinal surgery in the prone position; operations involving extracorporeal circulation; and neck, nasal, or sinus surgery may increase the risk of serious postoperative visual complications.

Corneal Abrasion

Although the most common ocular complication of general anesthesia is corneal abrasion,[136] the incidence varies widely, depending on the perioperative circumstances. In a prospective study, Cucchiara and Black[137] found a 0.17% incidence of corneal abrasion in 4,652 neurosurgical patients whose eyes were protected, whereas Batra and Bali[136] one decade earlier reported a 44% incidence of corneal abrasion when eyes were left unprotected and partly open. A variety of mechanisms can result in corneal abrasion, including damage caused by the anesthetic mask, surgical drapes, and spillage of solutions. During intubation of the trachea, moreover, the end of plastic watch bands or hospital identification cards clipped to the laryngoscopist's vest pocket can injure the cornea. Ocular injury may also occur from loss of pain sensation, obtundation of protective corneal reflexes, and decreased tear production during anesthesia. Therefore, it may be prudent to tape the eyelids closed immediately after induction, and during mask ventilation and laryngoscopy. In addition to taping the eyelids closed, applying protective goggles and instilling petroleum-based ointments into the conjunctival sac may provide protection. Disadvantages of ointments include occasional allergic reactions; flammability, which may make their use undesirable during surgery around the face and contraindicated during laser surgery; and blurred vision in the early postoperative period. The blurring and foreign-body sensation associated with ointments may actually increase the incidence of postoperative corneal abrasions if they trigger excessive rubbing of the eyes while the patient is still emerging from anesthesia. Moreover, halothane absorption into paraffin-based ointments can damage the cornea, and even water-based (methylcellulose) ointments may be irritating and cause scleral erythema. It would seem prudent, therefore, to close the eyelids with tape during general anesthesia for procedures away from the head and neck. For certain procedures on the face, ocular occluders or tarsorrhaphy may be indicated. Special attention should also be devoted to frequent checking of the eyes during procedures on a prone patient.

Patients with corneal abrasion usually complain of a foreign-body sensation, pain, tearing, and photophobia. The pain is typically exacerbated by blinking and ocular movement. It is wise to have an ophthalmologic consultation immediately. Treatment typically consists of the prophylactic application of antibiotic ointment and patching the injured eye shut. Although permanent sequelae are possible, healing usually occurs within 24 hours.

Chemical Injury

Spillage of solutions during skin preparation may result in chemical damage to the eye. The FDA has reported serious corneal damage from eye contact with Hibiclens, a 4% chlorhexidine gluconate solution formulated with a detergent. Again, with meticulous attention to detail, this misadventure is preventable. Treatment consists of liberal bathing of the eye with balanced salt solution to remove the offending agent. After surgery, it may be desirable to have an ophthalmologist examine the eye to document any residual injury or lack thereof.

Photic Injury

Direct or reflected light beams may permanently damage the eye. For patients undergoing nonocular laser surgery, the potential for serious injury to the cornea or retina from certain laser beams requires that the patient's eyes be protected with moist gauze pads and metal shields, and that operating room personnel wear protective glasses. These goggles must be appropriately tinted for the specific wavelength they are intended to block. Clear goggles may be worn when working with the carbon dioxide laser, whereas for work with the argon, Nd: YAG, or Nd: YAG-KTP (potassium titanyl phosphate) laser, the goggles must be tinted orange, green, and orange-red, respectively.

Mild Visual Symptoms

After anesthesia, transient, mild visual disturbances such as photophobia or diplopia are common. Blurred vision in the early postoperative period may reflect residual effects of petroleum-based ophthalmic ointments or ocular effects of anticholinergic drugs administered in the perioperative period (see "Corneal Abrasion").

In contrast, the complaint of postoperative visual loss is rare and is cause for alarm. Several of the following conditions may be associated with visual loss after anesthesia and surgery, and should be included in the differential diagnosis: hemorrhagic retinopathy, retinal ischemia, retinal artery occlusion, ischemic optic neuropathy, cortical blindness, and acute glaucoma.

Hemorrhagic Retinopathy

Retinal hemorrhages that occur in otherwise healthy people secondary to hemodynamic changes associated with turbulent emergence from anesthesia or protracted vomiting are termed *Valsalva retinopathy*. Fortunately, these venous hemorrhages are usually self-limiting and resolve completely in a few days to a few months.

Because no visual changes occur unless the macula is involved, most cases are asymptomatic. However, if bleeding into the optic nerve occurs, resulting in optic atrophy, or if the hemorrhage is massive, permanent visual impairment may ensue. In some instances of massive hemorrhage, vitrectomy may offer some improvement.

Retinal venous hemorrhage has also been described after injections of local anesthetics, steroids, or saline into the lumbar epidural space, and these cases have been summarized by Purdy and Ajimal.[138] The patients all received large injections (≥ 40 mL) into the epidural space, and they subsequently developed blurry vision or headaches. On funduscopic examination, retinal hemorrhage was consistently observed. Eight of the nine patients described had complete recovery. It is believed that the hemorrhage is produced by rapid epidural injection, which causes a sudden increase in intracranial pressure. This increase in cerebrospinal fluid pressure causes an increase of retinal venous pressure, which may cause retinal hemorrhages. It is possible that obesity, hypertension, coagulopathies, pre-existing elevated cerebrospinal fluid pressure (as seen in pseudotumor cerebri), and such retinal vascular diseases as diabetic retinopathy may be risk factors. Caution is recommended when injecting drugs or fluid into the epidural space; a slow injection rate and using the minimal volume necessary to accomplish the desired objective are strongly recommended.

Retinal Ischemia

Retinal bleeding may also originate from the arterial circulation. This bleeding may be associated with extraocular trauma. Funduscopic examination shows cotton-wool exudates, and this condition is known as *Purtscher retinopathy*. Purtscher retinopathy should be ruled out when a trauma patient complains of postanesthetic visual loss. This condition is associated with a poor prognosis, and most patients sustain permanent visual impairment.

Retinal ischemia or infarction may also result from direct ocular trauma secondary to external pressure exerted by an ill-fitting anesthetic mask, especially in a hypotensive setting, and from embolism during cardiac surgery, or from the intraocular injection of a large volume of sulfur hexafluoride or other gases in the presence of high concentrations of nitrous oxide. It may also result from increased ocular venous pressure associated with impaired venous drainage or elevated IOP.

The importance of carefully positioning patients and scrupulously monitoring external pressure on the eye cannot be overemphasized, especially when the patient is in the prone or jackknife position. When the head is dependently positioned, venous pressure may be elevated. If external pressure is applied to the globe from improper head support, perfusion pressure to the eye is likely to be reduced. An episode of systemic hypotension in this setting could further decrease perfusion pressure and thereby decrease intraocular blood flow, resulting in possible retinal ischemia.

It is imperative that a padded or foam headrest be used for procedures done with patients in the prone position. The patient's eyes must be in the opening of this headrest and they must be checked at frequent intervals for pressure. If the patient's head is too large to fit properly into the headrest, a pin head-holder should be used. During some spine procedures, a steep head-down position may be used to decrease venous bleeding and enhance surgical exposure. This position, in combination with deliberate hypotension and infusion of large quantities of crystalloid, may increase the risk of compromising the ocular circulation. It seems prudent to avoid combining these three risk factors to any significant degree.

Central retinal arterial occlusion and branch retinal arterial occlusion are important, and frequently preventable, causes of postoperative visual loss. Cases have occurred following spinal, nasal, sinus, or neck surgery, as well as after coronary artery bypass graft (CABG) surgery. In addition to external pressure on the eye, causes can include emboli from carotid plaques or other sources, as well as vasospasm or thrombosis after radical neck surgery complicated by hemorrhage and hypotension, and after intranasal injection of α-adrenergic agonists. Several cases have followed intra-arterial injections of corticosteroids or local anesthetics in branches of the external carotid artery, with possible retrograde embolization to the ocular blood supply.[139] Mabry[140] suggested that the needle must be positioned intra-arterially to produce retrograde flow into the branches of the ophthalmic artery, and the perfusion pressure must be overcome during the injection. Therefore, when injecting in the nasal and sinus areas, topical vasoconstrictors should be applied to decrease the size of the vascular bed, and a small (25-gauge) needle on a low-volume syringe should be used to minimize injection pressure. Moreover, because some cases have followed injections of corticosteroids combined with other drugs, it is believed that this practice may predispose to formation of drug crystals and therefore should be discouraged.

In cases of central retinal arterial occlusion, funduscopic examination discloses a pale, edematous retina and a cherry-red spot. Platelet-fibrin, cholesterol, calcific, or crystalloid emboli may be found in narrowed retinal arterioles. Computed tomography (CT) and magnetic resonance imaging (MRI) studies are negative.

Prevention is much more successful than treatment. It may be possible to apply ocular massage (contraindicated if glaucoma is a possibility) to dislodge an embolus to more peripheral sites, and intravenous acetazolamide and 5% carbon dioxide inhalation have been used to increase retinal blood flow. The prognosis, however, is typically poor, and approximately 50% of patients with central retinal arterial occlusion eventually have optic atrophy.

Ischemic Optic Neuropathy

Ischemic optic neuropathy in the nonsurgical setting is the most common cause of *sudden* visual loss in patients older than 50 years of age, and it may be either arteritic or nonarteritic. Our discussion is limited to postoperative ischemic optic neuropathy and contrasts the similarities and differences between anterior ischemic optic neuropathy and posterior ischemic optic neuropathy. Because of a perceived increase in the incidence of postoperative visual loss since the mid-1990s, the Committee on Professional Liability of the ASA established the Postoperative Visual Loss Database on July 1, 1999, to better identify associated risk factors so these tragic complications might be prevented in the future.[141] Because the incidence of postoperative vision loss after spine surgery in the prone position may be as high as 1%, it would seem prudent to discuss this potential complication preoperatively with the patient during the informed consent process.

Anterior Ischemic Optic Neuropathy

Although the multifactorial pathophysiology of anterior ischemic optic neuropathy has not been completely established, it is believed to involve temporary hypoperfusion or nonperfusion of the vessels supplying the anterior portion of the optic nerve, although intra-axonal edema and disturbed autoregulation to the optic nerve head may also play a role.[139] Coexisting systemic disease, especially involving the cardiovascular system and (to a lesser extent) the endocrine system, is common in patients in whom anterior ischemic optic neuropathy develops. Male gender also strongly predominates. Other risk factors for postoperative anterior ischemic optic neuropathy include CABG and other thoracovascular operations, as well as spinal surgery. Although massive bleeding, anemia, and hypotension are commonly described intraoperative risk factors, a retrospective survey of surgeons who perform spinal fusion surgery disclosed that hypotension and anemia were equally prevalent in patients in whom ischemic optic neuropathy developed and in those in whom it did not.[142] Other possible risk factors are increased IOP or orbital venous pressure. Although emboli may also play a role, anterior ischemic optic neuropathy is not usually caused by emboli because emboli preferentially lodge in the central retinal artery rather than in the short posterior ciliary arteries that supply the anterior optic nerve.

Increased IOP caused by extrinsic compression of the eye decreases retinal blood flow that can produce both retinal and optic nerve injury. Moreover, increased IOP can result from large infusions of crystalloid when the head is steeply dependent, as during many spinal operations.[143] Increased orbital venous pressure results in a decreased perfusion pressure gradient to the optic nerve head. Interestingly, one patient who had ischemic optic neuropathy despite perioperative normotension had marked facial edema after surgery of protracted duration.[143]

Similarly, a study in cardiac surgery patients revealed that increases in IOP correlated with the degree of hemodilution and the use of crystalloid priming solution.[144] Patients with anterior ischemic optic neuropathy were more likely to have significant weight gain within 24 hours of open heart surgery, again suggesting the role of elevated ocular venous pressure in impeding blood flow to the optic nerve.

According to Roth and Gillesberg,[139] a complex interaction of factors such as ocular venous pressure, hemodilution, hypotension, release of endogenous vasoconstrictors, and individual risk factors such as atherosclerosis and aberrant optic nerve circulation may be implicated in the development of anterior ischemic optic neuropathy. Therefore, specific recommendations for preventative strategies are elusive. Clearly, however, external pressure on the eyes must be meticulously avoided. It also seems prudent to minimize time in the prone position when the head is notably dependent. In patients with pre-existing cardiovascular disease, significant hypertension, or glaucoma, it seems advisable to maintain systemic blood pressure as close to baseline as possible.[139]

Patients with anterior ischemic optic neuropathy typically have painless visual loss that may not be noted until the first postoperative day (or possibly later), an afferent pupillary defect, altitudinal field defects, and optic disc edema or pallor. MRI or CT initially shows enlargement of the optic nerve. However, optic atrophy is detected by MRI later.

The prognosis for anterior ischemic optic neuropathy varies but is often grim. Although there is no recognized treatment for anterior ischemic optic neuropathy, Williams et al.[145] reviewed the various therapies that may be instituted. These include intravenous acetazolamide, furosemide, mannitol, and steroids. Maintaining the head-up position could be helpful if increased ocular venous pressure is operative. Surgical optic nerve sheath fenestration or decompression is not only ineffective, but may actually be harmful.[146]

Posterior Ischemic Optic Neuropathy

The posterior optic nerve has a less luxuriant blood supply than the anterior optic nerve. In contrast to anterior ischemic optic neuropathy, relatively few cases have been reported after CABG, and posterior ischemic optic neuropathy appears to be less related to coexisting cardiovascular disease. As with anterior ischemic optic neuropathy, male patients outnumber female patients four to one. Many cases have been associated with surgery involving the neck, nose, sinuses, or spine. In approximately one third of cases reported, facial edema has been noted.[139] Approximately 11% of cases were associated with cardiopulmonary bypass procedures.

Posterior ischemic optic neuropathy is produced by reduced oxygen delivery to the retrolaminar part of the optic nerve. Most likely, compression of the pial vessels (supplied by small collaterals from the ophthalmic artery) or embolic phenomena produce ischemia.[139]

An hypoxic insult in this region results in a slower development of ischemic damage so a symptom-free period often precedes the loss of vision. In some patients, the onset of symptoms may be delayed several days. Typical findings include an afferent pupillary defect or nonreactive pupil. Disc edema is not a feature of posterior ischemic optic neuropathy because of its retro-orbital position. CT scan in the early postoperative period may reveal enlargement of the intraorbital portion of the optic nerve. Bilateral blindness is more common with posterior ischemic optic neuropathy than with anterior ischemic optic neuropathy, possibly indicating involvement of the optic chiasm. Concomitant disease of the eye or ocular blood supply may be related to posterior ischemic optic neuropathy.[139] Some cases may show partial improvement spontaneously, but often no improvement is noted. Steroids may be considered for treatment. Preventive strategies are as outlined for anterior ischemic optic neuropathy.

A review of the first 6 years of cases submitted to the ASA Postoperative Visual Loss Registry found that spinal surgery patients at greatest risk for ischemic optic neuropathy and visual compromise include those with predisposing patient-specific factors, surgery exceeding 6 hours' duration, and blood loss of more than a liter.[147] In the 83 reported cases, there was no causative evidence of traumatic eye injury from edema or direct pressure on the globe. Mean blood pressures and hematocrits varied widely among those who developed postoperative blindness. However, 34% of cases had the lowest mean arterial blood pressure or systolic blood pressure ≥40% below baseline, and in only 6% of cases were the mean arterial or the systolic pressures <20% below baseline. The ASA practice advisory for perioperative visual loss associated with spine surgery concludes that there is no established "transfusion threshold" and that deliberate intraoperative hypotension during surgery has not been proven as contributory to postoperative loss of vision.[148] The consultants and specialty society members, however, expressed concern about the use of deliberate hypotension in high-risk patients and recommended that the use of this technique be determined on a case-by-case basis.

Cortical Blindness

Brain injury rostral to the optic nerve may cause cortical blindness. The impairment is produced by damage to the visual path beyond the lateral geniculate nucleus or the visual cortex in the occipital lobe. Similar to anterior ischemic optic neuropathy, cortical blindness is a significant concern in patients undergoing CABG, and systemic disease is often present. Emboli and sustained, profound hypotension are common causes. Other events implicated in the pathophysiology include cardiac arrest, hypoxemia, intracranial hypertension, exsanguinating hemorrhage, vascular occlusion, thrombosis, and vasospasm.

Differential diagnostic features include a normal optic disc on fundoscopy and normal pupillary responses. There is, however, loss of optokinetic nystagmus with normal eye motility. CT and MRI are helpful in delineating the extent of brain infarction associated with cortical blindness. Occipital lesions are frequently bilateral and CT findings typically indicate posterior cerebral artery thrombosis, basilar artery occlusion, posterior cerebral artery branch occlusion, or watershed infarction. Lesions after CABG often include the parieto-occipital area.

Whereas most cases of ischemic optic neuropathy do not improve significantly or completely, visual recovery from cortical blindness in previously healthy patients may be considerable but prolonged. Preventive strategies include maintenance of adequate systemic perfusion pressure and, in cardiac surgery, minimizing manipulation of the aorta, meticulous removal of air and particulate matter during valvular procedures, and use of an arterial line filter in selected patients during bypass.

Acute Glaucoma

Although topical application of such mydriatic drugs as atropine and scopolamine is contraindicated in patients with known, chronic glaucoma, the systemic use of anticholinergics in usual premedicating doses is safe for glaucomatous eyes. The use of an atropine–neostigmine combination for reversal of neuromuscular blockade is also safe in patients with glaucoma. Topical ophthalmic medications that are being administered to control glaucoma should be continued through the perioperative period.

Acute angle-closure glaucoma typically occurs spontaneously but has been reported, albeit rarely, after both spinal and general anesthesia. Acute angle-closure glaucoma caused by pupillary block is a serious, multifactorial disease. Risk factors include genetic predisposition, shallow anterior chamber depth, increased lens thickness, small corneal diameter, female gender, and advanced age. One study[149] explored possible precipitating events in at-risk patients and found no evidence that the type of anesthetic agent, the duration of surgery, the volume of parenteral fluids, or the intraoperative blood pressure were related to the development of acute angle-closure glaucoma.

Despite its seriousness, acute angle-closure glaucoma may be difficult to recognize. However, physicians should be knowledgeable about this potential complication because diagnostic delay may detrimentally affect visual outcome and cause permanent optic nerve damage. Fazio et al.[150] recommended that the preoperative evaluation include a thorough ocular history and a penlight examination to detect a shallow anterior chamber. Those patients considered at risk should then undergo a preoperative ophthalmic evaluation and perioperative miotic therapy. After surgery, these patients should be scrupulously watched for red eye or a fixed dilated pupil, as well as for complaints of pain and blurred vision. Acute glaucoma is a true emergency, and ophthalmologic consultation should be secured immediately to acutely decrease IOP with systemic and topical therapy. The intense periorbital pain typically described by these patients is an important aid in differential diagnosis.

Postcataract Ptosis

Ptosis after cataract surgery is not uncommon, and multiple factors have been implicated in its etiology.[151,152] These include the presence of a pre-existing ptosis, injection of anesthetic solution into the upper lid when performing facial nerve block, retrobulbar injection, injection of peribulbar anesthesia through the upper eyelid at the 12 o'clock position, ocular compression or massage, the eyelid speculum, placement of a superior rectus bridle suture with traction on the superior rectus–levator complex, creation of a large conjunctival flap, prolonged or tight patching in the postoperative period, and postoperative eyelid edema. Feibel et al.[151] believed that the development of postcataract ptosis is multifactorial and that no single aspect of cataract surgery is the sole contributor. More recently, Taylor et al.[152] used MRI immediately after diagnosis of diplopia in four patients who received peribulbar block. They found peribulbar edema consistent with direct local anesthetic-induced myotoxicity after presumed inadvertent intramuscular injection. Although local anesthetics are clearly myotoxic, the local anesthetic injection cannot be isolated as the primary factor because postsurgical ptosis is also seen in patients undergoing surgery with general anesthesia.

References

1. Eye Diseases Prevalence Research Group: Prevalence of age-related macular degeneration in the United States. Arch Ophthalmol 2004; 122: 564
2. Hebert LE, Scherr PA, Bienias JL et al: Alzheimer disease in the US population: Prevalence estimates using the 2000 Census. Arch Neurol 2003; 60: 119
3. Wimo A, Winblad B: Health economical aspects of Alzheimer disease and its treatment. Psychogeriatrics 2001; 1: 189
4. Bruce RA: Ocular anatomy, Anesthesia for Ophthalmology. Edited by Bruce RA, McGoldrick KE, Oppenheimer P. Birmingham, Aesculapius, 1982, p 3
5. Teng C, Gurses-Ozden R, Liebmann JM et al: Effect of a tight necktie on intraocular pressure. Br J Ophthalmol 2003; 87: 946
6. Stoelting RK: Circulatory changes during direct laryngoscopy and tracheal intubation: Influence of duration of laryngoscopy with or without prior lidocaine. Anesthesiology 1977; 47: 381

7. Duncalf D, Foldes FF: Effect of anesthetic drugs and muscle relaxants on intraocular pressure, Anesthesia in Ophthalmology. Edited by Smith RB. Boston, Little Brown, 1973, p 21

8. Garde JF, Aston R, Endler GC et al: Racial mydriatic response to belladonna preparations. Anesth Analg 1978; 57: 572

9. Watcha MF, Chu FC, Stevens JL et al: Effects of halothane on intraocular pressure in anesthetized children. Anesth Analg 1990; 71: 181

10. Thompson MF, Brock-Utne JG, Bean P et al: Anaesthesia and intraocular pressure: A comparison of total intravenous anaesthesia using etomidate with conventional inhalational anaesthesia. Anaesthesia 1982; 37: 758

11. Yoshikawa K, Murai Y: Effect of ketamine on intraocular pressure in children. Anesth Analg 1971; 50: 199

12. Corssen G, Hoy JE: A new parenteral anesthetic—CI581: Its effect on intraocular pressure. J Pediatr Ophthalmol 1967; 4: 20

13. Peuler M, Glass DD, Arens JF: Ketamine and intraocular pressure. Anesthesiology 1975; 43: 575

14. Ausinsch B, Rayburn RL, Munson ES et al: Ketamine and intraocular pressure in children. Anesth Analg 1976; 55: 773

15. Ausinsch B, Graves SA, Munson ES et al: Intraocular pressure in children during isoflurane and halothane anesthesia. Anesthesiology 1975; 42: 167

16. Duncalf D, Weitzner SW: Ventilation and hypercapnia on intraocular pressure in children. Anesth Analg 1963; 43: 232

17. Litwiller RW, Difazio CA, Rushia EL: Pancuronium and intraocular pressure. Anesthesiology 1975; 42: 750

18. Lincoff HA, Breinin GM, DeVoe AG et al: Effect of succinylcholine on the extraocular muscles. Am J Ophthalmol 1957; 44: 440

19. Pandey K, Badolas RP, Kumar S: Time course of intraocular hypertension produced by suxamethonium. Br J Anaesth 1972; 44: 191

20. Kelly RE, Dinner M, Turner LS et al: Succinylcholine increases intraocular pressure in the human eye with the extraocular muscles detached. Anesthesiology 1993; 79: 948

21. Miller RD, Way WL, Hickey RF: Inhibition of succinylcholine-induced increased intraocular pressure by nondepolarizing muscle relaxants. Anesthesiology 1968; 29: 123

22. Meyers EF, Krupin T, Johnson M et al: Failure of nondepolarizing neuromuscular blockers to inhibit succinylcholine-induced increased intraocular pressure: A controlled study. Anesthesiology 1978; 48: 149

23. Verma RS: "Self-taming" of succinylcholine-induced fasciculations and intraocular pressure. Anesthesiology 1979; 50: 245

24. Meyers EF, Singer P, Otto A: A controlled study of the effect of succinylcholine self-taming on IOP. Anesthesiology 1980; 53: 72

25. Stoelting RK: Blood pressure and heart rate changes during short duration laryngoscopy for tracheal intubation: Influences of viscous or intravenous lidocaine. Anesth Analg 1978; 57: 197

26. Smith RB, Babinski M, Leano N: Effect of lidocaine on succinylcholine-induced rise in IOP. Can Anaesth Soc J 1979; 26: 482

27. Grover VK, Lata K, Sharma S et al: Efficacy of lignocaine in the suppression of the intraocular pressure response to suxamethonium and tracheal intubation. Anaesthesia 1989; 44: 22

28. Jampolsky A: Strabismus: Surgical overcorrections. Highlights Ophthalmol 1965; 8: 78

29. Dell R, Williams B. Anaesthesia for strabismus surgery: a regional survey. Br J Anaesth 1999; 82: 761

30. Berler DK: Oculocardiac reflex. Am J Ophthalmol 1963; 12(56): 954

31. Alexander JP: Reflex disturbances of cardiac rhythm during ophthalmic surgery. Br J Ophthalmol 1975; 59: 518

32. Mirakur RK, Clarke RSJ, Dundee JW et al: Anticholinergic drugs in anaesthesia: A survey of their present position. Anaesthesia 1978; 33: 133

33. Massumi RA, Mason DT, Amsterdam EA et al: Ventricular fibrillation and tachycardia after intravenous atropine for treatment of bradycardias. N Engl J Med 1972; 287: 336

34. McGoldrick KE: Transient left bundle branch block during local anesthesia. Anesthesiol Rev 1981; 8(6): 36

35. Moonie GT, Rees DI, Elton D: Oculocardiac reflex during strabismus surgery. Can Anaesth Soc J 1964; 11: 621

36. Steward DJ: Anticholinergic premedication for infants and children. Can Anaesth Soc J 1983; 30: 325

37. Nachman RL, Esterly NB: Increased skin permeability in preterm infants. J Pediatr 1971; 79: 628

38. Ellis EP, Esterdahl M: Echothiophate iodide therapy in children: Effect upon blood cholinesterase levels. Arch Ophthalmol 1967; 77: 598

39. Meyers EF: Cocaine toxicity during dacryocystorhinostomy. Arch Ophthalmol 1980; 98: 842

40. Gay GR, Loper KA: Control of cocaine-induced hypertension with labetalol (letter). Anesth Analg 1988; 67: 92

41. Lansche RK: Systemic effects of topical epinephrine and phenylephrine. Am J Ophthalmol 1966; 49: 95

42. Brown MM, Brown GC, Spaeth GL: Lack of side effects from topically administered 10% phenylephrine eye drops: A controlled study. Arch Ophthalmol 1980; 98: 487

43. Jones FL, Eckberg NL: Exacerbation of asthma by timolol. N Engl J Med 1979; 301: 170

44. Kim JW, Smith PH: Timolol-induced bradycardia. Anesth Analg 1980; 59: 301

45. Shavitz SA: Timolol and myasthenia gravis. JAMA 1979; 242: 1612

46. Bailey PL: Timolol and postoperative apnea in neonates and young infants. Anesthesiology 1984; 61: 622

47. Vinker S, Kaiserman I, Waitman DA, Blackman S, Kitai E. Prescription of ocular beta-blockers in patients with obstructive pulmonary disease: does a central electronic medical record make a difference? Clin Drug Investig 2006; 26: 495.

48. Stinson TW, Donlon JV: Interaction of SF6 and air with nitrous oxide. Anesthesiology 1979; 51: S16

49. Wolf GL, Capriano C, Hartung J: Effects of nitrous oxide on gas bubble volume in the anterior chamber. Arch Ophthalmol 1985; 103: 418

50. Chang S, Lincoff HA, Coleman DJ et al: Perfluorocarbon gases in vitreous surgery. Ophthalmology 1985; 92: 651

51. Marcus EN, Gayer S, Anderson DR: Medical evaluation of patients before ocular surgery (editorial). Am J Ophthalmol 2003; 136: 338

52. Schein OD, Katz J, Bass EB et al: The value of routine preoperative medical testing before cataract surgery. N Engl J Med 2000; 342: 168

53. Hall DL, Steen WH, Drummond JW et al: Anticoagulants and cataract surgery. Ophthalmic Surg 1988; 19: 221

54. Charles S, Rosenfeld PJ, Gayer S: Medical consequences of stopping anticoagulants prior to intraocular surgery or intravitreal injections. Retina 2007; 27(7): 813

55. Feitl ME, Krupin T: Retrobulbar anesthesia. Ophthalmol Clin North Am 1990; 3: 83

56. Katz J, Feldman MA, Bass EB et al: Risks and benefits of anticoagulant and antiplatelet medication use before cataract surgery. Ophthalmology 2003; 110: 1784

57. Vicenzi MN, Meislitzer T, Heitzinger B et al: Coronary artery stenting and noncardiac surgery: a prospective outcome study. Br J Anaesth 2006; 96: 686

58. Mauermann WJ, Rehfeldt KH, Bell MR, Lowson SM: Percutaneous coronary interventions and antiplatelet therapy in the perioperative period. J Cardiothorac Vasc Anesth 2007; 21: 436

59. Bayes J: A survey of ophthalmic anesthetists on managing pacemakers and implanted cardiac defibrillators. Anesth Analg 2006; 103: 1615

60. Stoller GL: Ophthalmic surgery and the implantable cardioverter defibrillator. Arch Ophthalmol 2006; 124: 123

61. Bhananker SM, Posner KL, Cheney FW et al: Injury and liability associated with monitored anesthesia care: A closed claims analysis. Anesthesiology 2006; 104: 228

62. Gayer S: Key components of risk associated with ophthalmic anesthesia. Anesthesiology 2006; 105: 859

63. McGoldrick KE: Ocular pathology and systemic diseases: Anesthetic implications, Anesthesia for Ophthalmic and Otolaryngologic Surgery. Edited by McGoldrick KE. Philadelphia, WB Saunders, 1992, p 210

64. Leaming DV: Practice styles and preferences of ASCRS members: 2002 survey. J Cataract Refract Surg 2003; 29: 1421

65. Guise PA: Sub-Tenon anesthesia: A prospective study of 6000 blocks. Anesthesiology 2003; 98: 964

66. Gayer S, Flynn HW Jr: Sub-Tenon's injection for local anesthesia in posterior segment surgery (discussion). Ophthalmology 2000; 107: 46

67. The Joint Commission on Accreditation of Healthcare Organizations: Universal protocol for preventing wrong site, wrong procedure, wrong person surgery. Accessed October 19th, 2007. http://www.jointcommission.org/PatientSafety/UniversalProtocol

68. Wainwright AC: Positive pressure ventilation and the laryngeal mask airway in ophthalmic anaesthesia. Br J Anaesth 1995; 75: 249

69. Lamb K, James MFM, Janicki PK: The laryngeal mask airway for intraocular surgery: Effects on intraocular pressure and stress responses. Br J Anaesth 1992; 69: 143

70. Thomson KD: The effect of the laryngeal mask airway on coughing after eye surgery under general anesthesia. Ophthalmic Surg 1992; 23: 630

71. Knapp H: On cocaine and its use in ophthalmic and general surgery. Arch Ophthalmol 1884; 13: 402

72. Atkinson WS: Retrobulbar injection of anesthetic within the muscular cone. Arch Ophthalmol 1936; 16: 494

73. Gayer S: Ophthalmic anesthesia: More than meets the eye, American Society of Anesthesiologists Refresher Courses in Anesthesiology. Edited by Schwartz AJ. Philadelphia, Lippincott Williams & Wilkins, 2006, p 55

74. Korneef L: The architecture of the musculofibrous apparatus in the human orbit. Acta Morphol Neerl Scand 1977; 15: 35

75. Ripart J, Lefrant J, de la Coussaye J et al: Peribulbar versus retrobulbar anesthesia for ophthalmic surgery. Anesthesiology 2001; 94: 56

76. Capó H, Roth E, Johnson T et al: Vertical strabismus after cataract surgery. Ophthalmology 1996; 103: 918

77. Ripart J, Lefrant J, Lalourcey L et al: Medial canthus (caruncle) single injection periocular anesthesia. Anesth Analg 1996; 83: 1234

78. Katsev DA, Drews RC, Rose BT: An anatomic study of retrobulbar needle path length. Ophthalmology 1989; 96: 1221

79. Waller SG, Taboada J, O'Connor P: Retrobulbar anesthesia risk: Do sharp needles really perforate the eye more easily than blunt needles? Ophthalmology 1993; 100: 506

80. Unsold R, Stanley JA, DeGroot J: The CT topography of retrobulbar anesthesia. Graefes Arch Clin Exp Ophthalmol 1981; 217: 125

81. Liu C, Youl B, Moseley I: Magnetic resonance imaging of the optic nerve in extremes of gaze. Implications for the positioning of the globe for retrobulbar anesthesia. Br J Ophthalmol 1992; 76: 728

82. Gayer S, Denham D, Alarakhia K et al: Ocular decompression devices: Liquid mercury balloon versus the tungsten powder balloon. Am J Ophthalmol 2006; 142: 500

83. Birch A, Evans M, Redembo E: The ultrasonic localiazation of retrobulbar needles during retrobulbar block. Ophthalmology 1995; 102: 824
84. Grizzard WS, Kirk NM, Pavan PR et al: Perforating ocular injuries caused by anesthesia personnel. Ophthalmology 1991; 98: 1011
85. Miller-Meeks MJ, Bergstrom T, Karp KO: Prevalent attitudes regarding residency training in ocular anesthesia. Ophthalmology 1994; 101: 1353
86. Gayer S, Kumar C: Ultrasound-guided orbital blocks, Perioperative Diagnostic and Interventional Ultrasound. Edited by Harmon D, Frizelle HP, Sandhu NS, Griffin M. Philadelphia, Elsevier, 2007, p 123
87. Chang J-L, Gonzalez-Abola E, Larson CE: Brain stem anesthesia following retrobulbar block. Anesthesiology 1984; 61: 789
88. Nicoll JMV, Acharya PA, Ahlen K et al: Central nervous system complications after 6000 retrobulbar blocks. Anesth Analg 1987; 66: 1298
89. Swan KC: New drugs and techniques for ocular anesthesia. Trans Am Acad Ophthalmol Otolaryngol 1956; 60: 368
90. Gayer S, Cass GD: Sub-Tenon techniques should be one option among many. Anesthesiology 2004; 100: 196
91. Niemi-Murola L, Krootila K, Kivisaari R et al: Localization of local anesthetic solution by magnetic resonance imaging. Ophthalmology 2004; 111: 342
92. Guise PA: Sub-Tenon anesthesia: A prospective study of 6,000 blocks. Anesthesiology 2003; 98: 964
93. Frieman BJ, Friedberg MA: Globe perforation with sub-tenon's anesthesia. J Ophthalmol 2001; 131: 520
94. Ruschen H, Bremner FD, Carr C: Complications after sub-Tenon's eye block. Anesth Analg 2003; 96: 273
95. Ripart J, Metge L, Prat-Pradal D et al: Medial canthus single-injection episcleral (sub-Tenon) anesthesia: Computed tomography imaging. Anesth Analg 1998; 87: 42
96. Quantock C, Goswami T: Death potentially secondary to sub-Tenon's block. Anaesthesia 2007; 62: 175.
97. Palte H, Gayer S: Death after a sub-Tenon's block. Anaesthesia 2007; 62: 531
98. Bardocci A, Lofoco G, Perdicaro S et al: Lidocaine 2% gel versus lidocaine 4% unpreserved drops for topical anesthesia in cataract surgery: A randomized controlled trial. Ophthalmology 2003; 110: 144
99. Eggeling P, Pleyer U, Hartman C et al: Corneal endothelial toxicity of different lidocaine concentrations. J Cataract Refract Surg 2000; 26: 1403
100. Netland PA, Harris A: Color Doppler ultrasound measurements after topical and retrobulbar epinephrine in primate eyes. Invest Ophthalmol Vis Sci 1997; 38: 2655
101. Brown SM, Coats DK, Collins MLZ et al: Second cluster of strabismus cases after periocular anesthesia without hyaluronidase. J Cataract Refract Surg 2001; 27: 1876
102. Hamada S, Devys JM, Xuan TH, et al.: Role of hyaluronidase in diplopia after peribulbar anesthesia for cataract surgery. Ophthalmology 2005; 112(5): 879
103. Strouthidis NG, Sobha S, Lnaigan L, Hammond CJ: Vertical diplopia following peribulbar anesthesia: The role of hyaluronidase. J Pediatr Ophthalmol Strabismus 2004; 41: 25
104. Kirsch RE: Further studies on the use of digital pressure in cataract surgery. Optimal length of time for application of digital pressure. Arch Ophthalmol 1957; 58: 641
105. Jay WM, Aziz MZ, Green K: Effect of intraocular pressure reducer on ocular and optic nerve blood flow in phakic rabbit eyes. Acta Ophthalmologica 1986; 64: 52
106. Downs JB: Has oxygen administration delayed appropriate respiratory care? Fallacies regarding oxygen therapy. Respir Care 2003; 48: 611
107. Hug CC: MAC should stand for maximum anesthesia caution, not minimal anesthesiology care (editorial). Anesthesiology 2006; 104: 221
108. Norregaard JC, Schein OD, Bellan L et al: International variation in anesthesia care during cataract surgery: Results from the International Cataract Surgery Outcomes Study. Arch Ophthalmol 1997; 115: 1304
109. Eichel R, Goldberg I: Anaesthesia techniques for cataract surgery: A survey of delegates to the Congress of the International Council of Ophthalmology, 2002. Clinical and Exper Ophthalmol 2005; 33: 469
110. Rosenfeld SI, Litinsky SM, Snyder DA et al: Effectiveness of monitored anesthesia care in cataract surgery. Ophthalmology 1999; 106: 1256
111. Fung D, Cohen MM, Stewart S, Davies A: What determines patient satisfaction with cataract care under topical local anaesthesia and monitored sedation in a community hospital setting? Anesth Analg 2005; 100: 1644
112. Gayer S: Rethinking anesthesia strategies for patients with traumatic eye injuries: Alternatives to general anesthesia. Curr Anesth Crit Care 2006; 17: 191
113. Scott IU, McCabe CM, Flynn HW Jr, Gayer S et al: Local anesthesia with intravenous sedation for surgical repair of selected open globe injuries. Am J Ophthalmol 2002; 134: 707
114. Boscia F, La Tegola MG, Columbo G et al: Combined topical anesthesia and sedation for open-globe injuries in selected patients. Ophthalmology 2003; 110: 1555
115. Casson WR, Jones RM: Vecuronium induced neuromuscular blockade. Anaesthesia 1986; 41: 354
116. Ginsberg B, Glass PS, Quill T et al: Onset and duration of neuromuscular blockade following high-dose vecuronium administration. Anesthesiology 1989; 71: 201
117. Konchiergeri HN, Lee YE, Venugopal K: Effect of pancuronium on intraocular pressure changes induced by succinylcholine. Can Anaesth Soc J 1979; 26: 479
118. Libonati MM, Leahy JJ, Ellison N: The use of succinylcholine in open eye surgery. Anesthesiology 1985; 62: 637
119. McGoldrick KE: The open globe: Is an alternative to succinylcholine necessary? (editorial). J Clin Anesth 1993; 5: 1
120. de Boer H, Driessen JJ, Marcus MA, Kerkkamp H et al: Reversal of rocuronium-induced (1.2 mg/kg) neuromuscular block by sugammadex: A multi-center dose-finding and safety study. Anesthesiology 2007; 107: 239
121. Kopman AF: Sugammadex: A revolutionary approach to neuromuscular antagonism (editorial). Anesthesiology 2006; 104: 631
122. Baumgarten RK, Reynolds WJ: Priming principle and the open eye-full stomach. Anesthesiology 1985; 63: 561
123. France NK, France TD, Wordburn JD Jr, Burbank DP. Succinylcholine alteration of the forced duction test. Ophthalmology 1980; 87: 1282
124. Lerman MD, Eustis S, Smith DR: Effect of droperidol pretreatment on postanesthetic vomiting in children undergoing strabismus surgery. Anesthesiology 1986; 65: 322
125. Brown RE, James DG, Weaver RG et al: Low-dose droperidol versus standard-dose droperidol for prevention of postoperative vomiting after pediatric strabismus surgery. J Clin Anesth 1991; 3: 306
126. Gan TJ, Meyer TA, Apfel CC, et al. Society of Ambulatory Anesthesia guidelines for the management of postoperative nausea and vomiting. Anesth Analg 2007; 105: 1615
127. Watcha MF, Simeon RM, White PF et al: Effect of propofol on the incidence of postoperative vomiting after strabismus surgery in pediatric outpatients. Anesthesiology 1991; 75: 204
128. Munro HM, Riegger LQ, Reynolds PI et al: Comparison of the analgesic and emetic properties of ketorolac and morphine for paediatric outpatient strabismus surgery. Br J Anaesth 1994; 72: 624
129. Seaberg RR, Freeman WR, Goldbaum MH et al: Permanent postoperative vision loss associated with expansion of intraocular gas in the presence of a nitrous oxide-containing anesthetic. Anesthesiology 2002; 97: 1309
130. Dallinger S, Findl O, Strenn K et al: Age dependence of choroidal blood flow. J Am Geriatr Soc 1998; 46: 484
131. Langham ME, Grebe R, Hopkins S et al: Choroidal blood flow in diabetic retinopathy. Exp Eye Res 1991; 52: 167
132. Recchia FM, Brown GC. Systemic disorders associated with retinal vascular occlusion. Curr Opin Ophthalmol 2000; 11: 462
133. Roth S, Thisted RA, Erickson JP et al: Eye injuries after nonocular surgery: A study of 60,965 anesthetics from 1988–1992. Anesthesiology 1996; 85: 1020
134. Gild WA, Posner KL, Caplan RA et al: Eye injuries associated with anesthesia. Anesthesiology 1992; 76: 204
135. Lee LA, Posner KL, Domino KB et al: Injuries associated with regional anesthesia in the 1980s and 1990s: A Closed Claims analysis. Anesthesiology 2004; 101: 143
136. Batra YK, Bali M: Corneal abrasions during general anesthesia. Anesth Analg 1977; 56: 363
137. Cucchiara R, Black S: Corneal abrasion during anesthesia and surgery. Anesthesiology 1988; 69: 978
138. Purdy EP, Ajimal GS: Vision loss after lumbar epidural steroid injection. Anesth Analg 1988; 86: 119
139. Roth S, Gillesberg I: Injuries to the visual system and other sense organs, Anesthesia and Perioperative Complications, 2nd ed. Edited by Benumof JL, Saidman LJ. St. Louis, Mosby, 1999, p 377
140. Mabry RL: Visual loss after intranasal corticosteroid injection. Arch Otolaryngol 1981; 107: 484
141. Lee LA: Postoperative visual loss data gathered and analyzed. ASA Newsletter 2000; 64: 25
142. Myers MA, Hamilton SR, Bogosian AJ et al: Visual loss as a complication of spinal surgery. Spine 1997; 22: 1325
143. Dilger JA, Tetzlaff JE, Bell GR et al: Ischemic optic neuropathy after spinal fusion. Can J Anaesth 1998; 45: 63
144. Shapira OM, Kimmel WA, Lindsey PS et al: Anterior ischemic optic neuropathy after open heart operations. Ann Thorac Surg 1996; 61: 660
145. Williams EL, Hart WM, Tempelhoff R: Postoperative ischemic optic neuropathy. Anesth Analg 1995; 80: 1018
146. The Ischemic Optic Neuropathy Decompression Trial Research Group: Optic nerve decompression surgery is not effective and may be harmful. JAMA 1995; 273: 625
147. Lee LA, Roth S, Posner KL et al: The American Society of Anesthesiologists Postoperative Visual Loss Registry: Analysis of 93 spine surgery cases with postoperative visual loss. Anesthesiology 2006; 105: 652
148. American Society of Anesthesiologists Task Force on Perioperative Blindness: Practice advisory for perioperative visual loss associated with spine surgery: A report by the American Society of Anesthesiologists Task Force on Perioperative Blindness. Anesthesiology 2006; 104: 1319
149. Drance SM: Angle-closure glaucoma among Canadian Eskimos. Can J Ophthalmol 1973; 8: 252
150. Fazio DT, Bateman JB, Christensen RE: Acute angle-closure glaucoma associated with surgical anesthesia. Arch Ophthalmol 1985; 103: 360
151. Feibel RM, Custer PL, Gordon MO: Postcataract ptosis: A randomized, double-masked comparison of peribulbar and retrobulbar anesthesia. Ophthalmology 1993; 100: 660
152. Taylor G, Devys JM, Heran F, Plaud B. Early exploration of diplopia with magnetic resonance imaging after peribulbar anaesthesia. Br J Anaesth 2004; 92: 899

CHAPTER 52 ■ THE RENAL SYSTEM AND ANESTHESIA FOR UROLOGIC SURGERY

MARK STAFFORD-SMITH, ANDREW SHAW, RONALD GEORGE, AND HOLLY MUIR

KEY POINTS

1 Renal filtration and reabsorption are susceptible to alterations by surgical illness and anesthesia. Autoregulation of renal blood flow (RBF) is effective over a wide range of mean arterial pressures (50 to 150 mm Hg). Autoregulation of urine flow does not occur, but a linear relationship between mean arterial pressure above 50 mm Hg and urine output is observed.

2 Renal medullary blood flow is low (2% of total RBF) but central to the kidneys' ability to concentrate urine. During periods of reduced RBF, the metabolically active medullary thick ascending limb may be especially vulnerable to ischemic injury.

3 The physiological response to surgical stress invokes intrinsic mechanisms for sodium and water conservation. Renal cortical vasoconstriction causes, a shift in perfusion toward juxtamedullary nephrons, a decrease in glomerular filtration rate, and retention of salt and water result.

4 The stress response may induce a decrease in RBF and glomerular filtration rate, causing afferent arteriolar vasoconstriction. If this situation is not reversed, ischemic damage to the kidney may result in acute renal failure (ARF).

5 Anesthetic-induced reductions in RBF have been described for many agents but are usually clinically insignificant and reversible. Likewise, anesthetic agents have not been shown to interfere with the renal response to physiologic stress.

6 Overall, there are no conclusive comparative studies demonstrating superior renal protection or improved renal outcome with general versus regional anesthesia.

7 Isolated ARF carries a mortality of up to 60% in surgical patients, with acute tubular necrosis being the cause of ARF in most of these patients.

8 Surgical patients with nondialysis-dependent chronic kidney disease are at higher risk of developing end-stage renal disease. The single most reliable predictor of postoperative renal dysfunction is preoperative renal insufficiency.

9 Maintaining adequate intravascular volume and hemodynamic stability with aggressive management of kidney hypoperfusion is a basic principle of anesthetic care to prevent acute kidney injury.

10 Urologic patients are often elderly, have numerous comorbidities, and require critical evaluation prior to any urologic procedure.

11 Absorption of irrigating solution during procedures for transurethral resection of the prostate is ubiquitous but can reach levels that become serious and even life-threatening. Knowledge of specific concerns relevant to the different irrigating solutions, and vigilance of the anesthesiologist to factors that minimize absorption, recognition of signs and symptoms of transurethral resection of the prostate syndrome, and appropriate treatments are key to favorable outcomes with this procedure.

12 The advent of minimally invasive techniques and technological innovation, including robotics, is changing many high-risk urologic surgeries (e.g., radical prostatectomy, radical nephrectomy) so that they are becoming moderate or minimal risk procedures.

13 Combined epidural-general anesthetic techniques may offer advantages for accelerated recovery, improved analgesia, and even better outcomes, but these techniques must be conducted with respect for other perioperative issues, including thromboprophylaxis for prevention of deep venous thrombosis.

14 As urologic surgeries evolve, the anesthesiologist is being asked to identify candidates and facilitate fast-track anesthetic techniques for procedures and patients not previously considered eligible for such treatment.

INTRODUCTION AND CONTEXT

The kidney plays a central role in implementing and controlling a variety of homeostatic functions, including excreting metabolic waste products in the urine, while keeping extracellular fluid volume and composition constant. Renal dysfunction can occur as a direct result of surgical or medical disease, prolonged reduction in renal oxygen delivery, nephrotoxin insult, or a combination of these three factors. The first part of this chapter reviews renal physiology and pathophysiologic states as they relate to anesthetic practice, and then addresses strategies for recognizing and managing patients at risk for renal failure. The second part describes current urologic procedures and their attendant anesthetic management issues.

RENAL ANATOMY AND PHYSIOLOGY

Gross Anatomy

The two normal *kidneys* are reddish-brown organs and are approximately 10 cm long, 5 cm wide, and 2.5 cm thick. They are ovoid in outline, but the medial margin is deeply indented and concave at its middle, (Fig. 52-1). where a wide, vertical cleft (the hilus) transmits structures entering and leaving the kidney. The *hilus* lies at approximately the level of the first lumbar vertebra. The kidneys lie in the paravertebral gutters, behind the peritoneum, with the right kidney lying slightly lower than the left one because of the presence of the liver. At its upper end, the ureter has dilated to give rise to the *renal pelvis*, which passes through the hilus into the kidney proper. There it is continuous with several short funnel-like tubes (calyces) that unite it with the renal parenchyma. The renal blood vessels lie anterior to the pelvis of the kidney, but some branches may pass posteriorly. Renal pain sensation is conveyed back to spinal cord segments T10 through L1 by sympathetic fibers. Sympathetic innervation is supplied by preganglionic fibers from T8 to L1. The vagus nerve provides parasympathetic innervation to the kidney, and the S2 to S4 spinal segments supply the ureters.

The kidneys are enclosed by a thick, fibrous capsule, itself surrounded by a fatty capsule that fills the space inside the loosely applied renal fascia. The developing kidney is first formed in the pelvis and then ascends to its final position on the posterior abdominal wall. During its ascent the kidney receives blood supply from several successive sources, such that an accessory renal artery from the aorta may be found entering the lower pole of the kidney. When first formed, the rudimentary kidneys are close together and may fuse to give rise to a horseshoe kidney. This organ is unable to ascend, held in place by the inferior mesenteric artery, and thus when present it remains forever a pelvic organ.

The *bladder* is located in the retropubic space and receives its innervation from sympathetic nerves originating from T11 to L2, which conduct pain, touch, and temperature sensations, whereas bladder stretch sensation is transmitted via

ANESTHESIA FOR SURGICAL SUBSPECIALTIES

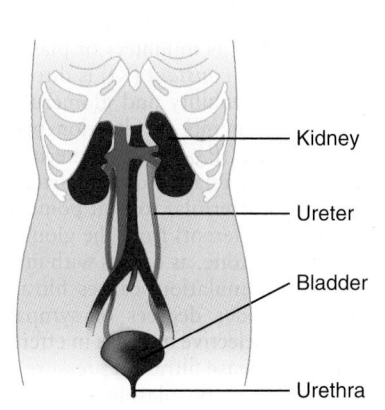

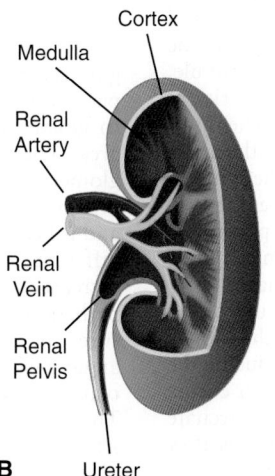

FIGURE 52-1. The gross anatomy (**A**) and internal structure of the genitourinary system and kidney. Internal organization of the kidney includes cortex and medulla regions and the vasculature (**B**). The nephron is the functional unit of the kidney (**C**). Plasma filtration occurs in the glomerulus (**D**); 20% of plasma that enters the glomerulus passes through the specialized capillary wall into Bowman capsule and enters the tubule to be processed and generate urine. PCT, proximal convoluted tubule, DCT, distal convoluted tubule. (From http://www.incontinenceaid.com/files/images/Urinary_system_components.jpg [A]; B; http://www.pathology.vcu.edu/education/PathLab/ pages/renalpath/rpsrhome.htm from Lecture 1 (modified with permission) [C];

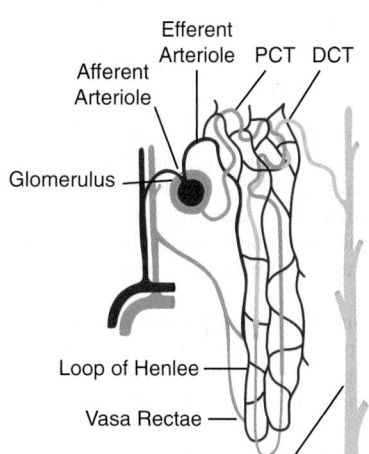

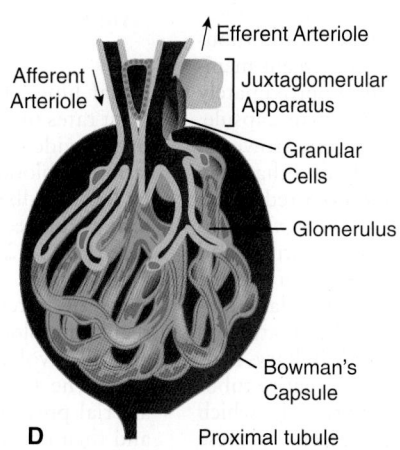

parasympathetic fibers from segments S2 to S4. Parasympathetics also provide the bladder with most of its motor innervation.

The *prostate, penile urethra,* and *penis* also receive sympathetic and parasympathetic fibers from the T11 to L2 and S2 to S4 segments, respectively. The pudendal nerve provides pain sensation to the penis via the dorsal nerve of the penis. Sensory innervation of the *scrotum* is via cutaneous nerves, which project to lumbosacral segments, whereas testicular sensation is conducted to lower thoracic and upper lumbar segments.

Ultrastructure

Inspection of the cut surface of the kidney reveals the paler *cortex,* adjacent to the capsule, and the darker, conical pyramids of the renal *medulla* (Fig. 52-1). The pyramids are radially striated and are covered with cortex, extending into the kidney as the renal columns. *Collecting tubules* from each lobe of the kidney (pyramid and its covering of cortex) discharge urine into the calyceal system via renal papillae at the entrance of each pyramid into the calyx proper. These collecting tubules originate deep within the radial striations (medullary rays) of the kidney and convey urine formed in the structural units of the kidneys, the *nephrons.* The parenchyma of each kidney contains approximately 1×10^6 tightly packed nephrons, each one consisting of a tuft of capillaries (the *glomerulus*) invaginated into the blind, expanded end (glomerular corpuscle) of a long tubule that leaves the renal corpuscle to form the proximal convoluted tubule in the cortex. This leads into the straight tubule, which loops down into the medullary pyramid (*loop of Henle*) and thence back to the cortex to become continuous with the distal convoluted tubule. This then opens into a collecting duct that is common to a number of nephrons, and passes through the pyramid to enter the lesser calyx at the papilla. It is in these parts of the nephron (proximal tubule, loop of Henle, distal tubule and collecting duct) that urine is formed, concentrated, and conveyed to the ureters. The distal convoluted tubule comes into very close contact with the afferent glomerular arteriole, and the cells of each are there modified to form the *juxtaglomerular apparatus,* a complex physiological feedback control mechanism contributing in part to the precise control of intra- and extrarenal hemodynamics that is a hallmark feature of the normally functioning kidney.

As is the case for the renal tubules, the vasculature of the kidney is highly organized. The renal artery enters the kidney at the hilum and then divides many times before producing the arcuate arteries that run along the boundary between cortex and outer medulla. Interlobular arteries branch from arcuate arteries toward the outer kidney surface, giving rise as they pass through the cortex to numerous afferent arterioles, each leading to a single glomerular capillary tuft. The barrier where filtration from the vascular to tubular space within the glomerulus occurs is highly specialized and includes fenestrated negatively charged capillary endothelial cells and tubular epithelial cells (podocytes) separated by a basement membrane. Normally, selective permeability permits approximately 25% of the plasma elements to pass into Bowman capsule; only cells and proteins >60 to 70 kDa cannot cross. However, abnormalities of this barrier can occur with diseases that may permit filtration of much larger proteins and even red blood cells; these changes manifest as the *nephrotic syndrome* (proteinuria >3.5 g/24 hr) or *glomerulonephritis* (hematuria and proteinuria). The glomerular capillaries exit Bowman capsule and merge to form the efferent arteriole and peritubular capillaries that nourish the tubules. The renal vasculature is unusual in having this arrangement of two capillary beds joined in series by arterioles. Blood supply to the entire tubular system comes from the glomerular efferent arteriole, which branches into an extensive capillary network. Some of these peritubular capillaries, the *vasa recta,* descend deep into the medulla to parallel the loops of Henle. The vasa recta then return in a cortical direction with the loops, join other peritubular capillaries, and empty into the cortical veins.

Correlation of Structure and Function

Because renal tissue makes up only 0.4% of body weight but receives 25% of cardiac output, the kidneys are by far the most highly perfused major organs in the body, and this facilitates plasma filtration at rates as high as 125 to 140 mL/min in adults. The functions of the kidney are many and varied, including waste filtration, endocrine and exocrine activity, immune and metabolic function, and maintenance of physiological homeostasis. As well as tight regulation of extracellular solutes such as sodium, potassium, hydrogen, bicarbonate, and glucose; the kidney also generates ammonia and glucose and eliminates nitrogenous and other metabolic waste including urea, creatinine, and bilirubin. Finally, circulating hormones secreted by the kidney influence red blood cell generation, calcium homeostasis, and systemic blood pressure.

The kidney fulfills its dual roles of waste excretion and body fluid management by filtering large amounts of fluid and solutes from the blood and secreting waste products into the tubular fluid. Filtration and reabsorption are affected by comorbid disease, surgery, and anesthesia and are the focus of the next section.

Glomerular Filtration

Production of urine begins with water and solute filtration from plasma flowing into the glomerulus via the afferent arteriole. The *glomerular filtration rate* (GFR) is a measure of glomerular function expressed as milliliters of plasma filtered per minute. The *ultrafiltration constant* (Kf) is directly related to glomerular capillary permeability and glomerular surface area. The two major determinants of filtration pressure are glomerular capillary pressure (P_{GC}) and glomerular oncotic pressure (π_{GC}). P_{GC} is directly related to renal artery pressure and is heavily influenced by arteriolar tone at points upstream (afferent) and downstream (efferent) from the glomerulus. An increase in afferent arteriolar tone, as occurs with intense sympathetic or angiotensin II stimulation, causes filtration pressure and GFR to fall. Milder degrees of sympathetic or angiotensin activity cause a selective increase in efferent arteriolar tone, which tends to increase filtration pressure and GFR. The π_{GC} is directly dependent on plasma oncotic pressure. Afferent arteriolar dilatation enhances GFR by increasing glomerular flow, which in turn elevates glomerular capillary pressure.

Autoregulation of Renal Blood Flow and Glomerular Filtration Rate

Renal blood flow *autoregulation* maintains relatively constant rates of renal blood flow (RBF) and glomerular filtration over a wide range of arterial blood pressure. Renal autoregulation of blood flow and filtration is accomplished primarily by local feedback signals that modulate glomerular arteriolar tone to protect the glomeruli from excessive perfusion pressure (Fig. 52-2).

In health, autoregulation of RBF is effective over a wide range of systemic arterial pressures. Several mechanisms for regulating blood flow to the glomeruli have been described, and all involve modulation of afferent glomerular arteriolar tone. The *myogenic reflex theory* holds that an increase in arterial pressure causes the afferent arteriolar wall to stretch and then constrict (by reflex); likewise, a decrease in arterial

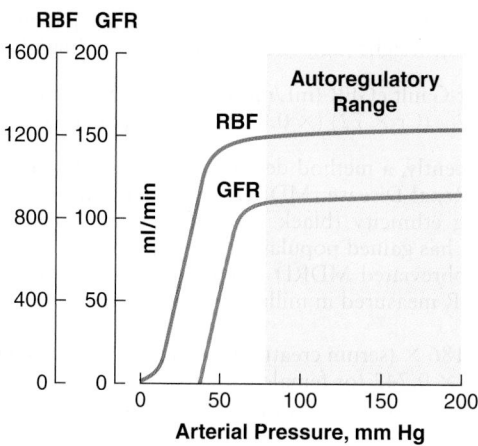

FIGURE 52-2. Renal blood flow (RBF) autoregulation maintains RBF and glomerular filtration rate (GFR) relatively constant with changes in systolic blood pressure from about 80 to 200 mm Hg. (From http://www2.kumc.edu/ki/physiology/course/two/ 2_8.htm.)

pressure causes reflex afferent arteriolar dilatation. The other proposed mechanism of RBF autoregulation is a phenomenon called *tubuloglomerular feedback*, which is also responsible for autoregulation of GFR.

Tubuloglomerular feedback allows the composition of distal tubular fluid to influence glomerular function through actions involving the juxtaglomerular apparatus. When RBF falls, the concomitant decrease in GFR results in less chloride delivery to the juxtaglomerular apparatus, which causes the afferent arteriole to dilate. Glomerular flow and pressure then increase, and GFR returns to previous levels. Chloride also acts as the feedback signal for control of efferent arteriolar tone. When GFR falls, declining chloride delivery to the juxtaglomerular apparatus triggers release of *renin*, which ultimately causes the formation of *angiotensin II*. In response to angiotensin, efferent arteriolar constriction increases glomerular pressure, which increases glomerular filtration. It is important to realize that autoregulation of urine flow does not occur and that above a mean arterial pressure of 50 mm Hg there is a linear relationship between and mean arterial pressure and urine output.

Tubular Reabsorption of Sodium and Water

Active, energy-dependent reabsorption of sodium begins almost immediately as the glomerular filtrate enters the proximal tubule. Here, an adenosine triphosphatase pump drives the sodium into tubular cells while chloride ions passively follow. Glucose, amino acid, and other organic compound reabsorption is strongly coupled to sodium in the proximal tubule. Normally, the proximal tubule reabsorbs two thirds of the filtered sodium, but no active sodium transport occurs in the loop of Henle until the medullary thick ascending limb is reached. Cells of the medullary thick ascending limb are metabolically active in their role of reabsorbing sodium and chloride, and have a high oxygen consumption compared with the thin portions of the descending and ascending limbs.

Reabsorption of water is a passive, osmotically driven process tied to the reabsorption of sodium and other solutes. Water reabsorption also depends on peritubular capillary pressure; high capillary pressure opposes water reabsorption and tends to increase urine output. The proximal tubule reabsorbs approximately 65% of filtered water in an isosmotic fashion with sodium and chloride. The descending limb of the loop of

Henle allows water to follow osmotic gradients into the renal interstitium. However, the thin ascending limb and medullary thick ascending limb are relatively impermeable to water and play a key role in the production of concentrated urine. Only 15% of filtered water is reabsorbed by the loop of Henle; the remaining filtrate volume flows into the distal tubule. There, and in the collecting duct, water reabsorption is controlled entirely by *antidiuretic hormone* (ADH) secreted by the pituitary gland. Conservation of water and excretion of excess solute by the kidneys would be impossible without the ability to produce concentrated urine. This is accomplished by establishing a hyperosmotic medullary interstitium and regulation of water permeability of the distal tubule and collecting duct via the action of ADH.

ADH increases the water permeability of the collecting ducts and allows for passive diffusion of water (under considerable osmotic pressure) back into the circulation. The posterior pituitary gland releases ADH in response to an increase in either extracellular sodium concentration or extracellular osmolality. In addition, ADH release can be triggered by an absolute or relative reduction in intravascular fluid volume. The arterial baroreceptors are activated when hypovolemia leads to a decrease in blood pressure, whereas atrial receptors are stimulated by a decline in atrial filling pressure. Both of these circulatory reflex systems stimulate release of ADH from the pituitary and cause retention of water by the kidney in an effort to return the intravascular volume toward normal. ADH also causes renal cortical vasoconstriction when it is released in large amounts, such as during the physiologic stress response to trauma, surgery, or other critical illness. This induces a shift of RBF to the hypoxia-prone renal medulla.

The Renin-Angiotensin-Aldosterone System. *Renin* release by the afferent arteriole may be triggered by hypotension, increased tubular chloride concentration, or by sympathetic stimulation. Renin enhances *angiotensin II* production, which in turn induces renal efferent arteriolar vasoconstriction. Angiotensin II also promotes ADH release from the posterior pituitary, sodium reabsorption by the proximal tubule, and aldosterone release by the adrenal medulla. *Aldosterone* stimulates the distal tubule and collecting duct to reabsorb sodium (and water), resulting in intravascular volume expansion. Sympathetic nervous system stimulation may also directly cause release of aldosterone. This leads to renal cortical vasoconstriction, a decrease in GFR, and salt and water retention.

Renal Vasodilator Mechanisms. Opposing the saline retention and vasoconstriction observed in stress states are the actions of *atrial natriuretic peptide* (ANP), *nitric oxide,* and the renal *prostaglandin* system. ANP is released by the cardiac atria in response to increased stretch under conditions of volume expansion. Both natriuresis and aquaresis increase as ANP blocks reabsorption of sodium in the distal tubule and collecting duct. ANP also increases GFR, causes systemic vasodilatation, inhibits the release of renin, opposes production and action of angiotensin II, and decreases aldosterone secretion.[1,2] Likewise, nitric oxide produced in the kidney opposes the renal vasoconstrictor effects of angiotensin II and the adrenergic nervous system, promotes sodium and water excretion, and participates in tubuloglomerular feedback.[3]

Prostaglandins are produced by the kidney as part of a complex system that modulates RBF and opposes the actions of ADH and the renin-angiotensin-aldosterone system.[4] Stress states, renal ischemia, and hypotension stimulate the production of renal prostaglandins through the enzymes phospholipase A_2 and cyclooxygenase. Prostaglandins produced by cyclooxygenase activity cause dilatation of renal arterioles (antiangiotensin II), whereas their distal tubular effects result in an increase in sodium and water excretion (anti-ADH and aldosterone). The renal prostaglandin system is important in maintaining RBF and sodium and water excretion during times of high physiologic stress and poor renal perfusion.[4]

Clinical Assessment of the Kidney

Most agree that measures such as urine output correlate only poorly with perioperative renal function[1]; however, much about the kidneys can be learned from knowing how effectively they clear circulating substances, and inspection of the urine (i.e., urinalysis).

Renal Function Tests

Filtration is the most clinically assessed kidney function. As a key indicator of disease, knowledge of limited filtration capacity is important to guide drug dosing for agents cleared by the kidneys and helps with preoperative risk stratification. Also, acute declines in filtration capacity also indicate kidney injury and predict a more complicated clinical course.[2] *Glomerular filtration rate,* as previously mentioned, refers to the plasma volume filtered per unit time by the kidneys, and normal values range from 90 to 140 mL/min. Normal GFRs are related to patient age, size, and gender. In general, GFR declines 10% per decade after age 30 and is approximately 10 mL/min higher in men than women. A GFR below 60 mL/min is considered impaired, and values lower than 15 mL/min are often associated with uremic symptoms and may require dialysis.

An "ideal" substance used to assess GFR through clearance from the circulation must have specific properties, including a steady supply, free filtration, and no tubular reabsorption or excretion; ideally, it is also cheap and easy to measure. Unfortunately, the perfect ideal substance is yet to be identified. The "gold standard" GFR tools involve expensive and cumbersome measurements (e.g., inulin, ^{51}Cr-EDTA or ^{99}Tc-DTPA clearance), while the most practical and inexpensive test involves an imperfect "ideal" substance, *creatinine*. However, despite creatinine's limitations, its relatively steady supply from muscle metabolism, modest tubular secretion, and proven usefulness in numerous clinical settings make it the most used renal filtration marker currently available. Although more ideal substances and other "early biomarkers" of acute kidney injury (AKI) are being evaluated as clinical tools, current candidates (e.g., cystatin C[3,4]) have yet to replace creatinine.

Estimates of GFR (eGFR) can be made by determining *creatinine clearance* (CrCl) from urine and blood creatinine tests. In stable, critically ill patients, 2-hour urine collections are sufficient to calculate CrCl,[5] using the following formula:

$$CrCl \ (mL/min) = U_{Cr} \ (mg/dL) \times V \ (mL)/P_{Cr} \ (mg/dL) \times time \ (min)$$

where U_{Cr} = urine creatinine, V = total volume of urine collected, P_{Cr} = plasma creatinine, time = collection time.

However, if patient characteristics are known GFR can also be estimated from a single steady-state serum creatinine value. Notably, predictive formulas are developed using data from stable (nonsurgical) populations, and factors such as fluid shifts, hemodilution, and hemorrhage may add an "unsteadiness" to perioperative estimates of GFR using serum creatinine.

Nonetheless, serum creatinine remains, so far, an unsurpassed perioperative tool, particularly to reflect *trends* of change in renal filtration and to predict outcome, even during the perioperative period.[6–8] Of the predictive formulas, the Cockroft-Gault equation is one of the oldest and most durable.[9] The Cockroft-Gault equation uses patient gender, age (years), weight (kg), and serum creatinine (mg/dL):

Cockroft-Gault eGFR (mL/min) = (140 − age) × weight (kg)/ (Cr × 72) (× 0.85 for female patients)

More recently, a method developed from the Modification of Diet in Renal Disease (MDRD) study that adds other factors including ethnicity (black vs. nonblack) to Cockroft-Gault equation has gained popularity.[10]

An abbreviated MDRD formula is available that can estimate GFR measured in milliliters per minute per 1.73 m²:

GFR = 186 × (serum creatinine − mg/dL)$^{-1.154}$ × (age)$^{-0.203}$ (× 0.742 for female patients) (× 1.210 for black patients)

However, even a detailed MDRD eGFR under ideal conditions sometimes correlates poorly with a gold standard-determined GFR, with more than a 30% error in 10% of patients, and 2% deviating more than 50%.[10]

Some consensus definitions for significant perioperative renal dysfunction exist. For example, the Society of Thoracic Surgeons defines postoperative renal failure as either a new requirement for dialysis or a rise in serum creatinine to >2.0 mg/dL involving at least a 50% increase in serum creatinine above baseline.[11] Another definition requires a creatinine rise of >25% or 0.5 mg/dL (44 μmol/L) within 48 hours.[12] The Acute Dialysis Quality Initiative Group definition for critically ill patients grades acute renal failure by an acute creatinine rise of 50% as *risk*, 100% as *injury*, or 200% as *failure* (the RIFLE criteria).[13] Notably, serum creatinine does not usually rise significantly until GFR rates fall below 50 mL/min, so preoperative serum creatinine may be normal in patients even with some degree of renal dysfunction (Fig. 52-3).

Blood urea nitrogen (BUN) is sometimes used to assess renal function, but possesses few of the characteristics of an ideal substance. Tubular urea transport changes with some conditions (e.g., dehydration), and urea generation can be highly variable, particularly during the postoperative period (i.e., catabolic state). In addition, hemodilution (e.g., cardiopulmonary bypass [CPB]) may affect circulating BUN levels.

Urinalysis and Urine Characteristics. Urine inspection can reveal abnormal cloudiness, color, and unexpected odors. Detailed descriptions of urine examination are available[14]; therefore, only a summary is provided here. Cloudy urine is due to suspended elements such as white or red blood cells and/or crystals. Lightly centrifuged urine sediment will normally contain 80 ± 20 mg of protein per day and up to two red blood cells per high-power field (400×); higher levels of red blood cells or protein reflect abnormal kidney function. Urine protein electrophoresis can differentiate proteinuria from a glomerular (filtering), tubular (reuptake), overflow (supply that saturates the reuptake system), or tissue (e.g., kidney inflammation) abnormality.[15] In contrast, color changes reflect dissolved substances; this occurs most commonly with dehydration, but other causes include food colorings, drugs, and liver disease (e.g., bilirubin). Unusual odors are less common but can also be diagnostic (e.g., maple syrup urine disease). Chromogenic "dipstick" chemical tests can determine urine pH and provide a semiquantitative analysis of protein, blood, nitrites, leukocyte esterase glucose, ketones, urobilinogen and bilirubin. In addition, microscopy can identify crystals, cells, tubular casts, and bacteria.

Urine *specific gravity* (the weight of urine relative to distilled water) normally ranges between 1.001 and 1.035, and can be used as a surrogate for osmolarity (normal 50 to 1,000

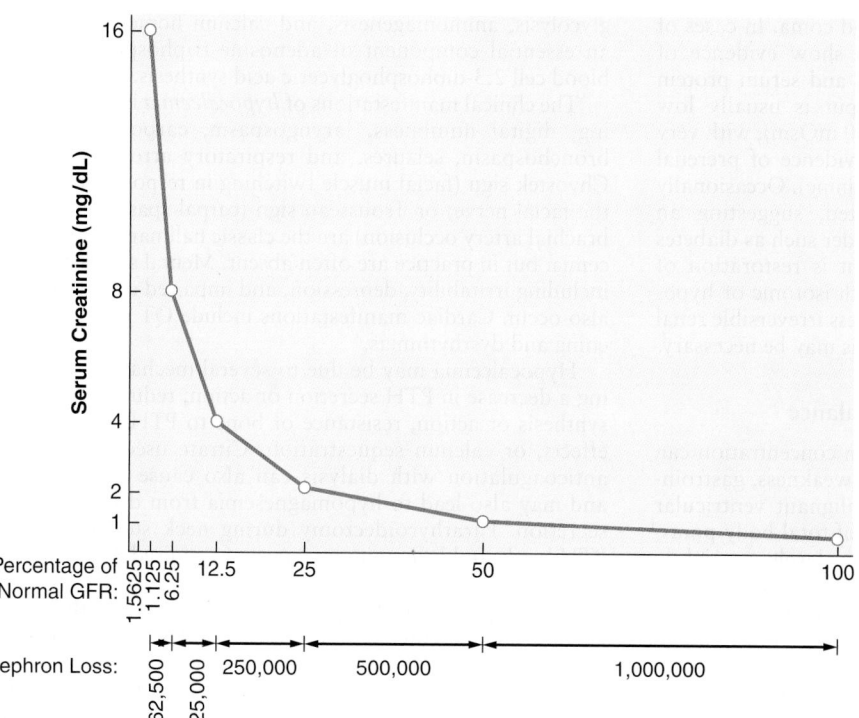

FIGURE 52-3. The nonlinear relationship between changes in renal filtration and serum creatinine level means that a large reduction (e.g., 75%, 120 to 30 mL/min) in glomerular filtration rate (GFR) may be associated with a modest rise in serum creatinine. Proportional reductions in GFR and (approximate) nephron loss (x axis) have an inverse logarithmic relationship with serum creatinine concentration (y axis). (Modified from Faber MD, Kupin WL, Krishna G et al: Acute Renal Failure: The differential diagnosis of ARF, 3rd edition. Edited by Lazarus JM, Brenner BM. New York, Churchill Livingstone, 1993, p 133.)

mOsm/kg), with 1.010 reflecting a specific gravity similar to that of plasma. High specific gravity (>1.018) implies preserved renal concentrating ability, unless high levels of glucose, protein, or contrast dye injection have raised specific gravity without significantly changing osmolarity.

Although poor urine output (e.g., <400 mL urine/24 hr) may reflect hypovolemia or impending *prerenal* renal failure, a majority of perioperative renal failure episodes develop in the absence of oliguria.[1] The normal response to hypovolemia is renal solute retention; fluid and electrolyte retention produces a concentrated urine with a low sodium content (<20 mEq/L). In contrast, impaired concentrating ability due to AKI causes urine to approach plasma osmolarity (isosthenuria) with a higher sodium content (>40 mEq/L). The kidneys' ability to retain electrolytes is also reflected in the *fractional excretion of sodium* (FE$_{Na}$), a test that uses a spot sample of urine and blood to compare sodium and creatinine excretion; this test can be useful to distinguish hypovolemia and renal injury:

$$FE_{Na} = U_{Na}/P_{Na} \times P_{Cr}/U_{Cr} \times 100$$

where U$_{Na}$ = urine sodium, P$_{Na}$ = plasma sodium, U$_{Cr}$ = urine creatinine, and P$_{Cr}$ = plasma creatinine.

FE$_{Na}$ <1% implies that sodium is being normally conserved while values above 1% are consistent with acute tubular necrosis.

PERIOPERATIVE NEPHROLOGY

Pathophysiology

Altered renal function can be thought of as a clinical continuum ranging from the normal compensatory changes seen during stress to frank renal failure. Clinically, there is considerable overlap between compensated and decompensated renal dysfunctional states. The kidney under stress reacts in a predictable manner to help restore intravascular volume and maintain blood pressure. The sympathetic nervous system reacts to trauma, shock, or pain by releasing norepinephrine, which acts much like angiotensin II on the renal arterioles. Norepinephrine also activates the renin-angiotensin-aldosterone system and causes ADH release. The net result of modest activity of the stress response system is a shift of blood flow from the renal cortex to the medulla, avid sodium and water reabsorption, and decreased urine output. A more intense stress response may induce a decrease in RBF and GFR by causing afferent arteriolar constriction. If this extreme situation is not reversed, ischemic damage to the kidney may result, and acute renal failure may become clinically manifest.

Electrolyte Disorders

Disorders of Sodium Balance

Hyponatremia is the most commonly occurring electrolyte disorder[16,17](see also Chapter 14). Symptoms rarely occur unless sodium values are <125 mmol/L, and these include a spectrum ranging from anorexia, nausea, and lethargy to convulsions, dysrhythmias, coma, and even death due to osmotic brain swelling.[18–20] Hyponatremia may occur in the setting of an expanded, normal, or contracted extracellular fluid volume, and volemic status and urinary sodium concentration are key markers in differentiating the large number of potential causes of hyponatremia. If water excess is a reason for hyponatremia, dilute urine (sodium >20 mmol/L) is expected. Conversely, avid renal sodium retention (urine sodium <20 mmol/L) suggests sodium loss as a cause. If hyponatremia is acute, the risk of neurologic complications is higher, and cautious treatment is indicated to prevent cerebral edema and seizures. This should be accomplished with intravenous hypertonic saline and furosemide to enhance water excretion and prevent sodium overload.

Hypernatremia (serum sodium >145 mmol/L) is generally the result of sodium gain or water loss, most commonly the latter. Dehydration of brain tissue can cause symptoms ranging from confusion to convulsions and coma. In cases of hypernatremia, laboratory studies often show evidence of hemoconcentration (increased hematocrit and serum protein concentrations). In addition, urine output is usually low (<500 mL/day) and hyperosmolar (>1,000 mOsm), with very low urinary sodium concentration and evidence of prerenal failure (elevations of BUN and serum creatinine). Occasionally the urine is not maximally concentrated, suggesting an osmotic diuresis or an intrinsic renal disorder such as diabetes insipidus. The primary goal of treatment is restoration of serum tonicity, which can be achieved with isotonic or hypotonic parenteral fluids and/or diuretics unless irreversible renal injury is present, in which situation dialysis may be necessary.

Disorders of Potassium Balance

Even minor variations in serum potassium concentration can lead to symptoms such as skeletal muscle weakness, gastrointestinal ileus, myocardial depression, malignant ventricular dysrhythmias, and asystole. Nearly 98% of total body potassium is intracellular. Circulating potassium levels are tightly controlled via renal and gastrointestinal excretion and reabsorption, but potassium also moves between the intra- and extracellular compartments under the influence of insulin and β_2-adrenoceptors. In the kidney, 70% of potassium reabsorption occurs in the proximal tubule and another 15 to 20% in the loop of Henle. The collecting duct is responsible for potassium excretion under the influence of aldosterone.

Hypokalemia may be due to a net potassium deficiency or transfer of extracellular potassium to the intracellular space. Notably, total body depletion may exist even with normal extracellular potassium levels (e.g., diabetic ketoacidosis). Causes of hypokalemia include extrarenal loss (e.g., vomiting, diarrhea), renal loss (impaired processing due to drugs, hormones, or inherited renal abnormalities), potassium shifts between the extra- and intracellular spaces (e.g., insulin therapy), and, occasionally, inadequate intake. Clinical manifestations of hypokalemia include electrocardiogram (ECG) changes (flattened T waves"no pot, no T," U waves, prodysrhythmic state) and skeletal muscle weakness. Hypokalemia treatment involves supplementation with intravenous or oral potassium; however, overly rapid potassium intravenous administration should be avoided because it can cause hyperkalemic cardiac arrest.

If a patient has *hyperkalemia* (elevated serum potassium level >5.5 mEq/L), it is important to consider the duration of the condition as chronic hyperkalemia is far better tolerated than an acute rise. Other than laboratory artifacts (e.g., hemolysed sample), causes of hyperkalemia include abnormal kidney excretion, abnormal cellular potassium release, or abnormal distribution between the intra- and extracellular space.

Disorders of Calcium, Magnesium, and Phosphorus

Most of a grown adult's 1 to 2 kg of calcium is in bone (98%), with the remaining 2% existing in one of three forms: ionized, chelated, or protein-bound. Normal serum calcium values range between 8.5 and 10.2 mg/dL, but only the ionized fraction (50%) is biologically active and precisely regulated. Ionized extracellular calcium concentration (iCa^{++}) is controlled by the combined actions of parathyroid hormone (PTH), calcitonin, and vitamin D, and further modulated by dietary and environmental factors. Hypocalcemia due to reduced serum protein levels is physiologically unimportant. Extracellular magnesium represents only 0.3% of total (mainly intracellular) stores, making normal serum levels (1.6 to 2.2 mg/dL) a poor reflection of total body magnesium. Phosphorus is a major intracellular anion that plays a role in regulation of glycolysis, ammoniagenesis, and calcium homeostasis and is an essential component of adenosine triphosphate and red blood cell 2,3-diphosphoglyceric acid synthesis.

The clinical manifestations of *hypocalcemia* include cramping, digital numbness, laryngospasm, carpopedal spasm, bronchospasm, seizures, and respiratory arrest. A positive Chvostek sign (facial muscle twitching in response to tapping the facial nerve) or Trousseau sign (carpal spasm induced by brachial artery occlusion) are the classic hallmarks of hypocalcemia, but in practice are often absent. Mental status changes, including irritability, depression, and impaired cognition, may also occur. Cardiac manifestations include QT interval shortening and dysrhythmias.

Hypocalcemia may be due to several mechanisms, including a decrease in PTH secretion or action, reduced vitamin D synthesis or action, resistance of bone to PTH or vitamin D effects, or calcium sequestration. Citrate used for regional anticoagulation with dialysis can also cause hypocalcemia and may also lead to hypomagnesemia from decreased PTH secretion. Parathyroidectomy during neck surgery reduces PTH levels and is a common cause of acquired hypoparathyroidism.

Clinical symptoms of *hypercalcemia* correlate with its acuity and include constipation, nausea and vomiting, drowsiness, lethargy, weakness, stupor, and coma. Cardiovascular manifestations may include hypertension, shortened QT interval, heart block, and other dysrhythmias. The most frequent causes of hypercalcemia are primary hyperparathyroidism and malignancy. Other causes include thiazide (increased renal calcium reabsorption) or lithium (inhibits PTH release) therapy and rarer medical conditions including granulomatous disease, thyrotoxicosis, and multiple endocrine neoplasia types I and II.

Hypomagnesemia (<1.6 mg/dL) may sometimes be asymptomatic, but clinically important problems can and do manifest, including neuromuscular, cardiac, neurologic, and related electrolytic (hypokalemia and hypocalcemia) abnormalities. Causes of hypomagnesemia can be divided in four broad categories: decreased intake, gastrointestinal loss, renal loss, and redistribution. Nutritional hypomagnesemia can result from malabsorption syndromes in patients receiving parenteral nutrition, and it is also present in 25% of alcoholics. Redistribution occurs with acute pancreatitis, administration of catecholamines, and in "hungry bone syndrome" after parathyroidectomy.[10] Magnesium can be supplemented orally or via the parenteral route.

Clinical manifestations of *hypermagnesemia* (>4 to 6 mg/dL) are serious and potentially fatal. Minor symptoms include hypotension, nausea, vomiting, facial flushing, urinary retention, and ileus. In more extreme cases, flaccid skeletal muscular paralysis, hyporeflexia, bradycardia, and bradydysrhythmias, respiratory depression, coma, and cardiac arrest may occur. Hypermagnesemia generally occurs in two clinical settings: compromised renal function (GFR <20 mL/min) and excessive magnesium intake (e.g., excessive intravenous therapy in preeclampsia). Although mild hypermagnesemia in the setting of normal renal function can be treated with supportive care and withdrawal of the cause, in some cases dialysis is necessary.

Hypophosphatemia is clinically more important than hyperphosphatemia and can result in symptoms including muscle weakness, respiratory failure, and difficulty in weaning critically ill patients from mechanical ventilation when serum levels are <0.32 mmol/L. In addition, low phosphate levels may diminish oxygen delivery to tissues and rarely cause hemolysis. Hypophosphatemia can result from intracellular redistribution (from catecholamine therapy), from inadequate intake or absorption secondary to alcoholism or malnutrition, or from increased renal or gastrointestinal losses.[11]

Intravenous and oral supplementation can be used to treat hypophosphatemia.

Hyperphosphatemia (>5 mg/dL) is generally related to accompanying hypocalcemia although increased phosphate levels may also lead to calcium precipitation and decreased intestinal calcium absorption.[12,13] Significantly elevated serum phosphate levels are most commonly due to reduced excretion from renal insufficiency but can also result from excess intake or redistribution of intracellular phosphorus. Treatment of chronic hyperphosphatemia includes dietary phosphate restriction and oral phosphate binders.

Acid-Base Disorders

The primary determinant of serum pH is the balance between plasma bicarbonate (HCO_3^-) concentration and the PCO_2 in the extracellular space. Acid-base homeostasis involves tight regulation of HCO_3^- and $PaCO_2$. Primary extracellular pH derangements due to abnormal bicarbonate reabsorption and proton (H^+) elimination by the kidney lead to metabolic acidosis or alkalosis, while factors that abnormally affect respiratory drive influence $PaCO_2$, leading to respiratory acidosis or alkalosis. Because combined problems are often seen in perioperative critically ill patients, an approach to both "pure" and "mixed" acid-base disorders is presented here.

Metabolic Acidosis

The *anion gap* (AG) represents the total serum concentration of unmeasured anions and can be calculated as $AG = (Na^+ + K^+) - (HCO_3^- + Cl^-)$. It allows differentiation of the causes of metabolic acidosis into normal AG (8 ± 4) and increased AG (>16 mmol/L) varieties. Conditions that cause an increase in negatively charged ions other than bicarbonate and chloride (e.g., lactate, salicylate) increase the AG. In contrast, non-AG metabolic acidosis results from renal or gastrointestinal HCO_3^- loss and is associated with high chloride levels (hyperchloremic metabolic acidosis). The usual compensatory response to all types of metabolic acidosis is hyperventilation, which leads to a partial pH correction toward normal. Winter's formula predicts expected $PaCO_2$ for a metabolic acidosis as follows: $PaCO_2 = (1.5 \times HCO_3^-) + 8$.

Metabolic Alkalosis

Metabolic alkalosis is a common primary acid-base disturbance associated with increased plasma HCO_3^-. Increased extracellular HCO_3^- is due to a net loss of H^+ and/or addition of HCO_3^-. The most common cause of metabolic alkalosis is gastrointestinal acid loss due to vomiting or nasogastric suctioning; the resulting hypovolemia leads to secretion of renin and aldosterone and enhanced absorption of HCO_3^-. Thiazides and loop diuretics both induce a net loss of chloride and free water and can cause a volume "contraction" alkalosis.

Respiratory Acidosis

If the lungs fail to eliminate CO_2, hypercapnia and respiratory acidosis result, characterized by increased $PaCO_2$ and decreased blood pH. Acute and chronic causes can be differentiated by examining arterial pH, $PaCO_2$, and HCO_3^- values. In the early phase of respiratory acidosis, increased $PaCO_2$ stimulates renal generation and secretion of H^+. The kidneys continue to adapt to the increased pH through greater titratable acid excretion (e.g., ammonium) and HCO_3^- generation. Therefore, acute respiratory acidosis is characterized by an elevated $PaCO_2$, acidemia, and a relatively normal HCO_3^-. In contrast, chronic respiratory acidosis is associated with an elevated

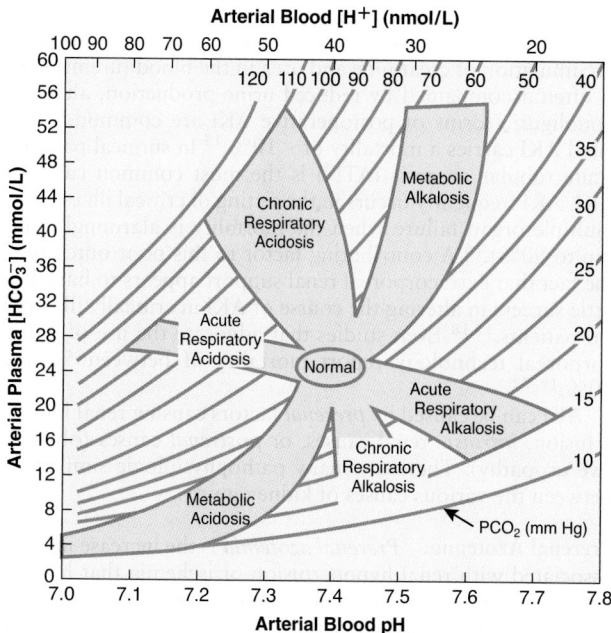

FIGURE 52-4. Acid-base map. Plotting the PCO_2 and H^+ (from the arterial blood gas) against plasma HCO_3^- (from the serum chemistry panel) for a patient can identify simple acid-base disorders. When mixed disorders exist, values may fall outside the shaded areas. (From DuBose TD Jr: Acid-Base Disorders, Brenner & Rector's The Kidney, B.M. Brenner (ed.) 7th edition. Philadelphia, WB Saunders, 2004, p 938, with permission.)

HCO_3^- (often accompanied by a relatively normal pH) due to renal compensation.

Respiratory Alkalosis

Increased minute ventilation is the primary cause of respiratory alkalosis, characterized by decreased $PaCO_2$ and increased pH. Patients with acute, uncompensated respiratory alkalosis have normal plasma HCO_3^-. In chronic respiratory alkalosis, renal compensation leads to decreased plasma HCO_3^-. The causes of respiratory alkalosis relate to abnormal respiratory drive from stimulants or toxins (e.g., salicylate, caffeine, nicotine, progesterone), central nervous system abnormalities (e.g., anxiety, stroke, increased intracranial pressure), pulmonary abnormalities (e.g., pulmonary embolism, pneumonia), mechanical hyperventilation, or systemic conditions such as liver failure and sepsis.

Mixed Acid-Base Disorders

It is not uncommon for a metabolic derangement to coexist with a respiratory derangement, particularly in intensive care patients. A general approach to the diagnosis of mixed acid-base disorders requires a step-wise approach that begins with a focused history and physical examination. An arterial blood gas and a concurrent serum chemistry panel (including Na^+, K^+, Cl^-, and total CO_2 concentrations) should also be obtained, and use of an acid-base map may help differentiate simple from mixed disorders (Fig. 52-4).

Acute Kidney Conditions

Acute Kidney Injury

Acute kidney injury (AKI) is now the preferred term for an acute deterioration in renal function. It is associated with a decline in glomerular filtration and results in inability of the kidneys to excrete nitrogenous and other wastes. This manifests as an accumulation of creatinine and urea in the blood (uremia) and is often accompanied by reduced urine production, although nonoliguric forms of postoperative AKI are common.[14] Isolated AKI carries a mortality of <10%.[15] In surgical patients, acute tubular necrosis (ATN) is the most common cause of AKI. AKI frequently occurs in the setting of critical illness with multiple organ failure when the mortality is alarmingly high (up to 90%).[16] A contributing factor to this poor outcome is the fact that extracorporeal renal support appears to have had little success in altering the course of AKI in critically ill surgical patients.[17,18] Even studies that advocate the use of extracorporeal technology report mortality of between 50 and 70%.[19–22]

AKI can be caused by *prerenal* factors causing renal hypoperfusion, *intrinsic* renal causes, or *postrenal* causes (obstructive uropathy). There are many pathophysiologic similarities between the various causes of kidney injury.

Prerenal Azotemia.   *Prerenal azotemia* is the increase in BUN associated with renal hypoperfusion or ischemia that has not yet caused renal parenchymal damage. The metabolically active cells of the medullary thick ascending limb of the loop of Henle are especially vulnerable to hypoxic damage because of their relatively high oxygen consumption.[23] AKI ensues when necrosis of tubular cells releases debris into the tubules, causing flow obstruction, increased tubular back pressure, and leak of tubular fluid. Often, prerenal AKI is precipitated in patients with pre-existing renal vasoconstriction (e.g., volume depletion, heart failure or sepsis) by nephrotoxin exposure or further reductions in cardiac output.[24]

Intrinsic Acute Kidney Injury. The term *intrinsic* not only implies a primary renal cause of AKI, but also includes AKI due to ischemia, nephrotoxins, and renal parenchymal diseases. ATN remains the most common ischemic lesion and represents an extension of prerenal azotemia, whereas cortical necrosis may follow a massive renovascular insult such as prolonged suprarenal aortic clamping or renal artery embolism. Nephrotoxins often act in concert with hypoperfusion or underlying renal vasoconstrictive states to damage renal tubules or the microvasculature. Several common nephrotoxins, some of which are difficult to avoid in a hospitalized patient population, are listed in Table 52-1.

Postrenal Acute Kidney Injury (Obstructive Uropathy). Downstream obstruction of the urinary collecting system is the least common pathway to established AKI, accounting for <5% of cases.[25] Because it is easy to treat, however, it is extremely important to exclude with a renal ultrasound examination. The obstructing lesion may occur at any level of the collecting system, from the renal pelvis to the distal urethra. Intraluminal pressure rises and is eventually transmitted back to the glomerulus, thereby reducing glomerular filtration pressure and rate.

Nephrotoxins and Perioperative Acute Kidney Injury

Nephrotoxin exposure is a common occurrence in hospitalized patients and frequently plays a role in the cause of AKI in this population. Nephrotoxins may take the form of drugs, nontherapeutic chemicals, heavy metals, poisons, and endogenous compounds (Table 52-1). The nephrotoxins most likely to contribute to renal dysfunction/failure in the perioperative period are certain antimicrobial and chemotherapeutic-immunosuppressive agents, radiocontrast media, nonsteroidal anti-inflammatory drugs (NSAIDs), and the endogenous heme pigments myoglobin and hemoglobin. These diverse groups of renal toxins share a common pathophysiologic characteristic: they disturb either renal oxygen delivery or oxygen utilization and thereby promote renal ischemia.

Antimicrobial and chemotherapeutic-immunosuppressive agents are effective because they are cellular toxins. When these drugs are filtered, reabsorbed, secreted, and eventually excreted by the kidney, toxic concentrations in renal cells can be reached. The aminoglycoside antibiotics and amphotericin B are particularly difficult to avoid because they are effective antimicrobials, with few available alternatives. Their effect can be additive with other nephrotoxic factors causing impairment of kidney function. Hypovolemia, fever, renal vasoconstriction, and concomitant therapy with other nephrotoxic agents should be avoided wherever possible. Electrolyte disorders such as hypercalcemia, hypomagnesemia, hypokalemia, and metabolic acidosis can further enhance nephrotoxic damage to the kidney.

Cyclosporin A and tacrolimus are indispensable components of many immunosuppressive drug regimens, but in combination with other nephrotoxins and clinical factors, they can cause acute and exacerbate chronic kidney injury in transplant recipients.[21]

Radiocontrast media poses a threat to the renal function of patients with diabetic nephropathy, pre-existing renal vasoconstriction (heart failure, hypovolemia), or renal insufficiency.[22] Radiocontrast dye has effects on renal function that develop 24 to 48 hours after exposure and peak at 3 to 5 days. Measures that may prevent AKI or lessen the severity of renal damage include prehydration, smaller contrast doses, and judicious

---

TABLE 52-1

NEPHROTOXINS COMMONLY FOUND IN THE HOSPITAL SETTING

■ EXOGENOUS	■ ENDOGENOUS
Antibiotics (Aminoglycosides, cephalosporins, amphotericin B, sulfonamide, tetracyclines, vancomycin)	Calcium (hypercalcemia)
	Uric acid (hyperuricemia and hyperuricosuria)
Anesthetic agents (Methoxyflurane, enflurane)	Myoglobin (rhabdomyolysis)
Nonsteroidal anti-inflammatory drugs	Hemoglobin (hemolysis)
(Aspirin, ibuprofen, naproxen, indomethacin, ketorolac)	Bilirubin (obstructive jaundice)
Chemotherapeutic–immunosuppressive agents	Oxalate crystals
(Cisplatinum, cyclosporin A, methotrexate, mitomycin, nitrosoureas, tacrolimus)	Paraproteins
Contrast media	

withholding of other nephrotoxins, such as NSAIDs. Elective surgery should be postponed until the effects of the dye have resolved. The idea that pretreatment with N-acetylcysteine can prevent radiocontrast nephropathy in patients with renal insufficiency[23] has now largely been abandoned.

NSAIDs produce reversible inhibition of prostaglandin synthesis and are well-known nephrotoxins.[24] Except in cases of massive overdose, NSAIDs produce renal dysfunction only in patients with coexisting renal hypoperfusion or vasoconstriction. Advanced age, hypovolemia, end-stage hepatic disease, heart failure, sepsis, chronic renal insufficiency, and major surgery are risk factors for development of NSAID-induced AKI.[25]

Myoglobin and hemoglobin are both capable of causing AKI in critically ill surgical patients. Myoglobin seems to be a more potent nephrotoxin than hemoglobin because it is more readily filtered at the glomerulus and can be reabsorbed by the renal tubules, where it chelates nitric oxide and thus induces medullary vasoconstriction and ischemia.[26] Hypovolemia and acidemia potentiate the toxicity of both pigments. Reduced intravascular volume causes a decrease in RBF and GFR, which results in a smaller volume of tubular fluid with a relatively higher concentration of pigment. There is also evidence suggesting that pigment precipitation inside the tubular lumen is enhanced under acidotic conditions and that tubular obstruction plays a role in the pathogenesis of AKI.[26,27]

Preventive treatment of pigment-induced AKI is directed at increasing RBF and tubular (urine) flow while correcting any existing acidosis. These goals may be accomplished by expanding the intravascular fluid volume with crystalloid infusion, stimulating an osmotic diuresis with mannitol, and increasing the urine pH with intravenous bicarbonate therapy.[28] Adequate systemic resuscitation from shock is a prerequisite if AKI is to be avoided, especially in massive crush injuries and electrical burns. Forced mannitol-alkali diuresis is indicated as the second step in the preventive treatment of myoglobinuria, with urine flow rates of up to 300 mL/hr and a urine pH of >6.5 advocated for patients with massive crush injuries.[28]

The nephrotoxicity of volatile agents remains controversial. Inhalation anesthetics such as enflurane, isoflurane, and sevoflurane can generate free fluoride ions during their metabolism, which (when levels are >50 μM/L) may cause polyuric AKI by interfering with tubular concentrating ability. However, peak fluoride levels during administration of these agents seldom reach toxic levels, and there are few reports describing volatile agent-induced nephrotoxicity.[29] The potential of sevoflurane-induced nephrotoxicity has been related to the production of compound A during prolonged, low fresh gas flow, sevoflurane anesthesia.[30] Although there are insufficient data to conclude that sevoflurane-induced kidney injury occurs in the human population, even during low gas flow anesthesia, it is probably prudent to maintain a fresh gas flow of at least 2 L/min formation during sevoflurane anesthesia.[31]

Chronic Kidney Disease

Patients with nondialysis-dependent chronic kidney disease (CKD) are at increased risk of developing *end-stage renal disease* (ESRD). ESRD is the term used to describe a clinical syndrome characterized by renal dysfunction that would prove fatal without renal replacement therapy. These patients have GFRs <25% of normal. Lesser degrees of renal dysfunction may be categorized as chronic renal insufficiency (25 to 40% of normal GFR) or decreased renal reserve (60 to 75% of normal GFR). Patients with decreased renal reserve are often asymptomatic and frequently do not have elevated blood levels of creatinine or urea. Established renal insufficiency results

in patently abnormal serum creatinine and BUN values, but nocturia (due to reduced concentrating ability) may be the only symptom.

The *uremic syndrome* represents an extreme form of chronic renal failure, which occurs as the surviving nephron population and GFR decrease below 10% of normal. It results in inability of the kidney to perform its two major functions: regulation of the volume and composition of the extracellular fluid and excretion of waste products. Water balance in ESRD becomes difficult to manage because the number of functioning nephrons is too small either to concentrate or to fully dilute the urine. This results in failure both to conserve water and to excrete excess water. Patients with uremic syndrome often require frequent or continuous dialysis.

Life-threatening hyperkalemia may occur in CKD because of slower-than-normal potassium clearance. Situations predisposing patients with renal failure to hyperkalemia are presented in Table 52-2. Derangements in calcium, magnesium, and phosphorus metabolism are also commonly seen in CKD (Table 52-3).

Metabolic acidosis occurs in two forms in ESRD: a hyperchloremic, normal AG acidosis and a high AG acidosis from inability to excrete titratable acids. Both render patients susceptible to an endogenous acid load such as may occur in shock states, hypovolemia, or with an increase in catabolism.

Cardiovascular complications of the uremic syndrome are primarily due to volume overload, high renin-angiotensin activity, autonomic nervous system hyperactivity, acidosis, and electrolyte disturbances. Hypertension due to extracellular fluid volume expansion, autonomic factors, and hyperreninemia is an almost universal finding in ESRD. Together with volume overload, acidemia, anemia, and possibly the presence

TABLE 52-2

FACTORS CONTRIBUTING TO HYPERKALEMIA IN CHRONIC RENAL FAILURE

■ POTASSIUM INTAKE

Increased dietary intake
Exogenous IV supplementation
Potassium salts of drugs
Sodium substitutes
Blood transfusion
Gastrointestinal hemorrhage

■ POTASSIUM RELEASE FROM INTRACELLULAR STORES

Increased catabolism, sepsis
Metabolic acidosis
β-Adrenergic blocking agents
Digitalis intoxication (Na-K-ATPase inhibition)
Insulin deficiency
Succinylcholine

■ POTASSIUM EXCRETION

Acute decrease in GFR
Constipation
Potassium-sparing diuretics
Angiotensin-converting enzyme inhibitors (decreased aldosterone secretion)
Heparin (decreased aldosterone effect)

IV, intravenous; Na-K-ATPase, Na-K-adenosine triphosphatase; GFR, glomerular filtration rate.

TABLE 52-3

THE UREMIC SYNDROME

■ WATER HOMEOSTASIS

Extracellular fluid expansion

■ ELECTROLYTE AND ACID-BASE

Hyponatremia
Hyperkalemia
Hypercalcemia or hypocalcemia
Hyperphosphatemia
Hypermagnesemia
Metabolic acidosis

■ CARDIOVASCULAR

Heart failure
Hypertension
Pericarditis
Myocardial dysfunction
Dysrhythmias

■ RESPIRATORY

Pulmonary edema
Central hyperventilation

■ HEMATOLOGIC

Anemia
Platelet hemostatic defect

■ IMMUNOLOGIC

Cell-mediated and humoral immunity defects

■ GASTROINTESTINAL

Delayed gastric emptying, anorexia, nausea, vomiting,
  hiccups, upper gastrointestinal tract inflammation/
  hemorrhage

■ NEUROMUSCULAR

Encephalopathy, seizures, tremors, myoclonus
Sensory and motor polyneuropathy
Autonomic dysfunction, decreased baroreceptor
  responsiveness, dialysis-associated hypotension

■ ENDOCRINE-METABOLISM

Renal osteodystrophy
↓ Glucose intolerance
Hypertriglyceridemia, ↑ atherosclerosis

of high-flow arteriovenous fistulae created for dialysis access, hypertension may contribute to the development of myocardial dysfunction and heart failure. Pericarditis may occur secondary to uremia or dialysis, with pericardial tamponade developing in 20% of the latter group.[32] Pulmonary problems associated with CKD are limited to changes in lung water and control of ventilation. Pulmonary edema and restrictive pulmonary dysfunction are commonly seen in patients with renal failure and are usually responsive to dialysis. Hypervolemia, heart failure, reduced serum oncotic pressure, and increased pulmonary capillary permeability are relevant factors in the development of pulmonary edema. Chronic metabolic acidosis may also be responsible for the hyperventilation seen in

patients with ESRD, but increased lung water and poor pulmonary compliance can also stimulate hyperventilation.

The anemia of CKD occurs as a result of reduced levels of erythropoietin, red cell damage, ongoing gastrointestinal blood loss, and iron or vitamin deficiencies. Platelet dysfunction may aggravate blood loss, but it is responsive to dialysis, cryoprecipitate administration, and desmopressin acetate (or DDAVP). Acquired defects in both cellular and humoral immunity probably account for the high prevalence of serious infections (60%) and high mortality from sepsis in CKD (30%).

Drug Prescribing in Renal Failure

If a drug depends solely on the kidney for clearance, then a simple approach to prescribing might involve a calculated percentage reduction in drug dosage that matches the reduction in GFR. Although GFR can be accurately measured, an estimated clearance derived from serum creatinine is usually adequate for these purposes. Unfortunately, clearance of most medications involves a more complex combination of both hepatic and renal function, and drug level measurement or algorithms for specific drugs are often recommended.

AKI may affect absorption of a drug. For example, a reduced first-pass effect through the gastrointestinal tract and liver is associated with increased serum levels of oral beta-blockers and opioids in patients with AKI. Also, an increase in the volume of distribution is seen in most patients with chronic kidney disease due to increased plasma volume and decreased plasma protein binding. However, plasma protein binding is highly variable, with acidic drugs having reduced binding and basic agents (e.g., amide local anesthetics) having increased binding. Importantly, for drugs with less binding, "normal" drug levels may reflect dangerously high active (unbound) drug levels. For example, therapeutic phenytoin levels are typically reported as being in the range of 10 to 20 mg/mL normally, but 4 to 10 mg/mL in cases of renal failure. Finally, hepatic metabolism of drugs is difficult to predict in the setting of renal failure because some hepatic enzymes are inhibited whereas others are induced, and accompanying liver disorders may alter the relationship of drug clearance with GFR.

Anesthetic Agents in Renal Failure

❺ With the exception of methoxyflurane and possibly enflurane, anesthetic agents do not directly cause renal dysfunction or interfere with the normal compensatory mechanisms activated by the stress response. The nephrotoxicity of methoxyflurane appears to be due to its metabolism, which results in release of the fluoride ions believed responsible for the renal injury.[33] It has been suggested that renal, not hepatic, metabolism of methoxyflurane may be responsible for generating fluoride ions locally that contribute to nephrotoxicity.[34] Enflurane nephrotoxicity may also occur[35] but is of minor clinical importance, even in patients with pre-existing renal dysfunction. Although direct anesthetic effects on the kidney are usually not harmful, indirect effects may combine with hypovolemia, shock, nephrotoxin exposure, or other renal vasoconstrictive states to produce renal dysfunction. If the chosen anesthetic technique causes a protracted reduction in cardiac output or sustained hypotension that coincides with a period of intense renal vasoconstriction, renal dysfunction or failure could result. This is true for either general or regional ❻ anesthesia. There are no comparative studies demonstrating superior renal protection or improved renal outcome with general versus regional anesthesia.

Significant renal impairment may affect the disposition, metabolism, and excretion of the commonly used anesthetic agents. Inhalation anesthetics are, of course, an exception to the rule that drugs with central nervous system activity (which generally are lipid-soluble) must be converted to more hydrophilic compounds by the liver before being excreted by the kidney. The water-soluble metabolites of agents that are not inhaled may accumulate in renal failure and display prolonged pharmacodynamic effects if they possess even a small percentage of the pharmacologic activity of the parent drug. Drugs that are eliminated unchanged by the kidneys (e.g., certain nondepolarizing muscle relaxants, the cholinesterase inhibitors, many antibiotics, digoxin) have a prolonged elimination half-life when given to patients with kidney failure. Many drugs used in anesthesia are highly protein-bound and may demonstrate exaggerated clinical effects when protein binding is reduced by uremia.

Induction Agents and Sedatives

Sodium thiopental serves as a good illustrative example of how reduced protein binding in CKD may affect the clinical use of an anesthetic agent. Burch and Stanski[36] showed that the free fraction of an induction dose of thiopental is almost doubled in patients with renal failure. This accounts for the exaggerated clinical effects of thiopental in these patients and explains the need for a substantial reduction in the induction dose of this agent in uremic patients when compared with patients with normal renal function.

Ketamine is less extensively protein-bound than thiopental, and renal failure appears to have less influence on its free fraction. Redistribution and hepatic metabolism are largely responsible for termination of the anesthetic effects, with <3% of the drug excreted unchanged in the urine. Norketamine, the major metabolite, has one-third the pharmacologic activity of the parent drug and is further metabolized before it is excreted by the kidney.[37]

Etomidate, although only 75% protein-bound in normal patients, has a larger free fraction in patients with ESRD.[38] The decrease in protein binding does not seem to alter the clinical effects of an etomidate anesthetic induction in patients with renal failure.

Propofol undergoes extensive, rapid hepatic biotransformation to inactive metabolites that are renally excreted. Its pharmacokinetics appear to be unchanged in patients with renal failure,[39] and there are no reports of prolongation of its effects in ESRD.

The benzodiazepines, as a group, are extensively protein-bound. CKD increases the free fraction of benzodiazepines in the plasma, and this potentiates their clinical effect. Certain benzodiazepine metabolites are pharmacologically active and have the potential to accumulate with repeated administration of the parent drug to anephric patients. For example, 60 to 80% of midazolam is excreted as its (active) α-hydroxy metabolite,[40] which accumulates during long-term infusions in patients with renal failure.[40] AKI appears to slow the plasma clearance of midazolam, whereas repeated diazepam or lorazepam administration in CKD may carry a risk of active metabolite-induced sedation. Alprazolam is one of the few drugs related to anesthesia practice that has undergone pharmacodynamic studies in patients with CKD. Schmith et al.[41] found that when decreased protein binding and increased free fraction of alprazolam are taken into account, patients with CKD are actually more sensitive to its sedative effects than healthy persons.

Dexmedetomidine is a relatively new sedative agent primarily metabolized in the liver. Volunteers with renal impairment receiving dexmedetomidine experienced a longer-lasting sedative effect than subjects with normal kidney function. The most likely explanation is that less protein binding of dexmedetomidine occurs in subjects with renal dysfunction.[42]

Opioids

Single-dose studies of the pharmacokinetics of morphine in renal failure demonstrate no alteration in its disposition. However, chronic administration results in accumulation of its 6-glucuronide metabolite, which has potent analgesic and sedative effects.[43] There is also a decrease in protein binding of morphine in ESRD, which mandates a reduction in its initial dose. Meperidine is remarkable for its neurotoxic, renally excreted metabolite (normeperidine) and is not recommended for use in patients with poor renal function. Hydromorphone is metabolized to hydromorphone-3-glucuronide, which is excreted by the kidneys. This active metabolite accumulates in patients with renal failure and may cause cognitive dysfunction and myoclonus.[44] Codeine also has the potential for causing prolonged narcosis in patients with renal failure and cannot be recommended for long-term use.[43]

Fentanyl appears to be a better choice of opioid for use in ESRD because of its lack of active metabolites, unchanged free fraction, and short redistribution phase.[45] Small-to-moderate doses, titrated to effect, are well tolerated by uremic patients.

Alfentanil has been shown to have reduced protein binding but no change in its elimination half-life or clearance in ESRD and is extensively metabolized to inactive compounds.[46] Therefore, caution should be exercised in administering a loading dose, but the total dose and infusion dose should be similar to those for patients with normal renal function. The free fraction of sufentanil is unchanged in ESRD; however, its pharmacokinetics are variable, and it has been reported to cause prolonged narcosis.[47]

Remifentanil is rapidly metabolized by blood and tissue esterases to a weakly active (about 4,600 times less potent) μ-opioid agonist and renally excreted metabolite, remifentanil acid. Renal failure has no effect on the clearance of remifentanil, but elimination of the principal metabolite, remifentanil acid, is markedly reduced. However, the clinical implications of this metabolite are likely limited.[48]

Muscle Relaxants

Muscle relaxants are the most likely group of drugs used in anesthetic practice to produce prolonged effects in ESRD because of their dependence on renal excretion (Table 52-4). Only succinylcholine, atracurium, *cis*-atracurium, and mivacurium appear to have minimal renal excretion of the unchanged parent compound. Most nondepolarizing muscle relaxants must be either hepatically excreted or metabolized to inactive forms in order to terminate their activity. Some muscle relaxants have renally excreted, active metabolites that may contribute to their prolonged duration of action in patients with ESRD. Although the following discussion focuses on the pharmacology of individual muscle relaxants, coexisting acidosis and electrolyte disturbances, as well as drug therapy (e.g., aminoglycosides, diuretics, immunosuppressants, magnesium-containing antacids), may alter the pharmacodynamics of muscle relaxants in patients with renal failure.[49]

Succinylcholine has a long history of use in CKD that has been somewhat confused by conflicting reports of plasma cholinesterase activity in renal failure.[50,51] Provided the serum potassium concentration is not dangerously elevated, its use can be justified as part of a rapid-sequence induction technique because its duration of action in ESRD is not significantly prolonged. Use of a continuous infusion of succinylcholine, however, is more problematic because the major metabolite, succinylmonocholine, is weakly active and excreted by the kidney.

NONDEPOLARIZING MUSCLE RELAXANTS IN RENAL FAILURE

■ DRUG	■ % RENAL EXCRETION	■ HALF-LIFE (hr) NORMAL/ESRD	■ RENALLY EXCRETED ACTIVE METABOLITE	■ USE IN ESRD
d-Tubocurarine	60	1.4–2.2	–	Avoid
Metocurine	45–60	6/11.4	–	Avoid
Pancuronium	30	2.3/4–8	+	Avoid
Gallamine	>85	2.5/6–20	+	Avoid
Pipecuronium	37	1.8–2.3/4.4	+	Avoid
Doxacurium	30	1.7/3.7	–	Avoid
Vecuronium	30	0.9/1.4	+	Avoid infusion
Rocuronium	30	1.2–1.6/1.6–1.7	–	Variable duration
Atracurium/*cis*-atracurium	<5	0.3/0.4	–	Normal
Mivacurium	<7	2 min/2 min	–	Duration 1.5 × normal
Rapacuronium	<12	0.5/0.5	++	Normal single dose

ESRD, end-stage renal disease.

Concern about the increase in serum potassium levels after succinylcholine administration (0.5 mEq/L in normal subjects) implies that the serum potassium should be normalized to the extent possible in patients with renal failure, but clinical experience has shown that the acute small increase in potassium following administration of succinylcholine is generally well tolerated in patients with *chronically* elevated serum potassium levels. Use of the long-acting muscle relaxants doxacurium, pancuronium, and pipecuronium might also be questioned in patients with known renal insufficiency. In a single-dose study of doxacurium, Cook et al.[52] demonstrated an increased elimination half-life, reduced plasma clearance, and prolonged duration of effect in patients with renal failure. Similar findings have been reported for the pharmacokinetics of pipecuronium.

Intermediate-acting muscle relaxants (atracurium, *cis*-atracurium, vecuronium, and rocuronium) have a distinct advantage in ESRD because of their shorter duration. The risk of a clinically significant, prolonged block is much reduced. Atracurium and its derivative, *cis*-atracurium, undergo enzymatic ester hydrolysis and spontaneous nonenzymatic (Hoffman) degradation with minimal renal excretion of the parent compound. Their elimination half-life, clearance, and duration of action are not affected by renal failure,[53] nor have they been reported to cause prolonged clinical effects in ESRD. These characteristics strongly support their use in patients with renal disease. One potential concern is that an atracurium metabolite, laudanosine, may causes seizures in experimental animals and may accumulate with repeated dosing or continuous infusion.[54] However, this has not been realized in intensive care patients with renal failure receiving prolonged infusions of atracurium. Consistent with its greater potency and lower dosing requirements, *cis*-atracurium metabolism results in lower laudanosine blood levels than does atracurium in ESRD patients.

The pharmacokinetics of vecuronium were initially reported as unchanged in renal failure, but it was later demonstrated that its duration of action was prolonged as a result of reduced plasma clearance and increased elimination half-life.[53] In addition, the active metabolite, 3-desmethylvecuronium, was shown to accumulate in anephric patients receiving a continuous vecuronium infusion who subsequently had prolonged neuromuscular blockade. An intubating dose would be expected to last approximately 50% longer in patients with ESRD.[55]

Rocuronium, a rapid-onset muscle relaxant, has a pharmacokinetic profile in normal subjects similar to that of vecuronium.[56] Single-dose pharmacokinetic studies in patients with renal failure have reported conflicting results. Szenohradszky et al.[57] reported that renal failure increased the volume of distribution and elimination half-life of rocuronium, but had no effect on its clearance. Cooper et al.[58] found that its clearance was reduced and the duration of block was widely variable in patients with renal failure, although the mean duration of relaxation and spontaneous recovery was not statistically different from that in control subjects.

The short-acting muscle relaxant mivacurium is enzymatically eliminated by plasma pseudocholinesterase at a somewhat slower rate than succinylcholine. Low pseudocholinesterase activity correlates with slower recovery from a bolus dose of mivacurium in anephric patients.[51] The maintenance infusion dose has been reported to be both lower[59] and similar[60] to that in normal control subjects.

The pharmacokinetics of the clinically available anticholinesterases are affected by renal failure.[61] They have a prolonged duration of action in ESRD because of their heavy reliance on renal excretion. The anticholinergic agents atropine and glycopyrrolate, used in conjunction with the anticholinesterases, are similarly excreted by the kidney. Therefore, no dosage alteration of the anticholinesterases is required when antagonizing neuromuscular blockade in patients with reduced renal function.

Diuretic Drugs: Effects and Mechanisms

Fluid overload occurs when salt or water intake exceeds renal and extrarenal losses and is characterized by increased total body water, and usually sodium. Fluid overload may be evenly distributed among the body compartments (e.g., congestive heart failure), or the interstitial space may be increased while the circulating blood volume may be normal or even decreased (e.g., posttraumatic or postoperative third-space fluid shifts). Edema results when Starling forces favor passage of fluid into the interstitial space. A variety of chronic medical conditions (congestive heart failure, renal failure, or hepatic cirrhosis) can lead to fluid overload and edema that may even require surgery to be delayed for treatment to reduce operative risk. The first line of therapy for fluid overload that includes all body compartments involves

Diuretic Sites of Action

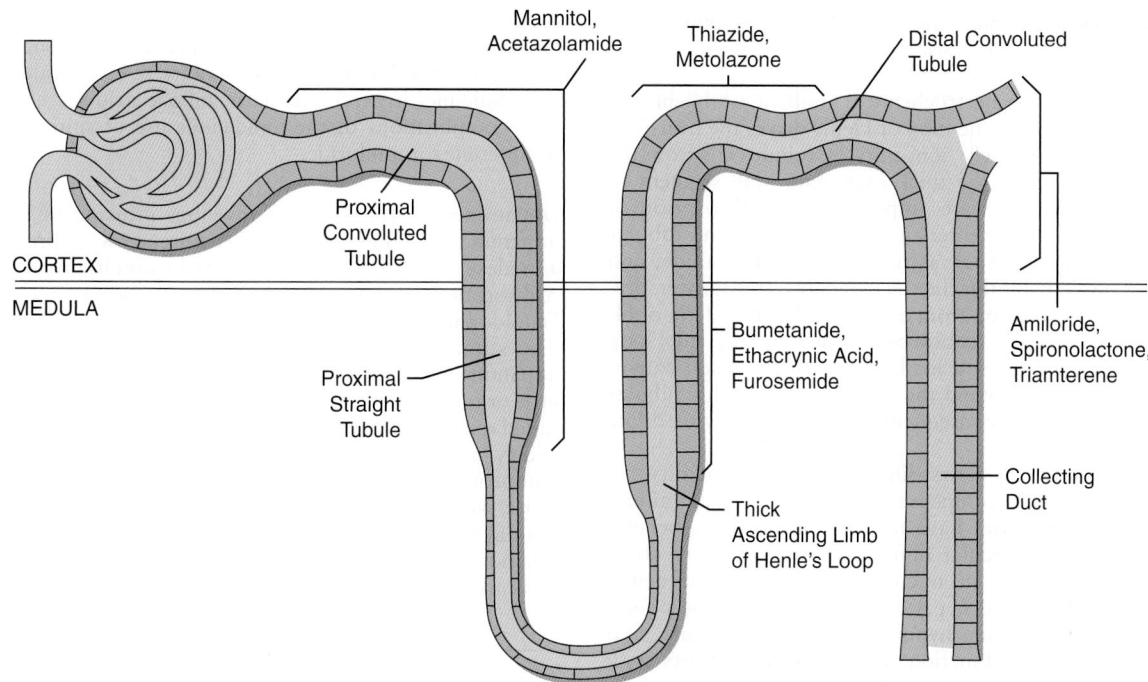

FIGURE 52-5.   Site of action of commonly available diuretics. (From Mende CW: Current issues in diuretic therapy. Hosp Pract 1990; 25(Suppl 1): 15, with permission.)

restriction of salt and water ingestion; however, diuretic therapy is often indicated.

The Physiologic Basis of Diuretic Action

Diuretics are typically grouped according to their site and mechanism of action (Fig. 52-5). Under normal conditions, kidney function assures that <1% of the filtered Na^+ load enters the urine (i.e. the fractional excretion of Na^+ (FENa) is <1%). The Na^+/K^+ ATPase pump on the basolateral surface (blood side) of renal tubular cells is primarily responsible for active pumping of Na^+ out of cells into blood in exchange for K^+. This pump causes a net movement of positive charge out of the cell (2 K^+ in, for every 3 Na^+ out) creating an electrochemical gradient that also causes Na^+ to enter the luminal (urine) side of the cell. Renal tubular cells in different portions of the nephron have different luminal "systems" to allow this Na^+ influx. These systems are the sites of action where the different diuretics work.

Proximal Tubule Diuretics.   In the proximal tubule, a specialized luminal transporter exchanges protons (H^+) for sodium ions; the result is sodium reabsorption and acidification of the urine. The excreted H^+ combines with bicarbonate (HCO_3^-) in the tubule to form carbonic acid: $H^+ + HCO_3^- \rightarrow H_2CO_3$. Carbonic acid converts to water (H_2O) and carbon dioxide (CO_2) in a reaction catalyzed by carbonic anhydrase: $H_2CO_3 \rightarrow H_2O + CO_2$. The same enzyme, carbonic anhydrase, allows this reaction to occur in reverse within tubular cells, converting H_2CO_3 to HCO_3^- and H^+, generating more H^+ for countertransport with Na^+, and releasing bicarbonate that passes into the circulation. Carbonic anhydrase inhibitors are drugs that inhibit this enzyme; the net effect of these agents is that sodium and bicarbonate, that would otherwise have been reabsorbed, remain in the urine and result in an alkaline diuresis.

Although patients may develop a metabolic acidosis when taking these agents, compensatory processes in the tubules accommodate the effects of carbonic anhydrase inhibitors so that their long-term use rarely causes this problem. However, these agents can be useful, for example, with contraction alkalosis from aggressive diuresis with loop diuretics (see later discussion); administration of these drugs can reduce $PaCO_2$ and improve PaO_2 for patients with little accompanying change in blood pH. Specific uses for carbonic anhydrase inhibitors include the treatment of mountain sickness, open-angle glaucoma, and to increase respiratory drive in patients with central sleep apnea.[62,63]

Osmotic Diuretics.   Substances such as mannitol that are freely filtered at the glomerulus but poorly reabsorbed by the renal tubule will cause an osmotic diuresis. In the water-permeable segments of the proximal tubule and loop of Henle, fluid reabsorption occurs and filtered mannitol is concentrated. Eventually oncotic pressure in the tubular fluid resists further fluid reabsorption. Mannitol also draws water from cells into the plasma and effectively increases RBF.

Mannitol has been widely used, especially for the prophylaxis of acute renal failure. In select patient populations, such as cadaveric kidney transplant recipients, it has been found to be effective.[64] However, in a controlled trial of mannitol prophylaxis in patients with mild chronic renal failure, it was less effective than hydration alone for prevention of contrast-associated nephropathy.[65] Although animal studies showed initial promise, apart from AKI prophylaxis in kidney transplantation there is no clear evidence that mannitol is effective either for the prevention or treatment of AKI.[66] As mannitol shifts water between fluid compartments, there can be effects on plasma and intracellular electrolyte concentrations, including hyponatremia and hypochloremia and intracellular increases in K^+ and H^+. Patients with normal renal function quickly correct these changes, but patients with renal impairment may develop significant circulatory overload with hemodilution and pulmonary edema, hyperkalemic metabolic acidosis, central nervous system depression, and even severe hyponatremia requiring urgent hemodialysis.[67]

Loop Diuretics. The electrochemical gradient established by the Na^+/K^+ ATPase in the loop of Henle drives the transport of 1 Na^+, 1 K^+, and 2 Cl^- ions into the tubule cells from the tubular fluid. Because the thick ascending limb segment of the loop of Henle is water-impermeable, reabsorption of solute concentrates the interstitium and dilutes the tubular fluid. Loop diuretics, such as furosemide, bumetanide, and torsemide, directly inhibit the electroneutral transporter, preventing salt reabsorption from occurring. Because 25% of filtered NaCl is normally reabsorbed in the loop of Henle, loop diuretics cause a large salt load to pass to the distal convoluted tubule that is beyond the extra reserve of this tubular segment to reabsorb; consequently, large volumes of dilute urine ensue.

Loop diuretics are a first-line therapeutic modality for treatment of acute decompensated congestive heart failure. Although loop diuretics have no proven mortality benefit, they reduce left ventricular filling pressures and very effectively relieve the symptoms of congestion, pulmonary edema, extremity swelling, and hepatic congestion. Adverse effects of loop diuretics include hypokalemia, hyponatremia, and also acute kidney dysfunction. Heart failure patients with atrial fibrillation may also be prescribed digitalis, which in combination with furosemide, can lead to hypokalemia-induced dysrhythmias. Loop diuretics, especially furosemide, may cause ototoxicity particularly in patients with renal insufficiency.[68]

Distal Convoluted Tubule Diuretics. Distal convoluted tubule diuretics, such as thiazides (e.g., hydrochlorothiazide) and metolazone, act in the early part of this segment to block the NaCl cotransport mechanism across apical plasma membranes. Because the distal tubule is relatively water-impermeable, net NaCl absorption causes urinary dilution. Clinically, distal convoluted tubule diuretics are used for the treatment of hypertension (often as sole therapy), volume overload disorders, and to relieve the symptoms of edema in pregnancy.

Adverse reactions associated with distal tubule diuretics include electrolyte disturbances and volume depletion. Hydrochlorothiazide specifically has been associated with a number of other side effects including pancreatitis, jaundice, diarrhea, and aplastic anemia.

Distal (Collecting Duct) Acting Diuretics. Unlike in the more proximal nephron segments, NaCl absorption in the collecting duct cells is not electroneutral. That is, a net electrical gradient is maintained both by the Na^+/K^+ ATPase Na^+ ion channels and in the luminal membranes. As a result, the tubule lumen is negatively charged with respect to the blood. This normally causes K^+ secretion into the tubular lumen through K^+-specific ion channels. Distal K^+-sparing diuretics (e.g., amiloride and triamterene) directly inhibit luminal Na^+ entry, blocking this mechanism, and resulting in a K^+ "sparing" effect. In addition, H^+ secretion is inhibited.

A second class of distal-acting, potassium-sparing diuretics is the competitive aldosterone antagonists (e.g., spironolactone and eplerenone). Ordinarily, the mineralocorticoid hormone aldosterone is released by the body in response to angiotensin II or hyperkalemia. Aldosterone normally stimulates Na^+ reabsorption and K^+ excretion by the collecting duct. Inhibition of the aldosterone effect by these drugs causes a mild natriuresis and K^+ retention. Distal K^+-sparing agents are used primarily for K^+-sparing diuresis (e.g., in patients with volume overload receiving digitalis or with hypokalemic

alkalosis). In addition, these drugs are especially useful in treating disorders involving secondary hyperaldosteronism, such as cirrhosis with ascites. Spironolactone treatment has been shown to improve survival over volume overload and left ventricular dysfunction or heart failure.[69] Hyperkalemia and hyperkalemic, hyperchloremic metabolic acidosis are significant complications of the injudicious use of spironolactone, triamterene, or amiloride.

Dopaminergic Agonists. Intravenous infusion of low-dose dopamine (1 to 3 μg/kg/min) is natriuretic owing primarily to a modest increase in the GFR and reduction in proximal Na^+ reabsorption mediated by dopamine type 1 (DA_1) receptors.[70] Fenoldopam is a selective DA_1 receptor agonist with little cardiac stimulation. At higher doses, the pressor response to dopamine is beneficial in patients with hypotension, but it has little or no renal effect in critically ill or septic patients.[70,71] So-called renal-dose dopamine for the treatment of AKI, although widely used, has not been demonstrated to have significant renoprotective properties in numerous studies[72–74] and can cause worsened splanchnic oxygenation, impaired gastrointestinal function, impaired endocrine and immunologic system function, blunting of ventilatory drive, and increased risk of postcardiac surgery atrial fibrillation.[75–77]

High-Risk Surgical Procedures

Cardiac Surgery

❼ Cardiac operations requiring CPB can be expected to result in renal dysfunction or failure in up to 7% of patients.[78,79] There are numerous risk factors associated with the development of postoperative AKI in this population (Fig. 52-6).[80] Interestingly, patients with preoperative CKD appear to tolerate surgery and CPB remarkably well.[81] Renal ischemia-reperfusion and toxin exposure are considered to be the two primary pathogenetic mechanisms involved in AKI. Renal risk factors contributing through these mechanisms include preoperative **❽** left ventricular dysfunction, duration of CPB, pulse pressure hypertension[82] and aprotinin therapy.[83]

Although some retrospective studies suggest "beating heart" off pump coronary artery bypass grafting lowers renal risk compared with the traditional CPB techniques,[84] randomized studies have been inconclusive. However, despite the fact that pulsatile CPB suppresses plasma renin activity, postoperative renal function in patients with normal kidneys undergoing pulsatile or nonpulsatile CPB is equivalent.

Numerous agents have been used intraoperatively without success in attempts to protect the kidney during cardiac surgery. Mannitol use during CPB is partly aimed at avoiding hemoglobin-induced AKI, by promoting urine flow and reducing renal cell swelling. Dopamine is infused at low doses (<5 μg/kg/min) as a renal vasodilator without benefit. Costa et al.[85] administered low-dose dopamine during CPB to patients with preoperative renal dysfunction and were able to induce a saluresis without affecting GFR or protecting the kidney from ischemic injury. Dopexamine improved creatinine clearance and systemic oxygen delivery in one cardiac surgery study,[86] but a systemic review of 21 randomized, controlled trials failed to confirm benefit.[87] Other studies examining the renal protective effects of fenoldopam, ANP, and insulinlike growth factor-1 in this population have not shown a consistently protective effect.

Noncardiac Surgery

Several common noncardiac surgical procedures can compromise previously normal renal function. Emergency surgery has

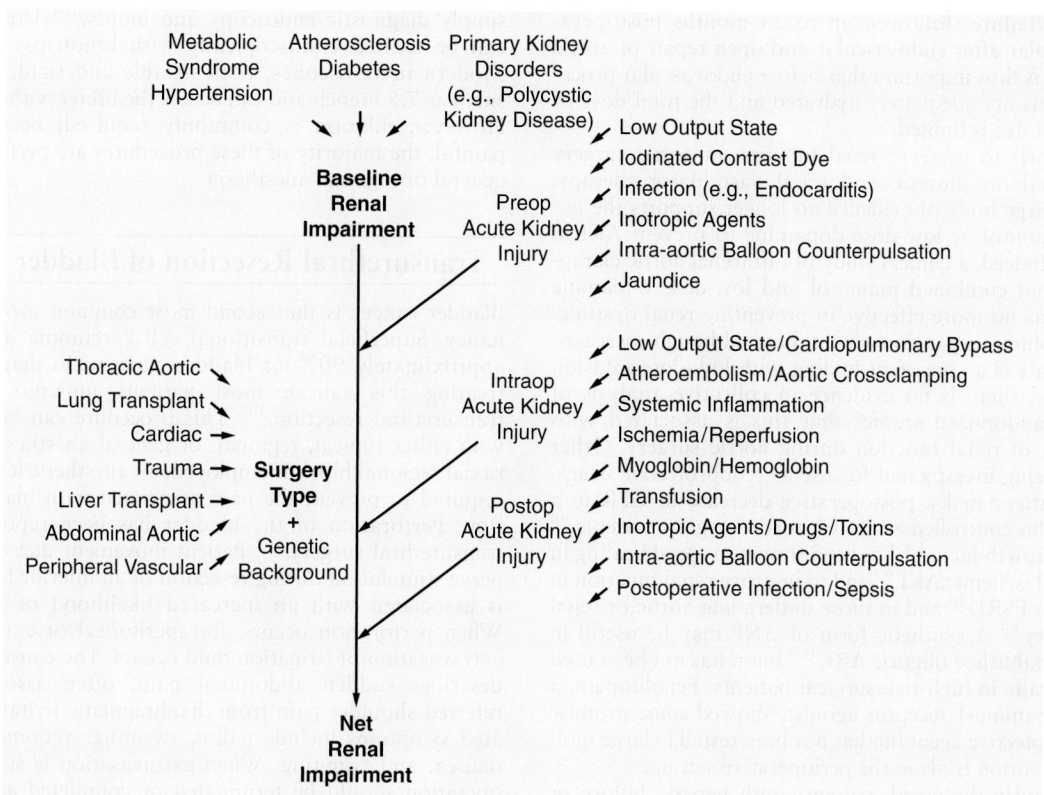

FIGURE 52-6.   Clinical risk factors that predict perioperative acute kidney injury and renal dysfunction. Preop, preoperative; Intraop, intraoperative; Postop, postoperative.

been reported as a risk factor for AKI, with trauma surgery figuring as a prominent subgroup of emergency procedures.[88] ATN is the typical renal lesion associated with trauma, and it may be produced by a number of ischemic mechanisms. Most often, hypovolemic shock, pigmenturia, multiple organ failure, or exogenous nephrotoxins are responsible for sequential or simultaneous insults to the kidney. AKI that develops in the trauma patient may be characterized by an early, oliguric picture related to inadequate volume resuscitation, or by a later, sometimes nonoliguric syndrome associated with multiple organ failure, nephrotoxin exposure, or sepsis. The outcomes of these two posttraumatic AKI scenarios are dramatically different. The early form is associated with high mortality rates, whereas only 20 to 30% of patients will die in the case of nonoliguric AKI.[89] Not surprisingly, trauma victims with pre-existing renal insufficiency experience much higher mortality than previously healthy patients.[90]

Preventing AKI in patients presenting for emergency surgery begins with proper management of intravascular volume depletion and shock. Restoring euvolemia and maintaining cardiac output, systemic oxygen delivery, and RBF can often obviate renal vasoconstriction. Urine flow, once established, is maintained at ≥0.5 mL/kg/hr. Invasive hemodynamic monitoring may be required to guide intraoperative management of ongoing cardiovascular instability due to surgical manipulation, blood loss, fluid shifts, and anesthetic effects. Intraoperative transesophageal echocardiography provides excellent assessment of left and right ventricular function, as well as guidance of fluid resuscitation. Nephrotoxin exposure should be kept to a minimum in the unstable trauma victim. Radiocontrast media, NSAIDs, and myoglobin pose the greatest threat to this patient group. There is no place for either furosemide or mannitol therapy in the early, resuscitative

phase of trauma management, except in the case of head injury with elevated intracranial pressure or when massive rhabdomyolysis is suspected.

Vascular surgery requiring aortic clamping has deleterious effects on renal function regardless of the level of clamp placement. Suprarenal clamping results in an attenuated ATN-like lesion.[91] Infrarenal clamping causes a smaller, short-lived reduction in GFR and is associated with a lower risk of AKI, whereas surgery involving the thoracic aorta has a 25% incidence of AKI.[92] Two major predictors of AKI following aortic surgery are pre-existing renal dysfunction and perioperative hemodynamic instability.[93] Olsen et al.[94] reported in a large series of patients undergoing abdominal aortic aneurysm repair that the overall incidence of AKI was 12%. Patients who had emergency surgery for ruptured aneurysm had a very high incidence of hemodynamic instability, and AKI developed in 26%; in contrast, elective aortic surgery was associated with good hemodynamic control and a 4% incidence of renal failure. Atheromatous renal artery emboli and prolonged aortic clamp time may contribute to ischemic renal injury in these patients.

The endovascular approach (endostent) to major aortic surgery has recently gained popularity.[95] The etiology of renal dysfunction after endovascular and open repair of aortic aneurysm is multifactorial (renal ischemia, atheroembolism, hemodynamic instability). Although hemodynamic changes during endovascular procedures on the aorta may be less dramatic than those accompanying open repair, the prevalence of renal complications appears to be similar. During endovascular procedures, patients may be exposed to substantial amounts of radiocontrast dye, which can exacerbate postoperative renal dysfunction, especially in those with pre-existing renal insufficiency. The long-term incidence of renal insufficiency/failure (followed up to 24 months postoperatively) is similar after endovascular and open repair of aortic aneurysm. It is thus important that before endovascular procedures, patients are adequately hydrated and the total dose of radiocontrast dye is limited.

Most efforts to preserve renal function in aortic surgery have centered on diuretic and renal vasodilator therapy, although a large body of evidence no longer supports the use of either mannitol or low-dose dopamine to prevent AKI in this setting. Indeed, a clinical study of infrarenal aortic clamping found that combined mannitol and low-dose dopamine treatment was no more effective in preventing renal dysfunction than volume expansion with saline. Although increased urine flow rate is a consistent finding with low-dose infusion of dopamine, there is no evidence in collective analysis of numerous randomized studies that this is associated with preservation of renal function during aortic surgery. Other agents are being investigated for use as renoprotective drugs. Nifedipine attenuated a postoperative decrease in GFR in a small, placebo-controlled study of aortic surgery patients.[96] Insulinlike growth factor-1 has been shown to speed healing in experimental ischemic AKI,[97] and to improve renal function in patients with ESRD[98] and in those undergoing aortic or renal artery surgery.[99] A synthetic form of ANP may be useful in managing established oliguric ARF,[100] but it has not been used prophylactically in high-risk surgical patients. Fenoldopam, a selective dopamine-1 receptor agonist, showed some promise as a renal protective agent but has not been tested in large multicenter prevention trials in the perioperative setting.

As previously discussed, patients with hepatic failure or cholestatic jaundice are particularly susceptible to renal dysfunction. When the serum conjugated bilirubin exceeds 8 mg/dL, endotoxins from the gastrointestinal tract are absorbed into the portal circulation, causing intense renal vasoconstriction. Intravenous mannitol and/or oral administration of bile salts in the preoperative period may limit renal dysfunction in patients with cholestatic jaundice. This probably accounts for the high incidence of AKI after liver transplantation and biliary surgery. Renal dysfunction/failure may occur in up to two thirds of liver transplant recipients.[101] Many liver transplant candidates have overt hepatorenal syndrome, renal dysfunction, and presumably underlying renal vasoconstriction. When such patients are exposed to intraoperative hemodynamic instability, massive transfusion, and nephrotoxins, AKI frequently follows.[102]

ANESTHESIA FOR URINARY TRACT DISEASE

Cystourethroscopy and Ureteral Procedures

10 Like all surgical specialties, urologic surgery is embracing technological advances and the philosophy that surgical goals can be safely achieved using less-invasive approaches (e.g., smaller or no incisions, less trauma). More urologic procedures are being completed endoscopically with instruments passed along the urinary tract. Examination of the lower urinary tract, once done exclusively with rigid scopes, is more often performed in offices with flexible endoscopes. Flexible endoscopy is relatively painless and can usually be completed with topical anesthesia to the urethra. For the group of patients who cannot tolerate flexible cystoscopy in the office, mild sedation in a more monitored setting is usually sufficient to provide adequate patient and surgical conditions.[103]

Ureteroscopy, a simple extension of cystoscopy into the upper urinary tract using a flexible or rigid scope, can facilitate treatment of upper urinary tract malignancies, strictures, or simply diagnostic endoscopy and biopsy.[104] Ureteric calculi can be treated endoscopically with lithotripsy or laser.[105] Modern ureteroscopes, both flexible and rigid, measure as small as 7.5 French and can access the ureter without dilation. However, dilation is commonly required; because this is painful, the majority of these procedures are performed using general or regional anesthesia.

Transurethral Resection of Bladder Tumors

Bladder cancer is the second most common urologic malignancy. Superficial transitional cell carcinoma accounts for approximately 90% of bladder cancers. In diagnosing and treating this cancer, most patients undergo endoscopic transurethral resection.[106] This procedure can be performed with either topical, regional, or general anesthesia. If a neuraxial regional block is employed, an anesthetic level to T10 is required to prevent the pain associated with bladder distention. Perforation of the bladder has been reported during transurethral surgery.[107] Patient movement due to obturator nerve stimulation during resection of an inferior lateral tumor is associated with an increased likelihood of perforation. When perforation occurs, intraperitoneal or extraperitoneal extravasation of irrigation fluid occurs. The conscious patient describes sudden abdominal pain, often associated with referred shoulder pain from diaphragmatic irritation. Associated symptoms include pallor, sweating, abdominal rigidity, nausea, and vomiting. When extravasation is suspected, the operation should be terminated or completed as quickly as possible. Small perforations are rarely of clinical significance and typically managed with urinary catheter drainage and postoperative antibiotics. Even large perforations can heal with urinary catheter drainage alone, but some require placement of a percutaneous drain. If perforation results in accumulation of large amounts of intraperitoneal irrigating fluid, particularly if the solution is sterile water, this condition can be life-threatening. Open laparotomy for drainage and bladder perforation repair is recommended in these cases.[108]

Lasers for Use in Urology

Since the first demonstration of its effectiveness in 1966,[109] laser therapy is now employed to treat a multitude of urologic problems, including condyloma acuminatum of the external genitalia and urethra, ureteral stricture or bladder neck contracture, interstitial cystitis, benign prostatic hypertrophy, ureteral calculi, and superficial carcinoma of the penis, bladder, ureter, and renal pelvis[104] (see Chapter 8). Compared with traditional surgical techniques, laser surgery reduces blood loss, decreases postoperative pain, and produces less tissue denaturation, a process that reduces risk of tumor implantation.

The biological effect of a laser depends on wavelength, energy density, and tissue absorbtion.[109,110] Absorption is the most important laser-tissue interaction. Absorbed laser radiation is converted to heat; depending on the amount of heat, the results are coagulation or vaporization of tissue.[111] The common lasers used for urology proceedures the carbon dioxide (CO_2) laser, the argon laser, the neodymium-doped: yttrium-aluminum-garnet (Nd:YAG) crystal laser, the potassium-titanyl-phosphate (KTP) crystal laser, and the holmium laser. The CO_2 laser is a high-power, continuous wave laser that produces intense heat with vaporization, but has minimal tissue penetration and is unable to penetrate water. Thus its use is limited to treating cutaneous lesions of the external genitalia. The argon laser is poorly absorbed by water, but selectively absorbed by hemoglobin and melanin, making it useful for procedures in the bladder requiring coagulation of bleeding. A widely used laser in urologic surgery, the Nd:YAG laser,[104] emits light at a wavelength that is poorly absorbed by water and body pigments and therefore can penetrate tissues deeply, producing deep tissue penetration via protein denaturation with minimal vaporization.[106] It can be used in water or urine without loss of effectiveness and is delivered with a fiberoptic laser delivery system for endourologic surgery. The KTP laser is a derivative of the Nd:YAG laser,[111] with a wavelength that is strongly absorbed by hemoglobin and therefore penetrates vascular tissue only a few micrometers. Without the presence of hemoglobin, the depth of penetration increases dramatically beyond the direct visual control of the surgeon.[111] It is extremely effective in treating urethral strictures and bladder neck contractures. Lastly, the holmium laser emits light in a series of rapid pulses and produces a cutting effect by the vaporization of tissue water.[106] Application of the holmium laser to a urinary stone generates an immediate buildup of steam, causing fragmentation of the stone.[111]

As with all aspects of anesthesia, safety issues assume paramount importance during laser surgery. Damage to the eye is the potential injury that requires the greatest attention because both direct and reflected laser energy can cause corneal or retinal injury.[112] Personnel in surgical suites with operating lasers should be equipped with protective goggles or lenses of the appropriate optical density and wavelength for the laser in use. Patients may wear protective lenses if awake, and if they are under a general anesthetic their eyes should be taped closed and covered with wet eye-pads or laser-specific shields.[113] Thermal injuries or inadvertent ignition of surgical drapes are avoidable if the laser is placed in the "standby" mode when not in operation and is activated only by the surgeon. Vaporization of condyloma acuminatum tissue produces a plume of smoke that contains active human papilloma virus particles.[114] However the risk of transmission of a viral infection to operating room personnel is low.[115] To avoid inhalation of infectious agents, all operating room personnel involved in laser procedures for genital lesions should wear protective high-efficiency laser masks that prevent small particles from being inhaled. Perhaps most importantly, a smoke evacuation system should prevent atmospheric contamination by removing the laser plume from the operating room.[116]

Extracorporeal Shock Wave Lithotripsy

In the United States, the prevalence of urolithiasis is 10 to 15%.[117] This disease is 3 times more common in men than in women, with a peak age incidence in the third to fourth decade of life. Since 1980, when extracorporeal shock wave lithotripsy (SWL) became available, it has been the leading modality for the treatment of urinary calculi. Currently, only 5% of all urinary calculi require open surgical procedures. SWL has the advantages of being a minimally invasive technique that is performed on an outpatient basis and is associated with minimal perioperative morbidity and a significant reduction in anesthetic needs.[117]

Technical Aspects of Shock Wave Lithotripsy

Lithotripters have four main components: an energy source, focusing device, coupling medium, and multiplane stone localization system (Fig. 52-7A). The original, first-generation lithotripter was the Dornier HM-3 (Dornier MedTech, Munich, Germany), which required the patient to be placed in a hydraulically supported gantry chair and immersed in a water bath (Fig. 52-7B). Its energy source is a spark plug generator that creates an explosive impact and transmits high pressures (shock waves) to the water when discharged. An ellipsoidal

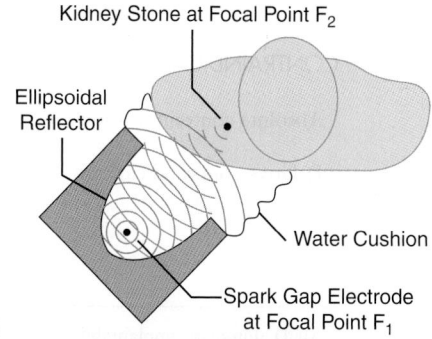

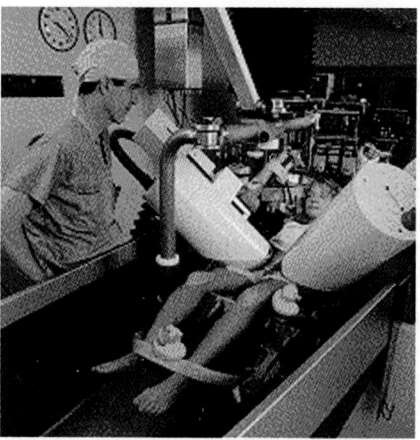

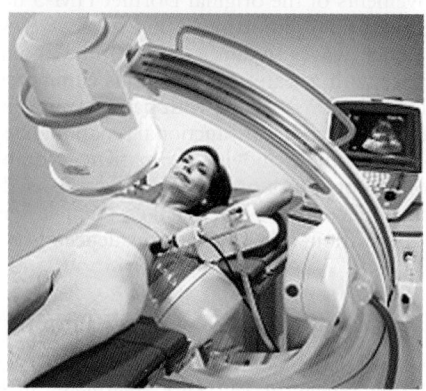

FIGURE 52-7. **A.** The principle of lithotripsy that causes comminution (fragmentation) of kidney stones involves the focused delivery of energy from a generated shock wave at a renal calculus. **B.** First-generation lithotripters such as the Dornier HM3 require seating the patient in a gantry chair, which is then lowered into a water bath. **C.** The physiologic consequences of full immersion are avoided using second- and third-generation lithotriptors, which instead achieve air-free contact to transmit their shock wave by direct application of a small water-filled drum or cushion with a silicone membrane to the skin. (From http://www.math.iupui.edu/m261vis/l itho.html [A]; http://www.geocities.com/hotsprings/villa/5556/history.html [B]; http://www.murtiindahsentosa.com/sections/view.php?id=34 [C].)

reflector aims the shock waves at a focal point. The patient's position in the tub is adjusted, aided by two fluoroscopes, so the calculus is centered in these beam paths.

Lowering a patient into a water bath during lithotripsy has a number of physiologic consequences. Immersion causes peripheral venous compression that increases central blood volume. Increases in central venous pressure (CVP) and pulmonary capillary wedge pressure are directly related to depth

TABLE 52-5

CONTRAINDICATIONS TO EXTRACORPEAL SHOCK WAVE LITHOTRIPSY

Absolute contraindications	Bleeding disorder or anticoagulation
	Pregnancy
Relative contraindications	Large calcified aortic or renal artery aneurysms
	Untreated urinary tract infection
	Obstruction distal to the renal calculi
	Pacemaker, AICD, or neurostimulation implant
	Morbid obesity

AICD, automatic implantable cardioverter-defibrillator

of immersion. Despite increased venous return, some immersed patients experience hypotension as a result of vasodilatation from the warm water.[118] Water in the lithotripter tub should be maintained in the temperature range of 35.8 to 37.5°C, and temperature monitoring should be used in every patient.[119] Respiratory effects of immersion and extrinsic pressure on the upper abdomen and thorax include a decrease in vital capacity, tidal volume, and functional reserve capacity. Continuous monitoring of hemodynamics and oxygenation should be used in all patients undergoing SWL. In high-risk patients, immersion should be achieved in a gradual fashion or the procedure should be performed with minimal immersion so only the shock wave entry site is covered with water.

Improvements of the original Dornier HM-3 have led to a second generation of lithotripters (Fig. 52-7C). Newer devices generate shock waves within a "shock tube" coupled to the body surface with a water cushion. This eliminates the water bath and problems associated with patient immersion. Newer lithotripter tables are multifunctional, enabling cystoscopy to be performed without moving the patient. Notably, second-generation lithotriptors are not as effective as the Dornier HM-3; their decreased power makes them less effective at stone fragmentation, and thus the prevalence of retreatment is higher.[117]

Complications of Shock Wave Lithotripsy

Absolute and relative contraindications to SWL are listed in Table 52-5. A review of 142 SWL treatments in pacemaker-dependent patients found a low (<1%) incidence of major pacemaker complications, with only one pacemaker deprogrammed during the treatment period.[120] Patients with pacemakers are acceptable candidates for lithotripsy provided that certain precautions are taken, including (1) preoperative determination of the type of pacemaker and its functional status; (2) availability of a programming device in the operating room, along with a person skilled in its use; (3) availability of an alternative pacing device; and (4) positioning of the patient so the pacemaker is not in the shock wave path. Patients with an automatic implantable cardioverter-defibrillator should have the defibrillator deactivated during lithotripsy.[121]

Cardiac dysrhythmias are observed in 80% of patients treated with first-generation lithotripters. The electrical discharge preceding each shock wave has been postulated to result in the premature electrical stimulation of the atria.[122] Most lithotripters are equipped with ECG-gated triggering to reduce the risk of ventricular fibrillation from an *R-on-T-wave phenomenon*. Electrocardiographic gating allows shock waves to be delivered only milliseconds after the R wave during the period of cardiac refractoriness. Regardless of the cause of the dysrhythmia, ECG gating limits the rate of shock wave delivery, and some practitioners recommend that all treatments first

be attempted by using a nonsynchronized mode of lithotripter operation.

Lithotripsy causes self-limited hematuria in nearly all patients, including some irreversible renal parenchymal injury that ultimately forms a region of scar. Notably, SWL is not typically associated with permanent renal dysfunction. However, subcapsular hematoma is seen in 0.5% of patients after lithotripsy.

External petechia and soft-tissue swelling are often apparent, especially in thin patients. Patients sometimes complain of flank pain, which may be severe for several days. As fractured calculus fragments pass down the urinary tract, up to 10% of patients have significant colic, occasionally requiring hospitalization and opioid analgesics.

Lung tissue is especially prone to SWL injury. Hemoptysis and pulmonary contusions have been reported.[123] Small adults and children are more prone to lung injury because of the close proximity of the lungs to the kidney. Lungs of small patients can be shielded by foam padding during the treatment to help prevent this complication. Radiation and auditory exposure of anesthesiology personnel during SWL appear to be safe with proper precautions.[124]

Anesthetic Techniques for Shock Wave Lithotripsy

New-generation SWL revolutionized the standard of treatment of urinary calculi. Shock wave propagation through the skin and viscera are responsible for the pain experienced during SWL. The majority of second- and third-generation lithotriptors require monitored anesthesia care with intravenous sedation and analgesia. The exception to this rule is pediatric patients, who for the most part require a general anesthetic.

Anesthesia for lithotripsy using the Dornier HM-3 typically has been either neuraxial block or general anesthesia. General anesthesia offers the advantages of controlling patient ventilation, rapid induction of anesthesia, and quicker recovery from anesthesia, compared with epidural anesthesia. However, patients have to be positioned in the lithotripter chair while unconscious, increasing the risk of peripheral nerve injuries. With spinal or epidural anesthesia, the patient is awake and cooperative during immersion, which allows simplifying patient positioning. Regional anesthetic techniques for this procedure require a sensory level of T6.

With second- and third-generation lithotriptors, monitored anesthesia care and sedative-analgesic combinations provide good treatment conditions and are associated with a high degree of patient satisfaction. Local anesthetic infiltration or topical application of local anesthetic has been used successfully during lithotripsy alone and with minimal systemic analgesia.[103,125] Remifentanil provides rapid analgesia and recovery with infusions of 0.025 to 0.1 μg/kg/min; however, it may not expedite discharge from hospital any faster than intermittent intravenous bolus dose fentanyl and propofol.[126,127]

ANESTHESIA FOR PROSTATIC SURGERY

Benign Prostatic Hyperplasia

Benign prostatic hyperplasia (BPH) is a frequent cause of lower urinary tract symptoms in older men.[128] The etiology is not known. The clinical symptoms of BPH (also known as *prostatism*) are not simply the result of mechanical obstruction of urine flow. Age-related detrusor dysfunction, an androgen-related phenomenon, plays an additional significant role.[129] BPH is the most common benign tumor in men and is characterized by an increased number of epithelial and stromal cells in the periurethral area of the prostate.[130] The prostate is a pear-shaped gland that surrounds the urethra at the base of the bladder (Fig. 52-8). The hypertrophied prostate surrounds and compresses the prostatic (proximal) urethra, causing obstruction that often produces urinary retention. The transitional zone, which only accounts for 5 to 10 % of prostatic glandular tissue in young men, is the region that hypertrophies to cause BPH.[129] BPH is responsible for the majority of urinary symptoms in men, and one third of male octogenarians will have to undergo prostatic surgery.[131]

Transurethral Resection of the Prostate

Transurethral resection of the prostate (TURP), the current gold standard surgical treatment for BPH,[132] accounts for most of the surgical BPH procedures.[106] After cystoscopy to rule out concomitant disease and evaluate the size of the prostate gland, the resectoscope, a specialized instrument with an electrode capable of both coagulating and cutting tissue, is introduced into the bladder, and the tissue protruding into the prostatic urethra is resected.[133] To facilitate clear vision of the surgical field, continuous irrigation is required. The irrigation fluid serves to distend the operative site and removes dissected tissue and blood.

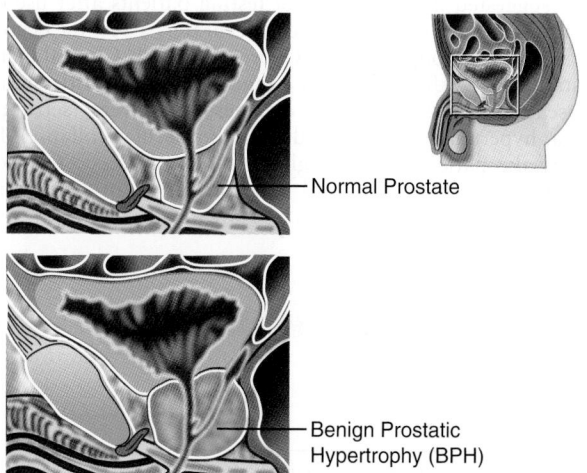

— Normal Prostate

— Benign Prostatic Hypertrophy (BPH)

FIGURE 52-8.   The prostate is normally a pear-shaped gland that surrounds the urethra as it exits the base of the bladder. Hyperplasia of prostatic stromal and epithelial cells is common in middle-aged and elderly men, leading to benign prostatic hypertrophy, which is associated with numerous symptoms including urinary hesitancy, frequent urination, and increased risk of urinary tract infections and urinary retention. (From http://www.nytimes.com/imagepages/2007/08/01/health/adam/18005BPH.html.)

If the irrigating fluid infusion pressure exceeds venous pressure during a TURP procedure, the lush venous plexus of the prostate may allow intravascular absorption of irrigating fluid.[106] Intravascular absorption of large volumes of irrigating fluid occasionally occurs and may result in perioperative complications unique to minimally invasive endoscopic surgery.

Irrigating Solutions for Transurethral Resection of the Prostate

The ideal safe irrigating fluid for use during TURP is one that would be isotonic, nonhemolytic, and nontoxic, not metabolized, and excreted rapidly if absorbed. In addition, surgical properties of such a fluid would include being nonelectrolytic to disperse the electrical current, transparent to allow clear visibility, and inexpensive, given the large volume that is necessary.[134] A multitude of candidate irrigating solutions have been evaluated for TURP, but all have limitations (Table 52-6).

Despite many ideal features, hypotonicity makes distilled water an unacceptable irrigating solution if intravascular absorption is possible. Distilled water has an osmolality of 0 mOsm/L, and when absorbed in large quantities, causes dilutional hyponatremia, intravascular hemolysis, hemoglobinemia and renal failure.[135] Distilled water is no longer used for TURP procedures, but is used for transurethral procedures without the possibility of absorption, such as cystoscopy.

Nearly isotonic solutions (moderate hypotonicity is maintained for visual qualities) used in modern TURP procedures include balanced electrolyte solutions (e.g., Ringer lactate), sorbitol (3.5%), mannitol (5%), glycine (1.5%), urea (1%), and glucose (2.5 to 4%). Because each of these solutions has its own perioperative complication profile, it is important that the anesthesiologist is aware of the irrigating solution used for TURP procedures at their institution (Table 52-6). Significant absorption of any irrigating solution can cause overhydration and volume overload, and all but the balanced salt solutions also cause dilutional hyponatremia. The conductivity of balanced electrolyte solutions such as Ringer lactate interferes with electrocautery and disperses electrical current from the resectoscope, potentially posing a risk to patient and surgeon. Sorbitol and glucose cause significant hyperglycemia if absorbed. Glycine, a nonessential amino acid, is normally metabolized by oxidative transformation into ammonia.[136] Depressed mental status and coma lasting 24 to 48 hours postoperatively, related to hyperammonemia, has been reported following TURP procedures using glycine irrigating solution, presumably from glycine metabolism.[136,137] Glycine has also been attributed a role in negative hemodynamic changes observed during TURP irrigation.[138]

Visual disturbances, including blurred vision and transient blindness, have also been reported following TURP procedures with glycine irrigation fluid, likely due to a peripheral mechanism, such as brainstem or cranial nerve inhibition.[139,140] Physical findings in these patients included sluggish or nonreactive pupils, suggesting a neurologic pathway disturbance rather than cerebral edema.[140] An inhibitory retinal action of glycine could be responsible for the transient blindness seen in these patients.[140] Glycine has structural similarities to aminobutyric acid, an inhibitory spinal cord and retina neurotransmitter.

Transurethral Resection of the Prostate Syndrome

TURP syndrome is a general term used to describe the symptoms that occur with excess absorption of irrigating solutions, primarily related to water intoxication, including mental confusion, nausea, hypertension, bradycardia, and visual disturbances. The principal components are respiratory distress resulting from

TABLE 52-6

PROPERTIES OF COMMONLY USED IRRIGATING SOLUTIONS FOR TRANSURETHRAL RESECTION PROCEDURES

■ SOLUTION	■ OSMOLALITY (mOsm/L)	■ ADVANTAGES	■ DISADVANTAGES
Distilled water	0	Improved visibility	Hemolysis Hemoglobinemia Hemoglobinuria Hyponatremia
Glycine (1.5%)	200	Less likelihood of TURP syndrome	Transient postoperative visual syndrome Hyperammonemia Hyperoxaluria
Sorbitol (3.3%)	165	Same as glycine	Hyperglycemia, possible lactic acidosis Osmotic diuresis
Mannitol (5%)	275	Isosmolar solution Not metabolized	Osmotic diuresis Possibility of acute intravascular volume expansion

TURP, transurethral resection of the prostate.
Adapted from Krongrad A, Droller MJ: Complications of transurethral resection of the prostate, Urologic Complications: Medical and Surgical, Adult and Pediatric, 2nd edition. Edited by Marshall FF. St. Louis, Mosby–Year Book, 1990, p 305, with permission.

rapid volume expansion, dilution of effective osmoles by the electrolyte-free (hypotonic) irrigating fluid, and symptoms related to the type of irrigating solution used.[134,141,142]

Typically, an irrigation solution infusion rate of 300 mL/min is required during TURP procedures for optimal visualization by the surgeon.[106] Factors that predict the amount of irrigation fluid absorption during a TURP procedure include the number and size of open venous sinuses (i.e., blood loss implies potential for irrigation absorption), duration of resection, hydrostatic pressure of the irrigating fluid, and venous pressure at the irrigant-blood interface.[143] Some absorption is to be expected, and rates are typically 20 mL/min but can reach as high as 200 mL/min.[142] Acute hemodynamic changes associated with intravascular volume expansion may exceed hemodynamic reserve, particularly for individuals with cardiac disease. Early symptoms associated with TURP syndrome are mostly related to acute intravascular volume expansion, independent of changes to serum osmolality and sodium.[142] Initial hypertension and bradycardia from acute volume overload may evolve into left heart failure, pulmonary edema, and even cardiovascular collapse.[144] With the continued absorption

of hypotonic irrigation fluid, cerebral edema as a consequence of dilutional hyponatremia may develop. Rapid change, as opposed to a specific low threshold serum sodium concentration, is responsible for most of the signs and symptoms of TURP syndrome (Table 52-7).[134]

To avoid excessive fluid absorption, procedural guidelines include limiting resection time to <1 hour, and suspending the irrigating fluid bag no more than 30 cm above the operating table at the beginning and 15 cm in the final stages of resection.[143,145] In addition, avoidance of hypotonic intravenous fluids and treatment of regional anesthesia-induced hypotension with judicious use of intravenous vasopressor agents rather than intravenous fluids should be considered. It has been suggested that breathalyzer testing patients after use of ethanol-labeled irrigating fluid can accurately assess the degree of fluid absorption during TURP procedures.[146] Clinical manifestations of TURP syndrome range from mild (restlessness, nausea, shortness of breath, dizziness) to severe (seizures, coma, hypertension, bradycardia, cardiovascular collapse). In the awake patient with a regional block, a classic triad of symptoms has been described that consists of an increase in

TABLE 52-7

SIGNS AND SYMPTOMS OF ACUTE HYPONATREMIA

■ SERUM Na$^+$ (mEq/L)	■ CNS CHANGES	■ ECG CHANGES
120	Confusion Restlessness	Possible widening of QRS complex
115	Somnolence Nausea	Widened QRS complex Elevated ST segment
110	Seizures Coma	Ventricular tachycardia or fibrillation

CNS, central nervous system; ECG, electrocardiogram.
Adapted from Jensen V: The TURP syndrome. Can J Anaesth 1991; 38: 90, 1991, with permission.

TABLE 52-8

TREATMENT OF THE TRANSURETHRAL RESECTION SYNDROME

Ensure oxygenation and circulatory support.
Notify surgeon and terminate procedure as soon as possible.
Consider insertion of invasive monitors if cardiovascular instability occurs.
Send blood to laboratory for evaluation of electrolytes, creatinine, glucose, and arterial blood gases.
Obtain 12-lead electrocardiogram.
Treat mild symptoms (with serum Na^+ concentration >120 mEq/L) with fluid restriction and loop diuretic (furosemide).
Treat severe symptoms (if serum Na^+ <120 mEq/L) with 3% sodium chloride IV at a rate <100 mL/hr.
Discontinue 3% sodium chloride when serum Na^+ >120 mEq/L.

both systolic and diastolic pressures associated with an increase in pulse pressure, bradycardia, and mental status changes.[134,147]

When neurologic or cardiovascular complications of TURP procedures are recognized, prompt intervention is necessary (Table 52-8). First, the surgeon should be informed of the patient's status change so the procedure can be completed or terminated as quickly as possible. The hallmark of patient treatment is to restore extracellular tonicity. Although the traditional recommended rate of serum sodium correction is 0.5 mEq/L/hr, this is for chronic hyponatremia and no established rate for correction of acute hyponatremia exists. Symptomatic patients with serum sodium concentrations <120 mEq/L should have their extracellular tonicity corrected with hypertonic saline. Sodium chloride in a 3% solution should be infused at a rate no greater than 100 mL/hr. Serum electrolytes should be followed closely and the hypertonic saline discontinued when the patient is asymptomatic or serum sodium concentration exceeds 120 mEq/L. Treatment with hypertonic saline has been associated with development of demyelinating central nervous system lesions (central pontine myelinolysis) due to rapid increases in plasma osmolality, and this approach should be reserved for patients with severe, life-threatening symptoms.[148] The demyelination is the result of excessive shrinkage of brain cells after rapid hydration with hyperosmolar solution as the brain cells have extruded important osmoles to compensate for the chronic hypotonicity. Notably, reports of demyelination after correction of acute symptomatic hyponatremia are rare, and there are no reports of demyelination after treatment of acute TURP syndrome.[142]

Other Complications of Transurethral Resection of the Prostate

Typically, blood loss during a resection is 2 to 4 mL/min.[143] The open venous sinuses are the most likely site of bleeding. Blood loss is very difficult to assess because of mixing with the irrigating fluid. With prolonged resections, serial hemoglobin levels and the patient's vital signs should be evaluated to guide the need for transfusion.[147] The incidence of intraoperative blood transfusion is approximately 2.5%.

Abnormal bleeding after TURP occurs in fewer than 1% of resections.[143] Thromboplastin, a thrombogenic stimulant found in high concentrations in prostate cancer cells, can rarely trigger disseminated intravascular coagulation.[147] Another cause of post-TURP bleeding is release of prostatic tissue plasminogen activators. These factors convert plasminogen to plasmin,

causing fibrinolysis. Treatment of these conditions is supportive and may include transfusion of coagulation factors and platelets.[149]

Surgical perforation of the prostatic capsule occurs in 2% of TURP procedures, usually resulting in extraperitoneal fluid extravasation.[147,150] Awake patients often complain of pain localized to the lower abdomen and back. This complication occurs more commonly during transurethral bladder tumor resection; management of this problem is discussed in an earlier section of this chapter.

Fever related to TURP procedures suggests bacteremia secondary to spread of bacteria through open prostatic venous sinuses. Hypothermia can complicate TURP procedures: body temperature decreases approximately 1°C/hr of surgery, and shivering occurs in 16% of patients who receive room-temperature irrigation fluids. Hypothermia does not develop if irrigation solutions are warmed to body temperature.[151]

Anesthetic Techniques for Transurethral Resection of the Prostate

Regional anesthesia, most commonly spinal block, has long been considered the anesthetic technique of choice for TURP.[152] Neuraxial block allows the patient to remain awake, which can facilitate early diagnosis of TURP syndrome and enable diagnosis of bladder perforation (shoulder pain due to diaphragmatic irritation by blood or fluid). Regional anesthesia may also decrease blood loss compared with general anesthesia.[153,154] Additionally, the need for analgesics is increased approximately fourfold after general anesthesia compared with regional anesthesia.[155] The lower CVP associated with regional anesthesia may actually increase the absorption of irrigation fluid.[156] Local anesthesia has been used for TURP procedures in patients with small-to-moderate size prostate glands, with limited success.[157]

Because many patients having prostate surgery are elderly, consideration should be given to prevention of postoperative cognitive dysfunction.[158] A prospective study comparing cognitive function after TURP using general versus spinal anesthesia found a significant impairment in both groups at 6 hours after surgery, but no differences between approaches at any time in the first 30 days after surgery.[159] The incidence of perioperative myocardial ischemia in patients undergoing transurethral surgery, assessed by Holter monitoring, increases following TURP surgery, but this also appears unaffected by choice of anesthesia.[160] Thus, choice of anesthetic technique for TURP procedures should be tailored to the individual and can be performed safely with either general or regional anesthesia.[161]

Morbidity and Mortality after Transurethral Resection of the Prostate

The majority of patients undergoing TURP are elderly and have numerous comorbidities. Since its introduction, and despite the steadily aging population and similar amounts of tissue being resected, the 30-day mortality following TURP has gradually declined, from 5% in the 1930s, 1.3% in 1974, to a low of 0.2%.[162–166] Mortality following TURP surgery is most commonly related to cardiac and respiratory comorbidities.[106]

A multicenter, randomized clinical trial comparing TURP with "watchful waiting" in patients with moderately symptomatic BPH showed that the majority (91%) of men had no complication during the first 30 days after surgery.[167] This study challenged previous less rigorous observations that TURP frequently leads to incontinence and impotence, as the incidence of these two complications was not significantly greater in the TURP group compared with those randomized to watchful waiting. The most common complications encountered were need for urinary recatheterization (4%), prostatic capsule perforation (2%), and hemorrhage requiring transfusion (1%).[167] There were no deaths following TURP in the first 30 postoperative days and a similar 3-year mortality rate as the watchful waiting group.

The Future of Transurethral Resection of the Prostate

The rate of TURP procedures has declined, largely because of the development of nonoperative strategies for BPH management.[129] Current medical strategies include separate or combined use of α_1-adrenergic antagonists that reduce dynamic urethral obstruction, and 5-α reductase inhibitors that block conversion of testosterone to reduce prostate hypertrophy.[129,168]

Less-invasive surgical treatments for BPH have also been developed including balloon dilatation, intraprostatic stents, transurethral incision, needle ablation, or vaporization of the prostate, and laser prostatectomy.[106,168] These procedures may be preferable for elderly patients with significant comorbidities because they can usually be performed on an outpatient basis, and decrease or avoid the risk of TURP syndrome.[169] Despite these other surgical options, TURP has not been displaced as the best treatment for BPH, particularly in highly symptomatic patients and those with recurrent urinary tract infections related to incomplete bladder emptying.[170] TURP has evolved into a safer operation while maintaining its efficacy.[132]

Surgery for Prostate Cancer

Radical Retropubic Prostatectomy

Prostate cancer is the most common cancer in men. In 2007, an estimated 218,900 cases of prostate cancer were diagnosed in the United States, with approximately 27,050 deaths from the disease. Radical prostatectomy remains the best therapeutic intervention for prostate cancer in men under age 65. Advances in surgical techniques for radical prostatectomy continue to improve outcomes and reduce the complexity of the anesthetic care for these procedures. The traditional approach has been open radical retropubic prostatectomy (ORRP). This procedure, involving a transverse abdominal incision, is often associated with blood loss exceeding 1,000 mL. Anesthetic technique and monitor selection needs to be tailored toward intravascular volume assessment and employing adjuncts that may help limit the volume of blood loss and reduce the need for blood transfusion.

Monitoring for radical prostatectomy should be dictated by patient comorbidities and anticipated blood loss. Notably, urine flow, a traditional monitor of intravascular volume, will be interrupted. CVP monitoring may be helpful, both to follow intravascular volume changes and provide access for rapid transfusion. An arterial line provides continuous blood pressure monitoring and the possibility of serial hemoglobin assessment. However, invasive monitors may be unnecessary for a procedure involving a healthy patient and a surgeon whose average blood loss is predictably low.

Avoidance of red blood cell transfusion is a goal for all surgical procedures. Transfusion of red blood cells may be associated with adverse outcomes such as immunologic and infectious complications and impaired immune response, which may predispose to cancer recurrence. It can also add significant expense to care delivery.[171]

Acute normovolemic hemodilution is a technique that reduces the need for transfusion in this patient population.[172] Preoperative erythropoietin therapy adds additional benefit but significantly increases cost. The use of cell salvage also reduces transfusion with this surgery, but controversy remains concerning the risk of tumor seeding.[173]

Choice of anesthetic technique may affect blood loss. Although disputed by some, reduced blood loss has been reported with spinal anesthesia[174] and combined general/epidural anesthesia[175] when compared with general anesthesia alone. The presumed mechanism for lower blood loss with regional block is reduced venous pressure in the prostatic venous plexus due to vasodilation.

Optimal patient positioning for this procedure is a hyperextended supine position. The patient's iliac crests are positioned over the break in the operating table, which is then extended to create a maximal distance between the iliac crest and the rib cage. The patient is then tilted to a head down (Trendelenberg) position to achieve an operative field that is parallel to the floor. Hyperextension of the back theoretically may increase the risk of nerve and back injuries, particularly for patients with spinal stenosis.[176] Additionally, this position could increase the potential for venous air embolism.[177] The head-down position can also contribute to ventilatory difficulties and venous pooling in the head and neck, which may be problematic for tracheal extubation and maintenance of airway patency, particularly with significant blood loss and crystalloid resuscitation. A number of cases of rhabdomyolysis have been reported with this position, often complicated by acute renal failure.[176]

Improved postoperative pain management can also lead to better patient outcomes and overall satisfaction. Both spinal and epidural regional anesthesia techniques have been demonstrated to reduce postoperative narcotic requirements, reduce postoperative nausea and vomiting, improve postoperative respiratory function, speed return of bowel function, and decrease time to first ambulation.[178,179] Some have reported good results simply with careful attention and a multimodal approach to pain management.[180,181] Adjuncts such as magnesium, gabapentin, and nonsteroidal anti-inflammatory agents help to reduce narcotic requirements.[182] Bladder catheter pain is often a significant source of discomfort with this procedure. Agents such as oxybutynin are helpful in treating this source of pain, and overall their use leads to significant reduction in analgesia requirements.[183]

Perineal Prostatectomy

An alternate open surgical approach to prostatectomy is radical perineal prostatectomy (RPP). This approach is suitable when sampling of the pelvic nodes is not required. It has several advantages over ORRP, including shorter operative time, better margin positive and biochemical recurrence rate, decreased blood loss and need for transfusion, reduced postoperative pain, and shorter convalescence.[184] However, positioning for this approach poses significant anesthetic challenge as patients are in an exaggerated lithotomy position. In addition to increased risk for nerve and muscle injuries, ventilatory mechanics are adversely affected, with dynamic and static compliance significantly impaired; peak, plateau, and mean airway pressures increased; and physiological dead space/tidal volume ratio and total inspiratory work of breathing increased by 11.1% and 33.7%, respectively. Arterial oxygen tension is typically decreased; however, no significant differences are seen in end-tidal or arterial carbon dioxide tension.[185] Although the exaggerated lithotomy is the optimal surgical position for the obese patient, ironically the respiratory consequences may make it impossible to maintain adequate ventilation in such patients. Hence, it is recommended to assess the adequacy of ventilation for a brief period before proceeding with surgical incision. Blood loss is typically significantly reduced compared with ORRP, but the need for CVP and/or arterial line should still be guided by patient comorbidities. Although the surgical site for this approach ideally would be amenable to spinal or epidural anesthesia, the position is so poorly tolerated by the patient and the ventilatory alterations are so profound that general anesthesia is often indicated.

Laparoscopic and Robotic Prostatectomy

12 In recent years considerable attention has been paid to the development and evolution of laparoscopic techniques for urologic cancer surgery. The laparoscopic radical prostatectomy (LRP) was first described in 1997 by Schuessler at al.[186] Since the original description, technological refinements have continued, including the introduction of robot assistance, leading to improved operative visualization with the anticipation of improved outcomes. A major impetus in the development of minimally invasive prostate cancer techniques has been patient satisfaction and quality of life. Shorter convalescence with a more rapid return to normal activity and shorter urinary catheter duration can be achieved with LRP. Additional potential benefits of LRP are decreased blood loss and magnification of the operative field. Most operative bleeding during radical prostatectomy is venous, which CO_2 insufflation theoretically tamponades by increased intra-abdominal pressure. The 10 to $15\times$ magnification afforded by laparoscopy provides better intraoperative visual detail, facilitating vesicourethral anastomosis and, it is hoped, further reducing the risk of blood loss and transfusion.

The initial report of LRP by Schuessler et al.[186] involved nine procedures performed through an intraperitoneal approach in antegrade fashion. Average operative time was 9.4 hours and there were three complications, namely cholecystitis, thrombophlebitis associated with pulmonary embolism, and small bowel hernia into a trocar site. In a more recent large series, average estimated blood loss for LRP varied from 290 to 380 mL, with an overall transfusion rate of 2.6 to 5.3%.[187] LRP is associated with decreased duration of postoperative urinary catheterization, decreased analgesic requirements, and decreased time to complete convalescence, when compared with open prostatectomy procedures.[188] Cost comparisons between standard robotic radical prostatectomy (RRP) and LRP have yielded variable results. One study reported a cost advantage with LRP compared with RRP when operating room expenses and hospitalization costs were evaluated.[189] In another U.S.-based study, LRP was found to be more expensive than ORRP largely because of an increase in operating room time and equipment expenses.[190] LRP is associated with a complication rate of 17.1%, including major (3.7%) and minor complications (14.6%), with reoperation required in 3.7% of patients. Conversion from LRP to open RRP occurs in a small number of cases (1.2%). Complication rates and duration of surgery decrease as the surgeon gains experience with the technique.

Potential anesthetic complications for LRP include standard concerns for laparoscopic procedures. Extended surgical times coupled with high abdominal insufflation pressures and the head-down position can sometimes compromise ventilation. The addition of positive end-expiratory pressure can be of benefit.[191]

Because blood loss with LRP is minimal, monitoring decisions based on hemorrhage concerns with ORRP are replaced by selection of monitors focused primarily on patient comorbidities. Anesthetic adaptations to longer surgery times include innovative approaches using continuous infusion of short-acting agents to facilitate faster emergence from general anesthesia. Fast-tracking techniques can be used with LRP; in one series, a reduction from 6.7 to 3.6 days was achieved.[192] Length of stay can be reduced with attention to temperature control, using forced air warming and warming insufflated gas to maintain normothermia, use of short-acting anesthetic agents, minimizing opioid administration, addressing postoperative nausea and vomiting, and reducing insufflation pressures from 15 to 12 mm Hg (to facilitate earlier return of bowel function). Curiously, postoperative pain with ORRP and LRP approaches to radical prostatectomy are similar, with the overall analgesic needs for both approaches being short-lived.[193]

Robotic prostatectomy currently accounts for approximately 10% of radical prostatectomies performed in the United States, although it is anticipated that this rate will increase. The da Vinci robotic system is currently the prevalent technology in this field. Robotic systems (Intuitive Surgical Inc., Sunnyvale, CA) typically have three components: (1) a surgeon console, (2) a patient-side cart, and (3) an image-processing or insufflation stack. The surgeon controls three or four robotic arms while sitting at the console away from the operating table. The three-dimensional view from the endoscope is projected on the console at $610\times$ magnification. The surgeon's thumb and forefinger control the movements of the robotic arms in the patient's abdomen. Foot pedals control diathermy and other energy sources. Motion scaling is a process that eliminates tremor, allowing very smooth and precise movements. Motion scaling significantly enhances the surgeon's precision using this technology.[194]

Since 2000, a surgical team from Detroit has performed >2,000 robotic prostatectomies, and this group is considered an innovator in this field. Describing their first 1,100 cases, Menon et al.[195] reported operative times of 70 to 160 minutes and an estimated blood loss of 50 to 150 mL, with no need for blood transfusions. Remarkably, 95% of the patients were discharged within 24 hours. Total continence was achieved in 96% of patients at 6 months. Robotic devices for prostate surgery require a large capital investment (purchase and maintenance).

Additional time is often required for operating room setup to use the robot. There is also an extended learning curve in using this device with longer operating times. In addition, costs are high as the laparoscopic instruments used by the master-slave robot require replacement after a defined number of procedures.[196] Currently, there are no randomized controlled trials comparing the surgical results to justify these expenses.

Anesthetic concerns for RRP are largely similar to those of other laparoscopic approaches. Longer procedures related to the initial learning curve requires careful attention to positioning, fluid management, and temperature control.[197] Patients are in a head-down, low lithotomy position that puts them at risk for brachial plexus and lower extremity injury. When maintenance of head-down position and high abdominal insufflation pressures continues for ≥4 hours, the patient is at high risk for airway edema. A careful evaluation should be done before tracheal extubation, which may include a trial over a tube changer.

ANESTHESIA FOR OTHER UROLOGIC CANCER SURGERY

Radical Nephrectomy

Renal cell carcinoma is the most common malignancy of the kidney and accounts for 2.6% of all malignancies in the United States. Approximately 85 to 90% of solid renal masses are renal cell carcinoma. Surgical excision remains the mainstay of treatment for renal cell carcinoma as this tumor is refractory to nonsurgical therapies (chemotherapy and radiation). Radical nephrectomy involves excision of the kidney, perinephric fat, surrounding fascia, and when indicated, the ipsilateral adrenal gland. Partial nephrectomy (nephron-sparing surgery) is used for smaller lesions, bilateral tumors, or inpatients with morbidities that put them at risk for further decline in renal function. The disease has a peak incidence at age 60. Thus, coronary artery disease and chronic obstructive pulmonary disease are comorbidities often seen in this patient population.[198] It can also be associated with a paraneoplastic phenomenon with anemia, hypercalcemia, and hypertension.

There has been significant evolution of radical nephrectomy surgical technique in the last decade with the introduction of laparoscopic radical nephrectomy (LRN) and hand-assisted laparoscopic radical nephrectomy (HALRN). Both of these approaches offer advantages over the traditional open radical nephrectomy (ORN). The HALRN technique is a modification of the traditional LRN, which offers some added potential advantages. HALRN shortens operative times, facilitates dissection, and allows intact extraction of the tumor without sacrificing the advantages of the laparoscopic approach, including reduced postoperative pain and shorter recovery.[199]

The three surgical approaches for ORN involve flank, subcostal, or thoracoabdominal incisions. All of these approaches are associated with significant postoperative pain and each has specific risks for surgical complications such as pneumothorax and splenic injury (for left-sided tumors).

Approximately 5 to 10 % of right-sided tumors extend into the inferior vena cava, and some even extend into the right atrium, requiring cardiopulmonary bypass for surgical resection.[200] Because these tumors are friable, a venous filter is always placed on the venous return catheter of the bypass circuit, to avoid obstruction of the oxygenator and minimize tumor embolization. Transesophageal echo is a valuable tool in the management of these procedures, and can sometimes identify when pulmonary artery tumor embolization has occurred.

As with the minimally invasive radical prostatectomy techniques, laparoscopic nephrectomy approaches offer the benefits of a faster recovery and return to work, reduced postoperative pain, reduced intraoperative blood loss, and better cosmetic outcome.[201]

In a single-center comparison, Baldwin et al.[202] reported similar operative times for LRN versus HALRN versus ORN procedures, but there were major differences among groups in terms of estimated blood loss (125 vs. 410 vs. 467 mL), analgesic requirements (22.9 vs. 42.1 vs. 97.7 mg of morphine), time to oral intake (7.3 vs. 9.2 vs. 54 hours), and length of hospital stay (1.3 vs. 2.6 vs. 3.75 days), respectively. Translated into total cost of hospital stay, these observations leaned in favor of the laparoscopic techniques. In another study of cost comparison between operative techniques, ORN proved to be 1.2 times as costly as LRN.[203] In this study a newer, less-invasive technique, computed tomography-guided percutaneous cryoablation, was also evaluated, and was 2.2 to 2.7 times less expensive than ORN. This option has the advantage of less patient morbidity and shorter hospital stay; however, its efficacy remains under investigation.

A primary concern in the anesthetic management for ORN is attention to fluid management and the potential for significant blood loss. Good intravenous access is essential, and the use of CVP and arterial line should be guided by patient comorbidities. Patients undergoing ORN are prone to hemodynamic instability not only from blood loss but from compression of the inferior vena cava. This can occur from positioning in the lateral flexed position or to compression of the vena cava by the surgeons or surgical retractors. In patients with evidence of tumor extension into the right atrium, insertion of a pulmonary artery catheter may be contraindicated. Patients having ORN often experience significant postoperative pain, and use of multimodal therapies including epidural analgesia may be helpful.

When planning for postoperative epidural analgesia, it is important to know what is planned for postoperative deep venous thrombosis (DVT) prophylaxis. All patients with cancer are at a high risk for DVT and pulmonary embolus, although DVT rates for patient with renal cell carcinoma are less that those seen in cancer patients overall (1.5% vs. 10 to 20%). Risk factors include a large surgical blood loss, long operating time, and pre-existing dysrhythmia. It has been proposed that pneumatic compression boots are appropriate DVT prophylaxis for radical nephrectomy and that intermittent subcutaneous heparin may not be necessary unless other major risk factors exist.[204] If regional anesthesia is planned for postoperative pain management and an anticoagulant is planned for DVT prophylaxis, the American Society of Regional Anesthesia guidelines should be followed.[205]

Anesthesia for the LRN procedures should involve all the usual considerations for laparoscopic surgery. As with other minimally invasive surgeries, there is opportunity to reduce length of stay for HALRN and LRN if fast-track strategies are employed intraoperatively and in the immediate postoperative period. Primary factors affecting length of stay are postoperative pain, nausea and vomiting, ileus, organ dysfunction, and fatigue. Anesthesia using short-acting agents, careful attention to fluid management, a multimodal approach to pain management with a goal of minimizing opioid requirements, and administration of prophylactic antiemetics coupled with early feeding and mobilization, have been shown to shorten length of hospital stay as compared with traditional approaches.[206]

As is typical with urologic surgeries, positioning is challenging for radical nephrectomy and puts the patient at significant risk for complications such as nerve injury (both upper and lower extremity), back pain, and/or rhabdomyolysis. A careful inspection of the patient's position at the start of surgery and at regular intervals throughout is essential.[207]

Radical Cystectomy

Bladder cancer is the second most common urologic malignancy. It is a disease that increases in incidence with increasing age. A majority of patients present with superficial tumor, although as many as 20 to 40% will develop more invasive disease. Radical cystectomy with pelvic node dissection is the gold standard for treatment of muscle-invasive bladder carcinoma. It is an aggressive surgery that is often performed in elderly patients with significant comorbidities.

The perioperative complication and 30-day mortality rate are as high as 28 and 4.5%, respectively. A review over a 12-year period (1993 to 2005) indicated a decline in 30-day mortality rate to as low as 0.8%, largely attributed to improvement in anesthesia and surgical techniques, but the perioperative complication rate (27.3%) did not change significantly.[208] Average blood loss for the procedure ranges between 560 and 3,000 mL. Transfusion is common. Hospital length of stay for this procedure is typically long, but also varies considerably between centers.

Anesthetic care for radical cystectomy should focus on preoperative assessment and patient optimization because these patients often are elderly and have multiple comorbidities. Intraoperative technique and monitoring should be individualized by patient. When selecting monitoring tools, in addition to considering comorbidities, any plan should permit assessment of intraoperative volume status. As with radical prostatectomy, urine output is lost early in the procedure as a measure of volume status. Usually a large midline incision is used and the patients experience significant insensible and evaporative fluid loss. Additionally, one should anticipate the possibility of significant blood loss and the need for transfusion. Large-bore intravenous access will be required. CVP monitoring or the use of a noninvasive cardiac output monitor may help guide fluid replacement. An arterial line offers the

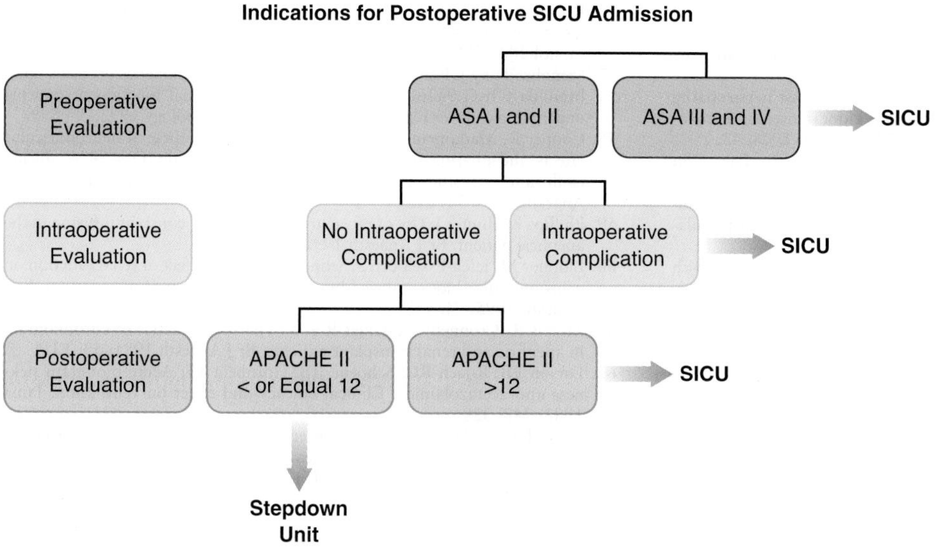

Indications for Postoperative SICU Admission

FIGURE 52-9. Algorithm to assess the need for postoperative surgical intensive care (SICU) admission based on preoperative American Society of Anesthesiologists classification, intraoperative course, and postoperative APACHE II score. (From Dahm P, Tuttle-Newhall JE, Yowell CW et al: Indications for surgical intensive care unit admission of postoperative urologic patients. Urology 2000; 55: 334, with permission.)

advantage of easy blood pressure monitoring in high-risk patients and a method for obtaining serial samples for hematocrit measurement.

Although there is no contraindication to the use of regional anesthesia, radical cystectomy is usually performed under general anesthesia because of the long duration of surgery. Combined epidural/general anesthesia is a good option, and there has been some suggestion that the combined technique is associated with lower intraoperative blood loss.[209] However, few studies have compared outcomes with epidural and/or general anesthesia for these cases. One small, randomized, controlled study looked at the use of general anesthesia compared with combined general/epidural anesthesia with postoperative analgesia either without the use of the epidural or using patient-controlled epidural analgesia (PCEA). In this cohort of 30 patients, when compared with the other two groups there was a significant reduction in dynamic pain scores and an earlier time to first bowel movement in the general/epidural/PCEA group, and reduced postoperative urinary catecholamine excretion. These investigators also reported better postoperative mobilization and a subjective report of less fatigue in the general/epidural/PCEA group. In this very small study there was no difference in length of stay among groups.[210] Although epidural analgesia is good for pain management, its use should not hinder thromboprophylaxis, as DVT is the most common medical complication in this patient population. Unlike with the other laparoscopic approaches to urologic surgery, fast-tracking strategies including the use of short-acting anesthesia agents have not proven beneficial. Thoughtful management of postoperative analgesia using a multimodal approach always has a role in major surgery and often needs to be managed by the anesthesiologist.

In recognition of the high mortality and complication rates seen with radical cystectomy, many patients are monitored immediately postoperatively in an intensive care unit (ICU). With improved anesthesia and surgery techniques, this may not always be necessary. One study demonstrated that 84.4% of patients admitted to ICU after major urologic surgery had an uneventful course, with 62.2% staying <24 hours and only 21% had a prolonged stay (>47 hours).[211] Age, operating time, and blood loss were not associated with an increased rate of active ICU-specific treatment. As ICU resources become more limited, automatic admission by type of procedure may need to be revisited across all surgical fields. Risk stratification can be applied to patients having cystectomy when deciding on appropriate arrangements for postoperative care. (Fig. 52-9).

References

1. Alpert RA, Roizen MF, Hamilton WK et al: Intraoperative urinary output does not predict postoperative renal function in patients undergoing abdominal aortic revascularization. Surgery 1984; 95: 707
2. Conlon PJ, Stafford-Smith M, White WD et al: Acute renal failure following cardiac surgery. Nephrol Dial Transplant 1999; 14: 1158
3. Levin A: Cystatin C, serum creatinine, and estimates of kidney function: searching for better measures of kidney function and cardiovascular risk. Ann Intern Med 2005; 142: 586
4. Grubb A, Bjork J, Lindstrom V et al: A cystatin C-based formula without anthropometric variables estimates glomerular filtration rate better than creatinine clearance using the Cockcroft-Gault formula. Scand J Clin Lab Invest 2005; 65: 153
5. Sladen RN, Endo E, Harrison T: Two-hour versus 22-hour creatinine clearance in critically ill patients. Anesthesiology 1987; 67: 1013
6. Bloor GK, Welsh KR, Goodall S et al: Comparison of predicted with measured creatinine clearance in cardiac surgical patients. J Cardiothorac Vasc Anesth 1996; 10: 899
7. Gowans EM, Fraser CG: Biological variation of serum and urine creatinine and creatinine clearance: ramifications for interpretation of results and patient care [see comments]. Ann Clin Biochem 1988; 25: 259
8. Morgan DB, Dillon S, Payne RB: The assessment of glomerular function: creatinine clearance or plasma creatinine? Postgrad Med J 1978; 54: 302
9. Cockcroft DW, Gault MH: Prediction of creatinine clearance from serum creatinine. Nephron 1976; 16: 31
10. Levey AS, Bosch JP, Lewis JB et al: A more accurate method to estimate glomerular filtration rate from serum creatinine: A new prediction equation. Modification of Diet in Renal Disease Study Group. Ann Intern Med 1999; 130: 461
11. Ferguson TB, Jr., Dziuban SW, Jr., Edwards FH et al: The STS National Database: current changes and challenges for the new millennium. Committee to Establish a National Database in Cardiothoracic Surgery, The Society of Thoracic Surgeons. Ann Thorac Surg 2000; 69: 680
12. Barrett BJ, Parfrey PS: Prevention of nephrotoxicity induced by radiocontrast agents. N Engl J Med 1994; 331: 1449
13. Bellomo R, Ronco C, Kellum JA et al: Acute renal failure—definition, outcome measures, animal models, fluid therapy and information technology needs: the Second International Consensus Conference of the Acute Dialysis Quality Initiative (ADQI) Group. Crit Care 2004; 8: R204
14. Greenberg A: Primer on Kidney Diseases, 4th edition. Philadelphia, Elsevier Saunders, 2005
15. Stafford-Smith M: Antifibrinolytic agents make alpha1- and beta2-microglobulinuria poor markers of post cardiac surgery renal dysfunction. Anesthesiology 1999; 90: 928
16. Anderson RJ, Chung HM, Kluge R, Schrier RW: Hyponatremia: a prospective analysis of its epidemiology and the pathogenetic role of vasopressin. Ann Intern Med 1985; 102: 164
17. Verbalis JG: Hyponatremia: epidemiology, pathophysiology, and therapy. Curr Opin Nephrol Hypertens 1993; 2: 636
18. Arieff AI: Hyponatremia, convulsions, respiratory arrest, and permanent brain damage after elective surgery in healthy women. N Engl J Med 1986; 314: 1529
19. Arieff AI, Ayus JC, Fraser CL: Hyponatraemia and death or permanent brain damage in healthy children. Bmj 1992; 304: 1218
20. Ayus JC, Wheeler JM, Arieff AI: Postoperative hyponatremic encephalopathy in menstruant women. Ann Intern Med 1992; 117: 891

21. Wilkinson A, Cohen D: Renal failure in the recipients of nonrenal solid organ transplants. J Am Soc Nephrol 1999; 10: 1136

22. Rudnick M, Feldman H: Contrast-induced nephropathy: what are the true clinical consequences? Clin J Am Soc Nephrol 2008; 3: 263

23. Alonso A, Lau J, Jaber B et al: Prevention of radiocontrast nephropathy with N-acetylcysteine in patients with chronic kidney disease: a meta-analysis of randomized, controlled trials. Am J Kidney Dis 2004; 43: 1

24. Taber S, Mueller B: Drug-associated renal dysfunction. Crit Care Clin 2006; 22: 357, viii

25. Huerta C, Castellsague J, Varas-Lorenzo C, Garcia Rodriguez L: Non-steroidal anti-inflammatory drugs and risk of ARF in the general population. Am J Kidney Dis 2005; 45: 531

26. Oh K, Lee H, Lee J et al: Reversible renal vasoconstriction in a patient with acute renal failure after exercise. Clin Nephrol 2006; 66: 297

27. Melli G, Chaudhry V, Cornblath D: Rhabdomyolysis: an evaluation of 475 hospitalized patients. Medicine (Baltimore) 2005; 84: 377

28. Singh D, Chander V, Chopra K: Rhabdomyolysis. Methods Find Exp Clin Pharmacol 2005; 27: 39

29. Eichhorn J, Hedley-Whyte J, Steinman T et al: Renal failure following enflurane anesthesia. Anesthesiology 1976; 45: 557

30. Eger En, Gong D, Koblin D et al: Dose-related biochemical markers of renal injury after sevoflurane versus desflurane anesthesia in volunteers. Anesth Analg 1997; 85: 1154

31. Conzen P, Kharasch E, Czerner S et al: Low-flow sevoflurane compared with low-flow isoflurane anesthesia in patients with stable renal insufficiency. Anesthesiology 2002; 97: 578

32. Gunukula S, Spodick D: Pericardial disease in renal patients. Semin Nephrol 2001; 21: 52

33. Crandell W, Pappas S, Macdonald A: Nephrotoxicity associated with methoxyflurane anesthesia. Anesthesiology 1966; 27: 591

34. Kharasch E, Hankins D, Thummel K: Human kidney methoxyflurane and sevoflurane metabolism. Intrarenal fluoride production as a possible mechanism of methoxyflurane nephrotoxicity. Anesthesiology 1995; 82: 689

35. Mazze R, Calverley R, Smith N: Inorganic fluoride nephrotoxicity: prolonged enflurane and halothane anesthesia in volunteers. Anesthesiology 1977; 46: 265

36. Burch P, Stanski D: Decreased protein binding and thiopental kinetics. Clin Pharmacol Ther 1982; 32: 212

37. Gan T: Pharmacokinetic and pharmacodynamic characteristics of medications used for moderate sedation. Clin Pharmacokinet 2006; 45: 855

38. Carlos R, Calvo R, Erill S: Plasma protein binding of etomidate in patients with renal failure or hepatic cirrhosis. Clin Pharmacokinet 1979; 4: 144

39. Kirvela M, Olkkola K, Rosenberg P et al: Pharmacokinetics of propofol and haemodynamic changes during induction of anaesthesia in uraemic patients. Br J Anaesth 1992; 68: 178

40. Vinik H, Reves J, Greenblatt D et al: The pharmacokinetics of midazolam in neonatal and renal failure patients. Anesthesiology 1983; 59: 390

41. Schmith V, Piraino B, Smith R, Kroboth P: Alprazolam in end-stage renal disease. II. Pharmacodynamics. Clin Pharmacol Ther 1992; 51: 533

42. De Wolf A, Fragen R, Avram M et al: The pharmacokinetics of dexmedetomidine in volunteers with severe renal impairment. Anesth Analg 2001; 93: 1205

43. Chan G, Matzke G: Effects of renal insufficiency on the pharmacokinetics and pharmacodynamics of opioid analgesics. Drug Intell Clin Pharm 1987; 21: 773

44. Babul N, Darke A, Hagen N: Hydromorphone metabolite accumulation in renal failure. J Pain Symptom Manage 1995; 10: 184

45. Murphy E: Acute pain management pharmacology for the patient with concurrent renal or hepatic disease. Anaesth Intensive Care 2005; 33: 311

46. Davis P, Stiller R, Cook D et al: Effects of cholestatic hepatic disease and chronic renal failure on alfentanil pharmacokinetics in children. Anesth Analg 1989; 68: 579

47. Wiggum D, Cork R, Weldon S et al: Postoperative respiratory depression and elevated sufentanil levels in a patient with chronic renal failure. Anesthesiology 1985; 63: 708

48. Pitsiu M, Wilmer A, Bodenham A et al: Pharmacokinetics of remifentanil and its major metabolite, remifentanil acid, in ICU patients with renal impairment. Br J Anaesth 2004; 92: 493

49. Szenohradszky J, Caldwell J, Wright P et al: Influence of renal failure on the pharmacokinetics and neuromuscular effects of a single dose of rapacuronium bromide. Anesthesiology 1999; 90: 24

50. Ryan D: Preoperative serum cholinesterase concentration in chronic renal failure. Clinical experience of suxamethonium in 81 patients undergoing renal transplant. Br J Anaesth 1977; 49: 945

51. Cook D, Freeman J, Lai A et al: Pharmacokinetics of mivacurium in normal patients and in those with hepatic or renal failure. Br J Anaesth 1992; 69: 580

52. Cook D, Freeman J, Lai A et al: Pharmacokinetics and pharmacodynamics of doxacurium in normal patients and in those with hepatic or renal failure. Anesth Analg 1991; 72: 145

53. Della Rocca G, Pompei L, Coccia C et al: Atracurium, cisatracurium, vecuronium and rocuronium in patients with renal failure. Minerva Anestesiol 2003; 69: 605, 612

54. Fahey M, Rupp S, Canfell C et al: Effect of renal failure on laudanosine excretion in man. Br J Anaesth 1985; 57: 1049

55. Lynam D, Cronnelly R, Castagnoli K et al: The pharmacodynamics and pharmacokinetics of vecuronium in patients anesthetized with isoflurane with normal renal function or with renal failure. Anesthesiology 1988; 69: 227

56. Robertson E, Driessen J, Booij L: Pharmacokinetics and pharmacodynamics of rocuronium in patients with and without renal failure. Eur J Anaesthesiol 2005; 22: 4

57. Szenohradszky J, Fisher D, Segredo V et al: Pharmacokinetics of rocuronium bromide (ORG 9426) in patients with normal renal function or patients undergoing cadaver renal transplantation. Anesthesiology 1992; 77: 899

58. Cooper R, Maddineni V, Mirakhur R et al: Time course of neuromuscular effects and pharmacokinetics of rocuronium bromide (Org 9426) during isoflurane anaesthesia in patients with and without renal failure. Br J Anaesth 1993; 71: 222

59. Phillips B, Hunter J: Use of mivacurium chloride by constant infusion in the anephric patient. Br J Anaesth 1992; 68: 492

60. Blobner M, Jelen-Esselborn S, Schneider G et al: Effect of renal function on neuromuscular block induced by continuous infusion of mivacurium. Br J Anaesth 1995; 74: 452

61. Morris R, Cronnelly R, Miller R et al: Pharmacokinetics of edrophonium in anephric and renal transplant patients. Br J Anaesth 1981; 53: 1311

62. Larson EB, Roach RC, Schoene RB, Hornbein TF: Acute mountain sickness and acetazolamide. Clinical efficacy and effect on ventilation. Jama 1982; 248: 328

63. White DP, Zwillich CW, Pickett CK et al: Central sleep apnea. Improvement with acetazolamide therapy. Archives of Internal Medicine 1982; 142: 1816

64. Better OS, Rubinstein I, Winaver JM, Knochel JP: Mannitol therapy revisited (1940–1997). Kidney Int 1997; 52: 886

65. Solomon R, Werner C, Mann D et al: Effects of saline, mannitol, and furosemide to prevent acute decreases in renal function induced by radiocontrast agents. N Engl J Med. 331(21):1416; 1994; 331: 1416

66. Conger JD: Interventions in clinical acute renal failure: what are the data? Am J Kidney Dis 1995; 26: 565

67. Borges HF, Hocks J, Kjellstrand CM: Mannitol intoxication in patients with renal failure. Arch Intern Med 1982; 142: 63

68. Gallagher KL, Jones JK: Furosemide-induced ototoxicity. Ann Intern Med 1979; 91: 744

69. Pitt B, Zannad F, Remme WJ et al: The effect of spironolactone on morbidity and mortality in patients with severe heart failure. Randomized Aldactone Evaluation Study Investigators. N Engl J Med 1999; 341: 709

70. Jose PA, Felder RA: What we can learn from the selective manipulation of dopaminergic receptors about the pathogenesis and treatment of hypertension? Curr Opin Nephrol Hypertens 1996; 5: 447

71. Bellomo R, Cole L, Ronco C: Hemodynamic support and the role of dopamine. Kidney Int Suppl 1998; 66: S71

72. Marik PE: Low-dose dopamine: a systematic review. Intensive Care Med 2002; 28: 877

73. Kellum JA, M Decker J. Use of dopamine in acute renal failure: a meta-analysis. Crit Care Med 2001; 29: 1526

74. Prins I, Plotz FB, Uiterwaal CS, van Vught HJ: Low-dose dopamine in neonatal and pediatric intensive care: a systematic review. Intensive Care Med 2001; 27: 206

75. Holmes CL, Walley KR: Bad medicine: low-dose dopamine in the ICU. Chest 2003; 123: 1266

76. Argalious M, Motta P, Khandwala F et al: "Renal dose" dopamine is associated with the risk of new-onset atrial fibrillation after cardiac surgery. Crit Care Med 2005; 33: 1327

77. Denton MD, Chertow GM, Brady HR: "Renal-dose" dopamine for the treatment of acute renal failure: scientific rationale, experimental studies and clinical trials. Kidney Int 1996; 50: 4

78. Abel RM, Buckley MJ, Austen WG et al: Etiology, incidence, and prognosis of renal failure following cardiac operations. Results of a prospective analysis of 500 consecutive patients. J Thorac Cardiovasc Surg 1976; 71: 323

79. Swaminathan M, Shaw A, Phillips-Bute B et al: Trends in acute renal failure associated with coronary artery bypass graft surgery in the United States. Crit Care Med 2007; 35: 2286

80. Filsoufi F, Rahmanian P, Castillo J et al: Early and late outcomes of cardiac surgery in patients with moderate to severe preoperative renal dysfunction without dialysis. Interact Cardiovasc Thorac Surg 2008; 7: 90

81. Bechtel J, Detter C, Fischlein T et al: Cardiac surgery in patients on dialysis: decreased 30-day mortality, unchanged overall survival. Ann Thorac Surg 2008; 85: 147

82. Aronson S, Fontes M, Miao Y, Mangano D: Risk index for perioperative renal dysfunction/failure: critical dependence on pulse pressure hypertension. Circulation 2007; 115: 733

83. Mangano D, Tudor I, Dietzel C: The risk associated with aprotinin in cardiac surgery. N Engl J Med 2006; 354: 353

84. Hix J, Thakar C, Katz E et al: Effect of off-pump coronary artery bypass graft surgery on postoperative acute kidney injury and mortality. Crit Care Med 2006; 34: 2979

85. Costa P, Ottino G, Matani A et al: Low-dose dopamine during cardiopulmonary bypass in patients with renal dysfunction. J Cardiothorac Anesth 1990; 4: 469

86. Berendes E, Mollhoff T, Van Aken H et al: Effects of dopexamine on creatinine clearance, systemic inflammation, and splanchnic oxygenation in patients undergoing coronary artery bypass grafting. Anesth Analg 1997; 84: 950

87. Renton MC, Snowden CP: Dopexamine and its role in the protection of hepatosplanchnic and renal perfusion in high-risk surgical and critically ill patients. Br J Anaesth 2005; 94: 459

88. Novis BK, Roizen MF, Aronson S, Thisted RA: Association of preoperative risk factors with postoperative acute renal failure. Anesth Analg 1994; 78: 143

89. Stene J: Renal failure in the trauma patient. Crit Care Clin 1990; 6: 111

90. Cachecho R, Millham F, Wedel S: Management of the trauma patient with pre-existing renal disease. Crit Care Clin 1994; 10: 523

91. Myers B, Miller D, Mehigan J et al: Nature of the renal injury following total renal ischemia in man. J Clin Invest 1984; 73: 329

92. Godet G, Fleron M, Vicaut E et al: Risk factors for acute postoperative renal failure in thoracic or thoracoabdominal aortic surgery: a prospective study. Anesth Analg 1997; 85: 1227

93. Svensson L, Coselli J, Safi H et al: Appraisal of adjuncts to prevent acute renal failure after surgery on the thoracic or thoracoabdominal aorta. J Vasc Surg 1989; 10: 230

94. Olsen P, Schroeder T, Perko M et al: Renal failure after operation for abdominal aortic aneurysm. Ann Vasc Surg 1990; 4: 580

95. Svensson L, Kouchoukos N, Miller D et al: Expert consensus document on the treatment of descending thoracic aortic disease using endovascular stent-grafts. Ann Thorac Surg 2008; 85: S1

96. Antonucci F, Calo L, Rizzolo M et al: Nifedipine can preserve renal function in patients undergoing aortic surgery with infrarenal crossclamping. Nephron 1996; 74: 668

97. Ding H, Kopple J, Cohen A, Hirschberg R: Recombinant human insulin-like growth factor-I accelerates recovery and reduces catabolism in rats with ischemic acute renal failure. J Clin Invest 1993; 91: 2281

98. Vijayan A, Franklin S, Behrend T et al: Insulin-like growth factor I improves renal function in patients with end-stage chronic renal failure. Am J Physiol 1999; 276: R929

99. Franklin S, Moulton M, Sicard G et al: Insulin-like growth factor I preserves renal function postoperatively. Am J Physiol 1997; 272: F257

100. Allgren R, Marbury T, Rahman S et al: Anaritide in acute tubular necrosis. Auriculin Anaritide Acute Renal Failure Study Group. N Engl J Med 1997; 336: 828

101. Yalavarthy R, Edelstein C, Teitelbaum I: Acute renal failure and chronic kidney disease following liver transplantation. Hemodial Int 2007; 11 Suppl 3: S7

102. Lopez Lago A, Fernandez Villanueva J, Garcia Acuna J et al: Evolution of hepatorenal syndrome after orthotopic liver transplantation: comparative analysis with patients who developed acute renal failure in the early postoperative period of liver transplantation. Transplant Proc 2007; 39: 2318

103. Monk T: Clinical applications of monitored anaesthesia care. Minim Invasive Ther 1994; 3: 17

104. Smith J: Urologic Laser Surgery, Campbell's Urology, 6th Edition. Edited by Walsh P, Retik A, Stamey T, Vaughn E. Philadelphia, WB Saunders, 1992, pp 2923

105. Gettman M, Segura J: Indications and outcomes of ureteroscopy for urinary stones, Urinary stone disease: The practical guide to medical and surgical management. Totowa, NJ, , Humana Press, 2004

106. Fitzpatrick J: Minimally invasive and endoscopic management of benign prostatic hyperplasia, Campbell-Walsh Urology, 9th edition. Edited by Wein A, Kavoussi L, Novick A et al. Philadelphia, Saunders Elsevier, 2007, p 2803

107. Smith R: Complications of transurethral surgery, Complications of Urologic Surgery, 2nd Edition. Edited by Smith R, Ehrlich R. Philadelphia, WB Saunders, 1990, pp 355

108. Dorotta I, Basali A, Ritchey M et al: Transurethral resection syndrome after bladder perforation. Anesth Analg 2003; 97: 1536

109. Gross AJ, Herrmann TR: History of lasers. World J Urol 2007; 25: 217

110. Malloy T, Wein A: Complications of lasers in urology, Urologic complications: Medical and Surgical, adult and pediatric, 2nd Edition. Edited by Marshall F. St. Louis Mosby-Year Book, 1990, pp 411

111. Teichmann HO, Herrmann TR, Bach T: Technical aspects of lasers in urology. World J Urol 2007; 25: 221

112. Widder RA, Severin M, Kirchhof B, Krieglstein GK: Corneal injury after carbon dioxide laser skin resurfacing. Am J Ophthalmol 1998; 125: 392

113. Recommended practices for laser safety in practice settings. AORN J 2004; 79: 836, 841

114. Gloster HM, Jr., Roenigk RK: Risk of acquiring human papillomavirus from the plume produced by the carbon dioxide laser in the treatment of warts. J Am Acad Dermatol 1995; 32: 436

115. Wisniewski PM, Warhol MJ, Rando RF et al: Studies on the transmission of viral disease via the CO2 laser plume and ejecta. J Reprod Med 1990; 35: 1117

116. Smith JP, Moss CE, Bryant CJ, Fleeger AK: Evaluation of a smoke evacuator used for laser surgery. Lasers Surg Med 1989; 9: 276

117. Pearle M, Lotan Y: Urinary lithiasis: Etiology, epidemiology, and pathogenisis, Campbell-Walsh Urology, 9th Edition. Edited by Wein A, Kavoussi L, Novick A, Partin A, Peters C. Philadelphia, Saunders Elsevier, 2007, pp 1363

118. Abbott MA, Samuel JR, Webb DR: Anaesthesia for extracorporeal shock wave lithotripsy. Anaesthesia 1985; 40: 1065

119. Malhotra V: Hyperthermia and hypothermia as complications of extracorporeal shock wave lithotripsy. Anesthesiology 1987; 67: 448

120. Drach GW, Weber C, Donovan JM: Treatment of pacemaker patients with extracorporeal shock wave lithotripsy: experience from 2 continents. J Urol 1990; 143: 895

121. Chung MK, Streem SB, Ching E et al: Effects of extracorporeal shock wave lithotripsy on tiered therapy implantable cardioverter defibrillators. Pacing Clin Electrophysiol 1999; 22: 738

122. Gravenstein D: Extracorporeal shock wave lithotripsy and percutaneous nephrolithotomy. Anesthesiol Clin North America 2000; 18: 953

123. Malhotra V, Rosen RJ, Slepian RL: Life-threatening hypoxemia after lithotripsy in an adult due to shock-wave-induced pulmonary contusion. Anesthesiology 1991; 75: 529

124. Bush WH, Jones D, Gibbons RP: Radiation dose to patient and personnel during extracorporeal shock wave lithotripsy. J Urol 1987; 138: 716

125. Demir E, Kilciler M, Bedir S et al: Comparing two local anesthesia techniques for extracorporeal shock wave lithotripsy. Urology 2007; 69: 625

126. Medina HJ, Galvin EM, Dirckx M et al: Remifentanil as a single drug for extracorporeal shock wave lithotripsy: a comparison of infusion doses in terms of analgesic potency and side effects. Anesth Analg 2005; 101: 365, table of contents

127. Burmeister MA, Brauer P, Wintruff M et al: A comparison of anaesthetic techniques for shock wave lithotripsy: the use of a remifentanil infusion alone compared to intermittent fentanyl boluses combined with a low dose propofol infusion. Anaesthesia 2002; 57: 877

128. Berry SJ, Coffey DS, Walsh PC, Ewing LL: The development of human benign prostatic hyperplasia with age. J Urol 1984; 132: 474

129. Connolly SS, Fitzpatrick JM: Medical treatment of benign prostatic hyperplasia. Postgrad Med J 2007; 83: 73

130. Roehrborn C, McConnell J: Benign prostatic hyperplasia: Etiology, pathophysiology, epidemiology, and natural history, Campbell-Walsh Urology, 9th Edition. Edited by Wein A, Kavoussi L, Novick A et al. Philadelphia, Saunders Elsevier, 2007, pp 2727

131. Richmann M, Bruskewitz R: Evaluation of benign prostatic hyperplasia, Management of urologic disorders. Edited by Brahnson R. London: Wolfe, 1994, pp 12

132. Lynch M, Anson K: Time to rebrand transurethral resection of the prostate? Curr Opin Urol 2006; 16: 20

133. Freiha F, Deem S, Pearl R: Urology: Transurethral resection of the protate (TURP), Anesthesiologist's manual of surgical procedures. Edited by Jaffe R, Samuels S. New York, Raven Press, 1994, pp 553

134. Jensen V: The TURP syndrome. Can J Anaesth 1991; 38: 90

135. Marx GF, Orkin LR: Complications associated with transurethral surgery. Anesthesiology 1962; 23: 802

136. Roesch RP, Stoelting RK, Lingeman JE et al: Ammonia toxicity resulting from glycine absorption during a transurethral resection of the prostate. Anesthesiology 1983; 58: 577

137. Hoekstra PT, Kahnoski R, McCamish et al: Transurethral prostatic resection syndrome–a new perspective: encephalopathy with associated hyperammonemia. J Urol 1983; 130: 704

138. Hahn RG, Sikk M: Glycine loading and urinary oxalate excretion. Urol Int 1994; 52: 14

139. Ovassapian A, Joshi CW, Brunner EA: Visual disturbances: an unusual symptom of transurethral prostatic resection reaction. Anesthesiology 1982; 57: 332

140. Barletta JP, Fanous MM, Hamed LM: Temporary blindness in the TUR syndrome. J Neuroophthalmol 1994; 14: 6

141. Agin C: Anesthesia for transurethral prostate surgery, Anesthesia for urologic surgery. Edited by Lebowitz P. Boston: Brown, 1993, pp 25

142. Gravenstein D: Transurethral resection of the prostate (TURP) syndrome: a review of the pathophysiology and management. Anesth Analg 1997; 84: 438

143. Hatch PD: Surgical and anaesthetic considerations in transurethral resection of the prostate. Anaesth Intensive Care 1987; 15: 203

144. Hahn RG, Stalberg HP, Ekengren J, Rundgren M: Effects of 1.5% glycine solution with and without 1% ethanol on the fluid balance in elderly men. Acta Anaesthesiol Scand 1991; 35: 725

145. Rippa A: Transurethral resection of the prostate: Aids and accessories, Smith's textbook of endourology. Edited by Smith A. St. Louis, Quality Medical, 1996, pp 1190

146. Hahn RG, Larsson H, Ribbe T: Continuous monitoring of irrigating fluid absorption during transurethral surgery. Anaesthesia 1995; 50: 327

147. Krongrad A, Droller M: Complications of transurethral resection of the prostate, Urologic complications: Medical and surgical, adult and pediatric, 2nd Edition. Edited by Marshall F. St. Louis, Mosby-Year Book, 1990, pp 305

148. Black R: Disorders of plasma sodium and plasma potassium, Intensive care medicine, 2nd Edition. Edited by Rippe J, Irwin R, Alpert J, Dalen J. Boston, Little, Brown, 1991, pp 794

149. Ansell J: Acquired bleeding disorders, Intensive Care Medicine, 2nd Edition. Edited by Rippe J, Irwin R, Alpert J, Dalen J. Boston, Little, Brown, 1991, pp 1013

150. Mebust WK, Holtgrewe HL, Cockett AT, Peters PC: Transurethral prostatectomy: immediate and postoperative complications. a cooperative study of 13 participating institutions evaluating 3,885 patients. 1989. J Urol 2002; 167: 999; discussion 1004

151. Allen TD: Body temperature changes during prostatic resection as related to the temperature of the irrigating solution. J Urol 1973; 110: 433

152. Raj P, Gesund P, Phero J: Rationale and choice for surgical procedures, Clinical practice of regional anesthesia. Edited by Raj P. New York, Churchill Livingstone, 1991, pp 197

153. Mackenzie AR: Influence of anaesthesia on blood loss in transurethral prostatectomy. Scott Med J 1990; 35: 14

154. McGowan SW, Smith GF: Anaesthesia for transurethral prostatectomy. A comparison of spinal intradural analgesia with two methods of general anaesthesia. Anaesthesia 1980; 35: 847

155. Bowman GW, Hoerth JW, McGlothlen JS et al: Anesthesia for transurethral resection of the prostate: spinal or general? AANA J 1981; 49: 63

156. Gehring H, Nahm W, Baerwald J et al: Irrigation fluid absorption during transurethral resection of the prostate: spinal vs. general anaesthesia. Acta Anaesthesiol Scand 1999; 43: 458

157. Sinha B, Haikel G, Lange PH et al: Transurethral resection of the prostate with local anesthesia in 100 patients. J Urol 1986; 135: 719

158. Newman S, Stygall J, Hirani S et al: Perioperative cognitive dysfunction after non-cardiac surgery: A systematic review. Anesthesiology 2007; 106: 572

159. Chung FF, Chung A, Meier RH et al: Comparison of perioperative mental function after general anaesthesia and spinal anaesthesia with intravenous sedation. Can J Anaesth 1989; 36: 382

160. Windsor A, French GW, Sear JW et al: Silent myocardial ischaemia in patients undergoing transurethral prostatectomy. A study to evaluate risk scoring and anaesthetic technique with outcome. Anaesthesia 1996; 51: 728

161. Reeves MD, Myles PS: Does anaesthetic technique affect the outcome after transurethral resection of the prostate? BJU Int 1999; 84: 982

162. Mebust WK, Holtgrewe HL, Cockett AT, Peters PC: Transurethral prostatectomy: immediate and postoperative complications. A cooperative study of 13 participating institutions evaluating 3,885 patients. J Urol 1989; 141: 243

163. Melchior J, Valk WL, Foret JD, Mebust WK: Transurethral prostatectomy: computerized analysis of 2,223 consecutive cases. J Urol 1974; 112: 634

164. Perrin P, Barnes R, Hadley H, Bergman RT: Forty years of transurethral prostatic resections. J Urol 1976; 116: 757

165. Fuglsig S, Aagaard J, Jonler M et al: Survival after transurethral resection of the prostate: a 10-year followup. J Urol 1994; 151: 637

166. Matani Y, Mottrie AM, Stockle M et al: Transurethral prostatectomy: a long-term follow-up study of 166 patients over 80 years of age. Eur Urol 1996; 30: 414

167. Wasson JH, Reda DJ, Bruskewitz RC et al: A comparison of transurethral surgery with watchful waiting for moderate symptoms of benign prostatic hyperplasia. The Veterans Affairs Cooperative Study Group on Transurethral Resection of the Prostate. N Engl J Med 1995; 332: 75

168. Kutikov A, Guzzo TJ, Malkowicz SB: Clinical approach to the prostate: an update. Radiol Clin North Am 2006; 44: 649, vii

169. Watson G: Lasers, Smith's textbook of endourology. Edited by Smith A. St. Louis, Quality Medical, 1996, pp 78

170. Fitzpatrick JM, Kasidas GP, Rose GA: Hyperoxaluria following glycine irrigation for transurethral prostatectomy. Br J Urol 1981; 53: 250

171. Hebert PC, Wells G, Blajchman MA et al: A multicenter, randomized, controlled clinical trial of transfusion requirements in critical care. Transfusion Requirements in Critical Care Investigators, Canadian Critical Care Trials Group. N Engl J Med 1999; 340: 409

172. Monk TG: Acute normovolemic hemodilution. Anesthesiol Clin North America 2005; 23: 271

173. Waters JH, Lee JS, Klein E et al: Preoperative autologous donation versus cell salvage in the avoidance of allogeneic transfusion in patients undergoing radical retropubic prostatectomy. Anesth Analg 2004; 98: 537, table of contents

174. Salonia A, Crescenti A, Suardi N et al: General versus spinal anesthesia in patients undergoing radical retropubic prostatectomy: results of a prospective, randomized study. Urology 2004; 64: 95

175. Dunet F, Pfister C, Deghmani M et al: Clinical results of combined epidural and general anesthesia procedure in radical prostatectomy management. Can J Urol 2004; 11: 2200

176. Roth JV: Bilateral sciatic and femoral neuropathies, rhabdomyolysis, and acute renal failure caused by positioning during radical retropubic prostatectomy. Anesth Analg 2007; 105: 1747

177. Memtsoudis SG, Malhotra V: Catastrophic venous air embolism during prostatectomy in the Trendelenburg position. Can J Anaesth 2003; 50: 1084

178. Maestroni U, Astesana L, Ferretti S et al: Postoperative analgesia by epidural infusion of ropivacaine and fentanyl versus intravenous administration of morphine in patients undergoing radical retropubic prostatectomy: results of a prospective study. Arch Ital Urol Androl 2007; 79: 7

179. Gupta A, Fant F, Axelsson K et al: Postoperative analgesia after radical retropubic prostatectomy: a double-blind comparison between low thoracic epidural and patient-controlled intravenous analgesia. Anesthesiology 2006; 105: 784

180. Ben-David B, Swanson J, Nelson JB, Chelly JE: Multimodal analgesia for radical prostatectomy provides better analgesia and shortens hospital stay. J Clin Anesth 2007; 19: 264

181. Hohwu L, Akre O, Bergenwald L et al: Oral oxycodone hydrochloride versus epidural anaesthesia for pain control after radical retropubic prostatectomy. Scand J Urol Nephrol 2006; 40: 192

182. Tauzin-Fin P, Sesay M, Delort-Laval S et al: Intravenous magnesium sulphate decreases postoperative tramadol requirement after radical prostatectomy. Eur J Anaesthesiol 2006; 23: 1055

183. Tauzin-Fin P, Sesay M, Svartz L et al: Sublingual oxybutynin reduces postoperative pain related to indwelling bladder catheter after radical retropubic prostatectomy. Br J Anaesth 2007; 99: 572

184. Martis G, Diana M, Ombres M et al: Retropubic versus perineal radical prostatectomy in early prostate cancer: eight-year experience. J Surg Oncol 2007; 95: 513

185. Choi SJ, Gwak MS, Ko JS et al: The effects of the exaggerated lithotomy position for radical perineal prostatectomy on respiratory mechanics. Anaesthesia 2006; 61: 439

186. Schuessler WW, Schulam PG, Clayman RV, Kavoussi LR: Laparoscopic radical prostatectomy: initial short-term experience. Urology 1997; 50: 854

187. Rassweiler J, Seemann O, Schulze M et al: Laparoscopic versus open radical prostatectomy: a comparative study at a single institution. J Urol 2003; 169: 1689

188. Bhayani SB, Pavlovich CP, Hsu TS et al: Prospective comparison of short-term convalescence: laparoscopic radical prostatectomy versus open radical retropubic prostatectomy. Urology 2003; 61: 612

189. Guillonneau B, Rozet F, Cathelineau X et al: Perioperative complications of laparoscopic radical prostatectomy: the Montsouris 3-year experience. J Urol 2002; 167: 51

190. Anderson JK, Murdock A, Cadeddu JA, Lotan Y: Cost comparison of laparoscopic versus radical retropubic prostatectomy. Urology 2005; 66: 557

191. Meininger D, Byhahn C, Mierdl S et al: Positive end-expiratory pressure improves arterial oxygenation during prolonged pneumoperitoneum. Acta Anaesthesiol Scand 2005; 49: 778

192. Gralla O, Haas F, Knoll N et al: Fast-track surgery in laparoscopic radical prostatectomy: basic principles. World J Urol 2007; 25: 185

193. Guazzoni G, Cestari A, Naspro R et al: Intra- and peri-operative outcomes comparing radical retropubic and laparoscopic radical prostatectomy: results from a prospective, randomised, single-surgeon study. Eur Urol 2006; 50: 98

194. Murphy D, Challacombe B, Khan MS, Dasgupta P: Robotic technology in urology. Postgrad Med J 2006; 82: 743

195. Menon M, Tewari A, Peabody JO et al: Vattikuti Institute prostatectomy, a technique of robotic radical prostatectomy for management of localized carcinoma of the prostate: experience of over 1100 cases. Urol Clin North Am 2004; 31: 701

196. Guillonneau B: What robotics in urology? A current point of view. Eur Urol 2003; 43: 103

197. Phong SV, Koh LK: Anaesthesia for robotic-assisted radical prostatectomy: considerations for laparoscopy in the Trendelenburg position. Anaesth Intensive Care 2007; 35: 281

198. Whalley DG, Berrigan MJ: Anesthesia for radical prostatectomy, cystectomy, nephrectomy, pheochromocytoma, and laparoscopic procedures. Anesthesiol Clin North America 2000; 18: 899, x

199. Nelson CP, Wolf JS, Jr.: Comparison of hand assisted versus standard laparoscopic radical nephrectomy for suspected renal cell carcinoma. J Urol 2002; 167: 1989

200. Chan F, Ngan Kee WD, Low JM: Anesthetic management of renal cell carcinoma with inferior vena caval extension. J Clin Anesth 2001; 13: 585

201. Dunn MD, Portis AJ, Shalhav AL et al: Laparoscopic versus open radical nephrectomy: a 9-year experience. J Urol 2000; 164: 1153

202. Baldwin DD, Dunbar JA, Parekh DJ et al: Single-center comparison of purely laparoscopic, hand-assisted laparoscopic, and open radical nephrectomy in patients at high anesthetic risk. J Endourol 2003; 17: 161

203. Link RE, Permpongkosol S, Gupta A et al: Cost analysis of open, laparoscopic, and percutaneous treatment options for nephron-sparing surgery. J Endourol 2006; 20: 782

204. Pettus JA, Eggener SE, Shabsigh A et al: Perioperative clinical thromboembolic events after radical or partial nephrectomy. Urology 2006; 68: 988

205. Horlocker TT, Wedel DJ, Benzon H et al: Regional anesthesia in the anticoagulated patient: defining the risks (the second ASRA Consensus Conference on Neuraxial Anesthesia and Anticoagulation). Reg Anesth Pain Med 2003; 28: 172

206. Recart A, Duchene D, White et al: Efficacy and safety of fast-track recovery strategy for patients undergoing laparoscopic nephrectomy. J Endourol 2005; 19: 1165

207. Practice advisory for the prevention of perioperative peripheral neuropathies: a report by the American Society of Anesthesiologists Task Force on Prevention of Perioperative Peripheral Neuropathies. Anesthesiology 2000; 92: 1168

208. Novotny V, Hakenberg OW, Wiessner D et al: Perioperative complications of radical cystectomy in a contemporary series. Eur Urol 2007; 51: 397; discussion 401

209. Ozyuvaci E, Altan A, Karadeniz T et al: General anesthesia versus epidural and general anesthesia in radical cystectomy. Urol Int 2005; 74: 62

210. Brodner G, Van Aken H, Hertle L et al: Multimodal perioperative management–combining thoracic epidural analgesia, forced mobilization, and oral nutrition–reduces hormonal and metabolic stress and improves convalescence after major urologic surgery. Anesth Analg 2001; 92: 1594

211. Dahm P, Tuttle-Newhall JE, Yowell CW et al: Indications for surgical intensive care unit admission of postoperative urologic patients. Urology 2000; 55: 334

CHAPTER 53 ■ ANESTHESIA FOR ORTHOPAEDIC SURGERY

TERESE T. HORLOCKER AND DENISE J. WEDEL

ANESTHESIA FOR SURGICAL SUBSPECIALTIES

KEY POINTS

1. Orthopaedic surgery is well suited to neuraxial and peripheral regional anesthetic techniques. Improved surgical outcomes have increased their popularity.
2. The frequency of neurologic injuries following scoliosis correction is approximately 1%, with half of these resulting in partial or complete paraplegia. Neurophysiologic monitoring and the wake-up test are often used to monitor spinal cord integrity.
3. Orthopaedic procedures are frequently associated with significant blood loss. The anesthesiologist must be proficient at blood salvage techniques, induced hypotension, and normovolemic hemodilution to decrease blood loss and transfusion requirements.
4. Visual changes, including blindness, may occur following major spine surgery.
5. Orthopaedic surgical procedures on the upper extremities are well suited to regional anesthetic techniques.
6. Proper positioning for orthopaedic procedures is paramount to providing optimal surgical conditions, as well as avoiding potential stretch and compression injuries.
7. Neuraxial and peripheral continuous blockade improve surgical outcome, including increased joint range of motion and decreased hospital stay, following total knee replacement.
8. Orthopaedic patients are at high risk for thromboembolic complications, with the highest risk reported among hip fracture patients.
9. Regional anesthetic techniques reduce the risk of thromboembolism. However, they do not currently replace the need for pharmacologic prophylaxis.

Surgical procedures involving bone, muscle, and related soft tissues require similar monitoring, regardless of the anesthetic techniques and/or the patient's age. Many orthopaedic surgical procedures lend themselves to the use of regional anesthesia. Regional anesthetic techniques allow intraoperative surgical anesthesia and postoperative analgesia, creating a further subspecialty within orthopaedic anesthesia. Another seemingly trivial but vitally important part of orthopaedic anesthesia is patient positioning. Experience and knowledge in positioning the patient are required to produce optimal surgical conditions and avoid potential injuries. Likewise, because orthopaedic procedures are frequently associated with major blood loss, the orthopaedic anesthesiologist must be experienced in techniques that decrease these risks, must be able to use intraoperative hypotension and blood salvage techniques, and must be able to manage transfusion-related complications.

Patients undergoing major orthopaedic surgery are also at risk for venous thromboembolism. Knowledge of the current pharmacologic and mechanical methods of thromboprophylaxis is required to prevent the occurrence of these thromboembolic complications, while potential interactions between anticoagulants and anesthetic drugs or regional anesthetic techniques must be thoroughly understood to reduce the risk of perioperative bleeding and neurologic injury for expanding hematomas.

Knowledge of specific orthopaedic surgical techniques, including duration, extent, predicted blood loss, and associated complications (including nerve injury), is invaluable for providing optimal patient care. Orthopaedic surgical patients usually require early mobilization and rehabilitation, both of which can be expedited by appropriate selection of anesthetic techniques and management of postoperative analgesia.

1375

PREOPERATIVE ASSESSMENT

The anesthesiologist's preoperative assessment is crucial to the formulation and execution of the anesthetic plan. The patient must be evaluated for pre-existing medical problems, previous anesthetic complications, potential airway difficulties, and considerations relating to intraoperative positioning.

Progression of cardiac symptoms and exercise tolerance in patients with a history of *coronary artery disease* may be difficult to assess because of the limitations in mobility induced by the underlying orthopaedic condition. As a result, pharmacologic functional cardiovascular testing may be warranted. Overall, patients undergoing orthopaedic procedures are considered at intermediate risk for cardiac complications perioperatively. Perioperative cardiac morbidity may be decreased by the initiation of β-blockade.[1]

Many patients undergoing orthopaedic surgery have *rheumatoid arthritis*. Systemic manifestations of this disease include pulmonary, cardiac, and musculoskeletal involvement. Particularly significant to the anesthesiologist is involvement of the cervical spine, temporomandibular joint, and larynx. Rheumatoid involvement of the cervical spine may result in limited neck range of motion, which interferes with airway management. Atlantoaxial instability, with subluxation of the odontoid process, can lead to spinal cord injury during neck extension. Patients with rheumatoid arthritis are often receiving chronic steroid therapy and may require perioperative steroid replacement.

The patient's medications should be reviewed and the patient specifically instructed which medications to continue until the time of surgery. Specifically, antihypertensive medications and chronic opioid therapy should *not* be discontinued. The patient should also be queried regarding the use of hemostasis-altering drugs; many patients are instructed by their surgeon to begin thromboprophylaxis with aspirin or warfarin preoperatively.

Preoperative evaluation should include a focused *physical examination*. Patients should be assessed for limitation in mouth opening or neck extension, adequacy of thyromental distance, and state of dentition. The heart and lungs should be auscultated. In addition, the site of proposed site of needle placement for regional anesthesia should be assessed for evidence of infection and anatomic abnormalities or limitations. A brief neurologic examination, with documentation of any pre-existing deficits, is crucial. At this time, the patient should also be evaluated for any potential positioning difficulties related to arthritic involvement of other joints or body habitus.

Hemoglobin and creatinine values are determined for all patients undergoing major procedures; other laboratory and imaging studies are performed as indicated by preoperative medical conditions. Ideally, the patient should undergo a preoperative educational session in which the surgical procedure, anesthetic/analgesic options, and the postoperative rehabilitative plan are described.

SELECTION OF ANESTHETIC TECHNIQUE

Many orthopaedic surgical procedures, because of their localized peripheral site, lend themselves to regional anesthetic techniques. Neural structures may be blocked at the peripheral nerve, plexus, or neuraxial level. Regional anesthetics offer several advantages over general anesthetics among these patients, including enhanced rehabilitation, more rapid hospital dismissal, improved postoperative analgesia, decreased incidence of nausea and vomiting, less respiratory and cardiac depression, improved perfusion via sympathetic block,

reduced blood loss, and decreased risk of thromboembolism. It is important to explain these benefits and encourage regional anesthesia when appropriate. The specific regional technique and local anesthetic solution used depend on a variety of factors, including duration of surgery, duration of postoperative analgesia, degree of sensory/motor block required to allow rehabilitation/ambulation, and indication for postoperative sympathectomy. Likewise, any patient who has an absolute contraindication to regional anesthesia (patient refusal, infection at the site of needle placement, systemic coagulopathy) is a candidate for general anesthesia. Importantly, a contraindication often may exist for neuraxial blockade, but more distal peripheral techniques remain appropriate. For example, a femoral nerve catheter may be maintained in the setting of thromboprophylaxis with low-molecular-weight heparin (LMWH), while an epidural catheter should be removed prior to initiation of LMWH therapy. The relative risks and benefits of regional and general anesthesia are discussed in the following sections.

SURGERY TO THE SPINE

Spinal Cord Injuries

Spinal injury occurs at a rate of 11,000 cases per year. Approximately half of these are at the cervical level. The examination of a person with a suspected spinal cord injury begins with a prompt neurologic examination and a rapid assessment for possible injury to other systems. Cervical injuries are frequently associated with head injury, thoracic fractures with pulmonary and cardiovascular injury, and lumbar fractures with abdominal and long-bone injuries. The patient should be examined immediately for signs of respiratory insufficiency, airway obstruction, rib fractures, and chest wall or facial trauma.

Serial neurologic examination is necessary to assess function of the spinal cord above the level of the fracture. The fifth cervical segment is perhaps the most important in providing clinical evidence of cervical spinal injury. This segment controls motor function of the deltoid, biceps, brachialis, and brachioradialis muscles. If these muscles are flaccid, the fifth cervical nerve is involved, and there will be partial diaphragmatic paralysis. A complete lesion at the fourth cervical segment is not compatible with survival unless artificial respiration is initiated. Spinal shock occurs acutely and results in complete cessation of spinal cord functions below the level of the lesion. This results in flaccid paralysis, loss of visceral and somatic sensation, and paralytic ileus. Vasopressor reflexes are also lost. Spinal shock may persist from a few days to 3 months.

Surgical treatment of spinal cord injuries is based on the presence or absence of neurologic function and the radiographic evaluation of vertebral displacement and instability. Patients with unstable spines who are not quadriplegic or paraplegic may become so during transport or positioning for surgery.

Tracheal Intubation

Airway management is critical in patients with cervical spinal cord injury. The most common cause of death with acute cervical spinal cord injury is respiratory failure. All patients with severe trauma or head injuries should be assumed to have an unstable cervical fracture until proven otherwise radiographically. During transport, the patient should be moved on a spine board with the neck immobilized to prevent further injury. Awake fiberoptic-assisted intubation may be necessary, with general anesthesia induced only after voluntary upper and lower extremity movement is confirmed. Blind nasotracheal intubation may be used if there is no evidence of facial or basal skull fractures. In a truly emergent situation, oral intubation with direct laryngoscopy is the usual approach. The trachea should be intubated with minimum flexion or extension of the neck.

Respiratory Considerations

Ventilatory impairment increases with higher levels of spinal injury. A high cervical lesion that includes the diaphragmatic segments (C4 to C5) results in respiratory failure, and death occurs unless artificial pulmonary ventilation is used. Lesions between C5 and T7 cause significant alterations in respiratory function, owing to the loss of abdominal and intercostal support. The indrawing of flaccid thoracic muscles during inspiration produces paradoxical respirations, resulting in a vital capacity reduction of 60%. Inability to cough and effectively clear secretions results in atelectasis and infection.

Cardiovascular Considerations

During spinal shock, there is loss of sympathetic vascular tone below the injury. If the cardioaccelerator fibers (T1 through T4) are damaged, bradycardia results. Therefore, hemorrhagic shock may not produce a compensatory tachycardia in these patients; the rate may remain at 40 to 60 beats per minute. Monitoring of central venous or pulmonary artery pressures may be necessary for fluid management in a patient with a high cervical lesion. Autonomic instability should be treated with vasoconstrictors, vasodilators, and positive chronotropic drugs as needed.

Succinylcholine-Induced Hyperkalemia

Hyperkalemia may develop after administration of succinylcholine to a patient with spinal cord injury. The amount of potassium released depends on the extent of the patient's motor deficit. It is considered safe to administer succinylcholine for the first 48 hours. After that time, there is a proliferation of acetylcholine receptors in muscle, and they become supersensitive to depolarizing muscle relaxants.[2] The increases in serum potassium are maximal between 4 weeks and 5 months after spinal injury. Serum potassium levels may increase from normal to as high as 14 mEq/L, causing ventricular fibrillation or cardiac arrest. Therefore, succinylcholine should be avoided in all spinal cord-injured patients after 48 hours. There are no contraindications to the nondepolarizing agents.

Temperature Control

Disruption of the sympathetic pathways carrying temperature sensation, and subsequent loss of vasoconstriction below the level of injury, causes spinal cord-injured patients to be poikilothermic. Maintenance of normal temperature can be achieved by applying exogenous heat to the skin, increasing ambient air temperature, warming intravenous fluids, and humidifying gases.

Maintaining Spinal Cord Integrity

All patients with spinal cord trauma should be considered to have compromised spinal cords, and an important component of anesthetic management is the preservation of spinal cord blood flow. Blood pressure and intravascular volume should be maintained within normal levels to ensure adequate spinal cord perfusion pressure. Sustained hypotension may worsen neurologic deficits. Hyperventilation should be avoided because hypocarbia decreases spinal cord blood flow. These considerations, as well as spinal cord monitoring, are discussed in detail later in this chapter.

Autonomic Hyperreflexia

After recovery from spinal shock, 85% of patients exhibit autonomic hyperreflexia when there has been complete cord transection above T5. The syndrome, which can also occur with injuries at lower levels, is characterized by severe paroxysmal hypertension with bradycardia (baroreceptor reflex), dysrhythmias, and cutaneous vasoconstriction below, and vasodilation above, the level of the injury. The episode is typically precipitated by distention of the bladder or rectum, but can be induced by any noxious stimulus. Many patients with spinal injuries and autonomic hyperreflexia will report characteristic headaches with bladder distention. The lack of supraspinal inhibition allows the sympathetic outflow below the lesion to react to the stimulus unopposed. If autonomic hyperreflexia occurs, it should be treated by removal of the stimulus, deepening anesthesia, and administration of direct-acting vasodilators. Untreated, the hypertensive crisis may progress to seizures, intracranial hemorrhage, or myocardial infarction.

Scoliosis

Scoliosis is a deformity of the spine resulting in lateral curvature and rotation of the vertebrae, as well as deformity of the rib cage (Fig. 53-1). The incidence of scoliosis predominantly reflects the incidence of idiopathic scoliosis, which represents 75 to 90% of cases. The remaining 10 to 25% of cases are associated with neuromuscular diseases and congenital abnormalities, including congenital heart disease, trauma, and mesenchymal disorders. The severity of scoliosis is defined by the angle of scoliosis, or *Cobb angle*. Surgical correction is performed for Cobb angles >50 degrees, with the intent of *halting*, not reversing, progression of respiratory and cardiac dysfunction. Likewise, quality of life is improved, but only modestly.[3]

Pulmonary Considerations

Scoliosis has profound effects on the respiratory and cardiovascular systems (Fig. 53-2). In patients with untreated scoliosis, respiratory failure and death usually occur by 45 years of age. Vital capacity appears to be a reliable prognostic indicator of perioperative respiratory reserve. Postoperative ventilation will most likely be required for patients with a vital capacity <40% of predicted. Although the long-term effect of scoliosis repair is to halt the decline in respiratory function, pulmonary function acutely deteriorates for 7 to 10 days after surgery.

The primary abnormality in gas exchange is ventilation–perfusion maldistribution, which contributes to hypoxemia. However, hypercapnia develops with increasing age as compensatory mechanisms fail. Prolonged hypoxia, hypercapnia, and pulmonary vascular constriction may result in irreversible pulmonary vascular changes and pulmonary hypertension. In general, the prognosis of scoliosis associated with neuromuscular disease is worse than that of idiopathic scoliosis. These patients frequently need postoperative ventilatory support.

Cardiovascular Considerations

Cardiovascular function is also affected in patients with scoliosis. At autopsy, these patients exhibit right ventricular hypertrophy and hypertensive pulmonary vascular changes. Prolonged alveolar hypoxia due to hypoventilation and ventilation–perfusion mismatch eventually causes irreversible vasoconstriction and pulmonary hypertension. Scoliosis is also associated with congenital heart conditions, including mitral valve prolapse, coarctation of the aorta, and cyanotic heart disease, suggesting a common embryonic insult or collagen defect.

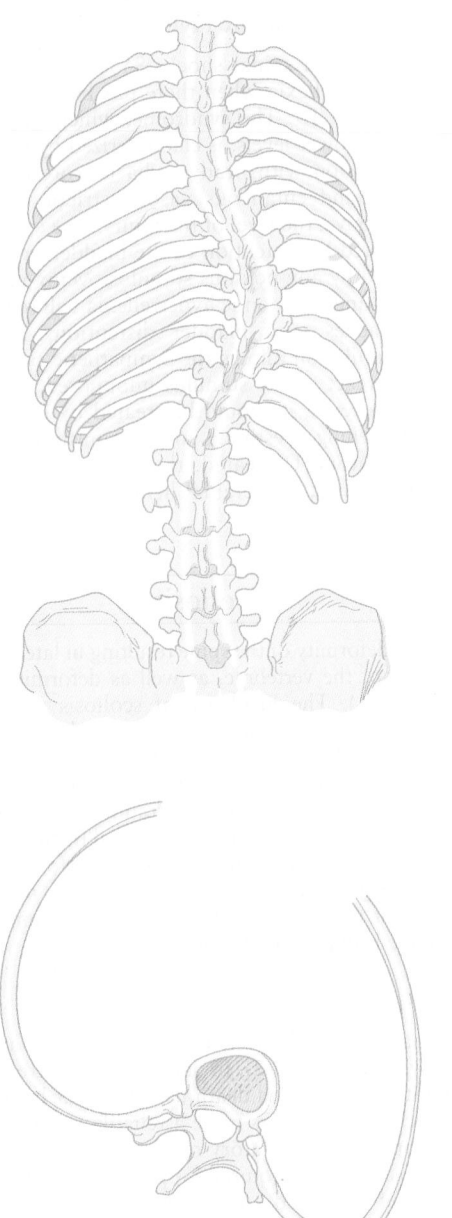

FIGURE 53-1. Deformity of the vertebrae and rib cage in scoliosis. Primary curvature occurs most frequently in the thoracic and lumbar regions. The vertebral bodies are wedge-shaped, and the posterior angles of the ribs are shallow on the side of concavity. On the convex side, the rib angles are more acute. (Reprinted from Horlocker TT, Cucchiara RF, Ebersold MJ: Vertebral column and spinal cord surgery, Clinical Neuroanesthesia. Edited by Cucchiara RF, Michenfelder JD. New York, Churchill Livingstone, 1990, p 325, with permission.)

Surgical Approach and Positioning

The prone position is used for the posterior approach to the spine. Pressure points should be carefully padded. An orthopaedic frame, such as the Jackson table or Wilson frame, can be used to free the chest and abdomen. In correct prone positioning for thoracolumbar spine surgery, the head is turned, the neck is slightly flexed, and the arms are anteriorly flexed and abducted to reduce tension on the brachial plexus (Fig. 53-3). Alternatively, the head may remain in the neutral position, supported by a foam headrest or a skull holder with pins. If only one arm is abducted, the head should be laterally

rotated toward the ipsilateral arm to prevent stretch injury to the brachial plexus. Because rotation of the neck in patients with cervical spondylosis may alter carotid or vertebral circulation and compromise the spinal cord, patients should be evaluated for neck pain or neurologic symptoms with neck rotation before surgery. The chest and iliac crest are supported by chest rolls or other supports to leave the abdomen free. Breasts should be positioned medially to avoid traumatic injury. The dependent ear and eye should be checked frequently during surgery to avoid injury and ischemia. Necrosis of the dependent ear cartilage may occur if the pinna is doubled back on itself. Eyes should be taped closed to avoid corneal abrasion, which occurs in the dependent eye with a frequency of 0.17%.

The anterior approach to the thoracolumbar spine is achieved with the patient in the lateral position, usually with the convexity of the curve uppermost. Removal of one or more ribs may be necessary for adequate surgical exposure. Likewise, placement of a double-lumen endotracheal tube, with collapse of the lung on the operative side may be required for surgery above T8. Thus, the thoracolumbar approach for anterior spinal fusion may be associated with more postoperative respiratory insufficiency than posterior fusion because of lung and diaphragmatic manipulation.

Combined anterior and posterior spinal procedures yield higher union rates and greater correction in patients undergoing scoliosis correction. It remains unclear whether these two major procedures should be performed on the same day or whether the posterior fusion should be delayed to allow the patient to recover from the anterior (first) procedure. Furthermore, the actual timing of the second procedure remains controversial. Although the degree of correction and the arthrodesis rates are similar for one- or two-stage procedures, the morbidity and number of complications, such as increased blood loss and transfusion requirements, decreased nutritional parameters, and longer hospital stays, may be increased for staged procedures.[4] However, these results are not consistent.[5] Because the risk of significant complications is present with either same-day or staged anterior–posterior fusion, prospective studies are needed to clarify this issue.

Anesthetic Management

The primary aim of preoperative evaluation of patients with scoliosis is to detect the presence and extent of cardiac or pulmonary compromise. Respiratory reserve is assessed by exercise tolerance, vital capacity, and arterial blood gases. Cardiac studies are performed as indicated to optimize preoperative cardiovascular status. A brief neurologic examination will document pre-existing neurologic deficits. Finally, cervical mobility and upper airway anatomy are assessed to discover any potential airway or positioning difficulties.

Anesthetic considerations for surgical correction of scoliosis by *spinal fusion and instrumentation* include management of a patient in the prone position, hypothermia secondary to a long procedure with an extensive exposed area, and replacement of blood and fluid losses, which may be extensive.[6] More recently, attention has been focused on the maintenance of spinal cord integrity, the prevention and treatment of venous air embolism (VAE), and reduction of blood loss through hypotensive anesthetic techniques.

Adequate hemodynamic monitoring and venous access are essential in management of patients undergoing spinal fusion and instrumentation. The radial artery is cannulated for direct blood pressure measurement and assessment of blood gases. A central venous catheter is helpful in evaluating fluid and fluid management, and can be used to aspirate air if VAE occurs. Patients with evidence of pulmonary hypertension, or severe coexistent cardiovascular or pulmonary disease, may require a pulmonary artery catheter.

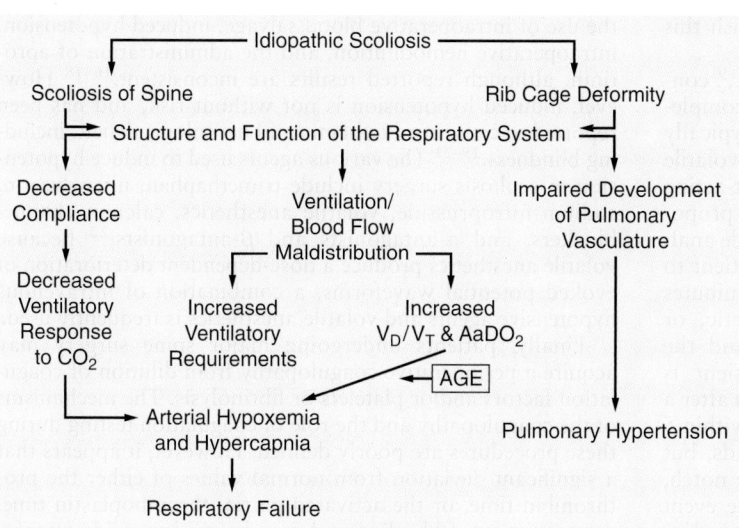

FIGURE 53-2. The factors in idiopathic scoliosis that contribute to respiratory function abnormalities and failure. VD, dead space volume; V_T, tidal volume; $AaDO_2$, alveolar to arterial oxygen gradient (Reprinted from Kafer ER: Respiratory and cardiovascular functions in scoliosis. Bull Eur Physiopathol Respir 1977; 13: 299, with permission.)

Degenerative Vertebral Column Disease

Spinal stenosis, spondylosis, and spondylolisthesis are all forms of degenerative vertebral column disease. It is not unusual for more than one of these degenerative changes in the spine to occur concomitantly, leading to a more rapid progression of neurologic symptoms and the need for surgical intervention.

Surgical Approach and Positioning

Cervical laminectomy is performed in the prone, lateral, or sitting position, whereas thoracolumbar laminectomy is usually performed prone. Considerations for positioning a prone patient have been previously discussed (see also Chapter 30). Patients undergoing cervical laminectomy should be assessed before surgery for cervical range of motion and the presence of neurologic symptoms during flexion, extension, or rotation. Fiberoptic-assisted intubation may be necessary in patients with severely limited cervical movement. With the anterior approach, the surgical incision approximates the anterior border of the sternocleidomastoid muscle, and is therefore near critical anatomic structures. Lateral retraction of the carotid artery may endanger blood flow to the brain, particularly in the elderly patient.[7] Retraction of the esophagus and trachea medially may cause pharyngeal laceration, laryngeal edema, and recurrent laryngeal nerve paralysis. Cerebrospinal fluid leaks and trauma to the vertebral artery have also been reported.

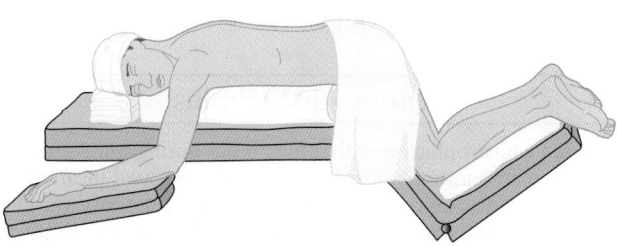

FIGURE 53-3. Prone position. The head is turned with the dependent ear and eye are protected from pressure. Chest rolls are in place, the arms are brought forward without hyperextension, and the knees are flexed. (Reprinted from Horlocker TT, Cucchiara RF, Ebersold MJ: Vertebral column and spinal cord surgery, Clinical Neuroanesthesia. Edited by Cucchiara RF, Michenfelder JD. New York, Churchill Livingstone, 1990, p 325, with permission.)

The use of the sitting position for cervical laminectomy has become increasingly popular. Blood flows away from the site of operation, producing a clear operative field and better surgical exposure. In this position, the patient sits with head, arms, and chest supported. The patient must be carefully positioned and the dependent areas must be padded to prevent compression injuries to nerves and skin. Extreme cervical flexion may obstruct the airway. Hypotension can be minimized by gradual attainment of the sitting position. A disadvantage of the sitting position is the increased occurrence of VAE. Although the incidence of VAE in sitting posterior fossa cases is 40%, the incidence is only 5 to 25% in sitting cervical spine procedures.[8] This decreased incidence may alter the need for a central venous pressure catheter.

Anesthetic Management

Either general or neuraxial anesthesia may be safely administered for relatively uncomplicated lower thoracic and lumbar spine surgery. However, general anesthesia is preferred for essentially all thoracic and cervical procedures because of the high spinal level that would be required with a regional technique. The advantages of regional anesthesia include a reduction in blood loss and improved operating conditions by contraction of the epidural vasculature. Both spinal and epidural techniques have been described. Epidural catheters may be placed under direct vision by the surgeon to provide intraoperative anesthesia and postoperative analgesia. Likewise, the accessibility of the dural sac facilitates intrathecal reinjection by the surgeon for extended procedures. Despite these considerations, most spine surgery is performed under general anesthesia. General anesthesia ensures airway access, is associated with greater patient acceptance, and can be used for prolonged operations. Succinylcholine should be avoided if there are progressive neurologic deficits.

Spinal Cord Monitoring

Paraplegia is one of the most feared complications of major spine surgery. The incidence of neurologic injuries associated with scoliosis correction is 1.2%, with partial or complete paraplegia occurring in half the cases. When patients awaken paraplegic, neurologic recovery is unlikely, although immediate removal of instrumentation improves the prognosis. It is therefore essential that any intraoperative compromise of spinal cord function be detected as early as possible and reversed immediately. The two methods developed to accomplish this are the wake-up test and neurophysiologic monitoring.

The *wake-up test,* first described by Vauzelle et al.,[9] consists of the intraoperative awakening of patients after completion of spinal instrumentation. Surgical anesthesia is typically provided with a balanced technique of nitrous oxide, a volatile drug, and opioids, although use of opioids with a short-acting volatile anesthetic (e.g., sevoflurane), or an infusion of propofol, is also possible. The opioids are important to provide analgesia while the patient is awake and to permit the patient to tolerate the endotracheal tube. During the 30 to 45 minutes before intraoperative wake-up, the volatile anesthetic, or propofol, and muscle relaxants are discontinued and the patient is allowed to gradually awaken. The patient is addressed by name and asked to move both hands, and after a positive response, both feet. Patients usually respond within 5 minutes. If there is satisfactory movement of the hands, but not the feet, the distraction on the rod is released one notch, and the wake-up test repeated. Although recall of the event occurs in only 0 to 20% of patients and is rarely viewed as unpleasant,[10] it is important to describe to the patient before surgery what will transpire so anxiety will be minimized should the patient be fully aware during the wake-up. It is extremely rare for a patient who was neurologically intact when awakened during surgery to have a neurologic deficit on completion of the procedure. However, certain hazards of the wake-up test do exist and include recall, pain, air embolism, dislocation of spinal instrumentation, and accidental tracheal extubation or removal of intravenous and arterial lines.

An adjunct or alternative to the wake-up test is neurophysiologic monitoring (see also Chapter 39). Somatosensory stimulation follows the dorsal column pathways of proprioception and vibration: pathways supplied by the posterior spinal artery. Accordingly, the motor pathway, which is supplied by the anterior spinal artery, is not addressed by monitoring somatosensory evoked potentials (SSEP). High concentrations of inhaled agents cannot be used when monitoring SSEP. Motor evoked potentials (MEP), in contrast, monitor motor pathways but are technically more difficult to use. Muscle relaxants cannot be used in patients having MEP monitoring. If both SSEP and MEP are to be monitored during spine surgery, one might consider providing anesthesia with an ultra short-acting opioid infusion with a low-dose inhaled anesthetic, and monitoring of the electroencephalogram to minimize the potential for intraoperative awareness. It is of critical importance to note that postoperative paraplegia has occurred in at least one patient with preserved intraoperative SSEPs.[11] The combined use of MEPs and SSPEPs may increase the early detection of spinal cord ischemia.[12]

Acute alterations in SSEP amplitude or latency signify spinal cord compromise and may be the result of direct trauma, ischemia, compression, or hematoma. If changes occur, it is recommended that surgery be discontinued, blood pressure returned to normal or 20% above normal, and volatile agents decreased or discontinued. Arterial blood gases may be drawn to rule out a metabolic derangement. If the waveform does not return to normal, the surgeon should release distraction on the cord. A wake-up test is often performed at this time to definitely exclude neurologic deficits. In addition to neural injury, SSEPs are altered by volatile anesthetics, hypercarbia, hypoxia, hypotension, and hypothermia.[13,14]

Blood Loss

❸ Most of the blood loss in spinal instrumentation and fusion occurs with decortication and is proportional to the number of vertebral levels decorticated.[15] Blood loss and transfusion requirements may be reduced through proper positioning and the use of intraoperative blood salvage, induced hypotension, intraoperative hemodilution, and the administration of aprotinin, although reported results are inconsistent.[16–18] However, induced hypotension is not without risk, and has been reported to cause cord ischemia and neurologic deficit, including blindness.[19–21] The various agents used to induce hypotension in scoliosis surgery include trimethaphan, nitroglycerin, sodium nitroprusside, volatile anesthetics, calcium channel blockers, and α-antagonists and β-antagonists.[22] Because volatile anesthetics produce a dose-dependent deterioration of evoked potential waveforms, a combination of intravenous hypotensive agents and volatile anesthetics is frequently used.

Finally, patients undergoing major spine surgery may acquire a perioperative coagulopathy from dilution of coagulation factors and/or platelets or fibrinolysis. The mechanisms of the coagulopathy and the role of coagulation testing during these procedures are poorly defined. However, it appears that a significant deviation from normal values of either the prothrombin time, or the activated partial thromboplastin time, are predictive of bleeding and may be used to guide transfusion therapy.[23] Although a variety of pharmacologic interventions, including administration of recombinant factor VIIa and aprotinin, have been reported to prevent and/or treat severe bleeding during spine surgery, their use remains controversial and unproven by well-designed studies.[24]

Another rare cause of bleeding during spine surgery is trauma to the aorta, vena cava, or iliac vessels. Unexplained hypotension or signs of hypovolemia without obvious blood loss should alert the anesthesiologist to this possibility.

Visual Loss After Spine Surgery

❹ Unilateral and bilateral blindness have been reported in case reports and small series after spine surgery.[19–21] The diagnoses included optic neuropathy, retinal artery occlusion, and cerebral ischemia. Most cases were associated with complex instrumented fusions.[20] Although no definitive risk factors have been identified, many cases were associated with significant (prolonged) intraoperative hypotension, anemia, large intraoperative blood loss, and prolonged surgery.[21] However, these conditions are present during many major spine procedures without visual sequelae. Therefore, actual risk factors remain unidentified at this time (see Chapters 4 and 39).

The American Society of Anesthesiologists Visual Loss Registry[25] reported that ischemic optic neuropathy was the most common cause of visual loss after spine surgery, and accounted for 83 of 93 spine surgery cases. Most patients were relatively healthy. Blood loss of ≥1,000 mL, or anesthetic duration of 6 hours or longer, was present in 96% of the cases. As a result, it is recommended that, the risk of visual loss should be considered in the preoperative discussion for patients undergoing lengthy spine surgery in the prone position.

Venous Air Embolus

VAE is a catastrophic event that may occur during spine surgery. The large amount of exposed bone and the elevated location of the surgical incision relative to the heart predispose to VAE. The use of capnography, mass spectrometry, and precordial Doppler are noninvasive, yet effective, in detecting VAE. VAE can occur in all positions associated with laminectomies because the wound is above the cardiac level. Incidences of VAE (defined by aspiration of air through a central venous catheter) in patients undergoing neurosurgical procedures in the sitting, supine, prone, and lateral positions are 25, 18, 10, and 8%, respectively.[8] The actual incidence of VAE in spine surgery is unknown; however, poor neurologic recovery is often reported.[26] The presenting sign is often unexplained hypotension and an increase in the end-tidal nitrogen concentration, or a precipitous fall in the end-tidal CO_2 concentration. The anesthesiologist, therefore, should be aware of the possibilities of VAE because prompt diagnosis and treatment increase patient survival. If VAE is suspected, the wound should be irrigated with saline, nitrous oxide discontinued, and vasopressors administered. Massive embolism may necessitate turning the patient supine and initiating cardiopulmonary resuscitation.

Postoperative Care

Most patients undergoing posterior spinal fusion can be extubated immediately after the operation if the procedure was relatively uneventful and preoperative vital capacity values were acceptable. Residual opioid or muscle relaxant may lead to hypoventilation or apnea, especially in patients with an associated neuromuscular disease. Some patients who have experienced considerable blood loss and who have received large amounts of intravenous fluids, particularly if they were prone, may have severe facial edema that renders immediate tracheal extubation unwise. Aggressive postoperative pulmonary care, including incentive spirometry, is necessary to avoid atelectasis and pneumonia. Continued hemorrhage in the postoperative period is another concern. Careful monitoring of systemic and central venous pressures, urine output, and wound drainage is essential. Neurologic status must also be monitored closely for deterioration.

Postoperative analgesia is typically provided by systemic opioids. However, wound instillation with local anesthetic or injection of intrathecal morphine is associated with improved pain scores and decreased side effects in the early postoperative period.[27,28]

Epidural and Spinal Anesthesia After Major Spine Surgery

Previous spine surgery has been considered to represent a relative contraindication to the use of regional anesthesia. The presence of postoperative spinal stenosis or other degenerative changes in the spine or pre-existing neurologic symptoms may preclude the use of regional anesthesia in these patients. Likewise, many of these patients experience chronic back pain and are reluctant to undergo epidural or spinal anesthesia, fearing exacerbation of their pre-existing back complaints. Finally, postoperative anatomic changes make needle or catheter placement more difficult and complicated after major spine surgery; needle insertion can be accomplished only at non-fused segments.

Spread of epidural local anesthetic following spine surgery may be affected by adhesions, producing an incomplete or "patchy" block. Obliteration of the epidural space may increase the incidence of dural puncture and make subsequent epidural blood patch placement impossible. Several retrospective studies have demonstrated that epidural anesthesia may be successfully performed in patients with previous spine surgery; however, successful catheter placement was possible on the first attempt in only 50% of patients, even with an experienced anesthesiologist. In addition, although adequate epidural anesthesia was eventually produced in 40 to 95% of patients, there appeared to be a higher incidence of traumatic needle placement, inadvertent dural puncture, and unsuccessful epidural needle or catheter placement, especially if spinal fusion extended to L5 through S1.[29–31]

Spinal anesthesia may produce a more reliable block and cause less trauma than epidural anesthesia. Although needle placement may be more difficult or traumatic in these patients,

the spread of local anesthetic in the subarachnoid space and quality of block would not be affected. A spinal anesthetic may be more desirable after spine surgery because the technique does not depend on a subjective loss of resistance, but instead has a definite end point—the presence of cerebrospinal fluid.

A study in 2005 examined the overall success and neurologic complication rates among 937 patients with spinal stenosis or lumbar disc disease undergoing neuraxial block, 207 (22%) of whom had previously undergone spine surgery, although the majority were simple laminectomies or discectomies.[32] Success rates did not differ between patients who had previous surgery and those who had undergone a spine procedure. Ten patients experienced new or progressive neurologic deficits when compared with preoperative findings. Although the majority of the deficits were related to surgical trauma or tourniquet ischemia, the neuraxial technique was the primary cause in four patients. Although it appears that patients with spinal stenosis or lumbar disc disease may undergo successful neuraxial block without a significant increase in neurologic complications, neurologic complications may occur after uneventful block.[32,33]

SURGERY TO THE UPPER EXTREMITIES

❺ Orthopaedic surgical procedures to the upper extremity are well suited to regional anesthetic techniques. In addition to intraoperative anesthesia, brachial plexus and peripheral nerve blocks may be used in the treatment and prevention of reflex sympathetic dystrophy. Continuous catheter techniques provide postoperative analgesia and allow early limb mobilization. Conversely, although the benefits of regional anesthesia in this patient population are well established, orthopaedic surgical procedures often involve peripheral nerves with pre-existing deficits, such as ulnar nerve transposition and carpal tunnel release. In addition, the operative site may be adjacent to neural structures, as with total shoulder arthroplasty or fractures of the proximal humerus. The decision to perform regional anesthesia in a patient with pre-existing neurologic deficits or who is at risk for perioperative neurapraxia should be made on an individual basis after discussion with the patient and surgeon. Meticulous regional anesthetic technique with appropriate use of local anesthetic solutions and vasoconstrictors, careful patient positioning, and serial postoperative neurologic examinations may reduce the incidence of neurologic dysfunction.

Local anesthetic selection is based on the duration and degree of sensory or motor block required. Although prolonged blockade of the lower extremities interferes with ambulation and therefore delays outpatient discharge, persistent upper extremity block is not a contraindication to hospital dismissal. However, the patient should be informed of the anticipated duration of analgesia during the postoperative visit and instructed to protect the blocked extremity until block resolution.

Surgery to the Shoulder and Upper Arm

Reconstructive shoulder surgery, including total shoulder arthroplasty and rotator cuff repair, presents unique management and positioning considerations to the anesthesiologist. For example, 4% of patients undergoing total shoulder arthroplasty have a documented postoperative neurologic deficit, including 3% of patients with injury to the brachial plexus. The level of injury is at the level of the nerve trunks, which is the level at which an interscalene block is performed, making it impossible to determine the etiology of the nerve injury (surgical vs.

anesthetic). Most of these nerve injuries represent a neurapraxia; 90% resolve in 3 to 4 months.[34] In addition, nerve injury often occurs in association with upper extremity trauma. Radial nerve palsy is identified in up to 18% of patients with humeral shaft fractures, whereas injury to the axillary nerve and brachial plexus is associated with proximal humerus fractures. However, the significant incidence of neurologic deficits demonstrates the importance of clinical examination before regional anesthetic techniques in these patients.

Surgical Approach and Positioning

⑥ Surgical procedures to the upper arm and shoulder are typically performed with the patient in the "beach chair" position. The patient's head, neck, and hips must be secured to prevent additional lateral movement. The head and neck must remain firmly supported by the operating table and secured in a neutral position; excessive rotation or flexion of the head away from the operative side results in stretch injury to the brachial plexus. Care also must be taken to avoid pressure on the eyes and ears. All airway connections should be tightened and possibly reinforced with tape because after surgical draping, access to the patient's face and airway is limited.

A tourniquet cannot be used during proximal upper extremity surgical procedures, and significant blood loss may occur. Therefore, arterial cannulation may be helpful for direct blood pressure measurement and monitoring of intraoperative hemoglobin concentrations during total shoulder arthroplasty and reduction of humeral fractures. In theory, VAE may occur during surgical procedures to the shoulder because the operative site is higher than the heart.

Anesthetic Management

Surgery to the shoulder and humerus may be performed under regional or general anesthesia.[35] With careful positioning and appropriate sedation, interscalene or supraclavicular blockade alone can provide excellent surgical anesthesia (Table 53-1). However, general anesthesia or a combination of regional and general anesthesia is often chosen because of limited access to the patient's airway during these surgical procedures. Interscalene brachial plexus block may be performed before surgical incision or after postoperative upper extremity neurologic function has been determined. Severe hypotension and bradycardia (i.e., Bezold-Jarisch reflex) have been reported in awake, sitting patients undergoing shoulder surgery under an interscalene block. The cause is presumed to be stimulation of intracardiac mechanoreceptors by decreased venous return, producing an abrupt withdrawal of sympathetic tone and enhanced parasympathetic output. This effect results in bradycardia, hypotension, and syncope. The frequency is decreased when prophylactic beta-blockers are administered.[36] Although preoperative interscalene block reduces the intraoperative requirement of volatile anesthetic and opioids, and in theory provides pre-emptive analgesia, postoperative evaluation of neurologic function will not be possible until block resolution.

Interscalene block should be performed with caution in patients with a pre-existing brachial plexopathy because of the risk of perioperative exacerbation of neurologic deficits. The ipsilateral diaphragmatic paresis and 25% loss of pulmonary function produced by interscalene block also contraindicates this block in patients with severe pulmonary disease.[37] The reduction in pulmonary function is present for the duration of the interscalene block.

Surgery to the Elbow

Although use of general anesthesia is appropriate, surgical procedures to the distal humerus, elbow, and forearm are commonly performed using regional anesthetic techniques. Infraclavicular and supraclavicular approaches to the brachial plexus are the most reliable and provide consistent anesthesia to the four major nerves of the brachial plexus: median, ulnar, radial, and musculocutaneous. However, the small but definite risk of pneumothorax associated with supraclavicular and infraclavicular blocks usually makes this approach unsuitable for outpatient procedures. Typically, the pneumothorax occurs 6 to 12 hours after hospital discharge; therefore, a postoperative

TABLE 53-1

REGIONAL ANESTHETIC TECHNIQUES FOR UPPER EXTREMITY SURGERY

■ BRACHIAL PLEXUS TECHNIQUE	■ LEVEL OF BLOCKADE	■ PERIPHERAL NERVES BLOCKED	■ SURGICAL APPLICATIONS	■ COMMENTS
Axillary	Peripheral nerve	Radial, ulnar, median; musculocutaneous unreliably blocked	Surgery to forearm and hand, less used for procedures about the elbow	Unsuitable for proximal humerus or shoulder surgery; patient must be able to abduct the arm to perform
Infraclavicular	Cords	Radial, ulnar, median, musculocutaneous, axillary	Surgery to elbow, forearm, and hand	Catheter site (near coracoid process) easy to maintain; no risk of hemo-, pneumothorax
Supraclavicular	Distal trunk-proximal cord	Radial, ulnar, median, musculocutaneous, axillary	Surgery to midhumerus, elbow, forearm, and hand	Risk of pneumothorax, unsuitable for outpatient procedures; phrenic nerve paresis in 30% of cases
Interscalene	Upper and middle trunks	Entire brachial plexus, although inferior trunk (ulnar nerve) not blocked in 15–20% of cases	Surgery to shoulder, proximal/middle humerus	Phrenic nerve paresis in 100% of patients for block duration; unsuitable for patients unable to tolerate 25% reduction in pulmonary function

Duration of block performed with long-acting local anesthetic (bupivacaine or ropivacaine) is 12 to 20 hours; intermediate-acting agents (lidocaine or mepivacaine) will resolve after 4 to 6 hours.

chest radiograph is not helpful. Although chest tube placement is advised for pneumothorax >20% of lung volume, the lung may also be re-expanded with a small Teflon catheter under fluoroscopic guidance, eliminating the need for hospital admission. The axillary approach to the brachial plexus eliminates the risk of pneumothorax and reliably provides adequate anesthesia for surgery near the elbow.[38]

Surgery to the Wrist and Hand

Surgery to the distal forearm, wrist, and hand may be performed under general or regional anesthesia. Brachial plexus block provides comprehensive and consistent regional anesthesia for the distal upper extremity, and can be used for outpatients.[39] Although the brachial plexus may be successfully blocked at several sites, the interscalene approach is seldom used for wrist and hand procedures because incomplete anesthesia of the ulnar nerve is noted in 15 to 30% of patients. In addition, although the supraclavicular approach results in blockade of all four major nerves, the risk of pneumothorax reduces its suitability for outpatient procedures. Therefore, the axillary approach is most commonly used for surgical procedures to the forearm, wrist, and hand.

Minor hand procedures such as carpal tunnel release, reduction of phalanx fractures, and superficial wound debridements may require only local infiltration or peripheral blockade at the midhumeral, elbow, or wrist level. Inflation of an upper arm tourniquet in these patients causes significant discomfort in 45 to 60 minutes and limits the duration of the surgical procedure. Intravenous regional anesthesia (Bier block) using a double tourniquet permits more extensive surgery and longer tourniquet times than distal peripheral block, but does not provide postoperative analgesia.

Continuous Brachial Plexus Anesthesia

Overall, there are early, but no long-term, benefits with a single-injection regional anesthetic technique compared with a general anesthetic. However, placement of an indwelling perineural catheter results in more substantial and lasting benefits, including avoidance of hospital admission/readmission, decreased opioid-related side effects and sleep disturbance, and improved rehabilitation.[40,41] Thus, anesthetic management of patients undergoing elbow surgery is focused on *postoperative* analgesia, rather than *intraoperative* anesthesia to improve perioperative outcomes. Brachial plexus catheters may be inserted using interscalene, infraclavicular, and axillary approaches. After surgery, the catheters may be left indwelling for 4 to 7 days without adverse effects. A continuous infusion of dilute local anesthetic solution, such as bupivacaine 0.125%, prevents vasospasm and increases circulation after limb replantation or vascular repair. More concentrated solutions result in complete sensory block and allow early joint mobilization after painful surgical procedures to the elbow. Ambulatory (at-home) applications provide superior analgesia with fewer side effects than conventional systemic analgesic therapy.[40]

SURGERY TO THE LOWER EXTREMITIES

Although orthopaedic procedures to the lower extremity may be performed under both general and regional anesthesia, the ability to provide superior postoperative analgesia, rapid postoperative rehabilitation, and reduced cost of medical care may result from thoughtfully implemented regional anesthetic and analgesic techniques.[42,43]

Multiple studies demonstrate significantly reduced intraoperative blood loss during total hip arthroplasty completed under central neuraxial blockade compared with general anesthesia.[44]. Likewise, postoperative pulmonary thromboembolism (PTE) from deep venous thrombosis (DVT) is an important cause of morbidity and mortality in orthopaedic surgical patients. Historical investigations reported a decreased incidence of DVT and PTE in patients whose surgery was conducted under regional anesthesia.[45,46] However, these patients did not receive pharmacologic thromboprophylaxis. The potential benefit of regional anesthesia in reducing thromboembolic complications is discussed later in this chapter.

Surgery to the Hip

More than 200,000 total hip replacements are performed annually in North America. Patients undergoing surgical procedures to the hip for arthritic conditions typically are elderly and often have pre-existing medical conditions that may affect perioperative outcome. In addition, because hospital costs appear to be directly related to the length of hospital stay, anesthetic techniques associated with improved recovery and reduced complications may decrease the total hospital costs among these patients.[42,43]

Surgical Approach and Positioning

The lateral decubitus position is frequently used to facilitate surgical exposure for total hip arthroplasty, whereas the fracture table is often used for repair of femur fractures. In transferring the patient from the supine to lateral decubitus position, care must be taken to maintain the head and shoulders in a neutral position. The patient is supported while the position is secured with hip rests or other mechanical devices. The dependent arm is abducted and placed on a padded arm rest; a rolled towel or wrapped intravenous fluid bag is placed in the axilla to avoid compression of the brachial plexus and vascular structures. The upper arm is placed on a padded over-arm board.

Positioning on the fracture table (Fig. 53-4) also requires adequate personnel to move the patient, with one person

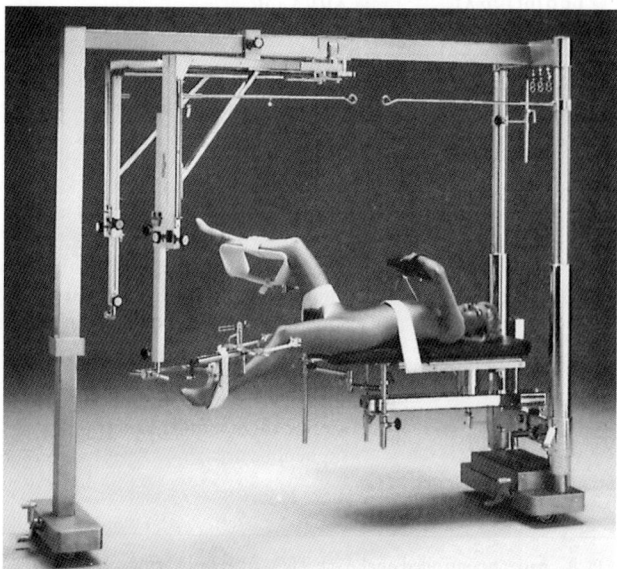

FIGURE 53-4.   The fracture table. The patient must be moved carefully with continuous traction on the fractured limb. The ipsilateral arm is positioned on an arm board or sling without stretching the brachial plexus. (Courtesy of Midmark Corporation, Versailles, OH.)

assigned to apply traction to the fractured limb. The fracture table affords two advantages: maintenance of traction on the fractured extremity, allowing manipulation for closed reduction and fixation, and access to the fracture site for radiography in several planes. The patient must be carefully monitored for hemodynamic changes during positioning, whether under regional or general anesthesia. Care must be taken to pad the perineal post before positioning the patient's pelvis. Usually, the arm ipsilateral to the fractured hip is placed on an arm board or in a sling to keep it from obstructing the fluoroscopic view.

Anesthetic Technique

Regional anesthetic techniques are well suited to procedures involving the hip. Central neuraxial blockade, including spinal and epidural blockade, is commonly used to provide intraoperative anesthesia. Both hypobaric and isobaric spinal anesthetic solutions are effective. Adequate intravenous hydration before placing the neuraxial block protects against a precipitous drop in blood pressure that can occur secondary to sympathetic blockade and peripheral vasodilation. Placement of an epidural catheter allows prolonged anesthesia as well as postoperative analgesia. More recently, both single-dose and continuous lumbar plexus techniques have been performed to provide postoperative analgesia in patients undergoing major hip surgery. Single-injection techniques are associated with short-term improvements in analgesia (approximately 6 hours) and a modest decrease in blood loss.[47]. However, prolonged analgesia with continuous psoas compartment block was associated with decreased postoperative pain, fewer episodes of cognitive dysfunction, decreased ileus, and facilitated hospital discharge.[43] The lumbar plexus block also contributes to the intraoperative anesthetic, allowing decreased dosing of volatile agents, opioids, and/or spinal anesthetic solutions (Table 53-2).

Blood Loss

Regional anesthetic techniques reduce blood loss in patients undergoing hip surgery. Deliberate hypotension can also be used with general anesthesia as a means of reducing surgical blood loss and has been recommended when the benefits can be expected to outweigh the risks.[48] Diltiazem, nitroprusside with and without captopril, beta-blockers, and nitroglycerin have also been used to induce hypotension.

Total Knee Arthroplasty

More than 300,000 total knee arthroplasties are performed annually in North America. Patients undergoing total knee arthroplasty experience significant postoperative pain. Failure to provide adequate analgesia impedes aggressive physical therapy and rehabilitation, which is critical to maintaining joint range of motion and potentially delays hospital dismissal. Thus, the anesthesiologist must devise a plan for not only intraoperative anesthesia, but also postoperative analgesia.

Surgical *anesthesia* for operative procedures on the knee in which a tourniquet will be used requires blockade of all four nerves (femoral, lateral femoral cutaneous, obturator, and sciatic nerves) innervating the leg. Although it is possible to perform major knee surgery under peripheral nerve blocks, more often a femoral three-in-one or lumbar plexus (psoas) block is combined with a spinal or general anesthetic. This is less difficult technically, reduces the amount of local anesthetic (and associated systemic toxicity), and provides postoperative analgesia for 12 to 24 hours. Continuous lumbar plexus techniques, with or without supplemental sciatic block, allow for prolonged postoperative analgesia. The routine performance of a sciatic block remains controversial. From investigations that did not include a sciatic block, it is apparent that block-

---

TABLE 53-2

LUMBOSACRAL TECHNIQUES FOR MAJOR LOWER EXTREMITY SURGERY

■ PERIPHERAL TECHNIQUE	■ AREA OF BLOCKADE	■ DURATION OF BLOCKADE[a]	■ PERIOPERATIVE OUTCOMES[b]
Lumbar Plexus Femoral	Femoral, partial lateral femoral cutaneous, and obturator	12–18 hr	Improved analgesia and joint range of motion, decreased hospital stay compared with PCA; fewer technical problems, less urinary retention and hypotension than epidural analgesia (TKA)
Fascia iliaca	Femoral, partial lateral femoral cutaneous, obturator, and sciatic (S1)		Improved analgesia and joint range of motion compared with PCA (TKA)
Psoas compartment	Complete lumbar plexus; occasional spread to sacral plexus or neuraxis		Reduced morphine consumption, pain at rest compared with PCA (TKA, THA); reduced blood loss (THA); analgesia equivalent to continuous femoral block (TKA)
Sciatic	Posterior thigh and leg (except saphenous area)	18–30 hr	Supplemental sciatic required (TKA); proximal approaches allow block of posterior femoral cutaneous nerve (TKA)

PCA , patient-controlled analgesia; TKA, total knee arthroplasty; THA, total hip arthroplasty.
[a]Duration of block performed with long-acting local anesthetic (bupivacaine or ropivacaine); intermediate-acting agents (lidocaine or mepivacaine) will resolve after 4 to 6 hours.
[b]Outcomes most marked in patients who receive a continuous lumbar plexus catheter with infusion of 0.1 to 0.2% bupivacaine or ropivacaine at 6 to 12 mL/hr for 48 to 72 hours.
From Horlocker TT: Anesthesia and pain management, Revision Hip and Knee Arthroplasty. Edited by Berry DJ, Trousdale RT, Dennis D, et al. 2008 Philadelphia, Lippincott Williams & Wilkins, with permission.

ade of the sacral plexus is crucial to some, but not all, patients undergoing major knee sugery.[49–51]

Regional anesthetic techniques that can be used for surgical procedures about the knee include neuraxial and peripheral leg blocks. Spinal anesthesia can be accomplished with hyperbaric or isobaric solutions, although the latter are favored by most orthopaedic anesthesiologists. Injection of hyperbaric solutions often results in a higher level of sensory and motor blockade than needed for the surgical procedure, with subsequent earlier offset of anesthesia. Epidural blockade offers the advantage of a continuous catheter technique that can be continued into the postoperative period. These procedures are often associated with significant postoperative pain, particularly when continuous-motion machines are applied to the affected joint.

The supine position optimizes surgical exposure during knee arthroscopy or arthroplasty, lower extremity amputations, and procedures to the tibia and fibula. Care must be taken to cushion the extremities and bony prominences.

Postoperative Analgesia After Major Joint Replacement

7 Pain after total joint replacement, particularly total knee arthroplasty, is severe. Traditionally, postoperative analgesia following total joint replacement was provided by either intravenous patient-controlled analgesia or epidural analgesia. However, each technique has distinct advantages and disadvantages. For example, opioids do not consistently provide adequate pain relief and often cause sedation, constipation, nausea and vomiting, and pruritus. Epidural infusions containing local anesthetics (with or without an opioid) provide superior analgesia but are associated with hypotension, urinary retention, motor block limiting ambulation, and spinal hematoma secondary to anticoagulation.[52] Numerous reports have documented that single dose and continuous peripheral nerve techniques that block the lumbar plexus (fascia iliaca, femoral, psoas compartment blocks), with or without sciatic nerve blockade, can be used with success for patients having total joint replacement.[42,43,49,51–60]

Several studies have also demonstrated that unilateral peripheral block provides a quality of analgesia and surgical outcomes similar to that of continuous epidural analgesia, but with fewer side effects.[54–56] These reports suggest that continuous peripheral techniques may be the optimal analgesic method following total joint arthroplasty. Appreciation of the indications, benefits, and side effects associated with both conventional and novel analgesic approaches is paramount to maximizing rehabilitative efforts and improving patient satisfaction.

The use of peripheral or neuraxial regional anesthetic techniques and a combination of opioid and nonopioid analgesic agents for breakthrough pain results in superior pain control, attenuation of the stress response, and decreases opioid requirements. Multimodal analgesia is a multidisciplinary approach to pain management with the aim of maximizing the positive aspects of the treatment while limiting the associated side effects. Because many of the negative side effects of analgesic therapy are opioid-related (and dose-dependent), limiting perioperative opioid use is a major principle of multimodal analgesia. Anti-inflammatory medications and acetaminophen are valuable adjuvants to systemic opioids. The addition of nonopioid analgesics reduces opioid use, improves analgesia, and decreases opioid-related side effects.

Knee Arthroscopy and Anterior Cruciate Ligament Repair

Outpatient knee surgery may be performed under a variety of anesthetic techniques. Traditionally, neuraxial or general anes-

thesia is used. Because diagnostic knee arthroscopy is a relatively minor procedure that may be performed under local anesthesia with sedation, the performance of a single-dose or continuous lower extremity block is probably not warranted in the majority of patients. The optimal anesthetic technique would allow rapid operating suite turnover and patient recovery, excellent operating conditions, and minimal side effects. Unfortunately, each approach is associated with advantages and disadvantages. For example, concerns over transient neurologic symptoms propelled a search for an alternative to intrathecal lidocaine; to date, its reliable sensory and motor block (of limited duration) have not been duplicated. Bupivacaine has a low incidence of transient neurologic symptoms. However, the time to hospital discharge following administration of low-dose bupivacaine (5 to 7.5 mg) with fentanyl (10 μg) may be as long as 3 hours. Conversely, general anesthesia is associated with nausea and vomiting, side effects prevalent in the patient population undergoing knee arthroscopy. Evidence has failed to demonstrate a clinically significant difference in patient outcome with respect to anesthetic technique.[61] Patient preference may also have a significant impact on selection of anesthetic technique.

Repair of the anterior cruciate ligament (ACL) is also performed as an outpatient procedure. However, the surgery is more extensive than knee arthroscopy, and postoperative pain may be significant. The anesthetic considerations are similar to those of diagnostic knee arthroscopy, with the additional need to provide substantial analgesia. Although few data exist on the use of lower extremity blocks for patients undergoing ACL repair, an early study suggests that lumbar plexus block (combined with a spinal or sciatic block) dramatically reduces postoperative opioids requirements and opioid-related side effects.[62] In a comprehensive evaluation of analgesia following ACL, Williams et al.[63] reported that femoral catheters reliably maintain pain scores below the moderate-to-severe pain threshold for the first 4 days after ACL reconstruction. Selected patients may be discharged home with an indwelling femoral catheter to provide sustained pain relief for 48 hours.[64] Thus, for outpatient procedures, the complexity/ duration of the surgical procedure will determine the usefulness of peripheral blocks compared with neuraxial or general anesthesia.

Hospital discharge criteria generally include successful oral intake, ambulation, and voiding by the patient. Thus, patients who have undergone a neuraxial technique will not be discharged until complete block resolution (although the requirement to void is somewhat controversial).

Intra-Articular Injection

Intra-articular injections of local anesthetics, opioids, or combinations have become routine for perioperative pain management after arthroscopic knee surgery. A number of reports enthusiastically recommend the use of this technique; however, the results remain conflicting.[65,66] Comparison of reports is difficult because of variability in underlying anesthetic techniques, different dosages and concentrations of local anesthetic, and lack of control groups. The safety of injecting large volumes of intra-articular bupivacaine has been ascertained,[67] and side effects are rare after intra-articular doses of morphine. Because these techniques are simple and low risk and seem to afford pain relief under some conditions, they will likely be continued.

Surgery to the Ankle and Foot

Innervation of the foot is provided by the femoral nerve (via the saphenous nerve) and by the sciatic nerve (via the posterior tibial, sural, and deep and superficial peroneal nerves).[50] Therefore, central neuraxial blockade and peripheral nerve blocks at

ANESTHETIC TECHNIQUES FOR COMMON FOOT AND ANKLE OPERATIONS

	■ SURGICAL PROCEDURE	■ REGIONAL TECHNIQUE	■ COMMENTS
Forefoot[a]	Hallux valgus	Metatarsal, ankle, popliteal blockade	Sural nerve block not necessary for surgery
	Amputations	Ankle, popliteal blockade	Popliteal blockade is the technique of choice in the presence of infection or swelling
Midfoot[a]	Transmetatarsal amputations	Popliteal, ankle blockade	—
Hindfoot[a]	Ankle arthroscopy	Spinal, epidural, or general anesthesia	Operation typically requires good muscle relaxation for manipulation; thigh tourniquet
	Achilles tendon repair	Spinal, epidural, or popliteal blockade	Spinal or epidural anesthesia whenever thigh tourniquet is required
	Triple arthrodesis	Spinal or epidural	Neuraxial technique preferred for bone graft harvesting; popliteal blockade for postoperative analgesia

[a]Femoral or saphenous block required if the incision extends to the medial aspect of the foot or ankle.
From Hadzic A, Vloka JD: Anesthesia for ankle and foot surgery. Tech Reg Anesth Pain Manage 1990; 3: 113, with permission.

the upper leg, knee, or ankle are appropriate regional anesthetic techniques for foot surgery. The selection of the regional technique is based on the surgical site, use of a calf or thigh tourniquet, degree of weight bearing/ambulation, and the need for postoperative analgesia. For example, inflation of a thigh tourniquet for longer than 15 to 20 minutes necessitates a general or neuraxial anesthetic, regardless of surgical site. Common surgical procedures and considerations regarding the choice of regional technique are discussed in Table 53-3.[68]

The distal surgical site and the ability to block the pain pathways at multiple sites give regional anesthesia an advantage over general anesthesia for surgery to the ankle and foot. Peripheral blockade avoids the cardiovascular and respiratory side effects, as well as the urinary retention associated with neuraxial and general anesthesia. Often, patients undergoing lower extremity peripheral techniques may be discharged directly from the operating room to the outpatient nursing station, reducing recovery time and charges. The use of long-acting local anesthetics and the addition of epinephrine or clonidine allow prolongation of postoperative analgesia. Mepivacaine and lidocaine may be more appropriate in the ambulatory setting, where fast-onset and reliable surgical anesthesia is essential. Placement of an indwelling catheter is the standard for major foot and ankle surgery and allows for superior and prolonged analgesia with minimal opioid-related side effects.[69]

Prolonged peripheral or plexus blockade provides excellent pain relief, however, the risk of accidental nerve trauma in an anesthetized extremity is theoretically higher outside the hospital environment. The patient should be informed of the risks and instructed in appropriate care of the extremity. Patients who are unable or unwilling to comply with recommended medical care may not be good candidates for regional anesthesia techniques and/or should be fully recovered before discharge. In all cases, a follow-up telephone call on the first postoperative day should include questions concerning residual areas of neural blockade or altered neural function, such as paresthesias. Any patient concerns regarding the anesthetic or surgery should also be discussed. Patients with indwelling plexus or peripheral catheters should be queried regarding the presence of residual block, signs of local anesthetic toxicity, and catheter migration.[64,69]

MICROVASCULAR SURGERY

Microvascular surgery includes both *replantation*, the reattachment of a completely severed body part, and *revascularization*, the re-establishment of blood flow through a severed body part. Most replantation surgery involves the upper extremity. Anesthetic management in microvascular surgery includes maintenance of blood flow through microvascular anastomoses, positioning considerations associated with a long surgical procedure during which the patient must lie completely still, and replacement of blood and fluid losses, which may be extensive.

Maintenance of blood flow through microvascular anastomoses is paramount to limb or graft viability. Blood flow may be improved by increasing the perfusion pressure, preventing hypothermia, and using vasodilators and sympathetic blockade. Microvascular perfusion pressure depends on both adequate intravascular volume and oncotic pressure. Blood loss during microvascular surgery is typically continual and insidious. Unrecognized bleeding and migration of intravascular fluid into the third space reduce microvascular perfusion pressure, and must be corrected. However, overzealous use of crystalloid results in generalized edema, including the replanted body part, whereas excessive transfusion of blood products increases blood viscosity and therefore decreases flow. Evidence suggests that use of phenylephrine to support blood pressure does not jeopardize blood flow to the tissue being replanted.[70] Rheologically, the oxygen-carrying capacity of blood is optimized with a hematocrit of 30%. Arterial cannulation allows frequent assessment of hemoglobin levels and acid-base status, as well as direct blood pressure measurement.

Body temperature is also a determinant of blood flow. Hypothermia not only results in peripheral vasoconstriction, but causes sympathetic activation, shivering, increased oxygen demand, a leftward shift of the oxygen–hemoglobin dissociation curve, and altered coagulation. Therefore, hypothermia must be prevented in microvascular surgical patients. The operating room temperature should be increased to 21°C, intravenous solutions should be warmed,[71] and the patient should be covered with a forced-air warming blanket.

The use of vasodilators has also been studied in the treatment of perioperative vasospasm. Local anesthetics and papaverine, applied topically, may be used to provide relaxation of vascular smooth muscle in the intraoperative setting.[72] All the volatile anesthetics are potent vasodilators and can increase tissue blood flow 200 to 300%, even at typical expired anesthetic concentrations. Direct-acting vasodilating agents, such as sodium nitroprusside, trimethaphan, and hydralazine, produce vasodilation but do not prevent vasospasm because of direct surgical stimulation. Nitroprusside has been shown to reduce perfusion in a microvascular free flap.[70] In addition, the volatile anesthetics and intravenous agents may also result in hypotension and decreased microvascular perfusion pressure. Regional anesthetic techniques provide sympathectomy and vasodilation to the proximal (innervated) segment of an extremity, but have no effect on vasospasm in the replanted (denervated) tissue. Antithrombotics (heparin), fibrinolytics (streptokinase, urokinase, low-molecular-weight dextran), and smooth muscle relaxants (papaverine, local anesthetics) are also used to preserve blood flow in microvascular anastomoses.

Microvascular surgery may be performed under regional or general anesthesia, or both. Regional anesthesia has several advantages over general anesthesia. The sympathectomy associated with local anesthetic blockade results in vasodilation and increased blood flow. A single-injection regional anesthetic technique may be of insufficient duration for many microvascular procedures. However, placement of an indwelling catheter (epidural, plexus, or peripheral) provides extended intraoperative anesthesia and continuous postoperative analgesia. General anesthesia ensures airway access and reduces the possibility of patient movement during critical surgical events. A combination of general and continuous regional anesthesia allows prolonged intraoperative anesthesia and postoperative analgesia, reduces the amount of inhalation agent, and increases the patient's acceptance of lengthy surgical procedures. However, regardless of anesthetic technique, conditions that stimulate vasospasm or vasoconstriction, such as pain, hypotension, and hypovolemia, must be avoided. Whether administration of a vasopressor with vasoconstrictive qualities or addition of epinephrine to local anesthetic solutions may decrease anastomotic blood flow is controversial.[70]

PEDIATRIC ORTHOPAEDIC SURGERY

Pediatric patients present with a variety of orthopaedic conditions, including congenital deformities, traumatic injuries, infections, and malignancies (see also Chapter 45). Anesthetic management of the pediatric orthopaedic patient involves not only the usual pediatric patient considerations, such as airway management, fluid replacement, and maintenance of body temperature, but also the unique concerns associated with orthopaedic surgery. Coexisting neuromuscular conditions, such as arthrogryposis or myelomeningocele, may predispose pediatric orthopaedic patients to latex allergy and malignant hyperthermia.

Orthopaedic procedures may be performed with children anesthetized with regional, general, or a combination of anesthetic techniques. The patient's age, operative site and positioning, and surgical duration are important factors in selection of an anesthetic. Children older than 7 years of age may tolerate a primary regional anesthetic technique, whereas younger children may benefit from a general or combination regional/general anesthesia. Neural blockade may be initiated after induction of general anesthesia and before surgical incision to provide possible preemptive analgesia, or, on completion of the surgical procedure, to extend the duration of postoperative analgesia. Often, regional anesthetic procedures are technically easier to perform on children because the relative lack of subcutaneous tissue facilitates identification of bony and vascular landmarks as well as spread of local anesthetic solutions. The advantages of regional anesthesia in children are similar to those in adults and include earlier ambulation and hospital discharge, decreased incidence of nausea and vomiting, and prolonged postoperative analgesia.

Surgical procedures to the lower extremity may be safely and successfully performed under caudal, epidural, and spinal anesthesia.[73] However, the anatomic differences between the pediatric and adult spine and spinal cord must be appreciated.[74] In addition, femoral, lateral femoral cutaneous, and sciatic nerve blocks allow prolonged anesthesia and analgesia to the blocked extremity, but often require additional intraoperative supplementation with intravenous or inhalation agents.[75]

Upper extremity procedures may be performed with any of the anesthetic techniques previously described for adults. The superficial location of the brachial plexus, decreased neural diameter, and rapid diffusion of local anesthetics contribute to the high success rate, which approaches 100%.[76] Blockade of the brachial plexus is usually accomplished with perivascular, sheath, or nerve stimulator techniques in children younger than 7 years of age because elicitation of paresthesias is regarded as uncomfortable (and therefore unacceptable) by the younger pediatric patients. Intravenous regional (Bier) block is particularly useful in the pediatric population for limited procedures such as closed reduction of forearm fractures.

OTHER CONSIDERATIONS

Anesthesia for Nonsurgical "Closed" Orthopaedic Procedures

Many orthopaedic procedures requiring anesthesia are carried out in areas other than the operating room. These include cast and dressing changes in pediatric patients, pin removal, hip and shoulder relocation, closed reduction of fractures, and joint manipulations. Although some of the minor procedures require only light sedation, those procedures involving bone and joint manipulation usually require a full anesthetic intervention. It is critically important that patients undergoing these procedures are managed with the same careful attention afforded those scheduled for a standard operating room. Regional anesthesia, usually with a short-acting local anesthetic, can be a good choice for these procedures.

Tourniquets

Tourniquets are often used to minimize blood loss and provide a bloodless operating field. Appropriate selection of tourniquet cuff size and inflation pressure is paramount in reducing the risk of neuromuscular injury related to tourniquet ischemia. The cuff should be large enough to comfortably circle the limb to ensure circumferentially uniform pressure. The point of overlap should be placed 180 degrees from the neurovascular bundle because there is some area of decreased compression at the overlap point. The width of the inflated cuff should be more than half the limb diameter.

Opinions differ as to the pressure required in tourniquets to prevent bleeding. In general, a cuff pressure 100 mm Hg above a patient's measured systolic pressure is adequate for the thigh, and 50 mm Hg above systolic pressure is adequate for the arm, with the understanding that if hypertensive episodes occur, the cuff pressure should be increased. Bleeding from the surgical site after cuff inflation may rarely be due to inadequate occlusion of the major arterial inflow, which is corrected by cuff reapplication and use of the proper degree of inflation. Bleeding during tourniquet inflation is more commonly due to intramedullary blood flow in the long bones, particularly in the skeletally immature patient, and to small arterial vessels between the two bones of distal extremities. Overinflation of the tourniquet does *not* resolve these problems. Likewise, the duration of safe tourniquet inflation is unknown. Recommendations range from 30 minutes to 4 hours. Five minutes of intermittent perfusion between 1- and 2-hour inflations, followed by repeated exsanguination through elevation and compression, *may* allow more extended use, although this remains controversial.[77,78]

Damage to underlying vessels, nerves, and skeletal muscles has been reported following tourniquet inflation.[79] Injury is a function of both inflation pressure and duration of inflation.[80,81] Direct pressure from the cuff is more damaging than the ischemia distally.[80,82] Arterial spasm, venous thrombosis, and nerve injury are all demonstrable after several hours. Clinical examination, electromyography, and effluent blood analysis all show completely reversible changes for inflations of 1 to 2 hours, which is the basis for the recommendation of this period as the safe duration for tourniquet use; longer inflation times are associated with prolonged or irreversible changes in neurologic and/or muscular function.[78,83]

Transient systemic metabolic acidosis and increased arterial carbon dioxide levels have been demonstrated after tourniquet deflation, and do not cause deleterious effects in healthy patients.[84,85] Measurable changes include a 10 to 15% increase in heart rate, a 5 to 10% increase in serum potassium, and a rise of 1 to 8 mm Hg in carbon dioxide tension in blood. Prolonged inflation or the simultaneous release of two tourniquets may produce clinically significant acidosis, particularly in patients with an underlying acidosis of other causes. Tourniquet release has also been associated with cerebral embolic phenomena.[86]

When a pneumatic tourniquet is used with regional anesthetic techniques, some patients complain of dull, aching pain or become restless, even though seemingly adequate analgesia exists for the operation itself. Patient discomfort usually appears approximately 45 minutes after the tourniquet is inflated and becomes more intense with time. No satisfactory explanation for its genesis has been found. Current explanations involve pain transmission through both A delta and C fibers, and its modulation in the dorsal horn synapses. The C (slow pain) fibers recover faster as the block wanes. Analogous phenomena may be observed at the same time point during general anesthesia. Evidence of lightening anesthesia (increase in blood pressure and pulse rate) may appear even though the same concentrations of anesthetic are being delivered.[87,88] The definitive treatment for tourniquet pain is release of the tourniquet. Relief of pain is prompt and complete. During surgery, however, opioids and hypnotics are usually effective.

Fat Embolus Syndrome

Fat embolus syndrome (FES) is associated with multiple traumatic injuries and surgery involving long-bone fractures.[89] Risk factors include male gender, age (20 to 30 years), hypovolemic shock, intramedullary instrumentation, rheumatoid arthritis, total hip arthroplasty using the technique of cementing femoral stems designed for press-fit application, and bilateral total knee surgery. The incidence of FES in isolated long-bone fractures is 3 to 4%, and the mortality rate associated with this condition is significant, ranging from 10 to 20%.

Clinical and laboratory signs of FES have been classified by Gurd[90] as major or minor (Table 53-4), with a diagnosis requiring at least one major and four minor criteria, as well as the exclusion of other posttraumatic causes of hypoxemia. Major signs of the syndrome include the presence of axillary

or subconjunctival petechiae, significant hypoxemia, central nervous system depression in excess of that expected because of the level of hypoxemia, and pulmonary edema. Classified as minor signs are tachycardia, hyperthermia, retinal fat emboli on funduscopic examination, urinary fat globules, an unexplained decrease in hematocrit or platelets, an increased erythrocyte sedimentation rate, and fat globules in the sputum. Symptoms usually occur 12 to 40 hours after the injury and can range from mild dyspnea to frank coma. Decreased arterial oxygen tension is the most consistent abnormal laboratory value. Fulminant episodes can occur within hours of the traumatic injury, causing severe hypoxemia, respiratory failure, and severe neurologic impairment. Disseminated intravascular coagulation can also occur in conjunction with FES.

Not all trauma patients who have demonstrated evidence of fat emboli fit the criteria for diagnosis of FES. Two theories are hypothesized to explain the mechanism of this syndrome: the mechanical theory and the biochemical theory. The mechanical theory proposes that long-bone trauma results in release of fat droplets that enter the vascular system through torn veins. These droplets are transported to the pulmonary vascular bed where they act as microemboli. The biochemical theory can be divided into two mechanisms: toxic and obstructive. The toxic mechanism proposes that free fatty acids released at the time of trauma directly affect pneumocytes in the lung and cause adult respiratory distress syndrome. This effect would be enhanced by the trauma-induced release of catecholamines, which would result in further mobilization of free fatty acids. The obstructive theory hypothesizes that an unspecified chemical event at the site of the fracture releases mediators that affect lipid solubility, resulting in coalescence of lipids and consequent embolization. Some or all these theories may play a role in development of FES. Other predisposing or aggravating factors such as shock, hypovolemia, sepsis, or disseminated intravascular coagulation may be required to trigger the conversion of fat emboli to FES.

Appropriate treatment of FES requires early recognition of the syndrome, reversal of possible aggravating factors such as hypovolemia, early surgical stabilization of fracture sites, and aggressive respiratory support. Corticosteroid therapy is controversial but may be beneficial. Other pharmacologic interventions, including heparin and dextran, have not been shown to be effective in treating FES.

TABLE 53-4

CRITERIA FOR DIAGNOSIS OF FAT EMBOLUS SYNDROME[a]

■ MAJOR

Axillary/subconjunctival petechiae
Hypoxemia (PaO_2 <60 mm Hg; FIO_2 <0.4)
Central nervous system depression (disproportionate to hypoxemia)
Pulmonary edema

■ MINOR

Tachycardia (>110 beats/min)
Hyperthermia
Retinal fat emboli
Urinary fat globules
Decreased platelets/hematocrit (unexplained)
Increased erythrocyte sedimentation rate
Fat globules in sputum

[a]Diagnosis of fat embolus syndrome requires at least one sign from the major and four signs from the minor criteria categories.
From Gurd AR: Fat embolism: An aid to diagnosis. J Bone Joint Surg Br 1970; 52: 732, with permission.

TABLE 53-5

VENOUS THROMBOEMBOLISM PREVALENCE AFTER MAJOR ORTHOPAEDIC SURGERY

	■ DEEP VENOUS THROMBOSIS[a]		■ PULMONARY EMBOLISM	
■ PROCEDURE	■ TOTAL (%)	■ PROXIMAL (%)	■ TOTAL (%)	■ FATAL (%)
Total hip replacement	42–57	18–36	0.9–28	0.14–2.0
Total knee replacement	41–85	5–22	1.5–10	0.1–1.7
Hip fracture surgery	46–60	23–30	3–11	2.5–7.5

[a]Total or proximal deep venous thrombosis prevalence based on the use of mandatory venography in prospective randomized clinical trials in which patients received either prophylaxis or a placebo.
From Geerts WH, Pineo GF, Heit JA et al: Prevention of venous thromboembolism: The seventh ACCP conference on antithrombotic and thrombolytic therapy. Chest 2004; 126(3 Suppl): 338S, with permission.

Methyl Methacrylate

Methyl methacrylate is an acrylic bone cement used during arthroplastic procedures. Insertion of this cement is associated with sudden onset of hypotension in some patients. This hypotension has been attributed to absorption of the volatile monomer of methyl methacrylate, embolization of air and bone marrow during femoral reaming, lysis of blood cells and marrow induced by the exothermic reaction, and conversion of methyl methacrylate to methacrylate acid. Adequate hydration and maximizing inspired oxygen concentration minimize the hypotension and hypoxemia that can accompany cementing of the prosthesis. Because air can be entrained during this procedure, nitrous oxide should be discontinued several minutes before this point.

Venous Thromboembolism

8 Venous thromboembolism is a major cause of death after surgery or trauma to the lower extremities. Without prophylaxis, venous thrombosis develops in 40 to 80% of orthopaedic patients, and 1 to 28% show clinical or laboratory evidence of pulmonary embolism. Fatal pulmonary embolism occurs in 0.1 to 8% of patients[91] (Table 53-5). The incidence of fatal pulmonary embolism is highest in patients who have undergone surgery for hip fracture. Although fatal pulmonary embolism may be the most common preventable cause of hospital death, many physicians fail to use prophylaxis appropriately because of concern about bleeding complications from anticoagulation. Effective thromboprophylaxis requires knowledge of clinical risk factors in individual patients, such as advanced age, prolonged immobility or bed rest, prior history of thromboembolism, cancer, pre-existing hypercoagulable state, and major surgery. In many patients, multiple risk factors may be present, and the risks are cumulative. After identification of the risk of thromboembolism, an assessment may be made regarding the risks and benefits of physical or pharmacologic techniques used to prevent thromboembolism.

Antithrombotic Prophylaxis

Thromboprophylaxis is based on identification of risk factors. Guidelines for antithrombotic therapy, including selection of pharmacologic agent, degree of anticoagulation desired, and duration of therapy continue to evolve.[91] Recommendations from the Seventh American College of Chest Physicians in 2004 are based on prospective randomized studies that assess the efficacy of therapy, using contrast venography or fibrinogen leg scanning to diagnose asymptomatic thrombi (Table 53-6). For patients undergoing major joint replacement, administration of LMWH, warfarin, or fondaparinux is recommended. Similar recommendations are made for patients with acute spinal cord injury. Conversely, other orthopaedic patients are considered low risk, and no pharmacologic prophylaxis is warranted. The need for *routine* thromboprophylaxis with LMWH or warfarin following total joint replacement has been questioned.[92]

Neuraxial Anesthesia and Analgesia in the Patient Receiving Antithrombotic Therapy

9 Several studies show a decrease in the incidence of both DVT and PTE in patients undergoing hip surgery under epidural[44–46] and spinal[93–95] anesthesia. Similar findings have been reported for knee surgery performed under epidural anesthesia.[96,97] Proposed mechanisms for this effect include (1) rheologic changes resulting in hyperkinetic lower extremity blood flow, reducing venous stasis and preventing thrombus formation; (2) beneficial circulatory effects from epinephrine added to the local anesthetic solutions; (3) altered coagulation and fibrinolytic responses to surgery under central neural blockade, resulting in a decreased tendency for blood to clot and better fibrinolytic function[98]; (4) the absence of positive-pressure ventilation and its concomitant effects on circulation; and (5) direct local anesthetic effects such as decreased platelet aggregation. It is important to note that most of the studies examining the value of epidural and spinal anesthesia in preventing DVT and PTE involved patients who were not receiving currently recommended pharmacologic prophylaxis. In addition, despite the reduction in thromboembolism in the presence of a neuraxial block, the risk of thromboembolism remains significant, and pharmacologic thromboprophylaxis is required.

The more recent introduction of more efficacious anticoagulants and antiplatelet agents has further increased the complexity of patient management. Anesthesiologists must balance the risk of thromboembolic and hemorrhagic complications. The actual incidence of neurologic dysfunction resulting from hemorrhagic complications associated with neuraxial blockade is unknown; however, the incidence cited in the literature is estimated to be less than 1 in 150,000 epidural and less than 1 in 220,000 spinal anesthetics.[99] The frequency of spinal hematoma is increased in patients who receive perioperative anticoagulation[100] and potentially in patients with spinal stenosis or other vertebral column pathology.[33]

Spinal hematoma was considered a rare complication of neuraxial blockade until the introduction of LMWH as a thromboprophylactic agent in the 1990s. The calculated incidence (approximately 1 in 3,000 epidural anesthetics), along with the catastrophic nature of spinal bleeding (only 30% of

TABLE 53-6

ANTITHROMBOTIC REGIMENS TO PREVENT THROMBOEMBOLISM IN ORTHOPAEDIC SURGICAL PATIENTS

■ HIP AND KNEE ARTHROPLASTY AND HIP FRACTURE SURGERY

- LMWH[a] started 12 hr before surgery or 12–24 hr after surgery, or 4–6 hr after surgery at half the usual dose and then increasing to the usual high-risk dose the following day
- Fondaparinux (2.5 mg started 6–8 hr after surgery)
- Adjusted-dose warfarin started preoperatively or the evening after surgery (INR target, 2.5; INR range, 2.0–3.0)
- Intermittent pneumatic compression is an alternative option to anticoagulant prophylaxis in patients who have a high risk of bleeding

■ SPINAL CORD INJURY

- LMWH once primary hemostasis is evident
- Intermittent pneumatic compression is an alternative option when anticoagulation is contraindicated early after the injury
- During the rehabilitation phase, conversion to adjusted-dose warfarin (INR target, 2.5; INR range, 2.0–3.0)

■ ELECTIVE SPINE SURGERY

- Routine use of thromboprophylaxis, apart from early and persistent mobilization, not routinely recommended for patients without additional risk factors

■ KNEE ARTHROSCOPY

- Routine use of thromboprophylaxis, apart from early and persistent mobilization, not routinely recommended

LMWH, low-molecular-weight heparin; INR, international normalized ratio.
[a]Use with caution in patients receiving neuraxial anesthesia/analgesia. Enoxaparin and dalteparin are LMWH approved by the U.S. Food and Drug Administration.
From Geerts WH, Pineo GF, Heit JA et al: Prevention of venous thromboembolism: the Seventh ACCP Conference on Antithrombotic and Thrombolytic Therapy. Chest 2004; 126: 338S, with permission.

patients had good neurologic recovery),[33,101] warranted an alternate approach to analgesic management following total hip and knee replacement. Although psoas compartment and femoral catheters are suitable (if not superior) alternatives to neuraxial infusions, there are no investigations that examine the frequency and severity of hemorrhagic complications following plexus or peripheral blockade in anticoagulated patients. All cases of major bleeding (significant decreases in hemoglobin and/or blood pressure) associated with nonneu-

raxial techniques occurred after psoas compartment or lumbar sympathetic blockade and have involved heparin, LMWH, warfarin, and thienopyridine derivatives. These cases suggest that significant blood loss, rather than neural deficits, may be the most serious complication of nonneuraxial regional techniques in the anticoagulated patient. Additional information is needed to make definitive recommendations. The current information focuses on neuraxial blocks and anticoagulants (Table 53-7).[102] Conservatively, these neuraxial guidelines

TABLE 53-7

NEURAXIAL ANESTHESIA AND ANALGESIA IN THE ORTHOPAEDIC PATIENT RECEIVING ANTITHROMBOTIC THERAPY

■ LMWH

Needle placement should occur 10–12 hr after a dose. Indwelling neuraxial catheters are allowed with once (but not twice daily) dosing of LMWH. In general, it is optimal to place/remove indwelling catheters in the morning and administer LMWH in the evening to allow normalization of hemostasis to occur prior to catheter manipulation.

■ WARFARIN

Adequate levels of all vitamin K-dependent factors should be present during catheter placement and removal. Patients chronically on warfarin should have normal INR prior to performance of regional technique. Monitor prothrombin time and INR daily. Remove catheter when INR <1.5.

■ FONDAPARINUX

Neuraxial techniques are not advised in patients who are anticipated to receive fondaparinux perioperatively.

■ NONSTEROIDAL ANTI-INFLAMMATORY DRUGS

No significant risk of regional anesthesia-related bleeding is associated with aspirin-type drugs. However, for patients receiving warfarin or LMWH, the combined anticoagulant and antiplatelet effects may increase the risk of perioperative bleeding. In addition, other medications affecting platelet function such as the thienopyridine derivatives and glycoprotein IIb/IIIa platelet receptor inhibitors should be avoided.

LMWH, low-molecular-weight heparin; INR, international normalized ratio.
Adapted from Horlocker TT, Wedel DJ, Benzon H et al: Regional anesthesia in the anticoagulated patient: defining the risks (the second ASRA Consensus Conference on Neuraxial Anesthesia and Anticoagulation). Reg Anesth Pain Med 2003; 28: 172.

may be applied to plexus and peripheral techniques. However, this may be more restrictive than necessary.

References

1. Eagle KA, Berger PB, Calkins H et al: American College of Cardiology. American Heart Association. ACC/AHA guideline update for perioperative cardiovascular evaluation for noncardiac surgery–executive summary: A report of the American College of Cardiology/American Heart Association Task Force on Practice Guidelines (Committee to Update the 1996 Guidelines on Perioperative Cardiovascular Evaluation for Noncardiac Surgery). J Am Coll Cardiol. 2002; 39: 542
2. Biebuyck JF, Martyn JA, White DA et al: Up-and-down regulation of skeletal muscle acetylcholine receptors: Effects on neuromuscular blockers. Anesthesiology 1992; 76: 822
3. Howard A, Donaldson S, Hedden D et al: Improvement in quality of life following surgery for adolescent idiopathic scoliosis. Spine 2007; 32: 2715
4. Ferguson RL, Hansen MM, Nicholas DA et al: Same-day versus staged anterior-posterior spinal surgery in a neuromuscular scoliosis population: The evaluation of medical complications. J Pediatr Orthop 1996; 16: 293
5. McDonnell MF, Glassman SD, Dimar JR II et al: Perioperative complications of anterior procedures on the spine. J Bone Joint Surg Am 1996; 78: 839
6. Winkler M, Marker E, Hetz H: The peri-operative management of major orthopaedic procedures. Anaesthesia 1998; 53(Suppl 2): 37
7. Sloan TB, Ronai AK, Koht A: Reversible loss of somatosensory evoked potentials during anterior cervical spinal fusion. Anesth Analg 1986; 65: 96
8. Albin MS, Chang JL, Babinski M et al: Intracardiac catheters in neurosurgical anesthesia. Anesthesiology 1979; 50: 67
9. Vauzelle C, Stagnara P, Jouvinroux P: Functional monitoring of spinal cord activity during spinal surgery. Clin Orthop 1973; 93: 173
10. Pathak KS, Brown RH, Nash CL et al: Continuous opioid infusion for scoliosis fusion surgery. Anesth Analg 1983; 62: 841
11. Ginsburg HH, Shetter AG, Raudzens PA: Postoperative paraplegia with preserved intraoperative somatosensory evoked potentials. J Neurosurg 1985; 63: 296
12. Schwartz DM, Auerbach JD, Dormans JP et al: Neurophysiological detection of impending spinal cord injury during scoliosis surgery. J Bone Joint Surg Am 2007; 89: 2440
13. Burke D, Hicks RG: Surgical monitoring of motor pathways. J Clin Neurophysiol 1998; 15: 194
14. Pathak KS, Ammadio M, Kalamchi A et al: Effects of halothane, enflurane, and isoflurane on somatosensory evoked potentials during nitrous oxide anesthesia. Anesthesiology 1987; 66: 753
15. Nuttall GA, Horlocker TT, Santrach PJ et al: Predictors of blood transfusions in spinal instrumentation and fusion surgery. Spine 2000; 25: 596
16. Copley LA, Richards BS, Safavi FZ et al: Hemodilution as a method to reduce transfusion requirements in adolescent spine fusion surgery. Spine 1999; 24: 219
17. Murray DJ, Forbes RB, Titone MB et al: Transfusion management in pediatric and adolescent scoliosis surgery: Efficacy of autologous blood. Spine 1997; 22: 2735
18. Brodsky JW, Dickson JH, Erwin WD et al: Hypotensive anesthesia for scoliosis surgery in Jehovah's Witnesses. Spine 1991; 16: 304
19. Dilger JA, Tetzlaff JE, Bell GR et al: Ischaemic optic neuropathy after spinal fusion. Can J Anaesth 1998; 45: 63
20. Myers MA, Hamilton SR, Bogosian AJ et al: Visual loss as a complication of spine surgery. A review of 37 cases. Spine 1997; 22: 1325
21. Warner ME, Warner MA, Garrity JA et al:. The frequency of perioperative vision loss. Anesth Analg 2001; 93: 1417
22. Patel NJ, Patel BS, Paskin S et al: Induced moderate hypotensive anesthesia for spinal fusion and Harrington-rod instrumentation. J Bone Joint Surg Am 1985; 67: 1384
23. Horlocker TT, Nuttall GA, Dekutoski MB et al: The accuracy of coagulation tests during spinal fusion and instrumentation. Anesth Analg 2001; 93: 33
24. Lentschener C, Cottin P, Bouaziz H et al: Reduction of blood loss and transfusion requirement by aprotinin in posterior lumbar spine fusion. Anesth Analg 1999; 89: 590
25. Lee LA, Roth S, Posner KL et al: The American Society of Anesthesiologists Postoperative Visual Loss Registry: Analysis of 93 spine surgery cases with postoperative visual loss. Anesthesiology 2006; 105: 652
26. Horlocker TT, Wedel DJ, Cucchiara RF: Venous air embolism during spinal instrumentation and fusion in the prone position [letter]. Anesth Analg 1992; 75: 152
27. Bianconi M, Ferraro L, Ricci R et al: The pharmacokinetics and efficacy of ropivacaine continuous wound instillation after spine fusion surgery. Anesth Analg 2004; 98: 166
28. France JC, Jorgenson SS, Lowe TG et al: The use of intrathecal morphine for analgesia after posterolateral lumbar fusion: A prospective, double-blind, randomized study. Spine 1997; 22: 2272
29. Daley MD, Rolbin SH, Hew EM et al: Epidural anesthesia for obstetrics after spinal surgery. Reg Anesth 1990; 15: 280
30. Crosby ET, Halpern SH: Obstetric epidural anaesthesia in patients with Harrington instrumentation. Can J Anaesth 1989; 36: 693
31. Hubbert CH: Epidural anesthesia in patients with spinal fusion. Anesth Analg 1985; 64: 843
32. Hebl JR, Horlocker TT, Schroeder DR: Neurologic complications after neuraxial anesthesia or analgesia in patients with pre-existing spinal stenosis or lumbar disc disease. Reg Anesth Pain Med 2005; 29: A89
33. Moen V, Dahlgren N, Irestedt L: Serious complications after central neuraxial blockade in Sweden 1990–1999. Anesthesiology 2004; 101: 950
34. Lynch NM, Cofield RH, Silbert PL et al: Neurologic complications after total shoulder arthroplasty. J Shoulder Elbow Surg 1996; 5: 53
35. Conn RA, Cofield RH, Byer DE et al: Interscalene block anesthesia for shoulder surgery. Clin Orthop 1987; 216: 94
36. Liguori GA, Kahn RL, Gordon J et al.: The use of metoprolol and glycopyrrolate to prevent hypotensive/bradycardic events during shoulder arthroscopy in the sitting position under interscalene block. Anesth Analg 1998; 87: 1320
37. Urmey WF, Talts KH, Sharrock NE: One hundred percent incidence of hemidiaphragmatic paresis associated with interscalene brachial plexus anesthesia as diagnosed by ultrasonography. Anesth Analg 1991; 72: 498
38. Schroeder LE, Horlocker TT, Schroeder DR: The efficacy of axillary block for surgical procedures about the elbow. Anesth Analg 1996; 83: 747
39. Davis WJ, Lennon RL, Wedel DJ: Brachial plexus anesthesia for outpatient surgical procedures on an upper extremity. Mayo Clin Proc 1991; 66: 470
40. Ilfeld BM, Morey TE, Wright TW et al: Interscalene perineural ropivacaine infusion: A comparison of two dosing regimens for postoperative analgesia. Reg Anesth Pain Med 2004; 29: 9
41. Ilfeld BM, Wright TW, Enneking FK et al: Total elbow arthroplasty as an outpatient procedure using a continuous infraclavicular nerve block at home: A prospective case report. Reg Anesth Pain Med 2006; 31: 172
42. Horlocker TT, Kopp SL, Pagnano MW et al: Analgesia for total hip and knee arthroplasty: A multimodal pathway featuring peripheral nerve block is superior to parenteral and neuraxial techniques. J Am Acad Orthop Surg 2006; 14: 126
43. Hebl JR, Kopp SL, Ali MH et al: A comprehensive anesthesia protocol that emphasizes peripheral nerve block markedly improves patient care and facilitates early discharge after total hip and knee arthroplasty. J Bone Joint Surg Am 2005; 87: 63
44. Sculco TP: Global blood management in orthopaedic surgery. Clin Orthop 1998; 357: 43
45. Modig J, Borg T, Karlstrom G et al: Thromboembolism after total hip replacement: Role of epidural and general anesthesia. Anesth Analg 1983; 62: 174
46. Modig J, Borg T, Bagge L et al: Role of extradural and of general anaesthesia in fibrinolysis and coagulation after total hip replacement. Br J Anaesth 1983; 55: 625
47. Stevens RD, Van Gessel E, Flory N et al: Lumbar plexus block reduces pain and blood loss associated with total hip arthroplasty. Anesthesiology 2000; 93: 115
48. Rosberg B, Fredin H, Gustafson C: Anesthetic techniques and surgical blood loss in total hip arthroplasty. Acta Anaesthesiol Scand 1982; 26: 189
49. Pham Dang C, Gautheron E, Guilley J et al: The value of adding sciatic block to continuous femoral block for analgesia after total knee replacement. Reg Anesth Pain Med 2005; 30: 128
50. Enneking FK, Chan V, Gregor J et al: Lower extremity peripheral nerve blocks: Essentials of our current understanding. Reg Anesth Pain Med 2005; 30: 4
51. Ben-David B, Schmalenberger K, Chelly JE: Analgesia after total knee arthroplasty: Is continuous sciatic blockade needed in addition to continuous femoral blockade? Anesth Analg 2004; 98: 747
52. Choi PT, Bhandari M, Scott J, Douketis J: Epidural analgesia for pain relief following hip or knee replacement. Cochrane Database of Systematic Reviews. (3):CD003071, 2003
53. Allen HW, Liu SS, Ware PD et al: Peripheral nerve blocks improve analgesia after total knee replacement surgery. Anesth Analg 1998; 87: 93
54. Capdevila X, Barthelet Y, Biboulet P et al: Effects of perioperative analgesic technique on the surgical outcome and duration of rehabilitation after major knee surgery. Anesthesiology 1999; 91: 8
55. Singelyn FJ, Deyaert M, Joris D et al: Effects of intravenous patient-controlled analgesia with morphine, continuous epidural analgesia, and continuous three-in-one block on postoperative pain and knee rehabilitation after unilateral total knee arthroplasty. Anesth Analg 1998; 87: 88
56. Singelyn FJ, Gouverneur JM: Postoperative analgesia after total hip arthroplasty: i.v. PCA with morphine, patient-controlled epidural analgesia, or continuous "3-in-one" block? A prospective evaluation by our acute pain service in more than 1,300 patients. J Clin Anesth 1999; 11: 550
57. Chelly JE, Greger J, Gebhard R et al: Continuous femoral blocks improve recovery and outcome of patients undergoing total knee arthroplasty. J Arthroplasty 2001; 16: 436
58. Kaloul I, Guay J, Cote C et al: The posterior lumbar plexus block and the 3-in-1 femoral nerve block provide similar postoperative analgesia after TKR. Can J Anesth 2004; 51: 45
59. Ganapathy S, Wasserman RA, Watson JT et al: Modified continuous 3-in-1 block for postoperative pain after TKA. Anesth Analg 1999; 99: 1197
60. Capdevila X, Macaire P, Dadure C et al: Continuous psoas compartment block for postoperative analgesia after total hip arthroplasty: New landmarks, technical guidelines, and clinical evaluation. Anesth Analg 2002; 94: 1606

61. Horlocker TT, Hebl JR: Anesthesia for outpatient knee arthroscopy: Is there an optimal technique? Reg Anesth Pain Med 2003; 28: 58

62. Matheny JM, Hanks GA, Rung GW et al: A comparison of patient-controlled analgesia and continuous lumbar plexus block after anterior cruciate ligament reconstruction. Arthroscopy 1993; 9: 87

63. Williams BA, Kentor ML, Vogt MT et al: Reduction of verbal pain scores after anterior cruciate ligament reconstruction with 2-day continuous femoral nerve block: A randomized clinical trial. Anesthesiology 2006; 104: 315

64. Klein SM, Greengrass RA, Gleason DH et al: Major ambulatory surgery with continuous regional anesthesia and a disposable infusion pump. Anesthesiology 1999; 91: 563

65. Stein C, Comisel K, Haimeri E et al: Analgesic effect of intraarticular morphine after arthroscopic knee surgery. N Engl J Med 1991; 325: 1123

66. Hughes DG: Intra-articular bupivacaine for pain relief in arthroscopic surgery. Anaesthesia 1985; 40: 821

67. Reuben SS, Sklar J: Pain management in patients who undergo outpatient arthroscopic surgery of the knee. J Bone Joint Surg Am 2000; 82: 1754

68. Hadzic A, Vloka JD: Anesthesia for ankle and foot surgery. Tech Reg Anesth Pain Manage 1999; 3: 113

69. Ilfeld BM, Morey TE, Wang RD et al: Continuous popliteal sciatic nerve block for postoperative pain control at home: a randomized, double-blinded, placebo-controlled trial. Anesthesiology 2002; 97: 959

70. Banic A, Krejci V, Erni D et al: Effects of sodium nitroprusside and phenylephrine on blood flow in free musculocutaneous flaps during general anesthesia. Anesthesiology 1999; 90: 147

71. Bird TM, Strunin L: Anaesthetic considerations for microsurgical repair of limbs. Can Anaesth Soc J 1984; 31: 51

72. Geter RK, Winters RR, Puckett CL: Resolution of experimental microvascular spasm and improvement in anastomotic patency by direct topical agent application. Plast Reconstr Surg 1986; 77: 105

73. Yaster M, Maxwell LG: Pediatric regional anesthesia. Anesthesiology 1989; 70: 324

74. Dalens B: Regional anesthesia in children. Anesth Analg 1989; 68: 654

75. Wedel DJ: Femoral and lateral femoral cutaneous nerve block for muscle biopsies in children. Anesth Analg 1989; 14: S63

76. Wedel DJ, Krohn JS, Hall J: Brachial plexus anesthesia in pediatric patients. Mayo Clin Proc 1991; 66: 583

77. Sapega A, Heppenstall RB, Chance B et al: Optimizing tourniquet application and release times in extremity surgery. J Bone Joint Surg Am 1985; 67: 303

78. Horlocker TT, Hebl JR, Gali B et al: Anesthetic, patient and surgical risk factors for neurologic complications following prolonged total tourniquet time during total knee arthroplasty. Anesth Analg 2006; 102: 950

79. Hamilton WK, Sokoll MD: Tourniquet paralysis. JAMA 1967; 199: 37

80. Patterson S, Klenerman L: The effect of pneumatic tourniquets on ultrastructure of skeletal muscle. J Bone Joint Surg Br 1979; 61: 178

81. Hurst LN, Weinglein O, Brown WF et al: The pneumatic tourniquet: A biomechanical and electrophysiological study. Plast Reconstr Surg 1981; 67: 648

82. Miller SH, Price G, Buck D et al: Effects of tourniquet ischemia and postischemic edema on muscle metabolism. J Hand Surg 1979; 4: 547

83. Heppenstall RB, Balderston R, Goodwin C: Pathophysiologic effects distal to a tourniquet in the dog. J Trauma 1979; 19: 234

84. Kadoi Y, Ide M, Saito S et al: Hyperventilation after tourniquet deflation prevents an increase in cerebral blood flow velocity. Can J Anaesth 1999; 46: 259

85. Bourke DL, Silberberg MS, Ortega R et al: Respiratory responses associated with release of intraoperative tourniquets. Anesth Analg 1989; 69: 541

86. Della Valle CJ, Jazrawi LM, Di Cesare PE et al: Paradoxical cerebral embolism complicating a major orthopaedic operation: A report of two cases. J Bone Joint Surg Am 1999; 81: 108

87. Valli H, Rosenberg PH: Effects of three anaesthetic methods on haemodynamic responses connected with the use of thigh tourniquets in orthopaedic patients. Acta Anaesthesiol Scand 1985; 29: 142

88. Hagenouw RPM, Bridenbaugh PO, van Egmond J et al: Tourniquet pain: A volunteer study. Anesth Analg 1986; 65: 1175

89. Parisi DM, Koval K, Egol K: Fat embolism syndrome. Am J Orthop 2002; 31: 507

90. Gurd AR: Fat embolism: An aid to diagnosis. J Bone Joint Surg Br 1970; 52: 732

91. Geerts WH, Pineo GF, Heit Jam Bergqvist D et al: Prevention of venous thromboembolism: The seventh ACCP conference on antithrombotic and thrombolytic therapy. Chest 2004; 126(3 Suppl): 338S

92. Callaghan JJ, Dorr LD, Engh GA et al: Prophylaxis for thromboembolic disease. J Arthroplasty 2005; 20: 273

93. Thorburn J, Louden JR, Vallance R: Spinal and general anaesthesia in total hip replacement: Frequency of deep vein thrombosis. Br J Anaesth 1980; 52: 1117

94. Donadoni R, Baele G, Devulder J et al: Coagulation and fibrinolytic parameters in patients undergoing total hip replacement: Influence of the anaesthesia technique. Acta Anaesthesiol Scand 1989; 33: 588

95. Davis FM, Laurenson VG, Gillespie WJ et al: Deep vein thrombosis after total hip replacement: A comparison between spinal and general anaesthesia. J Bone Joint Surg Br 1989; 71: 181

96. Sharrock NE, Haas SB, Hargett MJ et al: Effects of epidural anesthesia on the incidence of deep-vein thrombosis after total knee arthroplasty. J Bone Joint Surg Br 1991; 73: 502

97. Nielsen PT, Jorgensen LN, Albrecht-Beste E et al: Lower thrombosis risk with epidural blockade in knee arthroplasty. Acta Orthop Scand 1990; 61: 29

98. Simpson PJ, Radford SG, Forster SJ et al: The fibrinolytic effects of anaesthesia. Anaesthesia 1982; 37: 3

99. Tryba M: Epidural regional anesthesia and low molecular heparin: Pro [in German]. Anasthesiol Intensivmed Notfallmed Schmerzther 1993; 28: 179

100. Vandermeulen EP, Van Aken H, Vermylen J: Anticoagulants and spinal-epidural anesthesia. Anesth Analg 1994; 79: 1165

101. Horlocker TT, Wedel DJ: Neuraxial block and low molecular weight heparin: Balancing perioperative analgesia and thromboprophylaxis. Reg Anesth Pain Med 1998; 23: 164

102. Horlocker TT, Wedel DJ, Benzon H et al: Regional anesthesia in the anticoagulated patient: Defining the risks (the second ASRA consensus conference on neuraxial anesthesia and anticoagulation). Reg Anesth Pain Med 2003; 28: 172

CHAPTER 54 ■ TRANSPLANT ANESTHESIA

MARIE CSETE AND KATHRYN GLAS

ANESTHESIA FOR SURGICAL SUBSPECIALTIES

KEY POINTS

1 Brain death is declared when the clinical picture is consistent with irreversible cessation of all brain function.

2 The mainstay of donor management is maintenance of euvolemia, oxygenation, perfusion, and normothermia.

3 Donor organs once considered marginal are increasingly used for kidney, liver, lung, and heart transplantation because of severe organ shortages.

4 Living kidney donors must be healthy and without significant cardiopulmonary, neurologic, or psychiatric disease, diabetes, obesity, or hypertension.

5 Immune suppression is associated with severe, life-threatening infections (including recurrent hepatitis after liver transplantation), increased risk of tumors, and progressive vascular disease.

6 Renal transplant recipients are often anemic, with hyperdynamic cardiac indices.

7 For renal transplantation, the major anesthetic consideration is maintenance of renal blood flow. Typical hemodynamic goals during transplant are systolic pressure >90 mm Hg, mean systemic pressure >60 mm Hg, and central venous pressure >10 mm Hg.

8 Patients with end-stage liver disease have multisystem dysfunction with common cardiac, pulmonary, and renal compromise because of their liver disease.

9 Liver transplantation is traditionally described in three phases: dissection, anhepatic, and neohepatic, with reperfusion.

10 Intraoperative management of lung transplant patients should focus on fluid and ventilatory strategies designed to minimize acute lung injury and primary graft dysfunction.

11 Maintenance of normal preload and afterload is critical in patients with a left ventricular assist device to ensure maximal device function.

12 Heart transplant patients are at risk for right ventricular dysfunction of the donor heart if the recipient presented with pulmonary hypertension.

13 For all transplant recipients, antibiotic, antiviral, antifungal, and immune suppression regimens should be disrupted as little as possible in the perioperative period.

Transplantation is a growth industry in developed countries, and is increasingly performed worldwide. About 100,000 patients are on solid-organ transplant waiting lists in the United States. As transplant waiting lists grew, organ donation did not keep pace to meet demand. Consequently, living-related organ donation is increasingly common, although this is also insufficient to meet the need. Increasingly, use of donor organs once considered marginal is on the rise, complicating the anesthetic management of organ recipients. The transplant community has also responded to the disparity between need

and availability of organs by re-examining the scoring systems that prioritize recipients for transplantation. For example, kidneys from deceased donors are currently not allocated in a national, integrated system, and the kidney allocation practices may soon change in an attempt to equalize waiting times across the country, reduce organ waste, and provide organs for patients with longest expected life spans after transplant.

The United Network of Organ Sharing (UNOS; www. unos.org) is an important source of information related to organ transplantation for patients and for physicians. UNOS was created by the 1984 National Organ Transplant Act to operate the organ procurement and transplant network for efficient and equitable distribution of donated organs. To address local concerns and optimize organ allocation, the United States is divided into 11 regions for purposes of organ distribution, each with its own regional review board. Within each region, organ procurement organizations coordinate organ retrieval for local transplant centers. A second important source of transplant statistics is the Scientific Registry of Transplant Recipients (www.ustransplant.org). U.S. centers performed 27,527 transplants in 2005, and almost 200,000 Americans are living with transplanted organs.

Anesthesiologists are involved in the care of organ donors, perioperative management of transplant recipients, and, in major transplant centers, anesthesiologists with special expertise actively participate in the preoperative assessment and optimization of patients for major organ transplant procedures. Solid-organ transplantation is also a critical component of many anesthesia training programs.

ANESTHETIC MANAGEMENT OF ORGAN DONORS

Brain-Dead Donors

Brain-dead, heart-beating donors present challenging management issues because collected experience in a single center is usually small. Brain death is declared when the clinical picture is consistent with irreversible cessation of all brain function.[1] Legal and medical brain death criteria differ from state to state, but all require cessation of both cerebral and brainstem function. Physicians involved in the transplant recipient process should not be involved in declaration of brain death of the donor. Potentially reversible causes of coma or unresponsiveness must be ruled out (hypothermia, hypotension, drugs, toxins) before declaration of brain death. Flat electroencephalogram is consistent with brain death. Brain-dead donors are unresponsive to sensory stimuli and have no brainstem reflexes, including ventilatory drive with apnea testing. Transcranial Doppler and traditional or isotope angiography are used to confirm the clinical examination and lack of blood flow to the brain.[2] Brain-dead patients may have intact spinal reflexes, and so may require neuromuscular blockade during organ procurement.

Brain death is associated with hemodynamic instability, hormonal chaos, systemic inflammation, and oxidant stress, all of which may negatively impact donor organ function.[3] Just after brain death, adrenergic surges can cause ischemia and ischemia-reperfusion injuries. Recent studies of head trauma patients suggest that the onset of brain death is associated with a transient period of hypotension with increased cardiac index and tissue perfusion. During this period, vasoactive drugs administered to increase blood pressure can cause rapid circulatory deterioration.[4] This period precedes the autonomic storm associated with herniation of the brain, and emphasizes the wide dynamic swings in molecular mediators and hemodynamics after brain death. The timing of therapies to support hemodynamics is difficult as catecholamine storm is often followed quickly by pituitary failure. Once pituitary failure ensues, hormone therapy may help stabilize patients hemodynamically and therefore extend the donor pool.[5] However, only some,[6,7] but not all,[8] studies suggest that hormone therapy of the donor improves graft function. Cardiac graft function is likely improved by donor hormone therapy.[9] A typical regimen is tri-iodothyronine (4 μg intravenously then 3 μg/hr); methylprednisolone, 15 mg/kg intravenously every 24 hours; desmopressin, 1 U then 0.5 to 4 U/hr to maintain systemic vascular resistance (SVR) at 800 to 1,200 dyne/s/cm[5] (and reduce

the polyuria of diabetes insipidus); and insulin infusion to maintain blood glucose 120 to 180 mg/dL.[10] Other medications that should be available for the donor operation are broad-spectrum antibiotics, mannitol and loop diuretics, heparin, and norepinephrine.

Anesthetic management during organ harvest is guided by the needs of the procurement teams, who may come from several centers, and have discrepant requests, depending on the organs procured. UNOS has created a resource for managing organ donors, in an effort to improve donor care, and therefore the function of donated organs.[a]

The mainstay of donor management is maintenance of euvolemia; therefore, central venous pressure (CVP) monitoring is standard. CVP is maintained at 6 to 12 mm Hg, and when pulmonary artery (PA) catheters are used to assess cardiac function, pulmonary capillary wedge pressure is maintained at <12 mm Hg. The goals of volume and hormonal therapies are to minimize the use of vasopressors as use of high-dose dopamine is associated with renal graft failure.[8] Efforts should be made to maintain serum sodium levels below 155 mmol/L; higher levels are associated with poor liver graft function.[11] Generally, packed cells are used to maintain hematocrit of 30%, and fresh-frozen plasma (FFP) to maintain the international normalized ratio (INR) <1.5, although these practices are not evidence-based. Surgeons procuring the lungs will want to keep CVP low, and diuretics may be requested just prior to collection of the lungs, whereas surgeons procuring kidneys usually want high filling pressures. Obviously, the job of the anesthesiologist is to maintain donor oxygenation, perfusion, and normothermia, but the precise end points of therapy require coordination and communication with the various procurement teams. Generally arterial pCO_2 is maintained at 30 to 35 mm Hg. Transport of ventilated patients often requires positive end-expiratory pressure (PEEP) valves attached to the Ambu bag to maintain oxygenation of the donor. Peak airway pressures should be kept below 30 mm Hg.

Prior to lung removal, surgeons will perform bronchoscopy. An adapter, such as the Portex fiberoptic bronchoscopic swivel adapter (SIMS Portex, Inc., Keene, NH), facilitates ventilation during the procedure. Glucocorticoids are usually administered, and on occasion, prostaglandin E_1 is requested to improve circulation of the lung preservation solution. Surgical techniques have been developed to allow three recipients from one thoracic donor: two single lung transplants and a heart transplant.[12] The heart is removed first, leaving a small cuff of left atrium attached to the lungs. The harvesting team will ask for systemic heparinization just prior to exsanguination and excision. Cardioplegia is administered, the heart stops ejecting, and the heart is removed. The trachea is transected and the lungs are removed en bloc for later separation.

Donor lungs are more susceptible to injury in brain-dead patients before procurement than are other organs, likely from contusion, aspiration, or edema with fluid resuscitation. Consequently, many multiorgan donors do not meet the current strict criteria for lung donors. These criteria are listed in Table 54-1. A recent review published by the Pulmonary Council of the International Society for Heart and Lung Transplantation discusses the evidence (or lack thereof), for these criteria.[13] Lungs once considered marginal are being used increasingly because of this severe shortage of donor lungs. Exclusion of donors based on arterial blood gas[14] or chest roentgenogram (CXR)[13] (Table 54-1) is based on small single-center trials. With experience, lung transplantation using donors outside these boundaries does not negatively impact the recipient, and most centers rely on bronchoscopy to determine lung suitability for transplantation.[15]

---

[a]See the Critical Pathway for the adult or Pediatric Organ Donor at http://www.unos.org/resources/donorManagement.asp?index=2.

TABLE 54-1

IDEAL DECEASED LUNG DONOR

Age younger than 55 years
ABO compatibility
Clear chest radiograph
PaO_2 >300 on FIO_2 1.0, PEEP 5 cm H_2O
Tobacco history <20 pack-years
Absence of chest trauma
No evidence of aspiration or sepsis
Negative sputum Gram stain
Absence of purulent secretions at bronchoscopy

PEEP, positive end-expiratory pressure.
Adapted from www.unos.org.

Sputum Gram stains and cultures are routinely obtained on all lung donors. A positive Gram stain does not seem to impact outcome; however, organisms on bronchoalveolar lavage are associated with decreased survival.[16] One study suggested that evidence of aspiration seen on bronchoscopy, bilateral pulmonary infiltrates, or persistent purulent secretions are criteria for donor exclusion.[17] There is also uniform agreement that advanced donor age (>55 years) together with long ischemic time (>6 hours) are associated with poor transplant outcome. In addition to the usual hematologic criteria, donor-recipient compatibility is based on height and/or total lung capacity.

Mortality on the heart transplant waiting list is 15%, compounded by a donor "yield" of only 42%, prompting a consensus conference in 2002 to improve evaluation and utilization of cardiac donor organs.[18] The ideal heart donor is <50 years old and is hemodynamically stable. Presence of major chest trauma, cardiac disease, active infection, prolonged cardiac arrest, malignancy, human immunodeficiency virus or hepatitis, or intracardiac injections moves the donor from ideal to marginal status. Overall health status of the donor prior to determination of brain death can facilitate a directed laboratory evaluation. Electrocardiogram (ECG) is often abnormal in the setting of brain injury/death, and further evaluation with transthoracic echocardiography is often necessary. Cardiac catheterization is sometimes requested in older donors and those with significant personal or family history of coronary artery disease. In recipients with pulmonary hypertension, younger donors, short ischemic time, low donor inotrope requirement, and oversized organs are preferred.

③ A shortage of available donors has led to increased use of marginal donors and separate alternate transplant lists for recipients willing to accept marginal donors. Increased risk of primary graft dysfunction (PGD) is the main reason for avoiding marginal donors. Marginal donors are typically used for patients who do not meet the standard recipient criteria, with advanced age most often the reason for alternative listing. The most common donor factors that lead to marginal status are abnormal hepatitis screening tests, left ventricular dysfunction, or coronary artery disease. In selected recipients, these kinds of marginal donors can be used without increasing the incidence of PGD.[19]

Donation After Cardiac Death

The criteria for death of donation after cardiac death (DCD) donors (previously called non–heart-beating donors) are distinct from those of brain-dead donors. DCD donors typically have severe whole-brain dysfunction but have electrical activity in the brain. Death is defined by cessation of circulation and

respiration. Life support measures are used to control the timing of death and organ procurement, to maximize the function of organs from these donors. Based in part on a study by the Institute of Medicine,[20] the American Society of Anesthesiologists (ASA) developed a reference document for management of DCD patients[b] but every hospital must develop its own protocols reflecting local constraints. Optimally, end-of-life care is provided by the same medical team responsible for the care of the patient in the intensive care unit (ICU).[21] Anesthesiologists do not necessarily have to be involved in DCD donor management, even when withdrawal of care occurs in the operating room (OR). The main principles for institutional guidelines are outlined in the ASA report and include the following: The decision to withdraw care must be made prior to and independent of any discussion about organ donation. Suitable DCD donors are those in whom death is anticipated within 1 to 2 hours of withdrawal of life support. Informed consent is required for organ donation and for any preorgan recovery procedures such as drug administration or vascular cannulation. A plan for the donor's care should be in place if the patient does not die within the anticipated time frame. Circulation and respiration must be absent for 2 minutes before the start of organ recovery. Generally when organ recovery is started more than 5 minutes after respiratory and circulatory arrest, the donated organ quality is compromised. Obviously, detailed protocols for interactions with family members of the donor, transplant teams, organ procurement organizations, and OR personnel must be established before DCD is considered.

According to the Organ Procurement and Transplantation Network, the number of organs retrieved from DCD donors is increasing, with 647 DCD donors providing 1,366 transplanted organs in 2006 (Fig. 54-1). The benchmark set by the Department of Health and Human Services is 6,000 organs transplanted from DCD donors in 2013. Kidneys are most commonly recovered from DCD donors, but increasingly livers and islets, and even lungs, are being recovered.[22–24] The University of Wisconsin has been a leader in DCD donation, and a substantial percentage of their grafts are recovered from DCD donors. Furthermore, they developed tools to help centers with less experience in identifying appropriate DCD donors.[25] Pediatric DCD donors have also been sources of good-quality grafts.[26] Although DCD donors extend the donor pool, they are associated with increased complications, decreased graft survival, and increased cost of transplantation.[27] Optimal medical (anticoagulants and vasodilators) and surgical (flush, preservation solution) approaches to DCD are not yet optimized, so that protocols for DCD will change depending on research progress.[28]

Living Kidney Donors

④ Safety and comfort are the primary considerations in the care of living donors. Living donors must be healthy and without significant cardiopulmonary, neurologic, or psychiatric disease, diabetes, obesity, or hypertension. Renal function must be normal, with no history of renal stones or proteinuria. Historically, open nephrectomy is being progressively replaced by laparoscopic donor nephrectomy, which is easier on the donor in terms of comfort and hospital length of stay. For open nephrectomy, the patient is positioned in the lateral decubitus position with the bed flexed to expose and arch the flank. After the open procedure, donors usually require postoperative patient-controlled opioid analgesia for at least a day. Donors are generally managed with general anesthesia, but epidural

[b]http://www.asahq.org/clinical/OrganDonationsamplepolicy.pdf.

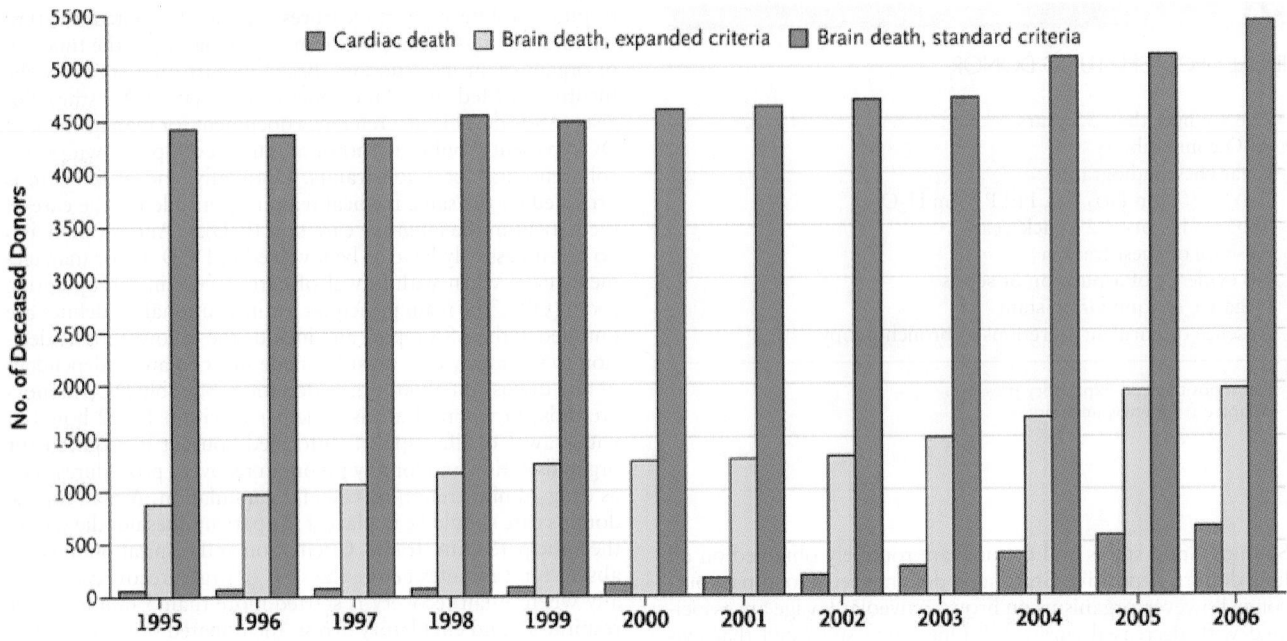

FIGURE 54-1.   Distribution of deceased organ donors in the United States, 1995–2006. Data from the Organ Procurement and Transplantation Network.

and combined epidural-spinal techniques (supplemented with intravenous propofol) have also been used successfully.[29]

Probably because of a learning curve with laparoscopic donor nephrectomies, longer anesthetics (and therefore longer period of reduced renal perfusion) have been blamed for a greater compromise of postoperative renal function after laparoscopic donation than after open nephrectomy.[30] Both anesthetics and insufflation of the peritoneum with CO_2 decrease renal blood flow so that fluid repletion is important to maintaining renal perfusion. For this reason, patients undergoing the laparoscopic procedure often receive more fluids than open nephrectomy donors.[31] A reasonable protocol is to administer crystalloid at 10 mL/kg/hr above calculated losses and to maintain urine output at about 100 mL/hour[32]; however, local protocols may titrate fluids to a CVP end point. Nitrous oxide is contraindicated for laparoscopic donor nephrectomy because bowel distention can impede the surgery.[33] For patient comfort, central venous lines are generally placed after induction of anesthesia.

Donor nephrectomy should be an uncomplicated procedure and donor tracheas can be extubated in the OR. Patient-controlled analgesia is common after donor surgery. Some centers admit donors to a step-down or medical ICU for a day after surgery, but the total hospital stay is usually only 2 to 4 days. Bladder catheters are removed on postoperative day 1. Patients should be advised that full recovery (i.e., feeling normal) takes 4 to 6 weeks. Complications after living donor nephrectomy include atelectasis of the lungs, pneumothorax, dysrhythmias, wound pain or infection, urinary tract infection, and mental status changes.[34] Fortunately, perioperative mortality is rare but cannot be denied as a possible outcome during preoperative patient discussions.[35]

Living Liver Donors

Left lobe liver donation is usually done in the context of parent-to-child donation. Although left lateral segmentectomy is a big operation, it is generally well tolerated (Fig. 54-2). Nonetheless, living liver donors must be healthy, and without a history or risk for thromboembolic disease. By comparison, donor right lobectomy needed for adult-to-adult liver transplantation is a major procedure and carries significant risk (Fig. 54-3). Mortality of right liver resection for donation is estimated at 0.3 to 1%.[36] Significant morbidity has been reported for this surgery, including air embolism, atelectasis, and pneumonia,[37] and biliary tract damage. An estimated 3.2% of donors in experienced centers suffer major complications.[38]

Large liver resections may require virtually complete hepatic venous exclusion (cross-clamping of the hepatic pedicle usually without cava clamping). Not unexpectedly, venous return falls by about 50%. Without the collaterals developed by patients with chronic liver disease, normal donors may experience significant hypotension when the hepatic pedicle is cross-clamped. Blood pressure is maintained largely through reflex increases in endogenous vasopressin and norepinephrine levels.[39] For these reasons, volume loading is reasonable prior to clamping. However, some authors argue that blood loss is reduced if the CVP is low during resections.[40,41] Sufficiently powered studies to prove that the benefits of low CVP (reduced transfusion requirements) outweigh risks (renal compromise, air embolism) are unlikely to be performed, and institutional practices vary widely. If vasopressors are needed, vasopressin and norepinephrine are reasonable choices to enhance normal endogenous reflexes. Isovolemic hemodilution has been reported to reduce allogeneic red cell requirements in major hepatic resections.[42] At experienced centers, blood loss is usually <1 L, with 20 to 40% of donors requiring transfusion.[43–45] Blood salvage is useful, and some centers offer autologous donation programs for donors; both can reduce the need for allogeneic blood transfusions.[46] Transesophageal echocardiography (TEE), if expertise is available, is ideal and may obviate central lines placement. Most donor tracheas can be extubated safely in the OR. Hypothermia is a preventable reason for not extubating in the OR.

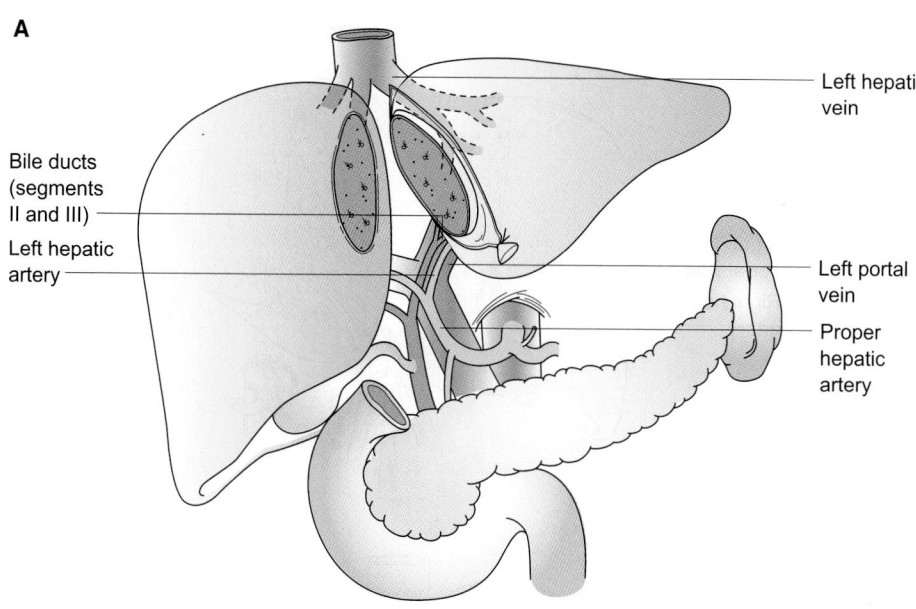

A

Left hepatic vein

Bile ducts (segments II and III)

Left hepatic artery

Left portal vein

Proper hepatic artery

FIGURE 54-2. Left lateral segment (segments II and III) living donor transplantation. **A.** Donor operation. **B.** Recipient operation complete.

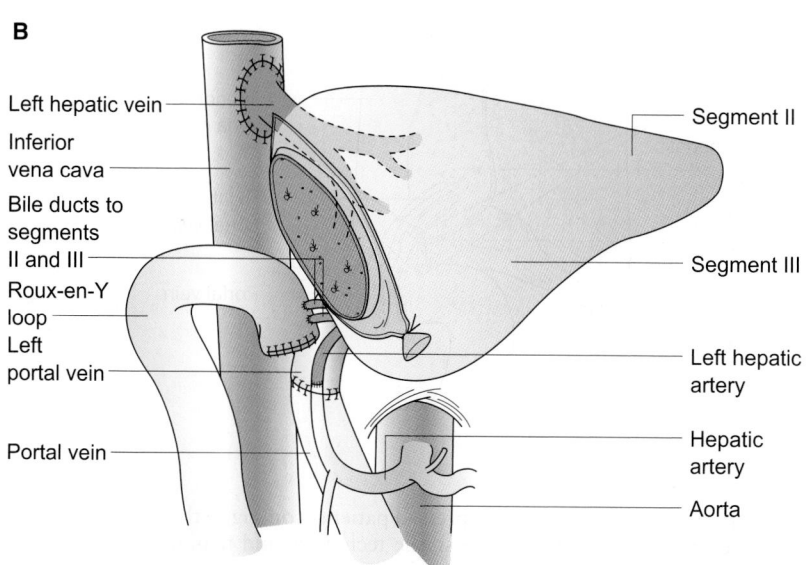

B

Left hepatic vein

Inferior vena cava

Bile ducts to segments II and III

Roux-en-Y loop

Left portal vein

Portal vein

Segment II

Segment III

Left hepatic artery

Hepatic artery

Aorta

ANESTHESIA FOR SURGICAL SUBSPECIALTIES

Postoperative pain management in these patients is a matter of controversy (see Chapter 57). Some institutions successfully place epidural catheters, providing excellent analgesia without reported complications. However, with right liver resection, INR rises significantly after surgery, peaking a few days after surgery along with a fall in platelet counts, just when the catheter is usually removed.[47,48] For this reason, many centers will not place epidural catheters in right liver donors, and rely on intravenous patient-controlled analgesia to manage postoperative pain. Laparoscopic liver resection of left liver grafts is a recent innovation[49] also recently applied to living right lobe donation.[50]

Living Lung Donors

Since 1998, UNOS has recorded 467 living donor lung transplants, but the practice seems to be declining in the United States, with only 6 in the past 3 years. Living donor lobar lung transplantation is typically reserved for critically ill recipients who are unlikely to survive until a brain-dead donor organ is available. Given this, as in all living donors, the inherently coercive conditions imposed on donors with a relationship to

the recipient must be balanced by staged consent, allowing donors numerous chances to review the procedure and withdraw from the donation process. Selection criteria for living lung donors are listed in Table 54-2.[51] No donor mortality has

TABLE 54-2

LIVING LUNG DONOR CRITERIA

Member of recipient's extended family
Age 18–55 years
No prior thoracic surgery on donor side
Good general health
Taller than recipient preferred
ABO compatible
FVC and FEV$_1$ >85% predicted
PO$_2$ >80 mm Hg on room air
No chronic viral diseases
Normal electrocardiogram and echocardiogram
Normal stress test in donors older than 40 years old

FVC, forced vital capacity; FEV$_1$, forced expiratory volume in 1 second. Adapted from www.unos.org.

FIGURE 54-3.   Right lobe (segments V to VIII) living donor transplantation. **A.** Donor operation. **B.** Recipient operation completed.

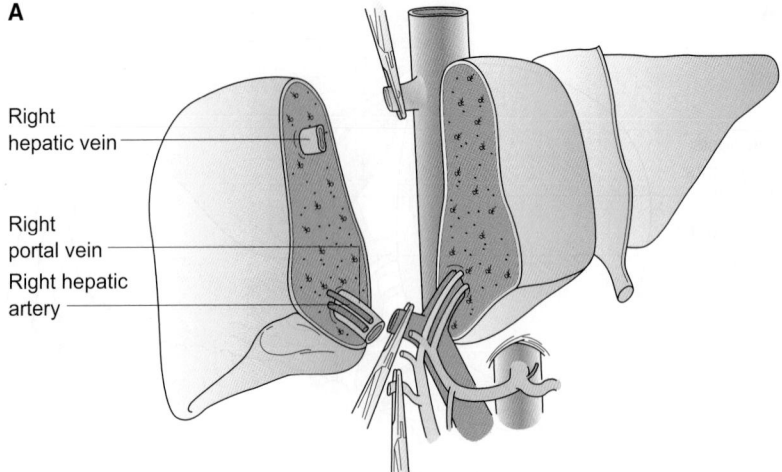

Right
hepatic vein

Right
portal vein

Right hepatic
artery

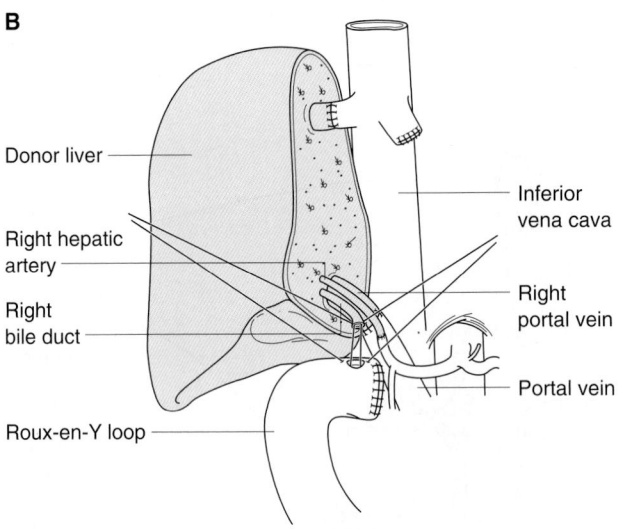

Donor liver

Right hepatic
artery

Right
bile duct

Roux-en-Y loop

Inferior
vena cava

Right
portal vein

Portal vein

been reported to date, and morbidity remains low. If two donors are used for one recipient, scheduling difficulties are considerable: The surgical procedure is performed in three ORs simultaneously, one for each donor and the recipient. Donors are generally managed with general anesthesia and epidural analgesia.

IMMUNOSUPPRESSIVE DRUGS

Pharmacologic suppression of the immune response to allografts is associated with major side effects. Considerable variability in intestinal absorption, and genetic and induced differences in metabolism of these drugs, and changing requirements with aging, all mandate individualization of immunosuppressive regimens. Immunosuppressed patients who are undertreated can reject a donor organ. All immunosuppression regimens carry major risks: infection, malignancy, and progressive vascular disease. Immunosuppression regimens differ considerably from center to center, and anesthesiologists must communicate with the transplant team to obtain the schedule and dose of immunosuppressive agents used for each patient. It is particularly important to review drug regimens with transplant coordinators when posttransplant patients are scheduled for surgery because the transplant team needs information about peak and trough drug levels that may not be accessible on the hospital record.

Immune-suppressed patients coming to the OR deserve special attention to sterile technique and maintenance of antibiotic/antifungal/antiviral regimens during the perioperative period. Complications of immunosuppression are summarized in Table 54-3.

TABLE 54-3

COMPLICATIONS OF CHRONIC IMMUNE SUPPRESSION

■ SYSTEM	■ COMPLICATION
Central nervous system	Lowered seizure threshold
Cardiovascular	Diabetes
	Hypertension
	Hyperlipidemia
	Atherosclerosis
Renal/electrolyte	Decreased glomerular filtration rate
	Hyperkalemia
	Hypomagnesemia
Hematologic/immune	Increased risk of infections
	Increased risk of malignancy
	Pancytopenia
Endocrine/other	Osteoporosis
	Poor wound healing

Calcineurin Inhibitors

The modern transplant era began with the introduction of the calcineurin inhibitor, *cyclosporine*, into clinical practice. Calcineurin inhibitors are still a mainstay of immunosuppression for solid-organ transplant recipients. *Tacrolimus* (FK-506) has been particularly important for kidney transplant recipients because of its potency in preventing acute rejection (within 6 months of transplantation), long-term graft survival, and relative lack of side effects compared with historic regimens.[52] Inhibition of calcineurin, among other effects, modifies NFAT (nuclear factor of activated T cells) and frees nuclear factor-kappa B to translocate to the nucleus, where it enhances transcription of T-cell interleukin-2 (IL-2).[53] These drugs, then, inhibit T-lymphocyte differentiation and cytokine elaboration.

Calcineurin is involved in diverse cellular processes in addition to immune function; therefore, inhibition of calcineurin has many significant side effects. These include hypertension (often requiring therapy), hyperlipidemia, ischemic vascular disease (including in heart recipients), diabetes, and nephrotoxicity.[54] Cyclosporine causes acute nephropathy, which is usually reversible with drug cessation, but chronic renal damage from cyclosporine is a more refractory problem[55]; hence, the introduction of cyclosporine-sparing immunosuppressive regimens. Ischemic cardiac disease is the leading cause of death of kidney transplant recipients, in part because of underlying disease that preceded transplantation, but calcineurin inhibitors can exacerbate risk factors for coronary artery disease.[56] It is important to note that end-stage liver disease (ESLD) does not confer protection from coronary artery disease, and liver transplant patients are also at risk for progression of ischemic cardiac disease after transplantation. Central neurologic side effects are also common with calcineurin inhibitors, and tacrolimus-induced polyneuropathy was recently reported.[57] Most side effects are dose-related, and patients typically require ongoing dosage adjustment after transplantation. Tacrolimus is metabolized by cytochrome P450 3A4 and causes its up-regulation.[58] When immunosuppression is interrupted by surgery or when multiple potentially interacting drugs are used, tacrolimus trough levels should be reassessed.

Cyclosporine may rarely prolong the action of pancuronium.[59,60] Cyclosporine increases minimum alveolar concentration in rats, but similar studies have not been reported in humans.[61] To switch from oral to intravenous dosing of cyclosporine, usually about one-third the oral dose is used. Usual doses of tacrolimus are 0.15 to 0.3 mg/kg/day given in two doses. To switch from oral to intravenous tacrolimus, a starting dose of about one-tenth the oral dose can be used.

Corticosteroids

Corticosteroids disrupt expression of many cytokines in T cells, antigen-presenting cells, and macrophages. These drugs are used both for maintenance immunosuppression and in pulse dosing for acute rejection. Especially for children, corticosteroid-sparing regimens are increasingly popular because growth is negatively affected by steroids and because the drugs are generally not tolerated well. Well-known side effects are hypertension, diabetes, hyperlipidemia, weight gain (including Cushingoid features), and gastrointestinal ulceration (see Chapter 49). Patients receiving chronic steroid therapy do not necessarily require large doses of perioperative steroids to cover their stress response, especially for small or local surgical procedures.[62] Again, communication with the transplant service is important in determining steroid coverage that least impacts the delicate balance of immunosuppression. Steroids are generally withheld during liver transplantation in recipients with hepatitis C, because of concern that they contribute to hepatitis C recurrence.[63]

Monoclonal and Polyclonal Antibodies

OKT3 antibody is directed against a component of the T-cell receptor complex and affects immunosuppression by blocking T-cell function. Acute administration of OKT3 in awake patients (especially first administration) may result in generalized weakness, fever, chills, and some hypotension. More severe hypotension, bronchospasm, and pulmonary edema have been reported.[64] Formulations of OKT3 may require syringe filtering before administration.

"Humanized" antibodies are used with increasing frequency. These are antibodies engineered to contain human constant regions in the immunoglobulin protein, so that patients do not develop an antimouse immunologic response against a purely mouse antibody. Muromonab-CD3 is a humanized form of OKT3, usually used for acute rejection. Basiliximab and daclizumab are newer humanized antibodies. These antibodies are both directed against a portion of the IL-2 receptor and work by blocking IL-2–mediated T-cell activation. Gastrointestinal upset is the most commonly cited side effect of these drugs. However, basiliximab has been implicated in causing pulmonary edema in young renal transplant patients.[65]

Polyclonal antibodies (directed against more than one protein epitope) include *antithymocyte globulin*, used to deplete T cells from the circulation. Side effects include serum sickness (treatable with plasmapheresis),[66] leukopenia and thrombocytopenia, and fever.

Tolerance of organ grafts without pharmacologic immunosuppression is possible using combined bone marrow and solid-organ transplants, with marrow and the solid organ derived from the same donor,[67] obviously not possible in many patients now. Nonetheless, patients with marrow chimerism who tolerate their grafts[68] can provide insights into transplant immunology that may lead to novel cellular and pharmacologic approaches to immunosuppression.

Other Immunosuppressive Drugs

mTOR (*mammalian target of rapamycin*) *inhibitors* are often used in combination with calcineurin inhibitors to decrease the complications of dose-related side effects ("calcineurin-sparing regimens") such as nephrotoxicity.[69] TOR is involved in complex signaling processes that promote synthesis of proteins, including several that regulate cellular proliferation. Thus, mTOR inhibitors such as rapamycin (sirolimus) are antiproliferative, used both in immunosuppression and increasingly in cancer therapies. Similar to cyclosporine and tacrolimus, sirolimus is metabolized in liver via P450CYP3A isoenzymes, but coadministration of sirolimus and a calcineurin inhibitor does not increase calcineurin inhibitor drug requirements. In fact, the combination may be synergistic.[70] Diltiazem raises the plasma concentration of sirolimus.[58] Sirolimus use is associated with poor wound healing.[71]

Azathioprine is hydrolyzed in blood to 6-mercaptopurine, a purine analog and metabolite with the ability to incorporate into DNA during the S phase of the cell cycle. Because DNA synthesis is a necessary prerequisite to mitosis, azathioprine exerts an antiproliferative effect. Antiproliferative drugs rely on the fact that immune activation implies explosive proliferation of lymphocytes. Side effects occur because other proliferating cells (gastrointestinal tract, bone marrow) are also affected. Repression of bone marrow cell cycling can cause pancytopenia. Cardiac arrest and severe upper airway edema are rare complications.[72] The intravenous dose is about half the oral dose.

TABLE 54-4

COMMON CAUSES OF RENAL FAILURE IN ADULT RENAL
TRANSPLANT RECIPIENTS

■ DIAGNOSIS	■ % OF PATIENTS ON LIST
Type 2 diabetes	21.7
Hypertensive nephrosclerosis	19.4
Retransplant/graft failure	8.7
Polycystic kidney disease	5.9
Type 1 diabetes	5.0
Focal glomerular sclerosis	4.7
Systemic lupus erythematosus	2.9
Chronic glomerulonephritis	2.9
Malignant hypertension	2.6
Immunoglobulin A nephropathy	2.4

Adapted from unos.org.

Mycophenolate mofetil is metabolized into a molecule that inhibits purine synthesis. It too can cause leukopenia and thrombocytopenia as side effects, as well as red cell aplasia,[73] and mycophenolate mofetil is teratogenic.[74] The usual oral dose is 1 to 1.5 g 2 times a day.

RENAL TRANSPLANTATION

Preoperative Considerations

In 2006 in the United States, 17,093 kidney transplants were performed, 38% from living donors. More than 5,000 patients were added to U.S. renal transplant waiting lists that year, so that more than 70,000 patients were listed at year's end, and mortality on the waiting list was 7%.[c] An enormous variety of diseases are treated with renal transplants (Table 54-4). Many of these underlying diagnoses are also risk factors for coronary artery disease, so preoperative evaluation is focused on cardiovascular function.

About half the mortality of patients on dialysis is due to heart failure,[75] and cardiovascular complications are a leading cause of death after renal transplantation. Therefore, cardiovascular risk factor modification is imperative before and after transplantation.[76] Obesity by itself is not a risk factor for renal graft dysfunction, but does contribute to lower survival after transplantation; malnourished, underweight patients are also at substantial increased risk of death after transplantation.[77] Renal transplant recipients are often anemic, with hyperdynamic cardiac indices. Patients older than 50 years (with or without risk factors for coronary disease) are generally screened with exercise or pharmacologic cardiac stress tests. The interval at which these studies are repeated in patients listed for transplantation varies from center to center. Peripheral vascular disease should also be assessed. Pulmonary function tests (PFTs) should be reviewed by anesthesiologists prior to transplantation (see Chapter 11). PFTs are particularly important in type I diabetics who often present with reduced lung volumes and diffusing capacity. The precise cause of abnormal PFTs in these patients is not known, but recent clinical studies suggest that long-term normoglycemia after kidney/pancreas transplantation is associated with improved

pulmonary function.[78] Hypercoagulable states are common in patients with renal disease and deserve detailed evaluation so that they can be managed perioperatively.[79]

All solid-organ transplant patients are screened for tumors (mammography, Pap test, colonoscopy, prostate-specific antigen) and infection (dental evaluation, viral serologies). Patients should have good control of their diabetes before transplantation and have an evaluation for psychiatric stability and social support. Severe heart, lung, or liver disease, most malignancies, and active or untreatable infections such as tuberculosis are exclusion criteria for renal transplantation.

Dialysis-dependent patients should be dialyzed before surgery. Cadaveric grafts can be safely transplanted after 24 hours of cold ischemia time, and potentially after 36 hours, allowing scheduling of preoperative dialysis. With preoperative dialysis, severe hyperkalemia during surgery is unusual.

Intraoperative Protocols

Renal transplantation is generally done under general anesthesia. Small studies have suggested good outcomes with epidural anesthesia[80] but concerns over uremic platelet dysfunction and residual heparin from preoperative dialysis have limited use of regional anesthesia for kidney transplantation. Rapid-sequence induction is indicated in diabetic patients with gastroparesis[81] (preceded by oral sodium bicitrate). Anemic, hyperdynamic patients may have higher dose requirements for induction agents such as propofol.[82] Rocuronium is useful for patients in whom rapid-sequence induction is indicated, but the duration of block is variable in patients with end-stage renal disease (ESRD).[83] Similarly, plasma clearance of rapacuronium is reduced with renal failure, but titration of dose to neuromuscular blockade monitoring end points prevents delayed recovery.[84] Before incision, antibiotics are given. A central venous catheter (usually triple lumen) is placed for CVP monitoring and drug administration, and a bladder catheter is placed.

Incision is usually in the lower right abdomen to facilitate placement of the graft in the iliac fossa. The recipient iliac artery and vein are used for graft vascularization, followed by connection of the ureter to the recipient bladder. If the kidney is too large for the iliac fossa, it can be positioned in the retroperitoneal space; iliac vessels may be used for anastomoses, or the aorta and inferior vena cava may be required.

The major anesthetic consideration is maintenance of renal blood flow. No data are available to determine whether inhaled versus intravenous techniques are better at preserving (graft) renal flow. Similarly, the choice of inhaled gas has not been shown to significantly impact posttransplant renal function.[85] Hypertensive renal transplant patients often require antihypertensive drugs perioperatively. Calcium channel blockers have been best studied for renal protection of cyclosporine-treated hypertensive transplant patients, but after surgery, angiotensin-converting enzyme inhibitors and α-blockers may be as effective as calcium channel blockers.[86] Typical hemodynamic goals during transplant are systolic pressure >90 mm Hg, mean systemic pressure >60 mm Hg, and CVP >10 mm Hg. These goals are usually achievable without vasopressors, using isotonic fluids and adjustment of anesthetic doses. Hemodynamic management varies widely from center to center, so that close communication between surgeon and anesthesiologist is imperative. If rapid resuscitation of intravascular volume depletion is needed, low-molecular-weight hydroxyethyl starch is generally recommended by nephrologists and does not compromise coagulation if <33 mL/kg are given.[87] Neuromuscular blockade is safely accomplished with cis-atracurium.

Once the first anastomosis is started, diuresis is initiated (both mannitol and furosemide are often given). Heparin and verapamil should also be available in the OR, and in some centers, anesthesiologists are asked to administer the first doses of immunosuppression. A kidney graft is defective in concentrating urine and reabsorbing sodium, so attention to electrolytes is important. For patients with diabetes, intraoperative administration of insulin to normalize blood glucose has not been formally studied for improving outcome. However, more recent studies in ICU patients suggest that outcome is significantly improved when glucose is tightly controlled,[88] and tighter glucose control after kidney transplant is associated with less rejection[89] although cause and effect here are difficult to interpret. Nonetheless, tight blood glucose control (80 to 110 mg/dL) is a reasonable anesthetic goal during renal transplantation.

Transfusion is rarely required in the OR, although renal transplant patients are often anemic coming to surgery (and may be receiving erythropoietin). Because of immunosuppression, if cytomegalovirus (CMV)-negative patients receiving a CMV-negative organ are to receive transfusion, CMV-negative blood is preferred. Leukocyte filters are also effective in preventing CMV transmission but are probably inferior to CMV-negative blood.[90] For crystalloid, Plasmalyte is superior to either Ringer lactate or normal saline in maintaining acid-base balance in patients with ESRD.[91] Dopamine was once commonly used for maintaining renal function during kidney transplants, and small studies show improved renal plasma flow and urine output with low-dose dopamine in the early posttransplant period.[92] However, reviews of the literature suggest that dopamine does not reliably improve renal function in this setting, and should not be used.[93] The selective DA1 agonist, fenoldopam, is used to preserve renal function during kidney transplantation in some centers[94] but is expensive and has not been extensively studied. The entire surgery should take about 3 hours.

Most surgical complications of renal transplantation are not recognized in the OR. The common postoperative complications are ureteral obstruction and fistulae, vascular thromboses, lymphoceles, wound complications,[95] and bleeding. Rare complications from self-retaining retractors are bowel perforation and femoral neuropathy.[96] Patient-controlled analgesia is a good choice for postoperative pain management. Nonsteroidal anti-inflammatory agents are contraindicated. Kidney transplant recipients are generally discharged from the hospital within a week of surgery.

Increasingly, extended criteria donors (ECDs) are used for kidney transplantation. Any donor over age 60 is considered an ECD donor. Donors over 50 years old are considered ECD if they have a history of hypertension, creatinine >1.5 mg/dL, or cause of death was cerebrovascular accident.[97] DCD donors are also an ECD category. ECD donors affect the scheduling of transplantation as minimization of cold ischemia times is essential. No data on intraoperative function of ECD kidneys have been published, but it is reasonable to anticipate that good graft function is delayed compared with that of standard criteria donor grafts.

In children, the most common causes of ESRD requiring transplantation are congenital (largely anatomic developmental anomalies). Only 15% of pediatric transplants, though, are performed for children <2 years of age.[98] Kidney size mismatch can complicate the surgery in small children. Adult donor kidneys may have to be placed in the retroperitoneum of small children. Although chronic peritoneal dialysis may help expand the abdominal volume,[99] attention to peak inspiratory pressures at closure is important, and increased pressures should be reported to the surgical team. Pediatric renal transplantation is associated with somewhat lower rates of success than adult transplantation, with vascular thromboses of the grafts more common in younger children.

LIVER TRANSPLANTATION

Preoperative Considerations

In the United States, 128 centers perform liver transplants, with highly variable volumes, and only a few programs perform more than 200 adult transplants per year. However, the number of transplants performed in a given center is only a small percentage of patients evaluated for liver transplantation. Anesthesiologists should be consulted about liver transplant recipients ideally as part of a team approach to assessing candidacy for transplantation and to help optimize recipient preparation prior to transplant. Patients with ESLD have multisystem dysfunction with cardiac, pulmonary, and renal compromise because of their liver disease, and multiorgan dysfunction at the time of transplantation is not uncommon (Table 54-5). Furthermore, 60% of wait-listed patients are age 50 to 64 years, and 12.3% are more than 65 years old. Common liver diagnoses leading to transplantation are shown in Table 54-6.

In an effort to minimize deaths on the liver transplant waiting list with objective factors, the national system for allocation of donor livers was changed in February 2002. Adult recipients are prioritized for transplantation by severity of illness, using the MELD (model for ESLD) score, which was originally developed to predict survival of patients with liver disease independent of liver transplantation[100]:

$$MELD\ Score = 0.957 \times Log_e\ (creatinine\ in\ mg/dL)$$
$$+ 0.378 \times Log_e\ (total\ bilirubin\ in\ mg/dL)$$
$$+ 1.12 \times Log_e\ (INR)$$
$$+ 0.643$$

Pediatric patients are prioritized for transplant using the pediatric ESLD score (PELD):

$$PELD\ Score = (0.463[age^d] - 0.687$$
$$\times Log_e\ [albumin\ g/dL]$$
$$+ 0.480 \times Log_e\ [total\ bilirubin\ mg/dL]$$
$$+ 1.857 \times Log_e\ [INR]$$
$$+ 0.667\ [growth\ failure^e]) \times 10$$

Patients with acute liver failure (Status 1) are given priority for donor livers, then the patients with the highest MELD score and appropriate blood group are next. Ongoing analysis of the MELD/PELD score as predictors of transplant survival suggests that this new scoring system helps minimize death on the waiting list, but difficulty balancing between transplanting the sickest patients and transplanting too sick patients means this system will evolve.

Renal failure is common in patients undergoing liver transplantation. Serum creatinine levels are not extremely useful in capturing renal function in patients with liver disease; even a small increase in serum creatinine in these patients suggests significant renal dysfunction; hence, the use of creatinine in MELD. Ongoing evaluation of MELD/PELD scores of wait-listed patients is mandated, with the sickest patients requiring the most frequent laboratory studies to update scores.

Difficult decisions about patient candidacy are common in evaluating liver transplant candidates. Several are discussed here to highlight the need for regular involvement of a transplant anesthesiologist in the candidacy evaluation process. Patients with ESLD generally have very low SVR, high cardiac

---

d<1 year old} = 1; > year old = 0.
e>2 SD below mean for age} = 1; ≤2SD below median for age} = 0.

TABLE 54-5

MULTISYSTEM COMPLICATIONS OF END-STAGE LIVER DISEASE

SYSTEM	CONSEQUENCE
Central nervous system	Fatigue
Encephalopathy (confusion to coma)	Blood–brain barrier disruption and intracranial hypertension (acute liver failure)
Pulmonary	Hypoxemia/hepatopulmonary syndrome
Respiratory alkalosis	
Pulmonary hypertension	Reduced right heart function
Cardiovascular	
Reduced systemic vascular resistance	Hyperdynamic circulation
Diastolic dysfunction	
Prolonged QT interval	
Blunted responses to inotropes	
Blunted responses to vasopressors	
Diabetes	
Gastrointestinal	
Gastrointestinal bleeding from varices	
Ascites	
Delayed gastric emptying	
Hematologic	
Decreased synthesis of clotting factors	Risk of massive surgical bleeding
Hypersplenism (pancytopenia)	
Impaired fibrinolytic mechanisms	
Renal	
Hepatorenal syndrome	Impaired renal excretion of drugs
Hyponatremia	
Endocrine	
Glucose intolerance	
Osteoporosis	Fracture susceptibility
Nutritional/metabolic	Muscle wasting and weakness
Other	
Poor skin integrity	
Increased volume of distribution for drugs	
Decreased citrate metabolism	Calcium requirement with rapid FFP infusion

FFP, fresh-frozen plasma.

TABLE 54-6

DIAGNOSES LEADING TO LIVER TRANSPLANTATION IN ADULTS

PATHOLOGY	DIAGNOSES
Hepatocellular disease	Hepatitis C
	Laennec cirrhosis (alcoholic)
	Combined HCV/Laennec cirrhosis
	Autoimmune hepatitis
	Cryptogenic (idiopathic) cirrhosis
	Hepatitis B
	Small hepatocellular carcinoma (usually with other hepatocellular disease)
	Nonalcoholic steatohepatitis
Cholestatic disease	Primary biliary cirrhosis
	Primary sclerosing cholangitis
Acute liver failure	Viral (unknown)
	Acute hepatitis viruses (A,B,C)
	Drug-induced liver failure
	Wilson disease

HCV, hepatitis C virus.

index, and increased mixed venous oxygen saturation. Liver disease is not protective against coronary artery disease. Most patients are screened for cardiac problems using dobutamine stress echocardiography,[101] adenosine stress tests, or cardiac positron emission tomography. If renal function permits, patients with evidence of significant coronary lesions usually require cardiac catheterization to identify stenoses amenable to angioplasty preoperatively. Patients with severe coronary artery disease are generally not candidates for liver transplantation. Significant aortic stenosis also presents a difficult dilemma pretransplant.[102] Because cardiac surgery is considered risky in a patient with ESLD, patients with aortic stenosis can be treated with valvuloplasty before liver transplantation. Then, after the liver graft is stable, aortic valve replacement can be considered. Similarly, patients with left ventricular outflow tract obstruction can be treated before surgery to improve cardiac function during transplantation.[103]

Echocardiography is also used to screen patients for portopulmonary hypertension and intracardiac shunts. Systolic PA pressure estimates are made by capturing the maximum velocity of regurgitant flow across the tricuspid valve, and using this velocity in the Bernoulli equation for the pressure gradient between right ventricle and right atrium ($\Delta P = 4V^4$). If moderate-to-severe pulmonary hypertension (estimated systolic PA pressure >50 mm Hg) is suggested, right heart catheterization is needed for direct pressure measurements.[104] Multiple case reports and small retrospective reviews demonstrate that patients with portopulmonary hypertension are at substantial risk of perioperative death. There is general agreement that mean PA pressure >50 mm Hg is an absolute contraindication to liver transplantation. Patients with PA pressures between 35 and 50 mm Hg and pulmonary vascular resistance >250 dynes/s/cm^{-5} are also likely at increased risk. Efforts to lower PA pressure before transplantation pay off and considerably reduce the risk of transplantation.[105] Epoprostenol is the usual first-line therapy for portopulmonary hypertension and is effective in lowering PA pressures significantly in many patients,[66] but requires home intravenous delivery in the United States. Sildenafil is also useful for treatment of portopulmonary hypertension[106] and, increasingly, the mixed endothelin antagonist, bosentan.[107] Right heart dysfunction that does not reverse after treatment of primary pulmonary hypertension is considered a contraindication to liver transplantation.[108] Intracardiac shunting imposes a risk of paradoxical embolization, and nonsurgical correction of patent foramen ovale preoperatively is also worth consideration.

PFTs are often abnormal in ESLD, with most patients showing reduced diffusion capacity for carbon monoxide. Hepatopulmonary syndrome (severe hypoxemia due to liver disease), once a contraindication to transplantation, is now an indication for transplantation as it is often reversible with good graft function.[109] If hepatopulmonary syndrome is severe and completely unresponsive to oxygen, transplantation is risky because the immediate perioperative period may be complicated by frank graft hypoxia and failure. Fortunately, most patients with hepatopulmonary syndrome have some element of physiologic ventilation-perfusion mismatch, are oxygen-responsive, and with this "room to move" can be safely transplanted.

As for other solid-organ transplants, major infection and malignancy may exclude patients from consideration for transplantation. Several centers, though, have good experience transplanting patients with human immunodeficiency virus, and infected patients who require liver transplants should be referred to these centers.[110]

Intraoperative Procedures

Management of liver transplant patients has progressed substantially in the last 5 years with collected experience of transplant teams, such that intraoperative extubation of some patients is routine in busier centers. Nonetheless, intensive preparation for surgery is important because it is difficult to predict which patients are at risk for massive blood loss. We place invasive lines and monitors after induction of general anesthesia. Rapid-sequence induction of general anesthesia is indicated because patients with ESLD often have gastroparesis[111] in addition to increased intra-abdominal pressure from ascites. We place two arterial catheters, one in the left radial and one in the right femoral artery. PA catheters or continuous echocardiography are used for monitoring volume status, and TEE is particularly useful for patients with cardiac lesions undergoing transplantation[112] (see Chapter 28). At least two large-bore (9 Fr) catheters are placed for rapid intravenous infusions. In many centers, anesthesiologists also place percutaneous lines specifically for use in venovenous bypass, if necessary.[113,114] Bladder catheters and nasogastric tubes are placed in all patients. A rapid infusion system with the ability to deliver at least 500 mL/min of warmed blood is primed and in the room. Before surgical incision, blood product availability is confirmed and some blood products are in the room and checked (routinely 10 U red cells and 10 U FFP). Normothermia, essential for optimal hemostasis, is maintained with fluid warmers and convective air blankets over the legs and over the upper body.

9 Liver transplantation is traditionally described in three phases: dissection, anhepatic, and neohepatic, with reperfu-

sion of the graft marking the start of the neohepatic phase. During the dissection phase of surgery, blood loss may be high. The major anesthetic goals of this phase are correction of coagulopathies and maintenance of intravascular volume for renal protection. Some centers advocate low CVP management of liver transplant patients to reduce blood loss,[115] but this technique may be harmful in patients with higher MELD scores.[116]

Coagulation Management

Similar to other surgical procedures, FFP is used to maintain INR ≤1.5 in patients with anticipated or ongoing bleeding. Rapid infusion of FFP implies rapid infusion of citrate, which can quickly lead to ionized hypocalcemia. Infusion of $CaCl_2$, adjusted to ionized Ca^{2+} levels, is better at maintaining constant Ca^{2+} levels than are intermittent boluses. Platelet transfusion has traditionally been used to maintain platelet count higher than 50,000/mm^3; however, recent data suggest that platelet transfusion is detrimental to graft and patient survival.[117] Importantly, we find that maintaining fibrinogen >150 mg/dL with cryoprecipitate is critical for hemostasis. Cell-saver blood may also be used to limit allogeneic transfusions, although generally not in patients with hepatocellular carcinoma.

In addition to complex coagulopathies of ESLD, many patients with liver disease have a superimposed hypercoagulable state (see Chapter 16). For example, patients with autoimmune liver diseases may have antiphospholipid antibodies. So, in addition to monitoring discrete parts of the coagulation profile to guide transfusion therapies, it is important to look at a measure of whole-blood clotting. Many centers use thrombelastography[118]; others use bedside Lee-White clotting times. Using these tests, normal or hypernormal whole clotting in the presence of high INR, low platelets (and usually elevated D-dimers) should be taken as a caution that the patient may have a clinically significant hypercoagulable state. Under these circumstances, our approach is to maintain transfusion therapies as noted previously and to avoid pharmacologic procoagulant drugs. For the majority of patients with synthetic dysfunction, thrombocytopenia, and hypofibrinogenemia, whole-blood clotting is delayed. In these patients, many centers supplement transfusion therapy with antifibrinolytic agents. Considerable center-dependent variation in use and dosing of antifibrinolytics makes generalizations difficult. The majority of adult patients in our center receive ε-aminocaproic acid (EACA; 5 g load and 1 g/hr infusion) to support hemostasis during surgery.[119] Other centers use considerably less drug, less often. Many centers, particularly in Europe, use aprotinin routinely during liver transplantation,[120] but several case reports of fatal pulmonary embolism associated with aprotinin use[121] have made many U.S. centers shy away from the drug or use very low doses. Fibrinolysis acutely worsens immediately after reperfusion to varying degrees, depending largely on the amount of tissue plasminogen activator released from the graft.[122] A (re)bolus of EACA (again, doses are highly variable) is helpful to maintain hemostasis once this postreperfusion exacerbation of fibrinolysis is documented.

Activated factor VII (NovoSeven, Novo Nordisk, Copenhagen, Denmark) is approved in Europe and appears to be a safe hemostatic agent during liver transplantation.[123] When this drug is given, INR rapidly normalizes,[124] even though the amount of circulating clotting factors does not change. In our center, acute NovoSeven administration is used for surgical hemostasis for placement of intracranial pressure (ICP) monitors in patients with acute liver failure and for selected patients undergoing liver transplantation with difficult red cell cross-matches. It is also used for Jehovah's Witness patients[125] and for particularly complex liver transplants,[126] but its expense and incomplete understanding of the potential for thrombosis has limited widespread use for liver transplantation.

Perioperative renal dysfunction is a major challenge in liver transplantation, with hypovolemia and anesthetic-induced reduction of renal blood flow. Creatinine levels may grossly underestimate the degree of renal dysfunction, especially in ESLD patients with significant muscle wasting.[127] Hepatorenal syndrome (HRS) is a functional renal disorder associated with liver disease, categorized as type 1 (acute severe decompensation, creatinine >2.5 mg/dL), which is usually fatal, and type 2 (chronic, moderate renal failure with creatinine >1.5 and glomerular filtration rate <40 mL/min). More recent evidence suggests that albumin may play a role in preventing and treating HRS in the setting of spontaneous bacterial peritonitis.[128] In addition, large-volume (>5 L) drainage of ascites with incision is paracentesis and should be accompanied by albumin therapy to prevent renal decompensation, with recommended albumin doses of 6 to 8 g/L of ascites drained.[129] Terlipressin (available in Europe) and other vasoconstrictors may be useful for HRS because they relieve splanchnic vasodilatation, but terlipressin must be used with caution in patients with heart disease. Norepinephrine may improve renal function in patients with type 1 HRS,[130] and the α_1-agonist, midodrine, is useful for improving renal function in some patients.[131] No prospective trials have been done to support use of one vasopressor over another during transplantation, and intraoperative pharmacologic renal support is largely guided by the hepatology literature. Dopamine is not useful for preserving renal function during liver transplantation. The most important consideration is to ensure adequate volume replacement before instituting diuresis in the OR.

The *anhepatic phase* begins when the liver is functionally excluded from the circulation. Historically, the vena cava is clamped above (suprahepatic anastomosis) and below (infrahepatic anastomosis) the liver, the portal vein and hepatic artery are clamped. With complete cava cross-clamp, venous return falls by 50 to 60%, often resulting in hypotension. Venovenous bypass (VVB) may be used to increase venous return and therefore, blood pressure, increase renal and gut perfusion pressures, and decompress portal pressures for a better surgical field. VVB is rarely used in our center as most patients can be managed without VVB using volume loading and vasopressors as needed. VVB carries potential complications, including arm lymphedema, air embolism, and vascular injury, and its benefit is limited when anhepatic times are short.[132] Surgical modifications to preserve caval flow (piggyback technique)[133] help preserve blood pressure, and obviate the need for VVB.

Reperfusion of the graft is the most treacherous time of the liver transplant. Communication between the surgical and anesthesia teams is essential in preparing for reperfusion. Caval clamps are removed first, and the integrity of the caval anastomoses are assured. Caval reperfusion is usually hemodynamically well tolerated. However, portal vein reperfusion often results in hemodynamic instability. The original descriptions of reperfusion syndrome emphasized (often severe) hypotension and bradycardia with portal reperfusion.[134] Now, with flushing techniques that precede reperfusion and changes in preservation solution, bradycardia is less common. Typically, reperfusion is associated with hypotension (further drop of already low SVR and increase in CO), which may or may not require treatment.

Our preparation for reperfusion is to give sodium bicarbonate just before unclamping (25 to 50 mEq) to meet the acid load from the graft, or treat severe acidosis during the anhepatic period with *tris*-hydroxymethyl aminomethane (THAM) infusion.[135] Importantly, we administer 500 mg of $CaCl_2$ precisely at the time of portal reperfusion to counteract the effects of potassium on the heart. If, despite these preparations, T waves (ECG) become elevated, the same treatment is repeated. Some anesthesiologists prefer to treat ECG changes only after they are diagnosed. Lidocaine, atropine, and norepinephrine are also available at the time of reperfusion in case of ventricular dysrhythmias, bradyarrhythmias, and severe hypotension. Hepatic artery unclamping is usually hemodynamically uncomplicated.

Recent human studies suggest the utility of other interventions to blunt reperfusion injury at the time of portal unclamping. Methylene blue (1 to 1.5 mg/kg bolus) reduces hemodynamic instability after reperfusion.[136] Methylene blue is thought to mediate its effects by scavenging reactive oxygen species and nitric oxide. On the other hand, a recent study suggests that inhaled nitric oxide (iNO) given during transplantation has significant acute benefits (decreased hepatocyte apoptosis) and promotes recovery of the graft including earlier elaboration of coagulation factors.[137]

Neohepatic Period

Calcium is not required after reperfusion so that one early indication of graft metabolic function is the lack of a calcium requirement even when FFP is infused rapidly. Usually within 30 minutes, the base deficit improves with graft metabolism of citrate and lactate. Within the first hour, the CO decreases (after an acute increase after portal reperfusion) and SVR increases as the graft metabolizes vasoactive substances. In addition, the graft appearance should be noted. It should have a smooth edge, no evidence of engorgement, and bile is made in the first half-hour after reperfusion. Often, renal function improves after reperfusion, probably because of graft metabolism of renal vasoconstrictors. Similar to kidney transplantation, ECD grafts are increasingly used to reduce wait-list mortality.[138] For livers, the major classes of ECD donors are advanced age, steatosis, DCD, and split grafts,[139] as well as donors with extended hospital stays.[140] These grafts are often slow to function metabolically in the OR. For these and other classes of ECD livers, cold ischemia times should be limited, which can significantly impact the OR schedule.

During the neohepatic period, biliary anastomoses are completed and sources of surgical bleeding are corrected. Drains are placed and the abdomen is closed. Fast-tracking protocols for liver transplant patients are common in experienced centers.[141]

Pediatric Liver Transplantation

Indications for pediatric liver transplantation differ considerably from that of adults, with biliary atresia the most common (43%). Inherited metabolic diseases are the indication for 13% of pediatric liver transplants.[142] Portopulmonary hypertension is rare in children but biliary atresia is associated with atrial septal defects and situs inversus.[142] Children younger than 1 year of age with inherited liver disease are often very small for age. In small children, a radial artery catheter and at least one large (18-g) peripheral intravenous line are placed after induction of anesthesia. Surgeons may place tunneled central lines before incision, useful for postoperative administration of drugs as well as CVP monitoring during surgery. Children with previous Kasai operations for biliary atresia may have massive bleeding during dissection because of adhesions. Small children receiving large grafts may have respiratory compromise with abdominal closure. Because hepatic artery thrombosis is a more common complication in children than adults, some centers choose to have INR at the end of surgery in the 1.8 to 2 range. Hepatic artery thrombosis is generally recognized to be a technical issue related to the small diameter of arteries in children,[143] and intraoperative reanastomosis may be required if flow is inadequate through the artery. Aortic cross-clamping may be required for these anastomoses. Biliary complications are also common in pediatric transplant recipients, especially those receiving adult left lateral segment grafts, and hepatic artery thrombosis is a significant contributor to biliary complications.[144]

Acute Liver Failure

Anesthetic considerations for both adults and children with acute liver failure are focused on protection of the brain (see Chapter 39). Patients with acute or fulminant hepatic failure may have a rapidly progressive course of elevated ICP, leading to herniation and death. ICP monitoring is useful in managing these patients but risks intracranial bleeding. Vasodilating anesthetics, including all inhaled agents, should be avoided, especially without ICP monitoring. In our experience, pentothal infusion is a good maintenance anesthetic, and acute rises in ICP can be managed with etomidate. Patients may come to the OR who are receiving N-acetylcysteine, a glutathione donor. Mannitol is used for osmotherapy to an end point of 310 mOsm/L and hyperventilation is also commonly used to manage ICP. Hypothermia is also considered brain-protective in patients with acute liver failure.[145] Hypertonic saline is also useful in some patients.[146] When antihypertensive therapy is required, labetalol does not cause significant cerebral vasodilation in these patients.[147] Acute cerebral vasodilatation often accompanies reperfusion. Management of intracranial hypertension and cerebral edema is based on very small studies of patients with acute liver failure and on adaptations of studies directed at control of intracranial hypertension in other settings, discussed in Chapter 39.

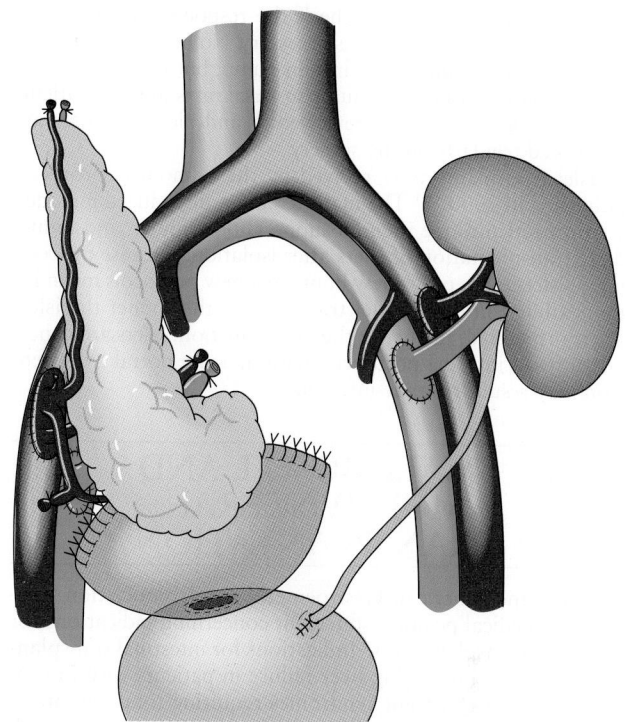

FIGURE 54-4. Pancreas/kidney transplantation performed with drainage of the pancreatic exocrine secretions urinary bladder (bladder drainage).

PANCREAS AND ISLET TRANSPLANTATION

The majority of pancreas transplants (about 75%) are done as simultaneous pancreas/kidney transplants from a single deceased donor (Figs. 54-4 and 54-5). Pancreata grafted in these procedures have the best long-term survival, compared with grafts done after kidney transplantation or independent pancreas grafts. Independent pancreas grafts are usually performed for patients with type I diabetes who have frequent metabolic complications (hypoglycemia) but preserved renal function. Living donor partial pancreas grafts are not commonly performed, with the largest ongoing experience at the University of Minnesota.[148] Living donor pancreatectomy is also now performed laparoscopically.[149]

The preoperative assessment of pancreas transplant recipients focuses on the end-organ complications of diabetes (reviewed in Chapter 44). Monitoring will depend on cardiac status, but generally patients do not require PA catheters and have been evaluated for risk of intraoperative cardiac complications as part of the transplant workup. Nonetheless, cardiovascular disease is present in many patients undergoing pancreas transplantation.

The major difference between pancreas transplantation and other procedures is that strict attention to control of blood glucose is indicated to protect newly transplanted beta cells from hyperglycemic damage. No formula for controlling blood glucose has emerged as a standard of intraoperative management. In general, if adult patients arrive with glucose >250 mg/dL, 10 U of insulin can be given intravenously, followed by an infusion of insulin. The infusion starting rate varies, depending on the initial blood glucose level. Once blood glucose levels are controlled (<150 mg/dL), intravenous 5% dextrose (about 100 mL/hr) should also be infused as the insulin infusion is continued. The

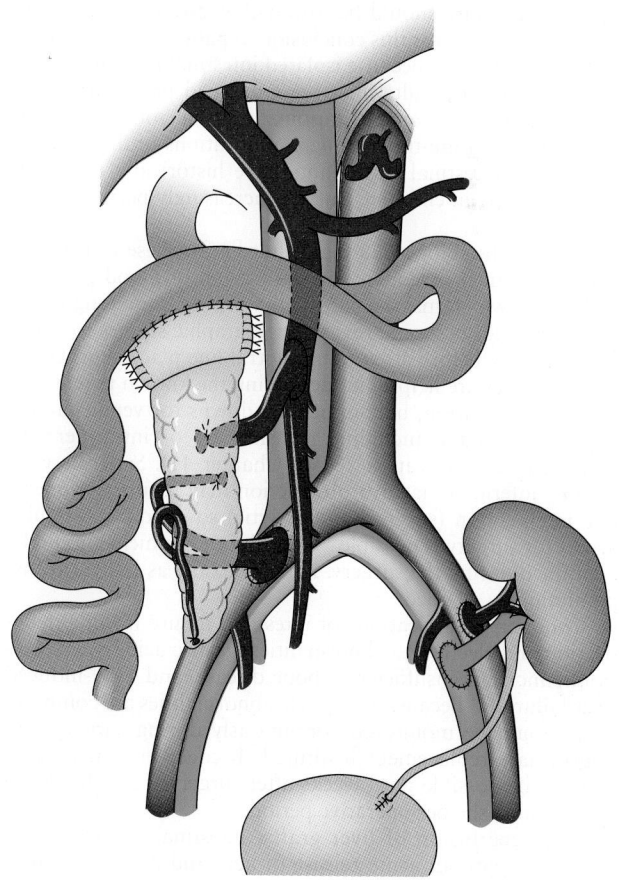

FIGURE 54-5. Pancreas/kidney transplantation performed with drainage of the pancreatic exocrine secretions into the proximal jejunum (enteric drainage).

most important issue is to check the response to insulin frequently and adjust infusions as necessary. No literature exists for a patient with an implanted insulin pump, but it seems reasonable to continue to use the pump at basal rates in these patients as long as its operation is reviewed[150] and blood glucoses are monitored regularly during surgery.

Islet transplants were revived by the Edmonton protocol, published in 2000.[151] The major changes introduced included a glucocorticoid-free immunosuppression regimen and immediate transplantation of islets after isolation. Because processing of islets takes only a few hours, the new protocols mean little flexibility in timing islet transplants—the sooner the islets are transplanted, the better they will function. Islets are generally infused into the portal circulation; acute portal hypertension may result from the infusion.

SMALL BOWEL AND MULTIVISCERAL TRANSPLANTATION

In 2003, the American Gastroenterological Association published a medical position statement concerning indications for intestinal transplantation.[f] Indications for intestinal transplantation include impending liver failure in patients with intestinal failure (or short-gut syndromes requiring total parenteral nutrition [TPN]), frequent severe dehydration in patients with intestinal failure, and severe complications of central lines for TPN (sepsis, thrombosis of central veins). Patients who develop liver failure from TPN for intestinal failure are candidates for combined liver-intestine transplantation. In these cases, liver failure should be irreversible, and biopsy findings are often required for this conclusion in patients without overt ESLD,[152] especially because isolated intestinal transplantation may have better results than the combined procedure.[153] In general, intestinal transplantation should be considered only in patients with life-threatening complications of their intestinal failure. Intestinal transplants have historically been performed mostly in children, but are increasingly performed for adult recipients.

For anesthesiologists, a major hurdle for these transplants is line placement adequate for transfusion of blood products and fluids, which may be substantial during these long cases. Anesthesiologists should review angiographic studies to determine patency before attempting central line placement. Ultrasound devices are helpful in identifying the known patent vessels for cannulation, but surgical cutdowns for venous access may be necessary, including transhepatic or intraoperative renal vein catheterization[154] (see Chapter 41). Superior vena cava or inferior vena cava obstruction may require preoperative intervention (surgical and/or lytic) so adequate vascular access for surgery is possible.[155] Antibiotic regimens should be continued during the surgery. Nitrous oxide, as in liver transplantation, is avoided.

Common complications of intestinal failure include dehydration and electrolyte abnormalities, gastric acid hypersecretion, pancreatic insufficiency, bone disease, and TPN-induced liver failure.[156] Because electrolyte abnormalities are common, they should be monitored continuously during surgery and appropriate replacement instituted. Because enteral feeding will not be possible until weeks after surgery, TPN should be continued in the perioperative period.

Like reperfusion of liver grafts, intestinal reperfusion is associated with an acute release of acid and potassium from

the graft. Anticipatory bicarbonate and $CaCl_2$ administration is used to counteract the effects of acid and potassium on the heart. After reperfusion, coagulopathy may worsen, usually managed by reassessment of INR, fibrinogen and platelet counts, and correction with blood products.

LUNG TRANSPLANTATION

Lung transplantation is now accepted therapy for end-stage pulmonary and pulmonary vascular disease, building on successful case series from the early 1980s.[157,158] UNOS reports >16,000 lung transplant procedures since 1988, but >5,000 patients have died awaiting transplant during this time because of the shortage of suitable organs. The Registry of the International Society for Heart and Lung Transplantation lists chronic obstructive pulmonary disease, idiopathic pulmonary fibrosis, cystic fibrosis (CF), and α_1-antitrypsin deficiency as the most common indications for lung transplantation.[159]

Surgical options for lung transplantation are single lung transplant, en bloc double, or sequential double transplants, and heart-lung transplantation. The International Society for Heart and Lung Transplantation registry for 2007 indicates an increase in double-lung transplants over the past 10 years, with a relatively stable number of single-lung transplants,[159] a trend likely related to recent reports of improved 1-year survival after double-lung transplantation. Single and sequential double-lung transplants can be performed without cardiopulmonary bypass (CPB), although CPB is often used, especially for recipients with pulmonary hypertension. Bilateral lung transplantation is most commonly used in patients with associated pulmonary vascular disease and CF-related bronchiectasis, although its use is increasing in chronic obstructive pulmonary disease and idiopathic pulmonary fibrosis recipients. Single-lung transplantation for emphysema gained favor based on good short-term outcomes, with the added advantage of leaving a donor lung for another recipient. Lung transplant centers vary in applying single- or double-lung transplant to different diagnoses, and the better procedure based on recipient preoperative status and diagnosis is still debated.[160] Double-lung transplantation, however, is generally indicated in the presence of pulmonary infection (CF), severe bullous emphysema, and primary pulmonary hypertension.

Recipient Selection

International Guidelines for the Selection of Lung Transplant Candidates were updated in 2006 by consensus agreement of several thoracic societies (summarized in Table 54-7).[159] In general, patients should be considered for lung transplantation if they exhibit decline in pulmonary function despite maximal medical therapy. Contraindications to lung transplantation are based on their impact on long-term survival. Absolute and relative contraindications are listed in Table 54-7. Patients with significant cardiac disease can be considered for heart-lung transplantation, but are not candidates for isolated lung transplant.[159] A new Lung Allocation System has been in use since May 2005.[159] Candidates are now given a Lung Allocation score to determine their wait-list status, instead of the prior method that relied heavily on waiting time on the transplant list. The new system weighs net benefit of transplant and clinical urgency.

As for other transplants, patients are screened for malignancy (mammography, Pap test, and colonoscopy). PFTs, left and right heart catheterization, and transthoracic echocardiography are routinely used for evaluating recipients. Lung transplantation has not been advocated for acute disease processes, such as acute respiratory distress syndrome. Specific age limits

---

[f]http://www.guideline.gov/summary/summary.aspx?ss=15&_id=3795&nbr=3021#s23.

TABLE 54-7

LUNG RECIPIENT SELECTION GUIDELINES

■ GENERAL INDICATIONS

End-stage lung disease
Failed maximal medical treatment of lung disease
Age within limits for planned transplant
Life expectancy <2–3 yr
Ability to walk and undergo rehabilitation
Sound nutritional status (70–130% of ideal body weight)
Stable psychosocial profile
No significant comorbid disease

■ DISEASE-SPECIFIC INDICATIONS

COPD	FEV_1 <25% of predicted value after bronchodilators and/or $PaCO_2$ = 55 mm Hg and/or pulmonary hypertension (especially with cor pulmonale) Chronic O_2 therapy
Cystic fibrosis	FEV_1 <30% predicted Hypoxemia, hypercapnia, or rapidly declining lung function Weight loss and hemoptysis Frequent exacerbations, especially young females Absence of antibiotic-resistant organisms
Idiopathic pulmonary fibrosis	Vital capacity <60–65% of predicted Resting hypoxemia Progression of disease despite therapy (steroids)
Pulmonary hypertension	NYHA functional status class III or IV, despite prostacyclin therapy Mean right atrial pressure <15 mm Hg Mean pulmonary artery pressure <55 mm Hg Cardiac index <2 L/min/m²
Eisenmenger syndrome	NYHA class III or IV, despite optimal therapy
Pediatric	NYHA class III or IV Disease unresponsive to maximal therapy Cor pulmonale, cyanosis, low cardiac output

COPD, chronic obstructive pulmonary disease; FEV_1, forced expiratory volume in 1 second; NYHA, New York Heart Association.

were recommended in the past; however, current guidelines list age >65 years as a relative contraindication only. One change from 1998 guidelines is the elimination of Eisenmenger syndrome as an indication for lung transplantation because small studies showed no survival benefit. CF is associated with complex pulmonary infections and colonization with microbial flora that can negatively impact transplant outcomes.[161,162] However, with the exception of patients colonized with *Burkholderia cepacia*, most CF patients can be successfully transplanted despite chronic bacterial infections.[163]

Preanesthetic Considerations

Medical evaluation prior to listing a patient for transplantation encompasses many specialties. Unfortunately, anesthesiologists are not always included in this process. If the patient has been on the waiting list for an extended period, it is important to review laboratory and functional data since the original transplant workup, which may not reflect current status. It is critical to confirm ABO compatibility of donor and recipient prior to surgery. By definition, lung transplant candidates have poor pulmonary status and are frequently receiving multiple therapies including oxygen, inhaled bronchodilators, steroids, and vasodilators. These medications should be continued in

the perioperative period. Because short ischemic times are necessary for optimal organ function, the procedure must be done as soon as a lung becomes available, precluding delay of cases for full stomachs.

Although transplant patients are understandably anxious, they also have minimal pulmonary reserve, and sedation must be given carefully under monitored conditions. After determining oxygen saturation, slow, incremental dosing of a short-acting benzodiazepine (0.25 to 1.0 mg midazolam) is used for anxiolysis. Narcotic premedication must be given with extreme care in hypercarbic patients. Premedication with a combination of metoclopramide, histamine-2 antagonists, and a nonparticulate antacid is usually warranted. Many patients are not able to rest supine or in Trendelenburg position for placement of central venous lines. Placement of large-bore peripheral intravenous and arterial access is usually adequate for initiation of the anesthetic, with central access placed after induction. Placement of a PA catheter with continuous cardiac output and mixed venous oxygenation (MvO_2) monitoring provides both rapid assessment of cardiopulmonary changes, and minimizes the fluid administration necessary for frequent cardiac output determinations. Epidural catheters are placed preoperatively at some centers, especially in patients who are believed unlikely to require CPB. (It is not always possible, however, to determine need for CPB preoperatively.) The

American Society for Regional Anesthesia consensus statement on regional anesthesia in the anticoagulated patient[164] states that there is currently insufficient evidence to determine the risk of neuraxial hematoma in patients receiving neuraxial anesthesia and full systemic anticoagulation. Another option is to place the epidural in the early postoperative period, after coagulopathies are corrected. The epidural can be placed using light sedation during weaning from mechanical ventilation, allowing better neurologic monitoring and pain control prior to tracheal extubation.

Intraoperative Management

Single-Lung Transplantation

Lung transplant recipients tend to be chronically intravascularly volume-depleted, and anesthetic induction can be associated with hypotension. Restriction of anesthetic doses because of hypotension has been associated with awareness in this patient population. Intraoperative bispectral index monitoring was associated with a fivefold reduction in the risk of awareness in this population.[165] Because fluid restriction is beneficial for postoperative management, small fluid boluses and slow induction with etomidate and narcotics is prudent. These patients remain intubated for hours to days postoperatively, so that a fast-track anesthetic technique is unnecessary. A balanced technique combining narcotic and inhalation anesthetics or benzodiazepines is preferred. Muscle relaxation can be maintained with any non–histamine-releasing agent. Nitrous oxide is rarely an anesthetic option because of bullous emphysematous disease, pulmonary hypertension, or intraoperative hypoxemia.

Lung isolation, preferably with a double-lumen endotracheal tube, is necessary for single and bilateral sequential lung transplantation. The double-lumen endotracheal tube facilitates suctioning of secretions and improved deflation of the operative lung during the initial dissection. A bronchial blocker is more easily dislodged with surgical manipulation, may not provide isolation of the right upper lobe, and requires repositioning midsurgery in the case of a bilateral sequential procedure. Left-sided endotracheal tubes are preferred because of ease of positioning in the left mainstem bronchus.

10 Fluid restriction and lung ventilation strategies designed to protect the lung allograft are indicated as these patients are at increased risk for acute lung injury and pulmonary edema. Management of acute lung injury includes use of small tidal volumes and oxygenation techniques using PEEP and lowest acceptable FIO_2 settings.[166] Fluid restriction recommendations are based on data showing that elevated CVP are associated with increased mortality after lung transplantation.[167] Intermittent fluid boluses to maintain CVP <7 cm H_2O and use of vasoactive drugs to maintain hemodynamic parameters is recommended. Lung recipients are susceptible to development of pulmonary hypertension and right ventricular (RV) dysfunction or failure during single-lung ventilation. Optimizing oxygenation and ventilation does not always improve RV function, and vasodilator and/or inotropic support may be required. Inhaled nitric oxide (iNO) is another option for improving respiratory and RV status (see later discussion).

During single-lung ventilation, hypoxemia is common. Strategies to improve oxygenation and ventilation are the same as those discussed in Chapter 56. Newer anesthesia machines with pressure-controlled ventilation have diminished the need for ICU ventilators during the operative procedure. Although an ICU ventilator can provide improved oxygenation and ventilation, it does not allow concomitant use of inhalation anesthetics, an option available on the newer anesthesia machines. CPB is indicated during lung transplantation if adequate oxygenation cannot be maintained despite ventilatory and pharmacologic maneuvers and PA clamping by the surgeons. Inability to ventilate or development of RV dysfunction is also an indication for CPB.

A single-lung transplant can be performed via posterolateral thoracotomy. If the surgeon is concerned about possible need for CPB, then the patient must be positioned to allow rapid access to either the aorta and right atrium, or the femoral artery and vein. This can be accomplished via either anterior thoracotomy with partial sternotomy, or posterolateral thoracotomy with decreased angulation of the hips to allow access to the femoral vessels. Determination of operative side is based on preoperative ventilation-perfusion studies and prior thoracic surgeries. The lung with poorer function is typically the one replaced.

After pneumonectomy, the surgeon will size the donor vascular tissue to the recipient vessels, and sequentially anastomose the atrial/pulmonary vein patch, bronchus, and pulmonary artery. The lung is kept cool with ice in the surgical field until reperfusion. Circulation is restored to the donor lung, suture lines are checked for hemostasis, and then ventilation is begun. Systemic hypotension can occur during reperfusion, but is usually not as significant as that with liver graft reperfusion. Hyperkalemia is also not a common reperfusion complication. Studies have shown that Perfadex, a low-molecular-weight dextran solution, improves early graft function and is now used widely for preservation during procurement.[168] However, there can be reperfusion injury to the lung presenting as pulmonary edema. PEEP is useful in this scenario. Bronchoscopy to suction secretions and blood is recommended to improve ventilation and oxygenation and to examine bronchial suture lines.

Intraoperative TEE has become a valuable tool in the assessment of lung transplant patients. A comprehensive TEE examination should be performed after induction of anesthesia with attention focused on biventricular function, presence of valvular regurgitation, patent foramen ovale or atrial septal defect, and pulse wave Doppler flow patterns in the pulmonary veins. Significant RV dysfunction, valvular regurgitation, or intra-atrial shunt may lead the surgeon to plan the operation with CPB. TEE can be helpful in monitoring RV function during initial clamping of the PA for a procedure done without CPB. After reperfusion, another comprehensive TEE examination should be performed. Pulmonary vein anastomotic obstruction can be diagnosed with careful Doppler examination of the pulmonary venous inflow (see Chapter 28). Because this condition leads to a high incidence of acute graft failure, rapid diagnosis and treatment in the OR is beneficial.

At the completion of the procedure, the patient should be evaluated for exchange of the double-lumen endotracheal tube to a large (8-mm internal diameter or larger) single-lumen endotracheal tube. Significant oropharyngeal edema or high PEEP requirement justifies leaving the double-lumen tube in place for 24 hours to allow improvement in clinical status prior to endotracheal tube exchange.

Double-Lung Transplantation

Bilateral lung transplant is performed in the supine position via the clamshell incision. The arms can be suspended on a padded bar above the patient or tucked at the sides. These cases can also be performed with sternotomy. En bloc double-lung transplant requires CPB, and a single-lumen endotracheal tube is sufficient. Bilateral sequential transplantation requires lung isolation, preferably via a double-lumen endotracheal tube. Bilateral sequential transplant is now the preferred procedure because a tracheal anastomosis is unnecessary, and there is less surgical bleeding. Most centers electively institute CPB for this procedure in the presence of preoperative pulmonary hypertension, and urgent CPB for indications previously discussed. Serial implantation implies longer ischemic time for the second lung, which does not adversely affect outcome. The clamshell incision is extensive and can cause significant postoperative pain. Thoracic epidurals are often used to provide pain relief.

Pediatric Lung Transplantation

The Registry of the International Society for Heart and Lung Transplantation Pediatric Report was last published in 2006.[169] Pediatric lung transplantation has remained at a steady level for the past 6 years, with adolescents continuing to account for the majority of the procedures. The most common diagnoses are CF, congenital heart disease, and primary pulmonary hypertension. Congenital heart disease is the most common indication in infants. Overall survival is similar for pediatric and adult populations. There now appear to be age-related survival differences, with infants doing better than adolescents, but overall, survival is improving. Patients receiving bilateral lung transplants have a better outcome than those receiving single lungs. Only 634 pediatric lung transplants are reported in the UNOS database, and 93 of these are living donor lobar lung transplantations. A recent evaluation of patients with CF listed and/or receiving lung transplantation showed that only 1% of the patients showed a survival benefit from surgery, a remarkably poor result.[170] However, quality of life still appears improved by lung transplantation in patients with CF. Given these recent data, the role of lung transplantation for treatment of CF deserves further study to determine optimal age, pretransplant diagnosis, status, and firm indicators. Most pediatric patients receive double-lung transplantation with CPB. Single-lung procedures are reserved for larger adolescents with CF. A single-lumen endotracheal tube is adequate. The clamshell incision is used. Central and arterial access are necessary for perioperative monitoring.

Primary Graft Dysfunction

The etiology of PGD is not yet clearly defined, and is certainly multifactorial. This disease process is a major cause of post-transplant morbidity, summarized in in-depth reviews.[171,172] PGD is graded on a scale of 0 to 3, with time after reperfusion indicated as a T score. The diagnosis is not applicable for dysfunction starting >72 hours after reperfusion. Grade 3 is defined as: PaO_2/FiO_2 <200 with radiographic infiltrates consistent with pulmonary edema. Grade 3 PGD is associated with statistically increased 30-day mortality.[171] The most recent working group summary indicates that type of procedure, presence of hepatic dysfunction, and increased risk of postoperative bleeding due to pleural adhesions, and/or prior surgery require more investigation as possible risk factors for the development of PGD. The only clear risk factor identified in the review was the presence of primary pulmonary hypertension. CPB does not appear to be an independent risk factor. Anesthetic management has also not emerged as a risk factor for PGD.

To date there are no data to support a link between transfusion and lung allograft PGD.[171] However, data are limited on transfusion during lung transplantation, in contradistinction to the large amounts of data on transfusion requirements during kidney or liver transplantation. Wang et al.[173] and Oto et al.[174] determined that patients undergoing double-lung transplants, procedures with CPB, or those with Eisenmenger syndrome or CF had increased transfusion requirements during lung transplantation. Further study is needed to determine whether transfusion negatively impacts lung transplant outcomes. The transplant literature does not show a correlation between fluid management in the OR and outcome, although fluid restriction and management of these patients as if they have acute lung injury is probably prudent. Severe, life-threatening PGD has been successfully managed with extracorporeal membrane oxygenation (ECMO).[175]

Inhaled Nitric Oxide

iNO therapy is used to decrease pulmonary vascular resistance and improve oxygenation (see Chapter 56). NO has an extremely short duration of action in vivo, rapidly inactivated by reacting with heme, producing methemoglobin. Because iNO is preferentially delivered to ventilated areas, vascular relaxation in these areas leads to improved blood flow, and hence improvements in ventilation-perfusion mismatch and improved oxygenation. Rapid inactivation of iNO in the pulmonary vasculature prevents systemic vasorelaxation and resulting systolic hypotension.

Some anesthesiologists use iNO routinely for lung transplantation,[176] while others believe the potential adverse side effects mean its use should be more restricted.[177] Proponents argue that use of iNO in the recipient, and possibly even the donor, takes advantage of immunomodulatory and antimicrobial activities of NO that reduce recipient lung injury.[178] Opponents argue that iNO use should be limited to the population at risk for needing CPB during lung transplantation, and to patients with reperfusion injury. They cite risks of methemoglobinemia, NO-metabolite related lung injury, and decreased sensitivity of exhaled NO monitoring as a diagnostic tool for acute lung rejection. Although small studies have suggested a prophylactic role for iNO, a randomized, placebo-controlled trial demonstrated no benefit.[179] A randomized clinical trial of 30 patients undergoing double-lung transplant at an institution with high usage of CPB showed no benefit of prophylactic iNO in prevention of pulmonary edema.[180]

NO may mediate other clinically beneficial effects. NO activates guanylate cyclase in platelets to attenuate platelet aggregation and adhesion.[181] iNO can decrease pulmonary vascular resistance, improve oxygenation, decrease inflammatory response to surgery or trauma, impede microbial growth, and have an effect limited only to the pulmonary system. Its use in successful management of lung transplant patients is well documented.[182,183]

Heart-Lung Transplant (Adult and Pediatric)

Heart-lung transplantation is the least common intrathoracic transplant procedure. UNOS lists 961 total procedures to date in the United States, with 167 pediatric recipients. Fewer than 100 procedures have been performed per year worldwide since 2001. Bilateral sequential lung transplant has largely replaced heart-lung transplantation, and improved pharmacologic management of pulmonary hypertension and RV failure obviates the need for the heart-lung procedure. As indications for lung transplantation have evolved to replace heart-lung transplant for diagnoses such as primary pulmonary hypertension and CF, congenital heart disease and acquired heart disease are increasingly common indications for heart-lung transplantation.[184] Most pediatric heart-lung transplants are currently being performed for children aged 11 to 17 years. The use of this procedure for CF is rapidly diminishing, leaving pulmonary vascular disease as the main indication for pediatric heart-lung transplantation.[185] Anesthetic management of these patients is similar to that of isolated heart or lung transplant patients. Because a tracheal anastomosis is performed, a single-lumen endotracheal tube is adequate. The endotracheal tube is either removed or withdrawn above the suture line during CPB to facilitate the tracheal anastomosis. Inotropes may be needed for RV dysfunction immediately after bypass. Pulmonary reperfusion injury can also occur, requiring management of acute lung injury as described for lung transplantation.

HEART TRANSPLANTATION

Since Christian Barnard performed the first successful heart transplant in South Africa in 1967, the procedure has become accepted practice for treatment of heart failure recalcitrant to medical therapy. Over 42,000 individuals have received heart transplants in the United States since 1988. Unfortunately, almost 8,000 patients died while waiting for a donor during that time. Currently, more than 2,600 patients await heart transplants. Overall 1-year survival has improved from 74% in the early 1980s to 87% currently. The 5-year survival for primary transplantation is currently 72%.[g]

Left Ventricular Assist Devices

The Randomized Evaluation of Mechanical Assistance for the Treatment of Congestive Heart Failure (REMATCH) trial demonstrated better survival and quality of life for end-stage heart failure patients than medical management alone.[186] Anesthesiologists will see more heart failure patients for both initial device placement and perioperative management of left ventricular assist devices (LVADs) for patients undergoing additional surgical procedures. A number of reviews are available for further information on management issues.[187,188] A brief summary of key considerations is included here. The devices vary in significant ways, and it is important to understand the specific management issues of the device in place or being placed. Variations include flow pattern (pulsatile or nonpulsatile), requirement for anticoagulation (none, aspirin, Coumadin), filling pattern (fill-to-empty or various other modes), power source (battery or alternating current), potential for electromagnetic interference, and impact of dysrhythmias and defibrillation on the device. Acetone-containing products and Betadine should be avoided near these devices as they can damage the cannula or drive lines.

⓫   LVAD pump flow is affected by intravascular volume and afterload. Failure to maintain adequate preload or normal afterload will result in decreased LVAD flow and hypotension because of low functional cardiac output. An individual familiar with the device in use should be present to assist with trouble-shooting device management if the clinician does not have sufficient experience. Patients presenting for initial device placement are in various stages of decompensated heart failure and need invasive monitoring with an arterial line and either PA catheter or central venous line. TEE is indicated to evaluate for valvular pathologies or intracardiac shunts that complicate LVAD placement. TEE examination is repeated after device placement to confirm cannula placement and flow.[189] These patients will likely need intensive inotropic support until institution of CPB and device placement. Many clinicians advocate standard placement of TEE, plus possibly central venous access for perioperative management of these patients for noncardiac surgery to ensure adequate volume status and for determination and infusion of inotropes or vasodilators to optimize forward flow by maintaining normal afterload and preload.

LVADs are being placed as rescue therapy, bridge to transplant, and destination therapy. Most patients will show significant hemodynamic improvement with an LVAD, but some patients require support of the right ventricle as well via a biventricular assist device. The Tandem Heart (Cardiac Assist Inc, Pittsburgh, PA) is a percutaneous ventricular assist device usually placed in a cardiac catheterization laboratory. The indications are short-term hemodynamic support for patients in cardiogenic shock or temporary support of a patient undergoing high-risk percutaneous intervention. The left-sided cannula is advanced from the femoral vein into the left atrium by puncturing the interatrial septum. The ABIOMED options (ABIOMED, Inc., Danvers, MA) are commonly used for postcardiotomy failure via direct cannulation. The chest is left open, and the

cannulas can be left in place for up to 2 weeks. The Thoratec device (Thoratec Corporation, Pleasanton, CA) is an implanted device that can be used for long-term biventricular support. The Heartmate devices (Thoratec) are currently approved as therapy for patients with intractable heart failure who are not candidates for transplantation (destination therapy).

The most common diagnoses leading to transplantation are ischemic and idiopathic dilated cardiomyopathies. Less common diagnoses include valvular heart disease, retransplant, and congenital heart disease.[190] Because of the limited availability of donor organs, technologies that can extend the life of patients waiting for donors have developed. Forty percent of recent recipients were receiving intravenous inotropic support and 27% were receiving mechanical support, including intra-aortic balloon counterpulsation or LVAD. In addition, cardiac resynchronization therapy (CRT) has been shown to reduce morbidity and mortality in patients with LV systolic dysfunction, prolonged QRS duration and New York Heart Association (NYHA) Class III or IV heart failure despite optimal pharmacologic therapy.[191] Many patients presenting for heart transplantation have had a CRT device placed as part of their management, frequently with implantable cardioverter-defibrillator capability as well. (See Appendix for further discussion of these therapies and perioperative device management.) Totally implantable artificial hearts are not currently in clinical use; however, their development is an active area of research. Heterotopic heart transplantation has been virtually abandoned.

Recipient Selection

In 1996, the five-year survival for chronic heart failure (CHF) was reported to be <30%.[192] Progress in modeling heart failure to better predict the mode of death (Seattle Heart Failure Model) may allow better design of therapies to improve this poor survival.[193] Medical therapy of CHF has improved dramatically in the last decade. Pharmacologic options include angiotensin-converting enzyme inhibitors, beta-blockers (specifically carvedilol), diuretics, and digoxin. Cardiac resynchronization therapy can also improve symptoms, exercise tolerance, and quality of life in properly selected patients,[194] although long-term survival data are not available. More than 5 million Americans have CHF, with the incidence increasing with age. Of these, only about 3,000 per year are listed for heart transplantation.

Consensus guidelines for selection of patients for heart transplantation were last published in 1993[195] with some recent modifications.[196,197] Patients referred for transplant evaluation should have NYHA Class III or IV heart failure despite optimal medical therapy. Surgical correction of coronary artery disease or valvular heart disease should be considered prior to listing. Patients with severe mitral regurgitation and low ejection fraction should be considered for mitral valve repair instead of transplantation as survival is better than with transplantation.[197] Most candidates have severe LV systolic dysfunction; however, transplantation is occasionally indicated for treatment of refractory angina, unmanageable dysrhythmias, or diastolic heart failure.

Prognosis in patients with CHF has been linked to functional capacity. Maximal exercise testing with oxygen uptake (VO_2) is an excellent method to determine functional capacity.[197] In patients on a stable medical regimen, maximal VO_2 <10 mL/kg/min is associated with a poor prognosis. Patients with VO_2 >10 mL/kg/min have a better 1-year prognosis with medical therapy than transplantation. Patients with Holter monitor evidence of asymptomatic, significant ventricular ectopy should be considered for transplantation to reduce the risk of sudden death.

Pulmonary hypertension is associated with increased perioperative mortality, so that severe, irreversible pulmonary hypertension is a contraindication to transplant. Right heart catheterization is performed to determine transpulmonary gradient (the difference between mean PA pressure and pulmonary capillary wedge pressure) and pulmonary arteriolar resistance. Transpulmonary gradient >12 mm Hg indicates significant pathology. Pulmonary arteriolar resistance (the ratio of transpulmonary gradient to cardiac output, expressed as Wood units) >2.5 also indicates a high risk of perioperative RV failure. Patients with elevated transpulmonary gradient or pulmonary arteriolar resistance require a trial with sodium nitroprusside, prostacyclin, dobutamine, or milrinone in an attempt to decrease pulmonary resistance. Patients unresponsive to these therapies are often considered too high a risk for transplantation, and may be candidates for LVAD insertion as definitive therapy or bridge to transplant.

Contraindications to cardiac transplantation include significant noncardiac diseases. Because immunosuppressive agents have renal and hepatic side effects, the presence of intrinsic renal or hepatic disease increases perioperative risk of organ dysfunction or failure. Some patients with multiorgan disease can be considered for combined heart-kidney or heart-liver transplantation. Patients with forced expiratory volume in 1 second (FEV_1) <50% predicted despite optimal management of CHF are at increased risk for ventilatory failure and respiratory infections posttransplant. The presence of significant atherosclerosis is a contraindication because of the increased perioperative morbidity and mortality from atheroembolic phenomenon.

Preanesthetic Considerations

Donor heart function worsens with donor cold ischemia times above 6 hours. For this reason, timing of transplantation depends on when the donor surgery can be done, frequently during night hours. Preoperative evaluation and preparation of the patient must be expeditious. Close communication between the donor and recipient teams facilitates optimal use of donor organs with minimal ischemia times. Optimally, the recipient heart is excised as soon as the donor heart arrives at the recipient hospital. Induction of anesthesia and surgical incision of the recipient begin when the donor team has evaluated the donor and made the final determination that the organ is acceptable. Timing decisions are based on distance and time necessary to transport the donor organ, as well as time it will take to prepare the recipient. History of prior sternotomy or difficult airway can increase recipient preparation time.

When evaluating the recipient, a few issues need special attention: nothing by mouth status, level of cardiovascular support (inotropic infusions, chronic medications for heart failure, presence of LVAD), and presence of hemodynamic monitoring lines or antiarrhythmic devices, such as pacemaker, CRT device, or defibrillator. Antiarrhythmic devices need to be interrogated and reprogrammed to a mode that will not be affected by electrocautery interference. Because of the emergency nature of these cases, it is common that the patient has recently eaten, and rapid-sequence induction may be necessary. Patients are frequently taking angiotensin-converting enzyme inhibitors that could increase the risk of intraoperative hypotension, or Coumadin that can increase risk of bleeding. Vasopressin infusions can be beneficial for treatment of angiotensin-converting enzyme inhibitor-induced hypotension, and FFP should be ordered if the INR is elevated. If cardiac status has deteriorated recently, the patient may be receiving infusions of inotropes, such as dobutamine or milrinone. On occasion, patients are receiving chronic dobutamine or milrinone therapy as outpatients. If patients have had multiple

central lines, ultrasound evaluation of the central vessels may be helpful to determine vessel patency. Recent chest films and laboratory studies must be reviewed to assess pulmonary, hepatic, and renal compromise associated with CHF.

Many anesthetic management issues related to the heart transplant patient are similar to those for open-heart surgeries (see Chapter 41). The notable differences are strictest attention to sterility and immunosuppression, poorer hemodynamic status of transplant candidates, and issues related to early donor heart function and denervation. The surgical team will request antibiotics specific to donor and recipient infection patterns, and immunosuppressive medications are often given prior to incision.

Placement of the PA catheter prior to anesthetic induction is favored by many centers. continuous cardiac output-MvO$_2$ PA catheters are useful because they provide continuous assessment of CO and MvO$_2$. If the patient cannot lie flat for central line placement, cautious induction can proceed but arterial catheters should always be used for blood pressure monitoring during induction. Large-bore intravenous access is necessary for administration of resuscitation medications if no central line is present during induction. Inotropes should be readily available prior to induction. Dobutamine, epinephrine, milrinone, norepinephrine, dopamine, vasopressin, and phenylephrine have all been used effectively in the perioperative management of heart transplant patients.

Presence of an LVAD or prior sternotomy increases the length and the risks associated with the procedure. Aprotinin reduces allogeneic transfusion requirements in patients undergoing repeat sternotomy.[198] Aprotinin has also been used extensively for high-risk procedures, such as LVAD insertion. Where possible, old medical records should be reviewed to determine if the patient had prior aprotinin exposure. Aprotinin is a foreign protein, and its use is associated with anaphylaxis if re-exposure occurs within 6 months.[199] If aprotinin has been used recently, or exposure is uncertain, the test dose should not be administered until the surgeons are ready to rapidly institute CPB for management of hemodynamic collapse. Aprotinin is not currently readily available in the United States and either EACA or tranexamic acid can be used as an antifibrinolytic agent. Four units of blood should be immediately available prior to sternotomy for all repeat procedures. CMV status of the donor and recipient is needed to determine whether CMV-negative packed red blood cells should be ordered. Products are typically irradiated. Availability of FFP, platelets, and cryoprecipitate should be confirmed at the start of the procedure.

Intraoperative Management

Anesthetic induction in patients with poor ventricular function can be complicated by hemodynamic instability. Instituting or increasing inotrope infusions can be beneficial in these cases. Choice of anesthetic technique should be focused on minimizing cardiovascular complications. High-dose narcotic techniques have been used for induction and management of cardiac transplant patients for many years with good results.[200] Balanced anesthetic techniques, using lower doses of narcotics and inhalation anesthetics, can be used as well.[201] Neuromuscular blockade with a nondepolarizing agent is recommended. Hypotension may not respond to ephedrine or phenylephrine, and inotrope use should be rapidly instituted or increased if response to phenylephrine is inadequate.

A comprehensive TEE examination should be performed after induction of anesthesia and after weaning from CPB. The native heart can be monitored prior to CPB for changes in ventricular function or an increase in valvular regurgitation. Early diagnosis of deterioration can facilitate rapid therapy and hemodynamic stability. The risk of intracardiac thrombus is increased in the recipient heart. The left atrium and ventricle should be carefully examined. Manipulation of the heart is minimized prior to aortic cross-clamping if thrombus is noted.

Incision is via median sternotomy for orthotopic heart transplantation. After initiation of CPB, the recipient heart is excised, except for the left atrial tissue encompassing the pulmonary veins. In the classic approach, the atria are transected at the grooves. The biatrial approach totally excises both atria, mandating bicaval anastomosis. The biatrial approach is preferred in pediatric recipients. A recent meta-analysis revealed a clinically relevant benefit of the bicaval technique, so it is likely that this technique will be performed more frequently.[202]

Heparin dosing is similar to that for other CPB procedures. Cannulation of the aorta is performed high along the ascending aorta, near the aortic arch. The superior and inferior vena cavae are cannulated individually. By encircling the cavae with tourniquets, all blood flow is directed through the cannula in to the bypass circuit, and the surgical field is bloodless. Prior to resection of the native heart, the PA catheter should be withdrawn from the surgical field. The catheter can be readvanced after removal of the superior caval cannula. Maintenance of CPB and weaning from CPB are associated with the same issues as for other cardiac surgical procedures. Ischemic time for the donor heart starts with aortic cross-clamp during the harvest, and ends with removal of the cross-clamp from the recipient aorta. Air should be evacuated prior to weaning from CPB.

Prior to weaning from CPB, the heart is re-evaluated with TEE, with attention to ventricular and valvular function. Intracardiac shunts should be ruled out. Because the donor heart is denervated, normal physiologic feedback loops controlling inotropy and chronotropy are lost. Isoproterenol is used frequently for its direct effects on cardiac β-receptors, to increase graft heart rate. Use of temporary epicardial pacing is sometimes needed until isoproterenol has had adequate time to reach maximal effect. (Vasoactive drug effects in heart transplantation are reviewed in Table 54-8.) Residual atrial tissue may continue to have electrical activity, seen clinically as two P waves on ECG. The native P wave has no physiologic effects on the donor heart.

Inotrope selection for weaning from CPB is similar to other cardiac surgical procedures (see Chapter 41). Special consideration should be given to recipients with preoperative pulmonary hypertension, donor hearts with long ischemic times, or those that are deemed marginal. The risk of donor right heart failure is increased in these cases. The donor right heart is not accustomed to high pulmonary resistance, and may fail acutely. Therapy for graft right heart failure is similar to therapy for right heart failure in other cardiac cases. The goal is to improve contractility and decrease pulmonary vascular resistance. If intravenous agents do not facilitate weaning from CPB, iNO and inhaled prostacyclin (iloprost) have been shown to be beneficial in this population.[203–206]

Pediatric Heart Transplantation

UNOS reports over 5,000 pediatric heart transplants performed since 1988; 60% are performed in children <1 year, or >11 years old. The pretransplant diagnosis was congenital heart disease or idiopathic/viral cardiomyopathy in 75% of these patients. In the United States, retransplantation an increasing indication. ECMO is used as a bridge to transplant at some centers, although it is acknowledged to be only a short-term option.[207] Even though ECMO is the therapeutic choice for circulatory support in most pediatric cardiac patients, some pediatric patients (mostly adolescents) benefit from placement of a ventricular assist device.[208]

Preoperative evaluation focuses on cardiopulmonary status and the particulars of the cardiac physiology in congenital heart disease patients (see Chapter 41) Palliative procedures may have been performed prior to transplant, and reoperation increases surgical risk. Central venous catheters and intra-arterial catheters are placed routinely, although frequently after induction. After an inhalation induction, anesthetic management frequently involves high-dose narcotics and intermittent benzodiazepines.

Marginal donors are, not surprisingly, also being used for pediatric heart grafts including size mismatches of over 3 times recipient body weight, high donor inotrope requirement, prolonged ischemic time, and ABO mismatch.[209–211] Although ABO incompatible transplantation is contraindicated in the adult population, it is more successful in infant recipients.[212,213] Hyperacute rejection does not occur because of the immaturity of the immune system and absence of antibodies to various antigens, including blood group antigens. For ABO

TABLE 54-8

EFFECT OF DENERVATION ON CARDIAC PHARMACOLOGY

■ SUBSTANCE	■ RECIPIENT	■ MECHANISM
	EFFECT ON	
Digitalis	Normal increase of contractility, minimal effect on atrioventricular node	Direct myocardial effect, denervation
Atropine	None	Denervation
Adrenaline	Increased contractility Increased chronotropy	Denervation hypersensitivity
Noradrenaline	Increased contractility Increased chronotropy	Denervation No neuronal uptake
Isoproterenol	Normal increase in contractility, normal increase in chronotropy	
Quinidine	No vagolytic effect	Denervation
Verapamil	Atrioventricular block	Direct effect
Nifedipine	No reflex tachycardia	Denervation
Hydralazine	No reflex tachycardia	Denervation
Beta-blocker	Increased antagonist effect	Denervation

Reprinted with permission from Deng MC: Cardiac transplantation. Heart 2002; 287: 177.

mismatched grafts, recipient isohemagglutinin titers are obtained pretransplantation, then plasma exchange is performed during CPB. Four-year follow-up data show similar morbidity and mortality compared with ABO-compatible recipients. Furthermore, waiting list survival is improved because of expansion of the donor pool.

Management of the Transplant Patient for Nontransplant Surgery

As the population of transplant recipients increases, the incidence of elective or emergent nontransplant surgery in this group will also increase. These patients cannot always return to the transplant facility for surgery, so anesthesiologists outside transplant centers will encounter transplant patients.[214]

For solid-organ recipients, evaluation of patients is centered on function of the grafted organ. In renal and liver transplant patients, the level of renal dysfunction will often determine choice of drugs, particularly neuromuscular blockers, and dose modification of drugs dependent on renal excretion such as antibiotics. Table 54-9 lists medications that can cause renal dysfunction when administered to a patient receiving immunosuppressive agents. A major consideration for renal transplant recipients is maintenance of renal perfusion with adequate volume replacement. Thus, CVP monitoring is useful for preventing prerenal damage to transplanted kidneys, but CVP lines must be placed using strict aseptic technique. It is important to note that signs of infection may be masked in transplant patients. Failing, rejecting, or reinfected liver grafts are often accompanied by deterioration of renal function. Protection of the kidneys is a central part of anesthesia plans, and CVP or TEE is useful to guide fluid replacement, especially in cases in which large fluid shifts are anticipated.

For all transplant recipients, antibiotic, antiviral, antifungal, and immune suppression regimens should be disrupted as little as possible in the perioperative period. The types of infection to which transplant recipients changes over time with donor-derived and hospital-acquired infections predominating in the first posttransplant month. Infections acquired by transplant patients in months 2 to 6 versus later after transplantation are also distinct, and these patterns should guide surgical prophylaxis and perioperative diagnostic procedures. Infectious disease specialists are important consults in preoperative transplant patients. A study of solid-organ transplant patients who developed appendicitis highlights the risks of infection in this population: Transplant recipients are likely to have more complications and longer hospital stays.[215] Complications of immune suppression are reviewed in Table 54-3, and important drug interactions with calcineurin inhibitors in Table 54-10.[214] Significant intraoperative fluid shifts can cause acute decrease in

TABLE 54-9

DRUGS THAT MAY CAUSE RENAL DYSFUNCTION WHEN COADMINISTERED WITH CALCINEURIN INHIBITORS

Amphotericin	Cotrimoxazole
Cimetidine	Vancomycin
Ranitidine	Tobramycin
Melphalan	Gentamicin
Nonsteroidal anti-inflammatory drugs	

Adapted with permission from Kostopanagiotou G, Smyrniotis V, Arkadopoulos N et al: Anesthetic and perioperative management of adult transplant recipients in non-transplant surgery. Anesth Analg 1999; 89: 613.

TABLE 54-10

DRUGS AFFECTING CYCLOSPORINE OR TACROLIMUS BLOOD LEVELS

■ INCREASE BLOOD LEVELS	■ DECREASE BLOOD LEVELS
Bromocriptine	Carbamazepine
Chloroquine[a]	Octreotide[a]
Cimetidine[b]	Phenobarbital
Clarithromycin	Phenytoin
Cotrimoxazole	Rifampin
Danazol	Ticlopidine
Erythromycin	
Fluconazole	
Itraconazole	
Ketoconazole	
Metoclopramide	
Nicardipine	
Verapamil	

[a]Reported with cyclosporine; may not interact with tacrolimus.
[b]May not interact with cyclosporine.

cyclosporine or tacrolimus blood levels, and in these cases, consideration should be given to repeat testing of drug levels during the day of surgery.[214] Nonsteroidal anti-inflammatory medications should be avoided for a number of reasons. First, many patients have underlying renal dysfunction related to immunosuppressive agents. Second, the risk of gastrointestinal hemorrhage is increased in patients already at risk for gastritis from chronic steroids.

Patients who present for surgery with signs of acute rejection or infection may benefit from delay of surgery to optimize status. Both rejection and infection in the face of surgery are associated with increased risk of morbidity and mortality.[214] Regional and general anesthetic techniques have been used successfully in posttransplant patients. In addition to the standard ASA monitors, invasive monitors should be used if warranted based on surgical procedure and general health status of the patient. Invasive monitoring is not indicated solely on the basis of prior transplantation. Nasal intubation should be avoided because of the potential risk for infection presented by nasal flora.

Virtually all liver diseases can recur in grafted livers, including autoimmune diseases, fatty liver, and hepatitis C. The degree of liver dysfunction from recurrent disease should be evaluated with hepatologists and by using standard laboratory tests.

For lung transplant recipients with a tracheal anastomosis, denervation has occurred below the level of the suture line and the cough reflex is diminished or absent. These patients are at increased risk of retained secretions and pneumonia, and have an increased airway hyperreactivity and bronchospasm. Because most lung transplants are now being done with bronchial instead of tracheal anastomoses, the risk of tracheal suture line stenosis or disruption with manipulation are markedly diminished. Advantages of regional anesthetic techniques in lung transplant patients include minimization of airway manipulation and decreased infectious risk.

Comparison of preoperative PFT, arterial blood gas, and CXR results with prior studies can help diagnose acute infection or rejection: Significant decreases in FEV_1, vital capacity, and total lung capacity and an obstructive pattern may indicate acute rejection. Arterial blood gas in the presence of rejection will show an increased A—a gradient from stable baseline gases, along with perihilar infiltration on CXR. However, rejection and infection can be difficult to distinguish clinically. If the patient is suspected of having an active pulmonary process, consultation with pulmonary medicine for a possible diagnostic bronchoscopy should be considered prior to surgery.

Transplanted hearts are denervated, impacting perioperative management significantly. The transplanted heart cannot respond to indirect acting agents, such as ephedrine and even dopamine, or to peripheral attempts to induce hemodynamic changes, such as carotid massage, Valsalva maneuver, or laryngoscopy. Beta effects of epinephrine and norepinephrine are exaggerated in heart transplant recipients (vs. alpha effects). Isoproterenol is the mainstay of chronotropic therapy in these patients. ECG analysis may show two P waves, one from the native atrium and one from the implanted atrium. The native P wave will not conduct to the implanted heart, and these nonconducted P waves should not be confused with complete heart block. Isoproterenol should be available as an inotrope and chronotrope. Dobutamine can also be helpful; norepinephrine and epinephrine should be reserved for refractory cardiogenic shock. Because the denervated heart does not reflexly compensate for hemodynamic changes induced by regional anesthetics, general anesthesia is usually preferred.

Preoperative evaluation of heart transplant recipients should focus on cardiac functional status. Significant rejection will present with symptoms of heart failure. All heart transplant patients should be evaluated with ECG and transthoracic echocardiography prior to surgery. New findings should be discussed with the cardiology consultant to determine need for stress-testing or myocardial biopsy. Invasive monitors should be placed only when warranted by the clinical status and surgical procedure. Use of either TEE or CVP monitoring can be helpful in managing fluid resuscitation and inotropic support.

References

1. A definition of irreversible coma. Report of the Ad Hoc Committee of the Harvard Medical School to Examine the Definition of Brain Death. JAMA 1985; 205: 337
2. Hevesi Z, Lopukhin SY, Giuditta A et al: . Supportive care after brain death for the donor candidate. Int Anesthesiol Clin 2006; 4: 21
3. Nijboer WN, Schuurs TA, van der Hoeven JAB et al: Effect of brain death and donor treatment on organ inflammatory response and donor organ viability. Curr Opin Organ Transpl 2004; 9: 110
4. Belzberg H, Shoemaker WC, Wo CCJ et al: Hemodynamic and oxygen transport patterns after head trauma and brain death: Implications for management of the organ donor. J Trauma 2007; 63: 1032
5. Novitzky D, Cooper DK, Rosendale JD et al: Hormonal therapy of the brain-dead organ donor: Experimental and clinical studies. Transplantation 2006; 82: 1396
6. Salim A, Vassiliu P, Velmahos GC et al: The role of thyroid hormone administration in potential organ donors. Arch Surg 2001; 136: 1377
7. Rosendale JD, Kauffman HM, McBride MA et al: Aggressive pharmacologic donor management results in more transplanted organs. Transplantation 2003; 75: 482
8. Kutsogiannis DJ, Pagliarello G, Doig C, Ross H, Shemie SD: Medical management to optimize donor organ potential: review of the literature. Can J Anesth 2006; 53: 820
9. Phongsamran PV: Critical care pharmacy in donor management. Prog Transplant 2004; 14: 105
10. Maximizing use of organs recovered from the cadaveric donor: Cardiac recommendations. Consensus Conference Report, Crystal City, VA, March 28–29, 2001. Circulation 2002; 106: 836
11. Figueras J, Busquets J, Grande L et al: The deleterious effect of donor high plasma sodium and extended preservation in liver transplantation: a multivariate analysis. Transplantation 1993; 61: 410
12. Todd TR, Goldberg M, Koshal A et al: Separate extraction of cardiac and pulmonary grafts from a single donor. Ann Thorac Surg 1988; 46: 356
13. Harjula A, Baldwin JC, Starnes VA et al: Proper donor selection for heart-lung transplantation. The Stanford experience. J Thorac Cardiovasc Surg 1987; 94: 874
14. Orens JB, Boehler A, Perrot M et al: A review of lung transplant donor criteria. J Heart Lung Transplant 2003; 22: 1183
15. Bhorade SM, Vigneswaran W, McCabe MA, Garrity ER: Liberalization of donor criteria may expand the donor pool without adverse consequence in lung transplantation. J Heart Lung Transplant 2000; 19: 1200
16. Studer SM, Orens JB: Cadaveric donor selection and management. Semin Respir Crit Care Med 2006; 27: 492
17. Sekine Y, Waddell TK, Matte-Martyn A et al: Risk quantification of early outcome after lung transplantation: Donor, recipient, operative, and post-transplant parameters. J Heart Lung Transplant 2004; 23: 96
18. Maximizing use of organs recovered from the cadaveric donor: Cardiac recommendations. Consensus Conference Report, Crystal City, VA, March 28–29, 2001. Circ 2002; 106: 836
19. Lima B, Rajagopal K, Petersen R et al: Marginal cardiac allografts do not have increased primary graft dysfunction in alternate list transplantation. Circulation 2006; 114(Suppl I): I-27
20. Committee on Non-Heart-Beating Transplantation II: The Scientific and Ethical Basis for Practice and Protocols, Division of Health Care Services, Institute of Medicine: Non-heart-beating organ transplantation: Practice and protocols. Washington, DC: National Academy Press, 2000
21. Van Norman GA: Another matter of life and death: What every anesthesiologist should know about the ethical, legal, and policy implications of the non-heart-beating cadaver organ donor. Anesthesiology 2003; 98: 763
22. Moon JI, Nishida S, Butt F et al: Multi-organ procurement and successful multi-center allocation using rapid en bloc technique from a controlled non-heart-beating donor. Transplantation 2004; 77: 1476
23. Steen S, Sjoberg T, Pierre L et al: Transplantation of lungs from a non-heart-beating donor. Lancet 2001; 357: 825
24. Nunez JR, Varela A, del Rio F et al: Bipulmonary transplants with lungs obtained from two non-heart-beating donors who died out of hospital. J Thorac Cardiovasc Surg 2004; 127: 297
25. Lewis J, Peltier J, Nelson H et al: Development of the University of Wisconsin donation after cardiac death evaluation tool. Prog Transplant 2003; 13: 265
26. Abt P, Kashyap R, Orloff M et al: Pediatric liver and kidney transplantation with allografts from DCD donors: A review of UNOS data. Transplantation 2006; 82: 1708
27. Saidi RF, Elias N, Kawai T et al: Outcome of kidney transplantation using expanded criteria donors and donation after cardiac death. Am J Transplant 2007; 7: 2769
28. Fung JJ, Eghtesad B, Patel-Tom K: Using livers from donation after cardiac death donors—A proposal to protect the true Achilles heel. Liver Transplant 2007; 13: 1633
29. Haberal M, Emirolu R, Arslan G et al: Living-donor nephrectomy under combined spinal-epidural anesthesia. Transplantation 2002; 34: 2448
30. Vats HS, Rayhill SC, Thomas CP: Early postnephrectomy donor renal function: laparoscopic versus open procedure. Transplantation 2005; 79: 609
31. Bergman S, Feldman LS, Carli F et al: Intraoperative fluid management in laparoscopic live-donor nephrectomy: challenging the dogma. Surg Endosc 2004; 18: 1625
32. Biancofiore G, Amorese G, Lugli D et al: Laparoscopic live donor nephrectomy: The anaesthesiologist's perspective. Eur J Anaesthesiol 2004; 21: 74
33. El-Galley R, Hammontree L, Urban D et al: Anesthesia for laparoscopic donor nephrectomy: is nitrous oxide contraindicated? J Urol 2007; 178: 225
34. Blohme I, Fehrman I, Norden G: Living donor nephrectomy. Complication rates in 490 consecutive cases. Scand J Urol Nephrol 1992; 26: 149
35. Starzl TE: Living donors: Con. Transpl Proc 1987; 19: 174
36. Schemmer P, Mehrabi A, Friess H et al: Living related liver transplantation: The ultimate technique to expand the donor pool? Transplantation 2005; 80: S138
37. Ayanoglu HO, Ulukaya S, Yuzer Y, Tokat Y: Anesthetic management and complications in living donor hepatectomy. Transplant Proc 2003; 35: 2970
38. Hwang S, Lee S-G, Lee Y-J et al: Lessons learned from 1,000 living donor liver transplantations in a single center: How to make living donation safe. Liver Transplant 2006; 12: 920
39. Eyraud D, Richard O, Borie DC et al: Hemodynamic and hormonal responses to the sudden interruption of caval flow: Insights from a prospective study of hepatic vascular exclusion during major liver resections. Anesth Analg 2002; 95: 1173
40. Smyrniotis V, Kostopanagiotou G, Theodoraki K, Tsantoulas D, Contis JC: The role of central venous pressure and type of vascular control in blood loss during major liver resections. Am J Surg 2004; 187: 398
41. Chen C-L, Chen Y-S, deVilla VH et al: Minimal blood loss living donor hepatectomy. Transplantation 2000; 69: 2580
42. Johnson LB, Plotkin JS, Kuo PC: Reduced transfusion requirements during major hepatic resection with use of intraoperative isovolemic hemodilution. Am J Surg 1998; 176: 608
43. Niemann CU, Roberts JP, Ascher NL, Yost CS: Intraoperative hemodynamics and liver function in adult-to-adult living donor livers. Liver Transpl 2002; 8: 1126
44. Cammu G, Troisi R, Cuomo O et al: Anaesthetic management and outcome in right-lobe living liver-donor surgery. Eur J Anaesthesiol 2002; 19: 93
45. Lentschener C, Ozier Y: Anaesthesia for elective liver resection: Some points should be revisited. Eur J Anaesthesiol 2002; 19: 788
46. Lutz JT, Valentin-Gamazo C, Gorlinger K, Malago M, Peters J: Blood transfusion requirements and blood salvage in donors undergoing right hepatectomy for living related liver transplantation. Anesth Analg 2003; 96: 351

47. Schumann R, Zabala L, Angelis M et al: Altered hematologic profiles following donor right hepatectomy and implications for perioperative analgesic management. Liver Transpl 2004; 110: 363

48. Matot I, Scheinin O, Eid A, Jurim O: Epidural anesthesia and analgesia in liver resection. Anesth Analg 2002; 95: 1179

49. Soubrane O, Cherqui D, Scatton O et al: Laparoscopic left lateral sectionectomy in living donors: safety and reproducibility of the technique in a single center. Ann Surg 2006; 244: 815

50. Koffron AJ, Kung R, Baker T, Fryer J, Clark L, Abecassis M: Laparoscopic-assisted right lobe donor hepatectomy. Am J Transplant 2006; 6: 2522

51. Barr ML, Belghiti J, Villamil FG et al: A report of the Vancouver Forum on the care of the live organ donor: lung, liver, pancreas, and intestine data and medical guidelines. Transplantation 2006; 81: 1373

52. Vicenti F: A decade of progress in kidney transplantation. Transplantation 2004; 77: S52

53. Dumont FJ: FK506, an immunosuppressant targeting calcineurin function. Curr Med Chem 2000; 7: 731

54. Heisel O, Heisel R, Balshaw R, Keown P: New onset diabetes mellitus in patients receiving calcineurin inhibitors: A systematic review and meta-analysis. Am J Transplant 2004; 4: 583

55. Bobadilla NA, Gamba G: New insights into the pathophysiology of cyclosporine nephrotoxicity: a role of aldosterone. Am J Physiol Renal Physiol 2007; 293: F2

56. Risaliti A, Baccarani U, Vianello V et al: Cardiovascular and metabolic complications after liver transplantation: Neoral-versus tacrolimus-based immunosuppression. Transplant Proc 2001; 33: 3684

57. De Weerdt A, Claeys KG, De Jonghe P et al: Tacrolimus-related polyneuropathy: Case report and review of the literature. Clin Neurol Neurosurg 2008; 110(3): 291–294.

58. Tsunoda SM, Aweeka FT: Drug concentration monitoring of immunosuppressive agents: focus on tacrolimus, mycophenolate mofetil and sirolimus. BioDrugs 2000; 14: 355

59. Sidi A, Kaplan RF, Davis RF: Prolonged neuromuscular blockade and ventilatory failure after renal transplantation and cyclosporine. Can J Anaesth 1990; 37: 543

60. Crosby E, Robblee JA: Cyclosporine-pancuronium interaction in a patient with a renal allograft. Can J Anaesth 1998; 35: 300

61. Niemann CU, Stabernack C, Serkova N et al: Cyclosporine can increase isoflurane MAC. Anesth Analg 2002; 95: 930

62. Thomason JM, Girdler NM, Kendall-Taylor P et al: An investigation into the need for supplementary steroids in organ transplant patients undergoing gingival surgery. A double-blind, split-mouth, cross-over study. J Clin Periodontol 1999; 26: 577

63. Kato T, Gaynor JJ, Yoshida H et al: Randomization trial of steroid-free induction versus corticosteroid maintenance among orthotopic liver transplant recipients with hepatitis C virus: Impact on hepatic fibrosis progression at one year. Transplantation 2007; 84: 829

64. Wilde MI, Goa KL: Muromonab CD3: A reappraisal of its pharmacology and use as prophylaxis of solid organ transplant rejection. Drugs 1996; 51: 865

65. Bamgbola FO, Del Rio M, Kaskel FJ, Flynn JT: Non-cardiogenic pulmonary edema during basiliximab induction in three adolescent renal transplant patients. Pediatr Transplant 2003; 7: 315

66. Lundquist AL, Chari RS, Wood JH et al: Serum sickness following rabbit antithymocyte-globulin induction in a liver transplant recipient: case report and literature review. Liver Transpl 2007; 13: 647

67. Scandling JD, Busque S, Dejbakhsh-Jones S et al: Tolerance and chimerism after renal and hematopoietic cell transplantation. N Engl J Med 2008; 358: 362

68. Alexander SI, Smith N, Hu M et al: Chimerism and tolerance in a recipient of a deceased-donor liver transplant. N Engl J Med 2008; 358: 369

69. Neuhaus P, Klupp J, Langrehr JM: mTOR inhibitors: An overview. Liver Pollard 2001; 7: 473

70. Barten MJ, Streit F, Boeger M et al: Synergistic effects of sirolimus with cyclosporine and tacrolimus: Analysis of immunosuppression on lymphocyte proliferation and activation in rat whole blood. Transplantation 2004; 77: 1154

71. Augustine JJ, Bodziak KA, Hricik DE: Use of sirolimus in solid organ transplantation. Drugs 2007; 67: 369

72. Jungling AS, Shangraw RE: Massive airway edema after azathioprine. Anesthesiology 2000; 92: 888

73. Engelen W, Verpooten GA, Van der Planken M et al: Four cases of red blood cell aplasia in association with the use of mycophenolate mofetil in renal transplant patients. Clin Nephrol 2003; 60: 119

74. Perez-Aytes A, Ledo A, Boso V et al: In utero exposure to mycophenolate mofetil: a characteristic phenotype? Am J Med Genet A 2008; 146: 1

75. Hunter K: Anesthesiology in renal and pancreas transplantation. Curr Opin Organ Transpl 2003; 8: 243

76. Aker S, Ivens K, Guo Z, Grabensee B, Heering P: Cardiovascular complications after renal transplantation. Transplant Proc 1998; 30: 2039

77. Chang SH, Coates PT, McDonald SP: Effects of body mass index at transplant on outcomes of kidney transplantation. Transplantation 2007; 84: 981

78. Dieterle CD, Schmauss S, Arbogast H et al: Pulmonary function in patients with type 1 diabetes before and after simultaneous pancreas and kidney transplantation. Transplantation 2007; 83: 566

79. Bunnapradist S, Danovitch GM: Evaluation of adult kidney transplant candidates. Am J Transplant 2007; 7: 2333

80. Akpek EA, Kayhan Z, Donmez A, Moray G, Arslan G: Early postoperative renal function following renal transplantation surgery: Effect of anesthetic technique. J Anesth 2002; 16: 114

81. Reissell E, Taskinen MR, Orko R, Lindgren L: Increased volume of gastric contents in diabetic patients undergoing renal transplantation: Lack of effect with cisapride. Acta Anaesthesiol Scand 1992; 36: 736

82. Goyal P, Puri GD, Pandey CK, Srivastva S. Evaluation of induction doses of propfol: comparison between end stage renal disease and normal renal function patients. Anaesth Intensive Care 2002; 30: 584

83. Robertson EN, Driessen JJ, Vogt M, De Boer H, Scheffer GJ: Pharmacodynamics of rocuronium 0.3 mg kg(−1) in adult patients with and without renal failure. Eur J Anaesthesiol 2005; 22: 929

84. Fisher DM, Dempsey GA, Atherton DP et al: Effect of renal failure and cirrhosis on the pharacokinetics and neuromuscular effects of rapacuronium administered by bolus followed by infusion. Anesthesiology 2000; 93: 1384

85. Teixeira S, Costa G, Costa F et al: Sevoflurane versus isoflurane: does it matter in renal transplantation? Transplant Proc 2007; 39: 2486

86. Olyaei AJ, deMattos AM, Bennett WM: A practical guide to the management of hypertension in renal transplant recipients. Drugs 1999; 58: 1011

87. Ragaller MJ, Theilen H, Koch T: Volume replacement in critically ill patients with acute renal failure. J Am Soc Nephrol 2001; 17: S33

88. Van den Berghe G, Wouters P, Weekers F et al: Intensive insulin therapy in critically ill patients. N Engl J Med 2001; 345: 1359

89. Ganji MR, Charkhchian M, Hakemi M et al: Association of hyperglycemia on allograft function in the early period after renal transplantation. Transplant Proc 2007; 39: 852

90. Nichols WG, Price TH, Gooley T, Corey L, Boeckh M: Transfusion-transmitted cytomegalovirus infection after receipt of leukoreduced blood products. Blood 2003; 101: 4195

91. Hadimioglu N et al: Effect of different crystalloid solutions on acid-base balance and early kidney function after kidney transplantation. Anesth Analg, in press, 2008

92. Dalton RSJ, Webber JN, Cameron C et al: Physiologic impact of low-dose dopamine on renal function in the early post renal transplant period. Transplantation 2005; 79: 1561

93. Schenarts PJ, Sagraves SG, Bard MR et al: Low-dose dopamine: a physiologically based review. Curr Surg 2006; 63: 219

94. Sorbello M, Morello G, Paratore A et al: Fenoldopam vs dopamine as a nephroprotective strategy during living donor kidney transplantation: preliminary data. Transplant Proc 2007; 39: 1794

95. Parada B, Figueiredo A, Mota Am Furtado A: Surgical complications in 1000 renal transplants. Transplant Proc 2003; 35: 1085

96. Noldus J, Graefen M, Huland H: Major postoperative complications secondary to use of the Bookwalter self-retaining retractor. Urology 2002; 60: 964

97. Ojo AO: Expanded criteria donors: process and outcomes. Semin Dial 2005; 18: 463

98. Giessing M, Muller D, Winkelmann B et al: Kidney transplantation in children and adolescents. Transplant Proc 2007; 39: 2197

99. Healey PJ, McDonald R, Waldhausen JH, Sawin R, Tapper D: Transplantation of adult living donor kidneys into infants and small children. Arch Surg 2000; 135: 1035

100. Freeman RB Jr, Wiesner RH, Harper A et al: UNOS/OPTN Liver Disease Severity Score, UNOS/OPTN Liver and Intestine, and UNOS/OPTN Pediatric Transplantation Committees: The new liver allocation system: Moving toward evidence-based transplantation policy. Liver Transpl 2002; 8: 851

101. Plotkin JS, Benitez RM, Kuo PC et al: Dobutamine stress echocardiography for preoperative cardiac risk stratification in patients undergoing orthotopic liver transplantation. Liver Transpl Surg 1998; 4: 253

102. Pollard RJ, Sidi A, Gibby GL, Lobato EB, Gabrielli A: Aortic stenosis with end-stage liver disease: Prioritizing surgical and anesthetic therapies. J Clin Anesth 1998; 10: 253

103. Paramesh AS, Fairchild RB, Quinn TM et al: Amelioration of hypertrophic cardiomyopathy using nonsurgical septal ablation in a cirrhotic patient prior to liver transplantation. Liver Transpl 2005; 11: 236

104. Kim WR, Krowka MJ, Plevak DJ et al: Accuracy of Doppler echocardiography in the assessment of pulmonary hypertension in liver transplant candidates. Liver Transpl 2000; 6: 453

105. Ashfaq M, Chinnakotla S, Rogers L et al: The impact of treatment of portopulmonary hypertension on survival following liver transplantation. Am J Transplant 2007; 7: 1258

106. Makisalo H, Koivusalo A, Vakkuri A, Hockerstedt K: Sildenafil for portopulmonary hypertension in a patient undergoing liver transplantation. Liver Transpl 2004; 10: 945

107. Hoeper MM, Halank M, Marx C et al: Bosentan therapy for portopulmonary hypertension. Eur Respir J 2005; 25: 502

108. Ramsay MA: Portopulmonary hypertension and hepatopulmonary syndrome, and liver transplantation. Int Anesthesiol Clin 2006; 44: 69

109. Pastor CM, Schiffer E: Therapy insight: hepatopulmonary syndrome and orthotopic liver transplantation. Nat Clin Pract Gastroenterol Hepatol 2007; 4: 614

110. Roland ME, Stock PG: Liver transplantation in HIV-infected recipients. Semin Liver Dis 2006; 26: 273

ANESTHESIA FOR SURGICAL SUBSPECIALTIES

111. Verne GN, Soldevia-Pico C, Robinson ME, Spicer KM, Reuben A: Autonomic dysfunction and gastroparesis in cirrhosis. J Clin Gastroenterol 2004; 38: 72

112. Aniskevich S, Shine TS, Feinglass NG, Stapelfeldt WH: Dynamic left ventricular outflow tract obstruction during liver transplantation: The role of transesophageal echocardiography. J Cardiothorac Vasc Anesth 2007; 21: 577

113. Budd JM, Isaac JL, Bennett J, Freeman JW: Morbidity and mortality associated with large-bore percutaneous venovenous bypass cannulation for 312 orthotopic liver transplantations. Liver Transpl 2001; 7: 1338

114. Planinsic RM, Nicolau-Raducu R, Caldwell JC, Aggarwal S, Hilmi I: Transesophageal echocardiography-guided placement of internal jugular percutaneous venovenous bypass cannula in orthotopic liver transplantation. Anesth Analg 2003; 97: 648

115. Massicotte L, Lenis S, Thibeault L et al: Effect of low central venous pressure and phlebotomy on blood product transfusion requirements during liver transplantations. Liver Transplant 2006; 12: 117

116. Schroeder RA, Collins BH, Tuttle-Newhall E et al: Intraoperative fluid management during orthotopic liver transplantation. J Cardiothorac Vasc Anesth 2004; 18: 438

117. de Boer MT, Christensen MC, Asmussen M et al: Impact of intraoperative transfusion of platelet and red blood cells on survival after liver transplantation. Anesth Analg 2008; 106: 32

118. Kang Y: Thromboelastography in liver transplantation. Semin Thromb Hemost 1995; 21(Suppl 4): 34

119. Quach T, Tippens M, Szlam F et al: Quantitative assessment of fibrinogen cross-linking by epsilon aminocaproic acid in patients with end-stage liver disease. Liver Transpl 2004; 10: 123

120. Molenaar IQ, Legnani C, Groenland TH et al: Aprotinin in orthotopic liver transplantation: Evidence for a prohemostatic, but not a prothrombotic, effect. Liver Transpl 2001; 7: 896

121. Sopher M, Braunfeld M, Shackleton C et al: Fatal pulmonary embolism during liver transplantation. Anesthesiology 1997; 87: 429

122. Porte RJ, Bontempo FA, Knot EA et al: Systemic effects of tissue plasminogen activator-associated fibrinolysis and its relation to thrombin generation in orthotopic liver transplantation. Transplantation 1989; 47: 978

123. Meijer K, Hendriks HG, De Wolf JT et al: Recombinant factor VIIa in orthotopic liver transplantation: Influence on parameters of coagulation and fibrinolysis. Blood Coagul Fibrinolysis 2003; 14: 169

124. Surudo T, Wojcicki M, Milkiewicz P et al: Rapid correction of prothrombin time after low-dose recombinant factor VIIA in patients undergoing orthotopic liver transplantation. Transplant Proc 2003; 35: 2323

125. Jabbour N, Gagandeep S, Peilin AC et al: Recombinant human coagulation factor VIIa in Jehovah's Witness patients undergoing liver transplantation. Am Surg 2005; 71: 175

126. Niemann CU, Behrends M, Quan D et al: Recombinant factor VIIa reduces transfusion requirements in liver transplant patients with high MELD scores. Tranfus Med 2006; 16: 93

127. Sherman DS, Fish DN, Teitelbaum I: Assessing renal function in cirrhotic patients: Problems and pitfalls. Am J Kidney Dis 2003; 41: 269

128. Sort P, Navasa M, Arroyo V et al: Effect of intravenous albumin on renal impairment and mortality in patients with cirrhosis and spontaneous bacterial peritonitis. N Engl J Med 1999; 341: 403

129. Runyon BA: Management of adult patients with ascites caused by cirrhosis. Hepatology 1998; 27: 264

130. Duvoux C, Zandirenas D, Hezode C et al: Effects of noradrenalin and albumin in patients with type 1 hepatorenal syndrome: A pilot study. Hepatology 2002; 36: 374

131. Moreau R, Lebrec D: The use of vasoconstrictors in patients with cirrhosis: Type I HRS and beyond. Hepatology 2006; 43: 385

132. Grande L, Rimola A, Cugat E et al: Effect of venovenous bypass on perioperative renal function in liver transplantation: Results of a randomized, controlled trial. Hepatology 1996; 23: 1418

133. Steib A, Saada A, Clever B: Orthotopic liver transplantation with preservation of portocaval flow compared with venovenous bypass. Liver Transpl Surg 1997; 3: 518

134. Aggarwal S, Kang Y, Freeman JA et al: Postreperfusion syndrome: Hypotension after reperfusion of the transplanted liver. J Crit Care 1993; 8: 154

135. Nahas GG, Sutin KM, Fermon C et al: Guidelines for the treatment of acidaemia with THAM. Durgs 1998; 55: 191

136. Koelzow H, Gedney JA, Baumann J, Snook NJ, Bellamy MC: The effect of methylene blue on the hemodynamic changes during ischemia reperfusion injury in orthotopic liver transplantation. Anesth Analg 2002; 94: 824

137. Lang JD Jr, Teng X, Chumley P et al: Inhaled NO accelerates restoration of liver function in adults following orthotopic liver transplantation. J Clin Invest 2007; 117: 2583

138. Barshes NR, Horwitz IB, Franzini L, Vierling JM, Goss JA: Waitlist mortality decreases with increased use of extended criteria donor liver grafts at adult liver transplant centers. Am J Transplant 2007; 7: 1265

139. Foster R, Zimmerman M, Trotter JF: Expanding donor options: Marginal, living, and split donors. Clin Liver Dis 2007; 11: 417

140. Cameron Am, Ghobrial RM, Yersiz H et al: Optimal utilization of donor grafts with extended criteria. Ann Surg 2006; 243: 748

141. Findlay JY, Jankowski CJ, Vasdev GM et al: Fast track anesthesia for liver transplantation reduces postoperative ventilation time but not intensive care unit stay. Liver Transpl 2002; 8: 670

142. Bennett J, Bromley P: Perioperative issues in pediatric liver transplantation. Int Anesthesiol Clin 2006; 44: 125

143. McDiarmid SV: Current status of liver transplantation in children. Pediatr Clin North Am 2003; 50: 1335

144. Kling K, Lau H, Colombani P: Biliary complications of living related pediatric liver transplant patients. Pediatr Transpl 2004; 8: 178

145. Jalan R, Olde Damink SW, Deutz NE, Hayes PC, Lee A: Moderate hypothermia in patients with acute liver failure and uncontrolled intracranial hypertension. Gastroenterology 2004; 127: 1338

146. Murphy N, Auzinger G, Bernel W, Wendon J: The effect of hypertonic sodium chloride on intracranial pressure in patients with acute liver failure. Hepatology 2004; 39: 464

147. Lidofsky SD, Bass NM, Prager MC et al: Intracranial pressure monitoring and liver transplantation for fulminant hepatic failure. Hepatology 1992; 16: 1

148. Sutherland DE, Gruessner AC: Long-term results after pancreas transplantation. Transplant Proc 2007; 39: 2323

149. Horgan S, Galvani C, Gorodner V et al: Robotic distal pancreatectomy and nephrectomy for living donor pancreas-kidney transplantation. Transplantation 2007; 84: 934

150. Mokshagundam SPL: Perioperative management of diabetes mellitus. Crit Care Nurs Q 2004; 27: 135

151. Shapiro AM, Lakey JR, Ryan EA et al: Islet transplantation in seven patients with type 1 diabetes mellitus using a glucocorticoid-free immunosuppressive regimen. N Engl J Med 2000; 343: 230

152. Langnas AN: Advances in small-intestine transplantation. Transplantation 2004; 77: S75

153. Fishbein TM: The current state of intestinal transplantation. Transplantation 2004; 79: 175

154. Goldman LJ, Santamaria ML, Gamez M: Anaesthetic management of a patient with microvillus inclusion disease for intestinal transplantation. Paediatr Anaesth 2002; 12: 278

155. Mims TT, Fishbein TM, Feierman DE: Management of a small bowel transplant with complicated central venous access in a patient with asymptomatic superior and inferior vena cava obstruction. Transplant Proc 2004; 36: 388

156. Goulet O, Ruemmele F, Lacaille F, Colomb V: Irreversible intestinal failure. J Pediatric Gastroenterol Nutr 2004; 38: 250

157. Reitz BA, Wallwork JL, Hunt SA et al: Heart-lung transplantation. Successful therapy for patients with pulmonary vascular disease. N Engl J Med 1982; 306: 557.

158. Toronto Lung Transplant Group: Unilateral lung transplantation for pulmonary fibrosis. N Engl J Med 1986; 314: 1140

159. Trulock EP, Christie JD, Edwards LB et al: Registry of the International Society for Heart and Lung Transplantation: Twenty-fourth Offical Adult Lung and Heart-Lung Transplantation Report—2007. J Heart Lung Transplant 2007; 26: 782

160. Reitz BA, Wallwork JL, Hunt SA: Heart-lung transplantation. Successful therapy for patients with pulmonary vascular disease. N Engl J Med 1982; 306: 557

161. Trulock ET, Edwards LB, Taylor DO et al: The registry of the International Society for Heart and Lung transplantation: Twentieth official adult lung and heart-lung transplant report—2003. J Heart Lung Transplant 2003; 22: 625

162. Weill D, Keshavjee S: Lung transplantation for emphysema: Two lungs or one. J Heart Lung Transplant 2001; 20: 739

163. Hadjiliadis D, Steele MP, Chapparo C et al: Survival of lung transplant patients with cystic fibrosis harboring panresistant bacteria other than Burkholderia cepacia, compared with patients harboring sensitive bacteria. J Heart Lung Transplant 2007; 26: 834

164. Horlocker TT, Wedel DJ, Benzon H et al: Regional anesthesia in the anticoagulated patient: Defining the risks (the second ASRA consensus conference on neuraxial anesthesia and anticoagulation). Reg Anesth Pain Med 2003; 28: 172

165. Myles PS, Leslie K, Forbes A et al: Bispectral index monitoring to prevent awareness during anaesthesia: the B-Aware randomised controlled trial. Lancet 2004; 363: 1757

166. Wiedemann HP, Wheeler AP, Bernard GR et al: Comparison of two fluid-management strategies in acute lung injury. N Engl J Med 2006; 354: 2564

167. Pilcher DV, Scheinkestel CD, Snell GI et al: A high central venous pressure is associated with prolonged mechanical ventilation and increased mortality following lung transplantation. J Thoracic Cardiovasc Surg 2005; 129: 912

168. Oto T, Griffiths AP, Rosenfeldt F et al: Preservation solutions in lung transplantation: Outcomes from Perfadex, Papworth, and Euro-Collins Solutions. Ann Thorac Surg 2006; 82: 1842

169. Waltz DA, Boucek MM, Edwards LB et al: Registry of the International Society for Heart and Lung Transplantation: Ninth Offical Pediatric Lung and Heart-Lung Transplantation Report-2006. J Heart Lung Transplant 2006; 25: 904

170. Liou TG, Adler FR, Cox DR, Cahill BC: Lung transplantation and survival in children with cystic fibrosis. N Engl J Med 2007; 357: 2143

171. Barr ML, Kawut SM, Whelan TP et al: Report of the ISHLT Working Group on Primary Lung Graft Dysfunction Part IV: Recipient-Related Risk Factors and Markers. J Heart Lung Transplant 2005; 24: 1468

172. Christie JD, Carby M, Bag R et al: Report of the ISHLT Working Group on Primary Lung Graft Dysfunction Part II: Definition. A Consensus Statement

of the International Society for Heart and Lung Transplantation. J Heart Lung Transplant 2005; 24: 1454

173. Wang YW, Kurichi JE, Blumenthal NP et al: Multiple variables affecting blood usage in lung transplantation. J Heart Lung Transplant 2006; 25: 533

174. Oto T, Rosenfeldt F, Rowland M et al: Extracorporeal Membrane Oxygenation After Lung Transplantation: Evolving Techniques Improves Outcomes. Ann Thorac Surg 2004; 78: 1230

175. Lang JD, Lell W: Pro: Inhaled nitric oxide should be used routinely in patients undergoing lung transplantation. J Cardiothorac Vasc Anesth 2001; 15: 785

176. McQuitty CK: Con: Inhaled nitric oxide should not be used routinely in patients undergoing lung transplantation. J Cardiothorac Vasc Anesth 2001; 15: 790

177. Meyer KC, Love RB, Zimmerman JJ: The therapeutic potential of nitric oxide in lung transplantation. Chest 1998; 113: 1360

178. Griffiths MJD, Evans TW: Inhaled nitric oxide therapy in adults. N Engl J Med 2005; 353: 2683

179. Perrin G, Roch A, Michelet P et al: Inhaled nitric oxide does not prevent pulmonary edema after lung transplantation measured by lung water content. Chest 2006; 129: 1024

180. Beghetti M, Sparling C, Cox PN et al: Inhaled NO inhibits platelet aggregation and elevates plasma but not intraplatelet cGMP in healthy human volunteers. Am J Physiol Heart Circ Physiol 2003; 285: H637

181. Cornfield DN, Milla CE, Haddad IY et al: Safety of inhaled nitric oxide after lung transplantation. J Heart Lung Transplant 2003; 22: 903

182. Hoehn T, Huebner J, Paboura E et al: Effect of therapeutic concentrations of nitric oxide on bacterial growth *in vitro*. Crit Care Med 1998; 26: 1857

183. Trulock EP, Christie JD, Edwards LB et al: Registry of the International Society for Heart and Lung Transplantation: Twenty-fourth Official Adult Lung and Heart-Lung Transplantation Report—2007. J Heart Lung Transplant 2007; 26: 782

184. Aurora P, Boucek MM, Christie J et al: Registry of the International Society for Heart and Lung Transplantation: Tenth Official Pediatric Lung and Heart/Lung Transplantation Report—2007. J Heart Lung Transplant 2007; 26: 1223

185. Rose EA, Gelijns AC, Moskowitz AJ et al: Long-term use of a left ventricular device for end-stage heart failure. N Engl J Med 2001; 345: 1435

186. Stone ME, Soong W, Krol M, Reich D: The anesthetic considerations in patients with ventricular assist devices presenting for noncardiac surgery: A review of eight cases. Anesth Analg 2002; 95: 42

187. Nicolosi A, Pagel PS: Perioperative considerations in the patient with a left ventricular assist device. Anesthesiology 2003; 98: 565

188. Chumnanvej S, Wood MJ, MacGillivray TE, Vidal Melo MF: Perioperative echocardiographic examination for ventricular assist device implantation. Anesth Analg 2007; 105: 583

189. Taylor DO, Edwards LB, Boucek MM et al: Registry of the International Society for Heart and Lung Transplantation: Twenty-fourth Official Adult Heart Transplant Report—2007. J Heart Lung Transplant 2007; 26: 769

190. McAlister FA, Ezekowitz J, Hooton N et al: Cardiac resynchronization therapy for patients with left ventricular systolic dysfunction- A systematic review. JAMA 2007; 297: 2502

191. Levy D, Larson MG, Vasan RS et al: The progression from hypertension to congestive heart failure. JAMA 1996; 275: 1557

192. Mozaffarian D, Anker SD, Anand I et al: Prediction of mode of death in heart failure: The Seattle Heart Failure Model. Circulation 2007; 116: 392

193. Seidl K, Rameken M, Vater M, Senges J: Cardiac resynchronization therapy in patients with chronic heart failure. Am J Cardiovasc Drugs 2002; 2: 219

194. Hunt SA: 24th Bethesda conference: Cardiac transplantation. J Am Coll Cardiol 1993; 22 (Suppl 1): 1

195. Deng MC: Cardiac transplantation. Heart 2002; 287: 177

196. Frantz RP, Olson LJ: Recipient selection and management before cardiac transplantation. Am J Med Sci 1997; 314: 139

197. Levy JH, Pifarre R, Schaff HV et al: A multicenter, double-blind, placebo-controlled trial of aprotinin for reducing blood loss and the requirement for donor-blood transfusion in patients undergoing repeat coronary artery bypass grafting. Circulation 1995; 92: 2236

198. Dietrich W, Spath P, Ebell A, Richter JA: Prevalence of anaphylactic reactions to aprotinin: analysis of two hundred forty-eight reexposures in heart operations. J Thor Cardiovasc Surg 1997; 113: 194

199. Hensley FA, Martin DE, Larach DR, Romanoff ME: Anesthetic management for cardiac transplantation in North America—1986 survey. J Cardiothorac Anesth 1987; 1: 429

200. Demas K, Wyner J, Mihm FG, Samuels S: Anaesthesia for heart transplantation. A retrospective study and review. Br J Anaesth 1986; 58: 1357

201. Schnoor M, Schafer T, Luhmann D, Sievers HH: Bicaval versus standard technique in orthotopic heart transplantation: A systematic review and meta-analysis. J Thorac Cardiovasc Surg 2007; 134: 1322

202. Sablotzki A, Czeslick E, Schubert S et al: Iloprost improves hemodynamics in patients with severe chronic cardiac failure and secondary pulmonary hypertension. Can J Anesth 2002; 49: 1076

203. Ardehali A, Hughes K, Sadeghi A et al: Inhaled nitric oxide for pulmonary hypertension after heart transplantation. Transplantation 2001; 72: 638

204. Mosquera I, Crespo-Leiro MG, Tabuyo T et al: Pulmonary hypertension and right ventricular failure after heart transplantation: Usefulness of nitric oxide. Transplant Proc 2002; 34: 166

205. Rajek A, Pernerstorfer T et al: Inhaled nitric oxide reduces pulmonary vascular resistance more than prostaglandin E(1) during heart transplantation. Anesth Analg 2000; 90: 523

206. Burch M, Aurora P: Current status of paediatric heart, lung, and heart-lung transplantation. Arch Dis Child 2004; 289: 386

207. Fynn-Thompson F, Almond C: Pediatric ventricular assist devices. Pediatr Cardiol 2007; 28: 149

208. Boucek MM, Mathis CM, Kanakriyeh MS et al: Donor shortage: use of the dysfunctional donor heart. J Heart Lung Transplant 1993; 12 (6 Pt 2): S186

209. De Begona JA, Gundry SR, Razzouk AJ et al: Transplantation of hearts after arrest and resuscitation. Early and long term results. J Thorac Cardiovasc Surg 1993; 106: 1196

210. Morgan JA, John R, Park YK et al: Successful outcome with extended allograft ischemic time in pediatric heart transplantation. J Heart Lung Transplant 2005; 1: 58

211. West LJ, Pollock-Barziv SM, Dipchand AI et al: ABO-incompatible heart transplantation in infants. N Engl J Med 2001; 344: 793

212. Rao JN, Hasan A, Hamilton JRL et al: ABO-incompatible heart transplantation in infants: The Freeman Hospital experience. Transplantation 2004; 77: 1389

213. Kostopanagiotou G, Smyrniotis V, Arkadopoulos N et al: Anesthetic and perioperative management of adult transplant recipients in nontransplant surgery. Anesth Analg 1999; 89: 613

214. Fishman JA: Infection in solid-organ transplant recipients. N Engl J Med 2007; 357: 2601

215. Savar A, Hiatt JR, Busuttil RW: Acute appendicitis after solid organ transplantation. Clin Transplant 2006; 20: 78

SECTION VIII ■ PERIOPERATIVE AND CONSULTATIVE SERVICES

SECTION VIII PSYCHIATRIC AND
CONSULTATIVE SERVICES

CHAPTER 55 ■ POST ANESTHESIA RECOVERY

MICHAEL A. FOWLER AND BRUCE D. SPIESS

PERIOPERATIVE AND CONSULTATIVE SERVICES

KEY POINTS

❶ The postoperative planning begins with the preoperative evaluation and formation of an intraoperative anesthetic plan. The type of anesthetic (i.e., inhalation technique, total intravenous anesthetic, sedation, local, regional) influences the type and length of postanesthesia care unit (PACU) recovery.

❷ The level of PACU care depends on the type/approach of surgery, type of anesthetic, intraoperative course of events, as well as patient pre-existing and evolving comorbidities. Typical recovery settings include inpatient recovery, ambulatory recovery (phase 1 for more intensive needs and phase 2 for less intensive needs), short stay (23-hour admit), and recovery from specific procedures (i.e., computed tomography, magnetic resonance imaging, invasive radiology, cardiac, pediatric, and radiation procedures).

❸ The transfer of care to a PACU nurse includes assuring that the patient has had appropriate monitoring applied, admission vital signs were taken, a direct and thorough report received that allows for rapid evaluation should complications arise, as well as a nurse capable of handling the acuity of the patient's medical/surgical problems.

❹ Postoperative analgesia should be individualized to requirements and expectations. A multimodal approach includes the appropriate use of nonsteroidal anti-inflammatory drugs, narcotics, adjuncts, regional and local anesthetics, as well as anxiety relief and appropriate emotional support.

❺ Discharge criteria should be tailored to the individual patient's underlying disease, recovery course, and postdischarge level of care.

❻ The cardiac risks during the postoperative stay include myocardial ischemia, which may be minimized with beta-blockers, analgesia, nitrates, supplemental oxygen, adequate circulating volume, oxygen-carrying capacity, heart rate control, and an understanding of hypercoagulable states.

❼ The respiratory risks of a patient must take into account the preoperative respiratory disease status. Residual anesthetics, opioids, and sedatives all impair responsiveness to increasing CO_2 and decreasing O_2 levels. Pain itself can decrease respiration/minute ventilation, leading to CO_2 retention and hypoxia. Supplemental O_2 application alone does not guarantee hypoxemia will not occur.

❽ The evaluation of a patient's ability to void may be affected by type of surgery (i.e., genitourinary surgery, hernia repairs) or type of anesthetic (i.e., regional, neuraxial, or opioids).

❾ Relative hypovolemia should be evaluated and managed in PACU based on the patient's comorbidities, preoperative status (i.e., bowel preparation, postdialysis), type and duration of surgery, blood loss, and urine output.

❿ Glycemic monitoring and control should persist as a continuum from intraoperative management. Good glycemic control may help with fighting infection, may improve wound healing, and may result in better surgical outcomes. Hypoglycemia occurs because of nothing by mouth status, intraoperative administration of insulin, as well as the patient using programmable insulin pumps.

⓫ Hypothermia can lead to an increased length of stay in PACU, lethargy, decreased minute ventilation, decreased strength, and increased cardiac demand. It is important to assure that the patient is dry and insulated. The use of air warming blankets, warming mats, and intravenous fluid warmers all minimize hypothermia.

⑫ Many elderly patients experience a varied degree of post-operative confusion, delirium, or cognitive dysfunction in the PACU. Many pediatric patients also experience post-emergence, delirium leading to increased length of stay in the PACU.

⑬ Postoperative nausea and vomiting is a major cause of patient discomfort and dissatisfaction, as well as an aspiration risk and causes prolonged PACU stay.

POSTANESTHESIA RECOVERY

Each patient recovering from an anesthetic has circumstances that require an individualized problem-oriented approach. Postanesthesia recovery must continue to lead; to adapt to meet the needs of the changing perioperative landscape, advances in technology, changing surgical techniques; and to respond to improved evidence-based research. Dissemination of anesthesia services beyond the perisurgical arena has brought changes and greater demands on recovery units.

Standards for Postanesthesia Care

The ASA House of Delegates approved Standards for Postanesthesia Care on October 12, 1988. These standards were last amended on October 27, 2004.[30]

VALUE AND ECONOMICS OF POSTANESTHESIA CARE UNIT

The quality of postanesthesia care is composed of many variables such as tracking of complications, time per patient spent in recovery, overall clinical outcomes, and patient satisfaction. The value of postanesthesia care is a measure of the quality of care provided compared with the amount of resources spent per patient outcome. The postanesthesia care unit (PACU) helps to use resources efficiently by having trained staff that routinely care for postsurgical patients, thereby recognizing/preventing complications, and by having physicians instituting appropriate and timely therapies.

The actual cost of PACU care incorporates costs of staffing, space, and hardware (resource utilization). Triage and discharge policies affect both how many admissions occur and what resources each admission consumes. Nurse staffing continues to be the largest direct cost in the PACU. The mix of nursing staff, experience of nurses, staffing ratios, and the complexity and duration of PACU stay affect the overall personnel cost per admission. The level of monitoring provided affects the capital expenditure for equipment, and disposable items account for operating expenditures. The patient acuity mix also determines needs for staffing and equipment such as ventilators, additional monitors, intravenous pumps, and patient-controlled analgesia pumps. The type of physician coverage—such as dedicated coverage versus on-demand coverage—can affect response time, efficiency of care, costs, and patient outcomes. Routine (perhaps unnecessary) postoperative diagnostic testing and routine therapies increase cost per patient. Routine testing and therapies may unnecessarily add to staffing resources required per patient without widespread demonstrated benefit to patient care.

Cost comparisons between institutions are difficult because charges and cost factors vary widely across institutions, in different regions of the United States, and between countries. They constantly change over time. Regulatory requirements, standards of care, medical-legal climates, and institutional requirements vary greatly between regions and even between facilities in the same locale. It is difficult to establish cost-effectiveness goals of a single PACU because of the differing requirements of individual patients having the same procedures. This difference can be the result of levels of patient comorbidities, level of procedure complexity, surgeon, type of anesthetic, as well as patient perception and expectations. These are just some of the factors that can determine the type of care needed postoperatively. Continued pressures from many fronts to contain costs and maximize cost-effectiveness force each surgical facility to continually evaluate the value of its PACU care to each individual patient.

PACU directors are challenged to optimize clinical results while minimizing expenditures. Innovative PACU practices should guarantee safe care, minimize cost, and fulfill regulatory and institutional requirements. Medical professionals (physicians, nursing, and support staff) must work in concert to identify practices that are wasteful versus those that have proven yield/benefit. The impact of many PACU-proposed interventions on clinical outcome is not easily substantiated by controlled scientific analysis. Useless testing, unnecessary or unjustifiable therapy, and inappropriate PACU admissions should be eliminated. However, using a more expensive therapy may generate real savings by decreasing additional therapies, testing, admissions, or length of stay. Another important element essential for patient safety and efficiency in the PACU is communications with the intraoperative anesthesiology service. Communication is perhaps the least expensive tool in medicine and the one most universally proven to be involved in human error events. Utilization of PACU resources is directly related to anesthetic duration and technique. In one study, 22.1% of 37,000 patients had a minor anesthesia-related event or complication that prolonged PACU stays and consumed PACU resources.[1] Another study showed how postoperative adverse events affects the amount of nursing resources needed in the PACU.[2] Close coordination between the PACU and the anesthesiology service should reduce the frequency and impact of such events.

Improvements in care might create an opportunity to shorten the length of stay in the PACU, but realized change is frequently reduced by transportation delays, persistence of pain or nausea, waiting for space, or surgeon discharge delays.[3] Cost-saving measures in other areas may also increase the cost of PACU care; for example, fast-tracking to discharge to home rather than to a hospital bed. The cost savings of not occupying a hospital bed is offset by an increase in PACU stay and therefore greater consumption of PACU resources.[4] The savings may be a cost savings for the patient and beneficial for the facility as a whole but at a greater expense to the PACU. True savings are realized when operational changes yield a decrease in expenditures for staff, supplies, or equipment. For example, patients who are able to bypass the PACU creates a savings opportunity only if paid nursing hours are reduced or if more surgical cases are covered with the same hours. With **❶** the use of less invasive surgical techniques combined with innovative anesthetic techniques, such as regional anesthetics, shorter PACU stays can result in real savings opportunities. However, the areas of scheduling, clerical, or maintenance tasks must not consume excess staffing hours, without savings realized. Finally, trimming costs could entail an increase in risk. Clearly, no one wants that to happen. Differentiating between cost-effective postanesthesia care and unsafe practice remains a matter of constant professional judgment and debate daily in most PACUs.

LEVELS OF POSTOPERATIVE/ POSTANESTHESIA CARE

With increasing demand to reduce health care costs, care must be taken to provide the most appropriate care for each patient. As anesthesia services expand to cover a variety of patient types in ever-increasing areas outside the operating room, selecting the correct type of recovery is essential. For the many differing anesthesia areas ranging from inpatient surgery, ambulatory surgery, to off-site procedures, the level of postoperative care that a patient requires is determined by the degree of underlying illness and the duration and type of anesthesia and surgery. These factors are used to assess the risk of postoperative complications. Less-invasive surgeries or procedures combined with shorter-duration anesthetic regimens facilitate high levels of arousal and minimal cardiovascular or respiratory depression at the end of surgery.

Using a less intensive postanesthesia setting for selected patients can reduce costs for a surgical procedure and allow the facility to divert scarce PACU resources to patients with greater needs. Alert patients are more satisfied when spared the unnecessary assessments in interventions of PACU care. Amenities such as recliners, reading material, television, music, and food improve perceptions (emotional satisfaction) without affecting quality or safety. Earlier reunion with family or visitors in the low-intensity setting is desirable assuming that postoperative care is safe and appropriate.

Creation of separate PACUs for inpatients, ambulatory, or off-site patients is one possible way to streamline PACU care for appropriately triaged patients. Phase I recovery would be reserved for more intense recovery and would require more one-on-one care for staff. Phase II recovery should be less intensive and is appropriate for patients after less invasive procedures requiring less attention from nursing while recovering. If separation of different phases of care is not possible, then providing the appropriate level of monitoring and coverage to the degree of postoperative impairment achieves similar results in a single PACU area. However, care equal to a full-intensity PACU must always be available, given the incidence of complications after anesthesia and surgery.[5] As the aging population generates an increase in the complexity of surgical care in the face of tighter control of resources, maintaining appropriate PACU capacity and safety by observing applicable PACU guidelines and standards will be increasingly important.[6,7]

POSTANESTHETIC TRIAGE

Patients must be carefully evaluated to determine which level of care is appropriate. Triage should be based on clinical condition, length/type of procedure and anesthetic, and the potential for complications that require intervention. Alternatives to PACU care must be used in a nondiscriminatory fashion. Arbitrary criteria based on age, American Society of Anesthesiologists (ASA) classification, ambulatory versus inpatient versus off-site procedure status, or type of insurance should not be used for determining the level of recovery care. An individual patient undergoing a specific procedure or anesthetic should receive the same appropriate level of postoperative care whether the procedure is performed in a hospital operating room, an ambulatory surgical center, an endoscopy room, an invasive radiology suite, or an outpatient office. If doubt exists

about a patient's safety in a lower intensity setting, the patient should be admitted to a higher level of care for recovery. Patient safety should always be favored regardless of the cost.

After superficial procedures using local infiltration, minor blocks, or sedation, patients can almost always recover with less intensive monitoring and coverage. Healthy patients undergoing more extensive procedures (e.g., hernia repairs, arthroscopic procedures, minor orthopaedic procedures) under local, plexus, or peripheral nerve blockade might also bypass phase I recovery and go directly to phase II. The increasing use of continuous peripheral nerve catheters for surgery has shortened PACU time and can eliminate many hospital admissions.[8] Innovative anesthetic techniques, advanced surgical techniques, and use of bispectral index monitoring help facilitate fast-track postoperative care.[9]

SAFETY IN THE POSTANESTHESIA CARE UNIT

The PACU medical director (every PACU should have medical oversight) must ensure the PACU environment is as safe as possible for both patients and staff. Beyond usual safety policies, maintain staffing and training to ensure appropriate coverage and skill mix are available to deal with unforeseen crises. Incidence of adverse events in the PACU correlates with nursing workload and staff availability.[2] Ideally, all staff should have PACU certification, and staffing ratios should never fall below acceptable standards.[7] Less skilled or training staff must be appropriately supervised, and a sufficient number of certified personnel must always be available to handle worst-case scenarios.

The PACU staff protects patients who are temporarily incompetent and preserves patients' rights to observance of advanced directives and to informed consent for additional procedures. The staff is obligated to optimize each patient's privacy, dignity, and to minimize the psychological impact of unpleasant or frightening events. Observance of procedures for hand-washing, sterility, and infection control should be strictly enforced.[10] Medical directors must safeguard against potential for personal assault of patients during recovery such as unwarranted restraints and procedures without consent. Access to the PACU should be strictly controlled.

The PACU environment must also be safe for professionals. Air handling should guarantee that personnel are not exposed to unacceptable levels of trace anesthetic gases, although trace gas monitoring is not necessary. Ensure that staff members receive appropriate vaccinations, including that for hepatitis B. Practitioners must adhere to policies for radiation safety, infection control, disposal of sharps, universal precautions for blood-borne diseases, and safeguarding against exposure to pathogens such as methicillin-resistant *Staphylococcus,* vancomycin-resistant *Enterococcus, Clostridium difficile,* or tuberculosis. Always keep masks, gloves, gowns, eye protection, and appropriate particulate respiratory equipment easily accessible. Following current infection control policies and guidelines are essential for patient and staff safety. Ensure that sufficient help is available to avoid injury while lifting and positioning patients or while dealing with emergence situations. Compulsive documentation and clear delineation of responsibility protect staff against unnecessary medicolegal exposure.

ADMISSION TO THE POSTANESTHESIA CARE UNIT

Every patient admitted to a PACU should have heart rate, rhythm, systemic blood pressure, airway patency, peripheral oxygen saturation, ventilatory rate/character, and level of pain recorded and periodically monitored.[6] Assessment with periodic recording every 5 minutes for the first 15 minutes and every 15 minutes thereafter is a minimum. Document temperature, level of consciousness, mental status, neuromuscular function, mental status, degree of nausea on admission/discharge, and more frequently if appropriate, are also minimum standards of care. Every patient should be continuously monitored with a pulse oximeter and at least a single-lead electrocardiogram (ECG). Extra leads, particularly precordial V3-6, are appropriate if left ventricular ischemia is likely. Capnography is necessary for patients receiving mechanical ventilation or those at risk for compromised ventilatory function. Transduction and recorded output from invasive monitors such as central venous, systemic, or pulmonary arterial catheters must be accomplished. Diagnostic (laboratory) testing should be ordered only for specific indications.

Anesthesiology personnel should manage the patient until a PACU nurse secures admission vital signs, attaches appropriate monitors, and care is transferred with a complete report to the nursing staff. A succinct but thorough report that includes sufficient information to allow rapid evaluation and intervention for postoperative complications must be legibly recorded using a standardized format printed on the PACU record (Table 55-1). Documentation of the time and amount of all neuromuscular relaxants, respiratory depressant medications, and reversal agents should be standard. Outlined orders, specific therapeutic end points, and, most importantly, how to contact the responsible anesthesiologist all must be transmitted. The anesthesiologist should never transfer responsibility to PACU personnel until the patient's airway status, ventilation,

and hemodynamics are appropriate for the caregivers to whom he or she entrusts the patient's care. Leaving a patient in the hands of someone unfamiliar or incapable of adequately handling the acuity of the medical situation in a rush to perform "the next case" may constitute abandonment of care. Check the function of indwelling cannulae, intravenous catheters, and monitors before leaving.

POSTOPERATIVE PAIN MANAGEMENT

Relief of surgical pain with minimal side effects is a major goal during PACU care and a top priority for patients.[6,11–13] Periodically assess and document level of pain throughout recovery. The Joint Commission for Accreditation of Health Organizations has mandated that a numerical pain scale be used with periodic recording and an acceptable score for discharge. Inadequate postoperative analgesia is a major source of preoperative fear/dissatisfaction for surgical patients. In addition to improving comfort, analgesia reduces sympathetic nervous system response, thereby avoiding hypertension, tachycardia, and dysrhythmias. In hypovolemic patients the sympathetic nervous system activity may well mask relative hypovolemia. Administration of analgesics can precipitate hypotension in an apparently stable patient, especially if direct or histamine-induced vasodilation occurs. It is important to assess a tachycardic patient with low or normal blood pressure who complains of pain carefully before giving analgesics that might precipitate or accentuate hypotension.

TABLE 55-1

COMPONENTS OF A POSTANESTHESIA CARE UNIT ADMISSION REPORT

◼ PREOPERATIVE HISTORY/PROCEDURES

- Medication allergies or reactions
- Pertinent earlier surgical procedures
- Underlying medical illness
- Chronic medications
- Acute problems (e.g., ischemia, acid-base status, dehydration)
- Premedications (e.g., antibiotics and time given, β-adrenergic blockers, antiemetics)
- Preoperative pain control (e.g., nerve blocks, adjunct medications, narcotics)
- Preoperative pain assessment (chronic and acute pain scores)
- NPO status

◼ INTRAOPERATIVE FACTORS

- Surgical procedure
- Type of anesthetic
- Type and difficulty of airway management
- Relaxant/reversal status
- Time and amount of opioids administered
- Type and amount of intravenous fluids administered
- Estimated blood loss
- Urine output
- Unexpected surgical or anesthetic events
- Intraoperative vital sign ranges
- Intraoperative laboratory findings
- Drugs given (e.g., steroids, diuretics, antibiotics, vasoactive medications, antiemetics)

◼ ASSESSMENT AND REPORT OF CURRENT STATUS

- Airway patency
- Ventilatory adequacy
- Level of consciousness
- Level of pain
- Heart rate and heart rhythm
- Endotracheal tube position
- Systemic pressure
- Intravascular volume status
- Function of invasive monitors
- Size and location of intravenous catheters
- Anesthetic equipment (e.g., epidural catheters, peripheral nerve catheters)
- Overall impression

◼ POSTOPERATIVE INSTRUCTIONS

- Expected airway and ventilatory status
- Acceptable vital sign ranges
- Acceptable urine output and blood loss
- Surgical instructions (e.g., positioning, wound care)
- Anticipated cardiovascular problems
- Orders for therapeutic interventions
- Diagnostic tests to be secured
- Therapeutic goals and end points before discharge
- Location of responsible physician

NPO, nothing by mouth.

The actual degree of postoperative pain can be difficult to establish. Severity of pain varies among surgical procedures and anesthetic techniques. Staff members are relatively ineffective at quantifying level of discomfort. Patients are able to communicate despite having received sedative hypnotic drugs. Furthermore, patients may be impaired in their communication abilities coming into the hospital or may be affected by the entire medical experience, and thereby may be afraid to express their needs. Inexperienced nurses overestimate a patient's pain, whereas more experienced nurses tend to underestimate the pain.[14] Either error leads to inappropriate treatment. Use of a numeric pain scale yields more reliable results but requires that a patient be willing to communicate. A wide divergence can exist between a patient's cognitive perception of pain and sympathetic nervous system response, related to psychological, cultural, and cardiovascular differences among individuals. Some patients perceive severe pain with minimal sympathetic nervous system activity, whereas others exhibit hypertension and tachycardia with minimal complaint of discomfort. The best measure of analgesia is the patient's perception. Heart rate, respiratory rate and depth, sweating, nausea, and vomiting all may be signs of pain but their absence or presence is not in itself reliable as a measure of the presence of pain.

Careful identification of patient subgroups, assessment of individual analgesic requirements, and implementation of a planned, multimodal approach will provide seamless pain control through and beyond the PACU interval.[15] In a study of postoperative pain in 10,008 ambulatory patients, only 5.3% related severe pain in the PACU and 1.7% in the discharge area (Fig. 55-1). However, a much higher percentage of patients relate that moderate-to-severe pain recurs after discharge.[16,17] To avoid masking signs of an unrelated condition or a surgical complication, ascertain that the nature and intensity of pain are appropriate for the surgical procedure. The central nervous system (CNS) signs of hypoxemia, acidemia, or cerebral hypoperfusion often mimic those of pain, especially during emergence. Administration of parenteral analgesics or sedatives can acutely worsen hypoventilation, airway obstruction, or hypotension, causing sudden deterioration. Evaluating orientation, the level of arousal, and cardiovascular or pulmonary status usually identifies such patients.

Surgical pain can be effectively treated with intravenous opioids as part of a planned analgesic continuum that begins prior to the induction of surgical anesthesia and continues throughout the postoperative course. Sufficient analgesia is the end point, even if large doses of opioids are necessary in tolerant patients. Short-acting opioids are useful to expedite discharge and minimize nausea in ambulatory settings,[18] although duration of analgesia can be a problem. During intravenous titration of opioids, assess for incremental respiratory or cardiovascular depression. Disadvantages of intramuscular administration include larger dose requirements, delayed onset, and unpredictable uptake in hypothermic patients. Oral and transdermal analgesics have a limited role in the PACU but are helpful for ambulatory patients after PACU discharge. Rectal analgesics are sometimes useful in small children.

Perioperative use of cyclooxygenase-2 inhibitors has decreased because of adverse cardiovascular events. These events have led to the withdrawal of most of this class of drug with the exception of celecoxib, which has shown to reduce opioid requirements and the incidence of opioid adverse events.[19] The concerns surrounding the negative cardiac side effects have made the overall appropriateness of this therapy more complicated. Nonselective nonsteroidal anti-inflammatory drugs such as ibuprofen or acetaminophen are also effective, especially when administered orally before surgery. Preoperative administration likely augments the overall level of analgesia rather than offering a substantial pre-emptive advantage.[20] Ketorolac is an effective analgesic and anti-inflammatory

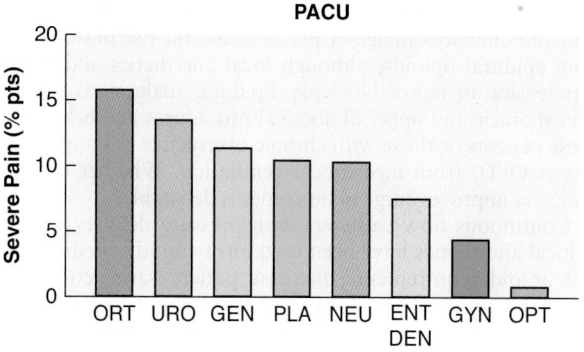

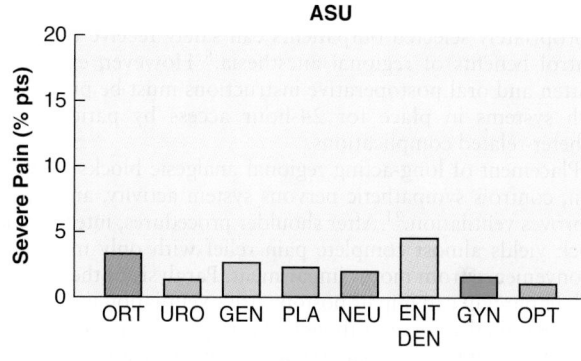

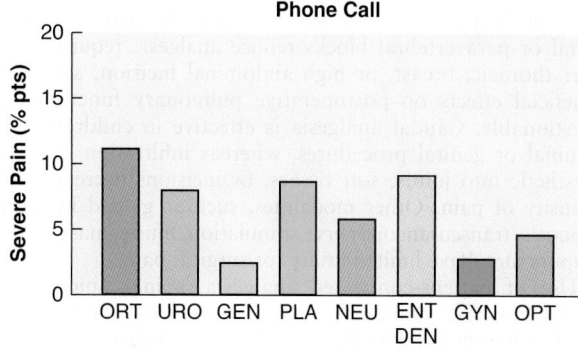

FIGURE 55-1. Percentage of patients experiencing severe pain in the postanesthesia care unit (PACU), the ambulatory surgery unit (ASU), and during phone call follow-up at 24 hours. ORT, orthopedics; URO, urology; GEN, general; PLA, plastics; NEU, neurology; ENT, ear, nose, throat; DEN, dental; GYN, gynecology; OPT, ophthalmology. (Reprinted from Chung F, Ritchie E, Su J: Postoperative pain in ambulatory surgery. Anesth Analg 1997; 85: 808, with permission.)

that lowers opioid requirements, although the possibility of hemorrhage due to its antiplatelet properties can limit its use. Ketorolac might also decrease ischemic events in patients with coronary artery disease through analgesic and antiplatelet actions. Use of clonidine to supplement analgesia is effective but can cause hypotension. Agonist–antagonist analgesics offer little advantage. Interventions such as repositioning, reassurance, or extubation also help minimize discomfort.

Other analgesic modalities provide pain relief in and beyond the PACU.[21] Intravenous opioid loading in the PACU is important for smooth transition to intravenous patient-controlled analgesia. Injection of opioids into the epidural or subarachnoid space during anesthesia or in the PACU yields prolonged postoperative analgesia in selected patients.[22,23] Nausea and pruritus are troubling side effects, and immediate or delayed ventilatory depression can occur related to vascular uptake and cephalad spread in cerebrospinal fluid. Nausea should resolve with antiemetics, whereas pruritus and ventilatory depression often respond to naloxone infusion. Addition of local anesthetic or clonidine enhances analgesia and decreases the risk of side effects from epidural opioids, although local anesthetics add risk of hypotension or motor blockade. Epidural analgesia is effective after thoracic and upper abdominal procedures and helps wean obese patients or those with chronic obstructive pulmonary disease (COPD) from mechanical ventilation. Whether epidural analgesia improves surgical outcomes is debatable.

Continuous flow catheters with pressure delivery systems of local anesthetics have been used intrawound to reduce pain and opioid requirements, increase patient satisfaction, and reduce length of hospital stay.[24] These same delivery systems have been safely used with continuous peripheral nerve catheters for in hospital as well as outpatient use.[25,26] With the use of ultrasound-guided techniques for catheter placement, appropriately selected outpatients can safely receive the pain control benefits of regional anesthesia.[8] However, extensive written and oral postoperative instructions must be provided, with systems in place for 24-hour access by patients for catheter-related complications.

Placement of long-acting regional analgesic blocks reduces pain, controls sympathetic nervous system activity, and often improves ventilation.[21] After shoulder procedures, interscalene block yields almost complete pain relief with only moderate inconvenience from motor impairment. Paralysis of the ipsilateral diaphragm can impair postoperative ventilation in patients with marginal reserve, although the impact is small in most patients.[27] Suprascapular nerve block might be an alternative to avoid this potentially serious side effect. Percutaneous intercostal or paravertebral blocks reduce analgesic requirements after thoracic, breast, or high abdominal incision, although beneficial effects on postoperative pulmonary function are questionable. Caudal analgesia is effective in children after inguinal or genital procedures, whereas infiltration of local anesthetic into joints, soft tissues, or incisions decreases the intensity of pain. Other modalities, such as guided imagery, hypnosis, transcutaneous nerve stimulation, music, massage, or acupuncture, have limited utility for surgical pain.

Use of patient-controlled analgesia, spinal opioids, or neural blockade mandates anticipation of risk beyond the PACU. One should plan for extended postoperative analgesia before induction of surgical anesthesia, and then orient the anesthetic and PACU care toward that plan. These plans should be in agreement with the patient, surgeon, and anesthesiologist. If one analgesic modality proves inadequate, take particular care when implementing a second technique.

Fear, anxiety, and confusion often accentuate postoperative pain during recovery, especially after general anesthesia. Titration of an intravenous sedative such as midazolam attenuates this psychogenic component, although analgesic requirements may increase slightly because benzodiazepines interact with γ-aminobutyric acid receptors. It is important to distinguish between requirements for analgesia and for anxiolysis. Opioids are poor sedatives and anxiolytics, whereas benzodiazepines are poor analgesics. However, when opioid dose appears larger than what might be anticipated as what the patient should require, one should consider the possibility that anxiety is playing a large role in the dysphoric event in the PACU.

DISCHARGE CRITERIA

When possible before discharge from postoperative care, each patient should be sufficiently oriented to assess his or her physical condition and be able to summon assistance. Airway reflexes and motor function must be adequate to maintain patency and prevent aspiration. One should ensure that ventilation and oxygenation are acceptable, with sufficient reserve to cover minor deterioration in unmonitored settings. Blood pressure, heart rate, and indices of peripheral perfusion should be relatively constant for at least 15 minutes and appropriately near baseline. Achieving normal body temperature is not an absolute requirement, but there should be resolution of shivering. Acceptable analgesia must be achieved and vomiting appropriately controlled. Patients should be observed for at least 15 minutes after the last intravenous opioid or sedative is administered to assess peak effects and side effects. If regional anesthetics have been administered, longer observation could be appropriate. One should monitor oxygen saturation for 15 minutes after discontinuation of supplemental oxygen to detect hypoxemia and then assess likely complications of surgery (e.g., bleeding, vascular compromise, pneumothorax) or of underlying conditions (e.g., hypertension, myocardial ischemia, hyperglycemia, bronchospasm). One should also document a brief neurologic assessment of orientation, eye signs, facial symmetry, and extremity movement and review results of diagnostic tests. If these generic criteria cannot be met, postponement of discharge or transfer to a specialized unit is advisable. There is no demonstrable benefit from a mandatory minimum duration of PACU care.

Scoring systems such as the Modified Aldrete Score or Postanesthesia Discharge Scoring System (Table 55-2) are two commonly used systems for patient assessment and attempt to simplify and standardize patient discharge criteria. Fixed PACU discharge criteria must be used with caution because variability among patients is tremendous. Scoring systems that quantify physical status or establish thresholds for vital signs are useful for assessment but cannot replace individual evaluation.[28,29] Ideally, each patient should be evaluated for discharge by an anesthesiologist using a consistent set of criteria, considering the severity of underlying disease, the anesthetic and recovery course, and the level of care at the destination (Table 55-2). A plan for the continued management of likely postdischarge symptoms such as pain, nausea, headache, dizziness, drowsiness, and fatigue must be made prior to discharge.[17]

CARDIOVASCULAR COMPLICATIONS

The purpose of this section is not to entirely review all the possible cardiovascular events that might beset a patient in the PACU, rather it is to help the reader decide what events might be unique to the PACU. In the PACU, some reflexes previously blunted by general anesthetics, sedatives, and opioids return toward baseline revealing an unexpected cardiovascular compromise. Perhaps the two most common types of patients to encounter troubles will be the patient with coronary artery disease and the patient with congestive heart failure. In the PACU it is a rare event for a patient to complain, de novo, of anginal type chest pain. The patients have significant blood opioid levels, and endorphins may be high because of the operation. The anesthetic makes the sensorium dulled and dysfunctional. The first sign of myocardial ischemia may well be hypotension. The most common sign of myocardial ischemia is tachycardia. Tachycardia is very often a reaction to, not the cause of, myocardial ischemia. That does not mean that all tachycardia heralds myocardial ischemia, but in a patient who seems at risk for coronary artery disease, new-onset tachycardia that is not caused by pain should be taken seriously. The ECG may show classic ST-T wave elevation or depression depending on lead placement and area of ischemia. But the lack of ST-T wave elevation does not rule out coronary artery disease. Transmural myocardial infarctions

TABLE 55-2

TWO MOST COMMONLY USED POSTANESTHESIA CARE UNIT DISCHARGE CRITERIA SYSTEMS

■ MODIFIED ALDRETE SCORING SYSTEM	■ POSTANESTHETIC DISCHARGE SCORING SYSTEM
Respiration 2 = Able to take deep breath and cough 1 = Dyspnea/shallow breathing 0 = Apnea	**Vital signs** 2 = BP + pulse within 20% preop baseline 1 = BP + pulse within 20–40% preop baseline 0 = BP + pulse >40% preop baseline
O_2 saturation 2 = Maintains SpO_2 >92% on room air 1 = Needs O_2 inhalation to maintain O_2 saturation >90% 0 = O_2 saturation <90% even with supplemental oxygen	**Activity** 2 = Steady gait, no dizziness or meets preop level 1 = Requires assistance 0 = Unable to ambulate
Consciousness 2 = Fully awake 1 = Arousable on calling 0 = Not responding	**Nausea and vomiting** 2 = Minimal/treated with PO medication 1 = Moderate/treated with parenteral medication 0 = Severe/continues despite treatment
Circulation 2 = BP ± 20 mm Hg preop 1 = BP ± 20–50 mm Hg preop 0 = BP ± 50 mm Hg preop	**Pain** Controlled with oral analgesics and acceptable to patient: 2 = Yes 1 = No
Activity 2 = Able to move four extremities voluntary or on command 1 = Able to move two extremities 0 = Unable to move extremities	**Surgical bleeding** 2 = Minimal/no dressing changes 1 = Moderate/up to two dressing changes required 0 = Severe/more than three dressing changes required
Score ≥9 for discharge	Score ≥9 for discharge

BP, blood pressure; PO, oral.

outside the PACU show no ECG diagnostic changes 10 to 30% of the time. So the clinician must be especially suspicious of a series of hemodynamic changes in a person at risk for coronary artery disease. Early intervention with nitrates, opioids, beta-blockers, and even anticoagulants may save a life. Cardiology should be involved to gain immediate and timely access to the cardiac catheterization laboratory or for angiolytic drug therapy. Involvement and communication with the surgical service must be immediate and decisions especially as to anticoagulation and lytic therapy should be made among several services in consultation. Thus, cardiac ischemia in the PACU may manifest subtly!

Congestive heart failure is epidemic in our ever-aging population. The outpatient cardiology services have an expanding armamentarium of new inotropic/vasodilator therapy, devices, and interventions that allow patients to compensate for their congestive heart failure. One should know not only the ejection fraction but the activities of daily living, exercise tolerance, and other risk indices. The ejection fraction is only an estimate of the fractional shortening of the myocardial actin and myosin fibrils. Although it is a useful estimate of severity of impairment, one is struck by how stable some patients may be with a large dilated heart contracting at a 15% ejection fraction. They are compensated but have little reserve. The potential problems of bleeding, volume shifts, and respiratory compromise in the PACU could quickly cause decompensation. There are also no absolute numbers with regard to fluid restriction. The usage of transesophageal echocardiography revolutionized cardiac anesthesia. It, along with surface echo, may be of great use in the PACU. Within a very few minutes a puzzling hypotensive situation might be explained by an echocardiogram. In the fast-paced dynamic environment of the PACU, placing a pulmonary artery (PA) catheter may give useful information, but may also take valuable time away

from patient triage and treatment. The ECG allows rapid viewing of myocardial contractility, regional wall motion, volume status, and valvular dysfunction.

The PACU has in the recent history taken on a new role in some hospitals. Cardiac surgical care is pushing toward "early extubation" or "fast tracking." In years past, especially when a "cardiac anesthetic" involved very large dosages of semisynthetic opioids that obligated patients to ≥24 hours of ventilation, the intensive care unit (ICU) was the standard place for all postoperative heart patients. Today, there is no such entity as a cardiac anesthetic. Balanced anesthetic techniques are used most often. Those who write about early extubation have pushed the limits from 24 hours all the way to extubation of patients on the operating table. Series are available with few if any reintubation catastrophes or events when this technique is practiced with good teams. The natural extension is to establish some highly specialized PACUs that function as step-down or short-term ICUs. In a study of 85 prospective patients[31] undergoing "off-pump" coronary artery bypass graft procedures, the patients were extubated in 12 ± 2 minutes after the chest was closed. They were then taken to a special part of the PACU where they were monitored for a number of hours (up to 480 minutes in some situations). Patients were then either discharged to the cardiac floors or sent to an ICU. Of the 85 patients in this study, only 4 failed the PACU stay and had to be admitted to an ICU. Bradycardia was the cause for failure in three cases and one there was one case of myocardial infarction. Two patients later returned to the ICU from the cardiac ward; there was one case of atrial fibrillation and another case of myocardial infarction. During the same time 304 patients who were not undergoing off-pump coronary artery bypass graft surgery were admitted to the cardiac ICU. The cost for PACU stay was $5,140.00 less than for an ICU-admitted patient. Although this study seems quite favorable, the two groups of patients were not comparable.

Studies from the mid-to-late 1990s looking at high-risk vascular and thoracic surgery patients showed that they could each be adequately cared for in an adequately staffed and prepared PACU.[32] The conclusion was that a hospital could well improve its patient throughput by putting more resources into expanded PACU care and not so much into ICU services. Several nursing reviews are available to give input as to how to structure such new units.[33,34]

Anesthesiology services are in increased demand throughout most hospitals. The PACU will likely need to prepare to care for those patients or to staff "ectopic" sites. In the evoked potential laboratories, for example, ablation procedures for dysrhythmias and the newer "mini-Maze" procedures may require care in the PACU. Automated implantable defibrillators are placed in hybrid suites, operating rooms, or catheterization laboratories. Now there is the possibility of percutaneous valve replacements as well as some hybrid and percutaneous coronary revascularization procedures. If these patients require deep sedation or general anesthesia, the patient will also require PACU care.

The cardiac patient is the common patient today. The new procedures and pressure to ever streamline operating room care is pressuring the PACU to become more and more a cardiac mini-ICU. The smart PACU medical director and hospital administrator will see that with targeted resources, patients may well be safely cared for in a more cost-effective manner with quicker throughput by using a PACU approach.

POSTOPERATIVE PULMONARY DYSFUNCTION

Mechanical, hemodynamic, and pharmacologic factors related to surgery and anesthesia impair ventilation, oxygenation, and airway maintenance.[35] Heavy smoking, obesity, sleep apnea, severe asthma, and COPD increase the risk of postoperative ventilatory events.[36] Preoperative pulmonary function testing has limited predictive value for postoperative complications,[37] perhaps with the exception of postoperative bronchospasm in smokers.[38]

Inadequate Postoperative Ventilation

In PACU patients, mild respiratory acidemia is expected; thus elevated PaCO$_2$ does not necessarily indicate inadequate postoperative ventilation. Inadequate ventilation should be suspected when (1) respiratory acidemia occurs coincident with tachypnea, anxiety, dyspnea, labored ventilation, or increased sympathetic nervous system activity; (2) hypercarbia reduces the arterial pH below 7.30; or (3) PaCO$_2$ progressively increases with a progressive decrease in arterial pH.

Inadequate Respiratory Drive

During early recovery from anesthesia, residual effects of intravenous and inhalation anesthetics blunt the ventilatory responses to both hypercarbia and hypoxemia. Sedatives augment depression from opioids or anesthetics and reduce the conscious desire to ventilate (a significant component of ventilatory drive).

Hypoventilation and hypercarbia can evolve insidiously during transfer and admission to the PACU. Although effects of intraoperative medications are usually waning, the peak depressant effect of an intravenous opioid given just before transfer occurs in the PACU. Coincident depression of medullary centers that regulate the sympathetic nervous system can blunt signs of acidemia or hypoxemia such as hypertension, tachycardia, and agitation, concealing hypoventilation. Patients might communicate lucidly and even complain of pain while experiencing significant opioid-induced hypoventilation. A balance must be struck between an acceptable level of postoperative ventilatory depression and a tolerable level of pain or agitation. Patients with abnormal CO$_2$/pH responses from morbid obesity, chronic airway obstruction, or sleep apnea are more sensitive to respiratory depressants.[39] Risk for apnea after anesthesia in preterm infants depends on type of anesthetic, postconceptual age, and preoperative hematocrit. Preterm infants should be monitored for at least 12 hours (see Chapter 44). Children with active or recent upper respiratory infection are more prone to breath-holding, severe cough, and arterial desaturations below 90% during recovery, especially if they have a history of reactive airway disease or secondhand smoke exposure or have undergone intubation and/or airway surgery.[40] If hypoventilation from opioids is excessive, forced arousal and careful titration (20 to 40 μg at a time) of intravenous naloxone reverses respiratory depression without affecting analgesia. Flumazenil (0.1 mg titrated to effect up to 1.5 mg) directly reverses depressant effects of benzodiazepines on ventilatory drive but is usually unnecessary.

The abrupt diminution of a noxious stimulus (e.g., tracheal extubation, placement of a postoperative block) may promote hypoventilation or airway obstruction by altering the balance between arousal from discomfort and depression from medication. Intracranial hemorrhage or edema sometimes presents with hypoventilation, especially after posterior fossa craniotomy. Bilateral carotid body injury after endarterectomy can ablate peripheral hypoxic drive. Chronic respiratory acidemia from COPD alters CNS sensitivity to pH and makes hypoxic drive dominant, but hypoventilation from supplemental oxygen rarely occurs.

Increased Airway Resistance

High resistance to gas flow through airways increases work of breathing and CO$_2$ production. If inspiratory muscles cannot generate sufficient pressure gradients to overcome resistance, alveolar ventilation fails to match CO$_2$ production and progressive respiratory acidemia occurs.

In postoperative patients, increased upper airway resistance is caused by obstruction in the pharynx (posterior tongue displacement, change in anteroposterior and lateral dimensions from soft tissue collapse), in the larynx (laryngospasm, laryngeal edema), or in the large airways (extrinsic compression from hematoma, tumor, or tracheal stenosis). Weakness from residual neuromuscular relaxation[41] or myasthenia gravis can contribute, but it is seldom the primary cause of airway compromise. If the airway is clear of vomitus or foreign bodies, simple maneuvers such as improving the level of consciousness, lateral positioning, chin lift, mandible elevation, or placement of an oropharyngeal or nasopharyngeal airway usually relieve obstruction. A nasopharyngeal airway is better tolerated when the patient has functional gag reflexes. Acute extrinsic upper airway compression (e.g., an expanding neck hematoma) must be relieved.

During emergence, stimulation of the pharynx or vocal cords by secretions, blood, foreign matter, or extubation can generate laryngospasm.[42] Laryngeal constrictor muscles occlude the tracheal inlet and reduce gas flow. Patients who smoke or are chronically exposed to smoke have irritable airway conditions, have copious secretions, or have undergone upper airway surgery are at higher risk.[35,40] Laryngospasm can usually be overcome by providing gentle positive pressure (10 to 20 mm Hg continuous) in the oropharynx by mask with 100% O$_2$. Prolonged laryngospasm is relieved with a small

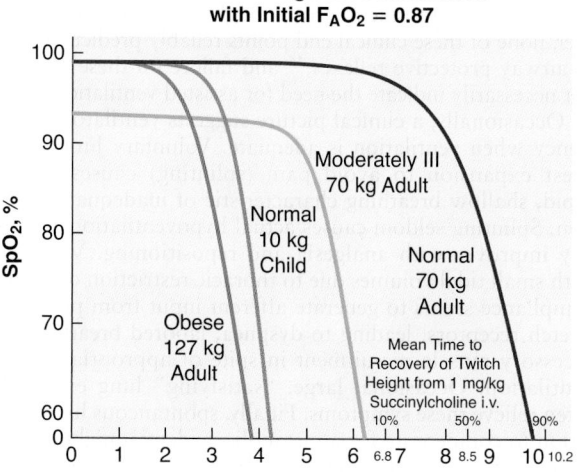

FIGURE 55-2. Rate of SpO2 decline after onset of apnea. (Reprinted from Benumof JL, Dagg R, Benumof R: Critical hemoglobin desaturation will occur before return to an unparalyzed state following 1 mg/kg intravenous succinylcholine. Anesthesiology 1997; 87: 979, with permission.)

dose of succinylcholine (e.g., 0.1 mg/kg) or deepening sedation with propofol. An intubating dosage of succinylcholine should not be used to break postoperative laryngospasm, especially if the alveolar partial pressure of oxygen (PaO2) is decreased by hypoventilation. As little as 5 to 10 mg of succinylcholine will do the job. Unless assisted ventilation is provided, declining PaO2 causes serious hypoxemia before spontaneous ventilation resumes[43] (Fig. 55-2). If the functional residual capacity (FRC) is abnormally reduced, the decreased volume of O_2 available in the lungs accelerates the development of hypoxemia. Severe laryngeal obstruction can occur secondarily because of hypocalcemia after parathyroid excision.

Soft-tissue edema worsens airway obstruction, especially in children and adults recovering from procedures on the neck. Nebulized vasoconstrictors help somewhat, but steroids have little effect acutely. Patients with C1 esterase inhibitor deficiency can develop severe angioneurotic edema after even slight trauma to the airway. Pathologic airway obstruction (e.g., severe edema, epiglottitis, retropharyngeal abscess, encroaching tumors) might require emergency tracheal intubation, but airway manipulation is dangerous because minor trauma from intubation attempts can convert a marginal airway into a total obstruction. Sedatives or muscle relaxants used to facilitate intubation can worsen obstruction by compromising the patient's volitional efforts to maintain the airway and by eliminating spontaneous ventilation. Equipment and personnel necessary for emergency cricothyroidotomy or tracheostomy should be available. Needle cricothyroidotomy using a 14-gauge intravenous catheter or a commercially available kit permits oxygenation and marginal ventilation until the airway is secured, especially if jet ventilation with 100% oxygen is used.

Reduction of cross-sectional area in small airways increases overall airway resistance because resistance varies inversely with the fourth power of radius during laminar flow and with the fifth power during turbulent flow. Pharyngeal or tracheal stimulation from secretions, suctioning, aspiration, or a tracheal tube can trigger a reflex constriction of bronchial smooth muscle in emerging patients with reactive airways. Histamine release precipitated by medication or allergic reactions also increases airway smooth muscle tone. Decreased radial traction on small airways reduces cross-sectional area in patients with COPD or with

decreased lung volume secondary to obesity, surgical manipulation, excessive lung water, or splinting. Preoperative spirometric evidence of increased airway resistance predicts an increased risk of postoperative bronchospasm.[38] Smokers and patients with bronchospastic conditions are at highest risk.[44] If ventilatory requirements are increased by warming, hyperthermia, or work of breathing, high flow rates convert laminar flow to higher-resistance turbulent flow. Prolonged expiratory time or audible turbulent air flow (wheezing) during forced vital capacity expiration often unmasks subclinical airway resistance. (Resistance is higher during expiration because intermediate-diameter airways are compressed by positive intrathoracic pressure.) High airway resistance does not always cause wheezing because flow might be so impeded that no sound is produced. Signs of increased resistance mimic those of decreased pulmonary compliance. Spontaneously breathing patients exhibit accessory muscle recruitment, labored ventilation, and increased work of breathing with either condition. Mechanically ventilated patients exhibit high peak inspiratory pressures.

The treatment of small airway resistance is directed at an underlying etiology. One must eliminate laryngeal or airway stimulation. Patients often respond to their pre-existing regimen of albuterol, pirbuterol, or salmeterol inhalers. Levalbuterol or metaproterenol nebulized in oxygen resolves postoperative bronchospasm with minimal tachycardia. Nebulized racemic epinephrine effectively relaxes smooth muscle, but side effects of tachycardia and flushing can be seen. Similarly, one can nebulize isoproterenol. Intramuscular or sublingual terbutaline can be added. Administration of steroid therapy offers little acute improvement, but may prevent later recurrence. Bronchospasm that is resistant to β_2-sympathomimetic medication may improve with an anticholinergic medication such as atropine or ipratropium. If bronchospasm is life-threatening, an intravenous epinephrine infusion yields profound bronchodilation. Increased small airway resistance caused by mechanical factors (e.g., loss of lung volume, retained secretions, pulmonary edema) usually does not resolve with bronchodilators. Restoration of lung volume with incentive spirometry or deep tidal ventilation increases radial traction on small airways. Reducing left ventricular filling pressures might relieve airway resistance caused by increased lung water, although interstitial fluid accumulation can persist. Also, extended contraction of airway smooth muscle obstructs venous and lymphatic flow, leading to airway wall edema that resolves slowly.

Decreased Compliance

Reduced pulmonary compliance accentuates the work of breathing. In the extreme, low compliance causes progressive respiratory muscle fatigue, hypoventilation, and respiratory acidemia. Parenchymal changes also affect compliance. Reduction of FRC leads to small airway closure and distal lung collapse, requiring greater energy expenditure to re-expand the lung. Pulmonary edema increases the lung's weight and inertia and elevates surface tension by interfering with surfactant activity, making expansion more difficult. Pulmonary contusion or hemorrhage interferes with lung expansion, as do restrictive lung diseases, skeletal abnormalities, intrathoracic lesions, hemothorax, pneumothorax, or cardiomegaly. Obesity affects pulmonary compliance, especially when adipose tissue compresses the thoracic cage or increases intra-abdominal pressure in supine or lateral positions. Extrathoracic factors such as tight muscles of the chest or abdominal dressings and gas in the stomach or bowel reduce compliance. Most notably after intra-abdominal laparoscopic procedures, retained CO_2 may impair diaphragm movement. The CO_2 has the capability to dissecting into the thorax creating either a pneumothorax or pneumomediastinum, which is usually a self-limited event as the CO_2 is relatively rapidly absorbed. There is usually no need for chest tube intervention. An intra-abdominal tumor, hemorrhage, ascites, bowel obstruction, or pregnancy impairs diaphragmatic excursion and reduces compliance.

Work of breathing is improved by resolving problems that reduce compliance. Allowing patients to recover in a semisitting (semi-Fowler) position reduces work of breathing. Incentive spirometry and chest physiotherapy help restore lung volume, as does positive end-expiratory pressure (PEEP) or continuous positive airway pressure (CPAP). In patients with COPD and highly compliant lungs, positive airway pressure might force the rib cage and diaphragms toward their excursion limits, accentuating inspiratory muscular effort.

Neuromuscular and Skeletal Problems

Postoperative airway obstruction and hypoventilation are accentuated by incomplete reversal of neuromuscular relaxation. Residual paralysis compromises airway patency, ability to overcome airway resistance, airway protection, and ability to clear secretions.[45] In the extreme, paralysis precludes effective spontaneous ventilation. Intraoperative use of shorter-acting relaxants might decrease the incidence of residual paralysis but does not eliminate the problem. Marginal reversal can be more dangerous than near-total paralysis because a weak, agitated patient exhibiting uncoordinated movements and airway obstruction is more easily identified. A somnolent patient exhibiting mild stridor and shallow ventilation from marginal neuromuscular function might be overlooked, allowing insidious hypoventilation and respiratory acidemia or regurgitation with aspiration to occur. PACU staff should be aware of patients who have received nondepolarizing muscle relaxants but no reversal agents because they often exhibit low levels of residual paralysis.[46] Safety of techniques designed to avoid reversal of short- and intermediate-duration relaxants has not been substantiated, and reversal of nondepolarizing relaxants is recommended.[6] The selective relaxant binding agent, γ-cyclodextrins (i.e., Sugammadex), is a promising reversal drug that can avoid the side effects of other anticholinesterases and anticholinergics.[47] Patients with neuromuscular abnormalities such as myasthenia gravis, Eaton-Lambert syndrome, periodic paralysis, or muscular dystrophies exhibit exaggerated or prolonged responses to muscle relaxants. Even without relaxant administration, these patients can exhibit postoperative ventilatory insufficiency. Medications potentiate neuromuscular relaxation (e.g., antibiotics, furosemide, propranolol, phenytoin), as does hypocalcemia or hypermagnesemia.

Diaphragmatic contraction is compromised in some postoperative patients, forcing more reliance on intercostal muscles and reducing the ability to overcome decreased compliance or increased ventilatory demands. Impairment of phrenic nerve function from interscalene block, trauma, or thoracic and neck operations can "paralyze" one or rarely both diaphragms.[27] Adequate ventilation will normally be maintained with only one diaphragm, and marginal ventilation by external intercostal muscles alone. However, with high work of breathing, muscle weakness, or increased ventilatory demands, a nonfunctional diaphragm impairs minute ventilation. Thoracic spinal or epidural blockade interferes with intercostal muscle function and reduces ventilatory reserve, especially in patients with COPD. Abnormal motor neuron function (e.g., Guillain-Barré syndrome, cervical spinal cord trauma), flail chest, or severe kyphosis or scoliosis can cause postoperative ventilatory insufficiency.

Simple tests help assess mechanical ability to ventilate. The ability to sustain head elevation in a supine position, a forced vital capacity of 10 to 12 mL/kg, an inspiratory pressure more negative than –25 cm H_2O, and tactile train-of-four assessment imply that strength of ventilatory muscles is adequate to sustain ventilation and to take a large enough breath to cough. However, none of these clinical end points reliably predicts recovery of airway protective reflexes,[46] and failure on these tests does not necessarily indicate the need for assisted ventilation.

Occasionally, a clinical picture suggests ventilatory insufficiency when ventilation is adequate. Voluntary limitation of chest expansion to avoid pain (splinting) causes labored, rapid, shallow breathing characteristic of inadequate ventilation. Splinting seldom causes actual hypoventilation and usually improves with analgesia and repositioning. Ventilation with small tidal volumes due to thoracic restriction or reduced compliance seems to generate afferent input from pulmonary stretch receptors, leading to dyspnea, labored breathing, and accessory muscle recruitment in spite of appropriate minute ventilation. Occasional large, "satisfying" lung expansions often relieve these symptoms. Finally, spontaneous hyperventilation to compensate for a metabolic acidemia might generate tachypnea or labored breathing, which is mistaken for ventilatory insufficiency.

Increased Dead Space

Ventilation of unperfused dead space or of poorly perfused alveoli with high ventilation/perfusion ($\dot{V}/\dot{Q}$) ratios is less effective in removing CO_2. Expansion of dead space volume or reduction of tidal volume increases the fraction of each breath wasted in dead space ($\dot{V}_D/\dot{V}_T$) and the amount of CO_2 from the previous exhalation that is rebreathed. A proportionally larger increase in total minute ventilation is required to meet any increase in CO_2 production. Patients with high $\dot{V}_D/\dot{V}_T$ are at greater risk for postoperative ventilatory failure.

Occasionally, an acute increase in dead space contributes to respiratory acidemia in postoperative patients. Although upper airway dead space is reduced after tracheal intubation and tracheostomy, excessive tubing volume or valve reversal in breathing circuits promotes rebreathing of CO_2. PEEP or CPAP elevates physiologic dead space, especially in patients with high pulmonary compliance. Pulmonary embolization with air, thrombus, or cellular debris increases physiologic dead space, although impact on CO_2 excretion is often compensated by accelerated minute ventilation from hypercarbic and hypoxic drives or reflex responses. Decreased cardiac output can transiently increase $\dot{V}_D/\dot{V}_T$ by decreasing perfusion to well-ventilated, nondependent lung. Irreversible increases in dead space occur if adult respiratory distress syndrome (ARDS) related to sepsis, transfusion-related acute lung injury, or hypoxia destroys pulmonary microvasculature. Dead space may appear high if an inhalation interrupts the previous exhalation and spent alveolar gas is retained. This "gas trapping" occurs when high airway resistance lengthens the time required to exhale completely, or if improper inspiration/expiration ratios or high ventilatory rates are used during mechanical ventilation.

Increased Carbon Dioxide Production

Carbon dioxide production varies directly with metabolic rate, body temperature, and substrate availability. During anesthesia, CO_2 production falls to approximately 60% of the normal 2 to 3 mL/kg/min as hypothermia lowers metabolic activity and neuromuscular relaxation reduces tonic muscle contraction. Therefore, during recovery, metabolic rate and CO_2 production can increase by 40%. Shivering, high work of breathing, infection, sympathetic nervous system activity, or rapid carbohydrate metabolism during intravenous hyperalimentation accelerates CO_2 production. Malignant hyperthermia generates CO_2 production many times greater than normal, which rapidly exceeds ventilatory reserve and causes severe respiratory and metabolic acidemia. Even mild increases of CO_2 production can precipitate respiratory acidemia if low compliance, airway resistance, or neuromuscular paralysis interferes with ventilation. With the exception of adjusting hyperalimentation, improving work of breathing, reducing shivering, or treating hyperthermia, there is little yield from addressing CO_2 production in PACU patients.

Inadequate Postoperative Oxygenation

Systemic arterial partial pressure of oxygen (PaO_2) is the best indicator of pulmonary oxygen transfer from alveolar gas to pulmonary capillary blood. Arterial hemoglobin saturation monitored by pulse oximetry yields less information on alveolar-arterial gradients and is not helpful in assessing impact of hemoglobin dissociation curve shifts or carboxyhemoglobin.[48] Evaluation of metabolic acidemia or mixed venous oxygen content yields insight into peripheral oxygen delivery and utilization. Adequate arterial oxygenation does not mean that cardiac output, arterial perfusion pressure, or distribution of blood flow will maintain tissue oxygenation. Sepsis, hypotension, anemia, or hemoglobin dissociation abnormalities can generate tissue ischemia despite adequate oxygenation.

In postoperative patients, the acceptable lower limit for PaO_2 varies with individual patient characteristics. A PaO_2 below 65 to 70 mm Hg causes significant hemoglobin desaturation, although tissue oxygen delivery might be maintained at lower levels. Maintaining PaO_2 between 80 and 100 mm Hg (saturation 93 to 97%) ensures adequate oxygen availability. Little benefit is derived from elevating PaO_2 above 110 mm Hg because hemoglobin is saturated and the amount of additional oxygen dissolved in plasma is negligible. During mechanical ventilation, a PaO_2 above 80 mm Hg with 0.4 FIO_2 and 5 cm H_2O PEEP,[48] CPAP or spontaneous breathing trial usually predicts sustained adequate oxygenation after tracheal extubation.

Strong inspiratory efforts against an obstructed airway decrease FRC and promote negative-pressure pulmonary edema. Small airway occlusion from compression, retained secretions, or aspiration leads to distal hypoventilation and hypoxemia, as does main stem intubation. Pneumothorax or hemothorax also reduce lung volume.

Conservative measures that restore lung volume often improve oxygenation. If possible, patients should recover in a semisitting position to reduce abdominal pressure on the diaphragms. Pain with ventilation encourages shallow breathing, so analgesia helps maintain FRC, especially with upper abdominal or chest wall incisions. Deep ventilation, cough, chest physiotherapy, and incentive spirometry seem to help expand FRC, mobilize secretions, and accustom a patient to incisional discomfort, but actual efficacy is debated.[51,52] For serious postoperative reduction of FRC, positive pressure is effective. CPAP (5 to 7 cm H_2O) can be delivered by face mask for several hours until factors promoting loss of lung volume resolve. If hypoxemia is severe or patient acceptance of mask CPAP is poor, tracheal intubation is usually required. Intubation for delivery of CPAP does not mandate positive-pressure ventilation. Ventilatory requirements should be assessed independently, considering $PaCO_2$, arterial pH, and work of breathing. Usually, 5 to 10 cm H_2O of CPAP or PEEP improves PaO_2 without risking hypotension, increased intracranial pressure, or barotrauma. If PaO_2 does not improve, one must re-evaluate the etiology. An occasional patient with ARDS or pulmonary contusion might require expiratory pressures in excess of 10 cm H_2O for improved oxygenation.

Tracheal intubation eliminates normal expiratory resistance and the "physiologic PEEP" (2 to 5 cm H_2O) that helps maintain lung volume during spontaneous ventilation. Exposing an intubated trachea to ambient pressure may cause a gradual reduction in FRC. Healthy, slender patients will often tolerate short periods of intubation without positive pressure, but generally it is prudent to use 5 cm H_2O CPAP for intubated postoperative patients.

Distribution of Ventilation

Loss of dependent lung volume commonly causes $\dot{V}/\dot{Q}$ mismatching and hypoxemia. A reduction in FRC decreases radial traction on small airways, leading to collapse and distal atelectasis that can worsen for 36 hours after surgery.[49] Reduced ventilation in dependent lung is particularly damaging because gravity directs pulmonary blood flow to dependent areas. Obese patients sustain large decreases in FRC during surgery. Older patients normally exhibit some airway closure at end expiration, and those with COPD have more severe closure that is exacerbated by small reductions in FRC. Retraction, packing, manipulation, or peritoneal insufflation during upper abdominal surgery reduces FRC, as does compression from leaning surgical assistants.[50] Prone, lithotomy, or Trendelenburg positions are disadvantageous, especially in obese patients. Right upper lobe collapse secondary to partial right main stem intubation is a frequently overlooked cause. During one-lung anesthesia, the weight of unsupported mediastinal contents, pressure from abdominal contents on the dependent diaphragm, and lung compression all reduce dependent lung volume. Gravity and lymphatic obstruction promote interstitial fluid accumulation and further $\dot{V}/\dot{Q}$ mismatching. This "down lung syndrome" may appear as unilateral pulmonary edema on the chest film.

Postoperatively, acute pulmonary edema from overhydration, ventricular dysfunction, airway obstruction, or increased capillary permeability (e.g., including transfusion-related acute lung injury, drug reactions) leads to hypoxemia by interfering with both $\dot{V}/\dot{Q}$ matching and diffusion of oxygen.

Distribution of Perfusion

Poor distribution of pulmonary blood flow also interferes with $\dot{V}/\dot{Q}$ matching and oxygenation. Flow distribution is primarily determined by hydrodynamic factors (PA and venous pressures, vascular resistance), which are affected by gravity, airway pressure, lung volume, and cardiac dynamics. Flow distribution is modulated by hypoxic pulmonary vasoconstriction (HPV), which diverts flow away from air spaces that exhibit low PaO_2. In postoperative patients, position affects oxygenation if gravity forces blood flow to areas with reduced ventilation. For example, placing a poorly ventilated lung in a dependent position can reduce PaO_2. Postoperative changes in PA pressure, airway pressure, and lung volume also have complex effects on blood flow distribution that can adversely affect $\dot{V}/\dot{Q}$ matching. Residual inhalation anesthetics, vasodilators, and sympathomimetics directly affect vascular tone and HPV, partially explaining larger alveolar-arterial oxygen gradients after general anesthesia. (Changes in distribution of ventilation also contribute.) Patients with liver cirrhosis exhibit poor $\dot{V}/\dot{Q}$ matching caused by small arteriovenous shunts that form throughout their lungs. Circulating endotoxin impairs HPV, contributing to hypoxemia in septic patients.

In the PACU, few interventions are useful to improve $\dot{V}/\dot{Q}$ matching by changing the distributions pulmonary blood flow. Maintain PA and airway pressures within an acceptable range. When possible, avoid placing an atelectatic or diseased lung in a dependent position. Placing poorly ventilated parenchyma in a nondependent position could improve $\dot{V}/\dot{Q}$ matching, but positioning a diseased lung in an "up" position may promote drainage of purulent material into the unaffected lung. Avoiding vasodilatory medications may improve PaO_2 but benefits from the medication usually outweigh drawbacks of impaired HPV.

Inadequate Alveolar PaO_2

Postoperative hypoxemia is occasionally caused by a global reduction of PaO_2, usually from inadequate ventilation, and marked increase in $PaCO_2$ (see the alveolar gas equation in Chapter 11). Hypoventilation must be severe to cause hypoxemia based on the alveolar gas equation. Complete apnea or airway obstruction by a foreign body, soft-tissue edema, or laryngospasm as well as very high small airway resistance all lead to rapid depletion of alveolar oxygen, and precludes effective ventilation. If cessation of ventilation does occur, the rate of PaO_2 decline varies with age, body habitus, degree of underlying illness, and initial PaO_2[43] (Fig. 55-3). Hypoxemia might also occur if opioids or residual anesthetic levels severely depress ventilatory drives. Partial airway obstruction does not usually reduce PaO_2, especially when patients are receiving supplemental oxygen. Increasing the oxygen content of the FRC with supplemental oxygen safeguards against hypoxemia from hypoventilation or airway obstruction, and eliminates the use of the pulse oximeter as a monitor of hypoventilation. Rarely, excessive concentrations of other gases reduce PaO_2. After general anesthesia, rapid outpouring of nitrous oxide displaces alveolar gas and can lower PaO_2 if a patient is hypoventilating or breathing ambient air, but this "diffusion hypoxia" would usually occur before PACU admission. Volume displacement of oxygen could also occur during severe hypercarbia in a patient breathing ambient air, although acidemia is often a greater problem.

Reduced Mixed Venous PO_2

Systemic venous partial pressure of oxygen ($P\bar{v}O_2$) is affected by arterial oxygen content, cardiac output, distribution of peripheral blood flow, and tissue oxygen extraction. If arterial oxygen content decreases or tissue extraction increases, $P\bar{v}O_2$ falls. The lower the $P\bar{v}O_2$ in blood that is shunted or flows through low $\dot{V}/\dot{Q}$ units, the greater the reduction of PaO_2. Blood with a low $P\bar{v}O_2$ also extracts larger volumes of oxygen from alveolar gas, amplifying the effect of hypoventilation or airway obstruction on PaO_2. Very low $P\bar{v}O_2$ increases the risk of resorption atelectasis in poorly ventilated alveoli. In postoperative patients, shivering, infection, and hypermetabolism lower $P\bar{v}O_2$ by increasing peripheral oxygen extraction. Low cardiac output and hypotension also lower $P\bar{v}O_2$ by decreasing tissue oxygen delivery. Supplemental oxygen reduces the impact of low $P\bar{v}O_2$ on alveolar oxygen extraction and on arterial oxygenation.

Obstructive Sleep Apnea

Obstructive sleep apnea (OSA) is a syndrome in which patients exhibit a period of partial or complete obstruction of the upper airway. This obstruction in turn interrupts sleep patterns, resulting in daytime hypersomnolence, decreased ability to concentrate, increased irritability, as well as aggressive and distractible behavior in children. The airway obstruction may cause episodic oxygen desaturation, hypercarbia, and possibly lead to cardiac dysfunction. It is estimated that 9% of women and 24% of men in the United States show disordered breathing while asleep, and 2% of women and 4% of men show overt symptoms of OSA.[53] These numbers are likely to increase as the population ages and become increasingly obese. In May 2003, the ASA Task Force on Perioperative Management of Patients with Obstructive Sleep Apnea issued guidelines based on the ASA scoring system for OSA and classifying patients as having mild, moderate, or severe OSA based on the apnea-hypopnea index.[54]

The perioperative management of the OSA patient must start preoperatively with a well-planned anesthetic taking into account the type, location, and recovery of surgery. Postoperative management concerns include analgesia, oxygenation, patient positioning, and monitoring. Regional anesthesia with minimal sedation is best for recovery versus increased use of opioids. Supplemental oxygen should be used immediately postoperatively. Patients who use CPAP or noninvasive positive-pressure ventilation should continue to use these therapies. Positioning should be used to minimize the patients' ability to obstruct the airway, which can be limited based on the type of surgery. Adult OSA patients show improvement in apnea-hypopnea index scores while in lateral, prone, and sitting positions compared with supine. With regard to monitoring, there is agreement among the consultants on the task force that pulse oximetry should be used until the patients' oxygen saturation remains above 90% on room air while sleeping. The use of telemetry for monitoring pulse oximetry, ECG, or ventilation can be beneficial in reducing adverse postoperative events and should be used on a patient need basis. With increasing studies in the area of OSA, the increased standardization of information regarding this patient population will lead to greater evidence-based treatment and supported clinical care.

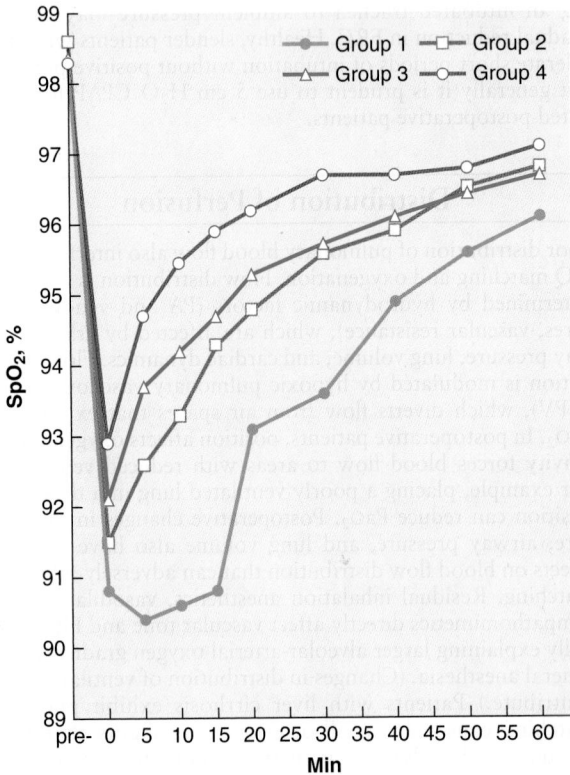

FIGURE 55-3. SpO2 versus postanesthesia care unit time in patients spontaneously ventilating in room air after general anesthesia (Group 1, 0 to 1 year of age; group 2, 1 to 3 years; group 3, 3 to 14 years; group 4, 14 to 58 years). (Reprinted from Xue FS, Huang YG, Tong SY et al: A comparative study of early postoperative hypoxemia in infants, children, and adults undergoing elective plastic surgery. Anesth Analg 1996; 83: 709, with permission.)

Anemia

Preoperative hematocrit and intraoperative hemorrhage determine a patient's red cell mass and oxygen-carrying capacity after surgery. Reduction of hematocrit caused by dilution has less impact. The hematocrit at which oxygen delivery becomes insufficient to match tissue needs varies with cardiac reserve, oxygen consumption, hemoglobin dissociation, PaO_2, and blood flow distribution. The actual level at which shock, lack of tissue oxygen delivery, occurs is known as the *critical DO_2* level. For animals and humans who have normal myocardial function and are euvolemic, critical DO_2 requires at least 3 to 3.5 g/dL hemoglobin concentration. Of course, hemoglobin this low may not be an appropriate transfusion trigger. However, it does illustrate the large excess of hemoglobin available to meet metabolic O_2 demands. Each patient has a minimum hematocrit below which tissues use inefficient anaerobic metabolism, generating a lactic acidemia. Patients with vascular disease are at increased risk of vital organ ischemia as hematocrit falls. Recent works from the ASA and the cardiac anesthesia/surgery societies (Society of Thoracic surgeons and Society of Cardiovascular Anesthesiologists) have published guidelines for transfusion and blood management. It is well accepted now that patients who are stable, not bleeding, and euvolemic can tolerate a hemoglobin of 6.0 g/dL. Transfusion may be of some benefit between 6 and 8 g/dL and it is rarely of use above 10 g/dL. Furthermore, transfusion of red cells to assist in weaning a patient from the ventilator has been shown to make the weaning process prolonged and/or make it far more difficult to remove the patient from the ventilator.

Supplemental Oxygen

The incidence of hypoxemia in postoperative patients is high. In PACU patients placed on room air, 30% of patients younger than 1 year of age, 20% aged 1 to 3 years, 14% aged 3 to 14 years, and 7.8% of adults had hemoglobin saturations fall below 90%, with many falling below 85%[55] (Fig. 55-3). Clinical observation and assessment of cognitive function do not accurately screen for hypoxemia, so monitoring with oximetry is essential throughout the PACU admission.[56] One cannot predict which patients will become hypoxemic or when hypoxemia will occur. Patients with lung disease or obesity, those recovering from thoracic or upper abdominal procedures, and those with preoperative hypoxemia are at increased risk.[57] Postoperative hypoxemia occurs in children, especially those with respiratory infections or chronic adenotonsillar hypertrophy. Hypoxemia occurs frequently after regional anesthesia.[23]

Supplemental oxygen should be administered only to patients at high risk of hypoxemia or with low SpO_2 readings (Table 55-3). However, some recommend supplemental oxygen be administered in the PACU during initial recovery and perhaps during transport to the PACU.[6] Supplemental oxygen does not address underlying causes of hypoxemia in postoperative patients, its use does not guarantee that hypoxemia will not occur, and it is likely to mask hypoventilation.[58] Although oxygen might cause minor mucosal drying, routine humidification is of little benefit unless intubation bypasses natural humidification. Oxygen apparatus can increase the risk of corneal abrasion during emergence.

Perioperative Aspiration

During anesthesia, depression of airway reflexes places patients at risk for intraoperative pulmonary aspiration that may manifest in the PACU, or for aspiration during recovery.

TABLE 55-3

COMMON OXYGEN DELIVERY SYSTEMS WITH CORRELATING O_2 FLOW RATES TO DELIVERED FiO_2 RANGES

SYSTEM	O_2 FLOW RATE (L/min)	FiO_2
Nasal cannula	1	0.21–0.24
	2	0.23–0.28
	3	0.27–0.32
	4	0.31–0.36
	5	0.35–0.40
	6	0.39–0.44
Simple mask	5	0.30–0.40
	8	0.40–0.60
Partial rebreathing mask	10	0.50–0.65
Nonrebreathing mask	10–15	0.60–near 1.00

Pulmonary morbidity from perioperative aspiration varies with the type and volume of the aspirate. Although aspiration of gastric contents is most widely feared, surgical patients also experience other aspiration syndromes.

Aspiration of clear oral secretions during induction, face mask ventilation, or emergence is common and usually insignificant. Cough, mild tracheal irritation, or transient laryngospasm are immediate sequelae, although large-volume aspiration predisposes to infection, small airway obstruction, or pulmonary edema. Aspiration of blood secondary to trauma, epistaxis, or airway surgery generates marked changes on the chest radiograph that are out of proportion with clinical signs. Aspirated "sterile" blood causes minor airway obstruction but is rapidly cleared by mucociliary transport, resorption, and phagocytosis. Massive blood aspiration or aspiration of clots obstructs airways, interferes with oxygenation, and leads to fibrinous changes in air spaces and to pulmonary hemochromatosis from iron accumulation in phagocytic cells. Secondary infection is a threat, especially if tissue or purulent matter is also aspirated.

Aspiration of food, small objects, pieces of teeth, or dental appliances causes persistent cough, diffuse reflex bronchospasm, airway obstruction with distal atelectasis, or pneumonia. Complications are often localized and treated with antibiotics and supportive care once the foreign matter is expelled or removed. Secondary thermal, chemical, or traumatic airway injury from aspirated objects can occur. Of course, complete upper airway or tracheal obstruction by an aspirated object is a life-threatening emergency.

Aspiration of acidic gastric contents during vomiting or regurgitation causes chemical pneumonitis characterized initially by diffuse bronchospasm, hypoxemia, and atelectasis.[59] The morbidity increases directly with volume and inversely with the pH of the acidic aspirate. Aspiration of partially digested food worsens and prolongs pneumonitis, especially if vegetable matter is present. Food particles mechanically obstruct airways and are a nidus for secondary bacterial infection. In serious cases, epithelial degeneration, interstitial and alveolar edema, and hemorrhage into air spaces rapidly progresses to ARDS with high-permeability pulmonary edema. Destruction of pneumocytes, decreased surfactant activity, hyaline membrane formation, and emphysematous changes can follow, leading to $\dot{V}/\dot{Q}$ mismatching and reduced compliance. Destruction of microvasculature increases pulmonary vascular resistance and dead space ventilation.

The incidence of serious aspiration is relatively low in PACU patients, but the risk is still significant. Frequency of postoperative vomiting remains high, especially if gas has accumulated in the stomach. Protective airway reflexes such as cough, swallowing, and laryngospasm are suppressed by depressant medications such as inhalation anesthetics, barbiturates, and opiates, so observe carefully patients with decreased levels of consciousness. Persisting effects of laryngeal nerve blocks or topical local anesthetics used to reduce airway irritability decrease postoperative airway protection, as does residual sedation. Reflexes are also impaired by residual neuromuscular paralysis.[46,60] Patients can sustain airway patency and spontaneous ventilation, pass a head lift test, have a tactile train-of-four T4/T1 ratio >0.7, and still have impaired airway reflexes from residual paralysis. The T4/T1 ratio should exceed 0.9 before reflexes are completely competent.[60] Risk of aspiration also increases if reversal is omitted. Hypotension, hypoxemia, or acidemia cause both emesis and obtundation, increasing aspiration risk.

Preventing aspiration is critical because effective therapy is limited.[61] For patients at high risk, preoperative administration of nonparticulate antacids such as sodium citrate increases the pH of gastric fluid without excessively increasing volume. Avoid particulate antacids. Histamine type 2 receptor blockers such as famotidine or ranitidine reduce the volume and increase the pH of gastric secretions. Metoclopramide increases gastroesophageal sphincter tone and accelerates gastric emptying. Inserting a nasogastric tube is often ineffective to remove particulate matter and interferes with gastroesophageal sphincter integrity.

In the PACU, vigilance against aspiration is important. Trendelenburg position might promote regurgitation but aids in airway clearance if regurgitation or vomiting occurs. Head elevation in unconscious patients should be avoided because it creates a gravitational gradient from pharynx to lung. High-risk patients should not have the trachea extubated until airway reflexes are restored. That being said, even though a patient is awake and able to follow commands he or she may well still have depressed gag reflex for some considerable number of hours after surgery/anesthesia. The introduction of opioids and other sedatives may well turn a situation of relatively good airway protection into one of potential aspiration. Aspiration of acidic fluid can still occur around an inflated tracheal tube cuff, so frequently monitor the upper airway for secretions or vomitus. One should avoid cuff deflation until extubation because the rigid tube impairs laryngospasm, swallowing, and other protective reflexes. The pharynx should use suction completely and the trachea extubated at end inspiration with positive airway pressure to promote expulsion of material trapped below the cords but above the inflated cuff. Observation is essential after extubation because airway reflexes might be temporarily impaired. Anatomic distortion in the airway from soft-tissue trauma or surgical intervention interferes with airway protection. Mandibular fixation makes expulsion of vomitus, blood, or secretions difficult, so have equipment for release of mandibular fixation available and ensure patients demonstrate cognitive and physical ability to clear the airway before the trachea is extubated.

Discovery of gastric secretions in the pharynx mandates immediate lateral head positioning (assuming cervical spine integrity) and suction of the airway. If airway reflexes are compromised, tracheal intubation is often appropriate. After intubation, the trachea is suctioned through the tracheal tube before positive-pressure ventilation; this avoids widely disseminating aspirated material into distal airways. Instillation of saline or alkalotic solutions is not recommended. Assessing the pH of tracheal aspirate is useless because buffering is immediate. Checking pharyngeal aspirate pH is more accurate but of little practical value. Suspicion that aspiration has occurred mandates 24 to 48 hours of monitoring for development of aspiration pneumonitis. If the likelihood of aspiration is small

in an ambulatory patient, outpatient follow-up can be done, assuming hypoxemia, cough, wheezing, or radiographic abnormalities do not appear within 4 to 6 hours. The patient should receive explicit instructions to contact a medical facility at the first appearance of malaise, fever, cough, chest pain, or other symptoms of pneumonitis. If likelihood of aspiration is high, the patient should be admitted to the hospital. Observation includes serial temperature checks, white blood cell counts with differential, chest radiograph, and blood gas determination. Chest physiotherapy, incentive spirometry, and restarting medications for pre-existing pulmonary conditions minimize the loss of lung volume, $\dot{V}/\dot{Q}$ mismatching, and infection. Fluffy infiltrates may appear on the chest radiograph any time within 24 hours. Hypoxemia might develop quickly or evolve insidiously as injury progresses, so frequent pulse oximetry monitoring is important.

If hypoxemia, increased airway resistance, consolidation, or pulmonary edema evolves, the patient should be supported with supplemental oxygen, PEEP, or CPAP. Mechanical ventilation may be necessary. Steroids yield no improvement and may increase the risk of bacterial super infection. Bacterial infection does not always follow aspiration, so prophylactic antibiotics merely promote colonization by resistant organisms. If bacterial infection is apparent, institute antibiotic therapy based on culture results. If cultures are equivocal, use broad-spectrum antibiotics with coverage for Gram-negative rods and anaerobes, including *Bacteroides fragilis*. Overall therapy is similar to that for ARDS. Pulmonary edema from increased capillary permeability should not be treated with diuretics unless high filling pressures or hypervolemia exist.

POSTOPERATIVE RENAL COMPLICATIONS

Ability to Void

8 The ability to void should be assessed because opioids and autonomic side effects of regional anesthesia interfere with sphincter relaxation and promote urine retention. Urinary retention is common after urologic, inguinal, and genital surgery, and retention frequently delays discharge.[3] Observation after these surgeries is needed to determine if inability to urinate is a possible surgical complication. Neither the patient nor staff can accurately estimate bladder volume through sensation or palpation. Avoid the archaic practice of "straight catheterization," unless indicated. An ultrasonic bladder scan helps assess bladder volume before discharge. It is reasonable to discharge selected ambulatory patients from the facility and inpatients to a floor before they void.[6,62,63] When inpatients are transferred prior to voiding, ensure urination can be monitored to avoid complications from urinary retention. Give ambulatory patients who are discharged without voiding a specific time interval in which to void (i.e., 10 to 12 hours after discharge). If retention persists, the patient must contact a health care facility. High return rates after urologic procedures are related to urinary retention.[64]

Renal Tubular Function

Analysis of urine yields information about postoperative renal tubular function. Urine color is not useful for assessing concentrating ability, but it does assist recognition of hematuria, hemoglobinuria, or pyuria. Urine osmolarity (reflecting the number of particles in solution) is a more reliable index of tubular function than specific gravity, which is affected by molecular weight of solutes. An osmolarity >450 mOsm/L indicates intact tubular concentrating ability. A urine sodium concentration far below or a potassium concentration above serum concentrations also indicates tubular viability, as does acidification or alkalinization of urine. Osmolarity, electrolyte, and pH values close to those in serum may indicate poor tubular function or acute tubular necrosis.

Inorganic fluoride released during metabolism of certain inhalation anesthetics can cause a transient reduction of tubular concentrating ability after long anesthetics. Higher fluoride levels cause renal tubular necrosis. Interaction of sevoflurane with dry carbon dioxide absorbents (often found in first cases or peripheral locations) generates compound A, a vinyl ether that degrades to release inorganic fluoride. Although transient impairment of protein retention and concentrating ability may occur, use of sevoflurane does not seriously affect renal function.

Oliguria

9 Oliguria (≤ 0.5 mL/kg/hr) occurs frequently during recovery and usually reflects an appropriate renal response to hypovolemia. The stress response of surgery also increases antidiuretic hormone (ADH), which can lead to decreased urine output. However, decreased urine output might indicate abnormal renal function. The acceptable degree and duration of oliguria vary with baseline renal status, the surgical procedure, and the anticipated postoperative course. In patients without catheters, one should assess interval since last voiding, and bladder volume to help differentiate oliguria from inability to void. One should check indwelling urinary catheters for kinking, for obstruction by blood clots or debris, and for the catheter tip being positioned above the urinary level in the bladder, and aggressively evaluate oliguria if intraoperative events could jeopardize renal function (e.g., aortic cross-clamping, severe hypotension, possible ureteral ligature, massive transfusion). Systemic blood pressure must be adequate for renal perfusion, based on preoperative pressures. Administration of desmopressin for hematologic purposes seldom affects postoperative urinary output. After urine is sent for electrolyte and osmolarity determinations, a 300 to 500 mL intravenous crystalloid bolus helps assess whether oliguria represents a renal response to hypovolemia. If output does not improve, consider a larger bolus or a diagnostic trial of furosemide, 5 mg intravenously. Furosemide increases urine output if oliguria reflects tubular resorption of fluid. Patients receiving chronic diuretic therapy might require a diuretic effect to maintain postoperative urine output.

Persistence of oliguria despite hydration, adequate perfusion pressure, and a furosemide challenge increases the likelihood of acute tubular necrosis, ureteral obstruction, renal artery or vein occlusion, or inappropriate ADH secretion. Cystoscopy, intravenous pyelography, angiography, or radionuclide scanning may help clarify renal status. Osmotic or loop diuretics may be useful to attenuate renal damage. The use of low-dose dopamine or dobutamine has not proven to improve renal function. Fenoldopam used perioperatively has shown to reduce the risk of acute kidney injury for select high-risk cardiac surgical patients.[65] Consultation with a nephrologist is prudent.

Polyuria

Relying on high postoperative urinary output to gauge intravascular volume status or renal viability can be misleading. Profuse urine output often reflects generous intraoperative fluid administration, but osmotic diuresis caused by hyperglycemia and glycosuria is another common cause, particularly if glucose-containing crystalloid solutions are infusing.

Polyuria might also reflect intraoperative diuretic administration. However, sustained polyuria (4 to 5 mL/kg/hr) can indicate abnormal regulation of water clearance or high-output renal failure, especially if urinary losses compromise intravascular volume and systemic blood pressure. Diabetes insipidus occurs secondary to intracranial surgery, pituitary ablation, head trauma, or increased intracranial pressure. A urine specific gravity of ≤ 1.005 and a urine osmolality <200 mOsm/kg are the hallmark of diabetes insipidus. A random plasma osmolality is generally >285 mOsm/kg. Diagnostic or therapeutic administration of vasopressin is useful.

METABOLIC COMPLICATIONS

Postoperative Acid-Base Disorders

Categorization of postoperative acid-base abnormalities into primary and compensatory disorders is difficult because rapidly changing pathophysiology can often generate multiple primary disorders.

Respiratory Acidemia

Respiratory acidemia is frequently encountered in PACU patients because anesthetics, opioids, and sedatives promote hypoventilation by depressing CNS sensitivity to pH and $PaCO_2$. In awake, spontaneously breathing patients with adequate analgesia, hypercarbia and acidemia are usually mild ($PaCO_2$ 45 to 50 mm Hg, pH 7.36 to 7.32). Deeply sedated patients exhibit more profound acidemia unless supplemental ventilation is administered. Patients with residual neuromuscular paralysis, increased airway resistance, or decreased pulmonary compliance might not sustain adequate ventilation despite an intact CNS drive, especially if CO_2 production is elevated by fever, shivering, or hyperalimentation. The kidneys require hours to generate a compensatory metabolic alkalosis, so compensation for acute postoperative respiratory acidemia is limited.

Symptoms of respiratory acidemia include agitation, confusion, ventilatory dissatisfaction, and tachypnea. Sympathetic nervous system response to low pH causes hypertension, tachycardia, and dysrhythmias. Respiratory acidemia caused by CNS depression often produces less intense signs of sympathetic nervous system activity. In patients with head injury, intracranial tumors, or cerebral edema, respiratory acidemia increases cerebral blood flow and intracranial pressure. At very low pH, catecholamines cannot interact with adrenergic receptors, so heart rate and blood pressure decrease precipitously. Treatment consists of correcting the imbalance between CO_2 production and alveolar ventilation. Raising the level of consciousness by the judicious reversal of opioids or benzodiazepines improves ventilatory drive. It is important to ensure that the patient does not have increased airway resistance or residual neuromuscular blockade. If spontaneous ventilation cannot maintain CO_2 excretion, tracheal intubation and mechanical ventilation are necessary. Reducing CO_2 production by controlling fever or shivering may be helpful.

Metabolic Acidemia

Evaluation of acute postoperative metabolic acidemia is relatively straightforward (Table 55-4). Occasionally, ketoacidosis occurs in diabetic patients. During ketoacidosis, serum glucose levels are elevated and ketones are detectable in blood or urine. Patients with renal failure or renal tubular acidosis usually exhibit a preoperative metabolic acidemia. Large volumes of saline infusions during surgery can generate a mild hyperchloremic, metabolic acidemia, but use of lactated Ringer

TABLE 55-4

CAUSES OF ACIDEMIA

Normal anion gap acidosis
  GI loss of bicarbonate
    Diarrhea
    Urinary diversion
    GI fistulas or drains
  Renal loss of bicarbonate
    Renal tubular acidosis
    Renal insufficiency
    Recovery phase of ketoacidosis
Increased anion gap acidosis
  Ketoacidosis (diabetic, alcoholic, severe cachexia)
  Lactic acidosis (seizures, neuroleptic malignant syndrome,
    MH, severe asthma, pheochromocytoma, cardiogenic
    shock, hypovolemia, severe anemia, regional ischemia,
    sepsis, hypoglycemia)
Respiratory acidosis

GI, gastrointestinal; MH, malignant hyperthermia.

solution avoids this problem.[66] Rarely, a patient manifests acidemia from toxic ingestion of aspirin or methanol. Once these unusual causes are excluded, postoperative metabolic acidemia almost always represents lactic acidemia secondary to insufficient delivery or utilization of oxygen in peripheral tissues. Peripheral hypoperfusion is often caused by low cardiac output (hypovolemia, cardiac failure, dysrhythmia) or peripheral vasodilation (sepsis, catecholamine depletion, sympathectomy). Arteriolar constriction from hypothermia or pressor administration reduces tissue perfusion and induces abnormal blood flow distribution. Hypoxemia, severe anemia, impaired hemoglobin dissociation, CO poisoning, and inability to use oxygen in the mitochondria (cyanide or arsenic poisoning) also generate lactic acidemia.

A spontaneously breathing patient will increase minute ventilation in response to metabolic acidemia and quickly generate a respiratory alkalosis to compensate for metabolic acidemia. However, general anesthetics and analgesics suppress this ventilatory response. The sympathetic response to acute postoperative metabolic acidemia is often milder than the response to respiratory acidemia because hydrogen and bicarbonate ions cross the blood–brain barrier with more difficulty than CO_2. Treatment consists of resolving the condition causing accumulation of metabolic acid. For example, ketoacidosis is treated with intravenous potassium, insulin, and glucose. Improving cardiac output or systemic blood pressure will reduce lactic acid production, as will rewarming. If conditions causing lactate accumulation are improved and acidemia is mild, renal excretion of hydrogen ions will restore normal pH. For severe or progressive acidemia, intravenous bicarbonate or calcium gluconate helps restore pH.

Respiratory Alkalemia

Pain or anxiety during emergence causes hyperventilation and acute respiratory alkalemia. Excessive mechanical ventilation also generates respiratory alkalemia, especially if hypothermia or paralysis has decreased CO_2 production. Pathologic causes of "central" hyperventilation include sepsis, cerebrovascular accident, or paradoxic CNS acidosis (an imbalance of bicarbonate concentration across the blood–brain barrier caused by prolonged hyperventilation). Acute respiratory alkalemia can generate confusion, dizziness, atrial dysrhythmias, and abnormal cardiac conduction. Alkalemia decreases cerebral blood flow, causing hypoperfusion and even stroke in patients with

cerebrovascular disease. If the alkalemia is severe, reduced serum ionized calcium concentration precipitates muscle fasciculation or hypocalcemic tetany. Very high pH depresses cardiovascular, CNS, and catecholamine receptor functions. Metabolic compensation for acute respiratory alkalemia is limited because time constants for bicarbonate excretion are large. Treatment necessitates reducing alveolar ventilation, usually by administering analgesics and sedatives for pain and anxiety. Rebreathing of CO_2 has little application in the PACU.

Metabolic Alkalemia

Metabolic alkalemia is rare in PACU patients unless vomiting, gastric suctioning, dehydration, alkaline ingestion, or potassium-wasting diuretics caused an alkalemia that existed before surgery. Excessive intraoperative bicarbonate administration causes postoperative metabolic alkalemia, but alkalemia from metabolism of lactate or citrate usually does not appear within the first 24 hours. Respiratory compensation through retention of CO_2 is rapid but limited because hypoventilation eventually causes hypoxemia. Hydration and correction of hypochloremia and hypokalemia allow the kidney to excrete excess bicarbonate.

Glucose Disorders and Control

❿ Tight glucose control has been recommended to reduce morbidity in a variety of postsurgical patients. The control of glucose in diabetic and nondiabetic patients has shown to reduce complications and hospital length of stay and improve patient outcomes. However, the potential for hypoglycemia and coma should not be discounted. Insulin therapy should be based on serum glucose levels. Urine glucose measurements should be reserved to assess osmotic diuresis and estimate renal transport thresholds by comparison with serum levels.

Hyperglycemia

Glucose infusions and stress responses commonly elevate serum glucose levels after surgery. For most patients during anesthesia, glucose should not be included in maintenance intravenous solutions. Moderate postoperative hyperglycemia (150 to 250 mg/dL) resolves spontaneously and has little adverse effect in the nondiabetic patient. Higher glucose levels cause glycosuria with osmotic diuresis and interfere with serum electrolyte determinations. Severe hyperglycemia increases serum osmolality to a point that cerebral disequilibrium and hyperosmolar coma occur. Type I diabetic patients are at risk for ketoacidosis. Potassium replacement and serial blood glucose determinations are essential.

Hypoglycemia

Hypoglycemia in the PACU can be caused by endogenous insulin secretion or by excessive or inadvertent insulin administration. Serious postoperative hypoglycemia is rare and easily treated with intravenous 50% dextrose followed by glucose infusion. Either sedation or excessive sympathetic nervous system activity masks signs and symptoms of hypoglycemia after anesthesia. Diabetic patients and especially patients who have received insulin therapy intraoperatively must have serum glucose levels measured to avoid the serious problems related to hypoglycemia.

Electrolyte Disorders

Hyponatremia

Postoperative hyponatremia occurs if free water is infused intravenously during surgery or if sodium-free irrigating solution is absorbed during transurethral prostatic resection or hysteroscopy. Accumulation of serum glycine or its metabolite, ammonia, might exacerbate symptoms. Free water retention is also caused by inappropriate ADH secretion, prolonged labor induction with oxytocin, or respiratory uptake of nebulized droplets. Theoretically, excessive infusion of isotonic saline leads to excretion of hypertonic urine, desalination, and iatrogenic hyponatremia. Symptoms of moderate hyponatremia include agitation, disorientation, visual disturbances, and nausea, whereas severe hyponatremia causes unconsciousness, impaired airway reflexes, and CNS irritability that progress to grand mal seizures. Therapy includes intravenous normal saline and intravenous furosemide to promote free water excretion. Infusion of hypertonic saline may be useful for severe hyponatremia, in which diligence not to increase serum sodium by 0.5 mEq/hr is needed to avoid CNS lesions or pulmonary edema. Monitor serum sodium concentration and osmolarity.

Hypokalemia

Postoperative hypokalemia is often inconsequential but might generate serious dysrhythmias, especially in patients taking digoxin. A potassium deficit caused by chronic diuretic therapy, nasogastric suctioning, or vomiting often underlies hypokalemia. Urinary and hemorrhagic losses, dilution, and insulin therapy generate acute hypokalemia that worsens during respiratory alkalemia. Excess sympathetic nervous system activity, infusion of calcium, or β-mimetic medications exacerbates effects of hypokalemia. Adding potassium to peripheral intravenous fluids often restores serum concentration, but concentrated solutions infused through a central catheter may be necessary. So often practitioners think 10 to 30 mEq of potassium will bring the patient back to normal. Potassium is an intracellular ion and a plasma potassium deficit is indicative of a far greater intracellular deficit. It is the intracellular-to-extracellular ratio that may well be important, and rapid changes can contribute to as many dysrhythmias as can mild hypokalemia alone.

Hyperkalemia

A high serum potassium level raises the suspicion of spurious hyperkalemia from a hemolyzed specimen or from sampling near an intravenous catheter containing potassium or banked blood. Postoperative hyperkalemia occurs after excessive potassium infusion or in patients with renal failure or malignant hyperthermia. Acute acidemia exacerbates hyperkalemia. Treatment with intravenous insulin and glucose acutely lowers potassium, whereas intravenous calcium counters myocardial effects.

Calcium and Magnesium

Although underlying parathyroid disease or massive fluid replacement reduces total body and ionized calcium, symptomatic hypocalcemia seldom occurs in the PACU. A rare patient might exhibit upper airway obstruction from hypocalcemia after parathyroid excision. Reduction of the ionized fraction by acute alkalemia may cause myocardial conduction and contractility abnormalities, decreased vascular tone, or tetany. Transfusion of blood containing chelating agents (e.g., citrate) rarely causes symptomatic hypocalcemia. Administration of calcium chloride or calcium gluconate to hypocalcemic patients improves cardiovascular dynamics.

Magnesium plays a key role in restoration of neuromuscular function after surgery and in maintenance of cardiac rhythm and conduction. Hypermagnesemia is rare because the kidneys are effective at excreting excessive magnesium. Obstetric patients who have been receiving magnesium for tocolysis or control of severe pregnancy-induced hypertension can present postoperatively hyporeflexive, and at higher serum levels show prolonged atrioventricular conduction or complete heart block. Treatment entails intravenous calcium and diuretics.

MISCELLANEOUS COMPLICATIONS

Incidental Trauma

Each patient admitted to the PACU should be carefully evaluated for traumatic complications. Discovery of a complication necessitates careful documentation, notification of physicians responsible for extended care, consultation with specialists, and follow-up.

Ocular Injuries and Visual Changes

Corneal abrasion caused by drying or inadvertent eye contact during face mask ventilation or intubation is a common intraoperative eye injury. The incidence of this type of injury in a nonophthalmic patient is estimated to be between 0.034 and 0.17%, with the higher incidence related to prone or lateral positioning.[67] Corneal injury can occur during emergence in the PACU from patients rubbing their eyes, if a rigid oxygen face mask rides up on the eye, or if the eye is rubbed with a pulse oximeter probe and from eye make-up (particularly mascara) being rubbed in the eyes. Abrasions cause tearing, decreased visual acuity, pain, and photophobia. Fluorescein staining aids diagnosis. Abrasions usually heal spontaneously within 72 hours without scarring, but severe injury can cause cataract formation and impair vision. There is no standard treatment for corneal abrasions, but symptomatic treatment includes artificial tears, topical antibiotics, topical analgesics, and eye closure.

Visual acuity is often impaired after anesthesia. Autonomic side effects of medications impair accommodation, and residual ocular lubricant clouds vision. Impairment of retinal perfusion by ocular compression generates postoperative visual disturbances ranging from loss of acuity to permanent blindness.[68,69] Ischemic optic atrophy can also occur in the absence of external compression.[70] Risk of blindness is higher after long procedures in the prone position, as well as in patients with vascular disease, pre-existing hypertension, diabetes, and sickle cell anemia. A significant percentage of postoperative patients suffer deficits in acuity unrelated to ocular trauma, some of whom require permanent refractive adjustment.[71] Anesthesiologists should be alert for visual impairment and check acuity when assessing patients at higher risk for ischemic optic atrophy.

Hearing Impairment

Hearing impairment after anesthesia and surgery is relatively common.[72] Although impairment is often subclinical, patients sometimes experience decreased auditory acuity, tinnitus, or roaring. Incidence of detectable hearing impairment is particularly high after dural puncture for spinal anesthesia (8 to 16%), and varies with needle size, needle type, and patient age. Impairment can be unilateral or bilateral and usually resolves spontaneously. Hearing loss also occurs after general anesthesia for both noncardiac and cardiac surgery, and is often related to disruption of the round window or tympanic membrane rupture. Eustachian tube inflammation and otitis secondary to endotracheal intubation can also impact hearing.

Oral, Pharyngeal, and Laryngeal Injuries

Laryngoscope blades, surgical instruments, rigid oral airways, and dentition can all cause trauma of oral soft tissues. Lip, tongue, or gum abrasions are treated with an ice pack and analgesia. Penetrating injuries caused by tissue entrapment between teeth and rigid devices may require topical antibiotics. After a traumatic tracheal intubation, hematoma or edema might cause partial upper airway obstruction. Nebulized racemic epinephrine often improves stridor more quickly than steroids. Dental damage can occur during airway manipulations or during emergence if a patient bites on a rigid oral airway or forcefully clenches his or her teeth. Document tooth or dental appliance damage, obtain a dental consultation, and observe for signs of foreign body aspiration.[73]

Sore throat and hoarseness after tracheal intubation occur in 20 to 50% of patients, depending on the degree of trauma during laryngoscopy and oropharyngeal suctioning, the duration of intubation, and the type of endotracheal tube. Mucosal irritation also presents as an unquenchable dryness in mouth and throat. The use of local anesthetic ointments to lubricate endotracheal tubes may cause additional mucosal irritation. Topical viscous lidocaine attenuates irritation from nasogastric tubes but may increase risk of aspiration during recovery. In children, the severity of postextubation laryngeal edema or tracheitis varies with age, intubation duration, and degree of trauma or tube movement. Most recover with cool mist therapy, but nebulized racemic epinephrine and dexamethasone may be needed in more severe cases. Laryngoscopy and intubation can also cause hypoglossal, lingual, or recurrent laryngeal nerve damage, vocal cord evulsion, desquamation of laryngeal or tracheal mucosa, edema or ulceration, and tracheal perforation. Postoperative sore throat and dysphagia also occurs without intubation, related to use of laryngeal mask airways,[74] oral airways, trauma from suctioning, or drying from unhumidified gases. Neck and jaw soreness is commonly seen after face mask anesthetics.

Nerve Injuries

Nerve injuries caused by improper positioning during anesthesia generate serious long-term complications (see Chapter 30).[75] Spinal cord injury can be caused by positioning for intubation or by hematoma accumulation after placement of neuraxial anesthetics. Peripheral nerve compression during general or regional anesthesia sometimes causes permanent sensory and motor deficits, as do stretch injuries from hyperextension of an extremity.[76] Any bruising or skin breakdown noted postoperatively should prompt evaluation for underlying nerve damage. Many postoperative neuropathies have no identifiable cause. This is particularly true for ulnar neuropathy, which may be related to subtle positioning problems, pre-existing impairment, or sensitivity of the nerve to ischemia.[77] Every complaint of nonsurgical pain, numbness, or weakness from a postoperative patient should be carefully evaluated. In the event of neuropathic weakness, electromyographic studies may determine the location of the lesion and possible reversibility of the nerve deficit. Sensory neuropathies rarely last longer than 5 days and should be referred to a neurologist if the deficit exceeds this time or if it progresses.[78]

Postdural puncture headache may first occur in the PACU, although most appear within 24 to 48 hours. Headache is more frequent after difficult subarachnoid anesthetics with multiple attempts and after dural puncture during attempted epidural placement. Subarachnoid air bubbles from loss-of-resistance testing may contribute. In the PACU, treatment is supportive with hydration, analgesics, and positioning. In severe cases, early intervention with the definitive treatment of epidural blood patch might be considered. Nerve injury secondary to needle contact or intraneuronal injection during placement of regional anesthesia is rare but does occur.[76,79] In one study, 6.3% of 4,767 patients experienced paresthesia during placement of spinal anesthesia, but only 0.126% had persisting symptoms.[80] In the PACU, patients often complain of pain, focal numbness, residual paresthesia, or dysesthesia. Symptoms are usually transient. Administer analgesia, reassure the patient, document findings, and follow for the possibility of an evolving neurologic deficit.

During recovery from spinal anesthesia, some patients exhibit lower extremity discomfort, buttock pain, and other signs of sacral or lumbar neurologic irritation. This problem is more common in obese patients, after procedures in lithotomy position, and after spinal anesthesia with 5% lidocaine.[79] Symptoms are transient and treated supportively. Rarely, a patient exhibits headache and meningeal signs caused by chemical meningitis after injection of a spinal drug that is contaminated or outside the acceptable pH range.

Soft-Tissue and Joint Injuries

If pressure points are improperly padded, soft-tissue ischemia and necrosis occur, especially with lateral or prone positioning. Prolonged scalp pressure causes localized alopecia, whereas entrapment of ears, breasts, genitalia, or skin folds causes inflammation or necrosis. Regional ischemia from major arterial compression is rare. Thermal, electrical, or chemical burns from cautery equipment, preparatory solutions, or adhesives also occur. Extravasation of intravenous medications or fluids can cause sloughing, localized chemical neuropathy, or compartment syndromes. Excessive joint or muscle extension leads to postoperative backache, joint pain, stiffness, and even joint instability. After regional anesthesia, extremities must be properly secured and padded to prevent nerve injury.

Skeletal Muscle Pain

Postoperative muscle pain is caused by many intraoperative factors. Prolonged lack of motion or unusual muscle stretch during positioning often contributes to muscle stiffness and aching. Postoperative myalgia has been reported to range between 5 and 83% of patients after the use of succinylcholine,[81] while the pathogenesis of this myalgia remains unclear.[79,82] Acute myalgia also occurs after administration of other relaxants and in patients receiving no relaxant. Delayed-onset muscle fatigue can appear days after surgery and resolves spontaneously.

Hypothermia and Shivering

Although intraoperative temperature maintenance is a goal, patients still exhibit postoperative hypothermia. During anesthesia, heat is redistributed and also is lost by evaporation during skin preparation, by humidification of dry gases in the airway, and by radiation and convection from the skin and wound. Temperature reduction is accelerated by cold intravenous fluids and low ambient temperatures. The thermoregulatory threshold, below which humans actively regulate body temperature, is decreased during general anesthesia and is less effective under anesthesia. Ability to maintain body temperature is also compromised because paralysis and anesthesia impair shivering and thermoregulatory vasoconstriction, and because nonshivering thermogenesis is ineffective in adults. Rate of heat loss is similar during general or regional anesthesia, but rewarming is slower after regional anesthesia because residual vasodilation and paralysis impede heat generation and retention. Cachectic, traumatized, or burned patients experience greater temperature reduction, as do infants because of a low ratio of body mass-to-surface area.

Hypothermia complicates and prolongs care in the PACU.[83] Average PACU stay is increased by 40 to 90 minutes for hypothermic patients.[84] Postoperative hypothermia increases sympathetic nervous system activity with increased epinephrine and norepinephrine levels,[85] elevates peripheral vascular resistance, and decreases venous capacitance. Risk of myocardial ischemia[86] and dysrhythmia from mechanical myocardial stimulation is increased. Vasoconstriction interferes with the reliability of pulse oximetry and intra-arterial pressure monitoring. Hypoperfusion jeopardizes marginal tissue grafts and promotes tissue hypoxia and metabolic acidemia. The higher affinity of hemoglobin compromises oxygen unloading to hypothermic tissues. Platelet sequestration, decreased platelet function, and reduced clotting factor function contribute to coagulopathy. Moderate hyperglycemia occurs, cellular immune responses are compromised, and postoperative infection rates increase.[87] A decrease in the minimal alveolar concentration of inhalation anesthetics (5 to 7% per 1°C cooling) accentuates residual sedation. Low perfusion and impaired biotransformation might increase the duration of neuromuscular relaxants and sedatives. Moderate hypothermia (28 to 32°C) is associated with cardiac dysrhythmias. Severe hypothermia (≤28°C) interferes with cardiac rhythm generation and impulse conduction. On ECG, the PR, QRS, or QT intervals lengthen, and J waves appear. Spontaneous ventricular fibrillation occurs at temperatures <28°C.

During emergence, hypothalamic regulation generates shivering to increase endogenous heat production.[88] Shivering increases the risk of incidental trauma, disrupts medical devices, and interferes with ECG and pulse oximetry monitoring. Oxygen consumption and CO_2 production can increase 200%. Associated increases in minute ventilation and cardiac output might precipitate ventilatory failure in patients with limited reserve or myocardial ischemia in those with coronary artery disease.[86] Shivering is accentuated by tremors related to emergence from inhalation anesthesia. Tremors exhibit clonic and tonic components, and likely reflect decreased cortical influence on spinal cord reflexes.

Restoration of normothermia is an important goal during recovery. Supplemental oxygen should be instituted and forced-air warming devices are most useful for treating hypothermia. Intravenous fluids and blood should be warmed. For most patients, shivering from mild-to-moderate hypothermia is uncomfortable but self-limited, and needs no treatment other than rewarming and reassurance. Many medications have been recommended to suppress shivering, but meperidine is most efficacious in conjunction rewarming.[6] Fentanyl has also been used with patients in whom meperidine is contraindicated. Withholding reversal of relaxants in ventilated, sedated patients attenuates shivering but increases rewarming time. If temperature is near normal (>96 to 97°F) and shivering is resolved, transfer from PACU to an inpatient floor or a discharge area is acceptable.

Hyperthermia

Hyperthermia is relatively uncommon in the PACU. Occasionally, a patient exhibits short-lived hyperthermia from close draping or aggressive intraoperative heat preservation. Postoperative fever sometimes reflects a pre-existing infection (e.g., sinusitis, upper respiratory or urinary tract infection) or an infection exacerbated by the surgical procedure (e.g., resection of infected tonsils or appendix, abscess drainage, urinary tract manipulation). Elevated temperature might indicate a drug or transfusion reaction. Muscarinic blocking agents such as atropine interfere with cooling and might contribute to fever, but they are seldom the cause in adults. Other hypermetabolic states such as thyroid storm must be considered. High fever occurs with malignant hyperthermia, but signs such as tachycardia, muscle rigidity, dysrhythmia, hyperventilation, and acidemia establish the diagnosis first.

Ambient cooling, chest physiotherapy, incentive spirometry, and antipyretics are usually sufficient to treat postoperative fever. One should withhold offending medications or blood products if a drug or transfusion reaction is suspected and notify the physician responsible for extended care to ensure postdischarge evaluation. Therapy for thyroid storm or malignant hyperthermia is well described elsewhere.

Persistent Sedation

Approximately 90% of patients regain consciousness within 15 minutes of admission to the PACU; unconsciousness persisting for a greater period is considered prolonged.[89] Even a highly susceptible patient should respond to a stimulus within 30 to 45 minutes after a reasonably conducted anesthetic. In a patient with prolonged sedation, research the level of preoperative responsiveness to uncover intoxication with drugs and alcohol or pre-existing mental dysfunction. One should note the time and amount of preoperative and intraoperative sedative medications, and review any unusual intraoperative events. The rate and character of spontaneous ventilation helps judge residual opioid effect. Physical assessment should include a tactile stimulus such as a light skin pinch, which elicits greater arousal than verbal stimulation, perhaps because sensory input is amplified through the reticular activating system. Diagnostic value of pupillary response is low.

Residual sedation from inhalation anesthetics might cause prolonged unconsciousness, especially after long procedures, in obese patients, or when high concentrations are continued through the end of surgery. Prolonged sedation is less likely after anesthesia with low solubility agents such as sevoflurane or desflurane. Premedications that have sedative effects (e.g., diphenhydramine, hydroxyzine, promethazine, droperidol, lorazepam, midazolam, meclizine, and scopolamine) contribute to postoperative somnolence. Sedation from intraoperative opioid or sedative administration is dose-related. Opioids are the only drugs that cause bradypnea; thus, regardless of what other drug effects, if the respiratory rate is <14 to 16, then opioids are clearly affecting the patient's level of consciousness. To assess sedation from opioids, one can administer low-dose intravenous naloxone (0.04-mg increments every 2 minutes, up to 0.2 mg). With careful titration, respiratory depression and sedation can be reversed without dangerous reversal of analgesia. If unconsciousness is related to residual opioid effects, ventilatory rate and arousal will increase with ≤0.2 mg of intravenous naloxone, unless a patient has received a massive opioid overdose.

Flumazenil (0.2 mg intravenously per minute to a total of 1.0 mg), a competitive benzodiazepine antagonist, differentiates sedation from midazolam and diazepam, although duration of action is short. Risk of inducing seizures must be considered in reversing chronic benzodiazepine users. Neither naloxone nor flumazenil should be used as a routine element of postoperative care.[6] Pharmaceutic reversal should be reserved for specific indications in individual patients. Administration of intravenous physostigmine (0.5 to 1 mg) counteracts but does not reverse sedation caused by inhalation anesthetics, other sedatives, and anticholinergics. If administration of naloxone, flumazenil, or physostigmine does not improve the level of consciousness, unconsciousness is most likely not related to reversible residual anesthetic medications. However, it is still possible that an unrecognized, preoperative overdose with depressant oral drugs (i.e., anticholinergic and antihistamines) is responsible.

Profound residual neuromuscular paralysis rarely might mimic unconsciousness by precluding any motor response to stimuli. This phenomenon could occur after gross overdosage, if reversal agents are omitted, in patients with unrecognized neuromuscular disease, or with phase II blockade from succinylcholine use in a patient with pseudocholinesterase deficiency. Observation of purposeful motion, spontaneous ventilation, or reflex muscular movement eliminates residual paralysis as an explanation. CNS depression secondary to intravenous local anesthetic toxicity or inadvertent subarachnoid injection can mimic postoperative coma. Children who were exhausted before surgery are often difficult to arouse after anesthesia, especially if sleep patterns are disrupted by emergency surgery at night. Hypothermia below 33°C impairs consciousness and increases the depressant effect of medications. Core temperatures below 30°C can cause fixed pupillary dilation, areflexia, and coma. A serum glucose level will eliminate severe hypoglycemia or hyperglycemic hyperosmolar coma as causes. Suspicion that unresponsiveness is caused by hypoglycemia indicates an immediate empiric trial of intravenous 50% dextrose. Hyposmolar states (<260 mOsm/L) such as acute hyponatremia (Na <125 mEq/L) are ruled out by checking serum electrolyte and osmolarity. Arterial blood gas analysis reveals CO_2 narcosis ($PaCO_2 >200$ to 250 mm Hg) as well as carboxyhemoglobin levels for carbon monoxide poisoning. A patient may also be feigning unresponsiveness or having a hysterical reaction that presents as unconsciousness.

If a diagnosis remains elusive, consult a neurologist for a thorough neurologic evaluation. Occasionally, unresponsiveness reflects subclinical grand mal seizures secondary to delirium tremens or an underlying seizure disorder. Cerebral anoxia from hypoperfusion or prolonged profound hypoxemia must be considered. In injured patients or those recovering from intracranial surgery, evaluate for unrecognized head trauma, intracerebral hemorrhage, or increased intracranial pressure. Patients sometimes awaken very slowly after long intracranial procedures.[90] Cerebral thromboembolism is another possibility in patients who have undergone internal jugular or subclavian cannulation. Patients with atrial fibrillation, carotid bruits, or hypercoagulable states are also at increased risk of thromboembolism. Paradoxic air or fat embolism through a right-to-left intracardiac shunt should be considered. After cardiac, proximal major vascular, or invasive neck surgery, risk of postoperative stroke ranges from 2.2 to 5.2%.[91] Postoperative cerebrovascular accidents in other patients are rare, showing a 0.03 to 0.08% incidence in the fourth decade but increasing to 3 to 4% by the eighth decade, and usually become evident after the PACU interval.[92]

Altered Mental Status

Recovering patients sometimes exhibit inappropriate mental reactions, ranging from lethargy and confusion to physical combativeness and extreme disorientation.

Emergence Reactions

Aside from the disturbance to staff and other patients, a stormy emergence reaction has significant medical consequences. The risk of incidental trauma increases, including contusion or fracture, corneal abrasion, and sprains from struggling. Thrashing jeopardizes suture lines, orthopaedic fixations, vascular grafts, drains, tracheal tubes, and vascular catheters. Agitated patients manifest high levels of sympathetic nervous system tone, tachycardia, and hypertension. Less appreciated is the risk of injury to PACU staff struggling to protect a combative patient.

For a short period after regaining consciousness, some patients appear unable to appropriately process sensory input. Most exhibit somnolence, slight disorientation, and sluggish mental reactions that rapidly clear. Others experience wide emotional swings such as weeping or escalating resistance to positioning and restraint. Predicting which patients will have adverse psychological reactions is difficult. Emergence delirium, which is prevalent in children and young adults, is difficult to predict preoperatively and does not appear to be related to specific types of anesthesia.[93] In young children, anxiety is heightened by parental separation. Heightened anxiety seems to be the one consistent factor in predicting emergence delirium.[94]

Many therapies have been tried to prevent or stop emergence delirium in pediatric patients without much success; however, the use of dexmedetomidine has shown promise in reducing this phenomenon without increasing time to extubate or time to discharge.[95] Ketamine and propofol have also been used with some success.[96] Very young children may react inappropriately to sound when hearing acutely improves after myringotomies. Patients with mental retardation, psychiatric disorders, organic brain dysfunction, or hostile preoperative interactions manifest those problems after surgery. Inability to speak secondary to oral fixation or tracheal intubation generates frustration or fear that exaggerates emergence reactions. Ethnic, cultural, and psychological characteristics play some role. A language barrier or a new postoperative hearing impairment accentuates an emergence reaction because input from PACU staff might not be understood. The incidence of stormy emergence is probably higher after procedures with high emotional significance. Recall of intraoperative events can generate severe panic and anxiety during emergence.[97] In patients who abuse alcohol, opioids, cocaine, or other illicit drugs, intoxication or withdrawal can elicit bizarre emergence behavior. Disorientation, paranoia, and combativeness occur after use of scopolamine as a premedication or antiemetic, which can be treated with intravenous physostigmine. Ketamine or droperidol can cause dysphoria and hallucination, although acute reactions are rare. Etomidate contributes to restlessness.

Pain amplifies agitation, confusion, and aggressive behavior during emergence[98]; therefore, it is helpful to ensure adequate postoperative analgesia early in the PACU course. Urinary urgency or gastric distention from trapped gas generates discomfort and agitation, as do tight dressings, painful phlebotomy, and poor positioning. Endotracheal or nasogastric tubes and urinary catheters are also uncomfortable. Check for unusual pain sources such as corneal abrasion, entrapment of body parts, infiltrated vascular catheters, or small devices left beneath a patient. Nausea, dizziness, and pruritus are distressing during emergence. Some patients struggle to move from a supine into a more comfortable semisitting or lateral position, especially those with gastroesophageal reflux, pulmonary congestion, or obesity. Emerging patients often resist physical restraint. Residual paralysis elicits agitation or uncoordinated motions that make a patient appear disoriented and combative. Observation of weakness or a peculiar flapping nature of voluntary motion helps in the diagnosis. However, patients can appear fully recovered by head lift and train-of-four monitoring but still perceive impaired swallowing, visual acuity, and sense of strength.[99]

Combativeness, confusion, or disorientation might reflect respiratory dysfunction. Moderate hypoxemia often presents with clouded mentation, disorientation, and agitation resembling that caused by pain. Respiratory acidemia elicits profound agitation, although acidemia caused by ventilatory center depression generates less agitation because higher CNS functions are also depressed. Hypercarbia is more likely to cause lethargy or somnolence. Limitation of inspiratory volume by chest dressings, gastric distention, or splinting causes a vague dissatisfaction with lung inflation similar to air hunger. This also occurs during mechanical ventilation with low delivered volumes and is probably mediated by stretch receptors in the lung. Inability to generate a forceful cough or clear secretions causes distress, as well as high work of breathing. Interstitial pulmonary edema elicits symptoms of air hunger before airway flooding occurs. Agitation can be profound, even with adequate ventilation and oxygenation.

Metabolic abnormalities interfere with lucidity. Lactic acidemia causes anxiety and mild disorientation; acute hyponatremia clouds the sensorium; and hypoglycemia causes first agitation and then diminished responsiveness. Seizure activity might mimic agitation and combativeness. Seizures should be higher in the differential diagnosis in patients with epilepsy, head trauma, and chronic alcohol or cocaine abuse. Cerebral hypoperfusion can produce disorientation, agitation, and combativeness, which can be seen after head trauma or space-occupying lesions. Action such as increasing the mean arterial pressure might be required to assure cerebral perfusion pressure.

There are few interventions that prevent "stormy" emergence reactions.[94] Altered mental status is treated supportively because most emergence reactions disappear within 10 to 15 minutes. Verbal reassurances that surgery is completed and that the patient is doing well are invaluable. One should use the patient's name frequently with reassurance of well-being, and stress the time and location. When practical, one should allow patients to choose their own position and provide adequate analgesia. In selected cases, parenteral sedation relieves fear or anxiety and smoothes emergence. Identifying whether a patient is reacting to pain or to anxiety is important. Benzodiazepines and barbiturates are ineffective analgesics, whereas opioids are poor sedatives. One should not administer sedative or analgesic medications if altered mental status might reflect a physiologic abnormality such as hypoxemia, hypoglycemia, hypotension, or acidemia, and use restraints only if a patient's or staff's safety is jeopardized.

Delirium and Cognitive Decline

A high percentage of elderly patients (5 to 50%) experience some degree of postoperative confusion, delirium, or cognitive decline.[100,101] Patients exhibit fluctuations in level of consciousness and orientation, or deterioration of memory, mental functions, and acquisition of new information. The problem may be related to exacerbation of central cholinergic insufficiency by narcotics, sedatives, or anticholinergics. However, stress of surgery, fever, pain, emesis, sleep deprivation, and loss of routine undoubtedly contribute. Presence of pre-existing dementia, cognitive abnormalities, organic brain syndrome, or hearing and visual impairment predicts postoperative delirium, as does evidence of physical infirmity such as high ASA physical status or lack of stress response to surgery. Cognitive dysfunction also occurs at lower incidence (15% greater than control) in younger patients, more frequently resolves within 3 months, and may be related to inactivity during recuperation.[102] Although signs often appear on the first to third postoperative day, onset is sometimes evident in the PACU.

Overall, recovery of cognitive function is slower in the elderly.[103] Because older patients are often skilled at concealing declining capabilities, careful assessment of preoperative capabilities helps identify deficits that affect postoperative status. Postoperative lethargy, clouded sensorium, or delirium sometimes reflects an acute physiologic change. Hyperosmolarity from hyperglycemia or hypernatremia as well as hyponatremia can alter consciousness. Cerebral fluid shifts with decreased mentation occur in patients on dialysis and after rapid correction of severe dehydration. Patients receiving atropine premedication or chronic meperidine therapy might exhibit anticholinergic-induced delirium. Disorientation or clouded sensorium can reflect chronic use of psychogenic drugs, premedication with long-acting sedatives, or unrecognized intoxication. Life-threatening conditions such as seizures, hypoxemia, hypoglycemia, hypotension, acidemia, or cerebrovascular accident sometimes present with confusion, disorientation, inability to vocalize, or reduced level of consciousness, especially if earlier premonitory signs and symptoms are misinterpreted.

Postoperative Nausea and Vomiting

Postoperative nausea and vomiting (PONV) continues to be a significant challenge to be avoided after many types of anesthetics. Not only is PONV considered by many patients the most unpleasant aspect following an anesthetic, many describe this as their greatest fear of subsequent anesthetics.[104] Patients are often more concerned about PONV than pain or other risks associated with anesthesia and surgery. In addition to patients' dissatisfaction with nausea and vomiting, there exist medical risks (increased abdominal pressure, increased central venous pressure, aspiration of gastric contents, sympathetic nervous system response with increasing blood pressure and heart rate as well as parasympathetic responses producing bradycardia and hypotension). PONV represents a significant burden to be avoided due to patient satisfaction and safety as well as the economic impact of prolonged PACU stays and unanticipated admissions.

The incidence of PONV varies with many potential causes. Patients often experience nausea and emesis after discharge from the PACU which may coincide with increased oral intake or waning effect of antiemetics. Surgeries associated with a higher risk of PONV are eye procedures, peritoneal or intestinal irritation, ear-nose-throat procedures especially with middle ear manipulation, dental and cosmetic procedures. Patient groups at increased are those with a previous history of PONV or motion sickness, menstruating females, children over the age of two, obesity, and nonsmokers.[105] Perioperative factors that may increase the incidence include no PO intake (starvation, dehydration), autonomic imbalance, pain, and the effects of anesthetics on the chemotactic center.

Incidence of PONV is lower following regional rather than general anesthesia especially with a decreased use of opioids.[106] The use of nonopioid analgesics may reduce the frequency of emesis while providing adequate pain control. Induction agents such as propofol and barbiturates are associated with reduced incidence compared to etomidate and ketamine. A total intravenous anesthetic (TIVA) technique with propofol greatly reduces PONV incidence compared to a pure inhalation anesthetic. There is little significant difference among inhalation agents, although sevoflurane and desflurane might generate slightly higher rates of nausea. The choice of anticholinergic reversal agents may be a contributing factor but remains unclear to what degree.

Several interventions have been evaluated and can be implemented to reduce the incidence of PONV. The use of meclizine 25 mg preoperatively for patients predisposed to motion sickness can be effective. Prophylaxis with 5-HT3 receptor antagonists (i.e., ondansetron) prior to emergence significantly reduces incidence and is cost effective. Dexamethasone also has antiemetic effects and can be used effectively with other prophylactic agents. Hydration is effective, easy and cost effective. The use of droperidol prophylaxis has decreased due to a black box warning with prolonged QT on EKG, but still remains an effective rescue method in select patients with EKG monitoring. Rescue with nonselective antihistamines (i.e., promethazine) is effective but caution is advised in patients where increased sedation can be problematic such as children and obstructive sleep apnea. Acupuncture and acupressure can provide relief but due to provider proficiency, patient acceptance and proven efficacy compared to antiemetic medications, these methods are less frequently used.[107] More serious causes of nausea and vomiting such as hypotension, hypoxia, hypoglycemia, increased intracranial pressure, or gastric bleeding should be considered prior to treatment.

References

1. Bothner U, Georgieff M, Schwilk B: The impact of minor perioperative anesthesia-related incidents, events, and complications on postanesthesia care unit utilization. Anesth Analg 1999; 89: 506
2. Cohen MM, O'Brien-Pallas LL, Copplestone C et al:. Nursing workload associated with adverse events in the postanesthesia care unit. Anesthesiology 1999; 91: 1882

3. Pavlin DJ, Rapp SE, Polissar NL et al: Factors affecting discharge time in adult outpatients. Anesth Analg 1998; 87: 816
4. Song D, Chung F, Ronayne M et al: Fast-tracking (bypassing the PACU) does not reduce nursing workload after ambulatory surgery. Br J Anaesth 2004; 93: 768
5. Hines R, Barash PG, Watrous G et al: Complications occurring in the postanesthesia care unit: A survey. Anesth Analg 1992; 74: 503
6. American Society of Anesthesiologists Task Force on Postanesthetic Care: Practice guidelines for postanesthetic care: A report by the American Society of Anesthesiologists Task Force on Postanesthetic Care. Anesthesiology 2002; 96: 742
7. Sullivan EE: Standards of perianesthesia nursing practice 2002. J Perianesth Nurs 2002; 17: 275
8. Swenson JD, Bay N, Loose E, et al: Outpatient management of continuous peripheral nerve catheters placed using ultrasound guidance: An experience in 620 patients. Anesth Analg 2006; 103: 1436
9. Apfelbaum JL, Walawander CA, Grasela TH, et al: Eliminating intensive postoperative care in same-day surgery patients using short-acting anesthetics. Anesthesiology 2002; 97: 66
10. Pittet D, Stephan F, Hugonnet S et al: Hand-cleansing during postanesthesia care. Anesthesiology 2003; 99: 530
11. Macario A, Weinger M, Carney S et al: Which clinical anesthesia outcomes are important to avoid the perspective of patients. Anesth Analg 1999; 89: 652
12. Strassels SA, Chen C, Carr DB: Postoperative analgesia: Economics, resource use, and patient satisfaction in an urban teaching hospital. Anesth Analg 2002; 94: 130
13. Apfelbaum JL, Chen C, Mehta SS et al: Postoperative pain experience: Results from a national survey suggest postoperative pain continues to be undermanaged. Anesth Analg 2003; 97: 534
14. Rundshagen I, Schnabel K, Standl T et al: Patients' vs nurses' assessments of postoperative pain and anxiety during patient- or nurse-controlled analgesia. Br J Anaesth 1999; 82: 374
15. American Society of Anesthesiologists Task Force on Acute Pain Management: Practice guidelines for acute pain management in the perioperative setting: An updated report by the American Society of Anesthesiologists Task Force on Acute Pain Management. Anesthesiology 2004; 100: 1573
16. Chung F, Ritchie E, Su J: Postoperative pain in ambulatory surgery. Anesth Analg 1997; 85: 808
17. Wu CL, Berenholtz SM, Pronovost PJ et al: Systematic review and analysis of postdischarge symptoms after outpatient surgery. Anesthesiology 2002; 96: 994
18. Peng PW, Sandler AN: A review of the use of fentanyl analgesia in the management of acute pain in adults. Anesthesiology. 1999; 90: 576
19. Ekman EF, Wahba M, Ancona F: Analgesic efficacy of perioperative celecoxib in ambulatory arthroscopic knee surgery: A double-blind, placebo-controlled study. Arthroscopy 2006; 22: 635
20. Moiniche S, Kehlet H, Dahl JB: A qualitative and quantitative systematic review of preemptive analgesia for postoperative pain relief: The role of timing of analgesia. Anesthesiology 2002; 96: 725
21. White PF: The role of non-opioid analgesic techniques in the management of pain after ambulatory surgery. Anesth Analg 2002; 94: 577
22. Gwirtz KH, Young JV, Byers RS, et al: The safety and efficacy of intrathecal opioid analgesia for acute postoperative pain: Seven years' experience with 5,969 surgical patients at indiana university hospital. Anesth Analg 1999; 88: 599
23. de Leon-Casasola OA, Lema MJ: Postoperative epidural opioid analgesia: What are the choices? Anesth Analg 1996; 83: 867
24. Baig MK, Zmora O, Derdemezi J et al: Use of the ON-Q pain management system is associated with decreased postoperative analgesic requirement: Double blind randomized placebo pilot study. J Am Coll Surg 2006; 202: 297
25. Capdevila X, Pirat P, Bringuier S, et al: Continuous peripheral nerve blocks in hospital wards after orthopedic surgery: A multicenter prospective analysis of the quality of postoperative analgesia and complications in 1,416 patients. Anesthesiology 2005; 103: 1035
26. Ilfeld BM, Enneking FK: Continuous peripheral nerve blocks at home: A review. Anesth Analg 2005; 100: 1822
27. Casati A, Fanelli G, Cedrati V et al: Pulmonary function changes after interscalene brachial plexus anesthesia with 0.5% and 0.75% ropivacaine: A double-blinded comparison with 2% mepivacaine. Anesth Analg 1999; 88: 587
28. Aldrete JA: The post-anesthesia recovery score revisited. J Clin Anesth 1995; 7: 89
29. White PF, Song D: New criteria for fast-tracking after outpatient anesthesia: A comparison with the modified Aldrete's scoring system. Anesth Analg 1999; 88: 1069
30. Standards for Postanesthesia Care (Approved by House of Delegates on October 12, 1988 and last amended on October 27, 2004). Available at: www.asahq.org/publicationsAndServices/standards/36.pdf
31. Noiseux N, Bracco D, Prieto I et al: Do patients after off-pump coronary artery bypass grafting need the intensive care unit? A prospective audit of 85 patients. Interact Cardiovasc Thorac Surg 2008; 7: 32
32. Schweizer A, Khatchatourian G, Hohn L et al: Opening of a new postanesthesia care unit: Impact on critical care utilization and complica-

tions following major vascular and thoracic surgery. J Clin Anesth 2002; 14: 486
33. Heland M, Retsas A: Establishing a cardiac surgery recovery unit within the post anaesthesia care unit. Collegian. 1999; 6: 10
34. Baltimore JJ. Perianesthesia care of cardiac surgery patients: A CPAN review. J Perianesth Nurs 2001; 16: 246
35. Rose DK, Cohen MM, Wigglesworth DF et al: Critical respiratory events in the postanesthesia care unit, patient, surgical, and anesthetic factors. Anesthesiology 1994; 81: 410
36. Schwilk B, Bothner U, Schraag S et al: Perioperative respiratory events in smokers and nonsmokers undergoing general anaesthesia. Acta Anaesthesiol Scand 1997; 41: 348
37. Ballantyne JC, Carr DB, deFerranti S, et al: The comparative effects of postoperative analgesic therapies on pulmonary outcome: Cumulative meta-analyses of randomized, controlled trials. Anesth Analg 1998; 86: 598
38. Warner DO, Warner MA, Offord KP et al: Airway obstruction and perioperative complications in smokers undergoing abdominal surgery. Anesthesiology 1999; 90: 372
39. Strauss SG, Lynn AM, Bratton SL et al: Ventilatory response to CO_2 in children with obstructive sleep apnea from adenotonsillar hypertrophy. Anesth Analg 1999; 89: 328
40. Tait AR, Malviya S, Voepel-Lewis T et al: Risk factors for perioperative adverse respiratory events in children with upper respiratory tract infections. Anesthesiology 2001; 95: 299
41. D'Honneur G, Lofaso F, Drummond GB, et al: Susceptibility to upper airway obstruction during partial neuromuscular block. Anesthesiology 1998; 88: 371
42. Asai T, Koga K, Vaughan RS: Respiratory complications associated with tracheal intubation and extubation. Br J Anaesth 1998; 80: 767
43. Benumof JL, Dagg R, Benumof R: Critical hemoglobin desaturation will occur before return to an unparalyzed state following 1 mg/kg intravenous succinylcholine. Anesthesiology 1997; 87: 979
44. Warner DO, Warner MA, Barnes RD, et al: Perioperative respiratory complications in patients with asthma. Anesthesiology 1996; 85: 460
45. Berg H, Roed J, Viby-Mogensen J, et al: Residual neuromuscular block is a risk factor for postoperative pulmonary complications. A prospective, randomised, and blinded study of postoperative pulmonary complications after atracurium, vecuronium and pancuronium. Acta Anaesthesiol Scand 1997; 41: 1095
46. Debaene B, Plaud B, Dilly MP et al: Residual paralysis in the PACU after a single intubating dose of nondepolarizing muscle relaxant with an intermediate duration of action. Anesthesiology 2003; 98: 1042
47. de Boer HD, Driessen JJ, Marcus MA et al: Reversal of rocuronium-induced (1.2 mg/kg) profound neuromuscular block by sugammadex: A multicenter, dose-finding and safety study. Anesthesiology 2007; 107: 239
48. Stoller JK, Kester L: Respiratory care protocols in postanesthesia care. J Perianesth Nurs 1998; 13: 349
49. Rothen HU, Sporre B, Engberg G et al: Airway closure, atelectasis and gas exchange during general anaesthesia. Br J Anaesth 1998; 81: 681
50. Karayiannakis AJ, Makri GG, Mantzioka A et al: Postoperative pulmonary function after laparoscopic and open cholecystectomy. Br J Anaesth 1996; 77: 448
51. Thomas JA, McIntosh JM: Are incentive spirometry, intermittent positive pressure breathing, and deep breathing exercises effective in the prevention of postoperative pulmonary complications after upper abdominal surgery? A systematic overview and meta-analysis. Phys Ther 1994; 74: 3
52. Overend TJ, Anderson CM, Lucy SD et al: The effect of incentive spirometry on postoperative pulmonary complications: A systematic review. Chest 2001; 120: 971
53. Young T, Palta M, Dempsey J et al: The occurrence of sleep-disordered breathing among middle-aged adults. N Engl J Med 1993; 328: 1230
54. Gross JB, Bachenberg KL, Benumof JL, et al: Practice guidelines for the perioperative management of patients with obstructive sleep apnea: A report by the American Society of Anesthesiologists Task Force on Perioperative Management of Patients with Obstructive Sleep Apnea. Anesthesiology 2006; 104: 1081
55. Xue FS, Huang YG, Tong SY, et al: A comparative study of early postoperative hypoxemia in infants, children, and adults undergoing elective plastic surgery. Anesth Analg 1996; 83: 709
56. Moller JT, Johannessen NW, Espersen K, et al: Randomized evaluation of pulse oximetry in 20,802 patients: II. perioperative events and postoperative complications. Anesthesiology 1993; 78: 445
57. Xue FS, Li BW, Zhang GS, et al: The influence of surgical sites on early postoperative hypoxemia in adults undergoing elective surgery. Anesth Analg 1999; 88: 213
58. Moller JT, Wittrup M, Johansen SH: Hypoxemia in the postanesthesia care unit: An observer study. Anesthesiology 1990; 73: 890
59. Ng A, Smith G: Gastroesophageal reflux and aspiration of gastric contents in anesthetic practice. Anesth Analg 2001; 93: 494
60. Eriksson LI, Sundman E, Olsson R, et al: Functional assessment of the pharynx at rest and during swallowing in partially paralyzed humans: Simultaneous videomanometry and mechanomyography of awake human volunteers. Anesthesiology 1997; 87: 1035
61. Practice guidelines for preoperative fasting and the use of pharmacologic agents to reduce the risk of pulmonary aspiration: Application to healthy

patients undergoing elective procedures: A report by the American Society of Anesthesiologist Task Force on Preoperative Fasting. Anesthesiology 1999; 90: 896

62. Mulroy MF, Salinas FV, Larkin KL et al: Ambulatory surgery patients may be discharged before voiding after short-acting spinal and epidural anesthesia. Anesthesiology 2002; 97: 315

63. Marshall SI, Chung F: Discharge criteria and complications after ambulatory surgery. Anesth Analg 1999; 88: 508

64. Twersky R, Fishman D, Homel P: What happens after discharge? Return hospital visits after ambulatory surgery. Anesth Analg 1997; 84: 319

65. Cogliati AA, Vellutini R, Nardini A, et al: Fenoldopam infusion for renal protection in high-risk cardiac surgery patients: A randomized clinical study. J Cardiothorac Vasc Anesth 2007; 21: 847

66. Waters JH, Gottlieb A, Schoenwald P, et al. Normal saline versus lactated Ringer's solution for intraoperative fluid management in patients undergoing abdominal aortic aneurysm repair: An outcome study. Anesth Analg 2001; 93: 817

67. Moos DD, Lind DM: Detection and treatment of perioperative corneal abrasions. J Perianesth Nurs 2006; 21: 332

68. Myers MA, Hamilton SR, Bogosian AJ et al: Visual loss as a complication of spine surgery. A review of 37 cases. Spine 1997; 22: 1325

69. Warner ME, Warner MA, Garrity JA et al: The frequency of perioperative vision loss. Anesth Analg 2001; 93: 1417

70. Williams EL, Hart WM Jr, Tempelhoff R: Postoperative ischemic optic neuropathy. Anesth Analg 1995; 80: 1018

71. Warner ME, Fronapfel PJ, Hebl JR, et al: Perioperative visual changes. Anesthesiology 2002; 96: 855

72. Sprung J, Bourke DL, Contreras MG et al: Perioperative hearing impairment. Anesthesiology 2003; 98: 241

73. Warner ME, Benenfeld SM, Warner MA et al: Perianesthetic dental injuries: Frequency, outcomes, and risk factors. Anesthesiology 1999; 90: 1302

74. Brimacombe J, Holyoake L, Keller C, et al: Pharyngolaryngeal, neck, and jaw discomfort after anesthesia with the face mask and laryngeal mask airway at high and low cuff volumes in males and females. Anesthesiology 2000; 93: 26

75. Practice advisory for the prevention of perioperative peripheral neuropathies: A report by the American Society of Anesthesiologists Task Force on Prevention of Perioperative Peripheral Neuropathies. Anesthesiology 2000; 92: 1168

76. Cheney FW, Domino KB, Caplan RA et al: Nerve injury associated with anesthesia: A closed claims analysis. Anesthesiology 1999; 90: 1062

77. Warner MA, Warner DO, Matsumoto JY et al: Ulnar neuropathy in surgical patients. Anesthesiology 1999; 90: 54

78. Warner MA: Perioperative neuropathies. Mayo Clin Proc 1998; 73: 567

79. Auroy Y, Benhamou D, Bargues L, et al: Major complications of regional anesthesia in France: The SOS regional anesthesia hotline service. Anesthesiology 2002; 97: 1274

80. Horlocker TT, McGregor DG, Matsushige DK et al: A retrospective review of 4,767 consecutive spinal anesthetics: Central nervous system complications. perioperative outcomes group. Anesth Analg 1997; 84: 578

81. Schreiber JU, Mencke T, Biedler A, et al: Postoperative myalgia after succinylcholine: No evidence for an inflammatory origin. Anesth Analg 2003; 96: 1640

82. Bettelli G: Which muscle relaxants should be used in day surgery and when. Curr Opin Anaesthesiol 2006; 19: 600

83. Sessler DI: Complications and treatment of mild hypothermia. Anesthesiology 2001; 95: 531

84. Lenhardt R, Marker E, Goll V, et al: Mild intraoperative hypothermia prolongs postanesthetic recovery. Anesthesiology 1997; 87: 1318

85. Sun LS, Adams DC, Delphin E, et al: Sympathetic response during cardiopulmonary bypass: Mild versus moderate hypothermia. Crit Care Med 1997; 25: 1990

86. Frank SM, Fleisher LA, Breslow MJ, et al: Perioperative maintenance of normothermia reduces the incidence of morbid cardiac events. A randomized clinical trial. JAMA 1997; 277: 1127

87. Ammori JB, Sigakis M, Englesbe MJ et al: Effect of intraoperative hyperglycemia during liver transplantation. J Surg Res 2007; 140: 227

88. De Witte J, Sessler DI: Perioperative shivering: Physiology and pharmacology. Anesthesiology 2002; 96: 467

89. Zelcer J, Wells DG: Anaesthetic-related recovery room complications. Anaesth Intensive Care 1987; 15: 168

90. Schubert A, Mascha EJ, Bloomfield EL et al: Effect of cranial surgery and brain tumor size on emergence from anesthesia. Anesthesiology 1996; 85: 513

91. Wong GY, Warner DO, Schroeder DR, et al: Risk of surgery and anesthesia for ischemic stroke. Anesthesiology 2000; 92: 425

92. Kim J, Gelb AW: Predicting perioperative stroke. J Neurosurg Anesthesiol 1995; 7: 211

93. Vlajkovic GP, Sindjelic RP: Emergence delirium in children: Many questions, few answers. Anesth Analg 2007; 104: 84

94. Voepel-Lewis T, Malviya S, Tait AR: A prospective cohort study of emergence agitation in the pediatric postanesthesia care unit. Anesth Analg 2003; 96: 1625

95. Isik B, Arslan M, Tunga AD et al: Dexmedetomidine decreases emergence agitation in pediatric patients after sevoflurane anesthesia without surgery. Paediatr Anaesth 2006; 16: 748

96. Abu-Shahwan I, Chowdary K: Ketamine is effective in decreasing the incidence of emergence agitation in children undergoing dental repair under sevoflurane general anesthesia. Paediatr Anaesth 2007; 17: 846

97. Schwender D, Kunze-Kronawitter H, Dietrich P et al: Conscious awareness during general anaesthesia: Patients' perceptions, emotions, cognition and reactions. Br J Anaesth 1998; 80: 133

98. Lynch EP, Lazor MA, Gellis JE et al: The impact of postoperative pain on the development of postoperative delirium. Anesth Analg 1998; 86: 781

99. Kopman AF, Yee PS, Neuman GG: Relationship of the train-of-four fade ratio to clinical signs and symptoms of residual paralysis in awake volunteers. Anesthesiology 1997; 86: 765

100. Cook DJ, Rooke GA: Priorities in perioperative geriatrics. Anesth Analg 2003; 96: 1823

101. Zakriya KJ, Christmas C, Wenz JFS et al: Preoperative factors associated with postoperative change in confusion assessment method score in hip fracture patients. Anesth Analg 2002; 94: 1628

102. Johnson T, Monk T, Rasmussen LS, et al: Postoperative cognitive dysfunction in middle-aged patients. Anesthesiology 2002; 96: 1351

103. Dodds C, Allison J: Postoperative cognitive deficit in the elderly surgical patient. Br J Anaesth 1998; 81: 449

104. Kerger H, Turan A, Kredel M, et al: Patients' willingness to pay for antiemetic treatment. Acta Anaesthesiol Scand 2007; 51: 38

105. Sinclair DR, Chung F, Mezei G: Can postoperative nausea and vomiting be predicted? Anesthesiology 1999; 91: 109

106. Williams BA, Kentor ML, Vogt MT, et al: Economics of nerve block pain management after anterior cruciate ligament reconstruction: Potential hospital cost savings via associated postanesthesia care unit bypass and same-day discharge. Anesthesiology 2004; 100: 697

107. Lee A, Done ML: The use of nonpharmacologic techniques to prevent postoperative nausea and vomiting: A meta-analysis. Anesth Analg 1999; 88: 1362

PERIOPERATIVE AND CONSULTATIVE SERVICES

CHAPTER 56 ■ CRITICAL CARE MEDICINE

MIRIAM M. TREGGIARI AND STEVEN DEEM

KEY POINTS

1 Simple and inexpensive interventions in the intensive care unit (ICU), such as the utilization of checklists and strict attention to aseptic technique during central venous catheterization, can result in substantial improvements in patient outcomes.

2 Administration of high-dose corticosteroids to patients presenting with traumatic brain injury is associated with 20% increase in the relative risk of death.

3 Administration of thrombolytic therapy to patients presenting within 3 hours of onset of acute ischemic stroke results in improved neurologic outcome.

4 Patients who are resuscitated from cardiac arrest by ventricular fibrillation have improved neurologic outcome and possibly reduced mortality when treated with mild therapeutic hypothermia (32 to 34°C) for 12 to 24 hours after hospital admission.

5 In patients with severe sepsis or septic shock, activated protein C is associated with a 6% absolute 28-day mortality reduction, and early goal-directed therapy, targeting a central venous oxygen saturation >70% in the first 6 hours after admission to the emergency department, has been associated with an even greater reduction in mortality.

6 Separation from mechanical ventilation in patients who are recovering from respiratory failure is accelerated by respiratory therapy-driven protocols and daily trials of spontaneous breathing.

7 Ventilation with low tidal volumes (6 mL/kg) in patients with acute lung injury and acute respiratory distress syndrome reduces mortality, compared with traditional tidal volumes (12 mL/kg).

8 Red blood cell transfusion in the ICU should be restricted (transfusion threshold hemoglobin <7g/dL) with the possible exception of patients with a diagnosis of active bleeding, early septic shock, acute myocardial infarction or unstable angina, or with primarily neurologic or neurosurgical problems.

9 Nurse-driven sedation protocols and daily interruption of sedative infusions reduce the duration of mechanical ventilation and ICU length of stay.

10 The incidence of ventilator-associated pneumonia can be reduced with strict hand washing during patient care and semirecumbent positioning of the patient. Antibiotic therapy of ventilator-associated pneumonia should use a "deescalating" strategy, and can be limited to an 8-day course in uncomplicated cases.

ANESTHESIOLOGISTS AND CRITICAL CARE MEDICINE

Critical Care Medicine (CCM) evolved as a specialty nearly simultaneously in Europe and North America, but has followed strikingly different models in regards to the involvement of anesthesiologists. The first intensive care unit (ICU) in Europe may have been located in Denmark in the 1950s, and concurrently the first critical care physician, or "intensivist," may well have been an anesthesiologist.[1] Anesthesiologists continued to play a defining role in the development of CCM in most of Europe, Australia, New Zealand, Japan, and elsewhere, and comprise the majority of intensivists in many countries around the world today. In North America anesthesiologists were also integral to the development of CCM as a specialty. However, in contrast to other countries, anesthesiologists in the United States have played an ever-diminishing role in the specialty, and today comprise a small minority of the intensivist workforce.[2]

Although it has been suggested that the first ICU in North America was established at Johns Hopkins in 1923 to care for postoperative neurosurgical patients, it was not until the late 1950s and early 1960s that true multidisciplinary ICUs began to appear. The driving forces behind ICU development included advances in surgical techniques, polio epidemics that resulted in widespread respiratory failure, and later, the recognition of the acute respiratory distress syndrome (ARDS). Anesthesiologists played a natural role in the evolution of ICUs, given their familiarity with surgical resuscitation and mechanical ventilation. Early on, however, the concept of intensivists did not exist, and patients were often managed by their primary physician (be it surgeon or internist) and nurses, with formal or informal consultation given by specialists, including anesthesiologists.

In the early 1960s, the first CCM training program was established at the University of Pittsburgh under the direction of an anesthesiologist, Peter Safar. At this point, the concept of intensivist was born; as defined by Dr. Safar, the qualities and qualifications of such an individual should include inquisitiveness, thoughtfulness, a high level of motivation, action orientation, diplomacy, and scientific training. In the late 1960s, a group including Dr. Safar and another anesthesiologist, Ake Grenvik, was instrumental in inaugurating the Society of Critical Care Medicine (SCCM). Anesthesiologists working through SCCM were instrumental in developing the board certification process for CCM, and in 1986 the first CCM certification examination was administered by the American Board of Anesthesiology.[3] From the 1960s until the present, numerous anesthesiologists have made important contributions to the development of the specialty, to critical care-related research, and to improvements in the care of critically ill patients. However, as of 2007 only about 1,200 anesthesiologists had completed the certification process in CCM in the United States,[4] and anesthesiologists comprised only about 5% of practicing intensivists (personal communication 2004, American Board of Anesthesiology).

Anesthesiology and Critical Care Medicine: The Future

Although it seems certain that anesthesiologists will continue to play an important role in CCM worldwide, in the United States anesthesiology is currently at a crossroads in regard to its continued involvement in CCM. There are several forces that will shape the evolution of the specialty of CCM as a whole, and the contribution that anesthesiologists will make to this evolution: (1) increasing evidence that intensivists increase the quality of care and improve outcomes; (2) business/economic factors, whereby employers, insurers, and hospitals recognize the cost savings associated with intensivists in the ICU, as exemplified by the Leapfrog Initiative (further discussed in the following section; and (3) the aging population and increasing demand for critical care services, which will result in a shortage of intensivists starting in 2007 that will grow to a >20% deficit by the year 2020, given current training levels (Table 56-1).[2]

Given these observations, it is clear that opportunities for careers in CCM will be amply available in the coming years. Anesthesiology as a specialty would seem ideally suited to

TABLE 56-1

LEAPFROG INTENSIVE CARE UNIT (ICU) PHYSICIAN STAFFING (IPS) STANDARD

Hospitals fulfilling the IPS Standard will operate adult and/or pediatric ICUs that are managed or co-managed by intensivists who:
1. Are present during daytime hours and provide clinical care exclusively in the ICU and,
2. At other times can—at least 95% of the time,
   i. return ICU pages within 5 minutes and
   ii. arrange for a FCCS-certified[a] nonphysician effector to reach ICU patients within 5 minutes.

[a]Fundamental Critical Care Support (course training to prepare non-intensivists to manage the first 24 hours of critical illness, sponsored by the Society of Critical Care Medicine).
From http://www.leapfroggroup.org/about_us/leapfrog-factsheet.

help satisfy the increasing demand for intensivists. Anesthesiologists are hospital-based; have sound fundamental training in physiology, pharmacology, invasive procedures, and monitoring; and have excellent historical and concurrent role models for the anesthesiologist as intensivist. However, economic and lifestyle incentives have recently dissuaded anesthesiology trainees from pursuing further training and careers in CCM. Critical care services are currently not reimbursed at rates commensurate with surgical anesthesia, and critical care practice is accurately perceived as more time-consuming and the workload is more unpredictable than an operating room-based practice. However, these factors may change in the coming years, as reimbursement for surgical anesthesia and critical care services equalize and the lifestyle constraints associated with critical care are moderated by creative organizational strategies, including the use of physician extenders and other mechanisms for reducing the "24-7" workload. Lastly, the increase in the anesthesiology residency training requirement to include 4 months of intensive care may imbue trainees with a greater interest in CCM as a career choice.

As previously stated, anesthesiology in the United States is at a crossroads; with the proper imagination, emphasis, support and training, the specialty can reassert itself as a leader in the field of CCM. The alternative is that the percentage of anesthesiologists involved in CCM will continue to decline and anesthesiology will become little more than a historical footnote in this field.

Critical Care Medicine: A Systems and Evidence-Based Approach

Critical care encompasses all disciplines of medicine. It is clearly beyond the scope of a single chapter to provide detailed coverage of all aspects of critical illness, including physiology, pathophysiology, and management of disease. In addition, many critical care issues are commonly encountered by anesthesiologists who practice solely in the operating room, and are covered in detail elsewhere in this text. Thus, this chapter will focus on topics that are relatively unique to the ICU, on therapeutic approaches, and on practices for which strong evidence exists, particularly when supported by randomized controlled trials. Where appropriate, the level of evidence supporting treatment regimens will be graded according to commonly accepted methodology (Table 56-2).[5]

PERIOPERATIVE AND CONSULTATIVE SERVICES

PROCESS OF CARE IN THE INTENSIVE CARE UNIT

The method by which care is delivered may affect outcomes as much or more than the specific interventions employed. For example, care delivery models that reduce errors and encourage utilization of evidence-based practices may have a profound effect on outcomes, in addition to reducing costs. A single adverse event in the ICU may cost as much as $4,000, and increase length of stay by 1 day.[6] Additional data suggest that implementation of evidence-based practices in the ICU is not consistent, and that more uniform implementation could save up to approximately 200,000 lives per year in the United States.[7]

As advances in medical and surgical therapeutics have increased the complexity of care for an aging and increasingly ill population of patients, it has become increasing clear that the involvement of intensivists in the management of the critically ill is desirable. Several studies have suggested that mortality and other intermediate end points such as ICU length of stay can be reduced when "high-intensity" physician staffing models that mandate management or comanagement by intensivists are used.[8] These studies, as summarized in a meta-analysis by Pronovost et al.[8] and further supported by two cohort studies,[9,10] have provoked a reconsideration of the ideal staffing model for ICUs in the United States, particularly among the business community.

The Business Roundtable, a national association of chief executive officers of Fortune 500 companies, formed the Leapfrog Group in 1999. The Leapfrog Group is a coalition of over 150 purchasers and providers of health care benefits, including large companies such as General Motors, Motorola, and Merck, and insurers such as Aetna. The stated goal of the Leapfrog Group is to improve health care, in particular by reducing deaths due to medical error. To accomplish this

mission, the group formulated the Leapfrog Initiative, which includes a series of "safety standards" that health care providers (largely hospitals) should strive for if they are to provide care for Leapfrog Group employees. Prompted by the data associating intensivists with improved outcomes, the Leapfrog Initiative included an ICU Physician Staffing standard that promotes the continuous involvement of intensivists in the care of critically ill patients (Table 56-1).[11] Less than 10% of hospitals met this standard prior to its publication, and a recent survey suggests that there has been little improvement in compliance since then.[12,13] Reported barriers to implementation of the Leapfrog Initiative include lack of ICU directors, cost, loss of control and continuity in patient care, and loss of income.[13] However, according to recent estimates there will be considerable cost savings as a result of Leapfrog Initiative implementation. Hopefully, this will provide additional impetus to widespread adoption of these practices.[14]

In addition to improved ICU staffing, other simple interventions in the process of care have been shown to improve outcomes. These include efforts to reduce errors of omission by utilizing checklists,[15] and by explicitly outlining daily goals of care during rounds.[16] Such efforts incur little or no cost, may incur substantial benefits, but are severely underused in the United States at present.

NEUROLOGIC AND NEUROSURGICAL CRITICAL CARE

Neuromonitoring

Several neuromonitoring devices are useful in the ICU setting for assessing pathophysiologic processes and adjusting therapy (see Chapter 39). The following discussion will be limited to transcranial Doppler ultrasonography, brain tissue oxygenation, and microdialysis. Other neurologic monitors are discussed elsewhere.

Transcranial Doppler Ultrasonography

Transcranial Doppler ultrasonography (TCD) measures mean, peak systolic, and end-diastolic flow velocities, and indirectly estimates cerebral blood flow (CBF). TCD can be used as a tool to identify vasospasm in patients with subarachnoid hemorrhage (SAH) or traumatic brain injury (TBI). Despite some technical limitation due to the quality of the bone window and the fact that increased velocity needs to be interpreted either in the context of vasospasm or hyperdynamic flow patterns, TCD remains a valuable monitoring device to follow trends over time. In patients with TBI, flow velocities are depressed, and impaired autoregulation and vascular reactivity are common. In these patients, monitoring of TCD and jugular venous oxygen saturation (SjO_2) (see later discussion) may be used to define the optimum cerebral perfusion pressure (CPP) level.[17] Patients with SAH are at high risk of cerebral vasospasm, and serial TCD can monitor changes in blood velocities detecting occurrence of ischemic flow patterns (see later discussion).

Brain Tissue Oxygenation

Brain tissue oxygen pressure ($PbrO_2$) measurements are performed by introducing a small, oxygen-sensitive catheter into the brain tissue. The device monitors a very local area of the brain tissue, and this technique is increasingly used for evaluation of cerebral oxygenation (normal $PbrO_2$ values: 25 to 30 mm Hg).[18] Monitoring may be performed in relatively undamaged parts of the brain or, preferably, in the penumbra region of an intracerebral lesion.[19] Various studies have shown that an increase in intracranial pressure (ICP) and a decrease in CPP or arterial oxygenation, and hyperventilation may result in decreased $PbrO_2$. This monitoring modality is helpful in detecting intraoperative brain hypoxia during episodes of hyperventilation.[20] In patients with TBI, ischemic episodes defined as $PbrO_2$ <10 mm Hg for longer than 15 minutes in the first week after the injury were found to be associated with unfavorable neurologic outcome, and a $PbrO_2$ = 0 mm Hg, not responding to an oxygen challenge, is compatible with brain death.[21] A $PbrO_2$ of ≤15 mm Hg should be considered as a threshold to initiate treatment (level III evidence).[22] CPP >60 mm Hg has been identified as the most important factor determining sufficient brain tissue oxygenation. Studies have demonstrated improvement in $PbrO_2$ after red blood cell transfusion,[23] during barbiturate coma,[24] and after decompressive hemicraniectomy.[25] However, only one study has shown a favorable effect on outcome with the use of $PbrO_2$ monitoring.[26]

Microdialysis

Microdialysis uses a probe as an interface to the brain to continuously monitor the chemistry of a small focal volume of the cerebral extracellular space. This method uses internally perfused semipermeable membrane probes, which allow neurochemical water-soluble substances to be collected outside the brain for further analysis. Substances that can be measured include: (1) energy-related metabolites such as lactate, pyruvate, glucose, adenosine, xanthine; (2) neurotransmitters: glutamate, aspartate, γ-aminobutyric acid; (3) markers of tissue damage and inflammation: glycerol, electrolytes and cytokines; and (4) exogenous substances such as drugs.[27] This monitoring modality thus provides insight into the bioenergetic status of the brain. Increased lactate, decreased glucose, and an elevated lactate/glucose ratio indicate accelerated anaerobic glycolysis. This metabolic pattern commonly occurs with cerebral ischemia or hypoxia, and increased glycolysis in this setting is associated with a poor outcome. Extracellular excitatory amino acids such as glutamate may provide a marker for secondary brain insults, as indicated by elevation during periods of hypoxia and intracranial hypertension. However, metabolism can be altered without changes of cerebral oxygenation, and may not correlate with high ICP or low CPP.[28] In addition, lack of equilibration with the extracellular space may introduce sampling error. Microdialysis catheters should be placed in the tissue at risk in patients with SAH, in the right frontal region in patients with nonfocal traumatic brain injury, while in patients with focal injury one catheter should be placed in the penumbra and a second placed in uninjured tissue.[29]

Diagnosis and Management of Common Types of Neurologic Failure

Traumatic Brain Injury

TBI is the leading cause of death from blunt trauma, with an incidence of approximately 10 per 100,000 per year. Twenty percent of deaths occur in patients between the ages of 5 and 45 years. TBI is the leading cause of death in this age group. The most powerful predictors of poor outcome from TBI are age >55 years, poor pupillary reactivity, a low postresuscitation Glasgow Coma Scale (GCS) score, hypotension, hypoxia, and an unfavorable intracranial diagnosis as established by computed tomography (CT) scan. In addition, early hyperglycemia (>200 mg/dL) is a reliable independent predictor of poor outcome.

The GCS (see Chapter 36) is the most widely used clinical measure of injury severity in patients with TBI. The advantages of this scale are that it provides an objective method of measuring consciousness, it has high intra- and interrater reliability across observers with a wide variety of experience, and it has an excellent correlation with outcome. However, the GCS is unmeasurable in up to 25 to 45% of the patients at admission, and is inaccurate when only the partial score is used, such as in patients with endotracheal intubation, whose verbal response cannot be assessed. TBI qualifies as severe when the GCS is ≤8 after cardiopulmonary resuscitation. The predictive value of the GCS at admission is about 69% for good neurologic outcome and 76% for unfavorable outcome. After 7 days these figures approximate 80% for both favorable and unfavorable outcome.[30]

Examination of the pupils can predict neurologic outcome. When both pupils are dilated and unreactive, the likelihood of poor neurologic outcome or death is as high as 90 to 95%. When both pupils are reactive, the likelihood of poor neurologic outcome is approximately 30 to 40%, while the probability of good outcome is 50 to 70%.

Hypotension is a strong predictor of poor outcome in TBI. Chesnut et al.[31] reported that there was a 15-fold increased risk of mortality in patients with early hypotension and an 11-fold increase in mortality in patients with late hypotension.

Radiologic imaging is important in the diagnosis and in the assessment of the prognosis of patients with TBI. Based on the CT scan, TBI can be classified according to the severity of the intracranial lesion, as follows: *diffuse injury I* (no visible intracranial pathology), *diffuse injury II* (cisterns are present with midline shift 0 to 5 mm; no high or mixed density lesion >25 mL), *diffuse injury III* (swelling; cisterns are compressed or absent with midline shift 0 to 5 mm; no high or mixed density lesion >25 mL), *diffuse injury IV* (shift; midline shift >5 mm; no high or mixed density lesion >25 mL), evacuated mass lesion (any lesion surgically evacuated), and nonevacuated mass lesion (high or mixed density lesion >25 mL; not surgically evacuated). The CT classification of TBI is correlated with neurologic outcome, with diffuse injury I having a 38% rate of unfavorable (death, vegetative or severe disability) outcome, increasing to a 94% rate in patients with a grade IV diffuse injury. In addition, it should be noted that about one third to one half of the patients show no lesion at admission and develop new lesions secondarily, which is associated with substantially worse neurologic outcome.

The goal of resuscitation in traumatic and other types of brain injury is to prevent continuing cerebral insult after a primary injury has already occurred. The extent of the primary cerebral injury is usually determined by the mechanism of the trauma, the cause, and the duration of cerebral ischemia. A primary insult is often associated with intracranial hypertension and systemic hypotension, leading to decreased cerebral perfusion and brain ischemia. Concomitant hypoxemia aggravates brain hypoxia, especially in the presence of hyperthermia, which increases brain metabolic demand. The combined effect of these factors leads to secondary brain injury characterized by excitotoxicity, oxidative stress, and inflammation. The resulting cerebral ischemia may be the single most important secondary event affecting outcome following a cerebral insult. Prevention of secondary injury is the main goal of resuscitative efforts.

Traumatized areas of the brain manifest impaired autoregulation, with increased dependency of CBF on perfusion pressure, and disruption of the blood–brain barrier. If space-occupying lesions or edema is present, these will contribute to reduced brain compliance, leading to increased ICP and a consequent deleterious effect on CBF. The rationale for attempting to optimize CPP arises from the fact that cerebral regions surrounding the primary lesion may be close to the ischemic threshold.

TABLE 56-3

INTENSIVE CARE UNIT MANAGEMENT OF PATIENTS WITH SEVERE TRAUMATIC BRAIN INJURY

Basic principles applied to all patients, assuming initial surgical management	<ul><li>Head elevation 30–45°[a]</li><li>CPP 50–70</li><ul><li>Euvolemia, vasopressors as needed</li></ul><li>ICP <20 mm Hg</li><ul><li>Mannitol, hypertonic saline</li><li>CSF drainage</li></ul><li>$SaO_2 \geq 95\%$; $PaCO_2$ 35–40 mm Hg</li><li>Temperature ≤37°C</li><li>Glucose <180 mg/dL[b]</li><li>Sedation and analgesia</li><li>Early enteral nutrition</li><li>Seizure, stress ulcer, and DVT prophylaxis</li></ul>
Refractory intracranial hypertension. Consider one or all of these interventions, depending on individual circumstances	<ul><li>Optimized hyperventilation with SjO_2 and/or $PbrO_2$ monitoring</li><li>Barbiturate coma</li><li>Mild therapeutic hypothermia (33–35°C)</li><li>Decompressive craniectomy</li></ul>

CPP, cerebral perfusion pressure; ICP, intracranial pressure; CSF, cerebrospinal fluid DVT, deep venous thrombosis.
[a]Unless contraindicated by spine injury, hemodynamic instability or otherwise.
[b]Consider intensive control (glucose <110 mg/dL).[147]

Therefore, the goals of neuroresuscitation are oriented at restoration of CBF by maintenance of adequate CPP, reduction of ICP, evacuation of space-occupying lesions, initiation of therapies for cerebral protection, and avoidance of hypoxia.

Unfortunately, the ICU treatment of TBI is hindered by a lack of rigorous, randomized controlled trials to prove benefit, or lack thereof, for many of the management strategies used today. Thus, treatment is based largely on pathophysiologic principles and uncontrolled trials (level III evidence or less). A general guideline for management of patients with severe TBI appears in Table 56-3. The basic principles of management of acute TBI include osmotherapy (see Chapter 36), sedation, hyperventilation, hypothermia, corticosteroids, and antiseizure prophylaxis.

Sedation of neurologically impaired patients should typically be achieved with short-acting sedatives to allow for frequent assessment of neurologic examination.[32] Although no studies have investigated the effect of sedation on outcome, a common practice is to provide sedation with propofol or benzodiazepines in patients following TBI. Both agents have favorable effects on cerebral oxygen balance, although propofol is more potent in this regard. Undesirable effects of sedatives include a reduction in cerebral perfusion pressure due to hemodynamic depression, or in the case of ketamine, an increase in CBF accompanied by a simultaneous increase in ICP.

Propofol rapidly penetrates the central nervous system (CNS) and has rapid elimination kinetics. Despite the induction of systemic hypotension, propofol decreases cerebral metabolism, resulting in a coupled decline in CBF with consequent decrease in ICP. The favorable pharmacologic and neurophysiologic profile of propofol has led to its widespread use in neurointensive care, and high-dose propofol has been advocated as a substitute for barbiturate therapy in patients with refractory intracranial hypertension. However, prolonged (>24 hours), high-dose (>80 μg/kg/min) propofol administration has been associated with lactic acidosis, cardiac failure, and death ("propofol infusion syndrome") in children and adults with TBI.[33] Thus, the use of high-dose propofol to control refractory intracranial hypertension is not recommended,

and barbiturates should be considered if ICP is not controlled by moderate doses of propofol.

The mechanisms by which barbiturates exert their cerebral protective effect appear to be mediated by a reduction in ICP via alteration in vascular tone, reduction of cerebral metabolic rate, and inhibition of free radical peroxidation. Although barbiturates are effective at reducing ICP, their routine use in TBI does not appear beneficial, and may in fact result in excess mortality in patients with diffuse brain injury (level II evidence).[34,35] This effect may in part relate to the profound cardiovascular depressant effects of barbiturates. Based on one small randomized trial, barbiturates do appear to reduce mortality in patients with refractory high ICP (level II evidence).[36] Thus, high-dose barbiturate therapy may be considered in hemodynamically stable severe TBI patients with intracranial hypertension refractory to maximal medical and surgical ICP-lowering therapy. In some patients barbiturates may induce cerebral hypoxia by reducing CBF in excess of metabolism, and therefore SjO_2 monitoring should be considered during barbiturate therapy.

Although neuromuscular blockade may result in a fall in ICP, the routine use of neuromuscular blockade is discouraged as its use has been associated with a longer ICU course, a higher incidence of pneumonia, and a trend toward more frequent sepsis without any improvement in outcome.

Hyperventilation effectively reduces ICP by reducing CBF. However, the role that hyperventilation should play in routine management of TBI is not clear. Primarily, this is related to concerns that hyperventilation may lead to critically low CBF, resulting in worsening cerebral ischemia.[37] In small randomized trials, prophylactic hyperventilation has not proven to be beneficial in TBI.[38] In contrast, it has been proposed that "optimized hyperventilation" in the presence of "luxury perfusion" (excess CBF) may increase global cerebral oxygen metabolism and help normalize global cerebral glucose extraction. Cruz[39] reported that an optimized hyperventilation strategy resulted in a reduction in mortality compared with CPP management in concurrent matched control patients, although this was not a randomized trial (level III evidence). Based on the available evidence, prolonged or prophylactic hyperventilation should be avoided after severe TBI, especially in the first 24 hours after the injury. Hyperventilation may be necessary for brief periods to reduce intracranial hypertension refractory to sedation, osmotic therapy, and cerebrospinal fluid drainage, and should be guided by SjO_2 and/or $PbrO_2$.[22] A marked fall in either of these values suggests a harmful effect of hyperventilation, and that it should be reduced or discontinued.

Experimentally, hypothermia causes a reduction in cerebral metabolism by decreasing all cell functions, both related to neuronal electric activity and those responsible for cellular integrity. In addition, mild hypothermia has been shown to decrease the release of substrates associated with tissue injury such as glutamate and aspartate. A meta-analysis of eight randomized trials of the use of mild hypothermia (33 to 35°C) in patients with TBI, and including 748 patients, indicated that despite a marginal improvement in poor neurologic outcome, there was no mortality advantage and there was an increased risk of pneumonia.[40] Therefore, there is insufficient evidence to provide recommendations for the use of moderate hypothermia in patients with TBI. In patients with TBI, mild therapeutic hypothermia should be differentiated from spontaneous hypothermia, which indeed carries a poor prognosis and is characterized by markedly abnormal brain metabolic indices. On the other hand, immediate rewarming of TBI patients with spontaneous hypothermia may further worsen outcome.[41]

Use of corticosteroids to reduce posttraumatic inflammatory injury in TBI has been advocated for 30 years or more, but without convincing evidence of benefit. However, a large, prospective, randomized trial in 2004 confirmed that corticosteroids in this setting are harmful. This CRASH study randomized over 10,000 patients presenting with acute TBI to receive high-dose methylprednisolone, or placebo, for 48 hours after hospital admission. Methylprednisolone administration was associated with an approximately 20% increase in the relative risk of death at 2 weeks in the entire cohort, and detriment was evident across subgroups divided by severity and type of injury (level I evidence).[42] Thus, high-dose corticosteroids should not be administered as therapy for acute TBI.[22]

Older animal studies have shown a neuroprotective effect of magnesium sulfate by limiting the extent of secondary brain injury. However, a recent randomized controlled trial of approximately 500 TBI patients, blindly assigned to receive high-dose continuous intravenous magnesium or placebo within 8 hours of injury for a duration of 5 days, did not observe an improvement in 6-month neurologic and cognitive function in patients receiving the active drug, and might even have a negative effect in the treatment of TBI.[43]

Antiseizure prophylaxis is not recommended for preventing posttraumatic late seizures. Anticonvulsants may be used to prevent early posttraumatic seizures within 7 days following head trauma. However, the evidence does not indicate that prevention of early seizures improves outcome following TBI.[44]

Finally, it should be noted that use of albumin as fluid replacement therapy in patients with TBI has been associated with increased mortality in a subgroup analysis of a randomized controlled trial comparing saline and albumin.[45]

Subarachnoid Hemorrhage

The incidence of SAH varies from 7.5 to 12.1 cases per 100,000 population. SAH is most commonly caused by the rupture of an intracranial aneurysm. Other causes of SAH include trauma, vertebral and carotid artery dissection, dural and spinal arteriovenous malformations, mycotic aneurysms, sickle cell disease, cocaine abuse, coagulation disorders, and pituitary apoplexy. SAH is associated with considerable morbidity and mortality, with only one third of the patients suffering from SAH being functional survivors. The leading causes of death and disability

are the direct effect of the initial bleed, cerebral vasospasm, and rebleeding. The report of the Cooperative Study of Intracranial Aneurysms and SAH estimated that 33% of the patients would die before receiving medical attention. Another 27% would either die during hospitalization or become severely disabled, leaving only about 30% to survive without major disability.[46,47] Severity of the initial bleed is the most important determinant of SAH outcome.

At the time of aneurysm rupture, there is a critical reduction in CBF because of an increase in ICP toward arterial diastolic values. The persistence of a no-flow pattern is associated with acute vasospasm and swelling of perivascular astrocytes, neuronal cells, and capillary endothelium. After SAH, injury to the posterior hypothalamus may stimulate release of norepinephrine (NE) from the adrenal medulla and sympathetic cardiac efferent nerves. The release of NE has been associated with ischemic changes in the subendocardium (neurogenic stunned myocardium), cardiac dysrhythmias, and pulmonary edema.

In survivors of the initial bleed, emphasis has been placed on early aneurysm securing with either surgery or interventional neuroradiology (coiling). Approximately 10 to 23% of unsecured aneurysms will rebleed in the first 2 weeks, most within the first 6 to 12 hours after the initial hemorrhage, and rebleeding is associated with mortality approximating 80%. Early aneurysm occlusion substantially reduces the risk of this complication. With the improvement of the operative management, delayed complications have become increasingly important causes of death and disability.

Cerebral vasospasm after SAH, consisting of intracerebral arterial narrowing, is identified by angiography in up to 60% of patients, and is correlated with the amount and location of subarachnoid blood. A reduction in CBF associated with vessel narrowing is ultimately responsible for the appearance of *delayed ischemic neurologic deficits (DINDS)*. DINDS occur in approximately one third of patients suffering from SAH. In a systematic review of the literature, Dorsch[48] found an overall death rate of 31% (vs. 17% in patients without vasospasm), permanent deficits in 35%, and good outcome in 34% of the patients who developed symptomatic vasospasm. DINDS typically present as alteration in consciousness and/or transient focal neurologic deficits that rarely occur within the first 3 days after aneurysm rupture, typically peak in 7 to 10 days, and resolve over 10 to 14 days. If severe, vasospasm can result in cerebral infarction and persistent neurologic deficits, which contribute to considerable long-term morbidity.

TCD has been used to identify and quantify cerebral vasospasm on the basis that velocity profiles increase as the diameter of the vessel decreases. Changes in measured velocities over time may be more reliable than absolute values in predicting symptomatic vasospasm. Velocities >200 cm/s have been associated with a high risk of infarction but there is a poor correlation between the TCD velocities and angiographic findings, especially for the posterior circulation.

The calcium channel blocker nimodipine (60 mg orally every 4 hours for 21 days) is recognized as effective prophylaxis for cerebral vasospasm and improvement in neurologic outcome (reduction of cerebral infarction and poor outcome) and mortality from cerebral vasospasm in patients suffering from SAH (level I evidence).[49] Although angiographic studies do not demonstrate a difference in the frequency of vasospasm compared with a placebo-treated group, the benefits of nimodipine have been attributed to a cytoprotective effect related to the reduced availability of intracellular calcium and improved microvascular collateral flow. No other pharmacologic therapies, with the exception of statins, have proven effective to prevent or treat cerebral vasospasm in clinical trials. A pilot study of simvastatin (80 mg)[50] and a phase II trial of pravastatin (40 mg)[51] for 2 weeks after SAH demonstrated improved outcomes through an improvement of vasospasm-related delayed ischemic deficits. The phase II trial suggested a reduction in the occurrence and duration of severe vasospasm,[51] and a reduction in unfavorable outcomes at the 6-month follow-up with pravastatin compared with placebo.[52] Although very promising, larger phase III trials are necessary to confirm the benefits of statins and the optimal dose and duration of administration.

Hypervolemic/hypertensive and hemodilution ("triple-H") therapy is one of the mainstays of treatment for cerebral ischemia associated with SAH-induced vasospasm despite the lack of evidence for its effectiveness, especially for its prophylactic use.[53] The rationale for this therapy is that hypovolemia is present because of blood loss, and also induced by hypothalamic dysfunction and secretion of natriuretic peptides. Volume expansion is therefore considered beneficial to optimize the patient's hemodynamic profile. The rationale for hypertension derives from the concept that a loss of cerebral autoregulation associated with vasospasm results in pressure-dependent CBF. Finally, hemodilution is a consequence of hypervolemic therapy and is thought to optimize the rheologic properties of the blood and thereby improve microcirculatory flow. There is no consensus with regard to the goals of therapy and it is unclear which component of this therapy is necessary or sufficient to treat vasospasm. Common complications of treatment are pulmonary edema and myocardial ischemia. Because the blood–brain barrier may be disrupted, aggravation of vasogenic edema or hemorrhagic infarction has also been described.[54]

Interventional neuroradiology with the use of balloon angioplasty can reverse or improve vasospasm-induced neurologic deficits. Patients treated within 6 to 12 hours after the development of ischemic symptoms have better results than those receiving delayed intervention. The risks of angioplasty include intimal dissection, vessel rupture, ischemia, and infarction.

Hydrocephalus is another cause of neurologic dysfunction after SAH, occurring in 25% of patients surviving the hemorrhage. The presence of blood in the ventricular system obstructs ventricular drainage and cerebrospinal fluid absorption sites (subarachnoid villi). Ventricular drainage is usually successful in improving neurologic symptoms due to hydrocephalus. A minority of patients will require a permanent ventriculoperitoneal shunt. Seizures occur in 13% of patients with SAH and are more common in patients with a neurologic deficit; thus, prophylactic anticonvulsant therapy is recommended.

A relatively common complication after SAH (10 to 34%) is hyponatremia. Hyponatremia usually develops several days after the hemorrhage and is attributed to two main causes: (1) a syndrome of inappropriate antidiuretic hormone, which is associated with euvolemia or mild hypervolemia, and an excess of free water, or (2) cerebral "salt wasting," which is marked by depletion of sodium and water. The differentiation of these two entities can be difficult but is theoretically important, in that syndrome of inappropriate antidiuretic hormone is treated by free water restriction and cerebral salt wasting with volume expansion and sodium administration. Thus, assessment of intravascular volume status along with the fraction of sodium excreted is a key component when deciding on the treatment regimen for hyponatremia associated with SAH. Other medical complications of SAH include pneumonia, neurogenic pulmonary edema and acute lung injury, sepsis, gastrointestinal (GI) bleeding, deep venous thrombosis, and pulmonary embolism.

Acute Ischemic Stroke

Although evidence indicates that the incidence of stroke has declined over the past 30 years, stroke remains one of the leading causes of disability and death in the United States. More than half of strokes can be attributed to a thrombotic mechanism or local occlusion due to atherosclerosis or cardioembolism.[55] Other major causes of stroke are embolism, lacunar infarct, cerebellar infarction, and hemorrhage. Unusual causes of stroke such as carotid artery dissection or infective endocarditis should be considered in younger patients without apparent risk factors. Transient ischemic attacks may precede stroke and thus should be considered as a warning sign. The prognosis of stroke patients varies depending on the size of the lesion. In patients with acute ischemic stroke, the duration of coma appears to be the most important predictor of outcome and successful therapy.

Rapid clot lysis and restoration of circulation have been proposed as measures to limit the extent of brain injury and improve outcome after stroke. In accordance with the American Heart Association guidelines, systemic thrombolysis using intravenous alteplase (rt-PA) at a dose of 0.9 mg/kg of body weight (maximum dose, 90 mg) with 10% of the dose administered as a bolus and the rest infused over 1 hour should be provided within 3 hours of symptom onset (level I evidence).[56] Thrombolytic therapy has been shown to recanalize both the carotid and the vertebrobasilar arteries in 21 to 93% of cases, when provided within 3 hours after the onset of symptoms, and to improve 24-hour and 3-month neurologic or functional outcome, but not mortality. A placebo-controlled study provided evidence of a sustained benefit at 1 year from systemic thrombolysis in patients with acute ischemic stroke. The overall rate of recurrent stroke was 6.6% and the transient ischemic attack rate 3.3% at 1 year. Regional or local intra-arterial administration of a thrombolytic agent within 6 hours of symptom onset demonstrated a high recanalization rate, but a potential limitation to the use of intra-arterial treatment is the time required to mobilize a team to perform angiography (level II evidence). Trials investigating the use of intravenous thrombolytics within 6 hours after the onset of symptoms failed to observe a benefit of thrombolysis but lend support to the known benefit of treatment within the first 3 hours of stroke onset. Even within the 3-hour window the benefits of rt-PA appear to be greater the sooner the treatment is started.[57]

There is no evidence that intra-arterial thrombolysis is superior or inferior to intravenous administration. Intravenous streptokinase is not indicated for the management of ischemic stroke (level I evidence).

Concerns persist regarding the safety of rt-PA therapy for acute ischemic stroke, primarily related to hemorrhage. The symptomatic intracerebral hemorrhage rate has been reported to be around 5 to 6%, and is greater than in patients receiving thrombolytic therapy for management of myocardial ischemia (level I evidence).[58] Patients receiving systemic rt-PA should not receive aspirin, heparin, warfarin, ticlopidine, or other antithrombotic or antiplatelet-aggregating drugs within 24 hours of treatment (level I evidence).

Unfractionated heparin (UFH) and low-molecular-weight heparin (LMWH) have not been shown to prevent progression or reduce the rate of stroke recurrence when administered within 48 hours of the acute event, and therefore their use is not recommended (level I evidence). In general, heparin is only recommended for early secondary prophylaxis in patients with suspected cardiac embolism. Aspirin (160 to 325 mg/day) has been shown to reduce the risk of early recurrent ischemic stroke when given within 48 hours of stroke onset, but increases the risk of hemorrhagic stroke. The routine use of low-dose aspirin has been recommended as a secondary prevention after the first few weeks. The frequency of deep venous thrombosis in acute stroke is reduced by anticoagulants, especially LMWH, but not by antiplatelet agents. However, it is unclear if the frequency of pulmonary embolism is also reduced.

The majority of patients with acute ischemic stroke present with severe arterial hypertension. If intracerebral hemorrhage is excluded, treatment of hypertension should be delayed since reduction of the perfusion pressure could compromise the viable brain surrounding the ischemia (ischemic penumbra). However, severe hypertension (systolic blood pressure >220 mm Hg, or mean arterial blood pressure of >130 mm Hg, or diastolic >120 mm Hg) should be controlled because of increased risk of hemorrhagic transformation in anticoagulated patients or after thrombolysis. Although there is no evidence for an optimal level of blood pressure, there is general consensus that the systolic pressure should not be lowered below 150 to 160 mm Hg. If the event is accompanied by raised ICP due to cerebral edema, the principles of treatment of raised ICP previously discussed with regard to TBI similarly apply. Cytotoxic brain edema usually occurs 24 to 96 hours after acute ischemic stroke, and osmotherapy constitutes the basis of ICP reduction. Steroids are of no value in the treatment of ischemic stroke. Because hyperglycemia is associated with poor outcome in ischemic stroke, tight glucose control has been recommended. However, a randomized trial of glucose-potassium and insulin infusion failed to demonstrate a mortality benefit at 90 days from targeting normoglycemia.[59]

Space-occupying middle cerebral artery (malignant middle cerebral artery syndrome) and cerebellar infarctions have a high mortality rate and, in selected cases in which signs of intractable intracranial hypertension are present, hemicraniectomy or decompressive surgery of the posterior fossa, respectively, could be life-saving and improve outcome.[60] Surgery seems to be less beneficial in patients presenting with aphasia, in patients older than 50 years, and in patients undergoing delayed surgery (>24 hours after presentation).

Anoxic Brain Injury

Anoxic brain injury most commonly occurs as a result of cardiac arrest. Of patients who survive their initial cardiac arrest, in-hospital mortality ranges from approximately 50 to 90%, and a high percentage of survivors suffer brain injury with significant long-term disability. The pathophysiology of anoxic brain injury is multifactorial and includes excitatory neurotransmitter release, accumulation of intracellular calcium, and oxygen free radical generation. Unfortunately, pharmacologic therapies aimed at several of these pathways, including barbiturates, benzodiazepines, corticosteroids, calcium channel antagonists, and free radical scavengers, have failed to improve the outcome of anoxic brain injury.

A strong experimental literature supports a role for mild therapeutic hypothermia in anoxic brain injury. Two prospective, randomized trials of mild hypothermia (temperature 32 to 34°C) in survivors of out-of-hospital ventricular fibrillation have provided some encouragement for survivors of cardiac arrest.[61,62] Hypothermia was associated with a relative increase in favorable neurologic outcome (moderate disability or less) of 40 to 50%, and in one study was also associated with relative 6-month reduction of mortality by approximately 25% (level II evidence).[61] Thus, mild therapeutic hypothermia should be routinely applied to comatose survivors of out-of-hospital cardiac arrest due to ventricular fibrillation; it should also be considered in other scenarios, including in-hospital cardiac arrest and cardiac arrest due to asystole and pulseless electrical activity. Hypothermia is also currently recommended in neonatal hypoxic encephalopathy. Studies are investigating the efficacy of prehospital induction of hypothermia in out-of-hospital cardiac arrest.[63]

CARDIOVASCULAR AND HEMODYNAMIC ASPECTS OF CRITICAL CARE

Principles of Monitoring and Resuscitation

Shock states are associated with impairment of adequate oxygen delivery resulting in decreased tissue perfusion and tissue hypoxia. It is important to emphasize that global hemodynamic monitoring may not reflect regional perfusion, or the peripheral tissue energy status. Occasionally, despite increased cardiac output and oxygen delivery, peripheral tissues suffer from hypoxia due to blood flow maldistribution, and uncoupling between oxygen delivery and oxygen utilization from mitochondrial dysfunction and energetic failure.

Invasive monitoring in shock states provides insight into the circulatory status, organ perfusion, tissue microcirculation, and cellular metabolic status of the critically ill patient. Hemodynamic monitoring ranges from the simple monitoring of electrocardiogram and pulse oximetry, to continuous measurement of arterial pressure via an arterial catheter, to monitoring of cardiac filling pressures with central venous or pulmonary artery catheters, to cardiac echocardiography. Several experimental monitoring devices detecting microenvironmental conditions at the tissue level are under continuous investigation.

Functional Hemodynamic Monitoring

Pulmonary Artery Catheter

The pulmonary artery catheter (PAC) measures hemodynamic indices including central venous pressure (CVP), pulmonary artery pressure and occlusion pressure (PaOP), cardiac output (thermodilution method), systemic and pulmonary vascular resistances, and mixed venous oxygen saturation (SvO$_2$), and provides data for deriving oxygenation variables (oxygen delivery [DO$_2$], consumption [VO$_2$], and extraction [O$_2$ER]). The information provided by the PAC may assist in the differentiation of cardiogenic and noncardiogenic circulatory and respiratory failure, and help guide fluid, inotropic, and vasopressor therapy.

Despite the theoretical benefits of the PAC, there are few data to support a positive effect on mortality or other substantive outcome variables. In a retrospective analysis using propensity scores, Connors et al. suggested that the use of the PAC within 24 hours following ICU admission was associated with increased mortality, length of stay and health care costs in postoperative patients.[64] Vieillard-Baron et al.[65] suggested that right heart catheterization may be associated with increased mortality, but after adjustment for the use of vasopressors there was no increased mortality associated with the use of the PAC. As a consequence of these studies questioning the benefits of the PAC, the frequency of use of the PAC has substantially decreased in the management of patients with cardiogenic shock and in other ICU settings.[66] A randomized controlled trial assigning patients with shock, ARDS, or both, to receive a PAC, or not, did not find any differences in mortality, organ system failures, renal support, and use of vasoactive agents between the two groups.[67] Similarly, there was no benefit to therapy directed by PAC over standard therapy in elderly, high-risk surgical patients requiring intensive care.[68] More recently a trial conducted in a large cohort of approximately 1,000 ARDS patients assigned to receive PAC- or central venous catheter-guided therapy did not find any survival or organ function differences between the two groups, but twice as many catheter-related complications (mostly dysrhythmias) in PAC-monitored patients.[69] These results, combined with those of previous studies, do not support the routine use of the PAC for the management of acute lung injury or septic shock.

Some, or all, of the following factors may be responsible for the observed lack of benefit associated with PAC use: (1) device or procedure-related complications, (2) inaccurate data, (3) fundamentally incorrect assumptions about the meaning of the measured data, (4) inappropriate decisions resulting from misinterpretation of the data, and (5) harmful effects of well-intended therapies. As an example of factor 3, there is increasing evidence that central venous and PA pressures do not predict the hemodynamic response to intravenous fluid administration in normal subjects or patients with shock.[70,71] As an example of factor 5, the ability to increase DO_2 with fluid resuscitation and inotropic therapy in patients with septic shock identifies a better prognosis. This observation led to a therapeutic strategy known as *supraphysiologic resuscitation* to defined end points (cardiac index >4.5 L/min, DO_2 >600 mL/m^2/min, and VO_2 >170 mL/m^2/min) in patients with septic and surgical/trauma-related shock. However, a large, randomized, prospective study found that this approach was associated with increased mortality in patients with septic shock.[72] As a result, supraphysiologic resuscitation has generally fallen out of favor, although it is still used in some centers. However, this example shows how information derived from the PAC can lead to patient harm, despite the best of intentions.

In summary, although the PAC remains a commonly used tool in CCM, the evidence supporting its benefit is scant. A 1997 consensus conference on the use of the PAC concluded that the catheter should be used only when noninvasive methods are not available to provide the information required.[73] The PAC may be most useful as a tool to allow interpretation of the relationship between cardiac output and the peripheral demand for oxygen and to direct therapy accordingly, rather than as a measure of intravascular volume status. Clearly, further research is necessary to establish the utility, if any, of the PAC in critically ill patients.

A somewhat less invasive and less costly alternative to placing a PAC for the measurement of SvO_2 is to measure central venous oxygen saturation ($ScvO_2$) via a fiberoptic central venous catheter. $ScvO_2$ is typically approximately 5 mm Hg higher than SvO_2, but appears to correlate well with SvO_2 during changes in hemodynamic status.[74] Targeting an $ScvO_2$ >70% as a component of early goal-directed therapy in patients with septic shock has been associated with a reduction in mortality.[75]

Arterial Pressure Waveform Analysis

In addition to static pressure measurements such as CVP and PaOP, dynamic indicators of preload include respiratory variation in systolic pressure and pulse pressure, both of which can be derived from the analysis of the waveform generated by a peripherally placed arterial catheter. In addition, techniques for deriving stroke volume, cardiac output, and intrathoracic blood volume have become available. These techniques present a less invasive and perhaps superior approach to hemodynamic monitoring of critically ill patients.

The variation in systolic blood pressure and pulse pressure during positive pressure ventilation is highly predictive of the response to intravascular fluid administration in both normal subjects and critically ill patients. During positive-pressure ventilation there is an inspiratory reduction in right ventricular stroke volume from decreased venous return and a subsequent reduction in left ventricular end-diastolic volume appearing during the expiratory phase of the respiratory cycle. Therefore, the left ventricular stroke volume varies cyclically with ventilation, and is paralleled by a similar variation in systolic blood pressure and pulse pressure; these effects are exaggerated during absolute and relative hypovolemia. Systolic and pulse pressure variation are superior predictors of fluid responsiveness (compared with static measures such as CVP and PaOP) in patients with a variety of critical illnesses, including septic shock, acute lung injury, and following cardiac surgery.[76]

Analysis of the systemic arterial pulse contour allows derivation of cardiac output after initial calibration using an indicator-dilution technique. Two commercially available devices use either lithium (injected through a peripheral intravenous line; LiDCO, LiDCO Group Plc, London, UK), or thermal dilution (injected through a central venous catheter; PiCCO, Pulsion Medical Systems AG, Munich, Germany) for initial calibration. Cardiac output derived using pulse contour analysis correlates well with thermodilution cardiac output in a variety of conditions, and has the advantage of providing continuous measurement without necessitating the placement of a PAC. The PiCCO device also allows for measurement of intrathoracic blood volume using transpulmonary thermodilution; the latter may be a more accurate reflection of preload than static central pressure measurements.

Echocardiography

An even less invasive hemodynamic monitoring tool is echocardiography (see Chapter 28). Transthoracic and transesophageal echocardiography provide accurate diagnostic information with regard to right and left ventricular function, valve function, pericardium anatomy, traumatic vascular injury, and pulmonary embolism (direct and indirect signs). Transesophageal echocardiography can also be used to assess volume status or preload via measurement of left ventricular end-diastolic volume and/or area. The major limitation of echocardiography is that it does not provide continuous monitoring, is associated with high initial cost, and requires a high standard of training and experience.

Transesophageal Doppler sonography using a small probe in a large nasogastric tube (6 mm) monitors descending aortic flow velocity continuously and allows noninvasive monitoring of cardiac output. The disadvantages of this technique are that it is inaccurate if not positioned correctly, ideally at an angle with the aorta of 45 degrees (minimal error in flow measurement), and that it does not measure the supra-aortic output or the aortic cross-sectional area, which is determined using a nomogram and assumed to remain constant throughout the systole.[77] Two cases of intrabronchial displacement of the probe have been reported.

Although the role of echocardiography in routine critical care management remains undefined, it has been suggested that this technique can replace pulmonary arterial catheterization in the ICU without adversely affecting outcomes.[78]

Definition and Types of Circulatory Failure

The common denominator of shock is circulatory instability characterized by severe hypotension and inadequate tissue perfusion (see Chapter 36). Shock states are classified according to the primary cause of circulatory failure. *Distributive* or *vasodilatory* shock results from a reduction in systemic vascular resistance, often associated with an increased cardiac output, whereas *cardiogenic* (left or right cardiac failure) and *hypovolemic* shock are low cardiac output states usually characterized by increased peripheral resistance. The most common forms of shock encountered in the ICU are cardiogenic, septic, and hypovolemic shock. Despite extensive research and aggressive management, the mortality from shock remains staggeringly high; approximately 35 to 40% of patients die within 28 days of the onset of septic shock, and the mortality rate is 70 to 80% for patients with cardiogenic shock. The mortality from hypovolemic shock is highly variable and depends on the cause and the rapidity of recognition and treatment.

Cardiogenic Shock

The initiating event in cardiogenic shock is a primary pump failure. Heart failure may result from extensive myocardial infarction, cardiomyopathy, dysrhythmias, mechanical complications (mitral regurgitation, ventricular septal defect), tamponade, and so forth. The pathophysiologic characteristics include reduction in contractility, usually accompanied by dilatation of cardiac cavities and venous congestion. Absence of pulmonary congestion at initial clinical evaluation does not exclude a diagnosis of cardiogenic shock by predominant left ventricular failure and is not associated with a better prognosis. The onset of pump failure is associated with two compensatory mechanisms: a reflex vasoconstriction in systemic vessels causing an increase in left ventricular workload and myocardial oxygen demand, and a redistribution of blood volume toward the heart and the lungs. However, cardiogenic shock developing within 36 hours of an acute myocardial infarction has been associated with variably decreased systemic vascular resistances, possibly mediated by the presence of a systemic inflammatory response.

Several studies demonstrated that the incidence and severity of left ventricular failure complicating acute myocardial infarction were directly related to the extent of ventricular mass necrosis. Consequently, therapy should minimize myocardial oxygen demand and raise oxygen delivery to the ischemic area. This goal is complicated by the fact that many resuscitative approaches to correct hypotension (preload augmentation, inotropes and vasopressors; see below) increase myocardial oxygen consumption. In patients without hypotension, pharmacologic vasodilatation using nitrates or sodium nitroprusside may reduce myocardial oxygen consumption and improve ventricular ejection by reducing left ventricular afterload, and possibly produce a shift of blood from the lungs to the periphery by reducing venous tone. B-type natriuretic peptide (nesiritide) and fenoldopam have similar effects, and have an additional beneficial diuretic effect.[79] When pharmacologic interventions are not sufficient to restore hemodynamic stability, the use of mechanical support with the insertion of intra-aortic balloon pump counterpulsation and ventricular assist devices can help unload the ventricles.

In patients with myocardial infarction, coronary reperfusion can be achieved with thrombolysis or, preferably, primary percutaneous coronary intervention. A randomized trial comparing emergency revascularization with primary percutaneous coronary intervention or coronary artery bypass surgery to a regimen of thrombolysis did not demonstrate a mortality difference at 30 days. However, at 6 months and 1 year, there was a significant mortality reduction with emergency revascularization in patients under the age of 75 years.[80] The use of primary percutaneous coronary intervention in patients younger than 75 years with an acute ST elevation myocardial infarction complicated by cardiogenic shock who can be treated within 18 hours of the onset of shock is a grade A recommendation.

Septic Shock

Septic shock is a form of distributive shock associated with the activation of the systemic inflammatory response, and is usually characterized by a high cardiac output, low systemic vascular resistance, hypotension, and regional blood flow redistribution, resulting in tissue hypoperfusion. Distributive shock can also be associated with pancreatitis, burns, fulminant hepatic failure, multiple traumatic injuries, toxic shock syndrome, anaphylaxis and anaphylactoid reactions, and drug or toxin reactions, including insect bites, transfusion reactions, and heavy metal poisoning. In patients with systemic infections, the physiologic response can be staged on a continuum from a systemic inflammatory response syndrome, to sepsis, severe sepsis, and septic shock (Table 56-4). The hemodynamic profile of septic shock is influenced by several sepsis-induced physiologic changes including hypovolemia and vasodilation, in addition to cardiac depression. Sepsis is associated with a global decrease in cardiac contractility, and echocardiographic measurements of the left ventricle size demonstrate an inability of the ventricle to dilate in septic patients.[81]

TABLE 56-4

DEFINITIONS OF SEPSIS AND ORGAN FAILURE

Clinical evidence of infection
Infection: Microbial phenomenon characterized by an inflammatory response to the presence of microorganisms or the invasion of normally sterile tissue by those organisms.
Bacteremia: The presence of viable bacteria in the blood.
Systemic inflammatory response syndrome (SIRS): Systemic inflammatory response to a variety of severe clinical insults. The response is manifested by two or more of the following conditions:
Core temperature <36°C or >38°C
Tachycardia >90 beats/min
Tachypnea >20 breaths/min while breathing spontaneously, or PaCO$_2$ <4.3 kPa
White blood count >12,000 cells/mm^3, <4000 cells/mm^3, or >10% immature forms
Sepsis: The systemic response to infection. This systemic response is manifested by three or more of the conditions described above (SIRS) and presented clinical or microbiological evidence of infection.
Severe sepsis: Sepsis associated with organ dysfunction, hypoperfusion, or hypotension. Hypoperfusion and perfusion abnormalities may include, but are not limited to, lactic acidosis, oliguria, or an acute alteration in mental status.
Septic shock: Sepsis with hypotension, despite adequate fluid resuscitation, along with the presence of perfusion abnormalities that may include, but are not limited to, lactic acidosis, oliguria, or an acute alteration in mental status. Patients who are taking inotropic or vasopressor agents may not be hypotensive at the time that perfusion abnormalities are measured.
Sepsis-induced hypotension: A systolic blood pressure of <90 mm Hg or a reduction of >40 mm Hg from baseline in the absence of other causes for hypotension.
Multiple organ dysfunction syndrome: Presence of several altered organ functions in an acutely ill patient such that homeostasis cannot be maintained without intervention.

From American College of Chest Physicians/Society of Critical Care Medicine Consensus Conference: Definitions for sepsis and organ failure and guidelines for the use of innovative therapies in sepsis. Crit Care Med 1992; 20: 864, with permission.

In endotoxemia and sepsis, metabolic needs are increased and the ability of the tissues to extract and use oxygen may be impaired. Thus, a metabolic acidosis may be present despite normal levels of oxygen transport. A decrease in cellular O$_2$ extraction capacity may result from factors other than hypoperfusion, such as direct cellular damage by toxins and/or mediators or maldistribution of blood flow. The impact of impaired perfusion on organ function depends on individual susceptibility to hypoxia. The intestinal mucosa is particularly vulnerable to ischemia. The GI tract has been implicated as the "motor" of multiple-organ dysfunction syndrome (MODS) and "splanchnic resuscitation" has been advocated as a central objective in patients with septic shock. Intramucosal pH and PCO$_2$ monitoring has been proposed as a technique to assess the splanchnic metabolic state.

Although hypoperfusion is the dominant cause of lactic acidosis in sepsis, various degrees of intermediary metabolic alterations may contribute to the increased lactate production independent of perfusion. Normally, lactate is cleared by the liver metabolic activity via the Cori cycle. Subsequently, with the development of liver perfusion impairment this organ may turn to a net lactate producer. Furthermore, the increase in the rate of glucose metabolism may also occur because of inhibition of the step-limiting enzyme, pyruvate dehydrogenase, for pyruvate to enter the Krebs cycle. An increase in the relative proportion of inactive to active enzyme results in pyruvate accumulation and lactate production.

MODS refers to the presence of altered organ function in an acutely ill patient such that homeostasis cannot be maintained without intervention.[82] The exact pathophysiology of MODS is not yet fully understood, although alterations in systemic hemodynamics, organ perfusion, and tissue microcirculation resulting in tissue hypoxia play a role in initiating and maintaining the syndrome. MODS accounts for most deaths in the ICU.

Although organ failure only qualifies a dichotomous event that is either present or absent, organ dysfunction represents a continuum of physiologic derangements. Different severity scores have been proposed to quantify the range of severity of MODS.[83] One scoring system assigns increasingly high values based on markers of increasing respiratory, renal, cardiovascular, hepatic, hematologic, and CNS dysfunction.

Based on the cause, MODS can be classified as either primary or secondary. Primary MODS is the result of a well-defined insult in which a primary organ dysfunction occurs early and can be directly attributable to the insult itself. (e.g., ARDS due to pulmonary contusion). Secondary MODS represents an abnormal host response (e.g., ARDS in patients with sepsis) and is the result of a systemic inflammatory response initiated by a primary insult involving another organ system.

Clinical Management of Shock/Circulatory Failure Based on Hemodynamic Parameters

The mainstay of treatment of hemodynamic instability is correction of hypotension and restoration of regional blood flow with intravascular volume expansion and vasopressors and/or inotropes. Adequacy of regional perfusion is usually assessed by evaluating indices of organ function, including myocardial ischemia, renal dysfunction (urine output and renal function tests), arterial lactate levels as an indicator of anaerobic metabolism, CNS dysfunction as indicated by abnormal sensorium, and hepatic parenchymal injury by liver function tests. However, these functional assessments of satisfactory organ perfusion may not allow rapid adjustments in therapy compared with more direct continuous monitoring of global and/or regional perfusion. Therefore, additional end points of treatment consist of mean arterial pressure and DO_2, or some surrogate of the latter (SvO_2 or $ScvO_2$).

Updated recommendations from the Surviving Sepsis Campaign, an international initiative aiming at improving outcome in patients with severe sepsis, propose a number of interventions (bundles) to guide management of patients with septic shock (Table 56-5).[84]

TABLE 56-5

SURVIVING SEPSIS CAMPAIGN: GUIDE TO MANAGEMENT OF PATIENTS WITH SEVERE SEPSIS OR SEPTIC SHOCK

- Initiation of early goal-directed resuscitation during the first 6 hours after onset of sepsis
- Blood cultures to identity causative organisms before starting antibiotic therapy, and prompt imaging studies performed identify potential source of infection
- Administration of empiric broad-spectrum antibiotics within 1 hour of diagnosis, and reassessment of appropriate therapy on availability of microbiology results
- Control of source of infection
- Administration of either crystalloid or colloids as choice for fluid resuscitation
- Fluid challenge to achieve adequate filling pressures, and reduction of rate of fluids with rising filling pressure and no improvement in tissue perfusion
- Use of norepinephrine or dopamine as first-line vasopressors for a target mean arterial pressure ≥65 mm Hg
- Use of vasopressin at fixed rate as an adjunct to catecholamines
- Use of low dopamine for renal protection not recommended
- Consideration for dobutamine in low cardiac output states despite fluid resuscitation
- Targeting supranormal values of oxygen delivery is not recommended
- Stress-dose steroid therapy for septic shock if blood pressure is poorly responsive to fluid and vasopressors
- Use of recombinant activated protein C in patients at high risk of death
- Targeting a hemoglobin of 7–9 g/dL in the absence of tissue hypoperfusion, coronary artery disease, or acute hemorrhage
- Appropriate use of fresh-frozen plasma and platelets
- Use of low tidal volume, limitation of inspiratory plateau pressure, and application of at least a minimal amount of positive end-expiratory pressure for ALI patients
- Elevation of the head of the bed to a semirecumbent position unless contraindicated
- Avoidance of routine use of pulmonary artery catheter in patients with ALI
- Use a conservative fluid strategy for patients with ALI who are not in shock
- Use of protocols for ventilation weaning and sedation/analgesia, with daily sedation interruption if using continuous infusion sedation
- Avoidance of neuromuscular blockade
- Glucose control, targeting blood glucose levels <150 mg/dL
- Equivalence of continuous veno-veno hemofiltration and intermittent hemodialysis
- Use of bicarbonate to correct arterial pH above 7.15 is not recommended
- Use of deep vein thrombosis and stress ulcer prophylaxis with H_2 blockers or proton pump inhibitors is recommended
- Consideration of limitation of life support when appropriate

ALI, acute lung injury.
Adapted from Dellinger RP, Levy MM, Carlet JM et al: Surviving Sepsis Campaign: International guidelines for management of severe sepsis and septic shock: 2008. Crit Care Med 2008; 36: 296.

Management of Hypotension with Fluid Replacement Therapy

Intravascular volume expansion is the first line of therapy in all forms of shock. Clinical indicators of the response to a fluid challenge (bolus fluid therapy of 250 to 1,000 mL crystalloids over 5 to 15 minutes) are heart rate, blood pressure, and urine output as well as invasively acquired measures including CVP, PaOP, systolic and pulse pressure variation, and cardiac output. An increase in cardiac output following volume expansion unmasks an absolute or relative hypovolemic state (preload dependency). Lack of change or a decrease in cardiac output following volume expansion suggests a euvolemic status, volume overload, or cardiac failure.

The choice of crystalloids versus colloids for volume expansion has been debated for decades, without clear resolution.[85,86] A multicenter, randomized, double-blind trial compared the effect of fluid resuscitation with albumin or saline on mortality in ICU patients.[87] The study indicated that use of either 4% albumin or normal saline for fluid resuscitation resulted in similar outcomes at 28 days (level II evidence). Another randomized study in 537 patients with severe sepsis compared volume resuscitation with hetastarch versus Ringer lactate. Although there was no difference in mortality between groups, patients randomized to receive hetastarch had a higher risk of renal failure and the need for renal replacement therapy.[88]

Management of Shock with Vasopressors/Inotropes

If patients remain persistently hypotensive despite volume expansion and markers of adequate preload, the use of vasopressors is indicated. Pharmacologic agents include adrenergic agonists with inotropic and vasoconstrictor effects (NE, dopamine, dobutamine, epinephrine, and phenylephrine), and other vasoconstrictors that are vasopressin and nitric oxide synthase inhibitors.

Norepinephrine. NE increases systemic arterial pressure, with variable effects on cardiac output and heart rate. This effect is mainly mediated by α- and β-adrenergic receptor agonism. Studies comparing the hemodynamic and splanchnic effects of NE with dopamine in patients with sepsis indicate that NE improves organ perfusion by an increase in systemic vascular resistance and oxygen consumption accompanied by a decrease in lactate levels, while dopamine acts largely by increasing cardiac performance, with an unfavorable effect on the oxygen delivery and consumption relationship.[89,90]

A concern that NE may compromise renal perfusion has led to some hesitancy to use this drug; however, the majority of available evidence suggests that NE improves renal function in volume-resuscitated, hypotensive patients with septic shock. It is worth noting that the combination of excessively high doses of NE with inadequate effective plasma volume expansion may reduce organ perfusion and should be avoided.

In summary, provided adequate fluid replacement therapy, NE restores perfusion pressure, improves organ function, and corrects splanchnic ischemia in hypotensive patients. Because of its favorable hemodynamic profile, NE is the drug of first choice in the management of septic shock.[89,90] In addition, in the only large, prospective evaluation of vasopressor therapy for septic shock, NE administration was associated with a reduction in mortality compared with dopamine or epinephrine, although this was not a randomized or blinded trial (level III evidence).[91]

Dopamine. Dopamine raises mean arterial pressure by increasing cardiac output and, less so, systemic vascular resistance. Dopamine does not have selective dopaminergic effects on renal blood flow, but rather improves urine output by either by improving overall hemodynamics, a direct diuretic effect, or by decreasing the release of antidiuretic hormone via baroreceptor responses.[89] Further, a large randomized trial and a meta-analysis comparing low-dose dopamine with placebo in critically ill patients found no differences in either renal function tests or survival, and the use of low-dose dopamine is therefore not recommended (level II evidence).[92] In addition, dopamine may have detrimental effects on the splanchnic circulation. Marik and Mohedin[90] showed that dopamine increased splanchnic oxygen consumption, which was not compensated by an increase in oxygen delivery and therefore resulted in increased oxygen debt, and suggested that dopamine might redistribute flow within the intestinal wall and ultimately reduce mucosal blood flow. Lastly, the response to receptor activation by dopamine administration is highly unpredictable at any dopamine dosage. In patients with septic shock, even low doses of dopamine have consistent inotropic effects and, despite an increased oxygen transport, dopamine may adversely affect gastric mucosal perfusion.

Dobutamine. Dobutamine is a β_1- and β_2-receptor agonist that demonstrates potent inotropic and chronotropic effects, and mild peripheral vasodilatation, with the ultimate effect of increasing oxygen delivery and consumption. Dobutamine is the drug of choice in patients with circulatory failure primarily due to cardiac pump failure (cardiogenic shock). However, dobutamine should not be used as first-line single therapy when hypotension is present. In patients with septic shock, dobutamine may be useful in the presence of impaired cardiac contractility with resulting inadequate cardiac output and oxygen delivery. Several studies show that dobutamine alone or added to standard vasopressor regimens increases both oxygen delivery and consumption in septic and elderly septic patients.[93] In patients with septic shock, the combination of NE plus dobutamine resulted in increased gastric mucosal perfusion compared with NE alone.[94] Other studies comparing the effects of NE plus dobutamine versus epinephrine or dopamine alone suggested an improved balance between oxygen delivery and consumption with the combination therapy.

Despite these physiologic benefits of dobutamine in septic shock, detrimental effects have been observed when therapy is oriented to supranormal cardiac output, DO_2 and VO_2 in critically ill patients, as discussed previously.[72] Based on this and other studies, the use of aggressive strategies such as high-dose dobutamine to drive cardiac index above a predefined supraphysiologic level is not recommended as routine therapy in the critically ill patient (grade A recommendation). In contrast, a clinical trial of early goal-directed therapy during the first 6 hours of septic shock to maintain central venous oxyhemoglobin saturation ($ScvO_2$) of $\geq 70\%$ with volume resuscitation, packed red blood cell transfusion to a hematocrit of 30% and, if not sufficient, with dobutamine up to 20 $\mu g/kg/min$, demonstrated a 16% absolute reduction in 28-day mortality compared with standard therapy (level II evidence).[75] It is not clear whether the observed benefits of early goal-directed therapy were because of the early initiation of treatment, achievement of the goal end points, or specific elements of treatment (e.g., blood transfusion or dobutamine). However, this early approach of increasing oxygen delivery in septic shock patients by targeting an indicator of supply/demand relationship is substantially different from the supraphysiologic resuscitation in general ICU populations previously described.

In summary, dobutamine treatment is the first line of treatment in patients with shock and decreased cardiac contractility and performance. In patients with septic shock, dobutamine may be useful as second-line agent, after adequate fluid resuscitation and if introduction of vasopressors has not restored sufficient levels of oxygen delivery, reflected by an $ScvO_2$ of $>70\%$ (which approximates a mixed venous oxygen saturation, SvO_2, of $>65\%$) and increased lactate clearance. However, further corroborating data are necessary to determine the true benefits of early optimization of oxygen delivery. Targeting supranormal levels of oxygen delivery and consumption is not recommended.

Epinephrine.   Epinephrine increases cardiac index by increasing contractility and heart rate, and also increases systemic vascular resistance. The response to stepwise dose increments of epinephrine on hemodynamic variables confirms that this drug is a strong inotropic agent even in patients with septic shock, and increases mean arterial blood pressure, cardiac output, DO_2, and VO_2. Epinephrine also increases VO_2 via activation of metabolic pathways.

In patients with septic shock, epinephrine may reduce splanchnic perfusion despite an increase in global hemodynamic and oxygen transport.[95,96] In addition, epinephrine therapy consistently increases plasma lactate levels in septic shock. Whether this reflects a reduction in vital organ perfusion with resulting anaerobic metabolism, increased production consequent to a thermogenic effect in skeletal muscle, or reduced clearance remains to be defined. However, epinephrine treatment at best brings no additional benefit to other catecholamine therapy in the management of patients with septic shock.

Vasopressin.   Vasopressin is a potent vasoconstrictor when administered in low doses to patients in shock, particularly those with distributive shock due to sepsis or hepatic failure, or with circulatory failure following cardiopulmonary bypass.[97] This may be in part related to a relative deficiency of vasopressin in these settings. Vasopressin may also be useful in resuscitation from cardiac arrest, particularly if due to asystole, and is offered as an option in the current ACLS algorithm for treatment of ventricular fibrillation (level II evidence).[98]

Vasopressin administration during shock typically results in dramatically increased systemic blood pressure, with either no effect or a mild decrease in cardiac output, little change in heart rate, and no effect on pulmonary vascular resistance. Although vasopressin has the potential to reduce mesenteric and renal blood flow, it does not appear to do so when administered at a low dose during vasodilatory shock.[99,100] In addition, vasopressin and its analogs have been show to improve urine output in the hepatorenal syndrome, supporting a positive effect of vasopressin on renal blood flow in vasodilatory states. Small clinical trials of vasopressin or vasopressin analogues (terlipressin) have consistently demonstrated a catecholamine sparing effect of vasopressin.[101,102]

Preliminary data from a randomized trial of over 700 patients comparing NE alone with NE plus vasopressin (VASST trial) at 0.03 U/min showed no mortality differences, although some possible benefits were seen in patients receiving doses of NE <15 μg/min.[84] Based on these data, the Surviving Sepsis Campaign suggests that vasopressin at the dose of 0.03 U/min may be added to NE with the expectation that the effect on blood pressure will be similar to that produced by NE. The experts also propose that epinephrine should be the first-choice alternative agent in septic shock that is poorly responsive to NE or dopamine.

Additional Treatment Considerations for Critically Ill Patients with Septic Shock

Activated Protein C.   Clinical or subclinical manifestations of intravascular disseminated coagulation and consumption coagulopathy (increase in D dimers, decreased protein C, thrombocytopenia, and increased prothrombin time) are present in essentially all patients with septic shock. The activation of protein C is thought to be an important mechanism for modulating sepsis-induced consumption coagulopathy. Activated protein C works as an antithrombotic agent by inactivating factors Va and VIIIa. Activated protein C also facilitates clot lysis by inhibiting plasminogen activator inhibitor 1. In patients with

sepsis, inflammatory cytokines (tumor necrosis factor-α, interleukin-1β) down-regulate two key components of the protein C activation complex, thrombomodulin and the endothelial cell protein C receptor resulting in decreased protein C activation. In addition, activated protein C inhibits the generation of inflammatory cytokines from monocytes and reduces the expression of adhesion receptors and inflammatory mediators from the endothelium. The rationale for replacing activated protein C relates to its anticoagulant and profibrinolytic properties, which interrupt the consumption coagulopathy and are particularly effective at preventing microvascular thrombosis. Drotrecogin-alfa, a human recombinant activated protein C, administered intravenously for 96 hours at the rate of 24 μg/kg/hr to patients with severe sepsis, has been investigated in a large randomized trial.[103] The study showed a 6.1% absolute 28-day mortality reduction (30.8 vs. 24.7%). Given the risk of drug-induced bleeding, activated protein C is approved only in patients with severe sepsis and high risk of death as indicated by an APACHE II score >25 (level II evidence).

Corticosteroids.   Although high-dose corticosteroids for the treatment of septic shock are of no benefit, lower doses, on the order of hydrocortisone 200 to 300 mg/day, can reduce dependency on vasopressors and expedite the resolution of shock, but they do not confer a mortality benefit (level I evidence).[104,105] A cosyntropin stimulation test prior to initiating steroid therapy is not considered necessary to identify patients with relative adrenal insufficiency, as the effects of corticosteroids are similar irrespective of the test results. This issue is discussed in depth in the Endocrinology section of this chapter.

Treatment of Infection.   Identifying the source of the infection, source control, and early initiation of appropriate antibiotic therapy are critical priorities in addition to hemodynamic support. Appropriate cultures should always be obtained before antimicrobial therapy is initiated. At least two blood cultures (one drawn percutaneously and one from drawn through vascular access device) and respiratory, urine, cerebrospinal fluid, and wounds or fluid collection should be obtained (grade D recommendation). Diagnostic studies should be performed promptly to assist in the identification of the source of infection and the causative organism, especially for foci amenable to source control measures (e.g., abscess drainage; grade E recommendation). Empiric antibiotic therapy should be started as soon as possible, within 1 hour of recognition of sepsis, after appropriate culture collection (level II evidence). Initial empiric therapy should be broad enough and include one or more drugs that have activity against the likely pathogens and which penetrate into the presumed site of infection. After antibiotic susceptibility testing is available, restriction of the number of antibiotics and narrowing the spectrum of antimicrobial treatment is appropriate. For a more detailed discussion and specific sites of infection, please refer to the "Nosocomial Infections."

ACUTE RESPIRATORY FAILURE

Acute respiratory failure is characterized by a derangement in pulmonary gas exchange or an imbalance between the work of breathing and respiratory muscle capacity, and is usually accompanied by hypoxemia and/or hypercapnia. Indeed, in some cases respiratory failure may be caused by "nonrespiratory" issues; for example, coma that results in the inability to protect the airway. Acute respiratory failure is a relatively common phenomenon; depending on the type of ICU, the majority of patients may be mechanically ventilated at any given time, and virtually all critically ill patients are mechanically ventilated for some portion of their ICU stay. Suffice it to say that the treatment of acute respiratory failure is primarily supportive and typically necessitates supplemental oxygen, and often mechanical ventilation with or without airway intubation. Acute respiratory therapy typically resolves when the initiating condition is adequately treated. The following subsections discuss basic principles of mechanical ventilation, some of the more challenging types of respiratory failure, and potential therapeutic approaches to respiratory failure.

Principles of Mechanical Ventilation

Mechanical ventilation in the ICU is provided through the application of positive pressure to the airway; commonly a preset tidal volume (volume control) or inspiratory pressure (pressure control) and rate are provided, and any breathing that the patient does above this set minute ventilation is either supported (continuous mandatory ventilation) or not (intermittent mandatory ventilation). However, beyond this simplest level ICU ventilators have become increasingly powerful and complex, and are high-flow capacity, microprocessor-based systems that offer multiple modes of ventilation and computer-compatible monitoring or control. Thus, ventilatory modes used today include pressure support ventilation, volume support ventilation, pressure-regulated volume control, high-frequency ventilation, proportional assist ventilation, and airway pressure-release ventilation. In reality, despite strong regional, local, and individual biases, there is little evidence to suggest that the mode of mechanical ventilation contributes significantly to any major outcome measure, and the choice of mode is at this point is largely one of clinician preference. Thus, this discussion will not dwell on specific modes of ventilation.

Mechanical ventilation has been traditionally considered supportive therapy that is applied until the initiating cause of respiratory failure improves sufficiently such that the patient can breathe without assistance. However, mechanical ventilation may be injurious in certain settings. Traditionally, tidal volumes of 10 to 15 mL/kg have been routinely used to ventilate patients in the ICU. The use of such supraphysiologic tidal volumes (normal resting tidal volumes are 5 to 7 mL/kg) evolved from the observation that the use of smaller-sized volumes was associated with the development of atelectasis and hypoxemia in anesthetized patients in the operating room. However, in certain patients, large tidal volumes can result in cardiovascular compromise, barotrauma, ventilator-induced (or ventilator-associated; VALI) lung injury and excess mortality, as discussed later.

Positive-pressure ventilation results in increased intrathoracic pressure, which reduces venous return, and in turn results in reduced cardiac output and blood pressure. In addition, positive-pressure ventilation can result in alveolar overdistension and alveolar rupture, which manifests as pneumothorax and pneumomediastinum (barotrauma). Both of these effects are amplified in patients with obstructive lung disease (asthma and COPD). In these patients, limitation of expiratory flow leads to air trapping and the development of intrinsic positive end-expiratory pressure, or auto-PEEP. Air trapping results in alveolar overdistension and increases the risk of barotrauma, and auto-PEEP can contribute substantially to increased intrathoracic pressure and cardiovascular depression. Auto-PEEP cannot be detected without holding exhalation for a prolonged interval (expiratory pause) with both inspiratory and expiratory ventilator valves closed; thus, auto-PEEP may not be appreciated unless actively sought.

The development of air trapping and auto-PEEP leads to significant morbidity and mortality in patients with obstructive lung disease. Thus, the ventilatory strategy in these patients should focus on prolongation of expiratory time by limiting

minute ventilation by using low tidal volumes (≤6 to 8 mL/kg) and a low rate (8 to 12 breaths per minute), and by reducing the inspiratory time of the respiratory cycle. Low minute ventilation is often associated with hypercapnia and respiratory acidosis (permissive hypercapnia); however, this does not appear to be harmful, and the benefits of reduced air trapping and auto-PEEP far outweigh any possible detriment. In order to decrease inspiratory time, the inspiratory flow rate must increase, and this results in increased peak airway pressure. However, most of the peak pressure is dissipated in the endotracheal tube and large airways, and more importantly, end-expiratory, static or plateau, and mean airway pressures will fall with increased expiratory time. In order to accomplish these goals, deep sedation is often required, and rarely neuromuscular blockade must be used. The adoption of this type of ventilatory strategy in the 1980s and 1990s was associated with a dramatic reduction in mortality from acute, severe asthma and respiratory failure, from as high as 23% to <5% (level IV evidence).[106]

In contrast to barotrauma, ventilator-induced lung injury or VALI refers to microscopic injury to the lung due to overdistention and cyclic reopening of alveoli. VALI has been well demonstrated in numerous experimental models, and is histologically similar to the features seen in acute lung injury of other causes, with diffuse alveolar damage and increased microvascular permeability.[107] In addition, VALI is associated with the systemic release of inflammatory mediators that may contribute to multiple organ failure. Clinically, patients thought to be at risk for VALI are those with abnormally low recruitable lung volumes, in particular those with acute lung injury (ALI) and ARDS. Thus, a "lung-protective" ventilatory strategy using low tidal volume ventilation has been proven to save lives when applied to patients with ALI/ARDS (see later discussion).

In summary, although tidal volumes of 10 to 12 mL/kg may still be indicated for some patients, in most cases an initial tidal volume of 8 mL/kg is probably appropriate, and volumes as low as 4 mL/kg may be appropriate in some cases. In addition, because lung volumes correlate with height rather than weight, tidal volume selection should be based on predicted, or ideal body weight, rather than actual weight to avoid lung overdistention.

Although mechanical ventilation generally implies airway intubation, noninvasive positive pressure ventilation (NPPV) or CPAP can be delivered via a tight-sealing nasal or full-face mask. NPPV is applied using either standard ICU ventilators (typically set to pressure support or pressure control modes, with or without PEEP), or specially designed ventilators that deliver CPAP or bilevel positive airway pressure. These dedicated noninvasive ventilators generate high gas flow, can cycle between a high inspiratory pressure and a lower expiratory pressure, and can sense and respond to patient inspiratory effort. Originally developed for home ventilation in patients with obstructive sleep apnea and chronic respiratory failure, newer models are targeted for use in the ICU and incorporate monitoring packages that allow assessment of delivered tidal volumes and respiratory patterns. However, there is no evidence that the type of ventilator used for NPPV affects patient outcome, and the choice of equipment is typically based on availability and familiarity.

NPPV compared with standard therapy has been associated with improved outcomes in a variety of causes of respiratory failure, including cardiogenic pulmonary edema, COPD, and ALI in immunosuppressed patients (level II evidence).[108,109] Improved outcomes include the avoidance of endotracheal intubation, a reduction in complications associated with intubation including ventilator-associated pneumonia, and reduced mortality. However, NPPV is not without risk, and has been associated with a higher rate of myocardial infarction in patients with cardiogenic pulmonary edema and increased mortality in patients with respiratory failure after extubation.[110,111] Therefore, NPPV is best and most safely used when patient characteristics are ideal, including an awake, cooperative patient (with the exception of rapidly reversible obtundation due to high PCO_2), a low risk for regurgitation and aspiration of gastric contents, and a high likelihood that the process resulting in respiratory failure is rapidly reversible. Further research including larger, randomized trials of NPPV, is necessary to better define the particular subgroups of patients who will benefit from this approach.

Weaning from mechanical ventilation is better termed *liberation* or *separation* from ventilation, as weaning implies that ventilation must be gradually withdrawn in order to allow respiratory muscle and patient adaptation to the process. In reality, separation from mechanical ventilation is more a function of the resolution of the cause of respiratory failure, rather than the technique used to withdraw ventilatory support. This is supported by a study showing that daily trials of unassisted ventilation ("T-piece trials") resulted in more rapid separation from ventilation than other more gradual approaches, particularly intermittent mandatory ventilation weaning (level I evidence).[112] In addition, so-called weaning parameters are inadequate predictors of the success or failure of withdrawal of ventilatory support and add little to routine management. Thus, the process of separation from mechanical ventilation is expedited when respiratory therapy-driven protocols are used that focus on daily assessment of the ability to breathe without assistance, assuming improvement of the inciting process, adequate oxygenation, and hemodynamic stability (grade A recommendation).[113] Once the patient can breathe comfortably for 30 to 120 minutes without support, the trachea can be extubated, assuming that there are not other precluding factors such as airway abnormalities and coma.

Acute Lung Injury and Acute Respiratory Distress Syndrome

ALI and ARDS are syndromes of acute, hypoxemic respiratory failure marked pathologically by diffuse alveolar damage, with resulting increased lung permeability and diffuse alveolar edema.[114] ARDS can occur as a result of direct injury to the lung (e.g., aspiration or pneumonia) or in association with extrapulmonary infection (sepsis) or injury (e.g., multiple trauma). ARDS and diffuse alveolar damage are associated with an inflammatory cell infiltration of the lung, increased systemic markers of inflammation, and progression through exudative, fibroproliferative, and fibrotic phases of injury over days to weeks.

In order to better standardize the definition of ARDS for epidemiologic and research purposes, in 1994 a joint American-European conference proposed criteria for characterizing ARDS according to the severity of gas exchange abnormality.[115] Despite some controversy, these criteria have been generally accepted (Table 56-6).[114] Thus, ALI is identical to ARDS in all aspects except for the ratio of PaO_2 to FIO_2 (P/F ratio) at the time of diagnosis. The rationale for characterizing ALI/ARDS according to gas exchange abnormality was that this might allow identification of patients at lower and higher risk of death. However, this does not appear to be the case, as evidence suggests that the P/F ratio is not a risk factor for mortality in ARDS, and mortality in ARDS and ALI appear to be similar.[116]

ALI/ARDS is highly prevalent in the ICU population. A prospective, multicenter study of ICUs in France found that patients with ALI/ARDS comprised approximately 9% of all ICU patients and approximately 40% of all patients with hypoxemic respiratory failure.[117] Of predisposing factors, sepsis carries the highest risk (approximately 30%) and is the most common cause of ALI/ARDS. Mortality associated with ARDS has fallen substantially over the past 20 years, and is currently in the 30 to 40% range overall. However, ARDS

TABLE 56-6

CONSENSUS CRITERIA FOR THE DIAGNOSIS OF ACUTE LUNG INJURY (ALI) AND ACUTE RESPIRATORY DISTRESS SYNDROME (ARDS)

1. Identifiable cause
2. Acute onset
3. Hypoxemia[a]
4. Diffuse, bilateral radiographic opacities
5. PaOP ≤18, or no clinical evidence of left atrial hypertension

PaOP, pulmonary artery occlusion pressure and occlusion pressure.
[a]ALI: PaO_2/FIO_2 ratio ≤300; ARDS: PaO_2/FIO_2 ratio ≤200.
Adapted from Bernard GR, Artigas A, Brigham KL et al: Report of the American-European consensus conference on ARDS: Definitions, mechanisms, relevant outcomes and clinical trial coordination. The Consensus Committee. Intensive Care Med 1994; 20: 225.

---

mortality varies greatly with the population of patients studied; for example, ARDS mortality in trauma patients is in the 10 to 15% range, whereas mortality in medical ICU patients is as high as 60%. Moreover, patients with ARDS continue to die primarily as a result of associated conditions (e.g., sepsis, multiple organ failure), and uncommonly die of hypoxemia per se.

Clinically, ARDS and ALI are characterized by reduced static thoracic (lung and chest wall) compliance and severe impairment of gas exchange, including high intrapulmonary shunt and dead space fraction. These mechanics and gas exchange abnormalities create a challenge in terms of optimizing mechanical ventilation, as maintenance of adequate oxygenation and CO_2 elimination are both problematic. In addition, although the P/F ratio does not appear to predict mortality, high dead space fraction does, and may reflect the extent of pulmonary vascular injury.[118] Pulmonary hypertension often develops as the syndrome progresses, and can complicate hemodynamic management.

Although ALI/ARDS appears to be a diffuse process by chest radiograph, lung opacification is surprisingly heterogeneous when the lung is imaged by CT. Areas of dense opacification are frequently confined to the posterior, dependent portion of the lung, leaving a small, relatively normal, recruitable volume available for ventilation. This low recruitable lung volume has been termed the *baby lung*, and has important implications for ventilatory management in ARDS, as discussed later.[107]

The treatment of ALI/ARDS is largely supportive, and includes aggressive treatment of inciting events, avoidance of complications, and mechanical ventilation. In regard to the latter, it is critical that tidal volumes and static ventilatory pressures are minimized in order to avoid further injury to the remaining relatively uninjured lung (VALI). A large, randomized prospective trial found that a strategy that used tidal volumes of ≤6 mL/kg and maintained static (plateau) airway pressure at ≤30 cm H_2O resulted in a relative mortality reduction of 22% when compared with a control group ventilated with tidal volumes of 12 mL/kg (level I evidence).[119] This approach was corroborated in a similar, smaller trial.[120] This is the only intervention that has been unequivocally proven to reduce mortality in patients with ARDS.

Because ARDS is marked by high intrapulmonary shunt, hypoxemia is relatively unresponsive to oxygen therapy. Thus, strategies to recruit collapsed lung are necessary. This is most commonly achieved by using PEEP. The optimal balance between PEEP and FIO_2 has been long debated, but at this point there is no strong evidence to favor either a "high PEEP, low FIO_2" versus a "minimal PEEP, high FIO_2" strategy (level II evidence).[121] Other maneuvers to promote recruitment of lung include the use of intermittent high-level end expiratory pressure or "sigh" breaths, pressure-controlled ventilation, inverse ratio ventilation (prolonged inspiratory time), prone positioning, and high-frequency ventilation. Prone positioning has been studied in three randomized controlled trials of patients with ARDS and ALI; although none of these trials found a significant mortality reduction with prone position, the most recent of the three suggests that mortality may be reduced with longer duration of prone positioning.[122–124] In addition, although each of the aforementioned interventions has been temporally associated with improved oxygenation, none have been convincingly shown to result in significant outcome differences when compared with standard approaches (level II and III evidence).

Inhaled nitric oxide also variably and transiently improves oxygenation in ALI/ARDS by improving blood flow to ventilated alveoli. However, several randomized prospective trials have failed to show any relevant long-term outcome benefits associated with inhaled nitric oxide administration to patients with ALI/ARDS (level I evidence).[125,126] Inhaled nitric oxide may still be useful as "rescue" therapy in selected patients with severe, refractory hypoxemia, although its benefits in this setting have not been rigorously tested.

Given that ALI/ARDS are marked by high permeability pulmonary edema, it is intuitive that administration of excessive fluids be avoided. To take this a step further, a randomized controlled trial found that a conservative fluid management strategy that emphasized diuresis resulted in improved oxygenation, more ventilator-free days, and days not in the ICU, but no significant difference in mortality compared with liberal fluid management (level I evidence).[127] Other promising interventions to facilitate reduction of lung water in ALI and ARDS include coadministration of albumin with furosemide,[128] and administration of inhaled β-agonists to promote sodium transport across the alveolar epithelium (level II evidence).[129] Multiple therapies have been tested in an effort to halt the inflammatory and proliferative phases of injury, with mixed success. Corticosteroid administration early in the course of ARDS is of no benefit or even harmful. However, administration during the fibroproliferative phase (day 3 and beyond) has been associated with reduced mortality in one small randomized trial and smaller case series and cohort studies.[130] A large study randomized patients between days 7 and 28 of ARDS onset to methylprednisolone versus placebo.[131]

Although there was no difference in 28-day mortality in the intention-to-treat analysis, patients with ARDS between 7 and 14 days' duration appeared to benefit, while those with ARDS for more than 14 days appeared to suffer harm. Furthermore, the group receiving methylprednisolone had more ventilator-free days and shock-free days at day 28, in addition to improved oxygenation and respiratory system compliance. Thus, it appears that patients with ARDS may benefit from corticosteroid treatment within a narrow time window, but further study is necessary before strong conclusions can be drawn.

ACUTE RENAL FAILURE

Acute renal failure (ARF) is reported to occur in 1.5 to 24% of critically ill patients. Unfortunately, the true incidence is difficult to pinpoint because of variability in patient populations and the use of multiple diagnostic criteria. In 2004 a consensus group proposed standard criteria for the diagnosis of renal risk, injury, and failure, which have been subsequently validated in several studies.[132,133] These criteria are expected to improve the ability to identify, study, and treat renal failure in the ICU.[133]

Despite these caveats regarding the diagnosis of ARF, the incidence appears to be fairly stable over the past 20 years.[134] Moreover, the hospital mortality associated with ARF requiring dialysis has remained approximately 60% for nearly 5 decades.[134,135] This is discouraging when one considers reductions in mortality in association with other organ failures over the same time interval. The reasons for the lack of improvement in outcome are unclear, but likely include insensitive means for identifying patients with incipient renal failure, and lack of effective preventive and therapeutic measures.

In the ICU, ARF occurs from prerenal causes and tubular injury (acute tubular necrosis) in most cases.[134] The initial evaluation of ARF should focus on identifying easily correctable causes; thus, urine sodium concentration and fractional excretion of sodium can help identify prerenal azotemia, urinalysis can identify possible glomerulonephritis or interstitial nephritis, and ultrasonography can rule out postrenal or obstructive sources of ARF (Table 56-7). In azotemic patients who have received diuretics, the fractional excretion of urea

TABLE 56-7

URINALYSIS, URINE CHEMISTRIES, AND OSMOLALITY IN ACUTE RENAL FAILURE

	▪ HYPOVOLEMIA	▪ ACUTE TUBULAR NECROSIS	▪ ACUTE INTERSTITIAL NEPHRITIS	▪ GLOMERULONEPHRITIS	▪ OBSTRUCTION
Sediment	Bland	Broad, brownish granular casts	WBCs, eosinophils, cellular casts	RBCs, RBC casts	Bland or bloody
Protein	None or low	None or low	Minimal but may be ↑ with NSAIDs	Increased, >100 mg/dL	Low
Urine Na$^+$, mEq/L^a	<20	>30	>30	<20	<20 (Acute) <40 (days)
Urine osmolality, mOsm/kg	>400	<350	<350	>400	<350
FENa$^+$, %^{b}	<1	>1	Varies	<1	<1 (Acute) >1 (days)

WBCs, white blood cells; RBCs, red blood cells; NSAIDs, nonsteroidal anti-inflammatory drugs.
^{a}The sensitivity and specificity of urine sodium of <20 in differentiating prerenal azotemia from acute tubular necrosis are 90% and 82%, respectively.
^{b}FENa$^+$: Fractional excretion of sodium is the urine to plasma (U/P) of sodium divided by U/P of creatinine ×100. The sensitivity and specificity of fractional excretion of sodium of <1% in differentiating prerenal azotemia from acute tubular necrosis are 96% and 95%, respectively.
Adapted from Singri N, Ahya SN, Levin ML: Acute renal failure. JAMA 2003; 289: 747, with permission.

may be more sensitive than the fractional excretion of sodium in detecting a prerenal cause.[136]

In incipient and established ARF, supportive care is the rule, with the focus on maintenance of euvolemia, avoidance of renal toxins, adjustment of medication doses, and monitoring of electrolytes and acid base status. Pharmacologic approaches to the prevention and treatment of ARF have been uniformly disappointing; these include low-dose dopamine[92] (level II evidence), anaritide (recombinant atrial natriuretic peptide; level I evidence), and diuretics. A large cohort study suggested that diuretic administration in early ARF may lead to increased mortality, although this was not corroborated in a second cohort study (level III evidence).[137,138] Nonetheless, diuretics should be administered with caution in early ARF and in response to defined physiologic problems such as hypervolemia or hyperkalemia until higher level of evidence showing benefit and safety is available.[139] In the specific setting of contrast-induced nephropathy, prophylactic administration of N-acetyl cysteine and sodium bicarbonate, particularly in combination, to patients with pre-existing renal disease appears to be of benefit in preventing nephropathy and improving other outcomes.[140,141]

Although hemodialysis (renal replacement therapy; RRT) is typically considered a supportive measure in ARF, recent interest has focused on the potential for RRT to improve renal recovery and reduce mortality. Research on RRT in the ICU has focused on the type and intensity or dose of dialysis; the timing of initiation of RRT is also of interest, but has not been rigorously studied in this setting.

The intensity of RRT is determined by both the frequency of treatment and the degree of solute clearance per time. Increased intensity of dialysis improves outcome in patients with end-stage renal disease, and recent studies suggest similar benefits in ARF. Daily dialysis has been associated with reduced mortality and faster recovery of renal function compared with alternate-day dialysis in ARF (level II evidence).[142] Likewise, increased clearance during continuous RRT (CRRT) is also associated with reduced mortality (level I evidence).[143]

CRRT (including continuous venovenous hemofiltration and hemodialysis) has long been known as a useful technique when hemodynamic instability is present; in contrast to intermittent hemodialysis, effective solute removal is possible with CRRT in the presence of arterial hypotension. Given these considerations regarding dialysis dose, the routine use of CRRT in order to increase the intensity of dialysis in ARF has been proposed as a means of improving outcome. Despite this theoretical advantage to CRRT, several studies, including a relatively large, multicenter, randomized study found no survival benefit to CRRT compared with intermittent hemodialysis.[144] Thus, the weight of evidence supports an increased intensity of dialysis, using either daily standard hemodialysis, CRRT, or extended daily hemodialysis ("slow dialysis"), but does not support one technique over another.

ENDOCRINE ASPECTS OF CRITICAL CARE MEDICINE

Glucose Management in Critical Illness

Hyperglycemia is commonly encountered in critically ill patients, and occurs in both diabetics and nondiabetics. Hyperglycemia results primarily because of increased glucose production and insulin resistance caused by inflammatory and hormonal mediators that are released in response to injury. Hyperglycemia may also be aggravated by various therapeutic and supportive interventions, including the use of corticosteroids and total parenteral nutrition. Although the risks of hyperglycemia for patients with diabetes who are ketosis-

prone have long been appreciated, mounting evidence suggests that hyperglycemia is detrimental to critically ill patients in a broader sense. Hyperglycemia is associated with increased risk of postoperative infection (wound and otherwise) and poor outcome in patients with stroke or traumatic brain injury.[145] In addition, the blood glucose level is a risk factor for mortality in diabetic patients admitted with acute myocardial infarction.[146]

Strict glycemic control in critically ill patients has been advocated as leading to multiple outcome benefits. This is based largely on evidence from a single, randomized trial in surgical patients that found that intensive insulin therapy (goal glucose <110 mg/dL) reduced ICU mortality by approximately 50% compared with more conventional therapy (goal glucose <215).[147] The benefit was most pronounced in patients who were in the ICU for more than 5 days. Intensive insulin therapy reduced multiple organ failure, blood stream infection, the need for dialysis, and the incidence of polyneuropathy. However, a subsequent study by the same investigators in medical ICU patients found no mortality benefit to intensive insulin therapy in the intention-to-treat analysis.[148] A new large trial in patients with sepsis was terminated early for an excess risk of hypoglycemia in the tight glycemic control group. The study was unable to detect any mortality difference; however, this finding should be interpreted cautiously because of the premature trial termination for safety concerns.[88] These data, combined with negative results from other studies, have diminished the enthusiasm for intensive insulin therapy with tight glycemic control in the ICU at this time.

Adrenal Function in Critical Illness

The stress response to injury includes an increase in serum cortisol levels in most critically ill patients.[149] However, adrenal insufficiency may also occur in critically ill patients for several reasons, including inhibition of adrenal stimulation or corticosteroid synthesis by drugs or cytokines, and direct injury to or infection of the pituitary or adrenal glands.[150] Thus, adrenal insufficiency has been reported to occur with increased frequency in critically ill patients with trauma, burns, sepsis, and other conditions in comparison with the general population.

The diagnosis of adrenal insufficiency in critical illness is complicated by limitations of commonly used tests of adrenal function. Cortisol is highly protein-bound, and serum proteins, including albumin, are commonly depressed in critically ill patients. A study found that although total serum cortisol levels are low in critically ill patients with hypoproteinemia, free cortisol levels are elevated.[151] This suggests that earlier reports that used total serum cortisol levels in critically ill patients may have overestimated the incidence of adrenal insufficiency. However, until free cortisol assays are more widely available, the diagnosis of adrenal insufficiency in critical illness must be based on clinical suspicion and total cortisol levels.

In addition to absolute adrenal insufficiency (low baseline cortisol and poor response to corticotropin administration/stimulation) a condition of relative adrenal insufficiency (defined as an increase in serum cortisol of ≤9 μg/dL in response to corticotropin independent of the baseline cortisol level) has been described in patients in septic shock and with other illnesses. Thus, low-normal baseline cortisol levels, high baseline cortisol levels, and a poor response to corticotropin are all predictors of increased mortality.[152,153]

Although high-dose corticosteroids for the treatment of septic shock are of no benefit, evidence suggests that lower doses, on the order of hydrocortisone 200 to 300 mg/day, can reduce dependency on vasopressors and shorten the duration of shock, but do not appear to confer a mortality benefit (level II evidence).[104,105] A randomized study of 499 patients found no mortality benefit of corticosteroid administration to patients with septic shock, even in those patients with relative adrenal insufficiency.[105] Thus, the administration of corticosteroids to patients in septic shock or with relative adrenal insufficiency is not recommended in the absence of more compelling evidence.

Thyroid Function in Critical Illness

Measures of thyroid function, including levels of thyrotropin (TSH), T_3, and T_4 are deranged in the majority of critically ill patients. Depression of T_3 occurs within hours of injury or illness, and can persist for weeks. TSH levels may be normal initially, but fall to inappropriately low levels as illness progresses. T_4 levels are also often low, but can be normal or high. Low hormone levels may occur for a variety of reasons, including altered binding and metabolism early in the course of illness and depressed neuroendocrine function with more prolonged courses. In addition, certain drugs, in particular dopamine, can depress thyroid function through central mechanisms.[154] Low thyroid hormone levels, particularly for T_3, correlate with the severity of illness and are associated with an increased risk of death.[149]

It is controversial as to whether the observed abnormalities in thyroid hormones represent an appropriate response to illness or true hypothyroidism; thus, the terms *euthyroid sick syndrome* or *nonthyroidal illness* have been coined to describe thyroid function abnormalities in critical illness.[155] Furthermore, it is not clear whether replacement of thyroid hormones is indicated or beneficial in critical illness. T_3 administration to brain-dead organ donors appears to improve hemodynamic stability (level IV evidence), although randomized trials found minimal or no benefit to T_3 or T_4 administration in patients undergoing cardiopulmonary bypass and cardiac surgery (level II evidence).[156] Large, randomized prospective trials are necessary to define the role of routine thyroid hormone supplementation in nonthyroidal illness.

Importantly, true hypothyroidism may be present in the critically ill patient, particularly in the geriatric population, and should be considered in the face of refractory shock, adrenal insufficiency, unexplained coma, and prolonged, unexplained respiratory failure. True hypothyroidism is marked by an elevation of TSH (usually >25 mU/L) in the face of a low T_4 level.

Somatotropic Function in Critical Illness

Growth hormone (GH) levels are low in prolonged critical illness, and it has been conjectured that deficiencies of GH and insulinlike growth factor-1 contribute to the muscle wasting seen in acute illness.[149] However, although small trials have found that GH administration can attenuate muscle catabolism in critical illness, a large, randomized prospective trial found that administration of large doses of GH to critically ill patients resulted in increased mortality (level I evidence).[157] Thus, GH administration during critical illness cannot be advocated at this time, although further exploration of the benefits of smaller doses of GH may be warranted.

ANEMIA AND TRANSFUSION THERAPY IN CRITICAL ILLNESS

Most patients admitted to the ICU are anemic at some point in their hospital stay, and more than one third of them will receive transfused blood.[158,159] Importantly, both anemia (hemoglobin [Hb] <9 g/dL) and the amount of transfused blood are independently associated with mortality.[158,159] However, this association does not denote cause and effect, particularly for anemia, which may just be a marker of the severity of illness.

The cause of anemia in critical illness is multifactorial and is related to blood loss from the primary injury or illness, iatrogenic blood loss due to daily blood sampling, and nutritional deficiencies.[160] Given that approximately 13% of ICU patients may have iron, folate, or vitamin B_{12} deficiencies, these parameters should be checked prior to blood transfusion.

Treatment of anemia in critical illness is the source of considerable debate. In unstressed subjects, severe anemia (Hb ≤5 g/dL) is amazingly well tolerated because of physiologic compensations that maintain oxygen delivery and extraction. However, it has long been assumed that critically ill patients have less efficient compensatory mechanisms and reduced physiologic reserve, and thereby require a higher Hb concentration than unstressed individuals. Historically, this has translated to a transfusion threshold at an Hb concentration of approximately 10 g/dL. However, a large, randomized, prospective trial or transfusion requirements in critically ill adults (the TRICC study) found that 30-day mortality was not affected when a restrictive transfusion threshold (Hb <7 g/dL) was used (level II evidence).[161] A similar trial in pediatric patients found no mortality difference between restrictive and liberal transfusion strategies, suggesting that a restrictive strategy is safe in critically ill children.[162] These data strongly suggest that routine transfusion of critically ill patients is not necessary and may be harmful unless the Hb concentration is below 7 g/dL. Unfortunately, despite the TRICC study, there is considerable heterogeneity in transfusion thresholds in ICUs both in the United States[158] and in Canada.[163]

There are multiple possible reasons for the persistence of a high transfusion threshold in the ICU. Although the TRICC study included a broad spectrum of critically ill patients, some groups were excluded (active bleeding) or underrepresented (neurologic or neurosurgical injury). Furthermore, although a retrospective analysis of the TRICC data suggested that patients with coronary artery disease did not benefit from more liberal transfusion unless they had unstable angina or acute myocardial infarction, concern remains about the tolerance for anemia in this group of patients. Lastly, Hb is an important determinant of oxygen delivery (DO_2), and transfusion is an integral component of goal-directed therapeutic strategies that aim to optimize DO_2 in early shock states.[75] In the absence of these possible exclusions (active bleeding, acute neurologic injury, active myocardial ischemia, or the early resuscitation of septic shock) restriction of blood transfusion to a threshold of <7.0 g/dL should be considered the standard of care and as potentially life saving.

Prevention of anemia in critical illness is an appealing alternative to transfusion. One simple and potentially cost-saving approach is to reduce the volume and frequency of blood draws in the ICU. As noted earlier, iatrogenic blood loss is a major factor in the development of anemia of critical illness. Another potential approach is the administration of recombinant erythropoietin and iron. A study found that administration of recombinant erythropoietin to critically ill patients on day 3 of ICU stay and every week thereafter reduced transfusion requirements significantly, without affecting mortality or other outcome variables (level I evidence).[164] However, a subsequent study with a lower recommended transfusion threshold found no reduction in blood transfusion in association with erythropoietin administration (level I evidence).[165] Interestingly, there was a reduction in mortality in trauma patients who received erythropoietin compared with placebo. This may reflect nonerythropoietic effects of this agent given the lack of effect on blood transfusion. Given the high cost of erythropoietin, it is not a cost-effective alternative at this time for general use in critical care.

PERIOPERATIVE AND CONSULTATIVE SERVICES

NUTRITION IN THE CRITICALLY ILL PATIENT

Critical illness can lead to hypermetabolic states, and if nutritional support is inadequate or delayed, patients are at immediate risk of malnutrition. Poor nutritional status is associated with increased mortality and morbidity. Therefore, appropriate nutrition is an important aspect of critical care and adequate nutritional support should be considered a standard of care; the American College of Chest Physicians recommends that the daily caloric intake be based on the patient's ideal body weight (25 kcal/kg or 27.5 kcal/kg in the presence of systemic inflammatory response syndrome), of which 15 to 20% should be represented by proteins (1.5 to 2 g/kg/day).

Patient metabolic requirements should be established early after ICU admission and enteral feeding tolerance evaluated without delay (within 24 hours of admission). A small randomized trial indicated that early enteral nutrition (EN) initiated within 4.4 hours after ICU admission resulted in less organ dysfunction than delayed feeding (36.5 hours after ICU admission; level II evidence).[166] Feeding intolerance due to high gastric residual volume can be improved by the administration of gastric prokinetic agents, and positioning the tube postpyloric. However, a systematic review comparing gastric versus postpyloric feeding did not suggest a clinical benefit from postpyloric tube feeding with regard to pneumonia, ICU length of stay, and mortality.[167] There is some suggestion that intermittent enteral feeding as opposed to a continuous feeding regimen is more likely to allow reaching the enteral calories goal earlier.[168]

Most of the trials evaluating parenteral nutrition (PN) do not demonstrate any favorable impact on outcome (level II evidence). Evidence suggests that EN is associated with lower infection risk and that PN is associated with increased rates of complications and death. Animal studies show that endotoxin-induced ischemia can be prevented by early EN, and adding EN to PN has favorable effects on bacterial translocation and nitrogen balance, independent of total energy and proteins intake. Therefore, EN is preferred over PN whenever possible because of its lower cost and less frequent complications.[169] Although not rigorously investigated, PN is preferable to no nutrition in patients who cannot tolerate enteral feedings. However, it is unclear how long of a delay in initiating PN is acceptable, assuming that EN is contraindicated or not tolerated despite vigorous attempts. Overall, strategies to optimize delivery of EN (starting at the target rate, use of a feeding protocol with a higher threshold of gastric residuals volumes, use of motility agents, and use of small bowel feeding) and minimize the risks of EN (elevation of the head of the bed) should be considered. There are no studies that demonstrate a benefit from the use of supplemental PN in patients unable to tolerate adequate EN.[169] Increasing attention has been drawn to supplemental PN for patients who, despite all attempts, remain unable to tolerate adequate EN for longer than 3 to 5 days.[170] Strategies that maximize the benefit and minimize the risks of PN (hypocaloric dose, withholding lipids, and the use of intensive insulin therapy to achieve glycemic control) should be considered. However, studies are needed to confirm that the benefits of aggressive early nutrition outweigh the risks inherent to the administration of PN.

Complications associated with enteral feedings include aspiration of gastric feeding, diarrhea, and fluid and electrolyte imbalance. To prevent aspiration with gastric feeding, the head of the patient's bed should be raised 30 to 45 degrees during feeding; jejunal access can be considered in patients with recurrent tube feeding aspiration. Diarrhea is a common complication during enteral feeding associated with many potential causes, including medications (antibiotics or sorbitol-containing products), altered bacterial flora (*Clostridium difficile*), formula composition (including osmolality), infusion rate, hypoalbuminemia, bacterial contamination of the enteral fluid, and the patient's related conditions. To prevent or reduce diarrhea all potential etiologies should be considered and corrected. Exchanging a polymeric formula with fiber with a more expensive elemental amino acid diet may improve feeding tolerance. Among special formulations, immunonutrition has been hypothesized to influence infectious morbidity and mortality in critically ill patients via a beneficial effect on GI immunologic function. Use of viable probiotics could provide enhancement in immune activity as measured by plasma levels of immunoglobulin G and A.[171] Specific enteral formulations, particularly those with high concentrations of branch chain amino acids (isoleucine, leucine, valine), arginine, glutamine, nucleotides, or omega-3 fatty acids, have been suggested to improve mortality and decrease infectious complications in burn and postoperative cancer patients.[172] The Canadian clinical practice guideline for nutrition support in critically ill patients, however, discourages the use of arginine-containing products.[173] A glutamine-enriched formula should be considered for patients with severe burns and trauma, and is associated with reduced infection. A meta-analysis indicates that immune-enhancing diets may be beneficial for elective surgical patients but have no demonstrated benefit and may be deleterious in critically ill patients (level II evidence).[174] Use of products with fish oils, borage oils, and antioxidants should be considered for patients with ARDS. A meta-analysis suggests that the administration of supplemental antioxidant micronutrients (selenium, zinc, vitamins A, C, and E) is associated with increased survival.[175]

SEDATION OF THE CRITICALLY ILL PATIENT

Critically ill patients are often deeply sedated, in part because of concerns for patient comfort, but also because of potential benefits afforded by a reduction in the sympathoadrenal response to injury. Additionally, complications associated with undersedation include ventilator dyssynchrony, patient injury, agitation, anxiety, stress disorders and, possibly, unplanned extubation.

Several studies have tempered the enthusiasm for deep sedation in the ICU. In a prospective cohort study, Kollef et al.[176] observed that patients who received continuous infusions of sedatives had nearly twice the duration of mechanical ventilation compared with patients not receiving continuous intravenous sedation (level III evidence). Furthermore, the implementation of nurse-driven sedation protocols that discourage the use of continuous infusions has been demonstrated to reduce the duration of mechanical ventilation, the ICU length of stay, and the requirement for tracheostomy (level I evidence).[177] In a randomized trial of critically ill patients receiving continuous sedative and analgesic drug infusions, daily interruption of these infusions was effective in reducing the length of mechanical ventilation and length of ICU stay (level I evidence).[178] Beyond longer duration of mechanical ventilation, other complications are associated with oversedation, such as excessive cardiovascular and respiratory depression, and infection.[179]

The depth of sedation may also play a role in long-term outcomes after discharge from the ICU and hospital. Patients admitted to the ICU are at risk of developing symptoms of posttraumatic stress disorders and of experiencing delusional memories. The extent of ICU recall is a function of the extent of sedation. Factual ICU recall has been associated with more wakefulness during mechanical ventilation, while recall of delirious memory during critical illness was associated with posttraumatic stress disorders symptoms.[180,181] Approximately two thirds of ICU patients have amnesia for the entire ICU course, and high-dose sedative is associated with lack of recall.[182]

Kress et al.[183] followed up long-term psychological effects in those subjects who were enrolled in a daily sedative interruption trial. Although the loss to follow-up was nonnegligible and the design was exploratory in nature, the study suggested that daily interruption of sedation might have been protective for subsequent development of posttraumatic stress disorders, or at least did not result in adverse psychological outcomes (level III evidence). Several factors such as interindividual variability, changes over time, severity of disease, intensity of painful stimuli, drug interactions, and organ dysfunction, influence the analgesic and sedative needs of ICU patients. Therefore, it is important to titrate medications according to established therapeutic goals and re-evaluate the sedation requirements frequently. Several scales are available to assess sedation levels over time. The most commonly used are the Ramsay sedation scale, the sedation-agitation scale, and the Richmond agitation-sedation scale. Common features to all of these scales are the grading of sedation over different depths and allowance for indicators of agitation. There is no evidence that one scale is superior to another at this time, although the Richmond agitation-sedation scale is the one that has been more rigorously and prospectively validated for reliability and validity.[184] A two-dimensional scale allows distinction between arousal (eye response) and muscular activity, and might be more sensitive to differentiate sedation depths.[185]

Confusion and agitation are common in ICU patients and could have unfavorable consequences on patient outcome. Patients experiencing agitation have been reported to have a higher incidence of major complications, higher admission to rehabilitation centers, and increase duration of hospital stay. Agitation is also a predictive factor for mortality. Agitation needs to be distinguished from delirium, which is relatively common in ICU patients and equally associated with increased length of stay, morbidity, and mortality.[186] Delirium can be difficult to diagnose in ICU patients as features of delirium, such as altered status of consciousness, are shared with several disorders typical of ICU patients. The distinguishing characteristics of delirium include acute onset and fluctuating course, inattention, disorganized thinking, and altered level of consciousness. An ICU delirium diagnostic scale (CAM-ICU scale) has been proposed and is a valid instrument to diagnose delirium in the ICU.[187]

Nonpharmacologic and pharmacologic means can be used to provide comfort and safety to ICU patients. The former include communication, frequent reorientation, maintenance of a day-night cycle, noise reduction, and ensuring ventilation synchrony. Pharmacologic agents include hypnotics-anxiolytics, opioids, and antipsychotics. Hypnotics most commonly used are propofol, midazolam, and lorazepam; each of these drugs has its own particular advantages, but there are insufficient data at this time to suggest a difference in relevant patient outcomes among them. A prospective, randomized, non-blinded trial compared a continuous infusion of lorazepam, midazolam, and propofol in trauma patients.[188] Midazolam appeared to be the most titratable drug, with the lowest incidence of over- and undersedation. Lorazepam was the most cost-effective choice for sedation despite the observation that oversedation occurred twice as often with lorazepam than with propofol or midazolam. A meta-analysis including 27 randomized trials comparing propofol versus midazolam suggested that tracheal extubation occurred earlier with the use of propofol for patients who were ventilated for a duration of shorter than 36 hours.[189] However, no differences were found with regard to the ICU length of stay or mortality. Greater levels of hypotension and elevated triglyceride levels were observed with the use of propofol. Since then, an open label randomized trial found that continuous infusion of propofol was associated with shorter length of mechanical ventilation and ICU stay compared with intermittent lorazepam administration.[190] Adverse effects unique to hypnotic-anxiolytic drugs

include a hyperosmolar acidosis caused by the diluent mixed with lorazepam (propylene glycol), and the potentially lethal "propofol infusion syndrome" (previously discussed).[33] Both of these complications can be avoided by minimizing the administered dose of the respective agent.

Dexmedetomidine, a unique sedative agent that is an α_2-adrenergic receptor agonist, provides sedation without inducing coma, has some analgesic effect, and has little effect on respiratory drive. Dexmedetomidine has been effectively used as a single agent or in combination with other drugs in ICU patients. However, dexmedetomidine is costly, it is currently approved by the Food and Drug Administration for use for only up to 24 hours, and there is insufficient evidence to recommend its routine use at the current time.[191] A trial of prolonged (>5 days) administration of dexmedetomidine compared with lorazepam conducted in critically ill patients indicated that patients receiving dexmedetomidine had a smaller number of days experiencing coma or delirium and were more likely to be on target level of sedation.[192] However, the study was unable to detect any differences in duration of mechanical ventilation or ICU length of stay.

Morphine and fentanyl are the most commonly used opioids to provide analgesia in the ICU. Morphine should be avoided in patients with renal failure due to active metabolites that accumulate in the presence of impaired renal elimination.

Delirium in the ICU is commonly treated with antipsychotic agents such as haloperidol, olanzapine, quetiapine, and risperidone. However, none of these agents has been proven effective for the treatment of ICU-associated delirium in a randomized, placebo-controlled trial, and it is not clear that the newer agents, although more expensive, are more effective than haloperidol.

Neuromuscular blockade may be occasionally indicated in ICU patients with severe TBI or respiratory failure, but routine use is discouraged because of concerns that this practice may predispose to critical illness polyneuropathy and myopathy (see "Acquired Neuromuscular Disorders in Critical Illness"), and because of an increased risk of nosocomial pneumonia in patients receiving these agents.

In summary, sedation and analgesia should be provided in the ICU population to ensure patient comfort and safety. In establishing treatment algorithms, analgesia should be prioritized over sedation. Titration and assessment of analgesia and sedation should be an integral part of ICU monitoring so that over- and undersedation can be avoided. The establishment of nurse-guided sedation protocols and daily interruption of sedation has been shown to be effective in reducing the length of mechanical ventilation and ICU stay.

COMPLICATIONS IN THE INTENSIVE CARE UNIT: DETECTION, PREVENTION, AND THERAPY

Nosocomial Infections

Nosocomial infections are a major source of morbidity and mortality in critically ill patients. At some level, nosocomial infections are unavoidable and occur because of the nature of intensive care: patients are critically ill with altered host defenses; they require invasive devices (e.g., endotracheal tubes, intravascular catheters) for support, monitoring, and therapy that provide portals of entry for infectious organisms; and they receive therapies that increase the risk of infection (glucocorticoids, PN). On the other hand, many nosocomial infections are preventable, with relatively simple interventions.[193] This became more financially relevant in the United States in 2008 when the Center for Medicare and Medicaid Services ceased reimbursing hospitals for preventable complications, one of which includes catheter-related urinary tract infection.

Several types and sources of infections are relatively unique to ICU care and should be included in the differential diagnosis when signs suggestive of infection arise. These infections include sinusitis, ventilator-associated pneumonia, intravascular catheter-associated bacteremia, catheter-associated urinary tract infection, and invasive fungal infection.

Sinusitis

Radiographic sinusitis is common in critically ill patients with indwelling oral and nasal tubes. Sinusitis associated with nasal intubation confers a greater risk than with oral intubation, occurring in approximately 95% and 25% of patients with nasal and oral tubes after 1 week of intubation, respectively.[194] Approximately 10% of radiographically diagnosed sinusitis is infected as determined by quantitative cultures, although the incidence may be much higher. Bacterial sinusitis was responsible for 16% of fevers of unknown origin in a surgical ICU.[195] The organisms cultured from sinuses represent those that are responsible for other nosocomial infections, particularly *ventilator-associated pneumonia* (VAP), *Staphylococcal* species, enteric Gram-negative bacteria, and nonlactose fermenting Gram-negative rods such as *Pseudomonas* and *Acinetobacter*. Bacterial sinusitis may predispose to the development of VAP, possibly because of microaspiration of infected secretions.

Prevention of sinusitis should focus on efforts to improve sinus drainage, including semirecumbent positioning and avoidance of nasal tubes. Bacterial sinusitis should be considered in patients with unexplained fever and leukocytosis. If radiographic sinusitis is documented, any nasal tubes should be removed, and nasal irrigation and short-term administration of nasal decongestants should be considered. If the patient is severely ill, broad-spectrum antibiotic coverage should be considered. If these maneuvers do not result in resolution of signs and symptoms of infection in 2 to 3 days, and in the absence of infection elsewhere, otolaryngologic consultation and consideration of sinus drainage procedures should be undertaken.

Ventilator-Associated Pneumonia

Endotracheal intubation and mechanical ventilation increase the risk of nosocomial pneumonia; thus the term *ventilator-associated pneumonia*, or VAP. The likelihood of developing VAP increases with the duration of mechanical ventilation, although the incremental risk may fall over time from a high of 3% per day in the first week of intubation/ventilation, to 1% per day after 15 days in the ICU.[196] The quoted incidence of VAP depends on the criteria used to diagnose pneumonia (clinical vs. invasive technique). As discussed later, traditional clinical criteria are likely both insensitive and nonspecific, and may lead to a falsely high or low incidence of VAP.[197] Given this caveat, studies that solely or primarily relied on invasive techniques to diagnose VAP suggest an incidence >15% at 1 week of ICU stay and >20% at 2 weeks.[196]

Although the mortality in patients with VAP ranges between 30 and 70%, the attributable mortality, the number of patients who die because of VAP rather than with VAP, is more difficult to pinpoint. This may be because of differences in the type of ICU, patient factors, diagnostic techniques across studies, or differences in the virulence of the causative pathogens. Thus, some investigators have been unable to find any mortality attributable to VAP, whereas others have suggested an attributable mortality >40%.[198]

VAP can be categorized as "early-onset," occurring within the first 48 to 72 hours of intubation/ventilation, or "late-onset," occurring thereafter. Early-onset VAP is generally caused by organisms such as *Hemophilus influenza*, *Streptococcus pneumoniae*, methicillin-sensitive *Staphylococcus aureus*, and other relatively antibiotic-sensitive oral flora that enter the trachea around the time of intubation. Late-onset VAP is associated with more virulent and antibiotic-resistant organisms such as methicillin-resistant *S. aureus*, *Pseudomonas aeruginosa*, and *Acinetobacter*. In general, early-onset organisms are associated with zero or low attributable mortality, whereas late-onset organisms, particularly *Pseudomonas* and *Acinetobacter* species, are associated with high mortality.[198]

There are a number of interventions that can reduce the incidence of VAP, some of which are relatively simple and inexpensive, and others of which are more costly and/or associated with some risk. The simplest and least expensive and yet very effective interventions are strict hand washing between patients, and semirecumbent positioning of the patient (head height at 30 degrees or greater from horizontal; level II evidence). These practices should be rigorously applied in all ICUs (granted that semirecumbent positioning is not possible in all patients).

A somewhat more controversial subject involves the use of prophylaxis to prevent GI bleeding. As mentioned earlier, acid-suppression therapies have been associated with an increased risk of VAP because they allow bacterial overgrowth in the stomach. Further, the risk of significant GI bleeding is very low in the ICU, even in high-risk patients (those with coagulopathy or on mechanical ventilation). Thus, GI prophylactic therapy should be reserved for only these high-risk patients, and sucralfate should be considered as an alternative agent to acid-suppressive regimens despite its potentially reduced effectiveness.

Somewhat more expensive interventions to reduce VAP that may be useful in certain patients include subglottic suctioning and oscillating beds.[199] Intermittent subglottic suctioning using specially designed tracheal tubes has been shown to reduce the incidence of VAP in several small studies (level II evidence). However, these tubes are more expensive than conventional tracheal tubes, and their cost-effectiveness has not been established, particularly if their use is instituted in all intubated patients. Oscillating beds have been shown to reduce the incidence of VAP in surgical populations and patients with neurologic injury (level II evidence). However, these beds are very costly and cannot be recommended for routine use.[199] Given that gastric and oropharyngeal colonization with resistant organisms appears to be a risk factor for the development of VAP, intervention to "decontaminate" these sites have been investigated. Selective digestive decontamination (SDD) typically involves the application of a mix of nonabsorbable antimicrobial agents, such as polymyxin, amphotericin, and aminoglycoside, in paste form to coat the oropharynx, and as an elixir applied orally and via a nasogastric tube to decontaminate the GI tract, with or without the concomitant administration of systemic antibiotics. SDD does reduce the incidence of VAP, and has been associated with variable mortality reduction in some studies (level II evidence). SDD is also associated with the development of antibiotic resistance, and concerns regarding the long-term impact of resistance has limited the widespread adoption of SDD.[199] However, more limited oral decontamination with chlorhexidine appears to reduce VAP rates without leading to excess antibiotic resistance.[200]

An additional and important approach to reduce the overall mortality from VAP involves refinement of the diagnostic process and limitation of antibiotic therapy to avoid the development of antibiotic resistance. As mentioned earlier, an invasive diagnostic strategy is likely more accurate than traditional clinical criteria to diagnose VAP. Invasive strategies typically involve collection of bronchial-alveolar specimens using lavage or protected brushes, and then quantitating bacterial growth in the laboratory. Thus, VAP is diagnosed only when bacteria are seen within bronchoalveolar cells microscopically, or when bacterial growth exceeds specific thresholds ($\geq 10^4$ CFU/mL for bronchoalveolar lavage and $\geq 10^3$ CFU/mL for protected brush specimens). Specimens have typically been obtained bronchoscopically, although newer data suggest that specimens obtained by direct aspiration through the tracheal tube are comparable to bronchoscopic specimens. Quantitation of bacterial growth, rather than the "invasiveness" of the technique, is more important (level II evidence).[201] The important adjunct to this diagnostic approach is that although antibiotics may be started at the time clinical criteria for pneumonia are met and quantitative cultures are sent, they are stopped if the threshold values for VAP are not reached.

A study of invasive versus noninvasive strategies to diagnose and treat VAP found that the invasive approach resulted in a mortality reduction at 14 days and a trend toward mortality reduction at 28 days (level II evidence).[197] In addition, the invasive strategy was associated with less multiple organ failure and reduced antibiotic use. Surprisingly, the invasive strategy did not result in a reduced incidence of emergence of resistant bacteria, although the incidence of *Candida* growth was reduced. Another study did not confirm the benefits found in the previous study and also had several methodologic weaknesses.[202] Thus, the data favor the use of an invasive strategy to diagnose VAP when and if possible.

It is clear that delay in treatment of nosocomial infections, including VAP, is associated with increased mortality. Thus, treatment should not be delayed pending diagnostic evaluation; rather treatment should be started after culture specimens are sent if the clinical suspicion of VAP is high. Antibiotics can then be narrowed in spectrum or discontinued depending on the results from quantitative cultures after 48 to 72 hours. This approach is known as "de-escalating therapy" and is designed to both ensure adequate antibiotic treatment up front, but avoid overuse of antibiotics in the long run.[198] Antibiotic selection should be predicated on hospital bacterial growth and resistance patterns. In general, for patients with early-onset VAP, antibiotics can be relatively narrow in spectrum and limited to a single agent; for late-onset VAP, broader spectrum antibiotics should be initiated and include agents from two different classes directed toward resistant Gram-negative organisms, and in many cases an agent directed against methicillin-resistant *S. aureus* (Table 56-8).

The optimal duration of antibiotic therapy for VAP is not well defined. A moderately sized, prospective, randomized trial found that 8 days of antibiotic therapy was comparable for treatment of VAP in terms of mortality and recurrent infections, and resulted in more antibiotic-free days (level II evidence).[203] However, patients who had VAP caused by nonlactose fermenting Gram-negative rods (including *Pseudomonas*) had a higher infection recurrence rate if they received an initial 8-day course of therapy. It is unclear whether intermediate courses of therapy would have avoided infection recurrence. Thus, it is reasonable to choose an 8-day course of therapy for many patients with VAP; however, if there is an inadequate early clinical response or infection with nonlactose fermenting Gram-negative rods, a longer course should be considered.

Intravascular Catheter-Associated Bacteremia

Intravascular catheter-associated bacteremia as strictly defined by the Center for Disease Control (CDC) includes the following criteria: (1) clinical suspicion of catheter-related infection (including low likelihood of infection elsewhere) plus, (2) positive culture of blood drawn from the catheter or of a segment of catheter plus, (3) matching positive blood culture drawn from another site, preferably by direct venotomy or arterial puncture. Given this strict definition, the incidence of catheter-associated bacteremia is <5% in most studies. However, the

TABLE 56-8

EMPIRIC THERAPY OF VENTILATOR-ASSOCIATED PNEUMONIA

■ COMMON ORGANISMS	■ ANTIBIOTICS
Early-Onset VAP	
Enteric Gram-negative rods • *Escherichia coli* • *Enterobacter* species • *Proteus* species • *Klebsiella* species • *Hemophilus influenzae* • Methicillin-sensitive *Staphylococcus aureus* (MRSA) • *Streptococcus pneumoniae*	β-Lactam/β-lactamase inhibitor combination, *or* second generation cephalosporin, *or* fluoroquinolone
Late-Onset or Severe Early-Onset VAP	
Above, plus: • *Pseudomonas aeruginosa* • *Acinetobacter* species • Methicillin-resistant *Staphylococcus aureus*	β-Lactam/β-lactamase inhibitor combination, *or* third or fourth generation cephalosporin, *or* fluoroquinolone *plus* aminoglycoside, *or* second, structurally unrelated agent with antipseudomonal activity *plus*, vancomycin or linezolid[a]

VAP, ventilator-associated pneumonia.
[a]If likelihood of MRSA is high.

incidence of bacteremia is affected by several factors, including the conditions and technique of insertion, type and location of catheter, and the duration of catheterization, and can vary widely. The attributable mortality of catheter-associated bacteremia is approximately 11%, which is much lower than that for primary bacteremia or bacteremia associated with another site of infection.[204]

Catheter infection is more likely when placement occurs under emergency conditions, and is reduced by the use of strict aseptic technique with full barrier precautions. This includes preinsertion hand washing, full gown and gloves, and the use of a large barrier drape.[205] In addition, skin cleansing with chlorhexidine is more effective than other agents. Attention to these practices can dramatically reduce catheter-related infection (level I evidence).[206,207] These simple interventions should be considered as standards of care and are recommended by the CDC.

Catheter-related infection and bacteremia increase with the duration of catheterization, particularly for durations of >2 days. However, routine catheter replacement at 3 or 7 days does not reduce the incidence of infection, and results in increased mechanical complications. Thus, routine guidewire exchange of catheters is not recommended.

Catheters coated with either antiseptics (chlorhexidine and silver sulfadiazine) or antibiotics (rifampin and minocycline) reduce bacterial colonization of catheters but have not been consistently shown to reduce bacteremia or other morbidities.[208] Antimicrobial-coated catheters are relatively expensive and their cost-effectiveness has not been sufficiently defined to recommend their widespread utilization. Thus, the CDC recommends the use of antimicrobial-coated catheters in patients when the expected duration of catheterization will be >5 days, particularly if the local rate of catheter-related infection is high.[209] Ultimately, a key component of strategies to reduce catheter-related infection is to limit the duration of insertion. The need for continued central venous catheterization should be reviewed daily.[206,207]

Catheter-related infection is insertion site-dependent, increasing in frequency from subclavian to internal jugular to femoral vein sites, respectively. Thus, the subclavian site should be used when possible if the duration of catheterization is predicted to be longer than 2 days.[205] Infection appears to be less likely for arterial than venous catheters.

Catheter-related venous thrombosis occurs commonly and is associated with an increased risk of infection. Routine flushing of catheter ports with heparin reduces both the incidence of thrombosis and infection (level II evidence).[205]

Organisms commonly responsible for catheter-related bacteremia include *Staphylococcus epidermidis* and *aureus*, enteric Gram-negative bacteria, *Pseudomonas aeruginosa* and *Acinetobacter*, and occasionally *Enterococcal* species. Note that although coagulase-negative *Staphylococci* are commonly isolated from blood cultures in the ICU, they are likely responsible for true infection in a minority of cases.[210] When catheter-related bacteremia is confirmed, the offending catheter should be removed and appropriate antibiotics continued for a minimum of 7 days; longer courses should be considered for *S. aureus* bacteremia given the predilection for this organism to cause endocarditis. Suspected catheter-related infections can be addressed by sending screening cultures drawn through the catheter and from a peripheral site; guidewire exchange of the catheter with culture of the intracutaneous segment and tip can also be considered. A strong suspicion of catheter-related bacteremia should trigger the institution of broad-spectrum antibiotic coverage, including coverage for methicillin-resistant *Staphylococcal* species and nonlactose fermenting Gram-negative rods until culture results return, with subsequent de-escalation of therapy. Similar to VAP, early appropriate antibiotic coverage of catheter-related

bacteremia will likely reduce mortality, although this has not been systematically studied.

Urinary Tract Infection

The urinary tract is the second most common source of infection in the ICU, with infections occurring in up to one third of patients. The incidence of urinary tract infection (UTI) increases with the duration of bladder catheterization.[193,211] The responsible organisms are similar to those causing other nosocomial infections, and include *Staphylococcal* species, *Enterococcus*, enteric Gram-negative bacteria, and nonlactose fermenting Gram-negative bacteria such as *Pseudomonas*. Bacteriuria is associated with bacteremia about 5% of the time. Similar to other ICU acquired infections, UTIs are associated with increased mortality, although the attributable mortality is not clear.

Prevention of ICU-acquired UTI includes careful hand washing, use of aseptic technique during catheter insertion, and minimization of catheterization duration. The use of silver-alloy and antibiotic-coated catheters may also reduce the incidence of UTI, although the evidence is insufficient at this point to recommend their general use.[212]

Invasive Fungal Infections

Invasive fungal infection in nonneutropenic patients is caused by *Candida* species in most cases, is increasingly common in the ICU population, and accounts for 5 to 10% of all blood stream infections in the ICU.[204,213] In addition, although fungal infection is not usually associated with pneumonia in a general ICU population, studies suggest that *Aspergillus* may be a common cause of VAP in patients with varying degrees of immunosuppression.[214] Other than neutropenia, risk factors for *Candida* blood stream infection include the presence of central venous catheters, uremia and dialysis-dependent renal failure, and administration of PN, multiple broad-spectrum antibiotics, and steroids. In addition, colonization of multiple sites by *Candida* is a risk factor for the development of fungemia.[215] The attributable mortality from *Candida* blood stream infection is high, approaching 40%, and mortality appears to be much higher in medical versus surgical ICU patients. Invasive *Candida* infection is also associated with increased duration of mechanical ventilation and ICU and hospital length of stay.

In addition to simple blood stream infection, *Candida* species are associated with UTI, postoperative peritonitis, and disseminated blood-borne infection. *Candida* is frequently cultured from the urine of catheterized patients, and candiduria is associated with the development of blood stream infection. True *Candida* peritonitis is also difficult to separate from contamination of culture specimens, but given that the mortality associated with *Candida* peritonitis is approximately 50%, treatment is warranted if clinical signs suggest infection. Disseminated blood-borne infection can result in endophthalmitis, endocarditis, hepatic, and pulmonary abscesses. It is likely to occur when initial treatment of candidemia is delayed and is associated with a high mortality. Lastly, although *Candida* is frequently grown from sputum cultures, true *Candida* pneumonia is unlikely. However, sputum colonization is a risk factor for blood stream infection.

Prevention of invasive *Candida* infection involves avoidance of risk factors, including limitation of intravascular catheterization, PN, and antibiotic administration. Prophylactic therapy with fluconazole is effective at reducing the risk of invasive *Candida* infection in high-risk patients, but this strategy has been studied most extensively in the neutropenic population. Prophylactic fluconazole appears to increase the incidence of invasive infection with more resistant species, such as *C. glabrata* and *krusei*; thus, prophylactic therapy should be reserved for only the highest risk patients.[216]

Candida grows slowly in blood culture medium, and invasive infection can be indolent, making diagnosis of invasive candidiasis difficult. Thus, a high level of suspicion for invasive *Candida* infection in critically ill patients is necessary, particularly in patients with multiple risk factors, including multiple site colonization. "Pre-emptive" therapy should be considered in patients with a high likelihood of invasive *Candida* infection while awaiting blood culture results, as delay in treatment is associated with increased mortality. Unfortunately, many cases of invasive candidiasis are identified only at autopsy.[213]

Documented *Candida* blood stream infection should be treated aggressively, with therapy started promptly (or pre-emptively, as previously described), and continued for at least 2 weeks after the last positive blood culture. An ophthalmologic examination is warranted in patients with documented or suspected blood stream infection, as patients with endophthalmitis may require longer courses of therapy. Intravascular catheters that are potential sources of blood stream infection should be removed.

It is not clear that routine treatment of candiduria is warranted, as candiduria often clears without treatment or with discontinuation of the bladder catheter. In addition, candiduria often recurs after initially successful antifungal therapy.[216] However, if candiduria is associated with signs of systemic infection, antifungal treatment should be considered; a similar approach can be taken when *Candida* is cultured from the peritoneal space.

Organisms sensitive to fluconazole cause the majority of invasive *Candida* infections in the ICU, and fluconazole is the first-line treatment given its reasonable efficacy and limited toxicity. Infections caused by resistant organisms such as *C. glabrata* and *C. krusei* may respond to newer-generation azoles such as voriconazole, although there are limited data on these agents at present. Caspofungin is another new antifungal agent with broad-spectrum activity and seemingly limited toxicity that is a reasonable alternative for infection due to resistant species. Amphotericin B is generally reserved for refractory, life-threatening infections due to its toxicity.[216]

Stress Ulceration and Gastrointestinal Hemorrhage

Gastric mucosal breakdown with resulting gastritis and ulceration ("stress ulceration") can lead to GI bleeding in the ICU. Clinically significant GI bleeding is that which results in hemodynamic instability and/or a sudden fall in hematocrit that results in blood transfusion. The incidence of clinically significant stress-related GI bleeding is <5% in high-risk patients, and <1% for low-risk patients.[217] The major risk factors for stress-related GI bleeding are mechanical ventilation and coagulopathy; secondary risk factors include renal failure, thermal injury, and possibly head injury, although the latter two factors have not been recently evaluated.[217–219] EN may protect against significant GI bleeding.[219]

Agents used to prevent stress ulceration and GI bleeding include methods to suppress acid production (H$_2$ blockers and proton pump inhibitors) and cytoprotective agents (sucralfate). However, the agent of choice—and whether any prophylaxis is beneficial or indicated—is somewhat controversial for the following reasons: (1) Although ranitidine was shown to be more effective than sucralfate in preventing clinically significant GI bleeding in high-risk patients in a large, randomized prospective trial (level I evidence), the incidence of bleeding with both agents was quite low (1.7 vs. 3.8%).[220] Furthermore, a meta-analysis suggests that neither ranitidine nor sucralfate is superior to placebo in reducing clinically important bleeding.[221] (2) Acid suppression may favor gastric colonization with enteric flora, which may in turn increase the risk of nosocomial pneumonia. Multiple small, randomized trials suggested a higher incidence of

VAP when ranitidine was compared with sucralfate, and in the large trial mentioned here, there was a trend toward increased VAP in the ranitidine group (level II evidence).[3] It appears that stress ulcer prophylaxis is more widely used than necessary, is often administered to low-risk patients, and results in an overall cost that may be higher than the benefit. Thus, although stress ulcer prophylaxis, predominantly with ranitidine, is commonly used in critically ill patients, the utility of this intervention is unclear.

Proton pump inhibitors (PPIs) are very effective at suppressing gastric acid production and have been shown to be as effective as ranitidine and cimetidine at reducing stress ulcer-related bleeding in the ICU. In addition, PPIs may be more effective than ranitidine in preventing rebleeding due to stress ulceration (level II evidence).[222] However, PPIs cannot be recommended for routine use as prophylactic agents because of insufficient data and cost considerations. In addition, PPIs have the potential to increase the risk of VAP, given their effective suppression of gastric acid secretion.

Venous Thromboembolism

Venous thromboembolism (VTE) occurs frequently in critically ill patients, with incidences of deep venous thrombosis (DVT) of 10 to 30% and of pulmonary embolism (PE) of 1.5 to 5%. However, the reported incidence varies widely depending on study design, tests used to detect DVT, and the patient population studied. Virtually all critically ill patients have one or more risk factors for VTE; risk factors can be grouped according to their importance as described by Anderson and Spencer[223] (Table 56-9). Determination of VTE risk is important in that it will help in choosing prophylactic therapy and in determining the level of suspicion for VTE in individual patients.

TABLE 56-9

RISK FACTORS FOR VENOUS THROMBOEMBOLISM

Strong risk factors (odds ratio >10)
  Fracture (hip or leg)
  Hip or knee replacement
  Major trauma
  Spinal cord injury
Moderate risk factors (odds ratio 2–9)
  Arthroscopic knee surgery
  Central venous lines
  Chemotherapy
  Congestive heart or respiratory failure
  Hormone replacement therapy
  Malignancy
  Oral contraceptive therapy
  Paralytic stroke
  Pregnancy/postpartum
  Previous venous thromboembolism
  Thrombophilia
Weak risk factors (odds ratio <2)
  Bed rest >3 days
  Immobility due to sitting (e.g., prolonged car or air travel)
  Increasing age
  Laparoscopic surgery (e.g., cholecystectomy)
  Obesity
  Pregnancy/antepartum
  Varicose veins

From Anderson FA Jr, Spencer FA: Risk factors for venous thromboembolism. Circulation 2003; 107: I9, with permission.

In addition to classic lower extremity DVT, upper extremity DVT occurs with increased frequency in the ICU population. This is directly associated with the use of central venous catheters in the subclavian and internal jugular sites. Upper extremity DVT can result in PE in up to two thirds of cases, with occasional fatalities. Catheter-related thrombosis is also associated with increased risk of catheter-associated infection and bacteremia. Finally, upper extremity DVT is associated with considerable long-term morbidity, particularly related to postthrombotic syndrome.[224]

The literature supporting prophylactic measures to prevent VTE in the ICU population is relatively poor, and marked by small, heterogeneous studies. In addition, studies supporting VTE prophylaxis in the ICU generally show differences only in intermediate end points, such as asymptomatic DVT, with no differences in the incidence of PE or death. This is particularly true for VTE prophylaxis in patients with traumatic injury, and makes evidence-based recommendations for prophylaxis difficult. Finally, the risks of VTE prophylaxis, including heparin-induced thrombocytopenia and bleeding, must be weighed when considering prophylaxis in the ICU population. Nonetheless, it is generally agreed that high-risk patients without contraindications should receive prophylaxis with LMWH, and that patients with low-to-moderate risk should receive low-dose UFH (Table 56-9). Patients with contraindications to LMWH or UFH should probably receive prophylaxis with mechanical devices (serial compression devices), although there is no compelling evidence to suggest that they are effective in the ICU population.[225] Fondaparinux has not been studied in critically ill patients, and there is no evidence to support the preventive placement of vena cava filters in the critically ill. To reduce central venous catheter-associated thrombosis and infection, catheter tips should be positioned in the superior vena cava and catheters should be flushed with a dilute heparin solution (level II evidence). Heparin bonding of catheters may also reduce local thrombosis. Importantly, it should be recognized that the incidence of VTE in patients receiving pharmacologic prophylaxis remains substantial, ranging between 5 and 30% depending on the therapy and population studied.

Given the high incidence of asymptomatic DVT in critically ill patients, a high index of suspicion for VTE must be maintained in the ICU. However, despite the high incidence of DVT, routine screening studies for DVT do not appear to improve clinical outcomes in the ICU. Thus, VTE should be considered in critically ill patients in the face of relatively nonspecific findings, such as unexplained tachycardia, tachypnea, fever, asymmetric extremity edema, and gas exchange abnormalities, including high dead space ventilation. Compression Doppler ultrasonography is the most commonly used test for diagnosis of DVT, and has good positive and negative predictive value compared with contrast venography[226]; helical chest CT has supplanted radionuclide ventilation-perfusion scanning as the primary test for the diagnosis of PE.[227,228] CT scanning can also be extended to include the extremities to diagnose DVT. However, ventilation-perfusion scanning and/or pulmonary angiography may have utility in specific circumstances, including in the presence of renal insufficiency (concerns about contrast-induced nephrotoxicity) or equivocal results on CT scan. In addition, pulmonary angiography may be the test of choice when the likelihood of PE is high and anticoagulation is contraindicated, necessitating immediate placement of a vena cava filter. Although low D dimer levels have a high negative predictive value in ruling out venous thromboembolism in outpatients, this test appears to have less utility in the ICU setting because of the frequent occurrence of high levels in critically ill patients.[229]

The mainstay of treatment for VTE is heparin, which should be started prior to confirmatory studies if clinical suspicion is high. LMWH may be superior to UFH in efficacy with compa-

rable rates of bleeding for the treatment of VTE (level II evidence); the choice of drug should be based on clinical circumstances and availability. The advantage of UFH in the ICU population is its titratability and rapid reversibility, which may be desirable in patients at high risk for bleeding. In patients with PE and hemodynamic instability, thrombolytic therapy should be considered if not contraindicated. Although the data supporting thrombolytic therapy for treatment of PE are limited, patients with massive PE and/or shock are likely to benefit from thrombolysis; patients with more subtle signs of instability, including right ventricular dilation, may also benefit.[230]

For patients who have contraindications to anticoagulation or who have recurrent PE despite anticoagulation, vena cava filters can be placed in the superior vena cava or inferior vena cava, depending on DVT location. Ultimately, given the long-term thrombotic complications associated with these devices, patients with vena cava filters should be anticoagulated when no longer contraindicated. Another attractive option is to place a retrievable vena cava filter and remove it once anticoagulation can be started.[230] The time frame for safe removal varies with filter type; they can remain permanently if necessary.

Acquired Neuromuscular Disorders in Critical Illness

Neuromuscular abnormalities developing as a consequence of critical illness can be found in the majority of patients in the ICU for a week or more. The spectrum of illness ranges from isolated nerve entrapment with focal pain or weakness, to disuse muscle atrophy with mild weakness, to severe myopathy and/or neuropathy with associated severe, prolonged weakness. Although various studies have attempted to distinguish neuropathic from myopathic syndromes, resulting in a bewildering list of associated acronyms, it is likely that there is considerable overlap between the two in terms of risk factors, presentation, and prognosis.[231]

Prospective studies have shown that 25 to 36% of patients receiving intensive care are weak by clinical evaluation; electrodiagnostic studies (nerve conduction and electromyography) suggest that neuromuscular abnormalities are present in 42 to 47% of patients in the ICU for 7 days or more, and in 68 to 100% of patients with sepsis or the systemic inflammatory response syndrome. In addition to sepsis, factors strongly associated with the development of ICU-acquired neuromuscular abnormalities include duration of illness and hyperglycemia. Although corticosteroid and neuromuscular blocking drug administration have also been associated with ICU-acquired neuromuscular abnormalities, these agents do not consistently appear as risk factors, and their ultimate role in the pathogenesis of this problem is as yet undefined.[232]

ICU-acquired neuromuscular abnormalities can result in severe weakness with flaccid quadriplegia that lasts for weeks or months, and likely prolong the duration of mechanical ventilation, ICU stay, and hospitalization, and provide a significant impediment to long-term functional recovery from critical illness.[233,234] In addition, acquired weakness in the ICU may be a significant contributor to ICU and hospital mortality.

Prevention of acquired neuromuscular disorders in the ICU centers on avoidance or minimization of contributory risk factors, including high-dose steroids, prolonged neuromuscular blockade, and hyperglycemia. In regard to the latter, the only prospectively proven intervention for prevention of polyneuropathy as defined by electrophysiologic testing is tight glycemic control using intensive insulin therapy (goal glucose <110 mg/dL).[147,235] In addition, rigorous hand washing and infection control procedures, semirecumbent positioning, careful aseptic technique and barrier protection for central venous catheter placement, and lung protective ventilation will likely result in a reduction in the incidence and ramifications of ICU-acquired neuromuscular abnormalities.

The diagnosis of ICU-acquired neuromuscular abnormalities should be entertained in all critically ill patients with unexplained weakness; electrodiagnostic studies can help confirm the diagnosis and rule out other, potentially treatable causes of weakness such as Guillain-Barré syndrome. Muscle biopsy is confirmatory in cases of myopathy, but is not warranted outside of research settings. Unfortunately, no treatment for ICU-acquired neuromuscular abnormalities has been identified; avoidance of potentially contributing agents and aggressive physical therapy are warranted. Discharge planning should include the potential need for long-term nursing and rehabilitative care.

References

1. Berthelsen PG, Cronqvist M: The first intensive care unit in the world: Copenhagen 1953. Acta Anaesthesiol Scand 2003; 47: 1190
2. Angus DC, Kelley MA, Schmitz RJ, White A et al: Caring for the critically ill patient. Current and projected workforce requirements for care of the critically ill and patients with pulmonary disease: can we meet the requirements of an aging population? JAMA 2000; 284: 2762
3. Spielman FJ: Critical care medicine: Anesthesiology steps forward. Bull Anesth Hist 2003; 21: 12
4. Kummer HB: Is the U.S. the odd one out? An international perspective on Anesthesiologist-Intensivists. American Society of Anesthesiologists Newsletter 2004; 68: 8
5. Sackett DL: Rules of evidence and clinical recommendations on the use of antithrombotic agents. Chest 1989; 95: 2S
6. Kaushal R, Bates DW, Franz C et al: Costs of adverse events in intensive care units. Crit Care Med 2007; 35: 2479
7. Pronovost PJ, Rinke ML, Emery K et al: Interventions to reduce mortality among patients treated in intensive care units. J Crit Care 2004; 19: 158
8. Pronovost PJ, Angus DC, Dorman T et al: Physician staffing patterns and clinical outcomes in critically ill patients: a systematic review. JAMA 2002; 288: 2151
9. Treggiari MM, Martin DP, Yanez ND et al: Effect of intensive care unit organizational model and structure on outcomes in patients with acute lung injury. Am J Respir Crit Care Med 2007; 176: 685
10. Nathens AB, Rivara FP, MacKenzie EJ et al: The impact of an intensivist-model ICU on trauma-related mortality. Ann Surg 2006; 244: 545
11. Manthous CA. Leapfrog and critical care: evidence and reality-based intensive care for the 21st century. Am J Med 2004; 116: 118
12. Angus DC, Shorr AF, White A et al: Critical care delivery in the United States: distribution of services and compliance with Leapfrog recommendations. Crit Care Med 2006; 34: 1016
13. Kahn JM, Matthews FA, Angus DC et al: Barriers to implementing the Leapfrog Group recommendations for intensivist physician staffing: a survey of intensive care unit directors. J Crit Care 2007; 22: 97
14. Pronovost PJ, Needham DM, Waters H et al: Intensive care unit physician staffing: financial modeling of the Leapfrog standard. Crit Care Med 2006; 34: S18
15. Hales BM, Pronovost PJ: The checklist—a tool for error management and performance improvement. J Crit Care 2006; 21: 231
16. Pronovost P, Berenholtz S, Dorman T et al: Improving communication in the ICU using daily goals. J Crit Care 2003; 18: 71
17. Chan KH, Miller JD, Dearden NM et al: The effect of changes in cerebral perfusion pressure upon middle cerebral artery blood flow velocity and jugular bulb venous oxygen saturation after severe brain injury. J Neurosurg 1992; 77: 55
18. Haitsma IK, Maas AI: Advanced monitoring in the intensive care unit: brain tissue oxygen tension. Curr Opin Crit Care 2002; 8: 115
19. Longhi L, Pagan F, Valeriani V et al: Monitoring brain tissue oxygen tension in brain-injured patients reveals hypoxic episodes in normal-appearing and in peri-focal tissue. Intensive Care Med 2007; 33: 2136
20. Ibanez J, Vilalta A, Mena MP et al: [Intraoperative detection of ischemic brain hypoxia using oxygen tissue pressure microprobes]. Neurocirugia (Astur) 2003; 14: 483; discussion 490
21. Smith ML, Counelis GJ, Maloney-Wilensky E et al: Brain tissue oxygen tension in clinical brain death: a case series. Neurol Res 2007; 29: 755
22. Guidelines for the management of severe traumatic brain injury. J Neurotrauma 2007; 24 Suppl 1: S1
23. Smith MJ, Stiefel MF, Magge S et al: Packed red blood cell transfusion increases local cerebral oxygenation. Crit Care Med 2005; 33: 1104
24. Thorat JD, Wang EC, Lee KK et al: Barbiturate therapy for patients with refractory intracranial hypertension following severe traumatic brain injury: Its effects on tissue oxygenation, brain temperature and autoregulation. J Clin Neurosci 2008; 15: 143

25. Stiefel MF, Heuer GG, Smith MJ et al: Cerebral oxygenation following decompressive hemicraniectomy for the treatment of refractory intracranial hypertension. J Neurosurg 2004; 101: 241
26. Stiefel MF, Spiotta A, Gracias VH et al: Reduced mortality rate in patients with severe traumatic brain injury treated with brain tissue oxygen monitoring. J Neurosurg 2005; 103: 805
27. Johnston AJ, Gupta AK: Advanced monitoring in the neurology intensive care unit: microdialysis. Curr Opin Crit Care 2002; 8: 121
28. Peerdeman SM, Girbes AR, Polderman KH, Vandertop WP: Changes in cerebral interstitial glycerol concentration in head-injured patients; correlation with secondary events. Intensive Care Med 2003; 29: 1825
29. Bellander BM, Cantais E, Enblad P et al: Consensus meeting on microdialysis in neurointensive care. Intensive Care Med 2004; 30: 2166
30. Thatcher RW, Cantor DS, McAlaster R et al: Comprehensive predictions of outcome in closed head-injured patients. The development of prognostic equations. Ann N Y Acad Sci 1991; 620: 82
31. Chesnut RM, Marshall SB, Piek J et al: Early and late systemic hypotension as a frequent and fundamental source of cerebral ischemia following severe brain injury in the Traumatic Coma Data Bank. Acta Neurochir Suppl (Wien) 1993; 59: 121
32. Mirski MA, Muffelman B, Ulatowski JA et al: Sedation for the critically ill neurologic patient. Crit Care Med 1995; 23: 2038
33. Cremer OL, Moons KG, Bouman EA et al: Long-term propofol infusion and cardiac failure in adult head-injured patients. Lancet 2001; 357: 117
34. Schwartz ML, Tator CH, Rowed DW et al: The University of Toronto head injury treatment study: a prospective, randomized comparison of pentobarbital and mannitol. Can J Neurol Sci 1984; 11: 434
35. Ward JD, Becker DP, Miller JD et al: Failure of prophylactic barbiturate coma in the treatment of severe head injury. J Neurosurg 1985; 62: 383
36. Eisenberg HM, Frankowski RF, Contant CF et al: High-dose barbiturate control of elevated intracranial pressure in patients with severe head injury. J Neurosurg 1988; 69: 15
37. Robertson CS, Valadka AB, Hannay HJ et al: Prevention of secondary ischemic insults after severe head injury. Crit Care Med 1999; 27: 2086
38. Muizelaar JP, Marmarou A, Ward JD et al: Adverse effects of prolonged hyperventilation in patients with severe head injury: a randomized clinical trial. J Neurosurg 1991; 75: 731
39. Cruz J: The first decade of continuous monitoring of jugular bulb oxyhemoglobin saturation: management strategies and clinical outcome. Crit Care Med 1998; 26: 344
40. Henderson WR, Dhingra VK, Chittock DR et al: Hypothermia in the management of traumatic brain injury. A systematic review and meta-analysis. Intensive Care Med 2003; 29: 1637
41. Clifton GL, Miller ER, Choi SC et al: Hypothermia on admission in patients with severe brain injury. J Neurotrauma 2002; 19: 293
42. Roberts I, Yates D, Sandercock P et al: Effect of intravenous corticosteroids on death within 14 days in 10,008 adults with clinically significant head injury (MRC CRASH trial): randomised placebo-controlled trial. Lancet 2004; 364: 1321
43. Temkin NR, Anderson GD, Winn HR et al: Magnesium sulfate for neuroprotection after traumatic brain injury: a randomised controlled trial. Lancet Neurol 2007; 6: 29
44. Temkin NR, Dikmen SS, Wilensky AJ et al: A randomized, double-blind study of phenytoin for the prevention of post-traumatic seizures. N Engl J Med 1990; 323: 497
45. Myburgh J, Cooper J, Finfer S et al: Saline or albumin for fluid resuscitation in patients with traumatic brain injury. N Engl J Med 2007; 357: 874
46. Kassell NF, Torner JC, Jane JA et al: The International Cooperative Study on the Timing of Aneurysm Surgery. Part 2: Surgical results. J Neurosurg 1990; 73: 37
47. Kassell NF, Torner JC, Haley EC, Jr et al: The International Cooperative Study on the Timing of Aneurysm Surgery. Part 1: Overall management results. J Neurosurg 1990; 73: 18
48. Dorsch NW: Cerebral arterial spasm—a clinical review. Br J Neurosurg 1995; 9: 403
49. Barker FG, 2nd, Ogilvy CS: Efficacy of prophylactic nimodipine for delayed ischemic deficit after subarachnoid hemorrhage: a metaanalysis. J Neurosurg 1996; 84: 405
50. Lynch JR, Wang H, McGirt MJ et al: Simvastatin reduces vasospasm after aneurysmal subarachnoid hemorrhage: results of a pilot randomized clinical trial. Stroke 2005; 36: 2024
51. Tseng MY, Czosnyka M, Richards H et al: Effects of acute treatment with pravastatin on cerebral vasospasm, autoregulation, and delayed ischemic deficits after aneurysmal subarachnoid hemorrhage: a phase II randomized placebo-controlled trial. Stroke 2005; 36: 1627
52. Tseng MY, Hutchinson PJ, Czosnyka M et al: Effects of acute pravastatin treatment on intensity of rescue therapy, length of inpatient stay, and 6-month outcome in patients after aneurysmal subarachnoid hemorrhage. Stroke 2007; 38: 1545
53. Treggiari MM, Walder B, Suter PM, Romand JA: Systematic review of the prevention of delayed ischemic neurological deficits with hypertension, hypervolemia, and hemodilution therapy following subarachnoid hemorrhage. J Neurosurg 2003; 98: 978
54. Shimoda M, Oda S, Tsugane R, Sato O: Intracranial complications of hypervolemic therapy in patients with a delayed ischemic deficit attributed to vasospasm. J Neurosurg 1993; 78: 423

55. van der Worp HB, van Gijn J: Clinical practice. Acute ischemic stroke. N Engl J Med 2007; 357: 572

56. Tissue plasminogen activator for acute ischemic stroke. The National Institute of Neurological Disorders and Stroke rt-PA Stroke Study Group. N Engl J Med 1995; 333: 1581

57. Hacke W, Donnan G, Fieschi C et al: Association of outcome with early stroke treatment: pooled analysis of ATLANTIS, ECASS, and NINDS rt-PA stroke trials. Lancet 2004; 363: 768

58. Adams HP, Jr., Brott TG, Furlan AJ et al: Guidelines for thrombolytic therapy for acute stroke: a supplement to the guidelines for the management of patients with acute ischemic stroke. A statement for healthcare professionals from a Special Writing Group of the Stroke Council, American Heart Association. Circulation 1996; 94: 1167

59. Gray CS, Hildreth AJ, Sandercock PA et al: Glucose-potassium-insulin infusions in the management of post-stroke hyperglycaemia: the UK Glucose Insulin in Stroke Trial (GIST-UK). Lancet Neurol 2007; 6: 397

60. Vahedi K, Hofmeijer J, Juettler E et al: Early decompressive surgery in malignant infarction of the middle cerebral artery: a pooled analysis of three randomised controlled trials. Lancet Neurol 2007; 6: 215

61. Hypothermia after Cardiac Arrest Study Group. Mild therapeutic hypothermia to improve the neurologic outcome after cardiac arrest. N Engl J Med 2002; 346: 549

62. Bernard SA, Gray TW, Buist MD et al: Treatment of comatose survivors of out-of-hospital cardiac arrest with induced hypothermia. N Engl J Med 2002; 346: 557

63. Kim F, Olsufka M, Longstreth WT, Jr et al: Pilot randomized clinical trial of prehospital induction of mild hypothermia in out-of-hospital cardiac arrest patients with a rapid infusion of 4 degrees C normal saline. Circulation 2007; 115: 3064

64. Connors AF, Jr., Speroff T, Dawson NV et al: The effectiveness of right heart catheterization in the initial care of critically ill patients. SUPPORT Investigators. JAMA 1996; 276: 889

65. Vieillard-Baron A, Girou E, Valente E et al: Predictors of mortality in acute respiratory distress syndrome. Focus On the role of right heart catheterization. Am J Respir Crit Care Med 2000; 161: 1597

66. Carnendran L, Abboud R, Sleeper LA et al: Trends in cardiogenic shock: report from the SHOCK Study. The Should we emergently revascularize Occluded Coronaries for cardiogenic shock? Eur Heart J 2001; 22: 472

67. Richard C, Warszawski J, Anguel N et al: Early use of the pulmonary artery catheter and outcomes in patients with shock and acute respiratory distress syndrome: a randomized controlled trial. JAMA 2003; 290: 2713

68. Sandham JD, Hull RD, Brant RF et al: A randomized, controlled trial of the use of pulmonary-artery catheters in high-risk surgical patients. N Engl J Med 2003; 348: 5

69. Wheeler AP, Bernard GR, Thompson BT et al: Pulmonary-artery versus central venous catheter to guide treatment of acute lung injury. N Engl J Med 2006; 354: 2213

70. Kumar A, Anel R, Bunnell E et al: Pulmonary artery occlusion pressure and central venous pressure fail to predict ventricular filling volume, cardiac performance, or the response to volume infusion in normal subjects. Crit Care Med 2004; 32: 691

71. Michard F, Boussat S, Chemla D et al: Relation between respiratory changes in arterial pulse pressure and fluid responsiveness in septic patients with acute circulatory failure. Am J Respir Crit Care Med 2000; 162: 134

72. Hayes MA, Timmins AC, Yau EH et al: Elevation of systemic oxygen delivery in the treatment of critically ill patients. N Engl J Med 1994; 330: 1717

73. Pulmonary Artery Catheter Consensus conference: consensus statement. Crit Care Med 1997; 25: 910

74. Reinhart K, Kuhn HJ, Hartog C, Bredle DL: Continuous central venous and pulmonary artery oxygen saturation monitoring in the critically ill. Intensive Care Med 2004; 30: 1572

75. Rivers E, Nguyen B, Havstad S et al: Early goal-directed therapy in the treatment of severe sepsis and septic shock. N Engl J Med 2001; 345: 1368

76. Michard F, Teboul JL: Predicting fluid responsiveness in ICU patients: a critical analysis of the evidence. Chest 2002; 121: 2000

77. Baillard C, Cohen Y, Fosse JP et al: Haemodynamic measurements (continuous cardiac output and systemic vascular resistance) in critically ill patients: transoesophageal doppler versus continuous thermodilution. Anaesth Intensive Care 1999; 27: 33

78. Vieillard-Baron A, Prin S, Chergui K et al: Hemodynamic instability in sepsis: bedside assessment by doppler echocardiography. Am J Respir Crit Care Med 2003; 168: 1270

79. Silver MA, Horton DP, Ghali JK, Elkayam U: Effect of nesiritide versus dobutamine on short-term outcomes in the treatment of patients with acutely decompensated heart failure. J Am Coll Cardiol 2002; 39: 798

80. Hochman JS, Sleeper LA, Webb JG et al: Early revascularization in acute myocardial infarction complicated by cardiogenic shock. SHOCK Investigators. Should We Emergently Revascularize Occluded Coronaries for Cardiogenic Shock. N Engl J Med 1999; 341: 625

81. Vieillard Baron A, Schmitt JM, Beauchet A et al: Early preload adaptation in septic shock? A transesophageal echocardiographic study. Anesthesiology 2001; 94: 400

82. American College of Chest Physicians/Society of Critical Care Medicine Consensus Conference: definitions for sepsis and organ failure and guidelines for the use of innovative therapies in sepsis. Crit Care Med 1992; 20: 864

83. Marshall JC, Cook DJ, Christou NV et al: Multiple organ dysfunction score: a reliable descriptor of a complex clinical outcome. Crit Care Med 1995; 23: 1638

84. Dellinger RP, Levy MM, Carlet JM et al: Surviving Sepsis Campaign: International guidelines for management of severe sepsis and septic shock: 2008. Crit Care Med 2008; 36: 296

85. Wilkes MM, Navickis RJ: Patient survival after human albumin administration. A meta-analysis of randomized, controlled trials. Ann Intern Med 2001; 135: 149

86. Cochrane Injuries Group Albumin Reviewers. Human albumin administration in critically ill patients: systematic review of randomised controlled trials. BMJ 1998; 317: 235

87. Finfer S, Bellomo R, Boyce N et al: A comparison of albumin and saline for fluid resuscitation in the intensive care unit. N Engl J Med 2004; 350: 2247

88. Brunkhorst FM, Engel C, Bloos F et al: Intensive insulin therapy and pentastarch resuscitation in severe sepsis. N Engl J Med 2008; 358: 125

89. Martin C, Papazian L, Perrin G et al: Norepinephrine or dopamine for the treatment of hyperdynamic septic shock? Chest 1993; 103: 1826

90. Marik PE, Mohedin M: The contrasting effects of dopamine and norepinephrine on systemic and splanchnic oxygen utilization in hyperdynamic sepsis. JAMA 1994; 272: 1354

91. Martin C, Viviand X, Leone M, Thirion X: Effect of norepinephrine on the outcome of septic shock. Crit Care Med 2000; 28: 2758

92. Bellomo R, Chapman M, Finfer S et al: Low-dose dopamine in patients with early renal dysfunction: a placebo-controlled randomised trial. Australian and New Zealand Intensive Care Society (ANZICS) Clinical Trials Group. Lancet 2000; 356: 2139

93. Shoemaker WC, Appel PL, Kram HB: Hemodynamic and oxygen transport effects of dobutamine in critically ill general surgical patients. Crit Care Med 1986; 14: 1032

94. Duranteau J, Sitbon P, Teboul JL et al: Effects of epinephrine, norepinephrine, or the combination of norepinephrine and dobutamine on gastric mucosa in septic shock. Crit Care Med 1999; 27: 893

95. Meier-Hellmann A, Reinhart K, Bredle DL et al: Epinephrine impairs splanchnic perfusion in septic shock. Crit Care Med 1997; 25: 399

96. Levy B, Bollaert PE, Charpentier C et al: Comparison of norepinephrine and dobutamine to epinephrine for hemodynamics, lactate metabolism, and gastric tonometric variables in septic shock: a prospective, randomized study. Intensive Care Med 1997; 23: 282

97. Holmes CL, Patel BM, Russell JA, Walley KR: Physiology of vasopressin relevant to management of septic shock. Chest 2001; 120: 989

98. Wenzel V, Krismer AC, Arntz HR et al: A comparison of vasopressin and epinephrine for out-of-hospital cardiopulmonary resuscitation. N Engl J Med 2004; 350: 105

99. Patel BM, Chittock DR, Russell JA, Walley KR: Beneficial effects of short-term vasopressin infusion during severe septic shock. Anesthesiology 2002; 96: 576

100. Dunser MW, Mayr AJ, Ulmer H et al: Arginine vasopressin in advanced vasodilatory shock: a prospective, randomized, controlled study. Circulation 2003; 107: 2313

101. Albanese J, Leone M, Delmas A, Martin C: Terlipressin or norepinephrine in hyperdynamic septic shock: a prospective, randomized study. Crit Care Med 2005; 33: 1897

102. Cartotto R, McGibney K, Smith T, Abadir A: Vasopressin for the septic burn patient. Burns 2007; 33: 441

103. Bernard GR, Vincent JL, Laterre PF et al: Efficacy and safety of recombinant human activated protein C for severe sepsis. N Engl J Med 2001; 344: 699

104. Annane D, Sebille V, Charpentier C et al: Effect of treatment with low doses of hydrocortisone and fludrocortisone on mortality in patients with septic shock. JAMA 2002; 288: 862

105. Sprung CL, Annane D, Didier K et al: Hydrocortisone therapy for patients with septic shock. N Engl J Med 2008; 358: 111

106. Feihl F, Perret C: Permissive hypercapnia. How permissive should we be? Am J Respir Crit Care Med 1994; 150: 1722

107. Moloney ED, Griffiths MJ: Protective ventilation of patients with acute respiratory distress syndrome. Br J Anaesth 2004; 92: 261

108. Nava S, Carbone G, DiBattista N et al: Noninvasive ventilation in cardiogenic pulmonary edema: a multicenter randomized trial. Am J Respir Crit Care Med 2003; 168: 1432

109. International Consensus Conferences in Intensive Care Medicine: noninvasive positive pressure ventilation in acute respiratory failure. Am J Respir Crit Care Med 2001; 163: 283

110. Esteban A, Frutos-Vivar F, Ferguson ND et al: Noninvasive positive-pressure ventilation for respiratory failure after extubation. N Engl J Med 2004; 350: 2452

111. Mehta S, Jay GD, Woolard RH et al: Randomized, prospective trial of bilevel versus continuous positive airway pressure in acute pulmonary edema. Crit Care Med 1997; 25: 620

112. Esteban A, Frutos F, Tobin MJ et al: A comparison of four methods of weaning patients from mechanical ventilation. Spanish Lung Failure Collaborative Group. N Engl J Med 1995; 332: 345

113. MacIntyre NR, Cook DJ, Ely EW, Jr et al: Evidence-based guidelines for weaning and discontinuing ventilatory support: a collective task force facilitated by the American College of Chest Physicians; the American Association for Respiratory Care; and the American College of Critical Care Medicine. Chest 2001; 120: 375S

114. Schuster DP: What is acute lung injury? What is ARDS? Chest 1995; 107: 1721
115. Bernard GR, Artigas A, Brigham KL et al: Report of the American-European consensus conference on ARDS: definitions, mechanisms, relevant outcomes and clinical trial coordination. The Consensus Committee. Intensive Care Med 1994; 20: 225
116. Bersten AD, Edibam C, Hunt T, Moran J: Incidence and mortality of acute lung injury and the acute respiratory distress syndrome in three Australian States. Am J Respir Crit Care Med 2002; 165: 443
117. Roupie E, Lepage E, Wysocki M et al: Prevalence, etiologies and outcome of the acute respiratory distress syndrome among hypoxemic ventilated patients. SRLF Collaborative Group on Mechanical Ventilation. Societe de Reanimation de Langue Francaise. Intensive Care Med 1999; 25: 920
118. Nuckton TJ, Alonso JA, Kallet RH et al: Pulmonary dead-space fraction as a risk factor for death in the acute respiratory distress syndrome. N Engl J Med 2002; 346: 1281
119. The Acute Respiratory Distress Syndrome Network. Ventilation with lower tidal volumes as compared with traditional tidal volumes for acute lung injury and the acute respiratory distress syndrome. N Engl J Med 2000; 342: 1301
120. Villar J, Kacmarek RM, Perez-Mendez L, Aguirre-Jaime A: A high positive end-expiratory pressure, low tidal volume ventilatory strategy improves outcome in persistent acute respiratory distress syndrome: a randomized, controlled trial. Crit Care Med 2006; 34: 1311
121. Brower RG, Lanken PN, MacIntyre N et al: Higher versus lower positive end-expiratory pressures in patients with the acute respiratory distress syndrome. N Engl J Med 2004; 351: 327
122. Gattinoni L, Tognoni G, Pesenti A et al: Effect of prone positioning on the survival of patients with acute respiratory failure. N Engl J Med 2001; 345: 568
123. Guerin C, Gaillard S, Lemasson S et al: Effects of systematic prone positioning in hypoxemic acute respiratory failure: a randomized controlled trial. JAMA 2004; 292: 2379
124. Mancebo J, Fernandez R, Blanch L et al: A multicenter trial of prolonged prone ventilation in severe acute respiratory distress syndrome. Am J Respir Crit Care Med 2006; 173: 1233
125. Taylor RW, Zimmerman JL, Dellinger RP et al: Low-dose inhaled nitric oxide in patients with acute lung injury: a randomized controlled trial. JAMA 2004; 291: 1603
126. Sokol J, Jacobs SE, Bohn D: Inhaled nitric oxide for acute hypoxic respiratory failure in children and adults: a meta-analysis. Anesth Analg 2003; 97: 989
127. Wiedemann HP, Wheeler AP, Bernard GR et al: Comparison of two fluid-management strategies in acute lung injury. N Engl J Med 2006; 354: 2564
128. Martin GS, Moss M, Wheeler AP et al: A randomized, controlled trial of furosemide with or without albumin in hypoproteinemic patients with acute lung injury. Crit Care Med 2005; 33: 1681
129. Perkins GD, McAuley DF, Thickett DR, Gao F: The beta-agonist lung injury trial (BALTI): a randomized placebo-controlled clinical trial. Am J Respir Crit Care Med 2006; 173: 281
130. Meduri GU, Headley AS, Golden E et al: Effect of prolonged methylprednisolone therapy in unresolving acute respiratory distress syndrome: a randomized controlled trial. JAMA 1998; 280: 159
131. Steinberg KP, Hudson LD, Goodman RB et al: Efficacy and safety of corticosteroids for persistent acute respiratory distress syndrome. N Engl J Med 2006; 354: 1671
132. Bellomo R, Kellum JA, Ronco C: Defining and classifying acute renal failure: from advocacy to consensus and validation of the RIFLE criteria. Intensive Care Med 2007; 33: 409
133. Bellomo R, Ronco C, Kellum J et al: Acute renal failure-definition, outcome measures, animal models, fluid therapy, and information technology needs: The Second International Consensus Conference of the Acute Dialysis Quality Initiative (ADQI) Group. Critical Care 2004; 8: R204
134. Singri N, Ahya SN, Levin ML: Acute renal failure. JAMA 2003; 289: 747
135. Uchino S, Kellum JA, Bellomo R et al: Acute renal failure in critically ill patients: a multinational, multicenter study. JAMA 2005; 294: 813
136. Carvounis CP, Nisar S, Guro-Razuman S: Significance of the fractional excretion of urea in the differential diagnosis of acute renal failure. Kidney Int 2002; 62: 2223
137. Mehta RL, Pascual MT, Soroko S, Chertow GM: Diuretics, mortality, and nonrecovery of renal function in acute renal failure. JAMA 2002; 288: 2547
138. Uchino S, Doig GS, Bellomo R et al: Diuretics and mortality in acute renal failure. Crit Care Med 2004; 32: 1669
139. Ho KM, Sheridan DJ: Meta-analysis of frusemide to prevent or treat acute renal failure. Bmj 2006; 333: 420
140. Briguori C, Airoldi F, D'Andrea D et al: Renal Insufficiency Following Contrast Media Administration Trial (REMEDIAL): a randomized comparison of 3 preventive strategies. Circulation 2007; 115: 1211
141. Marenzi G, Assanelli E, Marana I et al: N-acetylcysteine and contrast-induced nephropathy in primary angioplasty. N Engl J Med 2006; 354: 2773
142. Schiffl H, Lang SM, Fischer R: Daily hemodialysis and the outcome of acute renal failure. N Engl J Med 2002; 346: 305
143. Ronco C, Bellomo R, Homel P et al: Effects of different doses in continuous veno-venous haemofiltration on outcomes of acute renal failure: a prospective randomised trial. Lancet 2000; 356: 26
144. Vinsonneau C, Camus C, Combes A et al: Continuous venovenous haemodiafiltration versus intermittent haemodialysis for acute renal failure in patients with multiple-organ dysfunction syndrome: a multicentre randomised trial. Lancet 2006; 368: 379

145. McCowen KC, Malhotra A, Bistrian BR: Stress-induced hyperglycemia. Crit Care Clin 2001; 17: 107
146. Malmberg K, Norhammar A, Wedel H, Ryden L: Glycometabolic state at admission: important risk marker of mortality in conventionally treated patients with diabetes mellitus and acute myocardial infarction: long-term results from the Diabetes and Insulin-Glucose Infusion in Acute Myocardial Infarction (DIGAMI) study. Circulation 1999; 99: 2626
147. van den Berghe G, Wouters P, Weekers F et al: Intensive insulin therapy in the critically ill patients. N Engl J Med 2001; 345: 1359
148. van den Berghe G, Wilmer A, Hermans G et al: Intensive insulin therapy in the medical ICU. N Engl J Med 2006; 354: 449
149. van den Berghe G, de Zegher F, Bouillon R: Clinical review 95: Acute and prolonged critical illness as different neuroendocrine paradigms. J Clin Endocrinol Metab 1998; 83: 1827
150. Cooper MS, Stewart PM: Corticosteroid insufficiency in acutely ill patients. N Engl J Med 2003; 348: 727
151. Hamrahian AH, Oseni TS, Arafah BM: Measurements of serum free cortisol in critically ill patients. N Engl J Med 2004; 350: 1629
152. Annane D, Sebille V, Troche G et al: A 3-level prognostic classification in septic shock based on cortisol levels and cortisol response to corticotropin. JAMA 2000; 283: 1038
153. Lipiner-Friedman D, Sprung CL, Laterre PF et al: Adrenal function in sepsis: the retrospective corticus cohort study. Crit Care Med 2007; 35: 1012
154. van den Berghe G, de Zegher F, Lauwers P: Dopamine and the sick euthyroid syndrome in critical illness. Clin Endocrinol (Oxf) 1994; 41: 731
155. De Groot LJ: Dangerous dogmas in medicine: the nonthyroidal illness syndrome. J Clin Endocrinol Metab 1999; 84: 151
156. Bennett-Guerrero E, Jimenez JL, White WD et al: Cardiovascular effects of intravenous triiodothyronine in patients undergoing coronary artery bypass graft surgery. A randomized, double-blind, placebo-controlled trial. Duke T3 study group. JAMA 1996; 275: 687
157. Takala J, Ruokonen E, Webster NR et al: Increased mortality associated with growth hormone treatment in critically ill adults. N Engl J Med 1999; 341: 785
158. Corwin HL, Gettinger A, Pearl RG et al: The CRIT Study: Anemia and blood transfusion in the critically ill—current clinical practice in the United States. Crit Care Med 2004; 32: 39
159. Vincent JL, Baron JF, Reinhart K et al: Anemia and blood transfusion in critically ill patients. JAMA 2002; 288: 1499
160. Rodriguez RM, Corwin HL, Gettinger A et al: Nutritional deficiencies and blunted erythropoietin response as causes of the anemia of critical illness. J Crit Care 2001; 16: 36
161. Hebert PC, Wells G, Blajchman MA et al: A multicenter, randomized, controlled clinical trial of transfusion requirements in critical care. Transfusion Requirements in Critical Care Investigators, Canadian Critical Care Trials Group. N Engl J Med 1999; 340: 409
162. Lacroix J, Hebert PC, Hutchison JS et al: Transfusion strategies for patients in pediatric intensive care units. N Engl J Med 2007; 356: 1609
163. Hutton B, Fergusson D, Tinmouth A et al: Transfusion rates vary significantly amongst Canadian medical centres. Can J Anaesth 2005; 52: 581
164. Corwin HL, Gettinger A, Pearl RG et al: Efficacy of recombinant human erythropoietin in critically ill patients: a randomized controlled trial. JAMA 2002; 288: 2827
165. Corwin HL, Gettinger A, Fabian TC et al: Efficacy and safety of epoetin alfa in critically ill patients. N Engl J Med 2007; 357: 965
166. Kompan L, Kremzar B, Gadzijev E, Prosek M: Effects of early enteral nutrition on intestinal permeability and the development of multiple organ failure after multiple injury. Intensive Care Med 1999; 25: 157
167. Marik PE, Zaloga GP: Gastric versus post-pyloric feeding: a systematic review. Crit Care 2003; 7: R46
168. MacLeod JB, Lefton J, Houghton D et al: Prospective randomized control trial of intermittent versus continuous gastric feeds for critically ill trauma patients. J Trauma 2007; 63: 57
169. Zaloga GP: Parenteral nutrition in adult inpatients with functioning gastrointestinal tracts: assessment of outcomes. Lancet 2006; 367: 1101
170. Bistrian BR, McCowen KC: Nutritional and metabolic support in the adult intensive care unit: key controversies. Crit Care Med 2006; 34: 1525
171. Alberda C, Gramlich L, Meddings J et al: Effects of probiotic therapy in critically ill patients: a randomized, double-blind, placebo-controlled trial. Am J Clin Nutr 2007; 85: 816
172. Heyland DK, Cook DJ, Guyatt GH: Does the formulation of enteral feeding products influence infectious morbidity and mortality rates in the critically ill patients? A critical review of the evidence. Crit Care Med 1994; 22: 1192
173. Heyland DK, Schroter-Noppe D, Drover JW et al: Nutrition support in the critical care setting: current practice in Canadian ICUs—opportunities for improvement? JPEN J Parenter Enteral Nutr 2003; 27: 74
174. Heyland DK, Novak F, Drover JW et al: Should immunonutrition become routine in critically ill patients? A systematic review of the evidence. JAMA 2001; 286: 944
175. Heyland DK, Dhaliwal R, Suchner U, Berger MM: Antioxidant nutrients: a systematic review of trace elements and vitamins in the critically ill patient. Intensive Care Med 2005; 31: 327
176. Kollef MH, Levy NT, Ahrens TS et al: The use of continuous i.v. sedation is associated with prolongation of mechanical ventilation. Chest 1998; 114: 541

177. Brook AD, Ahrens TS, Schaiff R et al: Effect of a nursing-implemented sedation protocol on the duration of mechanical ventilation. Crit Care Med 1999; 27: 2609

178. Kress JP, Pohlman AS, O'Connor MF, Hall JB: Daily interruption of sedative infusions in critically ill patients undergoing mechanical ventilation. N Engl J Med 2000; 342: 1471

179. Schweickert WD, Gehlbach BK, Pohlman AS et al: Daily interruption of sedative infusions and complications of critical illness in mechanically ventilated patients. Crit Care Med 2004; 32: 1272

180. Jones C, Griffiths RD, Humphris G, Skirrow PM: Memory, delusions, and the development of acute posttraumatic stress disorder-related symptoms after intensive care. Crit Care Med 2001; 29: 573

181. Weinert CR, Sprenkle M: Post-ICU consequences of patient wakefulness and sedative exposure during mechanical ventilation. Intensive Care Med 2008; 34: 82

182. Samuelson K, Lundberg D, Fridlund B: Memory in relation to depth of sedation in adult mechanically ventilated intensive care patients. Intensive Care Med 2006; 32: 660

183. Kress JP, Gehlbach B, Lacy M et al: The long-term psychological effects of daily sedative interruption on critically ill patients. Am J Respir Crit Care Med 2003; 168: 1457

184. Ely EW, Truman B, Shintani A et al: Monitoring sedation status over time in ICU patients: reliability and validity of the Richmond Agitation-Sedation Scale (RASS). JAMA 2003; 289: 2983

185. Weinert C, McFarland L: The state of intubated ICU patients: development of a two-dimensional sedation rating scale for critically ill adults. Chest 2004; 126: 1883

186. Ely EW, Shintani A, Truman B et al: Delirium as a predictor of mortality in mechanically ventilated patients in the intensive care unit. JAMA 2004; 291: 1753

187. Ely EW, Inouye SK, Bernard GR et al: Delirium in mechanically ventilated patients: validity and reliability of the confusion assessment method for the intensive care unit (CAM-ICU). JAMA 2001; 286: 2703

188. McCollam JS, O'Neil MG, Norcross ED et al: Continuous infusions of lorazepam, midazolam, and propofol for sedation of the critically ill surgery trauma patient: a prospective, randomized comparison. Crit Care Med 1999; 27: 2454

189. Walder B, Elia N, Henzi I et al: A lack of evidence of superiority of propofol versus midazolam for sedation in mechanically ventilated critically ill patients: a qualitative and quantitative systematic review. Anesth Analg 2001; 92: 975

190. Carson SS, Kress JP, Rodgers JE et al: A randomized trial of intermittent lorazepam versus propofol with daily interruption in mechanically ventilated patients. Crit Care Med 2006; 34: 1326

191. Coursin DB, Maccioli GA: Dexmedetomidine. Curr Opin Crit Care 2001; 7: 221

192. Pandharipande PP, Pun BT, Herr DL et al: Effect of sedation with dexmedetomidine vs lorazepam on acute brain dysfunction in mechanically ventilated patients: the MENDS randomized controlled trial. JAMA 2007; 298: 2644

193. Vincent JL: Nosocomial infections in adult intensive-care units. Lancet 2003; 361: 2068

194. Rouby JJ, Laurent P, Gosnach M et al: Risk factors and clinical relevance of nosocomial maxillary sinusitis in the critically ill. Am J Respir Crit Care Med 1994; 150: 776

195. van Zanten AR, Dixon JM, Nipshagen MD et al: Hospital-acquired sinusitis is a common cause of fever of unknown origin in orotracheally intubated critically ill patients. Crit Care 2005; 9: R583

196. Cook DJ, Walter SD, Cook RJ et al: Incidence of and risk factors for ventilator-associated pneumonia in critically ill patients. Ann Intern Med 1998; 129: 433

197. Fagon JY, Chastre J, Wolff M et al: Invasive and noninvasive strategies for management of suspected ventilator-associated pneumonia. A randomized trial. Ann Intern Med 2000; 132: 621

198. Hoffken G, Niederman MS: Nosocomial pneumonia: the importance of a de-escalating strategy for antibiotic treatment of pneumonia in the ICU. Chest 2002; 122: 2183

199. Collard HR, Saint S, Matthay MA: Prevention of ventilator-associated pneumonia: an evidence-based systematic review. Ann Intern Med 2003; 138: 494

200. Chlebicki MP, Safdar N: Topical chlorhexidine for prevention of ventilator-associated pneumonia: a meta-analysis. Crit Care Med 2007; 35: 595

201. Wood AY, Davit AJ, 2nd, Ciraulo DL et al: A prospective assessment of diagnostic efficacy of blind protective bronchial brushings compared to bronchoscope-assisted lavage, bronchoscope-directed brushings, and blind endotracheal aspirates in ventilator-associated pneumonia. J Trauma 2003; 55: 825

202. Canadian Critical Care Trials Group. A randomized trial of diagnostic techniques for ventilator-associated pneumonia. N Engl J Med 2006; 355: 2619

203. Chastre J, Wolff M, Fagon JY et al: Comparison of 8 vs 15 days of antibiotic therapy for ventilator-associated pneumonia in adults: a randomized trial. JAMA 2003; 290: 2588

204. Renaud B, Brun-Buisson C: Outcomes of primary and catheter-related bacteremia. A cohort and case-control study in critically ill patients. Am J Respir Crit Care Med 2001; 163: 1584

205. Polderman KH, Girbes AR: Central venous catheter use. Part 2: infectious complications. Intensive Care Med 2002; 28: 18

206. Berenholtz SM, Pronovost PJ, Lipsett PA et al: Eliminating catheter-related bloodstream infections in the intensive care unit. Crit Care Med 2004; 32: 2014

207. Pronovost P, Needham D, Berenholtz S et al: An intervention to decrease catheter-related bloodstream infections in the ICU. N Engl J Med 2006; 355: 2725

208. McConnell SA, Gubbins PO, Anaissie EJ: Do antimicrobial-impregnated central venous catheters prevent catheter-related bloodstream infection? Clin Infect Dis 2003; 37: 65

209. O'Grady NP, Alexander M, Dellinger EP et al: Guidelines for the prevention of intravascular catheter-related infections. Am J Infect Control 2002; 30: 476

210. Ringberg H, Thoren A, Bredberg A: Evaluation of coagulase-negative staphylococci in blood cultures. A prospective clinical and microbiological study. Scand J Infect Dis 1991; 23: 315

211. Di Filippo A, De Gaudio AR: Device-related infections in critically ill patients. Part II: Prevention of ventilator-associated pneumonia and urinary tract infections. J Chemother 2003; 15: 536

212. Johnson JR, Kuskowski MA, Wilt TJ: Systematic review: antimicrobial urinary catheters to prevent catheter-associated urinary tract infection in hospitalized patients. Ann Intern Med 2006; 144: 116

213. Eggimann P, Garbino J, Pittet D: Epidemiology of Candida species infections in critically ill non-immunosuppressed patients. Lancet Infect Dis 2003; 3: 685

214. Meersseman W, Lagrou K, Maertens J et al: Galactomannan in bronchoalveolar lavage fluid: a tool for diagnosing aspergillosis in intensive care unit patients. Am J Respir Crit Care Med 2008; 177: 27

215. Verduyn Lunel FM, Meis JF, Voss A: Nosocomial fungal infections: candidemia. Diagn Microbiol Infect Dis 1999; 34: 213

216. Eggimann P, Garbino J, Pittet D: Management of Candida species infections in critically ill patients. Lancet Infect Dis 2003; 3: 772

217. Cook DJ, Fuller HD, Guyatt GH et al: Risk factors for gastrointestinal bleeding in critically ill patients. Canadian Critical Care Trials Group. N Engl J Med 1994; 330: 377

218. Metz CA, Livingston DH, Smith JS et al: Impact of multiple risk factors and ranitidine prophylaxis on the development of stress-related upper gastrointestinal bleeding: a prospective, multicenter, double-blind, randomized trial. The Ranitidine Head Injury Study Group. Crit Care Med 1993; 21: 1844

219. Cook D, Heyland D, Griffith L et al: Risk factors for clinically important upper gastrointestinal bleeding in patients requiring mechanical ventilation. Canadian Critical Care Trials Group. Crit Care Med 1999; 27: 2812

220. Cook D, Guyatt G, Marshall J et al: A comparison of sucralfate and ranitidine for the prevention of upper gastrointestinal bleeding in patients requiring mechanical ventilation. Canadian Critical Care Trials Group. N Engl J Med 1998; 338: 791

221. Messori A, Trippoli S, Vaiani M et al: Bleeding and pneumonia in intensive care patients given ranitidine and sucralfate for prevention of stress ulcer: meta-analysis of randomised controlled trials. Bmj 2000; 321: 1103

222. Morgan D: Intravenous proton pump inhibitors in the critical care setting. Crit Care Med 2002; 30: S369

223. Anderson FA, Jr., Spencer FA: Risk factors for venous thromboembolism. Circulation 2003; 107: I9

224. Joffe HV, Goldhaber SZ: Upper-extremity deep vein thrombosis. Circulation 2002; 106: 1874

225. Geerts W, Selby R: Prevention of venous thromboembolism in the ICU. Chest 2003; 124: 357S

226. Kearon C, Ginsberg JS, Hirsh J: The role of venous ultrasonography in the diagnosis of suspected deep venous thrombosis and pulmonary embolism. Ann Intern Med 1998; 129: 1044

227. Goldhaber SZ, Elliott CG: Acute pulmonary embolism: part I: epidemiology, pathophysiology, and diagnosis. Circulation 2003; 108: 2726

228. Anderson DR, Kahn SR, Rodger MA et al: Computed tomographic pulmonary angiography vs ventilation-perfusion lung scanning in patients with suspected pulmonary embolism: a randomized controlled trial. JAMA 2007; 298: 2743

229. Kollef MH, Zahid M, Eisenberg PR: Predictive value of a rapid semiquantitative D-dimer assay in critically ill patients with suspected venous thromboembolic disease. Crit Care Med 2000; 28: 414

230. Goldhaber SZ, Elliott CG: Acute pulmonary embolism: part II: risk stratification, treatment, and prevention. Circulation 2003; 108: 2834

231. Deem S: Intensive-care-unit-acquired muscle weakness. Respir Care 2006; 51: 1042; discussion 1052

232. Stevens RD, Dowdy DW, Michaels RK et al: Neuromuscular dysfunction acquired in critical illness: a systematic review. Intensive Care Med 2007; 33: 1876

233. Herridge MS, Cheung AM, Tansey CM et al: One-year outcomes in survivors of the acute respiratory distress syndrome. N Engl J Med 2003; 348: 683

234. Deem S, Lee CM, Curtis JR: Acquired neuromuscular disorders in the intensive care unit. Am J Respir Crit Care Med 2003; 168: 735

235. Hermans G, Wilmer A, Meersseman W et al: Impact of intensive insulin therapy on neuromuscular complications and ventilator dependency in the medical intensive care unit. Am J Respir Crit Care Med 2007; 175: 480

CHAPTER 57 ■ ACUTE PAIN MANAGEMENT

STEPHEN M. MACRES, PETER G. MOORE, AND SCOTT M. FISHMAN

PERIOPERATIVE AND CONSULTATIVE SERVICES

KEY POINTS

1. The inadequate relief of postoperative pain has adverse physiologic effects that can contribute to significant morbidity and mortality, resulting in the delay of patient recovery and return to daily activities.

2. The pain pathway is not "hardwired" and nociceptive input is not passively transmitted from the periphery to the brain. Tissue injury tends to fuel neuroplastic changes within the nervous system, which results in both peripheral and central sensitization.

3. In order for pre-emptive analgesia to be successful, three critical principles must be adhered to: (1) the depth of analgesia must be adequate enough to block all nociceptive input during surgery, (2) the analgesic technique must be extensive enough to include the entire surgical field, and (3) the duration of analgesia must include both the surgical and postsurgical periods.

4. The various opioid analgesics available today have distinct pharmacologic differences that we can credit to their intricate interaction with the three main opioid receptors mu, delta, and kappa. The opioid receptors are members of a G protein-coupled (guanosine triphosphate regulatory proteins) receptor family, which signals via a second messenger such as cyclic-adenosine monophosphate or an ion channel.

5. The therapeutic benefit of nonsteroidal anti-inflammatory drugs is believed to be mediated through the inhibition of cyclo-oxygenase enzymes, types 1 and 2, which convert arachidonic acid to prostaglandins.

6. Short-term use of parecoxib and valdecoxib in patients following coronary artery bypass surgery is associated with an increased risk of thromboembolic events. The authors, therefore, do not recommend prescribing a cyclo-oxygenase 2 inhibitor for patients with a known history of coronary artery disease or cerebrovascular disease.

7. The five variables associated with all modes of patient-controlled analgesia include: (1) bolus dose, (2) incremental (demand) dose, (3) lockout interval, (4) background infusion rate, and (5) 1- and 4-hour limits. A typical patient-controlled analgesia regimen in an otherwise healthy adult would be an incremental dose of 1 to 2 mg of morphine with an 8- to 10-minute lockout. The authors do not recommend a background infusion of opioid in the opioid-naive patient.

8. *Epidural analgesia* is a critical component of multimodal perioperative pain management and improved patient outcome. Meta-analyses investigating the efficacy of epidural analgesia found epidural analgesia to be superior to systemically administered opioids.

9. Continuous peripheral nerve block has proven to be an effective technique for postoperative pain management, which is superior to opioid analgesia with fewer opioid-related side effects and rare neurologic and infectious complications.

10. Should a perioperative nerve injury occur, it is incumbent on the physician to determine which combination of anesthetic, surgical, and patient risk factors are involved in any nerve injury and to not assume a priori that the regional anesthetic is the culprit.

11. The opioid-dependent patient is often identified just moments prior to surgery and the anesthesia team needs to be innovative. The anesthesiologist needs to be flexible enough to tailor an individual anesthetic that incorporates a multimodal approach, combining regional anesthesia with general anesthesia and nonopioid coanalgesics with opioid analgesics. Opioids remain the mainstay of perioperative pain management, and an adequate dose of opioid needs to be maintained to avoid precipitating withdrawal symptoms.

12. The key components to establishing a successful perioperative pain management service begins with an institutional commitment to support the service. The team must be built around a physician leader with training and experience in pain medicine. There must be other anesthesiologists available to support the service.

There are approximately 75 million surgical procedures performed each year in the United States and more than half are performed in the inpatient setting. Appropriate management of acute perioperative pain using multimodal or balanced analgesia is therefore crucial.

In 1992 clinical practice guidelines were promulgated by the Agency for Health Care Policy and Research, which provided guidelines for physicians for the treatment of acute pain.[1] Soon thereafter the American Society of Anesthesiologists developed treatment guidelines for acute postoperative pain, which have been updated and amended as of 2004.[2] Despite significant advances in our knowledge and treatment of acute pain and dissemination of these guidelines, significant deficits continue to persist and the management of acute postoperative pain is still less than optimal.

① The inadequate relief of postoperative pain has adverse physiologic effects that can contribute to significant morbidity and mortality, resulting in the delay of patient recovery and return to daily activities.[3] In addition, poor postoperative pain control contributes to patient dissatisfaction with the surgical experience and may have adverse psychological consequences.[4] Poorly managed postoperative pain can also increase the incidence of persistent postoperative pain conditions. Because aggressive treatment of acute postoperative pain is considered to be so beneficial, the Joint Commission on Accreditation of Healthcare Organizations has declared that "pain is the fifth vital sign" and all institutions seeking accreditation from this group must develop pain management programs.

ACUTE PAIN DEFINED

Acute pain has been defined as "the normal, predicted, physiological response to an adverse chemical, thermal, or mechanical stimulus."[5] Generally, acute pain resolves within 1 month. However, poorly managed acute pain that might occur following surgery can produce pathophysiologic processes in both the peripheral and central nervous systems that have the potential to produce chronicity.[4] Acute pain-induced change in the central nervous system is known as *neuronal plasticity*. This can result in sensitization of the nervous system resulting in allodynia and hyperalgesia. Surgical procedures that can be associated with chronic painful conditions include amputation of a limb, lateral thoracotomy, inguinal herniorrhaphy, abdominal hysterectomy, saphenous vein stripping, open cholecystectomy, nephrectomy, and mastectomy.[4]

ANATOMY OF ACUTE PAIN

The nociceptive pathway is an afferent (Fig. 57-1) three-neuron dual ascending (e.g., anterolateral and dorsal column medial lemniscal pathways) system, with descending modulation (Fig. 57-2) from the cortex, thalamus, and brainstem.[6] Nociceptors are free nerve endings located in skin, muscle, bone, and connective tissue with cell bodies located in the dorsal root ganglia. The first-order neurons that make up the dual ascending system have their origins in the periphery as A delta

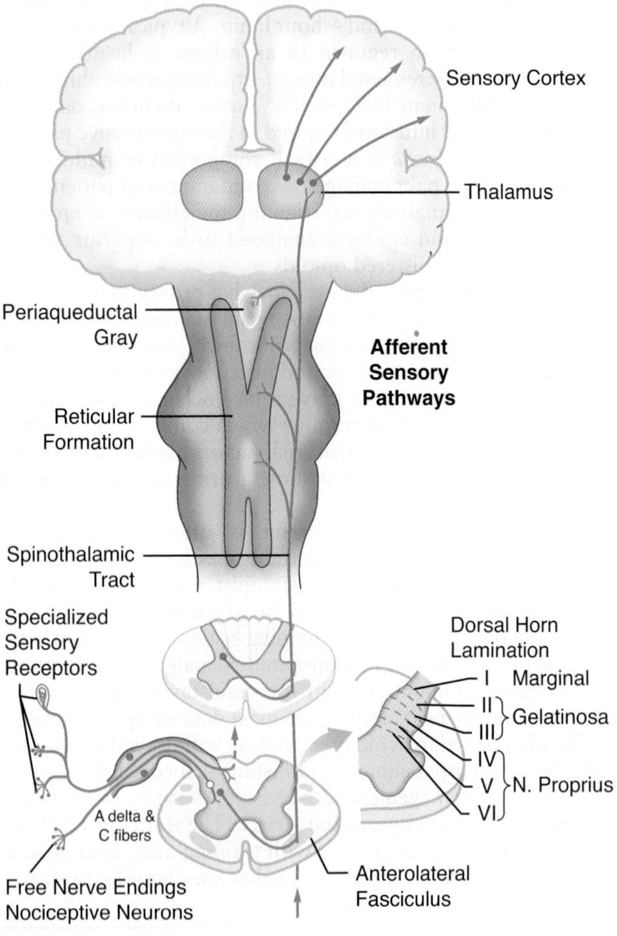

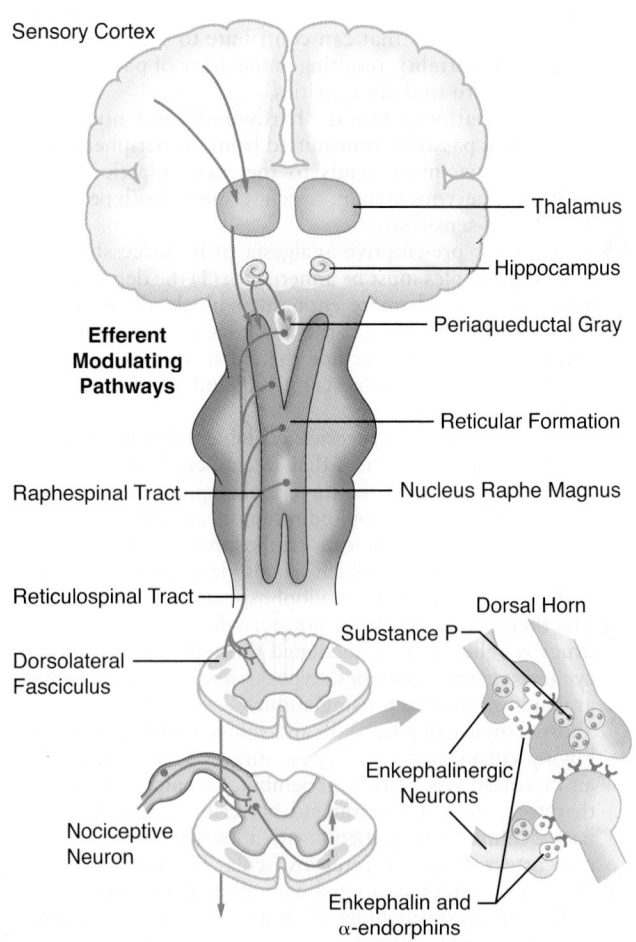

FIGURE 57-1. Afferent nociceptive pathway.

FIGURE 57-2. Efferent pathways involved in nociceptive regulation.

TABLE 57-1

PRIMARY AFFERENT NERVES

■ FIBER CLASS[a]	■ VELOCITY	■ EFFECTIVE STIMULI
Aβ (myelinated) (12–20 μ dia)	Group II (>40–50 m/sec)	Low-threshold mechanoreceptors Specialized nerve endings (pacinian corpuscles)
Aδ (myelinated) (1–4 μ dia)	Group III (10 < × < 40 m/sec)	Low-threshold mechanical or thermal High-threshold mechanical or thermal Specialized nerve endings
C (unmyelinated) (0.5–1.5 μ dia)	Group IV (<2 m/sec)	High threshold thermal, mechanical, and chemical Free nerve endings

[a]Aβ/Aδ/C is the Erlanger-Gasser classification and refers to axon size; II/III/IV is the Lloyd-Hunt classification and is defined on conduction velocity in muscle afferents. Because of the relationship between size and state of myelination with conduction velocity, these designations are often used interchangeably.
From Warfield CA, Bajwa ZH, eds. Principles and Practice of Pain Medicine, 2e, New York: McGraw Hill, 2004, p14.

and polymodal C fibers (Table 57-1). A delta fibers transmit "first pain," which is described as sharp or stinging in nature and is well localized. Polymodal C fibers transmit "second pain," which is more diffuse in nature and is associated with the affective and motivational aspects of pain. First-order neurons synapse on second-order neurons in the dorsal horn primarily within laminas I, II, and V, where they release excitatory amino acids and neuropeptides (Figs. 57-3 and 57-4). Some fibers can ascend or descend in Lissauer's tract prior to terminating on neurons that project to higher centers. Second-order neurons consist of nociceptive-specific and wide dynamic-range (WDR) neurons. Nociceptive-specific neurons are located primarily in lamina I, respond only to noxious stimuli, and are thought to be involved in the sensory-discriminative aspects of pain. WDR neurons are predominately located in laminae IV, V, and VI, respond to both nonnoxious and noxious input, and are involved with the affective-motivational component of pain. Axons of both nociceptive-specific and WDR neurons ascend the spinal cord via the dorsal column-medial lemniscus and the anterior lateral spinothalamic tract to synapse on third-order neurons in the contralateral thalamus, which then project to the somatosensory cortex where nociceptive input is perceived as pain (Fig. 57-1).

Pain Processing

❷ A key development in our understanding of pain processing is that the pain pathway is not "hardwired" and nociceptive input is not passively transmitted from the periphery to the brain.[7] Tissue injury tends to fuel neuroplastic changes within the nervous system, which results in both peripheral and central sensitization. Clinically this can manifest as *hyperalgesia*, which is defined as an exaggerated pain response to a normally painful stimulus, and *allodynia*, which is defined as a painful response to a typically nonpainful stimulus[7] (Fig. 57-5).

The four elements of pain processing include: (1) transduction, (2) transmission, (3) modulation, and (4) perception (Fig. 57-6). *Transduction* is the event whereby noxious thermal, chemical, or mechanical stimuli are converted into an action potential. *Transmission* occurs when the action potential is conducted through the nervous system via the first-, second-, and third-order neurons, which have cell bodies located in the dorsal root ganglion, dorsal horn, and thalamus, respectively. *Modulation* of pain transmission involves altering afferent neural transmission along the pain pathway. The dorsal horn of the spinal cord is the most common site for modulation of the pain pathway, and modulation can involve either *inhibition* or *augmentation* of the pain signals.[6] Examples of *inhibitory* spinal modulation include: (1) release of inhibitory neurotransmitters such as γ-amino butyric acid (GABA) and glycine by intrinsic spinal neurons, and (2) activation of descending efferent neuronal pathways from the motor cortex, hypothalamus, periaqueductal gray matter, and the nucleus raphe magnus, which results in the release of norepinephrine, serotonin, and endorphins in the dorsal horn. Spinal modulation, which results in *augmentation* of pain pathways, is manifested as central sensitization, which is a consequence of

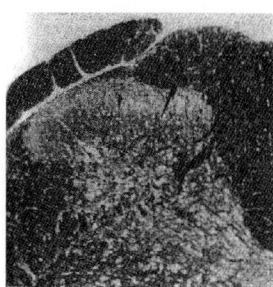

Spinal Lamination

Aβ
A∂
C

☐ Marginal Layer   ☐ Subst Gelatinosa   ☐ N. Proprius
   Lam I   Lam II   Lam III, IV, V, VI

☐ Motor Horn   ☐ Central Canal
   Lam VII, VIII, IX   Lam X

FIGURE 57-3. Schematic showing the Rexed lamination (right) and the approximate organization of the approach of the afferent to the spinal cord (left) as they enter at the dorsal root entry zone and then penetrate into the dorsal horn to terminate in laminae I and II (A/C) or penetrate more deeply to loop upward to terminate as high as the dorsum of lamina III (Aβ). Inset in lower left shows histologic appearance of the left dorsal quadrant, and large, myelinated axons. From Warfield CA, Bajwa ZH, eds. Principles and Practice of Pain Medicine, 2nd ed., McGraw Hill Medical Publishing Division.

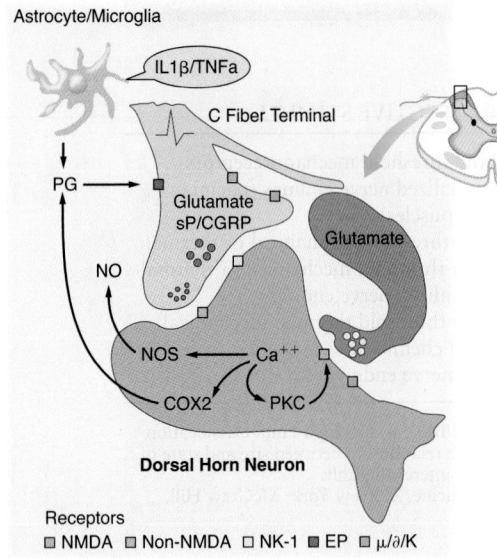

Receptors
☐ NMDA ☐ Non-NMDA ☐ NK-1 ■ EP ☐ μ/∂/K

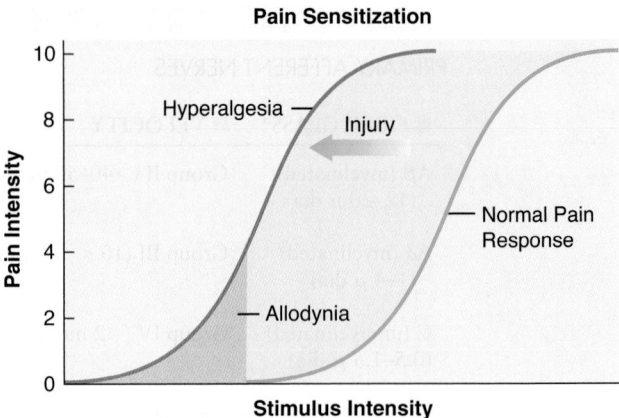

FIGURE 57-5.   Pain sensitization. (Obtained with permission from Dave Klemm, http:www.georgetown.edu/dml/facs/graphics/index.htm)

FIGURE 57-4.   Schematic summarizing the organization of dorsal horn systems that contribute to the processing of nociceptive information. 1) Primary afferent C fibers release peptide (e.g. substance P (sP), calcitonin gene-related peptide (CGRP), and so on) and excitatory amino acid (glutamate) products. Small dorsal root ganglion (DRG) cells, as well as some postsynaptic elements contain nitric oxide synthase (NOS) and are able upon depolarization, to release NO (nitric oxide). 2) Peptides and excitatory amino acids evoke excitation in second-order neurons. For glutamate, direct monosynaptic excitation is mediated by non-N-methyl-D-aspartate (NMDA) receptors (ie., acute primary afferent excitation of WDR neurons is not mediated by the NMDA or neurokinin 1 (NK-1) receptor). 3) Interneurons excited by afferent barrage induce excitation in second-order neurons via an NMDA receptor. This leads to a marked increase in intracellular Ca^{2+} and the activation of kinases and phosphorylating enzymes. Prostaglandins (PG) generated by cyclooxygenase-2 (COX-2) and NO by NOS are formed and released. These agents diffuse extracellulary and facilitate transmitter release (retrograde transmission) from primary and non-primary afferent terminals, either by a direct cellular action (eg. NO) or by an interaction with a specific class of receptors (eg. EP receptors for prostanoids). 4) Non-neuronal sources of prostaglandins may include activated astrocytes and microglia that are stimulated by circulating cytokines, which are released secondary to peripheral nerve injury and inflammation. Terminal excitability can be altered by activation of a variety of receptors located on the sensory terminal, including those for, μ, δ, and κ opioids. From: Warfield CA, Bajwa ZH eds. Principles and Practice of Pain Medicine, 2nd edition., McGraw Hill Medical Publishing Division.

FIGURE 57-6.   The four elements of pain processing: transduction, transmission, modulation, and perception. 5HT, serotonin; NE, norepinephrine; NMDA, N-methyl-D-asparate; NSAIDs, nonsteroidal anti-inflammatory drugs; CCK, cholecystokin; NO, nitric oxide.

neuronal plasticity. The phenomenon of "wind-up" is a specific example of central plasticity that results from repetitive C-fiber stimulation of WDR neurons in the dorsal horn. *Perception* of pain is the final common pathway, which results from the integration of painful input into the somatosensory and limbic cortices. Generally speaking, traditional analgesic therapies have only targeted pain *perception*. A *multimodal approach* to pain therapy should target all four elements of the pain processing pathway.

CHEMICAL MEDIATORS OF TRANSDUCTION AND TRANSMISSION

Tissue damage following surgical procedures leads to the activation of small nociceptive nerve endings and local inflammatory cells (e.g., macrophages, mast cells, lymphocytes, and platelets) in the periphery. Antidromic release of substance P and glutamate from small nociceptive afferents results in vasodilation, extravasation of plasma proteins, and stimulation of inflammatory cells to release numerous algogenic substances (Table 57-2 and Fig. 57-7). This chemical milieu will both directly produce pain transduction via nociceptor stimu-

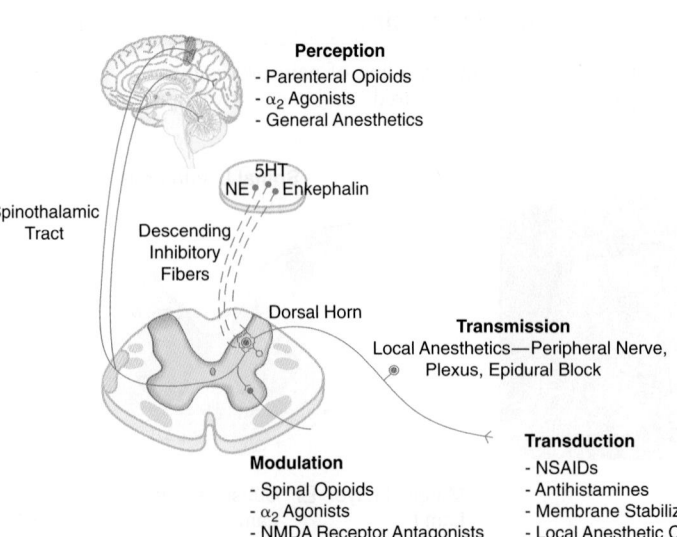

TABLE 57-2

ALGOGENIC SUBSTANCES

■ SUBSTANCE	■ SOURCE	■ EFFECT
Bradykinin	Macrophages and plasma kininogen	Activates nociceptors
Serotonin	Platelets	Activates nociceptors
Histamine	Platelets and mast cells	Produces vasodilation, edema and pruritus
		Potentiates the response of nociceptors to bradykinin
Prostaglandin	Tissue injury and cyclo-oxygenase pathway	Sensitize nociceptors
Leukotriene	Tissue injury and lipooxygenase pathway	Sensitize nociceptors
Excess H$^+$ ions	Tissue injury and ischemia	Increases pain and hyperalgesia associated with inflammation
Cytokines (e.g., interleukins and tissue necrosis factor)	Macrophages	Excite and sensitize nociceptors
Adenosine	Tissue injury	Pain and hyperalgesia
Neurotransmitters (e.g., glutamate and substance P)	Antidromic release by peripheral nerve terminals following tissue injury	Substance P activates macrophages and Mast cells
		Glutamate activates nociceptors
Nerve Growth Factor	Macrophages	Stimulates mast cells to release histamine and serotonin
		Induces heat hyperalgesia
		Sensitizes nociceptors

Data derived from Dougherty PM, Raja SN. Neurochemistry of Somatosensory and Pain Processing. In: Benzon HT, Raja SN, Molloy RE, et al. eds. Essentials of Pain Medicine and Regional Anesthesia: Elsevier, Churchill Livingstone; 2005:7.

lation as well as facilitate pain transduction by increasing the excitability of nociceptors. *Peripheral sensitization* of polymodal C fibers and high-threshold mechanoreceptors by these chemicals leads to *primary hyperalgesia*, which by definition is an exaggerated response to pain at the site of injury.

As is the case in the periphery, the dorsal horn of the spinal cord contains numerous transmitters and receptors involved in pain processing. Three classes of transmitter compounds integral to pain transmission include: (1) the excitatory amino acids glutamate and aspartate, (2) the excitatory neuropeptides substance P and neurokinin A, and (3) the inhibitory amino acids glycine and GABA. The various pain receptors include: (1) the NMDA (*N*-methyl-D-aspartate), (2) the AMPA

(α-amino-3-hydroxy-5-methylisoxazole-4-proprionic acid), (3) the kainate, and (4) the metabotropic (Fig. 57-8).

The AMPA and kainate receptors, which are sodium channel-dependent, are essential for fast synaptic afferent input. On the other hand, the NMDA receptor, which is calcium channel-dependent, is only activated following prolonged depolarization of the cell membrane. Release of substance P into the spinal cord will remove the magnesium block on the channel of the NMDA receptor giving glutamate free access to the NMDA receptor. Repetitive C-fiber stimulation of WDR neurons in the dorsal horn at intervals of 0.5 to 1.0 Hz can precipitate the occurrence of wind-up and *central sensitization* (Fig. 57-9). This leads to *secondary hyperalgesia*, which, by

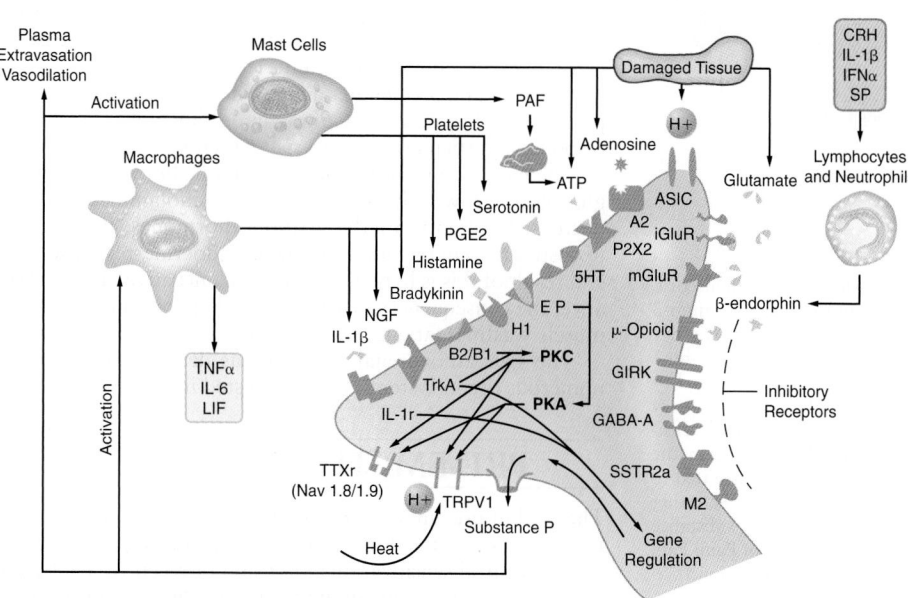

FIGURE 57-7. Schematic of the neurochemistry of somatosensory processing at peripheral sensory nerve endings. From: Benzon HT, Raja SN, Molloy RE et al., eds: Essentials of Pain Medicine and Regional Anesthesia, 2e, Elsevier, Churchill Livingstone; 2005: 8.

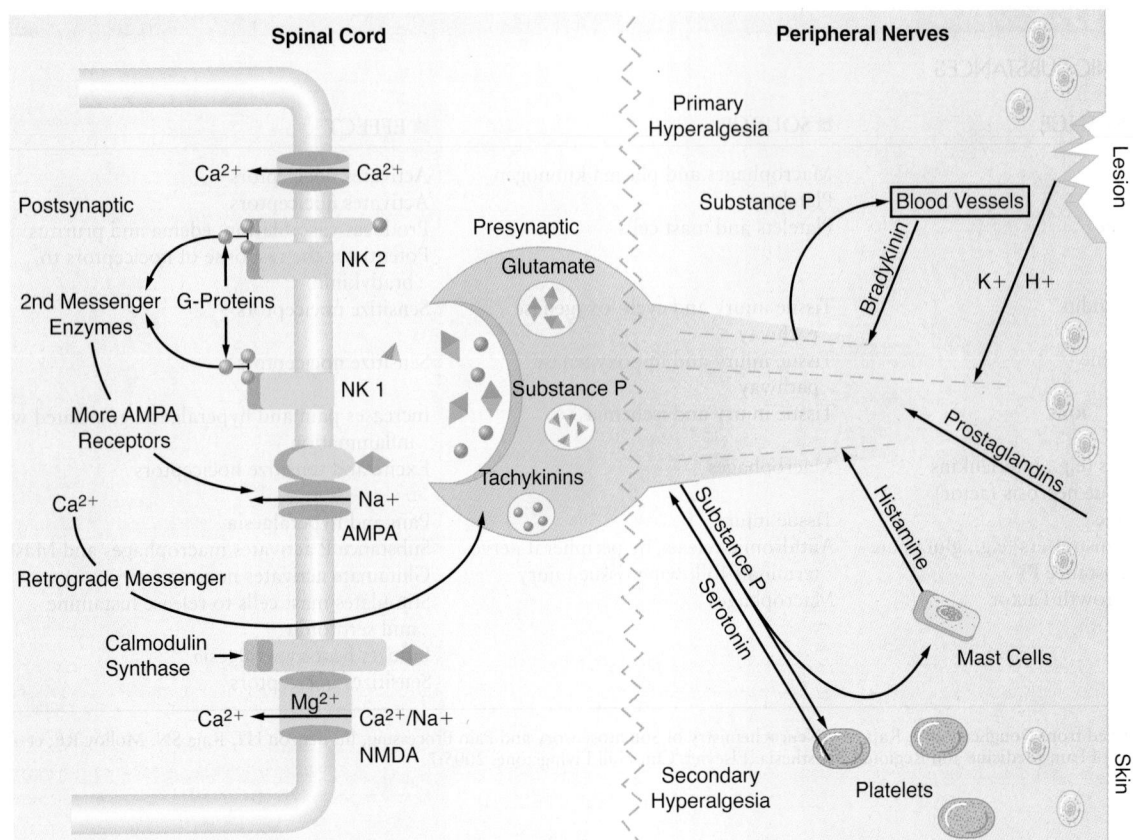

FIGURE 57-8. Schematic representation of peripheral and spinal mechanism involved in neuroplasticity. Primary hyperalgesia results from tissue release of toxic substances. These toxic substances spread to adjacent tissues, prolonging the hyperalgesic state (secondary hyperalgesia). As C fiber terminals increase in frequency of release of neurotransmitters, such as glutamate, substance P, tachykinins, brain-derived neurotrophic factor, and calcitonin gene-related peptide, the effects of these neurotransmitters are summated, resulting in prolonged depolarizations of second-order neurons ("wind-up"). Function changes at the second-order neuron occur as a result of neurotransmitter binding to postsynaptic receptors, which results in activity-dependent plasticity of the spinal cord. AMPA, α-amino-3 hydroxy-5-methyl-4-isoxazole propionic acid; NK, neurokinin; NMDA, N-methyl-D-asparate.

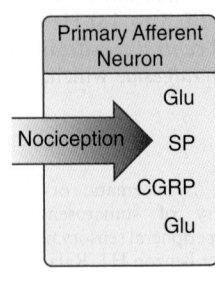
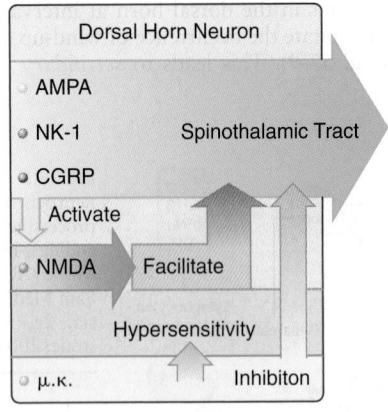

FIGURE 57-9. Primary nociceptive transmission in the spinal cord. Primary afferent nociceptive input is transmitted via α-amino-3 hydroxy-5-methyl-4-isoxazole propionic acid (AMPA), neurokinin-1 (NK1), and calcitonin gene-related peptide (CGRP) synapses, whose signals work their way to the thalamus. Glutaminergic (N-methyl-D-asparate; NMDA) synapses do not participate significantly in primary nociceptive transmission, but instead play a crucial role in spinal sensitization. Accordingly, even after complete NMDA blockade in the spinal cord, primary afferent nociceptive information is transmitted to the thalamus. NMDA antagonists thus have an antihyperalgesic rather than an analgesic effect in the spinal cord. Glu, glutamate; SP, substance P. (Reprinted from International Association for the Study of Pain: Pain Control Updates. IASP Newletter 2005; 13(2): 3, with permission.)

definition, is an increased pain response evoked by stimuli outside the area of injury.

THE SURGICAL STRESS RESPONSE

Although similar, postoperative pain and the surgical stress response are not the same. Surgical stress causes release of cytokines (e.g., interleukin-1, interleukin-6, and tumor necrosis factor-α) and precipitates adverse neuroendocrine and sympathoadrenal responses, resulting in detrimental physiological responses, particularly in high-risk patients.[4]

The increased secretion of the catabolic hormones cortisol, glucagon, growth hormone, and catecholamines and the decreased secretion of the anabolic hormones, insulin, and testosterone, characterize the neuroendocrine response. The end result of this is hyperglycemia and a negative nitrogen balance, the consequences of which include poor wound healing, muscle wasting, fatigue, and impaired immunocompetency.

The sympathoadrenal response has detrimental effects on numerous organ systems; these are listed in Table 57-3.[8]

PRE-EMPTIVE ANALGESIA

The goal of pre-emptive analgesia is to prevent NMDA receptor activation in the dorsal horn, which causes wind-up, facilitation, central sensitization expansion of receptive fields, and long-term potentiation, all of which can lead to a chronic pain

TABLE 57-3

CONSEQUENCES OF POORLY MANAGED ACUTE PAIN

Cardiovascular	Tachycardia, hypertension, and increase in cardiac work load
Pulmonary	Respiratory muscle spasm (splinting), decrease in vital capacity, atelectasis, hypoxia, and increased risk of pulmonary infection
Gastrointestinal	Postoperative ileus
Renal	Increased risk of oliguria and urinary retention
Coagulation	Increased risk of thromboemboli
Immunologic	Impaired immune function
Muscular	Muscle weakness and fatigue. Limited mobility can increase the risk of thromboembolism
Psychological	Anxiety, fear, and frustration results in poor patient satisfaction

Data derived from Joshi GP, Ogunnaike BO: Consequences of inadequate postoperative pain relief and chronic persistent postoperative pain. Anesthesiol Clin North Am 2005; 23: 21; Rowlingson JC: Update on acute pain management. International Anesthesia Research Society Review Course Lectures 2006; 95; and Kehlet H: Multimodal approach to control postoperative pathophysiology and rehabilitation. Br J Anaesth 1997; 78: 606.

state.[7] Although the use of pre-emptive analgesia is certainly enticing, its clinical benefit in humans has received mixed reviews. In order for pre-emptive analgesia to be successful, three critical principles must be adhered to: (1) the depth of analgesia must be adequate enough to block all nociceptive input during surgery, (2) the analgesic technique must be extensive enough to include the entire surgical field, and (3) the duration of analgesia must include both the surgical and postsurgical periods. Patients with pre-existing chronic pain tend to respond poorly to pre-emptive techniques because of pre-existing sensitization of the nervous system.

STRATEGIES FOR ACUTE PAIN MANAGEMENT

The majority of postoperative pain is nociceptive in character, but there are a small percentage of patients who can experience neuropathic pain postoperatively. It is critical to recognize this fact because patients with neuropathic pain are at increased risk of progressing to a chronic pain state. Neuropathic pain is a result of accidental nerve injury secondary to cutting, traction compression, or entrapment.[4,9] Clinical features may include continuous burning, paroxysmal shooting, or electric pain with associated allodynia, hyperalgesia, and dysesthesias. There can be a delay in the onset of the pain, and it can follow a nonder-matomal distribution. Surgical procedures that are a relatively high risk for neuropathic pain include limb amputations, breast surgery, gallbladder surgery, thoracic surgery, and inguinal her-nia repair.[4] Nociceptive pain responds best to opioids, non-steroidal anti-inflammatory drugs (NSAIDs), para-aminophe-nol agents, and regional anesthesia techniques.[10] Neuropathic pain, on the other hand, may benefit from the addition of the nonopioid analgesic adjuvants such as the NMDA receptor antagonists, α_2-agonists, and the α_2-δ subunit calcium channel ligands, which will be discussed in detail.

Strategies for acute pain management should also consider the sex of the patient as sex differences appear to exist for pain perception as well as response to opioid analgesics. Evidence suggests that women experience more pain following surgery than men, and therefore require more morphine to achieve a similar level of pain relief.[11]

ASSESSMENT OF ACUTE PAIN

The need for assessment of the patient in pain is illustrated by the postoperative patient who is said to be relatively pain-free, but who, on inspection, is lying almost completely still in bed. Too often, such a patient has had a recent cursory evaluation that included the traditional verbal analog score (VAS) 0–10 scale ("on a scale of zero to ten, with zero being no pain and ten being the worst pain you can imagine, how much pain are you in" from which the patient reported a low VAS score of 1/10) (Fig. 57-10). The treating team took that as reassuring information and moved along. No one asked the patient about pain with movement, breathing, moving bowels, and so forth, all potentially important functional goals for the postoperative course that may be undermined by untreated pain.

A variety of well-studied pain measurement scales exist that can be helpful yet are not definitive. Unidimensional instru-ments such as the familiar numerical pain scale already men-tioned, the visual analog scale, and the "faces" (Fig. 57-10) pain rating scale can provide some degree of guidance about a patient's experience of pain, but all of these are completely subjective and are open to wide variation between subjects and within subjects at different times.

Multidimensional instruments, such as the McGill Pain Questionnaire or the Brief Pain Inventory provide a broader pic-ture of a patient's experience, but are usually more cumbersome to administer and, in the end, suffer the same limitations as all other attempts to measure pain. A number of tools to assess cancer-related and noncancer chronic pain have been advanced and validated.[12] Most of these focus on persistent background pain and do not help identify intermittent or breakthrough pain. Several assessment scales specifically address breakthrough or episodic pain. The Breakthrough Pain Questionnaire was intro-duced by Portenoy and Hagen to assess breakthrough pain in cancer patients, and has also been studied in patients with acute noncancer pain, for which it can offer a picture of both break-through and background pain states.[13]

Ultimately, we are left with a maxim first attributed to Dr. John Bonica, the father of pain medicine: "Pain is what a patient says it is." The best way to begin assessing a patient's pain is to *ask* about it and *listen* to the answers. Attempts to reduce the experience to finite details may lead to failure to ask the right questions, distance us from our patients, focus us away from the whole person, and potentially miss golden diag-nostic clues that could lead to effective interventions.

Effective treatment of acute pain requires assessment as well as vigilant reassessment to determine if the primary goals are met, adversity has occurred, or changes are necessary. Acute pain may be viewed as breakthrough, intermittent, or background in nature (Table 57-4). The assessment process for each of these is relatively similar and will help to resolve the related condition into broad pathophysiologic groups such as cancer versus noncancer, and nociceptive versus neuropathic, or mixed pain states. Such an approach supports a rational

TABLE 57-4

THREE CLASSES OF ACUTE PAIN

1. Breakthrough: Pain that escalates above a persistent background pain.
2. Transitory and Intermittant: Pain that is episodic in the absence of background pain.
3. Background: Pain that is persistent but may vary over time.

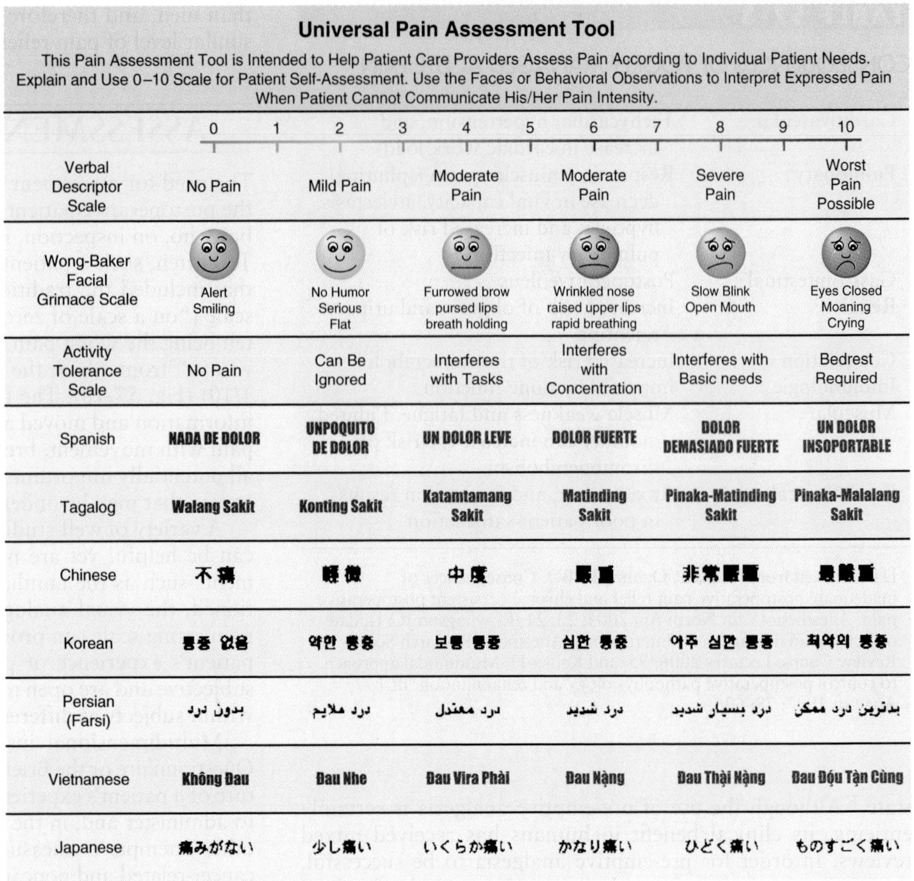

FIGURE 57-10. Linear verbal analog score and faces pain assessment tool.

Universal Pain Assessment Tool

This Pain Assessment Tool is Intended to Help Patient Care Providers Assess Pain According to Individual Patient Needs. Explain and Use 0–10 Scale for Patient Self-Assessment. Use the Faces or Behavioral Observations to Interpret Expressed Pain When Patient Cannot Communicate His/Her Pain Intensity.

	0	1	2	3	4	5	6	7	8	9	10
Verbal Descriptor Scale	No Pain		Mild Pain		Moderate Pain		Moderate Pain		Severe Pain		Worst Pain Possible
Wong-Baker Facial Grimace Scale	Alert Smiling		No Humor Serious Flat		Furrowed brow pursed lips breath holding		Wrinkled nose raised upper lips rapid breathing		Slow Blink Open Mouth		Eyes Closed Moaning Crying
Activity Tolerance Scale	No Pain		Can Be Ignored		Interferes with Tasks		Interferes with Concentration		Interferes with Basic needs		Bedrest Required
Spanish	NADA DE DOLOR		UN POQUITO DE DOLOR		UN DOLOR LEVE		DOLOR FUERTE		DOLOR DEMASIADO FUERTE		UN DOLOR INSOPORTABLE
Tagalog	Walang Sakit		Konting Sakit		Katamtamang Sakit		Matinding Sakit		Pinaka-Matinding Sakit		Pinaka-Malalang Sakit
Chinese	不痛		略微		中度		嚴重		非常嚴重		最嚴重
Korean	통증 없음		약한 통증		보통 통증		심한 통증		아주 심한 통증		최악의 통증
Persian (Farsi)	بدون درد		درد ملایم		درد معتدل		درد شدید		درد بسیار شدید		بدترین درد ممکن
Vietnamese	Không Đau		Đau Nhẹ		Đau Vừa Phải		Đau Nặng		Đau Thật Nặng		Đau Đớn Tận Cùng
Japanese	痛みがない		少し痛い		いくらか痛い		かなり痛い		ひどく痛い		ものすごく痛い

process for developing a useful differential diagnosis and approaches. Table 57-5 lists the common features of pain that are usually reviewed during the assessment for acute pain. A thorough physical examination must also be performed with particular attention to the neurologic examination, which may offer clues to aberrant neural processing. Such neurologic findings may indicate nerve injury, alerting the astute clinician to a neuropathic rather than a nociceptive pain state that requires a different analgesic approach.[14] A provocative physical examination may include examination of the affected areas with maneuvers that may provoke pain such as range of motion testing, walking, and cough. The benefits of provoca-

tive testing must outweigh the associated suffering incurred by the patient. Medical imaging is also a common part of the acute pain workup. Overemphasis on imaging data should, however, be avoided as this can potentially lead to misinterpretation of the patient's underlying pain syndrome.

OPIOID ANALGESICS

❹ Opioids are the mainstay for the treatment of acute postoperative pain, and morphine is the "gold-standard." The various opioid analgesics available today have distinct pharmacologic differences that we can credit to their intricate interaction with the three main opioid receptors: mu, delta, and kappa. The opioid receptors are members of a G protein-coupled (guanosine triphosphate regulatory proteins) receptor family, which signals via a second messenger such as cyclic adenosine monophosphate or an ion channel. In the ascending pain pathway opioid receptors are located in three areas that include: (1) the periphery, following inflammation; (2) the spinal cord dorsal horn; and (3) supraspinally in the brainstem, thalamus, and cortex. Mu opioid receptors are also found in the periaqueductal grey, the nucleus raphe magnus, and the rostral ventral medulla, which constitutes the descending inhibitory pain pathway. The three primary mechanisms of action for opioid analgesia at the level of the spinal cord, include: (1) inhibition of calcium influx presynaptically, which results in depolarization of the cell membrane and decreased release of neurotransmitters and neuropeptides into the synaptic cleft; (2) enhancing potassium efflux from the cell postsynaptically, which results in hyperpolarization of the cell and a decrease in pain transmission, and (3) activation of a descending inhibitory pain circuit via inhibition of GABAergic transmis-

TABLE 57-5

FEATURES OF PAIN COMMONLY ADDRESSED DURING ASSESSMENT

Onset of pain
Temporal pattern of pain
Site of pain
Radiation of pain
Quality (character) of pain
Intensity (severity) of pain
Exacerbating factors (what makes the pain start or get worse?)
Relieving factors (what prevents the pain or makes it better?)
Response to analgesics (including attitudes and concerns about opioids)
Response to other interventions
Associated physical symptoms
Associated psychological symptoms
Interference with activities of daily living

sion in the brainstem. Peripheral opioid receptors, which mediate analgesia, are located on primary afferent neurons. Activation of these receptors inhibits the release of pronociceptive and proinflammatory substances like substance P, which accounts for the analgesic and anti-inflammatory effects. The "broad-spectrum" opioid, methadone, has NMDA receptor antagonist properties and inhibits the reuptake of serotonin and norepinephrine, which may make it useful in the treatment of neuropathic pain.

There is great diversity in the available routes of administration of opioid analgesics. Table 57-6 is a list of relevant pharmacokinetic data. Table 57-7 offers equianalgesic dosing guidelines for the various opioids. The reader is referred to the section "Perioperative Pain Management of the Opioid-Dependent Patient" for a complete discussion of incomplete cross-tolerance between the different opioids and dosing considerations.

Common opioid-induced side effects include sedation, nausea and vomiting, respiratory depression, and constipation. Less common side effects include confusion, urinary retention, dizziness, and myoclonus. Tolerance rarely develops to the constipating effects of the opioids. Alvimopan, a peripherally acting mu receptor antagonist that has negligible systemic absorption, attenuates opioid-induced constipation and shortens postoperative ileus and length of hospital stay.[15] Opioid-induced hyperalgesia (OIH) is a relatively rare phenomenon whereby patients who are receiving opioids suddenly and paradoxically become more sensitive to pain despite continued treatment with opioids. Evidence suggests that OIH is more likely to develop following high doses of phenanthrene opioids such as morphine.[16] Changing the opioid to a phenyl piperidine derivative such as fentanyl may thwart OIH. There is also evidence that coadministration of an NMDA receptor antagonist can abolish opioid-induced tolerance and OIH.[16]

Morphine is the prototype opioid and is the "gold standard" to which all other analgesics are compared. Although the plasma half-life of the drug is approximately 2 hours its analgesic duration of action is closer to 4 to 5 hours. Morphine undergoes hepatic glucuronidation to morphine-6-glucuronide and morphine-3-glucuronide, both of which are cleared by the kidney. Morphine-6-glucuronide is an active metabolite of morphine and is thought to be responsible for most of the analgesia associated with chronic dosing of the drug. Morphine-3-glucuronide, on the other hand, is considered to be devoid of analgesic activity. With chronic dosing these metabolites can accumulate and can be particularly problematic in patients with renal failure. Dosing adjustment is therefore necessary and monitoring of side effects is important. Morphine-6-glucuronide contributes to side effects such as drowsiness, nausea and vomiting, coma, and respiratory depression. Morphine-3-glucuronide, on the other hand, is thought to cause agitation, myoclonus, delirium, and hyperalgesia.

Hydromorphone is a semisynthetic opioid that has 4 to 6 times the potency of morphine. It is available for oral, rectal, parenteral, and neuraxial administration. Whereas the oral bioavailability of the drug is reported to be 20 to 50%, its bioavailability via the subcutaneous route is 78%, making it the ideal drug for long-term subcutaneous administration in the opioid-tolerant patient. Like morphine, hydromorphone is biotransformed in the liver. The active metabolites are dihydromorphine and dihydroisomorphine and the inactive metabolite is hydromorphone-3-glucuronide. Although hydromorphone has traditionally been the preferred opioid for patients with acute pain and impaired kidney function, evidence suggests that hydromorphone-3-glucuronide can accumulate in those with renal failure and may contribute to side effects such as neuroexcitation and cognitive impairment. Opioid-related side effects such as nausea, vomiting, sedation, cognitive impairment, and pruritus are reported to be less intense with hydromorphone vis-à-vis morphine. In fact, the

incidence of pruritus following neuraxial administration of hydromorphone is reported to be approximately 5% versus the 11 to 77% range reported for neuraxial morphine.[17]

Fentanyl, a synthetic opioid chemically related to the phenylpiperidines, is a relatively selective mu receptor agonist, which is considered to be 80 times the potency of morphine following intravenous administration. It is extensively metabolized in the liver to norfentanyl and other inactive metabolites, which are excreted in the urine and bile. Fentanyl is therefore suitable for patients in renal failure. The drug is available for intravenous, subcutaneous, transdermal, transmucosal, and neuraxial administration. The transdermal administration of fentanyl using iontophoresis (Ionsys™, Janssen-Cilag LTD) is a novel on-demand drug delivery system that does not require venous access.

Sufentanil, alfentanil, and *remifentanil* are analogues of fentanyl that have analgesic effects similar to those of morphine and the other mu receptor agonists. *Sufentanil* is approximately 1,000 times the potency of morphine and is primarily used in the operating room either intravenously or neuraxially.[18] Like fentanyl, sufentanil is very lipophilic, and although their pharmacokinetic and pharmacodynamic profiles are similar, sufentanil has a smaller volume of distribution and shorter elimination half-life.[18] The high intrinsic potency of sufentanil makes it an excellent choice for epidural analgesia in the opioid-dependent patient.[19] *Alfentanil* is approximately 10 times the potency of morphine and, like sufentanil, is used primarily in the operating room either intravenously or neuraxially. *Remifentanil* is an ultra–short-acting synthetic opioid. The potency of the drug is approximately equal to that of fentanyl. Remifentanil is rapidly degraded by tissue and plasma esterases, which accounts for its incredibly short terminal elimination half-life of 10 to 20 minutes.[18] Rapid clearance and lack of accumulation make this a very desirable opioid in the operative setting. One disadvantage, however, is that discontinuation of a remifentanil infusion results in rapid loss of analgesia. There is also evidence to suggest that remifentanil infusions may be associated with the development of opioid-induced hyperalgesia. Further studies are clearly needed to better define this phenomenon.

Meperidine, a phenylpiperidine, is a synthetic mu opioid receptor agonist with a short half-life. The drug is recommended for the short-term management of acute pain only and has absolutely no role in the management of chronic pain. The drug is biotransformed by the liver to normeperidine, a potentially neurotoxic metabolite, which has a 12- to 16-hour half-life. Repetitive dosing of meperidine can cause accumulation of normeperidine, which may precipitate tremulousness, myoclonus, and seizures. It is therefore recommended that the total daily intravenous dose in an otherwise healthy adult without renal or central nervous system disease should not exceed 600 mg/day and should not be administered for longer than 48 hours.[20] We do not recommend administration of meperidine as an intravenous patient-controlled analgesia (PCA). The drug is contraindicated in patients receiving monoamine oxidase inhibitors as this may precipitate a syndrome characterized by muscle rigidity, hyperpyrexia, and seizures.

Methadone is a relatively inexpensive synthetic opioid considered to be a broad-spectrum opioid because it is a (1) mu receptor agonist, (2) NMDA antagonist, and (3) inhibitor of monoamine transmitter reuptake, making it potentially useful for the treatment of neuropathic pain. The drug is well absorbed from the gastrointestinal tract with a reported bioavailability of approximating 80%. The drug is extensively metabolized in the liver by the cytochrome P450 (CYP450) system to inactive metabolites, which are cleared in the bile and urine; unlike morphine, it is generally not necessary to adjust the dosage of methadone in patients with renal insufficiency. Methadone has an elimination half-life of 22 hours, and following a single dose the duration of analgesia is

TABLE 57-6

OPIOID ANALGESIC PHARMACOKINETICS

DRUG	ONSET OF EFFECT	PEAK EFFECT	DURATION OF EFFECT	ELIMINATION T ½	VD (L/kg)	PROTEIN BINDING (%)	METABOLISM PATHWAY	ACTIVE METABOLITES	MAJOR EXCRETION PATHWAY
Alfentanil	Immediate	1.5–2 min	<10 min	1.5–1.85 hr	0.4–1	92%	Liver	—	Urine
Codeine	Oral: 10–30 min, IV: 15 min	0.5–1 hr	Oral: 4–6 hr, IV: 5 hr	2.5–3 hr	—	—	Liver	Morphine	Urine
Fentanyl injection	IV: immediate, IM: 7–8 min	—	IV: 0.5–1 hr, IM: 1–2 hr	3.65 hr	4	Alters with increasing ionization	Liver	—	Urine
Fentanyl transdermal	—	24–72 hr	72 hr	≈17 hr	6	Decreases with increasing ionization	Liver: CYP3A4	—	Urine
Fentanyl transmucosal	—	—	—	7 hr	4	80%–85%	Liver: CYP3A4	—	Urine
Hydromor-phone	IM/Subcutaneous: 15 min Oral: 30 min	0.5–1 hr	IR: 4–5 hr, ER: 24 hr, IM/ Subcutaneous: 4–5 hr	IR: 2.3 hr, ER: 18.6 hr IM/Subcutaneous: 2.6 hr	≈4	8%–20%	Liver: glucuronidation	—	Urine
Levorphanol	IM: 15–30 min	Oral: 1 hr	2–4 hr	IV: 11–16 hr	IV: 10–13	40%	—	—	—
Meperidine	—	—	—	3–6 hr (parent), < 20 hr (normeperidine)	—	60%–80%	Liver	Normeperidine	—
Methadone	Parenteral: 10–20 min Oral: 30–60 min	—	4 hr	8–59 hr	2–6	85%–90%	Liver primarily CYP3A4 and to lesser extent CYP2D6	—	Urine and fecal
Morphine sulfate	IM/Subcutaneous: 10–30 min	Epidural: 10–15 min, Oral: 1 hr	Subcutaneous/IM: 4–5 hr	1.5–2 hr	1–6	20%–35%	Liver: glucuronidation	Morphine 6 glucuronide	Urine
Oxycodone	Within 60 min	—	IR: 3–4 hr CR[a]: 12 hr	IR: 3.2 hr, CR: 4.5 hr	2.6	45%	Liver: somewhat involves CYP2D6	Noroxycodone and oxymorphone	Urine
Oxymorphone	Parenteral: 5–10 min	—	Parenteral: 3–6 hr	1.3 hr	≈3	—	Liver	—	Urine
Propoxyphene	—	2–2.5 hr	—	6–12 hr (parent), 30–36 hr (norpropoxyphene)	—	80%	Liver	Norpropoxyphene	Urine
Remifentanil	Rapid	—	—	10–20 min	0.35	70%	Hydrolysis by esterases	—	Urine
Sufentanil	IV: immediate, Epidural: 10 min[b]	—	Epidural: 1.7 hr	2.7 hr	—	91%–93%, 79% in neonates	Liver and small intestine	—	Urine
Tramadol	—	—	2 hr (tramadol), 3 hr (M1, active metabolite)	6.3 hr (tramadol), 7.4 hr (M1, active metabolite)	2.6–2.9	20%	Liver: CYP2D6 and CYP3A4	O-desmethyl-tramadol (M1) via CYP2D6	Urine

IV, intravenous; CT, cytochrome; IR, immediate release; ER, extended release; IM, intramuscularly. Adapted with permission from Drug Facts and Comparisons, Wolter Kluwer Health.

TABLE 57-7

OPIOID EQUIANALGESIC DOSING

■ DRUG	■ IV/IM/SQ	■ ORAL (mg)
Morphine (MS Contin)	10 mg	30
Hydromorphone (Dilaudid)	1.5–2 mg	6–8
Hydrocodone (Vicodin)	NA	30–45
Oxymorphone (Opana IR and ER)	1 mg	10
Oxycodone (Percocet, Oxycontin)	10–15 mg	20
Levorphanol (Levo-Dromoran)	2 mg	4
Fentanyl	100 μg	NA
Meperidine (Demerol)	100 mg	300
Codeine	100 mg	200
Methadone	The conversion ratio for methadone is variable. Please see Table 57-8.	

IV, intravenous; IM, intramuscular; SQ, subcutaneous; IR, immediate release; ER, extended release.
Data derived from Carroll IR, Angst MS, Clark JD: Management of perioperative pain in patients chronically consuming opioids. Reg Anesth Pain Med 2004; 29: 576; Toombs JD, Kral LA: Methadone treatment for pain states. Am Fam Phys 2005; 71: 1353; Hadi I, Morley-Forster PK, Dain S et al: Brief review: Perioperative management of the patient with chronic non-cancer pain. Can J Anaesth 2006; 53: 1190.

approximately 3 to 6 hours. With repetitive dosing, however, methadone can accumulate and slow tissue release into the blood stream can result in a long elimination half-life of up to 128 hours and duration of analgesia of 8 to 12 hours. This long half-life explains the potential risk for cumulative toxicity, and therefore the importance of monitoring for side effects such as excessive sedation and confusion following the initiation of an around-the-clock dosing regimen.

Finally, opioid rotation is a very useful technique to restore analgesic sensitivity in the highly tolerant patient, and methadone is a common choice for opioid rotation. Because cross-tolerance is incomplete, the calculated equianalgesic dose of any new opioid is always lower than expected. One must be particularly cautious, however, when converting from morphine to methadone as the morphine/methadone equianalgesic ratio appears to be curvilinear; whereas the morphine-to-methadone conversion ratio is 3:1 at morphine doses of <100 mg/day, the ratio is 20:1 at morphine doses of >1,001 mg/day (Table 57-8). Methadone is principally metabolized by the CYP3A4 subtype enzyme of the cytochrome P450 system and to a lesser extent by the CYP1A2 and CYP2D6 subtypes. Consequently, there is the potential for numerous drug interactions with methadone, as shown in Table 57-9. Whereas

inhibition of methadone metabolism will theoretically provoke toxicity, induction of methadone metabolism could potentially precipitate inadequate analgesia or even withdrawal symptoms. Frequent adjustments of the methadone dosage may therefore be required if medications are added to or eliminated from a patient's drug regimen. A rare side effect associated with methadone is a pause-dependent dysrhythmia associated with bradycardia, QT prolongation, and Torsades de point.

Buprenorphine is a potent semisynthetic opioid that is derived from thebaine. The drug is classified as a mixed agonist-antagonist and partial mu receptor agonist with an analgesic potency 25 to 50 times greater than that of morphine. Buprenorphine is a lipophilic opioid with moderate intrinsic activity and a high affinity for the mu opioid receptor, with a half-life for dissociation from the receptor of 166 minutes compared with 7 minutes for fentanyl. The drug is metabolized by the gut and the liver and has a half-life of about 3 hours, but this bears little connection to the rate of disappearance of its clinical effects because of its avid binding to the mu receptor, as previously noted. The drug can be delivered by various routes of administration include: intravenous, intramuscular, neuraxial, subcutaneous, sublingual, and transdermal. Buprenorphine is also an excellent alternative for the treatment of acute pain in

TABLE 57-8

CONVERSION RATIOS FROM MORPHINE TO METHADONE

■ DAILY CHRONIC ORAL MORPHINE DOSE[a]		■ CONVERSION RATIO ORAL MORPHINE: ORAL METHADONE	
<100 mg	(e.g., 90 mg po morphine)	3:1	(e.g., 30 mg po methadone)
100–300 mg	(e.g., 300 mg po morphine)	5:1	(e.g., 60 mg po methadone)
300–600 mg	(e.g., 600 mg po morphine)	10:1	(e.g., 60 mg po methadone)
600–800 mg	(e.g., 720 mg po morphine)	12:1	(e.g., 60 mg po methadone)
800–1,000 mg	(e.g., 900 mg po morphine)	15:1	(e.g., 60 mg po methadone)
>1,000 mg	(e.g., 1,200 mg po morphine)	20:1	(e.g., 60 mg po methadone)

PO, by mouth.
[a]When converting from morphine to methadone use the table with caution. There is considerable variation from one individual to another. It is recommended that a clinician well versed in chronic pain therapy perform this task.
Data derived from Toombs JD, Kral LA: Methadone treatment for pain states. Am Fam Phys 2005; 71: 1353; Drug, Facts and Comparisons. St. Louis, MO, Wolters Kluwer Health, 2008; Ayonrinde OT, Bridge DT: The rediscovery of methadone for cancer pain management. Med J Austr 2000; 173: 536.

TABLE 57-9

METHADONE DRUG INTERACTIONS

■ CLINICAL SIGNIFICANCE	■ INCREASE METHADONE CONCENTRATION/EFFECTS	■ DECREASE METHADONE CONCENTRATION/EFFECTS
Documented clinical effects	Ciprofloxacin (Cipro), diazepam (Valium), ethanol (acute use), fluconazole (Diflucan), urinary alkalinizers	Amprenavir (Agenerase), efavirenz (Sustiva), nelfinavir (Viracept), nevirapine (Viramune), phenobarbital, phenytoin (Dilantin), rifampin (Rifadin), ritonavir (Norvir), urinary acidifiers
Documented enzyme effects	Cimetidine (Tagamet), fluoxetine (Prozac)	Carbamazepine (Tegretol)
Clinical effects uncertain	Omeprazole (Prilosec), quinidine, paroxetine (Paxil)	
Predicted interaction	Delavirdine (Rescriptor), grapefruit juice or fruit	Ethanol (chronic use)
No current clinical evidence	Ketoconazole (Nizoral), macrolide antibiotics (erythromycin, clarithromycin [Biaxin], troleandomycin [TAO]), tricyclic antidepressants, verapamil (Calan)	

Information derived from Raja SN, Dougherty PM: Anatomy and Physiology of Somatosensory and Pain Processing, Essentials of Pain Medicine and Regional Anesthesia, 2nd edition. Edited by Benzon HT, Raja SN, Molloy RE et al. Philadelphia, Elsevier, Churchill Livingstone, 2005, p 1; Rowlingson JC: Update on acute pain management. International Anesthesia Research Society Review Course Lectures 2006: 95; Power I: Recent advances in postoperative pain therapy. Br J Anaesth 2005; 95: 43; Weinbroum AA: A single small dose of postoperative ketamine provides rapid and sustained improvement in morphine analgesia in the presence of morphine-resistant pain. Anesth Analg 2003; 96: 789; Sveticic G, Gentilini A, Eichenberger U et al: Combinations of morphine with ketamine for patient-controlled analgesia: A new optimization method. Anesthesiology 2003; 98: 1195.

the patient who cannot tolerate morphine secondary to allergy or other sensitivity. In humans, buprenorphine is reported to have a ceiling effect for respiratory depression but not for analgesia. Buprenorphine is reported to have anti-inflammatory effects and therefore may be efficacious when administered intra-articularly. Investigators[21] have demonstrated that buprenorphine will significantly prolong the analgesic effects of a peripheral nerve block when 0.3 mg of the drug is combined with 40 mL of a local anesthetic mixture consisting of 1% mepivacaine, 0.2% tetracaine, and epinephrine 1:200,000.

NONOPIOID ANALGESIC ADJUNCTS

The *NSAIDs* are among the most commonly used drugs in the world because of their anti-inflammatory, analgesic, and antipyretic effects (Table 57-10). The therapeutic benefit of NSAIDs is believed to be mediated through the inhibition of cyclo-oxygenase (COX) enzymes, types 1 and 2, which convert arachidonic acid to prostaglandins. COX-1 is the constitutive enzyme that produces prostaglandins, which are important for general "house-keeping" functions such as gastric protection and hemostasis. COX-2, on the other hand, is the inducible form of the enzyme that produces prostaglandins that mediate pain, inflammation, fever, and carcinogenesis. Prostaglandin E_2 is the key mediator of both peripheral and central pain sensitization. Peripherally, prostaglandins do not directly mediate pain; rather, they contribute to hyperalgesia by sensitizing nociceptors to other mediators of pain sensation such as histamine and bradykinin.[22] Centrally, prostaglandins enhance pain transmission at the level of the dorsal horn by (1) increasing the release of substance P and glutamate from first-order pain neurons, (2) increasing the sensitivity of second-order pain neurons, and (3) inhibiting the release of neurotransmitters from the descending pain-modulating pathways.

NSAIDs have proved effective in the treatment of postoperative pain. In addition, they are opioid-sparing and can significantly decrease the incidence of opioid-related side effects such as postoperative nausea and vomiting and sedation.[23] Unlike the opioids, NSAIDs exhibit a "ceiling effect" with respect to maximum analgesic effects. Parenteral NSAIDs such as ketorolac are commonly employed as part of a multimodal approach for acute perioperative pain management. The optimal dose of ketorolac for postoperative pain control is 15 to 30 mg intravenously every 6 to 8 hours not to exceed 5 days. The dose should be decreased in patients with renal failure.

Despite the benefits of NSAIDs in the perioperative period they are not without some significant side effects. Platelet dysfunction, gastrointestinal ulceration, and an increased risk of nephrotoxicity are several reasons why the nonselective NSAIDs may be avoided in the perioperative period. The risk of nephrotoxicity is increased in patients with hypovolemia, congestive heart failure, and chronic renal insufficiency.[22] The COX-2 selective inhibitors were developed in an attempt to minimizing their side effects. Three COX-2–specific inhibitors celecoxib (Celebrex), rofecoxib (Vioxx), and valdecoxib (Bextra) have recently been available in the United States. Unfortunately, the latter two have been removed from the market because of concerns about adverse cardiovascular risks. Celecoxib is the only COX-2–specific inhibitor currently available in the United States for acute postoperative pain. The recommended oral loading dose is a 400 mg followed by 200 mg orally every 12 hours for several days. Parecoxib (Dynastat) is an injectable COX-2–specific inhibitor that is available only in Europe for the treatment of moderate-to-severe postoperative pain. The recommended dose of the drug in Europe is 40 mg intravenously or intramuscularly initially followed by 20 to 40 mg every 4 to 6 hours not to exceed 80 mg/day. Unlike the nonselective NSAIDs, however, COX-2–specific inhibitors offer the potential advantages of a reduced incidence of gastrointestinal ulceration and they do not inhibit platelet function. Because prostaglandins play a crucial role in renal function

TABLE 57-10

NONOPIOID ANALGESICS (ADULT DOSING GUIDELINES)

■ DRUG	■ ROUTE	■ HALF-LIFE (hr)	■ DOSE (mg)	■ COMMENTS
Para-aminophenols				
Acetaminophen	po	2	500–1,000 mg q4–6 hr Maximum daily dose (MDD) in the healthy adult is 4,000 mg.	Hepatotoxicity can occur in chronic alcoholics receiving therapeutic doses.
Salicylates				
Acetylsalicylic acid	po	0.25	500–1,000 mg q4–6 hr MDD is 4,000 mg in the healthy adult.	Salicylic acid has a $T_{1/2}$ 2–3 hr @ low doses and >20 hr at higher doses. Because of the risk of Reyes syndrome avoid the use of aspirin in children <12 years old.
Diflunisal	po	8–12	500 mg q8–12 hr Loading dose (LD) = 1,000 mg	Decrease the dose in the elderly to 500–1,000 mg/day
Choline magnesium trisalicylate	po	9–17	1,000–1,500 mg q12 hr	Unlike aspirin does not increase bleeding time. MDD = 2,000–3,000 mg
NSAID's				
Propionic acids				
Ibuprofen	po	2	400 mg q4–6 hr	MDD is 2,400 mg
Naproxen	po	12–15	250 mg q6–8 hr	LD = 500 mg. MDD = 1,500 mg
Ketoprofen	po	2.1	25–50 mg q6–8 hr	MDD = 300 mg
Oxaprozin	po	42–50	600 mg q12–24 hr	MDD = 1,200 mg
Indolacetic acids				
Indomethacin	po	2	25 mg q8–12 hr	MDD = 200 mg
Sulindac	po	7.8	150 mg q12 hr	MDD = 400 mg. Active metabolite has a half-life of 16 hr
Etodolac	po	7.3	300–400 mg q8–12 hr	MDD = 1,000 mg
Pyrrolacetic acids				
Ketorolac	IV	6	30 mg initially followed by 15–30 mg q6–8 hr not to exceed 5 days.	MDD = 120 mg. Hypovolemia should be corrected prior to administration. Decrease the dose in the elderly (>65 years of age) and in renal failure.
Phenylacetic acids				
Diclofenac potassium	po	2	50 mg q8 hr	MDD = 150 mg
Enolic acids (Oxicams)				
Meloxicam	po	15–20	7.5–15 mg q24 hr	
Piroxicam	po	50	20–40 mg q24 hr	
Naphthylalkanone				
Nabumetone	po	22.5	500–750 mg q8–12 hr	LD = 1,000 mg. MDD = 2,000 mg. Active metabolite has half-life = 22.5 hr
COX-2 inhibitor				
Celecoxib	po	11	100–200 mg q12 hr	LD = 400 mg. MDD = 400 mg. Avoid this drug in patients allergic to sulfonamides.

PO, by month; COX-2, cyclooxygenase.
Data derived from Principles of Analgesic Use in the Treatment of Acute Pain and Cancer Pain, fifth edition. Glenview, IL, American Pain Society, 2003; Drug, Facts and Comparisons. St. Louis, MO, Wolters Kluwer Health, 2008.

through their affect on blood flow, natriuresis and glomerular filtration, traditional NSAIDs and the COX-2 inhibitors can cause fluid retention and hypertension.

Short-term use of parecoxib and valdecoxib in patients following coronary artery bypass surgery is associated with an increased risk of thromboembolic events.[24]

The authors, therefore, do not recommend prescribing a COX-2 inhibitor for patients with a known history of coronary artery disease or cerebrovascular disease. Both COX-1 and COX-2 play significant roles in bone fusion following fracture, and the use of the traditional NSAIDs has been found to inhibit the healing process, particularly following lumbar spinal fusion surgery. The effect of COX-2 inhibitors on bone fusion following orthopaedic procedures continues to be controversial, and no recommendations can be made at this time. NSAIDs and COX-2–selective inhibitors should not be administered to patients with known hypersensitivity to the drugs or to patients with Samters triad (aka aspirin triad), which is a medical condition consisting of asthma, aspirin insensitivity, and nasal polyposis. Finally, avoid celecoxib and valdecoxib in patients with allergic-type reactions to sulfonamides.

The *para-aminophenol* derivative acetaminophen (aka paracetamol) has both analgesic and antipyretic properties, similar to aspirin, but is devoid of any anti-inflammatory effects. The mechanism of action of the drug is considered to be inhibition of a putative central cyclooxygenase, COX-3, that results in decreased production of prostaglandins in the CNS. In addition there may be modulation of descending inhibitory serotoninergic pathways and the drug may act on the opioidergic system and NMDA receptors. Acetaminophen is devoid of many of the side effects generally associated with the NSAIDs, such as gastrointestinal ulceration, impaired platelet function, adverse cardiorenal effects, and impairment of bone fusion following orthopaedic procedures. Acetaminophen is opioid-sparing and can be used in conjunction with an NSAID as part of a multimodal analgesic program. In adults, 2 g of oral acetaminophen is equivalent to 200 mg of celecoxib.[25]

Propacetamol is the intravenous prodrug formulation of paracetamol and is a popular adjuvant for perioperative pain control in Europe. The drug has the disadvantage that it must be reconstituted prior to administration. Two grams of propacetamol is equivalent to 1 g of paracetamol. Fortunately, a ready-to-use intravenous formulation of paracetamol (Perfalgan) has been released in Europe.[26] The intravenous formulation of acetaminophen would be a useful addition to our analgesic regimen; however, at the time of this writing, it is not yet available in the United States.

The *NMDA receptor antagonists* such as ketamine and dextromethorphan may be useful analgesic adjuncts. Excitatory neurotransmitter stimulation of the NMDA receptor is believed to be involved in the development and maintenance of several phenomena including: (1) persistent postoperative pain, (2) hypersensitivity, wind-up and allodynia, (3) opioid-induced tolerance, and (4) OIH. Low-dose ketamine (0.25- to 0.5-mg intravenous bolus followed by an infusion of 2 to 4 μg/kg/min) can provide significant analgesia and is opioid-sparing. The mechanism of action of ketamine is NMDA receptor blockade, but in addition the drug interacts with opioidergic, cholinergic, and monoaminergic receptors and blocks sodium channels.[27]

NMDA receptor antagonists may act synergistically when combined with an opioid. The ideal intravenous PCA morphine-ketamine combination ratio is 1:1 with an 8-minute lockout.[28] A double-blind study, however, demonstrates that the combination of ketamine (1 mg/mL) with morphine (1 mg/mL) administered as an intravenous PCA to patients following major abdominal surgery does not significantly improve pain relief.[29] In patients with morphine-resistant pain, however, the combination of 250 μg/kg of ketamine plus 15 μg/kg of morphine has been reported to provide significant analgesia.[27] Results are promising, but more studies will certainly be required to clearly define the role of ketamine for postoperative analgesia.

Dextromethorphan, the d-isomer of the codeine analogue levorphanol, is a noncompetitive NMDA receptor antagonist that has been used for many years as an antitussive. Dextromethorphan does not have a direct analgesic affect; rather, analgesia is likely mediated by its NMDA receptor antagonism. The drug can be administered orally, intravenously, and intramuscularly. There is a sustained-release suspension available that contains dextromethorphan, 30 mg/5 mL, and is marketed as Delsym™ (Adams Respiratory Therapeutics). Following oral administration the drug is metabolized to dextrorphan, which is the metabolite that accounts for most of the side effects, the most common of which is nausea and vomiting. Because the intravenous administration of large doses can lead to hypotension and tachycardia, the intramuscular route may be the preferred route of delivery. Dextromethorphan has been shown to both inhibit secondary hyperalgesia following peripheral burn injury and cause a reduction in temporal summation of pain. The preoperative administration of 150 mg of oral dextromethorphan can reduce the PCA morphine requirements of patients undergoing abdominal hysterectomy, and the preincisional administration of 120 mg of intramuscular dextromethorphan provides pre-emptive analgesia in patients undergoing elective upper abdominal surgery. Finally, a randomized double-blind placebo-controlled study[30] has demonstrated that dextromethorphan dosed 200 mg orally every 8 hours (e.g., 2 hours prior to surgery then 8 hours and 16 hours thereafter) can provide a modest reduction in morphine consumption following knee surgery.

The α_2-adrenergic agonists clonidine (half-life, 9 to 12 hours) and dexmedetomidine (half-life, 2 hours) may be administered perioperatively to provide analgesia, sedation, and anxiolysis. The presynaptic activation of α_2-receptors that results in the decreased release of norepinephrine is believed to mediate analgesia. Whereas clonidine is a selective partial agonist for the α_2-adrenoreceptor, dexmedetomidine is super selective for the receptor. Their respective α_2/α_1 binding ratios are 220:1 for clonidine versus 1,620:1 for dexmedetomidine. Analgesia is mediated supraspinally (locus coeruleus), spinally (substantia gelatinosa), and peripherally. Dexmedetomidine is reported to have greater affinity for the 2A subtype of the receptor, which may account for the drug's superior analgesic properties vis-à-vis clonidine. Clonidine can be administered orally, transdermally, intravenously, and neuraxially for perioperative pain management. Premedication with 5 μg/kg of oral clonidine in patients undergoing knee surgery can decrease the use of PCA morphine and decrease the incidence of postoperative nausea and vomiting. In addition the combination of oral clonidine, 3 to 5 μg/kg with 0.2 mg/24 hours of transdermal clonidine can decrease postoperative PCA morphine requirement by 50% following prostatectomy surgery. In a double-blind placebo-controlled study, investigators demonstrated that addition of 25 μg of intrathecal clonidine to a bupivacaine (15 mg) morphine (250 μg) spinal anesthetic cocktail, for total knee arthroplasty, could reduce postoperative morphine use and improve VAS pain scores at 24 hours.[31] Clonidine in doses of 0.5 to 1 μg/kg may enhance the efficacy and increase the duration of local anesthetics in peripheral nerve blockade. In addition, the intra-articular use of clonidine can be beneficial. Side effects include sedation, hypotension, and bradycardia if the dose exceeds 150 μg as part of a peripheral nerve block.

Dexmedetomidine is the D-enantiomer of medetomidine. It is a highly selective α_2-agonist that does not interact with the GABA-mimetic system and therefore does not depress the respiratory drive.[32] Other advantages include analgesia, titratable sedation (e.g., "cooperative sedation"), and anxiolysis. In addition, the centrally mediated reduction in sympathetic tone is reported to have a cardioprotective effect, particularly in high-risk patients undergoing vascular surgery. There is a low incidence of bradycardia and hypotension, which can be treated with atropine, ephedrine, or volume infusion.[32] Dexmedetomidine is a useful adjunct to both opioid and nonopioid analgesics as part of a multimodal analgesic protocol. Combining the drug with ketamine and opioids can obviate the respiratory depressant effects of the latter and the psychomimetic effects of the former.[33] Although the recommended dose of dexmedetomidine is a loading dose of 1 μg/kg intravenously over 10 minutes followed by an infusion of 0.2 to 0.7 μg/kg/hr,[32] infusions as high as 5 to 10 μg/kg/hr have been reported by some authors for use as a total intravenous anesthetic with favorable results.[34] A dexmedetomidine infusion (0.2 to 0.7 μg/kg/hr) combined with peripheral nerve blockade may provide superb analgesia, anxiolysis, and sedation during prolonged procedures.

The α_2-δ *subunit calcium channel ligands*, (e.g., gabapentin and pregabalin) are effective analgesics not only for the treatment of neuropathic pain syndromes but also for the treatment of postoperative pain. Furthermore, when these drugs are combined with an NSAID, the combination has been shown to be synergistic in attenuating the hyperalgesia associated with peripheral inflammation. Gabapentin prevents the development of central excitability and is antihyperalgesic. Meta-analysis of the analgesic effects of gabapentin suggests that it should be part of any multimodal analgesic regimen for perioperative pain management.[35] In a double-blinded, randomized, placebo-controlled study,[36] gabapentin was administered as a 1,200-mg oral dose 1 to 2 hours prior to surgery in patients scheduled to undergo elective arthroscopic anterior cruciate ligament repair. Advantages of this regimen included a 50% reduction in postoperative morphine consumption and improved early knee flexion following surgery. In another double-blind placebo-controlled study,[37] patients undergoing abdominal hysterectomy reported superior postoperative analgesia following the administration of gabapentin 1 to 2 hours preoperatively. The recommended adult dose of gabapentin as part of a multimodal pain regimen for postoperative pain management is 900 mg orally 1 to 2 hours prior to surgery.[38]

Pregabalin is another analogue of GABA that may be useful for the treatment of perioperative pain. Side effects associated with these drugs include somnolence, dizziness, confusion, and ataxia. The available data suggest these drugs may be useful analgesics but further investigation is needed to better define useful drug combinations and dosing regimens.

The *local anesthetic* lidocaine has been shown to be analgesic, antihyperalgesic, and anti-inflammatory following intravenous administration.[39] The perioperative infusion of lidocaine has been shown to not only improve postoperative analgesia in patients recovering from laparoscopic colectomy, but it also can decrease postoperative opioid requirements, attenuate postoperative ileus, and accelerate time to discharge from the hospital.[39] Further studies are certainly warranted to establish both the safety and efficacy of this novel approach.

The *glucocorticoids* are well known for their analgesic, anti-inflammatory, and antiemetic effects.[40] Inhibition of cytosolic phospholipase A_2 upstream from the lipoxygenase and COX enzymes in the prostaglandin cascade most certainly accounts for both their anti-inflammatory and analgesic effects by inhibiting leukotriene and prostaglandin production.[40] The mechanism of the antiemetic effect of the corticosteroids is less clearly understood but appears to be centrally mediated.[41] Although corticosteroids are well recognized as effective analgesics following oral surgery, the analgesic benefits following general surgery, orthopaedic surgery, and back surgery have had mixed reviews. Results from a recent study[41] suggest that the combination of dexamethasone (8 mg intravenously) and gabapentin (800 mg orally) administered 1 hour prior to varicocele surgery improves postoperative analgesia and decreases the incidence of postoperative nausea and vomiting. Side effects associated with the use of corticosteroids include gastrointestinal upset, impairment of the immune system, and delayed wound healing; however, because of the small doses used perioperatively, corticosteroids are considered to be relatively safe.[40] Future studies will better define the role of corticosteroids in perioperative pain management.

METHODS OF ANALGESIA

Patient-Controlled Analgesia

PCA is any technique of pain management that allows the patients to administer their own analgesia on demand. We will highlight some important aspects of PCA as a complete review of PCA is beyond the scope of this chapter; we refer the reader to the comprehensive review by Macintyre[42] on this topic. In the United States the most commonly used drugs are morphine, hydromorphone, and fentanyl. Hydromorphone is recommended as an alternative in renal failure; however, fentanyl might be a better choice as it has no active metabolites. Meperidine is not recommended for use in an intravenous PCA secondary to accumulation of its potentially toxic metabolite normeperidine.

The five variables associated with all modes of PCA include: (1) bolus dose, (2) incremental (demand) dose, (3) lockout interval, (4) background infusion rate, and (5) 1- and 4-hour limits.[42] A typical PCA regimen in an otherwise healthy adult would be an incremental dose of 1 to 2 mg of morphine with an 8- 10-minute lockout (Table 57-11). The authors do not recommend a background infusion of opioid in the opioid-naive patient. A background infusion should be reserved for the patient with chronic malignant or nonmalignant pain who is opioid-tolerant or in patients with persistent pain who have failed a trial of incremental PCA dosing. In the elderly the dose of the PCA should be decreased. The relative risk factors for use of an opioid PCA are listed in Table 57-12. If more than two risk factors exist, you may want to avoid using a PCA in the standard dosing regimen and administer opioids only as needed.

TABLE 57-11

USUAL INTRAVENOUS OPIOID PATIENT-CONTROLLED ANALGESIA REGIMENS IN THE OPIOID-NAIVE ADULT PATIENT

OPIOID	DEMAND DOSE	LOCKOUT (min)	BASAL INFUSION
Morphine	1–2 mg	6–10	0–2 mg/hr
Hydromorphone	0.2–0.4 mg	6–10	0–0.4 mg/hr
Fentanyl	20–50 μg	5–10	0–60 μg/hr
Sufentanil	4–6 μg	5–10	0–8 μg/hr
Tramadol	10–20 mg	6–10	0–20 mg/hr

Data derived from Macintyre PE: Safety and efficacy of patient-controlled analgesia. Br J Anaesth 2001; 87: 36; Grass JA: Patient-controlled analgesia. Anesth Analg 2005; 101(Suppl): S44.

RELATIVE RISK FACTORS ASSOCIATED WITH THE USE OF PATIENT-CONTROLLED ANALGESIA

Pulmonary disease
Obstructive sleep apnea
Renal or hepatic dysfunction
Congestive heart failure
Closed head injury
Altered mental status
Lactating mothers

Opioid-related side effects include nausea and vomiting, pruritus, sedation, and confusion. Consensus guidelines for the treatment of nausea and vomiting include prescribing various combinations of dopamine antagonists, serotonin antagonists, and glucocorticoids.[43] Pruritus can be ameliorated with the use of diphenhydramine, hydroxyzine, or a low dose of an opioid antagonist (e.g., naloxone) or mixed agonist-antagonist (e.g., nalbuphine). Excessive sedation may respond to a change in the opioid; however, use of a multimodal analgesic technique, which incorporates the use of a regional anesthetic (e.g., epidural or peripheral nerve blockade), an NSAID, acetaminophen, or other nonopioid analgesics such as an NMDA receptor antagonist or an α_2-δ subunit calcium channel ligand, will have an opioid-sparing effect, which should attenuate opioid induced sedation.

Neuraxial Analgesia

Although opioid analgesics have been prescribed to patients for many centuries, the exact mechanism of action was not completely understood until 1971 when the opioid receptor was discovered. Within 5 years time, Yaksh reported that morphine could produce spinally mediated analgesia in a rat model. Soon thereafter in 1979 and 1981, respectfully, Wang and then Onofrio reported significant pain relief following the neuraxial administration of morphine in patients with severe cancer-related pain. Since these discoveries, the intrathecal administration of opioids and the epidural administration of opioids plus a local anesthetic has produced significant comfort for our patients.

Epidural analgesia is a critical component of multimodal perioperative pain management and improved patient outcome. Meta-analysis investigating the efficacy of epidural analgesia found epidural analgesia to be superior to systemically administered opioids.[44] The efficacy of an epidural technique is determined by numerous factors that can include: (1) catheter incision site congruency, (2) choice of analgesic drugs, (3) rates of infusion, (4) duration of epidural analgesia, and (5) type of pain assessment (rest vs. dynamic).[44] Ideally, the epidural catheter is positioned congruent with the surgical incision (Fig. 57-11). Thoracic epidural catheter placement is recommended for both thoracic and upper abdominal surgical procedures because of the observed improvement in coronary artery blood flow, attenuation of pulmonary complications, and the reduction in the duration of postoperative ileus. Combining a local anesthetic plus an opioid in the epidural

FIGURE 57-11. Dermatome guide for placement of epidural catheters.

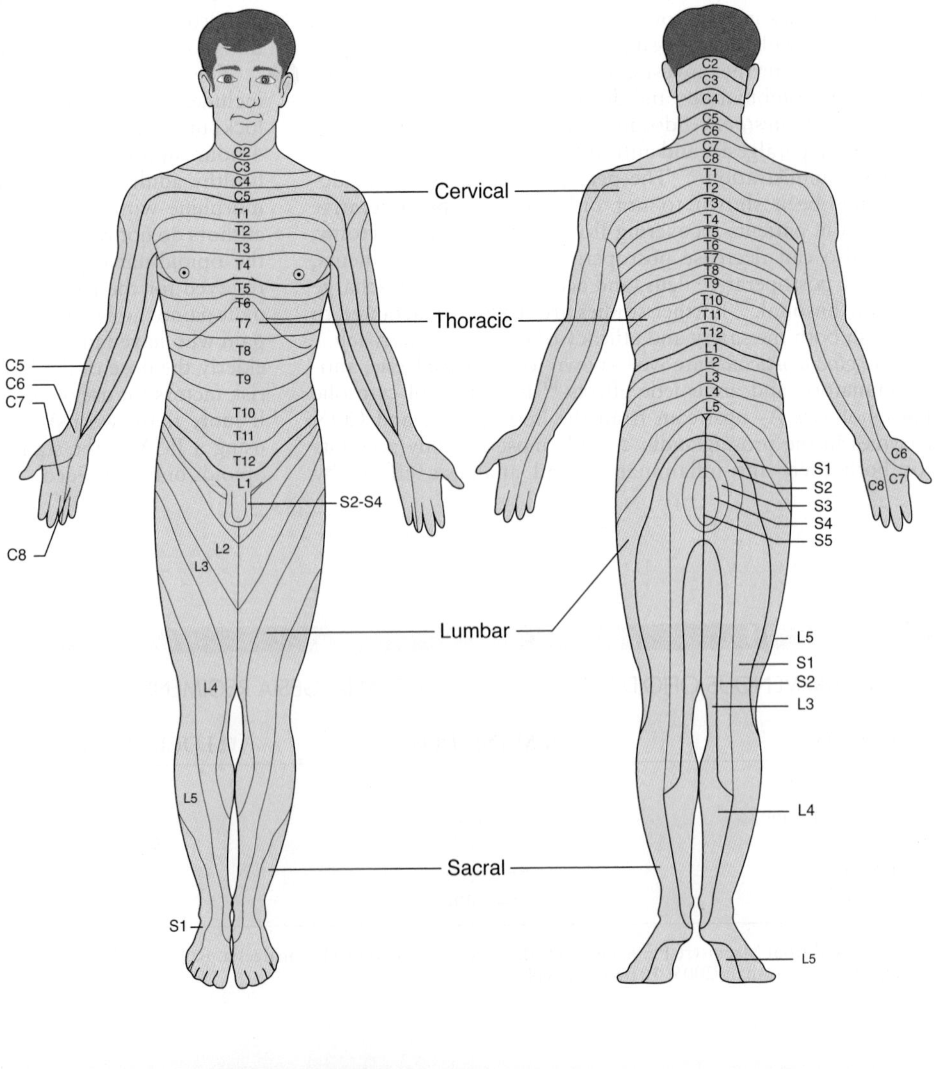

space is believed to have a synergistic effect.[44] The optimal duration of epidural analgesia has not been determined, but recommendations are that the infusion be continued for at least 2 to 4 days. Other than analgesia, epidural infusions lasting <24 hours do not appear to offer any clear cardiovascular advantages.

Epidurally administered opioids have the distinct advantage of producing analgesia without causing significant sympatholytic effect or motor blockade. Analgesia occurs by way of a *spinal mechanism* and through a *supraspinal mechanism* following systemic adsorption. The spinal mechanism occurs following diffusion of the drug into the spinal fluid, and is determined by meningeal permeability. Opioids with intermediate lipophilicity (e.g., hydromorphone, alfentanil, meperidine) have the ability to easily move between the aqueous and lipid regions of the arachnoid membrane and therefore have high meningeal permeability, which potentially confers higher bioavailability in the spinal cord. However, in a comprehensive review of the topic Bernards et al.[45] concluded that morphine has greater bioavailability in the spinal cord than alfentanil, fentanyl, and sufentanil.

In general, the epidural administration of hydrophilic opioids tends to have a slow onset, long duration, and a mechanism of action that is primarily spinal in nature. The epidural administration of lipophilic opioids, on the other hand, have a quick onset, short duration, and a mechanism of action that is primarily supraspinal, secondary to rapid systemic uptake. However, the data are controversial and the site of action of lipophilic opioids such as fentanyl may primarily be determined by the mode of administration.[46] Bolus administration of fentanyl appears to have a segmental analgesic effect whereas epidural infusion of fentanyl appears to have a nonsegmental (systemic) effect. There are some data, however, that suggest that there can be significant spinal mechanisms of action of the lipophilic opioids, particularly with the thoracic epidural infusion of fentanyl. In the opioid-tolerant patient taking >250 mg/day of oral morphine, sufentanil may be considered to be the epidural opioid of choice because of its high intrinsic activity.

As previously mentioned, local anesthetic-opioid combinations are the most common form of epidural infusion because the combination is considered to be synergistic.[44] Local anesthetics have the unique ability to block the stress response by blocking afferent input to the spinal cord. Although bupivacaine plus fentanyl may be the most common combination, bupivacaine plus morphine makes more sense from a bioavailability point of view. Hydromorphone plus bupivacaine also makes very good sense as this combination has all the advantages of a hydrophilic opioid with excellent meningeal permeability but less risk of pruritus. Remember, epidural infusions may consist of just a hydrophilic opioid if the patient cannot tolerate side effects from the local anesthetic or if the epidural is incongruent with the surgical incision. Likewise, an epidural infusion may consist simply of a local anesthetic if the patient cannot tolerate opioid-related side effects, provided that the epidural is correctly placed and is congruent with the surgical incision. Table 57-13 contains epidural dosing guidelines.

TABLE 57-13

GUIDELINES FOR ADULT EPIDURAL CATHETER DOSING REGIMEN[a]

■ CATHETER PLACEMENT	■ SURGICAL DERMATOME		
	Lumbar (e.g., total knee arthroplasty or lower extremity bypass surgery)	Low thoracic (e.g., exploratory laparotomy, xiphopubic incision)	Mid-to-high thoracic (e.g., thoracotomy, sternotomy)
Lumbar T$_{12}$-Caudal	Catheter congruent with incision! Bupivacaine 0.05–0.1% or Ropivacaine 0.1–0.2% with Fentanyl 2–5 μg/mL or morphine 0.1 mg/mL or hydromorphone 0.02 mg/mL	Catheter/incision incongruency! [c]May consider Bupivacaine or Ropivacaine with a hydrophilic opioid. *This is not ideal!* [d]Hydrophilic opioids are required! 1. Morphine 0.1 mg/mL or 2. Hydromorphone 0.02 mg/mL	Not Applicable
Low thoracic T$_8$-T1$_{12}$	Not Applicable	Catheter congruent with incision! Bupivacaine 0.05–0.1% or Ropivacaine 0.1–0.2% with Fentanyl 2–5 μg/mL or morphine 0.1 mg/mL or hydromorphone 0.02 mg/mL	Catheter/incision incongruency! [c]May consider Bupivacaine or Ropivacaine with an opioid but *this is not ideal!* Lipophilic Fentanyl 2–5 μg/mL. *This is not the ideal opioid!* [d]Hydrophilic opioids are a better choice! 1. Morphine 0.1 mg/mL or 2. Hydromorphone 0.02 mg/mL
Mid-to-high thoracic T$_4$-T$_8$	Not Applicable	Not Applicable	Catheter Congruent with incision! Bupivacaine 0.05–0.1% or Ropivacaine 0.1–0.2% with Fentanyl 2–5 μg/mL or morphine 0.1 mg/mL or hydromorphone 0.02 mg/mL

[a]Rate of infusion, 2–10 mL/hr. Recommended adult dose for epidural bupivacaine. Do not exceed 400 mg/24 hr!
[b]May consider Clonidine 2 μg/mL in the epidural. Remember hypotension, bradycardia, and sedation are common at doses greater than 14 μg/hr.
[c]Local anesthetic efficacy is diminished with catheter/incision incongruency!
[d]Hydrophilic opioids provide a broad band of analgesia! Morphine is the gold-standard. Epidural hydromorphone may cause less pruritus.

PERIOPERATIVE AND CONSULTATIVE SERVICES

Adjuvant medications, which may enhance analgesia, include clonidine and ketamine. Clonidine (2 μg/mL) can be combined with an opioid and a local anesthetic and is usually infused at a rate of 5 to 20 μg/hr. Side effects that limit its clinical usefulness include hypotension, bradycardia, and sedation. An epidural infusion consisting of ropivacaine 0.2%, fentanyl 5 μg/mL, and clonidine 2 μg/mL infused at a rate of 3 to 7 mL/hr following a total knee arthroplasty has been reported to cause no significant sedation in this dosage range.[47] The safety of epidurally administered ketamine has not been determined, and routine use cannot be recommended at this time.

A novel approach to postoperative pain control is extended-release epidural morphine (Depodur). The system consists of morphine encapsulated within a liposome delivery system, which provides controlled release of morphine for up to 48 hours. Double-blinded studies indicate that the epidural administration of liposomal morphine has proven to be efficacious in the treatment of postoperative pain associated with total hip arthroplasty, total knee arthroplasty, and cesarean section. Depodur is only approved for lumbar epidural administration.

Intrathecal analgesia with a variety of drugs is a widely accepted practice for the treatment of both acute and chronic pain. Rathmell et al.[48] have thoroughly reviewed the role of intrathecal analgesia for acute pain. Opioid analgesics are the most commonly administered drugs for this purpose, including morphine, hydromorphone, meperidine, methadone, fentanyl, and sufentanil. Their distribution within the intrathecal space following administration is complex. Hydrophilic opioids (e.g., morphine) penetrate the spinal cord and bind to specific pre- and postsynaptic receptors within the dorsal horn. They traverse the dura slowly, bind to epidural fat poorly, and slowly enter the plasma. They tend to have a slow onset of action, long duration, and provide a broad band of analgesia. Delayed respiratory depression is more common with hydrophilic opioids secondary to rostral spread.[48] Lipophilic opioids (e.g., fentanyl), on the other hand, tend to bind to nonspecific receptors in the white matter. They rapidly cross the dura and are quickly sequestered into epidural fat and swiftly enter the systemic circulation. As a general rule lipophilic opioids tend to have a rapid onset of action, short duration, and a narrow band of analgesia. Delayed respiratory depression is less of a problem with the lipophilic opioids. Other side effects associated with intrathecal opioids include nausea and vomiting, urinary retention, and pruritus. The incidence of pruritus with intrathecal hydromorphone is reported to be significantly less than with morphine (refer to Table 57-14 for dosing guidelines).

Other useful analgesic additives include the α_2-agonists, NSAIDs, NMDA receptor antagonists, acetylcholinesterase inhibitors, adenosine, epinephrine, and benzodiazepines. The α_2-agonists alter pain transmission by binding to pre- and postsynaptic receptors within the dorsal horn of the spinal cord. Evidence suggests that intrathecal clonidine is synergistic with spinal local anesthetics, prolongs sensory and motor blockade, and causes less urinary retention than intrathecal morphine.[48] Intrathecal clonidine does not cause respiratory depression or pruritus. Intrathecal doses of 150 μg, however, are reported to increase the incidence of hypotension, bradycardia, and nausea[48] (refer to Table 57-15 for additional dosing recommendations). Anecdotal reports suggest that the neuraxial administration of an NSAID, either accidentally or intentionally, is both safe and effective. Further investigation for the treatment of postoperative pain is required of the role of intrathecal NSAIDs, as well as the acetylcholinesterase inhibitors, NMDA receptor antagonists, adenosine, and benzodiazepines.

Peripheral Nerve Blockade

Single-injection peripheral nerve blockade has been shown to provide pain control that is superior to opioids with fewer side effects.[49] Single-injection techniques are limited in duration but continuous peripheral nerve block (CPNB) techniques can extend the benefits of peripheral nerve blockade well into the postoperative period. CPNB has proven to be an effective technique for postoperative pain management; it is superior to opioid analgesia with fewer opioid related side effects[50] and rare neurologic and infectious complications.[51] The benefits of CPNB in the ambulatory setting include prolonged postoperative analgesia, facilitated discharge from the hospital, fewer opioid-related side effects, and greater patient satisfaction.[52] Finally, CPNB has proven to be an extraordinarily useful technique in the austere and remote environment of the battlefield by providing site-specific and opioid-sparing analgesia for the wounded soldier. Tables 57-16 and 57-17 present indications and contraindications for specific peripheral nerve blocks. Table 57-18 has recommended dosing regimen of CPNB.

The Brachial Plexus

Above the Clavicle. The *interscalene block* is the ideal peripheral nerve block for painful orthopaedic and vascular procedures performed on the shoulder and upper arm, but is a poor choice for forearm and hand surgery as the ulnar nerve is

---

TABLE 57-14

INTRATHECAL ANALGESIA DOSING GUIDELINES[a]

■ SURGICAL PROCEDURE	■ INTRATHECAL DRUG DOSE
Labor analgesia	Sufentanil 2.5–5.0 μg
Cesarean section (C-section)	Morphine 100 μg. The addition of clonidine 60 μg is synergistic and can increase the duration of spinal analgesia after C-section but also increases intraoperative sedation.
Outpatient knee arthroscopy	Fentanyl 10–25 μg will improve intraoperative analgesia without prolonging postoperative motor blockade.
Total knee arthroscopy	Morphine 200–300 μg
Total hip arthroplasty	Morphine 100–200 μg
Thoracotomy and major abdominal surgery	Morphine 500 μg. The incidence of side effects such as nausea and vomiting, urinary retention, and pruritus increase significantly with doses >300 μg.

[a]NOTE: 50–100 μg of intrathecal hydromorphone approximates 100–200 μg of intrathecal morphine.
Data derived from Principles of Analgesic Use in the Treatment of Acute Pain and Cancer Pain, fifth edition. Glenview, IL, American Pain Society, 2003; Rathmell JP, Lair TR, Nauman B: The role of intrathecal drugs in the treatment of acute pain. Anesth Analg 2005; 101(5 Suppl): S30.

TABLE 57-15

INTRATHECAL ANALGESIA OTHER DOSING GUIDELINES

■ INTRATHECAL DRUG	■ DOSING	■ COMMENTS
Clonidine	15–45 μg improves the quality of spinal blockade in outpatient surgery.	Side effects increase significantly at intrathecal doses >150 μg.
Epinephrine	0.1–0.6 mg Dose related increase 1. Return of motor function 2. Return of micturition	Not recommended for outpatient surgery
Neostigmine	6.25–50 μg Dose related increase: 1. Motor blockade 2. Time for resolution of the block 3. Nausea and vomiting	Further studies of the appropriate intrathecal dose that optimizes analgesia while minimizing side effects are warranted.

Data derived from Rathmell JP, Lair TR, Nauman B: The role of intrathecal drugs in the treatment of acute pain. Anesth Analg 2005; 101(5 Suppl): S30; Liu SS, McDonald SB: Current issues in spinal anesthesia. Anesthesiology 2001; 94: 888.

TABLE 57-16

BRACHIAL PLEXUS BLOCKADE

■ PERIPHERAL NERVE BLOCK	■ INDICATIONS	■ CONTRAINDICATIONS	■ COMMENTS
Interscalene	Total shoulder arthroplasty, and hemiarthroplasty Open rotator cuff repair Open anterior reconstruction Open reduction, internal fixation (ORIF) and joint fusion.	Refusal by the patient, infection, or hematoma in the vicinity of the block, allergy to local anesthetics, and progressive neuropathy or lesion of unknown etiology. In the anticoagulated patient follow the recommendations set forth for neuraxial blockade until practice guidelines for peripheral nerve blocks are promulgated.	Catheter techniques are useful for painful surgeries such as shoulder arthroplasty. Meier's or Borgeat's modification to Winnie's approach may be the preferred catheter technique. Ultrasound-guided techniques may shorten onset time and decrease complications.
Supraclavicular	Provides anesthesia to the entire upper extremity with a single injection of local anesthetic.	See above	Pneumothorax (PTX) is a risk with the classic approach. Winnie's *perivascular approach* and the *plumb bob approach* can minimize but not totally eliminate the risk of PTX. Ultrasound guidance has the potential of significantly decreasing the risk of PTX.
Infraclavicular	This approach is ideally suited for surgery on the distal upper arm, the entire forearm, wrist, and hand.	See above Also: chest deformities and healed but dislocated fractures of the clavicle.	Catheter techniques are beneficial and relatively easy to perform. Ultrasound guidance can significantly improve the safety and effectiveness of this block.
Axillary	Surgery distal to the elbow: Arteriovenous fistula, Colles fracture, Dupytrens contracture release, wrist fusion and ORIF.	See above	Separate blockade of the musculocutaneous and intercostobrachial nerves are usually necessary. Catheter techniques can be useful. Consider ultrasound guidance.
Midhumeral	Surgery on the: forearm, wrist and hand	See above	When you need adequate blockade of the radial nerve (e.g., wrist surgery) consider this block over the axillary approach.

TABLE 57-17

LUMBAR AND SACRAL PLEXUS BLOCKADE

■ PERIPHERAL NERVE BLOCK	■ INDICATIONS	■ CONTRAINDICATIONS	■ COMMENTS
Lumbar plexus	Total knee reconstruction and joint replacement surgery. Anterior and posterior cruciate ligament repair. Patellar tendon or fracture repair. May be combined with sciatic nerve block for hip surgery.	Refusal by the patient, infection, or hematoma in the vicinity of the block, allergy to local anesthetics, and progressive neuropathy or lesion of unknown etiology. In the anticoagulated patient follow the recommendations set forth for neuraxial blockade until practice guidelines for peripheral nerve blocks are promulgated.	Catheter techniques are very useful in painful techniques such as cruciate ligament grafting or joint replacement surgery. Excellent blockade of femoral, obturator, and lateral femoral cutaneous nerves. A true 3-in-1 block.
Femoral nerve	Total knee arthroplasty (TKA) Antereior cruciate ligament repair, femoral neck fractures, and saphenous vein stripping. Muscle biopsies involving the ventral, medial, or lateral thigh.	See above	Good choice for TKA. May be combined with a sciatic nerve block for TKA. Catheter techniques can be useful. Ultrasound guidance confirms placement of the needle tip between the fascia iliaca and the iliopsoas muscle.
Sciatic nerve	Above-the-knee amputation. Combine with a lumbar plexus block. Ankle joint replacement. Ankle arthrodesis. Calcaneal osteotomy. Achilles tendon repair.	See above	Numerous approaches have been described. The *parasacral approach* is the most cephalad. The *infragluteal parabiceps approach* is useful. Catheter techniques are useful for prolonged analgesia. Ultrasound guidance can confirm needle placement in the subgluteal space.
Popliteal fossa	Below-the-knee amputation. Combine with a saphenous nerve block. *Ankle surgery:* triple arthrodesis, arthroscopy, and Achilles tendon repair. *Foot surgery:* bunion surgery and transmetatarsal amputation.	See above	Lateral and posterior approaches have been described. Catheter insertion following ambulatory foot surgery can provide prolonged analgesia. Ultrasound guidance is very useful. Use "seesaw" sign.

TABLE 57-18

RECOMMENDED DOSING REGIMEN OF LOCAL ANESTHETICS FOR CONTINUOUS PERIPHERAL NERVE BLOCKADE

■ CATHETER	■ AGENT	■ RATE OF INFUSION	■ PCA BOLUS (mL)	■ LOCKOUT (min)
Interscalene Infraclavicular	Ropivacaine 0.2% or bupivacaine 0.15–0.2%	5–8 mL/hr	2–4	15–20
Femoral Popliteal	Ropivacaine 0.2% or bupivacaine 0.15–0.2%	5–10 mL/hr — 5–8 mL/hr	5–10 2	30–60 15–20
Paravertebral	Ropivacaine 0.2% Bupivacaine 0.25% with 1:400,000 epinephrine	0.1–0.2 mL/kg/hr 0.1 mL/kg/hr	— —	— —

PCA, patient-controlled analgesia.
Data derived from Karmakar MK, Chui PT, Joynt GM et al: Thoracic paravertebral block for management of pain associated with multiple fractured ribs in patients with concomitant lumbar spinal trauma. Reg Anesth Pain Med 2001; 26: 169; Liu S: Update in use of continuous perineural catheters for postoperative analgesia. IARS 2006 Review Course Lectures. Anesth Analg Suppl 2006: 64.

commonly spared. It is the most cephalad approach to the brachial plexus and was originally described by Winnie in 1970.[52a] In his now-classic description, the plexus is approached at the C6 level (cricoid cartilage) where the roots of the brachial plexus (C5 through T1) pass between the anterior and middle scalene muscles in the interscalene groove. The direction of the needle is medial, dorsal, and caudad with the needle entry approximately 60 degrees from the sagittal plane. A motor response to the biceps, deltoid, or pectoralis major muscle has been shown to be an acceptable end point when performing an interscalene block with a neurostimulation. An important caveat is that if you produce a diaphragmatic or trapezius muscle contraction while performing the block, your block needle is respectfully either too anterior (phrenic nerve stimulation) or too posterior (spinal accessory nerve stimulation) to the interscalene groove.

This block is easily performed using ultrasound guidance with a posterior in-plane approach and the transducer positioned in an axial oblique plane. The needle tip can be advanced under real time and positioned near the nerve roots between the middle and anterior scalene muscles. A recent study has confirmed that regardless of motor response, as long as the needle tip is positioned between the two most lateral nerve structures you will achieve a successful blockade of the plexus.[53] Your end point for injection of local anesthetic has now become real-time observation of hydrodissection and not motor stimulation.

Single-injection interscalene blockade for shoulder surgery reduces postoperative VAS pain scores, total opioid consumption, postoperative nausea and vomiting, time for request of first dose of analgesic, time to discharge, and unplanned hospital admissions.[54] Interscalene blockade provides postoperative analgesia, which is superior to subacromial bursae blockade, suprascapular, nerve blockade, infusion of intra-articular local anesthetic, and parenteral opioids. To extend the period of postoperative analgesia, continuous catheter techniques have been successfully employed in both the inpatient and outpatient settings. In a randomized placebo-controlled study of patients undergoing total shoulder arthroplasty, investigators concluded that continuous nerve blockade with 0.2% ropivacaine provided potent analgesia that improved postoperative shoulder mobility and shortened the time to discharge.[55]

The *supraclavicular approach* to the brachial plexus provides anesthesia to the entire upper extremity with a single injection of local anesthetic. The supraclavicular approach is carried out at a point where the plexus is reduced to its fewest component parts, the superior, middle, and inferior trunks, as they pass under the clavicle and over the first rib. An important landmark is the subclavian artery, which is often palpable in the supraclavicular fossa. The nerves of the brachial plexus lie in a cephaloposterior relationship to the artery at this level. When performing the block with a peripheral nerve stimulator, stimulation of the middle trunk (hand twitch) is reported to be associated with the highest success rates.

In the now "classic" Kulenkampff description,[55a] needle insertion is 1 cm above the midpoint of the clavicle in a plane that is parallel to the patient's head and neck. This approach requires the elicitation of multiple paresthesias and multiple injections. Unfortunately, the incidence of pneumothorax has been reported to be as high as 0.5 to 5% with this technique. With the introduction of ultrasound-guided supraclavicular blockade, however, the safety of this approach has improved dramatically. Real-time imaging of the needle tip in order to optimize its position not only decreases the risk of pneumothorax but increases the quality and shortens the onset time of the block.[56] The optimal position of the needle tip when performing this block with ultrasound guidance is reported to be in the corner bordered by the subclavian artery medially, the first rib inferiorly, and the divisions of the brachial plexus

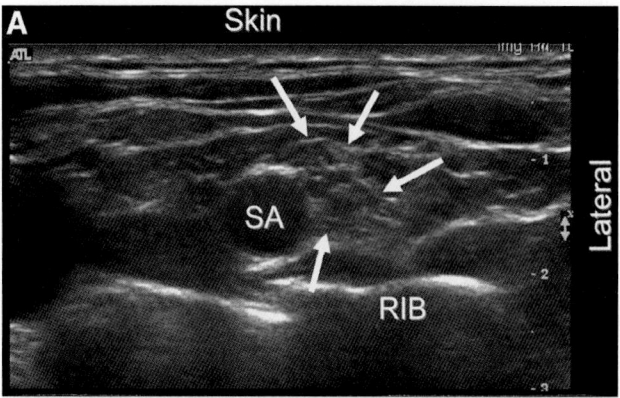

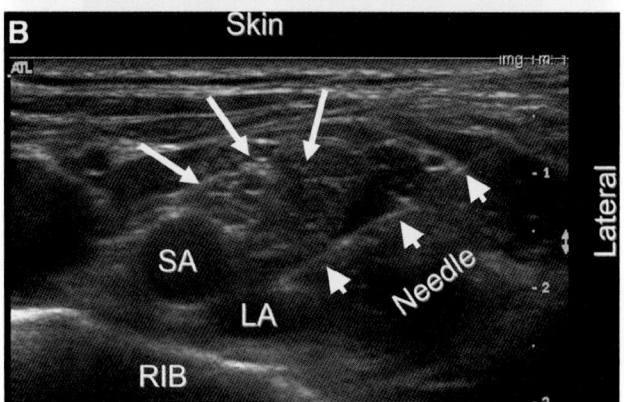

FIGURE 57-12. Ultrasound-guided supraclavicular nerve block. SA, subclavian artery; LA, local anesthetic. (Reprinted from Soares LG, Brüll R, Lai J et al Eight ball, corner pocket: The optimal needle position for ultrasound-guided supraclavicular block. Reg Anesth Pain Med 2007; 32: 2, with permission.)

superiorly and laterally.[57] Administration of local anesthetic at this location allows the brachial plexus to be displaced superiorly (Fig. 57-12) and a dense block sets up within minutes.[57] Although the supraclavicular approach is amenable to continuous catheter techniques, the literature on this subject is meager.

Below the Clavicle. The *infraclavicular block* is ideally suited for surgical procedures below the midhumerus[58] such as the hand, wrist, forearm, or elbow. The block targets the brachial plexus at the level of the cords where it is in close proximity to the axillary artery.[59] Unfortunately, the popularity of this approach has been less than enthusiastic because of unreliable surface landmarks and the potential risks of pneumothorax and vascular puncture. Ultrasound guidance has dramatically improved both the safety and efficacy of the infraclavicular approach and success rates are reported to be in the 90 to 100% range.[60] Ideal positioning is reported to be with the arm abducted to 110 degrees, externally rotated, and the elbow flexed 90 degrees.[58] With this positioning, the plexus lies closer to the surface, facilitating ultrasound visualization, and the block is performed with relative ease. The needle puncture is made at the apex of the deltopectoral groove in the sagittal plane. Because this is a deep block, visualization of individual cords may be challenging so the axillary artery becomes an important landmark. The optimal injection site is cranioposterior and adjacent to the axillary artery.[61] This area is closest to all three cords and potentially optimizes local anesthetic spread. A prospective randomized trial[59] comparing ultrasound-guided infraclavicular blockade, with and without neu-

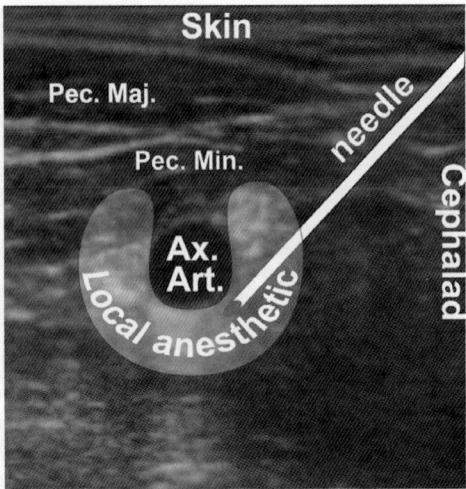

FIGURE 57-13. Ultrasound-guided infraclavicular nerve block. Ultrasonic anatomy, initial needle position, and desired U-shaped anesthetic distribution. Pec. Maj., pectoralis major muscle; Pec. Min., pectoralis minor muscle; Ax. Art., axillary artery. (Reused with permission from Dingemans et al: Neurostimulation in ultrasound guided infraclavicular block. Anesth Analg 2007; 104: 1274.)

rostimulation, has confirmed that the "U-shaped" distribution of local anesthetic around the posterior, medial, and lateral aspects of the axillary artery will reliably produce complete blockade of the brachial plexus (Fig. 57-13). The authors conclude that infraclavicular blockade is more rapidly performed and a block of better quality is achieved when you use local anesthetic spread as your end point for injection as opposed to neurostimulation.

A recent large-scale study documented the analgesic benefit and favorable safety profile of single-injection infraclavicular nerve blockade.[62] Placement of continuous infraclavicular nerve catheters has the advantage of providing prolonged analgesia for several days following surgery. Benefits include improved pain scores, decreased opioid requirements, less sedation, and less sleep disturbance with continuous infraclavicular nerve blockade.[63] The block can be performed with the arm *abducted* or *adducted* position. This flexibility in positioning can be advantageous particularly in the trauma patient who has significant pain and limited mobility. Placement of continuous infraclavicular catheters provides the advantage of a secure point of insertion that will not dislodge easily with patient movement. It is also relatively easy to keep clean and sterile particularly if the patient is to be discharged home with the catheter in situ to be removed at a latter date.

The Lumbar Plexus

Posterior Approach (Psoas Compartment Block). The lumbar plexus is formed from the ventral rami of the L1-4 spinal nerve roots, with a small contribution from T12 in some patients. The plexus lies within the substance of the psoas muscle in between the anterior and posterior masses and gives rise to the femoral (saphenous), obturator, lateral femoral cutaneous, ilioinguinal, iliohypogastric, and genitofemoral nerves. The nerves provide sensory innervation to the abdomen and groin, the anterior, lateral, and medial aspects of the thigh, the knee joint, and the medial part of the calf. Motor innervation is supplied to the abdominal muscles, the hip flexors, thigh adductors, and the quadriceps muscles. Numerous posterior and anterior approaches for lumbar plexus blockade (LPB) have been described[64] and the block is indicated for major surgeries of the hip and knee.

The posterior approach to the lumbar plexus reliably blocks the femoral, lateral femoral, and obturator nerves.[65]

The block is performed with the patient in the lateral decubitus position usually with the operative side in the uppermost (independent) position. The advantage of this position is that the block can be combined with a sciatic nerve block. The disadvantage, however, is the increased risk of epidural spread. When combined with sciatic nerve blockade, virtually any surgical procedure can be performed on the lower extremity. Although ultrasound-guided LPB has been described in the literature, it has not been studied extensively. Unfortunately, the depth of the plexus in adults may make ultrasound guidance both difficult and unreliable and preclude its use; however, in children ultrasound-guided LPB may prove to be efficacious.[66]

LPB alone and combined with sciatic nerve blockade has been safely and effectively used in the outpatient setting for knee arthroscopy. For more painful and invasive procedures such as total knee arthroplasty (TKA), total hip arthroplasty (THA), and anterior cruciate ligament repair (ACL), however, the benefit of LBP for postoperative pain management becomes even more evident. When compared with epidural analgesia there is a reduced requirement for urinary catheter insertion, and the risk of epidural hematoma formation secondary to postoperative anticoagulation is nearly eliminated. Continuous LPB with a catheter technique is reported to provide optimal analgesia both at rest and during physiotherapy following total hip arthroplasty and may provide opioid-free analgesia following both total knee arthroplasty and total hip arthroplasty.[67]

Complications are associated with the placement of sciatic and psoas compartment blocks therefore extreme care should be exercised if you choose to place these blocks. The incidence of sciatic nerve injury following total knee arthroplasty, unrelated to regional anesthesia technique, is reported to be in the range of 0.2 to 2.4%.[68] Risk factors include valgus deformity ($\geq$10 degrees), tourniquet time $\geq$120 minutes, pre-existing neuropathy, and postoperative bleeding.[68] Sciatic nerve blockade can mask these complications. Intermittent bolusing of the sciatic catheter (e.g., discontinuous catheter technique) allows neurologic examination between boluses. Complications associated with the placement of a psoas compartment block includes epidural spread, spinal anesthesia, systemic toxicity, unilateral sympathectomy, renal subscapular hematoma, and neurologic injury.[69] Psoas compartment blockade should be avoided in the anticoagulated patient.[69]

Anterior Approach (Femoral Nerve Block). The femoral nerve is formed from the posterior divisions of the ventral rami of L2-4 and is the largest terminal branch of the lumbar plexus. The nerve emerges from the lower lateral border of the psoas muscle and passes beneath the inguinal ligament in the groove between the iliacus and psoas muscles. In the inguinal region the nerve is covered by two fascial layers, the fascia lata and fascia iliaca, and whereas the fascia lata separates the subcutaneous tissue from the muscle and vessels, the fascia iliaca completely envelopes both the iliopsoas muscle and the femoral nerve,[70] physically separating the nerve from the femoral artery and vein. Although the nerve can be visualized with ultrasound, both above and below the inguinal ligament it is ideally visualized at the level of the inguinal crease, and at this level, the nerve is positioned approximately 0.5 cm lateral to the femoral artery.[70] The nerve provides motor innervation to the quadriceps femoris, sartorius, and pectineus muscles as well as sensory innervation to the anterior thigh and knee and the medial aspect of the lower extremity terminating as the saphenous nerve.

In 1973 Winnie and colleagues[70a] described a paravascular approach to femoral nerve blockade as a "3-in-1" technique suggesting that the fascial sheath that surrounds the femoral nerve acts as a conduit to reliably anesthetize the femoral, obturator, and lateral femoral cutaneous nerves. In reality, the obturator nerve is commonly spared.

Since the original description several anterior approaches to femoral nerve blockade have been described and the needle insertion site varies considerably. Needle insertion at the inguinal (femoral) crease (2 to 4 cm below the inguinal ligament) immediately lateral to the femoral pulse results in a 100% success rate for surgical anesthesia when using a peripheral nerve stimulator technique. With the patient in the supine position, a 2-inch (50-mm) insulated short bevel needle is advanced at a 60-degree angle in a posterior and cephalad direction. Quadriceps stimulation (patellar "snap") elicited at 0.3 to 0.5 mA confirms the ideal needle position, and local anesthetic can be incrementally injected with periodic aspiration to avoid intravascular injection.

Another very successful approach to femoral nerve blockade is the fascia iliaca compartment block. The injection site is distant from any neurovascular structures and therefore does not require neurostimulation to be successful.[69] The block has been described in both children and adults and is reported to be more successful than the three-in-one block. Continuous peripheral nerve catheter placement is reported to be faster with the fascia iliaca approach.[69] Ultrasound-guided femoral nerve blockade has also been described.[70] Care must be taken to place the tip of the needle within the space between the fascia iliaca and the iliopsoas muscle lateral to the femoral artery (Fig. 57-14). Local anesthetic can then be injected under real time and hydrodissection can be directly observed. In combination with ultrasound guidance, the fascia iliaca approach has been successfully used for the placement of continuous peripheral nerve catheters in the outpatient setting.[52]

Femoral nerve blockade is tremendously effective for postoperative pain control following arthroscopic reconstruction of the anterior cruciate ligament with *patellar tendon autograft*. Single-injection femoral nerve blockade improves postoperative pain control, delays the time to first request for an analgesic, and provides analgesia superior to intra-articular ropivacaine. Unfortunately, femoral nerve blockade alone is an inadequate block for anterior cruciate ligament reconstruction with *hamstring autograft* because of postoperative pain in the sciatic nerve distribution. A combination of femoral nerve blockade and sciatic nerve blockade is necessary in this case. In addition, continuous catheter techniques can prolong analgesia well into the postoperative period. Femoral nerve blockade alone or in combination with sciatic nerve blockade provides superior pain control and a reduction in unanticipated hospital admissions when used for more invasive and complex outpatient knee surgeries such as high osteotomy, multiple ligament reconstruction, and meniscal reconstruction. A meta-analysis concludes that femoral nerve blockade is as effective as epidural analgesia following total knee arthroplasty.[71] Femoral nerve blockade provides site-specific analgesia and is an integral part of any multimodal analgesic regimen following major knee surgery.

Saphenous nerve blockade is frequently combined with a lateral popliteal block or sciatic block for procedures involving the lower leg. The saphenous nerve is the only branch of the lumbar plexus below the knee and is the largest sensory terminal branch of the femoral nerve. The nerve provides sensory innervation to the medial, anteromedial, and posteromedial parts of the knee, leg, and medial malleolus and, in some people, the medial aspect of the large toe. Several approaches have been described at the level of the patella and medial malleolus. The paravenous approach is based on the close relationship of the saphenous vein and nerve at the level of the tibial tuberosity. Ultrasound-guided saphenous nerve blockade deep to the sartorius muscle near the adductor canal has also been described in the literature and this may prove to be a useful approach.[72]

Sacral Plexus

The sciatic nerve originates from the sacral plexus and is derived from the ventral rami of the fourth lumbar to the third sacral nerve roots. The three major components of the sciatic nerve include the tibial and common peroneal nerves and the posterior femoral cutaneous nerve to the thigh. The sciatic nerve provides sensory, motor, and some sympathetic innervation to the lower extremity and, its blockade in combination with an LPB, can provide complete anesthesia and postoperative analgesia for lower extremity surgery. Numerous proximal and distal techniques, using anterior, posterior, and lateral approaches to the sciatic nerve with the patient in the supine, prone lateral, and lithotomy positions, have been described. Patient comfort is a key factor in determining the preferred approach. *Proximal* sciatic nerve blockade is often combined with a psoas compartment block or a femoral nerve block for procedures on the lower extremity including total hip arthroplasty, total knee arthroplasty, and anterior cruciate ligament, as previously discussed. In addition, the combination of a femoral and sciatic nerve block is also indicated for complex outpatient knee surgeries, above- and below-the-knee amputations, and ankle and foot surgery.

Following foot and ankle surgery sciatic nerve blockade provides safe, effective, and long-lasting postoperative analgesia. The infragluteal parabiceps approach offers distinct advantages over the more traditional approaches as the approach relies on easily palpable soft-tissue landmarks. Inversion of the foot following nerve stimulation at <0.4 mA is the preferred evoked motor response because inversion is found to be associated with a more rapid onset and complete blockade. Unfortunately, single-shot proximal sciatic nerve blockade with a long-acting local anesthetic can only provide analgesia for 10 to 20 hours. Continuous proximal sciatic nerve blockade has been successfully applied for foot and ankle surgery and below-the-knee amputation. Continuous parasacral sciatic nerve blockade has been described in patients undergoing complex lower extremity surgery including total knee arthroplasty, osteotomy, above-the-knee amputation, osteosarcoma resection, and other procedures on the leg. The advantage of this approach is complete anesthesia of all three branches of the sciatic nerve.

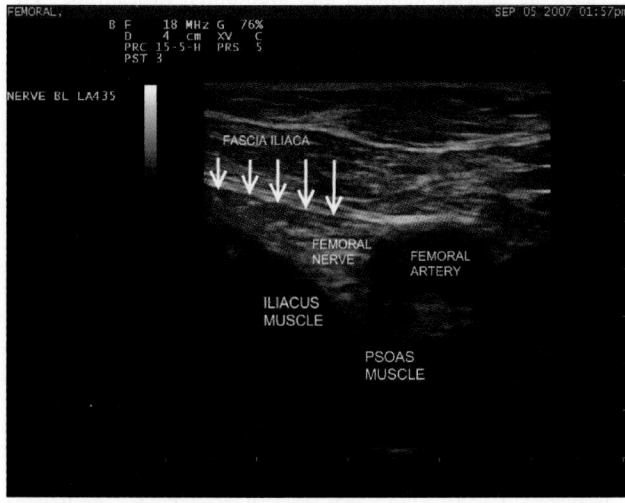

FIGURE 57-14. Ultrasound-guided femoral nerve blockade: Short axis ultrasound image of the infrainguinal structures. Femoral nerve blockade can be performed with a needle approach that is either in-plane or out-of-plane. The needle tip must be positioned within the space between the fascia iliaca and the iliopsoas muscle before local anesthetic is injected in order to achieve a successful block of the femoral nerve.

PERIOPERATIVE AND CONSULTATIVE SERVICES

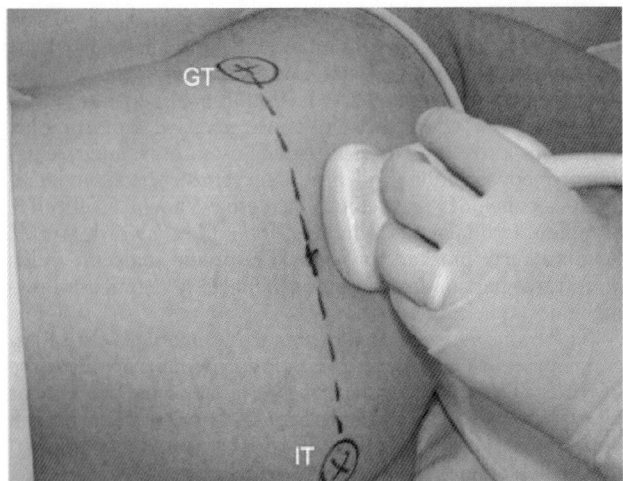

FIGURE 57-15.   Ultrasound-guided sciatic nerve blockade. Ultrasound transducer positioned transverse in the infragluteal region. GT, greater trochanter; IT, ischial tuberosity. (Reprinted from Chan VW, Nova H, Abbas S et al: Ultrasound examination and localization of the sciatic nerve. Anesthesiology 2006; 104: 310, with permission.)

Ultrasound guidance provides real-time visualization and high-quality images of the sciatic nerve. Using a curved 2- to 5-MHz (megahertz) transducer, very good-quality images of the sciatic nerve have been described in the gluteal, infragluteal, and proximal thigh locations[73] (Figs. 57-15 and 57-16). Successful ultrasound-guided blockade of the sciatic nerve within the subgluteal has also been described with the hyperechoic nerve being easily imaged with a 2- to 5-MHz transducer at the level of the greater trochanter and ischial tuberosity.[74] Ultrasound-guided subgluteal blockade with a stimulating catheter has also been described in children undergoing various lower extremity surgical procedures.[75] The authors describe excellent postoperative analgesia and patient satisfaction.

Distal sciatic nerve blockade is typically performed in the popliteal fossa using a lateral or posterior approach. In the adult patient, the block is preferably performed at least 100 mm superior to the popliteal crease cephalad to the bifurcation

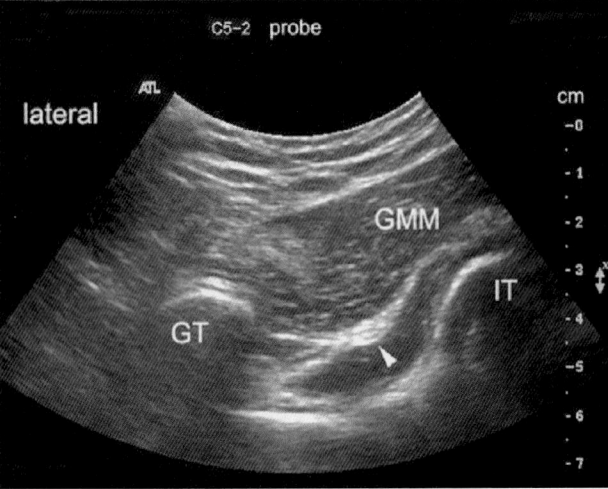

FIGURE 57-16.   Ultrasound image of the sciatic nerve. The *arrow* points to the sciatic nerve. GT, greater trochanter; GMM, gluteus maximus muscle; IT, ischial tuberosity. (Reprinted from Chan VW, Nova H, Abbas S et al: Ultrasound examination and localization of the sciatic nerve. Anesthesiology 2006; 104: 311, with permission.)

of the sciatic nerve into the tibial and common peroneal nerves. When using neurostimulation as the end point for injection of local anesthetic, inversion of the foot is the ideal motor response that best predicts complete sensory blockade. The popliteal approach to sciatic nerve blockade typically spares the posterior cutaneous nerve to the thigh, thus preserving hamstring function. This approach therefore has the added benefit of being less restrictive on ambulation, which is useful following ambulatory surgery. The block provides superior analgesia for foot and ankle surgery and is often paired with a saphenous nerve block for surgeries involving the medial aspect of the leg and foot. Compared with subcutaneous local anesthetic infiltration and ankle blockade, popliteal sciatic nerve blockade provides significantly longer postoperative analgesia and has a high degree of patient satisfaction. Ultrasound guidance significantly improves the accuracy of needle placement through real-time imaging of the nerve and potentially improves efficacy.[76] The image of the sciatic nerve in the popliteal space will vary depending on the type of transducer used, but the linear 5- to 12-MHz transducer provides the highest resolution image.[76] With the posterior approach and a short axis (transverse cross-sectional) view, active or passive dorsiflexion of the foot can produce external rotation of the sciatic nerve, which facilitates its identification. Real-time visualization of circumferential spread of local anesthetic around the nerve with ultrasound guidance will not only decrease the failure rate but it will expedite block onset compared with conventional techniques, reduce complications, and provide greater patient satisfaction.[76]

Continuous popliteal sciatic nerve blockade can significantly extend the duration of superb postoperative analgesia and has been successfully implemented in both the inpatient and outpatient settings. Pain-related sleep disruption is less, and hospital length of stay is shorter. Risks associated with at-home perineural infusions of local anesthetic include catheter site infection, nerve injury, and catheter migration with subsequent local anesthetic toxicity. Complications are relatively rare.[52,77]

Paravertebral blockade (PVB) can provide segmental analgesia for numerous surgical procedures including thoracotomy, mastectomy, nephrectomy, cholecystectomy and rib fractures, spinal surgery, and video-assisted thorascopic surgery, as well as inguinal and abdominal procedures. The paravertebral space (PVS) does not actually exist but is considered to be a potential space created by fluid distention of the tissues.[78] The PVS is defined anteriorly by the parietal pleura, posteriorly by the costotransverse ligament, superiorly by the occiput, inferiorly by the alar of the sacrum, and medially by the vertebral body, intervertebral disc, and the intervertebral foramen. Laterally, the PVS is contiguous with the intercostal space.[78] The PVS contains the anterior and posterior ramus of the spinal nerve root and the white and grey rami communicantes. Injection of local anesthetic into this potential space will therefore produce a dense sensory and sympathetic block resulting in unilateral segmental analgesia.[2] Generally speaking, PVB is performed at the thoracic level. When performed in the lumbar region it is better known as a *psoas compartment block* and when performed at the cervical level it is referred to as a *deep cervical plexus block*.[78]

Blind percutaneous PVB can be performed with the patient in the seated, prone, or lateral decubitus position. The block is administered with either a spinal needle or a Tuohy needle and multiple- and single-injection and catheter techniques have been described. Needle insertion is 2.5 cm lateral to the superior aspect of the spinous process (paramedial line) and advanced perpendicular to the skin in all planes until it contacts the transverse process, which is at a depth of about 2 to 5 cm in the adult. The needle is "walked" off the transverse process superiorly or inferiorly and advanced no more than 1 to 1.5 cm into the PVS. Loss of resistance to air or saline may be used but it has an indistinct end point. However, nerve stimulation and ultrasound both have the potential to facilitate needle placement. Although single-level (T4) and multilevel (C7-T6) blocks can be performed, four injections can provide a more reliable loss of sensation than a single injection.[79] The recommended bolus dose of bupivacaine, to be distributed over single or multiple levels, is 1.5 mg/kg (0.3 mL/kg of 0.5% bupivacaine) not to exceed 150 mg total dose. The addition of epinephrine 1:400,000 to 1:200,000 can prolong the blockade and serves to facilitate detection of intravascular injection. Ropivacaine 0.5% may be a safer alternative to bupivacaine, and besides it has been shown to have a more rapid onset, a broader initial spread, and a longer duration of action. The recommended dose for an infusion is 0.1 mL/kg/hr of 0.25% bupivacaine or 0.1 to 0.2 mL/kg/hr of 0.2% ropivacaine.[80] Complications include hypotension, vascular puncture, pleural puncture, pneumothorax, and epidural or intrathecal trespass. The risk of pleural puncture can be decreased with the assistance of sonographic guidance to identify the transverse process. Likewise, the risk of pleural puncture can be decreased when the paravertebral catheter is placed percutaneously under direct visualization of the parietal pleura by the surgeon or the anesthesiologist prior to closure of a thoracotomy incision.[81]

The advantages of PVB include lower postoperative VAS pain scores, a reduction in postoperative opioid consumption, and, therefore, less opioid-induced postoperative nausea and vomiting, less pain with movement, and shorter hospital stays. Continuous PVB compares favorably with thoracic epidurals for postthoracotomy analgesia. Continuous PVB provides analgesia that is equivalent to thoracic epidural blockade but without the side effects of hypotension, postoperative nausea and vomiting, and urinary retention[82] and may therefore be a reasonable alternative to a thoracic epidural catheter for postoperative analgesia.

Miscellaneous Regional Anesthesia Techniques

The *rectus sheath block* (RSB) is a regional anesthetic technique for use in adults to provide relaxation of the anterior abdominal wall during laparotomy. The RSB has been described in both adults and children and can provide effective postoperative analgesia for both umbilical and midline surgical incisions. The block is performed by depositing local anesthetic in the potential space between the rectus abdominis muscle and the posterior rectus sheath. Traditionally the RSB has relied on a "blind" technique using a short bevel needle with an end point for injection defined as a loss of resistance or an audible "pop." Complications associated with the block include intraperitoneal injection of local anesthetic, perforation of the bowel, and puncture of a mesenteric vessel. Ultrasound-guided RSB has been described in both the pediatric and adult populations and real-time imaging of the optimal needle position will eliminate or at least minimize the uncertainty and potential complications associated with the "blind" technique.

The *transversus abdominis plane* block is very similar to the RSB in that it anesthetizes neural afferents that supply the anterior abdominal wall. This block can provide adequate postoperative analgesia in patients undergoing major abdominal surgery. It is performed by injecting local anesthetic into the transversus abdominis plane via the triangle of Petit, which is defined by the latissimus dorsi muscle posteriorly, the external oblique muscle anteriorly, and the iliac crest caudally. This is a blind approach that uses a "double-pop" technique to advance the needle into the appropriate fascial plane. Fortunately, the transversus abdominis plane block can be performed using ultrasound guidance[83] and, as is the case with the RSB, potentially increasing the success rate of the block while decreasing complications.

Placement of a *continuous wound catheter* is a relatively simple and sometimes effective technique in which the surgeon places a catheter into the wound at the end of surgery and a local anesthetic infusion is begun. Appropriate placement of the catheter in the preperitoneal space, rather than the subcutaneous space, is required for adequate analgesia. Local anesthetics may inhibit the first and second stages of wound healing, so routine use may not be recommended.[84] Further study of this promising modality is recommended.

The *continuous intra-articular infusion* of local anesthetic plus opioid following joint surgery can be very effective. The one major disadvantage to this technique is the potential for larger wound effusions and the increased risk for infection with a catheter in place. An alternative to this technique is the *periarticular soft-tissue injection* of local anesthetic combined with an NSAID (e.g., ropivacaine and ketorolac) combined with an intra-articular catheter for 24 hours.[85] The technique appears to be safe and effective, and the risk of infection is minimized by removing the catheter on postoperative day 1.

Continuous Peripheral Nerve Blockade Caveats

Interest in CPNB increased following the Food and Drug Administration warning in 1997 on the risk of spinal hematoma in patients who received epidural placement and low-molecular-weight heparin concurrently.[86] Although bleeding complications can be associated with the placement of CPNB catheters, the actual risks related to this technique are not well defined. Hemorrhagic complications, rather than neurologic deficits, appear to be the predominant risk associated with the performance of peripheral nerve blockade in the anticoagulated patient.[87] Major hemorrhage can occur following performance of psoas compartment blockade (e.g., LPB) and lumbar sympathetic blockade.[87] Special risk seems likely in any patient who may be anticoagulated perioperatively.

Practice-based guidelines for the performance of *neuraxial techniques* in the anticoagulated patient are available online at the American Society of Regional Anesthesia (ASRA) Web site at http://www.asra.com/consensus-statements and are based on the recommendations set forth in the consensus statement by Horlocker et al.[87] At the time of this publication, however, no consensus statement has been promulgated by the society, outlining practice guidelines for the performance of *peripheral nerve blocks* in anticoagulated patients. Until performance guidelines are developed for the performance of peripheral nerve blockade in the anticoagulated patient, Horlocker et al.[87] recommend a conservative approach by adapting the guidelines set forth by ASRA for the performance of neuraxial blockade, which they acknowledge may be overly restrictive.

Despite the fact that a sustained-released morphine is currently available for epidural use, the routine application of timed-release formulations of local anesthetic and opioids for both neuraxial and peripheral analgesia is remote. The argument for their use is simplicity and prolonged analgesia; however, once administered, there is no turning off and the dose cannot be titrated to effect nor can it be turned off so a neurovascular check of the patient can be performed. Continuous catheter systems may be cumbersome and potentially more expensive but they are titratable and they can be turned on and off as appropriate and they can be intermittently bolused when indicated.

COMPLICATIONS FROM REGIONAL ANESTHESIA

The opinion of some is that regional anesthesia is safer than general anesthesia may be because regional anesthesia has been associated with reduced postoperative mortality secondary to thromboembolic phenomenon and myocardial infarction and provides superior postoperative analgesia.[88,89]

Nonetheless, data from the American Society of Anesthesiologists Closed Claims Project database suggests that the comparative safety of regional anesthesia in comparison to general anesthesia cannot be accurately determined. In a review of Closed Claims data, however, death is more common with claims involving general anesthesia and permanent-disabling and nondisabling temporary injuries are more often associated with regional anesthesia.[90] Serious complications associated with the performance of regional anesthesia include cardiac arrest, radiculopathy, cauda equina syndrome, and paraplegia. Fortunately, the incidence of severe anesthesia-related complications are rare (<0.1%); however, the incidence of cardiac arrest and neurologic complications are higher following spinal anesthesia than after all other types of regional procedures. The incidence of cardiac arrest following spinal anesthesia is 6.4 ± 1.2 per 10,000 versus 1.0 ± 0.4 per 10,000 for other forms of regional anesthesia. The incidence of neurologic injury after spinal anesthesia (6 ± 1 per 10,000 cases) is greater than all other regional techniques (e.g., epidural, peripheral nerve block and intravenous regional anesthesia) combined (1.6 ± 0.5 per 10,000 cases).

Should a perioperative nerve injury occur, it is incumbent on the physician to determine which combination of anesthetic, surgical, and patient risk factors are involved in any nerve injury and not assume a priori that the regional anesthetic is the culprit. The risk factors for nerve injury are listed in Table 57-19. *Patient risk factors* for perioperative nerve injury may include any pre-existing systemic neuropathy (e.g., diabetes mellitus) or drug-induced neuropathy (e.g., vincristine or *cis*-platin). Risk factors for ulnar nerve injury include male sex, prolonged hospitalization, increasing age, extremes of body habitus, and diabetes. Diabetics, for exam-

ple, have a decreased requirement for local anesthetic yet an increased risk for local anesthetic-induced nerve injury. This phenomenon has been described as the "double-crush" syndrome and proposes that axons injured at one site have an increased susceptibility to injury distally. Interestingly enough, in spite of this risk, regional anesthesia has been safely performed on patients with pre-existing ulnar neuropathy who underwent ulnar nerve transposition.[91] See Chapters 21 (local anesthetics), 37 (spinal and epidural anesthesia), and 38 (peripheral nerve blockade) for additional details on the reported complications of regional anesthesia.

PERIOPERATIVE PAIN MANAGEMENT OF THE OPIOID-DEPENDENT PATIENT

Although this discussion will focus on the patient with chronic pain syndromes, these strategies for perioperative pain management are easily adaptable to other opioid-dependent populations. Chronic pain is defined as "pain without apparent biological value that has persisted beyond the normal tissue healing time usually taken to be three months" (International Association for the Study of Pain) and "pain of a duration or intensity that adversely affects the function or well-being of the patient" (American Society of Anesthesiologists). Chronic pain is often associated with anxiety and depression, which may require treatment with various anxiolytics, antidepressants, anticonvulsants, antiarrhythmics, and skeletal muscle relaxants in addition to opioids. Symptoms unique to chronic pain include tight musculature, limited range of motion, and lack of energy, sleep disturbance, irritability, and social withdrawal. Associated psychiatric diagnoses may include hypochondriasis and psychosis.

Over the past decade, the percentage of patients with chronic pain for whom chronic opioids have been prescribed has increased dramatically. Although the goal of opioid therapy for chronic pain is improvement of pain, function, and quality of life, unacceptable opioid side effects and concerns about adverse hormonal effects and immune modulation from long-term exposure can cause patients to abandon therapy. In addition, long-term opioid use results in physical dependence, the potential for withdrawal symptoms on abrupt discontinuation of the opioid, and the development of tolerance and OIH.

Physical dependence is a "physiological state of adaptation to a specific psychoactive substance characterized by the emergence of a *withdrawal syndrome* during abstinence, which may be relieved in total or in part by readministration of the substance." Opioid *withdrawal* is characterized by an increased sympathetic and parasympathetic response that results in hypertension, tachycardia, diaphoresis, abdominal cramping, and diarrhea. Clinical experience suggests that patients are considered to be *physically dependent* on an opioid if they have been receiving the equivalent of 30 mg of intravenous morphine daily for a period of at least 2 to 4 weeks, and therefore failure to provide adequate amounts of opioids perioperatively will precipitate withdrawal symptoms. *Tolerance* is a rightward shift of the dose-response curve and by definition is "a state in which an increased dosage of a psychoactive substance is needed to produce a desired effect." Escalating doses of opioid may also be explained by an underlying progression of the disease state or by the development of OIH. Tolerance can be innate or acquired. Innate tolerance is a genetically predetermined sensitivity to a drug, whereas acquired tolerance can have a pharmacokinetic, learned, or pharmacodynamic basis. Pharmacokinetic tolerance involves a diminution in the effects of a drug because of changes in distribution and metabolism usually

TABLE 57-19

RISK FACTORS FOR NERVE INJURY DURING THE PERFORMANCE OF REGIONAL ANESTHESIA

■ VARIABLES	■ RISK FACTORS
Patient	Body habitus
	Pre-existing neurologic disorder (e.g., diabetes mellitus or patients who have received chemotherapy in the recent past)
	Male gender
	Advanced age
Surgical	Direct surgical trauma or stretch
	Prolonged tourniquet time
	Hematoma
	Infection
	Tightly applied casts or surgical dressings
	Patient positioning
Regional anesthesia	Mechanical injury from the needle or catheter
	Chemical neurotoxicity from the local anesthetic
	Ischemic injury to the nerve

Data derived from Neal JM, Hebl JR, Gerancher JC et al: Brachial plexus anesthesia: Essentials of our current understanding. Reg Anesth Pain Med 2002; 27: 402; Horlocker TT: Complications of regional anesthesia. IARS 2004 Review Course Lectures. Anesth Analg Suppl 2004: 56; Ben-David B: Complications of peripheral blockade. Anesthesiol Clin North Am 2002; 20: 457; Hebl JR, Horlocker TT, Pritchard DJ: Diffuse brachial plexopathy after interscalene blockade in a patient receiving cisplatin chemotherapy: The pharmacologic double crush syndrome. Anesth Analg 2001; 92: 249.

secondary to enzyme induction of the cytochrome 450 system, which results in accelerated metabolism. Learned tolerance refers to compensatory behavior that masks intoxication. Pharmacodynamic tolerance refers to neuroadaptive changes that occur following chronic exposure to opioids, which may involve receptor desensitization secondary to receptor down-regulation, internalization, and uncoupling of opioid receptors from G proteins. Opioids exhibit *cross-tolerance* to each other but the degree of cross-tolerance varies widely and is often incomplete.[92] Clinicians use incomplete cross-tolerance to their advantage to restore analgesic sensitivity in highly tolerant patients through opioid rotation.[92] Because cross-tolerance is incomplete, analgesia is restored with the new opioid at >50% below the predicted equianalgesic dose.[92] It must be stressed that the development of tolerance or physical dependence in no way implies that the patient is addicted to an opioid. *Addiction* is a biopsychosocial disease characterized by dysfunctional behavior that involves craving, compulsive use, loss of control, and the continued use of a drug in spite of adverse consequences. Finally, addiction should not be confused with *pseudoaddiction*, which, by definition, describes the patient who has behavioral features of addiction secondary to undertreatment of the pain syndrome. Pseudoaddiction is usually diagnosed retrospectively because once the dose of opioid is increased, pain resolves and aberrant behavior abates.

The onus for the identification of the opioid-dependent patient rests with the surgical team, the preoperative evaluation staff, and the anesthesia team assigned to the case.[93] Ideally the patient and the health care team will formulate a perioperative pain management plan prior to surgery, and the chronic pain service, if available, should be consulted. Often, however, the opioid-dependent patient is identified just moments prior to surgery and the anesthesia team needs to be innovative. The anesthesiologist needs to be flexible enough to tailor an individual anesthetic that incorporates a multimodal approach, combining regional anesthesia with general anesthesia and nonopioid coanalgesics with opioid analgesics. Opioids remain the mainstay of perioperative pain management, and an adequate dose of opioid needs to be maintained to avoid precipitating withdrawal symptoms (Table 57-20).

Preoperative management of the patient involves determining the patients "baseline" opioid requirement, and on the day of surgery the patient should be instructed to take the normal opioid dose. If for some reason the patient neglects to take the opioid on the day of surgery, the anesthesiologist can administer an equivalent dose preoperatively. During the preinduction period the dose of fentanyl, morphine, or hydromorphone administered for sedation can be 25 to 50% higher than the dose used in the opioid-naive patient. Patients prescribed transdermal fentanyl patches are usually instructed to maintain their fentanyl patch into the operating room and this can serve as their baseline opioid requirement. Occasionally, however, in the case of major surgery, in which the risk of major blood loss or sepsis is a significant, patients may be instructed to discontinue their transdermal patch, and an intravenous fentanyl infusion can be initiated to maintain adequate plasma concentrations. Patients maintained on methadone should continue their baseline dose throughout the perioperative period. In the United States methadone is available for both oral and intravenous administration. The reader is reminded that patients receiving >200 mg of methadone per day can develop a prolonged QT interval, which places them at risk for Torsades de pointe. It is therefore recommended that a baseline electrocardiogram be obtained for comparison. Patients who are maintained on the partial opioid agonist buprenorphine may continue to receive the drug for postoperative pain control, and either morphine or methadone may be adminis-

tered to supplement analgesia if required. Full antagonists (e.g., naloxone and naltrexone) and the partial agonists-antagonists (e.g., nalbuphine, pentazocine, and butorphanol) should be avoided because they will precipitate withdrawal symptoms in opioid-dependent patients.

Intraoperative management of the opioid-dependent patient requires the prudent use of fentanyl, morphine, or hydromorphone in order to provide effective intraoperative anesthesia, postoperative analgesia, and to prevent opioid withdrawal. This requires the administration of the patients' baseline opioid requirement plus their intraoperative require-

---

TABLE 57-20

SUGGESTED GUIDELINES FOR PERIOPERATIVE PAIN MANAGEMENT IN THE OPIOID-TOLERANT PATIENT

■ PREOPERATIVE

1. Evaluation: Evaluation should include early recognition and high index of suspicion.
2. Identification: Identify factors such as total opioid dose requirement and previous surgery/trauma resulting in undermedication, inadequate analgesia, or relapse episodes.
3. Consultation: Meet with addiction specialists and pain specialists with regard to perioperative planning.
4. Reassurance: Discuss patient concerns related to pain control, anxiety, and risk of relapse.
5. Medication: Calculate opioid dose requirement and modes of administration; provide anxiolytics or other medications as clinically indicated.

■ INTRAOPERATIVE

1. Maintain baseline opioids (oral, transdermal, intravenous).
2. Increase intraoperative and postoperative opioid dose to compensate for tolerance.
3. Provide peripheral neural or plexus blockade; consider neuraxial analgesic techniques when clinically indicated.
4. Use nonopioids as analgesic adjuncts.

■ POSTOPERATIVE

1. Plan preoperatively for postoperative analgesia; formulate primary strategy as well as suitable alternatives.
2. Maintain baseline opioids.
3. Use multimodal analgesic techniques.
4. Patient-controlled analgesia: Use as primary therapy or as supplementation for epidural or regional techniques.
5. Continue neuraxial opioids: intrathecal or epidural analgesia.
6. Continue continuous neural blockade.

■ AFTER DISCHARGE

7. If surgery provides complete pain relief, opioids should be slowly tapered, rather than abruptly discontinued.
8. Develop a pain management plan before hospital discharge. Provide adequate doses of opioid and nonopioid analgesics.
9. Arrange for a timely outpatient pain clinic follow-up or a visit with the patient's addictionologist.

Data derived from Mitra S, Sinatra RS: Perioperative management of acute pain in the opioid-dependent patient. Anesthesiology 2004; 101: 212.

PERIOPERATIVE AND CONSULTATIVE SERVICES

ments secondary to surgical stimulation. Exact opioid dosing guidelines do not exist but because of receptor down-regulation secondary to chronic opioid administration, opioid doses may need to be increased 30 to 100% vis-à-vis the opioid-naive patient. Because of receptor down-regulation an alternative opioid may be useful in this setting. Opioid rotation takes advantage of the fact that the new opioid will bind a different opioid receptor subtype and be metabolized differently. Following the cancer pain model, the dose of the new opioid is <50% of the calculated equianalgesic dose because of incomplete cross-tolerance.[92] Although the alternative opioid may be administered for several days postoperatively, prudence dictates that a physician or pharmacist well versed in pain management convert the patient to the appropriate oral opioid regimen for discharge from the hospital.

The optimal intraoperative dose of opioid varies considerably from patient to patient; therefore, monitoring intraoperative vital signs such as heart rate, pupil size, and respiratory rate can be useful and allows the clinician to avoid the negative consequences of overdosing or underdosing the patient with opioid. Reversing neuromuscular blockade toward the end of a general anesthetic and allowing the patient to breathe spontaneously can be a prudent technique. Patients with a respiratory rate >20 breaths per minute and significantly dilated pupils require additional opioid. Titrating fentanyl, morphine, or hydromorphone to a respiratory rate of 12 to 14 breaths per minute and a moderately miotic pupil is recommended. It is also recommend that patients who are receiving chronic methadone therapy may receive an additional intraoperative dose of 0.1 mg/kg intravenously, which can be titrated to hemodynamic effect and pupillary response.

Postoperative management of the opioid-dependent patient can be very challenging. Ideally, the optimal amount of opioid has been administered to the patient during the intraoperative period, allowing them to emerge from anesthesia comfortably sedated and pain-free. On arrival to the recovery room, intravenous opioids may be administered on an "as-needed" basis; however, initiation of an intravenous PCA opioid with both a basal and incremental (bolus) dose will minimize the risk of breakthrough pain. The recommended basal infusion should equate to the patient's hourly preoperative oral opioid dose requirement as this will avoid precipitating withdrawal symptoms, and the bolus dose, as calculated from the background infusion, is the 1-hour dose of the background infusion. For example, a patient taking 90 mg of oral morphine per day equates to 30 mg of intravenous morphine per day, which can be administered as a basal morphine infusion of 1.25 mg/hr. The bolus dose would be equivalent to 1.25 mg with a lockout interval of 6 to 10 minutes. Basal infusions are not required for patients who are maintained on their transdermal fentanyl patches as these provide adequate basal analgesia. Therefore, a fentanyl PCA with a bolus dose and an appropriate lockout interval is all that is required. Patients recovering from same-day surgery will be initially treated with intravenous doses of opioids in the recovery room; however, they can be quickly transitioned to an oral regimen consisting of their baseline opioid requirement plus an appropriate amount of short-acting opioid for breakthrough pain consistent with the invasiveness of the surgery.

Nonopioid coanalgesics are opioid-sparing and should be part and parcel of any multimodal perioperative pain management regimen in the opioid-dependent patient. Low-dose ketamine is highly recommended. A bolus dose of 0.25 to 0.5 mg/kg followed by an infusion of 2 to 4 μg/kg/min is reported to enhance analgesia in this population of patients. The preoperative administration of acetaminophen, a COX-2 inhibitor, an α_2-δ subunit calcium channel ligand, and α_2-agonists may also be particularly beneficial in the perioperative pain management of these patients.

Regional anesthesia is highly recommended in this patient population. Peripheral nerve blockade as a single-injection technique or as a continuous catheter can be very useful. Likewise, if indicated epidural analgesia should be part and parcel of the multimodal pain regimen for these patients. During the perioperative period, however, the epidural and systemic requirements for morphine have been reported to increase three- to fourfold. Epidural infusions that have been recommended include a combination of either fentanyl (2 to 5 μg/mL), morphine (0.1 to 0.2 mg/mL), or hydromorphone (0.02 to 0.04 mg/mL) combined with a local anesthetic such as bupivacaine (0.05 to 0.2%) or ropivacaine (0.1 to 0.2%). Switching to an opioid with high intrinsic efficacy may be useful. A combination of sufentanil (2 μg/mL) with 0.1% bupivacaine has been shown to be quite efficacious in an opioid-tolerant patient refractory to the analgesic effects of epidural morphine. The neuraxial administration of opioid is usually a very small fraction of the patient's baseline opioid requirement. Notwithstanding the fact that patients obtain excellent analgesia from the epidural, opioid serum levels and supraspinal receptor binding may not be totally adequate at preventing opioid withdrawal symptoms. It may therefore be necessary for the patient to receive at least part of their baseline opioid dose either orally or intravenously (PCA) to prevent opioid withdrawal symptoms. A physician well versed in chronic pain management and comfortable in the equianalgesic dosing of opioids via different routes of administration should therefore be involved in the care of the patient. Careful monitoring of the patient for excessive sedation or respiratory depression is mandatory, and caregivers in the recovery room and on the postsurgical units should be alerted to the potential risk for respiratory depression when parenteral and neuraxial opioids are combined.

ORGANIZATION OF PERIOPERATIVE PAIN MANAGEMENT SERVICES

There is a growing recognition in the health care industry that the undertreatment of pain is a widespread problem that cuts across all phases of patient care. The effective management of pain is a crucial component of good perioperative care and recovery from surgery. Unrelieved pain and inadequate pain relief have detrimental physiological and psychological effects on patients by slowing recovery and creating burdens for patients and their families, and by increasing costs to the health care system. Although the acute postoperative pain service plays an integral role in the pain management of the surgical patients, there are considerable barriers that challenge the establishment and/or effectiveness of acute pain teams in managing patients across the continuum of care. There is good evidence that the overall incidence of moderate-to-severe pain in surgical patients is about 25 to 40% despite the availability of pain treatment.[94] A major obstacle to the establishment of postoperative pain services is its cost in a privatized health system wherein limited reimbursement for postoperative care discourages the establishment of a service. The value of an acute pain service apart from its benefit for patient care also comes from the added value of reducing hospital costs by improving surgical outcome and by facilitating patient recovery and early discharge.[95] While providing direct patient care along previous lines such as the management of continuous epidural and regional catheter infusions and other modalities, the perioperative pain management service must also play a leading role in patient education and the education of other physicians, nurses, and caregivers to ensure their competence in effectively assessing, managing and meeting a patient's needs. The success of a perioperative pain management team can be established not only in the context of the direct patient care that the team provides, but also through its role in educating other health care professionals and service as physician leaders responsible for setting clinical standards and practice guidelines in the health care system.

⑫ The key components to establishing a successful perioperative pain management service begins with an institutional commitment to support the service. The team must be built around a physician leader with training and experience in pain medicine. There must be other anesthesiologists available to support the service. The institutional must support the service, which may be manifest through support of a nurse coordinator or the availability of a pharmacist to consult on the many pharmaceutical issues that arise in patients on preoperative medications that may conflict with the perioperative pain management plan. The perioperative pain management chief is responsible for the development and implementation of clinical pathways and protocols that are effective across the continuum. These protocols must include pain assessment tools that are adopted across the continuum of care by all caregivers.

Although it is convenient to regard postoperative pain primarily as acute pain caused by tissue injury associated with surgery, this may exclude other important factors that contribute to a patient's suffering following surgery. Acute postsurgical pain can also be caused by prolonged patient positioning or pressure effects from prolonged immobility. Many patients presenting for elective surgery may also suffer chronic pain from underlying illness or injury (e.g., degenerative diseases or malignancy) that may contribute significantly to the intensity of the postoperative pain experienced by the patient. Postoperative pain remains a substantial problem that is often masked by a patient's acceptance of pain as a natural consequence of surgery. Other common patient barriers include cultural and language barriers, stoicism and/or opiophobia, and personal experience or the experiences of friends and relatives. For these reasons, postoperative pain management begins preoperatively with patient education to alleviate the attendant anxiety, apprehension, and fear of surgery, to understand the patient's fears and concerns, and to come to an agreement with the patient that pain control is an expected goal of care. Education is also the key to changing attitudes of other caregivers to more effectively treat their patient's pain. In developing a perioperative pain service it is important to bear in mind that the importance of effective perioperative pain management extends well beyond the mere establishment of dedicated personnel but must also encompass a leadership role in transforming the institutional culture to elevate the relief of pain and suffering to its place as a primary goal of patient care.[96]

SPECIAL CONSIDERATIONS IN THE PERIOPERATIVE PAIN MANAGEMENT OF CHILDREN

Acute pain management in children undergoing surgery or invasive procedures offers several specific and unique challenges for the anesthesiologist. The challenges include the importance of the child's parents and siblings relative to their child's responses to the operative environment, unavoidable preoperative fear and anxiety in the child, developmental and communication issues, difficulties in evaluating pain and the effectiveness of treatment, and the patient's reaction to pain, surgery, and the environment manifest as active crying and screaming resistance to care. These problems all summate to emphasize the importance of a holistic approach to pain management that focuses on family-centered care wherein significant efforts are made to reduce preoperative stress and anxiety and to engage the parents

in gaining the cooperation of the child.[97] There is also good evidence that the level of preoperative anxiety and stress adversely impacts postoperative pain and recovery from surgery. A number of methods can be used to reduce preoperative anxiety in children. They include preoperative parental education and counseling about the operative experience,[98] distraction techniques including videos and music, hand-held video games, game-playing with the support of the family and/or child life specialists, and parental presence coupled with oral midazolam (0.5 mg/kg) administration to ease anxiety associated with the transition to the induction of anesthesia. As parental behavior and attitudes can be major determinants of a child's behavior during the inhalational induction of anesthesia, the anesthesiologist is obliged to counsel and inform parents as to the importance of modulating their fear and anxiety should they want to be present during anesthetic induction.

Effective pain management in the postoperative period depends on effective assessment and the precision of the evaluation tools used to measure pain intensity.[99] A child's responses to pain may be variable and unpredictable because of the age and development, verbal communication skills, fear and anxiety, withdrawal, prior experiences, parental presence or absence, and parent's reactions to the care.[100] A comprehensive approach to assessment that employs multiple assessment tools including behavioral responses offers the best option to assessment. The use of visual analogue "faces" pain scales referenced to the appropriate cultural identity of the patient can be useful in assessing postoperative pain severity. There is some question as to the value of parental or practitioner evaluation of a child's pain intensity relative to the visual analogue scale, but parents play a key role in the assessment and management of their child's pain in the postoperative period, particularly when their child is reluctant to communicate or suffers from a cognitive disorder.[101]

Nonparenteral Analgesics

Nonopioid Analgesics

The use of nonopioid analgesics administered orally or by rectal suppository are important adjuvant analgesic therapies under a wide variety of circumstances. Nonparenteral administration of acetaminophen either by oral administration (10 to 20 mg/kg) often given with oral midazolam (0.5 mg/kg) as a component of preoperative sedation or by rectal suppository (20 to 40 mg/kg) after induction of anesthesia provides excellent supplemental analgesia and may be more effective than when it is given by parenteral administration. Acetaminophen can be used across a wide spectrum of surgical procedures and may be sufficient for outpatient procedures. Although the short-term use of the NSAIDs (e.g., ibuprofen and ketorolac) are equipotent with acetaminophen and can be used with safety, the overall convenience and fewer side effects of acetaminophen have favored its use in children. Oral clonidine (4 μg/kg) given as a preoperative medication has also been used with good effect for sedation and postoperative pain management in children undergoing adenotonsillectomy. The greater degree of postoperative sedation with clonidine relative to other analgesics may limit its universal acceptance.

Opioid Analgesics

Codeine in combination with acetaminophen is commonly used with good effect for the management of moderate postoperative pain in the ambulatory patient.[102] The atypical opioid tramadol (3 mg/kg) has also been used as an oral preparation, usually in combination with midazolam (0.5 mg/kg) prior to the induction of anesthesia in children undergoing adenotonsillectomy. Oral tramadol can also be used for postoperative analgesia in children undergoing oral or dental procedures.[103] Intranasal sufentanil (0.2 μg/k) can also be used to manage preoperative anxiety and postoperative analgesia in children and may be more effective than oral tramadol.[103]

Patient-Controlled Analgesia

PCA is established as an important postoperative pain management tool in adults and is increasingly used in older children to good effect.[104,105] There are safety concerns with use of PCA in children that mandate a high level of surveillance with respect to the functioning of the equipment and careful patient monitoring that may be a limitation to its use in infants. PCA by proxy is a safety risk as there is no complete assurance that parents will be competent in assessing the intensity of their child's pain or be able to regulate the bolus dosages in order to avoid opioid overdosage.[106]

Epidural Neuraxial Analgesia

The use of epidural neuraxial analgesia either as a single-shot technique or continuous catheter technique has become a key component of the perioperative pain management plan for infants and young children undergoing abdominal, urologic, or orthopaedic procedures.[107] The use of a single-shot "kiddy" caudal using a local anesthetic with morphine is effective in relieving pain associated with minor procedures in the outpatient setting. Although the overall morbidity is low, there is serious risk associated with epidural analgesia in children related to the systemic toxicity of the local anesthetic and the need to place the epidural under general anesthesia. The risk of irreversible cardiac toxicity, although primarily associated with the use of bupivacaine, can also occur with the ropivacaine and levobupivacaine at an incidence of about 30 to 50% relative to bupivacaine. The risks are increased in children with hepatic dysfunction or when large volumes of local anesthetic are injected into the epidural space through a small, sharp, immobile needle. In the rare event that cardiac toxicity occurs, the anesthesiologist must be prepared to initiate chest compressions and lung ventilation to minimize the risk of anoxic injury and immediately start an intravenous bolus infusion of 20% intralipid (1 to 2 mL/kg) followed by a continuous infusion (0.25 to 0.5 mL/kg/min) until normal cardiac rhythm and the circulation is restored.[108] Although the use of lipid emulsions can be successful in reversing cardiac arrest, their immediate availability does not excuse the anesthesiologist from taking all precautions to prevent systemic injection or absorption when performing the procedure.

Peripheral Nerve Blocks in Children

The introduction of small stimulating needles and ultrasound imaging along with long-acting local anesthetics and continuous catheter techniques in selected cases has resulted in an increase in the use of peripheral nerve blocks in children undergoing orthopaedic extremity procedures.[109] The use of stimulating needles permits the anesthesiologist to place the injection after the child is anesthetized.[110] As the child is unresponsive, it is important that the initial injection meets no resistance in order to avoid intraneural injection. Combined ilioinguinal and iliohypogastric nerve blocks performed under ultrasound guidance to reduce the volume of the injection have gained increasing interest for effective pain management in children undergoing inguinal herniorrhaphy.[111]

CONCLUSION

In October 2000, the U.S. Congress designated the decade beginning January 1, 2001, as the Decade of Pain Control and Research. The onus is on dedicated health care professionals to provide our patients with the best care possible when it comes to pain and suffering, which applies directly to the perioperative state. Accomplishing this requires integration of information and systems from disparate disciplines within medicine. It challenges physicians to acquire a patient-focused perspective that spans the mind-body spectrum of the perioperative experience. In doing so, clinicians will be challenged to construct systems within hospitals to support such endeavors but will be able to show objective and meaningful outcomes with positive benefits to patients and to health care organizations. The cost of ignoring pain and suffering has been widely cited to be in the billions of dollars each, but the cost in suffering is immeasurable. Anesthesiology has led the way in improving the overall pain care of the surgical patient and is positioned to lead medicine into a new era in which perioperative pain management is better, safer, more assured, and consistently available at the highest levels to all.

References

1. United States Agency for Health Care Policy and Research. Acute pain management operative or medical procedures and trauma. Rockville, MD, US Dept of Health and Human Services Public Health Service Agency for Health Care Policy and Research, 1992
2. American Society of Anesthesiologists Task Force on Acute Pain Management. Practice guidelines for acute pain management in the perioperative setting: An updated report by the American Society of Anesthesiologists Task Force on Acute Pain Management. Anesthesiology 2004; 100: 1573
3. Wu CL, Naqibuddin M, Rowlingson AJ et al: The effect of pain on health-related quality of life in the immediate postoperative period. Anesth Analg 2003; 97: 1078
4. Joshi GP, Ogunnaike BO: Consequences of inadequate postoperative pain relief and chronic persistent postoperative pain. Anesthesiol Clin North Am 2005; 23: 21
5. Carr DB, Goudas LC: Acute pain. Lancet 1999; 353: 2051
6. Raja SN, Dougherty PM: Anatomy and physiology of somatosensory and pain processing, Essentials of Pain Medicine and Regional Anesthesia, 2nd edition. Edited by Benzon HT, Raja SN, Molloy RE et al: Philadelphia, Elsevier, Churchill Livingstone, 2005, p 1
7. Wilder-Smith OH, Arendt-Nielsen L: Postoperative hyperalgesia: its clinical importance and relevance. Anesthesiology 2006; 104(3): 601
8. Rowlingson JC: Update on Acute Pain Management. International Anesthesia Research Society Review Course Lectures 2006: 95
9. Amid PK: Causes, prevention, and surgical treatment of postherniorrhaphy neuropathic inguinodynia: triple neurectomy with proximal end implantation. Hernia 2004; 8(4): 343
10. Taylor DR: Improving outcomes in acute pain management: Optimizing patient selection. *Medscape Neurol Neurosurg* 2004; 6(2)
11. Cepeda MS, Carr DB: Women experience more pain and require more morphine than men to achieve a similar degree of analgesia. *Anesth Analg* 2003; 97(5): 1464
12. Caraceni A, Cherny N, Fainsinger R et al: Pain measurement tools and methods in clinical research in palliative care: recommendations of an Expert Working Group of the European Association of Palliative Care. *J Pain Symptom Manage* 2002; 23(3): 239
13. Portenoy RK, Bennett DS, Rauck R et al: Prevalence and characteristics of breakthrough pain in opioid-treated patients with chronic noncancer pain. *J Pain* 2006; 7(8): 583
14. Bennett M: The LANSS Pain Scale: the Leeds assessment of neuropathic symptoms and signs. *Pain* 2001; 92(1-2): 147
15. Viscusi ER, Goldstein S, Witkowski T et al: Alvimopan, a peripherally acting mu-opioid receptor antagonist, compared with placebo in postoperative ileus after major abdominal surgery: results of a randomized, double-blind, controlled study. *Surg Endosc* 2006; 20(1): 64
16. Angst MS, Clark JD: Opioid-induced hyperalgesia: a qualitative systematic review. *Anesthesiology* 2006; 104(3): 570
17. Sarhill N, Walsh D, Nelson KA: Hydromorphone: pharmacology and clinical applications in cancer patients. *Support Care Cancer* 2001; 9(2): 84
18. Mahajan G, Fishman SM: Major opioids in pain management, *Essentials of Pain Medicine and Regional Anesthesia*. Edited by Benzon H, Raja SN, Molloy RE, Liu S, Fishman SM. Philadelphia, Elsevier Churchill Livingstone, 2005, pp. 94

19. Mitra S, Sinatra RS: Perioperative management of acute pain in the opioid-dependent patient. *Anesthesiology* 2004; 101(1): 212

20. APS: *Principles of Analgesic Use in the Treatment of Acute pain and Cancer pain.* Fifth ed. American Pain Society, 2003

21. Candido KD, Winnie AP, Ghaleb AH et al: Buprenorphine added to the local anesthetic for axillary brachial plexus block prolongs postoperative analgesia. *Reg Anesth Pain Med* 2002; 27(2): 162

22. Katz JA: NSAIDs and COX-2 Selective Inhibitors, *Essentials of Pain Medicine and Regional Anesthesia, 2nd edition.* Edited by Benzon R, Molloy, Liu, Fishman S: Elsevier Churchill Livingston, 2005, pp. 141

23. Marret E, Kurdi O, Zufferey P, Bonnet F: Effects of nonsteroidal antiinflammatory drugs on patient-controlled analgesia morphine side effects: meta-analysis of randomized controlled trials. Anesthesiology 2005; 102(6): 1249

24. Nussmeier NA, Whelton AA, Brown MT et al: Complications of the COX-2 inhibitors parecoxib and valdecoxib after cardiac surgery. N Engl J Med 2005; 352(11): 1081

25. White PF: The changing role of non-opioid analgesic techniques in the management of postoperative pain. Anesth Analg 2005; 101(5 suppl): S5

26. Power I: Recent advances in postoperative pain therapy. Br J Anaesth 2005; 95(1): 43

27. Weinbroum AA: A single small dose of postoperative ketamine provides rapid and sustained improvement in morphine analgesia in the presence of morphine-resistant pain. *Anesth Analg* 2003; 96(3): 789

28. Sveticic G, Gentilini A, Eichenberger U et al: Combinations of morphine with ketamine for patient-controlled analgesia: a new optimization method. *Anesthesiology* 2003; 98(5): 1195

29. Reeves M, Lindholm DE, Myles PS et al: Adding ketamine to morphine for patient-controlled analgesia after major abdominal surgery: a double-blinded, randomized controlled trial. *Anesth Analg* 2001; 93(1): 116

30. Wadhwa A, Clarke D, Goodchild CS, Young D: Large-dose oral dextromethorphan as an adjunct to patient-controlled analgesia with morphine after knee surgery. *Anesth Analg* 2001; 92(2): 448

31. Sites BD, Beach M, Biggs R et al: Intrathecal clonidine added to a bupivacaine-morphine spinal anesthetic improves postoperative analgesia for total knee arthroplasty. *Anesth Analg.* Apr 2003; 96(4): 1083

32. Gerlach AT, Dasta JF: Dexmedetomidine: an updated review. *Ann Pharmacother* 2007; 41(2): 245

33. Ebert T, Maze M: Dexmedetomidine: another arrow for the clinician's quiver. *Anesthesiology* 2004; 101(3): 568

34. Ramsay MA, Luterman DL: Dexmedetomidine as a total intravenous anesthetic agent. *Anesthesiology* 2004; 101(3): 787

35. Hurley RW, Cohen SP, Williams KA et al: The analgesic effects of perioperative gabapentin on postoperative pain: a meta-analysis. *Reg Anesth Pain Med* 2006; 31(3): 237

36. Menigaux C, Adam F, Guignard B et al: Preoperative gabapentin decreases anxiety and improves early functional recovery from knee surgery. *Anesth Analg* 2005; 100(5): 1394

37. Turan A, White PF, Karamanlioglu B et al: Gabapentin: an alternative to the cyclooxygenase-2 inhibitors for perioperative pain management. *Anesth Analg* 2006; 102(1): 175

38. Kong VK, Irwin MG: Gabapentin: a multimodal perioperative drug? *Br J Anaesth* 2007; 99(6): 775

39. Kaba A, Laurent SR, Detroz BJ et al: Intravenous lidocaine infusion facilitates acute rehabilitation after laparoscopic colectomy. *Anesthesiology* 2007; 106(1): 11; discussion 15

40. Buvanendran A, Kroin JS: Useful adjuvants for postoperative pain management. *Best Pract Res Clin Anaesthesiol* 2007; 21(1): 31

41. Koc S, Memis D, Sut N: The preoperative use of gabapentin, dexamethasone, and their combination in varicocele surgery: A randomized controlled trial. *Anesth Analg* 2007; 105: 1137

42. Macintyre PE: Safety and efficacy of patient-controlled analgesia. *Br J Anaesth* 2001; 87(1): 36

43. Gan TJ, Meyer T, Apfel CC et al: Consensus guidelines for managing postoperative nausea and vomiting. *Anesth Analg* 2003; 97(1): 62

44. Block BM, Liu SS, Rowlingson AJ et al: Efficacy of postoperative epidural analgesia: a meta-analysis. JAMA 2003; 290(18): 2455

45. Bernards CM, Shen DD, Sterling ES et al: Epidural, cerebrospinal fluid, and plasma pharmacokinetics of epidural opioids (part 1): differences among opioids. *Anesthesiology* 2003; 99(2): 455

46. Ginosar Y, Riley ET, Angst MS: The site of action of epidural fentanyl in humans: the difference between infusion and bolus administration. *Anesth Analg* 2003; 97(5): 1428

47. Forster JG, Rosenberg PH: Small dose of clonidine mixed with low-dose ropivacaine and fentanyl for epidural analgesia after total knee arthroplasty. *Br J Anaesth* 2004; 93(5): 670

48. Rathmell JP, Lair TR, Nauman B: The role of intrathecal drugs in the treatment of acute pain. *Anesth Analg* 2005; 101(5 Suppl): S30

49. Sites BD, Beach M, Gallagher JD et al: A single injection ultrasound-assisted femoral nerve block provides side effect-sparing analgesia when compared with intrathecal morphine in patients undergoing total knee arthroplasty. *Anesth Analg* 2004; 99(5): 1539

50. Richman JM, Liu S, Courpas G et al: Does Continuous Peripheral Nerve Block Provide Superior Pain Control to Opioids? A Meta-Analysis. *Anesth Analg* 2006; 102: 248

51. Capdevila X, Pirat P, Bringuier S et al: Continuous peripheral nerve blocks in hospital wards after orthopedic surgery: a multicenter prospective analysis of the quality of postoperative analgesia and complications in 1,416 patients. *Anesthesiology* 2005; 103(5): 1035

52. Swenson JD, Bay N, Loose E et al: Outpatient management of continuous peripheral nerve catheters placed using ultrasound guidance: an experience in 620 patients. *Anesth Analg* 2006; 103(6): 1436

52a. Winnie AP. Interscalene brachial plexus block. Anesth Analg 1970; 49: 455

53. Sinha SK, Abrams JH, Weller RS: Ultrasound-guided interscalene needle placement produces successful anesthesia regardless of motor stimulation above or below 0.5 mA. *Anesth Analg* 2007; 105(3): 848

54. Hadzic A, Williams BA, Karaca PE et al: For outpatient rotator cuff surgery, nerve block anesthesia provides superior same-day recovery over general anesthesia. *Anesthesiology* 2005; 102(5): 1001

55. Ilfeld BM, Vandenborne K, Duncan PW et al: Ambulatory continuous interscalene nerve blocks decrease the time to discharge readiness after total shoulder arthroplasty: a randomized, triple-masked, placebo-controlled study. *Anesthesiology* 2006; 105(5): 999

55a. Kulenkampf D. Anesthesia of the brachial plexus (German). *Zentralbl Chir* 1911; 38: 1337

56. Perlas A, Chan VW, Simons M: Brachial plexus examination and localization using ultrasound and electrical stimulation: a volunteer study. *Anesthesiology* 2003; 99(2): 429

57. Soares LG, Brull R, Lai J, Chan VW: Eight ball, corner pocket: the optimal needle position for ultrasound-guided supraclavicular block. *Reg Anesth Pain Med* 2007; 32(1): 94

58. Bigeleisen P, Wilson M: A comparison of two techniques for ultrasound guided infraclavicular block. *Br J Anaesth* 2006; 96(4): 502

59. Dingemans E, Williams SR, Arcand G et al: Neurostimulation in ultrasound-guided infraclavicular block: a prospective randomized trial. *Anesth Analg* 2007; 104(5): 1275

60. Sandhu NS, Capan LM: Ultrasound-guided infraclavicular brachial plexus block. *Br J Anaesth* 2002; 89(2): 254

61. Sauter AR, Smith HJ, Stubhaug A et al: Use of magnetic resonance imaging to define the anatomical location closest to all three cords of the infraclavicular brachial plexus. *Anesth Analg* 2006; 103(6): 1574

62. Sandhu NS, Manne JS, Medabalmi PK, Capan LM: Sonographically guided infraclavicular brachial plexus block in adults: a retrospective analysis of 1146 cases. *J Ultrasound Med* 2006; 25(12): 1555

63. Ilfeld BM, Morey TE, Enneking FK: Infraclavicular perineural local anesthetic infusion: a comparison of three dosing regimens for postoperative analgesia. *Anesthesiology* 2004; 100(2): 395

64. Awad IT, Duggan EM: Posterior lumbar plexus block: anatomy, approaches, and techniques. Reg Anesth Pain Med 2005; 30(2): 143

65. Kaloul I, Guay J, Cote C, Fallaha M: The posterior lumbar plexus (psoas compartment) block and the three-in-one femoral nerve block provide similar postoperative analgesia after total knee replacement. *Can J Anaesth* 2004; 51(1): 45

66. Kirchmair L, Enna B, Mitterschiffthaler G et al: Lumbar plexus in children. A sonographic study and its relevance to pediatric regional anesthesia. *Anesthesiology* 2004; 101(2): 445

67. Becchi C, Al Malyan M, Coppini R et al: Opioid-free analgesia by continuous psoas compartment block after total hip arthroplasty. A randomized study. *Eur J Anaesthesiol* 2007; 1

68. Horlocker TT, Cabanela ME, Wedel DJ: Does postoperative epidural analgesia increase the risk of peroneal nerve palsy after total knee arthroplasty? *Anesth Analg* 1994; 79(3): 495

69. Capdevila X, Coimbra C, Choquet O: Approaches to the lumbar plexus: success, risks, and outcome. *Reg Anesth Pain Med* 2005; 30(2): 150

70. Gray AT, Collins AB, Schafhalter-Zoppoth I: An introduction to femoral nerve and associated lumbar plexus nerve blocks under ultrasound guidance. *Tech Reg Anesth Pain Mgmt* 2004; 8(4): 155

70a. Winnie AP, Ramamurthy S, Durrani Z. The inguinal paravascular technic of lumbar plexus anesthesia: The "3-in-1 block. Anesth Analg 1973; 52: 989

71. Fowler SJ, Symons J, Sabato S, Myles PS: Epidural analgesia compared with peripheral nerve blockade after major knee surgery: a systematic review and meta-analysis of randomized trials. *Br J Anaesth* 2008; 100(2): 154

72. Krombach J, Gray AT: Sonography for saphenous nerve block near the adductor canal. *Reg Anesth Pain Med* 2007; 32(4): 369

73. Chan VW, Nova H, Abbas S et al: Ultrasound examination and localization of the sciatic nerve: a volunteer study. *Anesthesiology* 2006; 104(2): 309, discussion 305A

74. Karmakar MK, Kwok WH, Ho AM et al: Ultrasound-guided sciatic nerve block: description of a new approach at the subgluteal space. *Br J Anaesth* 2007; 98(3): 390

75. van Geffen GJ, Gielen M: Ultrasound-guided subgluteal sciatic nerve blocks with stimulating catheters in children: a descriptive study. *Anesth Analg* 2006; 103(2): 328

76. Marhofer P, Chan VW: Ultrasound-guided regional anesthesia: current concepts and future trends. *Anesth Analg.* May 2007; 104(5): 1265

77. Zaric D, Boysen K, Christiansen J et al: Continuous popliteal sciatic nerve block for outpatient foot surgery—a randomized, controlled trial. *Acta Anaesthesiol Scan* 2004; 48(3): 337

78. Richardson J: Paravertebral anesthesia and analgesia. *Can J Anesth* 2004; 51(6): R1

79. Naja ZM, El-Rajab M, Al-Tannir MA et al: Thoracic paravertebral block: influence of the number of injections. *Reg Anesth Pain Med* 2006; 31(3): 196

80. Karmakar MK, Chui PT, Joynt GM, Ho AM: Thoracic paravertebral block for management of pain associated with multiple fractured ribs in patients with concomitant lumbar spinal trauma. Reg Anesth Pain Med 2001; 26(2): 169

81. Cook E, Downs C: Analgesia after thoracotomy: The role of the extrapleural paravertebral catheter. *Austr Anaesth* 2005: 103

82. Evans H, Steele SM, Nielsen KC et al: Peripheral nerve blocks and continuous catheter techniques. Anesthesiol Clin North Am 2005; 23(1): 141

83. Hebbard P, Fujiwara Y, Shibata Y, Royse C: Ultrasound-guided transversus abdominis plane (TAP) block. *Anaesth Intensive Care* 2007; 35(4): 616

84. Brower MC, Johnson ME: Adverse effects of local anesthetic infiltration on wound healing. *Reg Anesth Pain Med* 2003; 28: 233

85. Venditoli PA, Makinen P, Drolet P et al: A Multimodal Analgesia Protocol for Total Knee Arthroplasty. *J Bone Joint Surg* 2006; 88-A(2): 282

86. Horlocker TT, Wedel DJ: Neuraxial block and low-molecular-weight heparin: balancing perioperative analgesia and thromboprophylaxis. *Reg Anesth Pain Med* 1998; 23(6 Suppl 2): 164

87. Horlocker TT, Wedel DJ, Benzon H et al: Regional anesthesia in the anticoagulated patient: defining the risks (the second ASRA Consensus Conference on Neuraxial Anesthesia and Anticoagulation). *Reg Anesth Pain Med* 2003; 28(3): 172

88. Rodgers A, Walker N, Schug S et al: Reduction of postoperative mortality and morbidity with epidural or spinal anaesthesia: results from overview of randomised trials. *BMJ* 2000; 321(7275): 1493

89. Tuman KJ, McCarthy RJ, March RJ et al: Effects of epidural anesthesia and analgesia on coagulation and outcome after major vascular surgery. *Anesth Analg* 1991; 73(6): 696

90. Cheney FW: High-severity injuries associated with regional anesthesia in the 1990's. *Am Soc Anesthesiol Newsletter* 2001; 65(6): 6

91. Hebl JR, Horlocker TT, Sorenson EJ, Schroeder DR: Regional anesthesia does not increase the risk of postoperative neuropathy in patients undergoing ulnar nerve transposition. *Anesth Analg* 2001; 93(6): 1606

92. Pasternak GW: Incomplete cross tolerance and multiple mu opioid peptide receptors. *Trends Pharmacol Sci* 2001; 22(2): 67

93. Carroll IR, Angst MS, Clark JD: Management of perioperative pain in patients chronically consuming opioids. *Reg Anesth Pain Med* 2004; 29(6): 576

94. Dolin SJ, Cashman JN, Bland JM: Effectiveness of acute postoperative pain management: I. Evidence from published data. *Br J Anaesth* 2002; 89(3): 409

95. Stadler M, Schlander M, Braeckman M et al: A cost-utility and cost-effectiveness analysis of an acute pain service. *J Clin Anesth* 2004; 16(3): 159

96. Berry PH, Dahl JL: The new JCAHO pain standards: implications for pain management nurses. *Pain Manag Nurs* 2000; 1(1): 3

97. Kain ZN, Mayes LC, Caldwell-Andrews AA et al: Preoperative anxiety, postoperative pain, and behavioral recovery in young children undergoing surgery. *Pediatrics* 2006; 118(2): 651

98. Wright KD, Stewart SH, Finley GA, Buffett-Jerrott SE: Prevention and intervention strategies to alleviate preoperative anxiety in children: a critical review. *Behav Modif* 2007; 31(1): 52

99. Voepel-Lewis T, Malviya S, Tait AR et al: A comparison of the clinical utility of pain assessment tools for children with cognitive impairment. *Anesth Analg* 2008; 106(1): 72

100. Taylor EM, Boyer K, Campbell FA: Pain in hospitalized children: A prospective cross-sectional survey of pain prevalence, intensity, assessment and management in a Canadian pediatric teaching hospital. *Pain Res Manag* 2008; 13(1): 25

101. Franck LS, Allen A, Oulton K: Making pain assessment more accessible to children and parents: can greater involvement improve the quality of care? *Clin J Pain* 2007; 23(4): 331

102. Moir MS, Bair E, Shinnick P, Messner A: Acetaminophen versus acetaminophen with codeine after pediatric tonsillectomy. *Laryngoscope* 2000; 110(11): 1824

103. Bayrak F, Gunday I, Memis D, Turan A: A comparison of oral midazolam, oral tramadol, and intranasal sufentanil premedication in pediatric patients. *J Opioid Manag* 2007; 3(2): 74

104. Butkovic D, Kralik S, Matolic M et al: Postoperative analgesia with intravenous fentanyl PCA vs epidural block after thoracoscopic pectus excavatum repair in children. *Br J Anaesth* 2007; 98(5): 677

105. Saudan S, Habre W, Ceroni D et al: Safety and efficacy of patient controlled epidural analgesia following pediatric spinal surgery. *Paediatr Anaesth* 2008; 18(2): 132

106. Wuhrman E, Cooney MF, Dunwoody CJ et al: Authorized and Unauthorized ("PCA by Proxy") Dosing of Analgesic Infusion Pumps: position statement with clinical practice recommendations. *Pain Manag Nurs* 2007; 8(1): 4

107. Ecoffey C: Pediatric regional anesthesia—update. *Curr Opin Anaesthesiol* 2007; 20(3): 232

108. Corman SL, Skledar SJ: Use of lipid emulsion to reverse local anesthetic-induced toxicity. *Ann Pharmacother* 2007; 41(11): 1873

109. Ganesh A, Rose JB, Wells L et al: Continuous peripheral nerve blockade for inpatient and outpatient postoperative analgesia in children. *Anesth Analg* 2007; 105(5): 1234

110. DeVera HV, Furukawa KT, Matson MD et al: Regional techniques as an adjunct to general anesthesia for pediatric extremity and spine surgery. *J Pediatr Orthop* 2006; 26(6): 801

111. Weintraud M, Marhofer P, Bosenberg A et al: Ilioinguinal/iliohypogastric blocks in children: where do we administer the local anesthetic without direct visualization? *Anesth Analg* 2008; 106(1): 89

112. Dougherty PM, Raja SN: Neurochemistry of Somatosensory and Pain Processing, *Essentials of Pain Medicine and Regional Anesthesia*. Edited by Benzon HT, Raja SN, Molloy RE, Liu SS, Fishman SM: Elsevier, Churchill Livingstone, 2005, pp. 7

113. Kehlet H: Multimodal approach to control postoperative pathophysiology and rehabilitation. *Br J Anaesth* 1997; 78(5): 606

114. Fine P: The diagnosis and treatment of breakthrough pain. New York, Oxford American Pain Library, 2008

115. Foley KM: Acute and Chronic Cancer Pain Syndromes, *Oxford Textbook of Palliative Medicine*. Edited by Doyle D, Hanks G, Cherny N, Calman K: Oxford University Press, 2004, 298

116. Toombs JD, Kral LA: Methadone treatment for pain states. *Am Fam Phys* 2005; 71(7): 1353

117. Hadi I, Morley-Forster PK, Dain S et al: Brief review: Perioperative management of the patient with chronic non-cancer pain [Article de synthese court: Prise en charge perioperatoire des patients souffrant de douleur chronique non cancereuse. *Can J Anaesth* 2006; 53(12): 1190

118. Drugs, Facts and Comparisons: Wolters Kluwer Health, 2008

119. Ayonrinde OT, Bridge DT: The rediscovery of methadone for cancer pain management. *Med J Austr* 2000; 173(10): 536

120. Grass JA: Patient-controlled analgesia. *Anesth Analg* 2005; 101(5 Suppl): S44

121. Paech MJ, Pavy TJ, Orlikowski CE et al: Postcesarean analgesia with spinal morphine, clonidine, or their combination. *Anesth Analg* 2004; 98(5): 1460

122. Liu SS, McDonald SB: Current issues in spinal anesthesia. *Anesthesiology* 2001; 94(5): 888

123. Meier G, Bauereis C, Maurer H, Meier T: [Interscalene plexus block. Anatomic requirements—anesthesiologic and operative aspects]. *Anaesthesist*. May 2001; 50(5): 333

124. Borgeat A, Dullenkopf A, Ekatodramis G, Nagy L: Evaluation of the lateral modified approach for continuous interscalene block after shoulder surgery. *Anesthesiology*. Aug 2003; 99(2): 436

125. Marhofer P, Greher M, Kapral S: Ultrasound guidance in regional anesthesia. *Br J Anaesth* 2005; 94(1): 7

126. Schafhalter-Zoppoth I, Younger SJ, Collins AB, Gray AT: The "seesaw" sign: improved sonographic identification of the sciatic nerve. *Anesthesiology* 2004; 101(3): 808

127. Liu S: Update in use of continuous perineural catheters for postoperative analgesia. IARS 2006 Review Course Lectures. *Anesth Analg Suppl* 2006: 64

128. Neal JM, Hebl JR, Gerancher JC, Hogan QH: Brachial plexus anesthesia: Essentials of our current understanding. *Reg Anesth Pain Med* 2002; 27(4): 402

129. Horlocker TT: Complications of Regional Anesthesia. IARS 2004 Review Course Lectures. *Anesth Analg Suppl* 2004: 56

130. Ben-David B: Complications of peripheral blockade. *Anesthesiol Clin North Am* 2002; 20(3): 457

131. Hebl JR, Horlocker TT, Pritchard DJ: Diffuse brachial plexopathy after interscalene blockade in a patient receiving cisplatin chemotherapy: the pharmacologic double crush syndrome. *Anesth Analg* 2001; 92(1): 249

CHAPTER 58 ■ CHRONIC PAIN MANAGEMENT

HONORIO T. BENZON, ROBERT W. HURLEY, AND TIMOTHY R. DEER

KEY POINTS

1 A delta and C fibers, under normal conditions, transmit nociceptive (pain) information to the spinal cord from their free nerve endings in the periphery. In chronic pain conditions, the A beta fibers, which normally transmit nonnoxious information, also participate in nociceptive transmission.

2 Most randomized studies on the efficacy of epidural steroid injections show temporary relief of radicular pain. Studies on thermal rhizotomy of the medial branches, for relief of facet syndrome, show benefit that lasts 3 to 12 months. This relief avoids the usage of addicting opioids.

3 Neuraxial local anesthetics and methylprednisolone, when performed 3 to 4 times during the acute stage of herpes zoster, may prevent the development of postherpetic neuralgia. Postherpetic neuralgia is mostly managed pharmacologically, although interventional techniques may be used in resistant cases.

4 Antidepressants are effective in neuropathic pain syndromes but their use is limited because of their side effects. Anticonvulsants are effective in most neuropathic pain syndromes. Their favorable side effect profile makes them the first line of treatment for these syndromes.

5 Complex regional pain syndrome that does not respond to nerve blocks and physical therapy may respond to spinal cord stimulation.

6 Opioids are the mainstay for cancer pain management. Opioids are effective in postherpetic neuralgia and painful diabetic neuropathy, especially when combined with an anticonvulsant.

7 The majority of pain secondary to cancer is effectively managed pharmacologically with opioids, anticonvulsants, and antidepressants. Neurolysis of the visceral sympathetic system for pain secondary to abdominal or pelvic cancer relieves pain, decreases opioid consumption, and improves the patients' quality of life.

8 Most of the studies on percutaneous disc decompression are case series. The use of intradiscal electrothermal therapy is supported by a randomized control study.

9 Vertebroplasty and kyphoplasty are indicated for vertebral compression fractures; studies show their efficacy at long-term follow-up.

10 Spinal cord stimulation is effective in patients with failed back syndrome and radicular symptoms and in complex regional pain syndromes. Case series show its efficacy in treating peripheral ischemia.

11 Intrathecal drug delivery systems are valuable options in patients in whom opioids are ineffective at high doses or cause unacceptable side effects. To prevent the development of intrathecal granulomas, high concentrations of the opioid should be avoided, the catheter should be positioned in the lumbar thecal sac, and there should be conscientious follow-up of patients.

ANATOMY, PHYSIOLOGY, AND NEUROCHEMISTRY OF SOMATOSENSORY PAIN PROCESSING

Primary Afferents and Peripheral Stimulation

A variety of mechanical, thermal, or chemical stimuli can result in the sensation and perception of pain. Information about these painful or noxious stimuli is carried to higher brain centers by receptors and neurons that are distinct from those that carry innocuous somatic sensory information. The mammalian somatosensory system is subserved by four groups of afferent fibers differentiated by their anatomy, rate of transmission, and sensory modality transduced (Table 58-1).

The first group, the heavily myelinated large-diameter A alpha (Aα) fibers, have specialized terminals incorporated within muscle spindles, Golgi tendon organs, and joints. These fibers and their respective end organs transduce proprioceptive information. The second group, the heavily myelinated large-diameter A beta (Aβ) fibers, have specialized encapsulated nerve endings including the Meissner, Pacinian, and Ruffini corpuscles and the Merkel disk, which transduce innocuous or low-threshold mechanical stimulation. Aα fibers do not ordinarily participate in signaling pain sensations to the central nervous system. However, the activation of Aβ and, possibly, Aα fibers has been invoked as a part of the mechanism for the production of pain relief by transcutaneous electrical nerve stimulators, which may implicate their role in pain signal processing.[1] As well, it is becoming increasingly apparent that in chronic pain states, these fibers may indeed participate in pain signaling by adopting a "phenotype" similar to that of a C fiber (vide infra).[2]

The next groups of fibers represent the specialized sensory neurons that respond to actual or potential tissue damage, the *nociceptors*. The lightly myelinated medium-diameter A delta (Aδ) fibers and the unmyelinated small-diameter C fibers have free nerve endings that transduce noxious or high-threshold thermal, mechanical, and chemical stimulation. Unlike receptors in the first two groups (Aα and Aβ), the Aδ and C fibers respond to stimulation of their receptive fields in a characteristic manner with slow adaptation and residual firing following the withdrawal of the stimulus. Although these two fiber groups respond similarly to stimulation, they mediate different aspects of pain sensation. The rapidly conducting Aδ fibers mediate the "first" pain or *epicritic pain*, which is well localized and is characterized as sharp or prickling. The slowly conducting C fibers mediate the "second" pain or *protopathic pain*, which temporally follows the epicritic pain and is poorly localized or diffuse and is characterized as burning or dull.[3] The majority of Aδ and C nociceptors are polymodal and therefore are responsible for the transduction of noxious stimuli of different modalities. Nociceptive nerve endings are also located in muscle, the fascia, and adventitia of blood vessels, the knee joint, the dura, and viscera. Recent evidence suggests that sensory transduction in the skin can include mediation by nonneural skin cells including keratinocytes and epithelial cells. These cells are thought to directly participate in touch and thermal sensation and are believed to communicate with the nerve ending through paracrine transmission.[4] Chemical mediators of pain are numerous. These mediators come from sources intrinsic to the neuron, including various neurotransmitters such as serotonin and substance P, and extrinsic to the nervous system, including substances from inflammatory/immune cells and red blood cells such as prostaglandins, kinins, cytokines, chemokines, and adenosine triphosphate that are released following injury to the tissue.

The primary afferent peripheral (distal) terminals express a variety of specific transducer channels that are sensitive over a range of stimulus intensities. When they are activated by the appropriate stimulus (thermal, chemical, or mechanical) these channels activate voltage-sensitive cation channels (NaV and CaV) and initiate an action potential.

Although the sensory modalities may appear quite disparate at first glance, there are similarities. The cloning and characterization of the "capsaicin" receptor of the transient receptor potential (TRP) family of cation channels has expanded the field immensely[5] (Table 58-2). Members of this molecular family transduce thermal, mechanical, and chemical information in the periphery. The capsaicin receptor named *TRP vanilloid 1* (TRPV1), which responds not only to capsaicin and other vanilloid compounds but is also activated by acid and heat, provides an excellent example of the integration of multiple sensory modalities within a single neuron and is localized to nociceptors.[5] Furthermore, acidic environments can lower the activation threshold of the channel to heat stimuli. Therefore, the TRPV1 receptor may represent an important therapeutic target in inflammatory (acidic) pain conditions.

TABLE 58-1

PRIMARY AFFERENT FIBERS AND THEIR FUNCTION

■ MODALITY	■ RECEPTOR	■ FIBER TYPE	■ CONDUCTION VELOCITY AND DIAMETER	■ RATE OF ADAPTATION	■ FUNCTION
Proprioceptive	Golgi and Ruffini endings, muscle spindle afferents	Aα	70–120 m/s 15–20 microns	Slow and rapid	Muscle tension, length and velocity
Mechanosensitive	Meissner, Ruffini, Pacinian corpuscles and Merkel disc	Aβ	40–70 m/s 5–15 microns	Rapid (slow–Merkel)	Touch, flutter, motion, pressure, vibration
Thermoreceptive	Free nerve endings	Aδ	10–35 m/s 1–5 microns	Slow	Innocuous cold
	Free nerve endings	C	0.5–1 m/s <1 micron	Slow	Innocuous warmth
Nociceptive	Free nerve endings	Aδ	10–35 m/s 1–5 microns	Slow	Sharp pain
	Free nerve endings	C	0.5–1 m/s <1 micron	Slow	Burning pain

TABLE 58-2

MECHANOSENSORY AND THERMOSENSORY TRANSDUCTION CHANNELS FOUND IN MAMMALS

■ NAME	■ FAMILY	■ PHYSICAL MODALITY	■ ADDITIONAL ACTIVATORS	■ TEMPERATURE RANGE (°C)	■ NEURONAL EXPRESSION
TRPA1	TRPA	Thermal, mechanical	Icillin, calcium, isothiocyanates	<18	C-fibers
TRPC1	TRPC	Mechanical	Receptor-operated	NA	Aβ, Aδ
TRPM8	TRPM	Thermal	Menthol, Icillin	<28	C fibers
TRPV1	TRPV	Thermal, osmotic	Capsaicin, protons, endocannabinoids, diphenyl compounds	>42	C, Aδ, and keratinocytes
TRPV2	TRPV	Thermal, osmotic, mechanical	Diphenyl compounds	>52	Aβ, Aδ, keratinocytes
TRPV3	TRPV	Thermal	Camphor, carvacrol, diphenyl	>34–39	C fibers, keratinocytes
TRPV4	TRPV	Thermal, osmotic	Polyunsaturated fatty acids, epoxyeicosatrienoic acid	>27–34	Aδ, C, keratinocytes, merkel cells
ASIC1	DEG/ENaC	Mechanical	Protons	NA	Aβ, Aδ, C
ASIC2	DEG/ENaC	Mechanical	Protons	NA	Aβ, Aδ
ASIC3	DEG/ENaC	Mechanical	Protons	NA	Aβ, Aδ
TREK-1	Potassium channel	Thermal, mechanical	Lipids, protons	NA	Aβ, Aδ, C

Adapted from Lumpkin EA, Caterina MJ: Mechanisms of sensory transduction in the skin. Nature 2007; 445: 858.

Mice lacking the TRPV1 receptor are deficient in their response to thermal but not mechanical or other noxious stimuli.[6] These data suggest that this member of the family of TRP channels may play a role in the integration of noxious chemical and thermal stimuli while having relatively little to do with mechanical transduction. Although mechanical transduction has been less well characterized than either thermal or chemical nociceptive transduction, there is evidence of mechanically activated channels in the *degenerins* family of the nematode *Caenorhabditis elegans*. In mammals, studies have provided evidence that the transduction channel is a complex of degenerin and the epithelial Na+ channel[7] and may have a role in the transduction of mechanical stimuli in humans. More recently, a mechanosensitive stretch-inactivated channel has been localized to small-diameter sensory neurons.

Neurochemistry of Peripheral Nerve and the Dorsal Root Ganglion

The nociceptive primary afferents, the Aδ and C fibers, represent the principal target of pharmacologic manipulation by the physician treating pain. Glutamate receptors, as well as opioid, substance P, somatostatin, and vanilloid receptors, have been identified on the peripheral endings of these nerve fibers. Although the transmission of acute nociceptive information is primarily by the Aδ and C fibers, a subset of the Aδ and C fibers are "thermoreceptors" that transduce innocuous cold and warm information, respectively. The cell bodies of primary afferents, regardless of the structure they innervate, make up the *dorsal root ganglia* (DRG) located just outside the spinal cord within the bony foramen.

Primary afferent activation results in a postsynaptic excitatory event in the spinal cord. Glutamate is the primary neurotransmitter serving this function. Acute activation events are mediated by the AMPA-type (α-amino-3-hydroxy-5-methyl-4-isoxazole propionic acid) glutamate receptor present on the dorsal horn neurons. This receptor produces a robust, but short-lasting depolarization of the postsynaptic membrane by increasing sodium conductance and augmenting the activation of the NMDA-type (N-methyl-D-aspartate) glutamate receptor. In addition to glutamate, populations of primary afferents contain and corelease a variety of neuropeptides including substance P, calcitonin gene-related peptide, adenosine triphosphate, adenosine, galanin, and somatostatin and growth factors including brain-derived nerve growth factor.[8]

Neurobiology of the Spinal Cord and Spinal Trigeminal Nucleus

Primary afferent fibers enter the gray matter of the spinal cord through the *dorsal root entry zone* and innervate the spinal cord. The majority of heavily myelinated primary afferent fibers (Aα, Aβ) carrying sensory information, including tactile, pressure, and vibratory sense, enter in dorsal roots, traverse across the top of the dorsal horn of the spinal cord (Lissauer's tract), and ascend ipsilaterally within the dorsal column and provide collateral branches into the gray matter of the dorsal horn. The small-diameter lightly myelinated and the small-diameter unmyelinated fibers transmitting temperature and nociceptive information enter Lissauer's tract and innervate the gray matter of the spinal cord. Unlike the heavily myelinated fibers, these fibers may also ascend rostrally or descend caudally through Lissauer's tract before they innervate adjacent spinal levels.

The gray matter of the spinal cord is made up of synaptic terminations of primary afferents and the second-order neurons that form the first stage of processing and integration of sensory information. The gray matter of the spinal cord is

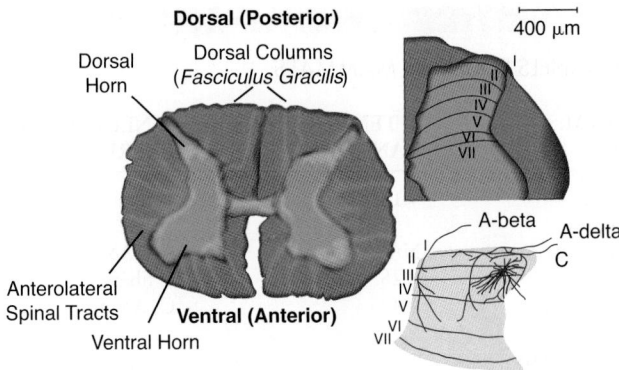

FIGURE 58-1. Anatomy: Histologic sections and schematic diagrams of the spinal dorsal horn. The histologic section at **left** is from the lumbar segment of the spinal cord. It is labeled to show the relationship between the major spinal somatosensory structures. The histologic section at **right** is from the rat lumbar spinal cord. The *outer heavy lines* show the boundary of the spinal gray matter while the *inner heavy lines* show the boundaries of Rexed's laminae. These boundaries are established by the histologic characteristics of each zone, and the layers are identified by the Roman numerals. The drawing at the **bottom** illustrates the pattern of primary afferent innervation to the nonhuman primate spinal dorsal horn. The large myelinated (A-beta) fibers segregate to the dorsal aspect of an entering root and then track medially in the dorsal horn and terminate in layers III to V. The small myelinated (A-delta) fibers and C fibers that carry nociceptive information segregate ventrally in the entering roots, course laterally in the dorsal horn, and then largely terminate in the superficial layers (I and II) of the dorsal horn. Adapted from Raja SN, Dougherty PM, Anatomy and physiology of somatosensory and pain processing, Essentials of Pain Medicine and Regional Anesthesia, 2nd edition. Edited by Benzon HT, Raja SN, Molloy RE, Liu SS, Fishman SM. Philadelphia, Elsevier-Churchill Livingstone, 2005, pp 3, with permission.

divided into 10 laminae based on histologic appearance. The dorsal horn includes laminae I to VI and represents the primary sensory complement of the spinal cord (Fig. 58-1). The ventral horn, including laminae VII to IX and lamina X, is involved in somatic motor and autonomic function, respectively. *Somatic* C-fiber nociceptive afferents endings primarily terminate in the laminae I and II of the same and/or one to two adjacent spinal segments from which they entered from the periphery, whereas *visceral* C-fiber nociceptive afferents can terminate in the dorsal horn more than five segments rostrally or caudally. They not only terminate in laminae I, II, V, X ipsilaterally and also in laminae V and X contralaterally. Therefore, visceral afferents have a wider branching pattern and the nociceptive information they transmit is less localizable to a particular area of the body.

In addition to the primary afferent endings, neurons of the descending pathways and local interneurons also innervate the superficial dorsal horn (laminae I and II). The outer marginal layer or lamina I contains interneurons and cells that send axonal projections to the brainstem and midbrain structures. The substantia gelatinosa or lamina II also contains excitatory and inhibitory interneurons but fewer projection neurons. Laminae III and IV contain interneurons and the second-order neurons that make up the dorsal column pathways relaying nonnociceptive sensory and proprioceptive information. Laminae IV to VI contain interneurons and a modest portion of nociceptive projection neurons that distribute input to the brainstem and thalamus.

Nociceptive somatic input is primarily transmitted by second-order lamina I, IV, and V projection neurons as the contralateral spinothalamic tract (STT) pathway traveling to numerous brainstem regions and the thalamus.[9] There is a nociceptive visceral processing area in laminae III, IV, V, VII, and X.

The visceral nociceptive input is relayed by second-order neurons whose axons travel within the dorsal column. Like the fibers transmitting nonnoxious sensory information, these fibers remain uncrossed until relayed with the crossed medial lemniscal fibers to the thalamus. The visceral pain information transmitted by the ventral STT is likely originating from cells also receiving somatic nociceptive input. Nociceptive and nonnociceptive sensory information from the head, neck, and dura transmitted via the trigeminal nerve innervates the dorsal horn of the spinal trigeminal nucleus in the caudal medulla. The organization and neurotransmitter complement of the spinal trigeminal nucleus is similar to that of the spinal dorsal horn.

Neurobiology of Ascending Pathways

Dorsal Column Tracts

The dorsal column contains the axons of second-order spinal cord projection neurons in addition to the ascending axons of primary afferent neurons relaying touch, pressure, and vibratory sensation. Second-order dorsal column cells in the central visceral processing region of the spinal cord around laminae X also respond to noxious visceral stimulation and converge on some of the thalamic cells receiving nociceptive information from the skin and other somatic structures.

Spinothalamic Tract (STT)

STT neurons are the primary relay cells providing nociceptive input from the spinal cord to supraspinal levels. The axons of STT cells cross the midline of the spinal cord through the anterior white commissure and ascend primarily in the contralateral lateral and anterolateral tracts. The axons of STT cells terminate primarily in the posterior complex of the thalamus including the ventral posterior lateral and ventral posterior medial nuclei. Nonnoxious sensory input from the same body region converges on the same target thalamic neurons providing somatotopic encoding for localization of the input onto the cortical representation of the specific body region, allowing the ability to locate the source of the nociceptive input. The STT cells receiving noxious somatic input are predominantly situated in lamina I and the lateral aspect of the dorsal horn in laminae IV to V.[9] However, other STT neurons are scattered throughout the deep dorsal horn, intermediate region including lamina X, and even in lamina VII of the ventral horn. These STT cells receive both somatic and visceral nociceptive information.

Spinobulbar Pathways

Major ascending lateral axonal projections relaying information about noxious stimuli terminate in the reticular formation of the ventrolateral medulla. This spinal projection pathway traverses brainstem regions containing catecholaminergic neurons, including the locus coeruleus and A7 nuclei of the dorsolateral pontine tegmentum (DLPT). These catecholaminergic neurons are involved in multiple functions, including modulation of nociceptive transmission through the spinal cord via descending inhibitory input. Connections between the rostral ventromedial medulla (RVM) and the catecholamine cells of the pons and brainstem serotonergic cells also play a role in descending modulation of noxious transmission in the spinal cord.[10] Spinobulbar pathways relaying information about pain also terminate in the parabrachial nucleus, periaqueductal gray (PAG), the RVM, and midline midbrain reticular formation.[11]

Spinohypothalamic, Limbic, and Cortical Connections

Pain is a sensory experience but also has an affective component to the perception of noxious stimuli. Pain can provoke fear, anxiety, and depression, resulting in autonomic responses including increased heart rate and blood pressure as well as the endocrine stress response. These responses to noxious stimuli are thought to be mediated by the spinohypothalamic and spinoamygdalar pathways. In addition to their affective function, these regions are also thought to be involved in antinociception. Ascending axonal projections of these pathways arise predominantly from the spinal cord laminae I and X.

Neurobiology of Descending Pathways

The primary components of this descending pain inhibition system, but certainly not all-inclusive, is the "triad" of the PAG, the RVM, and the DLPT.[11] The PAG is an important site for the production of antinociception following electrical or chemical activation, or the injection of opioid receptor agonists. The endogenous opioid enkephalin is present within this nucleus, and opioid receptors of each subtype are present in this region. The PAG provides dense projections to the RVM, the locus coeruleus, and A7.[12] Although each of these regions has direct projections to the spinal cord, it has been proposed that their projections to the RVM are important components in the modulation of nociception. Chemical or electrical inactivation of the RVM results in the attenuation of the antinociceptive effects produced by the activation of these midbrain structures.[13] Although the RVM can function as a relay nucleus in the production of antinociception by more cephalad midbrain structures including the PAG, it also has a primary role in the suppression of nociceptive transmission at the level of the spinal cord. The suppression of nociceptive reflex behavior is thought to be mediated by the axons of RVM neurons that descend within the dorsolateral funiculus and terminate bilaterally in laminae I, II, V, VI, and VII of the spinal cord. Anatomic studies have shown that these axons terminate coincident with interneurons of the dorsal horn that are related to nociceptive transmission.[14] Consistent with the anatomic terminations of the RVM axons, physiological studies have shown that stimulation of the RVM results in the inhibition of a population of nociceptive-specific neurons within the dorsal horn, as well as selective inhibition of the nociceptive responses of wide-dynamic range neurons.[15] The neurotransmitters found in the RVM neurons include enkephalin, γ-aminobutyric acid (GABA), glutamate, and substance P.[16] The DLPT is also an important component of spinal cord nociceptive modulation. It contains all of the noradrenergic neurons that project to the RVM and the spinal cord, and electrical stimulation of the DLPT sites produces spinal cord α_2-adrenergic receptor–mediated analgesia.[17]

Neurobiology of Supraspinal Structures Involved in Higher Cortical Processing

Higher cortical centers play a role in the perception of painful stimuli as well as the integration of the sensory-discriminative and affective components of the noxious stimulation. The localization of the neural structures involved in this perception and integration is still in its adolescence. The development of positron emission tomography and functional magnetic resonance imaging (MRI) technologies has moved this research forward. These imaging technologies produce indirect evidence of neural activity related to pain stimulation. They look for areas of increased blood flow as an indicator of regions of increased activity resulting from the stimulation. The primary and secondary somatosensory cortex, the anterior cingulate gyrus, the insula, and the prefrontal cortex appear to be involved in the higher processing of somatic and visceral

pain.[18] As the primary and secondary cortexes are known to be somatosensory processing regions, the imaging studies are consistent with a sensory-discriminative role of these structures. The insula and frontal cortex may contribute to memory and learning of events related to painful stimuli. The anterior cingulate cortex is thought to be involved in the analysis of the emotional significance of the painful input. Finally, the lentiform nucleus and cerebellum may be involved in the learning of self-protective reflexive motor responsiveness to painful input.

Transition from Acute to Persistent Nociception

Pain sensation is unique among the somatosensory modalities in that it does not rapidly adapt to prolonged stimulation as do the other sensory modalities, such as fine touch. In fact, continued stimulation may produce greater noxious sensation or reduce the stimulus threshold or intensity that is necessary for the appreciation of the sensation as noxious. For instance, previously innocuous thermal or mechanical stimulation may be perceived as painful following a prior noxious stimulus. For example, warm water of the shower or the light touch of the towel across sunburned skin produces a painful sensation that may persist for a few minutes following the stimulation. This is termed *allodynia*. Another example of an altered pain state that may follow an acute injury is that of *hyperalgesia*, in which a previously noxious stimulus is perceived as more painful. The sensation of increased intensity of noxious stimulation at the site of the injury is the result of the sensitization of the peripheral nociceptors.

Persistent C fiber, but not Aβ fiber, primary afferent activation of lamina I and lamina V, as occurs with tissue injury and inflammation, has been shown to enhance the response to subsequent stimulation and augment the size of the receptive field of the respective dorsal horn neuron. Therefore, afferent input from adjacent dermatomal areas now produces neuronal excitation. Furthermore, nonnoxious stimulation becomes increasingly able to activate these neurons. This general phenomenon has come to be termed *wind-up* or *central sensitization*.[19] It is these physiological effects that are believed to underlie the allodynia and hyperalgesia produced by persistent noxious stimulation or tissue injury. This persistent input will lead to cellular damage and migration of inflammatory cells including macrophages and neutrophils into the peripheral tissue. This leads to the release of histamine, bradykinin, prostaglandins, cytokines, growth factors, protons, and peptides that activate or sensitize receptors on the peripheral nociceptor. Activation of these receptors results in depolarization and, under these conditions, spontaneous afferent activity. This activation is thought to explain the allodynia and hyperalgesia observed surrounding the site of injury.

In addition to the alteration of the chemical milieu surrounding the primary afferent distal terminal that results from injury or persistent high-intensity stimulation, axonal sprouting and the formation of neuroma may occur. The neuroma may have an altered complement of ion channels including an up-regulation of sodium channels or a down-regulation of potassium channels that has the net result of increasing neuronal excitability and increasing nociceptive transmission. It has been shown that, following nerve damage, an increase in the expression of sodium channels occurs in the neuroma and the DRG. Numerous sodium channels exist on primary afferents; NaV1.8 and 1.9 subtypes are primarily found on C-fiber DRG cells. Genetic "knock-down" or removal of the NaV1.8 channel had no effect on baseline pain thresholds; however, it reversed nerve injury evoked nociception.[20] Also following nerve damage, potassium currents have been shown to be reduced, suggesting a reduction in these channels contributing to spontaneous nociceptive activity. Consistent with this notion, it has been observed that potassium channel antagonists increase and potassium channel agonists decrease ectopic firing after peripheral nerve injury.[21] Neuromas of injured primary afferents have altered sensitivity to a number of humoral factors, including cytokines, prostaglandins, and catecholamines. These factors are released from a variety of cell types including inflammatory cells and neuronal support cells. Cytokines directly activate the nerve and neuroma through receptors that become expressed in the membrane after the nerve injury. A molecule that has been shown to have a prominent role following nerve damage is tumor necrosis factor subunit *alpha* (TNF-α).[22] Shortly after injury, TNF-α decreases potassium conductance, increasing neuronal excitability, while the long-term changes may be produced through the activation of second messenger systems, resulting in altered protein production. Application of TNF-α to the peripheral nerve results in hyperalgesia while systemic delivery of antibodies to TNF-α or TNF-α–binding protein reduces neuropathic pain.

Prostaglandins are also released from inflammatory cells following nerve and tissue damage. They can enhance the opening of Nav1.8 channels by acting though receptors on the afferent terminal. Nerve growth factor is also released from glial and inflammatory cells after nerve damage, resulting in sprouting of postganglionic sympathetic efferents into the site of injury. The up-regulation of α_1-adrenergic receptors has been demonstrated in animals with nerve injuries.[23] Stimulation of the postganglionic axons results in the release of catecholamines and excites the injured axon and DRG of the injured axon via α-adrenergic receptors.

Although acute noxious stimuli are transmitted to the spinal cord via Aδ and C fibers, the presence of allodynia is thought to be mediated by the activation large-diameter Aβ fibers through what has been termed a *phenotypic* switch.[2] Prior to this peripheral injury, the Aβ fibers, unlike the C fibers, do not express substance P. However, following injury these fibers were able to express this neuropeptide.[24] These data therefore implicate Aβ fibers in the transmission of noxious peripheral stimulation and provide further support for the involvement of somatic Aβ fibers in at least some form of the allodynic pain states. Furthermore, the blockade of Aβ fibers results in a reduction in light-touch evoked allodynia.[25] This phenotypic switch of Aβ fibers may represent another avenue for therapeutic intervention; however, the difficulty will be in differentiating between those Aβ fibers involved in noxious versus nonnoxious sensory information.

MANAGEMENT OF COMMON PAIN SYNDROMES

Low Back Pain: Radicular Pain Syndromes

The common causes of low back pain include radiculitis/radiculopathy from herniated disc or spinal/foraminal stenosis, facet syndrome, and internal disc disruption. Myofascial pain syndrome also causes back pain, whereas sacroiliac joint syndrome and piriformis syndrome cause mostly buttock pain but can present as low back pain or radiculitis. Radicular symptoms of pain, paresthesias, and numbness in a typical dermatomal distribution in the presence of objective signs of weakness, diminished reflexes, and positive straight-leg raise are secondary to pathology or dysfunction of the sensory spinal nerve roots and dorsal root ganglia. Low back pain, with or without radicular pain, is mostly due to lesions of the intervertebral discs and degenerative spinal disorders. Other causes include spinal metastasis, vertebral body fractures, infections, abdominal aortic aneurysm, and chronic pancreatic lesions.

Low back and radicular pain secondary to a herniated disc is due to mechanical nerve root compression and the subsequent inflammatory process. The presence of a herniated disc does not necessarily result in pain. Up to 36% of the general population[26,27] and up to 53% of pregnant women[28] can have an asymptomatic herniated disc. Follow-up studies on patients with a herniated disc show spontaneous regression without treatment, absence of symptoms in the presence of more abnormalities, and partial or complete resolution with treatment that includes medications, bed rest, physical therapy, traction, or epidural steroids.[29,30] If symptomatic, the patient usually presents with low back pain and radicular symptoms that include paresthesias as well as numbness and weakness in the distribution of the involved nerve root. Radicular pain typically travels along a narrow band and has a sharp, shooting, and lancinating quality. Gait disturbances, loss of sensation, reduced muscle strength, and diminished reflexes involve the appropriate affected dermatomal distribution.

Inflammation in the spinal canal secondary to a herniated disc plays an important role in the causation of back and radicular pain. Herniated nucleus pulposus results in local release of cytokines and other inflammatory mediators that cause a chemical radiculitis. High levels of phospholipase A_2 activity were noted from human disc samples removed at surgery from patients with symptomatic radiculopathy. Increased levels of the inflammatory cytokines interleukins-6 and -8 were noted from disc material taken from patients with known disc disease.[31] The application of disc material onto spinal nerve roots can induce functional and morphologic changes in the nerves. Disc cells express TNF-α, which, when applied to spinal nerve roots, causes similar changes to those seen after application of disc material; selective inhibition of TNF-α may reduce the intraneural edema.[32] The intravenous administration of infliximab, a TNF-α inhibitor, in patients with disc herniation and radicular pain results in reduced pain scores. Etanercept, another TNF-α inhibitor, has also shown promise as an effective treatment for lumbosacral radicular syndrome. However, a double-blind, placebo-controlled study showed that one intradiscal injection of 1.5 mg of etanercept in a pain-generating disc did not reduce the pain scores or disability scores of patients with chronic discogenic pain or lumbosacral radiculopathy.[33]

Epidural steroid injections (ESIs) may be useful to treat some forms of low back pain because of their anti-inflammatory effect,[34] related to inhibition of phospholipase A_2 activity. In addition, steroids have a local anesthetic and antinociceptive effect. The local application of methylprednisolone blocks transmission of C fibers but not the Aβ fibers. Three prospective, randomized, and controlled studies have demonstrated short-term efficacy of ESIs for treatment of lumbar spine radiculopathy[35-37] and two studies have not.[38,39] A sixth study demonstrated less leg pain and sensory deficit with ESI, but the incidence of surgery was the same between the steroid and the control groups.[40] For cervical ESIs, the few studies that have been done are mostly descriptive and their results were the same as in lumbar ESIs, that is, transient relief from the injections. The transient efficacy of the ESIs lasted no more than 3 months.[35-37] These transient effects were noted by the Therapeutics and Technology Assessment Subcommittee of the American Academy of Neurology,[41] which recommended against the routine use of ESIs. This recommendation has to be viewed against the natural history of patients with herniated disc and spinal stenosis as these patients seem to do well over time with conservative management. The transient relief provided by ESIs may minimize the need for potent anti-inflammatory medications or opioids and reduce the incidence

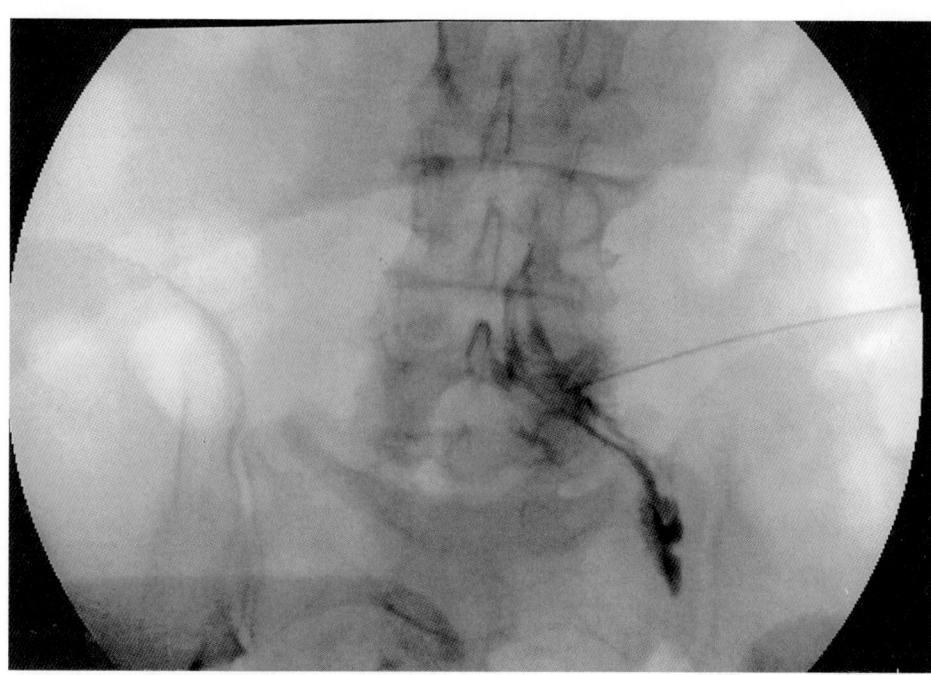

FIGURE 58-2.   Right L5 transforaminal epidural injection. Note the spread of the contrast medium proximally into the lateral epidural space and distally along the nerve root.

of drug-related side effects. ESIs should be a component, and not the sole modality, of the conservative management of radicular pain.

A transforaminal approach can be employed to deposit steroid in the anterolateral epidural space where the herniated disc is located, through the intervertebral foramina, and distally along the nerve root (Fig. 58-2). Prospective, randomized studies[42–44] on transforaminal ESIs show the same results as with the interlaminar approach, that is, short-term efficacy of the injection. A study by Riew et al.[42] demonstrated that when patients had the transforaminal ESI, fewer needed surgery after the treatment. The transforaminal approach has a better rationale than the interlaminar approach, and studies[45,46] that compared the two approaches show better efficacy with the transforaminal approach.

It is advisable that fluoroscopy be used in ESIs to assure insertion of the needle at the affected vertebral level and document and follow the flow of the contrast medium (and the drug). Reassessment should be carried out 2 to 3 weeks after the initial injection. The use of multiple ESIs in a patient, with a short interval between injections, is not advised. If there is no response to an initial injection, it can be repeated once as some patients require a second injection before they respond. If there is partial response, up to three injections can be performed.[47]

The complications of ESI may be due to the technique or from the injected drug, as well as the vehicle and additives. Complications related to the technique include needle trauma, vasospasm, and infection. Glucocorticoids reduce the hypoglycemic effect of insulin and interfere with blood glucose control in patients with diabetes mellitus. Insulin sensitivity may be impaired, there may be no change in the HbA1C levels, or the blood glucose can be increased for 1 week after ESIs. A single dose of 80 mg of methylprednisolone can suppress plasma cortisol levels and the ability to secrete cortisol in response to synthetic corticotropin for up to 3 weeks. Epidural triamcinolone, 80 mg, can suppress serum cortisol and corticotropin levels for up to 7 days after injection. The median recovery to normal levels occurs within 1 month after the last injection, and full recovery is at 3 months.

Injury to the brain or spinal cord can follow treatment with transforaminal ESIs.[48,49] The cerebral/cerebellar events can be ascribed to trauma to the vertebral artery, vasospasm from the injected steroid or dye, or embolism of the particulate steroid via the vertebral artery.[50,51] The spinal cord injuries can be ascribed to injury to the radicular artery accompanying the nerve root, spasm of the radicular artery from the injected dye or steroid, embolism of the particulate steroid, or from proximal intraneural spread of the injectate. The injection of contrast medium through a radicular artery that passed to the spinal cord or the anterior spinal artery has been demonstrated. The occurrence of adverse events at the lumbar level has been ascribed to intra-arterial injection into an abnormally low-lying artery of the Adamkiewicz. These adverse events have also been described after injection of local anesthetic or dye, without steroid.[51] The use of computed tomography (CT), instead of fluoroscopy, does not assure avoidance of the adverse events.

Huntoon[52] noted that the vertebral, ascending cervical, and deep cervical arteries supply segmental medullary vessels and that the ascending and deep cervical arteries are within 2 mm of the path of insertion of the needle for cervical transforaminal ESIs. The proximity of these arteries to the site of needle placement makes these blood vessels vulnerable to trauma or unintentional sites of injection of the steroid. Occlusion of the vessels occurs from the particulate steroids. Methylprednisolone acetate has the largest particle size, betamethasone the smallest particles, and triamcinolone acetonide is in between[51] (Fig. 58-3). Dexamethasone has no identifiable particles. Dexamethasone appears to be ideal for transforaminal ESIs; however, it is easily washed out from the epidural space, and studies on its efficacy are only preliminary.[53] The following steroids are recommended for ESIs: (1) methylprednisolone, triamcinolone, or betamethasone for interlaminar injections; (2) betamethasone (preferably) or triamcinolone for lumbar transforaminal injections; and (3) dexamethasone for cervical transforaminal injections.

There have been several prospective, randomized controlled studies on the efficacy of surgery in relieving back pain secondary to herniated disc or spinal stenosis. It appears that

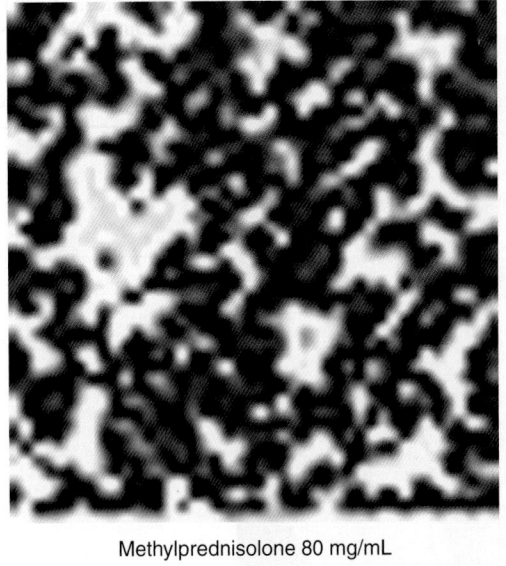

Methylprednisolone 80 mg/mL

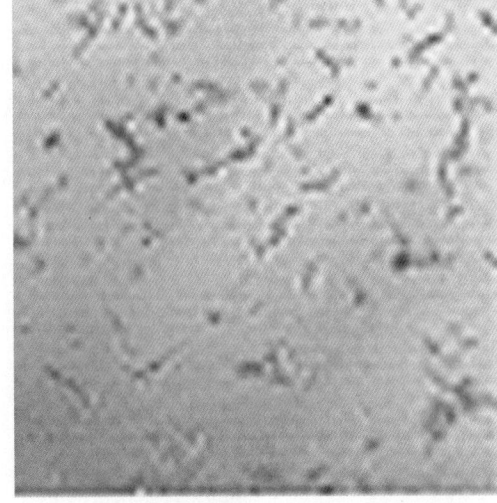

Betamethasone sodium
phosphate/betamethasone
acetate (Celestone Soluspan®)

Methylprednisolone 40 mg/mL

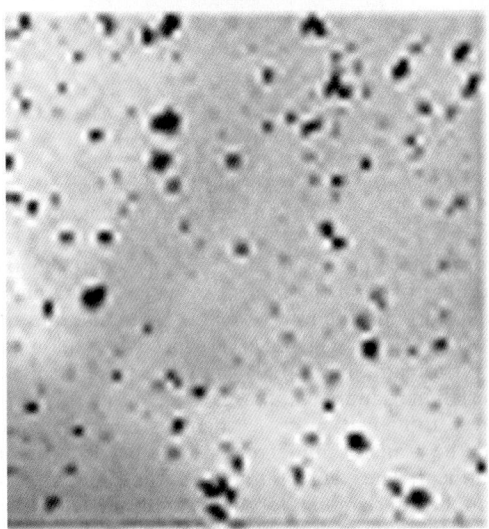

Betamethasone sodium
phosphate/betamethasone
B   acetate (Betamethasone repository)

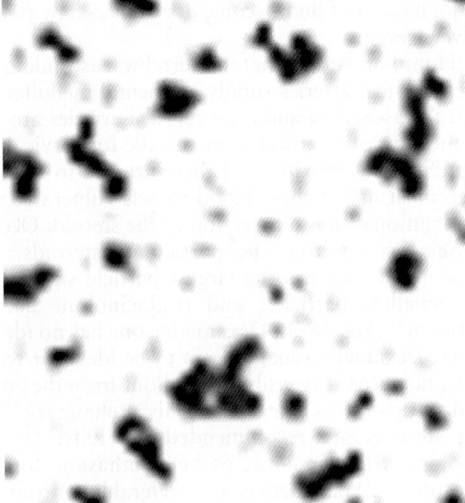

A   Triamcinolone 40 mg/mL

FIGURE 58-3. (A) Typical microscopic appearances of methylprednisolone, 80 mg/mL and 40 mg/mL, and triamcinolone 40 mg/mL. The particles are amorphous in appearance. (B) The particles of commercial betamethasone (Celestone Soluspan) are rodlike and lucent, while those of the compounded betamethasone (betamethasone repository) are amorphous. (*Continued*)

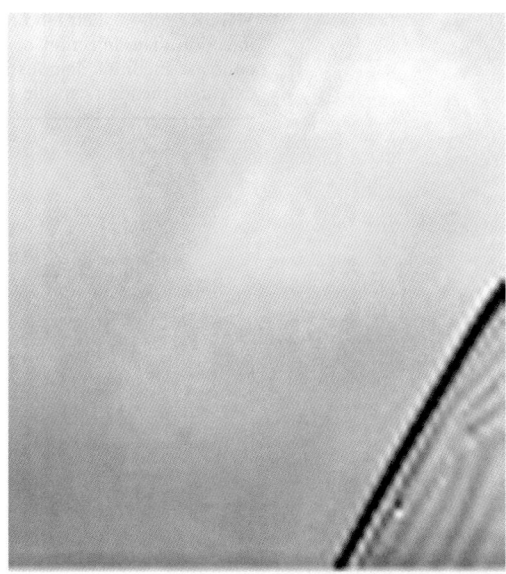

Dexamethasone

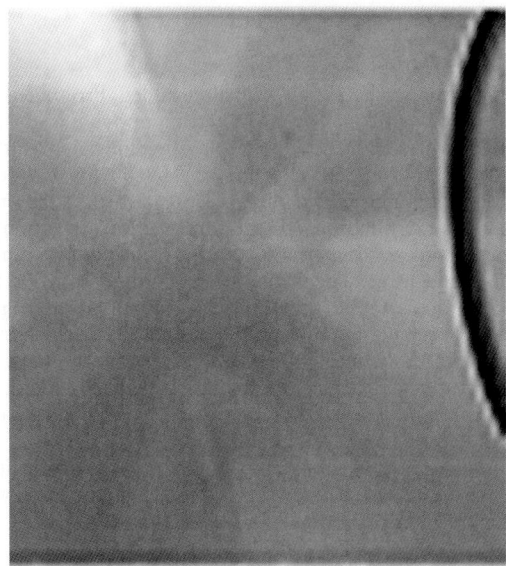

C   Betamethasone Sodium Phosphate

FIGURE 58-3. (*Continued*)   (C) Note that dexamethasone is pure liquid. (From Benzon HT, Chew TL, McCarthy R et al: Comparison of the particle sizes of the different steroids and the effect of dilution: A review of the relative neurotoxicities of the steroids. Anesthesiology 2007; 106: 331, with permission.)

surgery for herniated disc produces only short-term relief, whereas the long-term results are comparable with those with conservative management.[54] For spinal stenosis, surgery is associated with greater improvements in most outcome measures.

Low Back Pain: Facet Syndrome

Patients with low back pain secondary to facet problems have pain in the low back that radiates to the ipsilateral posterior thigh and usually ends at the knee. On physical examination there is paraspinal tenderness and reproduction of pain with extension-rotation maneuvers of the back. The diagnosis of facet syndrome is arrived at by a combination of the patient's history, physical examination findings, and a positive response to diagnostic medial branch blocks or facet joint injections (Fig. 58-4). For medial branch blocks, some investigators rec-

ommend the use of local anesthetics with different durations of effect (e.g. lidocaine and bupivacaine) and to correlate the duration of relief with the known duration of effect of the drug.

Some patients may have a prolonged response to facet joint injections, that is, up to 3 to 6 months. If the patient has a prolonged response it is best to wait for recurrence of the pain. If the relief is short-lived, especially after medial branch blocks, then thermal radiofrequency (RF) rhizotomy of the medial branches should be performed. Overall, randomized controlled studies have shown improvements after thermal RF of the lumbar medial branches that lasted 3 to 12 months (Table 58-3).[55–60] With regard to cervical facet syndrome, two controlled studies on thermal RF of the cervical medial branches have shown different results. Lord et al.[61] showed better results after RF (return to work and relief of pain) while Stovner et al.[62] showed no difference between the RF and sham procedures.

Buttock Pain: Sacroiliac Joint Syndrome and Piriformis Syndrome

The pain of sacroiliac joint syndrome is located in the region of the affected sacroiliac joint and the medial buttock. The pain may radiate to the groin, posterior thigh, and occasionally below the knee. Physical examination usually reveals tenderness over the sacroiliac sulcus, reduction in the joint mobility, and reproduction of the pain when the affected sacroiliac joint is stressed. The most commonly used tests for sacroiliac joint dysfunction include the FABER Patrick, Gaenslen, Yeoman, sacroiliac shear, and Gillet tests. The FABER Patrick and the Yeoman tests do not rule out hip pathology while the Yeoman and the shear tests are more specific for sacroiliac joint syndrome. Pain on three of the tests in addition to the patient's symptoms and physical examination findings and a positive response to sacroiliac joint injection are adequate to make the diagnosis of sacroiliac joint syndrome.

The treatments for sacroiliac joint syndrome include physical therapy, manipulation, intra-articular steroid injections (Fig. 58-5), radiofrequency denervation, and surgical fusion of the joint. Physical therapy and chiropractic manipulations are used extensively for the treatment of sacroiliac joint disease; however, there is no large outcome study validating their use. Intra-articular injections of steroid (40 to 80 mg of methylprednisolone or other depot steroid) and local anesthetic into the sacroiliac joint results in a few months of pain relief; no prospective controlled studies support their use.

Local anesthetic blockade of the medial branch of the dorsal rami of L5 and the lateral branches of the dorsal rami of S1 to S3 can be performed initially or when the relief from the sacroiliac joint injection is temporary. The medial branch of the dorsal ramus of L5 is located at the medial aspect of the transverse process of L5 and the sacral ala. The lateral branches are located at the lateral borders of the respective sacral foramina.[63] Relief from the local anesthetic block may last weeks to months when combined with physical therapy. Thermal radiofrequency lesioning of the lateral branches is performed for a more lasting relief. Studies show the efficacy of monopolar thermal RF lesioning of the lateral branches in 60 to 70% of patients for approximately 6 months.[63,64] To improve the efficacy of thermal RF, a bipolar strip lesion is created wherein two needles are placed 4 to 6 mm apart and a contiguous lesion is created.[65] Bipolar RF strip lesions at the lateral dorsal S1 to S3 periforaminal areas appear to be effective in relieving sacroiliac joint pain[66] (Fig. 58-6). Another technique for denervating the sacroiliac joint is the creation of bipolar RF strip lesions along the dorsal border of the sacroiliac joint in a leapfrog manner.[67] In this "leapfrog" technique, two needles are used at 4 to 6 mm distance to create a bipolar

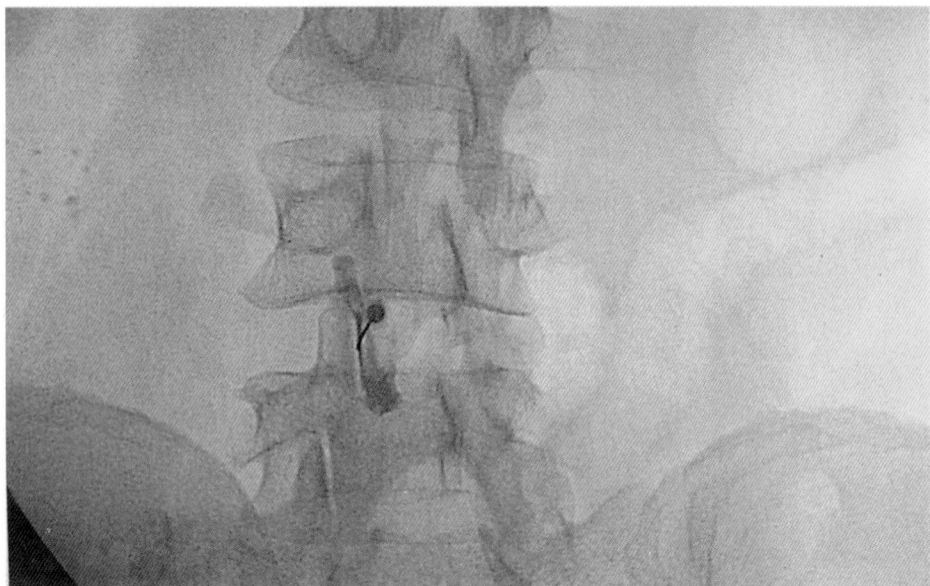

FIGURE 58-4. Left L4-5 facet joint injection. The injection of 5 mL of contrast medium demonstrates the extent of the joint capsule.

"strip" lesion. The lower needle is moved cephalad to the other needle and another RF lesion is created. The process is repeated, creating a strip RF lesion along the joint.

Piriformis Syndrome

Piriformis syndrome, another pain syndrome that originates in the buttock, comprises 5 to 6% of patients referred for the treatment of back and leg pain. It occurs after trauma, surgery, and infection, or from anatomic abnormalities wherein the piriformis muscle is split and one of the components of the sciatic nerve runs between the "two" split muscles.[68] Patients with piriformis syndrome complain of buttock pain with or without radiation to the ipsilateral leg. The buttock pain usually extends from the sacrum to the greater trochanter of the femur whereas irritation of the sciatic nerve results in a but-

tock pain that radiates to the ipsilateral leg. Prolonged sitting, as in driving or biking, or when getting up from a sitting position aggravates the pain. There may be tenderness in the buttock, a spindle-shaped mass may be felt in the buttock, and tenderness may be felt in the area of the piriformis on rectal and pelvic examinations. The pain is aggravated by hip flexion, adduction, and internal rotation. Neurologic examination is usually negative. There may be leg numbness when the sciatic nerve is irritated; the straight-leg test may be normal or limited. Three signs confirm the presence of piriformis syndrome[68]: (1) *Pace sign* wherein there is pain and weakness on resisted abduction of the hip in a patient who is seated, that is, the hip is flexed; (2) *Lasègue sign* wherein there is pain on flexion, adduction, and internal rotation of the hip in a patient who is supine (note that some clinicians call pain on straight-leg raise the Lasègue sign also); and (3) *Freiberg sign* wherein

---

TABLE 58-3

RANDOMIZED, CONTROLLED STUDIES ON RADIOFREQUENCY DENERVATION OF THE MEDIAL BRANCHES (FACET NERVES)

■ STUDY (REF. NO.)	■ STUDY POPULATION	■ RESULTS
King and Lagger (55)	RF of the posterior primary ramus vs. RF of the area of maximum tenderness vs control group (stimulation but no RF)	At 6 mo: 27% response rate for RF of primary ramus, 50% for RF of area of maximal tenderness, 0% in control group
Gallagher et al. (56)	Patients previously had good or equivocal response to facet joint injections randomized to RF or sham	Significantly better results noted in RF group at 1 and 6 mo
Sanders and Zuurmund (57)	Patients had ≥50% relief after intra-articular lidocaine, randomized to RF of medial branch vs. intra-articular RF	At 3 mo: improvements in both groups
van Kleef et al. (58)	Patients had favorable response to MBB, randomized to RF or sham	Better results noted in the RF group at 3 mo (60 vs. 25%) and at 1 yr (47 vs. 12.5%)
Leclaire et al. (59)	Patients had relief after intra-articular injection, randomized to RF or sham	At 1 mo: improvements in Roland-Morris scores in the RF group
van Wijk et al. (60)	Patients responded to intra-articular injection, randomized to RF or sham	At 3 mo: ≥50% relief in 62% (RF group) vs. 39% (sham)

RF, radiofrequency; MBB, medial branch block.
From Benzon HT: Outcomes, efficacy, and complications of the treatment of back pain, Raj's Practical Management of Pain, 4th edition. Edited by Benzon HT, Rathmell J, Wu C et al. Phildelphia, Mosby Elsevier, 2008, p 1242, with permission.

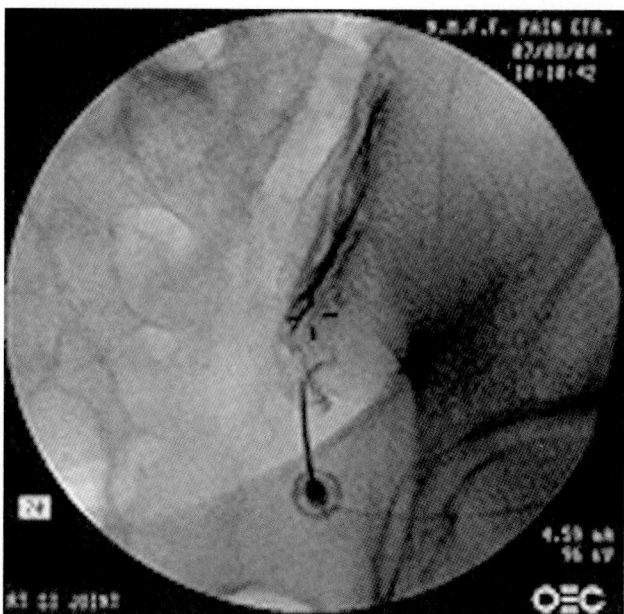

FIGURE 58-5.   Sacroiliac joint injection. Note the spread of the contrast medium along the joint. (From Benzon HT, Nader A: Hip, sacroiliac joint, and piriformis injections, Raj's Practical Management of Pain, 4th edition. Edited by Benzon HT, Rathmell J, Wu C et al. Philadelphia, Mosby Elsevier, 2008, p 1070, with permission.)

there is pain on forced internal rotation of the extended thigh. Note that the piriformis is an abductor of the flexed thigh an external rotator of the extended hip. The diagnosis of piriformis syndrome is made on clinical grounds. Electromyography may detect myopathic and neuropathic changes including a delay in the H-reflex with the affected leg in a flexed, adducted, and internally rotated (FAIR) position as compared with the same H-reflex in the normal anatomic position.[69] The CT of the soft tissues of the pelvis may show an enlarged piriformis muscle or abnormal uptake by the muscle and the MRI confirms the enlarged piriformis muscle.

The treatments of piriformis syndrome include physical therapy combined with medications including muscle relaxants, anti-inflammatory drugs, and analgesics to reduce the spasm, inflammation, and pain. Local anesthetic and steroid injections into the piriformis muscle may break the pain/muscle spasm cycle. Although blind injections can be done, more specific techniques involve identification of the piriformis muscle with muscle electromyography, guidance of CT, a nerve stimulator, or combined fluoroscopy-nerve stimulator guidance.[68] If relief from the local anesthetic does not last, then the piriformis muscle is injected with 100 units of botulinum toxin A in 2- to 3-mL of local anesthetic. The reported complications of botulinum toxin injection include brachial plexopathy, polyradiculoneuritis, and local psoriasiform dermatitis, so precautions should be followed to assure injection of the botulinum toxin into the belly of the piriformis muscle.

Myofascial Pain Syndrome and Fibromyalgia

Myofascial pain syndrome is a painful regional syndrome characterized by the presence of an active trigger point in a skeletal muscle. Manipulation of the trigger point by digital pressure or by penetration by a needle induces a twitch response, which can be felt as a palpable taut band. The essential criteria for diagnosis of myofascial pain syndrome include (1) palpable taut band, (2) exquisite spot tenderness of a nodule in the taut band, (3) pressure on the tender nodule that induces pain that the patient recognizes as an experienced pain pattern, and (4) painful limitation to full passive range of motion for the affected muscle. The confirmatory observations include (1) visual or tactile identification of local twitch response induced by needle penetration of a tender nodule, (2) pain or altered sensation (in the zone of reference distribution expected from a trigger point in that muscle) on compression of a tender nodule, and (3) electromyographic demonstration of spontaneous electrical activity characteristic of active loci in the tender nodule of a taut band.

The management of myofascial pain syndrome includes repeated applications of a cold spray over the trigger point in line with the involved muscle fibers, followed by gentle massage of the trigger point and stretching of the affected muscle. Another treatment is local anesthetic injection or dry needling of the trigger point. Dry needling may be as effective as local anesthetic injection; however, the local anesthetic makes the procedure less painful. Several injections at 1- to 3-week intervals, followed by physical therapy, may result in a long-term benefit. Botulinum toxin injections have been recommended but the results of clinical studies have not been uniform.[70,71] Beneficial physical therapy includes improving posture, body mechanics, relaxation techniques, trigger point massage, postisometric relaxation, and reciprocal inhibition.

Fibromyalgia

The American College of Rheumatology criteria for classification of fibromyalgia[72] requires only two components: a history of widespread pain for at least 3 months and allodynia to digital pressure at 11 or more of 18 anatomically defined tender points. The 18 locations are the following:

- Bilateral occiput, at the suboccipital muscle insertion
- Bilateral low cervical, at anterior aspect of intertransverse spaces between C5 and C7
- Bilateral trapezius, at midpoint of the upper border
- Bilateral supraspinatus, at its origin above scapular spine near the border
- Bilateral second rib, just lateral to the costochondral junctions on upper surface
- Bilateral lateral epicondyle, 2 cm distal to the epicondyle
- Bilateral glutei, at the upper outer quadrant of the buttock
- Bilateral greater trochanter, posterior to the trochanter
- Bilateral knee, medial fat pad proximal to the joint line

The tender point of fibromyalgia syndrome is different from the trigger point of myofascial pain syndrome in that the former is symmetrically widespread in the body, not necessarily located in muscles, and does not refer pain. The anatomic location of the tenderness at the fibromyalgia syndrome tender points is deep to the skin in a variety of soft-tissue structures such as skeletal muscles, ligaments, and bursae.

The objectives of fibromyalgia syndrome treatment are to reduce pain, improve sleep, restore physical function, maintain social interaction, and re-establish emotional balance. To achieve these goals, patients need a combination of social support, education, physical modalities, and medication. Physical modalities include heat therapy in the form of a hot bath, hot water bottles, electric heat pads, or sauna. The pharmacologic management of fibromyalgia syndrome includes an analgesic, specifically tramadol,[73] an antidepressant such as duloxetine,[74] an anticonvulsant such as pregabalin[75] and a sedative to improve the sleep pattern of the patients. Duloxetine and pregabalin have sedative effects, which is beneficial in this group of patients.

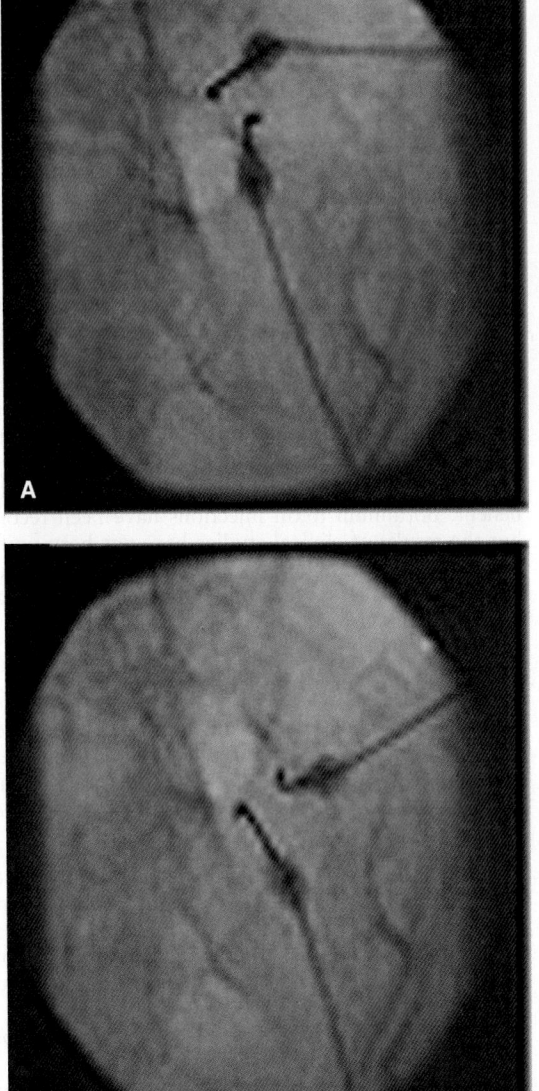

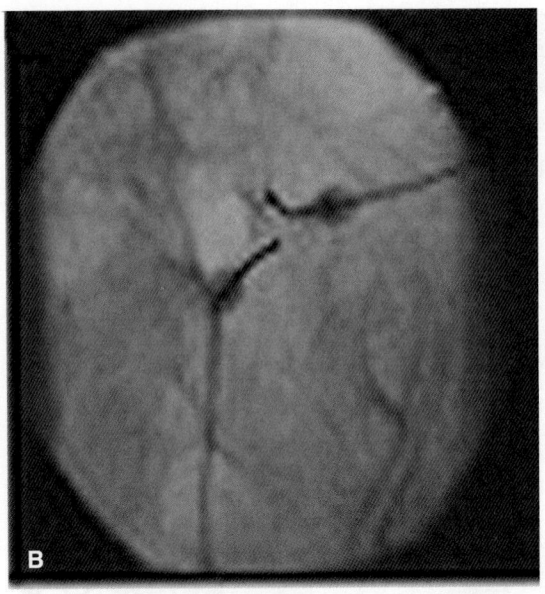

FIGURE 58-6. (**A**) Right S1 lateral branch rhizotomy with needles at the 12 and 2 o'clock positions. (**B**) Right S1 lateral branch rhizotomy with needles at the 2 and 4 o'clock positions, (**C**) Right S1 lateral branch rhizotomy with needles at the 4 and 6 o'clock positions. (From Burham RS, Yasui Y: An alternative method of radiofrequency neurotomy of the sacroiliac joint: A pilot study of the effect on pain, function, and satisfaction. Reg Anesth Pain Med 2007; 32: 12, with permission.)

NEUROPATHIC PAIN SYNDROMES

Herpes Zoster and Postherpetic Neuralgia

Some patients with acute herpes zoster have a prodrome of dermatomal pain before the skin eruptions. The pain of acute herpes zoster is usually moderate in severity and can be managed with analgesics, and the pain usually subsides with healing of the rash. Ten percent to 15% of the patients develop postherpetic neuralgia (PHN), or pain that persists >3 months after resolution of the rash; the incidence rises to 30 to 50% in the elderly. The risk factors for the development of PHN include increased pain during the acute stage, greater severity of the skin lesion, older age, and the presence of a prodrome. The use of antiviral drugs acyclovir, famciclovir, or valacyclovir has been shown to hasten the healing of the rash, reduce the duration of viral shedding, and decrease the increase of PHN.

Most of the studies on the efficacy of neuraxial and peripheral nerve blocks, performed during the acute stage of herpes zoster, were either retrospective or case series. More recent prospective, randomized, and controlled studies provide conflicting results. A study in which epidural methylprednisolone and bupivacaine was compared with acyclovir and prednisolone showed the epidural steroid group to have less pain (1.6 vs. 22%) and less allodynia (4 vs. 12%) at 1 year.[76] Another study in which standard therapy with oral antiviral medications and analgesics was compared with standard therapy and epidural methylprednisolone and bupivacaine noted less pain in the epidural group (48 vs, 58%) at 1 month but not at 3 months (21 vs. 28%).[77] The difference between the two studies is that only one epidural injection was performed in the study that showed no long-term beneficial effect of epidural steroid compared with two to four injections in the study that showed benefit with epidural steroid injections. To be effective in preventing PHN, the blocks are preferably done within 2 to 4 weeks of the onset of rash.[78]

The mainstay of treatment for PHN is pharmacologic management that includes anticonvulsants, opioids, and antidepressants. Although the antidepressants have been found to be effective,[79] their use is precluded by the frequent occurrence of side effects.[80] The side effects include anticholinergic effects such as tachycardia, dry mouth, constipation, and prostatism in the elderly. Amitriptyline was widely used in the past but nortriptyline is now preferred because it is equally effective and better tolerated. Opioids were initially thought to be not as effective, but later studies[81,82] found them to be efficacious. Tramadol, a norepinephrine and serotonin reuptake inhibitor and a μ-opioid agonist, titrated to a maximum daily dose of 400 mg a day, is effective in PHN.[83]

Anticonvulsants are also indicated in the management of PHN. Gabapentin, at daily dosages of 1,800 to 3,600 mg, was proven effective in two large clinical trials.[84,85] There were improvements in daily pain scores and improvements in the quality of life, in sleep, and in mood of the patients. Pregabalin, an anticonvulsant similar to gabapentin, is also effective in PHN.[86,87] The side effects of the drugs include somnolence, dizziness, and peripheral edema. The combination of gabapentin and controlled-release morphine was noted to result in better pain relief at lower daily dosages for the two drugs compared with each drug given alone.[88]

Based on efficacy, that is, numbers needed to treat, antidepressants are the first choice for neuropathic pain syndromes, followed by opioids, tramadol, and gabapentin/pregabalin.[89] If quality of life, side effects, prevention of addiction, and regulatory issues area to be considered with pain relief, then gabapentin/pregabalin are the first drugs of choice. This is followed by tramadol, opioids, and the tricyclic antidepressants.[89] For the allodynia that accompanies the PHN, lidocaine patch is recommended. Up to a maximum of three patches can be applied daily, at 12 hours a day; it should be noted that it may take up to 2 weeks before the patient notices some improvement.

Interventional techniques are available if medications do not control the pain of PHN. Intrathecal methylprednisolone, 60 mg in lidocaine, given once a week for 4 times, was noted to be more effective in relieving PHN compared with intrathecal lidocaine or no treatment.[90] The cerebrospinal fluid levels of interleukin-8, a marker of inflammation, decreased by >50% in the intrathecal methylprednisolone group and this correlated with the duration of global pain relief. It should be noted that epidural methylprednisolone does not offer as good a salutary effect as intrathecal administration.[91] Other interventional techniques for PHN are spinal cord stimulation and intrathecal alcohol. When a spinal cord stimulator was placed in 28 patients with intractable PHN for 2 years, long-term pain relief was achieved in 23 patients (82%) and the median pain score decreased from 9 to 1.[92] The improvements were confirmed by inactivation, followed by activation of the spinal cord stimulator at quarterly intervals. In a case series of six patients, pain was relieved by alcohol neurolysis of the spinal thoracic dermatomes affected by the herpes zoster.[93]

Diabetic Painful Neuropathy

Neuropathies secondary to diabetes can be classified into generalized neuropathies and focal/multifocal neuropathies. Peripheral neuropathy may be present in approximately 65% of patients with insulin-dependent diabetes, most commonly distal symmetric polyneuropathy followed by median nerve mononeuropathy at the wrist and visceral autonomic neuropathy. The incidence of diabetic neuropathy increases with duration of diabetes, age, and degree of hyperglycemia[94]; neuropathies generally develop after persistence of hyperglycemia for several years. The pathophysiology of diabetic neuropathy includes the polyol pathway, microvascular, and glycosylation end-product theories.[95] In the polyol pathway theory, high nerve glucose concentrations result from high blood glucose levels. The glucose is converted to sorbitol via the polyol pathway and fructose levels are also elevated. High sorbitol and fructose levels leads to a decrease in sodium/potassium adenosine triphosphatase activity and activation of the aldose reductase leads to decrease levels of nitric oxide and glutathione, which buffer against oxidative injury. The decrease in nitric oxide results in inhibition of vasodilation, contributing to chronic ischemia.[94] In the microvascular theory, capillary basement membrane thickening and endothelial cell hyperplasia lead to neuronal ischemia and infarction. In the glycosylation end-product theory, chronic hyperglycemia leads to generation and deposition of advanced glycosylation end products within and around peripheral nerves and interfere with axonal transport. Neurotrophic factors are essential for repair of nerve structure and function after an injury. Low levels of nerve growth factor and insulin-like growth factors, which are essential for repair of nerve structure and function after an injury, correlate with severity of diabetic neuropathy in animal models. Increased activity of voltage-dependent calcium channels and sodium channel dysfunction has been demonstrated in diabetic neuropathy.[94,95]

Chronic sensorimotor distal polyneuropathy is the most common type of diabetic neuropathy. The symptoms include burning pain, deep aching pain, electrical or stabbing sensations, paresthesias, and hyperesthesias; the symptoms are usually worse at night. The lower limbs are usually involved with loss of sensation to vibration, pressure, pain, and temperature, as well as absent ankle reflexes. Signs of peripheral autonomic dysfunction may be present and include a warm or cold foot, distended dorsal foot veins, dry skin, and calluses under pressure bearing areas.

The management of diabetic painful neuropathy (DPN) includes tight control of the patient's blood glucose and pharmacologic therapy. The anticonvulsants gabapentin and pregabalin appear to be effective in the management of DPN, with the efficacy of gabapentin enhanced by the addition of controlled-release morphine.[88] The tricyclic antidepressants are also effective in DPN whereas the selective serotonin reuptake inhibitors are not as effective. The antidepressant duloxetine appears to be effective[96] and, together with its favorable side effect profile compared with the tricyclics, is now widely used in treatment of DPN. Finally, the opioids and tramadol are also effective in the treatment of DPN.[97,98] The NMDA receptor antagonists such as dextromethorphan provide relief but only at high doses.[99]

Complex Regional Pain Syndrome

There are two types of complex regional pain syndrome (CRPS). CRPS type I was originally termed reflex sympathetic dystrophy, whereas CRPS type II represents causalgia. The risk factors for the development of CRPS include previous trauma, nerve injury (for causalgia), previous surgery, work-related injuries, and female sex. The signs and symptoms of CRPS include spontaneous pain, hyperalgesia, allodynia, plus trophic, sudomotor, vasomotor abnormalities, and finally, active and passive movement disorders. There is typically a discrepancy between the severity of the symptoms and intensity of the inciting injury. The clinical features of CRPS type II are the same as in CRPS type I except there is a preceding nerve injury in CRPS II. The International Association for the Study of Pain (IASP) has proposed standardized diagnostic consensus-based criteria for CRPS.[100] Studies on the validity of the IASP criteria suggest that patients should have (1) at least one symptom in each of the following general categories: sensory (hyperesthesia-increased sensitivity to a sensory stimulation), vasomotor (temperature abnormalities or skin color changes), sudomotor-fluid balance (sweating abnormalities or edema), or motor (decreased range of movement, weakness, tremor, or neglect); and (2) at least one sign within two or more of the following categories: sensory (allodynia or hyperalgesia), vasomotor (objective temperature abnormalities or skin color changes), sudomotor-fluid balance (sweating abnormalities or objective edema), or motor (objective decreased range of motion, weakness, tremor or neglect).

The primary treatment for CRPS includes sympathetic blocks, physical therapy, and oral medications. Intravenous regional anesthesia with bretylium and lidocaine or ketorolac may also be employed. Pharmacologic therapy for CRPS includes gabapentin[101] and memantine, an NMDA-blocker.[102] The initial dose of memantine is 5 mg daily, titrated up to a maximum dose of 15 mg twice a day. If the patient does not respond to these treatments, spinal cord stimulation can be entertained.[103]

Human Immunodeficiency Virus Neuropathy

Symptomatic neuropathy occurs in 10 to 35% of patients who are seropositive for human immunodeficiency virus (HIV), and pathologic abnormalities exist in almost all patients with end-stage AIDS. The sensory neuropathies associated with HIV include distal sensory polyneuropathy, the more common neuropathy related to the viral infection, and antiretroviral toxic neuropathy (ATN) secondary to the treatment. The clinical features of HIV sensory neuropathy typically include painful allodynia and hyperalgesia. The onset is gradual and most commonly involves the lower extremities. The neuropathy and dysesthesia progress from the distal to the more proximal structures. There is minimal subjective or objective motor involvement and this is generally limited to the intrinsic muscles of the foot. There may be a diminution or loss of ankle reflexes in addition to the sensory findings.

The treatment of HIV sensory neuropathy is symptomatic and includes optimization of the patient's metabolic and nutritional status. Cessation or dose reduction of treatment with nucleoside reverse transcriptase inhibitors may improve the symptoms of ATN. The anticonvulsants, particularly lamotrigine (300 mg/day), can be effective therapy for HIV sensory neuropathy as well as ATN.[104,105] Gabapentin is also effective at doses of 1,200 to 3,600 mg/day.[106]

Phantom Pain

Nearly all patients with amputated extremities experience nonpainful phantom sensations and phantom pain, or painful sensation referred to the *phantom limb*, occurs in as many as 80% of amputees. The onset of pain may be immediate but commonly occurs within the first few days following amputation. Approximately 50% of patients experience a decrease of their pain with time, whereas the other 50% report no change or an increase in pain over time. Phantom pain is not felt all the time, only a few days in a month. Phantom pain is caused by both peripheral and central factors. Peripheral mechanisms include neuromas, an increase in C-fiber activity, and sodium channel activation. Central mechanisms include abnormal firing of spinal internuncial neurons and supraspinal involvement secondary to the development of new synaptic connections in the cerebral cortex.

Numerous prophylactic measures have been undertaken in an attempt to reduce the incidence of phantom limb pain, including perioperative epidural infusions of opioids and local anesthetics or clonidine[107–109] and continuous brachial plexus

blockade with memantine, an NMDA antagonist.[110] The treatment of phantom limb pain includes pharmacologic and nonpharmacologic measures. Pharmacologic treatments include the use of opioids; gabapentin, an NMDA antagonist; and the empirical use of antidepressants. The nonpharmacologic measures include transcutaneous electrical nerve stimulation, spinal cord stimulators, and biofeedback.

CANCER PAIN

Significant pain is present in up to 25% of patients with cancer who are in active treatment and in up to 90% of patients with advanced cancer. The pain of cancer can be somatic, visceral, or neuropathic. The etiology and characteristics of these pain syndromes are different and they require different treatments. Somatic pain tends be responsive to opioids, nonsteroidal anti-inflammatory drugs (NSAIDs), or cyclooxygenase 2 inhibitors, and is amenable to treatment with neural blockade. Visceral pain responds to sympathetic blocks, and neuropathic pain is responsive to anticonvulsants, opioids, tricyclic antidepressants, or combinations of these drugs.

Management of cancer pain should be multifaceted and include the following: (1) antineoplastic treatment, (2) pharmacologic management, (3) interventional management, (4) behavioral and psychological management, and ultimately (5) hospice care. Pharmacologic therapies include opioids, antidepressants, anticonvulsants, NSAIDs, corticosteroids, oral local anesthetics, and topical analgesics. Continuous intravenous opioid infusions can be infused during the later stages of life. Interventional treatments include neurolytic sympathetic blocks and intrathecal opioids; vertebroplasty or kyphoplasty is performed for vertebral compression syndromes.

Opioids are the mainstay of treatment for cancer pain as approximately 70 to 95% of patients are responsive positively when appropriate guidelines are followed.[111] Neurolytic blocks and intrathecal opioids should be considered when pharmacologic agents are not completely effective at maximum tolerated dosages.

Neurolytic Blocks for Visceral Pain from Cancer

Celiac Plexus Block

The celiac plexus innervates all of the abdominal viscera including the liver, pancreas, gallbladder, stomach, spleen, kidneys, intestines, and adrenal glands. Unaffected structures include the left side of the colon and the pelvic viscera. The plexus contains two large ganglia that receive sympathetic fibers from the greater, lesser, and least splanchnic nerves. It also receives parasympathetic fibers from the vagus nerve. The splanchnic nerves are located retroperitoneally at the level of the T12 and L1 vertebrae, and the celiac plexus are anterior to the crura of the diaphragm and surrounds the abdominal aorta and the celiac and superior mesenteric arteries.

Blockade of the celiac plexus can be achieved by the classic retrocrural approach, anterocrural approach, or by neurolysis of the splanchnic nerves.[112] For the procedure, the tip of the needle is directed toward the upper third of the body of L1 for the retrocrural approach and the lower third of the body of L1 for an anterocrural approach (Fig. 58-7).[113] In the retrocrural approach, the tip of the needle is advanced approximately 0.5–1 cm anterior to the anterior border of L1. In anterocrural or transaortic approach, the tip of the needle is advanced through the aorta on the left side until blood can no longer be aspirated through the needle. For splanchnic nerve block, the tip of the needle is placed at the anterior portion of the T12 vertebral

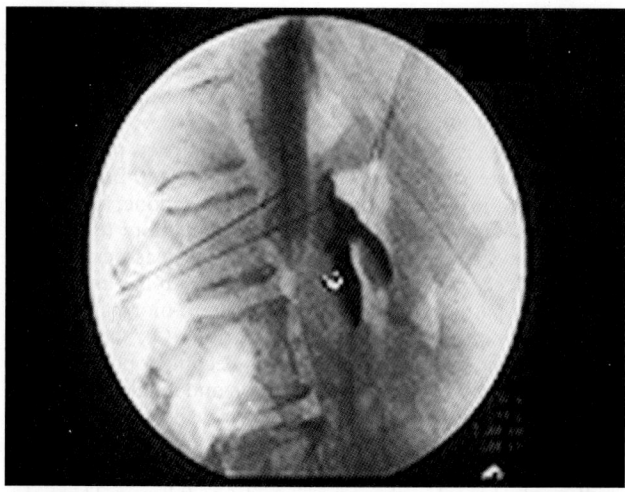

FIGURE 58-7. Retrocrural versus anterocrural approaches to neurolysis of the celiac plexus. Note that the tip of the needle is in the upper third of L1 and about 1 cm beyond the border of the vertebral body for the retrocrural technique; the spread of the contrast medium is cephalad. In contrast, the tip of the needle is the lower third of L1 and about 3 cm beyond the border of the vertebral body for the anterocrural technique; the spread of the contrast medium is caudad and in front of the aorta (*arrow*). (From de Leon-Casasola OA: Neurolysis of the sympathetic axis for cancer pain management, Raj's Practical management of Pain, 4th edition. Edited by Benzon HT, Rathmell J, Wu C et al. Philadelphia, Mosby Elsevier, 2008, p 918, with permission.)

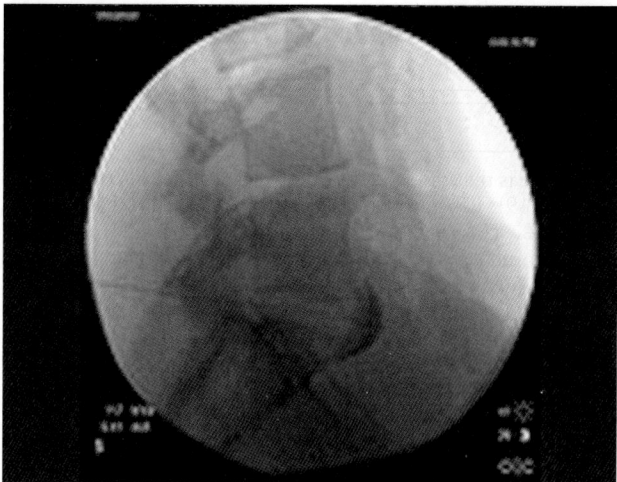

FIGURE 58-8. Transdiscal positioning of the needle at L5-S1 for superior hypogastric plexus block, lateral view. (From de Leon-Casasola OA: Neurolysis of the sympathetic axis for cancer pain management, Raj's Practical Management of Pain, 4th edition. Edited by Benzon HT, Rathmell J, Wu C et al. Philadelphia, Mosby Elsevier, 2008, p 922, with permission.)

body. There appears to be no differences in efficacy between the three approaches.[112] Fluoroscopy is needed in the performance of the procedure. CT allows visualization of the diaphragm and aorta, and is used in the transabdominal approach when patients cannot tolerate the prone position. Some clinicians perform an initial diagnostic block with a local anesthetic while others proceed immediately to a neurolytic block as the results of the diagnostic and neurolytic blocks may not be the same. Better results are usually seen with local anesthetics because of better spread (phenol is viscous) and its absorption may relieve pain. Fifty percent alcohol or 6 to 10% phenol is employed for the neurolytic block. The dosages of the neurolytic agents are 30 to 40 mL for the retrocrural and anterocrural approach, and 10 to 15 mL on each side for splanchnic nerve blockade.[113] Possible complications from the celiac plexus block are orthostatic hypotension, interscapular back pain, retroperitoneal hematoma, reactive pleurisy, hiccups, hematuria, transient diarrhea, abdominal aortic dissection, transient motor paralysis, and paraplegia. The paraplegia and transient motor paralysis may be due to spasm of the lumbar segmental arteries that perfuse the spinal cord, direct vascular or neurologic injury, or retrograde spread to the nerve roots or spinal cord.

The efficacy of celiac plexus neurolysis in relieving pain from cancer of the upper abdomen has been noted in one prospective study[114] and three randomized, controlled trials.[112,115,116] The end points of the studies were lower pain scores, less opioid consumption with lower incidence of side effects, and equal or better quality of life. Better results are achieved when there is better spread of the injectate.[117] A meta-analysis of 21 retrospective studies in 1,145 patients concluded that adequate-to-excellent pain relief was achieved in 89% of the patients during the first 2 weeks following the block[118] and partial-to-complete pain relief continued in 90% of the patients at the 3-month interval.

Superior Hypogastric Plexus Block

Superior hypogastric plexus is indicated for pelvic pain secondary to cancer and chronic nonmalignant conditions.[119,120] The plexus is located in the retroperitoneum, bilaterally extending from the lower third of the fifth lumbar vertebra to the upper third of the first sacral vertebra. For blockade of the plexus, the patient is placed in the prone position and two 7-cm needles are inserted, under fluoroscopy, in a medial and caudal direction until the tips lay anterolateral to the L5-S1 intervertebral disc space. Alternatively, a single needle can be used through a transdiscal approach (Fig. 58-8). After injection of contrast medium, 6 to 8 mL of local anesthetic is used for a diagnostic block while phenol or alcohol is employed for neurolysis. The complications are minimal and include nerve root blockade secondary to retrograde spread of the injectate. Neurolytic superior hypogastric plexus block is effective in reducing pelvic pain secondary to cancer and in decreasing opioid consumption.[119–121]

Ganglion Impar Block

Pain in the perineal area associated with malignancies can be treated with neurolysis of the ganglion impar (Walther's ganglion). The ganglion impar is a solitary retroperitoneal structure located anteriorly to the sacrococcygeal junction. Visceral afferents innervating the perineum, distal rectum, anus, distal urethra, vulva, and distal third of vagina converge at the ganglion. For the procedure, the patient is usually prone and a 22-gauge spinal needle, bent 1 inch from its hub to form a 30-degree angle, is inserted under local anesthesia through the anococcygeal ligament and directed along the midline to reach the sacrococcygeal junction. In the transsacrococcygeal approach,[122] a 20-gauge, 1.5-inch needle is inserted through the sacrococcygeal ligament until the tip of the needle is just anterior to the anterior portion of the sacrum. Four to 8 mL of local anesthetic is used for diagnostic block and 8 to 10% phenol or 50% alcohol is used for neurolysis. Prospective non-controlled studies document that ganglion impar block can provide complete or partial pain relief in most patients with perineal pain secondary to cancer.

PHARMACOLOGIC MANAGEMENT

Opioids

Morphine is the standard for opioid therapy of cancer pain (see Chapter 19). It has a variable oral bioavailability between 10 and 45%. The metabolites of morphine include morphine-6-glucuronide, which causes additional analgesia, and morphine-3-glucuronide, which can cause adverse effects (Table 58-4). Controlled-release preparations are available, one of which has the added advantage of a short onset of action. The *numbers needed to treat*, or NNT, is the number of patients who take the treatment before one shows a ≥50% reduction in their pain. Lower numbers imply better efficacy of the drug. The *numbers needed to harm*, or NNH, refers to the number of patients who need to take the drug before one drops out because of side effects. An ideal drug is one with a low NNT and a high NNH. The NNT for 10 mg of morphine for postoperative pain is 2.9[123] and its NNH is 9.1. Hydromorphone, a μ-receptor agonist, is 3 to 5 times more potent than morphine when given orally and 5 to 7 times more potent when given parenterally. Its 3- to 4-hour duration of analgesic effect is similar to that of morphine. Pruritus, sedation, nausea, and vomiting occur less frequently compared with morphine. Its metabolite, hydromorphone-3-glucoronide, lacks analgesic property but possesses properties similar to that of morphine-3-glucuronide. Meperidine has numerous undesirable side effects including anticholinergic effects, high lipophilicity, which induces drug-seeking behavior, and the metabolite normeperidine, which is a central nervous system stimulant. Meperidine has a poor and variable oral absorption, a short duration of action (2 to 3 hours), and is 8 to 10 time less potent than morphine.

Methadone has a 60 to 95% bioavailability, high potency, and a long duration of action. It has ideal characteristics that include the lack of an active metabolite, additional salutary effects such as NMDA receptor antagonist and serotonin reuptake inhibitor, and it is inexpensive. Its potency compared with morphine ranges from 1:1 to 1:4. It has a long and unpredictable half-life of 8 to 80 hours that makes it difficult to achieve steady-state plasma concentrations, increasing the risk of accumulation and the need for careful and individualized dosing. It is ideal in patients with renal failure because it does not accumulate in these patients. In 2006, the Food and Drug Administration issued an *alert advisory* regarding the hazards of death, narcotic overdose, and cardiac dysrhythmias associated with methadone. The cardiac rhythm abnormalities include QT prolongation and Torsade de pointes.[124] Most reports are based on high-dose maintenance (>120 mg) for the treatment of addiction; however, such occurrences have also been reported with lower dosages. QT prolongation can occur when methadone is given with concomitant drugs that inhibit cytochrome P450.

Oxycodone is mainly a prodrug. That is, it acts primarily by being converted by the enzyme cytochrome P450 2D6 to oxymorphone (a μ-opioid agonist) and noroxycodone, an inactive metabolite. Oxycodone has a high bioavailability (60%) and does not have hazardous metabolites. It is also associated with a low incidence of itching and hallucinations. It has an NNT of 2.5 in neuropathic pain[125]; the oxycodone-to-morphine ratio is 1:1.5. The controlled-release preparation (OxyContin) has good analgesic characteristics but has become a popular drug for abuse. Addicts crush the preparation and inhale the powder or inject a solution of the drug into their veins. Buprenorphine is a partial agonist at the μ-receptor, a κ-antagonist, and a weak δ-agonist. It has a rapid onset (30 minutes) when given orally and a long duration of action of 6 to 9 hours. There also have been increased reports of abuse of the drug.

The weak opioids include codeine, hydrocodone, propoxyphene, and tramadol. Codeine is transformed via the enzyme cytochrome P450 2D6, and has an NNT of 16.7.[123] Approximately 9% of whites do not have the enzyme and do not experience analgesia from codeine. Children <12 years of age lack maturity of the enzyme and cannot convert the drug to morphine, experiencing the drug's side effects with minimal analgesia.[126] Hydrocodone reaches peak serum concentrations within 1 to 2 hours and has a half-life of 2.5 to 4 hours. An additive effect is noted when ibuprofen is combined with hydrocodone. Propoxyphene, a synthetic opioid structurally related to methadone, has an NNT of 7.7 for 65 mg and 2.8 for 130 mg. The d-isomer, dextropropoxyphene, is a noncompetitive NMDA antagonist. The serious side effects associated with propoxyphene include seizures, cardiac dysrhythmias, and heart block. Its active metabolite, norpropoxyphene, has a weak opioid activity and may cause convulsions. The maximum dose is 400 mg/day; its perceived increased safety profile has led to overdoses in the past. The Food and Drug Administration issued a warning in 1987 wherein it recommended a reduction of the dose of the drug. In 2005, the British authorities ordered a gradual withdrawal of the drug from their market because of increased reports of overdoses from the drug.

Tramadol is an opioid agonist and a monoaminergic drug. It has a bioavailability of 80 to 90%, has a low abuse potential, low incidence of constipation, and a minimal risk of fatal respiratory depression that is possibly limited to patients with severe renal failure. It has a dose-dependent efficacy with

---

TABLE 58-4

SELECTED OPIOIDS: ORAL BIOAVAILABILITY, HALF-LIVES, DURATION OF ACTION, AND METABOLITES

■ OPIOID	■ AVAILABILITY (%)	■ HALF-LIFE (hr)	■ DURATION (hr)	■ METABOLITES
Morphine	10–45	2–3	4–5	M6G, M3G
Oxycodone SR (OxyContin, Purdue Pharma)	60–80	4.5	12	Oxymorphone Noroxycodone
Oxymorphone (Opana ER, Endo Pharmaceuticals)	10	9 ± 3	12	O3G 6-OH-oxymorphone
Hydromorphone	24	2.3	3–4	H3G
Methadone	60–95	8–80 (27)	6–8	

M6G, morphine-6-glucuronide; M3G, morphine-3-glucuronide; O3G, oxymorphone-3-glucuronide; H3G, hydromorphone-3-glucuronide.
From Cortazzo MH, Fishman SM: Major opioids and chronic opioid therapy, Raj's Practical Management of Pain, 4th edition. Edited by Benzon HT, Rathmell J, Wu C et al. Phildelphia, Mosby Elsevier, 2008, p 606, with permission.

NNTs of 8.5 for 50 mg, 5.3 for 75 mg, 4.8 for 100 mg, and 2.9 for 150 mg.[123] The maximum dose of tramadol is 400 to 500 mg/day.

The oral equianalgesic doses of morphine 10 mg intravenously or 30 mg orally are (1) 200 mg of codeine, (2) 30 mg of hydrocodone, (3) 20 to 30 mg of oxycodone, (4) 130 mg of propoxyphene, and (5) 120 mg of tramadol. Opioid rotation or substitution, wherein one opioid is changed with another to improve analgesia and decrease side effects, implies knowledge of the equianalgesic dosages of the different opioids.

There is considerable public concern regarding the effect of opioids on driving performance. It appears that cancer patients receiving chronic, stable doses of morphine, up to 290 mg, have minimal or no impairment of their driving abilities.[127] Patients receiving stable doses of transdermal fentanyl over 2 weeks show no significant psychomotor impairment when compared with volunteers.[128] Patients who have their opioid dose increased by >30% over a period of 2 days show worsening of their cognitive performance.[129] Patients receiving stable dose of opioids can probably drive, and those who are starting to take opioids and those who had a recent increase in their dose should be warned about the hazards of driving.

Opioids are used mostly for cancer pain, with long-acting opioids supplemented by short-acting ones for breakthrough pain.[130] Opioid monotherapy in cancer pain is rarely successful and adjuvants are usually added for increased efficacy. The use of opioids for treatment of neuropathic pain has been controversial but recent studies show them to be effective, although at higher doses.[81–83] Because of controversial issues associated with the use of opioids, such as addiction, aberrant behaviors, and regulatory issues, opioids are often a second-line drug for neuropathic pain. The combination of a gabapentin and an opioid has been shown to result in better analgesia, fewer side effects, and lower doses of each drug.[88] Combination therapy is now commonly practiced in the treatment of neuropathic pain. When considering the use of opioids for treatment of low back pain, it should be noted that while individual studies show the efficacy of opioids in low back pain, a meta-analysis did not show reduced pain when compared with a placebo or a nonopioid control group.[131] Opioids may be efficacious for the short-term relief of acute low back pain, in addition to NSAIDs and muscle relaxants, but the long-term efficacy of opioids ($\geq$16 weeks) is unclear; antidepressants are preferred for treatment of chronic low back pain.[132] When treating fibromyalgia, only tramadol or a tramadol/acetaminophen combination has been shown to be more effective than placebo. Opioids are usually not effective in pain secondary to spinal cord injury, although intravenous alfentanil has been shown to be better than placebo.

Antidepressants

Tricyclic antidepressants (TCAs) are thought to have several mechanisms for their analgesic effects. These include a serotonergic effect (interference with serotonin reuptake and alteration of serotonin binding to receptors in neural tissue),[133] a noradrenergic effect (includes interaction with α-receptors),[134] an opioidergic effect,[135] blockade of the NMDA receptor complex,[136] inhibition of the uptake of adenosine,[137] and blockade of sodium and calcium channels.[138] TCAs have also been shown to have an anti-inflammatory effect in animal models of pain. The NNTs of antidepressants are comparable with those of opioids and anticonvulsants. Antidepressants also inhibit the histaminic, cholinergic muscarinic, and nicotinic receptors resulting in sedation, dry mouth, and urinary retention. TCAs, specifically amitriptyline and nortriptyline, have been shown to be effective in PHN.[79,80] As stated in "Neuropathic Pain Syndromes," nortriptyline and amitriptyline are both effective

in PHN, with nortriptyline having fewer side effects. For DPN, amitriptyline and desipramine appear to be equally effective.[139] Clomipramine appears to be effective in DPN and in painful mononeuropathy and polyneuropathy. Amitriptyline may be effective in the relief of pain after stroke.[140]

In addition to their antidepressant action, the serotonin and norepinephrine receptor inhibitors (SNRIs) have an antinociceptive effect. For example, venlafaxine and duloxetine have been shown to have an analgesic effect in a nerve constriction model of neuropathic pain.[141] SNRIs block the reuptake of serotonin and norepinephrine, with duloxetine having increased selectivity for serotonin. Duloxetine is effective in DPN and fibromyalgia and has a good safety profile for long-term use.[96,142,143] Although their side effects are less, SNRIs are less effective than TCAs in the management of pain.

TCAs have a NNT of 2.1 to 2.8 for treatment of PHN, 1.3 to 3.4 for DPN, and 1.7 for central pain. The overall NNT for SNRIs is 15.3, and 5 for paroxetine. The side effects of antidepressants include cholinergic effects such as dry mouth, sedation, and urinary retention. Accidental or intentional overdose can lead to fatal dysrhythmias. TCAs are more likely to cause weight gain compared with SNRIs. TCAs impair driving ability during the first week of treatment or during dose escalation, but shortly thereafter driving performance returns to baseline.[144] No impairment of driving ability apparently occurs with SNRIs. Other sedating medications should not be prescribed when TCAs are used. Poor neonatal adaptation has been reported in children of women who received TCAs or SNRIs during their pregnancy. The NNHs are 5 to 11 for TCAs and 21 to 24 for SNRIs, showing the better tolerability of the serotonin reuptake inhibitors. Recommended doses for the commonly used antidepressants are in shown in Table 58-5.

Anticonvulsants

Neuropathic pain is associated with changes in sodium and calcium channel subunit expression resulting in functional changes. In chronic nerve injury, there is redistribution and alteration of subunit compositions of sodium and calcium channels resulting in spontaneous firing at ectopic sites along the sensory pathway. Sodium channel blockers inhibit spontaneous activities at neuromas, DRG, and at the dorsal horn of the spinal cord. Anticonvulsants block sodium channels, explaining their efficacy in neuropathic pain syndromes. Other anticonvulsants act on ion channel systems, including GABA$_A$ receptor agonists (topiramate and felbamate), GABA$_A$

TABLE 58-5

DOSAGES (mg/day) OF THE COMMONLY USED ANTIDEPRESSANTS AND ANTICONVULSANTS[a]

■ ANTIDEPRESSANTS	■ ANTICONVULSANTS
Amitriptyline: 10–300	Gabapentin: 900–3,600, tid
Doxepin: 30–300	Lamotrigine: 50–150
Nortriptyline: 50–150	Mexiletine: 300–1,350, tid
Desipramine: 25–300	Oxcarbazepine: 300–900, bid
Fluoxetine: 5–40	Pregabalin: 150–600, bid
Paroxetine: 20–40	Topiramate; 50–200, bid
Venlafaxine: 37.5– 300	
Duloxetine: 60–120 once daily or bid	

tid, three times a day; bid, twice a day; od,
[a]Note: Unless indicated, dosing is once a day. Start with smallest possible dose and titrate to efficacy or side effects.

transaminase blockers (vigabatrin), $GABA_A$ transport blockers (tiagabine), and glutamate receptor antagonists (felbamate and topiramate).The other drugs directly block calcium channels (lamotrigine), T-type calcium channels (topiramate and zonisamide) and α_2-delta subunits (gabapentin and pregabalin).

Randomized controlled studies demonstrate the efficacy of the anticonvulsants in the following neuropathic pain syndromes: (1) trigeminal neuralgia—carbamazepine and lamotrigine; (2) PHN—gabapentin and pregabalin; (3) DPN—gabapentin, pregabalin, topiramate; (4) HIV polyneuropathy—lamotrigine and gabapentin; (5) phantom limb pain—gabapentin; (6) spinal cord injury pain—amitriptyline and gabapentin; (7) central poststroke pain—lamotrigine; (8) Guillain-Barré syndrome—gabapentin; and (9) mixed neuropathic pain—gabapentin and valproic acid.[145]

Gabapentin is an effective drug in neuropathic pain (PHN, DPN, and spinal cord injury [SCI]), has few side effects, and lacks drug-drug interactions. Its median effective dose is 900 to 1,800 mg/day. Pregabalin shares the same mode of action as gabapentin but with an improved linear pharmacokinetic profile. It has been shown to be effective in PHN, DPN, and spinal cord injury pain. The maximum dose of pregabalin is 600 mg/day in patients with creatinine clearance >60 mL/min or 300 mg in patients with clearance of 30 to 60 mL/min.

Lamotrigine has been shown to be effective in HIV polyneuropathy, pain from spinal cord injury, and central poststroke pain.[104,105] The most common side effect is rash and its use is limited by the risk of Stevens-Johnson syndrome. Topiramate is not effective in DPN but is effective in migraine prophylaxis, similar to divalproex. Oxcarbazepine is similar in chemical structure to carbamazepine and noted to be effective in trigeminal neuralgia with few side effects[146]; its analgesic effect is fast and pain relief maybe noted within 24 to 48 hours. The recommended doses of the commonly used anticonvulsants are in Table 58-5.

The side effects of anticonvulsants include dizziness, fatigue, somnolence, weight gain, peripheral edema (gabapentin and pregabalin); rash (lamotrigine); paresthesia, cognitive effects, weight loss (topiramate); hyponatremia and low thyroid concentrations (oxcarbazepine).

For peripheral neuropathic pain, the drugs with the lowest NNT are the TCAs, followed by opioids and the anticonvulsants gabapentin and pregabalin. If pain relief is the only criteria, then the recommended drugs in order of efficacy are TCA > opioids ≥ tramadol ≥ gabapentin/pregabalin. However, if the criteria for efficacy are based on pain relief and quality of life, then the recommended order of drugs are gabapentin/pregabalin > tramadol > opioids > TCA.[89] Finnerup et al.[89] consider gabapentin/pregabalin as the first-line drug for neuropathic pain, and opioids and tramadol as the second- or third-line drugs. The SNRIs with their efficacy and fewer side effects may replace TCAs in the future. The combination of gabapentin and morphine in the treatment of neuropathic pain (PHN and DPN) appears to be more effective than either drug alone. Gilron et al.[88] showed better analgesia at lower doses for each drug than either drug as a single agent. The mean maximal tolerated dose of morphine and gabapentin is significantly lower with the combination (34 mg of morphine and 1,705 mg of gabapentin) than in the treatment with each as a single agent (45 mg of morphine and 2,207 mg of gabapentin).

Lidocaine Patch, Mexiletine, and Intravenous Lidocaine

The lidocaine patch 5% (Lidoderm, Endo Pharmaceuticals, Inc., Chadds Ford, PA) delivers lidocaine locally at the site of neuropathic pain generation, limiting its systemic effects and reducing its interactions with other concomitantly administered medications; analgesia is by local sodium channel blockade and not by its systemic effects. The patch contains 700 mg of lidocaine inside an adhesive. It is recommended that a maximum of three patches be applied for a maximum of 12 hours per day. Most patients experience pain relief within a few days of application.[147] The occurrence of a delayed response in some patients led to the recommendation that there be a 2-week trial period.[148] Some patients continue to experience relief between patch applications while others have pain when the patch is removed. For this reason, clinicians recommend using the patch for 16 to 18 hours in these patients. The absorption of lidocaine is limited; only about 3% of the total dose applied is absorbed systemically.[149] The maximum plasma lidocaine concentration is usually achieved on the second day of 12 hours per day of patch application and is significantly lower than concentrations that are cardiotoxic.[150] Clinical experience with the lidocaine patch has shown that it can be used effectively for patients with PHN[147,148,151] as well as patients with myofascial pain, low back pain, osteoarthritis, and diabetic and nondiabetic polyneuropathy. However, few good research studies exist to verify the efficacy of the patch.

Mexiletine is oral lidocaine. Its efficacy is similar to that of intravenous lidocaine, although a favorable response to intravenous lidocaine does not necessarily mean a similar response to mexiletine. The median recommended dose of mexiletine is 600 mg per day. Intravenous lidocaine infusions are sometimes used for resistant neuropathic pain syndromes. The median recommended dose of intravenous lidocaine infusions is 5 mg/kg given over 30 minutes. A meta-analysis has shown intravenous lidocaine to be superior to placebo and equal to morphine, gabapentin, and amitriptyline for neuropathic pain.[152] The beneficial effect was noted to be more consistent in patients with peripheral pain secondary to trauma and diabetes and central pain.

Based on original studies, review articles, and meta-analyses publications, the recommended drugs for several different chronic pain syndromes are listed in Table 58-6.

TABLE 58-6

RECOMMENDED DRUGS FOR CHRONIC PAIN SYNDROMES

■ POSTHERPETIC NEURALGIA	■ DIABETIC PAINFUL NEUROPATHY	■ SPINAL CORD INJURY	■ FIBROMYALGIA	■ HUMAN IMMUNODEFICIENCY VIRUS
Pregabalin	Duloxetine	Pregabalin/	Duloxetine	Lamotrigine
Gabapentin	Pregabalin	Gabapentin	Tramadol	Gabapentin
Opioid	Gabapentin	Lamotrigine	Pregabalin	
Antidepressants	Antidepressants	IV lidocaine		
Tramadol		Mexilitine (±)		
Lidoderm patch (allodynia)				

INTERVENTIONAL TECHNIQUES

Because of their particular knowledge, training, and technical expertise, anesthesiologists are well suited to perform invasive procedures for the treatment of chronic pain. However, before initiating these procedures it is important that the anesthesiologist complete a thorough course of study and training in interventional pain therapies. Completing a pain fellowship and becoming board-certified in pain management is recommended. The complications from some of these procedures can be dire, such as discitis, worsening neuropathy, and paraplegia. The treating physician must be able to fully understand the indications for the procedures, recognize complications that may result, and be prepared to appropriately address these complications.

Discography

The symptoms of discogenic pain are nonspecific and include nonradicular back pain that is worse in the sitting position. The pain is provoked by bending and may involve the buttocks, hip, groin, and thighs. The neurologic examination is usually normal including the straight-leg raise. The MRI may show a high-intensity zone on the T2 sagittal images, indicating an annular tear. Treatments include stabilization, exercise training, back education, activity modification, and epidural steroid injections.

The American Society of Interventional Pain Physicians has recommended guidelines on when to perform discography.[153] Some of the indications include: (1) evaluation of abnormal discs to assess the extent of abnormality or correlation of the abnormality with clinical symptoms, (2) the assessment of patients with persistent severe symptoms in whom diagnostic tests have failed to reveal which suspected disc is the source of pain, (3) assessment of discs before fusion to determine which discs within the proposed fusion segment are symptomatic, and (4) confirmation of a contained disc herniation or investigation of contrast distribution pattern before intradiscal procedures. The procedure can be performed on an outpatient basis with fluoroscopic guidance, under light sedation. Antibiotic prophylaxis is recommended and may be administered either intradiscally or intravenously.[154] The specifics of the technique are discussed in textbooks or an atlas of pain medicine. Nonionic contrast is injected into the disc, preferably with a controlled injection system with pressure readout. The patient is asked to rate his or her pain on a 0 to 10 scale before and during injection, and whether the pain is *concordant*, that is, similar to the pain for which the patient is being seen. The suggested end points for injection include (1) pain severity of 5/10 or greater that lasts at least 30 seconds, (2) intradiscal pressure of 80 to 100 psi, or (3) a total of 3.5 mL of contrast medium has been injected.[155] Anteroposterior and lateral images are taken to record the distribution of contrast medium and whether the contrast leaked outside the disc through a fissure in the annulus fibrosis. Functional discography involves the insertion of a catheter and injection of a local anesthetic followed by observation of the patient's response (Fig. 58-9). After recovery, the patient is sent for postdiscography CT scan, preferably within 4 hours of the discography.

Discitis is the most feared complication of discography. The incidence of discitis without prophylactic antibiotics is approximately 0.25% and is considerably decreased with prophylactic antibiotic use.[156] The diagnosis of discitis includes worsening back pain the week after discography, and elevated erythrocyte sedimentation rate and C-reactive protein that usually peaks 53 weeks after the procedure. The most common causative organism in discitis is *Staphylococcus aureus*.

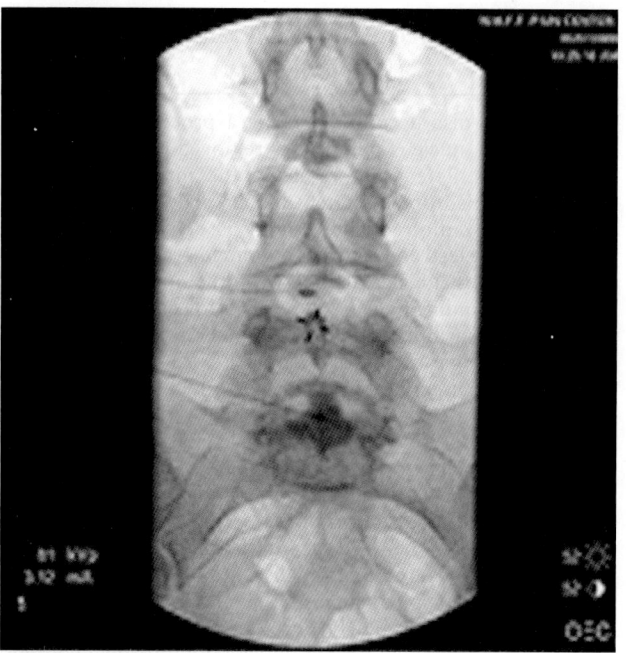

FIGURE 58-9. Functional discography at L4-5 and L5-S1 vertebral levels. A small amount of local anesthetic is injected through the catheter and the patient's response is observed. (Photograph courtesy of David R. Walega, MD.)

Intradiscal Electrothermal Therapy

Intradiscal electrothermal therapy (IDET) is a procedure wherein a thermal resistance catheter is placed percutaneously in the posterolateral portion of the disc. Heat causes the collagen of the annulus fibrosis to contract. The intervertebral disc is avascular so the heat does not travel as easily or dissipate quickly.[157] IDET is performed with a technique similar to discography including the use of prophylactic antibiotic, fluoroscopy, positioning, monitoring, and sedation. The needle is inserted contralateral to the lesion. The flexible electrode is advanced through the introducer until it assumes a circumferential position either between the nucleus pulposus and the annulus fibrosis, or within the annulus fibrosis. The portion between the proximal and distal radio-opaque markers of the catheter should cover the posterior wall of the annulus and as much a portion of the lateral walls as possible. The electrode is gradually heated to 90°C, if tolerated, and maintained for 4 minutes. If the patient cannot tolerate 90°C, heating is performed at 85 or 80°C for 5 minutes. The heating is stopped and the catheter repositioned if the patient has radicular pain. An increase in pain may be experienced but it usually subsides the following week. The patient rests for 1 to 3 days after the procedure, limits sitting or walking, and wears a corset for 6 to 8 weeks. A gradual increase in activity is encouraged, after which the patient is involved in a physical therapy program. The complications of IDET include catheter kinking or breakage, nerve root injury, nondermatomal leg pain, dural puncture, infection, bleeding, cauda equina syndrome, and spinal cord damage.[158]

The efficacy of IDET has been shown in a meta-analysis[159] and in a randomized study that showed improvements in outcome measures such as pain, physical function, and disability.[160] A review comparing IDET and surgical fusion in patients with intractable discogenic low back pain showed similar improvements in both groups.[161]

Percutaneous Disc Decompression (Nucleoplasty)

Percutaneous disc decompression is a procedure wherein a portion of the nucleus pulposus is removed or coagulated. It has been postulated that reducing the intradiscal volume results in a disproportionately higher drop in pressure. In nucleoplasty, radiofrequency energy is delivered through a percutaneous electrode creating a voltage gradient within the disc. A plasma field is created between the tip of the electrode and the surrounding nucleus pulposus. Molecular bonds of the nucleus pulposus break and the disc material is vaporized into low-molecular gases that are removed through the percutaneous needle. Discography may be performed prior to nucleoplasty to help decide which disc is involved. In contrast to IDET, the temperature created by nucleoplasty is in the 40 to 70°C range. The contraindications to percutaneous disc decompression include (1) a large, noncontained disc herniation, sequestration, or extrusion; (2) free fragments; (3) herniation greater than one-third the sagittal diameter of the spinal canal; (4) equivocal results from discography; (5) tumor, infection, fracture; (6) spinal stenosis, spinal instability; (7) cauda equina syndrome or newly developed signs of neurologic deficit; (8) patients who cannot understand informed consent; and (9) uncontrolled coagulopathy and bleeding disorders.[162]

The patient preparation, antibiotic prophylaxis, monitoring, and positioning are similar to discography and IDET. An electrode is passed through the introducer needle and advanced to the interface between the annulus and the nucleus pulposus. Tissue ablation and coagulation are performed with each pass. Six channels ("passes") are usually made through the nucleus, vaporizing a total of 1 cm^3 of intradiscal volume and causing a significant drop in intradiscal pressure.[163] Postoperatively, the patient's activity should be restricted. The complications are similar to those with discography and IDET. Complications that are specific to nucleoplasty include probe tip fracture when it is forced against an endplate. The efficacy of nucleoplasty is less well documented when compared with IDET. Prospective uncontrolled studies show nucleoplasty to be beneficial, with good short-term results in the majority of patients. One study revealed that pain relief was noted in 79 to 82% of the patients at the initial follow-up, with relief in 53 to 79% at 1-year follow-up.[164] Percutaneous disc decompression can also be attained with a percutaneous disc probe wherein disc material is removed with radiofrequency energy or thermal heat.

Vertebroplasty and Kyphoplasty

Vertebroplasty and kyphoplasty are percutaneous interventional modalities to treat vertebral compression fractures (VCF), a condition usually secondary to osteoporosis in elderly patients. Most VCFs are asymptomatic, incidentally noted on a chest x-ray, and usually occurring at the thoracolumbar junction. There may be no history of trauma; minor activities such as bending, coughing, and lifting objects have been associated with the development of VCFs. The pain can be severe and debilitating. Patients with symptomatic VCFs have decreased vertebral body height, kyphosis, and decreased mobility that may result in atelectasis, pneumonia, and deep venous thrombosis. Most VCFs are asymptomatic although pain may be experienced with bending, lifting, prolonged sitting or standing, or when the patient attempts to stand from a seated position. The pain is usually a deep back pain and there may be intercostal neuralgic symptoms or radiculitis and paravertebral muscle spasm. Pain is relieved by bed rest and the recumbent position. Radiography shows osteopenia or decreased bone mass and bone densitometry

shows decreased bone density. MRI is the imaging modality of choice.

Vertebroplasty involves the injection of polymethylmethacrylate (PMMA) into the affected vertebral body; kyphoplasty involves the insertion of a balloon prior to the injection of the cement. These procedures lead to restoration of some of the decreased vertebral height, improved strength of the vertebral body, and decreased stress placed on the adjacent vertebrae. Vertebroplasty is usually performed under fluoroscopic guidance, although a combination of fluoroscopy and CT guidance has been described. After administration of prophylactic antibiotic, vertebral body access is obtained through a uni- or bipedicular approach. Some physicians perform venography prior to injection of PMMA to show venous drainage and confirm needle placement into the bony trabeculae. The entire vertebral body does not have to be filled with cement to achieve pain relief as there is no correlation between volumes of cement injected and pain reduction.[165] Usually, 2 to 6 mL of cement is enough for the procedure (Fig. 58-10). The patient remains supine for 3 to 5 hours after the procedure for assessment of neurologic status and observation for the occurrence of bleeding and hematomas. The procedure can be done on an outpatient basis. A CT scan is usually performed afterward for assessment of cement distribution and the occurrence of complications such as bleeding and leakage of the cement. Kyphoplasty involves the percutaneous introduction of a balloon into the vertebral body, inflation of the balloon, then filling the balloon with PMMA that is more viscous than that used for vertebroplasty.

The complications of percutaneous vertebral augmentation include leakage of the cement and complications related to the procedure. The factors that contribute to cement leakage include the level of injection, severity of fracture, and the amount of cement injected. Although some leakage of cement is common, severe clinical sequelae occur in a small percentage of patients. Pulmonary embolism may result from leakage of cement into the paravertebral veins and bone marrow, or embolism of fat particles. Neurologic complications include radiculopathy, spinal claudication, and paraplegia.

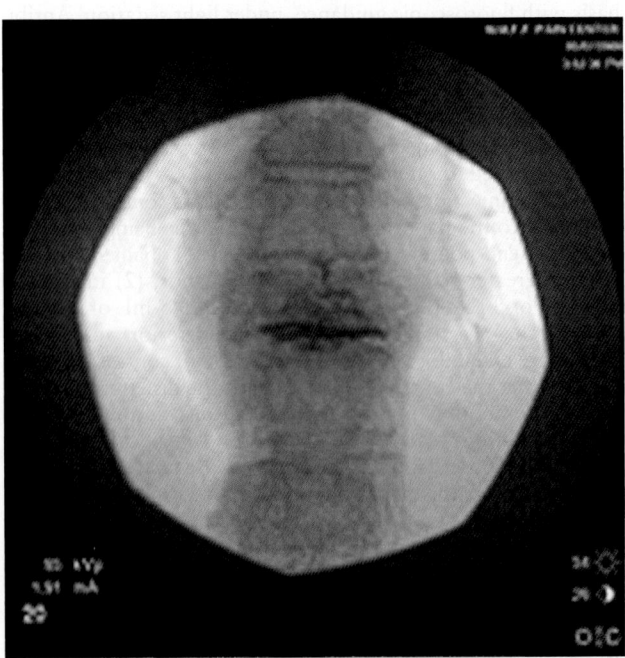

FIGURE 58-10.   Vertebroplasty at T10 vertebral level. A total of 5 mL of cement was injected.

Radiculopathy occurs from leakage of the cement into the neural foramen. Kyphoplasty is associated with a lower rate of cement extravasation because of the higher viscosity of the PMMA that is used, the lower injection pressure employed, and the inflatable bone trap that seals pathways for cement leakage.[166] Complications related to the procedure include infection, bleeding, and allergic reactions from the PMMA or contrast medium.

Kyphoplasty decreases pain and restores vertebral height. Pain is reduced by 50 to 60% after vertebroplasty. Partial or complete relief is seen within the first 3 days after the procedure and improvements in pain, physical, and mental functions remain at long-term follow-up. A nonrandomized prospective study compared percutaneous vertebroplasty with conservative treatment.[167] The patients who had vertebroplasty noted a reduction in pain, improvement in physical function, and reduction or stoppage of analgesic medications. These changes were not noted in the control group. Follow-up of patients after vertebroplasty noted lower pain scores at a 5-year follow-up.[168]

Kyphoplasty is associated with a greater restoration of vertebral height compared with vertebroplasty. Studies show a reduction in pain scores at the 1-year follow-up as well as an increase in physical activities[169] and an increase in the height of the vertebra from 65% before the procedure to 90% after the procedure.[170,171] A follow-up study of 300 patients noted a decrease in the patients' pain scores, improvement in the patients' emotional and mental status, and an increase in their physical and social functions.[172] No significant cement leaks or perioperative complications were noted.

Spinal Cord Stimulation

10 The analgesic effect of spinal cord stimulation (SCS) involves the *gate control theory* wherein it has been hypothesized that SCS increases the input of the large nerve fibers, thus closing the "gate" at the substantia gelatinosa of the dorsal horn of the spinal cord. SCS may alter the local neurochemistry at the dorsal horn, and there may be a decrease of the hyperexcitability of the wide dynamic neurons. It is correlated with increased levels of the inhibitory neurotransmitter GABA and a decrease of the excitatory neurotransmitters glutamate and aspartate.[173,174] In ischemic pain, the analgesia may be secondary to alteration of the sympathetic tone with restoration of a favorable oxygen supply-and-demand balance. Placement of the permanent stimulator is preceded by a trial period of 5 to 7 days to confirm its efficacy (Fig. 58-11).

Appropriate indications for SCS implantation include (1) patients with a diagnosis amenable to the therapy, for example, failed back surgery syndrome or neuropathic pain syndromes; (2) patients who have failed conservative therapy; (3) patients who have had a trial that has demonstrated pain relief; and (4) patients who have had significant psychological issues ruled out.[175] Many patients with chronic pain have some depressive symptoms. Implantation should be avoided in patients with major psychological disorders. There appears to be a high correlation between several items on some psychological tests and a favorable response to trial stimulation.[176] The recommended selection criteria for SCS placement in patients with neuropathic pain are (1) a confirmed diagnosis of neuropathic pain; (2) chronicity of >6 months; (3) failed trials of polypharmacy including anticonvulsants, antidepressants, and/or opioids; (4) the lemniscate pathway (spinal connection to painful site) is preserved so that stimulation-induced paresthesias can be felt; and (5) absence of contraindications, such as infection or nociceptive pain syndromes.[177] Complications include nerve and spinal cord injury, infection, hematoma, and lead breakage or migration.

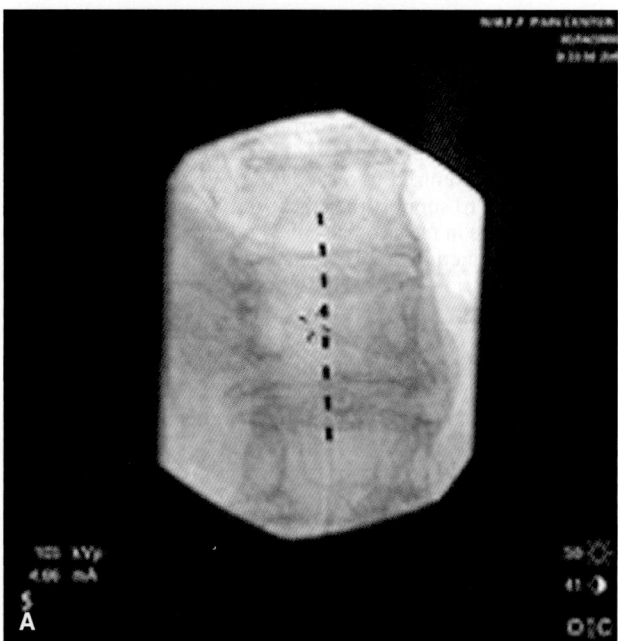

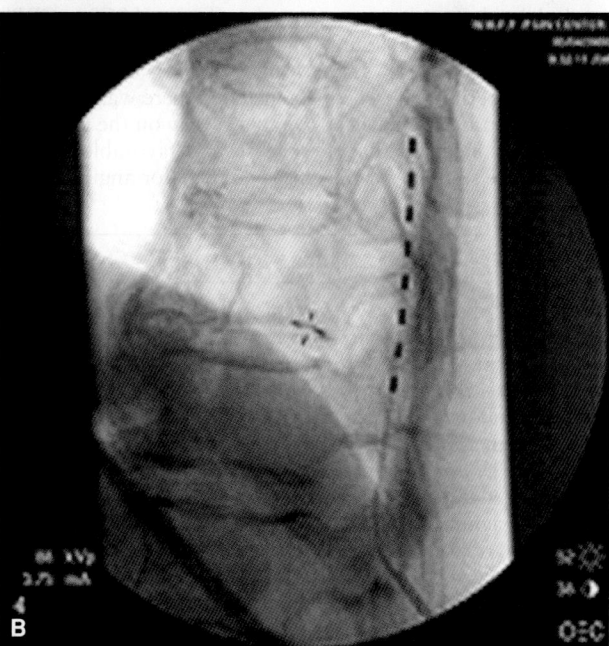

FIGURE 58-11. Anteroposterior (**A**) and lateral (**B**) views of a spinal cord stimulator placed over the T11 to T12 vertebral levels. The stimulator was placed for peripheral ischemia.

Studies that have looked into the efficacy of SCS for chronic pain often lack a randomized control group; they have ambiguous entry criteria, few outcome measures, and inadequate follow-up. Although the main indication for use of SCS in the United States is failed back surgery syndrome, it is a treatment of peripheral ischemia in Europe. A meta-analysis concluded that there was insufficient evidence to draw conclusions,[178] but several case series,[179,180] a prospective randomized study,[181] and review articles generally support the efficacy of SCS.[182,183] In the randomized study,[181] patients who were candidates for repeat laminectomy were randomized to either SCS or surgery. At the 6-month follow-up, 67% (10 of 15 patients) of patients who had reoperation crossed over to SCS, compared with only

17% (2 of 12 patients) of the SCS group who crossed over to reoperation. At the 3-year follow-up, SCS continued to have better outcomes compared with surgery. Overall, 47% of patients in the SCS group achieved ≥50% pain relief compared with 12% in the reoperation group ($p < 0.01$). The patients randomized to reoperation used significantly more opioids than those randomized to SCS. Thus, it appears there is sufficient evidence to support the efficacy of SCS for treating failed back syndrome in terms of sustained long-term pain relief with medication reduction, improvement in quality of life, increased patient satisfaction, increased ability to return to work, minimal side effects, cost-effectiveness compared with alternative therapies, and reversibility of the technique.[184]

Studies that examined the efficacy of SCS in CRPSs consist of a retrospective study,[185] case series[186,187] and a prospective randomized controlled study.[188] In the randomized controlled study,[188] patients with a 6-month history of CRPS of the upper extremity had either SCS or physiotherapy. At the 6-month follow-up, patients who were treated with SCS had a significantly greater reduction in pain, and a significantly higher percentage of patients graded their relief as much improved in terms of global perceived effect. However, there were no clinically significant improvements in functional status. A literature review[189] concluded that SCS is a powerful tool in the management of CRPS and a meta-analysis[183] concluded that a grade A level of evidence supports the efficacy of SCS in CRPS. For peripheral ischemia and angina, most of the published literature consists of case series. A meta-analysis on the efficacy of SCS for peripheral ischemia concluded there was a grade A level of supportive evidence,[190] and a review on the treatment of angina concluded that, despite several favorable reports, there is little support for the efficacy of SCS for angina.[191]

Intrathecal Pumps

Intrathecal drug delivery systems (IDDSs) are a valuable option in patients in whom oral or transdermal opioids are ineffective at reasonable doses, or cause unacceptable side effects. The main indications for IDDS are patients with cancer pain, followed by pain of spinal origin, with the majority of pumps placed in the United States for failed back surgery syndrome. A combination of opioid and baclofen has been administered in patients who have had a significant spinal cord injury or significant spasm as a part of the clinical picture. Intrathecal drug infusion allows the drug to be directly deposited near the spinal cord receptors, bypassing the blood–brain barrier. By enabling direct access to opioid receptors, an equianalgesic dose is markedly diminished compared with alternative routes. These lower doses result in a marked decrease in side effects and adverse events. Spinal opioids not only interact with the opioid receptors, spinal delivery also results in adenosine release in the cerebrospinal fluid.[192]

Several factors should be considered before instituting IDDS (Table 58-7).[193] Once the patient meets the necessary criteria, a trial period is recommended before an intrathecal pump is permanently placed. A trial can be performed intrathecally or through the epidural space, by a single shot, intermittent bolus, or a continuous infusion; the trial is usually with morphine; and can be performed on an inpatient or outpatient basis. Opioids alone may not be adequate to treat neuropathic or mixed pain syndromes. A survey showed that only 65% of patients had acceptable results when morphine was used as the sole agent.[194] The majority of physicians used other drugs as additives to morphine or changed to an alternate opioid such as hydromorphone.

A 2000 consensus conference on the proper use of intrathecal medications recommended morphine as a first-line agent.[195] A repeat consensus conference in 2003 resulted in an algorithm

TABLE 58-7

QUESTIONS TO CONSIDER BEFORE INTRATHECAL PUMP PLACEMENT

Are the pain complaints related to an objective physiological diagnosis?

Have less invasive therapies been tried or considered?

Is the patient's life expectancy 3 months or greater?

Is the patient's function limited by the pain symptoms?

Is the patient psychologically stable? Is there uncontrolled psychosis, severe depression, intractable anxiety, or significant personality disorders?

Is the patient compliant with other treatment recommendations?

Does the patient have any contraindications to pump placement such as bacteremia, bleeding disorders, or localized infection?

Has an acceptable trial been performed to document adequate pain response and controllable side effects?

Is the patient aware of the expectations of the procedure?

Is the patient agreeable to permanent pump placement despite the risks of the procedure and the long-term risks of the drugs to be infused?

From Deer TR: Intrathecal drug delivery: Overview of the proper use of infusion agents, Raj's Practical Management of Pain, 4th edition. Edited by Benzon HT, Rathmell J, Wu C et al. Phildelphia, Mosby Elsevier, 2008, p 947, with permission.

that is often used as a guide for patients with intrathecal pumps.[190] The revised algorithm recommends morphine and hydromorphone as acceptable first-line agents. If either morphine or hydromorphone does not produce relief, or cause side effects, then either one drug is switched to the other first-line drug if the patient has primary nociceptive pain, or clonidine or bupivacaine is added for patients with primary neuropathic or mixed pain syndromes. Ziconotide was not included in the 2003 consensus algorithm but a prospective, randomized, double-blind study published after the conference showed the efficacy of intrathecal ziconotide in patients with pain secondary to cancer and AIDS.[197] The panel of experts met again 2007 and included ziconotide as a first-line drug[198] (Fig. 58-12). Fentanyl was moved to a second-line agent because the more hydrophilic agents cause intractable side effects, and because of its apparent granuloma-sparing property and its widespread use and identified safety.

Complications

Complications of IDDS include infection, bleeding, respiratory depression, pump malfunction, catheter failure, hormonal dysfunction including decreased testosterone levels and small gonads, peripheral edema, and formation of an inflammatory mass. Low testosterone levels are managed with transdermal or injectable testosterone; the patient should undergo a prostate examination and have serum testosterone and prostate-specific antigen levels determined before the testosterone therapy. Peripheral edema should be treated with diuretics, compression stockings, extremity elevation, and rotation of the infused drug. If it occurs, an inflammatory mass is a noninfectious reaction that is usually located at the catheter tip. A consensus panel in 2006 recommended avoidance of morphine at concentrations of >20 mg/mL or hydromorphone >10 mg/mL as these drugs are associated with a known concentration-dependent risk of granuloma formation[199] (Table 58-8). In addition, the panel recommended positioning the tip in the lumbar thecal sac, and an attentive follow-up of the patients.

2007 POLYANALGESIC ALGORITHM FOR INTRATHECAL THERAPIES

	(a)		(b)		(c)
Line #1:	Morphine	⟷	Hydromorphone	⟷	Ziconotide

	(d)		(e)		(f)
Line #2:	Fentanyl	⟷	Morphine/Hydromorphone + Ziconotide	⟷	Morphine/Hydromorphone + Bupivacaine/Clonidine

	(g)		(h)
Line #3:	Clonidine	⟷	Morphine/Hydromorphone/Fentanyl Bupivacaine +/Clonidine + Ziconotide

	(i)		(j)
Line #4:	Sufentanil	⟷	Sufentanil + Bupivacaine +/Clonidine + Ziconotide

	(k)
Line #5:	Ropivacaine, Buprenophine, Midazolam Meperidine, Ketorolac

Line #6:	***Experimental Drugs***
	Gabapentin, Octreotide, Conpeptide, Neostigmine, Adenosine, XEN2174, AM336, XEN, ZGX 160

FIGURE 58-12. Recommended algorithm for intrathecal polyanalgesic therapies, 2007. Line 1: Morphine (a) and ziconotide (c) are approved by the Food and Drug Administration of the United States for intrathecal analgesic use and are recommended for first-line therapy for nociceptive, mixed, and neuropathic pain. Hydromorphone (b) is recommended based on clinical widespread usage and apparent safety. Line 2: Because of its apparent granuloma-sparing effect and because of its wide apparent use and identified safety, fentanyl (d) has been upgraded to a line 2 agent by the consensus conference when the use of the more hydrophilic agents of line 1 (a,b) result in intractable supraspinal side effects. Combinations of opioid + ziconotide (e) or opioid + bupivacaine or clonidine (f) are recommended for mixed and neuropathic pain and may be used interchangeably. When admixing opioids with ziconotide, pay attention to the guidelines for admixing ziconotide with other agents. Line 3: Clonidine (g) alone or opioids such as morphine/hydromorphone/fentanyl with bupivacaine and/or clonidine mixed with ziconotide (h) may be used when agents in line 2 fail to provide analgesia or side effects occur when these agents are used. Line 4: Because of its proven safety in animals and humans and because of its apparent granuloma-sparing effects, Sufenta alone (i) or mixed with bupivacaine and/or clonidine plus ziconotide (j) is recommended in this line. The addition of clonidine, bupivacaine, and/or ziconotide is to be used in patients with mixed or neuropathic pain. In patients facing end of life, the panelists thought that midazolam and octreotide should be tried when all other agents in lines 1 through 4 have failed. Line 5: These agents (k), although not experimental, have little information about them in the literature; use is recommended with caution and obvious informed consent regarding the paucity of information regarding the safety and efficacy of their use. Line 6: Experimental agents (l) must only be used experimentally and with appropriate independent review board-approved protocols. (From Deer T, Krames ES, Hassenbusch SJ et al: Polyanalgesic consensus conference 2007: Recommendations for the management of pain by intrathecal (intraspinal) drug delivery: Report of an interdisciplinary expert panel. Neuromodulation 2007; 10: 300, with permission.)

TABLE 58-8

CONCENTRATIONS AND DOSES OF INTRATHECAL AGENTS RECOMMENDED BY THE POLYANALGESIC CONSENSUS PANELISTS, 2007

▪ DRUG	▪ MAXIMUM CONCENTRATION	▪ MAXIMUM DOSE/DAY
Morphine	20 mg/mL	15 mg
Hydromorphone	10 mg/mL	4 mg
Fentanyl	2 mg/mL	No known upper limit
Sufentanil	50 μg/mL (not available for compounding)	No known upper limit
Bupivacaine	40 mg/mL	30 mg
Clonidine	2 mg/mL	1.0 mg
Ziconotide	100 μg/mL	19.2 μg (Elan recommendations)

From Deer T, Krames ES, Hassenbusch SJ et al: Polyanalgesic consensus conference 2007: Recommendations for the management of pain by intrathecal (intraspinal) drug delivery: Report of an interdisciplinary expert panel. Neuromodulation 2007; 10: 300, with permission.

References

1. Melzack R: Prolonged relief of pain by brief, intense transcutaneous somatic stimulation. Pain 1975; 1: 357
2. Neumann S, Doubell TP, Leslie T et al: Inflammatory pain hypersensitivity mediated by phenotypic switch in myelinated primary sensory neurons. Nature 1996; 384: 360
3. Fields HL: Pain Syndromes in Neurology. London, Butterworths, 1990
4. Lumpkin EA, Caterina MJ: Mechanisms of sensory transduction in the skin. Nature 2007; 445: 858
5. Caterina MJ, Schumacher MA, Tominaga M et al: The capsaicin receptor: A heat-activated ion channel in the pain pathway. Nature 1997; 389: 816
6. Caterina MJ, Leffler A, Malmberg AB et al: Impaired nociception and pain sensation in mice lacking the capsaicin receptor. Science 2000; 288: 306
7. Suzuki H, Kerr R, Bianchi L et al: In vivo imaging of C. elegans mechanosensory neurons demonstrates a specific role for the MEC-4 channel in the process of gentle touch sensation. Neuron 2003; 39: 1005
8. Honda CN, Lee CL: Immunohistochemistry of synaptic input and functional characterizations of neurons near the spinal central canal. Brain Res 1985; 343: 120
9. Willis WD, Kenshalo DR, Leonard RB: The cells of origin of the primate spinothalamic tract. J Comp Neurol 1979; 188: 543
10. Clark FM, Proudfit HK: The projections of noradrenergic neurons in the A5 catecholamine cell group to the spinal cord in the rat: anatomical evidence that A5 neurons modulate nociception. Brain Res 1993; 616: 200
11. Basbaum AI, Fields HL: Endogenous pain control systems: brainstem spinal pathways and endorphin circuitry. Annu Rev Neurosci 1984; 7: 309
12. Bajic D, Proudfit HK: Projections of neurons in the periaqueductal gray to pontine and medullary catecholamine cell groups involved in the modulation of nociception. J Comp Neurol 1999; 405: 359
13. Gebhart GF: Recent developments in the neurochemical bases of pain and analgesia. NIDA Res Monogr 1983; 45: 19
14. Basbaum AI, Clanton CH, Fields HL: Three bulbospinal pathways from the rostral medulla of the cat: an autoradiographic study of pain modulating systems. J. Comp. Neurol 1978; 178: 209
15. Duggan AW, Griersmith BT: Inhibition of the spinal transmission of nociceptive information by supraspinal stimulation in the cat. Pain 1979; 6: 149
16. Antal M, Petko M, Polgar E et al: Direct evidence of an extensive GABAergic innervation of the spinal dorsal horn by fibres descending from the rostral ventromedial medulla. Neuroscience 1996; 73: 509
17. Clark FM, Proudfit HK: The projection of noradrenergic neurons in the A7 catecholamine cell group to the spinal cord in the rat demonstrated by anterograde tracing combined with immunocytochemistry. Brain Res 1991; 547: 279
18. Peyron R, Laurent B, Garcia-Larrea L: Functional imaging of brain responses to pain. A review and meta-analysis (2000). Neurophysiol Clin 2000; 30: 263
19. Woolf CJ: Evidence for a central component of post-injury pain hypersensitivity. Nature 1983; 306: 686
20. Lai J, Gold MS, Kim CS et al: Inhibition of neuropathic pain by decreased expression of the tetrodotoxin-resistant sodium channel, NaV1.8. Pain 2002; 95: 143
21. Munro G, Dalby-Brown W: Kv7 (KCNQ) channel modulators and neuropathic pain. J Med Chem 2007; 50: 2576
22. Mulleman D, Mammou S, Griffoul I et al: Pathophysiology of disk-related sciatica. I. Evidence supporting a chemical component. Joint Bone Spine 2006; 73: 151
23. Novakovic SD, Levinson SR, Schachner M et al: Disruption and reorganization of sodium channels in experimental allergic neuritis. Muscle Nerve 1998; 21: 1019
24. Basbaum AI: Spinal mechanisms of acute and persistent pain. Reg Anesth Pain Med 1999; 24: 59
25. Torebjork HE, Lundberg LE, LaMotte RH: Central changes in processing of mechanoreceptive input in capsaicin-induced secondary hyperalgesia in humans. J Physiol (Lond) 1992; 448: 765
26. Boden SD, Davis DO, Dina TS et al: Abnormal magnetic-resonance scans of the lumbar spine in asymptomatic subjects. A prospective investigation. J Bone Joint Surg (Am) 1990; 72: 403
27. Jensen MC, Brant-Zawadzki MN, Obuchowski N et al: Magnetic resonance imaging of the lumbar spine in people without back pain. N Eng J Med 1994; 331: 69
28. Weinreb JC, Wolbarsht LB, Cohen JM et al: Prevalence of lumbosacral intervertebral disc abnormalities in MR images of pregnant and asymptomatic nonpregnant women, Radiology 1989; 170: 125
29. Teplick JG: Spontaneous regression of herniated nucleus pulposus. Am J Radiol 1985; 145: 371
30. Borenstein DG, O'Mara JW, Boden SD et al: The value of magnetic resonance imaging of the lumbar spine to predict low back pain in asymptomatic subjects: A seven-year follow-up study. J Bone Joint Surg (Am) 2001; 83: 1306
31. Burke JG, Watson RWG, McCormack D et al: Intervertebral discs which cause low back pain secrete high levels of proinflammatory mediators. J Bone Joint Surg (Br) 2002; 84: 196

32. Olmarker K, Rydevik B: Selective inhibition of tumor necrosis factor-alpha prevents nucleus induced thrombus formation, intraneural edema, and reduction of nerve conduction velocity: possible implications for future pharmacologic treatment strategy of sciatica. Spine 2001; 26: 863
33. Cohen SP, Wenzell D, Hurley RW et al: A double-blind placebo-controlled, dose-response pilot study evaluating intradiscal ethanercept in patients with chronic discogenic low back pain or lumbosacral radiculopathy. Anesthesiology 2007; 107: 99
34. Benzon HT: Epidural steroid injections for low back pain and lumbosacral radiculopathy. Pain 1986; 24: 277
35. Dilke TFW, Burry HC, Grahame R: Extradural corticosteroid injection in management of lumbar nerve root compression. Br Med J 1973; 2: 635
36. Arden NK, Price C, Reading I et al: WEST Study Group: A multicentre randomized controlled trial of epidural corticosteroid injections for sciatica: the WEST study. Rheumatology 2005; 44: 1399
37. Wilson-MacDonald J, Burt G, Griffen D et al: Epidural steroid injection for nerve root compression. A randomized, controlled trial. J Bone Joint Surg (Br) 2005; 87: 352
38. Snoek W, Weber H, Jorgensen B: Double blind evaluation of extradural methylprednisolone for herniated lumbar discs. Acta Orthop Scand 1977; 48: 635
39. Cuckler JM, Bernini PA, Wiesel SW et al: The use of epidural steroids in the treatment of lumbar radicular pain. J Bone Joint Surg (Am) 1985; 67: 63
40. Carette S, Leclaire R, Marcoux S et al: Epidural corticosteroid injections for sciatica due to herniated nucleus pulposus. N Engl J Med 1997; 336: 1634
41. Armon C, Argoff CA, Samuels J et al: Assessment: Use of epidural steroid injections to treat radicular lumbosacral pain. Neurology 2007; 68: 723
42. Riew KD, Yin Y, Gilula L et al: The effect of nerve-root injections on the need for operative treatment of lumbar radicular pain. A prospective, randomized, controlled, double-blind study. J Bone Joint Surg (Am) 2000; 82: 1589
43. Karppinen J, Malmivaara A, Kurunlahti M et al: Periradicular infiltration for sciatica: A randomized controlled trial. Spine 2001; 26: 1059
44. Ng L, Chaudhary N, Sell P: The efficacy of corticosteroids in periradicular infiltration for chronic radicular pain: A randomized, double-blind, controlled trial. Spine 2005; 30: 857
45. Kraemer J, Ludwig J, Bickert U et al: Lumbar epidural perineural injection: a new technique Eur Spine J 1997; 6: 357
46. Thomas E, Cyteval C, Abiad L et al: Effect of transforaminal versus interspinous corticosteroid injection in discal radiculalgia—a prospective, randomized, double-blind study. Clin Rheumatol 2003; 22: 299
47. Abram SE: Treatment of lumbosacral radiculopathy with epidural steroids. Anesthesiology 1999; 91: 1937
48. Rathmell JP, April C, Bogduk N: Cervical transforaminal injection of steroids. Anesthesiology 2004; 100: 1959
49. Rathmell JP, Benzon HT: Transforaminal injection of steroid: Should we continue? [editorial]. Reg Anesth Pain Med 2004; 29: 397
50. Tiso RL, Cutler T, Catania JA et al: Adverse central nervous system sequelae after selective transforaminal block: the role of corticosteroids. Spine J 2004; 4: 468
51. Benzon HT, Chew TL, McCarthy R et al: Comparison of the particle sizes of the different steroids and the effect of dilution: A review of the relative neurotoxicities of the steroids. Anesthesiology 2007; 106: 331
52. Huntoon MA: Anatomy of the cervical intervertebral foramina: vulnerable arteries and ischemic neurologic injuries after transforaminal epidural injections. Pain 2005; 117: 104
53. Dreyfuss P, Baker R, Bogduk N: Comparative effectiveness of cervical epidural steroid injections with particulate and non-particulate corticosteroid preparations for cervical radicular pain. Pain Med 2006; 7: 237
54. Benzon HT: Studies on diagnostic injections and surgery for low back pain: Problems, advances, and opportunities. Anesth Analg 2007; 105: 1523
55. King JS, Lagger R: Sciatica viewed as referred pain syndrome. Surg Neurol 1976; 5: 46
56. Gallagher G, Petriccione di Vadi PL, Vedley JR: Radiofrequency facet joint denervation in the treatment of low back pain: a prospective, controlled double-blind study to assess its efficacy. Pain Clinic 1994; 7: 193
57. Sanders M, Zuurmund WW: Percutaneous intra-articular lumbar facet joint denervation in the treatment of low back pain: A comparison with percutaneous extra-articular lumbar facet denervation. Pain Clinic 1999; 11: 329
58. van Kleef M, Barendse GA, Kessels A et al: Randomized trial of radiofrequency lumbar facet denervation for chronic low back pain. Spine 1999; 24: 1937
59. Leclaire R, Fortin L, Lambert R et al: Radiofrequency facet joint denervation in the treatment of low back pain: a placebo-controlled clinical trial to assess efficacy. Spine 2001; 26: 1411
60. van Wijk RM, Geurtz JW, Wynne HJ et al: Radiofrequency denervation of lumbar facet joints in the treatment of chronic low back pain: a randomized, double-blind, sham lesion-controlled trial. Clin J Pain 2005; 21: 335
61. Lord SM, Barnsley L, Wallis BJ et al: Percutaneous radio-frequency neurotomy for chronic cervical zygapophyseal-joint pain. N Engl J Med 1996; 335: 1721
62. Stovner LJ, Kolstad F, Helde G: Radiofrequency denervation of facet joints C2-C6 in cervicogenic headache: a randomized, double-blind sham-controlled study. Cephalalgia 2004; 24: 821

63. Yin W, Willard F, Carreiro J et al: Sensory stimulation guided sacroiliac joint radiofrequency neurotomy: technique based on neuroanatomy of the dorsal sacral plexus. Spine 2003; 28: 2419

64. Cohen SP, Abdi S: Lateral branch blocks as a treatment for sacroiliac joint pain: a pilot study. Reg Anesth Pain Med 2003; 28: 113

65. Pino CA, Hoeft MA, Hofsess C et al: Morphologic analysis of bipolar radiofrequency lesions: Implications for treatment of the sacroiliac joint. Reg Anes Pain Med 2005; 30: 335

66. Burnham RS, Yasui Y: An alternate method of radiofrequency neurotomy of the sacroiliac joint: A pilot study of the effect on pain, function, and satisfaction. Reg Anesth Pain Med 2007; 32: 12

67. Ferrante FM, King LF, Roche EA et al: Radiofrequency sacroiliac joint denervation for sacroiliac joint syndrome. Reg Anesth Pain Med 2001; 26: 137

68. Benzon HT, Katz JA, Benzon HA et al: Piriformis syndrome: Anatomic considerations, a new injection technique, and a review of the literature. Anesthesiology 2003; 98: 1442

69. Fishman LM, Zybert PA: Electrophysiologic evidence of piriformis syndrome. Arch Phys Med Rehabil 1992; 73: 359

70. Wheeler AH, Goolkasian P, Gretz SS: A randomized, double-blind, prospective pilot study of botulinum toxin injection for refractory, unilateral, cervicothoracic, paraspinal, myofascial pain syndrome. Spine 1998; 23: 1662

71. Ferrante FM, Bearn L, Rothrock R et al: Evidence against trigger point injection technique for the treatment of cervicothoracic myofascial pain with botulinum toxin type A. Anesthesiology 2005; 103: 377

72. Wolfe F, Smythe HA, Yunus MB et al: The American College of Rheumatology 1990 Criteria for the Classification of Fibromyalgia. Arthritis Rheum 1990; 33: 160

73. Russell IJ, Kamin M, Bennett RM et al: Efficacy of tramadol in treatment of pain in fibromyalgia. J Clin Rheumatol 2000; 6: 250

74. Arnold LM, Rosen A, Pritchett YL et al: A randomized, double-blind, placebo-controlled trial of duloxetine in the treatment of women with fibromyalgia with or without major depressive disorder. Pain 2005; 119: 5

75. Crofford LJ, Rowbotham MC, Mease PJ et al: Pregabalin for the treatment of fibromyalgia syndrome: results of a randomized, double-blind, placebo-controlled trial. Arthritis Rheum 2006; 52: 1264

76. Pasqualucci A, Pasqualucci V, Galla F et al: Prevention of postherpetic neuralgia: acyclovir and prednisolone versus epidural local anesthetic and methylprednisolone. Acta Anaesthesiol Scand 2000; 44: 910

77. van Wijck AJM, Opstelten W, Moons KGM et al: The PINE study of epidural steroids and local anaesthetics to prevent postherpetic neuralgia randomized controlled trial. Lancet 2006; 367: 219

78. Winnie AP, Hartwell PW: Relationship between time of treatment of acute herpes zoster with sympathetic blockade and prevention of post-herpetic neuralgia: Clinical support for new theory of the mechanism by which sympathetic blockade provides therapeutic benefit. Reg Anesth 1993; 18: 277

79. Max MB: Thirteen consecutive well-designed randomized trials show that antidepressants reduce pain in diabetic neuropathy and postherpetic neuralgia. Pain Forum 1995; 4: 248

80. Wu CL, Raja SN: An update on the treatment of postherpetic neuralgia. J Pain 2008; 9: S19

81. Watson CPN, Babul N: Efficacy of oxycodone in neuropathic pain: A randomized trial in postherpetic neuralgia. Neurology 1998; 50: 1837

82. Raja SN, Haythornthwaite JA, Papagallo M et al: Opioids versus antidepressants in postherpetic neuralgia: A randomized placebo-controlled trial. Neurology 2002; 59: 1015

83. Boureau F, Legallicier P, Kabir-Ahmadi M: Tramadol in postherpetic neuralgia: A randomized, double-blind, placebo-controlled trial. Pain 2003; 323

84. Rowbotham MC, Harden N, Stacey B et al: Gabapentin for the treatment of postherpetic neuralgia: A randomized, controlled trial. JAMA 1998; 280: 1837

85. Rice ASC, Maton S: Postherpetic Neuralgia Study group: Gabapentin in postherpetic neuralgia: A randomized, double-blind, placebo-controlled study. Pain 2001; 94: 215

86. Dworkin RH, Corbin AE, Young JP et al: Pregabalin for the treatment of postherpetic neuralgia: a randomized, placebo-controlled trial. Neurology 2003; 60: 1274

87. Freynhagen R, Strojek K, Griesing T et al: Efficacy of pregabalin in neuropathic pain evaluated in a 12-week, randomised, double-blind, multicentre, placebo-controlled trial of flexible- and fixed-dose regimens. Pain 2005; 115: 254

88. Gilron I, Bailey JM, Tu D et al: Morphine, gabapentin, or their combination for neuropathic pain. New Engl J Med 2005; 352: 1324

89. Finnerup NB, Otto M, McQuay HJ et al: Algorithm for neuropathic pain treatment: An evidence based proposal. Pain 2005; 118: 289

90. Kotani N, Kushikata T, Hashimoto H et al: Intrathecal methylprednisolone for intractable postherpetic neuralgia. N Engl J Med 2000; 343: 1514

91. Kikuchi A, Kotani N, Sato T et al: Comparative therapeutic evaluation of intrathecal versus methylprednisolone for long-term analgesia in patients with intractable postherpetic neuralgia. Reg Anesth Pain Med 1999; 24: 287

92. Harke H, Gretenkort P, Ladleif HU et al: Spinal cord stimulation in posthereptic neuralgia and in acute herpes zoster. Anesth Analg 2002; 9: 694

93. Lauretti GR, Trevelin WR, Frade LCP et al: Spinal alcohol neurolysis for intractable thoracic postherpetic neuralgia after test bupivacaine spinal analgesia. Anesthesiology 2004; 101: 244

94. Kelkar P: Diabetic neuropathy. Semin Neurol 2005; 25: 168

95. Williams KA, Hurley RW, Lin EE et al: Neuropathic pain syndromes, Raj's Practical Management of Pain, 4th edition. Edited by Benzon HT, Rathmell J, Wu CL et al. Philedelphia, Mosby Elsevier, 2008, p 427

96. Goldstein DJ, Lu Y, Detke MJ et al: Duloxetine vs. placebo in patients with painful diabetic neuropathy. Pain 2005; 116: 109

97. Watson CP, Moulin D, Watt-Watson J et al: Controlled-release oxycodone relieves neuropathic pain: a randomized controlled trial in painful diabetic neuropathy. Pain 2003; 105: 71

98. Gimbel JS, Richards P, Portenoy RK: Controlled-release oxycodone for pain in diabetic neuropathy: a randomized controlled trial. Neurology 2003; 60: 927

99. Sang CN, Booher S, Gilron I et al: Dextromethorphan and memantine in painful diabetic neuropathy and postherpetic neuralgia: efficacy and dose-response trials. Anesthesiology 2002; 96: 1053

100. Stanton-Hicks M, Jänig W, Hassenbusch S et al: Reflex sympathetic dystrophy: Changing concepts and taxonomy. Pain 1995; 63: 127

101. van de Vusse AC, Stomp-van den Berg SG, Kessels AH et al: Randomised controlled trial of gabapentin in complex regional pain syndrome type 1. BMC Neurol 2004; 29: 4

102. Sinis N, Birbaumer N, Gustin S et al: Memantine treatment of complex regional pain syndrome. A preliminary report of six cases. Clin J Pain 2007; 23: 237

103. Grabow TS, Tella PK, Raja SN: Spinal cord stimulation for complex regional pain syndrome: an evidence-based medicine review of the literature. Clin J Pain 2003; 19: 371

104. Simpson DM, Olney R, McArthur JC et al: A placebo-controlled trial of lamotrigine for painful HIV-associated neuropathy. Neurology 2000; 5411: 2115

105. Simpson DM, McArthur JC, Olney R et al: Lamotrigine Neuropathy Study HIV Team: Lamotrigine for HIV-associated painful sensory neuropathies: a placebo-controlled trial. Neurology 2003; 609: 1508

106. Hahn K, Arendt G, Braun JS et al: German Neuro-AIDS Working Group: A placebo-controlled trial of gabapentin for painful HIV-associated sensory neuropathies. J Neurol 2004; 251: 1260

107. Bach S, Noreng MF, Tjellden NU: Phantom limb pain in amputees during the first 12 months following limb amputation, after preoperative lumbar epidural blockade. Pain 1988; 33: 297

108. Nikolajsen L, Ilkjaer S, Christensen JH et al: Randomised trial of epidural bupivacaine and morphine in prevention of stump and phantom pain in lower-limb amputation. Lancet 1997; 350: 1353

109. Morey TE, Giannoni J, Duncan E et al: Nerve sheath catheter analgesia after amputation. Clin Orthop Relat Res 2002; 397: 281

110. Schley M, Topfner S, Wiech K et al: Continuous brachial plexus blockade in combination with the NMDA receptor antagonist memantine prevents phantom pain in acute traumatic upper limb amputees. Eur J Pain 2007; 11: 299

111. Foley KM: Treatment of cancer pain. N Engl J Med 1985; 313: 84

112. Ischia S, Ischia A, Polati E, Finco G: Three posterior percutaneous celiac plexus block techniques: a prospective randomized study in 61 patients with pancreatic cancer pain. Anesthesiology 1992; 76: 534

113. de Leon-Casasola OA: Neurolysis of the sympathetic axis for cancer pain management, Raj's Practical Management of Pain. 4th edition. Edited by Benzon HT, Rathmell J, Wu C et al. Philadelphia, Mosby Elsevier 2008: 917

114. Ventafridda GV, Caraceni AT, Sbanotto AM et al: Pain treatment in cancer of the pancreas. Eur J Surg Oncol 1990; 16: 1

115. Mercadante S: Celiac plexus block versus analgesics in pancreatic cancer pain. Pain 1993; 52: 187

116. Wong G, Schoeder DR, Carns PE et al: Effect of neurolytic celiac plexus block on pain relief, quality of life, and survival in patients with unresectable pancreatic cancer. JAMA 2004; 291: 1092

117. De Cicco M, Matovic M, Bortolussi R et al: Celiac Plexus Block: Injectate spread and pain relief in patients with regional anatomic distortions. Anesthesiology 2001; 94: 561

118. Eisenberg E, Carr DB, Chalmers TC: Neurolytic celiac plexus block for treatment of cancer pain: a meta-analysis. Anesth Analg 1995; 80: 290

119. Plancarte R, Amescua C, Patt RB et al: Superior hypogastric plexus block for pelvic cancer pain. Anesthesiology 1990; 73: 236

120. de Leon-Casasola OA, Kent E, Lema MJ: Neurolytic superior hypogastric plexus block for chronic pelvic pain associated with cancer. Pain 1993; 54: 145

121. Plancarte R, de Leon-Casasola OA, El-Helaly M et al: Neurolytic superior hypogastric plexus block for chronic pelvic pain associated with cancer. Reg Anesth 1997; 22: 562

122. Wemm KJ, Sabersky L: Modified approach to block the ganglion impar (ganglion of Walther). Reg Anesth 1995; 20: 544

123. McQuay HJ, Moore RA: An evidence-based resource for pain relief. Oxford: Oxford University Press, 1988

124. Krantz MJ, Lewkowicz L, Hays H et al: Torsade de pointes associated with very high dose methadone. Ann Intern Med 2002; 137: 501

125. Sindrup SH, Jensen TS: Efficacy of pharmacological treatments of neuropathic pain. An update and effect related to mechanism of drug action. Pain 1999; 83: 389

126. Williams DG, Patel A, Howard RF: Pharmacogenetics of codeine metabolism in an urban population of children and its implications for analgesic reliability. Br J Anaesth 2002; 89: 839

PERIOPERATIVE AND CONSULTATIVE SERVICES

127. Vainio A, Ollila J, Matikainen E et al: Driving ability in cancer patients receiving long-term morphine analgesia. Lancet 1995; 346: 667
128. Sabatowski R, Schwalen S, Rettig K et al: Driving ability under long-term treatment with transdermal fentanyl. J Pain Symptom Manage 2003; 25: 38
129. Bruera E, Macmillan K, Hanson J et al: The cognitive effects of the administration of narcotic analgesics in patients with cancer pain. Pain 1989; 39: 13
130. Ballantyne JC, Mao J: Opioid therapy for chronic pain. N Engl J Med 2003; 349: 1943
131. Martell BA, O'Connor PG, Kerns RD et al: Systematic review: opioid treatment for chronic back pain: prevalence, efficacy, and association with addiction. Ann Int Med 2007; 146: 116
132. Schnitzer TJ, Ferraro A, Hunsche E et al: A comprehensive review of clinical trials on the efficacy and safety of drugs for the treatment of low back pain. J Pain Symptom Manage 2004; 28: 72
133. Tura B, Tura SM: The analgesic effect of tricyclic antidepressants. Brain Res 1990; 518: 19
134. Gray AM, Pache DM, Sewell RD: Do alpha$_2$-adrenoreceptors play a role in the antinociceptive mechanism of action of antidepressant compounds? Eur J Pharmacol 1999; 378: 161
135. Gray AM, Spencer PS, Sewell RD: The involvement of the opioidergic system in the antinociceptive mechanism of action of antidepressant compounds. Br J Pharmacol 1998; 124: 669
136. Reynolds IJ, Miller RJ: Tricyclic antidepressants block N-methyl-D-aspartate receptors: similarities to the action of zinc. Br J Pharmacol 1988; 95: 95
137. Pareek SS, Chopde CT, Desai PA Thakur: Adenosine enhances analgesic effect of tricyclic antidepressants. Indian J Pharmacol 1994; 26: 159
138. Song J-H, Ham S-S, Shin Y-K et al: Amitriptyline modulation of Na$^+$ channels in rat dorsal root ganglion neurons. Eur J Pharmacol 2000; 401: 297
139. Max MB, Lynch SA, Muir J et al: Effects of desipramine, amitriptyline, and fluoxetine on pain in diabetic neuropathy. N Engl J Med 1992; 326: 1250
140. Leijon G, Boivie J: Central post-stroke pain—a controlled trial of amitriptyline and carbamazepine. Pain 1989; 36: 27
141. Bomholt SF, Mikkelsen JD, Blackburn-Munro G: Antinoceptive effects of the antidepressants amitriptyline, duloxetine, mirtazapine and citalopram in animal models of acute, persistent and neuropathic pain. Neuropharmacology 2005; 48: 252
142. Rashkin J, Pritchett YL, Wang F et al: A double-blind, randomized multicenter trial comparing duloxetine with placebo in the management of diabetic peripheral neuropathic pain. Pain Med 2005; 6: 346
143. Arnold LM, Rosen A, Pritchett YL et al: A randomized, double-blind, placebo-controlled trial of duloxetine in the treatment of women with fibromyalgia with or without major depressive disorder. Pain 2005; 119: 5
144. Ramaekers JG: Antidepressants and driver impairment: empirical evidence from a standard on-the-road test. J Clin Psychiatr 2003; 64: 20
145. Sang CN, Hayes KS: Anticonvulsant medications in neuropathic pain. Textbook of Pain. 5th edition. Edited by McMahon SB, Kaltzenburg M. New York, Elsevier-Churchill-Livingstone, 2006, pp 499
146. Zakrewska JM, Patsalos PN: Oxcarbazepine: a new drug in the management of intractable trigeminal neuralgia. J Neurol Neurosurg Psychiatr 1989; 52: 472
147. Rowbotham MC, Davies PS, Fields HL: Topical lidocaine gel relieves postherpetic neuralgia. Ann Neurol 1995; 37: 246
148. Katz NP, Gammaitoni AR, Davis MW et al: Lidocaine patch 5% reduces pain intensity and interference with quality of life in patients with postherpetic neuralgia: an effectiveness trial. Pain Med 2002; 3: 324
149. Campbell BJ, Rowbotham M, Davies PS et al: Systemic absorption of topical lidocaine in normal volunteers, patients with post-herpetic neuralgia, and patients with acute herpes zoster. J Pharm Sci 2002; 91: 1343
150. Benowitz NL, Meister W: Clinical pharmacokinetics of lignocaine. Clin Pharmacokinet 1978; 3: 177
151. Rowbotham MC, Davies PS, Verkempinck C et al: Lidocaine patch: double-blind controlled study of new treatment method for postherpetic neuralgia. Pain 1996; 65: 39
152. Tremont-Lukats IW, Challapalli V, McNicol ED et al: Systemic administration of local anesthetics to relieve neuropathic pain: a systematic review and meta-analysis. Anesth Analg 2005; 101: 1738
153. Boswell MV, Shah RV, Everett CR et al: Interventional techniques in the management of chronic spinal pain: Evidence-based practice guidelines. Pain Physician 2005; 8: 1
154. Rathmell JP, Lake T, Ramundo MB: Infectious risks of chronic pain treatments: Injection therapy, surgical implants, and intradiscal techniques: Reg Anesth Pain Med 2006; 31: 346
155. Derby R, Lee SH, Kim BJ et al: Pressure-controlled lumbar discography in volunteers without low back symptoms. Pain Med 2005; 6: 213
156. Cohen SP, Larkin TM, Barna SA et al: Lumbar discography: A comprehensive review of outcome studies, diagnostic accuracy, and principles. Reg Anesth Pain Med 2005; 30: 163
157. Saal JA, Saal JS: Intradiscal electrothermal therapy for the treatment of chronic discogenic low back pain. Clin Sports Med 2002; 21: 167
158. Cohen SP, Larkin T, Abdi S et al: Risk factors for failure and complications of intradiscal electrothermal theapy: A pilot study. Spine 2003; 28: 1142
159. Appleby D, Andersson G, Totta M: Meta-analysis of the efficacy and safety of intradiscal electrothermal therapy (IDET). Pain Med 2006; 7: 308
160. Pauza KJ, Howell S, Dreyfuss P et al: A randomized, placebo-controlled trial of intradiscal electrothermal therapy for the treatment of discogenic low back pain. Spine J 2004; 4: 27
161. Andersson GB, Mekhail NA, Block JE: Treatment of intractable discogenic low back pain. A systematic review of spinal fusion and intradiscal electrothermal therapy (IDET). Pain Physician 2006; 9: 237
162. Singh V, Derby R: Percutaneous lumbar disc decompression. Pain Physician 2006; 9: 139
163. Chen Y, Lee S, Chen D: Intradiscal pressure study of percutaneous disc decompression with nucleoplasty in human cadavers. Spine 2003; 28: 661
164. Singh V, Piryani C, Liao K: Role of percutaneous disc decompression using coblation in managing chronic discogenic low back pain: A prospective, observational study. Pain Physician 2005; 7: 419
165. Cotton A, Dewatre F, Cortet B et al: Percutaneous vertebroplasty for osteolytic metastases and myeloma: effects of the percentage of lesion filing and the leakage of methylmethacrylate at clinical followup. Radiology 1996; 200: 525
166. Philips FM, Wetzel FT, Leiberman I et al: An *in vivo* comparison of the potential for extravertebral cement leak after vertebroplasty and kyphoplasty. Spine 2002; 27: 2173
167. Diamond TH, Champion B, Clark WA: Management of actue osteoporotic vertebral fractures: a nonrandomized trial comparing percutaneous vertebroplasty with conservative therapy. Am J Med 2003; 114: 257
168. Perez-Higueras A, Alvarez L, Rossi RE et al: Percutaneous vertebroplasty: long term clinical and radiological outcome. Neuroradiology 2002: 44: 950
169. Ledlie JT, Renfro MJ: Balloon kyphoplasty: One year outcomes in vertebral body height restoration, chronic pain, and activity levels. J Neurosurg 2003: 98: 21
170. Garfin SR, Yuan HA, Reiley MA: Kyphoplasty and vertebroplasty for the treatment of painful osteoporotic compression fractures. Spine 2001; 26: 1511
171. Fourney DR, Schomer DF, Nader R et al: Percutaneous vertebroplasty and kyphoplasty for painful vertebral body fractures in cancer patients. J Neurosurg 2003; 98: 21
172. Coumans JV, Reinhardt MK, Lieberman IH: Kyphoplasty for vertebral compression fractures: 1 year clinical outcomes from a prospective study. J Neurosurg 2003; 99: 44
173. Oakley J, Prager J: Spinal Cord Stimulation: Mechanism of action. Spine 2002; 22: 2574
174. Linderoth B, Foreman R: Physiology of spinal cord stimulation: review and update. Neuromodulation 1999; 3: 150
175. Burchiel KJ, Anderson VC, Wilson BJ et al: Prognostic factors of spinal cord stimulation for chronic back and leg pain. Neurosurgery 1995; 36: 1101
176. Olson KA, Bedder MD, Anderson VC et al: Psychological variables associated with outcome of spinal cord stimulation trials. Neuromodulation 1998; 1: 6
177. Puig MM: When does chronic pain become intractable and when is pharmacological management no longer appropirate? The pain specialist's perspective. J Pain Sympt Manage 2006; 31: S1
178. Turner JA, Loeser JD, Bell KG: Spinal cord stimulation for chronic low back pain: a systematic literature synthesis. Neurosurgery 1995; 37: 1088
179. Barolat G, Oakley J, Law J et al: Epidural spinal cord stimulation with a multiple electrode paddle lead is effective in treating low back pain. Neuromodulation 2001; 2: 59
180. Burchiel KJ, Anderson VC, Brown FD et al: Prospective, multicenter study of spinal cord stimulation for the relief of chronic back and extremity pain. Spine 1996; 21: 2786
181. North RB, Kidd DH, Farrokhi F et al: Spinal cord stimulation versus repeated lumbosacral spine surgery for chronic pain: a randomized controlled trial. Neurosurgery 2005; 51: 106
182. North R, Wetzel T: Spinal cord stimulation for chronic pain of spinal origin. Spine 2002; 22: 2584
183. Taylor RS: Spinal cord stimulation in complex regional pain syndrome and refractory neuropathic back and leg pain/failed back surgery syndrome: Results of a systematic review and meta-analysis. J Pain Sympt Manage 2006; 31: S13
184. Van Buyten JP: Neurostimulation for chronic neuropathic back pain in failed back surgery syndrome. J Pain Symptom Manage 2006; 31: S25
185. Bennett D, Alo K, Oakley J et al: Spinal cord stimulation for complex regional pain syndrome I (RSD): A retrospective multicenter experience from 1995–1998 of 101 patients. Neuromodulation 1999; 3: 202
186. Calvillo O, Racz G, Didie J et al: Neuroaugmentation in the treatment of complex regional pain syndrome of the upper extremity. Acta Orthopeadica Belgica 1998; 1: 57
187. Oakley J, Weiner R: Spinal cord stimulation for complex regional pain syndrome: A prospective study of 19 patients at two centers. Neuromodulation 1999; 1: 47
188. Kemler MA, Barendse GA, van Kleef M et al: Spinal cord stimulation in patients with chronic reflex sympathetic dystrophy. N Engl J Med 2000; 343: 618
189. Stanton-Hicks M: Spinal cord stimulation for the management of complex regional pain syndromes. Neuromodulation 1999; 3: 193
190. Ubbink DTh, Vermeulen H: Spinal cord stimulation for critical leg ischemia: A review of effectiveness and optimal patient selection. J Pain Sympt Manage 2006; 31: S30

191. Buchser E, Durrer A, Albrecht E: Spinal cord stimulation for the management of refractory angina pectoris. J Pain Sympt Manage 2006; 31: S36

192. Eisenach JC, Hood DD, Curry R et al: Intrathecal but not intravenous opioids release adenosine from the spinal cord. Pain 2004; 5: 64

193. Deer TR: Intrathecal drug delivery systems: an overview of the proper use of infusion agents, Raj's Practical Management of Pain. 4th edition. Edited by Benzon HT, Rathmell J, Wu C et al. Philadelphia, Mosby Elsevier, 2008, pp 945

194. Hassenbusch SJ, Portenoy RK: Current practices in intraspinal therapy—a survey of clinical trends and decision making. J Pain Symptom Manage 2000; 20: S4

195. Bennett G, Burchiel K, Buchser E et al: Clinical guidelines for intraspinal infusion: a report of an expert panel. PolyAnalgesic Consensus Conference 2000. J Pain Symptom Manage 2000; 20: S37

196. Hassenbusch SJ, Portenoy RK, Cousins M et al: Polyanalgesic Consensus Conference 2003: an update on the management of pain by intraspinal drug delivery—report of an expert panel. J Pain Symptom Manage 2004; 27: 540

197. Staats P, Yearwood T, Charapata SG et al: Intrathecal ziconotide in the treatment of refractory pain in patients with cancer or AIDS: A randomized controlled trial. JAMA 2004; 291: 63

198. Deer T, Krames ES, Hassenbusch SJ et al: Polyanalgesic consensus conference 2007: Recommendations for the management of pain by intrathecal (intraspinal) drug delivery: Report of an interdisciplinary expert panel. Neuromodulation 2007; 10: 300

199. Hassenbusch S, Burchiel K, Coffey RJ et al: Management of intrathecal catheter-tip inflammatory masses: A consensus statement. Pain Med 2002; 3: 313

PERIOPERATIVE AND CONSULTATIVE SERVICES

CHAPTER 59 ■ CARDIOPULMONARY RESUSCITATION

CHARLES W. OTTO

KEY POINTS

1 Brain adenosine triphosphate is depleted after 4 to 6 minutes of no blood flow. It returns nearly to normal within 6 minutes of starting effective cardiopulmonary resuscitation (CPR).

2 Through living wills and other instruments, patients have begun placing limitations on medical treatment to include do not resuscitate orders.

3 The major components of resuscitation from cardiac arrest are airway, breathing, circulation, drugs, and electrical therapy (ABCDE).

4 Two theories for the mechanism of blood flow during closed-chest compression have been suggested, cardiac pump and thoracic pump.

5 Myocardial perfusion is 20 to 50% of normal, whereas cerebral perfusion is maintained at 50 to 90% of normal.

6 CPR has limited success, with only approximately 40% of victims being admitted to the hospital and 10% surviving to discharge.

7 The adequacy of closed-chest compression is usually judged by palpation of a pulse in the carotid or femoral vessels.

8 End-tidal carbon dioxide also has been found to be an excellent noninvasive guide to the adequacy of closed-chest compressions.

9 Effective uninterrupted chest compressions and defibrillation, if appropriate, should take precedence over medications.

10 After vasopressors, the drugs most likely to be of benefit during CPR are those that help suppress ectopic ventricular rhythms.

11 Ventricular fibrillation is the most common electrocardiogram pattern found during witnessed sudden cardiac arrest in adults.

12 Untreated ventricular fibrillation is a time-sensitive model with three phases: electrical, circulatory, and metabolic.

13 Arrest is less likely to be a sudden event and more likely related to progressive deterioration of respiratory and circulatory function in the pediatric age group.

Treatment of cardiac and respiratory arrest is an integral part of anesthesia practice. The American Board of Anesthesiology indicates in its *Booklet of Information* that the "clinical management and teaching of cardiac and pulmonary resuscitation" are some of the activities that define the specialty of anesthesiology. The cardiopulmonary physiology and pharmacology that form the basis of anesthesia practice are applicable to treating the victim of cardiac arrest. However, there is specialized knowledge relating to blood flow, ventilation, and pharmacology under the conditions of a cardiac arrest that must be understood to maintain leadership of the modern cardiopulmonary resuscitation (CPR) team. This chapter concentrates on those aspects of CPR that are different from the more common circumstances requiring cardiovascular support (e.g., shock, dysrhythmias).

HISTORY

Anesthesiologists have contributed many of the elements of modern CPR and continue to be active investigators and teachers in the field. Discoveries leading to current CPR practice have a long history recorded in many famous works.[1,2] The earliest reference may be the Bible story of Elisha breathing life back into the son of a Shunammite woman (II Kings 4: 34). In 1543, Andreas Vesalius described tracheotomy and artificial ventilation.[3] William Harvey's manual manipulation of the heart is well known. Early teaching of resuscitation was organized by the Society for the Recovery of Persons Apparently Drowned, founded in London in 1774. The combined techniques of modern CPR developed primarily from the fortuitous assemblage of innovative clinicians and researchers in Baltimore in the 1950s and early 1960s. Building on the long history of contributions from around the world, these investigators laid the framework for current CPR practice. In the late 1950s, mouth-to-mouth ventilation was established as the only effective means of artificial ventilation.[4–7] The internal defibrillator was developed in 1933,[8] but it was not applied successfully until 1947.[9] It was another decade before general use was made possible by the development of external cross-chest defibrillation.[10,11] Despite these advances, widespread resuscitation from cardiac arrest was not possible until Kouwenhoven et al.[12] described success with closed-chest cardiac massage in a series of patients. The final major component of modern CPR was added in 1963, when Redding and Pearson[13] described the improved success obtained by administering epinephrine or other vasopressor drugs.

SCOPE OF THE PROBLEM

Cardiovascular disease remains the most common cause of death in the industrialized world. Although cardiovascular mortality has been declining in the United States since the mid-1960s, >35% of all deaths are due to cardiovascular causes.[14] Of the 860,000 annual cardiovascular deaths, approximately half are related to coronary artery disease, the majority are sudden deaths and 70% occur out of the hospital or in hospital emergency departments. Thus, CPR teaching and research tend to focus on myocardial ischemia as the primary cause of cardiac arrest. However, anesthesiologists are more likely than other practitioners to deal with causes other than myocardial infarction. CPR is symptomatic therapy, aimed at sustaining vital organ function until natural cardiac function is restored. The details of effective resuscitation technique are important. However, search for a remediable cause of the arrest must not be lost in excessive attention to mechanics.

Brain adenosine triphosphate (ATP) is depleted after 4 to 6 minutes of no blood flow. It returns nearly to normal within 6 minutes of starting effective CPR. Studies in animals suggest that good neurologic outcome may be possible from 10- to 15-minute periods of normothermic cardiac arrest if good circulation is promptly restored.[15,16] In clinical practice, the severity of the underlying cardiac disease is the major determining factor in the success or failure of resuscitation attempts. Of those factors under control of the rescuers, poor outcomes are associated with long arrest times before CPR is begun, prolonged ventricular fibrillation (VF) without definitive therapy, and inadequate coronary and cerebral perfusion during cardiac massage. CPR begun by bystanders can more than double survival.[17] However, bystanders provide CPR only 25 to 30% of the time in sudden cardiac arrest. Optimum outcome from VF is obtained only if basic life support is begun within 4 minutes of arrest and defibrillation applied within 8 minutes.[18] The importance of early defibrillation has been known for some time and is emphasized in CPR practice.[19,20] What is not as well recognized is the tendency to interrupt chest compressions frequently during a resuscitation attempt. Studies of emergency medical systems suggest that chest compressions are performed for <50% of the time during a typical out-of-hospital resuscitation, being interrupted for pulse checks, intubations, starting intravenous catheters, defibrillation attempts, and moving the victim.[21] Because blood flow falls rapidly with cessation of compressions and resumes slowly with reinstitution of compressions, these interruptions undoubtedly contribute to the poor survival rates.

With an effective rapid-response emergency medical system, initial resuscitation rates of 40% and survival to hospital discharge of 10 to 15% are possible after out-of-hospital arrests[18,20] although the median reported survival to discharge with any first recorded rhythm is 6.4%.[22] Rates for survival to discharge from in-hospital arrest are about 18% in adults and 27% in children.[23] Within the hospital, the operating room is the location where CPR has the highest rate of success. Cardiac arrest occurs approximately 7 times for every 10,000 anesthetics.[24] The cause for the arrest is anesthesia-related, approximately 4.5 times for every 10,000 anesthetics, but mortality from these arrests is only 0.4 per 10,000 anesthetics. Thus, resuscitation is successful approximately 90% of the time in anesthesia-related cardiac arrests.

ETHICAL ISSUES: DO NOT RESUSCITATE ORDERS IN THE OPERATING ROOM

Institution of CPR is standard medical care when an individual is found to be apparently dead. In more recent years, terminally ill patients have become increasingly concerned about inappropriate application of life-sustaining procedures, including CPR. Through living wills and other instruments, patients have begun placing limitations on medical treatment to include do not resuscitate (DNR) orders. Such requests are generally accepted, even welcomed, by health care workers. However, the operating room is one area of the hospital where DNR orders continue to cause ethical conflicts between medical personnel and patients.[25,26] There are ethically sound arguments on both sides of the issue as to whether DNR orders should be upheld in the operating room.

The patient's right to limit medical treatment, including refusing CPR, is firmly established in modern medical practice based on the ethical principle of respect for patient autonomy. A terminally ill patient can reject heroic measures such as resuscitation and still choose palliative therapy. If a surgical intervention will ameliorate symptoms or cure a problem that improves quality of life, there is no reason to withhold this treatment. During surgery, the patient reasonably may want to maintain the DNR status to avoid heroic measures that serve only to prolong death. Operative intervention increases the risk of cardiac arrest, and the patient may not want the burden of surviving in a worse condition than preoperatively. Thus, the time that the DNR order provides the greatest protection against unwanted intervention is during surgery. The possibility of death under anesthesia may be viewed as especially peaceful.

Despite these rather strong arguments for treating a DNR status in the operating room the same way it is treated elsewhere in the hospital, most operating room personnel are at least a little uneasy caring for these patients. Many surgeons require that DNR orders be suspended during the perioperative period or assume consent to surgery includes such suspension. There are multiple reasons for the reluctance to accept DNR status during surgery and anesthesia. Approximately 75% of cardiac arrests in the operating room are related to a surgical or anesthetic complication, and resuscitative attempts are highly successful.[24] Ethically, surgeons and anesthesiologists feel responsible for what happens to patients in the operating room: primum non nocere (first, do no harm). Although the physicians are highly diligent in monitoring and managing changes in the patient's status, complications and arrests do occur. Honoring a DNR order under these circumstances is frequently viewed as failure to treat a reversible process, and hence, tantamount to killing. This is an ethically sound view if the cause of arrest is readily identifiable and easily reversible, and if treatment is likely to allow the patient to fulfill the objectives of coming to surgery.[25]

Institutionally, these ethical conflicts should be addressed by adoption of clear policies by hospitals.[27] For the individual patient, conflicts can be resolved by communication among the patient, family, and caregivers. A mutual decision can often be reached to suspend or severely limit a DNR order in the perioperative period if the patient understands the special circumstances of perioperative arrest, that interventions are brief and usually successful, and that the physicians support the patient's goals in coming to surgery and values in desiring not to prolong death. Many interventions commonly used in the operating room (mechanical ventilation, vasopressors, antidysrhythmics, blood products) may be considered forms of resuscitation in other situations. The only modalities that are not routine anesthetic care are cardiac massage and defibrillation. Therefore, the specific interventions included in a DNR status must be clarified with specific allowance made for methods necessary to perform anesthesia and surgery.

COMPONENTS OF RESUSCITATION

3 The major components of resuscitation from cardiac arrest are airway, breathing, circulation, drugs, and electrical therapy (ABCDE). Traditionally, these have been divided into basic life support (BLS) for those elements that can be performed without additional equipment—basic airway management, rescue breathing, and manual chest compressions—and advanced cardiac life support (ACLS), encompassing all the cognitive and technical skills necessary for resuscitation. The standard American Heart Association (AHA) algorithm for adult basic life support is shown in Figure 59-1. Recent advances in resuscitation, such as public-access automatic external defibrillators (AEDs), have tended to blur the lines between BLS and ACLS. Each of the components involved in resuscitation will be reviewed separately, followed by a discussion of combining the elements for the best outcome.

AIRWAY MANAGEMENT

The problem of airway obstruction by the tongue in the unconscious patient is familiar to the anesthesiologist. The techniques used for airway maintenance during anesthesia are applicable to the cardiac arrest victim. The primary method recommended to the public is the same "head tilt–chin lift" method commonly employed in the operating room.[28] The head is extended by pressure applied to the brow while the mandible is pulled forward by pressure on the front of the jaw, lifting the tongue away from the posterior pharynx. The "jaw thrust" maneuver (applying pressure behind the rami of the mandible) is an effective alternative. Properly inserted oropha-ryngeal or nasopharyngeal airways can be useful before intubation, recognizing the danger of inducing vomiting or laryngospasm in the semiconscious victim. Tracheal intubation provides the best airway control, preventing aspiration and allowing the most effective ventilation. However, it should not be performed until adequate ventilation (preferably with supplemental oxygen) and chest compressions have been established. A number of alternative airways designed for blind placement have been described and the laryngeal mask airway and the esophageal-tracheal (see Chapter 29) Combitube have been recommended for use during cardiac arrest by individuals who are not skilled laryngoscopists.[29] When other methods of establishing an airway are unsuccessful, translaryngeal ventilation or tracheotomy by cricothyroid puncture may be necessary.

Foreign Body Airway Obstruction

In 2004, unintentional choking or suffocation accounted for 5,891 deaths in the United States (approximately 0.2% of all deaths) and 725 of the victims were <1 year old.[14] Airway occlusion by a foreign object must be considered in any victim who suddenly stops breathing and becomes cyanotic and unconscious. It occurs most commonly during eating and is usually due to food, especially meat, impacting in the laryngeal inlet, at the epiglottis or in the vallecula. Sudden death in restaurants from this cause is frequently mistaken for myocardial infarction, leading to the label "cafe coronary." Poorly chewed pieces of food, poor dentition or dentures, and elevated blood alcohol levels are the most common factors contributing to choking. The signs of total airway obstruction are the lack of air movement despite respiratory efforts and the inability of the victim to speak or cough. Cyanosis, unconsciousness, and cardiac arrest follow quickly. Partial airway obstruction will result in rasping or wheezing respirations accompanied by coughing. If the victim has good air movement and is able to cough forcefully, no intervention is indicated. However, if the cough weakens or cyanosis develops, the patient must be treated as if there were complete obstruction.

Mothers and friends have been pounding on the backs of choking victims for centuries. In 1974, Heimlich[30] proposed abdominal thrusts as a better method of relieving airway obstruction and, in 1976, Guildner et al.[31] reported that sternal thrusts were just as effective. Subsequently, there were multiple studies of these maneuvers. In clinical practice, Redding[32] observed that no maneuver was always successful and that each occasionally was successful when another had failed. To minimize confusion from teaching multiple techniques (especially to the lay public), the AHA has elected to emphasize the abdominal thrust maneuver (with chest thrusts as an alternative for the pregnant and massively obese).[29] This recommendation is made on the twofold premise that the abdominal thrust is at least as effective as other techniques and that teaching one method simplifies education.

For the awake victim, abdominal thrusts are applied in the erect position (sitting or standing). The rescuer reaches around the victim from behind, placing the fist of one hand in the epigastrium between the xiphoid and umbilicus. The fist is grasped with the other hand and pressed into the epigastrium with a quick upward thrust. In the unconscious, thrusts are applied by kneeling astride the victim, placing the heel of one hand in the epigastrium and the other on top of the first hand. Care must be taken to ensure the xiphoid is not pushed into the abdominal contents and that the thrust is in the midline. Sternal thrusts are valuable in the massively obese or in women in advanced pregnancy. In the erect victim, the chest is encircled from behind as in the abdominal maneuver but the

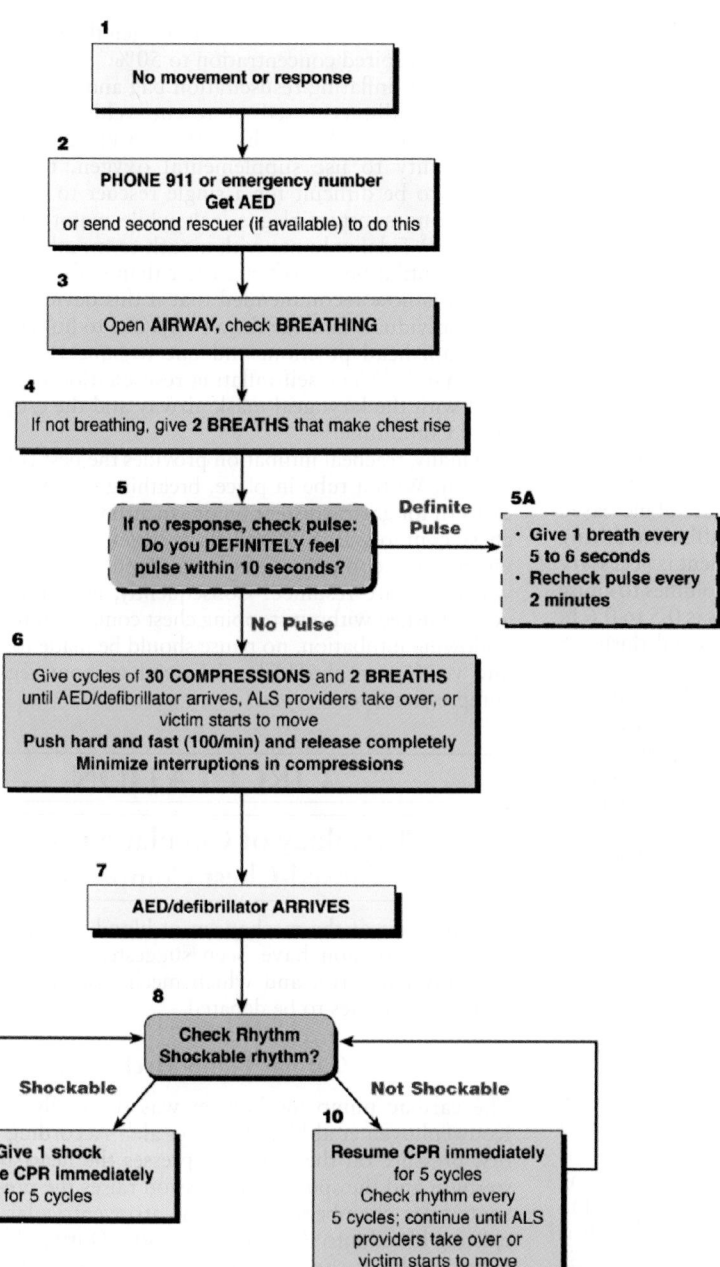

FIGURE 59-1. Adult basic life support (BLS) health care provider algorithm. AED, automatic external defibrillator; CPR, cardiopulmonary resuscitation; ALS, advanced life support. (From 2005 American Heart Association Guidelines for cardiopulmonary resuscitation and emergency cardiovascular care. Circulation 2005; 112(Suppl IV): IV, with permission.)

PERIOPERATIVE AND CONSULTATIVE SERVICES

fist is placed in the midsternum. For the unconscious, thrusts are applied from the side of the supine victim with a hand position the same as for external cardiac compression. Back blows are applied directly over the thoracic spine between the scapulae. They must be delivered with force. Placing the victim in a head-down position (e.g., leaning over a chair) may help move the obstruction into the pharynx.

Whatever technique is used, each individual maneuver must be delivered as if it will relieve the obstruction. If the first attempt is unsuccessful, repeated attempts should be made because hypoxia-related muscular relaxation may eventually allow success. Complications of thrust maneuvers include laceration of the liver and spleen, gastric rupture, fractured ribs, and regurgitation.

In the unconscious victim, manual dislodgement of the obstruction should be tried only if solid material can be seen obstructing the airway. The finger-sweep maneuver is done by inserting a finger along the buccal mucosa, attempting to dislodge the object laterally. If unsuccessful, grasping the object

under direct visualization with a Magill forceps or ordinary instrument (e.g., ice tongs) may be used. Care must be taken not to push the foreign body deeper into the larynx. Blind finger sweeps or grasping with instruments are rarely successful and may cause damage to tonsils or other tissue. Finally, if the object cannot be dislodged, a cricothyroidotomy can be lifesaving.

VENTILATION

The standard approach to the unresponsive victim is to follow opening the airway with ventilation (Fig. 59-1). When ventilation is provided in the rescue setting, mouth-to-mouth or mouth-to-nose ventilation is the most expeditious and effective method immediately available. Although inspired gas with this method will contain approximately 4% carbon dioxide and only approximately 17% oxygen (composition of exhaled air), it is sufficient to maintain viability.

Physiology of Ventilation During Cardiopulmonary Resuscitation

In the absence of an endotracheal tube, the distribution of gas between the lungs and stomach during mouth-to-mouth or mask ventilation will be determined by the relative impedance to flow into each (i.e., the opening pressure of the esophagus and the lung-thorax compliance). It is likely that esophageal opening pressure during cardiac arrest is no more than that found in anesthetized individuals (approximately 20 cm H_2O), and lung-thorax compliance is likely reduced. To avoid gastric insufflation, inspiratory airway pressures must be kept low.

Insufflation of air into the stomach during CPR leads to gastric distention, impeding ventilation and increasing the risk of regurgitation and gastric rupture. Avoiding gastric insufflation requires that peak inspiratory airway pressures stay below esophageal opening pressure. Partial airway obstruction by the tongue and pharyngeal tissues is a major cause of increased airway pressure contributing to gastric insufflation during CPR. Meticulous attention to airway management is necessary during rescue breathing. Recommended tidal volumes to cause a noticeable rise in the chest wall in most adults is 0.5 to 0.6 L. Each rescue breath should be given over 1 second during a pause in chest compressions.

A useful adjunct for preventing gastric insufflation during positive-pressure ventilation without an endotracheal tube is cricoid pressure (Sellick maneuver).[33] Properly applied pressure to the anterior arch of the cricoid causes the cricoid lamina to seal the esophagus and can prevent air from entering the stomach at airway pressures up to 100 cm H_2O.[34] Pressure on the thyroid cartilage is useless. Cricoid pressure should be used during rescue breathing without an endotracheal tube, but this inevitably involves the need for an additional rescuer.

Techniques of Rescue Breathing

While maintaining an open airway with the head tilt–jaw lift technique, the hand on the forehead pinches the nose, the rescuer takes a normal breath and seals the victim's mouth with the lips and exhales, watching for the chest to rise, indicating effective ventilation. For exhalation, the rescuer's mouth is removed from the victim, and the rescuer listens for escaping air while taking a breath. When both hands are being used in the jaw thrust maneuver of opening the airway, the cheek is used to seal the nose. For mouth-to-nose ventilation, the rescuer's lips surround the nose and the victim's lips are held closed. In some patients, the mouth must be allowed to open for exhalation with this technique. Give one breath over 1 second, take a normal breath, and give a second breath over one second. During CPR in adults and one-rescuer CPR in children, a pause for two breaths should be made after each 30 chest compressions. When there are two rescuers with a child victim, a pause for two breaths should be made after each 15 compressions.[29]

Several adjuncts to ventilation are available. An oropharyngeal airway with mouthguard and external extension mouthpiece has been used, but obtaining a good mouth seal is often difficult. Perhaps the most useful adjunct is a common mask, such as that used for anesthesia. The mask can be applied to the face and held in place with the thumbs and index fingers while the other fingers are used to apply jaw thrust. Breathing into the connector port of the mask provides ventilation. Mouth-to-mask ventilation may be more aesthetic than mouth-to-mouth ventilation and can be just as effective in trained hands. Masks are also available with one-way valves that direct the victim's exhaled gas away from the rescuer. Masks with integral nipple adapters are useful for pro-

viding supplemental oxygen. An oxygen flow of 10 L/min can raise the inspired concentration to 50%.

The self-inflating resuscitation bag and mask are the most common adjuncts used in rescue vehicles and hospitals. Although these devices have the advantages of noncontact and ability to use supplemental oxygen, they have been shown to be difficult for a single rescuer to apply properly, preventing substantial gas leak while maintaining a patent airway.[35] Tidal volumes with mouth-to-mouth and mouth-to-mask ventilation are often greater than with the resuscitation bag. It is now recommended that if this device is to be used, two individuals manage the airway: one to hold the mask and maintain head position, and one to squeeze the bag using both hands.[36] The self-inflating resuscitation bag can also be used with the laryngeal mask airway and the esophageal-tracheal Combitube.

Finally, tracheal intubation provides the best control of ventilation. With a tube in place, breathing can proceed without concern for gastric distention or synchronizing ventilation with chest compressions. Blood flow during CPR slows rapidly when chest compressions are stopped and recovers slowly when they are resumed. Consequently, intubation should be accomplished without stopping chest compressions, if possible. Following intubation, no pause should be made for ventilation and ventilation should be delivered without regard for the compression cycle.

CIRCULATION

Physiology of Circulation During Closed-Chest Compression

4 Two theories of the mechanism of blood flow during closed-chest compression have been suggested.[12,37] They are not mutually exclusive, and which mechanism predominates in humans continues to be debated.

Cardiac Pump Mechanism

The cardiac pump mechanism was originally proposed by Kouwenhoven et al.[12] and Jude et al.[38] According to this theory, pressure on the chest compresses the heart between the sternum and the spine. Compression raises the pressure in the ventricular chambers, closing the atrioventricular valves and ejecting blood into the lungs and aorta. During the relaxation phase of closed-chest compression, expansion of the thoracic cage causes a subatmospheric intrathoracic pressure, facilitating blood return. The mitral and tricuspid valves open, allowing blood to fill the ventricles. Pressure in the aorta causes aortic valve closure and coronary artery perfusion.

Thoracic Pump Mechanism

In 1976, Criley et al.[39] reported a patient undergoing cardiac catheterization who simultaneously developed VF and an episode of cough-hiccups. With every cough-hiccup, a significant arterial pressure was noted. This observation of self-administered "cough CPR" prompted further investigations on the mechanism of blood flow, and these studies produced the theory of a thoracic pump mechanism for blood flow during closed-chest compressions.[37] According to this theory, blood flows into the thorax during the relaxation phase of chest compressions in the same manner as that described for the cardiac pump mechanism. During the compression phase, all intrathoracic structures are compressed equally by the rise in intrathoracic pressure caused by sternal depression, forcing blood out of the chest. Backward flow through the venous system is prevented by valves in the subclavian and internal jugular veins, and by dynamic compression of the veins at the thoracic outlet by the increased intrathoracic pressure. Thicker, less compressible vessel walls prevent collapse on the arterial side, although arterial collapse will occur if intrathoracic pressure is raised enough.[40] The heart is a passive conduit with the atrioventricular valves remaining open during chest compression. Because there is a significant pressure difference between the carotid artery and jugular vein, blood flow to the head is favored. The lack of valves in the inferior vena cava results in less resistance to backward flow, and pressures in the arteries and veins below the diaphragm are nearly equal. This is consistent with the fact that there is little blood flow to organs below the diaphragm.[41,42]

It seems clear that fluctuations in intrathoracic pressure plays a significant role in blood flow during CPR. It is also likely that compression of the heart occurs under some circumstances. Factors that influence the mechanism probably include the compliance and configuration of the chest wall, size of the heart, force of the sternal compressions, duration of cardiac arrest, and other undiscovered factors. Which mechanism predominates varies from victim to victim and even during the resuscitation of the same victim.

Distribution of Blood Flow During Cardiopulmonary Resuscitation

Whatever the predominant mechanism, total body blood flow (cardiac output) is reduced to 10 to 33% of normal during experimental closed-chest cardiac massage. Similar severe reductions in flow are likely during clinical CPR in humans. Nearly all the blood flow is directed to organs above the diaphragm.[41,42] Myocardial perfusion is 20 to 50% of normal, whereas cerebral perfusion is maintained at 50 to 90% of normal. Abdominal visceral and lower extremity flow is reduced to 5% of normal. Total flow tends to decrease with time during CPR, but the relative distribution is not altered. Changes in CPR technique and the use of epinephrine may help sustain cardiac output over time.[42] Epinephrine improves flow to the brain and heart, whereas flow to organs below the diaphragm is unchanged or further reduced.

Gas Transport During Cardiopulmonary Resuscitation

During the low flow state of CPR, excretion of carbon dioxide (CO_2) (milliliters of CO_2 per minute in exhaled gas) is decreased from prearrest levels to approximately the same extent as cardiac output is reduced. This reduced CO_2 excretion is due primarily to shunting of blood flow away from the lower half of the body. The exhaled CO_2 reflects only the metabolism of the part of the body that is being perfused. In the nonperfused areas, CO_2 accumulates during CPR. When normal circulation is restored, the accumulated CO_2 is washed out, and a temporary increase in CO_2 excretion is seen.

Although CO_2 excretion is reduced during CPR, measurement of blood gases reveals an arterial respiratory alkalosis and a venous respiratory acidosis with a markedly elevated arteriovenous CO_2 difference.[43] The primary cause of these changes is the severely reduced cardiac output. Two factors account for the elevation of the venous partial pressure of CO_2 ($PvCO_2$). Buffering acid causes a reduction in serum bicarbonate so the same blood CO_2 content results in a higher $PvCO_2$. In addition, the mixed venous CO_2 content is elevated. When flow to a tissue is reduced, all the CO_2 produced fails to be removed and CO_2 accumulates, raising the tissue partial pressure of CO_2. This allows more CO_2 to be carried in each aliquot of blood and mixed venous CO_2 content increases. If flow remains constant, a new equilibrium is established in which all CO_2 produced in the tissue is

removed but at a higher venous CO_2 content and partial pressure. In contrast to the venous blood, arterial CO_2 content and partial pressure ($PaCO_2$) are usually reduced during CPR. This reduction accounts for most of the observed increase in arteriovenous CO_2 content difference. Even though venous blood may have an increased CO_2, the marked reduction in cardiac output with maintained ventilation results in efficient CO_2 removal.

Decreased pulmonary blood flow during CPR causes lack of perfusion to many nondependent alveoli. The alveolar gas of these lung units has no CO_2. Consequently, mixed alveolar CO_2 (i.e., end-tidal CO_2) will be low and correlate poorly with arterial CO_2. However, end-tidal CO_2 does correlate well with cardiac output during CPR. As flow increases, more alveoli become perfused, there is less alveolar dead space, and end-tidal CO_2 measurements rise.

Technique of Closed-Chest Compression

In an unconscious apneic patient, cardiac arrest must be assumed in the absence of a pulse in a major artery (carotid, femoral, axillary). Because a systolic pressure of approximately 50 mm Hg is necessary for a palpable pulse, some circulation may remain in the "pulseless" patient with primary respiratory arrest. Opening the airway and ventilation may be sufficient for resuscitation in such circumstances. Therefore, further search for a pulse should always be made following artificial ventilation and before beginning sternal compressions. Witnessed sudden collapse with unresponsiveness in an adult in the absence of seizure activity is nearly always dysrhythmic cardiac arrest and chest compressions should be started immediately.

Important considerations in performing closed-chest compressions are the position of the rescuer relative to the victim, the position of the rescuer's hands, and the rate and force of compression. The victim must be supine, the head level with the heart, for adequate brain perfusion. The victim must be on a firm surface. The rescuer should stand or kneel next to the victim's side. Compressions are performed most effectively if the rescuer's hips are on the same level, or slightly above the level of, the victim's chest.

Standard technique consists of the rhythmic application of pressure over the lower half of the sternum. The heel of one hand is placed on the lower sternum, and the other hand is placed on top of the first one. Great care must be taken to avoid pressing the xiphoid into the abdomen, which can lacerate the liver. Even with properly performed CPR, costochondral separation and rib fractures are common. Applying pressure on the ribs by improper hand placement increases these complications and risks puncturing the lung. Pressure on the sternum should be applied through the heel of the hand only, keeping the fingers free of the chest wall. The direction of force must be straight down on the sternum, with the arms straight and the elbows locked into position so the entire weight of the upper body is used to apply force. During relaxation, all pressure should be removed from the hands allowing the chest wall to recoil completely, but the hands should not lose contact with the chest wall.

The sternum must be depressed 4 to 5 cm in the average adult. Occasionally, deeper compressions are necessary to generate a palpable pulse. The duration of compression should be equal to that of relaxation, and the compression rate should be 100 times per minute. Push hard and push fast, minimizing interruptions in chest compressions. Allow a brief pause for two 1-second breaths after every 30 compressions. With an advanced airway in place, ventilations at a rate of 8 to 10 breaths per minute should be interposed between compressions without a pause.

Alternative Methods of Circulatory Support

6 As currently practiced, CPR has limited success, with only approximately 40% of victims being admitted to the hospital and 10% surviving to discharge. Despite the occasional success of prolonged resuscitation, standard CPR will sustain most patients for only 15 to 30 minutes. If return of spontaneous circulation has not been achieved in that time, the outcome is dismal. Recognition of these limits and improved understanding of circulatory physiology during CPR have led to several proposals for alternatives to the standard techniques of closed-chest compression. Most, but not all, are based on the thoracic pump mechanism of blood flow. The goals of the new methods are to provide better hemodynamics during CPR and thus improve survival and/or to extend the duration during which CPR can successfully support viability. Unfortunately, none of the alternatives has proved reliably superior to the standard technique.

Simultaneous Ventilation–Compression Cardiopulmonary Resuscitation and Abdominal Binding

According to the thoracic pump theory, elevation of intrathoracic pressure during chest compression should improve blood flow and pressure.[40] Initial studies with techniques that raise intrathoracic pressure (abdominal binding, simultaneous ventilation/compression) were encouraging because the increased aortic pressure suggested better myocardial and cerebral perfusion. Subsequent investigations demonstrated that right atrial pressure and intracranial pressure are elevated as much as, or more than, the arterial pressures. Thus, no improvement in myocardial or cerebral blood flow is found. Most important, survival from cardiac arrest is not improved when these techniques are compared with standard CPR in experimental animals or limited human trials.[44–46]

Interposed Abdominal Compression Cardiopulmonary Resuscitation

Interposed abdominal compression (IAC) is fundamentally different from abdominal binding. With this technique, an additional rescuer applies abdominal compressions manually during the relaxation phase of chest compression.[47] Abdominal pressure is released when chest compression begins. One large randomized trial of out-of-hospital cardiac arrest with IAC CPR found no improvement in survival compared with standard CPR,[48] but a subsequent in-hospital study demonstrated improved outcome.[49] The safety of IAC CPR has been established and is recommended as an alternative to standard CPR for in-hospital resuscitation. Further studies will be needed to establish out-of-hospital efficacy.

Load-Distributing Band Cardiopulmonary Resuscitation or Pneumatic Vest Cardiopulmonary Resuscitation

Following the description of "cough CPR" and the development of the thoracic pump theory, a pneumatic vest device was developed that would simulate the events of vigorous coughing.[50] The technique continues to be investigated with a number of modifications from the original method. Most active investigations use a circumferential chest-compression device composed of a pneumatically or electronically actuated constricting band and backboard. In a preliminary clinical study, aortic and coronary perfusion pressure was better with load-distributing band CPR than with standard CPR.[51] Additional studies are ongoing.

Active Compression–Decompression Cardiopulmonary Resuscitation

The newest proposed alternative technique developed from the anecdotal report of CPR performed with a plumber's helper applied to the anterior chest wall.[52] This suggested that active decompression of the chest wall might reduce intrathoracic pressure during the relaxation phase of chest compressions, leading to improved venous return, increased stroke volume with compression, and better blood flow. A suction device that can be applied to the chest wall to enable active compression and decompression was developed.[53] Hemodynamic studies in animals and humans with this technique have shown that coronary and cerebral perfusion may be somewhat improved with this method compared with standard CPR, although when epinephrine is used there is no difference between techniques.[53,54] Clinical trials of this technique have had mixed results, with four studies showing improved outcome and five showing no positive or negative effects. No survival benefit of active compression-decompression CPR over standard CPR was found in a meta-analysis of 10 trials involving 4,162 patients in the out-of-hospital setting and in a meta-analysis of 2 trials involving 826 patients in the in-hospital setting.[55]

Impedance Threshold Device

The impedance threshold device (ITD) is a valve that impedes air entry into the lungs during chest recoil of the relaxation phase of chest compressions, thus reducing intrathoracic pressure and increasing venous return to the thorax. Originally designed to be used with a cuffed endotracheal tube and active compression-decompression CPR (during which it would act to further increase the venous return of active decompression),[56] it has recently been used with conventional CPR and tight-fitting face mask.[57] Randomized trials of out-of-hospital cardiac arrest comparing conventional CPR and the ITD with and without active compression-decompression CPR have shown improvement in short-term resuscitation.[56,58] Although improved long-term survival has not been demonstrated, the ITD may be a useful adjunct for professionals trained in its use.

Invasive Techniques

In contrast to the closed-chest techniques, two invasive methods have been able to maintain cardiac and cerebral viability during long periods of cardiac arrest. In animal models, open-chest cardiac massage and cardiopulmonary bypass (through the femoral artery and vein using a membrane oxygenator) can provide better hemodynamics, as well as better myocardial and cerebral perfusion, than closed-chest techniques.[59] Prompt restoration of blood flow and perfusion pressure with cardiopulmonary bypass can provide resuscitation with minimal neurologic deficit after 20 minutes of fibrillatory cardiac arrest in canines.[15] However, these techniques must be instituted relatively early (probably within 20 to 30 minutes of arrest) to be effective.[16,60] If open-chest massage is begun after 30 minutes of ineffective closed-chest compressions, survival is no better even though hemodynamics are improved.[61] The need to apply these maneuvers early in an arrest obviously limits the application. Before invasive procedures play a greater role in modern CPR, a method must be developed to predict, early in resuscitation, which patients will and will not respond to closed-chest compressions.

Assessing the Adequacy of Circulation During Cardiopulmonary Resuscitation

7 The adequacy of closed-chest compression is usually judged by palpation of a pulse in the carotid or femoral vessels. The

TABLE 59-1

CRITICAL VARIABLES ASSOCIATED WITH
SUCCESSFUL RESUSCITATION

■ VARIABLE	■ AMOUNT
Myocardial blood flow (mL/min/100 g)	>15–20
Aortic diastolic pressure (mm Hg)	>40
Coronary perfusion pressure (mm Hg)	>15–25
End-tidal carbon dioxide (mm Hg)	>10

palpable pulse primarily reflects systolic pressure. Cardiac output correlates better with mean pressure and coronary perfusion with diastolic pressure. In the femoral area, the palpable pulse is as likely to be venous as arterial. Despite these shortcomings, palpating the pulse remains the only monitor available during BLS.

Return of spontaneous circulation with an arrested heart greatly depends on restoring oxygenated blood flow to the myocardium. In experimental models, a minimum blood flow of 15 to 20 mL/min/100 g of myocardium has been shown to be necessary for successful resuscitation.[62] Obtaining such flow depends on closed-chest compressions developing adequate cardiac output and coronary perfusion pressure. Similar to the beating heart, coronary perfusion during CPR occurs primarily in the relaxation phase (diastole) of chest compressions. In 1906, Crile and Dolley[63] suggested that a critical coronary perfusion pressure was necessary for successful resuscitation. This concept has been confirmed in numerous other reports.[42,62–72] During standard CPR, critical myocardial blood flow is associated with aortic diastolic pressure exceeding 40 mm Hg. Because right atrial pressure can be elevated with some techniques, the aortic diastolic pressure minus the right atrial diastolic pressure is a more accurate reflection of coronary perfusion pressure. The critical coronary perfusion pressure is 15 to 25 mm Hg. When invasive monitoring is available during CPR, adjustments in chest compression technique and epinephrine should be used to ensure critical perfusion pressures are exceeded. Damage to the myocardium from underlying disease may preclude survival no matter how effective the CPR efforts. However, vascular pressures below critical levels are associated with poor results even in patients who may be salvageable (Table 59-1).

Although invasive pressure monitoring may be ideal, it is **8** rarely available during CPR. End-tidal CO_2 also has been found to be an excellent noninvasive guide to the adequacy of closed-chest compressions.[73] Carbon dioxide excretion during CPR with an endotracheal tube in place is flow-

dependent rather than ventilation-dependent. Because alveolar dead space is large in low-flow states, end-tidal CO_2 is very low (frequently <10 mm Hg). If blood flow improves with better CPR technique, more alveoli are perfused and end-tidal CO_2 rises (usually to >20 mm Hg with successful CPR). The earliest sign of return of spontaneous circulation is frequently a sudden increase in end-tidal CO_2 to >40 mm Hg. Within a wide range of cardiac outputs during CPR, end-tidal CO_2 correlates well with cardiac output,[74] coronary perfusion pressure,[75] and initial resuscitation.[76] End-tidal CO_2 correlates with survival in human CPR and can predict outcome.[77,78] Patients with end-tidal CO_2 <10 mm Hg will not be resuscitated successfully. In the absence of invasive monitoring, end-tidal CO_2 should be used to judge the effectiveness of chest compressions, whenever possible.[79] Attempts should be made to maximize the measured end-tidal CO_2 by alterations in technique or drug therapy. It should be remembered that sodium bicarbonate administration liberates CO_2 into the blood and causes a temporary increase in end-tidal CO_2. The elevation returns to baseline within 3 to 5 minutes of drug administration and end-tidal CO_2 monitoring can again be used for monitoring effectiveness of closed-chest compressions.

PHARMACOLOGIC THERAPY

This discussion of drug therapy is confined to the use of drugs during CPR attempts to restore spontaneous circulation. The use of drugs to support the circulation when there is mechanical cardiac function is discussed elsewhere (see Chapter 15 and 42). During cardiac arrest, drug therapy is secondary to other **9** interventions. Effective uninterrupted chest compressions and defibrillation, if appropriate, should take precedence over medications. Establishing intravenous access and pharmacologic therapy should come as soon as possible but after these critical interventions are established. Although vasopressors are firmly established as improving survival in animal models, there is no strong evidence that they improve survival in human cardiac arrest.[80] The most common drugs and the appropriate adult doses are shown in Table 59-2. The standard AHA algorithm for management of pulseless arrest is shown in Figure 59-2. In addition, the algorithms for the AHA protocols for bradycardia and tachycardia are included (Figs. 59-3 and 59-4).

Routes of Administration

The preferred route of administration of all drugs during CPR is intravenous. The most rapid and highest drug levels occur with administration into a central vein. However, peripheral

TABLE 59-2

ADULT ADVANCED CARDIAC LIFE SUPPORT DRUGS AND DOSES (INTRAVENOUS)

	■ DOSE	■ INTERVAL	■ MAXIMUM
Epinephrine	1 mg	Every 3–5 min	None
If dose fails, consider	3–7 mg	Every 3–5 min	None
Vasopressin	40 units	May replace 1st or 2nd dose of epinephrine	—
Amiodarone	300 mg	Repeat 150 mg in 5 min	2 g
Lidocaine	1–1.5 mg/kg	Repeat 0.5–0.75 mg/kg in 5 min	3.0 mg/kg
Atropine	1 mg	Every 3–5 min	0.04 mg/kg
Sodium bicarbonate	1 mEq/kg	As needed	Check pH

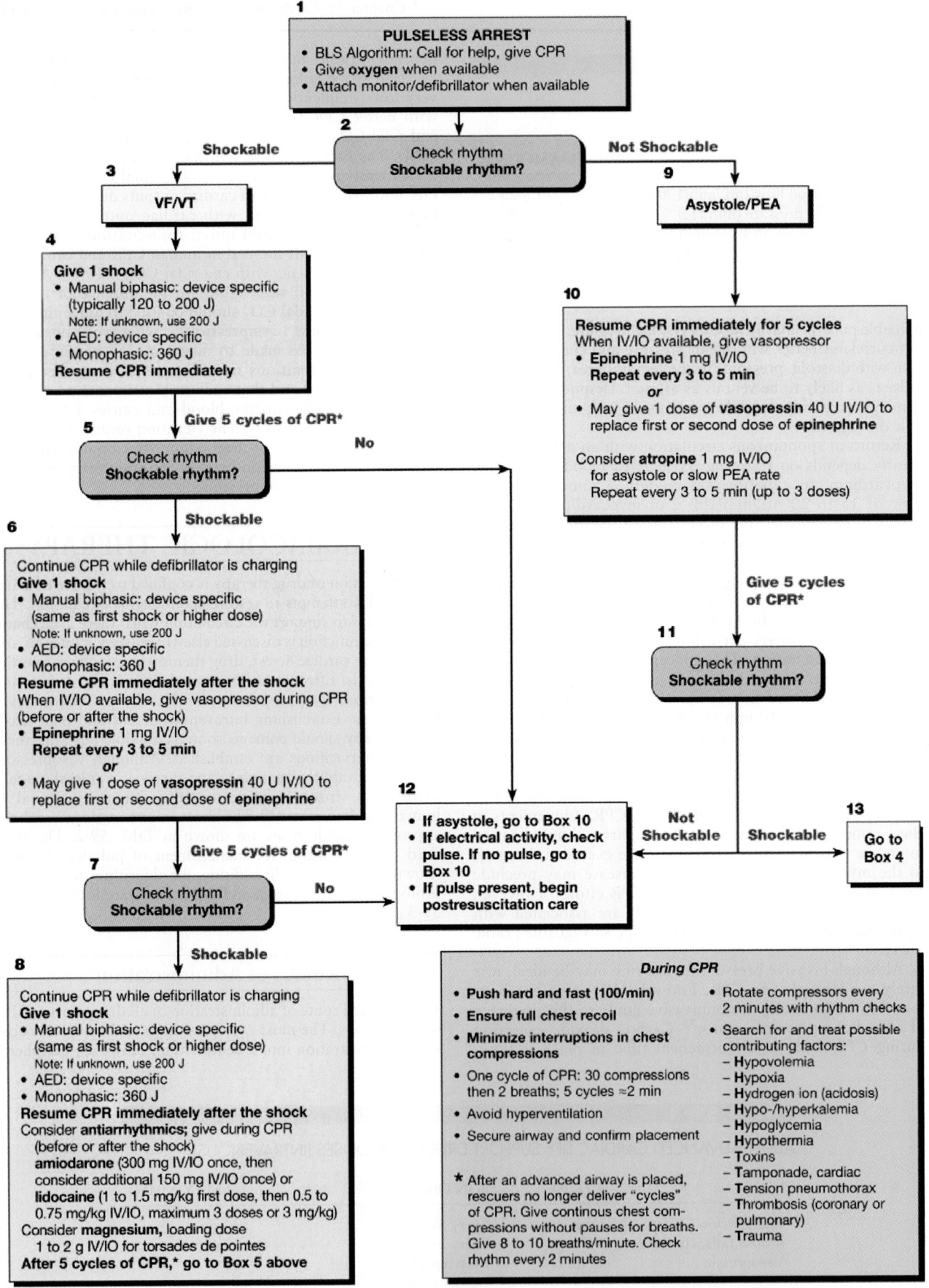

FIGURE 59-2. Adult advanced cardiac life support pulseless arrest algorithm. BLS, basic life support; CPR, cardiopulmonary resuscitation; VF, ventricular fibrillation; VT, ventricular tachycardia; PEA, pulseless electrical activity; AED, automatic external defibrillator; IV, intravenous(ly); IO, intraosseous(ly). (From 2005 American Heart Association Guidelines for cardiopulmonary resuscitation and emergency cardiovascular care. Circulation 2005; 112(Suppl IV): IV, with permission.)

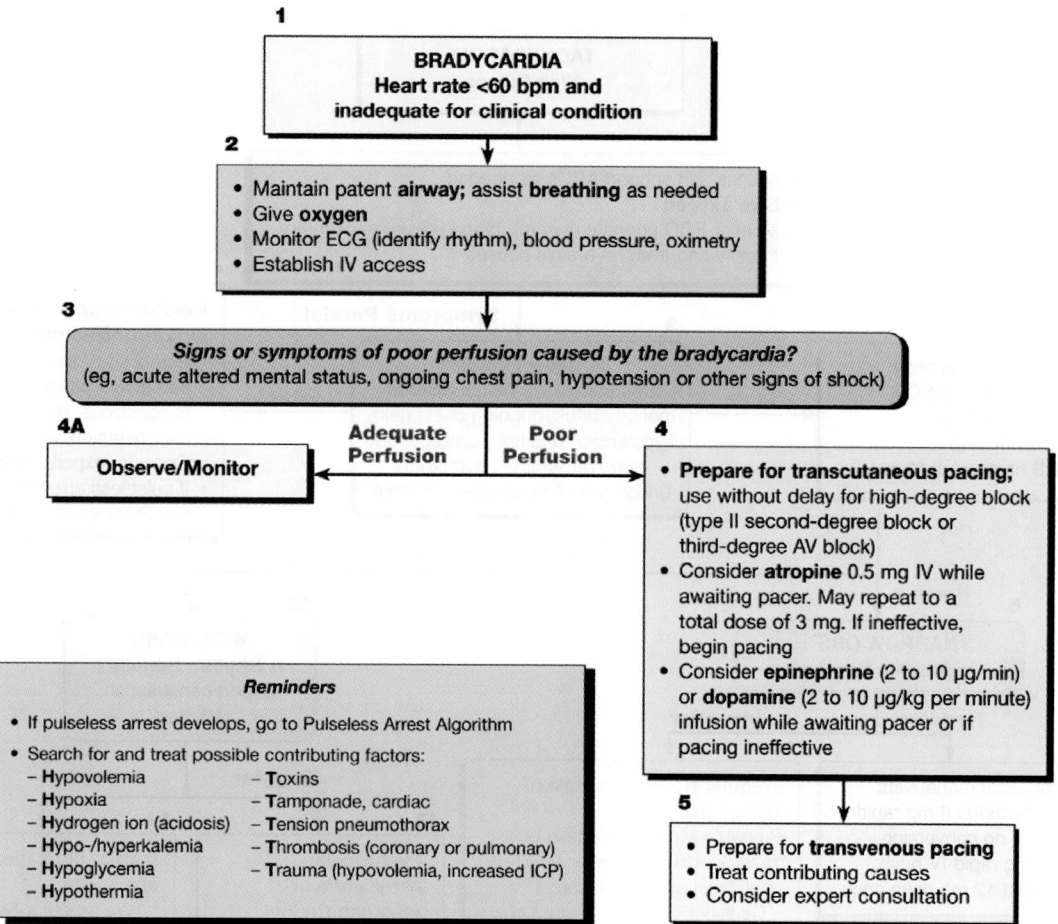

1

BRADYCARDIA
Heart rate <60 bpm and
inadequate for clinical condition

2
- Maintain patent **airway**; assist **breathing** as needed
- Give **oxygen**
- Monitor ECG (identify rhythm), blood pressure, oximetry
- Establish IV access

3
Signs or symptoms of poor perfusion caused by the bradycardia?
(eg, acute altered mental status, ongoing chest pain, hypotension or other signs of shock)

4A   Adequate Perfusion   Poor Perfusion   **4**

Observe/Monitor

- **Prepare for transcutaneous pacing;** use without delay for high-degree block (type II second-degree block or third-degree AV block)
- Consider **atropine** 0.5 mg IV while awaiting pacer. May repeat to a total dose of 3 mg. If ineffective, begin pacing
- Consider **epinephrine** (2 to 10 µg/min) or **dopamine** (2 to 10 µg/kg per minute) infusion while awaiting pacer or if pacing ineffective

5
- Prepare for **transvenous pacing**
- Treat contributing causes
- Consider expert consultation

Reminders
- If pulseless arrest develops, go to Pulseless Arrest Algorithm
- Search for and treat possible contributing factors:
  - Hypovolemia
  - Hypoxia
  - Hydrogen ion (acidosis)
  - Hypo-/hyperkalemia
  - Hypoglycemia
  - Hypothermia
  - Toxins
  - Tamponade, cardiac
  - Tension pneumothorax
  - Thrombosis (coronary or pulmonary)
  - Trauma (hypovolemia, increased ICP)

FIGURE 59-3.   Adult bradycardia algorithm. ECG, electrocardiogram; IV, intravenous(ly); AV, atrioventricular. (From 2005 American Heart Association Guidelines for cardiopulmonary resuscitation and emergency cardiovascular care. Circulation 2005; 112(Suppl IV): IV, with permission.)

intravenous administration is also effective. The antecubital and external jugular veins are the sites of first choice for starting an infusion during resuscitation because inserting a central catheter usually necessitates stopping CPR. Because of poor blood flow below the diaphragm during CPR, drugs administered in the lower extremity may be extremely delayed or may not reach the sites of action. Even in the upper extremity, drugs may require 1 to 2 minutes to reach the central circulation. Onset of action may be speeded if the drug bolus is followed by a 20- to 30-mL bolus of intravenous fluid. Intraosseous administration of fluids and medications is a good alternative to intravenous cannulation, allowing drug delivery similar to that of central venous administration. Commercial kits are available to facilitate intraosseous placement.

If intravenous access cannot be established, the endotracheal tube is an alternative route for administration of epinephrine, lidocaine, and atropine. (Sodium bicarbonate should not be given endotracheally.) The time to effect and drug levels achieved are inconsistent using this route during CPR, so the optimal dose of drug is unknown using this route. Better results may be obtained by administering 5- to 10-mL volumes. It is unclear whether deep injection is better than simple instillation into the endotracheal tube. In general, doses 2 to 2.5 times higher than the recommended intravenous dose should be administered when this route is used.

Catecholamines and Vasopressors

Mechanism of Action

Epinephrine has been used in resuscitation since the 1890s and has been the vasopressor of choice in modern CPR since the studies of Redding and Pearson[13,81] in the 1960s. The efficacy of epinephrine lies entirely in its α-adrenergic properties[69] (see Chapter 15). Peripheral vasoconstriction leads to an increase in aortic diastolic pressure, causing an increase in coronary perfusion pressure and myocardial blood flow.[42,82,83] All strong α-adrenergic drugs (epinephrine, phenylephrine, methoxamine, dopamine, norepinephrine), regardless of β-adrenergic potency, are equally successful in aiding resuscitation, as are strong nonadrenergic vasopressors (vasopressin, endothelin-1).[13,81,84,85] β-Adrenergic agonists without α activity (isoproterenol, dobutamine) are no better than placebo. α-Adrenergic blockade precludes resuscitation, whereas β-adrenergic blockade has no effect on the ability to restore spontaneous circulation.[66,67]

The β-adrenergic effects of epinephrine are potentially deleterious during cardiac arrest. In the fibrillating heart, epinephrine increases oxygen consumption and decreases the endocardial–epicardial blood flow ratio, an effect not seen with methoxamine. Myocardial lactate production in the fibrillating heart is unchanged after epinephrine administration during CPR, suggesting that the increased coronary blood flow does

PERIOPERATIVE AND CONSULTATIVE SERVICES

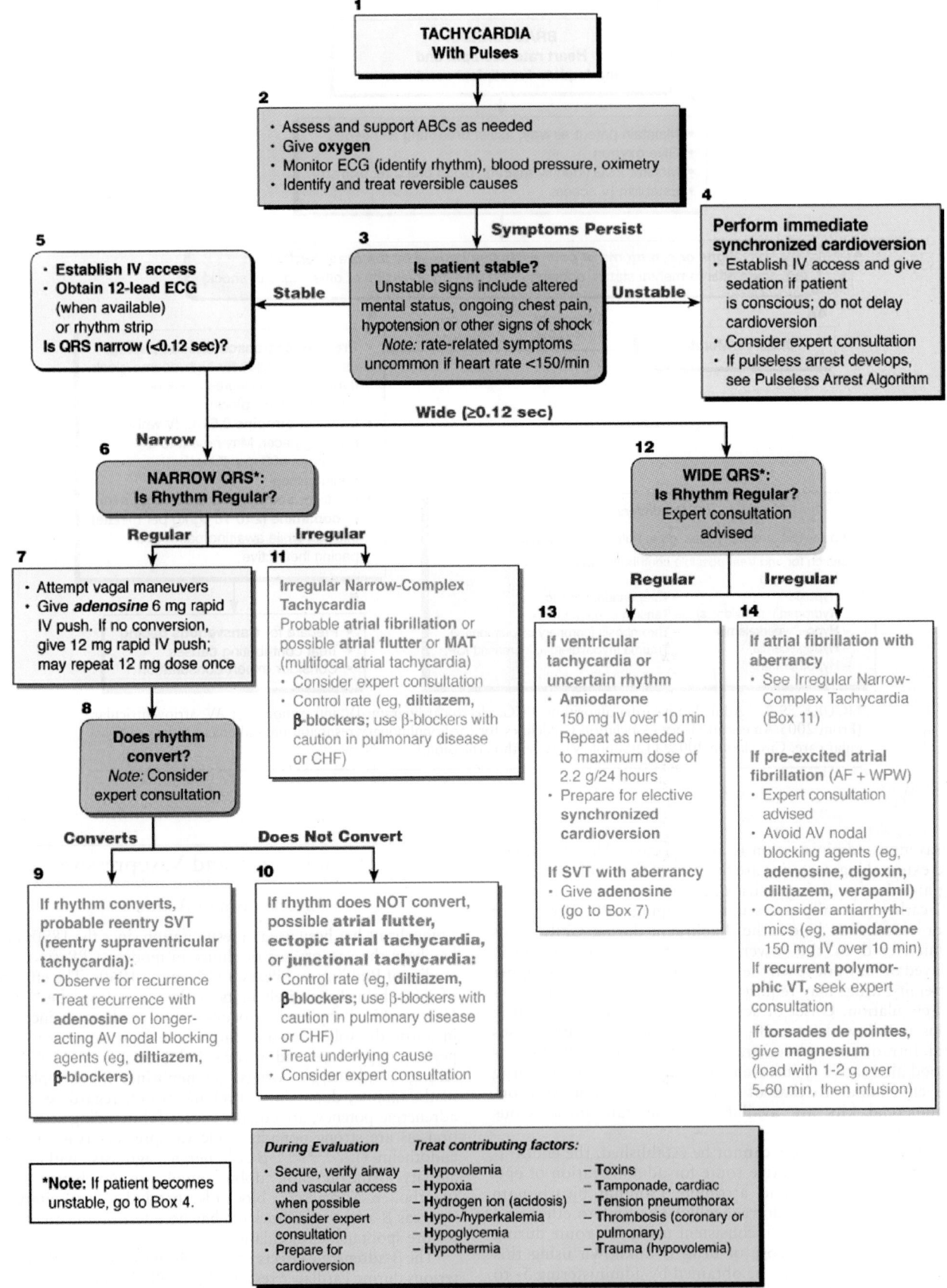

FIGURE 59-4.   Adult advanced cardiac life support tachycardia algorithm. ABCs, airway, breathing, and circulation; ECG, electrocardiogram; IV, intravenous(ly); CHF, congestive heart failure; SVT, supraventricular tachycardia. (From 2005 American Heart Association Guidelines for cardiopulmonary resuscitation and emergency cardiovascular care. Circulation 2005; 112(Suppl IV): IV, with permission.)

not improve the oxygen supply–demand ratio. Large doses of epinephrine increase deaths in swine early after resuscitation because of tachyarrhythmias and hypertension, an effect partially offset by metoprolol treatment. Despite these theoretical considerations, survival and neurologic outcome studies have shown no difference when epinephrine is compared with a pure α-agonist (methoxamine or phenylephrine) during CPR in animals[81,86] or humans.[87]

Epinephrine

When added to chest compressions, epinephrine helps develop the critical coronary perfusion pressure necessary to provide enough myocardial blood flow for restoration of spontaneous circulation. With invasive monitoring present during CPR, an arterial diastolic pressure of 40 mm Hg or coronary perfusion pressure of 20 mm Hg must be obtained with good chest-compression technique and/or epinephrine therapy (Table 59-1). In the absence of such monitoring, the dose of epinephrine must be chosen empirically. Since the studies of Redding and Pearson[13,81] in the 1960s, the standard intravenous dose used has been 0.5 to 1.0 mg. In the 1980s, animal studies suggested that higher doses of epinephrine in human CPR might improve myocardial and cerebral perfusion, and improve success of resuscitation. Case reports and a series of children with historical controls were published of return of spontaneous circulation when large doses (0.1 to 0.2 mg/kg) of epinephrine were given to patients who had failed resuscitation with standard doses.

Subsequent outcome studies have not demonstrated conclusively that higher doses of epinephrine will improve survival. Eight adult prospective randomized clinical trials involving >9,000 cardiac arrest patients have found no improvement in survival to hospital discharge or neurologic outcome, even in subgroups, when initial high-dose epinephrine (5 to 18 mg) is compared with standard doses (1 to 2 mg).[88–95] Some of the studies (and the cumulative data) suggest that there may be an improvement in immediate resuscitation with high-dose epinephrine. None of the studies found improvement in survival to hospital discharge. Retrospective studies of epinephrine dosing have suggested that higher doses may be associated with impaired postresuscitation cardiovascular function and worse neurologic outcome.[96,97] None of the prospective studies found lower survival or worse neurologic outcome with higher epinephrine dosing.

It should be noted that these outcome studies used high-dose epinephrine as initial therapy. High doses apparently are not needed early in most cardiac arrests and could be deleterious under some circumstances. The successful case reports were in patients who had failed conventional treatment. The high doses were given late in prolonged CPR when the vasculature may not be as responsive to catecholamines. Although the use of high-dose epinephrine as rescue therapy when standard doses have failed has not been rigorously studied, this may be its appropriate place in CPR practice. Current recommendations are to give 1 mg intravenously every 3 to 5 minutes in the adult. If this dose seems ineffective or to treat beta-blocker or calcium channel blocker overdose, higher doses (3 to 8 mg) may be considered.

Vasopressin

Arginine vasopressin is currently recommended as an alternative to either the first or second dose epinephrine in a dose of 40 units intravenous/intraosseous (see Chapter 15). Vasopressin is a naturally occurring hormone (antidiuretic hormone) that, when administered in high doses, is a potent non-adrenergic vasoconstrictor, acting by stimulation of smooth muscle V_1 receptors. It is usually not recommended for con-

scious patients with coronary artery disease because the increased peripheral vascular resistance may provoke angina. The half-life in the intact circulation is 10 to 20 minutes and longer than epinephrine during CPR. Animal studies have demonstrated that vasopressin is as effective as or more effective than epinephrine in maintaining vital organ blood flow during CPR. Repeated doses during prolonged CPR in swine were associated with significantly improved rates of neurologically intact survival compared with epinephrine and placebo. Postresuscitation myocardial depression and splanchnic blood flow reduction are more marked with vasopressin than epinephrine, but they are transient and can be treated with low doses of dopamine.[98] Clinical studies indicate that vasopressin is as effective as epinephrine, but have not definitively shown it to be superior. A small randomized, blinded study comparing vasopressin and standard-dose epinephrine in 40 patients with out-of-hospital VF found improved 24-hour survival with vasopressin, but no difference in return of spontaneous circulation or survival to hospital discharge.[99] A larger, clinical trial of 200 inpatients found no difference between the drugs in survival for 1 hour or to hospital discharge.[100] In this study, response times were short, indicating that CPR outcome achieved with both vasopressin and epinephrine in short-term cardiac arrest may be comparable. The hemodynamic effects of vasopressin, compared with epinephrine, are especially impressive during long cardiac arrests. Thus, vasopressin may find most use in CPR during prolonged duration resuscitation. A multicenter, randomized study of 1,186 patients comparing vasopressin 40 U and epinephrine 1 mg for the first two doses of vasopressor during resuscitation from out-of-hospital cardiac arrest found no overall difference in survival to hospital admission (36 vs. 31%) or discharge (10 vs. 10%).[101] However, in subgroup analysis, in patients presenting in asystole, there was a significant improvement in survival to hospital admission (29 vs. 20%) and discharge (4.7 vs. 1.5%). In those patients who did not resuscitate following two doses of study drug, approximately 60% received additional epinephrine. In these difficult-to-resuscitate patients, irrespective of presenting rhythm, those who received vasopressin followed by epinephrine had better outcomes than those who received epinephrine only, suggesting that the combination of the drugs may have advantages. Overall, evidence currently suggests that, like other potent vasopressors, vasopressin is equivalent to but not better than epinephrine for use during CPR.

Amiodarone and Lidocaine

After vasopressors, the drugs most likely to be of benefit during CPR are those that help suppress ectopic ventricular rhythms. Amiodarone and lidocaine are used during cardiac arrest to aid defibrillation when VF is refractory to electrical countershock therapy or when fibrillation recurs following successful conversion. Bretylium used to be included in this category but is no longer available for clinical use. Lidocaine, primarily an antiectopic agent with few hemodynamic effects, tends to reverse the reduction in VF threshold caused by ischemia or infarction. It depresses automaticity by reducing the slope of phase 4 depolarization and reducing the heterogeneity of ventricular refractoriness. Amiodarone is a pharmacologically complex drug with sodium, potassium, calcium, and α-adrenergic and β-adrenergic blocking properties that is useful for treatment of atrial and ventricular dysrhythmias. Amiodarone can cause hypotension and bradycardia when infused too rapidly in patients with an intact circulation.[102] This can usually be prevented by slowing the rate of drug infusion, or it can be treated with fluids, vasopressors, chronotropic agents, or temporary pacing. There are two randomized, blinded, placebo-controlled clinical trials in shock-resistant cardiac arrest victims demonstrating improved admission alive to hospital with amiodarone treatment, although there was no difference in survival to discharge.[103,104] Although weak, this is more evidence of efficacy than exists for lidocaine.

When VF or pulseless ventricular tachycardia is recognized, defibrillation should be attempted (Fig. 59-2). No antiarrhythmic agent has been shown to be superior to electrical defibrillation or more effective than placebo in the treatment of VF. Consequently, defibrillation should not be withheld or delayed to establish intravenous access or to administer drugs. When ventricular tachycardia or VF has not responded to or recurred following BLS, epinephrine, and defibrillation, amiodarone should be administered. In cardiac arrest, amiodarone is initially administered as a 300-mg rapid infusion. Supplemental infusions of 150 mg can be repeated as necessary for recurrent or resistant dysrhythmias to a maximum total daily dose of 2 g. (For dysrhythmias with an intact circulation, amiodarone is usually administered as 150 mg intravenously over 10 minutes, followed by 1 mg/min infusion for 6 hours and 0.5 mg/min thereafter.) Lidocaine is an alternative therapy in refractory fibrillation. To rapidly achieve and maintain therapeutic blood levels during CPR, relatively large doses are necessary. An initial bolus of 1 to 1.5 mg/kg should be given and additional boluses of 0.5 to 0.75 mg/kg can be given every 5 to 10 minutes during CPR up to a total dose of 3 mg/kg. Only bolus dosing should be used during CPR, but an infusion of 2 to 4 mg/min can be started after successful resuscitation.

Atropine

Atropine sulfate enhances sinus node automaticity and atrioventricular conduction by its vagolytic effects. Although atropine is frequently given during cardiac arrest associated with an electrocardiogram (ECG) pattern of asystole or slow pulseless electrical activity (PEA), neither animal nor human studies provide evidence that it actually improves outcome from asystolic or bradysystolic arrest.[105,106] The predominant cause of asystole and PEA is severe myocardial ischemia. Excessive parasympathetic tone probably contributes little to these rhythms during cardiac arrest in adults. Even in children, it is doubtful that parasympathetic tone plays a significant role during most arrests. Therefore, the most important treatment for asystole and PEA is effective chest compressions, ventilation, and epinephrine to improve coronary perfusion and myocardial oxygenation. However, cardiac arrest with these rhythms has a poor prognosis.[29] Because atropine has few adverse effects, it is recommended in arrest with asystole or PEA and refractory to epinephrine and oxygenation. The dose is 1.0 mg intravenously, repeated every 3 to 5 minutes up to a total of 0.04 mg/kg, which is totally vagolytic.[107] Full vagolytic doses may be associated with mydriasis, following successful resuscitation confounding neurologic examination. Occasionally, a sinus tachycardia following resuscitation may be the result of the use of atropine during CPR.

Sodium Bicarbonate

Although sodium bicarbonate was used commonly during CPR in the past, little evidence supports its efficacy. Use of sodium bicarbonate during resuscitation has been based on the theoretical considerations that acidosis lowers fibrillation threshold and impairs the physiologic response to catecholamines. But most studies have failed to demonstrate improved success of defibrillation or resuscitation with the use of bicarbonate.[108,109] The lack of effect of buffer therapy may be partially explained by the slow onset of metabolic acidosis during cardiac arrest. As measured by blood lactate or base deficit, acidosis does not become severe for 15 or 20 minutes of cardiac arrest.[43,110]

In contrast to the lack of evidence that buffer therapy during CPR improves survival, the adverse effects of excessive sodium bicarbonate administration are well documented. In the past, metabolic alkalosis, hypernatremia, and hyperosmolarity were common after administration of bicarbonate during resuscitation attempts.[110,111] These abnormalities are associated with low resuscitation rates and poor outcome. However, if sodium bicarbonate is given judiciously according to standard recommendations, no significant metabolic abnormalities should occur.

Intravenous sodium bicarbonate combines with hydrogen ion to produce carbonic acid that dissociates into CO_2 and water. The PCO_2 in blood is temporarily elevated until the excess CO_2 is eliminated through the lungs. Tissue acidosis during CPR is caused primarily by the low blood flow and accumulation of CO_2 in the tissues.[43] Therefore, concern has been expressed that the liberation of CO_2 by bicarbonate administration would only worsen the existing problem. This is of particular concern within myocardial cells and the brain. Carbon dioxide readily diffuses across cell membranes and the blood–brain barrier, whereas bicarbonate diffuses much more slowly. Thus, it is possible that sodium bicarbonate administration could result in a paradoxical worsening of intracellular and cerebral acidosis by further raising intracellular and cerebral CO_2 without a balancing increase in bicarbonate. Direct evidence for this effect has not been found. Use of clinically relevant doses causes no change in spinal fluid acid-base status or myocardial intracellular pH during bicarbonate administration.[112,113] Therefore, paradoxical acidosis from sodium bicarbonate therapy remains a concern primarily on theoretical grounds.

Current practice restricts the use of sodium bicarbonate primarily to arrests associated with hyperkalemia, severe preexisting metabolic acidosis, and tricyclic or phenobarbital overdose. It may be considered for use in protracted resuscitation attempts after other modalities have been instituted and failed. When bicarbonate is used during CPR, the usual dose is 1 mEq/kg initially with additional doses of 0.5 mEq/kg every 10 minutes. However, dosing of sodium bicarbonate should be guided by blood gas determination of acid-base status, whenever possible.

Calcium

With normal cardiovascular physiology, calcium increases myocardial contractility and enhances ventricular automaticity (see Chapter 10). Consequently, it has been advocated as a treatment for asystole and PEA. Early animal studies showed moderate success with calcium chloride in asphyxial arrest, although vasopressors were better.[13] In 1981, Dembo[114] reported dangerously high serum calcium levels (up to 18.2 mg/dL) during CPR and questioned the efficacy of calcium in cardiac arrest. Subsequently, several retrospective studies and prospective clinical trials during out-of-hospital cardiac arrest showed that calcium was no better than placebo in promoting resuscitation and survival from asystole or PEA.[115–118] Consequently, because of potentially deleterious effects, calcium is not recommended during CPR unless specific indications exist. Calcium may prove useful if hyperkalemia, hypocalcemia, or calcium channel blocker toxicity is present. There are no other indications for its use during CPR. When calcium is administered, the chloride salt is recommended because it produces higher and more consistent levels of ionized calcium than other salts. The usual dose is 2 to 4 mg/kg of the 10% solution administered slowly intravenously. Calcium gluconate contains one-third as much molecular calcium as does calcium chloride and requires metabolism of gluconate in the liver.

ELECTRICAL THERAPY

Electrical Pattern and Duration of Ventricular Fibrillation

⑪ Ventricular fibrillation is the most common ECG pattern found during witnessed sudden cardiac arrest in adults. The only consistently effective treatment is electrical defibrillation. The most important controllable determinant of failure to resuscitate a patient with VF is the duration of fibrillation.[119] Other important factors, such as underlying disease and metabolic status, are largely beyond the control of rescuers. The fibrillating heart has high oxygen consumption, increasing myocardial ischemia and decreasing the time to irreversible cell damage. The longer VF continues, the more difficult it is to defibrillate and the less likely is successful resuscitation.[60,120] If defibrillation occurs within 1 minute of fibrillation, CPR is unnecessary for resuscitation. Initial resuscitation success following out-of-hospital fibrillation and survival to hospital discharge are improved the earlier that defibrillation is accomplished.[19,121]

The coarseness of the fibrillatory waves on the ECG may reflect the severity and duration of the myocardial insult, and thus have prognostic significance.[122] However, the fibrillation amplitude seen on any one ECG lead varies with the orientation of that lead to the vector of the fibrillatory wave.[123] If the lead is oriented at right angles to the fibrillatory wave, a flat line can be seen. For this reason, the trace from a second lead or from a different position of paddle electrodes should always be inspected before a decision is made not to defibrillate. Low-*amplitude* fibrillatory waveforms are less likely to be associated with successful resuscitation and more likely to convert to asystole following defibrillation.[122] Similarly, low-*frequency* fibrillatory waveforms are associated with poor outcome, and the median frequency of the waveform correlates with myocardial perfusion during CPR and with success of defibrillation.[124,125] Multiple studies in animals and humans have shown that analysis of the VF waveform can predict, with varying reliability, the success of defibrillation attempts.[122,125–128] It is not yet clear whether such waveform analysis can predict success of resuscitation or direct modification of therapy prospectively. Catecholamines with β-adrenergic activity increase the vigor of fibrillation and the amplitude of the electrical activity, leading to the practice of administering epinephrine to make it "easier" to defibrillate. However, experimental work has shown that manipulation of the electrical pattern with epinephrine does not influence the success of defibrillation or reduce the energy needed for defibrillation.[120,129] Consequently, defibrillation should not be delayed for drug administration.

Defibrillators: Energy, Current, and Voltage

Defibrillators derive power from a line source of alternating current or an integral battery. The typical defibrillator consists of a variable transformer that allows selection of a variable voltage potential, an AC/DC converter to provide a direct current that is stored in a capacitor, a switch to charge the capacitor, and discharge switches to complete the circuit from capacitor to electrodes. Defibrillators are classified by the current waveform delivered: monophasic (current flows in one direction between electrodes) or biphasic (current reverses direction between electrodes during the shock). Until the past few years, the current waveform of most defibrillators was a monophasic damped half-sinusoid, although some delivered a monophasic truncated exponential waveform. Many of these monophasic defibrillators are still in use, although nearly all new defibrillators, including most AEDs, deliver either a biphasic truncated exponential waveform or a rectilinear biphasic waveform.

The AED is a device that monitors the ECG, recognizes VF, charges automatically, and gives a defibrillatory shock.[130] It has allowed the introduction of defibrillation into first-responder emergency medical system (EMS) networks and public access defibrillation because minimally trained individuals can incorporate defibrillation into BLS skills, improving survival in out-of-hospital arrest by reducing time to delivery of the first shock.[18–20,131] The algorithms these devices use to detect VF are accurate with nearly perfect specificity. They will not defibrillate a nonfibrillatory rhythm. Sensitivity rates are somewhat lower. They sometimes have trouble recognizing low-amplitude VF and can misinterpret pacemaker spikes as QRS complexes. Unfortunately, rhythm analysis can require up to 90 seconds during which chest compressions are not being given. This may adversely influence outcome in some circumstances.

Defibrillators have been developed that measure transthoracic impedance prior to the shock by passing a low-voltage current through the chest during the charge cycle.[132,133] Although not in clinical use, this technology allows current-based defibrillation by adjusting the delivered energy for the measured resistance permitting the use of low-energy shocks in appropriate patients and identification of victims needing higher energy.[134]

Defibrillation is accomplished by current passing through a critical mass of myocardium causing simultaneous depolarization of the myofibrils. However, the output of most defibrillators is indicated in energy units (joules or watt-seconds), not current (amperes). The relationships among energy, current, and impedance (resistance) are given by the following equations (standard units are indicated):

$$\text{Energy (joules)} = \text{Power (watts)} \times \text{Duration (seconds)} \quad (59\text{-}1)$$

$$\text{Power (watts)} = \text{Potential (volts)} \times \text{Current (amperes)} \quad (59\text{-}2)$$

$$\text{Current (amperes)} = \text{Potential (volts)}/\text{Resistance (ohms)} \quad (59\text{-}3)$$

$$\text{Current (amperes)} = \{\text{Energy (joules)}/[\text{Resistance (ohms)} \times \text{Duration (seconds)}]\}^{1/2} \quad (59\text{-}4)$$

From these equations, it can be determined that as the impedance between the paddle electrodes increases, the delivered energy will be reduced. Because internal resistance is low, the primary determinant of delivered energy will be transthoracic impedance. For consistency, the energy level indicated on most commercially available defibrillators is the output when discharged into a 50-ohm load. When transthoracic impedance is higher than that standard, actual delivered energy will be lower. Even at a constant delivered energy, Eq. 4 indicates that delivered current (the critical determinant of defibrillation) will be reduced as impedance increases. At high impedance and relatively low energy levels, current could be too low for defibrillation. Optimal success of defibrillation is obtained by keeping impedance as low as possible.

Transthoracic Impedance

Transthoracic impedance has been measured between 15 and 143 ohms in human defibrillation.[135] (see Chapter 10). The average transthoracic impedance in human defibrillation is 70 to 80 ohms. Many of the important factors in minimizing transthoracic impedance are under the control of the rescuers.

Resistance decreases with increasing electrode size, and studies suggest that optimal paddle size may be 13 cm in diameter.[136,137] For adults, handheld paddle electrodes and self-adhesive pad electrodes are most commonly 8 to 12 cm in diameter and work well in practice. Gel pads, electrode paste, or self-adhesive defibrillation/monitor pads specifically designed to conduct electricity in the defibrillation setting must be used.[136,137] When paste is used, it should be applied liberally to the paddle surface, especially the edges, to prevent burns and to obtain the maximum reduction in impedance. Transthoracic impedance is slightly, but significantly, higher during inspiration than during exhalation.[138] Air is a poor electrical conductor. Firm paddle pressure of at least 11 kg reduces resistance by improving paddle-to-skin contact and by expelling air from the lungs.[135] Resistance is probably of little clinical significance when reasonably proper technique and high-energy shocks are used. For lower energy shocks, great care should be taken to minimize resistance.

Adverse Effects and Energy Requirements

Repeated defibrillation with high energy in animals can be associated with dysrhythmias, ECG changes suggesting myocardial damage, and morphologic evidence of myocardial necrosis.[139,140] Whether similar injuries occur in humans is less certain. Slight elevations in creatine kinase MB fractions have been measured in patients following cardioversion with high energies.[141] A higher incidence of atrioventricular block has been observed in patients receiving high-energy shocks than in patients receiving low-energy shock.[142] It seems likely that high-energy shocks, especially if repeated at close intervals, may result in myocardial damage. However, if energy is too low, the delivered current may be insufficient for defibrillation, especially when transthoracic impedance is high. There appears to be little risk of significant myocardial injury with currently recommended energy levels.

Older studies using monophasic waveform defibrillators found a general relationship between body size and energy requirements for defibrillation. Geddes et al.[143] observed that the current that is necessary for defibrillation in animals increased with increasing body mass. Children need less energy than adults, perhaps as low as 0.5 J/kg,[144] although the recommended dose is 2.0 to 4.0 J/kg, similar to that for adults.[29] Clinically, over the size range of adults, weight variability is not clinically significant and other factors are more important.[145] Studies of out-of-hospital and in-hospital arrests have demonstrated equal success when using ≤200 J initial energy compared with administering all shocks at energies ≥300 J.[142,146] Both monophasic and biphasic waveforms are successful in terminating VF. Neither waveform has been associated with better return of spontaneous circulation or survival.

Prior to 2005, the AHA recommendation for defibrillation with monophasic waveform devices was to use a stacked shock approach with an initial shock or 200 J followed immediately by a second shock at 200 to 300 J if the first is unsuccessful, followed, if both fail, by a third shock at 300 to 360 J.[147] However, it was recognized that experimental studies demonstrated that the second and third shocks added limited incremental benefit and caused significant interruptions in chest compressions with possible reduced survival. Although optimal energy level is not known, expert consensus was that the 2005 Guidelines[29] should change the algorithm for applying shocks with monophasic defibrillators to a single shock of 360 J with immediate resumption of chest compressions (Fig. 59-2).

Termination of VF with biphasic shocks has occurred at lower energies than any of the monophasic waveforms.[148]

Selected energies of 150 to 200 J are generally effective with biphasic truncated exponential waveforms, and a selected energy of 120 J is effective with a rectilinear biphasic waveform. If the specific biphasic device being used has an indicated effective dose, the user should select that dose. If the effective dose for a biphasic device is unknown, a dose of 200 J may be selected. This dose may not be optimal but falls within the effective dose range of nearly all biphasic devices. As with the monophasic devices, a single shock should be delivered with immediate resumption of chest compressions. If additional shocks are necessary they may be given at the same or higher dose.

PUTTING IT ALL TOGETHER

Since the mid-1970s, CPR has become widely practiced, facilitated by the efforts of the AHA, the International Red Cross, the European Resuscitation Council, and many other organizations around the world. Specific guidelines for the teaching and practice of CPR are published periodically.[29,147] These guidelines were developed because numerous individuals with varying levels of expertise (laypersons, emergency personnel, nurses, and physicians) need to be trained if CPR is to be effective in saving lives. For training to be effective, a standardized approach is needed (Figs. 59-1 and 59-2). The organizations also develop and sponsor courses at different levels of complexity for teaching CPR. The two levels of CPR care are referred to as *basic life support* (BLS) for ventilation and chest compressions without additional equipment, and *advanced cardiac life support* (ACLS) for using all modalities available for resuscitation. Medical personnel need to be well versed in both levels of care. BLS is also appropriate for laypersons.

The AHA, in conjunction with the International Liaison Committee on Resuscitation, periodically coordinates an International Conference on CPR and emergency cardiac care, during which worldwide experts evaluate the scientific data regarding CPR. The recommendations resulting from the conference comprise the most complete compilation of guidelines for CPR practice.[29] International contributions to the most recent conferences produce similar CPR practices worldwide. However, no common infrastructure exists that allows adoption of true international guidelines for CPR. The algorithms for approaching the patient with cardiac arrest published in the guidelines are familiar to all physicians and are reproduced throughout this chapter.

CARDIOCEREBRAL RESUSCITATION

The AHA guidelines and algorithms are carefully researched using the best evidence and experts available. Nevertheless, in spite of multiple updates to guidelines for CPR practice and many courses for lay public and health care providers, survival rates are dismal and have remained stagnant for decades.[149] These poor outcomes may be attributable, at least in part, to the fact that standard CPR is being applied to two pathophysiologically distinct entities (respiratory arrest and cardiac arrest) and is not optimal care for either. In the former, arrest occurs because of hypoxemia and reoxygenating the blood by effective ventilation is mandatory for successful resuscitation. In the latter, arrest occurs because of cardiac dysrhythmia, usually with normal oxygenation, and attempts at ventilation during resuscitation, in fact, are harmful. Study of this problem led the University of Arizona CPR Research Group in 2003 to propose an alternative to standard CPR for treating victims of cardiac arrest.[150,151] This approach to the victim of

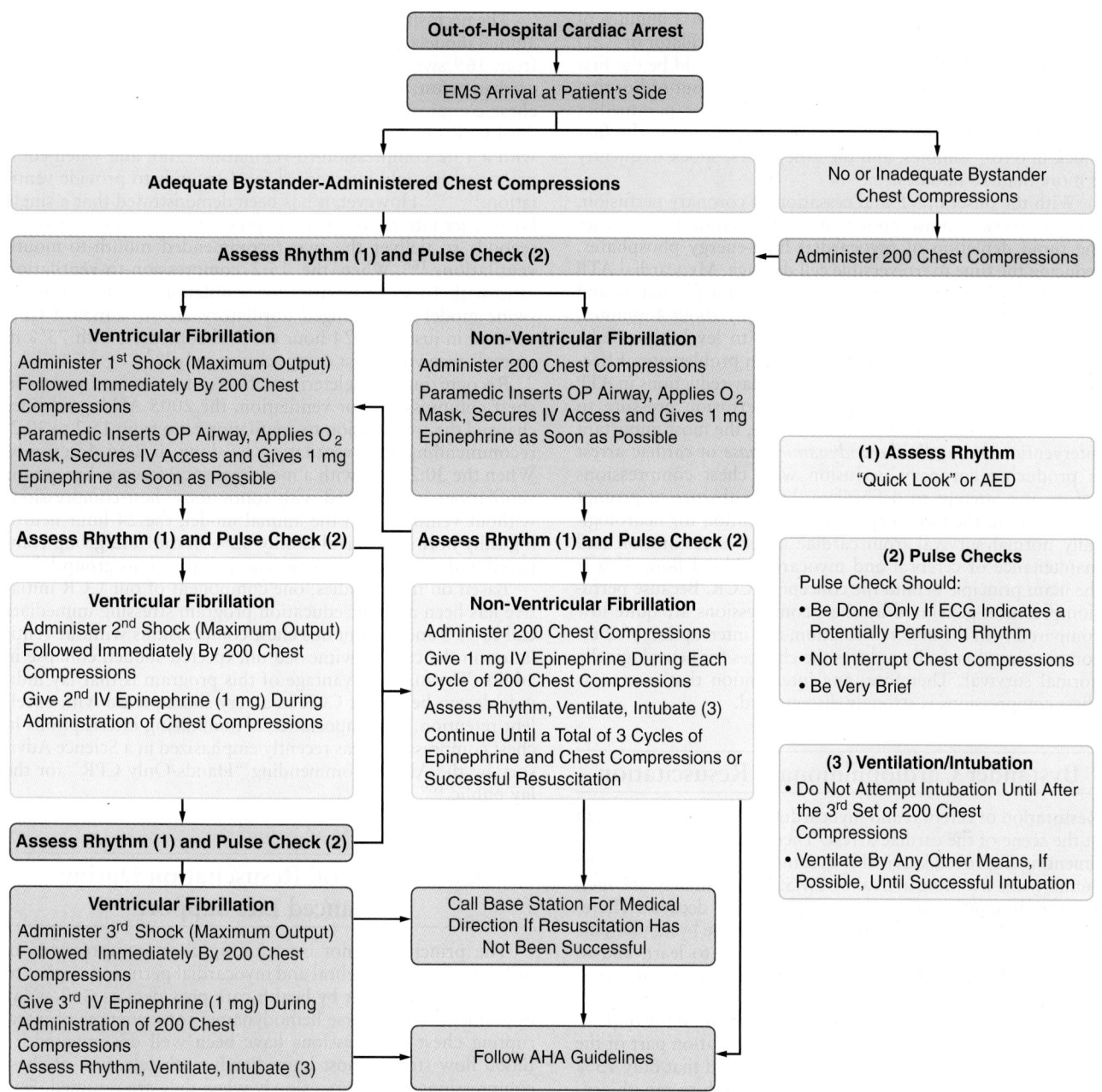

FIGURE 59-5. Cardiocerebral resuscitation algorithm. EMS, emergency medical system; OP, oropharyngeal; O₂, oxygen; IV, intravenous(ly); AHA, American Heart Association.

sudden cardiac death has been called *cardiocerebral resuscitation* (CCR) or *minimally interrupted cardiac resuscitation*. Although the nuances of the technique continue to evolve, the basic outline of CCR as practiced in Tucson is shown in the Figure 59-5. Some of the elements of CCR were incorporated in the 2005 AHA Guidelines but there are significant differences from the AHA pulseless arrest algorithm (Fig. 59-2).

Time-Sensitive Model of Ventricular Fibrillation

Weisfeldt and Becker[152] have described untreated VF as a time-sensitive model with three phases: electrical, circulatory and metabolic. The electrical phase occurs during the first 4 to 5 minutes of the arrest and early defibrillation is critical for success during this time. The hemodynamic phase follows for the next 10 to 15 minutes when perfusing the myocardium and

brain with oxygenated blood is critical. This is followed by what has been called the *metabolic phase,* when the ischemic injury to the heart is so great that it is not clear what interventions will be successful.

Prompt defibrillation during the *electrical phase* is when CPR has had the most dramatic effect and why public-access AED has proven beneficial. The longer VF continues, the more difficult it is to defibrillate and the less likely is successful resuscitation. AEDs have been employed successfully in many settings, including airplanes, airports, casinos, and in the community. The success of public access defibrillation was dramatically demonstrated by the results of installing AEDs in Chicago airports where, over the first 2 years, there was a 55% 1-year neurologically intact survival.[153] Similarly, when AEDs were installed in Las Vegas casinos and security personnel instructed in the use, there was a 53% survival to discharge

(74% in patients who received the shock within 3 minutes of collapse).[154] If an arrest is witnessed and a defibrillator or AED is immediately available, then defibrillation should be the first priority in resuscitation. However, in the usual out-of-hospital rescue with emergency medical technicians or paramedics doing the defibrillation, a rapid response is to apply the first shock in 6 to 7 minutes, and the time to first shock frequently is more than 10 minutes.

With the onset of VF and cessation of coronary perfusion, the high oxygen consumption of the fibrillating heart causes the rapid depletion of myocardial high-energy phosphates, reducing the time to irreversible cell damage. Myocardial ATP levels during VF correlate with the success of defibrillation and postdefibrillation contractile function.[155] By about 4 minutes, the ATP levels in the heart have fallen to levels that make restoration of normal contractile function problematic. Effective chest compressions help replete or delay reductions in ATP by generating an adequate coronary perfusion pressure to restore myocardial blood flow. Therefore, the most important intervention during the *hemodynamic phase* of cardiac arrest is producing coronary perfusion with chest compressions before any attempt to defibrillate. In the absence of prompt defibrillation, the most important intervention for neurologically normal survival from cardiac arrest is restoration and maintenance of cerebral and myocardial blood flow. This is the main principle behind the concept of CCR. Because perfusion pressures generated by chest compressions are quite low compared with the intact circulation, any interruption of chest compressions markedly reduces the chances for neurologically normal survival. Therefore, any intervention that interrupts chest compressions is strongly discouraged.

Bystander Cardiopulmonary Resuscitation

Restoration of cerebral and myocardial blood flow must begin at the scene of the cardiac arrest. There are many studies documenting improved survival if bystanders provide CPR to the victim while awaiting arrival of EMS. Unfortunately, the incidence of bystander CPR has been falling for 3 decades. Therefore, a focus of the CCR initiative is to increase bystander participation by making the intervention easier to learn and to perform. The reasons for bystander's reluctance to intervene are multiple but seem to be primarily (1) lack of training, (2) the complexity of the task, and (3) fear of harm. Many of these concerns focus on the mouth-to-mouth ventilation part of the CPR intervention.[156–158] One survey indicated that only 15% of lay persons would perform CPR with mouth-to-mouth ventilation on a stranger. When given the option of doing chest compressions only, 68% indicated they would perform CPR on a stranger.[158]

If the airway remains patent during CPR, chest compressions cause substantial air exchange. Early studies in anesthetized, paralyzed humans suggested that the airway would not remain open in the unconscious,[6,7] leading to the teaching that airway control and artificial ventilation must accompany chest compressions. However, there is considerable data to suggest that eliminating mouth-to-mouth ventilation early in the resuscitation of witnessed fibrillatory cardiac arrest is not detrimental to outcome and may improve survival. Data from the Belgian CPCR Registry has demonstrated that 14-day survival and neurologic outcome is the same if bystanders initiate full BLS or perform chest compressions only. Both are significantly better than if the bystanders only do mouth-to-mouth ventilation or attempt no CPR.[159,160] A recent Japanese study found better survival in victims who received bystander chest compression-only CPR than in those who received both chest compressions and mouth-to-mouth ventilation from bystanders.[161]

The necessity for ventilation during BLS has been studied in animal models. Since 1993, there are 6 studies containing data from 169 swine demonstrating that in prolonged fibrillatory cardiac arrest, neurologically intact survival is the same with chest compression-only resuscitation as with idealized standard CPR (as recommended by the 2000 AHA guidelines[147]) with a 15:2 compression-to-ventilation ratio, and when compressions are only interrupted for 4 seconds to provide ventilation.[162–165] However, it has been demonstrated that a single lay rescuer interrupts chest compressions for an average of 16 seconds to deliver the two recommended mouth-to-mouth ventilations.[166] When the 15:2 compression-to-ventilation ratio with 16-second pauses for ventilation was tested in the swine model of prolonged fibrillatory arrest, standard CPR resulted in just 13% 24-hour survival compared with 73% in animals receiving chest compressions only.[167]

Recognizing the deleterious effects of prolonged pauses in chest compressions for ventilation, the 2005 AHA guidelines changed the compression-to-ventilation ratio from 15:2 to 30:2, recommending that ventilation be done in 2 to 4 seconds. When the 30:2 ratio with a more realistic 16-second pause for ventilations is compared with continuous chest compressions without ventilation in the animal model, the 24-hour neurologically normal survival is only 42% in the 30:2 group compared with 70% in the continuous compressions group.[168]

Based on these studies, one component of our CCR initiative has been a public education program stressing immediate call to 911 and continuous chest compressions without ventilation in the case of witnessed unexpected sudden collapse in adults. The major advantage of this program is that lay individuals can be taught CCR in a very short period with excellent retention. The importance of minimizing interruptions in chest compressions was recently emphasized in a Science Advisory by the AHA recommending "Hands-Only CPR" for the lay public.[169]

Cardiocerebral Resuscitation During Advanced Life Support

The principle of not interrupting chest compressions in order to maintain cerebral and myocardial perfusion applies to resuscitation attempts by health care providers as well as lay bystanders. The adverse hemodynamic consequences of interrupting chest compressions have been well documented.[170] Blood flow stops almost immediately with cessation of chest compressions and returns slowly when they are resumed. Several compressions are necessary before perfusion pressures return to the levels obtained before compressions were stopped. This is particularly true for prolonged, repeated pauses for ventilation. But it is also relevant for the many other interruptions that occur during resuscitation: pulse checks, rhythm analysis, charging the defibrillator, stacked shocks, intubation, patient assessment, and intravenous line placement. Recent reports have documented that paramedics spend only about half the time during a resuscitation doing chest compressions, mostly because they are following the standard guidelines.[171,172]

Consequently, in CCR, the emphasis is that chest compressions are to be paused only when absolutely necessary, and then for the shortest time possible. Initial airway management consists of insertion of an oropharyngeal airway and providing oxygen by mask. Intravenous line placement should not require cessation of chest compressions. Pulse checks occur only during pauses for rhythm analysis. Rescue breaths or assisted ventilation/intubation are delayed until return of spontaneous circulation or until at least three cycles of compressions-rhythm analysis-shock are complete. The second rescuer's priorities are obtaining intravenous access, delivering drugs, and relieving the individual giving chest compressions. If there is time and resources for airway management, ventilation and intubation are encouraged to take place while chest compressions continue.

Once ventilation begins, rescuers must be aware of the potentially deleterious effects of positive-pressure ventilation.[173,174] Positive-pressure ventilation increases intrathoracic pressure reducing venous return, cardiac output, and coronary perfusion pressure and adversely effecting survival. These effects are amplified by the fact that physicians and paramedics often ventilate at rates that are many times the recommended 10 breaths per minute, even after extensive retraining.[171,173–175]

Rhythm Analysis and Defibrillation

As mentioned previously, after 4 to 5 minutes of VF, the myocardium is so depleted of high-energy phosphates that development of a normal contractile state is difficult, if not impossible. Therefore, immediate defibrillation during the circulatory phase is counterproductive, usually producing either asystole or pulseless electrical activity. In Seattle, it has been noted that patients who had CPR prior to defibrillation had a better survival and the improvement was all accounted for by better results in the group of patients in whom the response time was >4 minutes.[176] In a randomized trial of 200 out-of-hospital cardiac arrests in Oslo, there was a highly significant improvement in outcome if CPR was provided before defibrillation when the response time was >5 minutes.[177] Consequently, during CCR, resuscitation is initiated with 200 continuous chest compressions at a rate of 100/minute unless bystanders are already providing good chest compressions. Rhythm analysis and defibrillation, if indicated, follow. Pulse checks are done only during the period of rhythm analysis.

The interruption caused by stacked defibrillatory shocks was discussed previously. When combined with time for rhythm analysis and postshock pulse checks, this interruption may be unacceptably long or even fatal when an AED is in use instead of an experienced clinician interpreting the rhythm with a manual defibrillator.[178,179] The postshock pulse check detects a pulse in only 2.5% of the victims. The success rate of a single shock is between 70 and 85% with most monophasic waveform defibrillators and >90% with the newer biphasic waveform units. Recognizing these concerns, both CCR as well as the 2005 AHA Guidelines for CPR recommend a single shock at 360 J for monophasic defibrillators and at the manufacturer's recommended power for biphasic units, with immediate resumption of chest compressions.

In prolonged VF arrest, successful defibrillation almost always results in asystole or pulseless electrical activity, as indicated by the extremely small number of victims with a pulse following shocks. In fact, the standard laboratory model for pulseless electrical activity is prolonged VF followed by defibrillation, all without chest compressions. Immediately restarting chest compressions after defibrillation to provide coronary perfusion nearly always results in reversion to a perfusing rhythm.[150] This certainly suggests that the best chance for restoration of spontaneous circulation following defibrillation will be by immediately resuming chest compressions without waiting to check a pulse or reanalyze the ECG rhythm.

Cardiocerebral Resuscitation in Practice

In summary, CCR is an approach to the victim of cardiac arrest that maximizes the chances for restoring and maintaining cerebral and myocardial perfusion at levels that promote neurologically intact survival. For bystanders, it emphasizes activating the EMS system as soon as possible and providing continuous chest compressions until help arrives. Immediate defibrillation is encouraged if the collapse is witnessed and a defibrillator/AED is promptly available. If the collapse is not witnessed, 200 continuous chest compressions (100/minute) are performed before rhythm analysis and defibrillation. If a shockable rhythm exists, a single shock of 360 J monophasic (or the manufacturer's recommended dose biphasic) is administered and continuous chest compressions immediately resumed. Pulse checks are done only during rhythm analysis. Intravenous administration of drugs is encouraged as soon as possible but without interruption of continuous chest compressions.

Initial results of applying the CCR principles to EMS for out-of-hospital cardiac arrest are beginning to be reported. In rural Rock and Walworth counties in Wisconsin, in the 3 years preceding a change to CCR, there were 92 witnessed out-of-hospital adult cardiac arrests with an initially shockable rhythm, of whom 18 survived and 14 (15%) were neurologically intact. In a little over a year after instituting the new protocol, there were 33 witnessed out-of-hospital adult cardiac arrest with an initially shockable rhythm, of whom 19 survived and 16 (48%) were neurologically intact.[180] The results of the first 3 years of using CCR in these counties has now been reported with similar results. Of 89 witnessed out-of-hospital cardiac arrests, 42 (47%) survived and 35 (39%) were neurologically intact.[181] In two large metropolitan Arizona cities, Utstein-style data were collected on all out-of-hospital cardiac arrests (excluding trauma, drowning, and other noncardiac causes) before and after institution of minimally interrupted cardiac resuscitation by the EMS.[182] Among the 886 patients, survival to hospital discharge increased from 1.8 to 5.4% after CCR training and in the subgroup of 174 patients with witnessed cardiac arrest with VF, survival increased from 4.7 to 17.6%. These highly statistically significant results are encouraging that a significant improvement in outcome from sudden cardiac death is possible.

PEDIATRIC CARDIOPULMONARY RESUSCITATION

The principles of CPR discussed previously apply to the child in cardiac arrest. Arrest is less likely to be a sudden event and more likely related to progressive deterioration of respiratory and circulatory function in the pediatric age group. Airway and ventilation problems lead to asystole and PEA as the most common presenting rhythms. However, the consequences of myocardial and cerebral ischemia are the same as for the adult and the basic approach to the unresponsive victim is similar (Fig. 59-6). The specific anatomic and physiologic considerations necessary for the child will be familiar to anesthesiologists. The special circumstance of neonatal resuscitation has been discussed in other chapters.

The problem of airway management in the infant is well known to the anesthesiologist. Effective ventilation is especially critical because respiratory problems are frequently the cause for arrest. Mouth-to-mouth or mouth-to-nose and mouth (for infants) can be used as well as bag-valve-mask devices until intubation is possible. Cardiac compression in the infant is provided with two fingers on the midsternum or by encircling the chest with the hands and using the thumbs to provide compression. For the small child, compression can be provided with one hand on the midsternum.

The algorithm for pulseless arrest in the child is shown in Figure 59-7. Although defibrillation is less frequently necessary

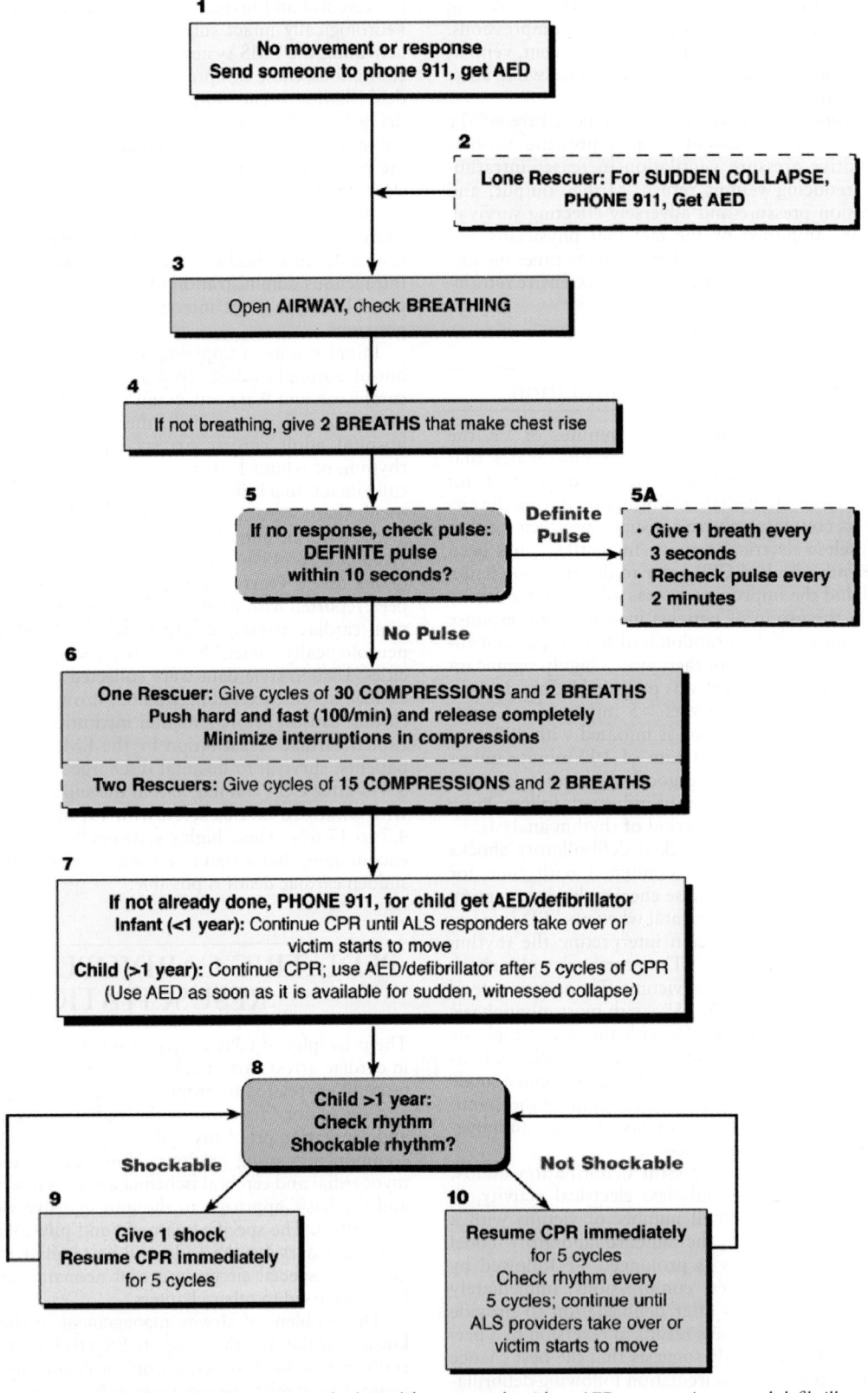

FIGURE 59-6.   Pediatric health care provider basic life support algorithm. AED, automatic external defibrillator; CPR, cardiopulmonary resuscitation; ALS, advanced life support. (From 2005 American Heart Association Guidelines for cardiopulmonary resuscitation and emergency cardiovascular care. Circulation 2005; 112(Suppl IV): IV, with permission.)

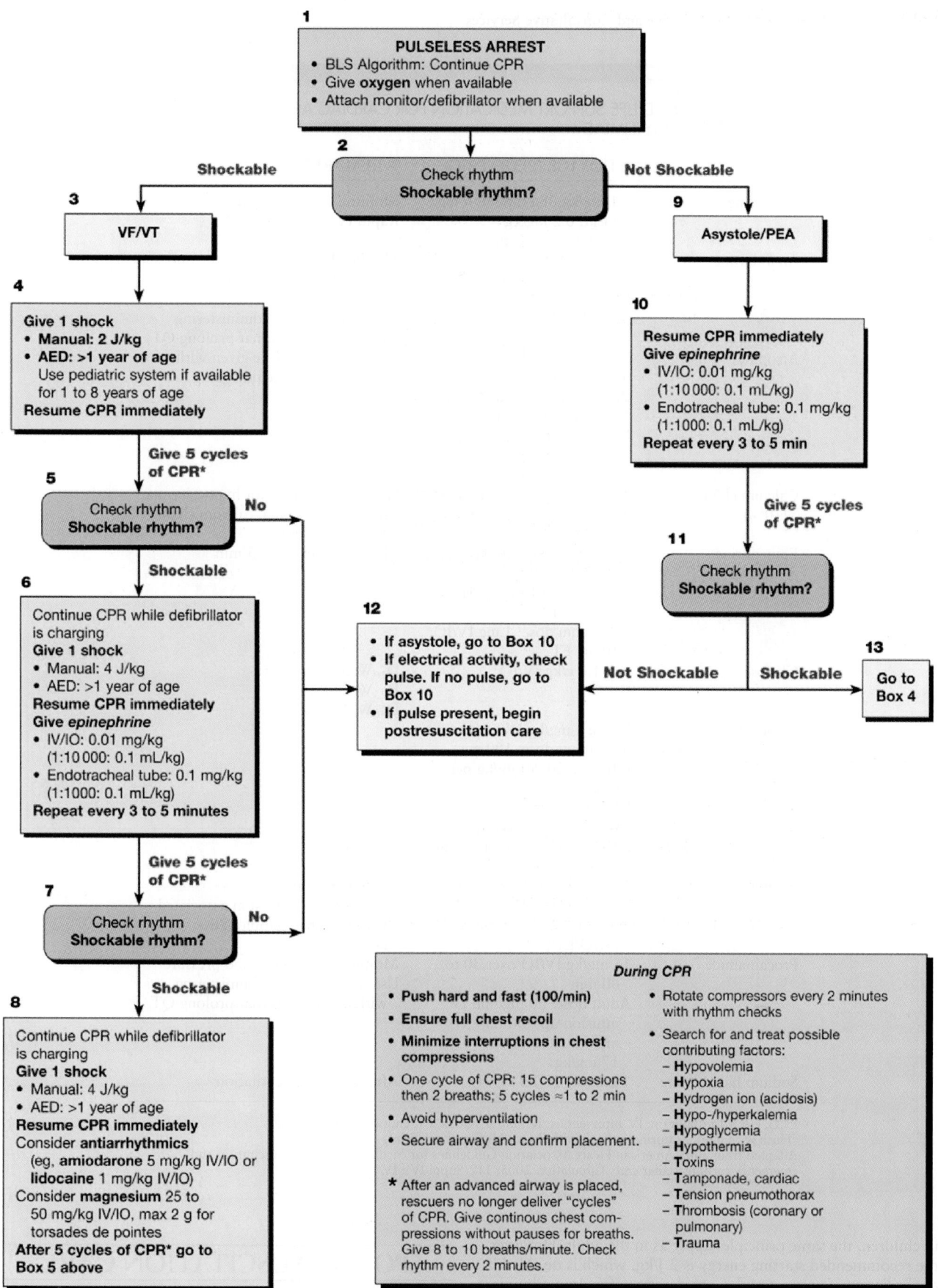

FIGURE 59-7.   Pediatric advanced life support pulseless arrest algorithm. BLS, basic life support; CPR, cardiopulmonary resuscitation; VF, ventricular fibrillation; VT, ventricular tachycardia; PEA, pulseless electrical activity; IV, intravenous(ly); IO, intraosseous(ly); AED, automatic external defibrillator. (From 2005 American Heart Association Guidelines for cardiopulmonary resuscitation and emergency cardiovascular care. Circulation 2005; 112(Suppl IV): IV, with permission.)

TABLE 59-3

PEDIATRIC ADVANCED LIFE SUPPORT MEDICATION FOR CARDIAC ARREST AND SYMPTOMATIC ARRHYTMIAS

■ DRUG	■ DOSAGE (PEDIATRIC)	■ REMARKS
Adenosine	0.1 mg/kg (maximum, 6 mg) Repeat: 0.2 mg/kg (maximum, 12 mg)	Monitor ECG during dose Rapid IV/IO bolus
Amiodarone	5 mg/kg IV/IO Repeat up to 15 mg/kg Maximum: 300 mg	Monitor ECG and blood pressure Adjust administration rate to urgency Use caution when administering with other drugs that prolong QT
Atropine	0.02 mg/kg IV/IO 0.03 mg/kg ET[d] Repeat once if needed Minimum dose: 0.1 mg Maximum single dose: Child, 0.5 mg Adolescent, 1.0 mg	Higher doses may be given with organophosphate poisoning
Calcium chloride (10%)	20 mg/kg IV/IO (0.2 mL/kg)	Give slow IV push for hypocalcemia, hypermagnesemia, calcium channel blocker toxicity
Epinephrine	0.01 mg/kg (0.1 mL/kg 1: 10,000) IV/IO 0.1 mg/kg (0.1 mL/kg 1: 1,000) ET[α] Maximum dose: 1 mg IV/IO; 10 mg ET	May repeat every 3–5 min
Glucose	0.5–1.0 g/kg IV/IO	$D_{10}W$: 5–10 mL/kg $D_{25}W$: 2–4 mL/kg $D_{50}W$: 1–2 mL/kg
Lidocaine	Bolus: 1 mg/kg IV/IO Maximum dose: 100 mg Infusion: 20–50 μg/kg per minute ET[α]: 2–3 mg/kg	—
Magnesium sulfate	25–50 mg/kg IV/IO over 10–20 min; faster in torsades Maximum dose: 2 g	—
Naloxone	≤5 years or ≤20 kg: 0.1 mg/kg IV/IO/ET[α] ≥5 y or >20 kg: 2 mg IV/IO/ET[α]	Use lower doses to reverse respiratory depression associated with therapeutic opioid use (1–15 μg/kg)
Procainamide	15 mg/kg IV/IO over 30 to 60 min Adult dose: 20 mg/min IV infusion up to total maximum dose of 17 mg/kg	Monitor ECG and blood pressure Use caution when administering with other drugs that prolong QT
Sodium bicarbonate	1 mEq/kg IV/IO slowly	After adequate ventilation

ECG, electrocardiogram; IV, intravenous; IO, intraosseous; ET, endotracheal.
[d]Flush with 5 mL of normal saline and follow with five ventilations.
Adapted from 2005 American Heart Association Guidelines for cardiopulmonary resuscitation and emergency cardiovascular care. Circulation 2005; 112(Suppl IV): IV.

in children, the same principles apply as in the adult. However, the recommended starting energy is 2 J/kg, which is doubled if defibrillation is unsuccessful. Considerations for drug administration are the same as for the adult, except that the interosseous route in the anterior tibia is particularly attractive option in small children. Drug therapy is similar to that of the adult but plays a larger role because electrical therapy is less often needed (Table 59-3). The pediatric algorithms for bradycardia and tachycardia are shown in Figures 59-8 and 59-9.

POSTRESUSCITATION CARE

The major factors contributing to mortality following successful resuscitation are progression of the primary disease and cerebral damage suffered as a result of the arrest. There is growing awareness that any cardiac arrest, even of brief duration, causes a generalized decrease in myocardial function similar to the regional hypokinesis seen following periods of regional

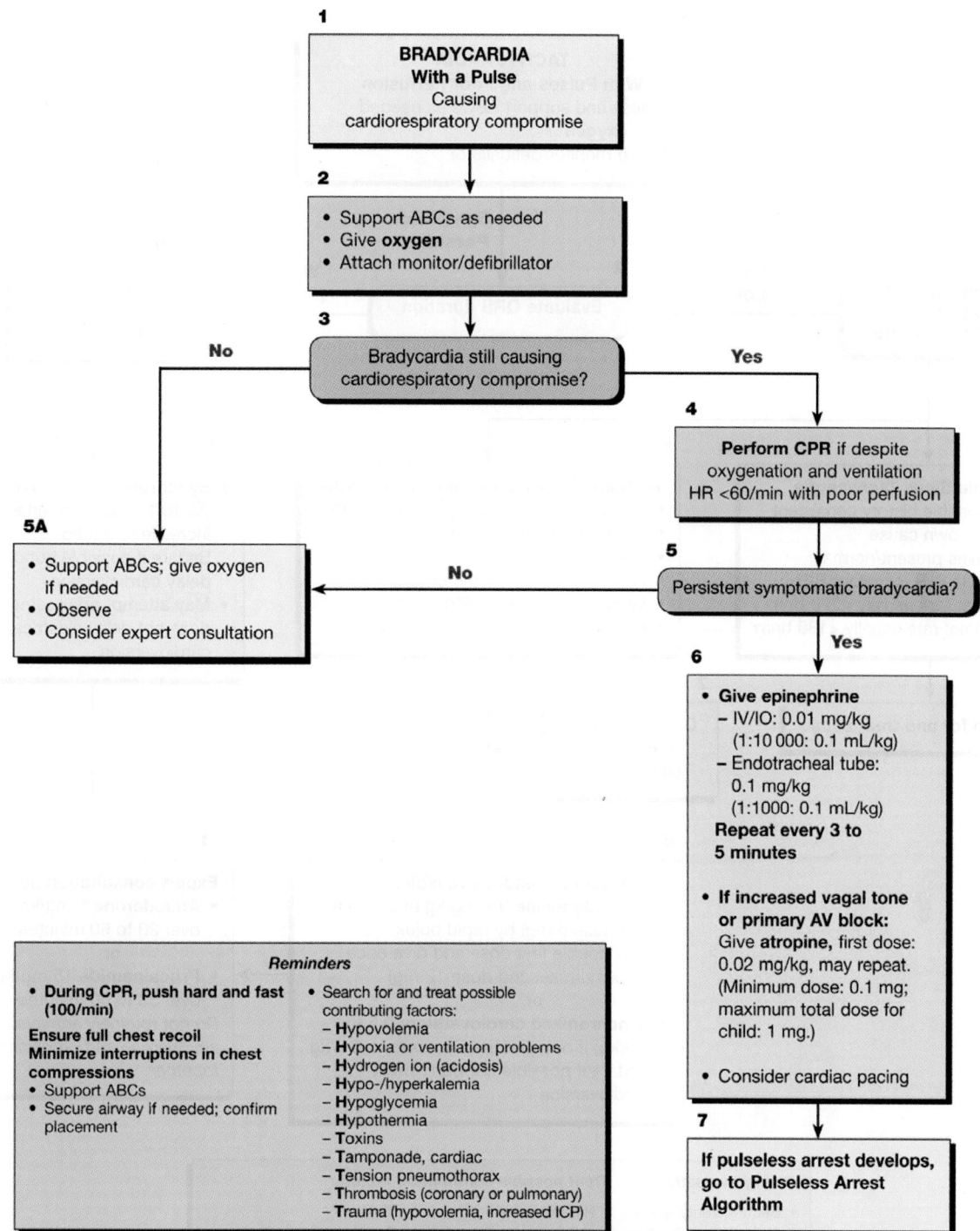

1

BRADYCARDIA
With a Pulse
Causing
cardiorespiratory compromise

2

- Support ABCs as needed
- Give **oxygen**
- Attach monitor/defibrillator

3

No ← Bradycardia still causing
cardiorespiratory compromise? → **Yes**

4

Perform CPR if despite
oxygenation and ventilation
HR <60/min with poor perfusion

5A

- Support ABCs; give oxygen
  if needed
- Observe
- Consider expert consultation

No ←— **5**

Persistent symptomatic bradycardia?

Yes

6

- **Give epinephrine**
  - IV/IO: 0.01 mg/kg
    (1:10 000: 0.1 mL/kg)
  - Endotracheal tube:
    0.1 mg/kg
    (1:1000: 0.1 mL/kg)
  Repeat every 3 to
  5 minutes

- **If increased vagal tone**
  or primary AV block:
  Give **atropine**, first dose:
  0.02 mg/kg, may repeat.
  (Minimum dose: 0.1 mg;
  maximum total dose for
  child: 1 mg.)

- Consider cardiac pacing

7

If pulseless arrest develops,
go to Pulseless Arrest
Algorithm

Reminders

- **During CPR, push hard and fast**
  (100/min)

Ensure full chest recoil
Minimize interruptions in chest
compressions
- Support ABCs
- Secure airway if needed; confirm
  placement

- Search for and treat possible
  contributing factors:
  – **H**ypovolemia
  – **H**ypoxia or ventilation problems
  – **H**ydrogen ion (acidosis)
  – **H**ypo-/hyperkalemia
  – **H**ypoglycemia
  – **H**ypothermia
  – **T**oxins
  – **T**amponade, cardiac
  – **T**ension pneumothorax
  – **T**hrombosis (coronary or pulmonary)
  – **T**rauma (hypovolemia, increased ICP)

FIGURE 59-8. Pediatric advanced life support bradycardia algorithm. ABCs, airway, breathing, and circulation; CPR, cardiopulmonary resuscitation; HR, heart rate; IV, intravenous(ly); IO, intraosseous(ly); AV, atrioventricular; ICP, intracranial pressure. (From 2005 American Heart Association Guidelines for cardiopulmonary resuscitation and emergency cardiovascular care. Circulation 2005; 112(Suppl IV): IV, with permission.)

ischemia. This is usually referred to as *global myocardial stunning* and can be mitigated with inotropic agents, if necessary. Active management following resuscitation appears to mitigate postischemic brain damage and improve neurologic outcome.[183] Although a significant number of patients have severe neurologic deficits following resuscitation, aggressive brain-oriented support does not seem to increase the proportion surviving in vegetative states. Most severely damaged victims die of multisystem failure within 1 to 2 weeks.

When flow is restored following a period of global brain ischemia, three stages of cerebral reperfusion are seen in the ensuing 12 hours. Immediately following resuscitation, there are multifocal areas of the brain with no reflow. Within 1 hour, there is global hyperemia followed quickly by prolonged global hypoperfusion. Elevation of intracranial pressure is unusual following resuscitation from cardiac arrest. However, severe ischemic injury can lead to cerebral edema and increased intracranial pressure in the ensuing days.

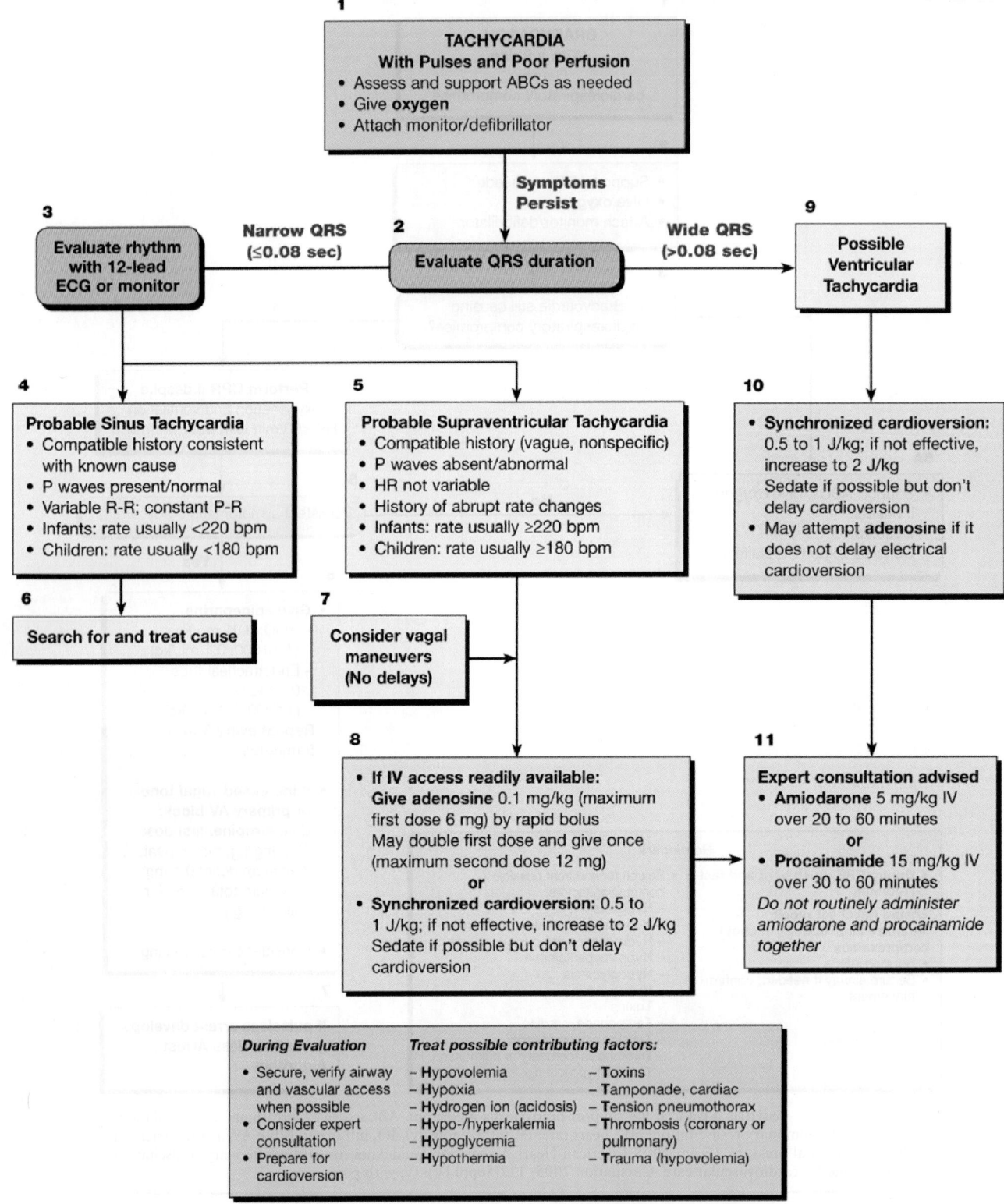

FIGURE 59-9.   Pediatric advanced life support tachycardia algorithm. ABCs, airway, breathing, and circulation; ECG, electrocardiogram; HR, heart rate; IV, intravenous. (From 2005 American Heart Association Guidelines for cardiopulmonary resuscitation and emergency cardiovascular care. Circulation 2005; 112(Suppl IV): IV, with permission.)

Postresuscitation support is focused on providing stable oxygenation and hemodynamics to minimize any further cerebral insult. A comatose patient should be maintained on mechanical ventilation for several hours to ensure adequate oxygenation and ventilation. Restlessness, coughing, or seizure activity should be aggressively treated with appropriate medications, including neuromuscular blockers, if necessary. Arterial PaO_2 should be maintained above 100 mm Hg, and hypocapnia ($PaCO_2$ <30 mm Hg) should be avoided. Blood volume should be maintained normal, and moderate hemodilution to a hematocrit of 30 to 35% may be helpful. A brief, 5-minute period of hypertension to mean arterial pressure of 120 to 140 mm Hg may help overcome the initial cerebral no reflow. This frequently occurs secondary to the effects of epinephrine given during CPR. Because cerebral autoregulation of blood flow is severely attenuated, both prolonged hypertension and hypotension are associated with a worsened outcome. Therefore, mean arterial pressure should be maintained at 90 to 110 mm Hg. Hyperglycemia during cerebral ischemia is known to result in increased neurologic damage. Although it is unknown if high serum glucose in the postresuscitation period influences outcome, it seems prudent to control glucose in the 100 to 150 mg/dL range. Specific pharmacologic therapy directed at brain preservation has not been shown to have further benefit. Some animal trials of barbiturates were promising, but a large multicenter trial of thiopental found no improvement in neurologic status when this drug was given following cardiac arrest.[183] Similar results were found with calcium channel blockers. Animal studies were encouraging, but a clinical trial found no improvement in outcome.[184]

In contrast to pharmacologic therapy, two more recent studies have demonstrated improved neurologic outcome when mild therapeutic hypothermia (32 to 34°C) was induced for 12 to 24 hours in cardiac arrest survivors who remained comatose after admission to the hospital.[185,186] Both investigations studied only patients whose initial rhythm was VF, and the larger of the trials included only witnessed arrests. Nevertheless, these are the first studies to document improved neurologic outcome with a specific postarrest intervention. The International Liaison Committee on Resuscitation now recommends "unconscious adult patients with spontaneous circulation after out-of-hospital cardiac arrest should be cooled to 32 to 34°C for 12 to 24 hours when the initial rhythm was ventricular fibrillation. Such cooling may also be beneficial for other rhythms or in-hospital cardiac arrest."

Prognosis

For the comatose survivor of CPR, the question of ultimate prognosis is important. One retrospective study demonstrated that the admission neurologic examination of comatose victims is highly correlated with the likelihood of awakening.[187] If there were no pupillary light response and no spontaneous eye movement, and if the motor response to pain were absent or extensor posturing, there was only a 5% chance the patient would ever awaken. A companion study demonstrated that the chance of ever awakening fell rapidly in the days following arrest.[188] If the patient was not awake by 4 days following arrest, the chance of ever awakening was 20%, and all those awakening had marked neurologic deficits. Most patients who completely recover show rapid improvement in the first 48 hours.

References

1. Wood Library Museum: Resuscitation: An Historical Perspective. Park Ridge, IL, Wood Library Museum, 1976

2. Brooks DK: Resuscitation: Care of the Critically Ill. London, Edward Arnold, 1986

3. Vesalius A: De Humani Corporis. Basel, Fabrica, 1543

4. Elam JO, Brown ES, Elder JD Jr: Artificial respiration by mouth to mask method: A study of the respiratory gas exchange of paralyzed patients ventilated by operator's expired air. N Engl J Med 1954; 250: 749

5. Gordon AS, Frye CS, Gittelson L et al: Mouth-to-mouth versus manual artificial respiration for children and adults. JAMA 1958; 167: 320

6. Safar P, Escarraga LA, Elam JO: A comparison of the mouth-to-mouth and mouth-to-airway methods of artificial respiration with the chest-pressure arm-lift methods. N Engl J Med 1958; 258: 671

7. Safar P: Failure of manual respiration. J Appl Physiol 1959; 14: 84

8. Hooker DR, Kouwenhoven WB, Langworthy OR: The effects of alternating current on the heart. Am J Physiol 1933; 103: 444

9. Beck CS, Pritchard WH, Feil HS: Ventricular fibrillation of long duration abolished by electric shock. JAMA 1947; 135: 985

10. Zoll PM, Linenthal AJ, Gibson W et al: Termination of ventricular fibrillation in man by an externally applied electric shock. N Engl J Med 1956; 254: 727

11. Kouwenhoven WB, Milnor WR, Knickerbocker GG et al: Closed-chest defibrillation of the heart. Surgery 1957; 42: 550

12. Kouwenhoven WB, Jude JR, Knickerbocker GG: Closed-chest cardiac massage. JAMA 1960; 173: 1064

13. Redding JS, Pearson JW: Evaluation of drugs for cardiac resuscitation. Anesthesiology 1963; 24: 203

14. Rosamond W, Flegal K, Furie K, et al: Heart Disease and Stroke Statistics 2008 Update. A Report From the American Heart Association Statistics Committee and Stroke Statistics Subcommittee. Circulation 2008; 117: e25

15. Angelos M, Safar P, Reich H: A comparison of cardiopulmonary resuscitation with cardiopulmonary bypass after prolonged cardiac arrest in dogs: Reperfusion pressures and neurologic recovery. Resuscitation 1991; 21: 121

16. Kern KB, Sanders AB, Janas W et al: Limitations of open-chest cardiac massage after prolonged, untreated cardiac arrest in dogs. Ann Emerg Med 1991; 20: 761

17. Wik L, Steen PA, Bircher HB: Quality of bystander cardiopulmonary resuscitation influences outcome after prehospital cardiac arrest. Resuscitation 1994; 28: 195

18. Weaver WD, Cobb LA, Hallstrom AP et al: Factors influencing survival after out-of-hospital cardiac arrest. J Am Coll Cardiol 1986; 7: 752

19. Eisenberg MS, Copass MK, Halstrom AP et al: Treatment of out-of-hospital cardiac arrest with rapid defibrillation by emergency medical technicians. N Engl J Med 1980; 302: 1379

20. Weaver WD, Hill D, Fahrenbruch CE et al: Use of the automatic external defibrillator in the management of out-of-hospital cardiac arrest. N Engl J Med 1988; 319: 661

21. Valenzuela TD, Kern KB, Clark LL, et al: Interruptions of chest compressions during emergency medical systems resuscitation. Circulation 2005; 112: 1259

22. Nichol G, Stiell IG, Laupacis A, et al: A cumulative meta-analysis of the effectiveness of defibrillator-capable emergency medical services for victims of out-of-hospital cardiac arrest. Ann Emerg Med 2005; 46: 512

23. Nadkarni VM, Larkin GL, Peberdy MA, et al: First documented rhythm and clinical outcomes from in-hospital cardiac arrest among children and adults. JAMA 2006; 295: 50

24. Olsson GI, Hallen B: Cardiac arrest during anaesthesia: A computer-aided study of 250,543 anaesthetics. Acta Anaesthesiol Scand 1988; 32: 653

25. Cohen CB, Cohen PJ: Do-not-resuscitate orders in the operating room. N Engl J Med 1991; 325: 1879

26. Walker RM: DNR in the OR: Resuscitation as an operative risk. JAMA 1991; 266: 2407

27. Margolis JO, McGrath BJ, Kussin PS et al: Do no resuscitate (DNR) orders during surgery: Ethical foundations for institutional policies in the United States. Anesth Analg 1995; 80: 806

28. Guildner CW: Resuscitation. Opening the airway: A comparative study of techniques for opening an airway obstructed by the tongue. JACEP 1976; 5: 588

29. 2005 American Heart Association Guidelines for Cardiopulmonary Resuscitation and Emergency Cardiovascular Care. Circulation 2005; 112(suppl 24): IV1–IV203

30. Heimlich HJ: Pop goes the cafe coronary. Emerg Med 1974; 6: 154

31. Guildner CW, Williams D, Subtich T: Airway obstructed by foreign material: The Heimlich maneuver. JACEP 1976; 5: 675

32. Redding JS: The choking controversy: Critique of evidence on the Heimlich maneuver. Crit Care Med 1979; 7: 475

33. Sellick BA: Cricoid pressure to control regurgitation of stomach contents during induction of anaesthesia. Lancet 1961; 2: 404

34. Salem MR, Wong AY, Fizzotti GF: Efficacy of cricoid pressure in preventing aspiration of gastric contents in paediatric patients. Br J Anaesth 1972; 44: 401

35. Harrison RR, Maull KI, Keenan RL et al: Mouth-to-mask ventilation: A superior method of rescue breathing. Ann Emerg Med 1982; 11: 74

36. Jesudian MCS, Harrison RR, Keenan RL et al: Bag-valve-mask ventilation: Two rescuers are better than one: Preliminary report. Crit Care Med 1985; 13: 122

37. Babbs CF: New versus old theories of blood flow during CPR. Crit Care Med 1980; 8: 191

38. Jude JR, Kouwenhoven WB, Knickerbocker GG: Cardiac arrest: Report of application of external cardiac massage on 118 patients. JAMA 1961; 178: 1063

39. Criley JM, Blaufuss AH, Kissel GL: Cough-induced cardiac compression: Self-administered form of cardiopulmonary resuscitation. JAMA 1976; 236: 1246

40. Rudikoff MJ, Maughan WL, Effrom M et al: Mechanisms of blood flow during cardiopulmonary resuscitation. Circulation 1980; 61: 345

41. Holmes HR, Babbs CF, Voorhees WD et al: Influence of adrenergic drugs upon vital organ perfusion during CPR. Crit Care Med 1980; 8: 137

42. Michael JR, Guerci AD, Koehler RC et al: Mechanisms by which epinephrine augments cerebral and myocardial perfusion during cardiopulmonary resuscitation in dogs. Circulation 1984; 69: 822

43. Weil MH, Rackow EC, Trevino R et al: Difference in acid–base state between venous and arterial blood during cardiopulmonary resuscitation. N Engl J Med 1986; 315: 153

44. Kern KB, Carter AB, Showen RL et al: Twenty-four-hour survival in a canine model of cardiac arrest comparing three methods of manual cardiopulmonary resuscitation. J Am Coll Cardiol 1986; 7: 859

45. Kern KB, Carter AB, Showen RL et al: Comparison of mechanical techniques of cardiopulmonary resuscitation: Survival and neurologic outcome in dogs. Am J Emerg Med 1987; 5: 190

46. Kirscher JP, Fine EG, Weisfeld ML et al: Comparison of prehospital conventional and simultaneous compression–ventilation cardiopulmonary resuscitation. Crit Care Med 1989; 17: 1263

47. Babbs CF, Tacker WA: Cardiopulmonary resuscitation with interposed abdominal compression. Circulation 1986; 74(Suppl 4): 37

48. Mateer JF, Stueven HA, Thompson BM et al: Pre-hospital IAC-CPR versus standard CPR: Paramedic resuscitation of cardiac arrests. Am J Emerg Med 1985; 3: 143

49. Sack JB, Kesselbrenner MB, Bregman D: Survival from in-hospital cardiac arrest with interposed abdominal counterpulsation during cardiopulmonary resuscitation. JAMA 1992; 267: 379

50. Niemann JT, Rosborough JP, Criley JM et al: Circulatory support during cardiac arrest using a pneumatic vest and abdominal binder with simultaneous high pressure airway inflation. Ann Emerg Med 1984; 13: 767

51. Timerman S, Cardoso LF, Ramires JA et al: Improved hemodynamic performance with a novel chest compression device during treatment of in-hospital cardiac arrest. Resuscitation 2004; 61: 273

52. Lurie KG, Lindo C, Chin J: CPR: The P stands for plumber's helper (Letter). JAMA 1990; 264: 1661

53. Cohen TJ, Tucker KJ, Lurie KG et al: Active compression–decompression. A new method of cardiopulmonary resuscitation. JAMA 1992; 267: 2916

54. Linder KH, Pfenniger EG, Lurie KG et al: Effects of active compression–decompression resuscitation on myocardial and cerebral blood flow in pigs. Circulation 1993; 88: 1254

55. Lafuente-Lafuente C, Melero-Bascones M: Active chest compression–decompression for cardiopulmonary resuscitation. Cochrane Database Syst Rev. 2004; CD002751

56. Plaisance P, Lurie KG, Payen D: Inspiratory impedance during active compression–decompression cardiopulmonary resuscitation: a randomized evaluation in patients in cardiac arrest. Circulation 2000; 101: 989

57. Aufderheide TP, Pirrallo RG, Provo TA et al: Clinical evaluation of an inspiratory impedance threshold device during standard cardiopulmonary resuscitation in patients with out of hospital cardiac arrest. Crit Care Med 2005; 33: 734

58. Plaisance P, Lurie KG, Vicaut E, et al: Evaluation of an impedance threshold device in patients receiving active compression–decompression cardiopulmonary resuscitation for out of hospital cardic arrest. Resuscitation 2004; 61: 265

59. DeBehnke DJ, Angelos MG, Leasure JE: Comparison of standard external CPR, open-chest CPR, and cardiopulmonary bypass in a canine myocardial infarct model. Ann Emerg Med 1991; 20: 754

60. Sanders AB, Kern KB, Atlas M et al: Importance of the duration of inadequate coronary perfusion pressure on resuscitation from cardiac arrest. J Am Coll Cardiol 1985; 6: 113

61. Kern KB, Sanders AB, Badylak SF et al: Long term survival with open-chest cardiac massage after ineffective closed-chest compression in a canine preparation. Circulation 1987; 75: 498

62. Ralston SH, Voorhees WD, Babbs CF: Intrapulmonary epinephrine during prolonged CPR: Improved regional blood flow and resuscitation in dogs. Ann Emerg Med 1984; 13: 79

63. Crile G, Dolley DH: Experimental research into resuscitation of dogs killed by anesthetics and asphyxia. J Exp Med 1906; 8: 713

64. Redding JS: Abdominal compression in cardiopulmonary resuscitation. Anesth Analg 1971; 50: 668

65. Pearson JW, Redding JS: Influence of peripheral vascular tone on cardiac resuscitation. Anesth Analg 1965; 44: 746

66. Yakaitis RW, Otto CW, Blitt CD: Relative importance of alpha and beta adrenergic receptors during resuscitation. Crit Care Med 1979; 7: 293

67. Otto CW, Yakaitis RW, Blitt CD: Mechanism of action of epinephrine in resuscitation from asphyxial arrest. Crit Care Med 1981; 9: 321

68. Ditchey RV, Winkler JV, Rhodes CA: Relative lack of coronary blood flow during closed-chest resuscitation in dogs. Circulation 1982; 66: 297

69. Otto CW, Yakaitis RW: The role of epinephrine in CPR: A reappraisal. Ann Emerg Med 1984; 13: 840

70. Sanders AB, Ewy GA, Taft TV: Prognostic and therapeutic importance of the aortic diastolic pressure in resuscitation from cardiac arrest. Crit Care Med 1984; 12: 871

71. Niemann JT, Criley JM, Rosborough JP et al: Predictive indices of successful cardiac resuscitation after prolonged arrest and experimental cardiopulmonary resuscitation. Ann Emerg Med 1985; 14: 521

72. Paradis NA, Martin GB, Rivers EP et al: Coronary perfusion pressure and the return of spontaneous circulation in human cardiopulmonary resuscitation. JAMA 1990; 263: 1106

73. Kalenda Z: The capnogram as a guide to the efficacy of cardiac massage. Resuscitation 1978; 6: 259

74. Weil MH, Bisera J, Trevino RP: Cardiac output and end tidal carbon dioxide. Crit Care Med 1985; 13: 907

75. Sanders AB, Atlas M, Ewy GA et al: Expired PCO_2 as an index of coronary perfusion pressure. Am J Emerg Med 1985; 3: 147

76. Sanders AB, Ewy GA, Bragg S et al: Expired PCO_2 as a prognostic indicator of successful resuscitation from cardiac arrest. Ann Emerg Med 1985; 14: 948

77. Sanders AB, Kern KB, Otto CW et al: End-tidal carbon dioxide monitoring during cardiopulmonary resuscitation: A prognostic indicator for survival. JAMA 1989; 262: 1347

78. Levine RL, Wayne MA, Miller CC: End-tidal carbon dioxide and outcome of out-of-hospital cardiac arrest. N Engl J Med 1997; 337: 301

79. Kern KB, Sanders AB, Raife J et al: A study of chest compression rates during cardiopulmonary resuscitation in humans: The importance of rate-directed compressions. Arch Intern Med 1992; 152: 145

80. Otto CW: Cardiovascular pharmacology II: The use of catecholamines, pressor agents, digitalis, and corticosteroids in CPR and emergency cardiac care. Circulation 1986; 74(Suppl 4): 80

81. Redding JS, Pearson JW: Resuscitation from ventricular fibrillation (drug therapy). JAMA 1968; 203: 255

82. Schleien CL, Dean JM, Koehler RC et al: Effect of epinephrine on cerebral and myocardial perfusion in an infant animal preparation of cardiopulmonary resuscitation. Circulation 1986; 73: 809

83. Schleien CL, Koehler RC, Gervais H et al: Organ blood flow and somatosensory-evoked potentials during and after cardiopulmonary resuscitation with epinephrine or phenylephrine. Circulation 1989; 79: 1332

84. Otto CW, Yakaitis RW, Redding JS et al: Comparison of dopamine, dobutamine, and epinephrine in CPR. Crit Care Med 1981; 9: 640

85. Lindner KH, Prengel AW, Pfenniger EG et al: Vasopressin improves vital organ blood flow during closed-chest cardiopulmonary resuscitation in pigs. Circulation 1995; 91: 215

86. Brillman JC, Sanders AB, Otto CW et al: A comparison of epinephrine and phenylephrine for resuscitation and neurologic outcome of cardiac arrest in dogs. Ann Emerg Med 1987; 16: 11

87. Silvast T, Saarnivaara L, Kinnunen A et al: Comparison of adrenaline and phenylephrine in out-of-hospital CPR: A double-blind study. Acta Anaesthesiol Scand 1985; 29: 610

88. Linder KH, Ahnefeld FW, Prengel AW: Comparison of standard and high-dose adrenaline in the resuscitation of asystole and electromechanical dissociation. Acta Anaesthesiol Scand 1991; 35: 253

89. Stiell IB, Hebert PC, Weitzman BN et al: High-dose epinephrine in adult cardiac arrest. N Engl J Med 1992; 327: 1045

90. Brown CG, Martin DP, Pepe PE et al: A comparison of standard-dose and high-dose epinephrine in cardiac arrest outside the hospital. N Engl J Med 1992; 327: 1051

91. Callaham M, Madsen CD, Barton CW et al: A randomized clinical trial of high-dose epinephrine and norepinephrine vs standard-dose epinephrine in prehospital cardiac arrest. JAMA 1992; 268: 2667

92. Choux C, Gueugniaud P-Y, Barbieux A et al: Standard doses versus repeated high doses of epinephrine in cardiac arrest outside the hospital. Resuscitation 1995; 29: 3

93. Gueugniaud P-Y, Mols P, Goldstein P et al: A comparison of repeated high doses and repeated standard doses of epinephrine for cardiac arrest outside the hospital. N Engl J Med 1998; 339: 1595

94. Lipman J, Wilson W, Kobilski S et al: High-dose adrenaline in adult in-hospital asystolic cardiopulmonary resuscitation: A double-blind randomized trial. Anaesth Intensive Care 1993; 21: 192

95. Sherman BW, Munger MA, Foulke GE et al: High-dose versus standard-dose epinephrine treatment of cardiac arrest after failure of standard therapy. Pharmacotherapy 1997; 17: 242

96. Rivers EP, Wortsman J, Rady MY et al: The effect of the total cumulative epinephrine dose administered during human CPR on hemodynamic, oxygen transport, and utilization variables in the postresuscitation period. Chest 1994; 106: 1499

97. Behringer W, Kittler H, Sterz F et al: Cumulative epinephrine dose during cardiopulmonary resuscitation and neurologic outcome. Ann Intern Med 1998; 129: 450

98. Prengel AW, Lindner KH, Keller A et al: Cardiovascular function during the postresuscitation phase after cardiac arrest in pigs: A comparison of epinephrine versus vasopressin. Crit Care Med 1996; 24: 2014

99. Lindner KH, Dirks B, Strohmenger HU et al: Randomized comparison of epinephrine and vasopressin in patients with out of hospital ventricular fibrillation. Lancet 1997; 349: 535

100. Stiell IG, Hebert PC, Wells GA et al: Vasopressin versus epinephrine for in hospital cardiac arrest: A randomized controlled trial. Lancet 2001; 358: 105

101. Wenzel V, Krismer AC, Arntz HR et al: A comparison of vasopressin and epinephrine for out-of-hospital cardiopulmonary resuscitation. N Engl J Med 2004; 350: 105

102. Kowey PR, Levine JH, Herre JM et al: Randomized, double-blind comparison of intravenous amiodarone and bretylium in the treatment of patients with recurrent hemodynamically destabilizing ventricular tachycardia or fibrillation. Circulation 1995; 92: 3255

103. Kudenchuk PJ, Cobb LA, Copass MK et al: Amiodarone for resuscitation after out of hospital cardiac arrest due to ventricular fibrillation. N Engl J Med 1999; 341: 871

104. Dorian P, Cass D, Schwartz B et al: Amiodarone as compared with lidocaine for shock-resistant ventricular fibrillation. N Engl J Med 2002; 346: 884

105. Stueven HA, Tonsfeldt DJ, Thompson BM et al: Atropine in asystole: Human studies. Ann Emerg Med 1984; 13: 815

106. Coon GA, Clinton JE, Ruiz E: Use of atropine for brady-asystolic prehospital cardiac arrest. Ann Emerg Med 1981; 10: 462

107. O'Rourke GW, Greene NM: Autonomic blockade and the resting heart rate in man. Am Heart J 1970; 80: 469

108. Guerci AD, Chandra N, Johnson E et al: Failure of sodium bicarbonate to improve resuscitation from ventricular fibrillation in dogs. Circulation 1986; 74(Suppl 4): 75

109. Federiuk CS, Sanders AB, Kern KB et al: The effect of bicarbonate on resuscitation from cardiac arrest. Ann Emerg Med 1991; 20: 1173

110. Bishop RL, Weisfeldt ML: Sodium bicarbonate administration during cardiac arrest: Effect on arterial pH, P_{CO_2}, and osmolality. JAMA 1976; 235: 506

111. Mattar JA, Weil MH, Shubin H et al: Cardiac arrest in the critically ill: II. Hyperosmolal states following cardiac arrest. Am J Med 1974; 56: 162

112. Sanders AB, Otto CW, Kern KB et al: Acid–base balance in a canine model of cardiac arrest. Ann Emerg Med 1988; 17: 667

113. Kette F, Weil MH, von Planta MS et al: Buffer agents do not reverse intramyocardial acidosis during cardiac resuscitation. Circulation 1990; 81: 1660

114. Dembo DH: Calcium in advanced life support. Crit Care Med 1981; 9: 358

115. Harrison EE, Amey BD: The use of calcium in cardiac resuscitation. Am J Emerg Med 1983; 1: 267

116. Stueven HA, Thompson BM, Aprahamian C et al: Use of calcium in prehospital cardiac arrest. Ann Emerg Med 1983; 12: 136

117. Stueven HA, Thompson BM, Aprahamian C et al: Calcium chloride: Reassessment of use in asystole. Ann Emerg Med 1984; 13: 820

118. Stueven HA, Thompson BM, Aprahamian C et al: Lack of effectiveness of calcium chloride in refractory asystole. Ann Emerg Med 1985; 14: 630

119. Kerber RE, Sarnat W: Factors influencing the success of ventricular defibrillation in man. Circulation 1979; 60: 226

120. Yakaitis RW, Ewy GA, Otto CW et al: Influence of time and therapy on ventricular defibrillation in dogs. Crit Care Med 1980; 8: 157

121. Weaver WD, Copass MD, Bufi D et al: Improved neurologic recovery and survival after early defibrillation. Circulation 1984; 69: 943

122. Weaver WD, Cobb LA, Dennis D et al: Amplitude of ventricular fibrillation waveform and outcome after cardiac arrest. Ann Intern Med 1985; 102: 53

123. Ewy GA, Dahl CF, Zimmermann M et al: Ventricular fibrillation masquerading as ventricular standstill. Crit Care Med 1981; 9: 841

124. Stewart AJ, Allen JD, Adgey AAJ: Frequency analysis of ventricular fibrillation and resuscitation success. Q J Med 1992; 306: 761

125. Brown CG, Griffith RF, Ligten PV et al: Median frequency—a new parameter for predicting defibrillation success rate. Ann Emerg Med 1991; 20: 787

126. Strohmenger HU, Lindner KH, Brown CG: Analysis of the ventricular fibrillation ECG signal amplitude and frequency parameters as predictors of countershock success in human. Chest 1997; 111: 584

127. Povoas HP, Weil MH, Tang W et al: Predicting the success of defibrillation by electrocardiographic analysis. Resuscitation 2002; 53: 77

128. Stromenger HU, Eftestol T, Sunde K et al: The predictive value of ventricular fibrillation electrocardiogram signal frequency and amplitude variables in patients with out-of-hospital cardiac arrest. Anesth Analg 2001; 93: 1428

129. Otto CW, Yakaitis RW, Ewy GA: Effects of epinephrine on defibrillation in ischemic ventricular fibrillation. Am J Emerg Med 1985; 3: 285

130. Cummins RO, Eisenberg MS, Bergner L et al: Sensitivity, accuracy and safety of an automatic external defibrillator: Report of a field evaluation. Lancet 1984; 1: 318

131. Cummins RO, Eisenberg MS, Graves JR et al: Automatic external defibrillators used by emergency medical technicians: A controlled clinical trial. Circulation 1985; 72(Suppl 3): 8

132. Kerber RE, Kouba C, Marines J et al: Advance prediction of transthoracic impedance in human defibrillation and cardioversion: Importance of impedance in determining the success of low energy shocks. Circulation 1984; 70: 303

133. Kerber RE, McPherson D, Charbonnier R et al: Automatic impedance-based energy adjustment for defibrillation: Experimental studies. Circulation 1985; 71: 136

134. Lerman BB, DeMarco JP, Haines DE: Current-based versus energy-based ventricular defibrillation: A prospective study. J Am Coll Cardiol 1988; 12: 1259

135. Kerber RE, Grayzel J, Hoyt R et al: Transthoracic resistance in human defibrillation: Influence of body weight, chest size, serial shocks, paddle size and paddle contact pressure. Circulation 1981; 63: 676

136. Connel PN, Ewy GA, Dahl CF et al: Transthoracic impedance to defibrillation discharge: Effect of electrode size and electrode-chest wall interface. J Electrocardiol 1973; 6: 313

137. Ewy GA, Taren D: Comparison of paddle electrode pastes used for defibrillation. Heart Lung 1977; 6: 847

138. Ewy GA, Hellman DA, McClung S et al: Influence of ventilation phase on transthoracic impedance and defibrillation effectiveness. Crit Care Med 1980; 8: 164

139. Dahl CF, Ewy GA, Warner ED et al: Myocardial necrosis from direct current countershock. Circulation 1974; 50: 956

140. Warner ED, Dahl CF, Ewy GA: Myocardial injury from transthoracic defibrillator countershock. Arch Pathol 1975; 99: 55

141. Ehsani A, Ewy GA, Sobel BE: Effects of electrical countershock on serum creatine phosphokinase (CPK) isoenzyme activity. Am J Cardiol 1976; 37: 12

142. Weaver WD, Cobb LA, Copass MK et al: Ventricular defibrillation: A comparative trial using 175-J and 320-J shocks. N Engl J Med 1982; 307: 1101

143. Geddes LA, Tacker WA, Rosborough JP et al: Electrical dose for ventricular defibrillation of large and small animals using precordial electrodes. J Clin Invest 1974; 53: 310

144. Gutgesell HP, Tacker WA, Geddes LA et al: Energy dose for defibrillation in children. Pediatrics 1976; 58: 898

145. Kerber RE, Sarnat W: Factors influencing the success of ventricular defibrillation in man. Circulation 1979; 60: 226

146. Kerber RE, Jensen SR, Gascho JA et al: Determinants of defibrillation: Prospective analysis of 183 patients. Am J Cardiol 1983; 52: 739

147. American Heart Association: Guidelines 2000 for Cardiopulmonary Resuscitation and Emergency Cardiovascular Care: International Consensus on Science. Circulation 2000; 102(8): I-1

148. Bardy GH, Marchlinski FE, Sharma AD et al: Multicenter comparison of truncated biphasic shocks and standard damped sine wave monophasic shocks for transthoracic ventricular defibrillation. Circulation 1996; 94: 2507

149. Rea TD, Eisenberg MS, Becker LJ et al: Temporal trends in sudden cardiac arrest: a 25-year emergency medical services perspective. Circulation 2003; 107: 2780

150. Ewy GA: Cardiocerebral resuscitation: the new cardiopulmonary resuscitation. Circulation 2005; 111: 2134

151. Ewy GA, Kern KB, Sanders AB et al: Cardiocerebral resuscitation for cardiac arrest. Am J Med 2006; 119: 6

152. Weisfeldt ML, Becker LB: Resuscitation after cardiac arrest: a 3-phase time-sensitive model. JAMA 2002; 288: 3035

153. Caffrey SL, Willoughby PJ, Pepe PE et al: Public use of automated external defibrillators. N Engl J Med 2002; 347: 1242

154. Valenzulea TD, Roe DJ, Nichol G et al: Outcomes of rapid defibrillation by security officers after cardiac arrest in casinos. N Engl J Med 2000; 343: 1206

155. Kern, KB, Garewal HS, Sanders AB et al: Depletion of myocardial adenosine triphosphate during prolonged untreated ventricular fibrillation: effect on defibrillation success. Resuscitation 1990; 20: 221

156. Ornato JP, Hallagan LF, McMahan SB et al: Attitudes of BCLS instructors about mouth-to-mouth resuscitation during the AIDS epidemic. Ann Emerg Med 1990; 19: 151

157. Brenner BE, Kauffman J: Reluctance of internists and medical nurses to perform mouth-to-mouth resuscitation. Arch Intern Med 1993; 153: 1763

158. Locke CJ, Berg RA, Sanders AB et al: Bystander cardiopulmonary resuscitation: Concerns about mouth-to-mouth contact. Arch Intern Med 1995; 155: 938

159. Bossaert L, Van Hoeyweghen R: The cerebral resuscitation study group: Bystander cardiopulmonary resuscitation (CPR) in out-of-hospital cardiac arrest. Resuscitation 1989; 17(Suppl): S55

160. Van Hoeyweghen RJ, Bossaert LL, Mullie A et al: Quality and efficiency of bystander CPR. Resuscitation 1993; 26: 47

161. Nagao K et al for the SOS-KANTO study group: Cardiopulmonary resuscitation by bystanders with chest compression only (SOS-KANTO): an observational study. The Lancet 2007; 369: 920

162. Berg RA, Kern KB, Sanders AB et al: Bystander cardiopulmonary resuscitation: Is ventilation necessary? Circulation 1993; 88: 1907

163. Berg RA, Wilcoxson D, Hilwig RW et al: The need for ventilatory support during bystander cardiopulmonary resuscitation. Ann Emerg Med 1995; 26: 342

164. Berg RA, Kern KB, Hilwig RW et al: Assisted ventilation does not improve outcome in a porcine model of single-rescuer bystander cardiopulmonary resuscitation. Circulation 1997; 95: 1635

165. Berg RA, Kern KB, Hilwig RW et al: Assisted ventilation during 'bystander' CPR in a swine acute myocardial infarction model does not improve outcome. Circulation 1997; 96: 4364

166. Assar D, Chamberlain D, Colquhoun M et al: Randomized controlled trials of staged teaching for basic life support: 1. skill acquisition at bronze stage. Resuscitation 2000; 45: 7

PERIOPERATIVE AND CONSULTATIVE SERVICES

167. Kern KB, Hilwig R, Berg RA et al: Importance of continuous chest compressions during cardiopulmonary resuscitation: improved outcome during a simulated single lay-rescuer scenario. Circulation 2002; 105: 645

168. Ewy GA, Zuercher M, Hilwig RW, et al: Improved neurological outcome with continuous chest compressions compared with 30: 2 compressions-to-ventilations cardiopulmonary resuscitation in a realistic swine model of out-of-hospital cardiac arrest. Circulation 2007; 116: 2525

169. Sayre MR, Berg RA, Cave DM et al: Hands-Only (Compression-Only) cardiopulmonary resuscitation: A call to action for bystander response to adults who experience out-of-hospital sudden cardiac arrest. A science advisory for the public from the American Heart Association Emergency Cardiovascular Care Committee. Circulation 2008; 117(16): 2162

170. Berg RA, Sanders AB, Kern KB et al: Adverse hemodynamic effects of interrupting chest compressions for rescue breathing during cardiopulmonary resuscitation for ventricular fibrillation cardiac arrest. Circulation 2001; 104: 2465

171. Wik L, Kramer-Johansen J, Myklebust H et al: Quality of cardiopulmonary resuscitation during out-of-hospital cardiac arrest. JAMA 2005; 293: 299

172. Valenzuela TD, Kern KB, Clark LL et al: Interruptions of chest compressions during emergency medical systems resuscitations. Circulation 2005; 112: 1259

173. Aufderheide TP, Sigudsson G, Pirrallo RG et al: Hyperventilation-induced hypotension during cardiopulmonary resuscitation. Circulation 2004; 109: 1960

174. Aufderheide TP, Lurie K: Death by hyperventilation: a common and life-threatening problem during cardiopulmonary resuscitation. Crit Care Med 2004; 32 (Suppl): S345

175. Milander MM, Hiscok PS, Sanders AB et al: Chest compression and ventilation during cardiopulmonary resuscitation: the effects of audible tone guidance. Acad Emerg Med 1995; 2: 708

176. Cobb LA, Fahrenbruch CE, Walsh TR et al: Influence of CPR prior to defibrillation in out-of-hospital ventricular fibrillation. JAMA 1999; 281: 1182

177. Wik L, Hansen TB, Fylling F et al: Delaying defibrillation to give basic cardiopulmonary resuscitation to patients with out-of-hospital ventricular fibrillation. JAMA 2003; 289: 1389

178. Berg RA, Hilwig RE, Kern KB et al: Automated external defibrillation versus manual defibrillation for prolonged ventricular fibrillation: lethal delays of chest compressions before and after countershocks. Ann Emerg Med 2003; 41: 458

179. Rea Td, Shah S, Kudenchuck PJ et al: Automated external defibrillators: To what extent does the algorithm delay CPR? Ann Emerg Med 2005; 46: 132

180. Kellum MJ, Kennedy KW, Ewy GA: Cardiocerebral resuscitation improves survival of patients with out-of-hospital cardiac arrest. Am J Med 2006; 119: 335

181. Kellum MJ, Kennedy KW, Barney R, et al: Cardiocerebral resuscitation improves neurologically intact survival of patients with out-of-hospital cardiac arrest. Ann Emerg Med 2008;52:253

182. Bobrow BJ, Clark LL, Ewy GA, et al: Minimally interrupted cardiac resuscitation by emergency medical services for out-of-hospital cardiac arrest. JAMA 2008; 299: 1158

183. Abramson NS, Safar P, Detre KM et al: Randomized clinical study of cardiopulmonary-cerebral resuscitation: Thiopental loading in comatose cardiac arrest survivors. N Engl J Med 1986; 314: 397

184. Brain Resuscitation Clinical Trial II Study Group: A randomized clinical study of a calcium-entry blocker (lidoflazine) in the treatment of comatose survivors of cardiac arrest. N Engl J Med 1991; 324: 1225

185. Holzer M: The Hypothermia After Cardiac Arrest Study Group: Mild therapeutic hypothermia to improve the neurologic outcome after cardiac arrest. N Engl J Med 2002; 346: 549

186. Bernard SA, Gray TW, Buist MD et al: Treatment of comatose survivors of out-of-hospital cardiac arrest with induced hypothermia. N Engl J Med 2002; 346: 557

187. Longstreth WT, Diehr P, Inui TS: Prediction of awakening after out-of-hospital cardiac arrest. N Engl J Med 1983; 308: 1378

188. Longstreth WT, Inui TS, Cobb LA et al: Neurologic recovery after out-of-hospital cardiac arrest. Ann Intern Med 1983; 98: 588

CHAPTER 60 ■ DISASTER PREPAREDNESS

MICHAEL J. MURRAY

KEY POINTS

1 The term *mass casualty* refers to a large number of injuries or deaths that occur in a short period and have the potential to exceed the capabilities of local facilities.

2 By having hospitals be prepared, the Joint Commission on Accreditation of Healthcare Organizations hopes to reduce the appeal to terrorists of using weapons of mass destruction as an effective means of warfare and to help communities better respond to natural disasters.

3 Community-wide emergency response plans are in place in some large cities, but the majority of metropolitan areas do not have such an organizational structure, and many hospitals and physicians are waiting for someone to take the first step in organizing such a response plan.

4 Whereas emergency preparedness is a way of life in many countries (e.g., Israel), it very much needs to become much more a part of life in the United States than it is today.

5 After the basics are established, the most important aspect of managing a mass casualty event, again whether it is natural, unintentional, or intentional, is having a command and control structure with which everyone is familiar.

6 As part of the emergency response, the health care system and its leaders must identify communication and information needs.

7 A medical disaster from the perspective of a health care organization is any unplanned event that is beyond the normal response resources of the entity and would require the response of outside resources and assistance for recovery.

8 The initial response to any disaster, whether natural, unintended, or terrorist-initiated, begins at the local level and involves firefighters, paramedics, and law enforcement agencies, especially if criminal activity is suspected.

9 The Federal Emergency Management Agency, now within the Department of Homeland Security, is the lead agency for management assistance to state and local governments, providing emergency relief to affected individuals and businesses, decontaminating affected areas, and helping to ensure public health safety.

10 Ideally, anesthesiologists or other health care providers who had an adequate supply of an opioid antagonist, such as naloxone, would have been readily available and present at the tragedy at the Nord-Ost Theater in Moscow in 2002 to manage both hostages and the terrorists themselves. Unfortunately, this was not the case.

11 The ideal biologic agent is one that has the greatest potential for adverse public health impact, generating mass casualties and with the potential for easy large-scale dissemination that could cause mass hysteria and civil disruption.

12 It is unlikely that an intensive care unit physician or anesthesiologist would be at the initial site of origin of a biologic attack, but it could happen. Most likely, physicians will become involved if the hospital at which they work ultimately provides care for a number of patients exposed to a biologic agent.

13 Treatment for cyanide toxicity is another problem for which anesthesiologists are quite familiar because of their use of nitroprusside, which, at high doses and for extended periods of time, also releases cyanide ions, which can poison the cellular respiration. Cyanide ions are normally metabolized by the rhodanese enzyme in the liver, which is a sulfur-requiring step that leads to the bioformation of methemoglobin.

MASS CASUALTY RESPONSE

Hurricane Katrina, 9/11, Sago mine, and SARS. These terms have entered our national consciousness, connoting vivid images of tragic circumstances. Although we cannot control or even predict the source of the next major disaster in the United States—it is far more likely to be Mother Nature and not an international terrorist who will be the force behind the destruction—we can control our preparedness and, therefore, our response to situations that result in mass casualties. As anesthesiologists, we have a responsibility not only to know our institution's disaster plan and our role therein, but also to prepare our family members and ourselves so that we do not become unintended victims of the next disaster.

❶ The term *mass casualty* refers to a large number of injuries or deaths that occur in a short period and have the potential to exceed the capabilities of local facilities. Mass-casualty incidents include naturally occurring as well as intentional or unintentional events (Table 60-1). Bombings or radiologic, biologic, and chemical attacks comprise the most likely intentional events, with industrial accidents, vehicle collisions, the collapse of stadiums or other public structures, and fires making up the most commonly encountered unintentional events.

Joint Commission on Accreditation of Healthcare Organizations

Following the events of September 11, 2001, and subsequent anthrax attacks, the Joint Commission on Accreditation of

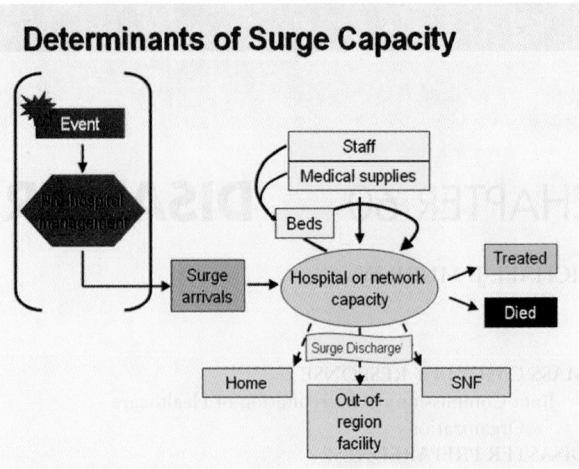

FIGURE 60-1. SNF: Skilled Nursing Facility. Published with permission: Nathaniel Hupert, MD, MPH, "Addressing Surge Capacity in a Mass Casualty Event" Web Conference, broadcast on October 26, 2004. Agency for Healthcare Research and Quality, Rockville, MD. Available at http://www.ahrg.gov/news/ulp/btsurgemass/.

Healthcare Organizations (JCAHO) published a white paper to help hospitals develop systems to create and sustain community-wide emergency preparedness.[1] Health care delivery in the United States over the last several years and decades, reflective of similar problems faced worldwide, has left the health care system underfunded, with limited resources[2] and ever-increasing demand, such that the surge capacity (Fig. 60-1) to handle major emergencies is limited.[3] Furthermore, despite the best efforts of the JCAHO and the American Hospital Association, as of 2004 only 9% of hospitals have tested their emer-
❷ gency preparedness as far as the components considered essential to an emergency response.[4] By having hospitals be prepared, the JCAHO hopes to reduce the appeal to terrorists of using weapons of mass destruction as an effective means of warfare and to help communities better respond to natural disasters. The JCAHO white paper focuses on three major areas:

1. Enlisting the community to develop the local response
2. Focusing on the key aspects of the system that prepare the community to mobilize to care for patients, protect its staff, and serve the public
3. Establishing the accountabilities, oversight, leadership, and sustainment of a community-preparedness system

The JCAHO guidelines are neither mandatory nor required by law, yet all hospitals aspire to acquire and maintain JCAHO accreditation. From that perspective, the white paper was an important step in helping prepare the medical community to deal with catastrophic events that could inundate the health care system. Anesthesiologists must be familiar with what their hospitals have done to comply with the JCAHO standards, in anticipation of what their roles may be in case of a mass casualty event.

Enlisting the Community to Develop the Local Response

In the past, the JCAHO required that hospitals test their disaster plans twice a year. Organizations often went through the motions without truly embracing the idea of planning for a catastrophe; even these minimal events did have benefit if the hospital was confronted with an actual disaster. However, with the Oklahoma City, the World Trade Centers, and the Pentagon bombings and the anthrax attacks of 2001 and 2002, the

---

TABLE 60-1

TYPES OF DISASTERS

■ **NATURAL**

Meterologic
Hurricanes
Tornados
Floods
Mudslides
Extreme heat or cold
Earthquakes
Forest fires

Geologic
Earthquakes
Tsunamis
Volcanic eruptions
Lahores

Biologic
Bacterial
Viral

■ **RESULTING FROM HUMAN ACTIVITY**

Unintentional
Airplane/train/bus crash
Boat sinking
Fire
Nuclear accident
Industrial accident
Building collapse/sports stadium disaster

Intentional
Bombing
Radiologic
Biologic
Chemical

TABLE 60-2

2004 EMERGENCY MANAGEMENT STANDARDS OF THE JOINT COMMISSION ON ACCREDITATION OF HEALTHCARE ORGANIZATIONS HOSPITAL ACCREDITATION STANDARDS ③

1. A management plan that addresses emergency management (Standards EC.4.10-4.110)
   - Four phases of emergency management activities
     - Mitigation
     - Preparedness
     - Response
     - Recovery
2. Hazard vulnerability analysis
   - Establish emergency procedures in response to a hazard vulnerability analysis
   - Define the organization's role with that of other community agencies
   - Notify external authorities of emergencies
   - Notify hospital personnel when emergency procedures are initiated
   - Assign available personnel to cover necessary positions
   - The following activities must be managed
     - Patient/resident activities
     - Staff activities
     - Staff/family support
     - Logistics of critical supplies
     - Security
     - Evacuation of the facility if necessary
     - Establish internal/external communication systems
     - Establish an orientation/education program
     - Monitor ongoing drills and real emergencies
     - Determine how an annual evaluation will occur
     - Provide alternate means of meeting essential building and utility needs
     - Identify radioactive and biologic isolation decontamination sites
     - Clarify alternate responsibility of personnel
3. Involved community-wide response
4. Re-establish and continue operations following a disaster

JCAHO recognized how deficient the plans of most hospitals were. By serendipity, prior to the events of 2001, the JCAHO had been reworking its disaster preparedness standards; their requirements were introduced in January 2002 and have been updated since then (Table 60-2). Central to these standards is the recognition that the initial response must occur on a local level. Communities and hospitals will have to be prepared to handle whatever they are confronted with during the first 24 to 72 hours after a disaster, as occurred following Hurricane Katrina on the Mississippi and Louisiana Gulf Coast. A better framework for integrating community resources and developing the means to deploy those resources is essential.

The aforementioned terrorist events of 2001 and 2002, the 2001 Houston flood, and the 2005 Hurricane Katrina experiences underscored the fact that health care provider organizations need to communicate more effectively with one another. There traditionally has been poor communication among law enforcement agencies, fire and rescue services, and emergency medical services. The medical community does no better in communicating with the public health community. They have different priorities: the medical community focuses on the individual, and public health personnel focus on the community at large. As is often the case, rarely have these five "agencies" come together to prepare a community-wide response, often expecting the local, state, or federal government to provide coordination. The experience in New Orleans underscores how

flawed those expectations were and are. There is a fundamental need to formalize an organization of community resources, of which hospitals and physicians are but one component.

Community-wide emergency response plans are in place in some large cities, but the majority of metropolitan areas do not have such an organizational structure, and many hospitals[4] and physicians are waiting for someone to take the first step in organizing such a response plan. The JCAHO, in publicizing its white paper, hopes to stimulate hospitals and hospital leadership to both initiate a discussion of the responsibility of "the community" in preparing a response and forge new partnerships in addressing this critical need. Progress has been made, but much more needs to be done.

New York City is one such place where a hospital association, the Greater New York Hospital Association, has taken a leadership role in forging a cross-disciplinary, cross-jurisdictional partnership to prepare an integrated response plan to any future disaster. New York City obviously has a vested interest in doing so. Not only New Yorkers, but the entire world watched the World Trade Center buildings collapse, and the anthrax attacks affected people in several states in addition to New York; these attacks received widespread media coverage.

Although the average layperson may conclude that the New York health care system responded adequately to the events of 9/11 and to the anthrax attacks, multiple lessons were learned, and the reality is that the health care system was not significantly challenged. New York City (as well as Oklahoma City with the bombing of the Federal Building on April 19, 1995) had a much higher fatality rate than is normal for mass casualties, in which the ratio of casualties to fatalities is typically between 5 and 10 to 1. In New York City and Oklahoma City, however, the ratio was reversed, with approximately 10 fatalities for every 1 casualty. In the post hoc analysis, multiple problems were identified, and the revised New York City disaster plan responded to these problems in anticipation of adequately addressing them in the future. Communications were one major problem that needed resolution. In New York City on 9/11, pilots in helicopters recognized shortly after the south tower collapsed that the north tower would also collapse, and they radioed that warning to rescuers on the ground 21 minutes before the building fell. The message was relayed to police over their radios, and most managed to escape. Unfortunately, firefighter radios used a different frequency and did not pick up the warning, and at least 121 firefighters died, a number that might have been attenuated if there had been better communication links between police and firefighters.[5] As the building fell, the entire telecommunications infrastructure in the area became nonfunctional. Communication throughout most of lower Manhattan had to take place person-to-person or with hand-delivered notes within and between hospitals.

The anthrax letters of October 2001 were the first bioterrorism attack in this country to which the Centers for Disease Control and Prevention (CDC) had to respond. Twenty-two cases were confirmed or suspected—11 inhalation and 11 cutaneous attacks—with 5 deaths. The first diagnosis of anthrax was made by a physician who suspected the disease; this was confirmed by a laboratory technician who had been trained in bioterrorism preparedness. But the general unfamiliarity of many health care professionals with biologic agents contributed to misdiagnoses and delayed treatment for some patients. Even when the diagnosis was made, personnel at hospitals and health care agencies were reluctant to notify others. After the Brentwood postal worker was diagnosed at a hospital in the District of Columbia and the case was reported to public health care officials, the latter did not immediately act to notify other area hospitals.[2] It seems incredible that, just months after the attacks on the World Trade Centers, people were still doubtful that the United States could be attacked with a biologic weapon.

4 Whereas emergency preparedness is a way of life in many countries (e.g., Israel), it very much needs to become much more a part of life in the United States than it is today. What we need to do as health care leaders is to call the first meeting to prepare a community response or, if a community response already exists, become familiar with the plan. Community planning needs to occur and the results of that planning need to be widely disseminated to as many potential partners in implementing the plan as possible.

Focusing on the Key Aspects of the System that Prepares the Community Health Care Resources to Mobilize to Care for Patients, Protect Its Staff, and Serve the Public

To respond to a mass casualty event, an emergency medical system must be able to assess and expand its surge capacity—that is, its ability to provide care for and transport countless numbers of patients to facilities with appropriate capacity, resources, and staff. To anticipate surge capacity, one must know the number and location of potential beds that are available for patients,[6] and what space is designated and available for triaging patients, decontaminating patients, and providing first aid and more comprehensive care. Because many emergency departments are already overwhelmed and because we have fewer hospitals today than we had 10 years ago, the U.S. health care system has less surge capacity. However, we need to be proactive, recognize that standards may change, and plan accordingly. Patients may be cared for in hallways, and decontamination may not even take place in the hospital. It may be best done outside the hospital, for example, near a loading dock or in an emptied parking lot between two fire trucks.

An attack with a biologic agent may test the system in other ways—not through an acute event with an overwhelming number of patients in just a few hours, but by the presence of an increasing number of patients, depending on the type of agent and the dispersal means, that expands almost exponentially over days.[3] In such an event, as occurred during the 1918 Spanish influenza epidemic, sports arenas may be converted to become improvised health care facilities (Fig. 60-2).

To preserve the functionality of the system, staff members must also protect themselves. In the Tokyo sarin attacks of 1995, several health care providers were contaminated with sarin when they cared for patients who had not been deconta-

minated,[7] thereby becoming patients themselves and further burdening the health care system. Similarly, in Canada and in several countries in Asia, in caring for patients with severe acute respiratory syndrome (SARS), not only did many health care providers become patients, but several became fatalities.[8] To maintain surge capacity, it is imperative that all health care providers recognize the importance of protecting themselves.

Also in these situations, one cannot forget about the patients for whom one is already caring. Patients who are well enough must be discharged immediately, but more critically ill patients may need to be moved to other hospitals. This may occur if a hospital is inundated with patients from a disaster, or as a result of the hospital being affected by the catastrophe, such as occurred in Houston during the 2001 flood[9] or in Florida in 2004 when some hospitals lost power and patients had to be transported elsewhere. Transferring patients to other hospitals is not necessarily easy, as evidenced by what happened in New Orleans after Hurricane Katrina. Independent of weather, though, other issues, such as availability of emergency transport vehicles, the number of patients who need to be transported, hospital access, and the viability of the highway infrastructure, may impede transfer. Whether it is an internal or external incident, hospitals need to have plans and agreements in place in anticipation of future emergencies.[10]

5 After the basics are established, the most important aspect of managing a mass casualty event, again whether it is natural, unintentional, or intentional, is having a command and control structure with which everyone is familiar.[11] In the Northridge earthquake in California in 1994, many health care providers coming into the hospital, which lacked electricity and which was severely damaged itself, had difficulty finding the command and control center so that efforts were not coordinated and were slow to be implemented.

Health care providers also need to be concerned not only about their personal safety, but about their psychological safety, and should have plans in place for their families, should the providers be required to stay at hospitals for an extended length of time.[12]

In addressing these issues, the public must be mobilized to participate in the response. Israelis are far more involved in their country's disaster management plan than is the average American.[13]

6 Finally, as part of the emergency response, the health care system and its leaders must identify communication and information needs. During the synagogue and business bombings in Istanbul, Turkey, in 2003,[14] the hospital at which most victims were admitted was ill-prepared to handle the information needs of multiple governments, their health care agencies, and their intelligence and law enforcement agencies.

Hospitals and health care providers must be able to manage not only the external, but also the internal communication needs of the hospital and must have a plan to address them, especially should any aspect of the system fail, as occurred at the World Trade Center site on September 11, 2001. Finally, one must test, learn, improve, and be ready to address deficiencies in the plan. JCAHO requires two drills annually, with one of them expected to be a community-wide drill.[15] These situations provide health care providers an opportunity to hone their skills and anticipate problems they might confront in the future in dealing with natural disasters and terrorist attacks.

Establishing the Accountabilities, Oversight, Leadership, and Sustainment of a Community Preparedness System

At this level, most of the responsibility for preparedness is with local, state, and federal governments and with hospitals and hospital organizations. As physicians, anesthesiologists should be familiar with the clinical competencies for emergency pre-

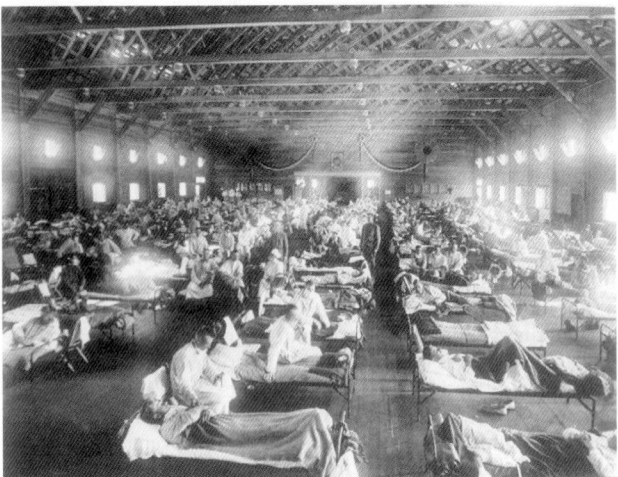

FIGURE 60-2. NCP 1603 - Emergency hospital during influenza epidemic, Camp Funston, Kansas. Courtesy of the National Museum of Health and Medicine, Armed Forces Institute of Pathology, Washington, D.C.

TABLE 60-3

TABLE 60-3

CLINICAL COMPETENCIES FOR CLINICIANS AND EMERGENCY PREPAREDNESS

Clinicians should be able to:
1. Describe their role in the emergency response
2. Respond to an emergency event within the emergency management system
3. Recognize an illness or injury as potentially resulting from exposure to weapons of mass destruction
4. Institute appropriate steps to limit the spread of the offending agent
5. Report identified cases or events through the public health care system
6. Initiate patient care within their professional skills[a]
7. Use reliable information sources
8. Provide reliable information to others
9. Communicate risks and actions to patients
10. Identify and manage expected stress anxiety
11. Participate in postevent feedback (after action report)

[a]Remain mindful of the fact that anyone can provide rudimentary first aid if that is what is needed in the situation.
Modified from Teachers of Preventive Medicine and Centers for Disease Control and Prevention: clinician competencies for emergency preparedness and bioterrorism.

TABLE 60-5

FATALITIES FROM NATURAL DISASTERS

■ NATURAL DISASTER	■ DATE OF OCCURRENCE	■ NUMBER OF FATALITIES
Bangladesh floods	November 12, 1970	300,000
Indian Ocean tsunami	December 26, 2004	155,000
Bam, Iran, earthquake	December 26, 2003	41,000
Galveston hurricane	September 8, 1900	6,000
Mount St. Helen volcanic eruption	May 18, 1980	57

paredness in bioterrorism developed through the Association of Teachers of Preventive Medicine in collaboration with the CDC (Table 60-3).[16]

DISASTER PREPAREDNESS

Over the last several years, a number of governmental and civilian agencies have become more involved and active in emergency preparedness (Table 60-4). A medical disaster from the perspective of a health care organization is any unplanned event that is beyond the normal response resources of the entity and would require the response of outside resources and assistance for recovery. However, the initial response is always local; it will take hours, if not days, to mobilize these resources. Hospitals, whether small or large, must be prepared to handle the initial influx of patients or casualties, obviously with a plan that focuses on any potential disaster that could occur in their area; for example, health care facilities on the Gulf Coast should be prepared for hurricanes, whereas those on the West Coast should be prepared for earthquakes (Table 60-1). Although we recognize the critical importance for planning for and preparing

to deal with the use of weapons of mass destruction, the reality is that we are much more likely to have to manage patients who are victims of natural and human-caused disasters, many of which will have profound effects on health care facilities. These are most often related to extreme weather, earthquakes, and industrial accidents (Table 60-1).[17]

Among weather-related events, tsunamis, hurricanes, tropical storms, and tornadoes are the most likely to wreak havoc, creating mass casualty situations (Table 60-5). Hurricane Katrina, which came ashore over Louisiana and Mississippi in 2005, killed 1,833 people in the United States, injured many more, left hundreds of thousands homeless, created more than $40 billion in insured losses alone, and severely compromised hospitals' and the government's ability to function.[18]

Although many die in such catastrophic events, the sequelae to survivors and the health care infrastructure are often unimaginable. The Indian Ocean tsunami of December 26, 2003, killed many health care workers and destroyed countless numbers of health care facilities. Survivors had to contend with lack of potable water, sanitation issues, rotting corpses, and incipient disease with a severely compromised health care system. Cholera, typhoid, and other communicable diseases were rampant in multiple countries. We in North America often assumed that the United States would do a better job, but our response to Hurricane Katrina demonstrated otherwise. Federal, state, and local disaster plans did not include provisions for keeping hospitals functioning during a large-scale emergency. The National Disaster Medical System was ill-prepared for providing medical care to patients who needed it. There was no coordinated system for recruiting, deploying, and managing volunteers.[19]

TABLE 60-4

WEB SITE ADDRESSES FOR DISASTER MANAGEMENT INFORMATION

■ ORGANIZATION	■ WEB SITE
Agency for Toxic Substance and Disease Registry	www.atsdr.cdc.gov
Centers for Disease Control and Prevention	www.cdc.gov
Centers for Disease Control and Prevention Emergency Preparedness and Response	www.bt.cdc.gov
Chemical, Biological, Radiological, and Nuclear Defense Information Analysis Center (CBRNIAC)	www.cbrniac.apgea.army.mil
Department of Defense, Defense Technical Information Center (DTC)	www.dtic.mil
National Oceanic and Atmospheric Administration	www.noaa.gov
National Disaster Medical System	http://hhs.gov.aspr.opeo.ndms.index.html
Pandemic Flu	Pandemicflu.gov/plan/panflureport5.html
U.S. Geologic Survey: Natural Hazards	http://www.usgs.gov/hazards/

PERIOPERATIVE AND CONSULTATIVE SERVICES

We should have been better prepared because we should have learned from past experiences. In the January 17, 1994, earthquake affecting Northridge, California, 8 of 91 acute care hospitals had to be evacuated. Six of the hospitals evacuated within the first day because of water damage and loss of electrical power. Two of the eight hospitals evacuated within 72 hours when major structural damage was found, despite the fact that initial inspections of the hospitals had not revealed significant damage. Both of these hospitals ultimately had to be demolished and rebuilt.[20] In 2001, Tropical Storm Allison stalled over Texas, dropping torrential rains that flooded Houston's bayous. Floodwaters filled Houston's Hermann Memorial Hospital with 5 feet of standing water, swamping the lower levels of the facility, which housed the hospital's emergency generators. The hospital lost electricity, its backup power source, running water, sewer services, and communications capabilities, and it had to evacuate 540 patients.[21] In response to this experience and in preparation for future storms, Houston's Memorial Hospital moved its generators off the first floor of the building and installed floodgates around the outside of the hospital. Yet, most hospitals in New Orleans, including Charity Hospital, had emergency generators on the first floor of their buildings when the levees failed 4 years later when Katrina hit New Orleans, and 9 of 11 generators were incapacitated by floodwaters.

Much can also be learned in preparing for disasters from a risk assessment of major earthquakes. The Marmara earthquake that struck northwest Turkey on August 17, 1999, killed approximately 16,000 people, injured 44,000 (many health care workers were killed or injured), and demolished most health care facilities. Patients had to be taken from Marmara to 35 hospitals outside the earthquake zone that were not affected. Of the thousands of injuries, many were to patients who were crushed and lay in the rubble for hours to days. Surprisingly, the time under the rubble did not correlate with morbidity and mortality. Most of these patients had amputations, but the incidence of renal failure did not increase as the time under the rubble increased.[22] Individuals involved in management of the disaster concluded that rescuers should try to find and uncover victims for at least 5 days after an earthquake.[22]

Casualties in earthquakes are from crush injuries, but some patients will also present with burn injuries. Obviously, the greatest likelihood of having to deal with patients with burns occurs when caring for victims of a fire, as evidenced from the Rhode Island nightclub fire on February 20, 2003, that killed 100 people immediately and left more than 200 injured. Anesthesiologists can learn important lessons from reviewing what happened with that fire. One of the greatest challenges faced by physicians and health care workers at the small community hospital that was only 2 miles away from the site of the fire was how to manage the airway of patients who had sustained burns. Physicians avoided using neuromuscular blockade when intubating the tracheas of patients with inhalation injuries; several patients had significant airway edema that may have made intubation difficult, if not impossible. Several patients were given local nerve blocks with small amounts of sedatives and were intubated awake.[23]

In situations in which area hospitals are completely destroyed or nonfunctional, the government may have to establish health care facilities, such as field hospitals,[24] or, if the city is coastal, bring in one of the Navy's hospital ships, as it did after the World Trade Center collapsed and after Hurricane Katrina.

Finally, health care facilities near large industrial complexes must anticipate chemical injuries, explosions, and fires. The Bhopal gas tragedy of December 3, 1984, is but one example. Methyl isocyanate gas leaked from a tank, killing approximately 3,800 people and injuring several thousand.[25] Four years later an independent investigation concluded that the tragedy could only have been the result of sabotage, when someone or some persons deliberately attached a water hose to the gas storage tank, initiating a massive chemical reaction.[25]

Role of Government

The initial response to any disaster, whether natural, unintended, or terrorist-initiated, begins at the local level and involves firefighters, paramedics, and law enforcement agencies, especially if criminal activity is suspected. Depending on the nature of the disaster, local passersby might also become involved, as is often the case. Fire departments are trained to deal with toxic chemicals and, depending on the size of the municipality, many have hazardous materials teams, which are trained to deal with chemical and toxic agent spills. Unfortunately, many other first responders may not have had such training and are at risk of becoming casualties themselves, as has happened several times in the past.

If the incident is more than local agencies can handle, not only from a government perspective but also from the hospital's perspective, then state emergency management systems are called into play. The governor of the state could call up the National Guard to provide medical decontamination, transportation, and other services.

Four years after the event, considerable controversy remains as to how city, state, and federal governments responded to Hurricane Katrina. Although many are quick to blame the federal government, the experience in Mississippi, compared with what occurred in Louisiana, underscores how important local and state resources are in handling disasters of such a magnitude.[19]

The federal government's actions in a disaster are predicated on multiple Presidential decision directives, many of which have been established following 9/11.[26] The Federal Bureau of Investigation has responsibility for domestic terrorism and crisis management, investigating and preparing documentation for any criminal proceedings that might be conducted within the judicial system. The Federal Emergency Management Agency (FEMA),[27] now within the Department of Homeland Security,[28] is the lead agency for management assistance to state and local governments, providing emergency relief to affected individuals and businesses, decontaminating affected areas, and helping to ensure public health safety. The National Response Framework, successor to the National Response Plan, was released by the Department of Homeland Security in January 2008.[29] The National Response Framework, which focuses on response and short-term recovery, articulates the doctrine, principles, and architecture by which the United States prepares for and responds to all-hazard disasters across all levels of government and all sectors of communities.[29]

In addition to FEMA and the Department of Homeland Security, the Department of Health and Human Services is committed to assisting practitioners, clinicians, and responders nationwide prepare for all public health emergencies.[30] The National Response Framework uses the National Disaster Medical System within the Department of Health and Human Services, Office of Preparedness and Response, under Emergency Support Function No. 8, Health and Medical Care, to support federal agencies in the management and coordination of the federal medical response to major emergencies and federally declared disasters.[30]

The National Disaster Medical System has three components—prehospital treatment, hospital evacuation, and in-hospital care. The prehospital treatment is provided by disaster medical assistance teams,[31] which are teams of about

40 individuals, including physicians, nurses, and paramedics, who are responsible for providing first aid, a casualty-clearing medical station, and field surgical intervention. As occurs with the National Guard, however, these activities take a minimum of 12 to 24 hours to organize and implement. The Department of Health and Human Services has a number of other specialized teams that help respond.

The Department of Defense is also in a position to assist with incidents of biologic or chemical terrorism, providing technical assistance, bomb disposal, decontamination, security, and other services to federal, state, and local authorities. The Department of Defense can assign a military support liaison officer who works with FEMA to coordinate interagency efforts between FEMA and the branches of the armed forces.[26]

While they are at their work sites during a disaster, anesthesiologists need to know that a number of local, state, and federal agencies are mobilizing to help them handle the situation, depending on the gravity and number of casualties. Anesthesiologists need to focus their activities on dealing with individual patients, as outlined later. Physicians who are geographically removed from the disaster but who want to volunteer can become a member of the National Disaster Medical System.[32]

The CDC has established a National Pharmaceutical Stockpile program, a national repository of antibiotics, chemical antidotes, life-support medications, intravenous administration and airway maintenance supplies, as well as medical/surgical items[33]; it consists of two phases. The first phase is the provision of eight separate, yet identical, prepackaged caches of medical materials, called 12-hour "push packages," that are deployed around the United States. If the incident requires a larger response, the second phase comes into play, in which vendor management inventories are deployed. These supplies are designed to arrive within 24 to 36 hours after the initial cache of materials arrives. Unfortunately, as with many of these initiatives, there are problems with the adequacy of the response plan.[34]

Role of Anesthesiologist in Managing Mass Casualties

It is probably difficult to anticipate every measure in which anesthesiologists could be asked to assist in managing mass casualty situations. For example, on October 26, 2002, terrorists held 750 hostages at the Nord-Ost Theater in Moscow. Many believe that the authorities instilled nebulized or volatile carfentanil into the air ducts of the opera house, thereby immobilizing the terrorists.[35] Unfortunately, because of the incapacitating effect of carfentanil, the hostages became victims too. Patients were transported from the theater to hospitals without treatment prior to transportation. Ideally, anesthesiologists or other health care providers who had an adequate supply of an opioid antagonist, such as naloxone, would have been readily available and present at the theater to manage both hostages and the terrorists themselves. Unfortunately this was not the case.

As unusual as this scenario is, anesthesiologists, depending on where they practice, may be called in to manage situations that are unimaginable by current standards. However, with their basic understanding of physiology and pharmacology, their airway skills, their fluid resuscitation expertise, and their ability to manage ventilators and to provide anesthesia in the field environment, in the emergency department, in the operating room, and in intensive care units (ICUs), anesthesiologists will be invaluable in managing the care of victims of mass casualties. In these mass casualty situations, many patients suffer burns, fractures, lacerations, soft tissue trauma, and amputations that will require triage, stabilization in the emergency department or in some other facility near the emergency department, and more definitive treatment in either the operating room or the ICU.

In caring for victims of previous industrial accidents and fires, appropriate management of the airway has been critical. Patients with large-area burns require establishment of intravenous access for provision of intravascular volume resuscitation. For patients with extensive soft-tissue and skeletal muscle damage, alkalinization of the urine with volume resuscitation and diuresis may be organ- and life-saving, depending on the event (burn vs. a crush injury—protocols for fluid resuscitation vary).

If chemical weapons have been used—again, depending on the severity of the injury—not only may tracheal intubation be required, but ventilator management may be necessary. The correct antidotes for managing patients who are victims of industrial chemical accidents or the use of chemical warfare agents will be discussed subsequently.

Radiation Injury

The greatest likelihood of dealing with patients who are exposed to ionizing radiation would come from a nuclear power plant or reactor accident and, in decreasing order of likelihood, from a terrorist action or detonation of a nuclear device (Table 60-6). Unfortunately, mishaps at power plants and testing facilities have occurred about once or twice a decade for the last 60 years, with Chernobyl being the best example. On April 26, 1986, workers at the Chernobyl nuclear power plant did not recognize or respond to evidence of malfunctioning in one of the reactors, with loss of cooling capacity and an explosion of the nuclear reactor.[36] Two workers died as a direct effect of the explosion, whereas those who remained in shielded areas survived unless they went to fight the fire, in which case they eventually died of radiation exposure. Short-term gamma and beta emissions from the explosion and subsequent gamma and beta radiation from the reactor core debris killed many more, with long-term health consequences affecting the entire community. Because the plant and city lacked an adequate evacuation plan, protective clothing, and respirators, the radioactive material that exploded into the atmosphere rained down for several hours and days, affecting many more workers and thousands of civilians. Primary sources of radiation were iodine 131 (^{131}I), strontium 90, and cesium 137. During the 24 hours following the explosion, 140,000 people were evacuated, and potassium iodide tablets were distributed to as many people as possible in the area. Two hundred thirty patients were subsequently hospitalized, with many patients succumbing to infections because of bone marrow suppression; among the patients in

TABLE 60-6

NUCLEAR THREATS[a]

Accident
    Nuclear power plants
    Reactors
Terrorist action
Detonation of a single nuclear bomb
Theater nuclear war
Strategic nuclear war

[a]In decreasing order of probability; the most likely is an accident involving a nuclear reactor and the least likely is a strategic nuclear war.

whom bone marrow transplantation was attempted, 17 died because of associated radiation burns. Oropharyngeal burns occurred in 28 patients. In all, radiation burns caused 21 deaths.

Over the next several years, the average radiation exposure around Chernobyl was 4 times normal because of residual ground contamination. Almost 2 decades later, the effects of Chernobyl continued to be felt in the immediate vicinity and in the area downwind from the reactor site.[36,37] The experience from Chernobyl should indicate the kind of injuries and results that anesthesiologists can anticipate when they encounter patients who have been involved in nuclear accidents: radiation burns, bone marrow suppression, and the destruction of the lining of the gastrointestinal (GI) tract, leading to GI bleeding with translocation of bacteria, infection, sepsis, septic shock, and death. The sequelae of infection and sepsis are best managed using the evidence-based medicine guidelines promulgated by 11 international groups in 2004.[38] As evidenced by the experiences in Chernobyl, the use of potassium iodide is indicated to protect the thyroid gland from taking up ^{131}I.

On March 28, 1979, at the Three Mile Island nuclear power plant, the number 2 nuclear reactor overheated and, because the pressure-relief valve failed to close, radioactive coolant was released into the containment facility.[39] As is often the case, numerous communication missteps occurred, which resulted in the release of inconsistent information to the general public, generating genuine fear among individuals living near the nuclear power plant. No biologic effects occurred as a result of the event, but many citizens experienced severe psychological sequelae.

On September 13, 1987, in Goiania, Brazil, a lead canister containing between 1,400 and 1,600 curies of cesium 137 was left in an abandoned building. Looters took and then opened the canister, and children played with the material. It contaminated 250 people, 4 of whom died; multiple individuals had short- and long-term health problems as a result.[40] Mitigation efforts required the removal of 6,000 tons of clothing, furniture, dirt, trees, and other materials.[41] Because of the possibility of exposure to ionizing radiation from nuclear power plants or other such facilities, the American Academy of Pediatrics recommends that at least two tablets of potassium iodide be available for all inhabitants within 10 miles of any nuclear power plant.[42]

Potential Sources of Ionizing Radiation Exposure

Everyone is exposed to radiation on an ongoing basis from cosmic radiation, radon, medical devices, and in multiple stores and factories. Even being a passenger on a commercial airline is associated with cosmic radiation exposure. A chest radiograph leads to 5 to 10 mrem of exposure, whereas a computerized tomographic scan can lead up to 5,000 mrem of exposure.[43]

Obviously, the greatest concern is the exposure to ionizing radiation that is unintentional, as occurred at the Chernobyl nuclear power plant, or is intentional. Intentional threats are the result of military conflict or terrorism; for example, in Hiroshima and Nagasaki in 1945. It is important to remember that, in Hiroshima, the bomb ("Little Boy") was only a 12.5-kiloton bomb, which killed an estimated 66,000 people and injured 69,000 more.[44] The bomb that fell at Nagasaki ("Fat Boy") was a 22-kiloton plutonium implosion-type bomb, which killed between 39,000 and 74,000 people, with 75,000 people sustaining severe injuries.[44] We learned in that experience that the majority of casualties are from the initial blast, from fire, and from the collapse of buildings. Radiation exposure subsequently killed many more. With any nuclear explosion, then, many individuals will be injured or killed from

building collapse or the thermal pulse. Patients could have burn, crush, or radiation injury or any combination thereof.

The United States detonation of a nuclear device in Japan had devastating effects. Detonating a nuclear device appeals to terrorists who want to inflict similar devastation. The 9/11 Commission recognized that failure to adequately safeguard the world's thermonuclear devices could lead to terrorists detonating a nuclear device in a major metropolitan area.[45] The Commission also expressed concern about the use of a "dirty bomb"—radionuclides such as cesium or strontium packed around explosive material. In 1987 Iraq tested a 1-ton dirty bomb, and in 1996 Islamic terrorists in Chechnya placed a bomb packed with cesium 137 in a Moscow park; the bomb did not explode.[46] Although explosion of a radiologic dispersion device remains the most likely event to take place in the future, terrorists could also target a nuclear power plant using commercial jets, munitions, or internal sabotage.

If any of these events were to occur, it is likely that patients would present with a combined injury syndrome, or injury from radiation and trauma.[47] Although blast, crush, or thermal injuries are readily apparent, the effects of ionizing radiation are usually not obvious. Individuals should be familiar with the various types of ionizing radiation, which include α-particles, β-particles, γ-rays, x-rays, and neutrons (Table 60-7).[48] It is also helpful to understand how radiation is measured (Table 60-8). Several methods take into account not only the decay rate of a radioactive isotope (becquerel [Bq] or a curie [Ci]), but also the dose absorbed, which is usually quantified as the amount absorbed by any type of tissue or material. The radiation-absorbed dose (rad) = 0.01 gray (Gy), which is the International System of Units (SI) for denoting the amount of energy deposited in joules per kilogram. One Gy equals 100 rad. A Sievert (Sv) is the SI unit for measurement of *human* exposure to radiation in joules per kilogram, with 1 Sv = 100 rem, or roentgen equivalent for man (rem).

TABLE 60-7

TYPES OF IONIZING RADIATION[a]

■ TERM	■ DEFINITION
α-Particle	A particle emitted from the nucleus of an atom; it contains 2 protons and 2 neutrons and is identical to the nucleus of a helium atom, without the electrons. Having a very large mass, α-particles have poor penetration and pose little hazard after external exposure but can produce tissue injury when inhaled or ingested.
β-Particle	A high-speed particle, identical to an electron, emitted from the nucleus of an atom.
γ-Rays	A form of ionizing radiation having no mass, γ-rays are emitted from nuclei. Like visible light, γ-rays are made of photons. γ-Rays have significant penetrance and are the most important external radiation hazard after a radiation disaster.
X-rays	Like γ-rays, x-rays have no mass; their energy is emitted from electrons.
Neutrons	A powerful but uncommon type of radiation, emitted only after a nuclear detonation; neutrons are highly destructive, producing 10 times more tissue damage than γ-rays.

[a]Ionizing radiation is a high-frequency, low-amplitude form of radiation that interacts significantly with biologic systems.

TABLE 60-8

RADIATION EXPOSURE TERMS

TERM	DEFINITION
Bq	The SI measurement of radioactivity, defined as decay events per second. 1 Bq = 1 disintegration per second
Ci	The traditional measure of radioactivity, as measured by radioactive decay. 1 Ci = 2.7×10^{10} disintegrations per second
rad	The energy deposited by any type of radiation to any type of tissue or material. 1 rad = 0.01 gray
Gy	The SI unit for the energy deposited by any type of radiation, in joules per kilogram. 1 Gy = 100 rad
rem	The unit of human exposure to radiation, roentgen equivalent for man. 1 rem = 0.01 Sievert
Sv	The SI unit for measurement of *human* exposure to radiation, in joules per kilogram. 1 Sv = 100 rem

Bq, becquerel; SI, the International System of Units; Ci, curie; rad, radiation-absorbed dose; Gy, gray; rem, roentgen equivalent human; Sv, Sievert.

In a nuclear accident or catastrophe, patients could be radiated by x-rays, γ-rays, or β-particles. They could be contaminated with debris emitting ionized radiation or they could have inhaled or ingested gaseous radioactive material, and some of this material can become incorporated into tissue; for example, the thyroid may incorporate isotopes of iodine. Various factors affect the amount of radiation that an individual absorbs, including the distance from the source of radiation, the amount of shielding between the individual and the source, the duration of exposure, and the amount of radiation to which one is exposed. Human tissue will block α-particles (although, if inhaled, α-particles can penetrate up to 50 microns into the pulmonary epithelium material, leading to the development of lung cancer) but will not stop β-particles or γ-rays. β-particles can be stopped by aluminum shields, but γ-rays can penetrate even concrete walls, but not lead. Therefore, lead is required to shield an individual from both γ-rays and x-rays.

The most likely injury from ionizing radiation is to those tissues that have the greatest turnover rate; that is, the sensitivity of tissues to radiation is greatest for lymphoid, greater than gastrointestinal (GI), greater than reproductive, greater than dermal, greater than bone marrow, greater than nervous system tissue. Ionizing radiation causes damage to lymphoid tissue and bone marrow. The thrombocytopenia, granulocytopenia, and GI injury lead to bleeding and bacterial translocation across the GI epithelium, the net result of which is hemorrhage and sepsis, the hallmarks of acute radiation syndrome.

Because ionizing radiation is invisible, individuals may appear normal or may present with nausea, vomiting, diarrhea, fever, hypotension, erythema, and central nervous system dysfunction. Patients who present with nausea, vomiting, diarrhea, and fever within minutes to hours are likely to have severe acute radiation syndrome. Hypotension, erythema, and central nervous system dysfunction will manifest later. "Short-term" effects such as these, however, may not appear until days to weeks after the exposure, depending on the amount of exposure (as little as 0.75 to 1.0 Gy), whereas hematopoietic syndrome (severe lymphoid and bone marrow suppression) results from exposure to 3 to 6 Gy and may lead to death within 8 to 50 days.[49] Long-term effects include thyroid cancer and psychologic injury, as has been documented many times in the past.

Management

Should a radiation disaster occur, it would be followed by a large coordinated local, state, and federal response, which, at the federal level, would include the Department of Homeland Security, the Department of Energy, the Department of Justice, FEMA, the Environmental Protection Agency, and the Nuclear Regulatory Commission.

Depending on the type of event, immediate evacuation of the area is of paramount importance. People who are not able to evacuate should seek a safe place within their homes or workplaces. The principles of disaster management always involve containment of emitting objects (avoid bringing patients with material that is emitting ionizing radiation to the hospital). Therefore, as part of the containment process—to the extent possible—patients should be decontaminated at the site of exposure. Those patients who have lethal radiation exposure should be declared expectant and should receive comfort care in the field.[49] Those patients who are going to be transported to a health care facility should remove their clothing and wash with warm soapy water to remove any radiation-emitting material. Rather than guess whether any radiation-emitting material is present—in the absence of having access to a Geiger counter—it is best to have all people who have potentially been exposed disrobe. In previous mass casualty situations, maintaining individuals' privacy has been a concern, but not one that is readily solved depending on the number of casualties. Care must be taken to isolate belongings and appropriately dispose of them, with the same consideration given to biologic fluids (e.g., saliva, blood, urine, or stool) as these substances may be contaminated with radioisotopes and may require special precautions when handling.

Potassium iodide can prevent radiation-induced thyroid effects but must be given as quickly as possible because it has little protective effect 24 hours after radiation exposure.[42] Other drugs under investigation for prophylaxis of radiation-induced injuries include vitamin E, 5-androstenediol, nitroxides,[50–52] and a new compound, HE2100, which is a naturally occurring synthetic adrenal steroid hormone that has been found to have protective effects against radiation injury in nonhuman primates.[53] Currently, though, treatment is largely supportive because these patients will develop, based on their acute exposure, acute radiation syndrome manifested by bleeding and sepsis.

Treatment guidelines for management of postirradiation sepsis have been developed and advocated by the military.[54] The use of granulocyte colony-stimulating factor may be of benefit.[46] Other treatments include oral and GI decontamination using nasopharyngeal lavage, oral lavage and brushing, early stomach lavage, or administration of an emetic and an osmotic laxative. Blocking agents include potassium iodide and strontium lactate. Mobilizing agents include ammonium chloride, calcium gluconate, and diuretics, which may enhance renal excretion. Chelation therapy has been recommended and includes the use of calcium DTPA (diethylene triamine pentaacetic acid) as an initial dose and then zinc DTPA.[55] The use of granulocyte macrophage colony-stimulating factor, thrombopoietin, and interleukin 11, though postulated, has not been proven to be of benefit. For individuals with a contaminated GI tract, selective decontamination may be helpful, but again, has not been demonstrated to be of benefit in this situation.[55]

BIOLOGIC DISASTERS

Although the threat of biologic warfare has existed for centuries, there has been heightened awareness of this threat in the United States following the anthrax attacks of 2001–2002. In 2003, the National Institutes of Health allocated $1.5 billion to biodefense research.

This heightened awareness of biologic terrorism is of benefit because it raises the consciousness of anesthesiologists about infectious disease epidemics that are not initiated by terrorist groups, that is, influenza, SARS, and West Nile virus. Influenza has killed more people in the 20th century than has any other infectious disease. Three large pandemics occurred during that century, including one in 1918 when an avian virus infected humans, creating the deadliest outbreak of disease in U.S. history. Between 25 and 50 million people, if not more, died, half of whom were otherwise healthy young adults. There were so many deaths in some communities that mass graves were dug to accommodate all the corpses.[56]

Epidemics

Influenza

The Spanish flu was caused by an influenza type A (there are three types of human influenza viruses: A, B, and C). Only subtypes of influenza A virus normally infect people: H1N1, H1N2, H3N2, H2N2, and now H1N5. Only influenza A viruses infect birds, although birds are natural hosts for all subtypes of influenza A virus. Typically, birds do not get sick when they are infected, but avian viruses can transform and infect humans, in which case a pandemic could result. Alternately, current human influenza A viruses could have antigenic drift or shift, in which case a virus for which there is already a vaccine could transform such that populations would not have immunity and another pandemic would develop. This was the case in 1957–1958 when the Asian flu (H2N2) caused some 70,000 deaths in the United States, and in 1968–1969 when the Hong Kong flu (H3N2) caused approximately 34,000 deaths in the United States.[57] The new pathogenic virus is usually detected several months in advance of major outbreaks, which allows sufficient time for the preparation of vaccines for entire populations. However, in the United States, there is currently a shortage of vaccines, a shortage that is unlikely to be resolved because of manufacturing liability issues, in which case the government must become more involved. However, as was found in the 1918–1919 influenza-pandemic, isolation and quarantine practices have a significant role to play in limiting the spread of the disease.[58] Such interventions are low cost and effective[59] but may be difficult to implement in the United States, where individual rights often have the priority.[60]

In addition, four antiviral drugs, including amantadine, rimantadine, zanamavir, and oseltamivir, have some benefit in treating patients with the flu. Resistance is already developing to oseltamivir,[61] which is unfortunate, because it, along with zanamavir, another neuraminidase inhibitor, has limited activity against avian flu anyway.[62] Amantadine and rimantadine, M2 ion channel-blocking drugs, are both partially effective (approximately 60% efficacy) against avian flu, but their widespread use for other viral diseases has infectious disease specialists concerned about the development of resistance.[62]

The World Health Organization (WHO) acknowledges that if there were to be another flu pandemic, it could kill up to 50 million people worldwide.[63] Anesthesiologists, because of their airway and ventilator management skills, will be involved in providing care for many of these patients.

Severe Acute Respiratory Syndrome

Of equal worry is a recurrence of SARS. This illness, caused by a coronavirus, first presented in February 2003, infecting thousands of people worldwide, almost 1,000 of whom died (almost a 10% fatality rate).[64] Health care workers were especially significantly at risk, because they were called on to manage the care of these patients in emergency departments, operating rooms, and ICUs. Because the virus is airborne and because some health care workers wore ineffective isolation equipment, such as standard face masks, some individuals inhaled virions, became sick, and died.[65] Entire hospitals had to be quarantined, with no individuals allowed to leave or enter for fear of spreading the virus. Although this quarantine seems draconian, the action of several governments in enforcing this strict quarantine was one of the most important ways in which the spread of the disease was limited. Treatment of SARS is currently supportive, with no definitive therapy. In 2004, several isolated cases were reported, but since December 2004, no further cases have been reported.[66] Much has been learned; perhaps most important has been the fact that we need an effective international system to monitor for emerging infectious diseases.[67]

Other Diseases

The West Nile virus, a mosquito-borne encephalitis, killed 87 of 2,432 infected people in 2004.[68] The death rate is relatively high, although the number of individuals infected is relatively small. The reason to highlight the West Nile virus is to underscore the importance of public health measures in controlling mosquito-borne diseases.

BIOLOGIC TERRORISM

History

Infectious agents have been used as biologic weapons since the dawn of history. Genghis Khan is reported to have used cats infected with fleas bearing the plague to destroy towns in his conquest of Asia. British forces distributed blankets that had been used by patients with smallpox to American Indians; the ensuing epidemic killed >50% of the indigenous people who were infected.[67] In World War II, Unit 731 of the Japanese military was reported to have dropped plague-infected fleas over populated areas of China, causing outbreaks of plague and killing several hundred thousand people.[67]

The ideal biologic agent is one that has the greatest potential for adverse public health impact, generating mass casualties and with the potential for easy large-scale dissemination that could cause mass hysteria and civil disruption.[69] Such a weapon should be relatively easy to produce, inexpensive, and highly infectious and contagious, resulting in widespread morbidity and mortality. To be effective, the target population must not have natural immunity, which is currently the case with diseases such as smallpox, for which we no longer routinely vaccinate individuals, except in the military and in high-risk public health areas. There are three categories of biologic weapons (Table 60-9). Category A agents are those that are highly contagious and fit all the characteristics of a relatively ideal biologic agent.

Smallpox

The last case of naturally occurring smallpox in the world was reported in 1977 in Somalia.[70] In 1978, two laboratory workers in the United Kingdom were infected with smallpox.[70] In 1980, the WHO announced that the world was free of this scourge. In 1972, routine vaccination for smallpox was discontinued in the United States.[70] It is precisely because of this lack of vaccination that people in the United States are at most risk for being the target of terrorists using smallpox as a

TABLE 60-9

BIOLOGIC AGENTS USED FOR WARFARE

■ CATEGORY A	■ CATEGORY B	■ CATEGORY C
Bacillus anthracis (anthrax)	*Coxiella burnetii* (Q fever)	Various equine encephalitic viruses
Variola major (smallpox)	*Vibrio cholerae* (cholera)	
Yersinia pestis (plague)	*Burkholderia mallei* (glanders)	
Clostridium botulinum (botulism)	Enteric pathogens (*Escherichia coli* 0157:H7, salmonella, shigella)	
Francisella tularensis (tularemia)	Cholera, cryptosporidium	
Viral hemorrhagic fever (Ebola, Lassa, Marburg, Argentine)	Various encephalitic viruses	
	Various biologic toxins	

biologic weapon. Forty percent to 80% of patients exposed to the smallpox virus will come down with the disease. Smallpox is highly infective, requiring only 10 to 100 organisms to infect an individual. The mortality rate is approximately 30% in unvaccinated people and as high as 50% if smallpox occurs in communities that have no native immunity against smallpox. The protective effect of the smallpox vaccine decreases with time, but even at 20 years after vaccination, those individuals who had previously received the vaccine have some protection.

When unvaccinated people are initially infected, they develop a prodrome of malaise, headache, and backache with the onset of fever to as high as 40°C. The fever decreases over the next 3 or 4 days, at which time a rash develops, which begins with macules that then progress to papules, and, in turn, vesicles, pustules, and scabs (Fig. 60-3). This is in contradistinction to chickenpox, in which the rash develops at the same time as the fever. Also unlike chickenpox, smallpox has a predilection for the distal extremities and face, although no part of the body is spared. Also, all lesions in a patient with smallpox are at the same stage, whereas chickenpox lesions are at multiple different stages so that the infected person will simultaneously have papules, vesicles, pustules, and scabs (Table 60-10). Most cases of smallpox are transmitted through

aerosolized droplets that are inhaled, but clothes and blankets that have come in contact with pustules, until the scab falls off, are infectious; the organism can be transmitted in this linen.

Smallpox has probably been present in humans since 10,000 BC. It is transmitted human-to-human and, if used as a bioterrorism agent, would likely be dispersed by aerosols in the environment with the hope that multiple humans would be infected and would transmit it to other humans. There is evidence that the former Soviet Union has developed transgenic smallpox viruses that are very infectious and for which the U.S. vaccine may not be completely protective. There are currently only two WHO-approved depositories of smallpox, at the CDC in Atlanta, Georgia, and at the Institute of Virus Preparations in Moscow, Russia. With the collapse of the Soviet Union, concern arose that some stores of smallpox made it into the hands of rogue countries that may have developed their own biologic weapons.

A look at how the WHO eradicated smallpox might be helpful in understanding how the United States has prepared to respond if smallpox is used as a biologic weapon. One must remember that, in the 18th century, 400,000 Europeans died each year of smallpox. Although only 1% of patients who survive smallpox become blind, the disease accounted for one

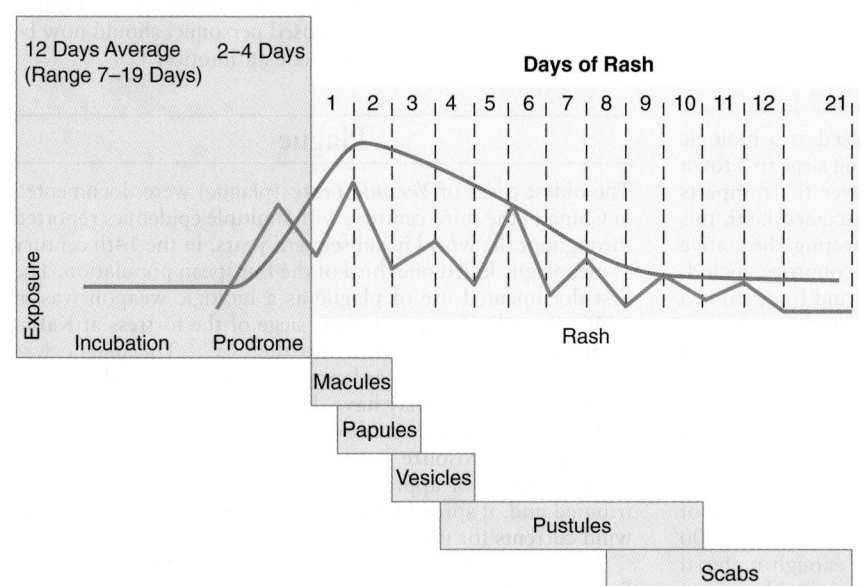

FIGURE 60-3. Fever, rash development, and viral shedding in smallpox. The *red line* shows body temperature and the *blue line* indicates viral shedding. From the Lancet, Vol 367, Moore ZS, Seward JF, Lane JM, Smallpox, 425–435, 2006 with permission from Elsevier.

TABLE 60-10

COMPARISON OF CHICKENPOX AND SMALLPOX

■ SIGN	■ CHICKENPOX	■ SMALLPOX
Fever	2–4 days before rash	Simultaneous with rash
Rash	All lesions have same-stage development	Lesions at various stages (papules, pustules, scabs all present)

third of all cases of blindness in Europe in the 19th century. In the 20th century, the WHO eradicated smallpox by identifying patients with smallpox and placing them in strict quarantine. Such patients can be readily identified because of the presence of smallpox lesions on the face. Not only were patients isolated, but all of their contacts were vaccinated because there is a 3- to 7-day window with the naturally occurring virus before the patient develops symptoms and signs of smallpox.[71]

Vaccination against smallpox is controversial. The vaccine is made from a live vaccinia virus developed in calf lymph, but the vaccine is not developed from an attenuated smallpox virus itself, but from a closely related virus. Smallpox is a member of the *orthopox* genus of the Poxviridae family of double-stranded DNA viruses that also contain cowpox, monkeypox, and vaccinia. In the event of a documented case of smallpox, the CDC has plans to quarantine the index case and then vaccinate immediate contacts and individuals within a certain geographic radius. Stockpiles of vaccines have been strategically placed throughout the United States for use in such an event, and the WHO has a stockpile of more than 200 million doses for use worldwide.[72] Vaccination takes place with a bifurcated needle dipped into the reconstituted vaccine, with the needle then jabbed 10 to 15 times into the dermis of the upper deltoid. Because of the side effects of smallpox vaccinations, people with immunologic disorders, eczema (active or with a history of severe eczema), and pregnant or nursing women will not be administered the vaccine. As of 2003, with the use of vaccination in the U.S. armed forces and for health care workers, the CDC has reported several nonserious adverse events, such as fever, rash, and malaise, and two cases of cardiomyopathy.[73] Because of these complications, no plan has been made to routinely vaccinate the U.S. population. The CDC and the state departments of health will implement their quarantine and vaccination plans should an index case or several cases (a cluster) occur.

Anthrax

Bacillus anthracis (anthrax) was probably used as a biologic weapon in the Middle Ages when troops laying siege to a town would catapult infected animal carcasses over the ramparts and into the inhabited areas. For reasons discussed later, this was not a particularly effective way of infecting the native population. During the 20th century, several countries, including the United States, Great Britain, Russia, and Iraq, studied ways to weaponize anthrax. Anthrax has appeal as a bioterrorism agent because, to be "weaponized," *B. anthracis* must be finely ground so that it readily aerosolizes and can get to and deposit in the terminal bronchioles and alveoli.[74] (Normally, if anthrax spores are inhaled, they clump in the nasal pharynx.) Inhalation anthrax, which occurred relatively rarely in the past, has an 80% fatality rate. One of the letters that was mailed in the anthrax attacks of 2001 contained 2 g of weapons-grade anthrax. With a median lethal dose of 1,000 spores, under optimum conditions this was enough material to infect 50 million individuals. Most countries that have

weaponized anthrax would either aerosolize it, using airplanes, or deliver it through a dispersion device mounted on top of a missile. The attacks in North America in 2001 and the accidental release of anthrax spores at a biologic facility in the city of Sverdlovsk in the former Soviet Union in 1979 are illustrative of the potential of anthrax as a weapon. In the United States, 5 of 11 patients died (50% mortality rate); in the former Soviet Union, 66 of 77 died (86% mortality rate).[75] The Aum Shinrikyo, a cult in Japan, also released anthrax spores in Tokyo in 1993. Fortunately, they used a nonpathogenic strain of anthrax and thus there were no casualties.[74] As demonstrated in 2001 in the United States, a smarter terrorist will be far more successful in using infectious weapons-grade anthrax. Such attacks, even if detected, create mass hysteria and greatly impact the public health care system.[76]

Anthrax is a Gram-positive, spore-forming bacillus that is transmitted to humans from contaminated animals, their byproducts, or carcasses. Spores may persist in soil for years. The disease is all but gone from North America, but it is still prevalent in many developing countries; herbivores, especially cattle, usually die within 24 to 48 hours of contracting the disease. These contaminated sources have such a large number of bacillus that humans, who are relatively resistant to infection, can be exposed and contract the disease.[77]

There are three primary types of anthrax infection: cutaneous, inhalation, and GI; 95% of cases are cutaneous. Infectious disease specialists worry most about inhalation anthrax, which worldwide usually affects 2,000 to 20,000 people per annum. People can be exposed through contact with animals in an agricultural setting or in an industrial setting (e.g., a rendering plant or leather tanning facility), or, as mentioned previously, in the production of biologic weapons.[78]

Anthrax has additional appeal to bioterrorists because inhalation anthrax is hard to detect. It manifests as an influenza-like disease with fever, myalgias, malaise, and a nonproductive cough with or without chest pain.[79] After a few days, the patient appears to get better, but then a couple days later, the patient becomes much sicker with dyspnea, cyanosis, hemoptysis, stridor, and chest pain. The most notable finding on a chest radiograph is a widened mediastinum. When a patient develops profound dyspnea, death ensues within 1 to 2 days. In the past, penicillin G was the treatment of choice but, because weaponized anthrax has been engineered to be resistant to penicillin G, ciprofloxacin or doxycycline is more commonly used. In the outbreaks in Florida, the District of Columbia, and New Jersey, contacts of infected patients or people exposed to the spores were treated with ciprofloxacin or doxycycline. Since these attacks, exposed personnel should now be vaccinated and receive prophylactic antibiotics.[80]

Plague

The oldest cases of *Yersinia pestis* (plague) were documented in China in the third century, with multiple epidemics reported throughout the world in subsequent years. In the 14th century alone, plague killed one third of the European population. The first documented use of plague as a biologic weapon was in 1346 when the Tartars, in their siege of the fortress at Kaffa, catapulted infected corpses into the city.[67] The plague was used by Unit 731 to infect large areas of China, and as many as 200,000 Chinese may have died. More recently, the United States and Russia have studied Y. *pestis* as a bioagent, examining ways to aerosolize it and ways to distribute it. *Yersinia pestis* is viable for approximately 60 minutes after being distributed, and if spread by an airplane, could remain viable on wind currents for up to 10 km from the dispersion site.

Yersinia pestis is a nonmotile, Gram-positive bacillus.[69] Rodents and fleas are its natural hosts, and they reinfect each other when fleas bite infected rodents or, because the soil can be contaminated, when rodents acquire the disease simply by digging in an infected area. Humans are an accidental host, and they usually acquire the disease from a flea bite, although rarely there can be direct inoculation of infected material into a person. Direct person-to-person transmission occurs with pneumonic plague.

There are two types of plague: bubonic and pneumonic. With bubonic plague, after a flea bite, there is a 2- to 6-day incubation period, with subsequent sudden onset of fever, chills, weakness, and headache. Intense painful swelling occurs in the lymph nodes, usually in the groin, axilla, and neck. This swelling (bubo) is typically oval in nature, 1 to 10 cm in diameter, and extremely tender. Up to 25% of patients will have pustules, papules, or skin lesions near this bubo. Without treatment, patients become septic and develop septic shock, with cyanosis and gangrene in peripheral tissues, leading to the "black death" descriptor that was used during the epidemics in Europe. As mentioned, material from these buboes is infective only if inoculated into human tissue. However, patients who have bubonic plague can seed their lungs, in which case they develop pneumonic plague. During coughing, they aerosolize Y. pestis, which is highly contagious. Mortality for either form of the disease is >50%. Diagnosis is made with a Gram stain or culture of organisms from blood, sputum, or buboes.

The treatment of choice is streptomycin, but chloramphenicol and tetracycline are acceptable alternatives. Patients with pneumonic plague should be cared for as one would manage the treatment of a patient with drug-resistant tuberculosis because the respiratory secretions are highly infectious.

Tests to help make the diagnosis efficaciously and quickly are urgently needed.[81] There was one formal and fixed whole-organism vaccine that has been removed from the market, but the U.S. government is continuing to attempt to develop vaccines to Y. pestis.[82]

Tularemia

Francisella tularensis (tularemia) has some similarities to anthrax and plague, but it is not nearly as dangerous. It was studied as a biologic weapon in the 20th century because it is highly infectious, requiring an inoculum of perhaps as small as only 10 organisms.[83] During World War II, tularemia developed in soldiers along the German-Russian front that was thought to be secondary to the use of F. tularensis as a biologic weapon. The fact that both armies were infected underscores one of the dangers of using infectious agents as biologic weapons. These agents are often dispersed with aerosols, and despite the best predictions, air currents are notoriously unpredictable; with shifting air currents, one's own troops could become infected. Unit 731 of the Japanese army also studied the use of F. tularensis as a biologic weapon, and the United States and Russia were known to have grown and stored large quantities of F. tularensis.

Francisella tularensis is a Gram-negative, pleomorphic rod.[69] There are several animal hosts, with the cotton-tailed rabbit being one of the most susceptible. Humans normally acquire F. tularensis with direct contact with an infected animal or from the bite of an infected tick or deer fly.[83] Occasionally, the ingestion of infected food or inhalation of a small amount of aerosol will initiate the disease. There are two strains of F. tularensis, Jellison A and B, with the B strain being relatively innocuous and, in North America the A strain being quite virulent. A patient will typically develop a cutaneous ulcer at the site of entry after contact with an animal. As few as 10 or 50 organisms can invade the body either through hair follicles or miniabrasions. The incubation period is 2 to 6 days, with swelling and ulceration at the site of entry. As the swelling continues, the skin eventually breaks, creating an ulcer, which develops a necrotic base that becomes black as it scars.

It is most likely that weaponized F. tularensis would be delivered from an aerosol disbursed from an airplane, in which case, following inhalation, there is a 3- to 5-day incubation period, with the onset of disease marked with fever, pharyngitis, bronchitis, pneumonia, pleuritis, and hilar lymphadenopathy. Mortality rate for pneumonic tularemia is 5 to 15%.[84]

The treatment of choice for tularemia is streptomycin, although gentamicin, tetracycline, and chloramphenicol have been used. Concern exists that the former Soviet Union, perhaps the United States, and perhaps terrorists have engineered F. tularensis to be resistant to a number of agents. Prophylaxis with streptomycin, ciprofloxacin, or doxycycline has been previously recommended for individuals exposed to the organism. A vaccine composed of an attenuated whole-organism strain was available but is no longer available. The U.S. Army Medical Research Institute of Infectious Diseases continues to work on developing vaccines to tularemia.[84]

Botulism

The first known work with *Clostridium botulinum* (botulism) as a biologic weapon was in World War II. Both the German and Japanese military and scientific communities experimented with C. botulinum. Unit 731 fed pure cultures of C. botulinum to Chinese captives, with devastating effects. Both the United States and former Soviet Union are known to have produced large quantities of C. botulinum toxin, as have Iraq, Iran, Syria, and North Korea. In fact, after the first Gulf War, Iraq admitted to having >19,000 liters of concentrated botulinum toxin, of which almost half were loaded on military weapons.[85] Nineteen thousand liters of botulinum toxin is enough to kill the world's population 3 times over. More recently, Aum Shinrikyo dispersed aerosols of botulinum toxin on three different occasions in Japan. Fortunately, their dispersal methods and the agent they chose were associated with multiple problems, and no one was injured. There is concern that a terrorist organization working with a rogue state may acquire and use C. botulinum as a bioterrorist weapon.

Botulism is a neuroparalytic disease caused by the toxin from C. botulinum. Unlike all the other bioterrorist agents mentioned previously, it is not caused by live organisms and therefore is not contagious. The organism from which botulinum toxin is derived is a Gram-positive spore that is an obligatory anaerobe widely distributed in nature in soil and in marine and agriculture products. Humans ingest C. botulinum without apparent effects. It is the toxin that produces toxicity. C. botulinum has seven distinct toxins and, once ingested or inhaled, the toxins are distributed in the bloodstream to the cholinergic receptor, where they block the release of acetylcholine by inhibiting the intracellular fusion of the acetylcholine vesicle to the membrane. Victims develop progressive weakness, a flaccid paralysis that begins in the extremities and progresses until the respiratory muscles are paralyzed. Of note, C. botulinum toxin is the most potent poison known to humans; the lethal dose is only 1 pg.[86]

The incubation period is between 2 hours and 8 days after the toxin is ingested or inhaled, but is most commonly between 12 and 36 hours.[87] As muscles become weak, the infection is manifest as diplopia, dysphonia, dysarthria, dysphagia, and eventually dyspnea and frank paralysis. Along with the effects on the skeletal muscular system caused by dysfunction of the nicotinic receptor, muscarinic blockade results in decreased salivation, ileus, and urinary retention. The toxin can be removed through gastric lavage and the use of cathartics and enemas. The treatment of patients includes the use of a trivalent antitoxin. Patients with profound respiratory embarrassment should have their trachea intubated for airway protection and mechanical ventilation. Without the use of antitoxin, it takes the patient 2 to 8 weeks to recover. From past experience, the mortality rate is thought to be 5 to 10%.

Hemorrhagic Fevers

A number of viral hemorrhagic fevers are listed as category A agents, including the arena viruses (e.g., Lassa fever), bunyaviruses (hanta), flaviviruses (dengue), and filoviruses (Ebola and Marburg). At least 18 viruses cause human hemorrhagic fevers, which form a special group of viruses characterized by viral replication in lymphoid cells, after which patients develop fever and myalgia, with an incubation of anywhere from 2 to 18 days, depending on the agent and the amount of agent that is inhaled or inoculated across the dermis. The hemorrhagic fevers encompass syndromes that vary from febrile hemorrhagic fever with edema to distributive shock, which rapidly leads to death. Both the United States and the former Soviet Union have experimented with and weaponized several of these viruses. Studies in nonhuman primates suggest that the agents are highly infectious, requiring only a few virions to produce illness.[87] As mentioned, several governments have weaponized hemorrhagic fever viruses, and the Aum Shinrikyo cult in Japan went to Africa in the 1990s to try to obtain an Ebola virus that they could weaponize. No known incidents have occurred in which these agents were used as a biologic weapon, but there is clear interest and potential for their use as weapons.

The viruses are single-stranded RNA viruses, which have a rodent or insect reservoir and are communicated to humans by inhalation of an aerosol or, as mentioned, contact with an infected animal or through a bite. Humans are not a reservoir for the virus. The diseases are contagious, and person-to-person transmission in Africa has been documented with several of these viruses.[84] As mentioned, the incubation period is within several days of contact or inhalation of the agent, at which time patients present with fever, myalgia, and evidence of capillary leak (peripheral or pulmonary edema), disseminated intravascular coagulation, and thrombocytopenia, which is one of the hallmarks of the illnesses. The fatality rate, depending again on the specific virus, is anywhere from 2 to 60%. There are no specific antiviral therapies for this class of viruses, but there have been anecdotal reports of ribavirin, interferon-α, and hyperimmune globulin as being protective; however, there is simply not enough experience to know with certainty.

A live attenuated virus vaccine exists for yellow fever, but there are none for any of the other agents. There is extensive ongoing testing for the development of vaccines for several of these most dangerous viruses.

The Role of the Anesthesiologist in Bioterrorism

12 It is unlikely that an ICU physician or anesthesiologist would be at the initial site of origin of a biologic attack, but it could happen. Most likely, physicians will become involved if the hospital at which they work ultimately provides care for a number of patients exposed to a biologic agent.[69] As in the previous situations, anesthesiologists could find themselves being involved with triage or in the emergency department, operating room, or ICU.[88] As suggested for several of these situations, airway management and ventilator management may

be critical, as be would the establishment of intravascular access and volume resuscitation. The use of neuromuscular blocking agents is not recommended in managing patients with suspected thermal injuries to the airway. However, anecdotal evidence from Asia indicates that, with infectious agents, health care workers are better protected if they use a neuromuscular blocking agent when intubating the trachea for the obvious reason that, when anesthesiologists intubate the trachea, they are less likely to be subjected to any aerosolized particles (S. F. Yim, personal communication, June 2003). Nonetheless, this argument is somewhat specious because, whenever dealing with a patient with a suspected contagious pulmonary disease such as anthrax, plague, hemorrhagic virus, tularemia, or drug-resistant tuberculosis, anesthesiologists must protect themselves by using 100% effective respiratory protection, going so far as to consider using an oxygen-rebreathing system.

Obviously, it is critical to rank the possibility that the patient has been exposed to a biologic agent high on your differential diagnosis if you are managing the index case or are caring for two or more patients with presenting signs and symptoms that are suggestive of the use of a biologic weapon. Unfortunately, as was demonstrated in the 2001–2002 anthrax cases, the ability of the average physician to diagnose and treat these infectious diseases is poor.[89] Members of the American Society of Anesthesiologists and its Committee on Trauma and Emergency Preparedness are working to develop a coordinated plan that would assist anesthesiologists if they were to be called to their hospital in the event of such an attack.[90]

The individual who is the point of contact for the index case should notify the hospital infectious disease specialist and the local and state health departments. Factors that might indicate the intentional release of a biologic agent would include unusual temporal or geographic clustering of cases, an uncommon age distribution, or a significant number of cases (more than one) of acute flaccid paralysis that might suggest exposure to botulinum toxin.

If anesthesiologists are called to the hospital to be involved in managing such a catastrophe, they must review basic decontamination and isolation techniques and, as previously discussed, must scrupulously follow those guidelines.

CHEMICAL AGENTS

Emergency management teams in the United States have traditionally prepared to respond to chemical spills and industrial accidents. Many communities have hazardous materials teams that respond to a chemical spill and exposure at an industrial or commercial site, and communities that have large industrial or chemical plants have emergency plans and systems in anticipation of an accident in their community. It is more difficult to prepare for accidents that involve derailments of railroad tank cars containing chemical agents, but in this circumstance, state and federal agencies respond in assisting local communities.

Before the last 20 years, it was unthinkable that chemical agents would be used by rogue states or terrorists, but much has changed. Dating back to antiquity, the use of chemical weapons has been scrupulously avoided—neither the Greeks nor Romans would use them. *Armis bella non venenis geri* (War is waged with weapons, not with poison) is a Roman condemnation of well poisoning.[91]

In the 20th century, during World War I, more than 1 million soldiers and civilians were injured by chemical agents, with more than 100,000 of them dying. In 1935, Italy invaded Abyssinia (Ethiopia) and, during that invasion, sprayed mustard gas from aircraft. When Japan invaded

China, they used mustard gas, phosgene, and hydrogen cyanide. In that same year, German chemical laboratories produced the first nerve agent, tabun. From 1963 through 1967, Egypt used phosgene and mustard agents in support of South Yemen during the civil war in that country. When Iraq attacked Iran in the 1980s, they used mustard gas and nerve agents. In all of these examples,[92] chemical agents were used by the military during armed conflict. In 1994 and 1995, the Japanese cult Aum Shinrikyo was the first terrorist group to use chemical agents, and now chemical agents must be considered any time one discusses terrorist use of weapons of mass destruction.[93] As outlined previously in this chapter, the cult had tried to use anthrax and botulinum spores and obtained specimens of hemorrhagic viruses for use as biologic weapons. They were not successful with any of these enterprises, but their use of sarin in Tokyo had major health care consequences and far-reaching ramifications. As a result of the attack, more than 5,000 persons required emergency medical evaluation, with approximately 1,000 of them likely exposed to the agent, resulting in at least 11 deaths.

Since then, and because of the events of September 11 and the anthrax attacks of 2001, the United States has had to prepare for the possibility that terrorists would use chemical weapons to attack this country. Chemical weapons make sense because they are relatively inexpensive, compared with conventional and nuclear weapons; they are relatively easy to use; and, when used against a population, create major fear and panic and incredible demands on health care systems.[92] Implementation of a well-planned attack would severely cripple a U.S. city and inflict considerable morbidity and mortality. A variety of chemical agents have been developed in the past, including the agents listed in Table 60-11.

Nerve Agents

Nerve agents are chemicals that affect nerve transmission by inhibiting acetylcholinesterase so that acetylcholine accumulates at the muscarinic and nicotinic acetylcholine receptor and within the central nervous system. Examples of nerve agents that anesthesiologists use on a regular basis are the carbamates, which include physostigmine, neostigmine, and pyridostigmine. Sevin is a carbamate compound that is an insecticide. Other anticholinesterases are the organophosphates, which include the insecticides malathion and diazinon, and the nerve agents. The management of organophosphate pesticide poisoning[94] is very similar to the management of nerve agent poisoning.

Nerve agents were developed by Germany before World War II but were not used in World War II. They include GA, GB, GD, GF, and VX in increasing potency and toxicity. These five agents are clear, colorless liquids that vaporize at room temperature and can then penetrate skin, clothing, or the epithelium of the lung or GI tract. As the agents bind to acetylcholinesterase, acetylcholine accumulates and the sequelae of excess acetylcholine become apparent.

With muscarinic site stimulation, patients experience airway, pupillary, and GI constriction; bradycardia; increased lacrimation and salivation; and diaphoresis. Nicotinic stimulation leads to tachycardia and hypertension at the preganglionic site and fasciculations, twitching, fatigue, and flaccid paralysis at the nicotinic acetylcholine receptor on the neuromuscular junction. Excess parasympathetic activity leads to miosis and loss of accommodation so that patients complain of blurred vision. Within the respiratory system, the increased parasympathetic activity leads to bronchospasm, dyspnea, and rhinorrhea. The agent on the skin will produce localized sweating, and fasciculations can be observed. Within the cardiovascular system, activity within the muscarinic system leads to bradycardia, and an increase in heart rate at the nicotinic site, preganglionic nodes. The net effect is difficult to anticipate; therefore, the patient's heart rate may be low, normal, or high. Within the GI tract, the increased parasympathetic activity leads to nausea, vomiting, diarrhea, and incontinence. This overall unopposed parasympathetic activity leads to a pneumonic of DUMBELS (diarrhea, urination, miosis, bronchorrhea and bronchoconstriction, emesis, lacrimation, and salivation).

The toxicity of the nerve agents depends on the compound delivered, the dose that is delivered, and the time that an individual is exposed to that dose. Toxicity of the compounds is shown in Table 60-11, where LCt_{50} is a measure of the concentration versus the time (Ct) of exposure. For example, a patient exposed to 10 mg/m^3 of an agent for 10 minutes would have a Ct of 100 mg/min/m^3. The same could be achieved by exposure to a concentration of 100 mg/m^3 for only 1 minute.

The treatment for nerve agent poisoning is one with which every anesthesiologist is familiar: atropine, a competitive muscarinic blocker. Atropine is administered at a dose of 2 to 6 mg or more and repeated every 5 to 10 minutes until secretions begin to decrease (the patient is not salivating) and ventilation is improved. In casualties with severe exposure, 15 to 20 mg would not be unusual, and some casualties have required more than a gram of atropine.[95]

Pralidoxime chloride (2-PAM-Cl) is the better long-term treatment because it reactivates acetylcholinesterase by removing the organophosphate compound. In severe organophosphate insecticide poisoning, continuous infusions of 2-PAM-Cl have been used with success.[96] However, a recent meta-analysis of human studies suggests that oxime therapy is of no benefit or may even be harmful.[97] The U.S. military travels with automatic injectors containing 2 mg of atropine and

---

TOXICITY OF NERVE AGENTS

	LCt$_{50}$ (mg/min/m^3)	LD$_{50}$ (mg/70 kg)
GA	400	1,000
GB	100	1,700
GD	70	50
GF	50	30
VX	10	10
Nerve		
	GA (tabun)	
	GB (sarin)	
	GD (soman)	
	GF	
	VX	
Pulmonary		
	Chlorine	
	Phosgene	
	Ricin	
Blood		
	AC (hydrogen cyanide)	
	CK (cyanogen chloride)	
Vesicants		
	H, HD (sulfur mustard)	
	HN$_1$, HN$_2$, HN$_3$ (nitrogen, mustard)	
	Lewisite (chlorovinyldichloroarsine)	

LCt$_{50}$, concentration versus time; LD$_{50}$, median lethal dose; GF, cyclosar.

600 mg of 2-PAM-Cl. These injectors are now available commercially.[98]

Treatment of exposure to pralidoxime chloride varies depending on the extent of exposure. With minimal exposure, as is often seen with brief exposure to the vapor of the nerve agent, people may complain of headache and tightness in the chest and may have miosis, rhinorrhea, and increased salivation. Individuals must be removed from further exposure, clothing must be removed, topical atropine must be instilled in the eye if eye pain is significant, and wet decontamination should take place in the event of liquid exposure. With moderate exposure, the same signs are present, but the patient demonstrates more severe rhinorrhea and complains of dyspnea and, on examination, there is evidence of bronchospasm and muscle fasciculations. Patients should now be treated intramuscularly with atropine and 2-PAM-Cl. Victims of casualty again must have their clothing removed, and, if they were exposed to liquid nerve agent, they need to go through a wet decontamination process. With severe exposure, the same symptoms are present, but now the person has severe respiratory compromise, flaccid paralysis, incontinence, convulsions, and dysrhythmias. The patient should receive aggressive treatment with atropine, along with intravenous or intramuscular injections of 2-PAM-Cl to a maximum of 1,500 mg, and should go through a wet decontamination process, with ventilatory assistance provided if necessary.

People who anticipate being exposed to a nerve agent should take pyridostigmine, a long-acting agent that binds with acetylcholinesterase, allowing the enzyme to spontaneously regenerate. It does not cross the blood–brain barrier and, if used, must be taken >30 minutes prior to exposure.

With nerve injury casualties—whether as the result of liquid or vapor exposure—decontamination is critical. It needs to be done as quickly as possible; the first step is to leave the area of exposure. As was commented on earlier in this chapter, health care and emergency workers in Japan became victims by standing unprotected in the subway cars in which liquid sarin and some vapor were present.[7] Patients should be decontaminated by removing their clothing and washing them with copious amounts of water in 5% hypochlorite (household bleach). The bleach is not as critical as is washing with copious amounts of water. Some emergency departments have plans in place to set up fire trucks side-by-side with a "chamber" established between the two trucks if a large number of casualties are expected. Individuals disrobe as they come into the chamber and are sprayed with water as they walk through the chamber to the other side.[99] Depending on the severity of the symptoms, they may then receive atropine, 2-PAM-Cl, and further treatment (e.g., assisted ventilation, benzodiazepines, and oxygen procedures).

Pulmonary Agents

The pulmonary or choking agents were probably the first chemicals to be used in warfare during World War I. On April 22, 1915, near Ypres, Belgium, the Germans released about 160 tons of chlorine gas from 6,000 pressurized cylinders along their lines while the wind blew toward the allied troops. The chlorine floated on huge clouds toward the allied lines and caused eye, nose, and throat burning. As it was inhaled, the gas created pulmonary edema and casualties began to cough up yellow-tinged pulmonary secretions. Approximately 5,000 soldiers died in that attack, and 2 days later in a second attack, another 500 soldiers died. In all, >15,000 men were wounded. By late 1915, chlorine was replaced by phosgene, which is more deadly than chlorine gas.[100] During World War II, no chemical weapons were used, but as mentioned previously, prior to the war the Germans discovered the chemical weapons known as nerve agents. After the war, both the Allies and the former Soviet Union used German chemists to develop their own chemical weapons programs.

The four primary pulmonary agents include chloropicrin, chlorine, phosgene, and diphosgene. Ricin can also be inhaled or it can be given parenterally; it will not be discussed here because Audi et al.[101] have provided an excellent review of the pathophysiology of this agent. Phosgene is a prototypical agent because, as stated, it is deadlier than any of the other compounds. Its chemical formula is $COCl_2$, with a molecular weight of 98 daltons and a boiling point of 8.2°C. It is a colorless gas and has an odor of recently cut hay at 22 to 28°C and normal pressure conditions. Because it has a vapor density of 3.4 units, it stays in the air for a long time, collecting in low-lying places. It is highly soluble in lipids and therefore can easily penetrate pulmonary epithelium and the cells lining the alveoli. Although it is very lipid-soluble, it reacts rapidly with water, forming hydrochloric acid and carbon dioxide. This reaction explains how it works: when phosgene reaches the alveoli, it produces hydrochloric acid, which is itself extremely toxic to tissues, causing a capillary leak and the development of acute lung injury, which progresses to acute respiratory distress syndrome. Depending on the amount of gas inhaled, hypoxia from a low FIO_2 would also complicate this picture. Immediately on exposure to phosgene, patients begin coughing because of the noxious nature of the gas; they also exhibit nausea, vomiting, choking, and chest tightness. After the initial exposure, depending on the amount of gas inhaled, the individual seems relatively free of abnormalities for the first 1 to 24 hours, but during this period, the pulmonary capillary membranes are being injured, with leakage of fluid into the alveoli.

Gas masks provide the best protection from exposure to phosgene. If gas masks are not available, individuals need to remove themselves from exposure as quickly as possible. For those individuals who inhale sufficient quantities of gas and then develop acute lung injury or acute respiratory distress syndrome, the management is similar to that of patients who develop this syndrome for other reasons. Anesthesiologists should feel relatively at ease in this situation because of their physiologic and pharmacologic experience in managing airways, ventilators, and hemodynamic monitoring to optimize care for patients with noncardiogenic pulmonary edema.

Blood Agents

The so-called blood agents, cyanogens, include hydrogen cyanide, hydrocyanic acid, cyanogen chloride, and arsine.[102] These agents are inhaled and release hydrogen cyanide, which impairs cytochrome oxidase and aerobic metabolism at the level of the mitochondria. At 22 to 27°C, hydrogen cyanide is a colorless liquid and can be taken up through the skin as a liquid or the gas can be inhaled. Its boiling point is 25.7°C, and it is difficult to use as a biologic weapon because it is so highly volatile, and therefore is not persistent. If this agent is released in an open area, high concentrations are hard to obtain. In a closed area, high lethal concentrations can be obtained readily. It is lethal because it interferes with cytochrome oxidase and cellular respiration. Oxygen can get to the tissue, but the uncoupled oxidative phosphorylation prevents effective usage of oxygen by the mitochondria. Patients quickly develop metabolic acidosis and all of the sequelae associated with cellular hypoxemia.

Patients who present with hydrogen cyanide exposure have a variety of symptoms, depending on the amount to which they were exposed, the root of the poisoning, and the exposure time. The patient will appear restless and tachypneic and will occasionally complain of headaches, palpitations, and dyspnea. As time progresses, depending on the severity of the inhalation, nausea, vomiting, convulsions leading to coma, and respiratory failure are manifest. If the hydrogen cyanide dosage is high, patients may not have any of these symptoms and may simply collapse within seconds to minutes of exposure, which would be followed within 1 to 2 minutes with convulsions and cardiac arrest.

Treatment for cyanide toxicity is another problem for which anesthesiologists are quite familiar because of their use of nitroprusside, which, at high doses and for extended periods, also releases cyanide ions, which can poison the cellular respiration. Cyanide ions are normally metabolized by the rhodanese enzyme in the liver, which is a sulfur-requiring step that leads to the bioformation of methemoglobin. However, there often is not enough sulfur present for rhodanese to operate efficiently; therefore, treatment involves the administration of sodium thiosulfate, with supportive care in the form of tracheal intubation, ventilation, 100% oxygen, and cardiac support with inotropes and vasopressors. If the number of casualties exceeds the means to care for them, mortality could be quite high.

Again, for the aforementioned reasons, terrorists would have difficulty using hydrogen cyanide as an effective chemical weapon to target large numbers of persons in civilian areas. This agent is mentioned primarily because of its historical interest and because of the possibility that it might be used in the future.

Vesicants

During World War I, not only were chlorine and phosgene used, but sulfur mustard was widely used on both sides of the conflict. Sodium mustard and related compounds such as nitrogen mustard, phosgene oxime, and lewisite are also known as "blister agents." This name is derived from the fact that when these compounds come into contact with skin, they produce burns and blisters. These compounds can also be inhaled, can inflict severe damage to the respiratory system and the eyes, and can produce multiple organ dysfunction syndrome. Vesicants are often used by warring factions to force enemy troops to wear protective equipment, which makes them less mobile and less able to fight efficiently.[102] Blister agents are colorless and almost odorless. However, if the temperature is high enough, an odor of rotten onions or mustard may be present.

Sulfur mustard is a bifunctional alkylating agent that contains two reactive chloroethyl moieties. These chloroethyl compounds are extremely reactive, which allows them to bind to other substances, such as nucleic acids, proteins, and nucleotides. Sulfur mustard readily penetrates clothing and infiltrates the skin and eyes. As it volatilizes, sulfur mustard can be inhaled or ingested through the GI tract. Depending on the amount of material to which an individual is exposed, symptoms of sulfur poisoning may not show up for 1 to 24 hours after the initial exposure occurs. By the time symptoms appear, most of the damage has already been done. Mild poisoning with sulfur mustard results in eye pain, with extensive tearing, erythema and inflammation of the skin, and irritation of the mucus membranes, with cough, sneezing, hoarseness, and so forth. Mild poisoning does not warrant any treatment other than supportive care, and will pass with time.

Exposure to larger amounts of sulfur mustard causes considerable dysfunction, incapacitating individuals, who require emergency medical care. Individuals lose their vision, as was common during World War I when soldiers were led around by one individual with good vision at the front of the line, followed by a chain of soldiers, each marching with one arm resting on the shoulder of the soldier in front of him. Nausea,

---

TABLE 60-12

ANESTHESIA AND MASS CASUALTIES

Treat injuries that are or will become life-threatening if untreated
Aim for anesthesia and surgery that are quick and effective
Expect perioperative deaths to occur
Understand that many patients are high risk
Realize that providing the usual standard of care is likely to be impossible
Provide drawover as typical inhalation anesthesia technique; no vaporizer necessary if TIVA is used

---

TIVA, total intravenous anesthesia.

---

vomiting, and diarrhea often develop, along with severe respiratory difficulty, because the same thing that happens to the skin can happen in the pulmonary epithelium.

A nuclear-biologic-chemical protective suit and gas mask provide the best protection against sulfur mustard. Decontamination for individuals who are exposed to this agent is identical to that following exposure to a nerve agent; that is, clothing is removed and the victim is washed with warm soapy water with or without 0.5% hypochlorite. Those patients who develop respiratory compromise are managed as they would be with the inhalation of a pulmonary agent.

CONCLUSION

It is difficult to anticipate the role anesthesiologists might play in managing patients who are victims of natural disasters or casualties of a terrorist attack with weapons of mass destruction. What is clear is that the anesthesiologists have the requisite training and experience to be of vital importance in managing such casualties. However, based on their training, they may not be emotionally prepared to manage these patients. Unlike in their normal practice, they may have to triage patients, accept the fact that the standard of care may be changed, and focus their efforts on interventions that will carry the greatest benefit for the greatest number of casualties (Table 60-12).

This process begins when anesthesiologists receive the call that a mass casualty has occurred or is about to occur. Anesthesiologists must first report to the command and control center and, although they most likely will work in the operating room, they could also be used in the triage area in the emergency department or in the ICU (Table 60-13). Of utmost

---

TABLE 60-13

POSSIBLE ROLES FOR ANESTHESIOLOGISTS ON REPORTING TO COMMAND AND CONTROL CENTER[a]

- Decontamination
- Triage
  - Dead
  - Expectant
  - Minor injury
  - To OR
  - To floor—stabilize
  - To ICU—to OR later
- Provide care in the OR
- Provide care in the ICU—burns, flail chest, traumatic amputation

---

OR, operating room; ICU, intensive care unit.
[a]May be difficult to reach; hospital may be secure.

importance is familiarity with the hospital's disaster plan. One must also develop one's own family care plan in anticipation of absence from the home for extended periods of time. Ensuring one's own safety through the appropriate use of protective devices to serve as barriers against radiologic, biologic, and chemical weapons is also of vital importance.

References

1. Health care at the crossroads. Strategies for creating and sustaining community-wide emergency preparedness systems. Oakbrook Terrace, IL, Joint Commission on Accreditation of Healthcare Organizations, 2003; 1

2. Chen L, Evans T, Anand S et al: Human resources for health: Overcoming the crisis. Lancet 2004; 364: 1984

3. Preparing for pandemic flu, Special Subcommittee on Aging, 109th Congress—2nd Session. Washington, DC, American Hospital Association, 2006, p 1

4. Niska RW, Burt CW: Emergency response planning in hospitals, United States: 2003–2004. Adv Data 2007; 1

5. Combs CD: Preparing Health Professionals for the Unthinkable. Washington, DC, Association of Academic Health Centers, 2003; 1

6. Kelen GD, Kraus CK, McCarthy ML et al: Inpatient disposition classification for the creation of hospital surge capacity: A multiphase study. Lancet 2006; 368: 1984

7. Okumura T, Suzuki K, Fukuda A et al: The Tokyo subway sarin attack: Disaster management, Part 3: National and international responses. Acad Emerg Med 1998; 5: 625

8. Cluster of severe acute respiratory syndrome cases among protected healthcare workers—Toronto, Canada, April 2003. MMWR Morb Mortal Wkly Rep 2003; 433

9. Copeland L: Houston drying out after deluge. USA Today June 13, 2001. (http://www.usatoday.com/weather/news/2001/2001-06-14-houston-allison.htm)

10. Castillo CJ: Mutual Aid Agreements for Public Assistance and Fire Management Assistance, 2005. (http://www.fema.gov/government/grant/pa/9523_6.shtm)

11. Tsai MC, Arnold JL, Chuang CC et al: Implementation of the Hospital Emergency Incident Command System during an outbreak of severe acute respiratory syndrome at a hospital in Taiwan, ROC. J Emerg Med 2005; 28: 185

12. Family Disaster Plan by the American Red Cross, and again another website, accessed today http://www.redcross.org/portal/site/en/menuitem.d229a5f06620c6052b1ecfbf43181aa0/?vgnextoid=bb2a1c99b5ccb110VgnVCM10000089f0870aRCRD&vgnextfmt=default

13. ASHTO. http://www.astho.org/pubs/IsraelReport.pdf. In: Association of State and Territorial Health Officials; 2007

14. Rodoplu U, Arnold J, Ersoy G: Terrorism in Turkey. Prehosp Disaster Med 2003; 18: 152

15. The Joint Commission is watching: Is your disaster response plan in order? Ed Manag 2004; 16: 73

16. Teachers of Preventive Medicine and Centers for Disease Control and Prevention: clinician competencies for emergency preparedness and bioterrorism. http://www.nycepce.org/info.htm

17. Moszynski P: Extreme weather affects half a billion people each year. BMJ 2007; 335: 321

18. Tropical Cyclone Report, Hurricane Katrina, 23–30 August 2005. Miami, FL, National Hurricane Center, 2005. (http://www.nhc.noaa.gov/pdf/TCR-AL122005_Katrina.pdf)

19. Public health response to Hurricanes Katrina and Rita—Louisiana, 2005. Morb Mortal Wkly Rep 2006; 55: 29

20. Schultz CH, Koenig KL, Lewis RJ: Implications of hospital evacuation after the Northridge, California, earthquake. N Engl J Med 2003; 348: 1349

21. Franco C, Toner E, Waldhorn R et al: Systemic collapse: Medical care in the aftermath of Hurricane Katrina. Biosecur Bioterror 2006; 4: 135

22. Sever MS, Erek E, Vanholder R et al: Lessons learned from the catastrophic Marmara earthquake: Factors influencing the final outcome of renal victims. Clin Nephrol 2004; 61: 413

23. Dacey MJ: Tragedy and response: The Rhode Island nightclub fire. N Engl J Med 2003; 349: 1990

24. Halpern P, Rosen B, Carasso S et al: Intensive care in a field hospital in an urban disaster area: Lessons from the August 1999 earthquake in Turkey. Crit Care Med 2003; 31: 1410

25. Bhopal Information Center: Chronology. http://www.bhopal.com/pdfs/chrono05.pdf

26. Military Support to Civil Authorities. Defense Do, ed.; 1993. (http://www.dtic.mil/whs/directives/corres/pdf/302501p.pdf)

27. FEMA (http://www.fema.gov/)

28. Homeland Security, Department of Homeland Security. (http://www.dhs.gov/xprepresp.)

29. The Department of Homeland Security. National Response Framework. (http://www.dhs.gov/xprepresp/committees/editorial_0566.shtm 2008.)

30. For Practitioners, Clinicians & Responders. (http://www.hhs.gov/disasters/discussion/responders/index.html

31. Mahoney LE, Whiteside DF, Belue HE et al: Disaster medical assistance teams. Ann Emerg Med 1987; 16: 354

32. Join the National Disaster Medical System Effort. (http://www.hhs.gov/aspr/opeo/ndms/join/index.html)

33. Esbitt D: The Strategic National Stockpile: Roles and responsibilities of health care professionals for receiving the stockpile assets. Disaster Manag Response 2003; 1: 68

34. Beaton RD, Oberle MW, Wicklund J et al: Evaluation of the Washington State National Pharmaceutical Stockpile dispensing exercise: Part I—Patient volunteer findings. J Public Health Manag Pract 2003; 9: 368

35. Dreyfus M: The war against terrorism collides with anesthesia. Anesthesiology News 2003; March, 46

36. Shibata Y, Yamashita S, Masyakin VB et al: 15 years after Chernobyl: New evidence of thyroid cancer. Lancet 2001; 358: 1965

37. Optimizing the international effort to study, mitigate and minimize the consequences of the Chernobyl disaster. In: United Nations General Assembly; 2005. (http://www.belarusembassy.org/chernobyl/355.pdf)

38. Dellinger RP, Carlet JM, Masur H et al: Introduction. Crit Care Med 2004; 32: S446

39. Collins DL: Human responses to the threat of or exposure to ionizing radiation at Three Mile Island, Pennsylvania, and Goiania, Brazil. Mil Med 2002; 167: 137

40. Collins DL, de Carvalho AB: Chronic stress from the Goiania ^{137}Cs radiation accident. Behav Med 1993; 18: 149

41. Case Study: Accidental Leakage of Cesium-137 in Goiania, Brazil, in 1987. (http://www.nbc-med.org/SiteContent/MedRef/OnlineRef/CaseStudies/csgoiania.html)

42. Radiation disasters and children. Pediatrics 2003; 111: 1455

43. American Academy of Pediatrics. Committee on Environmental Health: Risk of ionizing radiation exposure to children: A subject review. Pediatrics 1998; 101: 717

44. Total casualties, The Avalon Project at Yale Law School. The Atomic Bombings of Hiroshima and Nagasaki: Documents in Law, History, and Diplomacy. New Haven, CT, The Avalon Project at Yale Law School, 2002

45. The 9-11 Commission Report: Final Report of the National Commission on Terrorist Attacks Upon the United States, Official Government Edition. http://www.gpoaccess.gov/911/

46. Mongan P, Shields C, Via D: Threat of radiologic terrorism increases. Unfamiliar patient care and safety issues mandate preparedness. Anesthesia Patient Safety Foundation (APSF) Newsletter 2002; 17: 9

47. Manthous CA, Jackson WL Jr: The 9-11 Commission's invitation to imagine: a pathophysiology-based approach to critical care of nuclear explosion victims. Crit Care Med 2007; 35: 716

48. O'Neill K: The Nuclear Terrorist Threat, Washington, DC, Institute for Science and International Security, 1997. (http://www.isis-online.org/publications/terrorism/threat.pdf)

49. Koenig KL, Goans RE, Hatchett RJ et al: Medical treatment of radiological casualties: Current concepts. Ann Emerg Med 2005; 45: 643

50. Kumar KS, Srinivasan V, Toles R et al: Nutritional approaches to radioprotection: Vitamin E. Mil Med 2002; 167: 57

51. Mitchell JB, Krishna M: Nitroxides as radiation protectors. Mil Med 2002; 167: 49

52. Whitnall MH, Elliott EB, Landauer MR et al: Protection against gamma–irradiation and 5-androstenediol. Mil Med 2002; 167: 64

53. Stickney DR, Dowding C, Reading C et al: HE2100 and HE3204 protect Rhesus Macaques from chemotherapy or radiation-induced myelosuppression. J Clin Oncol 2004; 22: 6668

54. Brook I, Elliott TB, Ledney GD et al:. Management of postirradiation sepsis. Mil Med 2002; 167: 105

55. Reeves GI: Radiation injuries. Crit Care Clin 1999; 15: 457

56. Barry JM: Viruses of mass destruction. Fortune 2004; 74

57. CDC Resources for Pandemic Flu. Centers for Disease Control and Prevention. (http://www.cdc.gov/flu/Pandemic/)

58. Markel H, Lipman HB, Navarro JA et al: Nonpharmaceutical interventions implemented by US cities during the 1918–1919 influenza pandemic. JAMA 2007; 298: 644

59. Jefferson T, Foxlee R, Del Mar C et al: Physical interventions to interrupt or reduce the spread of respiratory viruses: systematic review. BMJ 2008; 336: 77

60. Gostin LO: Medical countermeasures for pandemic influenza: Ethics and the law. JAMA 2006; 295: 554

61. Moscona A: Oseltamivir resistance—disabling our influenza defenses. N Engl J Med 2005; 353: 2633

62. Jefferson T, Demicheli V, Rivetti D et al: Antivirals for influenza in healthy adults: systematic review. Lancet 2006; 367: 303

63. Enserink M: Influenza. WHO adds more "1918" to pandemic predictions. Science 2004; 306: 2025

64. Severe acute respiratory syndrome (ARDS). Current SARS situation. 2005. (www.cdc.gov/ncidod/sars/situation.htm)

65. Kamming D, Gardam M, Chung F: Anaesthesia and SARS. Br J Anaesth 2003; 90: 715

66. Zhong N, Zeng G: What we have learnt from SARS epidemics in China. BMJ 2006; 333: 389

67. Beeching NJ, Dance DA, Miller AR et al: Biological warfare and bioterrorism. BMJ 2002; 324: 336

68. West Nile Virus: Statistics, Surveillance, and Control. Centers for Disease Control and Prevention, 2004. (http://www.cdc.gov/ncidod/dvbid/westnile/surv&control.htm.)

69. Coursin DB, Ketzler JT, Kumar A et al: Bioterrorism may overwhelm medical resources. New and different patient safety challenges must be anticipated. Anesthesia Patient Safety Foundation (APSF) Newsletter 2002; 17: 4

70. Breman JG, Henderson DA: Diagnosis and management of smallpox. N Engl J Med 2002; 346: 1300

71. The World Health Organization Smallpox Eradication Programme. (http://choo.fis.utoronto.ca/fis/courses/lis2102/KO.WHO.case.html)

72. Moore ZS, Seward JF, Lane JM: Smallpox. Lancet 2006; 367: 425

73. From the Centers for Disease Control and Prevention. Smallpox vaccine adverse events among civilians—United States, January 24–February 18, 2003. JAMA 2003; 289: 1497

74. Inglesby TV, O'Toole T, Henderson DA et al: Anthrax as a biological weapon, 2002: Updated recommendations for management. JAMA 2002; 287: 2236

75. Kalamas AG: Anthrax. Anesthesiol Clin N Am 2004; 22: 533

76. Martin G: Anthrax: Lessons learned from the U.S. Capitol experience. Mil Med 2003; 168: 9

77. Swartz MN: Recognition and management of anthrax: An update. N Engl J Med 2001; 345: 1621

78. Dixon TC, Meselson M, Guillemin J et al: Anthrax. N Engl J Med 1999; 341: 815

79. Shafazand S, Doyle R, Ruoss S et al: Inhalational anthrax: Epidemiology, diagnosis, and management. Chest 1999; 116: 1369

80. Schmitt B, Dobrez D, Parada JP et al: Responding to a small-scale bioterrorist anthrax attack: Cost-effectiveness analysis comparing preattack vaccination with postattack antibiotic treatment and vaccination. Arch Intern Med 2007; 167: 655

81. Prentice MB, Rahalison L: Plague. Lancet 2007; 369: 1196

82. Plague. US Government, 2007. (http://www3.niaid.nih.gov/healthscience/healthtopics/plague.)

83. Zietz BP, Dunkelberg H: The history of the plague and the research on the causative agent Yersinia pestis. Int J Hyg Environ Health 2004; 207: 165

84. USAMRIID. 2007. (http://www.usamriid.army.mil/.)

85. Josko D: Botulin toxin: A weapon in terrorism. Clin Lab Sci 2004; 17: 30

86. Franz DR, Jahrling PB, Friedlander AM et al: Clinical recognition and management of patients exposed to biological warfare agents. JAMA 1997; 278: 399

87. Bhalla DK, Warheit DB: Biological agents with potential for misuse: A historical perspective and defensive measures. Toxicol Appl Pharmacol 2004; 199: 71

88. Baker DJ: Management of casualties from terrorist chemical and biological attack: A key role for the anaesthetist. Br J Anaesth 2002; 89: 211

89. Cosgrove SE, Perl TM, Song X et al: Ability of physicians to diagnose and manage illness due to category A bioterrorism agents. Arch Intern Med 2005; 165: 2002

90. Horton WG: COTEP Annual Meeting Panel: Well Prepared to Educate You. ASA Newsletter 2007; 71

91. Extracts from the report of the Secretary-General: chemical and bacteriological (biological) weapons and the effects of their possible use. United Nations, 1969. (http://www.unog.ch/80256EDD006B8954/(httpAssets)/83669D9CB 32C9F33C125718B0034C413/$file/Extract_UNSG-1969.pdf)

92. Evison D, Hinsley D, Rice P: Chemical weapons. BMJ 2002; 324: 332

93. de Jong RH: Nerve gas terrorism: A grim challenge to anesthesiologists. Anesth Analg 2003; 96: 819

94. Roberts DM, Aaron CK: Management of acute organophosphorus pesticide poisoning. BMJ 2007; 334: 629

95. Brennan RJ, Waeckerle JF, Sharp TW et al: Chemical warfare agents: Emergency medical and emergency public health issues. Ann Emerg Med 1999; 34: 191

96. Pawar KS, Bhoite RR, Pillay CP et al: Continuous pralidoxime infusion versus repeated bolus injection to treat organophosphorus pesticide poisoning: A randomised controlled trial. Lancet 2006; 368: 2136

97. Peter JV, Moran JL, Graham P: Oxime therapy and outcomes in human organophosphate poisoning: An evaluation using meta-analytic techniques. Crit Care Med 2006; 34: 502

98. FDA Approves Treatment for Nerve-Poisoning Agents for Use by Trained Emergency Medical Services Personnel. 2006. (http://www.fda.gov/bbs/topics/NEWS/2006/NEW01473.html)

99. Lake WA, Fedele PD, Marshall SM: Guidelines for mass casualty decontamination during a terrorist chemical agent incident. AMSSB-REN-HD-DI; 2000: 1. U.S. Army Soldier and Biological Chemical Command (SBCCOM) http://www.nlecbrne.com/pdf/guidelines_mass_causality_decon.pdf

100. Weapons of War: Poison Gas. firstworldwar.com. (www.firstworldwar.com/weaponry/gas.htm)

101. Audi J, Belson M, Patel M et al: Ricin poisoning: A comprehensive review. JAMA 2005; 294: 2342

102. Soldier and Biological Chemical Command (SBCCOM). 2003. (http://www.globalsecurity.org/military/agency/army/sbccom.htm)

PERIOPERATIVE AND CONSULTATIVE SERVICES

APPENDIX ■ ELECTROCARDIOGRAPHY

JAMES R. ZAIDAN AND PAUL G. BARASH

ELECTROCARDIOGRAM

LEAD PLACEMENT

	■ ELECTRODE	
	■ POSITIVE	■ NEGATIVE
BIPOLAR LEADS		
I	LA	RA
II	LL	RA
III	LL	LA
AUGMENTED UNIPOLAR		
aVR	RA	LA, LL
aVL	LA	RA, LL
aVF	LL	RA, LA
■ PRECORDIAL		
V_1	4 ICS–RSB	
V_2	4 ICS–LSB	
V_3	Midway between V_2 and V_4	
V_4	5 ICS–MCL	
V_5	5 ICS–AAL	
V_6	5 ICS–MAL	

THREE-LEAD SYSTEMS

■ BIPOLAR LEAD SYSTEM	■ ELECTRODE PLACEMENT	■ ECG LEAD[a]	■ ADVANTAGE
II	RA R–clavicle LA L–10th rib (midclavicular line) LL Ground	II (II)	Dysrhythmias
MCL 1	RA Ground LA L–clavicle LL V_1	III (V_1)	Dysrhythmias and conduction defects
CS 5	RA R–clavicle LA V_5 LL Ground	I (V_5)	Precordial ischemia
CB 5	RA R–scapula LA V_5 LL Ground	I (V_5)	Precordial ischemia and dysrhythmias

ECG, electrocardiogram; MCL, modified central lead; CB, central back; CS, central subclavian.
[a]Selected lead on monitor: ( ) = simulated ECG lead.

We wish to thank Dr. Malcom S. Thaler for graciously permitting reproduction of electrocardiographic tracings from his book, The Only EKG Book You'll Ever Need (Philadelphia, JB Lippincott, 1988).

THE NORMAL ELECTROCARDIOGRAM—CARDIAC CYCLE

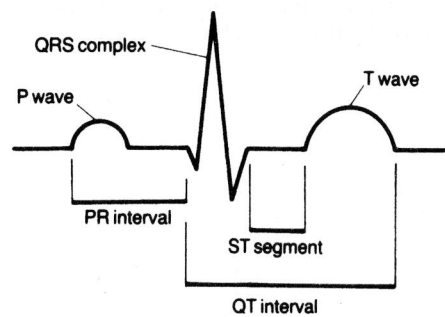

In this section the electrocardiogram (ECG) complex is divided into the atrial (PR interval) and ventricular (QT interval) components.

ASHMAN BEATS

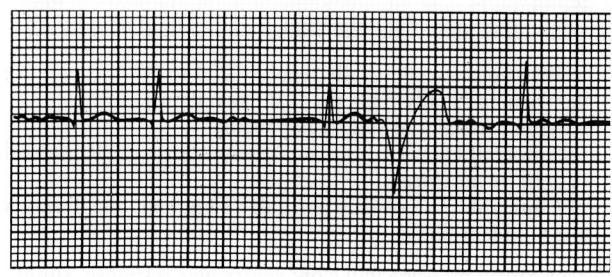

Rate: Variable.
Rhythm: Irregular.
PR interval: P wave may be present if supraventricular premature beat.
QT interval: QRS prolonged (>0.12 second) and altered, revealing bundle-branch pattern, most commonly right bundle. ST segment abnormal.

Note: Ashman beats are often confused with ventricular premature contractions. Ashman beats, usually seen with atrial fibrillation, have no compensatory pause and are a benign ECG finding, requiring no treatment.

ATRIAL FIBRILLATION

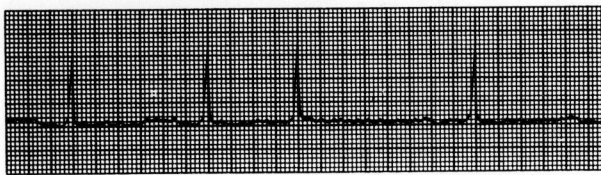

Rate: Variable (approximately 150 to 200 beats/min).
Rhythm: Irregular.
PR interval: No P wave, and PR interval not discernible.
QT interval: QRS normal.

Note: Must be differentiated from atrial flutter: (1) absence of flutter waves and presence of fibrillatory line, and (2) flutter usually associated with higher ventricular rates (>150 beats/min). Loss of atrial contraction reduces cardiac output (10 to 20%). Mural atrial thrombi may develop. Considered controlled if ventricular rate <100 beats/min.

ATRIAL FLUTTER

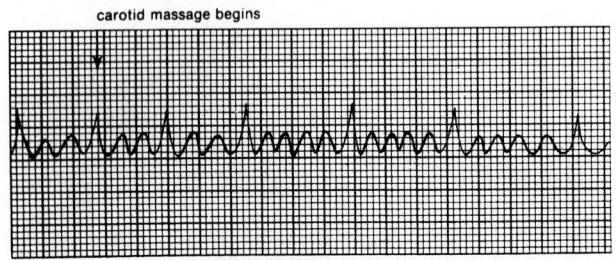

Rate: Rapid, atrial usually regular (250 to 350 beats/min); ventricular usually regular (<100 beats/min).
Rhythm: Atrial and ventricular regular.
PR interval: Flutter (F) waves are saw-toothed. PR interval cannot be measured.
QT interval: QRS usually normal; ST segment and T waves are not identifiable.

Note: Carotid massage will slow ventricular response, simplifying recognition of the F waves.

ATRIOVENTRICULAR BLOCK
(First-Degree)

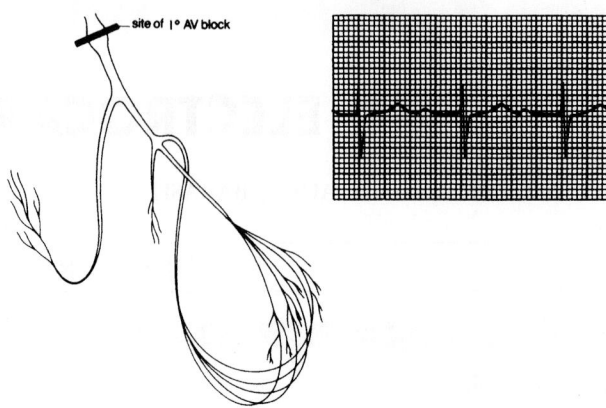

Rate: 60 to 100 beats/min.
Rhythm: Regular.
PR interval: Prolonged (>0.20 second) and constant.
QT interval: Normal.

Note: Usually clinically insignificant; may be early harbinger of drug toxicity.

ATRIOVENTRICULAR BLOCK
(Second-Degree), Mobitz Type I/Wenckebach Block

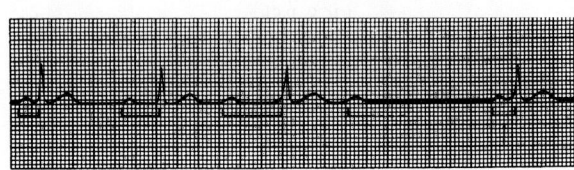

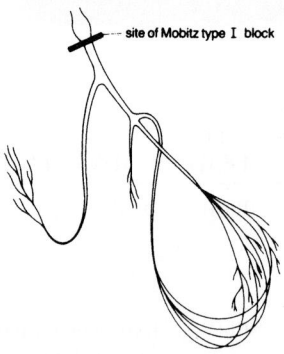

Rate: 60 to 100 beats/min.
Rhythm: Atrial regular; ventricular irregular.
PR interval: P wave normal; PR interval progressively lengthens with each cycle until QRS complex is dropped (dropped beat). PR interval following the dropped beat is shorter than normal.
QT interval: QRS complex normal but dropped periodically.

Note: Commonly seen (1) in trained athletes and (2) with drug toxicity.

ATRIOVENTRICULAR BLOCK
(Second-Degree), Mobitz Type II

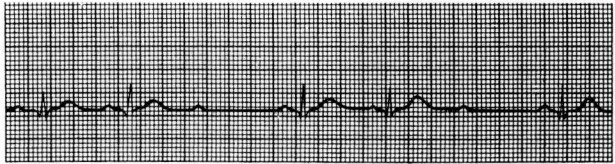

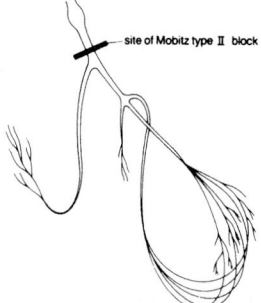

site of Mobitz type II block

Rate: <100 beats/min.

Rhythm: Atrial regular; ventricular regular or irregular.

PR interval: P waves normal, but some are not followed by QRS complex.

QT interval: Normal but may have widened QRS complex if block is at level of bundle branch. ST segment and T wave may be abnormal, depending on location of block.

Note: In contrast to Mobitz type I block, the PR and RR intervals are constant and the dropped QRS occurs without warning. The wider the QRS complex (block lower in the conduction system), the greater the amount of myocardial damage.

ATRIOVENTRICULAR BLOCK
(Third-Degree), Complete Heart Block

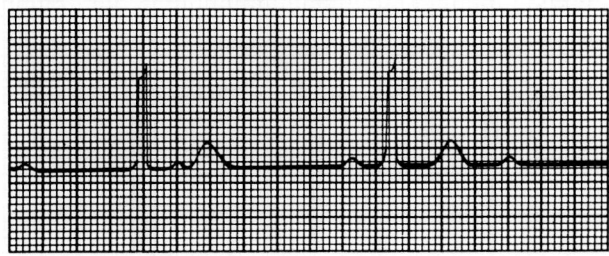

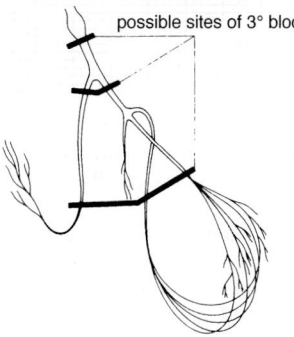

possible sites of 3° block

Rate: <45 beats/min.

Rhythm: Atrial regular; ventricular regular; no relationship between P wave and QRS complex.

PR interval: Variable because atria and ventricles beat independently.

QT interval: QRS morphology variable, depending on the origin of the ventricular beat in the intrinsic pacemaker system (atrioventricular junctional vs. ventricular pacemaker). ST segment and T wave normal.

Note: Immediate treatment with atropine or isoproterenol is required if cardiac output is reduced. Consideration should be given to insertion of a pacemaker. This block is seen as a complication of mitral valve replacement.

ATRIOVENTRICULAR DISSOCIATION

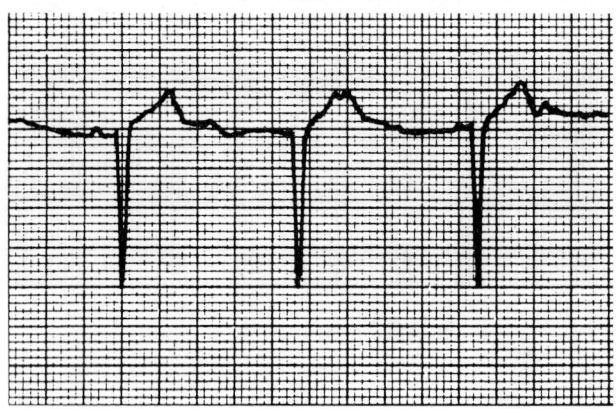

Rate: Variable.
Rhythm: Atrial regular; ventricular regular; ventricular rate faster than atrial rate; no relationship between P wave and QRS complex.
PR interval: Variable because atria and ventricles beat independently.
QT interval: QRS morphology depends on location of ventricular pacemaker. ST segment and T wave abnormal.

Note: Digitalis toxicity can present as atrioventricular dissociation.

BUNDLE-BRANCH BLOCK—RIGHT

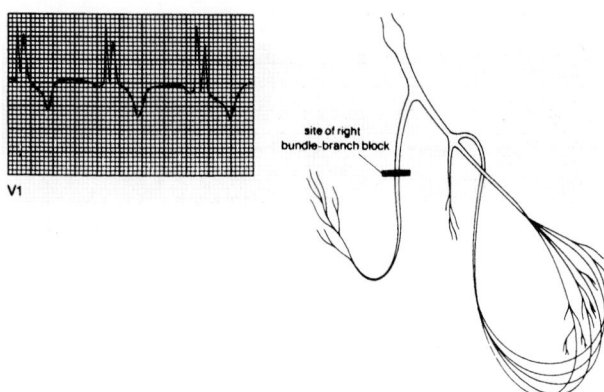

Rate: <100 beats/min.
Rhythm: Regular.
PR interval: Normal.
QT interval: Complete right bundle-branch block (RBBB) (QRS >0.12 second); incomplete RBBB (QRS = 0.10 to 0.12 second). Varying patterns of QRS complex; rSR (V_1); RS, wide R with M pattern. ST segment and T wave opposite direction of the R wave.

Note: In the presence of RBBB, Q waves may be seen with a myocardial infarction.

BUNDLE-BRANCH BLOCK—LEFT

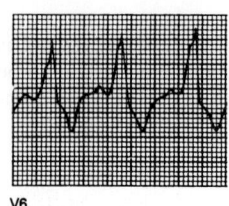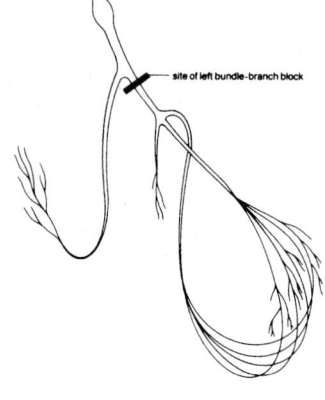

Rate: <100 beats/min.
Rhythm: Regular.
PR interval: Normal.
QT interval: Complete left bundle-branch block (LBBB) (QRS >0.12 second); incomplete LBBB.
(QRS = 0.10 to 0.12 second); Lead V_1 negative rS complex; I, aVL, V_6 wide R wave without Q or S component. ST segment and T-wave defection opposite direction of the R wave.

Note: LBBB does not occur in healthy patients and usually indicates serious heart disease with a poorer prognosis. In patients with LBBB, insertion of a pulmonary artery catheter may lead to complete heart block.

ELECTROLYTE DISTURBANCES

	■ ↓ Ca^{2+}	■ ↑ Ca^{2+}	■ ↓ K^+	■ ↑ K^+
Rate	<100 (beats/min)	<100 (beats/min)	<100 (beats/min)	<100 (beats/min)
Rhythm	Regular	Regular	Regular	Regular
PR interval	Normal	Normal/increased	Normal	Normal
QT interval QT decreased	Increased	Decreased	T flat U wave	T peaked

Note: Electrocardiogram (ECG) changes usually do not correlate with serum calcium. Hypocalcemia rarely causes dysrhythmias in the absence of hypokalemia. In contrast, abnormalities in serum potassium concentration can be diagnosed by ECG.

DIGITALIS EFFECT

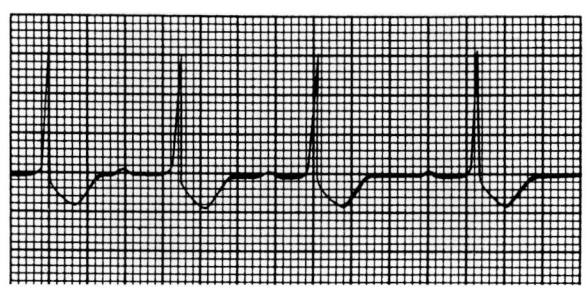

Rate: <100 beats/min.
Rhythm: Regular.
PR interval: Normal or prolonged.
QT interval: ST segment sloping ("digitalis effect").

Note: Digitalis toxicity can be the cause of many common dysrhythmias (e.g., premature ventricular contractions, second-degree heart block). Verapamil, quinidine, and amiodarone cause an increase in serum digitalis concentration.

CORONARY ARTERY DISEASE—MYOCARDIAL INFARCTION

■ ANATOMIC SITE	■ LEADS	■ ECG CHANGES	■ CORONARY ARTERY
Inferior	II, III, aVF	Q, ST, T	Right
Lateral	I, aVL, V_5–V_6	Q, ST, T	Left circumflex
Anterior	I, aVL, V_1–V_4	Q, ST, T	Left
Anteroseptal	V_1–V_4	Q, ST, T	Left anterior descending

ECG, electrocardiogram.

SUBENDOCARDIAL MYOCARDIAL INFARCTION

Persistent ST segment depression and/or T-wave inversion in the absence of Q wave. Usually requires additional laboratory data (e.g., isoenzymes) to confirm diagnosis.

TRANSMURAL MYOCARDIAL INFARCTION

Q waves seen on ECG useful in confirming diagnosis. Associated with poorer prognosis and more significant hemodynamic impairment; dysrhythmias frequently complicate course.

CORONARY ARTERY DISEASE—ISCHEMIA

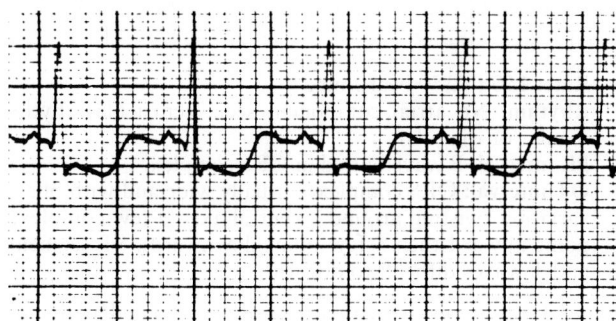

Rate: Variable.
Rhythm: Usually regular, but may show atrial and/or ventricular dysrhythmias.
PR interval: Normal.
QT interval: ST segment depressed; J-point depression; T-wave inversion; conduction disturbances. Coronary vasospasm (Prinzmetal) ST segment elevation.

Note: Intraoperative ischemia is usually seen in the presence of "normal" vital signs (e.g., ±20% of preinduction values).

PAROXYSMAL ATRIAL TACHYCARDIA

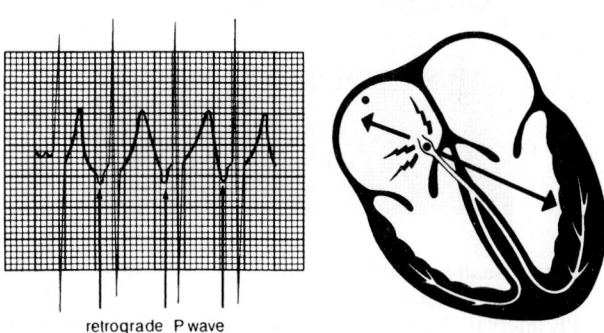

retrograde P wave

Rate: 150 to 250 beats/min.
Rhythm: Regular.
PR interval: Difficult to distinguish because of tachycardia obscuring P wave. P wave may precede, be included in, or follow QRS complex.
QT interval: Normal, but ST segment and T wave may be difficult to distinguish.

Note: Therapy depends on degree of hemodynamic compromise. In contrast to management of paroxysmal atrial tachycardia (PAT) in awake patients, synchronized cardioversion rather than pharmacologic treatment is preferred in hemodynamically unstable anesthetized patients.

PREMATURE ATRIAL CONTRACTION

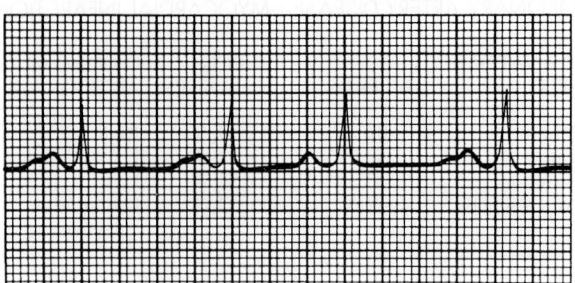

Rate: <100 beats/min.
Rhythm: Irregular.
PR interval: P waves may be lost in preceding T waves. PR interval is variable.
QT interval: QRS normal configuration; ST segment and T wave normal.

Note: Nonconducted premature atrial contraction (PAC) appearance similar to that of sinus arrest; T waves with PAC may be distorted by inclusion of P wave in the T wave.

PREMATURE VENTRICULAR CONTRACTION

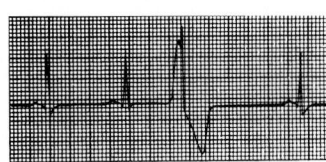

A

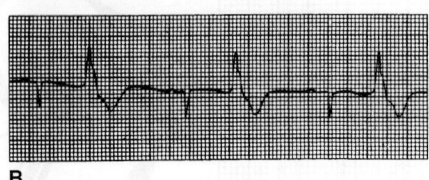

B

Rate: Usually <100 beats/min.
Rhythm: Irregular.
PR interval: P wave and PR interval absent; retrograde conduction of P wave can be seen.
QT interval: Wide QRS (>0.12 second); ST segment cannot be evaluated (e.g., ischemia); T wave opposite direction of QRS with compensatory pause (**A**). Bigeminy: every other beat a premature ventricular contraction (PVC) (**B**); trigeminy: every third beat a PVC. R-on-T occurs when PVC falls in the T wave and can lead to ventricular tachycardia or fibrillation.

Note: If compensatory pause is not seen following an ectopic beat, the complex is most likely supraventricular in origin.

SINUS TACHYCARDIA

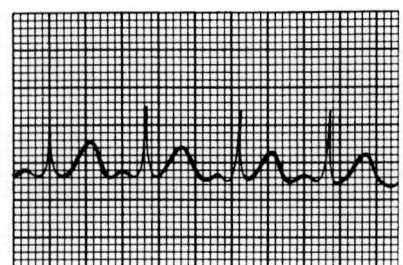

Rate: 100 to 160 beats/min.
Rhythm: Regular.
PR interval: Normal; P wave may be difficult to see.
QT interval: Normal.

Note: Should be differentiated from PAT. With PAT, carotid massage terminates dysrhythmia. Sinus tachycardia may respond to vagal maneuvers but reappears as soon as vagal stimulus is removed.

TORSADES DE POINTES

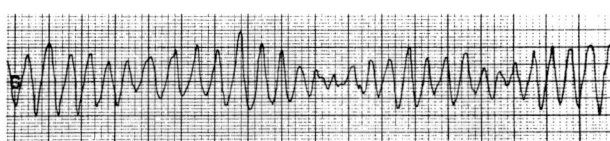

Rate: 150 to 250 beats/min.
Rhythm: No atrial component seen; ventricular rhythm regular or irregular.
PR interval: P wave buried in QRS complex.
QT interval: QRS complexes usually wide and with phasic variation twisting around a central axis (a few complexes point upward then a few point downward). ST segments and T waves difficult to discern.

Note: Type of ventricular tachycardia associated with prolonged QT interval. Seen with electrolyte disturbances (e.g., hypokalemia, hypocalcemia, and hypomagnesemia) and bradycardia. Administering standard antidysrhythmics (e.g., lidocaine, procainamide) may worsen torsades de pointes. Treatment includes increasing heart rate pharmacologically or by pacing.

VENTRICULAR FIBRILLATION

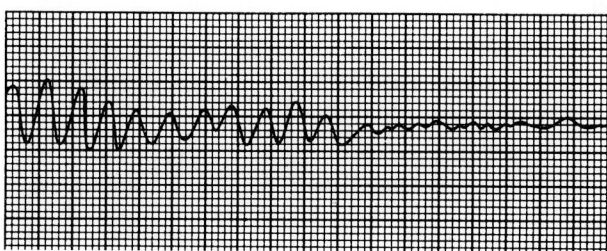

Rate: Absent.
Rhythm: None.
PR interval: Absent.
QT interval: Absent.

Note: "Pseudoventricular fibrillation" may be the result of a monitor malfunction (e.g., ECG lead disconnect). Always check for carotid pulse before instituting therapy.

VENTRICULAR TACHYCARDIA

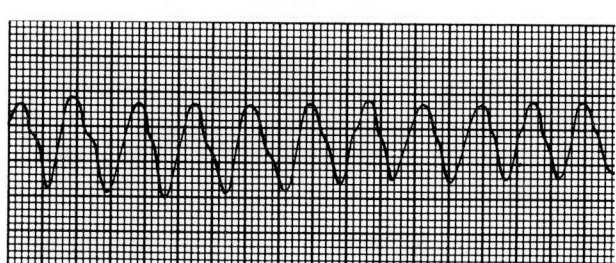

Rate: 100 to 250 beats/min.
Rhythm: No atrial component seen; ventricular rhythm irregular or regular.
PR interval: Absent; retrograde P wave may be seen in QRS complex.
QT interval: Wide, bizarre QRS complex. ST segment and T wave difficult to determine.

Note: In the presence of hemodynamic compromise, immediate DC synchronized cardioversion is required. If the patient is stable, with short bursts of ventricular tachycardia, pharmacologic management is preferred. Should be differentiated from supraventricular tachycardia with aberrancy (SVT-A). Compensatory pause and atrioventricular dissociation suggest a PVC. P waves and SR' (V_1) and slowing to vagal stimulus suggest SVT-A.

WOLFF-PARKINSON-WHITE SYNDROME

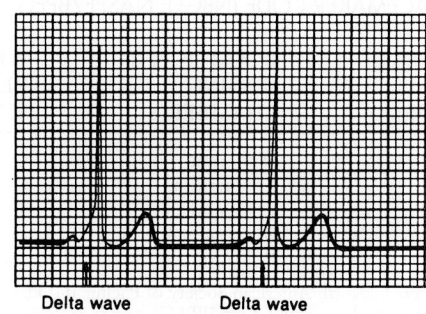

Delta wave   Delta wave

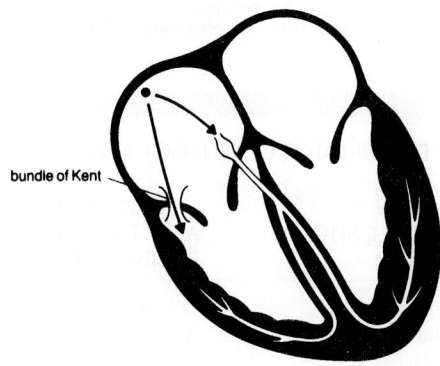

bundle of Kent

Rate: <100 beats/min.
Rhythm: Regular.
PR interval: P wave normal; PR interval short (<0.12 second).
QT interval: Duration (>0.10 second) with slurred QRS complex. Type A has delta wave, RBBB, with upright QRS complex V_1. Type B has delta wave and downward QRS-V_1. ST segment and T wave usually normal.

Note: Digoxin should be avoided in the presence of Wolff-Parkinson-White syndrome because it increases conduction through the accessory bypass tract (bundle of Kent) and decreases atrioventricular node conduction; consequently, ventricular fibrillation can occur.

GENERIC PACEMAKER CODE (NBG[a]): NASPE/BPEG REVISED (2002)

POSITION I, PACING CHAMBER(S)	POSITION II, SENSING CHAMBER(S)	POSITION III, RESPONSE(S) TO SENSING	POSITION IV, PROGRAMMABILITY	POSITION V, MULTISITE PACING
O = none A = atrium V = ventricle D = dual (A + V)	O = none A = atrium V = ventricle D = dual (A + V)	O = none I = inhibited T = triggered D = dual (T + I)	O = none R = rate modulation	O = none A = atrium V = ventricle D = dual (A + V)

[a]NBG: N refers to North American Society of Pacing and Electrophysiology (NASPE), now called the Heart Rhythm Society (HRS); B refers to British Pacing and Electrophysiology Group (BPEG); and G refers to generic.
From Practice advisory for perioperative management of patients with cardiac rhythm management devices: Pacemakers and implantable cardioverter-defibrillators. A report by the American Society of Anesthesiologists Task Force on Perioperative Management of Patients with Cardiac Rhythm Management Devices. Anesthesiology 2005; 103: 186, with permission.

GENERIC DEFIBRILLATOR CODE (NBG): NASPE/BPEG

POSITION I, SHOCK CHAMBER(S)	POSITION II, ANTITACHYCARDIA PACING CHAMBER(S)	POSITION III, TACHYCARDIA DETECTION	POSITION IV,[a] ANTIBRADYCARDIA PACING CHAMBER(S)
O = none A = atrium V = ventricle D = dual (A + V)	O = none A = atrium V = ventricle D = dual (A + V)	E = electrogram H = hemodynamic	O = none A = atrium V = ventricle D = dual (A + V)

NASPE, North American Society of Pacing and Electrophysiology; BPEG, British Pacing and Electrophysiology Group.
[a]For robust identification, position IV is expanded into its complete NBG code. For example, a biventricular pacing–defibrillator with ventricular shock and antitachycardia pacing functionality would be identified as VVE-DDDRV, assuming that the pacing section was programmed DDDRV. Currently, no hemodynamic sensors have been approved for tachycardia detection (position III).
From Practice advisory for perioperative management of patients with cardiac rhythm management devices: Pacemakers and implantable cardioverter-defibrillators. A report by the American Society of Anesthesiologists Task Force on Perioperative Management of Patients with Cardiac Rhythm Management Devices. Anesthesiology 2005; 103: 186, with permission.

EXAMPLE OF A STEPWISE APPROACH TO THE PERIOPERATIVE TREATMENT OF THE PATIENT WITH A CARDIAC RHYTHM MANAGEMENT DEVICE (CRMD)

PERIOPERATIVE PERIOD	PATIENT/CRMD CONDITION	INTERVENTION
Preoperative evaluation	Patient has CRMD	• Focused history • Focused physical examination
	Determine CRMD type (pacemaker, ICD, CRT)	• Manufacturer's CRMD identification card • Chest x-ray studies (no data available) • Supplemental resources[a]
	Determine whether patient is CRMD-dependent for pacing function	• Verbal history • Bradyarrhythmia symptoms • Atrioventricular node ablation • No spontaneous ventricular activity[b]
	Determine CRMD function	• Comprehensive CRMD evaluation[c] • Determine whether pacing pulses are present and create paced beats
Preoperative preparation	EMI unlikely during procedure	• If EMI unlikely, special precautions are not needed
	EMI likely: CRMD is pacemaker	• Reprogram to asynchronous mode when indicated • Suspend rate-adaptive functions[d]
	EMI likely: CRMD is ICD	• Suspend antitachyarrhythmia functions • If patient is dependent on pacing function, after pacing functions as above
	EMI likely: all CRMD	• Use bipolar cautery; ultrasonic scalpel • Temporary pacing and external cardioversion–defibrillation available
	Intraoperative physiologic changes likely (e.g., bradycardia, ischemia)	• Plan for possible adverse CRMD–patient interaction

EXAMPLE OF A STEPWISE APPROACH TO THE PERIOPERATIVE TREATMENT OF THE PATIENT WITH A CARDIAC RHYTHM MANAGEMENT DEVICE (CRMD) *(CONTINUED)*

▨ PERIOPERATIVE PERIOD	▨ PATIENT/CRMD CONDITION	▨ INTERVENTION
Intraoperative management	Monitoring	• Electrocardiographic monitoring per ASA standard • Peripheral pulse monitoring
	Electrocautery interference	• CT/CRP—no current through PG/leads • Avoid proximity of CT to PG/leads • Short bursts at lowest possible energy • Use bipolar cautery; ultrasonic scalpel
	Radiofrequency catheter ablation	• Avoid contact of radiofrequency catheter with PG/leads • Radiofrequency current path far away from PG/leads • Discuss these concerns with operator
	Lithotripsy	• Do not focus lithotripsy beam near PG • R wave triggers lithotripsy? Disable atrial pacing[e]
	MRI	• Generally contraindicated • If required, consult ordering physician, cardiologist, radiologists, and manufacturer
	RT	• PG/leads must be outside of RT field • Possible surgical relocation of PG • Verify PG function during/after RT course
	ECT	• Consult with ordering physician, patient's cardiologist, a CRMD service, or CRMD manufacturer
Emergency defibrillation–cardioversion	ICD: magnet disabled	• Terminate all EMI sources • Remove magnet to re-enable therapies • Observe for appropriate therapies
	ICD: programming disabled	• Programming to re-enable therapies or proceed directly with external cardioversion–defibrillation
	ICD: either of above	• Minimize current flow through PG/leads • PP as far as possible from PG • PP perpendicular to major axis PG/leads • To extent possible, PP in anterior–posterior location
	Regardless of CRMD type	• Use clinically appropriate cardioversion/defibrillation energy
Postoperative management	Immediate postoperative period	• Monitor cardiac R&R continuously • Backup pacing and cardioversion/defibrillation capability
	Postoperative interrogation and restoration of CRMD function	• Interrogation to assess function • Setting appropriate?[f] • Is CRMD an ICD?[g] • Use cardiology/pacemaker–ICD service if needed

ICD, internal cardioverter–defibrillator; CRT, cardiac resynchronization therapy; EMI, electromagnetic interference; ASA, American Society of Anesthesiologists; CT, cautery tool; CRP, current return pad; PG, pulse generator; MRI, magnetic resonance imaging; RT, radiation therapy; ECT, electroconvulsive therapy; PP, external cardioversion–defibrillation pads or paddles; R&R, rhythm and rate.

[a]Manufacturer's databases, pacemaker clinic records, cardiology consultation.

[b]With cardiac rhythm management device (CRMD) programmed WI at lowest programmable rate.

[c]Ideally, CRMD function assessed by interrogation, with function altered by reprogramming if required.

[d]Most times this will be necessary; when in doubt, assume so.

[e]Atrial pacing spikes may be interpreted by the lithotriptor as R waves, possibly inciting the lithotriptor to deliver a shock during a vulnerable period in the heart.

[f]If necessary, reprogram appropriate setting.

[g]Restore all antitachycardia therapies.

From Practice advisory for perioperative management of patients with cardiac rhythm management devices: Pacemakers and implantable cardioverter-defibrillators. A report by the American Society of Anesthesiologists Task Force on Perioperative Management of Patients with Cardiac Rhythm Management Devices. Anesthesiology 2005; 103: 186, with permission.

TREATMENT OF PACEMAKER FAILURE

▪ RATE	▪ POSSIBLE RESPONSE
Adequate to maintain blood pressure	1. Oxygen, airway control 2. Place magnet over pacemaker 3. Atropine if sinus bradycardia
Severe bradycardia and hypotension	1. Oxygen, airway control 2. Place magnet over pacemaker 3. Other types of pacing if magnet does not activate the pacemaker (transcutaneous, esophageal, or transvenous) 4. Atropine if sinus bradycardia 5. Isoproterenol to increase ventricular rate
No escape rhythm	1. Cardiopulmonary resuscitation 2. Place magnet over pacemaker 3. Other types of pacing if magnet does not activate the pacemaker (transcutaneous, esophageal, or transvenous) 4. Isoproterenol to increase ventricular rate

From Zaidan JR: Pacemakers, Cardiac, Vascular and Thoracic Anesthesia. Edited by Youngberg JA, Lake CL, Roizen MF et al. New York, Churchill Livingstone, 2000, with permission.

PACEMAKER TRACINGS ATRIAL PACING

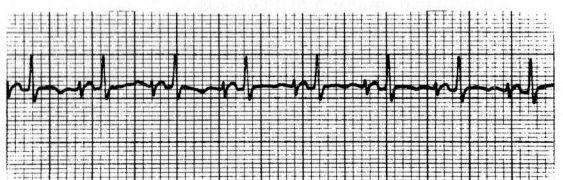

Atrial pacing as demonstrated in this figure is used when the atrial impulse can proceed through the atrioventricular (AV) node.[1] Examples are sinus bradycardia and junctional rhythms associated with clinically significant decreases in blood pressure.

VENTRICULAR PACING

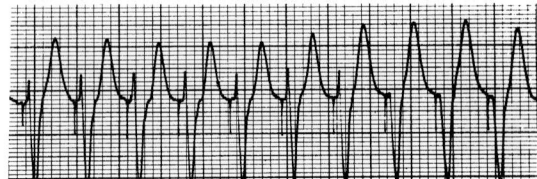

In this tracing ventricular pacing is evident by absence of atrial wave (P wave) and pacemaker spike preceding QRS complex. Ventricular pacing is employed in the presence of bradycardia secondary to AV block or atrial fibrillation.

DUAL-CHAMBER PACING

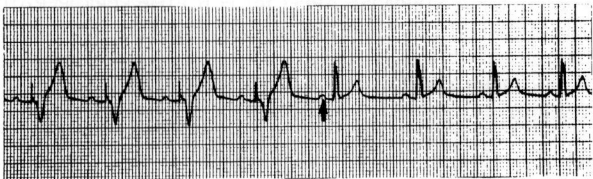

The dual-chamber (DDD) pacemaker (generator), one of the most commonly used, paces and senses both atrium and ventricle. In the first four beats, the P waves were not followed by a QRS complex within the programmed PR interval. Therefore, a ventricular pacing spike and a ventricular paced beat occurred. In the last four beats (after the *arrow* in the figure), atrial activity proceeded through the AV node in the allotted amount of time; therefore, ventricular pacing was inhibited.

ATRIAL ELECTROGRAM

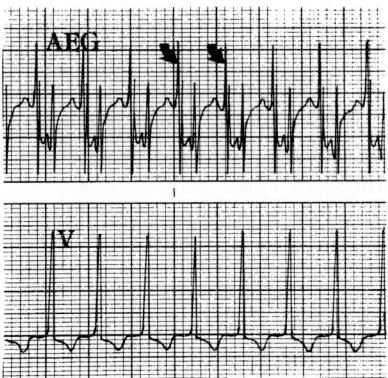

The atrial electrogram (AEG) is useful in differentiating various atrial dysrhythmias. The AEG is obtained from an intracardiac or esophageal lead if P waves are not clearly seen on the surface ECG. In this trace, the V lead does not have obvious P waves; however, the AEG reveals large P waves (*arrows*) that precede each QRS complex. Locate the QRS on the AEG by matching the R wave on the surface ECG to the AEG. The surface and AEG must be simultaneously recorded.

GUIDELINES FOR USING THE ELECTROCAUTERY

1. Electromagnet interference created by an electrocautery can cause a number of problems with pacemaker or ICD function including, but not limited to, reprogramming, inhibition, noise reversion mode, electrical reset, myocardial burns, increase in threshold, rate increment changes in rate adaptive pacemakers, and inappropriate sensing and charging in ICDs.[2,3]
2. When positioning the return plate of the electrocautery:
   a. Ensure it is located so the pacemaker or ICD is not between this return plate and the active electrode.
   b. Ensure the plane described by the return plate and the active electrode of the electrocautery is perpendicular to a plane described by the pacemaker or ICD and the pacemaker's electrodes.
3. Use the smallest current required to cut or coagulate.
4. Use the electrocautery in short bursts.
5. Avoid using the electrocautery within 6 inches of the device or leads.
6. Consider using the bipolar electrocautery or the ultrasonic scalpel[4,5] to minimize interference with pacemaker or ICD function.
7. Activating the electrocautery in the area of the pacemaker or ICD, even if the active electrode is not touching the patient, will cause interference.[6]
8. Do not use the electrocautery when an ICD is programmed to sense and deliver therapy.
9. Convert the ICD to no response either by programming or by using the magnet, depending on the manufacturer of the ICD, so the device will not deliver therapy secondary to misinterpretation of signals from the electrocautery as a dysrhythmia. These maneuvers will not change the program of a pacemaker that is incorporated into an ICD.
10. If desired, convert a pacemaker that does not have an ICD to the asynchronous mode so it is not inhibited by the electrocautery.
11. A magnet will not change bradycardia-related pacing parameters in the ICD.
12. ICDs must be programmed to respond to a magnet.

ICD, implanted cardioverter defibrillator.

ADDITIONAL ISSUES FOR PATIENTS WITH IMPLANTED CARDIOVERTER DEFIBRILLATORS

1. All ICDs have pacemakers incorporated into the circuitry.
2. Preoperative assessments should include those procedures that are standard for patients with heart disease.
3. Obtain a cardiology consult to help assess the patient, interrogate the ICD, program the device to no response, and program the device to respond to the magnet.
4. There is no particular anesthetic technique that is clearly right or wrong for a patient who has an ICD.
5. Apply patches for external defibrillation when the ICD is programmed to no response. Ensure these external patches are as far away as possible from the device and, if possible, not in the same plane as the device and electrodes.
6. Monitor as required for patient care. If monitoring with a pulmonary arterial catheter, discuss the issues of dislodgment of the ICD electrodes with the patient and cardiologist. Document in the chart your discussions and the logic supporting the necessity for a pulmonary arterial catheter. Maintain sterile technique, and consider administering antibiotics just before inserting central lines.
7. Continue antidysrhythmic agents until the time of surgery. Discuss with the cardiologist the necessity of administering an additional dose of an antidysrhythmic agent if the patient experiences an intraoperative dysrhythmia.
8. Intraoperative dysrhythmias:
   a. If the patient has a dysrhythmia, rule out and treat the usual intraoperative causes to prevent a recurrence.
   b. If the dysrhythmia continues and a magnet has been used to create the no-response mode, remove the magnet from the ICD and allow the ICD to charge and deliver a response.
   c. If the ICD has been programmed to the no-response mode, then either quickly reprogram the ICD to deliver a response or proceed directly to external defibrillation.
   d. If external defibrillation or cardioversion is required, apply the defibrillator paddles in an anterior-posterior position, if possible, and deliver the shock at a level sufficient to terminate the dysrhythmia.
   e. External pacing might be required if the pacemaker/ICD is damaged with the shock.
9. Monitor the patient's ECG and be prepared to deliver an external defibrillation when transporting the patient to and from the operating room.
10. Interrogate and reprogram the ICD when the patient has entered the postoperative care unit.

ICD, implanted cardioverter defibrillator; ECG, electrocardiogram.

References

1. Epstein AE, DiMarco JP, Ellenbogen KA et al: ACC/AHA/HRS 2008 Guidelines for Device-Based Therapy of Cardiac Rhythm Abnormalities. A report of the American College of Cardiology/American Heart Association Task Force on Practice Guidelines (Writing Committee to Revise the ACC/AHA/NASPE 2002 Guideline Update for Implantation of Cardiac Pacemakers and Antiarrhythmia Devices). Circulation 2008; 117: e350
2. Levine P: Evaluation and management of pacing system malfunctions, Cardiac Pacing and ICDs, 4th edition. Edited by Ellenbogen KA, Ward MA. Boston, Blackwell Publishing, 2005
3. Atlee JL, Bernstein AD: Cardiac rhythm management devices (part II): Perioperative management. Anesthesiology 2001; 95: 1492
4. Nandalan SP, Vanner RG: Use of the harmonic scalpel in a patient with a permanent pacemaker. Anaesthesia 2001; 94: 710
5. Ozeren M, Dogan OV, Duzgun C et al: Use of an ultrasonic scalpel in the open-heart reoperation of a patient with pacemaker. Eur J Cardiothorac Surg 2002; 21: 761
6. Stevenson WG, Chaitman BR, Ellenbogen KA et al, for the Subcommittee on Electrocardiography and Arrhythmias of the American Heart Association Council on Clinical Cardiology, in collaboration with the Heart Rhythm Society: Clinical assessment and management of patient with implanted cardioverter-defibrillators presenting to nonelectrophysiologists. Circulation 2004; 110: 3866